CLINICAL ANESTHESIA

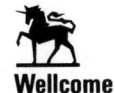

CLINICAL ANESTHESIA

Second Edition

Edited by

Paul G. Barash, M.D.

Professor and Chairman, Department of Anesthesiology
Associate Dean for Clinical Affairs
Yale University School of Medicine
Chief, Department of Anesthesiology
Yale–New Haven Hospital
New Haven, Connecticut

Bruce F. Cullen, M.D.

Professor
University of Washington School of Medicine
Anesthesiologist-in-Chief, Department of Anesthesiology
Harborview Medical Center
Seattle, Washington

Robert K. Stoelting, M.D.

Professor and Chairman, Department of Anesthesia
Indiana University School of Medicine
Indianapolis, Indiana

With 98 Contributors

J. B. LIPPINCOTT COMPANY   Philadelphia

Acquisitions Editor: Mary K. Smith
Editorial Assistant: Anne Geyer
Indexer: Maria Coughlin
Cover and Text Designer: Susan Blaker
Production Manager: Janet Greenwood
Production: P. M. Gordon Associates
Compositor: Achorn Graphic Services, Inc.
Printer/Binder: Courier Westford, Inc.

Second Edition

3   5   6   4   2

Library of Congress Cataloging-in-Publication Data

Clinical anesthesia / edited by Paul G. Barash, Bruce F. Cul-
    len, Robert K. Stoelting : with 98 contributors. — 2nd ed.
        p.   cm.
    Includes bibliographical references and index.
    ISBN 0–397–51160–4
    1. Anesthesiology.   2. Anesthesia.   I. Barash, Paul G.
II. Cullen, Bruce F.   III. Stoelting, Robert K.
    [DNLM: 1. Anesthesiology.   WO 200 C6398]
RD81.C58   1992
617.9′6—dc20
DNLM/DLC
for Library of Congress   92–11553
                                              CIP

For All Students of Anesthesiology

CONTRIBUTORS

Stephen E. Abram, MD
Professor of Anesthesiology
Medical College of Wisconsin
Milwaukee, Wisconsin

J. Jeff Andrews, MD
Associate Professor of Anesthesiology
Department of Anesthesiology
The University of Texas Medical Branch at Galveston
Galveston, Texas

Jeffrey Askanazi, MD
Associate Professor of Anesthesiology
Albert Einstein College of Medicine
Director of Research
Department of Anesthesiology
Division of Critical Care Medicine
Montefiore Medical Center
Bronx, New York

Michael J. Avram, PhD
Associate Professor of Anesthesia
Northwestern University School of Medicine
Research Consultant
Department of Veterans Affairs
Lakeside Medical Center
Affiliated Professional Staff
Northwestern Memorial Hospital
Chicago, Illinois

Max T. Baker, PhD
Assistant Professor
Department of Anesthesia
University of Iowa Hospitals and Clinics
Iowa City, Iowa

Steven J. Barker, PhD, MD
Associate Professor and Acting Chairman
Department of Anesthesiology
University of California, Irvine
Irvine, California

Audrée A. Bendo, MD
Assistant Professor
Department of Anesthesiology
State University of New York Health Science Center at
    Brooklyn
Brooklyn, New York

Arnold J. Berry, MD
Associate Professor of Anesthesiology
Department of Anesthesiology
Emory University School of Medicine
Emory University Hospital
Atlanta, Georgia

Frederic A. Berry, MD
Professor of Anesthesiology and Pediatrics
Department of Anesthesiology
University of Virginia Medical Center
Charlottesville, Virginia

David R. Bevan, MB, MRCP, FFARCS
Professor and Head
Department of Anaesthesia
University of British Columbia
Department Head
Department of Anaesthesia
Vancouver General Hospital
Vancouver, British Columbia

Morris Brown, MD
Associate Professor of Anesthesiology
Wayne State University School of Medicine
Chairman
Department of Anesthesiology
Sinai Hospital of Detroit
Detroit, Michigan

F. Peter Buckley, MB, FFARCS
Associate Professor
Department of Anesthesiology
University of Washington School of Medicine
Medical Director
Pain and Toxicity Research Program
Fred Hutchinson Cancer Research Center
Seattle, Washington

Rod K. Calverley, MD, FRCP(C)
Clinical Professor of Anesthesiology
University of California, San Diego
Attending Anesthesiologist
University of California, San Diego Medical Center
Department of Veterans Affairs Medical Center
San Diego, California

Frederick W. Campbell, III, MD
Professor and Vice-Chairman
Department of Anesthesiology
The Medical College of Pennsylvania
Philadelphia, Pennsylvania

Randall L. Carpenter, MD
Assistant Clinical Professor of Anesthesiology
University of Washington
Staff Anesthesiologist
Virginia Mason Hospital
Seattle, Washington

Frederick W. Cheney, MD
Professor of Anesthesiology
University of Washington
Director of Respiratory Care Services
University of Washington Medical Center
Seattle, Washington

Edmond Cohen, MD
Assistant Professor of Anesthesiology
Mount Sinai School of Medicine of the City University of
    New York
Assistant Attending in Anesthesiology
Mount Sinai Medical Center
New York, New York

D. Ryan Cook, MD
Professor of Anesthesiology and Pharmacology
University of Pittsburgh Medical Center
Director of Anesthesiology
Children's Hospital of Pittsburgh
Pittsburgh, Pennsylvania

James E. Cottrell, MD
Professor and Chairman
State University of New York Health Science Center at
    Brooklyn
College of Medicine
Professor and Chairman
University Hospital
Brooklyn, New York

Benjamin G. Covino, MD*
Professor and Chairman
Department of Anaesthesia
Harvard Medical School
Professor and Chairman
Department of Anesthesia
Brigham and Women's Hospital
Boston, Massachusetts

Stephen F. Dierdorf, MD
Professor of Anesthesia
Indiana University School of Medicine
Indianapolis, Indiana

* Deceased.

François Donati, PhD, MD, FRCPC
Associate Professor of Anesthesia
McGill University
Anaesthetist
Royal Victoria Hospital
Montréal, Québec

Jan Ehrenwerth, MD
Professor of Anesthesiology
Yale University School of Medicine
Attending Anesthesiologist
Yale–New Haven Hospital
New Haven, Connecticut

John H. Eichhorn, MD
Professor and Chairman
Department of Anesthesiology
The University of Mississippi School of Medicine
Chairman of Anesthesiology
The University of Mississippi Medical Center
Jackson, Mississippi

James B. Eisenkraft, MD
Professor of Anesthesiology
Mount Sinai School of Medicine of the City University of
    New York
Attending Anesthesiologist
Mount Sinai Medical Center
New York, New York

John E. Ellis, MD
Assistant Professor of Anesthesia and Critical Care
University of Chicago
Division of Biological Sciences
Pritzker School of Medicine
Chicago, Illinois

Norig Ellison, MD
Professor of Anesthesia
University of Pennsylvania School of Medicine
Anesthesiologist
Hospital of the University of Pennsylvania
Philadelphia, Pennsylvania

Robert Feinstein, MD, PhD
Assistant Professor
Department of Anesthesiology
Washington University School of Medicine
Chief Anesthesiologist
Barnes West County Hospital
St. Louis, Missouri

Richard H. Fine, MD
Assistant Professor of Anesthesia
Cornell University Medical School
Assistant Attending Anesthesiologist
New York Hospital–Cornell Medical Center
New York, New York

Mieczyslaw Finster, MD
Professor of Anesthesiology, Obstetrics and Gynecology
College of Physicians and Surgeons
Columbia University
Attending Anesthesiologist
Presbyterian Hospital
New York, New York

Leonard Firestone, MD
Associate Professor
Department of Anesthesiology/Critical Care Medicine
University of Pittsburgh School of Medicine
Chief, Cardiac Anesthesia
Presbyterian University Hospital
Pittsburgh, Pennsylvania

Susan Firestone, MD
Associate Professor
Department of Anesthesiology/Critical Care Medicine
University of Pittsburgh
Children's Hospital of Pittsburgh
Pittsburgh, Pennsylvania

Jeffrey E. Fletcher, PhD
Associate Professor of Anesthesiology and Biochemistry
Hahnemann University
Philadelphia, Pennsylvania

Arthur S. Foreman, MD
Assistant Professor
Department of Anesthesiology
Wake Forest University Medical Center
Bowman Gray School of Medicine
North Carolina Baptist Hospital
Winston-Salem, North Carolina

Robert J. Fragen, MD
Professor of Clinical Anesthesia
Northwestern University Medical School
Attending Staff
Northwestern Memorial Hospital
Chicago, Illinois

Simon Gelman, MD, PhD
Professor and Chairman
Department of Anesthesiology
The University of Alabama at Birmingham
University Hospital
Birmingham, Alabama

Hugh C. Gilbert, MD
Assistant Professor of Clinical Anesthesia
Northwestern University Medical School
Senior Attending Anesthesiologist
The Evanston Hospital
Evanston, Illinois

Bruce S. A. Gillies, MS, MD
Acting Assistant Professor
Director of Transplant Anesthesia
University of Washington School of Medicine
Seattle, Washington

George J. Graf, MD
Clinical Assistant Professor of Anesthesiology
University of California, Los Angeles
School of Medicine
Attending Anesthesiologist
Department of Anesthesiology and Internal Medicine
Cedars-Sinai Medical Center
Los Angeles, California

J. David Haddox, DDS, MD
Director, Division of Pain Medicine
Department of Anesthesiology
Emory University School of Medicine
Director, The Center for Pain Medicine
The Emory Clinic
Atlanta, Georgia

Ronald A. Harrison, MD
Associate Professor of Clinical Anesthesia
Northwestern University Medical School
Attending Staff Physician
Northwestern Memorial Hospital
Chicago, Illinois

John Hartung, PhD
Research Associate Professor
Departments of Anesthesiology and Pharmacology
State University of New York Health Science Center at
   Brooklyn
Brooklyn, New York

Robert J. Hudson, MD, FRCPC
Associate Professor of Anesthesia
Faculty of Medicine
University of Manitoba
Attending Anesthetist
St. Boniface General Hospital
Winnipeg, Manitoba

Cindy W. Hughes, MD
Assistant Professor of Anesthesiology
Albany Medical College and Hospital
Albany, New York

Anthony D. Ivankovich, MD
The William Gottschalk, MD Professor and Chairman
Department of Anesthesiology
Rush Medical College
Rush–Presbyterian–St. Luke's Medical Center
Chicago, Illinois

Ira S. Kass, PhD
Associate Professor
Departments of Anesthesiology and Pharmacology
State University of New York Health Science Center at
   Brooklyn
Brooklyn, New York

Jonathan D. Katz, MD
Associate Professor of Clinical Anesthesiology
Yale University School of Medicine
Attending Anesthesiologist
St. Vincent's Medical Center
Bridgeport, Connecticut

Hoshang J. Khambatta, MD
Associate Professor of Clinical Anesthesiology
College of Physicians and Surgeons
Columbia University
Associate Attending
Columbia Presbyterian Medical Center
New York, New York

Harry G. G. Kingston, MB, BCh, FFARCS
Professor of Anesthesiology
Oregon Health Sciences University
Clinical Director
Department of Anesthesiology
Oregon Health Sciences Hospital
Portland, Oregon

Donald A. Kroll, MD, PhD
Associate Clinical Professor
Department of Anesthesiology
University of California, Los Angeles
School of Medicine
Attending Physician
UCLA Medical Center
Los Angeles, California

Carol L. Lake, MD
Professor of Anesthesiology
University of Virginia Health Sciences Center
Charlottesville, Virginia

Donald H. Lambert, MD, PhD
Associate Professor of Anesthesia
Harvard Medical School
Director
Clinical Anesthesia Research
Brigham and Women's Hospital
Boston, Massachusetts

C. Philip Larson Jr., MD
Professor of Anesthesia and Neurosurgery
Stanford University School of Medicine
Stanford, California

Noel W. Lawson, MD
Professor of Anesthesiology
University of Missouri Health Sciences Center
Columbia, Missouri

Jerrold H. Levy, MD
Associate Professor of Anesthesiology
Emory University School of Medicine
Division of Cardiothoracic Anesthesia and Critical Care
The Emory Clinic
Atlanta, Georgia

Wen-Shin Liu, MD
Professor of Anesthesiology
Northeastern Ohio Universities College of Medicine
Rootstown, Ohio
Staff Anesthesiologist
Timken Mercy Medical Center
Canton, Ohio

Timothy R. Lubenow, MD
Assistant Professor
Department of Anesthesiology
Rush Medical College
Rush–Presbyterian–St. Luke's Medical Center
Chicago, Illinois

Philip D. Lumb, MB, BS
Professor and Chairman
Department of Anesthesiology
Professor of Surgery
Albany Medical College
Anesthesiologist-in-Chief
Co-director, Surgical ICU
Albany Medical Center Hospital
Albany, New York

David C. Mackey, MD
Consultant and Instructor in Anesthesiology
Mayo Medical School
Attending Anesthesiologist
St. Luke's Hospital
Jacksonville, Florida

Tuula Manner, MD, PhD
Visiting Research Fellow
Albert Einstein College of Medicine
Montefiore Medical Center
Bronx, New York

John T. Martin, MD
Professor Emeritus
Department of Anesthesiology
Medical College of Ohio at Toledo
Honorary Staff Member
Medical College Hospital
Toledo, Ohio

Robert J. McCarthy, PharmD
Associate Professor
Department of Anesthesiology
Rush Medical College
Rush–Presbyterian–St. Luke's Medical Center
Chicago, Illinois

Kathryn E. McGoldrick, MD
Professor of Anesthesiology
Yale University School of Medicine
Attending Anesthesiologist
Medical Director, One Day Surgery
Yale–New Haven Hospital
New Haven, Connecticut

Charles H. McLeskey, MD
Associate Professor and Director of Academic Affairs
Department of Anesthesiology
University of Colorado Health Sciences Center
Denver, Colorado

Roger S. Mecca, MD
Assistant Clinical Professor
Yale–New Haven Hospital
New Haven, Connecticut
Chairman, Department of Anesthesiology
Danbury Hospital
Danbury, Connecticut

John R. Moyers, MD
Professor of Anesthesia
University of Iowa
College of Medicine
University of Iowa Hospitals and Clinics
Iowa City, Iowa

Michael F. Mulroy, MD
Staff Anesthesiologist
Virginia Mason Medical Center
Seattle, Washington

Michael R. Murphy, MD
Associate Professor of Anesthesiology
Emory University School of Medicine
Co-deputy Chief of Anesthesiology
Crawford Long Hospital of Emory University
Atlanta, Georgia

Steven Neustein, MD
Assistant Professor of Anesthesiology
Mount Sinai School of Medicine
Assistant Attending
Mount Sinai Medical Center
New York, New York

William D. Owens, MD
Mallinckrodt Professor and Head of Anesthesiology
Washington University School of Medicine
Anesthesiologist-in-Chief
Barnes Hospital
St. Louis Children's Hospital
St. Louis, Missouri

Nathan Leon Pace, MD
Professor of Anesthesiology
Adjunct Professor of Bioengineering
University of Utah
Attending Staff
University Hospital
Salt Lake City, Utah

Hilda Pedersen, MB, CLB, FFARCS
Professor of Clinical Anesthesiology
Department of Anesthesiology
College of Physicians and Surgeons
Columbia University
Attending Anesthesiologist
The Presbyterian Hospital
New York, New York

Lawrence L. Priano, MD, PhD
Associate Professor of Anesthesiology
Oregon Health Sciences University
Portland, Oregon

Donald S. Prough, MD
Professor and Chairman
Department of Anesthesiology
The University of Texas Medical Branch at Galveston
Galveston, Texas

James J. Richter, MD, PhD
Director
Department of Anesthesiology
Hartford Hospital
Hartford, Connecticut

Christine S. Rinder, MD
Assistant Professor of Anesthesiology
Yale University School of Medicine
Attending Physician
Yale–New Haven Hospital
New Haven, Connecticut

Michael F. Roizen, MD
Professor and Chairman
Department of Anesthesia and Critical Care
University of Chicago
Division of the Biological Sciences
Pritzker School of Medicine
University of Chicago Hospitals and Clinics
Chicago, Illinois

Stanley H. Rosenbaum, MD
Professor of Anesthesiology, Medicine, and Surgery
Yale University School of Medicine
Attending Physician
Yale–New Haven Hospital
New Haven, Connecticut

Henry Rosenberg, MD
Professor and Chairman
Department of Anesthesiology
Hahnemann University
Chairman, Department of Anesthesiology
Hahnemann University Hospital
Philadelphia, Pennsylvania

Alan C. Santos, MD
Assistant Professor of Anesthesiology, Obstetrics and
  Gynecology
State University of New York at Stony Brook School of
  Medicine
Director, Obstetrical Anesthesiology
University Hospital
Stony Brook, New York

Mark S. Scheller, MD
Associate Professor of Anesthesiology
University of California, San Diego
Anesthesiologist
University of California, San Diego Medical Center
La Jolla, California

Alan Jay Schwartz, MD, MS Ed
Professor and Chairman
Department of Anesthesiology
The Medical College of Pennsylvania
Philadelphia, Pennsylvania

David T. Seitman, MD
Assistant Professor of Anesthesiology
Hahnemann University
Staff Anesthesiologist
Hahnemann University Hospital
Philadelphia, Pennsylvania

Björn Skeie, MD
Senior Attending
Department of Anesthesiology
Riks Hospitalet
University of Oslo
Norway

Howard S. Smith, MD
Instructor in Clinical Anesthesiology
Albany Medical College
Attending Anesthesiologist
Albany Medical Center
Albany, New York

Theodore C. Smith, MD
Professor of Anesthesiology
Loyola University
Chief of Anesthesiology
Edward A. Hines Jr. Veterans Affairs Hospital
Maywood, Illinois

Linda C. Stehling, MD
Former Professor
State University of New York Health Sciences Center at
    Syracuse
Medical Consultant
Blood Systems Inc.
Scottsdale, Arizona

Wendell C. Stevens, MD
Professor and Chairman
Department of Anesthesiology
Oregon Health Sciences University
Oregon Health Sciences University Hospital
Portland, Oregon

M. Christine Stock, MD
Associate Professor of Anesthesiology
Assistant Professor of Internal Medicine
Staff Anesthesiologist
Emory University Hospital
Atlanta, Georgia

Stephen J. Thomas, MD
Associate Professor of Anesthesiology
Cornell University School of Medicine
Vice Chairman, Department of Anesthesiology
New York Hospital–Cornell Medical Center
New York, New York

Kevin K. Tremper, PhD, MD
Professor and Chair
Department of Anesthesiology
University of Michigan
Chairman
Department of Anesthesiology
University of Michigan Medical Center
Ann Arbor, Michigan

Russell A. Van Dyke, PhD
Director, Anesthesia Research
Henry Ford Hospital
Detroit, Michigan

Jeffery S. Vender, MD, FCCM
Associate Professor of Clinical Anesthesia
Northwestern University Medical School
Chief of Anesthesiology
Director of Medical-Surgical Intensive Care
Evanston Hospital Corp.
Evanston, Illinois

Bernard V. Wetchler, MD
Director, Department of Anesthesiology
Medical Director, Ambulatory SurgiCare
The Methodist Medical Center of Illinois
Clinical Professor and Chief, Division of Anesthesia
University of Illinois College of Medicine at Peoria
Peoria, Illinois

K. C. Wong, MD, PhD
Professor and Chairman of Anesthesiology
Professor of Pharmacology
University of Utah School of Medicine
Salt Lake City, Utah

Doreen L. Wray, MD
Instructor in Anesthesiology
Assistant Attending Anesthesiologist
The New York Hospital–Cornell University Medical
    Center
New York, New York

James R. Zaidan, MD
Professor of Anesthesiology
Deputy Chairman for Education
Emory University School of Medicine
Chief of Anesthesiology
Grady Memorial Hospital
Atlanta, Georgia

Gary P. Zaloga, MD
Professor of Anesthesia and Medicine
Bowman Gray School of Medicine
Wake Forest University
Attending Physician, Critical Care
North Carolina Baptist Hospital
Winston-Salem, North Carolina

PREFACE

As we celebrate the 150th anniversary of the administration of the first ether anesthetic by Dr. Crawford Long, anesthesiology continues to have a significant impact on the practice of medicine. Our specialty is visible not only in the operating room, but also throughout the hospital, ambulatory facilities, and even the homes of patients who receive ambulatory pain therapy. This scope of practice challenges the practitioner to maintain clinical competency in the face of a virtual explosion of medical knowledge.

As in the first edition of *Clinical Anesthesia*, our primary goal is to develop a textbook that supports efficient, rapid acquisition of the information it contains. Our colleagues have been extraordinarily helpful in identifying new subject areas that have become essential components of contemporary anesthesia practice. In addition, they have offered constructive comments to guide us in making the text even more relevant to the resident and veteran practitioner. This textbook not only contains new areas of knowledge; it also amplifies traditional subject areas that are an integral part of clinical practice.

As a result, approximately 40% of the second edition of *Clinical Anesthesia* represents new chapters and significant revisions of the remaining chapters. The book is organized into six major parts to facilitate communication. These are "Introduction to Anesthesia Practice," "Basic Principles of Anesthesia Practice," "Basic Principles of Pharmacology in Anesthesia Practice," "Preparing for Anesthesia," "Management of Anesthesia," and "Postanesthesia and Consultant Practice." Four new chapters have been added to this edition. "Contemporary Anesthesia Practice and Quality Assurance" examines the elements of academic and private practice as well as issues related to quality assurance. "Cancer Therapy and Its Anesthetic Implications" focuses on modern cancer therapy and its importance to anesthetic practice; this significant new contribution highlights the importance of the toxic effects of chemotherapy, radiation, and biologic modalities on an appropriate anesthetic management plan. "Anesthesia Outside the Operating Room" emphasizes those diagnostic (e.g., MRI, CT scan) and thera-

peutic procedures that require the presence of the anesthesiologist at remote locations in the hospital. "Anesthesia for Organ Transplantation" concentrates on the anesthetic management of the donor and recipient for various organ transplant operations. Furthermore, it highlights the anesthetic challenge of the transplant recipient for non–transplant-related surgical procedures.

To allow for more comprehensive coverage, we have devoted separate chapters to the topics "Parenteral Nutrition" and "Fluids and Electrolytes." Also, because of recent emphasis on pain management, we now have separate chapters on "Management of Acute Postoperative Pain" and "Chronic Pain Management." Finally, to maintain a fresh approach, seven chapters have new primary contributors. Thus, we have remained true to the goals established for the first edition: to encompass significant new areas of knowledge as well as traditional subject areas, with emphasis on rapidly accessible information.

As in the first edition, we encouraged our contributors to develop clinically relevant themes and to prioritize various clinical options. Occasionally this results in some redundancy, as well as some disagreement; however, this also represents the realities of the consultant practice of anesthesiology.

Finally, we wish to express our gratitude to the individual contributors whose hard work and dedication expedited the development and production of this edition. We also thank our secretaries, Gail Norup, Deanna Walker, and Karen Frymoyer, each of whom gave unselfishly of her time to facilitate the editorial process. Thanks to our colleagues at the J. B. Lippincott Company, who have continued to demonstrate their commitment to excellence in medical publishing: Mary K. Smith, Medical Editor; Anne Geyer, Assistant Editor; and Janet Greenwood, Production Manager. We also thank Peggy M. Gordon and her staff of production editors.

Paul G. Barash, M.D.
Bruce F. Cullen, M.D.
Robert K. Stoelting, M.D.

PREFACE TO THE FIRST EDITION

The discovery and application of anesthesia has been the single most important contribution of American medicine to mankind. The major achievements of modern surgery would not have taken place without the accompanying vision of the pioneers of anesthesiology. Yet anesthesia was originally considered a technique with little scientific merit, and anesthesiology did not become a distinct academic discipline until 100 years after Dr. Crawford Long administered the first ether anesthetic.

Today, the boundaries of anesthesiology extend far beyond the operating room. As a consequence, the information needs of both the veteran practitioner and the resident in the specialty have increased dramatically, and a comprehensive reference for our discipline must now encompass significant new areas of knowledge as well as the traditional subject areas. Just as important, however, is the accessibility of the information. A truly modern textbook must support efficient, *rapid* use if it is to meet the demands of those in practice or training today. It has been the goal of the editors of *Clinical Anesthesia* to create such a comprehensive, usable book in a single volume.

The table of contents shows how we have attempted to meet this goal. The book begins with a discussion of the development of anesthesia—we have a proud heritage, and this chapter eloquently describes the exciting events that form the history of our specialty. Each of the subspecialties is discussed in subsequent chapters, with the scientific basis of each subject described in proximity to the clinical aspects. In addition, there are numerous chapters not found in traditional anesthesia textbooks. For example, the impact of modern genetics is discussed in the chapter entitled "Pharmacogenetics." Because environmental hazards continue to be a topic of great concern, "Hazards of Working in the Operating Room" eloquently examines the relationship of the anesthesiologist to the operating room setting and documents the importance of the OR environment to physical and mental well-being. This is complemented by a subsequent chapter, "Electrical Safety," which details the protection of both the patient and the operating room staff. The dilemmas confronting the anesthesiologist in the management of the elderly patient are addressed in the chapter "Anesthesia for the Geriatric Patient," which focuses on the implications of the aging process in clinical practice.

Certain topics require amplification because of their impact on daily practice. Orthopaedics, the genitourinary system, and the gastrointestinal system merit the greater detail found in separate chapters. Finally, certain areas that are clinically relevant but problematic are also presented. These include the positioning of the patient, the allergic response, and the special considerations arising with the traumatized patient.

The contributors of all these chapters form a remarkable blend of 86 outstanding authorities from 48 institutions. They have provided us with a truly nationwide perspective on our specialty. Each of them, whether up and coming or long-established, is a physician actively involved in the advancement of anesthesiology.

As editors, we have tried to envision the specialty of the future, and we feel that the presentation of the material should be unique. In this regard, we chose not to contribute chapters in our own areas of expertise. Instead, we extended our energies in the editorial process, in developing themes to be used in individual chapters, encouraging contributors to prioritize various clinical options, integrating each of the chapters within appropriate sections of the book, and, finally, avoiding the duplication so often seen in multi-authored volumes. On occasion, however, we felt it important to have some redundancy, and even disagreement, in the management of a given clinical problem, because this in fact reflects the realities of consultant practice of anesthesiology.

The editors wish to acknowledge and express their gratitude to a number of individuals whose hard work not only expedited this book, but also added quality and authority to its pages: first, each of the contributors, who not only completed their chapters in a timely fashion, but also offered numerous suggestions which we feel will enhance the value of *Clinical Anesthesia* to the resident and practitioner; next, our secretaries, Gail Norup, Sue Perkins, and Deanna Walker, whose unflagging devotion to the project was a continued source of support; and finally, a special word of thanks is due to our colleagues at the J. B. Lippincott Company: Susan Gay, Executive Editor; Richard Winters, Basic Books Editor; Carol Florence, Production Manager; and Jody DeMatteo and Janet Greenwood, Production Editors. Their vision and constructive comments continually demonstrated their commitment to the highest standard of medical publishing.

Paul G. Barash, M.D.
Bruce F. Cullen, M.D.
Robert K. Stoelting, M.D.

PREFACE TO THE FIRST EDITION

CONTENTS

I

INTRODUCTION TO ANESTHESIA PRACTICE

1

Rod K. Calverley
Mark Scheller*

Anesthesia as a Specialty: Past, Present, and Future

As the body of medical knowledge relevant to anesthesiology expands at a rapid pace, students and residents sometimes confine their studies to material that they believe will be immediately applicable in the operating room or the examination hall. By limiting their reading so narrowly, they fail to learn that it is only by knowledge of the past that we can appreciate our present situation and anticipate future developments. This chapter is not designed to be "commercially" valuable as a means to satisfy examiners; it has been created to help the reader understand important elements of our history, to learn how anesthesiology came to its present situation, and to recognize some of the forces that will shape both the immediate future and the more distant days to follow.

A reading of history overcomes an unfortunate tendency to accept the practice of anesthesia as having always been just what it was on the day of one's introduction to the specialty. To do so is to ignore the achievements of those who discovered all that is known and whose energies brought anesthesiology to its present attractive position. We have received a magnificent endowment from our predecessors—machines, drugs, and techniques that we use to bring comfort to our patients every day.

This chapter provides an overview of selected elements of our history to illustrate several important segments of the evolution of anesthesia, including the development of anesthetic agents, regional techniques, anesthesia machines, monitoring equipment, and endotracheal devices. This review of technical and pharmacologic landmarks is followed by a discussion of the development of North American and British professional practice and professional societies. The chapter closes with a look ahead, an attempt to forecast the future of anesthesiology.

SURGERY BEFORE INHALATIONAL ANESTHESIA

Before the introduction of anesthesia with diethyl ether, many surgeons believed that pain was, and would always be, an inevitable consequence of surgery. In those "dark"

*Mark Scheller is the author of the final section, "The Future of Anesthesiology."

days, many patients approached surgery as though facing execution, an often appropriate assessment of uncontained risks, including pain, hemorrhage, shock, and postoperative infection. While awaiting even a minor elective procedure, patients often put their estate and personal affairs in order in the anticipation that their wealth would soon be passed on to the next of kin. Curiously, as there was little that could be done to alleviate pain, and, as pain seemed an inevitable component of injury and most disease, philosophers ennobled pain as "providential." Scholars, debating issues from the comfort of their couches, assessed the courage of less fortunate persons before declaring that the ability to withstand pain ranked among the noble virtues. In ancient as well as in modern times, there is truth to the aphorism, "The easiest pain to bear is someone else's."

The Roman writer Celsus encouraged "pitilessness" as an essential character of the surgeon, an attitude that prevailed for centuries. Although some surgeons confessed that they found elements of their work intensely disturbing, most became inured to their patients' agony. Medical students emulated their teachers and often omitted to record any appraisal of the patient's distress while taking notes of the operations that they witnessed. Even the authors of leading surgical texts often ignored surgical pain as a topic of discussion. Just before the advent of anesthesia, Robert Liston's 1842 edition of *Elements of Surgery* contained detailed descriptions of elective and emergency procedures on the extremities, head and neck, breast, and genitals, but neglected a significant discussion of any technique to make the patient comfortable. In Liston's time, pain was considered primarily a symptom of importance in differential diagnosis.

Before the discovery of surgical anesthesia, Europeans attempted to relieve pain by hypnosis, by the ingestion of alcohol, herbs, and extracts of botanical preparations, and by the local application of pressure or ice. The topical anesthetic created by chewing coca leaves was known only to the Incas of South America before Pizarro's conquest. A Japanese physician, Seishu Manaoke, may have used drugs to render surgery painless in 1835, but before 1846 Western surgeons could only offer their patients oral concoctions of opium in wine or whiskey and the hollow promise of hasty surgery. As late as 1839 the French surgeon Louis Velpeau said, "To obviate pain in operations is a chimera which it is today no longer permissible to seek after."[1] Within a decade, his gloomy pronouncement was reversed. Velpeau became an enthusiastic supporter of anesthesia and pronounced it the most important discovery yet achieved.

ANESTHETIC ANTECEDENTS

Historic chronologies frequently memorialize the date of a discovery and relate the event to the actions of one person; it is, however, inappropriate to view the development of anesthesiology from such a confined perspective. William T. G. Morton is honored as the man who, in Boston, on October 16, 1846, showed the world that ether could work, but his historic public demonstration succeeded through the prior efforts of less celebrated men who made Morton's triumph possible.

Morton's demonstration of ether caught the world's attention in part because it took place in a public arena, the surgical amphitheater of a public institution, the Massachusetts General Hospital. Surgical amphitheaters, and the charitable hospitals of which they were a part, were then a relatively recent addition to American medical teaching. During the early 19th century, large hospitals had been erected in North America and Europe as an expression of the evolving social philosophy of the time. The privileged of the community accepted a responsibility to attempt to provide shelter and medical care for the sick and injured of the poorer classes. As a result, large numbers of patients could be attended in a single location. Their medical care, however, was often of an indifferent and uncertain nature. The course of the patient's disease might be observed by medical students who "walked the wards" informally but who would not yet profit from the techniques of bedside instruction that William Osler and his late 19th century colleagues brought to American medical practice. A few students might act as "dressers" to established surgeons, but most students only observed surgery when they sat or stood on the benches of the amphitheater where the poor underwent operations in public.

Medical school curricula were nonstandardized and highly variable. The most pronounced disparities were observed among American proprietary medical schools as a consequence of the influence of contending philosophies of medical care, which included homeopathy, hydropathy, allopathy, and eclectic healing—all vying for a dominant role in therapeutics. As a result, Americans were accustomed to hearing of new claims that assured a cure. Experimental procedures received attention that might be denied in more orthodox medical societies. As a consequence, nitrous oxide and ether, chemicals discovered in Europe, whose general properties were already known on both sides of the Atlantic, found their historic application in America.

A lost opportunity to discover anesthesia occurred two decades before the demonstration of ether in Boston. An English physician searched intentionally in 1823 and 1824 for an inhaled anesthetic to relieve the pain of surgery. Henry Hill Hickman (1800–1830) might have succeeded if he had used either of the drugs whose actions were later discovered in America, but the mice and dogs he studied inhaled neither ether nor nitrous oxide but high concentrations of carbon dioxide. Carbon dioxide has some anesthetic properties, as shown by the absence of response to an incision in the animals of Hickman's study, but carbon dioxide is not an appropriate clinical anesthetic. Hickman's concept was magnificent; his choice of agent, regrettable. His work was ignored both by surgeons and by the scientists of the Royal Society. Despite Hickman's earnest efforts, his research was never appreciated during his brief life. Ironically, a contemporary member of the Royal Society, Sir Humphry Davy, was familiar with the analgesic qualities of another inhaled gas, nitrous oxide. If Davy had encouraged Hickman, the younger man might have repeated his study with a more appropriate agent. Surgical anesthesia might then have been celebrated as a British rather than an American discovery.

EARLY USE OF ETHER AND NITROUS OXIDE

The first inhaled agents that would have a place in anesthesia were of different origins but had found a similar application as drugs for social entertainment in the years immediately before their use as anesthetics.

Diethyl Ether

Diethyl ether had been known for centuries. Although it may have been compounded first by an 8th century Arabian philosopher, Jabir ibn Hayyam, or by Raymond Lully, an alchemist of the 13th century, it was certainly known in the 16th century to both Valerius Cordus and Paracelsus, who prepared it by distilling sulfuric acid (oil of vitriol) with fortified wine to produce an "oleum vitrioli dulce" (sweet oil of vitriol). Paracelsus observed that it caused chickens to fall asleep and awaken unharmed. He must have been aware of its analgesic qualities, because he reported that it could be recommended for use in painful illnesses, but there is no record that his suggestion was followed. In 1540, Valerius Cordus recommended it as a medication to be taken in wine for the relief of whooping cough and other respiratory diseases.

For three centuries thereafter, this simple compound remained a therapeutic agent with only occasional use. Some of its properties were examined by distinguished British scientists, including Robert Boyle, Isaac Newton, and Michael Faraday, but without sustained interest. Its only routine application came as an inexpensive "recreational drug" among the poor of Britain and Ireland, who sometimes drank an ounce or two of ether when taxes made gin prohibitively expensive. An American variation of this practice was conducted by groups of medical students who held ether-soaked towels to their faces at nocturnal "ether frolics."

Nitrous Oxide

Nitrous oxide was inhaled from gas-tight bags by celebrants seeking an exhilarating experience. It was not used as frequently as was ether because it was more complex to prepare and was awkward to store. It was commonly produced by heating ammonium nitrate in the presence of iron filings. The evolved gas was passed through water to eliminate toxic oxides of nitrogen before being stored.

Nitrous oxide was first prepared in 1773 by Joseph Priestley (1733–1804), an English clergyman and scientist, who ranks among the great pioneers of chemistry. During his years of study, Priestley prepared and examined several gases, including nitrous oxide, ammonia, sulfur dioxide, oxygen, carbon monoxide, and carbon dioxide. Most of his work consisted primarily of scientific observation, but he also created the first carbonated beverage by charging water with carbon dioxide.

Even though his discovery of nitrous oxide would be sufficient to give Priestley a place in the history of anesthesia, he is also remembered for his recognition of the pure gas now known as oxygen. Priestley heated mercuric oxide to release a gas that caused greater beauty and intensity of a flame and that allowed a mouse to survive longer when breathing it than would be expected if the jar were filled with air. He identified many properties of the new gas, but, handicapped by his adherence to the phlogiston theory of combustion, termed it *dephlogisticated air*. It is a remarkable reflection of Priestley's genius that within a few months, he isolated both oxygen and nitrous oxide, the only pure gases still used routinely in anesthesia.

Other contributions might have followed if Priestley's career had remained undisturbed, but in 1791 his home, scientific apparatus, and library were burned by a mob angered by his sympathies for the revolution in France. He later left England and emigrated to Pennsylvania, where his friends and correspondents included three great American revolutionaries: Benjamin Franklin, John Adams, and Thomas Jefferson.

If the French Revolution was to result in an interruption of Joseph Priestley's research, its effect on a French scientist of exceptional genius was catastrophic. Antoine Lavoisier (1743–1794) examined Priestley's work with gases, recognized the fallacy of the phlogiston theory, and dispelled its confusion. He named Priestley's vital gas *oxygen*. Lavoisier later proved that respiration was equivalent to combustion as the oxygen inhaled into the lungs combined with carbon and hydrogen to produce carbon dioxide and water. Lavoisier erroneously believed that the process took place in the lungs. He might have overcome that error and extended his understanding of chemistry and physiology even further, but he was imprisoned on trivial charges during the Reign of Terror. Lavoisier went to the guillotine on May 8, 1794, after a sham trial during which Robespierre, the president of the tribunal, snarled, "The republic has no need for chemists."

Priestley's preparation of nitrous oxide drew the attention of other investigators on both sides of the Atlantic Ocean. A physician and chemist of New York, Samuel Latham Mitchell, recognized some of the cerebral effects of nitrous oxide while performing research on the influences of gases as factors in the transmission of disease. Although his conclusion that nitrous oxide might be a contagious influence in epidemics was erroneous, his comments on nitrous oxide were among the reports that would stimulate the attention of Thomas Beddoes and Humphry Davy of the Pneumatic Institute in Bristol, England.

At the end of the 18th century in England, there was a strong interest in the salubrious effects of mineral waters and healthful airs. This led to the development of spas, which were sought out by people of society. Particular waters and gases were believed to prevent and treat disease. A dedicated interest in the potential use of gases as remedies for scurvy, tuberculosis, and other diseases led Thomas Beddoes (1760–1808) to open his Pneumatic Institute close to the small spa of Hotwells, in the city of Bristol, where he hired Humphry Davy to conduct research projects.

Humphry Davy (1778–1829) was a young man of ability and drive. He performed a brilliant series of investigations of several gases but focused much of his attention on nitrous oxide, which he and his associates inhaled through face masks designed for the Institute by James Watt, the distinguished inventor of the steam engine. Davy used this equipment to measure the rate of uptake of nitrous oxide and its effect on respiration and other central nervous system actions. These results were combined with research on the physical properties of the gas in a 580-page book published in 1800, *Nitrous Oxide*. This impressive treatise is now best remembered for a few incidental observations: Davy's comments that nitrous oxide transiently relieved a severe headache, obliterated a minor headache, and briefly quenched an aggravating toothache. The most frequently quoted passage was a casual entry, "As nitrous oxide in its extensive operation appears capable of destroying physical pain, it may probably be used with advantage during surgical operations in which no great effusion of blood takes place."[2]

Although Davy did not pursue this prophecy—perhaps because he was set on a career in basic research—he did use nitrous oxide to entertain the young men of quality who visited the Pneumatic Institute, including Dr. Peter Mark Roget, later to become the author of *Roget's Thesaurus*, and two poets, Samuel Taylor Coleridge and the poet Laureate, Robert Southey, who, after inhaling nitrous oxide, was said to exclaim that the atmosphere of the highest of all possible heavens must be composed of this gas. After one of these episodes, Davy coined the persisting sobriquet for nitrous oxide, "laughing gas."

Following Davy's researches, the only application of nitrous oxide for the next four decades was to produce hilarity and uninhibited behavior at parties and public entertainments. Nitrous oxide capers and ether frolics would eventually introduce the concept of inhaling a vapor for the transient relief of pain to the first Americans to experiment with surgical anesthesia, William E. Clarke of Rochester, New York, and Crawford W. Long of Jefferson, Georgia.

An anesthesia text written by Henry Lyman in 1881 provides evidence that William E. Clarke gave the first ether anesthetic in Rochester, New York, in January 1842. From techniques learned as a chemistry student in 1839, Clarke entertained his companions with nitrous oxide and ether. Lyman reported, ". . . Clarke diligently propagated this convivial method among his fellow students. Emboldened by these experiences, in January, 1842, having returned to Rochester, he administered ether, from a towel, to a young woman named Hobbie, and one of her teeth was then extracted without pain by a dentist named Elijah Pope."[3] Another indirect reference to Clarke's anesthetic suggested that it was believed that her unconsciousness was due to hysteria. Clarke was advised to conduct no further anesthetic experiments. Regrettably, no statements by Clarke, Pope, or Miss Hobbie have been found.

Crawford W. Long (1815–1878)

There is no doubt that 2 months later, on March 30, 1842, Crawford Williamson Long did give ether with a towel for surgical anesthesia in Jefferson, Georgia. His patient, James M. Venable, was a young man who already knew ether's exhilarating effects, for he reported in a certificate that he had previously inhaled it frequently and was fond of its use. Venable had two small tumors on his neck but refused to have them excised, because he dreaded the cut of the knife. Knowing that Venable was familiar with ether's action, Dr. Long proposed that ether might alleviate pain and gained his patient's consent to proceed. After inhaling ether from the towel, Venable reported that he was unaware of the removal of the tumor. In determining the world's first fee for anesthesia, Long settled on a surgical charge of $2.00, plus $0.25 for the ether.[4]

As a rural physician with a very limited surgical practice, Crawford Long had few opportunities to give ether anesthesia, but he did conduct the first comparative trial of an anesthetic. He wished to prove that insensibility to pain was caused by ether and was not simply a reflection of the individual's pain threshold or the result of self-hypnosis. When ether was withheld during amputation of the second of two toes, his patient reported great pain and proclaimed a strenuous preference for ether.

For Long to gain an unrivaled position as the discoverer of anesthesia, all that remained for him to do would have been to announce his historic work in the medical literature. Long, however, remained silent until 1849, when ether anesthesia was already well known. He explained that he practiced in an isolated environment and had few opportunities for surgical or dental procedures. From our perspective it is difficult to understand why he was so reluctant to publish his work. This remarkable man might have changed the course of the history of medicine, but, because of his failure to publish, the public introduction of anesthesia was achieved by more assured and bolder persons.

The Crucial Experiment

In contrast to the limited opportunities for surgery presented to rural practitioners in the mid-19th century, urban dentists regularly met patients who refused restorative treatment for fear of the pain that would be inflicted by the dentist. From a dentist's perspective, pain was not so much life-threatening as it was livelihood-threatening. A few dentists searched for new techniques of effective pain relief. Pasteur's yet-to-be-delivered aphorism, that chance only favors the prepared mind, would have provided an apt description of one of these men, Horace Wells, of Hartford, Connecticut. Wells recognized what others had ignored, the analgesic potential of nitrous oxide.

Horace Wells (1815–1848)

Horace Wells' great moment of discovery came on December 10, 1844, when he attended a lecture-exhibition by an itinerant "scientist," Gardner Quincy Colton,[4a] who prepared nitrous oxide and encouraged members of the audience to inhale the gas. Wells observed that a young man, Samuel Cooley (later Colonel Cooley of the Connecticut militia), was unaware that he had injured his leg while under the influence of nitrous oxide. Sensing that nitrous oxide might also relieve the pain of dental procedures, Wells contacted Colton and boldly proposed an experiment. The following day, Colton gave Wells nitrous oxide before a fellow dentist, William Riggs, extracted a tooth. When Wells awoke, he claimed that he had not felt any pain and declared the experiment a great success. Colton taught Wells to prepare nitrous oxide, which the dentist administered with success in his practice. His apparatus probably resembled that used by Colton. The patient placed a wooden tube in his mouth through which he rebreathed nitrous oxide from a small bag filled with the gas.

A few weeks later, in January 1845, Wells attempted a public demonstration in Boston at the Harvard Medical School. He had planned to anesthetize a patient for an amputation, but, when the patient refused surgery, a dental anesthetic for a medical student was substituted. Wells, perhaps influenced by a large and openly critical audience, began the extraction without an adequate level of anesthesia, and the trial was judged a failure.

The exact circumstances of Wells' lack of success are not known. His less than enthusiastic patient may have refused to breathe the anesthetic. Alternatively, Wells might have lost part of his small supply of nitrous oxide, which could have happened if the patient involuntarily removed his lips from the mouthpiece or if the patient's nostrils were not held shut. It might be that Wells did not know that nitrous oxide lacks sufficient potency to serve predictably as an anesthetic without supplementation. In any event, the student cried out, and Wells was jeered by his audience. The disappointment disturbed him deeply, and, although he continued his dental practice for some time, his life became unsettled. While profoundly distressed, Wells committed suicide in 1848. Despite his personal failure, Wells remains an important pioneer of anesthesia, for he was the first person to recognize the anesthetic qualities of the only 19th century drug still in routine use, nitrous oxide.

William Thomas Green Morton (1819–1868)

Another New Englander, William Thomas Green Morton, briefly shared a dental practice with Horace Wells in Hartford. Wells's daybook shows that he gave Morton a course of instruction in anesthesia, but Morton apparently moved to Boston without paying for his lessons. In Boston, Morton continued his interest in anesthesia and, after learning from Charles Jackson that ether dropped on the skin provided analgesia, began experiments with inhaled ether. After anesthetizing a pet dog, he became confident of his skills and anesthetized patients in his dental office. Encouraged by that success, Morton gained an invitation to give a public demonstration in the Bullfinch amphitheater of the Massachusetts General Hospital.

The diethyl ether that Morton was to use would prove to be much more versatile than nitrous oxide. Professor Nicholas Greene has made a detailed examination of social and medical circumstances surrounding the discovery of anesthesia.[5] Greene has demonstrated that before the invention of the hollow needle and an awareness of aseptic technique, the only class of potential anesthetics that could offer a prompt, profound, and temporary action were the inhaled drugs. Of the available drugs, ether was a superb first choice. Bottles of liquid ether were easily transported, and the volatility of the drug permitted effective inhalation. The concentrations required for surgical anesthesia were so low that patients did not become hypoxic when breathing air. It also possessed what would later be recognized as a unique property among all inhaled anesthetics: the quality of providing surgical anesthesia without causing respiratory or cardiovascular depression. These properties, combined with a slow rate of induction, gave the patient a great margin of safety when physicians were attempting to master the new art of administering an inhaled anesthetic.

Pain Put to Sleep

On Friday, October 16, 1846, William T. Morton secured permission to provide an anesthetic to Edward Gilbert Abbott before the surgeon, John Collins Warren, excised a vascular lesion from the left side of Abbott's neck. Morton was late in arriving, so Warren was at the point of proceeding when Morton entered. The dentist had been obliged to wait for an instrument-maker to complete his inhaler (Fig. 1-1). It consisted of a large glass bulb containing a sponge soaked with colored ether and a spout, which was to be placed in the patient's mouth. An opening on the opposite side of the bulb allowed air to enter and to be drawn over the ether-soaked sponge with each breath.

The conversations of that morning were not accurately

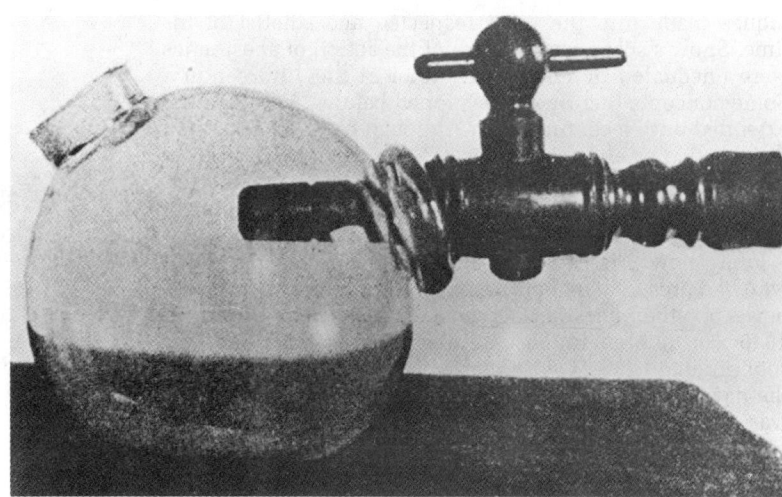

Figure 1-1. Morton's ether inhaler (1846).

recorded; however, popular accounts state that the surgeon responded testily to Morton's apology for his tardy arrival by remarking, "Sir, your patient is ready." Morton directed his attention to his patient and first conducted a very abbreviated preoperative evaluation. He inquired, "Are you afraid?" Abbott responded that he was not and took the inhaler in his mouth. After a few minutes, Morton is said to have turned to the surgeon to respond, "Sir, your patient is ready." Gilbert Abbott later reported that he was aware of the surgery but had experienced no pain. At the moment that the procedure ended, Warren turned to his audience and announced, "Gentlemen, this is no humbug."[6] Oliver Wendell Holmes soon suggested the term *anaesthesia* to describe the state of temporary insensibility.

What would be recognized as America's greatest contribution to 19th century medicine had been realized, but the immediate prospect was clouded by subterfuge and argument. Some weeks passed before Morton admitted that the active component of the colored fluid that he had called "Letheon" was the familiar drug, diethyl ether. Morton, Wells, Jackson, and their supporters soon became caught up in a contentious, protracted, and fruitless debate over priority for the discovery.

When the details of Morton's anesthetic technique became public knowledge, the information was transmitted by train, stagecoach, and coastal vessels to other North American cities and by ship to the world. Anesthetics were performed in Britain, France, Russia, South Africa, Australia, and other countries almost as soon as surgeons heard the welcome news of the extraordinary discovery. Even though surgery could now be performed with "pain put to sleep," the frequency of operations did not rise rapidly. Several years would pass before anesthesia was even universally recommended. Many American surgeons believed that anesthesia was not appropriate for all procedures in all classes of patients, but the "American invention" excited interest everywhere.

BRITISH CONTRIBUTIONS

Although Americans discovered inhalation anesthesia, British doctors initiated most of the noteworthy advances of the following decades. In the years after James Y. Simpson discovered chloroform anesthesia, John Snow, Joseph T. Clover, and Frederic Hewitt were earnest advocates of improved anesthetic care. Their publications directed the at-

tention of the medical profession to significant advances and earned greater respect for the emerging discipline of anesthesia. In succession, Snow, Clover, and Hewitt were each the leading London anaesthetist* of the day and gave anesthetics to members of the royal family. Their work not only established the principle that the administration of anesthetics was an appropriate activity for a medical doctor but also encouraged the understanding in Britain and the Commonwealth that anesthetics could be administered only by physicians.

J. Y. Simpson Champions Chloroform

James Young Simpson, a successful obstetrician of Edinburgh, Scotland, had been among the first to use ether for the relief of the pain of labor. He became dissatisfied with ether and sought a more pleasant, rapid-acting anesthetic. He and a few junior associates conducted a bold search for a new inhaled anesthetic by inhaling samples of several volatile chemicals collected for Simpson by British apothecaries.

David Waldie suggested chloroform, which had first been prepared in 1831. Simpson and his friends inhaled it at a dinner party in Simpson's home on the evening of November 4, 1847. They promptly fell unconscious from self-induced anesthesia. They awoke delighted at their success. Simpson quickly set about encouraging chloroform anesthesia. Within 2 weeks, he had dispatched his first account of its use to the Lancet. Although Simpson introduced chloroform with celerity, boldness, and enthusiasm and was later to become a vocal defender of the use of anesthesia for women in labor, he gave few anesthetics himself. His goal was simply to improve a patient's comfort during his operative or obstetric activities.

John Snow, The First Anesthesiologist

John Snow (1813–1858) was the first physician to undertake detailed clinical and pharmacologic studies of ether, chloroform, and other anesthetics. His mastery of clinical tech-

---

*Nineteenth century "anaesthetists" in America became 20th century "anesthesiologists," but their British and Canadian counterparts (unchallenged by competition from nurses) remained "anaesthetists." The author of this chapter has adhered to this distinction.

niques made him the most respected anaesthetist of his time. Snow's scholarly analyses of the action of anesthetics were unequaled by any other author of the 19th century. Some concepts that Snow developed before 1852 were not extended until a century later. Although he never restricted his practice solely to anesthesia, Snow is rightfully recognized as the first anesthesiologist, because he was a masterful clinician and dedicated investigator. Many elements of his work warrant detailed review.

John Snow (Fig. 1-2) was already a respected physician who had presented papers on physiologic subjects when the news of ether anesthesia reached England in December 1846. He took an interest in anesthetic practice and was soon invited to work with many of the leading surgeons of the day. He was not only facile at providing anesthesia but was also a remarkably keen observer. His innovative description of the stages or degrees of ether based on the patient's responsiveness was not improved upon for 70 years.

He soon realized the inadequacies of ether inhalers into which the patient rebreathed through a mouthpiece. After practicing anesthesia for only 2 weeks, Snow designed the first of his series of ingenious ether inhalers. His best-known apparatus featured unidirectional valves within a malleable, well-fitting mask of his own design, which closely resembles the form of a modern face mask (Fig. 1-3). The facepiece was connected to the vaporizer (Fig. 1-4) by a breathing tube, which Snow deliberately designed to be wider than the human trachea so that even rapid respirations would not be impeded. A metal coil within the vaporizer ensured that the patient's inspired breath was drawn over a large surface area to promote the uptake of ether. The device also incorporated a warm water bath to maintain the volatility

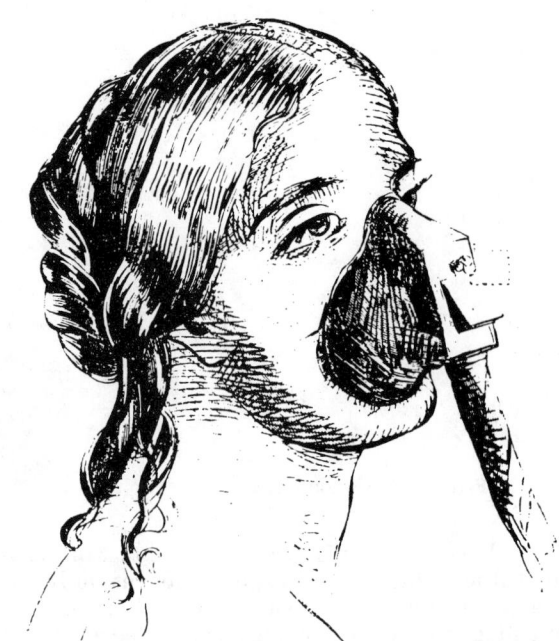

Figure 1-3. John Snow's face mask (1847). The expiratory valve can be tilted to the side to allow the patient to breathe air.

of the agent. Snow did not attempt to capitalize on his creativity; he closed his account of its preparation with the very generous observation, "there is no restriction respecting the making of it."[7]

The following year, John Snow introduced a chloroform inhaler; he had recognized the versatility of the new agent and came to prefer it in his practice. At the same time, he initiated what was to become an extraordinary series of experiments that were remarkable in both their scope and in the manner in which they anticipated sophisticated research performed a century later. Snow realized that successful anesthetics must not only abolish pain but also prevent movement. He anesthetized several species of animals with varying concentrations of ether and chloroform to determine the concentration required to prevent movement in response to a sharp stimulus. Despite the limitations of the technology of 1848, this element of his work anticipated the concept of minimum alveolar concentration (MAC).[8]

He assessed the anesthetic action of a large number of potential anesthetics, and, although he did not find any to rival chloroform or ether, he determined a relationship between solubility, vapor pressure, and anesthetic potency that was not fully appreciated until after World War II. He also created an experimental closed circuit device in which the subject (Snow himself) breathed oxygen while the exhaled carbon dioxide was absorbed by potassium hydroxide.

Snow's investigations were not confined to anesthesia. His memory is also respected by specialists in infectious and tropical diseases for his proof through an epidemiologic study in 1854 that cholera was transmitted by water. At that time, before the development of microbiology by Louis Pasteur and Robert Koch, most physicians in North America and Europe attributed the mysterious recurring epidemics of cholera to the contagion of "fecalized air." For many years, however, Snow had believed that since the disease affected the gastrointestinal tract, the causative agent must be ingested rather than inhaled. In 1854, he found an oppor-

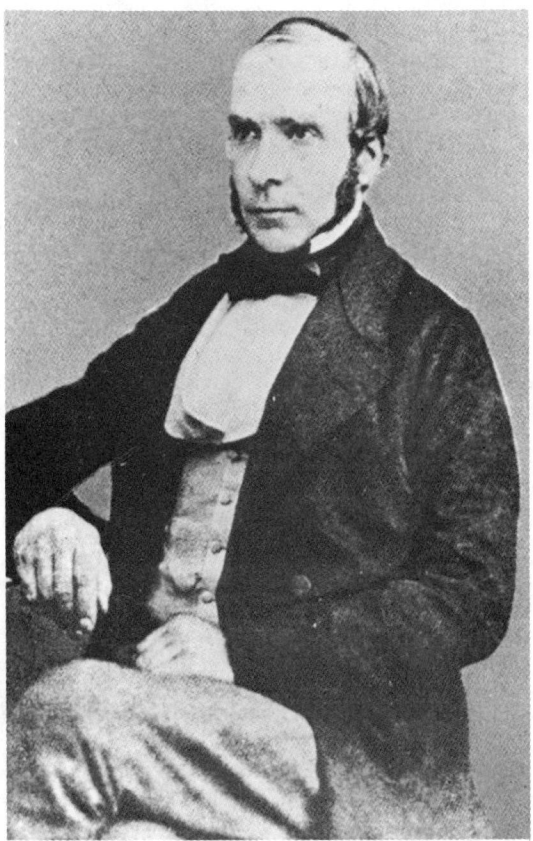

Figure 1-2. John Snow, the first anesthesiologist.

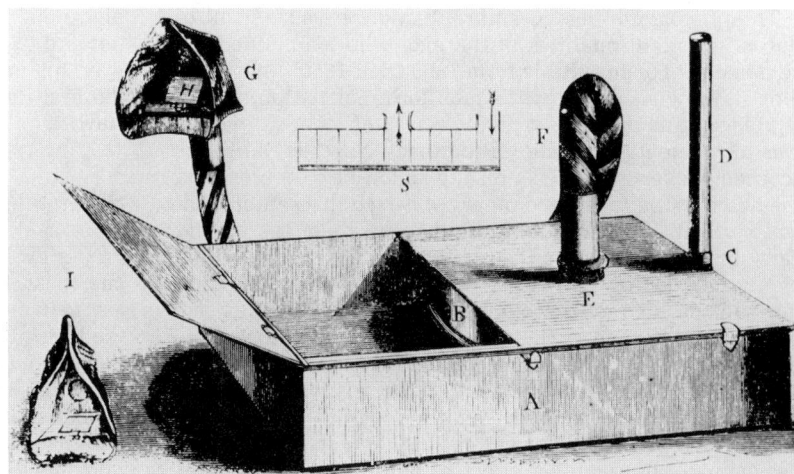

Figure 1-4. John Snow's ether inhaler (1847). The ether chamber (*B*) contained a spiral coil so that the air entering through the brass tube (*D*) was saturated by ether before ascending the flexible tube (*F*) to the face mask (*G*). The ether chamber rested in a bath of warm water (*A*).

tunity to prove his thesis when cholera visited his section of London and caused the deaths of more than 500 people near his residence. Snow determined that the water supply for these persons had been the Broad Street pump. He prepared what would come to be appreciated as the first epidemiologic survey to prove his contention. With that information, he was able to encourage the parish authorities to remove the pump handle so that residents were obliged to find other sources of water. The prompt resolution of the epidemic was attributed to his action.

One hundred years later, in a unique celebration commemorating Snow's action, the public house at the site of the Broad Street pump was named "The John Snow" to mark Snow's role as a pioneer of epidemiology. It is located at 39 Broadwick Street and is among the most popular pubs of Soho; it is visited by pilgrim-physicians from many countries. Whether John Snow would have approved of this unique memorial is uncertain, for he abstained from spirits except for medicinal and experimental purposes.

Snow was a highly respected clinician and author as well as investigator. These qualities are reflected in his books, *On the Inhalation of the Vapour of Ether* (1847) and *On Chloroform and other Anaesthetics* (1858), which was almost completed when he died of a stroke at the age of 45. His books have been reprinted by the American Society of Anesthesiologists.

His opinions were respected not only by his medical contemporaries but were also sought out by prominent people with an interest in science. Queen Victoria's consort, Prince Albert, interviewed John Snow before he was called to Buckingham Palace at the request of the Queen's obstetrician to give chloroform for the Queen's last two deliveries. During the monarch's labor, Snow gave analgesic doses of chloroform on a folded handkerchief, a technique that was soon termed *chloroform à la reine*. Victoria had abhorred the pain of labor and enjoyed the relief that chloroform provided; she wrote in her journal, "Dr. Snow gave that blessed chloroform and the effect was soothing, quieting and delightful beyond measure."[9] After the monarch's positive opinion became known, an ongoing debate over the appropriateness of the use of anesthesia in labor was abruptly quenched. Four years later, Snow was to give a second anesthetic to the Queen, who was again determined to have chloroform. Snow's daybook states that by the time he arrived, Prince Albert had begun the anesthetic and had given his wife "a little chloroform." This may be the only time in history that a Queen had a Prince as her anaesthetist.

Joseph Thomas Clover (1825–1882)

Joseph Clover was the leading anaesthetist of London after the death of John Snow in 1858. Clover was a talented clinician and facile inventor, but he never performed research or wrote to the extent achieved by Snow. If he had written a text, he might be better remembered, but most physicians have little knowledge of Clover beyond identifying the familiar photograph in which he is seen anesthetizing a seated man while palpating his patient's pulse (Fig. 1-5).

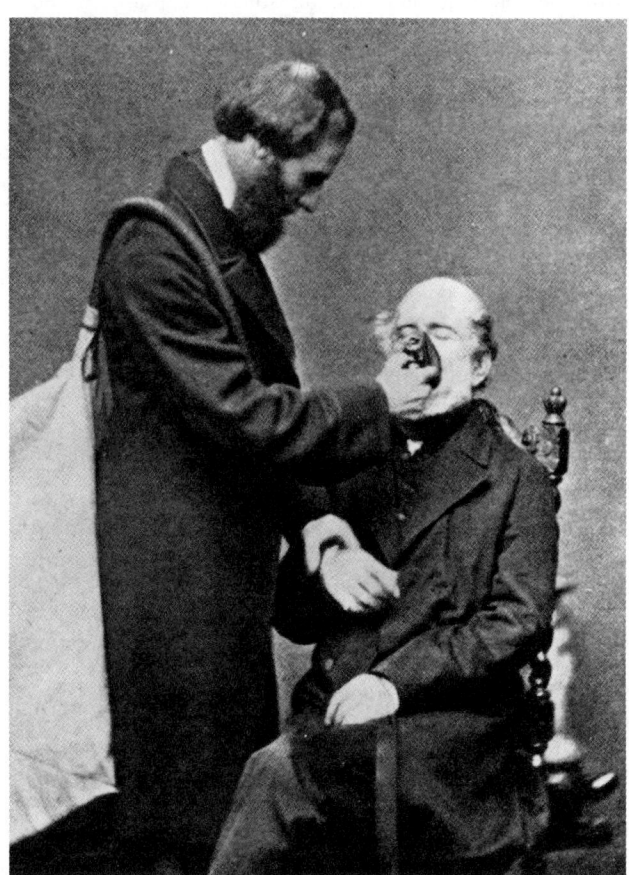

Figure 1-5. Joseph Clover anesthetizing a patient with chloroform and air passing through a flexible tube from a Clover bag.

The photograph deserves our attention, because it introduces important qualities of the man who maintained the advancement of anesthesia from 1860 until 1880. Anesthesiologists now accept Clover's monitoring of the pulse as a simple routine of prudent practice but in Clover's time this was a contentious issue. Prominent Scottish surgeons scorned Clover's emphasis on the action of chloroform on the heart. Baron Lister and others preferred that senior medical students give anesthetics and urged them to "strictly carry out certain simple instructions, among which is that of never touching the pulse, in order that their attention may not be distracted from the respiration."[10] Lister also counseled, "it appears that preliminary examination of the chest, often considered indispensable, is quite unnecessary, and more likely to induce the dreaded syncope, by alarming the patients, than to avert it."[11] Little progress in anesthesia could come from such reactionary statements. In contrast, Clover had observed the effect of chloroform on animals and urged other anaesthetists to monitor the pulse at all times and to discontinue the anesthetic temporarily if any irregularity or weakness was observed in the strength of the pulse. He earned a loyal following among London surgeons, who accepted him as a dedicated specialist.

Clover was the first anaesthetist to administer chloroform in known concentrations through his construction of the Clover bag, which is seen over his shoulder in Figure 1-5. He filled it by pumping air from a bellows over a warmed evaporating vessel containing a known volume of liquid chloroform to obtain a 4.5% concentration of chloroform in air. The apparatus had inspiratory and expiratory valves of ivory supported by springs. A flap valve in the face mask permitted the dilution of the anesthetic with air. In 1868, Clover reported no deaths among 1802 applications of his device, but he later reviewed a fatality in searching detail. He attributed the death to his undetected error in calculating the volume of air diluting the chloroform.[12] After 1870, Clover favored a nitrous oxide–ether sequence. The portable anesthesia machines that he designed were in popular use for decades after his death.

In Figure 1-5, Clover projects the image of attentiveness, but there is no evidence of the resuscitative equipment, which he also had available, to control the airway. In that regard, Clover was exceptional, for he practiced at a time when other anaesthetists could only administer gases and vapors but lacked any means to care for the patient if any difficulty occurred. Clover's prudence and foresight allowed him to anticipate potential problems and to be ready to respond rapidly when a complication threatened his patient. In that regard, he was an exemplary model for the modern anesthesiologist.

Clover was very facile in maintaining the airway. He was the first to urge the now universal practice of thrusting the patient's jaw forward to overcome obstruction of the upper airway by the tongue. Despite the limitation of working before the first endotracheal tube was used in anesthesia, Clover published a landmark case report in 1877. His patient had a tumor of the mouth that obstructed the airway completely once the anesthetic was begun. Clover averted disaster by inserting a small curved cannula of his own design through the cricothyroid membrane. The anesthetic was continued through the cannula until the tumor was excised. Clover, the model of the prepared anesthesiologist, remarked, "I have never used the cannula before although it has been my companion at some thousands of anaesthetic cases."[13]

Every element of Clover's records and his published accounts reflect a consistent dedication to patient safety coupled with a prudent ability to anticipate potential difficulties and to prepare an effective response beforehand. In that way, his manner was very much like that of his successor, the first English anaesthetist to be knighted, Sir Frederick Hewitt.

Sir Frederick Hewitt (1857–1916)

Frederick Hewitt gained the first of his London hospital anesthesia appointments in 1884. He earned a reputation as a superb and inventive clinician and came to be considered the leading British practitioner of the next 30 years. Hewitt engineered modifications of portable ether and nitrous oxide inhalers and, recognizing that nitrous oxide and air formed a hypoxic mixture, designed the first anesthetic apparatus to deliver oxygen and nitrous oxide in variable proportions. He also was influential in ensuring that anesthesia was taught in all British medical schools. His book, *Anaesthetics and Their Administration*, which first appeared in 1893 and continued through five editions, is considered the first true textbook of anesthesia.

Hewitt's most famous patient was King Edward VII, whose coronation in 1902 was canceled when the monarch's life was threatened by an appendiceal abscess. Hewitt anesthetized the King by mask while the surgeon, Frederick Treves, drained the abscess. Hewitt accepted the greater responsibility by anesthetizing an obese, bearded, febrile, dehydrated man with a well-developed and protracted affection for alcohol and tobacco. Following the patient's recovery and coronation, both men were honored, but at different levels. Although the reasons for the awarding of honors by the court are not announced, readers wonder why the surgeon was knighted and Hewitt received a lesser honor then but was eventually knighted 7 years later.

In 1908, Hewitt developed an important appliance that would assist all anesthesiologists in managing an obstructed upper airway. He called his oral device an *air-way*. After several modifications, and with the hyphen now deleted, all anesthesiologists insert airways routinely.

19TH CENTURY ANESTHESIA IN AMERICA

American anesthesiologists of the second half of the 19th century failed to achieve the lasting recognition gained by their British colleagues. Several factors contributed to this disparity. Snow, Clover, and Hewitt were men of such genius that they would have been exceptional in any period of history. They all had mastered the demands of chloroform, an agent that demanded greater skill in its administration than did diethyl ether, which remained the dominant anesthetic in America, where the provision of anesthesia was often a service relegated to medical students, junior house officers, nurses, and nonprofessionals. The subordinate status of anesthesia was even reflected in American art. Thomas Eakins's great studies, "The Gross Clinic" of 1876 and "The Agnew Clinic" of 1889, both present the surgeon as the focus of attention, while the person administering the anesthetic is found among the supporting figures.

In that period, however, Americans led the revival of nitrous oxide. Gardner Q. Colton, the "professor" who had first demonstrated the use of nitrous oxide to Horace Wells, developed the Colton Dental Association after he returned from the California gold rush. In several eastern cities he opened offices equipped with nitrous oxide generators and, perhaps profiting from Wells's unhappy experience, larger breathing bags of 30 l capacity. By 1869, his advertisements carried the intriguing slogan "31½ Miles Long." Colton had asked each patient to sign his name to a scroll, which then contained the names of 55,000 patients who had experienced painless extractions of teeth without hazard. He proposed that if this great number of patients were to march past in single file, the line would be extended for 31½ miles.[14]

Colton gave brief exposures of nitrous oxide undiluted with air or oxygen, which raised concern that the gas was acting as an asphyxiant. The following year a Chicago surgeon, Edmund Andrews, experimented with an oxygen–nitrous oxide mixture and proved that nitrous oxide does not cause anesthesia by depriving the brain of oxygen. While the oxygen–nitrous oxide mixture was safer, he identified a handicap to its use which was unique to that time when anesthetists attended many patients in their homes. The large bag was conspicuous and awkward to carry as he walked along busy streets. He observed that "[i]n city practice, among the higher classes, however, this is no obstacle as the bag can always be taken in a carriage, without attracting attention."[15] Four years later, Andrews was delighted to report the availability of liquefied nitrous oxide compressed under 750 lb of pressure, which allowed a supply sufficient for three patients to be carried in a single cylinder. Despite Andrews's early enthusiasm, few American surgeons relied on nitrous oxide until it was used in combination with regional anesthesia, the last important contribution to inhaled anesthetic practice achieved in the late 19th century.

REGIONAL ANESTHESIA

Several 19th century physicians experimented with the local application of drugs to relieve pain. In 1853, Alexander Wood invented the hollow metal needle in order to inject morphine directly into a painful area. Morphine did not act locally but relieved pain only by its systemic action, but the invention of the needle would allow the successful administration of another locally acting alkaloid three decades later.

Cocaine, an extract of the coca leaf, was the first effective local anesthetic. Its property of numbing mucous membranes and exposed tissues had been known for centuries in Peru, where folk surgeons performing trephinations chewed coca leaves and allowed their saliva to fall onto the surfaces of the wound. This was a unique situation in anesthesia; there are no other instances in which both the operator and his patient routinely shared the effects of the same drug. After Albert Niemann refined the active alkaloid and named it *cocaine*, it was used in experiments by a few investigators. It was noted that cocaine provided topical anesthesia and even produced local insensibility when injected, but these observations were not applied in clinical practice before 1884, when the significance of the action of cocaine was realized by Carl Koller, a Viennese surgical intern.

Carl Koller (1857–1944)

Carl Koller appreciated what others had failed to recognize because of his past experience and his ambition to practice ophthalmology at a time when many operations on the eye were still being performed without anesthesia. Almost four decades after the discovery of ether, general anesthesia by mask still had several limitations. The anesthetized patient could not cooperate with his surgeon. The anesthesiologist's

apparatus interfered with surgical access. More important, the high incidence of vomiting following the administration of either chloroform or ether threatened extrusion of internal contents of the globe with the risk of the permanent loss of sight. At that time, surgical incisions on the globe were left unclosed; fine ophthalmic sutures were not yet available.

While he had been a medical student, Koller had worked in a Vienna laboratory in a search for a topical anesthetic that would overcome the limitations of general anesthesia. Unfortunately, the suspensions of morphine, chloral hydrate, and other drugs that he had used had been ineffectual.

In 1884, his friend, Sigmund Freud, became interested in the cerebral stimulating effects of cocaine and gave Koller a small sample in an envelope, which he placed in his pocket. When the envelope leaked, a few grains of cocaine stuck to Koller's finger, which he casually licked with his tongue. It became numb. Koller realized that he had found the object of his search. That same afternoon, he dashed to the laboratory where he had worked as a student and made a suspension of the cocaine crystals. He and Gustav Gartner, a laboratory associate, observed its anesthetic effect on the eyes of a frog, a rabbit, and a dog before they dropped the solution onto their own corneas. To their amazement, their eyes were insensitive to the touch of a pin.[16]

Carl Koller could not afford to attend the Congress of German Ophthalmologists in Heidelberg on September 15, 1884, but, after his paper was read by a friend, a revolution in ophthalmic surgery and other surgical disciplines was underway. Within the next year, more than 100 articles supporting the use of cocaine appeared in European and American medical journals. Despite this gratifying success, Koller was not able to pursue his goal of gaining a residency position in Vienna. After a duel provoked by an anti-Semitic slur, Koller left Austria and, after studying briefly in Holland and Britain, emigrated in 1888 to New York, where he practiced ophthalmology for the remainder of his career.

American surgeons quickly developed new applications for cocaine. Its efficacy in anesthetizing the nose, mouth, larynx, trachea, rectum, and urethra was described in October 1884. The next month, the first reports were published of its subcutaneous injection. In December 1884, two young surgeons, William Halsted and Richard Hall, described blocks of the sensory nerves of the face and arm. Richard Hall may have been the first person to undergo dental surgery under local anesthesia when Halsted blocked his mandibular nerve. Halsted also performed a block of the brachial plexus under direct vision following a dissection of the plexus. As a consequence of their self-experimentation, both men became addicted to cocaine. Cocaine addiction was an ill-understood but frequent problem in the late 19th century, when it was easily obtained and was offered in scores of patent medicines that were readily available.

Spinal Anesthesia

In 1885, Leonard Corning, a neurologist who had observed Hall and Halsted performing nerve blocks, coined the expression "spinal anaesthesia." Corning wanted to assess the action of cocaine not for surgery, but as a specific therapy for neurologic problems. After first assessing its action in a dog, producing a blockade of rapid onset that was confined to the animal's rear legs, he administered cocaine to a man "addicted to masturbation." He received a proportionally larger dose, but the blockade had a much slower onset. Although Corning does not refer to the escape of cerebrospinal fluid in either case, it is likely that the dog had a spinal anesthetic and that the man had an epidural anesthetic. No therapeutic benefit was described, but Corning closed his account and his attention to the subject by suggesting that cocainization might in time be "a substitute for etherization in genito-urinary or other branches of surgery."[17]

Fourteen years passed before spinal anesthesia was performed for a surgical operation. In the interval, Heinrich Quincke of Kiel, Germany, described lumbar puncture. He proposed that the technique was most safely performed at the level of the third or fourth lumbar interspace, because an entry at that level would be below the termination of the spinal cord. Quincke's technique was used for the first deliberate cocainization of the spinal cord in 1899 by August Bier, a surgical colleague of Quincke. Six patients received small doses of cocaine intrathecally, but, because several of the patients cried out during surgery and some vomited and had postoperative headaches, Bier felt it necessary to conduct a clinical experiment.

Professor Bier permitted his assistant, Dr. Hildebrandt, to perform a lumbar puncture, but, after the needle penetrated the dura, Hildebrandt could not fit the syringe to the needle and a large volume of the professor's spinal fluid escaped. They were at the point of abandoning the study when Hildebrandt volunteered to be the subject of a second attempt. They had an astonishing success. Twenty-three minutes later, Bier noted: "A strong blow with an iron hammer against the tibia was not felt as pain. After 25 minutes: Strong pressure and pulling on a testicle were not painful."[18] They celebrated their success with wine and cigars. That night, both developed violent headaches, which they attributed at first to their celebration. Bier's headache was relieved after 9 days of bedrest. The house officer did not have the luxury of continued rest; Bier reported that Hildebrandt "felt very poor the next morning but with great physical effort he was able to do his work, which consisted mainly in operating and dressing of wounds."[19] Bier believed that their headaches were caused by the loss of large volumes of cerebrospinal fluid and urged that this be avoided if possible. The high incidence of complications following lumbar puncture with wide-bore needles and the toxic reactions attributed to cocaine explain Bier's later loss of interest in spinal anesthesia.

Surgeons in several other countries soon started practicing spinal anesthesia. Many of the observations found in their descriptions are still relevant. The first series from France of 125 cases was published by Theodor Tuffier, who later counseled that the solution should not be injected before cerebrospinal fluid was seen. The initial American report was by Dr. Rudolph Matas of New Orleans, whose first patient developed postanesthetic meningismus, a then-frequent complication that was overcome by the use of sterile gloves as advocated by Halsted and the hermetically sealed sterile solutions recommended by E. W. Lee of Philadelphia.

During 1899, Dudley Tait and Guidlo Caglieri of San Francisco performed experimental studies in animals and therapeutic spinals for orthopaedic patients.[20] They encouraged the use of fine needles to lessen the escape of cerebrospinal fluid and urged that the skin and deeper tissues be infiltrated beforehand with local anesthesia, as had been urged earlier by William Halsted and the foremost advocate of infiltration anesthesia, Carl Ludwig Schleich of Berlin. An early American specialist in anesthesia, Ormond Goldan, published an anesthesia record appropriate for recording the course of "intraspinal cocainization" in 1900. In the same year, Heinrich Braun learned of a newly described extract of the adrenal gland, epinephrine, which he used to prolong the action of local anesthetics with great success. Braun developed several new nerve blocks, coined the term *conduction anesthesia*, and is remembered by European writers as the "father of conduction anesthesia." Braun was the first person to use procaine, which, along with stovaine, was one of the first synthetic local anesthetics produced to reduce the toxicity of cocaine. Further advances in spinal anesthesia followed the introduction of these and other synthetic local anesthetics.

Before 1907, several anesthesiologists had been disappointed to observe that their nerve blocks were incomplete. Most believed that the drug spread solely by local diffusion before incomplete nerve blocks were investigated by Arthur Barker, a London surgeon.[21] Barker constructed a glass tube shaped to follow the curves of the human spine and used it to demonstrate the limited spread of colored solutions that he had injected through a T-piece in the lumbar region. Barker applied this observation to use solutions of stovaine made hyperbaric by the addition of 5% glucose, which worked in a more predictable fashion. After the injection was complete, Barker placed his patient's head on pillows to contain the anesthetic below the nipple line. Lincoln Sise acknowledged Barker's work in 1935 when he introduced the use of hyperbaric solutions of pontocaine. John Adriani advanced the concept further in 1946 when he used a hyperbaric solution to produce "saddle block" or perineal anesthesia. Adriani's patients were obliged to remain in the seated position for almost a minute after injection while the drug descended to bathe the sacral nerves.

Tait, Jonnesco, and other early masters of spinal anesthesia used a cervical approach for thyroidectomy and thoracic procedures, but this radical approach was supplanted in 1928 by the lumbar injection of hypobaric solutions of "light" nupercaine by G. P. Pitkin in America and E. Etherington-Wilson of Britain 5 years later. Although hypobaric solutions are now virtually limited to patients in the jackknife position, their former use for thoracic procedures demanded skill and precise timing. The enthusiasts of hypobaric anesthesia devised formulas to attempt to predict the time in seconds needed for a warmed solution of hypobaric nupercaine to spread in patients of varying size from its site of injection in the lumbar area to the level of the fourth thoracic dermatome. At this time, the patient was suddenly tipped head down so that the drug would not involve the innervation of the diaphragm and larynx. Among the accepted risks of the hypobaric technique was a prompt and total sympathetic blockade, which occurred so predictably that wise clinicians advised their residents, "Don't bother taking the blood pressure! I know that it will be down." Even the most expert practitioners of this now-abandoned approach identified some limitations. Etherington-Wilson observed that cranial surgery under spinal anesthesia should be left in the hands of an expert.

The recurring problem of inadequate duration of single-injection spinal anesthesia led a Philadelphia surgeon, William Lemmon, to report an apparatus for continuous spinal anesthesia in 1940.[22] Lemmon's procedure began with the patient in the lateral position. The spinal tap was performed with a malleable silver needle, which was left in position. As the patient was turned supine, the needle was positioned through a hole in the mattress and table. Additional injections of local anesthetic could be performed as required. Lemmon's malleable silver needles also found a less cumbersome and more common application in 1942 when Waldo Edwards and Robert Hingson encouraged the use of Lemmon's needles for continuous caudal anesthesia in obstetrics.

After his military service, the Mayo Clinic's Edward

Tuohy introduced two important modifications of the continuous spinal technique. He developed the now-familiar Tuohy needle as a means of improving the ease of passage of lacquered silk ureteral catheters through which he injected incremental doses of local anesthetic.[23] In 1949, Martinez Curbelo of Havana, Cuba, used Tuohy's needle and a ureteral catheter to perform the first continuous epidural anesthetic. Silk and gum elastic ureteral catheters were difficult to sterilize and sometimes caused infections before they were superseded by disposable plastic catheters.

Epidural Anesthesia

Deliberate single-injection peridural anesthesia had been practiced occasionally for decades before continuous techniques brought it greater popularity. At the beginning of the 20th century, two French clinicians experimented independently with caudal anesthesia. The neurologist, Jean Athanase Sicard, applied the technique for a nonsurgical purpose, the relief of back pain. Fernand Cathelin used caudal anesthesia as a less dangerous alternative to spinal anesthesia for hernia repairs. He wrote a thesis on epidural anesthesia in which he demonstrated the upper limit of the epidural space in the neck of a dog after injecting a solution of India ink into its caudal canal.

The lumbar approach was first used for multiple paravertebral nerve blocks before the Pagés-Dogliotti single-injection technique became accepted. The technique is identified with both men, as they worked separately. Captain Fidel Pagés prepared an elegant demonstration of segmental single-injection peridural anesthesia in 1921, but his paper appeared only in a Spanish military journal.[24] Pagés died in the line of duty before he could prepare additional reports. Ten years later, Achille M. Dogliotti of Turin, Italy, wrote a classic study that made the epidural technique well known.[25] Whereas Pagés used a tactile approach to identify the epidural space, Dogliotti identified it by the loss-of-resistance technique still taught today.

Nerve Block of the Extremities

Surgery on the extremities lent itself to other regional anesthesia techniques. At first, they were often combined with general anesthesia. In 1902, Harvey Cushing coined the phrase "regional anesthesia" for his technique of blocking either the brachial or sciatic plexus under direct vision during general anesthesia in order to reduce anesthesia requirements and provide postoperative pain relief.[26] Fifteen years before his publication, a similar approach had been energetically advanced to reduce the stress and shock of surgery by George Crile, who was another dedicated advocate of the use of regional and infiltration techniques during general anesthesia.

An intravenous technique of applying procaine peripherally was described in 1908 by August Bier, the surgeon who had pioneered spinal blockade. Bier injected procaine into a vein of the upper limb between two tourniquets. Even though the technique is termed the Bier block, it was not used for many decades until it was reintroduced 55 years later by Mackinnon Holmes, who modified the technique by exsanguination before applying a single cuff. Holmes used lidocaine, the very successful amide local anesthetic synthesized in 1943 by Lofgren and Lundquist of Sweden.

Several investigators achieved upper extremity anesthesia by percutaneous injections of the brachial plexus. In 1911, based on his intimate knowledge of the anatomy of the axillary area, Hirschel promoted a "blind" axillary injection. In the same year, Kulenkampff described a supraclavicular approach in which the operator sought out paresthesias of the plexus while keeping the needle at a point superficial to the first rib and the pleura. The risk of pneumothorax with Kulenkampff's approach led Mulley to attempt blocks more proximally by a lateral paravertebral approach, the precursor of what is now popularly known as the Winnie block. An excellent historic review of brachial plexus anesthesia is presented in Alon Winnie's text, Plexus Anesthesia.

Textbooks of Regional Anesthesia

Heinrich Braun wrote the earliest text of local anesthesia, which appeared in its first English translation in 1914. Although many books appeared in the next decade, one text dominated the American market for 20 years after 1922. This classic was Gaston Labat's Regional Anesthesia. When Labat arrived from France to begin a brief period of service as a surgeon with a special interest in regional anesthesia at the Mayo Clinic, he was already familiar with writing on the subject, as he had served as a coeditor of Pauchet's French text on regional anesthesia. Labat soon took a permanent position at the Bellevue Hospital in New York, where he worked with Hippolite Wertheim and an eager younger anesthesiologist from the University of Wisconsin, Emery Rovenstine. They formed the first American Society for Regional Anesthesia. Rovenstine developed the first American clinic for the treatment of chronic pain. He and his associates refined techniques of therapeutic injections for the relief of pain, an important component in the treatment provided in a modern pain clinic.

The development of the multidisciplinary pain clinic was one of the many contributions to anesthesiology made by John J. Bonica, a renowned teacher of regional techniques. During his periods of military, civilian, and university service, John Bonica formulated a series of improvements in the management of patients with chronic pain. His classic 1500-page text, The Management of Pain, now in its second edition, is regarded as a classic of the literature of anesthesia. Bonica was also a pioneer in the development of obstetric anesthesia. He served with extraordinary dedication to establish, almost single-handedly, 24-hour coverage for the obstetric patients of his hospital. When he wrote a text of obstetric anesthesia, it was not only directed to practitioners serving in well-equipped institutions but was also designed to help anesthesiologists serving in the less-privileged countries. As the first American President of the World Federation of Societies of Anaesthesiologists, Bonica received honors from the professional societies of many nations for his advancement of regional and obstetric anesthesia in all countries.

ANESTHESIA EQUIPMENT

The Anesthesia Machine

During the past few decades, the anesthesia machine has grown to become one of the most imposing objects in the operating room. Physicians who practiced anesthesia with just a "rag and bottle" would be amazed to observe modern techniques in which fresh gas flows are metered precisely before a predetermined fraction is diverted through a calibrated vaporizer. The gas and vapor mixture then enters a circuit where it may be humidified and warmed en route to the patient. Ventilators permit the mechanical control of respiration. Automated monitors continuously flash numeric and oscilloscopic signals to reflect the well-being of the patient and the performance of the apparatus. A deviation in any of several monitored variables may excite a strident alarm.

Modern medical practice demands that the patient be attended in a well-equipped surgical suite. In the 19th century, however, medical services were often provided in the patient's home. With the exception of the devices created by John Snow, Joseph Clover, Edmund Andrews, Paul Bert, and a few others, almost every early practitioner carried his simple pieces of equipment in a coat pocket, and, if a manufactured mask was not available, they learned to fabricate a substitute from household objects such as a towel, a newspaper, or a Derby hat. At that time, patient monitoring was limited to the observation of physical signs. Since chloroform was known to be hazardous in excessive concentrations, a series of cunningly contrived chloroform inhalers were used in Britain and Europe after 1867. After 1870, a few practitioners favored the use of tiny metal containers of compressed nitrous oxide and oxygen, but the application of the technique was limited by the cost of renting the cylinders and purchasing the gases. The cylinders had originally been designed to receive illuminating gas for theatrical companies, who created a spotlight, the "limelight," by directing the light of a flame through a cylinder of lime. Early anesthetists followed the practice of theatrical personnel, who had to have both hands free to direct the spotlight by placing the cylinders on the floor and controlling flow by simple foot-operated valves. Anesthesiologists did not have multistaged reducing valves, so the gas escaped at cylinder pressure to be collected in a reservoir bag from which the patient breathed.

Late in the 19th century free-standing anesthesia machines were manufactured in America and in Europe. Three American dentist-entrepreneurs, Samuel S. White, Charles Teter, and Jay Heidbrink, developed the first series of American instruments to use compressed cylinders of nitrous oxide and oxygen. Before 1900 the S. S. White Company modified Hewitt's apparatus and marketed its continuous-flow machine, which was refined by Teter in 1903. Heidbrink added reducing valves in 1912. In the same year other important developments were initiated by physicians. Water-bubble flow meters, introduced by Frederick Cotton and Walter Boothby of Harvard University, allowed the proportion of gases and their flow rate to be approximated. The Cotton and Boothby apparatus was transformed into a practical portable machine by James Tayloe Gwathmey of New York, who demonstrated it at a 1912 Medical Congress in London. The Gwathmey machine caught the attention of a London anaesthetist, Henry E. G. "Cockie" Boyle, who acknowledged his debt to the American when he incorporated Gwathmey's concepts in the first of the series of "Boyle" machines that were marketed by Coxeter and British Oxygen Corporation. During the same period in Lubeck, Germany, Heinrich Draeger and his son, Bernhaard, adapted compressed gas technology, which they had originally developed for mine rescue apparatus, to manufacture ether and chloroform-oxygen machines.

In the years after World War I, several American manufacturers continued to bring forward widely admired anesthesia machines. Some companies were founded by dentists, including Heidbrink and Teter. Karl Connell and Elmer Gatch were surgeons. Richard von Foregger was an engineer who was very receptive to clinicians' suggestions for additional features of his machines. Elmer McKesson became one of the country's first specialists in anesthesiology in 1910 and developed a series of gas machines. In an era of inflammable anesthetics, McKesson carried nonflammable nitrous oxide anesthesia to its therapeutic limit by performing inductions with 100% nitrous oxide and thereafter adding small volumes of oxygen. If the resultant cyanosis became too profound, McKesson depressed a valve on his machine that flushed a small volume of oxygen into the circuit. Even though his techniques of primary and secondary saturation with nitrous oxide are no longer used, the oxygen flush valve is part of McKesson's legacy.

The machines reflected the practices and dogma of the times in which they were designed. For many years a Yale physiologist, Yandell Henderson, argued that hypocapnia produced shock in the anesthetized patient, while hypercapnia was beneficial. As a consequence of Henderson's advocacy of elevated arterial concentrations of carbon dioxide, many early machines were designed to promote rebreathing and were often equipped with accessory cylinders of carbon dioxide.

Carbon Dioxide Absorbers

The first use of carbon dioxide absorbers in anesthesia came in 1906 from the work of Franz Kuhn, a German surgeon. His use of cannisters developed for mine rescues by Draeger was a bold innovation, but his circuit had unfortunate limitations: exceptionally narrow breathing tubes and a large dead space, which might explain its very limited use. The device was ignored. A few years later, the first American machine with a carbon dioxide absorber was independently fabricated by Dennis Jackson.

While working as a physiologist and pharmacologist in St. Louis, Missouri, in 1915, Dennis Jackson (1878–1979) developed an early technique of carbon dioxide absorption that permitted the use of a closed anesthesia circuit. His laboratory was located in an area heavily laden with coal smoke; Jackson reported that the apparatus allowed him the first breaths of absolutely fresh air he had ever enjoyed in St. Louis. He used solutions of sodium and calcium hydroxide to absorb carbon dioxide. The complexity of the apparatus limited its use in hospital practice, but his pioneering work in this field encouraged Ralph Waters to introduce a simpler device using soda lime granules 9 years later.

Ralph Waters (1882–1979) positioned a soda lime cannister between a face mask and an adjacent breathing bag to which was attached the fresh gas flow. As long as the mask was held against the face, only small volumes of fresh gas flow were required and no valves were needed.

When Waters made his first "to-and-fro" device, he was attempting to develop a specialist practice in anesthesia in Sioux City, Iowa, and was achieving only limited financial success. Waters believed that his device had advantages for both the clinician and the patient.[27] Economy of operation was an important advance at a time when private patients and insurance companies were reluctant to pay not only for professional services but even for the drugs and supplies that had been purchased by the anesthesiologist. Waters estimated that his new cannister would reduce his costs for gases and soda lime to less than $.50 per hour. Waters's apparatus was very portable. The cannister was easy to carry to the patient's home and, in any setting, prevented the pollution of the operating environment with the malodorous vapors of the anesthetics then used. His report recognized other advantages. The patient's body heat was conserved. The inspired gases were automatically humidified.

Finally, he stated that his clinical observations showed that there was no need for carbon dioxide rebreathing as advocated by Yandell Henderson.

An awkward element of Waters's device was the position of the cannister by the patient's face. Brian Sword overcame this limitation in 1930 with a circle system that featured unidirectional valves and an in-circuit carbon dioxide absorber (Fig. 1-6).[28] The circle system popularized by Sword nearly 60 years ago remains the most common North American anesthesia circuit.

Concern over the resistance to gas flow within the circuit caused by sticking inspiratory and expiratory valves led to modifications of equipment in Canada and Britain. Daniel Revell of Victoria, British Columbia, introduced the Revell Circulator, whose spinning blades kept the gases moving continuously around the circle system at a rate that eliminated valve-induced resistance to respiration.[29]

A second valveless device, the Ayre T-piece has found wide application in the management of intubated patients. Phillip Ayre practiced anesthesia when the limitations of equipment for pediatric patients produced what he termed "a protracted and sanguine battle between surgeon and anaesthetist with the poor unfortunate baby as the battlefield."[30] In 1937, Ayre introduced his valveless T-piece to reduce the effort of breathing in neurosurgical patients, but the T-piece found a much broader application in cleft palate repairs. This ingenious, lightweight, valveless, nonrebreathing method has passed through more than 100 modifications for a variety of special situations. A significant alteration was Gordon Jackson Rees's modification, which permitted improved control of ventilation by substituting a breathing bag on the outflow limb for the simple expiratory tube of the original T-piece that was periodically obstructed by the anesthesiologist's thumb to produce inspiration at what could be an erratic rate.[31]

Another method to reduce the amount of equipment near the patient is that provided by the coaxial circuit of the Bain-Spoerel apparatus.[32] This lightweight tube-within-a-tube has served very well in many circumstances since its Canadian innovators at the University of Western Ontario described it in 1972, but, as in other situations, the Bain-Spoerel circuit has not been the first application of coaxial circuitry in anesthesia. Some late 19th century inhalers, including Hewitt's 1890 chloroform apparatus, used a tube-within-a-tube to lead air into the vaporizer and then back within a smaller tube to the patient.

A second precursor of the modern coaxial circuit was that developed during World War II by Richard Salt and Edgar Pask for tests undertaken by the Royal Air Force of different types of life jackets. This work was prompted by the loss of airmen who had "ditched" without injury in the waters off England and whose drowned bodies were discovered face down, even though they were wearing a life jacket. Their flotation devices had failed to hold their faces above water once they lost consciousness from hypothermia. In order to mimic the motions of an unconscious person, Dr. Pask was given ether anesthesia while intubated, then placed in a swimming pool while wearing one of a series of experimental jackets. While the breathing circuit was several yards in length, its coaxial construction prevented rebreathing. Even if the jacket failed and his body sank, the coaxial circuit continued to perform safely as the expiratory valve was above water at the level of the anesthesia machine. Once the Pask-Salt experiments were completed, the coaxial circuit passed from use until other applications in clinical anesthesia were recognized by Drs. Bain and Spoerel.

Flow Meters

As closed and semiclosed circuit anesthesia became practical, there was a need to measure gas flow with greater accuracy. Wet flow meters were replaced with dry bobbins and ball-bearing flow meters, which, although they did not leak or spill, could cause inaccurate measurements if they adhered to the wall of the surrounding glass column. In 1910 M. Neu had been the first to apply rotameters in anesthesia for the administration of nitrous oxide and oxygen, but his machine was not a commercial success, perhaps because of the great cost of nitrous oxide in Germany at that time. Rotameters designed for use in German industry were first employed in 1937 by Richard Salt in Britain, but, as World War II approached, the Englishman was denied access to these sophisticated flow meters. After World War II rotameters became a standard of British anesthesia machines, while most American equipment still feature nonrotating floats. Metrication of gas flow in liters per minute was not uniformly displayed on all American machines until more than a decade after World War II. Many anesthesiologists still in practice learned to calculate gas flows in gallons per hour.

Vaporizers

Uncalibrated glass vaporizers could be used with confidence for the administration of ether but were inadequate for more potent agents. Skilled practitioners gave ethyl chlo-

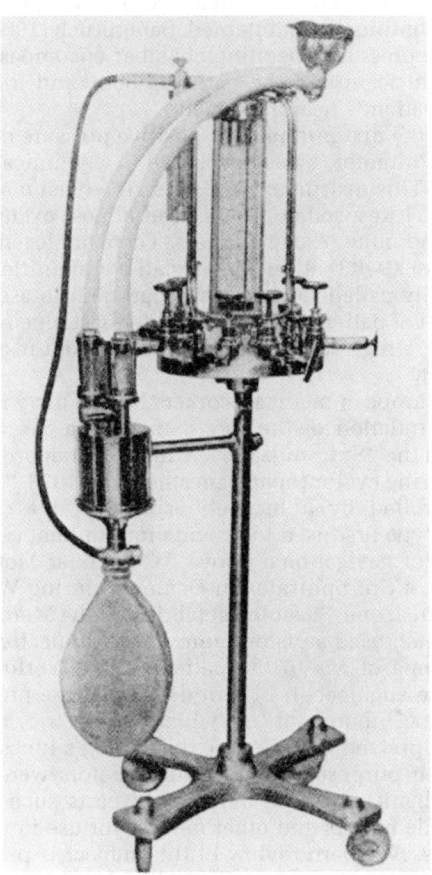

Figure 1-6. Brian Sword's closed circle anesthesia machine (1930).

ride and chloroform with safety, but their success was built upon their clinical expertise. Their approach was based primarily on subjective observations that were difficult to communicate to neophytes. When the inspired concentration of a potent anesthetic was unknown, the art of a smooth induction was a greater challenge.

This was particularly true for halothane; an excessive rate of administration produced lethal degrees of cardiovascular depression. The clinical introduction of halothane after 1956 might have been thwarted except for a fortunate coincidence: the prior development of calibrated vaporizers. Two types of calibrated vaporizers designed for the administration of other anesthetics had become available in the half decade before halothane was marketed. The initial prompt acceptance of the drug was in part due to the clinician's ability to provide it in carefully titrated concentrations.

The first of these was the copper kettle vaporizer, which had been developed by Lucien Morris at the University of Wisconsin in response to Ralph Waters's desire to give chloroform in carefully controlled concentrations.[33] Morris achieved this by passing a metered flow of oxygen through a vaporizer chamber that contained a porex disk to separate the oxygen into tiny bubbles, which became fully saturated with anesthetic vapor as they percolated through the liquid. The concentration of the anesthetic inspired by the patient could be easily calculated through knowledge of the vapor pressure of the anesthetic, the gas flow through the vaporizer, and the total volume of gas from all sources entering the anesthesia circuit. Although experimental models of Morris's vaporizer used a water bath to maintain stability, the excellent thermal conductivity of copper was substituted in later models to maintain a more stable vapor pressure—a suggestion that Dr. Morris recognized was first proposed by John Snow in January 1847. When first marketed, the copper kettle did not feature a thermometer to indicate changes in the temperature (and vapor pressure) of the liquid. Shuh-Hsun Ngai proposed the addition of a thermometer, a suggestion that was later incorporated in all vaporizers of that class.

Copper kettle (Foregger Company) and Vernitrol (Ohio Medical Products) vaporizers were universal vaporizers—a property that remained a distinct advantage as newer anesthetics were marketed. They could be charged with any anesthetic liquid, and, provided that the vapor pressure and temperature were known, the inspired concentration could be calculated quickly and with confidence. This feature gave an advantage to American investigators of newer anesthetics, for they were not dependent on the construction of an agent-specific vaporizer.

Halothane was first marketed in Britain, where an effective temperature-compensated, agent-specific vaporizer had recently been placed in clinical use. It had been developed for obstetric analgesia, as many women were delivered at home by midwives who needed a safe portable machine with which to give their patients an inhaled analgesic. The TECOTA (TEmperature COmpensated Trichloroethylene Air) vaporizer had been created by two engineers who had become frustrated by a giant corporation's unresponsiveness to their proposals and had set about starting a new company, Cyprane Limited. The TECOTA featured a bimetallic strip composed of brass and a nickel-steel alloy—two metals with different coefficients of expansion. As the anesthetic vapor cooled, the strip moved away from an orifice, thereby permitting more fresh gas to enter the vaporizing chamber. This maintained an unchanging inspired concentration of anesthetic despite changes in temperature and, as a consequence, vapor pressure. After their TECOTA vaporizer was accepted by the Central Midwives Board, their company soon gained a much greater success by adapting their technological advance to create the "Fluotec," the first of a series of agent-specific "tec" vaporizers for use in the operating room. All major manufacturers now offer a similar instrument.

Ventilators

Mechanical ventilators are now an integral part of the anesthesia machine. Patients are ventilated during general anesthesia by electrical or gas-powered devices that are simple to control yet sophisticated in their function. These now casually employed devices were created by men and women of many countries who were responding to a variety of clinical problems.

The history of mechanical positive pressure ventilation begins with attempts to resuscitate animals or humans by a pump or bellows attached to a mask or tracheal tube, but these experiments had no place in anesthetic care for many years. At the beginning of the 20th century, several other modalities were explored before intermittent positive pressure machines evolved.

One of these processes began as a result of the first thoracic surgeons being frustrated by the collapse of the lungs when they opened the pleura of spontaneously breathing patients. Between 1900 and 1910, sophisticated artificial environments were created in which the thoracic patient's lungs were kept in an inflated position by utilizing one of two ambitious alternatives: the positive and negative pressure techniques. Brauer (1904) and Murphy (1905) placed the patient's head and neck in a box in which positive pressure was continually maintained. Sauerbruch (1904) created a negative pressure operating chamber encompassing both the surgical team and the patient's body and from which only the patient's head projected.

In 1907 the first intermittent positive pressure device, the Draeger "Pulmotor," was developed to rhythmically inflate the lungs. This instrument and later American models such as the E & J Resuscitator were used almost exclusively by firemen and mine rescue workers. There are legends dating from before 1940 that, in some small communities, doctors occasionally called for the fire department to assist in the ventilation of patients who had suddenly stopped breathing in the operating room. Most hospitals lacked resuscitation equipment.

A few European medical workers had an early interest in rhythmic inflation of the lungs. In 1934 a Swedish team developed the "Spiropulsator," which C. Crafoord modified for use during cyclopropane anesthesia by 1938.[34] Its action was controlled by a magnetic control valve called the *flasher*, a type first used to provide intermittent gas flow for the lights of navigational buoys. When Trier Morch could not obtain a Spiropulsator in Denmark during World War II, this Danish anesthesiologist fabricated the Morch "Respirator," which used a piston pump to rhythmically deliver a fixed volume of gas to the patient. After World War II a motorcycle engineer in Britain developed the prototype of the Blease "Pulmoflator" in which an electric motor provided compressed air to inflate the patient's lungs. In those days, when purpose-built miniature motors were unavailable, mechanics adapted automotive parts such as windshield blade motors and other devices for use in their early ventilators. A superb review of this subject is provided by William Mushin and Leslie Rendell-Baker in *Thoracic Anaesthesia Past and Present* (reprinted by The Wood Library Museum, 1991).

A major stimulus to the development of ventilators in Europe came in 1952 as a consequence of a devastating epidemic of poliomyelitis that struck Copenhagen, Denmark. The only effective therapy for bulbar paralysis that could be provided was manual ventilation by a tracheostomy with devices such as Waters's "to-and-fro" circuit, but this was successful only through the continuous efforts of scores of volunteers. Danish medical students served in relays to ventilate paralyzed patients. The Copenhagen crisis stimulated a broad European interest in the development of portable ventilators in anticipation of a time when poliomyelitis might strike again.

At this time, the practice in North American hospitals was to place polio patients with respiratory involvement in "iron lungs"—large metal cylinders that encased the body below the neck. Inspiration was caused by intermittent negative pressure created by an electric motor acting on a piston-like device occupying the foot of the chamber. After an epidemic, as many as 10 or 12 iron lungs might be operated in a single room.

One now-distinguished consultant recalls that he became irrevocably committed to the development of better ventilators as an intern when he found himself alone with a dozen patients in iron lungs at the moment of a power failure. Before help arrived, he was exhausted by repeated urgent circuit of the room as he manually pumped the lever of each iron lung for a few life-sustaining breaths. His frantic efforts were rewarded by his helpless patients, who whispered their appreciation, "Way . . . to go . . . Wally!" Then they lay apneic until he could once again give them another mechanical breath.

Many early American ventilators were adaptations of respiratory-assist machines originally designed for the delivery of aerosolized drugs for respiratory therapy. Two of these employed the Bennett and Bird "flow-sensitive" valves. The Bennett valve was designed during World War II when a team of physiologists at the University of Southern California encountered difficulties in separating inspiration from expiration in an experimental apparatus for positive pressure breathing designed for high-altitude aviators. An engineer, Ray Bennett, visited their laboratory, observed their problem, and resolved it with a mechanical flow-sensitive automatic valve. A second valving mechanism was later designed by an aeronautical engineer, Forrest Bird, whose Bird ventilators still find wide usage.

The use of the Bird and Bennett valves gained an anesthetic application when the gas flow from the valve was directed into a plastic or glass jar containing a breathing bag or bellows as part of an anesthesia circuit. These "bag-in-bottle" devices mimicked the action of the anesthesiologist's hand as the gas flow compressed the bag, providing positive pressure inspiration. Passive exhalation was promoted by the descent of a weight on the bag or bellows. The function of the components of some of the first machines to use these principles could be examined with ease through clear plastic, whereas now they are hidden in the interior of the instrument. It is currently possible to operate an anesthesia machine with a ventilator for years without becoming aware of the principles that direct its action and protect against malfunction.

Operating Room Monitors

The use of equipment to promote the safety of patients in the operating room has evolved since 1900. Early clinicians concentrated on physical signs—the patient's color, the briskness of capillary refill, the dilation and position of the pupil, the regularity and depth of respiration, as well as the force and regularity of the pulse. These signs were subjective and difficult to teach and required experience to interpret.

Two American surgeons, George W. Crile and Harvey Cushing, developed a strong interest in measuring blood pressure during anesthesia. Both men wrote thorough and detailed examinations of blood pressure monitoring; however, Cushing's contribution is better remembered because he was the first American to apply the Riva Rocci cuff, which he saw while visiting Italy. Cushing introduced the concept in 1902 and had blood pressure measurements recorded on anesthesia records.[26] These improved records were the successor to those that Cushing and a colleague at Harvard Medical School, Charles Codman, had first used in 1894 in their attempt to assess the course of the anesthetics they administered as students.

Anesthesiologists began to auscultate blood pressure after 1905 when Nicholai Korotkoff, a surgeon-in-training in St. Petersburg, Russia, gave an abbreviated report of the sounds that he heard distal to the Riva Rocci cuff as it was deflated. Although his one-paragraph account does not explain why he came to listen over a normal vessel—a novel approach now used universally for the clinical measurement of blood pressure—it may be that his commitment to vascular surgery caused him to auscultate vessels in the assessment of masses that might be vascular and would, therefore, produce a bruit. Perhaps he happened to have his stethoscope positioned over a vessel as a cuff was deflated and fortuitously heard sounds never appreciated before. Cuffs and stethoscopes are now often replaced by automated blood pressure devices, which first appeared in 1936 and which operate on an oscillometric principle. The recent development of inexpensive microprocessors has promoted the routine use of these automatic cuffs in clinical settings. A detailed review of other elements of cardiovascular monitoring can be found in Leslie Geddes's *Cardiovascular Devices and Their Applications*.

Anesthesiologists routinely auscultate breath and heart sounds with precordial or esophageal stethoscopes. The first precordial scope was believed to have been used by S. Griffith Davis at Johns Hopkins University.[35] He adapted a technique favored by Harvey Cushing in the animal laboratory in which dogs with surgically induced valvular lesions had stethoscopes attached to their chest wall so that medical students might listen to bruits characteristic of a specific malformation. Davis's technique was forgotten but was rehabilitated by Robert Smith, an energetic pediatric anesthesiologist in Boston. A Canadian contemporary, Albert Codesmith, of the Hospital for Sick Children, Toronto, soon became frustrated by the repeated dislodging of the chest piece under the surgical drapes and fabricated his first esophageal stethoscope from urethral catheters and Penrose drains. His brief report heralded its clinical role as a monitor of both normal and adventitious respiratory and cardiac sounds.[36] An additional benefit was that the stethoscope could serve as a monitor to protect against the risk of disconnection of the patient from the anesthesia circuit. The patient's survival could depend on an alert anesthesiologist's recognition of the sudden disappearance of breath sounds.

Anesthesia Machine Monitors

The introduction of safety features was coordinated by the American National Standards Institute (ANSI) Committee Z79, which was sponsored from 1956 until 1983 by the American Society of Anesthesiologists (ASA). Since 1983 representatives from industry, government agencies, and health care professions have met on Committee F29 of the American Society for Testing and Materials. They establish voluntary standards that become the accepted national standards for the safety of anesthesia equipment.

Ralph Tovell (1901–1967) led the way in urging standards during World War II while he was the Senior Army Consultant in Anesthesiology in Europe. Tovell found that supplies dispatched to field hospitals might not fit their anesthesia machines, since there were four different dimensions for connectors, tubes, masks, or breathing bags. As Tovell observed, "when a sudden need for accessory equipment arose, nurses and corpsmen were likely to respond to it by bringing parts that would not fit."[37] Although Tovell's reports did not gain an immediate response, two anesthesiologists, Vincent Collins and Hamilton Davis, took up his concern and formed the ANSI Committee Z79.

One of the Committee's most active members, Leslie Rendell-Baker, has prepared an interesting account of its domestic and international achievements.[38] Ralph Tovell, an early member, encouraged all manufacturers to select a uniform orifice of 22 mm for all adult and pediatric face masks and to make every endotracheal tube connector 15 mm in diameter so that the Z79-designed mask-tube elbow adapter would fit every mask and endotracheal tube connector. Through the tenacity of purpose and determination of ASA members on Committee Z79, the anxieties encountered by Tovell and his military colleagues of World War II have been overcome.

Several other advances were introduced by the Z79 Committee, including nontoxic tracheal tubes, which often bear a Z79 mark. The Committee also mandated touch identification of oxygen flow control at Calverley's suggestion, which reduced the risk of the wrong gas being selected before internal mechanical controls prevented the selection of an hypoxic mixture.[39] These devices were helpful only if the gas in the line was oxygen. Pin indexing reduced the hazard of attaching the wrong cylinder in the place of oxygen. Diameter indexing of connectors prevented similar errors. For many years, however, mistakes committed by plumbers or technicians in reassembling hospital oxygen supply lines led to a series of tragedies before polarographic oxygen analyzers were added to the inspiratory limb of the anesthesia circuit.

Patient Monitors

Safer machines only assured the clinician that an appropriate gas mixture was delivered to the patient. As the practice of anesthesia evolved from simply the administration of an anesthetic to the assumption of professional responsibility for the care of patients during and after surgery, other monitors were required that would give an early warning of hazardous conditions before the patient suffered irrevocable damage. Every anesthesiologist who has remained in practice during the past 30 years has witnessed a great series of advances in monitoring with the advent of clinically employable forms of electrocardiography (ECG), arterial blood gas analysis, mass spectrometry, computer-processed electroencephalography, and oximetry.

Electrocardiography

Electrocardiography became practical with Willem Einthoven's application of the string galvanometer in 1903. Within two decades, Thomas Lewis had described its role in the diagnosis of disturbances of cardiac rhythm, while James

Herrick and Harold Pardee had drawn attention to the changes produced by myocardial ischemia. After 1928, cathode ray oscilloscopes were available, but the risk of explosion owing to the presence of inflammable anesthetics forestalled the introduction of the ECG into routine anesthetic practice until after World War II. The tiny screen of the heavily shielded "bullet" oscilloscope displayed only 3 seconds of data, but that information came to be highly prized. In some hospitals, priorities were established to determine where the expensive monitor was to be used. When an assistant was dispatched to bring the "bullet" scope, everyone knew that a major anesthetic enterprise was about to begin.

Arterial Blood Gas Analysis

Before 1955, the estimation of the tension of gases of the blood was a delicate activity performed best by skilled research technicians who conducted their intricate art in laboratories far removed from the operating room. Within a few years, however, the contributions of Astrup, Siggaard-Anderson, Stow, Bradley, Severinghaus, and Clark brought radical improvements in patient care through the creation of rapidly responding electrodes. Time-consuming multistaged analyses gave way to instruments whose complex functions were automated to a degree that allowed them to be operated at any hour. Many practitioners recall the historic impact of arterial blood gas analysis on their professional practice as information of vital importance returned to the clinician within minutes.

The series of discoveries that led to the clinical application of arterial blood gas analysis have been brilliantly recounted in two volumes by Poul Astrup and John Severinghaus, *The History of Blood Gases, Acids and Bases* and its companion from the International Anesthesiology Clinics series, Volume 25, Number 4, *History of Blood Gas Analysis*. They report how the Danish poliomyelitis epidemic of 1952 was not only responsible for an increased interest in mechanical ventilation, but also stimulated research in arterial carbon dioxide tension measurements to determine the adequacy of manual and mechanical ventilation. Both books captivate the reader and should be enjoyed by all students of anesthesiology.

Mass Spectrometry

Although arterial blood gas determinations could be performed within minutes, anesthesiologists have recognized a need for breath by breath measurement of respiratory and anesthetic gases. After 1954, infrared absorption techniques gave immediate displays of the exhaled concentration of carbon dioxide. Clinicians quickly learned to relate abnormal concentrations of carbon dioxide to threatening situations such as the inappropriate placement of an endotracheal tube in the esophagus, abrupt alterations in pulmonary blood flow, and other factors. Infrared techniques have been supplanted by mass spectrometers that display not only carbon dioxide but also the inspired and expired concentrations of other gases and anesthetic vapors. Mass spectrometry had only industrial applications before Albert Faulconer of the Mayo Clinic first used it to monitor the concentration of an exhaled anesthetic in 1954.

Electroencephalography

Faulconer was also a pioneer in the use of the electroencephalograph (EEG) in anesthesia. In 1946 Faulconer and a colleague, John W. Pender, began to work with an exceptionally gifted neurologist, Reginald Bickford, in studies of the effects of a variety of anesthetics on the EEG.[40] They related changes in anesthetic depth to alterations in the pattern of the EEG tracing and even extended their observations to include the hyperbaric administration of nitrous oxide and oxygen. Immediate application of their observations was limited by the technology of that time, but, after moving to the University of California, San Diego, Bickford returned to his interest in anesthesia as a practical application of the computer-generated Compressed Spectral Array, which he had been instrumental in developing. Bickford maintains an active involvement in anesthetic applications of the processed EEG more than 40 years after he and his Mayo Clinic colleagues first took up this study.

Pulse Oximetry

The pulse oximeter is the most recent addition to the anesthesiologist's array of routine monitors. This application of the optical measurement of oxygen saturation in tissues has been, by John Severinghaus's assessment, of exceptional importance. In a fine history of pulse oximetry, Severinghaus states, "Pulse oximetry is arguably the most important technological advance ever made in monitoring the well-being and safety of patients during anesthesia, recovery, and critical care."[41]

Severinghaus wrote that although research in this area began in 1932, its first practical application came during World War II. An American physiologist, Glen Millikan, responded to a request from British colleagues in aviation research. Millikan set about preparing a series of devices to improve the supply of oxygen that was provided to pilots flying at high altitude in unpressurized aircraft. In order to monitor oxygen delivery and to prevent the pilot from succumbing to an unrecognized failure of the oxygen supply, Millikan created an oxygen-sensing monitor worn on the pilot's earlobe, and coined the name oximeter to describe its action. Before his tragic death in a climbing accident in 1947, Millikan had begun to assess anesthetic applications of oximetry.

For the next three decades, oximetry was rarely used by anesthesiologists, and then primarily in research studies such as those of Faulconer and Pender. Recent refinements of oximetry by a Japanese engineer, Takuo Aoyagi, led to a new departure, the development of pulse oximetry. As Severinghaus recounted the episode, Aoyagi had attempted to eliminate the changes in a signal caused by pulsatile variations when he realized that this fluctuation could be used to measure both the pulse and oxygen saturation. Severinghaus observed this was "a classic example of the adage that 'one man's noise is another man's signal'."[42]

Intubation in Anesthesia

All anesthesiologists are expected to be adept in the art of endotracheal intubation. They are assisted in this complex task by a variety of instruments that allow them to intubate the trachea of patients with severe anatomic abnormalities that would have been beyond the skill of all but the most expert (or fortunate) practitioner of past decades. The development of techniques and instruments for intubation ranks among the major advances in the history of the specialty. We are supported by a magnificent heritage of innovation and discovery that has come to us through the efforts of scores of persons, of whom only a few are remembered through the eponyms attached to the Guedel airway, Magill forceps, and Macintosh blade.

The landmark advances in intubation form a fascinating history filled with episodes of brilliant observation, forgotten or unappreciated invention, rediscovery, and clinical advance. When possible, the first discoverer of an instrument will be identified, but in other instances, the person who successfully brought it into regular use will receive greater attention. Although most of the achievements related to intubation have been realized in this century, a few date from Victorian times.

19th Century Intubation

The first endotracheal tubes were developed for the resuscitation of the newborn and victims of drowning but were not used in anesthesia until 1878. Although John Snow and others had already anesthetized patients by means of a tracheostomy, the first use of elective oral intubation for an anesthetic was undertaken by a Scottish surgeon, William Macewan. He had practiced passing flexible metal tubes through the larynx of a cadaver before attempting the maneuver on an awake patient with an oral tumor at the Glasgow Royal Infirmary, on July 5, 1878.[43] Since topical anesthesia was not yet known, the experience must have demanded fortitude on the part of Macewan's patient, because his airway was unanesthetized. Once the tube was correctly positioned, an assistant gave a chloroform anesthetic through the tube, and the patient soon stopped coughing. Macewan's interest in intubation of the trachea was only transient. Even though he performed successful awake intubations on at least two other patients with severe obstructions of the upper airway, one due to infection and the other to the too-rapid ingestion of a hot potato, he abandoned the practice following an unusual fatality. His last patient had been intubated while awake but had removed the tube before the anesthetic could begin. The patient later died while receiving chloroform by mask.

Joseph O'Dwyer (1841–1898). Although there was a sporadic interest in endotracheal anesthesia in Edinburgh and other European centers, a contemporary American surgeon is remembered for his extraordinary dedication to the advancement of tracheal intubation. Joseph O'Dwyer had witnessed the distressing death by asphyxiation of children with diphtheria and sought an alternative to the multilation of a hasty tracheotomy. In 1885, O'Dwyer designed a series of metal laryngeal tubes, which he inserted between the vocal cords of children during a diphtheretic crisis. His humanitarian efforts were applauded by colleagues. Three years later, O'Dwyer designed a second rigid tube with a conical tip that occluded the larynx so effectively that it could be used for artificial ventilation when applied with the bellows and T-piece tube of George Fell's apparatus.[44] The Fell-O'Dwyer apparatus was used during thoracic surgery by Rudolph Matas of New Orleans, who was so pleased with it that he predicted, "The procedure that promises the most benefit in preventing pulmonary collapse in operations on the chest is . . . the rhythmical maintenance of artificial respiration by a tube in the glottis directly connected with a bellows."[45] This principle would be occasionally rediscovered by other surgeons for several decades before Matas's prophetic description would become routine.

Franz Kuhn (1866–1929). After O'Dwyer's death, the outstanding pioneer of tracheal intubation was Franz Kuhn, a surgeon of Kassel, Germany. From 1900 until 1912, Kuhn wrote a series of fine papers and a classic monograph, "Die perorale Intubation," which were not well known in his lifetime but have since become widely appreciated.[46] Kuhn described techniques of oral and nasal intubation that he performed with flexible metal tubes similar to the coiled tubing often used for the spout of metal gasoline cans. Kuhn's tubes were introduced over a curved metal stylet and directed toward the larynx with his left index finger (Fig. 1-7). While he was aware of the subglottic cuffs that had been used briefly by Victor Eisenmenger, Franz Kuhn preferred to seal the larynx by positioning a supralaryngeal flange near the tube's tip before packing the pharynx with gauze. His writings reflect a mastery of intubation techniques unequaled for many years.

Kuhn's work might have had a much more immediate impact if it had been translated into English. Many of his principles were only appreciated after they had been rediscovered by others. His patients were made more comfortable through the use of topical cocaine, a practice that he was the first to use. He was among the first to recommend an inhalation technique through a large tube over the continuous insufflation of gases through narrow tubes that failed to protect the airway. He was the first to suggest that tracheal secretions or blood could be suctioned from the airway through a flexible catheter. He recommended the nasal route for long-term intubation, because a nasal tube was more easily tolerated and did not require a dental guard to prevent it from being crushed by the teeth of a restless patient. Kuhn even monitored the patient's breath sounds continuously through a monaural earpiece that was connected to an extension of the endotracheal tube by a narrow rubber tube.

Early Laryngoscopes

Intubation of the trachea by palpation was an uncertain and sometimes traumatic act. Even though the use of a mirror for indirect laryngoscopy antedated Macewan's intubations, the technique could not be adapted for use in anesthesia. For some years, many surgeons believed that it would be anatomically impossible to visualize the vocal cords di-

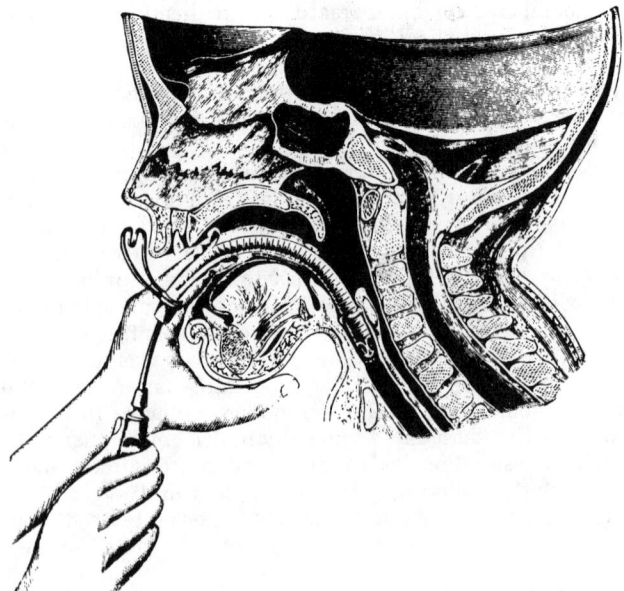

Figure 1-7. Kuhn's endotracheal tube. The tube and introducer were guided to the trachea by the fingers of the operator's left hand.

rectly. This misapprehension was overcome in 1895 by Alfred Kirstein in Berlin who devised the first direct-vision laryngoscope.[47] Kirstein was motivated by a friend's report that a patient's trachea had been accidentally intubated during esophagoscopy. Kirstein promptly fabricated a hand-held instrument that at first resembled a shortened cylindrical esophagoscope. He soon substituted a semicircular blade that opened inferiorly. Kirstein could now examine the larynx while standing behind his seated patient, whose head was placed in an attitude approximating the "sniffing position" later recommended by Ivan Magill. Although Alfred Kirstein's "autoscope" was not used by anesthesiologists, it was the forerunner of all modern laryngoscopes.

Endoscopy was refined by Chevalier Jackson in Philadelphia, who designed a U-shaped laryngoscope by adding a hand grip that was parallel to the blade. The Jackson blade has remained a standard instrument for endoscopists but was not favored by anesthesiologists. Two laryngoscopes that closely resembled modern L-shaped instruments were designed in 1910 and 1913 to facilitate intubation by two American surgeons, Henry Janeway and George Dorrance, but neither instrument achieved lasting use despite their excellent designs.

These clever innovations may have failed to capture wide attention because intubating laryngoscopes lacked a wide market at a time when there were fewer than 100 anesthesiologists active in the United States. Many of these practitioners had never attempted intubation and might never learn the skill. Even after 1940, it was routine in some hospitals to call a laryngologist to the operating room for every intubation while the attending anesthesiologists confined their attention to providing the anesthetic. In time, however, all anesthesiologists would learn the skills of atraumatic nasal and oral intubation by using the instruments and techniques developed by a few British and North American specialists.

Sir Ivan Magill (1888–1986). The most distinguished pioneer of endotracheal intubation was a self-trained British anaesthetist, Ivan (later Sir Ivan) Magill.[48] In 1919, when serving in the Royal Army as a general medical officer with no special interest in anesthesia, Magill was assigned to a military hospital near London that received large numbers of men with maxillofacial injuries. Although previously untrained in anesthesia, Magill accepted an assignment in the anesthesia service, where he was joined by another neophyte anaesthetist, Stanley Rowbotham.[49] They attended casualties disfigured by severe facial injuries who underwent repeated restorative operations that would be successful only if the surgeon, Harold Gillies, had almost unrestricted access to the face and airway. Some patients were formidable challenges, but both men became competent quickly and, because they were adept and able to appreciate the significance of fortuitous observations, soon extended the scope of early oral and nasal endotracheal anesthesia.

Magill's and Rowbotham's expertise with blind nasal intubation began after they learned to soften the semirigid insufflation tubes that they passed through the nose after the nostril had been dilated with a series of lubricated tubes. Even though they originally planned to position the tips of the tubes in the posterior pharynx only, the slender tubes sometimes passed directly into the trachea. Stimulated by these chance experiences, Magill developed techniques of deliberate nasotracheal intubation and, as an aid to manipulating the catheter tip, devised the Magill angulated forceps in 1920, which are still manufactured according to Magill's original design of 71 years ago.

They continued to practice anesthesia after they were released from military service. Some time later, Magill set out to develop a wide-bore tube that could be curved into a form resembling the contours of the upper airway but that would also resist kinking. In a hardware store he found several sizes of mineralized red rubber tubing which he cut, beveled, and smoothed to produce tubes that clinicians in all countries would come to call "Magill tubes." His tubes remained the standard for universal use for more than 40 years, until rubber products were replaced with inert plastics. Magill also rediscovered the advantages of cocainization of the airway, a technique that he perfected in developing his mastery of awake blind nasal intubation.

Magill's success in performing awake blind nasal intubation of the trachea excited the curiosity of other anesthetists. Magill shared his principles at meetings attended by the few specialists in anesthesia, but, since his colleagues were also his competitors for the limited private practice opportunities available in London, he sometimes omitted a pertinent point from his review. As a consequence, few members of his audience could match his success.

A few determined men visited Magill to study his craft. He carefully pointed out the advantages of a tube of the correct length and the appropriateness of the "sniffing position," which he described as placing the patient's head in the posture of a man standing before his open bedroom window sniffing the morning air. They marveled at his dexterity and speed at passing the tube, not always realizing that the patient had received topical cocaine before entering the induction area.

Magill soon allowed his small secrets to become public knowledge, but few colleagues ever matched his control of the airway until muscle relaxants were introduced. Throughout his distinguished and long career, he continued to create new devices, to the advantage of all concerned. His other innovations included endotracheal tubes with T-piece connectors for children, an L-shaped laryngoscope, a tracheoscope, and a wire-tipped endobronchial tube for thoracic surgery. The "Magill Circuit," now catalogued as the Mapleson A Circuit, was noted for its simplicity and economy. After a distinguished career, Magill was knighted for his services to anesthesiology. Until his death in his 99th year on November 28, 1986, Sir Ivan Magill was universally recognized as the master of British anesthesiology.

Arthur Guedel (1883–1956). Arthur Guedel's name is linked to the Guedel airway, but his classic device is only one of several important contributions made by this self-trained pioneer of American anesthesia.[50] The cuffed endotracheal tube is another reflection of his genius. In 1926, unaware of the prior work of Eisenmenger and Dorrance, Guedel began a series of experiments that would lead to the reintroduction of the cuffed tube. His goal was to combine the safety of endotracheal anesthesia with the economy of the closed-circuit technique, which had been recently refined by his friend, Ralph Waters.

Guedel transformed the basement of his Indianapolis home into a small laboratory, where he subjected each step of the preparation and application of his cuffs to a vigorous review.[51] He fashioned cuffs from the rubber of dental dams, condoms, and surgical gloves that were glued onto the outer wall of tubes. Using animal tracheas donated by the family butcher as his model, he considered whether the cuff should be positioned above, below, or at the level of the vocal cords. He recommended that the cuff be positioned just below the vocal cords. In that position, it not only sealed the airway and reduced the risk of the tube becoming dislodged but also prevented the accumulation of fluid below the cords but above the cuff, in a position where it might be impossible to remove by suctioning before extubation. Ralph Waters later recommended that cuffs be constructed of two layers of soft rubber cemented together along the edge so that a ruptured cuff might be readily replaced. The detachable cuffs were first manufactured by Waters's children, who earned money for college by selling the cuffs to the Foregger Company.

Guedel demonstrated the safety and utility of his cuff in his hospital. He filled the mouth of an anesthetized and intubated patient with water and showed that the cuff sealed the airway. Even though this exhibition was successful, he searched for a more dramatic technique to capture the attention of an audience unfamiliar with the advantages of intubation. He reasoned that if the cuff prevented water from entering the trachea of an intubated patient, it should also prevent an animal from drowning, even if it were to be submerged under water.

In order to encourage others to use endotracheal techniques, Guedel prepared the first of several "dunked dog" demonstrations (Fig. 1-8). An anesthetized and intubated

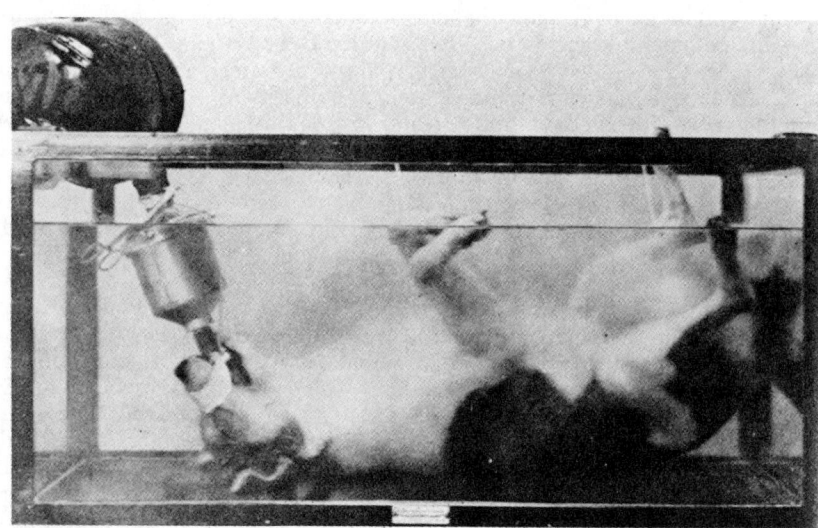

Figure 1-8. "The dunked dog." Arthur Guedel demonstrated the safety of endotracheal intubation with a cuffed tube by submerging his anesthetized pet, Airway, in an aquarium while the animal breathed an ethylene-oxygen anesthetic through an underwater Waters's "to and fro" anesthesia circuit.

dog, Guedel's own pet, Airway, was immersed in an aquarium. After the demonstration was completed, the anesthetic was discontinued and the animal removed from the water. Airway awoke promptly, shook water over the onlookers, then exited the hall to the applause of the audience. With this novel demonstration, the cuffed tube gradually gained wide use.

Endobronchial Tubes

Talented observers can recognize a therapeutic opportunity when presented with what at first appears to be only a complication. This principle was demonstrated in 1931 by an episode at the University of Wisconsin. After a patient experienced an accidental endobronchial intubation, Ralph Waters realized that a very long cuffed tube could be used to ventilate the dependent lung while the upper lung was being resected.[52] On learning of his friend's success with intentional one-lung anesthesia, Arthur Guedel proposed an important modification for chest surgery, the double-cuffed single-lumen tube, which was introduced by Emery Rovenstine. These tubes could be positioned easily, which was a definite advantage over the best-known alternative, bronchial blockers, which had to be inserted by a skilled bronchoscopist.

Following World War II, several double-cuffed single-lumen tubes were used for thoracic surgery, but after 1953, these were supplanted by double-lumen endobronchial tubes. The double-lumen tube that is currently used was designed by Frank Robertshaw of Manchester, England, and is prepared in both right- and left-sided versions. Robertshaw tubes were first manufactured from mineralized rubber but are now made of extruded plastic, a technique refined by David Sheridan. Sheridan was also the first person to embed centimeter markings along the side of all endotracheal tubes—a safety feature that has reduced the risk of the tip of the tube being incorrectly positioned within the trachea.

Miller and Macintosh Laryngoscopes

Early practitioners of tracheal intubation were frustrated by laryngoscopes that were cumbersome, were ill designed for prevention of dental injury, and offered only a very limited exposure of the larynx. Before the introduction of muscle relaxants, intubation of the trachea was often a severe challenge. It was in that period, however, that two blades were invented, that have become the classic models of the straight and curved laryngoscope. Robert Miller of San Antonio, Texas, and Robert Macintosh of Oxford University created blades that have maintained lasting popularity.

Both blades appeared within 2 years. In 1941, Miller brought forward a slender, predominantly straight blade with a slight curve near the tip to ease the passage of the tube through the larynx. Although Miller's blade was a refinement, the technique of its use was identical to that of earlier models, as the epiglottis was lifted to expose the larynx.[53] The Macintosh blade was unique in that the tip of the blade passed in front of the epiglottis.

The event that promoted the invention of the Macintosh blade was a routine tonsillectomy, an operation that was performed at that time without intubation. Years later, Sir Robert Macintosh wrote a note to describe the circumstances of its discovery in an appreciation of the career of Mr. Richard Salt, the Chief Technician of his department, who had constructed the blade. Sir Robert recalled, "A Boyle-Davis gag, a size larger than intended, was inserted

for tonsillectomy, and when the mouth was fully opened the cords came into view. This was a surprise since conventional laryngoscopy, at that depth of anaesthesia, would have been impossible in those pre-relaxant days. Within a matter of hours, Salt had modified the blade of the Davis gag and attached a laryngoscope handle to it; and streamlined, (after testing several models), the end result came into widespread use."[54] Sir Robert's observation of widespread use was an understatement; more than 800,000 Macintosh blades have been produced, and many special-purpose versions have been marketed.

The variations of the Macintosh blade are representative of the diversity of equipment now available for intubation of the trachea. Prisms and fiberoptic bundles provide anesthesiologists with images beyond the expectations of early masters of tracheal intubation. Multiple special-purpose plastic tubes have overcome the limitations of the metal and rubber products used two decades ago. Through the efforts of our predecessors, we have gained a vital skill—the ability to perform intubation of the trachea safely.

DRUGS IN ANESTHESIA

The Evolution of Inhaled Anesthetics

The first inhaled anesthetics were chemicals of simple preparation that had had prior application before their anesthetic action was discovered. Thoughout the second half of the 19th century, many compounds were examined for their anesthetic potential, but these random searches uniformly ended in failure. The pattern of fortuitous discovery that brought nitrous oxide, diethyl ether, and chloroform forward between 1844 and 1847 continued for decades. The next inhaled anesthetics to be used routinely, ethyl chloride and ethylene, were also discovered as a result of unexpected observations.

Ethyl chloride and ethylene were first formulated in the 18th century, and both had been tested as anesthetics in Germany soon after the discovery of ether's action but were then ignored for decades. Ethyl chloride retained some use as a topical anesthetic and counterirritant, because it was so volatile that the skin "froze" after ethyl chloride was sprayed on it. Its rediscovery came after 1894, when a Swedish dentist used this technique to "freeze" a dental abscess. Carlson was surprised to discover that his patient suddenly, but briefly, lost consciousness. Ethyl chloride became a commonly used inhaled anesthetic in several countries. Because of its rapid action, it remained in routine use and was particularly favored for pediatric inductions until approximately 1960, when its inflammability caused it to be banned from operating rooms.

The rediscovery of ethylene in 1923 also came from an unlikely observation. After it was learned that ethylene gas had been used in Chicago greenhouses to inhibit the opening of carnation buds, it was speculated that a gas that put flowers to sleep might also have an anesthetic action on humans. Arno Luckhardt was the first to publish a clinical report, in February 1923, but within a month two other independent studies were presented, by Isabella Herb in Chicago and W. Easson Brown in Toronto. Ethylene was not a very successful anesthetic because it was explosive. It also had a particularly unpleasant smell that, even though it could be partially disguised with the use of oil of orange or a cheap perfume, is still recalled with distaste by older patients and operating room personnel. A final limitation was its low potency. It had to be administered in high concentrations. Ethylene was abandoned 10 years later when cyclopropane was introduced.

There was even a fortuitous element in the discovery of cyclopropane's anesthetic action in 1929.[55] W. Easson Brown and Velyien Henderson had previously shown that propylene had desirable properties as an anesthetic when freshly prepared, but, after storage in a steel cylinder, it partially deteriorated to create a toxic material that produced nausea and cardiac irregularities in humans. Henderson, a professor of pharmacology at the University of Toronto, later suggested to a chemist, George Lucas, that the toxic product be identified. After Lucas found cyclopropane in the tank, the chemist prepared a sample, which he administered in a low concentration with oxygen to two kittens that had been placed in a bell jar. The animals fell asleep quietly and, after their removal from the chamber, recovered rapidly. The investigators saw that rather than being a toxic contaminant, cyclopropane was a very potent anesthetic. After its effects in other animals were studied and cyclopropane proved stable after storage, human experimentation began. Henderson was the first volunteer; George Lucas followed. They arranged a public demonstration in which Frederick Banting, already a Nobel laureate for his discovery of insulin, was anesthetized in the presence of a group of physicians. Despite this promising beginning, further research was abruptly halted for an illogical reason. It was argued that since there had been three anesthetic deaths in Toronto under ethyl chloride, no clinical trials of cyclopropane would be allowed despite its apparent safety. Rather than abandon the study, Velyien Henderson encouraged an American friend, Ralph Waters, to use cyclopropane at the University of Wisconsin. The Wisconsin group investigated the drug thoroughly and reported their clinical success in 1933. The slow pace of their studies was due to the extreme paucity of research funding during the Great Depression.

By coincidence, external interference also frustrated the clinical trials of the first anesthetic to be created deliberately from a pharmacologist's knowledge of structure-activity relationships. In 1930, Chauncey Leake and MeiYu Chen performed successful laboratory trials of vinethene (divinyl ether) but were thwarted in its further development by a professor of surgery at the University of California, San Francisco. Ironically, Canadians, who had lost cyclopropane to Wisconsin, learned of vinethene from Leake and Chen in California and conducted the first human study in 1932 at the University of Alberta, Edmonton.

All potent anesthetics of this period were explosive except for chloroform, whose hepatic and cardiac toxicity limited its use in America. Anesthetic explosions were a rare but devastating risk to both the anesthesiologist and the patient. To reduce the danger of explosion during the incendiary days of World War II, many British anesthesiologists turned to trichlorethylene, a noninflammable anesthetic of limited application; it decomposed to release phosgene when warmed in the presence of soda lime. By the end of that great conflict, the first of another class of noninflammable anesthetics was being prepared for laboratory trials. After another decade, fluorinated hydrocarbons would revolutionize inhalation anesthesia.

Fluorinated Anesthetics

Fluorine, the lightest and one of the more reactive halogens, produces exceptionally stable bonds that, although sometimes created with explosive force, resist separation by chemical or thermal means. For that reason, many early attempts to fluorinate hydrocarbons in a controlled manner were frustrated by the extreme chemical activity of fluorine. In 1930, the first commercial application of fluorine chemistry was made in the production of a refrigerant, Freon. This was followed by the first attempt to prepare a fluorinated anesthetic, by Harold Booth and E. May Bixby in 1932. Although their drug, monochlorodifluoromethane, was devoid of anesthetic action, as were all other drugs produced by other investigators during that decade, their report accurately forecast future developments; it began, "A survey of the properties of 166 known gases suggested that the best possibility of finding a new noncombustible anesthetic gas lay in the field of organic fluoride compounds. Fluorine substitution for other halogens lowers the boiling point, increases stability, and generally decreases toxicity."[56]

The secret demands of the Manhattan Project for refined uranium 235 were the next impetus to an improved understanding of fluorine chemistry. Researchers learned that the isotopes of uranium might be separated from uranium oxide through the creation of an intermediate compound, uranium hexafluoride. Part of this work was undertaken by Earl T. McBee of Purdue University, who had a long-standing interest in the fluorination of hydrocarbons. McBee also held a grant from the Mallinckrodt Chemical Works, a manufacturer of ether and cyclopropane, to prepare new fluorinated compounds, which were to be tested as anesthetics. By 1945, the Purdue team had created minute amounts of 46 fluorinated ethanes, propanes, butanes, and an ether.

The value of these chemicals might never have been appreciated, however, if Mallinckrodt had not also provided financial support for pharmacology research at Vanderbilt University. At that time, the Vanderbilt anesthesia department was unique in that its first chairman was a pharmacologist, Benjamin Robbins, who could assess the drugs more effectively than could any other anesthesiologist of that period. Robbins tested McBee's compounds in mice and selected the most promising for evaluation in dogs. Although none of these compounds found a place as an anesthetic, Robbins's conclusions on the effects of fluorination, bromination, and chlorination in his landmark report of 1946 encouraged later studies that would prove to be successful.[57]

A team at the University of Maryland under Professor of Pharmacology John C. Krantz, Jr investigated the anesthetic properties of dozens of hydrocarbons over a period of several years; only one hydrocarbon, ethyl–vinyl ether, entered clinical use in 1947. Because it was inflammable, Krantz requested that it be fluorinated. In response, Julius Shukys prepared several fluorinated analogues. One of these, trifluorethyl vinyl ether, or fluroxene, became the first fluorinated anesthetic. Fluroxene was marketed from 1954 until 1974. As the drug was marginally inflammable, fluroxene had already been supplanted by more potent agents when it was withdrawn as a consequence of the delayed discovery of the action of a metabolite that was toxic to lower animals. Fluroxene is important not only for its historic interest as the first fluorinated anesthetic but also as a reminder of the importance of the continual surveillance of a drug's action—a process in which all clinicians play a significant role each day.[58]

While American researchers were conducting a rather random search for new anesthetics, a British team of researchers was applying a more direct approach. In 1951, Charles Suckling, a chemist of Imperial Chemical Industries (ICI) who already had an expert understanding of fluorination, was asked to create a new anesthetic. Suckling began by asking anaesthetists to describe the properties of an ideal anesthetic; he learned from this inquiry that his search must consider several limiting factors, including the volatility, noninflammability, stability, and high potency of the compounds. Within 2 years, Charles Suckling created halothane. As a reflection of the degree of planning that he carried out beforehand, halothane, the most successful of all fluorinated anesthetics, was among the first six compounds synthesized.

The limited number of chemicals produced for testing reflected Suckling's expert knowledge of the pharmacology of halogens and his ability to appreciate important physical relationships that apply to all anesthetics. His achievement was an extension of a principle that had been recognized in 1939 by his superior, James Ferguson, which Ferguson later learned had first been considered by John Snow in 1848. The principle was to relate the opioid actions of known anesthetics along a thermodynamic scale—the ratio of the partial pressure producing anesthesia over the saturated vapor pressure of the drug at the temperature of the experiment. The resulting ratios fall within a very narrow range, as opposed to the more than 200-fold variations seen when anesthetics are graphed by the inspired concentration required for anesthesia.[59]

Suckling verified halothane's purity by the new technique of gas chromatography. He determined that it had an anesthetic action by reversibly anesthetizing meal worms and houseflies, and forwarded it to a pharmacologist, James Raventos, along with Suckling's accurate prediction, based on Ferguson's principles, of the concentration that would be required for anesthesia during testing in higher animals. After Raventos completed a favorable review, halothane was offered to Michael Johnstone, a respected anesthesiologist of the nearby city of Manchester, England, who recognized its great advantages over the other anesthetics available in 1956.

Halothane was followed in 1960 by methoxyflurane, an anesthetic that was popular until 1970. At that time, a rare dose-related nephrotoxicity following methoxyflurane anesthesia was found to be due to the action of inorganic fluoride, a metabolite released by the enzymatic cleavage of a monofluoro carbon bond. As a consequence of that observation and a persisting concern that rare cases of hepatitis following anesthesia might be due to a metabolite of halothane, the search for newer inhaled anesthetics focused on the stability of the molecule and its resistance to metabolic degradation.

Two fluorinated anesthetics more recently accepted for clinical use are enflurane and its isomer, isoflurane, which were synthesized by Ross Terrell in 1963 and 1965, respectively. Because enflurane was much easier to manufacture, it preceded isoflurane, but its applications were restricted after it was shown to be a marked cardiovascular depressant and to have convulsant properties in some situations. Isoflurane was nearly abandoned because of difficulties in its purification, but after this problem was overcome by Louise Speers, a series of successful trials was published in 1971. The release of isoflurane for clinical use was delayed for more than half a decade by calls for increased testing in lower animals, owing to an inappropriately raised concern that the drug might be a carcinogen. As a consequence, isoflurane was more thoroughly assessed before being offered to anesthesiologists than any other drug heretofore used in anesthesia. The era when an anesthetic could be introduced following a single fortuitous observation has given way to a cautious program of assessment and reassessment before a new drug such as desflurane can be used in routine practice.

Intravenous Anesthetics

Less than three decades after 1628, when William Harvey described the circulation of the blood, the first intravenous (iv) administration of a drug was undertaken by two leaders of 17th century science. In 1657, Sir Christopher Wren and his assistant, Robert Boyle, ligated a dog's vein, pierced it with a quill, and infused an opium-containing solution, which, they observed, caused the animal to become stuporous. Although they made no practical application of that observation, there is a fragmentary account that 8 years later, Sigasmund Elsholtz made the first successful iv injection of opium into a patient with the goal of producing anesthesia. No further work was reported until the mid-19th century, when several inventors prepared hollow metal needles and glass syringes. Two decades later, a French surgeon, Pierre Cyprien Oré, experimented with iv injections of chloral hydrate in animals before initiating a small clinical series. He reported his work with great enthusiasm, but, because chloral hydrate caused prolonged unconsciousness, his technique was not followed by others. In 1909, a German, Ludwig Burkhardt, produced surgical anesthesia by injecting the volatile anesthetics, chloroform and ether, iv. Seven years later, Elisabeth Bredenfeld of Switzerland reported the use of iv morphine and scopolamine. These attempts failed to show a significant improvement over inhaled techniques. None of the drugs had an action that was both sufficiently prompt and abbreviated.

The first barbiturate, barbital, was synthesized in 1903 by Fischer and von Mering. Phenobarbital and all other immediate successors of barbital had very protracted action and, thus, found little use in anesthesia. After 1929, oral pentobarbital was used as a sedative before surgery, but when the drug was given in higher concentrations for its anesthetic effect, long periods of unconsciousness followed. The first short-acting oxybarbiturate was hexobarbital (Evipal), which was used clinically in 1932.

Hexobarbital was enthusiastically received in Britain and America because its abbreviated induction times were unrivaled by any other technique. A London anaesthetist, Ronald Jarman, found that it had a dramatic advantage over inhalation inductions for minor procedures. Jarman developed the "falling arm" sign of anesthesia, described by Terence Steen. Immediately before induction, the patient was instructed to raise one arm above him while Jarman injected hexobarbital into a vein of the opposite forearm. As soon as the upraised arm fell, indicating the onset of anesthesia, the surgeon was permitted to make the incision. Steen observed that the list of cases was completed at an astonishing pace. Although today this technique would be recognized as unsafe, it was welcomed in 1933. Patients were also pleased by barbiturate anesthesia, because the onset of its action was so abrupt that many patients awoke unable to believe they had been anesthetized.*

---

* Soon after Evipal was introduced, Robert Macintosh administered it to Sir William Morris, the manufacturer of the Morris Garages (MG) automobiles. Macintosh secured a result that later changed the course of anesthesia in Great Britain.[60] When Morris awoke, he glanced at his watch and inquired as to why the operation had been postponed. On learning that his surgery was completed, he was amazed by this "magic experience," which he contrasted with his vivid recollections of the terror of undergoing a mask induction as a child in a dentist's office. So impressed was Morris (later Viscount Nuffield) with the quality of anesthetic he had received that he insisted, over the objections of Oxford's medical establishment, on endowing a university department of anesthe-

Even though hexobarbital's prompt action had a dramatic effect on the conduct of anesthesia, it was soon replaced by two thiobarbiturates. In 1932, Donalee Tabern and Ernest H. Volwiler of the Abbott Company synthesized thiopental (Pentothal) and thiamylal (Surital). The sulfated barbiturates proved to be much more potent and rapid acting than their oxybarbiturate analogues. Thiopental was first given to a patient at the University of Wisconsin in March 1934, but the successful introduction of thiopental into anesthetic practice was due to the energy of John S. Lundy and his colleagues at the Mayo Clinic, who began their intense and protracted assessments of thiopental during June 1934.

When first introduced, thiopental was often given in repetitive increments as the primary anesthetic for protracted procedures. Its hazardous side-effects came to be appreciated over time. At first, its depression of respiration was sometimes monitored by the simple expedient of placing a wisp of cotton over the nose and observing its motion. Only a few skilled practitioners were prepared to pass an endotracheal tube if the patient stopped breathing. These men also realized that thiopental without supplementation did not suppress airway reflexes, and they therefore encouraged topical anesthesia of the airway beforehand. The cardiovascular depressant effects were appreciated only later. When the powerful vasodilating effect of thiopental caused a series of fatalities among hypovolemic military casualties in the early stages of World War II, fluid replacement came to be used more aggressively, whereas thiopental was given with greater caution.

Muscle Relaxants

Many anesthesiologists regard the introduction of curare as the most important advance in anesthesia since the discovery of ether's action in 1846. Men and women who practiced without muscle relaxants recall the terror they felt when a premature attempt to intubate the trachea under cyclopropane caused persisting laryngospasm. Before 1942, abdominal relaxation was possible only if the patient tolerated high concentrations of an inhaled anesthetic, which might lead to immediate and persisting problems, a profound respiratory depression, and a protracted recovery.

Curare and the drugs that followed it transformed anesthesia profoundly. Before this time, endotracheal anesthesia was an art reserved for the expert; now it became a skill that all anesthesiologists could acquire. Intubation of the trachea could be taught in a deliberate manner, as the neophyte could fail on a first attempt without placing the patient in a hazardous situation. Abdominal relaxation could be attained with light planes of anesthesia induced by inhaled agents or by a combination of iv agents providing "balanced anesthesia." The sedated and paralyzed patient could now undergo the major physiologic trespasses of cardiopulmo-

nary bypass and deliberate hypothermia, or might receive long-term respiratory support after surgery.

The curares are alkaloids prepared from plants native to equatorial rainforests. The refinement of the harmless sap of several species of vines into toxins that were lethal only when injected was an extraordinary triumph introduced by paleopharmacologists in loincloths. Their discovery was the more remarkable, because it was independently repeated in South America, Africa, and Southeast Asia. These jungle tribesmen on three separate continents also achieved nearly identical methods of delivering the toxin by darts, which, after being dipped in curare, maintained their potency indefinitely until they were propelled through blowpipes to strike the flesh of monkeys and other animals of the treetops.

Europeans observed (and a few suffered) the actions of curare during explorations of South America. Some specimens of the drug were taken back to Europe. In 1780, the Abbe Felix Fontana determined that although curare had no action upon a nerve and spared the heart, it destroyed the irritability of voluntary muscles.[61] Early in the 19th century, the action of curare was examined by Squire Waterton, Francis Sibson, and Sir Benjamin Brodie in British experiments. They showed that animals injected with curare would recover unharmed if artificial ventilation were maintained. Waterton recognized that curare might have a role in the treatment of tetanus but did not have an opportunity to test his hypothesis. Seventy years after Fontana's study, Claude Bernard used curare to identify the neuromuscular junction. For the next 60 years, it was used only in the physiology laboratory, where animals were paralyzed, intubated, and ventilated.

Curare was first used in surgery in 1912, but the report was ignored for decades. Arthur Lawen, a physiologist/physician of Leipzig, had used curare in his laboratory before producing abdominal relaxation at a light level of anesthesia in a surgical patient. His report, written in German, was not appreciated for decades, nor could it have been until his fellow clinicians learned the skills of intubation of the trachea and controlled ventilation of the lungs.

Curare remained a curiosity of laboratory practice. In 1938, Richard and Ruth Gill returned to New York from South America with 11.9 kg of crude curare they had collected near their Ecuadorian ranch for the Merck Company. The Gills' motivation for this unusual expedition was a mixture of personal and altruistic goals. Some months before, while on a visit to the United States from Ecuador, Richard Gill had been told by Dr. Walter Freeman that he had multiple sclerosis. Freeman mentioned that curare could have a therapeutic role in the management of spastic disorders. When the Gills returned to America with a large supply of crude curare, they were initially disappointed to learn that Merck's researchers had lost interest, but they were later able to share some of it with E. R. Squibb & Co. The pharmaceutical company offered a semirefined curare to two groups of American anesthesiologists, who assessed its action but soon abandoned their studies when it caused total respiratory paralysis in two patients and the death of laboratory animals.

Curare entered clinical medicine through the actions of midwestern psychiatrists. In 1939 A. R. McIntyre refined a portion of Gill's curare. A. E. Bennett of Omaha, Nebraska, first injected it into children with spastic disorders and, after observing no persisting benefit, next gave it to psychiatric patients about to receive Metrazol, a shock treatment that was a precursor to electroconvulsive therapy. Curare

sia for the university as a precondition of his support for a postgraduate medical center.

In 1937, Sir Robert Macintosh became Oxford's first professor of anesthesiology and led the growth of the first university department in Europe from the first fully endowed Chair of Anaesthesia in the world. Fifty years later, on July 24, 1987, when the Nuffield Department of Anaesthetics celebrated its Golden Jubilee, Sir Robert greeted alumni who had returned from scores of countries. Morris's "magic experience" of barbiturate anesthesia had led to a result beyond his imagining—the creation of one of the world's most distinguished anesthesia centers.

was termed a "shock absorber" because it eliminated seizure-induced fractures. By 1941, other groups of psychiatrists were following this practice and even used neostigmine as an occasional antidote when the action of curare was too protracted.

Some months later, Harold Griffith, the chief anaesthetist of the Montreal Homeopathic Hospital, learned of Bennett's successful use of curare and resolved to try it in anesthesia. Griffith was already a master of cyclopropane anesthesia and was among Canada's foremost pioneers of tracheal intubation. He was much better prepared than most of his contemporaries to attend to complications that might follow an excessive response. On January 23, 1942, Griffith and his resident, Enid Johnson, anesthetized and intubated the trachea of a young man before injecting curare early in the course of his appendectomy. Satisfactory abdominal relaxation was obtained as the surgery proceeded without incident. Griffith and Johnson's report of the successful use of curare in their series of 25 patients launched a great revolution in anesthetic care.[62]

The successful use of curare prompted several pharmacologic studies that led to the introduction of other nondepolarizing and depolarizing relaxants. Gallamine and decamethonium were synthesized by 1948. Metubine, a relaxant "rediscovered" in the past decade, was first used clinically in the same year. The most successful depolarizing relaxant, succinylcholine, was prepared by the Nobel laureate Daniel Bovet in 1949 and was in wide international use before historians noted that the drug was much older and that earlier investigators had not observed its primary action. In 1906, Hunt and Taveaux had prepared succinylcholine and other choline esters, which they had injected into rabbits to observe their effects on the heart. If the rabbits had not been paralyzed with curare, the depolarizing action of succinylcholine might have been known decades earlier.

Research in relaxants was rekindled in 1960, when researchers became aware of the action of maloetine, a relaxant from the Congo basin, which was remarkable in that it had a steroidal nucleus. Investigations of maloetine led to pancuronium and vecuronium. As these drugs have provided new avenues for investigation, the pace of research has accelerated.

Newer Drugs

During the first two decades following World War II, other classes of drugs were developed. Anesthesiologists learned a new vocabulary as words were coined to describe the actions of novel compounds. "Lytic cocktails," "dissociative anesthesia," and "neuroleptanalgesia" became common expressions. Intravenous mixtures concocted from a succession of analgesics and anxiolytics produced a state of euphoria, tranquility, and indifference when provided with care, or profound respiratory depression when presented carelessly. "Dissociative" anesthesia was a neologism invented in 1966 by Guenter Corrsen and Edward Domino to describe the trance-like state of profound analgesia produced by ketamine. "Neuroleptanalgesia" was pioneered by Juan de Castro, a Belgian anesthesiologist, who performed the first clinical investigations of many compounds synthesized under the direction of Paul Janssen.

Although many pharmacologists are remembered for the introduction of a single drug, since 1953 Paul Janssen has brought more than 60 agents forward from among 70,000 chemicals created in his laboratory. His products have had profound effects on disciplines as disparate as parasitology

and psychiatry. The pace of productive innovation in Janssen's research laboratory has been astonishing. Chemical R4263 (fentanyl), synthesized in 1960, was followed only a year later by R4749 (droperidol). Although the fixed combination (Innovar) in which they were introduced in America is now less popular, new relatives of fentanyl, such as sufentanil and alfentanil, are in common use.

THE EVOLUTION OF THE PROFESSIONAL ANESTHESIOLOGIST

The preceding segments of this survey have provided an overview of the evolution of many of the drugs, instruments, and techniques used in anesthesia. As this armamentarium began to expand at the beginning of the 20th century, a few men and women of vision recognized that a distinct body of knowledge was being created and sought to encourage its growth by forming organizations to foster their common interests. In time, regional societies grew to attract national and, in some cases, international representation. The charter members of these societies, most of whom were entirely self-trained, pressed for recognition of the need for formal training in anesthesiology at both the undergraduate and postgraduate levels. Ralph Waters and a few other anesthesiologists gained university posts, where they performed studies in collaboration with pharmacologists and physiologists. Their basic research extended the range of articles appearing in the first journals of anesthesia, which had begun publication after World War I. With the development of a body of knowledge unique to anesthesia and with the recognition of the talents of able physicians, anesthesiology slowly became recognized as a separate specialty in clinical practice and as an appropriate discipline for research. As a consequence, a separate organization that was granted powers to establish examinations for the specialty, the American Board of Anesthesiology, was formed in 1938. By 1991 over 20,000 anesthesiologists had been conferred "Board-certified" status.

The Beginnings of Specialization

One of the first physicians to declare himself a specialist in anesthesia was Sydney Ormond Goldan of New York, who published seven papers in 1900, including an early description of the use of cocaine for spinal anesthesia. After studying Goldan's early career, Raymond Fink recognized in him some of the qualities of many modern anesthesiologists: "He was brimful of enthusiasm for anesthesia, an excellent communicator and a prolific writer, a gadgeteer and the owner of several patents of anesthesia equipment."[63] At a time when some surgeons considered that spinal anesthesia did away with their need for an anesthesiologist, Goldan was particularly bold in his written opinions. He called for equality between surgeon and anesthesiologist and was among the first to state that the anesthesiologist had a right to establish and collect his own fee. Goldan regarded the anesthesiologist as being more important than the surgeon to the welfare of the patient. His forthright pronouncements may not have been well received, for he was not listed among the nine founding members of the Long Island Society of Anesthetists when the nation's first specialty society was founded on October 6, 1905, with annual dues of $1.00.

After 1911, the annual fee rose to $3.00 when the Long Island Society became the New York Society of Anesthetists. Although the new organization still carried a local title, it drew members from several states and, by 1915, had a membership of 70 physicians. A second society with roots in the Midwest merged in 1912 as the brief-lived American Association of Anesthetists, which, by 1915, became the Interstate Association of Anesthetists. Most of the approximately 100 professional anesthesiologists in America belonged to both medical societies.

Two years later, several specialists volunteered to serve with American forces in France. Major James T. Gwathmey, the highest ranking American anesthesiologist, taught his British counterparts the advantages of his anesthesia machine and, as the result of his service in France, gained an international audience for the first American text, Gwathmey and Baskerville's *Anesthesia*. Captain Arthur Guedel from Indianapolis gained the title of "the motorcycle anesthetist" because he dashed between hospitals to supervise orderlies and nurses whom he had trained to give anesthetics to the thousands of casualties evacuated from the war front.

Francis Hoeffer McMechan (1879–1939)

Accounts of the dramatic experiences of American, British, and Canadian military anesthesiologists were collected by a remarkable man, Dr. Francis Hoeffer McMechan, who reported them in the quarterly anesthesia supplements of the American Journal of Surgery, which he later republished as "The American Yearbook of Anesthesia and Analgesia." Francis McMechan had been a practicing anesthesiologist in Cincinnati until 1911, when he suffered a severe first attack of rheumatoid arthritis, which was to leave him confined to a wheelchair. Despite this limitation, McMechan, with the assistance of his devoted wife, Laurette, became a strong force in the development of anesthesia.[64] He supported himself through editing the Quarterly Supplement from 1914 until August 1922, when he became editor of the first journal devoted to anesthesia, "Current Researches in Anesthesia and Analgesia," the precursor of "Anesthesia and Analgesia," the oldest journal of the specialty. As well as fostering the organization of the International Anesthesia Research Society in 1925, Francis and Laurette McMechan became international ambassadors of American anesthesia. With Laurette's assistance, Dr. McMechan was able to travel and lecture in Britain, Europe, Cuba, Australia, and New Zealand before his death in 1939. After his passing, Ralph Waters wrote a fine appreciation of McMechan's contributions in a note entered on the inside cover of my copy of McMechan's first "American Yearbook of Anesthesia," "Frank McMechan revived anesthesia in America in the 20th century and left it for others to carry on."

Ralph M. Waters (1883–1979)

Ralph Waters ranks among the most respected founding fathers of academic anesthesiology.[65] After completing his internship in 1913, he entered medical practice in Sioux City, Iowa, and, because he liked to give anesthetics, gradually limited his practice until, by 1916, his work was completely limited to anesthesia. His personal experience and extensive reading were supplemented by the only postgraduate training available—a 1-month course conducted in Ohio by E. I. McKesson. At that time, the custom of becoming a self-proclaimed specialist in medicine and surgery was not uncommon. Ralph Waters, who was frustrated by low standards and who would eventually have a great influence on establishing both anesthesia residency training and the formal examination process, recalled that before 1920, "The

requirements for specialization in many midwestern hospitals consisted of the possession of sufficient audacity to attempt a procedure and persuasive power adequate to gain the consent of the patient or his family."[66]

In his effort to improve anesthetic care, Waters exchanged correspondence with Dennis Jackson and other scientists. He lectured regularly at medical meetings both before and after he moved to Kansas City in 1925 with the goal of gaining an academic post at the University of Kansas, but the department of surgery did not support his proposal. The larger city did allow him to expand his concept of the outpatient surgical facility, the "Downtown Surgical Clinic," which featured one of the first postanesthetic recovery rooms. He continued in private practice until 1927.

Erwin Schmidt, professor of surgery at the University of Wisconsin's new medical school, encouraged Dean Charles Bardeen to recruit Waters. In accepting the first American academic position in anesthesia, Waters described four objectives that have been adopted by all other academic departments. His goals were: "(1) to provide the best possible service to patients of the institution; (2) to teach what is known of the principles of Anesthesiology to all candidates for their medical degree; (3) to help long-term graduate students not only to gain a fundamental knowledge of the subject and to master the art of administration, but also to learn as much as possible of the effective methods of teaching; (4) to accompany these efforts with the encouragement of as much cooperative investigation as is consistent with achieving the first objectives."[67]

Ralph Waters' personal and professional qualities impressed many talented young men and women who sought residency posts in his department. He encouraged his residents to initiate research interests. They joined enthusiastically in studies with two pharmacologists Waters had known previously, Arthur Loevenhart and Chauncey Leake, as well as others with whom he became associated in Madison, Arthur Tatum, W. J. Meek, and H. R. Hathaway. Clinical concerns were also pursued. Anesthesia records were entered on punch cards and coded to form a data base that was used to analyze departmental activities.

Morbidity and mortality meetings, now a requirement of all training programs, originated in Madison. They were attended by all members of the department and by distinguished visitors from other cities. As a consequence of their critical reviews of the conduct of anesthesia and its outcome, responsibility for a tragedy passed from the patient to the physician. In former times, a practitioner could complain, "The patient did not take a good anesthetic." Alternatively, he might attribute the death to "status lymphaticus," of which Arthur Guedel, a master of sardonic humor, observed, "Certainly status lymphaticus is at times a great help to the anesthetist. When he has a fatality under anesthesia with no other cleansing explanation he is glad to recognize the condition as an entity."[68] Through the instruction received from Ralph Waters and his colleagues, anesthesiologists in training learned to accept responsibility for their actions by realizing that the fault lay not with the patient, but with the anesthesiologist's assessment or actions.

The University of Wisconsin became a popular destination for visiting specialists. In 1929, Ralph Waters helped organize the Anesthesia "Travel Club," whose members were leading American or Canadian teachers of anesthesia. Each year one member was the host for a group of 20 to 40 anesthesiologists who gathered for a program of informal discussions. There were demonstrations of new innovations for the operating room and laboratory, which were all subjected to what is remembered as a "high spirited, energetic, critical review." Even during the lean years of the Great Depression, international guests visited occasionally. To Geoffrey Kaye of Australia, Torsten Gordth of Sweden, Robert Macintosh and Michael Nosworthy of England, and others, Waters's department was always the "Mecca of anesthesia." It became the model for other academic departments in Europe, South America, and Asia.

Ralph Waters trained 60 residents during the 22 years he was "The Chief." From 1937 onward, the alumni, who called themselves the "Aqualumni" in his honor, returned for an annual professional and social reunion. Thirty-four "Aqualumni" took academic positions, and, of these, 14 became chairmen of departments of anesthesia. They maintained Waters's professional principles and encouraged teaching careers for many of their own graduates. Sixty years after Waters arrived in Madison, more than 80 chairmen or former chairmen of academic departments could trace their professional lineage back to Ralph Waters. Each of the 114 departments of anesthesia with residency programs in the United States has faculty members who were trained in a department led by a 2nd, 3rd, 4th, or 5th generation professional descendant of Ralph Waters. Charles Bardeen, the Dean who had recruited him in 1927, once recognized Waters's enduring legacy when he observed, "Ralph Waters was the first person the University hired to put people to sleep, but, instead, he awakened a world-wide interest in anesthesia."

Ralph Waters energetically supported the growth of physician anesthesia organizations. He supported Paul Wood's drive to give the pre-eminent New York Society of Anesthetists a title reflecting its national role. In 1936, the American Society of Anesthetists was formed, with annual dues of $5.00. A few years later, the officers of the American Society of Anesthetists were challenged by Dr. M. J. Seifert, who wrote, "An Anesthetist is a technician and an Anesthesiologist is the specific authority on anesthesia and anesthetics. I cannot understand why you do not term yourselves the American Society of Anesthesiologists?"[69] Ralph Waters was declared the first President of the newly named American Society of Anesthesiologists in 1945. In that year, when World War II ended, 739 of 1977 ASA members were in the armed forces. In the same year, the Society's first Distinguished Service Award was presented to Paul M. Wood for his tireless service to the specialty, one element of which can be examined today in the extensive archives of anesthesiology preserved in the Society's excellent Wood Library–Museum in Park Ridge, Illinois.

Women in Anesthesia

Female Physicians

The first woman physician of modern times, Elizabeth Blackwell, graduated in 1849. For some years this courageous lady was followed by only a few others, but many women entered the profession as medical colleges for women were established. Although it is not possible to determine when the first anesthetic was given by a female physician, a woman was the first American resident in anesthesia. Mary A. Ross of the University of Iowa was awarded her certificate on June 5, 1923. When Dr. Ross entered the speciality, other women physicians were already among its leaders. Before the beginning of the 20th century, Mary Botsford and Isabella Herb had been among the first Americans to become specialists in anesthesia. Both women were highly regarded as clinicians and were influential in the formation of professional societies.

Botsford is believed to be the first woman to establish a practice as a specialist in anesthesia. In 1897 she became anesthesiologist to a children's hospital in San Francisco. Following her example, several other California women doctors joined the specialty. She later received the first academic appointment in anesthesia in the western United States when she became Clinical Professor of Anesthesia at the University of California, San Francisco. She was active in medical affairs and became a leader of state and national anesthesia organizations. Botsford served as the president of the Associated Anesthetists of the United States and Canada.

Isabella Herb trained in anesthesia at the Augustana Hospital in Chicago before working as an anesthesiologist at the Mayo Clinic from 1900 until 1904. After further study in Europe, she became an Associate Professor of Rush Medical College and Chief Anesthetist at the Presbyterian Hospital, Chicago, where she established a widely respected clinical department. Her colleagues elected her to positions of leadership in both the American Medical Association and anesthesia societies. One of Dr. Herb's residents and colleagues was Huberta Livingstone. Livingstone was among the first to use positive pressure ventilation, which she described in several of the 150 articles she wrote between 1928 and 1952.

After World War II, other female anesthesiologists gained international respect. Kathleen Belton was a superb pediatric specialist. In 1948, while working in Montreal, Belton and her colleague, Digby Leigh, wrote the classic text, *Pediatric Anesthesia*. At the same time, another pediatric anesthesiologist, Margot Deming, was the Director of Anesthesia at the Children's Hospital of Philadelphia. Pediatric anesthesia also figured in the career of Doreen Vermeulen-Cranch, who had earlier initiated thoracic anesthesia in the Netherlands and, together with the surgeon, Boerema, pioneered hypothermic anesthesia. In 1958, the University of Amsterdam appointed Dr. Vermeulen-Cranch to the first Chair of Anesthesia in Europe. In 1990 Betty P. Stephenson became the first female president of the American Society of Anesthesiologists. For many years, the emerging discipline of obstetric anesthesia was led in America by Gertie F. Marx, who was the second woman to receive the ASA's Distinguished Service Award in 1988.

Obstetric anesthesia also figured prominently in the career of the first female anesthesiologist to receive the ASA Distinguished Service Award. After encountering severe financial and professional frustrations while serving as Director of the Division of Anesthesia at Columbia University, Virginia Apgar turned to obstetric anesthesia in 1949. She dedicated a decade of her multifaceted career to the assessment and support of mothers and their newborn infants.

One of the earliest expressions of her concern was the Apgar score. She formulated it during an informal morning conference immediately after a medical student requested a method of evaluating the newborn's need for resuscitative support. Although it was created in a few minutes, the Apgar score was substantiated by careful study before it was published in 1952. It has since found universal application as a method of neonatal assessment during the first minutes after delivery. After the Apgar score was accepted, Virginia Apgar continued her research and, with her associates, Norman James and Duncan Holladay, was among the first to recognize the impact of acidosis and hypoxia on the newborn.[70]

Nurse Anesthetists

Anesthesiology evolved slowly as an American medical specialty in part because of the presence of a second group of anesthesia care providers, nurse anesthetists. During the last decades of the 19th century, small communities were often served by a single physician, who was obliged to assign a nurse to "drop" ether under his direction. In larger towns, most doctors practiced independently and would not necessarily welcome being placed in what they perceived to be the subordinate role of anesthetist while their competitor enhanced his surgical reputation and collected the larger fee. Many American surgeons recalled the simple techniques they had practiced as junior house officers and regarded the administration of any anesthetic as a technical art that could be left to a nurse in any circumstance. Some hospitals preferred to pay a salary to an anesthetist while reducing their deficit from the fees charged for anesthesia. The most compelling argument to be advanced in favor of nurse anesthesia was that of skill: a trained nurse who administered anesthetics every working day was to be preferred to a physician who practiced this skill rarely.

Religious communities of the Roman Catholic Church played a major role in building hospitals in the western United States as the railways expanded. Sisters entering their order first trained in metropolitan hospitals before traveling to isolated communities. Many joined small classes in hospital-based schools of nurse anesthesia. This author, and tens of thousands of members of my and earlier generations, received our first anesthetic under the skilled care of a nun.

By the first years of this century, the surgeons of many surgical clinics preferred nurse anesthesia and personally trained the most able candidates they could recruit. The Mayo brothers' personal anesthetist was Alice Magaw. George W. Crile relied on the skills of Agatha Hodgins. During World War I, Agatha Hodgins, Geraldine Gerrard, Ann Penland, and Sophie Gran were among the more than 100 nurse anesthetists who attended many thousands of American and Allied casualties in France. Several became instructors of civilian schools of nurse anesthesia on their return from military service.

The extraordinary demands of wartime service were repeated during World War II. The nation had a desperate lack of trained physicians; at the beginning of 1940, the American Board of Anesthesiologists had recognized only 87 Diplomates. Scores of nurses and young physicians were selected each year for abbreviated training. The "90 day wonders" served with distinction in arduous conditions. After the end of hostilities, many members of both professional groups elected to remain in anesthesia, a specialty into which they had been catapulted in an abrupt and involuntary fashion. In July, 1991, the American Association of Nurse Anesthetists (AANA) reported 24,681 members.

ANESTHESIA IN CANADA

The development of anesthesia as a speciality in Canada is in many ways comparable to the American experience; the major difference is that only physicians are allowed to administer anesthetics. Only in recent decades has there been a requirement that the physician giving the anesthetic have formal training. The progress of the specialty in Canada has been closely linked to its growth in America, particularly in its earliest years. The first meeting of a short-lived Canadian Society of Anaesthetists on June 1–3, 1921, was a joint gathering with both the Interstate Association of Anesthetists and the New York Society of Anesthetists. William Webster of Winnipeg, the author of the first text by a Canadian, The Science and Art of Anesthesia, became the first president; Wesley Bourne of Montreal, who would later become the only Canadian to serve as president of the ASA, was the Secretary-Treasurer. Seven years later, the infant organization disappeared, only to re-emerge in 1943 as the Canadian Anaesthetists Society (CAS). A detailed history of Canadian anesthesia is being prepared by Professor Emeritus Roderick Gordon.[71]

Although there were three 1-year training positions as "Senior Interne" before World War II, dozens of Canadian physicians entering medical service took short courses in Montreal, Toronto, and Quebec City and remained in specialist practice thereafter. Norman Parks was assigned to a British plastic surgery unit and, like Ivan Magill before him, returned with an incomparable mastery of intubation that amazed all those he trained at The Hospital for Sick Children, Toronto.

For many years, any physician with sufficient temerity could announce that he was a "specialist," but in 1939, a process of certification was begun by the Royal College of Physicians and Surgeons (Canada), which has been superseded by the creation of the higher demands of a fellowship examination. Canadian specialists in anesthesia are obliged to complete a residency equal in length to those undertaken by surgical specialists before entering an examination process assumed to be as demanding as that of any other specialty. These requirements have gained the Canadian specialist a status equal to that of all other medical and surgical specialists.

In mid-1991, the Canadian Anaesthetists Society had 1,566 active and Canadian Associate members and 392 student members. Since Canada's population is approximately one-tenth that of the United States, the representation of anesthesiologists in the population is nearly equal. In July, 1991, the American Society of Anesthesiologists reported a total of 27,962 members, of whom 18,346 held active memberships and 4,595 were resident members.

THE SCOPE OF MODERN ANESTHESIOLOGY

This overview of the development of anesthesiology could be extended almost indefinitely by an exploration of each of the anesthetic subspecialty areas, but an assessment of its present situation can be undertaken in a simple fashion by considering the areas in which anesthesiologists are involved in hospital and university service. A comparable tour could be undertaken in any university training department.

The operating room and obstetric delivery suite remain the central interest of most members of the specialty. Aside from being the location where the techniques described previously find regular application, service in these areas brings anesthesiologists into regular contact with new departures in pharmacology and bioengineering.

After surgery, patients are transported to the postanesthesia care unit or recovery room, an area that is now considered the anesthesiologist's hospital ward. Fifty years ago, most patients returned immediately to their own bed to be attended by a junior nurse, who lacked the skills or equipment to intervene when complications occurred. After the experiences of World War II had taught anesthesiologists the value of centralized care, anesthesiologists and the nursing staff worked together to manage complex problems. Recovery rooms were soon mandated for all hospitals. By 1960, patients requiring several days of intensive medical and nursing management were often attended in a curtained corner of the recovery room. In time, drawn curtains gave way to partitions and the relocation of those areas as intensive care units. The principles of resuscitative and supportive care established by anesthesiologists were expanded in the growth of critical care medicine. From the operating room or intensive care unit, anesthesiologists make their rounds as they attend patients requiring an expert's support in controlling acute or chronic pain. At other locations within the hospital and in the classrooms and laboratories of the university campus, anesthesiologists teach undergraduates and residents and explore unproven hypotheses that may bring further progress to anesthesiology.

THE FUTURE OF ANESTHESIOLOGY*

As we have seen, the face of anesthesiology has changed remarkably in the 50 years since the beginning of World War II. Like most other medical specialties, anesthesiology has progressed primarily by quantum leaps made possible by numerous lesser technical and theoretical advancements, many of which have been directly attributable to the scientists working in industry. Examples that readily come to mind are the discoveries and applications of halothane and synthetic opioids. At the same time, however, as it was not possible to separate the social, political, and economic exigencies of the past 50 years from scientific advancement, so too will it be necessary to examine these forces when anticipating the future.

Much of what anesthesiologists do today would not seem unusual to anesthesiologists of 50 years ago. Although anesthesiologists have expanded the scope of their practice to include intensive care work and pain management, the primary focus of anesthesiology is still to provide a motionless surgical field and maintain optimal physiologic function during surgical procedures.

Clearly, the surgical procedures performed today are vastly different from those of 50 years ago, and it is likely that the surgical procedures in which anesthesiologists will find themselves participating 50 years from now will bear little resemblance to those of today. Specifically, the field of transplant surgery will expand tremendously. Not only will virtually all organs be subject to allograft replacement, but microsurgical techniques will make possible transplantation of genetically engineered tissue to cure many medical conditions such as Parkinson's disease or Huntington's chorea. It is quite likely that mental illnesses such as schizophrenia, depression, or addiction may be treated by surgical transplantation of cultured tissues, producing either natural products such as neurotransmitters or synthetically created drugs. These transplanted tissues may also act to remove substances from the microenvironment or process these substances in some way as to effect therapeutic change. These approaches are just starting to be pursued but will likely occupy a greater place in mid-21st century practice.

Microprocessor advances may make exogenous reinervation of skeletal muscle a distinct possibility in the near fu-

ture. These procedures would require surgical implantation of electrodes in various muscle groups connected to processing units in some way controlled by the patient. This has already been somewhat accomplished by applying external stimulating electrodes to lower extremity muscle groups to produce artificial gain in paraplegic patients.

Another possibility for anesthetic administration may arise if therapeutic applications for anesthetics are discovered. For example, anesthetic agents toxic only to viruses (or other infectious agents) could play a part in the treatment of acute infectious illnesses but require, of course, the administration of an anesthetic. Similarly, might there be mental disorders effectively treated or controlled acutely by anesthetic administration? There is already some precedent for immediately anesthetizing patients undergoing acute-myocardial infarction to rest the myocardium and allow for expeditious management of clot lysis or angioplasty.

Nuclear war, even conducted on a limited scale, could potentially adversely affect progress in many areas of human endeavor; this would be likely to include anesthesiology. Even if the researchers or their institutions were not directly harmed, progress could be indirectly halted by forcing resources to be channeled exclusively to patient care. All medical specialties could similarly be affected. Many have pointed out for over a decade that the only possible rational treatment of such an epidemic is prevention, and physicians from all specialties in both the Soviet Union and the United States have participated in efforts to educate the political and general population as to the possible global devastation of even limited nuclear war. Physicians in general and anesthesiologists in particular may be able to influence proliferation or use policies by virtue of their current economic and, hence, political power.

However horrible the thought of nuclear war, the reality facing us in the next 50 years is that the probability of nuclear war occurring is greater than zero. In anticipation of this, anesthesiologists will need to be involved in research detailing the logistics and effects of anesthetic administration in patients suffering from radiation poisoning, radiation burns, and other diseases unique to the aftermath of nuclear explosions. This area has not yet been explored by anesthesiologists but could potentially yield invaluable information if nuclear war were to occur.

It is unlikely that anesthesiologists will need to organize on an international scale for the purposes of changing international or national law regarding the regulation of anesthesiology in the foreseeable future. What will become vitally important to the preservation of anesthesiology as a medical specialty within the United States are organized national and state lobbies that inform anesthesiologists about pending legislation and amass funds to support candidates whose views are consistent with the tenets that (1) anesthesiology is the practice of medicine, which requires *medical training*; (2) as physicians, anesthesiologists must be allowed free access to hospitals' medical staffs; and (3) as physicians, anesthesiologists must be allowed to prescribe the conduct of anesthetics free from regulation by administrators or other nonanesthesiologist physicians.

Anesthesiologists have not built a positive public image over the last 50 years. As an example, the head of the Health Care Financing Administration, who controls virtually all governmental medical spending, once made the public statement that "anesthesiologists don't even say hello to their patients." This demonstrates how awareness about anesthesiology is lacking, even among other physicians. These public attitudes will need to be challenged if anesthesiologists are to remain independent medical practitioners and

---

*This section was contributed by Mark S. Scheller, M.D., Assistant Professor of Anesthesiology at the University of California, San Diego.

not become simply employees of the hospital akin to technicians and nurses. To the extent that anesthesiologists will organize and support and educate candidates for national and state office, anesthesiologists will have a chance of existing as independent practitioners. If their efforts fall short, it is likely that their services will become the property of others.

A strongly related issue relating to services rendered by anesthesiologists is that of compensation for those services. Third-party payers such as health plans, county, state, and even the federal government have (unfairly) targeted anesthesiologists as physicians who will have to accept payment based on whatever political or economic cost-cutting plan happens to be popular, with little regard for quality of care. At the extreme, these payers would prefer to simply employ the physician or contract directly with the physician's employer, that is, the hospital. Hospital-based physicians such as anesthesiologists, pathologists, and radiologists are clearly the most vulnerable, because the third-party payers, hospital administrators, and, perhaps more sadly, the public believe that these physicians are strictly technicians and therefore employable as such. The patient/physician relationship thus changes to a patient/hospital relationship or a patient/health plan relationship. The economic implications of this to those employed are obvious, as the hospital, like any business, would be attempting to turn a profit on physician services. Anesthesiologists have been somewhat protected by their relatively high cost of malpractice insurance and liability exposure, which has made them, as a group, unattractive for hospitals or health plans to employ directly. If this changes, either because of legislation limiting liability or because it will ultimately be more lucrative for the hospital or health plan to assume the liability of the physician, economic remuneration for anesthesiologists' services will be greatly curtailed. If this occurs on a widespread basis, other physicians such as surgeons and internists will very likely find themselves in the midst of similar arrangements. Again, firm and constant political pressure at the national and state level will be the anesthesiologist's major defensive weapon of the next half century.

Changes will undoubtedly occur in the education of anesthesiologists. The American Board of Anesthesiology has increased the anesthesiology residency requirement to 4 years from 3 years following graduation from medical school. The educational requirements for anesthesiologists in the next 50 years will depend to a great extent upon their success in remaining independent practitioners, and on supply and demand in the marketplace. If they are successful and if the demand for anesthesiologists' services continues to remain high, it is almost certain that the educational requirements for board certification will increase. At the extreme, this would result in anesthesiology training programs accepting only physicians board certified in another specialty such as internal medicine or pediatrics. There are already precedents for this in the medical and surgical subspecialties.

On the other hand, if nonphysician practitioners are successful in winning concessions from government agencies with regard to the scope of their practices and liability, the educational requirements for anesthesiologists may actually need to expand to include areas traditionally taught in nursing school. This would be primarily a defensive maneuver by anesthesiologists to demonstrate that their training is over and above that of nonphysician practitioners and not merely of a different focus, as has been the contention of some. The politics involved are obviously difficult to predict, but it is not outside the realm of possibilities that future practitioners would need to be duly certified in both disciplines.

Research done by anesthesiologists in the next five decades will be more closely aligned with the needs of industry and other medical specialties. Simply performing physiology experiments on normal animals or humans will be neither fundable nor interesting. Academic anesthesiology departments have traditionally performed poorly in securing significant national grant support compared with medicine or surgery departments. As funding becomes tighter, as it inevitably will, anesthesiologists will be forced to compete with other medical specialists and basic scientists for funds. This will force physician researchers to gain additional training, such as a doctoral degree. The anesthesiologist with advanced training will be in a unique position to adequately design and monitor experiments requiring the administration of an anesthetic. At the present time, the effects of anesthesia *per se* are frequently either ignored or poorly controlled by nonanesthesiologist investigators.

Tackling problems such as acquired immunodeficiency syndrome (AIDS), Alzheimer's disease, coronary artery disease, and cancer will become bigger priorities for anesthesiologist researchers if they are to survive the funding wars. Another avenue to secure funding, however, will be through liaisons with private industry. Competition in the marketplace will force entrepreneurs to have new products evaluated as quickly as possible in an ever more regulated society. Anesthesiologists will find themselves taking products from the laboratory to the operating room for evaluation more frequently in the years to come.

Monitoring of the patient will also become more rigorous. If there is any question or worry about a patient's well-being or status during an anesthetic, monitoring is by definition inadequate. With the recent widespread availability of noninvasive and reliable measures of oxygenation (pulse oximetry), ventilation, and anesthetic depth (end-tidal gas analysis), it is clear that "beat to beat" or "breath to breath" monitoring capabilities are a new standard of practice. With this new technology, however, comes the problem of accurately recording the ever-increasing amount of data. This problem will be solved quickly with completely automated recordkeeping. Advances in artificial intelligence, speech recognition, and data storage and retrieval will make manual recordkeeping obsolete within 15 years. All information about a patient will be instantly accessible by the anesthesiologist and permanently recorded. These systems will become as familiar to the anesthesiologist of the 21st century as clipboards are to present-day practitioners.

Noninvasive measures of tissue well-being will evolve quickly. For example, edema formation, particularly in the lungs and brain, but probably in other organs as well, is, at the present time, recognized too late in its course. Likewise, currently, we have only limited abilities to recognize local tissue ischemia, substrate deficiency, or other metabolic disturbance. On-line, noninvasive measurement techniques, which will probably require technology we cannot yet imagine, may be a reality by the year 2040.

Our understanding of the etiology, function, and treatment of pain has evolved very slowly over the last 50 years. The rather recent discoveries of the participation of specific spinal pathways in the expression of pain may be the quantum leap upon which a more complete appreciation of the physiology of pain can be built. If this is so, it is conceivable that pain as it relates to surgery or disease could be of historic interest midway into the 21st century. Research along a number of very different lines will need to intersect to eventually make this happen. Presumably, drugs with the potential to selectively block the propagation of afferent pain impulses might be developed, or, alternatively, methods of interfering with afferent pain impulses at more central locations will need to be refined (e.g., gating). At the present time, the complete understanding and control of pain is perhaps the greatest scientific challenge facing anesthesiologists.

It is likely that the number of scientific and technical breakthroughs or innovations in the next 50 years will exceed that of the previous 50 years by orders of magnitude, as a direct result of the burgeoning worldwide demand for biomedical products. These advances will affect every clinical specialty, anesthesiology included.

In the near future, newer drugs will be developed, such as volatile anesthetics with very low blood:gas solubility ratios, which will be used as nitrous oxide is used today. In fact, with the introduction of these agents, nitrous oxide will permanently be dropped from the pharmacopoeia of the anesthesiologist. Likewise, extremely short-acting non-depolarizing muscle relaxants will be used routinely within 15 years and will completely displace succinylcholine. Although fentanyl, alfentanil, and sufentanil will serve us well to the end of this century and perhaps a bit beyond, they too will be replaced by even shorter-acting, more potent compounds with no side-effects such as rigidity, nausea, hypotension, or pruritis. Along with these drugs, our understanding and ability to apply kinetic principles to clinical practice will increase, such that we will be able to deliver truly predictable iv anesthetics. It is likely that the anesthesia machine of the 21st century will have calibrated dispensers for all available iv anesthetic agents, muscle relaxants, and vasoactive drugs built into them, much as present-day machines have vaporizers attached. These delivery systems would be interfaced directly with physiologic data, including on-line plasma or possibly tissue levels of drug, and would require little or no hands-on attention.

The manipulation of gene expression in eukaryotic organisms may be a reality in the next 50 years. Thus, it may be possible to implant genes that can be turned on and off in humans. These genes could code for proteins that would either act directly at some site, for example, beta-endorphin, or the genes could code for proteins that would assemble compounds from normal cellular pools of components or from substances introduced by the anesthesiologist. For example, it may be possible to induce a state of prolonged hibernation (? anesthesia) by turning on a gene that produces a peptide hibernation factor. Hibernation factors have already been isolated and shown to include hibernation-like states in nonhibernating animals.

As artificially produced human insulin and erythropoietin will change clinical practice during the remainder of this century, so too will artificial blood components be an advance of the next century. All clotting factors, platelets, and oxygen-carrying compounds will be produced in the laboratory and be commercially available.

A mission to Mars is planned for the mid-21st century. The length of interplanetary trips, that is, years, will initially necessitate the availability of surgical and hence anesthetic capabilities on board the spacecraft. This alone will open an entirely new area of scientific inquiry within the field of anesthesiology.

Acknowledgment. The authors wish to express their appreciation to Professor Leslie Rendell-Baker for his review of the historical elements of this chapter while Dr. Calverley was on military duty in Southwest Asia.

REFERENCES

1. Duncum BM: The Development of Inhalation Anaesthesia, p 86. London, Oxford University Press, 1947
2. Davy H: Researches Chemical and Philosophical Chiefly Concerning Nitrous Oxide or Dephlogisticated Nitrous Air, and Its Respiration, p 533. London, J Johnson, 1800
3. Lyman HM: Artificial Anaesthesia and Anaesthetics, p 6. New York, William Wood, 1881
4. Long CW: An account of the first use of sulphuric ether by inhalation as an anaesthetic in surgical operations. South Med Surg J 5:705, 1849
4a. Smith GB, Hirsch NP: Gardner Quincy Colton: Pioneer of nitrous oxide anesthesia. Anesth Analg 72:382, 1991
5. Greene NM: A consideration of factors in the discovery of anesthesia and their effects on its development. Anesthesiology 35:515, 1971
6. Duncum BM: The Development of Inhalation Anaesthesia, p 110. London, Oxford University Press, 1947
7. Snow J: On the Inhalation of the Vapour of Ether, p 23. London, J Churchill, 1847
8. Snow J: On Chloroform and Other Anesthetics, pp 58–74. London, J Churchill, 1858
9. Journal of Queen Victoria. In Strauss MB (ed): Familiar Medical Quotations, p 17. Boston, Little, Brown & Co, 1968
10. Duncum BM: The Development of Inhalation Anaesthesia, p 540. London, Oxford University Press, 1947
11. Duncum BM: The Development of Inhalation Anaesthesia, p 538. London, Oxford University Press, 1947
12. Calverley RK: J. T. Clover: A giant of victorian anaesthesia. In Rupreht J, van Lieburg MJ, Lee JA, Erdmann W (eds): Anaesthesia: Essays on its History, p 21. Berlin, Springer-Verlag, 1985
13. Clover JT: Laryngotomy in chloroform anesthesia. Br Med J 1:132, 1877
14. Colton Dental Association (advertisement from the Public Ledger and Transcript, Philadelphia, December 4, 1869, Reynolds Historical Library, University of Alabama in Birmingham)
15. Andrews E: The oxygen mixture, a new anaesthetic combination. Chicago Medical Examiner 9:656, 1868
16. Becker HK: Carl Koller and cocaine. Psychoanal Q 32:332, 1963
17. Corning JL: Spinal anaesthesia and local medication of the cord. NY Med J 42:485, 1885
18. Bier AKG: Experiments in cocainization of the spinal cord, 1899. In Faulconer A, Keys TE (trans): Foundations of Anesthesiology, p 854. Springfield, Illinois, Charles C Thomas, 1965
19. Bier AKG: Experiments in cocainization of the spinal cord, 1899. In Faulconer A, Keys TE (trans): Foundations of Anesthesiology, p 855. Springfield, Illinois, Charles C Thomas, 1965
20. Tait D, Caglieri G: Experimental and clinical notes on the subarachnoid space. JAMA 35:6, 1900
21. Lee JA: Arthur Edward James Barker, 1850–1916; British pioneer of regional anaesthesia. Anaesthesia 34:885, 1979
22. Lemmon WT: A method for continuous spinal anesthesia: A preliminary report. Ann Surg 111:141, 1940
23. Tuohy EB: Continuous spinal anesthesia: Its usefulness and technic involved. Anesthesiology 5:142, 1944
24. Pages F: Metameric anesthesia, 1921. In Faulconer A, Keys TE (trans): Foundations of Anesthesiology, p 927. Springfield, Illinois, Charles C Thomas, 1965
25. Fink BR: History of local anesthesia. In Cousins MJ, Bridenbaugh PO (eds): Neural Blockade, p 12. Philadelphia, JB Lippincott, 1980
26. Cushing H: On the avoidance of shock in major amputations by cocainization of large nerve trunks preliminary to their division: With observations on blood-pressure changes in surgical cases. Ann Surg 36:321, 1902
27. Waters RM: Clinical scope and utility of carbon dioxide filtration in inhalation anesthesia. Curr Res Anesth Analg 3:20, 1923
28. Sword BC: The closed circle method of administration of gas anesthesia. Curr Res Anesth Analg 9:198, 1930
29. Revell DG: An improved circulator for closed circle anesthesia. Can Anaesth Soc J 6:104, 1959
30. Obituary of T. Philip Ayre. Br Med J 280:125, 1980

31. Rees GJ: Anaesthesia in the newborn. Br Med J 2:1419, 1950
32. Bain JA, Spoerel WE: A stream-lined anaesthetic system. Can Anaesth Soc J 19:426, 1972
33. Morris LE: A new vaporizer for liquid anesthetic agents. Anesthesiology 13:587, 1952
34. Mushin WW, Rendell-Baker L: The Principles of Thoracic Anaesthesia Past and Present, p 89. Springfield, Illinois, Charles C Thomas, 1953
35. Shephard DAE: Harvey Cushing and anaesthesia. Can Anaesth Soc J 12:431, 1965
36. Codesmith A: An endo-esophageal stethoscope. Anesthesiology 15:566, 1954
37. Tovell RM: Problems in supply of anesthetic gases in the European theater of operations. Anesthesiology 8:303, 1947
38. Rendall-Baker L: History of standards for anesthesia equipment. In Rupreht J, van Lieburg MJ, Lee JA, Erdmann W (eds): Anaesthesia: Essays on Its History, pp 161–165. Berlin, Springer-Verlag, 1985
39. Calverley RK: A safety feature for anaesthesia machines: Touch identification of oxygen flow control. Can Anaesth Soc J 18:225, 1971
40. Faulconer A, Pender JW, Bickford RG: The influence of partial pressure of nitrous oxide on the depth of anesthesia and the electro-encephalogram in man. Anesthesiology 10:601, 1949
41. Severinghaus JC, Honda Y: Pulse oximetry. Int Anesthesiol Clin 25(4):212, 1987
42. Severinghaus JC, Honda Y: Pulse oximetry. Int Anesthesiol Clin 25(4):206, 1987
43. Macewan W: Clinical observations on the introduction of tracheal tubes by the mouth instead of performing tracheotomy or laryngotomy. Br Med J 2:122–124, 163–165, 1880
44. Mushin WW, Rendall-Baker L: The Principles of Thoracic Anaesthesia Past and Present, pp 44–45. Springfield, Illinois, Charles C Thomas, 1953
45. Mushin WW, Rendall-Baker L: The Principles of Thoracic Anaesthesia Past and Present, p 44. Springfield, Illinois, Charles C Thomas, 1953
46. Kuhn F: Nasotracheal intubation (trans): In Faulconer A, Keys TE (eds): Foundations of Anesthesiology, pp 677–680. Springfield, Illinois, Charles C Thomas, 1965
47. Hirsch NP, Smith GB, Hirsch PO: Alfred Kirstein, pioneer of direct laryngoscopy. Anaesthesia 41:42, 1986
48. Thomas KB: Sir Ivan Whiteside Magill, KCVO, DSc, MB, BCh, BAO, FRCS, FFARCS (Hon), FFARCSI (Hon), DA. A review of his publications and other references to his life and work. Anaesthesia 33:628, 1978
49. Condon HA, Gilchrist E: Stanley Rowbotham, twentieth century pioneer anaesthetist. Anaesthesia 41:46, 1986
50. Calverley RK: Arthur E Guedel (1883–1956). In Rupreht J, van Lieburg MJ, Lee JA, Erdmann W (eds): Anaesthesia: Essays on Its History, pp 49–53. Berlin, Springer-Verlag, 1985
51. Calverley RK: Classical file. Surv Anesth 28:70, 1984
52. Gale JW, Waters RM: Closed endobronchial anesthesia in thoracic surgery: Preliminary report. Curr Res Anesth Analg 11:283, 1932
53. Miller RA: A new laryngoscope. Anesthesiology 2:317, 1941
54. Macintosh RR: Richard Salt of Oxford, anaesthetic technician extraordinary. Anaesthesia 31:855, 1976
55. Lucas GHW: The discovery of cyclopropane. Curr Res Anesth Analg 40:15, 1961
56. Calverley RK: Fluorinated anesthetics: I. The early years. Surv Anesth 29:170, 1986
57. Robbins BH: Preliminary studies of the anesthetic activity of the fluorinated hydrocarbons. J Pharmacol Exp Therap 86:197, 1946
58. Calverley RK: Fluorinated anesthetics: II. Fluroxene. Surv Anesth 30:126, 1987
59. Suckling CW: Some chemical and physical factors in the development of Fluothane. Br J Anaesth 29:466, 1957
60. Macintosh RR: Modern anaesthesia, with special reference to the chair of anaesthetics in Oxford. In Rupreht J, van Lieburg MJ, Lee JA, Erdmann W (eds): Anaesthesia: Essays on Its History, pp 352–356. Berlin, Springer-Verlag, 1985
61. Knoefel PK: Felice Fontana: Life and Works, pp 284–285. Trento, Societa de Studi Trentini, 1985
62. Griffith HR, Johnson GE: The use of curare in general anesthesia. Anesthesiology 3:418, 1942
63. Fink BR: Leaves and needles: The introduction of surgical local anesthesia. Anesthesiology 63:77, 1985
64. Seldon TH: Francis Hoeffer McMechan. In Volpitto PP, Vandam LD (eds): Genesis of American Anesthesiology, pp 5–20. Springfield, Illinois, Charles C Thomas, 1982
65. Bamforth BJ, Siebecker KL: Ralph M. Waters. In Volpitto PP, Vandam LD (eds): Genesis of American Anesthesiology, pp 51–68. Springfield, Illinois, Charles C Thomas, 1982
66. Waters RM: Pioneering in anesthesiology. Postgrad Med 4:265, 1968
67. Waters RM: Pioneering in anesthesiology. Postgrad Med 4:267, 1968
68. Guedel AE: Inhalation Anesthesia: A fundamental Guide, p 129. New York, Macmillan, 1937
69. Little DM Jr, Betcher AM: The Diamond Jubilee 1905–1980, p 8. Park Ridge, Illinois, American Society of Anesthesiologists, 1980
70. Calmes SH: Development of the Apgar score. In Rupreht J, van Lieburg MJ, Lee JA, Erdmann W (eds): Anaesthesia: Essays on Its History, pp 45–48. Berlin, Springer-Verlag, 1985
71. Gordon RA: A capsule history of anaesthesia history in Canada. Can Anaesth Soc J 25:75, 1978

2

John H. Eichhorn

Contemporary Anesthesia Practice and Quality Assurance

The organization and execution of anesthesia practice in the 1990s is evolving very rapidly. Beyond basic and clinical research, new medications, and new equipment, a great many forces are directly affecting anesthesia practice. Entities and influences that may have been poorly explained during anesthesia training play a major role in the daily lives of all anesthesiologists. The traditional practice of passing down by word of mouth understandings about, for example, practice arrangements is no longer adequate. Further, recent years have seen dramatic developments in areas such as quality assurance (QA), risk management, and defined standards of care. Quality assurance, also referred to as *quality improvement,* is intended to help optimize care. In the past, risk management was largely concerned with minimizing potential legal and financial liability and related compensation or insurance costs. It has evolved into a larger understanding that could be considered prospective QA in that its goal is to identify and prevent clinical problems before they occur. Nontraditional, prospective endeavors such as these have assumed a significant role in defining, guiding, and shaping modern anesthesia practice. This chapter outlines the content and impact of these new forces and then shifts to some practical considerations of operating room management from an anesthesiologist's perspective and, finally, to some of the issues faced by an anesthesiologist who is deciding how to practice.

PREREQUISITES

Before programs are established and effective QA, risk management, and organizational efforts can be implemented in an anesthesia department or group, several fundamental prerequisites must be in place.

The Credentialing Process and Clinical Privileges

The process of credentialing of health care professionals has been the focus of considerable recent attention, in part the result of very rare incidents of untrained persons—imposters—infiltrating the health care system. The more common situation, however, involves health professionals who fail to disclose adverse past experiences. There has been some justified publicity concerning physicians who lose their licenses sequentially in several states and simply move on each time to start practice again elsewhere.

The patient-physician relationship also has changed radically in recent years, with a concomitant increase in suspicion directed toward the medical profession. There is now a pervasive public perception that physicians are inadequately policed, particularly by their own professional organizations. As a result, intense public and political pressure has been brought to bear on various law-making bodies, regulatory and licensing agencies, and health care institution administrations to discover and purge both (1) fraudulent, criminal, and deviant health care providers, and (2) incompetent or simply poor-quality practitioners whose histories show sufficient poor patient outcomes to attract attention, usually through malpractice suits. Identifying incompetence is a valid component of QA and risk management efforts. Verification of appropriate education, training, and experience on the part of a candidate for a position giving anesthesia care is one component of prospective risk management. Such verification assumes special importance in light of the legal doctrine of vicarious liability, which can be described as follows: if an individual, group, or institution hires an anesthesia provider or even simply approves of that person (e.g., as by granting clinical privileges), then those involved in the decision may later be held liable in the courts, along with the individual, for the individual's actions. This would be especially true if it were later discovered that the offending practitioner's past adverse outcomes had not been adequately investigated during the credentialing process.

Out of these various concerns has arisen the sometimes cumbersome process of obtaining state licenses to practice, and of obtaining hospital privileges. It is somewhat analogous to passing through screening and metal detection devices at airports, which is tolerated by the individual in the interest of the safety of all. The stringent credentialing process is intended both to protect patients and to safeguard the integrity of the medical profession.

There are checklists of the requirements for the granting of medical staff privileges by hospitals.[1,2] In addition, there has been the recent development of a national data bank and reporting system administered by the federal government. It is a central repository of licensing and credentials information about physicians. Any adverse situation involving a physician, particularly instances of substance abuse, malpractice litigation, or the revocation, suspension, or limitation of that physician's license to practice medicine or to hold hospital privileges, must be reported (via the state board of medical registration/licensure) to the National Practitioner Data Bank. It is a statutory requirement that all applications for hospital staff privileges be cross-checked against the national data bank. The potential medicolegal liability for failing to do so is staggering.

It is critically important that the documentation for the credentialing process for each anesthesia practitioner be complete. Privileges to administer anesthesia must be officially granted and delineated in writing.[1] This can be straightforward—and there are good models offered by the American Society of Anesthesiologists[3] (ASA)—or it can be more complex to accommodate institutional needs or desires for identifying those anesthesia practitioners deemed qualified to practice in designated subspecialty areas within anesthesia such as cardiac, infant/pediatric, obstetric, intensive care, or pain management. Specific documentation of the process of granting or renewing clinical privileges is required and, unlike some other records, the documentation would be protected as confidential peer review information under the Federal Health Care Quality Improvement Act of 1986. A related 1988 U.S. Supreme Court decision questioning this confidentiality involved a case that occurred in 1981. The subsequent 1986 federal law is constructed so that it still applies now, even in light of the 1988 decision.

After the initial granting of clinical privileges to practice anesthesia, anesthesiologists must periodically renew their privileges within the institution or facility (e.g., annually or biannually).There are moral, ethical, and societal obligations on the part of the privilege-granting entity to take this process seriously. It is a central component of large-scale QA and risk management within health care. State licensing bodies often become aware of problems with health professionals very late in the evolution of the difficulties. An anesthesia provider's peers in the hospital or facility are much more likely to notice untoward developments as they first appear. However, privilege renewals are often essentially automatic and receive little of the necessary attention. Judicious checking of renewal applications and awareness of relevant peer review information is absolutely necessary. The physicians or administrators responsible for evaluating staff members and reviewing their practices and privileges may be justifiably concerned about retaliatory legal action by a staff member who is censured or denied privilege renewal. Accordingly, such evaluating groups must be thoroughly objective (totally eliminating any hint of political or financial motives) and must have documentation that the staff person who would be censured or denied renewal is in fact practicing below the standard of care. Court decisions have found liability by a hospital or its medical staff group or both when the incompetence of a staff member was known or should have been known and was not acted upon.[2]

A major issue today in the granting of clinical privileges, especially in procedure-oriented specialties such as anesthesiology, is whether it is reasonable to continue the common practice of "blanket" privileges. This process in effect authorizes the practitioner to attempt any treatment or procedure normally considered within the purview of the applicant's medical specialty. These considerations may have profound political and economic implications within medicine, such as which type of surgeon should be doing carotid endarterectomies or lumbar diskectomies. More important, however, is whether the practitioner being evaluated is qualified to do everything traditionally associated with the specialty. Specifically, should the granting of privileges to practice anesthesia automatically approve the practitioner to handle pediatric cardiac cases, critically ill newborns (such as a 2-day-old infant with a large diaphragmatic hernia), ablative pain therapy (such as an alcohol celiac plexus block under fluoroscopy), high-risk obstetric cases, and so forth? This question raises the issue of procedure-specific or limited privileges. The QA and risk management considerations in this question are weighty if inexperienced or insufficiently qualified practitioners are allowed or expected, because peer or scheduling pressures, to undertake major challenges for which they are not prepared. The likelihood of complications will be higher and the difficulty of defending the practitioner against a malpractice claim in the event of catastrophe will be significantly increased.

There is no clear answer to the question of procedure-specific credentialing and granting of privileges. Ignoring issues of qualifications has clear negative potential. On the other hand, stringent procedure-specific credentialing is impractical in smaller groups, and in larger groups allows many small "fiefdoms" to spring up, with a consequent further atrophy of the clinical skills outside of the practitioner's specific areas. Each anesthesia department or group needs to address these issues. At the very least, the common practice of every applicant for privileges checking off every line on the printed list of anesthesia procedures should be reviewed.

Policy and Procedure

Important to the QA process is the creation and use of a complete departmental or institutional anesthesia policy and procedure manual. Maintaining this manual may be tiresome, but a good manual can be extraordinarily valuable, providing crucial information on, for example, emergency procedures. Some suggestions for the content of this compendium exist,[4] but, at minimum, there must be organizational and procedural elements.

The organizational elements include a chart of organization and responsibilities that is not just a call schedule but a clear explanation of who is responsible for what functions and what areas of the department and when, with attendant details such as expectations for the practitioner's presence within the institution at designated hours, telephone availability, pager availability, the maximum permissible distance from the institution, and so forth. Sadly, these issues often are only considered after a disaster has occurred that involved miscommunication and the mistaken belief by one or more people that someone else should or would take care of a problem.

Also included in the organizational component of policy and procedure is a clear explanation of the orientation and check-out procedure for new personnel, continuing medical requirements and opportunities, the mechanisms for evaluating personnel and for communicating this evaluation to them, disaster plans (or reference to a separate disaster manual or protocol), QA activities of the department, and the format for statistical record keeping (number of procedures, types of anesthetics given, types of patients anesthetized, number and types of invasive monitoring procedures, number and type of responses to emergency calls, and the like).

The procedural component of policy and procedure gives both handy practice tips and specific outlines of proposed courses of action for particular circumstances; it also stores little-used but valuable information. Frequently, reference is made to the statements, guidelines, and standards appearing in the back of the ASA's Directory of Members. Also included are references to or specific protocols for the areas mentioned in the Joint Commission on Accreditation of Healthcare Organizations (JCAHO) standards[5]: preanesthetic evaluation, immediate preinduction re-evaluation, safety of the patient during the anesthetic period, release of the patient from any postanesthesia care unit (PACU), recording of all pertinent events during anesthesia, recording of postanesthesia visits, guidelines defining the role of anesthesia services in hospital infection control, and guidelines for safe use of general anesthetic agents. Other appropriate topics include the following:

1. Recommendations for preanesthesia apparatus check-out, such as from the U.S. Food and Drug Administration (FDA).
2. Guidelines for minimal monitoring of an infant, child, or adult in the PACU.
3. Procedures for transporting patients to the OR, PACU, or ICU.
4. Policy on ambulatory surgical patients—screening, use of regional anesthesia, discharge home.
5. Policy on same-day admissions.
6. Policy on recovery room admission and discharge.
7. Policy on ICU admission and discharge.
8. Policy on physicians responsible for writing orders in recovery room and ICU.
9. Policy on informed consent.
10. Policy on the participation of patients in clinical research.
11. Guidelines for the support of cadaver organ donors and its termination.
12. Guidelines on environmental safety, including pollution with trace gases and electrical equipment inspection, maintenance, and hazard prevention.
13. Procedure for change of personnel during an anesthetic.
14. Procedure for the introduction of new equipment, drugs, or clinical practices.
15. Procedure for epidural and spinal narcotic administration and subsequent patient monitoring (e.g., type, minimum time).
16. Procedure for initial treatment of cardiac or respiratory arrest.
17. Policy for handling patient's refusal of blood or blood products, including the mechanism to obtain a court order to transfuse.
18. Procedure for the management of malignant hyperthermia.
19. Procedure for the induction and maintenance of barbiturate coma.
20. Procedure for the evaluation of suspected pseudocholinesterase deficiency.
21. Protocol for responding to an adverse anesthetic event.

Individual departments may add to the above suggestions as dictated by their specific needs. A thorough, carefully conceived policy and procedure manual is a valuable tool. Many of the components are intended to mandate or encourage practices that will prevent untoward events (e.g., unfamiliarity with a new anesthesia machine when called "stat" for an emergency case), will help the management of crises (e.g., malignant hyperthermia), or will encourage communication in difficult situations (e.g., refusal of blood). The manual should be reviewed and updated as needed but at least annually, with a particularly thorough review preceding each JCAHO inspection. Each member of a group or department should review the manual at least annually and sign off in a log indicating familiarity with current policies and procedures.

Meetings and Case Discussion

There must be regularly scheduled departmental meetings. Although didactic lectures and continuing education meetings are valuable and necessary, there also must be regular opportunities for open clinical discussion about interesting and problem cases. Also, the JCAHO requires that there be at least monthly meetings at which risk management and QA activities are "documented and reported."[5] Whether these meetings are called case conferences, morbidity and mortality conferences, or deaths and complications, the entire department or group should gather for an interchange of ideas. More recently these gatherings have been called QA meetings. An open review of departmental statistics should be done, including all complications, even those that may appear trivial. Unusual patterns of small events may point toward a larger or systematic problem, especially if they are more frequently associated with one individual practitioner.

A problem case presented at the departmental meeting might be an overt accident (very rarely), a near accident ("critical incident"), or an untoward outcome of unknown origin. Honest but constructive discussion, even of an anesthetist's technical deficiencies or lack of knowledge, should take place in the spirit of the QA process. The classic question, "What would you do differently next time?", is a good way to start the discussion. There may be situations in which inviting the surgeon or the internist involved in a specific case would be advantageous. The opportunity for each type of provider to hear the perspective of another discipline not only is inherently educational but also can promote communication and cooperation in future potential problem cases.

Records of these meetings must be kept for accreditation purposes, but the enshrining of overly detailed minutes (potentially subject to discovery by a plaintiff's attorney at a later date) may inhibit true educational and corrective interchanges about untoward events.

Support Staff

The last fundamental prerequisite is for support staff. Even independent practitioners rely in some measure on facilities, equipment, and services provided by the organization maintaining the anesthetizing location. In large, well-organized departments, reliance on support staff is often very great. The need for adequate staff to execute the necessary duties and the inadvisability of scrimping on critical support personnel to cut costs is obvious. What is often overlooked, however, is a process analogous to that of credentialing and privileges for anesthesiologists, although at a slightly different level. The people expected to provide clinical anesthesia practice support must be qualified and must at all times understand what they are expected to do and how to do it. It is singularly unfortunate to realize only after an anesthesia catastrophe has occurred that basic details of simple work assignments were routinely ignored.

QUALITY ASSURANCE

How to assure quality in any activity has been of interest for centuries. Treatises were written in ancient Rome about how best to guarantee the production of uniform and consistently high-quality wine.

A necessary first step is deciding what "quality" is in the context of the product or activity being considered. In business, particularly in the manufacture of mass-produced items, the concept has taken root that product quality must be controlled. Quality control in manufacturing—and we may take as random examples the manufacture of automobiles, stereo components, or cookies—considers how close the manufacturing process came to producing an item whose physical and functional characteristics match those specified by the research and development, engineering, design, and marketing personnel.

In classic quality control in manufacturing, it is accepted that some of the items produced by the manufacturing process will be defective. There is an acknowledged error rate. The goal of the activity is to find out the rate of appearance of the defective product and then to adjust the manufacturing process to lower this rate to an acceptable level. A very small sample of the product—typically less than 1%—is tested to see if it meets the manufacturer's specifications, and a fundamental assumption is then made: that the sample is representative of the entire production run, and that statistics for the defect rate of the sample can be extrapolated to the entire output of the production process. Interesting logistical questions arise when the error rate is unacceptably high or an essential characteristic is unacceptable in a small sample. Does this mean that the entire batch or all the items made since the last acceptable check should be discarded or recalled? Often, more testing, both of a larger sample and of a more exhausting nature, is ordered before difficult decisions are made. The analogies to QA in medical care are clear. If a small-sample review of anesthesia records revealed a number of cases of lip lacerations associated with intubation by one particular practitioner, then all that provider's anesthesia charts would be retrieved for a more thorough review.

A contrasting situation exists in some manufacturing sectors. If either the manufacturer's business philosophy or the nature of the product demands perfection, then the sample fraction must become unity and every item made, or the entirety of every batch, must be evaluated and tested. Any defective product is recycled for correction or discarded, and it is believed that the product shipped is as close to perfect as possible.

As service industries gained prominence in the world economy in the past half-century, it was only logical that the concepts of quality control would be applied to these types of businesses and their activities as well. Because it is much more difficult to define quality in regard to a service than in regard to a manufactured product, and because so much more of the human element is involved, it became apparent that it was essentially impossible to control the quality of services rendered in the same way that a manufacturing process could be controlled. Acknowledging this, those involved shifted the emphasis to trying prospectively to "assure" the quality of the service rather than to control it by sampling or by universal testing/review after the fact. Thus was born the QA process in the service sector.

The analogy in the service sector to freedom from manufacturing defects in the business sector is a matter of considerable interest and has led to the concept of "outcome" as a central component of the QA process. A good outcome of the act of rendering a service is the best equivalent of a correctly manufactured product. Although in some situations it may seem intuitively obvious, there is intense debate about what constitutes a good outcome from the rendering of a service. In medical care, it may be reassuring a worried patient or family member, curing (or preventing) disease, relieving pain, prolonging life (for a day or decades), or even avoiding the complications of potentially dangerous procedures.

Medical care, like many activities, has three essential components:

1. *Structure*—the material and the plans used to carry out the activity.
2. *Process*—what is actually done, and how.
3. *Outcome*—the result of applying process to structure to obtain a result.

Early QA efforts focused almost exclusively on structure and process, and only relatively recently did QA activities in medical care begin to focus on outcome. This is because evaluating, testing, and analyzing the outcome of medical care is difficult. It is much easier to walk down a hospital corridor counting fire extinguishers, testing electrical outlets, or checking that all the proper forms and logs are filled out. Because this type of QA activity was for many years associated with hospital inspections and usually involved the preparation of voluminous reports, many medical care providers developed a negative attitude about QA, finding it a bureaucratic annoyance that obstructed them in their daily tasks. Fortunately, a great deal has changed in this area. The QA process described here, because of its direct and indirect involvement with the outcome of anesthesia care, is relevant to the modern practice of anesthesia.

QA may still evoke negative attitudes from anesthesia providers. As a group, anesthesia providers tend to be action oriented and even impatient, and the review process and attendant paperwork may clash with those characteristics. Some anesthesia providers may feel threatened, and feel that "Big Brother" is watching over their shoulder, prepared to discipline them. This is not the intention of the QA process. The QA process does involve cooperation by all providers and some work by a few. However, the specific major benefits far outweigh the minor investment of energy. In addition to the intangible satisfaction of learning by objective evaluation that patients are receiving good care, everyone involved in the process is continually educated by the constant flow of information and material. Further, there are tangible benefits. The examination of the details of practice uncovers previously unavailable or buried information that can be used to improve the ease and efficiency of practice. Also, with objective documentation that the outcome of the care rendered has become excellent, there may even be financial benefits, such as a reduction in medical malpractice insurance premiums, as has happened for the large majority of American anesthesiologists in the recent past.

Defining Quality

Defining quality in medical care is problematic. Outcome is the main focus, but many component elements contribute to the ultimate outcome. There have been debates about the degree to which outcome reflects quality, and consequent cautions against focusing too narrowly on the outcome of medical care alone.[6,7] Also, there have been debates as to whether only the medical practitioner's performance should be considered in assessing the quality of medical care, or whether the role of the health care system and the actions of the patients themselves should also be included.[8] Because factors beyond those controlled by practitioners may play a central role in the ultimate outcome, the logical conclusion is to assess the impact of all potential influences on the outcome of medical care. Good or acceptable quality of care will vary among patients because the specific needs of each patient vary. Goals must be individualized. However, this may make screening for quality in very large numbers of patients much more difficult to construct and execute.[9] A current, popular definition of the quality of medical care invokes the concept that medical care rendered to a patient should increase the likelihood of a desirable outcome for the individual patient while decreasing the probability of any undesirable outcome. Thus, the best quality medical care optimizes the likelihood of a desirable patient outcome.

The fundamental goal of optimizing outcome is particularly pertinent to anesthesia care because surgical anesthesia is facilitative rather than therapeutic. There is no "cure rate" that would allow comparison of different medications, for example. In light of this, and building on the dictum *primum, non nocere*, it is possible to understand why there has evolved in both the medical and lay communities the expectation that anesthesia care should never cause any patient injury. Further, this expectation has been encouraged by the suggestion that the nature of intraoperative anesthesia care is uniquely amenable to the absolute minimization of anesthesia-related adverse patient outcome.[10] Therefore, while significant discussion of "quality" in anesthesia has occurred for some time,[11] the current focus clearly is on the identification and avoidance of anesthesia-related complications.

The Mechanism of Quality Assurance

The traditional QA construct[12] consists of assessing quality by objective means (measurements whenever possible) that are well documented, and then working to assure the best possible quality by reinforcing and rewarding high-quality performance and, conversely, solving any problems discovered and improving poor-quality performance.

The fundamental QA process has two parts: (1) monitoring the target activity to see what the quality of performance is, and (2) helping to resolve problems discovered. When it is suspected that quality is suboptimal, the QA process has four steps: (1) problem identification, (2) problem analysis and evaluation, (3) problem resolution, and (4) follow-up monitoring to be sure the resolution was effective.

Problem identification involves data acquisition and consequent examination for patterns, trends, or specific incidents. Problem evaluation can be as simple as a case conference discussion within the department or as complex as seeking an outside evaluation from recognized experts, including even a formal peer review evaluation of the hospital or anesthesia department. Problem resolution, by definition, involves change. Some new policy, procedure, privilege, knowledge, habit, or attitude must be applied to the identified problem. Follow-up is intended not only to verify that the problem has in fact been resolved, but also to monitor for recurrence or mutation of the original issue.

Elements Covered by Quality Assurance

While outcome is considered the most important component of care, structure and process are intertwined in producing outcome and have themselves characteristics worthy of attention by the QA system.

The structural elements in anesthesia practice include things such as the policy and procedure manual described earlier, and, classically, the apparatus involved in rendering care. The practice of anesthesia depends heavily on equipment and supplies. Purchase of these and the maintenance and servicing of anesthesia equipment are central to high-quality anesthesia care. Specific programs for QA of anesthesia equipment have been developed.[13] Conducting a QA audit to study whether functioning suction is in place prior to induction of general anesthesia is a good example of QA involving structure.

The element of process in anesthesia simply refers to how the practice is carried out. A good example of a QA issue would be whether or not the ASA standards for basic intraoperative monitoring are being observed during the administration of anesthesia. This might be the subject of a one-time investigation, a periodic audit, or a continual ongoing review. Multiple other examples also illustrate the process issue. Is there a full surgical workup on the chart before the patient arrives in the OR? Is there a complete, separate preanesthetic evaluation? Is the anesthesia machine checked out according to protocol at the beginning of the workday and prior to each case? Most of these points involve documentation, and concern has been expressed that this type of QA activity assesses writing ability rather than the quality of anesthesia care. The fact is, documentation has become central in medical care. There are multiple medicolegal cases in which the adage, "If you didn't write it down, you didn't do it," has determined the outcome of a trial. Accordingly, the process element of QA in medical care should focus simultaneously on both the action and its documentation. Note, however, that wide latitude must be given in considering whether process goals in QA have been accomplished. One practitioner reviewing charts for a QA evaluation might write a note in the medical record quite differently from what is entered. If the note as written is reasonably complete and communicative, the assessor must set aside issues of personal style in favor of avoiding needless confrontation with its author. Rarely is the letter of the prescribed process nearly as important as the spirit of compliance with full documentation.

The outcome element of care has become the greatest focus of attention. The JCAHO now uses a list of anesthesia outcomes as QA "indicators" (see below) as part of its routine inspection protocol. Because operative anesthesia is facilitative, anesthesia outcome traditionally has been associated with the absence of complications. Complications can be as simple as deviation from prearranged plans (discharge home of a same-day-surgery patient at 5 P.M. rather than 2 P.M.) or as serious as death or permanent grave central nervous system damage from unrecognized hypoventilation causing hypoxemia and cardiac arrest, with an entire spectrum of intermediate events in between. Anesthesia outcome does not always have to be considered in terms of complications. Patient satisfaction is a valid indicator. Doing an appropriate survey and being able to report that the day after outpatient surgery, 87% of patients were pleased with their anesthetics, is a very useful anesthesia QA activity.

Whether outcome in medical care is necessarily correlated or even likely to be correlated with structure and process has been debated.[14-16] A good outcome (particularly the absence of complications from an anesthetic) may result from poor performance of a procedure or sloppy care with inadequate or inappropriate equipment. Therefore, maximally effective QA efforts in medicine must include examination of all three central elements: structure, process, and outcome.

Implementation of a Quality Assurance Program

Any anesthesia department or group initiating or significantly restructuring a QA program should first investigate what types of programs already exist in the institution or area. Particularly within a hospital, there may be established mechanisms in place for meeting the various reporting requirements, both with regard to the hospital and the requisite outside agencies (most often the state board for medical licensing/registration). Any new system should be compatible with and also tap into, or at least interface with, available communication mechanisms. Because the only logical way to manage a genuine QA program today is with a computerized data base, it may be possible to connect hard-wire links from the anesthesia data base computer to the offices or agencies requiring reports and thus minimize paperwork and bother when filing QA reports.

The anesthesia department or group must decide what baseline statistics, before the QA information is considered, are to be kept. This will depend on the nature of the department and the interests of the members. Large academic departments with ongoing clinical research projects will likely record permanently in their own records as much demographic information about the patient as is available on the anesthesia chart (including a list of associated medical conditions), the CPT-4 procedure code (and possibly the ICD-9 diagnosis code), medications used, and perhaps even some representative vital signs. Groups not planning to search the data base for clinical research projects may decide that such information need not be recorded. In both cases, the data base program could likely be coupled with or driven by a computerized billing program that may already be in place and functional. Once fundamental decisions are made, this first part of the computerized system should be constructed. This may challenge a programming-facile member of the anesthesia department, but often is simpler with the help of a hired professional programmer familiar with such tasks. There are several commercially available prepackaged programs specifically intended for anesthesia information management and QA. While potentially time-saving and useful, often they need to be modified to accommodate the specific needs or characteristics of the department, thus negativing some of the advertised ease and cost savings.

Initially the terminology of QA often seems foreign to medical practitioners. Consequently, they tend either to ignore the process or to assume it is cumbersome and complex, and thus to be avoided. Implementation of a QA program involves three main issues: (1) Selection of indicators. Indicators are simply the events or characteristics looked for in the QA data collection. (2) Establishment of performance criteria where necessary. Criteria are the expected or acceptable rates of appearance of the indicators. (3) Creation of a data collection system that examines the clinical activity in question and looks for appearance of the indicators.

Indicators

Indicators are simply the events, good or bad, looked for during the review of clinical care (either in medical records or in summaries prepared by providers of the care). Indicators are sometimes called *monitors*; but it is incorrect to refer to them as "criteria." Indicators are whatever the QA system is organized to find out about. If there is a perceived problem with patients arriving in the OR without complete surgical workups, then an indicator such as "History and Physical complete" can be added to an ongoing QA screening process or can be the subject of a special QA audit for a sufficient amount of time to yield a thorough understanding of the situation. A common process indicator might be, "Anesthesia machine check-out recorded." Indicators may be positive, such as for data collected at the postoperative visit having the indicators: "Patient states satisfied with anesthetic," or "Patient denies memory for procedure." Most commonly in anesthesia, however, indicators are related to adverse outcomes or adverse events that would have caused untoward outcomes if not caught and corrected (critical incidents)—in other words, complications. Because high-quality anesthesia care is in large part defined in the minds of many as the absence of complications, the majority of anesthesia QA is related to identifying and studying complications and then reducing their incidence.

Lists of anesthesia indicators based on outcomes largely interpreted to be adverse have been published.[17,18] Figure 2-1 is a sample audit form with a long list of anesthesia indicators. It is offered as an example and not necessarily a prototype. Such a list may not be best for all departments or groups, each of which must develop a list of indicators appropriate to the specific characteristics of the institution or facility. General indicators can be as simple as "case canceled" or "more than two attempts to start an IV," or as grave as "anesthesia-caused death." Airway indicators might range from "chipped tooth" to "esophageal intubation—recognized" or "accidental extubation." Vital sign indicators include significant or dangerous deviations from normal or acceptable. Apparatus indicators could include "breathing system disconnection during mechanical ventilation." Organ system indicators are many and varied. Samples are "myocardial ischemia," "aspiration," "postoperative nausea and vomiting," "significant atelectasis," "grossly abnormal blood gas values," or "neurologic change after anesthesia." All these are valid, but merely examples. Considerable thought is required to establish a thorough yet manageable list of indicators that an anesthesiology department wishes to examine in its QA system. One specific indicator, such as failed regional block, might or might not be part of a continuous, permanent set of indicators that are always being studied or tracked (the generic screening process described below). If not, the suggestion of a problem might cause it to be moved onto such a list, either permanently or for a specified period of time or number of cases. The permanent list must be comfortable for those using it. It may have fewer than ten items in one setting and more than 100 in another. The JCAHO has had many iterations of an anesthesia outcome indicator list. Table 2-1 is the most recent version. It is essentially guaranteed that JCAHO inspectors will be looking for QA data along these lines. However, creating a QA mechanism that can track an indicator is more important than the sheer number of indicators tracked. Major complications will very rapidly be widely known in all but the largest anesthesia departments, and therefore departments often focus many QA indicators on complications that either have been identified as problems or that tend to be routinely overlooked.

Criteria

Once indicators are chosen, quantitative criteria need to be established where appropriate (for almost all the indicators). The intended use of the word *criteria* in classic QA concerns the establishment of performance criteria—what is the minimum acceptable rate of the appearance of a "good" indicator (e.g., complete workup on the chart preop-

QUALITY ASSURANCE REPORT FORM

Department of Anesthesiology
CLINICAL QUALITY ASSURANCE PEER REVIEW AUDIT
(Return form with anesthesia record to OR desk.
Do not make copies. Do not attach to patient record.)

Date _____   Pre op: [ ] Complete
OR# _____ Other OR(s) attended _____   [ ] Completed in OR (e.g., labs)
Operation _____   (as posted)   [ ] Incomplete (explain below)
ASA Class _____   [ ] Made by another anesthetist
                                             [ ] Plan changed (exlain below)

Anesthetic [ ] General   [ ] Regional   [ ] MAC
Anesthesiologist _____ Anesthesiology Resident _____
Surgeon _____   Surgery Resident _____
Recovery Room Nurse _____ Discharge:[ ] ONR [ ] ICU [ ] Ward [ ] Home

[ ] NO UNTOWARD EVENTS   [ ] UNTOWARD EVENTS (check below)

OR RR Airway   OR RR Respiratory
__ __ Chipped tooth/loosened tooth __ __ Post op ventilatory assistance
__ __ Stridor, Laryngospasm, Obstruction   (unplanned)
__ __ Failed rapid sequence induction __ __ Significant Hypoxemia/hypercapnia
__ __ Nose bleed or other trauma of airway __ __ Pneumothorax
__ __ Inability to intubate by route __ __ Inappropriate bronchial
          originally planned   intubation
__ __ Esophageal intubation   __ __ Aspiration-respiratory
__ __ Lip trauma   distress syndrome
__ __ Accidental extubation   __ __ Reintubation (other than accidental
                                              extubation)
       CV   __ __ Bronchospasm
__ __ Death
__ __ Cardiac arrest   Miscellaneous
__ __ Significant Hypertension (sustained __ __ Other (desribe below)
          >30% above preop systolic) __ __ Hyperpyrexia >38 C
__ __ Significant Hypotension (sustained __ __ Hypothermia <34 C (uninduced)
          <30% below preop diastolic) __ __ Wrong medication/dose given
__ __ Significant Bradycardia (30% below   (describe below)
          preop or that associated with __ __ Drug reaction (allergic/adverse)
          hypotension)   __ __ Intravascular line problem
__ __ Significant Tacycardia (30% above __ __ Delayed or erroneous lab report/other
          preop or that associated with __ __ Nausea and vomiting
          hypertension)   __ __ Equipment failure (explain below)
__ __ Myocardial ischemia/MI suspected __ __ Pain medication delayed/inadequate
__ __ Congestive heart failure/pulmonary edema
__ __ Dysrhythmia associated with one or Regional (including pain therapy)
          more of above   __ __ Pain unresponsive to block
                                    __ __ Failed block, inadequate block
       Discharge planning   __ __ Toxic reaction
__   Unplanned outpatient admission __ __ Excessive block (high spinal)
__   Unplanned transfer to ICU   __ __ Wet tap (epidural)
__   Unplanned return to OR
__   Unscheduled ONR   Neurological
__   > 3 hr. stay in RR   __ __ Prolonged neuromuscular block
__   Delayed waiting for M.D. to evaluate __ __ Prolonged sedation
__   Delayed waiting for X-ray   __ __ Peripheral nerve injury
__   Delayed waiting for Room   __ __ Stroke
__   Delayed for medical reasons __ __ Recall
__   Other delay (explain below) __ __ Seizure
                                    __ __ Other damage (explain below)

For each of the above, describe briefly on back

Event 1 [ ] OR   [ ] RR

A) Cause of Event

_____
_____
_____

B) Treatment of Event

_____
_____
_____

C) Result of Treatment

_____
_____

Figure 2-1. Prototype anesthesia quality assurance audit form with a lengthy list of indicators.[18] The form is completed by the primary anesthesia provider and is used as the basis for generic screening in a large anesthesia department. Note the "peer review" heading, placed in an attempt to ensure that the document is considered peer review material in the medicolegal sense. (Reproduced with permission of Jerry A. Cohen, M.D., Department of Anesthesiology, University of Florida College of Medicine, Gainesville, Florida.)

TABLE 2-1. JCAHO Anesthesia Indicators

1. Patients diagnosed with a central nervous system (CNS) complication occurring during procedures involving anesthesia administration or within 2 postprocedure days of its conclusion, subcategorized by American Society of Anesthesiologists Physical Status (ASA-PS) class, patient age, and CNS *vs.* non-CNS-related procedures.
2. Patients developing a peripheral neurologic deficit during procedures involving anesthesia administration or within 2 postprocedure days of its conclusion.
3. Patients with an acute myocardial infarction during procedures involving anesthesia administration or within 2 postprocedure days of its conclusion, subcategorized by ASA-PS class, patient age, and cardiac *vs.* noncardiac procedures.
4. Patients with a cardiac arrest during procedures involving anesthesia administration or within 24 postprocedure hours of its conclusion, excluding patients with required intraoperative cardiac arrest, subcategorized by ASA-PS class, patient age, and cardiac *vs.* noncardiac procedures.
5. Patients with an unplanned respiratory arrest during procedures involving anesthesia administration or within 24 postprocedure hours of its conclusion.
6. Death of patients during procedures involving anesthesia administration or within 48 postprocedure hours of its conclusion, subcategorized by ASA-PS class and patient age.
7. Unplanned admission of patients to the hospital within 1 postprocedure day following outpatient procedures involving anesthesia administration.
8. Unplanned admission of patients to an intensive care unit within 1 postprocedure day of procedures involving anesthesia administration.
9. Patients with a discharge diagnosis of fulminant pulmonary edema developed during procedures involving anesthesia administration or within 1 postprocedure day of its conclusion.
10. Patients diagnosed with an aspiration pneumonitis occurring during procedures involving anesthesia administration or within 2 postprocedure days of its conclusion.
11. Patients developing a postural headache within 4 postprocedure days following procedures involving spinal or epidural anesthesia administration.
12. Patients experiencing a dental injury during procedures involving anesthesia care.
13. Patients experiencing an ocular injury during procedures involving anesthesia care.

Reproduced with permission from Joint Commission on the Accreditation of Healthcare Organizations: AMH/91: Accreditation Manual for Hospitals. Chicago, Joint Commission on the Accreditation of Healthcare Organizations, 1990.

eratively) or the maximum acceptable for a "bad" indicator (*e.g.*, chipped tooth from intubation). These criteria are functionally group standards, but it is strongly advisable from a medicolegal standpoint to avoid that particular label, in order to minimize confusion with the concept of standard of care.

Examples of criteria include, "No more than 4% of same-day surgery patients should require admission to the hospital for anesthesia-related causes," "there should be fewer than 2% accidental wet taps during attempts at epidural catheter placement," and "fewer than 0.2% of general anesthesia patients should require emergency reintubation in the PACU." Obviously, for many indicators of major complications, the desirable and sought-after criterion will be "none." Some indicators do not lend themselves easily to absolute criteria. It may be difficult to specify, for example, an acceptable number of patients having diastolic blood pressures more than 30% below baseline if that particular vital sign change is an indicator chosen for audit or tracking. In such situations, it is better to study the indicator through the QA system long enough to get good statistics on the appearance of the indicator. Once a baseline rate is determined, this indicator can be evaluated over time for changes, and, if desired, numerical criteria can be established against which to compare the performance of the group of practitioners as a whole, a subgroup, or an individual anesthesia provider.

Once indicators and criteria are in place, the QA system is ready to gather data from review of clinical activities.

Input Data

The source of the input data for the QA system and the method of its collection are among the most significant issues of the entire process.

The first of the two main purposes of QA, the quality monitoring function, requires a significant data base. It can be debated whether it is adequate in anesthesia practice to sample a fraction of the anesthesia cases done and make this the QA data base. There are proposed QA systems that focus exclusively on reported problems. Because the number of cases with acknowledged problems will be small in comparison with the total number of cases done, the sample fraction of cases will be small and quite skewed, simply because only problem cases will be reviewed. Other systems call for a review of a fraction of routine cases (cases in which no major problem was obvious on the surface) and then extrapolate the rate of appearance of indicators to the entire body of anesthetics administered in that institution or facility. The traditional and most thorough QA system, however, involves review of each and every case done. This is called *generic screening* or *occurrence screening*.

With regard to the other main purpose of QA, there are many sources of potential problem identification, the most obvious being from within the anesthesia department—by word of mouth, from cases discussed at rounds or conferences, from incident reports, and through the QA process itself in the form of the information discovered through the data-gathering mechanism established. Other sources of identification of problems with anesthesia care may become apparent. Within the hospital these sources might include surgical colleagues, cases discussed at surgical rounds, record room generic screens (particularly valuable in identifying complications that are noted only after the routine postoperative visit on the day after surgery), the hospital QA or risk management office (especially if incident reports are filed here), or the nursing service. Outside the hospital, sources might include professional associates, information learned at meetings, and material in the anesthesia literature. A key feature of the data collection system is that it must be decided whether the reporting mechanism to the departmental QA system will be used to record critical incidents—events, that, if not recognized and corrected in time, would have led to an untoward patient outcome. If so, specific assurances of anonymity or freedom from possible retribution must be built into the process or no events will be reported. Finally, it must be decided if all cases done in the department will become part of the QA data base. If so, this is classic generic screening—looking at each and every case, not just a sample, for the appearance of the indicators selected. Generic screening is always a component of fully actualized QA systems. It is the best source of initial clinical data input into a medical QA system.

Who should do the actual generic screening is a key question in QA data acquisition. In anesthesia practice there are two fundamental choices. One way is to have the practitioner who administered the anesthetic or was directly involved with the case provide the data, usually by filling out a form or making a computer entry at the completion of the anesthetic. The other way is to rely on the completeness of the anesthesia chart and subsequent related records and have a trained chart reviewer retrospectively study the chart and then make the appropriate data entry. Neither way is necessarily better than the other. Each department or group establishing a QA system must evaluate the unique aspects of that practice and choose accordingly. For example, departments with computerized automated anesthesia records likely will choose the simple option of adding a final customized screen to the information management system sequence and have the computer abstract what relevant information it can (e.g., variation of vital signs from baseline), with the practitioner entering the remainder in response to screen prompts.

The generic screen is constructed to note the appearance of the agreed-upon indicators. If one of the indicators is "unintentional intraoperative temperature below 34°C," the practitioner or reviewer first notes "yes" or "no" in response to the prompt asking whether the temperature was measured. If "yes," then omitting any further entry means no temperature that low. If "yes" is checked for low temperature, a space or field allows the entry of the lowest temperature value and a brief note as to the reason. All this could be done at the end of the case or any time thereafter. In one large study of anesthesia care, 18% of over 12,000 patients had at least one *intraoperative* event noted that qualified as the appearance of a QA indicator.[19] If an indicator studied is "admission to the PACU for longer than four hours," then this datum can only be captured if (1) the practitioner who administered the anesthetic comes back later and notes how long the patient was in the PACU, or (2) PACU personnel enter the information in some assigned manner, or (3) a retrospective reviewer notes the times recorded in the medical record. For indicators such as "myocardial ischemia," if the data are collected by a chart reviewer, that person must be able to read, "ST down, TNG started" and understand the implication and record it correctly. These examples illustrate some common issues in implementation of a QA data collection system.

Generic screening interacts with the QA mechanism in two separate ways. First, generic screening can discover otherwise subtle problems. If one practitioner has a higher than expected incidence of some small but definite problem such as lip lacerations associated with use of a specific laryngoscope blade, correctly executed generic screening should reveal this problem and trigger the traditional four-step QA protocol within the department that calls for change as resolution. There may also follow, for example, a detailed prospective study specifically of the relationship of blade choice to lip trauma for either that practitioner, a subset of the group, or all anesthesia providers. Second, in contrast to the surveillance screening generating unexpected information, the process can be used to look specifically to see if something suspected is true. For example, if in one month a hospital report revealed that two ambulatory surgical patients who happened to be anesthetized by one provider required admission to the hospital for severe postoperative nausea, the generic screening process could be used to look at that anesthetist's record retrospectively (and prospectively, if indicated) for all incidents of postoperative nausea for that one provider, or among all patients receiving a particular medication, or whatever. Thus, in summary, identification of a clinical problem can come *from* the generic

screening process identifying the unexpected or (coming from another source) can be taken *to* the process, which is then used to study the suspected problem. Both situations lead eventually to intervention and subsequent resolution of the problem.

A central issue in generic screening QA data collection involves the "self-reporting" mentality. Will anesthesia providers be honest in recording on the QA form or the anesthesia chart minor problems, complications, or "near accidents" that caused no readily identifiable adverse outcome? If a practitioner working alone accidently intubates the esophagus, immediately recognizes it, and immediately replaces the endotracheal tube correctly in the trachea, with no untoward effect visible, will this be recorded? Many anesthesiologists agree that the situation should be noted, but others believe it is quite common and benign, not worthy of mention. Issues of individual personality are also involved. One key point is the use to which the QA data will be put once collected. QA data can be used to create "provider profiles," records of the number of times a practitioner was associated with the appearance of QA indicators, whether complications or simply observations. Thus, the fact that provider X intubated the esophagus, however transiently, would in the example be documented in that person's permanent file. Some may argue that this is both appropriate and valuable because if there is a pattern, the provider can be advised of it and thus seek training or experience to overcome an apparent weakness or bad habit. Clearly, provider X must be informed of all this in a friendly and nonthreatening manner. If, however, such provider profile information is used in an adverse fashion (e.g., evaluation for promotion or salary increase, or even for disciplinary action), there would be incomplete reporting of nonobvious problems or situations. This is a difficult area, and it must be handled delicately wherever it appears. Constructively approached, it is possible to achieve complete self-reporting and to use this information as the source of QA input data in whichever of the two capture mechanisms is chosen.

Deciding which of the two basic mechanisms for capture of the raw QA data to use is often difficult. In an ideal world, each anesthesia practitioner would follow up each case with completion of some form of data record, either on paper, by filling out a form, or electronically, by making a keyboard entry. Further, this same person would follow up and make small additional entries following discharge from the PACU, after the postoperative visit, and even at the time of discharge from the hospital. The realities of life being what they are, however, it is very difficult to imagine both the inclination and the ability to achieve complete cooperation from a group of anesthesia providers. Simply getting a QA form filled out at the end of each case would constitute a victory. Because QA activities are now routinely extended at a minimum to cover the patients' stay in the PACU (Fig. 2-2), some institutions and facilities have supplemental capture mechanisms. These usually are put into effect at the time of PACU discharge or even discharge from the hospital (from either inpatient or outpatient care) and involve the primary care providers, usually the nurses who have cared for the patient. Such a mechanism, although more achievable than requiring the anesthesia provider to maintain responsibility for data capture up to the time of hospital discharge, is equally unrealistic. Accordingly, the alternative is to stress strongly to all providers the necessity for completeness of the anesthesia record, and then to have an employee in the department or group retrospectively review the anesthesia chart and related records for indicators. This

UNIVERSITY OF CHICAGO
DEPARTMENT OF ANESTHESIA and CRITICAL CARE

NOT PART OF PATIENT MEDICAL RECORD

FOR DEPARTMENT QUALITY
ASSURANCE PURPOSES ONLY

DO NOT DUPLICATE
please complete a form for each patient by filling in all appropriate information and depositing with
billing sheets in appropriate slot

CONFIDENTIAL ANESTHESIA & CRITICAL CARE UNEXPECTED EVENT REPORT FORM

IMMEDIATE, POSTOPERATIVE PERIOD (PAR)

PATIENT NAME   UNIT NUMBER   DATE

A. INADEQUATE P.A.R. SCORE (<6)   **B. RESPIRATORY**
1. [ ] Oversedation   1. [ ] Aspiration
2. [ ] Inadequate reversal of neuromuscular blockade   2. [ ] Reintubation
3. [ ] Unexpected disorientation   3. [ ] Hypoventilation
4. [ ] Other_____   4. [ ] Inadequate ABG's
                                             5. [ ] Other_____

C. CARDIOVASCULAR (requiring therapy)
1. [ ] Dysrythmia   5. [ ] Bradycardia
2. [ ] Hypotension   6. [ ] Myocardia Ischemia
3. [ ] Hypertension   7. [ ] Cardiac Arrest
4. [ ] Tachycardia   8. [ ] Other_____

D. CNS   **E. REGIONAL**
1. [ ] Obtundation   1. [ ] Nerve Injury
2. [ ] Stroke   2. [ ] Prolonged Block
3. [ ] Other_____   3. [ ] Other_____

F. GENERAL (requiring therapy)
1. [ ] Nausea
2. [ ] Vomiting
3. [ ] Oliguria/ Anuria
4. [ ] Other_____

G. DRUG REACTION
Drug_____   Therapy_____
Outcome_____

H. TRANSFUSION REACTION
Symptoms_____   Therapy_____
Outcome_____

I. MISC.
Events_____
_____

J. UNSCHEDULED ADMISSION_____   **K. NO UNEXPECTED EVENTS NOTED**_____

Figure 2-2. Prototype PACU anesthesia quality assurance Unexpected Event Report Form. Note that it is not part of the medical record and is designated as being for QA purposes only. (Reproduced with permission of the Department of Anesthesia and Critical Care, University of Chicago.)

employee might be a former anesthesia provider seeking part-time work, or a nonprofessional office worker (with backup immediately available to answer questions) who is trained to screen the anesthesia records for the appearance of indicators. If this type of system is chosen, efficiency might be maximized if the QA screener reviewing the charts one by one is simultaneously involved in the billing process. Also, this type of system is interpreted as the most acceptable by the anesthesia providers because they do not complete the QA data entry for each case. Thus, because the reporting and review requirements will be met with a minimum of annoyance, the anesthesia practitioners' energy can be devoted to using the results of the QA process rather than to the mere generation of statistics. Whichever data capture mechanism best meets the needs and desires of the individual group or department, the result should be a continuously flowing stream of information into a process aimed at improving the quality of practice.

Output from the Quality Assurance Process

Because the resolution of clinical problems identified or confirmed through the QA process involves change, there must be a process for implementing the change and then verifying that it has produced the desired result. Many larger anesthesiology departments have a QA committee that is charged with carrying out the classic four-step process of problem identification, evaluation, resolution, and follow-up monitoring. In smaller groups there may be one or two staff people who are responsible for QA, or the chief of service may do it as part of his or her job. It would be this committee or person who would initiate some additional QA activity after an appropriate interval of time to examine the effect of changes in policy, procedure, protocols, equipment, and the like. This could be as simple as watching the generic screening results for a change in the rate of appearance of the indicator of concern. In other circumstances, special studies or audits may be initiated to verify that the change implemented has caused the intended effect in clinical results. For such things as the availability and use of specific pieces of equipment or the preanesthetic check-out of the machine, some QA representative may need to make and record observations in the operating suite. This is not the most popular activity for the person doing it or for those being observed, but at least the department members know that attention is being given to issues of concern in a sincere attempt to improve care.

It is critical to provide feedback to members of the group or department about the results of QA activity. Those responsible for the system must document all QA activities; this makes the subsequent reporting and inspection processes much easier. Also, the QA documentation should be shared in some manner with the anesthesia providers, who ultimately are the data source for the QA system. It is very frustrating to staff to extend efforts to cooperate with QA data gathering and then not get any information back from the system. This situation reinforces the negative impression that QA is a waste of time and merely accumulates masses of useless statistics that nobody cares about anyway.

After the necessary data analysis, the QA results should be shared at regular and frequent intervals in some detail with the staff. If there are no indicators showing an incidence above the numeric criteria, it should be strongly reinforced to the staff that they are doing a good job. If problems are identified, the proposed solutions and the follow-up should be discussed thoroughly. The group may not need to know the details of a specific untoward situation involving one provider, but the staff should know that constructive QA activity is taking place. The success of the QA program depends on this responsiveness and communication by the QA system and those responsible for it.

Quality Assurance Models

A generic QA program based on many of the most traditional understandings in QA has been outlined in the foregoing sections. Wide variations on this basic theme have been successfully implemented in different institutions.

One very specific and extremely comprehensive QA model from a large academic anesthesia department is based on "adverse patient outcomes" (APOs) as indicators in the QA process. An extensive generic screening form with a long list of intraoperative and postoperative indicators (see Fig. 2-1) must be completed by the anesthesiology resident doing each anesthetic and then the form returned by that resident to one of the departmental offices. A corrected OR schedule is used as the master checklist allowing verification that forms were received for each and every patient anesthetized in the institution. A departmental secretary seeks out and reminds residents of the need to complete a form if there is none received for a specific case, although the intention is for the form to be completed immediately at the conclusion of the OR and PACU components of the anesthetic care. Forms listing APOs are separated and reviewed by the departmental QA officer, who categorizes the findings (avoidable vs. unavoidable event, appropriate vs. inappropriate treatment, and so on) using detailed definitions established by the QA system. About 10% of the cases are labeled "severe" (e.g., cardiac arrest/death, myocardial infarction, new congestive heart failure, significant hypoxemia for more than 3 minutes, aspiration, neurologic complication, any permanent injury) and are flagged for further review. The findings for all cases, major and minor, are entered into a computerized data base and compared with all past information in an analysis for possible evidence of trends, either for the specific provider or the department as a whole. Additional data, such as from the hospital QA or utilization review committees is added and, if indicated, the anesthesia provider involved is interviewed. Then, in a traditional manner, the QA officer and departmental committee proceed with problem evaluation, resolution, and follow-up. The system has extensive documentation built into its structure, and all required statistics and reporting, including back to the department itself, "fall out" automatically.

An alternate anesthesia QA mechanism, the *clinical competence model*,[20] has been publicized by the ASA's Committee on Peer Review.[3] This model cites three principles: (1) peer review should be used to determine a practitioner's competence, (2) the best indication of competence is outcome, and (3) people make mistakes, and one error does not necessarily imply incompetence. Competence is judged by error analysis, which in turn is based on the ideas that competence or the lack of it is reflected in errors made and that incompetent practitioners have patterns of errors that differ markedly from those of competent practitioners. The data gathering does not depend on generic screening, but rather on required reporting of "any event that might be related to anesthesia management" by the provider(s) involved or anyone else anywhere in the institution who discovers an event that might be relevant in this process. All such forms submitted to the QA committee are stripped of all identifying information and copies are circulated to members of the QA committee for evaluation decisions regarding the event: (1) relationship to anesthesia care, (2) grading with a "negative outcome score" (0–10, "no sequelae"–"death"), (3) identity and classification of the errors committed (Table 2-2), (4) conclusions with explanations and references, and (5) recommendations for future prevention. With the provider (theoretically) still anonymous, the QA committee prepares a report based on a synthesis of error analysis decisions of its members, and that report goes to the entire department. Only after its approval will the report be associated with the individual practitioner involved, and the report becomes a part of that practitioner's permanent file. The report contributes to the practitioner's "error profile," the components of which are shown in Table 2-3. In addition to the application of the minimum performance levels, this profile is compared with the aggregate departmental profile to see if the individual practitioner has more errors than his or her peers. If so, this points the way to another need for problem resolution related to the specific individ-

TABLE 2-2. Clinical Competence Quality Assurance Model Error Analysis

Management Areas

Airway
Behavior
  Violation of bylaws, rules,
    regulations, or procedures
  Unprofessional conduct
  Substance abuse
Circulatory
Central and peripheral nervous
  system
Drug action
  Inhalation agents
  Intravenous agents
    Relaxants
    Opioids
    Sedative-hypnotics
  Local anesthetics
  Allergic reaction
  Cardiovascular drugs
  Drug interaction
Electrical
Endocrine
Hematologic
  Anemia
  Transfusion
  Coagulation
Hepatic
Instrumentation
  Invasive monitors
  Noninvasive monitors
Intravenous infusion
Metabolic
  Fluid and electrolyte
  Malignant hyperthermia
Pulmonary (lung function)
  Oxygenation
  Parenchymal
  Ventilation
Positive injury
Regional technique
Renal
Thermoregulation

Genesis of Error

This category is designed to provide insight into why human errors occur. The classifications used to describe the etiology of human errors are listed here:

Inadequate knowledge
  Didactic
  Experience
Inadequate data
  Failure to seek data
  Collection of irrelevant data
Disregard for data
  Failure to recognize a pattern
  Failure to accept a conclusion
Lack of an alternative plan

Nature of Error

None = an unavoidable circumstance
Mechanical = failure of a device
Human = related to formulation or execution of a decision
  Judgmental = errors occurring when "the action taken is the action intended"; these errors constitute faulty decision processes (*e.g.,* mask anesthesia in "full stomach" situation)
  Technical = errors occurring when "the action taken is not the action intended" (*e.g.,* syringe swap); such errors involve mistakes in the execution of a decision
  Vigilance = errors associated with a lack of adequate general attention (*e.g.,* iv infiltration)

Reproduced with permission from Vitez TS: A model for quality assurance in anesthesiology. J Clin Anesth 2:280, 1990.

TABLE 2-3. Clinical Competence Quality Assurance Model Error Profile for Anesthesia Providers

Comparative Elements

1. Frequency of anesthesia-related events
2. Average negative outcome score
3. Number of errors per event
4. Area of clinical management
5. Nature of errors
6. Genesis of errors

Minimal Performance Levels

1. Anesthetizes ASA I and II patients without negative outcome score >6
2. Institutes appropriate life-sustaining actions in life-threatening situations
3. Displays insight when involved in an important error

Reproduced with permission from Vitez TS: A model for quality assurance in anesthesiology. J Clin Anesth 2:280, 1990.

ual. In the study, an average anesthesia provider made one to two "important" errors per year with a negative outcome score 2–3 (escalation of care) with an average of one to two errors per event. The limitations of semivoluntary self-reporting and the reliance on input from outside the anesthesia department were noted, but it was maintained that the large majority of relevant occurrences were captured in the data base with this system. The clinical competence QA model differs from traditional models in that it truncates certain components and expands others. Again, individual departments and groups must examine the available alternative methods to conduct QA and synthesize them into a program most appropriate to the particular setting and practice.

Whatever model is chosen or constructed, the goal of QA is universal: the optimization of the quality of anesthesia care through the identification of strengths and weaknesses or problems in anesthesia practice and the appropriate reinforcement and resolution, respectively, thereof. Properly implemented, a comprehensive QA program will be minimally intrusive and will pay handsome dividends. Although it is impossible to document scientifically, there exist very strong impressions that the growth and development of widespread anesthesia QA efforts in the mid- to late 1980s were an integral component of the recent general improvement in anesthesia safety and the quality of anesthesia care.

RISK MANAGEMENT

Because risk management is inextricably intertwined with quality assurance, the goal is, at least in part, similar: optimization of care. For the same reasons as outlined for QA, in risk management anesthesia practice focuses on reducing or eliminating the likelihood of anesthesia-caused or anesthesia-related complications (particularly the large fraction of problems caused by human error). Where risk management goes beyond QA is in helping to put in place structure and process that will minimize the impact of an adverse anesthesia event on the patient, the anesthesia provider, and the medical care system. Some components of risk management may at first appear defensive. If such efforts promote better quality care in an attempt to avoid complications, they are very useful. Beyond its primary goal of optimizing care, risk management offers a significant ability to reduce liability exposure. It is true. Unfortunately, it is necessary to be aware of the medicolegal system and the existence of the malpractice crisis. Although there are strong suggestions that the medicolegal crunch of astronomically high settlements and awards with consequent skyrocketing malpractice insurance premiums is lessening in the early 1990s, it has also been maintained that this is merely a cycle that will inevitably reverse itself.[21] Whichever is true, it must be recognized that some attitudes and procedures in risk management are influenced by the characteristics of the medicolegal system and the insurance industry. Further, case precedents have revealed certain characteristics that make the defense of anesthesia providers against unwarranted charges of malpractice more difficult. Theoretically, legal defensive issues ("defensive medicine") should not influence health care practices. However, the potentially devastating emotional and financial impact of a malpractice lawsuit on a practitioner—even a suit with no merit at all—is significant enough to justify awareness of and application of proven risk management strategies intended to minimize the likelihood of malpractice claims.

Risk management concepts have traditionally been associated with the economic aspects of business or professional activity. It began with the insurance industry recognizing "risk": certain activities predictably lead to insurance claims requiring payment. As a result, efforts were made to (1) plan to pay for the loss and (2) try to reduce the likelihood and/or magnitude of loss (and consequent cost). Thus, there was an attempt to control or "manage" the known risk. Regarding anesthesia, it was clear that data "demonstrate that anesthetic mishaps, although relatively few in number, present considerable risk of loss in the areas of hospital cost, human suffering, and the integrity of the medical profession," and, as a result, providers "have developed formal programs to systematically identify and control risks that may lead to patient injury or financial loss."[22] Financial loss usually means settlements and judgments associated with malpractice claims and suits. The emphasis of medical risk management is focused on the prevention of any loss-generating untoward incident or outcome. However, a key traditional component is the effort to limit financial loss once an incident has occurred. A common impression is that the hospital or insurance company risk manager is the person to call as soon as an accident or injury is identified. Although this is true, there also needs to be a shift in perception to the fact that prevention is the primary and damage control a secondary part of the process.

Classic risk management involves the same four steps as the QA process: problem identification, evaluation, resolution (with change), and follow-up (with monitoring for impact of the resolution and recurrence of the problem). A large-scale example that has affected anesthesia practice illustrates these ideas. After notification from the malpractice insurer of perceived excessive anesthesia-caused losses, the newly created Risk Management Committee of the Harvard Medical School Department of Anaesthesia reviewed the available literature and all the anesthesia-related claims and incidents for 1976–1986 from the department's malpractice insurer. Considering the substantive identifiable problems, the committee generated a list of subject categories into which problems and incidents were classified. In order of perceived magnitude, the list of identified areas associated with problems and incidents included (1) minimal monitoring during anesthesia (by far the most frequent issue) and in the postanesthetic recovery period, (2) anesthetizing loca-

tions outside traditional ORs, (3) equipment standards, including preanesthetic equipment check-out, (4) equipment maintenance and servicing, (5) record keeping, and (6) preoperative and postoperative visits by anesthesia personnel. This list then became the basis of a comprehensive program to attempt to devise strategies to improve clinical practice associated with each of the identified areas. Because preventable intraoperative catastrophe accounted by far for the greatest cost, a program to help prevent these accidents was given first priority. In an attempt to give earlier warning of untoward intraoperative developments to anesthesia providers and thus increase the likelihood of the correct diagnosis and treatment before patient injury resulted, mandatory standards for intraoperative monitoring were developed.[10] This effort at the time applied to one institution and seemed potentially to be of general interest to most anesthesiologists, but it was first publicly offered and evaluated essentially as an example of a new application of the risk management process.[23] There had been extensive problem identification, evaluation, and then resolution through change. Further work along the same lines led to other standards concerning other topics on the original list of identified subject areas associated with problems and incidents.[24] After an interval, the follow-up component of the classic risk management process led to an evaluation of the potential impact of the original Harvard monitoring standards.[25] Overall, this large-scale example shows the application of risk management techniques that first stress prevention of untoward events and also include but go far beyond the traditional emphasis on financial loss.

In recent years, risk management has assumed increasing significance within the practice of medicine. Among the reasons are (1) the so-called malpractice crisis, which heightened awareness of risk management among anesthesia practitioners because of intense interest and activity on the part of hospital administrations and malpractice insurance carriers; (2) the major emphasis on containment of the cost of medical care, which has caused thorough critical review of many traditionally accepted practices, with particular attention to outcome of care; and (3) great emphasis by both regulators and the public on the quality of medical care and, again, particularly on outcome, which has led to analysis of events at the most basic level in the medical care delivery system. These three points tend to spotlight any adverse outcome of care, regarding both specific instances and trends.

Adverse outcome of anesthesia care spans a spectrum. The most severe untoward results in anesthesia are among the worst in all of medicine, rivaled in impact only by those in obstetrics. Anesthetists must be constantly aware that anesthesia accidents have the potential to cause great harm. Until the late 1980s, anesthesiologists accounted for about 3% of American physicians and correspondingly generated about 3% of the number of malpractice claims filed. These 3% of claims, however, accounted for about 11% of the total indemnity (dollars paid or set aside for future payment) for medical malpractice cases. Serious untoward results in anesthesia tend to have lasting impact (death or permanent injury), which is very unfortunate and very expensive. The causes of untoward anesthesia outcome are presented elsewhere. Foremost in such discussions is the issue of preventability. Although there is debate about what fraction of adverse incidents might be prevented, it is an inescapable conclusion from study of the literature and from knowledge of current cases that a significant majority of major untoward results (anesthesia accidents) are preventable. There have been many thoughtful discussions of specific clinical strategies and practices for avoiding adverse outcome from anesthesia, including some labeled (probably incorrectly) as dealing with risk management.[26] Consideration of specific monitoring equipment, anesthesia teaching techniques, and case analysis methods is valuable but is only one small component of a comprehensive risk management program in anesthesia. Such a program must cover all relevant aspects of practice. Genuine risk management in anesthesia emphasizes the creation of optimum conditions of structure and process and optimum preparation, awareness, and skill of the anesthesia practitioners. This will help both to prevent complications and to minimize their impact when they occur.

COMPONENTS OF ANESTHESIA RISK MANAGEMENT

The prerequisites for QA cited at the opening of this chapter apply equally to risk management. The risk management implications of the failure of an anesthesia department or hospital to investigate and verify the credentials of and grant appropriate privileges to a new anesthesiologist are major and obvious. Even if the anesthesia provider who becomes the target of a malpractice suit is not an employee of the group or hospital, both will likely be named as co-defendants in the legal action if there is even the slightest hint of any unknown past problems or if the practitioner is attempting clinical activities for which he or she may not be qualified. Similarly obvious from a risk management standpoint is the need for departmental meetings and meaningful case discussions. Likewise, the need for the appropriate qualifications and training of the support staff is clear; if a technician mishandles a piece of equipment out of ignorance, thereby causing or contributing to an anesthesia accident, the anesthesiologists and the facilities will automatically be sued also. The risk management utility of policy and procedure efforts parallel the QA desire to minimize untoward anesthesia outcome. Standards of practice are a component of this effort.

Standards of Practice and Regulatory Agencies

The *standard of care* is the conduct by and skill of a prudent practitioner that can be expected all the time by a reasonable patient. This is a very important medicolegal concept because a bad medical result due to failure to meet the standard of care is malpractice. How to establish exactly what is the applicable standard of care has been discussed for a long time. Courts have traditionally relied on medical experts knowledgeable about the point in question to give opinions as to what is the standard of care and if it has been met in an individual case. This type of standard is somewhat different from the standards followed by various authoritative bodies regarding, for example, the color of gas hoses connected to an anesthesia machine or the inability to open simultaneously two vaporizers on that machine. However, ignoring the equipment standards and tolerating what would be considered an unsafe situation is a violation of the standard of care. Promulgated standards such as the various safety codes and anesthesia machine specifications rapidly become the standard of care because patients (through their attorneys, if there has been an untoward event) expect the authoritative published standards to be observed by the prudent practitioner.

Anesthesiology may be the medical specialty that is most involved with published standards of care. It has been suggested that the nature of anesthesia practice (having certain central critical functions relatively clearly defined and common to all situations and with an emphasis on technology) makes it the most amenable of all the fields of medicine to the use of published standards.[27] The original intraoperative monitoring standards were part of a classic risk management effort. The ASA adopted its own set of basic intraoperative monitoring standards in 1986 (Table 2-4). This document includes clear specification for the presence of personnel during an anesthetic episode and for continual evaluation of oxygenation, ventilation, circulation, and temperature. The rationale for these monitoring standards[27] simply involves the fact that it was felt that functionally mandating certain behaviors oriented toward providing the maximum possible warning of threatening developments during an anesthetic should help minimize intraoperative catastrophic patient injury. These ASA monitoring standards very quickly became part of the accepted standard of care in anesthesia practice. This means they have two important risk management implications. First, in the best spirit of risk management (problem identification, evaluation, resolution), they contribute to the effort to optimize care. Second, they carry profound medicolegal implications: a catastrophic accident occurring while the standards are being actively ignored is very difficult to defend in the consequent malpractice suit, whereas an accident that occurs during well-documented full compliance with the standards will automatically have a strong defense because the standard of care was being met. Several states in the United States have made compliance with these ASA standards mandatory under state regulations or even statutes. Various malpractice insurance companies offered discounts on malpractice insurance policy premiums for compliance with these standards, something quite natural to insurers because they are familiar with the idea of managing known risks to help minimize financial loss to the company. The ASA monitoring standards have been widely emulated in other medical specialties and even in fields outside of medicine. Although there are definite parallels in these other efforts (such as in obstetrics and gynecology), no other area has a structure quite as amenable to the applications of published standards as does anesthesia practice.

Many of the same risk management questions that led to the intraoperative monitoring standards have close parallels in the immediate postoperative period in the PACU. With many of the same elements of thinking, the ASA in 1988 adopted standards for postanesthesia care (Table 2-5). There was consideration of and collaboration with the very detailed standards of practice for PACU care published by the American Society of Post Anesthesia Nurses. The risk management implications of these sets of standards are the same as for the intraoperative monitoring standards.

A slightly different situation exists with regard to the standards for conduct of anesthesia in obstetrics. Originally passed by the ASA in 1988 as standards, in the same manner as the other ASA standards, there were eventually some questions from the ASA membership as to whether they reflected a realistic and desirable standard of care. Accordingly, the obstetric anesthesia standards were downgraded in 1990 to "guidelines" (Table 2-6), specifically to remove the mandatory nature of the document. The intention is to eventually draft new obstetric anesthesia standards. However, until there can be agreement as to what should be prescribed as the standard of care, the medicolegal imperative of published standards has been temporarily set aside.

TABLE 2-4. ASA Standards for Basic Intraoperative Monitoring

**Approved by House of Delegates of the American Society of Anesthesiologists
on October 21, 1986, and last amended on October 23, 1990,
effective January 1, 1991**

These standards apply to all anesthesia care although, in emergency circumstances, appropriate life support measures take precedence. These standards may be exceeded at any time based on the judgement of the responsible anesthesiologist. They are intended to encourage high quality patient care, but observing them cannot guarantee any specific patient outcome. They are subject to revision from time to time, as warranted by the evolution of technology and practice. This set of standards addresses only the issue of basic intra-operative monitoring, which is one component of anesthesia care. In certain rare or unusual circumstances, (1) some of these methods of monitoring may be clinically impractical, and (2) appropriate use of the described monitoring methods may fail to detect untoward clinical developments. Brief interruptions of continual† monitoring may be unavoidable. *Under extenuating circumstances, the responsible anesthesiologist may waive the requirements marked with an asterisk (*); it is recommended that when this is done, it should be so stated (including the reasons) in a note in the patient's medical record.* These standards are not intended for application to the care of the obstetrical patient in labor or in the conduct of pain management.

STANDARD I

Qualified anesthesia personnel shall be present in the room throughout the conduct of all general anesthetics, regional anesthetics, and monitored anesthesia care.

OBJECTIVE

Because of the rapid changes in patient status during anesthesia, qualified anesthesia personnel shall be continuously present to monitor the patient and provide anesthesia care. In the event there is a direct known hazard, *e.g.,* radiation, to the anesthesia personnel which might require intermittent remote observation of the patient, some provision for monitoring the patient must be made. In the event that an emergency requires the temporary absence of the person primarily responsible for the anesthetic, the best judgement of the anesthesiologist will be exercised in comparing the emergency with the anesthetized patient's condition and in the selection of the person left responsible for the anesthetic during the temporary absence.

STANDARD II

During all anesthetics, the patient's oxygenation, ventilation, circulation and temperature shall be continually evaluated.

OXYGENATION

OBJECTIVE

To ensure adequate oxygen concentration in the inspired gas and the blood during all anesthetics.

METHODS

1. Inspired gas: During every administration of general anesthesia using an anesthesia machine, the concentration of oxygen in the patient breathing system shall be measured by an oxygen analyzer with a low oxygen concentration limit alarm in use.*
2. Blood oxygenation: During all anesthetics, a quantitative method of assessing oxygenation such as pulse oximetry shall be employed.* Adequate illumination and exposure of the patient is necessary to assess color.*

VENTILATION

OBJECTIVE

To ensure adequate ventilation of the patient during all anesthetics.

METHODS

1. Every patient receiving general anesthesia shall have the adequacy of ventilation continually evaluated. While qualitative clinical signs such as chest excursion, observation of the reservoir breathing bag and auscultation of breath sounds may be adequate, quantitative monitoring of the CO_2 content and/or volume of expired gas is encouraged.
2. When an endotracheal tube is inserted, its correct positioning in the trachea must be verified by clinical assessment and by identification of carbon dioxide in the expired gas.* End-tidal CO_2 analysis, in use from the time of endotracheal tube placement, is encouraged.
3. When ventilation is controlled by a mechanical ventilator, there shall be in continuous use a device that is capable of detecting disconnection of components of the breathing system. The device must give an audible signal when its alarm threshold is exceeded.
4. During regional anesthesia and monitored anesthesia care, the adequacy of ventilation shall be evaluated, at least, by continual observation of qualitative clinical signs.

CIRCULATION

OBJECTIVE

To ensure the adequacy of the patient's circulatory function during all anesthetics.

METHODS

1. Every patient receiving anesthesia shall have the electrocardiogram continuously displayed from the beginning of anesthesia until preparing to leave the anesthetizing location.*
2. Every patient receiving anesthesia shall have arterial blood pressure and heart rate determined and evaluated at least every five minutes.*
3. Every patient receiving general anesthesia shall have, in addition to the above, circulatory function continually evaluated by at least one of the following: palpation of a pulse, auscultation of heart sounds, monitoring of a tracing of intra-arterial pressure, ultrasound peripheral pulse monitoring, or pulse plethysmography or oximetry.

BODY TEMPERATURE

OBJECTIVE

To aid in the maintenance of appropriate body temperature during all anesthetics.

METHODS

There shall be readily available a means to continuously measure the patient's temperature. When changes in body temperature are intended, anticipated or suspected, the temperature shall be measured.

†Note that "continual" is defined as "repeated regularly and frequently in steady rapid succession" whereas "continuous" means "prolonged without any interruption at any time."

Reprinted with permission of the American Society of Anesthesiologists, 515 Busse Highway, Park Ridge, Illinois 60068–3189.

TABLE 2-5. ASA Standards for Postanesthesia Care

**Approved by House of Delegates of the American Society of Anesthesiologists
on October 12, 1988, and last amended on October 23, 1990**

These Standards apply to postanesthesia care in all locations. These Standards may be exceeded based on the judgement of the responsible anesthesiologist. They are intended to encourage high-quality patient care, but cannot guarantee any specific patient outcome. They are subject to revision from time to time as warranted by the evolution of technology and practice. *Under extenuating circumstances, the responsible anesthesiologist may waive the requirements marked with an asterisk (*); it is recommended that when this is done, it should be so stated (including the reasons) in a note in the patient's medical record.*

STANDARD I

All patients who have received general anesthesia, regional anesthesia, or monitored anesthesia care shall receive appropriate postanesthesia management.

1. A Postanesthesia Care Unit (PACU) or an area which provides equivalent postanesthesia care shall be available to receive patients after surgery and anesthesia. All patients who receive anesthesia shall be admitted to the PACU **except** by specific order of the anesthesiologist responsible for the patient's care.
2. The medical aspects of care in the PACU shall be governed by policies and procedures which have been reviewed and approved by the Department of Anesthesiology.
3. The design, equipment and staffing of the PACU shall meet requirements of the facility's accrediting and licensing bodies.
4. The nursing standards of practice shall be consistent with those approved in 1986 by the American Society of Post Anesthesia Nurses (ASPAN).

STANDARD II

A patient transported to the PACU shall be accompanied by a member of the anesthesia care team who is knowledgeable about the patient's condition. The patient shall be continually evaluated and treated during transport with monitoring and support appropriate to the patient's condition.

STANDARD III

Upon arrival in the PACU, the patient shall be re-evaluated and a verbal report provided to the responsible PACU nurse by the member of the anesthesia care team who accompanies the patient.

1. The patient's status on arrival in the PACU shall be documented.
2. Information concerning the preoperative condition and the surgical/anesthetic course shall be transmitted to the PACU nurse.
3. The member of the Anesthesia Care Team shall remain in the PACU until the PACU nurse accepts responsibility for the nursing care of the patient.

STANDARD IV

The patient's condition shall be evaluated continually in the PACU.
1. The patient shall be observed and monitored by methods appropriate to the patient's medical condition. Particular attention should be given to monitoring oxygenation, ventilation and circulation. During recovery from all anesthetics, a quantitative method of assessing oxygenation such as pulse oximetry shall be employed in the initial phase of recovery.* This is not intended for application during the recovery of the obstetrical patient in whom regional anesthesia was used for labor and vaginal delivery.
2. An accurate written report of the PACU period shall be maintained. Use of an appropriate PACU scoring system is encouraged for each patient on admission, at appropriate intervals prior to discharge, and at the time of discharge.
3. General medical supervision and coordination of patient care in the PACU should be the responsibility of an anesthesiologist.
4. There shall be a policy to assure the availability in the facility of a physician capable of managing complications and providing cardiopulmonary resuscitation for patients in the PACU.

STANDARD V

A physician is responsible for the discharge of the patient from the PACU.
1. When discharge criteria are used, they must be approved by the Department of Anesthesiology and the medical staff. They may vary depending upon whether the patient is discharged to a hospital room, to the ICU, to a short stay unit, or home.
2. In the absence of the physician responsible for the discharge, the PACU nurse shall determine that the patient meets the discharge criteria. The name of the physician accepting responsibility for discharge shall be noted on the record.

Reprinted with permission of the American Society of Anesthesiologists, 515 Busse Highway, Park Ridge, Illinois 60068–3189.

From a risk management perspective, this makes the guidelines no less valuable, because the intent of optimizing care through the avoidance of complications is no less operative. Further, in the event of the need to defend against a malpractice claim in this area, it is clear from this sequence of events that the exact standard of care is debatable and not yet finally established.

In the same manner that additional standards followed both the original monitoring standards and the ASA monitoring standards, additional sets of published practice standards in anesthesiology are likely to be forthcoming.

Another type of related document is called a *practice parameter*. This has many of the same elements as a standard of practice but is more intended to guide judgment in addition to directing the details of specific procedures. A good example of a set of practice parameters comes from the cardiologists and addresses the indications for cardiac catheterization. Beyond the details of the minimum standards for carrying out the procedure, these practice parameters set

forth algorithms and guidelines for helping to determine under what circumstances to perform it. It is likely that there will be some type of analogous effort to develop practice parameters in anesthesiology. One obvious example would be parameters for the insertion of a pulmonary artery catheter preoperatively. Understandably, third-party payers with a strong desire to limit the costs of medical care have great interest in practice parameters as potential vehicles for helping to eliminate "unnecessary" procedures. How this type of document is developed in anesthesiology, what its impact on specifying and determining the standard of care (especially medicolegally) will be, and how it is accepted by practitioners all remain to be seen.

The other type of standards associated with medical care are those of the Joint Commission on the Accreditation of Healthcare Organizations, the best-known medical care quality regulatory agency. As noted earlier, these standards were for many years concerned largely with structure (e.g., gas tanks chained down) and process (e.g., documentation

TABLE 2-6. ASA Guidelines for Conduction Anesthesia in Obstetrics

**Approved by House of Delegates of the American Society of Anesthesiologists
on October 12, 1988, and last amended on October 23, 1990,**

These guidelines apply to the use of major conduction anesthesia administered to the parturient during labor and delivery. These guidelines may be exceeded based on the judgement of the responsible anesthesiologist. They are intended to encourage high-quality patient care, but cannot guarantee any specific patient outcome. They are subject to revision from time to time as warranted by the evolution of technology and practice.

GUIDELINE I

Major conduction anesthesia (lumbar or caudal epidural, subarachnoid or bilateral lumbar sympathetic block) shall be initiated and maintained only in locations in which appropriate resuscitation equipment and drugs are immediately available to manage procedurally related problems (e.g. hypotension, respiratory depression, convulsions, and myocardial depression).

Resuscitation equipment shall include: sources of oxygen and suction, equipment to maintain an airway and perform endotracheal intubation, and a means to provide positive pressure ventilation. Drugs and equipment for cardiopulmonary resuscitation shall be immediately available.

GUIDELINE II

Major conduction blocks in obstetrics shall be initiated and maintained by or under the direction of a physician with appropriate privileges.

Physicians must be approved through the institutional credentialing process to administer or supervise the administration of obstetric anesthesia and must be qualified to manage procedurally related complications.

GUIDELINE III

Major conduction anesthesia should not be administered until the patient has been examined, and the fetal status and progress of labor evaluated by a qualified physician who is readily available to supervise the labor and to deal with any obstetric complications that may arise.

GUIDELINE IV

An intravenous infusion shall be established before initiation and maintained throughout the duration of major conduction block.

GUIDELINE V

A qualified individual shall monitor continually* the parturient's oxygenation, ventilation, and circulation.

Anesthetic techniques, drugs, and maternal vital signs shall be documented in the medical record.

GUIDELINE VI

Qualified personnel, other than the anesthesiologist attending the mother, should be immediately available to assume responsibility for resuscitation of the depressed newborn.

The primary responsibility of the anesthesiologist is to provide care to the mother. If the anesthesiologist is also requested to provide brief assistance in the care of the newborn, the benefit to the child must be compared to the risk of temporarily leaving the mother.

GUIDELINE VII

All patients recovering from major conduction anesthesia shall receive appropriate postanesthesia care.
1. A Postanesthesia Care Unit shall be available to receive patients. The design, equipment and staffing shall meet requirements of the facility's accrediting and licensing bodies.
2. When the PACU is not available, equivalent postanesthesia care shall be provided in a suitable location.

GUIDELINE VIII

A physician with appropriate privileges shall remain in the facility to manage anesthetic complications until the patient is accepted by the PACU or equivalent area.

GUIDELINE IX

There shall be a policy to assure the availability in the facility of a physician capable of managing anesthetic complications and providing cardiopulmonary resuscitation for patients in the PACU.

*Note that "continual" is defined as "repeated regularly and frequently in steady rapid succession" whereas "continuous" means "prolonged without any interruption at any time."
Reprinted with permission of the American Society of Anesthesiologists, 515 Busse Highway, Park Ridge, Illinois 60068–3189.

---

complete), but in recent years they have been expanded to include QA activities and reviews of the outcome of care. JCAHO standards also focus on credentialing and privileges, verification that anesthesia services are of uniform quality throughout an institution, the qualifications of the director of the service, continuing education, and basic guidelines for anesthesia care (need for preoperative and postoperative evaluations, documentation, and so forth). Full JCAHO accreditation is usually for 3 years. Even the best hospitals and facilities receive some citations of problems or deficiencies that are expected to be corrected, and an interim report of efforts to do so is required. If there are enough problems, accreditation can be conditional for 1 year, with a complete reinspection at that time. JCAHO inspections involve a great deal of work in the preparation for them, but because the standards are reasonable and do promote high-quality care, the majority of this work is highly constructive and of benefit to the institution and its medical staff.

Another type of regulatory agency is the peer review organization. Professional standards review organizations (PSROs) were established in 1972 as utilization review/quality assurance overseers of the care of federally subsidized patients (Medicare and Medicaid). Despite their efforts to deal with quality of care, these groups were seen by all involved as primarily interested in cost containment. A variety of negative factors led to the PSROs being replaced in 1984 with the peer review organization (PRO).[28] There is a PRO in each state, most being associated with a state medical association. The objectives of a PRO include 14 statements related to hospital admissions (including to shift care to an outpatient basis as much as possible) and five related to quality of care (including to reduce avoidable deaths and avoidable postoperative or other complications). The PROs comprise full-time support staff and physician reviewers paid as consultants or directors. Ideally, PRO monitoring will discover suboptimal care, and this will lead to specific recommendations for improvement in quality. There is a perception that quality of care efforts are hampered by the lack of realistic objectives and also that these PRO groups, like others before them, will largely or entirely function to limit the cost of health care services.[28]

Aside from the as yet unrealized potential for quality improvement efforts, the most likely interaction between the local PRO and an anesthesia provider will surround a request for perioperative admission of a patient whose care is mandated to be outpatient surgery. This frequently will also be a risk management issue. If the anesthesiologist feels, for example, that either (1) preoperative admission for treatment to optimize cardiac, pulmonary, diabetic, or other medical status or (2) postoperative admission for monitoring of labile situations such as uncontrolled hypertension will reduce clear anesthetic risks for the patient, then an application to the PRO for approval of admission must be made and vigorously supported. All too often, however, such issues surface a day or so prior to the scheduled procedure in a preanesthesia screening clinic or even in a preoperative holding area outside the OR on the day of surgery. This will continue to occur until anesthesia providers educate their constituent surgeon community as to what types of associated medical conditions may disqualify a proposed patient from the outpatient (ambulatory) surgical schedule. If adequate notice is given by the surgeon, such as at the time an elective case is booked for the OR, then the patient can be seen far enough in advance by an anesthesiologist to allow appropriate planning.

In the circumstance of the first knowledge of a questionable patient coming 1 or 2 days before surgery, the anesthesiologist can try to have the procedure postponed, if possible and reasonable, or can undertake the time-consuming task of multiple telephone calls to get the surgeon's agreement, get PRO approval, and make the necessary arrangements. As neither alternative is particularly attractive, especially from administrative and reimbursement perspectives, there may be a strong temptation to "let it slide" and try to deal with the patient as an outpatient even though this may be questionable from the risk management viewpoint. In almost all cases, it is likely that there would be no adverse result. However, the patient would be exposed to an avoidable risk. Both because of the workings of probability and because of the inevitable tendency to let sicker and sicker patients slip by as the lax practitioners repeatedly "get away with it" and are lulled into a false sense of security, sooner or later in a long series of such situations, there will be an unfortunate outcome or some preventable major morbidity or even mortality.

It is even worse when the first contact with a questionable ambulatory patient is immediately preoperatively on the day of surgery. There may be intense pressure from the patient, the surgeon, or the OR administrator and staff to proceed with a case for which the anesthesia practitioner believes the patient is poorly prepared. The arguments made regarding patient inconvenience and anxiety are valid. However, they should not outweigh the best medical interests of the patient. Although this is a point in favor of screening all outpatients prior to the day of surgery, the anesthetist facing this situation on the day of operation should state clearly to all concerned the reasons for postponing the surgery, stressing the issue of avoidable risk and then help with alternative arrangements (including, if necessary, dealing with the PRO).

Potential liability exposure is the other side of risk management. Particularly regarding questions of postoperative admission of ambulatory patients who have been unstable in some worrisome manner, it is an extremely poor defense against a malpractice claim to state that the patient was discharged home only later to suffer a complication because the PRO deemed that operative procedure outpatient and not inpatient surgery. As bureaucratically annoying as it may be, it is a prudent risk management strategy to admit the patient if there is any legitimate question, thus minimizing the chance for complications, and later haggle with the PRO or directly with the involved third-party payer.

Anesthesia Equipment: Maintenance and Records

Problems with anesthesia equipment have been discussed for some time.[29-31] (See Chapter 25.) However, compared to human error, overt equipment failure very rarely causes intraoperative critical incidents[32] or deaths resulting from anesthesia care.[33] Aside from the obvious human errors involving misuse of or unfamiliarity with the equipment, when the rare equipment failure does occur, it appears that correct maintenance and servicing of the apparatus almost always could have prevented the failure.

In the rare situation of an anesthesia equipment failure which, if undetected, would lead to patient injury, the monitoring prescribed by the standards should detect the untoward development. An appropriate response from the anesthesia provider (which may even mean completely detaching the patient from the anesthesia delivery system and ventilator and ventilating with a hand resuscitator bag until a new anesthesia machine can be secured) will prevent patient injury. However, there always remains the possibility of damage to a patient from equipment failure. Efforts to minimize these equipment failures are basic to practice and must be maintained.

Programs for anesthesia equipment maintenance and service have been outlined.[13] A distinction is made between failure due to progressive deterioration of equipment—which should be preventable because it is observable and should provoke appropriate action—and catastrophic failure, which often cannot practically be predicted. Preventive maintenance for mechanical parts is critical and involves periodic performance checks every 4–6 months. Also, an annual safety inspection of each anesthetizing location and the equipment itself is necessary. For equipment service, an excellent mechanism is a relatively elaborate cross-reference system to identify both the device needing service and the mechanism to secure the needed maintenance or repair.

Equipment-handling principles are straightforward. Prior to purchase, it must be verified that a proposed piece of equipment meets all applicable standards, which will usually automatically be true when dealing with recognized major manufacturers. Upon arrival, electrical equipment must be checked for absence of hazard (especially leakage current) and compliance with applicable electrical standards. Complex equipment such as anesthesia machines and ventilators should be assembled and checked out by a representative from the manufacturer or manufacturer's agent. There are potential adverse medicolegal implications of relatively untrained personnel certifying a particular piece of equipment as functioning within specification, even if they do it perfectly. It is also very important to involve the manufacturer's representative in pre- and in-service training for those who will use the new equipment. Also upon arrival, a sheet or section in the master equipment log must be created with the make, model, serial number, and in-house identification number for each individual piece of capital equipment. This not only allows immediate identification of any equipment involved in a future recall or product alert but also serves as the permanent repository of the record of every problem, problem resolution, maintenance, and servicing occurring until that particular piece is "scrapped." This log must be kept up to date at all times. There have been rare but frightening examples of potentially lethal problems with anesthesia machines leading to product alert notices requiring immediate identification of certain equipment and its service status.

Who should maintain and service major anesthesia equipment has been widely debated. There are significant risk management implications. Equipment setup and check-out have been mentioned. After that, some groups or departments rely on factory service representatives for all attention to equipment, while others engage independent service contractors, and still other (often larger) departments have access to personnel (engineers or technicians) in their institution or department or in a separate bioengineering/medical engineering department within the facility. Needs and resources differ. The single underlying principle is clear: the persons doing preventive maintenance and service must be qualified. Anesthesia practitioners may wonder how they can assess these qualifications. The best way is to unhesitatingly ask pertinent questions about the education, training, and experience of those involved, including asking for references and speaking to supervisors and managers responsible for those doing the work. Whether an engineering technician who spent a week at a course at a factory can perform the most complex repairs depends on a variety of factors that can be investigated by the practitioners ultimately using the equipment in the care of patients. Failure to be involved in this oversight manner exposes the practitioner to increased liability in the event of an untoward outcome associated with improperly maintained or serviced equipment.

In addition to preventive maintenance and servicing, there must be adequate day-to-day clinical attention to equipment. In this era of great emphasis on cost containment, it seems that anesthesia technicians are a popular target for budget cutters. It is false economy to reduce the number of personnel below that genuinely needed to retrieve, clean, sort, disassemble, sterilize, reassemble, store, and distribute the wherewithal of daily anesthesia practice. Inadequate attention to all these steps truly creates "an accident waiting to happen." An improperly installed canister of carbon dioxide absorbent is only one of many possible examples of potential dangers from inadequate routine technical support.

The period of time after which anesthesia equipment becomes obsolete and should or must be replaced is another question difficult to answer. Replacement of obsolete anesthesia machines and monitoring equipment is a key element of a risk modification program.[34] Ten years is often cited as an estimated useful life for an anesthesia machine. Anesthesia machines considerably more than 10 years old do not meet certain of the safety standards now in force for new machines (such as vaporizer lockout and fresh gas ratio protection, included in gas machine standards in 1979) and, unless extensively retrofitted, do not incorporate the new technology, which advanced very rapidly during the 1980s, much of it directly referable to the effort to prevent untoward incidents. Further, it appears that technology of this type will continue to advance and to appear in the equipment. Some anesthesia equipment manufacturers, anxious to minimize their own potential liability, have refused to support (with parts and service) some of the oldest of their pieces, particularly gas machines, still in use. Such "disowning" of equipment by its own manufacturer is a strong message to practitioners that the equipment must be replaced as soon as possible.

Should a piece of equipment fail, it must be removed from service and a replacement substituted. Groups or departments are obligated to have sufficient backup equipment to cover any reasonable incidence of failure. The equipment removed from service must be clearly marked with a prominent label (so it is not returned into service by a well-meaning technician or practitioner) containing the date, time, person discovering, and the details of the problem. The responsible personnel must be notified so they can remove the equipment, make an entry in the log, and initiate the repair. As indicated in the protocol for response to an adverse event, a piece of equipment involved or suspected in an anesthesia accident must be immediately sequestered and not touched by anybody—particularly not by any equipment service personnel. If a severe accident occurred, it may be necessary for the equipment in question to be inspected at a specific later time by a group consisting of qualified representatives of the manufacturer, the service personnel, the plaintiff's attorney, the insurance companies involved, and the practitioner's defense attorney. Also, major equipment problems may, in some circumstances, reflect a pattern of failure due to a design or manufacturing fault. These problems should be reported to the Medical Device Problem Reporting system of the U.S. FDA *via* the Device Experience Network (telephone 1-800/638-6725).[35] This system accepts voluntary reports from users and requires reports from manufacturers when there is knowledge of a medical device being involved in a serious incident.

Informed Consent

The recent trend of the essentially automatic additional charge of lack of informed consent when there is a malpractice suit resulting from an anesthesia catastrophe has propelled this issue to the forefront of anesthesia risk management.

There is a fundamental legal principle that a patient has the right to exercise control over his or her own body and must therefore consent to proposed treatments or procedures.[36] The issue of treatment rendered in the absence of any consent at all (for whatever reason, but usually due to gross misunderstandings) involves potential claims by the patient of assault and battery. This is relatively rare and much less likely to involve anesthesia providers than is the issue of informed consent. Informed consent is obtained by discussing the potential risks and benefits of a proposed treatment or procedure and any available alternatives, and then ascertaining that the patient (or the patient's agent, in the case of a child or an incompetent person) understands and agrees to what is being proposed.

Some residual debate may still exist regarding whether there needs to be separate informed consent for the anesthesia for a planned surgical operation or whether consent to the operation implies consent for the anesthesia. In many practice settings now, anesthesia providers obtain a separate informed consent because there are wholly separate, identifiable material risks associated with the anesthetic independent of the surgery. It is inadequate to expect the surgeon to fully discuss the anesthetic and, particularly, any special implications for anesthesia of the patient's medical condition. Anesthesia providers do not do the surgery and cannot obtain a genuine informed surgical consent. Similarly, surgeons are not anesthesiologists and do not have the training and experience to discuss the plans and risks of the anesthesia care.

The question always arises as to what risks should be disclosed to the patient when obtaining informed consent for anesthesia. There must be a balance between giving enough information to allow a reasonable decision and frightening the patient with a long list of extremely rare but potentially severe complications, the latter making a trusting, friendly doctor-patient working relationship very difficult. In the past, the standard was disclosure of risks that any reasonable physician would think appropriate. This doctrine has been significantly altered over time to that involving the "reasonable person" (patient) and now centers on the concept of material risk. A material risk "is one which the physician knows or ought to know would be significant to a reasonable person in the patient's position of deciding whether or not to submit to a particular medical treatment or procedure."[36] Legal precedents stating that *all* risks must be disclosed to the patient in order to obtain informed consent were subsequently modified with the qualification that there need not be disclosure of every conceivable, remotely possible complication whose severity or incidence is "negligible." This balances the patient's right to know with fairness to physicians, thus avoiding unrealistic and unnecessary burdens on practitioners.

When the issue of informed consent for anesthesia arises, it usually involves questions about the occurrence of rare but devastating complications such as severe neurologic damage or death. Whether the risk of these complications is considered negligible in a legal context remains to be determined. Therefore, there is no firm guideline as to whether it is wise to tell all patients that general anesthesia might lead to anoxic brain damage or death or that regional anesthesia could cause permanent paralysis. It is possible, however, to state that all anesthesia procedures have some risks, including risks of injury and death, just as riding in a car or crossing the street has risks. The vast majority of patients can identify with this analogy and are not threatened by it. Questions as to specific complications prompted by this statement, of course, should be answered. Statistics can be cited to give a perspective. Again, patients understand when told that the risk of death or grave injury from an anesthetic for a healthy patient is far less than that from riding in an automobile during the normal course of a year. Any special risks attendant on the patient's medical or surgical condition should be discussed in more detail. Some patients state that they do not want to hear about risks. A reasonable attempt to make the patient understand why the discussion is important should be undertaken, and then a comment about the patient's desire not to be informed should be entered into the anesthesia note in the chart.

Consent is a state of mind achieved through the establishment of an understanding between people. It is not an act such as the signing of one's name. Many anesthesia practitioners ask patients to sign a consent form that bears a long list of potential complications and any specific additional risks for that particular patient. This is an accepted, reasonable practice. However, both anesthetist and patient must understand that no matter what the form says, it does not release the anesthesia provider from liability. The form is one way to document that an informed consent discussion took place, but it does not limit the patient's right to later make a claim in the event of an accident. Whether the form is used or a note is written in the patient's chart (or both), there must be a clear record (created after the discussion) that a discussion took place and that informed consent was obtained. Verbal consent alone is not enough when there is a later question.

In certain life-threatening emergency circumstances, it may be necessary to administer anesthesia without consent. Case law recognizes this, and the requirements outlined are necessarily modified. In such an event, it is advisable to write a note in the chart as soon as possible about the necessity of proceeding, and it is also advisable to notify the hospital administrator or legal counsel about the situation.

Obtaining informed consent must not be a perfunctory bureaucratic irritation. It is an integral component of the anesthetist-patient relationship. It essentially forces communication and discussion of important issues. Further, it was noted that it is routine for plaintiffs' attorneys to charge lack of informed consent in virtually any case of an unexpected poor patient outcome. Although the charge cannot be avoided, careful attention to the principles detailed here should allow successful defense against such claims. (See also Chapter 5.)

Record Keeping

One of the greatest problems in medical risk management and medicolegal issues is inadequate documentation in the medical record. A great many anesthesia malpractice cases have been lost, even when there probably was no malpractice, because of incomplete or illegible anesthesia records. The anesthesia chart is the cornerstone of all the information about an anesthetic case for risk management purposes. The old dictum, "If you didn't write it down, it didn't happen," is still very much applicable in a medicolegal sense. The best anesthetic care cannot be defended or even referred to if there is no clear record that such care took place. "If the record hardly exists, . . . it is tantamount to an outright confession, in the eyes of the law, to careless practice."[37] (See also Chapter 5.)

In many cases of malpractice claims against anesthesiologists, the documentation of the preanesthetic evaluation frequently is weak or inadequate. The guiding principles regarding what should be documented are very simple. The practitioner should record all the information necessary for another anesthesia provider to pick up the chart and quickly obtain a complete enough picture to safely and intelligently conduct the anesthetic. One good way to think of it is for the anesthetist doing the evaluation to project him/herself into the role of picking up the chart and then include everything he/she would want to see. Further, the preoperative evaluation should contain some evidence of the thinking associated with the evaluation. Assigning an ASA patient classification is a start. Recording any unusual or dangerous conditions and how these influence plans and risks is mandatory. In all cases, some type of statement about the anesthetic plan (or possible alternatives if the plan is not final) is necessary. It is unfortunate but true that the best possible care may not appear so in the record without some appropriate effort to document what went into that care. Even when thorough notes are written, it is of no help if they cannot be read. All notes must be dated and timed, and made as legible as humanly possible.

Aside from the potential legal uses, an excellent way of approaching the record is to try to do two things: (1) create a legible record of "all pertinent events" (required by JCAHO[5]) and of the perianesthetic period and (2) have a compendium of all the salient features (history, allergies, chronic medications, acute medications, positioning, monitoring used, reasons for special monitoring, events, and the patient's responses to these and all factors) in as complete a manner as you would like to see them were you to be the next person, new to the patient, to give anesthesia. Virtually all facilities in which anesthesia is given have a preprinted form that facilitates accomplishment of these goals. The form should be readily legible, should be easy to use, should encourage completeness, and should be reviewed frequently by those using it to see if revision would improve it.

There exist computer-driven devices that will automatically maintain intraoperative anesthesia records.[38-40] Noninvasive or invasive monitors may be connected to these computers so that vital signs, FIO_2, expired volume and ventilation rate, SaO_2, and $ETCO_2$ are automatically recorded (often with no possibility to edit) at preset time intervals. Sensors that would automatically record gas flows and volatile agents and infusions used are being developed. Other drugs and fluids given, blood lost, and events noted can be input by the anesthesia provider using a touchscreen, keyboard, light pen, or even eventually voice. These instruments will automatically record the time of the entry, even if its operator states in the entry that an event or action took place at some past time. There are significant risk management implications. Proponents of these devices state that the technology allows more time to focus on the patient and that a genuinely complete record of vital signs will give a truer picture of events and trends. In addition to being inherently interesting, this should aid in evaluation of poor outcome, usually by demonstrating the absence of untoward intraoperative events. Further, it will demonstrate the wide range of normal vital signs that often is "smoothed out" on handwritten records. Some downside risks are hypothesized: automatic sampling may miss trends by picking up and recording transient major variations and may even record erroneous, grossly incorrect values because of mechanical or electrical artifact, thus exposing the anesthetist later to unjustified accusations in the event of a poor outcome. Acceptance and utilization of this technology will depend on the resolution of this typical risk-benefit ratio question and the ability to both justify and meet the significant capital cost of these instruments.

Keeping any anesthetic record involves a few basics. Medications and vital signs should be recorded as contemporaneously as possible and should be entered first when there are many things to record, such as immediately after induction. Descriptive information, important as it is, can wait. During the maintenance phase of the anesthetic, vital signs should be recorded at least every 5 minutes. Numerical values from instruments such as the pulse oximeter, capnograph, spirometer, mass spectrometer, and any other monitoring devices should be recorded at appropriate intervals. It is inadequate only to note that these or other devices were used. The generated information must be recorded both for reference (during or after the case) and to prove that the anesthetist was aware of what transpired during the anesthetic.

Postoperative documentation is very important in anesthesia risk management. Aside from the fact that it is a JCAHO requirement to see patients in follow-up, it is simply good anesthesia care. It also broadens and deepens the relationship with the patient, which is necessarily transient, thus making less likely misunderstanding or misplaced hostility about the outcome of the surgery. Leaving a positive impression can be a key element, for example, in avoiding being named a co-defendant in a malpractice action against the surgeon. More important, however, is the opportunity to discover any complications or issues with the patient. Assuming the vast majority of these will be minor, they can be dealt with on the spot, thus eliminating any chance that they will grow out of proportion if neglected. It is reasonable to ask patients what they remember about the operative experience (not directly whether they had recall during general anesthesia), if they were hoarse, if the intravenous (iv) line hurt, and so forth, while also examining the chart and patient for more serious problems. The patients' responses should be entered into a postoperative note, along with some comment about current status (including vital signs) and the anesthetist's assessment, such as, "No apparent postanesthetic complications. Appears to be doing well."

In case of an adverse event, with or without patient injury, a complete account of facts and, when appropriate, impressions should go on the chart as soon as possible. An important caution is that an entry so made must not be influenced by the heat of the moment, by guilt, or by the desire to suggest blame or innocence on the part of any individual. It may be wise to seek advice from an objective person, perhaps a coworker not involved in the case, while recording the account of the event. Most important, the existing record must not be changed. No matter what is on it, the actual record is better than an altered one. No matter how excellent the anesthetic care may have been, alteration of the record guarantees the inability to defend against any charges, however unjustified they might be. If there is need to explain, elaborate, or fill in gaps in the record, it should be done as soon as practical via a dated and timed amendment note in the patient chart. The contents of such a note must be carefully thought out, and it is potentially advantageous for this note to be written in the presence of an objective witness.

Additional benefits in risk management efforts accrue from complete and legible anesthetic records. Certain of the necessary and desirable activities of both risk management and QA depend on the ability to retrieve and compile data about the anesthetic practice of both individuals and a group or department as a whole.

Response to an Adverse Event

Even the most careful, skillful anesthesia providers who understand and apply proven risk management principles will likely be involved in a major anesthesia accident. Precisely because such an event is so rare, almost no one is prepared for it. It is probable that the involved personnel will have no relevant past experience regarding what to do. Although an obvious resource is another anesthetist who has had some exposure or experience, there may not be one of these either.

The appropriate immediate response to an accident is straightforward and logical. Unfortunately, however, the personnel involved in a significant untoward event may be so surprised or shocked that logic temporarily is absent. There have been cases of major intraoperative accidents in which the responsible anesthesia provider was so stunned upon realizing what had happened that he or she became nonfunctional or, worse, left the room before help arrived.

Help must be called the moment anyone recognizes a major anesthetic complication has occurred or is occurring. A sufficient number of people to deal with the situation must be assembled immediately. For example, if an esophageal intubation goes unrecognized long enough during the induction of general anesthesia to cause a cardiac arrest (likely a failure to apply the principles of the monitoring standards), the immediate need is for enough skilled personnel to make the correct diagnosis and replace the tube into the trachea while simultaneously conducting the resuscitative efforts. Whether the anesthetist apparently responsible for the complication should direct the immediate remedial actions will depend on the people involved and the situation. In such a circumstance, it would be wise for a senior or supervising anesthesiologist to evaluate quickly the appropriateness of the behavior and actions of the involved party and decide whether that person should be asked (tactfully) to step back and allow the responding personnel to take over.

Consider an alternative scenario: an anesthesiologist recognizes an evolving or impending major complication and, out of embarrassment, refuses to call for help. This course of action is illogical and dangerous. However strong the feelings of pride and fear, they themselves are indicators of impaired judgment, and the anesthesiologist must put aside such feelings in the interest of the patient. Delay while trying to fix a significant problem alone so that no one will know could turn an embarrassing but remediable situation into one more serious or even fatal to the patient.

The primary anesthesia providers should usually concentrate on continuing patient care and documenting what they did and are doing. The anesthesiologist responsible for directing activities in that clinical area, having responded to the call for help, will become the "incident supervisor." This person assumes overall responsibility while the primary personnel and others (as needed) care for the patient. The supervisor directs the process of immediate prevention of recurrence of the event, ongoing investigation, and general documentation.

In all circumstances, anesthesia equipment and supplies in use at the time of the untoward event, whether thought to be materially involved or not, should initially be sequestered under lock and key. It is imperative that nothing be altered in any way or discarded. There may be reluctance, for example, to take an anesthesia machine out of service. This is mandatory, however, until it is agreed upon by all involved that the equipment is not material to the accident investigation and can be inspected and returned to service, or that it is material and plans are made for further investigation. Anesthesia malpractice cases have been lost because no one thought in time to save the endotracheal tube that was plugged with thick secretions, thus causing the impaired ventilation.

Immediately following a nonfatal accident, comprehensive evaluation and care of the patient should be carried out thoroughly and efficiently. Close association and communication with the surgeon at that time and throughout subsequent events will be extremely valuable. Further, there should be no hesitation at all to call consultants immediately. Often a cardiologist, neurologist, neurosurgeon, or nephrologist can offer constructive suggestions that might improve the patient's prognosis. It is very unfortunate when such requests are delayed and the consultant is later forced to state that the practitioner might have had a better chance to save the patient if only something different had been done immediately after the incident.

As soon as this comprehensive care is underway, it is necessary for the personnel directly involved, often *via* the incident supervisor or anesthesia chief, to notify the facility administrator or risk manager. This person may in turn choose to notify the facility's malpractice insurance carrier. If different, the anesthesiologist's malpractice insurer should be called. Depending on the nature of the incident, the risk manager and the insurers may suggest their involvement from the very first contact with the family. If there is an involved surgeon of record, he or she probably will first notify the family, but the anesthetist and others (risk manager, insurance loss control officer, or even legal counsel) might appropriately be included at the outset. Full disclosure of facts as they are best known, with no confessions, opinions, speculation, or placing of blame, is the best presentation throughout all dealings with the family and patient. Any attempt to conceal, withhold, or shade the truth will later confound an already difficult situation. Comfort and support should be offered, including, if appropriate, the services of facility personnel such as clergy, social workers, and counselors.

The primary anesthesia provider and any others involved must document relevant information about the incident in the medical record. As noted, existing entries in the record must not be changed. Instead, an amendment note is written if needed, with careful explanation of why amendment is necessary, particularly stressing explanations of professional judgments involved. Only known facts are stated. No judgments about causes or responsibility and no judgmental terms should appear. The same guidelines hold true for the filing of the incident report in the facility, which should be done as soon as is practical. Further, all discussions with the patient or family should be carefully documented in the medical record.

Follow-up after the immediate handling of the incident will involve the primary anesthesia providers but should again be directed by a senior supervisor, who may or may not be the same person as the incident supervisor on the scene at the time of the event. The follow-up supervisor verifies the adequacy and coordination of ongoing care of the patient and facilitates communication among all involved, especially with the risk management and QA personnel. Final decisions about the sequestered equipment need to be made. If it is suggested that the equipment was involved in the accident, a plan is outlined. Lastly, it is necessary to verify that adequate postevent documentation is taking place.

Unpleasant as it is to contemplate, it is better to have a plan ahead of time and the knowledge to execute it in the event of a major accident. Vigorous immediate intervention at the time of and following an incident may improve the outcome for all concerned.

OPERATING ROOM MANAGEMENT

An OR suite is a minisociety with various constituent groups, social dynamics, and tensions determining the tone, pace, and flow of events. The three key groups are the anesthesia providers, the surgeons, and the OR staff (which usually comprises nursing and support personnel). As difficult as it may occasionally seem, it is possible and important for these three groups not only to get along, but also to constructively work together to create a friendly and efficient work environment that promotes high-quality patient care. It is difficult to outline more than the most general points regarding OR management because there is an extremely wide spectrum of OR types, from the largest inner-city teaching hospitals to the smallest free-standing ambulatory surgery specialty centers, with each particular facility having its own individual needs and characteristics.

Organization

Because both the anesthesia and surgical arms of the OR triangle often involve physicians who are not employees of the institution, there usually is not one central authority to which all the personnel involved in the functioning of an OR must answer. Even when the physicians are employees, they report through their chiefs of service to the chief of the medical staff, who likely is not the hospital administrator. Therefore, even before one considers the relationships between anesthesiologists and surgeons, there is a natural division between the physicians and the OR staff. In this milieu, the anesthesia providers often find themselves in the middle of the group of the triangle, trying to balance the needs and demands of both the OR staff and the surgeons with what is possible and desirable from an anesthesia standpoint. This balancing act is part of the art of anesthesia practice.

Anesthesia practitioners and surgeons have a symbiotic relationship. Without surgeons, there is no need for anesthesia services, and without anesthesia providers, surgeons cannot work. In most circumstances, both specialists recognize this and also the common goals of needing and wanting surgery performed in an expeditious, safe manner. One of the large organizational sticking points can involve the age-old question, who is in charge of the OR? Often there is no real answer because the interrelationships in the OR environment are so many and so complex. Some institutions do, however, have a position that carries the title, Medical Director of the OR. The implications to surgeons of an anesthesiologist in that position, and *vice versa*, are potentially contentious enough so that some institutions simply abandoned that title. There does need to be some dispute-resolving and policy-setting authority, however. If there is no medical director with authority to make decisions, and to make those decisions stick, then the authority usually resides with the OR committee. When there are major policy and financial decisions to be made, this committee becomes a microcosm political system that lobbies and campaigns for votes. No matter what it is called or how it is structured, there will be a forum for this type of activity in every OR in which standard tactics of diplomacy and negotiation will be carried out regularly.

Lines of authority parallel lines of responsibility. Who has hiring and firing power over whom and who pays whom will determine a great deal about how the organization of an individual OR works. A classic example involves perfusionists for cardiac surgery. In some circumstances they are employed by the hospital, in others by the cardiac surgeons, in a few cases by the anesthesiologists, and occasionally by no one in that they function as completely independent contractors almost with a separate department unto themselves. The organizational implications of each of the different scenarios is relatively clear regarding the standard issues of determining work and call schedules, policy and procedure for bypass operations, equipment purchases, and so forth. Each institution develops its own tradition, often by trial and error, or by default based on the abundance or scarcity of various resources, including the perfusionists themselves. In some cases the system that evolves never works well, or does initially and then deteriorates over time. At this juncture, one of the other constituent components of the OR environment that has been "out of power" steps forward and offers to take (or seizes) control of the perfusionists. Then the cycle begins anew, under new management, and the process starts again. This is essentially healthy because an OR that has no cycles or problems and runs like a finely tuned machine because of a very strong central authority often is an unappealing work place. There is significant intensity and consequent stress working in an OR simply because of the nature of surgery and its implications for the human condition. This is little appreciated by outsiders, who may be influenced by the drama of surgery but know very little of what actually goes on, and also little appreciated by those who do work there because to them it appears routine—until they stop and reflect for a moment. Therefore, an effort to create a maximally collegial work environment will pay many significant dividends for all involved.

Other issues involving lines of responsibility can greatly affect the daily functioning of the OR. Very often the OR staff consists of hospital or facility employees. It may be perceived that the hospital is more concerned with limiting the cost of salaries than providing as many personnel as the OR supervisor, the surgeons, and the anesthesia providers believe is necessary for optimal function of the OR. The topic of adequate nursing and technical support staffing frequently is a never-ending discussion with the hospital administration. If there are genuine issues that cannot be resolved, it is not unreasonable in the appropriate settings for the anesthesiologists, for example, to contribute some of their practice income to hire the additional anesthesia technicians that are needed to better and more quickly provide the needed equipment and turn over ORs between cases. Similarly, surgeons who find the availability of scrub techs or nurses limited can pool resources to fund positions of this type from their practice income. This spirit of support and cooperation for the ultimate benefit of all would be both refreshing and most productive.

A central issue for the anesthesia providers in an OR is who among them will be the primary organizational person to interact with the OR. In situations where all the anesthesia providers are independent contractors who make independent arrangements with surgeons to provide services, there may be a titular "chief of anesthesia" who, by default, becomes the contact person. Larger groups or departments that function as a single entity and make their own assignments of personnel often have a clinical director, whose job it is to be the contact person with the system and to speak for the anesthesia department on OR organizational matters. Usually there is one anesthesiologist supervising the schedule or running the board daily in the OR for the group. One of the virtues of this person usually being the clinical director (as opposed to rotating the responsibility among all the anesthesiologists) is that he or she likely has a greater understanding on a day-to-day basis of the resources and demands of an anesthesia service. An additional benefit is that a comparative level of consistency in the application of policies, particularly regarding the scheduling of cases, can be more easily achieved. One of the most frustrating things to both surgeons and OR staff is inconsistency and unpredictability of decision-making from the anesthesia department. A patient that may be deemed unacceptable for surgery by anesthesiologist X running the schedule on Monday might well be considered, in exactly the same condition, a routine preop by anesthesiologist Y on Tuesday. Some differences of opinion are unavoidable, but the more there are, the more difficult OR life becomes for the surgeons and the OR staff. Without stifling individual practice styles and philosophies, some measure of consistency applied to similar situations, whether through the clinical director or not, will facilitate OR function considerably.

The availability of the resources to administer anesthesia is another component of OR organization. Usually there is an anesthesia work room that is staffed, maintained, and run by the anesthesia service and that contains all the supplies and equipment unique to anesthesia practice. Most of this is chosen and ordered by the anesthesia providers, either from a hospital or facility budget or paid for by the practice revenue. There must be coordination with the OR staff as to who will be responsible for the routine items that are not necessarily unique to anesthesia, such as syringes and needles, iv fluids, and pulmonary artery catheters. An important goal is the avoidance of duplication and waste. Decisions as to what brands of supplies to buy and major equipment purchases for the anesthesia side of the OR usually reside with the OR committee or its equivalent.

Scheduling Cases

Anesthesia providers need to be involved in the scheduling of OR cases in their institution or facility. In some circumstances, the booking office and the associated clerical personnel will reside within the department of anesthesia. More often, however, this function is part of the OR staff's responsibility, most likely under the direct control of the OR supervisor. In this case, there must be a clear mechanism for input from the anesthesia providers into the case scheduling process, both on a daily basis and from the policy management aspect. This is important even in situations in which all the anesthesia providers are independent contractors and not really associated in any way. In such situations, the titular chief of anesthesia should be the person to coordinate schedules to guarantee after-hours coverage and to help plan for program changes, such as the addition of a new group of surgeons to the hospital staff.

When there is an anesthesia department that functions as a cohesive unit, its chairman, clinical director, or appointed representative will be the person who meets with the OR supervisor and surgeons as necessary to establish policies regarding the scheduling of OR cases. There are as many different ways to do this as there are operating suites. Most hospitals and facilities have evolved traditions that attempt to meet the needs of their particular OR. Nevertheless, OR scheduling remains one of the most difficult aspects of medical practice. Acknowledging that it will be impossible to satisfy everyone all the time, the anesthesia department should attempt to smooth the process as much as possible by listening sympathetically to the surgeons' desires and considering the OR staff's ability to provide rooms, equipment, and personnel, and then attempting to establish a schedule of anesthesia services and coverage to mesh realistically with the other two groups.

Regarding scheduling, surgeons are basically divided into two groups—the large majority, who want early-morning operating time for elective cases, and the others, who will operate essentially any time they can get their cases scheduled and do not understand why the OR cannot run full tilt 24 hours a day, 7 days a week. Neither group can be fully accommodated, and therein is generated the need for extensive compromise. The anesthesia providers approaching this need as calmly and with as little confrontation as possible will facilitate the compromise process considerably. There will always be some element of politics involved in the decisions regarding which surgeons get to operate when, particularly if the OR uses block time instead of open scheduling. The goal of the anesthesia department is to be as neutral as possible while being realistic about what can be accomplished regarding the number of rooms open and the length of the operating day.

Even in small operating suites, case scheduling will be greatly facilitated by some type of computerized scheduling system. Organization is simpler and much faster than if a large ledger book is used. Juggling cases from room to room and trying various possibilities is much simpler with a computer than erasing and rewriting handwritten entries. Personnel or equipment conflicts can be instantly identified. Also, most systems of this type will produce reports and statistics automatically. One extremely valuable component of many such programs is automatic assignment of projected case duration based on historical precedent. If Dr. X or service Y has an 8-hour block on a given day and wants to book four cases, the scheduling program determines what procedures are to be done (such as by CPT-4 code) and refers to previous cases for information on OR time. The program then automatically assigns a projected length for each of the cases booked. If the computer concludes that the first three cases will consume the entire available block of time, it will not accept the fourth case into that room's schedule on that day. Once the surgeons' initial resistance is overcome and they get in the habit of either making more realistic time estimates for themselves or accepting those from the computer, the scheduling process becomes much smoother and there are far fewer days when disputes arise with the anesthesia and OR staffs in midafternoon about whether or not the last case scheduled can actually be done.

In general, many variables contribute to the scheduling process. The nature of the institution and the patient population served have a great impact. An ambulatory surgery center in an upscale suburban neighborhood doing mostly cosmetic plastic surgery can schedule OR cases of fairly predictable length and complexity well in advance and be relatively certain that the vast majority of patients will appear in appropriate condition, ready to go, on the appointed day. On the other hand, a large inner-city teaching hospital serving a largely indigent population and receiving mostly acute problems and trauma patients will find it very difficult to schedule the OR much more than a day in advance, if that. In the latter circumstance, maximal cooperation and flexibility from the anesthesia department (within the limitations of available resources) is mandatory to accommodate the surgeons' requests and the OR staff's ability to do cases. These are two extreme examples from the ends of the spectrum. Most situations are somewhere in between. In all circumstances, however, open communication and honest discussion among the three principal groups involved in OR scheduling about realistic requests and realistic estimates of what is possible are key to the smooth functioning of the OR. It is very important to overcome "us versus them" attitudes in the OR. Surgeons may be perceived by anesthesia providers as having totally unrealistic expectations or demands for operating time. Anesthesiologists may be perceived by surgeons as arbitrarily canceling or refusing to do cases in an attempt to avoid work. This contentious atmosphere need not prevail. If each of the three groups involved in OR scheduling tries hard to understand the positions and thinking of the other two and realizes that all must work together toward a common goal—safe, efficient, expedient patient care—then the OR need not be the most difficult working environment in the hospital.

Scheduling Personnel

Except in the most unusual circumstances, scheduling anesthesia providers is a continual juggling act. Even with independently contracting individuals who make themselves available on lists at various hospitals and depend on surgeons (or OR staff people acting at the direction of surgeons) to contact them directly regarding availability and consequent scheduling, there are time conflicts and, conversely, unwanted idle time. When departments or groups accept responsibility for providing anesthesia services for an OR suite, they must be sure that on any given day there are enough providers (and supervisors, if that is the mode of practice) to staff the rooms scheduled. Ideally, a department or group would hire enough people so that there would always be a surplus above and beyond the minimum number needed to run regular rooms during the day and cover the call schedule. Even if there were enough providers to hire, too many people with no clinical activity may be seen as an economic disadvantage in many groups. Therefore, often there is an attempt to have just the right number of providers available, which may work well until someone is out with a family problem or an extended illness. In academic departments, anesthesia attending faculty and residents may be assigned nonclinical time intended for research, teaching, and administration. These people may provide a buffer to help deal with day-to-day variations in the number of people available to work in the OR, but repeated pulling of academic personnel into clinical service quickly undermines the academic programs of a teaching department and leads to resignations that eventually eliminate what buffer of extra people existed. Accordingly, those responsible for scheduling anesthesia personnel must try as hard as possible to anticipate both reasonable needs and available personnel far enough in advance (at least 6 months) to hire accordingly.

Again, there are as many different types of situations as there are places to have them. Each operating suite evolves its own system. There must be very close coordination between the responsible anesthesia person and the OR supervisor as to how many ORs can be used on any given day and how late in the afternoon or evening they can be open. Inevitably, some cases take longer than planned, and emergency cases are booked during the day, leading to the need to run more rooms than anticipated at the end of the afternoon and into the evening. The anesthesia providers who are thus required to stay late, whether or not they are being paid overtime, may accept such a situation as a matter of course occasionally, but not routinely. These practitioners become exhausted and also resentful—of being "abused" in general and of the time away from their outside lives, homes, and families in particular. If the practice environment is such that there almost always are rooms that run significantly late, it is a worthwhile investment to have additional anesthesia personnel on late call who come in fresh at noon or 1 P.M. with the intention of giving lunch breaks and then staying into the evening until all the scheduled cases from the day are finished and there has been a good start on the add-ons, which will then be completed by the anesthesia call personnel.

Scheduling after-hours anesthesia coverage is similarly difficult. In this consideration, the variation among institutions and facilities is greater still. Whether or not anesthesia residents, CRNAs, and attending staff need to take in-hospital call overnight depends on the nature of the institution and work load. Major referral centers for high-risk obstetrics and trauma, for example, need primary providers in-house 24 hours a day and, if these are residents or CRNAs, also need the attending staff to supervise them. In other settings, primary providers may be in-house, with the attending staff taking call from home, or both may take call from home (assuming home is close enough to guarantee arrival in the OR within some agreed-upon interval, such as 30 minutes in the case of a stat cesarean section). The number of people needed for call is always a question. Should the call team be staffed for the minimum, average, or maximum expected load? Often the easiest solution is to anticipate an average load and acknowledge that there will be some idle time unused and other times when the need will outstrip the available personnel and an effort to get more help in that unusual circumstance must be made. Of course, if that circumstance becomes commonplace rather than unusual, the number of providers on call must be increased.

There are important medicolegal concerns. In a small community hospital, for example, if there are three anesthesiologists on staff who do their own cases with no CRNAs involved, they likely will agree that each will cover every third weekend, with the other two being off call and not obligated to the OR. If that one anesthesiologist is administering an anesthetic and cannot safely leave the room and another emergency patient arrives in the OR suite with a major acute problem, what should happen? If the other two anesthesiologists are legitimately unavailable and unreachable, should the anesthesiologist in the OR abandon the anesthetized patient to tend to the emergency patient? There is no easy answer. Those on the scene at the time must assess the relative risks and benefits and make hard choices. This example illustrates the difficulties of trying to provide call coverage to deal with all possible contingencies in the OR.

A related scheduling question is that of anesthesia providers who have worked overnight while on call and whether they should work in the OR the following day. Again, the individual practice environment will largely dictate the answer. If call almost never means a long night's work that leaves the practitioner fatigued and stressed in the morning, it is reasonable for a provider to be scheduled in the OR the following day, with the understanding that on the rare occasion when there has been all-night activity, that practitioner will be dismissed as early in the morning as possible. Alternatively, if the calls usually do involve extensive night work, there should be no assignment for the next morning. In the rare circumstance that the provider is able to sleep the night, then he or she is an unexpected extra helper the next day for as long as needed. Common sense and reason guide this thinking. In the same vein, even if there is no indication that fatigue could have played a role, should an anesthesia catastrophe occur with a provider who was up all the previous night, the defense of the resultant malpractice suit would be extraordinarily difficult.

PRACTICE ARRANGEMENTS

There is no limit to the number of possible types of practice arrangements within the specialty of anesthesiology. Teaching hospitals with anesthesiology residency programs constitute only a very small fraction of the total number of institutions and facilities requiring anesthesia services. These academic departments tend to be among the largest, but the aggregate fraction in academic practices out of the entire anesthesiologist population is also small. It is interesting, however, that most residents finishing their training have almost exclusively been exposed only to academic anesthesiology. Accordingly, finishing residents often are comparatively unprepared to evaluate and enter the anesthesiology job market.

Specialty certification by the American Board of Anesthesiology (ABA) is likely the goal of the vast majority of anesthesia training graduates. Whereas some finishing residents who know they are eventually headed for private practice start out their attending careers as junior faculty in academic departments in order to obtain some experience as a supervisor, and also to have the opportunity to prepare for and take the ABA examinations in the nurturing and protected academic environment with which they are familiar, most do not. The newly trained resident who accepts a practice position immediately should take into account the need to become ABA certified and to build in to his or her new practice arrangement the stipulation that there will be time and consideration for this goal. The hectic and unsettling period of embarking on a new career, possibly also moving one's home and family, and getting acclimated to both a new professional and financial environment may potentially inhibit optimum performance on important examinations, written and oral. The possibilities of avoiding disruption may be comparatively limited, but awareness of the problem can help lead to the forging of arrangements that will maximize the probability of success on the examinations.

Academic Practice

For those that do choose to stay in academic practice, the first question is whether to consider staying at one's training institution. There is an old adage about the devil you know being preferable to the devil you don't know. However, fear of the unknown should not inhibit investigation of all possibilities. Perusal of the classified advertisements in the major anesthesiology journals and the recruiting letters coming into training programs usually reveals many academic departments seeking new junior faculty. Aside from obvious personal preference issues, such as area of the country, size of city, and climate, there are a number of specific characteristics of academic anesthesia departments that can be used as screening questions:

How big is the department? Junior faculty can get lost in very big departments and may be treated as little better than glorified senior residents. On the other hand, the availability of subspecialty service opportunities and significant resources for research and educational activities can make large departments extremely attractive. In smaller academic departments, there may be fewer resources, but the likelihood of being accepted quickly as a valued, contributing member of the teaching faculty (and research team, if appropriate) may be higher. In very small departments, there may be so many expectations, projects, and involvements that it could potentially be overwhelming. This may not be the case at all, but the issue deserves investigation.

What exactly is expected of the junior faculty? If teaching one resident class every other week is standard, the candidate must enthusiastically accept that assignment and the attendant preparation. Similarly, if it is expected that the junior faculty will by definition be actively involved in publishable research, then specific plans for projects amenable to the candidate must be made. In such situations, clear stipulations about startup research funding and nonclinical time to carry out the projects must be obtained. Particularly important is determining what the anticipation is concerning grant funding because it can be a rude shock to realize that projects will suddenly halt, for example, after 2 years if extramural funding has not been secured.

What are the prospects for advancement? Most new junior faculty directly out of residency start with medical school appointments as instructors unless there is something in their background qualifying them to be assistant professors immediately. It is wise to understand from the beginning what it takes in that department and medical school to facilitate academic advancement. There may be more than one

track, in the sense that the tenure track is usually dependent more on published research, while the clinical or teaching track considers more one's value in patient care and as a clinical educator. The criteria for promotion may be clearly spelled out by the institution as to number of papers needed, involvement and recognition at various levels, grants submitted and funded, and the like, or the system may be less rigid and depend more on the department chairman's evaluation and recommendation. In either case, careful inquiry prior to accepting the position can avoid later surprise and disappointment.

Lastly, how much does it pay? Traditionally, academic anesthesiologists have not earned as much as those in private practice. There is now a significant amount of activity and attention concerning reimbursement of anesthesiologists, and it is difficult to predict exactly the future income for any anesthesia practice situation. However, all of the forces influencing payment for anesthesia care may well lead to a significant lessening of the traditional income differential between academic and private practice. This is not a small issue, because anesthesiologists justifiably can expect to live reasonably well. Income is also a valid consideration both because anesthesiologists are frequently at least 30 years old before they finish training and are thus starting somewhat behind their age-mates in lifetime earnings, and also because many physicians still have substantial educational loans to repay when finally finishing residency. The compensation arrangements in academic practice vary widely in structure. In certain cases a faculty member is exclusively an employee of the institution, which bills and collects for the patient care rendered by the faculty member and then pays a negotiated amount that constitutes the faculty person's entire income. Under other arrangements the faculty can bill and collect for their clinical work. Some institutions have a (comparatively small) academic salary from the medical school for being on the faculty, but many do not, and, of these, some channel variable amounts of money into the academic practice (so-called Part A payments) in recognition of teaching and administration. This salary from the medical school, if extant, is then supplemented by the practice income. Usually the faculty will be members of some type of group (either for the anesthesia department alone or the entire faculty as a whole) that bills and collects and then distributes the practice income to the faculty under an arrangement that must be examined by the candidate. An important corollary issue is that of the source of the salaries of the department's primary anesthesia providers—residents and, in some cases, CRNAs. While often the hospital pays at least for some of these, arrangements vary, and it is important to ascertain whether the faculty practice income is also expected to cover the cost of the primary providers.

Private Practice

Some residents finish their anesthesia training never having seen a private practice anesthesia setting or even talked to an anesthesiologist who has been in private practice. These candidates are at a disadvantage and are ill-equipped to seek a position in private practice. Rotations to a private practice hospital in the third year of the anesthesia residency could greatly help in this regard, but not all residency programs offer such opportunities. In that case, it is necessary for the finishing resident who is certain about going into private practice to find and use educational opportunities such as meetings and workshops on career development and also mentors from the private sector who can be a great wealth of useful information.

Armed with as much information as possible, the resident must make a fundamental initial decision between independent individual practice and a position with a group that bills and collects as one unit (either a sole proprietorship, a partnership, or a corporation). Independent practice usually first involves attempting to secure clinical privileges at a number of hospitals or facilities in the area in which one chooses to live. This is not always easy, and has been the subject of many antitrust suits in recent years. Then the anesthesiologist makes it known to the respective surgeon communities that he or she is available to render anesthesia services and waits until there is a request from a surgeon or OR for his or her services. The anesthesiologist obtains the requisite financial information from the patient and then either individually bills and collects for services rendered or employs a service to do the billing and collection for a percentage of the fee. How much of the needed equipment and supplies is provided by the hospital and how much by the independent anesthesiologist varies widely. If an anesthesiologist spends considerable time in one operating suite, he or she may purchase an anesthesia machine exclusively for personal use and move it from room to room as needed. It is impractical today to move a fully equipped anesthesia machine from hospital to hospital on a day-to-day basis. Among the features of this style of practice are the collegiality and relationships of a genuine private practice based on referrals and also the ability to decide independently how much of the time one wants to be available to work. The downside is the potential unpredictability of the demand for service, although if the practitioner is located in an area with only a small number of anesthesia providers, this likely would not be a problem.

When seeking a position with a private group, the applicant will search for potential practice opportunities through word of mouth, recruiting letters sent to the training program supervisor, journal advertisements, and placement services (either commercial or professional, such as that provided at the ASA's annual meeting). Some of the screening questions are the same as for an academic position, but there must be even more emphasis on the exact details of the clinical expectations and the financial arrangements. Some residents finish residency and, even more so fellowship training, very highly skilled in complex, difficult anesthesia procedures. They may be surprised to find that in some private practice situations, the juniormost anesthesiologist in a group setting must wait some time, perhaps even years, before being eligible to do open heart anesthesia, for example, and in the meantime will mostly be assigned routine, less challenging anesthetics. This is not always the case, but the applicant must investigate thoroughly to be certain that the opportunity satisfies the desire for professional challenge.

Financial arrangements in private group practices are many and varied. Some groups are only loose organizational alliances of independent practitioners who bill and collect separately and rotate clinical assignments and call for mutual convenience. Many groups also act as a fiscal entity. There are many possible variations on this theme. Almost always, new junior members start out as employees of the group for a probationary interval before being considered for full membership or partnership. There have been enough instances of established groups abusing this arrangement that the ASA includes in its fundamental Statement of Pol-icy the proviso, "Exploitation of anesthesiologists by other anesthesiologists is improper."[3] The statement goes on to say that after a reasonable trial period, income should reflect services rendered. Some groups have a history of demanding excessively long trial periods during which the junior anesthesiologist's income is artificially low, and then denying partnership and terminating the relationship, to employ a new probationer and start the cycle over again. Accordingly, new junior staff attempting to join groups should have all such arrangements spelled out carefully in an agreement drafted by an expert representing the anesthesiologist.

CONCLUSION

The topics covered in this chapter are rarely covered in the formal curricula of residency programs and review courses. There is a great deal of folklore in these areas, some of which is repeated here. Conditions have changed greatly in anesthesia practice in recent years, and these areas have much greater importance for modern anesthesia practitioners.

QA and risk management are here to stay. The evolution of health care practice will continue to focus more and more attention on these activities. In anesthesia practice in particular, poor patient outcome will be less and less tolerated by the public, insurers, regulators, inspectors, plaintiffs' attorneys, the media, and the anesthesia profession itself. The primary goal of both QA and risk management is the best possible quality of anesthesia care. For the reasons outlined, this means the absolute minimization of anesthesia-related complications. There will be a low but irreducible minimum rate of adverse events in anesthesia practice because humans are involved. However, rigorous application of all the principles of QA and risk management outlined here will help achieve that absolute minimum occurrence of adverse events. Significant improvements in anesthesia care have occurred and further progress is both possible and probable.

The considerations of OR management and practice arrangements give some very basic guidance for anesthesia personnel. Because of the wide spectrum of variation in both, those interested in these areas must creatively extrapolate from the basics to their own individual circumstances, and forge ahead.

REFERENCES

1. Gilbert B: Relating quality assurance to credentials and privileges. In Chapman-Cliburn G (ed): Risk Management and Quality Assurance: Issues and Interactions, p 79. Chicago, Joint Commission on the Accreditation of Hospitals, 1986
2. Peters JD, Fineberg KS, Kroll DA et al: Anesthesiology and the Law. Ann Arbor, Health Administration Press, 1983
3. American Society of Anesthesiologists: Peer Review in Anesthesiology, 1991. Park Ridge, Illinois, ASA, 1991
4. American Society of Anesthesiologists: Peer Review in Anesthesiology, 1991, p 109. Park Ridge, Illinois, ASA, 1991
5. Joint Commission on the Accreditation of Healthcare Organizations: AMH/91: Accreditation Manual for Hospitals. Chicago, JCAHO, 1990
6. Lohr KN, Schroeder SA: A strategy for quality assurance in medicine. N Engl J Med 322:707, 1990
7. Epstein AM: The outcomes movement: Will it get us where we want to go? N Engl J Med 323:266, 1990
8. Donabedian A: The quality of care: How can it be assessed? JAMA 260:1743, 1988

9. Steffen GE: Quality medical care: A definition. JAMA 260:56, 1988

10. Eichhorn JH, Cooper JB, Cullen DJ et al: Standards for patient monitoring during anesthesia at Harvard Medical School. JAMA 256:1017, 1986

11. Grundy BL, Gravenstein JS (eds): The Quality of Care in Anesthesia. Springfield, Illinois, Charles C Thomas, 1982

12. Council on Medical Service: Guidelines for quality assurance. JAMA 259:2572, 1988

13. Duberman S, Wald A: An integrated quality control program for anesthesia equipment, p 105. In Chapman-Cliburn G (ed): Risk Management and Quality Assurance: Issues and Interactions. Chicago, Joint Commission on the Accreditation of Hospitals, 1986

14. Duberman SM: Quality Assurance in the Practice of Anesthesia, 1986. Park Ridge, Illinois, American Society of Anesthesiologists, 1986

15. Schroeder SA: Outcome assessment 70 years later: Are we ready? N Engl J Med 316:160, 1987

16. The Challenge of Quality (special issue). Inquiry 25(1):1, 1988

17. Miller CL: An anesthesia QA program. QRC Advisor 3(8):1, 1987

18. Cohen JA: A quality assurance program for anesthesiology. Scientific exhibit, IARS, March 1988

19. Cooper JB, Cullen DJ, Nemeskal R et al: Effects of information feedback and pulse oximetry on the incidence of anesthesia complications. Anesthesiology 67:686, 1987

20. Vitez TS: A model for quality assurance in anesthesiology. J Clin Anesth 2:280, 1990

21. Keats AS: Anesthesia mortality in perspective. Anesth Analg 71:113, 1990

22. Holzer JF: Current concepts in risk management. In Pierce EC, Cooper JB (eds): Analysis of anesthetic mishaps. Int Anesthesiol Clin 22(2):91, 1984

23. Hornbein TF: The setting of standards of care. JAMA 256:1040, 1986

24. Eichhorn JH, Cooper JB, Cullen DJ et al: Anesthesia practice standards at Harvard: A review. J Clin Anesth 1:56, 1988

25. Eichhorn JH: Prevention of intraoperative anesthesia accidents and related severe injury through safety monitoring. Anesthesiology 70:572, 1989

26. Pierce EC (ed): Risk Management in Anesthesia. Int Anesthesiol Clin 27(3), 1989

27. Eichhorn JH: Are there standards for intraoperative monitoring? Adv Anesth 5:1, 1988

28. Dans PE, Weiner JP, Otter SE: Peer review organizations: Promises and potential pitfalls. N Engl J Med 313:1131, 1985

29. Rendell-Baker L (ed): Problems with Anesthesia and Respiratory Therapy Equipment. Int Anesthesiol Clin 20(3), 1982

30. Spooner RB, Kirby RR: Equipment-related anesthetic incidents. In Pierce EC, Cooper JB (eds): Analysis of Anesthetic Mishaps. Int Anesthesiol Clin 22(2):133, 1984

31. Cooper JB, Newbower RS, Kitz RJ: An analysis of major errors and equipment failures in anesthesia management: Considerations for prevention and detection. Anesthesiology 60:34, 1984

32. Cooper JB, Newbower RS, Long CD et al: Preventable anesthesia mishaps: A study of human factors. Anesthesiology 49:399, 1978

33. Lunn JN, Mushin WW: Mortality Associated with Anaesthesia. London, Nuffield Provincial Hospitals Trust, 1982

34. Pierce EC: Risk modification in anesthesiology. In Chapman-Cliburn G (ed): Risk Management and Quality Assurance: Issues and Interactions [A special publication of the Quality Review Bulletin]. Chicago, Joint Commission on the Accreditation of Hospitals, 1986

35. HHS Publication No. (FDA) 85-4196. Food and Drug Administration, Center for Devices and Radiologic Health, Rockville, Maryland, 1985

36. Peters JD, Fineberg KS, Kroll DA et al: Anesthesiology and the Law. Ann Arbor, Health Administration Press, 1983

37. Lunn JN: The role of the anaesthetic record. In Lunn JN (ed): Epidemiology in Anesthesia, p 136. London, Edward Arnold, 1986

38. Gravenstein JS, Newbower RS, Ream AK, Smith NT (eds): The Automated Anesthesia Record and Alarm Systems. Boston, Butterworths, 1987

39. Whitcher C: Advantages of automated record keeping. In Gravenstein JS, Holzer JF (eds): Safety and Cost Containment in Anesthesia, p 208. Boston, Butterworths, 1988

40. Eichhorn JH: Disadvantages of automated record keeping. In: Gravenstein JS, Holzer JF (eds): Safety and Cost Containment in Anesthesia, p 223. Boston, Butterworths, 1988

3

Nathan Leon Pace

Research Design and Statistics

INTRODUCTION

We anesthesiologists live submerged in an ocean of numbers. Each day in the operating room we record, tabulate, graph, and contemplate numbers. Our medical journals are replete with numbers that we are supposed to understand. These numbers include weights, lengths, pressures, volumes, flows, concentrations, counts, temperatures, rates, currents, energies, and forces. For 30 years, our anesthesia journals have exhorted the researcher to collect, analyze, and interpret these numbers more carefully.[1-3] The analysis and interpretation of these numbers require the use of statistical techniques; the design of the experiment to acquire these numbers is also part of statistical competence. The need for these statistical techniques is not an intellectual affectation but is mandated by the nature of our universe, which is both ordered and random at the same time.

The word "stochastic," strange sounding but currently very popular in scientific circles, means random, chancy, chaotic. . . . The stochastization of the world . . . means the adoption of a point of view wherein randomness or chance or probability is perceived as a real, objective and fundamental aspect of the world. It refers as well to the utilization of those methods of the theory of mathematical statistics and probability which are intended to reduce the chaos of the single unpredictable event to a less wild and more predictable pattern. The "opposite" of stochastic is deterministic; but we have learned to live simultaneously in a world that is both stochastized and deterministic. . . .[4]

The elements of randomness are ubiquitous in the operating room. For example, the anesthesiologist knows that the greater the inhaled concentration of halothane, the greater the effect; a sufficiently high concentration will anesthetize the patient; even higher concentrations will kill. Yet, for any individual patient, only a guess can be made in advance as to the necessary concentration to produce anesthesia. If everything was known about the function of the body, then possibly the desired anesthetic concentration could be predicted. Instead, we must rely on minimum alveolar anesthetic concentration (MAC), which characterizes the expected required halothane concentration for a group of patients. It allows only an initial guess as to the amount required for any individual patient.

Historians of science have differing opinions about the relative lateness of the emergence of the concept of probability in the development of mathematics. When it did emerge, the laws of probability were formulated to help gamblers in Renaissance Italy increase their winnings at dice and cards. Continuing since then, new statistics have been created to solve practical problems. In the 19th century, regression and correlation were originated by Francis Galton to aid in understanding biologic inheritance. At the beginning of this century, William Sealy Gosset worked for the Guinness Brewery in Dublin, Ireland; he developed the Student's *t* test to understand variations in strains of barley in order to make the best brew. The greatest statistician of the 20th century, Ronald Fisher, developed the analysis of variance to help produce better agricultural crops. Even studies in anesthesia have inspired new statistics; for example, the National Halothane Study prompted new advances in the analysis of frequency tables. The continuing development of statistical techniques is manifest in the increasing use of more sophisticated research designs and statistical tests in anesthesia journal articles.[5]

Many anesthesiologists have an aversion to mathematics and statistics; this aversion impedes their willingness to use numeric skills. The greater the time elapsed from training, the greater the decrease in such skills.[6] Yet, if any physician is to be a practitioner of scientific medicine, he or she must read the language of science in order to be able to independently assess and interpret the scientific report, and, without exception, the language of the medical report is increasingly statistical. Readers of the anesthesia literature, whether in a community hospital or a university environment, cannot and should not depend on the editors of journals to banish all errors of statistical analysis and interpretation. This chapter briefly scans the elements of experimental design, study execution, data collection, statistical analysis, and interpretation of results.

DESIGN OF RESEARCH STUDIES

The investigator should view himself or herself as an experimenter and not as a naturalist. The naturalist literally or figuratively goes out into the field ready to capture and report the numbers that flit into view; this is a worthy activity, typified by the case report. Case reports engender interest, suspicion, doubt, wonder, and, one hopes, the desire to experiment; however, the case report is not sufficient evidence to advance scientific medicine. The experimenter attempts to constrain and control, as much as possible, the environment in which he or she collects numbers to test a hypothesis. Yet, the investigator may be enticed to function as a naturalist. Marvelous advances in technology and instrumentation have provided the medical researcher with ingenious devices to collect more and more numbers about previously unmeasured and unmeasurable biologic events. It is tempting to simply turn these devices on and use them to collect numbers, hoping that serendipity will bless this mindless number gathering. However, thought must be invested in research design before numbers are harvested. Discovery will not come by fatuously applying statistical tests one after another to a pile of numbers until the right way of extracting information is found.

In undertaking a research project, the investigator is implicitly accepting the statistical concept that the results in a group of subjects can be applied to an individual subject. Especially as applied to the therapy of disease, this idea has engendered controversy for centuries.[7] On the one side is the contention that the individuality of each person demands that the therapy of disease be unique. Proponents would argue as follows: "The probabilities and results of a research report may not apply to an individual patient. For the individual patient, a treatment is either a failure or a success. A patient cannot be four fifths alive, but is either alive or dead. Treatment should be individualized to each patient. Any type of therapy which might be possibly and plausibly beneficial should be allowed."

On the other side is the position that no therapeutic agent can be employed with discrimination unless the general efficacy of the agent has been confirmed in analogous cases. Although it admits that each patient is distinct and that therapy should be adapted to the circumstances, this position accepts the difficulty of choosing wisely in a stochastic world. *The most likely therapy to benefit a patient will be that which is supported by experimental evidence.* This chapter espouses this latter point of view.

Sampling

Two words of great importance to statisticians are "population" and "sample." In statistical language, each has a specialized meaning. Instead of referring only to the count of individuals in a geographic or political region, population refers to any target group of things (animate or inanimate) in which there is interest. For anesthesia researchers, a typical target population would be mothers in the first stage of labor or head trauma victims undergoing craniotomy. A target population could also be cell cultures, isolated organ preparations, or hospital bills. A sample is a subset of the target population. Samples are taken because of the impossibility of observing the entire population; it is generally not affordable, convenient, or practical to examine more than a relatively small fraction of the population. Nevertheless, the researcher wishes to generalize from the results of the small sample group to the entire population.

Although the subjects of a population are alike in at least one way, these population members are generally quite diverse in other ways. Since the researcher can only work with a subset of the population, he or she hopes that the sample of subjects in the experiment is representative of the

population's diversity. Head injury patients can have open or closed wounds, a variety of coexisting diseases, or normal or increased intracranial pressure. These subgroups within a population are called strata. Often the researcher wishes to increase the sameness or homogeneity of the target population by further restricting it to only a few strata; perhaps only closed and not open head injuries will be included. Restricting the target population to eliminate too much diversity must be balanced against the desire to have the results be applicable to the broadest possible population of patients. The researcher should clearly identify the target population; regrettably, this is often overlooked.

The best hope for a representative sample of the population would be realized if every subject in the population had the same chance of being in the experiment; this is called random sampling. If there are several strata of importance, random sampling from each stratum would be appropriate. Unfortunately, in most clinical anesthesia studies researchers are limited to using those patients who happen to show up at their hospitals; this is called convenience sampling. Convenience sampling is also subject to the nuances of the surgical schedule, the good will of the referring physician and attending surgeon, and the willingness of the patient to cooperate. At best, the convenience sample is representative of patients at that institution, with no assurance that these patients are similar to those elsewhere. Convenience sampling is also the rule in studying new anesthetic drugs in volunteers; such studies are typically performed on healthy, young students. Arguments about the definition of the population and the adequacy of the sampling can challenge the validity of a published study.

The researcher must define the conditions to which the sample members will be exposed. Particularly in clinical research, one must decide whether these conditions should be rigidly standardized or whether the experimental circumstances should be adjusted or individualized to the patient. In anesthetic drug research, should a fixed dose be given to all members of the sample or should the dose be adjusted to produce an effect or to achieve a specific end point? Standardizing the treatment groups by fixed doses simplifies the research work. There are risks to this standardization, however: (1) a fixed dose may produce excessive numbers of side-effects in some patients, (2) a fixed dose may be therapeutically insufficient in others, and (3) a treatment standardized for an experimental protocol may be so artificial that it has no broad clinical relevance, even if demonstrated to be superior.

Control Groups

Even if a researcher is studying only one experimental group, the results of the experiment are usually not interpreted solely in terms of that one group but are also contrasted and compared with other experimental groups. Examining the effects of a new drug on blood pressure during anesthetic induction is important, but what is more important is comparing those results with the effects of one or more standard drugs commonly used in the same situation. Where can the researcher obtain this comparative data? There are several possibilities: (1) each patient could receive the standard drug under identical experimental circumstances at another time; (2) another group of patients receiving the standard drug could be studied simultaneously; (3) a group of patients could have been studied previously with the standard drug under similar circumstances; and (4) literature reports of the effects of the drug under related but not necessarily identical circumstances could be used. Under the first two possibilities, the patient either serves as his or her own control (self-control) or there is a so-called parallel control group. The second two possibilities are examples of the use of historical controls.

Since historical controls often already exist, they are convenient and seemingly cheap to use. Unfortunately, the history of medicine is littered with the debris of therapies enthusiastically accepted on the basis of comparison with past experience but later found to be worthless. A classic example was operative ligation of the internal mammary artery for the treatment of angina pectoris. There is now firm empirical evidence that studies using historical controls usually show a favorable outcome for a new therapy, whereas studies with concurrent controls, i.e., parallel control group or self-control, usually fail to show a benefit.[8] Nothing seems to increase the enthusiasm for a new treatment as much as the omission of a concurrent control group. If the outcome with an old treatment is not studied simultaneously with the outcome of a new treatment, one cannot know if any differences in results are a consequence of the two treatments, or of unsuspected and unknowable differences between the patients, or of other changes over time in the general medical environment. One possible exception would be in studying a disease that is uniformly fatal (100% mortality) over a very short time.

Random Allocation of Treatment Groups

Having accepted the necessity of an experiment with a control group, the question arises as to the method by which each subject should be assigned to the predetermined experimental groups. Should it depend on the whim of the investigator, the day of the week, the preference of a referring physician, the wish of the patient, the assignment of the previous subject, the availability of a study drug, a hospital chart number, or some other arbitrary criterion? All such methods have been used and are still used, but all can ruin the purity and usefulness of the experiment. It is important to remember the purpose for sampling: by exposing a small number of subjects from the target population to the various experimental conditions, one hopes to make conclusions about the entire population. Thus, the experimental groups should be as similar as possible to each other in reflecting the target population; if the groups are different, this introduces a bias into the experiment. Although randomly allocating subjects of a sample to one or another of the experimental groups requires additional work, this principle prevents selection bias by the researcher, minimizes (but cannot always prevent) the possibility that important differences exist among the experimental groups, and disarms the critics' complaints about research methods.

Originally, random allocation was performed by rolling die or by using a random number table; today, computer programs can create the random allocation scheme. There are many nuances to the actual process of random allocation. Generally it is desirable to have roughly equal numbers of patients or subjects in each treatment group; this maximizes the capacity to distinguish between treatments. If the experimenter desires to constrain equal numbers of patients to be assigned to each treatment group within each stratum, a separate random allocation scheme is prepared for each stratum. In multicenter trials, each center is usually considered a stratum and is randomized independently. Another concern in allocating patients and subjects to treatment groups is temporal change. There is usually a learning curve

in the adeptness of research skills; application of experimental conditions and collection of research data are less proficient with the initial subjects of a study. In addition, the experimental units—be they patients, rats, or cell cultures—may change with time. For example, in the recruitment of patients, there may be a number of consecutive patients whose health is better or worse than typical. With simple randomization, it is possible that a chance run of treatment assignments to one treatment group could occur; this might create bias in the baseline characteristics of patients of the various treatment groups. It is usually desirable to divide the total number of subjects into equal-sized subgroups, also known as blocks; within each block there is a balancing of the numbers assigned to each treatment group. This is named blocked randomization. Although random allocation does not guarantee that the experimental groups are alike, there is no better strategy for attempting to do so.

Blinding

Blinding refers to the masking from the view of patient and experimenter the experimental group to which the subject has been or will be assigned. In clinical trials, the necessity for blinding starts even before a patient is enrolled in the research study. There is good evidence that, if the process of random allocation is accessible to view, the referring physicians, the research team members, or both are tempted and will be tempted to manipulate the entrance of specific patients into the study to influence their assignment to a specific treatment group; they do so having formed a personal opinion about the relative merits of the treatment groups and desiring to get the "best" for someone they favor. This creates bias in the experimental groups.

Each subject should remain, if possible, ignorant of the assigned treatment group after entrance into the research protocol. The patient's expectation of improvement, a placebo effect, is a real and useful part of clinical care. But when studying a new treatment, one must ensure that the fame or infamy of the treatments does not induce a bias in outcome by changing patient expectations. Such a study, in which the subject is unaware of the treatment given, is called single blind. A researcher's knowledge of the treatment assignment can bias his or her ability to administer the research protocol and to observe and record data faithfully; this is true for clinical, animal, and in vitro research. If the treatment group is known, those who observe data cannot trust themselves to impartially and dispassionately record the data. A double-blind study, in which both subject and data collector are ignorant of the treatment group, is the best way to test a new therapy.

Ethics of Alternative Therapies

Enrolling patients into a randomized controlled trial can engender considerable physician anxiety because it requires the admission and discussion of uncertainty. "The randomized clinical trial highlights the conflict of having to say, 'We don't know,' rather than the more familiar, 'I think this is the best thing to do.' "[9] Also, considerable debate on ethics has ensued since the realization of the absolute superiority of the randomized controlled trial. These arguments usually revolve around the perceived conflict between the physician's ethical imperative to do the "best" for each patient and the need for random allocation of patients to both old and new therapies. Since there is usually some preliminary evidence to suggest the superiority of the new therapy, it is argued that the patient must be given that therapy to which the physician's affection and allegiance have been attracted. Of course, this preliminary evidence has not been confirmed by definitive therapeutic trials. What is required to resolve these qualms is the candor to recognize that, in spite of one's personal opinions about the comparative merits, a randomized controlled clinical trial is the only ethical way to solve conflicting claims about which the expert medical community is genuinely uncertain.

Types of Research Design

Ultimately, research design consists of choosing what subjects to study, what experimental conditions and constraints to enforce, and which observations to collect at what intervals. A few key features in this research design largely determine the strength of scientific inference on the collected data. These key features allow the classification of research reports. This classification exposes the variety of experimental approaches and reveals strengths and weaknesses of the same design applied to many research problems (Table 3-1).

The first distinction is between longitudinal and cross-sectional studies. The former has as an object the study of changes over time, whereas the latter describes a phenomenon at a certain point in time. "Generally, longitudinal designs require patient follow-up, documentation of intervening events, and analysis of a series of measurements. These features are less important in cross-sectional studies, so that other kinds of problems—such as errors of measurement, the interpretation of transient effects, and definitions of disease states—become relatively more prominent."[10] Reporting the frequency with which certain drugs are used during anesthesia is a cross-sectional study, whereas investigating the hemodynamics of different drugs during anesthesia is a longitudinal one.

Longitudinal studies are next classified by the method with which the research subjects are selected. These methods for choosing research subjects can be either prospective or retrospective; these two approaches are also known as cohort (prospective) or case-control (retrospective). A prospective study assembles groups of subjects by some input characteristic that is thought to change an output characteristic; a typical input characteristic would be the primary drug used for anesthetic induction, e.g., alfentanil or sufentanil. A retrospective study gathers subjects by an output characteristic; an output characteristic is the status of the

subject after an event, e.g., the occurrence of a myocardial infarction. A prospective (cohort) study would be one in which a group of patients undergoing heart surgery was divided in two groups, given two different anesthetic inductions (alfentanil or sufentanil), and followed for the development of a perioperative myocardial infarction. In a retrospective (case-control) study, patients who suffered a perioperative myocardial infarction would be identified from hospital records; a group of subjects of similar age, gender, and disease who did not suffer a perioperative myocardial infarction also would be chosen, and the two groups would then be compared for the relative use of the two anesthetic induction drugs (alfentanil or sufentanil). Retrospective studies are a primary tool of epidemiology. A case-control study can often identify an association between an input and output characteristic, but the causal link or relationship between the two is more difficult to specify.

Prospective studies are further divided into those in which the investigator performs a deliberate intervention and those in which the investigator merely observes. In a study of deliberate intervention, the investigator would choose several anesthetic maintenance techniques and compare the incidence of postoperative nausea and vomiting. If it was performed as an observational study, the investigator would observe a group of patients receiving anesthetics chosen at the discretion of each patient's attending anesthesiologist and compare the incidence of postoperative nausea and vomiting among the anesthetics used. Obviously, in this example of an observational study, there has been an intervention; an anesthetic has been given. The crucial distinction is whether the investigator controlled the intervention. An observational study may reveal differences among treatment groups, but whether such differences are the consequence of the treatments or of other differences among the patients receiving the treatments will remain obscure.

With the availability of large computer data bases of patient treatment information, some researchers have argued that observational studies can be performed by using advanced multivariable statistical techniques on these large data pools and that these observational studies will have equal merit with randomized controlled trials.[11] These suggestions include the claim that decisions about treatment efficacy are possible by such observational studies. Although such observational studies may be useful in suggesting hypotheses for further study, there are tremendous methodological problems that prevent the inferences of such an observational study from being generally accepted. The problems include (1) bias in assignment to treatment groups, (2) nonstandard definitions in the data base, (3) changing definitions over time, and (4) missing data.[12,13]

Studies of deliberate intervention are further subdivided into those with concurrent controls and those with historical controls. Concurrent controls are either a simultaneous parallel control group or a self-control study; historical controls include previous studies and literature reports. A randomized controlled trial is, thus, a longitudinal, prospective study of deliberate intervention with concurrent controls.

Although most of this discussion about experimental design has focused on human experimentation, the same principles apply and should be followed in animal experimentation. The randomized, controlled clinical trial is the most potent scientific tool for evaluating medical treatment; randomization into treatment groups is relied upon to equally weight the subjects of the treatment groups for baseline attributes that might predispose or protect the subjects from the outcome of interest.

TABLE 3-1. Classification of Biomedical Research Reports

I. Longitudinal studies
  A. Prospective (cohort) studies
    1. Studies of deliberate intervention
      a. Concurrent controls
        (1) Parallel control group
        (2) Self-control
      b. Historical controls
        (1) Previous experiments
        (2) Literature reports
    2. Observational studies
  B. Retrospective (case-control) studies
II. Cross-sectional studies

Hypothesis Formulation

Whether the research subjects are tissue preparations, animals, or people, the researcher is constantly faced with finding both similarities and differences among the diversities of a group of subjects. The researcher starts the work with some intuitive feel for the phenomenon to be studied. Whether stated explicitly or not, this is the biologic hypothesis; it is a statement of experimental expectations to be accomplished by the use of experimental tools, instruments, or methods accessible to the research team. An example would be the hope that isoflurane would produce less myocardial ischemia than fentanyl; the experimental method might be the electrocardiographic determination of ST segment changes. The biologic hypothesis of the researcher becomes a statistical hypothesis during research planning. In a statistical hypothesis, statements are made about the relationship among parameters of one or more populations. A parameter is a number describing a population; Greek letters are used to denote parameters. The statistical hypothesis can be established in a somewhat rote fashion for every research project, regardless of the methods, materials, or goals.

The most frequently used method of setting up the algebraic formulation of the statistical hypothesis is to create two mutually exclusive statements about some parameters determined from the study population (Table 3-2); estimates for the values for these parameters are acquired by sampling data. In the hypothetical example comparing isoflurane and fentanyl, ϕ_1 and ϕ_2 would represent the ST segment changes with isoflurane and with fentanyl. The null hypothesis is the hypothesis of no difference of ST segment changes between isoflurane and fentanyl. The alternative hypothesis is nondirectional, i.e., either $\phi_1 < \phi_2$ or $\phi_1 > \phi_2$; this is known as a two-tail alternative hypothesis. This is a more conservative alternative hypothesis than assuming that the inequality can only be either < or >. Only the conservative, nondirectional, two-tail tests are used in this chapter.

Logic of Proof

The statisticians Neyman and Pearson have provided the decision strategy used almost universally to choose between the null and alternative hypothesis. The decision strategy is similar to a method of indirect proof used in geometry called *reductio ad absurdum*. If a theorem cannot be proved directly, assume that it is not true; show that the falsity of this theorem will lead to contradictions and absurdities; thus, reject the original assumption of the falseness of the theorem. For statistics, the approach is to assume that the null hypothesis is true even if the goal of the experiment is to show that there is a difference. One examines the consequences of this assumption by examining the actual sample numbers obtained. This is done by calculating what are called sample test statistics; associated with a sample test

statistic is a probability. One also chooses the level of significance; the level of significance is the probability level considered too low to warrant support of the null hypothesis being tested. If sample values are sufficiently unlikely to have occurred by chance (i.e., the probability of the sample test statistic is less than the chosen level of significance), the null hypothesis is rejected; otherwise the null hypothesis is not rejected.

Since the statistics deal with probabilities, and not certainties, there is a chance that the decision concerning the null hypothesis is erroneous. These errors are best displayed in table form (Table 3-3); condition one and condition two could be different drugs, two doses of the same drug, or different patient groups. Of the four possible outcomes, two are clearly undesirable. The error of wrongly rejecting the null hypothesis (false positive) is called the Type I or alpha error. The experimenter should choose a probability value for alpha before collecting data; the experimenter decides how cautious to be about falsely claiming a difference. The most common choice for the value of alpha is 0.05. What are the consequences of choosing an alpha of 0.05? Assuming that there is, in fact, no difference between the two conditions and that the experiment is to be repeated 20 times, then during one of these experimental replications (5% of 20) a mistaken conclusion that there is a difference would be made. The probability of a Type I error depends on only two factors: the chosen level of significance, and the existence or nonexistence of a difference between the two experimental conditions. The smaller the chosen alpha, the smaller will be the risk of a Type I error. There is a trend recently for the research report to include the actual probability values of test statistics rather than just a statement of whether or not the alpha probability was or was not exceeded. This allows the reader to use his or her own judgment in deciding the plausibility or implausibility of the experimental result.

The error of failing to reject a false null hypothesis (false negative) is called a Type II or beta error. The power of a test is 1 minus beta. The probability of a Type II error depends on four factors. Unfortunately, the smaller the alpha, the greater the chance of a false-negative conclusion; this fact keeps the experimenter from automatically choosing a very small alpha. Second, the more variability there is in the populations being compared, the greater the chance of a Type II error. This is analogous to listening to a noisy

---

TABLE 3-2. Algebraic Statement of Statistical Hypotheses

H_0: $\phi_1 = \phi_2$ (Null hypothesis)
H_a: $\phi_1 \neq \phi_2$ (Alternative hypothesis)
ϕ_1 = Parameter sample 1 (*e.g.*, ST segment change with isoflurane)
ϕ_2 = Parameter sample 2 (*e.g.*, ST segment change with fentanyl)

TABLE 3-3. Errors in Hypothesis Testing: The Two-Way Truth Table

Conclusion from Observations (Sample Statistics)	Actual Situation/Reality (Population Parameters)	
	Conditions One and Two Equivalent	*Conditions One and Two Not Equivalent*
Conditions one and two equivalent*	Correct conclusion	False negative Type II error (beta error)
Conditions one and two not equivalent†	False positive Type I error (alpha error)	Correct conclusion

*Do not reject null hypothesis: Condition one = Condition two.
†Reject null hypothesis: Condition one ≠ Condition two.

radio broadcast; the more static there is, the harder it will be to discriminate between words. Next, increasing the number of subjects will lower the probability of a Type II error. The fourth and most important factor is the magnitude of the difference between the two experimental conditions. The probability of a Type II error goes from very high, when there is only a small difference, to extremely low, when the two conditions produce large differences in population parameters.

Sample Size Calculations

Discussion of hypothesis testing by statisticians has always included mention of both Type I and Type II errors, but usually the researcher has effectively ignored the latter. The practical importance of worrying about Type II errors reached the consciousness of the medical research community with the appearance of the much quoted report of Freiman et al.[14] This work showed that the majority of controlled clinical trials that claimed to find no advantage of new therapies compared with standard therapies in fact lacked sufficient statistical power to discriminate between the experimental groups, would have missed an important therapeutic improvement, and did not give the new therapies a fair test. There are four options for increasing statistical power: (1) raise alpha, (2) reduce population variability, (3) make the sample bigger, and (4) make the difference between the conditions greater. Under most circumstances, only the sample size can be varied. Sample size planning has become an important part of research design for controlled clinical trials; there are a variety of tables and formulas for these calculations that depend on specific research design circumstances.[15]

Data Collection and Data Management

The observations that are collected for anesthesia research are of all types and include demographics, physical examination, medical history, laboratory results, hemodynamic variables, questionnaires, and intraoperative events. There is a tendency for the researcher to try to collect all possible observations on the experimental subject for fear that some crucial item will be left out that will impair analysis; with the aid of computers, the amount of research data being collected per experiment does seem to be increasing. Yet, the biologic hypothesis and its associated statistical hypothesis should determine what to observe. There are real disadvantages to collecting excessive observations: (1) it costs more money, (2) it requires more research personnel, (3) data entry becomes more cumbersome, (4) there are more errors in data storage, (5) more data storage space is required, and (6) data analysis is bogged down by extraneous variables. Guidelines to follow in data collection include (1) confine the collected variables to those relevant to the study question; (2) establish explicit, rigid, totally unambiguous rules about where data are found and how they are recorded; (3) define precisely how non-numeric observations will be categorized and scored; (4) design and use a data collection record, also called a case record form, instead of collecting data on scratch paper; (5) do not expect observations in the hospital medical record to be consistently defined or consistently entered; (6) distinguish between a missing value and a zero value or an uncompleted

data field; and (7) make provision on the data collection record for the entry of unanticipated but relevant data. The investigator must continually check that the experimental protocol is not being violated. Murphy's law seems to apply to data collection. It is always more time consuming and more expensive than expected to collect data; there are also always more mistakes than expected in the data record.

Data collection is only one of several steps in the process of data management; next in the sequence are data entry, data editing, and data storage. All these steps are sequential operational components in the process of moving intact and incorruptible numbers from their collection point onward to statistical analysis. A failure at any step can ruin the basic integrity of the research protocol.

The second step in data management is entry of data into a permanent record, usually in a computer storage device. The use of electronic data processing has become ubiquitous in even small-scale research projects. A small, personal computer, as opposed to larger machines, allows the investigator greater flexibility and greater control over the data but also puts the burden of responsibility for hardware and software maintenance on him or her. After data entry, the data must be verified and edited for errors. Such errors may have been made during recording onto the case record form or may be transcription errors made during electronic entry; some entries are clearly illogical or impossible, whereas others are merely improbable. Once detected, some will be corrected by comparison with the case record form; other, probably erroneous, entries will remain, and difficult decisions about what efforts to make backtracking into other primary records must be made. Eventually, the validity of some entries will remain undecided, and these data will be rejected from analysis. The last stage in data management is data storage. There are four basic formats for electronic data storage: (1) text file, (2) spread sheet, (3) data base management system, and (4) statistical analysis software data storage. The choice of format depends on study size (number of patients and amount of data), computer resources (equipment, budget, personnel), and confidentiality considerations. Regardless of storage method, plans to back up the electronic data are crucial. The original electronic data record must be archived and only electronic copies used for statistical analysis.

Institutional Review Boards and the Federal Drug Administration

The liberation of survivors from Nazi concentration camps in 1945 and the discovery of the criminal experiments performed by some physicians on camp inmates shocked the world. The trial of some of these physicians prompted the Nuremburg Military Tribunal to enunciate a set of principles on permissible human experimentation. In 1964, the World Medical Association created the Declaration of Helsinki—recommendations concerning biomedical research in humans. Against this background of the Nazi camp medical murders and the statements of principles and guidelines at Nuremburg and Helsinki, media reports during the 1960s and 1970s of certain experiments in the United States created a furor and made medical experimentation a suspect activity. Scientists, such as the anesthesiologist Henry K. Beecher, reviewed research protocols and found many to be ethically deficient.[16] Beginning in the mid-1970s, laws were passed, commissions were established, and regulations were promulgated to control the ethical aspects of human research.

Biomedical research with human subjects is distinguished from clinical care by the focus of attention; during ordinary clinical care, the attention is on the individual patient; during research, the acquisition of knowledge describing a sample and generalizable to the population is pursued. Obviously, during research involving patients, clinical care must continue even as generalizable knowledge is acquired. Three ethical principles have been seen as fundamental to guide human behavior in clinical research: (1) respect for persons, (2) beneficence, and (3) clinical justice. Respect for people acknowledges the autonomy of each individual and demands his or her consent before beginning any treatment. Beneficence includes the classic prescription to do no harm and the obligation to maximize benefits. Justice requires that all people are treated fairly and that burdens and benefits are fairly shared. Vulnerable groups (the poor and minorities) must be particularly safeguarded from exploitation.

The application of these ethical principles during research proceeds from the fundamental premise that the investigator should not have sole responsibility for ensuring the fulfillment of ethical standards; disinterested outsiders, not involved with the research, should share the burden of this responsibility. By federal regulation, this responsibility is to be placed on a committee at the research institution or hospital; this committee is known generically as the Institutional Review Board.

During Institutional Review Board review, research proposals are judged for the presence of (1) good research design, (2) competent investigators, (3) a favorable balance of benefit to risk, (4) an adequate informed consent form and procedure, (5) equitable selection of research subjects, and (6) provision for compensation for injury. A good research design includes optimizing the sample size and using proper statistical techniques for analysis. Institutional Review Boards are required to perform an ongoing review of active research protocols at least yearly; there is great variation in the application of this review. Investigators are also required to maintain their research files and data sheets for at least 3 years following the completion of the project.

The Institutional Review Board is constituted and functions according to federal guidelines from the National Institutes of Health, Department of Health and Human Services, and it is subject to oversight by the federal government. Although the federal government only requires Institutional Review Board approval of federally funded research, at most universities, hospitals, and research institutions, Institutional Review Board review and approval have been mandated for all human research, regardless of the source of research funding. This requirement for approval of all human research is generally made by executive authority of the governing body of the research site in order to enforce similar standards and a consistency of approach. The Food and Drug Administration has its own set of regulations concerning human research with new drugs and new medical devices. These are essentially similar to those under which the Institutional Review Board have been established.

The investigator must work flexibly with the Institutional Review Board of his or her own institution to satisfy the slightly different requirements of different federal agencies and the local interpretations and implementations of the regulations. Penalties for failure to follow the Institutional Review Board procedure to obtain protocol approval and for violations of approved protocols can be very severe and can include prohibition of future federal research funding and of Institutional Review Board approval of future research protocols. Submission of manuscripts to scientific journals and of abstracts to scientific society meetings almost uniformly must be accompanied by a statement that human research projects have been reviewed by an Institutional Review Board and that informed consent has been obtained.

Animal Welfare

In the 1980s an outcry arose in the United States concerning the use of animals for research. Self-described animal activists and animal liberationists sought publicity, broke into laboratories, stole research animals, stole and destroyed research records, and made threats against medical researchers. The proclaimed goal of these individuals was to stop the use of animals in scientific investigation; some traditional animal organizations seem to have accepted, at least in part, the same goal of banning animal research. Some of the publicized experiments were described by the press as being subsidized sadism and baboon brain bashing. As a consequence, federal, state, and local legislative and regulatory action was intensified. Federal legislation and regulation have established a system of review for animal research that is comparable to that for the supervision of human research.

The Public Health Service has mandated that each institution doing research that it supports must establish an Institutional Animal Care and Use Committee (IACUC). The IACUC has jurisdiction over all research involving live vertebrate animals; nonvertebrates can be used without supervision. The U.S. Department of Agriculture has its own regulations concerning the use of animals for research; for the scientific investigator, the Public Health Service and U.S. Department of Agriculture regulations are both fulfilled by working with the IACUC. The IACUC is established by the authority of the chief executive of the institution; as with the Institutional Review Board, most institutions have chosen to require review of all live vertebrate animal research by the IACUC, regardless of funding source.

Every 6 months, the IACUC is charged with reviewing the institution's program for the humane care and use of animals and with inspecting the institution's animal facilities; a federal guide has been published that must be used for this evaluation. This guide is very specific concerning recommendations for physical restraint, multiple major surgical procedures, housing systems, minimal space allowances, and activity.

The IACUC reviews all live vertebrate animal research projects and may require protocol modification; without IACUC approval, research cannot be initiated. The following requirements are emphasized during IACUC review: (1) avoidance and minimization of animal pain, distress, and discomfort through the use of analgesia and anesthesia by qualified personnel; (2) appropriate euthanasia; (3) good living conditions; and (4) the availability of veterinary care for the animals. The investigator must work carefully to observe the approved research protocol, as the IACUC may suspend ongoing research projects for violations of their standards. With increasing frequency, research reports involving animals submitted to scientific journals and society meetings must be accompanied by a statement that animal research projects have been reviewed by an IACUC and that animal care conformed to humane guidelines.

PRINCIPLES AND APPLICATIONS OF STATISTICS

Statistics is a method for working with sets of numbers, a set being a group of objects. Statistics involves the description of number sets, the comparison of number sets with theoretical models, comparison between number sets, and the comparison of recently acquired number sets with those from the past. A typical scientific hypothesis asks which of two methods, X and Y, is better. A statistical hypothesis is formulated concerning the set of numbers collected for X and collected for Y. Statistics provides methods for deciding if the values of set X are different from the values of set Y. Statistical methods are necessary because there are three sources of variation in any data: biologic error, temporal error, and measurement error. These errors in the data cause difficulties in avoiding bias and in being precise. Bias keeps the true value from being known; precision deals with the problem of the data scatter. These statistical methods are relatively independent of the particular field of study. Regardless of whether the numbers in sets X and Y are systolic pressures, body weights, or serum chlorides, the approach for comparing sets X and Y is usually the same.

Statistical analysis consists of four broad phases: (1) initial data manipulation, (2) preliminary analysis, (3) definitive analysis, and (4) presentation of conclusions. Data manipulation begins by assembling the data into a form suitable for analysis, whether this is tables of numbers on paper or electronic files in a computer; it also includes examination of the data for problems such as logically inconsistent values or missing observations. During preliminary analysis, several statistical methods may be tried on the same data to clarify the structure of the data and to specify the direction for the more elaborate definitive analysis; simple tables and graphs are often helpful during preliminary analysis. Definitive analysis then provides the basis for conclusions. Considerable thought should be given to the final phase, which is the presentation of results in a lucid fashion adapted to the statistical competence of the listener and the reader; simpler methods consistent with data complexity are preferred.

Data Structure

Data collected in an experiment include the defining characteristics of the experiment and the values of events or attributes that vary over time or conditions. The former are called explanatory variables and the latter are called response variables. The researcher records his or her observations on data sheets or case record forms, which may be one to many pages in length, and assembles them together for statistical analysis. However, the data are most profitably assembled by placing them into a matrix or spread sheet form. Such a matrix reveals the data structure of the experiment (Table 3-4). All research observations must be in numeric form for statistical analysis. If first obtained as a code or as text, the research observation must be encoded as a number. This encoding of observations generally takes place as the data form is completed. The data structure includes the number of subjects, the grouping or classification of subjects, and the number and nature of variables measured on each individual. Most experiments have identifiable subjects on which a number of variables are recorded. Each row of the matrix is the data for only one subject. A subject is not necessarily a person or animal but might be a tissue

preparation or a laboratory instrument. For a large experiment, the data structure may include thousands of rows (subjects) and hundreds of columns (variables).

Each column of the matrix is a variable recorded for each subject. The columns include explanatory and response variables and a subject identification code. The subject identification code is necessary to always allow each row of the data matrix to be identified with its data sheets or case record form. One or more columns classify or group subjects together. Some grouping variables are part of the experimental plan. If a different dose of an opioid was given to five groups of subjects, the codes in the group column might be 1 to 5. There would be n_1 subjects receiving dose 1, n_2 receiving dose 2, and so on. Other grouping columns, which might include gender, age, and doses of accompanying drugs, reflect the variability of the experimental subjects. Explanatory variables, it is hoped, explain the systematic variations in the response variables. In a sense, the response variables are dependent on the explanatory variables.

Response variables are also called dependent variables. Response variables reflect the primary properties of experimental interest in the subjects. In our experiment with five doses of an opioid, variable 1 might be blood loss and variable 2 might be apnea duration. Research in anesthesiology is particularly likely to have repeated measurement variables, *i.e.*, a particular measurement recorded more than once for each individual. Systolic blood pressure (variable 3) and heart rate (variable 4) might be measured at Time 1, Time 2, and so forth after receiving the opioid test drug. Some variables can be both explanatory and response; these are called intermediate response variables. For example, in our hypothetical experiment with five doses of opioids, two other variables might be intraoperative maximum ST segment depression and postoperative death. One might analyze how ST segments depended on the dose of opioids; here, maximum ST segment depression is a response variable. Maximum ST segment depression might also be used as an explanatory variable to address the more subtle question of the extent to which the effect of an opioid dose on postoperative deaths can be accounted for by ST segment changes.

The mathematic characteristics of the possible values of a variable fit into five classifications (Table 3-5). Properly assigning a variable to the correct data type is essential for choosing the correct statistical technique. For interval variables, there is equal distance between successive intervals; the difference between 15 and 10 is the same as the difference between 25 and 20. Discrete interval data can only have integer values, *e.g.*, ages in years, number of live children, or papers rejected by a journal. Continuous interval data are measured on a continuum and can be a decimal fraction; for example, blood pressure can be described as accurately as desired, *e.g.*, 136, 136.1, or 136.14 mm Hg. The same statistical techniques are used for discrete and continuous data.

Categorical variables are derived by putting observations into two or more discrete categories; for statistical analysis, numeric values are assigned as labels to the categories. Dichotomous data allow only two possible values, *e.g.*, male versus female. Ordinal data have three or more categories that can logically be ranked or ordered; however, the ranking or ordering of the variable indicates only relative and not absolute differences between values; there is not necessarily the same difference between American Society of Anesthesiologists Physical Status score I and II as there is between III and IV. Although ordinal data are often treated as interval data in choosing a statistical technique, such

TABLE 3-4. Typical Data-Structure Matrix

	Explanatory Variables			Response Variables					
Subject ID	Group	Variable	Variable 1	Variable 2	Time 1 Variable 3	Time 1 Variable 4	Time 2 Variable 3	Time 2 Variable 4
× × ×	1	× × ×	× × ×	× × ×	× × ×	× × ×	× × ×	× × ×
× × ×	1	× × ×	× × ×	× × ×	× × ×	× × ×	× × ×	× × ×
× × ×	·	× × ×	× × ×	× × ×	× × ×	× × ×	× × ×	× × ×
× × ×	1	× × ×	× × ×	× × ×	× × ×	× × ×	× × ×	× × ×
× × ×	2	× × ×	× × ×	× × ×	× × ×	× × ×	× × ×	× × ×
× × ×	2	× × ×	× × ×	× × ×	× × ×	× × ×	× × ×	× × ×
× × ×	·	× × ×	× × ×	× × ×	× × ×	× × ×	× × ×	× × ×
× × ×	2	× × ×	× × ×	× × ×	× × ×	× × ×	× × ×	× × ×
× × ×	·	× × ×	× × ×	× × ×	× × ×	× × ×	× × ×	× × ×
× × ×	·	× × ×	× × ×	× × ×	× × ×	× × ×	× × ×	× × ×
× × ×	k	× × ×	× × ×	× × ×	× × ×	× × ×	× × ×	× × ×
× × ×	k	× × ×	× × ×	× × ×	× × ×	× × ×	× × ×	× × ×
× × ×	·	× × ×	× × ×	× × ×	× × ×	× × ×	× × ×	× × ×
× × ×	k	× × ×	× × ×	× × ×	× × ×	× × ×	× × ×	× × ×

analysis may be suspect; alternative techniques for ordinal data are available. Nominal variables are placed into categories that have no logical ordering. The eye colors blue, hazel, and brown might be assigned the numbers 1, 2, and 3, but it is nonsense to say that blue < hazel < brown.

Descriptive Statistics

After the experimental observations are double-checked and entered into the data matrix, there will be one or more sets of numbers. A typical hypothetical set could be A = [29, 32, 27, 28, 26, 27, 28, 29, 30, 32, 35, 31], representing a sample of ages of 12 residents in an anesthesia training program. Although the results of a particular experiment might be presented by repeatedly showing the entire set of numbers, there are concise ways of summarizing the information content of the set A into a few numbers. These numbers are called sample or summary statistics; summary statistics are calculated using the numbers of the sample. By convention,

the symbols of summary statistics are Roman letters. The two summary statistics most frequently used for interval variables are the central location and the variability, but there are other summary statistics. Other data types have analogous summary statistics.

Although the first purpose of descriptive statistics is to describe the sample of numbers obtained, there is also the desire to use the summary statistics from the sample to characterize the population from which the sample was obtained. For example, what can be said about the age of all anesthesia residents from the information in set A? The population also has measures of central location and variability that are called the parameters of the population; as previously mentioned, population parameters are denoted by Greek letters. Usually, the population parameters cannot be directly calculated, because data from all population members cannot be obtained. The beauty of properly chosen summary statistics is that they are the best possible estimators of the population parameters.

These sampling statistics can be used in conjunction with a theoretical probability distribution to provide additional descriptions of the sample and its population. A theoretical probability distribution is an algebraic equation, $f(x)$, which gives a theoretical percentage distribution of x. Each value of x has a probability of occurrence given by $f(x)$. The percentage is obviously $100 \cdot f(x)$. If $f(x)$ is summed or integrated for all possible values of x, the percentage must total 100% and the probability must total 1.0. The most important probability distribution is the normal or gaussian function:

$$f(x) = \frac{1}{\sqrt{2\pi\sigma^2}} \cdot e^{-(x-\mu)^2/2\sigma^2} \qquad (3\text{-}1)$$

There are two constants in the equation, μ and σ. The normal equation can be plotted and produces the familiar bell-shaped curve. Why are the mathematic properties of this curve so important to biostatistics? First, it has been empirically noted that when a biologic variable is sampled repeatedly, the pattern of the numbers plotted as a histogram resembles the normal curve; thus, most biologic data are said to follow or to obey a normal distribution. Second, if it is reasonable to assume that a sample is from a normal population, the mathematic properties of the normal equation can be used with the sampling statistic estimators of

TABLE 3-5. Data Types

Data Type	Definition	Examples
Interval		
Discrete	Data measured with an integer-only scale	Age, parity
Continuous	Data measured with a constant scale interval	Blood pressure, temperature
Categorical		
Dichotomous	Binary data	Mortality, gender
Nominal	Qualitative data that cannot be ordered or ranked	Eye color, drug category
Ordinal	Data ordered, ranked, or measured without a constant scale interval	ASA physical status score, pain score

the population parameters to describe the sample and the population. Third, a mathematic theorem (the Central Limit Theorem) allows the use of the assumption of normality for certain purposes, even if the population is not normally distributed.

Central Location

The three most common summary statistics of central location for interval variables are the arithmetic mean, the median, and the mode; these summary statistics are calculated for the hypothetical set A (Table 3-6). The *mean* is merely the average of the numbers in the data set. Statistical formulas use a summation notation that considerably reduces the ink needed to print mathematic equations. The summary notation for the arithmetic mean is given below:

$$\bar{x} = \Sigma x_i/n \qquad (3-2)$$

Capital sigma (Σ) is the summation operator; its purpose is to add up all values of x from x_1 to x_n; the sum is then divided by the count of individuals (n) in the sample. Being a summary statistic of the sample, the arithmetic mean is denoted by the Roman letter $\bar{x}$. If all values in the population could be obtained, then the population mean (μ) could be calculated:

$$\mu = \Sigma x_i/N \qquad (3-3)$$

Because these values cannot be obtained, the sample mean is the unbiased, consistent, minimum variance, sufficient estimator of the population mean; thus, $\bar{x} = \mu$, where μ is the population mean and N is the population count. The μ in the normal equation is the population mean.

The *median* is the middlemost number or the number that divides the sample into two equal parts. The median is obtained by first ranking the sample values from lowest to highest and then counting up halfway. The concept of ranking is used in nonparametric statistics. A virtue of the median is that it is hardly affected by a few extremely high or low values. The *mode* is the most popular number of a sam-

ple, i.e., the number that occurs most frequently. A sample may have ties for the most common value and be bi- or polymodal; these modes may be widely separated or adjacent. The raw data should be inspected for this unusual appearance. The mode is always mentioned in discussions of descriptive statistics but is rarely used in statistical practice.

Spread or Variability

Any set of interval data has variability unless all the numbers are identical. The range of ages from lowest to highest expresses the largest difference within set A. This spread, diversity, and variability can also be expressed in a concise manner. Variability is specified by calculating the deviation or deviate of each individual x_1 from the center (mean) of all the x_i's (see Table 3-6). Two derivatives of the deviate are used, the absolute deviate and the squared deviate. These individual deviates are totaled; the sum of the deviates is always zero, whereas the sum of either the absolute or the squared deviates is always positive unless all set values are identical. This sum is then divided by the number of individual measurements. The result is the average absolute deviation and the average squared deviation; they can be considered as average distances from data points to the center of the data. Whereas the mean absolute deviation is used very little, the average squared deviation is ubiquitous in statistics.

The concept of describing the spread of a set of numbers by calculating the average distance from each number to the center of the numbers applies to both a sample and a population; this average squared distance is called the *variance*. For a population, the variance is a parameter and is represented by σ^2:

$$\sigma^2 = \Sigma(x_i - \mu)^2/N \qquad (3-4)$$

As with the population mean, the population variance is not usually known and cannot be calculated. The sample has a sample variance, s^2, given below:

$$s^2 = \Sigma(x_i - \bar{x})^2/(n - 1) \qquad (3-5)$$

TABLE 3-6. Central Location and Variability of a Hypothetical Data Set of Anesthesia Resident Ages

Subject i	Age x_i	Mean $\bar{x}$	Deviation $(x_i - \bar{x})$	Absolute Deviation $\lvert x_i - \bar{x}\rvert$	Deviation Squared $(x_i - \bar{x})^2$
1	26	29.5	−3.5	3.5	12.25
2	27	29.5	−2.5	2.5	6.25
3	27	29.5	−2.5	2.5	6.25
4	28	29.5	−1.5	1.5	2.25
5	28	29.5	−1.5	1.5	2.25
6	29	29.5	−0.5	0.5	0.25
7	29	29.5	−0.5	0.5	0.25
8	30	29.5	+0.5	0.5	0.25
9	31	29.5	+1.5	1.5	2.25
10	32	29.5	+2.5	2.5	6.25
11	32	29.5	+2.5	2.5	6.25
12	35	29.5	+5.5	5.5	30.25
12	354	354.0	0.0	25.0	75.00

Sample median: 29
Sample mode: Polymodal
Sample mean: $\bar{x} = \Sigma x_i/n = 354/12 = 29.5$
Sample standard deviation: $s = (\Sigma(x_i - \bar{x})^2/(n - 1))^{0.5} = (75/11)^{0.5} = 2.61$
Sample standard error: $SE = s/(n)^{0.5} = 2.61/(12)^{0.5} = 0.75$

Statistical theory demonstrates that if the divisor in the formula for s^2 is $n - 1$ rather than n, the sample variance is an unbiased estimator of the population variance. While the variance is used extensively in statistical calculations, the units of variance are squared units of the original observations. The square root of the variance has the same units as the original observations; the square roots of the sample and population variances are called the sample and population standard deviations, s and σ, respectively. Along with μ, the population *standard deviation* is the other constant in the normal equation.

It was previously mentioned that most biologic observations appear to come from populations with normal or gaussian distributions. By accepting this assumption of a normal distribution, further meaning can be given to the sample summary statistics that have been calculated. This involves the use of the expression $x \pm k \cdot s$, where $k = 1$, 2, 3, *etc.* If the population from which the sample is taken is unimodal and roughly symmetric, then:

- $\bar{x} \pm 1 \cdot s$ encompasses roughly 68% of the sample and population members;
- $\bar{x} \pm 2 \cdot s$ encompasses roughly 95% of the sample and population members;
- $\bar{x} \pm 3 \cdot s$ encompasses roughly 99% of the sample and population members.

In our example of hypothetical resident ages (see Table 3-6), $29.5 \pm 1 \cdot 2.61$ includes 10 of 12 observations, $29.5 \pm 2 \cdot 2.61$ includes 11 of 12 observations, and $29.5 \pm 3 \cdot 2.61$ includes all 12 values. The standard deviation usually gives a fairly good approximation of the spread of the sample data.

Confidence Intervals

A confidence interval describes how likely it is that the population parameter is guessed by any particular sample statistic. Confidence intervals are a range of the form: parameter = summary statistic $\pm$ (confidence factor) $\cdot$ (precision factor).

The precision factor is derived from the sample itself, whereas the confidence factor is taken from a theoretical probability distribution and also depends on the specific confidence level chosen. For a sample of interval data taken from a normally distributed population for which confidence intervals are to be chosen for μ, the precision factor is called the *standard error of the mean* (SE) and is obtained by dividing the sample standard deviation by the square root of the sample size. The confidence factors are the same as those used for the dispersion or spread of the sample and are obtained from the normal distribution. The confidence interval is read as follows:

- $\bar{x} \pm 1 \cdot$ SE has roughly a 68% chance of containing the population mean;
- $\bar{x} \pm 2 \cdot$ SE has roughly a 95% chance of containing the population mean;
- $\bar{x} \pm 3 \cdot$ SE has roughly a 99% chance of containing the population mean.

For the example of Table 3-6, there is a 95% chance that 29.5 ± 1.5 years will include the mean age of the anesthesia residents in the population sampled. The coefficients given above for confidence intervals are not exact; the 95% interval should use the coefficient 1.96. But 1, 2, and 3 are easier to remember and use. These confidence intervals are also calculated, assuming that the population σ is known. In actuality, the sample s was substituted for σ. Strictly speaking, when σ is not known, the confidence factors should be taken from the t distribution, another theoretical probability distribution. These coefficients will be larger than those used above. This is usually ignored if the sample size is reasonable, for example, $n \geq 25$. Even when the sample size is only five or greater, the use of the coefficients 1, 2, and 3 is simple and sufficiently accurate for quick mental calculations of parameter confidence intervals.

Almost all research reports include the use of SE, regardless of the probability distribution of the populations sampled. This use is a consequence of the Central Limit Theorem previously mentioned; it is considered one of the most remarkable theorems in all of mathematics. The Central Limit Theorem states that the sample SE can always be used, if the sample size is sufficiently large, to specify confidence intervals on the population mean. These confidence intervals are calculated as described above. This is true even if the population distribution is so different from normal that the sample s cannot be used to characterize the dispersion of the population members. Only rough guidelines can be given for the necessary size of n; for interval data, certainly, $n = 25$ and above is large enough, and $n = 4$ and below is too small.

Although the standard error is discussed here in the section on Descriptive Statistics, it is really an inferential statistic. The standard deviation and standard error are mentioned together because of their similarities of computation and because of the confusion of their use in research reports. This use is most often of the form "mean $\pm$ number"; some confusion results from the failure of the author to specify whether the number after the $\pm$ sign is the one or the other. More important, the choice between using s and SE has become controversial; because SE is always less than s, it has been argued that authors seek to deceive by using SE to make the data look better than they really are. The choice is really simple. When describing the spread, scatter, or dispersion of the sample, use s; when describing the precision with which the population center is known, use SE.

Bivariate Data

Some of the data collected in an experiment seem to naturally pair off because of a relationship or dependency between two variables; these paired variables are known as (x, y) pairs, or bivariate data. Typical examples found in anesthesia journals are (time, plasma concentration) and (dose, effect). Regression and correlation constitute the statistical techniques for investigating such relationships. There are considerable computational similarities between the two, but the approaches are different. In *regression*, one variable (the x or independent variable) is considered as having been picked or specified; the analysis focuses on the variation of the y or dependent variable with changes in x. In *correlation*, there is no such distinction between a dependent and an independent variable; both x and y are considered dependent. If five doses of an opioid are administered and blood pressure is measured after each dose, regression analysis to describe the dose-response relationship is appropriate. If intracranial pressure and cerebral blood flow are measured simultaneously, correlation analysis is used to describe their interrelationship. Sometimes it is difficult to make the choice between the two methods; the formulas for both are easily applied, regardless of the source of the data. One of the distinctions between regression and correlation is in assumptions about the nature of x and y. In regression, x is considered a fixed or precisely known variable, whereas y is a random variable; in correlation, both x and y are random variables. From a practical point of view, x is never really a precisely known variable; however, as long as the uncertainty in the measurement of x is small, the usual regression analysis is used. There is also a distinction between regression and correlation concerning other assumptions necessary for interpretation. Regardless of these differences, experimenters most frequently apply both techniques to all data sets.

The concept of a model is used extensively in statistics. A model is a mathematical equation that expresses a relationship among variables and parameters; it is an algebraic expression of one's belief about the nature and relationship of experimental measurements. A model is held tentatively and is critically examined during analysis; if a model does not agree with the facts, i.e., the numbers of the sample, it is rejected. The idea of a model is inherent in linear regression analysis. *Linear regression* is the fitting of a straight line through a set of (x, y) pairs (Fig. 3-1). The assumption that such a straight line relationship exists between x and y is a model. The regression relationship is usually written $y = a + b \cdot x$, where b is the slope of the line and a is the intercept or intersection of the line at the y axis. Both a and b are summary statistics that are calculated from the sample; a and b are estimates of α, the population intercept, and β, the population slope, which are the parameters of the model. If all possible (x, y) pairs from the target population could be sampled, then α and β could be calculated directly. In the regression equation, y actually means the value of y predicted by the regression equation; this predicted y value is not necessarily a value of y actually measured in the sample. For this reason, statisticians write the equation as $\hat{y} = a + b \cdot x$, where $\hat{y}$ reads "the predicted y." This distinction is usually overlooked in biomedical research reports.

The most common but not the only method to calculate a and b is that of least squares. To any line drawn through the points of a data set, a vertical line can be drawn to connect every (x, y) pair with the regression line. The least squares regression line will have the property that the sum of the squared distances of all these vertical lines will be minimized. By differential calculus, equations for the unique determination of both a and b can be derived; these equations use the values of the (x, y) pairs of the sample

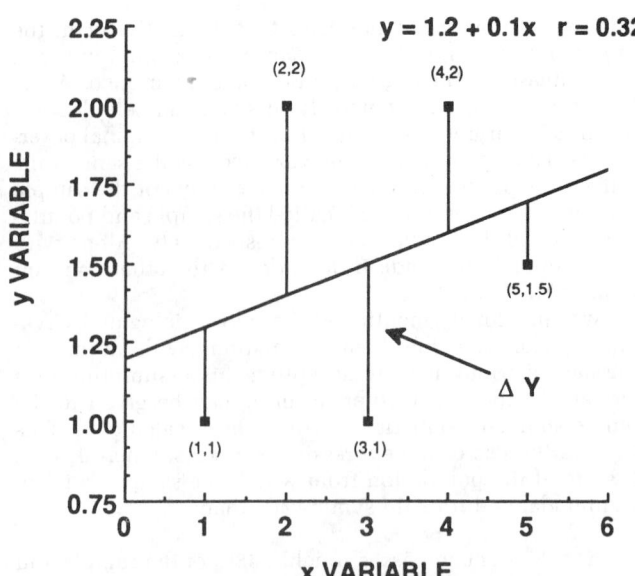

Figure 3-1. Descriptive regression analysis. Five hypothetical data points are plotted. The line fitted by least squares regression makes the sum of the squared vertical deviations of the observed points about the line as small as possible. For the pair (3,1), ΔY denotes the deviation.

(Table 3-7). Much as $\bar{x}$ is the central location of the x_i's, the linear regression line is a descriptive statistic for all the (x, y) points; it divides the points into approximately two equal groups. With the exception of a set of points whose x values are identical, a regression equation can always be calculated. The ability to calculate and plot a regression line does not necessarily imply that there is actually a relationship between x and y. The more nearly the regression line is either perfectly vertical or perfectly horizontal, the less important is the relationship between x and y. Also, even though the regression line can be extended beyond the minimum and maximum of the x values (see Fig. 3-1), this regression relationship may well have no biologic meaning outside the range of the sample; the intercept value describes the regression line but does not necessarily exist as a measured value.

TABLE 3-7. Descriptive Statistics for a Hypothetical Bivariate Data Set

x_i	y_i	$(x_i - \bar{x})$	$(x_i - \bar{x})^2$	$(y_i - \bar{y})$	$(y_i - \bar{y})^2$	$(x_i - \bar{x}) \cdot (y_i - \bar{y})$
1.0	1.0	−2.0	4.00	−0.5	0.25	+1.0
2.0	2.0	−1.0	1.00	+0.5	0.25	−0.5
3.0	1.0	0.0	0.00	−0.5	0.25	0.0
4.0	2.0	+1.0	1.00	+0.5	0.25	+0.5
5.0	1.5	+2.0	4.00	0.0	0.00	0.0
15.0	7.5	0.0	10.00	0.0	1.00	1.0

$\bar{x} = 15.0/5 = 3.0$ $\bar{y} = 7.5/5 = 1.5$ $n = 5$

$s_x = (10/4)^{0.5} = 1.58$ $s_y = (1/4)^{0.5} = 0.5$

$SE_x = 1.58/5^{0.5} = 0.71$ $SE_y = 0.5/5^{0.5} = 0.22$

Slope: $b = (\Sigma(x_i - \bar{x}) \cdot (y_i - \bar{y}))/(\Sigma(x_i - \bar{x})^2) = 1.0/10.0 = 0.1$

Intercept: $a = \bar{y} - b \cdot \bar{x} = 1.5 - 0.1 \cdot 3.0 = 1.2$

Equation: $y = 1.2 + 0.1x$

Correlation coefficient:

$r = [\Sigma(x_i - \bar{x}) \cdot (y_i - \bar{y})]/\{[\Sigma(x_i - \bar{x})^2] \cdot [\Sigma(y_i - \bar{y})^2]\}^{0.5}$

$= 1.0/(10.00 \cdot 1.00)^{0.5}$

$= 0.32$

Assuming that x and y are now random variables, the same hypothetical data can be used in calculations of correlation (see Table 3-7). The *correlation coefficient*, denoted r, is also known as the product moment correlation, or Pearson's coefficient of correlation. Inspection of the formula for r shows it to be a dimensionless ratio whose possible values extend from −1 to +1. There is a perfect correlation between x and y if r is either −1 or +1; for perfect correlation, all the points lie on the regression line. The intimate computational relationship between correlation and regression is shown by the relationship $b = r \cdot s_y/s_x$, where s_y and s_x are the standard deviations of y and x. If all (x, y) pairs of the target population were measured, the population correlation coefficient ρ could be calculated; r is the summary statistic estimate of ρ. Unless all the values of x in a sample are 0, r can always be calculated. There are certain cautions about the use of r. The correlation coefficient applies only to linear relationships. If r is 0, there is no linear relationship, but some other mathematic model may be appropriate. Most important is the warning that "correlation does not imply causation." Just because the height of skirts and the height of the stock market rise and fall together does not mean that one causes the other.

Proportions

Categorical binary data, also called enumeration data, provide counts of subject responses. Given a sample T of n subjects of whom x have a certain characteristic (e.g., death, female gender), a ratio of responders to the number of subjects can be easily calculated as $p = x/n$; this can also be expressed as a percentage, $100 \cdot p$. The ratio p is a descriptive or summary statistic of the sample T. Assume that n = 15 subjects and x = 10 deaths for sample T, then p = 10/15 = 0.67 and $100 \cdot p$ = 67%. If each subject who dies is given the score 1 and the others are given the score 0, the calculation of p is seen to be exactly the same as the calculation of $\bar{x}$ (Table 3-8); p is a measure of central location of the sample in the same way that $\bar{x}$ is. In the population from which the sample is taken, the ratio of responders to total subjects is a population parameter, denoted π; π is the measure of central location for the population. This population parameter, π, is not related to the geometry constant π = 3.1415926.... As with other data types, π is usually not known but must be estimated from the sample. The sample ratio p is the best estimate of π.

The probability of binary data is provided by the binomial distribution, another theoretical probability distribution. This distribution calculates the chance of x occurrences in a sample of n subjects from a population with an occurrence rate of π.

$$f(x) = (n!/(x! \cdot (n - x)!)) \cdot (\pi^x) \cdot ((1 - \pi)^{(n - x)}) \qquad (3\text{-}6)$$

If the π of a population is known, then the probability of the observed response rate p is easily calculated. For example, if there are 10 deaths in 15 subjects and the population death rate is 50% (π = 0.5), then the probability is:

$$(15!/(10! \cdot (15 - 10)!)) \cdot (0.5^{10}) \cdot ((1 - 0.5)^{(15-10)}) = 0.09$$

This would be expressed as follows: if the population death rate was 50%, then in a sample of 15 individuals, there would be about a 9% chance of finding 10 deaths.

TABLE 3-8. Central Location and Variability for Hypothetical Data Set of Patient Mortality

Subject i	Outcome* x_i	Mean p	Deviation $(x_i - p)$	Absolute Deviation $|x_i - p|$	Deviation Squared $(x_i - p)^2$
1	1	0.67	+0.33	0.33	0.11
2	1	0.67	+0.33	0.33	0.11
3	1	0.67	+0.33	0.33	0.11
4	1	0.67	+0.33	0.33	0.11
5	1	0.67	+0.33	0.33	0.11
6	1	0.67	+0.33	0.33	0.11
7	1	0.67	+0.33	0.33	0.11
8	1	0.67	+0.33	0.33	0.11
9	1	0.67	+0.33	0.33	0.11
10	1	0.67	+0.33	0.33	0.11
11	0	0.67	−0.67	0.67	0.44
12	0	0.67	−0.67	0.67	0.44
13	0	0.67	−0.67	0.67	0.44
14	0	0.67	−0.67	0.67	0.44
15	0	0.67	−0.67	0.67	0.44
15	10	10.00	0.00	5.00	3.33

Sample rate or proportion:
   $p = \Sigma x_i/n = 10/15 = 0.67$
Sample standard deviation:
   $s = (p \cdot (1 - p))^{0.5} = (0.67 \cdot (1 - 0.67))^{0.5} = 0.47$
or:
   $s = (\Sigma(x_i - p)^2/n)^{0.5} = (3.33/15)^{0.5} = 0.47$
Sample standard error of the proportion:
   $SE = (p \cdot (1 - p)/n)^{0.5} = s/(n)^{0.5} = 0.47/(15)^{0.5} = 0.12$

*Patient dead = 1; Patient not dead = 0.

Since the population π is not generally known, the experimenter usually wishes to estimate π by the sample statistic p and to specify with what confidence π is known. Although it is computationally involved, this can be done by using the binomial distribution; or, advantage may be taken of the Central Limit Theorem. As previously mentioned in discussing interval data, the sampling distribution of the mean of the binomial distribution resembles the normal distribution if n is sufficiently large. This may be said in another way: as n increases, the binomial and the normal probability distributions become increasingly similar; n is said to be sufficiently large if both $n \cdot p \geq 5$ and $n \cdot (1 - p) \geq 5$ are true. Even though the probability distribution of the population from which the sample was taken is not normally distributed, a sample standard deviation and standard error may be calculated analogously to that calculated for interval data (see Table 3-8).

$$\text{Sample Standard Deviation} = s = (p \cdot (1 - p))^{0.5} \quad (3\text{-}7)$$

$$\text{Sample Standard Error} = \text{SE} = s/n^{0.5} = (p \cdot (1 - p)/n)^{0.5} \quad (3\text{-}8)$$

The sample standard deviation is the best estimate of the population standard deviation $(\pi \cdot (1 - \pi))^{0.5}$; since the population is binomial and not normal, the properties of the normal distribution cannot be used to give estimates of the spread or variability of the sample and population. However, the sample standard error is exactly analogous to the sample standard error of the mean for interval data, except that it is a standard error of the proportion. Just as a 95% confidence limit of the mean was calculated, so may a confidence limit on the proportion be obtained. Using the data of 10 deaths in 15 subjects, the summary statistic $p = 10/15 = 0.67$. Since $15 \cdot 0.67 = 10$ and $15 \cdot (1 - 0.67) = 5$, then n is sufficiently large. The sample standard error is:

$$(0.67 \cdot (1 - 0.67)/15)^{0.5} = 0.12$$

The 95% confidence interval on π will be:

$$p \pm 2 \cdot \text{SE} = 0.67 \pm 2 \cdot 0.12 = 0.67 \pm 0.24$$

Thus, the best guess of the population death rate is 67%, and there is a 95% certainty that in the population sampled the death rate is in the range of 43–91%. The approximate nature of this calculation is reflected by the exact 95% confidence interval (36–86%) derived for these data from the binomial equation. Larger n's and p's closer to 0.5 will have even greater precision. This simple equation can be used by the reader when authors do not calculate confidence intervals on rates and proportions.

Display of Data and Statistics

The research report must justify its conclusions by displaying the raw data, summary statistics of the raw data (descriptive statistics), and statistical test results; the presentation of raw data is encouraged to allow the reader to perform his or her own numeric and statistical tests. Three display methods are available: (1) text descriptions, (2) tables, and (3) graphs. Text descriptions are most commonly used to cite descriptive and inferential statistics. Descriptive statistics include means, variances, standard deviations, standard errors, frequency counts (proportions), and linear regression equations. Any listing of the form "number

1" $\pm$ "number 2" must clarify whether "number 2" is a standard deviation or a standard error of the parameter. The listing of more than three to five data items and descriptive statistics in a text list is an awkward, difficult to read, and uninformative method of display. There are a variety of ways of listing inferential statistics; the most complete would include (1) null hypothesis, (2) statistical test, (3) value of test statistic, (4) degree(s) of freedom, and (5) associated probability value. The inclusion of this level of detail is cumbersome in text form; text listings of inferential statistics more commonly include only items (3)–(5). Without giving any detail (items 1–5), authors frequently make sweeping statements in the results section of their papers concerning the presence or absence of statistical significance for a list of variables. Unless the methods section of a paper is very clear, there will be confusion about the statistical test(s) used.

A table is a list with two or more adjacent columns characterized by descriptive headings. The use of tables is a very efficient way of displaying small raw data sets. Larger sets of raw data can be listed in a table by showing the number of subjects (frequency distribution) at each value or range of values. Tables are also used to display large numbers of means $\pm$ standard errors; generally, the table is organized with different experimental groups on each row, while each column represents a different variable or repeated measurement on the same variables.

Two or more proportions or rates are most commonly presented in table form. If the proportions or frequency data represent a comparison of classifications for the sample(s), a contingency table is used. In a contingency table, data are entered at each intersection of a row and column; each intersection is called a cell. The descriptive headings of the rows and of the columns cross-classify data into cells of subjects having similar characteristics. Contingency tables are described by the number of rows and columns they contain; a contingency table with three rows and three columns would be a 3-by-3 contingency table. Thus, in a 3-by-3 contingency table, there are nine cells. The data entered in a cell are either a count of subjects or the proportion of the total subjects having the property of the intersecting row and column. The investigator must specify whether a cell entry is a frequency count or a proportion.

Tables are preferred for descriptive statistics and larger data sets because they make possible a future analysis using the displayed summary statistics. Complete details of inferential statistics can also be presented in tabular form; there is no more efficient way of detailing an analysis of variance output. More commonly, in the anesthesia literature, inferential statistics in tables are limited to superscripted notations (e.g., *, #, ¶) of probabilities. Unfortunately, these superscripts with their footnoted explanations can be rather ambiguous in specifying the statistical test and statistical hypothesis being used for the probability value displayed.

A graph is a visual display of measured quantities (either raw data or summary statistics) by the combined use of geometric elements (a coordinate system, points, lines, or circles), text elements (numbers, symbols, words), and art elements (shading, colors, patterns). Graphs are most suitable for showing broad qualitative features of the data. The most common graph formats used in biomedical literature are the bar graph, scatter plot, and line plot. Bar graphs can be used to show large raw data sets as a frequency histogram and to allow group comparisons of summary statistics; vertical bar graphs are also known as column graphs. Scatter plots are used to display bivariate data ((x, y) pairs). Line plots can be used for either raw data or descriptive statistics. As with tables, inferential statistics are generally limited to notations of probability values. The text elements of a graph are available to list regression equations and correlation coefficients.

Inferential Statistics

There are two major areas of statistical inference: the estimation of parameters and the testing of hypotheses. The use of the SE to create confidence intervals is an example of parameter estimation. The testing of hypotheses or significance testing is the main focus of inferential statistics. Hypothesis testing allows the experimenter to use data from the sample to make inferences about the population. Statisticians have created formulas that use the values of the samples to calculate test statistics. Statisticians have also explored the properties of various theoretical probability distributions. Depending on the assumptions about how data are collected, the appropriate theoretical probability distribution is chosen as the source of critical values to accept or reject the null hypothesis; if the value of the test statistic calculated from the sample(s) is greater than the critical value, the null hypothesis is rejected. The critical value is chosen from the appropriate probability distribution after the magnitude of the Type I error is specified.

There are parameters within the equation that generate any particular theoretical probability distribution; for the normal probability distribution, the parameters are μ and σ. For the normal distribution, each set of values for μ and σ will generate a different shape for the bell-like normal curve. All theoretical probability equations contain one or more parameters and can also be plotted as curves; these parameters may be discrete (integer only) or continuous. Each value or combination of values for these parameters will create a different curve for the probability distribution being used. Thus, each theoretical probability distribution is actually a family of probability curves. Some parameters have been given the special name, degrees of freedom, and are represented by the letters m, n, p, and s.

Associated with the formula for computing a test statistic is a rule for assigning integer values to the one or more parameters called degrees of freedom. The number of degrees of freedom and the value for each degree of freedom depend on (1) the number of subjects, (2) the number of experimental groups, (3) the specifics of the statistical hypothesis, and (4) the type of statistical test. The correct curve of the theoretical probability distribution from which to obtain a critical value for comparison with the value of the test statistic is obtained with the values of the one or more degrees of freedom.

To accept or reject the null hypothesis, the following steps are performed: (1) confirm that experimental data conform to the assumptions of the intended statistical test; (2) choose a significance level (alpha); (3) calculate the test statistic; (4) determine the degrees of freedom; (5) find the critical value for the chosen alpha and the degrees of freedom from the appropriate theoretical probability distribution; (6) if the test statistic exceeds the critical value, reject the null hypothesis; and (7) if the test statistic does not exceed the critical value, do not reject the null hypothesis.

Interval Data

Parametric statistics are the usual choice in the analysis of interval data, both discrete and continuous. The purpose of such analysis is to test the hypothesis of a difference between population means. The population means are unknown and are estimated by the sample means. A typical example would be the comparison of the mean heart rates of patients receiving and not receiving atropine. Parametric test statistics have been developed by using the properties of the normal probability distribution and two related theoretical probability distributions, the t and the F distribution. In using such parametric methods, the assumption is made that the sample or samples is/are drawn from population(s) with a normal distribution. The parametric test statistics that have been created for interval data all have the form of a ratio. In general terms, the numerator of this ratio is the variability of the means of the samples; the denominator of this ratio is the variability among all the members of the samples. These variabilities are similar to the variances developed for descriptive statistics. The test statistic is, thus, a ratio of variabilities or variances. All parametric test statistics are used in the same fashion; if the test statistic ratio becomes large, the null hypothesis of no difference is rejected. The critical values against which to compare the test statistic are taken from tables of the three relevant probability distributions.

By definition, in hypothesis testing, at least one of the population means is unknown, but the population variance(s) may or may not be known. Parametric statistics can be divided into two groups according to whether or not the population variances are known. If the population variance is known, the test statistic used is called the z score; critical values are obtained from the normal distribution. In most scientific applications, the population variance is rarely known; the use of z score test statistics for interval data is not discussed further in this chapter.

t Test

An important advance in statistical inference came early in the 20th century with the creation of the Student's t test statistic and the t distribution, which allowed the testing of hypotheses when the population variance is not known. The most common use of the Student's t test is to compare the mean values of two populations. This use is further subdivided by a particular aspect of experimental design. If each subject has two measurements taken, for example, one before and one after a drug, the one sample or paired t test procedure is used; each control measurement taken before drug administration is paired with a measurement in the same patient after drug administration. Of course, this is a self-control experiment. This pairing of measurements in the same patient reduces variability and increases statistical power. There are two target populations in such an experiment: subjects before and subjects after the study drug. For purposes of statistical analysis, the problem is converted into a one-population test (Table 3-9). The difference d_i of each pair of values is calculated; $\bar{d}$ is a sample statistic estimator of δ. In our example, the target population has become the difference in values of blood pressure before and after a study drug; δ is the parameter of central location for this new population of blood pressure differences. Our null hypothesis is one of no drug effect, i.e., $\delta = 0$. In the formula for the Student's t statistic, the numerator is $\bar{d}$, whereas the denominator is the standard error of d (SE_d). All t statistics are created in this way; the numerator is the difference of two means, whereas the denominator is the standard error of the two means. If the difference between the two means is large compared with their variability, then the null hypothesis of no difference is rejected. The critical values for the t statistic are taken from the t probability distribution.

TABLE 3-9. Inferential Statistics for Hypothetical Paired Interval Data of Systolic Blood Pressure Before and After Treatment

Subject i	Control x_{i1}	Treated x_{i2}	Difference $d_i = x_{i2} - x_{i1}$	Deviation $(d_i - \bar{d})$	Deviation Squared $(d_i - \bar{d})^2$
1	190	170	−20	0	0
2	180	150	−30	−10	100
3	180	160	−20	0	0
4	170	170	0	+20	400
5	190	170	−20	0	0
6	160	170	+10	+30	900
7	200	150	−50	−30	900
8	190	160	−30	−10	100
8	1460	1300	−160	0	2400

H_0: $\delta = 0$
H_a: $\delta \neq 0$
$\bar{d} = \Sigma d_i/n = -160/8 = -20$
$s_d = (\Sigma(d_i - \bar{d})^2/(n - 1))^{0.5} = (2400/7)^{0.5} = 18.5$
$SE_d = s_d/(n)^{0.5} = 18.5/(8)^{0.5} = 6.55$
Paired t test $= t_{(df)} = (\bar{d} - 0)/SE_d$ df $= n - 1$
$t_{(7)} = -20/6.55 = -3.05$ Critical value $= t_{(0.05,7)} = 2.37$
Reject null hypothesis, since $|t_{(7)}| = 3.05 >$ critical value $= 2.37$

The t distribution is symmetric and bell-shaped but more spread out than the normal distribution. The t distribution has a single integer parameter; for a paired t test, the value of this single degree of freedom is the sample size minus one. There can be some confusion about the use of the letter t. It refers both to the value of the test statistic calculated by the formula $t_{(df)} = \bar{d}/SE_d$ and to the critical value from the theoretical probability distribution. The critical t value is determined by looking in a t table after a significance level is chosen and the degree of freedom is computed.

More commonly, measurements are taken on two separate groups of subjects. For example, one group receives blood pressure treatment, whereas no treatment is given to a control group. The number of subjects in each group might or might not be identical; regardless of this, in no sense is an individual measurement in the first group matched or paired with a specific measurement in the second group. An unpaired or two-sample t test is used to compare the means of the two groups (Table 3-10). The obvious null hypothesis of no difference between the groups is used; thus, the numerator of the t statistic is $\bar{x} - \bar{y}$. The denomina-

TABLE 3-10. Inferential Statistics for Hypothetical Unpaired Interval Data of Systolic Blood Pressure With and Without Treatment

Control x_i	Treated y_i	Deviation $(x_i - \bar{x})$	Squared Deviation $(x_i - \bar{x})^2$	Deviation $(y_i - \bar{y})$	Squared Deviation $(y_i - \bar{y})^2$
190	170	+7.5	56.25	+7.5	56.25
180	150	−2.5	6.25	−12.5	156.25
180	160	−2.5	6.25	−2.5	6.25
170	170	−12.5	156.25	+7.5	56.25
190	170	+7.5	56.25	+7.5	56.25
160	170	−22.5	560.25	+7.5	56.25
200	150	+17.5	306.25	−12.5	156.25
190	160	+7.5	56.25	−2.5	6.25
1460	1300	0.0	1150.00	0.0	550.00

H_0: $\mu_x = \mu_y$
H_a: $\mu_x \neq \mu_y$
$n_x = 8$ $\bar{x} = \Sigma x_i/n_x = 1460/8 = 182.5$
$n_y = 8$ $\bar{y} = \Sigma y_i/n_y = 1300/8 = 162.5$
$s_x = (\Sigma(x_i - \bar{x})^2/(n_x - 1))^{0.5} = (1150/7)^{0.5} = 12.8$
$s_y = (\Sigma(y_i - \bar{y})^2/(n_y - 1))^{0.5} = (550/7)^{0.5} = 8.9$
Pooled $s = s_p = \{[(n_x - 1) \cdot s_x^2 + (n_y - 1) \cdot s_y^2]/(n_x + n_y - 2)\}^{0.5}$
$\qquad = \{(7 \cdot 12.8^2 + 7 \cdot 8.9^2)/14\}^{0.5} = 11.0$
SE of difference $= SE_{(x-y)} = s_p \cdot (1/n_x + 1/n_y)^{0.5} = 11.0 \cdot (1/8 + 1/8)^{0.5} = 5.5$
Unpaired t test $= t_{(df)} = (\bar{x} - \bar{y})/SE_{(x-y)}$ df $= n_x + n_y - 2$
$t_{(14)} = (182.5 - 162.5)/5.5 = 3.63$ Critical value $= t_{(0.05,14)} = 2.15$
Reject null hypothesis, since $t_{(14)} = 3.63 >$ critical value $= 2.15$

tor requires extra work. It is necessary to assume that the population variance of x equals the population variance of y; under that assumption, a pooled estimate of s (s_p) can be calculated. The standard error of the difference of x and y is s_p divided by a weighted average of the count of subjects in x and the count of subjects in y. The degree of freedom for an unpaired t test is calculated as the sum of the subjects of the two groups minus two. As with the paired t test, if the t ratio becomes large, the null hypothesis is rejected.

Multiple Comparisons and Analysis of Variance

Experiments in anesthesia, whether they are with humans or with animals, are rarely limited to only one or two groups of data for each variable. It is very common to follow a variable longitudinally; heart rate might be measured five times before and during anesthetic induction. These are also called repeated measurement experiments; the experimenter will wish to compare changes between the initial heart rate measurement and those obtained during induction. The experimental design might also include several groups receiving different induction drugs, e.g., comparing heart rate across groups immediately after laryngoscopy by induction drug. Researchers have commonly handled these analysis problems with the t test. If heart rate is collected five times, these collection times could be labeled A, B, C, D, and E. Then, in a paired sense, A could be compared with B, C, D, and E; B could be compared with C, D, and E; and so forth. There are a total of ten possible pairings; thus, ten paired t tests could be calculated for all the possible pairings of A, B, C, D, and E. A similar approach can be used for comparing more than two groups for unpaired data.

The use of t tests in this fashion is inappropriate. In testing a statistical hypothesis, the experimenter sets the level of Type I error; this is usually chosen to be 0.05. When using many t tests, as in the example above, the chosen error rate for performing all these t tests is much higher than 0.05, even though the Type I error is set at 0.05 for each individual comparison. In fact, the Type I error rate for all t tests simultaneously, *i.e.*, the chance of finding at least one of the multiple t test statistics significant merely by chance, is given by the formula $\alpha = 1 - 0.95^k$. If 13 t tests are performed, the real error rate is 49%. This problem can be simulated by generating mock data on a computer; simply applying t tests over and over again to all the possible pairings of a variable will misleadingly identify statistical significance when there is, in fact, none.

TABLE 3-11. Inferential Statistics on Hypothetical Data with Three Groups: One-Way Analysis of Variance (Part I)

Subject Number	Group 1	Group 2	Group 3	Groups Combined
1	3	3	2	
2	5	0	1	
3	4	4	2	
4	2	3	3	
5	4	4	4	
6	3	1	4	
7	4	4	3	
8	7	1	6	
9	2	1	0	
10	6	6	4	
n	$10 = n_1$	$10 = n_2$	$10 = n_3$	$30 = N$
Σx_i	$40 = T_1$	$27 = T_2$	$29 = T_3$	$96 = G$
Σx_i^2	184	105	111	400
$\bar{x}$	4.0	2.7	2.9	
s	1.63	1.89	1.73	
SE	0.52	0.60	0.55	

H_0: $\mu_1 = \mu_2 = \mu_3$
H_a: $\mu_1 \neq \mu_2 \neq \mu_3$

The most versatile approach for handling comparisons of means among more than two groups is called *analysis of variance* and is frequently cited by the acronym ANOVA. Analysis of variance consists of rules for creating test statistics on means when there are more than two groups. These test statistics are called F ratios, after Ronald Fisher; the critical values for the F test statistic are taken from the F theoretical probability distribution that Fisher derived.

Suppose that data for three groups are obtained (Table 3-11). What can be said about the mean values of the three target populations? The null hypothesis for such comparisons is more complex, as it contains three identities. The F test is actually asking several questions simultaneously: Is group 1 different from group 2, is group 2 different from group 3, and is group 1 different from group 3? As with the t test, the F test statistic is a ratio; in general terms, the numerator expresses the variability of the mean values of the three groups, whereas the denominator expresses the average variability or difference of each sample value from the mean of all sample values. The formulas to create the test statistic (Table 3-12) are computationally elegant but

TABLE 3-12. Inferential Statistics on Hypothetical Data with Three Groups: One-Way Analysis of Variance (Part II)

Source	Sum of Squares	Degrees of Freedom	Mean Square
Between treatments	SST = 9.8	$k - 1 = 2$	SST/$(k - 1)$ = 9.8/2 = 4.90
Within treatments (error)	SSE = 83.0	$N - k = 27$	SSE/$(N - k)$ = 83.0/27 = 3.07
Total	S = 92.8	$N - 1 = 29$	

Sum of squares total = $S = \Sigma x_i^2 - G^2/N = 400 - 96^2/30 = 92.8$
Sum of squares between treatments = SST = $\Sigma(T_i^2/n_i) - G^2/N = [(40^2 + 27^2 + 29^2)/10] - 96^2/30 = 9.8$
Degree of freedom between treatments = $k - 1 = 3 - 1 = 2$
Sum of squares within treatments = SSE = $S - SST = 92.8 - 9.8 = 83.0$
Degree of freedom within treatments = $N - k = 30 - 3 = 27$
$F_{(2,27)}$ ratio = $[SST/(k - 1)]/[SSE/(N - k)] = 4.90/3.07 = 1.59$
Critical ratio = $F_{(2,27;0.05)} = 3.37$
Do not reject null hypothesis, since $F_{(2,27)} = 1.59 < F_{(2,27;0.05)} = 3.37$

are rather hard to appreciate intuitively. The F statistic has two degrees of freedom, denoted m and n; the value of m is a function of the number of experimental groups; the value for n is a function of the number of subjects in all experimental groups.

Enormous effort has been expended to develop different types of ANOVA. For example, there are at least three ANOVA techniques for analyzing repeated measurement data; these are the two-way ANOVA, the multivariate ANOVA (also known as MANOVA), and the maximum likelihood mixed-model ANOVA. Very complex experimental designs are difficult to analyze statistically without the flexibility of ANOVA methods for developing test statistics. The analysis of multigroup data is not necessarily finished after the ANOVAs are calculated. If the null hypothesis is rejected and it is accepted that there are differences among the groups tested, how can it be decided where the differences are? A variety of techniques are available to make what are called multiple comparisons after the ANOVA test is performed. These include tests by Bonferroni, Tukey, Scheffé, and Dunnett; there are also the Duncan and Newman-Keuls multiple range tests. All these multiple comparison tests tend to be variations on the t test statistic. The reader should refer to a text on statistics for a more comprehensive review of ANOVA.

Transformations, Robustness, and Nonparametric Tests

Most statistical tests depend on certain assumptions about the nature of the distribution of values in the underlying populations from which experimental samples are taken. For the parametric statistics, i.e., t tests and analysis of variance, it is assumed that the populations follow the normal distribution. There is a further assumption when dealing with samples from two or more populations. The variances of the populations are assumed to be equal and common; this is also described as homogeneity of variance. Usually, the experimenter cannot discern the population distributions of his or her data. However, for some data, there is experience or historical reasons to believe that these assumptions of a normal distribution and homogeneity of variance do not hold; some examples include proportions, percentages, and response times. Many other instances of poorly conditioned data exist. What should the experimenter do if he or she fears that the data are not normally distributed?

One possibility would be to engage a statistician to create new test statistics and new theoretical probability distributions. This would be expensive and inefficient; many years of work by many statisticians have been invested in the creation of parametric statistics. It is more desirable to use existing statistical techniques to save money and to avoid explaining these new methods to editors and readers. Another possibility would be to transform the data before analysis. In transforming data, a function is applied to a raw value; a common transformation is the use of logarithms. If the raw value is 10, the transformed value is log (10) or 1. These transformations can be thought of as changing the scale of measurement; it is as if the ruler by which a measure is obtained is stretched and compressed along its length. The most frequently used transformations are the logarithmic, the square root, the inverse sine function, and the reciprocal. Under appropriate circumstances, these transformations can be shown to create normally distributed data and/or homogeneity of variance. The usual parametric statistics can then be used with confidence. Using data transformations does have its complications. What is the inher-

ent meaning of these transformed data? How should model and population parameters (mean, standard deviation, slope) of transformed data be retransformed to the original scale of measurement after analysis? Data transformation is not as widely practiced now as it was several decades ago.

The experimenter might also choose to ignore the problem of non-normal data and inhomogeneity of variance, hoping that everything will work out. Such insouciance is actually a very practical and reasonable approach to the problem. Parametric statistics are called "robust" statistics; they stand up to much adversity. To a statistician, robustness implies that the magnitude of Type I errors is not seriously affected by ill-conditioned data. Parametric statistics are sufficiently robust that the accuracy of decisions reached by means of t tests and analysis of variance remains very credible, even for moderately severe departures from the assumptions.

A fourth possibility would be to use existing statistics that do not require any assumptions about probability distributions of the populations. Such statistics are known as nonparametric tests; they can be used whenever there is very serious concern about the shape of the data. Nonparametric statistics are also the tests of choice for ordinal data. The basic concept behind nonparametric statistics is the ability to rank or order the observations; nonparametric tests are also called order statistics. If there are sample values from two populations, all values are thrown into a common list and arranged or ranked in value from lowest to highest; each sample value is assigned the new value of its place in line or rank in the list. For each group, these rank values are summed. A test statistic is calculated that is a function of the rank sum and of the count of subjects for each group; if the test statistic is sufficiently large, the null hypothesis of no difference is rejected.

Most nonparametric statistics still require the use of theoretical probability distributions; the critical values that must be exceeded by the test statistic are taken from the binomial, normal, and chi-square distributions, depending on the nonparametric test being used. The nonparametric sign test, Mann-Whitney rank sum test, and Kruskal-Wallis one-way analysis of variance are analogous to the paired t test, unpaired t test, and one-way analysis of variance, respectively. The currently available nonparametric tests are not used more commonly because they do not adapt well to complex statistical models and because they are less able than parametric tests to distinguish between the null and alternative hypotheses if the data are, in fact, normally distributed. Using the data of Table 3-10, the probability of the hypothesis comparing the two groups is $p = 0.003$ by unpaired t test and $p = 0.009$ by the Mann-Whitney rank sum test. Statistical significance is detected by both tests but the nonparametric test is less powerful.

Regression and Correlation

After calculating a regression line, what inferences can be made about the regression equation? Recall that this calculation required the assumption of a model relating variables and model parameters and that the model needed re-examination during analysis. One of the crucial features of the least squares linear model is the slope of the straight line; the sample statistic b is an estimate of the population slope β. If the slope of the line is 0, there is no relationship between x and y and the model must be rejected. The most commonly performed statistical test during regression analysis compares b to a slope value of 0. Although no assumptions were required to calculate a regression equation, inferential statistics concerning regression assume that y is normally distributed and that the variability of y is the same regardless of the value of x; this latter property is called homoscedasticity. These assumptions are usually reasonable, even if the values of y are not quite normally distributed; the Central Limit Theorem also applies to regression analysis.

The test statistic for inferences about β is a t test (Table 3-13). Critical values are obtained from the t distribution; the degree of freedom is the sample size minus two. The numerator is the difference between the two estimates of the population slope, b minus 0. The denominator is the standard error of the sample slope b (SE_b); a previously unmentioned sample statistic is used to calculate this denominator. Similar to a sample standard deviation, the standard deviation from regression ($s_{y \cdot x}$) estimates deviations of sample points about the fitted regression line. Both the standard error of the intercept and SE_b are estimated by the use of $s_{y \cdot x}$. One cannot reject the null hypothesis of $\beta = 0$ in our hypothetical data set; thus, the model of a linear relationship must be abandoned. Even when this t test is significant, the data must often be examined more closely to confirm the model. This is most frequently done by examining the residuals. In regression analysis, residuals are the difference between the sample y and the predicted $\hat{y}$ for each (x, y) pair. Other inferential statistics include confidence limits on the slope b and on the values of $\hat{y}$ predicted by the regression equation.

Inferential statistics for correlation tend to be more complicated computationally. The assumptions are more rigorous also; in general, x and y must be bivariate normally distributed. However, these assumptions are not necessary for the most commonly used test on r, which is the null hypothesis that $\rho = 0$, i.e., the hypothesis of no dependency between x and y. This hypothesis is also tested by a t test statistic. As is clear in the hypothetical example (Table 3-13), the statistical test for $\beta = 0$ and for $\rho = 0$ gives identical results for both and they are, in fact, equivalent. This equivalence again shows the close ties between regression and correlation. The form of the test statistic for corre-

lation does give some additional insight into the effects of sample size on significance. Notice that t increases as n increases. Suppose that 100 points had been sampled with the same calculated r. Then the value of $t = (r^2/(1 - r^2))^{0.5} \cdot (n - 2)^{0.5} = (0.32^2/(1 - 0.32^2))^{0.5} \cdot 98^{0.5} = 3.34$. This value exceeds the critical value of $t_{(0.05,98)} = 1.99$.

In addition to deciding whether there is a statistically significant association between x and y, one should find the degree of this association. The square of r, the coefficient of determination, provides this measure of association. Roughly speaking, $100 \cdot r^2$ is the percent of the variation in y explained by the regression of y on x. For $r = 0.32$, $100 \cdot r^2$ is 10%. Thus, even though there is a significant relationship between x and y when 100 points are sampled, this relationship is very weak. Whenever an author reports a correlation coefficient, this strength of association can be mentally calculated by the reader; a remarkable number of the correlations reported to be significant have very weak associations between the two variables.

Contingency Tables

In a hypothetical experiment comparing performance on an examination, about 83% of the anesthesia faculty passed, whereas less than 38% of anesthesia residents passed (Table 3-14). Is this difference real? This question is also stated as whether there is a dependency or association between the rows and the columns of the 2-by-2 contingency table. There are a variety of statistical techniques to compare this pass/fail rate in the underlying populations of all anesthesia faculty and all anesthesia residents. This section discusses two test statistics: (1) the most commonly used, the chi-square test, and (2) the z score test based on an approximation to the normal distribution. These methods are used for both ordinal and nominal variables.

TABLE 3-13. Inferential Statistics for a Hypothetical Bivariate Data Set*

Regression

H_0: $\beta = 0$
H_a: $\beta \neq 0$
$s_{y \cdot x} = [\{[\Sigma(y_i - \bar{y})^2] - [\Sigma(x_i - \bar{x}) \cdot (y_i - \bar{y})]^2/[\Sigma(x_i - \bar{x})^2]\}/(n - 2)]^{0.5}$
$\quad = [(1 - 1/10)/3]^{0.5} = 0.55$
$SE_b = s_{y \cdot x}/(\Sigma(x_i - \bar{x})^2)^{0.5} = 0.55/(10)^{0.5} = 0.17$
$t_{(df)} = (b - 0)/SE_b = b/SE_b \qquad df = n - 2$
$t_{(3)} = 0.1/0.17 = 0.58 \qquad$ Critical value $t_{(0.05,3)} = 3.18$
Do not reject null hypothesis, since $t_{(3)} = 0.58 <$ critical value = 3.18

Correlation

H_0: $\rho = 0$
H_a: $\rho \neq 0$
$t_{(df)} = [r^2/(1 - r^2)]^{0.5} \cdot [n - 2]^{0.5} \qquad df = n - 2$
$t_{(3)} = [0.32^2/(1 - 0.32^2)]^{0.5} \cdot 3^{0.5} = 0.58 \quad$ Critical value $t_{(0.05,3)} = 3.18$
Do not reject null hypothesis, since $t_{(3)} = 0.58 <$ critical value = 3.18
Coefficient of determination = $r^2 = 0.32^2 = 0.10$

*The data set used is that given in Table 3-7.

TABLE 3-14. Contingency Table of Hypothetical Data Comparing Pass/Fail Rates on Standardized Board Examination for Anesthesia Personnel

	Pass	Fail	Total
Anesthesia residents	15 (37.5%)	25 (62.5%)	40
Anesthesia faculty	33 (82.5%)	7 (17.5%)	40
Total	48 (60.0%)	32 (40.0%)	80

Descriptive Statistics

$n_1 = 40 \qquad x_1 = 15 \qquad n_2 = 40 \qquad x_2 = 33$
$p_1 = x_1/n_1 = 15/40 = 0.375 \quad p_2 = x_2/n_2 = 33/40 = 0.825$

Inferential Statistics

H_0: $\pi_1 = \pi_2$
H_a: $\pi_1 \neq \pi_2$

$p_2 - p_1 = 0.825 - 0.375 = 0.45$
Combined proportion = $\bar{p} = (x_1 + x_2)/(n_1 + n_2)$
$\qquad = (15 + 33)/(40 + 40) = 0.6$
$SE_{(p2-p1)} = [\bar{p} \cdot (1 - \bar{p}) \cdot (1/n_1 + 1/n_2)]^{0.5}$
$\qquad = [0.6 \cdot (1 - 0.6) \cdot (1/40 + 1/40)]^{0.5} = 0.11$
Test statistic = $z = (|p_2 - p_1|)/SE_{(p2-p1)} = 0.45/0.11 = 4.11$
Corrected test statistic = $z_c = [|p_2 - p_1| - 0.5 \cdot (1/n_1 + 1/n_2)]/SE_{(p2-p1)}$
$\qquad = [0.45 - 0.5 \cdot (1/40 + 1/40)]/0.11$
$\qquad = 3.88$
Critical value = $z_{(0.05)} = 1.96$
Reject null hypothesis, since $z_c = 3.88 >$ critical value = 1.96

Just as the normal approximation of the binomial distribution was used for descriptive statistics of rates and proportions, a comparison of the relative frequencies of two groups can be created using the normal distribution if the sample sizes are sufficiently large. Under the assumption of null hypothesis, the frequencies of the two groups are identical, i.e., $\pi_1 = \pi_2$. The best estimate for the differences of the means of the two samples is the difference of the proportions, $p_1 = p_2$; $p_1 - p_2$ is a summary statistic that estimates the population parameter, $\pi_1 - \pi_2$. There is a standard error for $p_1 - p_2$, giving the precision with which $\pi_1 - \pi_2$ is known; this standard error uses a weighted average of p_1 and p_2.

$$SE(p_1 - p_2) = (p \cdot (1 - p) \cdot (1/n_1 + 1/n_2))^{0.5} \quad (3\text{-}9)$$

where

$$p = (n_1 \cdot p_1 + n_2 \cdot p_2)/(n_1 + n_2)$$

The *z score test* statistic is literally a ratio; the numerator consists of the difference between the means of the samples, whereas the denominator is the standard error of this difference.

$$z \text{ score} = \frac{|p_1 - p_2|}{SE(p_1 - p_2)} \quad (3\text{-}10)$$

If the difference in proportions increases ($|p_1 - p_2|$ larger), and/or if the precision of the difference decreases ($SE(p_1 - p_2)$ smaller), then the z score increases. The greater the z score, the greater the likelihood of a difference between the two populations from which samples were taken. If each of the quantities $n_1 \cdot p$, $n_1 \cdot (1 - p)$, $n_2 \cdot p$, $n_2 \cdot (1 - p)$ has a value greater than or equal to 5, the normal approximation may be used; these conditions are met in the hypothetical example (see Table 3-14). The critical values against which the z score test statistic is compared are found in the tables of the normal probability function; there is no degree of freedom for the z score test statistic or the normal probability curve. As with other test statistics, if the z score value exceeds the predetermined critical value, the null hypothesis is rejected. It has been discovered that the z score test statistic, being a continuous approximation of the discrete binomial distribution, slightly overestimates the probability of a difference; for this reason, a z score with a smaller numerator is used because it more closely approximates the exact probabilities:

$$\text{corrected } z \text{ score} = \frac{(|p_1 - p_2| - 0.5) \cdot (1/n_1 + 1/n_2)}{SE(p_1 - p_2)} \quad (3\text{-}11)$$

The chi-square test is a more frequently used alternative to the z score; it is also known as the Pearson chi-square statistic. When used with 2-by-2 contingency tables, it is equivalent to the z score test (Table 3-15). The chi-square test offers the advantage of being computationally simpler than the z score test and can also analyze contingency tables with more than two rows and two columns. The chi-square test statistic is a sum of ratios. For each cell of the contingency table, the observed value has been recorded. Using the assumption that there is no association between the rows and the columns, the expected value for each cell is the row total multiplied by the column total divided by the total number of subjects. For each cell, the squared difference between the observed and expected value divided by the expected value expresses the variability of the observed value away from the expected value. The test statistic is the sum of these difference ratios.

$$X^2_{(df)} = \Sigma((|\text{observed} - \text{expected}| - 0.5)^2/\text{expected}) \quad (3\text{-}12)$$

If the difference between observed and expected cell values grows larger, it is more likely that there is an association between the rows and columns. The critical values used with the chi-square test statistic are from the χ^2 or chi-square continuous theoretical probability distribution. A distinction must be made between the chi-square test statistic, which is denoted X^2, and the chi-square probability distribution, which is denoted χ^2. The χ^2 distribution has a single integer parameter or degree of freedom. The value of this degree of freedom is the product of the number of rows minus 1 times the number of columns minus 1. As with the z score, a continuity correction is used, and certain restrictions concerning cell size are recommended. For 2-by-2 tables, the smallest expected cell value should be at least 5, or the test statistic will be biased. The method shown in Table 3–15 can be used to calculate a chi-square statistic for any size contingency table. For 2-by-2 contingency tables, there is an even simpler formula for the calculation of the chi-square test statistic (Table 3-16).

There is a third alternative to the z score and chi-square

TABLE 3-15. Calculation of Chi-Square Test Statistic for Data Given in Table 3-14

	Observed Counts			Expected Counts		
	Pass	*Fail*	*Total*	*Pass*	*Fail*	*Total*
Residents	15	25	40	$48 \cdot 40/80 = 24$	$32 \cdot 40/80 = 16$	40
Faculty	33	7	40	$48 \cdot 40/80 = 24$	$32 \cdot 40/80 = 16$	40
Total	48	32	80	48	32	80

Inferential Statistics

$X^2_{(df)} = \Sigma[(|\text{observed} - \text{expected}| - 0.5)^2/\text{expected}]$
Degree of freedom = df = (rows − 1) · (columns − 1)

Degree of freedom = df = (2 − 1) · (2 − 1) = 1
$X^2_{(1)} = (|15 - 24| - 0.5)^2/24 + (|25 - 16| - 0.5)^2/16 + (|33 - 24| - 0.5)^2/24 + (|7 - 16| - 0.5)^2/16$
   $= (8.5)^2/24 + (8.5)^2/16 + (8.5)^2/24 + (8.5)^2/16 = 15.05$
Critical value = $\chi^2_{(0.05,1)} = 3.84$
Reject null hypothesis, since $X^2_{(1)} = 15.05 >$ critical value = 3.84

TABLE 3-16. Calculation of Chi-Square Test Statistic for Data Given in Table 3-14

	Observed Counts			Algebraic Notation		
	Pass	*Fail*	*Total*	*Pass*	*Fail*	*Total*
Residents	15	25	40	*a*	*b*	*a + b*
Faculty	33	7	40	*c*	*d*	*c + d*
Total	48	32	80	*a + c*	*b + d*	*n = a + b + c + d*

Inferential Statistics

$X^2_{(df)} = n \cdot (|a \cdot d - b \cdot c| - n/2)^2/((a + c) \cdot (b + d) \cdot (a + b) \cdot (c + d))$

Degree of freedom = df = (rows − 1) · (columns − 1)

Degree of freedom = df = (2 − 1) · (2 − 1) = 1

$X^2_{(1)} = 80 \cdot (|33 \cdot 25 - 7 \cdot 15| - 80/2)^2/((33 + 15) \cdot (7 + 25) \cdot (33 + 7) \cdot (15 + 25)) = 15.05$

Critical value = $\chi^2_{(0.05,1)} = 3.84$

Reject null hypothesis, since $X^2_{(1)} = 15.05 >$ critical value = 3.84

Cross product ratio = odds ratio = (a · d)/(b · c) = (33 · 25)/(7 · 15) = 7.86

test that is coming into greater use now that computations are cheap. It is known as the *Fisher exact test* and gives the exact probability of a 2-by-2 contingency table; the Fisher exact test uses the hypergeometric probability distribution, which is related to the binomial distribution. The Fisher test should be used if any expected cell value is less than five. As the total count of frequencies in a contingency table increases, the Fisher exact test and X^2 test give almost identical probabilities. In our example, the exact probability for Table 3-15 is p = 0.00008, whereas the probability for $X^2 = 15.05$ is p = 0.00010. That is truly a good approximation.

In the hypothetical example (see Table 3-14), the X^2 test statistic showed a statistically significant difference between the faculty and resident examination pass rate. A common mistake is to stop the analysis of contingency tables after testing for statistical significance. Although X^2 is excellent as a measure of the significance of association, it is not at all useful as a measure of the degree of association. The basic measure of association is the odds ratio or cross-product ratio (Table 3-16). If the odds ratio is one, there is no association between rows and columns; if the odds ratio is not one, there is an association or dependency between rows and columns. In the sample problem, the odds ratio shows that faculty members are over seven times more likely to pass the examination than residents. X^2 is a function of both the cell proportions and the total number of subjects, whereas the odds ratio is only a function of the cell proportions. If a large number of subjects are used, the X^2 test may reveal statistical significance, even when there is little dependency between rows and columns. The odds ratio is easily calculated and can be used to check the importance of a contingency table result.

Interpretation of Results

Scientific studies do not end with the statistical test. The experimenter must commit an opinion as to the generalizability of his or her work to the rest of the world. Even if there is a statistically significant difference, the experimenter must decide if this difference is medically or physiologically important. Statistical significance does not always equate with biologic relevance. The questions an experimenter should ask about the interpretation of results are highly dependent on the specifics of the experiment. Three examples are given. First, even small, clinically unimpor-

tant differences between groups can be detected if the sample size is sufficiently large. On the other hand, if the sample size is small, one must always worry that identified or unidentified confounding variables may explain any difference; as the sample size decreases, randomization is less successful in assuring homogenous groups. Second, if the experimental groups are given three or more doses of a drug, do the results suggest a steadily increasing or decreasing dose-response relationship? Suppose the observed effect for an intermediate dose is either much higher or much lower than that for both the highest and lowest dose; a dose-response relationship may exist, but some skepticism about the experimental methods is warranted. Third, for clinical studies comparing patient outcome from receiving different drugs, devices, and operations, are the patients, clinical care, and studied therapies sufficiently similar to those provided at other locations to be of interest to a wide group of practitioners? This last point is so important that it is now receiving editorial attention in anesthesia journals.[17] In comparing alternative therapies, the experimenter will have more or less confidence that a claim for a superior therapy is true, depending on the study design. The strength of the evidence concerning efficacy will be least for an anecdotal case report; next in importance will be a retrospective study, then a prospective series of patients compared with historical controls, and finally a randomized, controlled clinical trial. The greatest strength for a therapeutic claim is a series of randomized, controlled clinical trials confirming the same hypothesis.

RESOURCES FOR STATISTICAL METHODS: TEXTS, JOURNALS, SOFTWARE, AND STATISTICIANS

Many materials are available to guide both the researcher and the journal reader into the depths of simple and sophisticated statistics. There are journal articles that present specific recommendations concerning common statistical problems and research design goals.[18,19] Several journals are totally devoted to research methods and statistical analysis in biologic fields: *Statistics in Medicine* and *Controlled Clinical Trials* are clinically oriented, whereas *Biometrics* and *Biometrika* are journals for the professional statistician. Particularly interesting is a regular section in *Controlled*

Clinical Trials featuring an annotated bibliography of publications regarding statistics. Other authors have published reading lists with comments for self-education.[20] Besides the textbooks of statistical theory, there are many excellent textbooks of applied biomedical statistics at both introductory and intermediate levels (see Bibliography). A variety of monographs and texts address specific subjects including (1) regression analysis, (2) graphic display, (3) contingency table analysis, (4) experimental measurement, (5) multivariate analysis of variance, (6) research design and analysis, (7) the epidemiology of anesthetic practice, (8) the ethics of human experimentation, (9) confidence intervals, and (10) the application of statistics to clinical practice.

Unless the data sets become large, all the statistical tests described in this chapter can be done by manual calculation; hand-held scientific calculators can assist in this analysis and reduce computational errors. With the spread of computers into every laboratory and office, statistical software has made the process even more convenient. Also, more advanced statistical techniques are not computationally feasible without computer assistance. Whether data storage is on the investigator's desktop computer or in a large shared computer, the data can be moved electronically anywhere for statistical analysis. Traditionally, the analysis has been done by large, all-inclusive statistical software packages available only on mainframe and departmental computers; the most well known of these packages are SAS, BMDP, SPSS, MINITAB, and STAT80. The users' manuals for this software are not statistical textbooks, but the manuals do contain sample problems to help explain the software command language. These examples, which often involve rather advanced problems, can be followed in a "cookbook" fashion to analyze related problems. Besides the basic descriptive statistics available in most spread sheet packages, an increasing variety of statistical software is now available for the personal computer. Choosing from all this statistical wealth should be guided by (1) the types of analysis required, (2) the availability of computer hardware, (3) the number of subjects and number of variables, (4) the need for data management by the statistical software, (5) the experience of the user, (6) the production of finished reports consisting of merging of text, statistics, and graphics, and (7) the budget. Although programming errors in the software can generate erroneous computer output, these packages are increasingly free of "bugs."

Biostatisticians can make available the richness of better research design and advanced statistical techniques to every researcher. For large clinical trials, the participation of a biostatistician has become mandatory from the inception of research planning. Biostatisticians also provide trained data clerks, data storage facilities, and access to large statistical software packages. Unfortunately, most researchers do not have the budget to pay for this help on all projects, but they should attempt to get consultations on research design, analysis, and interpretation as new research areas are entered.

RESEARCH REPORTS: WRITING AND EDITING

When published scientific reports are evaluated for the correctness of their statistical techniques, the majority of papers are found to have errors in the application of the statistics. This is true for both general and specialty medical journals, including anesthesia journals.[21] These errors include all aspects of study design, analysis, and interpretation, the omission of pertinent study design details, and the presentation of results.[22] Although it is not possible to assess the seriousness of these statistical errors in misrepresenting and misinterpreting the experimental results, they should be viewed as severe offenses against the scientific method and not as trivial violations of unimportant and arbitrary rules. The ethical consequences of this misuse of statistics can be serious: (1) research subjects have been put at risk or have been inconvenienced for no benefit; (2) for future patients, inferior treatment may be chosen or superior treatment may be delayed; (3) resources have been squandered; and (4) each generation of researchers will copy the substandard statistical methods reported by their predecessors. The abolition of these usually unintentional statistical sins will require a long-term commitment of interest and effort.

For several decades, there has been a commonly accepted structure to the research report; this is the IMRAD format, i.e., Introduction, Methods, Results (and) Discussion. To further the standardization of the editorial process, editors of major biomedical journals have promulgated "uniform requirements" for manuscripts.[23] These uniform requirements ask that the experimental design and statistical methods be described with sufficient detail to enable another researcher who is given access to the raw data to verify the reported results. The editorial instructions for anesthesia journals generally give few specifics about the use of statistics. Although not all anesthesia journals have accepted the use of the uniform requirements, these requirements could be used profitably by an author preparing a manuscript for any journal.

The need for more explicit and detailed statistical guidelines for authors has been debated among professional statisticians. The 1988 revision of the uniform requirements prompted two North American statisticians to write guidelines amplifying the requirements on statistical reporting.[24] Another outstanding set of such guidelines has been published by four English medical statisticians.[25] An international *ad hoc* group has also formulated guidelines for a more structured and informative abstract for clinical research reports;[26] this proposed abstract format includes considerable detail on research design and statistical methods and has already been adopted by several journals.

RESEARCH REPORTS: READING

Medical journals are mainly written by medical school physicians. In addition to their obvious interest in improving medical care, authors may also be motivated by concerns about obtaining faculty tenure, establishing a reputation, and getting research grants. Regardless of these disparate motives, how should the clinician determine which articles are useful? As suggested previously, the anesthesiologist must have some basic skills and understanding of research design and statistics to be able to critique the research report; these skills can be acquired or refreshed through the study of texts and other publications. Yet, additional skills are required. There are tens of hundreds of thousands of words written each year in journal articles relevant to anesthesia. No one can read them all, even if reading to the exclusion of other activities; a physician will probably never have more time for journal reading than he or she already spends to peruse the literature. All that is possible is to learn to rapidly skip over most articles and concentrate on the few selected for their importance to the reader. Those few should be chosen by their relevance and credibility. Relevance is determined by the specifics of one's anesthetic practice. Credibility is a function of the merits of the research methods, the experimental design, and the statistical analysis; the more proficient one's statistical skills are, the more rapidly it is possible to accept or reject the credibility of a research article.

Six easily remembered appraisal criteria for clinical studies can be fashioned from the words WHY, HOW, WHO, WHAT, HOW MANY, and SO WHAT: (1) WHY: Is the biologic hypothesis clearly stated? (2) HOW: What is the research design? (3) WHO: Is the target population clearly defined? (4) WHAT: How was the therapy administered and the data collected? (5) HOW MANY: Are the test statistics convincing? and (6) SO WHAT: Is it clinically relevant to my patients? Although the statistical knowledge of most physicians is limited,[27] these skills of critical appraisal of the literature can be learned[28] and can tremendously increase the efficiency and benefit of journal reading.

FUTURE DEVELOPMENTS OF STATISTICS AND ANESTHESIOLOGY

What of the future? Research presentations, both oral and written, will continue to follow the trend of ever-increasing statistical rigor that has been evident for several decades. This statistical rigor will be obvious, both by the quantity of descriptive and test statistics that will be reported and by the complexity of the methods that will be used. More advanced statistical tests will provide greater power in understanding complex phenomena. This also suggests the prospect of even less comprehension of the scientific article by the typical journal reader. To counterbalance this complexity, better graphic data displays will become more common to provide an intuitive grasp of results. Newly published statistical concepts are already being incorporated into the journal articles of our specialty. Two examples illustrate these innovations.

New methods of physiologic monitoring, e.g., invasive blood pressure measurements, are being engineered and used in the operating room. To gain acceptance, these new measurements must have some reasonable agreement with measurements obtained simultaneously by a standard procedure. How should this assessment be performed? Traditionally, linear regression and correlation have been the statistical tools. In 1986 Bland and Altman pointed to serious errors in this method of analysis and suggested an alternative approach that emphasized analysis of bias and variability.[29] This is now known as measurement "comparison" methods as opposed to the older measurement "calibration" methods. Other statisticians have amplified their suggestions.[30] "Comparison" method analysis has been recommended by anesthesia journals.[31]

In anesthesiology journals, studies of new drugs and new therapies are numerous but generally include few patients. The ability to generate inferences about the benefits or hazards of new therapies is limited by the low power of each individual study. Traditionally, narrative summaries (review and medical intelligence articles) have synthesized inferences by combining the results of several studies. During the 1980s, methods for the statistical pooling of results from published studies have been created.[32] This is called *meta-analysis*; it offers a structured, quantitative way of accumulating evidence.[33] The journals of anesthesiology offer rich prospects for the use of meta-analysis.[34]

Statistics and probability will be increasingly used in the actual practice of anesthesia. As in all other areas of medicine, there is an "information explosion" in anesthesiology.

A new field, "medical informatics," has been created by those interested in the computer use and management of medical information; medical informatics includes research, education, and patient care. One of the creations of medical informatics has been medical expert systems; expert systems are computational tools designed to capture and make available the knowledge of experts. Some of the most noted expert systems have been designed for medical diagnosis, but there is also an expert system to provide advice for anesthetic management planning.[35] Statistical methods, including linear discriminant analysis, bayesian probability theory, and logistic regression, are used extensively, although not exclusively, in the design of some of these medical expert systems. Also applied are mathematic techniques called neural networks; these statistical type methods are being used to develop "smart" physiologic monitors and anesthesia machines.

A parallel development has been the use of formal decision analysis for medical applications. Using the tools of decision trees, Bayesian probability theory, sensitivity analysis, and utility assessment, decision analysis is a logically consistent way of reasoning and choosing therapy in the face of uncertainty. Although little has been developed for anesthesiology, there is some acceptance of decision analysis for other fields of medical practice.[36]

Statistical theory will continue to develop with great practical applications for medicine. Two examples are given here. Using inexpensive computers, computationally intensive methods will replace the use of theoretical probability distributions with massive numbers of calculations; a billion arithmetic operations might be used to analyze 500 data points. Smart statistical software will be developed that will provide (1) a computerized statistical reference source, (2) expert guidance for the use of statistical tests, and (3) an expert system to consult on the design and analysis of experiments.

One intent of this chapter is to present the scope of support that the discipline of statistics can provide to anesthesia research. Although an intuitive understanding of certain basic principles is emphasized, these basic principles are not necessarily simple and have been developed by statisticians with great mathematic rigor. Academic anesthesia needs more workers to immerse themselves in these statistical fundamentals; having done so, these statistically knowledgeable academic anesthesiologists will be prepared to improve their own research projects, to assist their colleagues in research, to efficiently seek consultation from the professional statistician, to strengthen the editorial review of journal articles, and to expound to the clinical reader the whys and wherefores of statistics. The clinical reader also needs to expend his or her own effort to acquire some basic statistical skills.

One of the originators of the use of statistics in medicine was Francis Galton; living from 1822 to 1911, he studied the inheritance of physical and mental characteristics. Galton believed that "The object of statistical science is to discover methods of condensing information concerning large groups of allied facts into brief and compendious expressions suitable for discussion."[37] Anesthesiologists would be well advised to accept Galton's insight.

REFERENCES

1. Editorial: Clinical investigation. Anesthesiology 12:114, 1951
2. Longnecker DE: Support versus illumination: Trends in medical statistics. Anesthesiology 57:73, 1982

3. Pace NL: Ever more statistics. Anesth Analg 64:561, 1985
4. Davis PJ, Hersh R: Descartes' Dream. The World According to Mathematics, p 18. San Diego, Harcourt Brace Jovanovich, 1986
5. Avram MJ, Shanks CA, Dykes MHM et al: Statistical methods in anesthesia articles: An evaluation of two American journals during two six-month periods. Anesth Analg 64:607, 1985
6. Berwick DM, Fineberg HV, Weinstein MC: When doctors meet numbers. Am J Med 71:991, 1981
7. Armitage P: Controversies and achievements in clinical trials. Controlled Clin Trials 5:67, 1984
8. Louis TA, Mosteller F, McPeek B: Timely topics in statistical methods for clinical trials. Annu Rev Biophys Bioeng 11:81, 1982
9. Taylor KM, Margolese RG, Soskolne CL: Physicians' reasons for not entering eligible patients in a randomized clinical trial of surgery for breast cancer. N Engl J Med 310:1363, 1984
10. Bailar JC III, Louis TA, Lavori PW, Polansky M: A classification for biomedical research reports. N Engl J Med 311:1482, 1984
11. Califf RM, Pryor DB, Greenfield JC Jr. Beyond randomized clinical trials: Applying clinical experience in the treatment of patients with coronary artery disease. Circulation 74:1191, 1986
12. Byar DP: Why data bases should not replace randomized clinical trials. Biometrics 36:337, 1980
13. Green SB, Byar DP: Using observational data from registries to compare treatments: The fallacy of omnimetrics. Stat Med 3:361, 1984
14. Freiman JA, Chalmers TC, Smith H Jr, Kuebler RR: The importance of beta, the type II error and sample size in the design and interpretation of the randomized control trial: Survey of 71 "negative" trials. N Engl J Med 299:690, 1978
15. Donner A: Approaches to sample size estimation in the design of clinical trials: A review. Stat Med 3:199, 1984
16. Beecher HK: Ethics and clinical research. N Engl J Med 274:1354, 1966
17. McPeek B: Inference, generalizability, and a major change in anesthetic practice. Anesthesiology 66:723, 1987
18. Glantz SA: Biostatistics: How to detect, correct and prevent errors in the medical literature. Circulation 61:1, 1980
19. Wallenstein S, Zucker CL, Fleiss JL: Some statistical methods useful in circulation research. Circ Res 47:1, 1980
20. Sacks ST, Glantz SA: Introduction to biostatistics: An annotated bibliography for medical researchers. West J Med 139:723, 1983
21. DerSimonian R, Charette LJ, McPeek B, Mosteller F: Reporting on methods in clinical trials. N Engl J Med 306:1332, 1982
22. Vaisrub N: Manuscript review from a statistician's perspective. JAMA 253:3145, 1985
23. International Committee of Medical Journal Editors: Uniform requirements for manuscripts submitted to biomedical journals. N Engl J Med 324:424, 1991
24. Bailar JC III, Mostellar F: Guidelines for statistical reporting in articles for medical journals: Amplifications and explanations. Ann Intern Med 108:266, 1988
25. Altman DG, Gore SM, Gardner MJ, Pocock SJ: Statistical guidelines for contributors to medical journals. Br Med J 286:1489, 1983
26. Ad Hoc Working Group for Critical Appraisal of the Medical Literature: A proposal for more informative abstracts of clinical articles. Ann Int Med 106:598, 1987
27. Wulff HR, Andersen B, Brandenhoff P, Guttler F: What do doctors know about statistics? Stat Med 6:3, 1987
28. Bennett KJ, Sackett DL, Haynes RB et al: A controlled trial of teaching critical appraisal of the clinical literature to medical students. JAMA 257:2451, 1987
29. Bland JM, Altman DG: Statistical methods for assessing agreement between two methods of clinical measurement. Lancet 1:307, 1986
30. Chinn S: The assessment of methods of measurement. Stat Med 9:351, 1990
31. LaMantia KR, O'Connor T, Barash PG: Comparing methods of measurement: An alternative approach. Anesthesiology 72:781, 1990
32. Sacks HS, Berrier J, Reitman D et al: Meta-analyses of randomized control trials. N Engl J Med 316:450, 1987
33. Boissel J-P, Blanchard J, Panak E et al: Considerations for the meta-analysis of randomized clinical trials: Summary of a panel discussion. Controlled Clin Trials 10:254, 1989
34. Pace NL: Prevention of succinylcholine myalgias: A meta-analysis. Anesth Analg 70:477, 1990
35. Miller PL: Critiquing anesthetic management: The "ATTENDING" computer system. Anesthesiology 53:362, 1983
36. Kassirer JP, Moskowitz AJ, Lau J, Pauker SG: Decision analysis: A progress report. Ann Intern Med 106:275, 1987
37. Galton F: Quotation. In Strauss MB (ed): Familiar Medical Quotations, p 569. Boston, Little, Brown, and Company, 1968

BIBLIOGRAPHY

General Biostatistical Textbooks

Introductory

Colton T: Statistics in Medicine. Boston, Little, Brown and Company, 1974
Dawson-Saunders B, Trapp RG: Basic and Clinical Biostatistics. San Mateo, Appleton & Lange, 1990
Glantz SA: Primer of Biostatistics. New York, McGraw-Hill, 1981
Matthews DE, Farewell VT: Using and Understanding Medical Statistics, 2nd revised ed. Basel, Karger, 1988
Mattson DE: Statistics. Difficult Concepts, Understandable Explanations. St Louis, CV Mosby, 1981
Phillips JL Jr: Statistical Thinking, 2nd ed. San Francisco, WH Freeman, 1982

Intermediate

Cox DR, Snell EJ: Applied Statistics: Principles and Examples. New York, Chapman and Hall, 1981
Hacking I: The Emergence of Probability: A Philosophical Study of Early Ideas about Probability, Induction and Statistical Inference. Cambridge, Cambridge University Press, 1975
McCullagh P, Nelder JA: Generalized Linear Models. New York, Chapman and Hall, 1983
Mood AM, Graybill FA, Boes DC: Introduction to the Theory of Statistics, 3rd ed. New York, McGraw-Hill Book Company, 1974
Searle SR: Linear Models. New York, John Wiley & Sons, 1971
Snedecor GW, Cochran WG: Statistical Methods, 7th ed. Ames, Iowa, State University Press, 1980
Winer BJ: Statistical Principles in Experimental Design, 2nd ed. New York, McGraw-Hill, 1971

Monographs and Specialized Textbooks

Animal Care

Public Health Service, National Institutes of Health: Guide for the Care and Use of Laboratory Animals (NIH Publication No. 85-23). Washington DC, Government Printing Office, 1985

Confidence Intervals

Gardner MJ, Altman DG: Statistics with Confidence: Confidence Intervals and Statistical Guidelines. London, British Medical Journal, 1989

Contingency Table Analysis

Fienberg SE: The Analysis of Cross-Classified Categorical Data. Cambridge, MIT Press, 1977
Fleiss JL: Statistical Methods for Rates and Proportions, 2nd ed. New York, John Wiley & Sons, 1981
Freeman DH: Applied categorical data analysis. New York, Marcel Dekker Inc, 1987

Epidemiology

Lunn JN: Epidemiology in Anaesthesia: The Techniques of Epidemiology Applied to Anaesthetic Practice. Baltimore, Edward Arnold, 1986

Ethics of Human Experimentation

Beecher HK: Research and the Individual: Human Studies. Boston, Little, Brown and Company, 1970
Greenwald RA, Ryan MK, Mulvihill JE (eds): Human Subjects Research: A Handbook for Institutional Review Boards. New York, Plenum Press, 1982
Levine RJ: Ethics and Regulation of Clinical Research. Baltimore, Urban & Schwarzenberg, 1986

Experimental Measurement

Barford NC: Experimental Measurements: Precision, Error and Truth, 2nd ed. New York, John Wiley & Sons, 1985

Graphic Display

Cleveland WS: The Elements of Graphing Data. Monterey, Wadsworth Advanced Books and Software, 1985
Schmid CF: Statistical Graphics: Design Principles and Practices. New York, John Wiley & Sons, 1983
Tufte ER: The Visual Display of Quantitative Information. Cheshire, Graphics Press, 1983

Meta-analysis

Hedges LV, Olkin I: Statistical Methods for Meta-analysis. New York, Academic Press, 1985
Light RJ, Pillemer DB: Summing Up: The Science of Reviewing Research. Cambridge, Harvard University Press, 1984

Multivariate Analysis of Variance

Afifi AA, Clark V: Computer-Aided Multivariate Analysis. New York, Van Nostrand Reinhold Company, 1984

Morrison DF: Multivariate Statistical Methods, 2nd ed. New York, McGraw-Hill, 1976
Tabachnick BG, Fidell LS: Using Multivariate Statistics. New York, Harper & Row, 1982

Nonparametric Analysis

Krauth J: Distribution-Free Statistics: An Application-Oriented Approach. Amsterdam, Elsevier, 1988

Regression Analysis

Draper N, Smith H: Applied Regression Analysis, 2nd ed. New York, John Wiley & Sons, 1981
Edwards AL: An introduction to linear regression and correlation. San Francisco, WH Freeman, 1976

Research Design

Feinstein AR: Clinical Biostatistics. St Louis, CV Mosby, 1977
Gore SM, Altman DG: Statistics in Practice. Devonshire, Torquay, 1982
Iber FL, Riley WA, Murray PJ: Conducting Clinical Trials. New York, Plenum Medical Book Company, 1987
Marks RG: Analyzing Research Data: The Basics of Biomedical Research Methodology. Belmont, California, Lifetime Learning Publications, 1982
Marks RG: Designing a Research Project: The Basics of Biomedical Research Methodology. Belmont, California, Lifetime Learning Publications, 1982
Silverman WA: Human Experimentation: A Guided Step into the Unknown. New York, Oxford University Press, 1985

Statistics and Clinical Practice

Kronick DA: The Literature of the Life Sciences: Reading, Writing, Research. Philadelphia, ISI Press, 1985
Ingelfinger JA, Mosteller F, Thibodeau LA, Ware JH: Biostatistics in Clinical Medicine. New York, Macmillan, 1983
Sackett DL, Haynes RB, Tugwell P: Clinical Epidemiology. Boston, Little, Brown and Company, 1985

4

Arnold J. Berry
Jonathan D. Katz

Hazards of Working in the Operating Room

Anesthesia personnel spend long hours, in fact, a majority of their waking day, in an environment that is filled with many potential hazards—the operating room. This setting is unlike the usual work place in that in addition to potential exposure to vapors from chemicals, to ionizing radiation, and to infectious agents, there is the psychological stress resulting from the constant vigilance required for quality care of patients and from the interactions with other members of the surgical and operating room teams. Although some physical hazards, such as fires and explosions from flammable anesthetic agents, are no longer a concern, occupational illnesses, such as alcohol and drug abuse, are now well recognized as significant within the anesthesia community. Some hazards, such as exposure to trace levels of waste anesthetic gases, have been extensively studied, whereas others, like suicide, have been recognized but not adequately pursued. Only within the past 20 years have epidemiologic surveys been conducted to assess the health of anesthesia personnel. In general, the potential health risks to those working in the operating room may be significant, but with awareness of the problems and the use of proper precautions, they are not formidable.

PHYSICAL HAZARDS

Anesthetic Gases

Although the inhalation anesthetics, diethyl ether, nitrous oxide, and chloroform, were first used in the 1840s, the biologic effects of occupational exposure to these agents were not investigated for many years. There were early reports in the German literature of headaches and fatigue in personnel who had been exposed to chloroform and ether in the operating rooms. In 1949, Werthmann reported three persons who had fatigue, headaches, memory loss, and electrocardiographic abnormalities with chronic exposure to ether.[1] Not until the 1960s were studies of the effects of chronic environmental exposure to anesthetics undertaken. At the time of these studies, it was estimated that over 60,000 anesthesiologists, nurse anesthetists, and operating room nurses and technicians, 100,000 dentists and dental assistants, and 50,000 veterinarians and their employees worked in environments with potential exposure to anesthetic gases.[2,3]

Reports on the effects of chronic environmental exposure to anesthetics have included epidemiologic surveys, in vitro studies, cellular research, and studies in laboratory animals and humans. These reports have addressed the areas of fertility and spontaneous abortion; incidence of congenital malformations; mortality rate, incidence of cancer, hematopoietic diseases, liver disease, and neurologic disease; and psychomotor and behavioral changes produced by anesthetic exposure. There have been many reviews of these earlier studies.[4-8] In the following section, relevant reports are reviewed to provide an understanding of the current evidence in each of these areas. Also, suggested standards for waste anesthetic gas levels in the operating room are reviewed. Scavenging systems for the reduction of anesthetic concentrations in the operating room are discussed in Chapter 25.

Anesthetic Levels in the Operating Room

Early investigators established that significant levels of ether were present in the operating room when the open drop technique was used, but the first report of occupational exposure to modern anesthetics was by Linde and Bruce in 1969.[9] They sampled air at various distances from the pop-off valve of anesthesia machines and noted an average concentration of halothane of 10 parts per million (ppm) and of nitrous oxide of 130 ppm (parts per million is a volume-per-volume unit of measurement; 10,000 ppm equals 1%). These investigators found from 0 to 12 ppm of halothane in end-expired air samples taken from 24 anesthesiologists after work. Others reported similar levels of halothane around semiclosed and non–rebreathing circuits and showed that the environmental levels could be reduced significantly with the use of scavenging equipment.[10] Higher concentrations of nitrous oxide (1100 to 9700 ppm) were found in the work spaces of anesthesiologists when 5 l min^{-1} flows were used to deliver a 60% concentration to the patient.[11]

In spite of the characteristic odors of volatile anesthetics, smell is not a reliable method for detecting trace levels of halothane in operating room air. Only 50% of volunteers could detect 33 ppm of halothane by smell, and 75% could not detect 15 ppm.[12]

In a criteria document initially published in 1977,

the National Institute for Occupational Safety and Health (NIOSH) proposed standards of less than 25 ppm nitrous oxide (time-weighted average during use) and 0.5 ppm for halogenated anesthetics, or 2.0 ppm (1-hour ceiling) for halogenated agents when used alone.[13] Methods for reducing and monitoring waste gases in the operating room have been suggested.[5,14-17] Through the use of scavenging equipment, equipment maintenance procedures, altered anesthetic work practices, and efficient operating room ventilation systems, the environmental anesthetic concentration can be reduced more than tenfold. Monitors to detect leaks in the high- and low-pressure systems of anesthetic machines, contamination due to faulty anesthetic technique, and scavenging system malfunction should be incorporated in programs to ensure reduced occupational exposure. Environmental levels of anesthetics can be measured using instantaneously collected samples, continuous air monitoring, or time-weighted averages. Methods and equipment for these monitoring techniques have been well described.[5,15,16]

With appropriate care, environmental levels of anesthetics in the operating room can be reduced to comply with those suggested by NIOSH. In a survey conducted in Ontario hospitals, the level of exposure to halogenated anesthetics was within the published standard, but nitrous oxide concentrations exceeded 25 ppm in many operating rooms.[18] When improved scavenging devices and routine equipment maintenance were instituted, nitrous oxide levels were reduced. A similar situation was documented through a survey of operating rooms in four Glasgow hospitals.[19] This emphasizes that despite the use of scavenging devices, there is a need for continued monitoring of anesthetic levels in the operating room and routine attention to equipment maintenance.

The waste anesthetic concentrations in operating rooms where routine scavenging is performed are less than those noted prior to the 1960s and are often less than those found in the only studies conducted to assess the effects of occupational exposure. This raises the questions of whether chronic exposure to these low levels of waste anesthetic gases actually constitutes a significant occupational hazard and whether results from studies performed in "unscavenged" operating rooms are applicable to current practice.

Epidemiologic Studies

Epidemiologic surveys were among the first studies to suggest the possibility of a hazard resulting from trace levels of anesthetics. Although epidemiologic studies may be useful in assessing problems of this type, they have the potential for errors associated with the collection of data and their interpretation. In his review on the potential of trace anesthetic gases to produce disease, Ferstandig outlined the design strategies necessary for valid epidemiologic studies.[4] First, there should be an appropriate control group for the cohort being studied. Second, the use of questionnaires to obtain personal medical information may be misleading, since individuals may knowingly or unknowingly give incorrect information. The use of medical records provides more reliable data. Third, retrospective epidemiologic studies rely on recorded or remembered data. In prospective studies, the anticipated, significant information can be collected temporally. Fourth, cause-and-effect relationships cannot be documented by epidemiologic data unless all other possible etiologies can be ruled out or other lines of evidence are used for substantiation. Fifth, most epidemiologic studies use a p of 0.05 for determination of statistical significance. Walts et al, in reviewing one epidemiologic

study, argued that this level of statistical significance is too high.[20] Since a false-positive conclusion may have profound implications, even a p level of 0.01 may be too large for epidemiologic data. Sixth, percentage increases in the incidence of disease are sometimes reported. Large changes in percentage may imply clinical significance, even when the findings are not statistically significant. Few epidemiologic studies on the effects of occupational exposure to waste anesthetic gases fulfill these criteria.

Reproductive Outcome. Vaisman, in 1967, surveyed 303 Russian anesthesiologists (193 men and 110 women) by questionnaire.[21] The majority used diethyl ether and nitrous oxide in their practice without scavenging waste anesthetic gases. These anesthesiologists reported a high incidence of headache, irritability, and increased fatigability. There were 18 spontaneous abortions among the 31 pregnant women in the survey. Although this was an extremely small study and there was no control population, Vaisman concluded that these occurrences were caused by factors in the working environment, including chronic exposure to anesthetics, a high level of emotional stress, irregular work hours, and an excessive workload.

After the early study by Vaisman, others began to perform epidemiologic surveys to assess the effects of trace anesthetics on reproductive outcome. One of the largest studies was conducted by an *Ad Hoc* Committee of the American Society of Anesthesiologists (ASA).[2] Questionnaires were sent to 49,585 operating room personnel who had potential exposure to waste anesthetic gases (members of the ASA, the American Association of Nurse Anesthetists, the Association of Operating Room Nurses, and the Association of Operating Room Technicians). A nonexposed group of 23,911 from the American Academy of Pediatrics and the American Nurses' Association served as controls. The Committee concluded that there was an increased risk of spontaneous abortion and congenital abnormalities in children of women who worked in the operating room and an increased risk of congenital abnormalities in offspring of unexposed wives of male operating room personnel. Several reviews have identified inconsistencies in the data comparing exposed and unexposed groups and within groups. Expected levels of anesthetic exposure did not correlate with reproductive outcome.[4,5,20,22]

A Swedish study clearly demonstrates the inaccuracies encountered in such studies when using mailed questionnaires.[23] Women working at one hospital were surveyed to determine the relationship between anesthetic exposure and spontaneous abortion rate and the confounding effects of age, smoking habits, and work site during the first trimester of pregnancy. All spontaneous abortions in the exposed group were accurately documented in the responses to the questionnaire, but a review of hospital records revealed that one third of spontaneous abortions went unreported in the unexposed group. When verified data were analyzed, there was no statistically significant difference between reproductive outcome in the exposed and nonexposed groups.

The ASA commissioned a group of epidemiologists and biostatisticians to evaluate the many epidemiologic surveys that had been published in the literature to provide an assessment of the conflicting data.[6] The group used the relative risk (the ratio of the rate of disease among those exposed to that found in those not exposed) as a measure of the strength of the association between exposure to the operating room environment and several disease processes. In considering studies on spontaneous abortion and congenital abnormalities in offspring of anesthesia personnel, the data

TABLE 4-1. Epidemiologic Studies of Spontaneous Abortion Among Females

| Reference | Exposed Population* | Control | Rate of Spontaneous Abortion (per 100 Cases) | | Relative Risk† |
			Exposed	Control	
Cohen et al[24]	Operating room nurses (n = 67)	General duty nurses (n = 92)	30	9	3.4‡
	Anesthetists (n = 50)	Nonanesthetist MDs (n = 81)	38	10	3.7‡
Knill-Jones et al[25]	Anesthetists (n = 563)	Nonanesthetist MDs (n = 828)	18	15	1.2‡
Rosenberg & Kirves[26]	Operating room nurses (n = 124) Nurse anesthetists (n = 58)	Nurses (n = 75) ICU nurses (n = 48)	20	11	1.7‡
ASA Ad Hoc Committee[2]	MD anesthetists (n = 1059)	Pediatricians (n = 639)	17	9	1.9‡
	Nurse anesthetists (n = 7136)	General nurses (n = 6560)	17	15	1.1
	Operating room nurses/technicians (n = 12,272)	General nurses (n = 6560)	20	15	1.3‡
Axelsson & Rylander[23]	Operating room personnel (n = 288)	Hospital personnel (n = 322)	15	11	1.2

*n = the number of responders in the survey.
†Incidence in exposed group versus incidence in control group.
‡Statistically significant with p < 0.05.

from all but five studies were excluded from analysis because of errors in study design or statistical analysis.[2,23-26] The relative risk of spontaneous abortion for female physicians working in the operating room was 1.4 and 1.3 for female nurses (a relative risk of 1.3 represents a 30% increase in risk when compared with the risk of the control population). The increased relative risk for congenital abnormalities was of borderline statistical significance for exposed physicians only. In considering these findings, Mazze and Lecky[27] noted that the epidemiologic studies assessing the association of cigarette smoking and lung cancer have established a value for relative risk of 8–12 for men in the United States. The high relative risks found in smoking studies contrast with the values of less than 2 in most of the well-designed reproductive studies among those working in the operating room environment (Table 4-1). Relative risks of less than 2–3 may occur solely from incorrect classification of subjects. Although Buring et al[6] found a statistically significant relative risk of spontaneous abortion and congenital abnormalities in women working in the operating room, the relative risk was small compared with other more well-documented environmental hazards. They also point out that duration and level of anesthetic exposure were not measured in any of the studies and that other factors, such as stress, infections, and radiation exposure, were not considered.

Retrospective surveys of large numbers of women who worked during pregnancy indicate that negative reproductive outcomes may be related to job-associated conditions other than exposure to trace anesthetic gases. In a Canadian study, the ratio of observed to expected late spontaneous abortions (16 to 28 weeks) was increased in operating room nurses as well as radiology technicians and employees in agriculture and horticulture.[28] Analysis of the data from health workers demonstrated an increased risk of abortion associated with specific work requirements and conditions:

lifting heavy weights more than 15 times a day, other physical effort, working 46 or more hours a week, and changing shift work.

The majority of the existing epidemiologic data purporting to show a cause-and-effect relationship between trace anesthetic gas exposure in the operating room and reproductive complications is fraught with problems. There appears to be a slight increase in the relative risk of spontaneous abortion and congenital abnormalities in offspring of female physicians working in the operating room. Whether this is attributable to anesthetic exposure cannot be determined from this type of investigation. Well-designed surveys of large numbers of personnel and appropriate control groups are necessary for definitive answers. The routine use of scavenging techniques has lowered environmental anesthetic levels in the operating room and may make it more difficult to prove any adverse effects using epidemiologic data.

Mortality and Nonreproductive Diseases. One of the first surveys enumerating causes of death among anesthesiologists was reported by Bruce et al in 1968.[29] The authors compared the death rates of members of the ASA from 1947 to 1966 with those for American males and male policy holders of a large insurance company. There was a higher death rate among male anesthesiologists from malignancies of the lymphoid and reticuloendothelial tissues and from suicide, but a lower death rate from lung cancer and coronary artery disease.

In a subsequent prospective study, Bruce et al compared the causes of death in ASA members during the years 1967–1971 with those of males insured by one company.[30] The overall death rate for ASA members was lower than for the controls, and contrary to the previous results, there was no increase in death rates from malignancies of lymphoid and reticuloendothelial tissues. The authors concluded that their data provided no evidence to support the speculation that lymphoid malignancies were an occupational hazard for anesthesiologists.

Because of the interest in the effect of trace anesthetics on the health of operating room personnel, NIOSH and an *Ad Hoc* Committee of the ASA agreed to a national study to address the problem[2] (data on reproductive outcomes from this study were reviewed above). In 1972, the two groups planned a two-phase study, with the initial survey being conducted primarily in 1973 and a second phase planned for 1978. Data from the first questionnaire did not permit the investigators to prove a direct cause-effect relationship between trace concentrations of anesthetic gases and any demonstrated health hazards. By the time of the second survey, it was hoped that the introduction of scavenging and other techniques would reduce the levels of waste anesthetic gases in the operating room. If a lower incidence of health problems was demonstrated in the second phase, it could more safely be assumed that waste anesthetic gases were the causative agents. Because NIOSH believed that it had sufficient information to incriminate waste anesthetic gases as a health hazard after the initial study, it withdrew its support of the planned second phase of the study, and the follow-up survey was never conducted.[31]

The national study conducted by the ASA found no differences in cancer rates between males exposed and those not exposed to trace concentrations of anesthetic gases.[2] For women who responded to the survey, there was an approximately 1.3-fold to twofold increase in the occurrence of cancer in the exposed group, resulting predominantly from an increase in leukemia and lymphoma. The analysis of Buring *et al* of these data confirmed an increase in relative risk of cancer in exposed women (1.4) but attributed the increase solely to cervical cancer (2.8).[6] They also noted that the ASA study did not assess the effect of confounding variables, such as sexual history or smoking, that may have contributed to the findings. It is doubtful that the carcinogenic effect of anesthetics would be sex-related, and the conflicting results for men and women, especially in light of the low statistical significance of the data, cast doubt that anesthetics were the causative agents.

The data from the ASA *Ad Hoc* Committee noted a statistical increase in hepatic disease for female anesthesiologists, female nurse anesthetists, and male anesthesiologists but not for other exposed groups.[2] Again, it is difficult to explain why male anesthetists did not experience the same consequences from exposure to trace anesthetic gases as their female nurse anesthetist counterparts. Although the investigators tried to exclude infectious hepatitis as a cause of hepatic disease, hepatitis B is asymptomatic in approximately 50% of infected individuals. At the time that this survey was conducted, the serum markers to identify hepatitis B had not been elucidated. From the information collected for this study, it cannot be determined whether the hepatic disease was caused by anesthetic exposure or by hepatitis B or another viral infection acquired from frequent exposure to blood.

In a survey of mortality among British physicians from 1951–1971, the overall mortality rate and incidence of death caused by ischemic heart disease, chronic bronchitis, and lung cancer were lower for anesthesiologists than the average for all medical specialists.[32] There was a slightly increased risk of other cancers (107% of expected) because of cancer of the pancreas in anesthesiologists. These mortality data were confirmed when applied to members of the ASA in a survey published in 1979.[33] ASA membership lists from 1954, 1959, 1967, and 1976 were obtained, so that the population studied included those exposed to both older anesthetics and to halogenated volatile agents. Mortality from all causes in anesthesiologists remained below that of the general population since 1954. Specifically, there was no evidence for an increased rate of cancer or hepatic or renal disease.

Epidemiologic studies are useful tools to assess adverse effects of the operating room environment, including exposure to many substances, only one of which is waste anesthetic gases. The data from epidemiologic surveys can, at best, suggest relationships but can never prove cause-and-effect associations between exposure to some condition or substance and a disease process. In this chapter, other physical and emotional factors in the operating room environment are explored. It must be realized that all of these have an impact on operating room personnel. The individual also brings hereditary, nutritional, and psychological factors that interact with the environment and may play a role in any disease process.

There are shortcomings in many surveys that attempt to assess the effects of waste anesthetic gases, and these have resulted in conflicting conclusions. Overall, there appears to be some evidence that the operating room environment produces a slight increase in the rate of spontaneous abortion and cancer in women anesthesiologists and nurses.[6] There is also a statistically significant increase in liver disease in both men and women, but this is consistent with the proven risk of infectious hepatitis among operating room personnel (see Infection Hazards below). Overall mortality rates remain lower in anesthesiologists than for the general population and for other medical specialists.

Laboratory Studies

Concurrent with the epidemiologic studies, investigators have been active in the laboratory assessing the effects of anesthetic agents on cell, tissue, and animal models. It is hoped that this work will provide the scientific evidence linking anesthetics to the adverse effects that have been reported in the epidemiologic surveys.

Cellular Effects. At clinically useful concentrations, volatile anesthetics interfere with cell division in a reversible manner, possibly owing to a reduction in oxygen uptake by mitochondria.[34] There have been no cellular studies to indicate that trace levels of volatile anesthetics have a similar effect.

Nitrous oxide administered in clinically useful concentrations affects hematopoietic and neural cells. After exposure to 0.8 atm nitrous oxide for 30 minutes, liver methionine synthetase activity decreased by more than 50% in mice.[35] Although 0.05 atm of nitrous oxide did not affect methionine synthetase activity after 4 hours, exposure to 1100 ppm for 8–22 days produced a significant reduction in enzyme activity. Nitrous oxide oxidizes the cobalt atom of vitamin B_{12} from an active to inactive state, which inhibits methionine synthetase. This prevents the conversion of methyltetrahydrofolate to tetrahydrofolate, which is required for DNA synthesis.[35] This suggests that inhibition of methionine synthetase in patients and abusers who are exposed to high concentrations of nitrous oxide may result in anemia and polyneuropathy, but chronic exposure to trace levels does not appear to produce these effects.[36,37]

Many studies have been performed in animals to assess the carcinogenicity of anesthetics. Corbett's pilot work indicated that isoflurane produced hepatic neoplasia when administered to mice during gestation and early life.[38] A subsequent well-controlled study failed to reproduce these results.[39] Other studies in mice and rats found no carcinogenic effect of halothane, nitrous oxide, or enflurane.[40-42] In an attempt to simulate environmental exposure to waste anesthetics, rats were exposed to low levels of halothane and nitrous oxide for 7 hours per day, 5 days per week, for 104 weeks.[40] This degree of exposure produced no effect on body weight, behavior, survival, or incidence of tumors.

Several investigators have used the Ames bacterial assay system for studying the mutagenicity of anesthetics.[43-45] This assay is popular in evaluating carcinogens because it is rapid, inexpensive, and has a high true-positive rate when compared with other in vivo tests.[46] Halothane, enflurane, methoxyflurane, isoflurane, and urine from patients anesthetized with these agents were not mutagenic using this assay.[43,44] Urine from individuals working in scavenged or unscavenged operating rooms was also negative for mutagens using this bacterial system for analysis.[45]

There have been reports of structural changes in cells brought about by prolonged exposure of animals to subclinical levels of anesthetics. Chang and Katz reviewed a series of relevant studies from their laboratory.[47] Exposure to halothane, 10–500 ppm, for 4–8 weeks produced ultrastructural changes in hepatic, renal, and neuronal tissue. Changes included the degeneration of the mitochondria, endoplasmic reticulum, and bile canaliculi in hepatocytes. The extent of the changes cannot be ascertained from these reports, and since control animals were not used, the effects of tissue preparation and other factors are unknown. It is also possible that the ultrastructural changes were reversible and resulted from the administration of the xenobiotic.[48] There is no proof that there is a relationship between anesthetic exposure, cellular ultrastructural changes, and functional abnormalities.

Reproductive Outcome. Because of the suggestion from epidemiologic data that occupational exposure to waste anesthetic gases resulted in an increase in spontaneous abortion and congenital abnormalities in children of female operating room personnel, numerous studies have been performed in laboratory animals to assess reproductive outcome. In one report that suggested anesthetics have an adverse effect, Coate et al exposed male and female rats to combinations of halothane and nitrous oxide for 60 days prior to mating.[49] The anesthetic levels used in this experiment were similar to those found in unscavenged operating rooms. Exposed females had decreased ovulation and implantation efficiency, especially in the groups receiving higher concentrations of anesthetics. There were no major teratologic effects. Chromosomal aberrations were observed in both bone marrow and spermatogonial cells in the male rats.

Prolonged exposure of pregnant rats to 1000 ppm nitrous oxide resulted in smaller litter size, increased frequency of fetal resorption, and reduced fetal crown-rump measurements.[50] Lower concentrations of nitrous oxide had no effect on reproductive outcome. Similarly, daily exposure of mice to 4000 ppm isoflurane before and during pregnancy produced no adverse effect on their litters.[51]

Sperm collected from men working in operating rooms where scavenging devices were used showed no morphologic changes when compared with specimens from physicians who practiced in other environments.[52] Low concentrations of nitrous oxide also fail to alter spermatogenesis in the mouse.[53] Analysis of sister chromatid exchanges is another method of assessing the mutagenic effect of anesthetics. Nitrous oxide and volatile anesthetic agents did not increase the sister chromatid exchange values in hamster ovary cells.[54] When this test was performed on lymphocytes taken from nurses before and during training as anesthetists, there was no indication of mutagenicity for the anesthetics in current use.[55]

The majority of animal experiments fail to demonstrate alterations in female or male fertility or reproduction with exposure to subanesthetic concentrations of the currently used anesthetic agents. It is important to realize that data from laboratory investigations in animals may not be directly applicable to humans. There is little from the animal studies to confirm that the slight increase in relative risk of spontaneous abortions and congenital abnormalities in children of female operating room personnel is caused by exposure to trace amounts of anesthetic gases. Although it is easy to measure and quantify the levels of anesthetic in the operating room air, it is harder to measure and assess the effect of other possible factors, such as stress, alterations in working schedule, and fatigue.

Effects of Trace Anesthetic Levels on Psychomotor Skills

When individuals working in the operating room are exposed to trace concentrations of anesthetics, do the low levels interfere with the psychomotor skills required for providing quality care? Several studies have been conducted to attempt to clarify the effects of low concentrations of anesthetics. Student volunteers were exposed to 500 ppm nitrous oxide with or without 15 ppm halothane in air for 4 hours and were then given tests of perceptual, cognitive, and motor skills.[56] After exposure to halothane and nitrous oxide, their performance was impaired on four of 12 tests; exposure to nitrous oxide alone produced decreased performance on only one test. A subsequent study assessed the effect of nitrous oxide (500, 50, or 25 ppm) alone or with halothane (10, 1.0, or 0.5 ppm) by using psychomotor tests.[57] After exposure to the highest concentrations of nitrous oxide and halothane, subjects' performance declined on four of the seven tests. Interestingly, there was a decrease in ability in six of seven tests after exposure to the same level of nitrous oxide alone. Exposure to the lowest concentrations studied, 25 ppm nitrous oxide and 0.5 ppm halothane, produced no effects in this group as measured by this battery of tests. These investigators suggested that attempts be made to lower anesthetic concentrations in the operating room air to levels no higher than those which were without effect in their study.

Other investigators have found no effect on psychomotor test performance after exposure to trace concentrations of halothane or nitrous oxide.[58] The reasons for difference in outcome between studies are unclear.

Recommendations of the National Institute for Occupational Safety and Health

In 1970, the Occupational Safety and Health Act was legislated by Congress, and created NIOSH, the federal agency responsible for assuring that workers have a safe and healthy working environment. The agency was to meet these goals through the conduct and funding of research, through education of employers and employees about occupational illnesses, and through establishing occupational health standards. A second federal agency, the Occupational Safety and Health Administration (OSHA), was responsible for enacting job health standards, investigating work sites to detect violation of standards, and enforcing the standards by citing violators.[31,59] In 1977, NIOSH published a criteria document that recommended that waste anesthetic exposure should not exceed 2 ppm of halogenated anesthetic agents when used alone, or 0.5 ppm of a halogenated agent and 25 ppm of nitrous oxide.[13] In addition, it stated that operating room employees should be advised of the potential harmful effects of anesthetics. The guidelines proposed that annual medical and occupational histories be obtained from all personnel and that any abnormal outcomes of pregnancies should be documented. The publication also included information on scavenging procedures and equipment and methods for monitoring concentrations of waste anesthetic gases in the air. For the NIOSH criteria document to become a federal standard, the proposal would have to be published in the *Federal Register*, and following a public hearing, OSHA would finalize the text of the standard to be adopted. At present, NIOSH's criteria document has not gone through this process. The NIOSH recommendations are still included in a publication summarizing occupational and health standards.[60]

It is interesting to examine the rationale given for the selection of NIOSH's standards for waste anesthetic gases. According to the criteria document, "Based on the available health information a safe level of exposure to the halogenated agents cannot be defined. Since a safe level of occupational exposure to halogenated anesthetic agents cannot be established by either animal or human investigations, NIOSH recommends that exposure be controlled to levels no greater than the lowest level detectable using the sampling and analysis techniques recommended by NIOSH in this document."[13] Based on this, the recommendations for halogenated agents were set for 2 ppm. The recommendations for nitrous oxide were based on the studies of Bruce, who noted that after exposure to levels of 25 ppm nitrous oxide with 0.5 ppm halothane, there was no impairment of subjects' performance on psychomotor tests.[57]

In view of the conflicting scientific data, it is reasonable to ask what is an acceptable exposure level for waste anesthetic gases. Although it may be difficult to be certain of a threshold concentration below which chronic exposure is "safe," it is prudent to institute scavenging techniques and anesthetic practices that reduce waste anesthetic levels in the operating room environment without compromising patient safety. Monitoring of the operating room air for nitrous oxide and halogenated agents at regular intervals is a necessary part of any program to ensure the adequacy of machine servicing, to prevent leakage of anesthetics from improper seals and fittings, and to confirm appropriate practice techniques. The implementation of a well-designed program with periodic assessment should result in environmental levels of waste gases within the limits suggested by NIOSH.

Chemicals

Methylmethacrylate

Methylmethacrylate is commonly used to cement prostheses to bone or to repair bone defects. The cardiovascular effects of methylmethacrylate in patients have been thoroughly studied and reviewed, but there are fewer data on the effects of occupational exposure. OSHA has established an 8-hour, time-weighted average allowable exposure of 100 ppm. Factory workers exposed to methylmethacrylate complained of respiratory, cutaneous, and genitourinary problems after exposure to levels lower than those allowed by OSHA.[61] When the Ames test was used to assess the mutagenic potential of methylmethacrylate, it was found that the compound alone was toxic to the bacteria, but when methylmethacrylate was incubated with a rat liver enzyme metabolizing system, mutagenesis was induced.[62]

When methylmethacrylate is prepared to be used in the operating room, concentrations up to 90 ppm have been measured during the period required for polymerization. Scavenging devices for venting methylmethacrylate vapor have been described[63] and are now commercially available. With the use of these venting devices, peak concentrations of the vapor can be decreased by 75%.

Allergic Reactions

In addition to concerns about toxic effects of methylmethacrylate vapor and waste anesthetic gases, allergic reactions to these substances have been reported. Occupational asthma after exposure to methylmethacrylate in orthopedic operating rooms has been described in at least two cases.[64,65] One anesthesiologist developed asthma 8–12 hours after administering enflurane to his patients.[66]

A thoroughly documented case report of an anesthesiologist who developed recurrent hepatitis after exposure to and challenge with halothane was interpreted to indicate that halothane was a sensitizing agent in some individuals.[67] Repeated bouts of hepatitis in this anesthesiologist were attributed to hypersensitivity reactions rather than to a direct toxic effect of halothane.

Radiation

Occupational radiation exposure in anesthesia practice has had only limited study.[9] Anesthesiologists received an average of 13 mrem (milliroentgen equivalent, man) per week, which was well below the acceptable limit, at the time, of 100 mrem per week.[9] Since anesthesia personnel are now requested to care for patients in many areas of the hospital, there are numerous situations in which radiation exposure may occur. Diagnostic radiographs are taken in the operating room, postanesthetic care unit, and intensive care units. Some patients undergoing diagnostic or therapeutic procedures such as angiography, angioplasty, biliary dilation, extracorporeal shock wave lithotripsy, or radiation therapy may require care by anesthesiologists. Anesthesia personnel may also be exposed to radionuclides given to patients for diagnostic procedures or for therapy.

Hospital personnel have generally been uninformed about the effects of radiation exposure. Oncogenesis, teratogenesis, and long-term genetic effects may occur with sufficiently high or frequent doses of radiation. For policies on radiation safety, regulatory agencies divide workers into two classes: those who are only occasionally exposed to radiation (i.e., anesthesia personnel) and radiation workers whose normal duties require them to be in areas with large potential exposure.[68] The nonoccupational limit of exposure is set at less than 500 mrem per year. Implementation of radiation protection policies that include education and monitoring programs can reduce maximum exposure to this limit.[69]

Technologic advances in imaging equipment and radiation handling have reduced the risk of radiation exposure for most hospital personnel. Measurements of radiation doses to radiologists and nursing personnel provide a worse case example for estimating radiation exposure to anesthesiologists involved in the care of patients having diagnostic and therapeutic procedures.[70-75] These studies documented only minimal exposure levels that were well within the recommended limits.

Radiation exposure should be monitored with film badges or pocket dosimeters in anesthesia personnel at risk. Monthly documentation of exposure allows for recognition of personnel with high levels of exposure so that their work practices can be evaluated and reassignment to work areas with less radiation exposure can be considered. Educational programs on the effects of radiation and techniques for preventing exposure are important parts of radiation safety programs.

Noise Pollution

A potential health hazard that is virtually uncontrolled in the modern operating room is noise pollution. Noise pollution is quantified by determining both the intensity of the sound in decibels (db) and the duration of the exposure. OSHA has established a maximum level for safe noise exposure of 90 db for 8 hours.[60] Furthermore, each increase in noise of 5 db halves the permissible exposure time, so that 100 db is acceptable for only 2 hours per day. The maximum allowable exposure in an industrial setting is 115 db.

The noise level that we routinely endure in our daily practice is surprisingly close to what constitutes a health hazard.[76] Continuous background noise at a level of 75–90 db is produced by ventilators, suction equipment, music, and conversation. Superimposed on this are such sporadic and unexpected noises as dropped equipment and monitor alarms. Resultant noise levels frequently exceed those of a freeway and even of a rock and roll band.

The predictable results of excessive exposure to noise are well documented in the literature of industrial hygiene.[77] At the very least, noise pollution is an important factor in decreased worker productivity. At higher noise levels, workers are likely to show signs of irritability and demonstrate evidence of stress, such as elevated blood pressure. Ultimately, hearing loss ensues.

Maintaining Vigilance

The work performed by an anesthesiologist is intricate and includes a number of complex tasks. These entail both precise psychomotor and cognitive responses involved in monitoring and interpreting large volumes of complicated clinical data. Fundamental to successfully performing these functions is the ability to maintain long periods of attention, or "vigilance."[78] Gaba has stated that "Vigilance is thus a necessary, but not sufficient condition for averting (anesthetic) accidents."[79] The seal of the American Society of Anesthesiologists bears as its only motto, "Vigilance" (Fig. 4-1), and the official motto of the Australian Society of Anaesthetists is "*Vigila et Ventila.*" These mottoes serve as formal recognition of the critical importance of this function.

Several components of the vigilance task deserve attention. First, it is important to recognize that this particular function may be repetitive and monotonous. However, there are major differences that distinguish the vigilance task from other monotonous tasks, such as production line sorting or assembling, and promote the early onset of boredom in the former. One is the unpredictable nature and timing of the changes in the parameters being monitored. The individual is unable to establish his or her own pace but rather

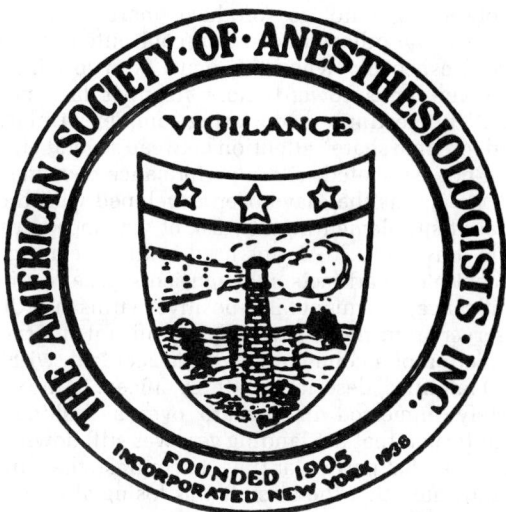

Figure 4-1. Official Seal of the American Society of Anesthesiologists. "VIGILANCE" has always been recognized as the most critical of the tasks of the anesthesiologist.

must respond to the cues from the monitors. Lack of automaticity is also a detriment, because the task does not fully occupy the anesthesiologist's mental activity but neither does it leave him or her free to perform other mental functions. And last, the task is complex, requiring visual attention as well as manual dexterity, and the ability to perform a vigilance task varies inversely with the complexity of that task.[80]

Vigilance tasks are generally performed at the level of 90% accuracy.[81] Obviously, in a setting where the stakes are as high as that of anesthesia, this leaves an unacceptable margin of error. In fact, human error, in part resulting from lapses in attention, accounts for a large proportion of the estimated 2000 preventable deaths and serious injuries resulting from anesthetic mishaps in the United States annually.[82] The current profusion of monitoring, alarm, and automation devices represents one avenue of effort to incrementally improve this performance factor. It is crucial for practitioners to recognize that this instrumentation may enhance their practice but will not replace scrupulous personal attention.

A number of factors at work in the operating room environment may serve to diminish the ability of the operator to perform the task of vigilance.[83] Obvious factors are sleep loss and fatigue. Several studies have documented the deleterious effect of sleep loss and fatigue on work efficiency.[84-86] Additionally, they have detrimental effects upon such cognitive tasks as monitoring and accurate clinical decision making.[87,88] Performance does not return to normal levels until 24 hours of rest and recovery have occurred. An interesting phenomenon is the "end-spurt," in which previously deteriorated performance shows improvement when the subject realizes that the task is 90% completed.[89] The converse undoubtedly also occurs, a "let-down" with additional deterioration in performance when the procedure is unexpectedly prolonged.

Poor design in the monitor displays and the various other sources of information input can adversely affect the vigilance task. Engineering details, such as signal frequency and signal strength, as well as the mode of presentation of the input, significantly influence the operator's ability to maintain the task of vigilance. For example, if the signal rate is slow, observers tend to produce more false-positive alarms.[90] On the other hand, when confronted with a fast event rate, especially when the signal is of low intensity, the observer tends toward more frequent false-negative findings.[91] Interestingly, monitoring complex displays and the need to "time share" attention between several vigilance tasks are not associated with a performance decrement.[92]

Even the alarms that have been developed with the specific goal of supplementing the task of vigilance have considerable drawbacks.[93] Alarms used in the operating room are susceptible to artifacts and transients (true readings of no significance). Frequent false-positive alarms may distract the observer from more clinically significant information. One depiction of a commercial airline accident, with more than 150 fatalities, describes all three officers in the cockpit completely immersed in concern over a flashing light, which indicated that the landing gear was still down, a trivial concern at that particular time. In contrast, the altimeter, which indicated that the aircraft was losing altitude, went unnoticed until too late. Analogous situations occur in the operating room; therefore it is not unusual for frequently distractive alarms to be inactivated.[94]

Noise may have a detrimental influence on the observer who is attempting to perform a vigilance task. In general, various intrusive noises, such as loud talking, excessive clanging of instruments, and "broadband" noise, are all associated with decrements in performance.[95] On the other hand, certain types of background music produce the least decrement in vigilance.[96]

Exposure to trace anesthetic gases may adversely affect the performance of the vigilance task. Several studies have shown decreases in performance of various psychomotor functions after prolonged exposure to trace anesthetic gases.[97,98] However, others have failed to corroborate these findings and have suggested that a tolerance to these adverse effects develops in individuals who are exposed to them on a daily basis.[99]

Ergonomics

A fertile area for research and development lies within the discipline of ergonomics, the consideration of the human-machine interface. The configuration of the typical machinery in most anesthetic locations is the end product of a series of add-ons to existing equipment (Fig. 4-2). In fact, the basic "anesthesia machine" in use today, on which all these embellishments and monitors are hung, is a direct descendant of Boyle's original apparatus.

However, this historical evolution of equipment has not produced an optimal product by ergonomic standards. A sample of poor equipment design is the usual placement of electrocardiogram (ECG) and O_2/CO_2 monitors on a shelf above the flow meters. This places the display well above the visual field of a tall and seated or a short and standing anesthesiologist (Fig. 4-2).[100]

Probably worse than inappropriate placement of visual displays in the vertical plane is the positioning of machinery and displays out of the view of the anesthesiologist in the horizontal plane. In McIntyre's study of this problem, he reported situations in which the machine was squarely at the back of the anesthesiologist as he or she viewed the patient (Fig. 4-3).[101]

This problem appears to be getting worse. In recent years, there has been almost universal application of oximeters and real-time gas analyzers at all anesthetizing locations. It is not unusual to have four or more analog displays, along with digital readouts and alarms, attached to each machine.

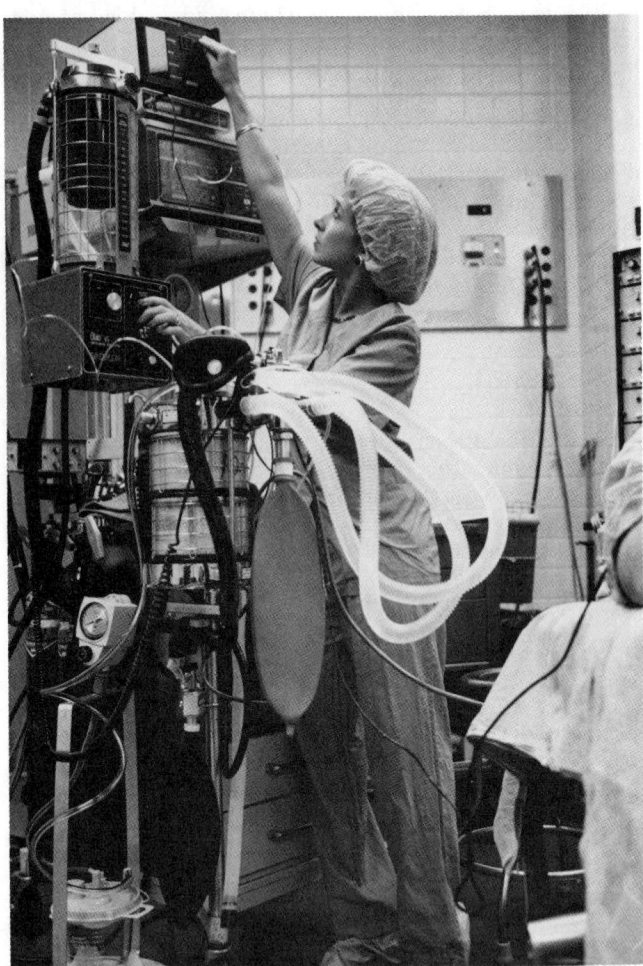

Figure 4-2. An example of an older anesthesia machine with modern "add-on" monitors and alarms. When he or she is sitting, the anesthesiologist is unable to see or reach any of the monitors on the top shelf of the machine. Even when the anesthesiologist is standing, extraordinary efforts must be taken to visualize the display on the pulse oximeter and blood pressure monitor. (Courtesy of Alexandra Pousoula Pappas.)

These are usually add-ons to the existing equipment and often are mounted on top of a vacant shelf or cart surface.

Such deficiencies in equipment design seriously diminish an anesthesiologist's ability to successfully complete his or her myriad tasks. Especially vulnerable are the capabilities to respond to a critical incident and to sustain complex monitoring tasks. One example of the impediment created by such haphazard placement of equipment is distraction of the anesthesiologist's attention. Indeed, nearly half of the anesthesiologist's time is spent with his or her attention diverted away from the patient-surgeon field.[102] In this circumstance, unnecessary energy is expended to perform routine work and fatigue occurs prematurely.[103]

Any factor that requires the expenditure of excessive energy to perform a given task contributes to fatigue and produces a predictable decrement in performance.[104] Even the most trivial aspect of an operator's performance plays a significant role over the course of time. For example, if the anesthesiologist must make frequent, rapid changes in observation from a dim distant to a bright nearby screen, the continuous muscular activity required for pupil dilation and constriction and lens accommodation promotes fatigue.

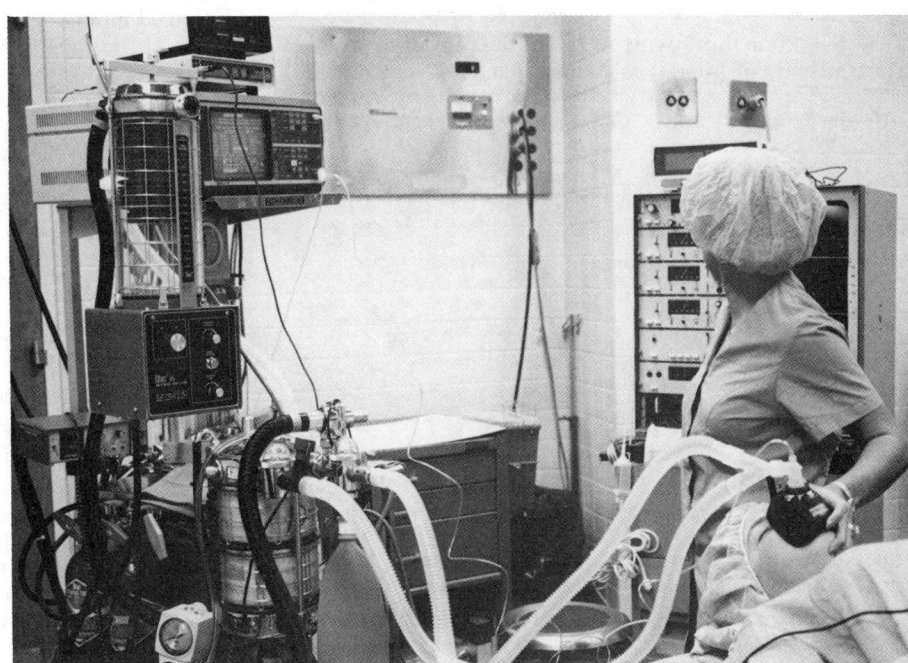

Figure 4-3. In order to view the display of the electrocardiogram and the transduced arterial and central blood pressures, the anesthesiologist must turn fully 180 degrees from the patient-surgical field. (Courtesy of Alexandra Pousoula Pappas.)

Excessive energy expenditure need not be entirely physical. As we monitor more functions in the operating room and we are required to process more data during the course of a surgical procedure, we are expending increasingly larger amounts of mental work. The mental work varies directly with the difficulty encountered in extracting the information from the various displays competing for the attention of the anesthesiologist. Sustained mental alertness hastens fatigue, and fatigue adversely affects vigilance.

The importance of the people-system interface has long been recognized by industry. In fact, design and engineering standards for certain military installations and for applications in the aerospace industry are analogous, in many ways, to requirements in the operating room.[105] With this in mind, attempts have been made to modernize anesthetic equipment to meet ergonometric standards.[106,107] Most promising is the application of microprocessors to enhance the integration of data from various sources and to provide trend information as well as "intelligent" warnings of potential difficulties.[108] There is also progress in the application of computer technology to servocontrol systems that will introduce automation into the delivery of anesthetics.[109,110]

Work Hours and Night Call

A less subtle determinant of fatigue, well known to all clinicians, relates to "on-call" schedules and work hours. For practicing anesthesiologists, 10–12 hour work days are not at all unusual. Emergency and on-call coverage is usually tacked onto the end of one of these days, resulting in a 24–32 hour shift.

A survey of anesthesia residents showed that the average work week was 69 hours and that administration of anesthesia for 7 or more hours without a break was common.[111] Not surprisingly, fatigue was often experienced and many thought it contributed to the commission of an error.

Several studies have substantiated the claim that fatigue or continuous wakefulness has a deleterious effect on performance of complex cognitive tasks such as monitoring and vigilance.[84,112,113] What is particularly troubling is the suggestion that this deterioration in psychomotor functioning may contribute directly to anesthetic mishaps. In a survey of serious anesthetic-related accidents, fatigue was one of the two major sources of human error (confusion with anesthetic equipment was the other).[114] Together, these two sources of error accounted for more than 96% of the lethal or near-lethal human errors reported. Similarly, in Cooper et al's critical incidence analysis of anesthetic mishaps, fatigue was among the most frequently reported associated factors contributing to these potentially serious incidents.[115] This problem obviously deserves more attention.

An additional area of concern is the potential effect of sleep deprivation and chronic fatigue on health and psychosocial adjustment.[116] Work schedules that thoroughly disrupt circadian rhythms are associated with impaired health, emotional problems, and a decline in performance. Manpower considerations in all but the largest practices prohibit the utilization of a "night float system," which is probably the best scheduling plan for late night coverage. Fortunately, most anesthesiologists work in a situation that provides enough recuperative time (24 hours) after a day and night on-call to avoid circadian disruption and the associated risk of chronic sleep deprivation and its complications.

National attention has been focused on the problem of fatigue by the well-publicized Libby Zion case.[117] A large portion of this claim hinged on the allegation that fatal, avoidable mistakes were made by exhausted, unsupervised house officers. Various medical organizations and state legislatures have identified the problem of sleep deprivation among physicians. Several specialty boards have ratified policies that limit the number of work hours for their resident physicians. The State of New York has already instituted regulations that prohibit resident physicians from working more than 24 consecutive hours. It is expected that similar laws will be adopted in other states.

TABLE 4-2. Factors Involved in the Successful Transmission of Infectious Agents, Bacteria, and Viruses

1. A source of infectious particles, usually from patients or personnel who are carriers
2. The stability of the pathogen in the physical environment
3. The numbers of infectious particles in the vehicle of transmission
4. The infectivity of the agent
5. The appropriate vector or medium for transmission
6. A portal of entry in a susceptible host

INFECTION HAZARDS

Anesthesia personnel are at risk for acquiring infections from both patients and other personnel (Table 4-2). Viral infections reflecting their prevalence in the community are the most significant threat to health care workers. Most commonly, these are spread through the respiratory route, and unfortunately, this mechanism is the most difficult to control effectively with environmental alterations. Blood-borne pathogens such as hepatitis and human immunodeficiency virus (HIV) are serious infections, but transmission can be prevented with mechanical barriers blocking portals of entry or, in the case of hepatitis B, by producing immunity by vaccination. Hospital-acquired bacterial infections are uncommon in workers who do not have compromised immune systems.

Respiratory Viruses

Respiratory viruses, which are responsible for many community-acquired infections, are usually transmitted by two routes. Small-particle aerosols produced by coughing, sneezing, or talking may propel viruses over large distances. The influenza and measles viruses are spread in this way. The second mechanism requires close person-to-person contact. Transmission can occur when large droplets produced by coughing or sneezing contaminate the donor's hands or an inanimate surface, and subsequently the virus is transferred to the oral, nasal, or conjunctival mucous membranes of a susceptible individual by self-inoculation. Rhinovirus and respiratory syncytial virus are spread by this process.

Influenza Viruses

Because of the ease of viral transmission and infection, community epidemics of influenza are common, with large outbreaks occurring annually. The influenza virus contains RNA and is classified into two types, A or B, based on antigens associated with the viral envelope. Acutely ill patients shed virus through small-particle aerosols by coughing or sneezing for as long as 5 days after the onset of symptoms. Respiratory isolation precautions can be used for the duration of the clinical illness in an attempt to prevent spread to susceptible individuals. Because of their contact with nasopharyngeal secretions, anesthesiologists may play a role in the spread of influenza virus in hospitals.[118]

Influenza rarely produces significant morbidity in healthy health care workers but may result in high rates of absenteeism. Hospital staff who have patient contact should be immunized annually with the inactivated (killed virus) influenza virus vaccine.[119] Antigenic variation of influenza viruses occurs over time so that new viral strains are selected for inclusion in each year's vaccine. Vaccination programs for personnel should be conducted in October or November, since the number of cases of influenza in the community begins to increase in December. During hospital outbreaks of influenza A, amantadine may be effective in preventing nosocomial infection in unvaccinated hospital personnel.[119] Amantadine has not been useful for prophylaxis against influenza B. Because of possible morbidity as a result of influenza in hospitalized patients with chronic illnesses, it is recommended that during community epidemics, elective hospital admissions and surgery should be limited. If surgery is necessary in a patient with influenza, data from an animal model suggest that general anesthesia results in no increase in respiratory morbidity.[120]

Respiratory Syncytial Virus

During periods when respiratory syncytial virus is prevalent in the community (usually late December through February), many hospitalized infants and children may carry the virus. Large numbers of virus are present in respiratory secretions of infected children, and viable virus can be recovered for up to 6 hours on contaminated environmental surfaces.[121] Infection of susceptible individuals occurs by self-inoculation when respiratory syncytial virus in secretions is transferred to the hands, which then contact the mucous membranes of the eyes or nose. Although most children have been exposed to respiratory syncytial virus early in life, immunity is not permanent and reinfection is common.

Respiratory syncytial virus is shed for approximately 7 days after infection. Hospitalized patients with the virus should be isolated in a single room or in a unit with other infected patients, but during seasonal outbreaks large numbers of patients may make isolation impractical. Careful hand washing between contacts with patients and use of gowns and gloves are recommended to prevent spread of the disease.[122] Controlled studies have demonstrated that use of masks and goggles reduced respiratory syncytial virus infection in pediatric hospital personnel.[123]

Rhinovirus

Rhinovirus infections are probably the most common of all acute infections and are the cause of approximately one third of common colds. The transmission of this virus usually requires close personal contact. Large numbers of virus are shed in nasal secretions, with lower concentrations in saliva. Successful transmission probably results from self-inoculation by touching the mucous membranes of the nose or eyes with hands that have been directly contaminated. Airborne spread appears to be less likely. There are over 100 antigenically different rhinoviruses; therefore an individual may expect to experience multiple infections over a lifetime.

Thorough handwashing may be effective in preventing transmission of rhinovirus. Iodine-containing solutions, sodium hypochlorite, 70% ethyl alcohol, and activated glutaraldehyde are effective disinfectants for contaminated surfaces. Vaccine development is in progress, but researchers are pessimistic about having a vaccine in the near future because of the large number of antigenic types of rhinoviruses.

Herpes Viruses

Varicella-zoster virus (VZV), herpes simplex virus Types 1 and 2, and cytomegalovirus (CMV) are members of the Herpetoviridine family. Close personal contact is required for transmission of all the herpes viruses except for VZV, which is spread by direct contact or small-particle aerosols. After the primary infection with herpes viruses, the organism becomes latent and may reactivate at a later time. Most individuals in the United States have been infected with all of the herpes viruses by middle age. Therefore, nosocomial transmission is uncommon except in the pediatric population and in immunosuppressed patients.

Varicella-Zoster Virus

Varicella-zoster virus produces both chickenpox and herpes zoster (shingles). Chickenpox is a common childhood disease and is the second most frequently reported infectious disease in the United States. Although the infection is usually uncomplicated in healthy children, VZV infection in adults may be associated with major morbidity or death. Infection during pregnancy may result in fetal death or rarely in congenital defects. Health care workers with active VZV infection are a risk, since they may transmit the virus to other personnel or to hospitalized immunocompromised patients.

After the primary infection, VZV remains latent in dorsal root or extramedullary cranial ganglia. Herpes zoster results from reactivation of the VZV infection and produces a painful vesicular rash in the innervated dermatome. Anesthesiologists working in pain clinics may be called upon to care for patients who have discomfort from herpes zoster.

Varicella-zoster virus is highly contagious, and the Centers for Disease Control estimates that the period of communicability is from 1 to 2 days prior to the onset of the rash through the first 5 to 6 days after its appearance.[124] The majority of adults in the United States have protective antibodies to VZV and are immune to new infection. One survey of hospital health care workers found that all of those aged 36 years and over had VZV antibodies, whereas 7.5% of those younger were susceptible.[125] Anesthesia personnel should be questioned about prior varicella infection, and individuals with a negative or unknown history of such infection should be serologically tested. Employees with negative titers should be restricted from caring for patients with active VZV infection and should consider immunization with live, attenuated varicella vaccine. Susceptible personnel who are exposed to individuals with VZV infection are candidates for varicella zoster immune globulin, which is most effective when administered within 96 hours after exposure. The Centers for Disease Control recommends that potentially susceptible hospital personnel with significant VZV exposure should not have direct patient contact from the 10th to the 21st day after exposure.[124] Personnel without VZV immunity should be reassigned to alternative locations so that they do not care for patients who have active VZV infections.

Herpes Simplex

Herpes simplex infection is quite common in adults. After viral entry through the mucous membranes of the mouth, the primary infection with herpes simplex virus Type 1 is usually clinically inapparent but may involve severe oral lesions, fever, and adenopathy. In healthy individuals, the primary infection subsides and the virus persists in a latent state within the sensory nerve ganglion innervating the site of infection. Any of several mechanisms can reactivate the virus to produce recurrent infection, which manifests in the vicinity of the primary lesion, frequently as herpes labialis.

A second herpes simplex virus, Type 2, is usually associated with infections below the waist and is spread by sexual contact. Newborns may become infected with herpes simplex virus Type 2 during vaginal delivery from the mother's genital infection.

Herpes simplex virus Type 1 is probably spread by self-inoculation after contact with contaminated oral secretions. Asymptomatic individuals can unknowingly transmit herpes simplex virus Type 1, since the virus has been isolated from oral secretions of 5% of some populations. The fingers of health care personnel may be inoculated by direct contact with body fluids carrying either herpes simplex virus Type 1 or 2.

Herpetic Whitlow. Herpetic infection of the finger, herpetic paronychia or herpetic whitlow, is an occupational hazard for anesthesia personnel.[126,127] The infection usually begins at the portal of viral entry, a site on the distal finger where the integrity of the skin has been broken. Initially, there is itching and pain at the site of infection, followed by the appearance of a vesicle surrounded by erythema (Fig. 4-4). There may be associated constitutional symptoms such as fever, malaise, and lymphadenopathy. Satellite vesicles appear near the primary lesion over several days. Within 3 weeks, the throbbing pain lessens, and the lesions begin to heal. A diagnosis of herpes simplex infection can be made by demonstrating multinucleated giant epithelial cells or nuclear inclusion bodies in smears (Tzanck's technique) taken from a vesicle. Although the process may resemble a bacterial paronychia, treatment should be conservative and surgical drainage is not indicated.[128]

To prevent herpes simplex virus infections of the hands, anesthesia personnel should wear gloves when in contact with patients' oral secretions such as during endotracheal intubation and extubation, pharyngeal suctioning, and insertion of nasogastric tubes.[129] Skin and wound precautions should be followed when caring for patients with herpes simplex virus Type 2 genital infections. Anesthetists who have active herpetic whitlow may infect susceptible pa-

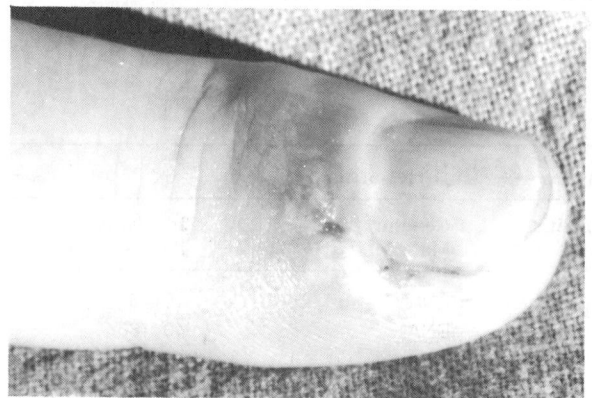

Figure 4-4. Herpetic whitlow on the index finger near the site of minor trauma in the cuticle. Erythema surrounds the blister formed from the coalescence of individual vesicles. (Reproduced with permission from Orkin FK: Herpetic whitlow. In Orkin FK, Cooperman LH (eds): Complications in Anesthesiology, p 709. Philadelphia, JB Lippincott, 1983.)

tients, and a decision must be made as to whether an infected individual should be allowed to participate in direct patient care. Use of acyclovir, an antiviral drug that inhibits replication, of herpes simplex virus Types 1 and 2 may shorten the course of primary cutaneous viral infection.

Cytomegalovirus

Cytomegalovirus infection commonly occurs during childhood, and most individuals develop antibodies to CMV following the initial infection, which may be clinically inapparent. Following this, there are intermittent periods of virus excretion even in the presence of high levels of circulating antibody. Transmission of CMV probably occurs through close contact with an individual excreting the virus, although CMV has been isolated from environmental surfaces that have been contaminated with infected secretions. It is unlikely that aerosols or small droplets play a role in CMV transmission.

Primary or recurrent CMV infection during pregnancy results in fetal infection in up to 2.5% of occurrences. Congenital CMV syndrome may be found in up to 10% of infected infants. Thus, although CMV infection usually does not result in morbidity in healthy adults, it may have significant sequelae in pregnant women.

The two major reservoirs of CMV infection within the hospital include infected infants and immunocompromised patients such as those who have undergone organ transplants or those on oncology units. Although there is some evidence that workers in day-care centers may be at risk for acquiring CMV from infected children,[130] studies of employees at a pediatric hospital[131] and nurses in renal transplant units[132] indicate that CMV infection is not an occupational risk. It appears that routine infection control procedures such as handwashing after patient contact and use of gloves to avoid touching body fluids are sufficient to prevent CMV infection in health care workers.[133] There is no evidence to indicate that it is necessary to reassign pregnant women from patient care areas in which they may have contact with CMV-positive patients.

Rubella

Outbreaks of rubella, or German measles, in hospital personnel have resulted in significant loss in employee working time, employee morbidity, and cost to the hospital.[134,135] Although the majority of adults in the United States are immune to rubella, up to 20% of women of child-bearing age are still susceptible. Rubella infection during the first trimester of pregnancy is associated with congenital malformations or fetal death.

Serologic testing for antibody is the only specific indicator of immunity, since patient history has been shown to be unreliable.[136] A live attenuated rubella virus vaccine is available to produce immunity in susceptible adults. Many hospitals require employees to document immunity to rubella by serologic testing. Susceptible women of childbearing age and all personnel who might transfer rubella to pregnant patients or workers should be vaccinated.[137]

Measles

Since the introduction of the measles vaccine in the United States in 1963, the incidence of the disease decreased significantly. In spite of this, there have been recent outbreaks among unvaccinated preschool-aged children and among older children who have had vaccine failures. Transmission of measles has been documented in medical facilities with both patient-to-patient spread and patient-to-health care worker transmission.[138]

Health care workers are at increased risk for acquiring measles from patients.[139] The Centers for Disease Control recommends that medical personnel have adequate immunity to measles, as documented by one of the following: evidence of two live vaccinations for measles, records of physician-diagnosed measles, or serologic evidence of measles immunity. Susceptible individuals born in or after 1957 should receive two doses of the live measles vaccine at the time of employment.[139]

Viral Hepatitis

Although many viruses may produce hepatitis, the most common types of viral hepatitis are Type A or infectious hepatitis, Type B or serum hepatitis, and non-A, non-B hepatitis. The viruses responsible for Type A, Type B, and one form of non-A, non-B (Type C) hepatitis have been clearly defined (Table 4-3). Delta hepatitis, caused by an incomplete virus, only occurs in individuals infected with the hepatitis B virus. Of these, the greatest risks of occupational transmission to anesthesia personnel are associated with Type B and non-A, non-B hepatitis.

TABLE 4-3. Viral Hepatitis

Hepatitis Virus	Genetic Material	Incubation Period (days)	Transmission	Chronic Hepatitis	Chronic Carrier State
A	RNA	15–45	Fecal-oral	No	No
B	DNA	40–180	Parenteral, venereal, perinatal, blood transfusion	5–10%	Adult 5–10% Infant 70–90%
C	RNA	15–150	Parenteral, blood transfusion	50%	Yes
D	RNA (requires hepatitis B virus infection)	21–50	Parenteral, blood transfusion	Coinfection < 5% Superinfection > 75%	Yes

Hepatitis A

About 20–40% of viral hepatitis in adults in the United States is caused by the Type A virus, a picornavirus containing RNA. Hepatitis A is usually a self-limited illness, and no chronic carrier state exists. Spread is predominantly by the fecal-oral route, and outbreaks are usually found in institutions or other closed groups where there has been a breakdown in normal sanitary conditions. Hospital personnel do not appear to be at increased risk for hepatitis A because the majority of patients with this form of hepatitis are rarely hospitalized. Also, at the time that a patient with hepatitis A becomes jaundiced, there is little fecal excretion of the virus. In spite of this, until a viral etiology has been ruled out, jaundiced patients who are hospitalized should be placed on enteric precautions.

Occasional hospital outbreaks of hepatitis A have occurred when patients were admitted during the prodromal stage of the infection.[140] The use of gloves and meticulous handwashing during contact with feces or contaminated linens or clothing should be adequate to prevent viral spread to hospital personnel.[141] Anesthesia personnel exposed to patients with hepatitis A should receive immune globulin within 2 weeks of the exposure to reduce the likelihood of infection.[142]

Hepatitis B

Hepatitis B is a significant occupational hazard for anesthesiologists and other medical personnel who are in contact with blood and blood products.[143] The prevalence (a proportion of persons who have or have had the condition at the time of the survey) of hepatitis B in the general population of the United States is 3–5%, and the carrier rate is 0.2% to 0.9% based on serologic screening. Surveys conducted in the United States and several other countries demonstrate a significantly increased prevalence of serologic markers indicating prior hepatitis B infection in anesthesiologists and anesthesia personnel (Table 4-4).[144-152] The range of seropositive findings in anesthesia personnel in various locations

TABLE 4-5. Patterns of Serologic Markers of Hepatitis B Virus Infection

Stage of Infection	HBsAg	Anti-HBc	Anti-HBs
Early acute hepatitis B or chronic carrier state	+	−	−
Acute* or chronic hepatitis B	+	+	−
Recovery from acute* or chronic hepatitis B	−	+	+
Distant hepatitis B virus infection, early recovery stage of hepatitis B*, or chronic carrier state	—	+	−
Distant hepatitis B virus infection or after immunization with hepatitis B vaccine	−	−	+

* Anti-HBc of IgM type should be present.

probably reflects the prevalence of hepatitis B carriers in the referral population for the area. Within the United States, the prevalence of hepatitis B markers in anesthesia personnel varied from 19% in one multicenter study[145] to 49% in the anesthesia department of an inner-city hospital.[147] It appears that the risk of hepatitis B infection begins early during the period of training when patient contact is initiated, and it continues throughout practice in physicians and hospital personnel who are in contact with blood and blood products.

Acute hepatitis B infection resolves without significant hepatic damage in about 90% of cases. Less than 1% of acutely infected patients develop fulminant hepatitis. The remaining 10% of infected individuals become chronic carriers of the hepatitis B virus (i.e., serologic evidence demonstrated for more than 6 months). Within 2 years, half of the chronic carriers resolve their infection without significant hepatic impairment. Chronic active hepatitis is found most commonly in those individuals with chronic viral infection for more than 2 years. Chronic active hepatitis may progress to cirrhosis, and chronic hepatitis B virus carriers have an increased risk of hepatocellular carcinoma. The Centers for Disease Control estimates that 300,000 persons in the United States, including 12,000 health care workers, are infected with hepatitis B virus annually.[142] Acute and chronic sequelae of occupationally acquired hepatitis B result in the death of 250 medical personnel each year.

The diagnosis and classification of the stage of hepatitis B virus infection can be made on the basis of serologic testing (Table 4-5). Hepatitis B surface antigen (HBsAg) is detectable in the serum within 3 to 4 weeks after infection with hepatitis B virus.[154] At this time, the patient is asymptomatic but is capable of infecting others with hepatitis B virus. Within 8 to 12 weeks after infection, symptoms of hepatitis and jaundice occur, and liver function test findings are elevated. With resolution of acute hepatitis B, HBsAg disappears from the serum and is followed by the appearance of antibody to the surface antigen (anti-HBs). Anti-HBs is the antibody that confers lasting immunity against subsequent hepatitis B virus infections. During the "window" period in which HBsAg has declined to undetectable levels and anti-HBs is not measurable, antibody to the core antigen (anti-HBc) is detectable. With resolution of hepatitis B virus infection, anti-HBc and anti-HBs persist, but after many years one of these antibodies may no longer be detectable in the serum. Chronic hepatitis B virus carriers are likely to have HBsAg and anti-HBc present in serum samples.

TABLE 4-4. Prevalence of Hepatitis B Seropositivity in Anesthesia Personnel

Reference	Study Population	Prevalence
Denes et al[143]	MDs at AMA meeting	17%
Berry et al[144]	MDs and non-MD anesthetists in one U.S. department	23%
Berry et al[145]	MDs and non-MD anesthetists in four U.S. Departments	19%
Berry et al[146]	Residents in seven U.S. departments	13%
Fyman et al[147]	NY inner-city hospital	49%
Malm et al[148]	Anesthetists in teaching hospitals in Vancouver, Canada	12%
Chernesky et al[149]	Anesthetists in Ontario, Canada	17%
Siebke and Degre[150]	MD and non-MD anesthesia personnel in Norway	4%
Carstens et al[151]	South African anesthetists	18%
Sinclair et al[152]	Anesthetists in Oxford, UK	3%
Janzen et al[153]	Anesthesia personnel at Medical School of Hannover (West Germany)	31%

Hepatitis B virus transmission in the community takes place through sexual contact, close personal contact (as occurs in institutions), shared use of needles and syringes for intravenous drug use, and perinatally from infected mother to newborn. Anesthesia personnel are at risk for occupationally acquired hepatitis B virus infection as a result of accidental percutaneous or permucosal contact with blood or body fluids from patients carrying the virus. Several patient groups with a very high prevalence of hepatitis B virus carriers have been identified and include immigrants from endemic areas, users of illicit parenteral drugs, homosexual males, and individuals on hemodialysis.[142] Hepatitis B virus carriers are frequently not identified during hospitalization because the clinical history and routine preoperative laboratory tests may be insufficient for diagnosis.[155] Percutaneous exposure (usually an accidental needle stick) with blood carrying hepatitis B virus may result in infection in up to 30% of occurrences. Hepatitis B virus can be found in saliva, but transmission appears unlikely after permucosal contact with infected oral secretions.[156] Hepatitis B virus is a hardy virus that may be infectious for at least 1 week when there is contact with dried blood on environmental surfaces.[157]

Hepatitis B Vaccines

Use of hepatitis B vaccine is the primary strategy to prevent occupational transmission of hepatitis B virus to anesthesia personnel and other health care workers at increased risk.[142] Administration of three doses of vaccine in the deltoid muscle results in the production of protective antibodies (anti-HBs) in more than 90% of healthy hospital workers.[158,159] The first hepatitis B vaccine available for use in the United States was composed of HBsAg prepared from the plasma of chronic hepatitis B virus carriers. Because the population from whom plasma was taken for preparation of the vaccine was also at high risk for acquired immunodeficiency syndrome (AIDS), there was concern that the virus responsible for AIDS might be transmitted through this vaccine. Extensive serologic, virologic, and epidemiologic evaluations found no evidence that AIDS was transmitted by the plasma-derived vaccine.[160] Two other hepatitis B vaccines are now available in the United States. Both are composed of HBsAg that has been produced by recombinant technology.[161] These recombinant vaccines are safe and provide effective immunity to hepatitis B virus.[162] Hospitals and/or anesthesia departments should have policies for screening and counseling personnel about their risk of acquiring hepatitis B virus infection and should make vaccination available for susceptible individuals.[142]

To ensure adequate postvaccination immunity, serologic testing of vaccinees for anti-HBs should take place within 6 months after the last dose of vaccine. Nonresponders may develop protective antibodies with additional vaccine doses.[163] Vaccine-induced antibodies decline over time, with maximum titers after vaccination correlating directly with duration of antibody persistence.[163] The Centers for Disease Control states that for vaccinated adults with normal immune status, routine booster doses are not necessary for at least 7 years after vaccination.[142] Surveillance programs are continuing to assess the need for booster doses after longer intervals.

When susceptible, nonvaccinated anesthesia personnel have documented exposure to a contaminated needle or to blood from a HBsAg-positive patient, postexposure prophylaxis with hepatitis B immune globulin is recommended.[142] Hepatitis B immunoglobulin is prepared from human plasma that contains a high anti-HBs titer and provides temporary, passive immunity.

Non-A, Non-B Hepatitis

Acute non-A, non-B hepatitis is diagnosed by clinical and laboratory evidence of hepatitis without a history of other causes of hepatocellular injury and negative serologic findings for hepatitis A and B. Although non-A, non-B hepatitis is often thought of as a transfusion-associated infection, sporadic parenteral transmission accounts for 20–40% of all reported cases of acute viral hepatitis in the United States. Centers for Disease Control surveillance demonstrates that only about 6% of cases of non-A, non-B hepatitis are attributed to blood transfusions, whereas 42% are associated with intravenous drug use. Only 2% occur in health care workers from occupational exposure.[164] In the United States, it is estimated that up to 5% of the population may be non-A, non-B hepatitis carriers.

Researchers have now identified a virus, hepatitis C virus, as one agent responsible for parenterally transmitted non-A, non-B hepatitis and have cloned its genome.[165] An immunoassay for detection of IgG antibodies to a hepatitis C viral antigen has been developed.[166] In one study, anti-hepatitis C virus testing has confirmed that this virus is the cause of approximately 60% of cases of transfusion-transmitted non-A, non-B hepatitis, but there appears to be at least one other currently unidentified virus capable of producing this disease.[167] Studies of blood donors and the recipients who developed non-A, non-B hepatitis indicate that using the current assay, anti-hepatitis C virus is not detectable until almost 6 months after transfusion and 4 months after onset of hepatitis.[168] Therefore, patients with acute or chronic non-A, non-B hepatitis who are negative for anti-hepatitis C virus may have hepatitis C virus infection but be seronegative at the time, or they may have another viral or nonviral etiology for the hepatitis.

It appears that hepatitis C virus is transmitted through blood like hepatitis B virus, but further investigation is needed. A limited study suggests that the risk of hepatitis C virus infection through routine personal contact is not high.[169] Non-A, non-B hepatitis after an accidental needle stick in health care workers has been documented.[170,171] Until other protective strategies are available, anesthesia personnel should use barrier and needle stick precautions with patients with non-A, non-B hepatitis, as is done with patients with other blood-borne infections.

Pathogenic Human Retroviruses

The agent that produces AIDS is the human immunodeficiency virus (HIV-1), one of several pathogenic human retroviruses.[172,173] HIV-1 is a member of the human T-cell lymphotrophic viruses (HTLVs) and was initially designated as HTLV-III.[172] HTLV-I was the first human retrovirus to be discovered and has been documented as a cause of adult T-cell leukemia/lymphoma. This highly aggressive malignancy occurs in about 1 of 80 HTLV-I infected patients after a latency period of approximately 20 years. HTLV-I has been found in intravenous drug users and female prostitutes in the United States and has been isolated in the country's blood supply. Serologic studies indicate that the virus is endemic in parts of Japan, the Caribbean, and Africa.

HTLV-II, like HTLV-I, appears to cause a form of leukemia. Serologic testing indicates that it is present in groups of intravenous drug users and female prostitutes in some areas of the United States. The epidemiology of HTLV-I and HTLV-II has not been well defined. Transmission appears to be through blood or from male to female during sexual intercourse. Occupational transmission to health care workers has not been studied, but since it is a blood-borne infection, this cannot be ruled out.

A second virus, HIV-2, produces an AIDS-like syndrome in parts of western Africa. The epidemiologic pattern of HIV-2 spread is predominantly through heterosexual activity, with almost equal numbers of infected men and women. The only reported cases of HIV-2 infection in the United States have been in individuals who came from or had contact with residents of Africa.

Human Immunodeficiency Virus-1 Infection and AIDS

Current estimates suggest that up to 1 million individuals in the United States are infected with HIV-1. The initial infection presents clinically as a mononucleosis-like syndrome with lymphadenopathy and rash. Within weeks, antibody to the virus may be detected by the enzyme-linked immunosorbent assay (ELISA) or the more specific Western blot test. Viral genetic material is quickly incorporated into cells of the host after infection. Although the patient then has an asymptomatic period, monocyte-macrophage cells are a reservoir for the virus throughout the body and CD4+ T cells harbor the virus in the blood. During this chronic phase, HIV-1 continues to infect host cells. Based on studies of homosexual men, half of infected individuals develop AIDS within 8 years of infection.[174] Finally, there is a recrudescence of viral replication and impaired immunity, resulting in opportunistic infections and malignancies.[175] According to Centers for Disease Control data, from 1981 through February 1991, there have been over 165,000 cases of AIDS in the United States, resulting in a fatality rate of 63% in adults and 51% in children.[176]

Human immunodeficiency virus Type 1 is spread by sexual contact, perinatally from infected mother to neonate, and through infected blood (transfusion or shared needles) and blood products.[177] Investigation of AIDS patients with no recognized risk factors indicates no evidence for additional modes of transmission.[178] Although the virus can be found in saliva, tears, and urine, these body fluids have not been implicated in viral transmission.[177] Exposure categories of adults that account for the highest percentage of AIDS cases include male homosexual/bisexual contact, intravenous drug use, heterosexual contact with an HIV-infected individual, or receipt of an infected blood transfusion, blood component, or tissue.[176]

All HIV-infected patients may not be identified as such by initial or presenting diagnosis. Six percent of patients cared for in one urban hospital emergency department had HIV infection, with 63% of those being unrecognized.[179] Surveillance at 26 sentinel hospitals in 21 United States cities indicated an overall rate of HIV-1 seroprevalence in inpatients and outpatients of 1.3% and a range of 0.1–7.8%.[180]

Risk of Occupational Human Immunodeficiency Virus Infection

Although there are several modes of transmission for HIV-1 infection in the community, the most important source of HIV for health care workers is blood.[181] Prospective studies by the Centers for Disease Control[182] and the National Institutes of Health[183] indicate that the risk of occupationally acquired HIV infection in health care workers is low. As of December 1990, there were 24 reported cases of documented seroconversion in health care workers following occupational exposure to HIV. Additionally, there are reports of 16 health care workers in whom HIV infection was thought to be occupationally acquired but there was no documented seroconversion after a specific exposure. Percutaneous exposure, such as through an accidental needle stick, is the most frequent mechanism for HIV transmission to health care workers and results in infection in one of every 200 occurrences.[184] Mucous membrane and cutaneous exposures are less efficient and probably represent a lower risk. No prospective studies have been conducted specifically in anesthesiologists to assess the risks of occupationally acquired HIV infection.

Because of the tasks they perform, anesthesia personnel are frequently exposed to blood and body fluids. Results of a questionnaire completed by anesthesia personnel indicated a high rate of blood contact during insertion of vascular catheters, arterial punctures, and set-up of blood for transfusion.[185] The authors of this report suggest that 98% of the contacts with blood could have been prevented by the proper use of gloves. In a study of reported needle stick injuries in employees at a university hospital, Jagger et al noted that the greatest percentage of such incidents resulted from needles on disposable syringes and the lowest percentage from intravenous catheter stylets.[186] A third of the injuries were related to recapping of needles. In another series, anesthesiologists were the physician group with the second highest frequency of reported needle punctures, 4 per 100 persons per year.[187]

When operating room personnel were observed during approximately 1300 consecutive surgical procedures, knowledge of patients' HIV infection or high-risk status did not affect the documented rate of personnel exposure to blood.[188] The authors concluded that preoperative testing of patients for HIV infection would be unlikely to reduce health care workers' exposure to blood.

Postexposure Treatment and Prophylactic Zidovudine

When personnel have been exposed to patients' blood or body fluids, the incident should be reported to the employer immediately. The Centers for Disease Control recommends that the exposed worker and the source individual be tested for serologic evidence of HIV and hepatitis B virus infection.[189] Current local laws must be consulted in determining policies for testing individuals, and confidentiality should be maintained at all times. The employee should be retested periodically for HIV antibodies for a minimum of 6 months after exposure, although most infected persons are expected to undergo seroconversion within the first 6 to 12 weeks after exposure. During this period, the exposed employee should follow Centers for Disease Control recommendations for preventing transmission of HIV to family members and patients.

Some investigators have advocated the use of prophylactic, postexposure administration of zidovudine (AZT) as a possible means of preventing HIV infection after occupational exposure.[190] This was based on two lines of evidence: zidovudine has been an effective treatment for extending the duration and quality of life of patients with HIV infection, and in laboratory studies it was useful in altering the course of acute retroviral infections. The Centers for Disease Control has stated that "data from animal and human studies are inadequate to establish the efficacy or safety of zidovudine for prophylaxis after occupational exposure to HIV."[189] Zidovudine is not approved for use prophylactically after occupational exposure, and since it may produce significant side-effects and toxicities, it is suggested that informed consent be obtained from employees who choose to use it in this manner. There are case reports that

TABLE 4-6. Universal Precautions

1. All needles, blades, and sharp instruments should be handled to prevent accidental injuries, and all should be considered potentially infected. Disposable sharp items should be placed in puncture-resistant containers located as close as practical to the area in which they are used. Needles should not be recapped, bent, broken, or removed from disposable syringes prior to placing them in appropriate disposable containers.
2. Gloves should be worn when touching mucous membranes or open skin of all patients. When the possibility exists of exposure to blood, body fluids, or items soiled with these, gloves should be used. With some procedures such as endoscopy when aerosolization or splashes of blood or secretions are likely to occur, masks, eye coverings, and gowns are indicated. Gloves and body coverings should be removed and disposed of properly after patient contact.
3. Frequent handwashing, especially between patient contact and after removal of gloves, should be encouraged. If hands are accidentally contaminated with blood or other body fluids, they should be washed as soon as possible.
4. Ventilation devices for resuscitation should be available at appropriate locations to prevent the need for emergency mouth-to-mouth resuscitation.
5. Health-care workers who have exudative lesions or weeping dermatitis should not participate in direct patient care activities until the condition resolves.

From Guidelines from Centers for Disease Control, References 181, 184, and 192

demonstrate that zidovudine failed to prevent HIV infection when given after accidental exposure.[191]

Universal Precautions

The Centers for Disease Control has formulated recommendations, or universal precautions, for preventing transmission of blood-borne infections (including HIV and hepatitis B virus) to health care workers.[181,184,192] The guidelines are based on the epidemiology of hepatitis B as a worst case model for transmission of blood-borne infections and current knowledge of the epidemiology of HIV.

The Centers for Disease Control strategies for infection control describe appropriate handling of blood, body fluids, and items soiled with these. In many instances, patients who are capable of transmitting blood-borne infections are not identified,[179] and therefore universal precautions should be used during *all* patient contact. The Centers for Disease Control guidelines are summarized in Table 4-6. Although exposure to blood carries the greatest risk of occupationally related transmission of HIV and hepatitis B virus, the Centers for Disease Control states that universal precautions also apply to semen, vaginal secretions, human tissues, and the following body fluids: cerebrospinal, synovial, pleural, peritoneal, pericardial, and amniotic.[192] Universal precautions do not apply to feces, nasal secretions, sputum, sweat, tears, urine, and vomitus, unless they contain visible blood.[192] The categorization of risk of transmission is based on epidemiologic surveys of health care workers, but proof of transmission through many of these body fluids is unknown. Although universal precautions do not apply to saliva, general infection control practice recommends use of gloves when a health care worker is in contact with mucous membranes and oral fluids, such as during endotracheal intubation and pharyngeal suctioning.

Observational surveys of health care workers indicate that in many instances universal precautions are not being followed.[179] Reasons given by personnel include lack of time and that protective gear or equipment interfered with their technical abilities. Although many health care workers were trained before the introduction of universal precautions, the procedures can be incorporated into routine practice without undue difficulty. There is now direct evidence that implementation of universal precautions decreases the number of exposure incidents that result in worker contact with patient blood and body fluids.[193]

The Occupational Safety and Health Administration has proposed standards to protect employees from occupational exposure to blood-borne pathogens.[194] After finalization and publication of this standard, employers will be required to comply with the federal regulations. This will involve providing essential protective equipment, educational activities, and medical follow-up of personnel at risk for occupational exposure to blood-borne pathogens.

Slow Viruses

Creutzfeldt-Jakob disease, caused by a slow virus, may be unsuspected in patients presenting with dementia. The risk of transmission to hospital personnel seems low, but the long period from the time of infection until the onset of symptoms makes epidemiologic surveillance difficult.[195] Care must be taken in handling specimens from patients with suspected Creutzfeldt-Jakob disease. Gloves should be used to prevent contact with spinal fluid, blood, or tissue specimens. Careful hand washing is essential. Use of ethylene oxide, steam sterilization, or disinfection with 0.5% sodium hypochlorite or iodine is effective for eradication of the virus from equipment.

Tuberculosis

Although the incidence of tuberculosis in the United States had been declining, there was an increase in reported cases in 1986.[196] This reversal in the decline of new cases of tuberculosis is in part due to the prevalence of the disease in individuals with HIV infection. Most infected patients are treated on an outpatient basis, but undiagnosed patients with the disease may be hospitalized for work-up for pulmonary pathology. Hospital personnel are especially at risk for infection from unrecognized cases.[197,198] Tuberculosis may not be suspected until a routine culture report is returned or it may not be recognized until an autopsy is performed. Some of the high-risk groups for tuberculosis include (1) individuals with HIV infection, (2) personal contacts of persons with tuberculosis, (3) persons from countries with a high prevalence of tuberculosis, and (4) alcoholics and intravenous drug users.[199]

Tuberculous infection is transmitted through viable bacilli in sputum and aerosolization of sputum by coughing. Respiratory isolation should be used for hospitalized patients with tuberculosis until they are confirmed as nontransmitters by sputum examination that demonstrates no bacilli.[200,201] Chemotherapy is the most effective means to prevent spread of tuberculous infection. Elective surgery should be postponed until infected individuals have had an adequate course of chemotherapy.[200] Disposable anesthesia breathing circuits or sterilization of equipment is necessary when managing patients with untreated tuberculous infection. The Centers for Disease Control recommends that face masks, designed to filter out particles 1–5 μ in diameter, be worn by health care workers when in proximity with patients who are infectious and during procedures such as endotracheal suctioning that are likely to produce aerosolized droplets.[201]

Personnel who may have been infected by an unrecognized contagious tuberculous patient should be followed by skin testing. Persons who have recently converted their skin test and personnel with negative skin test findings who have high-risk contacts with infected patients should be counseled on the need for isoniazid therapy. Routine periodic screening of employees for tuberculosis should be included as part of a hospital's employee health policy.

Viruses in Laser Plumes

The laser is commonly being used for vaporizing carcinomatous and viral tumors. Use of lasers is associated with several hazards, both to patients and to operating room personnel. Risks include thermal burns, eye injuries, electrical hazards, and fires and explosions. Additionally, there is now evidence that the laser plumes resulting from tissue vaporization contain toxic chemicals such as formaldehyde. Clinical and laboratory studies have demonstrated that when the carbon dioxide laser is used to treat verrucae (papilloma and warts), intact viral DNA could be recovered from the plume.[202] Scientists at the Center for Devices and Radiological Health used an *in vitro* model to demonstrate that viable viruses can be found in plumes produced by both carbon dioxide and argon laser vaporization of a virus-loaded culture plate.[203]

To protect operating room personnel from exposure to the viral and chemical content of the laser plume, it is recommended that the tubing from a smoke evacuator be held within 2 inches of the tissue being vaporized.[204] This will effectively remove the particulate material in the plume by trapping it in the filter of the evacuator. Although high filtration masks have been suggested for use by operating room personnel, these may not be effective if improper fit results in leakage around the masks.[205,206]

Recent concern over occupationally acquired hepatitis B and AIDS has resulted in heightened attention to the use of infection control procedures in anesthesia practice. Current strategies for reducing the spread of blood-borne infectious agents are based on the use of physical barriers such as gloves, gowns, masks, and eye glasses and immunologic protection using active or passive immunization. These barrier mechanisms are also effective in preventing transmission of other pathogens. It is essential to have regular educational programs for all employees who are at risk for occupationally acquired infections. There should be a system in place in every hospital for maintaining immunization records and for follow-up of workers with accidental exposures.

EMOTIONAL CONSIDERATIONS

Stress

Among the potential health hazards of working in the operating room, stress is well recognized.[207] However, despite this wide recognition, there is very little objective information specifically directed toward understanding the nature of job-related stress among anesthesiologists.

The problem of stress has been studied in air traffic controllers,[208,209] and this may provide some close analogies to help understand the problem and relate it to anesthesiologists. This context also permits refining definitions, as the general concept of stress can be obscure. It may be helpful to consider the concept of *stress*, as used in engineering—the objective demands placed on an individual—and *strain*—the subjective response to these demands. Psychological *stress* occurs when an individual must deal with a situation in which his or her typical response pattern promises to be inadequate, and the consequences of not responding appropriately will be serious. The *strain* on an individual is a direct result of the stresses in conjunction with variables such as experience, aptitude, skills, age, and personality. The response of an individual to these stresses and strains is a consequence of defense mechanisms, which serve to alter the individual's perception of the situation, and coping mechanisms, which attempt to modify the objective nature of the situation.

What are the conditions in anesthesiologists' workplaces that account for the stress in their professional life? Many of these conditions are shared by both anesthesiologists and air traffic controllers, including an excessive workload, the process of making difficult decisions, night duty, fatigue, increasing reliance on technology, and interpersonal tensions.[210,211] Those areas that are specific to the practice of anesthesiology are the anesthetic induction, overlapping areas of responsibility with the surgeon, and dealing with the critically ill or dying patient.

It is not surprising to note that the process of inducing anesthesia produces a great deal of stress in the practitioner. Although this observation is self-evident to any anesthesiologist, documentation is limited. Two reports have demonstrated changes in heart rate[212] and blood pressure[213] in the anesthesiologist during the anesthetic induction. Individual observations from these studies included cardiac arrhythmias (premature ventricular contractions), ischemic changes on the electrocardiogram, and a blood pressure elevation to as high as 193/137 mm Hg.

Interpersonal relationships impose a unique set of demands that may serve as stressors to the anesthesiologist. In most locations within a hospital or clinic setting (e.g., radiology department, pathology laboratory, or during evaluation and treatment as a consultant), the direct responsibility for a patient is temporarily transferred to the consulting physician. The operating room is probably the only arena where two coequal physicians simultaneously share ultimate responsibility for the well-being of a patient.[214] To many anesthesiologists and surgeons, the overlapping of realms of responsibility produces the highest degree of stress in their clinical practices.

The level of training and degree of experience play a role in determining the amount of strain perceived by an anesthesiologist. It has been shown that an inverse relationship exists between the duration of clinical experience and the level of anxiety[215] and hemodynamic changes[212] occurring in the anesthesiologist during the anesthetic induction.

Stress on the job is unavoidable and to a certain degree is desirable. Several factors determine the nature of the individual anesthesiologist's response to stress. Commonly employed defense mechanisms include denial, intellectualization, reaction formation, and repression. Humor, denial, displacement of affect (anger), and projection are examples of coping mechanisms that are frequently utilized. The success of these defense and coping mechanisms depends on the degree of the individual's personal integrity, the range of his or her defense repertory, and the level of his or her coping abilities. To a large extent, personality characteristics dictate which defense and coping mechanisms are employed and how successfully they function.

Several studies have focused on personality characteristics, some identifiable prior to entrance to medical school, that appear to predispose the individual to maladaptive responses to stress.[216,217] Prominent among these traits is the obsessive-compulsive, dependent character structure. These individuals typically manifest pessimism, passivity, self-doubt, and feelings of insecurity, and commonly they respond to stress by internalizing anger and becoming hypochrondriacal and depressed. In work reported by Vaillant, undergraduate students who demonstrated these characteristics were more likely than controls to have their medical careers disrupted by alcoholism or drug abuse, psychiatric illness, and marital disturbances.[217]

It is crucial to remember that stress on the job is a two-sided coin and may produce either a decrease or improvement in job performance. Only when the magnitude of the stress exceeds the individual's threshold do his or her defenses become exaggerated and inappropriate. It is this situation that gives rise to maladaptive behavior and the personal and professional deterioration that can lead to disorders such as drug addiction.

Substance Use, Abuse, and Addiction

Illicit drug use and the risk of addiction are ever-increasing concerns in Western society. It has been estimated that as many as 22 million Americans have experimented with cocaine and 4–5 million are regular users of cocaine. Drugs have now become a $110 billion per year habit for Americans. In addition, estimates of the prevalence of alcoholism in the population run as high as 10%.

Epidemiology

The abuse of drugs by physicians has gained considerable media attention and notoriety. However, recognition of the problem of substance abuse among physicians is not new. In the first edition of The Principles and Practice of Medicine, edited by Sir William Osler and published in 1892, it is stated: "The habit [morphia] is particularly prevalent among women and physicians who use the hypodermic syringe for the alleviation of pain, as in neuralgia or sciatica."[218] Two years later, Mattison commented: "It is a fact—striking though sad—that more cases of morphinism are met with among medical men than in all other professions combined."[219]

Whether or not substance abuse is more prevalent among physicians than the general population is a subject worthy of debate. There is a large body of literature that attempts to support the notion that drug problems are more frequent among physicians.[220-222] The reported figure for drug and/or alcohol addiction among physicians varies from 10–40%.[223,224] Certainly, the lower estimate is not far out of line with that estimated for the adult population at large. However, if drug addiction alone is examined, the reported incidence of 1–2% among physicians is 30–100 times that seen in the general public.[225]

The data from which these estimates are drawn are notoriously difficult to collect and interpret. Bias in reporting technique alone can account for extremes in under- or over-estimating the actual prevalence of this disease.[226] In her extensive review of the English-language literature, Brewster finally concluded, "no one really knows how many practicing physicians are having problems with alcohol and other drugs."[225]

Reliable documentation exists that substance abuse is a significant problem among physicians and specifically among anesthesiologists.[227] At the present time, there are more addictive diseases among anesthesiologists than among any other medical specialists.[224] To some observers, addiction represents the primary occupational hazard for the specialty of anesthesiology.

These conclusions are drawn from a number of studies that examine the problem from various vantage points. One of the most easily accessed and frequently quoted sources of information on drug abuse comes from statistics on the number of individuals who are in drug treatment programs. However, there are major flaws inherent in this system of data collection. Before a physician is entered into any treatment program, he or she must first recognize that he or she has a drug problem. Unfortunately, denial is typically the first and most tenaciously maintained defense mechanism for the physician–substance abuser.

Even after recognizing that a drug-related problem exists, physicians are less likely than the population in general to seek professional assistance.[228] Again, denial plays a major role in this reluctance to undergo counseling or therapy. Medical students learn early in their education to employ denial mechanisms to enable them to endure long, sleepless nights and the personal shortcomings that inevitably must be faced in clinical medicine. These well-developed denial mechanisms encourage the physician-addict to conclude that his or her problem is minor and that self-treatment is possible. Physicians typically enter programs for treatment only after they have reached the end stages of their illness.

With these caveats in mind, it is still informative to look at the statistics pertaining to the number of anesthesiologists who are involved in treatment programs for drug-related illness. Probably the most extensive experience comes from the Medical Association of Georgia Disabled Doctors' Program.[224] Their study population includes 1000 disabled physicians, 920 of whom were treated for chemical dependency. One hundred and twenty-one of these patients were anesthesiologists (12%), although anesthesia accounts for only 3.9% of the American physician population. Even more troubling is the fact that anesthesia residents constitute 33.7% of the resident population in their treatment group, despite their representation as only 4.6% of the American resident population. Anesthesia residents have a 7.4 times excess representation in this treatment population.

Another approach to uncovering the prevalence of drug abuse among anesthesiologists is the directed survey. As with the statistics drawn from the drug treatment programs, there are major weaknesses inherent in this form of data collection. Most obvious is the willingness of the respondent to honestly and completely detail his or her experience in an area as sensitive as drug abuse.

One of the most extensive surveys was conducted by Ward et al.[229] They reported on the results of a questionnaire completed by 247 American anesthesia training programs. Sixty-four percent of the respondents identified at least one of their personnel as an abuser of drugs. In ten programs (4%), there were five or more such individuals identified during the 10-year study period (1970–1980). The overall incidence of suspected abuse was 1.3%, and confirmed abuse was 1.1%. The two most favored chemicals for abuse were reported to be meperidine and fentanyl, with a definite tendency toward the latter in the most recent half-decade of the study. This preference had previously been observed by Talbott, who had treated 105 fentanyl addicts among the 125 anesthesiologists admitted to his facility at the time.[230]

TABLE 4-7. Number of Drug and Alcohol Abusers Among Clinical Personnel in Gravenstein's Survey of Selected Academic Departments*

Year	Total Personnel	Drug Abusers	Alcoholics	Total
1974	358	3	3	6
1975	443	4	2	6
1976	583	5	5	10
1977	641	5	3	8
1978	763	13	1	14
1979	814	11	3	14

*Of concern is the increasing prevalence of drug abusers noted in the more recent years of the survey.

Reproduced with permission from Gravenstein JS, Kory WP, Marks RG: Drug abuse by anesthesia personnel. Anesth Analg 62:467, 1983

Similar results were obtained by Menk et al[231] and Gravenstein et al.[232] In Gravenstein's study, questionnaires regarding substance abuse were completed by chairmen of academic anesthesia departments, clinical personnel from these departments, and a group of third-year medical students. Seventy-six percent of the responding chairmen reported that one or more of their staff members had been affected by substance abuse during the period of study (1974–1979). Overall, 1–2% of the anesthesia personnel suffered from substance abuse and required some action from the chairman (Table 4-7).

Drug Addiction As a Disease

What accounts for this disproportionally high incidence of drug addiction among anesthesiologists? In order to answer this, it is best to view drug addiction as a psychosocial, biogenetic disease.[233] As such, the addiction (1) is a primary condition (not a symptom), (2) is associated with specific anatomic and physiologic changes, (3) has a set of recognizable signs and symptoms, (4) has a predictable, progressive course (if left untreated), and (5) has established etiologies.

It is important to recognize that the causative factors in this disease process involve genetics as well as the environment. The disease results from a dynamic interplay between a susceptible host and a "favorable" environment. Vulnerability in the host is an important factor. What constitutes an instigating exposure to a drug in one individual may have absolutely no effect on another. Unfortunately, there is no good predictive tool to identify the susceptible individual until he or she gets the disease.

There are causative factors specific to the specialty of anesthesiology. These include job stress, an orientation toward self-medication, lack of external recognition and self-respect, the availability of addicting drugs, and a susceptible premorbid personality.[234]

Self-prescription is commonly seen as a prelude to more extensive drug abuse and addiction. Similarly, recreational use of drugs may proceed to drug dependence, with the drug used for recreation usually becoming the primary drug of dependence.[235] Of concern is the increasing recreational use of drugs among younger physicians and medical students and the choice of more potent drugs with enhanced potential for addiction, such as cocaine and the newer synthetic opioids, fentanyl and sufentanil.[236] As a result, recreational drug use is becoming a leading source of impairment among younger physicians.[237]

The general public's image of the anesthesiologist frequently falls short of that of other physicians. In a report from Australia, only 66% of the patients knew that anesthesiologists needed medical qualifications, and less than 10% could remember their anesthesiologist's name.[238] It is even more distressing when coworkers in the medical field fail to recognize the special skills and contributions of anesthesiologists. In another study from Australia, only 83% of hospital nurses knew that anesthesiologists had to be medically qualified.[239]

Positive reinforcement and a sense of a job "well done" are important components of job satisfaction.[240] It is more difficult for the anesthesiologist than the surgeon to achieve recognition from patients and medical colleagues for a successful outcome. The Rodney Dangerfield syndrome—"I don't get no respect"—has been cited by several authors as an instigating factor in drug experimentation.[234]

Anesthesiologists work in a climate in which a large quantity of powerful psychoactive drugs is freely available. From the experience of the United States Army in Vietnam, it is apparent that when there is easy access to narcotics, alcohol use declines in favor of use of opiates.[241] As each new synthetic opioid becomes available for clinical use, it also becomes the drug of choice of abusing anesthesiologists. Currently, fentanyl is seen most frequently as the abused drug, but sufentanil is rapidly increasing in popularity.[230]

Since availability of drugs does play a role in the onset of this disease, it is logical that programs to better audit the distribution of drugs within the operating room setting should be a valuable preventive measure. Two university-affiliated anesthesiology departments have published their protocols for better controlling the distribution of these medications.[242,243] Talbott et al acknowledge that the strategies advocated within the anesthesia community are better than those of our colleagues in other medical specialties.[224] However, these are mainly limited to academic centers and require wider dissemination to be effective.

There is an apparent link between behavior prior to entering medical school and subsequent development of drug abuse.[244] At least one study examining personality profiles of anesthesiologists revealed a disturbingly high proportion with a predisposition toward maladaptive behavior.[245] Talbott et al have observed that many of the anesthesia residents in their treatment program specifically chose the specialty of anesthesiology because of the known availability of powerful drugs.[224] It is apparent that residency selection committees must begin to screen for personality disorders as an important part of the admissions process.

The consequences of substance abuse are ultimately devastating to the practicing anesthesiologist. If left untreated, addiction is a fatal illness. In the study reported by Ward et al, among the 334 confirmed drug abusers, 27 died of "drug overdose," and in another three, "abuse was discovered at death."[229] Gravenstein et al reported seven deaths among 44 confirmed drug abusers.[232] In the Menk et al study, there were 14 drug-related deaths (18%) among the 79 drug abusers who had been re-enrolled in their anesthesiology residencies after treatment.[231]

Intentional or inadvertent drug-related death is, of course, only one of the potential consequences of substance abuse (Table 4-8). More common is a gradual and inexorable deterioration in professional, family, and social relationships. The substance abuser becomes increasingly withdrawn and isolated, first in his or her personal life, and ultimately in his or her professional existence. Every attempt is made to maintain a facade of normalcy at work, because discovery means isolation from the source of the abused drug. When

TABLE 4-8. Signs of Substance Abuse and Addiction

Social

Withdrawal from leisure activities, friends, family
Uncharacteristic or inappropriate behavior in social gatherings
Impulsive behavior, e.g., overspending, gambling
Domestic turmoil, e.g., separation from spouse, child abuse, sexual problems
Change in behavior of spouse or children
Legal problems, e.g., arrest for driving while intoxicated

Health

Deterioration in personal hygiene
Accidents
Numerous health complaints; frequent need for medical attention for unrelated illnesses

Professional

Unreliability, e.g., missed appointments, inappropriate response to emergency calls, absences, poor record keeping
Complaints by patients or staff, subject of hospital gossip
Overprescription of medicines, excessive ordering of drugs from mail-order houses
Unstable employment history, e.g., several relocations
Working at a level below qualifications

Reproduced with permission from Spiegelman WG, Saunders L, Mazze RI: Addiction and anesthesiology. Anesthesiology 60:335, 1984

professional conduct is finally impaired such that it is apparent to the physician's colleagues, the disease is approaching its end stage.

In addition to the health hazards of drug addiction, there are significant legal and medicolegal considerations.[246] Each state has laws that detail the necessary steps for handling the drug-abusing physician. Most states require reporting such physicians to the licensing board and impose a criminal penalty upon those who knowingly fail to do so. Disciplinary action taken as a result of such a disability must also be reported to the National Practitioner Data Bank in order to be in compliance with federal law.

An interesting debate is emerging regarding the issue of compulsory drug testing of physicians.[247,248] Random drug testing protocols have already been established in various high-risk industries (nuclear, aviation) and the military. Several large teaching hospitals have announced their intention to initiate similar programs to test their staff physicians. Although many agree that this is a step in the right direction, questions remain about the legality and effectiveness of this approach.

A very aggressive program of detection and intervention is critical if careers and lives are to be saved. If left untreated, less than 30% of addicted physicians will be practicing in 10 years and some 10% will have died from their disease. On the other hand, physicians are generally highly motivated and high rehabilitation rates can be expected. Anesthesiologists appear to have a recovery rate approximating that of other physicians.[223] In the report of Ward et al, approximately 55% of the confirmed drug abusers underwent rehabilitation, and half of these were offered re-employment in their original departments.[229]

The anesthesiology department at the University of Pennsylvania has reported its policy for dealing with the problem of substance abuse.[249] It is important that an intervention process and referral arrangements be in place and that con-

frontation of suspected abusers be handled by trained individuals with appropriate skills.

Some controversy remains about the ultimate career path of the recovering addicted anesthesiologist. Prior to the reports by Talbott et al[224] and Ward et al,[229] most recovering addicts were discouraged from continuing their careers in anesthesiology. However, Talbott's, Ward's, and other encouraging reports during the 1980s provided optimism that these individuals could be successfully rehabilitated and safely returned to their practice of anesthesiology.

A more recent report by Menk and colleagues casts some doubt on the advisability of re-entry into the field for all anesthesiologists who have been treated for chemical dependency.[231] Among 79 opioid-addicted anesthesiology residents, there was a 66% (52 of 79) failure rate for successful rehabilitation and return to practice. Even more discouraging, there were 14 suicide or overdose deaths among those 79 returning trainees. Their conclusion is that redirection into another specialty is the safer course following rehabilitation.

Because of conflicting data, no firm recommendations can be made about re-entry into the practice of anesthesia after treatment. The ASA has published a sample chemical dependency policy for departments of anesthesiology.[250] This document describes the process of re-entry and provides a model for a re-entry contract that can be used when it is felt that a recovering anesthesiologist is ready to come back into practice.

Impairment

Substance abuse probably accounts for some 85% of the cases of impairment* among physicians.[251] Other factors that may lead to impairment include physical or mental illness and deterioration owing to the aging process. Some authorities include unwillingness or inability to keep up with current literature and techniques as a form of disability.

Data regarding the prevalence of these disabling disorders are more difficult to obtain than are those on drug abuse. Statistics derived from the admitting diagnoses to various psychiatric facilities indicate that close to 1% of those admitted are physicians.[252] In the order of increasing frequency, admission is required for organic psychoses, personality disorders, schizophrenia, neuroses, and affective disorders—particularly depression.[253]

It is not surprising that depression should figure prominently among the personality characteristics of emotionally impaired physicians. Indeed, many of the personality traits that are adaptive and assure success in the physician's world may also serve as risk factors for depression when exaggerated. These character traits include self-sacrifice, competitiveness, achievement orientation, denial of feelings, and intellectualization of emotions.[254] Two studies on alcoholic physicians provide some insight into this link between achievement orientation and emotional disturbance. Bissell and Jones reported that more than half of their group of alcoholic physicians graduated in the upper one third of their medical school class, 23% were in the upper one tenth, and only 5% were in the lower one third of their class.[255]

---

* An impaired physician is defined as one "whose performance as a professional person and as a practitioner of the healing arts is impaired because of alcoholism, drug abuse, mental illness, senility, or disabling disease."[248]

Similarly, a report on alcohol use in medical school demonstrated better first-year grades and higher scores on Part I—National Board of Medical Examiners among those students identified as alcohol abusers.[256] Alcohol abuse clearly does not enhance the learning process. Rather, the alcohol abuse is a manifestation of psychological disturbance resulting from excessive degrees of stress among some students who are most determined to have flawless records.

When all of these forms of impairment are considered, it is estimated that as many as 10% of practicing physicians are seriously impaired.[257] Fortunately, in recent years, most state legislatures and medical societies have formally recognized this problem and have enacted laws and formed committees that address the impaired physician. These programs are generally therapeutic and nonpunitive in nature. Ideally, the committees provide a nonthreatening environment for identification and intervention of the impaired physician. Only in cases in which a real risk to the public welfare exists and the involved physician is unwilling to voluntarily suspend practice and accept assistance is the license suspension power of the State Board of Medical Examiners exercised. Management protocols for dealing with the impaired physician are covered in a series of articles by Canavan.[258]

Suicide

Perhaps one of the most alarming of the occupationally associated hazards for anesthesiologists is the high rate of suicide.[29,30,33,260] The incidence is three to four times the suicide rate expected among a contemporary, otherwise comparable socioeconomic group and exceeds that of all but one or two other medical specialties.[259] A high incidence of suicide has also been observed among residents in anesthesiology training programs. A report from England has identified five deaths from suicide over a recent 5-year period in this group.[261] Their ratio of 1 suicide per 500 residents compares unfavorably with the approximately 1 suicide per 12,000 in the general U.S. population and 1 suicide in 4000 for physicians per year.[262]

Why should there be such a high rate of suicide among anesthesiologists? A partial explanation lies with the high degree of stress that is an integral part of the job. The relationship between generalized stress and suicide is not direct. But, clearly, in susceptible individuals, feelings of inability to cope resulting from overwhelming stress may give way to despair and suicide ideation.

Extensive personality profiles have been collected from suicide-susceptible individuals; these indicate characteristics such as high anxiety, insecurity, low self-esteem, impulsiveness, and poor self-control. It is disturbing to note that in Reeve's study of personality traits of a sample of anesthesiologists, some 20% manifested psychological profiles that reflected a predisposition to behavioral disintegration and attempted suicide when placed under extremes of stress.[245] His study raises the discomforting notion that "premorbid" personality characteristics that exist prior to entering speciality training are not being identified in the admissions process.[263,264]

One specific type of stress, that resulting from a malpractice lawsuit, may have a direct causative association with suicide among physicians in general and anesthesiologists in particular. An anecdotal report described, in tragic detail, the emotional deterioration and ultimate suicide of an experienced and previously healthy physician involved in a malpractice suit.[265] One study specifically identified the anesthesiologist involved in a lawsuit as being at particularly high risk for suicide.[266] In this report, four of 185 anesthesiologists being sued attempted or committed suicide.

Another potential etiologic basis for the observed high suicide rate is the high incidence of drug abuse found among anesthesia personnel.[231,232] Physicians who are impaired and whose privileges to practice medicine are removed by the licensing authority are at heightened risk of attempting suicide. Crawshaw et al reported eight successful and two near-miss suicide attempts among 43 physicians placed on probation for drug-related disability.[267] Other occupational factors that may contribute to the high incidence of suicide include isolation and lack of colleagues' support at work and the ready access to various means of carrying out the act of suicide.

REFERENCES

1. Werthmann H: Chronic ether intoxication in surgeons. Beitr Klin Chir 178:149, 1949 (Ger)
2. American Society of Anesthesiologists Ad Hoc Committee on the Effect of Trace Anesthetics on the Health of Operating Room Personnel: Occupational disease among operating room personnel: A national study. Anesthesiology 41:321, 1974
3. Cohen EN, Brown BW, Bruce DL et al: A survey of anesthetic health hazards among dentists. J Am Dent Assoc 90:1291, 1975
4. Ferstandig LL: Trace concentrations of anesthetic gases: A critical review of their disease potential. Anesth Analg 57:328, 1978
5. Lecky JH: Problems of trace anesthetic levels. In Orkin FK, Cooperman LH (eds): Complications in Anesthesiology, p 715. Philadelphia, JB Lippincott, 1983
6. Buring JE, Hennekens CH, Mayrent SL et al: Health experiences of operating room personnel. Anesthesiology 62:325, 1985
7. Vessey MP: Epidemiological studies of the occupational hazards of anaesthesia—A review. Anaesthesia 33:430, 1978
8. Spence AA, Knill-Jones RP: Is there a health hazard in anaesthetic practice? Br J Anaesth 50:713, 1978
9. Linde HW, Bruce DL: Occupational exposure of anesthetists to halothane, nitrous oxide and radiation. Anesthesiology 30:363, 1969
10. Whitcher CE, Cohen EN, Trudell JR: Chronic exposure to anesthetic gases in the operating room. Anesthesiology 35:348, 1971
11. Corbett TH: Retention of anesthetic agents following occupational exposure. Anesth Analg 52:614, 1973
12. Flemming DC, Johnstone RE: Recognition thresholds for diethyl ether and halothane. Anesthesiology 46:68, 1977
13. National Institute for Occupational Safety and Health (NIOSH): Criteria for a Recommended Standard . . . Occupational Exposure to Waste Anesthetic Gases and Vapors. Department of Health, Education, and Welfare (NIOSH) Publication No. 77–140. Cincinnati, Ohio
14. Lecky JH: The mechanical aspects of anesthetic pollution control. Anesth Analg 56:769, 1977
15. Whitcher C, Piziali RL: Monitoring occupational exposure to inhalation anesthetics. Anesth Analg 56:778, 1977
16. The American Society of Anesthesiologists Ad Hoc Committee on Effects of Trace Anesthetic Agents on Health of Operating Room Personnel: Waste Anesthetic Gases in Operating Room Air: A Suggested Program to Reduce Personnel Exposure. Park Ridge, American Society of Anesthesiologists
17. Lecky JH: Anesthetic pollution in the operating room: A notice to operating room personnel. Anesthesiology 52:157, 1980
18. Rajhans GS, Brown DA, Whaley DA et al: Evaluation of occupational exposure to waste anesthetic gases in Ontario hospitals. Ann Occup Hyg 33:27, 1989
19. Gray WM: Occupational exposure to nitrous oxide in four hospitals. Anaesthesia 44:511, 1989

20. Walts LF, Forsythe AB, Moore JG: Critique: Occupational disease among operating room personnel. Anesthesiology 42:608, 1975

21. Vaisman AL: Working conditions in surgery and their effect on the health of anesthesiologists. Eksp Khir Anesteziol 3:44, 1967

22. Fink BR, Cullen BF: Anesthetic pollution: What is happening to us? Anesthesiology 45:79, 1976

23. Axelsson G, Rylander R: Exposure to anaesthetic gases and spontaneous abortion: Response bias in a postal questionnaire study. Int J Epidemiol 11:250, 1982

24. Cohen EN, Bellville JW, Brown BW: Anesthesia, pregnancy, and miscarriage: A study of operating room nurses and anesthetists. Anesthesiology 35:343, 1971

25. Knill-Jones RP, Moir DD, Rodrigues LV et al: Anaesthetic practice and pregnancy: Controlled survey of women anaesthetists in the United Kingdom. Lancet 2:1326, 1972

26. Rosenberg P, Kirves A: Miscarriages among operating theatre staff. Acta Anaesthesiol Scand 53 (suppl):37, 1973

27. Mazze RI, Lecky JH: The health of operating room personnel. Anesthesiology 62:226, 1985

28. McDonald AD, McDonald JC, Armstrong B et al: Fetal death and work in pregnancy. Br J Ind Med 45:148, 1988

29. Bruce DL, Eide KA, Linde HW et al: Causes of death among anesthesiologists: A 20-year survey. Anesthesiology 29:565, 1968

30. Bruce DL, Eide KA, Smith NJ et al: A prospective survey of anesthesiologist mortality, 1967–1971. Anesthesiology 41:71, 1974

31. Mazze RI: Waste anesthetic gases and the regulatory agencies. Anesthesiology 52:248, 1980

32. Doll R, Peto R: Mortality among doctors in different occupations. Br Med J 1:1433, 1977

33. Lew EA: Mortality experience among anesthesiologists, 1954–1976. Anesthesiology 51:195, 1979

34. Jackson SH: Anesthetics and cell multiplication. Clin Anesth 11:75, 1975

35. Nunn JF, Sharer N: Inhibition of methionine synthetase by trace concentrations of nitrous oxide. Br J Anaesth 53:1099, 1981

36. Koblin DD, Watson JE, Deady JE et al: Inactivation of methionine synthetase by nitrous oxide in mice. Anesthesiology 54:318, 1981

37. Nunn JF, Sharer N: Serum methionine and hepatic enzyme activity in anaesthetists exposed to nitrous oxide. Br J Anaesth 54:593, 1982

38. Corbett TH: Cancer and congenital anomalies associated with anesthetics. Ann NY Acad Sci 271:58, 1976

39. Eger EI, White AE, Brown CL et al: A test of the carcinogenicity of enflurane, isoflurane, halothane, methoxyflurane and nitrous oxide in mice. Anesth Analg 57:678, 1978

40. Coate WB, Ulland BM, Lewis TR: Chronic exposure to low concentrations of halothane-nitrous oxide: Lack of carcinogenic effect in the rat. Anesthesiology 50:306, 1979

41. Baden JM, Mazze RI, Wharton RS et al: Carcinogenicity of halothane in Swiss/ICR mice. Anesthesiology 51:20, 1979

42. Baden JM, Egbert B, Mazze RI: Carcinogen bioassay of enflurane in mice. Anesthesiology 56:9, 1982

43. Baden JM, Brinkenhoff M, Wharton RS et al: Mutagenicity of volatile anesthetics: Halothane. Anesthesiology 45:311, 1976

44. Baden JM, Kelley M, Wharton RS et al: Mutagenicity of halogenated ether anesthetics. Anesthesiology 46:346, 1977

45. Baden JM, Kelley M, Cheung A et al: Lack of mutagens in urines of operating room personnel. Anesthesiology 53:195, 1980

46. Tennant RW, Margolin BH, Shelby MD et al: Prediction of chemical carcinogenicity in rodents from in vitro genetic toxicity assays. Science 236:933, 1987

47. Chang LW, Katz J: Pathologic effects of chronic halothane inhalation: An overview. Anesthesiology 45:640, 1976

48. Ross WT: Are effects of halothane on hepatocytes "pathologic"? Anesthesiology 47:76, 1977

49. Coate WB, Kapp RW, Lewis TR: Chronic exposure to low concentrations of halothane-nitrous oxide: Reproductive and cytogenetic effects in the rat. Anesthesiology 50:310, 1979

50. Vieura E, Cleaton-Jones P, Austin JC et al: Effects of low concentrations of nitrous oxide on rat fetuses. Anesth Analg 59:175, 1980

51. Mazze RI: Fertility, reproduction and postnatal survival in mice chronically exposed to isoflurane. Anesthesiology 63:663, 1985

52. Wyrobek AJ, Brodsky J, Gordon L et al: Sperm studies in anesthesiologists. Anesthesiology 55:527, 1981

53. Land PC, Owen EL: Nitrous oxide does not alter spermatogenesis in the mouse. Anesthesiology 53:S255, 1980

54. White AE, Takehisa S, Eger EI et al: Sister chromatid exchanges induced by inhaled anesthetics. Anesthesiology 50:426, 1979

55. Husum B, Wulf HC, Niebuhr E: Monitoring of sister chromatid exchanges in lymphocytes of nurse-anesthetists. Anesthesiology 62:475, 1985

56. Bruce DL, Bach MJ, Arbit J: Trace anesthetic effects on perceptual, cognitive and motor skills. Anesthesiology 40:453, 1974

57. Bruce DL, Bach MJ: Effects of trace anaesthetic gases on behavioural performance of volunteers. Br J Anaesth 48:871, 1976

58. Smith G, Shirley AW: A review of the effects of trace concentrations of anaesthetics on performance. Br J Anaesth 50:701, 1978

59. Geraci CL: Operating room pollution: Governmental perspectives and guidelines. Anesth Analg 56:775, 1977

60. NIOSH recommendations for occupational safety and health standard. MMWR 37(suppl no 5–7):1, 1988

61. Cromer J, Kronoveter K: A Study of Methylmethacrylate Exposure and Employee Health. Department of Health, Education, and Welfare Publication No. 77–119 (NIOSH). Washington DC, U.S. Government Printing Office, 1976

62. Poss R, Thilly WG, Kaden DA: Methylmethacrylate is a mutagen for Salmonella typhimurium. J Bone Joint Surg 61A:1203, 1979

63. Taylor G: A scavenging device for venting methylmethacrylate monomer vapor. Anesthesiology 41:612, 1974

64. Pickering CAC, Bainbridge D, Birtwistle IH et al: Occupational asthma due to methyl methacrylate in an orthopaedic theatre sister. Br Med J 292:1362, 1986

65. Lee CM: Unusual reaction to methyl methacrylate monomer. Anesth Analg 63:371, 1984

66. Schwettmann RS, Casterline CL: Delayed asthmatic response following occupational exposure to enflurane. Anesthesiology 44:166, 1976

67. Klatskin G, Kimberg DV: Recurrent hepatitis attributable to halothane sensitization in an anesthetist. N Engl J Med 280:515, 1969

68. National Council on Radiation Protection and Measurements. Radiation Protection for Medical and Allied Health Personnel. Report No 48. Washington DC, 1977

69. Laughlin JS: Experience with a sustained policy of radiation exposure control and research in a medical center. Health Phys 5:709, 1981

70. Giachino AA, Cheng M: Irradiation of the surgeon during pinning of femoral fractures. J Bone Joint Surg 62B:227, 1980

71. Poznanski AK, Kanellitsas C, Roloff DW et al: Radiation exposure to personnel in a neonatal nursery. Pediatrics 54:139, 1974

72. Kan K, Santen BC, Velthuyse HJM et al: Exposure of radiologists to scattered radiation during radiodiagnostic examinations. Radiology 119:455, 1976

73. Santen BC, Kan K, Velthuyse HJM et al: Exposure of radiologists to scattered radiation during angiography. Radiology 115:447, 1975

74. Burks J, Griffith P, McCormick K et al: Radiation exposure to nursing personnel from patients receiving diagnostic radionuclides. Heart Lung 11:217, 1982

75. Liu J, Edwards FM: Radiation exposure to medical personnel during iodine-125 seed implantation of the prostate. Radiology 132:748, 1979

76. Hodge B, Thompson JF: Noise pollution in the operating theatre. Lancet 335:891, 1990

77. National Institutes of Health Consensus Conference. Noise and hearing loss. Conn Med 54:385, 1990

78. Olmeda EL, Kirk RE: Maintenance of vigilance by non-task

related stimulation in the monitoring environment. Percept Mot Skills 44:715, 1977

79. Gaba DM, Maxwell M, DeAnda A: Anesthetic mishaps: Breaking the chain of accident evolution. Anesthesiology 66:670, 1987

80. Thackray RI, Bailey JP, Touchstone RM: The effect of increased monitoring load on vigilance performance using a simulated radar display. Ergonomics 22:529, 1979

81. Paget NS, Lambert TF, Sridhar K: Factors affecting an anaesthetist's work: Some findings on vigilance and performance. Anaesth Intensive Care 9:359, 1981

82. Cooper JB, Newbower RS, Kitz RJ: An analysis of major errors and equipment failures in anesthesia management: Considerations for prevention and detection. Anesthesiology 60:34, 1984

83. Weinger MB, Englund CE: Ergonomic and human factors affecting anesthetic vigilance and monitoring performance in the operating room environment. Anesthesiology 73:995, 1990

84. Friedman RL, Bigger JT, Kornfield DS: The intern and sleep loss. N Engl J Med 285:201, 1971

85. Morgan BB, Brown BR, Alluisi EA: Effects on sustained performance of 48 hours of continuous work and sleep loss. Hum Factors 16:406, 1974

86. Krueger GP: Sustained work, fatigue, sleep loss and performance: A review of the issues. Work & Stress 3:129, 1989

87. Denisco RA, Drummond JN, Gravenstein JS: The effect of fatigue on the performance of a simulated anesthetic monitoring task. J Clin Monit 3:22, 1987

88. Narang V, Laycock JRD: Psychomotor testing of on-call anesthetists. Anaesthesia 41:868, 1986

89. Catalano JF: Effect of perceived proximity to end of task upon end spurt. Percept Mot Skills 36:363, 1973

90. Mackworth JF: The effect of signal rate on performance in two kinds of vigilance task. Hum Factors 10:11, 1968

91. Guralnick MJ: Effects of event rate and signal difficulty on observing responses and detection measures in vigilance. J Exp Psychol 99:261, 1973

92. Gould JD, Schaffer A: The effects of divided attention on visual monitoring of multi-channel displays. Hum Factors 9:191, 1967

93. Stanford LM, McIntyre JWR, Nelson TM, Hogan JT: Affective responses to commercial and experimental auditory alarm signals for anesthesia delivery and physiological monitoring equipment. Int J Clin Monit Comput 5:111, 1988

94. McIntyre JWR: Ergonomics: Anaesthetists' use of auditory alarms in the operating room. Int J Clin Monit Comput 2:47, 1985

95. Davenport WG: Vigilance and arousal: Effects of different types of background stimulation. J Psychol 82:339, 1972

96. Wolf RH, Weiner FF: Effects of four noise conditions on arithmetic performance. Percept Mot Skills 35:928, 1972

97. Bruce DL, Bach MJ: Psychological studies of human performance as affected by traces of enflurane and nitrous oxide. Anesthesiology 42:194, 1975

98. Gamberale F, Svensson G: The effect of anaesthetic gases on the psychomotor and perceptual functions of anaesthetic nurses. Work Environ Health 11:108, 1974

99. Kortilla K, Pfaffli P, Linnoila M et al: Operating room nurses' psychomotor and driving skills after occupational exposure to halothane and nitrous oxide. Acta Anaesthesiol Scand 22:33, 1978

100. Kendall J: Vision considerations for the anesthesia machine operator. J Assoc Nurse Anesth 54:225, 1986

101. McIntyre JWR: Man-machine interface: The position of the anaesthesia machine in the operating room. Can Anaesth Soc J 29:74, 1982

102. Drui AB, Behm RJ, Martin WE: Predesign investigation of the anesthesia operational environment. Anesth Analg 52:584, 1973

103. Jerison HJ, Pickett RM: Vigilance: A review and reevaluation. Hum Factors 5:221, 1963

104. Childs JM, Halcomb CG: Effects of noise and response complexity upon vigilance performance. Percept Mot Skills 35:735, 1972

105. Human Engineering Design Criteria for Military Systems. U.S. Army Missile Command Standard MIL-STD-1472C

106. Boquet G, Bushman JA, Davenport HT: The anaesthetic machine—a study of function and design. Br J Anaesth 52:61, 1980

107. Calkins JM: Anesthesia equipment: Help or hindrance? In Stoelting RK, Barash PG (eds): Advances in Anesthesia, pp 377–406. New York, Gallagher Year Book Medical Publishers, 1985

108. Arnell WJ, Schultz DG: Computers in anesthesiology—a look ahead. Med Instrum 17:393, 1983

109. Smith NT, Quinn ML, Flick J: Automatic control in anesthesia: A comparison in performance between the anesthetist and the machine. Anesth Analg 63:715, 1984

110. Kraft HH, Lees DE: Closing the loop: How near is automated anesthesia? South Med J 77:7, 1984

111. Gravenstein JS, Cooper JB, Orkin FK: Work and rest cycles in anesthesia practice. Anesthesiology 72:737, 1990

112. Narang V, Laycock JRD: Psychomotor testing of on-call residents. Anaesthesia 41:868, 1986

113. Wallace-Barnhill GL, Florex G, Turndoff H et al: The effect of 24 hour duty on the performance of anesthesiology residents on vigilance, mood, and memory tasks. Anesthesiology 59:A460, 1983

114. McDonald JS, Peterson S: Lethal errors in anesthesiology. Anesthesiology 63:A497, 1985

115. Cooper JB, Newbower RS, Long CD et al: Preventable anesthesia mishaps: A study of human factors. Anesthesiology 49:399, 1978

116. McCall TB: The impact of long working hours on resident physicians. N Engl J Med 318:775, 1988

117. McCall TB: The Libby Zion case: One step forward or two steps backward? N Engl J Med 318:771, 1988

118. Hoffman DC, Dixon RE: Control of influenza in the hospital. Am Intern Med 87:725, 1977

119. Douglas RG: Prophylaxis and treatment of influenza. N Engl J Med 322:443, 1990

120. Tait AR, DuBoulay PM, Knight PR: Alterations in the course of and histopathologic response to influenza virus infections produced by enflurane, halothane, and diethyl ether anesthesia in ferrets. Anesth Analg 67:671, 1988

121. Hall CB, Douglas RG, Geiman JM: Possible transmission by fomites of respiratory syncytial virus. J Infect Dis 141:98, 1980

122. Leclair JM, Freeman J, Sullivan BF et al: Prevention of nosocomial respiratory syncytial virus infections through compliance with glove and gown isolation precautions. N Engl J Med 317:329, 1987

123. Agah R, Cherry JD, Garakian AJ, Chapin M: Respiratory syncytial virus (RSV) infection rate in personnel caring for children with RSV infections: Routine isolation procedure vs routine procedure supplemented by use of mask and goggles. Am J Dis Child 141:695, 1989

124. Centers for Disease Control: Varicella-zoster immune globulin for the prevention of chickenpox. Recommendations of the Immunization Practices Advisory Committee (ACIP). MMWR 33:84, 1984

125. McKinney WP, Horowitz MM, Battiola RJ: Susceptibility of hospital-based health care personnel to varicella-zoster virus infections. Am J Infect Control 17:26, 1989

126. Orkin FK: Herpetic whitlow. In Orkin FK, Cooperman LH (eds): Complications in Anesthesiology, p 706. Philadelphia: JB Lippincott, 1983

127. Juel-Jensen BE: Herpetic whitlow: An occupational risk. Anaesthesia 28:324, 1973

128. Rosato FE, Rosato EF, Plotkin SA: Herpetic paronychia—an occupational hazard of medical personnel. N Engl J Med 283:804, 1970

129. DeYoung GG, Harrison AW, Shapley JM: Herpes simplex cross infection in the operating room. Can Anaesth Soc J 15:394, 1968

130. Adler SP: Cytomegalovirus and child day care: Evidence for an increased infection rate among day-care workers. N Engl J Med 321:1290, 1989

131. Balcarek KB, Bagley R, Cloud GA, Pass RF: Cytomegalovirus infection among employees of a children's hospital: No evi-

dence for increased risk associated with patient care. JAMA 263:840, 1990

132. Balfour CL, Balfour HH: Cytomegalovirus is not an occupational risk for nurses in renal transplant or neonatal units: Results of a prospective surveillance study. JAMA 256:1909, 1986

133. Brady MT: Cytomegalovirus infections: Occupational risk for health professionals. Am J Infect Control 14:197, 1986

134. Edell TA, Howard C, Ferguson SW et al: Rubella in hospital personnel and patients—Colorado. MMWR 28:325, 1979

135. Polk BF, White JA, DeGirolami PC, Modlin JF: An outbreak of rubella among hospital personnel. N Engl J Med 303:541, 1980

136. Lerman SJ, Lerman LM, Nankervis GA, Gold E: Accuracy of rubella history. Am Intern Med 74:97, 1971

137. Advisory Committee on Immunization Practices: Rubella prevention. MMWR 33:301, 315, 1984

138. Davis R, Orenstein WA, Frank JA et al: Transmission of measles in medical settings: 1980 through 1984. JAMA 255:1295, 1986

139. Centers for Disease Control: Measles prevention: Recommendations of the Immunization Practices Advisory Committee (ACIP). MMWR 38 (no. S-9):1, 1989

140. Goodman RA, Carter CC, Allen JR et al: Nosocomial hepatitis A transmission by an adult patient with diarrhea. Am J Med 73:220, 1982

141. Favero MS, Maynard JE, Leger RT et al: Guidelines for the care of patients hospitalized with viral hepatitis. Ann Intern Med 91:872, 1979

142. Centers for Disease Control: Protection against viral hepatitis: Recommendations of the Immunization Practices Advisory Committee (ACIP). MMWR 39(no. RR-2):1, 1990

143. Denes AE, Smith JL, Maynard JE et al: Hepatitis B infection in physicians. Results of a nationwide seroepidemiologic survey. JAMA 239:210, 1978

144. Berry AJ, Isaacson IJ, Hunt D, Kane MA: The prevalence of hepatitis B viral markers in anesthesia personnel. Anesthesiology 60:6, 1984

145. Berry AJ, Isaacson IJ, Kane MA et al: A multicenter study of the prevalence of hepatitis B viral serologic markers in anesthesia personnel. Anesth Analg 63:738, 1984

146. Berry AJ, Isaacson IJ, Kane MA et al: A multicenter study of the epidemiology of hepatitis B in anesthesia residents. Anesth Analg 64:672, 1985

147. Fyman PN, Hartung J, Weinberg S, Stackhouse J: Prevalence of hepatitis B markers in the anesthesia staff in a large inner city hospital. Anesth Analg 63:433, 1984

148. Malm DN, Mathias RG, Turnbull KW et al: Prevalence of hepatitis B in anaesthesia personnel. Can Anaesth Soc J 33:167, 1986

149. Chernesky MA, Browne RA, Rondi P: Hepatitis B virus antibody prevalence in anesthetists. Can Anaesth Soc J 31:239, 1984

150. Siebke JC, Degre M: Prevalence of viral hepatitis in the staff in Norwegian anaesthesiology units. Acta Anaesthesiol Scand 28:549, 1984

151. Carstens J, Macnab GM, Kew MC: Hepatitis B virus infection in anaesthetists. Br J Anaesth 49:887, 1977

152. Sinclair ME, Ashby MW, Kurtz JB: The prevalence of serological markers for hepatitis B virus infection amongst anaesthetists in the Oxford region. Anaesthesia 42:30, 1987

153. Janzen J, Tripatzis I, Wagner U et al: Epidemiology of hepatitis B surface antigen (HBsAg) and antibody to HBsAg in hospital personnel. J Infect Dis 137:261, 1978

154. Ahtone J, Maynard JE: Laboratory diagnosis of hepatitis B. JAMA 249:2067, 1983

155. Linnemann CC, Hegg ME, Ramundo N, Schiff GM: Screening hospital patients for hepatitis B surface antigen. Am J Clin Pathol 67:257, 1977

156. Osterholm MT, Bravo ER, Crosson JT et al: Lack of transmission of viral hepatitis type B after oral exposure to HBsAg-positive saliva. Br Med J 2:1263, 1979

157. Bond WW, Favero MS, Peterson NJ et al: Survival of hepatitis B virus after drying and storage for one week. Lancet 1:550, 1981

158. Dienstag JL, Werner BG, Polk BF et al: Hepatitis B vaccine in health care personnel: Safety, immunogenicity and indicators of efficacy. Ann Int Med 101:34, 1984

159. Centers for Disease Control: Suboptimal response to hepatitis B vaccine given by injection into the buttock. MMWR 34:105, 1985

160. Francis DP, Feorino PM, McDougal S et al: The safety of the hepatitis B vaccine. Inactivation of the AIDS virus during routine vaccine manufacture. JAMA 256:869, 1986

161. Scolnick EM, McLean AA, West DJ et al: Clinical evaluation in healthy adults of a hepatitis B vaccine made by recombinant DNA. JAMA 251:2812, 1984

162. Brown SE, Stanley C, Howard CR et al: Antibody responses to recombinant and plasma derived hepatitis B vaccines. Br J Med 292:159, 1986

163. Hadler SC, Francis DP, Maynard JE et al: Long-term immunogenicity and efficacy of hepatitis B vaccine in homosexual men. N Engl J Med 315:209, 1986

164. Alter MJ, Hadler SC, Judson FN et al: Risk factors for acute non-A, non-B hepatitis in the United States and association with hepatitis C virus infection. JAMA 264:2231, 1990

165. Choo QL, Kuo G, Weiner AJ et al: Isolation of a cDNA clone derived from a bloodborne non-A, non-B viral hepatitis genome. Science 244:359, 1989

166. Kuo G, Choo QL, Alter JH et al: An assay for circulating antibodies to a major etiologic virus of human non-A, non-B hepatitis. Science 244:362, 1989

167. Mosley JW, Aach RD, Hollinger FB et al: Non-A, non-B hepatitis and antibody to hepatitis C virus. JAMA 263:77, 1990

168. Alter HJ, Purcell RH, Shih JW et al: Detection of antibody to hepatitis C virus in prospectively followed transfusion recipients with acute and chronic non-A, non-B hepatitis. N Engl J Med 321:1494, 1989

169. Everhart JE, DiBisceglie AM, Murray LM et al: Risk for non-A, non-B (type C) hepatitis through sexual or household contact with chronic carriers. Ann Intern Med 112:544, 1990

170. Mayo-Smith MF: Type non-A, non-B and type B hepatitis transmitted by a single needlestick. Am J Infect Control 15: 266, 1987

171. Ahtone J, Francis D, Bradley D, Maynard J: Non-A, non-B hepatitis in a nurse after percutaneous needle exposure. Lancet 1:1142, 1980

172. Gallo RC, Salahuddin SZ, Popovic M et al: Frequent detection and isolation of cytopathic retroviruses (HTLV-III) from patients with AIDS and at risk of AIDS. Science 224:500, 1984

173. Broder S: Pathogenic human retroviruses. N Engl J Med 318: 243, 1988

174. Lui KJ, Darrow WW, Rutherford GW: A model-based estimate of the mean incubation period for AIDS in homosexual men. Science 240:1333, 1988

175. Baltimore D, Feinberg MB: HIV revealed: Toward a natural history of the infection. N Engl J Med 321:1673, 1989

176. Centers for Disease Control: HIV/AIDS Surveillance Report, Rockville, Maryland, March 1991

177. Lifson AR: Do alternate modes for transmission of human immunodeficiency virus exist? A review. JAMA 259:1353, 1988

178. Castro KG, Lifson AR, White CR et al: Investigations of AIDS patients with no previously identified risk factors. JAMA 259:1338, 1988

179. Kelen GD, DiGiovanna T, Bisson L et al: Human immunodeficiency virus infection in emergency department patients: Epidemiology, clinical presentations, and risk to health care workers: The Johns Hopkins experience. JAMA 262:516, 1989

180. St. Louis ME, Rauch KJ, Petersen LR et al: Seroprevalence rates of human immunodeficiency virus infection at sentinal hospitals in the United States. N Engl J Med 323:213, 1990

181. Centers for Disease Control: Guidelines for prevention of transmission of human immunodeficiency virus and hepatitis B virus to health-care and public-safety workers. MMWR 38 (no. S-6):1, 1989

182. Marcus R, and the CDC Cooperative Needlestick Surveillance Group: Surveillance of health care workers exposed to blood from patients infected with the human immunodeficiency virus. N Engl J Med 319:1118, 1988

183. Henderson DK, Saah AJ, Zak BJ et al: Risk of nosocomial infection with human T-cell lymphotropic virus type III/lymphadenopathy-associated virus in a large cohort of intensively exposed health care workers. Am Int Med 104:644, 1986

184. Centers for Disease Control: Update: Acquired immunodeficiency syndrome and human immunodeficiency virus infection among health-care workers. MMWR 37:229, 1988

185. Kristensen MS, Sloth E, Jensen TK: Relationship between anesthetic procedure and contact of anesthesia personnel with patient body fluids. Anesthesiology 73:619, 1990

186. Jagger J, Hunt EH, Brand-Elnaggar J, Pearson RD: Rates of needle-stick injury caused by various devices in a university hospital. N Engl J Med 319:284, 1988

187. Mansour AM: Which physicians are at high risk for needlestick injuries? Am J Infect Control 18:208, 1990

188. Gerberding JL, Littel C, Tarkington A et al: Risk of exposure of surgical personnel to patients' blood during surgery at San Francisco General Hospital. N Engl J Med 322:1788, 1990

189. Centers for Disease Control: Public Health Service statement on management of occupational exposure to human immunodeficiency virus, including considerations regarding zidovudine postexposure use. MMWR 39(no. RR-1):1, 1990

190. Henderson DK, Gerberding JL: Prophylactic zidovudine after occupational exposure to the human immunodeficiency virus: An interim analysis. J Infect Dis 160:321, 1989

191. Lange JMA, Boucher CAB, Hollak CEM et al: Failure of zidovudine prophylaxis after accidental exposure to HIV-1. N Engl J Med 322:1375, 1990

192. Centers for Disease Control: Update: Universal precautions for prevention of transmission of human immunodeficiency virus, hepatitis B virus, and other bloodborne pathogens in health-care settings. MMWR 37:377, 1988

193. Wong ES, Stotka JL, Chinchilli VM et al: Are universal precautions effective in reducing the number of occupational exposures among health care workers? A prospective study of physicians on a medical service. JAMA 265:1123, 1991

194. Department of Labor, Occupational Safety and Health Administration: Occupational exposure to bloodborne pathogens: Proposed rule and notice of hearing. Fed Register 54:23042, 1989

195. Gajdusek DC, Gibbs CJ, Asher DM et al: Precautions in medical care of, and in handling materials from, patients with transmissible virus dementia (Creutzfeldt-Jakob disease). N Engl J Med 297:1253, 1977

196. Rieder HL, Cauthen GM, Kelly GD et al: Tuberculosis in the United States. JAMA 262:385, 1989

197. Kantor HS, Poblete R, Pusateri SL: Nosocomial transmission of tuberculosis from unsuspected disease. Am J Med 84:833, 1988

198. Ehrenkranz NJ, Kicklighter JL: Tuberculosis outbreak in a general hospital: Evidence for airborne spread of infection. Ann Intern Med 77:377, 1972

199. Centers for Disease Control: Screening for tuberculosis and tuberculous infection in high-risk populations, and the use of preventive therapy for tuberculous infection in the United States. MMWR 39(no. RR-8):1, 1990

200. Centers for Disease Control: Guidelines for Prevention of TB Transmission in Hospitals. Atlanta, U.S. Department of Health and Human Services, Public Health Service, HHS Publication No. (CDC) 82–8371, 1982

201. Centers for Disease Control: Guidelines for preventing the transmission of tuberculosis in health-care settings, with special focus on HIV-related issues. MMWR 39(no. RR-17):1, 1990

202. Garden JM, O'Banion MK, Shelnitz LS et al: Papillomavirus in the vapor of carbon dioxide laser-treated verrucae. JAMA 259:1199, 1988

203. Center for Devices and Radiological Health: Center scientists conduct study for viable viruses in common laser plumes. Med Devices Bull 8:3, 1990

204. Smith JP, Moss E, Bryant CJ, Fleeger AK: Evaluation of a smoke evacuator used for laser surgery. Lasers Surg Med 9:276, 1989

205. Pippin DJ, Verderame RA, Weber KK: Efficacy of face masks in preventing inhalation of airborne contaminants. J Oral Maxillofac Surg 45:319, 1987

206. Davis WT: Filtration efficiency of surgical face masks: The need for more meaningful standards. Am J Infect Control 19:16, 1991

207. McCue JD: The effects of stress on physicians and their medical practice. N Engl J Med 306:458, 1982

208. Crump JH: Review of stress in air traffic control: Its measurement and effects. Aviat Space Environ Med 50:243, 1979

209. Melton CE, Smith RC, McKenzie JM et al: Stress in air traffic personnel: Low density towers and flight service stations. Aviat Space Environ Med 49:724, 1978

210. Clarke TZ, Maniscalco WM, Taylor-Brown S et al: Job satisfaction and stress among neonatologists. Pediatrics 74:52, 1984

211. Mawardi BH: Satisfactions, dissatisfactions, and causes of stress in medical practice. JAMA 241:1483, 1979

212. Toung TJK, Donham RT, Rogers MC: The stress of giving anesthesia on the electrocardiogram (ECG) of anesthesiologists. Anesthesiology 61:A465, 1984

213. Azar I, Sophie S, Lear E: The cardiovascular response of anesthesiologists during induction of anesthesia. Anesthesiology 63:A76, 1985

214. Modell JH: Who is captain of the anesthesia ship? Arch Surg 121:753, 1986

215. Pinnock CA, Elling AE, Eastley RJ et al: Anxiety levels in junior anaesthetists during early training. Anaesthesia 41:258, 1986

216. Vaillant GE, Sobowale NC, McArthur C: Some psychological vulnerabilities of physicians. N Engl J Med 287:372, 1972

217. Vaillant GE, Brighton JR, McArthur C: Physician's use of mood-altering drugs. N Engl J Med 282:365, 1970

218. Osler W: The Principles and Practice of Medicine, p 1005. New York, D. Appleton & Co., 1892

219. Mattison JB: Morphinism in medical men. JAMA 23:186, 1894

220. Keeve JP: Physicians at risk: Some epidemiologic considerations of alcoholism, drug abuse and suicide. J Occup Med 26:503, 1984

221. American Medical Association Council on Mental Health: The sick physician: Impairment by psychiatric disorders, including alcoholism and drug dependence. JAMA 223:684, 1973

222. McAuliffe WE, Rohman M, Fishman P et al: Psychoactive drug use by young and future physicians. J Health Soc Behav 25:34, 1984

223. Spiegelman GS, Saunders L, Mazze RI: Addiction and anesthesiology. Anesthesiology 60:335, 1984

224. Talbott DG, Gallegos KV, Wilson PO et al: The Medical Association of Georgia's impaired physicians program. JAMA 257:2927, 1987

225. Brewster JM: Prevalence of alcohol and other drug problems among physicians. JAMA 255:1913, 1986

226. Jones RE: Do psychiatrists cover up addiction of physicians? Psychiatr Opinion 12:31, 1975

227. Arnold WP: Substance abuse and chemical dependence in Anesthesiology. ASA Newsletter 55:4, 1991

228. Talbott GD: Elements of the impaired physician program. J Med Assoc Ga 73:747, 1984

229. Ward CG, Ward GC, Saidman LJ: Drug abuse in anesthesia training programs. JAMA 250:922, 1983

230. Gallagher W: The looming menace of designer drugs. Discover Aug:24, 1986

231. Menk EJ, Baumgarten RK, Kingsley CP et al: Success of reentry into anesthesiology training programs by residents with a history of substance abuse. JAMA 263:3060, 1990

232. Gravenstein JS, Kory WP, Marks RG: Drug abuse by anesthesia personnel. Anesth Analg 62:467, 1983

233. Talbott GD: Alcoholism and other drug addictions: A primary disease entity. J Med Assoc Ga 75:490, 1986

234. Farley WJ, Talbott GD: Anesthesiology and addiction. Anesth Analg 62:465, 1983

235. Lewis DC: Doctors and drugs. N Engl J Med 315:826, 1986

236. McAuliffe WE, Rohman M, Santangelo S et al: Psychoactive

drug use among practicing physicians and medical students. New Engl J Med 315:805, 1986

237. McAuliffe WE: Nontherapeutic opiate addiction in health professionals: A new form of impairment. Am J Drug Alcohol Abuse 10:1, 1984

238. Burrow BJ: The patient's view of the anaesthetist in an Australian teaching hospital. Anaesth Intens Care 10:20, 1982

239. Salmon NS: The role of the anaesthetist as seen by nurses in training. Anaesthesia 38:801, 1983

240. Linn LS, Yager J, Cope D et al: Health status, job stress, and life satisfaction among academic and clinical faculty. JAMA 254:2775, 1985

241. Goodwin DW, Davis DH, Robins LN: Drinking amid abundant illicit drugs: The Vietnam case. Arch Gen Psychiatry 32:230, 1975

242. Moleski RJ, Easley S, Barash PG et al: Control and accountability of controlled substance administration in the operating room. Anesth Analg 64:989, 1985

243. Adler GR, Potts FE, Kirby RR et al: Narcotics control in anesthesia training. JAMA 258:3133, 1985

244. Moore RD: Youthful precursors of alcohol abuse in physicians. Am J Med 88:332, 1990

245. Reeve PE: Personality characteristics of a sample of anaesthetists. Anaesthesia 335:559, 1980

246. Arnold WP: Legal aspects of chemical dependence. ASA Newsletter. 55:9, 1991

247. Orentlicher D: Drug testing of physicians. JAMA 264:1039, 1990

248. Scott M, Fisher KS: The evolving legal context for drug testing programs. Anesthesiology 73:1022, 1990

249. Lecky JH, Aukburg SJ, Conahan TJ et al: A departmental policy addressing chemical substance abuse. Anesthesiology 65:414, 1986

250. American Society of Anesthesiologists Committee on Occupational Health of Operating Room Personnel: Chemical Dependence Guidelines for Departments of Anesthesiology. Park Ridge, Illinois, American Society of Anesthesiologists, 1991

251. Canavan DJ: The impaired physician program: The subject of impairment. Med Soc NJ 80:47, 1983

252. Roeske NCA: Stress and the physician. Psych Annals 11:245, 1981

253. Duffy JC, Litin EM: Psychiatric morbidity of physicians. JAMA 189:989, 1984

254. Bittker TE: Reaching out to the depressed physician. JAMA 236:1713, 1976

255. Bissell L, Jones R: The alcoholic physician: A survey. Am J Psychiatry 133:1142, 1976

256. Clark DC, Eckenfels EJ, Daugherty SR et al: Alcohol-use patterns through medical school. JAMA 257:2921, 1987

257. Council on Mental Health: The sick physician; impairment by psychiatric disorders, including alcoholism and drug dependence. JAMA 223:684, 1973

258. Canavan DI: The impaired physicians program. J Med Soc NJ 79:980, 1982

259. DeSole DE, Singer P, Aronson S: Suicide and role strain among physicians. Int J Soc Psychiatry 15:294, 1969

260. Cohen EN: Mortality among anesthesiologists. Anesthesiology 51:193, 1979

261. Helliwel PJ: Suicides amongst anaesthetists-in-training. Anaesthesia 38:1097, 1983

262. Council on Scientific Affairs: Results and implication of the AMA-APA physicians mortality project—Stage II. JAMA 257:2949, 1987

263. Crisp AH: Selection of medical students—is intelligence enough? J R Soc Med 77:35, 1984

264. Springman SR, Berry AJ, Cascorbi HF et al: What attributes do we want in anesthesia residents? Anesthesiology 65:107, 1986

265. Wohl S: Death by malpractice. JAMA 255:1927, 1986

266. Birmingham PK, Ward RJ: A high risk suicide group: The anesthesiologist involved in litigation. Am J Psychiatry 142:1225, 1985

267. Crawshaw R, Bruce JA, Eraker PL et al: An epidemic of suicide among physicians on probation. JAMA 243:1915, 1980

5

Donald A. Kroll
Frederick W. Cheney

Medicolegal Aspects of Anesthetic Practice

The legal aspects of medical practice have become increasingly important as the American public has turned to the courts for economic redress when their expectations of medical treatment are not met. Although the cost of liability insurance premiums for anesthesiologists is in the low to middle range of all specialists, the average cost of a professional liability policy in 1990 was about $20,000. There were wide geographic differences, with premiums ranging from under $10,000 in some states to over $60,000 in others for the same coverage. It is little consolation to the anesthesiologist that some other specialists, such as cardiac surgeons, vascular surgeons, orthopaedic surgeons, obstetricians, and neurosurgeons, have higher premiums.

The purpose of this chapter is to provide a background for the practitioner about how the legal system handles malpractice claims and the steps that should be taken when one is the target of a malpractice action. Risk management and liability insurance options are also discussed. More extensive texts are available for detailed information.[1]

THE TORT SYSTEM

Although physicians may become involved in the criminal law system in a professional capacity, they more commonly become involved in the legal system of civil laws. Civil law is broadly divided into *contract law* and *tort law*. A tort may be loosely defined as a civil wrongdoing, and negligence is one type of tort. The majority of medical malpractice lawsuits are pursued on the basis of negligence theories, but there are occasional cases where contract law theories are utilized. *Malpractice* actually refers to any professional misconduct, but its use in legal terms typically refers to professional negligence.

To be successful in a malpractice suit, the patient–plaintiff must prove four things:

Duty: that the anesthesiologist owed him or her a duty;
Breach of duty: that the anesthesiologist failed to fulfill his or her duty;
Causation: that a reasonably close causal relation exists between the anesthesiologist's acts and the resultant injury; and
Damages: that actual damage resulted because of the acts of the anesthesiologist.

Failure to prove any one of these four elements will result in a decision for the defendant–anesthesiologist.

DUTY

As a physician, the anesthesiologist establishes a duty to the patient when a doctor–patient relationship exists. When the patient is seen preoperatively, and the anesthesiologist agrees to provide anesthesia care for the patient, a duty to the patient has been established. In the most general terms, the duty the anesthesiologist owes to the patient is to adhere to the *standard of care* for the treatment of the patient. Because it is virtually impossible to delineate specific standards for all aspects of medical practice and all eventualities, the courts have created the *reasonable and prudent physician*. For all specialties, there is a national standard, which has displaced the local standard.

There are certain general duties that all physicians have to their patients, and breaching these duties may also serve as the basis for a lawsuit. One of these general duties is that of obtaining informed consent for a procedure. Consent may be written, verbal, or implied. Oral consent is just as valid, albeit harder to prove years after the fact, as written consent. Implied consent for anesthesia care may be present in circumstances in which the patient is unconscious or unable, for any reason, to give his or her consent, but where it is presumed that any reasonable and prudent patient would give consent if able.

Although there are exceptions to the requirement that consent be obtained, as a general rule, anesthesiologists should be sure to obtain consent whenever possible. Failure to do so exposes the anesthesiologist to possible prosecution for battery.

The requirement that the consent be *informed* is somewhat more opaque. The guideline is determining whether the patient received a fair and reasonable account of the proposed procedures and the risks inherent in these procedures. The duty to disclose risks is not limitless, but it does extend to those risks that are reasonably likely in any patient under the circumstances and to those that are reasonably likely in particular patients because of their condition.

Other general duties include the maintenance of medical records, the performance of an appropriate examination of the patient, and the use of consultations and referrals to other physician specialists. Although these duties are more applicable to the primary care specialties, anesthesiologists may be held liable for the failure to perform these general duties as they are applied to the specialty. For example, if an anesthesiologist performs a preoperative examination for another anesthesiologist or a CRNA and fails to provide adequate documentation in the medical record or to report a significant condition by direct consultation, he or she will be liable for any injury that results.

BREACH OF DUTY

In a malpractice action, expert witnesses will review the medical records of the case and determine whether the anesthesiologist acted in a reasonable and prudent manner in the specific situation and fulfilled his or her duty to the patient. If they find that the anesthesiologist either did something that should not have been done, or failed to do something that should have been done, then the duty to adhere to the standard of care has been breached, and the second requirement for a successful suit will have been met.

CAUSATION

Judges and juries are interested in determining whether the breach of duty was the *proximate cause* of the injury. If the odds are better than even that the breach of duty led, however circuitously, to the injury, then this requirement is met.

There are two common tests employed to establish causation. The first is the *"but for"* test, and the second is the *substantial factor* test. If the injury would not have occurred "but for" the action of the defendant–anesthesiologist, or if the act of the anesthesiologist was a substantial factor in the injury despite other causes, then proximate cause is established.

Although the burden of proof of causation ordinarily falls on the patient–plaintiff, it may, under special circumstances, be shifted to the physician–defendant under the doctrine of *res ipsa loquitur* (literally, "the thing speaks for itself"). Applying this doctrine requires proving that:

The injury is of a kind that typically would not occur in the absence of negligence;

The injury must be caused by something under the exclusive control of the anesthesiologist;

The injury must not be attributable to any contribution on the part of the patient;

The evidence for the explanation of events must be more accessible to the anesthesiologist than to the patient.

Because anesthesiologists render patients insensible to their surroundings and unable to protect themselves from injury, this doctrine may be invoked in anesthesia malpractice cases. All that needs to be proved is that the injury typically would not occur in the absence of negligence; the anesthesiologist is then put in the position of having to prove that he or she was not negligent.

DAMAGES

The law allows for three different types of damages. *General damages* are those such as pain and suffering that directly result from the injury. *Special damages* are those actual

damages that are a consequence of the injury, such as medical expenses, lost income, and funeral expenses. *Punitive damages* are intended to punish the physician for negligence that was reckless, wanton, fraudulent, or willful. Occasionally, *exemplary damages* are awarded to make an example of the case to prevent any other physician from doing the same thing. Determining the dollar amount of damages is the job of the jury, and the determination is usually based on some assessment of the plaintiff's condition versus the condition he or she would have been in had there been no negligence. Plaintiffs' attorneys generally charge a percentage of the damages, and will, therefore, seek to maximize the award given.

Because medical malpractice usually involves issues beyond the comprehension of lay jurors and judges, the court establishes the standard of care in a particular case by the testimony of *expert witnesses*. These witnesses differ from factual witnesses mainly in that they may give opinions. The trial court judge has sole discretion in determining whether a witness may be qualified as an expert. Although any licensed physician may be an expert, information will be sought regarding the witness's education and training, the nature and scope of the person's practice, memberships and affiliations, and publications. The purpose in gathering this information is not only to establish the qualifications of the witness to provide expert testimony, but also to determine the weight to be given to that testimony by the jury. In many cases, the success of a suit depends primarily on the stature and believability of the expert witnesses.

In certain circumstances, the standard of care may also be determined from published societal guidelines, written policies of a hospital or department, or textbooks and monographs. Some medical specialty societies have carefully avoided applying the term "standards" to their guidelines, in the hope that no binding behavior or mandatory practices have been created. In the past, the American Society of Anesthesiologists (ASA) has published a number of guidelines relating to the practice of anesthesia. In 1986, the ASA, for the first time, published "Standards for Basic Intra-operative Monitoring" (see the Appendix).[2] These standards have been updated several times since their initial adoption and are more binding than guidelines. Essentially, guidelines *should* be adhered to, and standards *must* be adhered to.

WHAT TO DO WHEN SUED

A lawsuit begins when the patient–plaintiff's attorney files a complaint and demand for jury trial with the court. The anesthesiologist is then served with the complaint and a summons requiring an answer to the complaint. Until this happens, no lawsuit has been filed. Insurance carriers must be notified immediately after the receipt of the complaint. The anesthesiologist will need assistance in answering the complaint, and there is a time limit placed on the response.

Specific actions at this point include:

Do not discuss the case with *anyone*, including colleagues who may have been involved, operating room personnel, or friends.

Never alter any records.

Gather together all pertinent records, including a copy of the anesthetic record, billing statements, and correspondence concerning the case.

Make notes recording all events recalled about the case. It may be necessary to review the medical record. Some attorneys will recommend that physicians establish a separate file for all documents pertinent to the case, making certain that the file is marked as confidential. Cooperate fully with the attorney provided by the insurer in answering the complaint.

If a physician believes that the attorney provided by an insurance carrier is not representing his or her interests fully, then one of several options may be exercised. The insurance company may be requested to provide another attorney, or the physician may consider retaining private counsel. If the estimated damage settlement is greater than the limits of the insurance coverage, the physician may be personally liable for the difference. A second reason to obtain private counsel is a potential impact on retaining the ability to practice. If there is a possibility that practice privileges will be limited or revoked, then there is reason enough to hire someone to represent the physician's interests independent of the malpractice claim. A third reason to retain separate counsel is lack of confidence in the attorney provided by the insurance carrier when an alternative cannot be provided. Because the physician will be working closely with the attorney, it is of some importance that the physician have confidence in his or her abilities.

The first task the anesthesiologist must perform with an attorney is to prepare an answer to the complaint. The complaint contains certain facts and allegations with which the defense may either agree or disagree. Denial of facts or allegations constitutes a *negative defense*. There may also be *affirmative defenses*, which, if proved, would exonerate the anesthesiologist even if the facts alleged in the complaint were true. For example, the statute of limitations may have run out before the complaint was filed, the patient may be alleged to have assumed the risk, or another physician might have contributed to the injury. Defense attorneys rely on the frank and totally candid observations of the physician in preparing an answer to the complaint. Physicians should be willing to educate their attorneys about the medical facts of the case, although most medical malpractice attorneys will be knowledgeable and medically sophisticated.

The next phase of the malpractice suit is called *discovery*. The purpose of discovery is the gathering of facts and clarification of issues in advance of the trial. Another purpose of discovery is to assess or harass the defendant to determine how good a witness he or she will make. This occurs at several points in the discovery process, and by several mechanisms.

The anesthesiologist will, in all likelihood, receive a written interrogatory, which will usually be filed through the defense attorney. Written interrogatories requesting factual information about training, experience, and qualifications are perfectly legitimate. However, if the anesthesiologist receives an interrogatory that appears to contain many irrelevant or personal questions, it is a good idea to consult with the defense attorney before spending time answering them. The interrogatory should be answered in writing, in consultation with the defense attorney, because carelessly or inadvertently misstated facts can become troublesome later.

Depositions are a second mechanism of discovery. The defendant–anesthesiologist will be deposed as a fact witness, and depositions will be obtained from other anesthesiologists who will act as expert witnesses. The defendant–anesthesiologist may be asked to suggest other anesthesiologists who will review the medical records. A nationally recognized expert in the area in question who is not a personal friend but agrees with the defense position may be very valuable. Generally speaking, an acquaintance

or a partner is not as believable as a stranger. Other than making a recommendation about who will serve as the expert for the defense, the defendant–anesthesiologist has little control over the selection of experts. However, the conduct of the defendant–anesthesiologist during deposition may have a profound impact on the outcome of the suit.

The anesthesiologist will be deposed by the plaintiff's attorney, not the defense attorney. Physicians may receive a subpoena demanding their presence at an inconvenient time or place in an attempt to harass them or make them angry. If this happens, the defense attorney will probably be able to take care of the matter for the physician. Most often, the arrangements for the deposition will be made amicably by both sides, and the deposition will occur at a place and time convenient for the anesthesiologist, typically in the defense attorney's office. As a general rule, it is best that physicians avoid having the deposition taken in their own offices, because the plaintiff's attorney will carefully note such things as the medical books on the shelves, the diplomas on the walls, and the general state of disarray of the office. Information may thus be provided that the plaintiff's attorney may find a way to use against the anesthesiologist. A second reason to avoid pleasant and familiar surroundings is that the physician will tend to lower his or her guard if comfortable and fall prey to certain common traps in deposition. *Despite the apparent informality of the deposition, the anesthesiologist must be constantly aware that what is said during the deposition carries as much weight as what would be said in court.*

The anesthesiologist should meet with his or her attorney prior to the deposition for the sole purpose of being coached on how to give the deposition. The defense attorney should be experienced in both taking and giving deposition testimony, and he or she should be able to advise anesthesiologists on what to expect and how to conduct themselves. There are some general guidelines to follow, and there may be specific points the attorney will ask the anesthesiologist to make during his or her testimony.

It is important to be factually prepared for the deposition. A review of notes, the anesthetic record, and the medical record is necessary. The defendant anesthesiologist will be asked some specific questions about the dates and places of medical training and whether he or she has published any articles or papers or written any chapters in textbooks. Physicians may also be asked details about their practice, the size of their group, or, possibly, details about their relationship to the hospital in which they practice. Defendant–anesthesiologists should be sure about these details, update their curriculum vitae, and be familiar with such information before the deposition.

For the deposition, the physician should dress conservatively and professionally, as appearance and image are very important. The opposition is assessing the physician to see how he or she will appear to a jury. Answers to questions should be brief and concise. Being evasive or hostile is not helpful. Answer only the question asked, and do not volunteer information. The plaintiff's attorney may pause for long periods after a question in an attempt to procure an expanded answer. Silence is awkward, and there is a natural tendency to say something during a pause. Physicians should avoid this temptation, and look to their attorney for clues about answers. If the defense attorney raises an objection, stop talking immediately, and allow the attorney to voice his or her objections. Most often, the physician will be expected to complete his or her answer after the objection, but the answer may be tempered somewhat by what the defense attorney is objecting to.

Occasionally, physicians will be asked leading questions that are impossible to answer without qualifications. In this case, the physician may qualify his or her answer but should avoid giving lengthy opinion answers. The defendant anesthesiologist is being deposed as a witness of facts, not opinions. Experts may give opinions, but the defendant should try to avoid doing so.

Another common ploy is to try to get a physician to admit something that is apparently benign but which opens up a line of questioning the attorney otherwise could not pursue. Questions about insurance coverage, personal assets, contractual relationships with the hospital, or anything else for which there is no obvious connection to the case are suspect. Physicians should not admit that there are any "definitive" or "authoritative" textbooks on which they rely in their practice, as doing so may make them responsible for everything that is said in the book, whether they agree with it or not. The defense attorney should advise the anesthesiologist on how to respond to this type of questioning. Do not underestimate the plaintiff's attorney, no matter how friendly or inept he or she may seem. Taking a deposition is a finely honed skill for which the plaintiff's attorney is much better trained and more experienced than the defendant–anesthesiologist. Physicians must not become cocky or overconfident and allow themselves to be led into a trap by relaxing their guard.

The best answers are those which are responsive to the question without volunteering additional information. The answers should be given in the simplest possible terms. Technical medical terms, medical jargon, pejorative terms, and slang should be avoided. Do not try to be humorous or make a joke, as these efforts do not translate well on paper. Court reporters will record exactly what is said, so it is important to speak clearly. Speaking slightly more slowly than normally will facilitate an accurate transcription and will also give the defense attorney the opportunity to interrupt if the physician is headed into unfriendly territory.

The plaintiff's attorney may try to intimidate the anesthesiologist or make him or her angry. This serves two purposes. First, the anesthesiologist may say something he or she will later regret. Second, if the attorney knows that the defendant–anesthesiologist is a volatile person, he or she will welcome the opportunity to make the defendant look foolish in front of a jury. Do not get angry or become emotional. Remember that the goal of the plaintiff's attorney in taking defendants' depositions is to try to get them to admit to facts that will be helpful to the plaintiff's case and to size them up for a possible courtroom trial. The defense attorney already knows what is going to be said and what the defense position will be. If the case against an anesthesiologist is weak or doubtful, a favorable performance in deposition will greatly reduce the likelihood of a jury trial and a high award. On the other hand, if there is a reasonably good case against the anesthesiologist, a poor deposition performance might make the plaintiff's attorney unwilling to consider settlement at all.

There will be depositions from expert witnesses, both for the plaintiff and for the defense. The anesthesiologist should work with his or her attorney to suggest questions and rebuttals. The better educated the attorney is about the medical facts, the reasons the anesthesiologist did what was done, and the alternative approaches, the better able he or she will be to conduct these expert depositions. The presence of the defendant–anesthesiologist during the depositions of plaintiff's experts may be crucial.

There will probably be much posturing, jockeying for position, and negotiating among the various attorneys involved in the case during the discovery phase. Anesthesiologists may find that they are in an adversarial relationship, not only with the plaintiff's attorney, but also with the hospital's attorney and the attorneys for other defendants. It is important not to personalize these procedures. Anesthesiologists must realize that the only issue of importance is getting out of the suit with the minimum dollar cost. If the case against them is without merit, it probably will be dropped early in the discovery process. Sometimes, lawsuits are filed by plaintiffs' attorneys before they have actually had the case reviewed by an expert. An example of this would be when the statute of limitations is about to run out at the time the attorney is consulted.

If there is some merit in the case but the damages are minimal, or if proof will be difficult, there will probably be a settlement offer. There is a high cost incurred by both plaintiffs and defendants in pursuing a malpractice claim up through a jury trial. Unless there is a strong probability of a large dollar award, reputable plaintiffs' attorneys are not likely to pursue the claim. Thus, even if physicians believe that they are totally innocent of any wrongdoing, they should not be offended or angered about settling of the case: this is solely a matter of money, not medicine. The only reason for physicians to fight the settlement of an unmeritorious claim early in the discovery process is if such a settlement will have some repercussions that affect their ability to practice or impose a financial burden on them.

A settlement may be offered because the claim is likely to be successful and to result in a larger award in the event of a jury trial. In this situation, the insurer presumes that the evidence will show that the insured anesthesiologist was negligent and is attempting to limit his or her losses. The insurer will be quite uninterested in whether the defendant–anesthesiologist wishes to settle. Fighting the settlement will probably not be advantageous. The best the physician may hope for is that his or her practice will not be affected, personal assets affected, or licensure questioned.

If a settlement is not reached during the discovery phase, a trial will occur. Only about 1 in 20 malpractice cases ever reaches the point of a jury trial, because both plaintiffs' and defendants' attorneys are aware of the strengths of the case, and it usually becomes clear during discovery whether the suit will be successful. Preparing for and conducting a jury trial is expensive for both sides, and there is, therefore, economic pressure to reach a settlement, especially for the side that is likely to lose. Only those cases in which both sides feel they can win, and which are likely to have significant financial impact, will proceed to trial.

The jurisdiction in which a case is tried, and the composition of the jury, may have a profound impact on the eventual outcome. Juries tend to become sympathetic to one side or the other during the trial. The more pathetic and helpless the patient–plaintiff, the more likely it is that the anesthesiologist will lose. Alternatively, the more reasonable and professional the physician seems, the more likely it is that he or she will win. Whether the jury trusts the physician and the defense side of the story depends on the physician's ability to communicate with the jury, his or her appearance, and the jury's belief in the physician's skills and competence.

The discussion of deposition testimony also applies to testimony in court, but there are a few additional points to consider during the trial. The members of the jury will not be as sophisticated medically as the attorneys who deposed the anesthesiologist during discovery. The anesthesiologist should review his or her discovery deposition. A tendency to overuse specific medical terms should be corrected by learning to explain answers in lay terms for the benefit of the jury. Do not underestimate the intelligence of the jury, however, because talking down to them will create an unfavorable impression. Physicians should pay attention to the jury as they speak and try to estimate whether the members of the jury are understanding the answers. It is best to speak clearly, using understandable terms. Physicians should be confident in their answers without seeming smug or pompous. If the answer to a question is not known, avoid guessing. If specific facts cannot be remembered, say so. Nobody expects total recall of events that may have occurred years before.

The defendant–physician should be present during the trial, even when not testifying, and should dress conservatively, neatly, and professionally. Displays of anger, remorse, relief, or hostility will hurt the physician in court. Unnecessary consultation with defense counsel while others are testifying creates a bad impression with the jury, but the defendant–anesthesiologist should not appear bored or disinterested. When giving testimony, the anesthesiologist must give clear answers to all questions asked. If a question is poorly phrased and imprecise, clarification should be requested. Defendant–physicians should answer only the question asked and should not volunteer information, except when it is necessary to qualify an answer. The physician should be able to give his or her testimony without using notes or documents. When it is necessary to refer to the medical record, it will be admitted into evidence. If there are misleading or damaging statements in the medical record, the defense attorney may have gone to great lengths to try to avoid having the record admitted in evidence; admitting any part of the record may lead to having to admit the entire record.

The anesthesiologist's goal is to convince the jury that he or she behaved in this case as any other competent and prudent anesthesiologist would have behaved. Specifying the reasons for selecting a procedure or technique or for excluding alternative methods will help the defendant–anesthesiologist, assuming that the reasons were valid. This is true even if the anesthesiologist disagrees with the expert who is testifying for the plaintiff. Creating the impression that there were several possible approaches, and that the defendant–anesthesiologist selected the one that was the best for the patient at the time, will tend to enhance credibility of the defense to a greater extent than trying to convince the jury that the defendant's decisions were based on 100% certainty, and, hence, that the opposing expert is 100% wrong.

It is important to keep in mind that *proof* in a malpractice case means only "more likely than not." The patient–plaintiff must "prove" the four elements of negligence, not to absolute certainty, but only to a probability greater than 50%. On the positive side, this means that the defendant–anesthesiologist must only show that his or her actions were, more likely than not, within an acceptable standard of care.

CAUSES OF SUITS

The principal cause of suits against anesthesiologists is patient injury. In a nationwide analysis of 1002 lawsuits against anesthesiologists conducted by the ASA Committee on Professional Liability, the leading injuries for which suit was filed were death (37%), nerve damage (15%), and brain damage (12%).[3] The causes of death and brain damage were predominantly inadequate ventilation, esophageal intuba-

tion, and other airway problems. Nerve damage not related to needle trauma from regional anesthesia or central venous catheter placement often occurs despite apparently adequate positioning.[4] (See Chapter 27.)

As death and brain damage are high-cost injuries, anesthesia practice is clearly a high-risk endeavor. Anesthesiologists use complex equipment, which can fail, and potent drugs, with which mistakes in dose or labelling can have disastrous consequences. Vigilance, which is the highest priority in anesthesia practice, is often difficult to maintain at all times of the day and night through long, tedious surgical procedures. The anesthesiologist is more likely to be the target of a suit if an untoward outcome occurs because the physician–patient relationships are usually tenuous at best. The patient rarely chooses the anesthesiologist, the preoperative visit is brief, and the anesthesiologist who sees the patient preoperatively may not actually anesthetize the patient. Communication between anesthesiologists and surgeons about complications is often lacking, and the tendency is for the surgeon to "blame anesthesia."

Supervision of nurse anesthetists is another endeavor that puts the anesthesiologist in a high-risk category. The more nurse anesthetists supervised by any one anesthesiologist, the greater the exposure to the possibility of patient injury. At the present time, there are no national standards as to the number of nurse anesthetists who can legally be supervised by one anesthesiologist. However, some professional liability insurance companies specify a staffing ratio of 1:2 or 1:3 and charge higher rates for supervision of more than this number. Anesthesiologists are liable, not only for nurse anesthetists they employ, but also for those they supervise who are employed by the hospital.

Because anesthesiologists are employed in the care of patients undergoing high-risk surgical procedures, they are often sued along with the surgeon in the case of an adverse outcome. This may occur even if the outcome was in no way related to the anesthetic care.

RISK MANAGEMENT

The primary goal of any risk management program is the prevention of patient injury. In the absence of a patient injury from anesthesia, the likelihood of a lawsuit is minimal. The nature of anesthetic practice, however, is such that some patient injury will inevitably occur. Therefore, the second phase of risk management is the practice of defensive medicine, the performance of which is hard to separate from good medicine.

The key factors in the prevention of patient injury are vigilance, up-to-date knowledge, and adequate monitoring.[5] Physiologic monitoring of cardiopulmonary function, combined with monitoring of equipment function, might be expected to reduce anesthetic injury to a minimum. Equipment monitors are designed to detect serious failure before patient injury results.

A study of closed malpractice claims by the ASA Committee on Professional Liability indicated that the use of end-tidal CO_2 monitoring and pulse oximetry will significantly reduce the incidence of brain damage and death.[6] Although everyone would agree that adequacy of oxygenation, ventilation, and circulation should be monitored during all anesthetics, the means may be subject to some controversy. Clearly, it is prudent to adhere to the ASA "Standards for Basic Intra-operative Monitoring" (see the Appendix).[2] Basically, these standards call for the presence of qualified anesthesia personnel in the room at all times and for monitoring of oxygenation, ventilation, and circulation. During general anesthesia, an oxygen analyzer and a pulse oximeter should be used, and there should be adequate illumination and exposure of the patient to assess blood oxygenation. The ASA standards call for monitoring of ventilation during anesthesia, which may include such qualitative clinical signs as chest excursion, observation of the reservoir breathing bag, and auscultation of breath sounds, with the use of quantitative devices such as end-tidal CO_2 monitors being encouraged. When an endotracheal tube is inserted, its correct position in the trachea must be verified by clinical assessment and the identification of CO_2 in the expired gas. The use of continuous end-tidal CO_2 analysis is encouraged. When a mechanical ventilator is in use, there should be a disconnect alarm with an audible signal. During regional anesthesia and monitored anesthesia care, the adequacy of ventilation should be evaluated by continual observation of the aforementioned qualitative clinical signs, and the assessment of oxygenation with pulse oximetry is mandatory.

In order to ensure adequacy of circulation, the standards call for continuous ECG monitoring, with arterial blood pressure and heart rate evaluated at least every 5 minutes. In addition, each patient should have circulatory function evaluated continually by at least one of the following: palpation of the pulse, auscultation of heart sounds, monitoring of intra-arterial pressure, or some other device such as a pulse oximeter. Body temperature should be monitored when changes are "intended, anticipated, or suspected." The ASA standards also call for pulse oximetry monitoring in the early stages of recovery from anesthesia.

In addition to Standards for Basic Intra-operative Monitoring, the ASA has published Standards for Pre-anesthesia Care and Post-anesthesia Care. These standards are less specific than those for intraoperative monitoring, but they should be scrupulously observed. The ASA Directory of Members should be reviewed yearly for any changes in ASA Standards of Practice. It would also be reasonable to review the ASA Guidelines published in the Directory.

It should be noted that, although membership in the ASA is not required for the practice of anesthesiology, expert witnesses will with virtual certainty hold any practitioner to the ASA standards. It also is possible that an individual anesthesiologist will be held to standards higher than those promulgated by the ASA by his or her professional liability insurer as a risk management strategy.

Another risk management tool is the use of checklists prior to each case, or at least daily, in an attempt to reduce equipment-related mishaps.[7-9]

The practice of "defensive medicine" includes making of preoperative and postoperative rounds, developing good patient relationships, and maintaining up-to-date practice habits. Informed consent should be documented with a general consent, which should include a statement to the effect that "I understand that all anesthetics involve risks of complications, serious injury, or, rarely, death from both known and unknown causes." In addition, there should be a note in the patient's record that the risks of anesthesia and alternatives were discussed, and that the patient accepted the proposed anesthetic plan. A brief documentation in the record that the common complications of the proposed technique were discussed is helpful. If it is necessary to change the agreed-on anesthesia plan significantly after the patient is premedicated or anesthetized, the reasons for the change should be documented in the record.

Good records can form a strong defense if they are adequate and can be disastrous if inadequate. The anesthesia record itself should be as accurate, complete, and neat as possible. The use of automated anesthesia records may be helpful in the defense of malpractice cases.[10] In addition to vital signs every 5 minutes, special attention should be paid to ensure that the patient's ASA classification, the monitors utilized, fluids administered, and doses and times of all administered drugs are accurately charted. As the principal causes of hypoxic brain damage and death during anesthesia are related to ventilation, all respiratory variables that are monitored should be documented accurately. It is important to note when there is a change of anesthesia personnel during the conduct of a case. Sloppy, inaccurate anesthesia records, enlarged and placed before a jury, can be quite damaging to the defense.

If a critical incident occurs during the conduct of an anesthetic, the anesthesiologist should document, in narrative form, in the patient's progress notes what happened, which drugs were used, the time sequence, and who was present. A catastrophic intra-anesthetic event cannot be summarized adequately in a small amount of space on the usual anesthesia record. The critical incident note should be written as soon as possible, while all details are still fresh in the anesthesiologist's mind. The report should be as consistent as possible with concurrent records, such as the anesthesia, operating room, recovery room, and cardiac arrest records. If inconsistencies exist, they should be explained in the critical incident note. Records should never be altered after the fact. If an error is made in recordkeeping, a line should be drawn through the error, leaving it legible, and the correction should be initialed and timed. Litigation is a lengthy process, and a court appearance to explain the incident to a jury may be years away, when memories have faded.

In the event of a sudden, unexpected intra-anesthetic cardiac arrest for which there is no readily apparent explanation, blood and urine should be obtained for drug screening. With the increasing frequency of surgery on an outpatient basis, some patients may be tempted to relieve their anxiety with the use of recreational drugs, which may interact adversely with drugs used for anesthesia.

If anesthetic complications occur, the anesthesiologist should be honest with both the patient and family about the cause. Whenever an anesthetic complication becomes apparent postoperatively, appropriate consultation should be obtained quickly, and the departmental or institutional risk management group should be notified. If the complication is apt to lead to prolonged hospitalization or permanent injury, the liability insurance carrier should be notified. The patient should be followed closely while in the hospital, with telephone follow-up, if indicated, after discharge. Also, the anesthesiologist and surgeon should be consistent in their explanations to the patient as to the cause of any complication.

Although it may seem obvious, it needs stressing that qualified anesthesia personnel should be in continuous attendance during the conduct of all anesthetics. The only exception should be those which lay people (i.e., judge and jury) can understand, such as radiation hazards or an unexpected life-threatening emergency elsewhere. Even then, provisions should be made for monitoring the patient adequately. Anesthetic complications occurring while anesthesia personnel are out of the room without urgent reason are indefensible and command high financial settlements or court awards. Adequate supervision of nurse anesthetists and residents, and good communication with surgeons when adverse anesthetic outcomes occur, are also important.

On a departmental level, an ongoing process of concurrent record review based on established standards of care criteria and anesthesia-related morbidity and mortality data should be reviewed regularly. A regular schedule of equipment maintenance and procedures to follow whenever equipment malfunction is suspected of contributing to patient injury should be established. If equipment malfunction is suspected to have contributed to a complication, the device should be impounded and examined by representatives of the hospital and the manufacturer. Extensive information on anesthesia departmental quality assurance activities is available in the Joint Commission on Accreditation of Health Organizations (JCAHO) guidelines and the ASA quality assurance manual.[11]

LIABILITY INSURANCE

Throughout the above discussion, there has been frequent reference to the role of the insurer in the defense of malpractice claims. Traditional malpractice coverage has been issued on an *occurrence* basis. As long as the anesthesiologist was insured at the time of the incident, coverage was provided continuously for that occurrence thereafter. This type of coverage was favorable for the physician, but insurers recognized the actuarial problem of being unable to predict the likelihood of a claim or the amount of expected losses. Most insurers no longer provide coverage on a per-occurrence basis and have replaced this type of policy with *claims made* coverage. With these policies, the anesthesiologist must be insured at the time of the loss and at the time of reporting. Typically, the insurance rates start at a lower level, then increase to the mature policy rate and level off. This arrangement makes coverage affordable to new specialists. The rates will vary with the limits of coverage, which are usually expressed as a pair of numbers indicating the limits in millions of dollars per occurrence and an annual total. For example, a policy for $0.5/1.5 million indicates that the limit is $500,000 for any single claim and that the total annual claims cannot exceed $1.5 million. Claims made coverage is typically available with limits of $0.5/1.5, $1/3, or $2/4 million. The usually recommended coverage is $1 million/3 million.

When purchasing coverage, it is important to know whether the policy is *assessable*. Assessability means that, if the yearly premium is not adequate to cover losses, the policy holder will be "assessed" an extra amount in subsequent years to make up the difference.

Because the anesthesiologist must be insured both at the time of the loss and at the time the loss is reported, a problem arises when one type of policy or company is converted to another policy or company. This problem has led to two types of conversion coverage. When the new company agrees to provide coverage for claims that occurred under the previous policy but have not yet been reported, it is said to provide "nose" coverage. If the old company provides such coverage, it is called "tail" coverage. Tail coverage also applies when the anesthesiologist leaves practice.

A third type of malpractice insurance is the *umbrella*, or excess coverage, policy. This type of coverage is applied only when the limits of the primary policy are exceeded. The intent of excess coverage is to protect the physician in the event of a catastrophic loss.

In addition to changing the types of malpractice insurance coverage available, insurers are instituting practice guidelines as conditions for insurability. Several companies will insure anesthesiologists only if certain minimal patient monitoring criteria are met. Anesthesiologists who contract with their insurers to follow such guidelines may be financially responsible for damages that occur when the guidelines are not followed.

ANTITRUST LAWS

Antitrust laws are becoming more important to anesthesiologists because of developments in three areas: (1) exclusive service contracts; (2) managed care medicine; and (3) the Health Care Quality Improvement Act.

Restraint of trade exists only when two or more legal entities interact anticompetitively by means of a contract, combination, or conspiracy. Furthermore, not all restraint of trade is "unreasonable." There are two tests that may be applied. The *per se* rule applies to situations where the activity is so likely to restrict competition, without any mitigating efficiency gains, that all one need prove is that the activity existed: there is no need to prove that any actual restraint occurred. Examples include such activities as price fixing and market allocations. Group boycotts and tying arrangements were formerly viewed as per se violations but are now generally considered under the *rule of reason*. Under rule of reason analyses, the plaintiff must show actual harm to competition, and the court will weigh the anticompetitive effect against the potentially legitimate purpose of the restraint. This analysis traditionally was applied for cases involving monopolies but has been extended to anticompetitive cases where the discriminatory behavior was based on public service or ethical norms, the so-called "patient care defense."[12] As the application of this type of analysis increases, so does the importance of determining proof of market power. Without market power, it is difficult to demonstrate harm caused by the actions of a single group.

EXCLUSIVE SERVICE CONTRACTS

There have been several antitrust cases involving group contracts with hospitals. In such actions, the excluded anesthesiologist alleges that the group has established an illegal monopoly by tying the provision of anesthesiology care within the hospital to membership in the group. The hospital alleges that only by establishing an exclusive contract may good patient care be assured. There have been two key considerations in these cases.

The first consideration is that a tying arrangement must exist. That is, it must be proved that the hospital requires patients who use its operating rooms to purchase anesthesiology services solely from the group. Even though the hospital is entitled to restrict access to its operating rooms to a limited number of anesthesiologists, no tying arrangement exists unless access is restricted to members of the group.

The second consideration is whether the hospital has market power. If it can be shown that the hospital has sufficient market power that the effect is forcing patients to select only from their group, then the per se rule against tying arrangements might apply. It would not be a sufficient defense that the restraint was adopted to improve patient care (a rule of reason approach).

MANAGED CARE MEDICINE: PPOs AND IPAs

Preferred provider organizations (PPOs) may be formed by brokers or entrepreneurs, payers, or providers. Of these different types, provider-sponsored PPOs are most at risk for antitrust problems, because they may be viewed as a horizontal arrangement among competing providers. If it is viewed as a joint venture, then it becomes a single legal entity, and no concerted activity can be shown.

Individual practice associations (IPAs) and other novel types of economic bargaining units have been formed to answer some of these problems for physician groups. Such groups will be analyzed under the same principles as a provider PPO. The IPA must be viewed as a bona fide joint venture that offers some new capabilities. The restraints in question must be reasonably related to the function of the joint venture, and the overall market power of the joint venture must not be so large as to be excessively anticompetitive.

ANTITRUST IMMUNITY: THE HEALTH CARE QUALITY IMPROVEMENT ACT

There are two main areas of antitrust immunity important to physicians. Because membership in a professional association may be sufficient evidence of concerted activity, and because professional associations are increasingly involved in lobbying activities, it is significant that lobbying efforts are protected. The *Noerr-Pennington doctrine*[12] exempts acts seeking to influence government action or legislation, even if their sole purpose is anticompetitive. It should be noted that efforts to influence private associations are not exempt. Thus, an advertising campaign designed to influence the passage of a law would be immune, but if the same campaign were designed to influence a JCAHO guideline, it would not be immune.

The second area of immunity is peer review activity under the *state action doctrine*.[13] The Health Care Quality Improvement Act of 1986 (HCQIA) was a direct result of an antitrust action involving hospital peer review activities. Under the state action doctrine, hospitals have a common law duty to exercise care in selecting qualified medical staffs. States regulate and supervise the process, and it therefore becomes immune. The state must actively supervise its policies, and the policies must be clearly articulated and expressed. These provisions may not always be clearly defined, and the landmark Patrick v. Burget case left open the potential for abuses, so the HCQIA attempts to define the conditions under which peer review is exempt. The act contains provisions that serve, not only to broaden the applicability of the state action doctrine to include all medical peer review, but also to specify standards of fairness for peer review. The other thing that the HCQIA did in an attempt to protect the public from incompetent physicians was to establish the National Practitioner Data Bank for Adverse Information on Physicians and Other Health Care Practitioners (NPDB).

THE NATIONAL PRACTITIONER DATA BANK

The NPDB established a nationwide information system that theoretically would allow licensing boards and hospitals a better means of detecting adverse information about physicians.[14] Simply moving into another state would no longer provide safe haven for incompetent physicians.

The NPDB requires input from four sources: medical malpractice payments, license actions by medical boards, clinical privilege actions taken by hospitals, and membership actions taken by societies if the society has formal peer review mechanisms. There has been a great deal of effort to establish a minimum reporting dollar value below which no report is necessary, but to date, any payment made on behalf of a physician in response to a written complaint or claim must be reported. Settlements made by cancellation of bills, or settlements made on verbal complaints, are not considered a reportable payment.

Once a report has been submitted, the physician is notified and has 60 days from the date the data bank processed the report to dispute the input. At this time, the reporting entity may correct the form or void it. Failing that, the physician has the option of putting a brief statement in the file or appealing to the U.S. Secretary of Health and Human Services, who may also either correct or void the form. Once it is entered, there is no means of purging the form.

The security of the data bank is protected by requiring legitimate inquirers to have an identification number. Hospitals are required to query the data bank at the time a physician initially requests staff privileges and at 2-year intervals, but they may query it at any time. State licensing boards also may make a query, and any health care entity that provides patient care may query as long as the entity has a formal peer review process. A plaintiff's attorney may query the data bank only when there is evidence that a hospital failed to make a mandatory query and the claim is made against the hospital. A practitioner may make a query about his or her file at any time.

Because mandatory data entry became effective September 1, 1990, it is too early to tell what impact the NPDB will have. Efforts to modify some of its provisions continue, and it is therefore likely that the details of mandatory reporting criteria will change.

SPECIAL SITUATIONS

Jehovah's Witnesses

It is important to recognize that patients have well-established rights, and that among these is the right to refuse specific treatments because of religious beliefs. In the case of Jehovah's Witnesses, the treatment refused is the administration of blood or blood products, a central part of their religious beliefs, which hold that they will be forbidden the pleasures of the afterlife if they receive blood or blood products. Thus, for them to receive a transfusion is a mortal sin, and many Jehovah's Witnesses would actually rather die in grace, as they see it, than to live with no possibility of salvation. Anesthesiologists recognize and respect these beliefs but are also cognizant that these convictions may conflict with the physicians' personal, religious or ethical codes.

Minor children of Jehovah's Witness parents represent a special group for consideration. Although the U.S. Supreme Court has upheld the right of an adult to become a martyr by refusing treatments based on religious convictions, no court has extended to parents the right to make their children martyrs. States have upheld the overriding interest in protecting children, and most states have provisions for the guarantee of access to medical treatment for children. This involves making the child a ward of the court for the purpose of rendering medical treatment. It must be stressed that obtaining a proper court order is of critical importance in the care of a minor child of Jehovah's Witness parents when the parents refuse to authorize a blood transfusion.

As a general rule, physicians are not obligated to treat all patients who apply for treatment in elective situations. It is well within the rights of a physician to decline to care for any patient who wishes to place burdensome constraints on the physician or unacceptably to limit the physician's ability to provide optimal care. When presented with the opportunity to provide elective care for a Jehovah's Witness, the physician may decline to provide any care or may limit, by mutual consent with the patient, his or her obligation to adhere to the patient's religious beliefs. If such an agreement is reached, it must be documented clearly in the medical record, and it is desirable to have the patient co-sign the note. Not all Jehovah's Witnesses have identical beliefs regarding blood transfusions or which methods of blood preservation or sequestration will be allowed. Some patients will not allow any blood that has left the body to be reinfused. Yet others will accept autotransfusion if their blood remains in constant contact with the body (via tubing). Therefore, it is important to reach a clear understanding of which techniques for blood preservation are to be used and to document this plan in the record.

Emergency medical care imposes greater constraints on the treating physician, as there is no opportunity to decline the care of a patient with an immediately life-threatening condition. If the patient is an adult and is conscious and mentally competent, then he or she has the right to refuse blood transfusion. The exceptions to patients' rights in this regard include pregnant women and adults who are the sole support of minor children. In these circumstances, the interests of the fetus in surviving may supersede the rights of the mother, as may the interests of the state in not being obligated to provide for the welfare of dependent children. In either case, obtaining a court order is the best plan if time permits. If the problem concerns blood products and there is insufficient time to obtain a court order, pregnant women should be given a transfusion to save the life of the fetus, but parents of minor children should not receive transfusions against their wishes unless the dependency of the children is obvious.

When the patient is a minor, it is important to ascertain the true wishes of the parents. Some parents know that a court order can be obtained and view this as a relief from the onerous burden of having to decide whether they are willing to let their child die. On the other hand, some parents are adamant that blood not be given, and there have been cases where children have been ostracized by their parents and religious community for having received a court-ordered transfusion. Reaching an understanding about the consequences for the child who receives a court-ordered transfusion is, therefore, vital for the determination of what risks will be taken before ordering a transfusion.

The procedure for obtaining a court order may vary, depending on the specific state laws. Typically, an order may be obtained over the telephone. The initial contact may be with a social worker who will put the physician in contact with a judge. Details of the case will be ascertained, and the judge will issue an informal order declaring the patient a ward of the court for the purposes of receiving medical treatment only. This call initiates the issue of a written order, which will arrive several days later. Although not a totally automatic procedure, it would be very rare for a judge to deny this order for a minor.

Anesthesiologists concerned about the care of Jehovah's Witnesses should familiarize themselves with the details of the procedure in their practice locations.

Impaired Physicians

Physicians may become impaired in their abilities to practice medicine skillfully and safely for a variety of reasons, but the most common impairment among anesthesiologists is chemical dependence (see Chapter 4). There are two primarily legal issues of importance: the first issue is the duty to report suspected substance abuse, and the second is the potential liability imposed by reporting.

There is considerable variability among the states in defining the *legal* responsibilities of a physician in reporting suspected substance abuse. In some states, the licensing authority must be notified, whereas in others, there is no requirement. The *ethical* mandate to limit or restrict the practice of impaired physicians is clearly established. Furthermore, vicarious liability for the acts of an incompetent or impaired physician may be imposed on physicians who either knew, or should have known, of the impairment. Because the hospitals that grant practice privileges may be vicariously liable for the acts of the physicians, and because the state has an inherent interest in protecting its citizens from incompetent medical care, it is likely that an impaired physician program of some sort currently exists for most practice locations. Because liability may be imposed for not reporting suspected chemical dependency, and because there is an ethical obligation to help the impaired physician, suspicions that a colleague is impaired should not be ignored.

Physicians are constitutionally protected by the same due process provisions as any other citizens. This has led to the fear that reporting the suspicion of an impairment, or acting as a member of an impaired physician committee in recommending restriction of privileges, may lead to a lawsuit for defamation, deprivation of livelihood, or restraint of trade. In most states, immunity from such prosecution is granted to groups or committees whose purpose is to review the quality of medical care and to physicians who provide information to such committees. There is, however, the provision that such individuals and groups are acting reasonably and without malice or for personal gain. The issue of immunity for peer review groups has been raised at the federal level, and it is likely that federal legislation will someday clarify the issues.

Acknowledgment. Portions of this chapter have been reproduced from the publication "Professional Liability and the Anesthesiologist" with the permission of the American Society of Anesthesiologists.

REFERENCES

1. Peters JD, Fineberg KS, Kroll DA et al: Anesthesiology and the Law. Ann Arbor, Health Administration Press, 1983
2. American Society of Anesthesiologists Directory of Members 1991, p 670
3. Cheney FW, Posner K, Caplan RA, Ward RJ: Standard of care and anesthesia liability. JAMA 261:1599, 1989
4. Kroll DA, Caplan RA, Posner K et al: Nerve injury associated with anesthesia. Anesthesiology 73:202, 1990
5. Gaba DM, Maxwell M, DeAnda A: Anesthetic mishaps: breaking the chain of accident evolution. Anesthesiology 66:670, 1987
6. Tinker JH, Dull DL, Caplan RA et al: Role of monitoring devices in prevention of anesthetic mishaps: a closed claims analysis. Anesthesiology 71:541, 1989
7. Petty C: The Anesthesia Machine, p 213. New York, Churchill Livingstone, 1987
8. Spooner RB, Kirby RR: Equipment-related anesthetic incidents. Int Anesthesiol Clin 22:133, 1984
9. US Food and Drug Administration: Anesthesia Apparatus Checkout Recommendations. Bethesda, August 1986
10. Kroll DA: The medicolegal aspects of automated anaesthesia records. Bailliere's Clin Anaesthesiol 4:237, 1990
11. Duberman S: Quality Assurance in the Practice of Anesthesiology. Park Ridge, American Society of Anesthesiologists, 1986
12. Gilmore DA: The antitrust implications of boycotts by health

care professionals: Professional standards, professional ethics and the First Amendment. Am J Law Med 14(2, 3):221, 1988

13. McDowell TN, Rainer JM: The state action doctrine and the local government antitrust act: The restructured public hospital model. Am J Law Med 14(2, 3):171, 1988

14. Johnson ID: Reports to the National Practitioner Data Bank. JAMA 265:417, 1991

APPENDIX
STANDARDS FOR BASIC INTRA-OPERATIVE MONITORING*

Approved by House of Delegates of the American Society of Anesthesiologists on October 21, 1986, and last amended on October 23, 1990

These standards apply to all anesthesia care although, in emergency circumstances, appropriate life support measures take precedence. These standards may be exceeded at any time based on the judgement of the responsible anesthesiologist. They are intended to encourage high quality patient care, but observing them cannot guarantee any specific patient outcome. They are subject to revision from time to time, as warranted by the evolution of technology and practice. This set of standards addresses only the issue of basic intra-operative monitoring, which is one component of anesthesia care. In certain rare or unusual circumstances, 1) some of these methods of monitoring may be clinically impractical, and 2) appropriate use of the described monitoring methods may fail to detect untoward clinical developments. Brief interruptions of continual† monitoring may be unavoidable. *Under extenuating circumstances, the responsible anesthesiologist may waive the requirements marked with an asterisk (*); it is recommended that when this is done, it should be so stated (including the reasons) in a note in the patient's medical record.* These standards are not intended for application to the care of the obstetrical patient in labor or in the conduct of pain management.

†Note that "continual" is defined as "repeated regularly and frequently in steady rapid succession" whereas "continuous" means "prolonged without any interruption at any time."

STANDARD I

QUALIFIED ANESTHESIA PERSONNEL SHALL BE PRESENT IN THE ROOM THROUGHOUT THE CONDUCT OF ALL GENERAL ANESTHETICS, REGIONAL ANESTHETICS AND MONITORED ANESTHESIA CARE.

OBJECTIVE

Because of the rapid changes in patient status during anesthesia, qualified anesthesia personnel shall be continuously present to monitor the patient and provide anesthesia care. In the event there is a direct known hazard, e.g., radiation, to the anesthesia personnel which might require intermittent remote observation of the patient, some provision for monitoring the patient must be made. In the event that an emergency requires the temporary absence of the person primarily responsible for the anesthetic, the best judgement of the anesthesiologist will be exercised in comparing the emergency with the anesthetized patient's condition and in the selection of the person left responsible for the anesthetic during the temporary absence.

STANDARD II

DURING ALL ANESTHETICS, THE PATIENT'S OXYGENATION, VENTILATION, CIRCULATION AND TEMPERATURE SHALL BE CONTINUALLY EVALUATED.

OXYGENATION

OBJECTIVE

To ensure adequate oxygen concentration in the inspired gas and the blood during all anesthetics.

METHODS

1. Inspired gas: During every administration of general anesthesia using an anesthesia machine, the concentration of oxygen in the patient breathing system shall be measured by an oxygen analyzer with a low oxygen concentration limit alarm in use.*

2. Blood oxygenation: During all anesthetics, a quantitative method of assessing oxygenation such as pulse oximetry shall be employed.* Adequate illumination and exposure of the patient is necessary to assess color.*

VENTILATION

OBJECTIVE

To ensure adequate ventilation of the patient during all anesthetics.

METHODS

1. Every patient receiving general anesthesia shall have the adequacy of ventilation continually evaluated. While qualitative clinical signs such as chest excursion, observation of the reservoir breathing bag and auscultation of breath sounds may be adequate, quantitative monitoring of the CO_2 content and/or volume of expired gas is encouraged.

2. When an endotracheal tube is inserted, its correct positioning in the trachea must be verified. Clinical assessment is essential and end-tidal CO_2 analysis, in use from the time of endotracheal tube placement, is encouraged.

3. When ventilation is controlled by a mechanical ventilator, there shall be in continuous use a device that is capable of detecting disconnection of components of the breathing system. The device must give an audible signal when its alarm threshold is exceeded.

4. During regional anesthesia and monitored anesthesia care, the adequacy of ventilation shall be evaluated, at least, by continual observation of qualitative clinical signs.

CIRCULATION

OBJECTIVE

To ensure the adequacy of the patient's circulatory function during all anesthetics.

---

* Reproduced with permission from American Society of Anesthesiologists Directory of Members 1991, p 670.

METHODS

1. Every patient receiving anesthesia shall have the electrocardiogram continuously displayed from the beginning of anesthesia until preparing to leave the anesthetizing location.*

2. Every patient receiving anesthesia shall have arterial blood pressure and heart rate determined and evaluated at least every five minutes.*

3. Every patient receiving general anesthesia shall have, in addition to the above, circulatory function continually evaluated by at least one of the following: palpation of a pulse, auscultation of heart sounds, monitoring of a tracing of intra-arterial pressure, ultrasound peripheral pulse monitoring, or pulse plethysmography or oximetry.

BODY TEMPERATURE

OBJECTIVE

To aid in the maintenance of appropriate body temperature during all anesthetics.

METHODS

There shall be readily available a means to continuously measure the patient's temperature. When changes in body temperature are intended, anticipated or suspected, the temperature shall be measured.

II

BASIC PRINCIPLES OF ANESTHESIA PRACTICE

6

James J. Richter

Mechanisms of General Anesthesia

General anesthesia is the result of reversible changes in neurologic function caused by drugs that modulate synaptic communication. Intravenous agents interfere with membrane protein receptors and volatile agents interact with the hydrophobic regions of membrane lipids and proteins. This chapter summarizes the major work that supports the neurophysiologic and molecular theories about the action of anesthetics.

Exhaustive reviews and critical analysis of the experimental evidence are available to satisfy the basic scientist or the anesthesiologist with research interests. Two recent volumes devoted to anesthetic mechanisms give thorough reviews of the many theories and approaches to mechanisms of action of anesthetics.[1,2] Dluzewski et al[3] focus on membrane actions of anesthetic molecules. These reviews[1,3] and their exhaustive bibliographies are good points of entry to the basic science literature. The intent of this chapter is to give a brief overview of the current theories of the mechanisms of both intravenous and volatile anesthetics, including a discussion concerning memory and amnesia.

The elements of general anesthesia that are frequently described include amnesia, analgesia, inhibition of noxious reflexes, and skeletal muscle relaxation.[4] Reversible changes in neurologic function cause loss of perception and reaction to pain, unawareness of immediate events, and loss of memory of those events.[5] The pharmacologic mechanisms for such reversible neurologic events include effects of drugs on synaptic communication and the physicochemical behavior of volatile hydrocarbons in biologic membranes.

SYNAPTIC COMMUNICATION

Discussion of synaptic communication begins by reviewing the work of Sherrington,[6] who established that communication between neurons occurs at synaptic junctions and is the physiologic basis for central nervous system (CNS) function. The classic explanation states that a chemical neurotransmitter is released from the presynaptic ending, traverses the synaptic cleft, and binds to a receptor on the postsynaptic membrane. When occupied by a neurotransmitter molecule, the receptor complex induces electrochemical changes in the postsynaptic cell. Figure 6-1 is a generalized scheme to illustrate the concept of synaptic function.

The neuropharmacologic basis for these concepts is reviewed by Cooper et al.[7]

Neurotransmitters can have either inhibitory or excitatory properties. Gamma-aminobutyric acid (GABA) is the major inhibitory neurotransmitter in the brain and glycine is the major inhibitory neurotransmitter in the spinal cord.[8-10] Glutamate is the major excitatory neurotransmitter in the brain.

DRUG-RECEPTOR INTERACTIONS

Drug-receptor interactions have been described for most of the intravenous drugs used in anesthesia practice. Neuromuscular blockers bind to receptors and modulate (inhibit) the function of acetylcholine (ACh) on the motor end-plates of skeletal muscle cells. It was well established in 1975 that opioids work by occupying opiate receptors in the brain and spinal cord. Analgesia results from the modulation of peptide function (endorphins and enkephalins), which are endogenous ligands for the opiate receptors.[5] Receptor mechanisms are recognized also for other drugs commonly used in intravenous anesthesia techniques, including benzodiazepines, barbiturates, and neuroleptic drugs.[4,9]

MODULATION OF GABA FUNCTION

Accumulating data support the concept that several aspects of anesthesia may result from modulation of GABA function. Intravenous drugs such as benzodiazepines and barbiturates,[4] and even inhalation drugs,[11] have been shown to enhance inhibitory tone mediated by GABA. The inhibitory properties of GABA, a major neurotransmitter in mammalian brain, have been deduced from data about the metabolic turnover and receptor binding of the compound. Some convulsive drugs work by inhibiting the synthesis of GABA.[8] The consequent decrease in tissue concentration of GABA results in a decreased inhibitory tone of upper motor neurons, which leads to myoclonic seizure activity.[8] Other convulsants, such as picrotoxin and bicuculline, are GABA antagonists and bind directly to GABA receptors. The antagonistic action of these drugs prevents the normal inhibitory influence of GABA and results in seizure activity.[8,9]

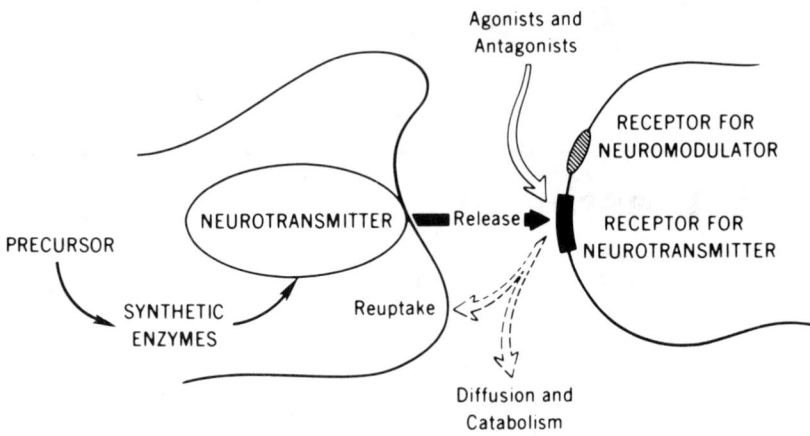

PRE-SYNAPTIC CELL   **POST-SYNAPTIC CELL**

Figure 6-1. Generalized schematic diagram of neurotransmitter function. (Reprinted with permission from Richter JJ: Current theories about the mechanisms of benzodiazepines and neuroleptic drugs. Anesthesiology 54:66, 1981.)

Systems other than motor activity are inhibited by the neurotransmitter function of GABA. Gillis et al[12] showed that GABA-mediated mechanisms are important in the CNS control of autonomic and cardiovascular function. Control of serotonin-releasing neurons may also be influenced by GABA.[13] In 1982 Antonaccio[14] suggested that GABA inhibits the flow of autonomic stimulation from the CNS. In 1987 Sample and DiMiccio[15] localized forebrain sites where GABA agonists and antagonists mediated cardiovascular function. They demonstrated that GABA-ergic centers in the brain stem modulate sympathetic tone and that GABA agonists depress sympathetic activity (blood pressure and heart rate). Their data suggest that sympathetic effects of GABA arise from sites in the caudal periventricular hypothalamus and that vagal effects of GABA arise from rostral periventricular hypothalamic regions.[15] Because the hypothalamus and limbic region of the brain are associated with emotional changes in humans, the authors speculate that decreased GABA-ergic tone may be responsible for cardiovascular changes that accompany emotional arousal.[15]

The potential role of GABA-mediated mechanisms in the control of sympathetic activity could be quite significant in the development of drugs useful in anesthesia practice. Certainly, the control of sympathetic activity is of central importance in the administration of general and regional anesthesia.

As a neurotransmitter, GABA mediates inhibition of neurons by binding to a receptor protein in postsynaptic membranes. Benzodiazepines bind to specific receptors that are contingent to the GABA receptor. The GABA–benzodiazepine receptor complex has been designated the GABA$_A$ receptor.[16] When occupied by drug molecules, the benzodiazepine receptor reacts allosterically with the adjacent GABA receptor in a fashion that enhances the inhibitory tone. The GABA$_A$ receptor causes neural inhibition by opening a transmembrane channel for conducting chloride ions.

Recent and exciting research has outlined much of the detail of the macromolecular structure and function of the GABA$_A$ receptor in membrane action.[16] Using bovine cerebral cortex, Sigel and Barnard[17] purified the receptor complex and Casalotti et al[18] identified alpha and beta subunits. The alpha subunit binds benzodiazepines and the beta subunit binds GABA. Schofield et al[16] have described the amino acid sequences of the alpha and beta subunits of the GABA$_A$ receptor. Although the receptor macromolecule is too large and complex for direct-sequencing studies, the amino acid sequences of peptide fragments were determined. Synthetic DNA probes were prepared to match the templates of the peptide amino acid chains. The synthetic DNA probes were then used to screen libraries of DNA from bovine brain. These steps allowed the identification of hybridizing clones of DNA where the probe DNA matched up with fragments of nucleic acids representing brain tissue. The resulting DNA was subsequently used to deduce the code and the amino acid sequence of the entire receptor macromolecule.

Analysis of the amino acid sequence of the receptor subunits yields information about the structural and functional details of the membrane proteins. Specific sequences of hydrophobic amino acids are identified as the transmembrane portion of the receptor. Branches of the protein that project into the intracellular and extracellular environments are also described (Fig. 6-2). In addition to the transmembrane structure, functional aspects of the receptor proteins begin to emerge from analysis of the amino acid sequence. A unique proline residue in the transmembrane portion of the protein causes a flexure in the structure that might change and thereby control the transport of chloride ion when neurotransmitters bind to the receptor portion of the macromolecule.

Furthermore, Schofield et al[16] have recognized remarkably similar domains in the structures of GABA$_A$ receptors and nicotinic receptors for acetylcholine (nAChR). Transmembrane portions of the two receptors have very similar amino acid sequences, as do some parts of the extracellular portions of the molecules. These structural similarities imply that common mechanisms are responsible for functional aspects of binding receptors and activation of ion channels across membranes. Schofield et al suggest that the structural similarities between GABA$_A$ and ACh receptors indicate that they may both belong to a "super family of chemically gated ion channel receptors."[18]

An elegant confirmation of the authenticity of the receptor structure is the synthesis and function of the GABA$_A$ complex in Xenopus oocyte membranes. Cloned DNA encoding the receptor structure was inserted into plasmids and in vitro transcription produced appropriate messenger RNA. Purified RNA was then injected into Xenopus oocytes that subsequently synthesized and inserted GABA$_A$ receptors into the cell membrane. With the intact GABA$_A$ receptor, the oocyte demonstrated an appropriate current response to GABA, indicating correct functional assembly of the membrane protein complex.[18]

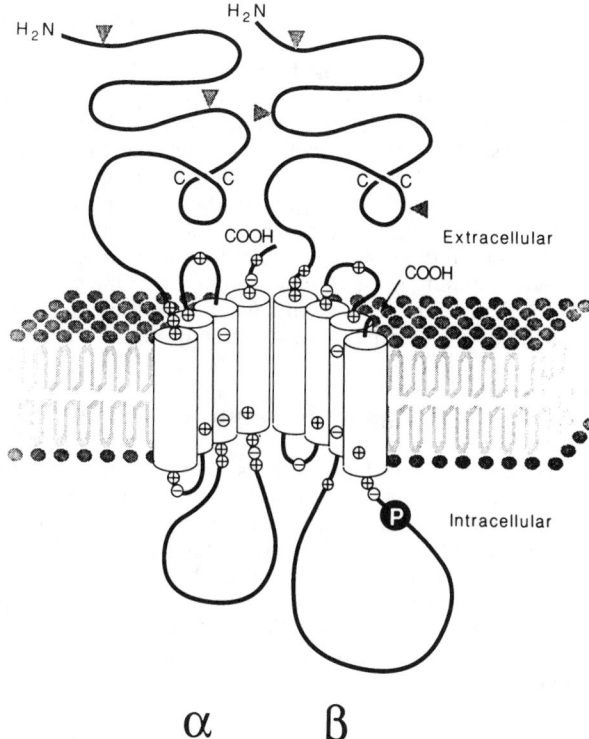

Figure 6-2. Schematic diagram of the GABA$_A$ receptor in the lipid matrix of a membrane. The binding site for GABA is the extracellular portion of the beta subunit. The binding site for benzodiazepines is the extracellular portion of the alpha subunit. The generalized structure may be similar for other types of membrane receptor complexes. (Reprinted with permission from Schofield PR, Darlison MG, Fugita N *et al:* Sequence and functional expression of the GABA$_A$ receptor shows a ligand-gated receptor super-family. Nature 328:221, 1987. © 1987 Macmillan Magazines Limited.)

Detailed explanations of membrane structure and function will provide a framework for the development of new and more specific drugs that will modulate synaptic communication and improve the specificity and safety of general anesthesia.

Benzodiazepines and GABA Function

It is well established that most properties of benzodiazepines result from drug-receptor interactions that modulate GABA function. The properties of benzodiazepines are (1) antianxiety, (2) anticonvulsant, (3) sedation, (4) centrally mediated muscle relaxation, and (5) amnesia. Costa and Guidotti[19] proposed that the anticonvulsant and sedative properties result from enhanced inhibitory effects of GABA caused by benzodiazepines bound to receptors that are contingent with, but separate from, GABA receptors.

The muscle relaxation and anti-anxiety properties of benzodiazepines have been attributed to glycinemimetic effects.[10] The drugs have been shown to bind to glycine receptors, mimicking the inhibitory tone of glycine neurotransmission in the brain stem and spinal cord.[9,10]

Benzodiazepine antagonists have been identified. An imidazobenzodiazepine, flumazenil, antagonizes the sedative and hypnotic effects of midazolam in human volunteers.[20]

During infusions to maintain constant plasma concentrations of midazolam, flumazenil promptly caused all seven subjects to become fully oriented within 2 minutes after administration.[20] The antagonist did not induce anxiety or agitation in the subjects. The antagonist data further support the concept of benzodiazepine-receptor interactions as the basis for pharmacologic activity of this class of drugs.

Barbiturates and GABA Function

Although barbiturates have been used much longer, it has only been since the discovery of benzodiazepine receptors that similar mechanisms have been demonstrated for barbiturate mechanisms. Receptors for barbiturates are adjacent to GABA receptors, and the barbiturate-occupied receptor is thought to enhance the inhibitory tone of GABA and thereby exert the anticonvulsant and sedative effects of these drugs.[21] Olsen has summarized the experimental data suggesting that a GABA receptor-ionophore complex of proteins exists in synaptic membranes, with associated receptors for benzodiazepines and barbiturates.[22] GABA-occupied receptors produce inhibitory actions by increasing membrane conductance to chloride ion. When associated receptors are occupied by benzodiazepine or barbiturate molecules, the chloride conductance is increased further, enhancing the effect of GABA.

Experimental evidence cited above suggests strongly that benzodiazepines and barbiturates modulate synaptic function by enhancing the inhibitory effects of GABA. There are, however, probably many other neurochemical mechanisms that might be involved in the pharmacologic mechanisms of sedative and hypnotic drugs. Richards and Strupinski have shown recently that pentobarbital depressed miniature end-plate synaptic potentials but did not change resting membrane potentials in guinea pig olfactory cortex neurons.[23] These investigators found no evidence for a GABA-mediated change in membrane potential from barbiturate action when they used drug concentrations that spanned the effective anesthetic range.[23] In a subsequent report, Pocock and Richards[24] described the inhibition of catecholamine release from bovine adrenal chromaffin cells by pentobarbital. Pentobarbital competitively inhibited the action of nicotinic agonists that stimulate release of catecholamines. They also showed that pentobarbital decreased calcium ion influx, and they speculated that such a mechanism could inhibit release of neurotransmitters, thereby causing CNS depression.[24] Both of these articles illustrate that the mechanisms of action of CNS-active drugs are much more complex and subtle than merely enhancing GABA-mediated inhibition.

Steroid Anesthetics and GABA Function

Steroid anesthetic molecules were shown to interact with the GABA receptor complex by Harrison et al in 1987.[25] In an experimental preparation of rat hippocampal neurons, they showed that steroid anesthetic molecules caused a marked prolongation of postsynaptic inhibitory currents mediated by GABA. In this preparation, synaptically released GABA normally binds to receptors and causes an increased chloride conductance in the postsynaptic membrane. The steroid molecules prolong this chloride conductance and thereby enhance the inhibitory actions of GABA. Whereas barbiturates and benzodiazepines bind to specific receptors contingent to the GABA receptor–chloride chan-

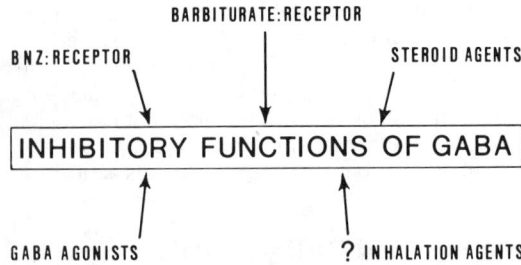

Figure 6-3. Drugs that modulate GABA. Several drugs used in anesthesia practice have been shown to depress some CNS functions by enhancing the inhibitory effects of this endogenous neurotransmitter.

nel complex of proteins, they have not identified such specific binding of steroid anesthetic molecules to membrane proteins. Specific binding of steroids might be masked from experimental detection by nonspecific interaction of the steroids with membrane sites. Nevertheless, this report[25] does strongly suggest that the mechanism of steroid-induced anesthesia may involve modulating GABA function.

Cheng and Brunner[26] have proposed that volatile anesthetics act by potentiating the inhibitory effects of GABA-mediated neurotransmission. Intravenously administered GABA does not induce general anesthesia or act as an anticonvulsant because the molecule does not cross the blood-brain barrier and is also subject to metabolic transformation. In 1981, however, Cheng and Brunner[26] described the use of a GABA analog that does induce general anesthesia. This report is strong evidence for a GABA-mediated mechanism as a central aspect of general anesthesia. It also suggests the possibility of synthesizing prospectively designed molecules that might be more specific anesthetics without undesirable side effects. Figure 6-3 is a summary of drugs that have been shown to modulate the inhibitory functions of GABA.

Peripheral Benzodiazepine Receptors

Although not yet directly linked with anesthetic agents, recent data on the existence and physiologic functions of peripheral benzodiazepine receptors may be a model for even more subtle communication between intracellular membranes that may have ultimate implications for mechanisms of anesthesia. The interactions of GABA receptors, benzodiazepines, and other drugs used in anesthesia have been described above. The benzodiazepine receptors are located in various anatomic regions of the brain and are considered "central" benzodiazepine receptors. In a review article, Verma and Snyder examined recent progress in the identification of a second category of peripheral-type benzodiazepine receptors,[27] and described a second class of benzodiazepine receptors with high concentrations in adrenal cortex renal tissue and liver. These peripheral-type receptors have marked differences in specificity for different classes of benzodiazepine-like compounds. Subcellular localization of the receptors is concentrated on outer mitochondrial membranes in adrenal, kidney, and liver preparations. The data suggest that endogenous ligands for these receptors may include porphyrins. The receptors and the ligands may be involved in indirect modulation of endocrine function and water and electrolyte balance in microenvironments. There are also data to suggest that arachidonic acid metabolites may be influenced by drugs that modulate the peripheral benzodiazepine receptors.

Verma and Snyder suggest that the subtle interactions of receptors on mitochondrial membranes implicate mechanisms of communication and control among intracellular membranes. The concept of cellular communication by neurotransmitters and other types of receptor mechanisms is now well known and thoroughly studied at the level of intercellular communication. Emerging data about peripheral benzodiazepine-type receptors may lead to studies of communication among intracellular membranes. One can speculate that intracellular mechanisms of communication may also ultimately prove to be manipulated by anesthetic drugs.

Neuroleptic Drugs and Dopamine Receptors

The effects of neuroleptic drugs (e.g., droperidol) are thought to result from interaction with dopaminergic receptors. Although the details are complex, the general concept is that neuroleptic drugs bind to receptors and modulate the neurotransmitter effects of dopamine.[28]

The common element in the mechanisms of intravenous anesthetic agents is the modulation of synaptic function that results from drug-receptor interactions as summarized in Table 6-1.

CURRENT THEORIES FOR MECHANISMS OF VOLATILE ANESTHETICS

Volatile agents probably cause general anesthesia by modulating synaptic function from within cell membranes rather than by direct binding to receptors in the fashion of intravenous agents. Miller reviews the major details of the theories of molecular mechanisms of action of anesthetics.[1,2] Because anesthesia can be produced by a wide range of chemically distinct compounds (e.g., inert gases, alcohols, volatile hydrocarbons, steroids, and so forth), it is unlikely that a unique "receptor" exists for anesthetic drugs. The potency of various anesthetic drugs has been correlated with their physical properties.[29] Lipid solubility and pressure reversal studies have characterized the physical theories about anesthetic action. Such studies have implicated the lipid matrix

TABLE 6-1. Summary of Drug-Receptor Interactions for Intravenous Agents Used to Produce General Anesthesia*

Class of Drugs	Receptor	Neurotransmitters Modulated
Narcotics	Opiate	Enkephalins
Muscle relaxants	Motor end-plate	Acetylcholine
Benzodiazepines	Benzodiazepine	GABA
Barbiturates	Barbiturate	GABA
Steroid anesthetics	Specific membrane site†	GABA
Neuroleptics	Dopaminergic	Dopamine

*Drug-receptor interactions modify normal physiologic processes caused by "endogenous ligands" or neurotransmitters.

†Specific membrane receptors for steroid molecules have not been identified.

Modified with permission from Richter JJ: Neuropharmacologic mechanisms of general anesthesia. In Barash PG (ed): Refresher Courses in Anesthesiology, vol 14, p 199. Philadelphia, JB Lippincott, 1986.

TABLE 6-2. Theories of Anesthetic Mechanisms

Experimental Observations	Molecular Theories	Neurophysiologic Effects
Lipid solubility/potency correlations	Meyer-Overton hypothesis	
Pressure reversal data	Membrane expansion Membrane disordering	Modulation of synaptic communication
Physicochemical changes of lipid bilayers	Lipid perturbation Lipid phase transitions Lipid protein interactions	
Luciferase inhibition	Direct protein actions	

Detailed explanations of the experimental data and the molecular theories are presented in review articles by Dluzewski *et al*[3] and Miller.[1]

of cell membranes as the most important site for the pharmacologic effects of anesthetics.[1] The various physical and chemical theories of anesthetic mechanisms are outlined in Table 6-2.

Neurophysiologic Effects of Volatile Anesthetics

Five steps of synaptic communication have been identified as possible sites for the action of anesthetics:[29]

1. Synthesis and transport of neurotransmitters.
2. Release of neurotransmitter from the presynaptic cell.
3. Removal of neurotransmitter from the synaptic cleft.
4. Binding of neurotransmitter to the postsynaptic receptor.
5. Electrochemical changes at the postsynaptic membrane.

Many observations have suggested that volatile anesthetics depress excitatory transmission regardless of the specific neurotransmitter. Sodium and chloride ion channels in postsynaptic membranes are affected by volatile agents.[30] There have been little data to suggest that volatile anesthetics affect the synthesis, release, or binding of neurotransmitters.[30]

Richards has suggested that general anesthesia results from the disruption of information transfer at a synaptic level of organization in the CNS.[31] Although basic processes of synaptic function are similar in all systems, the susceptibilities of various synaptic groups to volatile agents are different. Richards suggests that the specific nature of channel structure or of the activation mechanisms determines the sensitivity of each synapse to volatile agents.[31] In a brief review, Halsey notes that synapses in the region of the ventrobasal thalamus may be particularly sensitive to manipulation by volatile anesthetics.[32] However, a single brain region for the control of consciousness or the anesthetic state has not been identified. The brain stem reticular activating system has been implicated in the control of wakefulness, and a variety of anesthetics are known to alter the neurophysiologic activity of the region.[33] It is clear that there is no exclusive brain region for the pharmacologic control of consciousness or all of the CNS elements of general anesthesia.

Molecular Mechanisms of Volatile Anesthetics

The dominant theories of the molecular mechanisms by which volatile agents affect membrane function are based on the lipid solubility of the drugs and on experimental demonstrations of pressure reversal of anesthesia. An excellent detailed review appeared in 1983 by Dluzewski et al.[3]

All discussions of anesthetic mechanisms acknowledge the early observations of the Meyer-Overton lipid solubility theory.[1-3] The anesthetic potency of volatile agents correlates directly with the relative solubility of each drug.[29] The conclusion is that the primary molecular actions of anesthetics occur in the lipid portion of cell membranes. Potential membrane regions for anesthetic actions include hydrophobic areas of proteins and protein-lipid interface regions, as well as the phospholipid matrix.

Volume Expansion Theories

In the 1950s it was demonstrated that high pressures (100–200 atmospheres) reversed the anesthetic effects of several drugs.[1,34] The conclusion was that the high pressure could be compressing the volume of cell membranes. If membrane compression reverses anesthesia, the drugs could be causing anesthesia by increasing membrane volume at normal atmospheric pressure. Miller and colleagues[34,35] have generated considerable data to support the concept, and it has been expanded to a "critical-volume theory" for the mechanism of action of anesthetics.

Pressure reversal experiments have also led to a "multisite" expansion hypothesis from Halsey's laboratory.[36] Anesthetic potencies of drug mixtures were shown to be additive in some cases, but others were not additive. The interpretation of such data is consistent with the concept that general anesthesia is caused by membrane expansion at several types of molecular sites and that different drugs may be acting at different sites.[36] The studies included intravenous as well as inhalation drugs.[37] Halsey's summary of the concept describes several critical hydrophobic sites that are susceptible to expansion by different drugs. The sites of anesthetic action must have varying sensitivity to drugs. Such sites could include hydrophobic portions of proteins as well as membrane lipids.[36] Expansion of critical hydrophobic sites would modify protein activity and thereby modulate synaptic function.[30,36]

The effects of anesthetic agents on pressure-reversible binding of ACh to cholinergic membranes prepared from the electric eel have been studied.[34] Firestone et al[38] found that most agents did increase ACh binding, but the drug concentrations required were about four times greater than the amounts sufficient to cause signs of anesthesia (loss of righting reflex) in experimental animals. They further noted some paradoxical results: the most potent anesthetics did not have similar effects on the binding assay. They concluded that the electroplaque model does not reflect all of the properties of the unidentified CNS sites of action of anesthetics.[38]

Dodson and Miller[39] showed that anesthesia (loss of righting reflex in amphibians) could be reversed with pressure when anesthesia was produced by either an alcohol (octanol) or by a peptide, the leucine-enkephalin analogue BW831C. The octanol-induced anesthesia was unaffected by naloxone, but the peptide-induced anesthesia was reversed by the opiate antagonist. They interpret their data to reveal distinct sites for the action of the different anesthetic molecules.[38] Although the sites of action are different, they share the properties of hydrophobic environments and susceptibility to pressure reversal.

Theories About Fluidity of Membrane Lipids

In the lipid matrix of cell membranes, individual molecules have well-defined, limited motion that has been described as *fluidity*. Measured by physicochemical changes (e.g., order parameter) of probe molecules inserted into experimental membranes, changes in fluidity caused by anesthetics have been described by several investigators, including Trudell.[40] Such observations have suggested that anesthetics cause "disordered" (i.e., more fluid) motions of membrane lipids and possibly lateral separation of fluidity phases within membranes that indirectly alter protein behavior. However, it has also been argued that such fluid changes are caused by anesthetics only at very high concentrations (partial pressures).

In contrast, Ueda et al used a different manifestation of lipid fluidity to suggest that anesthetics weaken lipid-water interactions rather than lipid-lipid interactions.[41] They showed that halothane decreased the surface viscosity (i.e., increased the fluidity) of an artificial monolayer of phospholipid spread on a water surface.[41] Consequently, these investigators suggest, the primary effect of anesthetics is to weaken lipid-water interfaces. At this point there are no direct biologic models by which to relate the postulated effect to membrane functional changes.

Anesthetic-Protein Interactions

Franks and Lieb have described details of the effects of anesthetics on the enzyme luciferase, a soluble protein isolated from fireflies.[42-44] The enzyme activity is inhibited by clinically effective concentrations of anesthetics. They have shown that anesthetics appear to participate in competitive inhibition by preventing the substrate (luciferin) from binding to a specific site on the enzyme macromolecule.[42] They suggest that despite the structural and chemical diversity of general anesthetic agents, the drugs might act by preventing endogenous ligands from binding to specific protein sites.

Franks and Lieb have also shown that the luciferase model is consistent with the "cut-off" effect associated with certain types of anesthetics.[44] In a homologous series of some compounds (N-alkanes, H-alcohols), anesthetic potency stops at a specific point as larger molecules in the series are tested. The same cut-off effect is exhibited when homologous series of anesthetic compounds are tested for inhibition of luciferase activity. Franks and Lieb claim that the cut-off effect is a consequence of drug molecules binding to an amphiphilic protein site of fixed dimensions. The implication is that the critical site cannot accommodate molecules above a certain size, rendering such larger compounds ineffective as inhibitors of the enzyme (and therefore presumably ineffective as anesthetics at some structurally similar site of anesthetic action).[44]

Gibbons, Fonteh, and McBride have recently proposed that anesthetics may function by interacting with specific membrane-bound protein receptors such as lipid methyltransferases. Their model further suggests that products of lipid methyltransferase activity subsequently are responsible for biochemical and physiologic actions of anesthetic drugs.[45] Citing data that demonstrate that anesthetics affect lipid methylation, and describing the characteristics of receptor proteins and lipid interactions appropriate for a theory of anesthetic action, these authors propose a model that would describe the mechanism of action of both local and general anesthetic agents. Although their proposal is broad, they suggest that any acceptable theory of anesthetic action must include a role for major lipids of cell membranes and their membrane-bound enzymes. Additional work in this direction by Hasinoff and Davey has demonstrated that aliphatic alcohols with anesthetic actions can inhibit the membrane-bound enzyme cytochrome C oxidase. These authors attribute their findings to the effect of alcohols on the protein-phospholipid interface within the membrane structure supporting cytochrome C oxidase.[46]

Saturable Binding of Halothane

New evidence reported in 1987 by Evers et al[47] that rat brains have saturable binding sites for halothane may have dramatic effects on the future direction of research and theories of anesthetic mechanisms. So far in this chapter, proposed mechanisms of volatile anesthetics can be grouped into theories of nonspecific, general membrane perturbations (volume expansion, etc.) or direct effects of anesthetics on specific membrane proteins. Evers et al[47] presented data suggesting that specific membrane sites that become saturated with anesthetic molecules. By using nuclear magnetic resonance ^{19}F-NMR labeling of halothane, they measured both the brain concentration and the molecular environments of halothane in anesthetized rats. In vitro and in vivo experiments showed that brain tissue became saturated with halothane at inspired concentrations of 2.5%. Half-maximal brain concentration was observed with a 1.2% concentration of inspired halothane, which is the ED_{50} for halothane in rats.[47]

Specialized calculations from NMR spectroscopy data give information about the rotational motion of the labeled molecule (^{19}F-halothane) and thereby suggest features of the chemical environment of the labeled compound. Spin-lattice relaxation time and spin-spin relaxation time are indicators of molecular motion that can be determined from NMR spectroscopy data. Observations of these parameters exhibited by ^{19}F-halothane led the authors to suggest that brain halothane resides in two chemically distinct microenvironments. One site of brain halothane probably represents nonspecific accumulation in membrane lipids. The second site, however, represents halothane molecules that are relatively immobile, and therefore in an environment other than the lipid matrix. As noted by Evers et al, their data cannot distinguish between separate sites within membranes or between separate cell types altogether.[47] Nevertheless, this shows that the immobilized halothane binding becomes saturated at 2.5% inspired concentration and that the other site continues to accumulate halothane as a linear function of inspired concentration up to 4% (Fig. 6-4). The saturable location becomes 50% occupied by halothane at 1.2% inspired concentration, suggesting that occupancy of this site is associated with the anesthetic effect. Evers et al point out that the saturable, immobile halothane binding locus might represent drug interaction with a family of membrane proteins that shares similar macromolecular characteristics.[47]

In an editorial accompanying the report about NMR studies of halothane binding, Franks and Lieb comment about the potential significance of this approach to the study of anesthetic mechanisms.[48] They emphasize the surprising data of Evers et al showing that with the rapid induction of inhalation anesthesia, only a small amount of halothane

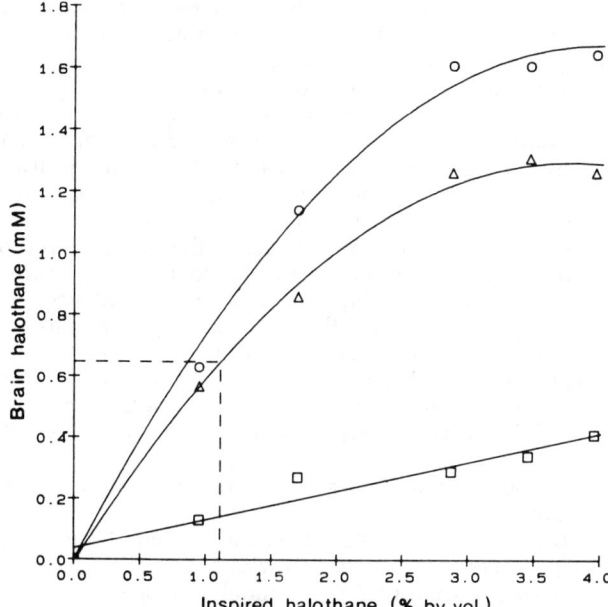

Figure 6-4. Halothane concentrations in brain as a function of inspired concentration. Total halothane concentration (○) was measured by NMR spectroscopy. The microenvironment that becomes saturated with "immobile" halothane is shown (△). Nonsaturable accumulation of more freely mobile halothane (□) is also illustrated. The saturable binding of halothane (△) at inspired concentrations that cause anesthesia might represent an important site for the molecular mechanism of anesthesia. (Reprinted with permission from Evers AS, Berkowitz BA, d'Avignon DA: Correlation between the anesthetic effect of halothane and saturable binding in brain. Nature 328:157, 1987. © 1987 Macmillan Magazines Limited.)

appears in the general lipid portion of membranes and that, in fact, most of the halothane is in a saturable environment, specialized at least to the point where the bound anesthetic molecules are relatively immobile. The implication is that the saturable site might be lipid-protein interface regions or direct-binding regions of membrane proteins.[45]

More recent data reported by Evers et al[49] and Lockhart et al[50] have failed to confirm a saturable binding site in the brain for volatile anesthetics. In a letter to *Nature*, Evers et al corrected the conclusions of their 1987 publication. Their more recent data showed that the brain concentration of halothane did not in fact become saturated at 2.5% inspired concentration.[49] Subsequently Lockhart and Eger reported that both halothane and isoflurane concentration in brain tissue paralleled the concentration in blood and demonstrated that there was no saturation above 3% inspired concentrations.[50] Lockhart et al[51] further demonstrated that an apparent saturation of brain concentration might have been related to depressed ventilation rather than to an actual difference in saturable binding sites.

Although the more recent data challenge the initial interpretation of differential binding sites in the brain, and therefore cast doubt on the implications of the 1987 work, the sequence of these publications illustrates the enormous difficulty investigators have with current techniques in establishing the mechanisms of action of volatile anesthetics. The physiologic variables of anesthetic effects on respiration and cardiovascular function must be controlled for, on the one hand, and on the other hand the technical difficulties of working with volatile agents in tissue, buffers, and analyt-

ical techniques remain significant impediments to this type of investigation.

Signal Transduction

"Signal transduction" is a term now used to describe membrane and intracellular consequences of membrane receptors that become occupied by their endogenous ligands. In the above discussion of synaptic communication, summarized in Figure 6-1, the effect of neurotransmitter binding to postsynaptic receptors was described as inducing electrochemical changes in the postsynaptic cell. Receptor-induced signal transduction includes functions of ion channels in membranes and intracellular second messenger systems that include G proteins. Considerable research is now appearing on the mechanisms of ion channel function, G protein second messenger function, and the effects of anesthetics, especially in the autonomic nervous system. It is quite possible that many of the theories of anesthetic action described earlier may ultimately be manifested in the effects of anesthetic drugs on both ion channel function and intracellular second messenger systems. Maze[52] reviewed the effects of anesthetic agents on ion channels in autonomic nervous system tissue. Nicotinic acetylcholine receptors activate sodium channel conductance in membrane systems. In autonomic tissue, beta$_1$ receptors influence the conductance of calcium ion, potassium ion, and chloride ion channels. Beta$_2$-adrenergic receptors, through a cAMP-mediated system, activate potassium conductance. Details of the membrane physiology of these ion channels and the effects of anesthetic agents and drugs on the systems are described by Maze.[52]

Towler and Evers[53] recently reviewed the effects of anesthesia on the intracellular second messenger system, focusing on G proteins. They pointed out that in addition to providing loss of consciousness and analgesia, anesthetic agents also block many autonomic system responses. The intracellular effects of anesthetics on ion channels and G protein functions in autonomic nervous systems may account for the autonomic effects of anesthetics, as well as provide an additional model for mechanisms by which anesthetics modulate the synaptic communication in areas of the brain that control consciousness and pain perception.[53] The biochemical details of intracellular events in autonomic tissue are described in these review articles.[52,53] Birnbaumer[54] has a detailed review of G proteins in signal transduction.

In the immediate future, research on mechanisms of anesthetic action will likely focus on the control of ion channels and intracellular second messenger systems. It is conceivable that molecular mechanisms such as lipid fluidization, volume expansion, and anesthetic effects on membrane-bound proteins may find physiologic expression in the modulation of ion channel function within membranes and intracellular communication by way of G proteins. This field of research is expected to generate significant new data on the intracellular mechanisms of anesthetic action.

Anesthesia and Amnesia

Amnesia, or the absence of awareness of stimuli and events, is an essential element of general anesthesia; however, clinical episodes and case reports of awareness during general anesthesia are not uncommon. It is estimated 1% to 3.8% of patients have some psychological manifestation of memory or recall during an anesthetic.[55,56] Robinson et al[57] reported a 2% incidence of intraoperative awareness during cardiac surgery with high-dose fentanyl, lorazepam, and isoflurane anesthesia. They speculated that supplemental doses of lorazepam might have prevented the awareness in those particular patients. Knowledge of the biochemical and physiologic mechanisms of memory and learning would allow the future development of anesthetics that could modulate more predictably the amnesia component of general anesthesia. Anesthesia and amnesia have been discussed in two reviews,[58,59] so only a brief summary is included here.

From a clinical point of view, the highest incidence of awareness during general anesthesia is associated with cesarean section and cardiac surgery.[55,56,59] Most prospective studies have not been able to document conscious recall when patients have been tested for memory of stimuli delivered during anesthesia. Eich et al[60] distinguished between the awareness of recall and the unconscious acquisition of learned behavior, but they were unable to demonstrate that either type of memory developed during a prospective study of patients receiving general anesthesia; however, Bennett et al[61] reported that patients do exhibit nonverbal behavior in response to intraoperative suggestions. Goldmann et al[62] have confirmed similar observations about patients exhibiting nonverbal manifestations of intraoperatively acquired suggestions.

The fundamental clinical dilemma is whether awareness occurs during otherwise adequate general anesthesia, or whether it is merely the consequence of inadequate or "too light" anesthesia. This issue reflects the most basic problem, which is the lack of definitive parameters for monitoring the depth of general anesthesia when muscle relaxants preclude movement as a clinical sign. The few prospective studies that reported that patients did learn nonverbal responses to intraoperative suggestions did not control for depth of anesthesia.[61] In 1987, Woo et al[63] reported "the lack of response to suggestion under controlled surgical anesthesia." Their subjects were divided in four groups, and all underwent the identical surgical procedure with identical anesthetic techniques in which depth was judged to be stable by vital signs, end-tidal anesthetic concentrations, and compressed spectral array of EEG signals.[63] Postoperative evaluation showed that none of the patients had conscious recall, nor did they have behavioral or emotional characteristics that might be attributed to acquiring subliminal intraoperative information.[63] The researchers conclude that awareness does not occur during adequately controlled depth of general anesthesia.

A 1987 editorial by Mori[64] offered exceptionally good insight into the difficulties of measuring physiologic indicators (EEG signals) that reflect the transition of brain functioning from awareness to unawareness. He defined depth of anesthesia as the "efficiency of performance of brain functions." He pointed out that slowing of EEG signals has only an empirical correlation with brain function and may not be sensitive enough to indicate the transition from awareness to unawareness. Mori stated that our present knowledge of EEG signals and neurophysiologic function of the cerebral cortex is still rather primitive.[64]

In a short, speculative article, Crick suggested a model for memory formation by subtle changes (e.g., phosphorylation) of synaptic proteins.[65] Schwartz and Greenberg[66] in 1987 reviewed the literature supporting Crick's generalized idea. The suggestion is that the short-term phase of memory is represented by synaptic events such as second messenger–mediated changes in synaptic ion channels or receptors

(membrane proteins). Long-term memory retention is thought to require durable changes in protein structure secondary to changes in gene expression.[66,67]

Lynch and Baudry proposed a calcium-activated mechanism for changes in synaptic protein structure and function that could be associated with memory formation.[68] Their proposal incorporated several observations about electrical activity and receptor function in hippocampus-to-cortex pathways.[59,68] It has been established that memory formation and retrieval involve pathways in the hippocampus of the human brain, with communication to the cerebral cortex for memory storage. During memory formation, intense electrical activity occurs in pathways of the hippocampus and cortex. Long-term potentiation (LTP) is a particular type of electrical activity that occurs in the hippocampus during memory formation. Lynch and Baudry have therefore suggested the following sequence of events as a hypothesis:[68]

1. Memory formation begins with electrical activity associated with LTP;
2. Binding of glutamate (an excitatory neurotransmitter) is increased in association with LTP;
3. Associated with LTP and initial glutamate binding is an intracellular release of calcium ion;
4. Within synaptic terminals, the free calcium activates a proteinase called calpain;
5. Activated calpain degrades a structural protein (fodrin) at the synaptic membrane; and
6. Changes in fodrin result in an ultrastructural change in the membrane that enables even further binding of glutamate.

According to this scheme, memory is associated with changes in the actual structure of synaptic membranes and consequent remodeling of the receptors exposed at the surface of the membranes (Fig. 6-5).

Further support for the concept of calcium-activated changes in synaptic proteins is emerging from current work on spectrin, a cytoskeletal protein found in erythrocytes and neurons.[69,70] A protein involved in the structure and shape of red blood cells, spectrin has been identified and studied in the brain tissue as well. In the red blood cell model, spectrin is a tetramer of two alpha and two beta subunits that binds to actin filaments and is attached to the membrane by interactions with membrane proteins (protein 4.1, ankyrin).[69] Two isoforms of brain spectrin with characteristics similar to the red blood cell protein, have been identified in nerve cell membranes. One of the spectrin types has been named *fodrin* (see above). It has been suggested that the protein lends structure to neural membranes and may be involved in the placement and movement of vesicles.[69]

Lynch and Baudry[70] reviewed evidence that calpain activation can result in partial degradation of cytoskeletal protein (spectrin), causing changes in the availability of receptors and the shape of red blood cell and platelet membranes. The blood cell phenomena are models for the proposed sequence of long-term potential changes releasing intracellular calcium, which activates calpain. Activated calpain could then break down brain spectrin, resulting in altered ultrastructure and receptor availability in synaptic membranes.[70]

It is also well established that cholinergic mechanisms are important in memory formation. Bartus et al have summarized the cholinergic hypothesis based on the effects of cholinergic drugs and on the measurements of cholinergic dysfunction in brain tissues of patients with Alzheimer's disease:[59,71]

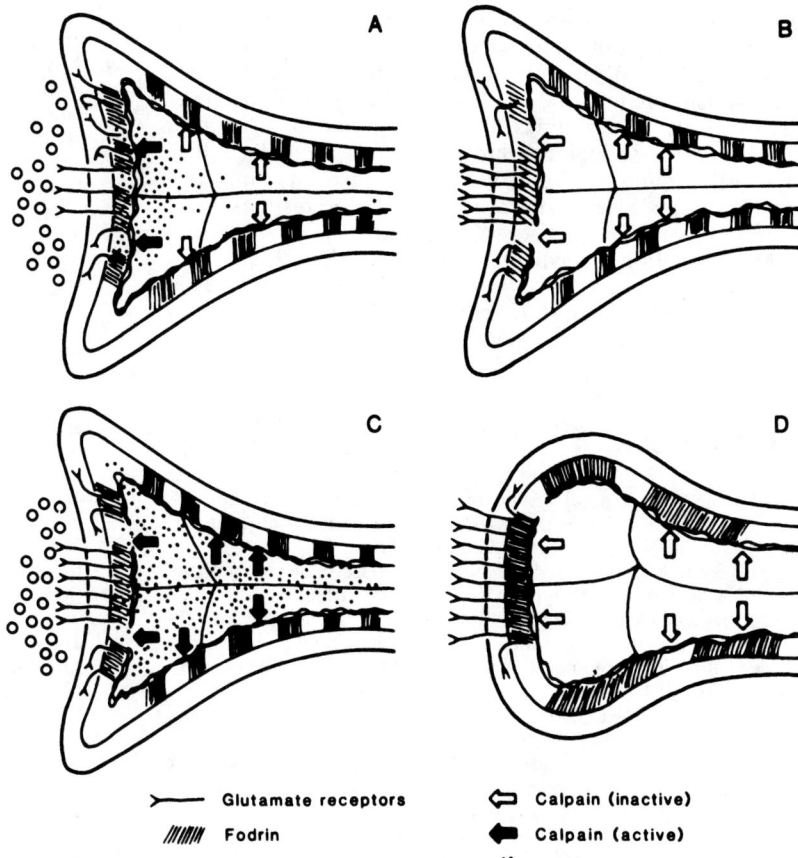

Figure 6-5. Proposed calcium-activated mechanism for changes in synaptic protein structure and function that could be associated with memory formation. Intracellular calcium activates calpain, an enzyme that degrades a membrane structural protein called fodrin. With partially degraded fodrin, glutamate receptors and membrane structure change. (Reprinted with permission from Lynch GA, Baudry M: The biochemistry of memory: A new and specific hypothesis. Science 224:1057, 1984. © 1984 by the American Association for the Advancement of Science.)

1. *Cholinergic markers.* The activity of choline acetyltransferase (CAT) is reduced in the brain tissue of patients with Alzheimer's disease. CAT is the enzyme that catalyzes the synthesis of ACh in presynaptic cells.
2. *Loss of cholinergic function at the neuronal level.* The density of postsynaptic cholinergic receptors decreases in brain tissue with normal aging.
3. *Pharmacologic evidence.* Scopolamine is a cholinergic drug well known to cause amnesia. The CNS effects of scopolamine can be reversed by physostigmine, an acetylcholinesterase inhibitor. Also, cholinemimetic drugs (e.g., arecoline) have been shown to improve the acquisition of memory in experimental situations.

The cholinergic hypothesis attributes the memory loss of Alzheimer's disease to a decrease in activity of cholinergic synapses in brain tissue. The hypothesis also suggests that cholinergic function is critical to learning, memory, and amnesia in general.[71] Arendash et al[72] have reported experiments that support the concept of cholinergic dysfunction as a key element in the neurochemical basis of Alzheimer's disease. Lesions to the nucleus basalis of Meynert result in neuropathologic and neurochemical changes after 14 months in rats that show cognitive deficits, suggesting a possible animal model for the study of cholinergic dysfunction in Alzheimer's disease.[72] A 1986 review article by Squire[73] described studies of memory and learning that focused on brain processes and systems at a "neuropsychological level of analysis." Obviously, cellular and molecular actions of anesthetics and amnesia-producing drugs are

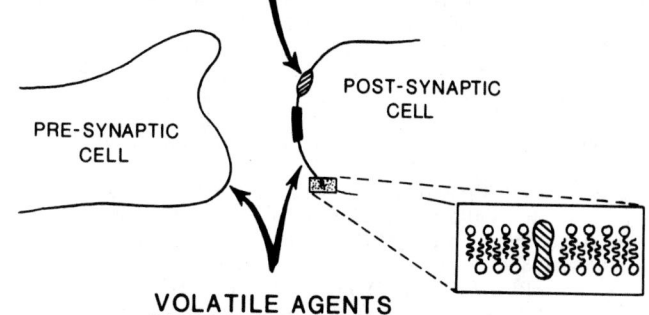

Figure 6-6. Diagram of the synaptic mechanisms of general anesthesia. Anesthesia results from the reversible modulation of synaptic communication between neurons. Most intravenous agents bind to receptors and influence the effects of neurotransmitters. Volatile agents influence membrane function by causing physicochemical changes within membrane lipids and proteins.

likely to influence neurophysiologic processes and the integrative functions of neuroanatomic regions in the brain.

Whereas the details of the current theories of memory mechanisms do not easily reconcile with the pharmacologic mechanisms of anesthetics, elements common to all aspects are in fact emerging. The broad, general principle is that synaptic communication is the basis of CNS function. Amnesia, analgesia, and control of sympathetic responses are features of anesthesia that result from drug-induced, reversible modulation of synaptic communication. Figure 6-6 summarizes anesthetic actions on synaptic activity. This discussion has been a simplistic overview of neuropharmacologic mechanisms of general anesthesia.

REFERENCES

1. Miller KW: General anaesthetics. In Feldman SA, Scun CF, Paton W (eds): Drugs in Anaesthesia: Mechanisms of Action, p 133. London, Edward Arnold, 1987
2. Roth SH, Miller KW (eds): Molecular and Cellular Mechanisms of Anesthetics, p 490. New York, Plenum, 1986
3. Dluzewski AR, Halsey MJ, Simmonds AC: Membrane interactions with general and local anaesthetics: A review of molecular hypotheses of anaesthesia. Molec Aspects Med 6:459, 1983
4. Richter JJ: Neuropharmacologic mechanisms of general anesthesia. In Barash PG (ed): Refresher Courses in Anesthesiology, vol 14, p 199. Philadelphia, JB Lippincott, 1986
5. Finck AD: Opiate receptors and endorphins: Significance for anesthesiology. In Hershey SG (ed): Refresher Courses in Anesthesiology, vol 7, p 103. Philadelphia, JB Lippincott, 1979
6. Sherrington CS: The Integrative Action of the Nervous System, p 80. New Haven, Yale University Press, 1986
7. Cooper JR, Bloom FE, Roth RH: The Biochemical Basis of Neuropharmacology. New York, Oxford University Press, 1978
8. Tapia R: Biochemical pharmacology of GABA in CNS. In Iverson LL, Iverson SD, Snyder SH (eds): Handbook of Psychopharmacology, vol 4. Amino Acid Transmitters, p 1. New York, Plenum Press, 1975
9. Richter JJ: Current theories about the mechanisms of benzodiazepines and neuroleptic drugs. Anesthesiology 54:66, 1981
10. Snyder SH, Enna SJ: The role of central glycine receptors in the pharmacologic actions of benzodiazepines. Adv Biochem Psychopharmacol 14:81, 1975
11. Cheng S-C, Brunner EA: Inducing anesthesia with a GABA analog, THIP. Anesthesiology 63:147, 1985
12. Gillis RA, DiMiccio JA, Williford DJ et al: Importance of CNS GABA-ergic mechanisms in the regulation of cardiovascular function. Brain Res Bull 5(suppl 2):303, 1980
13. Stein L, Wise CD, Beluzzi JD: Effect of benzodiazepines on central serotonergic mechanisms. Adv Biochem Psychopharmacol 14:29, 1975
14. Antonaccio MJ: GABA and inhibition of autonomic outflow: A central transmitter role. In Kalsner S (ed): Trends in Autonomic Pharmacology, vol 2, p 217. Baltimore, Urban and Schwarzenberg, 1982
15. Sample RHB, DiMiccio JA: Localization of sites in periventricular forebrain mediating cardiovascular effects of γ-aminobutyric acid agonists and antagonists in anesthetized cats. J Pharmacol Exp Ther 240:498, 1987
16. Schofield PR, Darlison MG, Fujita N et al: Sequence and functional expression of the GABA_A receptor shows a ligand-gated receptor super-family. Nature 328:221, 1987
17. Sigel E, Barnard EA: A gamma-aminobutyric acid/benzodiazepine receptor complex from bovine cerebral cortex. Improved purification with preservation of regulatory sites and their interactions. J Biol Chem 259:7219, 1984
18. Casalotti SO, Stephenson FA, Barnard EA: Separate subunits for agonist and benzodiazepine binding in the gamma-aminobutyric acid A receptor oligomer. J Biol Chem 261:15013, 1986
19. Costa E, Guidotti A: Molecular mechanisms in the receptor action of benzodiazepines. Annu Rev Pharmacol Toxicol 19:531, 1979
20. Lauven DM, Schwilden H, Stoeckel H et al: The effects of benzodiazepine antagonist Ro 15-1788 in the presence of stable concentrations of midazolam. Anesthesiology 63:61, 1985
21. Ho IK: Mechanism of action of barbiturates. Annu Rev Pharmacol Toxicol 21:83, 1981
22. Olsen RW: Drug interactions at the GABA receptor–ionophore complex. Annu Rev Pharmacol Toxicol 22:245, 1982
23. Richards CD, Strupinski K: An analysis of the action of pentobarbitane on the excitatory postsynaptic potentials and membrane properties of neurones in the guinea-pig olfactory cortex. Br J Pharmacol 89:321, 1986
24. Pocock G, Richards CD: The action of pentobarbitone on stimulus-secretion coupling in adrenal chromaffin cells. Br J Pharmacol 90:71, 1987
25. Harrison NL, Majewska M, Harrington JW et al: Structure-activity relationships for steroid interaction with the γ-aminobutyric acid_A receptor complex. J Pharmacol Exper Therap 241:346, 1987
26. Cheng S-C, Brunner EA: Effects of anesthetic agents on synaptosomal GABA disposal. Anesthesiology 55:34, 1981
27. Verma A, Snyder SH: Peripheral type benzodiazepine receptors. Annu Rev Pharmacol Toxicol 29:307, 1989
28. Seeman P, Titeler M, Tedesco J et al: Brain receptors for dopamine and neuroleptics. Adv Biochem Psychopharmacol 19:167, 1978
29. Firestone LL, Miller JC, Miller KW: Tables of physical and pharmacological properties of anesthetics. In Roth SH, Miller KW (eds): Molecular and Cellular Mechanisms of Anesthetics, p 453. New York, Plenum Medical, 1986
30. Judge SE: Effect of general anaesthesia on synaptic ion channels. Br J Anaesth 55:191, 1983
31. Richards CD: Actions of general anaesthetics on synaptic transmission in the CNS. Br J Anaesth 55:201, 1983
32. Halsey MJ: Anaesthetic mechanisms. Br J Hosp Med 36:445, 1986
33. Winters WD: Effects of drugs on the electrical activity of the brain: Anesthetics. Annu Rev Pharmacol Toxicol 16:413, 1976
34. Sauter JF, Braswell LM, Miller KW: Action of anesthetics and high pressure on cholinergic membranes. In Fink BR (ed): Progress in Anesthesiology. Vol 2. Molecular Mechanisms of Anesthesia, p 199. New York, Raven Press, 1980
35. Miller KW: The pressure reversal of anesthesia and the critical volume hypothesis. In Fink BR (ed): Progress in Anesthesiology. Vol 1. Molecular Mechanisms of Anesthesia, p 341. New York, Raven Press, 1975
36. Wardley-Smith B, Halsey MJ: Mixtures of inhalation and IV anaesthetics at high pressure. A test of the multi site hypothesis of general anaesthesia. Br J Anaesth 57:1248, 1985
37. Halsey MJ, Wardley-Smith B, Wood S: Pressure reversal of alphaxalone/alphadolone and methohexitone in tadpoles: Evidence for different molecular sites for general anaesthesia. Br J Pharmacol 89:299, 1986
38. Firestone LL, Sauter JF, Braswell LM et al: Actions of general anesthetics on acetylcholine-receptor-rich membranes from Torpedo californica. Anesthesiology 64:694, 1986
39. Dodson BA, Miller KW: Evidence for a dual mechanism in the anesthetic action of an opioid peptide. Anesthesiology 62:615, 1985
40. Trudell JR: A unitary theory of anesthesia based on lateral phase separation in nerve membranes. Anesthesiology 46:5, 1977
41. Ueda I, Hirakawa M, Arakawa K et al: Do anesthetics fluidize membranes? Anesthesiology 64:67, 1986
42. Franks NP, Lieb WR: Molecular mechanisms of general anesthesia. Nature 300:487, 1982
43. Franks NP, Lieb WR: Do general anesthetics act by competitive binding to specific receptors? Nature 310:599, 1984
44. Franks NP, Lieb WR: Mapping of general anaesthetic target sites provides a molecular basis for cut-off effects. Nature 316:349, 1985
45. Gibbons WA, Fonteh AN, McBride K: New criteria for, and a biochemical theory of, both general and local anaesthetics. Biochem Soc Trans 17:722, 1989

46. Hasinoff BB, Davey JP: The inhibition of a membrane-bound enzyme as a model for anaesthetic action and drug toxicity. Biochem J 258:101, 1989

47. Evers AS, Berkowitz BA, D'Avignon DA: Correlation between the anaesthetic effect of halothane and saturable binding in brain. Nature 328:157, 1987

48. Franks NP, Lieb WR: Neuron membranes: Anesthetics on the mind. Nature 328:113, 1987

49. Evers AS, Berkowitz BA, d'Aignon DA: Correlation between the anaesthetic effect of halothane and saturable binding in brain. Nature 341:766, 1989

50. Lockhart SH, Eger EI: Absence of abundant saturable binding sites for halothane or isoflurane in rabbit brain: Inhaled anesthetics obey Henry's law. Anesth Analg 71:70, 1990

51. Lockhart SH, Cohen Y, Yasuda N et al: Absence of abundant binding sites for anesthetics in rabbit brain: An in vivo NMR study. Anesthesiology 73:455, 1990

52. Maze M: Anesthesia and ion channel function in the autonomic nervous system. Int Anesthesiol Clin 27:248, 1989

53. Towler SC, Evers AS: Anesthesia and chemical second messenger generation in the adrenergic nervous system. Int Anesthesiol Clin 27:234, 1989

54. Birnbaum L: G Proteins in signal transduction. Annu Rev Pharmacol Toxicol 30:675, 1990

55. Mummaneni N, Rao TLK, Montoya A: Awareness and recall with high-dose fentanyl-oxygen anesthesia. Anesth Analg 59:948, 1980

56. Abuleish E, Taylor FH: Effect of morphine-diazepam on signs of anesthesia, awareness and dreams of patients under nitrous oxide for cesarean section. Anesth Analg 55:702, 1976

57. Robinson RJS, Boright WA, Ligier B et al: The incidence of awareness and amnesia for perioperative events, after cardiac surgery with lorazepam and fentanyl anesthesia. J Cardiothorac Anesth 1:524, 1987

58. Breckenridge JL, Aitkenhead AR: Awareness during anaesthesia: A review. Ann R Coll Surg 65:93, 1983

59. Richter JJ: Anesthesia, amnesia, and alchemy. Semin Anesth 6:128, 1987

60. Eich E, Reeves JL, Katz RL: Anesthesia, amnesia, and the memory/awareness distinction. Anesth Analg 64:1143, 1985

61. Bennett HL, Davis HS, Giannini JA: Non-verbal response to intraoperative conversation. Br J Anaesth 57:174, 1985

62. Goldmann L, Shah MV, Hebden MW: Memory of cardiac anaesthesia. Anaesthesia 42:596, 1987

63. Woo R, Seltzer JL, Marr A: The lack of response to suggestion under controlled surgical anesthesia. Acta Anaesthesiol Scand 31:567, 1987

64. Mori K: The EEG and awareness during general anaesthesia. Anaesthesia 42:1153, 1987

65. Crick F: Memory and molecular turnover. Nature 312:101, 1984

66. Schwartz JH, Greenberg SM: Molecular mechanisms for memory: Second messenger induced modifications of protein kinases in nerve cells. Annu Rev Neurosci 10:459, 1987

67. Goelet P, Castellucci VF, Shacher S et al: The long and the short of a long-term memory—a molecular framework. Nature 322:419, 1986

68. Lynch G, Baudry M: The biochemistry of memory: A new and specific hypothesis. Science 224:1057, 1984

69. Goodman SR, Zagon IS: Brain spectrin: Structure, location, and function. A symposium overview. Brain Res Bull 18:773, 1987

70. Lynch G, Baudry M: Brain spectrin, calpain and long-term changes in synaptic efficacy. Brain Res Bull 18:809, 1987

71. Bartus RT, Dean RL, Beer R et al: The cholinergic hypothesis of geriatric memory dysfunction. Science 217:408, 1982

72. Arendash GW, Millard WJ, Dunn AJ et al: Long-term neuropathological and neurochemical effects of nucleus basalis lesions in the rat. Science 238:952, 1987

73. Squire LS: Mechanisms of memory. Science 232:1612, 1986

7

Steven J. Barker
Kevin K. Tremper

Physics Applied to Anesthesia

INTRODUCTION

Applications of the laws of physics are seen in every aspect of anesthesiology. An understanding of some of these basic principles thus facilitates the study of anesthesiology and makes clinical practice more rewarding, enjoyable, and safe. Classical physics is not difficult to understand; it is only the mathematical modeling of physical laws that may become complex. In this chapter, we explain important principles both in words and in the language of mathematics. The latter will be kept as fundamental as possible, but without mathematics we cannot apply basic principles to the solution of practical problems. We assume only a knowledge of basic algebra and an understanding of derivatives.

Each physical principle will be illustrated with simple examples. We hope the reader will find these applications useful both for their own sake and as aids in clarifying the underlying physics. Some readers may wish to pass over the details of the more complex examples. These details are presented so that the interested reader can see complete derivations of solutions to physics problems. Previous texts and chapters aimed at physicians suffer from an almost phobic avoidance of mathematics, making physics seem unscientific or arcane. The only earlier physics text for anesthesiologists that we recommend is that of Macintosh and associates.[1]

It is traditional for physics texts or chapters to begin with a rather dull treatise on units and dimensions, running the risk of spoiling the reader's taste for the whole subject. Instead, we handle units and dimensions as they are needed with each topic, and hope this approach makes them more palatable by dilution.

CLASSICAL MECHANICS

Basic Principles: Newton's Second Law

The term "classical mechanics" is used by physicists to distinguish this field from both quantum mechanics and relativity. Classical mechanics describes the motions of all types of matter (solids, liquids, gases) acted on by various forces (gravity, electromagnetic fields, pressure). It becomes inaccurate for small bits of matter (e.g., atoms) and for very large objects (stars) or for those with velocities close to the speed of light. Classical mechanics is subdivided into the mechanics of solids (particles, rigid bodies, vibrations) and the mechanics of fluids (liquids and gases). The early history of classical mechanics is described nicely by Dugas.[2]

Most of classical mechanics is based on a single physical principle: Newton's second law of motion.[3] In its simplest terms, this law is given by the equation:

$$\mathbf{F} = m\mathbf{a} \tag{7-1}$$

where $\mathbf{F}$ is the force vector acting on mass m to produce the acceleration vector $\mathbf{a}$. Acceleration is the time derivative of the velocity vector $\mathbf{v}$; that is, it is the rate of change of velocity. Force and mass, although well understood intuitively, are not easily defined mathematically. Newton defined these terms using his law of motion in the form of Equation 7-1. Force and acceleration are vectors; that is, they have both magnitude and direction. Each is described by three numbers, such as the x, y, and z components in the Cartesian coordinate system. Mass is a scalar and is described by only one number.

Each time we encounter a new physical quantity in this chapter, we define its units in the Système International d'Unités (SI) or meters-kilograms-seconds system. English units and practical units, such as millimeters of mercury (mm Hg), may also be used. The SI unit of force is the newton (N), and the English unit is the pound (lb). (Note that the pound is a unit of force, not mass. This confusing usage is one of many reasons the English system is being replaced.) The SI unit of mass is the kilogram (kg), and the English unit is the slug. Acceleration has SI units of meters per second per second, abbreviated as m/s^2. The English units are ft/s^2. Equation 7-1 states that 1 N equals one $kg\text{-}m/s^2$.

There is frequent confusion between the terms units and dimensions, and the two words are often inappropriately interchanged. A dimension describes the measure by which a physical variable is expressed quantitatively. For example, length (L) is the dimension used to describe distance, height, and width. Units are specific ways of measuring a given dimension; meters, feet, furlongs, and light-years are examples of units of length. In mechanics, all dimensions can be expressed in terms of the three fundamental dimensions: mass (m), length (L), and time (t). In problems involving energy transport, a fourth dimension, temperature (T)

or heat, must be added. In Newton's second law, the dimensions of acceleration are L/t^2, and the dimensions of force are mL/t^2.

Another common source of confusion in mechanics arises from the terms *mass* and *weight*, particularly in the English system of units. Mass is the property of matter that resists being put into motion, as expressed in Equation 7-1. Weight is the force exerted by gravity (g) on a given mass. Weight is proportional to mass, with a proportionality constant on the earth's surface of 9.8 N/kg (32.2 lb/slug in English units). An object in outer space may have no weight, but its mass is the same as it is on the surface of the earth.

Mechanics of Particles

The simplest applications of Newton's second law involve known forces acting on particles, which are simply objects whose mass can be represented as being concentrated at one point. A particle's location at time t can be fully described by three numbers: the Cartesian coordinates x, y, and z. This may seem like an oversimplification in dealing with large objects, but Newtonian particle mechanics is accurate enough for virtually all problems of orbital mechanics. This includes predicting the trajectories of planets as well as of spacecraft.

We begin with the simplest of all particle problems, one-dimensional motion of a particle of mass m. Suppose the particle starts at $x = 0$ with velocity $v = 0$ at time $t = 0$ and is free to move in the x direction under the influence of a constant force F. The particle's position, which we are trying to find, is given by $x(t)$ at a given time t. Its velocity is $v = dx/dt$,* and its acceleration is:

$$a = \frac{dv}{dt} = \frac{d^2x}{dt^2} \tag{7-2}$$

If F is a constant, then Equation 7-1 reduces to:

$$F = m\frac{d^2x}{dt^2}$$

or

$$\frac{d^2x}{dt^2} = \frac{F}{m}$$

Because F/m is constant, we can integrate this equation twice with respect to time:

$$\frac{dx}{dt} = \frac{F}{m}t + A \tag{7-3}$$

$$x = \frac{1}{2}\frac{F}{m}t^2 + At + B$$

The two *boundary conditions* that $x = 0$ and $v = 0$ when $t = 0$ require that the integration constants A and B must both be zero (Equation 7-3). The solution to our simple one-dimensional problem is thus:

$$x = \frac{1}{2}\frac{F}{m}t^2 \tag{7-4}$$

*The symbol dx/dt means "the derivative of x with respect to time," and d^2x/dt^2 is the time derivative of dx/dt.

This solution by itself may not help us practice better anesthesia, but it illustrates the technique used for solving all problems in classical mechanics. First, we must write an *equation of motion* in the form of Equation 7-1, which requires a mathematical description of all the forces involved. Second, we must solve this equation to obtain an expression for the particle's location. Finally, we must use the specified boundary conditions (often the initial position and velocity) to assign values to the integration constants that arise in the second step. In complicated problems, steps 2 and 3 may consist of millions of calculations performed by a computer.

It is convenient to use the example above to introduce the concepts of momentum and kinetic energy. Newton defined momentum (**P**) as the product of an object's mass and its velocity, or:

$$\mathbf{P} = m\mathbf{v} \tag{7-5}$$

The dimensions of momentum are mL/t, and the SI units are kg-m/s. Note that the momentum **P** is a vector quantity, as is velocity **v**. Newton's second law can be rewritten in terms of momentum as:

$$\mathbf{F} = \frac{d\mathbf{P}}{dt} \tag{7-6}$$

In words, force equals the rate of change of momentum. The kinetic energy K of a particle is given by:

$$K = \frac{1}{2}mv^2 \tag{7-7}$$

The dimensions of energy are mL^2/t^2. The SI unit is the kg-m^2/s^2, which is called the *joule* (J). K is a scalar quantity: it has magnitude but no direction. This distinction between K and **P** is important when we consider systems of multiple particles. For example, two particles of equal mass and equal speed moving in opposite directions have a total momentum of zero because the vectors cancel. However, their total kinetic energy is twice that of either one. The total momentum of all the molecules of gas in a stationary box is zero, but the total energy is the sum of all the K's of the individual molecules. This total energy defines a new variable called temperature, to be discussed below.

Another important concept in mechanics is that of *work*, defined as force times the distance over which the force acts:

$$W = Fd \tag{7-8}$$

(Here F is the magnitude of the force rather than the force vector.) The dimensions of work are mL^2/t^2—the same dimensions as energy! Let us look back at the example of linear motion under a constant force. We found that in time t the particle reaches a velocity of $v = Ft/m$ and moves a distance of $\frac{1}{2}(F/m)t^2$, so the work done in that time is:

$$W = Fd = F \cdot \frac{1}{2}\frac{F}{m}t^2$$

$$= \frac{1}{2}\frac{F^2t^2}{m} = \frac{1}{2}m\left(\frac{Ft}{m}\right)^2 \tag{7-9}$$

$$= \frac{1}{2}mv^2$$

We have shown for this example that the work done on the particle is equal to the kinetic energy acquired by the particle. This statement is true for all forces, constant or not, and is a direct consequence of $F = ma$.*

Now that we understand work and kinetic energy, we introduce another form of energy, potential energy. The simplest illustration of this concept is gravitational potential energy. In a uniform gravitational field such as that at the earth's surface, the force of gravity on any object is proportional to its mass:

$$F = mg \qquad (7\text{-}10)$$

The gravitational constant g equals 9.8 N/kg (32.2 lb/slug) at the earth's surface. If we lift an object of mass m to a height z above its origin, we must do work given by:

$$W = Fd = mgz \qquad (7\text{-}11)$$

What happens to the energy represented by this amount of work? It is stored in the form of *gravitational potential energy*, which can be converted into kinetic energy simply by letting the mass fall back to its origin. That is, when the mass falls to $z = 0$, its acquired velocity will be such that the kinetic energy (K) equals the previous potential energy (U):

$$K = U$$
$$\tfrac{1}{2}mv^2 = mgz \qquad (7\text{-}12)$$
$$v = \sqrt{2gz}$$

The same result could be obtained by applying $F = ma$ directly to this problem.

Potential energy is thus a form of stored energy that can be exchanged for kinetic energy or used to do work. In systems in which energy cannot be lost in other forms, such as heat or radiation, the sum of the kinetic and potential energies will be constant:

$$\text{Total energy} = U + K = \text{constant} \qquad (7\text{-}13)$$

Potential energy can be found in many forms in the operating room. For example, a great deal of energy is stored in a cylinder filled with oxygen at a pressure of 2100 pounds per square inch (psi). Relatively little energy would be stored in the same cylinder filled with water at the same pressure. Why?

EXAMPLE 7-1. THE HARMONIC OSCILLATOR AND ARTERIAL PRESSURE MEASUREMENT

Now we shall use simple particle dynamics to investigate a problem of importance to all anesthesiologists: the interpretation of intra-arterial pressure waveforms. The moving particle discussed above was acted on by a constant force. Suppose instead that this particle is acted on by an oscillating external force given by:

$$F = A \sin (\omega t)$$

Furthermore, suppose the particle is tethered by a spring and its motions are resisted by a damper (Fig. 7-1). The

*In the case of a force that varies with x, the expression for work $W = Fd$ is replaced by the integral expression $W = \int F(x)\, dx$, where the limits of integration are given by the distance over which the force acts.

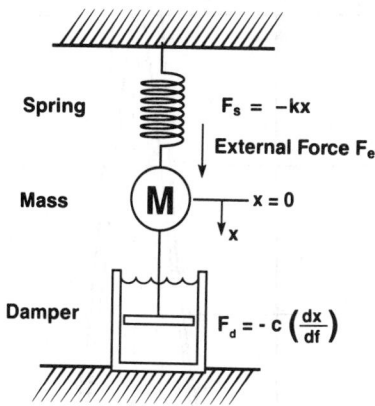

Figure 7-1. The forced simple harmonic oscillator. Mass *m* is acted on by driving force $F = A \sin (\omega t)$, spring force $F = -kx$, and damping force $F = -c(dx/dt)$.

spring force, assuming a linear *Hooke's Law* spring, is given by:

$$F_S = -kx$$

The damping force is assumed to be proportional to the particle velocity:

$$F_d = -c\left(\frac{dx}{dt}\right)$$

The spring and damping forces are both negative, because both forces tend to restore the particle to its equilibrium position at $x = 0$.

Now we can write the equation of motion ($\mathbf{F} = \mathbf{ma}$) for this system by summing the three forces:

$$A \sin (\omega t) - kx - c\left(\frac{dx}{dt}\right) = m\left(\frac{d^2x}{dt^2}\right)$$

or, by transposing the terms:

$$m\left(\frac{d^2x}{dt^2}\right) + c\left(\frac{dx}{dt}\right) + kx = A \sin (\omega t) \qquad (7\text{-}14)$$

This differential equation is called the *forced harmonic oscillator equation*. It is a second-order linear, ordinary differential equation. The solution is:

$$x(t) = D \sin (\omega t + \phi) \qquad (7\text{-}15)$$

where the motion amplitude D is given by:

$$D = \frac{A/k}{\sqrt{\left(1 - \dfrac{\omega^2}{\omega_0^2}\right)^2 + 4\,\zeta^2\,\omega^2/\omega_0^2}} \qquad (7\text{-}16)$$

In Equation 7-16, ω_0 is the *resonant angular* frequency, given by:

$$\omega_0 = \sqrt{\frac{k}{m}} \qquad (7\text{-}17)$$

*Angular frequency is related to ordinary frequency f by $\omega = 2\pi f$.

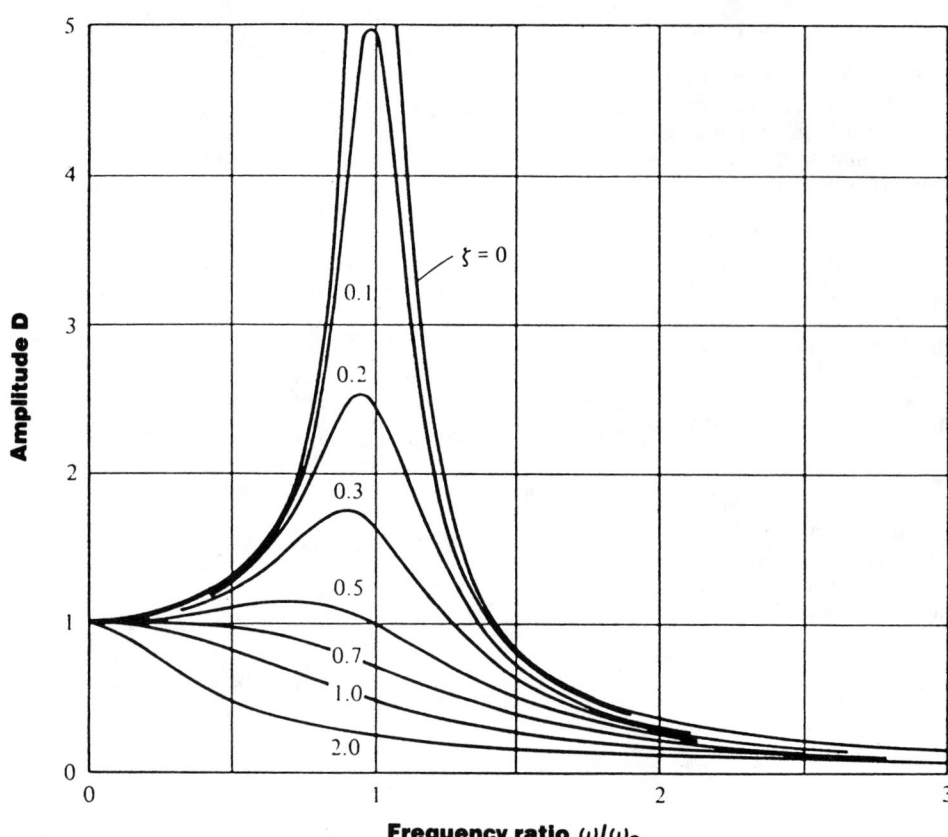

Figure 7-2. Amplitude D of the forced harmonic oscillator versus ratio of driving frequency ω to resonant frequency ω_0. Curves shown are for different values of damping coefficient ζ. Note that for $\zeta = 0.2$ (clinical transducer systems), the maximum amplification factor is greater than 2.

and ζ is the *damping coefficient*, given by:

$$\zeta = \frac{c}{\sqrt{2km}} \qquad (7\text{-}18)$$

The phase angle ϕ in Equation 7-15 is given by another expression that is not important to us here.

Figure 7-2 shows a series of plots of the motion amplitude D (Equation 7-16) as a function of the driving frequency ω for various values of the damping coefficient ζ. Note that if there is no damping ($\zeta = 0$), the amplitude of oscillation will become infinite when the driving frequency equals the resonant frequency. As the damping is increased, the amplification that occurs at resonance decreases. The *amplification ratio*, given by D/A, is approximately $1/(2\zeta k)$ at resonance (Equation 7-16).

How does this analysis relate to arterial waveforms? A good analogy exists between the forced harmonic oscillator and the commonly used arterial pressure monitoring system involving fluid-filled tubing and an extracorporeal transducer. The mass m of the oscillator represents the mass of the fluid in the pressure tubing (from cannula to transducer). The spring constant k represents the elasticity of the tubing itself and the compliance of the transducer diaphragm. The damping constant c is a measure of the friction in the system, which is mainly viscous friction from the fluid moving to and fro in the pressure tubing.

Using this forced oscillator model, we can characterize a catheter–transducer system by two quantities: the resonant frequency f_0 ($f_0 = \omega_0/2\pi$) and the damping coefficient ζ. Gardner has measured these quantities for various systems, and some of his results are presented in Table 7-1.[4] Typical clinical systems have damping coefficients of 0.2–0.3 and

resonant frequencies as low as 10 Hz. This implies a maximum amplification factor of about 2.0 at resonance (Fig. 7-2). If resonance occurs at 10 Hz (or 600 cycles per minute), we might expect that amplification will be insignificant. However, arterial pressure waveforms are not sinusoids. Fourier analysis, or representation of the waveforms as a sum of sinusoids, shows that they have significant energy at frequencies as high as ten times the heart rate. It is these *harmonics* that are amplified by the catheter-transducer system, producing severe distortion of the waveform. Depending on the shape and frequency of the *true* arterial waveform, this distortion can result in a 20–30% *overshoot* error in systolic blood pressure readings. Furthermore, the magnitude of the error is dependent on the heart rate (Equation 7-16), so that an error determined for a given patient may not remain constant.

What characteristics of the transducer system determine the f_0 and ζ values given in Table 7-1? Obviously, these are related to system mass, elasticity, and damping, as described above. A system with a longer length of fluid-filled tubing will have more mass and a lower resonant frequency f_0. Softer, more compliant tubing adds elasticity (lower spring constant k), which also lowers f_0. The presence of air bubbles in the tubing affects both f_0 and ζ. First, bubbles add elasticity in proportion to their total volume, thus lowering f_0. Also, large bubbles increase friction and thereby increase ζ. Both large and small bubbles must therefore be eliminated in order to obtain the f_0 and ζ values given in Table 7-1.

In the clinical setting, it is easy to determine the approximate resonant frequency of a transducer system. If the high-pressure flush is turned on and then rapidly turned off at a chart speed of 50 mm/s, the resulting tracing will oscillate

TABLE 7-1. Catheter–Tubing–Transducer System Characteristics*

No.	Description	Natural Frequency (Hz) f_0	Damping Coefficient ζ
1	5-Fr two-lumen pulmonary artery HP transducer; dyne diaphragm dome	9.5	0.32
2	5-Fr two-lumen pulmonary artery HP transducer; HP diaphragm dome	10.0	0.30
3	4-Fr two-lumen pulmonary artery (47 cm); Bell & Howell transducer and diaphragm dome	12.0	0.30
4	6-Fr two-lumen pulmonary artery HP transducer; no diaphragm dome	13.0	0.15
5	5-Fr two-lumen pulmonary artery HP transducer; no diaphragm dome	14.0	0.25
6	7-Fr four-lumen thermodilution pulmonary artery (#1)	14.5	0.20
7	CAP† 18-ga with 24″ pressure tubing	15.0	0.72
8	7-Fr pulmonary artery (#2) (see #6)	15.5	0.20
9	7-Fr pulmonary artery (#3) (see #6)	14.0	0.32
10	Vinca‡ + 84-inch pressure tube (#1)	16.0	0.10
11	Vinca + 84-inch pressure tube (#2) (see #10)	16.0	0.20
12	CAP 18-gauge direct	20.0	0.30
13	48″ pressure tubing direct	24.0	0.28
14	7-Fr pulmonary artery	25.0	0.15
15	Vinca + 24-inch PVC pressure tubing	38.0	0.10
16	Vinca + 48-inch PVC pressure tubing	45.0	0.13
17	Vinca + 24-inch polyethylene pressure tubing	48.0	0.14

*Unless otherwise specified, runs were made with Bentley Model 800 transducer without a diaphragm dome.

†CAP = 18-gauge CAP catheter–Sorenson.

‡Vinca = 2-inch, 18-gauge over-the-needle arterial catheter.

through several cycles at a frequency near ω_0. The damping coefficient can also be determined from the ratio of amplitudes of successive oscillations. Thus, the solution of a basic problem in particle mechanics has provided us with a quantitative method to evaluate the performance of catheter–transducer pressure-monitoring systems.

There are many intermediate and advanced texts on the mechanics of particles and rigid bodies.[5-8] In addition to looking at Newton's *In Principia*,[3] the historically inclined reader should see the works of Lord Kelvin.[9]

MECHANICS OF FLUIDS

The mechanics of fluids has numerous applications in physiology, anesthesiology, and critical care. Here we discuss some basic principles and illustrate these with applications related to anesthesia.

First of all, what is a fluid? By definition, a fluid is matter that deforms continuously when subjected to a shearing stress. Visualize two flat, parallel walls with a fluid contained between them (Fig. 7-3). If we exert a tangential (parallel to the surface) force on the upper wall while holding the lower wall stationary, we create a shearing stress in the fluid. Our definition says that the upper wall will continue to move, thereby deforming or *straining* the fluid, for as long as we exert the force. This behavior is in contrast to that of solid matter, which, when stressed in this way, will deform a given amount and reach a fixed equilibrium shape. The amount of deformation is referred to as a *strain*. In other words, shearing stress is related to strain in solids, whereas in fluids it is related to *rate of strain*. By this definition both

liquids and gases are fluids. The difference is that gases can be compressed by external pressure, whereas liquids are nearly incompressible. (In medicine, we often say "fluid" when what we really mean is "liquid." For example, "do you use air or fluid to test for loss of resistance when performing an epidural?" Air is a fluid, which makes this question irrational.)

There are numerous texts on the subject of fluid mechanics, and only a few will be cited here. The reader who wants a rigorous yet broad coverage at the intermediate to advanced level is referred to Landau and Lifshitz[10] or to Bat-

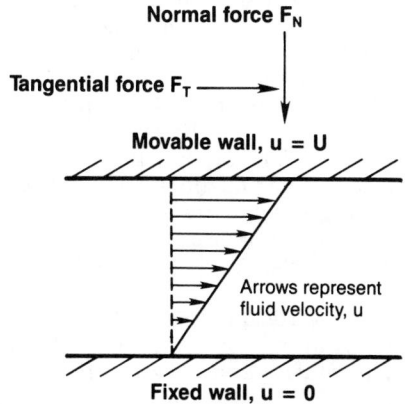

Figure 7-3. Flow between two parallel plane walls. The upper wall is moving to the right at speed *U;* the lower wall is stationary. *Arrows* represent fluid velocity vectors at points between the walls.

chelor.[11] Somewhat easier and more applied general texts include those of Streeter and Wylie[12] and Sabersky and Acosta.[13] For excellent and very readable coverage of viscous flows, we recommend Schlichting.[14] For the historically inclined, we suggest Sir Horace Lamb.[15] The best introductory text on compressible flows is that of Liepmann and Roshko,[16] and we also recommend Thompson[17] and Zucrow and Hoffman.[18]

Incompressible Fluids

We deal first with incompressible fluids, a term that refers, not only to liquids but also to gases in situations in which compressibility is not important. For example, the flow of air in and out of the lungs and through an anesthesia circuit can be considered incompressible for practical purposes, because the pressure variations in this flow are small relative to the total pressure of 1 atmosphere (atm). We have not yet defined the term *pressure*, and for this purpose we shall consider nonmoving fluids, the field of *hydrostatics*.

We defined a fluid as matter that deforms continuously as long as a shearing or tangential force is exerted. This means that if the fluid is not deforming, there can be no shear stress present. Therefore, a stationary fluid can have only *normal forces*, or forces applied perpendicular to plane areas such as those shown in Figure 7-3. If we divide this normal force by the area of the plane surface, we obtain the pressure. Pressure (p) is defined at a point by letting the area of the imaginary surface approach zero. Pressure thus has dimensions of force per area, or m/Lt^2. The SI unit of pressure is the newton per square meter, called the *pascal* (Pa). Because this is a rather small unit of pressure, we usually prefer kilopascals (kPa). The English unit of pressure is the pound per square foot (lb/ft²), although lb/in² (psi) is often used for convenience. Handy values to remember are that atmospheric pressure at sea level (called 1 *atmosphere of pressure*) equals 101.3 kPa, or 2116 lb/ft², or 14.69 lb/in².

To express Newton's second law in fluids, we define the *density* (ρ) as the mass per unit volume of fluid. The dimensions of density are mass per volume or m/L^3. The SI unit of density is kilograms per cubic meter and the English unit is slugs per cubic foot. Because liquids are nearly incompressible, their density is usually constant except for a dependence on temperature. The density of water at room temperature is 997.8 kg/m³ or 1.936 slugs/ft³. A more practical unit of density in liquids is the gram per cubic centimeter (g/cm³), because the density of water is very near 1.0 g/cm³.

The force exerted by gravity on an object is proportional to the object's mass, as shown in Equation 7-10: $F = mg$. The direction of this force is usually chosen as the $-z$ direction in a Cartesian system. The dimensions of g are force per mass, or L/t^2 (use Equation 7-1 to show that these dimensions are equivalent). At the earth's surface, g is equal to 9.8 N/kg or 9.8 m/s². If gravity is the only force acting on an object, we have from Equations 7-1 and 7-10: $mg = ma$, or $g = a$. Thus, any object in *free fall* near the earth's surface will fall with an acceleration of 9.8 m/s². For this reason, the gravitational constant g is also called the *acceleration of gravity*.

Consider now a vertical cylinder of liquid with a cross-sectional area (A) in the horizontal plane of 1 m² (see Fig. 7-4). The height of this cylinder is z, and the volume of fluid within it is $V = zA = z$ (because A = 1). Because ρ is the mass per unit volume of liquid, the total mass in the cylinder is $m = \rho V = \rho z$. The gravitational force on this mass

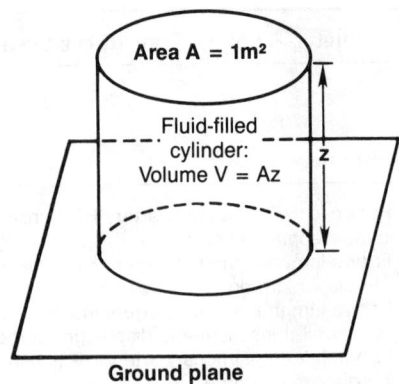

Figure 7-4. Hydrostatics of a fluid-filled cylinder resting on a horizontal plane (gravity directed downward). The cylinder has height z and cross-section $A = 1$ m². It is filled with incompressible fluid of density ρ.

(i.e., its weight) is just mg, or ρgz. If the cylinder is resting on its bottom surface as in Figure 7-4, this weight is balanced by the pressure force ρ acting on that surface. (Pressure force $= pA$; $A = 1$ in this case.) Thus the *balance of forces* in this statics problem is pressure force = weight, or:

$$p = \rho gz \qquad (7\text{-}19)$$

This equation is the basis of hydrostatics, the determination of pressures and forces in liquids at rest.

EXAMPLE 7-2. THE MANOMETER

A manometer is simply a vertical or inclined column of liquid used to measure an opposing pressure or force. Examples in medicine include the sphygmomanometer for blood pressure measurement and the water manometer for measurement of central venous or intracranial pressure. Equation 7-19 is a formula for manometer pressures. If the manometer contains mercury, the density ρ is 13,600 kg/m³ in SI units (13.6 g/cm³, or 13.6 times the density of water). The manometer pressure is then:

$$p\,[\text{Pa}] = 13{,}600 \times 9.8 \times z\,[\text{m}] = 1.333 \times 10^5 \times z\,[\text{m}]$$
$$(7\text{-}20)$$

We often use the millimeter of mercury (mm Hg), or *torr*, as a unit of pressure. If we convert meters to millimeters and pascals to kilopascals, Equation 7-20 becomes $p[\text{kPa}] = 0.1333\ z\,[\text{mm Hg}]$; that is, 1 mm Hg equals 0.1333 kPa (1 atm = 760 mm Hg = 101.3 kPa). Manometer pressures using any liquid can be calculated from Equation 7-19 by substituting the appropriate value for the density ρ.

We turn now to incompressible fluids in motion, or *incompressible fluid dynamics*. Newton's second law can appear complex in fluids because of the coordinate systems used and the various forces that exist. Fluid forces are usually divided into three categories: gravity, pressure, and friction. We have already shown that the gravity force per unit volume is ρg, acting in the vertical ($-z$) direction. Pressure forces in fluids are caused by *differences* in pressure, expressed mathematically as the negative of the pressure gra-

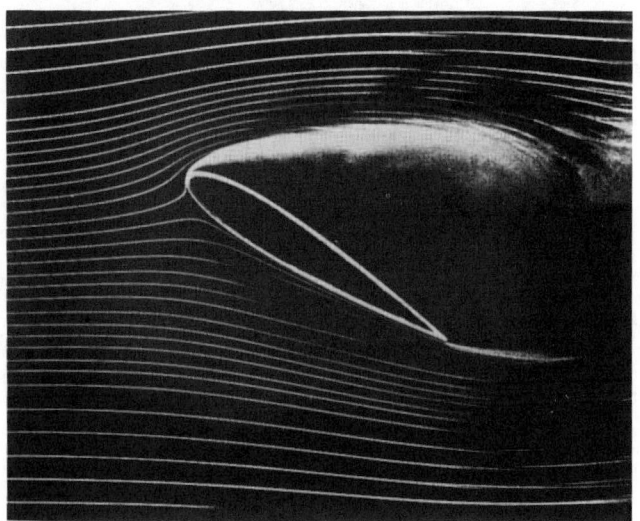

Figure 7-5. Streamlines of flow approaching an airfoil at a high angle of attack, illustrating separation of flow from the upper surface or *stall*.

dient.* If the fluid can move only in the x direction (one-dimensional motion), then the pressure gradient is simply dp/dx.

Before we examine friction (viscous) forces in fluids, let us consider flow of an *ideal* fluid, one which has zero viscosity. We define *streamlines* as lines in a moving fluid that are everywhere parallel to the velocity vector, as shown in Figure 7-5. For steady flow of an incompressible, inviscid fluid, the equation of motion yields:

$$p_0 = p + \tfrac{1}{2}\rho U^2 + \rho g z \qquad (7\text{-}21)$$

where p_0, called the *stagnation pressure*, is constant along streamlines. U is the magnitude of the fluid velocity. Even though there is no such thing as an inviscid fluid, this *Bernoulli equation* can be applied to many flows in which viscosity is not important.

EXAMPLE 7-3. FLOW THROUGH A VENTURI TUBE

Consider steady flow through a horizontal pipe of changing diameter as shown in Figure 7-6. Given the pressure p and velocity U at cross-section #1, find the values of p and U at cross-section #2.

We can neglect gravity in this problem because the pipe is horizontal. The Bernoulli equation therefore becomes:

$$p_1 + \tfrac{1}{2}\rho U_1^2 = p_2 + \tfrac{1}{2}\rho U_2^2 \qquad (7\text{-}22)$$

We also know that the volume of flow or *flux* (Q) at each cross-section must be the same, because no fluid is entering or leaving through the walls of the pipe. Fluid flux has SI units of cubic meters per second (dimensions L^3/t) and is

---

*In three dimensions, the pressure gradient ∇p is given by:

$$\nabla p = \frac{\partial p}{\partial x}\hat{X} + \frac{\partial p}{\partial y}\hat{Y} + \frac{\partial p}{\partial z}\hat{Z}$$

where $\hat{X}$, $\hat{Y}$, and $\hat{Z}$ are unit vectors.

---

given at each cross-section by the velocity U times the cross-sectional area A:

$$Q = U_1 A_1 = U_2 A_2 \qquad (7\text{-}23)$$

Now use Equation 7-23 to solve for u_2 in terms of u_1, and plug this expression into Equation 7-22, which we solve for $p_2 - p_1$:

$$p_2 - p_1 = \tfrac{1}{2}\rho U_1^2\left[1 - \left(\frac{A_1}{A_2}\right)^2\right] \qquad (7\text{-}24)$$

Note some features of this result. First, because A_1 is greater than A_2, the pressure falls as we enter the narrowing of the pipe. Second, for large A_1/A_2, the pressure drop is proportional to the square of the area ratio, or the fourth power of the diameter ratio. Finally, the pressure drop is proportional to the square of the velocity. We could just as easily make A_2 greater than A_1, in which case, p_2 would be greater than p_1. Thus, pressure falls as pipe diameter decreases and rises as pipe diameter increases. This last statement violates some people's intuition—pressure does not always fall in the direction of flow!

The *Venturi effect* of lower pressure in areas of smaller diameter and higher velocity has many practical applications. For example, it can contribute to airway closure in patients having chronic obstructive pulmonary disease by creating lower pressures in regions of narrowing where velocities are higher. As expiratory flow velocity increases, the Venturi effect moves the *equal pressure point*, the point at which the pressures inside and outside of an airway are equal, more distally into smaller airways. These smaller airways are less well tethered and hence more likely to collapse, particularly in the emphysematous patient. We could also solve Equation 7-24 for u_1 in terms of $p_1 - p_2$ and thus use the Venturi tube of Figure 7-6 as a flow meter; we can measure $p_1 - p_2$ with a simple liquid manometer.

The technique of jet ventilation (e.g., during rigid bronchoscopy) makes use of a principle related to the Venturi effect. The high-velocity, small-diameter jet *entrains* the surrounding gas and sets it into motion in the direction of the jet. As we travel downstream in the jet flow, more and more of the moving fluid is entrained fluid that came from the gas surrounding the initial jet. Hence the gas mixture (i.e., the oxygen fraction) of the downstream flow in the trachea can be considerably different (lower F_{IO_2}) than the mixture in the original jet at the orifice.

If fluids were inviscid, we could use Bernoulli's equation on every flow problem. However, friction exists in all real fluids and is manifested by the physical property called *viscosity*. This fluid property was defined by Newton using the flow geometry shown in Figure 7-3. The upper wall in the figure has surface area A, is moving with speed U, and

Cross-section #1:
Area A_1, Velocity U_1

Cross-section #2:
Area A_2, Velocity U_2

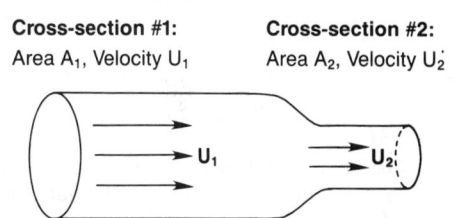

Figure 7-6. Flow into a contraction. At #1, the cross-sectional area is A_1 and the mean velocity is U_1; at #2, the area is A_2 and the mean velocity is U_2.

is separated from the lower wall by distance d. If the force required to move the upper wall is F and the local fluid velocity is u, then as Newton found,

$$F = \mu \frac{uA}{d} \qquad (7\text{-}25)$$

The force is directly proportional to velocity and area and inversely proportional to the distance between the parallel walls. The proportionality constant μ is called the *dynamic viscosity*. If we define *shear stress* τ as F/A in Equation 7-25 and replace u/d with the derivative of fluid velocity in the y direction, we obtain:

$$\tau = \mu \frac{du}{dy} \qquad (7\text{-}26)$$

Fluids that obey this linear relation between shear stress and rate of strain (du/dy) are called *Newtonian fluids*. From Equation 7-25, μ has dimensions of Ft/L^2, or m/Lt. The SI units of μ are kilogram per meter-second; the English units are slug per foot-second.

Viscosity is a function of temperature: it usually increases with rising temperature in gases and decreases in liquids. Here are some sample viscosity values (in kg/m-s):

air (20°C)	1.8×10^{-5}
water (20°C)	1.0×10^{-3}
SAE 30 motor oil (20°C)	0.26
glycerin (20°C)	1.5
blood (37°C)	$3\text{–}6 \times 10^{-3}$*

Now that we understand viscosity as a proportionality between shear stress and rate of strain, we consider a viscous flow of physiological importance: flow through a circular tube. The equation of motion for an incompressible, viscous fluid (called the *Navier-Stokes equation*) has a simple solution if we assume a straight, circular tube of infinite length (Fig. 7-7). We must also assume here that the flow is steady and *laminar*, a distinction we shall discuss below. Under these precise conditions, we can show that the flow velocity u at a distance r from the center of a tube of radius R is given by:

$$u(r) = -\frac{1}{4\mu} \frac{dp}{dx} (R^2 - r^2) \qquad (7\text{-}27)$$

The velocity is proportional to the pressure gradient dp/dx, is a maximum at the centerline ($r = 0$), and is zero at the wall of the tube ($r = R$). The shape of this velocity profile (Fig. 7-7) is that of a parabola. To find the volume flow or flux Q through the tube, we integrate this velocity over the cross-sectional area of the tube (velocity × area = volume flow). The result is called the Hagen-Poiseuille law of friction:

$$Q = \frac{\pi R^4}{8\mu} \left(-\frac{dp}{dx} \right) \qquad (7\text{-}28)$$

This famous *R to the fourth law* is often incorrectly applied in medicine, as we shall see below. Note that (1) flow is directly proportional to the pressure derivative along the

---

*The viscosity of blood depends on the shear rate, which means that blood is a non-Newtonian fluid.

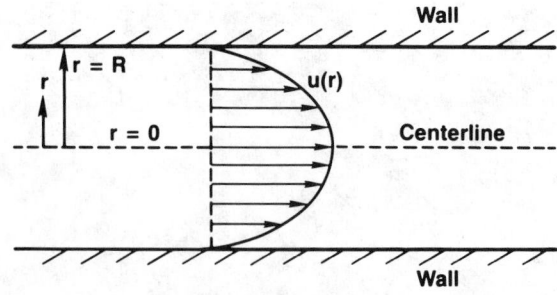

Figure 7-7. Poiseuille flow in a tube of circular cross-section. The tube radius is *R*; the fluid velocity at distance *r* from the centerline is $\mu(r)$. At the tube wall, $\mu(R) = 0$. *Arrows* represent velocity vectors within the tube.

tube; (2) it is proportional to the fourth power of the tube radius; and (3) it is inversely proportional to the viscosity.

EXAMPLE 7-4. FLOW THROUGH AN INTRAVENOUS CANNULA

Consider a 20-gauge (inside radius = 3.81×10^{-4} m) 2-in long (0.0508-m) cannula connected to a bag of normal saline at a height of 0.8 m above the end of the cannula. The viscosity of saline is near that of water: 1.0×10^{-3} kg/m-s. We neglect the pressure loss through the supply tubing, because its diameter is much greater than that of the cannula. The pressure at the upstream (proximal) end of the cannula is thus given by our manometer formula (Equation 7-19):

$$p = \rho gz = (1000 \text{ kg/m}^3)(9.8 \text{ m/s}^2)(0.8 \text{ m})$$
$$= 7840 \text{ Pa} = 7.84 \text{ kPa}$$

This pressure is actually relative to 1 atm (the pressure exerted on the upper surface of the saline solution), so we refer to it as a *gauge pressure*. The pressure derivative along the cannula is the pressure change divided by the cannula length:

$$dp/dx = (7840 \text{ Pa})/(0.0508 \text{ m}) = 1.54 \times 10^5 \text{ Pa/m}$$

We can apply the Hagen-Poiseuille law (Equation 7-28) to predict the flow Q:

$$Q = (3.142)(3.81 \times 10^{-4} \text{ m})^4/(8 \times 1.0 \times 10^{-3} \text{ kg/m-s})$$
$$\times (1.54 \times 10^5 \text{ Pa/m})$$
$$= 1.27 \times 10^{-6} \text{ m}^3/\text{s} = 1.27 \text{ cc/s} = 76 \text{ cc/min}$$

Comparing this value with experimental data, we find that the actual flow is about ⅔ of our prediction. Equation 7-28 assumes ideal conditions: a perfectly round, straight tube with a smooth entrance and walls, steady flow, and no turbulence (discussed below). This formula will usually underestimate friction and thereby overestimate flow by amounts that depend on the actual conditions.

The Hagen-Poiseuille law states that volume flow increases in direct proportion to pressure gradient. However, if we continue increasing the supply pressure in a Poiseuille flow, we eventually find that the actual flow is increasing more slowly than predicted. Experiments show that above a certain *critical velocity*, the flow will become *turbulent*. Turbulence is characterized by erratic, unsteady motion of fluid particles, with much mixing in directions perpendicular to the mean flow. This activity is in sharp contrast to laminar flow, in which fluid streamlines are steady, and there is very little mixing. The transition from laminar to turbulent flow usually occurs rather abruptly, so that any region of flow can be characterized as one or the other. In Figure 7-5, turbulent flow is illustrated by the rapid mixing of the smoke-lines above the airfoil.

Osborne Reynolds showed in 1883 that the transition from laminar to turbulent flow in a given flow geometry is determined by the value of the *Reynolds number*:[19]

$$Re = \frac{\rho UL}{\mu} \qquad (7\text{-}29)$$

where U and L are a characteristic velocity and length for the flow in question. Verify that this number is dimensionless; that is, all the units in Equation 7-29 cancel out. For the Poiseuille flow we have been considering, Re is given by $\rho UD/\mu$, where U is the mean velocity in the tube and D is the diameter. Reynolds showed that for tubes of any size, transition to turbulence occurs when Re reaches a value of about 2100. Once this transition has taken place, the Hagen-Poiseuille R to the fourth law is invalid. This is a common reason for the misuse of this law in medicine. In the 20-gauge cannula in the example above, Re at our predicted flow rate is 2111—equal roughly to the transition value of 2100. This is one reason the calculated flow through the cannula is higher than the experimental result. If disturbances are carefully minimized, much higher transition Reynolds numbers can be achieved, up to 100,000 in tube flow. However, most flows in physiologic or anesthetic applications are not low in disturbance levels.

The exact equations of motion have never been solved for any turbulent flow. We are therefore forced to rely on experimental data and semiempirical laws to predict turbu-

lent flow behavior. We consider again flow through a circular tube as an example. We wish to predict the frictional pressure loss through an intravenous cannula for Re values at which the flow is likely to be turbulent. First, we must express everything in nondimensional form, so that we can use experimental results obtained in tubes of different sizes. Because pressure has the same dimensions as density times velocity squared (see Equation 7-21), we can "normalize" the pressure drop per unit length of tube with the formula:

$$\frac{p_1 - p_2}{L} = \frac{\lambda}{D}\left(\frac{1}{2}\rho U^2\right) \qquad (7\text{-}30)$$

Here L is the length of the tube, D is its diameter, U is the mean velocity, and λ is called the *friction factor*. Note that λ is dimensionless.

According to Reynolds' principle of *dynamical similarity*, any dimensionless coefficient in an incompressible flow depends only on the flow geometry and the Reynolds number.[19] Thus the friction factor λ for flow through a circular tube depends only on Re. The relation, determined from experimental data, is shown in Figure 7-8. Also shown in this figure is the Hagen-Poiseuille friction law for laminar flow, which, when expressed in this form, is simply $\lambda = 64/Re$. It is often stated that friction in turbulent flow is proportional to velocity squared. Figure 7-8 shows that this statement is incorrect for the circular tube. Although pressure loss appears proportional to U^2 in Equation 7-30, the friction factor λ decreases with increasing velocity, so that friction varies, roughly as $U^{7/4}$ in this case.

As an example of a turbulent flow calculation, suppose we wish to increase the flow Q in the 20-gauge cannula

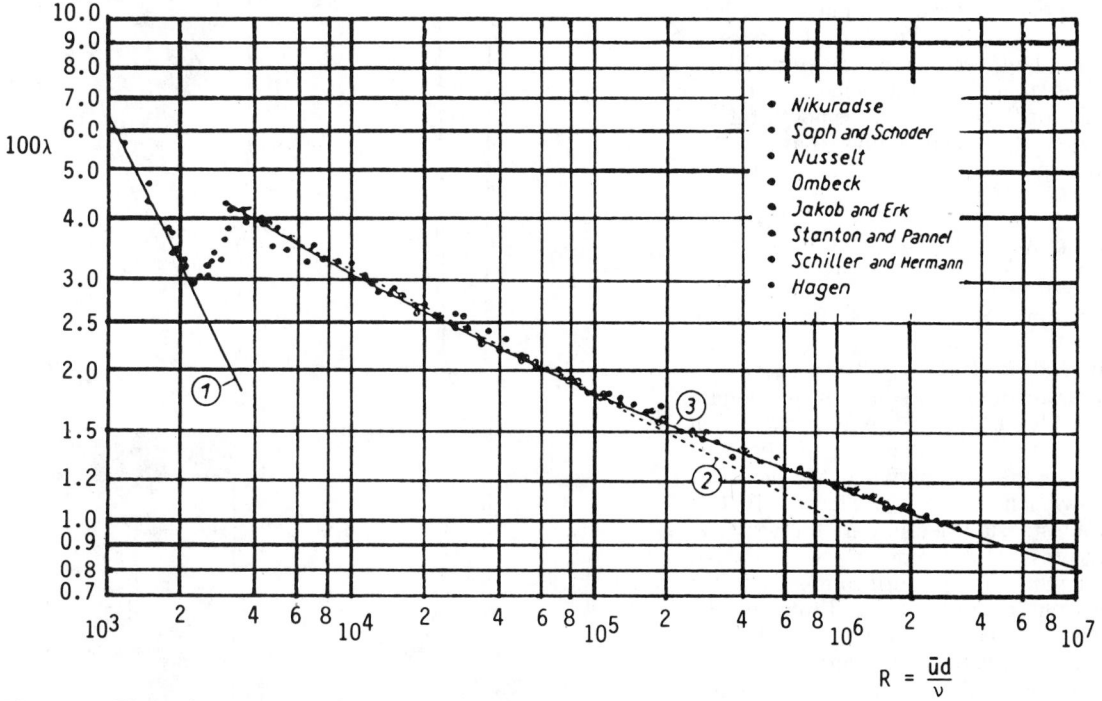

Figure 7-8. Friction factor λ versus Reynolds number (Re) for flow through a tube. Experimental data from several investigators are shown. *Curve 1:* Laminar friction predicted by Hagen-Poiseuille law ($\lambda = 64/Re$). *Curve 2:* Blasius' law for turbulent friction ($\lambda = 0.3164/Re^{0.25}$). *Curve 3:* Prandtl's universal law of turbulent friction. Curves 2 and 3 are purely empirical best-fit relations. (Reproduced with permission from Schlichting H: Boundary Layer Theory. New York, McGraw-Hill, 1968.)

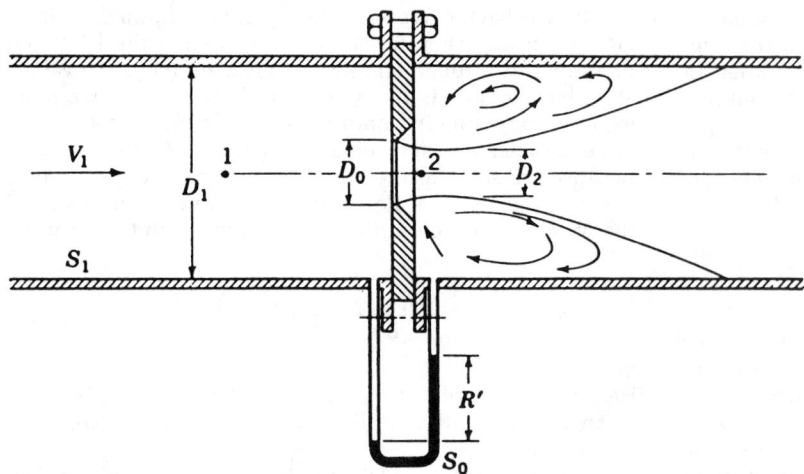

Figure 7-9. Schematic of a fixed-orifice flow meter. Orifice of diameter D_0 is located in tube of diameter D_1. The manometer height R' is related to the square of the flow rate Q (see text). Jet leaving orifice contracts to diameter D_2 (which is less than D_0); therefore, the discharge coefficient C_d is <1.

discussed above from 76 to 200 cc/min. The cross-section A of the cannula is 4.56×10^{-7} m², which means the required mean velocity ($U = Q/A$) is 7.31 m/s. This yields an Re (Equation 7-29) of 5570, well above the 2100 value for transition to turbulence. From Figure 7-8, we predict a friction factor of 0.037. Using this value of λ in Equation 7-30, we find a pressure loss through the cannula of 65.05 kPa, or 6.65 m of water! We must therefore increase the supply pressure by a factor of 8.3 to produce 2.6 times the original flow rate.

EXAMPLE 7-5. ORIFICE FLOW METERS

Most flow meters used in anesthesia are based on known relations between pressure and flow rate through an orifice, such as that depicted in Figure 7-9. The flow downstream of such an orifice is turbulent, because the transition Re for this flow geometry is less than 100. (Remember, the transition Re of 2100 is only for flow in straight, smooth tubes.) Using the same approach as in the tube flow, the flow Q is related to pressure loss ($p_1 - p_2$) by:

$$Q = C_d A \sqrt{\frac{2(p_1 - p_2)}{\rho}} \qquad (7\text{-}31)$$

As you might guess, the dimensionless *discharge coefficient* C_d is a function of the diameter ratio D_0/D_1 (Fig. 7-9) and Re. Here C_d is roughly 0.59 for $D_0/D_1 < 0.2$ and Re > 10^5.

If we measure the pressure loss across the orifice of Figure 7-9, Equation 7-31 provides a *fixed-orifice flow meter*; that is, the orifice area A is fixed, and the pressure loss is a measure of the flow. Another alternative is the *variable-orifice flow meter*, shown schematically in Figure 7-10. Gas flow meters used on anesthesia machines are the variable-orifice type. Here the pressure difference $p_1 - p_2$ is fixed by the weight of the bobbin, and the orifice area A varies according to the bobbin height in the tapered tube. As the flow through the meter increases, the pressure loss through the orifice (an annular space between the bobbin and the tube) increases, and the bobbin rises. As it rises, the orifice area increases because of the gradual widening of the tube, which in turn causes the pressure loss to decrease (Equation 7-31). An equilibrium is reached when the height of the bobbin is such that the pressure force on the bobbin is equal to its weight. Each value of bobbin height thus corresponds to a specific value of flow Q.

The only fluid property appearing in Equation 7-31 is the density ρ; therefore, the calibration of the flow meter should depend only on density. However, remember that at lower Reynolds numbers (*i.e.*, low flow rates through the meter), the discharge coefficient C_d also varies with Re, which in

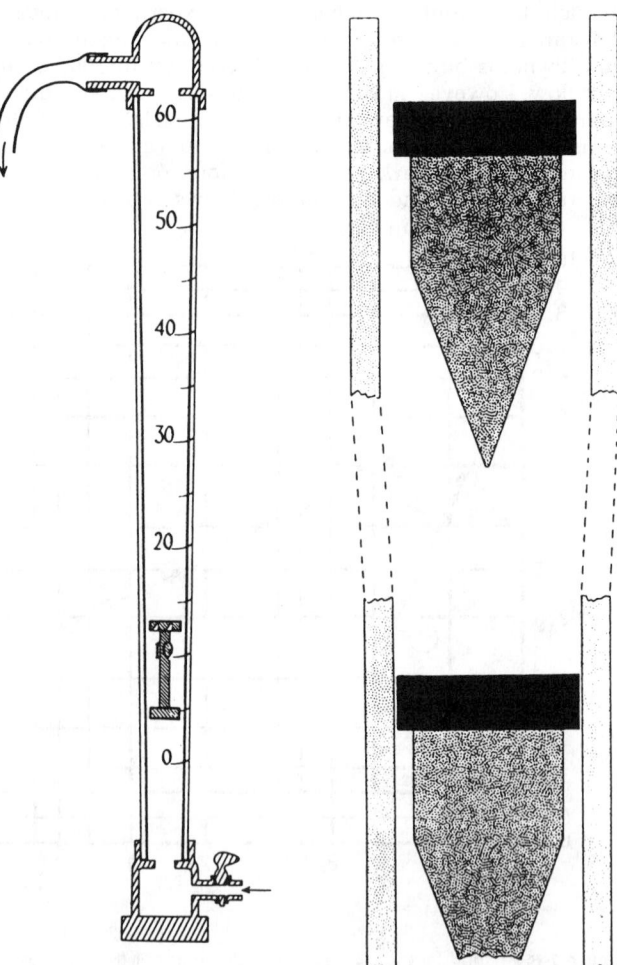

Figure 7-10. Schematic of a variable-orifice flow meter. Orifice area is proportional to bobbin height in tapered tube. (Reproduced with permission from Macintosh R (Sir), Mushin WW, Epstein HG: Physics for the Anesthetist. Springfield, Illinois, Charles C Thomas, 1958.)

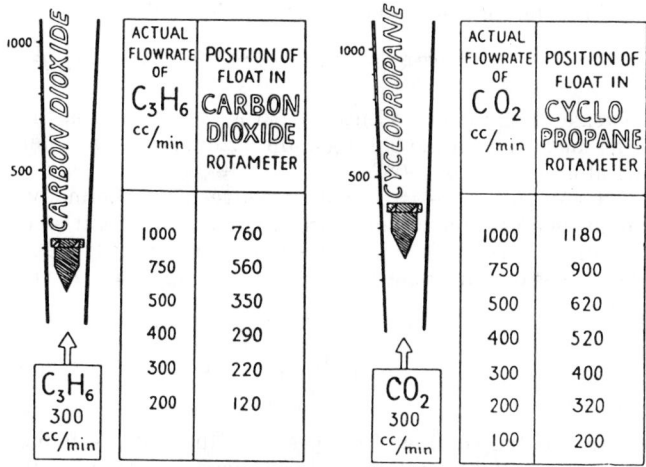

CARBON DIOXIDE	ACTUAL FLOWRATE OF C_3H_6 cc/min	POSITION OF FLOAT IN CARBON DIOXIDE ROTAMETER	CYCLOPROPANE	ACTUAL FLOWRATE OF CO_2 cc/min	POSITION OF FLOAT IN CYCLO PROPANE ROTAMETER
	1000	760		1000	1180
	750	560		750	900
	500	350		500	620
	400	290		400	520
	300	220		300	400
	200	120		200	320
C_3H_6 300 cc/min			CO_2 300 cc/min	100	200

Figure 7-11. Effects of passing C_3H_6 through a CO_2 flow meter and vice versa. The two gases have nearly the same density, but the viscosity of cyclopropane is 0.6 that of carbon dioxide. (Reproduced with permission from Macintosh R (Sir), Mushin WW, Epstein HG: Physics for the Anesthetist. Springfield, Illinois, Charles C Thomas, 1958.)

turn depends on the fluid viscosity μ. Thus, the meter calibration will depend on both density and viscosity at low flow rates but only on density at higher flow rates. A good example of this effect is seen with carbon dioxide and cyclopropane (Fig. 7-11). These gases have nearly the same density, but the viscosity of cyclopropane is 0.6 that of carbon dioxide. Thus, if we produce a flow of 1000 cc/min of CO_2 through a cyclopropane flow meter, the meter will indicate 1180 cc/min, a 12% error. However, if we reduce the flow of CO_2 to 100 cc/min (low flow, low Re), the meter will indicate 200 cc/min, or a 100% error.[1]

In our discussion of incompressible flow, we have emphasized the use of the Reynolds number because this dimensionless parameter enables us to compare flows of different physical scales. In this way, the results of an experiment done in a tube 1 cm in diameter can be used to predict flow behavior in a tube 0.01 cm in diameter. Equations that can be expressed with nondimensional coefficients, such as the discharge coefficient C_d in Equation 7-31, are universally applicable because dimensionless coefficients do not depend on the system of units used. Other dimensionless flow parameters become important in types of flows that we have not considered here. For example, in high-speed gas flows, we must consider the Mach number, which is the ratio of the flow velocity to the speed of sound.[16] In physiologic gas flows, Mach number is usually unimportant, and the fluid behaves as though it were incompressible.

Surface Tension: Law of Laplace

The interface between a liquid and a gas is called a *free surface*. The molecules of the liquid are attracted more strongly to one another than to the gas molecules, which means that energy (work) is required to move molecules from within the liquid to the free surface. This required energy per unit area of free surface has dimensions of *energy per area*, which is the same as force per length. This energy is therefore called the *surface tension* (σ) because it causes the surface to behave as though it were a membrane stretched under a tension σ. The surface tension is a function of the substances on both sides of the free surface and of the temperature. For example, the surface tension of an

air–water interface at 20°C is 0.073 N/m, whereas for a mercury–air interface it is 0.48 N/m.

Because surface tension causes a free surface to behave as a stretched membrane, any free surface that is curved will have a pressure jump across it. For a spherical drop of liquid of radius r, it is easy to show that the pressure inside the drop is greater than the pressure outside by $p_i - p_o = 2\sigma/r$. For a general surface that is curved in two directions with radii of curvature r_1 and r_2, the pressure change is given by the *law of Laplace*:

$$p_i - p_o = \sigma(1/r_1 + 1/r_2) \qquad (7\text{-}32)$$

This physical law is of more than academic interest to anesthesiologists; for example, it determines the pressure needed to open alveoli in the lung. If we think of the alveoli as small, liquid-lined spheres, the surface tension of the alveolar fluid accounts for about two-thirds of the normal recoil pressure tending to collapse the alveoli. (The remainder results from elastic forces within the tissues.) In a normal resting lung in which the alveoli are at atmospheric pressure, the intrapleural pressure required to prevent collapse is about -4 mm Hg. During deep inspiration, this negative intrapleural pressure reaches -12 to -18 mm Hg. Pulmonary surfactant, secreted by specialized alveolar cells, reduces the surface tension σ of the alveolar fluid by roughly a factor of 10, thus minimizing the alveolar pressure difference, as shown in Equation 7-32. In the absence of surfactant, the resting intrapleural pressure needed to prevent collapse would be -30 mm Hg.[20] This calculation explains why premature babies with inadequate surfactant develop severe respiratory distress syndrome, or *hyaline membrane disease*.

The law of Laplace also implies an inherent instability of alveoli. Suppose two nearby alveoli are connected to the same small airway and have the same exterior pressure p_o. If the two are of different radii, then, by Equation 7-32, the smaller alveolus will generate a larger inside pressure p_i, thereby forcing air into the larger alveolus and leading to the complete collapse of the smaller alveolus. This does not normally happen: as the alveolus becomes smaller, surfactant becomes more concentrated and further reduces the surface tension. Thus, the decrease in radius is offset by a corresponding decrease in σ in Equation 7-32, and alveolar stability is maintained.

Another important consequence of surface tension is the phenomenon of surface wetting and *capillarity*, the consequence of a three-way interface between liquid, gas, and solid such as shown in Figure 7-12. A drop of liquid resting on a solid surface surrounded by a gas is characterized by a specific *contact angle*, as shown. This angle θ is a function

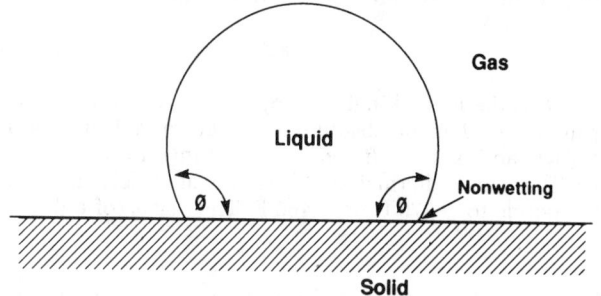

Figure 7-12. Contact-angle effects at a liquid–gas–solid interface. If $\theta < 90°$, the liquid *wets* the solid; if $\theta > 90°$, the liquid is nonwetting.

of all three substances involved in the interface. If θ is less than 90°, the liquid is said to *wet* the solid; if θ is greater than 90°, the liquid is termed *nonwetting*. For example, pure water is perfectly wetting to clean glass, having θ = 0°. On the other hand, mercury does not wet glass, as it has a contact angle of 130°. The surface tension at the contact interface results in the familiar capillary action, whereby a wetting liquid rises in a narrow tube and a nonwetting liquid becomes depressed. A balance of forces shows that the amount of capillary rise or depression (h) is given by:

$$h = 4\sigma \cos(\theta)/\rho g D \qquad (7\text{-}33)$$

where ρ is the liquid density and D is the diameter of the tube. Capillary action will cause a water-glass manometer to overestimate actual pressure and a mercury-glass manometer to underestimate it. The exact magnitude of these errors can be calculated from Equation 7-33.

Compressible Fluids: Thermodynamics

With incompressible fluids, pressure and velocity are the only variables needed to describe flow. Because velocity has three components (x, y, and z), we have a maximum of four variables. With compressible fluids, we must also consider temperature, density, and *heat*, which is defined below. The study of heat and its interactions with other variables comprises the subject of *thermodynamics*. Much of the original work in this field is described in the writings of Carnot[21] and Planck.[22] A very readable short text is that of Fermi.[23] Several intermediate and advanced texts also are available.[24-29]

Temperature and the Equation of State

Let us start with temperature: what is it? We already have an intuitive concept of temperature (T), but thermodynamics defines it precisely. According to the "zeroeth law of thermodynamics,"

> *There exists a variable of state, the temperature T. Two systems that are in thermal contact; i.e., separated by an enclosure that transmits heat, are in equilibrium only if T is the same in both.*[16]

In other words, equality of temperature is a condition two systems in thermal contact will reach if left alone long enough. Simple analysis shows that this *equilibrium* means that the average kinetic energy of the molecules in both systems is the same. Temperature is thus a measure of the mean kinetic energy of random molecular motions. We arbitrarily define an absolute temperature scale by:

$$E = \tfrac{1}{2} kT \qquad (7\text{-}34)$$

where E is the mean kinetic energy per degree of freedom* per molecule, T is the absolute temperature in degrees Kelvin (°K), and k is *Boltzmann's constant* (1.38×10^{-23} J/°K). There is no thermal kinetic energy at 0° Kelvin, which corresponds to −273°C or −460°F. The "size" of a degree

---

Degrees of freedom are modes of molecular motion that can carry kinetic energy. These modes can be translational, rotational, or vibrational. The number of degrees of freedom depends on the number of atoms in the gas molecule.

Kelvin is the same as a degree Centigrade, so that:

$$T(°K) = T(°C) + 273 \qquad (7\text{-}35)$$

The size of one degree Centigrade was chosen so that the difference between the boiling and freezing points of water at 1 atm pressure is 100°C.

For any gas, there is a relation between the thermodynamic state variables of pressure (p), density (ρ), and temperature (T). This relation is called an *equation of state*. An *ideal gas* is one that obeys the following simple equation of state:

$$pV = \frac{m}{M} RT \qquad (7\text{-}36)$$

where V is the volume of the gas, m is the mass, M is the molecular weight, and R is the *universal gas constant*: R = 8317 J/kg-mole-°K (8.317×10^7 erg/g-mole-°K in centimeter-gram-second units). The number of *gram-moles* (n) of a gas is defined as the mass in grams divided by the molecular weight. One mole of anything contains 6.023×10^{23} molecules (Avogadro's number). Equation 7-36 states that one mole of any ideal gas at atmospheric pressure and 0°C occupies the same volume, namely 22.4 l.

Equation 7-36 describes important features of ideal gas behavior. For any *isothermal* process, *i.e.*, a change in which T is held constant, the product pV is a constant (Boyle's law). For an *isobaric* process, where p is constant, the ratio V/T is constant (Charles' law). Although real gases do not obey Equation 7-36 exactly, it is usually a good approximation.

As an example, let's calculate the mass of oxygen (M = 32) in 1 m³ at atmospheric pressure (101.3 kPa) and room temperature (293°K). Solving Equation 7-36 for m:

$$\begin{aligned}
m &= MpV/RT \\
&= (32)(101.3 \times 10^3 \,\text{Pa})(1.0\,\text{m}^3)/ \\
&\quad (8317\,\text{J/kg-mole-°K})(293°K) \\
&= 1.33\,\text{kg}
\end{aligned}$$

By this same law, at 10 atm, our 1 m³ would contain 13.3 kg of oxygen. Perform this same calculation for an H-cylinder at 13,800 kPa (2000 lb/in²) and you will find that the cylinder contains 9 kg of oxygen.

When we have a mixture of more than one gas, say oxygen and nitrogen, the concept of *partial pressure* becomes important. The partial pressure of each gas is defined as the pressure that would be exerted if that gas alone occupied the entire volume at the same temperature. Dalton's law states that the pressure exerted by a mixture of gases is equal to the sum of the partial pressures of all the components present in the mixture. Partial pressures are additive, and they obey Equation 7-36 if the gases are ideal.

Work, Energy, Heat: The First Law of Thermodynamics

We have seen that work and energy are related in mechanics; now we will formulate this relation in gases. All matter has an internal *thermal energy* related to random molecular motions. This form of energy has been used above in the definition of temperature, and therefore it is a function of temperature. For a *calorically perfect gas*, the thermal energy e (per unit mass of gas) is given by:

$$e(T) = c_v T \qquad (7\text{-}37)$$

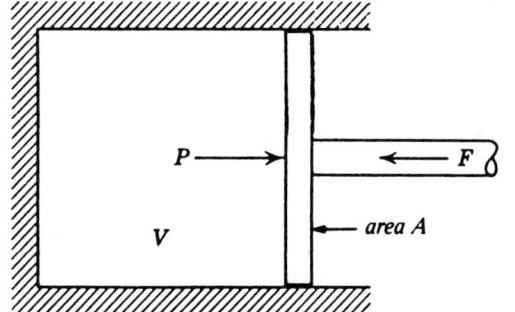

Figure 7-13. Piston and gas-containing cylinder. Force F applied to piston of area A is opposed by pressure P ($F = PA$) in gas having volume V.

where the constant c_v is called the *specific heat at constant volume*.

We now consider the work done by an expanding gas in Figure 7-13. The gas in the cylinder exerts a pressure p on a piston of area A, thus applying a force $F = pA$ to the piston. If the piston moves to the right by a small amount dx (dx is small so p remains constant), then the gas has performed an amount of work $dw = Fdx$ (work = force × distance). But $Fdx = pAdx$, and Adx is the change in the volume of the gas, dV. Therefore:

$$dw = Fdx = pAdx = pdV \qquad (7\text{-}38)$$

or the work done by a gas on its surroundings is equal to the pressure times the change in gas volume.

If the cylinder and piston in Figure 7-13 are thermally insulated, then no heat (which we are about to define) can get in or out, and the change in internal energy is equal to the work:

$$de = -dw = -pdV \qquad (7\text{-}39)$$

The minus sign is needed because dw is work done *by* the gas, which obviously results in a *decrease* in internal energy.

We now define *heat* as thermal energy that can pass through the cylinder walls if they are not well insulated, thus adding another term to our energy conservation equation:

$$de = dq - dw \qquad (7\text{-}40)$$

This is the first law of thermodynamics, which states that the increase in internal energy equals the heat absorbed by the gas minus the work done by the gas. Heat has the same dimensions as energy (mL^2/T^2) and is thus measured in joules. It is also often measured in calories: one calorie of heat will raise the temperature of 1 g of water from 14.5 to 15.5°C (1 cal = 4.185 J).

An adiabatic, or "isentropic," process is one in which there is no heat conduction ($dq = 0$), and changes are made slowly. If a gas expands or is compressed adiabatically, then $de = -dw = -pdV$. If that gas is also calorically perfect (Equation 7-37), then:

$$de = c_v \, dT = -pdV \qquad (7\text{-}41)$$

Combining Equation 7-41 with the equation of state (Equa-

tion 7-36), we find for an adiabatic process:

$$pV^\gamma = \text{constant} \qquad (7\text{-}42)$$

where $\gamma = (R/c_v) + 1$. If we define c_p as the specific heat at constant pressure, we find that $R = c_p - c_v$ and $\gamma = c_p/c_v$.

Why is this important? We know that as a gas expands, it cools. Now we can see the difference between an isothermal expansion (which is uncommon) and an adiabatic expansion (which is very common). In the isothermal case, $pV =$ constant, so if we double the volume, we halve the pressure. In the adiabatic case, using oxygen ($\gamma = 1.4$) as an example, doubling the volume multiplies the pressure by 0.38. The pressure drops more in an adiabatic expansion than in an isothermal one, which is obvious, because in the latter we must supply heat from the outside. In this same adiabatic volume doubling, the absolute temperature is reduced by a factor of 0.76. Thus, if we started at 20°C (293°K), we would finish at −51°C (222°K)!

Phase Changes

Matter can exist in three forms: solid, liquid, or gas. Many substances can exist in all three of these states, depending on the temperature and pressure. The different forms of the same material are called *phases*. The most familiar example is H_2O: it can exist as ice, water, or steam. We know that at 1 atm H_2O changes from solid to liquid at 0°C and from liquid to gas (steam) at 100°C.

What happens at pressures other than 1 atm? The easiest way to understand this is through a pressure versus volume graph, in which we plot *isotherms*, or lines of constant temperature. A family of such isotherms is shown in Figure 7-14. Consider first the isotherm labeled g, corresponding to the highest temperature. As the gas is compressed (decreasing volume V), pressure p increases smoothly and continuously, and the substance stays in its gaseous phase throughout. If our substance were an ideal gas, curve g would be a hyperbola ($pV =$ constant), as given by Equation 7-36. Now look at the isotherm labeled a, starting from the right at high volume and low pressure. As V decreases on this isotherm, p increases until we reach the area bounded by the dashed curve. At this point, some of the gas turns into liquid, so that we have both gas and liquid phases at the same temperature and pressure. The bottom of our container holds liquid, while the rest is still filled with gas,

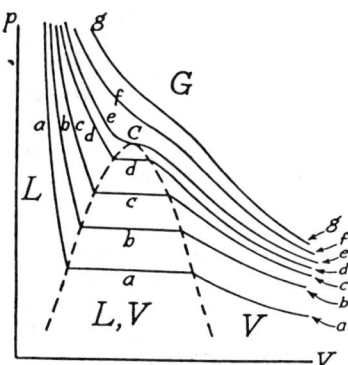

Figure 7-14. Isotherms on a pressure *versus* volume plot for a real gas. Region G: gas only is present; region V: vapor; region L, V: liquid and vapor in equilibrium; region L: liquid only. Isotherm e is at critical temperature.

TABLE 7-2. Critical Temperatures and Other Parameters for Common Substances

	Molecular Weight	Density at 20°C (g/ml)	Vapor Pressure at 20°C (mm Hg)	Latent Heat at 20°C (Cal/g)	Boiling Point (°C)	Critical Temp (°C)
Chloroform	119	1.49	160	64	61	260
Ethyl alcohol	46	0.79	44	220	78	240
Diethyl ether	74	0.71	440	87	35	190
Halothane	197	1.86	243	35	50.2	
Isoflurane	184.5	1.51*	239	41*	48.5	
Water	18	1.0	18	580	100	370
Carbon dioxide	44	0.00184	56 Atm.	35		31
Nitrous oxide	44	0.00184	51 Atm.	41	−89	36
Air	29	0.0012				−141
Oxygen	32	0.00133				−119
Nitrogen	28	0.00117				−147

*Values at 25°C.

which, in this liquid-gas equilibrium, is referred to as a *vapor*. As we continue to reduce the volume V, the pressure does not increase. Instead, we continue changing more of the substance from the gas to the liquid phase. As we move left on the isotherm in this region, visualize a steadily shrinking container filled more and more with liquid. When we reach the dashed curve on the left side of Figure 7-14, the whole container is filled with liquid, and there is no vapor left: we have *condensed* all the vapor to the liquid phase. As we further reduce volume, the pressure rises very steeply because we are now attempting to compress a liquid.

The area labeled *L,V* in Figure 7-14 is a region in which liquid and vapor exist together in equilibrium. As we increase temperature (move to higher isotherms on Fig. 7-14), this equilibrium region becomes smaller until, at the isotherm labeled *e*, it disappears. This temperature is called the *critical temperature*, T_c, and it is the highest temperature at which the substance can be liquified by any amount of pressure. In other words, in the isotherms above *e*, the substance stays in a gaseous phase at all pressures. Critical temperatures and other parameters for some common substances are shown in Table 7-2. Note that nitrous oxide has a T_c of 36°C, which means that at room temperature, N_2O can be liquified if we can apply the 51 atm of pressure required for the task. Oxygen, on the other hand, has a T_c of −119°C, which means that oxygen cannot be liquified at room temperature by any amount of pressure. When a substance is in the gaseous phase at a temperature at which it could be liquified by sufficient pressure, we call it a *vapor* (region V in Fig. 7-14). The same substance at any temperature above T_c is then referred to as a *gas* (region G in Fig. 7-14).

In any liquid-vapor equilibrium (region *L,V* in Fig. 7-14), there is only one value of pressure possible for a given temperature. This is called the *vapor pressure*, p_v, and it always increases with temperature. For example, the vapor pressure of water at 20°C is 2.4 kPa (18 mm Hg). At 37°C, p_v (H_2O) is 6.3 kPa (47 mm Hg), and at 100°C, it is 101.3 kPa or 1 atm. The temperature at which p_v equals 1 atm is called the *boiling point*. If we try to increase T further without raising the pressure, the liquid will rapidly change to vapor, or *boil*, until there is no liquid left. The boiling point of

nitrous oxide is −89°C. The vapor pressure versus temperature relations of some common substances are shown in Figure 7-15.

When we convert liquid to vapor at a constant temperature (moving to the right along an isotherm in the L,V region of Fig. 7-14), we increase the volume of our container while maintaining constant pressure. This means that the vapor is doing work on the environment ($dw = pdV$; Equation 7-38). By the first law of thermodynamics (Equation 7-40), we know that heat (dq) must be added to the vapor to accomplish this volume increase ($de = 0$ in this case, so $dq = dw$). The amount of heat that must be added per unit of mass vaporized is called the *latent heat of vaporization*. It is a function of the temperature and the substance being vaporized. For water at 20°C, the latent heat is 580 cal/g, while at 100°C, it is 540 cal/g. If the latent heat is not supplied by the surroundings, then it must come from the liquid itself, which is why open liquids become cooler as they evaporate. The rate of evaporative cooling is proportional to p_v (because higher p_v means faster evaporation) and the latent heat.

For the same reason, vaporizers for the volatile anesthetics tend to cool as they are used. They are therefore designed to conduct heat from the environment into the liquid to minimize the fall in liquid temperature. If the liquid temperature falls, the vapor pressure will decrease, as shown in Figure 7-15, thus reducing the amount of anesthetic being vaporized. Modern variable-bypass vaporizers are temperature compensated to correct for this effect, but older vaporizers such as the Copper Kettle and Vernitrol are not. During administration of ether by the open drop method (which few of us remember), it was common to see ice crystals forming on the mask—an excellent illustration of latent heat of vaporization.

EXAMPLE 7-6. OXYGEN AND NITROUS OXIDE STORAGE

Now that we thoroughly understand gases, vapors, and latent heat, let us consider the storage of a gas and a vapor: oxygen and nitrous oxide (Fig. 7-16). Oxygen is a gas at 20°C; it cannot be liquified by any amount of pressure be-

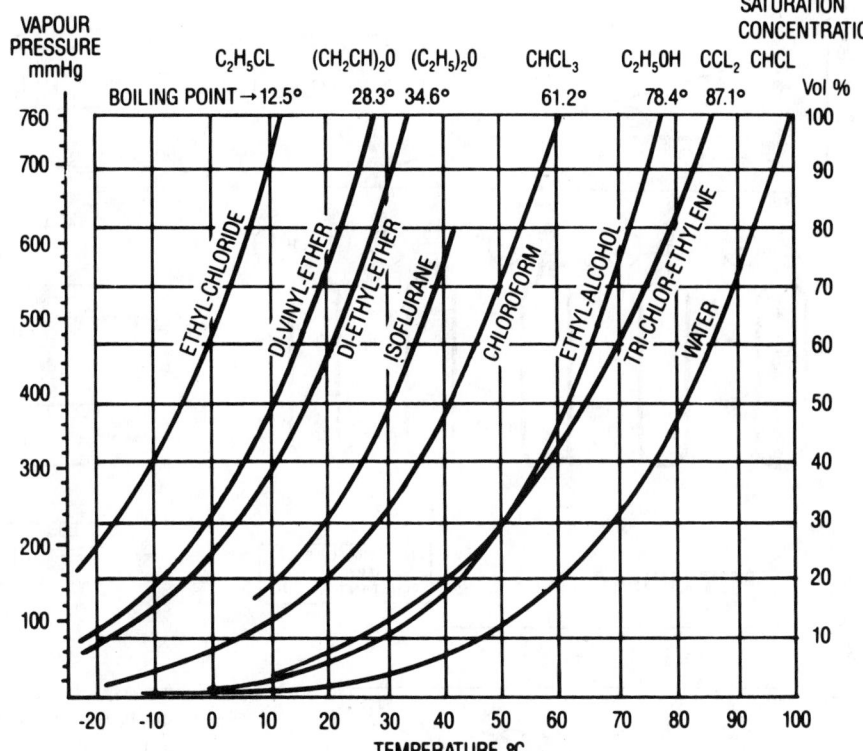

Figure 7-15. Vapor pressure *versus* temperature curves for volatile anesthetics and other liquids. The temperature at which P_v = 760 mm Hg is the boiling point.

cause it is above its critical temperature. Thus, when the oxygen cylinder is full at 136 atm (13,777 kPa or 2000 lb/in^2) of pressure, it contains twice as many grams of oxygen as it would at 68 atm and four times what it would contain at 34 atm. In other words, the oxygen follows ideal gas behavior: $pV = (m/M)RT$. In contrast, nitrous oxide is a vapor at 20°C; it can be liquified by a pressure of 51 atm (5166 kPa or 750 lb/in^2) at this temperature.

Consider a tank filled to the top with liquid nitrous oxide (Fig. 7-16). If we remove some N$_2$O from the tank, some of the remaining liquid will vaporize, and the tank will be filled partially with liquid and partially with vapor. The pressure in the tank will remain at 51 atm as long as any liquid remains; we are simply moving to the right along one of the L,V isotherms of Figure 7-14. When the pressure does begin to fall, it means there is no longer any liquid in the tank. Because the density of N$_2$O vapor at 51 atm and 20°C is less than one fourth the density of liquid N$_2$O, the tank is actually less than one fourth full before the pressure begins to fall. A pressure gauge is not a good indicator of how much N$_2$O is in a tank, but if the gauge reads less than 51 atm, the tank is nearly empty. There is one exception to this behavior: if we take N$_2$O from the tank very rapidly, the remaining liquid will be cooled by the effect of latent heat of vaporization. This cooling decreases the vapor pressure, thus lowering the tank pressure below 51 atm while there is still liquid remaining. Of course, the pressure would return to 51 atm as the tank warmed to room temperature again.

EXAMPLE 7-7. HALOTHANE STORAGE AND VAPORIZATION

How much halothane gas can we get from 1 ml of halothane liquid? Like nitrous oxide, halothane is a vapor at room temperature, but unlike N$_2$O, the vapor pressure of halo-

thane at 293°K is less than 1 atm (243 mm Hg, 32.4 kPa, 0.32 atm). This means that to vaporize all of the liquid halothane in a closed container, we must reduce the internal pressure to 0.32 atm. (Similarly, we had to raise the pressure in our N$_2$O tank to 51 atm in order to liquify the N$_2$O.) One milliliter of liquid halothane (293°K) has a mass of 1.86 g or 0.00186 kg. The molecular weight (M) of halothane is 197. The ideal gas law (Equation 7-36) tells us the volume occupied by this mass of halothane at the given pressure and temperature (SI units):

$$\begin{aligned}
V &= (m/M)RT/p \\
&= (0.00186/197)(8317) \times 293/32{,}400 \\
&= 7.10 \times 10^{-4} \text{ m}^3 = 710 \text{ ml}
\end{aligned}$$

One milliliter of liquid halothane becomes 710 ml of vapor at room temperature and p_v = 0.32 atm.

If we mix this 710 ml of halothane with oxygen to obtain a gas-vapor mixture with a total pressure of 1 atm, we must supply 0.68 atm (68.9 kPa, 517 mm Hg) of oxygen to make up the difference (see Dalton's law of partial pressure, above). The gas-vapor mixture will occupy a volume of 710 ml at a pressure of 1 atm and will consist of 1.86 g of halothane and 0.642 g of oxygen. (The last number is again from Equation 7-36.) We say that such a mixture consists of "⅓ halothane and ⅔ oxygen" because those are the proportions of their partial pressures and of the numbers of molecules of each species. Thus, if 100 ml of oxygen at 1 atm pass through a vaporizer and become fully saturated with halothane, the mixture that emerges will have a volume of 147 ml, and the partial pressures of halothane and oxygen will be 0.32 and 0.68 atm, respectively. Although we often say that the oxygen has "picked up" 47 ml of halothane vapor, the halothane actually occupies the entire 147 ml volume, as does the oxygen.

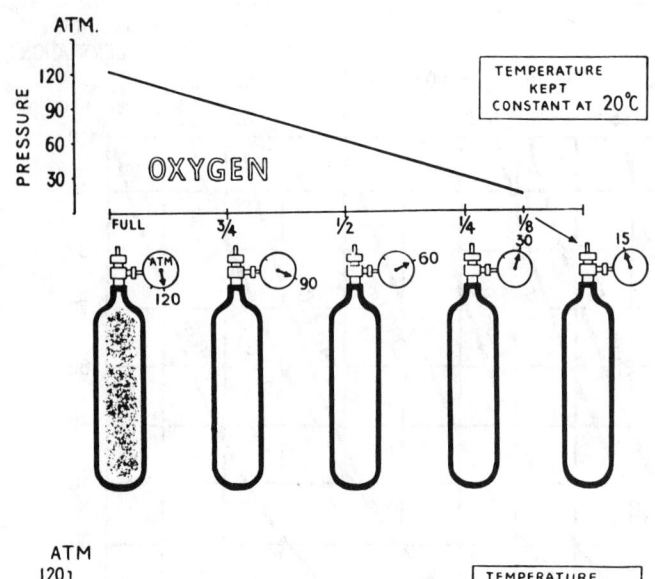

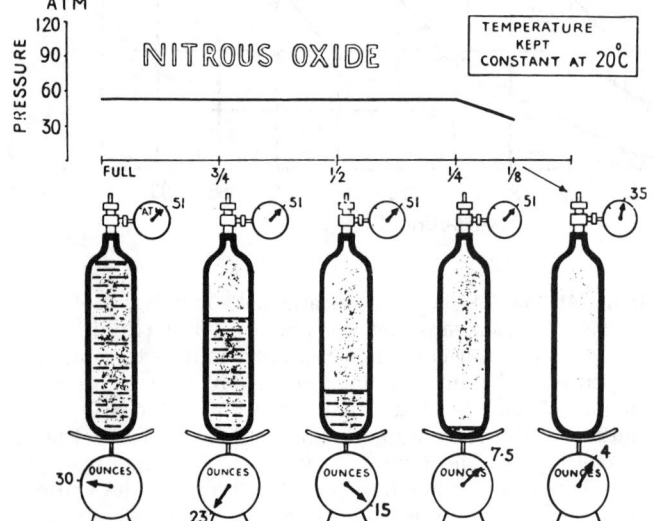

Figure 7-16. Pressure cylinders containing oxygen and nitrous oxide at 20°C. The oxygen is a gas at all pressures at this temperature; the pressure falls steadily as gas is removed. The nitrous oxide is liquefied at 51 atm pressure; as N_2O is removed from a full cylinder, the pressure remains constant until there is no more liquid in the cylinder. (Reproduced with permission from Macintosh R (Sir), Mushin WW, Epstein HG: Physics for the Anesthetist. Springfield, Illinois, Charles C Thomas, 1958.)

Sound Transmission and Doppler Effect

Sound waves are small perturbations in pressure, density, and velocity that propagate through all types of matter: solids, liquids, and gases. Sound waves cannot propagate through a vacuum. They are called *longitudinal waves* because the motions of the fluid particles are in the same direction as the wave propagation, as shown in Figure 7-17. By contrast, surface waves on the ocean are *transverse waves* because the particle motions are mostly perpendicular to the direction of wave propagation. In gases, if the changes in pressure and density are small relative to their mean values, then sound waves of all frequencies will propagate at the same speed. For an ideal gas, it is easy to show

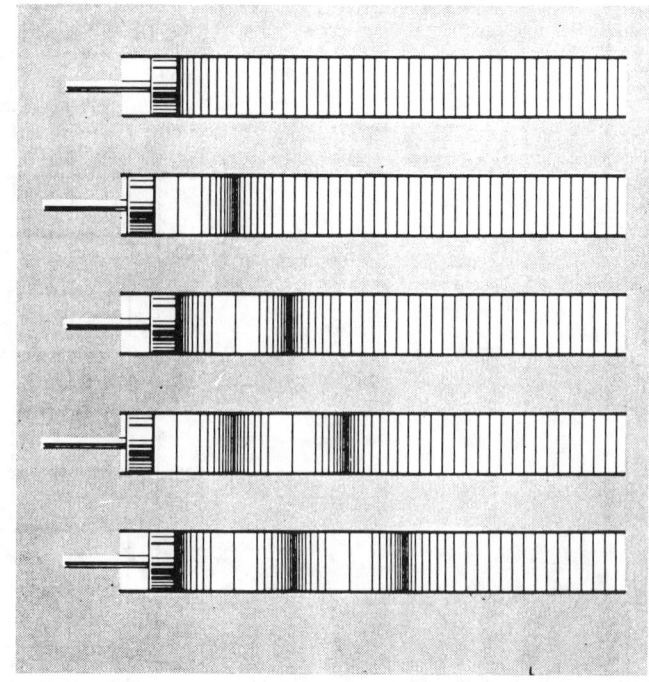

Figure 7-17. Sound waves generated by movement of a piston in a straight tube. The gas movement is in the same direction as the wave propagation, making this a "longitudinal wave."

that this *speed of sound* is given by:

$$a = \sqrt{\frac{\gamma p}{\rho}} \qquad (7\text{-}43)$$

We can use the ideal gas equation of state (Equation 7-36) to obtain another useful form of this expression:

$$pV = (m/M)RT \qquad (7\text{-}44)$$

$$p = (m/V)(R/M)T = \rho R'T$$

Here we have used the fact that m/V is the density ρ, and we have defined a new *gas constant* by $R' = R/M$. (R' is gas species dependent; it is not a universal constant.) Substituting Equation 7-44 into Equation 7-43, we have:

$$a = \sqrt{\frac{\gamma p}{\rho}} = \sqrt{\gamma R'T} \qquad (7\text{-}45)$$

In other words, the speed of sound in an ideal gas depends only on the gas properties γ and R' and the temperature T. For example, in air at room temperature ($M = 28.8$, $\gamma = 1.4$):

$$a = \sqrt{1.4 \times \frac{8317}{28.8} \times 293}$$
$$= 344 \text{ m/s} = 1129 \text{ ft/s} = 770 \text{ mi/h}$$

By comparison, at an altitude of 13,000 m (40,000 ft), the temperature is $-57°C$ (216°K), and the speed of sound is only 295 m/s (661 mi/h). Speeds of sound in some common substances are given in Table 7-3.

moving listener is:

$$f' = (a + v_0)/\lambda = f + v_0/\lambda = f + v_0 f/a$$
$$= f(1 + v_0/a) \tag{7-48}$$

Thus the listener's frequency increases by the factor $1 + v_0/a$. A listener moving toward the source at half the speed of sound hears a frequency 1.5 times that of a stationary listener. Similarly, a listener moving away from the source at this same speed will hear a frequency one half that of the stationary listener.

Now suppose the listener is stationary and the source is approaching at speed v_s. The wavefronts now have the pattern illustrated in Figure 7-18B, in which the wavefront labeled 1 was emitted when the source was at S1 and wavefront 2 was emitted when the source was at S2. The source is following the rightward-moving waves, so these waves become closer together. If the source frequency is f and the source speed is v_s, then during each vibration, the source moves a distance of v_s/f. (Remember, the time between vibrations is $1/f$.) Hence, each wavelength will be shortened by the distance v_s/f, so the wavelength at the listener is $\lambda' = a/f - v_s/f$. The waves themselves still travel at speed a, so the frequency heard by the stationary listener is:

$$f' = \frac{a}{\lambda'} = \frac{a}{(a - v_s)/f} = f\frac{a}{a - v_s}$$
$$= f\left(\frac{1}{1 - v_s/a}\right) \tag{7-49}$$

If the source is moving at half the speed of sound toward the listener, the apparent frequency will double. Yet when the listener is moving at the same speed toward a stationary source (Equation 7-48), the frequency increases by only 50%. What happens if the source is moving faster than the speed of sound in Equation 7-49? The answer is that the small perturbation analysis of linear acoustics is no longer valid. However, we can intuitively predict the result of these wavefronts piling on top of each other near the source: a sonic boom!

In the Doppler systems used in medicine, we have a slightly different geometry. Here the source is a stationary transducer, and the sound is reflected from a moving target (e.g., red blood cells), from which it returns to a stationary listener (the receiving transducer). This can be analyzed as a two-stage process, in which the "target" is first a moving listener to sound from a stationary source. The target then re-radiates this sound as a moving source transmitting to a stationary listener. The result is thus a combination of Equations 7-48 and 7-49:

$$f' = f\left(\frac{1 + v/a}{1 - v/a}\right) \tag{7-50}$$

Now if the target is moving toward the detector at half the speed of sound, the observed frequency f' will increase by a factor of three! Changes in the frequency of sinusoidal sound waves can be measured very precisely. The trained human ear can often detect a 1-Hz frequency change at 1000 Hz.

The Doppler principle thus provides an accurate way to measure the velocity of any moving object that reflects sound. If frequencies of 10 megaHertz (MHz) or more are used, objects as small as red blood cells will scatter enough sound for detection. The same principle can be applied to

TABLE 7-3. Speed of Sound in Various Media

Medium	Temperature (°C)	Speed m/s	ft/s
Air	20	344	1129
Air	0	331.3	1087
Hydrogen	0	1286	4220
Oxygen	0	317.2	1041
Water	15	1450	4760
Lead	20	1230	4030
Aluminum	20	5100	16,700
Copper	20	3560	11,700
Iron	20	5130	16,800
Extreme values			
Granite		6000	19,700
Vulcanized rubber	0	54	177

We determine the intensity of sound waves from the root–mean-square (rms) value of the pressure fluctuation p', which is used to calculate *sound pressure level*, or SPL. Because a wide range of intensities is common in everyday life, we use a logarithmic scale for SPL:

$$SPL = 20 \log\left(\frac{p'}{p_0}\right) \tag{7-46}$$

The units of this scale are called *decibels*, and the reference pressure p_0 is chosen as the lowest sound pressure detectable by the human ear. This hearing threshold, at a frequency of 2 kiloHertz (kHz; 1 kHz = 1000 cycles/s) is an rms pressure of 2×10^{-8} kPa (0.0002 dyne/cm²). Thus a sound pressure of 2×10^{-8} kPa corresponds to an SPL of zero decibels (0 db), because $p'/p_0 = 1$ and log (1) = 0. The threshold of pain is an SPL of about 120 db, a level that has been measured frequently at rock concerts. Prolonged exposure to an SPL greater than 90 db will eventually result in permanent hearing impairment. Note that 100 db is an rms pressure 100,000 times that of the hearing threshold.

In 1842, Christian Johann Doppler described how the color of a luminous body and the pitch of a sound source are changed by the relative motions of the source and observer or listener. This *Doppler effect* has many applications in modern medicine and is worthy of discussion here. If the source of sound is stationary (Fig. 7-18A) and is radiating sound of frequency f, the wavelength λ is given by:

$$\lambda = a/f \tag{7-47}$$

because the time between wavefronts is $1/f$ and these fronts are traveling at the speed of sound a. A listener moving toward this stationary source at speed v_0 (Fig. 7-18A) will be crossing more wavefronts per unit time than if he or she were standing still. The listener's velocity relative to the moving wavefronts is $a + v_0$, so the number of wavefronts crossed per unit time is:

$$f' = \frac{\text{relative velocity}}{\text{distance between waves}} = (a + v_0)/\lambda$$

Because the sound frequency for the stationary listener (Equation 7-47) is $f = a/\lambda$, the frequency f' heard by the

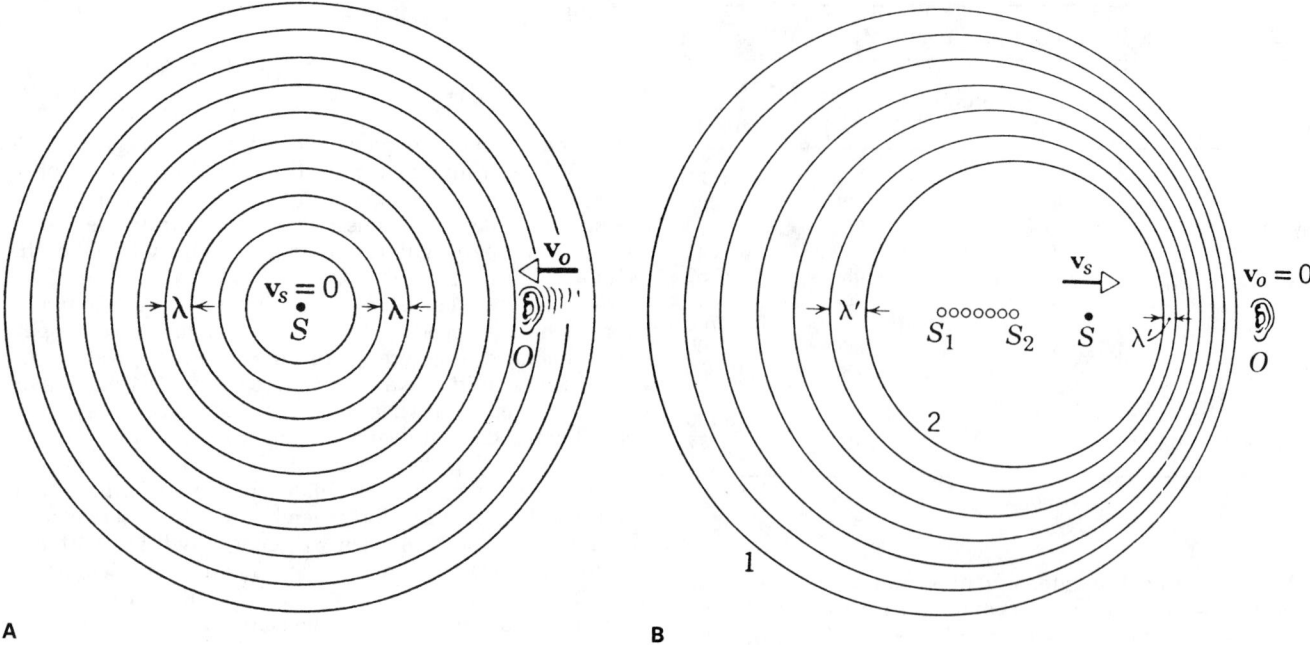

A   **B**

Figure 7-18. (*A*) A stationary source "S" of sound being heard by a moving listener "0." The wavefronts are concentric circles separated by a constant wavelength λ. (*B*) A moving source of sound being heard by a stationary listener. The circular wavefronts are not concentric, and the wavelength λ' depends on the direction from the source.

reflection of light, as in the laser Doppler velocimeters used to detect skin blood flow.

EXAMPLE 7-8. ECHOCARDIOGRAPHY

Modern echocardiography uses measurements of both the amplitude and frequency of reflected sound waves to image cardiac structures and blood flow velocity. Sound waves in the frequency range from 1 to 10 MHz are transmitted into the heart in short bursts from a piezoelectric transducer, which then "listens" to the reflected echoes between signal bursts. The speed of sound in the heart and surrounding tissues is a fairly constant 1540 m/s, so that the time of flight between the signal burst and the received echo can be used to derive the distance to the reflecting structure. Strong echoes come from large changes in tissue density; lung (low density) and bone (high density) will therefore reflect most of the sound waves and must be kept out of the signal path. The sound beam is a very narrow "searchlight" pattern, so that the exact direction of the reflecting structures is known. If the beam is aimed in a fixed direction and the echo strength is displayed versus the distance from the transducer and time, the result is called *M-mode* or one-dimensional ultrasound. Because M-mode looks in only one direction, it provides very limited information. On the other hand, it can sample roughly 1000 times per second, thus providing excellent time resolution of rapidly moving objects (*e.g.*, a mitral valve leaflet).

If we vary the direction of the ultrasound beam by sweeping it through an arc, we can develop a *two-dimensional* (*2-D*) *echocardiogram*, which shows the reflecting structures in an entire plane. The 2-D echo technique obviously shows us much more of the heart at a given time, but its time resolution is more limited in that it can produce only 15–100 pictures per second.[30-32] A recent development in 2-D echo technology is the addition of Doppler analysis.[33] Moving reflectors shift the frequency of the echo as derived

above (Equation 7-50), resulting in a change in color on the display screen.

HEAT TRANSPORT

As discussed above, heat is energy in the form of random molecular motions in matter. Heat transfer occurs from a point of higher temperature to one of lower temperature. Heat is transferred from one body to another by three mechanisms: conduction, convection, and radiation. Conduction requires that the two bodies be in contact; convection requires fluid motion; and radiation can take place through a vacuum.

Heat can be conducted through solids, liquids, and gases. Illustrations of heat conduction are usually chosen with an opaque solid as the conducting substance, because in such materials conduction is the only method by which heat can be transferred. The basic equation for one-dimensional heat conduction is Fourier's equation:

$$q = -KA\frac{dT}{dx} \qquad (7-51)$$

where

q = heat conduction rate in the x direction
(calories per second)
A = cross-sectional area for heat transport
dT/dx = temperature gradient (x component)
K = thermal conductivity of the conducting medium

The thermal conductivity K is relatively independent of temperature until the material changes phase. Conductivity decreases significantly as a substance changes from solid to liquid to gas, as shown in Table 7-4.[34]

For heat conduction through a layer of thickness Δx, the

TABLE 7-4. Thermal Conductivities

Material	K (W/ m-°K)
Solids	
Silver	429
Steel	15
Skin	0.37
Wool	0.04
Water	0.60
Air	0.026

Reproduced with permission from Incropera FP, De-Witt DP: Fundamentals of Heat and Mass Transfer, 2nd ed, p 752. New York, John Wiley & Sons, 1985.

rate of heat conduction is proportional to the temperature difference:

$$q = \frac{KA}{\Delta x}(T_1 - T_2) \qquad (7\text{-}52)$$

where T_1 and T_2 are the temperatures on either sides of a layer of thickness Δx. This one-dimensional, steady-state heat conduction equation can be applied to a series of thermal conducting layers as in Figure 7-19:

$$q = \frac{K_a A}{\Delta x_a}(T_1 - T_2) = \frac{K_b A}{\Delta x_b}(T_2 - T_3)$$
$$= \frac{K_c A}{\Delta x_c}(T_3 - T_4) \qquad (7\text{-}53)$$

The heat conduction q through layers a, b, and c must be equal. Solving each of these equations for the temperature difference and adding the equations produces the following result:

$$q = \frac{T_1 - T_4}{\dfrac{\Delta x_a}{K_a A} + \dfrac{\Delta x_b}{K_b A} + \dfrac{\Delta x_c}{K_c A}} \qquad (7\text{-}54)$$

Thermal Conducting Layers

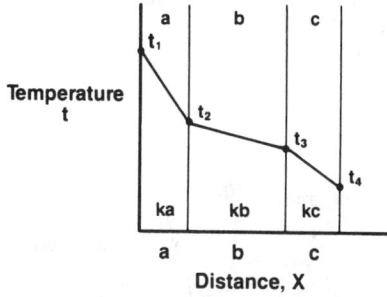

Figure 7-19. The temperature gradient for steady-state heat conduction through three layers, a, b, and c, with three different thermal conductivities, K_a, K_b, and K_c. Because of conservation of energy, the heat conducted through each layer will be equal; therefore, the temperature drop from T_1 to T_4 can be solved by writing Fourier's law of heat conduction for each layer and equating the amount of heat transferred, q. Note above that layer b has the highest thermal conductivity, as noted by the least rate of temperature decrease across that layer.

This equation can be used to determine the temperature drop across a series of thermal conducting layers, just as the voltage drop across a series of electrical resistors is calculated (discussed below). The term $\Delta x/kA$ is the *thermal resistance* of the layer. The mathematics becomes more complex as the geometry becomes three-dimensional instead of one-dimensional and as unsteady-state (time response to temperature changes) solutions are required.[34]

The heat transport associated with fluid motion is called *convective* heat transport. If the fluid motion is caused by the heat itself, this motion is called *natural convection*. Heating a fluid causes it to expand and rise, producing fluid motion and carrying heat with the motion. If the fluid motion is produced by an external energy source (a fan or a pump), it is called *forced convection*. The equation used to describe convective heat transport is similar to Fourier's equation for conduction:

$$q = hA(T_s - T_m) \qquad (7\text{-}55)$$

where T_s is the surface temperature, T_m is the moving fluid mean temperature, and A is the contact area.

Because convective heat transport occurs at a phase interface (i.e., solid-liquid, solid-gas, or liquid-gas), the thickness Δx is not easily measured, so it is incorporated into the heat-transfer coefficient h. The resistance attributable to convective heat transport $(1/hA)$ is thus similar to the conductive resistance $(\Delta x/kA)$. Because convective heat transport can involve complex geometric and fluid dynamic problems, the determination of h is a mixture of theoretical and empirical effort. Table 7-5 gives some example values.

Conductive and convective heat transport can be combined into an overall heat transport coefficient, U.[35,36] Below is an example of the use of this coefficient to describe the heating of water in a pot:

$$q = U(T_{air} - T_{water}) \qquad (7\text{-}56)$$

where

$$U = \frac{1}{\dfrac{1}{h_{air} A} + \dfrac{\Delta xa}{KaA} + \dfrac{1}{h_{water} A}}$$

and

h_{air} = convective heat transfer coefficient from air to pot
h_{water} = convective heat transfer coefficient from pot to water
ka = the thermal conductivity of pot, whose thickness is Δxa

Radiant heat energy is emitted by every body having a temperature greater than 0°K (-273°C). This does not mean that the amount of thermal radiation is always significant compared to the other forms of heat transfer. In most situations in which objects are below room temperature, thermal radiation is small. When the temperature of an object exceeds 500°C, radiation is usually the predominant mechanism of heat transport. Because thermal radiation is electromagnetic (see section below), it requires no medium for transport. The sun radiates energy at a temperature of 5000°C to the earth through 93,000,000 miles of vacuum.

All radiant energy hitting a surface is either absorbed, transmitted, or reflected. The fractional contributions of

TABLE 7-5. Typical Values of Convective Heat Transfer Coefficients, *h*

Process	*h* (W/m²-°K)
Natural convection	5–25
Forced convection	
Gases	25–250
Liquids	50–20,000
Convection with phase change	
Boiling or condensation	2500–100,000

Reproduced with permission from Incropera FP, DeWitt DP: Fundamentals of Heat and Mass Transfer, 2nd ed, p 8. New York, John Wiley & Sons, 1985.

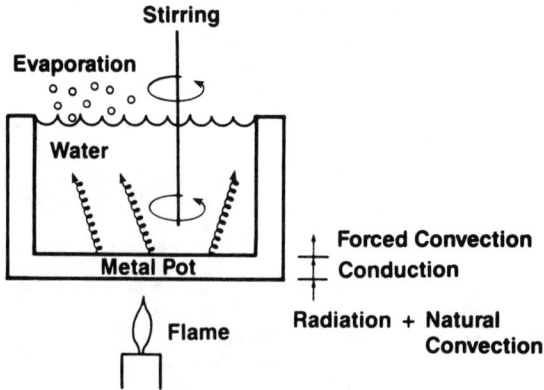

Figure 7-20. This illustration demonstrates that several types of heat transport are simultaneously involved in the process of heating a pot of water. The flame transmits heat to the metal pot by radiant heat transport and natural convection owing to the rising hot gases from the hot flame. Heat is transported through the metal bottom of the pot purely by conduction. The water within the pot is being stirred; therefore, the predominant mechanism of transport is forced convection. Finally, as the water is evaporating, it is being cooled by the latent heat vaporization of the water.

these three processes must total 1:

$$\alpha + \tau + \rho = 1 \qquad (7\text{-}57)$$

where

$$\alpha = \text{absorptivity}$$
$$\tau = \text{transmissivity}$$
$$\rho = \text{reflectivity}$$

These fractions usually vary with the wavelength of the radiant energy. If $\alpha = 1$, the object will gain the maximum possible amount of heat. Such an object is called a *black body*. By contrast, if all radiant energy is either reflected or transmitted (e.g., $\rho + \tau = 1$), the object will gain no heat.

The equation for radiant heat transfer to a black body ($\alpha = 1$) is called the Stefan-Boltzmann law:

$$q_{1,2} = \sigma \times A \times F_{1,2}(T_1^4 - T_2^4) \qquad (7\text{-}58)$$

where $q_{1,2}$ is the net heat transferred between objects 1 and 2 at temperatures T_1 and T_2, respectively, σ is the Stefan-Boltzmann constant (2×10^{-4} J/h-m² °K⁴ or 5.6×10^{-8} W/m² °K⁴), A is the area being irradiated, and $F_{1,2}$ is the *view factor*. The view factor is the fraction of the radiation from object 1 "seen" by object 2 and is a complex function of geometric considerations. Because radiant heat transport depends on temperature to the fourth power, we expect this form of heat transport to dominate at high temperature differences.

Figure 7-20 illustrates all three mechanisms of heat transport. In this example, water is being heated in a pot by a flame. The flame transfers heat to the pot by natural convection and by radiation. Heat is conducted through the metal of the bottom of the pot and then heats the water predominantly by forced convection because the water is being stirred. Ultimately, much of the heat transported into the water will be dissipated by the latent heat of vaporization of the water (see above for discussion of latent heat of vaporization).

Analyzing the heat transport to and from a patient in the operating room is a complex problem involving all these mechanisms of heat transport. To maintain a constant temperature, the patient must dissipate an amount of heat equal to his or her metabolic heat production. A 70-kg adult reading this chapter will generate approximately 85 kcal/h or the same as a 100-W light bulb (1 kcal/h = 1.16 W or 1.16 J/s).[37,38] Figure 7-21 illustrates the four mechanisms of heat loss for a patient in the operating room: conduction, convection, radiation, and latent heat vaporization. The following

example will illustrate how each mechanism participates in the dissipation of metabolic heat. It should be mentioned that many assumptions and approximations are made in attempting to model the real situation, and the accuracy of the calculations is dependent on the validity of these assumptions. For this reason, several assumptions will be made to demonstrate how these changes will affect the amount of heat loss by each mechanism.

EXAMPLE 7-9. HEAT LOSS FOR A PATIENT IN THE OPERATING ROOM

Mechanism 1. Heat Loss by Conduction

For a patient lying uncovered on an operating table, heat is lost by conduction through contact with the table itself. If the patient is covered with a blanket, heat will also be conducted through the blanket. The conductive heat loss will be calculated using Equation 7-51 for three conditions: the patient lying on a cold metal table, on an insulated table, and on a heating blanket.

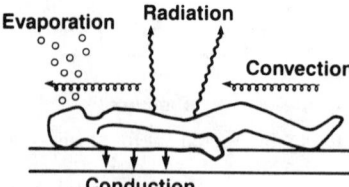

Figure 7-21. Schematic illustration of the major mechanisms of heat loss for a patient in the operating room. Although it is often written that 50% or more of heat loss is due to radiation, any of the four forms of heat loss illustrated above can be substantial, depending on the surrounding conditions. See the text for several example calculations for each mechanism of heat loss.

Heat Loss to the Table

Assuming the patient's skin temperature is 37°C, the table temperature is 20°C, the table thickness is 1 cm, and the body surface area (BSA) in contact is 0.5 m².

CASE 1. STEEL TABLE WITHOUT INSULATION:

$$q = (0.5 \text{ m}^2)\left(15 \frac{\text{W}}{\text{m°C}}\right)\left(\frac{37 - 20}{0.01 \text{ m}}\right)°\text{C}$$

$$q = 12{,}750 \text{ W!}$$

CASE 2. TABLE WITH 2 CM OF INSULATION. Insulation having a thermal conductivity of 0.04 W/m°C (e.g., wool, foam):

$$q = (0.5 \text{ m}^2)\left(0.4 \frac{\text{W}}{\text{m°C}}\right)\left(\frac{37 - 20}{0.02 \text{ m}}\right)°\text{C}$$

$$q = 170 \text{ W}$$

CASE 3. TABLE WITH A 1-CM HEATING BLANKET (37°C):

$$q = (0.5 \text{ m}^2)\left(0.60 \frac{\text{W}}{\text{m°C}}\right)\left(\frac{37 - 37}{0.01 \text{ m}}\right)°\text{C}$$

$$q = 0 \text{ W}$$

Conductive Heat Loss to 20°C Room When Covered

CASE 4. WOOL BLANKET OF 0.3-CM THICKNESS. The contact area is assumed to be 1 m²:

$$q = (1.0 \text{ m}^2)\left(0.04 \frac{\text{W}}{\text{m°C}}\right)\left(\frac{37 - 20}{0.003 \text{ m}}\right)°\text{C}$$

$$q = 227 \text{ W}$$

CASE 5. TWO WOOL BLANKETS WITH A 0.5-CM AIR SPACE BETWEEN THE PATIENT AND THE BLANKET. Using Equation 7-54:

$$q = \frac{(37 - 20)°\text{C}}{\dfrac{0.006 \text{ m}}{(0.5 \text{ m}^2)\left(0.04 \dfrac{\text{W}}{\text{m°C}}\right)} + \dfrac{0.005 \text{ m}}{(0.5 \text{ m}^2)\left(0.026 \dfrac{\text{W}}{\text{m°C}}\right)}}$$

$$q = 25 \text{ W}$$

Cases 4 and 5 assume that the outer surface of the blanket is maintained at 20°C.

The above calculations illustrate the dramatic dependence of conductive heat loss on the insulation of the patient and table. The skin temperature assumed (37°C) is too high for skin in contact with a cold operating table. Nonetheless, it is evident that even a small amount of good insulating material can dramatically reduce the heat loss to the operating table by conduction. Because air is a fluid, the analysis of heat transport from the patient (whether covered with a blanket or not) to the air involves convection, which will be discussed next.

Mechanism II. Heat Loss by *Convection*

Wherever the body surface is in contact with a fluid, natural or forced convection is involved. A standard operating room is ventilated with 10–15 room volume changes per hour. Reducing this to a linear air velocity for a standard-size operating room yields an air speed over the body of approxi-

mately 3 cm/s. Using this velocity, and assuming the patient to be a cylinder 30 cm in diameter, one can estimate the flow Reynolds number. This fluid dynamic effect on heat transport (forced convection) is then weighed against the heat transport from natural convection. The result of a fairly involved analysis is an estimate of a heat transfer coefficient (Equation 7-55) for the convective heat loss. (The details of this calculation are beyond the scope of this chapter, and readers are referred to engineering texts on the subject.[39,40]) This type of analysis predicts a natural convective heat transfer coefficient of approximately 4 W/m² °C, and a forced convective heat transfer coefficient of 1 W/m² °C. An increase in air velocity caused by patient or personnel movement would increase the forced convective heat transfer coefficient. A rule of thumb is that the heat transport will go up in proportion to the square root of the air velocity. Using this heat transfer coefficient, the heat loss by convection in our patient would be:

$$q = Ah(T_b - T_r)$$

CASE 6. ASSUMING THE PATIENT IS NOT COVERED. Assuming also that the patient has a temperature of 37°C and has an exposed area of 1 m²:

$$q = (1 \text{ m}^2)\left(4 \frac{\text{W}}{\text{m}^2 \text{°C}}\right)(37 - 20)°\text{C}$$

$$q = 68 \text{ W}$$

CASE 7. ASSUMING THE PATIENT IS COVERED WITH A BLANKET AS IN CASE 5. The blanket surface temperature (T_b) must be calculated. This is done by equating the heat conducted in (q_{in}) and convected out (q_{out}) of the blanket:

$$q_{in} = \frac{(37 - T_b)°\text{C}}{0.685 °\text{C/W}}$$

$$q_{out} = \frac{(T_b - 20)°\text{C}}{\left[\dfrac{1}{(1 \text{ m}^2)\left(4 \dfrac{\text{W}}{\text{m}^2 \text{°C}}\right)}\right]}$$

$$0.685 (T_b - 20) = 0.25(37 - T_b)$$

$$T_b = 24.5°\text{C}$$

With a blanket surface temperature of 24.5°C, the convective heat loss can be calculated:

$$q = (1 \text{ m}^2)\left(4 \frac{\text{W}}{\text{m}^2 \text{°C}}\right)(24.5 - 20)°\text{C}$$

$$q = 18 \text{ W}$$

Mechanism III. Radiant Heat Loss From a Patient in the Operating Room

Assuming the patient acts as a black body absorber ($\alpha = 1$), the following calculations can be made.

Heat Losses by Radiation (Stefan-Boltzmann Equation)

$$q = A\sigma(T_{body}^4 - T_{room}^4)$$

where

$$\sigma = 5.6 \times 10^{-8} \text{ W/m}^2 \text{ °K}^4$$

CASE 8. ASSUMING THE SKIN TEMPERATURE IS 37°C (310°K). If the room wall temperature is 20°C (293°K), and the BSA is 1 m²:

$$q = (1 \text{ m}^2)\left(5.6 \times 10^{-8} \frac{W}{\text{m}^2 \text{°K}^4}\right)(310^4 - 293^4)\text{°K}^4$$

$$q = 104 \text{ W}$$

CASE 9. ASSUMING THE SKIN TEMPERATURE IS 35°C (308°K):

$$q = (1 \text{ m}^2)\left(5.6 \times 10^{-8} \frac{W}{\text{m}^2 \text{°K}^4}\right)(308^4 - 293^4)\text{°K}^4$$

$$q = 91 \text{ W}$$

CASE 10. ASSUMING A BLANKET TEMPERATURE OF 24.5°C (297.5°K). The radiation from the blanket to the walls is:

$$q = (1 \text{ m}^2)\left(5.6 \times 10^{-8} \frac{W}{\text{m}^2 \text{°K}^4}\right)(297.5^4 - 293^4)\text{°K}^4$$

$$q = 26 \text{ W}$$

Mechanism IV. Heat Loss by Evaporation

Heat loss by evaporation in the form of perspiration is the body's predominant mechanism of cooling when its temperature is above 37°C. When the body becomes cold, the evaporative loss from the skin is minimized. Evaporative heat losses from the respiratory tract are a side effect of ventilation and therefore are an obligate heat loss. If a patient inspires 100% humidified gases at body temperature, there will be no heat loss from respiratory evaporation. However, as seen below, if the patient inspires dry gases, there can be a significant heat loss secondary to respiratory evaporation.

Heat Loss by Respiratory Evaporation (Latent Heat)

$$q = M \times LH$$

where

M = rate of water loss
LH = latent heat of vaporization of water (at 37°C)

Thus,

$$q = 0.580 \text{ kcal/g}$$

Assuming that the minute ventilation is 7 l/min, the inspired air is dry, and the expired air is 100% saturated at 37°C (34 mg of H_2O/l), the mass of water evaporated will be as follows.

$$
\begin{aligned}
M &= (7 \text{ l/min})(34 \text{ mg } H_2O/\text{l}) \\
&= 238 \text{ mg/min} \\
q &= (238 \text{ mg/min})(0.58 \text{ kcal/g})(10^{-3} \text{ g/mg}) \\
&= 0.138 \text{ kcal/min} = 8.3 \text{ kcal/h} \\
&= 9.6 \text{ W}
\end{aligned}
$$

The preceding examples illustrate the basic mechanisms of heat loss for a patient in the operating room. Each mechanism has been treated independently to simplify calculating the heat loss, but in reality, these processes are occurring in series and in parallel and therefore should be analyzed in that fashion (analogous to series and parallel resistors in an electrical circuit analysis; see below).

It is evident from these calculations that the heat loss by each mechanism can be altered dramatically by the assumed boundary conditions. Conduction to the table can be completely eliminated by a heating blanket, whereas convective and radiative losses can be substantially reduced by covering the patient with a blanket.[41,42] Finally, the loss by evaporation can be eliminated by using heated, humidified inspired gases. When heat loss in the operating room is discussed, it is generally stated that radiation is the predominant mechanism followed by convective and evaporative losses.[20,41-43] As can be seen from this example, there can be wide variation in heat loss by each mechanism, depending on the specific conditions. Radiation can be an important source of heat loss that is less controllable than some of the other losses. In the real situation, there are also potential heat losses from the surgical field by evaporation, convection, and radiation. Furthermore, the skin temperature will probably be somewhat less than body core temperature, and the patient will be well insulated from the operating table.[20,43] Some of these predicted heat losses will therefore be reduced, whereas an open surgical field will allow dramatic increases in evaporative and radiative heat losses.

MASS TRANSPORT AND KINETIC THEORY

Matter is transported by bulk flow, forced or natural convection, and molecular diffusion. This section will discuss molecular diffusion. The other two mechanisms, which are much more efficient, have been covered in previous sections.

Molecular Diffusion

Molecular diffusion is a process described by what is called the *kinetic theory*.[44] Kinetic theory assumes that all matter is composed of particles (atoms or molecules) that are in continuous, random motion that stops only when the temperature is lowered to absolute zero (0°K, −273°C). When kinetic theory is applied to gases, it assumes that the particles are small and that all collisions between particles and the walls of the container are completely elastic (i.e., no energy is lost). With these assumptions, the ideal gas laws discussed above can be derived from kinetic theory.

Diffusion occurs because of the random motion of fluid (gas or liquid) particles. In Figure 7-22A, the container is filled with particles of nitrogen. Because all the N's are in constant random motion, on the average equal numbers of particles will be going east and west. Consequently, the container is homogeneously filled with N's and there is no net transport of N's in either direction, in spite of the fact that diffusion of N's is occurring constantly in all directions. Now we add a second type of particle, which we call oxygen, on the west side of the container in Figure 7-22B. The O particles will be randomly moving east and west, but because, initially, there are no O's on the east side, there will be a net movement of O's from west to east. The opposite will happen with the N's that were initially on the east side until the N's and the O's are homogeneously filling the container. This is the process of molecular diffusion. For a net mass transport to take place in one direction, there must be a concentration difference or *gradient* in that direction. This net transport by diffusion in the presence of a concentration gradient is described by Fick's law of diffusion:[44]

$$J = D_{O,N} \frac{dC_O}{dx} \tag{7-59}$$

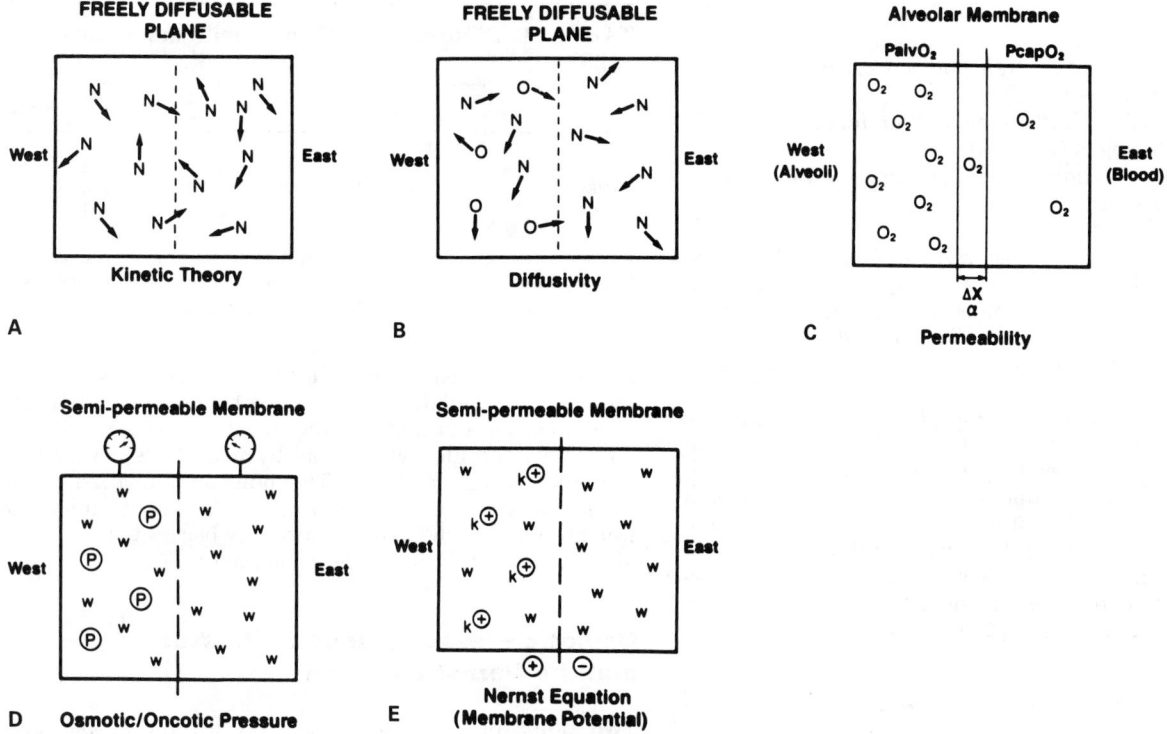

Figure 7-22. Aspects of diffusion. (*A*) A container filled with molecules N moving randomly. Because of random motion, the particles eventually will be homogeneously distributed throughout the container, and at any one time an equal number of particles will be passing through a plane (*dotted line*) in both directions. (*B*) A container similar to the one in *A* except that there are two types of molecules, N and O. Initially, the O molecules are all on the west side of the container. Because of the random motion of both the N's and the O's, an equal number of molecules will be moving in both directions. Because there initially are no O molecules on the east side of the container, there will be no O molecules moving from the east, and therefore there will be a net movement of O molecules from west to east until the container is homogeneously filled with both N's and O's throughout. This process of net movement of one type of molecule through space as a result of random motion is called *diffusion*. (*C*) A container divided into two sections by a permeable membrane of thickness Δ*x*. Oxygen molecules are in higher concentration on the west side, which represents an alveolus, than on the east side, which represents capillary blood. Because of the higher concentration on the west side, oxygen molecules will randomly diffuse eastward. The amount of oxygen in the membrane is related to the concentration of oxygen on the alveolar side and the solubility of the oxygen in the membrane material, α. If the capillary blood is flowing and continuously removing oxygen from the east side, there will be a continuous flux of oxygen molecules from the west side to the east side by diffusion. (*D*) A container similar to that shown in *B* except that the membrane dividing the east and the west sides of the container is semipermeable; that is, permeable to some components but not others. In the above container, the W's, which represent water, pass freely through the membrane and therefore are distributed homogeneously throughout the container. The membrane is not permeable to the P molecules, which represent protein, and which cannot diffuse freely through the membrane and therefore remain on the west side of the container. The water molecules diffuse randomly in both directions through the membrane, unaffected by the presence of the P molecules on the west side. For this reason, the water molecules try to distribute evenly throughout the entire container, thus producing more total molecules on the west side and resulting in a higher pressure, known as *osmotic pressure*. If the semipermeable membrane is a capillary wall and the osmotic pressure is produced by plasma proteins, this pressure is referred to as *oncotic pressure*. (*E*) A container similar to *D* except that the component on the west side of the container capable of passing through the membrane is a charged particle, K^+. The semipermeable membrane thus maintains a difference in charge concentrations between the west and east sides of the container. This potential difference maintained by the membrane can be calculated, if the difference in concentrations of the ions is known, by means of the Nernst equation (see Equation 7-61).

where

J = mass flux or net transport across a plane (molecules/s-cm^2)

$D_{O,N}$ = diffusivity (diffusion constant) for component O diffusing in N (cm^2/s)

dC_O/dx = concentration gradient of O in the x direction (molecules/cm^3/cm)

If component O were constantly removed as it reached the east side of the container, there would be a steady diffusion of O from the west to the east. In biologic systems, it is common that diffusion takes place through a membrane; e.g., oxygen diffusing through the alveolar cell wall and the pulmonary capillary wall into the blood stream. Oxygen diffuses from a high concentration (or partial pressure) in the alveoli to a low concentration in the blood stream. Concentration can be replaced by partial pressure if the solubility (the ratio of concentration to partial pressure) is entered into Fick's equation. (Solubility is discussed below.) In biologic systems, it is difficult to determine the actual partial pressure gradient through a membrane, so the partial pressure difference across the membrane is used. For oxygen diffusing in the lung (Fig. 7-22C):

$$J = \frac{\alpha D}{\Delta x}(\text{P}_{AO_2} - \text{Pcap}_{O_2}) \qquad (7\text{-}60)$$

where

D = diffusivity

α = solubility constant for oxygen

Δx = membrane thickness

P_{AO_2} = alveolar oxygen partial pressure

Pcap_{O_2} = pulmonary capillary oxygen partial pressure

In biologic systems, D, α, and Δx are combined and called the permeability constant P:

$$P = \frac{\alpha D}{\Delta x}$$

As shown in Equation 7-60 and Figure 7-22C, the rate of diffusion J of a substance through a membrane is directly proportional to the partial pressure difference, the solubility of the substance in the membrane, and the molecular diffusivity constant. It is inversely proportional to the thickness of the membrane. The molecular diffusivity D of a substance is inversely proportional to the square root of the molecular weight and directly proportional to the temperature.[44]

Molecular diffusion of gases through gases is a slow process; diffusion of gases through liquids is very slow; and the diffusion of gases through solids is extremely slow (Table 7-6).[34] For this reason, in sites where the body depends on molecular diffusion for transport, the distances are very short. For example, in oxygen delivery, diffusion is the only mechanism involved in transport from the alveolus to the blood and again from the tissue capillary wall to the mitochondria. These diffusion distances are 5–20 μm.

It is interesting that CO_2 has a slightly smaller diffusivity than O_2, even though it is often stated that CO_2 diffuses more quickly in the lung than oxygen. The diffusivity of CO_2 is lower because it is a larger molecule, but because its solubility in water is approximately 20 times that of oxygen, CO_2 has a larger permeability constant P for lung transport (Equation 7-60). The capacity of solubility to increase the

TABLE 7-6. Diffusivities of Oxygen and Carbon Dioxide at 25°C

	O$_2$	CO$_2$ cm^2/s
Air	0.21	0.16
Water	2.40×10^{-5}	2.0×10^{-5}
Rubber	2.1×10^{-6}	1.1×10^{-6}

Reproduced with permission from Incropera FP, DeWitt DP: Fundamentals of Heat and Mass Transfer, 2nd ed, p 777. New York, John Wiley & Sons, 1985.

permeability constant and thereby increase mass flux is used in *facilitated* diffusion, a process whereby a freely diffusible carrier substance in the membrane attaches to the diffusing molecule, which may by itself have a very low solubility in the membrane. The molecule plus carrier will have a lower diffusivity (because of the larger molecular weight) but a much larger permeability because of the effect of increased solubility in the membrane.

Osmotic Pressure, Oncotic Pressure, and the Nernst Equation

Two other phenomena involving diffusion of particles through membranes are important in biologic systems: diffusion through semipermeable membranes (osmotic pressure and oncotic pressure) and diffusion of charged substances through semipermeable membranes (Nernst equation and membrane potential).

In Figure 7-22C, if there is neither production nor consumption of either substance, equal concentrations on either side of the membrane will eventually result. What will happen if the membrane separating the two compartments is permeable to one type of particle but not to the other, as in Figure 7-22D? For example, let W represent water, which passes freely through the entire container and equilibrates. The P's represent protein molecules, to which the membrane is nonpermeable and which therefore remain on the west side of the container. Consequently, there are more total particles (W's and P's) on one side, which causes the pressure to be greater on that side of the membrane (see Dalton's law, under the section on Temperature and the Equation of State). This pressure difference is called the *osmotic pressure* and is related to the number of particles or moles of nonpermeable solute, i.e., the number of P's. When this principle is applied to the vascular space, whose capillary walls are permeable to water and electrolytes but not to plasma proteins, the pressure developed is referred to as *oncotic pressure*.

When a semipermeable membrane between solutions is permeable to one ion but not to the oppositely charged ion, a charge imbalance can be produced, as shown in Figure 7-22E. This imbalance produces a transmembrane potential difference, which can be calculated by the Nernst equation:[20]

$$\text{EMF (mV)} = -61 \log \frac{K^+ \text{(east)}}{K^+ \text{(west)}} \qquad (7\text{-}61)$$

Nerve cells use this diffusion mechanism to re-establish their transmembrane potential after depolarization and impulse transmission. The original concentration gradient between the inside and outside of the cell is produced by a sodium-potassium pump. This pump is an active process, pumping ions against a concentration gradient.

SOLUBILITY

Vapors and Gases

When a pure solid substance reaches its melting point, it becomes a liquid; when it reaches its boiling point, it becomes a vapor; and when it reaches its critical temperature, it becomes a gas. It is easy to distinguish a solid from a liquid from a vapor, but vapors and gases are not as easily distinguished. By definition, when a substance reaches its critical temperature, it is a gas. The difference between a vapor and a gas is that a vapor can be compressed at constant temperature into a liquid, whereas a gas cannot. (See the section above on thermodynamics.)

When a liquid is placed in a container, some of the molecules will evaporate, forming a vapor phase above the liquid. Eventually, an equilibrium state will be reached between molecules leaving and molecules entering the liquid phase. At this point, the pressure of the vapor is called the equilibrium vapor pressure, as discussed above (Table 7-2 and Fig. 7-15).

Solubility

When a pure liquid is enclosed in a container, the vapor above that liquid will produce a pressure (the vapor pressure at that temperature), which is also the total pressure. When a second vapor or gas is added to the container, it also will produce a pressure, and the sum of these pressures will be the total pressure (Dalton's law of partial pressures, discussed above). Some of the molecules of this second gas will dissolve in the primary liquid, and the amount dissolved is directly proportional to the partial pressure of the gas above the liquid. This proportionality is known as Henry's law of solubility:

$$P_i = H_{i,1} \times x_i \qquad (7\text{-}62)$$

where

P_i = partial pressure of substance i in the gas phase
$H_{i,1}$ = Henry's law constant for i in 1
x_i = mole fraction of i in the liquid phase

The Henry's law constant $H_{i,1}$ is specific for a solute (gas) and solvent (liquid) pair and is a function of temperature. Almost all gases and vapors become more soluble in liquids as temperature decreases; i.e., they become closer to being liquids themselves. The specific solubility constant depends on the molecular weight and size and the intermolecular forces between the solvent and solute molecules. These constants are determined experimentally. Because the partial pressure in the gas phase and the concentration in the liquid phase are directly proportional (Equation 7-62), it is common to express the concentration of a gas in a liquid in terms of its equilibrium partial pressure or tension.

In Henry's law the concentration of the solute is expressed in terms of mole fraction x_i, which is not convenient for medical calculations. Solubility coefficients may also be expressed in terms of the volume of gas that will dissolve in a given volume of liquid. The international scientific community uses the *Bunsen coefficient* (α), defined as the

TABLE 7-7. Ostwald Solubility Coefficients at 37°C

	Water	Blood	Oil	Muscle
Nitrogen	0.014	0.015	0.07	—
Nitrous oxide	0.47	0.47	1.4	1.1
Halothane	0.80	2.4	220	155
Enflurane	0.78	1.9	98	70
Forane	0.62	1.4	97	68

Reproduced with permission from Hill DW: Physics Applied to Anesthesia, 3rd ed, p 177. London, Butterworths, 1976.

volume of gas, corrected to standard temperature and pressure (0°C and 1 atm), which dissolves in a unit volume of liquid at the temperature concerned. A more useful way of expressing solubility for anesthetic practice is the *Ostwald solubility coefficient*, defined as the volume of gas that dissolves in a unit volume of liquid at the temperature concerned. In the Ostwald coefficient, the gas volume is not corrected to standard temperature and pressure. Table 7-7 lists the Ostwald coefficients for several anesthetic agents in clinically important material.[45]

Another way of describing solubility is in terms of the distribution of a substance between two phases. The *partition coefficient* is defined as the ratio of the amount of substance present in equal volumes of two phases at a stated equilibrium temperature. If one of the phases is gaseous, then the partition coefficient is the same as the Ostwald coefficient. The partition coefficient is most frequently used when the phases are both solid or liquid, such as oil-water or tissue-blood. The partition coefficient can be calculated as the quotient of the Ostwald (liquid-gas) coefficients for each of the liquid phases. For example, a tissue-blood partition coefficient may be obtained by dividing the Ostwald tissue-gas coefficient by the blood-gas coefficient: T/b = (T/g)/(b/g). Thus from Table 7-7, the muscle-blood coefficient for halothane would be 6/2.4 = 2.5.

It is said that solubility coefficients and partition coefficients are a function of temperature but not of pressure or concentration. This is not exactly true, for these coefficients do vary slightly over wide ranges of pressure. In the clinical range, however, we can assume that the coefficients are independent of pressure and concentration.

MEASUREMENT TECHNIQUES FOR OXYGEN, CARBON DIOXIDE, AND HEMOGLOBIN SATURATION

The assurance of adequate oxygenation and ventilation may be the most important aspect of monitoring critically ill and anesthetized patients. To this end, over the past 30 years several techniques have been developed to measure oxygen, carbon dioxide, and hemoglobin saturation. More recently, techniques have been developed for the continuous monitoring of oxygenation and ventilation. This section describes the theoretical principles on which these techniques are based.

Oxygen Measurement

Blood oxygen content is defined as the number of milliliters of oxygen contained in 100 ml of blood (volume%). Because oxygen is both dissolved in plasma and bound to hemoglobin, the calculation of oxygen content has two terms:

$$\text{Cao}_2 = (1.37 \times \text{Hb} \times \text{Sao}_2) + (0.003 \times \text{Pao}_2) \quad (7\text{-}63)$$

where the "a" refers to an arterial value and where

Hb = hemoglobin concentration (g/dl of blood)
Sao$_2$ = (oxyhemoglobin/total hemoglobin)
    × 100%, or the fractional hemoglobin saturation
1.37 = the number of milliliters of oxygen bound to 1 g
    of fully saturated hemoglobin
Pao$_2$ = arterial oxygen partial pressure
0.003 = the solubility coefficient of oxygen in plasma

Equation 7-63 contains three variables and two constants, the variables being Hb, Sao$_2$ and Pao$_2$. Hemoglobin can be estimated as one third of the hematocrit. To determine Cao$_2$, we must therefore be able to measure Sao$_2$ and Pao$_2$. For this reason, oxygen-measuring devices can be divided into two groups: those that measure oxygen partial pressure (Po$_2$) and those that measure hemoglobin saturation (Sao$_2$).

Oxygen partial pressure can be measured in the gas phase by polarographic electrode, paramagnetic analyzer, oxygen fuel cell, mass spectrometer, Raman scattering, or, most recently, the fluorescence-quenching "optode." Two of these methods, the polarographic electrode and the optode, can just as easily be used to measure oxygen tension in a liquid and therefore are used to measure the Po$_2$ of blood. The method most commonly used in medicine today is the polarographic *Clark* oxygen electrode. This device is composed of a platinum cathode and a silver anode in an electrolyte solution covered with an oxygen-permeable membrane (Fig. 7-23). When an electric potential is maintained between these electrodes, a current flows in proportion to the Po$_2$. Oxygen is consumed at the cathode according to the following reaction:

$$O_2 + 2H_2O + 4e^- \rightarrow 4OH^-$$

This electrode was developed by Leland Clark in 1956 and is currently used in all blood gas analyzers.[46] It is also used for the measurement of inspired oxygen tension and has been miniaturized to create an *in vivo* continuous Pao$_2$ monitor. Oxygen tension can also be measured at the heated skin surface with a Clark electrode, which continuously and noninvasively monitors oxygenation (transcutaneous Po$_2$).[47]

Recently, the phenomenon of fluorescence quenching by oxygen has been used to create new Po$_2$ measurement devices.[48,49] The ability of oxygen to absorb energy from excited states in certain fluorescent dyes and thus prevent this energy from being radiated as light is illustrated in Figure 7-24. In theory, a fluorescence-quenching probe is relatively simple, requiring only a fiberoptic light transmission path and the fluorescent dye. For this reason these devices can be made much smaller than Clark electrodes. Another theoretical advantage of the optode over the Clark electrode is that its sensitivity is highest at lower Po$_2$ values.

Hemoglobin Saturation Measurements

In the 1930s, Matthes used spectrophotometry to determine hemoglobin oxygen saturation. This method of measuring oxyhemoglobin concentration, known as *oximetry*, is based

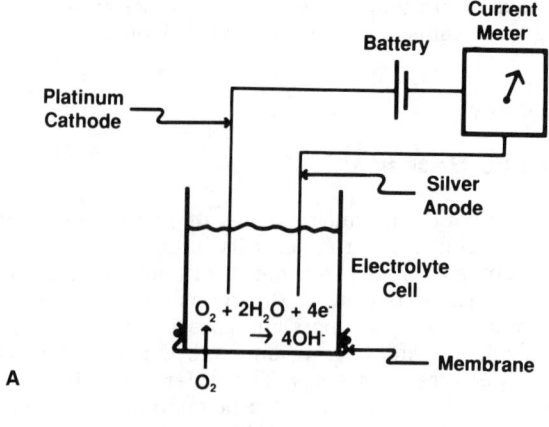

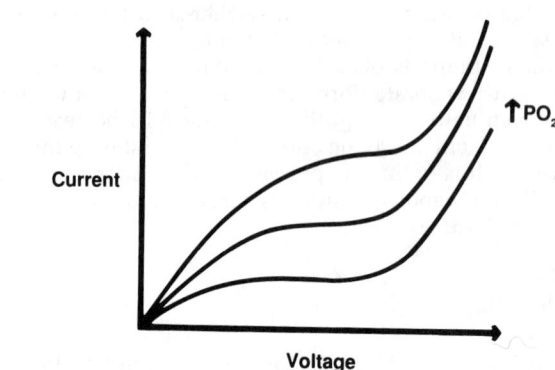

Figure 7-23. (*A*) Schematic of a Clark polarographic oxygen electrode. The circuit consists of a voltage source (battery) and a current meter connecting platinum and silver electrodes. The electrodes are immersed in an electrolyte cell. A membrane permeable to oxygen, but not to the electrolyte, covers one surface of the cell. Oxygen diffuses through the membrane and reacts at the platinum cathode with water to produce hydroxyl ions. The meter measures the current produced by the electrons consumed in the reaction at the cathode. (*B*) A plot (polarogram) of current produced as a function of the voltage between the two electrodes (polarizing voltage). In the range of 600 mV, there is a plateau in the polarogram that occurs at higher currents as the Po$_2$ in the cell is increased. Most polarographic oxygen electrodes use a 600-mV polarizing voltage to obtain a stable current at each Po$_2$.

on the *Lambert-Beer law*. This law relates the concentration of a solute in suspension to the intensity of light transmitted through the solution:

$$I_{\text{trans}} = I_{\text{in}}\, e^{-DC\alpha} \quad (7\text{-}64)$$

where

I_{trans} = intensity of transmitted light
I_{in} = intensity of incident light
D = distance light is transmitted through the liquid
C = concentration of solute (hemoglobin)
α = extinction coefficient of the solute
    (a constant for a given solute
    at a specified wavelength)

If a known solute is in a clear solution in a cuvette of known dimensions, the solute concentration may be calculated

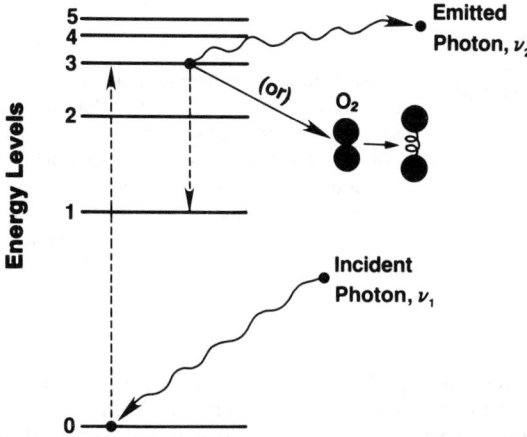

Figure 7-24. The fluorescence-quenching phenomenon. An electron of the fluorescent dye is excited to a higher energy level by an incident photon (ν_1). The excited electron can return to a lower energy level either by emitting a photon (ν_2) or by interacting with an oxygen molecule and raising the latter to a higher vibrational energy level. (Reproduced with permission from Tremper KK: Transcutaneous Po_2 measurement. Can Anaesth Soc J 31:664, 1984.)

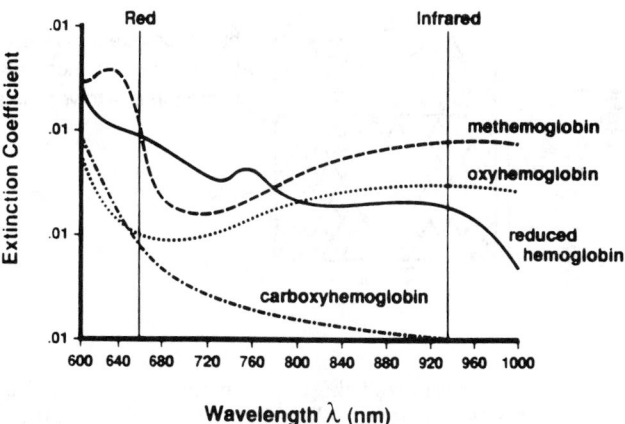

Figure 7-25. Transmitted-light absorbance spectra of four hemoglobin species: oxyhemoglobin, reduced hemoglobin, carboxyhemoglobin, and methemoglobin. (Reproduced with permission from Barker SJ, Tremper KK: Pulse oximetry: applications and limitations. Int Anesthesiol Clin 25:155, 1987.)

from measurements of the incident and transmitted light intensity at a known wavelength.

Laboratory oximeters use this principle to determine hemoglobin concentration by measuring the intensity of the light transmitted through a cuvette filled with a hemoglobin dispersion produced from lysed red blood cells. For Beer's law to be valid, both the solvent and the cuvette must be transparent at the wavelength used, the light path length must be known exactly, and no other absorbing species can be present in the solution. It is difficult to fulfill all of these requirements in clinical devices; therefore, each device theoretically based on Beer's law also requires empirical corrections to its calibration.

Adult blood usually contains four types of hemoglobin: oxyhemoglobin (O_2Hb), reduced hemoglobin (RHb), methemoglobin (MetHb), and carboxy-hemoglobin (COHb). The last two species exist in low concentrations except in pathologic conditions. The hemoglobin saturation can be defined in several ways. *Fractional saturation* (Sao_2) is defined as the concentration of oxyhemoglobin divided by the total hemoglobin.[50]

$$Sao_2 = \frac{O_2Hb}{Total\ Hb} \qquad (7\text{-}65)$$

A recently popularized definition of Sao_2 is that of *functional saturation*, defined as the concentration of oxyhemoglobin divided by the concentration of oxyhemoglobin plus reduced hemoglobin:

$$Func.\ Sao_2 = \frac{O_2Hb}{RHb + O_2Hb} \qquad (7\text{-}66)$$

In this definition, MetHb and COHb are ignored because they do not contribute to oxygen transport.

When oximetry is used to measure hemoglobin saturation, each wavelength of light will produce one equation (Equation 7-64) to solve for one unknown concentration. If either fractional or functional saturation is to be determined in the presence of significant concentrations of MetHb and

COHb, at least four wavelengths of light are required. Even though only two hemoglobin species appear in the definition of functional Sao_2 (Equation 7-66), four equations are required to solve for the four unknowns: RHb, O_2Hb, MetHb, and COHb. If there were two wavelengths at which both MetHb and COHb had zero absorbance while HbO_2 and RHb did not, then functional Sao_2 could be determined with a two-wavelength oximeter. Unfortunately, this is difficult in practice because of the behavior of the absorption coefficients, as seen in Figure 7-25.

Invasive *in vivo* oximeters can estimate hemoglobin saturation by analyzing light reflected from intact red cells. These devices use fiberoptics incorporated into catheters placed in the vascular space for continuous monitoring of mixed venous saturation in the pulmonary artery or arterial saturation in a major artery.[51] These reflectance oximeters use either two or three wavelengths. Because of extraneous reflectances in the vascular space from red cell membranes, vascular wall artifacts, and other blood constituents, empirical data have been required to calibrate these devices. Little is known about the effect of dyshemoglobins on these invasive oximeters. In an animal study of the effects of methemoglobinemia on the accuracy of pulmonary artery oximeters, the monitored mixed venous saturation values increased with rising MetHb levels in spite of decreasing values measured *in vitro* of mixed venous saturation and Po_2.[52] Because of their empirical calibration, it is difficult to predict *a priori* how dyshemoglobins will affect these invasive oximeters.

Over the past 40 years noninvasive oximeters have been developed for continuous monitoring of arterial hemoglobin saturation (Sao_2). These devices measure red and infrared light transmitted through a tissue bed, such as a finger or ear. In effect, they use the tissue as a cuvette containing the hemoglobin. There are several problems in estimating Sao_2 by this method. There are many absorbers in the light path other than arterial hemoglobin, including skin, soft tissue, and venous and capillary blood. The early oximeters eliminated the effect of tissue absorbance by first compressing the tissue to eliminate all the blood and using the absorbance of bloodless tissue as the zero point. Next, to obtain a signal that is related to arterial blood without interference by venous and capillary blood, the oximeter heated the tissue. Heating produced hyperemia beneath the sensor, which was

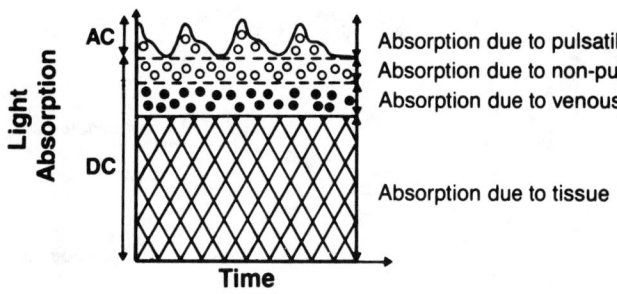

Figure labels:

AC — Absorption due to pulsatile arterial blood
Absorption due to non-pulsatile arterial blood
Absorption due to venous and capillary blood

DC — Absorption due to tissue

Figure 7-26. Schematic representation of the absorption of light by living tissue. Note that arterial blood (the AC component) is the only pulsatile component in the series of light absorbers. The DC component represents all the nonpulsatile absorbers. (Reproduced with permission from Tremper KK, Barker SJ: Pulse oximetry. Anesthesiology 70:104, 1989.).

assumed to "arterialize" the blood in that tissue bed. Devices of this type were developed during World War II for use in aviation research.[53] Later, in the 1950s, these oximeters were used in the operating room, where they detected significant arterial desaturation during routine anesthetics.[54] In spite of the utility recognized by early users, these oximeters were not clinically accepted because they were cumbersome to calibrate and apply and had the potential to burn tissue.[54]

Two technological advances and one bright idea in the late 1970s permitted the development of a new generation of noninvasive oximeters. The two technological advances were the development of small inexpensive light-emitting diodes (LEDs) as monochromatic light sources and of miniature microprocessors that could handle complex empirical algorithms. The bright idea was that of a Japanese engineer named Takuo Aoyagi, who found that the pulsatile component of light absorbance is sensitive chiefly to changes in SaO_2.[55] Because these new oximeters estimate SaO_2 by analyzing the pulsatile component of absorbance, which is assumed to represent only arterial blood, they are referred to as *pulse oximeters*.

Figure 7-26 illustrates the principle of a pulse-added absorber based on Beer's law. The baseline or DC component represents the absorbances of the tissue bed, including venous, capillary, and nonpulsatile arterial blood. The pulse-added or AC component is from the pulsatile arterial blood.

Pulse oximeters use two wavelengths of light: 660 nm (red) and 940 nm (infrared). The oximeter analyzes the AC component of absorbance at both wavelengths and produces a ratio of the pulse-added absorbances, which is empirically related to the SaO_2. Figure 7-27 is an example of a pulse oximeter calibration curve.[56] The actual curves used in commercial devices are developed from experimental studies in human volunteers. Note in Figure 7-27 that when the ratio of red to infrared absorbance is 1, the saturation is approximately 85%.

There are several technical limitations inherent in pulse oximeters. First, being two-wavelength devices, they can identify only two unknowns. This would be adequate to measure functional hemoglobin saturation if MetHb and COHb did not absorb red or infrared light at the wavelengths used. Unfortunately, as can be seen in Figure 7-25, MetHb and COHb do absorb at 660 and 940 nm and therefore if present will cause errors in the pulse oximeter reading. The magnitude of the effect of COHb on pulse oximeter values has been evaluated experimentally. It was noted that the pulse oximeter reads approximately the sum of O_2Hb plus COHb[57] because both O_2Hb and COHb are red, and they absorb red light similarly. The effect of MetHb on pulse oximeter readings has also been measured. It was found that as MetHb increased the pulse oximeter tended toward showing 85% saturation and eventually became almost in-

dependent of SaO_2.[52] This effect has been explained by the fact that MetHb is very dark and absorbs both red and infrared light. It causes a large pulsatile absorbance at both wavelengths and thus forces the ratio of red to infrared absorbance toward 1 (saturation of 85%).

Intravenous dyes can also affect the accuracy of pulse oximeters.[58,59] Scheller and associates[58] evaluated the effects of methylene blue, indigo carmine, and indocyanine green on pulse oximeters in human volunteers, finding that methylene blue causes a drop in the saturation reading to approximately 65% for 1 to 2 minutes. Indigo carmine produces a very small drop in the saturation reading, whereas indocyanine green has an intermediate effect.

There are three engineering problems in pulse oximeter design that may affect clinical use.[56] The first of these problems is light interference. The photodiodes used as light sensors cannot discriminate one wavelength of light from another. Therefore, the sensor does not know whether a light signal it receives is from the red LED, the infrared LED, or the room lights. This problem is solved by alternating the red and infrared LED. That is, the red LED is turned on first, and the photodiode produces a current resulting from the red LED plus the room lights. Next, the red LED is turned off and the infrared LED is turned on; the photodiode signal then represents the infrared LED and the room lights. Finally, both LEDs are turned off, and the photodiode measures a signal from just the room lights. This sequence is repeated 480 times per second. In this way the oximeter

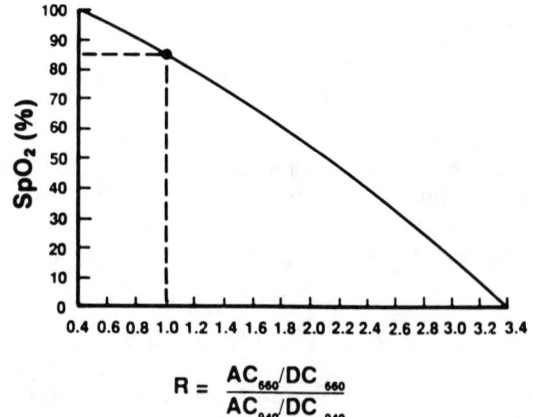

$$R = \frac{AC_{660}/DC_{660}}{AC_{940}/DC_{940}}$$

Figure 7-27. Calibration curve used by the oximeter to calculate arterial oxygen saturation (SaO_2) from the ratio (R) of the light absorbed (A) by the tissue being monitored. (Reproduced with permission from Severinghaus JW, Astrup PB: History of blood gas analysis: pulse oximetry. J Clin Monitoring 3:135, 1987.)

removes interference even in a quickly changing background of room light. However, some light sources can cause problems in spite of this clever design.

The other problems, which are difficult to overcome, are those of low signal-to-noise ratio and motion artifact. When a low pulse-added absorbance signal is seen by the photodetector, the pulse oximeter will amplify the signal and then estimate the saturation from the ratio of amplified absorbances. The pulse oximeter can thereby estimate saturation values from a wide range of patients with various pulse-added absorbance amplitudes. Unfortunately, as with a car radio, when a weak signal is amplified, the background noise (static) also is amplified. If it is amplified enough, it is possible that the pulse oximeter will analyze this noise signal and interpret it as a value of saturation. To prevent the oximeter from amplifying background noise and reporting false saturation values, the manufacturers incorporate cutoff values for a signal-to-noise ratio below which the device will display no saturation value. Some oximeters also display a low signal-strength error message. A similar problem is encountered when there is noise secondary to patient motion artifact. In this situation, the pulse oximeter may not be able to determine an appropriate ratio of absorbances.

One of the main clinical advantages of a pulse oximeter is that it does not require calibration. Indeed, a pulse oximeter cannot be calibrated, because the calibration curve is set in the factory using data gathered from a small number of adult volunteers. Therefore, it is important that these devices be tested to insure their accuracy under the conditions of actual clinical use. We have already discussed how dyshemoglobins, dyes, and motion artifact can alter the output of a pulse oximeter. Severinghaus and Naifeh evaluated the response of pulse oximeters from six manufacturers to an acute hypoxic plateau of 40 to 70% saturation in adult volunteers[60] and found significant variability between the various models in both response time and accuracy in determining the low saturation value. Sensors placed on the ears responded more quickly than finger sensors. The accuracies were in the range of ±5–10%, compared with the manufacturers' stated accuracies of ±2–3%.

Carbon Dioxide Measurement

The polio epidemic of the 1950s spurred the development of a rapid method for measuring the carbon dioxide tension in arterial blood ($Paco_2$). In 1958, Severinghaus presented the first blood gas analyzer using a Clark electrode for measuring Po_2 and a new Pco_2 electrode of his own design.[61] The Severinghaus Pco_2 device consists of a pH-sensitive glass electrode in an electrolyte cell surrounded by a CO_2-permeable membrane (Fig. 7-28). The CO_2 diffuses through the membrane into the cell and reacts with water to produce carbonic acid, which changes the pH within the cell. The pH electrode is then calibrated to measure Pco_2. This "secondary" sensing Pco_2 electrode is currently used in all blood gas analyzers. Like the oxygen electrode, the Severinghaus CO_2 electrode has been used to monitor carbon dioxide continuously from heated skin (transcutaneous Pco_2).[62]

In SI units the hydrogen ion concentration is given in nanomoles per liter, although it is more frequently expressed as the negative logarithm of the hydrogen ion concentration, in pH units. The pH is usually measured with a glass electrode, which, when placed in solution, will develop a voltage relative to a reference electrode that is proportional to the hydrogen ion concentration. This electrode

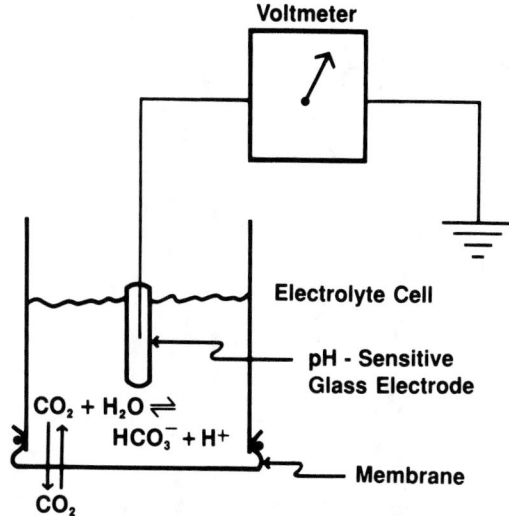

Figure 7-28. Schematic diagram of a Stow-Severinghaus Pco_2 electrode. It consists of a pH-sensitive glass electrode referenced to a silver–silver chloride electrode. The glass electrode is immersed in an electrolyte cell with a CO_2-permeable membrane covering on the surface. When CO_2 diffuses into the cell, it reacts with water, producing carbonic acid, and the pH electrode detects the acidity change.

will produce approximately 60 mV for each pH unit. As noted above, the CO_2 electrode (Fig. 7-28) incorporates a pH electrode as its sensing device. A pH-sensitive optode also has been developed using a dye whose fluorescence is quenched in the presence of hydrogen ions. This pH optode has also been employed to produce a CO_2 measuring device using the same secondary sensing principle as the Severinghaus CO_2 electrode.

RESPIRATORY GAS AND ANESTHETIC AGENT MEASUREMENT: INFRARED ABSORPTION AND RAMAN SCATTERING

Infrared Absorption

Beer's law, described earlier in the section on oximetry, may also be applied to the measurement of inspired and expired gases and vapors. Because it is a very rapid measurement technique (95% response time ≈ 300 ms), it is adequate for measuring real-time expired CO_2 waveforms (capnography).[63] The Severinghaus electrode described above is used in the blood gas machine because it can selectively measure the CO_2 partial pressure in the liquid or gas phase in the presence of the many constituents in blood, but its response time is too slow to be of use in capnography (95% response time >90 s).

For a molecule to absorb infrared light it must be both polyatomic and asymmetric. That means infrared light will not be useful in detecting symmetric molecules such as oxygen (O_2) or nitrogen (N_2) or individual atoms such as helium. The infrared radiation is absorbed because the frequency of the radiation is the same as the natural vibrational frequencies of the molecules. Absorption of the radiation increases the amplitude of that naturally occurring vibrational frequency. Figure 7-29 illustrates the infrared absorption peaks for various respiratory gases and anesthetic

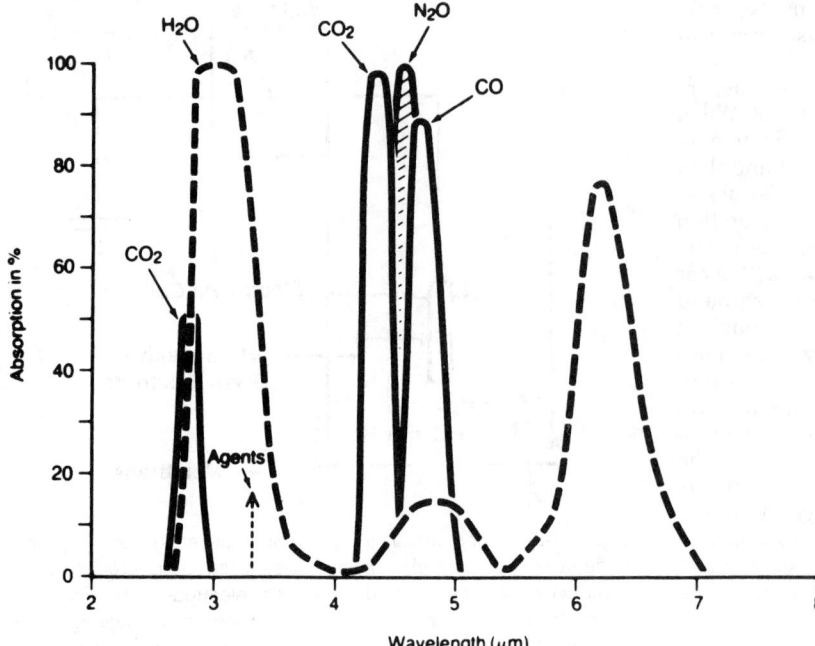

Figure 7-29. Absorption spectra for respiratory gases and anesthetic vapors in the red and infrared range. (Reproduced with permission from Gravenstein JS, Paulus DA, Hayes TJ: Capnography in Clinical Practice. Boston, Butterworths, 1989.)

vapors. Note that the CO_2 and N_2O peaks overlap. Capnometers used in the operating room must measure the concentrations of both N_2O and CO_2 so they may correct for the overlapping absorption.

For a more comprehensive description of the theory and design of capnometers, the reader is referred to the text by Gravenstein et al.[63] Although the development of accurate respiratory gas analyzers involves a substantial amount of engineering, the basic principle on which they measure concentrations is the same as Beer's law used in oximetry (Eq. 7-64).

Raman Scattering

When light of a specific energy strikes a substance, it is either transmitted, reflected, or absorbed. Devices based on Beer's law use light absorption to measure concentration. Another phenomenon, known as *Raman scattering*, may be used to identify molecules according to their light absorption and re-emission. Light in the visible and ultraviolet range may be absorbed by molecules of a substance, producing unstable vibrational and rotational energy states. Because these excited states are unstable, some of the absorbed energy is re-emitted, allowing the molecules to relax into their stable state. This Raman scattering occurs infrequently because most of the light passes directly through the gas sample without taking part in the absorption–re-emission phenomenon. If the intensity of the light is sufficiently great, the Raman scatter signal can be measured and used to identify the molecules within the gas sample. The signal is scattered light: it is emitted in all directions relative to the incident beam. The signal is of very low intensity relative to the incident beam, so it is best measured at right angles to the exciting beam of light.

The advantage of Raman scattering over infrared gas analyzers is that it requires only that the molecules be polyatomic (i.e., have at least one bond) and not be asymmetric. Therefore, Raman scattering can identify O_2 and N_2, whereas infrared analyzers cannot. A Raman analyzer may be able to identify all respiratory gases and vapors used in

anesthesia with the sole exception of helium. For a more comprehensive description of the technique, the reader is referred again to the text by Gravenstein et al.[63]

The only method available clinically that can measure all the above molecules and inert gas atoms is mass spectrometry, which is discussed later in this chapter.

ELECTRICITY, MAGNETISM, AND CIRCUITS

Much physiology is based on electrical phenomena, as is virtually all the modern technology that we apply to critical care. Electromagnetic waves are so important to us that they deserve special mention in Genesis: "Let there be light." One modern physicist paraphrased this quotation to read: "Let there be electricity and magnetism, and there is light!"[64] In this section we survey this field superficially but we hope with enough depth to provide some understanding of electromagnetics and its importance in medicine. Those interested in original sources can consult the republished works of Faraday,[65] Priestley,[66] Thompson,[67] and Maxwell,[68] who were pioneers in the field. Good histories of electrical science have been written by Meyer,[69] Benjamin,[70] and Bordeaux.[71] There are many modern texts of electricity and magnetism for the reader in need of more detail.[72-78] The subject of electrical safety is also discussed in Chapter 8.

Electrostatics: Charge and Fields

Benjamin Franklin (1706–1790) is credited with being the first to understand that there are two (and only two) types of electric charge, which he named *positive* and *negative*. His early experiments, in which glass and rubber rods were charged by being rubbed, led to the conclusion that "like charges repel and unlike charges attract." Franklin also realized that in some materials the charge is free to move within the material, whereas in others it is not. We call the former materials *conductors* and the latter *insulators* or *dielectrics*. Other experiments show that in metallic conductors, only the negative charges (electrons) are free to move, whereas the positive ones are immobile. In electrolyte conductors, both positive and negative charges can move.

In 1785 Coulomb determined that the force between two point charges is proportional to the magnitude of charge and the inverse square of the separating distance r, thus leading to *Coulomb's law*:

$$F = \frac{1}{4\pi\epsilon_0} \frac{q_1 q_2}{r^2} \qquad (7\text{-}67)$$

Here, q_1 and q_2 are the magnitudes of the two charges, and ϵ_0 is called the *permittivity constant*. The dimensions of the charge pose a problem, because charge was initially defined in two different ways. In one system (*electrostatic units or esu*), the dimensions are length × (force)$^{1/2}$, and the units of charge are *statcoulombs*. In the other system (*electromagnetic units or emu*), charge has dimensions of time × (force)$^{1/2}$, and the units are called *abcoulombs*. The conversion is one abcoulomb = 2.998×10^{10} statcoulombs. Along with most modern texts, we use the "rationalized emu," in which 1 rationalized coulomb (C) = 0.1 abcoulomb. In these units, the permittivity constant is $\epsilon_0 = 8.854 \times 10^{-12}$ C^2/N-m^2, and the charge of an electron is -1.60×10^{-19} C.

The electrostatic force exerted on any charged particle has a magnitude and a direction; that is, it is a vector. If we measure this force vector on a small "test charge," which we move around to determine the force everywhere in space, we can define an *electrostatic field* (or *electric field*). This field E is simply the vector force exerted on a unit charge at any point in space (x, y, z) and time (t). The force on any charged particle is proportional to its charge q and the field strength:

$$\mathbf{F} = q\mathbf{E} \qquad (7\text{-}68)$$

A related concept is that of *lines of force*,[69] which are everywhere parallel to the direction of the field vector. Lines of force between two point charges of opposite sign, called a *dipole*, are shown in Figure 7-30.

Suppose that two flat, parallel plates have equal and opposite charges and are separated by distance d, as shown in Figure 7-31. If the plates are large and closely spaced, the field between them will have uniform strength and direction. The force on a charged particle in that field is qE, and the work (W) required to move that particle from P_2 to P_1 is:

$$W = \text{force} \times \text{distance} = qEd \qquad (7\text{-}69)$$

We define the work required to move a unit charge from one point to another as the *potential difference* (V) between those two points. In our example, the potential difference is simply:

$$V = W/q = Ed \qquad (7\text{-}70)$$

Because field strength E has dimensions of force/charge (Equation 7-68), the dimensions of potential difference are (force × distance)/charge or work/charge. The SI unit of potential difference is the joule per coulomb or *volt*.

The strength of the field between the two plates in Figure 7-31 is directly proportional to the total charge Q on either plate. This means that V must also be proportional to Q (Equation 7-70), so that:

$$Q = CV \qquad (7\text{-}71)$$

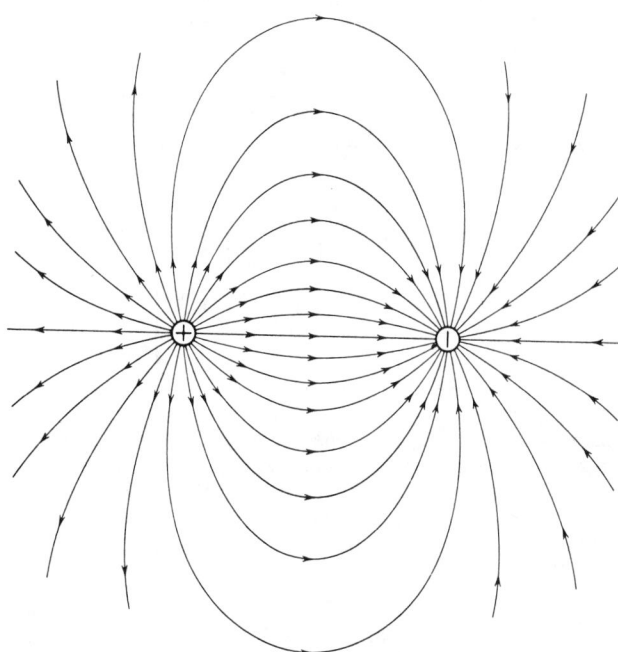

Figure 7-30. Electric lines of force from a dipole, or two point charges of equal strength and opposite sign. The lines are everywhere parallel to E, and they are more closely spaced where E is stronger.

The constant of proportionality (C) is called the *capacitance*, and the two plates form a *capacitor* (in older terminology, a *condenser*). The dimensions of capacitance from Equation 7-71 are charge^2/(force × distance), and the SI unit of capacitance is the coulomb per volt or *farad* (F). (A farad is such a large capacitance that we usually deal in the *microfarad*, μF, where 1 μF = 10^{-6}F.) The capacitance of the plates in Figure 7-31 is directly proportional to their area and inversely proportional to the distance between them. Think of a capacitor as something that accumulates charge in response to a potential difference. The mechanical analogue of a capacitor is a spring, which stores mechanical potential energy as the capacitor stores electrical potential energy.

Groups of capacitors are often combined in series or in parallel (Fig. 7-32A). In the parallel connection, the total accumulated charge is $Q = q_1 + q_2 + q_3$; the potential difference V is the same across all three capacitors, and

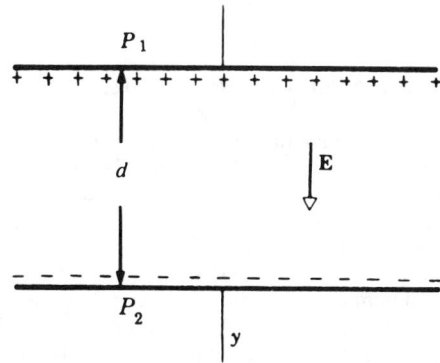

Figure 7-31. The parallel plate capacitor. Plates P_1 and P_2, separated by distance d, have equal and opposite charges distributed on them, resulting in a uniform electric field E between the plates.

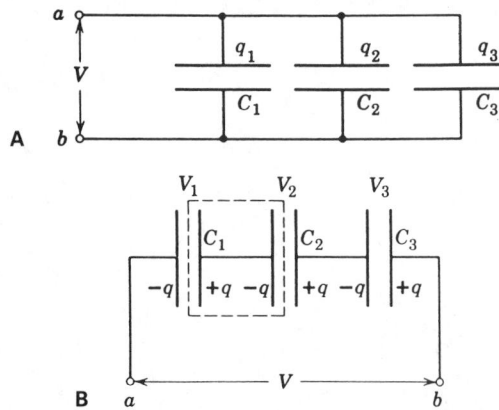

Figure 7-32. (*A*) Capacitors connected in parallel. The voltage *V* is the same across all three capacitors. (*B*) Capacitors in series. The charge on each capacitor must be the same (the net charge inside the dotted line must be zero). (Reproduced with permission from Halliday D, Resnick R: Physics, Part II. New York, John Wiley & Sons, 1962.)

therefore the total parallel capacitance (C_p) is simply the sum of the individual values:

$$C_p = C_1 + C_2 + C_3 \qquad (7\text{-}72)$$

In other words, capacitances in parallel are additive. This has important implications in the combination of leakage capacitances from several operating room devices, as we shall see below. In Figure 7-32B, a series connection, we note that the charge q on each capacitor must be the same. The potential differences across the three are not the same but are related by Equation 7-71:

$$V_1 = q/C_1, \qquad V_2 = q/C_2, \qquad V_3 = q/C_3$$

and, because potential differences in series are additive:

$$V = V_1 + V_2 + V_3$$
$$= q/C_1 + q/C_2 + q/C_3 = q[1/C_1 + 1/C_2 + 1/C_3]$$

The equivalent capacitance of the three is given by $V = q/C_s$, so:

$$1/C_s = 1/C_1 + 1/C_2 + 1/C_3 \qquad (7\text{-}73)$$

Capacitors in series combine reciprocally, so that the equivalent capacitance is less than the smallest capacitance in the chain.

Current, Resistance, and Circuits

A *battery* is an electrochemical device that generates a potential difference or *electromotive force* (EMF) between two points called *terminals*. If we connect the two battery terminals by a conductor, an electrical field will be set up within the conductor, causing charges to move. This flow of charge through the conductor is called an *electric current*, *I*, and it has dimensions of charge/time. The SI unit of current is the coulomb/second or *ampere* (A). Although the electrons in a metal conductor flow in the opposite direction of the electric field (because they are negatively charged), the current is defined to be in the same direction as the field, or in the

direction that positive charges would flow if they were free to move.

Now suppose we connect a particular conductor to several batteries having different EMF values. For most metals at constant temperature, we obtain a linear relation between the voltage and the current:

$$V = IR \qquad (7\text{-}74)$$

Equation 7-74 is called *Ohm's law*, and R is called *resistance*. Its dimensions are length/time (or force × length × time/charge^2), and the SI units are volts/amperes or *ohms*. Although it is valid for most metals, there are many materials that do not obey Ohm's law.

The *current density*, *J*, or current per unit cross-sectional area of conductor, has dimensions of charge/second/length^2, and SI units of amperes/meter^2. If A is the cross-sectional area of the conductor, then $J = I/A$. Another useful form of Ohm's law is:

$$E = \Omega J \qquad (7\text{-}75)$$

where E is electric field, J is current density, and Ω is the resistivity, which is a property of the conducting material rather than of a particular specimen. The Ω has units of ohm-meters and is related to R by:

$$R = \Omega L/A \qquad (7\text{-}76)$$

where L and A are the length and cross-section of the specimen, respectively. (To show that Equations 7-75 and 7-74 are equivalent, use $V = EL$, $I = JA$, and Equation 7-76 in Equation 7-74.) The resistivity values of common metals at room temperature are shown in Table 7-8. Note that the resistivity of metals increases with temperature (second column), whereas that of carbon decreases. Materials that develop extremely low resistivities at low temperatures are called *superconductors*. Low-temperature superconductors are used in magnetic resonance imaging (MRI) to generate the intense magnetic fields required (see below).

How much work per unit time, or *power*, is required to drive a current through a given resistance? The work done on a unit charge in moving it from point A to point B is the potential difference V between these points. The number of charges being moved per unit time is the current I. Therefore, the total work being done per unit time is the product of the two:

$$P = VI \qquad (7\text{-}77)$$

If we combine Equation 7-77 with Ohm's law, $V = IR$, we obtain two other important power relations:

$$P = I^2R, \qquad P = V^2/R \qquad (7\text{-}78)$$

Power has dimensions of force × distance/time, and the SI unit is the joule/sec or *watt* (W). Another common unit of power is the horsepower (1 hp = 746 W).

The power required to drive a current through a resistance is dissipated as heat. Any fixed resistance through which current flows will generate heat in proportion to the square of the current (Equation 7-78). For example, a resistance of 1 ohm carrying a current of 1 A will dissipate 1 W of power. The same resistance carrying 2 A will dissipate 4 W. In terms of common heat units, 1 W = 0.239 calorie/sec = 0.860 kCal/h.

TABLE 7-8. Properties of Metals as Conductors

	Resistivity (at 20°C), ohm-m	Temperature Coefficient of Resistivity,* α, per °C	Density g/cm³	Melting Point, °C
Aluminum	2.8×10^{-8}	3.9×10^{-3}	2.7	659
Copper	1.7×10^{-8}	3.9×10^{-3}	8.9	1080
Carbon (amorphous)	3.5×10^{-5}	-5×10^{-4}	1.9	3500
Iron	1.0×10^{-7}	5.0×10^{-3}	7.8	1530
Manganin	4.4×10^{-7}	1×10^{-5}	8.4	910
Nickel	7.8×10^{-8}	6×10^{-3}	8.9	1450
Silver	1.6×10^{-8}	3.8×10^{-3}	10.5	960
Steel	1.8×10^{-7}	3×10^{-3}	7.7	1510
Wolfram (tungsten)	5.6×10^{-8}	4.5×10^{-3}	19	3400

*This quantity, defined from

$$\alpha = \frac{1}{\rho} \frac{d\rho}{dT}$$

is the fractional change is resistivity ($d\rho/\rho$) per unit change in temperature. It varies with temperature, the values here referring to 20°C. For copper ($\alpha = 3.9 \times 10^{-3}$/°C), the resistivity increases by 0.39% for a temperature increase of 1°C near 20°C. Note that α for carbon is negative, which means that the resistivity *decreases* with increasing temperature.

Reproduced with permission from Halliday D, Resnick R: Physics, part II. New York, John Wiley & Sons, 1962.

EXAMPLE 7-10. ELECTROCAUTERY

Electrocautery uses the resistive or *joule* heating described above to generate high temperatures near a cauterizing electrode. High-frequency (10^5–10^6 Hz) electrical current is used to minimize the risk of ventricular fibrillation. The heat produced is I^2R (Eq. 7-78), and the local rate of heating is proportional to the square of the current density, J, as defined above. The value of J is far greater near the cauterizing electrode than in the surrounding tissue, because the current "spreads out" as it leaves the small electrode. (J falls as $1/r^2$, where r is the distance from the electrode.) Therefore, the tissue heating is significant only very near the electrode.

In a *unipolar* electrocautery system, the current from the single cauterizing electrode travels through the body and exits by means of the *grounding pad*, which makes good (*i.e.*, low-resistance) electrical contact with a large area of the skin. There are two factors that can cause skin burns in the area of the grounding pad. First, if only a small area of the pad is in actual contact with the skin, then J becomes large in this area. Second, if the ground pad is not well covered with conducting gel, it will make a high-resistance contact with the skin. Even though the contact area may be large and the current density small in this case, I^2R is increased (by increasing R), and a large burn can result. The electrocautery circuitry is designed to supply a fixed current no matter what the resistance between the electrode and ground. In cases of defective grounding pads, patients have been burned at ECG electrode sites and other grounding pathways. We know an anesthesiologist (SJB) who was burned while touching a patient with one hand and the anesthesia machine with the other.

In the *bipolar* electrocautery system, the current flows between two small electrodes that are held 1 mm or so apart in the tissue. This geometry not only reduces the risk of skin burns but is also less likely to cause unwanted tissue damage or to interfere with cardiac pacemakers. Bipolar devices are used exclusively in intracranial neurosurgery and are strongly recommended in all patients with pacemakers.

We have shown that capacitances connected in a parallel circuit are additive, whereas those in a series circuit combine reciprocally (Equation 7-72 and 7-73). Resistances connected in series (Fig. 7-33A) will be additive, because the same current I must pass through all three resistors:

$$V = IR_1 + IR_2 + IR_3 = I(R_1 + R_2 + R_3)$$
$$R_s = R_1 + R_2 + R_3 \tag{7-79}$$

For resistances connected in parallel (Fig. 7-33B), the voltage will be the same across all three:

$$I = I_1 + I_2 + I_3$$
$$= V(1/R_1 + 1/R_2 + 1/R_3) = V/R_p \tag{7-80}$$
$$1/R_p = 1/R_1 + 1/R_2 + 1/R_3$$

Resistances in parallel thus combine in the same way as capacitances in series.

The preceding discussion and examples of resistive circuits are valid whether the voltage supply is a direct current battery or an alternating current generator such as that of the commercial electricity supply. Alternating current implies a voltage that varies sinusoidally with time:

$$V(t) = A \sin(2\pi f t) \tag{7-81}$$

where A is an amplitude constant and f is the frequency (60 Hz in the United States; 50 Hz in Europe). When we speak of an "AC voltage," we usually mean the root-mean-square (rms) value of $V(t)$, which is equal to 0.707 times the peak value (A) for a sinusoidal waveform.

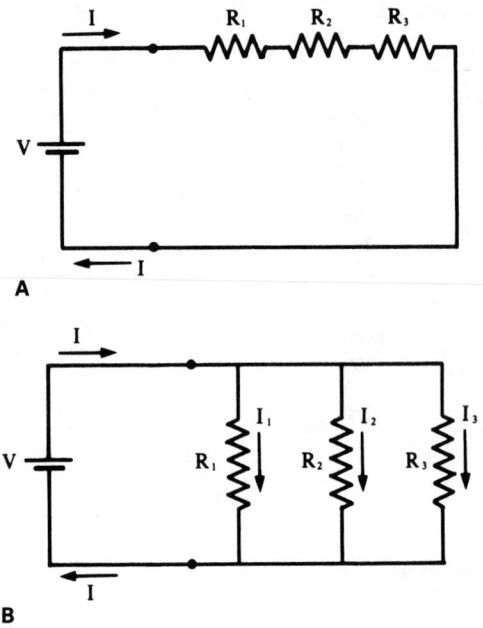

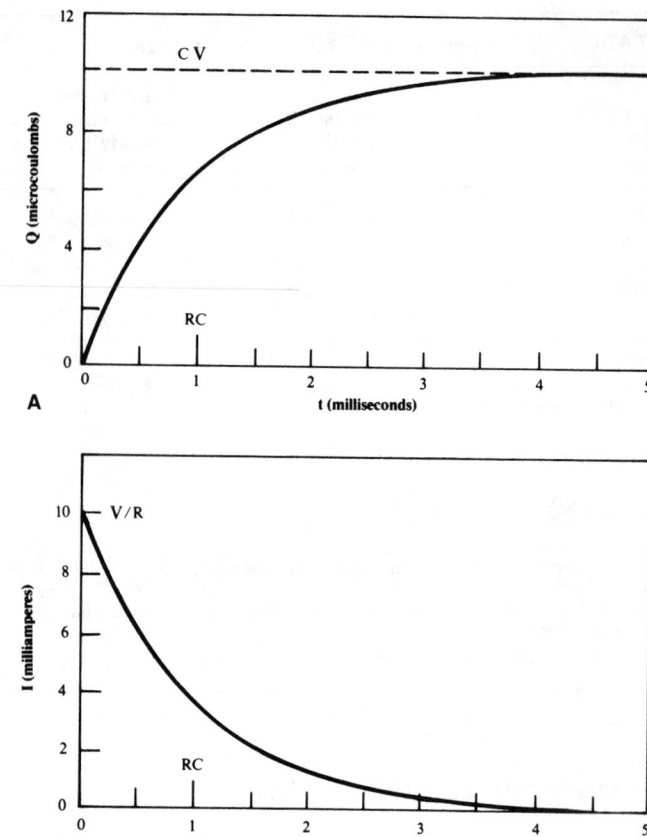

A

B

Figure 7-33. (A) Resistors connected in series to a source of EMF (V). The current I is the same through all three resistors. (B) Resistors connected in parallel. The voltage V is the same across all three resistors.

Figure 7-35. The RC circuit (R = 1000 ohms, C = 1 μF, V = 10 V), showing charge Q on the capacitor (A) and current I through the resistor (B) as functions of time t after switch closure. As t increases, Q approaches CV, and I approaches 0.

EXAMPLE 7-11. THE RC CIRCUIT

Let us consider a circuit involving both resistance and capacitance, an "RC circuit" (Fig. 7-34). When the switch is thrown from b to a at time $t = 0$, the battery will drive a current I through the resistor and thereby charge the capacitor. As charge Q builds up on the capacitor, the potential difference across it will increase ($V = Q/C$) until it is equal to the EMF from the battery. At this point the current will reach 0. At any time during this process the EMF from the battery equals the sum of the voltage change across the resistor and that across the capacitor (Q/C):

$$V = IR + Q/C \qquad (7\text{-}82)$$

The variables I and Q are related by $I = dQ/dt$. Thus we can rewrite Equation 7-82 as a differential equation for the charge Q:

$$R(dQ/dt) + Q/C - V = 0 \qquad (7\text{-}83)$$

The solution to this equation is:

$$Q = CV[1 - \exp(-t/RC)]$$

and

$$I = dQ/dt = (V/R)\exp(-t/RC) \qquad (7\text{-}84)$$

Figure 7-35 shows the charge Q and current I plotted versus time for R = 1000 ohms, C = 1.0 μF, and V = 10 V. At $t = 0$, the current is V/R, which is the value it would have if the capacitor were not present. At $t = RC$ (note that RC has the dimensions of time), Equation 7-84 yields:

$$I = (V/R)\exp(-1) = 0.37\ V/R$$

The quantity RC is called the RC time constant of the circuit, and it is the time required for the current to fall to 37% of its initial value. During the same period, the charge Q rises to 63% of its final value of CV. The RC time constant is analogous to the time constants used in any process that can be represented by an exponential function, such as the "wash-in time" of fresh gas introduced into an anesthesia circuit. In one time constant, an exponential quantity will change by 63% of the difference between its values at $t = 0$ and $t = \infty$ (Fig. 7-35). It will change by 86% in two time constants and by 95% in three time constants.

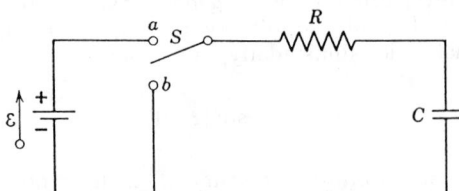

Figure 7-34. Schematic diagram of an RC circuit. Switch S moves from b to a at t = 0, which begins the charging of capacitor C through resistor R.

Magnetism

Observations of magnetic phenomena date back centuries, but it was Oersted[78] in 1820 who first noted that an electric current in a wire produces magnetic effects, namely, movement of a compass needle. Magnetic forces can be represented by a vector magnetic field **B**, also called the *magnetic induction*. If a particle carrying charge q moving at velocity **v** is deflected by a sideways force, we say that a magnetic induction or field is present. The magnetic deflecting force is proportional to the field strength, the charge, and the velocity of the particle. Mathematically, this magnetic force is given by:

$$\mathbf{F} = q\mathbf{v} \times \mathbf{B} \qquad (7\text{-}85)$$

The product indicated here is the vector product or *cross product* of the two vectors **v** and **B**. This is a vector of magnitude $vB \sin(\sigma)$, where σ is the angle between **v** and **B**, and direction perpendicular to both **v** and **B** (Fig. 7-36). Because the force is perpendicular to the velocity vector **v**, it is always at right angles to the direction of motion. Whereas only one direction is required to determine the electrostatic force (the direction of **E**), we need two directions (**v** and **B**) to determine the magnetic force.

From Equation 7-85, **B** has dimensions of force/charge/velocity. The SI unit of induction is the (newton/coulomb)/(meter/sec), called the *tesla* (T). Because 1 C/s is 1 A, the tesla is also equivalent to the newton/ampere-meter. An older unit of magnetic induction is the *gauss* (G) given by $1\ \text{T} = 10^4\ \text{G}$. The earth's magnetic induction is roughly 0.5 gauss in most parts of the United States. The direction of **B** is about 60° downward from horizontal, so the horizontal component is 0.2–0.3 G. The field generated in a magnetic resonance imager (MRI) is on the order of 1–2 T ($1\text{–}2 \times 10^4\ \text{G}$).

EXAMPLE 7-12. MASS SPECTROMETRY

The mass spectrometer determines the charge to mass ratio (q/m) of charged molecules or *ions* by making use of both magnetic and electric forces. For a particle acted on by both types of force, Equations 7-68 and 7-85 can be combined:

$$\mathbf{F} = q\mathbf{E} + q\mathbf{v} \times \mathbf{B} \qquad (7\text{-}86)$$

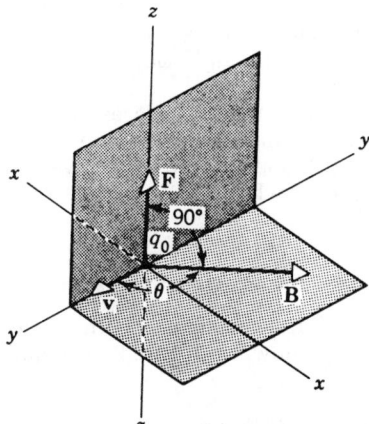

Figure 7-36. Vector relations between a charged particle's velocity **v**, the magnetic field **B**, and the magnetic force **F** acting on the particle.

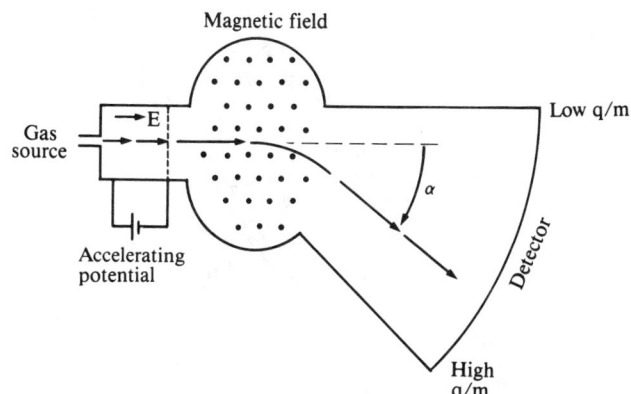

Figure 7-37. Schematic diagram of the mass spectrometer principle. Gas ions at left are accelerated by electric field **E**; their trajectories are then bent by magnetic field (shown directed out of the page). The deflection angle is proportional to the charge/mass ratio (q/m).

The mass spectrometer is able to identify ions by their characteristic q/m values and thus to determine how much of each species is present. As shown in Figure 7-37, the spectrometer first accelerates the ions through a known electric field **E**. Once accelerated, the particles pass through a magnetic field **B** oriented perpendicular to their direction of motion. The ions experience a sideways magnetic force given by Equation 7-86, and their trajectories bend. The sideways force is proportional to q, and the sideways acceleration is inversely proportional to m, so that the deflection angle α (Fig. 7-37) is a function of q/m. The angle α is measured by the detectors, and q/m is thus determined.

From Equation 7-85, we can also calculate the magnetic force exerted on a wire carrying a current through a magnetic field. If a length L of a wire carrying current I is placed in a field of strength B and direction perpendicular to the wire, it is easy to show that the force on the wire is:

$$F = ILB \qquad (7\text{-}87)$$

The direction of this force is perpendicular to both the wire and the field.

Just as a magnetic field exerts a force on a moving charged particle, any moving charge or electric current will itself generate a magnetic field. For a current I passing through a long, straight wire, the induction at a distance r from the wire is given by:

$$B = (\mu_0 I)/(2\pi r) \qquad (7\text{-}88)$$

The *permeability constant*, μ_0, is $4\pi \times 10^{-7}$ in SI units. The direction of the magnetic field is in a series of concentric circles around the wire, as specified by the *right-hand rule*. That is, if we grasp the wire with the right hand, the thumb pointing in the direction of the current, then the fingers will curl around the wire in the direction of **B**. With this rule and Equation 7-85, we can predict the direction of the magnetic force between two parallel wires carrying current in the same direction (Fig. 7-38). The two wires will attract each other with a force proportional to the product of the two currents. If the currents are in opposite directions, the wires will mutually repel. These facts were discovered by both Ampere and Oersted in 1820, and Equation 7-88 is a form of Ampere's law.

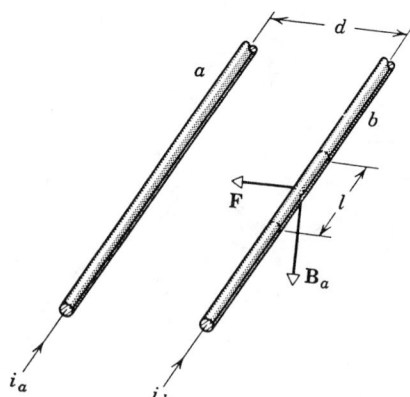

Figure 7-38. Two parallel wires *a* and *b* carrying currents i_a and i_b in the same direction. The magnetic field from wire *a* (**B_a**) is directed downward at wire *b*, causing a magnetic force **F** that attracts wire *b* toward wire *a*.

Magnetic Induction and Inductance

In 1831 Faraday[65] discovered another link between electricity and magnetism: a moving magnet will generate an electric current in a stationary wire (Fig. 7-39A). As long as this magnet is moving, a current will flow through the wire loop, causing a deflection of the galvanometer. If the direction of motion or the polarity of the magnet is reversed, the current will reverse. Similarly, in Figure 7-39B when the switch is closed and a current begins to flow through wire loop A, an *induced current* will flow through loop B until the current through A reaches a constant value. When this occurs, the induced current through B will fall to 0. In other words, it is the *rate of change* of the magnetic field that is responsible for the induced current in both cases.

The quantitative form of this physical law, called *Faraday's law of induction*, is the basis of function of all generators and transformers. A *generator* is simply an apparatus that moves loops of wire through a fixed magnetic field or *vice versa*—it does not matter which element is moving. An induced current is generated in the wires, and the energy required to turn the generator is thereby converted into electrical energy. The current generated can be AC or DC, depending on the switching connections to the moving wires. A *transformer* is an arrangement of two sets of wire coils that operates on the principle illustrated in Figure 7-39B.

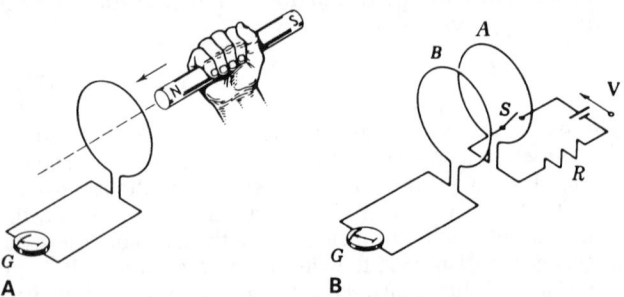

Figure 7-39. Current induced by a changing magnetic field (Faraday's law). (*A*) A magnet moving through a wire loop induces current through galvanometer G. (*B*) When switch S is thrown, the time-varying current through loop A causes a time-varying magnetic field in loops A and B, which induces a current in loop B. (Reproduced with permission from Halliday D, Resnick R: Physics, Part II. New York, John Wiley & Sons, 1962.)

The changing magnetic field caused by the varying current through the *primary coil* induces a current in the *secondary coil*. Because it is the rate of change of the magnetic field that induces current in the secondary coil, transformers function only for AC power. A transformer can change the voltage of an AC source while maintaining constant power ($P = VI$; Equation 7-77). The ratio of the secondary voltage to the primary voltage is equal to the ratio of the number of loops in the secondary and primary coils.

When a changing current passes through a coil of wire as in the primary coil of a transformer, the resulting varying magnetic field will also induce an EMF *in the same coil* that produces the field. This phenomenon is called *self-induction*, and the induced EMF always opposes the EMF that produced the original current. This self-induced EMF is proportional to the rate of change of the current through the coil:

$$V = L(dI/dt) \qquad (7\text{-}89)$$

The proportionality constant L is called the *inductance of the coil*. The SI unit of inductance is the volt-second/ampere, or *henry* (H). The henry is a rather large unit (like the farad in capacitance), so we commonly use the millihenry (10^{-3} H).

With the addition of inductance, we now have three types of *reactance* or voltage changes resulting from current:

Reactance Type (Units)	Symbol	Formula
Resistance (ohm):	⎓⋀⋀⋀⎓	$V = IR$
Capacitance (farad):	—⊢ ⊢—	$V = Q/C$
Inductance (henry):	⎓ᴕᴕᴕᴕᴕᴕᴕᴕ⎓	$V = L(dI/dt)$

Because current is the time derivative of charge ($I = dQ/dt$), the three reactances are proportional to charge and the first and second time derivatives. These formulas imply that the ratio of voltage to current in capacitors and inductors will depend on the frequency for alternating current. For a sinusoidally varying voltage of angular frequency ω, the voltage-current ratio (reactance) is given by:

Capacitive reactance:	$R_c = 1/\omega C$
Inductive reactance:	$R_L = \omega L$

$(7\text{-}90)$

Capacitive reactance thus decreases with increasing frequency, whereas inductive reactance increases. For a frequency of zero (DC source), the capacitive reactance is infinite (open circuit), while the inductive reactance is zero (short circuit).

EXAMPLE 7-13. THE *LR* CIRCUIT

If we combine all three reactances with a time-varying voltage source V(t) as shown in Figure 7-40, Ohm's law for this circuit is:

$$V(t) = L(d^2Q/dt^2) + R(dQ/dt) + Q/C \qquad (7\text{-}91)$$

Comparing this equation with Equation 7-14 for the forced harmonic oscillator problem, we see that they are essen-

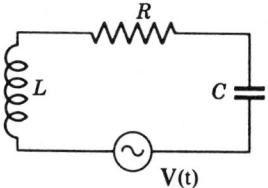

Figure 7-40. The LRC circuit. An oscillating source of EMF, V(t), drives current through inductance L, resistance R, and capacitance C.

tially the same. We can therefore draw an analogy between the mass-spring oscillator and the *LRC* circuit of Figure 7-40, in which displacement x is analogous to electrical charge Q. Mass m corresponds to inductance L; spring constant k corresponds to reciprocal capacitance 1/C; and friction c corresponds to resistance R. The solution for the *LRC* circuit shows the same resonance behavior (Equation 7-16; Fig. 7-2) as the mass-spring oscillator. This analogy between mechanics and electrical circuits is useful in studying many physical phenomena, such as the arterial pressure waveform discussed previously.

EXAMPLE 7-14. ELECTRICAL SAFETY AND ISOLATION TRANSFORMERS

The human body is not very tolerant of electrical current; in fact, as little as 50 μA (1 μA = 10^{-6} A) passing through the heart can cause ventricular fibrillation. Current delivered directly to the heart is called *microshock*, whereas current passing through the skin tissue or tissue remote from the heart is called *macroshock*. While a microshock current of 50 μA can cause the heart to fibrillate, the required macroshock is in the range of 0.1–2.5 A. Thus the distinction between the two is important in electrical safety. The threshold of sensation of a 60-Hz macroshock current is 300–500 μA; pain is felt at 1–2 mA (1 mA = 10^{-3} A). Sustained muscle contraction occurs at 8–20 mA, the "cannot let-go" current: above this value, a subject who grasps a "hot" wire will not be able to release it. Shocks also pose other hazards in the operating room: fires, tissue burns, nerve stimulation or damage, and pacemaker interference are only a few.[79-82] (See Chapter 8.)

Figure 7-41 illustrates the danger of macroshock from electrical equipment. Figure 41A depicts a 60-Hz power supply connected directly at points A and B to equipment shown as resistance R. Side B of the power supply is connected to *ground*, which is simply an infinite source (or sink) for electrons, always maintained at zero electrical potential. One side of the equipment circuitry is grounded (through point B), as is the metal case around the equipment. A grounded patient (or anesthesiologist) who touches a part of the equipment circuitry connected to side A of the power supply will receive a macroshock of as much as 120 V (the supply voltage). This will produce a current well above the "cannot let-go" value, even if the contact is with dry skin. The *line isolation monitor* (LIM) shown in Figure 7-41A would indicate a current of 120 mA in this case (see below).

The dangers of the circuit in Figure 41A led to the use of the *isolation transformer*, shown in Figure 41B. Side B of the power supply is still grounded, but the equipment power leads C and D are both ungrounded or *floating*. Nei-

ther lead makes contact with the equipment case, which is grounded. The isolation transformer creates a potential difference between leads C and D, but there is no potential between either C or D and ground. Thus the equipment receives power (current flows through R), but a grounded patient touching any part of the circuitry will not receive a macroshock. The LIM reads 0 current, because it does not

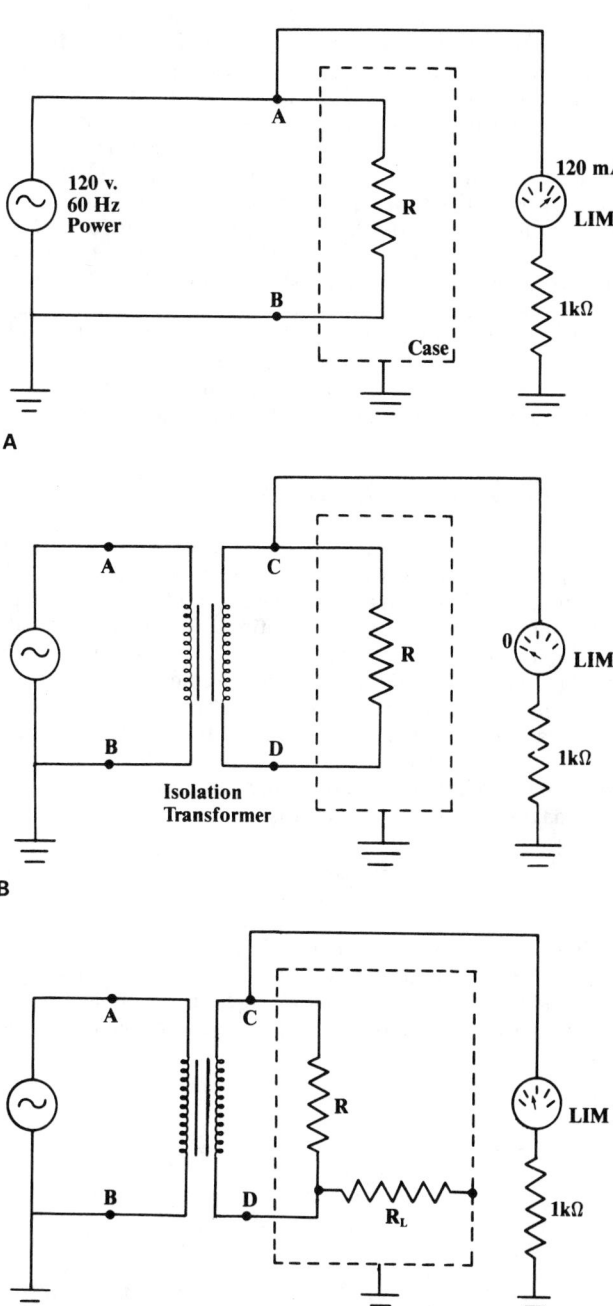

Figure 7-41. Electrical isolation and leakage currents. (A) No isolation: circuitry (R) is "hot" relative to electrical ground, resulting in serious macroshock hazard. The line isolation monitor (LIM) reads 120 mA. (B) Isolation: neither C nor D is "hot" relative to ground. The LIM reads 0. (C) Isolation with leakage in equipment (R_L): D is now partially grounded through R_L, making C "hot" relative to ground. The LIM reads leakage current inversely proportional to R_L.

complete a circuit between power leads C and D or between A and ground. The LIM tests the safety of all circuits connected to the transformer at C, D by indicating their degree of isolation from ground.

In practice, electrical circuits are never perfectly isolated from ground. There is always some capacitive coupling to ground—recall the parallel plate capacitor example discussed above (Fig. 7-31). Because capacitances connected in parallel are additive (Equation 7-72), the capacitive leakage from multiple devices will be cumulative. Faulty equipment may also have a resistive connection to ground or even a short-circuit to one side of the power supply (C or D). This is illustrated in Figure 7-41C by the *leakage* resistance R_L. The LIM now registers a leakage current, because it completes a circuit (through R_L) between C and D. In the operating room, the LIM actually monitors both sides of the power supply (C and D), and is usually set to trigger an alarm at a current of 2–4 mA. The LIM will not warn of leakage currents in the microshock range (50 μA). Additional precautions should therefore be taken with equipment that is in contact with the heart or major blood vessels (e.g., ECG measured through a central venous line). Blood is a fairly good electrical conductor, and leakage currents into large vessels must be considered microshock hazards.

Electromagnetic Waves

If we combine all of the above relations between **E**, **B**, I, and q, we obtain a set of four equations called Maxwell's equations.[68] These govern the behavior of all electromagnetic fields. Using Maxwell's equations, we can demonstrate the existence of electromagnetic waves of the type shown in Figure 7-42, in which the **E** and **B** fields are oriented at right angles to one another and both are perpendicular to the direction of wave propagation. This is called a *transverse electromagnetic wave*, and it propagates to the right in Figure 7-42 at the speed of light, c. The oscillating electric and magnetic fields are given by:

$$E = E_m \sin k(x - ct)$$
$$B = B_m \sin k(x - ct)$$
$$(7\text{-}92)$$

(k is called the *wavenumber* and is related to wavelength by $k = 2\pi/\lambda$.) Numerous experiments have determined c to be 2.9979×10^8 m/s (186,400 mi/s or 7.5 times around the earth's circumference in 1 s). Foucault measured c with

three-digit accuracy as early as 1862, using a rotating mirror apparatus.

There are important differences between electromagnetic waves and the sound waves discussed previously. The particle motions in sound waves are in the same direction as the wave propagation (longitudinal wave), whereas in electromagnetic waves both the **E** and **B** fields are perpendicular to the direction of propagation (transverse wave). Sound waves propagate only through matter, whereas electromagnetic waves will propagate through a vacuum without attenuation. The speed of light is about one million times that of sound in air. An observer moving relative to a sound source can measure a speed of sound that depends on his or her own motion, but the speed of light is the same to any observer in any frame of reference—this is the basic premise of Einstein's special theory of relativity.

Electromagnetic radiation spans a very wide frequency spectrum, as shown in Figure 7-43. Frequency and wavelength are related by $c = f\lambda$. The visible light spectrum is centered at a wavelength of 5.55×10^{-7} m. For historical reasons, three different units are used to describe light wavelengths:

1 micrometer (μm):	10^{-6} m
1 nanometer (nm):	10^{-9} m
1 angstrom (Å):	10^{-10} m

The visible light spectrum extends from 4300 Å (violet) to 6900 Å (red). The corresponding frequency range ($c = f\lambda$) is from 4.3 to 7×10^{14} Hz. Visible light covers a very small fraction of the total electromagnetic spectrum.

EXAMPLE 7-15. ELECTROMAGNETIC RADIATION IN THE OPERATING ROOM

Ampere's law (Equation 7-88) states that any electric current in a wire will create a magnetic field. If the current is oscillating, electromagnetic (EM) radiation will be emitted from the wire. This is the principle of all radio antennas. Maxwell's equations predict that the power radiated from a wire is proportional to the square of the frequency.[77] This has important implications for two sources of EM radiation in the operating room: the 60-Hz power supply and electrocautery. If the electrocautery current frequency is 500 kHz, then the relative efficiency of these two radiators is 7×10^7. That is, a given length of wire carrying a given current will emit

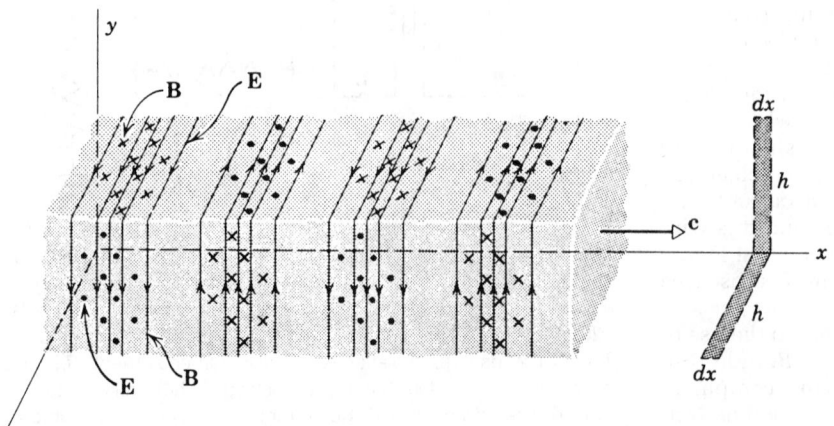

Figure 7-42. A transverse electromagnetic wave. The **E** field is in the z direction; the **B** field is in the y direction; and the wave propagates in the x direction at speed c.

Figure 7-43. The electromagnetic wave spectrum (frequency above, wavelength below). Visible light represents a small fraction of this spectrum. (Reproduced with permission from Halliday D, Resnick R: Physics, Part II. New York, John Wiley & Sons, 1962.)

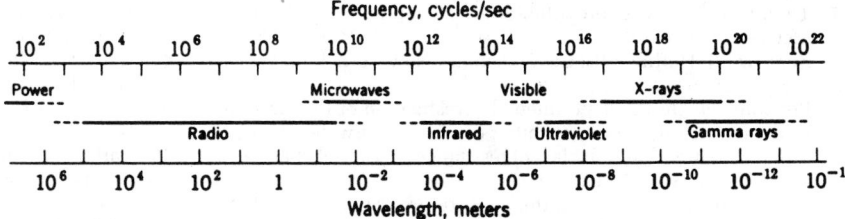

7×10^7 as much EM radiation at 500 kHz as it will at 60 Hz. Thus, although 60-Hz interference may be significant with unshielded ECG leads, it is relatively easy to eliminate from shielded circuits. On the other hand, electrocautery interference or *Bovie artifact* is a constant problem that may never be completely solved.

Ionizing Radiation

At the high-frequency end of the EM radiation spectrum in Figure 7-43, we see two forms of ionizing radiation: X-rays and gamma rays. These high-frequency EM waves are capable of removing electrons from their orbits and can cause cell injury, cell death, or oncogenesis. Gamma rays are commonly emitted by decaying radioactive nuclei, along with two other types of ionizing radiation: alpha and beta particles. Alpha particles are helium nuclei (two protons, two neutrons) and are relatively heavy and slow moving. Although they can injure tissue with prolonged exposure near a source, they do not travel far in air, and most are stopped by a sheet of paper. Beta particles are high-energy electrons emitted from unstable nuclei. They can damage tissue but are blocked by a thin sheet of almost any metal. Gamma rays are the most penetrating of the nuclear emissions; they can travel any distance through air and require lead or other heavy shielding to block them. Radiation not originating from nuclear decay can also be hazardous, as exemplified by the proton accelerators now used to treat cancer. High-energy X-rays and particle beams are not reliably blocked by lead aprons.

Ionizing radiation is quantified in four ways: activity, exposure, absorption, and biologic damage. The activity of a radioactive substance is simply the number of disintegrations per second and is measured in curies; $1 \text{ Ci} = 3.7 \times 10^{10}$ disintegrations/s. Exposure is a measure of radiation ionization at a particular location and is defined by the number of free electrons released from a kilogram of exposed air. The unit of exposure is the roentgen ($1 \text{ R} = 2.58 \times 10^{-4}$ C/kg of air). Absorption refers to the radiation energy dissipated in each kilogram of tissue, given in rads or grays ($1 \text{ rad} = 0.01 \text{ Gy} = 0.01$ J/kg). The biological damage, or *dose-equivalent*, depends on the type of radiation as well as the absorption; it equals absorption times a quality factor Q. The unit is the *rem*, or roentgen-equivalent-man. The maximum "safe" occupational whole-body radiation dose is now set at 5 rem/yr. For comparison, a patient having a chest radiograph receives 20–30 millirem (mrem), and the dose for a CT scan is about 1 rem per cross-section. The obligate radiation dose from cosmic rays at sea level in the United States is about 80 mrem/yr.[83-87]

Radiation exposure of operating room personnel depends on the source intensity or activity, the directionality of the radiation (e.g., for X-ray or proton beam), and the distance from the source. Radioactive substances, such as iridium implants, emit equally in all directions. The exposure is then directly proportional to the activity and inversely pro-

portional to the square of the distance from the source. In other words, the exposure 10 m from the source is 1% of that at 1 m. For X-rays, the exposure will depend on the direction as well as the distance from the source. In general, the back-scattered radiation (in the direction opposite that of the gun) is more intense than the forward-scattered radiation.

CONCLUSION

We have only scratched the surface of the fields discussed in this chapter, and there are many important fields of physics not even mentioned here. Concepts that start as simple as $\mathbf{F} = m\mathbf{a}$ can lead to considerable mathematical complexity when applied to practical problems, as we have seen. Although this complexity may discourage some readers, as physicians we should at least be familiar with the basic concepts and with the types of approaches used to apply these to the "real world." Only with some understanding of the mathematics of physics can we make use of the many physical analogies that apply to anesthesia. For example, how can we speak of the time constant of a circle system without knowing how a time constant is defined for an exponential process (such as the RC-circuit) or why such a process should occur? The more we know of basic physics, the better we shall be able to understand, practice, and teach anesthesiology.

REFERENCES

1. Macintosh R, Mushin WW, Epstein HG: Physics for the Anesthetist. Springfield, Ill, Charles C Thomas, 1958
2. Dugas R: A History of Mechanics. Switzerland, Editions du Griffon, 1955
3. Newton I: In Principia Mathematica. Translation by A Motte. Berkeley, University of California Press, 1934
4. Gardner RM: Direct blood pressure measurement—dynamic response requirements. Anesthesiology 54:227, 1981
5. Goldstein H: Classical Mechanics. Reading, Mass, Addison-Wesley, 1953
6. Lindsay R: Physical Mechanics. New York, Van Nostrand, 1961
7. Symon K: Mechanics. Reading, Mass, Addison-Wesley, 1960
8. Meriam JL: Statics and Dynamics. New York, John Wiley & Sons, 1978
9. Thompson W (Lord Kelvin): Principles of Mechanics. New York, Dover, 1962
10. Landau LD, Lifshitz EM: Fluid Mechanics. Reading, Mass, Addison-Wesley, 1959
11. Batchelor GK: Introduction to Fluid Dynamics. Cambridge, Cambridge University Press, 1970
12. Streeter VL, Wylie EB: Fluid Mechanics. New York, McGraw-Hill, 1979
13. Sabersky R, Acosta A: Fluid Flow. New York, Macmillan, 1971
14. Schlichting H: Boundary Layer Theory. New York, McGraw-Hill, 1968
15. Lamb H: Hydrodynamics. New York, Dover, 1945
16. Liepmann HW, Roshko A: Elements of Gas Dynamics. New York, McGraw-Hill, 1972

17. Thompson P: Compressible-fluid Dynamics. New York, McGraw-Hill, 1972

18. Zucrow MJ, Hoffman JD: Gas Dynamics. New York, John Wiley & Sons, 1976

19. Reynolds O: On the experimental investigation of the circumstances which determine whether the motion of water shall be direct or sinuous, and the law of resistance in parallel channels. Phil Trans R Soc 174:935, 1883

20. Guyton AC: Body temperature, temperature regulation, and fever. In Textbook of Medical Physiology, 6th ed, pp 104, 477, 886. Philadelphia, WB Saunders, 1981

21. Carnot S: Reflexions on the Motive Power of Fire. New York, Lillian Barber Press, 1986

22. Planck M: Treatise on Thermodynamics. New York, Dover, 1945

23. Fermi E: Thermodynamics. New York, Dover, 1936

24. Sabersky R: Elements of Engineering Thermodynamics. New York, McGraw-Hill 1957

25. Beattie JA, Oppenheim I: Principles of Thermodynamics. New York, Elsevier Publishing, 1979

26. Black WZ, Hartley JG: Thermodynamics. New York, Harper & Row, 1985

27. Guggenheim EA: Thermodynamics. New York, John Wiley & Sons, 1967

28. Lewis GN, Randall M: Thermodynamics. New York, McGraw-Hill, 1961

29. Sears FW: Thermodynamics: The Kinetic Theory of Gases, and Statistical Mechanics. Reading, Mass, Addison-Wesley, 1953

30. Riba A, Berger HJ: Echocardiography. In Glenn WWL, Baue AE, Geha AS, et al (eds): Thoracic and Cardiovascular Surgery, 4th ed. New York, Appleton-Century-Crofts, 1983

31. Gramiak R, Nanda NC: New Techniques in cardiac imaging with ultrasound: State of the art. Radiology 6:1, 1981

32. Popp RL, Rubenson DS, Tucker CR, French JW: Echocardiography: M-mode and two-dimensional methods. Ann Intern Med 93:844, 1980

33. Ludomirsky A, Huhta JC, Vick GW et al: Color Doppler detection of multiple ventricular septal defects. Circulation 74:1317, 1986

34. Incropera FP, DeWitt DP: Fundamentals of Heat and Mass Transfer, 2nd ed, pp 752, 777. New York, John Wiley & Sons, 1958

35. Incropera FP, DeWitt DP: Fundamentals of Heat and Mass Transfer, 2nd ed, pp 8, 66. New York, John Wiley & Sons, 1985

36. Bennett CO, Myers JE: Conduction and thermal conductivity. In Momentum, Heat and Mass Transport, p 242. New York, McGraw-Hill, 1962

37. Brown AC: Energy metabolism. In Ruch TC, Patton HD (eds): Physiology and Biophysics. Vol 3: Digestion, Metabolism, Endocrine Function and Reproduction, p 85. Philadelphia, WB Saunders, 1973

38. Brengelmann G: Temperature regulation. In Ruch TC, Patton HD (eds): Physiology and Biophysics. Vol 3: Digestion, Metabolism, Endocrine Function and Reproduction, p 105. Philadelphia, WB Saunders, 1973

39. Ruch TC, Patton HD: Free convection. In Physiology and Biophysics. Vol 3: Digestion, Metabolism, Endocrine Function and Reproduction, p 417. Philadelphia, WB Saunders, 1973

40. Edwards DK, Denny VE, Mills AF: Convective transfer rates. In Transfer Processes: An Introduction to Diffusion, Convection and Radiation, 2nd ed, p 140. Washington, DC, McGraw-Hill, 1979

41. Morley PK: Unintentional hypothermia in the operating room. Can Anaesth Soc J 33:516, 1986

42. Chang KS, Farrell RT, Snellen JW, King FG: Calorimetrical comparison of insulative properties of metalized plastic, clear polyethylene, and polyester blanket. Can Anaesth Soc J 31:690, 1984

43. Parbrook GD, Davis PD, Parbrook EO: Temperature. In Basic Physics and Measurement in Anesthesia, 2nd ed, p 119. New York, Appleton-Century-Crofts, 1986

44. Bird RB, Stewart WE, Lightfoot EN: Transport phenomena. In Diffusivity and Mechanisms of Mass Transport, p 495. New York, John Wiley & Sons, 1960

45. Hill DW: Physics Applied to Anaesthesia, 3rd ed, p 177. London, Butterworths, 1976

46. Clark LC: Monitor and control of blood and tissue oxygen tension. Trans Soc Artif Int Organs 2:41, 1956

47. Tremper KK: Transcutaneous PO_2 measurement. Can Anaesth Soc J 31:664, 1984

48. Barker SJ, Tremper KK, Hyatt J et al: Continuous fiberoptic arterial oxygen measurement in dogs. J Clin Monitoring 3:48, 1987

49. Optiz N, Lubbers DW: Theory and development of fluorescence-based optochemical oxygen sensors: Oxygen optodes. In Tremper KK, Barker SJ (eds): IAC Advances in Oxygen Monitoring, p 177. Boston, Little, Brown, 1987

50. Payne JP, Severinghaus JW (eds): Pulse oximetry, p xxi. Berlin, Springer-Verlag, 1986

51. Schweiss JF: Mixed venous hemoglobin saturation: Theory and applications. In Tremper KK, Barker SJ (eds): IAC Advances in Oxygen Monitoring, p 113. Boston, Little, Brown, 1987

52. Barker SJ, Tremper KK, Hyatt J, Zaccari J: Effects of methemoglobinemia on pulse oximetry and mixed venous oximetry. Anesthesiology 67:A171, 1987

53. Severinghaus JW, Astrup PB: History of blood gas analysis: Oximetry. Int Anesthesiol Clin 25:167, 1987

54. Stephen CR, Slater HM, Johnson AL, Sekelj P: The oximeter: A technical aid for the anesthesiologist. Anesthesiology 12:541, 1951

55. Severinghaus JW, Astrup PB: History of blood gas analysis: Pulse oximetry. J Clin Monitoring 3:135, 1987

56. Pologe J: Pulse oximetry: Technical aspects of machine design. Int Anesthesiol Clin 25:137, 1987

57. Barker SJ, Tremper KK: The effect of carbon monoxide inhalation on pulse oximetry and transcutaneous PO_2. Anesthesiology 66:667, 1987

58. Scheller MS, Unger RJ, Kelner MJ: Effects of intravenously administered dyes on pulse oximeter readings. Anesthesiology 65:550, 1986

59. Kessler MR, Eide T, Humayun B, Poppers PJ: Spurious pulse oximeter desaturation with methylene blue injection. Anesthesiology 65:435, 1986

60. Severinghaus JW, Naifeh KH: Accuracy of response of six pulse oximeters to profound hypoxia. Anesthesiology 67:551, 1986

61. Severinghaus JW, Bradley AF: Electrodes for blood PO_2 and PCO_2 determination. J Appl Physiol 13:515, 1958

62. Severinghaus JW: A combined transcutaneous PO_2–PCO_2 electrode with electrochemical HCO_3 stabilization. J Appl Physiol 51:1027, 1981

63. Gravenstein JS, Paulus DA, Hayes TJ: Capnography in Clinical Practice. Boston, Butterworths, 1989

64. Feynman RP, Leighton RB, Sands M: The Feynman Lectures on Physics. Reading, Mass, Addison-Wesley, 1966

65. Faraday M: Experimental Researches in Electricity. New York, Dover, 1966

66. Priestley J: The History and Present State of Electricity. New York, Johnson Reprint, 1966

67. Thompson JJ: Electricity and Matter. New York: Charles Scribner's Sons, 1904

68. Maxwell JC: A Treatise on Electricity and Magnetism. London, Oxford University Press, 1955

69. Meyer HW: A History of Electricity and Magnetism. Norwalk, Conn, Burndy Library, 1972

70. Benjamin P: A History of Electricity. New York, Arno Press, 1975

71. Bordeaux S: Volts to Hertz: The Rise of Electricity. Minneapolis, Burgess Publishing, 1982

72. Sears FW: Electricity and Magnetism. Reading, Mass, Addison-Wesley, 1958

73. Bleaney BI, Bleaney B: Electricity and Magnetism. London, Oxford University Press, 1976

74. Lorrain P, Carson DR: Electromagnetic Fields and Waves. San Francisco, WH Freeman, 1970

75. Rojansky V: Electromagnetic Fields and Waves. Englewood Cliffs, NJ, Prentice-Hall, 1971

76. Kip AF: Fundamentals of Electricity and Magnetism. New York, McGraw-Hill, 1968

77. Jackson JD: Classical Electrodynamics. New York, John Wiley and Sons, 1962

78. Halliday D, Resnick R: Physics, part II. New York, John Wiley and Sons, 1962

79. Bruner JMR: Hazards of electrical apparatus. Anesthesiology 28:396, 1967

80. Bruner JMR: Common abuses and failures of electrical equipment. Anesth Analg 51(5):810, 1972

81. Ward CS: On electrical safety. Anaesthesia 35(9):921, 1980

82. Titel JH, El Etr AA: Fibrillation resulting from pacemaker electrodes and electrocautery during surgery. Anesthesiology 29:845, 1968

83. Prasad KN: Human Radiation Biology. Hagerstown, MD, Harper and Row, 1974

84. Whalen JP, Balter S: Radiation Risks in Medical Imaging. Chicago, Year Book Medical Publishers, 1984

85. Noz ME, Maguire GQ: Radiation Protection in the Radiologic and Health Sciences. Philadelphia, Lea and Febiger, 1985

86. Meredith WJ, Massey JB: Fundamental Physics of Radiology. Chicago, Year Book Medical Publishers, 1977

87. Feldman KL (ed): Radiological quality of the environment in the United States, 1977. EPA 520/1–77–009. Washington, DC, US Environmental Protection Agency, Office of Radiation Programs

8

Jan Ehrenwerth

Electrical Safety

The myriad electrical and electronic devices in the modern operating room greatly improve patient care and safety. However, these devices also subject both the patient and the operating room personnel to risks. To combat this problem, these systems include specific safety features designed to reduce the risk of electrical shock. Nevertheless, it is incumbent on the anesthesiologist to have a thorough understanding of the basic principles of electricity and an appreciation of the concepts of electrical safety applicable to the operating room environment.

PRINCIPLES OF ELECTRICITY

A basic principle of electricity known as Ohm's law is represented by the equation

$$E = I \times R$$

where E = electromotive force (volts), I = current (amperes), and R = resistance (ohms). Ohm's law has been used as the basis for the physiologic equation where the blood pressure is equal to the cardiac output times the total peripheral resistance (BP = CO $\times$ TPR). In this case, the blood pressure in the vascular system is analogous to voltage, the cardiac output to current, and the peripheral resistance to the forces opposing the flow of electrons.

Electrical power is measured in units called *watts*. A watt is equal to the product of the voltage and the amperage and is defined by the formula

$$W = E \times I$$

The amount of electrical work done is measured in watts per unit of time. The watt-second (a joule, J) is a common designation for electrical energy expended in doing work. The energy produced by a defibrillator is measured in watt-seconds (or joules), and the kilowatt-hour is frequently used to measure very large quantities of electrical energy.

Wattage can be thought of not only as a measure of work done, but also as heat produced in any electrical circuit. Substituting Ohm's law in the formula

$$W = EI$$

yields

$$W = IR \times I \qquad \text{or} \qquad W = I^2R$$

Thus, wattage is equal to the square of the amperage times the resistance. Using these formulas, it is possible to calculate the number of amperes and the resistance of a given device if the wattage and the voltage are known. For example, a 60-watt light bulb operating on a household 120-volt circuit would require 0.5 ampere of current for operation. Rearranging the formula so that

$$I = W/E$$

we have

$$I = \frac{60 \text{ watts}}{120 \text{ volts}}$$

$$I = 0.5 \text{ ampere}$$

Using this in Ohm's law ($R = E/I$), the resistance can be calculated to be 240 ohms (Ω):

$$R = \frac{120 \text{ volts}}{0.5 \text{ ampere}}$$

$$R = 240 \text{ ohms}$$

It is obvious from the previous discussion that 1 volt of electromotive force flowing through a 1-ohm resistance will generate 1 ampere of current. Similarly, 1 ampere of current induced by 1 volt of electromotive force (EMF) will generate 1 watt of power.

Direct and Alternating Currents

Any substance that permits the flow of electrons is considered to be a conductor. Current is characterized by electrons flowing through a conductor. If the electron flow is always in the same direction, it is referred to as direct current (DC). If the electron flow reverses direction at a regular interval, it is termed alternating current (AC). Either of these types of current can be pulsed or continuous.[1]

The previous discussion of Ohm's law is accurate when applied to DC circuits. However, when dealing with AC circuits, the situation is more complex because the flow of the current is opposed by a more complicated form of resistance known as *impedance*.

Impedance

Impedance is defined as the sum of the forces that oppose electron movement in AC circuits and is designated by the letter Z. Impedance consists of resistance (ohms) but also takes into account capacitance as well as inductance. In actuality, when referring to AC circuits, Ohm's law is defined as

$$E = I \times Z$$

An insulator is a substance that opposes the flow of electrons and therefore has a high impedance to flow, whereas a conductor has a low impedance to electron flow.

In AC circuits, the capacitance and inductance can be important factors in determining the total impedance. Both capacitance and inductance are influenced by the frequency (cycles per second or Hertz, Hz) that the AC current reverses direction. The impedance is directly proportional to the frequency (f) times the inductance (IND):

$$Z \propto (f \times \text{IND})$$

and the impedance is inversely proportional to the product of the frequency (f) and the capacitance (CAP):

$$Z \propto \frac{1}{f \times \text{CAP}}$$

As the AC current increases in frequency, the net effect of both capacitance and inductance will increase. However, because impedance and capacitance are inversely related, total impedance will decrease as the product of the frequency and the capacitance increases. Thus, as frequency increases, impedance will fall, and more current will be allowed to pass.[2]

Capacitance

A capacitor consists of any two parallel conductors that are separated by an insulator (Fig. 8-1). A capacitor has the ability to store charge, and capacitance is the measure of that substance's ability to store charge. In a DC circuit, the capacitor plates are charged by a voltage source (i.e., a battery), and there is only a momentary current flow. The circuit is not completed, and there can be no further current flow unless a resistance is connected between the two plates and the capacitor is discharged.[3]

In contrast to DC circuits, a capacitor in AC circuits permits current flow even when there is no completed circuit. This is attributable to the nature of AC circuits, in which the current flow is constantly reversing itself. Because current flow results from the movement of electrons, the capacitor plates are alternately charged, first positive and then negative, with every reversal of the AC current direction. The consequence of this is an effective current flow as far as the remainder of the circuit is concerned, even though the circuit is not completed.[4]

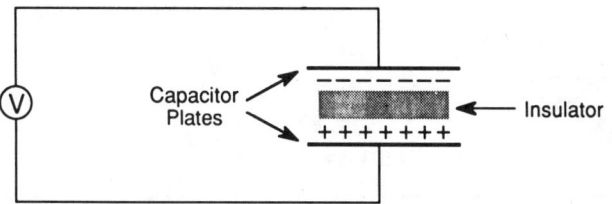

Figure 8-1. A capacitor consists of two parallel conductors separated by an insulator. The capacitor is capable of storing charge supplied by a voltage source.

Because the effect of capacitance on impedance varies directly with the AC frequency (Hz), the greater the AC frequency, the lower the impedance. Therefore, high-frequency currents (0.5–2 million Hz), such as those seen with electrosurgical units, will cause a marked decrease in impedance. As an example, a 20-million-ohm impedance in a 60-Hz AC circuit will be reduced to only a few hundred–ohm impedance when the frequency is increased to 1 million Hz.[5]

Electrical devices use capacitors for various beneficial purposes. There is, however, a phenomenon known as *stray capacitance*, which is defined as capacitance that was not designed into the system but is incidental to the construction of the equipment.[6] All AC-operated equipment produces stray capacitance. An ordinary power cord, for example, consisting of two insulated wires running next to each other, will generate significant capacitance simply by being plugged into a 120-volt circuit, even though the piece of equipment is not turned on. Another example of stray capacitance is found in electric motors. The circuit wiring in electric motors generates stray capacitance to the metal housing of the motor.[7] The clinical importance of capacitance is emphasized later in the chapter.

Inductance

Whenever electrons flow in a wire, a magnetic field is induced around the wire. If the wire is coiled repeatedly around an iron core, as in a transformer, the magnetic field can be very strong. Inductance is a property of AC circuits in which an opposing EMF can be generated electromagnetically in the circuit. The net effect of inductance is to increase impedance. Because the effect of inductance on impedance is also dependent on the AC frequency, increases in frequency will increase the total impedance. Therefore, the total impedance of a coil will be much greater than its simple resistance.[4]

Shock Hazards

Alternating and Direct Currents

Whenever an individual contacts an external source of electricity, an electrical shock is possible. An electrical current can stimulate skeletal muscle cells and thus can be used therapeutically in devices such as pacemakers or defibrillators. However, casual contact with an electrical current, whether AC or DC, can lead to injury or death. Although it takes approximately three times as much direct current as alternating current to cause ventricular fibrillation,[3] this by no means renders direct current harmless. Devices such as

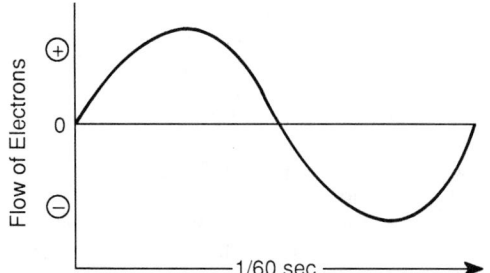

Figure 8-2. Sine wave flow of electrons in a 60-Hz alternating current.

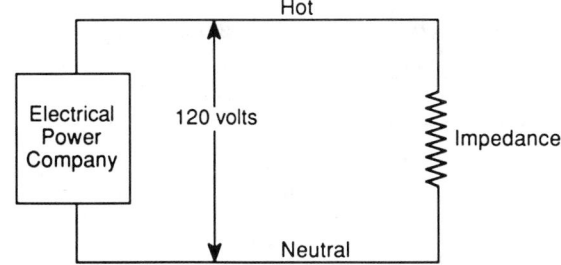

Figure 8-3. A typical AC circuit where there is a potential difference of 120 volts between the hot and neutral sides of the circuit. The current flows through a resistance, which in AC circuits is more accurately referred to as *impedance,* and then returns to the electrical power company.

an automobile battery or a DC defibrillator can be sources of DC shocks.

In the United States, utility companies supply electrical energy in the form of alternating currents of 120 volts at a frequency of 60 Hz.* (The 60 Hz refers to the number of times in 1 second that the current reverses its direction of flow.[8]) Both the voltage and the current waveforms form a sinusoidal pattern (Fig. 8-2).

In order to have the completed circuit necessary for current flow, a closed loop must exist, and there must be a voltage source to drive the current through the impedance. If current is to flow in the electrical circuit, there has to be a voltage differential or a drop in the driving pressure across the impedance. According to Ohm's law, if the resistance is held constant, then the greater the current flow, the larger the voltage drop must be.[9]

The power company attempts to maintain the line voltage constant at 120 volts. Therefore, by Ohm's law, the current flow is inversely proportional to the impedance. A typical power cord consists of two conductors. One, designated the "hot," carries the current to the resistance; the other, the "neutral," returns the current to the source. The potential between the two is effectively 120 volts (Fig. 8-3). The amount of current used by a given device is frequently referred to as the *load.* The load of the circuit is dependent on the impedance. A very high-impedance circuit allows only a small current flow and thus will have a small load. A very low-impedance circuit will draw a large current and is said to be a large load. A *short circuit* occurs when there is a zero impedance load with a very high current flow.[10]

Source of Shocks

In order to practice electrical safety, it is important for the anesthesiologist to understand the basic principles of electricity and to be aware of how electrical accidents can occur. Electrical accidents or shocks occur when a person becomes part of or completes an electrical circuit. Thus, in order to receive a shock, one must contact the electrical circuit at two points, and there must be a voltage source to drive the current (Fig. 8-4).

When an individual contacts a source of electricity, it can cause damage in two ways. First, the electrical current can disrupt the normal electrical function of cells. Depending

on its magnitude, the current can contract muscles, alter brain function, paralyze breathing, or disrupt normal heart function, leading to ventricular fibrillation. The second mechanism involves the dissipation of electrical energy throughout the body's tissues. An electrical current passing through any resistance raises the temperature of that substance. If enough energy is released, the temperature will rise sufficiently to cause a burn. Accidents involving household currents usually do not result in severe burns. On the other hand, in accidents involving very high voltages (*i.e.,* power transmission lines), severe burns are common.

Because current is the flow of electrical charges per unit of time, it is the amount of current (number of amperes) with which an individual comes in contact that determines the severity of the shock. For the purposes of this discussion, electrical shocks are divided into two categories. *Macroshock* refers to gross amounts of current coming into contact with a person that can cause harm or death. *Microshock* applies only to the electrically susceptible patient who has an external conduit that is in direct contact with the heart. This can be a pacing wire or a saline-filled catheter such as a central venous or pulmonary artery catheter. In the case

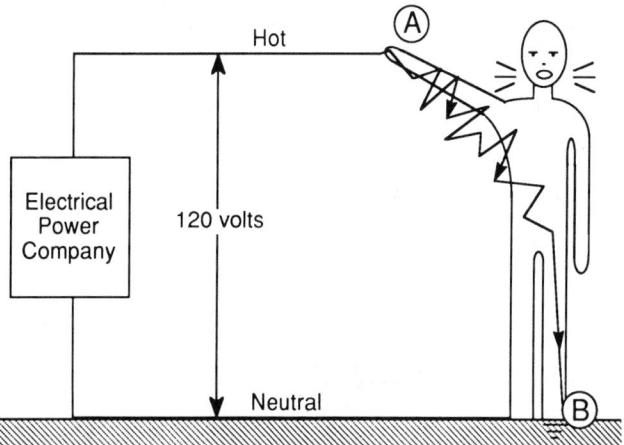

Figure 8-4. An individual can complete an electric circuit and receive a shock by coming in contact with the hot side of the circuit (Point A). This is because he or she is standing on the ground (Point B) and the contact point A and the ground point B provide the two contact points necessary for a completed circuit. The severity of the shock the individual receives is dependent on his or her skin resistance.

---

*The 120 volts of EMF and 1 ampere of current are the effective voltage and amperage in an AC circuit. This is also referred to as RMS, which stands for "root-mean-square." In fact, it takes 1.414 amperes of peak amperage in the sinusoidal curve to give an effective amperage of 1 ampere. Similarly, it takes 170 volts (120 × 1.414) at the peak of the AC curve to get an effective voltage of 120 volts.[8]

TABLE 8-1. Effects of a 60-Hz Current on an Average Human for a 1-Second Contact

Current*	Effect
Macroshock	
1 mA (0.001A)	Threshold of perception
5 mA (0.005A)	Accepted as maximum harmless current intensity
10–20 mA (0.01–0.02A)	"Let-go" current before sustained muscle contraction
50 mA (0.05A)	Pain, possible fainting, mechanical injury; heart and respiratory functions continue
100–300 mA (0.1–0.3A)	Ventricular fibrillation will start, but respiratory center remains intact
6000 mA (6A)	Sustained myocardial contraction, followed by normal heart rhythm; temporary respiratory paralysis; burns if current density is high
Microshock	
100 μA (0.1 mA)	Ventricular fibrillation
10 μA (0.01 mA)	Recommended maximum 60-Hz leakage current

*A = amperes; mA = milliamperes; μA = microamperes.

of the electrically susceptible patient, even minute amounts of current may cause ventricular fibrillation.

Table 8-1 shows the effects typically produced by various currents after a 1-second contact with a 60-Hz current. When an individual contacts a 120-volt household current, the severity of the shock will depend on his or her skin resistance, the duration of the contact, and the current density. Skin resistance can range from a few thousand to more than a million ohms. If a person with a skin resistance of 1000 ohms contacts a 120-volt circuit, he or she would receive 120 mA of current, which would probably be lethal. However, if that same person's skin resistance was 100,000 ohms, the current flow would be 1.2 mA, which would hardly be perceptible:

$$I = \frac{E}{R} = \frac{120 \text{ volts}}{1000 \text{ ohms}} = 120 \text{ mA}$$

$$\frac{120 \text{ volts}}{100,000 \text{ ohms}} = 1.2 \text{ mA}$$

The longer an individual is in contact with the electrical source, the more dire the consequences, because more energy will be released and more tissue damaged. Also, there will be a greater chance of ventricular fibrillation from excitation of the heart during the vulnerable period of the ECG cycle.

Current density is merely a way of expressing the amount of current that is applied per area of tissue. The diffusion of current in the body tends to be in all directions. The higher the current or the smaller the area to which it is applied, the higher the current density. In relation to the heart, a current of 100 mA (100,000 μA) is generally required to produce ventricular fibrillation when applied to the surface of the body. However, a current of only 100 μA (0.1 mA) is required to produce ventricular fibrillation when that minute current is applied directly to the myocardium through an instrument having a very small area, such as a pacing wire electrode. In this case, the current density is 1000-fold higher when applied directly to the heart and therefore requires only $^{1}/_{1000}$ as much energy to cause ventricular fibrillation. Therefore, the electrically susceptible patient can be electrocuted with currents well below 1 mA, which is the threshold of perception for humans.

The frequency at which the current reverses itself is also an important factor in determining the amount of current with which an individual can safely come into contact. Utility companies in the United States produce electricity at a frequency of 60 Hz because higher frequencies cause greater power loss through transmission lines, and lower frequencies cause a detectable flicker from light sources.[11] The "let-go" current is defined as that current above which sustained muscular contraction occurs so that an individual would be unable to let go of an energized wire. The let-go current for 60-Hz AC power is 10–20 mA,[10,12,13] whereas at a frequency of 1 million Hz, a current of up to 3 amperes (3000 mA) is generally regarded as safe.[3] It should be noted that very high-frequency currents do not excite contractile tissue; consequently, they do not cause cardiac dysrhythmias.

Therefore, it can be seen that for a completed circuit to exist, there must be a closed loop with a driving pressure to force a current through a resistance in accordance with Ohm's law, just as in the cardiovascular system there must be blood pressure to drive the cardiac output through the peripheral resistance. Figure 8-5 illustrates that a hot wire carrying a 120-volt pressure through the resistance of a 60-watt light bulb produces a current flow of 0.5 ampere. The voltage in the neutral wire is approximately 0, while the current in the neutral wire remains at 0.5 ampere. This correlates with our cardiovascular model, where a mean blood pressure drop of 80 mm Hg from the aortic root to the

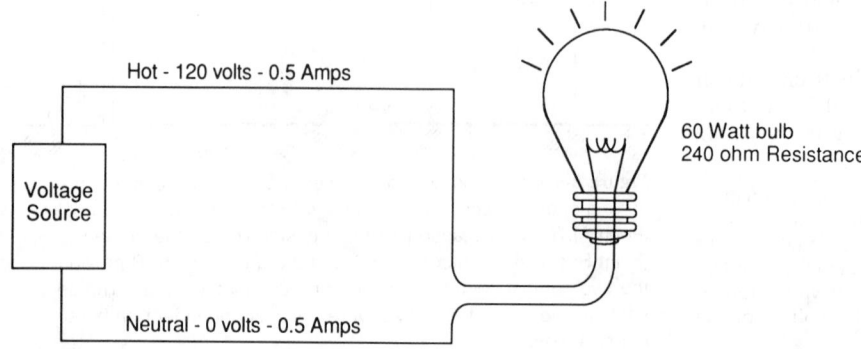

Hot - 120 volts - 0.5 Amps

Voltage Source

60 Watt bulb
240 ohm Resistance

Neutral - 0 volts - 0.5 Amps

Figure 8-5. A 60-watt light bulb has an internal resistance of 240 ohms and draws 0.5 ampere of current. The voltage drop in the circuit is from 120 in the hot wire to 0 in the neutral wire, but the current is 0.5 ampere in both the hot and the neutral wires.

right atrium forces a cardiac output of 6 l·min⁻¹ through a resistance of 13.3 peripheral resistance units. However, the flow (in this case, the cardiac output, or in the case of the electrical model, the current) is still the same everywhere in the circuit. That is, the cardiac output on the arterial side is the same as the cardiac output on the venous side.

GROUNDING

In order to understand electrical shock hazards and their prevention fully, one must have a thorough knowledge of the concepts of grounding. These concepts probably constitute the most confusing aspects of electrical safety, because the same term is used to describe several different principles. In electrical terminology, "grounding" is applied to two separate concepts: the grounding of electrical *power*, and the grounding of electrical *equipment*. Thus, the concepts that power can be grounded or ungrounded and it may supply electrical devices that are themselves grounded or ungrounded are not mutually exclusive. It is vital to understand this point as the basis of electrical safety (Table 8-2). While electrical *power* is grounded in the home, it is ungrounded in the operating room. In the home, electrical *equipment* may be grounded or ungrounded, but it should always be grounded in the operating room.

Electrical Power—Grounded

Electrical utilities universally provide power that is grounded (by convention, the earth ground potential is zero, and all voltages represent a difference between potentials). That is, one of the wires supplying the power to a home is intentionally connected to the earth. The utility companies do this as a safety measure to prevent electrical charges from building up in their wiring during electrical storms and to prevent the very high voltages used in transmitting power by the utility from entering the home in the event of an equipment failure in their high-voltage system.[3]

The power enters the typical home in the form of two wires that are attached to the main fuse or circuit breaker box at the service entrance. The "hot" wire supplies power to the "hot" distribution strip. The neutral wire is connected to the neutral distribution strip and to a service entrance ground (*i.e.*, a pipe buried in the earth) (Fig. 8-6).

TABLE 8-2. Differences Between Power and Equipment Grounding in the Home and the Operating Room*

	Power	Equipment
Home	+	±
Operating room	−	+

* + = grounded, − = ungrounded, ± = may or may not be grounded.

From the fuse box, three wires leave to supply the electrical outlets in the house. The "hot" wire is color-coded black and carries a voltage 120 volts above ground potential. The second wire is the neutral or white wire; the third wire is the ground wire, which is the green or bare wire. The ground and the neutral wires are attached at the same point in the circuit breaker box and then further connected to a cold water pipe (Figs. 8-7 and 8-8). Thus, this grounded power system is also referred to as a "neutral grounded power system." The black wire is not connected to the ground, as this would create a short circuit. Rather, it is attached to the "hot" (*i.e.*, 120 volts above ground) distribution strip on which the circuit breakers or fuses are located. From here, numerous branch circuits supply electrical power to the house. Each branch circuit is protected by a circuit breaker or fuse, which limits current to a specific maximum amperage. Most electrical circuits in the house are 15- or 20-ampere circuits. These typically supply power to the electrical outlets and lights in the house. Several higher-amperage circuits are also provided for devices such as an electric stove or an electric clothes dryer, which can draw from 30 to 50 amperes of current. The circuit breaker will interrupt the flow of current on the hot side of the line in the event of a short circuit or if the demand placed on that circuit is too high. For example, a 15-ampere branch circuit will be capable of supporting 1800 watts of power:

$$W = EI$$
$$W = 120 \text{ volts} \times 15 \text{ amperes}$$
$$W = 1800 \text{ watts}$$

Therefore, if two 1500-watt hair dryers were simultaneously plugged into one outlet, the load would be too great for a

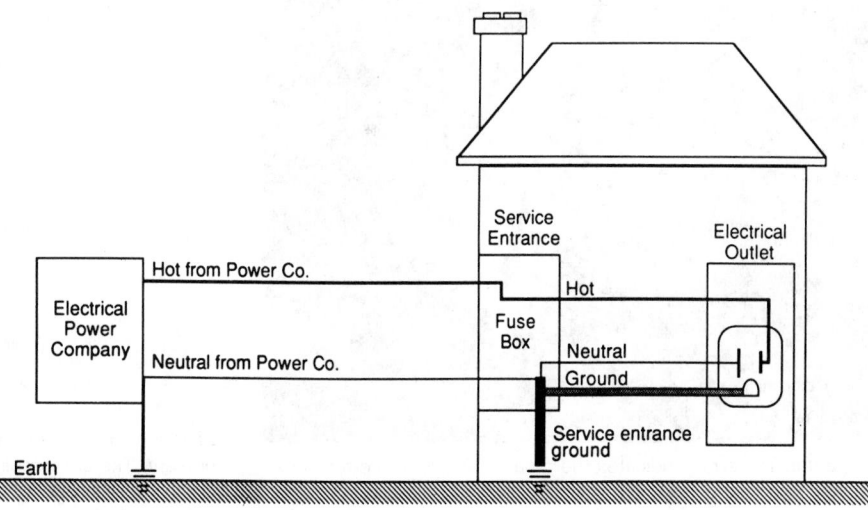

Figure 8-6. In a neutral grounded power system, the electrical company supplies two lines to the typical home. The neutral is connected to ground by the power company and is again connected to a service entrance ground when it enters the fuse box. Both the neutral and the ground wires are connected together in the fuse box at the neutral bus bar, which is also attached to the service entrance ground.

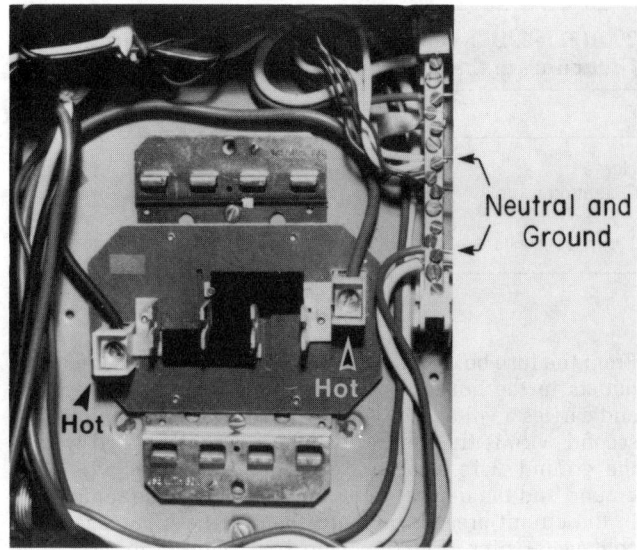

Figure 8-7. Inside a fuse box with the circuit breakers removed. The *arrowheads* indicate the hot wires energizing the strips where the circuit breakers are located. The *arrows* point to the neutral bus bar, where the neutral and ground wires are connected.

15-ampere circuit, and the circuit breaker would open or the fuse would melt. This is done to prevent the supply wires from melting and starting a fire. The amperage of the circuit breaker on the branch circuit is determined by the thickness of the wire that it supplies. If a 20-ampere breaker is used with wire rated for only 15 amperes, the wire could melt and start a fire before the circuit breaker would trip. It is important to note that a 15-ampere circuit breaker does not protect an individual from lethal shocks. The 15 amperes of current that will open the circuit breaker far exceed the 100–200 mA that will produce ventricular fibrillation.

The wires that leave the circuit breaker supply the electrical outlets and lighting for the rest of the house. In older homes, the electrical cable consists of two wires, a hot and a neutral, which supply power to the electrical outlets (Fig. 8-9). In newer homes, a third wire has been added to the electrical cable (Fig. 8-10). This third wire is either green or bare and serves as a ground wire for the power receptacle (Fig. 8-11). On one end, the ground wire is attached to the

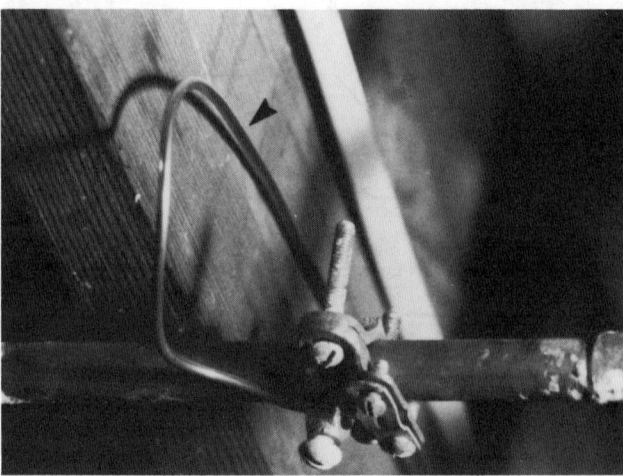

Figure 8-8. The *arrow* indicates the ground wire from the fuse box attached to a cold water pipe.

Figure 8-9. An older style electrical outlet consisting of only two wires (a hot and a neutral). There is no ground wire.

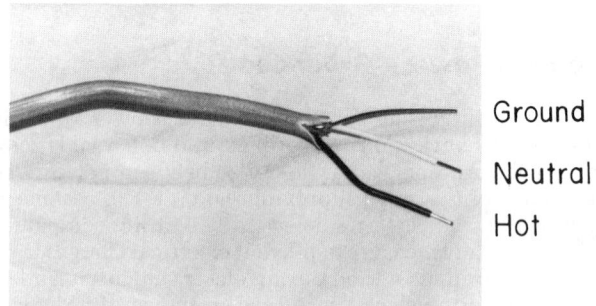

Figure 8-10. Modern electrical cable in which a third or ground wire has been added.

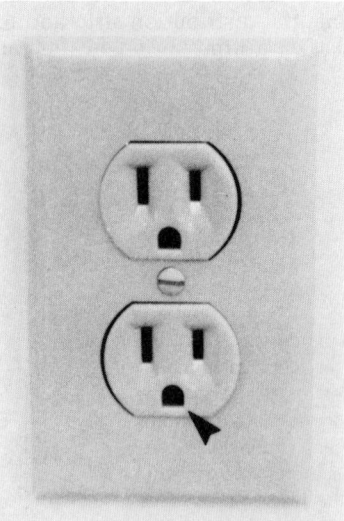

Figure 8-11. Modern electrical outlet in which a ground wire is present. The *arrow* points to the part of the receptacle where the ground wire connects.

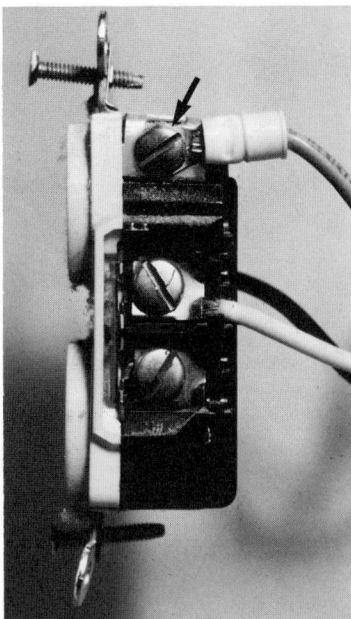

Figure 8-12. Detail of modern electrical power receptacle. The *arrow* points to the ground wire, which is attached to the grounding screw on the power receptacle.

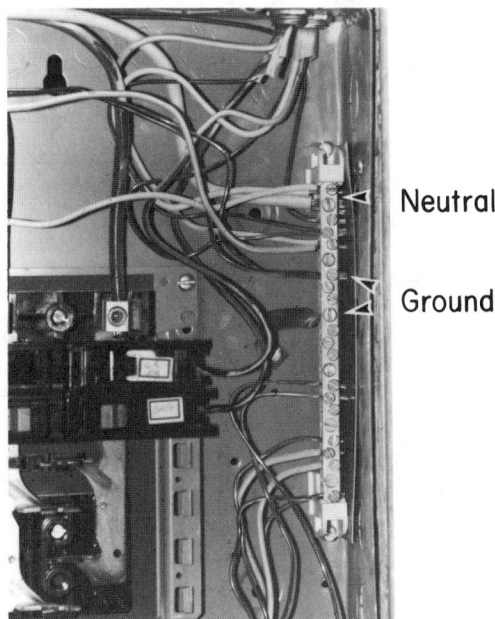

Figure 8-13. The ground wires from the power outlet are run to the neutral bus bar, where they are connected with the neutral wires (*arrowheads*).

electrical outlet (Fig. 8-12); on the other, it is connected to the neutral distribution strip in the circuit breaker box along with the white or neutral wires (Fig. 8-13).

It should be realized that in both the old and the new situations, the power is grounded; that is, a 120-volt potential exists between the black and the white wire and between the black wire and ground. In this case, the ground is the earth (Fig. 8-14). In modern home construction, there is still a 120-volt potential difference between the black and the white wire, as well as between the black wire and the equipment ground wire, which is the third wire, and between the black wire and the earth (Fig. 8-15).

A 60-watt light bulb can be used as an example to further demonstrate this point. Normally, the black and white wires are connected to the two wires of the light bulb socket, and throwing the switch will illuminate the bulb (Fig. 8-16).

Similarly, if the black wire is connected to one side of the bulb socket and the other wire from the light bulb is connected to the equipment ground wire, the bulb will still illuminate. If there is no equipment ground wire, the bulb will still light if the second wire is connected to any grounded metallic object such as a water pipe or a faucet. This illustrates the fact that the 120-volt potential difference exists, not only between the hot and the neutral wire, but also between the hot wire and any grounded object. Thus, in a grounded power system, the current will flow between the black wire and any conductor with an earth ground.

As previously stated, current flow requires a closed loop with a source of voltage. For an individual to get an electric shock, he or she must contact the loop at two points. Since we may be standing on ground or be in contact with an object that is referenced to ground, only *one* additional con-

Figure 8-14. Diagram of a house with older style wiring that does not contain a ground wire. A 120-volt potential difference exists between the hot and the neutral wire, as well as between the hot wire and the earth.

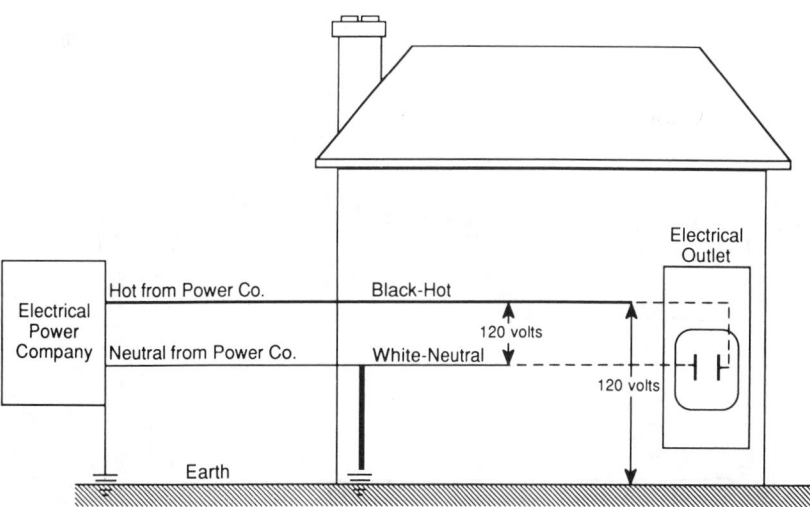

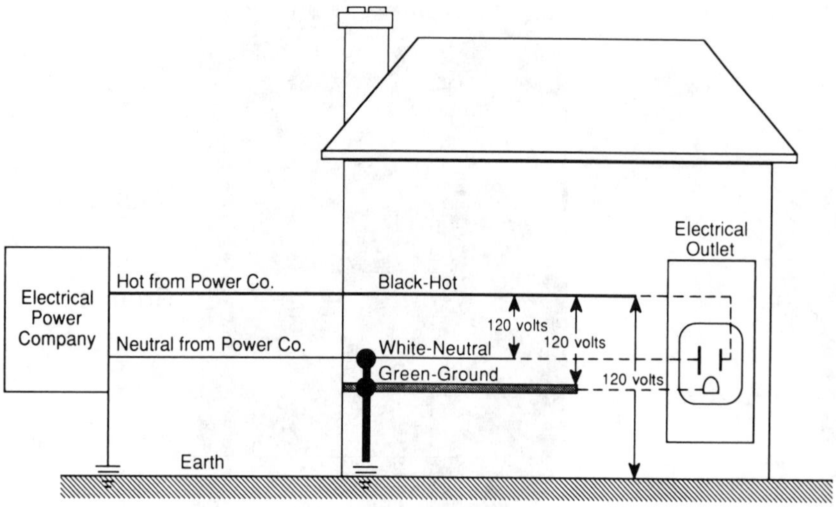

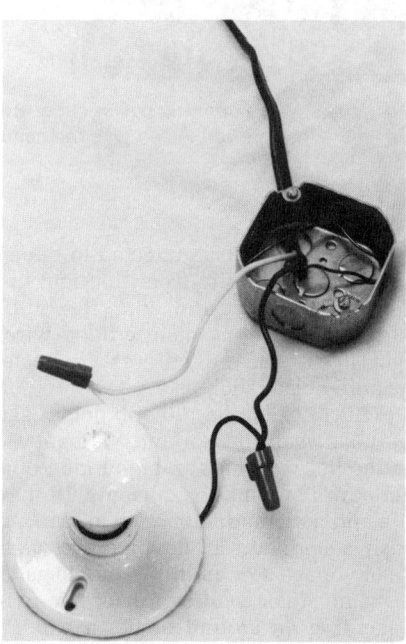

Figure 8-15. Diagram of a house with modern wiring in which the third or ground wire has been added. The 120-volt potential difference exists between the hot and neutral wires, the hot and the ground wires, and the hot wire and the earth.

tact point is necessary to complete the circuit and thus receive an electrical shock. An unfortunate and inherently dangerous consequence of grounded power systems is that an individual can receive an electric shock with only one additional contact point. Modern wiring systems have added the third wire, the equipment ground wire, as a safety measure to reduce the severity of a potential electrical shock. This is accomplished by providing an alternate low-resistance pathway through which the current can flow.

Over time, the insulation covering wires may deteriorate. It is then possible for a bare, hot wire to contact the metal case or frame of an electrical device. The case would then become energized and constitute a shock hazard to someone coming in contact with it. Figure 8-17 illustrates a typical short circuit, where the individual has come in contact with the hot case of an instrument. This picture illustrates the type of wiring found in older homes. There is no equipment ground wire, nor is the electrical apparatus equipped with a ground wire. Here, the individual completes the circuit and receives a severe shock. Figure 8-18 illustrates a similar example, except that now the equipment ground wire is part of the electrical distribution system. In this example, the equipment ground wire provides a pathway of low impedance through which the current can travel. Therefore, the majority of the current would travel through the ground wire, and, although the person may get a shock, it is not likely to be fatal.

Figure 8-16. A simple light bulb circuit in which the hot and neutral wires are connected with the corresponding wires from the light bulb fixture.

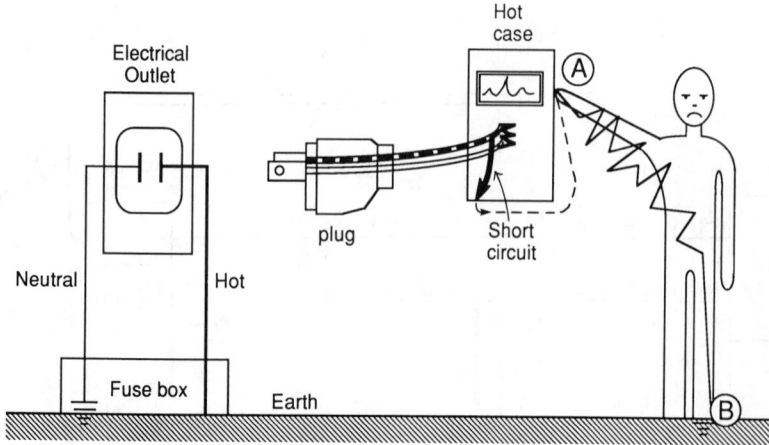

Figure 8-17. When a faulty piece of equipment without an equipment ground wire is plugged into an electrical outlet not containing a ground wire, the case of the instrument will become hot. If an individual touches the hot case (Point A) he will receive a shock, because he is standing on the earth (Point B) and completes the circuit. The current (*dashed line*) will flow from the instrument through the individual touching the hot case.

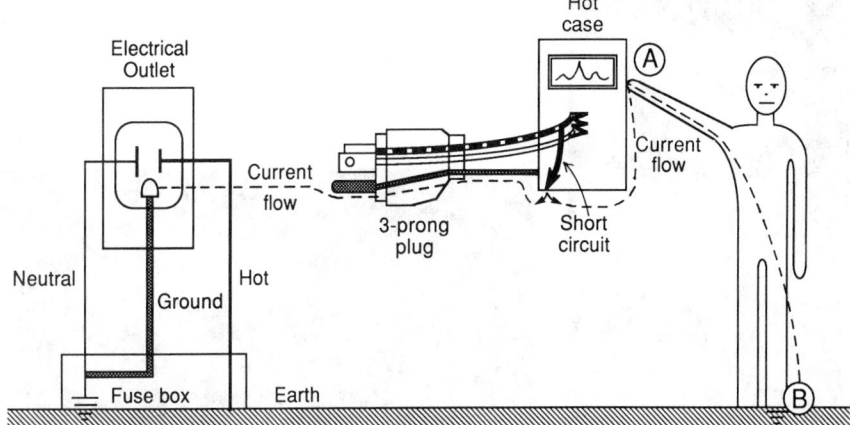

Figure 8-18. When a faulty piece of equipment containing an equipment ground wire is properly connected to an electrical outlet with a grounding connection, the current (*dashed line*) will preferentially flow down the low-resistance ground wire. An individual touching the case (Point A) and standing on the ground (Point B) will still complete the circuit; however, only a small part of the current will go through the individual.

The electrical power supplied to homes is always grounded. A 120-volt potential always exists between the hot conductor and the ground or earth. The third, or equipment ground, wire used in modern electrical wiring systems does not normally carry current. In the event of a short circuit, an electrical device with a three-prong plug (i.e., a ground wire connected to its case) will conduct the majority of the short-circuited or fault current through the ground wire and away from the individual. This provides a significant safety benefit to someone accidentally contacting the defective device. If a large enough fault current exists, the ground wire also will provide a means to complete the short circuit back to the circuit breaker or fuse, and this will either melt the fuse or trip the circuit breaker. Thus, in a grounded power system, it is possible to have either grounded or ungrounded equipment, depending on the age of the wiring and whether the electrical device is equipped with a three-prong plug containing a ground wire. Obviously, attempts to bypass the safety system of the equipment ground should be avoided. Devices such as a "cheater plug" (Fig. 8-19) should never be used, because they defeat the safety feature of the equipment ground wire.

Electrical Power—Ungrounded

The numerous electronic devices, along with power cords and puddles of saline-filled solutions on the floor in the operating room, tend to make it an electrically hazardous environment for both patients and personnel. Bruner and colleagues[14] found that 40% of electrical accidents in hospitals occurred in the operating room. The complexity of the electronic equipment in the modern operating room demands that electrical safety be a factor of paramount importance. In order to provide an extra measure of safety from gross electrical shock (macroshock), the power supplied to most operating rooms is ungrounded. In this ungrounded power system, the current is isolated from ground potential. The 120-volt potential exists only between the two wires of the isolated power system, but no circuit exists between the ground and either of the isolated power lines.

Supplying ungrounded power to the operating room requires the use of an isolation transformer (Fig. 8-20). This device uses electromagnetic induction to induce a current in the ungrounded or secondary winding of the transformer using energy supplied to the primary winding. There is no direct electrical connection between the power supplied by

the utility company on the primary side and the power induced by the transformer on the ungrounded or secondary side. Thus, the power supplied to the operating room is isolated from ground (Fig. 8-21). Because the 120-volt potential exists only between the two wires of the isolated circuit, neither wire is hot or neutral with reference to ground. In this case, they are simply referred to as line 1 and line 2 (Fig. 8-22). Using the example of the light bulb, if we connect both wires of the bulb socket to the two wires of the isolated power system, the bulb will illuminate. However, if we connect one of the wires to one side of the isolated power and the other wire to ground, the bulb will not illuminate. If the wires of the isolated power system are shorted together, it will trip the circuit breaker. In comparing the two systems, the standard grounded power has a direct connection to ground, whereas the isolated system

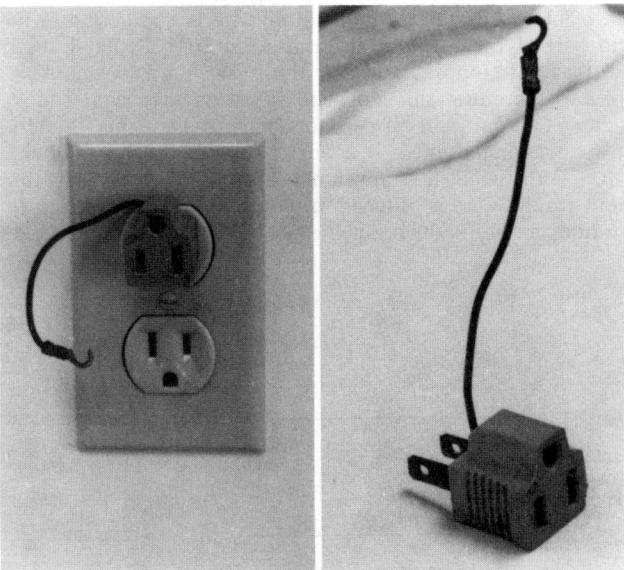

Figure 8-19. The right side of the figure illustrates a "cheater plug" that converts a three-prong power cord to a two-prong cord. The left side of the picture illustrates that the wire attached to the cheater plug is rarely connected to the screw in the middle of the outlet. This totally defeats the purpose of the equipment ground wire.

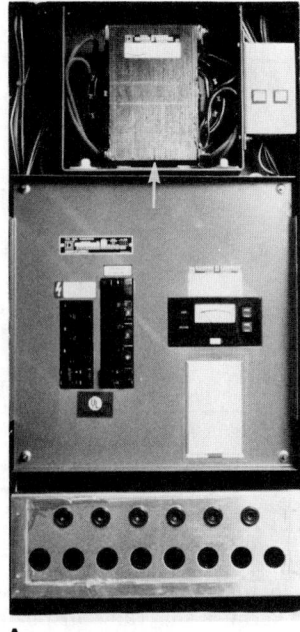
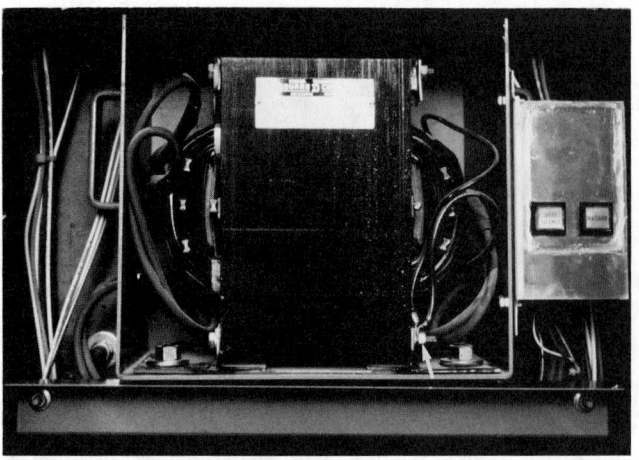

A   **B**

Figure 8-20. (*A*) Isolated power panel showing circuit breakers, LIM, and isolation transformer (*arrow*). (*B*) Detail of an isolation transformer with the attached warning lights. The *arrow* points to the ground wire connection on the primary side of the transformer. Note that no similar connection exists on the secondary side of the transformer.

imposes a very high impedance to any current flow to ground.

The added safety of this system can be seen in Figure 8-23. In this case, a person has come in contact with one side of the isolated power system (Point A). Since standing on ground (Point B) does not constitute a part of the isolated circuit, the individual does not complete the loop and will not receive a shock. This is because the ground is part of the primary circuit (solid lines) and he is contacting only one part of the isolated secondary circuit (striped lines). He does not complete either circuit (i.e., have two contact points); therefore, this does not pose an electrical shock hazard. Of course, if he contacts both lines of the isolated power system (an unlikely event), he would receive a shock.

If a faulty electrical appliance that has an intact equipment ground wire is plugged into a standard household outlet, and the home wiring has a properly connected ground wire, then the amount of electrical current that will flow through the individual is considerably less than what will flow through the low-resistance ground wire. Here, an individual would be fairly well protected from a serious shock. However, if that ground wire is broken, the individual may receive a lethal shock. No shock would occur if the same faulty piece of equipment were plugged into the isolated power system, even if the equipment ground wire were broken. Thus, the isolated power system provides a significant amount of protection from macroshock. Another feature of the isolated power system is that the faulty piece of equipment, even though it may be partially short-circuited, will not usually trip the circuit breaker. This is an important feature, because the faulty piece of equipment may be part of a life-support system for a patient.

It is important to note that even though the power is isolated from ground, the case or frame of all electrical equip-

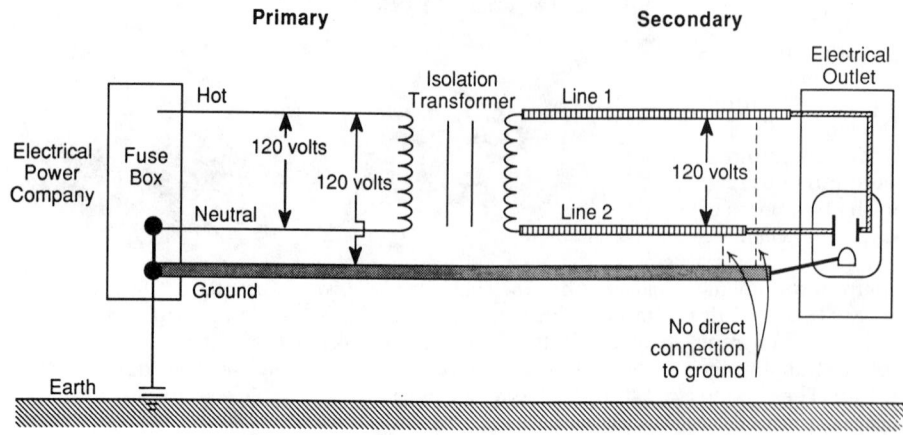

Figure 8-21. In the operating room, the isolation transformer converts the grounded power on the primary side to an ungrounded power system on the secondary side of the transformer. A 120-volt potential difference exists between line 1 and line 2. There is no direct connection from the power on the secondary side to ground. The equipment ground wire, however, is still present.

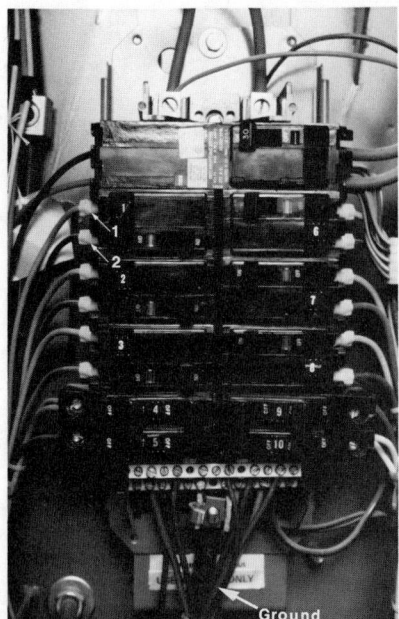

Figure 8-22. Detail of the inside of a circuit breaker box in an isolated power system. The *bottom arrow* points to ground wires meeting at the common ground terminal. *Arrows 1* and *2* indicate line 1 and line 2 from the isolated power circuit breaker. Neither line 1 nor line 2 is connected to the same terminals as the ground wires. This is in marked contrast to Figure 8-13, where the neutral and ground wires are attached at the same point.

ment is still connected to an equipment ground. The third wire (equipment ground wire) is necessary for a total electrical safety program.

Figure 8-24 illustrates a scenario involving a faulty piece of equipment connected to the isolated power system. This does not represent a hazard but merely converts the isolated power back to a grounded power system as exists outside the operating room. In fact, a *second* fault is necessary to create a hazard.

The previous discussion assumes that the isolated power system is perfectly isolated from ground. Actually, perfect isolation is impossible. All AC-operated power systems and electrical devices manifest some degree of capacitance. As previously discussed, electrical power cords, wires, and electric motors exhibit capacitive coupling to the ground

wire and metal conduits and ''leak'' small amounts of current to ground (Fig. 8-25). This so-called leakage current partially ungrounds the isolated power system. This current does not usually amount to more than a few milliamperes in an operating room, so an individual coming in contact with one side of the isolated power system would receive only a very small shock (1–2 mA). Although this amount of current would be perceptible, it would not be dangerous.

THE LINE ISOLATION MONITOR

The line isolation monitor (LIM) is a device that continuously monitors the integrity of an isolated power system. If a faulty piece of equipment is connected to the isolated power system, this will, in effect, change the system back to a conventional grounded system. Also, the faulty piece of equipment will continue to function normally. Therefore, it is essential that a warning system be in place to alert the personnel to the fact that the power is no longer ungrounded. The LIM continuously monitors the isolated power to ensure that it is indeed isolated from ground, and the device has a meter that displays a continuous indication of the integrity of the system (Fig. 8-26). As previously discussed, with perfect isolation, impedance would be infinitely high, and there would be no current flow in the event of a first-fault situation ($Z = E/I$; if $I = 0$, then $Z =$ infinity). Because all AC wiring and all AC-operated electrical devices have some capacitance, small ''leakage currents'' are present that partially degrade the system. The meter of the LIM will indicate (in milliamperes) the total amount of leakage in the system resulting from capacitance, electrical wiring, and any devices plugged into the isolated power system. (See Chapter 7.)

The reading on the LIM does *not* mean that current is actually flowing but merely indicates how much current would flow in the event of a first fault. The LIM is set to trigger an alarm at 2 or 5 mA, depending on the age and make of the system. Once this preset limit is exceeded, visual and audible alarms are triggered to indicate that the isolation from ground has been degraded beyond the predetermined limit (Fig. 8-27). This alarm does not necessarily mean that there is a hazardous situation, but rather that the system is no longer totally isolated from ground. It would in fact require a second fault to create a dangerous situation.

For example, if the LIM was set to trigger an alarm at 2 mA, using Ohm's law, the impedance for either side of the

Figure 8-23. A safety feature of the isolated power system is illustrated. An individual contacting one side of the isolated power system (Point A) and standing on the ground (Point B) will not receive a shock. In this instance, the individual is not contacting the circuit at two points and thus is not completing the circuit. Point A (*crosshatched lines*) is part of the isolated power system, and Point B is part of the primary or grounded side of the circuit (*solid lines*).

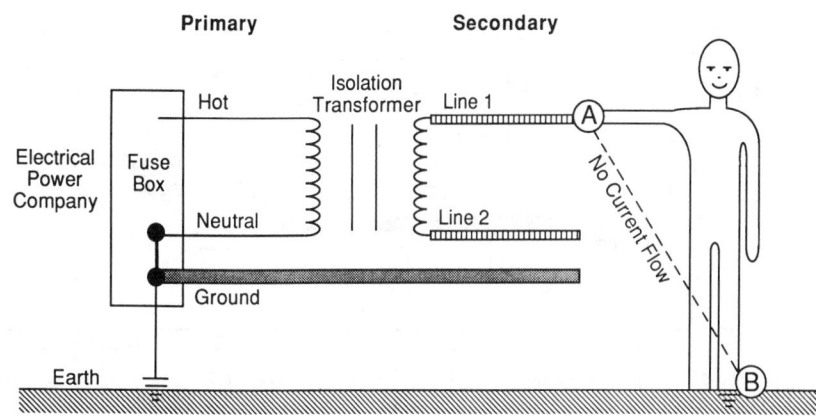

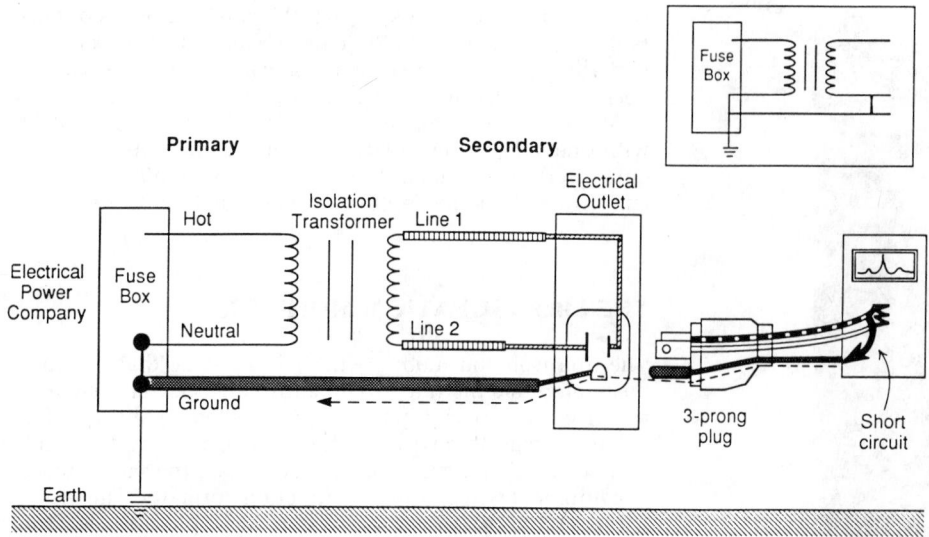

Figure 8-24. A faulty piece of equipment plugged into the isolated power system does not present a shock hazard. It merely converts the isolated power system into a grounded power system. The figure *insert* illustrates that the isolated power system is now identical to the grounded power system. The *dashed line* indicates current flow in the ground wire.

isolated power system would be 60,000 ohms:

$$Z = \frac{E}{I}$$

$$Z = \frac{120 \text{ volts}}{0.002 \text{ ampere}}$$

$$Z = 60,000 \text{ ohms}$$

Therefore, if either side of the isolated power system had less than 60,000 ohms impedance to ground, the LIM would alarm. This might occur in two situations. The first is when a faulty piece of equipment is plugged into the isolated power system. In this case, a true fault to ground exists with a short circuit of essentially zero impedance from one line to ground. Now the system would be converted to the equivalent of a grounded power system. This faulty piece of equipment should be removed and serviced as soon as possible. However, it could still be used safely if it was essential

for the care of the patient. It should be remembered that continuing to use this faulty piece of equipment would create the potential for a serious electrical shock. This would occur if a *second* faulty piece of equipment were simultaneously connected to the isolated power system.

The second situation involves connecting many perfectly normal pieces of equipment to the isolated power system. Although each piece of equipment has only a small amount of leakage current, if the total leakage exceeds 2 mA, the LIM will trigger an alarm. Assume that in the same operating room, there are 30 electrical devices each having 100 μA of leakage current. The total leakage current (30 × 100 μA) would be 3 mA. The impedance to ground would still be 40,000 ohms (120/0.003). The LIM alarm would sound, because the 2-mA set point has been violated. However, the system is still safe and represents a significantly different state than the first situation. For this reason, the newer LIMs are set to alarm at 5 mA instead of 2 mA.

The newest LIMs are referred to as third-generation moni-

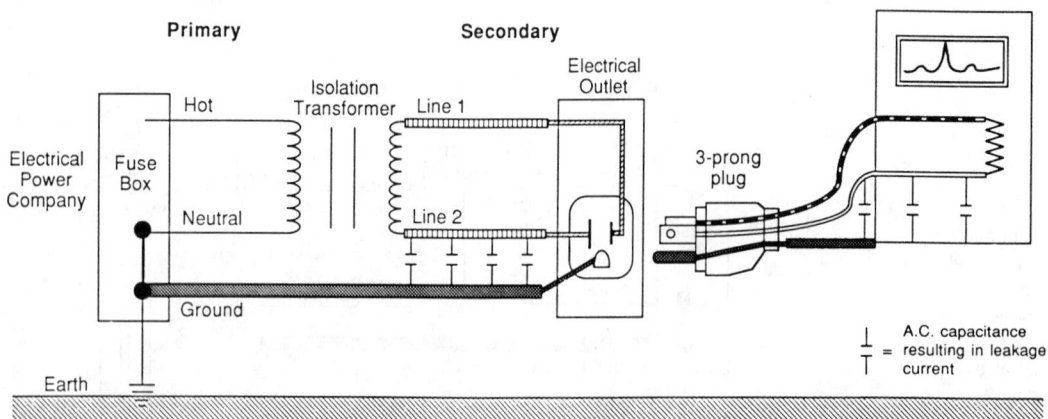

Figure 8-25. The capacitance that exists in AC power lines and AC-operated equipment results in small "leakage currents" that partially degrade the isolated power system.

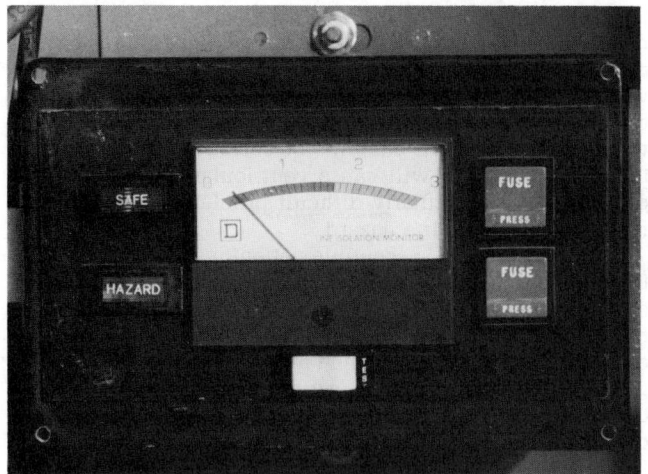

Figure 8-26. The meter of the line isolation monitor is calibrated in milliamperes. If the isolation of the power system is degraded such that more than 2 mA (5 mA in newer systems) of current could flow, the hazard light will illuminate, and a warning buzzer will sound. Note the button for testing the hazard warning system.

tors. The first-generation monitor, or static LIM, was unable to detect balanced faults. The second-generation, or dynamic LIM, did not have this problem but could interfere with physiological monitoring. Both of these monitors would trigger an alarm at 2 mA, which led to annoying "false" alarms. The third-generation LIM corrects the problems of its predecessors and has the alarm set at 5 mA.[15] Proper functioning of the LIM is dependent on having intact equipment ground wires as well as its own connection to ground. First- and second-generation LIMs could not detect the loss of the LIM ground connection. The third-generation LIM can detect this loss of ground to the monitor. In this case, the LIM alarm would sound and the red hazard light would illuminate, but the LIM meter would read 0. This

condition will alert the staff that the LIM needs repair. However, the LIM still cannot detect broken equipment ground wires. An example of the third-generation LIM is the Iso-Gard made by Square D Company.

The equipment ground wire is, again, a very important part of the safety system. If this wire is broken, a faulty piece of equipment that is plugged in will operate normally, but the LIM will not sound an alarm. A second fault could therefore cause a shock without any alarm from the LIM. Also, in the event of a second fault, the equipment ground wire provides a low-resistance path to ground for most of the fault current (see Fig. 8-24). The LIM will only be able to register leakage currents from pieces of equipment that are connected to the isolated power system and have intact ground wires.

GROUND FAULT CIRCUIT INTERRUPTER

The ground fault circuit interrupter (GFCI) is another popular device used to prevent individuals from receiving an electrical shock in a grounded power system. Electrical codes for most new construction require that a GFCI circuit be present in potentially hazardous areas such as bathrooms, kitchens, or outdoor electrical outlets. The GFCI may be installed as an individual power outlet (Fig. 8-28) or may be a special circuit breaker to which all the individual outlets are connected at a single point. The special GFCI circuit breaker is located in the main fuse box and can be distinguished by its red test button (Fig. 8-29).

Figure 8-5 demonstrates that the current flowing in the hot and the neutral wires is usually equal. The GFCI monitors both sides of the circuit for the equality of current flow, and if a difference is detected, the power is immediately interrupted. If an individual should contact a faulty piece of apparatus such that current was flowing through the individual, an imbalance in the two sides of the circuit would be created, which would be detected by the GFCI. Because the GFCI can detect very small current differences (in the

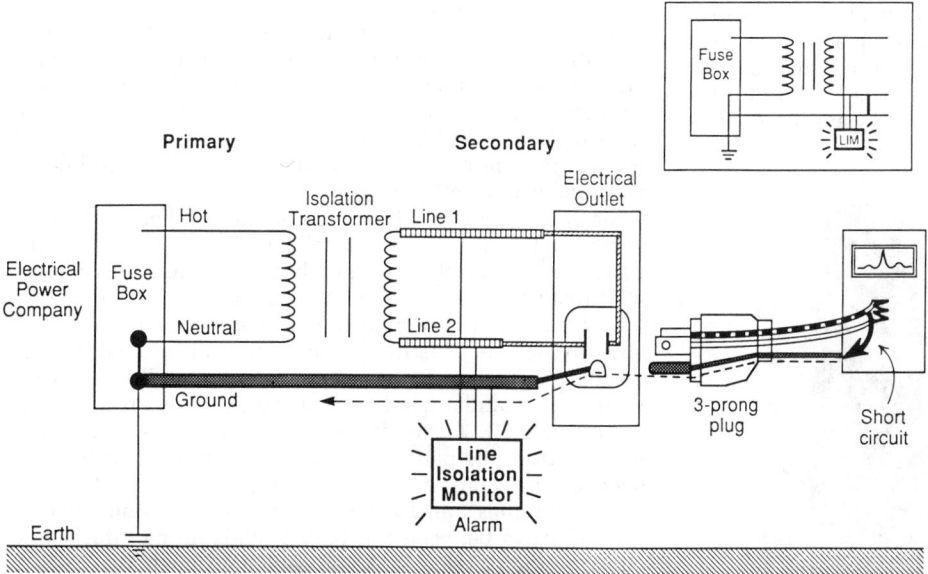

Figure 8-27. When a faulty piece of equipment is plugged into the isolated power system, it will markedly decrease the impedance from line 1 or line 2 to ground. This will be detected by the line isolation monitor, which will sound an alarm.

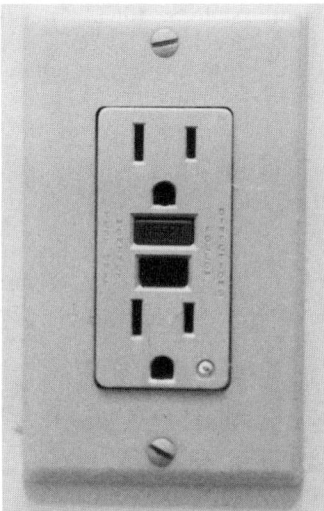

Figure 8-28. A ground fault circuit interrupter (GFCI) electrical outlet with integrated test and reset buttons.

range of 5 mA), the GFCI will open the circuit in a few milliseconds, thereby interrupting the current flow before a significant shock occurs. Thus, the GFCI provides a high level of protection at a very modest cost.

The problem with using a GFCI in the operating room is that it interrupts the flow of power. A defective piece of equipment could no longer be used, which might be a problem if it were of a life-support nature. Whereas if the same faulty piece of equipment was plugged into an isolated power system, the LIM would respond with an alarm, but the equipment could still be used.

MICROSHOCK

As previously discussed, the concept of macroshock concerns relatively large amounts of current applied to the surface of the body. The current is conducted through all the tissues in proportion to their conductivity and the area in a plane perpendicular to the current. Consequently, the *density* of the current (amperes per meter squared) that reaches the heart is considerably less than what is applied to the body surface. However, an electrically susceptible patient

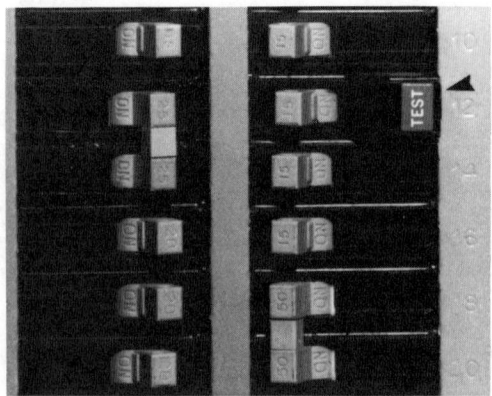

Figure 8-29. Special GFCI circuit breaker. The *arrowhead* points to the distinguishing red test button.

(*i.e.*, one who has a direct external connection to the heart) may be at risk from very small currents, and this is called *microshock*.[16] The catheter orifice or electrical wire with a very small surface area in contact with the heart produces a relatively large current density at the heart.[17] Stated another way, even very small amounts of current applied directly to the myocardium will cause ventricular fibrillation. Microshock is a particularly difficult problem because of the insidious nature of the hazard.

In the electrically susceptible patient, ventricular fibrillation can be produced by a current that is below the threshold of human perception, although the exact amount of current necessary to cause ventricular fibrillation in this type of patient is unknown. Whalen and colleagues were able to produce fibrillation with 20 μA of current applied directly to the myocardium of dogs.[18] Raftery and associates produced fibrillation with 80 μA of current in some patients.[19] Hull[20] used data obtained by Watson et al[21] to show that 50% of patients would fibrillate at currents of 200 μA. Because 1000 μA (1 mA) is generally regarded as the threshold of human perception with 60 Hz AC current, the electrically susceptible patient can be electrocuted with one tenth of normally perceptible currents. This is not only of academic interest, but also of practical concern, as many cases of ventricular fibrillation from microshock have been reported.[22-27]

The stray capacitance that is part of any AC-operated electrical instrument may result in significant amounts of charge build-up on the case of the instrument. An individual who simultaneously touches the case where this has occurred and the electrically susceptible patient may unknowingly cause a discharge to the patient that results in ventricular fibrillation. Once again, the equipment ground wire constitutes the principal protection against microshock for the electrically susceptible patient. In this case, the equipment ground wire provides a low-resistance path by which most of the leakage current is dissipated instead of being stored as a charge.

Figure 8-30 illustrates a situation involving a patient with a saline-filled catheter in the heart with a resistance of approximately 500 ohms. The ground wire with a resistance of 1 ohm is connected to the instrument case. A leakage current of 100 μA will divide according to the relative resistances of the two paths. In this case, 99.8 μA will flow through the equipment ground wire, and only 0.2 μA will flow through the fluid-filled catheter. This extremely small current does not endanger the patient. However, if the equipment ground wire was broken, the electrically susceptible patient would be at great risk, because all 100 μA of leakage current could flow through the catheter and cause ventricular fibrillation (Fig. 8-31).

Modern patient monitors incorporate another mechanism to reduce the risk of microshock for electrically susceptible patients. This mechanism involves electronically isolating all direct patient inputs from the power supply of the monitor by placing a very high impedance between the patient and any device. This limits the amount of internal leakage through the patient connection to a very small value. Currently, the standard is less than 10 μA. For instance, the output of an ECG monitor's power supply is electrically isolated from the patient by placing a very high impedance between the monitor and the patient's ECG leads.[6,28] Isolation techniques are designed to inhibit hazardous electrical pathways between the patient and the monitor while allowing the passage of the physiologic signal.

It must be remembered that the line isolation monitor is not designed to provide protection from microshock. The microampere currents involved in microshock are far below

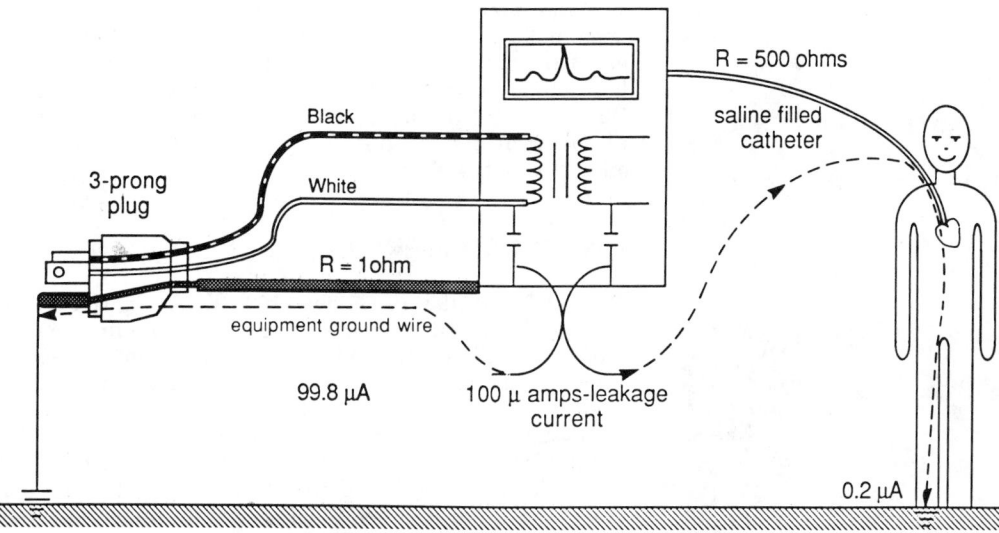

Figure 8-30. The electrically susceptible patient is protected from microshock by the presence of an intact equipment ground wire. The equipment ground wire provides a low-impedance path in which the majority of the leakage current (*dashed lines*) can flow.

the LIM's threshold of protection. In addition, the LIM does not register the leakage of individual monitors, but rather, it indicates the status of the total system. The LIM reading indicates the total amount of leakage current resulting from the entire capacitance of the system. This is the amount of current that would flow to ground in the event of a first-fault situation.

The essence of electrical safety is a thorough understanding of all the principles of grounding. As John Bruner states, "Grounding is neither safe nor unsafe. Its significance is dependent on what is grounded and in what context."[9] The objective of electrical safety is to make it difficult for electrical current to pass through people. For this reason, both the patient and the anesthesiologist should be isolated from ground as much as possible. That is, their resistance to cur-

rent flow should be as high as is technologically possible. In the inherently unsafe electrical environment of an operating room, several measures can be taken to help insure against contacting hazardous current flows. First, the grounded power provided by the utility company can be transformed to ungrounded power by means of an isolation transformer. The LIM will continously monitor the status of this isolation from ground, and warn that the isolation of the power (from ground) has been lost in the event a defective piece of equipment is plugged into the electrical system. In addition, the shock that an individual could receive from a faulty piece of equipment is determined by the capacitance of the system and is limited to a few milliamperes. Second, all equipment plugged into the isolated power system is equipped with an equipment ground wire that is attached to the case of the

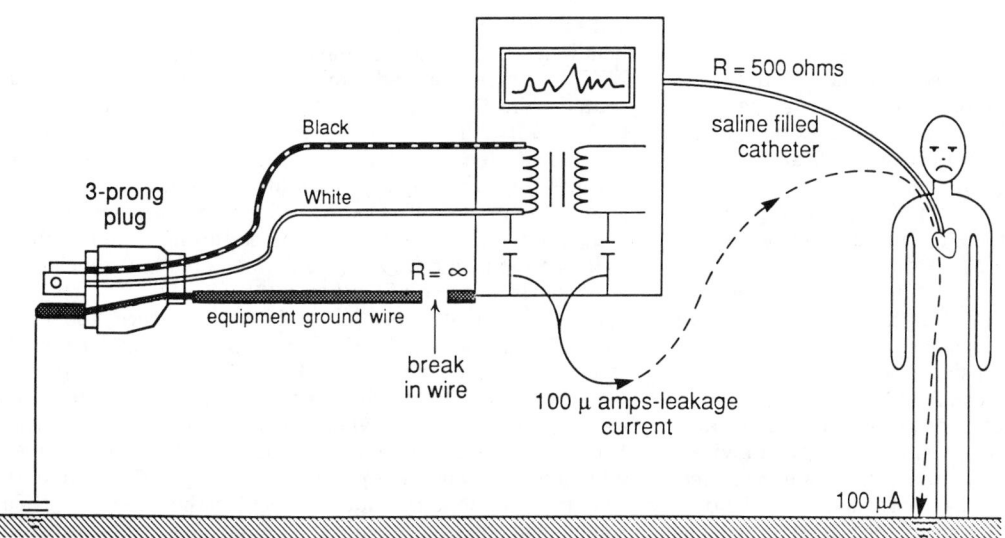

Figure 8-31. A broken equipment ground wire results in a significant hazard to the electrically susceptible patient. In this case, the entire leakage current can be conducted to the heart and may result in ventricular fibrillation.

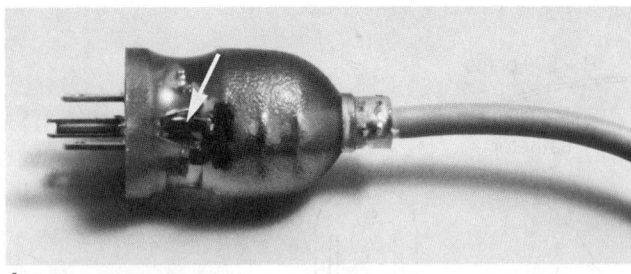

A

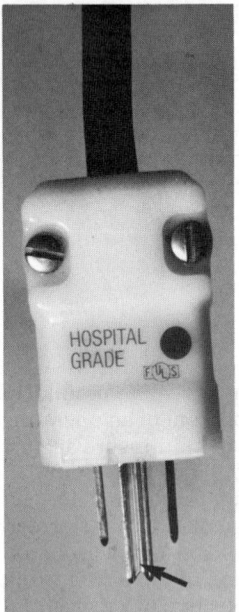

B

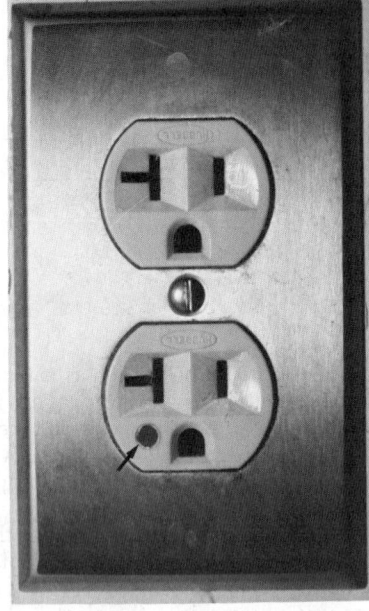

C

Figure 8-32. (*A*) A hospital grade plug that can be visually inspected. The *arrow* points to equipment ground wire whose integrity can be readily verified. (*B*) A hospital-grade plug that can be easily disassembled for inspection. Note that the prong for the ground wire (*arrow*) is longer than the hot or neutral prong, so that it is the first to enter the receptacle. (*C*) The *arrow* points to the green dot denoting a hospital-grade power outlet.

instrument. This wire provides an alternative low-resistance pathway enabling potentially dangerous currents to flow to ground. Thus, the patient and the anesthesiologist should be as insulated from ground as possible, and all electronic equipment should be grounded.

The equipment ground wire serves three functions. First, it provides a low-resistance path for fault currents to reduce the risk of macroshock. Second, it dissipates leakage currents that are potentially harmful to the electrically susceptible patient. Finally, it provides information to the LIM on the status of the ungrounded power system. If the equipment ground wire is broken, a significant factor in the prevention of electrical shock is lost. Additionally, the isolated power system will appear safer than it actually is because the LIM is unable to detect broken equipment ground wires.

Because power cord plugs and receptacles are subjected to greater abuse in the hospital than in the home, the Underwriters Laboratory has issued a strict specification for special *hospital-grade* plugs and receptacles (Fig. 8-32), which are marked by green dots.[29] The hospital-grade plug is one that can be visually inspected or easily disassembled to en-

sure the integrity of the ground wire connection. Molded opaque plugs are not acceptable. Edwards reported that out of 3000 nonhospital-grade receptacles installed in a new hospital building, 1800 (60%) were defective after 3 years.[30] When 2000 of the nonhospital-grade receptacles were replaced with ones of hospital grade, no failures occurred after 18 months of use.

ELECTROSURGERY

On that fateful day in October 1926 when Dr. Harvey W. Cushing first used an electrosurgical machine invented by Professor William T. Bovie to resect a brain tumor, the course of modern surgery and anesthesia was forever altered.[31] The ubiquitous use of electrosurgery today attests to the success of Professor Bovie's invention. However, this technology was not adopted without a cost. The widespread use of electrocautery has, at the least, hastened the elimination of explosive anesthetic agents from the operating room. In addition, as every anesthesiologist is aware, there are few things in the operating room that are immune to interference from the "Bovie." The high-frequency electrical energy generated by the electrosurgery unit (ESU) interferes with everything from the ECG signal to cardiac output computers, pulse oximeters, and even implanted cardiac pacemakers.[32]

The ESU operates by generating very high-frequency currents (radiofrequency range) of anywhere from 500,000 to more than 1 million Hz. Heat is generated whenever a current passes through a resistance. The amount of heat produced is proportional to the square of the current (I) and inversely proportional to the area (A) through which the current passes ($H = I^2/A$).[33] By concentrating the energy at the tip of the "Bovie pencil," the surgeon can produce either a cut or coagulation at any given spot. This very high-frequency current behaves quite differently from the standard 60-Hz AC current and can pass directly across the precordium without causing ventricular fibrillation.[33] This is possible because high-frequency currents have a low tissue penetration and do not excite contractile cells.

The large amount of energy generated by the ESU can pose other problems to the operator and the patient. Dr. Cushing became aware of one such problem. He wrote, "once the operator received a shock which passed through a metal retractor to his arm and out by a wire from his headlight, which was unpleasant to say the least."[34] The ESU cannot be operated safely unless the energy is properly routed from the unit through the patient and back to the unit. Ideally, the current generated by the active electrode is concentrated at the ESU tip, constituting a very small surface area. This energy has a high current density and is able to create enough heat to produce a therapeutic cut or coagulation. The energy then passes through the patient to a dispersive electrode of large surface area that returns the energy safely to the ESU (Fig. 8-33).

One unfortunate quirk in terminology concerns the return (dispersive) plate of the ESU. This plate, often mistakenly referred to as a "ground plate," is actually a dispersive electrode of large surface area that safely returns the generated energy to the ESU via a low current-density pathway. When inquiring whether the dispersive electrode has been attached to the patient, operating room personnel frequently ask "is the patient grounded?" Because the aim of electrical safety is to isolate the patient from ground, this expression not only is a misnomer but leads to confusion.

Because the area of the return plate is large, the current density is low; therefore, no harmful heat is generated, and

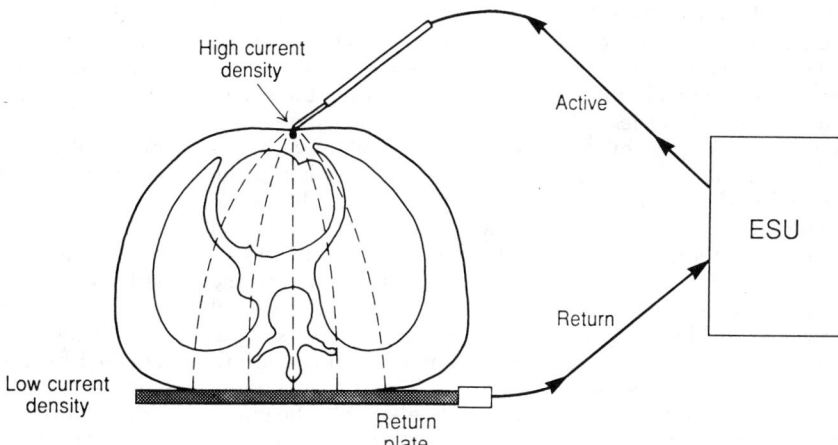

Figure 8-33. A properly applied ESU return plate. The current density at the return plate is low, resulting in no danger to the patient.

no tissue destruction occurs. In a properly functioning system, the only tissue effect is at the site of the active electrode that is held by the surgeon. Problems can arise if the electrosurgical return plate is improperly applied to the patient or if the cord connecting the return plate to the ESU is damaged or broken. In these instances, the high-frequency current generated by the ESU will seek an alternate return pathway. Anything attached to the patient, such as ECG leads or a temperature probe, can provide this alternate pathway. The current density at the ECG pad will be considerably higher than normal, because its surface area is much less than that of the ESU return plate. This may result in a serious burn at this alternate return site. Similarly, a burn may occur at the site of the ESU return plate if it is not properly applied to the patient or if it becomes partially dislodged during the operation (Fig. 8-34). That this is not merely a theoretical possibility is evidenced by the numerous case reports of patients who have received ESU burns.[35-40]

The original ESUs were manufactured with the power supply connected directly to ground by the equipment ground wire. These devices made it extremely easy for ESU current to return by alternate pathways. In fact, the ESU would continue to operate normally even without the return plate connected to the patient. In most modern ESUs, the power supply is isolated from ground in order to protect the patient from burns. It was hoped that by isolating the return pathway from ground, the only route for current flow would be by the return electrode. Theoretically, this would eliminate alternate return pathways and greatly reduce the incidence of burns.[5] However, Mitchell found two situations in which the current could return via alternate pathways, even with the isolated ESU circuit.[41] If the return plate were left either on top of an uninsulated ESU cabinet or in contact with the bottom of the operating room table, the ESU could operate fairly normally, and the current would return via alternate pathways. It will be recalled that the impedance is inversely proportional to the capacitance times the current frequency. The ESU operates at 500,000 to more than 1 million Hz, which greatly enhances the effect of capacitive coupling and causes a marked reduction in impedance. Therefore, even with isolated ESUs, the decrease in impedance allows the current to return to the ESU by alternate pathways. Additionally, the isolated ESU does not protect the patient from burns if the return electrode does not make proper contact with the patient. Although the isolated ESU does provide additional patient safety, it is by no means foolproof protection against patient burns.

Preventing patient burns from the ESU is the responsibility of all professional staff in the operating room. Not only the circulating nurse, but also the surgeon and the anesthesiologist must be aware of proper techniques and vigilant to potential problems. The most important factor is the proper application of the return plate. It is essential that the plate have the appropriate amount of electrolyte gel and an intact return wire. Reusable return plates must be properly cleaned after each use, and disposable plates must be

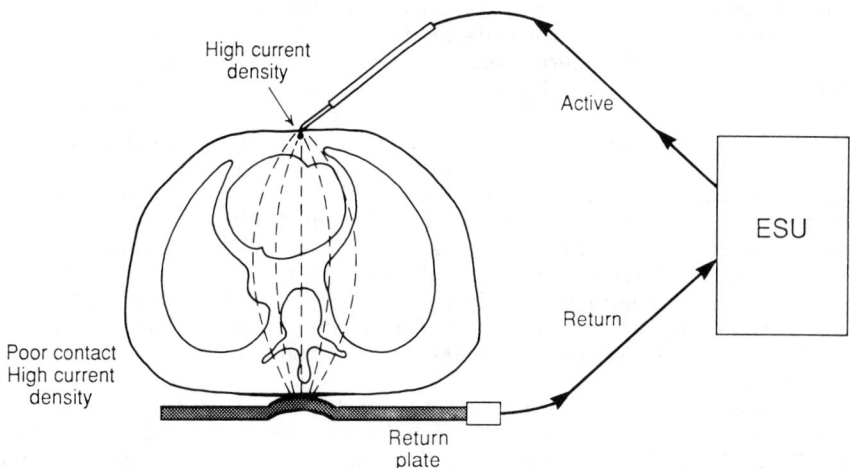

Figure 8-34. An improperly applied ESU return plate. Poor contact with the return plate results in a high current density and a possible burn to the patient.

checked to be certain the electrolyte has not dried out during storage. In addition, it is prudent to place the return plate as close as possible to the site of the operation. Electrocardiographic pads should be placed as far from the site of the operation as is feasible. Operating room personnel must be alert to the possibility that pools of flammable prep solutions such as ether and acetone can be ignited when using the ESU. If the ESU must be used on a patient with a demand pacemaker, the return electrode should be located below the thorax, and preparations for treating dysrhythmias should be available, including a magnet to convert the pacemaker to a fixed rate, a defibrillator, and an external pacemaker. The ESU has also caused other problems in patients with pacemakers, including reprogramming and microshock.[42,43] If the surgeon requests higher than normal power settings on the ESU, this should alert both the circulating nurse and the anesthesiologist to a potential problem. The return plate and cable must be inspected immediately to ensure that it is functioning and properly positioned. If this does not correct the problem, the return plate should be replaced. If the problem still remains, the entire ESU unit should be taken out of service. Finally, an ESU that is dropped or damaged must be removed immediately from the operating room and thoroughly tested by a qualified biomedical engineer. Following these simple safety steps will prevent most patient burns from the ESU.

The previous discussion concerned only unipolar units. There is a second type of ESU in which the current passes only between the two blades of a pair of forceps. This type of device is referred to as a bipolar ESU. Because the active and return electrodes are the two blades of the forceps, it is not necessary to attach another dispersive electrode to the patient unless a unipolar ESU is also being used. The bipolar ESU generates considerably less power than the unipolar unit and is used mainly for ophthalmic and neurologic surgery.[2]

In 1980, Mirowski et al reported the first human implantation of a device to treat intractable ventricular tachyarrhythmias.[44] This device, known as the automatic implantable cardioverter-defibrillator (AICD), is capable of sensing ventricular tachycardia and ventricular fibrillation and then automatically defibrillating the patient. In the last 10 years, thousands of patients have received AICD implants.[45,46] Because some of these patients may now present for noncardiac surgery, it is important that the anesthesiologist be aware of the potential problems.[47] The use of a unipolar ESU may cause electrical interference, which could be interpreted by the AICD as a ventricular tachyarrhythmia. This would trigger a defibrillation pulse to be delivered to the patient and would likely cause an actual episode of tachycardia or fibrillation. The patient with an AICD is also at risk for fibrillation during electroconvulsive therapy (ECT).[47] In both cases, the AICD should be disabled. This is accomplished by placing a donut pacemaker magnet over the device. A tone synchronous with the heartbeat will then be heard. The magnet is left in place until the tone becomes continuous, at which time the AICD is disabled and the magnet can be removed. The device can be reactivated by reversing the process. Also, an external defibrillator and a noninvasive pacemaker must be in the operating room whenever one is anesthetizing a patient with an AICD. If the anesthesiologist is unfamiliar with the operation of the AICD, someone experienced with the device should be available.

Electrical safety in the operating room is a matter of combining common sense with some basic principles of electricity. Once operating room personnel understand the importance of safe electrical practice, they are able to develop a heightened awareness of potential problems. All electrical equipment must undergo routine maintenance, service, and inspection to ensure that it conforms to designated electrical safety standards. Records of these test results must be kept for future inspection, because human error can easily compound electrical hazards. Starmer et al cite a case of a newly constructed laboratory where the ground wire was not attached to the receptacle.[48] In another study, Albisser and colleagues found a 14% (198/1424) incidence of improperly or incorrectly wired outlets.[49] Furthermore, potentially hazardous situations should be recognized and corrected before they become a problem. For instance, electrical power cords are frequently placed on the floor, where they can be crushed by various carts or the ansthesia machine. These cords could be located overhead or in an area of low traffic flow. Multiple-plug extension boxes should not be left on the floor where they can come in contact with electrolyte solutions. These could easily be mounted on a cart or the anesthesia machine. Pieces of equipment that have been damaged or have obvious defects in the power cord must not be used until they have been properly repaired. If everyone is aware of what constitutes a potential hazard, dangerous situations can be prevented with minimal effort.

CONDUCTIVE FLOORING

Conductive flooring was mandated for operating rooms where flammable anesthetic agents were being administered. The conductive floor was supposed to have a resistance of between 25,000 and 1 million Ω. This would minimize the build-up of static charges, which could cause a flammable anesthetic agent to ignite. The standards have been changed to eliminate the necessity for conductive flooring in anesthetizing areas where flammable agents are no longer used.

CONSTRUCTION OF NEW OPERATING ROOMS

A final area of concern to the anesthesiologist is the design of new operating room facilities. Frequently, an anesthesiologist is asked to consult with hospital administrators and architects in designing new operating rooms. In the past, a very strict electrical code was enforced because of the use of flammable anesthetic agents. This code included a requirement for isolated power systems and LIMs. In recent years, the National Fire Protection Association (NFPA) has revised its standard for health care facilities (NFPA 99-1984). These new standards no longer require isolated power systems or LIMs in areas designated for use of only nonflammable anesthetizing agents.[50,51] Although not mandatory, NFPA standards are usually adopted by local authorities when revising their electrical codes.

This change in the standard creates a dilemma. The NFPA 99-Standard for Health Care Facilities—1990 Edition mandates that "wet location patient care areas be provided with special protection against electric shock. . . ." Section 3-4.1.2.6 further states: "this special protection shall be provided by a power distribution system that inherently limits the possible ground fault current due to a first fault to a low value, without interrupting the power supply; or by a power distribution system in which the power supply is interrupted if the ground fault current does, in fact, exceed a value of 6 milliamperes."

The decision of whether to install isolated power hinges on two factors. The first is whether the operating room is considered a *wet location;* and, if so, whether an interruption of the power supply is tolerable. Where power interruption is tolerable, a GFCI is permitted as the protective means. However, the standards also state that "the use of an isolated power system (IPS) shall be permitted as a protective means capable of limiting ground fault current without power interruption."

Most people who have worked in an operating room would attest to its being a wet location. The blood, body fluids, and saline solutions spilled on the floor all contribute to making this a wet environment.[52] The cystoscopy suite serves as a good example.

Once the premise that the operating room is a wet location is accepted, then it must be determined if a GFCI can provide the means of protection. The argument against using GFCIs in the operating room is illustrated by the following example. Assume that during an open heart procedure, the cardiopulmonary bypass pump and the patient monitors are plugged into outlets on the same branch circuit. Also assume that during bypass, the circulating nurse plugs in a faulty headlight. If there is a GFCI protecting the circuit, the fault will be detected, and the GFCI will interrrupt all power to the pump and the monitors. This undoubtedly would cause a great deal of confusion and consternation among the operating room personnel and may place the patient at risk for injury. The pump would have to be operated manually while the problem was being resolved. In addition, the GFCI could not be reset (and power restored) until the headlight was identified as the cause of the fault and unplugged from the outlet. On the other hand, if the operating room was protected with an isolated power system and LIM, then the same scenario would cause the LIM to sound an alarm, but the pump and patient monitors would continue to operate normally. There would be no interruption of power, and the problem could be resolved without risk to the patient.

It should be realized that a GFCI is an active system. That is, a potentially hazardous current is already flowing and must be actively interrupted, whereas the isolated power system with LIM is designed to be safe during a first-fault situation. Thus, it is a passive system in that no mechanical action is required to activate the protection.[53]

It is likely that hospital administrators may want to eliminate isolated power systems in new operating room construction as a cost-saving measure. However, Lennon and Leonard,[54] Bruner and Leonard,[53] and Matjasko and Ashman[52] all advocate the retention of isolated power systems, and it is this author's opinion that not to do this would be a short-sighted and foolhardy measure. This is especially true because the cost of adding isolated power is estimated to be less than 1% of the cost of constructing an operating room.[53] Although not perfect,[55] the isolated power system and LIM do provide both the patient and the operating room personnel with a significant amount of protection in an electrically hazardous environment. Anesthesiologists need to be aware of this change and insist that new operating rooms be constructed with isolated power systems. The relatively small cost savings the alternative would represent does not justify the elimination of such a useful safety system, and the alternative of using GFCIs is not practical in the operating room environment.

REFERENCES

1. Bruner JMR: Hazards of electrical apparatus. Anesthesiology 28:396, 1967
2. Hull CJ: Electrical hazards in monitoring. Int Anesthesiol Clin 19:177, 1981
3. Leonard PF, Gould AB: Dynamics of electrical hazards of particular concern to operating-room personnel. Surg Clin North Am 45:817, 1965
4. Miller F: College Physics, 2nd ed, p 457. New York, Harcourt Brace & World, 1967
5. Uyttendaele K, Grobstein S, Svetz P: Monitoring instrumentation—isolated inputs, electrosurgery filtering, burns protection: What does it mean? Acta Anaesthesiol Belg 29:317, 1978
6. Leonard PF: Characteristics of electrical hazards. Anesth Analg 51:797, 1972
7. Taylor KW, Desmond J: Electrical hazards in the operating room, with special reference to electrosurgery. Can J Surg 13:362, 1970
8. Leonard PF: Apparatus and appliances current thinking. III. Alternating current, the isolation transformer, and the differential-transformer pressure transducer. Anesth Analg 45:814, 1966
9. Bruner JMR: Fundamental concepts of electrical safety. In Hershey SG (ed): ASA Refresher Courses in Anesthesiology, p 11. Philadelphia, JB Lippincott, 1974
10. Harpell TR: Electrical shock hazards in the hospital environment: Their causes and cures. Can Hosp 47:48, 1970
11. Buczko GB, McKay WPS: Electrical safety in the operating room. Can J Anaesth 34:315, 1987
12. Wald A: Electrical safety in medicine. In Skalak R, Chien S (eds): Handbook of Bioengineering, p 341. New York, McGraw-Hill, 1987
13. Dalziel CF, Massoglia FP: Let-go currents and voltages. AIEE Trans 75(2):49, 1956
14. Bruner JMR, Aronow S, Cavicchi RV: Electrical incidents in a large hospital: A 42 month register. JAAMI 6:222, 1972
15. Bernstein MS: Isolated power and line isolation monitors. BioMed Instrum Technol 24:221, 1990
16. Weinberg DI, Artley JL, Whalen RE, McIntosh HD: Electric shock hazards in cardiac catheterization. Circ Res 11:1004, 1962
17. Starmer CF, Whalen RE: Current density and electrically induced ventricular fibrillation. Med Instrum 7:158, 1973
18. Whalen RE, Starmer CF, McIntosh HD: Electrical hazards associated with cardiac pacemaking. Ann NY Acad Sci III:922, 1964
19. Raftery EB, Green HL, Yacoub MH: Disturbances of heart rhythm produced by 50-Hz leakage currents in human subjects. Cardiovasc Res 9:263, 1975
20. Hull CJ: Electrocution hazards in the operating theatre. Br J Anaesth 50:647, 1978
21. Watson AB, Wright JS, Loughman J: Electrical thresholds for ventricular fibrillation in man. Med J Aust 1:1179, 1973
22. Furman S, Schwedel JB, Robinson G, Hurwitt ES: Use of an intracardiac pacemaker in the control of heart block. Surgery 49:98, 1961
23. Noordijk JA, Oey FJI, Tebra W: Myocardial electrodes and the danger of ventricular fibrillation. Lancet 1:975, 1961
24. Pengelly LD, Klassen GA: Myocardial electrodes and the danger of ventricular fibrillation. Lancet 1:1234, 1961
25. Rowe GG, Zarnstorff WC: Ventricular fibrillation during selective angiocardiography. JAMA 192:947, 1965
26. Hopps JA, Roy OS: Electrical hazards in cardiac diagnosis and treatment. Med Electr Biol Eng 1:133, 1963
27. Mody SM, Richings M: Ventricular fibrillation resulting from electrocution during cardiac catheterization. Lancet 2:698, 1962
28. Leeming MN: Protection of the electrically susceptible patient: A discussion of systems and methods. Anesthesiology 38:370, 1973
29. Cromwell L, Weibell FJ, Pfeiffer EA: Biomedical Instrumentation and Measurements, 2nd ed, p 430. Englewood Cliffs, Prentice-Hall, 1980
30. Edwards NK: Specialized electrical grounding needs. Clin Perinatol 3:367, 1976
31. Goldwyn RM: Bovie: The man and the machine. Ann Plast Surg 2:135, 1979
32. Lichter I, Borrie J, Miller WM: Radio-frequency hazards with cardiac pacemakers. Br Med J 1:1513, 1965
33. Dornette WHL: An electrically safe surgical environment. Arch Surg 107:567, 1973

34. Cushing H: Electro-surgery as an aid to the removal of intracranial tumors. With a preliminary note on a new surgical-current generator by W. T. Bovie. Surg Gynecol Obstet 47:751, 1928

35. Meathe EA: Electrical safety for patients and anesthetists. In Saidman LJ, Smith NT (eds): Monitoring in Anesthesia, 2nd ed, p 497. Boston, Butterworths, 1984

36. Rolly G: Two cases of burns caused by misuse of coagulation unit and monitoring. Acta Anaesthesiol Belg 29:313, 1978

37. Parker EO: Electrosurgical burn at the site of an esophageal temperature probe. Anesthesiology 61:93, 1984

38. Schneider AJL, Apple HP, Braun RT: Electrosurgical burns at skin temperature probes. Anesthesiology 47:72, 1977

39. Bloch EC, Burton LW: Electrosurgical burn while using a battery-operated Doppler monitor. Anesth Analg 58:339, 1979

40. Becker CM, Malhotra IV, Hedley-Whyte J: The distribution of radiofrequency current and burns. Anesthesiology 38:106, 1973

41. Mitchell JP: The isolated circuit diathermy. Ann R Coll Surg Engl 61:287, 1979

42. Titel JH, El Etr AA: Fibrillation resulting from pacemaker electrodes and electrocautery during surgery. Anesthesiology 29:845, 1968

43. Domino KB, Smith TC: Electrocautery-induced reprogramming of a pacemaker using a precordial magnet. Anesth Analg 62:609, 1983

44. Mirowski M, Reid PR, Mower MM et al: Termination of malignant ventricular arrhythmias with an implanted automatic defibrillator in human beings. N Engl J Med 303:322, 1980

45. Crozier IG, Ward DE: Automatic implantable defibrillators. Br J Hosp Med 40:136, 1988

46. Elefteriades JA, Biblo LA, Batsford WP et al: Evolving patterns in the surgical treatment of malignant ventricular tachyarrhythmias. Ann Thorac Surg 49:94, 1990

47. Carr CME, Whiteley SM: The automatic implantable cardioverter-defibrillator. Anaesthesia 46:737, 1991

48. Starmer CF, McIntosh HD, Whalen RE: Electrical hazards and cadiovascular function. N Engl J Med 284:181, 1971

49. Albisser AM, Parson ID, Pask BA: A survey of the grounding systems in several large hospitals. Med Instrum 7:297, 1973

50. Kermit E, Staewen WS: Isolated power systems: Historical perspective and update on regulations. Biomed Tech Today 1(3):86, 1986

51. National Fire Protection Association: National Electric Code (ANSI/NFPA 70-1984). Quincy, Massachusetts, National Fire Protection Association, 1984

52. Matjasko MJ, Ashman MN: All you need to know about electrical safety in the operating room. In Barash PG, Deutsch S, Tinker J (eds): ASA Refresher Courses in Anesthesiology, 18:251. Philadelphia, JB Lippincott, 1990

53. Bruner JMR, Leonard PF: Electricity, safety and the patient, p 300. Chicago, Year Book Medical Publishers, 1989

54. Lennon RL, Leonard PF: Letter: A hitherto unreported virtue of the isolated power system. Anesth Analg 66:1049, 1987

55. Gilbert TB, Shaffer M, Matthews M: Electrical shock by dislodged spark gap in bipolar electrosurgical device. Anesth Analg 73:355, 1991

9 Gary P. Zaloga
Donald S. Prough

Fluids and Electrolytes

Trauma and surgery acutely alter the volumes and composition of the intracellular and extracellular spaces. Subsequent therapeutic infusion of fluids, primarily intended to replenish blood volume and maintain cardiac output, further alters compartmental volumes and composition. Both hypovolemia, which increases the risk of organ hypoperfusion and injury, and hypervolemia, which increases the risk of pulmonary edema, are potential hazards of perioperative fluid therapy. In addition to acute changes in intravascular, interstitial, and intracellular volume, surgical patients may develop potentially harmful disorders of the concentrations and total body content of important electrolytes. Precise perioperative management of fluids and electrolytes may minimize surgical morbidity and mortality.

PHYSIOLOGY

Body Fluid Compartments

Accurate replacement of fluid deficits necessitates an understanding of the distribution spaces of water, sodium, and colloid (Fig. 9-1). Total body water (TBW), the distribution volume of sodium-free water, approximates 60% of total body weight, or 42 liters in a 70-kg person. TBW consists of intracellular volume (ICV), which constitutes 40% of total body weight (28 liters in a 70-kg person), and extracellular volume (ECV), which constitutes 20% of body weight (14 liters). Plasma volume (PV), approximately 3 liters, equals about one fifth of ECV, the remainder of which is interstitial fluid (IF). Red cell volume, approximately 2 liters, is part of ICV.

The ECV contains most of the sodium in the body, with equal sodium concentrations ($[Na^+]$) in the PV and IF, *i.e.*, plasma $[Na^+]$ is approximately 140 mEq·l^{-1}; intracellular $[Na^+]$ is approximately 10 mEq·l^{-1}. The predominant intracellular cation is potassium, with the intracellular concentration ($[K^+]$) approximating 150 mEq·l^{-1}, in contrast to a $[K^+]$ in ECV of approximately 4.0 mEq·l^{-1}. Albumin, the most important oncotically active constituent of ECV, is unequally distributed in PV and IF and is virtually excluded from ICV. The serum concentration of albumin approximates 4.0 g·dl^{-1}; the IF concentration averages 1.0 g·dl^{-1}, but varies greatly among tissues. TBW is the distribution volume for sodium-free water; ECV is the distribution volume both for crystalloid solutions in which $[Na^+]$ is approximately 140 mEq·l^{-1} and for colloid, although the concentration of colloid usually is greater in the PV.

For example, assume that a 70-kg patient has suffered an acute blood loss of 2000 ml, approximately 40% of the predicted 5-liter blood volume. Further assume that 5% dextrose in water (D5W), lactated Ringer's solution, or 5% or 25% human serum albumin could be chosen to replace shed blood. The formula describing the effects of fluid infusion on PV is as follows:

$$\text{Expected PV increment} = \frac{\text{volume infused} \times \text{normal PV}}{\text{distribution volume}}$$

Rearranging the equation yields the following:

$$\text{Volume infused} = \frac{\text{expected PV increment} \times \text{distribution volume}}{\text{normal PV}}$$

To achieve restoration of blood volume using D5W (which distributes throughout TBW), it would be necessary to administer 28 liters:

$$28 \text{ liters} = \frac{2 \text{ liters} \times 42 \text{ liters}}{3 \text{ liters}}$$

where 2 liters is the desired PV increment, 42 liters = TBW in a 70-kg person, and 3 liters is the normal estimated PV.

If lactated Ringer's solution (which distributes throughout ECV) were chosen, a 2.0-liter PV increment would require infusion of approximately 9.3 liters:

$$9.3 \text{ liters} = \frac{2 \text{ liters} \times 14 \text{ liters}}{3 \text{ liters}}$$

where 14 liters = ECV in a 70-kg person.

If 5% albumin or 6% hetastarch, both of which exert oncotic pressure similar to or slightly greater than that of plasma, were infused, most of the volume initially would remain in the PV (the approximate distribution volume), perhaps attracting additional interstitial fluid intravascularly. Twenty-five percent human serum albumin, a hyperoncotic fluid, expands PV by approximately 400 ml for each

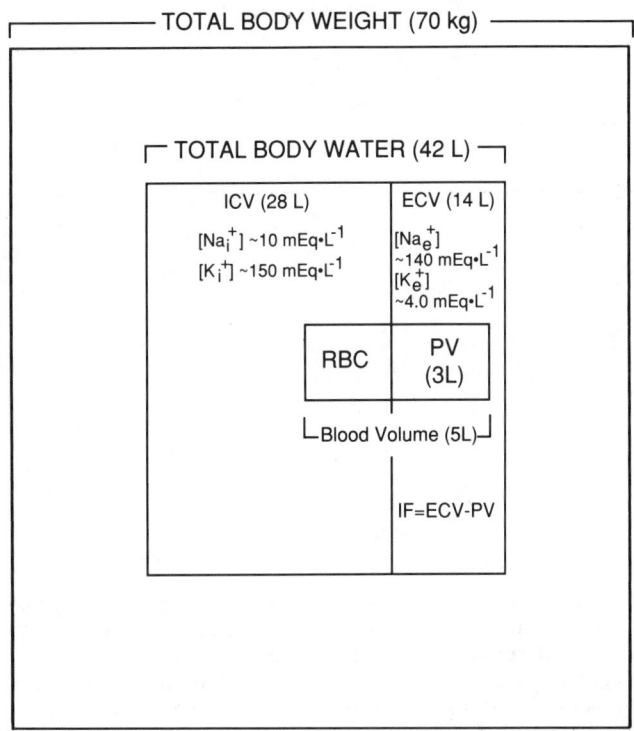

Figure 9-1. The distribution volume of water, approximately 60% of total body weight, includes both the extracellular (ECV) and intracellular volume (ICV). Sodium is distributed primarily in the extracellular volume (ECV). If capillary integrity is preserved, the concentration of colloid is higher in the plasma volume (PV) than in interstitial fluid (IF). $[Na_i^+]$ and $[Na_e^+]$ = intracellular and extracellular concentrations of sodium, respectively; $[K_i^+]$ and $[K_e^+]$ represent intracellular and extracellular concentrations of potassium.

100 ml infused, reflecting an additional 300-ml increment in PV due to translocation of interstitial fluid.

Regulation of Extracellular Fluid Volume

Afferent and Efferent Limbs of ECV Control

Both low-pressure and high-pressure receptors detect changes in blood volume and blood pressure. Because 85% of circulating blood volume resides within the highly compliant venous system, low-pressure intrathoracic volume receptors, located within the great veins, cardiac atria, and pulmonary capillaries, readily detect decreases in blood volume. High-pressure arterial receptors, found within the carotid sinuses, aortic arch, and intrarenal arterioles, are relatively insensitive to small changes in intravascular volume but respond to decreased perfusion pressure.

To preserve circulating blood volume and organ perfusion, afferent signals from volume and pressure receptors must be converted to efferent signals. In response to decreased renal perfusion pressure, intrarenal baroreceptors initiate renin release, which increases the production of angiotensin II and aldosterone, which in turn increase blood pressure, increase afferent glomerular arteriolar resistance, and enhance sodium reabsorption. Aldosterone also decreases salt loss in sweat. Activation of the sympathetic nervous system, secretion of antidiuretic hormone (ADH), and suppression of atrial natriuretic peptide (ANP) release also serve to increase systemic vascular resistance and conserve sodium and water during volume depletion. Thirst and salt-craving stimulate increased intake of water and sodium. Insufficiency or the use of pharmacologic antagonism of these systems may aggravate hypovolemia.

Renal adaptation to hypovolemia (and decreased cardiac output) occurs through three primary mechanisms: a reduc-

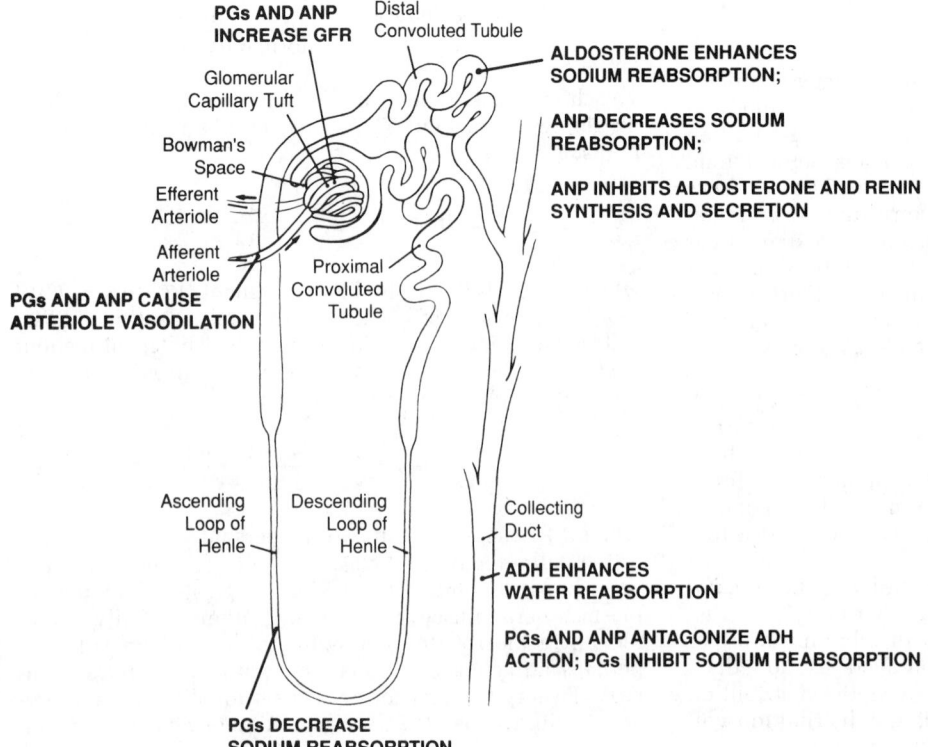

Figure 9-2. Important neuroendocrine modifiers of glomerular and tubular function include aldosterone, antidiuretic hormone (ADH), atrial natriuretic hormone (ANP), and the renal prostaglandins (PGs). The primary actions of the hormones affect afferent and efferent arteriolar resistance, glomerular permeability, and absorption and secretion of water and electrolytes in the loop of Henle, the distal convoluted tubule, and the collecting duct.

tion in renal blood flow (RBF), a reduction in glomerular filtration, and increased tubular reabsorption of sodium and water.[1] Initially, RBF is maintained (i.e., RBF is autoregulated) as perfusion pressure decreases by reductions in renal afferent arteriolar resistance. Further decreases in cardiac output may decrease the fraction of cardiac output delivered to the kidneys. Increases in renal vascular resistance redistribute blood flow from the kidneys in an attempt to preserve perfusion of other tissues.

As RBF decreases, the efferent arterioles constrict, primarily in response to angiotensin II and norepinephrine, thereby increasing the filtration fraction (FF), according to the equation:

$$FF = \frac{\left(\begin{array}{c}\text{afferent arteriolar plasma flow} - \\ \text{efferent arteriolar plasma flow}\end{array}\right)}{\text{afferent arteriolar plasma flow}} \times 100$$

Renal perfusion during acute hypovolemia is determined by the balance between renal vasoconstrictive factors (the renal sympathetic nerves, angiotensin II, and catecholamines) and vasodilatory mechanisms (intrinsic renal autoregulation and the renal vasodilatory effects of prostaglandins).[2] Although RBF autoregulates (remains constant over a wide range of perfusion pressures), autoregulation may be impaired or lost during severe, acute hypovolemia.[3,4] Renal sympathetic stimulation with secretion of alpha-adrenergic catecholamines[2] and angiotensin II increases renal vascular resistance. Hypovolemia also redistributes renal perfusion from outer cortical nephrons to inner cortical nephrons,[5] in which longer loops of Henle, which penetrate more deeply into the hypertonic renal medulla, are capable of greater sodium conservation.

To preserve PV, reabsorption of filtered water and sodium is enhanced by changes mediated by the hormonal factors ADH, ANP, and aldosterone (Fig. 9-2). Although a change in serum osmolality of only 1–2% significantly alters ADH secretion from the posterior pituitary, a 10–20% decrease in blood volume is necessary before ADH secretion increases (Fig. 9-3).[6] ADH acts primarily on the medullary collecting ducts and to a lesser extent on the cortical collecting tubules to increase water permeability, resulting in greater water reabsorption and the excretion of smaller volumes of more highly concentrated urine. Water excretion is further reduced in volume-depleted patients by impaired delivery of tubular fluid to distal nephron sites and by ADH-independent water reabsorption by the collecting ducts.

In contrast to increased secretion of ADH, ANP secretion is decreased during hypovolemia. ANP, released from the cardiac atria in response to increased atrial stretch, exerts vasodilatory effects and increases the renal excretion of sodium and water.[7-11] Many of the physiologic effects of ANP appear to be hemodynamically mediated, increasing the glomerular filtration rate (GFR) and resulting in diuresis.

In volume-depleted states, sodium conservation results both from decreased filtration of sodium (decreased GFR) and from increased tubular reabsorption of sodium. Aldosterone, the most important humoral regulator of sodium reabsorption, is produced by the adrenal cortex as the final product of a series of endocrine events. Hypoperfusion stimulates the release of renin from the granular cells of the juxtaglomerular apparatus. Renin catalyzes the conversion of angiotensinogen to angiotensin I. Angiotensin-converting enzyme converts angiotensin I to angiotensin II, and finally angiotensin II stimulates the adrenal cortex to synthesize and release aldosterone.[12-14] Acting primarily in the distal

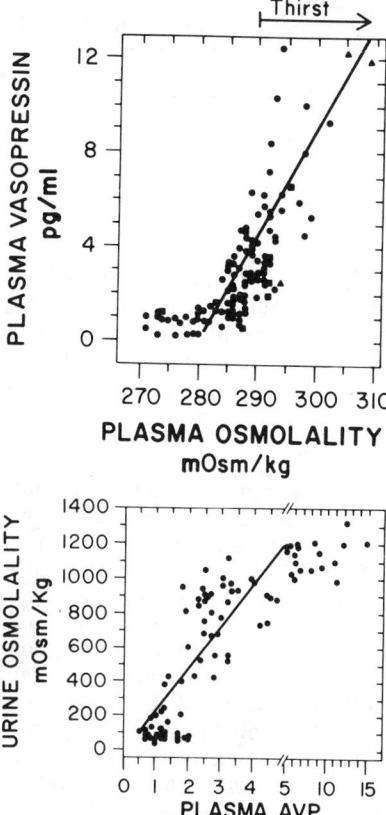

Figure 9-3. (*Top*) As plasma osmolality increases beyond a threshold of approximately 280 mOsm·kg^{-1}, plasma arginine vasopressin (antidiuretic hormone) progressively increases. (*Bottom*) As plasma concentrations of arginine vasopressin (AVP) increase, urinary osmolality progressively increases to reach a plateau of approximately 1200 mOsm·kg^{-1}. (Reproduced with permission from Hall J, Robertson G: Diabetes insipidus. In Kirby RR, Taylor RW (eds): Problems in Critical Care. vol 4. Endocrine Emergencies (GP Zaloga, guest ed), p 343. Philadelphia: JB Lippincott, 1990.)

tubules, high concentrations of aldosterone may reduce urinary excretion of sodium nearly to zero.

The kidney also contains large quantities of prostaglandin metabolites that appear to modulate changes in renal vascular tone and glomerular filtration produced by other hormones.[15] Vasodilator prostaglandins may play a crucial role in protecting the kidney from the effects of systemic vasoconstrictor hormones and for maintaining RBF during hypovolemia. The protective effect of endogenous renal prostaglandins may be lost if renal circulatory compromise develops in patients receiving nonsteroidal anti-inflammatory drugs.[16]

FLUID REPLACEMENT THERAPY

Maintenance Fluid Requirements

Water

In healthy adults, sufficient water is required to balance gastrointestinal losses of 100–200 ml·day^{-1}, insensible losses of 500–1000 ml·day^{-1} (half of which is respiratory and half cutaneous), and urinary losses of 1000 ml·day^{-1}. When deciding whether to replace urinary losses exceeding

TABLE 9-1. Maintenance Water Requirements

	$ml \cdot kg^{-1} \cdot h^{-1}$	$ml \cdot kg^{-1} \cdot day^{-1}$
1st–10th kg	4	100
11th–20th kg	2	50
21st–nth kg	1	20

1000 ml·day^{-1}, it is prudent to consider whether increased urinary output represents an appropriate physiologic response to ECV expansion or an inability to conserve salt or water. Two simple formulas are used interchangeably to estimate maintenance water requirements (Table 9-1).

Electrolytes

Renal sodium conservation is highly efficient, resulting in an average daily adult requirement of 75 mEq. However, normal kidneys can reduce sodium excretion to less than 10 mEq per day during chronic sodium depletion. Because the kidneys also efficiently excrete excess sodium, patients with normal cardiac and renal reserve may tolerate intravenous administration of sodium far in excess of normal daily requirements. Renal conservation and excretion of potassium is less efficient. Daily potassium requirements slightly exceed 40 mEq. Physiologic diuresis typically induces an obligate potassium loss of at least 10 mEq·l^{-1} of urine. Other electrolytes such as chloride, calcium, and magnesium require no short-term replacement, although they must be supplied during chronic intravenous fluid maintenance.

Combining the daily maintenance requirements for water, sodium, and potassium results in predicted maintenance intravenous fluid for healthy, 70-kg adults of 2500 ml·day^{-1} of a solution with a [Na$^+$] of 30 mEq·l^{-1} and a [K$^+$] of 15–20 mEq·l^{-1}. However, in practice, the [Na$^+$] in postoperatively administered fluids is typically 77 mEq·l^{-1}. Approximately one half of the volume of this fluid, colloquially termed "half-normal" saline, is sodium-free water. Intraoperatively, fluids containing free water are rarely employed in adults, largely because of the necessity for replacing losses of PV and IF, both of which are sodium rich.

Dextrose

Traditionally, glucose-containing intravenous fluids have been given in an effort to prevent hypoglycemia and limit protein catabolism. However, due to the hyperglycemic response associated with surgical stress, only infants and patients receiving insulin or drugs that interfere with glucose synthesis are at risk for hypoglycemia. Iatrogenic hyperglycemia can limit the effectiveness of fluid resuscitation by

inducing an osmotic diuresis and, in animals, may aggravate global and focal neurologic ischemic injury.[17-19] The clinical influence of hyperglycemia on neurologic injury in humans is less well defined. Although hyperglycemia is associated with worse outcome in both ischemic[20] and traumatic[21] brain injury, it is likely that the increase in blood glucose in patients is in fact a hormonally mediated accompaniment of more severe injury.[20] Sieber *et al* have concisely summarized the issue of intraoperative glucose administration by stating, "glucose administration is indicated during clinical situations where hypoglycemia is likely to occur."[22]

Surgical Fluid Requirements

Water and Electrolyte Composition of Fluid Losses

Surgical patients require replacement of PV and ECV losses secondary to wound or burn edema, ascites, and gastrointestinal secretions. Wound and burn edema and ascitic fluid are protein rich and contain electrolytes in concentrations similar to plasma. If ECV is adequate and renal and cardiovascular function are normal, all gastrointestinal secretions (Table 9-2) can be replaced using lactated Ringer's solution or 0.9% ("normal") saline. Substantial loss of gastrointestinal fluids requires replacement of other electrolytes (i.e., potassium, magnesium, phosphate). However, if cardiovascular or renal function is impaired, more precise replacement may require frequent assessment of serum electrolytes. Chronic gastric losses may produce hypochloremic metabolic alkalosis that can be corrected with 0.9% saline; chronic diarrhea may produce hyperchloremic metabolic acidosis that may be prevented or corrected by infusion of fluid containing bicarbonate or bicarbonate substrate (i.e., lactate).

Fluid Shifts During Surgery

Replacement of intraoperative fluid losses must compensate for the acute reduction of functional IF that accompanies trauma, hemorrhage, and tissue manipulation. This reduction, often called "third-space" loss,[23,24] is surprisingly extensive. Upper abdominal surgery not involving major hemorrhage is associated with a 15% decline in functional ECV, the reservoir available for physiologic repletion of PV in response to hypovolemia.[23] Otherwise healthy subjects undergoing gastric or gallbladder surgery demonstrate a decline in ECV of nearly 2 liters and an acute 13% decline in GFR when they receive no intraoperative sodium.[23] In contrast, patients who receive lactated Ringer's solution maintain ECV and increase GFR by 10%. In more extensive surgical procedures, the decrease in ECV is presumably much greater.

TABLE 9-2. Average Volumes and Electrolyte Composition of Gastrointestinal Secretions

Source	Volume (ml·day^{-1})	Na$^+$ (mEq·l^{-1})	K$^+$ (mEq·l^{-1})	Cl$^-$ (mEq·l^{-1})	HCO$_3^-$ (mEq·l^{-1})
Gastric	1500	60	10	130	—
Ileal	3000	140	5	104	30
Pancreatic	400	140	5	75	115
Biliary	400	140	5	100	35

For ethical reasons, there are no data describing acute changes in PV, IF, and ICV during acute, unresuscitated shock in humans. In response to mild hemorrhage, physiologic defenses rapidly reconstitute PV. In humans, hypovolemia has been associated with net transfer of IF to PV at a rate as great as 500 ml every 10 minutes.[25] In contrast, during prolonged experimental hemorrhagic shock, both sodium and water accumulate intracellularly.[26] Shock depletes energy stores and impairs cellular membrane function; shock-induced depletion of high-energy substrates contributes to cellular swelling[27] because sodium is pulled intracellularly by nondiffusible, intracellular, anionic solutes, primarily organic phosphates and proteins. Sodium, in turn, draws water along an osmotic gradient. Most investigators believe that shock-induced alterations in cellular membrane function and intracellular concentrations of sodium return to normal once systemic hemodynamic stability is restored. Patients studied during the first 10 days after resuscitation from massive trauma or sepsis in fact demonstrate a slight percentage decrease in ICV[28]; however, total body weight is increased in these patients as a consequence of a 55% increase in IF volume (Fig. 9-4).[28] As would be expected, because of the reduction of colloid oncotic pressure in trauma patients, the ratio of IF to blood volume is increased, in some patients exceeding 5:1.[28]

Based on estimates of the magnitude of the sequestration of fluid associated with extensive tissue manipulation, guidelines have been developed for replacement of third-spaces losses during high-risk surgical procedures. The simplest formula provides, in addition to maintenance fluids and replacement of estimated blood loss, 4 ml·kg^{-1}·h^{-1} for procedures involving minimal trauma, 6 ml·kg^{-1}·h^{-1} for those involving moderate trauma, and 8 ml·kg^{-1}·h^{-1} for those involving extreme trauma.[29]

Mobilization of Expanded Interstitial Fluid

An important corollary of IF expansion is the mobilization and return of accumulated fluid to the ECV and the PV, colloquially termed "deresuscitation" (Fig. 9-5). In most patients, mobilization occurs on approximately the third postoperative day, although it may occur sooner or later, depending on patient characteristics, the severity and duration of the initial insult, and the development of postoperative complications such as acute renal failure or sepsis. If the cardiovascular system and kidneys can effectively transport and excrete mobilized fluid, no important physiologic consequences follow. However, should the cardiovascular system be unable to accommodate the increase in intravascular

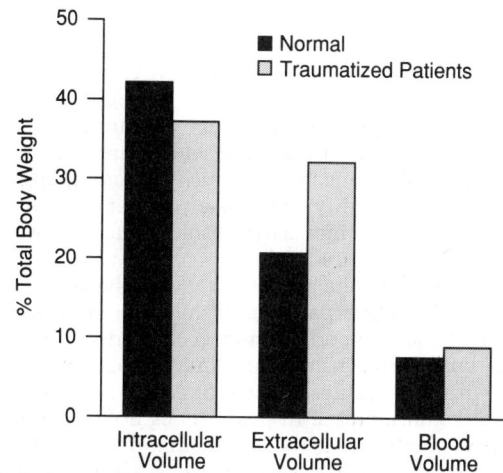

Figure 9-4. In comparison with normal individuals, patients recently subjected to severe trauma (fluid and blood requirements exceeding an average of 21 liters on the day of admission) have a slight decrease in intracellular volume (as percentage of body weight) and an increase in extracellular volume and blood volume. (Data redrawn with permission from Böck JC *et al:* Post-traumatic changes in effective colloid osmotic pressure on the distribution of body water. Ann Surg 210:398, 1989.)

volume or the kidneys be unable to increase urinary volume (*i.e.,* due to renal insufficiency or to stress-induced secretion of ADH), hypervolemia and pulmonary edema may occur.

COLLOIDS, CRYSTALLOIDS, AND HYPERTONIC SOLUTIONS

Physiology and Pharmacology

Intravenous fluids vary in oncotic pressure, osmolarity, and tonicity. Osmotically active particles attract water across semipermeable membranes until equilibrium is attained. The *osmolarity* of a solution, which quantifies the forces determining the distribution of water, refers to the number of osmotically active particles per *liter* of solution. In contrast, *osmolality* is a measurement of the number of osmotically active particles per *kilogram* of solvent.

The osmotic activity of body fluids, conventionally reported as *osmolality* (in mmol·kg^{-1}), can be estimated as

Figure 9-5. In the presence of untreated, prolonged hemorrhagic shock, the functional extracellular volume (ECV) is diminished by sequestration of sodium and water that is unavailable to the systemic circulation. During resuscitation, the interstitial fluid (IF) expands, as is frequently evident from accumulation of peripheral edema. During recovery, sodium and water from the expanded IF are returned to the plasma volume (PV), at which time they must be excreted by the kidneys. If the cardiovascular system and kidneys cannot adequately manage the mobilized fluid, pulmonary edema may result.

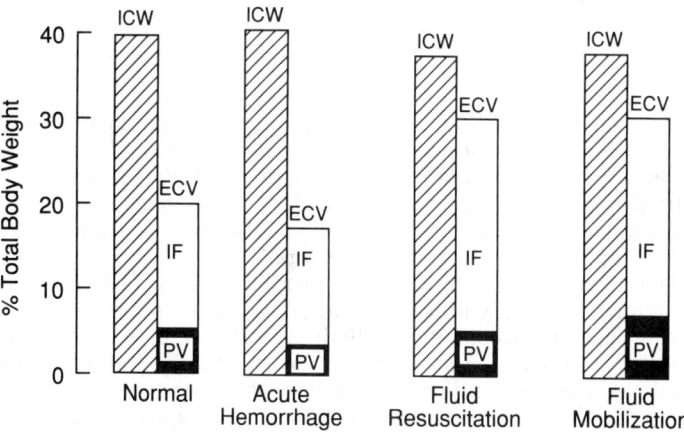

follows:

$$\text{Osmolality} = ([Na^+] \times 2) + (\text{Glucose} \div 18) + (\text{BUN} \div 2.3)$$

where $[Na^+]$ is expressed in $mEq \cdot l^{-1}$, serum glucose is expressed in $mg \cdot dl^{-1}$, and BUN is blood urea nitrogen expressed in $mg \cdot dl^{-1}$. Sugars, alcohols, and radiographic dyes that increase osmolality may falsely lower the calculated value, generating an increased "osmolal gap" between the calculated and measured values.

A hyperosmolar state occurs whenever the concentration of osmotically active particles is high. Thus, uremia (increased BUN) and hypernatremia (increased serum sodium) increase both serum osmolality and osmolarity. However, because urea distributes throughout TBW, an increase in BUN, unlike an increase in $[Na^+]$, does not cause *hypertonicity*. An osmotically active solute that does not distribute evenly throughout body water causes a shift of water into the compartment in which the solute is concentrated. Therefore, because sodium is largely restricted to the ECV, hypernatremia causes hypertonicity, *i.e.*, osmotically mediated redistribution of water from ICV to ECV. The term "tonicity" is also used colloquially to compare the osmotic pressure of a solution to that of plasma. A fluid in which the osmotic pressure is similar to that of plasma is termed isotonic. Hypotonic solutions exert lower osmotic pressures than plasma; hypertonic solutions exert higher osmotic pressures.

Although only a small proportion of the osmotically active particles in blood consist of plasma proteins, those particles are essential in determining the equilibrium of fluid between the interstitial and plasma compartments of ECV. Because systemic capillary beds are only semipermeable to plasma proteins, interstitial protein concentrations remain lower than plasma.

The reflection coefficient (σ) describes the permeability of capillary membranes to individual solutes, with 0 representing free permeability and 1.0 representing complete impermeability. The reflection coefficient for albumin ranges from 0.6 to 0.9 in various capillary beds. Because capillary protein concentration exceeds interstitial concentrations, the osmotic pressure exerted by plasma proteins (termed *oncotic pressure*) is higher than interstitial oncotic pressure and tends to preserve PV. The filtration rate of fluid from the capillaries into the interstitial space is the net result of a combination of forces, including the gradient from intravascular to interstitial colloid oncotic pressures and the hydrostatic gradient between intravascular and interstitial pressures. The net fluid filtration at any point within a systemic or pulmonary capillary is represented by Starling's law of capillary filtration (Fig. 9-6), as expressed in the equation:

$$Q = kA [(P_c - P_i) + \sigma(\pi_i - \pi_c)]$$

where Q = fluid filtration, k = capillary filtration coefficient (conductivity of water), A = the area of the capillary membrane, P_c = capillary hydrostatic pressure, P_i = interstitial hydrostatic pressure, σ = reflection coefficient for albumin, π_i = interstitial colloid oncotic pressure, and π_c = capillary colloid oncotic pressure.

The IF volume is determined by the relative rates of capillary filtration and lymphatic drainage; homeostatic mechanisms acutely accommodate limited amounts of excess fluid. P_c, the most powerful factor favoring fluid filtration, is determined by capillary flow, arterial resistance, venous resistance, and venous pressure.[30] Increased capillary fil-

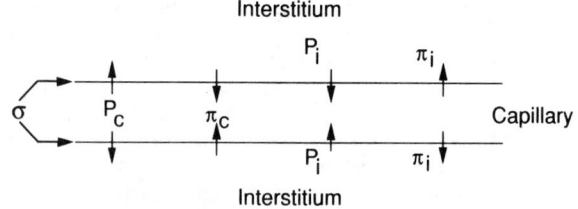

Figure 9-6. Movement of fluid between the capillaries and the interstitium is a function of hydrostatic pressure in the capillaries (P_c) and in the interstitium (P_i) and oncotic pressure in the capillaries (π_c) and in the interstitium (π_i). The permeability of the capillary membrane to albumin is described by the reflection coefficient, σ.

tration alters the balance of forces in the Starling equilibrium. Usually, the rate of water and sodium filtration exceeds protein filtration, resulting in preservation of π_c, dilution of π_i, and preservation of the oncotic pressure gradient, the most powerful factor opposing fluid filtration. When coupled with increased lymphatic drainage, preservation of the oncotic pressure gradient limits the accumulation of IF. Though IF contains less protein than plasma, the interstitium contains glycosaminoglycans and proteoglycans, which absorb fluid (Fig. 9-7). As increased IF decreases the concentrations of glycosaminoglycans and proteoglycans, fluid and protein drain more freely into the lymphatics.[31] If P_c is increased at a time when lymphatic drainage is maximal, then IF accumulates, forming edema. In chronic edematous states, IF pressure is reduced by enhanced lymphatic drainage through dilated lymphatic vessels.[32] The proteoglycans in the vascular basement membrane also help to maintain normal vascular permeability. Dilution of this proteoglycan matrix increases while dehydration of the interstitium reduces vascular permeability.[30]

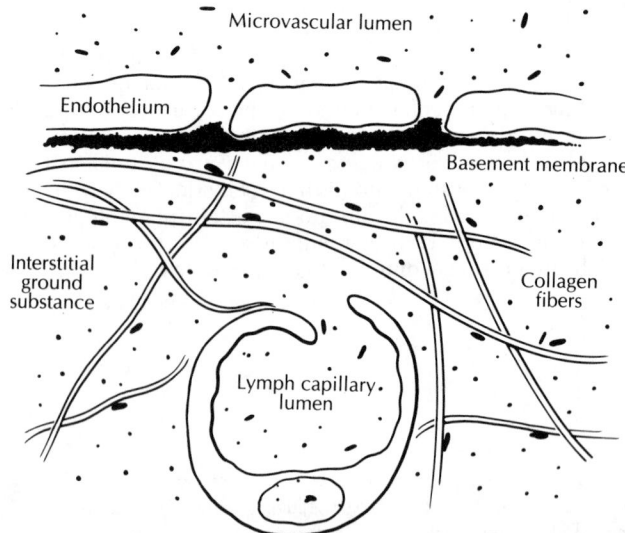

Figure 9-7. As fluid enters the interstitium from the microvascular lumen, most of it is absorbed by the interstitial ground substance, which includes proteoglycans and aminoglycosans. Free fluid enters the lymph capillary lumen for transport back to the circulation. (Reproduced with permission from Demling RH: Shock and fluids. In Chernow B, Shoemaker WC (eds): Critical Care: State of the Art, vol 7, p 308. Fullerton, California, Society of Critical Care Medicine, 1986.)

TABLE 9-3. Advantages and Disadvantages of Colloid *vs.* Crystalloid Intravenous Fluids

Solution	Advantages	Disadvantages
Colloid	Smaller infused volume Prolonged increase in plasma volume Minimal peripheral edema Lower intracranial pressure*	Greater expense Coagulopathy (dex. > HES) Pulmonary edema (capillary leak states) Decreased Ca^{2+} (alb.) Decreased GFR Osmotic diuresis (low molecular weight dextran)
Crystalloid	Less expense Greater urinary flow Replaces interstitial fluid	Short-lived hemodynamic improvement Peripheral edema Pulmonary edema*

*Conflicting data.

HES = hydroxyethyl starch; GFR = glomerular filtration rate

If membrane permeability is intact, fluids containing colloids such as albumin or hydroxyethyl starch preferentially expand PV rather than IF volume. Concentrated colloid-containing solutions (*i.e.*, 25% albumin) may exert sufficient oncotic pressure to translocate substantial volumes of IF into the PV. PV expansion unaccompanied by IF expansion offers apparent advantages: lower fluid requirements, less peripheral and pulmonary edema accumulation, and reduced concern about the cardiopulmonary consequences of later fluid mobilization.

However, exhaustive research has failed to establish the superiority of either colloid-containing or crystalloid-containing fluids.[33] Colloid solutions require a smaller initial infused volume, generate a more prolonged increase in PV, are associated with less peripheral edema, and, perhaps, are less likely to increase intracranial pressure (Table 9-3). Crystalloid is less expensive, tends to increase glomerular filtration, and more effectively replaces depleted IF. However, crystalloid fluids exert short-lived hemodynamic effects in comparison to colloid and, when used for massive resuscitation, invariably produce peripheral edema. Crystalloid solutions are also associated with pulmonary edema, usually as a result of increased left atrial pressure, perhaps in combination with a reduction of the gradient between π_c and pulmonary P_c. The disadvantages of colloid-containing fluids include greater expense, coagulopathy (especially with dextran), a reduction in ionized calcium (with albumin), impaired cross-matching (with dextran), a reduction in GFR, and osmotic diuresis (with low molecular weight dextran). Finally, in disease states associated with increased alveolar capillary permeability (*i.e.*, sepsis or the adult respiratory distress syndrome), infusion of colloid may aggravate pulmonary edema. If microvascular permeability increases (*i.e.*, σ decreases), as commonly occurs in response to injury, infection, or prolonged tissue hypoperfusion, the gradient between π_c and π_i diminishes. In the absence of an oncotic pressure gradient, the hydraulic gradient is unopposed and minimal increases in P_c can result in clinically important edema accumulation.

Although synthetic colloids are less expensive than albumin, one concern has been laboratory evidence of coagulopathy associated with large doses of hydroxyethyl starch.[34] However, 6.0% hydroxyethyl starch, used in recommended volumes, is not apparently associated with clinically important coagulopathy.[35-39] Gold *et al* randomly assigned 40 patients undergoing repair of abdominal aortic aneurysms to receive either 5.0% albumin or 6.0% hydroxyethyl starch in a dose of 1 $g \cdot kg^{-1}$ (approximately 1200 ml of the albumin solution or 1100 ml of the hydroxyethyl starch solution in a 70-kg adult).[35] All objective measurements of coagulation status at all intervals were comparable and were within normal limits. Blood loss, total fluid required, and subjective assessment of surgical bleeding were similar. The use of hydroxyethyl starch has also resulted in no evidence of coagulopathy in patients undergoing surgery for multisystem trauma,[36] major abdominal surgery,[37] and cardiac surgery.[38,39]

Part of the difficulty in defining the superiority of crystalloid or colloid fluids is directly attributable to the difficulty of defining comparable experimental end points (Table 9-4).[40,41] Because PV expansion persists longer after colloid administration, substantially greater quantities of crystalloid must be given to maintain comparable systemic hemodynamics. In general, to achieve comparable PV expansion, isotonic crystalloid must be infused in a volume at least fourfold greater than volumes of iso-oncotic colloid solutions. Infusion of 1000 ml of iso-oncotic colloid solutions significantly increases PV for at least 2 hours after infusion, whereas 1000 ml of lactated Ringer's solution produces a significantly smaller increase than iso-oncotic colloids 1 and 2 hours after administration.[42] The necessity for infusion of four times as much crystalloid as colloid, which reflects the normal 4:1 ratio of IF to PV, may be exaggerated in hypoproteinemic trauma patients, in whom the ratio may be much higher.[28]

More recently developed experimental models compare crystalloid and colloid solutions in specific, clinically modeled situations. Baum *et al*, comparing lactated Ringer's solution to 6.0% hydroxyethyl starch dissolved in 0.9% saline in animals infused with *E. coli* lipopolysaccharide, evaluated mesenteric blood flow, mesenteric oxygen delivery, ileal hydrogen ion concentration, and ileal and pulmonary extravascular water.[43] In that model, which mimics some aspects of clinical sepsis, clinically relevant doses of lactated Ringer's solution or 6.0% hydroxyethyl starch produced comparable effects on the critical end point of oxygen delivery while producing the expected differences in extravascular fluid accumulation. The efficacy with which various colloids restore oxygen transport after surgical hemorrhagic shock has been investigated in a more complex porcine model, consisting of temporary exteriorization of the small intestine accompanied by incremental hemorrhage and replacement.[44] Colloid solutions, in contrast to Ringer's acetate solution, produced superior restoration of

TABLE 9-4. Possible End Points for Comparison of Resuscitation Fluids

End Point	Advantages	Disadvantages
Equal volume	Simple calculation	Different acute effects and time course
Equal sodium load	Simple calculation	Different acute effects and time course
Equal preload (i.e., CVP, PAOP)	Simple, continuous measurement	Determined by multiple, simultaneously changing variables
Equal cardiac output	Simple measurement, easily repeated	Misleading if fluids differently affect hemoglobin concentration
Equal Do_2	Logical, physiologically appealing end point	Difficult calculation to perform frequently; calculated from two simultaneously changing variables
Equal Vo_2	Physiologically important variable	Difficult calculation to perform frequently; calculated from simultaneously changing variables

CVP = central venous pressure, PAOP = pulmonary artery occlusion pressure, Do_2 = systemic oxygen delivery, Vo_2 = systemic oxygen consumption.

Reproduced with permission from Prough DS, Johnston WE: Fluid resuscitation in septic shock: No solution yet. Anesth Analg 69:699, 1989.

cardiac output, oxygen delivery, and oxygen consumption. Although the results are intriguing, one possible interpretation is that an insufficient volume of Ringer's acetate was infused.

One of the most intriguing developments in colloid research is the possibility that pentafraction, the generic name attached to hydroxyethyl starch molecules of a specific size range (100,000–1,000,000 daltons), may actually counteract increases in capillary permeability associated with a variety of lesions, including myocardial ischemia,[45] scalded rat jejunum,[46] ischemic muscle,[47] and endotoxin-damaged lung.[48] In such models, fluid accumulation in injured tissue and permeability to protein are substantially reduced. If these data can be confirmed in clinical states associated with increased permeability, pentafraction may offer major therapeutic advantages in hypovolemic patients with sepsis or the adult respiratory distress syndrome.

Pulmonary Implications of Colloid Oncotic Pressure

Much of the acrimonious controversy regarding the merits of perioperative fluid therapy with either colloids or crystalloids stems from the perceived influence of the two types of fluids on the risk of pulmonary edema in patients who have diseases that increase pulmonary P_c, decrease π_c, or increase microvascular permeability (i.e., decrease σ). Some clinicians preferentially administer colloid solutions to reduce the risk of pulmonary edema. However, either crystalloid or colloid administration may precipitate pulmonary edema in patients who have valvular heart disease, decreased left ventricular compliance, or decreased left ventricular contractility (i.e., heart failure). Increased left atrial pressure increases filtration from PV into IF, and if fluid accumulates, into the alveoli. The peak increase in left atrial pressure after colloid infusion may be delayed and sustained because of the time-dependent shift of IF to PV as a consequence of increased π_c. Colloid-induced PV expansion redistributes slowly; if pulmonary edema develops, diuretic therapy is often required.

The administration of large volumes of crystalloid solutions dilutes serum protein concentrations, reduces π_c, and enhances interstitial accumulation of fluid. Hypoproteinemia has been associated with the development of pulmonary edema[49,50] and with increased mortality in critically ill patients.[51] However, increasing filtration of protein-poor fluid dilutes pulmonary π_i, increases P_i, and enhances lymphatic flow. These physiologic defenses must be overwhelmed before the accumulation of interstitial fluid results in clinically apparent pulmonary edema. The use of colloid-containing fluids that maintain π_c does not prevent pulmonary edema. Excessive colloid administration may even elevate pulmonary artery occlusion pressure (PAOP), thus reducing the gradient between π_c and PAOP.

There appear to be no important clinical differences in pulmonary function after administration of crystalloid or colloid solutions in the absence of hypervolemia.[52-57] Despite moderate experimental increases in microvascular permeability, Pearl et al found no differences between increases in extravascular lung water induced by colloid or crystalloid.[58] Uncomplicated hemorrhagic shock can be treated with either crystalloid or colloid without undue concern regarding pulmonary edema.[30] However, sustained, untreated hypoperfusion can result in increased microvascular permeability as a consequence of the initiation of a variety of tissue-injuring processes.[59] Shock-induced microvascular injury is associated with noncardiogenic pulmonary edema regardless of whether crystalloid or colloid is administered.

In surgical patients at risk for the development of pulmonary edema, pulmonary artery catheterization may facilitate management. If the σ for albumin is likely to be decreased, pulmonary fluid accumulation becomes highly dependent on pulmonary P_c; therefore PAOP should be maintained at the lowest practical level. However, if increased microvascular permeability occurs in conjunction with hypovolemia, administration of fluid to improve organ perfusion directly conflicts with the goal of minimizing pulmonary P_c. Theoretically, hemodynamic monitoring coupled with volume expansion with colloid should minimize edema formation. However, Virgilio et al found no correlation in surgical patients between intrapulmonary shunt fraction (Q_s/Q_t) and the π_c–PAOP gradient (Fig. 9-8).[56]

Implications of Crystalloid and Colloid Infusions for Intracranial Pressure

Because the cerebral capillary membrane, the blood-brain barrier, is highly impermeable to protein, clinicians have assumed that administration of colloid-containing solutions should increase intracranial pressure (ICP) less than crystalloid solutions. In fact, in rabbits subjected to isovolemic hemodilution with 6.0% hetastarch or lactated Ringer's solution, the Ringer's solution was associated with a significant increase in ICP and brain water; no significant changes occurred in animals that had received 6.0% hetastarch.[60] In dogs subjected to hemorrhagic shock in the presence of an intracranial mass lesion, resuscitation with 6.0% hetastarch resulted in a significantly lower ICP than did resuscitation with lactated Ringer's solution.[61] However, in both studies, the difference probably occurred because 6.0% hetastarch is dissolved in 0.9% saline ([Na^+] = 154 mEq·l^{-1}). In contrast to 0.9% saline, lactated Ringer's solution ([Na^+] = 130 mEq·l^{-1}) is slightly hyposmotic relative to serum.[47] In anesthetized rabbits subjected to plasmapheresis, a reduction in plasma osmolality of 13 mOsm·kg^{-1} (baseline value = 295 mOsm·kg^{-1}) increased cortical water content and ICP; a reduction in oncotic pressure from 20 to 7 mm Hg produced no significant change in either variable.[62] Subsequent studies in animals after forebrain ischemia[63] and cryogenic brain injury[64,65] also clearly indicate that oncotic pressure exerts little if any effect on brain water accumulation. A prolonged reduction in colloid oncotic pressure generates peripheral edema but not cerebral edema.[65]

Clinical Implications of Hypertonic Fluid Administration

An ideal alternative to conventional crystalloid and colloid fluids would be inexpensive, would produce minimal peripheral or pulmonary edema, and would generate sustained hemodynamic effects. In addition, the value for resuscitation of civilian or military trauma victims would be enhanced if the solution were effective even if administered in smaller volumes than conventional fluids.[66] Based on data gathered during the past decade, hypertonic, hypernatremic solutions appear to fulfill some of these criteria.

Although investigators have studied various hypertonic resuscitation solutions for much of this century,[67-74] current enthusiasm results from the work of Velasco et al.[75] They employed small volumes (6.0 ml·kg^{-1}) of 7.5% hypertonic saline as the sole resuscitative measure in lightly anesthetized dogs that had been subjected to sufficient hemorrhage (averaging 23 ± 2.1 ml·kg^{-1}) to reduce mean arterial pressure (MAP) to 45–50 mm Hg for 30 minutes. Hypertonic saline restored systolic blood pressure and cardiac output and increased mesenteric blood flow to greater than control values for 6 hours after resuscitation. All animals in a group that had undergone slightly greater hemorrhage survived after infusion of 4.0 ml·kg^{-1} of 7.5% saline.[75] Although post-treatment serum osmolality exceeded 330 mOsm·kg^{-1}, no animal showed adverse effects attributable to acute hypertonicity. The mechanism of hemodynamic improvement once was considered to be reflex systemic venoconstriction mediated by the arrival of a highly hypertonic mixture in the pulmonary circulation.[76,77] However, recent data suggest that the primary mechanism by which hyperosmotic saline increases venous return is by PV expansion.[78] The specific solute producing a hyperosmotic solution appears to be an

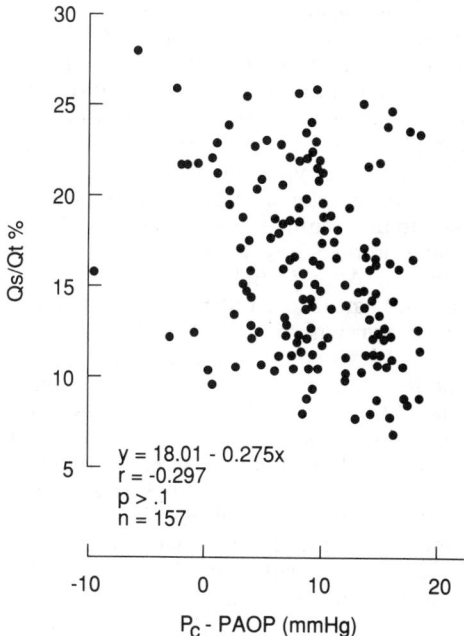

Figure 9-8. There is poor correlation between intrapulmonary shunt fraction (Q_s/Q_t%) and the difference between colloid oncotic pressure (COP) and pulmonary capillary wedge pressure (PCWP) in patients undergoing major surgical procedures. (Reproduced with permission from Virgilio RW *et al:* Balanced electrolyte solutions: Experimental and clinical studies. Crit Care Med 7:102, 1979.)

essential determinant of efficacy. In hemorrhaged, food-deprived rats, hyperosmotic sodium chloride produced 100% survival, in contrast to 78% survival in a group that received a glucose infusion of comparable osmolality.[79]

Although hyperosmotic saline solutions (usually 250–300 mEq·l^{-1} sodium) have been used for many years for burn resuscitation,[71,72] recent studies in animals and humans suggest that highly hyperosmotic (7.5% sodium chloride in 6.0% dextran 70)[80] or less hyperosmotic saline (250 mEq·l^{-1} sodium)[81] are of limited value. In sheep subjected to a scald burn of 40% of body surface area, resuscitation with hyperosmotic saline-dextran (4 ml·kg^{-1}) only transiently improved hemodynamics. The only apparent advantage over conventional isosmotic (0.9% saline) resuscitation was a slightly longer interval before additional fluid therapy was required.[80] In burned adults randomly assigned to receive lactated Ringer's solution or hyperosmotic saline to achieve comparable hemodynamic end points, the hyperosmotic solution did not decrease total fluid requirements, improve tolerance to feedings, or decrease edema accumulation.[81]

Hypertonic solutions exert favorable effects on cerebral hemodynamics, in part because of the reciprocal relationship between plasma osmolality and brain water.[62] ICP increases during resuscitation from hemorrhagic shock with lactated Ringer's solution but remains unchanged if 7.5% saline is infused in a sufficient volume to comparably improve systemic hemodynamics.[82,83] In anesthetized rabbits, hypertonic lactated Ringer's solution (252 mEq·l^{-1} [Na^+]) maintains a lower ICP than 0.9% saline after isovolemic hemodilution.[84] In hemorrhaged rats subjected to mechanical brain injury, brain water content in the injured hemisphere increases regardless of the resuscitation solution, but water content is lower in uninjured brain after resuscitation with a hyperosmotic solution.[85] In dogs with intracranial mass lesions, hypertonic solutions may also restore regional cerebral blood flow better than slightly hypotonic solutions.[86] However, recent data also suggest that differences between fluids of varying tonicity may become negligible if fluid resuscitation continues after immediate stabilization.[87]

Resuscitation with hyperosmotic solutions requires ongoing attention to maintenance of intravascular volume. Unfortunately, in most animal models, systemic hemodynamic improvement produced by hypertonic resuscitation has not been sustained. After initial improvement, both cerebral blood flow and cardiac output rapidly decline after single-dose resuscitation with either lactated Ringer's solution or hypertonic saline in pentobarbital-anesthetized dogs.[83] In a canine model of oleic acid–induced pulmonary edema, 7.5% saline (5.0 ml·kg^{-1} iv) produced prompt increases in cardiac output and systolic and diastolic pressures, but the improvement had largely disappeared 30 minutes after injection.[88] In experimental endotoxic shock, acute improvements in MAP, cardiac output, and left ventricular stroke work associated with a combination hypertonic/hyperoncotic solution had greatly diminished by 60 minutes after infusion, despite continued maintenance of PAOP with additional fluid.[89]

The transient effects of hypertonic saline administration represent a major obstacle to wider clinical application. Possible strategies that might prolong the therapeutic effects beyond 30–60 minutes include continued infusion of hypertonic saline, subsequent infusion of blood or conventional fluids, or addition of colloid to hypertonic resuscitation. Combined hyperoncotic/hypertonic saline solutions appear to exert more sustained effects. Jelenko and colleagues resuscitated burn patients by adding albumin to a solution containing 240 mEq·l^{-1} of sodium.[70] In hemorrhaged animals, adding 6.0% Dextran 70 to 7.5% saline increased the duration of hemodynamic improvement when compared with equal volumes of hypertonic saline, sodium bicarbonate, or sodium chloride/sodium acetate.[90] In traumatized patients, the combination of 6.0% Dextran 70 in 7.5% saline is as safe and effective as the initial intravenous infusion.[91]

Initial concerns regarding the adverse neurologic sequelae of hypertonic resuscitation appear to have been premature. First, the increment in serum sodium in response to addition of concentrated sodium is less than would be expected.[92] Second, patients tolerate acute increases in serum sodium to 155–160 mEq·l^{-1} without apparent harm.[91,93] Third, central pontine myelinolysis, which follows rapid correction of severe hyponatremia,[94,95] appears to be most likely after correction of chronic hyponatremia[96] and has not been observed in clinical trials of hypertonic resuscitation.[91] The least encouraging observations regarding hyperosmotic resuscitation involve models of uncontrolled hemorrhage,[97,98] in which hyperosmotic solutions increase bleeding and may adversely affect mortality.[98] However, hyperosmotic solutions may still offer superior prehospital restoration of blood pressure.[97]

The clinical efficacy of hypertonic resuscitation in comparison to conventional fluids remains unclear because most preclinical studies have compared the effects of single boluses of experimental and control fluids. Although such a design may duplicate acute field resuscitation after military or civilian trauma, routine fluid resuscitation rarely consists of a single bolus; rather, it continues until clinical signs indicate that no additional fluid is required. If single boluses of equal volumes of fluids of markedly differing tonicity are compared, the results of the comparison are predictable. Therefore, 6.0 ml·kg^{-1} of 0.9% saline should not be expected to produce hemodynamic effects equivalent to 6.0 ml·kg^{-1} of 7.5% saline. An attempt to simulate the clinical situation necessitates a choice among a variety of possible goals of resuscitation (Table 9-5). PAOP reflects the interaction of multiple variables, including blood volume, venous capacitance, and left ventricular afterload, diastolic compliance, and contractility. Consequently, comparison of two or more resuscitation regimens that alter more than one variable may generate misleading conclusions. For example, because hypertonic fluids reduce systemic vascular resistance, systolic ventricular ejection may improve, leading to decreased PAOP; theoretically, therefore, more fluid would be necessary to restore a filling pressure similar to that produced by a colloid solution. Conversely, if hypertonicity-

---

TABLE 9-5. Hypertonic Resuscitation Fluids: Advantages and Disadvantages

Solution	Advantages	Disadvantages
Hypertonic crystalloid	Inexpensive Promotes urinary flow Small initial volume Improved myocardial contractility Arteriolar dilation Reduced peripheral edema Lower intracranial pressure	Hypertonicity Precipitation of subdural hematoma Transient effect
Hypertonic crystalloid plus colloid (in comparison to hypertonic crystalloid alone)	More sustained hemodynamic response Reduced subsequent volume requirements	Added expense of colloid Coagulopathy (dex. > HES) Accelerated loss in capillary leak states Decreased Ca^{2+} (alb.) Renal failure (dextran) Osmotic diuresis Impaired cross-match (dextran) Hypertonicity

HES = hydroxyethyl starch

Reproduced with permission from Prough DS, Johnston WE: Fluid resuscitation in septic shock: No solution yet. Anesth Analg 69:699, 1989.

induced venoconstriction reduces the size of the capacitance bed, as suggested by Velasco et al,[75] a given blood volume should produce a greater PAOP. Therefore, the observation that hypertonic solutions do not reduce the volume of fluid required after the initial bolus may apply only if PAOP is used as the goal of resuscitation.

More physiologically sophisticated goals, also based on invasive monitoring, have been proposed. A predetermined level of systemic oxygen delivery (Do_2) is a theoretically attractive end point for resuscitation. It combines in a single term cardiac output (Q) and arterial oxygen content (Cao_2) according to the equation:

$$Do_2 = Q \cdot Cao_2 \cdot 10$$

where the factor 10 corrects Cao_2, usually measured in ml $O_2 \cdot dl^{-1}$, to $ml \cdot l^{-1}$.

However, because asanguineous fluid resuscitation both increases cardiac output and decreases hemoglobin concentration, the application of Do_2 as a goal poses practical difficulties. For example, cardiac output acutely increased 70% in response to infusion of hypertonic saline in animals with oleic acid–induced pulmonary edema.[88] Because the acute increase in cardiac output greatly exceeded the acute 12% decline in hemoglobin concentration, Do_2 increased. However, as the effects on cardiac output dissipated, the hemoglobin remained lower than preinfusion values, resulting in a small decline in Do_2 from preinfusion levels. Despite the straightforward arithmetic implications of simultaneous increases in cardiac output and decreases in Cao_2, many clinicians attempt to increase cardiac output (whether or not it is directly measured) as a goal during rapid volume expansion.

Will clinicians routinely use hypertonic or combination hypertonic/hyperoncotic fluids for resuscitation in the future? At present, there is no clear answer. Burn resuscitation is the only clinical situation in which hypertonic resuscitation solutions are commonly employed. Pending further preclinical work, the theoretical advantages of such fluids appear most attractive in the acute resuscitation of hypovolemic patients who have decreased intracranial compliance.

FLUID STATUS: ASSESSMENT AND MONITORING

Assessment of Hypovolemia and Tissue Hypoperfusion

Two contrasting methods are used to assess the adequacy of intravascular volume. The first, conventional clinical assessment, is appropriate for most patients; the second, goal-directed hemodynamic management, may be superior for high-risk surgical patients.

Preoperative Clinical Assessment

The ability to estimate the adequacy of intravascular volume is a critical skill. Unfortunately, clinical quantification of blood volume and ECV is difficult. An approximation begins with the recognition of settings in which deficits are likely, such as protracted gastrointestinal losses, bowel obstruction, bowel perforation, preoperative bowel preparation, chronic hypertension, chronic diuretic use, sepsis, burns, pancreatitis, and trauma.

The physical signs of hypovolemia are insensitive and nonspecific. However, suggestive evidence includes oliguria, supine hypotension, and a positive tilt test. Oliguria suggests the presence of hypovolemia, although hypovolemic patients may be nonoliguric and normovolemic patients may be oliguric because of renal failure or stress-induced endocrine responses. Supine hypotension implies a blood volume deficit exceeding 30%. However, arterial blood pressure within the normal range could represent relative hypotension in an elderly or chronically hypertensive patient. Substantial depletion of blood volume and organ hypoperfusion may occur despite an apparently normal blood pressure and heart rate.

In the tilt test, one of the traditional methods of assessing intravascular volume depletion, a positive response is defined as an increase in heart rate ≥ 20 beats$\cdot$min^{-1} and a decrease in systolic blood pressure ≥ 20 mm Hg when the subject assumes the upright position. However, a high incidence of false positive and false negative findings limits the value of the test. In general, classic studies[99] demonstrate that young, healthy subjects can withstand acute loss of 20% of blood volume while exhibiting only postural tachycardia and variable postural hypotension. Similar studies have not been performed in the elderly, those with autonomic dysfunction, those on chronic hypertensive therapy, and those who have reduced cardiovascular reserve. Twenty to 30% of elderly patients may demonstrate orthostatic changes in blood pressure despite normal blood volume.[100]

In an attempt to refine the traditional tilt test, Gotshall et al "tilted" normal and critically ill patients to 45 degrees while the legs were maintained in a horizontal position, and assessed responses using thoracic electrical bioimpedance, a noninvasive measurement of cardiac output.[101] In normal persons, as expected, heart rate and blood pressure did not change in the 45-degree head-up position, but cardiac index and stroke volume index significantly decreased, and systemic vascular resistance significantly increased.[101] Surprisingly, the heterogeneous group of critically ill patients exhibited no significant alterations in any variable.[101] In volunteers, Wong et al measured heart rate, blood pressure, and cardiac output using thoracic bioimpedance before and after withdrawing 500 ml of blood,[102] half of the blood volume depletion associated with a positive tilt test in normal individuals. Before blood withdrawal, standing produced a significant increase in heart rate (though less than 20 beats$\cdot$min^{-1}) and blood pressure; cardiac index and stroke volume index both decreased significantly. After blood withdrawal, heart rate increased an average of 21.5 beats$\cdot$min^{-1}, but blood pressure did not change. Changes in cardiac index and stroke volume index were comparable to the changes that occurred before blood withdrawal. Therefore, noninvasively measured cardiac index and stroke volume index during orthostatic challenge appear to offer little advantage over conventional assessment.

Orthostatic changes in filling pressure, coupled with assessment of the response to fluid infusion, may represent a more sensitive test of the adequacy of circulating blood volume. Amoroso et al examined changes in central venous pressure (CVP) as a function of position in a group of patients with chronic renal failure.[103] Baseline CVP, which averaged 0.1 cm H_2O, declined precipitously to a mean value of -9.7 cm H_2O when the patients assumed a 45-degree sitting posture. Infusion of fluid resulted in a small increase in the mean supine CVP to 2.3 cm H_2O but eliminated the marked postural decline in CVP.

Laboratory evidence that suggests hypovolemia or ECV depletion includes hemoconcentration, azotemia, low urinary sodium, metabolic alkalosis, and metabolic acidosis.

Hematocrit, a poor indicator of intravascular volume, changes in relationship to the magnitude of hemorrhage, the time elapsed since hemorrhage, and the volume of asanguineous replacement fluid. Hematocrit is virtually unchanged by acute hemorrhage; later, hemodilution occurs as fluids are administered or as fluid shifts from the interstitial to the intravascular space. If intravascular volume has been restored, hematocrit measurement will reflect red cell mass more accurately, and can be used to guide transfusion.

Both BUN and serum creatinine (SCr) may be increased if hypovolemia has been sufficiently prolonged. However, both measurements require careful interpretation. BUN, normally 8.0–20 mg·dl^{-1}, is increased by hypovolemia, high protein intake, gastrointestinal bleeding, or accelerated catabolism. Hepatic dysfunction decreases urea synthesis. Serum creatinine, a product of muscle catabolism, may be misleadingly low in elderly adults, in females, and in debilitated or malnourished patients. In contrast, in muscular or acutely catabolic patients, serum creatinine may exceed the normal range (0.5–1.5 mg·dl^{-1}) because of more rapid muscle breakdown. If the ratio of BUN:SCr exceeds the normal range (10–20), one should suspect dehydration or one of the individual factors that alter the serum concentration of the two metabolites. In prerenal oliguria, enhanced sodium reabsorption should reduce urinary sodium to ≤20 mEq·l^{-1} and enhanced water reabsorption should increase urinary concentration (i.e., urinary osmolality > 400; urine/plasma creatinine ratio > 40:1). However, the sensitivity and specificity of measurements of urinary sodium, osmolality, and creatinine ratios may be misleading in acute situations. Although hypovolemia does not generate metabolic alkalosis, ECV depletion is a potent stimulus for the maintenance of metabolic alkalosis. Severe hypovolemia may result in systemic hypoperfusion and lactic acidosis.

Intraoperative Clinical Assessment

Visual estimation, the simplest technique for quantifying intraoperative blood loss, assesses the amount of blood absorbed by gauze squares and laparotomy pads, and modifies the estimate depending on whether or not the sponges have been prerinsed in saline. An estimate of blood accumulation on the floor and surgical drapes and in the suction containers is then added. Both surgeons and anesthesia providers tend to underestimate losses, the magnitude of the error being directly proportional to the actual blood loss. Weighing blood-soaked gauze squares and laparotomy pads improves accuracy, but this tedious process is confounded by evaporation from the wet materials.

The adequacy of intraoperative fluid resuscitation during hemorrhagic shock cannot be ascertained by any single modality. Commonly measured clinical variables include heart rate, arterial blood pressure, urinary output, arterial oxygenation, and pH. Tachycardia is an insensitive, nonspecific indicator of hypovolemia. In patients receiving potent inhalational agents, maintenance of a satisfactory blood pressure implies adequate intravascular volume. Preservation of blood pressure, accompanied by a CVP of 6–12 mm Hg, more strongly suggests adequate replacement. During profound hypovolemia, indirect measurements of blood pressure may significantly underestimate true blood pressure. In patients undergoing extensive procedures, direct arterial pressure measurements are more accurate than indirect techniques and provide convenient access for obtaining arterial blood samples.

Urinary output usually declines precipitously during moderate to severe hypovolemia. Renal perfusion decreases after moderate hemorrhage in anesthetized mammals.[104]

Therefore, in the absence of glycosuria or diuretic administration, a urinary output of 0.5–1.0 ml·kg^{-1}·h^{-1} during anesthesia suggests adequate renal perfusion. Pulse oximetry is an unreliable indicator of decreased flow.[105] Arterial pH is an insensitive reflection of tissue perfusion since pH may decrease only in severe tissue hypoxia. Invasive measurement of cardiac output and PAOP may be more useful in patients with known cardiac disease or those who have recently sustained cardiac trauma (e.g., contusion).[106,107] However, cardiac output can be normal despite severely reduced regional blood flow. Mixed venous oxygenation, a sensitive indicator of poor systemic perfusion,[108] reflects average perfusion in multiple organs and cannot supplant regional monitors such as urinary output.

Goal-Directed Hemodynamic Management

No intraoperative monitor is sufficiently sensitive or specific to detect hypoperfusion in all patients. Moreover, certain postoperative surgical complications, such as acute renal failure, hepatic failure, and sepsis, may result from unrecognized, subclinical tissue hypoperfusion during the immediate perioperative period. Several important studies suggest that possibility.[109-112] Average cardiac output and Do$_2$ are greater in high-risk surgical patients who survive than in those who succumb to critical illness.[109,110,112] One key variable that appears to be highly associated with survival is a Do$_2$ ≥ 600 ml O$_2$·m^{-2}·min^{-1} (equivalent to a cardiac index of 3.0 l·m^{-2}·min^{-1}, a hemoglobin concentration of 14 g·dl^{-1}, and 98% oxyhemoglobin saturation). Therefore, Shoemaker et al adjusted hemodynamic therapy in high-risk surgical patients to achieve those hemodynamic values (including a Do$_2$ of 600 ml O$_2$·m^{-2}·min^{-1}).[111] In the first of two protocols they compared conventional management of a control surgical group that received conventional monitors, including a central venous pressure catheter, to goal-directed hemodynamic therapy. In the group treated by goal-directed management, survival was improved and complications were reduced.[111] In a second protocol, an additional control group received conventional monitoring supplemented by pulmonary artery catheterization without specific management guidelines. As in the first series, the protocol group that received goal-directed therapy had better survival and fewer complications.[111] The control group that underwent pulmonary artery catheterization but was managed without specific hemodynamic goals had a mortality complication rate equal to the group managed without a pulmonary artery catheter.[111] These data suggest that aggressive, goal-directed hemodynamic support in high-risk surgical patients reverses clinically inapparent hypoperfusion and as a consequence limits the mortality and morbidity secondary to that process. Similar management also appears to improve outcome in septic patients.[112] Confirmation, however, is essential before this concept can be recommended routinely.

ELECTROLYTES

Sodium

Physiologic Role

Increases or decreases in total body sodium, the principal extracellular cation and solute, tend to increase or decrease ECV and PV (Table 9-6). Because sodium is largely confined to ECV, disorders of sodium *concentration*, i.e., hypona-

TABLE 9-6. Physiologic Role of Electrolytes

Electrolyte	Roles
Sodium	Osmolality Extracellular volume Action potential
Potassium	Membrane potential Action potential
Calcium	Excitation-contraction Secretion Neurotransmission Mitosis Other structures requiring movement (*e.g.,* cilia) Second messenger Third messenger Enzyme activation Cardiac pacemaker activity Cardiac action potential Membrane structure Bone structure
Phosphorus	Stores energy (*i.e.,* ATP, creatine phosphate) Component of second messengers (*i.e.,* cAMP, phosphoinositides) Component of nucleic acids Component of membranes (*i.e.,* phospholipids) 2,3-diphosphoglycerate Protein phosphorylation Nicotinamide adenine dinucleotide phosphate (NADP) Urinary buffer
Magnesium	Enzyme cofactor (*i.e.,* sodium-potassium pump, Ca-ATPase, adenyl cyclase) Regulates slow calcium channels Regulates parathyroid gland secretion (calcium metabolism) Regulates end-organ sensitivity to parathyroid hormone and vitamin D Controls potassium movement into cells (Na–K ATPase) Membrane excitability Bone structure

TABLE 9-7. Regulation of Electrolytes

Electrolyte	Regulated by
Sodium	Aldosterone Atrial natriuretic peptide $[Na^+]$ altered by antidiuretic hormone, which affects water balance
Potassium	Aldosterone Epinephrine Insulin Intrinsic renal mechanisms
Calcium	Parathyroid hormone Vitamin D
Phosphorus	Primarily renal mechanisms Minor: Parathyroid hormone
Magnesium	Primarily renal mechanisms Minor: Parathyroid hormone, vitamin D

which, in the absence of adequate water intake, results in hypernatremia. In response to changes in plasma $[Na^+]$, changes in secretion of ADH can vary urinary osmolality from 50 to 1400 $mOsm \cdot kg^{-1}$ and urinary volume from 0.4 to 20 $l \cdot day^{-1}$ (see Fig. 9-3).

Hyponatremia

The signs and symptoms of hyponatremia depend on both the rate at which plasma $[Na^+]$ decreases and the severity of the decrease. Symptoms usually accompany $[Na^+] \leq 120$ $mEq \cdot l^{-1}$ (Table 9-8). Acute central nervous system (CNS) manifestations relate to brain overhydration. Although the blood-brain barrier (which separates blood from interstitial fluid) is poorly permeable to sodium, water equilibrates rapidly. Therefore, a decrease in plasma $[Na^+]$ promptly leads to an increase in both extracellular and intracellular brain water. The magnitude of brain swelling is limited by bulk movement of interstitial fluid into the cerebrospinal fluid and the loss of intracellular solutes,[113-115] including potassium and organic osmolytes (previously termed "idiogenic osmoles") such as taurine, phosphocreatine, myoinositol, glutamine, and glutamate.[116-118] Because the brain rapidly compensates for changes in osmolality, the symptoms of acute hyponatremia are considerably more severe than those of chronic hyponatremia at similar levels of plasma

tremia and hypernatremia, usually result from relative excesses or deficits, respectively, of water. The relationship between serum $[Na^+]$ (the primary solute that determines extracellular tonicity), serum potassium, and total body water is expressed by the equation:[113]

$$\text{Serum } [Na^+] = \frac{\text{total body sodium} + \text{total body potassium}}{\text{total body water}}$$

As one of the ions involved in the action potential, sodium also is essential for proper function of both neurologic and cardiac tissue.

Regulation of the quantity and concentration of sodium is accomplished primarily by the endocrine and renal systems (Table 9-7). *Total body sodium* is primarily regulated by aldosterone, which is responsible for renal sodium reabsorption in exchange for potassium and hydrogen.[12] In addition, when the cardiac atria are stretched, secretion of ANP increases renal sodium excretion and decreases PV.[8,10] *Sodium concentration* is primarily regulated by ADH, although ADH does not regulate sodium balance. Increased secretion of ADH in response to either osmotic or hemodynamic stimuli results in reabsorption of water by the kidneys and subsequent dilution of the plasma $[Na^+]$; inadequate ADH secretion results in renal free water excretion,

TABLE 9-8. Hyponatremia: Clinical Manifestations

Neurologic

Altered consciousness
Coma
Seizures
Cerebral edema

Gastrointestinal

Loss of appetite
Nausea
Vomiting

Muscular

Cramps
Weakness

[Na$^+$]. The symptoms of chronic hyponatremia probably relate to depletion of brain electrolytes. Cerebral edema is minimal if hyponatremia is chronic.[116,119] Once the brain has adapted by decreasing the intracellular concentrations of potassium and organic osmolytes, rapid correction of hyponatremia may lead to abrupt brain dehydration.

The occasional postoperative occurrence of hyponatremia, mental status changes, and seizures has been attributed historically to intravenous administration of hypotonic fluids and inappropriate secretion of ADH.[120] Prospective studies suggest that at least 4.0% of postoperative patients develop plasma [Na$^+$] < 130 mEq·l^{-1}.[121] Smaller females are most susceptible to rapid changes in sodium concentration in response to administration of hypotonic intravenous fluids. Administration of 200 ml·h^{-1} of sodium-free water to a 50-kg woman (in whom TBW would be estimated as 50% of body weight, or 25 liters) would reduce plasma [Na$^+$] by 1.0 mEq·l^{-1}·h^{-1}.[113] An 80-kg, muscular male, in whom TBW would be equal to 60% of body weight (48 liters), would require twice as rapid an infusion of sodium-free water to achieve similar dilution. In extreme cases, administration of hypotonic fluids to healthy, young women after surgery has resulted in severe neurologic symptoms and death secondary to transtentorial herniation.[122,123] A substantial proportion of postoperative patients, including pediatric patients, develop laboratory evidence of the syndrome of inappropriate ADH secretion (SIADH).[124] These patients develop impaired water excretion and are susceptible to hyponatremia. Although neurologic manifestations are relatively uncommon in postoperative hyponatremia, signs of hypervolemia are occasionally present.[121]

Careful attention to fluid and electrolyte balance in the postoperative period may minimize the occurrence of symptomatic hyponatremia. However, the actual relationship of hyponatremia and urinary volume to ADH secretion is unclear.[125] Many factors in addition to ADH influence perioperative water balance (Table 9-9).[126]

Hyponatremia is classified as factitious or true. Factitious hyponatremia occurs when hyperproteinemia or hyperlip-

idemia displaces water from plasma, thereby producing an apparently low plasma [Na$^+$]. Factitious hyponatremia occurs if protein concentrations are nearly twice normal or if hyperlipidemia is sufficiently severe to produce plasma lactescence. In such patients, serum osmolality is normal (Fig. 9-9). Although [Na$^+$] is conveniently reported in terms of mEq·l^{-1}, true [Na$^+$] is expressed per unit volume of plasma divided by the percentage of plasma that is comprised of water. Factitious hyponatremia requires no treatment.

True hyponatremia may be associated with normal, high, or low serum osmolality. In turn, hyponatremia with hypoosmolality is associated with a high, low, or normal total body sodium and PV. Hyponatremia ([Na$^+$] < 135 mEq·l^{-1}) with a normal or high serum osmolality results from the presence of a nonsodium solute, such as glucose or mannitol, which does not diffuse freely across cell membranes (see Fig. 9-9). The resulting osmotic gradient causes water to move from the ICV to the ECV, resulting in dilutional hyponatremia. In anesthesia practice, a common cause of hyponatremia associated with a normal osmolality is the absorption of large volumes of sodium-free irrigating solutions during transurethral resection of the prostate.[127,128] Although plasma [Na$^+$] is markedly reduced, plasma osmolality remains nearly normal because of the absorbed irrigant solute, whether that is mannitol, glycine, or sorbitol. Neurologic symptoms are minimal if mannitol is employed because the agent does not cross the blood-brain barrier and is excreted with water in the urine. In contrast, as glycine or sorbitol is metabolized, hyposmolality will gradually develop and cerebral edema may appear as a late complication.[128] Metabolism of glycine may also cause neurologic symptoms secondary to ammonia intoxication.[128]

A discrepancy exceeding 10 mOsm·kg^{-1} between the measured and calculated osmolality suggests either factitious hyponatremia or the presence of a nonsodium solute. Hyponatremia with a normal or elevated serum osmolality may also occur in renal insufficiency if excessive free water has been ingested or infused. Although an elevated BUN increases both measured and calculated osmolality, calculation of *effective* osmolality (2 [Na$^+$] + glucose ÷ 18) demonstrates true hypotonicity. BUN, included in the calculation of total osmolality, is excluded from the calculation of effective osmolality because it distributes throughout both ECV and ICV.

Hyponatremia with hyposmolality (see Fig. 9-9) is evaluated by assessing BUN, serum creatinine, total body sodium content, urinary osmolality, and urinary [Na$^+$]. Hyponatremia with increased total body sodium is characteristic of edematous states, *i.e.*, congestive heart failure, cirrhosis, nephrosis, and renal failure. The common denominator among these conditions is decreased effective circulating volume, usually accompanied by edema. Reduced urinary diluting capacity in patients with renal insufficiency can lead to hyponatremia when excess free water is given. Hyponatremia with low total body sodium content (hypovolemia) may occur in association with nonrenal or renal losses of sodium, in response to which volume-responsive ADH secretion sacrifices tonicity in order to preserve intravascular volume.

A third group of patients develop euvolemic hyponatremia associated with a relatively normal total body sodium and ECV. Although in such patients TBW is usually expanded by 2 to 3 liters, edema is rarely evident. Almost invariably due to SIADH, euvolemic hyponatremia is usually associated with excessive ectopic ADH secretion (as occurs with certain neoplasms), excessive hypothalamic-

---

TABLE 9-9. Hyponatremia: Perioperative Precipitating Factors

Drugs

Opioids
Diuretics
Antiemetics

Increased ADH

Hypovolemia
Nausea
Surgical stress
Pain

Excessive Water Administration

Hypotonic fluids
Hypotonic urologic irrigant

Impaired Renal Water Excretion

Increased proximal reabsorption (hypovolemia, blood loss)
Impaired urinary dilution (ascending loop of Henle)
Increased tubular water reabsorption

Reproduced with permission from Ayus JC, Arieff AL: Symptomatic hyponatremia: Making the diagnosis rapidly. J Crit Illness 5:847, 1990.

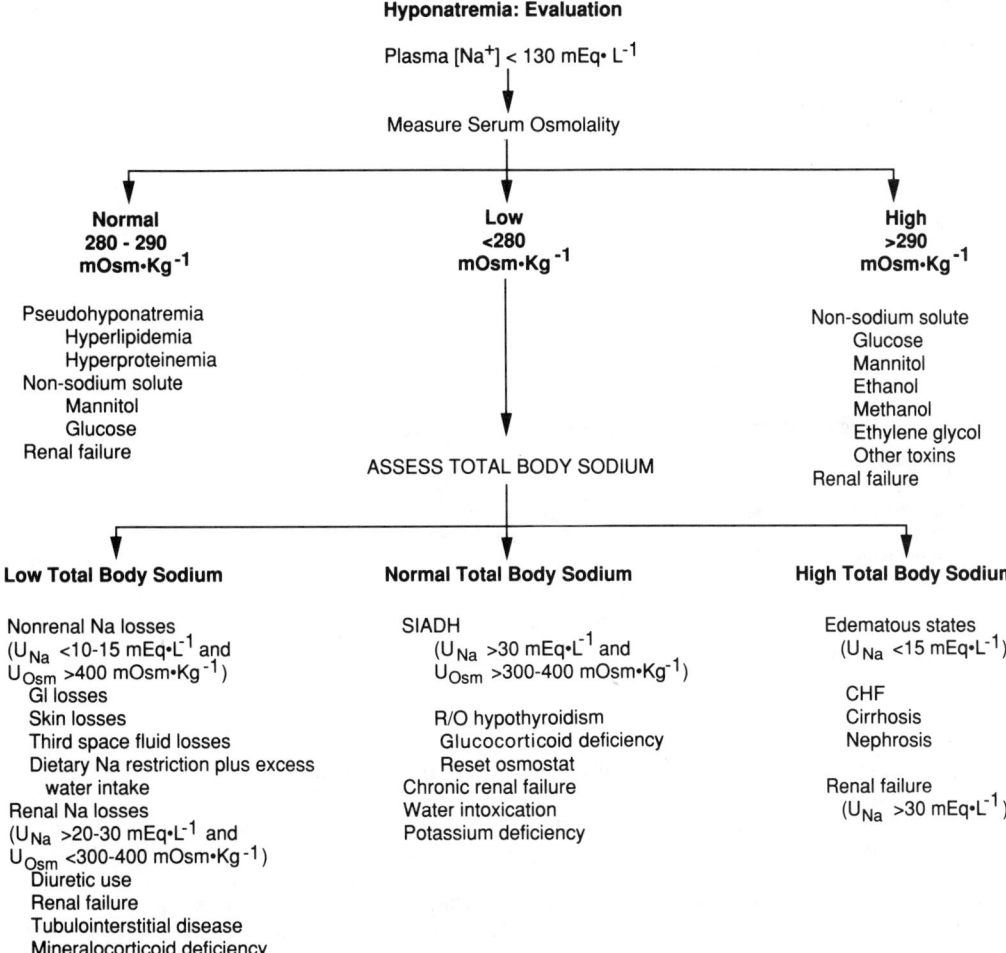

Figure 9-9. Hyponatremia is evaluated using the designated steps.

pituitary release of ADH (secondary to stress, pulmonary disease, CNS pathology, or endocrine abnormalities), exogenous ADH administration, pharmacologic potentiation of ADH action, or drugs that mimic the action of ADH in the renal tubules.

Treatment of hyponatremia associated with a normal or high serum osmolality requires reduction of the elevated concentrations of the responsible solute. Uremic, hyponatremic patients are treated by free water restriction or dialysis. Treatment of edematous (hypervolemic) hyponatremia patients necessitates restriction of both sodium and water (Fig. 9-10). Therapy is directed toward improving cardiac output and renal perfusion and using diuretics to inhibit sodium reabsorption. In patients with congestive heart failure, furosemide and an inhibitor of angiotensin-converting enzyme (ACE) may be particularly effective,[129] probably because the ACE inhibitor limits both the thirst and ADH release associated with angiotensin II.[113] In hypovolemic, hyponatremic patients, blood volume must be restored, usually by infusion of 0.9% saline, and excessive sodium losses must be curtailed. Correction of hypovolemia usually results in removal of the stimulus for ADH release, accompanied by a rapid water diuresis. If plasma [Na$^+$] increases too rapidly (a urinary output of 500 ml·h^{-1} will increase plasma [Na$^+$] by approximately 2 mEq·l^{-1}·h^{-1} in a 50-kg woman),[113] it may be necessary to administer sodium-free water to avoid the complications of excessively rapid cor-

rection.[130] Diuretics should be stopped or temporarily withheld. Patients who lose excessive sodium because of adrenal insufficiency may require administration of mineralocorticoids.

The cornerstone of SIADH management is free water restriction and elimination of precipitating causes. Water restriction, sufficient to decrease TBW by 0.5–1.0 l·day^{-1}, decreases ECV even if excessive ADH secretion continues. The resultant reduction in GFR enhances proximal tubular reabsorption of salt and water, thereby decreasing free water generation, and stimulates aldosterone secretion. It is important not to restrict fluid intake so much that adequate nutrition is impossible. As long as free water losses (i.e., renal, skin, gastrointestinal) exceed free water intake, serum [Na$^+$] will increase. Free water excretion can be increased by administering furosemide.

Neurologic symptoms or profound hyponatremia ([Na$^+$] < 115–120 mEq·l^{-1}) require more aggressive therapy. Hypertonic (3%) saline is most clearly indicated in patients who have seizures or patients who develop symptoms of water intoxication secondary to intravenous fluid administration. In such cases, 3% saline could be administered at a rate of 1–2 ml·kg^{-1}·h^{-1}, to increase plasma [Na$^+$] by 1–2 mEq·l^{-1}·h^{-1}; however, this treatment should not continue for more than a few hours to avoid excessively rapid correction.[114,131] In 25 children treated in this fashion, seizures were promptly terminated and there were no delayed neuro-

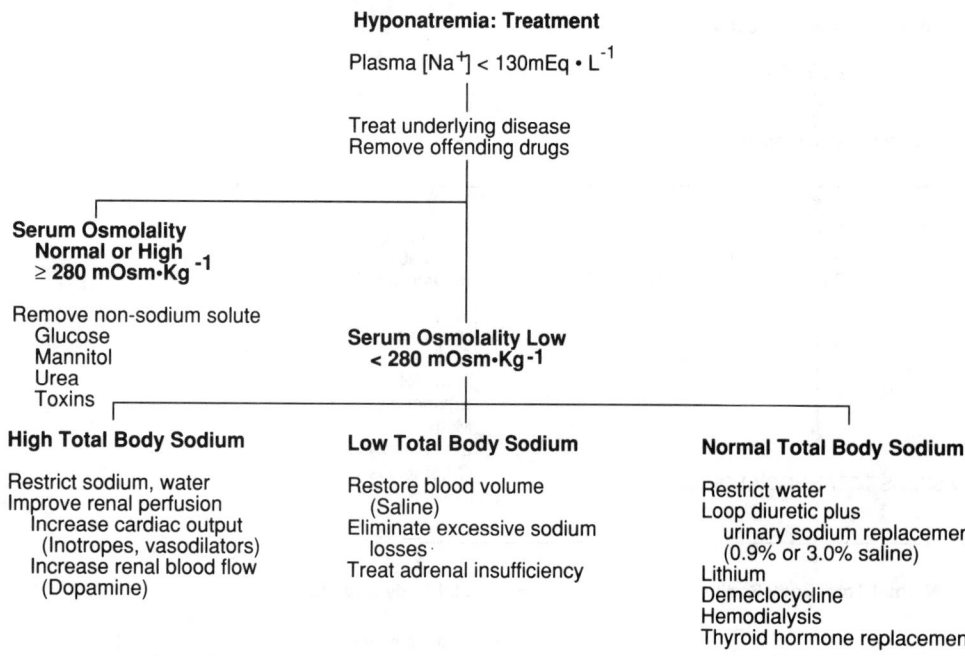

Figure 9-10. Hyponatremia is treated according to the etiology, the level of serum osmolality, and a clinical estimation of total body sodium.

logic sequelae.[132] Three percent saline alone will increase total body sodium as well as TBW; nevertheless, plasma [Na+] may only transiently increase, since ECV expansion results in rapid sodium excretion in the urine. Intravenous furosemide, combined with quantitative replacement of urinary sodium losses with 0.9% or 3.0% saline, can rapidly increase plasma [Na+], in part by increasing free water clearance.

Hyponatremia should be corrected cautiously. Although delayed correction may result in neurologic injury, inappropriately rapid correction also may result in permanent neurologic sequelae (*i.e.*, central pontine myelinolysis or the osmotic demyelination syndrome),[94-96,133] cerebral hemorrhage, or congestive heart failure. The symptoms of the osmotic demyelination syndrome vary from mild (transient behavioral disturbances or seizures) to severe (including pseudobulbar palsy and quadriparesis).[114,115,131,133,134] Within 3–4 weeks of the clinical onset of the syndrome, areas of demyelination are apparent on magnetic resonance imaging.[134,135] In rats, rapid correction of severe hyponatremia to normonatremic or hypernatremic levels results in severe demyelinating brain lesions; in contrast, rapid correction to mildly hyponatremic levels is associated with less severe pathology.[136] The rapidity of correction appears to be a critical factor in both clinical and experimental osmotic demyelination.[94,95,133] Greater chronicity of hyponatremia predisposes experimental animals to more severe demyelination.[96]

Initially, plasma [Na+] may be increased by 1–2 $mEq \cdot l^{-1} \cdot h^{-1}$; however, plasma [Na+] should not be increased more than 12 $mEq \cdot l^{-1}$ in 24 hours or 25 $mEq \cdot l^{-1}$ in 48 hours.[137-141] Hypernatremia should be avoided. Most patients in whom the osmotic demyelination syndrome is fatal have undergone correction of plasma [Na+] of more than 20 $mEq \cdot l^{-1} \cdot day^{-1}$.[133,138] Once the plasma [Na+] exceeds 120–125 $mEq \cdot l^{-1}$, water restriction alone is usually sufficient to normalize [Na+]. As acute hyponatremia is corrected, CNS signs and symptoms usually improve within

24 hours, although 96 hours may be necessary for maximal recovery.

Demeclocycline and lithium, though potentially toxic, have been used effectively to reverse SIADH in patients in whom the primary disease process is irreversible. Although better tolerated than lithium, demeclocycline may induce nephrotoxicity, a particular concern in patients with hepatic dysfunction. Hemodialysis is occasionally necessary in severely hyponatremic patients who cannot be adequately managed with drugs or hypertonic saline. Once hyponatremia has improved, careful fluid restriction is necessary to avoid recurrence of hyponatremia.

Hypernatremia

Because neurons are extremely vulnerable to dehydration, hypernatremia also produces neurologic symptoms, including alterations in the level of consciousness and seizures (Table 9-10).[6,142] Most hospitalized patients who

---

TABLE 9-10. Hypernatremia: Clinical Manifestations

Neurologic

Thirst
Weakness
Hyperreflexia
Seizures
Intracranial hemorrhage

Cardiovascular

Hypovolemia

Renal

Polyuria or oliguria
Renal insufficiency

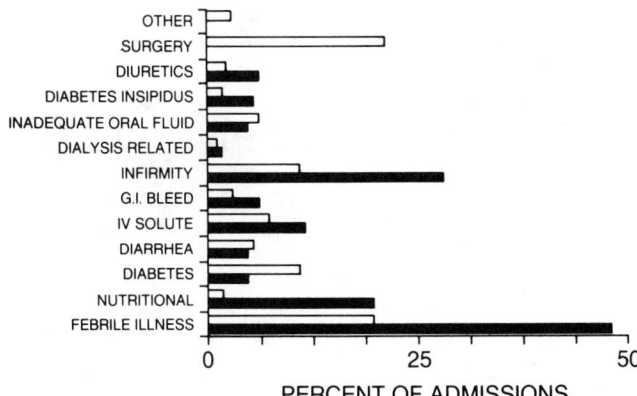

Figure 9-11. Primary (*open bars*) and associated (*solid bars*) causes leading to hypernatremia in 162 hospital admissions. The horizontal axis equals the percent of 162 admissions. GI = gastrointestinal, IV = intravenous. (Reproduced with permission from Snyder NA *et al*: Hypernatremia in elderly patients: A heterogeneous, morbid, and iatrogenic entity. Ann Intern Med 107:311, 1987.)

have hypernatremia also have severe associated illness (Fig. 9-11).[143] Because hypernatremia frequently results from diabetes insipidus or osmotically induced losses of sodium and water, many patients are hypovolemic or bear the stigmata of renal disease. Postoperative neurosurgical patients who have undergone pituitary surgery are at particular risk of developing transient or prolonged diabetes insipidus.[144,145] Polyuria may be present for only a few days within the first week of surgery, may be permanent, or may demonstrate a triphasic sequence: early diabetes insipidus, return of urinary concentrating ability, then recurrent diabetes insipidus.[146] The clinical consequences of hypernatremia are most serious at the extremes of age[143] and when hypernatremia develops abruptly. Brain shrinkage damages the delicate cerebral vessels, leading to subdural hematoma, subcortical parenchymal hemorrhage, subarachnoid hemorrhage, and venous thrombosis. Polyuria may cause bladder distention, hydronephrosis, and permanent renal damage.

By definition, hypernatremia ($[Na^+] > 150$ mEq·l^{-1}) indicates an absolute or relative water deficit and is always associated with hypertonicity. The TBW deficit can be estimated from the plasma $[Na^+]$ using the equation:

$$\text{TBW deficit} = (0.6)\,(\text{weight in kg}) - (140 \div \text{actual }[Na^+])\,(0.6)\,(\text{weight in kg})$$

Because hypovolemia accompanies most pathologic water loss, signs of hypoperfusion also may be present. In many patients, before the development of hypernatremia, an increased volume of hypotonic urine suggests an abnormality in water balance.[146,147]

Hypernatremic patients can be separated into three groups, based on clinical assessment of ECV (Fig. 9-12). The plasma $[Na^+]$ does not reflect total body sodium, which must be estimated based on signs of the adequacy of ECV. The next differential diagnostic decision to be made in polyuric patients, after assessing ECV, is between solute diuresis and diabetes insipidus. As extracellular $[Na^+]$ increases, intracellular water is shifted out of cells and ICV is depleted.

Treatment of hypernatremia produced by water loss consists of water replacement as well as repletion of associated deficits in total body sodium and other electrolytes (Table 9-11). Hypernatremia must be corrected slowly because of the risk of neurologic sequelae such as seizures or cerebral edema (Fig. 9-13).[143,148] The water deficit should be replaced over 24–48 hours, and the plasma $[Na^+]$ should not be reduced by more than 1–2 mEq·l^{-1}·h^{-1}. Reversible underlying causes should be treated. Hypovolemia should be corrected promptly with 0.9% saline. Once hypovolemia is corrected, water can be replaced orally or with intravenous hypotonic fluids, depending on the ability of the patient to tolerate oral hydration. In the occasional sodium-overloaded patient, sodium excretion can be accelerated using loop diuretics or dialysis, and diuresed or dialyzed volume can be replaced with hypotonic fluids.

Hypernatremia secondary to diabetes insipidus is managed according to whether the etiology is central or nephrogenic (see Table 9-11). Central diabetes insipidus requires replacement of ADH, with care taken to avoid water intoxication. The two most suitable agents for correcting central

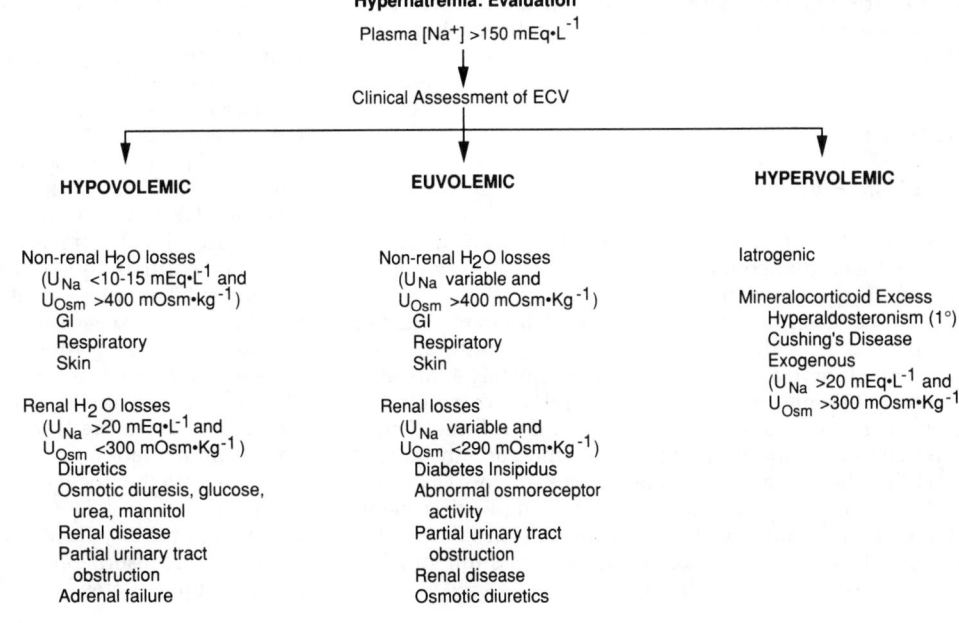

Figure 9-12. Severe hypernatremia is evaluated by first assessing extracellular volume (ECV). After patients are divided into hypovolemic, euvolemic, and hypervolemic groups, potential etiologic factors are diagnostically assessed.

Hypernatremia: Evaluation

Plasma $[Na^+] > 150$ mEq·L^{-1}

Clinical Assessment of ECV

HYPOVOLEMIC

Non-renal H$_2$O losses
(U$_{Na}$ <10-15 mEq·L^{-1} and
U$_{Osm}$ >400 mOsm·kg^{-1})
GI
Respiratory
Skin

Renal H$_2$O losses
(U$_{Na}$ >20 mEq·L^{-1} and
U$_{Osm}$ <300 mOsm·kg^{-1})
Diuretics
Osmotic diuresis, glucose,
urea, mannitol
Renal disease
Partial urinary tract
obstruction
Adrenal failure

EUVOLEMIC

Non-renal H$_2$O losses
(U$_{Na}$ variable and
U$_{Osm}$ >400 mOsm·Kg^{-1})
GI
Respiratory
Skin

Renal losses
(U$_{Na}$ variable and
U$_{Osm}$ <290 mOsm·Kg^{-1})
Diabetes Insipidus
Abnormal osmoreceptor
activity
Partial urinary tract
obstruction
Renal disease
Osmotic diuretics

HYPERVOLEMIC

Iatrogenic

Mineralocorticoid Excess
Hyperaldosteronism (1°)
Cushing's Disease
Exogenous
(U$_{Na}$ >20 mEq·L^{-1} and
U$_{Osm}$ >300 mOsm·Kg^{-1})

TABLE 9-11. Hypernatremia: Treatment

Sodium Depletion (Hypovolemia)

Hypovolemia correction (0.9% saline)
Hypernatremia correction (hypotonic fluids)

Sodium Overload (Hypervolemia)

Enhance sodium removal (loop diuretics, dialysis)
Replace water deficit (hypotonic fluids)

Normal Total Body Sodium (Euvolemia)

Replace water deficit (hypotonic fluids)
Control diabetes insipidus
  Central diabetes insipidus:
    DDAVP, 10–20 μg intransally; 2–4 μg sc
    Aqueous vasopressin, 5 U q 2-4 hours im or sc
    Chlorpropramide, 250–750 mg·day^{-1}
    Clofibrate, 500 mg q 6 hours
  Nephrogenic diabetes insipidus:
    Restrict sodium, water intake
    Thiazide diuretics

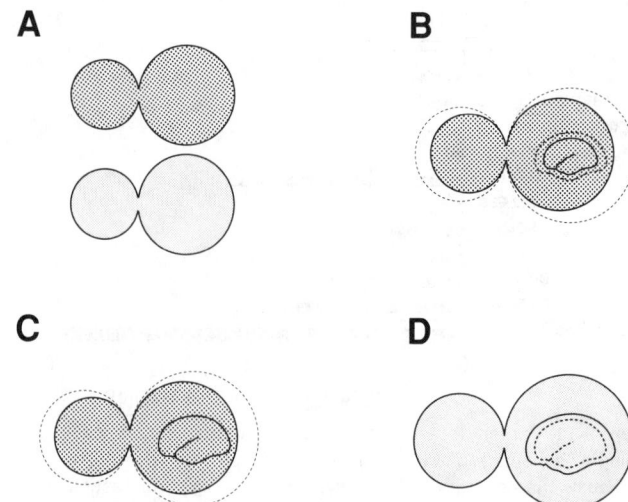

Figure 9-13. (A) The concentration of sodium is reflected in the intensity of the stippling: the upper figure, representing extracellular volume (smaller circle) and intracellular volume (larger circle), is more heavily stippled, *i.e.*, serum sodium is higher. (B) In response to an acute increase in serum sodium resulting from water, both intracellular and extracellular volume substantially decrease. The brain (schematically illustrated) shrinks in proportion to the reduction in intracellular volume in other tissues. (C) However, owing to the production of idiogenic osmoles, the brain rapidly restores its intracellular volume, despite the persistent reduction in intracellular volume in other tissues and in extracellular volume. (D) With excessively rapid correction of hypernatremia (the reduction in serum sodium is reflected in the decrease in the intensity of stippling), the brain expands to greater than its original size. The resulting increase in cerebral edema and intracranial pressure can cause severe neurologic damage. (Modified with permission from Feig PU: Hypernatremia and hypertonic syndromes. Med Clin North Am 65:285, 1981.)

diabetes insipidus are desmopressin (DDAVP) and aqueous vasopressin. DDAVP, given subcutaneously in a dose of 1–4 μg every 12–24 hours, is effective in the vast majority of patients. The medication can also be administered intranasally in a dose of 5–20 μg at 12–24 hour intervals. DDAVP lacks the vasoconstrictor effects of vasopressin and is less likely to produce abdominal cramping.[149-154] Incomplete ADH deficits (partial diabetes insipidus) often are effectively managed with pharmacologic agents that stimulate ADH release or enhance the renal response to ADH. The combination of chlorpropamide (100–250 mg·day^{-1}) and clofibrate or a thiazide diuretic has proven effective in patients who respond inadequately to either drug alone. Because the dose of chlorpropamide may be reduced if a thiazide is added, the combination reduces the risk of chlorpropamide-induced hypoglycemia. Chlorpropamide and thiazides may also be effective in treating disorders of the osmoreceptors. In nephrogenic diabetes insipidus, the renal collecting ducts are resistant to the action of ADH. Urinary water losses can be decreased by using salt and water restriction or thiazide diuretics to induce ECV contraction and enhance fluid reabsorption in the proximal tubules.

Potassium

Physiologic Role

Potassium, the predominant intracellular cation, normally has an intracellular concentration of 150 mEq·l^{-1} while the extracellular concentration is only 3.5–5.0 mEq·l^{-1}. Serum potassium concentration ([K$^+$]) is about 0.5 mEq·l^{-1} higher than plasma [K$^+$] due to cell lysis during clotting. Total body potassium in a 70-kg adult is approximately 4256 mEq, of which 4200 mEq is intracellular, 56 mEq is extracellular, and only 12 mEq is located in the plasma volume. Potassium plays an important role in cell membrane physiology, especially that of excitable membranes in the CNS and heart. Potassium is essential in maintaining resting membrane potentials and in generating action potentials (see Table 9-6). Thus, changes in extracellular potassium strongly influence excitation of cardiac tissue.

Total body potassium and potassium concentration are primarily regulated by three hormones: aldosterone, epinephrine, and insulin (see Table 9-7). Aldosterone increases renal reabsorption of sodium and renal excretion of potassium. Epinephrine and insulin are important regulators of the circulating potassium concentration. Secretion of either hormone results in an intracellular shift of potassium and provides an important mechanism for short-term prevention of hyperkalemia.

Potassium is also influenced independently by intrinsic renal mechanisms that regulate renal potassium excretion and are especially important in preventing chronic potassium overload. Assuming a plasma [K$^+$] of 4.0 mEq·l^{-1} and a normal GFR of 180 l·day^{-1}, 720 mEq of potassium is filtered daily. Most is reabsorbed; usually, only the amount ingested (normally 40–120 mEq·day^{-1}) is lost. Dietary potassium intake, unless greater than normal, can be excreted as long as GFR exceeds 8.0 ml·min^{-1}. In the proximal renal tubule, 50–70% of filtered potassium is passively reabsorbed. After secretion into the descending limb of the loop of Henle, potassium is subsequently reabsorbed from the medullary collecting ducts as part of a recycling loop.[155] Potassium excretion is primarily dependent on potassium secretion into the distal convoluted tubules and cortical collecting ducts, and is increased by aldosterone, hyperkalemia, high urinary flow rates, and the presence in luminal fluid of nonreabsorbable anions such as carbenicillin, phosphates, and sulfates.[156,157] Within the distal nephron, a magnesium-dependent sodium/potassium ATPase enzyme plays a critical role in potassium reabsorption.[158] Magnesium depletion impairs the activity of the enzyme, leading to renal potassium wasting.

Hypokalemia

The signs and symptoms of hypokalemia ($[K^+] < 3.0$ $mEq·l^{-1}$) reflect the diffuse effects of hypokalemia on cell membranes and excitable tissue. Hypokalemia causes muscle weakness and, when severe, may even cause paralysis (Table 9-12). The ratio of intracellular to extracellular potassium contributes to the resting potential difference across cell membranes and therefore to the integrity of cardiac and neuromuscular transmission. The resting membrane potential (E_m) is calculated from the Nernst equation:

$$E_m = -61 \log r [K_i] + 0.01 [Na_i]/r[K_e] + 0.01 [Na_e]$$

where $r = 1.5$ (the ratio of sodium to potassium actively transported by the ATPase pump), the subscripts i and e refer to intracellular and extracellular concentrations of sodium or potassium, respectively, and 0.01 is the relative membrane permeability of sodium and potassium. With chronic potassium loss, the ratio of intracellular to extracellular $[K^+]$ remains relatively stable; in contrast, acute redistribution of potassium from extracellular to intracellular spaces substantially changes E_m.

Cardiac rhythm disturbances are among the most dangerous complications of potassium deficiency. Acute hypokalemia causes hyperpolarization of the cardiac cell and may lead to ventricular escape activity, re-entrant phenomena, ectopic tachycardias, and delayed conduction. Despite the

---

TABLE 9-12. Hypokalemia: Clinical Manifestations

Cardiovascular

Dysrhythmias
  PVCs
  Tachycardia
ECG changes
  Widened QRS complex
  ST segment depression
  T wave depression
  U wave prominence
  First-degree AV block
Digitalis toxicity potentiation
Postural hypotension
Impaired pressor responses

Neuromuscular

Weakness
Rhabdomyolysis
Respiratory failure
Hyporeflexia
Confusion
Depression

Renal

Polyuria
Concentrating defect

Metabolic

Glucose intolerance
Potentiation of hypercalcemia, hypomagnesemia

---

long-standing concern of anesthesia personnel that preoperative chronic hypokalemia increases the incidence of intraoperative dysrhythmias, prospective studies fail to confirm that suspicion.[159]

Potassium depletion also induces defects in renal concentrating ability, resulting in polyuria and a reduction in GFR.[160-162] Potassium replacement improves GFR; however, the concentrating deficit may not improve for several months after treatment of hypokalemia. If hypokalemia is sufficiently prolonged, chronic renal interstitial damage may occur.

The plasma potassium concentration ($[K^+]$) poorly reflects total body potassium; hypokalemia may occur with normal, low, or high total body potassium stores. Ninety-eight percent of potassium is intracellular while only 2% is found in the ECV. Total body potassium approximates $50-55$ $mEq·kg^{-1}$ body weight. As a general rule, a chronic decrement of 1.0 $mEq·l^{-1}$ in the plasma $[K^+]$ corresponds to a total body deficit of approximately $200-300$ mEq. In uncomplicated hypokalemia, the potassium deficit exceeds 300 mEq if plasma $[K^+]$ is <3.0 $mEq·l^{-1}$ and 700 mEq if plasma $[K^+]$ is <2.0 $mEq·l^{-1}$.[163]

Hypokalemia may result from acute redistribution of potassium from the extracellular to intracellular space, in which case total body potassium will be normal, or from chronic depletion of total body potassium. Redistribution of potassium into cells occurs when the activity of the sodium-potassium ATPase pump is acutely increased by extracellular hyperkalemia or increased intracellular concentrations of sodium, as well as by insulin, carbohydrate loading (which stimulates release of endogenous insulin), beta$_2$ agonists, and aldosterone. Changes in acid-base balance also cause potassium redistribution. Both metabolic and respiratory alkalosis lead to decreases in plasma $[K^+]$.[153] Metabolic acidosis and respiratory acidosis tend to cause an increase in plasma $[K^+]$. However, organic acidoses (i.e., lactic acidosis, ketoacidosis) have little effect on $[K^+]$, whereas mineral acids cause significant cellular shifts. Acute hypokalemia is also associated with hypothermia; overzealous replacement of potassium during hypothermia has been associated with postrewarming hyperkalemia.[154]

Causes of chronic hypokalemia include those etiologies associated with renal potassium conservation (extrarenal potassium losses; low urinary $[K^+]$) and those with renal potassium wasting. A low urinary $[K^+]$ suggests inadequate dietary intake or extrarenal depletion (in the absence of recent diuretic use). Diuretic-induced urinary potassium losses are frequently associated with hypokalemia, secondary to increased aldosterone secretion, alkalemia, and increased renal tubular flow. Aldosterone does not cause renal potassium wasting unless sodium ions are present; i.e., aldosterone primarily controls sodium reabsorption, not potassium excretion. Renal tubular damage due to nephrotoxins such as aminoglycosides or amphotericin B may also cause renal potassium wasting.

Initial evaluation of hypokalemia includes a medical history (e.g., diarrhea, vomiting, diuretic or laxative use), physical examination (e.g., hypertension, cushingoid features, edema), measurement of serum electrolytes (e.g., magnesium), and arterial pH assessment. Twenty-four hour urinary excretion of sodium and potassium may permit distinction of extrarenal from renal causes. Plasma renin and aldosterone levels may be helpful in the differential diagnosis.

The treatment of hypokalemia consists of potassium repletion, correction of alkalemia, and removal of offending drugs (Table 9-13). Hypokalemia secondary only to acute

TABLE 9-13. Hypokalemia: Treatment

Correct Precipitating Factors

Alkalemia
Hypomagnesemia
Drugs

Mild Hypokalemia

($[K^+] > 2.0$ mEq·l^{-1})
Infuse KCl at rate ≤ 10 mEq·h^{-1}

Severe Hypokalemia

($[K^+] \leq 2.0$ mEq·l^{-1} or paralysis or ECG changes)
Infuse KCl at rate ≤ 40 mEq·h^{-1}
Continuously monitor ECG

TABLE 9-14. Hyperkalemia: Clinical Manifestations

Cardiovascular

Dysrhythmias
  Asystole
  Heart block
ECG changes
  Tall, peaked T waves
  Decreased P waves
  P-R prolongation
  Atrial asystole
  QRS widening

Neuromuscular

Paresthesias
Weakness
Paralysis
Confusion

redistribution may not require treatment. If total body potassium is decreased, oral potassium supplementation is preferable to intravenous replacement. Potassium is usually replaced as the chloride salt because coexisting chloride deficiency may limit the ability of the kidney to conserve potassium.

Potassium repletion must be performed cautiously (i.e., usually at a rate no greater than 10–20 mEq·h^{-1}) since the absolute deficit is unpredictable. The plasma $[K^+]$ and the ECG must be monitored during rapid repletion (>20 mEq·h^{-1}) to avoid hyperkalemic complications. Particular care should be taken in patients who have concurrent acidemia, type IV renal tubular acidosis, diabetes mellitus, or in those patients receiving nonsteroidal anti-inflammatory agents, ACE inhibitors, or beta blockers, all of which delay movement of extracellular potassium into cells.

Hypokalemia associated with hyperaldosteronemia (e.g., primary aldosteronism, Cushing's syndrome) usually responds favorably to reduced sodium intake and increased potassium intake. Spironolactone, an aldosterone antagonist, reduces urinary potassium losses in patients who have adrenal hyperplasia. Hypomagnesemia, if present, aggravates the effects of hypokalemia, impairs potassium conservation, and should be treated. Cyclo-oxygenase inhibitors such as aspirin can improve hypokalemia in patients with Bartter's syndrome. Potassium supplements or potassium-sparing diuretics should be given cautiously to patients who have diabetes mellitus or renal insufficiency, which limit compensation for acute hyperkalemia. In patients, such as those who have diabetic ketoacidosis, who are both acidemic and hypokalemic, potassium administration should precede correction of acidosis to avoid a precipitous decrease in plasma $[K^+]$ as pH increases.

Hyperkalemia

The clinical manifestations of hyperkalemia ($[K^+] > 5.0$ mEq·l^{-1}) primarily involve the neuromuscular and cardiovascular systems. The most lethal manifestations involve the cardiac conducting system and include dysrhythmias, conduction abnormalities, and cardiac arrest (Table 9-14). In anesthesia practice, the classic example of hyperkalemic cardiac toxicity is associated with the administration of succinylcholine to paraplegic or quadriplegic patients (Fig. 9-14).[164] If plasma $[K^+]$ is <6.0 mEq·l^{-1}, cardiac effects are negligible. As the concentration increases further, the electrocardiogram shows tall, peaked T waves, especially in the precordial leads. With further increases, the PR interval becomes prolonged, followed by a decrease in the amplitude of the P wave. Finally, the QRS complex widens into a pattern resembling a sine wave, as a prelude to cardiac standstill. Hyperkalemic cardiotoxicity is enhanced by hyponatremia, hypocalcemia, or acidosis. Because progression to fatal cardiotoxicity is unpredictable and often swift, the presence of hyperkalemic ECG changes mandates immediate therapy. The life-threatening cardiac effects usually require more urgent treatment than other manifestations of hyperkalemia. However, ascending muscle weakness appears when plasma $[K^+]$ approaches 7.0 mEq·l^{-1}, and may progress to flaccid paralysis, inability to phonate, and even respiratory arrest.[165]

Hyperkalemia may occur with normal, high, or low total body potassium stores. A deficiency of aldosterone, a major regulator of potassium excretion, leads to hyperkalemia in adrenal insufficiency and hyporeninemic hypoaldosteronism, a state associated with diabetes mellitus, renal insufficiency, and advanced age.[166] Because the kidneys excrete potassium, severe renal insufficiency commonly causes hyperkalemia (Table 9-15). Patients with chronic renal insufficiency can maintain normal plasma $[K^+]$ despite markedly decreased GFR because urinary potassium excretion depends on tubular secretion, not glomerular filtration. Nevertheless, potassium excretion becomes impaired when the GFR falls below 8 ml·min^{-1}.

Drugs are now the most common cause of hyperkalemia.[167] Drugs that may limit potassium excretion include nonsteroidal anti-inflammatory drugs,[168] ACE inhibitors, cyclosporin, and potassium-sparing diuretics such as triamterene. Drug effects most commonly occur in patients with other factors that predispose to hyperkalemia, such as diabetes mellitus, renal insufficiency, advanced age, or hyporeninemic hypoaldosteronism. ACE inhibitors are particularly likely to produce hyperkalemia in patients who have renal insufficiency[169] or severe congestive heart failure.[170]

In patients who have normal total body potassium, hyperkalemia may accompany a sudden shift of potassium from the ICV to the ECV because of acidemia, increased catabolism, or rhabdomyolysis. Pseudohyperkalemia, which occurs when potassium is released from cells in blood collection tubes, can be diagnosed by comparing serum and plasma K$^+$ levels from the same blood sample.

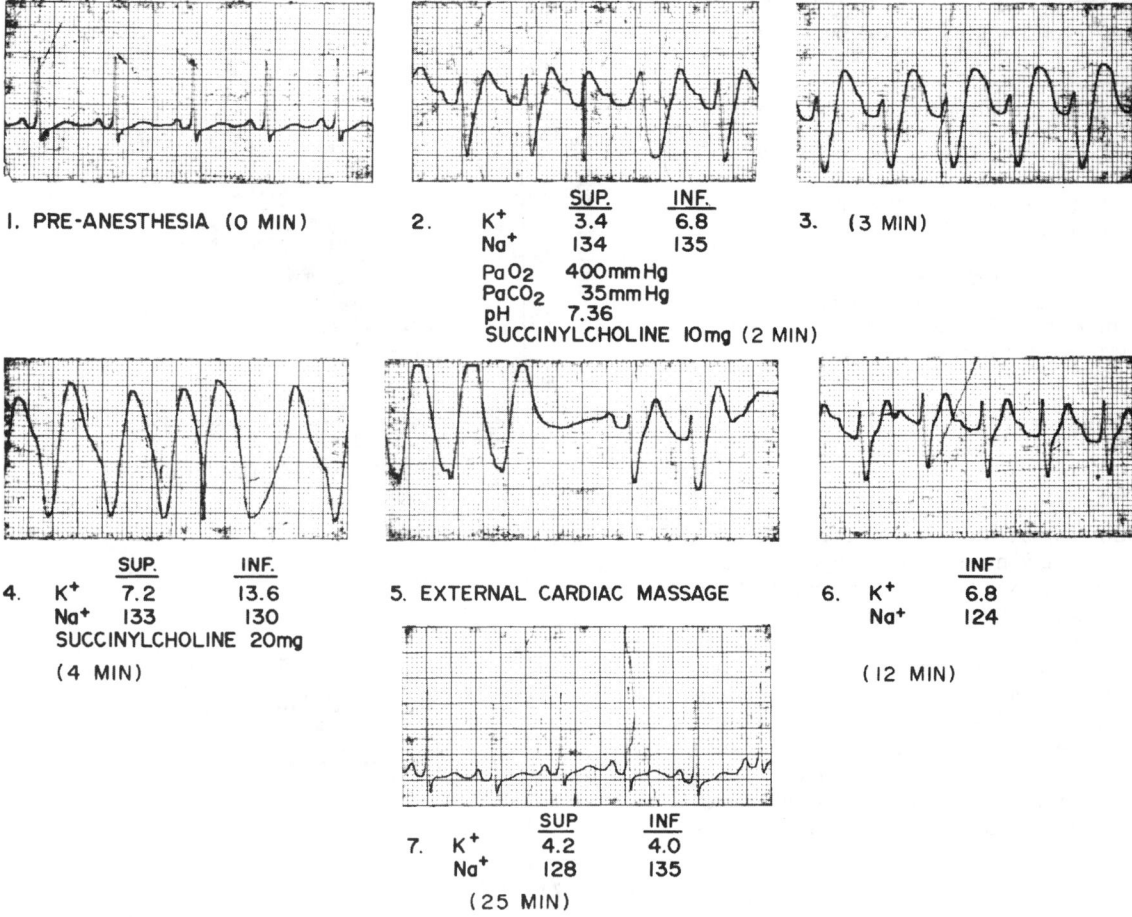

1. PRE-ANESTHESIA (0 MIN)

2.
	SUP.	INF.
K⁺	3.4	6.8
Na⁺	134	135

PaO_2 400 mm Hg
$PaCO_2$ 35 mm Hg
pH   7.36
SUCCINYLCHOLINE 10 mg (2 MIN)

3.   (3 MIN)

4.
	SUP.	INF.
K⁺	7.2	13.6
Na⁺	133	130

SUCCINYLCHOLINE 20 mg
(4 MIN)

5. EXTERNAL CARDIAC MASSAGE

6.
	INF.
K⁺	6.8
Na⁺	124

(12 MIN)

7.
	SUP	INF
K⁺	4.2	4.0
Na⁺	128	135

(25 MIN)

Figure 9-14. Electrocardiographic tracings in a traumatically paraplegic patient receiving succinylcholine. As succinylcholine-induced hyperkalemia supervenes, potassium in the inferior vena cava (INF) progressively increases, the T waves increase in amplitude, the QRS complex widens, and a "sine wave" ventricular tachycardia develops. After resuscitation, including external cardiac massage, potassium in both the superior vena cava (SUP) and INF gradually decreases and the electrocardiographic tracing returns to normal. (Reproduced with permission from Tobey RE: Paraplegia, succinylcholine and cardiac arrest. Anesthesiology 32:360, 1970.)

The treatment of hyperkalemia is aimed at eliminating the cause, reversing membrane hyperexcitability, and removing potassium from the body (Table 9-16). Mineralocorticoid deficiency can be treated with 9-alpha-fludrocortisone (0.025–0.10 mg·day⁻¹). Hyperkalemia secondary to digitalis intoxication may be resistant to therapy because attempts to shift potassium from the ECV to the ICV are often ineffective. In this situation, use of digoxin-specific antibodies has been successful.

Hyperexcitability can be antagonized by translocating potassium from the ECV to the ICV, removing excess potassium, or (transiently) by infusing calcium chloride to depress the membrane threshold potential. Acute alkalinization using sodium bicarbonate (50–100 mEq over 5–10 minutes in a 70-kg adult) transiently promotes movement of potassium from the ECV to the ICV. Bicarbonate can be administered even if pH exceeds 7.40; however, it should not be administered to patients with congestive cardiac failure or hypernatremia. Insulin, in a dose-dependent fashion, causes cellular uptake of potassium by increasing the activity of the sodium/potassium ATPase pump.[171] Insulin increases cellular uptake of potassium *best* when high insulin levels are achieved by intravenous injection of insulin.[172] Therefore, administration of 5–10 U of regular insulin intravenously, accompanied by 50 ml of 50% glucose, is an effective way to transiently reduce serum potassium.[173] Beta₂-adrenergic drugs also increase potassium uptake by skeletal muscle and reduce plasma [K⁺],[174-176] an action that may explain hypokalemia with severe, acute illness.[177] Beta₂ agonists have been used to treat hyperkalemia in a few specific settings.[178]

Rapid infusion of calcium chloride (one ampule of $CaCl_2$ over 3 minutes, or two to three ampules of 10% calcium

TABLE 9-15. Hyperkalemia: Etiology

Mineralocorticoid deficiency
Acute or chronic renal failure
Renal tubular dysfunction
Drugs
Translocation from ICV to ECV
Excess potassium intake
Insulin deficiency
Catecholamine insufficiency

TABLE 9-16. Severe Hyperkalemia:* Treatment

Reverse membrane effects
  Calcium (10–30 ml of 10% calcium gluconate IV over 10 min)
Transfer K^+ into cells
  Glucose and insulin (D10W + 5–10 U regular insulin per 25–50 g
    glucose)
  Sodium bicarbonate (1–2 ampules over 5–10 min)
Remove potassium from body
  Proximal or loop diuretics
  Potassium-exchange resins: sodium polystyrene sulfonate (Kay-
    exalate), 20–30 g po in 50 ml 70% sorbitol q 4 hours or
    50–100 g in 200 ml water, or 20% sorbitol by retention enema
  Hemodialysis (removes 25–50 mEq·h^{-1})
Monitor ECG and serum K^+ level

*[K^+] > 7.0 mEq·l^{-1} or ECG changes.

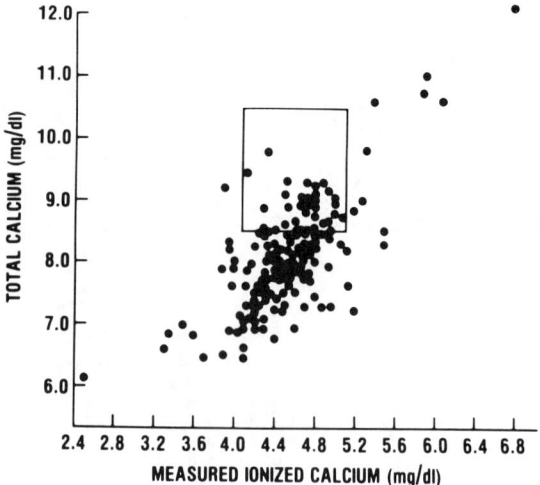

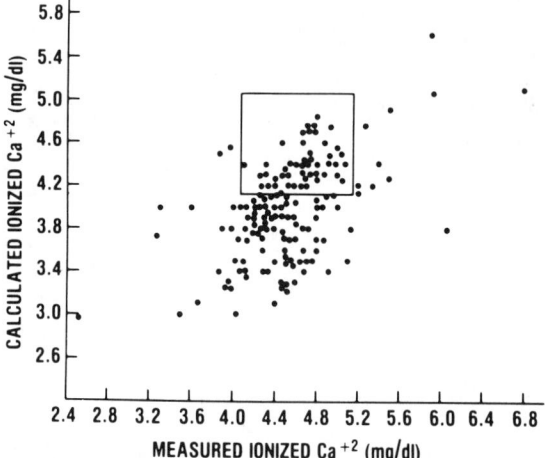

Figure 9-15. Total serum calcium and calculated ionized calcium concentrations are poor indicators of directly measured serum ionized calcium in critically ill surgical patients. (*Top*) Total serum calcium *vs.* measured serum ionized calcium in 156 surgical ICU patients. Despite apparent hypocalcemia, based on measurement of total calcium, many patients have normal ionized calcium. (*Bottom*) Calculated ionized calcium (using the McLean-Hastings nomogram) is frequently low in surgical ICU patients in whom measured ionized calcium is within the normal range. (Reproduced with permission from Zaloga GP *et al*: Assessment of calcium homeostasis in the critically ill surgical patient. Ann Surg 202:589, 1985.)

gluconate over 5 minutes) may buy time for definitive treatment. Calcium should be given cautiously if digitalis intoxication is likely. Potassium may be removed from the body by renal or gastrointestinal routes. Furosemide promotes kaliuresis in a dose-dependent fashion. Sodium polystyrene sulfonate resin (Kayexalate) exchanges sodium for potassium. Kayexalate can be given orally (30 g) or as a retention enema (50 g in 200 ml of 20% sorbitol). However, sodium overload and hypervolemia are potential risks. Because these temporizing measures are usually sufficient, emergency hemodialysis is rarely necessary. When used, hemodialysis may remove 25–50 mEq·h^{-1}. Peritoneal dialysis is less efficient.

Calcium

Physiologic Role

Calcium is a divalent cation found primarily in the extracellular fluid. The concentration of free calcium [Ca^{2+}] in the ICV approximates 100 nM, whereas the free [Ca^{2+}] in ECV is approximately 1 mM. Thus, the gradient between ECV and ICV is approximately 10,000 to 1. Circulating calcium consists of a protein-bound fraction (40%), a chelated fraction (10%), and an ionized fraction (50%), which is the physiologically active and homeostatically regulated component.[179] Attempts to correct total calcium measurements for albumin concentration are inaccurate in critically ill patients (Fig. 9-15).[180] Therefore, ionized calcium should be directly measured.[181]

Calcium serves vital cellular functions (see Table 9-6). In general, all movement that occurs in mammalian systems requires calcium. Essential for normal excitation-contraction coupling, calcium is also necessary for proper function of muscle tissue, ciliary movement, and mitosis. Calcium also is involved in contractile elements that are responsible for secretion in neural tissue (i.e., neurotransmission), enzyme secretion, and hormonal secretion from endocrine tissue. Cyclic AMP (cAMP) and phosphoinositides, which are major second messengers regulating cellular metabolism, function primarily through the regulation of calcium movement. Activation of numerous intracellular enzyme systems requires calcium. Important both for generation of the cardiac pacemaker activity and for generation of the cardiac action potential, calcium is the primary ion responsible for the plateau phase of the action potential.

Calcium also plays vital functions in membrane and bone structure.

Calcium is regulated through two primary hormones, parathyroid hormone (PTH) and vitamin D (see Table 9-7). Both of these hormones, secreted when circulating ionized [Ca^{2+}] decreases, result in the mobilization of calcium from bone, the reabsorption of calcium from the renal tubule, and the absorption of calcium from the intestine. Metabolites of vitamin D exert a major role in long-term control of circulating calcium. Vitamin D, after ingestion or manufacture of vitamin D in the skin under the stimulus of ultraviolet light, is 25-hydroxylated to calcidiol in the liver and then is 1-hydroxylated to calcitriol in the kidney. Calcitriol, the active metabolite, stimulates osseous calcium release, renal calcium reabsorption, and enteric calcium absorption. PTH and vitamin D can maintain a normal circulating [Ca^{2+}],

TABLE 9-17. Hypocalcemia: Clinical Manifestations

Cardiovascular	*Respiratory*
Dysrhythmias	Apnea
Digitalis insensitivity	Laryngeal spasm
ECG changes	Bronchospasm
QT prolongation	
ST prolongation	*Psychiatric*
T wave inversion	Anxiety
Heart failure	Dementia
Hypotension	Depression
	Psychosis
Neuromuscular	
Tetany	
Muscle spasm	
Papilledema	
Seizures	
Weakness	
Fatigue	

even in the absence of dietary calcium intake, by mobilizing calcium from bone.

Hypocalcemia

The hallmark of hypocalcemia, increased neuronal membrane irritability and tetany (Table 9-17), classically is demonstrated by eliciting Chvostek's or Trousseau's signs. In frank tetany, tonic contraction of respiratory muscles may lead to laryngospasm, bronchospasm, or respiratory arrest. Smooth muscle spasm can result in abdominal cramping and urinary frequency. Mental status alterations include irritability, depression, psychosis, and dementia. Hypocalcemia may impair cardiovascular function and has been associated with heart failure, hypotension, dysrhythmias, insensitivity to digitalis, and impaired beta-adrenergic action.

Hypocalcemia (ionized calcium < 4.0 mg·dl^{-1} or 1 mM) occurs as a result of failure of PTH or calcitriol action or because of calcium chelation or precipitation. Dietary calcium deficiency alone does not cause hypocalcemia; PTH and vitamin D maintain normocalcemia by mobilizing osseous stores. PTH deficiency can result from surgical parathyroid gland damage or removal, or from parathyroid gland suppression. Parathyroid gland suppression may occur during severe hypo- or hypermagnesemia. Burns, sepsis, and pancreatitis may suppress parathyroid function and interfere with vitamin D action. Vitamin D deficiency may result from lack of dietary vitamin D or vitamin D malabsorption in patients who lack sunlight exposure. Failure of renal hydroxylation occurs in some patients who have renal failure, sepsis, or rhabdomyolysis. Hyperphosphatemia-induced hypocalcemia may occur as a consequence of overzealous phosphate therapy, from cell lysis secondary to chemotherapy, or as a result of cellular destruction from rhabdomyolysis. Hyperphosphatemic hypocalcemia results from calcium precipitation and suppression of calcitriol synthesis. In massive transfusion, citrate may produce hypocalcemia by chelating calcium; however, decreases are usually transient and produce no cardiovascular effects. A healthy, normothermic adult who has intact hepatic and renal function can metabolize the citrate present in 20 units of blood within 1 hour without becoming hypocalcemic.[182] However, when citrate clearance is decreased (e.g., by hepatic or renal disease, hypothermia) and when blood transfusion rates are

rapid (e.g., $>0.5-2$ ml·kg^{-1}·min^{-1}), hypocalcemia and cardiovascular compromise may occur.

Reduced total serum calcium occurs in as many as 80% of critically ill and postsurgical patients.[179,180] However, fewer patients develop ionized hypocalcemia, including 15–20% of critically ill patients,[179-181] 20% of patients after cardiopulmonary bypass, and 30–40% after multiple trauma. However, the ionized hypocalcemia in these situations is clinically mild, associated with ionized serum calcium concentrations > 0.8 mM.

Formulas and nomograms that purport to correct calcium measurements for alterations of serum proteins and pH poorly predict directly measured ionized [Ca^{2+}], the best estimate of the adequacy of available calcium. When ionized [Ca^{2+}] cannot be measured directly, a 1 g·dl^{-1} change in serum albumin is said to correspond to an approximately 0.8 mg·dl^{-1} change in total serum calcium. Acute acidemia decreases protein-bound calcium (i.e., increases ionized calcium) whereas acute alkalemia increases protein-bound calcium (i.e., decreases ionized calcium).

The definitive treatment of hypocalcemia necessitates identification and treatment of the underlying cause (Table 9-18). Symptomatic hypocalcemia usually occurs when serum ionized [Ca^{2+}] is below 0.7 mM. The clinician should determine whether mild ionized hypocalcemia requires therapy, particularly in ischemic and septic states in which experimental evidence suggests that calcium may increase cellular damage.[183,184]

Unnecessary offending drugs should be discontinued. Hypocalcemia resulting from hypomagnesemia or hyperphosphatemia is treated by repletion or removal of magnesium or phosphate, respectively. Potassium and other electrolytes should be measured and abnormalities should be corrected. Hyperkalemia and hypomagnesemia potentiate hypocalcemia-induced cardiac and neuromuscular irritability. In contrast, hypokalemia protects against hypocalcemic tetany; therefore, correction of hypokalemia without correction of hypocalcemia may provoke tetany.

In anesthesia practice, it is particularly important that ionized hypocalcemia not be overtreated in patients recovering from cardiac surgery. Considerable evidence demonstrates that the administration of calcium after cardiac surgery only increases MAP,[185,186] actually attenuates the beta-adrenergic effects of epinephrine (Fig. 9-16),[185] and does not increase vasoconstriction produced by alpha agonists.[186] Calcium salts appear to confer no benefit to patients who otherwise require inotropic or vasoactive agents.[187]

The cornerstone of therapy for confirmed, symptomatic, ionized hypocalcemia ([Ca^{2+}] < 0.7 mM) is calcium administration. In patients who have severe hypocalcemia or hy-

TABLE 9-18. Hypocalcemia: Acute Treatment

Administer calcium
  IV: 10 ml 10% calcium gluconate* over 10 min as bolus, followed by 0.3–2 mg elemental calcium·kg^{-1}·h^{-1}
  Oral: 500–1000 mg elemental calcium q 6 hours
Administer vitamin D
  Ergocalciferol, 1200 μg·day^{-1} ($T_{1/2} = 30$ days)
  Dihydrotachysterol, 200–400 μg·day^{-1} ($T_{1/2} = 7$ days)
  1,25-dihydroxycholecalciferol, 0.25–1.0 μg·day^{-1} ($T_{1/2} = 1$ day)
Monitor ECG

*Calcium gluconate contains 93 mg elemental calcium per 10-ml vial; $T_{1/2} =$ half-life.

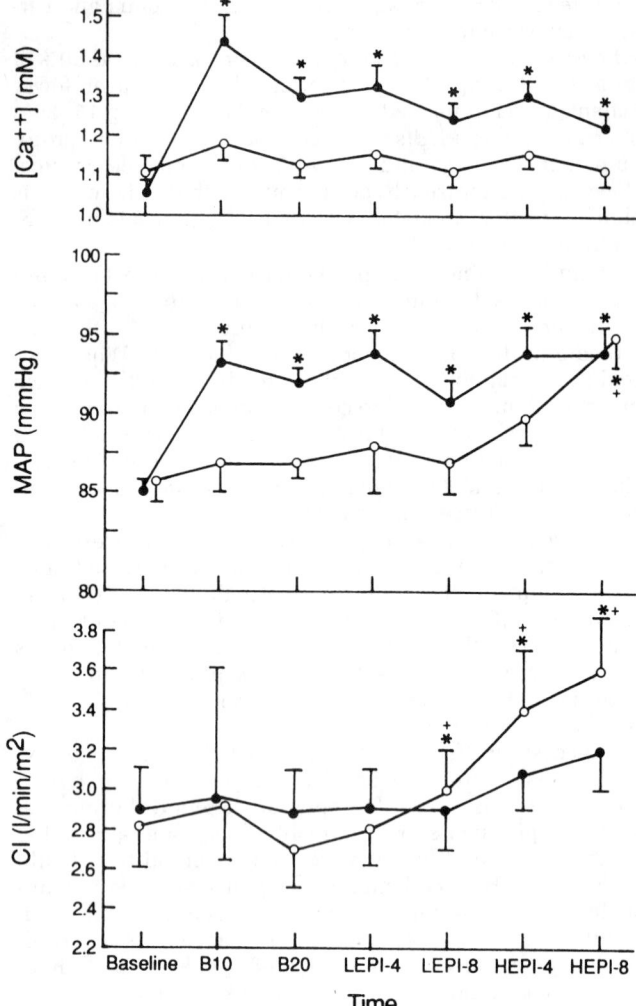

Figure 9-16. Effects of epinephrine infusion, with (*closed circle*) and without (*open circle*) simultaneous infusion of calcium chloride (10 mg·kg^{-1} bolus followed by 2 mg·kg^{-1}·h^{-1} infusion). In 12 adult patients on the first day after aortocoronary bypass surgery, calcium chloride significantly increased ionized calcium levels and mean arterial pressure (*$p < 0.05$ in comparison to baseline). Epinephrine was infused in a low dose (LEPI; 10 mg·kg^{-1}·min^{-1}) for 4 minutes and 8 minutes (LEPI-4 and LEPI-8, respectively) and in a high dose (HEPI; 30 mg·kg^{-1}·min^{-1}) for 4 and 8 minutes (HEPI-4 and HEPI-8, respectively). Infused alone, epinephrine significantly increased blood pressure and cardiac output in comparison to predrug (B20) data ($p < 0.05$). During the infusion of calcium chloride, epinephrine failed to significantly increase either mean arterial pressure (MAP) or cardiac index (CI). (Reproduced with permission from Zaloga GP *et al*: Calcium attenuates epinephrine's β-adrenergic effects in postoperative heart surgery patients. Circulation 81:199, 1990.)

pocalcemic symptoms, calcium should be administered intravenously. In emergency situations, in an averaged-sized adult, the "rule of 10's" advises infusion of 10 ml of 10% calcium gluconate (93 mg elemental calcium) over 10 minutes, followed by a continuous infusion of elemental calcium, 0.3–2 mg·kg^{-1}·h^{-1} (i.e., 3–16 ml·h^{-1} of 10% calcium gluconate for a 70-kg adult). Calcium salts should be diluted in 50–100 ml D5W (to limit venous irritation and thrombosis), should not be mixed with bicarbonate (to prevent pre-

cipitation), and must be given cautiously to digitalized patients because calcium increases the toxicity of digitalis compounds. The response to treatment can be monitored clinically by using Chvostek's and Trousseau's signs. Continuous ECG monitoring during initial therapy will detect cardiotoxicity (e.g., heart block, ventricular fibrillation). During calcium replacement, the clinician should monitor serum calcium, magnesium, phosphate, potassium, and creatinine. Once the ionized [Ca^{2+}] is stable in the range of 4–5 mg·dl^{-1} (1.0–1.25 mM), oral calcium supplements can substitute for parenteral therapy. Urinary calcium should be monitored in an attempt to avoid hypercalciuria (>5 mg·kg^{-1} per 24 hours) and urinary tract stone formation.

When supplementation fails to maintain serum calcium within the normal range, or if hypercalciuria develops, vitamin D may be added. Although the principal effect of vitamin D is to increase enteric calcium absorption, bone calcium resorption is also enhanced. When rapid changes in dosage are anticipated or an immediate effect is required (e.g., postoperative hypoparathyroidism), shorter-acting calciferols such as dihydrotachysterol may be preferable. The earliest vitamin D metabolite that is deficient should be administered first, to allow the body a chance to regulate activation of the vitamin to calcitriol and replenish other vitamin D metabolites. When the 1-hydroxylase enzyme is deficient, as in renal failure, it is best to administer calcitriol. Because the effect of the vitamin is not regulated, the dosages of calcium and vitamin D should be adjusted to raise the serum calcium into the low normal range.

Physiologic states and concurrently administered drugs may influence therapeutic results. Bone remineralization after initiation of therapy (e.g., after correction of hyperparathyroidism) may increase calcium requirements. Once remineralization is complete, a reduction in calcium or vitamin D may be necessary to avoid hypercalcemia. Malabsorption states impair vitamin D absorption more than calcium absorption; major dosage adjustments may be required as malabsorption is corrected. Calciferol requirements are increased in patients receiving bile acid sequestrants (e.g., cholestyramine), barbiturates, phenytoin, corticosteroids, and calciuric diuretics (e.g., furosemide). Requirements are decreased by hypocalciuric diuretics (e.g., thiazides).

Adverse reactions to calcium and vitamin D result in hypercalcemia and hypercalciuria. If hypercalcemia develops, calcium and vitamin D should be discontinued and appropriate therapy given. The toxic effects of vitamin D metabolites persist in proportion to their biologic half-lives (ergocalciferol, 20–60 days; dihydrotachysterol, 5–15 days; calcitriol, 2–10 days). Glucocorticoids antagonize the toxic effects of vitamin D metabolites.

Hypercalcemia

Although ionized calcium is best for detecting hypercalcemia, most patients with elevated total serum calcium concentrations will be hypercalcemic (unless a chelator is present). Most studies of hypercalcemia have defined hypercalcemia using total serum calcium values.

Hypercalcemia (total serum calcium > 10.5 mg·dl^{-1} or ionized calcium > 1.3 mM) causes a variety of pathophysiologic alterations (Table 9-19). Patients in whom total serum calcium is less than 11.5 mg·dl^{-1} are usually asymptomatic. Patients with moderate hypercalcemia (total serum calcium 11.5–13 mg·dl^{-1}) may show symptoms of lethargy, anorexia, nausea, and polyuria. Severe hypercalcemia (total serum calcium > 13 mg·dl^{-1}) is associated with more severe

TABLE 9-19. Hypercalcemia: Clinical Manifestations

Cardiovascular	*Urologic*
Hypertension	Nephrolithiasis
Heart block	Nephrocalcinosis
Digitalis sensitivity	Tubular dysfunction (polyuria)
	Azotemia
Neuromuscular	
	Gastrointestinal
Weakness	
Atrophy	Peptic ulcer disease
Hyporeflexia	Pancreatitis
Obtundation	Anorexia
Coma	

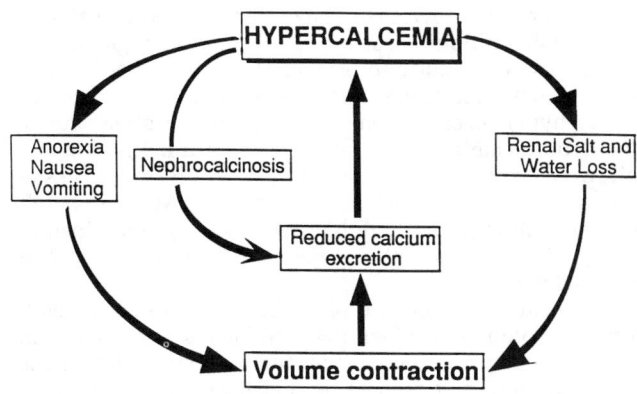

Figure 9-17. Hypercalcemia initiates a vicious cycle in which hypercalcemia itself reduces renal salt and water loss and anorexia, nausea, and vomiting, resulting in hypovolemia. The resulting volume contraction further reduces calcium excretion accentuating hypercalcemia. Nephrocalcinosis further reduces renal function and calcium excretion, and results in additional increments in serum calcium. (Reproduced with permission from Davis KD, Attie MF: Management of severe hypercalcemia. In Zaloga GP (guest ed): Endocrine Crises. Crit Care Clin 7:177, 1991.)

neuromyopathic symptoms, including muscle weakness, depression, impaired memory, emotional lability, lethargy, stupor, and coma.

Urinary concentrating ability deteriorates early in hypercalcemic patients. Hypercalcemia impairs renal excretory capacity for calcium by precipitating calcium salts within the renal parenchyma and by reducing RBF and GFR. Renal calcium salt precipitation (nephrocalcinosis) is irreversible. In response to hypovolemia, renal tubular reabsorption of sodium results in enhanced renal calcium reabsorption (Fig. 9-17). When hypercalcemia is severe, effective treatment is necessary to prevent progressive dehydration and renal failure leading to further increases in total serum calcium. Skeletal disease may occur secondary to direct osteolysis or humoral bone resorption. The cardiovascular effects of hypercalcemia include hypertension, arrhythmias, heart block, cardiac arrest, and digitalis sensitivity.

Hypercalcemia occurs when calcium enters the ECV more rapidly than the kidneys can excrete the excess. To compensate for increased gut absorption or bone resorption of calcium, renal excretion can readily increase from 100 to more than 400 mg·day^{-1}, and thus serve to maintain normocalcemia. Clinically, hypercalcemia most commonly results from an excess of bone resorption over bone formation, usually secondary to malignant disease, hyperparathyroidism, hypocalciuric hypercalcemia, thyrotoxicosis, granulomatous diseases, and immobilization. Hypercalcemia induced by malignant disease results from neoplastic bone destruction or from the secretion of humoral substances that stimulate bone resorption.[188-192] Although weakness, weight loss, and anemia associated with primary hyperparathyroidism may suggest malignancy, these may result simply from the primary disease process.[193] Hypercalcemia associated with granulomatous diseases (*i.e.*, sarcoidosis) results from the production of calcitriol by granulomatous tissue.[194,195]

The ionized [Ca^{2+}] provides the best diagnostic information. However, a fasting total serum calcium exceeding 10.5 mg·dl^{-1} is a reliable indicator of hypercalcemia. In hypoalbuminemic patients, total serum calcium can be estimated by assuming an increase of 0.8 mg·dl^{-1} for every 1 g·dl^{-1} of albumin concentration below 4.0 g·dl^{-1}. The development of hypercalcemia can be antagonized by coexisting disorders that cause hypocalcemia, such as pancreatitis, sepsis, or hyperphosphatemia.

Definitive treatment of hypercalcemia requires correction of underlying causes. However, as the diagnostic evaluation continues, temporizing therapy may be necessary to avoid complications and to relieve symptoms. Total serum calcium exceeding 14 mg·dl^{-1} represents a medical emergency associated with frequent complications.

General supportive treatment includes hydration, correction of associated electrolyte abnormalities, removal of offending drugs, dietary calcium restriction, and increased physical activity. Although gastrointestinal calcium absorption can be minimized by restricting calcium intake, no therapy increases gut calcium secretion. Because anorexia and antagonism by calcium of ADH action invariably lead to sodium and water depletion, infusion of 0.9% saline will dilute serum calcium, promote renal excretion, and can reduce total serum calcium by 1.5–3 mg·dl^{-1}.[196] Urinary output should be maintained at 200–300 ml·h^{-1}. As GFR increases, the sodium ion increases calcium excretion by competing with the calcium ion for reabsorption in the proximal renal tubules and loop of Henle. Furosemide further enhances calcium excretion by increasing tubular sodium. Patients who have renal impairment may require higher doses of furosemide. During saline infusion and forced diuresis, careful monitoring of cardiopulmonary status and electrolytes, especially magnesium and potassium, is required. Intensive diuresis and saline administration can achieve net calcium excretion rates of 2000–4000 mg per 24 hours, a rate eight times greater than saline alone, but still somewhat less than the rate of removal achieved by hemodialysis (*i.e.*, 6000 mg every 8 hours).

Bone resorption, the primary cause of hypercalcemia, can be minimized by mobilization and drug therapy. Calcitonin, which inhibits osteoclastic bone resorption and increases renal calcium clearance, is most effective in hypercalcemia states resulting from increased bone resorption (e.g., Paget's disease, malignant disease, and immobilization).[196] Calcitonin begins to reduce serum calcium within 1–2 hours following drug administration, with the maximal effect evident at 6–10 hours. Usually calcitonin reduces total serum calcium by only 1–2 mg·dl^{-1}.[197-199] After 24–48 hours of treatment, resistance to the hypocalcemic effects of calcitonin frequently develops, an effect that may be delayed by co-administration of glucocorticoids. Although calcitonin is relatively nontoxic, more than 25% of patients may not respond. Thus, calcitonin is unsuitable as a first-line drug during life-threatening hypercalcemia.

Mithramycin, a cytotoxic agent, lowers serum calcium primarily by inhibiting osteoclastic bone resorption, probably because of toxicity to osteoclasts.[200] Effective in most patients with malignant disease, mithramycin also improves hypercalcemia from other hyper-resorptive causes. The hypocalcemia effect, usually seen within 12–24 hours following a single intravenous dose of 25 $\mu g \cdot kg^{-1}$, peaks at 48–72 hours, and persists for 5–7 days.[201] Major toxic effects of mithramycin, more likely to occur in renal insufficiency, include thrombocytopenia, nephrotoxicity, and hepatotoxicity.

Etidronate disodium, a diphosphonate that inhibits both bone resorption and mineralization, lowers serum calcium in many patients with malignant tumors. Daily intravenous administration of etidronate normalizes serum calcium for up to 2 weeks in many patients with hypercalcemia caused by malignancy.[202-204] Often, however, mithramycin must be added.[204]

Hydrocortisone is effective in treating hypercalcemic patients with lymphatic malignancies, vitamin D or A intoxication, and diseases associated with production by tumor or granuloma of 1,25(OH)$_2$D or osteoclast-activating factor. Glucocorticoids rarely improve hypercalcemia secondary to malignancy or hyperparathyroidism, and may be little better than simple saline infusion.[205] Gallium nitrate, an antineoplastic drug now in clinical trials, lowers the serum calcium by inhibiting bone resorption. Infused over a 5-day period, gallium nitrate decreases the total serum calcium concentration in more than 75% of patients with hypercalcemia from malignant disease.[199-204] Indomethacin, a cyclo-oxygenase inhibitor that decreases prostaglandin production, can be occasionally effective in treating rare cases of hypercalcemia that result from excess prostaglandin production. Cyclo-oxygenase inhibitors are ineffective in most patients with hypercalcemia caused by malignancy.[206]

Phosphates, which lower serum calcium by causing deposition of calcium in bone and soft tissue, risk extraskeletal calcification of vital organs such as the kidneys and myocardium. Therefore, intravenous phosphates are rarely indicated in hypercalcemia. Because soft-tissue calcification is less likely if phosphates are given orally, the intravenous route should be reserved for patients with life-threatening hypercalcemia or patients in whom other measures have failed. The initial dose of intravenous phosphates should not exceed 50 mM within 8 hours. Patients treated with phosphates should be well hydrated. Ethylenediaminetetraacetic acid (EDTA) complexes with calcium and increases its excretion. Although effective in lowering serum calcium, the use of EDTA is limited by its nephrotoxicity. Slow calcium channel antagonists such as verapamil and nifedipine may also be useful in reversing hypercalcemia cardiotoxicity.[207]

Phosphate

Physiologic Role

Phosphorus, in the form of phosphate, is distributed in similar concentrations throughout intracellular and extracellular fluid. Eighty-five percent of phosphate is osseous and 15% is nonosseous. Phosphate circulates as the free ion (55%), complexed ion (33%), and in a protein-bound form (12%). Blood levels vary widely: the normal total serum phosphate level ranges from 2.7 to 4.5 mg·dl^{-1} in adults. Phosphates play a vital role in energy storage and are re-

sponsible for the primary energy bond in ATP and creatine phosphate. Therefore, severe phosphate depletion results in cellular energy depletion. Phosphorus is an essential element of second-messenger systems, including cAMP and phosphoinositides, and a major component of nucleic acids, phospholipids, and cell membranes. As part of 2,3-diphosphoglycerate, phosphate is important for off-loading oxygen from the hemoglobin molecule. Phosphorus also functions in protein-phosphorylation and acts as a urinary buffer (see Table 9-6).

Hypophosphatemia

Hypophosphatemia is characterized by low levels of phosphate-containing cellular components, including ATP, 2,3-diphosphoglycerate, and membrane phospholipids. Neurologic manifestations of hypophosphatemia include paresthesias, myopathy, encephalopathy, delirium, seizures, and coma (Table 9-20).[208,209] Hematologic abnormalities include dysfunction of erythrocytes, platelets, and leukocytes. Muscle weakness and malaise are common. Respiratory muscle failure[210-213] and myocardial dysfunction[214,215] are potential problems of particular concern to anesthesiologists. Serious life-threatening organ dysfunction may occur when the serum phosphate (PO$_4$) concentration falls below 1 mg·dl^{-1}.

Common in hospitalized patients[216,217] and postoperative or traumatized patients,[218,219] hypophosphatemia (PO$_4$ < 2.5 mg·dl^{-1}) is caused by three primary abnormalities in PO$_4$ homeostasis: an intracellular shift of PO$_4$, an increase in renal PO$_4$ loss, and a decrease in gastrointestinal PO$_4$ absorption. High carbohydrate intake, such as occurs with parenteral nutrition, stimulates insulin secretion, which in turn increases cellular PO$_4$ uptake. Carbohydrate-induced hypophosphatemia is the type most commonly encountered in hospitalized patients. Hypophosphatemia may also occur as catabolic patients become anabolic, and during medical management of diabetic ketoacidosis. Acute alkalemia secondary to respiratory or metabolic alkalosis increases intracellular consumption of PO$_4$ by increasing the rate of glycolysis. Hyperventilation to a Paco$_2$ of 20 mm Hg may reduce the serum PO$_4$ level by 2–3 mg·dl^{-1}.[220,221] Acute correction of respiratory acidemia may also result in severe hypophosphatemia.[216] In response to acute alkalemia, serum PO$_4$ frequently falls to 1–2 mg·dl^{-1}. Respiratory alkalosis probably explains the hypophosphatemia associated with gram-negative bacteremia and salicylate poisoning. Excessive renal loss of PO$_4$ explains the hypophosphatemia associated with hyperparathyroidism, hypomagnesemia, hypothermia, diuretic therapy, and renal tubular defects in PO$_4$ absorption. Excess gastrointestinal loss of PO$_4$ is most com-

---

TABLE 9-20. Hypophosphatemia: Clinical Manifestations

Cardiovascular	*Gastrointestinal*
Myocardial failure	Nausea, vomiting
	Anorexia
Neuromuscular	
Respiratory muscle failure	
Rhabdomyolysis	
Decreased level of consciousness	
Hyporeflexia	
Seizures	

TABLE 9-21. Hypophosphatemia: Treatment

Parenteral phosphate, 0.2 mM–0.68 mM·kg^{-1} (5–16 mg·kg^{-1}) over 12 hours
  Potassium phosphate (contains phosphate, 93 mg·ml^{-1})
  Sodium phosphate (contains phosphate, 93 mg·ml^{-1})
Oral phosphate
  Neutra-Phos (contains phosphate, 250 mg per capsule), 2 capsules b.i.d.–t.i.d.
  Phospho-Soda (Fleet) (contains phosphate, 129 mg·ml^{-1}), 5 ml b.i.d.–t.i.d.
  Potassium phosphate (contains phosphate, 125 mg per tablet), 4 tablets b.i.d.–t.i.d.

monly secondary to the use of PO_4-binding antacids or to malabsorption syndromes.

Measurement of urinary PO_4 aids in differentiation of hypophosphatemia due to renal losses from that due to excessive gastrointestinal losses or redistribution of PO_4 into cells. Extrarenal causes of hypophosphatemia cause avid renal tubular PO_4 reabsorption, reducing urinary PO_4 excretion to less than 100 mg·day^{-1}.[222]

Patients who have severe (<1 mg·dl^{-1}) or symptomatic hypophosphatemia require intravenous phosphate administration (Table 9-21).[208,209,223] In chronically hypophosphatemic patients, 0.2–0.68 mmol·kg^{-1} (5–16 mg·kg^{-1} elemental phosphorus) should be infused over 12 hours. The dosage is then adjusted as indicated by the serum PO_4 level, because the cumulative deficit in total body phosphate cannot be predicted accurately based on serum levels.[223] Phosphate should be administered cautiously to hypocalcemic patients because of the risk of precipitating more severe hypocalcemia. In hypercalcemic patients, PO_4 may cause soft-tissue calcification. Phosphorus must be given cautiously to patients with renal insufficiency because of impaired excretory ability. During treatment, close monitoring of serum PO_4, calcium, magnesium, and potassium levels is essential to avoid complications including hyperphosphatemia.[224] Oral therapy can be substituted for parenteral PO_4 once the serum PO_4 level exceeds 2.0 mg·dl^{-1}. Continued therapy with PO_4 supplements is required for 5–10 days in order to replenish body stores.

Hyperphosphatemia

The clinical features of hyperphosphatemia relate primarily to the development of hypocalcemia (see Table 9-17) and ectopic calcification.

Hyperphosphatemia (PO_4 > 5.0 mg·dl^{-1}) is caused by three basic mechanisms: inadequate renal excretion, increased movement of PO_4 to the ECV from the ICV, and increased PO_4 or vitamin D intake. Rapid cell lysis from chemotherapy, rhabdomyolysis, and sepsis can cause hyperphosphatemia, especially when renal function is impaired. Frequent iatrogenic causes of hyperphosphatemia include oral PO_4 supplements, PO_4 enemas, and overenthusiastic administration of PO_4 in diabetic ketoacidosis. Renal excretion of PO_4 remains adequate until the GFR falls below 20–25 ml·min^{-1}. Renal excretion of PO_4 is reduced in hypoparathyroid patients because of the loss of the phosphaturic effect of PTH.

Measurements of BUN, creatinine, GFR, and urinary PO_4 are helpful in the differential diagnosis of hyperphosphatemia. Normal renal function accompanied by high PO_4 excretion (>1,500 mg·day^{-1}) indicates increased PO_4 ex-

cretory requirements because of endogenous or exogenous oversupply. An elevated BUN, elevated creatinine, and low GFR suggest impaired renal excretion of PO_4. Normal renal function and PO_4 excretion less than 1,500 mg·day^{-1} suggest increased PO_4 reabsorption (*i.e.*, hypoparathyroidism).

Hyperphosphatemia is corrected by eliminating the cause of the PO_4 elevation and correcting the associated hypocalcemia and hyperphosphatemia. The serum concentration of PO_4 is reduced by restricting intake, increasing urinary excretion with saline and acetazolamide (500 mg every 6 hours), and increasing gastrointestinal losses by enteric administration of aluminum hydroxide (30–45 ml every 6 hours). Aluminum hydroxide absorbs PO_4 secreted into the bowel lumen and increases PO_4 loss even if no PO_4 is ingested. Hemodialysis and peritoneal dialysis are effective in removing PO_4 in patients who have renal failure.

Magnesium

Physiologic Role

Magnesium is an important, multifunctional, divalent cation located primarily in the intracellular space (intracellular magnesium ~ 2400 mg; extracellular magnesium ~ 280 mg). Approximately 50% of magnesium is located in bone, 25% is found in muscle, and less than 1% of total body magnesium circulates in the serum. Of the normal circulating total magnesium concentration (1.6–2.4 mEq·l^{-1} or 0.8–1.2 mmol·l^{-1} or 1.8–3.0 mg·dl^{-1}), there are three components: protein-bound (30%), chelated (15%), and ionized (55%), of which only ionized magnesium is active. A primary regulator or cofactor in many enzyme systems, magnesium is important for the regulation of the sodium-potassium pump, Ca-ATPase enzymes, adenyl cyclase, proton pumps, and slow calcium channels. Magnesium has been called an endogenous calcium antagonist, because regulation of slow calcium channels contributes to maintenance of normal vascular tone, prevention of vasospasm, and perhaps to prevention of calcium overload in many tissues. Because magnesium partially regulates PTH secretion and is important for the maintenance of end-organ sensitivity to both PTH and vitamin D, abnormalities in ionized magnesium concentration ($[Mg^{2+}]$) may result in abnormal calcium metabolism. Magnesium functions in potassium metabolism primarily through regulating sodium-potassium ATPase, an enzyme that controls potassium entry into cells, especially in potassium-depleted states, and controls reabsorption of potassium by the renal tubules. In addition, magnesium functions as a regulator of membrane excitability and serves as a structural component in both cell membranes and the skeleton.

Serum $[Mg^{2+}]$ is regulated primarily by intrinsic renal mechanisms, although PTH and vitamin D exert minor influences. While both magnesium and PO_4 are primarily regulated by intrinsic renal mechanisms, PTH exerts a greater effect on renal loss of PO_4.

Hypomagnesemia

The clinical features of hypomagnesemia ($[Mg^{2+}]$ < 1.7 mg·dl^{-1}), like those of hypocalcemia, are characterized by increased neuronal irritability and tetany (Table 9-22).[225,226] Symptoms are rare when the serum $[Mg^{2+}]$ is above 1.5–1.7 mg·dl^{-1}; most symptomatic patients have serum $[Mg^{2+}]$ less than 1.0 mg·dl^{-1}. Patients frequently complain of weakness, lethargy, muscle spasms, paresthesias, and depression.

TABLE 9-22. Hypomagnesemia: Clinical Manifestations

Cardiovascular	*Miscellaneous*
Heart failure	Dysphagia
Dysrhythmias	Anorexia
Coronary spasm	Nausea
Refractory ventricular fibrillation	Hypokalemia
	Hypocalcemia
Neuromuscular	
Latent or overt tetany	
Weakness	
Decreased level of consciousness	
Seizures	

When severe, hypomagnesemia may induce seizures, confusion, and coma. Cardiovascular abnormalities include coronary artery spasm, cardiac failure, dysrhythmias, and hypotension.

Magnesium may influence dysrhythmias by direct effects on myocardial membranes, by altering cellular potassium and sodium concentrations, by inhibiting cellular calcium entry, by improving myocardial oxygen supply and demand, by prolonging the effective refractory period, by depressing conduction, by antagonizing catecholamine action on the conducting system, and by preventing vasospasm.[227] Dysrhythmias following myocardial infarction may be related to hypokalemia and hypomagnesemia.[228,229] Consequently, administration of magnesium reduces the incidence of dysrhythmias and improves outcome after myocardial infarction.[230-233] Treatment of hypomagnesemia, which frequently occurs after cardiopulmonary bypass, decreases the incidence of ventricular dysrhythmias after heart surgery from 63% to 22%.[234] In addition, magnesium may be useful as treatment for torsades de pointes, even in normomagnesemic patients.[235] Because the sodium-potassium pump is magnesium dependent, hypomagnesemia increases myocardial sensitivity to digitalis preparations and may cause hypokalemia as a result of renal potassium wasting. Both severe hypomagnesemia and hypermagnesemia suppress PTH secretion and can cause hypocalcemia. Severe hypomagnesemia may also impair end-organ response to PTH.

Because magnesium is present in many foods, hypomagnesemia rarely results from inadequate dietary intake. The most common causes of hypomagnesemia are inadequate gastrointestinal absorption, excessive magnesium losses, or failure of renal magnesium conservation. Gastrointestinal disease can cause hypomagnesemia by decreasing absorption and increasing magnesium losses in intestinal secretions. Excessive magnesium loss is also associated with prolonged nasogastric suctioning, gastrointestinal or biliary fistulas, and intestinal drains. Renal magnesium wasting complicates a variety of systemic and renal diseases because of the inability of the renal tubule to conserve magnesium. Although hypomagnesemia is common in critically ill patients,[236] the incidence of serum hypomagnesemia probably underestimates the incidence of total body magnesium depletion.[237] Polyuria, whether secondary to ECV expansion or to pharmacologic[238,239] or pathologic diuresis, may also result in excessive urinary magnesium excretion. Various drugs and toxins, including aminoglycosides,[240] cisplatinum, cardiac glycosides, and diuretics, enhance urinary magnesium excretion and may cause hypomagnesemia. However, patients who have renal disease and reduced GFR

frequently develop magnesium retention. Hypoparathyroidism, though frequently associated with hypomagnesemia, appears to be a consequence rather than the cause. Intracellular shifts of magnesium as a result of thyroid hormone or insulin administration may also decrease serum $[Mg^{2+}]$.

Measurement of 24-hour urinary magnesium excretion is useful in separating renal from nonrenal causes of hypomagnesemia. Normal kidneys can reduce magnesium excretion to less than $1-2$ mEq·day^{-1} in response to magnesium depletion. Hypomagnesemia accompanied by high urinary excretion of magnesium ($>3-4$ mEq·day^{-1}) suggests a renal etiology for hypomagnesemia.

Magnesium deficiency is treated by the administration of magnesium supplements (Table 9-23). One gram of magnesium sulfate provides approximately 4 mmol (8 mEq, or 98 mg) of elemental magnesium. Mild deficiencies can be treated with diet alone. Daily magnesium requirements range from 0.3 to 0.4 mEq·kg^{-1}·day^{-1}, in addition to replacement of abnormal losses. Symptomatic or severe hypomagnesemia ($[Mg^{2+}] < 1.0$ mg·dl^{-1}) should be treated with parenteral magnesium: $1-2$ g ($8-16$ mEq) of magnesium sulfate as an intravenous bolus over the first hour, followed by a continuous infusion of $2-4$ mEq·h^{-1}. Therapy should be guided subsequently by the serum magnesium level. The rate of infusion should not exceed 1 mEq·min^{-1}, even in emergency situations, and the patient should receive continuous cardiac monitoring to avoid cardiotoxicity. Because magnesium exerts calcium antagonistic properties, blood pressure and cardiac function should be monitored. In experimental animals, magnesium infusion produces a dose-dependent decrease in systemic vascular resistance.[241] Hypertensive animals are more susceptible to its hypotensive effects.[242] Despite a demonstration of decreased cardiac function in open-chest dogs,[243] effects on myocardial contractility and blood pressure appear to be modest under clinical circumstances, although magnesium does tend to increase the cardiac index.[244]

During repletion, the patellar reflexes should be monitored frequently and magnesium withheld if they become suppressed. Repletion of systemic magnesium stores usually requires $5-7$ days of therapy. Once depleted magnesium stores have been replenished, all patients should receive daily maintenance doses of magnesium. Magnesium can be given orally, usually in a dose of $60-90$ mEq·day^{-1} of magnesium oxide (30% absorbed). Magnesium-containing antacids are poorly absorbed and the dosage is limited by diarrhea. Hypocalcemic, hypomagnesemic patients should receive magnesium as the chloride salt, because the sulfate ion can chelate calcium and further reduce the serum $[Ca^{2+}]$. Patients who have renal insufficiency have a diminished ability to excrete magnesium and require careful monitoring during therapy.

TABLE 9-23. Hypomagnesemia: Treatment

Intravenous Mg*: $8-16$ mEq bolus over 1 hour, followed by $2-4$ mEq·h^{-1} as continuous infusion
Intramuscular Mg*: 10 mEq q $4-6$ hours
Oral magnesium oxide: (35 mEq Mg per tablet), $2-3$ tablets b.i.d.–t.i.d.

*MgSO$_4$: 1 g = 8 mEq Mg. MgCl$_2$: 1 g = 10 mEq Mg.

TABLE 9-24. Hypermagnesemia: Clinical Findings

Clinical Findings	Serum Mg^{2+} Level $(mg \cdot dl^{-1})$
Normal	1.7–2.4
Therapeutic range (pre-eclampsia)	5–8
Hypotension	3–5
Deep tendon hyporeflexia	5
Somnolence	8.5
Respiratory insufficiency, deep tendon arreflexia	12
Heart block, respiratory paralysis	18
Cardiac arrest	24

Hypermagnesemia

Therapeutic hypermagnesemia is used to treat patients with premature labor, pre-eclampsia, and eclampsia. Because magnesium blocks the release of catecholamines from adrenergic nerve terminals and the adrenal gland, magnesium has been used to reduce the hypertensive response to tracheal intubation,[245] and to reduce the effects of catecholamine excess in patients with tetanus[246] and pheochromocytoma.[247] Other rarer causes of mild hypermagnesemia are hypothyroidism, Addison's disease, lithium intoxication, and familial hypocalciuric hypercalcemia.

Most cases of hypermagnesemia ($[Mg^{2+}] > 2.5$ mg·dl^{-1}) are iatrogenic in origin, resulting from the administration of magnesium-containing preparations, such as antacids, enemas, and parenteral nutrition formulas, especially to patients with impaired renal function. Hypermagnesemia antagonizes the release and effect of acetylcholine at the neuromuscular junction. The result is depressed skeletal muscle function and neuromuscular blockade. Magnesium potentiates the action of nondepolarizing muscle relaxants[248] and decreases potassium release in response to succinylcholine.[249] The clinical features of progressive hypermagnesemia are listed in Table 9-24.

The neuromuscular and cardiac toxicity of hypermagnesemia can be acutely, but transiently, antagonized by giving intravenous calcium (5–10 mEq) to buy time while more definitive therapy is instituted.[250] All magnesium-containing preparations must be stopped. Urinary excretion of magnesium can be increased by expanding ECV and inducing diuresis with a combination of saline and furosemide. In emergency situations and in patients with renal failure, magnesium may be removed by dialysis.

REFERENCES

1. Badr KF, Ichikawa I: Prerenal failure: A deleterious shift from renal compensation to decompensation. N Engl J Med 319: 623, 1988
2. Henrich WL, Anderson RJ, Berns AS et al: The role of renal nerves and prostaglandins in control of renal hemodynamics and plasma renin activity during hypotensive hemorrhage in the dog. J Clin Invest 61:744, 1978
3. Aukland K, Kirkebo A, Loyning E, Tyssebotn I: Effect of hemorrhagic hypotension on the distribution of renal cortical blood flow in anesthetized dogs. Acta Physiol Scand 87:514, 1973
4. Henrich WL, Pettinger WA, Cronin RE: The influence of circu-lating catecholamines and prostaglandins on canine renal hemodynamics during hemorrhage. Circ Res 48:424, 1981
5. Stone AM, Stahl WM: Renal effects of hemorrhage in normal man. Ann Surg 172:825, 1970
6. Hall J, Robertson G: Diabetes insipidus. In Kirby RR, Taylor RW (eds): Problems in Critical Care. Vol 4. Endocrine Emergencies (GP Zaloga, guest ed), p 342. Philadelphia, JB Lippincott, 1990
7. Salazar FJ, Romero JC, Burnett JC Jr et al: Atrial natriuretic peptide levels during acute and chronic saline loading in conscious dogs. Am J Physiol 251:R499, 1986
8. Needleman P, Greenwald JE: Atriopeptin: A cardiac hormone intimately involved in fluid, electrolyte, and blood-pressure homeostasis. N Engl J Med 314:828, 1986
9. Roy LF, Ogilvie RI, Larochelle P et al: Cardiac and vascular effects of atrial natriuretic factor and sodium nitroprusside in healthy men. Circulation 79:383, 1989
10. Cernacek P, Maher E, Crawhall JC, Levy M: Renal dose response and pharmacokinetics of atrial natriuretic factor in dogs. Am J Physiol 255:R929, 1988
11. Shenker Y: Atrial natriuretic hormone effect on renal function and aldosterone secretion in sodium depletion. Am J Physiol 255:R867, 1988
12. Laragh JH: The endocrine control of blood volume, blood pressure and sodium balance: atrial hormone and renin system interactions. J Hypertens Suppl 4:S143, 1986
13. Barajas L, Powers K: The structure of the juxtaglomerular apparatus (JGA) and the control of renin secretion: An update. J Hypertens 2(suppl 1):3, 1984
14. Briggs JP, Schnermann J: Macula densa control of renin secretion and glomerular vascular tone: Evidence for common cellular mechanisms. Renal Physiol 9:193, 1986
15. Scharschmidt LA, Lianos E, Dunn MJ: Arachidonate metabolites and the control of glomerular function. Fed Proc 42:3058, 1983
16. Murray MD, Brater DC: Adverse effects of nonsteroidal antiinflammatory drugs on renal function (editorial). Ann Intern Med 112:559, 1990
17. Lanier WL, Stangland KJ, Scheithauer BW et al: The effects of dextrose infusion and head position on neurologic outcome after complete cerebral ischemia in primates: Examination of a model. Anesthesiology 66:39, 1987
18. Lundy EF, Kuhn JE, Kwon JM et al: Infusion of five percent dextrose increases mortality and morbidity following six minutes of cardiac arrest in resuscitated dogs. J Crit Care 2:4, 1987
19. Pulsinelli WA, Kraig RP, Plum F: Hyperglycemia, cerebral acidosis, and ischemic brain damage. In Plum F, Pulsinelli W (eds): Cerebrovascular Diseases, p 201. New York, Raven Press, 1985
20. Longstreth WT Jr, Diehr P, Cobb LA et al: Neurologic outcome and blood glucose levels during out-of-hospital cardiopulmonary resuscitation. Neurology 36:1186, 1986
21. Lam AM, Winn HR, Cullen BF, Sundling N: Hyperglycemia and neurological outcome in patients with head injury. J Neurosurg, 75:545, 1991
22. Sieber FE, Smith DS, Traystman RJ, Wollman H: Glucose: A reevaluation of its intraoperative use. Anesthesiology 67:72, 1987
23. Roberts JP, Roberts JD, Skinner C et al: Extracellular fluid deficit following operation and its correction with Ringer's lactate: A reassessment. Ann Surg 202:1, 1985
24. Carrico CJ, Coln CD, Lightfoot SA et al: Extracellular fluid volume replacement in hemorrhagic shock. Surg Forum 14:10, 1963
25. Lundvall J, Länne T: Large capacity in man for effective plasma volume control in hypovolaemia via fluid transfer from tissue to blood. Acta Physiol Scand 137:513, 1989
26. Chiao JJ, Minei JP, Shires GT III, Shires GT: In vivo myocyte sodium activity and concentration during hemorrhagic shock. Am J Physiol 258:R684, 1990
27. Shires GT, Cunningham JN, Baker CR et al: Alterations in cellular membrane function during hemorrhagic shock in primates. Ann Surg 176:288, 1972

28. Böck JC, Barker BC, Clinton AG et al: Post-traumatic changes in effective colloid osmotic pressure on the distribution of body water. Ann Surg 210:395, 1989
29. Giesecke AH Jr, Egbert LD: Perioperative fluid therapy-crystalloids. In Miller R (ed): Anesthesia, vol 2, 2nd ed, p 1313. New York, Churchill Livingstone, 1986
30. Demling RH: Shock and fluids. In Chernow B, Shoemaker WC (eds): Critical Care: State of the Art, p 301. Fullerton, California, Society of Critical Care Medicine, 1986
31. Swabb EA, Wei J, Gullino PM: Diffusion and convection in normal and neoplastic tissues. Cancer Res 34:2814, 1974
32. Uhley HN, Leeds SE, Sampson JJ, Friedman M: Role of pulmonary lymphatics in chronic pulmonary edema. Circ Res 11:966, 1962
33. Rainey TG, English JF: Pharmacology of colloids and crystalloids. In Chernow B (ed): The Pharmacologic Approach to the Critically Ill Patient, 2nd ed, p 219. Baltimore, Williams & Wilkins, 1988
34. Stump DC, Strauss RG, Henriksen RA et al: Effects of hydroxyethyl starch on blood coagulation, particularly factor VIII. Transfusion 25:349, 1985
35. Gold MS, Russo J, Tissot M et al: Comparison of hetastarch to albumin for perioperative bleeding in patients undergoing abdominal aortic aneurysm surgery: A prospective, randomized study. Ann Surg 211:482, 1990
36. Shatney CH, Deepika K, Militello PR et al: Efficacy of hetastarch in the resuscitation of patients with multisystem trauma and shock. Arch Surg 118:804, 1983
37. Halonen P, Linko K, Myllyla G: A study of haemostasis following the use of high doses of hydroxyethyl starch 120 and dextran in major laparotomies. Acta Anaesthesiol Scand 31:320, 1987
38. Palanzo DA, Parr GV, Bull AP et al: Hetastarch as a prime for cardiopulmonary bypass. Ann Thorac Surg 34:680, 1982
39. Sade RM, Crawford FA Jr, Dearing JP, Stroud M: Hydroxyethyl starch in priming fluid for cardiopulmonary bypass. J Thorac Cardiovasc Surg 84:35, 1982
40. Prough DS, Johnston WE: Fluid resuscitation in septic shock: No solution yet. Anesth Analg 69:699, 1989
41. Dawidson I: Fluid resuscitation of shock: Current controversies (editorial). Crit Care Med 17:1078, 1989
42. Van den Broek WGM, Trouwborst A, Bakker WH: The effect of iso-oncotic plasma substitutes: Gelatine, dextran 40 (50 g/l) and the effect of Ringer's lactate on the plasma volume in healthy subjects. Acta Anaesth Belg 40:275, 1989
43. Baum TD, Wang H, Rothschild HR et al: Mesenteric oxygen metabolism, ileal mucosal hydrogen ion concentration, and tissue edema after crystalloid or colloid resuscitation in porcine endotoxic shock: Comparison of Ringer's lactate and 6% hetastarch. Circ Shock 30:385, 1990
44. Linko K, Makelainen A: Cardiorespiratory function after replacement of blood loss with hydroxyethyl starch 120, dextran-70, and Ringer's acetate in pigs. Crit Care Med 17:1031, 1989
45. Zikria BA, Subbarao C, Oz MC et al: Hydroethyl starch macromolecules reduce myocardial reperfusion injury. Arch Surg 125:930, 1990
46. Zikria BA, Subbarao C, Oz MC et al: A biophysical approach to capillary permeability. Surgery 105:625, 1989
47. Zikria BA, Subbarao C, Oz MC et al: Macromolecules reduce abnormal microvascular permeability in rat limb ischemia-reperfusion injury. Crit Care Med 17:1306, 1989
48. Schmitz M, Traber L, Toole J et al: Pentafraction reduces the lung lymph response to endotoxin (LPS). Anesthesiology 71:A174, 1989
49. Rackow EC, Falk JL, Fein IA et al: Fluid resuscitation in circulatory shock: A comparison of the cardiorespiratory effects of albumin, hetastarch, and saline solutions in patients with hypovolemic and septic shock. Crit Care Med 11:839, 1983
50. Rackow EC, Fein IA, Siegel J: The relationship of the colloid osmotic-pulmonary artery wedge pressure gradient to pulmonary edema and mortality in critically ill patients. Chest 82:433, 1982
51. Weil MH, Henning RJ, Puri VK: Colloid oncotic pressure: Clinical significance. Crit Care Med 7:113, 1979
52. Hauser CJ, Shoemaker WC, Turpin I, Goldberg SJ: Oxygen transport responses to colloids and crystalloids in critically ill surgical patients. Surg Gynecol Obstet 150:811, 1980
53. Lowe RJ, Moss GS, Jilek J, Levine HD: Crystalloid vs colloid in the etiology of pulmonary failure after trauma: A randomized trial in man. Surgery 81:676, 1977
54. Moss GS, Lowe RJ, Jilek J, Levine HD: Colloid or crystalloid in the resuscitation of hemorrhagic shock: A controlled clinical trial. Surgery 89:434, 1981
55. Moss GS, Siegel DC, Cochin A, Fresquez V: Effects of saline and colloid solutions in pulmonary function in hemorrhagic shock. Surg Gynecol Obstet 133:53, 1971
56. Virgilio RW, Rice CL, Smith DE et al: Crystalloid vs colloid resuscitation: Is one better? A randomized clinical study. Surgery 85:129, 1979
57. Gammage G: Crystalloid versus colloid: Is colloid worth the cost? Int Anesthesiol Clin 25:37, 1987
58. Pearl PG, Halperin BD, Mihm FG, Rosenthal MH: Pulmonary effects of crystalloid and colloid resuscitation from hemorrhagic shock in the presence of oleic acid-induced pulmonary capillary injury in the dog. Anesthesiology 68:12, 1988
59. Finn JC, Rosenthal MH: Pulmonary edema in trauma and critically ill patients. Semin Anesth 8:265, 1989
60. Tommasino C, Moore S, Todd MM: Cerebral effects of isovolemic hemodilution with crystalloid or colloid solutions. Crit Care Med 16:862, 1988
61. Poole GV Jr, Prough DS, Johnson JC et al: Effects of resuscitation for hemorrhagic shock on cerebral hemodynamics in the presence of an intracranial mass. J Trauma 27:18, 1987
62. Zornow MH, Todd MM, Moore SS: The acute cerebral effects of changes in plasma osmolality and oncotic pressure. Anesthesiology 67:936, 1987
63. Warner DS, Boehland LA: Effects of iso-osmolal intravenous fluid therapy on post-ischemic brain water content in the rat. Anesthesiology 68:86, 1988
64. Zornow MH, Scheller MS, Todd MM, Moore SS: Acute cerebral effects of isotonic crystalloid and colloid solutions following cryogenic brain injury in the rabbit. Anesthesiology 69:180, 1988
65. Kaieda R, Todd MM, Warner DS: Prolonged reduction in colloid oncotic pressure does not increase brain edema following cryogenic injury in rabbits. Anesthesiology 71:554, 1989
66. Maningas PA, DeGuzman LR, Tillman FJ et al: Small-volume infusion of 7.5% NaCl in 6% Dextran 70 for the treatment of severe hemorrhagic shock in swine. Ann Emerg Med 15:1131, 1986
67. Weed LH, McKibben PS: Experimental alteration of brain bulk. Am J Physiol 48:531, 1919
68. Wilson BJ, Jones RF, Coleman ST, Moyer CA: The effects of various hypertonic sodium salt solutions on cisternal pressure. Surgery 30:361, 1958
69. Baue AE, Tragus ET, Parkins WM: Effects of sodium chloride and bicarbonate in shock with metabolic acidosis. Am J Physiol 212:54, 1967
70. Jelenko C III, Williams JB, Wheeler ML et al: Studies in shock and resuscitation: I. Use of a hypertonic, albumin-containing fluid demand regimen (HALFD) in resuscitation. Crit Care Med 7:157, 1979
71. Monafo WW, Chuntrasakul C, Ayvazian VH: Hypertonic sodium solutions in the treatment of burn shock. Am J Surg 126:778, 1973
72. Monafo WW: The treatment of burn shock by the intravenous and oral administration of hypertonic lactated saline solution. J Trauma 10:575, 1970
73. Liang CS, Hood WB Jr: Mechanism of cardiac output response to hypertonic sodium chloride infusion in dogs. Am J Physiol 235:H18, 1978
74. Shackford SR, Sise MJ, Fridlund PH et al: Hypertonic sodium lactate versus lactated Ringer's solution for intravenous fluid therapy in operations on the abdominal aorta. Surgery 94:41, 1983

75. Velasco IT, Pontieri V, Rocha e Silva MR Jr, Lopes OU: Hyperosmotic NaCl and severe hemorrhagic shock. Am J Physiol 239:H664, 1980

76. Lopes OU, Pontieri V, Rocha e Silva MR Jr, Velasco IT: Hyperosmotic NaCl and severe hemorrhagic shock: Role of the innervated lung. Am J Physiol 241:H883, 1981

77. Younes RN, Aun F, Tomida RM, Birolini D: The role of lung innervation in the hemodynamic response to hypertonic sodium chloride solutions in hemorrhagic shock. Surgery 98:900, 1985

78. Schertel ER, Valentine AK, Rademakers AM, Muir WW: Influence of 7% NaCl on the mechanical properties of the systemic circulation in the hypovolemic dog. Circ Shock 31:203, 1990

79. Ljungqvist O, Boija PO, Ware J: The effect of hyperosmolar infusions on survival after hemorrhage. Acta Chir Scand 155:433, 1989

80. Onarheim H, Missavage AE, Kramer GC, Gunther RA: Effectiveness of hypertonic saline-dextran 70 for initial fluid resuscitation of major burns. J Trauma 30:597, 1990

81. Gunn ML, Hansbrough JF, Davis JW et al: Prospective, randomized trial of hypertonic sodium lactate versus lactated Ringer's solution for burn shock resuscitation. J Trauma 29:1261, 1989

82. Prough DS, Johnson JC, Poole GV Jr et al: Effects on intracranial pressure of resuscitation from hemorrhagic shock with hypertonic saline versus lactated Ringer's solution. Crit Care Med 13:407, 1985

83. Prough DS, Johnson JC, Stump DA et al: Effects of hypertonic saline versus lactated Ringer's solution on cerebral oxygen transport during resuscitation from hemorrhagic shock. J Neurosurg 64:627, 1986

84. Todd MM, Tommasino C, Moore S: Cerebral effects of isovolemic hemodilution with a hypertonic saline solution. J Neurosurg 63:944, 1985

85. Wisner DH, Schuster L, Quinn C: Hypertonic saline resuscitation of head injury: Effects on cerebral water content. J Trauma 30:75, 1990

86. Prough DS, Whitley JM, Taylor CL et al: Regional cerebral blood flow following resuscitation from hemorrhagic shock with hypertonic saline: Influence of a subdural mass. Anesthesiology 1991, 75:319, 1991

87. Whitley JM, Prough DS, Brockschmidt JK et al: Cerebral hemodynamic effects of fluid resuscitation in the presence of an experimental intracranial mass. Surgery 1991, 110:514, 1991

88. Johnston WE, Alford PT, Prough DS et al: Cardiopulmonary effects of hypertonic saline in canine oleic acid–induced pulmonary edema. Crit Care Med 13:814, 1985

89. Armistead CW Jr, Vincent JL, Preiser JC et al: Hypertonic saline solution–hetastarch for fluid resuscitation in experimental septic shock. Anesth Analg 69:714, 1989

90. Smith GJ, Kramer GC, Perron P et al: A comparison of several hypertonic solutions for resuscitation of bled sheep. J Surg Res 39:517, 1985

91. Vassar MJ, Perry CA, Holcroft JW: Analysis of potential risks associated with 7.5% sodium chloride resuscitation of traumatic shock. Arch Surg 125:1309, 1990

92. Spital A, Sterns RD: The paradox of sodium's volume of distribution: Why an extracellular solute appears to distribute over total body water. Arch Intern Med 149:1255, 1989

93. Shackford SR, Fortlage DA, Peters RM et al: Serum osmolar and electrolyte changes associated with large infusions of hypertonic sodium lactate for intravascular volume expansion of patients undergoing aortic reconstruction. Surg Gynecol Obstet 164:127, 1987

94. Norenberg MD, Leslie KO, Robertson AS: Association between rise in serum sodium and central pontine myelinolysis. Ann Neurol 11:128, 1982

95. Laureno R: Central pontine myelinolysis following rapid correction of hyponatremia. Ann Neurol 13:232, 1983

96. Norenberg MD, Papendick RE: Chronicity of hyponatremia as a factor in experimental myelinolysis. Ann Neurol 15:544, 1984

97. Mazzoni MC, Borgstrom P, Arfors KE, Intaglietta M: The efficacy of iso- and hyperosmotic fluids as volume expanders in fixed-volume and uncontrolled hemorrhage. Ann Emerg Med 19:350, 1990

98. Gross D, Landau EH, Klin B, Krausz MM: Treatment of uncontrolled hemorrhagic shock with hypertonic saline solution. Surg Gynecol Obstet 170:106, 1990

99. Shenkin HA, Cheney RH, Govons SR et al: On the diagnosis of hemorrhage in man: A study of volunteers bled large amounts. Am J Med Sci 208:421, 1944

100. Lipsitz LA: Orthostatic hypotension in the elderly. N Engl J Med 321:952, 1989

101. Gotshall RW, Wood VC, Miles DS: Modified head-up tilt test for orthostatic challenge of critically ill patients. Crit Care Med 17:1156, 1989

102. Wong DH, O'Connor D, Tremper KK et al: Changes in cardiac output after acute blood loss and position change in man. Crit Care Med 17:979, 1989

103. Amoroso P, Greenwood RN: Posture and central venous pressure measurement in circulatory volume depletion. Lancet 2:258, 1989

104. Vatner SF, Braunwald E: Cardiovascular control mechanisms in the conscious state. N Engl J Med 293:970, 1975

105. Lawson D, Norley I, Korbon G et al: Blood flow limits and pulse oximeter signal detection. Anesthesiology 67:599, 1987

106. Mangano DT: Monitoring pulmonary artery pressure in coronary-artery disease. Anesthesiology 53:364, 1980

107. Shah DM, Browner BD, Dutton RE et al: Cardiac output and pulmonary wedge pressure: Use for evaluation of fluid replacement in trauma patients. Arch Surg 112:1161, 1977

108. Scalea TM, Holman M, Fuortes M et al: Central venous blood oxygen saturation: An early, accurate measurement of volume during hemorrhage. J Trauma 28:725, 1988

109. Bland RD, Shoemaker WC, Abraham E, Cobo JC: Hemodynamic and oxygen transport patterns in surviving and nonsurviving postoperative patients. Crit Care Med 13:85, 1985

110. Bland RD, Shoemaker WC: Probability of survival as a prognostic and severity illness score in critically ill surgical patients. Crit Care Med 13:91, 1985

111. Shoemaker WC, Appel PL, Kram HB et al: Prospective trial of supranormal values of survivors as therapeutic goals in high-risk surgical patients. Chest 94:1176, 1988

112. Tuchschmidt J, Fried J, Astiz M et al: Supranormal oxygen delivery improves mortality in septic shock patients (abstr). Crit Care Med 19:S66, 1991

113. Sterns RH: The management of hyponatremic emergencies. Crit Care Clin 7:127, 1991

114. Berl T: Treating hyponatremia: Damned if we do and damned if we don't. Kidney Int 37:1006, 1990

115. Sterns RH: Neurological deterioration following treatment for hyponatremia. Am J Kidney Dis 13:434, 1989

116. Lien YH, Shapiro JI, Chan L: Effects of hypernatremia on organic brain osmoles. J Clin Invest 85:1427, 1990

117. Thurston JH, Hauhart RE, Nelson JS: Adaptive decreases in amino acids (taurine in particular), creatine, and electrolytes prevent cerebral edema in chronically hyponatremic mice: Rapid correction (experimental model of central pontine myelinolysis) causes dehydration and shrinkage of brain. Metab Brain Dis 2:223, 1987

118. Thurston JH, Sherman WR, Hauhart RE, Kloepper RF: Myoinositol: A newly identified nonnitrogenous osmoregulatory molecule in mammalian brain. Pediatr Res 26:482, 1989

119. Sterns RH, Thomas DJ, Herndon RM: Brain dehydration and neurologic deterioration after rapid correction of hyponatremia. Kidney Int 35:69, 1989

120. Deutsch S, Goldberg M, Dripps RD: Postoperative hyponatremia with the inappropriate release of antidiuretic hormone. Anesthesiology 27:250, 1966

121. Chung HM, Kluge R, Schrier RW, Anderson RJ: Postoperative hyponatremia: A prospective study. Arch Intern Med 146:333, 1986

122. Arieff AI: Hyponatremia, convulsions, respiratory arrest, and

permanent brain damage after elective surgery in healthy women. N Engl J Med 314:1529, 1986

123. Fraser CL, Arieff AI: Fatal central diabetes mellitus and insipidus resulting from untreated hyponatremia: A new syndrome. Ann Intern Med 112:113, 1990

124. Burrows FA, Shutack JG, Crone RK: Inappropriate secretion of antidiuretic hormone in a postsurgical pediatric population. Crit Care Med 11:527, 1983

125. Fieldman NR, Forsling ML, Le Quesne LP: The effect of vasopressin on solute and water excretion during and after surgical operations. Ann Surg 201:383, 1985

126. Ayus JC, Arieff AI: Symptomatic hyponatremia: Making the diagnosis rapidly. Women of childbearing age are most at risk for encephalopathy. J Crit Illness 5:846, 1990

127. Mitnick PD, Bell S: Rhabdomyolysis associated with severe hyponatremia after prostatic surgery. Am J Kidney Dis 16:73, 1990

128. Rothenberg DM, Berns AS, Ivankovich AD: Isotonic hyponatremia following transurethral prostate resection. J Clin Anesth 2:48, 1990

129. Packer M, Medina N, Yushak M: Correction of dilutional hyponatremia in severe chronic heart failure by converting-enzyme inhibition. Ann Intern Med 100:782, 1984

130. Oh MS, Uribarri J, Barrido D et al: Case report: Danger of central pontine myelinolysis in hypotonic dehydration and recommendation for treatment. Am J Med Sci 298:41, 1989

131. Sterns RH: Severe symptomatic hyponatremia: Treatment and outcome. A study of 64 cases. Ann Intern Med 107:656, 1987

132. Sarnaik AP, Meert K, Hackbarth R, Fleischmann L: Management of hyponatremic seizures in children with hypertonic saline: A safe and effective strategy. Crit Care Med 19:758, 1991

133. Sterns RH, Riggs JE, Schochet SS Jr: Osmotic demyelination syndrome following correction of hyponatremia. N Engl J Med 314:1535, 1986

134. Brunner JE, Redmond JM, Haggar AM et al: Central pontine myelinolysis and pontine lesions after rapid correction of hyponatremia: A prospective magnetic resonance imaging study. Ann Neurol 27:61, 1990

135. Miller GM, Baker HL Jr, Okazaki H, Whisnant JP: Central pontine myelinolysis and its imitators: MR findings. Radiology 168:795, 1988

136. Ayus JC, Krothapalli RK, Armstrong DL: Rapid correction of severe hyponatremia in the rat: Histopathological changes in the brain. Am J Physiol 248:F711, 1985

137. Ayus JC, Arieff AI: Symptomatic hyponatremia: Correcting sodium deficits safely. Extent of replacement may be more important than infusion rate. J Crit Illness 5:905, 1990

138. Cluitmans FH, Meinders AE: Management of severe hyponatremia: Rapid or slow correction? Am J Med 88:161, 1990

139. Narins RG: Therapy of hyponatremia. Does haste make waste? (editorial). N Engl J Med 314:1573, 1986

140. Berl T: Treating hyponatremia: What is all the controversy about? Ann Intern Med 113:417, 1990

141. Anderson RJ, Chung HM, Kluge R, Schrier RW: Hyponatremia: A prospective analysis of its epidemiology and the pathogenetic role of vasopressin. Ann Intern Med 102:164, 1985

142. Ober KP: Diabetes insipidus. Crit Care Clin 7:109, 1991

143. Snyder NA, Feigal DW, Arieff AI: Hypernatremia in elderly patients: A heterogeneous, morbid, and iatrogenic entity. Ann Intern Med 107:309, 1987

144. Black PM, Zervas NT, Candia GL: Incidence and management of complications of transsphenoidal operation for pituitary adenomas. Neurosurgery 20:920, 1987

145. Seckl JR, Dunger DB, Lightman SL: Neurohypophyseal peptide function during early postoperative diabetes insipidus. Brain 110:737, 1987

146. Verbalis JG, Robinson AG, Moses AM: Postoperative and post-traumatic diabetes insipidus. In Czernichow P, Robinson AG (eds): Diabetes Insipidus in Man. Front Hormone Res 13:247, 1985

147. Robertson GL: Differential diagnosis of polyuria. Annu Rev Med 39:425, 1988

148. Griffin KA, Bidani AK: How to manage disorders of sodium and water balance: Five-step approach to evaluating appropriateness of renal response. J Crit Illness 5:1054, 1990

149. Robinson AG: DDAVP in the treatment of central diabetes insipidus. N Engl J Med 294:507, 1976

150. Cobb WE, Spare S, Reichlin S: Neurogenic diabetes insipidus: Management with dDAVP (1-desamino-8-D-arginine-vasopressin). Ann Intern Med 11:183, 1978

151. Shucart WA, Jackson I: Management of diabetes insipidus in neurosurgical patients. J Neurosurg 44:65, 1976

152. Chanson P, Jedynak CP, Dabrowski G et al: Ultralow doses of vasopressin in the management of diabetes insipidus. J Crit Care Med 15:44, 1987

153. Adrogue HJ, Madias NE: Changes in plasma potassium concentration during acute acid-base disturbances. Am J Med 71:456, 1981

154. Koht A, Cerullo LJ, Land PC, Linde HW: Serum potassium levels during prolonged hypothermia. Anesthesiology 51: S203, 1979

155. Jamison RL: Potassium recycling. Kidney Int 31:695, 1987

156. Greger R, Gogelein H: Role of K^+ conductive pathways in the nephron. Kidney Int 31:1055, 1987

157. Wiegand CF, Davin TD, Raij L, Kjellstrand CM: Severe hypokalemia induced by hemodialysis. Arch Intern Med 141:167, 1981

158. Sweadner KJ, Goldin SM: Active transport of sodium and potassium ions: Mechanism, function, and regulation. N Engl J Med 320:777, 1980

159. Vitez TS, Soper LE, Wong KC, Soper P: Chronic hypokalemia and intraoperative dysrhythmias. Anesthesiology 63:130, 1985

160. Relman AS, Schwartz WB: The nephropathy of potassium depletion: A clinical and pathological entity. N Engl J Med 255:195, 1956

161. Schwartz WB, Relman AS: Effects of electrolyte disorders on renal structure and function. N Engl J Med 276:383, 1967

162. Torres VE, Young WF Jr, Offord KP, Hattery RR: Association of hypokalemia, aldosteronism, and renal cysts. N Engl J Med 322:345, 1990

163. Sterns RH, Cox M, Feig PU, Singer I: Internal potassium balance and the control of the plasma potassium concentration. Medicine 60:339, 1981

164. Tobey RE: Paraplegia, succinylcholine and cardiac arrest. Anesthesiology 32:359, 1970

165. Pollen RH, Williams RH: Hyperkalemic neuromyopathy in Addison's disease. N Engl J Med 263:273, 1960

166. Noth RH, Lassman MN, Tan SY et al: Age and the renin-aldosterone system. Arch Intern Med 137:1414, 1977

167. Rimmer JM, Horn JF, Gennari FJ: Hyperkalemia as a complication of drug therapy. Arch Intern Med 147:867, 1987

168. Tan SY, Shapiro R, Franco R et al: Indomethacin-induced prostaglandin inhibition with hyperkalemia: A reversible cause of hyporeninemic hypoaldosteronism. Ann Intern Med 90:783, 1979

169. Textor SC, Bravo EL, Fouad FM, Tarazi RC: Hyperkalemia in azotemic patients during angiotensin-converting enzyme inhibition and aldosterone reduction with captopril. Am J Med 73:719, 1982

170. Maslowski AH, Ikram H, Nicholls MG, Espiner EA: Haemodynamic, hormonal, and electrolytes responses to captopril in resistant heart failure. Lancet 1:71, 1981

171. Gavryck WA, Moore RD, Thompson RC: Effect of insulin upon membrane-bound ($Na^+ + K^+$)-ATPase extracted from frog skeletal muscle. J Physiol 252:43, 1975

172. DeFronzo RA, Felig P, Ferrannini E, Wahren J: Effect of graded doses of insulin on splanchnic and peripheral potassium metabolism in man. Am J Physiol 238:E421, 1980

173. Guerra S, Kitabchi AE: Comparison of the effectiveness of various routes of insulin injection: Insulin levels and glucose response in normal subjects. J Clin Endocrinol Metab 42:869, 1976

174. Clausen T: Adrenergic control of Na^+-K^+-homeostasis. Acta Med Scand Suppl 672:111, 1983

175. Struthers AD, Reid JL: Adrenaline causes hypokalaemia in man by beta-2 adrenoreceptor stimulation. Clin Endocrinol 20:409, 1984

176. Vincent HH, Boomsma F, Man in't Veld AJ et al: Effects of selective and nonselective β-agonists on plasma potassium and norepinephrine. J Cardiovasc Pharmacol 6:107, 1984

177. Brown MJ: Hypokalemia from beta 2-receptor stimulation by circulating epinephrine. Am J Cardiol 56:3D, 1985

178. Allon M, Dunlay R, Copkney C: Nebulized albuterol for acute hyperkalemia in patients on hemodialysis. Ann Intern Med 110:426, 1989

179. Zaloga GP, Chernow B: Hypocalcemia in critical illness. JAMA 256;1924, 1986

180. Zaloga GP, Chernow B, Cook D et al: Assessment of calcium homeostasis in the critically ill surgical patient: The diagnostic pitfalls of the McLean-Hastings nomogram. Ann Surg 202:587, 1985

181. Zaloga GP: Evaluation of bedside testing options for the critical care unit. Chest 97:185S, 1990

182. Rutledge R, Sheldon GF, Collins ML: Massive transfusion. Crit Care Clin 2:791, 1986

183. Malcolm DS, Holaday JW, Chernow B, Zaloga GP: Calcium and calcium antagonists in shock and ischemia. In Chernow B (ed): The Pharmacologic Approach to the Critically Ill Patient, 2nd ed, p 889. Baltimore, Williams & Wilkins, 1988

184. Zaloga GP, Chernow B: The multifactorial basis for hypocalcemia during sepsis: Studies of the parathyroid hormone-vitamin D axis. Ann Intern Med 107:36, 1987

185. Zaloga GP, Strickland RA, Butterworth JF IV et al. Calcium attenuates epinephrine's beta-adrenergic effects in postoperative heart surgery patients. Circulation 81:196, 1990

186. Butterworth JF IV, Strickland RA, Mark LJ et al: Calcium does not augment phenylephrine's hypertensive effects. Crit Care Med 18:603, 1990

187. Prielipp R, Zaloga GP: Calcium action and general anesthesia. Adv Anesth 8:241, 1991

188. Broadus AE, Mangin M, Ikeda K et al: Humoral hypercalcemia of cancer: Identification of a novel parathyroid hormone-like peptide. N Engl J Med 319:556, 1988

189. Mundy GR: Hypercalcemic factors other than parathyroid hormone-related protein. Endocrinol Metab Clin North Am 18:795, 1989

190. Stewart AF, Horst R, Deftos LJ et al: Biochemical evaluation of patients with cancer-associated hypercalcemia: Evidence for humoral and non-humoral groups. N Engl J Med 303:1377, 1980

191. Burtis WJ, Brady TG, Orloff JJ et al: Immunochemical characterization of circulating parathyroid hormone-related protein in patients with humoral hypercalcemia of cancer. N Engl J Med 322:1106, 1990

192. Davis KD, Attie MF: Management of severe hypercalcemia. Crit Care Clin 7:175, 1991

193. Mallette LE, Bilezikian JP, Heath DA, Aurbach GD: Primary hyperparathyroidism: Clinical and biochemical features. Medicine 53:127, 1974

194. Adams JS, Singer FR, Gacad MA et al: Isolation and structural identification of 1,25-dihydroxyvitamin D3 produced by cultured alveolar macrophages in sarcoidosis. J Clin Endocrinol Metab 60:960, 1985

195. Sandler LM, Winearls CG, Fraher LJ et al: Studies of the hypercalcaemia of sarcoidosis: Effect of steroids and exogenous vitamin D$_3$ on the circulating concentrations of 1,25-dihydroxy vitamin D$_3$. Q J Med 53:165, 1984

196. Hosking DJ, Gilson D: Comparison of the renal and skeletal actions of calcitonin in the treatment of severe hypercalcaemia of malignancy. Q J Med 53:359, 1984

197. Binstock ML, Mundy GR: Effect of calcitonin and glucocorticoids in combination on the hypercalcemia of malignancy. Ann Intern Med 93:269, 1980

198. Ralston SH, Gardner MD, Dryburgh FJ et al: Comparison of aminohydroxypropylidene diphosphonate, mithramycin, and corticosteroids/calcitonin in treatment of cancer-associated hypercalcemia. Lancet 2:907, 1985

199. Warrell RP Jr, Israel R, Frisone M et al: Gallium nitrate for acute treatment of cancer-related hypercalcemia: A randomized, double-blind comparison to calcitonin. Ann Intern Med 108:669, 1988

200. Kiang DT, Loken MK, Kennedy BJ: Mechanism of the hypocalcemic effect of mithramycin. J Clin Endocrinol Metab 48:341, 1979

201. Singer FR, Neer RM, Murray TM et al: Mithramycin treatment of intractable hypercalcemia due to parathyroid carcinoma. N Engl J Med 283:634, 1970

202. Hasling C, Charles P, Mosekilde L: Etidronate disodium in the management of malignancy-related hypercalcemia. Am J Med 82:51, 1987

203. Ryzen E, Martodam RR, Troxell M et al: Intravenous etidronate in the management of malignant hypercalcemia. Arch Intern Med 145:449, 1985

204. Warrell RP, Murphy WK, Schulman P et al: Gallium nitrate vs. etidronate for acute treatment of cancer-related hypercalcemia: A randomized double-blind study (abstr). Am Soc Bone Mineral Res 5(suppl 2):S271, 1990

205. Percival RC, Yates AJ, Gray RE et al: Role of glucocorticoids in management of malignant hypercalcemia. Br Med J 289:287, 1984

206. Brenner DE, Harvey HA, Lipton A, Demers L: A study of prostaglandin E2, parathormone, and response to indomethacin in patients with hypercalcemia of malignancy. Cancer 49:556, 1982

207. Zaloga GP, Malcolm D, Holaday J, Chernow B: Verapamil reverses calcium cardiotoxicity. Ann Emerg Med 16:637, 1987

208. Peppers MP, Geheb M, Desai T: Hypophosphatemia and hyperphosphatemia. Crit Care Clin 7:201, 1991

209. Zaloga GP: Phosphate disorders. In Kirby RR, Taylor RW (eds): Problems in Critical Care. Vol 4. Endocrine Emergencies (GP Zaloga, ed), p 416. Philadelphia, JB Lippincott, 1990

210. Newman JH, Neff TA, Ziporin P: Acute respiratory failure associated with hypophosphatemia. N Engl J Med 296:1101, 1977

211. Agusti AG, Torres A, Estopa R, Agustividal A: Hypophosphatemia as a cause of failed weaning: The importance of metabolic factors. Crit Care Med 12:142, 1984

212. Aubier M, Murciano D, Lecocguic Y et al: Effect of hypophosphatemia on diaphragmatic contractility in patients with acute respiratory failure. N Engl J Med 313:420, 1985

213. Varsano S, Shapiro M, Taragan R, Bruderman I: Hypophosphatemia as a reversible cause of refractory ventilatory failure. Crit Care Med 11:908, 1983

214. Fuller TJ, Nichols WW, Brenner BJ, Peterson JC: Reversible depression in myocardial performance in dogs with experimental phosphate deficiency. J Clin Invest 62:1194, 1978

215. O'Connor LR, Wheeler WS, Bethune JE: Effect of hypophosphatemia on myocardial performance in man. N Engl J Med 297:901, 1977

216. Laaban JP, Grateau G, Psychoyos I et al. Hypophosphatemia induced by mechanical ventilation in patients with chronic obstructive pulmonary disease. Crit Care Med 17:1115, 1989

217. Halevy J, Bulvik S: Severe hypophosphatemia in hospitalized patients. Arch Intern Med 148:153, 1988

218. Swaminathan R, Bradley P, Morgan DB, Hill GL: Hypophosphatemia in surgical patients. Surg Gynecol Obstet 148:448, 1979

219. England PC, Durari M, Tweedle DE et al: Postoperative hypophosphataemia. Br J Surg 66:340, 1979

220. Watchko J, Bifano EM, Bergstrom WH: Effect of hyperventilation on total calcium, ionized calcium, and serum phosphorus in neonates. Crit Care Med 12:1055, 1984

221. Mostellar ME, Tuttle EP Jr: Effects of alkalosis on plasma concentration and urinary excretion of inorganic phosphate in man. J Clin Invest 43:138, 1964

222. Lotz M, Zisman E, Bartter FC: Evidence for a phosphorus-depletion syndrome in man. N Engl J Med 278:409, 1968

223. Lentz RD, Brown DM, Kjellstrand CM: Treatment of severe hypophosphatemia. Ann Intern Med 89:941, 1978

224. Chernow B, Rainey TG, Georges LP, O'Brian JT: Iatrogenic

hyperphosphatemia: A metabolic consideration in critical care medicine. Crit Care Med 9:772, 1981

225. Zaloga GP, Roberts JE: Magnesium disorders. In Zaloga GP (guest ed.), Kirby RR, Taylor RW (eds): Problems in Critical Care. Vol 4. Endocrine Emergencies (GP Zaloga, ed), p 437. Philadelphia, JB Lippincott, 1990

226. Salem M, Munoz R, Chernow B: Hypomagnesemia in critical illness: A common and clinically important problem. Crit Care Clin 7:225, 1991

227. Dyckner T, Wester PO: Relation between potassium, magnesium and cardiac arrhythmias. Acta Med Scand Suppl 647: 163, 1981

228. Rasmussen HS, Aurup P, Hojberg S et al: Magnesium and acute myocardial infarction: Transient hypomagnesemia not induced by renal magnesium loss in patients with acute myocardial infarction. Arch Intern Med 146:872, 1986

229. Kafka H, Langevin L, Armstrong PW: Serum magnesium and potassium in acute myocardial infarction: Influence on ventricular arrhythmias. Arch Intern Med 147:465, 1987

230. Rasmussen HS, McNair P, Norregard P et al: Intravenous magnesium infusion in acute myocardial infarction. Lancet 1:234, 1986

231. Morton BC, Nair RC, Smith FM et al: Magnesium therapy in acute myocardial infarction—a double-blind study. Magnesium 3:346, 1984

232. Abraham AS, Rosenmann D, Kramer M et al: Magnesium in the prevention of lethal arrhythmias in acute myocardial infarction. Arch Intern Med 147:753, 1987

233. Rasmussen HS, Suenson M, McNair P et al: Magnesium infusion reduces the incidence of arrhythmias in acute myocardial infarction: A double-blind, placebo-controlled study. Clin Cardiol 10:351, 1987

234. Harris MN, Crowther A, Jupp RA, Aps C: Magnesium and coronary revascularization: Br J Anaesth 60:779, 1988

235. Tzivoni D, Banai S, Schuger C et al: Treatment of torsade de pointes with magnesium sulfate. Circulation 77:392, 1988

236. Chernow B, Bamberger S, Stoiko M et al: Hypomagnesemia in patients in postoperative intensive care. Chest 95:391, 1989

237. Fiaccadori E, Del Canale S, Coffrini E et al: Muscle and serum magnesium in pulmonary intensive care unit patients. Crit Care Med 16:751, 1988

238. Dyckner T, Wester PO: Intracellular magnesium loss after diuretic administration. Drugs 28:161, 1984

239. Ryan MP, Devane J, Ryan MF, Counihan TB: Effects of diuretics on the renal handling of magnesium. Drugs 28:167, 1984

240. Zaloga GP, Chernow B, Pock A et al: Hypomagnesemia is a common complication of aminoglycoside therapy. Surg Gynecol Obstet 158:561, 1984

241. James MF, Cork RC, Dennett JE: Cardiovascular effects of magnesium sulphate in the baboon. Magnesium 6:314, 1987

242. DiPette DJ, Simpson K, Guntupalli J: Systemic and regional hemodynamic effect of acute magnesium administration in the normotensive and hypertensive state. Magnesium 6:136, 1987

243. Friedman HS, Nguyen TN, Mokraoui AM et al: Effects of magnesium chloride on cardiovascular hemodynamics in the neurally intact dog. J Pharmacol Exp Ther 243:126, 1987

244. Mroczek WJ, Lee WR, Davidov ME: Effect of magnesium sulfate on cardiovascular hemodynamics. Angiology 28:720, 1977

245. James MF, Beer RE, Esser JD: Intravenous magnesium sulfate inhibits catecholamine release associated with tracheal intubation. Anesth Analg 68:772, 1989

246. James MF, Manson ED: The use of magnesium sulphate infusions in the management of very severe tetanus. Intensive Care Med 11:5, 1985

247. James MF: The use of magnesium sulfate in the anesthetic management of pheochromocytoma. Anesthesiology 62:188, 1985

248. Ghoneim MM, Long JP: The interaction between magnesium and other neuromuscular blocking agents. Anesthesiology 32:23, 1970

249. James MF, Cork RC, Dennett JE: Succinylcholine pretreatment with magnesium sulfate. Anesth Analg 65:373, 1986

250. Van Hook JW: Hypermagnesemia. Crit Care Clin 7:215, 1991

10

Howard Smith
Philip D. Lumb

Acid-Base Balance

Maintenance of the body's internal milieu is the major function of buffering systems, while oxygen transport and the successful preservation of aerobic metabolism are key components in maintaining cellular integrity. As normal aerobic metabolism is compromised or as the ratio of buffering elements is altered, disturbances in acid-base homeostasis occur. Therefore, this subject should be approached with good basic knowledge of simple definitions. The chapter presents definitions of the four types of acid-base disturbances, followed by some practical examples from the intensive care unit (ICU) and operating room.[1]

FUNDAMENTALS OF ACID-BASE BALANCE

Historically, knowledge of acid-base balance developed slowly and came from multiple sources.

The law of mass action recognizes that the ratio of the product of the ionized components to that of the un-ionized components of a solution at equilibrium is equal to a constant, K, or

$$K = \frac{[H^+]\,[A^-]}{[HA]} \qquad (10\text{-}1)$$

and that the dissociation of an acid can be expressed as:

$$HA = [H^+] + [A^-]. \qquad (10\text{-}2)$$

In 1908 Henderson rearranged Equation 10-1 for blood buffers:

$$[H^+] = \frac{K \cdot [HA]}{[A^-]} = K \cdot \frac{[H_2CO_3^-]}{[HCO_3^-]} \qquad (10\text{-}3)$$

In 1912 Sorensen established *puissance hydrogen* ("the power of hydrogen"), or pH, as the negative logarithm of the hydrogen ion concentration.

In 1916 Hasselbalch rearranged Equation 10-3 in the form of a negative logarithm:

$$pH = 6.1 + \log \frac{[HCO_3^-]}{[H_2CO_3]} \qquad (10\text{-}4)$$

This can be simplified to:

$$pH = 6.1 + \log \frac{[HCO_3^-]}{0.03 \times Paco_2} \quad \text{or} \quad \frac{Kidney}{Lung} \qquad (10\text{-}5)$$

where 6.1 = the pK_a of carbonic acid, and 0.03 is the solubility coefficient of carbon dioxide dissolved in blood.[1]

Most of the buffering action occurs within 1 pH unit of the pK of the buffering system. The most important intravascular buffering system is the carbonic acid–bicarbonate buffer pair, or:

$$pH = 6.1 + \log \frac{[HCO_3^-]}{0.03 \times Paco_2} \quad \text{or} \quad [H^+] = \frac{24 \times Pco_2}{[HCO_3^-]}$$

where 24 is derived from the numerical value of the Bunsen coefficient of carbon dioxide $\times$ $K_{H_2CO_3}$. Because its pK is 6.1, its buffering capacity at a pH of 7.4 is poor. The division of buffering between sodium bicarbonate and dissolved carbon dioxide leads to the commonly named metabolic and respiratory components of acid-base balance:

$$
\begin{array}{c}
Paco_2 \ (lungs) \\
\uparrow \\
CO_2 + H_2O \rightleftharpoons H_2CO_3 \rightleftharpoons H^+ + HCO_3^- \\
\downarrow \\
Kidney
\end{array}
$$

In 1920 van Slyke described a manometric method for the measurement of CO_2 content.[1] In 1922 Walter Hughes described the operation of a glass electrode for the measurement of pH, based on Sorenson's work in the early 1900s in which Sorenson noted a voltage differential between two sides of a thin glass membrane placed in fermenting beer and yeast cultures.[1]

In 1923 Bronsted defined an acid as a molecule capable of giving off a hydrogen ion, and a base as a molecule capable of taking up a hydrogen ion. William Stadie developed a functional electron tube voltmeter necessary for measurement of voltage changes across the glass membranes of the electrodes.

In 1948 Hastings and Singer defined buffer base, in the 1950s Astrup, Siggaard-Anderson, Engel, and Jorgensen defined and described base excess and standard bicarbonate, and in 1956 Clark developed the oxygen electrode. By the late 1950s, theory, experimentation, and technology had coalesced. Clinicians had the means to determine acid-base relationships and arterial oxygenation as routine procedures.

Today, major surgical operations of all kinds, especially thoracic and thoracoabdominal procedures, are performed with an indwelling arterial cannula. This is useful not only for monitoring blood pressure on a continuous basis, but also for immediate access to arterial blood to draw samples for determining a wide range of variables. The most commonly used values that bear directly on acid-base balance are Po_2, pH, Pco_2, bicarbonate, base excess, oxygen saturation (So_2), reduced hemoglobin, and total oxygen content. The blood-gas analyzers in clinical use perform all measurements at a temperature of 37°C, which is carefully maintained within the sample chamber. For this reason, correction of measured blood gas values to patient temperature has been regarded as an important clinical necessity. The Po_2, Pco_2, and pH of a blood sample are temperature dependent, and correction of Po_2 to patient temperature has been well described.[2] However, recent controversy about whether or not pH and Pco_2 values should be temperature corrected has arisen.[3] Because hemoglobin saturation is temperature independent, direct measurement of this variable, as with a CO-oximeter or a pulse oximeter, will give maximum information about oxygen transport. In cases in which saturation is not measured, Po_2 values can be temperature corrected by reference to a standard nomogram.[2] However, the clinician should decide independently whether or not to correct measured values for pH and Pco_2.[4] Cooling blood with a constant oxygen content increases the solubility of carbon dioxide in the blood, so that more carbon dioxide goes into solution, leaving less gaseous carbon dioxide. Therefore, Pco_2 decreases and pH increases. This observation is important in postoperative patient management in the ICU and postanesthesia care unit (PACU).

There may be marked temperature gradients in the body, leading to gross differences in pH and Pco_2. With alpha-stat management, the blood gases are analyzed at the usual 37°C, and those values are used to manage the patient. In pH-stat management, blood gases are measured in the same way but the results are reported corrected to the patient's body temperature at the time of sampling, using the previously mentioned nomograms. No universal agreement has been reached by clinicians on appropriate management techniques or measurement standardization.

At the hypothermic temperature used in cardiopulmonary bypass, maintaining a temperature-corrected Pco_2 of 40 mm Hg may result in excessive amounts of carbon dioxide dissolved in the blood. This causes hyperperfusion of the brain through the mechanism of hypercarbic dilation of the central vasculature. In addition, the clinician must realize that some of the aforementioned values are measured directly and others are calculated. The parameters directly measured by a blood gas analyzer are pH, Po_2, and Pco_2, from which is calculated the bicarbonate value. Only in the chemistry laboratory is the bicarbonate value directly measured clinically, usually when a blood sample is sent for electrolyte determination. Discrepancies between calculated and measured bicarbonate values may result from measurements made on samples that were not simultaneously obtained, from measurement errors, from arterial-venous differences (the blood drawn for determination of carbon dioxide content is usually venous, and venous bicarbonate is usually 2–3 mm Hg higher than arterial), or from changes in pK that may occur in critically ill patients (the

significance of these changes is controversial) (A. Aberman, unpublished observation).

Measurement of the total carbon dioxide contained in the blood is performed by acidifying the sample. As HCO_3^- is acidified, the reaction $H^+ + HCO_3^- \rightarrow H_2O + CO_2$ occurs. This releases the carbon dioxide dissolved in the blood, which, along with carbonic acid, represents approximately 5% of the total carbon dioxide, and the portion that is carried as HCO_3^- and comprises the remainder of carbon dioxide carried. The dissolved component is then measured or can be estimated by multiplying the $Paco_2$ by 0.03, the solubility coefficient for carbon dioxide in blood at 37°C.[5]

ACID-BASE CHEMISTRY

Hydrogen is the simplest element in nature. It consists of a one-proton nucleus with a single orbiting electron. A single proton without any associated electron is a hydrogen ion, H^+. In aqueous solutions, these ions do not exist independently but are bound to one or more water molecules.[6] According to the Bronsted-Lowry definition, an acid is a molecule that can act as a proton donor and a base is a molecule that can act as a proton acceptor. Therefore, if K is the dissociation constant for a specific set of conditions, described in Equations 10-1 and 10-3, the following obtain:

$$\text{Acid} \rightleftharpoons \text{Base} + H^+$$

$$\frac{[H^+] \times [\text{Base}]}{[\text{Acid}]} = K \quad \text{or} \quad [H^+] = K \times \frac{[\text{Acid}]}{[\text{Base}]}$$

Strong acids have high dissociation constants and freely dissociate from their corresponding weak bases, which have a low affinity for hydrogen ions.[6]

In 1969 Waddell and Bates questioned the rationale of changing from pH units (pH $= -\log [H^+]$) to the Système Internationale (SI) nomenclature, in which acidity is expressed as $[H^+]$ in $nmol \cdot l^{-1}$.[7] However, assessment of acidity in these terms (using the Henderson equation) yields the following:

$$[H^+] = \frac{24 \times Paco_2}{[HCO_3^-]} \quad \text{(Henderson equation)}$$

which simplifies the mathematics of acid-base chemistry. It is apparent from the Henderson equation that acid concentration, or $[H^+]$, is a function of two variables, Pco_2 and HCO_3^-. A normal arterial pH of 7.4 has an $[H^+]$ of 40 $nmol \cdot l^{-1}$. From pH 7.2 to 7.5, the curve of $[H^+]$ vs. pH is relatively linear, and for each change of 0.01 pH unit from 7.40, the $[H^+]$ can be estimated by a change of 1, e.g.,

$$\text{pH } 7.40 = 40 \text{ } nmol \cdot l^{-1}$$
$$\text{pH } 7.39 = 41 \text{ } nmol \cdot l^{-1}$$
$$\text{pH } 7.41 = 39 \text{ } nmol \cdot l^{-1}$$

A more accurate approximation can be achieved if at each increment of 0.1 pH unit the $[H^+]$ is estimated as 80% of the previous value for pH values above 7.0, and as 125% of the next highest value for pH values below 7.0, e.g.,

$$\text{pH } 7.0 = 100 \text{ } nmol \cdot l^{-1}$$
$$\text{pH } 6.9 = 125 \text{ } nmol \cdot l^{-1}$$
$$\text{pH } 7.1 = 80 \text{ } nmol \cdot l^{-1}$$
$$\text{pH } 6.8 = 125 \times 1.25 = 156.3 \text{ } nmol \cdot l^{-1}$$
$$\text{pH } 7.2 = 80 \times 0.8 = 64 \text{ } nmol \cdot l^{-1}$$

Buffering

Acute deviations in normal blood acid-base homeostasis are corrected by two processes, buffering and compensation. Buffering provides rapid correction of metabolic derangements by providing an available source of proton acceptors through a shift in the reaction,

$$H^+ + HCO_3^- \rightarrow H_2O + CO_2$$

Carbon dioxide is eliminated *via* the lungs and water through the kidneys. However, the process cannot effect clearance of protons (hydrogen ions) or bicarbonate, which requires renal excretion, a process recognized as compensation that is never complete. The respiratory system, through changes in ventilation and Pco_2, compensates for alterations in metabolic disturbances, while renal excretion of hydrogen ions and bicarbonate provides compensation for and correction of chronic respiratory and metabolic disturbances.

Buffering is the ability of a solution containing weak acid-base pairs to resist changes in pH when a strong acid or base is added. A buffer is defined as a substance within a solution that prevents extreme changes in free $[H^+]$.[6] A base, by accepting a hydrogen ion and forming a weak acid, prevents a change in the $[H^+]$ of the solution. Factors affecting the association or dissociation of H^+ from buffer pairs include the dissociation ionization constant (pK) for that pair and the H^+ concentration in the solution.[6] If the dissociation constants and one of the buffer pair ratios are known, the ratios of all other buffer pairs in the system may be calculated. This is the isohydric principle.

As recognized in the Henderson equation, $[H^+]$ and therefore pH are determined by two key variables, Pco_2 and the plasma bicarbonate concentration, $[HCO_3^-]$. If two of these three variables are known, the third can be calculated. The lungs regulate Pco_2 by changes in ventilation:

$$Paco_2 = \frac{\dot{V}co_2}{\dot{V}_A} \times K$$

where $\dot{V}co_2$ is carbon dioxide production per minute, $\dot{V}_A$ is minute alveolar ventilation, and K is a constant. The kidneys control $[HCO_3^-]$ by recapturing filtered HCO_3^- and by excreting a net nonvolatile or fixed acid load equal to the acid load added to body fluids by metabolism. This concept was alluded to earlier (Eq. 10-5) and underscores the importance of the symbiotic relationship between the lungs and kidneys in regulating acid-base homeostasis.

The determinants of Pco_2 and bicarbonate concentration are detailed in the following fashion:

$$Input \rightarrow Plasma\ CO_2\ tension \rightarrow Output$$

$Paco_2$ is affected by the rate of carbon dioxide production and the rate of alveolar ventilation. In the average adult, cellular processes generate roughly 15,000 mmol (range, 12,500–20,000 mmol) of net volatile carbon dioxide daily under resting conditions.[8] The rate of production may be markedly altered when energy requirements change.

Carbon Dioxide Transport

Carbon dioxide is the normal waste product of cellular aerobic metabolism, and it is transported from the tissues as bicarbonate ion or as carbamino compounds. Dissolved carbon dioxide and carbonic acid play a minor role. Approximately 5% of the carbon dioxide entering the blood remains in the plasma, with about 99.9% of the plasma carbon dioxide remaining in the dissolved state and 0.1% reacting with water to form H_2CO_3.[5]

Ninety-five percent of the carbon dioxide entering the blood enters red blood cells (RBCs). Approximately 30% is bound to the amino acids (predominantly histidine) in hemoglobin and other proteins to form carbamino compounds, and 65% is hydrolyzed to carbonic acid, a reaction catalyzed by the enzyme carbonic anhydrase.[5] Carbonic acid (H_2CO_3) rapidly dissociates at normal body temperatures and pH to hydrogen ion and bicarbonate. Following the concentration gradient, bicarbonate ions diffuse out of RBCs into the plasma in exchange for chloride. This process maintains cellular electrical neutrality and is called the Hamburger chloride shift.[5] The hydrogen ions combine with certain basic groups of hemoglobin in the RBC. The formation of carbamino groups and the hemoglobin buffering of hydrogen ions enhance oxygen release from hemoglobin (Bohr effect).[5] These mechanisms are reversed in the lungs, where the addition of oxygen to blood enhances the release of carbon dioxide from hemoglobin. By the transient conversion of carbon dioxide to plasma bicarbonate and carbamino compounds, these transport processes enable large amounts (up to 20,000 $mmol \cdot l^{-1}$) of metabolic carbon dioxide to be transported from peripheral tissues to the lungs with minimal changes in plasma carbon dioxide tension. The rate of carbon dioxide excretion from the lungs is related to alveolar ventilation. The partial pressure of carbon dioxide in alveolar and arterial blood is essentially the same because the alveolar capillary membrane does not significantly impede carbon dioxide diffusion. Therefore, under steady-state conditions the rate of carbon dioxide excretion equals the rate of carbon dioxide production. Regulation of carbon dioxide excretion is extremely efficient under normal conditions, as the respiratory control mechanisms in the central nervous system (CNS) are exquisitely sensitive. Increased $Paco_2$ may result from impaired ventilation (decreased carbon dioxide excretion) or increased carbon dioxide production. The latter may occur with exercise, hyperthermia, hyperthyroidism, stress or trauma, surgery, light anesthesia, or the use of carbohydrate as the predominant metabolic fuel.

$$Input \rightarrow Plasma\ [HCO_3^-] \rightarrow Output$$

Plasma $[HCO_3^-]$ is affected by the intravascular volume of bicarbonate distribution, the rate of H^+ input or output, the rate of net acid excretion or retention by the kidneys, the rate of H^+ or HCO_3^- loss *via* the gastrointestinal (GI) tract, and the availability of nonbicarbonate buffers.[9] Although the actual space for HCO_3^- distribution is the extracellular fluid (ECF), it is recognized that when bicarbonate is administered, H^+ comes out of cells and enters the ECF. Therefore, the effective space of HCO_3^- distribution is throughout total body water.

The kidneys' role in regulating $[HCO_3^-]$ is in recapturing of filtered bicarbonate and in excreting fixed or nonvolatile acid (hydrogen ion, H^+). The amount of H^+ secreted to recapture filtered bicarbonate is estimated from the glomerular filtration rate (180 $l \cdot day^{-1}$) multiplied by the plasma bicarbonate (about 24–25 $mEq \cdot l^{-1}$) and is approximately 4320–4500 $mEq \cdot day^{-1}$.[6] Hydrogen ions are secreted into the renal tubular lumen by an Na^+/H^+ antiporter and by an H^+–ATPase. Because of this secretion, both systems generate intracellular bicarbonate ions, which leave the cell *via* an $Na(HCO_3^-)_3$ co-transporter and Cl^-/HCO_3^- exchangers.[10] Bicarbonate reabsorption in the proximal tubule is stimulated by an increase in luminal bicarbonate concentration, luminal flow rate, angiotensin II, and hypercarbia; it is inhibited by an increase in peritubular bicarbonate concentration, hypocarbia, and parathyroid hormone.[11]

Acids and bases are present in the diet only in minor quantities, if at all. The fixed or nonvolatile acid load comes from endogenous acids. These may be derived from the oxidation of the sulfhydroxyl group of cysteine and methionine to form sulfuric acid, from hydrolysis of phosphoesters to form phosphoric acid, and from the incomplete breakdown of neutral carbohydrates, fats, and proteins to form organic acids.[6] Endogenous organic acids produced may be true end products of metabolism (e.g., uric acid, creatinine) or metabolic intermediates (e.g., beta-hydroxybutyric acid, lactic acid) that may be generated more rapidly than they can be converted to carbon dioxide and water.[12] An average adult produces endogenous net fixed acid averaging approximately $1–1.5$ $mEq \cdot kg^{-1} \cdot day^{-1}$, with values of $1.5–3$ $mEq \cdot kg^{-1} \cdot day^{-1}$ in infants and young children.[6] Therefore, the normally metabolizing cells of the average 70-kg adult produce $50–100$ $mmol \cdot day^{-1}$ of fixed or nonvolatile acid that enters the circulation.[6] This is an enormous amount compared to the plasma $[H^+]$. For example, 60 mmol of acid produced is 60 million nmol, or 100,000 times the usual amount of hydrogen ion in the ECF. (Normal body fluids have a total $[H^+]$ of 40 $nmol \cdot l^{-1}$, or 600 nmol H^+ in 15 liters of ECF.[13]) Fortunately, the kidneys eliminate $60–100$ nmol of H^+ every day, and thus a balance is achieved. But, as Pestana has pointed out, a daily production of 60 million nmol is a production of almost 700 $nmol \cdot sec^{-1}$.[13] Therefore, every second a little more than the total amount of H^+ in all of the ECF is produced.[13] Because roughly three times a normal concentration is the maximum compatible with life, every 3 seconds enough H^+ is produced to lead to death.[13] Clearly, a buffering system is essential to preserve life.

Common blood buffering agents that react with endogenous hydrogen ions include bicarbonate (about 50% buffering action), dibasic phosphate, hemoglobin (35%), other proteins, and bone.[12] In normothermia, bicarbonate and hemoglobin are the most important buffers. Plasma proteins are one-fourth as effective a buffer as hemoglobin. During hypothermia, the buffering capacity of bicarbonate to proteins is reversed. Blood is a very effective buffer. Paradoxically, blood is a better buffer *in vitro* than *in vivo* because in the body, blood is part of the larger pool of ECF, which has a lower buffer concentration per liter of fluid than does blood. The following example, described by Pestana, illustrates the effectiveness of blood buffers.[13]

If 100 mmol of HCl is added to 5 liters of blood *in vitro*, 100 mmol of H^+ is liberated, since HCl is a strong acid. If there were no buffers, the blood would now contain 20 mmol of $H^+ \cdot l^{-1}$ (20 million nmol), or 500,000 times the original amount of 40 $nmol \cdot l^{-1}$. Instead of the concentration going up from 40 to 20,000,000, it goes up only to 80, or double the original amount instead of 0.5 million times the original amount. The buffering capacity of the blood is backed up by the buffering capacity of the ECF and the cells. This reservoir of buffers may bear the major brunt of the buffering action when a sustained excessive load of H^+ depletes the ECF buffers. Secreted hydrogen ions may be buffered or remain free in the urine. (At a minimum physiologic urine pH, free H^+ in the urine amounts to less than 0.1 $nmol \cdot l^{-1}$.) Therefore, almost all the H^+ in urine is buffered. The minimum urine pH of about 4.5 (40,000 $nEq \cdot l^{-1}$) is generated with a maximum plasma to tubular fluid H^+ gradient $(1:1000)$. Hydrogen ions are buffered predominantly by ammonia (NH_3) to form ammonium (NH_4^+), and secondarily by titratable acid. NH_3 is generated in the renal tubular cells, mostly from glutamate. Metabolic acidosis enhances the net rate of ammonia excretion, primarily by increased ammonia production from glutamine. Goodman has reviewed the various mechanisms postulated to occur in this process.[14] Acidosis may activate phosphoenolpyruvate carboxykinase, enhancing gluconeogenesis and the eventual conversion of alpha-ketoglutarate to glucose. The diminished concentration of alpha-ketoglutarate may then stimulate a mitochondrial phosphate-dependent glutaminase (the enzyme that deaminates glutamine to glutamate).[14] This reaction is followed by deamination of glutamate to alpha-ketoglutarate by the enzyme glutamic dehydrogenase.

Titratable acid is the amount of H^+ present in the urine in combination with basic components of filtered buffer destined for excretion.[9] It can be measured by titrating urine with NaOH to a pH of 7.4 (the original plasma pH). The amount of NaOH needed (mEq) will equal the mEq of secreted H^+ in the tubular fluid that combined with phosphate or organic buffers. Most titratable acid is phosphate. At a pH of 7.40, 80% of this buffer is in the dibasic form, but with a maximally concentrated urine, virtually all the phosphate is excreted in the monobasic form. This process is limited by the amount of excreted $HPO_4^=$. Net acid excretion is the amount of H^+ removed from the body by kidney excretion per day. Bicarbonate ion lost from the body *via* urinary excretion generates the net addition of H^+ to body fluids. It is the sum of urinary ammonium and titratable acidity minus urinary bicarbonate.[9] If a 70-kg adult has a net acid excretion of 70 $mmol \cdot day^{-1}$, NH_4^+ excretion will contribute about 40 $mmol \cdot day^{-1}$ and titratable acid about 30 $mmol \cdot day^{-1}$.[9]

Critically ill patients exhibit primary or compensatory metabolic and respiratory acid-base disturbances that may contribute to death and morbidity. Frequent interventions are necessary to treat metabolic acidosis, metabolic alkalosis, respiratory acidosis, respiratory alkalosis, or mixed disorders and to limit the detrimental impact of these derangements. The following is a brief description of the pathophysiology and clinical implications of the four simple major acid-base disorders.

ACID-BASE DISORDERS

Metabolic Alkalosis

Metabolic alkalosis is caused by a primary increase in HCO_3^-. It is characterized by a pH >7.45 and a bicarbonate concentration >30 $mEq \cdot l^{-1}$. It is the most common acid-base disturbance in hospitalized patients. The body appears better able to tolerate acidosis than alkalosis. In a retrospective study, Hodgkin et al found that 51% of 13,430 arterial blood gas samples revealed metabolic alkalosis.[15] Wilson et al found that 12.5% of 1415 critically ill or injured patients had an arterial pH of 7.55 or higher.[16] Patients with a pH of 7.60–7.64 had a mortality of 65%, and those with a pH > 7.64 had an 80% mortality.[16] These patients usually had a mixed respiratory and metabolic alkalosis.

Fruits are the main dietary sources of alkali. They contain sodium and potassium salts of weak organic acids, and the anions of these salts are metabolized to carbon dioxide, leaving $NaHCO_3$ and $KHCO_3$ in the body.[1] The major source of bases is from metabolism of anionic amino acids (i.e., glutamate, aspartate) and oxidation of organic anions (i.e., citrate, lactate). These organic anions generate alkali by consuming H^+ that comes mostly from weak components of total body buffers. As an example,

$$CH_3\text{—}CHOH\text{—}COO^- + 3O_2 \xrightarrow[]{\overset{HA\quad A^-}{\rightleftharpoons}} 3CO_2 + 3H_2O$$
Lactate

A primary increase in plasma $[HCO_3^-]$ can occur by net loss of $[H^+]$ from the ECF and net addition of HCO_3^- or its precursors to the ECF, or by a loss of chloride in much greater amounts than the HCO_3^- loss from the ECF.[9] Roughly a third of the increase in $[HCO_3^-]$ is buffered by intracellular H^+ entering the ECF, primarily from phosphate and protein sources. A small amount of H^+ is derived from a slight increase in lactic acid production. The respiratory compensation in metabolic alkalosis appears extremely variable but may account for an increase in $PaCO_2$ of about 0.7 mm Hg for every 1 mEq increase in $[HCO_3^-]$.[17] In the surgical ICU population, this may delay separation from mechanical ventilatory assistance. Compensation is a slow process, taking days to weeks to accomplish. This mechanism therefore cannot be relied on to correct severe acute metabolic alkalosis.[17,18] With properly functioning kidneys the excess HCO_3^- will be lost in the urine, provided there are no mechanisms maintaining the metabolic alkalosis via increased HCO_3^- reabsorption. These mechanisms include volume depletion, chloride or severe potassium depletion, excess mineralocorticoid activity, and possibly hypercapnia.[9]

Metabolic alkalosis may be divided into two major groups: sodium chloride–responsive alkalosis (urinary Cl^- < 10 mmol·l^{-1}), such as occurs with vomiting, excessive gastric drainage, chloride-containing diarrheal stools, diuretic therapy, correction of chronic hypercapnia, and cystic fibrosis, and sodium chloride–unresponsive alkalosis (urinary Cl^- > 20 mmol·l$^-$), which may be associated with hyperaldosteronism, Cushing's syndrome, steroid therapy, Bartter's syndrome, and excess licorice intake. All may be accompanied by excess mineralocorticoid activity or severe potassium depletion.[9] Other causes include milk-alkali syndrome, alkali administration, massive transfusion of citrated blood, hypercalcemia (not from hyperparathyroidism), glucose ingestion after starvation, and high-dose penicillin therapy. The contribution of moderate potassium depletion to metabolic alkalosis maintenance is probably small because it is usually correctable without potassium repletion.[9] Metabolic alkalosis is associated with low levels of serum potassium and ionized calcium. Hypokalemia and alkalemia are associated with primary ventricular arrhythmias and may potentiate the toxicity of cardiac glycosides. Magnesium levels should be checked and supplemented if necessary. Additionally, metabolic alkalosis shifts the oxyhemoglobin dissociation curve to the left, impairing peripheral unloading of oxygen. With prolonged metabolic alkalosis, the accompanying increased pH in cerebrospinal fluid (CSF) may blunt the hypoxic ventilatory drive.

Treatment of metabolic alkalosis entails halting ongoing acid losses, if there are any, and halting gastric drainage or adding an H_2 receptor blocker to minimize H^+ loss. For mild to moderate metabolic alkalosis, a trial of NaCl or KCl may be attempted. If clinically warranted, a course of acetazolamide (Diamox) may be useful in causing a bicarbonaturia. For severe metabolic alkalosis, one of the four following procedures may be elected. (1) Dilute HCl, 0.05–0.20 mmol·l^{-1}, may be given slowly through a central vein at a rate not greater than 300–500 ml·h^{-1}.[37] One liter of 0.1N

HCl provides 100 mEq of H^+.[37] However, the solution must be prepared in the hospital pharmacy or ICU, and if it extravasates, it can cause skin necrosis or mediastinitis. (2) Arginine HCl may be given orally or via nasogastric tube but may cause hyperkalemia (300 ml of a 10% solution provides about 150 mEq of H^+ and can be given over 1 hour).[37] (3) Ammonium chloride may be used. It is a small molecule (molecular weight = 53 daltons) that is converted in the body to HCl. One liter of a 2% solution of ammonium chloride (400 mEq·l^{-1} of H^+) given over 8 hours should be well tolerated and produce a "safer" pH value in most instances. If it is given rapidly, at a rate greater than 150–200 mEq·h^{-1}, or if it is given to patients with liver dysfunction, it can cause ammonia toxicity.[37] (4) Hemodialysis may be instituted.

The bicarbonate concentration can be safely reduced by 8–12 mEq·l^{-1} over 12–24 hours.[37] The amount of acid in mEq needed can be calculated by multiplying the desired decrease in $[HCO_3^-]$, e.g., 8 mEq·l^{-1}, by half the body weight in kg to approximate the volume of distribution of administered acid as H^+.

Metabolic Acidosis

Metabolic acidosis is characterized by a pH < 7.35 and a bicarbonate < 20 mEq·l^{-1}. The plasma $[HCO_3^-]$ can be diminished by one of the three following methods: (1) the addition of strong acids to the body, (2) by the loss of HCO_3^- via the kidney or GI tract, or (3) by rapid dilution of the ECF with a nonbicarbonate solution.[9] The buffering defense to additional acid loads was discussed earlier. The respiratory compensation for metabolic acidosis is roughly a decrease of 1.2 mm Hg $PaCO_2$ for every 1 mEq decrease in $[HCO_3^-]$.[17] (All compensatory mechanisms are partial. Buffering systems are designed to provide temporary correction of acute abnormalities in acid-base balance; full correction requires restitution of normal homeostasis by elimination of fixed acid or base, or restoration of the buffer pool.) Respiratory compensation for metabolic acidosis occurs secondary to alveolar hyperventilation. Although this process begins rapidly, it may not reach steady state for 12–24 hours. Ultimately the kidneys must be involved to correct metabolic acidosis, as the lung cannot excrete fixed (nonvolatile) acid loads. The kidney's ability to increase net acid load excretion lags 12–24 hours behind the initial respiratory response and may not reach maximum value for up to 5 days. During severe metabolic acidosis, net acid excretion may increase to 600 mmol·day^{-1}, or more. This is accomplished predominantly by an increase in ammonium excretion, as only a limited increase in titratable acid excretion, largely mediated by phosphate, is seen. In severe diabetic keto-acidosis, renal acid excretion may approach 700–750 mmol·day^{-1}.[19]

For every molecule of acid made, a molecule of HCO_3^- disappears and an anion appears. Electrical or charge neutrality between positively charged and negatively charged ions must exist, and these unmeasured anions (e.g., proteins, sulfates, phosphates, lactate) account for a discrepancy between the charges of routinely measured substances. This discrepancy is referred to as the anion gap. It can be calculated using the following equation:

$$[Na^+] + [K^+] = [HCO_3^-] + [Cl^-] + [\text{unmeasured anions}].$$
$$AG = [Na^+] - [HCO_3^- + Cl^-]$$

A normal anion gap value is approximately 11 ± 3.[20]

Based on this definition, metabolic acidosis can be divided into anion gap metabolic acidosis and non-anion gap metabolic acidosis, depending on measured pH and summated ionic blood constituents. Anion gap metabolic acidosis is found in alcoholic ketoacidosis, diabetic ketoacidosis, lactic acidosis, starvation, nonketotic hyperosmolar coma, acute or chronic renal failure, and the ingestion of toxic doses of salicylates, paraldehyde, methanol, or ethylene glycol.[9] Non-anion gap metabolic acidosis may be seen in diarrhea, following small-bowel or pancreatic drainage or fistula procedures, following the use of anion exchange resins, following ureterosigmoidostomy, following a long or obstructed ileal loop conduit, following ingestion of $CaCl_2$ or $MgCl_2$, following treatment with carbonic anhydrase inhibitors, in renal tubular acidosis, in hyperparathyroidism, in hypoaldosteronism, in dilutional acidosis, following acid or sulfur ingestion, and following parenteral alimentation acidosis.[9]

During metabolic acidosis, when H^+ enters the cell, in order to maintain electrical neutrality, either (1) K^+ comes out of the cell, if the anion is nonpermeable to the cell (i.e., Cl^-, phosphates, sulfates, bicarbonate), or (2) the anion (A^-) is permeable to the cell and enters the cell with H^+ (i.e., lactic acid, ketone bodies). This distinction has significant implications, as illustrated in the following example. In the case of metabolic acidosis associated with a nonpermeable anion, hyperkalemia will ensue because K^+ must exit the cell to maintain electrical neutrality. In the situation associated with pure lactic acidosis, hyperkalemia is not a *sine qua non* because lactate is permeable to the cell.

One of the most important causes of metabolic acidosis with an increased anion gap is secondary to the net accumulation of lactic acid with a resultant fall in plasma $[HCO_3^-]$. This is termed *lactic acidosis*. Lactic acidosis is the end product of the anaerobic metabolism of glucose. It is the most frequent cause of organic acidosis in critically ill patients.

$$H^+ + H_3C-\overset{\overset{\displaystyle O}{\|}}{C}-\overset{\overset{\displaystyle O}{\|}}{C}-O- + NADH$$
$$\text{Pyruvate}$$

$$\approx H_3C-\overset{\overset{\displaystyle HO}{|}}{C}-\overset{\overset{\displaystyle O}{\|}}{C}-O- + NAD^+$$
$$\text{Lactate}$$

$$\text{Lactate} = (K_{eq})(\text{pyruvate})\left(\frac{NADH}{NAD^+}\right)(H^+)$$

where K_{eq} = equilibrium constant of the reaction.

From the above equation it can be seen that lactate concentration depends on three variables: pyruvate concentration, the redox state of the cell ($NADH^+/NAD^+$), and the pH ($[H^+]$).[12] During aerobic metabolism, pyruvate is oxidized to acetyl coenzyme A (acetyl CoA), which then enters the tricarboxylic acid cycle. Pyruvate needs to enter the mitochondrion, and intact mitochondrial function and functioning pyruvate dehydrogenase are also required for this to occur. Pyruvate may also follow different metabolic pathways ultimately to synthesize fat, amino acids, or glucose.[12] If none of the above occurs, then increased pyruvate may be converted to lactate, a metabolic dead end.

The average resting adult produces about 1400 mmol of lactic acid per day, predominantly from metabolism of skeletal muscle, RBCs, brain, and skin.[12] The lactic acid diffuses into the ECF, with a resultant change of $NaHCO_3^-$ to sodium lactate. The turnover is complete when hepatic oxidation of sodium lactate regenerates $NaHCO_3^-$.[12] This 1400 mmol of lactate-related proton flux dwarfs the daily net fixed acid load of 50–100 mmol.[12] Hepatic lactate clearance accounts for the major portion of total lactate clearance at rest. The kidneys also rid the body of lactate by urinary excretion, by gluconeogenesis, or by oxidation.[12]

Transformation of pyruvate to lactate allows anaerobic glycolysis to continue; otherwise it would be inhibited by pyruvate accumulation. Eventually the acidosis inhibits glycolysis by inhibiting the activity of the enzyme phosphofructokinase. Catecholamines may produce a lactic acidosis secondary to enhanced glycolysis; however, the lactate-pyruvate (L/P) ratio is unchanged or slightly decreased, whereas in lactic acidosis secondary to anaerobic metabolism, L/P is increased.

Blood lactate concentration is usually less than 2 $mmol \cdot l^{-1}$ and can be measured in most hospital laboratories either enzymatically, which takes hours, or by lactimetry, a rapid analysis that takes about the same amount of time as arterial blood gas analysis with result reporting. The lactate concentration depends on the lactate production and clearance. The value should be followed serially before interpretation and possible therapeutic action. For example, seizures can produce an acute lactic acidosis that is followed by a rapid clearance and spontaneous resolution. This situation does not require therapeutic alkali administration, but if the acute value had been interpreted in isolation, inappropriate therapy could have resulted. Serial quantitative increases in blood lactate levels are usually related to oxygen deficit and anaerobic metabolism. During shock, when lactic acid concentration increases from 2 to 8 $mmol \cdot l^{-1}$, the survival rate declines from 90% to 10%.[22]

Although bicarbonate therapy may increase lactate production, it is usually still warranted if metabolic acidosis is severe (i.e., pH < 7.2). Definitive therapy involves treatment of perfusion/oxygen deficit and therapeutic measures to combat specific causes of shock. Effective therapy is accompanied by a decline in lactate levels.

Cohen and Woods have classified lactic acidosis into two groups: Type A, secondary to tissue hypoxia with resultant anaerobic metabolism, and Type B, secondary to other causes.[21]

Type B lactic acidosis has been divided into three types: B_1, which is seen in various medical conditions (e.g., diabetes mellitus, hepatic disease, leukemia); B_2, seen following administration of drugs and toxins (e.g., phenformin) or parenteral nutrition with fructose/sorbitol; and B_3, seen in inherited disorders (e.g., methyl malonic acidemia).[21] Dichloroacetate stimulates the activity of pyruvate dehydrogenase, the enzyme involved in the conversion of lactate to pyruvate, and may be of therapeutic benefit in certain of these situations.

At pH levels < 7.25, some enzyme systems do not function properly and bicarbonate therapy may be indicated. Cardiovascular function and the response of the heart and peripheral vascular beds to catecholamines may be impaired. Severe metabolic acidosis may be associated with decreased cardiac contractility, peripheral vasodilation, catecholamine release, and a decreased threshold for ventricular fibrillation.[12] Additionally, the actions of bronchodilators on the airways of a severe asthmatic with significant metabolic acidosis may be reduced, and bicarbonate therapy may result in a dramatic decrease in airway resistance. This occurs only at very low pH values.

At low pH values bicarbonate therapy has a positive inotropic effect. Other reported effects of alkali administration include a left shift in the oxyhemoglobin dissociation curve, which improves central oxygen loading but impairs tissue unloading; paradoxical CSF acidosis; hypernatremia; cardiac arrhythmias; hyperosmolarity; and postresuscitation alkalosis.[12] Paradoxical CSF acidosis has been described by Posner and Plum[23] and is due to the following features of HCO_3^- administration. $NaHCO_3^+ \rightarrow Na^+ + HCO_3^- \rightarrow H_2O + CO_2$. The blood-brain barrier is impermeable to H^+ and HCO_3^-, but carbon dioxide equilibration is rapid. Therefore, following bicarbonate administration, rapid passage or equilibration of carbon dioxide across the blood-brain barrier creates CSF acidosis. HCO_3^- equilibration lags behind.[23] Factors affecting $P_{CSF}CO_2$ include the ratio between neural tissue production of carbon dioxide and the removal of carbon dioxide to the systemic circulation (dependent on local blood flow and the carbon dioxide gradient from CSF to systemic blood).[24] Also, HCO_3^- may inactivate simultaneously administered catecholamines.

Appropriate therapy for metabolic acidosis involves rapid restoration of hemodynamic stability and early correction of primary respiratory disorders. However, if bicarbonate therapy is required, calculation of the base requirement should be performed as indicated below. Full correction is never indicated because ongoing therapy should ameliorate the inciting event, and total correction initially leads rapidly to postresuscitation metabolic alkalosis, which may have serious consequences. An appropriate target pH for correction is 7.25. At pH 7.25, the $[H^+] = 55$ mmol$\cdot$l^{-1}. Substituting these values in the Henderson equation provides the following:

$$55 = 24 \times \frac{Paco_2}{Desired\ HCO_3^-}$$

Replacing $Paco_2$ with the value from the arterial blood gas measurement, the desired HCO_3^- can be calculated. The number of mEq of HCO_3^- to be administered can then be estimated as:

(Desired plasma [HCO_3^-]/Measured plasma [HCO_3^-])
$\times$ 50% Body weight (kg) [9]

The actual space of HCO_3^- distribution is the ECF, but when HCO_3^- is administered, H^+ comes out of cells and enters the ECF. Therefore, the effective space of HCO_3^- distribution is the total body water.

If the blood pH is less than 7.1, 80% of body weight can be used.[9] Alternatively, the base excess can be used to calculate the total base deficit (TBD). This method is commonly used by anesthesiologists and critical care physicians and is based on the amount of acid or base needed to titrate a blood gas sample from its measured pH back to a normal value of 7.40. This quantity can then be used to estimate the amount of alkali (or acid) needed to correct a patient's measured abnormality. This method has inherent inaccuracies (there are methods that attempt to correct these)[25] but is adequate to use for clinical purposes.

$$TBD = Base\ excess \times 0.2 \times Body\ weight\ (kg)$$

or for a measured base excess of -7 in a 70-kg adult, the following dose of bicarbonate would be recommended: $-7 \times 0.2 \times 70 = 98$. However, only 50% or less would be administered initially. Therefore, it would be appropriate to prescribe 50 mEq of $NaHCO_3$ (one ampule) and to repeat arterial blood gas measurements following administration and interim therapy to guide further treatment.

Hemodialysis is another mode of treatment of metabolic acidosis.

In cardiopulmonary arrest, it is now recommended that HCO_3^- therapy be withheld for at least 10 minutes and then given cautiously as clinically necessary, with blood gases used as a guide. This new stipulation is based on the observation that HCO_3^- administration during arrest may produce arterial respiratory alkalosis and venous respiratory acidosis,[26] apparently as a result of excess HCO_3^- administration and inadequate resuscitation and tissue cellular aerobic metabolism. This relationship occurs as follows:

$$H^+ + HCO_3^- \rightarrow H_2O + CO_2$$

However, because of abnormal pulmonary blood flow, carbon dioxide is poorly cleared by the lungs, leading to acute respiratory acidosis.[26] The carbon dioxide produced may also cause CSF acidosis and intracellular acidosis. Acidosis of myocytes with an increased Pco_2 may result in significant decreases in cardiac contractility.[26] Dissolved carbon dioxide rapidly diffuses across cell membranes, whereas HCO_3^- transport into cells is delayed.

Respiratory Acidosis

Primary respiratory acidosis is characterized by a pH < 7.35 and a $Paco_2 > 45$ mm Hg. This state occurs when minute alveolar ventilation is inadequate to maintain a normal carbon dioxide concentration. In cases of increased carbon dioxide production, an otherwise normal minute alveolar ventilation that does not also correspondingly increase will lead to elevated Pco_2. In mixed acid-base disturbances, respiratory acidosis is characterized by a Pco_2 that is significantly higher than one would expect from compensatory mechanisms correcting a primary alkalosis.

Respiratory acidosis is either acute, in which compensation by renal bicarbonate retention is minimal, or chronic, in which renal bicarbonate retention prevents a fall in pH. It occurs either from a decreased minute alveolar ventilation or from an increased production of carbon dioxide, or both. A reduction in minute alveolar ventilation may be due to an overall decrease in minute ventilation or to an increase in the amount of dead space ventilation (ventilation without associated perfusion). Reduction in total minute alveolar ventilation may occur secondary to central ventilatory depression or to an increased work of breathing. Increases in dead space ventilation occur with chronic obstructive lung disease, following pulmonary embolism, and in most forms of acute respiratory failure. Usually carbon dioxide production parallels metabolic oxygen consumption and the type of energy substrate provided for the patient. The most common situations in which carbon dioxide production is increased in the critically ill are hypermetabolic states (e.g., sepsis, pyrexia, multiple trauma) and during administration of excessive quantities of glucose calories in relation to nitrogen.

In simple acute respiratory acidosis, an elevated Pco_2 increases $[H^+]$ (about 80% of the increase in Pco_2 in mm Hg):

$$(CO_2 + H_2O \rightleftharpoons H_2CO_3 \rightleftharpoons H^+ + HCO_3^-)$$

The H^+ is buffered by nonbicarbonate buffers (97% are cellular buffers, primarily hemoglobin, but also phosphates, protein, and lactate; and 3% are from ECF proteins).[18] This process rapidly produces bicarbonate, but the quantity is very limited (usually $[HCO_3^-]$ is not more than 32 $mEq \cdot l^{-1}$).[12] There is no significant renal reabsorption of HCO_3^- by the kidney, and therefore simple acute respiratory acidosis can be rapidly corrected by increasing ventilation without fear of secondary acid-base problems developing because of this intervention.

A simple and rough approximation is that simple acute respiratory acidosis should have an HCO_3^- value between 24 and 32 $mEq \cdot l^{-1}$.[12] If respiratory acidosis exists with $HCO_3^- < 24$ $mEq \cdot l^{-1}$, a coexisting metabolic acidosis is likely.[12] If respiratory acidosis exists with $HCO_3^- > 32$ $mEq \cdot l^{-1}$, then either a chronic respiratory acidosis or coexisting metabolic alkalosis is a likely diagnosis.[12]

Acute Respiratory Acidosis:[18]

$$\Delta[HCO_3^-] = \frac{\Delta PaCO_2}{10} \pm 3$$

In simple chronic respiratory acidosis, the kidneys play a significant role by increasing bicarbonate reabsorption in addition to cell buffering. It is inappropriate to treat chronic respiratory acidosis by increasing ventilation to achieve a normal $PaCO_2$. Following this maneuver, the patient will retain the initial high $[HCO_3^-]$, and therapy will be ineffective and may be counterproductive.

Chronic Respiratory Acidosis:

$$\Delta[HCO_3^-] = \frac{3.0 - 4.0 \times \Delta PaCO_2}{10}$$

Respiratory Alkalosis

Primary respiratory alkalosis is characterized by a pH > 7.45 and $PaCO_2 < 35$ mm Hg. Primary respiratory alkalosis is commonly seen in critically ill patients and may be induced therapeutically by controlled hyperventilation to control elevated intracranial pressure (ICP) following head trauma and in other conditions associated with ICP elevations. Respiratory alkalosis occurs when minute alveolar ventilation exceeds systemic carbon dioxide production. Patients hyperventilate in response to pain or anxiety, but the response is transient. More commonly, respiratory alkalosis is a compensatory response to hypoxemia or CNS disease, or is an early sign of systemic sepsis (possibly as a response to increasing oxygen consumption) or of impending congestive heart failure. The sudden onset of hyperventilation in a previously normocarbic patient should prompt investigation with special attention to sepsis and metabolic acidosis (e.g., diabetic ketoacidosis). Also, the onset of congestive heart failure may be heralded by hyperventilation, in this case stimulated by J-receptor activation.

Intracellular buffers (99%) and plasma proteins (1%) supply H^+, which is released to decrease $[HCO_3^-]$.[18] Cellular metabolism is increased to raise lactate (about 10% of the 99%). This process is completed within minutes, after which rapid decreases in $PaCO_2$ can be tolerated. Again, similar to what occurs in respiratory acidosis, there is no significant renal participation in acute respiratory alkalosis, so it can be rapidly corrected. In chronic respiratory alkalosis, if the $PaCO_2$ is corrected to normal, the initial low HCO_3^- remains.

Acute Respiratory Alkalosis:[18]

$$\Delta[HCO_3^-] = \frac{2.0 - (2.5 \times \Delta PaCO_2)}{10}$$

In other words, the expected metabolic compensation for a primary acute respiratory alkalosis with a $PaCO_2$ of 20 mm Hg is a decrease in $[HCO_3^-]$ of 4–5 $mEq \cdot l^{-1}$.

Chronic Respiratory Alkalosis:[18]

$$\Delta[HCO_3^-] = \frac{5 \times \Delta PaCO_2}{10}$$

The expected metabolic compensation for a primary chronic respiratory alkalosis with the same $PaCO_2$ value of 20 mm Hg is a decrease in $[HCO_3^-]$ of 10 $mEq \cdot l^{-1}$.

In chronic respiratory alkalosis, the renal compensation to lower plasma $[HCO_3^-]$ occurs either as a decrease in the amount of HCO_3^- reabsorption, hence bicarbonaturia, or as a reduction in the HCO_3^- that is generated to buffer the usual daily acid load. As a rough guideline, pH values < 7.30 or > 7.50 are usually more likely to have an acute component than to be purely chronic.[5]

INTERPRETATION OF ARTERIAL BLOOD GAS VALUES

Assessing a patient's acid-base status from arterial blood gas values can be done without recourse to nomograms, by using the Henderson equation and knowing what compensatory responses can be expected. The following examples illustrate these principles.

Case 1

A 27-year-old man is seen on the neurosurgical service for management of an intracerebral hemorrhage. His trachea is intubated and his lungs are mechanically hyperventilated to decrease cerebral blood flow. Arterial blood gas values are as follows:

pH = 7.55
$PaCO_2$ = 28 mm Hg

At a pH of 7.55 the $[H^+]$ is approximately 28 $mEq \cdot l^{-1}$.
From the Henderson equation,

$$[H^+] = \frac{24 \times PaCO_2}{[HCO_3^-]}$$

$$28 = 24 \times \frac{28}{[HCO_3^-]}$$

$$HCO_3^- \approx 24 \ mEq \cdot l^{-1}$$

In acute respiratory disturbances with no metabolic component and in a pH range of 7.2–7.5, a rough guide is that the $PaCO_2$ in mm Hg equals $[H^+]$ in $nmol \cdot l^{-1}$. Therefore, in this case, with a $PaCO_2$ of 28 mm Hg, there should be 28 $nmol \cdot l^{-1}$ of H^+. This corresponds to a pH of about 7.55. Therefore, the patient has a pure primary respiratory alkalosis with no metabolic component.

Case 2

A 66-year-old woman is in the ICU following repair of an abdominal aortic aneurysm. Her trachea is intubated and the lungs are being mechanically ventilated. Arterial blood gas values are as follows:

pH = 7.20
$Paco_2$ = 28 mm Hg

The expected $[HCO_3^-]$, from simple substitution as before, reveals the following:

$$63 = 24 \times \frac{28}{HCO_3^-}$$

or

$$HCO_3^- \approx 11 \text{ mEq} \cdot l^{-1}$$

In this case, the $[HCO_3^-]$ is down 13 mEq·l^{-1} from a normal of 24. Therefore, it is anticipated that $Paco_2$ should be decreased 1.2 mm Hg × 13, or 16 mm Hg, from a normal of 40 mm Hg. The expected respiratory compensation for this would be 40 − 16 ≈ 24 mm Hg. Thus, the patient has a primary metabolic acidosis with roughly appropriate respiratory compensation.

Discussion. The management of all acute acid-base disturbances involves diagnosing the cause and instituting specific therapy directed toward the primary cause. The aim is to return to the patient's arterial blood gas values to baseline. Therefore, it is not practical to have a management algorithm. This is especially true for metabolic acidosis.

If the arterial blood gas values of the patient in Case 2 were from a 16-year-old patient with Type I diabetes in diabetic ketoacidosis, therapy would include fluid and insulin without bicarbonate administration. However, if the pH were much below 7.2, bicarbonate therapy would be advisable.

Case 3

A 53-year-old man on the surgical service is admitted to the ICU prior to surgical correction of an intestinal obstruction. A nasogastric tube is attached to intermittent low wall suction. The following arterial blood gas values are obtained:

pH = 7.6
$Paco_2$ = 55 mm Hg

At a pH of 7.6, the $[H^+]$ is approximately 24–25 mEq·l^{-1}.

$$24 = 24 \times \frac{55}{[HCO_3^-]}$$

or

$$[HCO_3^-] \approx 55 \text{ mEq} \cdot l^{-1}$$

This represents primary metabolic alkalosis. The $[HCO_3^-]$ is increased by 31 mEq·l^{-1} (from a normal of 24 to 55), so the $Paco_2$ would be anticipated to increase (0.7 mm Hg × 31 ≈ 22 mm Hg) to as high as 62 mm Hg with a concomitant hypoxemia. This is a primary metabolic alkalosis with partial respiratory compensation. Acid loss from the stomach can be minimized by placing this patient on an H$_2$ receptor antagonist. Gastric acid loss is decreased substantially even if the gastric pH is mildly increased from a pH of 1.0 to 3.0. (At a pH of 1.0, the $[H^+]$ in the stomach is about 100

mEq·l^{-1}, *versus* about 1 mEq·l^{-1} at pH 3.0.) A plasma HCO_3^- greater than 50 mEq·l^{-1} or if associated with persistent hypercarbia should definitely be treated with an exogenous acid load.

Case 4

A 78-year-old obese woman with a history of chronic obstructive pulmonary disease is on the surgical ward following cholecystectomy for acute cholecystitis. She has not been mobile and has been unable to cough effectively. A surgical intern, believing that if he could diminish her pain she would cough more effectively, gave her morphine sulfate intravenously. The following blood gas values were obtained on room air:

pH = 7.24
Pco_2 = 88 mm Hg

At a pH of 7.24, the anticipated $[H^+]$ is about 57 nmol·l^{-1}. To calculate the expected $[HCO_3^-]$, simple substitution as in the previous example reveals the following:

$$57 = 24 \times \frac{88}{[HCO_3^-]} \approx 37 \text{ mEq} \cdot l^{-1}$$

If this were a simple acute respiratory acidosis without any metabolic component, the expected $[H^+]$ would be 88 mEq·l^{-1} (corresponding to a pH of about 7.06). If there were a metabolic compensation, it would be an increase of about 5 mEq·l^{-1} (from 24 mEq·l^{-1} to 29 mEq·l^{-1}). The $[HCO_3^-]$ in this case is increased by 13 mEq·l^{-1}. Therefore, the patient has acute respiratory acidosis superimposed on chronic respiratory acidosis.

OXYGENATION

Normally, roughly 28% carbohydrates, 18% proteins, and 54% fat are fed into the tricarboxylic acid cycle, producing reducing equivalents that are fed into the electron transport chain in the mitochondria, which produces potential energy in the form of adenosine triphosphate (ATP). Oxygen is the terminal electron acceptor, with water and ATP being produced. Continued production of ATP is required for long-term cell survival. The critical level of oxygen required for oxidative phosphorylation to proceed normally *in vivo* is unknown, but it appears that the intramitochondrial Po_2 needed is only about 1 mm Hg or less.[2] Mitochondrial oxygen utilization accounts for about 90% of total cellular oxygen consumption, with much of the remainder used in reactions with mixed-function oxidase (e.g., tyrosine and tryptophan hydroxylase are used in the synthesis of catecholamines and serotonin, respectively), dioxygenases (e.g., prolyl and lysyl hydroxylase are used in the synthesis of collagen), the cytochrome P-450 system, and NADPH oxidase. If there is sufficient oxygen supply to the tissues, organic substrates are metabolized aerobically through the tricarboxylic acid cycle, and then ATP generation occurs in the mitochondria *via* the electron transport chain. The dramatic differences in the potential energy produced *via* aerobic *versus* anaerobic metabolism are illustrated below.

Glucose can yield 2820 kJ·mol^{-1} as heat during *in vitro* combustion.[2] *In vivo*, anaerobic metabolism of glucose yields 2 molecules of lactic acid + 2 moles ATP ≈ 67 kJ of energy, or 67 ÷ 2820 ≈ 2% of the total potential energy.[2]

Aerobic metabolism of glucose yields $(CO_2 + H_2O)$ + 38 moles ATP $\approx$ 1270 kJ of energy, or 1270 $\div$ 2820 $\approx$ 45% of the total potential energy.[2]

Oxygen delivery (Do_2) can be calculated as:

$$Do_2 = 10 \times CaO_2 \times Q \; (l \cdot min^{-1})$$

where Q is the cardiac output and CaO_2 is the arterial oxygen content.

$$CaO_2 = (1.39 \times [Hb] \times SaO_2) + (0.003 \times PaO_2)$$

where [Hb] = hemoglobin concentration, SaO_2 = arterial oxygen saturation, PaO_2 = the partial pressure of oxygen in arterial blood, and 1.39 = the stochiometric oxygen-binding capacity of the hemoglobin molecule. This value is variably reported in the literature, but 1.39 corresponds to the value commonly used in the software calculation packages available for many commercial analyzers. Normally, arterial blood has an oxygen content about 20 ml·dl^{-1} with an oxygen delivery of about 1 l·min^{-1} to the periphery. The venous blood returning to the right atrium still has about 750 ml of oxygen ~5 liters, or an oxygen content of 15 ml·dl^{-1}.[2] This yields a normal arterial − venous oxygen content difference of $(20 - 15) \approx 5$ ml O_2·dl^{-1}.[2] The following illustrates the partial pressure gradients of oxygen going from atmosphere to the inside of the mitochondria.

Total atmospheric pressure is 760 mm Hg, 20.9% of which is air. $P_{air}O_2 = 760$ mm Hg $\times$ 0.209 = 159 mm Hg.[27] After inhalation air becomes saturated with water vapor, so that the partial pressure of water vapor (47 mm Hg at 37°C) must be incorporated as follows:

$$P_{inspired\,gas}O_2 = (760 - 47) \times 0.209$$
$$= 713 \times 0.209 \approx 149$$

or about 150 mm Hg. The partial pressure of oxygen in alveolar blood (PAO_2) is about one-third less (~100 mm Hg) because of the equilibrium reached between the delivery of oxygen to the lung from normal ventilation *versus* the uptake of alveolar oxygen by pulmonary blood flow.[27] Thus, hypoventilation or an increased resting oxygen consumption will further lower PaO_2 below 100 mm Hg. Taking this into account ($PaCO_2$ reflecting ventilatory status), a simplified alveolar gas equation can be used to calculate PAO_2:

$$PaO_2 = FIO_2(PB - sat.\,H_2O\,vapor) - \frac{PaCO_2}{RER}$$

At a $PaCO_2$ of 40 mm Hg and a respiratory exchange ratio (RER) of 0.8,

$$PAO_2 = (760 - 47) \times 0.209 - \frac{40}{0.8}$$
$$\approx 100 \; mm \; Hg$$

Additionally, three other mechanisms minimally contribute to a further oxygen deficit of a few mm Hg between the alveolus and the pulmonary venous blood returning to the left atrium. A calculated PaO_2 of about 100 mm Hg drops a few more mm Hg to a PaO_2 in the high 90 mm Hg, owing to the following factors:

1. *Diffusion*. The RBC traverses the pulmonary capillary in about 0.75 second. In approximately 0.25 second oxygen transfer is complete, leaving 0.5 second of buffer or reserve time in a normal lung.[28] PaO_2 approaches (but never reaches)

PAO_2. Uptake of oxygen in the pulmonary capillary depends on oxygen diffusion through the alveolar-capillary membrane and the reaction of oxygen with hemoglobin. The former is proportional to the area of membrane involved, oxygen solubility in blood, and the driving pressure $[(P_1 - P_2) \rightarrow$ normally 60 mm Hg, or (100 mm Hg − 40 mm Hg)].[28] It is inversely proportional to the square of the molecular weight of oxygen and the thickness of the alveolar-capillary membrane (usually less than 0.5 μm).[28] Diffusion may also be affected by the rate of blood flow through the capillary and the volume of blood in the capillary.[28]

2. *Shunt*. Normally, shunt is from bronchial venous blood, thebesian veins, and the like and plays a very minor role. However, in some critically ill patients, the shunt value may increase dramatically and cause significant management problems. The derivation of the shunt equation and a discussion of ventilation-perfusion mismatch is addressed in Chapter 33.

3. *Ventilation-Perfusion (V/Q) Inequality*. The ideal V/Q ratio of 1.0 does not exist for the lung as a whole. V/Q is normally about 0.63 at the lung bases, with the ratio at the apex being about 3.3.[27] The overall value for the entire lung is roughly 0.85.[27] This normal V/Q inequality also contributes to a lower Po_2 in pulmonary venous blood than if the V/Q ratio were everywhere 1.0.

A further drop in Po_2 occurs in distal peripheral vascular beds, with an additional and significant decrement occurring across the capillary endothelial cells. Under normal circumstances the mixed venous blood returning to the heart has a Po_2 of 40 mm Hg and an So_2 of 75%.

As already mentioned, oxygen diffuses from the capillary into the cell and enters the mitochondrion, intramitochondrial Po_2 being about 1 mm Hg or less.

HYPOXEMIA

A resting PaO_2 more than 2 SD below the normal mean resting PaO_2 for a patient's age and FIO_2 may be considered to represent hypoxemia. One cause of hypoxemia that is of great concern to anesthesiologists is delivery of a low FIO_2 to the patient. Four other major causes of hypoxemia are:[27]

1. *Hypoventilation*—the only one of the four in which the alveolar-arterial gradient is normal.
2. *V/Q inequality*—accounts for the great majority of all cases of hypoxemia.
3. *Diffusion impairment* (e.g., severe pulmonary fibrosis)—caused by a thickened alveolar-capillary membrane, usually contributes to hypoxemia only in conditions of stress, as in exercise.
4. *Shunt*—the only one of the four that is refractory to oxygen administration. Shunt refers to alveoli that are perfused but not ventilated. This occurs when:
   a. alveoli are totally collapsed or atelectatic (referring to loss of alveolar volume). There are four major types of atelectasis:[29]
      (1) *Resorption atelectasis*—the most common; occurs by continued uptake of alveolar gas in the presence of tracheobronchial tree obstruction. Administration of 100% oxygen may exacerbate this process by removing intra-alveolar nitrogen, a prime alveolar "splint."[29]
      (2) *Passive atelectasis*—occurs secondary to intrathoracic space-occupying processes (pneumothorax, hydrothorax, and the like).[29]

(3) *Adhesive atelectasis*—occurs secondary to decreased alveolar surfactant; commonly seen in prematures.[29]

(4) *Cicatrization atelectasis*—occurs secondary to decreased pulmonary compliance with diminished elastic forces (e.g., pulmonary fibrosis).

b. Alveoli are filled with blood, pus, water, and so forth.

c. An anatomic shunt bypasses alveoli (e.g., intrapulmonary fistula).

d. Functional residual capacity (FRC) is much greater than closing capacity, so that the alveoli remain closed during normal tidal ventilation.

HYPOXIA

Inadequate tissue oxygenation is called tissue hypoxia. The four major kinds of hypoxia by cause are as follows:

1. *Anemic hypoxia*—caused by diminished oxygen-carrying capacity secondary to a decrease in the quantity or quality of hemoglobin.[5]
2. *Hypoxemic hypoxia*—occurs secondary to a low Pa_{O_2}.[5]
3. *Circulatory hypoxia*—occurs either from sluggish capillary blood (stagnant hypoxia) or from blood flow bypassing tissues (arteriovenous shunting).[5]
4. *Histotoxic hypoxia*—follows failure of proper cellular utilization of oxygen (e.g., cyanide poisoning).[5]

When oxygen supply to the mitochondria is adequate, NADH is reoxidized through the proton shuttle of the mitochondrial membrane. However, when oxygen supply to the mitochondria is inadequate, pyruvate reoxidizes NADH, resulting in excess lactate accumulation and a change in the cytosol redox state. During exercise this point has been called the anaerobic threshold. Persistent inadequate tissue oxygenation with resultant anaerobic glycolysis and metabolic acidosis leads to inability to produce enough energy to maintain normal cellular function. This leads to ionic imbalances and diminished cell-structural integrity. Because there are no significant stores of oxygen (roughly 1550 ml while a subject is breathing air),[2] there must be a constant supply of oxygen; even short periods of oxygen deprivation can produce an oxygen debt that must be repaid rapidly. In the normal state, oxygen utilization equals metabolic demand. Basal metabolic oxygen rate is about 3.5 ml $O_2 \cdot kg^{-1} \cdot min^{-1}$ and the lungs take in this amount of oxygen, with most of it binding to hemoglobin.[30] Normally, oxygen utilization equals oxygen delivery (cardiac output × arterial oxygen content) times oxygen extraction. Oxygen release and extraction are also influenced by the distribution of cardiac output and the P50 (the oxygen tension at 50% hemoglobin saturation). Mild acidosis generally has a beneficial effect on tissue oxygenation. An increased $[H^+]$ within the RBC diminishes the affinity of hemoglobin for oxygen, shifting the oxyhemoglobin dissociation curve to the right and enhancing peripheral oxygen unloading to tissues. However, increasing acidemia inhibits glycolysis and tends to deplete RBCs of various intermediate metabolites of glycolysis, especially 2,3-diphosphoglyceric acid (DPG). This may occur over 12–36 hours, and the depletion of 2-3 DPG with time may eventually offset the usual beneficial effects of acidosis on tissue oxygenation.[12,30]

Normally, oxygen utilization is independent of oxygen supply until oxygen delivery falls below about 10 ml $O_2 \cdot kg^{-1} \cdot min^{-1}$.[31] However, in various pathologic states the critical oxygen delivery, the level at which oxygen consumption becomes dependent on supply, may increase to about 21 ml $O_2 \cdot kg^{-1} \cdot min^{-1}$.[32] In these pathologic supply-dependent states, an increased oxygen delivery may be achieved by volume expansion, blood transfusion, or inotropic drugs, which in turn leads to increased oxygen utilization. Shoemaker et al found that a supranormal oxygen utilization (about 25% above normal) following resuscitation from shock was associated with increased survival.[33]

Decreased oxygen consumption during anesthesia may reflect reduced oxygen need, inadequate tissue oxygen delivery, or impaired cellular oxygen extraction. Waxman et al studied arterial blood lactate concentration pre-, intra-, and postoperatively in high-risk surgical patients.[34] Elevated lactate levels intraoperatively and in the postoperative period that occurred irrespective of anesthetic management correlated with an intraoperative oxygen deficit.[34] Lubarsky et al studied mixed venous oxygen saturation (Sv_{O_2}) in hemodynamically stable patients undergoing cardiac surgery.[35] They found normal to elevated values for Sv_{O_2} despite dramatic decreases in cardiac output, oxygen delivery, and oxygen consumption.[35] Based on their findings they suggested that anesthesia may cause a maldistribution of blood flow (similar to that proposed in septic shock) to account for a maintenance or elevation of Sv_{O_2} values despite inadequate tissue oxygenation.[35] The clinical relevance of following serial intraoperative lactate levels or attempting to achieve supranormal intraoperative oxygen utilization (as Shoemaker did in the postoperative period) is unknown at present.

Oxygen delivery concerns the transport of oxygen through conduits, the macrocirculation, but it does not yield information about the microcirculation, the amount of oxygen that actually diffuses into the mitochrondia, or the state of the cell and its ability to use oxygen in a normal fashion. Additionally, oxygen release and the distribution of cardiac output are unknowns. More work needs to be done to elucidate the mechanisms of aerobic metabolism. Attempts to modify each of these variables may be valuable, in order to learn more about their clinical significance.

Another extremely important variable, in addition to tissue oxygenation and the adequate supply of other cell nutrients, is flow. Flow is needed not only to supply cells with oxygen and nutrients but also to remove cellular waste products and is vital for long-term cell survival.

Weil and Shubin have categorized shock (inadequate tissue perfusion) into four major causes:[36]

1. *Hypovolemic*—due to inadequate circulatory volume (e.g., massive hemorrhage).
2. *Cardiogenic*—due to pump failure (e.g., extensive myocardial infarction).
3. *Distributive*—e.g., septic shock, anaphylactic shock.
4. *Obstructive*—e.g., massive pulmonary embolus, aortocaval compression.

This classification addresses problems of the macrocirculation, but the microcirculation and cellular ability to function normally are often involved. Work has been done on these so-called micro-aspects of inadequate flow, but their therapeutic relevance remains to be determined.

It appears that long-term exposure to low flow states (but above the threshold of viability) may lead to various cellular changes (including excess accumulation of lipid metabolites in the cell). This may cause the cell to enter a chronic vegetative state in which viability is maintained but cellular function is impaired; examples include the hibernating myocardium (heart)[38] or chronic penumbra (brain).[39] In such states it is conceivable that only those cellular processes crucial for basic cell survival remain intact, other cellular machinery having been shut down. Specialized cells may differentiate to some dormant progenitor cell state, equipped only to survive. Internal cellular derangements, membrane derangements, protein activation or inactivation, and repression or derepression of genetic material may contribute to such a phenomenon, which could play a role in organ failure in various different viscera.

Certain patients have supranormal oxygen delivery, apparently supply independent, but continue to deteriorate. In these cases the problem appears to be impaired oxygen utilization, inadequate for oxygen demand, and they represent a unique challenge. Many hypotheses have been proposed to explain these states; however, definitive explanations are not known. One widely held theory proposes a maldistribution of perfusion, with certain tissues adequately perfused and other tissues inadequately perfused. Arterial blood gases represent both a snapshot and global view. Unfortunately, clinically it is impossible to measure for each organ blood flow, vascular resistances, arterial and venous blood gases, and so forth. So although a "regional breakup" may be advantageous, currently only global arterial and mixed venous values are available clinically. However, these values should be followed serially and in longitudinal fashion in an attempt to construct trends that aid in patient management. Multiple snapshots should be collated to make a movie.

Other possible reasons for impaired cellular oxygen utilization despite apparently supply-independent physiology may include the buildup of cellular metabolites (e.g., adenosine), electron transport chain toxins or partial uncouplers, and oxygen radicals and mediators from platelets, neutrophils, macrophages, and complement activation; an impaired microcirculation (e.g., due to microemboli, endothelial damage, white cell or platelet plugs, intense vasoconstriction from thromboxane or neurohumoral loss of normal vasomotion); and increased distance between capillaries and cells (e.g., edema); decreased capillary density; shunts; and precapillary diffusion of oxygen.

Near infrared spectrometry to assess the state of cytochrome $a-a_3$ (niroscopy) and positron emission tomography may be important adjunctive tools in the future to better deal with these various physiological disturbances. A greater understanding of this pathophysiology and what events are primary phenomena versus secondary phenomena or epiphenomena will hopefully lead to better (or at least more rational) patient management.

OXYGEN CALCULATIONS

Arterial oxygen saturation (SaO_2) can be followed noninvasively in real time with a pulse oximeter or invasively with special oximetric catheters. To interpret oxygenation noninvasively or from arterial or mixed venous blood gas values, the FIO_2 delivered to the patient must be known. If a blood gas sample is being obtained, the FIO_2 should be recorded by the sampler and sent to the laboratory. Additionally, the patient's age, medical history, pulmonary history, smoking history, and so forth should be determined. The reason why blood gas values are wanted should be known, as should the current clinical circumstances (is the patient intubated, on continuous positive airway pressure or mechanical ventilation, and so forth), and recent resting baseline arterial

blood gas values determined when the patient was not acutely ill should be used for comparison. In the absence of this information, the interpretation of the results will be suspect and the direction of future therapeutic interventions hampered.

A major problem for most clinicians is the complexity of interpreting arterial blood gas values. In part, this complexity may have arisen from the novelty of the measurement and the desire to glean as much information as possible from the sample. The subsequent development of complex nomograms and the debate over whether or not to temperature correct samples have further confused the issue. The following estimations, based on physiologic phenomena described earlier in the chapter, should simplify this problem and allow rapid determination of the patient's oxygenation and ventilatory status.

Oxygen flows down concentration gradients from the atmosphere to the mitochondria. Logically it would be anticipated that as the FIO_2 is increased, PaO_2 and PAO_2 would also increase. The magnitude of the change reflected in the blood gas will be determined by the success of oxygen therapy in increasing PAO_2, the extent of impediments to diffusion between the alveolus and the capillary blood, and the degree of V/Q mismatch in the lungs. The normal alveolararterial difference in partial oxygen pressure ($D(A-a)O_2$) is less than 10 mm Hg. Therefore, if PAO_2 is calculated from the alveolar air equation, an approximation of PaO_2 can be derived easily.

The alveolar air equation states that $PAO_2 = FIO_2 \times$ (atmospheric pressure − saturated water vapor pressure at patient temperature) − $PaCO_2$/RQ, where RQ = respiratory quotient. RQ is also referred to as the RER (respiratory exchange ratio) and is the volume of carbon dioxide produced per minute divided by the volume of oxygen consumed per minute. The value depends on the predominant metabolic fuel, in the following fashion: when fat is predominant, RQ approximates 0.7; when carbohydrate is predominant, RQ approaches 1.0. The value has become available in many ICUs with the advent of direct, clinically available metabolic monitoring, but traditionally this value is reported as 0.8. In patients receiving 100% oxygen, the value will be closer to 1.0. With this information, the PAO_2 at sea level for a patient receiving 40% oxygen by mask can be calculated:

$$PAO_2 = (760 - 47) \times 0.4 - 40/0.8 = 713 \times 0.4 - 50$$
$$= 285 - 50 = 235$$

where 760 mm Hg = sea level barometric pressure, 47 mm Hg = saturated water vapor pressure at 37°C, and 40 = $PaCO_2$.

This value should be compared to the measured blood gas, and it may be assumed that a 1% intrapulmonary shunt is responsible for each 20 mm Hg change in $DA-aO_2$. Therefore, if the measured PaO_2 in this example is 50 mm Hg, the clinician should recognize that the patient has a pulmonary abnormality representing an approximate shunt of (378 − 50) ÷ 20, or 16%.

An even simpler approximation can be made if the following shorthand is used to estimate PaO_2:

$$FIO_2 = 0.21 \text{ to } 0.5: PaO_2 = FIO_2 \times 5 \times 100$$

e.g., for $FIO_2 = 0.4$, estimated $PaO_2 = 200$ mm Hg.

$$FIO_2 = 0.5 \text{ to } 1.0: PaO_2 = FIO_2 \times 6 \times 100$$

e.g., for $FIO_2 = 0.6$, estimated $PaO_2 = 360$ mm Hg.

From this estimate of Pa_{O_2}, the previous example is calculated as follows: measured Pa_{O_2} = 50 mm Hg on F_{IO_2} = 0.6; expected Pa_{O_2} = 6 × 0.6 × 100 = 360; measured Pa_{O_2} = 50; estimated D_{A-aO_2} = 360 − 50 = 310; estimated intrapulmonary shunt = 310 ÷ 20 = 16%.

The perceived abnormality should be compared with the situation that would exist if the patient were known to have chronic obstructive lung disease and the Pa_{O_2} had been measured on room air. In this instance the estimated Pa_{O_2} = (.21 × 5 × 100) = 105; measured Pa_{O_2} = 50; D_{A-aO_2} = 55; estimated shunt = 3%. Although an arterial oxygen tension of 50 mm Hg is abnormal, the clinical and measurement conditions surrounding the result make a significant difference to the way in which the clinician responds therapeutically.

Another important therapeutic challenge is to regulate mechanical ventilation in an attempt to control Pa_{CO_2} through alveolar ventilation. Although a trial-and-error approach is commonly employed to determine ultimate settings, there is much to be gained by anticipating the Pa_{CO_2} for any ventilator setting. A number of approaches may be used to derive this information: the approach described below builds on common physiologic principles.

1. Carbon dioxide regulation depends on effective alveolar ventilation and, to a lesser extent, on normal V/Q relationships throughout the lungs.

2. Tidal volume (V_T) is divided into the portions that ventilate the physiologic dead space (V_D) and the total alveolar space (V_A). Because in normal tissue, carbon dioxide diffuses 20 times more rapidly than oxygen, V/Q mismatch has less effect on P_{CO_2} than on P_{O_2}. However, this should not be interpreted to mean that carbon dioxide clearance is not a serious problem in critically ill patients. Indeed, the reverse is true, and many patients die with terminal hypercarbia rather than terminal hypoxemia.

3. In the physiologic range, carbon dioxide clearance is linearly related to minute alveolar ventilation, with a doubling of effective ventilation equaling a 50% reduction in Pa_{CO_2}.

4. Normal physiologic dead space equals the patient's weight in pounds, and the normal dead space to tidal volume ratio (V_D/V_T) is 1:3. Additionally, if it is assumed that an individual breathes 12–16 times per minute to maintain a Pa_{CO_2} of 40 mm Hg, then the following relationships can be approximated for a 70-kg (150-lb) patient:

V_D = 150 ml
V_A = 300 ml
V_T = 450–500 ml
Minute ventilation = 7.0 l·min^{-1} (500 × 14)
Minute alveolar ventilation = 4.2 l·min^{-1} (300 × 14)

Additionally, the following relationships can be assumed for mechanically ventilated patients:

V_D will be reduced 30–50% secondary to intubation or tracheostomy. Traditionally, V_T is increased to reduce dyspnea and improve patient/ventilator harmony. A commonly used V_T is 12–15 ml·kg^{-1}. The compliance of the ventilator circuitry can be assumed to be 3–4 ml per cm H_2O inflation pressure. With this information, the following can be inferred from a typical clinical example.

Example

The patient is a 70-kg male victim of a motor vehicle accident who has suffered a closed head injury. If all other considerations are controlled (e.g., concerns of resuscitation and hemodynamic stability, and the like), what are the anticipated ventilator settings required to produce an initial Pa_{CO_2} of 25 mm Hg? The following assumptions are made. The patient is intubated without incident, and appropriate muscle relaxation and sedation are provided to ensure delivery of mechanical ventilation without asynchrony. (Use of sedatives in this situation is controversial, and carefully planned therapeutic and diagnostic plans must be formulated before independent therapy is initiated in the emergency department, operating room or ICU.) V_T is set at 12 ml·kg^{-1}, or 850 ml, and the patient is set to receive 12 breaths per minute with an F_{IO_2} of 0.5. The peak inflation pressure (PIP) is noted to be 20 cm H_2O. What are the anticipated arterial blood gases on these settings?

From the preceding discussion, Pa_{O_2} and Pa_{CO_2} can be evaluated as follows:

$$\text{Predicted } Pa_{O_2} = 0.5 \times 5 = 250 \text{ mm Hg}$$

The Pa_{CO_2} can be predicted in the following manner:

$$V_D = 150 - (150 \times 0.3) = 105 \text{ ml}$$
$$V_A = (850 - [105 + 80]) \times 12 = 7.9 \text{ l·min}^{-1}$$

where V_D = 150 ml, 0.3 = reduction in anatomic dead space following intubation, and 80 ml = compliance of ventilator tubing at 20 cm H_2O PIP. From the preceding discussion, normal V_A = 4.2 l·min^{-1}. Therefore, it is anticipated that the patient will have a Pa_{CO_2} between 20 and 25 mm Hg, based on the assumption that alveolar ventilation has been increased by approximately 85% and that the Pa_{CO_2} should be reduced proportionately (if alveolar ventilation is doubled, Pa_{CO_2} will be halved), or a Pa_{CO_2} of approximately 23 mm Hg. Obviously, V/Q characteristics will modify these results, but it is likely that they will be a reasonable approximation of the measured values in an otherwise healthy individual; certainly if a major discrepancy is revealed, further investigation is warranted to identify its source. This exercise provides a good check on ventilator function, and no discrepancy should remain uninvestigated.

Another useful and simple calculation can be performed from the previously described relationships to predict whether or not a change in F_{IO_2} is acceptable and whether any changes in observed blood gas values are consistent with the change. This is predicated on the assumption that Pa_{CO_2}, V/Q mismatch, and the D_{A-aO_2} will remain constant for the duration of the measurement. Under these conditions, how will the Pa_{O_2} change in the following situation?

Pa_{O_2} = 180 mm Hg
F_{IO_2} = 0.4

The F_{IO_2} is changed to 0.21; what is the anticipated Pa_{O_2}? With an F_{IO_2} of 0.4, the predicted Pa_{O_2} is 200 mm Hg; at F_{IO_2} = 0.21, it is 105 mm Hg. The following relationship is then proposed:

$$180 \div 200 = x \div 105$$

where x is the new Pa_{O_2} on F_{IO_2} of 0.21.

$$x = 95 \text{ mm Hg}$$

These approximations provide the clinician with a simple tool to evaluate therapeutic prerogatives in the management of complex situations in the operating room and ICU.

CONCLUSIONS

This chapter has focused on issues of acid-base balance that are of primary concern to the clinician. Although the discussion is somewhat abbreviated, it remains true that the practitioner is unlikely to manage patients effectively if complex nomograms or significant calculations outside the range of mental or pocket calculator approximations made at the bedside are required to utilize information obtained from routine arterial blood gas determinations. (Mixed venous values have not been dealt with specifically, although all manipulations are applicable if new baseline values are assumed.) Aerobic metabolism depends on an uninterrupted delivery of oxygen to metabolically active tissues. Local oxygen and carbon dioxide concentration gradients and metabolic conditions will determine the unique environment of specific organs or regions. The variables measured and discussed in acid-base balance provide both a snapshot of the acute global environment through the arterial blood gas values of Pao_2, $Paco_2$, and pH_a, and a chronic view if the total bicarbonate is studied. Careful integration of the information presented in this chapter with discussions on pulmonary pathophysiology and available therapeutic options (including mechanical ventilatory support and its anticipated benefits) will provide mechanisms to evaluate patient requirements for and response to therapy.

REFERENCES

1. Lumb PD: Perioperative pulmonary physiology. In Sabiston DC, Spencer FC (eds): Gibbon's Surgery of the Chest, 4th ed, vol 1, p 17. Philadelphia, WB Saunders, 1983
2. Nunn JF: Applied Respiratory Physiology, 3rd ed. Boston, Butterworth, 1987
3. Ream AK, Reitz BA, Silverberg G: Temperature correction of Pco_2 and pH in estimating acid base status: An example of the emperor's new clothes? Anesthesiology 56:41, 1982
4. Williams JJ, Marshall BE: A fresh look at an old question. Anesthesiology 56:1, 1982
5. Shapiro BA, Harrison RA, Walton JR: Clinical Application of Blood Gases, 3rd ed. Chicago, Year Book Medical Publishers, 1982
6. Cohen JJ: Disorders of hydrogen ion metabolism. In Early LE, Gottschalk CE (eds): Strauss and Welt's Diseases of the Kidney, 3rd ed, vol II. Boston, Little, Brown & Co, 1979
7. Waddell WJ, Bates RG: Intracellular pH. Physiol Rev 49:285, 1969
8. Astrup P, Jorgensen K, Siggaard-Anderson O, Engel K: The acid-base metabolism: A new approach. Lancet 1:1035, 1960
9. Kaehny WD, Gabow PA: Pathogenesis and management of metabolic acidosis and alkalosis. In Shrier RW (ed): Renal and Electrolyte Disorders, 2nd ed, p 115. Boston, Little, Brown & Co, 1980
10. Burckhardt G, Warnock DG: Mechanism of H^+ secretion in the proximal convoluted tubule. Semin Nephrol 10:93, 1990
11. Cogan MG: Regulation and control of bicarbonate reabsorption in the proximal tubule. Semin Nephrol 10:115, 1990
12. Narins RG, Krishna GG, Bresuler L et al: The metabolic acidoses. In Maxwell MH, Kleeman CR, Narins RG (eds): Clinical Disorders of Fluid and Electrolyte Metabolism, 4th ed, p 597. New York, McGraw-Hill, 1987
13. Pestana CC: Fluids and Electrolytes in the Surgical Patient, 4th ed. Baltimore, Williams & Wilkins, 1989
14. Goodman DA: Relationship of gluconeogenesis to ammonia production in the kidney. Isr J Med Sci 8:285, 1972
15. Hodgkin JE, Saeprono FF, Chen DM: Incidence of metabolic alkemia in hospitalized patients. Crit Care Med 8:725, 1980
16. Wilson RF, Gibson D, Percinel AK et al: Severe alkalosis in critically ill surgical patients. Arch Surg 105:197, 1972
17. Cohen JJ, Kassirer JP: Acid-Base, 1st ed. Boston, Little, Brown & Co, 1982
18. Kaehny WD: Pathogenesis and management of respiratory and mixed acid-base disorders. In Schrier RW (ed): Renal and Electrolyte Disorders. 2nd ed, p 159. Boston, Little, Brown & Co, 1980
19. Pitts RF: Physiology of the Kidney and Body Fluids, 3rd ed. Chicago, Year Book Medical Publishers, 1974
20. Rose BD: Clinical Physiology of Acid-Base and Electrolyte Disorders, 3rd ed. New York, McGraw-Hill Information Services, 1989
21. Cohen RD, Woods HF: Clinical and Biochemical Aspects of Lactic Acidosis. Oxford, England, Blackwell Scientific Publications, 1976
22. Weil MH, Afifi AA: Experimental and clinical studies on lactate and pyruvate as indicators of the severity of acute circulatory failure (shock). Circulation 41:989, 1970
23. Posner JB, Plum F: Spinal-fluid pH and neurologic symptoms in systemic acidosis. N Engl J Med 277:605, 1967
24. Plum F, Siesjo BK: Recent advances in CSF physiology. Anesthesiology 42:708, 1975
25. Severinghaus JW: Acid-base nomogram: A Barton-Copenhagen denlente. Anesthesiology 45:539, 1976
26. Weil MH, Rackow EC, Trevino R et al: Difference in acid-base state between venous and arterial blood during cardiopulmonary resuscitation. N Engl J Med 315:153, 1986
27. West JB: Ventilation/Blood Flow and Gas Exchange, 4th ed. London, Blackwell Scientific Publications, 1985
28. West JB: Respiratory Physiology: The Essentials, 3rd ed. Baltimore, Williams & Wilkins, 1985
29. Pare JA, Fraser RG: Synopsis of Diseases of the Chest. Philadelphia, WB Saunders, 1983
30. Finch CA, Lenfan C: Oxygen transport in man. N Engl J Med 286:407, 1972
31. Cain SM: Oxygen delivery and uptake in dogs during anemic and hypoxic hypoxia. J Appl Physiol 42:228, 1977
32. Mohsenifar Z, Goldbach P, Tashkin DP et al: Relationship between oxygen delivery and oxygen consumption in the adult respiratory distress syndrome. Chest 84:267, 1983
33. Shoemaker WC, Appel P, Bland R: Use of physiologic monitoring to predict outcome and assist in clinical decisions in critically ill post-operative patients. Am J Surg 146:43, 1983
34. Waxman K, Nolan LS, Shoemaker WC: Sequential perioperative lactate determination: Physiological and clinical implications. Crit Care Med 10:96, 1982
35. Lubarsky D, Kaufman BS, Sharnicks S, Turndorf H: The effects of induction of anesthesia on mixed venous and peripheral venous oxygen saturations. Anesth Analg 68:S172, 1989
36. Weil MH, Shubin H: Prepared reclassification of shock states with special reference to distributive defects. In Hinshaw LB, Cox BG (eds): The Fundamental Mechanisms of Shock. Adv Exp Med Biol 23:13, 1972
37. Kassirer JP, Hricik DE, Cohen JJ: Repairing Body Fluids: Principles and Practice. Philadelphia, WB Saunders Co, 1989
38. Rahmitoola SH: A perspective on the three large multicenter randomized clinical trails of coronary bypass surgery for chronic stable angina. Circulation 72 (suppl V) V:123, 1985
39. Jones TH, Morawetz RB, Cromwell RM, Marcoux FW et al: Threshold of focal cerebral ischemia in awake monkeys. J Neurosurg 54:773, 1981

11

Norig Ellison

Hemostasis and Hemotherapy

Bleeding as a result of a defect in hemostasis may have numerous etiologies ranging from congenital deficiencies of coagulation factors, through trauma, to iatrogenic causes such as surgery or thrombocytopenia secondary to cancer chemotherapy. During surgery, some bleeding is to be expected and is not necessarily a cause for concern; however, blood loss in excess of what would be expected at any stage in the procedure should be investigated. Furthermore, although the body's ability to seal off leaks in the circulatory system with a platelet plug or clot is essential, that ability to respond with rapid, localized hemostasis in a fluid medium is not without risk.

Whereas imbalance in one direction, such as deficiency in platelet number or Factor X concentration, leads to excessive bleeding, imbalance in the other direction leads to thrombosis. The problem of imbalance in the direction of excessive thrombosis formation has become more widely recognized in the past two decades. For example, whereas bleeding disorders associated with specific clinical entities such as dead fetus or hemolytic transfusion reaction have long been recognized, the recognition of a common denominator and use of the terms *disseminated intravascular coagulation* (DIC) are recent developments. It was not until 1972 that DIC first appeared as a separate heading in *Index Medicus*. Although DIC may be considered a "disease of medical progress" in that it is now being diagnosed more frequently because more critically ill patients are surviving for longer periods of time, an alternative explanation is that the entity is now well accepted and thus is just being recognized more readily and earlier.[1]

HEMOSTASIS

Normal Physiology

When a defect in the circulatory system develops, a primary hemostatic plug will form within 5 minutes of injury, requiring only interaction between the injured vessel and platelets (Fig. 11-1). The coagulation mechanism is not involved in the formation of the primary hemostatic plug, which is usually sufficient to stem the initial hemorrhage. However, fibrin formation is necessary for permanent hemostasis.[2] As a platelet plug forms, vasoactive substances, which are released from the platelets, produce vasoconstriction, a salutory effect in that decreasing the orifice that must be plugged will also decrease the leak. The formation of the definitive or secondary hemostatic plug, which will require an additional 1–2 hours, involves two more steps. First, a loose fibrin clot will be formed by the conversion of fibrinogen to fibrin through activation of the coagulation mechanism. Second, Factor XIII activation induces cross-polymerization of the loose fibrin to produce a firm, insoluble clot that in turn retracts into a firm, definitive hemostatic plug under the influence of platelets. Finally, fibrinolysis, a physiologic process, is activated to localize the clot and to remodel the area of injury as the endothelium regenerates.

The Blood Vessel

In the absence of such injury, the endothelium, which functions as a permeable barrier that prevents loss of colloid from the circulation, exerts multiple antithrombotic properties. First, on the luminal surface is heparan sulfate, which can weakly stimulate antithrombin III (AT-III) and provide an ideal localized surface for AT-III to act. Second, the vascular endothelial cell produces prostacyclin, which is both a potent vasodilator and an inhibitor of the hemostatic function of platelets. Third, the vascular endothelial membrane also contains a receptor, thrombomodulin, which forms a complex with thrombin to alter its activity radically.[3] Instead of forming a complex with Factor VIII to activate Factor Xa, or converting fibrinogen to fibrin, the thrombin–thrombomodulin complex converts protein C, a vitamin K–dependent physiologic anticoagulant, to its activated form. Active protein C inactivates Factor V and Factor VIII and regulates the release of tissue plasminogen activator. Once a definitive hemostatic plug has been formed, the vascular endothelial cells play a role in fibrinolysis by synthesizing tissue plasminogen activator, which appears to bind to fibrin and facilitates the action of fibrin-bound plasminogen, leading to clot lysis and healing.

Surgery cannot be performed without routinely creating multiple blood vessel defects. Although the spontaneous arrest of bleeding from ruptured vessels conveying blood under pressure involves autonomic mechanisms that are extremely complex in detail, the mechanical principles gov-

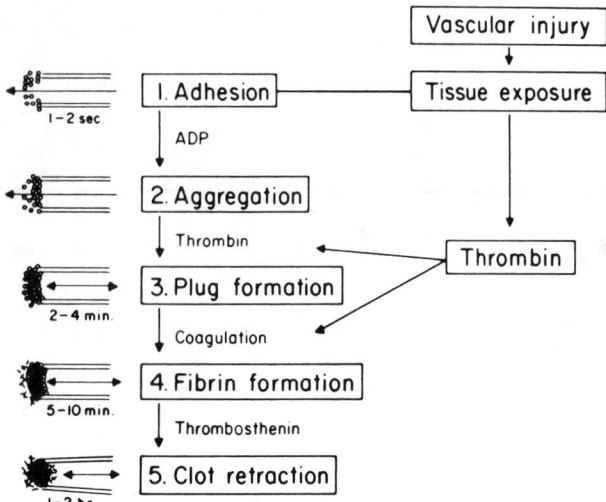

Figure 11-1. Formation of the primary and secondary (definitive) hemostatic plugs. (Reprinted with permission from Harker LA: Hemostasis Manual, p 4. Seattle, University of Washington Press, 1970.)

erning the laws of blood flow through such a defect are quite simple. Blood loss will continue as long as pressure within the vessel exceeds the pressure outside the vessel. Blood vessel mechanisms to arrest blood loss include (1) vasoconstriction to decrease the size of the defect; (2) anastomotic dilatation to shunt blood away from the defects; (3) bleeding into tissues to increase the extravascular pressure and decrease the intravascular-extravascular gradient; (4) increased permeability of the microcirculation to promote further increase in extravascular pressure as edema fluid

escapes from the blood vessels; (5) hemoconcentration, resulting from diminished plasma volume as fluid leaves the vascular compartment due to the increased permeability, to slow circulation and further reduce intravascular pressure; and (6) continual blood loss without replacement to produce sufficient hypotension to minimize or halt blood loss.[4] Finally, surgical ligation of the bleeding vessel will restore vascular integrity more quickly and completely in instances where these mechanisms would not suffice until irreparable harm had occurred.

Coagulation Mechanism

Because most blood vessels are less than 1 mm in diameter, and in vessels of this caliber platelets and coagulation factors play the major role in hemostasis, an efficient coagulation mechanism is essential to prevent bleeding. Figure 11-2 outlines the currently accepted theory of the coagulation scheme, and Table 11-1 lists the coagulation factors with some of their synonyms. By common consent, the suffix "a" is used to designate the activated form, and the numeral VI has not been assigned to another factor. Three factors (I, V, VIII) do not exist in an enzymatically active form. With the exception of Factors III and IV, all of the factors are plasma proteins.

Primary hemostasis, the formation of the platelet plug, is accompanied by activation of the coagulation mechanism or cascade, the end result of which is formation of the de-

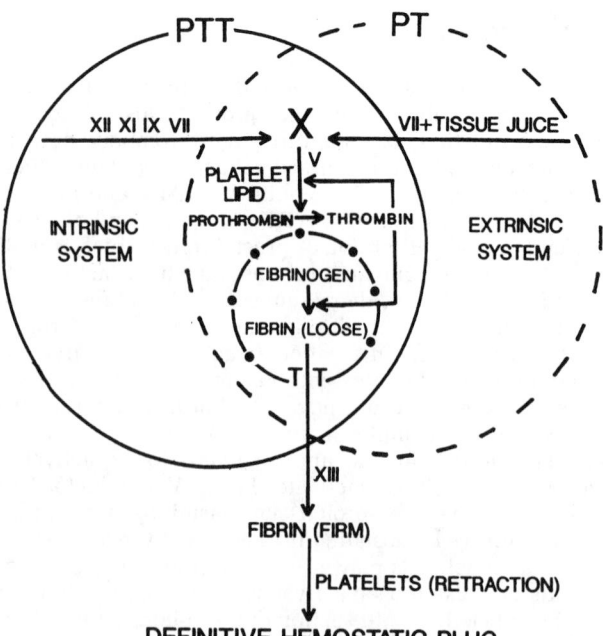

Figure 11-2. Schematic representation of the coagulation mechanism as measured *in vitro*. Factors involved in the PT, PTT, and the thrombin time are noted. (Adapted with permission from Morrison FS: Hemorrhagic complications in surgery. In Artz, Hardy [eds]: Management of Surgical Complications. Philadelphia, WB Saunders, 1978.)

TABLE 11-1. List of Coagulation Factors With Some of Their Synonyms

Factor	Synonym	Clinical Syndrome Caused by Deficiency
I	Fibrinogen	Yes
II	Prothrombin, prethrombin	Yes
III	Tissue factor, tissue thromboplastin	No
IV	Calcium	No
V	Labile factor, proaccelerin, plasma accelerator globulin (ac-G)	Yes
VI	No factor assigned to this numeral	
VII	Stable factor, proconvertin, auto-prothrombin I, serum prothrombin conversion acceleration (SPCA)	Yes
VIII	Antihemophilia globulin (AHG), antihemophilic factor (AHF), thromboplastinogen, platelet cofactor I, antihemophilic Factor A	Yes
IX	Plasma thromboplastin component (PTC), Christmas factor, auto-thrombin II, antihemophilic Factor B, platelet cofactor II	Yes
X	Stuart-Prower factor, auto-prothrombin C (or III)	Yes
XI	Plasma thromboplastin antecedent (PTA), Rosenthal syndrome, antihemophilic Factor C	mild
XII	Hageman factor, glass factor	No
XIII	Fibrin stabilizing factor (FSF), Laki-Lorand factor, fibrinase serum factor, urea-insolubility factor	Yes

Reprinted with permission from Ellison N: Coagulation evaluation and management. In Ream AK, Fogdall RP (eds): Acute Cardiovascular Management, p 773. Philadelphia, JB Lippincott, 1982.

finitive hemostatic plug. In the final common pathway, Factor X is activated by the end product of either the intrinsic or the extrinsic system. The complex sequence of events that leads up to activation of Factor X serves as a biologic amplifier, so that only a small stimulus is needed to initiate fibrin formation from fibrinogen. With a molecular weight of 340,000, fibrinogen conversion proceeds with thrombin splitting off two fibrinopeptides, A and B, which constitute about 3% of the fibrinogen molecule. Spontaneous polymerization of fibrin monomers into a loose fibrin net ensues and then, under the stimulus of Factor XIIIa, conversion of the loose fibrin net by covalent bonds into a more stable clot occurs. Finally, platelets induce retraction of the clot to form the definitive hemostatic plug.[3]

The concept of a rigid division of the coagulation cascade into an intrinsic and an extrinsic system is no longer valid. In fact, not only can Factor VIIa activate Factor IX, as indicated in Figure 11-3 but Factors IXa, Xa, thrombin, and XIIa can probably activate Factor VII. Clearly, both systems are necessary for effective hemostasis because patients with isolated deficiencies in either system do present with clinical bleeding syndromes. Activation of coagulation factors is surface-oriented, with platelet surfaces providing a protective environment that allows such activation to proceed unimpeded by the physiologic anticoagulants such as plasma AT-III.

Factor VIII is a complex consisting of von Willebrand's factor (Factor VIII:vWF) and Factor VIII:C. The latter is that property of normal plasma missing in patients with hemophilia; it is measured in the standard coagulation assays, and because of the presence of a procoagulant glycoprotein, can be identified by immunoassay. Factor VIII:vWF is a large polymeric glycoprotein that mediates platelet adhesion to a foreign surface such as collagen during formation of the primary hemostatic plug. It is also necessary for formation of the definitive hemostatic plug because Factor VIII:vWF regulates the production or release of Factor VIII:C. Although these two are non–covalently bound and closely associated in plasma, they are the products of different genes and have different immunologic properties.[5]

Platelets

Platelets have been called the keystone to the hemostatic arch because of their involvement in all phases of hemostasis. Not only are they the first nonvascular direct response of the body to bleeding but they are involved in activating the coagulation mechanism as well as in initiating clot retraction. The initial event in platelet activation is exposure of the platelet to an appropriate stimulus, which produces a shape change in the platelet from its natural disk form to a "spiny sphere." After the shape change is completed, platelet adhesion and platelet aggregation appear to develop simultaneously. Platelet adhesion is the affinity of platelets for nonplatelet surfaces, and platelet aggregation is the affinity of platelets for each other.

This phase of platelet activation culminates with the release reaction, during which the contents of cytoplasmic granules are released extracellularly and thromboxane A_2 is synthesized. The released substances include adenosine diphosphate (ADP), serotonin, platelet factor 4, catecholamines, and factors that modify vascular permeability and integrity. ADP is a potent aggregating agent, and its escape from platelets undergoing a release reaction causes more platelets to become activated. The released vasoactive substances stimulate contraction of the injured blood vessel. Platelets serve as a nidus for membrane-based coagulation reactions involved in the generation of thrombin and the formation of thrombin and actively participate in several steps of the coagulation cascade, as indicated in Figure 11-3. Platelet factor 3 is a property of lipoproteins within, and inseparable from, the platelet membrane. In contrast, platelet factor 4, which neutralizes heparin, can be recovered from plasma after platelet aggregation and is a protein present in the granular fraction of platelet homogenates. The activated platelet membrane acts as a surface upon which the macromolecular complexes of blood coagulants (IXa, VIII, X, Ca^{2+}, and Xa, V, Ca^{2+}) are assembled.

Platelets have also been reported to play a role in the activation of Factor XII in the presence of adenosine diphosphate and possibly to provide an alternative route bypassing

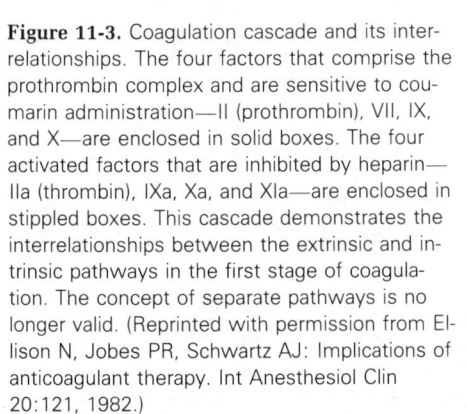

Figure 11-3. Coagulation cascade and its interrelationships. The four factors that comprise the prothrombin complex and are sensitive to coumarin administration—II (prothrombin), VII, IX, and X—are enclosed in solid boxes. The four activated factors that are inhibited by heparin—IIa (thrombin), IXa, Xa, and XIa—are enclosed in stippled boxes. This cascade demonstrates the interrelationships between the extrinsic and intrinsic pathways in the first stage of coagulation. The concept of separate pathways is no longer valid. (Reprinted with permission from Ellison N, Jobes PR, Schwartz AJ: Implications of anticoagulant therapy. Int Anesthesiol Clin 20:121, 1982.)

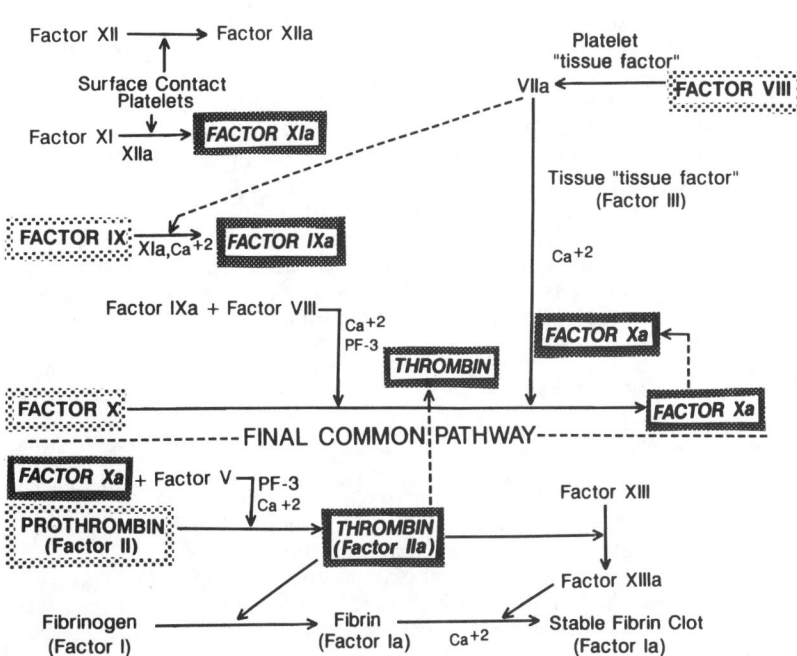

Factor XIIa by collagen-induced activation of Factor XI. This may explain why patients who are deficient in Factor XII and have markedly abnormal coagulation profiles do not bleed excessively. The final step in the sequence, clot retraction, is attributable to another platelet protein, thrombosthenin.

Fibrinolysis

There are several natural built-in checks to keep thrombus formation localized and to prevent the process from continuing to the point of complete intravascular thrombosis. These built-in checks include (1) rapid blood flow, producing dilution of coagulation factors below threshold levels; (2) clearance of activated coagulation factors by the liver and reticular endothelial system; and (3) blocking action of naturally occurring inhibitory plasma proteins such as AT-III on the action of thrombin. When the insult is overwhelming, the fibrinolytic system may be activated.

The fibrinolytic system digests fibrin to remodel the area of injury and prevent or reopen thrombotic occlusion of the vessel. A classic example of the ability of the fibrinolytic system to recanalize occluded vessels is presented in the study of Bedford and Wollman, who reported 100% recanalization of radial arteries in 20 patients following demonstrated total occlusion after radial artery catheters were removed.[6] Both the plasminogen and coagulation systems contain inactive profactors, activators, and inhibitors. The primary activator of the plasminogen system is tissue plasminogen activator, which selectively binds to fibrin and activates fibrin-bound plasminogen to plasmin, an event that tends to limit the extent of the fibrin formation. Plasmin is a serine protease that digests many substrates, including fibrinogen and Factors V and VIII. Ordinarily, upon escape from the fibrin surface, plasmin is rapidly inactivated by an extremely efficient inhibitor, alpha$_2$ antiplasmin.

The physiologic function of fibrinolysis is to localize fibrin deposition to the area of injury as well as to remove the secondary hemostatic plug during the course of healing. Recognized physiologic activators include vigorous exercise, anoxia, and stress in addition to the coagulation mechanism in which both Factor XIIa and thrombin can activate plasminogen to plasmin. The activation of the fibrinolytic system in response to the intravascular deposition of fibrin is, therefore, a normal defense mechanism.

The pathologic form of fibrinolysis represents a response to increased thrombogenesis and occurs in the setting of DIC. Rarely, pathologic fibrinolysis may occur in the absence of any obvious thrombogenic stimulus. In both types plasmin circulates intravascularly and digests not only fibrin but also fibrinogen and Factors V and VIII. Ordinarily, in vivo plasmin acts primarily on fibrin, breaking it down into successfully smaller fragments known as fibrin split products, which possess anticoagulant properties of their own by inhibiting polymerization of fibrin monomers.

Tests of Hemostasis

General Principles

The best means of detecting a hemorrhagic diathesis is a properly taken history. Especially important is information about the hemostatic response to a prior surgical procedure. Specific questions concerning dental extractions, for example, may suggest the need for further tests. Equally important is a detailed history of drug ingestion. Patients usually volunteer the information if they are taking anticoagulants when interviewed, but perhaps not if they have been taking aspirin or other nonsteroid anti-inflammatory drugs, which have a profound effect in low doses on platelet function. Ideally, these drugs should be withheld for at least 3 days prior to surgery to permit return toward normal of platelet function.[2,7]

The first step in the laboratory analysis of hemostasis is obtaining a blood specimen, which must be done with the same attention to detail as performing the test. Although the use of silicon needles and syringes has been advocated, disposable needles and plastic syringes are satisfactory. The venipuncture should be accurate and atraumatic to avoid introducing tissue fluid. One way to ensure this is to use a two-syringe technique in which the first syringe is discarded after collection of 2 ml, and a second syringe is attached to the indwelling needle to collect the sample. The second syringe size and additives will vary, depending on what tests are to be performed.

An alternate approach to obtaining a blood specimen is the use of indwelling arterial or central venous cannulas. These lines may contain heparin flush solutions, and the frequent contamination of samples with heparin has prompted many laboratories to proscribe samples for coagulation tests being obtained from such lines. This proscription is not necessary if samples are collected with the same attention to detail as is venipuncture collection. Withdrawing an adequate aliquot prior to collecting a sample is particularly important. Withdrawing twice the dead space from the line prior to collecting the sample will eliminate the chance of heparin contamination. Additionally, the use of indwelling catheters around which hemostasis has been secured will obviate the need for venipuncture, which should ideally be avoided in patients with a hemorrhagic diathesis who are already bleeding from previous venipuncture sites.[8]

An increasing number of mechanical devices are available to perform coagulation tests, with the end point being measured by electrical, magnetic, mechanical, or optical means. Whereas all these machines have the advantage of reducing human variability in a given test, they are more expensive except in large-volume laboratories where their use has resulted in more efficient processing of many samples and usually more rapidly available results.

One of the limiting factors on the value of any test is how fast the results will be available. For this reason, tests that can be performed in the operating room appeal to many. Table 11-2 lists the criteria that are desirable for a hemostasis testing device designed for use in the operating room.[9] The recent development of "point-of-care" tests of coagula-

---

TABLE 11-2. Characteristics of the Ideal Device for Testing Hemostasis in the Operating Room

Simple test procedures yield reproducible results
Equipment is compact, inexpensive, and operates quietly
Result is available quickly, even with abnormally prolonged time
Test is performed on whole blood rather than plasma
Test reagents are stable indefinitely
Test must not require prolonged attention away from operator's usual duties
Heparin concentration is linearly related to the test results (for open heart surgery)

Adapted with permission from Ellison N, Jobes DR, Schwartz AJ: Implications of anticoagulant therapy. Int Anesthesiol Clin 20:121, 1982.

tion may decrease the time of availability of test results so that they can influence treatment.[10] No one test or pair of tests is sufficient to make the diagnosis of a bleeding disorder.

Tests of Coagulation Mechanisms

The activated coagulation time, a modification of the whole blood coagulation time in which celite is added to promote maximal activation of Factor XII, is a test of the intrinsic system and the final common pathway. The automated activated coagulation time is widely used to monitor heparin therapy, especially in the operating room.[9] Normal values for the automated variation of the activated coagulation time as provided by the manufacturer are usually in the range of 90–120 seconds.

The partial thromboplastin time (PTT) evaluates the intrinsic system and final common pathway but eliminates the platelet variable by adding cephalin as a substitute for the platelet factor 3. The original test, when modified by the addition of kaolin to produce maximal contact activation, is called the activated PTT (aPTT). Normal values are less than 35 seconds. This test will detect deficiencies of coagulation factors below 25% of normal levels except for Factors VII and XIII.

The prothrombin time (PT), one of the oldest and most commonly performed tests of coagulation today, is used to monitor coumarin anticoagulation. The PT tests the extrinsic system in the same way that the aPTT tests the intrinsic system. Both the PT and aPTT, of course, test the final common pathway. One of the principal determinants of the PT is the strength of the thromboplastin suspension, which may vary greatly. For this reason, the use of control plasma and reporting both values are recommended in lieu of "per cent activity."[11] Prolongation of the PT or aPTT may be due to a coagulation factor deficiency or to a circulating anticoagulant. To differentiate these, the tests are repeated, with equal volumes of control plasma and patient plasma being compared with a 9:1 patient:control plasma. Continued prolongation in the former suggests the presence of an inhibitor, whereas shortening with the latter suggests that a coagulation factor deficiency in the patient is more likely.

The thrombin time bypasses all but the final stage of fibrin formation. Thrombin solution is prepared and diluted until the thrombin time of the controlled oxalated plasma usually falls into the range of 20–35 seconds. By diluting the thrombin suspension, this test can be made even more sensitive. Prolonged thrombin time is due to a fibrinogen level less than 90 mg·dl^{-1}, heparin or heparin-like anticoagulants that inhibit thrombin, or an abnormal fibrinogen. As with the PT, mixture of a patient's plasma with control plasma will confirm or disprove the presence of an anticoagulant.

Tests of Platelet Function

Again, a properly taken history is the first test. Common sites of bleeding due to platelet deficiency are reflected in easy bruising, epistaxis, gingival bleeding, and menorrhagia. Gastrointestinal bleeding and hematuria are less common, and other sites (e.g., joints) are rare.[2]

All platelet tests suffer from the same potential pitfall inherent in handling platelets, which tend to clump, fragment, and adhere to the sides of the collecting implements. To reduce the influence of this inherent platelet characteristic on test results, tissue damage and blood manipulation during collection must be minimized. Because most bleeding attributed to platelet problems is secondary to a reduc-

tion in platelet numbers, a platelet count should be the first test performed. The platelet count is a quantitative test only and does not measure platelet function. Counts can be performed with either light or phase microscopy, but electronic counters offer greater accuracy. Bleeding rarely occurs unless the platelet count decreases to less than 50,000–70,000 mm^3.

The Ivy bleeding time, the most widely accepted clinical test of platelet function, measures both quality and quantity. Inability to control the many variables has made the Duke earlobe method obsolete. These variables include the length and depth of incision, the venous pressure, and patient cooperation. For that matter, in children or uncooperative adults who may not keep their arms still, the Ivy bleeding time may be invalidated. The introduction of a disposable template, which produces an incision of standard depth and width, has also improved the reproducibility of the Ivy bleeding time.[11] A normal bleeding time is 3–8 minutes.

The platelet aggregometer is designed to measure this function spectrophotometrically. The aggregometer has provided much information about the physiology of platelets. Platelet-rich plasma and platelet-poor plasma are prepared from citrated plasma and used to standardize an aggregometer, with platelet-rich plasma representing 0% light transmission and platelet-poor plasma 100% transmission. Aliquots of 0.5 ml platelet-rich plasma are tested with various reagents. The amount of a given reagent required to produce the release reaction is a measure of how sensitive the platelets are.

Clot retraction is another function of platelets that can be grossly measured. When maintained at 37°C, a clot should begin to retract within 2–4 hours. Efforts to quantitate the degree of retraction have not been successful and the test remains a qualitative test, with the presence of any clot retraction being considered positive.

Tests of Fibrinolysis

A clot should not lyse while maintained at 37°C for up to 48 hours. Lysis may occur in less than 1 hour in the presence of fibrinolysis. Care must be taken, however, not to mistake the fragmentation of the weak, friable clot of hypofibrinogenemia for fibrinolysis. A fibrinogen level obviously helps in distinguishing these two possibilities. A confirmatory test of fibrinolysis is performed by mixing a clot from normal plasma with an equal volume of test plasma or serum. If a normal clot lyses within 24 hours in the test plasma, increased fibrinolytic activity is present.

Plasminogen activator, plasminogen, plasmin, and fibrinogen are all euglobulins and can be separated from water-soluble inhibitors by precipitation when diluted with water. Sampling is extremely important in this test because prolonged venostasis (e.g., tourniquet on too long) and trauma (e.g., excessive alcohol rub of the skin) stimulate the release of plasminogen activator. Platelets will prolong the euglobulin lysis time because of their antiplasmin activity; therefore platelet-poor plasma should be used in this test. A normal euglobulin lysis time is longer than 2 hours.

Fibrin(ogen) split products formed from the breakdown of either fibrin or fibrinogen cause coagulase-positive *Staphylococcus aureus* to become adherent to one another and to produce visible clumping in contrast to the smooth suspension usually seen when no clumping has occurred. Serial dilutions of fibrinogen standards and patient serum are prepared and mixed with the bacterial suspension to measure the lowest dilution where clumping is easily visualized as an end point. The comparison to standard fibrinogen dilution end points gives the final answer, which is expressed in $\mu g \cdot ml^{-1}$ fibrinogen equivalents, with values greater than 12 $\mu g \cdot ml^{-1}$ indicating active fibrinolysis.

Routine Evaluation

Again, a properly taken history is the best means of detecting a hemorrhagic diathesis, and together with a complete physical examination is the first and most important step in evaluating the hemostatic status of any patient. In patients who are poor historians or who have acquired a hemostatic defect since their last surgical experience, a history obtained regarding the hemostatic response to prior surgery is of little value. Rappaport has proposed performing screening tests of various levels, depending on the magnitude of the surgery contemplated.[12] Conversely, the concept that preoperative hemostasis tests should not be arbitrarily ordered has been advanced.[13] Nevertheless, a screening coagulation profile on any patient scheduled for major surgery as well as those whose history suggests a hemorrhagic diathesis is recommended. A useful profile includes a PT, aPTT, platelet count, fibrinogen level, and bleeding time. In the operating room, a baseline automated activated coagulation time is usually performed. Although the yield from such a profile may be low, the advantage of not having to include a pre-existing defect in the differential diagnosis of a bleeding disorder that occurs intraoperatively justifies the effort. With a negative history and a normal screening coagulation profile, this is a valid assumption. In addition, baseline values are available for comparison.

Figure 11-2 illustrates why no one test or pair of tests is sufficient to make an accurate diagnosis of a coagulopathy. While the aPTT and PT test both the intrinsic and extrinsic systems as well as the final common pathway, more refined mixing tests using plasma known to be deficient in Factor VIII, for example, are necessary before a definitive diagnosis of hemophilia A can be made. For that reason, a history of excessive bleeding must be given serious consideration and quantitative assays of at least the three hemophilia factors (VIII, IX, and XI) should be performed in such a patient to be certain that there is no pre-existing hemorrhagic diathesis.

Pathology

Congenital Defects

The relative frequency of congenital hemostatic deficiencies varies greatly, with estimates of von Willebrand's disease as high as 1% of the population compared with less than 100 cases of familial afibrinogenemia having been reported. Some of the latter are believed to have represented DIC because they were associated with a low platelet count.[1] The relative frequencies of the three hemophilias are 85% for Factor VIII, 14% for Factor IX, and 1% for Factor XI, with the incidence of classic hemophilia A, Factor VIII deficiency, reported to be as high as 1 per 10,000–25,000 live births. The remainder of the congenital defects are extremely rare.[3]

Factor VIII, for which the kinetics have best been worked out, will be discussed to illustrate the eight variables that determine the dose. *Patient size, initial level of the deficient factor,* and *potency of the preparation* are three obvious determinants. *Hemostatic level* of each factor varies greatly. Table 11-3 lists the coagulation factors and the minimum level (% of normal) of each necessary for surgical hemostasis. Even this is not complete, as evidenced by Table 11-4, which equates the recommended levels of Factor VIII with

surgical procedures. From this it can be seen that during the preoperative and convalescent periods Factor VIII levels should be maintained above 30% at all times. The *magnitude of the operation* influences the treatment mainly with respect to the duration of treatment—24-hour treatment or just one dose may be given in cases of minor dental surgery, whereas sustained levels above 30% are necessary in major orthopedic reconstruction for several weeks. The *half-life* of coagulation factors varies greatly, with Factor VIII levels at 10–12 hours, necessitating treatment at 8–12 hour intervals in contrast to von Willebrand's disease, in which treatment at 3-day intervals may suffice. *Redistribution* occurs out of the vascular space following the administration of all coagulation factors. The administration of any blood component results in a characteristic double exponential decay curve with the early rapid decrease due to redistribution. Again, for Factor VIII the extravascular distribution is twice the intravascular distribution, whereas for Factor VII extravascular distribution it is one half the intravascular distribution. The *metabolic rate* will affect the dose in that an increase of metabolism with a fever, for example, will decrease the half-life of the products.

Deficiencies of hemophilia A and von Willebrand's disease and their treatment are discussed as examples of a complete approach to these patients.

Hemophilia A. Factor VIII deficiency, hemophilia A, is transmitted as a sex-linked recessive trait, but in 25–30% of patients no family history of hemophilia can be obtained. There have been three dramatic breakthroughs in the management of patients with hemophilia.[3] The first was the isolation by Pool in 1964 in 3% of the original plasma volume of 30–60% of the Factor VIII originally present. Prior to this isolation, fresh frozen plasma was the only blood component available to treat hemophilia. This new component, cryoprecipitate, eliminated the volume constraints that previously plagued physicians and patients alike. The second breakthrough was the recognition that patients or their families could treat the patient at home at the first suggestion of a hemorrhage or on a regular schedule, a development that was made possible after the introduction of lyophylized plasma concentrates eliminated the need for storing frozen cryoprecipitate. In particular the management of hemarthrosis and limb hematomas is very effectively managed on a home treatment program. The major advantages of home programs are rapid treatment, which minimizes the crippling effects of hemorrhage, and economy of time and money by avoiding multiple trips to the clinic or hospitalizations and avoiding the need for repeated infusions that early treatment may obviate. Home treatment also effectively eliminated the chain that kept patients with hemophilia in close proximity to their treatment centers.

The third breakthrough was the development of regional hemophilia centers to provide total care. These centers contain hematologists with a special interest in the treatment of hemophilia, general and orthopaedic surgeons who are well versed in the care of these patients, and dentists, oral surgeons, and social workers. The intraoperative care of these patients is also greatly facilitated by anesthesiologists who have a similar special knowledge. Usually these patients, who have lived with this disease all their lives, are extremely knowledgeable and can educate physicians and nurses caring for them. Each program needs a coordinator who serves as the focal point for provision of care. The average patient with hemophilia will receive approximately 40,000–50,000 units of Factor VIII annually at a mean cost of $4000–5000. Today, in most states the financial burden

TABLE 11-3. Minimum Levels of Coagulation Factors and Platelets Necessary for Effective Hemostasis; Distribution and Fate of Clotting Factors After Transfusion Therapy; and Treatment Schedules

	Minimal Level for Surgical Hemostasis (% of normal)	Genetic Pattern in Congenital Deficiencies	In Vivo Half-Life (hours)	Therapeutic Agent	Dose (per kg body weight)	
					Initial	Maintenance
Factors						
I (Fibrinogen)	50–100	Autosomal recessive	72–144	Cryoprecipitate	Ppt from 100 ml	Ppt from 14–20 ml, once daily
II	20–40	Autosomal recessive	72–120	Plasma	10–15 ml	5–10 ml, once daily
V	5–20	Autosomal recessive	12–36	Fresh or frozen plasma	10–15 ml	10 ml, once daily
VII	10–20	Autosomal recessive	4–6	Plasma	5–10 ml	5 ml, once daily
VIII	30	Males affected Females carriers	10–18	Cryoprecipitate	Ppt from 70 ml	Ppt from 35 ml, twice daily
von Willebrand's	30	Autosomal dominant Variable penetrance		Plasma	10 ml	10 ml every 2–3 days
IX	20–25	Males affected Females carriers	18–36	Plasma or II, VII, IX, X concentrate	60 ml Variable	7 ml once daily
X	10–20	Autosomal recessive	24–60	Plasma	15 ml	10 ml, once daily
XI	20–30	Autosomal recessive	40–80	Plasma	10 ml	5 ml, once daily
XII	0	Autosomal recessive	?50–70	Plasma	5 ml	5 ml, once daily
XIII	1–3	Autosomal recessive	?72–120	Plasma	2–3 ml	None
Platelets	50,000–100,000 mm³			Platelet concentrate	1–2 units per desired 10,000 increment in count	

Ppt = precipitate

Adapted with permission from Ellison N: Coagulation evaluation and management. In Ream AK, Fogdall RP (eds): Acute Cardiovascular Management, p 733. Philadelphia, JB Lippincott, 1982.

has been eased greatly through the development of programs supported by the National Hemophilia Foundation or a state agency.

One unit of Factor VIII:C clotting activity is defined as the amount present in 1 ml of fresh normal, pooled plasma.[14] A concentrate of one unit of Factor VIII:C activity per milliliter (i.e., 100 units·dl⁻¹) is expressed as 100%, with the normal range being 60–140%. The practical way to plan treatment is based on the plasma volume, as follows:

$$\text{Initial dose before surgery} = 1\ PV$$

where PV = 1 unit of Factor VIII for each ml of plasma.

TABLE 11-4. Recommended Factor VIII Levels and Duration of Treatment for Certain Operations or Bleeding Conditions

	Factor VIII Level (Unit·ml⁻¹)	Treatment	
		Frequency (hours)	Duration (days)
Hemarthrosis	0.3	every 12	1
Dental (minor)	0.3	every 12	1
Dental (extraction)	0.3	every 8	1–2
All surgery	0.5	every 8	2–10

Maintenance dose = ½PV every 8 hours
    × postoperative day 1
    = ½PV every 12 hours × for 7–10 days
    = ¼PV every 12 hours × for 5–7 days

In theory, Factor VIII requirements could be reduced while maintaining desired levels if the concentrate were given by continuous infusion. Treatment routinely should start 1½ hours before surgery, and adequate plasma factor level goals should be confirmed before surgery. In recent years some patients have been discharged from the hospital to continue home treatment during further convalescence.

As in many disease states, treatment often carries complications. Because of the large number of donors to whom patients are exposed, acute hepatitis and chronic hepatitis have long been recognized as complications of treatment. This is probably true whether the patient receives the cryoprecipitate, where each bag comes from one donor, or the commercial lyophilized products prepared from plasma pools of 10,000 donors. However, some centers treat hemophiliacs who are only mildly deficient in Factor VIII or IX and all children less than 5 years old with cryoprecipitate or fresh frozen plasma in an attempt to decrease the incidence of hepatitis. Donors for commercial concentrates are all checked for hepatitis B surface antigen, but the tests lack sufficient sensitivity to detect 100%. Thus, small amounts of surface antigen can contaminate an entire plasma pool.

For that reason, hepatitis B vaccine should be administered to all patients with hemophilia. The risk of acquired immunodeficiency syndrome (AIDS) transmission is discussed below.

The development of antibodies or inhibitors, which is seen in 7–10% of patients, usually occurs in patients with severe hemophilia. In the case of "nonresponding inhibitors" that do not increase in titer when challenged by infusion of the antigen, merely increasing the level of Factor VIII will suffice to achieve hemostasis. In the case of a "responding inhibitor," the titer will increase 4–6 days after infusion and will remain elevated for months or even years. Attempts to treat these patients with porcine Factor VIII or plasmapheresis have not met with universal success. As improved fractionation has led to Factor IX concentrates that contain less activated factors, higher doses of Factor IX concentrate are required. For that reason, today activated Factor IX concentrates that have Factor VIII inhibitor bypassing activity are used. These products presumably work by bypassing the Factor VIII step in the coagulation cascade. A future alternative therapy may be porcine Factor VIII.

Von Willebrand's Disease. Von Willebrand's disease, a milder bleeding disorder than hemophilia A, is characterized by mucosal rather than visceral bleeding and is unique in that it involves both primary and secondary hemostasis. The disease is inherited either as an autosomal dominant (Types 1 and 2) or, rarely, as an autosomal recessive trait (Type 3). Type 1 involves a quantitative abnormality of Factor VIII:vWF, and Type 2 involves a qualitative abnormality. The former also have low levels of Factor VIII:C, whereas the latter may have normal levels. Type 3 involves markedly defective synthesis of Factor VIII and an autosomal recessive inheritance pattern resulting in a bleeding pattern similar to that seen in severe hemophilia. Recognition that Factor VIII is a complex consisting of two portions, Factor VIII:vWF and Factor VIII:C, has permitted a better understanding of the relationships between these two diseases. Whereas in hemophilia A only Factor VIII:C production is deficient in amount and quality, in von Willebrand's disease there is a decrement in both Factor VIII:C and Factor VIII:vWF. Infusion of Factor VIII concentrate in hemophilia will result in levels that peak at the conclusion of the infusion and demonstrate a half-life of 10–18 hours as they decrease. In contrast, infusion of plasma or cryoprecipitate in von Willebrand's disease produces peak levels of Factor VIII:C 48 hours after the conclusion of the infusion that are sustained for 72 hours. This response has prompted the recommendation to infuse plasma or cryoprecipitate the evening before surgery to permit the delayed response to occur. However, correction of the bleeding time, a manifestation of the primary hemostatic defect, lasts only 2–6 hours. To achieve both the increase in Factor VIII levels and the decrease in bleeding time, treatment with plasma or cryoprecipitate both the evening before and immediately before surgery is recommended. Repeat infusion of cryoprecipitate need be administered only at 24–48 hour intervals because of the sustained response.

In Type 2 von Willebrand's disease, in which Factor VIII:C levels are normal, often only a single treatment given in the immediate preoperative period may be required. Cryoprecipitate is the blood product of choice to be used to treat von Willebrand's disease because Factor VIII concentrate lacks Factor VIII:vWF. Factor VIII concentrates are also not used to raise Factor VIII:C levels because supplemental plasma infusion is still required to provide Factor VIII:vWF. 1-Deamino, 8-d-arginine vasopression (DDAVP) increases Factor VIII:C levels in normal individuals, in patients with hemophilia who are mildly deficient in Factor VIII, and especially in patients with von Willebrand's disease, Type 1. Intravenous administration is more effective than the intranasal route. Although it is not a form of treatment, it should be emphasized that aspirin ingestion by patients with von Willebrand's disease may markedly increase the hemostatic defects.

Acquired Defects

Defects in vascular integrity, deficiencies in coagulation factor levels, and quantitative or qualitative deficiencies in platelets constitute the possible etiologies of acquired defects of hemostasis. Within the framework of that classification, the following causes of defective hemostasis are discussed: (1) anti-coagulants; (2) liver failure; (3) massive transfusion; (4) DIC; and (5) thrombocytopenia.

Anticoagulants. Coumarin-like drugs inhibit production of prothrombin (Factor II) and Factors VII, IX, and X, which together are known as the prothrombin complex or vitamin K–dependent factors, whereas heparin inhibits the action of thrombin (Factor IIa), IXa, Xa, and XIa. Low doses of coumarin inhibit Factor VII, resulting in prolongation of the PT while the aPTT remains normal. Higher doses of coumarin produce depression of prothrombin and Factors VII, IX, and X in addition, resulting in prolongation of both PT and aPTT. Low doses of heparin inhibit Factor IXa initially, resulting in a prolonged aPTT and a normal PT. Higher doses affect thrombin, Factors Xa and XIa, also resulting in a prolongation of both PT and aPTT. The presence of heparin in the patient's blood can be confirmed by adding protamine to the patient's citrated plasma and assessing whether this improves the aPTT. Coumarin can also be measured in the patient's plasma, a technique especially valuable in suspected cases of surreptitious ingestion or "coumarin malingerers."

A rebound hypercoagulable state resulting in exacerbation of the original condition for which the anticoagulant was originally prescribed has been suggested as a theoretical hazard of anticoagulant neutralization. There are no reliable data on which this theory is based and, furthermore, in an emergency situation such gradual tapering is impossible. Cessation of anticoagulant therapy because of hemorrhage carries no greater risk of recurrent embolism than does elective discontinuation, nor does the manner of termination (gradual or abrupt) affect the incidence of thromboembolism.[10]

Although protamine is the only commercial antidote available for neutralizing heparin, protamine requirements remain a confused and controversial area. *In vitro*, protamine will retard clot formation and has been shown to impair platelet aggregation in response to adenosine diphosphate. This may explain the bleeding problem seen following excessive doses of protamine.[15] Recent reports of adverse responses (allergic reactions, pulmonary hypertension) on administration of protamine have alerted clinicians to the possibility of severe and potentially lethal complications.[16]

Bleeding following neutralization of heparin and not due to obvious inadequate surgical hemostasis may be caused by heparin rebound, which is defined as the recurrence of heparin effect in blood following laboratory-demonstrated adequate neutralization with protamine. Heparin rebound has been described as occurring up to 24 hours following heparin neutralization and is most likely to occur in the first 4–6 hours after neutralization. Although the occurrence of heparin rebound is probably a relatively rare event in the usual clinical setting, the diagnosis is easily made by means of an activated coagulation time and a protamine titration, and specific, simple treatment with protamine is readily available.[17]

The two methods available to neutralize coumarin are transfusion of blood or plasma or the administration of vitamin K. Vitamin K is the specific antidote for coumarin but will take at least 3–6 hours to have an effect in patients with normal liver function. Vitamin K, in doses of 2.5–50 mg, should be given orally or parenterally, depending on severity. Response to therapy should be monitored with serial prothrombin times to ensure a satisfactory response. Because the action of coumarin may last 4–5 days, it is advisable to follow the PT daily for that period. In the emergency situation, transfusion is required. Although transfusion produces immediate results, there is no formula available to predict the volume of blood or plasma required because the degree of depression of the patient's coagulation factors for a given PT, and the level of coagulation factors present in each unit of blood or plasma is extremely variable. Because the four vitamin K–dependent factors (II, VII, IX, and X) are all present in banked blood, administration of fresh whole blood or fresh frozen plasma is not necessary. Concentrates of the prothrombin complex are no longer recommended as an antidote for coumarin because as a pooled product, they carry a high risk of hepatitis and also contain thrombogenic material or activated clotting factors that may initiate DIC.

Liver Failure. In advanced cases of liver failure, bleeding may be caused by portal hypertension and mechanical factors such as esophageal varices or thrombocytopenia secondary to hypersplenism, excessive fibrinolysis, or decreased production of clotting factors. Thus, isolated or combined defects in vascular integrity or decreased levels of platelets or coagulation factors are all possible in these patients. The synthesis of clotting factors in the liver decreases in proportion to the loss of liver cells. For this reason the PT is a good prognostic indicator in patients with liver failure. Treatment of bleeding episodes associated with liver failure depends on an accurate diagnosis whenever possible and will vary from vitamin K administration or platelet transfusion to surgical decompression of the portal vein.

Factors I, V, and XI are produced in the liver as well as the four vitamin K–dependent factors (II, VII, IX, and X); therefore, vitamin K alone, even in massive doses, will not correct the deficiency seen in liver failure. Slight improvement following parenteral administration of vitamin K may be seen because of malabsorption of vitamin K owing to lack of bile salts. More often, clinically significant depression of fibrinogen is a feature of advanced liver disease or of increased fibrinolysis and DIC more than the result of decreased synthesis of coagulation factors.

One iatrogenic cause of bleeding owing to decreased production that may be seen in critically ill patients is the intestinal sterilization syndrome. The intestinal flora are a major source of vitamin K in humans. Patients who have their gastrointestinal tracts sterilized with high doses of antibiotic preoperatively lose this source of vitamin K. If they are maintained on intravenous fluids or receive a restricted diet without vitamin K–containing foods, their vitamin K stores will be depleted in approximately 1 week. This syndrome is easily diagnosed on the basis of history, the finding of an isolated prolonged PT, and the prompt response to vitamin K administration.[18]

Massive Transfusion. Ideally, therapy should be designed to treat a pathologic condition without producing another one. The need to correct an acute hypovolemic state with large volumes of blood, however, may produce a hemostatic defect inherent in bank blood. Factor VIII levels decrease by 50% after 2 days, but Factor V levels do not decrease to 50% for over 2 weeks. However, the remaining levels are well above the minimal hemostatic level for Factor V and usually for Factor VIII. Thus, deficiencies of these two factors are rarely a primary cause of bleeding. However, patients who require massive transfusions (defined as "> one blood volume within several hours") may develop diffuse microvascular bleeding, which is not surgically correctable. The hemostatic effectiveness of platelets decays rapidly over 5 days, and repeated studies have defined a dilutional thrombocytopenia as the cause of microvascular bleeding. Ciavarella et al additionally found out that fibrinogen levels <80 mg·dl^{-1} were associated with increased bleeding and advocated the use of whole blood in cases of massive transfusion (as previously discussed).[19,20] Nevertheless, the potential production of a qualitative or quantitative defect in platelets does not justify routine administration of platelets in massive transfusion.[17] It is not clear whether mild deficiencies of Factor V and VIII, which are insufficient to produce bleeding on their own, may possibly aggravate the bleeding seen in patients with thrombocytopenia.

Disseminated Intravascular Coagulation. DIC is a pathologic syndrome in which formation of fibrin thrombi, consumption of Factors V and VIII, loss of platelets, and activation of the fibrinolytic system suggest the presence of thrombin in the systemic circulation. The clinical findings of DIC may vary, with patients manifesting thrombotic, hemorrhagic, or mixed signs and symptoms. Furthermore, some patients with no clinical manifestations may have classic laboratory findings of DIC. Table 11-5 lists the potential causes of DIC.

The hemorrhagic component of the DIC spectrum is readily appreciated and has been characterized as a paradox

TABLE 11-5. Potential Causes of Disseminated Intravascular Coagulation Divided into Three Basic Mechanisms*

1. Cellular damage releasing into the bloodstream phospholipids, which are necessary for both the extrinsic and intrinsic systems of coagulation to function
   Examples: hemolytic transfusion reaction, malaria, trauma, extracorporeal circulation, near drowning
2. Endothelial damage resulting in activation of the intrinsic clotting system through exposure of blood to collagen
   Examples: viremia, heat stroke, meningococcemia, trauma, aortic aneurysm, shock, glomerulonephritis
3. Introduction of tissue factor into the bloodstream resulting in activation of the extrinsic clotting system
   Examples: neoplasms, leukemia, trauma and tissue injury, obstetric defibrination syndromes, extracorporeal circulation, burns, transplant rejection

*The difficulty in dividing cases of DIC into different categories is illustrated by the listing of trauma in all three categories. Trauma can damage cells, injure blood vessels and expose collagen, and introduce tissue factor into the bloodstream.

in that bleeding and thrombosis are occurring simultaneously and are further complicated by another paradox in that one of the recommended forms of treatment of the hemorrhage is the administration of an anticoagulant, heparin. The thrombotic component of the DIC spectrum, although obviously a necessary precursor of the hemorrhagic component, is less readily appreciated.

There is no one pathognomonic laboratory test for DIC. Colman and Robboy have established the following criteria.[21] In the absence of hepatic disease or blood transfusion, they use a screening triad of PT greater than 15 seconds, fibrinogen level less than 160 mg·dl^{-1}, and platelet count less than 150,000 mm^3. Abnormalities of all three indicate DIC. If results of two of these three tests are abnormal, then either the TT time or fibrinogen split products must be abnormal to confirm the laboratory diagnosis of DIC.[20] Although these criteria may sound straightforward, patients have frequently received at least a blood transfusion before the diagnosis is entertained. In that case, a high index of suspicion permits the diagnosis to be made on clinical grounds. Perhaps the *sine qua non* from the laboratory tests to support a diagnosis of DIC is a decrease in the platelet count. As a practical matter in a patient who presents with a typical clinical setting, in whom the platelet count and fibrinogen level are decreased, the diagnosis of DIC can be presumed until proved otherwise.

The differential diagnosis of primary *versus* secondary fibrinolysis must be considered, although the validity of differentiating primary and secondary fibrinolysis is now being questioned.[22] The conversion of plasminogen to plasmin as a defense mechanism (secondary fibrinolysis) to the intravascular deposition of fibrin would destroy fibrin or fibrinogen and Factors V and VIII. Both the consumption of platelets and coagulation factors and the presence of fibrinogen split products, which result from the plasmin degradation of fibrin or fibrinogen and possess anticoagulant properties of their own, will further aggravate the bleeding disorder. If differentiation of primary from secondary fibrinolysis is vital, a normal platelet count most likely suggests primary fibrinolysis. Certain disease states such as cirrhosis or prostatic surgery are also commonly associated with primary fibrinolysis.

DIC is never a primary disease state, nor will every patient who receives, for example, an incompatible blood transfusion develop DIC because of the natural defense mechanisms that facilitate elimination of thrombin within the vascular tree. Thus, in most cases of incompatible blood transfusion for example, the combination of rapid blood flow–dilution, hepatic–reticuloendothelial system clearance, and naturally occurring inhibitors will prevent DIC; however, in cases of stagnant blood flow such as shock, hepatic–reticuloendothelial system impairment such as hypoxemia, or when the insult is so overwhelming such as massive transfusion of ABO incompatible blood, DIC may develop.

The initial treatment of DIC is not heparin. The first goal of treatment should be correction of the primary disorder. This may be all that is necessary and DIC will be self-limited. In some patients with primary disorders such as septic shock or neoplasia, however, correction of the primary disorder may not be readily accomplished. Heparin therapy in these patients is designed to stop clot formation and thus to inhibit the continued consumption of coagulation factors and platelets so that they can reach normal levels. Heparin doses of 40–80 units·kg^{-1} are administered every 4–6 hours, the object being to prolong the whole blood coagulation time to two to three times normal. Ideally, this should produce sufficient anticoagulation to prevent clot formation but not produce bleeding. Monitoring heparin therapy with a whole blood coagulation time is recommended instead of the aPTT because the latter is more sensitive to depleted coagulation factors and the anticoagulant effects of fibrinogen split products and cannot distinguish between them and the effect of heparin.[21]

Heparin therapy is by no means universally accepted in the treatment of DIC, and the decision to employ heparin is not to be taken lightly. There is some disagreement that at best heparin therapy merely replaces one cause of bleeding with another and that theoretical grounds are not sufficient to justify the use of such a dangerous drug. We have been extremely reluctant to use heparin therapy in surgical patients, especially in patients with severe fibrinogenemia (less than 50 mg·dl^{-1}), an accompanying vasculitis, or local defect in vasculature.[1]

The most recent addition to the therapeutic regimen for DIC is cryoprecipitate. Although this blood product was originally developed for the treatment of hemophilia, a unit of cryoprecipitate contains one third of the fibrinogen in the plasma from which it is derived. There is less risk of hepatitis with cryoprecipitate than with fibrinogen, which is a pooled product that contains no Factor VIII. The use of cryoprecipitate will therefore increase levels of fibrinogen and Factor VIII, both of which are depressed in DIC. Fresh frozen plasma and platelet concentrates also may be required to treat other deficiencies.

Thrombocytopenia. Thrombocytopenia can occur in massive transfusion, liver failure, or DIC. Thrombocytopenia may also develop independently of these conditions because of decreased production, as in cases of aplastic anemia or in oncologic patients who are receiving chemotherapy or owing to increased destruction as in idiopathic thrombocytopenic purpura, which could well be called "immune" thrombocytopenic purpura.

The recommended cut-off below which elective surgery should not be performed in patients with thrombocytopenia ranges from 50,000–100,000 per mm^3.[23] Furthermore, if the bleeding time is less than twice the upper limit of normal and the platelet count is greater than 50,000 per mm^3, some authorities recommend surgery without prophylactic transfusion. This recommendation is based in part on the fact that bleeding due to thrombocytopenia is not rapid. When blood loss is rapid in the patient with thrombocytopenia, a significant bleeding lesion should be sought, and the repair of such a lesion requires more attention than increasing the platelet count. In fact, since transfused platelets would just be lost during the period of rapid blood loss, transfusion should always be delayed until a modicum of surgical hemostasis has been achieved.

HEMOTHERAPY

In the United States anesthesiologists administer over 50% of all blood products to patients, making this their most common non–pain-relieving therapeutic maneuver. Unfortunately, surveys suggest that many of these products are administered on the basis of protocol or habit.[23] As indications for transfusion become better defined, protocol-based therapy will become less common.[24]

Red Blood Cell *Versus* Whole Blood Administration

To increase oxygen-carrying capacity, red blood cells (RBCs) only are required. Ideally, therefore, only RBCs, formally referred to as "packed red blood cells," or PRBCs should be administered. Certainly that is the case in treating anemia, in which the administration of RBCs produces almost a twofold greater increase in the hemoglobin level than a similar volume of whole blood. In the surgical patient, however, especially one who is bleeding massively and losing plasma as well as RBCs, the use of whole blood seems logical.

The pressing need to provide Factor VIII concentrate to treat patients with hemophilia and platelet concentrates to treat oncology patients has led many blood banks to fractionate increasing amounts of blood. Mollison has questioned whether the current practice of fractionating approximately 80% of units will leave sufficient units of whole blood to satisfy the need in cases of massive transfusion.[25] Schmidt has outlined his practice as follows: preoperative orders to cross-match four or more units of blood are filled with whole blood; for three or fewer units, RBCs are prepared and supplemented as necessary by crystalloid solutions.[26] More recently it has been recommended that patients who lose more than 25% of their blood volume and are continuing to bleed should receive whole blood.[27]

What are the objections to using RBCs in surgical patients? Slow flow rate, inadequate volume replacement, and deficiency of coagulation factors are frequently mentioned. The major objection seems to be that because of the increased viscosity, the RBCs flow more slowly, especially through a microfilter. This objection can easily be overcome, however, by reconstitution with saline. In cases where rapid replacement of blood loss is required, some form of pressurized system is usually employed, and this will also markedly improve flow rate. The issue of volume replacement is also answered by reconstitution. The third major objection to the use of RBCs is that the level of plasma coagulation factors and platelets may decrease to the point that a hemorrhagic diathesis is produced, further complicating the bleeding. Because blood stored over 24 hours contains few viable platelets, the need for platelet concentrates to treat dilutional thrombocytopenia is not lessened by using whole blood in lieu of RBCs unless fresh whole blood is used. Logistically, a requirement for fresh whole blood cannot be met by most blood banks. Fresh frozen plasma may be required to correct a coagulation factor deficiency.

Fresh Frozen Plasma

In cases of liver failure, the administration of fresh frozen plasma, which contains all the clotting factors generally produced by the liver and is often prescribed in massive doses, has recently been questioned. The dramatic increase in the use of fresh frozen plasma in the United States may represent its use as a volume replacement solution, although it is not specifically required for this purpose.[28] Indeed, the role of fresh frozen plasma in the management of coagulopathy in patients receiving large volumes of stored blood is not well defined despite its widespread advocacy in these situations. A 1984 National Institutes of Health Consensus Development Conference reached the same conclusions.[29] Two large-scale prospective studies of massively transfused patients have failed to indicate that either the PT or the aPTT possess sufficient specificity to justify fresh frozen plasma administration. Therefore, rigid use of the outlined screening tests to determine when fresh frozen plasma is to be administered cannot be recommended. Again, laboratory tests must be correlated with the clinical picture to guide appropriate therapy. Roy *et al* demonstrated the futility of administration of fresh frozen plasma in nonbleeding patients on a prophylactic basis after a case of noncardiogenic pulmonary edema prompted an abrupt change in their use of fresh frozen plasma.[30] Similarly, the value of any pre-established fresh frozen plasma regimen (e.g., 1 unit fresh frozen plasma for every 3–6 units of RBCs) has not been proved effective. In summary, although fresh frozen plasma may be the most widely overprescribed blood product, the guidelines for the use of fresh frozen plasma based on current literature are necessarily vague. In view of the potential hazards of infection and severe pulmonary complications, the use of this product should be minimized.

Platelets

For the surgical patient who has not previously received platelet transfusions, administration of ABO-nonidentical platelets is acceptable. If the patient has received platelets previously and the desired increase in platelet count and decrease in bleeding time are not achieved with a platelet transfusion, alloimmunization to HLA antigens may be responsible. If HLA-matched platelets produce the desired results, this can definitely be assumed to be the case. In women of child-bearing potential who are Rh-negative, platelets from Rh-positive donors should be avoided whenever possible. Alternatively, Rh-immune globulin should be administered after the transfusion to reduce the risk of Rh sensitization.

One unit contains 5.5×10^{11} platelets and 1 unit·10 kg^{-1} should raise the platelet count to effective hemostatic levels.[23] Platelets should be administered as rapidly as the patient's cardiovascular system will permit because the peak post-transfusion increment determines the hemostatic effectiveness of the transfusion. Slow infusions of platelets are inappropriate. In the past decade the American Red Cross has increased its annual platelet processing almost tenfold. Much of this increase can be attributed to the demonstrable effectiveness of such transfusions in patients who are receiving chemotherapy for hematologic malignancy. More recently there has been an increased use of platelets in patients who are having open heart surgery. Studies to document the effectiveness of platelet transfusion in these patients are lacking.[31] What documentation should be sought? Ideally an increase in the platelet count at 1 hour and 24 hours and a decrease in the bleeding time should be documented. However, these measures are frequently not practical to obtain during the intraoperative period. Patients should receive platelet therapy only if they have excessive bleeding as a result of thrombocytopenia or thrombocytopathia.

Complications of Hemotherapy

Table 11-6 lists the potential complications of transfusion. The most severe complication of blood transfusion is an acute hemolytic transfusion reaction, something that can be avoided with a properly performed cross-match and meticulous clerical attention to detail to ensure that the correct

TABLE 11-6. Potential Side-Effects and/or Hazards of the Administration of Blood or Blood Components

1. Hemolytic transfusion reaction, immediate or delayed
2. Disease transmission
     Viral hepatitis
     Cytomegalovirus
     Other infections
3. Recipient alloimmunization
4. Graft vs host disease
5. Febrile reactions
6. Allergic reactions
     Angioedematous
     Anaphylactoid
7. Circulatory overload reactions
8. Bacterial contamination
9. Iron overload
10. Depletion of procoagulants and platelets
11. Microaggregates
12. Metabolic complications
     Hypothermia
     Citrate toxicity
     Acidosis
     Hypo-/or hyperkalemia

Reproduced with permission from Ellison N, Faust RJ: Complications of blood transfusions. In Benumof JL, Saidman LJ (eds): Anesthesia and Perioperative Complications. St. Louis, Mosby-Year Book, 1991.

unit of blood is administered to the correct patient. In addition, the chances of an acute hemolytic transfusion reaction are extremely small if ABO- and Rh-type specific blood is administered. Fever, nausea, shaking chills, and flank pain may herald the onset of an acute hemolytic transfusion reaction in the awake patient. Recognition of an acute hemolytic transfusion reaction in an anesthetized patient may be difficult. The onset of red urine due to free plasma hemoglobin in a patient whose bladder is catheterized or because of uncontrollable bleeding caused by DIC may be the first sign. Support of blood pressure as necessary to maintain renal blood flow and fluid and diuretic therapy to maintain urine flow are the mainstays of treatment. If renal shut-down occurs, hemodialysis may be necessary.

Other potential causes of acute hemolysis during transfusion include faulty blood warmers, concurrent infusion of nonisotonic solutions with osmotic lysis of RBCs, infusion under pressure (especially through a small needle), unrecognized paroxysmal nocturnal hemoglobinuria, glucose-6-phosphate dehydrogenase deficiency, sepsis, or the infusion of contaminated blood.[32]

Febrile reactions, the most common type of reaction, are defined as a temperature elevation of more than 1°C occurring in association with a transfusion, and they can be effectively prevented by the use of white blood cell–poor saline washed blood, RBCs, or microaggregate filtration. Although febrile reactions are relatively benign, differentiating them from an acute hemolytic transfusion reaction or sepsis at the time of presentation is a reason for stopping the transfusion.

Allergic reactions are the second most common reaction to blood transfusion and are usually easily treated with an antihistamine. Under general anesthesia, the appearance of hives in a patient receiving blood transfusion may be the only manifestation. Rarely, after the infusion of a few milliliters of blood, patients may develop respiratory distress, cyanosis, and shock. This usually occurs in IgA-deficient patients who have developed IgA antibodies. In addition to

discontinuing the transfusion, treatment with epinephrine is required.

Delayed hemolytic transfusion reactions occur in patients who have a compatible cross-match, but over a 4–21 day period the transfused RBCs are destroyed. The reactions are usually subclinical and only diagnosed when a positive Coombs' test and an antibody not present on a previous cross-match is subsequently detected.

Infection caused by viruses, bacteria, or spirochetes may be transmitted *via* blood transfusion. Hepatitis and AIDS are the two most feared diseases of this type. Hepatitis transfusion has been markedly decreased by the elimination of paid blood donors and the perfection of third-generation testing for hepatitis B surface antigen. However, estimates of hepatitis B infection are as high as 1:300 despite the availability of a screening test since 1971. Presumably these units are obtained from donors in the "window period" between infection and the development of serologic markers. Indeed, hepatitis B was the fourth most common cause of blood transfusion-associated death (26 of 355) in the decade of 1976–1985.[33]

Transmission of AIDS is the most feared complication, and although that fear has developed a healthy conservative approach to blood transfusion, the hysteria that has accompanied the recognition of transfusion-associated AIDS is regrettable. Recipients of blood products constitute 2% of AIDS cases.[34] Since the human immunodeficiency virus (HIV) is heat-sensitive, lyophilized concentrates of Factors VIII and IX can now be prepared using techniques that greatly decrease AIDS transmission. The development of tests for HIV antibody are another positive development. Unfortunately there is a "window" between infection and seropositivity that makes the test less than perfect.

The immunosuppressive nature of blood transfusion in decreasing renal homograft rejection has been well accepted since 1973; this is a beneficial effect.[34] More recently, early recurrence and poor prognosis in several forms of malignancy and increased risk of bacterial infection have been correlated with perioperative transfusion.[35] The logical suggestion that the need for blood suggested a more advanced cancer has been refuted by several studies involving colorectal, kidney, lung, and prostate cancer. This is more marked following whole blood transfusion than administration of RBCs, suggesting that a component of plasma is responsible for the changes that are clearly harmful.[32]

BLOOD SUBSTITUTES

Autologous blood is technically not a substitute for blood, but when blood is needed, predeposited autologous blood is absolutely the best substitute for homologous blood. Units may be collected weeks, or if frozen, months in advance for elective surgical procedures. Unfortunately, although the practice of predeposit autologous blood is increasing rapidly in the United States, much greater use is still possible. Fear of transfusion-associated AIDS (see further on) undoubtedly explains this increase and will be the major stimulus for a further increase.[36] Alternatively, acute isovolemic hemodilution and collection of 1–2 units of blood immediately before surgery can provide fresh whole blood for use toward the end of the operation. Intraoperative scavenging, washing, and subsequent infusion of blood collected intraoperatively is a third method of autologous blood transfusion.

Use of type-and-screen permits more efficient utilization of stored blood and is cost-effective. Type-and-screen denotes that the patient's blood that has been typed for A, B, and Rh antigens and screened for antibodies. A type-and-cross-match, in contrast to a type-and-screen, indicates that an homologous blood unit has been reserved for the patient and is unavailable to other patients, resulting in the possible loss of storage time if that blood is not used. Type-and-screen is used when the scheduled surgical procedure is unlikely to require transfusion of blood but is one for which blood should be available.

Crystalloid infusion to maintain normovolemia in a patient who is losing blood is a standard practice, and usually 2–4 ml of crystalloid must be infused for each milliliter of blood loss because of crystalloid's extravascular distribution. Crystalloid is administered until a predetermined hemoglobin level is achieved. Although a minimum hemoglobin level of 10 g·dl^{-1} was formerly used, there is now no uniform level.[37] The level is not the same for all patients or for all procedures.

Colloid may be used in lieu of crystalloid to replace blood loss and has the advantage that it may be used in a 1:1 ratio but has the disadvantage of being more expensive. In addition, some of these products contain vasoactive substances that may produce hypotension.[38] Plasma protein fraction and 5% and 25% albumin are blood products that have been heated to 60°C for 10 hours, which removes the risk of disease transmission. Hydroxyethyl starch and dextran are other colloids that stay largely within the vascular compartment.

A long-standing controversy in fluid management is the need for colloid administration. Does colloid administration increase survival or decrease morbidity in surgical patients? The number of studies on this subject is impressive, and the preponderance of evidence suggests that if sufficient crystalloid is administered, there are no important differences in the two groups. In particular, lung water accumulation and pulmonary edema are usually not increased when crystalloid is used. In cases of hypoproteinemia in which the body stores of protein are depleted, there may be a greater need for colloid administration.[39]

Artificial blood development would be a tremendous breakthrough. The current precarious balance between supply and demand would be obviated and the complications associated with homologous blood products avoided. Unfortunately, the current perfluro compound under limited investigation, Fluosol-DA, is not likely to gain widespread acceptance clinically because of its limited oxygen-carrying capacity. However, a genetically engineered hemoglobin is likely to be available soon.

SUMMARY

Effective hemostasis in the perioperative period rests on a triad of vascular integrity, platelets, and coagulation factors. A working knowledge of the normal hemostatic process, of the tests for hemostasis, and of the available blood products for treating deficiencies is essential. A high index of suspicion will permit the development of a hemostatic defect to be detected early and treatment to be started promptly. In this way, the effects of hemostatic defects will be minimized and outcome improved. In appropriate cases, the administration of blood, especially large volumes of blood, can be life-saving. Alternatively, injudicious administration of blood wastes a precious national resource and can even have fatal consequences. Intelligent individualization is necessary for each unit of blood or blood product administered to each patient.[40]

REFERENCES

1. Ellison N: Diagnosis and management of bleeding disorders. Anesthesiology 47:171, 1977
2. George JN, Shattil SJ: The clinical importance of acquired abnormalities of platelet function. N Engl J Med 234:27, 1991
3. Ellison N, Silberstein LE: Hemostasis in the perioperative period. In Stoelting RK, Barash PG, Gallagher TJ (eds): Advances in Anesthesia, vol. 3, p 67. Chicago, Year Book Medical Publishers, 1986
4. McFarlane RG: Symposium No. 27. Zoological Society of London. The Hemostatic Mechanism in Man and Other Animals. London, Academic Press, 1970
5. Ware AJ: Desmopression acetate in hemorrhagic conditions. In Ellison N, Jobes DR (eds): Effective Hemostasis in Cardiac Surgery, Orlando, Grune & Stratton (in press)
6. Bedford RF, Wollman H: Complications of percutaneous radial artery cannulation. Anesthesiology 38:228, 1973
7. Halonen P, Linko K, Wirtavuori K et al: Evaluation of risk factors in intraoperative bleeding tendency. Ann Chir Gynaecol 76:298, 1987
8. Palermo LM, Andrews RA, Ellison N: Avoidance of heparin contamination in coagulation studies drawn from indwelling lines. Anesth Analg 59:222, 1980
9. Jobes DR, Schwartz AJ, Ellison N et al: Monitoring heparin anti-coagulation and its neutralization. Ann Thorac Surg 31:161, 1981
10. Despotis GJ, Poler SM, Heerdt DM, Lappis DG: Evaluation of a portable coagulation monitor in cardiac surgical patients. Anesthesiology 73:A-502, 1990
11. Ellison N, Jobes DR, Schwartz AJ: Implications of anticoagulant therapy. Int Anesthesiol Clin 20:121, 1982
12. Rappaport SI: Preoperative hemostatic evaluation: Which tests, if any? Blood 61:229, 1983
13. Barber A, Green D, Galluzzo T et al: The bleeding time as a preoperative screening test. Am J Med 78:761, 1985
14. Pisciotto PT (ed): Blood Transfusion Therapy, A Physician's Handbook, 3rd ed. Arlington, Virginia, AABB, 1989
15. Ellison N, Edmunds LH Jr, Colman RW: Platelet aggregation following heparin and protamine administration. Anesthesiology 48:65, 1978
16. Morel DR, Zapol WM, Thomas SJ et al: C$_5$A and thromboxane generation associated with pulmonary vaso- and broncho-constriction during protamine reversal of heparin. Anesthesiology 66:597, 1987
17. Jobes DR, Ellison N: Effective hemostasis in the cardiac surgical patient: Current status. In Ellison N, Jobes DR (eds): Effective Hemostasis in Cardiac Surgery, pp 195–202. Philadelphia, W.B. Saunders, 1988
18. Alperin JB: Coagulopathy caused by vitamin K deficiency in critically ill, hospitalized patients. JAMA 258:1916, 1987
19. Ciavarella D, Reed DL, Counts RB et al: Clotting factor levels and the risk of diffuse microvascular bleeding in the massively transfused patient. Br J Haematol 67:365, 1987
20. Murray DJ, Olson J, Strauss R, Tinker JH: Coagulation changes during packed red blood cell replacement of major blood loss. Anesthesiology 69:839, 1988
21. Colman RW, Robboy SS: Postoperative disseminated intravascular coagulation. Urol Clin North Am 3:107, 1974
22. Marengo-Rowe AJ: Experts opine. Survey of Anesthesiology 37:377, 1986
23. Stehling LC, Ellison N, Faust RJ et al: A survey of transfusion practices among anesthesiologists. Vox Sang 52:60, 1987
24. Myhre EA: To treat the patient or to treat the surgeon? JAMA 265:97, 1991
25. Mollison PL: Summary of reports presented at the XVI Congress of the International Society of Blood Transfusion. Vox Sang 40:289, 1981
26. Schmidt PJ: Whole blood transfusion. Transfusion 24:368, 1984
27. Grindon AJ, Tomasulo PS, Bergin JJ et al: The hospital transfusion committee: Guidelines for improving practice. JAMA 253:540, 1985
28. Braunstein AH, Oberman HA: Transfusion of plasma components. Transfusion 24:281, 1984

29. Consensus Development Conference: Fresh frozen plasma. JAMA 253:551, 1985
30. Roy R, Stafford MA, Hudspeth AS, Meredith JW: Failure of prophylaxis with fresh frozen plasma after cardiopulmonary bypass. Anesthesiology 69:254, 1988
31. Consensus Development Conference: Platelet transfusion therapy. JAMA 257:1777, 1987
32. Ellison N, Faust RJ: Complications of blood transfusions. In Benumof JL, Saidman LJ (eds): Anesthesia and Perioperative Complications, pp 507–519. St. Louis, Mosby-Year Book, 1991
33. Sazama K: Report of three hundred fifty-five transfusion-associated deaths: 1976–1985. Transfusion 30:583, 1990
34. Alexander JW: Transfusion-induced immunomodulation and infection. Transfusion 31:195, 1991
35. Schriemer PA, Longnecker DE, Mintz PD: The possible immunosuppressive effects of blood transfusion in cancer patients. Anesthesiology 68:422, 1988
36. Toy PTCY, Strauss RG, Stehling LC et al: Predeposited autologous blood for elective surgery: A national multi-center study. N Engl J Med 360:517, 1987
37. Consensus Development Conference: Perioperative red cell transfusion. JAMA 260:2700, 1988
38. Ellison N, Behar M, MacVaugh HA III et al: Bradykinin, plasma protein fraction, and hypotension. Ann Thorac Surg 29:15, 1980
39. Rackow EC, Weil MH, MacNeil AR et al: Effects of crystalloid and colloid fluids on extravascular lung water in hypoproteinemic dogs. J Appl Physiol 62:2421, 1987
40. Ellison N, Silberstein LE: A commentary on three consensus development conferences on transfusion medicine. Anesth Clin North Am 8:609, 1990

12

B. Skeie   J. Askanazi

T. Manner   H. Khambatta

Parenteral Nutrition

Nutritional and electrolyte disturbances in surgical and intensive care patients correlate with increased morbidity and mortality rates. Recent advances in understanding these disturbances coupled with the introduction of new nutrient regimens and refinements in delivery methods have resulted in the development of nutritional and metabolic support as a major form of therapy. The goals for treatment include maintaining body tissue stores, prevention and correction for specific deficiencies, and use of synthetic nutrients to optimize organ function. Currently, a new generation of synthetic nutrients is available as solutions with modified amino acid composition (high branched-chain amino acids), altered fatty acid profile (medium-chain triglycerides, polyunsaturated fatty acids), and small molecular weight substrates such as ketones and ketoacids. These nutrient mixtures may lead to more specific metabolic support for specific diseases in the coming years.

The basic knowledge of the changes in body composition and metabolism in response to malnutrition, surgical stress, and injury, is important for the understanding and proper treatment of nutritional and electrolyte disturbances in surgical and intensive care patients and is therefore outlined first (see Chapter 9).

BODY COMPOSITION

Definitions

The body is composed of fat and lean body mass (LBM). The latter is subdivided into extracellular fluid, body cell mass (BCM), and extracellular supportive structures such as skeleton, cartilage, and tendons. The sum of the LBM and adipose tissue is equal to total body weight (TBW).

The fat functions as the energy storage area. It is a relatively anhydrous mass, with water representing only about 20% by weight, whereas in skeletal muscle total water content is 80% by weight. If total caloric intake and energy expenditure are equal, there is no reduction or gain of fat mass. Since fat provides 9.5 cal·g^{-1} and fat tissue is only 20% water, this is a very compact storage area. Metabolic use of fat results in only one eighth the amount of weight loss as compared with skeletal muscle, i.e., 2000 calories of fat or protein would be equal to the loss of 275 g of adipose tissue or 2500 g of skeletal muscle.

Extracellular mass consists of plasma, interstitial water, transcellular water (cerebrospinal fluid, pericardial fluid, and the fluid that is in the joint spaces), and the supporting structures such as skeleton, tendons, and cartilage.

BCM is the metabolically active portion of the LBM. It consists of skeletal muscle (60%), viscera (30%), and the cells of the supporting structure of the extracellular mass such as red blood cells and the cellular component of adipose tissue.

The standard 70-kg man contains 20 kg of fat and 50 kg of LBM that is equally divided by weight as extracellular fluid and BCM. These parameters vary with sex, body build, and age. Women tend to have decreased LBM and increased adipose tissue. The ratio of LBM to TBW also decreases with age. Very muscular individuals have a LBM:TBW ratio that is greater than normal.

These relationships remain constant as long as caloric intake equals expenditures. With excess caloric intake, there is an increase in the adipose tissue unless a vigorous exercise program is undertaken, in which circumstances an increase in skeletal muscle mass occurs if adequate protein is supplied. Excess energy is stored as fat; there are no storage deposits of protein, and glycogen can only be stored in limited amounts (900 kcal on average).

Body Composition Measurements

There are two major approaches to measuring body composition: (1) balance measurements, which only measure changes in amount of body constituents; and (2) direct body composition measurements, which measure the total amount of any constituent.[1]

Measurements of balance have been used mostly for nitrogen, sodium, potassium, calcium, phosphorus, energy, fat, and carbohydrate. Use of a defined enteral or parenteral diet greatly simplifies the problems of analysis of individual foods for nitrogen. Output of each constituent must be determined in urine, stool, vomitus, and all drainages. The common practice of measuring 24-hour urinary urea nitrogen level and adding a constant for other losses is sometimes useful for clinical evaluation of patients but is inadequate for research purposes.[2] Total nitrogen and all other elements under study, such as sodium, potassium, and phosphorus, should be analyzed in all samples.

Early methods used to perform direct measurement of body composition include underwater weighing to determine density and thereby estimate the LBM:fat ratio, and indicator dilution methods to compartmentalize the various water compartments. The latter methods use an indicator compound not normally present in the body that penetrates a known body water compartment. By dividing the amount administered by the concentration in plasma, the volume or space distribution of the indicator can be determined. The dye, T-1825, which binds to albumin, was introduced to measure plasma volume; sodium thiocyanate has been used to measure extracellular space; and antipyrine is used for TBW. The introduction of a variety of radioisotopes after World War II greatly extended the use of the indicator dilution method; plasma volume of the extracellular mass can now be measured by radioactive albumin; red blood cell mass can be measured by using radioactive chromium-tagged red blood cells; tritium can be used to measure total body water; and radioactive bromine can be used to measure the total extracellular water. Recently, potentially useful methods have been introduced; these include neutron activation analysis, which provides simultaneous measurements of whole body calcium, chloride, sodium, potassium, phosphorus, and nitrogen; and electrical conductance, which gives an estimation of the ratio of fat-free mass and LBM.[3]

Most of the methods for measuring changes in body composition are not available in the usual clinical setting. The clinical evaluation, based on history taking and physical examination, is probably almost as effective as objective measurement for body composition. Of particular importance are indications of weight loss, edema, anorexia, vomiting, diarrhea, and decreased food intake. Frequent measurements of body weight are probably the most important nutritional parameter clinically available. Large day-to-day changes in weight usually represent changes in the extracellular fluid, whereas long-term changes represent changes in BCM as well as fat. Additional useful clinical measurements are 24-hour values for urinary excretion of sodium, potassium, urea, and creatinine. These, together with accurate estimates of intake, can be used to calculate daily balance and serve as an approximation of the changes in extracellular fluid (sodium) and BCM (potassium and nitrogen). In addition, daily urine creatinine output permits calculation of the creatinine height index, which serves as an index of prior loss of BCM.[4]

Body Composition Changes in Acute Illness

Starvation

Complete starvation in the unstressed patient results in a loss of fat and LBM. With partial starvation the amount and proportion of the two compartments lost depend on both the amount and the composition of nutrients ingested. The rates of loss differ greatly for the three components of LBM: extracellular fluid, BCM, and extracellular structural components.

With nutrient intakes that are just below energy expenditure, losses of LBM and fat occur approximately in the proportion of 0.5:1.[5] During complete starvation, the ratio approximates 2.6:1 (Table 12-1).[6] Further, the composition of weight loss changes with duration even on a fixed nutrient intake. In the first few days, water losses are high when compared with fat and protein losses, and include the loss of water associated with glycogen depletion and a preferen-

TABLE 12-1. Tissue Composition of Weight Loss in Different Conditions

Condition	BCM (kg) Fat (kg)	Reference
Normal subjects		
Marginal intake	0.35–0.51	Calloway[5]
Fasting	2.6	
Postoperative		
Men	2.6	Kinney et al[6]
Women	1.7	Kinney et al[6]
Major injury	4.5	Kinney et al[6]

BCM = body cell mass.

Reprinted with permission from Insel J, Elwyn DH: Body composition. In Askanazi J, Starker PM, Weissman C (eds): Fluid and Electrolyte Management in Critical Care, p 1. Boston, Butterworths 1986.

tial loss of extracellular fluid.[7] This occurs because initially there is a diuresis and natriuresis secondary to an anti-antidiuretic hormone and antialdosterone effect because of the increased glucagon levels. However, the rate of water loss declines rapidly with time. The rate of fat loss declines less rapidly than that for protein, indicating conservation of LBM and a relative expansion of extracellular fluid with respect to BCM.[8] Although weight loss is more rapid during fasting than with balanced hypocaloric diets, the pattern of compartmental changes is very similar. As starvation progresses, adipose tissue and BCM continue to erode and extracellular fluid continues to increase relative to BCM. For example, a measured weight loss of 16% was associated with reductions in adipose tissue and BCM of 37% and 40%, respectively.[9] For this reason it is obvious that body weight does not adequately reflect the extent of BCM loss during malnutrition.

The relative expansion of extracellular fluid and blood volume that is seen during uncomplicated starvation or fasting is not due to renal failure or to decreases in plasma total protein or albumin levels, which are maintained at relatively normal levels during starvation and balanced hypocaloric diets. The relative extracellular fluid expansion stems from the failure of the extracellular fluid to contract during weight loss.[1] It has been hypothesized[8] that because there is no decrease in the size of the blood vessels in parallel with BCM during nutritional depletion, there should be no decrease in blood volume. If the processes that regulate the volume of the extravascular extracellular fluid in relation to blood volume continue to operate normally, these two compartments will remain at the usual size despite shrinkage of BCM and fat. If starvation is complicated by infection, hypoproteinemia, kidney failure, or other conditions, additional factors contribute independently to the relative and absolute expansion of extracellular fluid.

Effects of Carbohydrate Administration

When carbohydrate is administered alone in the complete absence of protein, there is an absolute and relative increase in the extracellular fluid. Kwashiorkor, a form of malnutrition, results from intake of little or no protein, with fairly adequate caloric levels derived mainly from carbohydrate. In this condition there is a marked expansion of extracellular fluid with pitting edema, ascites, and anasarca. One week of carbohydrate feeding can produce the fully developed kwashiorkor syndrome in an already undernourished child.[10]

In hospitalized patients it is routine to administer 2 liters of 5% dextrose as nutritional support. This regimen provides only 100 g·day^{-1} of glucose and results in a kwashiorkor-like syndrome if used for prolonged duration. Ingestion of 100 g·day^{-1} of glucose has been reported to result in marked retention of sodium when given to volunteers during a 6-day fasting period.[11] There was little effect on potassium losses; i.e., carbohydrate administration exacerbates the increased extracellular fluid/BMC that occurs during starvation. Combined glucose (100 g) and sodium chloride (4.5 g) ingestion (equivalent to 2 liters of 5% dextrose, 0.45 normal saline solution) has been found to completely abolish the sodium loss, whereas potassium loss exceeds that of a complete fast. Thus the use of 5% dextrose in saline results in a greater extracellular fluid/BCM ratio than total starvation.

Carbohydrate can increase the extracellular fluid when given in great excess even if protein is present. Volunteers receiving normal diets with an excess of carbohydrate equal to 1500 kcal·day^{-1} above energy requirements had an average weight gain in 7 days of 5.1 kg, much of which must be an expanded extracellular fluid.[12] Increased plasma glucose levels necessitate an increased extracellular fluid volume if isotonicity is to be maintained. Carbohydrate may also inhibit glucocorticoid production and thereby potentiate the effect of antidiuretic hormone on water and sodium retention.

Effects of Injury and Sepsis

At any given nutrient intake, injury increases the rate of loss of LBM; after elective operations weight loss occurs in the ratio of LBM:fat of 2:1. With severe injury the ratio rises to 4:1 (see Table 12-1).[7] Both surgical and accidental trauma have been shown to cause acute increases in the extracellular fluid compartment (third space).[13] These increases in extracellular fluid are grossly proportional to the degree of tissue injury and often necessitate the intravenous administration of large quantities of fluids during resuscitation and the perioperative period. Such fluids are not retained when administered to normal subjects but are retained when given to stressed patients. Several days following the injury, there is usually a diuresis of both sodium and water and the excess extracellular fluid is lost. This sudden drive of sometimes considerable fluid loads into the circulation may become hazardous if the patient's cardiac capacity is impaired. Failure to diurese suggests an underlying complication such as sepsis.

After initial resuscitation following injury, sepsis has been shown to be associated with a further increase in extracellular fluid volume and a decrease in serum sodium concentration. Several authors have reported that patients with sepsis are generally hyponatremic with an expanded extracellular fluid; as the sepsis resolves, they diurese and their serum sodium concentration increases. The more severe the infectious process, the more exaggerated the changes in the extracellular fluid. This phenomenon has been attributed to numerous factors, including expansion and dilution of extracellular fluid volume, fluid therapy, inappropriate antidiuretic hormone secretion, and salt losses resulting from sweating, vomiting, and diarrhea.[1] It seems clear that nutritional therapy cannot reverse the increased extracellular fluid volume in septic patients unless the sepsis is controlled.

Clinical Implications of Body Composition in Critically Ill Patients

Body composition changes in acutely ill patients can result from various combinations of starvation, metabolic and hormonal responses associated with injury or sepsis, carbohydrate administration, and other factors that may be less well defined. If an absolute increase in extracellular fluid is found, it suggests that the starvation has been of the kwashiorkor form or complicated by trauma or sepsis. In the critically ill patient prior loss of BCM as a result of protein–calorie insufficiencies will affect therapy. Recent weight losses of less than 10% of normal body weight may not require urgent nutritional treatment. Losses of 10–30% represent a serious complication, and failure to provide nutritional therapy will almost certainly interfere with recovery despite treatment that is optimum in other respects. Losses greater than 30% are life-threatening and can cause permanent damage to the musculoskeletal system. Nutritional therapy must be administered immediately, but with caution, because overfeeding in these conditions can cause life-threatening complications.[8]

An expanded extracellular fluid volume is generally considered undesirable. As outlined below, it is correlated with postoperative complications and undesirable effects on pulmonary and cerebral function.[14] Adequate nutrition will result in a relative decrease of the extracellular fluid when the water retention has occurred for nutritional reasons alone. If the expanded extracellular fluid results from trauma or sepsis, however, nutritional support alone may not be sufficient.

NUTRITION

General Principles

Metabolism

Energy Generation. By metabolism of carbohydrate, lipid, and protein, energy is released for mechanical work, synthesis, membrane transport, and thermogenesis. Glucose, amino acids, fatty acids, triglycerides, lactate, and ketones all, under different circumstances, play a role in energy generation. Glucose metabolism generally occurs along the glycolysis and the oxidative phosphorylation pathways. Anaerobic glycolysis produces a small amount of adenosine triphosphate (ATP) as compared with oxidative phosphorylation; however, it becomes important during anoxic and hypoxic conditions. Fatty acids and amino acids are metabolized aerobically and need slightly more oxygen per kilocalorie of energy generated than does glucose; this is true even during aerobic glucose metabolism.

Fuel Stores. To maintain adequate metabolism during periods of enhanced energy needs or reduced dietary intake, expenditure of endogenous tissue stores is required. The energy available from circulating substrates is negligible. Carbohydrate is stored as glycogen in liver and muscle. The average healthy adult stores 200–300 g of carbohydrate, which gives a total energy available of approximately 900 kcal. This can only fulfill energy requirements for 8–10 hours, and thus the glycogen stores become depleted within 24 hours. Fat contributes to about 15–30% of the body weight. The average 70-kg adult man has 15–20 kg adipose tissue, making the total available caloric storage from fat about 140,000 kcal. This constitutes 85% of the total body energy stores and is the major energy source during periods of prolonged starvation. Fat is stored as triglyceride.

Protein is present in lean body tissue, the major part in skeletal muscle and visceral organs. Fourteen to twenty percent of the body weight is protein, giving a total amount available of approximately 24,000 kcal. There is no protein whose sole function is energy storage, but during poor dietary intake protein can be oxidized for energy. Some degree of functional loss always accompanies the use of LBM for energy generation.

An individual's total caloric storage could potentially sustain life for about 4–5 months; however, functionally most persons would be at the point of death on burning about 140,000 kcal, or about 75% of the fat and 50% of the protein. This occurs in approximately 60 days during a complete fast.

Metabolic Responses to Fasting and Starvation. After the first day of starvation the carbohydrate stores are exhausted and fat and protein are expended to meet whole body energy needs. A wide variety of metabolic adaptations takes place if the starvation state continues. The metabolic changes in response to starvation are aimed primarily at conservation of fuel stores and reduction of the body's dependence on glucose.

Complete starvation of 1 week's duration without any intervening stress causes a progressive decrease in urinary nitrogen loss. The decrease is due to ketoadaptation; the liver starts to synthesize ketones from incoming fatty acids that are used for energy. In the absence of any significant carbohydrate intake, gluconeogenesis is the main source of glucose, resulting in protein breakdown as amino acids are converted to glucose. Most amino acids are glucogenic and can be converted to Krebs' cycle intermediates, which may then be converted to glucose *via* gluconeogenesis. In addition, as much as 20 g·day^{-1} of glucose can be synthesized from the glycerol that is released by hydrolysis of adipose tissue triglyceride. Other adaptive mechanisms include reduction in the rate of glucose utilization by tissues capable of using fat and changes in the insulin release affecting protein catabolism and gluconeogenesis. A decrease in resting energy expenditure occurs during a fast; this decrease appears to be an adaptive mechanism designed to minimize tissue losses.

Most tissues can oxidize fat as the primary fuel for energy requirements. Free fatty acids do not cross the blood–brain barrier and are not available to the brain as metabolic substrate. In the complete absence of glucose intake, the central nervous system progressively increases its use of ketones produced by the liver as an energy substrate.[15] In the absence of ketones, 100–150 g·day^{-1} of glucose is required, mainly derived through gluconeogenesis from amino acids provided by protein breakdown. Thus, use of ketones for fuel lowers the cerebral glucose requirements and spares protein breakdown that would otherwise be expended for gluconeogenesis.

Under normal steady-state conditions, nitrogen excretion equals dietary nitrogen intake (10–30 g·day^{-1}). Starvation of 1 week causes a progressive decrease in urinary nitrogen to 6–8 g·day^{-1}, which represents a loss of about one-half pound of lean tissue a day. Administration of 100 g of carbohydrates reduces the nitrogen losses to about 3–4 g·day^{-1}.[16] A protein-free diet with adequate carbohydrate can cut protein losses; however, this nitrogen-sparing effect of carbohydrate may not be entirely beneficial because it seems to result in a diffuse whole body expansion of the extracellular fluid compartment.

The healthy subject will adapt over 5–10 days by excreting less nitrogen during fasting. In the critically ill patient, however, the compensations do not occur readily. In addition there are the increased nitrogen requirements associated with tissue repair, synthesis of immune proteins, and the acute-phase reactants. These patients may also often have extrarenal nitrogen losses from gastrointestinal tract or direct tissue injury after trauma or from hemorrhage. Metabolic requirements during this condition are increased rather than decreased, as during a fast. The hyperglycemia seen in critically ill patients prevents the development of the ketotic, nitrogen-sparing state observed in starvation.

The respiratory quotient (RQ) is calculated from the carbon dioxide production divided by the oxygen consumption. The RQ of carbohydrate is 1.00, fat 0.71, and protein 0.82. Lipogenesis, the synthesis of fat from glucose, is associated with an RQ of approximately 8.0. A whole body RQ greater than 1.0 would imply net lipogenesis. Prolonged starvation is associated with a whole body RQ approaching 0.7 as fat and fat-derived fuels provide substrates for the major portion of the organism's energy needs. During refeeding, the RQ reflects the composition of the fuel being administered. If a hypertonic solution of glucose and amino acids is given, the RQ will rise from 0.7 to 1.0 or higher as glucose becomes the major fuel substrate and excess glucose is converted to fat (lipogenesis).

Metabolic Responses to Trauma and Surgical Stress. Cuthbertson divided the response to injury into three stages.[17] The shock phase is associated with an early period of weight gain due to fluid sequestration. The metabolic rate is depressed, body temperature is lowered, and the circulating blood volume is reduced. This is followed after a day or two by the catabolic phase (flow stage) with increased metabolic activity. In this stage body energy stores are mobilized to meet increased needs. Weight is lost as the retained fluid is mobilized; this is combined with a mobilization of fat and LBM. Maximal nitrogen loss generally occurs between the 4th and 8th days after injury. The nitrogen excretion is increased as a function of the severity of the trauma.[18] Kinney et al[19] found that multiple fractures resulted in a 10–20% increase in resting energy expenditure for 1–3 weeks, whereas infection produced increases of 15–50%. Extensive burns resulted in increases from 40–100% that lasted for several weeks. Uncomplicated elective operations did not increase resting energy expenditure (Fig. 12-1). The catabolic phase is followed by the anabolic or recovery phase.

The degree of the catabolic response depends on the severity and duration of the trauma or stress. After an uncomplicated surgical procedure in an otherwise healthy patient, the catabolic response persists for about 1 week with a net nitrogen loss. These mild nitrogen losses are well tolerated and readily replaced by subsequent oral feeding. By contrast, the fasting patient recovering from severe trauma or stress catabolizes considerable amounts of lean body tissue and fat.

The catabolic response can be viewed as a mobilization of body protein, fat, and carbohydrate stores to ensure adequate circulatory levels of substrate (glucose, fatty acids, and amino acids) when dietary intake is limited. The increased available amino acid pool occurs predominantly at the expense of skeletal muscle. These amino acids may be oxidized directly for fuel or used for gluconeogenesis; this process also makes more precursors available for synthesis of visceral protein and the proteins of tissue repair.

In response to injury gluconeogenesis is increased in the

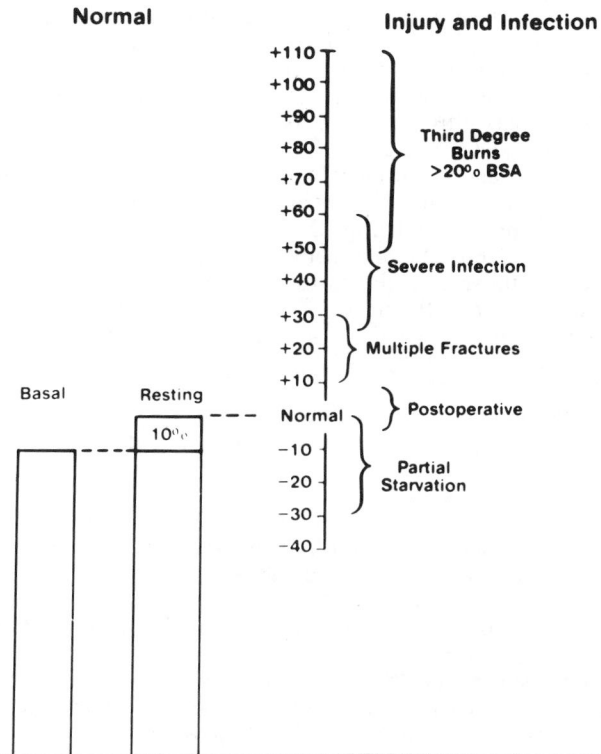

Figure 12-1. The effects of injury, sepsis, and nutritional depletion on resting energy expenditure. (Reprinted with permission from Kinney JM: The application of indirect calorimetry to clinical studies. In Kinney JM [ed]: Assessment of Energy Metabolism in Health and Disease, p 42. Columbus, Ross Laboratories, 1980.)

presence of high levels of glucose.[20] This hyperglycemia, referred to as the *diabetes of injury*, reflects the urgent nature of glucose requirements that the healing tissues require.[21] Fat is mobilized to obtain high circulating levels and is used for the energy needs of cardiac, skeletal, and respiratory muscles; this allows glucose to be spared for tissues that specifically require it, such as the central nervous system, the cellular immune system, and the healing wound. There is an increased body metabolism in response to trauma that is characterized by fever and enhanced oxygen consumption. The hormonal changes include an increased adrenal glucocorticoid, glucagon, and catecholamine release.[18]

Nutritional Requirements

Maintenance of the BCM and organ function requires a supply of water, energy, and all the 36 essential nutrients. The recommended enteral intake of these nutrients is presented in several sources,[22] and suggested allowances for intravenous intake are also presented. In this section the basic rules for estimating the normal requirements are outlined. In patients the requirements may vary greatly, depending on the type of disease and the organs involved. Specific nutritional support during metabolic stress and failure of vital organs (heart, lung, liver, brain, kidney) are discussed in a separate section.

Water. Normal individuals require about 1 ml of water for each ingested calorie, or about 2000–3000 ml·day^{-1} for adult subjects. When intake and output records are measured, water requirements are usually estimated as follows:

TABLE 12-2. Recommended Daily Basic Requirements per Kilogram Body Weight During Intravenous Nutrition

Element	Amount
Sodium	1–1.4 mmol
Potassium	0.7–0.9 mmol
Calcium	0.11 mmol
Phosphorus	0.15 mmol
Magnesium	0.04 mmol
Iron	0.25–1.0 μmol
Manganese	0.1 μmol
Zinc	0.7 μmol
Chloride	1.3–1.9 mmol
Fluoride	0.7 μmol
Iodide	0.015 μmol
Chromium	0.015 μmol
Molybdenum	0.003 μmol
Selenium	0.006 μmol

Adapted with permission from Shenkin A, Wretlind A: Parenteral nutrition. World Rev Nutr Diet 28:1, 1978.

500 ml (insensible loss) + urine output (ml) + nonurinary losses (ml) (e.g., enteral drainage).

Electrolytes, Minerals, and Trace Elements. Electrolytes should be tailored to the individual patient's need. For example, the patient with a metabolic alkalosis due to gastrointestinal losses may require more chloride and less acetate, and the patient with a chronic metabolic acidosis may require addition of lactate to the system. Similarly, calcium, potassium, magnesium, and trace element requirements may vary with the clinical setting. Guidelines for maintenance dose of electrolytes and trace elements are listed in Table 12-2. An outline of electrolyte balance and disturbances and their treatment is described in the section on Fluid and Electrolytes.

Energy. Caloric requirements should be predicted to prevent insufficient caloric intake as well as overfeeding. The basal caloric requirements can be calculated from the Harris-Benedict equation.[23] The equation is based on the patient's sex, age (A), height (H), and weight (W):

Female: $655 + 9.6(W) + 1.8(H) - 4.7(A) = \text{kcal·day}^{-1}$
Male: $66 + 13.7(W) + 5(H) - 6.8(A) = \text{kcal·day}^{-1}$

In clinical practice the caloric requirements usually are estimated on the basis of the patient's weight: 25–30 kcal·kg^{-1}·day^{-1}.

Depending on the clinical condition of the patient, the energy intake may be increased. If the patient has fever, the energy expenditure will increase by approximately 13% for each degree Celsius of body temperature above normal. Major surgery, sepsis, and burns increase energy expenditure. Intake must be adjusted upward if urinary and fecal calorie losses are increased. On the other hand, semistarvation, which is often seen in surgical patients, may reduce energy expenditure by as much as 30% (Fig. 12-2). In a nutritionally depleted patient, a greater intake than calculated expenditure is necessary for deposition of new tissue. For nutritional repletion, energy intake should exceed resting energy expenditure by 50%. For maintenance, only 20% above rest-

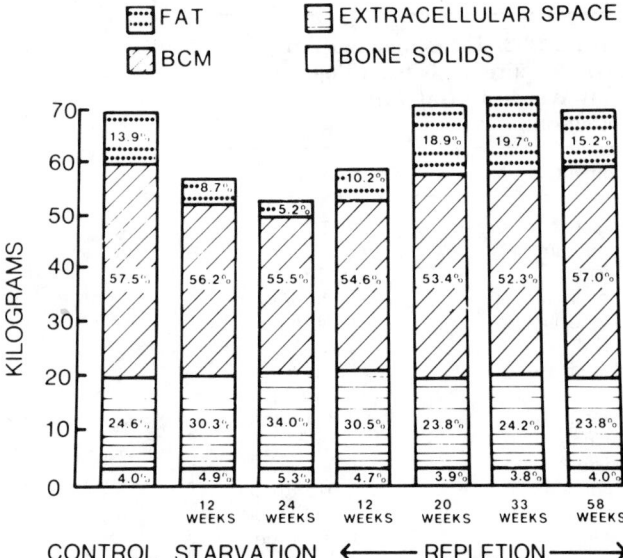

☐☐ FAT   ☐ EXTRACELLULAR SPACE
☐ BCM   ☐ BONE SOLIDS

Figure 12-2. Effects of 24 weeks of starvation followed by 58 weeks of repletion on body composition of active young men. Control energy requirements were estimated at 3490 kcal·day⁻¹. Energy intake during starvation averaged 1570 kcal·day⁻¹, 45% of the control level. Energy intake was restricted to an average of 2900 kcal·day⁻¹ for the first 12 weeks of repletion; subsequently, the subjects had free access to food. (Adapted with permission from Keys A, Brozek J, Henschel H *et al:* The Biology of Human Starvation. Minneapolis, University of Minnesota Press, 1950.)

ing energy expenditure is necessary. In the previously malnourished individual with more than 10% weight loss one should aim for repletion, whereas the previously healthy individual who is acutely ill requires maintenance only. Overfeeding, particularly with glucose, may lead to hypermetabolism, hepatic steatosis, and elevated carbon dioxide production.

Nonprotein Energy. Normally, carbohydrates contribute 40–60%, protein 10–15%, and fat 30–40% of the total energy intake. The amount of the protein intake used for energy varies because parts of the amino acids are used for protein synthesis. The body is more sensitive to protein intake than to total energy provision. Optimal nutritional support therefore first optimizes protein intake and then adds sufficient calories. The nonprotein calories can be provided by carbohydrates or fat. A minimum of approximately 500 kcal·day⁻¹ should be administered as glucose to supply carbohydrate for the brain, bone marrow, and injured tissue. On the other hand, at least 10% of the energy should be given as fat to provide sufficient essential fatty acids (linoleic and linolenic acid). The essential fatty acid deficiency syndrome has been reported in patients who received fat-free intravenous nutrition.

Once the minimal intake for glucose and fat is met, the additional nonprotein calories may be provided as either of these substrates. Total parenteral nutrition (TPN) systems have been described that provide nonprotein calories from 83% lipid/17% glucose to the traditional 100% glucose. The optimum balance of fat and glucose is not yet determined. TPN systems with 50% of nonprotein calories delivered as fat are as effective in maintaining nitrogen balance as those with 100% glucose and seem to minimize complications.

Protein. In healthy humans the normal ingestion is about 1 g of protein·kg⁻¹·day⁻¹. Losses of protein (nitrogen) occur through urine and stool. The adult human usually remains in zero nitrogen balance. With a daily protein intake of 70 g, the urinary nitrogen losses are about 9 g and fecal nitrogen losses are about 1–2 g.

To calculate the nitrogen balance, the nitrogen intake and nitrogen output must be determined. The nitrogen intake in grams is determined from the equation protein intake (g) = 6.25 × N(g). The total urinary nitrogen is 70–80% urea nitrogen under normal conditions, and because the latter is easily measured, the nitrogen output (g·day⁻¹) can be estimated as urea (g·day⁻¹) + 4 g. The equation for nitrogen balance is:

$$\text{N balance (g·day}^{-1}) = \text{N intake (g·day}^{-1}) - \text{N output (g·day}^{-1})$$

where

$$\text{N intake} = \text{protein intake}:6.25 \text{ (g·day}^{-1})$$
$$\text{N output} = \text{urea in urine} + 4 \text{ (g·day}^{-1})$$

Negative nitrogen balance is associated with resorption and positive nitrogen balance with deposition of cellular protoplasm. In healthy adults a nitrogen equilibrium is established when daily protein intake is about 0.6–1 g·kg⁻¹·day⁻¹. Surgical stress and possible postoperative complications increase nitrogen requirements, and protein intake has to be increased accordingly to prevent loss of cellular protoplasmic mass. As a simple guide to make up for the increased protein needs after major surgery and postoperative complications, protein must be increased in proportion to energy (calorie/nitrogen ratio) to about 100 kcal·g⁻¹ of nitrogen. For example if energy expenditure is estimated at 2000 kcal·day⁻¹, the nitrogen intake would be 2000/100 = 20 g N per day (× 6.25) = 130 g protein. Renal or hepatic failure will increase this ratio. Patients with malabsorption have an increased protein demand varying from 2–8 g·kg⁻¹·day⁻¹, depending on the severity of the disease. When a nutritional program is aimed at repleting LBM, protein intake must be increased above maintenance protein requirements.

Vitamins. The vitamins are important to normal metabolic functions. They are essential nutrients and therefore have to be supplied to the nutritional support regimen (Table 12-3).

TABLE 12-3. Maintenance Dose of Vitamins

Vitamin	Dose
Vitamin A	3300 IU
Vitamin D	200 IU
Vitamin E	10 IU
Vitamin C	100 mg
Thiamine	3 mg
Riboflavin	3.6 mg
Niacin	40 mg
Pyridoxine	4 mg
Biotin	60 μg
Folate	3 μg/kg
B₁₂	5 μg

Nutritional Failure

Malnutrition. Nutritional failure is associated either with protein depletion in the presence of adequate calories or with combined protein–calorie deficiency. In protein–calorie deficiency the food has adequate proportions of proteins but the total caloric intake is inadequate. Protein deficiency corresponds to kwashiorkor and combined protein–calorie deficiency corresponds to marasmus in their respective end-stage forms.

Protein depletion affects the protein content of all organs. The liver and gut are rapidly depleted, whereas the brain is affected less than other organs. In severe protein depletion the gut may be unable to tolerate or digest food, presumably because protein is needed to produce digestive enzymes. The skeletal muscle is most affected and may lose as much as 70% of its protein.

Protein–calorie depletion is a frequent finding in surgical patients as well as in the critically ill. Nutritional deficits are often unsuspected and remain unnoticed. Patients with malnutrition have been shown to be at an increased risk for infections and mechanical complications in the postoperative period, as outlined below. TPN can be used to correct the nutritional abnormalities and thus decrease the risk of perioperative morbidity and mortality with a shortening of the hospital stay.

Diagnosis of Malnutrition. An evaluation of the nutritional status is an important means of identifying the patient who needs nutritional intervention as well as assessing the efficacy of the nutritional support. The lack of a specific test for protein–calorie malnutrition makes the diagnosis difficult in many cases.

Nutritional assessment begins with a medical history and physical examination, including recording of height and weight. During the start of TPN weight should be measured daily.

Practical clinical tools of anthropometric measurement of body composition include the triceps skinfold thickness and midarm circumference. The former is an indicator of body fat, and the latter is an indicator of muscle and, thereby, of LBM. These are simple tests that can be quickly performed. Both measurements, however, have a wide range of normal values and are rather insensitive to early changes in nutritional status. Further, the tests are limited in that it is difficult to differentiate kwashiorkor from marasmus.

Dynamic nutritional assessment is performed using energy and nitrogen balance. Energy balance measurements, however, require calorimetry. Nitrogen balance requires careful collection of all drainage and excreta. In the clinical setting, nitrogen loss is usually estimated by measuring 24-hour urinary urea nitrogen excretion and adding correction factors for nonurea urinary nitrogen. The nitrogen balance provides an estimate of net protein degradation or synthesis. Creatinine excretion is directly related to muscle mass, and expected creatinine excretion can be calculated based on sex and height.[24] The creatinine/height index is a useful indicator of muscle mass.

Analysis of the visceral proteins synthesized in the liver includes measurement of serum albumin, transferrin, retinol-binding protein, and prealbumin. Albumin is distributed throughout the extracellular compartment so that changes in total body water influence the level of albumin independent of changes in nutritional status. There also exists a large exchangeable pool of albumin; the albumin half-time is approximately 21 days, and this limits its usefulness as a short-term indicator of efficacy of nutritional support. Serum albumin concentration appears to be most useful in the initial assessment of chronic malnutrition. Transferrin has a shorter half-life (approximately 8 days); however, it is also an acute-phase reactant and is affected by the status of iron stores. Retinol-binding protein and prealbumin turn over more rapidly, with half-lives of 12 and 36 hours, respectively. They may be potentially more sensitive and specific indicators of nutritional status, but their clinical usefulness has not yet been established. Decreased humoral and cellular immunity is a serious consequence of protein–calorie malnutrition. Total lymphocyte count and cutaneous reactivity are commonly used in the clinical setting. Sepsis and carcinoma, however, also cause anergy independent of nutritional status. This lack of specificity limits their use in the clinical setting.

There is today no single best indicator of nutritional status or the efficacy of nutritional support. The prognostic nutritional index[25] and the protein–energy malnutrition scale[26] attempt to develop more objective measures to predict outcome based on a combination of parameters; however, clinical judgment has been reported to be as good as any of the objective measurements in predicting morbidity and mortality.[27]

Nutritional Treatment

The first step in planning any nutritional regimen is to identify the need for intervention; the next step is to determine the route of delivery. The last step is to prescribe the amounts of macronutrients and micronutrients based on the clinical setting and nutritional assessment of the patient.

Indications. Critically ill patients are often in a hypercatabolic state and are at high risk of rapidly developing malnutrition, even though their premorbid nutritional status was adequate. The goal is to meet their increased nutritional requirements to minimize the loss of LBM and function during the catabolic phase. Patients with severe injury, major burns, or sepsis fall into this group. Patients with chronic diseases with or without gastrointestinal tract involvement often require intravenous nutrition. Patients with short gut syndrome, gastrointestinal fistula, severe malabsorption, or inflammatory bowel disease may require intravenous nutrition. Often, nutritional debilitation is seen in chronic diseases even though the gastrointestinal tract is not directly involved, for example, in patients with chronic renal failure. Malnutrition is common in patients with cancer. In the patient with malignancy who is about to undergo a surgical procedure, the risks of delaying the operation because of preoperative nutritional status and the benefit in terms of morbidity and mortality must be considered in each patient. Nutritional support improves patient tolerance to chemotherapy and radiation.[28,29] No significant long-term benefit, however, has been demonstrated to date.

For hepatic encephalopathy, renal failure, and hypercatabolic stress states, specific amino acid formulations have been developed in order to affect the specific metabolic derangements of each of these conditions. Their clinical use is outlined later in this chapter. Intravenous fat emulsions have also been proposed to alter the inflammatory profile of the lung *via* alterations in prostaglandin (PG) synthesis.[30] In addition to providing energy and essential micronutrients, nutritional therapy can be considered as specific pharmacologic therapy in these situations.

Enteral Route of Administration. Patients can be fed by either the enteral or the parenteral route or by a combination of the two. Intravenous feeding is an alternative to oral feeding and should be used only when the gastrointestinal tract is unavailable. When *ad libitum* food intake is negligible (less than 500 kcal·day^{-1}), enteral solutions are used to supply the total daily requirements. The solutions can be sipped or administered through a nasogastric feeding tube with a thin lumen.

Enteral solutions vary in composition, palatability, and cost. The formula ingredients are either premixed by the manufacturer or added together shortly before use. The two major groups of fixed-composition formulas are elemental and polymeric; the formulas prepared *de novo* are termed *modular*.

Elemental solutions consist of an easily digested and absorbed nitrogen source, a carbohydrate source requiring little amylase activity, and a small amount of fat in the form of medium-chain triglycerides or essential fatty acids. They provide all essential nutrients and most of them contain about 1 kcal·ml^{-1} of fluid.[31] Elemental formulas are generally used in patients who have maldigestion and malabsorption. The disadvantages of these formulas are that they are unpalatable and require tube feeding; they are hyperosmolar (500–900 mOsm·kg^{-1}), which may result in cramping and osmotic diarrhea if infused too rapidly; they are relatively high in carbohydrates, which in turn increases carbon dioxide production and ventilation; and they are expensive relative to polymeric solutions.

Polymeric solutions are indicated in patients with normal or near-normal gastrointestinal function. Their protein, carbohydrate, and fat are provided in high molecular weight forms. Many of the polymeric formulas are palatable and can be tolerated without tube feeding. They are less expensive and generally lower in osmolality than elemental solutions.

A modular formula is prepared by combining two or more ingredients to form the mixture. The type and amount of protein, carbohydrate, and fat, and the mineral and vitamin content can be adjusted to meet the needs of each patient. Modular solutions are thus prepared from available sources of protein, carbohydrate, fat, minerals, and proteins.[32] Alternatively, any one of the individual modules can be added to one of the complete formulas, which serves as a base solution. Modular formulas offer specific advantages in patients with cardiac failure, decreased pulmonary function, malabsorption, diabetes, and renal insufficiency.

The nutrition-depleted patient does not tolerate an adequate diet instantly; diarrhea almost always occurs. The first goal, therefore, is to provide volume and then slowly increase concentration until adequate nutrition is achieved without diarrhea. If an isotonic enteral formula is used, however, the initial infusion in most situations can be started at full strength if an appropriate slow speed is selected. The infusion rate is then advanced as tolerated. In practice, it appears helpful to administer enteral feeding as a slow, continuous infusion by using thin, mostly silicon-covered specific nasogastric tubes. To avoid pulmonary aspiration, feeding is usually stopped during night hours, and a slight head-up position is recommended during infusion. Considering these guidelines, enteral feeding is a realistic alternative even for intubated patients on ventilators.

Parenteral Nutrition. Intravenous nutrition may be given alone as TPN or as a supplement in some patients if oral or tube feeding may be possible but insufficient.

History. In 1913, Henriques and Anderson achieved the intravenous administration of a protein hydrolysate in a goat.[33] They were able to keep the goat in a positive nitrogen balance for 14 days. In the ensuing decades, a growing understanding and clinical awareness of the influence of nutritional status on the outcome following injury or surgery was seen.[33-36] Two major advances, however, opened the door to the clinical application of TPN. In 1960, Wretlind and Haakansson in Sweden developed a clinically usable fat emulsion.[37,38] In the United States in 1968, Wilmore and Dudrick reported their experience with central venous catheterization for the delivery of hypertonic dextrose solution.[39] They demonstrated that administration of intravenous nutrients exclusively could not only support life but also promote growth and development.

The last two decades have seen advancements in the understanding of the metabolic response to starvation and stress and refinements in methodology. A current interest in nutritional support is the attempt to differentiate various nutritional support solutions for different disease states.

Routes of Parenteral Administration. Parenteral nutrition can be delivered by central or peripheral vein. The subclavian, external, or internal jugular vein may be cannulated percutaneously and the central catheter placed with the tip in the superior vena cava. A subcutaneously implanted port or Hickman or Broviac type of Silastic catheter with a Dacron cuff placed *via* venotomy with subcutaneous tunneling may also be used for long-term therapy. This catheter may be inserted by venotomy *via* the cephalic, basilic, or external jugular vein.[40-43] The insertion of the percutaneous subclavian catheter is associated with a 5–7% incidence of significant mechanical complications such as pneumothorax and subclavian artery puncture.[44] The risk of infection, especially in septic and otherwise immunologically depleted patients, calls for careful monitoring of catheters. The advantage of routine replacement of catheters at 4- to 6-day intervals has not been clearly defined.

Short-term intravenous nutrition can be administered by peripheral vein. Lipids are then used as a substantial proportion of the nonprotein calories to reduce the irritability of the solution. An example of such a mixture would be 500 ml of a 20% fat emulsion, 1000 ml of 8.5% amino acid solution, and 1000 ml of 10% dextrose. This provides nearly 1800 kcal·day^{-1} when infused at 100 ml·h^{-1}. The final concentration of dextrose is less than 5%; hence the phlebitis rate is quite low and comparable with that observed with 5% dextrose and saline solution. The vein puncture site should be rotated every 2–3 days. In general, arteriovenous shunts or vascular fistulae are not recommended for administration of TPN.

Nutritional Program Components. In Table 12-4 a nutritional program is outlined based on a glucose–lipid system for an average 70-kg man who has lost 10 kg weight due to stress and illness. Formulas for nutrition for specific disease states are discussed below.

Nitrogen balance is influenced by both protein intake and total energy (calories) consumed. Optimal nutritional support first maximizes protein intake and then adds sufficient calories in the form of glucose and fat,[45] since positive nitrogen balance cannot be achieved by giving amino acids alone without calories. Nonprotein calories can reduce the nitrogen excretion, but only to a minimum level in the absence of protein intake.[46] The effects of nitrogen and energy intake

TABLE 12-4. Nutrient Regimen for the Standard 70-kg Man Following Weight Loss Aiming for Nutritional Repletion	
Regimen	**Content**
Nutrient Mixture	
Protein	110 g
Nonprotein calories	1000–2000
Distribution	50% glucose and 50% fat
Parenteral Solutions*	
1000 ml	11% amino acids
1000 ml	20% glucose
500 ml	20% fat emulsion

*The parenteral solutions can be mixed in one bag and infused over 24 hours at 100 ml·h^{-1}. Electrolytes, trace elements, and vitamins are added to the TPN mixture.

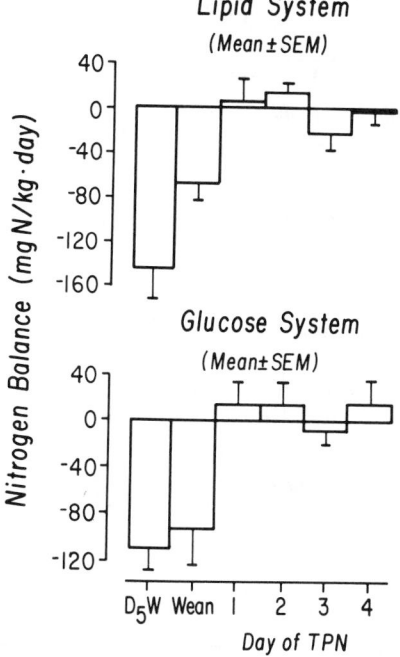

Figure 12-3. Nitrogen balance in subjects given two forms of nutritional support systems: a lipid-based system *vs* a glucose-based system. During administration of parenteral nutrition, nitrogen balance with both systems is equivalent. (Reprinted with permission from Nordenström J, Askanazi J, Elwyn DH *et al*: Nitrogen balance during total parenteral nutrition: Glucose *versus* fat. Ann Surg 197:27, 1983.)

on nitrogen balance, however, are not independent of one another; their interaction is complex. If nitrogen intake is adequate, zero nitrogen balance is achieved when caloric intake meets caloric expenditure. Similarly, increasing caloric intake above requirements increases nitrogen retention and results in net positive nitrogen balance.[47] During nutritional repletion there is a greater positive nitrogen balance in the beginning that declines as the BCM returns more to its prestarvation levels.

The large nitrogen loss that occurs during the first 6 days of fasting can be halved by daily ingestion of only 100 g of glucose.[11] The nitrogen-sparing effect of a relatively small (400 kcal·g^{-1}) caloric load occurs with carbohydrate only because fat does not produce the same suppression of nitrogen excretion during fasting.[47] When carbohydrate is administered in amounts of more than 600 kcal·day^{-1}, the nitrogen-sparing effects of fat and carbohydrate are equal,[48] while fat has only a small nitrogen-sparing effect in the absence of 600 kcal·day^{-1} of carbohydrates;[49,50] however, no differences in nitrogen balances have been detected in studies comparing groups receiving the nonprotein calories in form of glucose with those whose nonprotein calories were supplied as one-half fat and one-half glucose[51,52] (Fig. 12-3). When the lipid-based system is administered, a lesser calorigenic response and a decreased norepinephrine excretion have been found compared to the "glucose system."[53] A reduction in carbon dioxide production has also been observed in patients receiving "the lipid system."[54] Liver function tests have shown fewer abnormalities when lipid was used to replace one third of the glucose calories.[55] These studies provide evidence of the efficacy of 20% fat emulsion as a concentrated nutrient source that allows provision of calories without risks of overhydration, and with fewer demands on ventilation. Fat emulsions represent a logical alternative to glucose loading, especially in patients with an exaggerated caloric requirement and a diminished ability to clear exogenous glucose (e.g., in metabolic stress) as well as in those with hepatic or pulmonary dysfunction.

Delivery of Nutrients. Parenteral nutrients are mostly administered as a continuous infusion *via* the central route. Mixing of all the components for TPN in one mix ("three-in-one" system) before administration simplifies procedures for the nursing personnel and also obviously reduces the

risk of infection due to reduced manipulations with infusion sets and connections.

Complications. Complications of parenteral nutrition arise from technical problems associated with the maintenance of the intravenous catheter or from metabolic complications due to inappropriate provision nutrients. The most common metabolic complications are hyperglycemia and glucosuria, and frequent monitoring of glucose in urine and serum is important, particularly at the start of TPN. If glucose in serum is more than 250 mg·dl^{-1}, insulin is usually added to the TPN solution. Hyperglycemic hyperosmolar coma has been reported from infusion of the TPN solution, whereas hypoglycemia and shock may ensue with a sudden termination of TPN infusion. A frequent metabolic complication is hyperchloremic acidosis, which can be prevented by decreasing the ratio of chloride to acetate in the TPN.[56] Rapid infusion of amino acid solutions has been associated with nausea, headache, and a warm sensation. When the patient begins to become anabolic, large amounts of potassium and phosphate shift into the intracellular space; to avoid a deficit of these, supplementation is needed. Development of hepatic dysfunction has been reported in 10–15% of patients receiving long-term TPN. The reason for the TPN-associated deterioration in liver function is unclear. It has been suggested that fewer hepatic complications occur when part of the TPN glucose calories are replaced with fat.[55]

The mechanical catheter-related complications of TPN are outlined in Table 12-5. Of these complications, sepsis deserves special mention. The venous catheters are often in place for long periods, and the fluids used are ideal for

TABLE 12-5. Mechanical Complications of Total Parenteral Nutrition

Central Venous Catheter Placement

Malposition
Catheter embolism
Air embolism
Thrombosis and thromboembolism
Sepsis
Cardiac dysrhythmias
Myocardial perforation

Subclavian or Internal Jugular Venipuncture

Arterial puncture
Pneumothorax, hemothorax, chylothorax
Brachial plexus injury
Mediastinal hematoma

Peripheral Venipuncture

Pain
Hematoma
Thrombosis
Phlebitis
Extravasation

supporting growth of microorganisms. In a recent publication, an infection rate of 3.3% was reported for central catheters in general.[44] Strict antiseptic conditions should prevail during catheter placement, and the catheter should be used only for the infusion of TPN. The incidence of sepsis is increased with the use of multilumen catheters for TPN. In one study the frequency of sepsis was 14.6% for multilumen catheters compared with 3.2% for single-lumen catheters.[56]

Patient Monitoring. Table 12-6 gives guidelines for monitoring the patient for the development of infection or metabolic

TABLE 12-6. Suggested Monitoring Schedule During Total Parenteral Nutrition

Parameter	Suggested Frequency	
	Early	*After Stable*
Volume in (iv and oral)	Daily	Daily
Volume out (urine and drainage)	Daily	Daily
Body temperature	Daily	Daily
Urine S&A	4 Times daily	Twice daily
Electrolytes	Daily	Biweekly
BUN/creatinine	Biweekly	Biweekly
Ca^{2+}, PO_4^{2-}, Mg^{2+}	Biweekly	Weekly
CBC, platelets	Weekly	Weekly
Glucose	Daily	Biweekly
PT, PTT	Weekly	Weekly
Triglycerides, cholesterol	Weekly	Weekly
Liver profile	Biweekly	Weekly
ABGs, urine electrolytes, drainage analysis, blood cultures, serum insulin, ketones, plasma amino acids, plasma fatty acids	Weekly	Weekly
Weight	Biweekly	Biweekly

iv = intravenous; S&A = sugar and acetone; BUN = blood urea nitrogen; CBC = complete blood count; PT = prothrombin time; PTT = partial thromboplastin time; ABGs = arterial blood gases.

Reprinted with permission from Robin AR, Greig PD: Basic principles of intravenous nutritional support. Clin Chest Med 7:29, 1986.

complications. When the patient is stable and tolerating a particular regimen, most of those determinations can be performed less frequently.

Weight should be measured daily; acute changes reflect changes in water and sodium. Body weight changes may underestimate the degree of malnutrition because extracellular fluid does not change during malnutrition, and nutritional repletion may be associated with a diuresis and contraction of the extracellular compartment, so that early weight loss may occur, even though BCM is increasing.

If the patient becomes hyperglycemic (blood glucose > 250 mg·dl^{-1}), the infusion rate of glucose should be reduced[57] and insulin may be administered. The requirement for insulin often decreases rapidly when the patient's stress resolves and the patient shifts from the catabolic to the anabolic state. The need for insulin should be re-evaluated daily by close monitoring of blood and urinary glucose. The discontinuing of glucose–insulin mixtures should be done with caution to avoid hypoglycemia.

When the patient begins to become anabolic, additional supplementation of potassium and phosphate is needed as these shift into the intracellular space. Hypophosphatemia may reduce cardiac and muscle contraction, as well as central nervous system, red blood cell, and leukocyte functions.[58]

Specific Nutrient Support in Disease States

Liver Disease

Protein–calorie malnutrition is common in the patient with liver disease; therefore, nutritional support is an important part of the therapy. The protein component of the nutrition, however, presents a problem to the patient who suffers from hepatic insufficiency and consequently risks developing hepatic encephalopathy.

A number of metabolic alterations in liver disease affect design of a nutritional support regimen. Diminished degradation of circulating hormones and portal-systemic shunting may result in a persistent elevation of glucagon and insulin.[59,60] The increase in glucagon may be greater than insulin,[61] resulting in a decreased insulin:glucagon ratio and a catabolic state.[61] In addition to the tendency toward catabolism, there may also exist an energy deficit in liver failure owing to impaired utilization of carbohydrates and lipids.[61,62] The cirrhotic liver fails to store glucose as glycogen. The chronic hyperglucagonemia presumably results in depletion of glycogen. Increased lipolysis also lessens the requirement for glucose. Lipolysis liberates glycerol, which contributes to gluconeogenesis, and fatty acids, which are used directly or oxidized to ketones (although this latter pathway may be impaired). The increased lipolysis combined with a decreased metabolism of fatty acids leads to high blood levels of nonesterified fatty acids.[63] The tendency toward gluconeogenesis from amino acids from muscle breakdown would require an equal capacity for ureagenesis in order to prevent hyperammonemia. In addition to hyperammonemia caused by diminished ureagenic capacity, there is a shunting of ammonia of gut origin, resulting in persistent elevation of plasma ammonia concentrations with advancing liver disease.

A specific amino acid pattern is seen in hepatic failure. Amino acids that are dependent on hepatic metabolism show increases. The aromatic amino acids (e.g., tyrosine, tryptophan) levels are elevated.[64] Conversely, the branched-chain amino acids that are catabolized in the periphery (e.g., skeletal muscle) are decreased owing to the increased peripheral demand and utilization.[64,65]

The increased level of aromatic amino acids and a decreased level of branched-chain amino acids in plasma have been correlated with the presence of encephalopathy.[66] Members of the neutral amino acid group compete at the blood–brain barrier for a single transport system (termed the L-system) that mediates their entry across the blood–brain barrier.[67] In hepatic encephalopathy there may be a derangement of the blood–brain barrier,[68] which results in a selective increase in transport of the neutral amino acids. Within this group it is hypothesized that the transport of the aromatic amino acids is preferentially increased because of their elevated plasma levels as well as the decreased competition for the transport system due to decreased plasma branched-chain amino acids.[65,69] According to this theory, which is by no means generally accepted, a decrease in the branched-chain/aromatic amino acid plasma ratio would be responsible for an imbalance of central aminergic neurotransmitters. The aromatic amino acids (phenylalanine, tyrosine, tryptophan) are precursors of neurotransmitters, and an increase in brain concentrations of serotonin and false neurotransmitters has been found in hepatic encephalopathy.[66] The false neurotransmitters are produced locally in the brain and may replace the physiologic transmitters (dopamine, noradrenaline) at the synapse. It has become clear, however, that the brain or cerebrospinal fluid amino acid content cannot be predicted from plasma amino acid levels alone.[70] Although controversy continues, it seems that the ratio of branched-chain to aromatic amino acids is a good predictor of hepatic function but not of encephalopathy.[71] According to this hypothesis, ammonia does not exert a direct toxic effect but rather appears to contribute to the pathogenesis of hepatic encephalopathy indirectly through the brain metabolite glutamine, which may accelerate transport of aromatic amino acids across the blood–brain barrier.[72,73]

The administration of branched-chain amino acid–enriched solutions was originally advocated for patients with liver failure. The standard balanced amino acids used in nutrition contain 19–25% of their amino acids as branched-chain, whereas the branched-chain amino acid–enriched solutions have about 45% of the amino acids as branched-chain. The branched-chain amino acids are unique in their partial utilization as an energy source by tissues (primarily muscle), other than the liver.[74] At the same time NH_2 groups are formed from the branched-chain amino acids for the synthesis of alanine and glutamine. Alanine is released from muscle and used as substrate for gluconeogenesis by the liver (alanine–glucose cycle).[75] Glutamine is mainly used as an energy source by the intestine and the kidneys. In addition to their use as an energy source, the branched-chain amino acids have been found to play a role in the regulation of protein turnover; the branched-chain amino acids may decrease muscle breakdown[76] and promote protein synthesis in muscle[77] as well as in the liver.[78] The ketoacid analogues of the branched-chain amino acids seem to be more efficacious in this regard than the amino acids themselves.[79]

Given the above-mentioned properties, the branched-chain amino acid–enriched solutions offer advantages in hepatic failure. Promising reports of studies in dogs and monkeys clearly indicated that a branched-chain amino acid–enriched solution was superior to a commercially available amino acid mixture in achieving positive nitrogen balance and normalizing of neurologic symptoms.[70,80,81] Encouraged by these reports, numerous anecdotal studies

were published in which branched-chain amino acid infusions were found to be useful in patients with liver disease.[82,83] Subsequently more conflicting reports have been reported.[84-89] Patients in hepatic coma awoke as quickly in response to administration of branched-chain amino acids and hypertonic dextrose solution as they did in response to the conventional treatment with starvation and neomycin/lactulose therapy. In the studies in which fat was given as the principal energy source,[83,84] branched-chain amino acid–enriched solutions failed to show beneficial effects on hepatic encephalopathy. In the opinion of certain authors, the high lipid intake could possibly worsen the encephalopathy.[88]

There is evidence that patients with cirrhosis may be able to tolerate protein administered in a branched-chain amino acid–enriched form better than as conventional protein.[90] Two of the controlled studies have suggested improved survival in patients with liver disease when treated with branched-chain amino acid–enriched solutions.[87,88] However, patients treated with conventional amino acids also have improved survival,[89] which indicates that the nutritional support in itself may be responsible for the result.

As a conclusion, branched-chain amino acid–enriched solutions seem indicated in hepatic failure with encephalopathy to reduce the cerebral symptoms and to provide usable calories. It is still not clear, however, whether the in vitro effects on protein turnover and possible promotion of hepatic protein synthesis are of clinical importance.

Clinical experience of our group and others suggests beneficial effects of intravenous medium-chain triglycerides on liver function in patients with hepatic dysfunction. The observed benefits of medium-chain triglycerides are based on their rapid hydrolysis, noncarnitine–dependent metabolism, and nonsequestration in the reticuloendothelial system.[91] In hepatic failure, the endogenous synthesis of carnitine may be insufficient. Carnitine is normally both absorbed from the gut and synthesized by the liver from its precursor amino acids, methionine and lysine. Carnitine stores are known to be critically reduced in stressed and septic patients, during long-term TPN, and in preterm infants.[92]

Medium-chain triglycerides are not stored and are more likely to be oxidized. They induce higher rates of ketogenesis than long-chain triglycerides, thus providing a readily available source of energy for peripheral tissues.[93] In comparative studies, medium-chain triglycerides have proven to be equally effective as long-chain triglycerides in maintaining muscle protein synthesis, and they are associated with an increased rate of protein synthesis in the liver.

We have seen marked improvements in liver function tests and general well-being of patients with prevailing hepatic failure developed during long-term TPN.[94] Bilirubin levels and aminotransferases show the most prominent amelioration. The observed findings suggest a cytoprotective potential of medium-chain triglycerides in patients at high risk for liver failure.

Metabolic Stress

The response to injury and infection can be described as a mobilization of body protein, fat, and carbohydrate stores to provide normal or above-normal circulating levels of substrate (glucose, free fatty acids, and amino acids) in the absence of dietary intake. Injury increases the rate of loss of LBM at any given nutrient intake; after elective operations weight loss occurs in the ratio of 2 : 1 (LBM : fat); with severe injury the ratio rises to 4 : 1 (see Table 12-1). The persistence of gluconeogenesis, despite high serum concentrations of glucose, demonstrates the urgent nature of the need for glucose. Fat is mobilized to meet the energy needs of cardiac and skeletal muscle; this spares glucose for the tissues that specifically oxidize it, such as the central nervous system and the cellular immune system. This pattern, unlike that observed in fasting normal humans, does not respond easily to nutritional manipulation. As a result, hypertonic glucose doses are usually ineffective in these patients and may add additional stress by precipitating increases in oxygen consumption, carbon dioxide production, and noradrenaline excretion and by inducing hepatic complications. These findings do not indicate that glucose infusion is contraindicated in stressed patients; a certain amount of carbohydrate intake is essential to meet obligatory glucose requirements.[95] A nutritional regimen appropriate for a patient under metabolic stress would therefore consist of a relatively modest amount of glucose administered with amino acids and other essential nutrients. Fat emulsions appear preferential to glucose loading in patients with an exaggerated caloric requirement. The fat emulsion allows provision of calories without overhydration and hemodilution. It seems, therefore, that a regimen supplying nonprotein calories in the form of both glucose and fat may be particularly appropriate for the stressed patient. When fat is the main substrate available for oxidation, a relative decrease in tissue concentration or increased competition for available carnitine may lead to limitations in fat metabolism. The consequent lack of ketone bodies contributes to the tissue-energy depletion. In these circumstances, medium-chain triglyceride–based fat emulsions have been shown to be superior because of their strong ketogenic effects.[91]

The amino acid requirement is increased by sepsis or trauma. A plasma amino acid pattern resembling that seen in hepatic failure has been noted in patients with systemic sepsis. These findings led to investigations of the utility of branched-chain amino acid–enriched solutions for critically ill patients. In addition branched-chain amino acids can serve as energy substrates, promote the synthesis of muscle and visceral protein, and reduce the breakdown of muscle protein.[74,96-100] All these effects may be beneficial in states with metabolic stress to decrease catabolism.

Several animal and human studies have indicated beneficial effects of the use of branched-chain amino acid solutions in patients with metabolic stress.[101-105] Other studies, however, have not found any difference in nitrogen retention in normal (25%) and high (45%) branched-chain amino acid groups.[106-108] The overall conclusions from the controlled human studies are clouded by the variability of stress and the number of septic patients included. The studies showing promotion of nitrogen balance with enriched branched-chain amino acid solutions have not used a balanced substrate for nonprotein caloric support. Several investigators have shown that a balanced TPN regimen in which the nonprotein calories have been given as carbohydrates and lipids can lead to a positive nitrogen balance.[52,109] In one study no significant difference was found in nitrogen balance promotion when a 44.6% branched-chain amino acid solution was compared with a standard TPN regimen (19% branched-chain amino acid, carbohydrate:lipid ratio 7:3).[107] The lack of difference may be the result of an effective utilization of lipids as fuel source by both groups.[110]

The in vitro studies that have suggested a beneficial effect of the branched-chain amino acids in decreasing protein degradation have investigated muscle tissue from nonseptic animals. Preliminary results, however, suggest that the controls of muscle degradation may be different in septic animals than in normal ones,[111] and this may explain the marginal effects demonstrated with the branched-chain amino acids in septic patients. It has also been proposed that the most important property of the branched-chain amino acids in sepsis may be their apparent effect on hepatic protein synthesis, with improved synthesis of proteins involved in host defense.[112]

As a conclusion, the role of branched-chain amino acids in the support of the critically ill stressed patient remains unclear. Further studies of the control of protein synthesis in the stressed state and the effect of a balanced TPN on nitrogen balance have to be undertaken.

Respiratory Disease

The effects of nutrition on respiration involve respiratory drive, respiratory muscle function, and pulmonary parenchyma as well as metabolic demand. In general, nutritional support increases the respiratory workload by increasing metabolic demand and ventilatory drive, but it seems that improvements in respiratory muscle and lung function make up for the disadvantages, especially if nutrition is given over a longer period.

Malnutrition leads to deterioration of the respiratory muscles. Nutritional support can improve the function of respiratory muscles as positive nitrogen balance occurs,[113] but these improvements require time to have a discernible effect (from 2 to 3 weeks). Preliminary results from in vitro incubation studies suggest that branched-chain amino acids may markedly improve the reversal of muscle force that occurs with fatigue.[114] Malnutrition also has important effects on the pulmonary parenchyma by causing emphysema-like changes and indirectly by impairment of the immune function. It is not yet clear whether and to what extent these malnutrition-induced lesions on the pulmonary parenchyma can be reversed.[115] Surfactant production seems to be dependent on an adequate supply of certain dietary fats.

When hypertonic glucose is used as the sole source of nonprotein calories in TPN, a marked rise in carbon dioxide production occurs.[116,117] As substrates shift from fat oxidation to glucose oxidation, an increase in respiratory quotient occurs; if sufficient glucose is given, lipogenesis occurs with an additional rise in the level of carbon dioxide production.[118] This increase in ventilatory demand can lead to respiratory distress in patients with impaired lung function. Substitution of nonprotein calories by fat emulsions lowers the respiratory quotient and reduces minute ventilation and ventilatory demand.[54] Thus, administration of the nonprotein calories as a mixture of fat and carbohydrate is important in patients with pulmonary disease.

Recent investigations have indicated a specific role for branched-chain amino acids in the control of respiration. As mentioned earlier, amino acids have been shown to stimulate ventilatory responsiveness.[119,120] A series of investigations have demonstrated that solutions with high branched-chain amino acid content induce a larger decrease in arterial CO_2 tension and a more marked ventilatory response to CO_2 challenge as compared with conventional solutions.[121] A nocturnal infusion of branched-chain amino acids in normal volunteers significantly decreased the end-tidal CO_2 concentrations, corresponding to an increased respiratory drive and improved alveolar gas exchange during sleep.[122] In subsequent investigations, seven chronic renal failure patients on maintenance dialysis were investigated in a sleep laboratory. Initially, the patients studied were characterized by reduced sleep quality and decreased

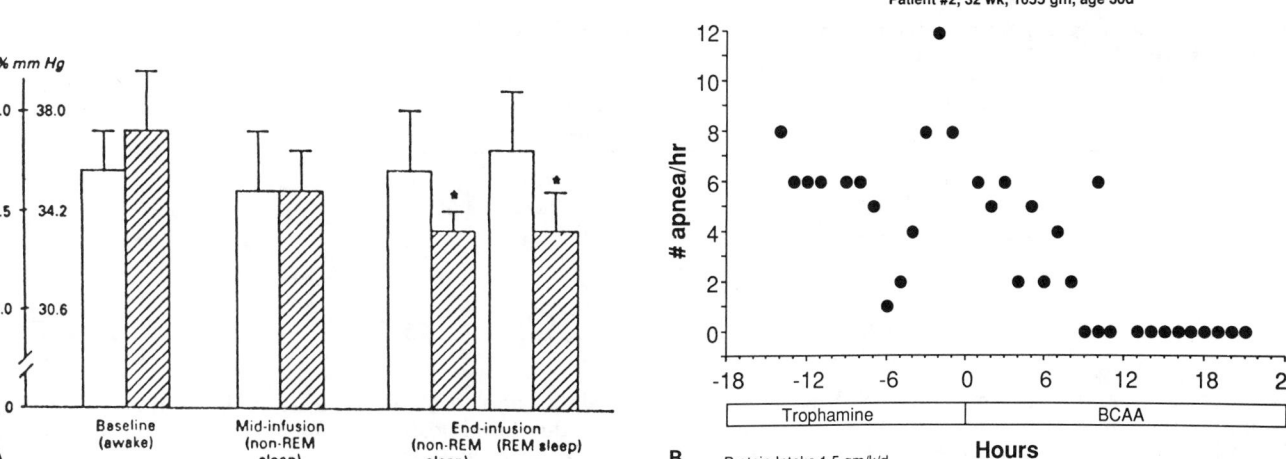

Figure 12-4. (A) End-tidal CO$_2$ during nocturnal infusion of saline (*open bars*) and of 4% BCAA (*shaded bars*) solution (mean ± SE). (Reprinted with permission from Söreide E, Skeie B, Kirvelä O *et al:* Branched-chain amino acid in chronic renal failure patients: Respiratory and sleep effects. Kidney Int 40:539, 1991.) (B) Apneic spells in a neonate (gestational age 32 weeks) before and after administration of branched-chain–enriched TPN. There is a significant reduction in the number of apneic spells associated with the change from standard amino acid solution (TrophAmine: BCAA 30%) to BCAA-enriched solution (BCAA 53%).

amount of rapid eye movement (REM) sleep. During infusion of branched-chain amino acids, the amount of REM sleep returned to normal, and the end-tidal CO$_2$ concentrations decreased significantly, both during REM and non-REM sleep (Fig. 12-4A).[123] This finding suggests that branched-chain amino acids, in addition to their respiratory stimulant actions, may also have advantageous effects on sleep disturbances.[124]

The mechanism for the respiratory stimulant actions of branched-chain amino acids is not known. The observed stimulation of ventilation in response to CO$_2$ challenge exceeds the expectations based on the change in metabolic rate,[120,121] which speaks against solely thermic effects. One hypothesis suggests that branched-chain amino acids may compete with other large neutral amino acids at the blood-brain barrier for the entry into the central nervous system. In particular, inhibition of the entry of tryptophan (a precursor of serotonin) may result in decreased production of serotonin, which has inhibitory influences on respiration.

Fats are also required as a source of essential fatty acids. These constitute two groups of polyunsaturated fatty acids, namely, linoleic and linolenic acids. These fatty acids constitute essential components of all cell membranes and are precursors of several groups of hormone-like substances, the prostaglandins, thromboxanes, and leukotrienes, which are collectively named eicosanoids.[125] Eicosanoids are intimately involved in a wide variety of physiologic functions, such as modulation of vasomotor tone, immune responses, and smooth muscle tone.[126] By altering the composition of dietary fats, metabolism of eicosanoids can be influenced to some extent. In cystic fibrosis promising results have been observed with administration of lipid emulsions, which have been attributed to an alteration in the prevailing imbalance in eicosanoid metabolism.[127] Clinically, the patients showed a marked thinning of secretions and improvements in lung function tests and exercise tolerance. Furthermore, recent investigations have suggested advantageous effects of fish oils in patients with chronic lung diseases. In animal studies, fish oils have reduced pulmonary hypertension in-

duced by chronic hypoxia and protected against vascular remodeling and lung fibrosis. They also reduce inflammatory responses, chiefly through decreased production of proinflammatory leukotrienes. Based on animal experiments, fish oils are suspected to benefit patients with cystic fibrosis or chronic obstructive lung disease. Future research will provide more information concerning the clinical potential of fish oils in these conditions.

Branched-Chain Amino Acids and Respiratory Problems in Preterm Infants. The stimulatory effects of branched-chain amino acids on respiration have evoked a further interest in their impact on the respiratory dysfunction in premature infants. Relatively limited and/or confusing data have been reported in the literature about the quantitative and qualitative requirements of protein in preterm babies. Obviously, sufficient protein must be supplied to preserve both normal tissue renewal (maintenance) and rapid growth (anabolism), and to support the needs associated with various catabolic conditions (e.g., sepsis, respiratory distress). In general, it is believed that positive nitrogen balance and appropriate weight gain may be achieved in a full-term infant by provision of approximately 2–2.5 g·kg^{-1}·day^{-1} of parenteral protein with adequate nonprotein nitrogen calories. The equivalent amount for a preterm is higher, about 2.7–3.5 g·kg^{-1}·day^{-1}.[128]

During the newborn period both mature and premature infants have limited enzymatic activities, resulting in decreased synthesis capacity of some amino acids. Histidine, cysteine, tyrosine, and taurine are considered essential for a newborn.[129,130] The amino acid profile in plasma has been found to change within hours following birth. A marked and rapid decline has been observed in the branched-chain amino acids, resembling a plasma profile of older infants and children with protein-calorie malnutrition. However, a later study has suggested that the lower branched-chain amino acid levels reflect increased utilization rather than malnutrition.[131]

Based on our previous studies with branched-chain

TABLE 12-7. Changes in Dynamic Compliance (Total) and Dynamic Compliance/kg in Premature Infants During Branched-Chain Amino Acid–Enriched (BCAA) Infusion (n = 10)

	Dynamic Compliance (Mean ± SE)	Dynamic Compliance/kg (Mean ± SE)
Day 1 (30% BCAA)	100.0%	100.0%
Day 2 (53% BCAA)	186.9% ± 24.2%*	186.9% ± 23.0%*
Day 3 (30% BCAA)	107.0% ± 5.2%†	106.2% ± 5.3%†

*p < 0.01 vs day 1.
†p < 0.01 vs day 2.

amino acids in adults, a pilot study has been performed examining the effects of these acids in premature infants. Ten babies received routine TPN (30% branched-chain amino acids), enriched TPN (53% branched-chain amino acids), and routine TPN (30% branched-chain amino acids) for three consecutive 24-hour periods. The mean total protein intake was 2.2 $g \cdot kg^{-1} \cdot day^{-1}$ for babies with a mean birth weight of 1503 g. During the study, no significant changes were seen in serial serum electrolytes, calcium, blood urea nitrogen, creatinine, hematocrit, or platelet values. Although plasma amino acids remained within normal range, significant elevations were observed in valine, leucine, and isoleucine after the higher dose of branched-chain amino acids. Pulmonary function tests revealed a significant improvement in compliance during branched-chain amino acid infusion but not in other parameters (Table 12-7). In four of ten infants who had significant apneic spells, there was a marked reduction in the number of apneic periods with enriched branched-chain amino acid administration (Fig. 12-4B). This result strongly supports the concept of the respiratory stimulatory actions of branched-chain amino acids and emphasizes the need for further investigations on the effects of nutritional interventions on various physiologic functions.

Cardiac Disease

The effect of nutrition on the myocardium is a twofold phenomenon. Nutrition has an acute effect on the myocardium; the choice of fuel has important implications for myocardial function and the myocardial tissue damage that occurs under stressed states. A second important effect of nutrition on the myocardium involves protein synthesis and degradation; the myocardium is not spared in starvation and stress conditions, and during catabolic states there is protein loss by the myocardium similar to protein loss by skeletal muscle throughout the body. The loss of protein occurring from the myocardium during starvation is restored during refeeding. The effect of nutrition on myocardial protein synthesis and degradation is important in the preoperative and postoperative periods.

Acute Nutritional Effects on the Myocardium. Cardiac muscle is capable of using a wide variety of substrates as sources of energy.[132-134] Glucose and plasma free fatty acids as well as lactate are the primary fuels, but pyruvate, ketone bodies, triglycerides, and to a lesser extent amino acids can all serve as sources of energy under varying conditions. Utilization of these substrates by the heart is a function of their plasma concentrations, availability of alternate competing substrates, mechanical activity of the heart, supply of oxygen, and plasma levels of certain hormones.

Under normal circumstances, oxidative phosphorylation accounts for almost all of the adenosine triphosphate produced. In a well-oxygenated heart all substrates are completely oxidized in the citric acid cycle. The importance of fatty acids in myocardial metabolism is well known. Their oxidation normally accounts for 60–70% of oxidative metabolism but may under some conditions account for as much as 100%.[135,136] Under most conditions free fatty acids are utilized in preference to carbohydrate. This is particularly true at high levels of cardiac work where fatty acids are the main substrate utilized.[134,137]

Although fatty acids appear to be the preferred fuel under most circumstances, glucose represents an important fuel for respiration in hypoxic hearts. Ischemia leads to a manifold increase in glucose transportation and anaerobic glycolysis. The glycolytic adenosine triphosphate production, however, is insufficient to maintain tissue concentrations of high-energy phosphates. In this situation, lactate becomes an important fuel. With enhancing arterial concentration, as much as 90% of myocardial energy needs can be provided by lactic acid, with a plateau occurring at blood concentrations of 4.5 $mmol \cdot 1^{-1}$.[138] Lactate may also be the preferred substrate in clinical conditions such as septic shock and postcardiac bypass state. During ischemia the oxidation of fatty acids sharply declines, and fatty acids are diverted to deposition as triglycerides.[139] The importance of this phenomenon is explained by the observations that high levels of fatty acids appear to increase myocardial oxygen consumption, to depress cardiac contractility, and to induce cardiac dysrhythmias.[140,141] The regulation of substrate utilization under various conditions is controlled by the glucose fatty acid cycle,[126] which adjusts substrate supply with regard to energy needs.

Physiologic studies over a 50-year period suggest that glucose, insulin, and potassium are beneficial to myocardial performance during conditions such as acute myocardial ischemia or during the perioperative period. In 1926, it was reported that insulin had positive inotropic effects on the isolated, beating turtle heart,[142] and diphtheritic myocarditis was reported to respond positively to dextrose and insulin administration in 1930.[143] The theoretical rationale behind glucose, insulin, and potassium treatment is manifold: raising the blood glucose level increases the rate of glucose utilization; an elevated insulin level stimulates transport of glucose as well as stabilizes cell membranes; and the addition of potassium should compensate for its loss from myocardium during hypoxemia and ischemia.[144,145] Infusion of glucose, insulin, and potassium also depresses the circulating levels of free fatty acids, which are liberated under stressful conditions.

Experimental data have demonstrated protective effects such as improved contractile function, augmented myocardial adenosine triphosphate provision, and preservation of function and structure of hypoxic myocardium with glucose, insulin, and potassium.[145,146] In line with animal studies, administration of glucose, insulin, and potassium in patients has been shown to stabilize ischemic myocardium;[147] to improve ventricular function;[148] to reduce the infarction size;[149] and to reduce hospital mortality in acute myocardial infarction.[150] Attention to serum levels of glucose and potassium is necessary during and following discontinuation of glucose, insulin, and potassium. Pulmonary ingestion, phlebitis, and hypoglycemia are not infrequent complications of the therapy.

Nutrition in Cardiac Cachexia. The undernourished state characteristic of severe heart disease is usually called *cardiac cachexia*.[151] There are two types of cardiac cachexia: the "classic" type, which occurs in patients suffering from severe heart failure, and the "nosocomial" type, which develops in the postoperative state when complications occur, preventing a resumption of normal eating after surgery. One third of patients with Class III or IV heart disease have been found to suffer from cardiac cachexia.[152] In hospitalized patients suffering from both types of cardiac cachexia, approximately one half have been found to have some degree of undernutrition diagnosed by serum albumin and anthropometric measurements.[153]

Patients with classic cardiac cachexia frequently complain of poor appetite, which is compounded by the prescription of unappealing diets. There may be drug-induced vitamin and mineral losses and often some degree of malabsorption. The body weight is frequently normal, but physical and biochemical examinations indicate chronic undernutrition. The nosocomial cachexia develops in days or weeks postoperatively because of complications; intake is sharply reduced and nutrient losses are excessive.

A profound difference in mortality and morbidity rates has been found between patients with cardiac disease who suffered from preoperative malnutrition and patients with good nutritional status.[154] It has been suggested that preoperative nutritional care could reduce myocardial complications following surgery and improve myocardial function.[155]

When the undernourished cardiac patient is scheduled for surgery, some researchers recommend a 2-week preoperative course of nutrition therapy.[153] Minimal recommended therapy in the classic form of cardiac cachexia is vitamin and mineral replacement; some patients may benefit from complete nutritional supplementation.

The branched-chain amino acids have been shown to exert some stimulatory actions on cardiac protein synthesis. This effect is primarily caused by leucine, which also inhibits protein degradation.[155] However, the beneficial effects of branched-chain amino acids on the myocardium appear to occur only under catabolic conditions, and no acute effects on muscle protein turnover could be obtained in cardiac patients with muscle wasting, *i.e.*, cardiac cachexia.[156] Some preliminary animal data suggest that branched-chain amino acids could preserve myocardial energy supply during ischemic conditions,[157] but more detailed studies are needed to understand the clinical implications.

Adequate cardiac levels of carnitine are necessary for oxidative metabolism of long-chain fatty acids. Carnitine transports long-chain fatty acids from the cytosol to the mitochondrial site of beta oxidation. It has been proposed that carnitine supplementation might benefit the myocardium during ischemic, stressed conditions owing to its prevention of intracellular accumulation of free fatty acids.[158] Hypoxia and ischemia obviously deplete cardiac stores of carnitine.[159] Carnitine deficiency has been suggested as an etiologic factor for cardiomyopathia, and administration of carnitine has improved myocardial function in cardiomyopathic animals.[160,161] Medium-chain triglycerides are not dependent on carnitine for oxidation and may thus be beneficial for cardiac patients.

Ingestion of a fatty meal may precipitate angina (postprandial angina). This occurs some hours after ingestion and can be avoided by continuous (intravenous or enteral) administration of nutrients. In particular, infusion of fat emulsions may produce negative inotropic effects on the heart.[30] In cardiac patients, a rapid infusion of intravenous fat emulsions has been shown to decrease cardiac output. This effect is absent if the infusion rate is decreased, which suggests vasomotor effects of intravenous fat emulsions, most likely mediated through changes in the production of prostaglandins.

Brain Injury

Development of irreversible brain tissue damage in brain ischemia is not always proportional to the degree of tissue oxygen deficiency. In experimental animal studies, raising the blood glucose level before a global ischemic insult increases brain damage.[162-164] This suggests that preischemic hyperglycemia may have contributed to the neurologic injury. Findings similar to those in animals have been described in patients with ischemic stroke.[165] In a retrospective study, blood glucose level on admission was significantly related to neurologic recovery after cardiac arrest, with a high blood glucose level on admission being associated with poor neurologic recovery.[166] The mechanism for glucose-mediated injury may be related to enhanced tissue lactic production, or the glucose may exert the effect by acting as an osmotic agent.[167] The results strongly suggest that hyperglycemia should be avoided in patients at risk for cerebral ischemia (during cardiopulmonary bypass, induced hypotension, cerebral vascular surgery, and head injury).

There is considerable controversy regarding glucose administration during intracranial surgery. The administration of $100-150$ g·day^{-1} of glucose produces protein sparing in starving individuals, decreases fat and protein mobilization during a short fast, and provides free water; it has therefore been advocated for patients undergoing general surgery.[168] In view of the risk of intraoperative ischemia and the experimental and clinical findings noted above, it may be prudent to avoid giving excessive amounts of glucose intraoperatively.[169] The same considerations apply for glucose infusion to patients with head injury. Sieber et al[170] found that intraoperative glucose infusion ($11-15$ g·hr^{-1}) produces glucose levels greater than 200 mg·dl^{-1}, which are the levels that have been associated with potentiation of ischemic neurologic damage. Similarly, the intensive care management of patients with head trauma should include avoidance of hyperglycemia.

Acute Renal Failure

Most patients with acute renal failure (ARF) have some degree of net protein breakdown and disordered fluid, electrolyte, or acid–base status. There is often excess total body water, azotemia, hyperkalemia, hyperphosphatemia, hypocalcemia, hyperuricemia, and a large anion-gap metabolic acidosis. The net protein degradation in ARF can be massive.[171] Patients are more likely to be catabolic when the ARF is caused by shock or sepsis. It is likely that the profound catabolic response of many patients with ARF may increase the risk of infection and delayed wound healing, prolong convalescence, and increase mortality. The net protein catabolism may accelerate the rate of rise in the plasma levels of potassium, phosphorus, nitrogenous metabolites, and acids.[172] The mechanisms for the catabolic effects of ARF are not well defined. The uremia *per se* may have potential catabolic effects, but other causes of wasting and malnutrition in ARF (e.g., anorexia and vomiting, underlying medical disorders, loss of nutrients during dialysis) clearly also contribute. The aim of nutritional therapy in ARF is to counter the increased protein breakdown and to maintain protein stores. This goal should be accomplished without an increase in the production of uremic toxins, e.g., without worsening azotemia. Ultimately, improved nutritional status in ARF patients should improve recovery, renal function, and survival.

Clinical studies performed in the 1960s suggested that amino acid therapy hastened recovery and lessened mortality in ARF.[173,174] Patients with ARF who received an essential amino acid solution and hypertonic glucose had an improved recovery of renal function but no significant improvement in overall hospital survival.[174] In a more recent study, three treatment regimens were compared: hypertonic dextrose alone; dextrose in combination with essential amino acids; and dextrose in combination with essential and nonessential amino acids.[171] No improvement was found in the recovery of renal function or in patient survival among the three groups, and the patients in the amino acid groups did not show an improvement in nitrogen balance. Increasing the nitrogen intake of patients with ARF does not seem to improve nitrogen balance.[175] It has been suggested that a different formulation of amino acids might be required for patients with ARF. Solutions with enhanced branched-chain amino acid content have been reported to reduce net protein catabolism in nonuremic patients. Further studies are needed to assess the high branched-chain amino acid solutions in ARF. However, in experimental ARF, amino acid solutions have been reported to increase the rapidity and severity of ARF and to increase the severity of postischemic ARF.[176,177] Lysine has recently been suggested to have nephrotoxic effects,[178] but it is unknown whether the lysine in standard amino acid solutions exerts a nephrotoxic effect in humans.

Another important factor in the nutritional therapy is the calorie intake. Adequate calorie intake in nonuremic patients is correlated with positive nitrogen balance and better outcome. Because the provision of adequate calories in many patients requires an infusion of 1–1.5 liters of fluid daily, an increased frequency of dialysis may be needed. Those patients undergoing dialysis usually tolerate standard amino acid solutions, but special attention should be given to monitoring fluid and electrolyte balance. Those who are not undergoing dialysis tolerate standard amino acid formulations poorly, and administration of an essential amino acid formulation with adequate amounts of carbohydrate may result in better utilization of endogenous urea by conversion to nonessential amino acids.[179]

Perioperative Nutritional Support

Preoperative Nutritional Support

There is a well-established relationship between the nutritional status of patients undergoing surgical procedures and the risk of perioperative morbidity and mortality.[4,6-8] Several studies have reported a decreased incidence of com-plications (sepsis, wound infections, pneumonia, and mortality) after preoperative nutritional support.[4,180-182] The impact on mortality and morbidity is unclear,[181,183-188] however, and the optimal duration of nutrition support and criteria for the use of preoperative TPN remain poorly defined. Some authors suggest that the patient's response to TPN in terms of weight, albumin, and so forth may be used as an indicator of appropriate timing of elective operation.[181] Patients who lost weight and showed a rise in serum albumin levels during 1 week of TPN were at a reduced risk for postoperative complications, whereas patients who responded with decreased serum albumin values and increased weight remained at high risk for postoperative complications and should be considered candidates for prolonged preoperative nutritional support.

Patients who are well nourished and require intravenous fluids for less than 5 days should receive conventional hypocaloric fluid therapy postoperatively. If the patient is depleted, TPN should be considered even if a return to an oral diet is anticipated within a few days. TPN should always be considered if the postoperative semistarvation period is likely to be greater than 4 or 5 days. In general, one should begin TPN early, based on this estimation, rather than waiting in anticipation of a return to gastrointestinal function.

Interactions Among Nutrition, Body Composition, and Perioperative Mortality and Morbidity

With nutritional depletion, the extracellular fluid compartment increases in relation to total body water.[12,189,190] It is clear that the regulation of albumin synthesis is sensitive to the patient's nutritional status,[191,192] but the relationship between serum albumin, protein synthesis, and body composition has not been well defined.

With nutritional repletion, as defined by positive nitrogen balance, it has been observed that the expected increases in albumin concentrations are not consistently seen. The relationship between serum albumin and nutritional status appears to be more dependent on changes in body composition than on protein synthesis.

Patients with anorexia nervosa are markedly protein-calorie depleted, but since this occurs on a balanced nutritional regimen (including protein), there is no absolute expansion of the extracellular fluid compartment. Under these conditions serum albumin levels tend to remain normal. In the healthy adult who is injured or has an acute septic episode, a marked degree of fluid resuscitation is required. This is accompanied by a fall in serum albumin, even though whole body protein status is fairly intact. This indicates that expanding extracellular fluid, rather than negative nitrogen balance, is the cause of the reduction in serum albumin. When parenteral nutrition is administered and albumin synthesis is increased, an expanded extracellular fluid prevents an increase in serum albumin concentration; the albumin simply diffuses through an enlarged fluid space. When the stress response and capillary leak diminish, however, the extracellular fluid compartment contracts; this contraction is associated with a return of serum albumin to normal levels.

Starker et al[193,194] used nitrogen balance to document the nutritional status of hospitalized patients during refeeding. Measurements of sodium balance were used to show alterations in the extracellular fluid. By examining concurrent changes in plasma levels of albumin, body weight, and sodium balance, the relation of albumin to the status of the extracellular fluid compartment, rather than to nitrogen balance, was established.[193] Patients were categorized as being

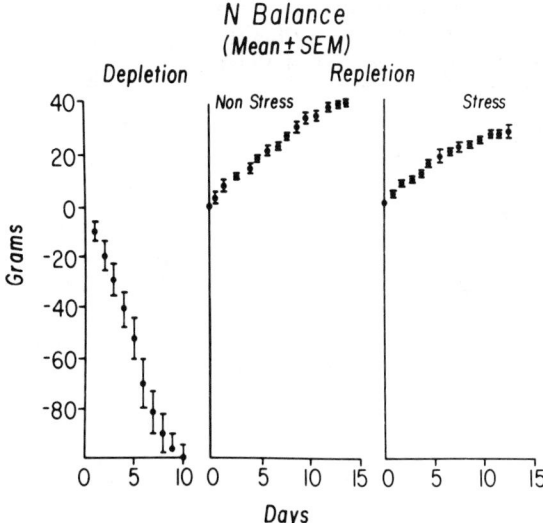

Figure 12-5. Changes in nitrogen (N) balance in stressed and unstressed patients. Both groups were in positive N balance. (Reprinted with permission from Starker PM, Gump FE, Askanazi J *et al:* Serum albumin levels as an index of nutritional support. Surgery 91:194, 1982.)

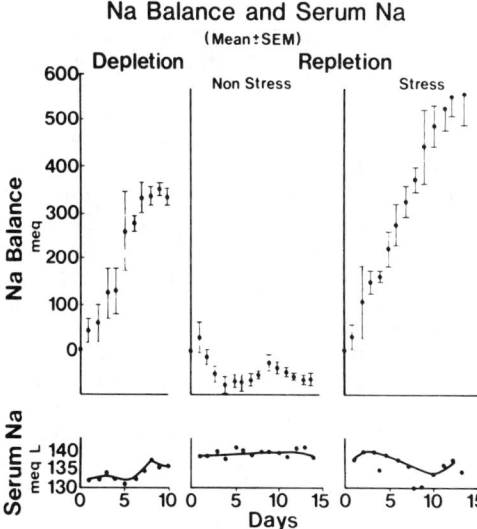

Figure 12-6. Alterations in sodium balance are shown. The stressed patients retain sodium, whereas the unstressed patients contract their extracellular fluid, as evidenced by a negative Na balance. (Reprinted with permission from Starker PM, Gump FE, Askanazi J *et al:* Serum albumin levels as an index of nutritional support. Surgery 91:194, 1982.)

either stressed or nonstressed; the stressed group consisted mostly of patients with active underlying infection. Figure 12-5 demonstrates that there was no significant difference in nitrogen balance between the stressed and the unstressed group. Figure 12-6 shows the changes in sodium balance and serum sodium concentrations. During nutritional depletion, sodium balance was positive. It appears that weight loss under hospital conditions does not necessarily reflect the loss of body tissue, since an expanded extracellular fluid compartment tends to mask the loss of body protein. During repletion, the nonstressed group displayed a negative sodium balance, whereas in the stressed group sodium balance was markedly positive. Thus there was a contraction of the extracellular fluid compartment during repletion in the nonstressed group.

Serum albumin levels are shown in Figure 12-7. There is a rise in serum albumin in the nonstressed group, whereas it falls during the first 2 weeks of repletion in the stressed group of patients. The response observed among the stressed group probably reflects an altered response of the fluid compartment to nutritional therapy. Many of the patients in this group had underlying infection or tumor. It is likely that one of these stresses played a part in the failure of this group to diurese and normalize the extracellular fluid.

It should be emphasized that these patients were in positive nitrogen balance and hence were in the anabolic state. Under these conditions, we would have expected albumin synthesis to increase.[192] In a study of patients who were in a poor nutritional state postoperatively, Shizgal[195] noted that one patient, who developed an intra-abdominal abscess, had a markedly greater extracellular fluid expansion than the other patients, indicating that nutritional depletion can exacerbate the expansion of the extracellular fluid seen in sepsis. Furthermore, ongoing sepsis can prevent normalization of the extracellular fluid despite nutritional support. This may have profound implications for patients, particularly those with respiratory and neurologic dysfunction. Larca *et al*,[196] studying patients who received nutritional support while on mechanical ventilation, demonstrated that

patients who had a rise in plasma protein levels in response to nutritional therapy could be weaned from a mechanical ventilator, whereas those whose plasma protein levels fell during TPN could not. Bryan-Brown *et al*[197] reported three cases in which cerebral edema, although unresponsive to conventional therapy, improved as a result of adequate nutritional support. Body composition changes in these patients demonstrate that the extracellular fluid returned to normal with adequate nutrition.

Starker *et al*[194] correlated changes in skeletal muscle composition with whole body electrolyte and nitrogen balance in order to establish the contribution made by skeletal muscle to changes in whole body fluid and electrolyte composi-

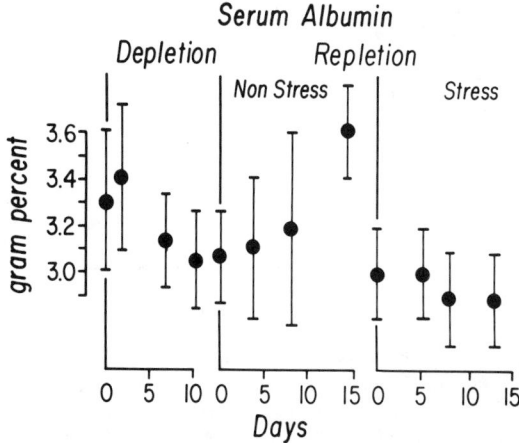

Figure 12-7. Serum albumin levels increase in relation to negative sodium balance and not in relation to nitrogen balance. (Reprinted with permission from Starker PM, Gump FE, Askanazi J *et al:* Serum albumin levels as an index of nutritional support. Surgery 91:194, 1982.)

tion during nutritional repletion. In this study, TPN was administered to ten patients for up to 25 days. Metabolic rate and balances of nitrogen, sodium, and potassium were measured daily. Muscle biopsies were taken prior to the administration of TPN, in the middle, and at the end of the nutritional regimen. Prior to the institution of parenteral nutrition, muscle concentrations of water, sodium, and chloride were higher than normal. With the administration of exogenous nutrients, all three declined. The calculated loss in muscle water, however, accounted for only about one half of the whole body changes. It would appear, then, that nutritional support results in a restoration of cell mass and a contraction of the extracellular fluid compartment (Fig. 12-8). The restoration of cell mass may occur primarily in muscle, but the contraction of the extracellular fluid must occur in other tissues. The contraction of the extracellular fluid is believed to occur in such tissues as the brain and the lung, thus resulting in the improvements in pulmonary and cerebral status observed in patients receiving nutritional support.

For patients undergoing an operation, the expansion of the extracellular fluid due to nutritional depletion may represent a serious risk factor. A study has correlated the postoperative course with the preoperative response to nutritional support.[180] Nutritionally depleted patients received an average of 1 week of TPN prior to major abdominal operation. Of the 16 patients who exhibited the characteristic response to early nutritional support, i.e., diuresis of the expanded extracellular fluid with a resultant loss of weight and rise in serum albumin, only one developed a complication in the postoperative period. The other 16 patients did not ex-

TABLE 12-8. Postoperative Complications Related to Response to Total Parenteral Nutrition

Complications	Group I (n = 16)	Group II (n = 16)	Group III (n = 16)
Mechanical			
Prolonged ventilatory support	0	4	0
Fistula	0	0	1
Wound dehiscence	0	1	0
Anastomotic leak	0	1	0
Total	0	6	1
Infections			
Sepsis	0	2	0
Pneumonia	1	3	0
Wound infection	0	3	1
Abscess	0	1	0
Total	1	9	1
Death (nutritionally related)	0	2	0
Total complications	1	15	2
Total number of patients developing complications*	1	9	2
Percent of patients developing complications	4.3	45	12.5

*$p < 0.01$ (Group I/Group II); $p < 0.05$ (Group II/Group III).

Reprinted with permission from Starker PM, LaSala PA, Askanazi J et al: The response to TPN: A form of nutritional assessment. Ann Surg 198:720, 1983, and Starker PM, LaSala PA, Askanazi J et al: The influence of preoperative TPN on morbidity and mortality. Surg Gynecol Obstet 162:569, 1986.

hibit this response to TPN. They retained additional fluid, gained weight, and showed a decrease in serum albumin levels. Eight of these patients developed a total of 15 postoperative complications (Table 12-8). In a follow-up study, Starker et al[181] demonstrated that patients who do not respond positively to TPN in 1 week will do so if TPN is maintained for 4–6 weeks, with a consequent reduction in the rate of mortality and morbidity (Group III in Table 12-8).

Postoperative Nutritional Support

A study by Askanazi et al[182] reviewed the effect of nutritional support on duration of hospitalization in patients undergoing radical cystectomy. Thirty-five patients were randomly assigned to receive either 5% dextrose solution plus electrolytes or TPN following an operation. The assigned nutritional regimen was continued for 1 week after the operation until oral intake resumed. The group receiving immediate postoperative TPN had a median duration of hospital stay of 17 days, while median hospital stay for the group receiving 5% dextrose solution was 24 days (Fig. 12-9). All other patient characteristics such as age, sex, stage/grade of tumor, and extent of preoperative radiotherapy were similar. These results demonstrated that immediate postoperative institution of nutritional support reduced hospitalization time following radical cystectomy and indicated that the routine use of 5% dextrose as postoperative nutrition should be re-evaluated.

Recently, there has been growing acceptance of the practice of immediate postoperative enteral feeding. It is well known that gradual atrophy of intestinal mucosa occurs within a few days if no enteral feeding is given. Aside from the detrimental effects on the motility and absorptive functions of the bowel, atrophy predisposes to translocation of

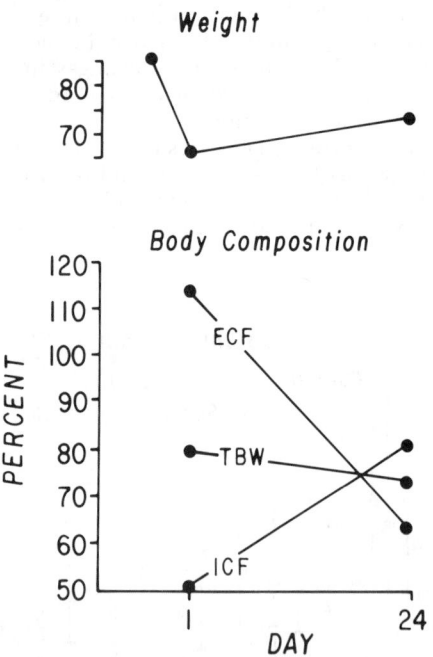

Figure 12-8. Changes in body weight (kg) and body composition (percent of predicted) during nutritional repletion in a patient with neurologic damage. The study demonstrates a reduction in extracellular fluid after the institution of nutritional support, which corresponds to an improvement in clinical condition. (Reprinted with permission from Bryan-Brown CW, Savitz MH, Elwyn DH et al: Cerebral edema unresponsive to conventional therapy in neurosurgical patients with unsuspected nutritional failure. Crit Care Med 1:125, 1973.)

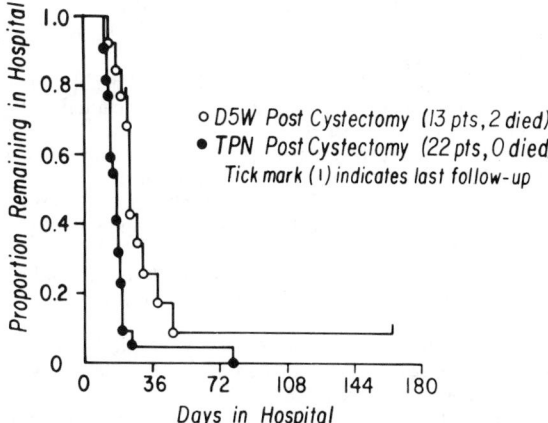

Figure 12-9. Length of hospital stay following radical cystectomy. In the group receiving immediate postoperative parenteral nutrition, median duration of hospitalization is reduced by 7 days. (Reprinted with permission from Askanazi J, Hensle TW, Starker PM et al: Effect of immediate postoperative nutritional support on length of hospitalization. Ann Surg 203:236, 1986.)

bacteria and their toxins across the intestinal wall to the portal circulation and to the liver, with subsequent deterioration of hepatic function or development of serious infectious complications.[198] Hence, it appears reasonable to utilize the enteral route as soon as possible to preserve villous function. Postoperatively the functioning of stomach and colon is impaired for 2–5 days, but the small intestine is able to accept nutrients as early as the day of the operation. Therefore, the common practice is to place the tip of feeding tube through the pyloric port into the jejunum. At first glucose or amino acid solutions are given at low concentrations, but during the next few days the feeding regimen can gradually be increased up to its full composition.

REFERENCES

1. Insel J, Elwyn DH: Body composition. In Askanazi J, Starker P, Weissman C (eds): Fluid and Electrolyte Management in Critical Care, p 3. Boston, Butterworths, 1986
2. Shaw SN, Elwyn DH, Askanazi J et al: Effects of increasing nitrogen intake on nitrogen balance and energy expenditure in nutritionally depleted adult patients receiving parenteral nutrition. Am J Clin Nutr 37:930, 1983
3. Heymsfield SB, Lichtman S, Baumgartner RN, et al: Body composition of humans: Comparison of two improved four-compartment models that differ in expense, technical complexity, and radiation exposure. Am J Clin Nutr 52:52, 1990
4. Blackburn GL, Bistrian BR, Miani BS et al: Nutritional and metabolic assessment of the hospitalized patient. JPEN 1:11, 1977
5. Calloway DH: Nitrogen balance of men with marginal intakes of protein and energy. J Nutr 105:914, 1975
6. Kinney JM, Long CL, Gump FE et al: Tissue composition of weight loss in surgical patients. Ann Surg 168:459, 1968
7. Keys A, Brozek J, Henschel H et al: The biology of human starvation. Minneapolis, University of Minnesota Press, 1950
8. Shizgal HM: Body composition and nutritional support. Surg Clin North Am 61:727, 1981
9. Viteri F, Behar M, Arroyave G et al: Clinical aspects of protein malnutrition. In Munro HN, Allison JB (eds): Mammalian Protein Metabolism, vol 2, p 235. New York, Academic Press, 1964
10. Gamble JL: Physiological information gained from studies on the life raft ration. Harvey Lect 42:247, 1946–1947
11. Schutz Y, Acheson K, Bessard T et al: Effects of a 7-day carbohydrate hyperalimentation on energy metabolism in healthy individuals. JPEN 6:351, 1982
12. Elwyn DH, Bryan-Brown CW, Shoemaker WC: Nutritional aspects of body water dislocations in postoperative and depleted patients. Ann Surg 182:76, 1975
13. Abrams JS, Deane RS, Davis HJ: Adverse effects of salt and water retention on pulmonary functions in patients with multiple trauma. J Trauma 13:788, 1973
14. Bursztein S, Elwyn DH, Askanazi J, Kinney JM (eds): Fuel utilization in normal, starving and pathological states. In Energy Metabolism, Indirect Calorimetry, and Nutrition, p 119. Baltimore, Williams & Wilkins, 1989
15. Owen OE, Morgan AP, Kemp HG et al: Brain metabolism during fasting. J Clin Invest 46:1589, 1967
16. Aoki TT, Muller WA, Brennan MF et al: Metabolic effects of glucose in brief and prolonged fasted man. Am J Clin Nutr 28:507, 1975
17. Cuthbertson DP: Post-shock metabolic response. Lancet 1:433, 1942
18. Bursztein S, Elwyn D, Askanazi J, Kinney JM (eds): Fuel utilization in normal, starving, and pathological states. In: Energy Metabolism, Indirect Calorimetry, and Nutrition, p. 119. Baltimore, Williams & Wilkins, 1989
19. Kinney JM, Duke JH Jr, Long CL et al: Tissue fuel and weight loss after injury. J Clin Pathol 4 (suppl 23):65, 1970
20. Long CL, Spencer JL, Kinney JM et al: Carbohydrate metabolism in man: Effect of elective operations and major surgery. J Appl Physiol 31:110, 1971
21. Chen RW, Postlethwart RW: The biochemistry of wound healing. Monogr Surg Sci 1:215, 1964
22. Recommended Dietary Allowances, 9th ed. Washington, DC, Nutritional Academy of Sciences, 1980
23. Blakburn GL, Bistrian BR, Miani BS et al: Nutritional and metabolic assessment of the hospitalized patient. JPEN 1:11, 1977
24. Kudsk KA, Sheldon GF: Nutritional assessment. In Fisher JE (ed): Surgical Nutrition, p 407. Boston, Little, Brown, 1983
25. Mullen JL, Buzby GP, Waldman MT et al: Prediction of greater morbidity and mortality by preoperative nutritional assessment. Surg Forum 30:80, 1979
26. Linn BS: A protein energy malnutrition scale (PEMS). Ann Surg 200:747, 1984
27. Baker JP, Detsky AS, Wesson DE et al: Nutritional assessment: A comparison of clinical judgment and objective measurements. N Engl J Med 306:969, 1982
28. Copeland EM, MacFayden BV, Lanzotti VF: Intravenous hyperalimentation as an adjunct to cancer therapy. Am J Surg 129:167, 1975
29. Daly JM, Hoffman K, Lieberman M et al: Nutritional support in the cancer patient. JPEN 14:244S, 1990
30. Skeie B, Askanazi J, Rothkopf MM et al: Intravenous fat emulsions and lung function. Crit Care Med 16:183, 1987
31. Heymsfield SB, Erbland M, Casper BS et al: Enteral nutritional support. Clin Chest Med 7:41, 1986
32. Smith JL, Heymsfield SB: Enteral nutritional support: Formula preparation from modular ingredients. JPEN 7:280, 1982
33. Henriques V, Anderson AC: Über parenteral Ernahring durch intravenous Injection. J Physiol Chem 23:31, 1977
34. Brunschwig AD, Clark DE, Corbin N: Symposium on abdominal surgery: Postoperative nitrogen loss and studies on parenteral nitrogen nutrition by means of casein digestion. Ann Surg 115:1091, 1942
35. Cuthbertson DP: Further observations on the disturbance of metabolism caused by injury, with particular reference to the dietary requirements of fracture cases. Br J Surg 23:505, 1936
36. Rhoads JE, Alexander CE: Nutritional problems of surgical patients. Ann NY Acad Sci 63:268, 1955
37. Schuberth O, Wretlind A: Intravenous infusion of fat emulsions, phosphatides and emulsifying agents. Clinical and experimental studies. Acta Chir Scand (Suppl) 278:1021, 1961
38. Wretlind A: Development of fat emulsions. JPEN 5:230, 1981

39. Wilmore DW, Dudrick SJ: Growth and development of an infant receiving all nutrients exclusively by vein. JAMA 203: 860, 1968

40. Starker PM, LaSala PA, Askanazi J: Placement of Broviac catheters for total parenteral nutrition. Surg Gynecol Obstet 156: 229, 1983

41. Heimbach DM, Ivey TD: Technique for placement of a permanent home hyperalimentation catheter. Surg Gynecol Obstet 143:635, 1976

42. Broviac JW, Cole JJ, Scribner BH: A silicone rubber atrial catheter for prolonged parenteral alimentation. Surg Gynecol Obstet 136:602, 1973

43. Hickman RO, Buckner D, Chift RA et al: A modified right atrial catheter for access to the venous system in marrow transplant recipients. Surg Gynecol Obstet 148:871, 1979

44. Rose SG, Pitsch RJ, Karrer FW, Moor BJ: Subclavian catheter infections. JPEN 12:511, 1988

45. Elwyn DH: Repletion of the malnourished patient. In Blackburn GL, Grant JP, Young VR (eds): Amino Acids: Metabolism and Medical Application, p 359. Boston, Wright PSG, 1983

46. Wolfe BM, Culebras JM, Sim AJ et al: Substrate interaction in intravenous feeding: Comparative effects of carbohydrate and fat on amino acid utilization in fasting man. Ann Surg 186: 518, 1977

47. Burstein S, Elwyn DH, Askanazi J, Kinney JM (eds): Nitrogen balance. In: Energy Metabolism, Indirect Calorimetry, and Nutrition, p 85. Baltimore, Williams & Wilkins, 1989

48. Munro HN: General aspects of the regulation of protein metabolism by diet and by hormones. In Munro HN, Allison JB (eds): Mammalian Protein Metabolism, vol 1, p 381. New York, Academic Press, 1964

49. Brennan MF, Fitzpatrick GF, Cohen KH et al: Glycerol: Major contributor to the short term protein sparing effect of fat emulsions in normal man. Ann Surg 182:386, 1975

50. Long JM III, Wilmore DW, Mason AD Jr et al: Effect of carbohydrate and fat intake on nitrogen excretion during total intravenous feeding. Ann Surg 185:417, 1977

51. Nordenström J, Askanazi J, Elwyn DH et al: Nitrogen balance during total parenteral nutrition: Glucose versus fat. Ann Surg 197:27, 1983

52. MacFie J, Smith RC, Hill GL: Glucose or fat as a nonprotein energy source. Gastroenterology 80:103, 1981

53. Nordenström J, Jeevanandam M, Elwyn DH et al: Increasing glucose intake during total parenteral nutrition increases norepinephrine excretion in trauma and sepsis. Clin Physiol 1:525, 1981

54. Askanazi J, Nordenström J, Rosenbaum SH et al: Nutrition for the patient with respiratory failure: Glucose versus fat. Anesthesiology 54:373, 1981

55. Meguid MM, Akahoshi M, Jeffers S et al: Amelioration of metabolic complications of conventional TPN: A prospective randomized study. Arch Surg 119:1294, 1984

56. Wolfe BM, Ryder MA, Nishikawa RA et al: Complications of parenteral nutrition. Am J Surg 152:93, 1986

57. Parsa MH, Habif DV, Ferrer JM et al: Intravenous hyperalimentation: Indications, technique and complications. Bull NY Acad Med 48:920, 1972

58. Knochel JP: Hypophosphatemia. West J Med 125:15, 1981

59. Sherwin R, Joshi P, Hendler R et al: Hyperglucagonemia in Laennec's cirrhosis. The role of portal-systemic shunting. N Engl J Med 290:239, 1974

60. Striebel JP, Holm E, Lutz H et al: Parenteral nutrition and coma therapy with amino acids in hepatic failure. JPEN 3:240, 1979

61. Soeters PB, Fisher JE: Insulin, glucagon, amino acid imbalance, and hepatic encephalopathy. Lancet 2:880, 1976

62. Bower RH, Fisher JE: Nutritional management of hepatic encephalopathy. In Draper HH (ed): Advances in Nutritional Research, vol 5, p 1. New York, Plenum Publishing, 1983

63. Fischer JE: Current concepts of pathogenesis of hepatic encephalopathy. In Preisig R, Bircher J (eds): The Liver, p 374. Bern, Edito Cantor Aulendorf, 1979

64. James JH, Freund H, Fischer JE: Amino acids in hepatic encephalopathy. Gastroenterology 77:421, 1979

65. Rosen HM, Yoshimura N, Hodgman JM et al: Plasma amino acid patterns in hepatic encephalopathy of differing etiology. Gastroenterology, 72:483, 1977

66. Fischer JE, Rosen HM, Ebeid AM et al: The effect of normalization of plasma amino acids on hepatic encephalopathy in man. Surgery 80:77, 1976

67. James JH, Fischer JE: Transport of neutral amino acids at the blood brain barrier. Pharmacology 22:1, 1981

68. Cangiano C, Cascino A, Fiaccadori F et al: Is the blood-brain barrier really intact in portal-systemic encephalopathy? Lancet 1:1367, 1981

69. James JH, Escourrou J, Fischer JE: Blood-brain neutral amino acid transport activity is increased after portacaval anastomosis. Science 200:1395, 1978

70. Smith AR, Rossi-Fanelli F, Ziparo V et al: Alterations in plasma and CSF amino acids, amines and metabolites in hepatic coma. Ann Surg 187:343, 1978

71. McCullough AJ, Czaja AJ, Jones JD et al: The nature and prognostic significance of serial amino acid determinations in severe chronic active liver disease. Gastroenterology 81:645, 1981

72. Fischer JE, Baldessarini RJ: False neurotransmitters and hepatic failure. Lancet 2:75, 1971

73. James JH, Cangiano C, Cardelli-Cangiano P et al: Glutamine linked hyperammonemia and neurotransmitter derangements in portal systemic shunting. Gastroenterology 78:1308, 1980

74. Skeie B, Gil K, Kvetan V et al: Branch-chain amino acids: Their metabolism and clinical utility. Crit Care Med 18:549, 1990

75. Felig P, Wahren J: Protein turnover and amino acid metabolism in the regulation of gluconeogenesis. Fed Proc 33:1092, 1974

76. Buse MG, Reid SS: Leucine: A possible regulator of protein turnover in muscle. J Clin Invest 56:1250, 1975

77. Chua B, Seihl DL, Morgan HE: Effect of leucine and metabolites of branched chain amino acids on protein turnover in heart. J Biol Chem 254:8358, 1979

78. Freund HR, James JH, Fischer JE: Nitrogen-sparing mechanisms of singly administered branched chain amino acids in the injured rat. Surgery 90:237, 1981

79. Sapir DG, Owen OE, Pozefsky T et al: Nitrogen-sparing induced by ketoanalogues of essential amino acids. J Clin Invest 53:70a, 1974

80. Fischer JE, Funovics JM, Aguirre A et al: The role of plasma amino acids in hepatic encephalopathy. Surgery 78:276, 1975

81. Smith AR, Rossi-Fanelli F, Freund H et al: Sulfur-containing amino acids in experimental hepatic coma in the dog and the monkey. Surgery 85:677, 1979

82. Okada A, Kamata S, Kim CW et al: Treatment of hepatic encephalopathy with BCAA-rich amino acid mixture. In Walser M, Williamson R (eds): Metabolism and Clinical Implications of Branched-Chain Amino and Ketoacids, p 447. New York, Elsevier/North Holland, 1987

83. Wahren JJ, Denis J, Desurmont P et al: Is intravenous administration of branched chain amino acids effective in treatment of hepatic encephalopathy? A multicenter study. Hepatology 3:475, 1983

84. Michel H, Pomier-Layrargues G, Duhamel O et al: Intravenous infusion of ordinary and modified amino acid solutions in the management of hepatic encephalopathy (controlled study of 30 patients). Gastroenterology 79:1038, 1979

85. Rossi-Fanelli F, Riggio O, Cangiano C et al: Branched-chain amino acids versus lactulose in the treatment of hepatic coma. A controlled study. Dig Dis Sci 27:929, 1982

86. Gluud C, Dejgaard A, Hardt F et al: Preliminary treatment results with balanced amino acid infusion to patients with hepatic encephalopathy. Scand J Gastroenterol 18 (suppl 86): 19, 1983

87. Fiaccadori F, Ghinelli F, Pedretti G et al: Branched chain amino acid enriched solutions in the treatment of encephalopathy: A controlled study. In Capocaccia L, Fischer JE, Rossi-Fanelli F (eds): Hepatic Encephalopathy in Chronic Liver Failure, p 311. New York, Plenum Press, 1984

88. Cerra FB, Cheung NK, Fischer JE et al: Disease-specific amino

acid infusion (F080) in hepatic encephalopathy: A prospective, randomized, double-blind, controlled trial. JPEN 9:288, 1985

89. Michel H, Bories P, Aubin JP et al: Treatment of acute hepatic encephalopathy in cirrhotics with a branched-chain amino acids enriched versus a conventional amino acids mixture. Liver 5:282, 1985

90. Marchesini G, Zoli M, Dondi C et al: Anticatabolic effect of branched-chain amino acid-enriched solutions in patients with liver cirrhosis. Hepatology 2:420, 1982

91. Bach AC, Storck D, Meraihi Z: Medium-chain triglyceride-based fat emulsions: An alternative supply in stress and sepsis. JPEN 12:82S, 1988

92. Tao RC, Yosimura NN: Carnitine metabolism and its application to parenteral nutrition. JPEN 4:469, 1980

93. Weissman C, Chiolero R, Askanazi J, Gil KM, Elwyn D, Kinney JM: Intravenous infusion of a medium-chain triglyceride enriched lipid emulsion. Cri Care Med 16:1183, 1988

94. Manner T, Katz DP, Haberek A, Shaw HL, Askanazi J, Kirvelä O: The effects of parenteral medium chain emulsion in a patient with liver function abnormalities: Submitted for publication

95. Liaw KY, Askanazi J, Michelson CB et al: Effect of postoperative nutrition on muscle high energy phosphates. Ann Surg 195:12, 1982

96. Sakamato A, Moldawer LL, Usui S et al: In vivo evidence for the unique nitrogen-sparing mechanism of branched-chain amino acid administration. Surg Forum 30:67, 1979

97. Odessey RK, Khairallah EA, Goldberg AL: Origin and possible significance of alanine production by skeletal muscle. J Biol Chem 249:7623, 1974

98. Blackburn GL, Moldawer LL, Usui S et al: Branched chain amino acid concentrations and metabolism during starvation, injury, and infection. Surgery 86:307, 1979

99. Freund HR, Yoshimura N, Fischer JE: The effect of branched chain amino acids and hypertonic glucose infusions on post injury catabolism in the rat. Surgery 87:401, 1980

100. Blackburn GL, Desai SP, Keenan RA et al: Clinical use of branched chain amino-acid enriched solutions in the stressed and injured patient. In Walser M, Williamson JR (eds): Metabolism and Clinical Implications of Branched Chain Amino and Ketoacids, p 521. New York, Elsevier/North Holland, 1981

101. Gimmon Z, Freund HR, Fischer JE: The optimal branched-chain to total amino acid ratio in the injury-adapted amino acid formulation. JPEN 9:133, 1985

102. Cerra FB, Upson D, Angelico R et al: Branched chains support postoperative protein synthesis. Surgery 92:192, 1982

103. Cerra FB, Mazuski J, Teasley K et al: Nitrogen retention in critically ill patients is proportional to the branched chain amino acid load. Crit Care Med 11:775, 1983

104. Desai SP, Bistrian BR, Moldawer LL et al: Plasma amino acid concentrations during branched-chain amino acid infusions in stressed patients. J Trauma 22:747, 1982

105. Echenique MM, Bistrian BR, Moldawer LL et al: Improvement in amino acid use in the critically ill patient with parenteral formulas enriched with branched chain amino acids. Surg Gynecol Obstet 159:223, 1984

106. Van Way CW, Moore EE, Allo M et al: Comparison of total parenteral nutrition with 25 percent and 45 percent branched chain amino acids in stressed patients. Ann Surg 51:609, 1985

107. Wounde PV, Morgan RE, Kosta JM: Addition of branched-chain amino acids to parenteral nutrition of stressed critically ill patients. Crit Care Med 14:685, 1986

108. Daly JM, Mihranian MH, Vehoe JE et al: Effects of postoperative infusion of branched chain amino acids on nitrogen balance and forearm muscle substrate flux. Surgery 94:151, 1983

109. Kirkpatrick JR, Dahn M, Lewis L: Selective versus standard hyperalimentation. A randomized prospective study. Am J Surg 141:116, 1981

110. Nanni G, Siegel JH, Coleman B et al: Increased lipid fuel dependence in the critically ill septic patient. J Trauma 24:14, 1984

111. Sax HC, Talamini MA, Fischer JE: Clinical use of branched chain amino acids in liver disease, sepsis, trauma and burns. Arch Surg 121:358, 1986

112. Bower RM, Muggia-Sullham M, Vallgren S et al: Branched chain amino acid-enriched solutions in the septic patient. Ann Surg 1:13, 1986

113. Goldstein S, Thomashow B, Askanazi J: Functional changes during nutritional repletion in patients with COPD. Clin Chest Med 7:141, 1986

114. Yamada H, Ohta Y, Kvetan V, et al: Diaphragm contractility and fatigue: Branched-chain amino acids vs. aminophylline. ACCP Chest 104S, 1990

115. Sahebjami H: Nutrition and the pulmonary parenchyma. Clin Chest Med 7:111, 1986

116. Askanazi J, Carpentier YA, Elwyn DH et al: Influence of total parenteral nutrition on fuel utilization in injury and sepsis. Ann Surg 194:40, 1980

117. Askanazi J, Rosenbaum SH, Hyman AL et al: Respiratory changes induced by the large glucose loads of total parenteral nutrition. JAMA 243:1444, 1980

118. Askanazi J, Elwyn DH, Silverberg PA et al: Respiratory distress secondary to a high carbohydrate load: A case report. Surgery 87:596, 1980

119. Weissman C, Askanazi J, Rosenbaum SH et al: Amino acids and respiration. Ann Intern Med 98:41, 1983

120. Askanazi J, Weissman C, LaSala P et al: Effect of protein on ventilatory drive. Anesthesiology 60:106, 1984

121. Takala J, Askanazi J, Weissman C et al: Changes in respiratory control induced by amino acid infusions. Crit Care Med 16:465, 1988

122. Kirvelä O, Thorpy M, Takala J et al: Respiratory and sleep patterns during nocturnal infusions of branched chain amino acids. Acta Anaesthesiol Scand 34:645, 1990

123. Söreide E, Skeie B, Kirvelä O et al: Branch-chain amino acid: A preliminary study on the effects on sleep and respiratory pattern in chronic renal failure patients on hemodialysis. Kidney Int, 40:539, 1991

124. Kimmel PL: Sleep apnea in end-stage renal disease. Semin Dialysis 4:52, 1991

125. Needleman P, Turk J, Jakschik BA et al: Arachidonic acid metabolism. Annu Rev Biochem 55:69, 1986

126. Voelkel NF, Stenmark KR, Westcott JY, Chang SW: Lung eicosanoid metabolism. Clin Chest Med 10:95, 1989

127. Askanazi J, Rothkopf MM, Rosenbaum SH, Ross E: Treatment of cystic fibrosis with long term home total parenteral nutrition. Nutrition 3:277, 1987

128. Hanning RM, Zlotkin SH: Amino acid and protein needs of the neonate: Effect of excess and deficiency. Semin Perinatol 13:131, 1989

129. Snyderman SE, Prose PH, Holt LE Jr: Histidine, an essential amino-acid for the infant. Am J Dis Child 98:65/459, 1959

130. Miller SA: Nutrition in the neonatal development of protein metabolism. Fed Proc 29:1497, 1970

131. Scott PH, Berger HM, Wharton BA et al: Growth velocity and plasma amino acids in the newborn. Pediatr Res 19:446, 1985

132. Newsholme EA, Leech AR: Biochemistry for the Medical Sciences. New York, John Wiley, 1983

133. Neely JR, Rovetto MJK, Oram JF: Myocardial utilization of carbohydrate and lipids. Prog Cardiovasc Dis 15:289, 1972

134. Carlsten A, Hallgren B, Jagenburg R et al: Myocardial metabolism of glucose, lactic acid, amino acids and fatty acids in healthy human individuals at rest and at different work loads. Scand J Clin Lab Invest 13:418, 1961

135. Wisneski JA, Gertz EW, Neese RA et al: Myocardial metabolism of free fatty acids. J Clin Invest 79:359, 1987

136. Most AS, Brachfeld N, Gorlin R et al: Free fatty acid metabolism of the human heart at rest. J Clin Invest 48:1177, 1969

137. Newsholme EA, Randle PJ: Regulation of glucose uptake by muscle. VII. Effects of fatty acids, ketone bodies, and pyruvate, and of alloxon-diabetes, hypophysectomi and adrenalectomy on the concentration of hexose phosphates, nucleotides and inorganic phosphate in perfused rat heart. Biochem J 93:641, 1964

138. Drake A, Haines JR, Noble MIM: Preferential uptake of lactate

by the normal myocardium in dogs. Cardiovasc Res 14:65, 1980

139. Opie LH: Metabolism of the heart in health and disease. Am Heart J 76:685, 1968

140. Mjos OD: Effect of free fatty acids on myocardial function and oxygen consumption in intact dogs. J Clin Invest 50:1386, 1971

141. Opie LH: Effect of fatty acids on contractility and rhythm of the heart. Nature 227:1055, 1970

142. Visscher MB, Muller EA: The influence of insulin upon the mammalian heart. J Physiol 62:341, 1926

143. Schwenther FF, Noel WW: Circulatory failure of diphtheria: Carbohydrate metabolism in diphtheria intoxication. Bull Johns Hopkins Hosp 46:259, 1930

144. Rogers WJ, Russell RO Jr, McDaniel HG et al: Acute effects of glucose-insulin-potassium infusion on myocardial substrates, coronary blood flow and oxygen consumption in man. Am J Cardiol 40:421, 1977

145. Apstein CS, Gravino FN, Handenschild CC: Determinants of a protective effect of glucose and insulin on the ischemic myocardium. Circ Res 52:515, 1983

146. Haider W, Benzer H, Schultz W et al: Improvement of cardiac preservation by preoperative high insulin supply. J Thorac Cardiovasc Surg 88:294, 1984

147. Rackley CE, Russell RO Jr, Rogers WJ et al: Myocardial metabolism in coronary artery disease. In Rackley CI, Russell RO Jr (eds): Coronary Artery Disease: Recognition and Management, p 261. Mt Kisco, NY, Futura, 1979

148. Gwata T, Edwards IR: Glucose, insulin, potassium (GIK) in the treatment of congestive cardiomyopathy. Cent Afr J Med 26:249, 1980

149. Whitlow PL, Rogers WJ, Smith LR et al: Enhancement of left ventricular function by glucose-insulin-potassium infusion in acute myocardial infarction. Am J Cardiol 49:811, 1982

150. Rogers WJ, Stanley AW, Breinig JB et al: Reduction of hospital mortality rate of acute myocardial infarction with glucose-insulin-potassium infusion. J Am Heart 92:441, 1976

151. Pittman JG, Cohen P: The pathogenesis of cardiac cachexia. N Engl J Med 271:403, 1964

152. Heymsfield SB, Bleier J, Wenger N: Detection of protein-calorie undernutrition in advanced heart disease. Circulation 56 (suppl III):102, 1977

153. Blackburn GL, Gibbons GW, Bothe A et al: Nutritional support in cardiac cachexia. J Thorac Cardiovasc Surg 73:480, 1977

154. Abel RM, Fischer JE, Buckley MJ et al: Malnutrition in cardiac surgical patients: Result of a prospective randomized evaluation of early postoperative total parenteral nutrition (TPN). Arch Surg 111:45, 1976

154. Lolley DM, Myers WO, Roy JR III et al: Clinical experience with preoperative myocardial nutrition management. J Cardiovasc Surg 26:236, 1985

155. Chua BHL, Siehl DL, Morgan HE: A role for leucine in the regulation of protein turnover in working rat hearts. Am J Physiol 239:E510, 1980

156. Morrison WL, Gibson NA, Rennie MJ: Skeletal muscle and whole body protein turnover in cardiac cachexia: Influence of branched-chain amino acid administration. Eur J Clin Invest 18:648, 1988

157. Schwalb H, Izhar U, Yaroslasky E et al: The effect of amino acids on the ischemic heart. J Thorac Cardiovasc Surg 98:551, 1989

158. Folts JD, Shug AL, Kohe JR et al: Protection of the ischemic myocardium with carnitine. Am J Cardiol 41:1209, 1978

159. Shug AL, Thompson JH, Folts JD et al: Changes in tissue levels of carnitine and other metabolites during myocardial ischemia and anoxia. Arch Biochem Biophys 187:25, 1978

160. Borum PR, Park JH, Law PK et al: Altered tissue carnitine levels in animals with hereditary muscular dystrophy. J Neurol Sci 38:113, 1978

161. Whitmer JT: L-carnitine treatment improves cardiac performance and restores high energy phosphate pools in cardiomyopathic Syrian hamster. Circ Res 61:396, 1987

162. Siemkowicz E, Gjedde A: Post-ischemic coma in rat: Effect of different preischemic blood glucose levels on cerebral metabolic recovery after ischemia. Acta Physiol Scand 110:225, 1980

163. Myers RE: Anoxic brain pathology and blood glucose. Neurology 26:345, 1976

164. Ginsberg MD, Welsh FA, Budd WW: Deleterious effect of glucose pretreatment on recovery from diffuse cerebral ischemia in the cat. I. Local cerebral blood flow and glucose utilization. Stroke 11:347, 1980

165. Pulsinelli WA, Levy DE, Sigsbee B et al: Increased damage after ischemic stroke in patients with hyperglycemia with or without established diabetes mellitus. Am J Med 74:540, 1983

166. Longstreth WT Jr, Inui TS: High blood glucose level on hospital admission and poor neurological recovery after cardiac arrest. Ann Neurol 15:59, 1984

167. Welsh FA, Ginsberg MD, Rider W et al: Deleterious effect of glucose pretreatment on recovery from diffuse cerebral ischemia in the cat. II. Regional metabolite levels. Stroke 11:355, 1980

168. Elwyn DH: Nutritional requirements of adult surgical patients. Crit Care Med 8:9, 1980

169. Seiber FE, Smith DS, Traystman RJ et al: Glucose: A re-evaluation of intraoperative use. Anesthesiology 67:72, 1987

170. Sieber F, Smith DS, Kupferberg J et al: Effects of intraoperative glucose on protein catabolism and plasma glucose levels in patients with supratentorial tumors. Anesthesiology 64:453, 1986

171. Feinstein EI, Blumenkrantz MJ, Healy H et al: Clinical and metabolic responses to parenteral nutrition in acute renal failure: A controlled double-blind study. Medicine 60:124, 1981

172. Kopple JD: Altered metabolic and nutritional status in acute renal failure. American Society for Parenteral and Enteral Nutrition, 11th Clinical Congress, New Orleans, p 27, 1987

173. Abel RM, Beck CH Jr, Abbott WM et al: Improved survival from acute renal failure after treatment with intravenous essential amino acids and glucose: Results of a prospective double-blind study. N Engl J Med 288:685, 1973

174. Toback FG: Amino acid enhancement of renal regeneration after acute tubular necrosis. Kidney Int 12:193, 1977

175. Feinstein EI, Kopple J, Silberman H et al: Total parenteral nutrition with high or low nitrogen intakes in patients with acute renal failure. Kidney Int 24:S319, 1983

176. Solez K, Stout R, Bendush B et al: Adverse effect of amino acid solutions in amino glycoside-induced renal failure in rabbits and rats. In Eliahou H (ed): Acute Renal Failure, p 241. London, Libbey and Co, 1982

177. Zager RA, Venkatachalam MA: Potentiation of ischemic renal injury by amino acid infusion. Kidney Int 24:620, 1983

178. Racusen LC, Whelton A, Solez K: Effects of lysine and other amino acids on kidney structure and function in the rat. Am J Pathol 120:436, 1985

179. Abel RM, Shih VE, Abbott WM et al: Amino acid metabolism in acute renal failure. Ann Surg 180:350, 1974

180. Starker PM, LaSala PA, Askanazi J et al: The response to TPN: A form of nutritional assessment. Ann Surg 198:720, 1983

181. Starker PM, LaSala PA, Askanazi J et al: The influence of preoperative TPN on morbidity and mortality. Surg Gynecol Obstet 162:569, 1986

182. Askanazi J, Hensle TW, Starker PM et al: Effect of immediate postoperative nutritional support on length of hospitalization. Ann Surg 203:236, 1986

183. Hadfield JIH: Preoperative and postoperative intravenous fat therapy. Br J Surg 52:291, 1965

184. Heatley RV, Williams RHP, Lewis MH: Preoperative intravenous feeding: Controlled trial. Postgrad Med J 55:541, 1979

185. Muller JM, Brewer V, Dienst C et al: Preoperative parenteral feeding in patients with gastrointestinal carcinoma. Lancet 1:68, 1982

186. Holter AR, Fischer JE: The effects of perioperative hyperalimentation on complications in patients with carcinoma and weight loss. J Surg Res 23:31, 1977

187. Mullen JL, Buzby GP, Matthews DC et al: Reduction of operative morbidity and mortality by combined preoperative and postoperative nutritional support. Ann Surg 192:604, 1980

188. Mullen JL: Consequences of malnutrition in the surgical patient. Surg Clin North Am 61:465, 1981

189. Barac-Nieto M, Spurr GB, Lotero H et al: Body composition during nutritional repletion of severely undernourished men. Am J Clin Nutr 32:981, 1979

190. Deo MG, Bhan AK, Ramalingaswami V: Metabolism of albumin and body fluid compartments in protein deficiency: An experimental study in the rhesus monkey. J Nutr 104:858, 1974

191. Morgan EH, Peters T Jr: The biosynthesis of rat serum albumin. V. Effect of protein depletion and refeeding on albumin and transferrin synthesis. J Biol Chem 246:3500, 1971

192. Skillman JJ, Rosenoer VM, Smith PC et al: Improved albumin synthesis in postoperative patients by amino acid infusion. N Engl J Med 295:1037, 1976

193. Starker PM, Gump FE, Askanazi J et al: Serum albumin levels as an index of nutritional support. Surgery 91:194, 1982

194. Starker PM, Askanazi J, LaSala PA et al: The effect of parenteral nutritional repletion on muscle water and electrolytes: Implications for body composition. Surg Gynecol Obstet 152:22, 1981

195. Shizgal HM: The effect of malnutrition on body composition. Surg Gynecol Obstet 152:22, 1981

196. Larca L, Greenbaum DM: Effectiveness of intensive nutritional regimes in patients who fail to wean from mechanical ventilation. Crit Care Med 10:297, 1982

197. Bryan-Brown CW, Savitz MH, Elwyn DH et al: Cerebral edema unresponsive to conventional therapy in neurosurgical patients with unsuspected nutritional failure. Crit Care Med 1:125, 1973

198. Deitch EA, Winterton J, MA L et al: The gut as a portal of entry for bacteremia: Role of protein malnutrition. Ann Surg 205:681, 1987

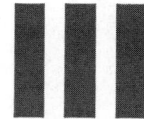

BASIC PRINCIPLES OF PHARMACOLOGY IN ANESTHESIA PRACTICE

13 Robert J. Hudson

Basic Principles of Clinical Pharmacology

About 30 years ago, Dr. E. M. Papper opened a symposium on inhalational anesthetics by emphasizing the importance of understanding the basic pharmacology of anesthetics:[1]

Clinical anaesthetists have administered millions of anaesthetics during more than a century with little precise information of the uptake, distribution, and elimination of inhalational and non-volatile anaesthetic agents. Considering how serious is the handicap of not knowing those fundamental and important facts about the drugs they have used so often, the record of success and safety in clinical anaesthesia is an extraordinary accomplishment indeed. It can in some measure be attributed to the accumulated experience and successful teaching of a highly developed sense of intuition from generation to generation of anaesthetists. It can also be attributed in part to the ability to learn by error after observing patients come uncomfortably close to injury and even to death.

In the last few years, however, sufficient fundamental information has become available to explain these clinical successes. The empirical process of giving an anaesthetic can be better understood because of the specific data provided by the studies reported in this symposium and by the work of others which has preceded them.

Understanding the principles of pharmacology and knowledge of the specific properties of individual drugs are probably even more important today. In the past few years, new anesthetics, opioids, and neuromuscular blockers have been introduced. We do not have the benefit of decades of experience with these new drugs, and so we must depend on carefully conducted investigations to provide the information needed to use them safely. As Dr. Papper wrote,

If the anaesthetist studies the pharmacology of these agents and understands their pharmacokinetic properties, he can with reasonable certainty predict which of these newer anaesthetic agents will hold promise for clinical utility . . . the clinician can spare his patients much danger and his own work many hardships if he is aware of the physicochemical and pharmacological [properties] of new agents.

Our patients are also changing. Many present for surgery with concomitant diseases that were once considered contraindications to anesthesia and surgery. Therefore, we must consider the impact of chronic diseases, and of the drugs used to treat those diseases, on the response to drugs administered during the perioperative period. Clearly, comprehensive knowledge of clinical pharmacology is a prerequisite to the practice of anesthesiology.

The first sections of this chapter discuss the biologic and pharmacologic factors that influence drug absorption, distribution, and elimination. The quantitative analysis of these processes is discussed in the section on pharmacokinetics. The next section presents the fundamentals of pharmacodynamics—those factors that determine the duration and intensity of pharmacologic effects. The application of pharmacokinetics and pharmacodynamics to clinical anesthesiology is then discussed. The final section briefly presents the mechanisms of drug interactions. Although specific properties of some drugs have been used to illustrate basic pharmacologic principles, detailed information regarding the pharmacology of drugs used in anesthesiology is presented in succeeding chapters.

TRANSFER OF DRUGS ACROSS MEMBRANES

Absorption, distribution, metabolism, and excretion of drugs require that they be transferred across cell membranes. Most drugs must also traverse cell membranes to reach their sites of action. Biologic membranes consist of a lipid bilayer with a nonpolar core and polar elements on the intracellular and extracellular surfaces of the membrane. Proteins are embedded in the lipid bilayer and are oriented similarly, with ionic, polar groups on the membrane surfaces and hydrophobic groups in the membrane interior. The nonpolar core hinders the passage of water-soluble molecules, so that only lipid-soluble molecules easily traverse cell membranes.

Transport Processes

Drugs can cross membranes either by passive processes or by active transport through the membrane. *Passive diffusion* occurs when a concentration gradient exists across a membrane. The rate of passive transfer is directly proportional to the magnitude of the concentration gradient and to the lipid solubility of the drug. The passage of water-soluble drugs is restricted largely to small aqueous channels through the membrane. These channels are generally so narrow that only molecules having molecular weights less than 200 daltons can pass through them. Capillary endothelial membranes, except those in the central nervous system (CNS), have larger aqueous channels that permit transfer of much larger molecules, such as albumin (molecular weight = 67,000 daltons). There are also large intercellular gaps in capillary endothelium. Because of these unique features, diffusion of drugs across capillary membranes outside the CNS is limited by blood flow, not by lipid solubility.[2]

Some drugs are transferred through cell membranes of hepatocytes, renal tubular, and other cells by *active transport*. This is an energy-requiring process that is both specific and saturable. Active transport can pump compounds across membranes against their concentration gradients. *Facilitated diffusion* shares some characteristics with active transport. It is also carrier-mediated, specific, and saturable, but does not require energy and cannot work against a concentration gradient.[2]

Effects of Molecular Properties

Most drugs are too large to pass through cellular membrane channels and must traverse the lipid component of membranes. Almost all drugs are either weak acids or weak bases, and are present in solution in both the ionized and non-ionized forms at physiologic pH. Generally, it is the non-ionized form that is more lipid soluble and able to traverse easily cell membranes. The non-ionized fraction of weak acids, such as salicylates and barbiturates, is greater at low pH values, so acidic drugs become more lipid soluble as pH decreases. The non-ionized fraction of weak bases like opioids and local anesthetics increases as the pH becomes more alkaline. The pK_a is the pH at which exactly 50% of a weak acid or base is present in each of the ionized and non-ionized forms. The closer the pK_a is to the ambient pH, the greater the change in the degree of ionization for a given change in pH. If there is a pH gradient across a membrane, drug will be trapped on the side that has the higher ionized fraction, because only the non-ionized drug is diffusible. This phenomenon is known as *ion trapping*. The total drug concentration is greater on the side of the membrane with the higher ionized fraction. However, at equilibrium, the concentration of non-ionized drug will be the same. In most situations, the range of pH values is too small to cause major changes in the degree of ionization. However, there are major pH changes in the upper gastrointestinal (GI) tract, which can affect drug absorption.

DRUG ABSORPTION

Except for intravenous (iv) injections, drugs must be absorbed into the circulation before they can be delivered to their sites of action. The manner in which drugs are absorbed is an important determinant of both the intensity and duration of drug action. Incomplete absorption limits the amount of drug reaching the site of action, reducing the peak pharmacologic effect. Rapid absorption is a prerequisite for rapid onset of action. In contrast, slow absorption permits a sustained duration of action because of the "depot" of drug at the absorptive site. The speed of absorption depends on the solubility and concentration of drug. All drugs must dissolve in water to reach the circulation. Consequently, drugs in aqueous solutions are absorbed faster than those in solid formulations, suspensions, or organic solvents, such as propylene glycol. A high concentration of drug facilitates absorption. Local blood flow also affects absorption. Increased circulation to the absorptive site increases the rate of absorption. Decreased blood flow secondary to hypotension, the use of vasoconstrictors, or other factors slows drug absorption.[2] Vasoconstrictors are often added to local anesthetics to delay absorption after subcutaneous injection. This prolongs the duration of action at the site of injection and lessens the chance of systemic toxicity.

Route of Administration

In general medical practice, drugs are most commonly administered orally. The advantages of oral administration are convenience, economy, and safety. Disadvantages include the requirement for a cooperative patient, incomplete absorption, and metabolism of the drug in the GI tract or liver before it reaches the systemic circulation.[2] In anesthesia, drugs are most frequently administered *via* the iv and inhalational routes. Both permit rapid attainment of the desired blood concentration of drug in a reasonably predictable manner.

Oral Administration

Drug absorption occurs mainly from the upper part of the small intestine, and, to a lesser extent, from the stomach. Absorption from the GI tract is highly variable because of the multiple factors involved. Tablets and capsules must disintegrate before the drug can dissolve in the GI lumen. The drug must then cross the lipid membranes of the GI epithelial cells before it can be absorbed into the portal circulation. The most important site of absorption of all drugs is the small intestine, because of the large surface area and anatomic characteristics of its mucosa. The non-ionized fraction of weak acids such as barbiturates is higher at low pH values, which would favor absorption from the stomach. However, the effect of pH on ionization of acidic drugs in the stomach is offset by the small surface area and thickness of the gastric mucosa and the rapidity of gastric emptying. Basic drugs are highly ionized at low pH, so they cannot cross the gastric mucosa and are "trapped" in the stomach. The more alkaline pH of the small intestine increases the non-ionized fraction of basic drugs such as opioids, which facilitates their absorption from this site.[2]

Once the drug has entered the portal circulation, it must pass through the liver before reaching the systemic circulation. A considerable proportion of certain drugs is metabolized during this initial pass through the liver, so that only a small fraction of the absorbed drug reaches the systemic circulation. This phenomenon is called the *first-pass effect*. Depending on the magnitude of this effect, the oral dose must be proportionately larger than the iv dose to achieve the same pharmacologic response.[3] Metabolism of some drugs by the GI mucosa may also contribute to the first-pass effect.[4]

Sublingual Administration

Drug absorbed from the oral mucosa passes directly into the systemic circulation, which eliminates the possibility of the first-pass effect. Because of the small surface area available for absorption, this route is efficacious only for non-ionized, highly lipid-soluble drugs, such as nitroglycerin.[2]

Rectal Administration

The first-pass effect is less evident after rectal administration because much of the drug is absorbed into the systemic circulation. Unfortunately, absorption from the rectum is often irregular and incomplete.[2]

Transcutaneous Administration

Only lipid-soluble drugs can penetrate intact skin sufficiently to produce systemic effects. Nitroglycerin ointment is probably the medication most commonly administered transcutaneously. Recently, sophisticated systems for transcutaneous delivery of drugs have been developed. They consist of an adhesive patch containing a reservoir of drug that is slowly released after the patch is applied to the skin. This produces a stable pharmacologic effect that can last for several days. Drugs currently administered in this fashion include scopolamine (for motion sickness), clonidine, and nitroglycerin. Transcutaneous administration of opioids for postoperative analgesia or treatment of chronic pain is under investigation.[5]

Intramuscular and Subcutaneous Injection

Absorption of drugs from subcutaneous tissue is relatively slow, which permits a sustained effect. Also, the rate of absorption can be altered by changes in the drug formulation. Examples of such manipulations are the various types of insulin, and the addition of vasoconstrictors to local anesthetic solutions.

Uptake of drugs after intramuscular injection is more rapid than after subcutaneous administration because of greater blood flow. Drugs in aqueous solution are very readily absorbed. The effect of drugs in nonaqueous solutions, such as diazepam in propylene glycol, is less predictable because of erratic absorption.[6]

Intravenous Injection

Intravenous injection bypasses absorption processes, so that therapeutic blood concentrations can be rapidly attained. This is especially advantageous when rapid onset of drug action is desired. It also facilitates titration of dosage to individual patients' responses. Unfortunately, the rapidity of onset also has its hazards. Should an adverse drug reaction or overdose occur, the effects are immediate and potentially severe.[2]

Inhalational Administration

Uptake of inhalational anesthetics from the pulmonary alveoli to the blood is exceedingly rapid because of the large total surface area of the alveoli and the fact that alveolar blood flow is almost equal to cardiac output. The low molecular weight and high lipid solubility of these drugs also facilitate their absorption from the alveoli.

Drugs are also given by inhalation when local endobronchial effects are desired. Inhaled bronchodilators are delivered directly to their site of action, minimizing the risk of adverse effects from high blood levels.

Intrathecal and Epidural Injection

Spinal anesthesia is produced by intrathecal injection of local anesthetics. Injection close to the sites of action in the spinal cord permits the use of very low doses, reducing the risk of adverse systemic drug effects. This advantage is lessened with epidural anesthesia, because a much greater total dose is required. The major disadvantage of these routes of injection is the expertise that they require.

Bioavailability

Bioavailability is defined as the fraction of the total dose that reaches the systemic circulation. Bioavailability is reduced by factors such as incomplete absorption from the GI tract, the first-pass effect, and poor absorption from the site of injection.

Even after iv injection, the bioavailability of drugs formulated in lipid suspensions may be less than 100%. These suspensions contain small lipid droplets similar to endogenous chylomicra. Some, but not all, of the drug diffuses from the lipid droplets into the plasma. These droplets are taken up by the liver and metabolized. Presumably, some of the drug is also metabolized before it is released back into the circulation. The bioavailability of the lecithin suspension of diazepam is 30% less than that of diazepam in propylene glycol, even with direct iv injection.[7]

DRUG DISTRIBUTION

After absorption or injection into the systemic circulation, drugs are distributed throughout the body. The initial pattern of distribution depends on regional blood flow. Highly perfused organs, such as the brain, heart, lungs, liver, and kidneys, receive most of the drug soon after injection. Delivery to muscle, skin, fat, and other tissues with lower blood flows is slower, and equilibration of distribution into these tissues may take several hours or even days.[2]

Capillary membranes are freely permeable in most tissues except the brain, so drugs quickly pass into the extracellular space. Subsequent distribution varies according to the physicochemical properties of the drug. The distribution of highly polar, water-soluble drugs such as the neuromuscular blockers is essentially limited to the extracellular fluid. Lipid-soluble drugs such as thiopental easily cross cell membranes and are therefore distributed much more extensively.[2]

Distribution of drugs into the CNS is unique. Brain capillaries do not have the large aqueous channels typical of capillaries in other tissues. Consequently, diffusion of water-soluble drugs into the brain is severely restricted. In contrast, distribution of highly lipid-soluble drugs into the CNS is limited only by cerebral blood flow. For more polar compounds, the rate of entry into the brain is proportional to the lipid solubility of the non-ionized drug.[2]

Drugs can accumulate in tissues because of binding to tissue components, pH gradients, or uptake of lipophilic drugs into fat. These tissue stores can act as reservoirs that prolong the duration of drug action, either in the same tissue or by delivery to the site of action elsewhere after reabsorption into the circulation.[2]

The degree of binding of drugs to plasma proteins and erythrocytes influences distribution to other tissues. Drugs that are highly bound to blood constituents cannot be distributed extensively because only free, unbound drug can cross capillary membranes.

Redistribution

The rapid entry and equally rapid egress of lipophilic drugs from richly perfused organs such as the brain and heart is referred to as *redistribution*. This phenomenon is illustrated by the events that follow an injection of thiopental. The brain concentration of thiopental peaks within 1 minute, because of high blood flow to the brain and the high lipid solubility of thiopental. As the drug is taken up by other, less well-perfused tissues, the plasma level rapidly decreases. This creates a concentration gradient from cerebral tissue to the blood, so that thiopental quickly diffuses back into the blood, where it is redistributed to the other tissues that are still taking up drug. Ultimately, adipose tissue takes up most of the drug because of the high lipid solubility of thiopental. However, recovery from a single dose of thiopental is dependent predominantly on redistribution of thiopental from the brain to muscle, because of the larger mass and greater perfusion of muscle compared to adipose tissue.[8,9]

A single moderate dose of thiopental (5–6 mg·kg^{-1}) has a very short duration of action because of redistribution. If repeated injections are given, the concentration of thiopental builds up in the peripheral tissues, and termination of drug action becomes increasingly dependent on the much slower process of drug elimination. Termination of the pharmacologic effects of other lipophilic drugs, such as fentanyl and its derivatives and propofol, is also governed by these factors.

Placental Transfer

Most drugs cross the placenta by simple diffusion, so thiopental and other lipid-soluble drugs with low molecular weights are most readily transferred. Highly polar, water-soluble compounds such as the neuromuscular blocking drugs do not cross the placenta to a significant extent. Fetal pH is slightly lower than maternal pH, and this difference increases with fetal distress. This pH gradient causes the ionized fraction of weak bases, such as opioids and local anesthetics, to be higher in the fetus. Therefore, the fetal total drug level may be higher than predicted from the maternal total drug level because of "ion trapping."[10] Different total drug concentrations can also be due to differences between mother and fetus in the extent of drug binding to plasma proteins and erythrocytes. However, regardless of the effects of pH and protein binding, the concentration of free, non-ionized drug will be the same on both sides of the placenta once equilibrium is reached. For most drugs, this is the most important form, because it has the most pharmacologic activity. Therefore, although ion trapping may increase total fetal drug levels, it is of little clinical significance.

DRUG ELIMINATION

Elimination is an inclusive term referring to all the processes that remove drugs from the body. Elimination occurs either by excretion of unchanged drug or by metabolism (biotransformation) and subsequent excretion of metabolites. The liver and the kidney are the most important organs for drug elimination. The liver eliminates drugs primarily by metabolism to less active compounds and, to a lesser extent, by hepatobiliary excretion of drugs or their metabolites. The primary role of the kidneys is the excretion of water-soluble, polar compounds. Drugs such as the nondepolarizing neuromuscular blockers d-tubocurarine and metocurine undergo renal excretion intact.[11] The kidneys are also the primary route for excretion of water-soluble metabolites of drugs that initially undergo hepatic biotransforma-

tion. Pulmonary excretion is the major route for elimination of anesthetic gases and vapors. Drugs can also be eliminated via tears, saliva, sweat, and breast milk, but these routes are quantitatively unimportant.

The term *drug clearance* describes the ability of an individual organ, or the whole body, to remove drug from the blood. Drug clearance is the theoretical volume of blood from which drug is completely removed in a given time interval. It is analogous to creatinine clearance, which quantitatively describes the ability of the kidneys to eliminate creatinine. Like creatinine clearance, drug clearance has units of flow, ml·min^{-1}. Many drugs are cleared by more than one means, and multiple elimination pathways are additive. As a result, total drug clearance is equal to the sum of the clearances of all of the elimination pathways.

Total drug clearance can be calculated with pharmacokinetic models of blood concentration *versus* time data. However, clearance by individual organs and the biologic factors influencing drug elimination cannot be estimated from blood concentration data alone. Additional data, such as the hepatic arteriovenous drug concentration difference or the rate of urinary excretion of the drug, are needed to determine the contribution of a specific organ to total drug clearance.

Hepatic Drug Clearance

Drug clearance by the liver is dependent on three biologic factors: (1) hepatic blood flow, (2) the intrinsic ability of the liver to irreversibly eliminate the drug from the blood, and (3) the degree to which the drug is bound to plasma proteins or other blood constituents. The interrelationships between these factors have been described with the venous equilibration model of hepatic drug clearance.[12-14] According to this model, drug in the liver cells is in equilibrium with drug in the blood leaving the liver. Therefore, the unbound concentration of drug in hepatic venous blood is equal to the unbound concentration in hepatocytes. The unbound drug within the liver is the drug that can be eliminated by biotransformation and biliary excretion.

The venous equilibration model is based on the assumptions that hepatic drug clearance is limited by delivery of drug to the liver, and that elimination is a first-order process.[13] By definition, "first order" means that a constant fraction of the drug is eliminated per unit of time. The fraction of the drug removed from the blood passing through the liver is the hepatic extraction ratio, E:

$$E = \frac{C_a - C_v}{C_a} \qquad (13\text{-}1)$$

where C_a is the mixed hepatic arterial-portal venous drug concentration and C_v is the mixed hepatic venous drug concentration. The total hepatic drug clearance, Cl_H, is:

$$Cl_H = Q \cdot E \qquad (13\text{-}2)$$

where Q is the hepatic blood flow. Therefore, hepatic clearance is a function of hepatic blood flow and the ability of the liver to extract drug from the blood perfusing the liver. The ability to extract drug depends on the activity of hepatic drug-metabolizing enzyme systems and other elimination processes, such as hepatobiliary excretion.

The concept of intrinsic clearance was developed to overcome the modifying effects of blood flow and drug binding in the blood on elimination processes.[13] Intrinsic clearance

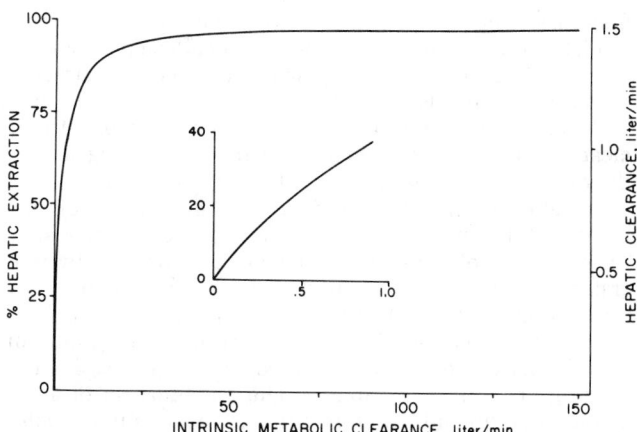

Figure 13-1. The relationship between hepatic extraction ratio, intrinsic clearance, and hepatic clearance at the normal hepatic blood flow of 1.5 l·min^{-1}. For drugs with high intrinsic clearance (>25 l·min^{-1}), increasing the intrinsic clearance has little effect on hepatic extraction and total hepatic clearance. The inset demonstrates the relationship at low values of intrinsic clearance on an expanded scale. (Reprinted with permission from Wilkinson GR, Shand DG: A physiologic approach to hepatic drug clearance. Clin Phamacol Ther 18:377, 1975.)

represents the overall ability of the liver to remove drug from the blood in the absence of any limitations imposed by blood flow or drug binding. The relationship of total hepatic drug clearance to the extraction ratio and intrinsic clearance, Cl_I, is:

$$Cl_H = Q \cdot E = Q \left(\frac{Cl_I}{Q + Cl_I} \right) \qquad (13\text{-}3)$$

The right-hand side of Equation 13-3 indicates that if intrinsic clearance is very high (many times larger than hepatic blood flow), then total hepatic clearance will approach hepatic blood flow. This is intuitively obvious. On the other hand, if intrinsic clearance is very small, hepatic clearance will be similar to intrinsic clearance. These relationships are shown in Figure 13-1.

The preceding discussion indicates that hepatic drug clearance and extraction are determined by two independent biologic variables, intrinsic clearance and hepatic blood flow. Changes in either will change hepatic clearance. However, the extent of the change depends on the initial intrinsic clearance.

If the inherent ability of the liver to eliminate a drug (intrinsic clearance) is doubled, then the extraction ratio will also increase, but not necessarily to the same extent. The extraction ratio and intrinsic clearance do not have a simple, linear relationship:

$$E = \frac{Cl_I}{Q + Cl_I} \qquad (13\text{-}4)$$

If the initial intrinsic clearance is small (in relation to hepatic blood flow), then the extraction ratio is also small, and Equation 13-4 indicates that doubling intrinsic clearance will produce an almost proportional increment in the extraction ratio, and, consequently, clearance. However, if intrinsic clearance is much greater than hepatic blood flow, a twofold change in intrinsic clearance has a negligible effect on the extraction ratio and drug clearance. In nonmathemat-

ical terms, high intrinsic clearance indicates efficient hepatic elimination. It is hard to enhance an already efficient process, whereas it is relatively easy to improve upon inefficient drug clearance due to low intrinsic clearance.

The effect of changes in hepatic blood flow also depends on the magnitude of intrinsic clearance (Figs. 13-2 and 13-3). If extraction and intrinsic clearance are high, a decrease in hepatic blood flow causes a small increase in the extraction ratio (see Fig. 13-2) that is insufficient to offset the effects of reduced hepatic flow (Eq. 13-4). Consequently, changes in hepatic blood flow produce virtually proportional changes in clearance of drugs with high extraction ratios (see Fig. 13-3). For a drug with a low intrinsic clearance, a decrease in hepatic blood flow is associated with a larger, almost proportional increase in the extraction ratio (see Fig. 13-2). This largely offsets the effects of changes in blood flow, so that clearance of drugs with low extraction ratios is essentially independent of hepatic blood flow (see Fig. 13-3).

Under some circumstances, binding of drugs to plasma proteins and other blood constituents can also affect hepatic drug clearance. Only free drug can enter hepatocytes and subsequently be eliminated. However, in many cases, the intrinsic ability of the liver to eliminate drugs is so high that free drug is reduced to very low concentrations early during passage through the liver. When this happens, more drug dissociates from binding sites, and some of this newly released drug is extracted. Therefore, two types of extraction can be described. If both free and bound drug can be eliminated, then extraction is *nonrestrictive*.[13] This applies to drugs having high extraction ratios, so their clearance is independent of the degree of binding in the blood.[13,15] If extraction is limited to the free drug, it is termed *restrictive*.[13] This situation is typical of drugs with low extraction ratios. Depending on the fraction of the drug that is bound, clearance of these drugs may be altered by changes in binding. If the free fraction is already very high, then a given absolute change in the degree of binding has a small relative

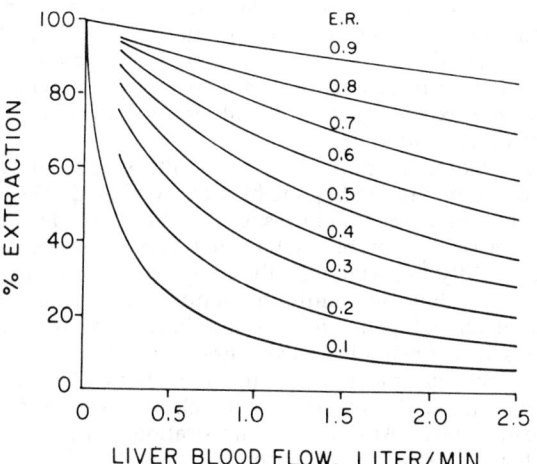

Figure 13-2. The effect of changes in hepatic blood flow on extraction of drugs with different extraction ratios. The extraction ratios at the normal hepatic blood flow of 1.5 l·min^{-1} are above the corresponding curves. (Reprinted with permission from Wood AJJ: Drug disposition and pharmacokinetics. In Wood M, Wood AJJ [eds]: Drugs and Anesthesia: Pharmacology for Anesthesiologists, p 27. Baltimore, Williams & Wilkins, 1990. After Wilkinson GR, Shand DG: A physiologic approach to hepatic drug clearance. Clin Pharmacol Ther 18:377, 1975.)

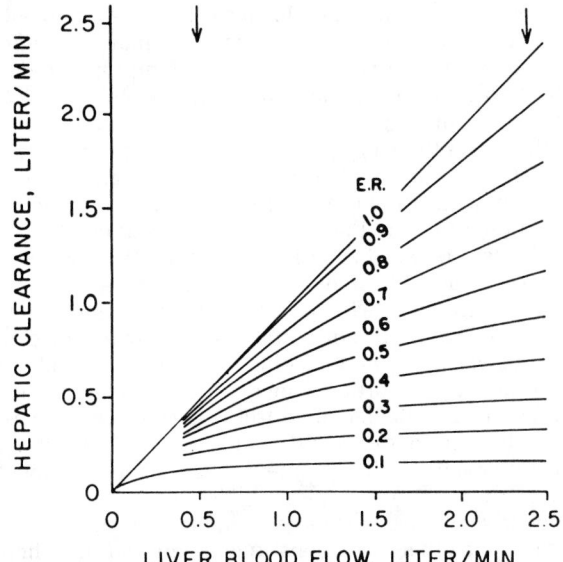

Figure 13-3. The effect of changes in hepatic blood flow on hepatic clearance of drugs with different extraction ratios. The extraction ratios for each curve at 1.5 l·min⁻¹ flow are indicated. The arrows indicate the normal physiologic range of hepatic blood flow. (Reprinted with permission from Wood AJJ: Drug disposition and pharmacokinetics. In Wood M, Wood AJJ [eds]: Drugs and Anesthesia: Pharmacology for Anesthesiologists, p 27. Baltimore, Williams & Wilkins, 1990. After Wilkinson GR, Shand DG: A physiologic approach to hepatic drug clearance. Clin Pharmacol Ther 18:377, 1975.)

effect on the free drug concentration, and clearance is minimally affected. In contrast, if the free fraction is low, the same absolute change in binding produces a greater relative change of the free drug concentration and results in a proportional change in extraction and drug clearance.

The ultimate extraction ratio reflects not only the intrinsic ability of the liver to eliminate a drug but also takes into account the influence of blood flow and drug binding. Drugs can be classified as having either high, intermediate, or low extraction ratios (Table 13-1). Comparing drugs with high versus low extraction ratios reveals easily discernible differences in disposition.[13]

A low extraction ratio is due to an intrinsic clearance that is small in relation to hepatic blood flow. Hepatic clearance of drugs with extraction ratios of 30% or less is independent of changes in liver blood flow but very sensitive to the liver's ability to metabolize the drug, which can vary as a result of pathologic conditions, inhibition or induction of drug-metabolizing enzymes, or interindividual differences. Increased intrinsic clearance causes a parallel increase in total hepatic clearance, which in turn decreases the elimination half-time. Decreased intrinsic clearance produces the opposite effects. After oral administration of a drug with a low hepatic extraction ratio, the first-pass effect is minimal; most of the drug reaches the systemic circulation, and variations in intrinsic clearance will not significantly change the bioavailability.[13]

For drugs with high extraction ratios (>70%), hepatic clearance is determined primarily by liver blood flow rather than by the activity of drug-metabolizing enzymes. Accordingly, clearance and elimination half-time will be affected by changes in hepatic blood flow but not by changes in metabolic activity. These drugs undergo considerable first-pass elimination, so their bioavailability after oral administration is small and is significantly affected by changes in intrinsic clearance.[13] Drugs with intermediate extraction ratios, between 30% and 70%, share characteristics with both the other groups. The relative importance of intrinsic clearance and hepatic blood flow in determining hepatic drug clearance varies according to extraction ratio.

The effect of the unbound drug concentration is complex because it depends on the magnitude of intrinsic clearance. Three classes of hepatic clearance can be defined by integrating the effects of drug binding in the blood and the extraction ratio (Fig. 13-4).[15] Clearance of drugs with high extraction ratios is *flow-limited*, because it depends only on hepatic perfusion and is not affected by changes in drug binding or intrinsic clearance. The combination of a low extraction ratio and a high free fraction results in *capacity-limited, binding-insensitive* clearance, which is affected by changes in intrinsic clearance but is not significantly influenced by binding or hepatic perfusion. Drugs with low extraction ratios and low free fractions have *capacity-limited, binding-sensitive* clearance, which is not greatly affected by changes in hepatic blood flow but depends on both intrinsic clearance and the free drug concentration. Elimination of drugs with intermediate extraction ratios and binding will be influenced by all three biologic factors—hepatic blood flow, intrinsic clearance, and the free drug concentration in the blood. The relative importance of these three factors cannot be predicted unless the extraction ratio and the unbound fraction in the blood are known.

Physiologic, Pathologic, and Pharmacologic Alterations in Hepatic Drug Clearance

At rest, approximately 30% of total cardiac output perfuses the liver. The hepatic artery provides roughly 25% of total hepatic flow, with the remainder supplied *via* the portal vein. Many physiologic and pathologic conditions alter hepatic blood flow, but there is little information regarding the effect of these changes in blood flow on hepatic drug clearance. The splanchnic circulation responds to a variety of stimuli, and splanchnic flow is often sacrificed to meet the demands of other tissues.

Moving from the supine to the upright position decreases

TABLE 13-1. Classification of Some Drugs Encountered in Anesthesiology According to Hepatic Extraction Ratios

Low	High
Diazepam	Alprenolol
Lorazepam	Bupivacaine
Methadone	Diltiazem
Phenytoin	Fentanyl
Theophylline	Ketamine
Thiopental	Lidocaine
	Meperidine
Intermediate	Metoprolol
	Morphine
Alfentanil	Naloxone
Methohexital	Nifedipine
Midazolam	Propofol
Vecuronium	Propranolol
	Sufentanil
	Verapamil

Drugs eliminated primarily by other organs are not included in this table.

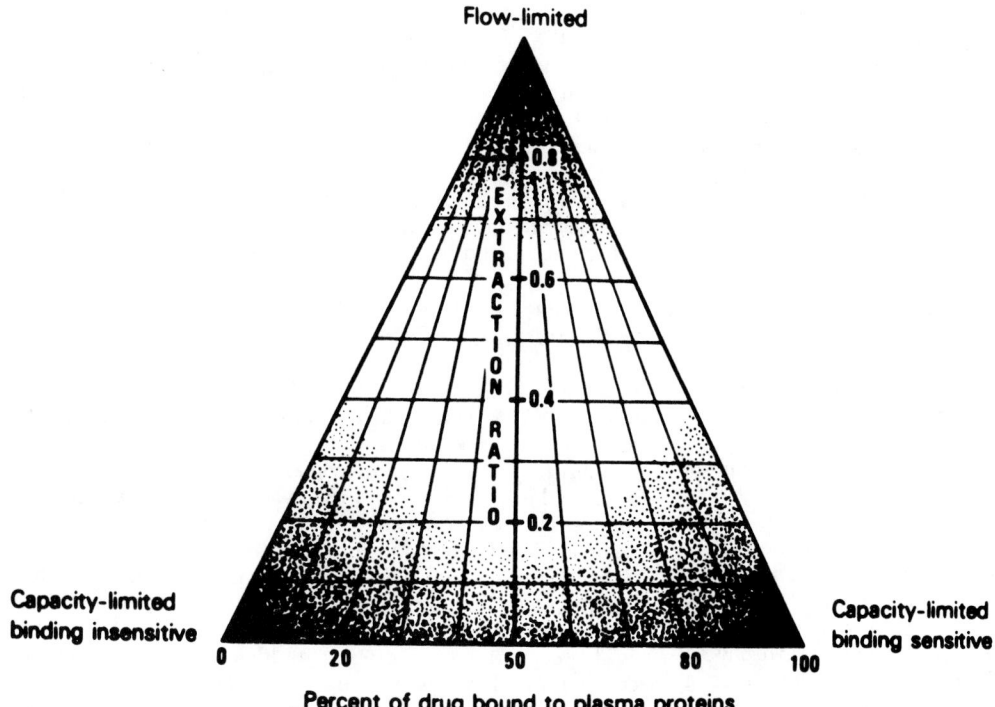

Figure 13-4. Classification of drugs according to the factors affecting hepatic drug clearance. The closer a drug comes to one of the apices of the triangle, the more its clearance will be affected by the factors indicated on the graph. (Reprinted with permission from Blaschke TF: Protein binding and kinetics of drugs in liver disease. Clin Pharmacokinet 2:32, 1977.)

cardiac output, which produces a reflex increase in systemic vascular resistance. The splanchnic circulation participates in this generalized vasoconstriction, which decreases hepatic blood flow by 30–40%.[14] The clearance of aldosterone, which has a high hepatic extraction ratio, is decreased in the upright position.[14] Postural changes probably also influence clearance of drugs with high hepatic extraction ratios, but this has not been systematically investigated.

Exercise, heat stress, and hypovolemia all decrease splanchnic blood flow in proportion to the associated increase in heart rate, which suggests that these responses are mediated by the sympathetic nervous system.[14] As expected, these conditions decrease clearance of indocyanine green, which has a high hepatic extraction ratio. In contrast, the clearance of antipyrine, a drug with a low extraction ratio, is not affected by these conditions.[16]

Pathologic decreases in cardiac output produce reflex splanchnic vasoconstriction, which in turn reduces hepatic blood flow. Congestive heart failure decreases liver blood flow in proportion to the reduction in cardiac output.[17] Clearance of lidocaine is reduced in patients with congestive cardiac failure.[18] During a continuous iv infusion, the steady-state blood level of a drug is inversely proportional to drug clearance. Consequently, if usual doses of lidocaine are given to patients with congestive heart failure, the incidence of lidocaine toxicity is increased. This demonstrates that decreased liver blood flow can produce clinically important changes in the clearance of lidocaine and other drugs with high hepatic extraction ratios. Marked reduction in hepatic blood flow can result in hepatocellular dysfunction. Therefore, severe congestive heart failure can decrease drug clearance by reducing both intrinsic clearance and hepatic blood flow.[19]

Regardless of its cause, cardiovascular collapse severely compromises both liver blood flow and hepatocellular function.[14] In experimental hemorrhagic shock, clearance of lidocaine was decreased by 40%, while hepatic blood flow declined by 30%.[20] The reduction in clearance was too large to be attributed to only decreased hepatic perfusion, implying a concomitant reduction in intrinsic clearance secondary to hepatic ischemia.

Liver disease can decrease drug clearance because of hepatocellular dysfunction, altered hepatic blood flow, or both.[14] Cirrhosis reduces the clearance of many drugs with high extraction ratios, including lidocaine,[18] meperidine,[21,22] and propranolol.[23] This is secondary to decreased hepatic perfusion, which can be due to reduced total liver blood flow, intrahepatic shunting, or extrahepatic shunting of portal venous blood.[14] Any shunting will greatly increase the bioavailability of drugs with high extraction ratios that are administered orally.[14] Cirrhosis also decreases the clearance of some drugs with low extraction ratios, such as diazepam,[24,25] because of impaired hepatocellular function, which decreases intrinsic clearance. Acute viral hepatitis reduces the clearance of drugs with both high (meperidine,[26] lidocaine[27]) and low (diazepam[24]) hepatic extraction ratios. These observations suggest that both acute and chronic liver disease affect hepatocellular function and hepatic perfusion in a parallel fashion. It follows that, as a general rule, the dose of any drug cleared by the liver should be reduced in the presence of hepatic disease.

Drugs that alter splanchnic hemodynamics will affect clearance of highly extracted drugs. Propranolol decreases hepatic blood flow, thus decreasing its own clearance[14] and the clearance of concomitantly administered lidocaine.[28] The volatile anesthetic agents halothane, enflurane, and isoflurane all decrease hepatic blood flow, although isoflurane does so to a lesser extent.[29,30] Intra-abdominal surgery causes a further decrease in hepatic perfusion.[29] Hypotension produced by spinal anesthesia reduces splanchnic blood flow.[31] In contrast to the volatile anesthetics, nitrous oxide, opioids, and barbiturates have little effect on hepatic blood flow.[14] Although they are potentially of great clinical importance, the effects of these hemodynamic alterations have not been thoroughly investigated. It is logical to assume that the clearance of drugs with high hepatic extraction ratios will be reduced during anesthesia and surgery.

Renal Drug Clearance

Although the kidneys can metabolize drugs, their major function in drug elimination is to excrete drugs, and metabolites produced elsewhere (primarily the liver), into the urine. The renal clearance of a drug is determined by the net effects of three processes: glomerular filtration, tubular secretion, and tubular reabsorption.[32,33]

Glomerular filtration is an inefficient means of drug elimination. The glomerular filtration rate is approximately 20% of renal plasma flow.[33] Consequently, even if none of the drug was bound to plasma proteins, only about 20% of the total amount in the plasma could be removed by glomerular filtration. Drug binding to plasma proteins and erythrocytes reduces the amount filtered, because only unbound drug can pass through the glomerular membrane into the renal tubule.[33] If a drug is neither secreted nor reabsorbed by the renal tubules, then renal drug clearance will be equal to glomerular clearance. Drugs and metabolites excreted in this fashion have low renal extraction ratios, and their renal clearance depends on the degree of binding to blood constituents. Therefore, protein binding is a major determinant of both hepatic and renal clearance of drugs with low extraction ratios.

Proximal renal tubular cells have two discrete mechanisms for secreting acidic and basic organic compounds.[32,33] These processes are carrier-mediated, so they are saturable. Drugs with similar physicochemical characteristics will compete for available carrier molecules and interfere with each other's secretion. Although this relationship has the potential to cause toxicity, it can also be advantageous. For example, probenecid is used to delay excretion of penicillin and prolong the duration of effective antimicrobial levels. If a drug is very avidly secreted by the tubular cells and not subsequently reabsorbed, it will have a high renal extraction ratio. Renal clearance of such drugs is largely determined by the magnitude of renal blood flow.[32] This is analogous to the importance of liver blood flow in the clearance of drugs with high hepatic extraction ratios.

Clearance of drugs filtered by the glomeruli or secreted by the proximal renal tubule may be decreased by subsequent reabsorption from the renal tubule. If this is extensive, the drug will have a very low renal extraction ratio and negligible renal clearance. Tubular reabsorption occurs by active, carrier-mediated transport that is similar to active secretion.[33] Drugs can also be reabsorbed into the circulation by passive diffusion across the tubular epithelium. The progressive reabsorption of water from the renal tubule facilitates passive reabsorption of drugs by creating a tubule-to-plasma concentration gradient for free drug. Consequently, oliguria can decrease renal drug clearance.[33] Passive reabsorption is determined by the lipid solubility and the degree of ionization of a drug. Highly lipophilic drugs like thiopental are almost completely reabsorbed and have virtually no renal clearance. For less lipophilic drugs, the degree of ionization is a major determinant of the extent of passive reab-

sorption because only the non-ionized drug readily diffuses across the renal tubular epithelium. Urine pH can range from 4.5 to 8.0, which can cause large changes in the ionized fraction of weak acids and bases, particularly if the pK_a is close to or within this range. Urine pH can be manipulated to increase renal clearance following overdoses. Alkalinizing the urine by iv injection of sodium bicarbonate increases the excretion of weak acids, such as phenobarbital and salicylates.[34] Renal excretion of basic drugs like amphetamines can be enhanced by acidifying the urine.

Physiologic, Pharmacologic, and Pathologic Alterations in Renal Drug Clearance

In the adult human, renal blood flow is approximately 1200 $ml\cdot min^{-1}$, so renal plasma flow is approximately 700 $ml\cdot min^{-1}$. About one fifth of the plasma is filtered by the glomerulus, resulting in an average glomerular filtration rate of 125 $ml\cdot min^{-1}$. Renal blood flow and glomerular filtration rate are autoregulated, so they remain fairly constant as long as mean arterial pressure is between 70 and 160 mm Hg.[35] Consequently, renal drug clearance is more constant than hepatic clearance, because renal blood flow is more closely autoregulated than hepatic blood flow.

The capacity for excreting endogenous and exogenous compounds depends on the number of functionally intact nephrons. Decreased glomerular filtration is accompanied by a parallel loss of renal tubular functions. Therefore, clearance of endogenous creatinine, which is essentially equivalent to the glomerular filtration rate, can be used to estimate overall renal function. It follows that renal drug clearance is proportional to creatinine clearance, even for drugs eliminated primarily by tubular secretion. This principle has been used to develop nomograms for reducing drug doses according to the creatinine clearance in the presence of renal dysfunction.[33,34] Many drugs, including lidocaine,[36] pancuronium,[37] and meperidine,[38] have pharmacologically active metabolites than are excreted by the kidneys. Therefore, both parent drugs and their metabolites can contribute to drug toxicity in patients with renal failure.

Renal function decreases progressively with age. By age 80 years, creatinine clearance is reduced by about 50%.[39] Creatinine is produced by metabolism of muscle creatine. Despite the age-related decrease in glomerular filtration rate, the serum creatinine concentration is not elevated in healthy elderly patients because skeletal muscle mass also decreases progressively with age. Therefore, even if the serum creatinine concentration is normal, renal clearance of drugs is reduced in elderly patients.

Many drugs encountered in anesthetic practice are eliminated primarily by the kidneys (Table 13-2). In the setting

---

TABLE 13-2. Drugs with Significant Renal Excretion Encountered in Anesthesiology

Aminoglycosides	Nadolol
Atenolol	Neostigmine
Cephalosporins	Pancuronium
Cimetidine	Penicillins
Digoxin	Pipecuronium
Doxacurium	Procainamide
d-Tubocurarine	Pyridostigmine
Edrophonium	Vecuronium
Metocurine	

of renal failure, doses of these drugs must be reduced to avoid adverse effects. In addition to renal disease, other pathologic processes can impair kidney function. Circulatory shock and severe congestive heart failure reduce renal flood flow, glomerular filtration, and, consequently, renal drug clearance.[32] Advanced hepatic cirrhosis also interferes with renal function,[32] and this combination, termed the *hepatorenal syndrome,* will reduce the elimination of virtually any drug.

DRUG METABOLISM

It is obvious that, unless tolerance* develops, termination of drug action depends on elimination of the drug and any pharmacologically active metabolites from the body. As discussed earlier, drugs must usually cross cell membranes to reach their sites of action. Consequently, most pharmacologically active compounds are lipid soluble to some extent. This property makes excretion of drugs difficult, because lipophilic compounds are readily reabsorbed from the gut and the distal renal tubule after hepatobiliary or renal excretion. Metabolism, or *biotransformation* of drugs to more polar, water-soluble compounds, facilitates the ultimate excretion of metabolites in the bile and urine. Therefore, the rate of biotransformation of drugs is a primary determinant of the duration and intensity of their pharmacologic effects. Teleologically, biotransformation can be regarded as a protective mechanism for preventing the accumulation and resultant toxic effects of various lipophilic compounds acquired from the environment.

Metabolites are usually less active pharmacologically than the parent drug. However, this is not always true. Many benzodiazepines have metabolites that have similar pharmacologic effects.[6] The biotransformation of codeine to morphine produces a metabolite that is more potent than the parent compound. Metabolites can also be toxic. The major metabolite of meperidine is normeperidine, which can cause seizures.[38] If metabolites are active or toxic, further biotransformation or excretion is required for termination of pharmacologic effect.

Metabolism of drugs and other exogenous compounds, known collectively as *xenobiotics,* occurs primarily in the liver. Other organs, including the kidneys, lungs, gut, and skin, also metabolize drugs. However, the contribution of these extrahepatic sites to biotransformation is quantitatively unimportant in most instances.

Biotransformation Reactions

The biochemical reactions responsible for biotransformation have classically been divided into two groups. Phase I reactions consist of processes that alter the molecular structure of xenobiotics by modifying an existing functional group of the drug, by adding a new functional chemical group to the compound, or by splitting the original molecule into two fragments. These changes in molecular structure result from either oxidation, reduction, or hydrolysis of the

*Tolerance is defined as decreasing pharmacologic effect with sustained exposure to a drug. It results in higher doses (or concentrations) being required to maintain a given effect. The mechanisms responsible for tolerance are diverse. They include adaptive or reflex responses to drug effects that alter the observed effects, as well as such mechanisms as alterations in the number or sensitivity of receptors.

parent compound. Phase II reactions consist of the coupling, or conjugation, of a variety of endogenous compounds to polar chemical groups. The polar functional group at which conjugation occurs is frequently the result of a previous Phase I reaction, hence the Phase I–Phase II nomenclature. However, not all drugs are eliminated by this sequential pathway of biotransformation. Oxidation of thiopental produces its major metabolite, thiopental carboxylic acid,[40] which undergoes renal excretion without undergoing further (Phase II) biotransformation. Morphine already has polar functional groups, so it can be directly conjugated to form its major metabolite, morphine glucuronide, without first undergoing a "Phase I" reaction.[41] Because of the many exceptions to the Phase I–Phase II sequence of biotransformation, the term "functionalization reactions" has been proposed as an alternative to "Phase I reactions" to describe those reactions that result in the creation or modification of functional chemical groups.[42] Similarly, Phase II reactions are often termed "synthetic" or "conjugation reactions."

Phase I Reactions

Phase I reactions either hydrolyze, oxidize, or reduce the parent compound. Hydrolysis is defined chemically as the insertion of a molecule of water into another molecule, which forms an unstable intermediate compound that subsequently splits apart. Thus, hydrolysis cleaves the original substance into two separate molecules. Hydrolytic reactions are the primary way amides, such as lidocaine and other amide local anesthetics, and esters, such as succinylcholine, are metabolized. Amide hydrolysis is catalyzed by amidases that are primarily located in the cytoplasm of hepatocytes.[43] Ester hydrolysis is catalyzed by esterases found in the liver and many other tissues; for example, the hydrolysis of succinylcholine by plasma pseudocholinesterase.[43]

Many drugs are biotransformed by oxidative reactions. Oxidations are defined as reactions that result in the removal of electrons from a molecule. The common element of most, if not all, oxidations is an enzymatically mediated reaction that inserts a hydroxyl ($-OH$) group into the drug molecule.[43] In some instances this produces a chemically stable, more polar hydroxylated metabolite. However, hydroxylation often creates unstable compounds that spontaneously split into separate molecules. Many different biotransformations are effected by this basic mechanism. Dealkylation (removal of a carbon-containing group), deamination (removal of nitrogen-containing groups), oxidation of nitrogen-containing groups, desulfuration, dehalogenation, and dehydrogenation all follow an initial hydroxylation.[43] It is evident that hydrolysis and hydroxylation are analogous processes. Both have an initial, enzymatically mediated step that produces an unstable compound that rapidly dissociates into separate molecules.

Some drugs are metabolized by reductive reactions, that is, reactions that add electrons to a molecule. In contrast to oxidations, where electrons are transferred from NADPH to an oxygen atom, the electrons are transferred to the drug molecule. Oxidative metabolism of xenobiotics requires oxygen, but reductive biotransformation is inhibited by oxygen, so it is facilitated when the intracellular oxygen tension is low.[44]

The Cytochrome P-450 System. The complex of enzymes and pigmented hemoproteins that catalyzes most oxidative and some reductive biotransformations is known collectively as the *cytochrome P-450 system.* This term is derived from the fact that the heme-containing pigments, when reduced by carbon monoxide, have an absorption spectrum with a peak at the 450 nm wavelength. This system is incorporated into the smooth endoplasmic reticulum of hepatocytes. Other tissues, including the kidneys, lungs, gut, and skin, also contain cytochrome P-450, but in much smaller amounts.[41] The endoplasmic reticulum is an intracellular network of tubules similar in ultrastructure to cellular membranes. When liver cells are homogenized, the fragments of the endoplasmic reticulum form vesicles called *microsomes* that can be separated from other cellular constituents by centrifugation. The cytochrome P-450 complex is capable of metabolizing hundreds of compounds, including endogenous substances such as steroids and biogenic amines, as well as drugs and other exogenous compounds acquired from the environment.[45] The cytochrome P-450 system oxidizes its substrates primarily by the insertion of an atom of oxygen in the form of a hydroxyl ($-OH$) group, while another oxygen atom is reduced to water. Because of these various properties, other terms have been used to describe the cytochrome P-450 complex, such as microsomal hydroxylase, mono-oxygenase, mixed-function oxidase, and polysubstrate mono-oxygenase.

The sequence of reactions involved in the oxidation of drugs and other substrates by the cytochrome P-450 system is shown in Figure 13-5. The drug molecule binds to the oxidized form of cytochrome P-450, designated as Fe^{3+} in Figure 13-5. This drug–cytochrome P-450 complex is then reduced by transfer of an electron from NADPH *via* the flavoprotein NADPH–cytochrome P-450 reductase.[46] The reduced drug–cytochrome complex then binds a molecule of oxygen. The reaction is completed with the addition of a second electron (e^-) and two hydrogen ions (H^+), which reduces one of the oxygen atoms to water while the drug is oxidized. The oxidized drug–cytochrome complex then dissociates, regenerating the oxidized form of cytochrome P-450. NADPH is regenerated by intermediary metabolism of carbohydrates.

Cytochrome P-450 is not a single entity. Rather, cytochrome P-450 is a superfamily of *isoenzymes*.[47] Isoenzymes are enzymes that catalyze similar reactions despite differences in their own molecular structures. In any given mammalian species, the number of cytochrome P-450 genes is currently estimated to be between 60 and over 200,[48] with more than 20 isoenzymes expressed.[46]

Cytochrome P-450 drug-metabolizing activity increases after exposure to various exogenous chemicals, including some drugs. Early research demonstrated two distinct patterns of altered drug-metabolizing enzyme activity after exposure to two different inducing agents, phenobarbital and polycyclic hydrocarbons. Consequently, compounds were originally classified as belonging to one of these two prototypic classes of cytochrome P-450 inducers.[49] However, this two-tiered classification is now known to be an oversimplification. There are "constitutive" forms of cytochrome P-450 that are involved in the metabolism of various endogenous compounds, such as steroids, thyroxine, prostaglandins, and biogenic amines. In addition to the constitutive forms, multiple isoenzymes can be induced by a wide variety of xenobiotics.[48] It has been suggested that there is the genetic capacity to produce hundreds of inducible isoenzymes of cytochrome P-450, and that the number and type of isoenzymes present at any time vary according to exposure to different xenobiotics. If this hypothesis is true, then induction of cytochrome P-450 isoenzymes would be analogous to the synthesis of specific immunoglobulins after exposure to different antigenic substances.[45]

After a single injection of phenobarbital, cytochrome P-450 activity peaks at 24 hours.[41] With continued exposure to an inducing agent, cytochrome P-450 increases until a new steady state is reached, usually within 3–5 days. The degree of enzyme induction is dependent on the dose of the inducing agent. After removal of the enzyme inducer, the amount of cytochrome P-450 decreases, with a half-time of approximately 24 hours. This appears to be the usual half-time for turnover of hepatic cytochrome P-450.[41]

The cytochrome P-450 system is able to protect the organism from the deleterious effects of accumulation of exogenous compounds because of its two fundamental characteristics—broad substrate specificity and the capability to adapt to exposure to different substances by induction of different isoenzymes.

Biotransformations can also be inhibited if different substrates compete for the drug-binding site on cytochrome P-450. The effect of two competing substrates on each other's metabolism depends on their relative affinities for the enzyme. Generally, metabolism of the compound with the lower affinity will be inhibited to a greater degree. This is the mechanism by which the H_2 receptor antagonist cimetidine inhibits the metabolism of many drugs, including meperidine, propranolol, and diazepam.[50-52] The newer H_2 antagonist ranitidine has a different structure and has been shown to cause fewer clinically significant problems related to decreased biotransformation.[53] Other drugs, including the calcium channel blockers verapamil and diltiazem, also bind to cytochrome P-450, and diltiazem inhibits oxidative drug metabolism in humans.[54] Because so many drugs are metabolized by the cytochrome P-450 system, it is likely that more clinically significant interactions affecting drug metabolism will become evident in the future.

Induction and inhibition of hepatic drug-metabolizing enzyme systems will result in changes in the intrinsic hepatic clearance of drugs. This is most important for drugs having low hepatic extraction ratios, because intrinsic clearance is the primary determinant of their hepatic clearance. Alterations in drug-metabolizing enzyme activity have little effect on drugs with high hepatic extraction ratios, because their clearance is primarily dependent on hepatic blood flow.

Phase II Reactions

Phase II reactions are also known as *conjugation* or *synthetic* reactions. The end products of these reactions result from the enzymatically mediated combination of various endogenous compounds with parent drugs or metabolites.[43]

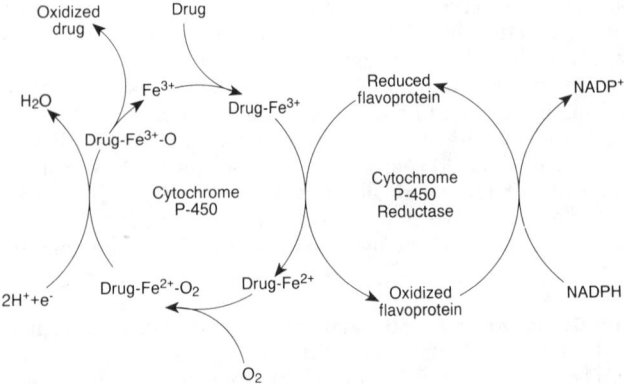

Figure 13-5. The cytochrome P-450 drug metabolizing system. See text for explanation.

Conjugation reactions can occur only at susceptible functional groups. Many drugs do not have a suitable functional group, and the site at which conjugation occurs is a result of a previous Phase I reaction. Other drugs, such as morphine, already have a functional group that can serve as a "handle" for conjugation, and they undergo these reactions directly.[41]

Various endogenous compounds can be attached to parent drugs or their Phase I metabolites to form different conjugation products. The endogenous substrates include glucuronic acid, acetate, and amino acids. Mercapturic acid conjugates result from the binding of exogenous compounds to glutathione. Other conjugation reactions produce sulfated or methylated derivatives of drugs or their metabolites. The enzymes that catalyze glucuronide conjugations are part of the drug-metabolizing complex that is bound to the endoplasmic reticulum.[43] The other enzymes are located in the cytoplasm.[43] Like the cytochrome P-450 system, the enzymes that catalyze Phase II reactions are inducible.[49]

Phase II reactions produce conjugates that are polar, water-soluble compounds. This facilitates the ultimate excretion of the drug *via* the kidneys or, to a lesser extent, by hepatobiliary secretion. Conjugates that enter the gut after hepatobiliary secretion may be hydrolyzed by bacterial or mucosal enzymes. This regenerates a more lipid-soluble drug moiety which can then be reabsorbed into the portal circulation and returned to the liver. This process is termed *enterohepatic circulation*, and it limits excretion of conjugates *via* the GI tract. Because not all of the reabsorbed drug is extracted by the liver, some will re-enter the systemic circulation, prolonging the duration of action of the drug.

Factors Affecting Biotransformation

Drug metabolism varies substantially between individuals. To a large extent, this variability stems from differences in the genes that control the numerous enzymes responsible for biotransformation. For most drugs, individual subjects' rates of metabolism are normally distributed. However, inherited differences in rates of biotransformation do not always conform to this type of unimodal distribution. Distinct subpopulations with different rates of elimination of some drugs have been identified. This results in a multimodal distribution of individual rates of metabolism, a phenomenon known as *polymorphism*. For example, different genotypes result in either normal, low, or (rarely) absent plasma pseudocholinesterase activity, accounting for the well-known differences in individuals' responses to succinylcholine, which is hydrolyzed by this enzyme.[55] Several acetylation reactions also exhibit polymorphism.[43]

Drug metabolism also varies with age. The fetus and neonate have less capacity for some biotransformations, especially those catalyzed by cytochrome P-450.[56,57] However, cytochrome P-450 activity increases dramatically in early infancy.[56,57] Neonates also have less capacity for conjugation reactions, especially glucuronidation.[56,57] This is the cause of "physiologic jaundice," which is due to impaired conjugation of bilirubin. Metabolism of some drugs may also be decreased in geriatric patients, although it is difficult to separate the effects of age *per se* from the effects of other factors, such as pathologic processes.[58,59]

Exposure to various foreign compounds can alter drug-metabolizing enzyme activity. Barbiturates, phenytoin, macrolide antibiotics, imidazole antifungal agents, and corticosteroids can cause drug interactions secondary to induction of hepatic drug-metabolizing enzymes.[49] Chronic ethanol consumption induces enzyme activity, but acute intoxication inhibits the biotransformation of some drugs.[60] Smoking increases the metabolism of many drugs secondary to enzyme induction by polycyclic hydrocarbons in tobacco smoke.[61]

Liver disease profoundly affects drug disposition. However, because of the normal variability in drug metabolism and differences in the severity and type of pathologic processes, it is often very difficult to demonstrate significant changes in patients with hepatic diseases. It is also difficult to separate the effects of altered biotransformation *per se* from other effects of liver disease, such as altered binding of drugs to plasma proteins and decreased liver blood flow. Nonetheless, hepatic disease has been shown to decrease the clearance of drugs with low hepatic extraction ratios,[15,62] which implies impaired biotransformation.

Congestive heart failure has been shown to decrease the metabolism of lidocaine and theophylline.[19] Renal failure has different effects on different biotransformation reactions. The rates of hydrolytic and acetylation reactions are decreased, but conjugations usually are not affected, and some oxidations may actually be enhanced.[63]

Effects of Anesthesia and Surgery on Biotransformation

Drug disposition is altered in the perioperative period. Although many other factors are probably also involved, biotransformation reactions are affected by anesthesia and surgery. In dogs anesthetized with halothane, the intrinsic hepatic clearance of propranolol is decreased, which implies that hepatic drug-metabolizing ability is impaired.[64] Animal studies indicate that halothane inhibits demethylation of aminopyrine in a dose-dependent fashion.[65] The same study showed that isoflurane is a less potent inhibitor, and that enflurane did not affect this biotransformation.

Many investigators have studied the effects of anesthesia and surgery on antipyrine clearance. Antipyrine, an antipyretic that is no longer used therapeutically, does not bind to plasma proteins, has a low hepatic extraction ratio, and is not cleared by the kidneys. Therefore, clearance of antipyrine is independent of changes in protein binding and hepatic blood flow and is solely dependent on the activity of hepatic drug-metabolizing enzymes. This permits the use of antipyrine clearance as an indicator of hepatic drug-metabolizing activity.[66] Clearance of antipyrine is generally increased after surgery conducted with a wide variety of general anesthetic techniques,[67-69] although there are exceptions to this rule. General anesthesia with enflurane does not appear to increase antipyrine clearance.[70] After operations lasting more than 4 hours, antipyrine clearance is decreased.[67] Presumably, major surgical trauma interferes with drug metabolism, although the precise mechanisms are not known. Antipyrine clearance is also increased after spinal anesthesia.[69] Therefore, general anesthesia is not a prerequisite for increased rates of biotransformation in the postoperative period, and other perioperative factors also affect drug metabolism. For example, the caloric source of iv nutritional regimens influences antipyrine clearance. It is decreased when the only caloric source is 5% dextrose, and increased when amino acids are substituted for dextrose.[71] Occupational exposure to halothane increased antipyrine clearance in anesthesiologists working in operating theaters without equipment for scavenging excess anesthetic gases.[72] The implications of this finding for operating room personnel are not known.

In addition to altered rates of biotransformation, other factors, such as decreased hepatic blood flow during surgery,[29,30] can affect drug elimination in the perioperative period. In many patients the magnitude of these changes is too small to cause any clinically evident problems. However, in some patients clinically significant changes in drug elimination will occur. Decreased drug clearance can result in higher concentrations of drugs and increase the risk of adverse effects, especially during and after prolonged surgery. The clinician must be vigilant in looking for signs of excessive pharmacologic effects and must tailor doses according to individual patients' responses. Increased drug clearance after surgery could theoretically decrease the effectiveness of usual doses of drugs, necessitating increased doses.

BINDING OF DRUGS TO PLASMA PROTEINS

After injection or ingestion, drugs are transported to their sites of action and to eliminating organs *via* the blood. Drugs are present in the blood in two fractions. Some is simply dissolved in plasma water; the rest is bound to various components of whole blood, such as plasma proteins and red blood cells. Usually only the total drug concentration is measured. However, knowledge of the degree of binding is critical to interpreting the therapeutic implications of the total drug concentration. If binding is decreased, then the free drug concentration will be higher for any given total drug concentration, increasing the risk of adverse effects.

Drug concentrations are usually measured in plasma or serum. Ideally, drug concentrations should be measured in whole blood, because drugs are transported in blood, not plasma, and drugs equilibrate between erythrocytes and plasma very quickly.[73] Unfortunately, measurement of total drug levels and drug binding in whole blood is technically much more difficult than in plasma, and very few investigators have directly measured whole blood binding. As a compromise, the blood:plasma concentration ratio can be used to estimate whole blood binding.

Drugs bind to plasma proteins in a reversible fashion that obeys the law of mass action:

$$[\text{unbound drug}] + [\text{protein}] \underset{k_2}{\overset{k_1}{\rightleftharpoons}} [\text{drug--protein complex}]$$

$$(13\text{-}5)$$

The rate constant of the forward (association) and reverse (dissociation) reactions are k_1 and k_2, respectively. These reactions are very rapid, having half-times of a few milliseconds.[74] Binding of drugs to blood constituents other than proteins, such as erythrocytes, proceeds in an analogous fashion. The equilibrium association constant, K_a, quantifies the affinity of drug-protein binding:

$$K_a = \frac{k_1}{k_2} = \frac{[\text{drug--protein complex}]}{[\text{unbound drug}] \times [\text{protein}]} \qquad (13\text{-}6)$$

Binding can also be described with the dissociation constant, K_d, which is the reciprocal of the association constant and is equal to k_2/k_1. The dissociation constant has units of moles·l^{-1}, and is the drug concentration at which 50% of the binding sites are occupied.[74] Equations 13-5 and 13-6 indicate that the degree of binding is dependent on the protein concentration, the affinity of the protein for the drug, and the unbound drug concentration, which in turn is dependent on the total drug concentration.

The extent of plasma drug binding can be expressed as the *percentage of drug bound*, which is the percentage of the total drug present that is bound to plasma proteins. Al-

ternatively, the *free fraction*, which is the percentage of drug not bound to plasma proteins, can be used. For example, approximately 83% of fentanyl is bound to plasma proteins. Therefore, the free fraction of fentanyl is about 17%.[75,76]

The degree of drug binding to plasma proteins is determined by one of two methods, equilibrium dialysis or ultrafiltration.[77] In equilibrium dialysis, drug-containing plasma is separated from a protein-free buffer by a membrane that is permeable to the drug but does not allow passage of protein molecules. After equilibration, the drug concentration on the protein-free side will be identical to the free drug concentration in the plasma. Ultrafiltration uses centrifugation to create a protein-free filtrate across a similarly semipermeable membrane. In both techniques, the drug concentration in the protein-free solution is measured, and the free fraction in plasma is then calculated. Protein binding is affected by many factors, including temperature and pH.[73,74] At high drug concentrations, binding sites become saturated and the free fraction increases.[74] There are also qualitative differences between species in plasma proteins that affect drug binding, and binding to purified human albumin may not correlate with binding in plasma.[73,74] Consequently, to provide clinically useful information, studies of drug binding must be conducted at physiologic temperature and pH with human plasma, and at concentrations within the usual therapeutic range.

Drug-protein binding has important pharmacologic implications, because only unbound drug can cross cell membranes to reach its sites of action. Also, free drug is more readily available for elimination. This has led to the frequently held misconception that drug bound to plasma proteins and other blood constituents is pharmacologically inert. This is not the case. As soon as unbound drug leaves circulation, the law of mass action dictates that some drug will dissociate from binding sites, which tends to restore the free drug concentration. This occurs almost instantaneously,[74] so that binding of drugs to plasma proteins creates a dynamic reservoir that buffers acute changes in the free drug concentration.

As discussed earlier, the rate of elimination of some drugs is dependent on the degree of protein binding. The extent of distribution of drugs throughout the body also depends on the degree of binding. At equilibrium, the proportion of drug in the body that is in extravascular sites is determined by the relative affinity of blood binding *versus* binding to other tissues. A drug that is highly bound to plasma proteins or erythrocytes cannot be extensively distributed. Exceptions to this rule are drugs that have even greater affinity for extravascular binding sites. Protein binding also affects drug action. Drug interactions may result from competition for the same binding site. These pharmacokinetic and pharmacodynamic consequences of altered drug-protein binding will be discussed in succeeding sections of this chapter.

Binding Proteins

Two plasma proteins are primarily responsible for drug binding: albumin and alpha$_1$-acid glycoprotein (AAG). Drugs also bind to other plasma proteins, such as globulins or lipoproteins, and to erythrocytes. Many drugs bind to more than one protein. For example, fentanyl and sufentanil bind to albumin, AAG, globulins, and also to red blood cells.[76]

Albumin comprises over half of the total plasma protein content and is the most important drug-binding protein. In addition to a wide range of drugs, including barbiturates,

TABLE 13-3. Drugs Binding to Alpha₁-Acid Glycoprotein

Alfentanil	Meperidine
Alprenolol	Methadone
Bupivacaine	Propranolol
Disopyramide	Quinidine
Etidocaine	Sufentanil
Fentanyl	Verapamil
Lidocaine	

TABLE 13-4. Plasma Protein Binding of Some Drugs Used in Anesthesiology

Class/Drug	Percent Bound	Reference
Cardiovascular Drugs		
Digoxin	20–30	149
Diltiazem	77–80	150
Esmolol	55	151
Nifedipine	96–98	150
Propranolol	89	100
Verapamil	84–91	150
Benzodiazepines		
Diazepam	97–99	152
Lorazepam	88–92	153
Midazolam	96	90
Intravenous Anesthetics		
Methohexital	73	154
Propofol	98	155
Thiopental	85	97
Local Anesthetics*		
Bupivacaine	95	156
Etidocaine	95	156
Lidocaine	70	156
Mepivacaine	80	156
Neuromuscular Blockers		
d-Tubocurarine	49–56	11, 157
Metocurine	65	11
Pancuronium	11–29	157, 158
Vecuronium	30	157
Opioids		
Alfentanil	92	76
Fentanyl	84	76
Meperidine	53–63	89
Methadone	60–90	159
Morphine	20–35	94, 159, 160
Sufentanil	92	76

* At nontoxic concentrations. At toxic plasma concentrations, binding of local anesthetic decreases, leading to a marked increase in the free drug concentration.

benzodiazepines, and penicillins, albumin binds endogenous compounds such as bilirubin. Many drugs bind to more than one site on the albumin molecule, and most drugs have one or perhaps two high-affinity (primary) binding sites and a variable number of secondary, low-affinity sites.[73] Studies with radioactively labeled drugs indicate that albumin has at least three discrete, high-affinity drug-binding sites.[78] Diazepam, digitoxin, and warfarin each bind to a different site. The sites at which other drugs bind to albumin and the affinity of the drug-albumin bond can be determined by using these three markers.[78] This permits prediction of the likelihood of one drug displacing another. Drugs that compete for the same binding site are more likely to displace one another than drugs that bind at different sites, and the drug with the lower affinity for the binding site will be more easily displaced.

Albumin is the major binding protein for organic acids, such as penicillins and barbiturates. Basic drugs also bind to albumin, but to a lesser extent. The primary binding protein for many basic drugs, such as propranolol, amide local anesthetics, and opioids, is AAG. Some drugs known to bind to AAG are listed in Table 13-3. Basic drugs also bind to lipoproteins and globulins. AAG is an acute phase reactant, and its plasma concentration increases in a variety of acute and chronic illnesses.

Factors Affecting Drug Binding

The physicochemical properties of drugs influence binding to plasma proteins. Organic acids bind preferentially to albumin, and basic drugs have a higher affinity for AAG. Generally, the greater the lipid solubility of a drug, the greater is the binding to plasma proteins. It is evident from Table 13-4 that water-soluble drugs, such as the neuromuscular blocking agents d-tubocurarine, pancuronium, and vecuronium, are bound to a lesser extent than lipid-soluble drugs, such as sufentanil and thiopental. This is also true for drugs that belong to the same class. The degree of binding of opioids parallels their lipid solubility. Morphine is the least bound, fentanyl and its derivatives are highly bound, and meperidine is intermediate in binding. Similarly, bupivacaine is bound to a greater extent than lidocaine.

Many physiologic and pathologic states result in quantitative and qualitative changes in the primary drug-binding plasma proteins, albumin and AAG. Drug binding may also be affected by acid-base disturbances that alter the degree of ionization of drugs and proteins, and by accumulation of endogenous compounds that compete for drug-binding sites.

Maternal and Neonatal Drug Binding

Binding of drugs in pregnancy and in the fetus or neonate has received much attention because of its impact on placental drug transfer. Pregnant women have reduced levels of albumin, and the binding of many organic acids, such as phenytoin, is decreased at term.[79-81] Thiopental, another organic acid, is widely used in obstetric patients for induction of anesthesia. However, unlike phenytoin, the free fraction of thiopental is not increased in patients undergoing cesarean section,[82] so that usual doses of thiopental do not result in excessive free drug levels. This is fortunate, because high free drug levels would increase the risk of side-effects and enhance placental transfer of the drug. The free fraction of diazepam, which binds primarily to albumin, is increased at term.[83] AAG levels are not changed during pregnancy.[83] However, the free fractions of lidocaine and propranolol are, nonetheless, increased at term.[83]

Neonates have decreased levels of albumin and levels of AAG that are only about one-third the adult level.[81,83,84] In addition to these quantitative differences, neonatal albumin may have less affinity for some drugs.[81,84] Consequently, the free fraction of many drugs, especially those that bind to AAG, is higher in the neonate than in the mother.[84] Although binding of many drugs is decreased in neonates, this does not affect the unbound concentration of drugs transferred across the placenta. Under near steady-state conditions, maternal and fetal free drug concentrations will be the same, although the total fetal level will be lower. Because the free drug is the more pharmacologically active species, the decrease in maternal plasma protein drug binding is of greater consequence as far as placental transfer of drugs is concerned. Obviously, decreased drug binding must be considered in neonatal therapeutics.[57]

Age and Sex

The plasma concentrations of the primary drug-binding proteins change with increasing age: albumin decreases slightly, while AAG tends to increase.[85-87] However, these changes are generally too small to produce clinically important effects on drug binding. The free fractions of lidocaine, meperidine, and propranolol, all of which bind to AAG, are not changed in the elderly.[85-89] Similarly, binding of drugs to albumin is minimally altered. The binding of midazolam does not change,[90] and diazepam binding may decrease slightly.[24,85,91] The typical magnitude of age-associated decreases in drug binding is illustrated by thiopental. The average free fraction of thiopental increases from about 18% in young adults to only 22% in geriatric patients.[92] Clinically significant changes in drug binding are much more likely to be due to various pathologic conditions than to the effects of age per se.

Studies comparing drug binding in men and women have generally not found any differences between the sexes. For example, the free fractions of diazepam, lidocaine, meperidine, phenytoin, and propranolol in men and women are similar.[83,86] This is not surprising, because the concentrations of albumin and AAG in men and women do not differ significantly.[83,86]

Hepatic Disease

The plasma albumin concentration is often decreased by liver disease. Drug binding may also be affected by qualitative changes in the albumin molecule that decrease affinity for drugs, and by accumulation of endogenous substances, such as bilirubin, that compete for drug-binding sites.[15] Although hepatic diseases vary widely in pathophysiology and severity, it is possible to make some generalizations regarding their impact on drug binding. The free fractions of drugs that bind primarily to albumin are increased. This is true for diazepam,[24,93] morphine,[94] and for the organic acids phenytoin[94] and thiopental.[95,96] The free fractions of basic drugs, such as lidocaine[27] and meperidine,[26] are not increased in patients with acute viral hepatitis, which suggests that drug binding to AAG is minimally affected by liver disease.

Renal Disease

Albumin levels tend to decrease in all types of renal disease. However, even when albumin levels are normal, binding of thiopental[97] and phenytoin[94] is decreased. The free fraction of phenytoin is correlated with both the albumin concentration and the severity of renal dysfunction.[94] This indicates that renal failure produces a qualitative defect of albumin that reduces its affinity for organic acids. Dialysis does not restore the affinity of albumin for thiopental or phenytoin.[94,97] The plasma protein binding of many other organic acids is also decreased in renal failure.[98]

The effect of renal disease on the binding of basic drugs depends on whether the drug binds primarily to albumin or to AAG, and on the type of renal disease. The free fraction of diazepam, which binds primarily to albumin, is increased in the nephrotic syndrome, renal failure, and after renal transplantation.[99] Similarly, binding of morphine is decreased in uremia.[94] Binding of other basic drugs varies according to the changes in AAG in different types of renal disease. Lidocaine binding increases in renal failure and after renal transplantation, conditions associated with increased AAG levels.[99] Likewise, propranolol binding is increased in patients with renal disease and elevated concentrations of AAG.[100] Lidocaine binding is not altered in nephrotic patients who have normal levels of AAG.[95]

Other Diseases

Patients with various inflammatory diseases, such as rheumatoid arthritis and Crohn's disease, have increased levels of AAG and, consequently, decreased free fractions of drugs that bind to this protein.[101,102] Malignant disease is also associated with elevated levels of AAG, and increased binding of lidocaine, propranolol, and other basic drugs has been demonstrated in patients with cancer. In contrast, albumin tends to decrease in patients with malignancies, which can decrease binding of acidic drugs.[102]

After acute myocardial infarction AAG levels double and remain elevated for about 3 weeks.[103] Consequently, the binding of lidocaine and propranolol is increased in these patients.[103,104]

Surgery and Trauma

The catabolic state that follows surgery and trauma decreases plasma albumin levels.[105] In contrast, the concentration of AAG increases after trauma[106] and surgery[107] and remains elevated for several weeks. These changes result in alterations in drug binding to plasma proteins after surgery and trauma. The free fraction of phenytoin increases after surgery, probably secondary to decreased levels of albumin, although the contemporaneous increase in free fatty acids may result in competition for binding sites.[105] The increase in AAG levels results in increased binding of basic drugs, such as lidocaine and propranolol, after trauma[106] and surgery.[108,109]

PHARMACOKINETIC PRINCIPLES

The concentration of a drug at its site or sites of action is a fundamental determinant of its pharmacologic effects. Because drugs are transported to and from their sites of action in the blood, the concentration at the active site is in turn a function of the concentration in the blood. Changes in drug concentration over time in the blood, at the site of action, and in other tissues are a result of complex interactions of various biologic factors with the physicochemical characteristics of the drug. Together, these factors determine the rate, extent, and pattern of drug absorption, distribution, metabolism, and excretion. The term *pharmacokinetics*, which is derived from the Greek words for "drug" and "moving," applies to the study of these factors. In its broadest sense, pharmacokinetics is the quantitative analysis of the relationship between the dose of a drug and the ensuing changes in drug concentration in the blood and other tissues.

Some early studies of the pharmacokinetics of iv and inhalational anesthetics used physiologic, or perfusion models. In these models, body tissues are classified according to similarities in perfusion and affinity for drugs.[110] Highly perfused tissues, including the brain, heart, lungs, liver, and kidneys, make up the vessel-rich group. Muscle and skin comprise the lean tissue group, and fat is considered as a separate group. The vessel-poor group, which has minimal effect on drug distribution and elimination, is composed of bone and cartilage.

Physiologic pharmacokinetic models made major contributions to understanding the factors influencing recovery from thiopental. They demonstrated that awakening after a single dose was primarily due to redistribution of thiopental from the brain to muscle and skin.[8,9] Distribution to other tissues and metabolism played minor roles. This fundamental concept, *redistribution*, also applies to other lipophilic drugs, such as fentanyl. Physiologic models have also contributed greatly to the understanding of the uptake and distribution of inhalational anesthetics.[111]

Physiologic pharmacokinetic models provide much insight into factors affecting drug action. They can predict the effects of physiologic changes, such as altered regional blood flows or reduced cardiac output, on drug distribution and elimination.[112] The disadvantage of perfusion-based models is their complexity. Verification of these models requires that drug concentrations be measured in many different tissues, which is rarely practical, and requires sophisticated mathematical analyses.[110] Because of these disadvantages, simpler pharmacokinetic models have been developed. In these models the body is envisaged as composed of one or more compartments. Drug concentrations in the blood are used to define the relationship between dose and the time course of changes of the drug concentration.[113] It is important to understand that the "compartments" that make up a compartmental pharmacokinetic model cannot be equated with the tissue groups used in physiologic pharmacokinetic models. Compartments are theoretical entities that are used to derive pharmacokinetic parameters, such as clearance, volume of distribution, and half-times. This provides a quantitative analysis of drug distribution and elimination.

Although compartmental models are simpler than physiologic pharmacokinetic models, they also have some disadvantages. For example, cardiac output is not a parameter of compartmental models. Therefore, compartmental models cannot be used to predict the effects of congestive heart failure on drug disposition. In spite of lacking such predictive capabilities, compartmental models can still quantify the effects of reduced cardiac output on the disposition of a drug if a group of patients with cardiac failure is compared to a group of normal subjects.

The discipline of pharmacokinetics is, to the despair of many, mathematically based. In the succeeding sections, the number of equations has been kept to the minimum required to develop the concepts needed to understand and interpret pharmacokinetic studies.

Pharmacokinetic Concepts

Rate Constants and Half-times

The disposition of most drugs follows *first-order* kinetics. A first-order kinetic process is one in which a constant fraction of the drug is removed during a finite period of time. This fraction is equivalent to the *rate constant* of the process. Rate constants are usually denoted by the letter k, and

have units of inverse time, such as min^{-1} or h^{-1}. If 10% of the drug is eliminated per minute, then the rate constant is $0.1\ min^{-1}$.

Because a constant fraction is removed per unit of time in first-order kinetics, the absolute amount of drug removed is proportional to the concentration of the drug. It follows that, in first-order kinetics, the rate of change of the concentration at any given time is proportional to the concentration present at that time. When the concentration is high, it will fall faster than when it is low. First-order kinetics apply not only to elimination processes but also to absorption and distribution of drugs.[113]

Rather than using rate constants, the rapidity of pharmacokinetic processes are often described with half-times—the time required for the plasma concentration to change by a factor of 2. Half-times are calculated directly from the corresponding rate constants with this simple equation:

$$t_{1/2} = \frac{\text{(natural logarithm of 2)}}{k} = \frac{0.693}{k} \quad (13\text{-}7)$$

Thus, a rate constant of $0.1\ min^{-1}$ translates into a half-time of 6.93 minutes. The half-time of any first-order kinetic process, including drug absorption, distribution, and elimination, can be calculated.

In theory, first-order processes, such as drug elimination, can never be completed because a constant fraction of the drug, not an absolute amount, is removed per unit of time. Therefore, first-order processes asymptotically approach completion. However, after five half-times, the process will be almost 97% complete (Table 13-5). For practical purposes, this is close enough to 100%, and can be considered as such.

Volumes of Distribution

The volume of distribution is the pharmacokinetic parameter that quantifies the extent of drug distribution. The physiologic factor that governs the extent of drug distribution is the overall capacity of tissues, relative to the capacity of the blood, for that drug. Overall tissue capacity for uptake of a drug is in turn a function of the total volume of the tissues into which a drug distributes and their average affinity for the drug. In compartmental pharmacokinetic models, drugs are envisaged as distributing into one or more "boxes," or compartments. These compartments cannot be equated with tissues. Rather, they are hypothetical entities that permit analysis of drug distribution and elimination.

The volume of distribution is an "apparent" volume because it represents the size of these hypothetical boxes, or compartments, that is necessary to explain the concentra-

TABLE 13-5. Elimination Half-times and Percentage of Drug Eliminated

Number of Elimination Half-Times	Percentage of Drug Remaining	Percentage of Drug Eliminated
0	100	0
1	50	50
2	25	75
3	12.5	87.5
4	6.25	93.75
5	3.125	96.875

tion of drug in a reference compartment, usually the so-called *central* or *plasma compartment*. The volume of distribution, *Vd*, relates the total amount of drug present to the concentration observed according to this equation:

$$Vd = \frac{\text{total amount of drug present}}{\text{concentration}} \quad (13\text{-}8)$$

Putting the arithmetic aside, this formula is logical. If a drug is extensively distributed, then the concentration will be lower, which equates to a larger volume of distribution. For example, if a total of 10 mg of drug is present and the concentration is 2 mg·l^{-1}, then the apparent volume of distribution is 5 liters. On the other hand, if the concentration was 4 mg·l^{-1}, then the volume of distribution would be 2.5 liters.

Simply stated, the apparent volume of distribution is a numeric index of the extent of drug distribution that does not have any relationship to the actual volume of any tissue or group of tissues. It may be as small as plasma volume, or, if overall tissue uptake is extensive, the apparent volume of distribution may greatly exceed the actual total volume of the body (Fig. 13-6). Because the volume of distribution is a mathematical approximation, it cannot be directly correlated with the anatomic and physiologic factors that influence drug distribution. Determination of the volume of distribution from a compartmental model does not provide any information regarding the tissues into which the drug actually distributes or the concentrations in those tissues. Despite these limitations, knowledge of the volume of distribution is often very useful. For example, if a drug has a larger apparent distribution volume than another drug with similar pharmacologic activity, then a larger loading dose will be required to "fill up the box" and achieve the same concentration. Various pathologic conditions also alter the volume of distribution, necessitating therapeutic adjustments.

Total Drug Clearance

In compartmental pharmacokinetic models, the ability of the system as a whole to irreversibly eliminate a drug is quantified by the *total drug clearance*. Drug clearance is the portion of the volume of distribution from which drug is completely removed in a given time interval. It is analogous to creatinine clearance, which measures the ability of the kidneys to eliminate creatinine; and, like creatinine clearance, drug clearance has units of flow. Multiple elimination pathways are additive, so that total drug clearance is the sum of the clearances of the various routes of elimination. Drug clearance is often corrected for weight or body surface area, in which case the units are ml·min^{-1}·kg^{-1} or ml·min^{-1}·m^{-2}, respectively.

Total drug clearance, *Cl*, can be calculated from the declining blood levels observed after an iv injection, as follows:

$$Cl = \frac{\text{dose}}{\text{area under the concentration } versus \text{ time curve}} \quad (13\text{-}9)$$

Again, this formula is intuitively logical. If a drug is rapidly removed from the plasma, its concentration will fall more quickly than the concentration of a drug that is less readily eliminated. This results in a smaller area under the concentration *versus* time curve, which equates to greater clearance.

There are limitations to the calculation of total drug clearance from pharmacokinetic models of concentration *versus* time data. If drug levels are measured in plasma, then only total *plasma* clearance can be derived, whereas drug elimination is actually a function of total *blood* clearance. The relative contribution of different organs to drug elimination cannot be determined from blood concentration data alone. Nonetheless, estimation of drug clearance with these models has made important contributions to clinical pharmacology. In particular, these models have provided a great deal of clinically useful information regarding altered drug elimination in various pathologic conditions.

Compartmental Pharmacokinetic Models

One-Compartment Model

In this model, the body is envisaged as a single homogeneous compartment. Drug distribution after injection is assumed to be instantaneous, so there are no concentration gradients within the compartment. The concentration can decrease only by elimination of drug from the system. The plasma concentration *versus* time curve for a hypothetical drug that instantly distributes throughout the body is shown in Figure 13-7. The initial plasma concentration is 10 μg·ml^{-1}, and the concentration decreases with time as a result of first-order elimination. With the concentration plotted on a logarithmic scale, then the concentration *versus* time curve becomes a straight line (see Fig. 13-7). The slope of this line is equal to the first-order elimination rate constant.

Immediately after injection, before any drug can be eliminated, the amount of drug present is equal to the dose. Therefore, by modifying Equation 13-8, the volume of distribution can be calculated:

$$Vd = \frac{\text{dose}}{\text{initial concentration}} \quad (13\text{-}10)$$

Although, for most drugs, the one-compartment model is an oversimplification, it does serve to illustrate the basic relationships between clearance, volume of distribution, and the elimination half-time. In the one-compartment

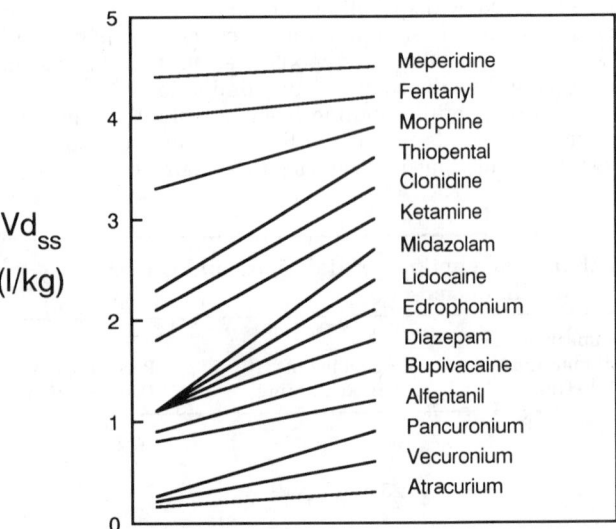

Figure 13-6. The volume of distribution for some drugs used in anesthesiology.

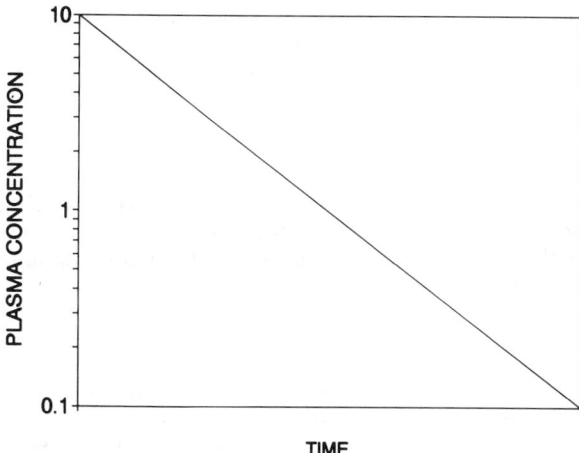

Figure 13-7. The plasma concentration, plotted on a logarithmic scale, *versus* time for a hypothetical drug exhibiting single compartment, first-order pharmacokinetics.

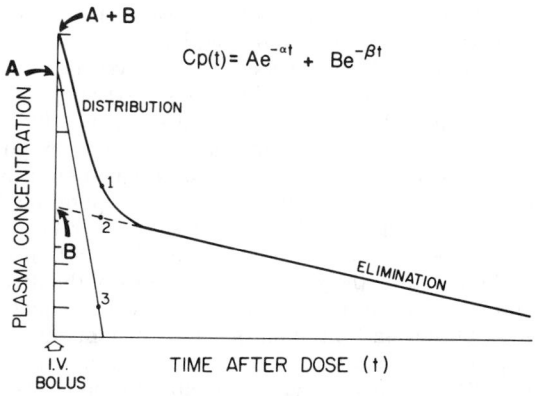

Figure 13-8. A schematic graph of the plasma concentration, on a logarithmic scale, *versus* time for a drug with a distribution phase preceding the elimination phase (two-compartment or biexponential kinetics). See text for explanation. (Reprinted with permission from Stanski DR, Watkins WD: Drug Disposition in Anesthesia, p 13. New York, Grune & Stratton, 1982.)

model, drug clearance, $\bar{Cl}$, is equal to the product of the elimination rate constant and the volume of distribution:

$$Cl = k \cdot Vd \qquad (13\text{-}11)$$

Combining Equations 13-7 and 13-11 yields:

$$Cl = \frac{0.693 \cdot Vd}{t_{1/2}}; \text{ thus: } t_{1/2} = \frac{0.693 \cdot Vd}{Cl} \qquad (13\text{-}12)$$

Therefore, the greater the clearance, the shorter the elimination half-time, which is easy to understand. Less obvious is the impact of the volume of distribution on the elimination half-time. It is easiest to understand if the physiologic correlate of a large volume of distribution is considered. A large volume of distribution reflects extensive tissue uptake of a drug, so that only a small fraction of the total amount of drug is in the blood and accessible to the organs of elimination. Consequently, the greater the volume of distribution, the longer the elimination half-time. For drugs that exhibit multicompartment pharmacokinetics, the relationships between clearance, volume of distribution, and the elimination half-time is not a simple linear one such as Equation 13-12. However, the same principles apply. All else being equal, the greater the clearance, the shorter the elimination half-time; the larger the volume of distribution, the longer the elimination half-time. Thus, the elimination half-time is dependent on two other variables, clearance and volume of distribution, that, respectively, characterize the extent of drug distribution and efficiency of drug elimination.

Two-Compartment Model

For many drugs, a graph of the logarithm of the plasma concentration *versus* time after an iv injection is similar to the schematic graph shown in Figure 13-8. There appear to be two discrete phases in the decline of the plasma concentration. The first phase after injection represents drug distribution and is characterized by a very rapid decrease in concentration. The rapid decrease in concentration during this "distribution phase" is largely due to passage of drug from the plasma into tissues. The distribution phase is followed by a slower decline of the concentration owing to drug elimination. Elimination also begins immediately after injection,

but its contribution to the drop in plasma concentration is initially masked by the much greater fall in concentration due to drug distribution.

To account for this biphasic behavior, one must consider the body to be made up of two compartments, a central (or plasma) compartment and a peripheral compartment (Fig. 13-9). In the two-compartment model, it is assumed that it is the central compartment into which the drug is injected and from which the blood samples for measurement of concentration are obtained, and that drug is eliminated only from the central compartment (see Fig. 13-9). Drug distribution within the central compartment is considered to be instantaneous. In reality, this last assumption cannot be true. However, drug uptake into some of the highly perfused tissues is so rapid that it cannot be detected as a discrete phase on the plasma concentration *versus* time curve.

Immediately after iv injection, all of the drug is in the central compartment. Simultaneously, three processes begin. Drug moves from the central to the peripheral compartment. This intercompartmental transfer is a first-order process, and its magnitude is quantified by the rate constant k_{12}. As drug builds up in the peripheral compartment, some passes back to the central compartment, a process characterized by the rate constant k_{21}. Drug is eliminated from the system *via* the central compartment. The elimination rate constant is k_e. The fall in the central compartment concentration following iv injection is a result of the net effects of these three processes.

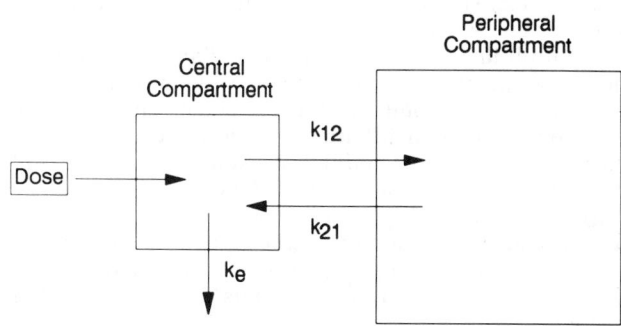

Figure 13-9. A two-compartment pharmacokinetic model. See text for explanation.

The distribution and elimination phases can be separated and then individually characterized by graphic analysis of the plasma concentration *versus* time curve, as shown in Figure 13-8. The elimination phase line is extrapolated back to time zero (the time of injection). At any time, the difference between the total concentration (indicated by point 1 on the graph) and the value on the extrapolated elimination phase line (indicated by point 2) is the corresponding value on the distribution phase line (point 3). This process is repeated at several times to construct the distribution phase line. In Figure 13-8, the zero time intercepts of the distribution and elimination lines are points A and B, respectively. The distribution and elimination rate constants are determined from the slopes of the two lines and are then used to calculate the distribution and elimination half-times. Therefore, at any time after an iv injection, the plasma concentration of drugs with two-compartment kinetics is equal to the sum of two exponential terms:

$$Cp_{(t)} = Ae^{-\alpha t} + Be^{-\beta t} \qquad (13\text{-}13)$$

where $Cp_{(t)}$ = plasma concentration at time t, A = intercept of the distribution phase line, α = rate constant of the distribution phase, B = intercept of the elimination phase line, β = rate constant of the elimination phase; and t = time. The first term characterizes the distribution phase and the second term characterizes the elimination phase. Immediately after injection, the first term is a much larger fraction of the total plasma concentration than the second term. After several distribution half-times, the value of the first term approaches zero, and the plasma concentration is essentially equal to the value of the second term.

In multicompartment models, the drug is initially distributed only within the central compartment. Therefore, the initial apparent volume of distribution is the volume of the central compartment. Immediately after injection, the amount of drug present is the dose, and the concentration is the extrapolated concentration at time $t = 0$, which is equal to the sum of the intercepts of the distribution and elimination lines. The volume of the central compartment, Vc, is calculated by modifying Equation 13-8:

$$Vc = \frac{\text{dose}}{\text{initial plasma concentration}} = \frac{\text{dose}}{A + B} \qquad (13\text{-}14)$$

The volume of the central compartment is important in clinical anesthesiology, because it is the pharmacokinetic parameter that determines the peak plasma concentration after an iv bolus injection. Hypovolemia, for example, might reduce the volume of the central compartment. If doses are not correspondingly reduced, the higher plasma concentrations will increase the incidence of adverse pharmacologic effects.

At equilibrium, the drug is distributed among the central and the peripheral compartment, and by definition, the concentrations in the compartments are equal. Therefore, the ultimate volume of distribution, termed the volume of distribution at steady-state (Vd_{ss}), is the sum of the central and peripheral compartment volumes. Extensive tissue uptake of a drug is reflected by a large volume of the peripheral compartment. Consequently, Vd_{ss} can greatly exceed the actual volume of the body. Vd_{ss} can be calculated directly from the intercepts and rate constants of the exponential equation.[114]

As in the single-compartment model, in multicompartment models the total drug clearance is equal to the dose divided by the area under the concentration *versus* time curve. This area, and hence clearance, can also be directly calculated from the intercepts and rate constants.[114]

Three-Compartment Model

After iv injection of some drugs, the initial, rapid distribution phase is followed by a second, slower distribution phase before the elimination phase becomes evident. Therefore, the plasma concentration is the sum of three exponential terms:

$$Cp_{(t)} = Pe^{-\pi t} + Ae^{-\alpha t} + Be^{-\beta t} \qquad (13\text{-}15)$$

where $Cp_{(t)}$ = plasma concentration at time t, P = intercept of the rapid distribution phase line; π = rate constant of the rapid distribution phase, A = intercept of the slower distribution phase line, α = rate constant of the slower distribution phase, B = intercept of the elimination phase line, β = rate constant of the elimination phase, and t = time. This triphasic behavior is explained by a three-compartment pharmacokinetic model (Fig. 13-10). As in the two-compartment model, the drug is injected into and eliminated from the central compartment. Drug is reversibly transferred between the central compartment and two peripheral compartments, which accounts for two distribution phases. Drug transfer between the central compartment and the more rapidly equilibrating, or "shallow," peripheral compartment is characterized by the first-order rate constants k_{12} and k_{21}. Transfer in and out of the more slowly equilibrating, "deep," compartment is characterized by the rate constants k_{13} and k_{31}.

The pharmacokinetic parameters of interest to clinicians, such as clearance, volumes of distribution, and distribution and elimination half-times, are determined by calculations analogous to those used in the two-compartment model. Accurate estimates of these parameters depend on accurate characterization of the measured plasma concentration *versus* time data. A frequently encountered problem is that the duration of sampling is not long enough to accurately define the elimination phase.[115] Similar problems arise if the assay cannot detect low concentrations of the drug. Whether a drug exhibits two- or three-compartment kinetics is of no clinical consequence. In fact, some drugs have two-compartment kinetics in some patients and three-compartment kinetics in others.[91,116] In selecting a pharmacokinetic model, the most important factor is that it accurately characterize the measured concentrations. Generally, the model with the smallest number of compartments or exponents that accurately reflects the data is used.

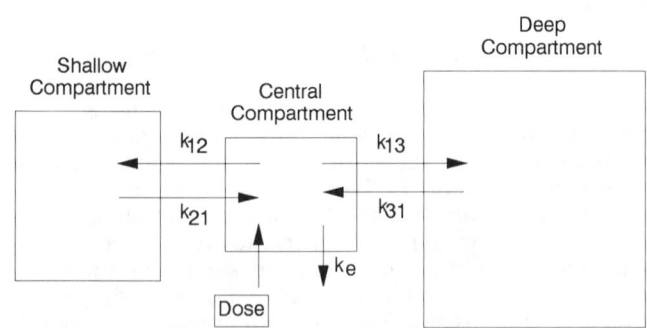

Figure 13-10. A three-compartment phamacokinetic model. See text for explanation.

Effects of Hepatic or Renal Disease on Pharmacokinetic Parameters

As discussed earlier, hepatic and renal disease affect not only the ability to eliminate drugs, but also often change binding of drugs to plasma proteins. Consequently, the effects of altered protein binding must be considered in addition to the effects of impaired organ function to fully understand the impact of hepatic or renal disease on pharmacokinetic variables.

The extent of drug distribution depends on the relative affinity of blood *versus* tissues for the drug. Therefore, if the free fraction in plasma increases, the volume of distribution must also increase. The magnitude of the change depends on the initial free fraction and volume of distribution. An increase in the free fraction will produce the greatest increase in the volume of distribution for drugs that are highly bound to plasma proteins and have small volumes of distribution. In contrast, changes in plasma protein binding of drugs with large volumes of distribution have minimal effects on the volume of distribution, because so little of the total amount of drug is in the plasma.[117]

In theory, a parallel change in tissue binding would cancel the effect of changes in plasma binding. However, this appears to be uncommon. Increased volumes of distribution of propranolol[118] and diazepam[24] associated with increased free fractions have been observed in patients with hepatic disease. Decreased binding of thiopental in patients with renal failure also increases the volume of distribution.[97]

The effect of altered protein binding on total drug clearance also depends on the initial magnitude of the clearance. Increases in the free fraction of drugs with low hepatic extraction ratios and drugs eliminated primarily by glomerular filtration cause a proportional increase in clearance. In contrast, altered protein binding has little effect on drugs with high hepatic or renal clearance.

The effect of an increased free fraction on the elimination half-time depends on the net effect on clearance and the volume of distribution.[117] The elimination half-time will increase if increased volume of distribution is the paramount change, or decrease if increased clearance predominates. The elimination half-time may not change if clearance and volume of distribution change in parallel fashion. The increase of the free fraction of thiopental in renal failure increases both clearance and volume of distribution to a similar extent. Consequently, the elimination half-time is unchanged.[97]

Diverse pathophysiologic changes preclude precise prediction of the pharmacokinetics of a given drug in individual patients with hepatic or renal disease. However, some generalizations can be made. Binding of drugs to albumin is decreased, so that doses of drugs given as an iv bolus, such as thiopental, must be reduced. In patients with hepatic disease, the elimination half-time of drugs metabolized or excreted by the liver will often be increased because of decreased clearance and, possibly, increased volume of distribution. Large doses of such drugs as benzodiazepines, opioids, and barbiturates may have a greatly prolonged duration of action and should be avoided. Recovery from small doses of drugs such as thiopental and fentanyl is largely due to redistribution, so recovery from conservative doses will be minimally affected. In patients with renal failure, similar concerns apply to the administration of drugs excreted by the kidneys. It is almost always better to underestimate a patient's dose requirement, observe the response, and give additional drug if necessary.

Nonlinear Pharmacokinetics

The physiologic and compartmental models that have been discussed thus far are based on the assumption that drug distribution and elimination are first-order processes. Therefore, their parameters, such as clearance and elimination half-time, are independent of the dose or concentration of the drug. However, the rate of elimination of a few drugs is dose dependent, or *nonlinear*.

The elimination of most drugs involves interactions with protein molecules, either enzymes of biotransformation reactions, or carried-mediated secretion. If sufficient drug is present, the capacity of the drug-eliminating systems can be exceeded. When this occurs, it is no longer possible to excrete a constant fraction of the drug present to the eliminating system. Consequently, the extraction ratio decreases as the concentration increases. Decreased extraction decreases total drug clearance. Phenytoin is a well-known example of a drug that exhibits nonlinear elimination. If the concentration is high enough to completely saturate the system, then a constant amount, as opposed to a constant fraction, of the drug is eliminated per unit of time. This is known as *zero-order* elimination. Ethanol is metabolized in a zero-order fashion at usual "therapeutic" concentrations. In theory, all drugs are cleared in nonlinear fashion. In practice, the capacity to eliminate most drugs is so great that this is rarely evident at usual or even toxic doses.

Nonlinear clearance has important clinical implications. The plasma concentration is the arithmetic product of clearance and the rate of administration. Therefore, the concentration will progressively increase unless the dose is adjusted. This sets up a positive-feedback loop whereby decreased extraction leads to even higher concentrations, which further decreases extraction and clearance, and so on. The other consequence of nonlinear clearance is that the elimination half-time gets progressively longer as the concentration increases. Clearance of thiopental is nonlinear at high concentrations.[119] This may be partly responsible for the delayed awakening of patients given thiopental for prophylaxis of neurologic complications during open-heart surgery.[120]

PHARMACODYNAMIC PRINCIPLES

In its broadest sense, *pharmacodynamics* can be defined as the study of the effects of drugs on the body. Classically, pharmacologic effects have been examined with dose-response studies. Advances in drug assay techniques and methods of data analysis have made it possible to define the relationship between the drug concentration and the associated pharmacologic effect *in vivo*. As a result, the term *pharmacodynamics* has acquired a more specific definition. It is now considered to be the quantitative analysis of the relationship between the drug concentration in the blood, or at the site of action, and the resultant effects of the drug on biochemical or physiologic processes.[112,121]

Dose-Response Relationships

Dose-response studies determine the relationship between increasing doses of a drug and the ensuing changes in pharmacologic effects. A schematic dose-response curve, beginning with a dose that produces a barely measurable effect, is shown in Figure 13-11A. There is a curvilinear relationship between dose and the intensity of response such that at

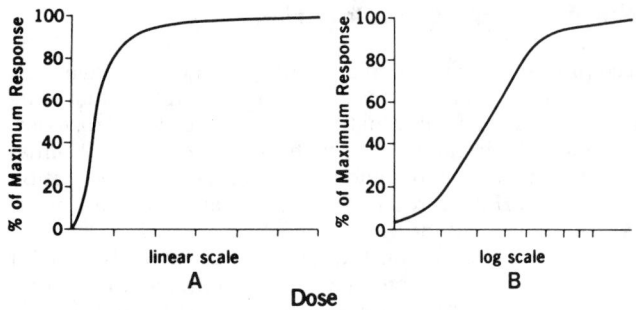

Figure 13-11. (A) A schematic curve of the effect of a drug plotted against dose, starting with a dose that produces a barely measurable response. (B) The same curve, replotted with dose on a logarithmic scale. This yields the familiar sigmoid-shaped dose-response curve, which is linear between 20% and 80% of the maximal effect. (Reprinted with permission from Stanski DR, Watkins WD: Drug Disposition in Anesthesia, p 39. New York, Grune & Stratton, 1982.)

near-maximal response, large increases in dose produce little change in effect. Usually the dose is plotted on a logarithmic scale (Fig. 13-11B), which expands the part of the curve where a small increase in dose produces a large change in response. Between 20% and 80% of the maximum effect, there is a linear relationship between the logarithm of the dose and the intensity of the response.

Dose-response curves provide information regarding four aspects of the relationship of dose and pharmacologic effect. The *potency* of the drug, that is, the dose required to produce a given effect, is determined. Potency is usually expressed as the dose required to produce a given effect in 50% of subjects, the ED50. The *slope* of the curve between 20% and 80% of the maximal effect indicates the rate of increase in effect as the dose is increased. The maximum effect is referred to as the *efficacy* of the drug. Finally, the *variability* in potency, efficacy, and the slope of the dose-response curve can be estimated.

Dose-response curves can be constructed with either single-dose or cumulative-dose techniques. In the former method, the effect of a single dose in each subject is measured. If a range of doses is administered to different subjects, the dose-response curve can be defined for the group as a whole. In the cumulative-dose technique, small, incremental doses are given and the effect is plotted against the cumulative dose. The two methods generally yield equivalent results. However, if the drug has a very short duration of action, the ED50 of a cumulative dose-response curve will be higher than the ED50 of a single-dose response curve, because the effects of the initial doses wane during the course of the study. This has been demonstrated for the short-acting nondepolarizing neuromuscular blockers.[122] Some drugs produce all-or-none, or quantal, responses. For example, after a dose of thiopental, a patient is either asleep or awake. Dose-response curves for these drugs must be constructed with the single-dose technique.

In anesthesiology, the usual therapeutic objectives are to rapidly achieve and then maintain a given pharmacologic effect, such as unconsciousness or neuromuscular blockade, for a finite period, and then to have rapid recovery. Attaining these objectives is made difficult by the wide range of individual patients' sensitivity to drugs. This variability in response is a result of differences between individuals in the relationship between drug concentration and pharmaco-

logic effect, superimposed upon differences in pharmacokinetics. Dose-response studies have the disadvantage of not being able to determine whether variations in pharmacologic response are due to differences in pharmacokinetics, pharmacodynamics, or both.

Concentration-Response Relationships

Ideally, the concentration of drug at its site of action should be used to define the concentration-response relationship. Unfortunately, these data are rarely available, so the relationship between the concentration of drug in the blood and pharmacologic effect is studied instead. This relationship is easiest to understand if the changes in pharmacologic effect that occur during and after an iv infusion of a hypothetical drug are considered (Fig. 13-12). If a drug is infused at a constant rate, the plasma concentration initially increases rapidly, and asymptotically approaches a steady-state level after approximately five elimination half-times have elapsed. The effect of the drug initially increases very slowly, then more rapidly, and eventually also reaches a steady state (see Fig. 13-12). When the infusion is discontinued, indicated by point C in Figure 13-12, the plasma concentration immediately decreases because of drug distribution and elimination. However, the effect stays the same for a short period, and then also begins to decrease. It is evident that there is a time lag between changes in plasma concentration and changes in pharmacologic response. Figure 13-12 also demonstrates that the same concentration can produce different responses if the concentrations in the plasma and at the site of action are changing. At points A and B in Figure 13-12, the plasma concentrations are the same, but the effects at each time differ. When the concentration is increasing, there is a concentration gradient from blood to the site of action. When the infusion is discontinued, the concentration gradient is reversed. Therefore, at the same plasma concentration, the concentration at the site of action is higher after, compared to during, the infusion. This is associated with a correspondingly greater effect.

In theory, there must be some degree of temporal disequilibrium between plasma concentration and drug effect for all drugs with extravascular sites of action. However, for some drugs, the time lag may be so short that it cannot be demonstrated. The magnitude of this temporal disequilibrium depends on several factors:

1. perfusion of the organ on which the drug acts,
2. the rate of diffusion or transport of the drug from the blood to the cellular site of action,

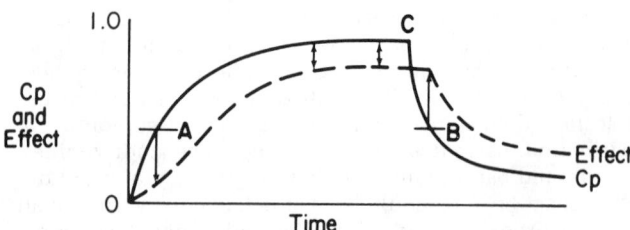

Figure 13-12. The changes in plasma drug concentration and pharmacologic effect during and after an intravenous infusion. See text for explanation. (Reprinted with permission from Stanski DR, Sheiner LB: Pharmacokinetics and pharmacodynamics of muscle relaxants. Anesthesiology 51:103, 1979.)

3. the tissue:blood partition coefficient of the drug,
4. the rate and affinity of drug-receptor binding, and
5. the time required for processes initiated by the drug-receptor interaction to produce the pharmacologic effect.

The consequence of this time lag between changes in concentration and changes in effects is that the plasma concentration will only have an unvarying relationship with pharmacologic effect under steady-state conditions. At steady state, by definition, the concentration in the plasma is in equilibrium with the concentrations in all tissues, including the site of action. Accordingly, the steady-state plasma concentration is directly proportional to the steady-state concentration at the site of action that is actually causing the observed pharmacologic effect. A plot of the logarithm of the steady-state plasma concentration *versus* percent maximal response will be identical in appearance to the dose-response curve shown in Figure 13-11*B*. From the concentration-response curve, the average steady-state plasma concentration producing 50% of the maximal response $(Cp_{ss}50)$ can be determined. Like the ED50, the $Cp_{ss}50$ is a measure of sensitivity to a drug, but the $Cp_{ss}50$ has the advantage of being unaffected by pharmacokinetic variability. Because it takes five elimination half-times to approach steady-state conditions, it is rarely practical to directly determine the $Cp_{ss}50$. For drugs that have long elimination half-times, the pseudoequilibrium that exists during the elimination phase can be used to approximate steady-state conditions, because the concentrations in plasma and at the site of action are changing very slowly.

From the foregoing discussion, it is evident that the onset and duration of pharmacologic effects depends not only on pharmacokinetic factors but also on the pharmacodynamic factors governing the degree of temporal disequilibrium between changes in concentration and changes in effect. The magnitude of the pharmacologic effect is a function of the amount of drug present at the site of action, so that increasing the dose will increase the peak effect. Larger doses have a more rapid onset of action because the rate at which drug is delivered to the site of action increases. The duration of action also increases because pharmacologically effective concentrations will be maintained for a longer time.

Integrated pharmacokinetic-pharmacodynamic models have been developed by several investigators.[121,123] These models fully characterize the relationships between time, dose, plasma concentration, and pharmacologic effect. This is accomplished by adding an "effect compartment" to a standard compartmental pharmacokinetic model. The effect compartment is sometimes referred to as the *biophase*. Transfer of drug between central (plasma) compartment and the effect compartment, or biophase, is assumed to be a first-order process, and the pharmacologic effect is assumed to be directly related to the concentration in the biophase. By quantifying the time lag between changes in plasma concentration and changes in pharmacologic effect, these models can also define the $Cp_{ss}50$, even if steady-state conditions have not been attained. These models have contributed greatly to our understanding of factors influencing the response to intravenous anesthetics,[124,125] opioids,[126,127] and nondepolarizing muscle relaxants[123,128,129] in man.

Dose-response and concentration-response relationships can be altered by many factors, such as interactions with other concomitantly administered drugs or pathologic conditions. They are also affected by the development of toler-ance to the drug's effects, which increases the ED50 and $Cp_{ss}50$. When tolerance develops after only a few doses of drug, it is usually referred to as *tachyphylaxis*.

Drug-Receptor Interactions

The biochemical and physiologic effects of many drugs, neurotransmitters, and hormones are due to the binding of these compounds to receptors, which initiates changes in cellular function. In addition to the well-known muscarinic and nicotinic cholinergic receptors, and alpha- and beta-adrenoceptors, there are specific receptors for histamine, serotonin, dopamine, eicosanoids, peptide hormones, endorphins and exogenous opiates, benzodiazepines, and calcium channel blockers, to name a few. Subtypes of many of these receptors have been characterized. In mammals, there are at least 85 distinct receptors for various endogenous and exogenous compounds.[130,131] Most receptors are protein molecules situated on the cell membrane, although some are located within the cell.

Binding of drugs to receptors, like the binding of drugs to plasma proteins, is generally reversible, and follows the law of mass action:

$$[drug] + [receptor] \rightleftharpoons [drug\text{-}receptor\ complex] \qquad (13\text{-}16)$$

The higher the concentration of free drug or unoccupied receptor, the greater the tendency for drug-receptor binding. Plotting the percentage of receptors occupied by a drug against the logarithm of the concentration of the drug yields a sigmoid curve, as shown in Figure 13-13.

It is often assumed that the percentage of the maximal effect observed at any given drug concentration is equal to the percentage of receptors occupied by the drug. However, this is not always the case. At the neuromuscular junction,

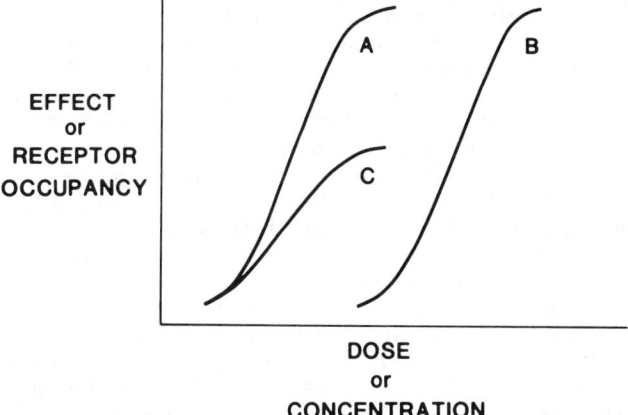

Figure 13-13. Schematic dose-response curves representing various conditions. Either dose or concentration is plotted on the *x*-axis, and either effect or the number of receptors occupied is plotted on the *y*-axis. Curve *A* is a typical dose-response curve. Curve *B* is a parallel rightward shift of the curve and represents a drug that is less potent than the drug depicted by curve *A* but that is a full agonist and thus capable of producing the same maximal effect. Curve *B* would also result if the drug used to generate curve *A* were studied in the presence of a competitive antagonist. Curve *C* is shifted to the right, with a reduction in slope and the maximal effect. This is the curve observed with partial agonists, and also when a full agonist (curve *A*) is studied in the presence of a noncompetitive antagonist.

only 20–25% of the postjunctional nicotinic cholinoceptors need to bind acetylcholine to produce contraction of all the fibers in the muscle.[132] Thus, 75–80% of the receptors can be considered "spare receptors." There are two important consequences of the presence of spare receptors. As indicated by Equation 13-16, the higher the concentration of unoccupied receptors, the greater the tendency to form the drug-receptor complex. Therefore, spare receptors permit near-maximal effects at very low concentrations of drugs or neurotransmitters.[133] The other corollary of the existence of spare receptors is that most of the receptors must be occupied by an antagonist before transmission is affected. This accounts for the "margin of safety" of neuromuscular transmission.[132]

The binding of drugs to receptors and the resulting changes in cellular function are the last two steps in the complex series of events between administration of the drug and production of its pharmacologic effects. These two processes contribute to the delay between changes in the plasma concentration of the drug and changes in the intensity of its effects.

Receptors are not static entities. Rather, they are dynamic cellular components that adapt to their environment. For example, administration of beta-adrenergic agonists leads to desensitization of beta-adrenoceptors. This occurs by "downregulation," which is the removal of receptors from the cell membrane, and also by alterations in the functional state of the receptor.[134] Administration of adrenoceptor antagonists increases the number of receptors.[134] Other hormones and various disease states also influence the number of adrenergic receptors.[134]

Agonists, Partial Agonists, and Antagonists

Drugs that bind to receptors and produce an effect are called *agonists*. Many drugs may be capable of producing the same maximal effect, although they may differ in potency. Agonists that differ in potency but bind to the same receptors will have parallel dose-response curves (curves *A* and *B* in Fig. 13-13). Differences in potency of agonists reflect differences in affinity for the receptor. *Partial agonists* are drugs that are not capable of producing the maximal effect, even at very high concentrations (curve *C* in Fig. 13-13).

Compounds that bind to receptors without producing any changes in cellular function are referred to as *antagonists*. Binding of agonists to receptors is inhibited by antagonists. *Competitive antagonists* bind reversibly to receptors, and their blocking effect can be overcome by high concentrations of an agonist. Therefore, competitive antagonists produce a parallel shift in the dose-response curve, but the maximum effect is not altered (see Fig. 13-13, curves *A* and *B*). *Noncompetitive antagonists* bind irreversibly to receptors. This has the same effect as reducing the number of receptors and shifts the dose-response curve downward and to the right, decreasing both the slope and the maximum effect (curves *A* and *C* in Fig. 13-13). The effect of noncompetitive antagonists is reversed only by synthesis of new receptor molecules.

The underlying mechanisms by which different compounds that bind to the same receptor act as agonists, partial agonists, or antagonists are not fully understood. Presumably, agonists produce a structural or functional alteration of the receptor molecule that initiates changes in cellular function. Partial agonists may produce a qualitatively different change in the receptor, while antagonists bind without producing a change in the receptor that results in altered cellular function.

CLINICAL APPLICATION OF PHARMACOKINETICS AND PHARMACODYNAMICS

In anesthesia, the usual therapeutic objectives are to rapidly produce pharmacologic effects, such as unconsciousness or muscle relaxation, to maintain the optimal intensity of these effects during the anesthetic, and to have the patient recover rapidly on conclusion of surgery. Knowledge of pharmacokinetic principles and of the pharmacokinetic and pharmacodynamic properties of the drugs used in anesthesiology makes it easier to attain these objectives. If the pharmacokinetics and the therapeutic concentration of a drug are known, then the average doses required to achieve and maintain the desired pharmacologic effect can be calculated. The steady-state plasma concentration (Cp_{ss}) is a function of the rate of infusion of the drug and drug clearance:

$$Cp_{ss} = \frac{\text{infusion rate}}{Cl}; \text{ thus: infusion rate} = Cp_{ss} \cdot Cl$$

(13-17)

Infusion of the drug for five elimination half-times is required to reach steady-state conditions. Therefore, for many of the iv agents used in anesthesia, it would take 24 hours or more to reach a stable plasma concentration by merely infusing the drug at a constant rate. This is obviously impractical, and it does not meet the first of the above-stated objectives.

The volume of distribution must be rapidly "filled up" by giving a loading dose to achieve a more rapid onset of action. The loading dose can be calculated by multiplying the volume of distribution (Vd) by the desired concentration:

$$\text{Loading dose} = Cp_{ss} \cdot Vd \qquad (13\text{-}18)$$

Almost all drugs, including those used in anesthesia, have multicompartment pharmacokinetic properties. Therefore, their initial volume of distribution, which is equal to the volume of the central compartment, gets progressively larger until the ultimate volume of distribution, the volume of distribution at steady state (Vd_{ss}), is reached. Consequently, the loading dose can vary according to specific therapeutic objectives.

A minimal loading dose is the amount of drug required to "fill up" the central compartment:

$$\text{Minimal loading dose} = Cp_{ss} \cdot Vc \qquad (13\text{-}19)$$

This rapidly achieves the desired concentration and effect, satisfying the first of the three therapeutic objectives. However, the concentration will decrease very quickly because of drug distribution and elimination, even if the loading dose is followed by an infusion, as calculated with Equation 13-17. This means that the desired effect will be maintained for a very short period.

A full loading dose can be defined as the amount of drug needed to provide the desired concentration once distribution has been completed. It is calculated as follows:

$$\text{Full loading dose} = Cp_{ss} \cdot Vd_{ss} \qquad (13\text{-}20)$$

Figure 13-14 demonstrates the plasma concentration profile if a full loading dose is followed by a maintenance infusion. The concentration is initially much higher than de-

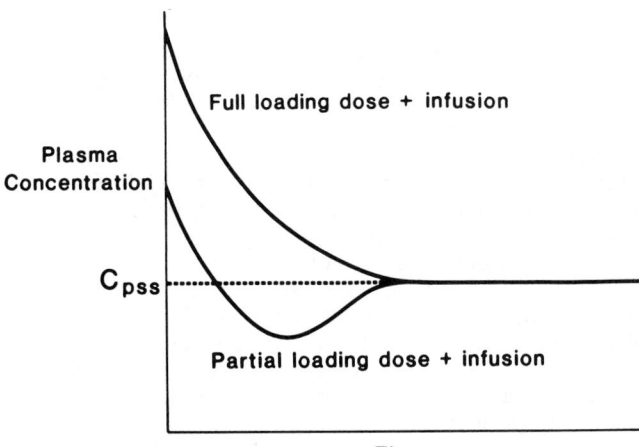

Figure 13-14. Plasma concentration *versus* time curves after administration of a full or partial loading dose, followed by a maintenance infusion at a constant rate (see Eqs. 13-17 and 13-20).

sired, and it eventually falls to the optimal concentration. The disadvantage of this combination is obvious. The high initial concentration may produce adverse effects, and there may still be a higher than optimal concentration at the conclusion of surgery, preventing rapid recovery.

As a compromise, a partial (more than the minimal, but less than the full) loading dose can be given. If this is followed by a maintenance infusion, the concentration will initially be higher than desired, and will then fall below the optimal concentration before increasing toward the steady-state value. Figure 13-14 demonstrates that the discrepancy between the desired and actual concentrations is less after the partial loading dose–infusion combination than with the full loading dose–maintenance infusion combination. The lower initial concentration is less prone to produce adverse effects, and there is also less likelihood of having an excessive concentration at the conclusion of the operation. Therefore, the partial loading dose–maintenance infusion combination comes closest to fulfilling the three therapeutic objectives. If the nadir of the concentration results in an inadequate effect, then a supplementary loading dose can be given. This principle can be extended by giving a minimal loading dose, followed by many progressively smaller supplementary doses, so that the concentration is close to the desired level virtually all the time.

Although the elimination half-time is often thought of as the most important pharmacokinetic parameter, it does not appear in Equations 13-17 to 13-20. The elimination half-time is not a truly fundamental pharmacokinetic parameter. It is a function of the compartmental volumes, the rate of equilibration between compartments, and total drug clearance. During most anesthetics, termination of pharmacologic effects depends more on *redistribution* of drugs from their sites of action to other tissues than on elimination of drugs from the body, especially for lipophilic agents. The ultimate elimination half-time of propofol may be 10 hours or more.[135] However, even after infusion of propofol for 18 hours, a rapid decrease in the blood concentration occurs on termination of the infusion.[136] This is due to uptake of propofol by peripheral tissues, which permits redistribution of propofol from the brain to those tissues. Sufentanil is more lipophilic than alfentanil, and simulations suggest that the concentration of sufentanil at its sites of action actually may decrease faster than the concentration of alfentanil under conditions typical of the vast majority of anesthetics.[137] Therefore, when drugs are administered for only a few hours, the elimination half-time is of limited usefulness in predicting the rapidity of recovery from lipophilic drugs, because redistribution will lower the plasma, and hence brain, concentration below pharmacologically active levels. Less lipophilic agents, such as neuromuscular blockers, are less extensively taken up by tissues, and the rate of recovery from these drugs more closely parallels their elimination half-times.

Systems for Administration of Intravenous Agents

Several studies comparing the traditional intermittent bolus injection of iv anesthetics and adjuvants with continuous infusions suggest that the latter method is preferable.[138] The pharmacologic effect is more stable, and often lower total doses are given when continuous infusions, titrated according to individual patients' requirements, are used.

The various systems available for administration of iv infusions are shown in Table 13-6, ranked according to increasing cost, complexity, and precision. With the use of iv sets with in-line graduated chambers, drugs can be injected into the chamber, diluted to an appropriate concentration, and infused at the desired rate. The flow rate is controlled either with a standard roller clamp or with the slightly more accurate gravity-driven flow controllers. Although these systems are simple, they are inherently imprecise because they are manually controlled and because the flow rate de-

TABLE 13-6. Delivery Systems for Intravenous Anesthetics

System	Advantages	Disadvantages
Intravenous set with graduated chamber	Inexpensive Widely available Ease of use	Inaccurate
Syringe pumps	Ease of use	Relatively low maximum flow rates
Volumetric pumps	Accuracy	More difficult to set up
"Smart" syringe pumps	Eliminate errors in converting dose to flow rate	Often not suitable for pediatric patients
Computer-assisted infusion systems	Dose based on desired plasma concentration, not an infusion rate	High cost—requires both a computer and an infusion pump

creases as the level of the fluid in the chamber decreases. Syringe pumps offer improved accuracy but often have relatively low maximum flow rates, typically 100 ml·h^{-1}. This disadvantage is overcome by volumetric infusion pumps, which are considerably more expensive.

"Smart" syringe pumps have recently been introduced. These devices allow the user to set the infusion rate in mass units per unit time, such as mg·kg^{-1}·h^{-1}, rather than setting a flow rate, such as ml·h^{-1}. The concentration of drug being infused is entered, either via a numeric keypad or by placing an agent-specific, magnetically encoded faceplate on the pump. The desired infusion rate, in mg·kg^{-1}·h^{-1}, or other similar units appropriate for the specific drug, are selected and the patient's weight is entered. A microprocessor uses this information to calculate the correct infusion flow rate for the desired dose. These devices eliminate the need to convert the desired dose from mass units per unit time to volume per unit time, thus eliminating one potential source of error.

Pharmacokinetic and pharmacodynamic principles have been used to develop computer-controlled drug infusion systems, which consist of a computer linked to a volumetric pump via a serial interface.[139,140] Pharmacokinetic parameters are entered into the programs, which use algorithms based on compartmental pharmacokinetic models to determine the infusion rates necessary to achieve and maintain the desired plasma concentration. The desired concentration is specified, and the software converts this into the flow rates required to rapidly give enough drug to "fill up" the central compartment as a loading dose. The software continuously updates the concentration predicted by the pharmacokinetic model, taking into account the drug already infused. Several times a minute, the infusion rate is adjusted to minimize the discrepancy between the predicted concentration and the desired concentration. If desired concentration is increased, the software gives a supplemental loading dose and calculates the infusion rates required to maintain the higher concentration. If the desired concentration is decreased, the software interrupts the infusion until the predicted concentration has decreased to the desired concentration. In a given patient, the actual plasma concentration and the predicted concentration will differ because of pharmacokinetic variability. However, this bias is generally constant for the duration of the vast majority of anesthetics.[140,141] Compared to manually controlled devices, these systems permit more rapid, precise, proportional changes of the plasma concentration of iv agents.

Computer-assisted infusion systems facilitate the usual therapeutic objectives in anesthesiology—rapid onset and maintenance of the optimal effect, followed by rapid recovery at the end of surgery. The major disadvantage of computer-assisted infusion systems is their high cost. Widespread clinical application of these systems will likely require demonstration of improved patient care and reduction in costs.

DRUG INTERACTIONS

If one takes into account premedication, perioperative antibiotics, iv agents used for induction or maintenance of anesthesia, inhalational anesthetics, opioids, muscle relaxants, and the drugs used to restore neuromuscular transmission, postoperative analgesics, ten or more drugs may be given for a relatively "routine" anesthetic. Consequently, thorough understanding of the basic mechanisms of drug interactions

and knowledge of specific interactions with drugs used in anesthesia is essential to the safe practice of anesthesiology. Indeed, anesthesiologists often deliberately take advantage of drug interactions. For example, reversal of nondepolarizing neuromuscular blockers is accomplished by giving cholinesterase inhibitors, such as edrophonium or neostigmine, which increases the concentration of acetylcholine at the nicotinic postjunctional receptors. Unfortunately, the concentration of acetylcholine is also increased at muscarinic receptors, leading to undesirable side-effects such as bradycardia, so an antimuscarinic agent, atropine or glycopyrrolate, is administered concomitantly. Therefore, the reversal of neuromuscular blockade involves interactions between three drugs at two different receptors. The basic principles of drug interactions, illustrated by a few examples, are covered in this section.

Drug interactions due to physicochemical properties can occur in vitro. Mixing acidic drugs, such as thiopental, and basic drugs, such as opioids or muscle relaxants, results in the formation of insoluble salts that precipitate out of solution.[142] Another type of in vitro reaction is the absorption of drugs by plastics. Examples include the uptake of nitroglycerin by polyvinylchloride infusion sets,[143] and the absorption of fentanyl by the apparatus used for cardiopulmonary bypass.[144]

Drugs can alter each other's absorption, distribution, and elimination. Absorption from the GI tract can be altered by drugs like ranitidine, which alters gastric pH,[53] and metoclopramide, which speeds gastric emptying.[145] Vasoconstrictors are added to local anesthetic solutions to prolong their duration of action at the site of injection and to decrease the risk of systemic toxicity from rapid absorption.

Drugs that compete for binding sites on plasma proteins have complex interactions.[73] Displacement of a drug from plasma proteins affects its distribution. The increase in the free drug concentration increases tissue uptake of the drug, increasing the volume of distribution. The extent of the effect on drug distribution depends on the fraction of the total drug in the body that is bound to plasma proteins. The change in distribution will be greatest when drugs with small volumes of distribution that are extensively bound to plasma proteins are displaced. Displacement of one drug by another may produce toxic free drug concentrations. When a steady state is re-established, the effect of decreased binding on total and free drug concentrations depends on the rate of clearance of the drug. For drugs with low extraction ratios, clearance varies with the degree of binding, and clearance will increase proportionately to the increase in free fraction. Therefore, when a steady state is re-established, the total drug concentration will be lower, but the free drug level will be the same as the level prior to displacement. Clearance of drugs with high extraction ratios is not restricted to the free fraction and is not affected by changes in binding. Consequently, when a new steady state is reached, the total drug concentration is unchanged, and the higher free drug level will persist. Adverse interactions are thus most likely to occur if the displaced drug has high (nonrestrictive) clearance, a small volume of distribution, and is extensively bound to plasma proteins.

As discussed earlier, drugs that inhibit or induce the enzymes that catalyze biotransformation reactions can affect clearance of other concomitantly administered drugs. Clearance can also be affected by drug-induced changes in hepatic blood flow. Drugs cleared by the kidneys and that have similar physicochemical characteristics compete for the transport mechanisms involved in renal tubular secretion.

Pharmacodynamic drug interactions fall into two broad classifications. Drugs can interact, either directly or indirectly, at the same receptors. Opioid antagonists *directly* displace opioids from opiate receptors. Cholinesterase inhibitors *indirectly* antagonize the effects of neuromuscular blockers by increasing the amount of acetylcholine at the motor end-plate, which displaces the blocking drug from the nicotinic receptor. Pharmacodynamic interactions can also occur if two drugs affect a physiologic system at different sites. Benzodiazepines and opioids, each acting on their own specific receptors, appear to interact synergistically to induce anesthesia.[146,147] Although receptors and mechanisms are not as well defined as for the benzodiazepine-opioid interaction, this is presumably how volatile anesthetics increase sensitivity to neuromuscular blocking drugs,[128] and also how premedication increases sensitivity to inhalational anesthetics.[148]

REFERENCES

1. Papper EM: The pharmacokinetics of inhalation anaesthetics: Clinical applications. Br J Anaesth 36:124, 1964
2. Benet LZ, Mitchell JR, Sheiner LB: Pharmacokinetics: The dynamics of drug absorption, distribution and elimination. In Gilman AG, Rall TW, Nies AS, Taylor P (eds): The Pharmacological Basis of Therapeutics, 8th ed, p 1. New York, Pergamon Press, 1990
3. Stanski DR, Watkins WD: Drug Disposition in Anesthesia, p 24. New York, Grune & Stratton, 1982
4. George CF: Drug metabolism by the gastrointestinal mucosa. Clin Pharmacokinet 6:259, 1981
5. Holley FO, van Steennis C: Postoperative analgesia with fentanyl: Pharmacokinetics and pharmacodynamics of constant-rate i.v. and transdermal delivery. Br J Anaesth 60:608, 1988
6. Greenblatt DJ, Shader RI, Abernethy DR: Current status of benzodiazepines. N Engl J Med 309:354, 410, 1983
7. Fee JPH, Collier PS, Dundee JW: Bioavailability of three formulations of intravenous diazepam. Acta Anaesthesiol Scand 30:337, 1986
8. Price HL, Kovnat PJ, Safer JN et al: The uptake of thiopental by body tissues and its relationship to the duration of narcosis. Clin Pharmacol Ther 1:16, 1960
9. Saidman LJ, Eger EI II: The effect of thiopental metabolism on duration of anesthesia. Anesthesiology 27:118, 1966
10. Brown WU Jr, Bell GC, Alper MH: Acidosis, local anesthetics and the newborn. Obstet Gynecol 48:27, 1976
11. Meijer DFK, Weitering JG, Vermeer GA et al: Comparative pharmacokinetics of d-tubocurarine and metocurine in man. Anesthesiology 51:402, 1979
12. Rowland M, Benet LZ, Graham GG: Clearance concepts in pharmacokinetics. J Pharmacokinet Biopharm 1:123, 1973
13. Wilkinson GR, Shand DG: A physiological approach to hepatic drug clearance. Clin Pharmacol Ther 18:377, 1975
14. Nies AS, Shand DG, Wilkinson GR: Altered hepatic blood flow and drug disposition. Clin Pharmacokinet 1:135, 1976
15. Blaschke TF: Protein binding and kinetics of drugs in liver diseases. Clin Pharmacokinet 2:32, 1977
16. Swartz RD, Sidell FR, Cucinell SA: Effects of physical stress on the disposition of drugs eliminated by the liver in man. J Pharmacol Exp Ther 188:1, 1974
17. Stenson RE, Constantino RT, Harrison DC: Interrelationships of hepatic blood flow, cardiac output, and blood levels of lidocaine in man. Circulation 43:205, 1971
18. Thomson PD, Melmon KL, Richardson JA et al: Lidocaine pharmacokinetics in advanced heart failure, liver disease, and renal failure in humans. Ann Intern Med 78:499, 1973
19. Benowitz NL, Meister W: Pharmacokinetics in patients with cardiac failure. Clin Pharmacokinet 1:389, 1976
20. Benowitz NL, Forsyth RP, Melmon KL et al: Lidocaine disposition kinetics in monkey and man: II. Effects of hemorrhage and sympathomimetic drug administration. Clin Pharmacol Ther 16:99, 1974
21. Klotz U, McHorse TS, Wilkinson GR et al: The effect of cirrhosis on the disposition and elimination of meperidine in man. Clin Pharmacol Ther 16:667, 1974
22. Neal EA, Meffin PJ, Gregory PB et al: Enhanced bioavailability and decreased clearance of analgesics in patients with cirrhosis. Gastroenterology 77:96, 1979
23. Wood AJJ, Kornhauser DM, Wilkinson GR et al: The influence of cirrhosis on steady-state blood concentrations of unbound propranolol after oral administration. Clin Pharmacokinet 3:478, 1978
24. Klotz U, Avant GR, Hoyumpa A et al: The effects of age and liver disease on the disposition and elimination of diazepam in adult man. J Clin Invest 55:347, 1975
25. Klotz U, Antonin KH, Brugel H et al: Disposition of diazepam and its major metabolite desmethyldiazepam in patients with liver disease. Clin Pharmacol Ther 21:430, 1977
26. McHorse TS, Wilkinson GR, Johnson RF et al: Effect of acute viral hepatitis in man on the disposition and elimination of meperidine. Gastroenterology 68:775, 1975
27. Williams RL, Blaschke TF, Meffin PJ et al: Influence of viral hepatitis on the disposition of two compounds with high hepatic clearance: Lidocaine and indocyanine green. Clin Pharmacol Ther 20:290, 1976
28. Branch RA, Shand DG, Wilkinson GR et al: The reduction of lidocaine clearance by dl-propranolol: An example of hemodynamic drug interaction. J Pharmacol Exp Ther 184:515, 1973
29. Gelman S: Disturbances in hepatic blood flow during anesthesia and surgery. Arch Surg 111:881, 1976
30. Gelman S, Fowler KC, Smith LR: Liver circulation and function during isoflurane and halothane anesthesia. Anesthesiology 61:726, 1984
31. Cooperman LH: Effects of anaesthetics on the splanchnic circulation. Br J Anaesth 44:967, 1972
32. Duchin KL, Schrier RW: Interrelationship between renal haemodynamics, drug kinetics, and drug action. Clin Pharmacokinet 3:58, 1978
33. Garrett ER: Pharmacokinetics and clearances related to renal processes. Int J Clin Pharmacol 16:155, 1978
34. Bjornsson TD: Nomogram for drug dosage adjustment in patients with renal failure. Clin Pharmacokinet 11:164, 1986
35. Guyton AC: Textbook of Medical Physiology, 5th ed, p 468. Philadelphia, WB Saunders, 1976
36. Collinsworth KA, Strong JM, Atkinson AJ et al: Pharmacokinetics and metabolism of lidocaine in patients with renal failure. Clin Pharmacol Ther 18:59, 1975
37. Miller RD, Agoston S, Booij LHDJ et al: The comparative potency and pharmacokinetics of pancuronium and its metabolites in anesthetized man. J Pharmacol Exp Ther 207:539, 1978
38. Szeto HH, Inturrisi CE, Houde R et al: Accumulation of normeperidine, an active metabolite of meperidine, in patients with renal failure or cancer. Ann Intern Med 86:738, 1977
39. Bennett WM: Geriatric pharmacokinetics and the kidney. Am J Kidney Dis 26:283, 1990
40. Stanski DR, Watkins WD: Drug Disposition in Anesthesia, p 76. New York, Grune & Stratton, 1982
41. Remmer H: The role of the liver in drug metabolism. Am J Med 49:617, 1970
42. Testa B, Jenner P: Novel drug metabolites produced by functionalization reactions: Chemistry and toxicology. Drug Metab Rev 7:325, 1978
43. Tucker GT: Drug metabolism. Br J Anaesth 51:603, 1979
44. de Groot H, Sies H: Cytochrome P-450, reductive metabolism, and cell injury. Drug Metab Rev 20:275, 1989
45. Nebert DW, Eisen HJ, Negishi M et al: Genetic mechanisms controlling the induction of polysubstrate monooxygenase (P450) activities. Annu Rev Pharmacol Toxicol 21:431, 1981
46. Guengerich FP: Enzymatic oxidation of xenobiotic chemicals. Crit Rev Biochem Mol Biol 25:97, 1990
47. Nebert DW, Nelson DR, Adesnik M et al: The P450 superfam-

ily: Updated listing of all genes and recommended nomenclature for the chromosomal loci. DNA 8:1, 1989

48. Gonzalez FJ, Nebert DW: Evolution of the P-450 gene superfamily: Animal-plant warfare, molecular drive and human genetic differences in drug oxidation. Trends Genet 6:182, 1990

49. Okey AB: Enzyme induction in the cytochrome P-450 system. Pharmacol Ther 45:241, 1990

50. Guay DRP, Meatherall RC, Chalmers JL et al: Cimetidine alters pethidine disposition in man. Br J Clin Pharmacol 18:907, 1984

51. Feely J, Wilkinson GR, Wood AJJ: Reduction of liver blood flow and propranolol metabolism by cimetidine. N Engl J Med 304:692, 1981

52. Klotz U, Reimann I: Delayed clearance of diazepam due to cimetidine. N Engl J Med 302:1012, 1980

53. Smith SR, Kendall MJ: Ranitidine versus cimetidine: A comparison of their potential to cause clinically important drug interactions. Clin Pharmacokinet 15:44, 1988

54. Carrum G, Egan JM, Abernethy DR: Diltiazem treatment impairs hepatic drug oxidation: Studies of antipyrine. Clin Pharmacol Ther 40:140, 1986

55. Whittaker M: Plasma cholinesterase variants and the anaesthetist. Anaesthesia 35:174, 1980

56. Besunder JB, Reed MD, Blumer JL: Principles of drug biodisposition in the neonate: A critical evaluation of the pharmacokinetic-pharmacodynamic interface. Clin Pharmacokinet 14:189, 261, 1988

57. Morselli PL: Clinical pharmacology of the perinatal period and early infancy. Clin Pharmacokinet 17(suppl 1):13, 1989

58. Durnas C, Loi C-M, Cusack BJ: Hepatic drug metabolism and aging. Clin Pharmacokinet 19:359, 1990

59. Woodhouse KW, James OFW: Hepatic drug metabolism and ageing. Br Med Bull 46:22, 1990

60. Lane EA, Guthrie S, Linnoila M: Effects of ethanol on drug and metabolite pharmacokinetics. Clin Pharmacokinet 10:228, 1985

61. Miller LG: Recent developments in the study of the effects of cigarette smoking on clinical pharmacokinetics and clinical pharmacodynamics. Clin Pharmacokinet 17:90, 1989

62. Williams RL, Mamelok RD: Hepatic disease and drug pharmacokinetics. Clin Pharmacokinet 5:528, 1980

63. Reidenberg MM: The biotransformation of drugs in renal failure. Am J Med 62:482, 1977

64. Reilly CS, Wood AJJ, Koshakji RP et al: The effect of halothane on drug disposition: Contribution of changes in intrinsic drug metabolizing capacity and hepatic blood flow. Anesthesiology 63:70, 1985

65. Wood M, Wood AJJ: Contrasting effects of halothane, isoflurane, and enflurane on in vivo drug metabolism in the rat. Anesth Analg 63:709, 1984

66. Vesell ES: The antipyrine test in clinical pharmacology: Conceptions and misconceptions. Clin Pharmacol Ther 26:275, 1979

67. Pessayre D, Allemand H, Benoist C et al: Effect of surgery under general anaesthesia on antipyrine clearance. Br J Clin Pharmacol 6:505, 1978

68. Duvaldestin P, Mazze RI, Nivoche Y et al: Enzyme induction following surgery with halothane and neurolept anesthesia. Anesth Analg 60:319, 1981

69. Loft S, Boel J, Kyst A et al: Increased hepatic microsomal enzyme activity after surgery under halothane or spinal anesthesia. Anesthesiology 62:11, 1985

70. Duvaldestin P, Mauge F, Desmonts JM: Enflurane anesthesia and antipyrine metabolism. Clin Pharmacol Ther 29:61, 1981

71. Pantuck EJ, Pantuck CB, Weismann C et al: Effects of parenteral nutrition regimens on oxidative drug metabolism. Anesthesiology 60:534, 1984

72. Duvaldestin P, Mazze RI, Nivoche Y et al: Occupational exposure to halothane results in enzyme induction in anesthetists. Anesthesiology 54:57, 1981

73. Wood M: Plasma drug binding—Implications for anesthesiologists. Anesth Analg 65:786, 1986

74. Koch-Weser J, Sellers EM: Binding of drugs to serum albumin. N Engl J Med 294:311, 526, 1976

75. McLain DA, Hug CC: Intravenous fentanyl kinetics. Clin Pharmacol Ther 28:106, 1980

76. Meuldermans WEG, Hurkmans RMA, Heykants JJP: Plasma protein binding and distribution of fentanyl, sufentanil, alfentanil and lofentanil in blood. Arch Int Pharmacodynam 257:4, 1982

77. Bowers WF, Fulton S, Thompson J: Ultrafiltration vs equilibrium dialysis for determination of free fraction. Clin Pharmacokinet 9(suppl 1):49, 1984

78. Sjoholm I, Ekman B, Kober A et al: Binding of drugs to serum albumin: XI. Mol Pharmacol 16:767, 1979

79. Chen S-S, Perucca E, Lee J-N et al: Serum protein binding and free concentration of phenytoin and phenobarbitone in pregnancy. Br J Clin Pharmacol 13:547, 1982

80. Dean M, Stock B, Patterson RJ et al: Serum protein binding of drugs during and after pregnancy in humans. Clin Pharmacol Ther 28:253, 1980

81. Notarianni LJ: Plasma protein binding of drugs in pregnancy and in neonates. Clin Pharmacokinet 18:20, 1990

82. Morgan DJ, Blackman GL, Paull JD et al: Pharmacokinetics and plasma binding of thiopental: II. Studies at cesarean section. Anesthesiology 54:474, 1981

83. Wood M, Wood AJJ: Changes in plasma drug binding and alpha$_1$-acid glycoprotein in mother and newborn infant. Clin Pharmacol Ther 29:522, 1981

84. Hill MD, Abramson FP: The significance of plasma protein binding on the fetal/maternal distribution of drugs at steady-state. Clin Pharmacokinet 14:156, 1988

85. Davis D, Grossman SH, Ketchell BB et al: The effects of age and smoking on the plasma protein binding of lignocaine and diazepam. Br J Clin Pharmacol 19:261, 1985

86. Verbeeck RK, Cardinal J-A, Wallace SM: Effect of age and sex on the plasma binding of acidic and basic drugs. Eur J Clin Pharmacol 27:91, 1984

87. Wallace S, Whiting B: Factors affecting drug binding in plasma of elderly patients. Br J Clin Pharmacol 3:327, 1976

88. Herman RJ, McAllister CB, Branch RA et al: Effect of age on meperidine disposition. Clin Pharmacol Ther 37:19, 1985

89. Holmberg L, Odar-Cederlof I, Nilsson JLG et al: Pethidine binding to blood cells and plasma proteins in old and young subjects. Eur J Clin Pharmacol 23:457, 1982

90. Greenblatt DJ, Abernethy DR, Locniskar A et al: Effect of age, gender, and obesity on midazolam kinetics. Anesthesiology 61:27, 1984

91. Greenblatt DJ, Allen MD, Harmatz JS et al: Diazepam disposition determinants. Clin Pharmacol Ther 27:301, 1980

92. Jung D, Mayersohn M, Perrier D et al: Thiopental disposition as a function of age in female patients undergoing surgery. Anesthesiology 56:263, 1982

93. Thiessen JJ, Sellers EM, Denbeigh P et al: Plasma protein binding of diazepam and tolbutamide in chronic alcoholics. J Clin Pharmacol 16:345, 1976

94. Olsen GD, Bennett WM, Porter GA: Morphine and phenytoin binding to plasma proteins in renal and hepatic failure. Clin Pharmacol Ther 17:677, 1975

95. Ghoneim MM, Pandya H: Plasma protein binding of thiopental in patients with impaired renal or hepatic function. Anesthesiology 42:545, 1975

96. Pandale G, Chaux F, Salvadori C et al: Thiopental pharmacokinetics in patients with cirrhosis. Anesthesiology 59:123, 1983

97. Burch PG, Stanski DR: Decreased protein binding and thiopental kinetics. Clin Pharmacol Ther 32:212, 1982

98. Reidenberg MM, Drayer DE: Alteration of drug-protein binding in renal disease. Clin Pharmacokinet 9(suppl 1):18, 1984

99. Grossman SH, Davis D, Kitchell BB et al: Diazepam and lidocaine plasma protein binding in renal disease. Clin Pharmacol Ther 31:350, 1982

100. Piafsky KM, Borga O, Odar-Cederlof I et al: Increased plasma protein binding of propranolol and chlorpromazine mediated by disease-induced elevations of plasma alpha$_1$-acid glycoprotein. N Engl J Med 299:1435, 1978

101. Jackson PR, Tucker GT, Woods HF: Altered plasma drug bind-

ing in cancer: Role of alpha$_1$-acid glycoprotein and albumin. Clin Pharmacol Ther 32:295, 1982

102. Zini R, Riant P, Barré J, Tillement J-P: Disease-induced variations in plasma protein levels. Implications for drug dosage regimens. Clin Pharmacokinet 19:147, 218, 1990

103. Routledge PA, Stargel WW, Wagner GS et al: Increased alpha$_1$-acid glycoprotein and lidocaine disposition in myocardial infarction. Ann Intern Med 93:701, 1980

104. Routledge PA, Stargel WW, Wagner GS et al: Increased plasma protein binding in myocardial infarction. Br J Clin Pharmacol 9:438, 1980

105. Elfstrom J: Drug pharmacokinetics in the postoperative period. Clin Pharmacokinet 4:16, 1979

106. Edwards DJ, Lalka D, Cerra F et al: Alpha$_1$-acid glycoprotein concentration and protein binding in trauma. Clin Pharmacol Ther 31:62, 1982

107. Fremstad D, Bergerud K, Haffner JFW et al: Increased plasma binding of quinidine after surgery: A preliminary report. Eur J Clin Pharmacol 10:441, 1976

108. Feely J, Forrest A, Gunn A et al: Influence of surgery on plasma propranolol levels and protein binding. Clin Pharmacol Ther 28:579, 1980

109. Holley FO, Ponganis KV, Stanski DR: Effects of cardiac surgery with cardiopulmonary bypass on lidocaine disposition. Clin Pharmacol Ther 35:617, 1984

110. Balant LP, Gex-Fabry M: Physiological pharmacokinetic modelling. Xenobiotica 20:1241, 1990

111. Eger EI II: Anesthetic Uptake and Action, p 79. Baltimore, Williams & Wilkins, 1974

112. Hull CJ: Pharmacokinetics and pharmacodynamics. Br J Anaesth 51:579, 1979

113. Gibaldi M, Perrier D: Pharmacokinetics, 2nd ed, p 45. New York, Marcel Dekker, 1982

114. Wagner JH: Linear pharmacokinetic equations allowing direct calculation of many needed pharmacokinetic parameters from the coefficients and exponents of polyexponential equations which have been fitted to the data. J Pharmacokinet Biopharm 4:443, 1976

115. Gibaldi M, Weintraub H: Some considerations as to the determination and significance of biologic half-life. J Pharm Sci 60:624, 1971

116. Hudson RJ, Stanski DR, Burch PG: Pharmacokinetics of methohexital and thiopental in surgical patients. Anesthesiology 59:215, 1983

117. Rowland M: Protein binding and drug clearance. Clin Pharmacokinet 9(suppl 1):10, 1984

118. Branch RA, James J, Read AE: A study of factors influencing drug disposition in chronic liver disease, using the model drug (+)-propranolol. Br J Clin Pharmacol 3:243, 1976

119. Stanski DR, Mihm FG, Rosenthal MH et al: Pharmacokinetics of high-dose thiopental used in cerebral resuscitation. Anesthesiology 53:169, 1980

120. Nussmeier NA, Arlund C, Slogoff S: Neuropsychiatric complications after cardiopulmonary bypass: Cerebral protection by a barbiturate. Anesthesiology 64:165, 1986

121. Holford NHG, Sheiner LB: Understanding the dose-effect relationship: Clinical application of pharmacokinetic-pharmacodynamic models. Clin Pharmacokinet 6:429, 1981

122. Fisher DM, Fahey MR, Cronnelly et al: Potency determination for vecuronium (Org NC45). Anesthesiology 57:309, 1982

123. Hull CJ, Van Beem H, McLeod K et al: A pharmacodynamic model for pancuronium. Br J Anaesth 50:1113, 1978

124. Stanski DR, Hudson RJ, Homer TD et al: Pharmacodynamic modelling of thiopental anesthesia. J Pharmacokinet Biopharm 12:223, 1984

125. Homer TD, Stanski DR: The effect of increasing age on thiopental disposition and anesthetic requirement. Anesthesiology 62:714, 1985

126. Scott JC, Ponganis KV, Stanski DR: EEG quantitation of narcotic effect: The comparative pharmacodynamics of fentanyl and alfentanil. Anesthesiology 62:234, 1985

127. Scott JC, Cooke JE, Stanski DR: Electroencephalographic quantitation of opioid effect: Comparative pharmacodynamics of fentanyl and sufentanil. Anesthesiology 74:34, 1991

128. Stanski DR, Ham J, Miller RD et al: Pharmacokinetics and pharmacodynamics of d-tubocurarine during nitrous oxide-narcotic and halothane anesthesia in man. Anesthesiology 51:235, 1979

129. Fisher DM, O'Keeffe C, Stanski DR et al: Pharmacokinetics and pharmacodynamics of d-tubocurarine in infants, children, and adults. Anesthesiology 57:203, 1982

130. Snyder SH: Drug and neurotransmitter receptors in the brain. Science 224:22, 1984

131. Birnbaumer L, Brown AM: G proteins and the mechanism of action of hormones, neurotransmitters, and autocrine and paracrine regulatory factors. Am Rev Respir Dis 141:S106, 1990

132. Waud BE, Waud DR: The margin of safety of neuromuscular transmission in the muscle of the diaphragm. Anesthesiology 37:417, 1972

133. Norman J: Drug-receptor reactions. Br J Anaesth 51:595, 1979

134. Lefkowitz RJ, Caron MG, Stiles GL: Mechanisms of membrane receptor regulation. N Engl J Med 310:1570, 1984

135. Sebel PS, Lowdon JD: Propofol: A new intravenous anesthetic. Anesthesiology 71:260, 1989

136. McMurray TJ, Collier PS, Carson IW et al: Propofol sedation after open heart surgery: A clinical and pharmacokinetic study. Anaesthesia 45:322, 1990

137. Shafer SL, Varvel JR: Pharmacokinetics, pharmacodynamics, and rational opioid selection. Anesthesiology 74:53, 1991

138. White PF: Clinical uses of intravenous anesthetic and analgesic infusions. Anesth Analg 68:161, 1989

139. Alvis JM, Reves JG, Govier AV et al: Computer-assisted infusions of fentanyl during cardiac anesthesia: Comparison with a manual method. Anesthesiology 63:41, 1985

140. Shafer SL, Siegel LC, Cooke JE et al: Testing computer-controlled infusion pumps by simulation. Anesthesiology 68:261, 1988

141. Ausems ME, Vujk J, Hug CC Jr et al: Comparison of a computer-assisted infusion versus intermittent bolus administration of alfentanil as a supplement to nitrous oxide for lower abdominal surgery. Anesthesiology 68:851, 1988

142. Cullen BF, Miller MG: Drug interactions in anesthesia: A review. Anesth Analg 58:413, 1979

143. Mutch WAC, Thomson IR: Delivery systems for intravenous nitroglycerin. Can Anaesth Soc J 30:98, 1983

144. Koren G, Goresky G, Crean P et al: Pediatric fentanyl dosing based on pharmacokinetics during cardiac surgery. Anesth Analg 63:577, 1984

145. Rawlins MD: Drug interactions and anaesthesia. Br J Anaesth 50:689, 1978

146. Vinik HR, Bradley EL Jr, Kissin I: Midazolam-alfentanil synergism for anesthetic induction in patients. Anesth Analg 69:213, 1989

147. Kissin I, Vinik HR, Castillo R, Bradley EL Jr: Alfentanil potentiates midazolam-induced unconsciousness in subanalgesic doses. Anesth Analg 71:65, 1990

148. Quasha AL, Eger EI II, Tinker JH: Determinations and applications of MAC. Anesthesiology 53:315, 1980

149. Mooradian AD: Digitalis: An update of clinical pharmacokinetics, therapeutic monitoring techniques and treatment recommendations. Clin Pharmacokinet 15:165, 1988

150. Echizen H, Eichelbaum M: Clinical pharmacokinetics of verapamil, nifedipine and diltiazem. Clin Pharmacokinet 11:425, 1986

151. Lowenthal DT, Porter RS, Saris SD et al: Clinical pharmacology, pharmacodynamics and interactions with esmolol. Am J Cardiol 56:14F, 1985

152. Mandelli M, Tognoni G, Garattini S: Clinical pharmacokinetics of diazepam. Clin Pharmacokinet 3:72, 1978

153. Greenblatt DJ: Clinical pharmacokinetics of oxazepam and lorazepam. Clin Pharmacokinet 6:89, 1981

154. Brand L, Mark LC, Snell MM et al: Physiologic disposition of methohexital in man. Anesthesiology 24:331, 1963

155. Kirkpatrick T, Cockshott ID, Douglas EJ, Nimmo WS: Pharma-

cokinetics of propofol (Diprivan) in elderly patients. Br J Anaesth 60:146, 1988

156. Tucker GT, Mather LM: Pharmacokinetics of local anaesthetic agents. Br J Anaesth 47:213, 1975

157. Duvaldestin P, Henzel D: Binding of tubocurarine, fazadinium, pancuronium, and Org NC45 to serum proteins in normal man and in patients with cirrhosis. Br J Anaesth 54:513, 1982

158. Wood M, Stone WJ, Wood AJJ: Plasma binding of pancuronium: Effects of age, sex, and disease. Anesth Analg 62:29, 1983

159. Säwe J: High-dose morphine and methadone in cancer patients. Clinical pharmacokinetic considerations of oral treatment. Clin Pharmacokinet 11:87, 1986

160. Patwardhan RV, Johnsson RJ, Hoyumpa A et al: Normal metabolism of morphine in cirrhosis. Gastroenterology 81:1006, 1981

14

Noel W. Lawson

Autonomic Nervous System Physiology and Pharmacology

Neither the old, nor the new by itself is interesting: the absolutely old is insipid, the absolutely new makes no appeal at all. The old in the new is what claims attention.

William Jones
(1842–1910)

Claude Bernard (1878–1979) stated that, "The constancy of the 'Milieu Interieur' is the condition of a free and independent existence." In 1932, Walter Cannon referred to the biologic responses necessary to maintain a steady state in the internal environment as homeostasis. Bernard suspected and Cannon proved that the autonomic nervous system (ANS) is in large measure responsible for maintaining constant conditions within the body.[1]

Anesthesiology is the practice of ANS medicine. The drugs that produce anesthesia also produce potent ANS side-effects. For example, most vasoactive drugs in clinical use either alter or mimic effects of the ANS. The greater part of our training and practice is spent acquiring skills in averting or utilizing the ANS side-effects of anesthetic drugs under a variety of pathophysiologic conditions. The success of any anesthetic undertaking depends upon how well we maintain homeostasis. The numbers that we generate and faithfully record during the course of anesthesia often reflect ANS function and homeostasis. Numbers, such as heart rate and blood pressure measurements, do not necessarily indicate the presence of surgical anesthesia.[2] A knowledge of the anatomy, physiology, and biochemistry of the ANS, particularly its junctional sites and receptors, is a prerequisite to an understanding of its pharmacology.

AUTONOMIC NERVOUS SYSTEM PURPOSE

The ANS includes that part of the central and peripheral nervous systems that is concerned with the involuntary regulation of cardiac muscle, smooth muscle, and glandular and visceral functions throughout the body. ANS activity refers to visceral reflexes that function essentially below the conscious level.[3] The term *autonomic* remains the best description of this ubiquitous nervous system, as opposed to automatic. ANS implies self-controlling, whereas automatic infers nonreflexic or intrinsic responses; however, the use of "autonomy" to describe this nervous system is also illusory. The ANS is exquisitely responsive to changes in somatic motor and sensory activities of the body.[4] The physiologic evidence of visceral reflexes as a result of somatic events is abundantly clear.[5] Psychosomatic disease is an expression of this connection and has long interested those concerned with disease related to emotional behavior. The ANS is therefore not as distinct an entity as the term suggests, since neither somatic nor ANS activity occurs in isolation.[6] The ANS organizes visceral support for somatic behavior and adjusts body states in anticipation of emotional behavior or responses to the stress of disease, *i.e.*, fight or flight.

Traditionally, the ANS has been viewed as strictly a peripheral, efferent (motor) system.[4] This concept is no longer tenable.[3,7,8] Afferent fibers from visceral structures are the first link in the reflex arcs of the ANS whether relaying visceral pain or changes in vessel stretch. Most ANS efferent fibers are accompanied by sensory fibers that are now commonly recognized as components of the ANS. The afferent components of the ANS cannot be as distinctively divided as can the efferent nerves.

Historically, many investigators have refused to classify any afferent fibers within the ANS because visceral sensory nerves are anatomically indistinguishable from somatic sensory nerves.[9,10] Visceral afferent pathways are like afferent somatic nerves in that they are unipolar. ANS efferents are bipolar (Fig. 14-1). Furthermore, afferent fibers that are anatomically aligned with ANS efferents do not differ by design, function, or drug response from somatic afferents.[11] In addition, both somatic and visceral sensory nerves are able to initiate ANS reflexes. However, the argument is functional rather than anatomic because visceral pain can be attenuated by sympathectomy. ANS afferent fibers that arise from the baroreceptors and chemoreceptors of the carotid arteries and aorta are carried by the glossopharyngeal (cranial nerve IX) and vagus (cranial nerve X) nerves to the medulla. These reflexes are important in the control of cardiac output and ventilation but do not involve any somatic nerve.[3] Four fifths of vagal nerve fibers are sensory.[6] The clinical importance of visceral afferent fibers is more closely associated with chronic pain management.

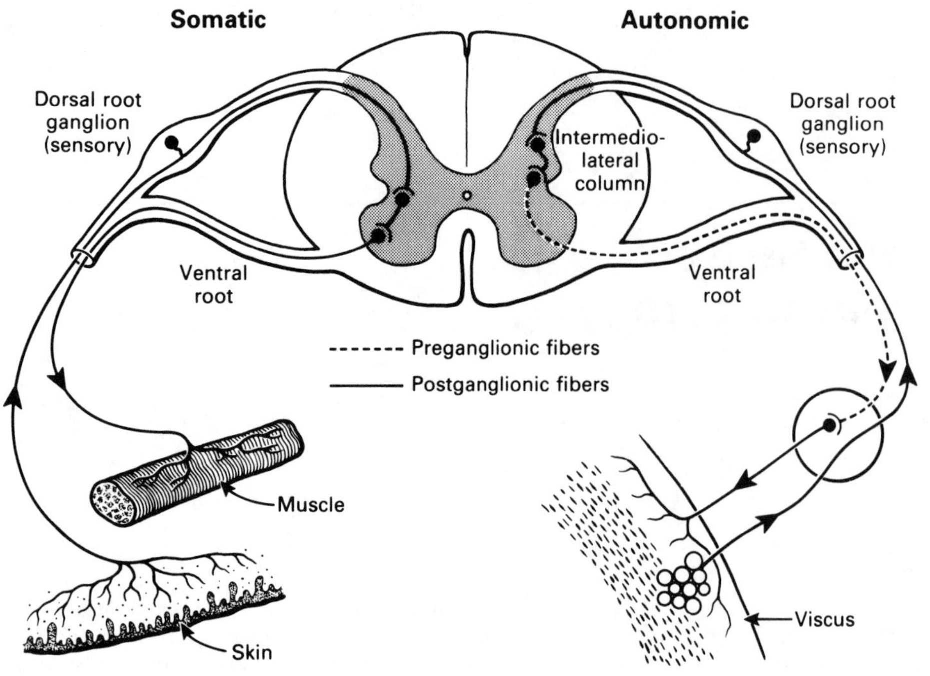

Figure 14-1. Comparison of somatic and autonomic reflex arcs. Somatic arcs are unipolar and autonomic arcs are bipolar.

FUNCTIONAL ANATOMY

From the anatomic, physiologic, and pharmacologic viewpoints, the ANS naturally falls into two divisions.[3] Willis in 1665 recognized the sympathetic nervous system (SNS) and carefully distinguished it from the vagus (L. wandering) nerve. He designated this ganglion chain the intercostal nerve. In 1732, Winslow studied the intercostal nerve and renamed it the grand sympathetic nerve. Stimulation or injury to one part of the body was accompanied by reactions in other organs, as though sympathetic relationships existed. It was in 1921 that Langley divided this nervous system into two parts. He retained the term *sympathetic* for the first part and introduced the term *parasympathetic* (parasympathetic nervous system, PNS) for the second. The term *autonomic nervous system* was adopted as a comprehensive name for both. Ordinarily, activation of the SNS produces expenditure of body energy, whereas stimulation of the PNS produces conservation or accumulation of resource.[7] Table 14-1 lists the complementary effects of SNS (adrenergic) and PNS (cholinergic) activity of organ systems.

Central Autonomic Organization

No purely central ANS or somatic centers are known, and extensive overlap of function occurs.[12] Integration of ANS activity occurs at all levels of the cerebrospinal axis. Efferent ANS activity can be initiated locally and by centers located in the spinal cord, brain stem, and hypothalamus. The cerebral cortex is the highest level of ANS integration. Fainting at the sight of blood is an example of this higher level of somatic and ANS integration. ANS function has also been successfully modulated through conscious,[13] intentional efforts demonstrating that somatic responses are always accompanied by visceral responses and *vice versa*.

The principal site of ANS organization is the hypothalamus. SNS functions are controlled by nuclei in the posterolateral hypothalamus. Stimulation of these nuclei results in a massive discharge of the sympathoadrenal system (Table 14-2). PNS functions are governed by nuclei in the midline and some anterior nuclei of the hypothalamus. Regulation of temperature is involved with the anterior hypothalamus. The supraoptic hypothalamic nuclei are involved in water metabolism and are anatomically and functionally associated with the posterior lobe of the pituitary (see the section on Interaction of Autonomic Nervous System Receptors).[1] This hypothalamic-neurohypophyseal connection represents a central ANS mechanism that affects the kidney by means of antidiuretic hormone. Long-term blood pressure control, reactions to physical and emotional stress, sleep, and sexual reflexes are regulated through the hypothalamus.

The medulla oblongata and pons are the vital centers of acute ANS organization. Together, they integrate momentary hemodynamic adjustments and maintain the sequence and automaticity of ventilation (Fig. 14-2). Integration of afferent and efferent ANS impulses at this central nervous system (CNS) level is responsible for the tonic activity exhibited by the ANS.[4,6] Control of peripheral vascular resistance and thus of blood pressure is a striking example of this tonic activity. Tonicity holds visceral organs in a state of intermediate activity that can either be diminished or augmented by altering the rate of nerve firing. The nucleus tractus solitarius, located within the medulla, is the primary area for relay of afferent chemoreceptor and baroreceptor information from the glossopharyngeal and vagus nerves. Increased afferent impulses from these two nerves inhibit peripheral SNS vascular tone, producing vasodilation, and increase efferent vagal tone, producing bradycardia. High spinal cord transection eliminates the medulla and results in severe hypotension.[8] Unwanted ANS side-effects of drugs may be produced at medullary sites and thus overshadow their desired peripheral effects.[14]

Reflex ANS centers within segments of the spinal cord are capable of producing complex, organized responses to afferent stimuli. Studies of patients with high spinal cord lesions show that a number of reflex changes are mediated at the spinal or segmental level. ANS hyper-reflexia is an

TABLE 14-1. Homeostatic Balance Between Adrenergic and Cholinergic Effects

Organ System	Response	
	Adrenergic	Cholinergic
Heart		
Sinoatrial node	Tachycardia	Bradycardia
Atrioventricular node	Increased conduction	Decreased conduction
His-Purkinje	Increased automaticity and conduction velocity	Minimal
Myocardium	Increased contractility, conduction velocity, automaticity	Minimal decrease in contractility
Coronary vessels	Constriction (alpha$_1$) and dilation (beta$_1$)	Dilation and constriction?*
Blood Vessels		
Skin and mucosa	Constriction	Dilation
Skeletal muscle	Constriction (alpha$_1$) > dilation (beta$_2$)	Dilation
Pulmonary	Constriction	? Dilation
Bronchial Smooth Muscle	Relaxation	Contraction
Gastrointestinal Tract		
Gallbladder and ducts	Relaxation	Contraction
Gut motility	Decreased	Increased
Secretions	Decreased	Increased
Sphincters	Constriction	Relaxation
Bladder		
Detrusor	Relaxes	Contracts
Trigone	Contracts	Relaxes
Glands		
Nasal	Vasoconstriction and reduced secretion	Stimulation of secretions
Lacrimal		
Parotid		
Submandibular		
Gastric		
Pancreatic		
Sweat Glands	Diaphoresis (cholinergic)	None
Apocrine Glands	Thick, odiferous secretion	None
Eye		
Pupil	Mydriasis	Miosis
Ciliary muscle	Relaxation for far vision	Contraction for near vision

*See the section on Interaction of Autonomic Nervous System Receptors.

example of spinal cord mediation of ANS reflexes without integration of function from higher inhibitory centers.[15,16]

Peripheral Autonomic Nervous System Organization

The peripheral ANS is the efferent (motor) component of the ANS and consists of two complementary parts: the SNS and the PNS. Most organs receive fibers from both divisions (Fig. 14-3). In general, activities of the two systems produce opposite but complementary effects (see Table 14-1). Actions of the two subdivisions are supplementary in some tissues such as the salivary glands. A few tissues, such as sweat glands and spleen, are innervated by only SNS fibers.

Although the anatomy of the somatic and ANS sensory pathways is identical, the motor pathways are characteristically different. The efferent somatic motor system, like somatic afferents, is composed of a single (unipolar) neuron with its cell body in the ventral gray matter of the spinal cord.[5] Its myelinated axon extends directly to the voluntary striated muscle unit. In contrast, the efferent (motor) ANS is a two-neuron (bipolar) chain from the CNS to the effector organ (see Fig. 14-1). The first neuron of both the SNS and PNS originates within the CNS but does not make direct contact with the effector organ. Instead, it relays the impulse to a second station known as an ANS ganglion, which contains the cell body of the second ANS (postganglionic) neuron. Its axon contacts the effector organ. Thus, the motor pathways of both divisions of the ANS are schematically a serial, two-neuron chain consisting of a preganglionic neuron and a postganglionic effector neuron (Fig. 14-4).

Preganglionic fibers of both subdivisions are myelinated with diameters of less than 3 μm.[3,4,6] Impulses are conducted at a speed of 3–15 m·s^{-1}. The postganglionic fibers are unmyelinated and conduct impulses at slower speeds of less than 2 m·s^{-1}. They are similar to unmyelinated visceral and somatic afferent C fibers (Table 14-3). Compared with the myelinated somatic nerves, the ANS conducts impulses at speeds that preclude its participation in the immediate phase of a somatic response.

Sympathetic Nervous System or Thoracolumbar Division

The efferent SNS is also referred to as the thoracolumbar nervous system. The origin of its preganglionic fibers provides the anatomic basis for this designation. Figure 14-3 demonstrates the distribution of the SNS and its innervation of visceral organs.

The preganglionic fibers of the SNS (thoracolumbar division) originate in the intermediolateral gray column of the twelve thoracic (T1–12) and the first three lumbar segments (L1–3) of the spinal cord. The myelinated axons of these nerve cells leave the spinal cord with the motor fibers to form the white (myelinated) communicating rami (Fig. 14-5). The rami enter one of the paired 22 sympathetic ganglia at their respective segmental levels. Upon entering the paravertebral ganglia of the lateral sympathetic chain, the preganglionic fiber may follow one of three courses: (1) synapse with postganglionic fibers in ganglia at the level of exit; (2) course upward or downward in the trunk of the SNS chain to synapse in ganglia at other levels; or (3) track for variable distances through the sympathetic chain and exit without synapsing to terminate in an outlying, unpaired, SNS collateral ganglion (Fig. 14-5). The adrenal gland is an exception to the rule. Preganglionic fibers pass directly into the adrenal medulla without synapsing in a ganglion (see Fig. 14-4). The cells of the medulla are derived from neuronal tissue and are analogous to postganglionic neurons.[4,6,12]

The sympathetic postganglionic neuronal cell bodies are located in ganglia of the paired lateral SNS chain or unpaired collateral ganglia in more peripheral plexus. Col-

TABLE 14-2. Hypothalamic Nuclei	
Anterior	**Posterior**
Paraventricular Nucleus	***Posterior Hypothalamus***
Oxytocin release	Increased blood pressure
Water conservation	Pupillary dilation
	Shivering
Medial Preoptic Area	Corticotropin
Bladder contraction	
Decreased heart rate	***Dorsomedial Nucleus***
Decreased blood pressure	Gastrointestinal stimulation
Supraoptic Nucleus	***Perifornical Nucleus***
Water conservation	Hunger
	Increased blood pressure
Posterior Preoptic and	Rage
Anterior Hypothalamic Area	
	Ventromedial Nucleus
Body temperature regulation	Satiety
Panting	
Sweating	***Mammillary Body***
Thyrotropin inhibition	Feeding reflexes
	Lateral Hypothalamic Area
	Thirst and hunger

lateral ganglia, such as the celiac and inferior mesenteric ganglia (plexus), are formed by the convergence of preganglionic fibers with many postganglionic neuronal bodies. SNS ganglia are almost always located closer to the spinal cord than to the organs they innervate. The sympathetic postganglionic neuron can therefore originate in either the paired lateral paravertebral SNS ganglia or one of the unpaired collateral plexus. The unmyelinated postganglionic fibers then proceed from the ganglia to terminate within the organs they innervate.

Many of the postganglionic fibers pass from the lateral SNS chain back into the spinal nerves, forming the gray (unmyelinated) communicating rami at all levels of the spinal cord (Fig. 14-5). They are distributed distally to sweat glands, pilomotor muscle, and blood vessels of the skin and

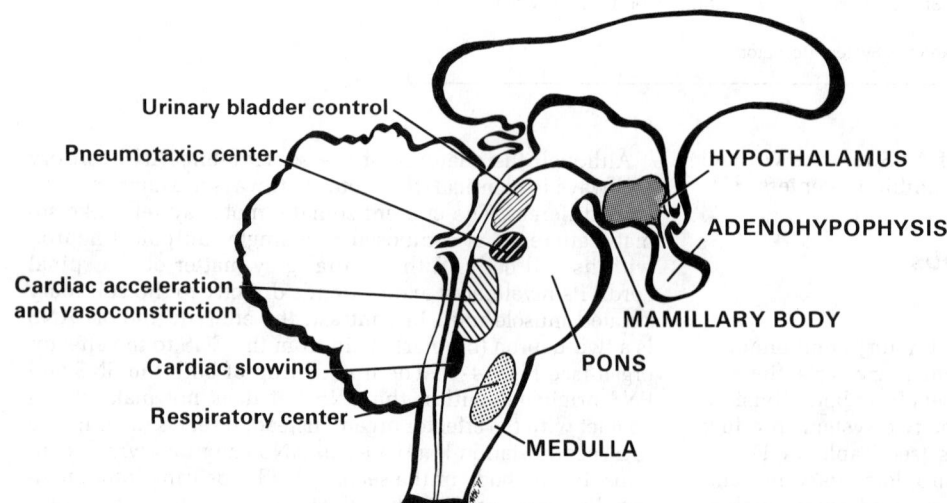

Figure 14-2. Central vital centers of the medulla oblongata and pons.

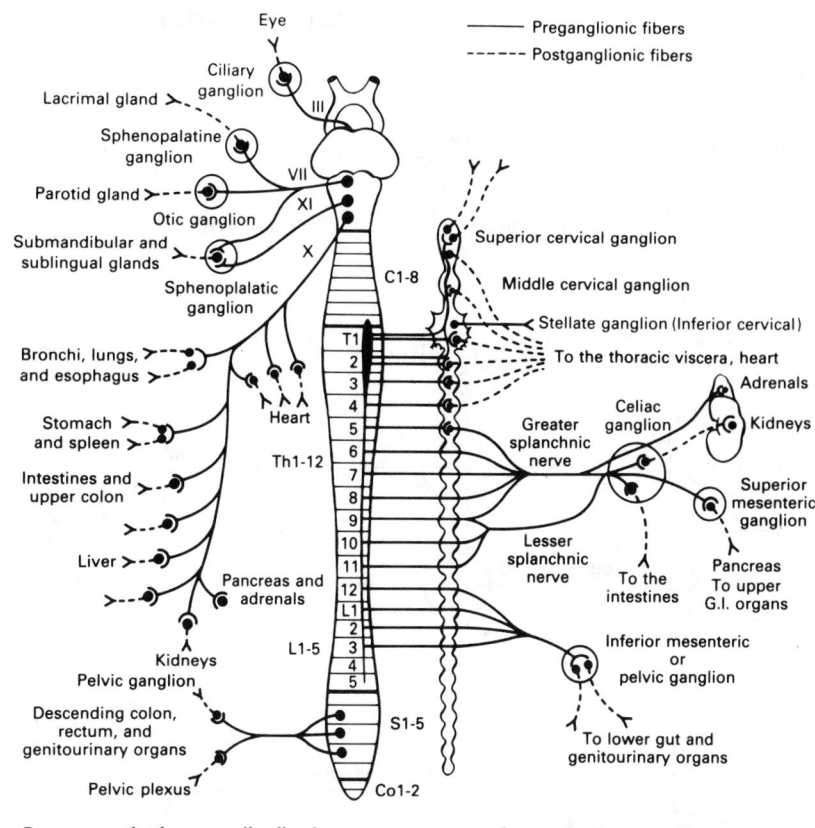

Figure 14-3. Schematic distribution of the craniosacral (parasympathetic) and thoracolumbar (sympathetic) nervous systems. Parasympathetic preganglionic fibers pass directly to the organ that is innervated. Their postganglionic cell bodies are situated near or within the innervated viscera. This limited distribution of parasympathetic postganglionic fibers is consistent with the discrete and limited effect of parasympathetic function. The postganglionic sympathetic neurons originate in either the paired sympathetic ganglia or one of the unpaired collateral plexus. One preganglionic fiber influences many postganglionic neurons. Activation of the sympathetic nervous system produces a more diffuse physiologic response rather than discrete effects.

muscle. These nerves are unmyelinated C type fibers (see Table 14-3) and are carried within the somatic nerves. Approximately 8% of the fibers in the average somatic nerve are sympathetic.[6]

The first four or five thoracic spinal segments generate preganglionic fibers that ascend in the neck to form three special paired ganglia. These are the superior cervical, middle cervical, and cervicothoracic ganglia. The last is known as the stellate ganglion and is actually formed by the fusion of the inferior cervical and first thoracic SNS ganglia. These ganglia provide sympathetic innervation of the head, neck, upper extremities, heart, and lungs. Afferent pain fibers also travel with these nerves, accounting for chest, neck, or upper extremity pain with myocardial ischemia.

Activation of the SNS produces a diffused physiologic response (mass reflex) rather than discrete effects. Function follows design. SNS postganglionic neurons outnumber the preganglionic neurons in an average ratio of 20:1 to 30:1.[4,5,17] One preganglionic fiber influences a larger number of postganglionic neurons, which are dispersed to many organs. In addition, the SNS response is augmented by the hormonal release of epinephrine from the adrenal medulla.

Parasympathetic Nervous System or Craniosacral Division

The PNS, like the SNS, has both preganglionic and postganglionic neurons. This division is sometimes called the craniosacral outflow because the preganglionic cell bodies originate in the brain stem and sacral segments of the spinal cord. PNS preganglionic fibers are found in cranial nerves

III (oculomotor), VII (facial), IX (glossopharyngeal), and X (vagus). The sacral outflow originates in the intermediolateral gray horns of the second, third, and fourth sacral nerves. Figure 14-3 shows the distribution of the PNS division and its innervation of visceral organs.

The vagus (cranial nerve X) nerve has the most extensive distribution of all the PNS, accounting for more than 75% of PNS activity.[6] The paired vagus nerves supply PNS innervation to the heart, lungs, esophagus, stomach, small intestine, proximal half of the colon, liver, gallbladder, pancreas, and upper portions of the ureters. The sacral fibers form the pelvic visceral nerves, or nervi erigentes. These nerves supply the remainder of the viscera that are not innervated by the vagus. They supply the descending colon, rectum, uterus, bladder, and lower portions of the ureters and are primarily concerned with emptying. Various sexual reactions are also governed by the sacral PNS. The PNS is responsible for penile erection, but SNS stimulation governs ejaculation.

In contrast to the SNS division, PNS preganglionic fibers pass directly to the organ that is innervated. The postganglionic cell bodies are situated near or within the innervated viscera and generally are not visible. The proximity of PNS ganglia to or within the viscera provides a limited distribution of postganglionic fibers. The ratio of postganglionic to preganglionic fibers in many organs appears to be 1:1 to 3:1 compared with the 20:1 found in the SNS system.[4,5] Auerbach's plexus in the distal colon is the exception, with a ratio of 8000:1. The fact that PNS preganglionic fibers synapse with only a few postganglionic neurons is consistent with the discrete and limited effect of PNS function.

BIPOLAR AUTONOMIC NERVES

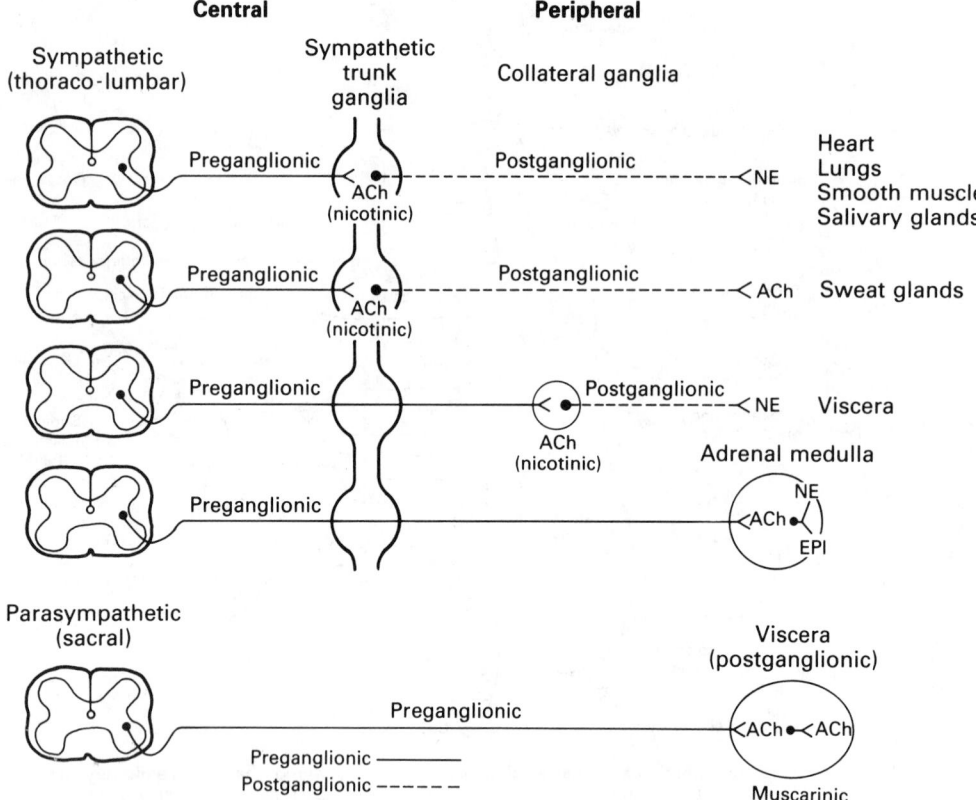

Figure 14-4. Schematic diagram of the efferent autonomic nervous system. Afferent impulses are integrated centrally and sent reflexly to the adrenergic and cholinergic receptors. Sympathetic fibers ending in the adrenal medulla are preganglionic, and acetylcholine (ACh) is the neurotransmitter. Stimulation of the chromaffin cells, acting as postganglionic neurons, releases epinephrine (EPI) and norepinephrine (NE).

For example, vagal bradycardia can occur without a concomitant change in intestinal motility or salivation. Mass reflex action is not a characteristic of the PNS. The effects of organ response to PNS stimulation are outlined in Table 14-1.

Autonomic Innervation

Heart. The heart is well supplied by the SNS and PNS. These nerves affect cardiac pumping in three ways: (1) by changing the rate (chronotropism); (2) by changing the strength of contraction (inotropism); and (3) by modulating coronary blood flow. The PNS cardiac vagal fibers approach the stellate ganglia and then join the efferent cardiac SNS fibers; therefore, the vagus nerve to the heart and lungs is a mixed nerve containing both PNS and SNS efferent fibers. The PNS fibers are distributed mainly to the sinoatrial and atrioventricular nodes and to a lesser extent to the atria. There is little or no distribution to the ventricles.[5,18] Therefore, the main effect of vagal cardiac stimulation to the heart is chronotropic. Vagal stimulation decreases the rate of sinoatrial node discharge and decreases excitability of the atrioventricular junctional fibers, slowing impulse conduction to the ventricles. A very strong vagal discharge can completely arrest sinoatrial node firing and block impulse conduction to the ventricles. Vagal stimulation or vagotonic drugs such as methacholine reduce the vulnerability of the heart to ventricular fibrillation, decrease the frequency of premature ventricular beats, and can abolish ventricular tachycardia (see the section on Interaction of Autonomic Nervous System Receptors).[19]

The physiologic importance of the PNS on myocardial contractility is not as well understood as that of the SNS. Cholinergic blockade can double the heart rate without altering contractility of the left ventricle. Vagal stimulation of the heart can reduce left ventricular maximum rate of tension development (dP/dT) and decrease contractile force by

TABLE 14-3. Classification of Nerve Fibers

Description of Nerve Fibers	Group		Diameter (μm)	Conduction Velocity (m·s⁻¹)
Myelinated somatic	A	Alpha α	20	120
		Beta β		
		Gamma γ		5–40 (pain fibers)
		Delta δ	3–4	5–40 (pain fibers)
		Epsilon ε	2	5
Myelinated visceral (preganglionic autonomic)	B		<3	3–15
Unmyelinated somatic	C		<2	0.5–2 (pain fibers)

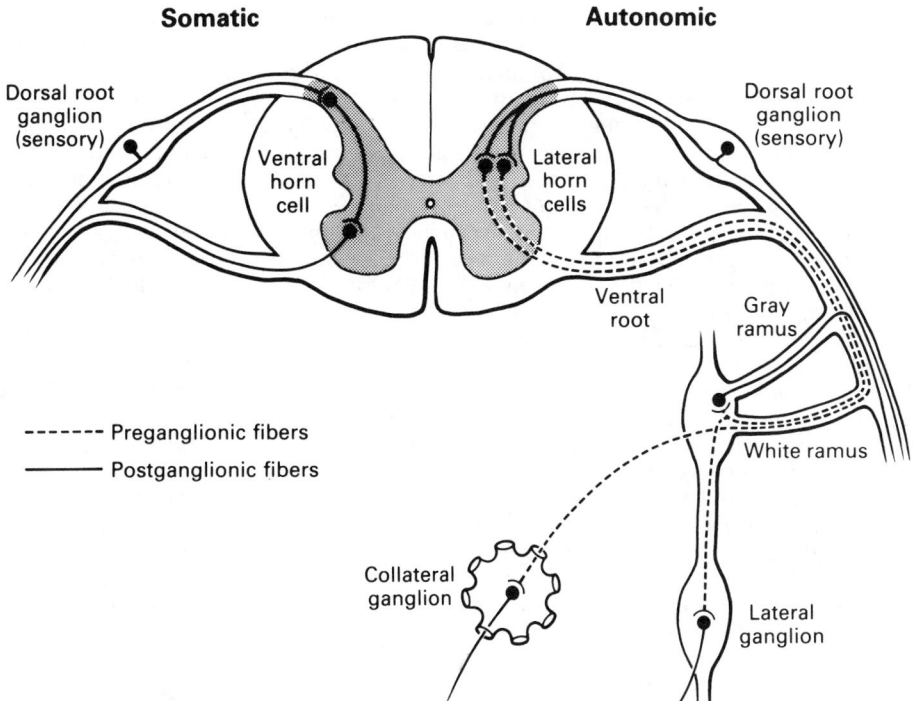

Figure 14-5. The spinal reflex arc of the somatic nerves is shown on the left. The different arrangements of neurons in the sympathetic system are shown on the right. Preganglionic fibers coming out through white rami may make synaptic connections following one of three courses: (1) synapse in ganglia at the level of exit; (2) course up or down the sympathetic chain to synapse at another level; or (3) exit the chain without synapsing to an outlying collateral ganglion.

as much as 10–20%. However, PNS stimulation is relatively unimportant in this regard compared with its predominant effect on heart rate.

The SNS has the same supraventricular distribution as the PNS, but with stronger representation to the ventricles. SNS efferents to the myocardium funnel through the paired stellate ganglia. The right stellate ganglion distributes primarily to the anterior epicardial surface and the interventricular septum.[20,21] Right stellate stimulation decreases systolic duration and increases heart rate. The left stellate ganglion supplies the posterior and lateral surfaces of both ventricles. Left stellate stimulation increases mean arterial pressure and left ventricular contractility without causing a substantial change in heart rate. Normal SNS tone maintains contractility approximately 20% above that in the absence of any SNS stimulation.[22] Therefore, the dominant effect of the ANS on myocardial contractility is mediated primarily through the SNS. Intrinsic mechanisms of the myocardium, however, can maintain circulation quite well without the ANS, as evidenced by the success of cardiac transplants[23,24] (see the section on Denervated Heart).

Early investigations, performed in anesthetized, open-chest animals, demonstrated that cardiac ANS nerves exert only slight effects on the coronary vascular bed; however, more recent studies on chronically instrumented, intact, conscious animals show considerable evidence for a strong SNS regulation of the small coronary resistance and larger conductance vessels.[25-27] This information is important, but the anesthesiologist must be careful to place this new information into context. As in the older studies, our patients are anesthetized and often have their thoraces open. The new studies refute the old concept that there is minimal ANS coronary influence but instead demonstrate that anesthesia minimizes the contribution of the ANS to the regulation of coronary blood flow as compared with in the conscious state. These data have already proved useful in anesthetizing patients during acute myocardial infarction.[28]

Different segments of the coronary arterial tree react dif-

ferently to various stimuli and drugs. Large conductance vessels, the primary location for atheromatous plaques, are found on the epicardial surface, whereas the small, precapillary resistance vessels are found within the myocardium. Normally, the large conductance vessels contribute little to overall coronary vascular resistance. Fluctuations in resistance primarily reflect changes in lumen size of the small, precapillary vessels. Blood flow through the resistance vessels is regulated primarily by the local metabolic requirements of the myocardium. The larger conductance vessels, however, can constrict markedly with neurogenic stimulation. Neurogenic influence also assumes a greater role in the resistance vessels when they become hypoxic and lose autoregulation. There is a strong interaction between SNS and PNS nerves in organs with dual, antagonistic innervation. The tone of the coronary arteries is under this interacting control in a manner that is only now becoming understood (see the section on Interaction of Autonomic Nervous System Receptors).[29]

Peripheral Circulation. The SNS nerves are by far the most important regulators of the peripheral circulation.[30] The PNS nerves play only a minor role in this regard.[6] PNS stimulation dilates vessels, but only in certain limited areas such as the genitals. SNS stimulation produces both vasodilation and vasoconstriction, with vasoconstrictor effects predominating. The effect is determined by the type of receptors on which the SNS fiber terminates (see section on Receptors). SNS constrictor receptors are distributed to all segments of the circulation. This distribution is greater in some tissues than in others. Blood vessels in the skin, kidneys, spleen, and mesentery have an extensive SNS distribution, whereas those in the heart, brain, and muscle have less SNS innervation. SNS stimulation of the coronary arteries may produce vasoconstriction or vasodilation, depending upon the predominant receptor activity at the time of stimulation (see Table 14-1). Vagal stimulation may also produce coronary vasoconstriction (see section on Beta-Adrenergic Receptors).[27] However, local autoregulatory factors usually have the predominant influence on coronary vascular tone.

Vascular tone is the sum of the muscular forces in the walls of blood vessels that oppose an increase in vessel diameter. Vasomotor tone denotes that portion of vascular tone controlled by the ANS vasomotor nerves. Thus, vascular tone can be influenced by local and circulating substances as well as by the vasomotor nerves. Blood vessels have differing sensitivities to the influence of local or neurogenic control. Arterioles and venules are under strong neurogenic control and have vasomotor tone. Local autoregulation is the predominant force at the precapillary and postcapillary sphincters.[31,32]

Basal vasomotor tone is maintained by impulses from the lateral portion of the vasomotor center in the medulla oblongata that continually transmits impulses through the SNS, maintaining partial arteriolar and venular constriction. Circulating epinephrine from the adrenal medulla has additive effects. This basal ANS tone maintains arteriolar constriction at near half-maximum diameter.[4] The arteriole, therefore, has the potential for either further constriction or dilation. If the basal tone were not present, the SNS could only effect vasoconstriction and not vasodilation.[6,33] The SNS tone in the venules produces little resistance to flow as compared with the arterioles and the arteries. The importance of SNS stimulation of veins is to reduce or increase their capacity. By functioning as a reservoir for approximately 80% of the total blood volume, small changes in venous capacitance produce large changes in venous return and, thus, cardiac preload.

Lungs. The lungs are innervated by both the SNS and PNS.[4] Postganglionic SNS fibers from the upper thoracic ganglia (stellate) pass to the lungs to innervate the smooth muscles of the bronchi and pulmonary blood vessels. PNS innervation of these structures is from the vagus nerve.

SNS stimulation produces bronchodilation and pulmonary vasoconstriction.[34] Little else has been proved conclusively about the vasomotor control of the pulmonary vessels other than that they adjust to accommodate the output of the right ventricle. The effect of stimulation of the pulmonary SNS nerves on pulmonary vascular resistance is not very great but may be quite important in maintaining hemo-dynamic stability during stress and exercise by balancing right and left ventricular output.[35,36] This response is probably mediated *via* the hypothalamus. Stimulation of the vagus nerve, on the other hand, produces almost no vasodilation of the pulmonary circulation. The recently described phenomenon of hypoxic pulmonary vasoconstriction appears to be a more important force in regulation of pulmonary blood flow.[37,38] Hypoxic pulmonary vasoconstriction, however, does not appear to be mediated through the ANS but rather is a local phenomenon capable of providing a faster adjustment to needs.

Both the SNS and the vagus nerve provide active bronchomotor control. SNS stimulation causes bronchodilation, whereas vagal stimulation produces constriction. PNS stimulation may also increase secretions of the bronchial glands. Vagal receptor endings in the alveolar ducts also play an important role in the reflex regulation of the ventilation cycle.[39] The lung has important nonventilatory activity as well. It serves as a metabolic organ that removes local mediators such as norepinephrine (NE) from the circulation and converts others, such as angiotensin I, to active compounds[40-43] (see section on Interaction with Other Regulatory Systems).

AUTONOMIC NERVOUS SYSTEM— NEUROTRANSMISSION

Transmission of excitation across the terminal junctional sites (synaptic clefts) of the peripheral ANS occurs through the mediation of liberated chemicals (Fig. 14-6). These chemical transmitters interact with a receptor on the end organ to evoke a biologic response. The ANS can be pharmacologically subdivided by the neurotransmitter secreted at the effector cell. Pharmacologic parlance designates the SNS and PNS as adrenergic and cholinergic, respectively. The terminals of the PNS postganglionic fibers release acetylcholine (ACh). With the exception of sweat glands, NE is the neurotransmitter released at the terminals of the sympathetic postganglionic fibers (see Fig. 14-4). The preganglionic neurons of both systems secrete ACh.

The terminations of the postganglionic fibers of both ANS subdivisions are anatomically and physiologically similar. The terminations are characterized by multiple branchings called terminal effector plexus, or reticula. These filaments surround the elements of the effector unit "like a mesh stocking."[44] Thus, one SNS postganglionic neuron, for example, can innervate some 25,000 effector cells, e.g., vascular smooth muscle.[12,17] The terminal filaments end in presynaptic enlargements called varicosities. Each varicosity contains vesicles, approximately 500 A in diameter, in which the neurotransmitters are stored (Fig. 14-6). The varicosities are also heavily populated with mitochondria, which relates to the increased energy (adenosine triphosphate) requirements of ACh and NE synthesis. The rate of synthesis depends on the level of ANS activity and is regulated by local feedback. The distance between the varicosity and the effector cell (synaptic or junctional cleft) varies from 100 A in ganglia and arterioles to as much as 20,000 A in large arteries. This distance determines the amount of transmitter required to stimulate and the time it takes to diffuse to the effector cell. The time for diffusion is directly proportional to the width of the synaptic gap. Depolarization releases the vesicular contents into the synaptic cleft by exocytosis.

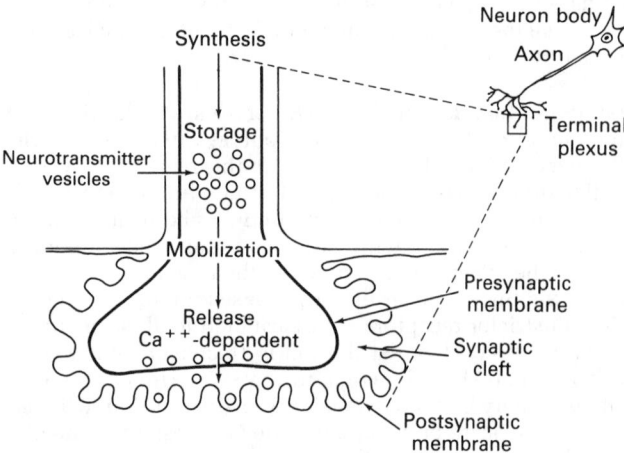

EFFECTOR CELL

Figure 14-6. The anatomy and physiology of the terminal postganglionic fibers of sympathetic and parasympathetic fibers are similar.

Parasympathetic Nervous System Neurotransmission

Synthesis

ACh is the neurotransmitter that mediates the PNS. It is formed in the presynaptic terminal by acetylation of choline with acetyl coenzyme A. This step is catalyzed by choline acetyl transferase (Fig. 14-7). ACh is then stored in a concentrated form in presynaptic vesicles containing about 10,000 molecules of ACh. A continual release of small amounts of ACh, called quanta, occurs during the resting state. Each quantum results in small changes in the electrical potential of the synaptic end plate without producing depolarization. These are known as miniature end-plate potentials. Arrival of an action potential causes a synchronous release of hundreds of quanta, resulting in depolarization of the end plate (see Fig. 14-6). Release of ACh from the vesicles is dependent on influx of calcium (Ca^{2+}) from the interstitial space.[45] Drugs that alter Ca^{2+} binding or influx may decrease ACh release and affect end-organ function.[46] ACh is not reused like NE, and therefore it must be synthesized constantly.

Metabolism

The ability of a receptor to modulate function of an effector organ is dependent upon rapid recovery to its baseline state after stimulation. For this to occur, the neurotransmitter must be rapidly removed from the vicinity of the receptor. In the case of ACh, removal occurs by rapid hydrolysis by acetylcholinesterase (Fig. 14-7). This enzyme is found in neurons, at the neuromuscular junction, and in various other tissues of the body. A similar enzyme, butyrocholinesterase (pseudocholinesterase or plasma cholinesterase), is also found throughout the body but only to a limited extent in nervous tissue. It does not appear to be physiologically important in termination of the action of ACh. Both acetylcholinesterase and pseudocholinesterase hydrolyze ACh as well as other esters (such as the ester-type local anesthetics), but they may be distinguished by specific biochemical tests.[19,47]

ACh is a quarternary ammonium compound that possesses a cationic moiety joined by a chain of two carbon atoms to an ester grouping. ACh binds to acetylcholinesterase at two sites. One site is specific for the positively charged quarternary ammonium moiety, the anionic site.

The other is specific for the esteratic moiety. These binding sites stereospecifically orient ACh correctly as the substrate for hydrolysis. The ester site forms a covalent bond with the enzyme, thus acetylating the enzyme that ruptures the ester linkage of ACh (see Fig. 14-7). The acetylated enzyme reacts with water to produce regenerated active enzyme and acetic acid. Thus, the products of ACh hydrolysis are free choline, acetic acid, and the enzyme regenerated for further use.

Sympathetic Nervous System Neurotransmission

The SNS is mediated peripherally by the catecholamines, epinephrine, and NE. NE is the exclusive neurotransmitter released from localized postganglionic, presynaptic vesicles. It is released directly into the site where it acts. The SNS fibers ending in the adrenal medulla are preganglionic, and ACh is the neurotransmitter (see Fig. 14-4). It interacts with the chromaffin cells in the medulla, causing the release of epinephrine and NE. The chromaffin cells take the place of the postganglionic neurons.[12,23] Stimulation of the sympathetic nerves to the adrenal medulla, however, causes the release of large quantities of a mixture of epinephrine and NE into the circulation to become neurotransmitter hormones. The greater portion of this hormonal surge is normally epinephrine.[6,12,48] Epinephrine and NE, when released into the circulation, are classified as hormones in that they are synthesized, stored, and released from the adrenal medulla to act at distant sites.

Hormonal epinephrine and NE have almost the same effects on effector cells as those caused by local direct sympathetic stimulation; however, the hormonal effects, although brief, last about ten times as long as those caused by direct stimulation.[4,49] Epinephrine has a greater metabolic effect than NE. It can increase the metabolic rate of the body by as much as 100%.[6] It also increases glycogenolysis in the liver and muscle with glucose release into the blood. These functions are all necessary to prepare the body for fight or flight.

The normal resting state of secretion by the adrenal medulla is about 0.02 $\mu g \cdot kg^{-1} \cdot min^{-1}$ of epinephrine and about 0.02 $\mu g \cdot kg^{-1} \cdot min^{-1}$ of NE.[6,48,49] Some of the overall vascular tone results from the basal resting secretion of the adrenal medulla in addition to the tone that is maintained directly

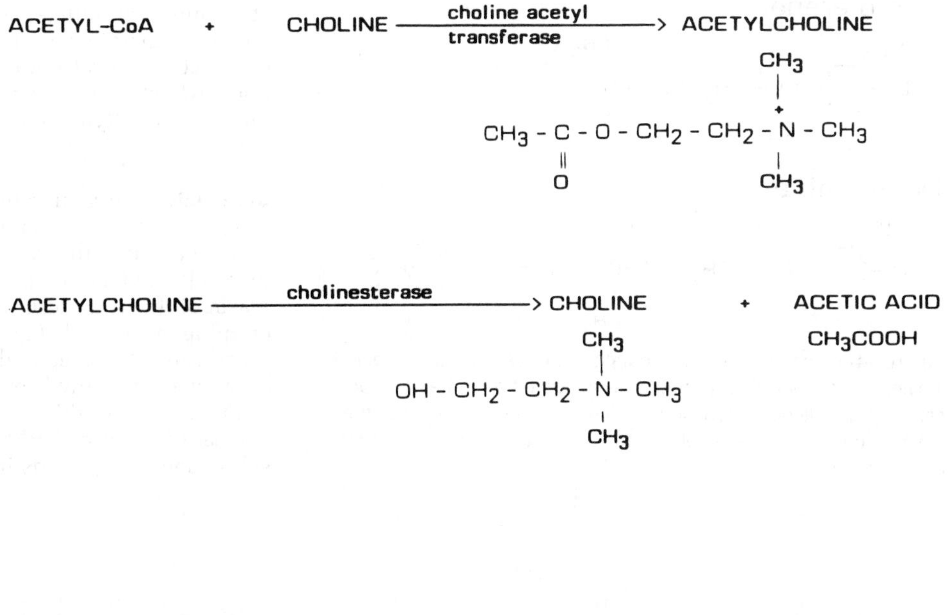

Figure 14-7. Synthesis and metabolism of acetylcholine.

through stimulation from central vasomotor centers in the medulla.

Catecholamines—The First Messenger

The endogenous catecholamines in humans are dopamine, NE, and epinephrine.[12,24] Dopamine is a neurotransmitter in the CNS. It is primarily involved in coordinating motor activity in the brain. In addition, it is the precursor of NE.[17] NE is synthesized and stored primarily in nerve endings of postganglionic SNS neurons. It is also synthesized in the adrenal medulla and is the chemical precursor of epinephrine. Stored epinephrine is located chiefly in chromaffin cells of the adrenal medulla. Eighty to eighty-five percent of the catecholamine content of the adrenal medulla is epinephrine and 15–20% is NE. The brain contains both noradrenergic and dopaminergic receptors, but circulating catecholamines do not cross the blood-brain barrier.[29] The catecholamines present in the brain are synthesized there. Endogenous catecholamines are unique in that several intermediates in the synthesis function as neurotransmitters.

A catecholamine is any compound of a catechol nucleus (a benzene ring with two adjacent hydroxyl groups) and an amine-containing side chain.[50] The chemical configuration of five of the more common catecholamines in clinical use is demonstrated in Figure 14-8. A true catecholamine must possess this basic structure. Catecholamines are often re-

TABLE 14-4. Sympathomimetic Drugs	
Adrenergic Amines	
Catecholamines	*Trade Name*
Epinephrine	Adrenalin
Norepinephrine	Levophed
Dopamine*	Inotropin
Dobutamine	Dobutrex
Dopexamine	
Isoproterenol	Isuprel
Noncatecholamines	
Metaraminol*†	Aramine
Mephentermine†	Wyamine
Ephedrine†	Ephedrine
Methoxamine	Vasoxyl
Phenylephrine	Neo-Synephrine
Nonadrenergics	
Xanthines	Aminophylline
Glucagon	Glucagon
Digitalis	Lanoxin
Calcium salts	
Naloxone	Narcan
Amrinone	Inocor

* Direct-acting catecholamine with some indirect action.

† Primarily indirect-acting with some direct action. Adrenergic amines produce sympathomimetic effects *via* adrenergic receptors. Nonadrenergics produce sympathomimetic effects exclusive of the adrenergic receptor.

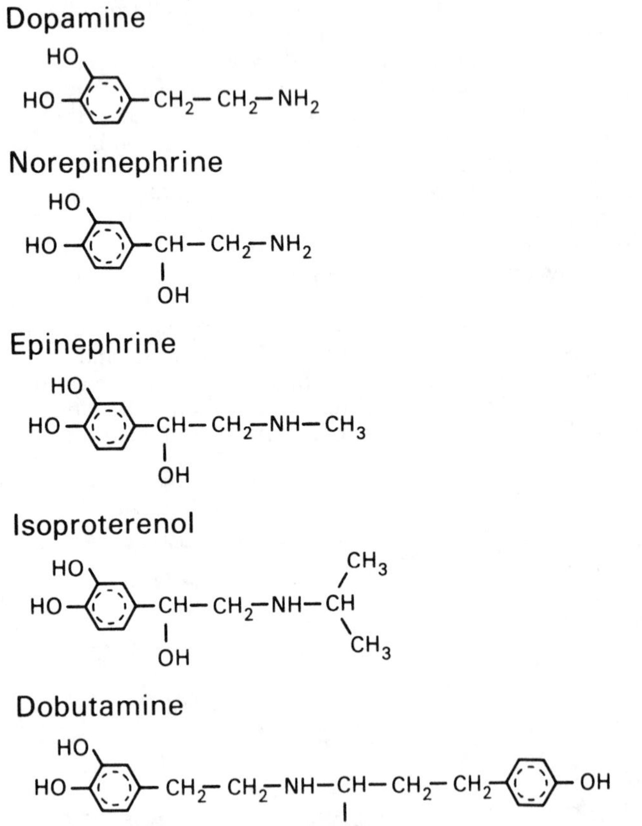

ferred to as adrenergic drugs because their effector actions are mediated through receptors specific for the SNS. Synthetic catecholamines can activate these same receptors because of their structural similarity. Drugs that produce sympathetic-like effects but lack the basic catecholamine structure are defined as sympathomimetics. All clinically useful catecholamines are sympathomimetics, but not all sympathomimetics are catecholamines (Table 14-4). In addition, not all sympathomimetic drugs are adrenergic. Many are capable of producing a sympathomimetic effect by acting at sites exclusive of adrenergic receptors.

The effects of endogenous or synthetic catecholamines on adrenergic receptors can be direct or indirect (Table 14-4).[51,52] Indirect-acting catecholamines have little intrinsic effect on adrenergic receptors but produce their effects by stimulating release of the stored neurotransmitter from SNS nerve terminals. Some synthetic and endogenous catecholamines stimulate adrenergic receptor sites directly, whereas others have a mixed mode of action. The actions of direct-acting catecholamines are independent of endogenous NE stores; however, the indirect-acting catecholamines are totally dependent on adequate neuronal stores of endogenous NE.

Synthesis. The main site of NE synthesis is in or near the postganglionic nerve endings.[3] Some synthesis does occur in vesicles near the cell body that pass to the nerve endings.[53] Phenylalanine or tyrosine is taken up into the axoplasm of the nerve terminal and synthesized into either NE or epinephrine.[6,12,17] Figure 14-9 demonstrates this synthesis cascade. Tyrosine hydroxylase catalyzes the conversion of tyrosine to dihydroxyphenylalanine. This is the rate-limiting step at which NE synthesis is controlled through feedback inhibition.[12,54,55] Dihydroxyphenylalanine and the subsequent compounds in this cascade are catecholamines.

Dopamine

Norepinephrine

Epinephrine

Isoproterenol

Dobutamine

Figure 14-8. The chemical configurations of five common catecholamines are shown. Sympathomimetic drugs differ in their hemodynamic effects largely because of differences in substitution of the amine group on the catechol nucleus (a benzene ring with two hydroxyl groups).

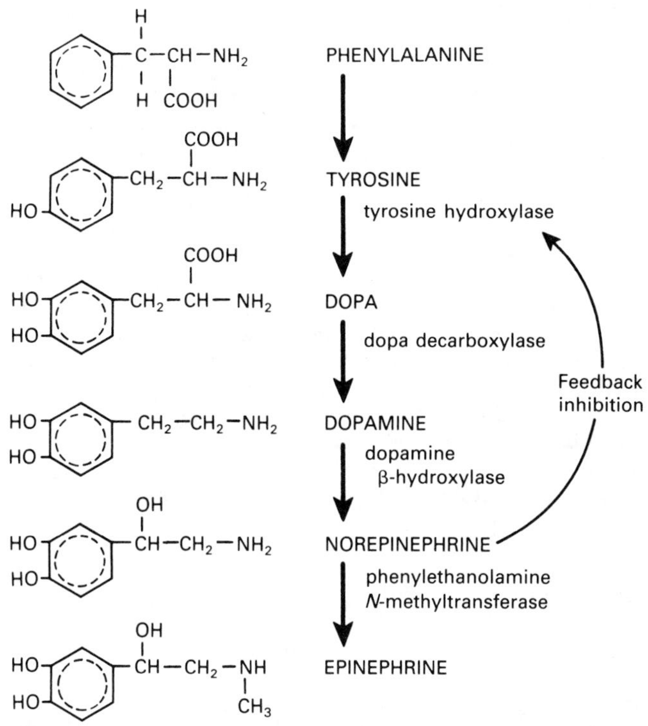

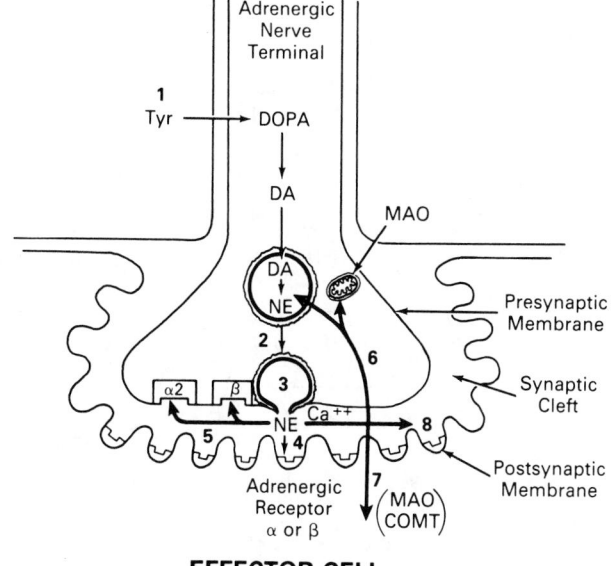

Figure 14-9. Schematic of the synthesis of catecholamines. The conversion of tyrosine to DOPA by tyrosine hydroxylase is inhibited by increased NE synthesis. Epinephrine is shown in these steps but is primarily synthesized in the adrenal medulla.

EFFECTOR CELL

Figure 14-10. Schematic of the synthesis and disposition of NE in adrenergic neurotransmission. (1) synthesis and storage in neuronal vesicles; (2) action potential permits calcium entry with (3) exocytosis of NE into synaptic gap. (4) Released NE reacts with receptor on effector cell. NE (5) may react with presynaptic alpha$_2$ receptor to inhibit further NE release or with presynaptic beta receptor to enhance reuptake of NE (6) (uptake 1). Extraneuronal uptake (uptake 2) absorbs NE into effector cell (7) with overflow occurring systemically (8). MAO = monoamine oxidase; COMT = catechol-O-methyltransferase; Tyr = tyrosine; DOPA = dihydroxyphenylalanine; NE = norepinephrine.

Dopamine is formed from dihydroxyphenylalanine by dihydroxyphenylalanine decarboxylase. Synthesis to this point occurs in the cytoplasm of the neuron. Dopamine then enters the storage vesicles. In the brain, synthesis stops at this point where dopamine is the neurotransmitter. The vesicles of peripheral postganglionic neurons contain the enzyme dopamine-beta-hydroxylase, which converts dopamine to NE. The adrenal medulla additionally contains phenylethanolamine-N-methyltransferase, which converts NE to epinephrine. This reaction takes place outside the medullary vesicles, and the newly formed epinephrine then enters the vesicle for storage (Fig. 14-10). All the endogenous catecholamines are stored in presynaptic vesicles and released on arrival of an action potential. Excitation-secretion coupling in sympathetic neurons is Ca^{2+}-dependent.[45,56]

Regulation. Increased SNS nervous activity, as in congestive heart failure or chronic stress, stimulates the synthesis of tyrosine hydroxylase and dopamine-beta-hydroxylase.[12,57] Glucocorticoids from the adrenal cortex pass through the adrenal medulla and stimulate an increase in phenylethanolamine-N-methyltransferase that methylates NE to epinephrine.[3]

The mechanism of NE release by nerve stimulation is not completely understood, but the release of NE is dependent upon depolarization of the nerve and an increase in calcium ion permeability. Calcium may cause microfilaments in the prejunctional membrane to contract and trigger exocytosis of NE granules.[45,55,56] This release is inhibited by colchicine and prostaglandin E$_2$, suggesting a contractile mechanism. Blockade of prostaglandin synthesis enhances NE release. NE inhibits its own release by stimulating presynaptic (pre-

junctional) alpha$_2$ receptors. Phenoxybenzamine and phentolamine, alpha receptor antagonists, increase the release of NE by blocking inhibitory presynaptic alpha$_2$ receptors (Fig. 14-11). Other receptors may also be important in NE regulation and are discussed later (see the section on Other Receptors).

Inactivation. As with the PNS, the ability of the adrenergic receptor to modulate function of the end organ is dependent on rapid recovery to its baseline state after stimulation. The neurotransmitter must, therefore, be rapidly inactivated. Unlike ACh, the catecholamines are removed from the synaptic cleft by three mechanisms (see Fig. 14-10).[12] These are (1) reuptake into the presynaptic terminals, (2) extraneuronal uptake, and (3) diffusion. Termination of NE at the effector site is almost entirely by reuptake of NE into the terminals of the presynaptic neuron (uptake 1). Once NE is back in the nerve terminal, it is stored in the varicosities for reuse. A small amount is deaminated in the cytoplasm of the neuron by monoamine oxidase to form dihydroxymandelic acid, which diffuses out of the nerve terminal and into the interstitial fluid. Uptake 1 is an active, energy-requiring, temperature-dependent process that can be inhibited pharmacologically.

The reuptake of NE in the presynaptic terminals is also a stereo-specific process. Structurally similar compounds (guanethidine, metaraminol) may enter the vesicles and displace the neurotransmitter. Tricyclic antidepressants and cocaine inhibit the reuptake of NE, resulting in high synaptic NE concentrations and accentuated receptor response. In addition, recent evidence suggests that NE reuptake is

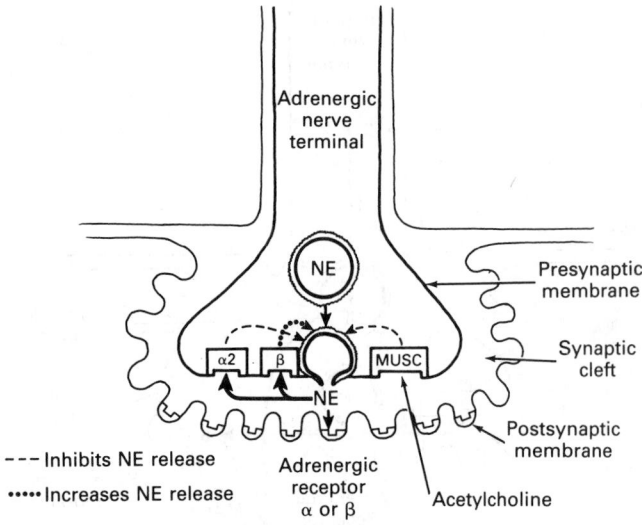

--- Inhibits NE release

····· Increases NE release

Effector Cell

Figure 14-11. This schematic demonstrates just a few of the presynaptic adrenergic receptors thought to exist. Agonist and antagonist drugs are clinically available for these receptors (see Table 14-5). The alpha$_2$ receptors serve as a negative feedback mechanism whereby NE stimulation inhibits its own release. Presynaptic beta stimulation increases NE uptake, augmenting its availability. Presynaptic muscarinic (MUSC) receptors respond to ACh diffusing from nearby cholinergic terminals. They inhibit NE release and can be blocked by atropine.

mediated by a presynaptic beta-adrenergic mechanism because beta blockade causes marked elevations of epinephrine and NE[58] (see Figs. 14-10 and 14-11), whereas alpha blockade does not. The clinical significance of this presynaptic beta-receptor is unknown at this time.

Extraneuronal uptake (uptake 2) is a minor pathway for inactivating NE. NE is taken up by effector cells and other extraneuronal tissues. The NE that is taken up by the extraneuronal tissue is metabolized by monoamine, oxidase and by catechol-O-methyltransferase to form vanillylmandelic acid (Fig. 14-12).[9,59] The minute amount of catecholamine that escapes uptake 1 and uptake 2 diffuses into the circulation (uptake 3),* where it is similarly metabolized in the liver and kidney. The importance of uptake 1 and uptake 2 is diminished when sympathomimetics are given exogenously. Epinephrine is inactivated by the same enzymes. Whereas uptake 1 is the predominant pathway for inactivation of the endogenous catecholamines, uptake 3 is the predominant pathway for catecholamines given exogenously and is clinically important. This accounts for the longer duration of action by exogenous catecholamines than that noted at the local synapse. The former is slow (liver metabolism) and the latter is fast (uptake 1).

The final metabolic product of the catecholamines is vanillylmandelic acid. Vanillylmandelic acid constitutes the major metabolite (80–90%) of NE found in the urine. Less than 5% of released NE appears unchanged in the urine.[9] The metabolic products excreted in the urine provide a gross estimate of SNS activity and can facilitate the clinical diagnosis of pheochromocytoma.

*Uptake 3 is used as a clinical term to describe uptake of exogenous drug administration.

RECEPTORS

The concept that receptors are the initial decoders of extracellular messengers has guided research on hormones and neurotransmitters for many years. An agonist is a substance that interacts with a receptor to evoke a biologic response. ACh and NE are the agonists of the ANS. An antagonist is a substance that interferes with the evocation of a response at a receptor site by an agonist. Receptors are therefore regarded as target sites on a cell that when activated by an agonist will lead to a response by the effector cell. Receptors have never been identified as precise anatomic structures; rather, their existence has been demonstrated biochemically and on the basis of biologic response.[24] Receptors are macromolecules that appear to be proteins and are located in the plasma membrane. Several thousand receptors have been demonstrated in a single cell.[12,60] The enormity of this network is realized when it is considered that some 25,000 single cells can be innervated by a single neuron.[17,61]

Cholinergic Receptors

ACh is the neurotransmitter at three distinct classes of receptors. These receptors can be differentiated by their anatomic location and their affinity to bind various agonists and antagonists.[62] ACh mediates the "first messenger" function of transmitting impulses in the PNS, the ganglia of the SNS, and the neuroeffector junction of striated, voluntary muscle (see Fig. 14-4). The receptors are referred to as choliceptive or cholinergic receptors. The PNS is often referred to as the cholinergic system.

Cholinergic receptors are further subdivided into muscarinic and nicotinic receptors because muscarine and nicotine stimulate them selectively.[3,19] However, both muscarinic and nicotinic receptors respond to ACh (see the section on Cholinergic Drugs). Muscarine, derived from the poisonous mushroom *Amantia muscaria*, stimulates cholinergic receptors at the postganglionic PNS junctions of cardiac and smooth muscle throughout the body. Muscarinic stimulation is characterized by bradycardia, decreased inotropism, bronchoconstriction, miosis, salivation, gastrointestinal hypermotility, and increased gastric acid secretion (see Table 14-1). Muscarinic receptors can be blocked by atropine without effect on nicotinic receptors (see the section on Cholinergic Drugs).

Muscarinic receptors are known to exist in sites other than PNS postganglionic junctions. They are found on the presynaptic membrane of sympathetic nerve terminals in the myocardium, coronary vessels, and peripheral vasculature (Fig. 14-11).[20,24] These are referred to as adrenergic muscarinic receptors because of their location; however, they are stimulated by ACh. Stimulation of these receptors inhibits release of NE in a manner similar to alpha$_2$ receptor stimulation.[27,63] Muscarinic blockade removes inhibition of NE release, augmenting SNS activity. Atropine, the prototypical muscarinic blocker, may produce sympathomimetic activity in this manner as well as vagal blockade. Neuromuscular blocking drugs that cause tachycardia are thought to have a similar mechanism of action.

ACh acting on presynaptic adrenergic muscarinic receptors is a very potent inhibitor of NE release.[20,58] The prejunctional muscarinic receptor may play an important physiologic role because several autonomically innervated tissues (e.g., the heart) possess ANS plexus in which the SNS and

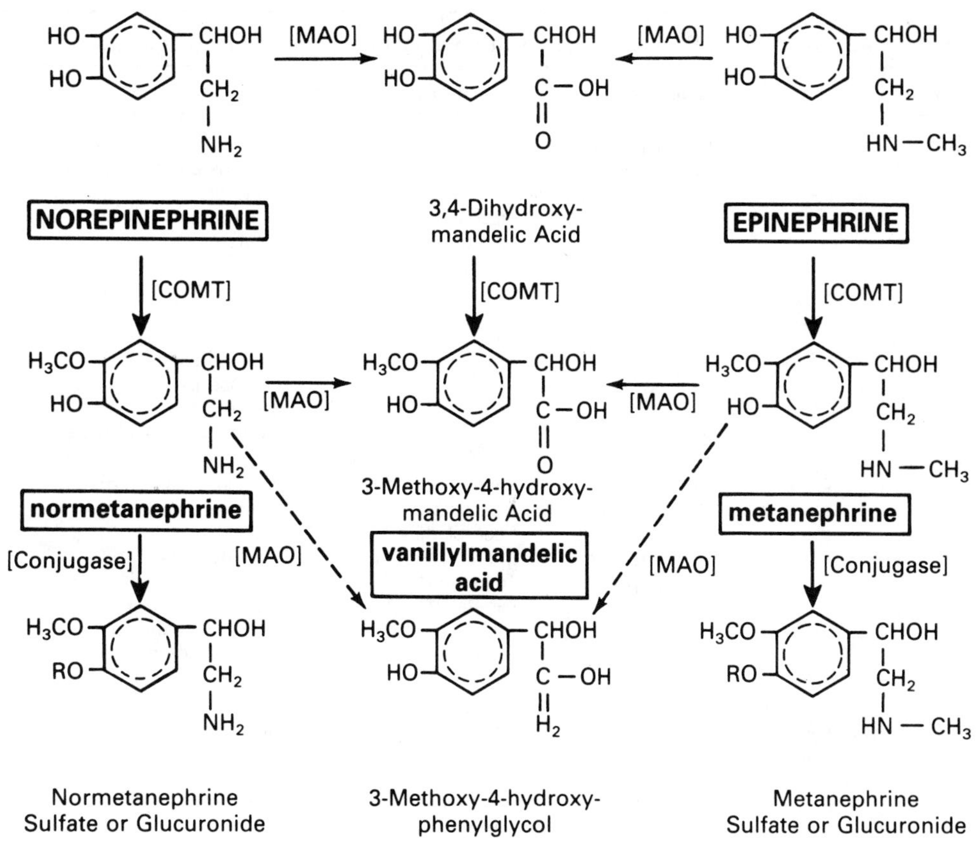

Figure 14-12. Catabolism of nor-epinephrine and epinephrine.

Normetanephrine
Sulfate or Glucuronide

3-Methoxy-4-hydroxy-
phenylglycol

Metanephrine
Sulfate or Glucuronide

PNS nerve terminals are closely associated.[19] In these plexus, ACh, released from the nearby PNS nerve terminals (vagus nerve), can inhibit NE release by activation of pre-synaptic adrenergic muscarinic receptors (Fig. 14-11).

Nicotinic receptors are found at the synaptic junctions of both SNS and PNS ganglia. Since both junctions are cholinergic, ACh or ACh-like substances such as nicotine will excite postganglionic fibers of both systems (see Fig. 14-4). Low doses of nicotine produce stimulation of ANS ganglia, whereas high doses produce blockade. This dualism is referred to as the nicotinic effect (see section on Ganglionic Drugs). Nicotinic stimulation of the SNS ganglia produces hypertension and tachycardia by causing the release of epinephrine and NE from the adrenal medulla. Adrenal hormone release is mediated by ACh in the chromaffin cells, which are analogous to postganglionic neurons (see Fig. 14-4).[6] A further increase in nicotine concentration produces hypotension and neuromuscular weakness as it becomes a ganglionic blocker. The cholinergic neuroeffector junction of skeletal muscle also contains nicotinic receptors, although they are not identical to the nicotinic receptors in ANS ganglia. For example, PNS transmission is not "all or nothing" as at the neuromuscular junction.[3] Postganglionic cholinergic transmission appears to be graded. The magnitude of response is related to the number of active units and their frequency of firing. Continuous, small amounts of ACh are released from the cholinergic nerve endings without nerve stimulation. This results in random, small, spontaneous depolarization of the postganglionic membrane known as miniature end-plate potentials. ACh is not taken up by the presynaptic nerve terminals and, in contrast to NE, must be continuously synthesized.

Adrenergic Receptors

Von Euler differentiated the physiologic effects of epinephrine and NE in 1946.[64] The adrenergic receptors were termed adrenergic or noradrenergic, depending on their responsiveness to epinephrine or noradrenaline (NE). The dissimilarities of these two drugs led Ahlquist in 1948 to propose two types of opposing adrenergic receptors, termed alpha and beta.[65] This postulation further implied that selective antagonism of these receptors was possible. The receptors can be classified according to the order of potency by which they are affected by SNS agonists and antagonists.[66] Receptors that respond with an order of potency of NE ≥ epinephrine > isoproterenol are called alpha receptors. Those responding with an order of potency of isoproterenol > epinephrine ≥ NE are called beta receptors (Table 14-5). The development of new agonists and antagonists with relatively selective activity allowed Lands to subdivide the beta receptors into and beta$_1$ and beta$_2$ in 1967.[67,68] Alpha receptors were subsequently divided into alpha$_1$ and alpha$_2$. The concept of relative selective activity arises from differential potencies among tissue groups to the same drug, such that two dose-response curves are obtained (Fig. 14-13). The sympathomimetic adrenergic drugs in current use differ from one another in their effects largely because of differences in substitution on the amine group, which influences the relative alpha or beta effect (see Fig. 14-8).[50] Figure 14-14 demonstrates the spectrum of actions of catecholamines on alpha and beta receptors, with methoxamine representing a pure alpha drug and isoproterenol a pure beta drug.

TABLE 14-5. Adrenergic Receptors: Order of Potency of Agonists and Antagonists

Receptor		Agonists*	Antagonists	Location	Action
Alpha$_1$	+ + + + + + + + + +	Norepinephrine Epinephrine Dopamine Isoproterenol	Phenoxybenzamine† Phentolamine† Ergot alkaloids† Prazosin Tolazoline† Labetalol†	Smooth muscle (vascular, iris, radial, ureter, pilomotor, uterus, trigone, gastrointestinal, and bladder sphincters) Brain Smooth muscle (gastrointestinal) Heart Salivary glands Adipose tissue Sweat glands (localized) Kidney (proximal tubule)	Contraction Vasoconstriction Neurotransmission Relaxation Glycogenolysis Increased force$^+$, glycolysis Secretion (K$^+$, H$_2$O) Glycogenesis Secretion Gluconeogenesis Na$^+$ reabsorption
Alpha$_2$	+ + + + + + + + + + + +	Clonidine Norepinephrine Epinephrine Norepinephrine Phenylephrine	Yohimbine Piperoxan Phentolamine† Phenoxybenzamine† Tolazoline† Labetalol†	Adrenergic nerve endings Presynaptic—CNS Platelets Adipose tissue Endocrine pancreas Vascular smooth muscle—? Kidney Brain	Inhibition norepinephrine release Aggregation, granule release Inhibition lypolysis Inhibition insulin release Contraction Inhibition renin release Neurotransmission
Beta$_1$	+ + + + + + + + + +	Isoproterenol† Epinephrine Norepinephrine Dopamine	Acebutolol Practolol Propranolol† Alprenolol† Metoprolol Esmolol	Heart Adipose tissue	Increased rate, contractility, conduction velocity Coronary vasodilation Lipolysis
Beta$_2$	+ + + + + + + + + + +	Isoproterenol* Epinephrine Norepinephrine Dopamine	Propranolol† Butoxamine Alprenolol Esmolol Nadolol Timolol Labetalol	Liver Skeletal muscle Smooth muscle (bronchi, uterus, vascular, gastrointestinal, detrusor, spleen capsule) Endocrine pancreas Salivary glands	Glycogenolysis, gluconeogenesis Glycogenolysis, lactate release Relaxation Insulin secretion Amylase secretion
DA$_1$	+ + + + + + + + + + +	Dopamine Epinephrine Apomorphine Metaclopramide	Haloperidol Droperidol Phenothiazines	Vascular smooth muscle Renal and mesentery	Vasodilation
DA$_2$	+ + +	Dopamine Bromocriptine	Domperidone	Presynaptic—adrenergic nerve endings	Inhibits norepinephrine release

* Listed in decreasing order of potency.

† Nonselective.

$^+$ Beta$_1$ = Adrenergic responses are greater.

Pluses indicate strength of potency.

Further studies have revealed not only subsets of the alpha and beta receptors but also the DA receptor.[31,69] These DA receptors have been identified in the CNS and in renal, mesenteric, and coronary vessels. The physiologic importance of these receptors is a matter of controversy because there are no identifiable peripheral DA neurons. Dopamine measured in the circulation is assumed to result from spillover from the brain.

Dopamine not only stimulates alpha and beta receptors in a dose-related manner but also dilates renal and mesenteric vessels, unlike the other catecholamines. This action has been found to be independent of alpha or beta blockade but is modified by DA antagonists such as haloperidol and phenothiazines.[30] Thus, the necessity of adding the DA receptor to the Ahlquist classification is explained. The DA receptor has also been subdivided according to action. There are three types of receptors (six subtypes) that respond to the catecholamines: alpha, beta, and DA. Table 14-5 lists the types, locations, and actions of adrenergic receptors now thought to exist.

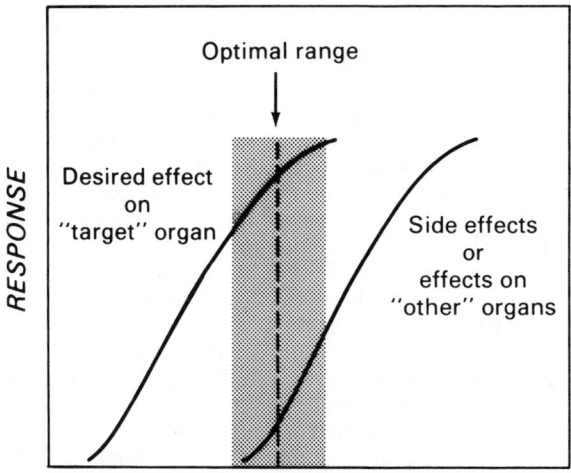

Figure 14-13. Relative dose-response relationship on target and other organs. Relative selectivity is illustrated by showing the relationship between two dose-response curves. The curve on the left represents the desired response of bronchodilation using a relatively selective beta$_2$ agonist. The unwanted effects on other organs that occur at higher doses are represented by the curve on the right. For example, an increased heart rate (beta$_1$ effect) may occur with higher doses of a relatively select beta$_2$ agonist. The *optimal range* is that concentration of drug that will give the maximal desired response with minimal effects on other organs. The size of the optimal range is dependent on the *therapeutic index,* or the distance between the two curves (see Chapter 3). These are usually established *in vitro* where drug concentration can be precisely controlled. For many cardiovascular drugs, the optimal range is small, and wide fluctuations in serum level of the drug are common; therefore, secondary or side-effects are often seen during drug therapy.

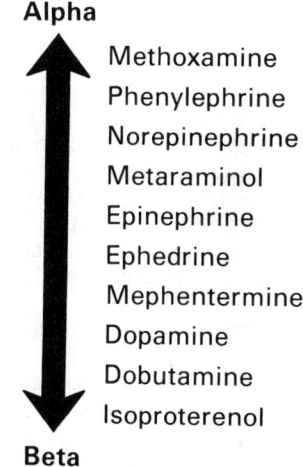

Figure 14-14. The differential effects of the catecholamines on adrenergic receptors range from the pure alpha drug, methoxamine, or the pure beta drug, isoproterenol. (Reprinted with permission from Lawson NW, Wallfisch HK: Cardiovascular pharmacology: A new look at the "pressors." In Stoelting RK, Barash PG, Gallagher TJ [eds]: Advances in Anesthesia, p. 195. Chicago, Year Book Publishers, 1986.)

Alpha-Adrenergic Receptors

Two classes of alpha receptors have been demonstrated, alpha$_1$ and alpha$_2$. The alpha$_1$-adrenergic receptors are found in the smooth muscle cells of the peripheral vasculature of the coronary arteries, skin, uterus, intestinal mucosa, and splanchnic beds (see Table 14-5).[30] The alpha$_1$ receptors serve as postsynaptic activators of vascular and intestinal smooth muscle as well as of endocrine glands. Their activation results in either decreased or increased tone, depending upon the effector organ. The response in resistance and capacitance vessels is constriction, whereas in the intestinal tract it is relaxation. There is now a large body of evidence documenting the presence of postjunctional alpha$_1$ adrenoreceptors in the mammalian heart. Alpha$_1$ adrenoreceptors have been shown to have a positive inotropic effect on cardiac tissues from most mammals studied, including humans.[52,70] Experimental work strongly supports the concept that enhanced myocardial alpha$_1$ responsiveness plays a primary role in the genesis of malignant arrhythmias induced by catecholamines during myocardial ischemia and reperfusion. Drugs possessing potent alpha$_1$ antagonist activity such as prazosin and phentolamine may provide significant antiarrhythmic activity. The clinical mechanism and significance of these findings are not yet clear.[71,72] However, there is no doubt that alpha$_1$-adrenergic antagonists prevent catecholamine-induced ventricular arrhythmias.[73,74] In contrast, studies of the effects of beta antagonists in experimental and clinical myocardial infarction have provided conflicting results, and any antiarrhythmic benefit from acute beta blockade in patients with myocardial infarction is far from certain.

The discovery of presynaptic alpha adrenoreceptors and their role in the modulation of norepinephrine transmission provided the stimulus for the subclassification of alpha receptors into alpha$_1$ and alpha$_2$ subtypes.[75,76] The successful cloning of genes for alpha$_1$ and alpha$_2$ receptors has provided unequivocal evidence for their separate identities and structures.[77] The alpha$_2$ receptors subsequently have been identified in both presynaptic and postsynaptic positions at the adrenergic neuroeffector junction. Recently, it has become apparent that the alpha$_2$ adrenoreceptors may be subdivided even further into as many as four possible subtypes.[78] Presynaptic alpha$_2$ adrenoreceptors have been clearly demonstrated in the CNS and ANS. Postsynaptic alpha$_2$ receptors have also been identified both inside and outside the ANS, which includes the pulmonary circulation.[79] Many actions have been attributed to the postsynaptic alpha$_2$ receptor, including arterial and venous vasoconstriction, platelet aggregation, inhibition of insulin release, inhibition of bowel motility, stimulation of growth hormone release, and inhibition of antidiuretic hormone release.

The central organization of autonomic control is quite complex. Alpha$_2$ receptors can be found in cholinergic pathways as well as in adrenergic pathways. They can significantly modulate parasympathetic activity as well. Current research implies that alpha$_2$ stimulation in parasympathetic pathways plays a role in the modulation of the baroreceptor reflex (increased sensitivity), vagal mediation of heart rate (bradycardia), bronchoconstriction, and salivation (dry mouth). On the other hand, cholinergic receptors can also be found in adrenergic pathways; thus muscarinic and nicotinic receptors have been found in pre- and postsynaptic locations, where they in turn modulate sympathetic activity (see Fig. 4-11). Maze speculates that although the functional role of the postsynaptic alpha$_2$ receptor in the CNS has not been well characterized, it is probable that the features that are so desirable to the anesthesiologist, such as sedation, anxiolysis, analgesia, and hypnosis, are mediated through this site.[74]

Stimulation of presynaptic alpha$_2$ receptors mediates inhibition of NE release into the synaptic cleft, serving as a negative feedback mechanism.[80] The central effects are primarily related to a reduction in sympathetic outflow with a concomitantly enhanced parasympathetic outflow (e.g., enhanced baroreceptor activity). This results in a decreased systemic vascular resistance, decreased cardiac output, decreased inotropic state in the myocardium, and decreased heart rate. The peripheral presynaptic alpha$_2$ effects are similar, and NE release is inhibited in postganglionic neurons. However, stimulation of postsynaptic alpha$_2$ receptors, like the alpha$_1$ postsynaptic receptor, affects vasoconstriction. The distinction between the postsynaptic alpha$_1$ and alpha$_2$ receptor effect on vascular smooth muscle is based on differences in order of potency for a series of agonists and antagonists[66-68] (see Table 14-5). NE acts on both alpha$_1$ and alpha$_2$ receptors. Thus, NE not only activates smooth muscle vasoconstriction (postsynaptic alpha$_1$ and alpha$_2$ receptors) but also stimulates presynaptic alpha$_2$ receptors and inhibits its own release.[58] Selective stimulation of the presynaptic alpha$_2$ receptor could produce a beneficial reduction of peripheral vascular resistance. Unfortunately, most known presynaptic alpha$_2$ agonists also stimulate the postsynaptic alpha$_2$ receptors, causing vasoconstriction. Blockade of alpha$_2$ presynaptic receptors, however, ablates normal inhibition of NE, causing vasoconstriction. Vasodilation occurs with the blockade of postsynaptic alpha$_1$ and alpha$_2$ receptors.

Beta-Adrenergic Receptors

The beta-adrenergic receptors, like the alpha receptor, have been subdivided into two categories.[67,68] The beta$_1$ receptors predominate in the myocardium, the sinoatrial node, the ventricular conduction system, and adipose tissue. Also, the beta$_1$ receptors mediate the effects of the sympathomimetic amines on myocardium. These receptors are equally sensitive to epinephrine and NE, which distinguishes them from the beta$_2$ receptors. Effects of beta$_1$ stimulation are outlined in Table 14-5.

The beta$_2$ receptors are located in the smooth muscle of the blood vessels in the skin, muscle, and mesentery, and in bronchial smooth muscle. Stimulation produces vasodilation and bronchial relaxation. The beta$_2$ receptors are more sensitive to epinephrine than NE.[30,81] The beta$_1$ receptors are suggested to be innervated receptors responding to neuronally released NE, whereas beta$_2$ receptors are "hormonal" receptors responding primarily to circulating epinephrine.

Dopaminergic Receptors

Dopamine was recognized in 1959 not only as a precursor in the synthesis of epinephrine and NE but also as an important neurotransmitter. DA receptors have been localized on blood vessels and postganglionic sympathetic nerves (see Table 14-5). There are two subdivisions of DA receptors. The DA$_1$ receptors are found on vascular smooth muscle and mediate vasodilation of the renal and mesenteric vessels. The DA$_2$ receptors, like the alpha$_2$ receptors, are presynaptic and inhibit NE release.[58,80] Stimulation of the presynaptic DA$_2$ receptor results in vasodilation.[82] Unlike the alpha$_2$ receptor, DA$_2$ receptors have not been found postsyn-

aptically.[83] Dopamine receptors have been identified in the hypothalamus, where they are involved in prolactin release, and they are also found in the basal ganglia, where they coordinate motor function.[84,85] Another central action of dopamine is to stimulate the chemoreceptor trigger zone of the medulla, producing nausea and vomiting. Dopamine antagonists such as haloperidol or droperidol are clinically effective in countering this action. There is evidence for existence of DA receptors in the esophagus, stomach, and small intestine. These receptors enhance secretions and diminish intestinal motility when stimulated.[86] Metoclopramide, a dopamine antagonist, is useful in aspiration prophylaxis by promoting gastric emptying.[87]

Defining specific DA receptors has been difficult because dopamine also exerts an effect on the alpha and beta receptors.[84,85] This effect is weak in the cardiovascular system. The action of DA receptors on adrenergic receptors is only 1/35 and 1/50 as potent as that of epinephrine and NE, respectively.[86,88,89]

Other Receptors

There are a number of receptors on the presynaptic sympathetic nerve ending in addition to the alpha$_2$ receptor and muscarinic receptor. These receptors, when activated, mediate inhibition of NE release in a manner similar to that of the alpha$_2$ presynaptic receptor. The clinical significance of these observations remains to be defined.

Adenosine Receptors

Adenosine produces inhibition of NE release.[58,80] The effect of adenosine is blocked by caffeine and other methylxanthines.[90,91] The physiologic and pharmacologic roles of adenosine-mediated inhibition of NE release are not clearly defined. The physiologic function of these receptors may be the reduction of sympathetic tone under hypoxic conditions when adenosine production is enhanced. As a consequence of reduced NE release, cardiac work would be decreased and oxygen demand reduced. Recently, adenosine has been effectively used to produce controlled hypotension.[92]

Serotonin

Serotonin (5-hydroxytryptamine) depresses the response of isolated blood vessels to SNS stimulation and decreases release of labeled NE in these preparations.[93] This inhibitory action of serotonin is antagonized by raising the external calcium ion concentration. Thus, serotonin may inhibit neuronal NE release by a mechanism that limits the availability of calcium ions at the nerve terminal.

Prostaglandin E$_2$, Histamine, and Several Opioids

Prostaglandin E$_2$, histamine, and several opioids have been reported to act on prejunctional receptor sites to inhibit NE release in certain sympathetically innervated tissue.[58] However, these inhibitory receptors are unlikely to play a physiologic role in limiting NE release because inhibitors of cyclo-oxygenase, histamine antagonists, and naloxone produce no increase in NE release.

Histamine acts in a manner similar to the neurotransmitters of the SNS.[94] It has membrane receptors specific for histamine, with the individual response being determined by the type of cell being stimulated. Two receptors for histamine have been determined. These have been designated

H_1 and H_2, for which it has been possible to develop specific agonists and antagonists. Stimulation of the H_1 receptors produces bronchoconstriction and intestinal contraction. The major role of the H_2 receptors is related to acid production by the parietal cells of the stomach; however, histamine is present in relatively high concentrations in the myocardium and cardiac conducting tissue, where it exerts positive inotropic and chronotropic effects while depressing dromotropism. The positive inotropic and chronotropic effects of histamine are H_2 receptor effects that are not blocked by beta antagonism. These effects are blocked by H_2 antagonists, such as cimetidine, which accounts for the occasional report of cardiovascular collapse following the use of cimetidine.[95] The negative dromotropic effect and that of coronary spasm caused by histamine are H_1 receptor effects.

Adrenergic Receptor Numbers or Sensitivity

The number or sensitivity of adrenergic receptors can be influenced by hormonal, genetic, and developmental factors.[67,68,96,97] Changes in the number of receptors alter the response to catecholamines. Alteration in the number of receptors is referred to as either up or down regulation.[98] As a rule, there is an inverse relationship between the ambient concentration of the catecholamines and the number of receptors.[99] Extended exposure of receptors to their agonists markedly reduces but does not ablate the biologic response to the agonist. This phenomenon has been demonstrated for a large number of hormones and drugs. There appears to be a reduction in numbers or sensitivity of beta receptors in hypertensive patients who also have elevated plasma catecholamine levels. Down regulation is reversible on termination of the agonist. Down regulation is the presumptive explanation for the lack of correlation between plasma catecholamine levels and the blood pressure elevation in patients with pheochromocytoma. Chronic use of beta agonists such as terbutaline, isoproterenol, or epinephrine for the treatment of asthma can result in tachyphylaxis because of down regulation in receptor numbers.[100] Even short-term use (1–6 hours) of beta-adrenergic agonists may cause down regulation of receptor numbers.

When blood and tissue levels of catecholamines are lowered, the number of receptor sites increases. Sympathetic denervation of an organ increases both alpha- and beta-adrenergic receptor concentrations. Chronic depletion of catecholamines in animal studies results in a 50–100% increase in beta receptors.[97] Likewise, chronic treatment of animals with the beta-adrenergic antagonist propranolol causes a 100% increase in the number of beta receptors.[101] This might account for the propranolol withdrawal syndrome. The discontinuation of beta antagonists leaves unopposed a greater number of sensitive beta receptors. This phenomenon may also account for the clonidine withdrawal syndrome.[102,103] Inhibition of vasodilation by antagonists, however, does not increase the sensitivity of alpha receptors to alpha agonists.[104] Receptor numbers and sensitivity should not be confused. Up or down regulation of receptor numbers may not alter the sensitivity of the receptor. Likewise, sensitivity may be increased or decreased in the presence of a normal population of receptors.

The pharmacologic factors affecting up or down regulation of the alpha and beta receptors are similar. Humoral influences known to regulate alpha receptor numbers include estrogen (up), progesterone (down), and thyroxine (up).[105] The effects of dopamine on receptor number and binding affinity remain largely unknown, but estrogen does increase dopamine receptor numbers centrally.[61]

MOLECULAR PHARMACOLOGY AND EFFECTOR RESPONSE

Receptors are only the first link in a series of reactions that summate in the cellular response. The beta-adrenergic receptor is the best delineated ANS receptor at the present time. This is largely because of the pioneering work of Sutherland, who revealed that for the beta receptor, cyclic adenosine monophosphate (cAMP) serves as the intracellular mediator of the first messenger—the catecholamines.[106-108] cAMP is often referred to as the *second messenger*. Recently, receptor complexes have been isolated that consist of distinctive components, each of which affect the cellular response.

The beta-adrenergic receptor consists of three distinct components: (1) a specific hormone receptor that interacts with the chemical messenger; (2) two regulatory proteins that bind guanosine triphosphate and regulate the interaction of the receptor protein with adenyl cyclase; and (3) the catalytic moiety of adenyl cyclase.[109] The guanine nucleotide regulatory components are important moderators of the receptor complex (Fig. 14-15). Both inhibitory (N_i) and stimulatory (N_s) components have been isolated. These appear to be two of a large group of guanine nucleotide regulatory proteins that may function in the coupling of various receptors to different physiologic effector systems.[110] These are referred to as G proteins because they bind guanine nucleotides. They act as transducers of information across cell membranes.[111] As such, they are important in modulating the response of the ANS or the effects of certain sympathomimetic drugs.

The receptor itself is actually a bifunctional protein situated on the superficial surface of the plasma membrane. It interacts specifically with a chemical messenger and then undergoes a conformational change to activate some other response mechanism. In the case of the beta receptor, this effector mechanism is the adenyl cyclase AMP system.[112]

The first messenger, the catecholamine, binds to the receptor and stimulates adenyl cyclase (Fig. 14-15). Adenyl cyclase catalyzes the conversion of adenosine triphosphate to cAMP, which, in cascade fashion, phosphorylates multiple cellular components, altering cellular function. The cellular response is tissue-specific. The positive inotropic and chronotropic actions of the catecholamines in the heart are the result of augmented cAMP concentrations that, in turn, enhance the mobilization and availability of ionized calcium within the myocardial cell. The transmembrane flux of calcium is also an important regulator of contractility in vascular smooth muscle. Here, however, beta receptor stimulation activates the adenyl cyclase system, but cellular components are activated that enhance removal of calcium from the cytosol, resulting in relaxation rather than contraction; therefore, drugs that augment cAMP levels have opposite effects in cardiac and smooth muscle.

The final mediator of the effects of beta receptor stimulation in cardiac muscle is Ca^{2+}. The concentration of Ca^{2+} in the cytosol during systole regulates not only strength of myocardial contraction but also ion fluxes across the sarcolemma and, therefore, impulse conduction. Cytosolic Ca^{2+} is derived from several cellular sources, including the sarcoplasmic reticulum and the superficial surface of the sarcolemma. Ca^{2+} derived from the sarcolemma enters *via* chan-

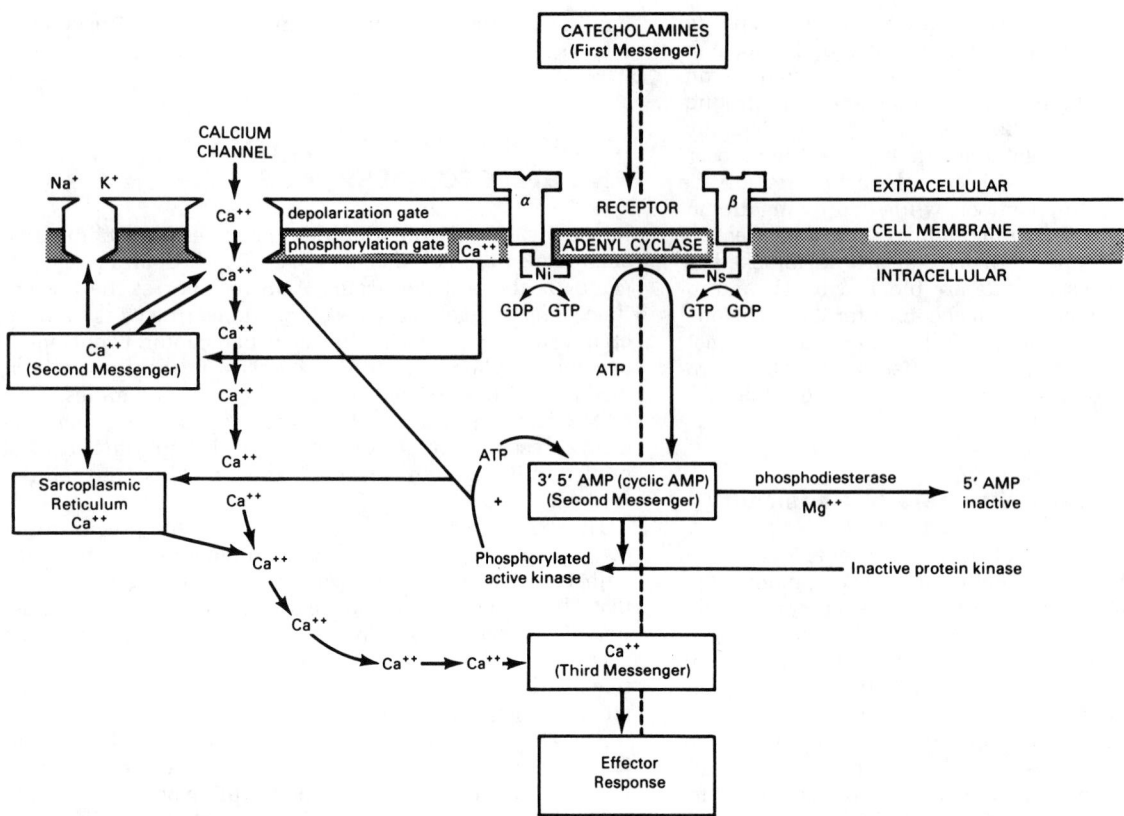

Figure 14-15. The putative cascade from the first messenger to effector response. The activated alpha receptor inhibits, whereas the activated beta receptor stimulates the enzyme adenyl cyclase, which catalyzes the conversion of adenosine triphosphate to the second messenger, cyclic adenosine monophosphate (cyclic AMP). Interactions of the receptor-enzyme complex are regulated by guanine nucleotide regulatory proteins (Ns, Ni). cAMP regulates many cellular functions, including opening of membrane Ca^{2+} channels, which allows the third messenger Ca^{2+} into the cell. Ca^{2+} channels are further regulated by an intracellular membrane-bound receptor, which is stimulated by BAY K 8644 and inhibited by the calcium-entry blockers nifedipine and verapamil. It is also postulated that in some tissues, alpha stimulation releases adjacent membrane-bound Ca^{2+}, which also acts as a second messenger, releasing more Ca^{2+}. Intracellular free Ca^{2+} is the third messenger, which is the final link in initiating the effector response. Nonadrenergic sympathomimetic drugs enhance the effector response by either stimulating the formation of cAMP (forskolin or glucagon inhibition of phosphodiesterase (xanthines)) or enhancing Ca^{2+} entry (BAY K 8644 [5]).

nels in the membrane called slow Ca^{2+} channels, so named because of their action potential characteristics. These membrane calcium channels are thought to be double-gated. The outer gate is dependent upon depolarization for Ca^{2+} influx, whereas phosphorylation of a cAMP–dependent protein kinase is necessary to open the inner gate. Beta receptor stimulation is therefore intimately involved in regulation of Ca^{2+} influx.[113] Increased cAMP activates myocardial sarcolemmal calcium channels, resulting in an increase in the rate and degree of tension development. Phosphorylation of components of the sarcoplasmic reticulum also enhances Ca^{2+} uptake and causes more rapid relaxation.[114] Augmented cAMP in cardiac nodal and conduction tissues increases the slope of diastolic depolarization (phase 4) and the rate of rapid depolarization (phase 0), effecting an increase in both heart rate and conduction.

Transmembrane calcium influx can be blocked at two points: (1) blockade of depolarization, and (2) inhibition of enzymatic reduction of adenosine triphosphate to cAMP. Beta blocking drugs interfere with agonist binding to the receptor and, therefore, the formation of cAMP. Verapamil, a calcium channel blocker, is thought to interact with a receptor on the inner surface of the sarcolemma, which regulates activation of the calcium channel. Thus, beta blockers and calcium channel blockers, working at different steps in the receptor cascade, have a final common pathway—the calcium channel. The potentiating effect of beta blockers and verapamil in humans is well known, and historically verapamil was originally thought to be a beta blocker.

The cellular responses to beta receptor activation cannot be totally ascribed to cAMP, however. Activation of sarcolemmal Ca^{2+} transport systems may occur directly by beta receptor stimulation. Increased cytosolic Ca^{2+} also results in activation of another intracellular second messenger called calmodulin.[115] A protein binds Ca^{2+} and activates a variety of enzymes and cellular processes via a calmodulin-dependent protein kinase. The result is enhanced contractility in cardiac muscle. In smooth muscle of blood vessels, esophagus, and ureters, the Ca^{2+}-calmodulin complex activates myosin kinase and increases tone. In this case, the

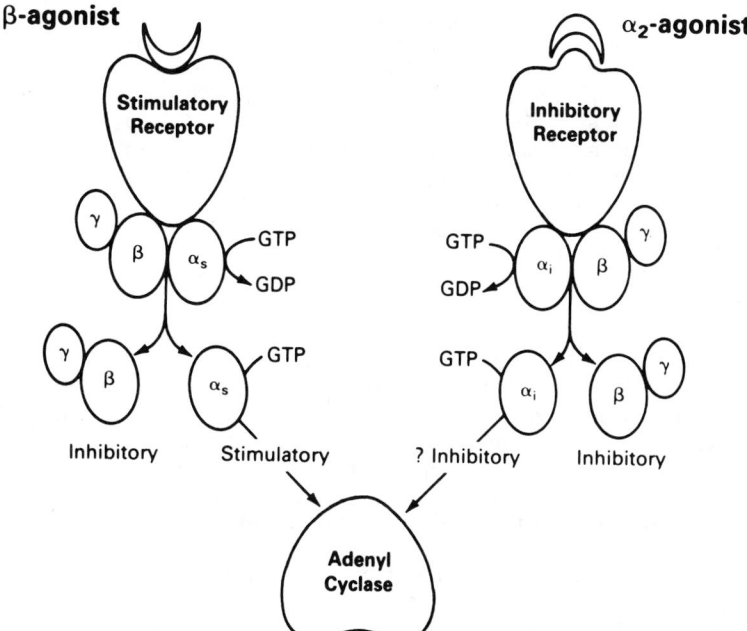

Figure 14-16. The molecular mechanisms involved in regulating the formation of cAMP are shown schematically. The beta-adrenergic agonist stimulates, whereas the alpha$_2$-adrenergic agonist inhibits the enzyme adenyl cyclase that catalyzes the formation of cAMP. Guanine-nucleotide–binding proteins influence the response not only by mediating the hormone-receptor interaction but also by modulating the coupling of the agonist-receptor complex to adenyl cyclase. (Reproduced with permission from Exton EH: Mechanisms involved in α-adrenergic phenomena. Am J Physiol 248:E633, 1985.)

primary trigger is *via* the alpha receptor, however, illustrating how the same second messenger can be activated by two different receptors and cause opposite physiologic effects in different organs (Fig. 14-16).

Other intracellular messengers have been proposed, but their physiologic roles are as yet incompletely characterized. Cyclic guanosine triphosphate may be important in mediating the relaxant effects of nitroglycerin and nitroprusside, but earlier suggestions that it mediates cholinergic or alpha-adrenergic responses are no longer accepted.[115,116] Hormones that use Ca^{2+} as an intracellular mediator, such as epinephrine and ACh, also appear to trigger changes in a family of membrane lipids.[117,118] Phosphatidyl inositol is acted on by a phosphatidyl inositol kinase and broken down to a series of lipid compounds with cellular activity. One of these, inositol triphosphate, appears to be important in triggering Ca^{2+} release from intracellular stores. The physiologic significance of the inositols is not well understood, but they appear to be important second messengers that may mediate cellular responses of the ANS.

Each signal must be transient in nature for the adenylate-cyclase system to be an effective modulator of cell activity. This is assured by the rapid hydrolysis of cAMP to inactive metabolites by phosphodiesterase enzymes. Three phosphodiesterases have been isolated and characterized.Their activity may be inhibited pharmacologically, resulting in elevated cAMP levels and a cellular response that mimics that of beta receptor stimulation.[119] These phosphodiesterases appear to be selectively inhibited by different drugs (see the section on Nonadrenergic Sympathomimetic Agents).

A similar enzyme second messenger system has not been substantiated for alpha receptors. In general, stimulation of alpha$_1$ receptors results in increased cytosolic Ca^{2+} levels and enhanced tone.[97] However, alpha$_1$ activation in gastrointestinal smooth muscle causes relaxation. In either case, the mechanism is thought to involve release of Ca^{2+} from the internal membrane surface adjacent to the alpha$_1$ receptor.[115] This event triggers the release of more Ca^{2+} from the sarcoplasmic reticulum. In blood vessels, the internal release of Ca^{2+} is responsible for the initial phasic contraction, which is succeeded by a slower tonic component that

is dependent upon extracellular Ca^{2+}. Calcium is regarded as the *third messenger*, but it may also function as a second messenger in mediating its own membrane flux (see Fig. 14-15).[120]

The transmembrane flux of Ca^{2+} is an important commonality in the function of both alpha and beta receptors.[24] Adequate ionized calcium is a prerequisite for the function of the catecholamines, regardless of either alpha or beta properties. The calcium messenger system promises to be one of the most exciting areas of clinical pharmacology of this decade. It has become evident that the Ca^{2+} messenger system is more complex than the cAMP messenger system. Rasmussen and Barret summarize the four major attributes of messenger Ca^{2+}: "(1) Calcium is a nearly universal messenger in animal cells; (2) it is a miniatory messenger in that excess cellular Ca^{2+} leads to cellular death; (3) it is a mercurial messenger in that its rise in concentration in the cell is transient even in those cells displaying a sustained response; (4) it is a synarchic messenger in that it nearly always regulates cell function in concert with other intracellular messengers, such as cAMP.[121,122]

Therefore, the response of a receptor to a catecholamine can be regulated by (1) the concentration of the catecholamine agonists, (2) the activity of phosphodiesterase, (3) factors affecting coupling of the receptor to the activated kinases, (4) receptor numbers and binding affinity, (5) and calcium availability.[61] All these factors can be medically manipulated, with the possible exception of receptor numbers. However, guanine nucleotides have been shown to quickly reverse alpha and beta receptor insensitivity owing to down regulation and may, one day, be available clinically.[24]

AUTONOMIC NERVOUS SYSTEM REFLEXES

The ANS reflex has been compared to the computer circuit.[123] This control system, as in all reflex systems, has (1) sensors, (2) afferent pathways, (3) CNS integration, and (4) efferent pathways to the receptors and efferent organs. Fine adjustments are made at the local level according to positive and negative feedback mechanisms. The baroreceptor is an example. The variable to be controlled (blood pressure) is sensed (carotid sinus), integrated (medullary vasomotor center), and adjusted through specific effector receptor sites. Drugs or disease can interrupt this circuit at any point. Beta blockers may attenuate the effector response, whereas an alpha agonist such as clonidine may alter both the effector and the integrator functions of blood pressure control[102] (see the section on Antihypertensives).

Baroreceptors

Several reflexes in the cardiovascular system help control arterial blood pressure, cardiac output, and heart rate. An examination of the cardiovascular ANS reflexes reveals an anachronism. The business of circulation is the production of blood flow. Yet, the most important controlled variable to which the sensors are attuned is blood pressure, a product of flow and resistance. "Nature, like the human engineer, finds it easier to measure pressure than flow."[124]

Etienne Marey noted in 1859 that the pulse rate is inversely proportional to the blood pressure, and this is known as Marey's law.[22] Subsequently, Hering, Koch, and others demonstrated that the alterations in heart rate evoked by changes in blood pressure were dependent on baroreceptors located in the aortic arch and the carotid sinuses. These pressure sensors react to alterations in stretch caused by blood pressure. Impulses from the carotid sinus and aortic arch reach the medullary vasomotor center by the glossopharyngeal and vagus nerves, respectively. Increased sensory traffic from the baroreceptors, caused by increased blood pressure, inhibits SNS effector traffic. The relative increase in vagal tone produces vasodilation, slowing of the heart rate, and a lowering of blood pressure.[125] Real increases in vagal tone occur when blood pressure exceeds normal limits.[123,126]

The arterial baroreceptor reflex can best be demonstrated by using the Valsalva maneuver as an example (Fig. 14-17). The Valsalva maneuver raises the intrathoracic pressure by forced expiration against a closed glottis. The arterial blood pressure rises momentarily as the intrathoracic blood is forced into the heart (preload).[17] Sustained intrathoracic pressure diminishes venous return, reduces the cardiac output, and drops the blood pressure. Reflex vasoconstriction and tachycardia ensue. Blood pressure returns to normal with release of the forced expiration, but then briefly "overshoots" because of the vasoconstriction and increased venous return. A slowing of the heart rate accompanies the overshoot in pressure, according to Marey's law.

The cardiovascular responses to the Valsalva maneuver require an intact ANS circuit from peripheral sensor to peripheral adrenergic receptors. The Valsalva maneuver has been used to identify patients at risk for anesthesia due to ANS instability (Fig. 14-17). This was once a major concern in patients receiving drugs that depleted catecholamines, such as reserpine. Dysfunction of the SNS is implicated if exaggerated and prolonged hypotension develops during the forced expiration phase (more than 50% from resting mean arterial pressure).[22,123] In addition, the overshoot at the end of the Valsalva maneuver is absent. Dysfunction of the PNS can be assumed if the heart rate does not respond appropriately to the blood pressure changes. The Valsalva maneuver may still be a valid clinical preoperative test for detecting the autonomic dysautonomia that accompanies several disease states, most commonly diabetes.

The ready availability of blood pressure and heart rate

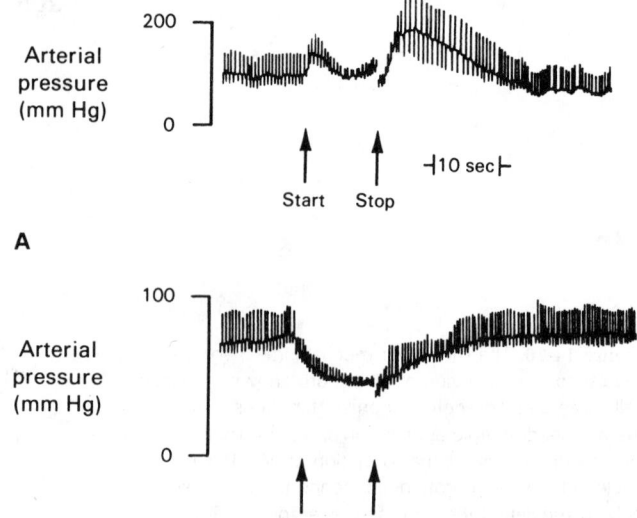

Figure 14-17. (A) The normal blood pressure response to the Valsalva maneuver is demonstrated. Pulse rate moves in a reciprocal direction according to Marey's law of the heart. (B) An abnormal Valsalva response is shown in a patient with C5 quadriplegia.

measurements serves to emphasize the importance of the arterial baroreceptors. However, venous baroreceptors may be more dominant in the moment-to-moment regulation of cardiac output. Baroreceptors in the right atrium and great veins produce an increase in heart rate when stretched by increased right atrial pressure.[31,127] Reduced venous pressure decreases heart rate. Unlike the arterial baroreceptors, venous sensors are not thought to alter vascular tone; however, venoconstriction is postulated to occur when atrial pressures decline.[128] Nevertheless, stretch of the venous receptors produces changes in heart rate opposite to those produced when the arterial pressure sensors are stimulated. The pressure receptors, arterial and venous, are separately monitoring two of the four major determinants of cardiac output—afterload and preload. Venous baroreceptors sample preload by the stretch of the atrium produced by venous pressure. Arterial baroreceptors survey resistance, or afterload, as reflected in the arterial pressure. Afterload and preload produce opposite effects on cardiac output; thus, one should not be surprised that the venous and arterial baroreceptors produce effects opposite those of a similar stimulus, pressure.

Bainbridge described the venous baroreceptor reflex and demonstrated that it can be abolished by vagal resection. Numerous investigators have confirmed the acceleration of the heart rate in response to volume.[22] However, the magnitude and direction of the heart rate response are dependent on the prevailing heart rate at the time of stimulation. The exact mechanism of the Bainbridge reflex remains in doubt and is a matter of controversy. It is of interest that the denervated, transplanted mammalian heart also accelerates in response to volume loading.[129] Heart rate, like cardiac output, can be adjusted to the quantity of blood entering the heart.[130,131]

Greene relates the Bainbridge reflex to the characteristic but paradoxical slowing of the heart seen with spinal anesthesia.[132] Blockade of the SNS levels of T1–4 ablates the efferent limb of the cardiac accelerator nerves. This source of cardiac deceleration is obvious, as the vagus nerve is unopposed. Close study, however, reveals that bradycardia during spinal anesthesia is more related to the development of arterial hypotension than to the height of the block. The primary defect in the development of spinal hypotension is a decrease in venous return. Theoretically, the arterial hypotension should reflexly produce a tachycardia through the arterial baroreceptors. Instead, bradycardia is more common. Greene feels that in the unmedicated person, the venous baroreceptors are dominant over the arterial. A reduced venous pressure therefore slows heart rate.[133] In contrast, humorally mediated tachycardia is the usual response to hypotension or acidosis from other causes.

Denervated Heart

Reflex modulation of the adrenergic agonists is best seen in the denervated transplant heart, which retains the recipient's innervated sinoatrial node and the donor's denervated sinoatrial node. Knowledge derived from these studies is assuming great importance not only because of the re-emergence of cardiac transplants on a national scale but also because we are treating an increasing population of patients whose intact hearts are being selectively denervated with adrenergic and calcium channel blockade.[134] Table 14-6 is a summary of drug effects on the transplanted heart.[129,135,136] It was derived from several sources, which were not always complete because the studies were limited by the delicate condition of the volunteer patients.[137-140] NE simultaneously activates alpha and beta receptors of the intact heart and vessels. NE infusion in the transplanted heart produces a slowing of the recipient's atrial rate through vagal feedback as the blood pressure rises. In the unmodulated donor heart, atrial rate increases. Methoxamine-induced hypertension and nitrite-induced hypotension fail to induce deceleration and acceleration of the donor atrial rate. The baroreceptors

are therefore not operant in the transplanted heart. Isoproterenol, a pure beta agonist, increases the discharge rate of both the recipient and donor node by direct action, with the donor rate near doubling that of the recipient node. Atropine accelerates the recipient's atrial rate, whereas no effect is seen on the donor rate, which now controls heart rate. Hypersensitivity to beta cardiac stimulation in denervated dog hearts has been demonstrated.[20] Whether or not this occurs in the human heart remains unclear. Patients who have undergone chemical sympathectomy with bretylium or guanethidine are known to be hyper-reactive to the usual doses of catecholamines. Beta blockade produces comparable slowing of the sinoatrial node of both recipient and donor. The exercise capability of the denervated heart is conspicuously reduced by beta blockade, presumably because of its reliance on circulating catecholamines. Propranolol has also been demonstrated to reduce the beta response to chronotropic effects of NE and isoproterenol in the transplanted heart. The cardiac output of the transplanted heart varies appropriately with changes in preload and afterload.

INTERACTION OF AUTONOMIC NERVOUS SYSTEM RECEPTORS

Recently, strong interactions have been noted between SNS and PNS nerves in organs that receive dual, antagonistic innervation. Release of NE at the presynaptic terminal is modified by the PNS. For example, vagal inhibition of left ventricular contractility is accentuated as the level of SNS activity is raised.[19] This interaction is termed *accentuated antagonism* and is mediated by a combination of presynaptic and postsynaptic mechanisms.[20] The coronary arteries present an example of this phenomenon and deserve special attention.

The myocardium and coronary vessels are abundantly supplied with adrenergic and cholinergic fibers.[141] Strong

TABLE 14-6. Drug Effects on the Denervated Heart

Drug	Sinus Rate Recipient	Sinus Rate Donor	Atrioventricular Conduction Velocity	Intraventricular Conduction Velocity	Blood Pressure	Cardiac Output	Systemic Vascular Resistance
Resting	Normal	↑ *	Normal	Normal	Normal	Normal or low	Normal
Exercise	↑	Slow ↑			↑	↑	
Atropine	↑	—	—				
Norepinephrine	↓	↑ ↑ *	↑	—	↑	— or ↑	↑ ↑
Methoxamine	↓	—			↑	↓	↑ ↑
Isoproterenol	↑	↑ ↑	↑		↓	↑ ↑	↓
Glucagon	↑	↑			—	↑	
Propranolol	↓	↓	↓	—	— or ↓	↓	↑
Amyl nitrite	↑	—			↓		↓
Digoxin							
Acute	↓	—	—*	—	—	— or ↑↑ †	
Chronic	↓	—	↓				
Quinidine	↑	↓ *	↓ *	↓			
Edrophonium	↓	—*	—*				
Increased preload		↑				↑ or ↓ †	

↑ = Increase; ↓ = Decrease; — = No change.
* = Opposite from normals.
† = Response depends on contractile state related to rejection.

Reprinted with permission from Lawson NW, Wallfisch HK: Cardiovascular pharmacology: A new look at the "pressors." In Stoelting RK, Barash PG, Gallagher TJ (eds): Advances in Anesthesia, p 195. Chicago, Year Book Medical Publishers, 1986.

activity of both alpha and beta receptors has been demonstrated in the coronary vascular bed. The predominant adrenergic receptor in the coronary arteries is the beta$_1$ receptor.[22,142] Normally, the tone of these arteries favors relaxation because tonic stimulation of these receptors by endogenous NE produces vasodilation (see Table 14-6). This action is like the vasodilation produced by stimulation of beta$_2$ receptors in peripheral vessels; however, exogenous NE, usually given in exponentially higher concentrations, causes coronary vasoconstriction and a reduction of blood flow, which can be reversed to vasodilation in the presence of alpha$_1$-adrenergic blockade. Selective stimulation of both the alpha$_1$ and postsynaptic alpha$_2$ receptors increases coronary vascular resistance, whereas selective alpha blockade eliminates this effect. Therefore, both beta$_1$ and alpha$_1$ adrenoreceptors are present on coronary arteries and accessible to NE from sympathetic nerves.[25,141]

The close anatomic proximity of the postganglionic vagal and SNS nerve endings in coronary arteries provides the morphologic basis for strong interaction.[19,32,66] SNS and PNS nerve terminals are found in such close proximity that transmitter from one can easily reach the other and affect transmitter release. In addition, the presynaptic adrenergic terminals of the myocardium and coronary vessels, like all blood vessels examined, contain muscarinic receptors.[33,58,143] Recent observations confirm that muscarinic agents and vagal stimulation, acting on the presynaptic, SNS muscarinic receptor, inhibit the release of NE in a manner similar to that of the presynaptic alpha$_2$ and DA$_2$ receptors (see Fig. 14-11). Conversely, blockade of the muscarinic receptors with atropine markedly augments the positive inotropic responses to catecholamines.[20] Suppression of NE release explains, in part, vagal-induced attenuation of the inotropic response to strong SNS stimulation (accentuated antagonism) and only a weak negative inotropic effect of vagal stimulation when there is low background SNS activity. This may also explain why vagal activity reduces the vulnerability of the myocardium to fibrillation during infusions of NE.

ACh may cause coronary spasm during periods of high SNS tone.[27,144] Inhibition of NE release by presynaptic adrenergic muscarinic receptors of the smooth muscle of coronary vessels would lessen the coronary relaxation normally produced by NE on the beta$_1$ receptor (see Fig. 14-11). In anesthetized dogs, the rate of NE outflow into the coronary sinus blood, evoked by cardiac SNS stimulation, is markedly diminished by simultaneous vagal efferent stimulation.[145,146] This action is known to be prevented by atropine, which also causes coronary vasodilation. Metacholine, a muscarinic parasympathomimetic agent, has been reported to cause coronary vasoconstriction.[147] However, it simultaneously reduces ventricular irritability by reducing NE release in myocardial fibers.[19]

The concept of accentuated antagonism has yet to be clearly defined because it is unusual for high SNS and PNS activity to coexist, except during anesthesia. The importance of accentuated antagonism in the intact, conscious human has yet to be demonstrated; however, it may explain the clinical observation that angina and myocardial infarction owing to coronary spasm in humans are not often related to cardiac work as is angina that is caused by sclerotic coronary disease. Attacks of angina usually occur at rest, often waking the patient from sleep. This diurnal variation also corresponds to the greatest activity of the PNS system. The mechanism by which coronary arterial spasm occurs remains unknown, but this continues to be an exciting area of investigation.

INTERACTION WITH OTHER REGULATORY SYSTEMS

The ANS is integrally related to several endocrine systems that ultimately summate to control blood pressure and regulate homeostasis. These include the renin-angiotensin system, antidiuretic hormone, glucocorticoids, and insulin.

Antidiuretic hormone or vasopressin is formed in the hypothalamus and released from nerve endings in the posterior pituitary gland. It causes vasoconstriction and increased reabsorption of water in the distal collecting ducts of the kidney. It therefore affects not only central blood volume but also plasma osmolality. The primary regulator of antidiuretic hormone release is plasma osmolality; however, several other stimuli may outweigh this control in stressful situations.[148] Release is also triggered by decreased central blood volume via low-pressure atrial receptors and hypotension via the carotid baroreceptors. Stress, pain, hypoxia, anesthesia, and surgery also stimulate release of antidiuretic hormone. Infusion of catecholamines may alter its release, but these effects appear to be mediated by the carotid baroreceptors. ANS drugs that induce hypotension or decreased cardiac filling may induce release of antidiuretic hormone and thus affect plasma osmolality.

Both alpha and beta receptors have been found in the endocrine pancreas and modulate insulin release (see Table 14-5). Beta stimulation increases insulin release, whereas alpha stimulation decreases it. The overall importance of this interaction is not entirely clear, but decreased glucose and potassium tolerance have been noted in subjects taking beta blocking drugs.[149,150]

The renin-angiotensin system is a complex endocrine system that modulates both blood pressure and water-electrolyte homeostasis (Fig. 14-18). Renin is a proteolytic enzyme contained within the cells of the juxtaglomerular apparatus of the renal cortex. When released, it acts on plasma angiotensinogen to form angiotensin I. Angiotensin I is then converted to angiotensin II by converting enzyme in the lung. Angiotensin II is a very powerful direct arterial vasoconstrictor. It also acts on the adrenal cortex to release aldosterone and on the adrenal medulla to release epinephrine. In addition to its direct effects on vascular smooth muscle, angiotensin II augments NE release via presynaptic receptors, thus enhancing peripheral SNS tone. A group of drugs called angiotensin-converting enzyme inhibitors act by interfering with the formation or function of angiotensin II. These drugs have been found very useful in the treatment of essential and renovascular hypertension and of congestive heart failure. Captopril, enalapril, and lisinopril inhibit the action of converting enzyme, thus preventing the conversion of angiotensin I to angiotensin II.[151-156] They have supplanted diuretics and beta blockers as first-line agents in the treatment of hypertension. Saralasin is a direct angiotensin II receptor antagonist that is useful as an antihypertensive drug but is not in common use.

Renin is released in response to hyponatremia, decreased renal perfusion pressure, and ANS stimulation via beta receptors on juxtaglomerular cells. Changes in sympathetic tone may thus alter renin release and affect homeostasis in a variety of ways. The mechanism of action of some antihypertensive agents is thought to involve alterations in activity of the renin-angiotensin system in parallel with the ANS.

The ANS is also intimately related to adrenocortical function. As outlined above, glucocorticoid release modulates phenylethanolamine-N-methyltransferase formation and thus synthesis of epinephrine. Glucocorticoids are also im-

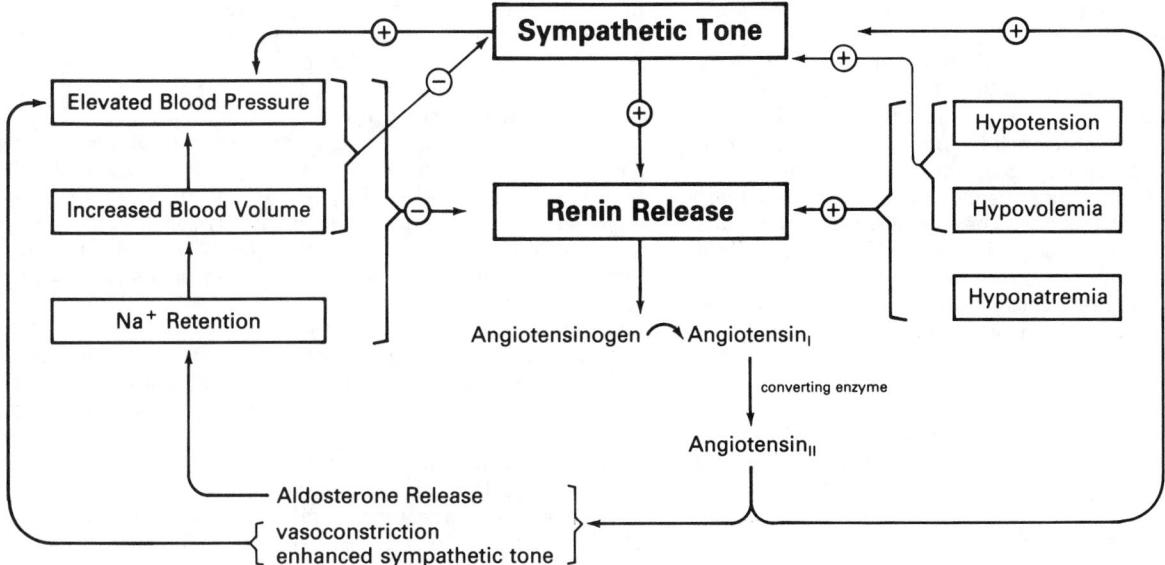

Figure 14-18. The interactions of the renin-angiotensin and sympathetic nervous systems in regulating homeostasis are shown schematically along with the physiologic variables that modulate their function. *Arrows* with a + represent stimulation, and those with a − represent inhibition. See text for details.

portant in regulating the response of peripheral tissues to changes in SNS tone. Thus, the ANS is intimately related to other homeostatic mechanisms.[1]

CLINICAL AUTONOMIC NERVOUS SYSTEM PHARMACOLOGY

The clinical application of ANS pharmacology is based on knowledge of ANS anatomy, physiology, and molecular pharmacology. Drugs that modify ANS activity can be classified by their (1) site of action, (2) mechanism of action, or (3) pathology for which they are most commonly used. Antihypertensive drugs are an example of the third category.

Site of Action

ANS drugs may be broadly categorized as working on the CNS or at peripheral nerve sites. This classification is a matter of degree because considerable functional overlap occurs. An example of classification by site relates to the ganglionic agonists or blocking agents.[7] ANS drugs can be further categorized as those that act at the postjunctional membrane and those acting postjunctionally. They can then be more specifically classified by the predominant receptor or receptors on which they act.

Mode of Action

ANS drugs may be broadly classified by mode of action according to their mimetic or lytic actions. This may also be termed agonist or antagonist. A sympathomimetic, such as ephedrine, mimics SNS sympathetic activity by stimulation of adrenergic receptor sites both directly and indirectly. Sympatholytic drugs cause dissolution of SNS activity at these same receptor sites. Beta receptor blockers are exam-

ples of sympatholytic drugs. The terms *parasympathomimetic* and *parasympatholytic* are self-explanatory and may be further divided by their site of action on the muscarinic or nicotinic receptors.

Several modes of ANS drug action become evident when one follows the cascade of neurotransmission. The mode is related to site. Drugs that act on prejunctional membranes may therefore (1) interfere with transmitter synthesis (alpha-methyl paratyrosine); (2) interfere with transmitter storage (reserpine); (3) interfere with transmitter release (clonidine); (4) stimulate transmitter release (ephedrine); or (5) interfere with reuptake of transmitter (cocaine). Drugs may also (6) modify metabolism in the neurotransmitter in the synaptic cleft (anticholinesterase). Drugs acting at postjunctional sites may (7) directly stimulate postjunctional receptors and (8) interfere with transmitter agonist at the postjunctional receptor.

The ultimate response of an effector organ to an agonist or antagonist depends on (1) the drug, (2) its plasma concentration, (3) the number of receptors in the effector organ, (4) binding by the receptor, and (5) reflex adjustments by the organism. This is the source of conflicting results for drugs used in differing clinical circumstances.

Ganglionic Drugs

SNS and PNS ganglia are pharmacologically similar in that transmission through these ANS ganglia is effected by ACh (see Fig. 14-4). Most ganglionic agonists and antagonists are not selective and affect SNS and PNS ganglia equally.[157] This nonselective property creates many undesirable and unpredictable side-effects, which have limited the clinical usefulness of this category of drug.

Agonists

There are essentially no clinically useful ganglionic agonists. Nicotine is the prototypical ganglionic agonist.[3] In low doses, it stimulates ANS ganglia and the neuromuscular junction of striated muscle. High doses produce ganglionic and neuromuscular blockade. Low-dose stimulation and high-dose blockade are referred to as nicotinic effects in describing any drug with similar effects. Most ganglionic agonists and antagonists produce their effects through their nicotinic effects. The protean side-effects of nicotinic stimulation render it useful only as an investigative tool.

Despite its lack of clinical usefulness, nicotine is widely used in the form of tobacco. The novice tobacco user can often describe the overlap of SNS and PNS side-effects of nicotinic stimulation, which appear as nausea and vomiting, tachycardia, bradycardia, diarrhea, and sometimes fainting as a result of high-dose ganglionic blockade.[19]

Antagonists

Drugs that interfere with neurotransmission at ANS ganglia are known as ganglionic blocking agents. Nicotine, in high doses, is the prototypical ganglionic blocking agent also; however, early stimulatory nicotinic activity can be blocked at the ganglia and muscle end plates with other ganglionic blockers and muscle relaxants, respectively, without blocking muscarinic effects.[158] Ganglionic blockers produce their nicotinic effects by competing, mimicking, or interfering with ACh metabolism. Hexamethonium, trimethaphan, and pentolinium produce a selective nondepolarizing blockade of neurotransmission at ANS ganglia without producing nicotinic neuromuscular blockade. They compete with ACh in the ganglia without stimulating the receptors. Decamethonium, a depolarizing muscle relaxant, selectively produces neuromuscular blockade in a manner similar to that of nicotine but possesses no ganglionic effect.[19] The depolarization produced is initially associated with increased excitability, but depolarization persists. The neuron, therefore, cannot be excited and block exists. d-Tubocurare (dTC), on the other hand, produces a competitive nondepolarizing block of both motor end plates and ANS ganglia. The action of motor paralysis predominates, but the concomitant ganglionic blockade at higher doses explains part of the hypotensive effect often seen with the use of dTC for muscle relaxation. Histamine release is the major hypotensive factor that is common to dTC and other ganglionic blockers. Anticholinesterase drugs may produce nicotinic type ganglionic blockade by competition with ACh as well as by persistent depolarization *via* accumulated ACh.

The overall effects of ganglionic blockers on particular organ systems depend on whether the ANS activity of the system is predominantly sympathetic or parasympathetic (see Table 14-1). The overall effect on peripheral vessels is vasodilation due to release from SNS ganglionic constrictor control. The effect on the gastrointestinal tract may produce ileus. Although these drugs have a paraganglionic effect, blockade of the SNS ganglia and vascular dilation are the properties for which they were first used. They were initially used to treat chronic hypertension, but their lack of selectivity and global side-effects curtailed their popularity. The introduction of drugs that produce vasodilation directly or by action on the SNS vasomotor center has made the ganglionic blockers obsolete. They continue to have limited acute use in anesthesia to produce controlled hypotension and to treat hypertensive crisis.

Trimethaphan is the only ganglionic blocker available in the United States. Trimethaphan produces blockade by competition with ACh for receptors, thus stabilizing the postsynaptic membrane. However, side-effects and rapid onset tachyphylaxis have markedly reduced its use in anesthesia.[159] The patient's pupils become fixed and dilated dur-

ing administration, which obscures eye signs, an important consideration for neurosurgery. In this regard, it is distinctly inferior to nitroprusside. The major advantage of trimethaphan is its short duration of action, which is the result of pseudocholinesterase hydrolysis.

Trimethaphan in mixed in a concentration of 500 mg in 250–500 ml of diluent. The dosage to produce a given blood pressure is extremely variable. A starting dose of 10–20 $\mu g \cdot kg^{-1} \cdot min^{-1}$ by infusor with invasive arterial monitoring is recommended. Doses higher than 1 g are not recommended because ganglionic blockade may persist, direct vasodilation develops, histamine is released, and nicotinic neuromuscular blockade may appear.

Pentolinium is a ganglionic blocking drug available in the United Kingdom.[158] Its mechanisms of action are similar to those of trimethaphan, but it is devoid of muscle relaxant properties. The main disadvantage of pentolinium is its relative lack of controllability compared with trimethaphan or nitroprusside. Pentolinium is given in intermittent intravenous doses after anesthesia and position are established. The dose is 2.5–10 mg, with the effect lasting up to 45 minutes. One fourth of the initial amount is repeated if needed. Pupillary dilation, as with trimethaphan, occurs. Hypotension and vasomotor instability may outlast the procedure.

Cholinergic Drugs

Cholinergic drugs may be classified by the following outline, which follows physiologic response and site of action. Neuromuscular transmission is discussed in detail in Chapter 19. Nicotinic agonists and antagonists have been discussed as ganglionic drugs.

 I. Cholinergic Drugs—Agonists[19]
  A. Nicotinic
   1. ANS ganglionic transmission
   2. Neuromuscular transmission
  B. Muscarinic
   1. Direct-acting
   2. Indirect-acting
 II. Cholinolytic Agents—Antagonists
  A. Nicotinic
   1. ANS ganglionic transmission
   2. Neuromuscular transmission
  B. Muscarinic

Muscarinic Agonists

The cholinomimetic muscarinic drugs act at sites in the body where ACh is the neurotransmitter of the nerve impulse. These drugs may be divided into three groups, the first two of which are direct muscarinic agonists.[160,161] The third group acts indirectly. These groups are choline esters (ACh, methacholine, carbamylcholine, bethanechol); alkaloids (pilocarpine, muscarine, arecoline); and anticholinesterases (physostigmine, neostigmine, pyridostigmine, edrophonium, echothiophate).

Direct Cholinomimetics. ACh has virtually no therapeutic applications because of its diffuse action and rapid hydrolysis by cholinesterase (see Fig. 14-7).[160] One may encounter the use of topical ACh (1%) drops during cataract extraction when a rapid miosis is desired. Systemic effects are not usually seen because of the rapidity of ACh hydrolysis.

Other choline esters have been synthesized, mostly deriv-

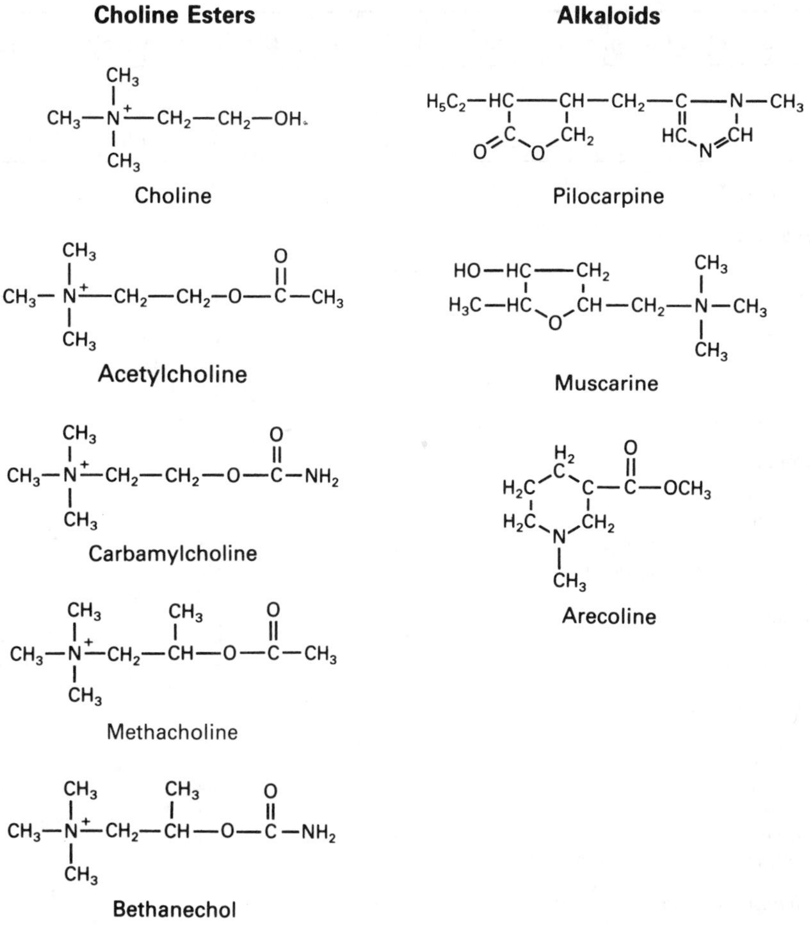

Choline Esters   **Alkaloids**

Choline

Pilocarpine

Acetylcholine

Muscarine

Carbamylcholine

Arecoline

Methacholine

Bethanechol

Figure 14-19. Chemical structures of direct-acting cholinomimetic esters and alkaloids.

atives of ACh, which possess more selective muscarinic activity than ACh. They differ from ACh in being more resistant to inactivation by cholinesterase and thus having a more prolonged and useful action. They also differ from ACh in their relative muscarinic and nicotinic activities.[161] The best studied of these drugs are methacholine, bethanechol, and carbamylcholine.[19] The chemical structures of ACh and these choline esters are shown in Figure 14-19. Their pharmacologic actions are compared to those of ACh in Table 14-7. These are not important drugs in anesthesiology, but they deserve discussion because anesthesiologists may encounter patients who are receiving them, and they may be useful in the postoperative period to alleviate cardiac tachydysrhythmias, urinary retention, and ileus.[162]

ACh is a quarternary ammonium compound that interacts with postsynaptic receptors, causing conformational membrane changes. This results in increased permeability to small ions and thus, depolarization. All the receptors translate the reversible binding of ACh into openings of discrete channels in excitable membranes, allowing Na^+ and K^+ ions to flow along their electromechanical gradients. Structure-activity relationships point to the presence of two important binding sites on the receptor, an esteractic site that binds the ester end of the molecule and an ionic site that binds the quarternary amine portion (see Fig. 14-7). Subtle changes in the structure of the compound can markedly alter the responses among different tissue groups. The degree of muscarinic activity falls if the acetyl group is replaced, but this confers a resistance to enzymatic hydrolysis. Carbamylcholine is synthesized by replacing the acetyl

group with carbamyl (Fig. 14-19). It possesses both muscarinic and nicotinic actions but is virtually resistant to esterase hydrolysis (Table 14-7). Bethanechol is also resistant to hydrolysis but possess mainly muscarinic activity. Betamethyl substitution produces methacholine, which is less resistant to hydrolysis but is primarily a muscarinic agonist.

Methacholine is destroyed by cholinesterase less rapidly than ACh and is potentiated by anticholinesterase drugs. Its muscarinic effects are predominantly cardiovascular. Methacholine slows the heart and dilates peripheral blood vessels. It is used to terminate supraventricular tachydysrhythmias, especially paroxysmal tachycardia, when other measures have failed. It also increases intestinal tone. Methacholine should not be given to patients with asthma. Hypertensive patients may also develop marked hypotension. Side-effects are those of PNS stimulation such as nausea, vomiting, and flushed sweating. Methacholine dosage is 100–200 mg orally or 10–25 mg subcutaneously. Overdose is treated with atropine.

Bethanechol has predominantly muscarinic actions that are relatively select for the gastrointestinal and urinary tracts. In usual doses it does not slow the heart or lower the blood pressure, as does methacholine. Bethanecol is of value in treating postoperative abdominal distention (nonobstructive paralytic ileus), gastric atony following bilateral vagotomy, congenital megacolon, nonobstructive urinary retention, and some cases of neurogenic bladder. The optimal oral dose is 30–60 mg daily in divided doses. It is not a parenteral drug. Precautions are as for methacholine.

The use of carbamylcholine has largely been supplanted

TABLE 14-7. Comparative Muscarinic Actions of Direct Cholinomimetic Agents

	Systemic				
	Acetylcholine	Methacholine	Carbamylcholine	Bethanechol	Pilocarpine
Esterase Hydrolysis	+ + +	+	0	0	0
Eye (Topical)					
Iris	+ +	+ +	+ + +	+ + +	+ + +
Ciliary	+ +	+ +	+ + +	+ + +	+ +
Heart					
Rate	− − −	− − −	−	−	?
Contractility	−	−	−	−	
Conduction	− −	− − −	−	−	
Smooth Muscle					
Vascular	− −	− − −	−	−	− −
Bronchial	+ +	+ +	+	+	+ +
Gastrointestinal motility	+ +	+ +	+ + +	+ + +	+ +
Gastrointestinal sphincters	− −	−	− − −	− − −	+ +
Biliary	+ +	+ +	+ + +	+ + +	+ +
Bladder					
detrusor	+ +	+ +	+ + +	+ + +	+ +
sphincter	− −	−	− − −	− − −	− −
Exocrine Glands					
Respiratory	+ + +	+ +	+ + +	+ +	+ + + +
Salivary	+ +	+ +	+ +	+ +	+ + + + +
Pharyngeal	+ +	+ +	+ +	+ +	+ + + +
Lacrimal	+ +	+ +	+ +	+ +	+ + + +
Sweat	+ +	+ +	+ +	+ +	+ + + + +
Gastrointestinal acid and secretions	+ +	+ +	+ +	+ +	+ + + +
Nicotinic Actions	+ + +	+	+ + +	−	+ + +

+ = Stimulation; − = Inhibition.

by better drugs because of its dual nicotinic and muscarinic effects. It is a long-acting agent because it is completely resistant to hydrolysis. Atropine will block its muscarinic actions but unmask its nicotinic effects. In this case, blood pressure will rise as sympathetic ganglia are stimulated and catecholamines released. Carbamylcholine is currently limited to use as topical ophthalmologic drops to produce miosis and for the treatment of wide-angle glaucoma.[160]

Direct-acting cholinomimetic alkaloids include muscarine, pilocarpine, and arecoline. They act at the same sites as ACh, and their effects are similar to those of ACh as described in Table 14-7. There are no uses for these drugs in anesthesiology. Pilocarpine is the only drug of this group used therapeutically in the United States. Its sole use is for the treatment of glaucoma, for which it is the standard. It is used as a topical miotic drug in ophthalmologic practice to reduce intraocular pressure in glaucoma. Pilocarpine has primary muscarinic effects with minimal nicotinic effects unless given systemically, in which case hypertension and tachycardia may result. Toxicity with topical application is rare.

Muscarine acts almost exclusively at muscarinic receptor sites, but it has no therapeutic application. Arecoline stimulates nicotinic receptors in addition to muscarinic receptors when given systemically. Its use has been limited to topical application in ophthalmology.

The benefits of muscarinic agonists must be carefully considered when one or more of their actions are likely to be dangerous (see Table 14-7). They are rarely given intravenously because of side-effects. Common side-effects are those of intense PNS stimulation, which include gastrointestinal cramping, hypotension, diaphoresis, salivation, diarrhea, and bladder pain.[19] Muscarinic agonists are particularly dangerous in patients with myasthenia gravis (who are receiving anticholinergics), bulbar palsy, cardiac disease, asthma, peptic ulcer, progressive muscular atrophy, or mechanical intestinal obstruction or urinary retention.[163]

Indirect Cholinomimetics. The indirect-acting cholinomimetic drugs are of greater importance to the anesthesiologist than are the direct-acting drugs. These drugs produce cholinomimetic effects indirectly as a result of inhibition or inactivation of the enzyme acetylcholinesterase, which normally destroys ACh by hydrolysis.[47] They are referred to as cholinesterase inhibitors or anticholinesterases. Table 14-8 lists therapeutic cholinesterase inhibitors and their major indications. Most of these drugs inhibit both acetylcholinesterase and pseudocholinesterase. Inhibition of acetylcholinesterase permits the accumulation of ACh transmitter in the synapse, resulting in intense PNS activity similar to that of the direct cholinomimetic agents. The action of ACh is therefore potentiated and prolonged. Their effects can be predicted from a knowledge of ANS pharmacology previously presented (see Table 14-7). Some of the acetylcholinesterase drugs (i.e., edrophonium) may also stimulate cholinergic receptors by direct action.[164] The accumulation of

TABLE 14-8. Cholinesterase Inhibitors

Drug	Trade Name	Route	Duration	Indications
Reversible				
Physostigmine	Eserine	Topical	6–12 hours	Glaucoma
Pyridostigmine	Mestinon Regonol	Oral, iv, im	4 hours	Myasthenia gravis Reversal of neuromuscular blockade
Neostigmine	Prostigmin	Oral, iv	4–6 hours	Myasthenia gravis Reversal of neuromuscular blockade
Edrophonium	Tensilon Enlon	iv	1–2 hours	Reversal of neuromuscular blockade Diagnosis of myasthenia gravis
Demecarium	Humorsol	Topical	3–5 days	Glaucoma
Ambenonium	Mytelase	Oral	4 hours	Myasthenia gravis
Nonreversible				
Echothiophate	Phospholine	Topical	3–14 days	Glaucoma
Isofluorophate		Topical	3–7 days	Glaucoma research
Malathion		Topical		Insecticide—relatively safe for mammals because of rapid hepatic metabolism
Parathion		Topical		Insecticide—highly toxic to higher animals; frequent accidental poisoning
Sarin (GB)	Nerve gas	Topical and gas		
Tabun	Nerve gas	Topical and gas		There are no indications for the use of nerve gas
Soman	Nerve gas	Topical and gas		

Note: Atropine should always be given prior to or with intravenous cholinesterase inhibitors and when only nicotinic effects are desired; muscarinic effects are dangerous when excessive.

ACh by the anticholinesterases potentially can produce all of the following: (1) stimulation of muscarinic receptors at ANS effect organs; (2) stimulation followed by depression of all ANS ganglia and skeletal muscle (nicotinic); and (3) stimulation with later depression of cholinergic receptor sites in the CNS. All of these effects may be seen with lethal doses of anticholinesterase drugs, but therapeutic doses only produce the first two.

Actions of therapeutic significance of the anticholinesterase drugs to the anesthesiologist concern the eye, the intestine, and the neuromuscular junction. The effects of anticholinesterases are useful in the treatment of myasthenia gravis, glaucoma, and atony of the gastrointestinal and urinary tracts. Acetylcholinesterase drugs are used routinely in anesthesia to reverse nondepolarizing neuromuscular block. A detailed discussion of their use for this purpose is covered in Chapter 19.

The most prominent pharmacologic effects of the anticholinesterase drugs are muscarinic. Their most useful actions are their nicotinic effects.[19] Muscarinic activity is evoked by lower concentrations of ACh than are necessary to produce the desired nicotinic effect. For example, the anticholinesterase, neostigmine, reverses neuromuscular blockade by increasing ACh concentration at the muscle end plate, a nicotinic receptor. Nicotinic reversal of neuromuscular blockade can usually be produced safely only when the patient has been protected by atropine or other muscarinic blockers. This prevents the untoward muscarinic effects of bradycardia, hypotension, bronchospasm, or intestinal spasm. Conversely, neuromuscular paralysis can be produced or increased if excessive anticholinesterase is used. Excess accumulation of ACh at the motor end plates produces a depolarization block similar to that produced by succinylcholine or nicotine. This is characteristic of the nicotine receptors.

Reversal of neuromuscular blockade in patients who have had bowel anastomosis was at one time a major controversy.

Some felt that the muscarinic effects of anticholinesterase drugs (hypermotility) increased the risk of anastomotic leakage[165,166] whereas others found no association between their use and subsequent breakdown.[167,168] National experience has favored the latter opinion.

The interactions between ACh, and the anticholinesterases are complex.[169] Anticholinesterase drugs inhibit hydrolysis of ACh by binding to either or both the anionic or esteratic sites of acetylcholinesterase, forming inhibitor-enzyme complexes that are more stable than ACh-enzyme complexes. These complexes prevent proper stereotactic access of ACh to the active enzyme sites; thus, hydrolysis is delayed, and ACh accumulates.

Clinically, anticholinesterase drugs may be divided into two types: the reversible and nonreversible cholinesterase inhibitors.[62,161] Reversible cholinesterase inhibitors delay the hydrolysis of ACh from 1 to 8 hours. Nonreversible drugs are so named because their inhibitory effects may last from days to weeks. The differences in duration of various anticholinesterases apparently depend on whether they inhibit the anionic or esteratic site of acetylcholinesterase.[164] Therefore the anticholinesterase drugs have also been pharmacologically subdivided. Drugs that inhibit the anionic site are called prosthetic, competitive inhibitors. Their action is due to competition between the anticholinesterase and ACh for the anionic site. These drugs tend to be short-acting. Edrophonium is an example of this type. Those drugs that inhibit the esteratic site are called acid-transferring inhibitors. These drugs include the longer acting neostigmine, pyridostigmine, and physostigmine. Thus, the differences in the mechanism of inhibition produced by prosthetic inhibitors (edrophonium) and acid-transferring inhibitors (neostigmine) account for the longer duration of action associated with the latter agents.

Most of the reversible cholinesterase inhibitors are quaternary ammonium compounds and do not cross the blood-brain barrier. Physostigmine is a tertiary amine that readily

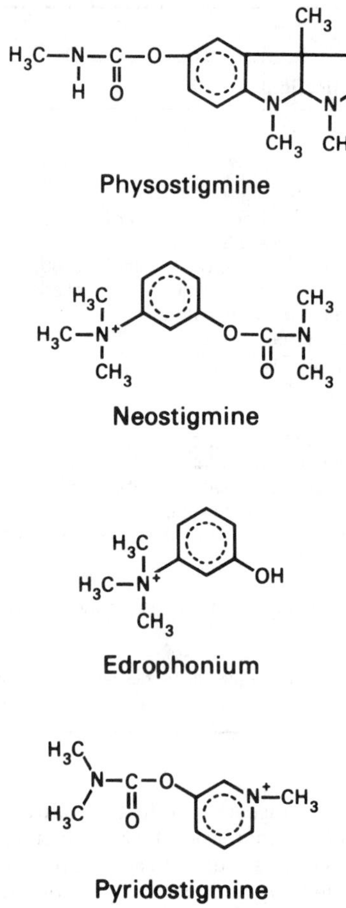

Figure 14-20. Structural formulas of clinically useful reversible anticholinesterase drugs. Physostigmine is a tertiary amine and crosses the blood-brain barrier. It is useful in treating the central anticholinergic syndrome.

passes into the CNS (Figure 14-20). It produces central muscarinic stimulation and, thus, is not used to reverse neuromuscular blockade but can be used to treat atropine poisoning. Conversely, atropine is used to treat physostigmine poisoning. Physostigmine has also been found to be a specific antidote in the treatment of postoperative delirium (see the section on Central Anticholinergic Syndrome).[19]

The irreversible cholinesterase inhibitors are mostly organophosphate compounds. These are also considered acid-transferring inhibitors, which form a phosphorylated enzyme resistant to attack by water. The phosphorylated enzyme cannot hydrolyze ACh to any measurable degree. In addition, the organophosphate compounds are highly lipid-soluble; they readily pass into the CNS and are rapidly absorbed through the skin. They are used as the active ingredient in potent insecticides and chemical warfare agents known as nerve gases. Table 14-8 lists some of these agents.

The only therapeutic drug of this group is echothiophate, which is available in the form of topical drops for the treatment of glaucoma. Its primary advantage is its prolonged duration of action. Topical absorption is variable but considerable. Echothiophate can remain effective for 2 or 3 weeks following cessation of therapy.[170] A history of use of echothiophate is important in avoiding prolonged action of succinylcholine, which requires pseudocholinesterase for its hydrolysis.

Organophosphate poisoning manifests all the signs and symptoms of excess ACh.[171] The antidote cartridges dispensed to troops to counter the effects of anticholinesterase nerve gases contain only atropine, which would effectively counter the muscarinic effects of the gas; however, atropine does little to counter the high-dose nicotinic muscle paralysis or the central ventilation depression that contributes to death from nerve gases. Treatment requires high doses of atropine, 35–70 $\mu g \cdot kg^{-1}$ intravenously every 3–10 minutes until muscarinic symptoms abate. Lower doses at less frequent intervals may be required for several days. Central ventilatory depression and nicotinic paralysis or weakness require respiratory support and specific therapy of the cholinesterase lesion. Pralidoxime has been reported to reactivate cholinesterase activity by hydrolysis of the phosphate enzyme complex. It is particularly effective with parathion poisoning and is the only cholinesterase reactivator available in the United States.[161]

Muscarinic Antagonists

Muscarinic antagonist refers to a specific drug action for which the term anticholinergic is widely used. Any drug that interferes with the action of ACh as a transmitter can be considered an anticholinergic agent. The term *anticholinergic* refers to a broader classification that would include the nicotinic antagonists already discussed.

Atropinic Drugs. Atropine, scopolamine, and glycopyrrolate are the most commonly used muscarinic antagonists used in anesthesia (Fig. 14-21). The use of antimuscarinic drugs for premedication is outlined in Chapter 19.

The actions of these drugs include inhibition of salivary, bronchial, pancreatic, and gastrointestinal secretions. Historically, atropine was introduced to anesthesia practice to prevent excessive secretions during ether anesthesia and to prevent vagal bradycardia during the administration of chloroform. Atropine-like drugs increase heart rate, relax bronchial and tracheal smooth muscle, and act as gastrointestinal relaxants.[172] Atropine and scopolamine also possess antiemetic action. Scopolamine skin patches are now used to control motion sickness and perhaps could be useful in controlling nausea on an outpatient basis.[173] Atropine, however, reduces the opening pressure of the lower esophageal sphincter, which theoretically increases the risk of passive regurgitation.[174] Atropinic drugs also produce dilation of the pupil (mydriasis) and paralysis of accommodation (cycloplegia).

Antimuscarinic agents do not inhibit transmission equally, and there are marked variations in sensitivity at different muscarinic sites owing to differences in penetration and affinities of the various receptors.[175] Differences in relative potency between the different antimuscarinics are outlined in Table 14-9. For example, glycopyrrolate produces less tachycardia than atropine and is a more potent antisialogogue. Antimuscarinics are also used to counter unwanted muscarinic actions of anticholinesterases when these are required for their nicotinic effect (see Chapter 19).

The antimuscarinic effects of the atropinic drugs are the result of competitive inhibition of ACh at the receptors of organs innervated by cholinergic postganglionic nerves. The antagonism can be overcome by sufficient concentrations of cholinomimetic drugs or anticholinesterases that increase ACh levels at the receptor site. This explains most of the therapeutic actions of atropinic drugs; however, they are neither purely antimuscarinic nor purely antagonist.[19]

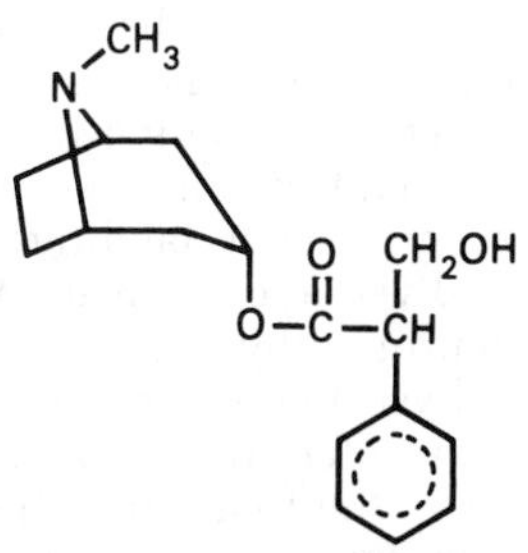

Figure 14-21. Structural formulas of the clinically useful antimuscarinic drugs.

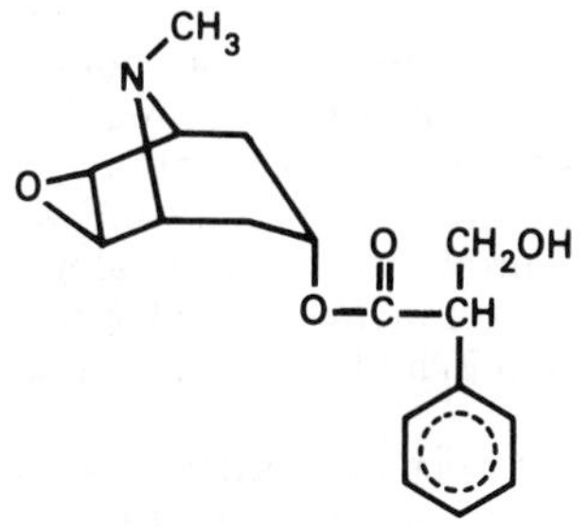

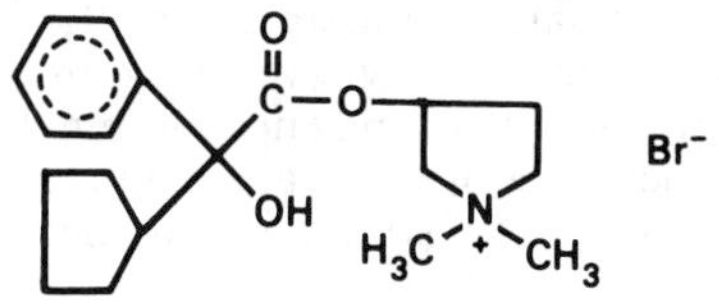

The belladonna alkaloids (atropine and scopolamine) also block ACh transmission to sweat glands, which, although they are cholinergic, are innervated by the SNS. Antimuscarinic agents produce antinicotinic actions at higher doses and result in important actions on CNS transmission that are pharmacologically similar to the postganglionic cholinergic function.[176] Atropine and scopolamine are tertiary amines (Fig. 14-21) and easily penetrate the blood-brain barrier and placenta. Glycopyrrolate is a quarternary amine that, like the reversible anticholinesterase drugs, does not easily penetrate these barriers. Glycopyrrolate, a synthetic

antimuscarinic, has gained popularity because it avoids the central effects of the other two drugs.

Atropine and scopolamine have notable CNS effects that are dissimilar. Scopolamine differs from atropine mainly in its central depressant effects, which produce sedation, amnesia, and euphoria. Such properties are widely used for premedication for cardiac patients in combination with morphine and a major tranquilizer. Atropine, as a premedicant, has slight effects on the CNS, including mild stimulation. Higher doses such as those given for reversal of muscle relaxants (1–2 mg) may produce restlessness, disorientation, hallucinations, and delirium (see the section on Central Anticholinergic Syndrome). Excessive stimulation may be followed by depression and paralysis of respiration. Atropine is closely related chemically to cocaine. Occasionally, scopolamine in low doses may cause restlessness and delirium. This syndrome is more frequently seen in the elderly and patients experiencing pain, e.g., in obstetric patients.

Atropine and scopolamine are noted to produce a paradoxical bradycardia when given in low doses. Scopolamine (0.1–0.2 mg) usually causes more slowing than atropine but also produces less cardiac acceleration at higher doses. The usual intramuscular premedicant doses of scopolamine cause either a decrease or no change in heart rate, which is another advantage of its use in cardiac anesthesia. The paradoxical bradycardia was once thought to be caused by an early central inhibition of the medullary cardioinhibitory center. However, this phenomenon occurs in animals that have had total vagotomy. Flacke and Flacke conclude that atropine must have a weak peripheral cholinergic agonist effect at low doses superceded by high-dose antimuscarinic effects.[19] Atropine may also produce sympathomimetic effects by blocking presynaptic muscarinic receptors found on adrenergic nerve terminals.[20,27,58] ACh stimulation of these receptors inhibits NE release, and blockade by atropine releases this inhibition (see the section on Cholinergic Receptors: Muscarinic).

The antimuscarinic drugs are used in anesthesia to diminish salivary and bronchial secretions during anesthesia, to protect heart rate from vagal inhibition, and to antagonize the muscarinic side-effects of anticholinesterases during reversal of muscle relaxants. Atropine is useful in increasing cardiac output with sinus bradycardia due to vagal stimulation if hypoxia is ruled out. It has many uses outside of anesthesia for the treatment of renal colic, gastrointestinal spasm, gastric secretion, and asthma.

Atropinic drugs are widely used in ophthalmology as mydriatics and cycloplegics. Atropine is contraindicated in patients with narrow-angle glaucoma. Pupillary dilation

TABLE 14-9. Comparison of Antimuscarinic Drugs

	Duration		CNS	GI Tone	Gastric Acid	Airway Secretions*	Heart Rate
	iv	*im*					
Atropine	15–30 minutes	2–4 hours	+ +	– –	–	–	+ + +‡
Scopolamine	30–60 minutes	4–6 hours	+ + +†	–	–	– – – –	– 0‡
Glycopyrrolate	2–4 hours	6–8 hours	0	– – –	– – –	– – –	+ 0

*Secretions may be reduced but inspissated.

†CNS effect often manifest as sedation before stimulation.

‡May decelerate initially.

thickens the peripheral part of the iris, which narrows the iridocorneal angle. Drainage of aqueous humor is impaired, and intraocular pressure increases. Doses of atropine used for premedication have little effect in this regard, whereas equal doses of scopolamine cause mydriasis. Prudence would dictate avoidance of either agent in patients with narrow-angle glaucoma. The need for antimuscarinic premedication is questionable in this situation.[174]

Atropine is best avoided where tachycardia would be harmful, as may occur in thyrotoxicosis, pheochromocytoma, or obstructive coronary artery disease. Theoretically, antimuscarinic drugs should benefit coronary spasm, but the benefit may be offset by the oxygen cost of the ensuing tachycardia. Atropine should be avoided in hyperpyrexial patients because it inhibits sweating.

Central Anticholinergic Syndrome. The belladonna alkaloids have long been known to produce undesirable side-effects ranging from stupor (scopolamine) to delirium (atropine). This syndrome has otherwise been called postoperative delirium and atropine toxicity. The central anticholinergic syndrome appears to involve the muscarinic receptor.[19] Biochemical studies have demonstrated abundant muscarinic ACh receptors in the brain that can be affected by any drug possessing antimuscarinic activity and capable of crossing the blood-brain barrier. Hundreds of drugs exist that meet these criteria with which this syndrome has been associated. Table 14-10 lists some of those drugs.[19,176] It is surprising that this syndrome is not more prevalent.

Patients receiving high doses of atropinic alkaloids rapidly develop dryness of the mouth, blurred vision with photophobia (mydriasis), hot and dry skin (flushed), and fever.[176] Mental symptoms range from sedation, stupor, and coma to anxiety, restlessness, disorientation, hallucinations, and delirium. Patients may have convulsions and ventilatory arrest if lethal poisoning has occurred. This is not the usual case encountered in anesthesiology. Although an alarming reaction may occur, fatalities are rare. Intoxication is usually short-lived and followed by amnesia. These reactions can be controlled by the intravenous injection of physostigmine.[177] Physostigmine is an anticholinesterase that, by virtue of being a tertiary amine, readily passes into the CNS to counter antimuscarinic activity. It should be given slowly in 1-mg doses, not exceeding 3 mg, to avoid producing peripheral cholinergic activity. Neostigmine, pyridostigmine, and edrophonium are not effective because they cannot pass into the CNS. Likewise, atropine is an effective antidote for physostigmine overdose.[19] The duration of physostigmine action may be shorter than that of the offending antimuscarinic agent and require repeated injection if symptoms recur. Physostigmine appears safe when used within dose recommendations and when indications are established. Central disorientation alone does not establish a diagnosis.[175] Peripheral signs of antimuscarinic activity should be present in addition to a central anticholinergic syndrome.

Physostigmine has been reported to reverse the CNS effects of many of the drugs listed in Table 14-10, including antihistamines, tricyclic antidepressants, and tranquilizers. Reversal of the sedative effects of opioids and benzodiazepines has also been reported.[178,179] However, anticholinesterase agents potentiate cholinergic synaptic transmission and increase neuronal activity, even if no receptor antagonist is present. Thus, arousal may not be a function independent of its cholinesterase activity, and claims that physostigmine is a nonspecific CNS stimulant may not be warranted

---

TABLE 14-10. Antimuscarinic Compounds Associated with Central Anticholinergic Syndrome

Belladonna Alkaloids

Atropine sulfate
Scopolamine hydrobromide

Synthetic and Natural Tertiary Amine Compounds

Dicyclomine (Bentyl)—antispasmodic with local anesthetic activity
Thiphenamil (Trocinate)—antispasmodic with local anesthetic activity
Procaine
Cocaine
Cyclopentolate (Cyclogyl) mydriatic

Quarternary Derivatives of Belladonna Alkaloids

Methscopolamine bromide (Pamine)—antispasmodic
Homatropine methylbromide—sedative, antispasmodic
Homatropine hydrobromide—ophthalmic solution—mydriatic

Synthetic Quarternary Compounds

Methantheline bromide (Banthine)
Propantheline bromide (Pro-Banthine)

Antihistamines

Chlorpheniramine (Ornade)
Diphenhydramine (Benadryl)

Plants

Deadly nightshade (atropine)
Bittersweet
Potato leaves and sprouts
Jimson or loco weed
Coca plant (cocaine)

Over-the-Counter

Asthma-Dor—atropine-like
Compoz—scopolamine sedation
Sleep Eze—scopolamine sedation
Sominex—scopolamine sedation

Antiparkinson Drugs

Benztropine (Cogentin)
Trihexphenidyl (Artane)
Biperiden (Akineton)
Ethopropazine (Parsidol)
Procyclidine (Kemadrin)

Antipsychotic Drugs

Chlorpromazine (Thorazine)
Thioriazine (Mellaril)
Haloperidol (Haldol)
Droperidol (Inapsine)
Promethazine (Phenergan)

Tricyclic Antidepressants
Amitriptyline (Elavil)
Imipramine (Tofranil)
Desipramine (Norpramine, Pertofrane)

Synthetic Opioids

Meperidine
Methadone

and could, in fact, be dangerous.[19] These phenomena require more study.

Adrenergic Drugs

Adrenergic Agonists

Since the isolation of epinephrine by Abel in 1899, the naturally occurring catecholamines and synthetic sympathomimetic amines have attracted considerable attention and enjoyed popular use as vasopressors. A vasopressor is a drug that is used to elevate arterial blood pressure above the existing level because the pressure is too low. Until recently, sympathomimetics were the most common means of treating shock, or the low output syndrome, because of the associated hypotension.[57] Elevation of arterial blood pressure has been repeatedly demonstrated to be an insufficient goal in the treatment of the low output syndrome.[31] The goal instead is to re-establish blood flow to vital organs. There is no definite evidence that the adrenergic amines increase survival from shock states, with the exception of epinephrine for anaphylaxis.[180] The outcome of cardiogenic shock treated with the "pressors" alone shows a mortality rate of 90% or higher.[181,182] The sympathetic amines do not remove the cause of the shock or hypotension; they are temporary drugs to be used only until more definite therapy is instituted or the pathologic process abates.

Today shock is simply defined as tissue perfusion inadequate to meet metabolic demands. Shock can be present with "normal" blood pressures, and hypotension can be produced without shock. Hence, blood pressure is no longer the *sine qua non* in defining shock.[31] However, we often remain mind-locked by our preoccupation with blood pressure as a goal of therapy. Jarish commented in 1928, "It is a source of regret that the measurement of flow is so much more difficult than the measurement of pressure. This has led to an undue interest in the blood pressure manometer. Most organs require flow and not pressure."

We have realized for over a century that the primary aim of cardiorespiratory monitoring is to determine the extent to which oxygen transport meets organ demands. Although blood pressure has been the historical gold standard for estimating perfusion, there is no correlation between blood pressure and oxygen transport[183] (Fig. 14-22). Oxygen transport is the product of the arterial oxygen content and cardiac output. Today it is much easier to measure flow using thermodilution. Flow used in this context refers to cardiac output:

$$DO_2 = CaO_2 \times CO$$

Oxygen transport correlates closely with cardiac output, since it is one of the two determinants of transport. Unfortunately, oxygen transport is not identical to cellular oxygen supply, which can be inadequate despite a normal or elevated oxygen transport because of maldistribution of blood flow to vital organs or an inability of the organs to utilize the oxygen.[183,184] Control of distribution remains an enigma.

The physiologic equation that expresses how cardiac output is generated states that the cardiac output is equal to the heart rate (HR) times the stroke volume (SV):

$$CO = HR \times SV$$

However, stroke volume is determined by three factors that can either be measured or calculated. These are (1) contrac-

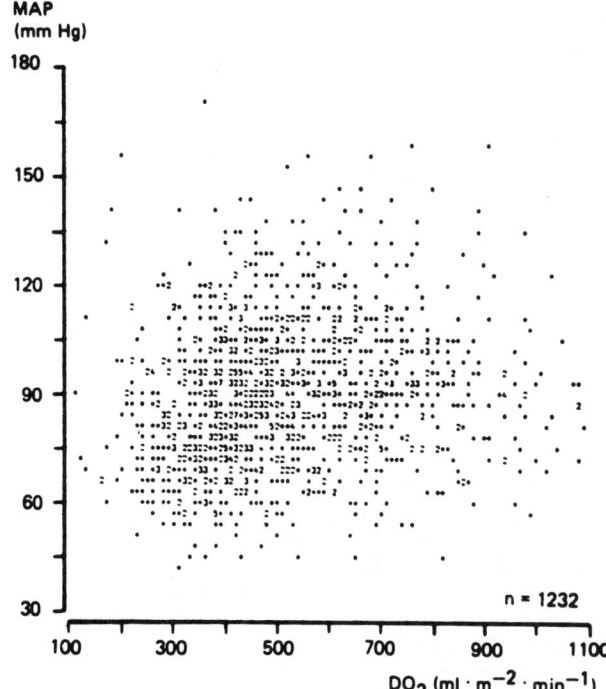

Figure 14-22. Correlation between mean arterial pressure (MAP) and O_2 delivery (DO_2) during the perioperative period in patients undergoing aorta bifemoral bypass grafting. (Reprinted with permission from Reinhart K: Principles and Practice of SvO_2 Monitoring, pp 121–124. London, Intensive Care World, King and Worth, Publishers, vol 5, no 4, Dec 1988.)

tility or the inotropic state of the myocardium, (2) preload, and (3) afterload. The physiologic determinants of cardiac output can therefore be expressed as

Cardiac output = Heart rate

$\times$ (inotropism : preload : afterload)

This equation is graphically depicted in Figure 14-23. This figure demonstrates that the biologic mechanisms that produce and regulate cardiac output are interdependent and cannot be divorced in the clinical situation. The relationships are so tight and dynamic that terms such as inotropism, preload, and afterload cannot be defined independently.

An inotropic agent is defined as one that influences the contractility of the myocardium negatively or positively. Adrenergic agonists are often selected to treat myocardial failure if they possess positive inotropic or chronotropic effects. Preload is clinically synonymous with the volume of venous return to the heart, which establishes cardiac output by the Frank-Starling mechanism. Preload may be increased either by the infusion of additional volume or by acute venoconstriction. Afterload is a measure of impedance to ventricular ejection, which is important to patients with impaired inotropism. In the absence of outlet obstruction, the clinical correlate of afterload to the left ventricle is the systemic vascular resistance. Ohm's law states that blood flow through any organ is directly related to the blood pressure gradient across that organ but is inversely proportional to the resistance. Indeed, afterload (resistance) is the only factor of the four major determinants of cardiac output that, if increased, will reduce cardiac output (flow)—Ohm's

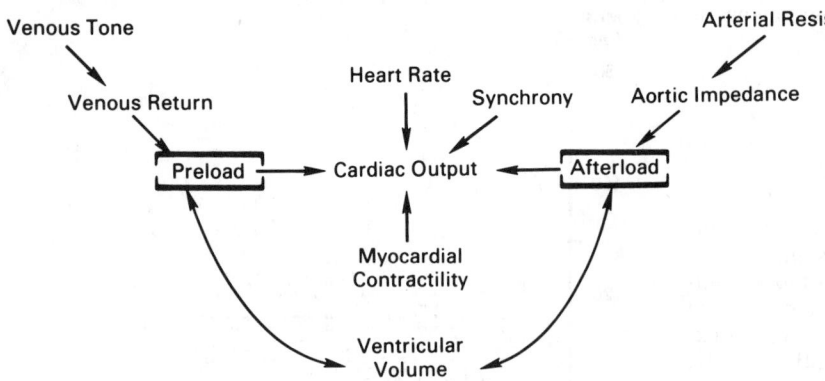

Figure 14-23. The four principal factors determining cardiac output are demonstrated. Synchrony of atrioventricular contraction is an additional factor becoming important with the development of cardiac dysrhythmias. (Reprinted with permission from Lawson NW, Wallfisch HK: Cardiovascular pharmacology: A new look at the "pressors." In Stoelting RK, Barash PG, Gallagher TJ (eds): Advances in Anesthesia, p 195, Chicago, Year Book Publishers, 1986.)

law revisited. Lusitropism is a factor in determining cardiac output but is not depicted in Figure 14-23. Lusitropism was coined to described abnormalities of myocardial relaxation or diastole as opposed to problems of inotropism. Some vasodilators such as nitroglycerin and some sympathomimetic "inodilators" are thought to improve cardiac function by promoting diastolic relaxation. Lusitropism is only now becoming understood. Lusitropic dysfunction may play a large role in many myocardial disease processes and may, in fact, precede inotropic dysfunction.[185]

Observation of the blood pressure alone does allow one to distinguish which factor was at fault for producing a low-flow state or which one was corrected.[51,52] The overriding importance attached to blood pressure in the past led to the indiscriminate use of vasopressors. Note in Figure 14-23 that blood pressure is not among the physiologic determinants of cardiac output. It is the product and not the etiology. Recognition of the importance of volume therapy brought an end to the "age of the vasopressor" and ushered in a more rational approach to vasoactive drugs used with adequate hydration. It is now apparent that the problems associated with the use of vasopressors were caused, in large part, by an insufficient understanding of clinical cardiovascular physiology and the inability to monitor critically ill patients. We can now selectively detect and manipulate the weak links in the chain of cardiovascular events that produce blood flow and oxygen transport rather than the mindless increase in blood pressure. The term vasopressor, once synonymous with vasoconstriction, has now become a generic term for several species of drugs which, by whatever means, increase cardiac output and may or may not increase blood pressure. Their uses in anesthesia include (1) maintenance of organ perfusion; (2) treatment of allergic reactions; (3) prolongation of the action of local anesthetics; and (4) for cardiopulmonary resuscitation.

Selection of Adrenergic Effect. The selection of vasoactive drugs requires a knowledge of both the hemodynamic disturbance and pharmacology of the available drugs. The principal hemodynamic effects include changes in heart rate (chronotropism), contractility (inotropism), myocardial conduction velocity (dromotropism), rhythm, and peripheral vascular dilation or constriction. The latter influences preload and afterload.

Most commonly used adrenergic amines activate both alpha and beta receptors (Table 14-11). The exceptions are phenylephrine and methoxamine, which are predominantly alpha agonists, and isoproterenol, which is exclusively a beta agonist. Each catecholamine has a distinctive effect, qualitatively and quantitatively, on the myocardium and peripheral vasculature. The relative effects of the adrenergic amines on inotropism, chronotropism, and arteriolar resistance vessels have long been recognized. Table 14-11 demonstrates the relative potencies of the adrenergic amines on

TABLE 14-11. Actions of Adrenergic Agonists

Sympatho-mimetics	Alpha$_1$	Alpha$_2$	Beta$_1$	Beta$_2$	DA$_1$	DA$_2$	Dose Dependence (Alpha, Beta, or DA)	Comments
Methoxamine	+ + + + +	?*	0	0	0		0	Vasoconstriction only
Phenylephrine	+ + + + +	?	±	0	0		+ +	Primarily vasoconstriction
Norepinephrine	+ + + + +	+ + + + +	+ + +	0	0		+ + +	Beta$_2$ effect *present* but not seen clinically
Metaraminol	+ + + + +	?	+ + +	0	0		+ + +	Releases norepinephrine
Epinephrine	+ + + + +	+ + +	+ + + +	+ +	0		+ + + +	
Ephedrine	+ +	?	+ + +	+ +	0		+ +	Direct and indirect
Mephentermine	0 to + +	?	+ + + +	+?	0		+ +	Cerebral stimulation
Dopamine	+ to + + + + +	?	+ + + +	+ +	+ + +	?	+ + + + +	
Dobutamine	0 to +	?	+ + + +	+ +	0		+ +	Inotropism greater than chronotropism
Dopexamine	0	0	+	+ + + +	+		+ +	
Prenalterol	+		+ + + +	+ +			+	
Isoproterenol	0	0	+ + + + +	+ + + + +	0		0	

*The clinical significance of the effects of agonism and antagonism is not yet known.

the various myocardial and arteriolar adrenergic receptors. This relative potency is often dose-dependent, adding still another variable.

The net effect of a sympathomimetic drug is usually defined as the algebraic sum of its relative action on the alpha, beta, and dopaminergic receptors.[52] This traditional pharmacologic statement requires further physiologic definition. For many years, the emphasis on catecholamines was focused almost entirely on their actions on the myocardium and on arteriolar resistance vessels. This was in keeping with the preoccupation with maintaining blood pressure. Changes in venous resistance contribute little to total vascular resistance and blood pressure. However, small changes in venous capacitance result in large changes in venous return because 60–70% of the circulating blood volume is in the venous circulation.[127] Venous return (preload) has repeatedly been demonstrated to be of paramount importance in supporting cardiovascular function, although the effect of the vasoactive amines on venous capacitance has largely been ignored.[186] The effect of the sympathomimetic amines on the venous circulation appears to be distributive in that acute venular constriction increases the central blood volume (preload), whereas dilation decreases venous return by the promotion of peripheral pooling.[187,188] The distributive effect of a catecholamine may be as important as its inotropic action and more important than its arteriolar effect.[43,189,190]

Zaimis[51] and Smith and Corbascio[52] reviewed the effect of catecholamines on the venous circulation, but until recently few data have become available. Further definition should elucidate some of the complex and confusing data in the literature generated when clinical observations are limited solely to adrenergic effects on the myocardium and arteriolar vasculature.

The catecholamines exert potent constrictor effects on the resistance and capacitance vessels in addition to their effects on capillary sphincters.[191,192] Intravenous and intra-arterial infusions of epinephrine in humans have been shown to cause marked constriction of the veins.[193] Arteriolar vasoconstriction precedes venoconstriction; however, stroke volume does not increase until the onset of venoconstriction.[128] Sharpey-Schafer and Ginsberg have concluded that the initial increase in cardiac output seen with the infusion of epinephrine is more an effect of increased preload than an arteriolar or direct cardiac effect.[194] NE produces a similar effect, but the onset of venoconstriction is slower.

Zimmerman et al[195] noted a differential ability of the amines to constrict veins. The data are expressed as the average percentage contribution of venous resistance to total change in vascular resistance (Table 14-12). Note in Table 14-11 that methoxamine and NE are considered equipotent alpha$_1$ arteriolar vasoconstrictors; however, these effects differ dramatically from their effects on venoconstriction in Table 14-12. Venoconstriction contributes little to the overall increase in total resistance with methoxamine, whereas NE produces a marked venoconstriction. The lack of venoconstrictor response to methoxamine has been demonstrated in humans.

Schmid et al[196] performed a similar study in humans and found similar results. Table 14-13 is the result of their study of the relative potencies of several catecholamines on resistance vs capacitance vessels. These data represent only the relative potencies of the amines within either resistance or capacitance vessels and are not a comparison of potency ratios between the two. Nevertheless, the data point out the marked differences between the agents. NE is the most potent amine with respect to arteriolar and venous con-

striction. Metaraminol is 1.5 times more potent than phenylephrine in constricting resistance vessels; however, phenylephrine is 1.5 times more effective in constricting capacitance vessels than metaraminol. NE proved to be 12 times more potent than metaraminol in constricting resistance vessels and 24 times more effective in constricting capacitance vessels.

Marino et al[197] reported the responses of resistance and capacitance vessels to catecholamines in humans on cardiopulmonary bypass. This is a unique method of examining hemodynamic drug response because flow rate (cardiac output) is fixed, excluding the myocardial effects of the drugs. Changes in resistance or capacitance are reflected as either changes in pressure or changes in reservoir volume, respectively. The alpha agonist phenylephrine produced a marked decrease in venous capacitance (venoconstriction). Arteriolar resistance increased also, but to a lesser degree, confirming the study by Schmidt et al. Isoproterenol reduced arteriolar and venous resistance in a manner similar to the alpha antagonist phentolamine. Surprisingly, dopamine produces significant venoconstriction at doses that have no direct arteriolar or cardiac effect, confirming studies of dopamine in animals.[190,198,199]

An in vitro study by DeMay and Vanhoutte[200] compared the effects of sympathetic agonists on rings of arterial and

TABLE 14-12. Average Percentages of Contributions of Increments in Venous Resistance to Increments in Total Resistance ($\Delta VR/\Delta TR \times 100$)

Agent	$\Delta VR/\Delta TR \times 100$
Norepinephrine	13.8
Tyramine	8.0
Metaraminol	7.2
Ephedrine	3.3
Mephentermine	1.9
Phenylephrine	1.8
Methoxamine	1.4

After Zimmerman BG, Abboud FN, Eckstein JW: Comparison of the effects of sympathomimetic amines upon venous and total vascular resistance in the foreleg of the dog. J Pharmacol Exp Ther 139:290, 1963, with permission.

TABLE 14-13. Relative Potencies of Several Sympathomimetic Amines in Humans with Respect to Constrictor Effects on Resistance Vessels and Capacitance Vessels

Resistance Vessels		Capacitance Vessels	
Drug	Relative Potency	Drug	Relative Potency
Norepinephrine	1.0000	Norepinephrine	1.0000
Metaraminol	0.0874	Phenylephrine	0.0570
Phenylephrine	0.0684	Metaraminol	0.0419
Tyramine	0.0148	Methoxamine	0.0068
Mephentermine	0.0049	Ephedrine	0.0025
Ephedrine	0.0020	Tyramine	0.0023
Methoxamine	0.0018	Mephentermine	0.0023

After Schmid PG, Eckstein JW, Abboud FM: Comparison of the effects of several sympathomimetic amines on resistance and capacitance vessels in the forearm of man. Circulation 34:III-209, 1966, with permission.

venous vessels from dogs. Their data were similar to the information in Table 14-13. NE was the most potent arterial and venous constrictor, and relative sensitivity of the arterioles to phenylephrine and methoxamine was also similar. Their data, however, indicated that methoxamine had greater venoconstrictor effect than that demonstrated in humans. Nevertheless, their study demonstrated that the differences in response between veins and arteries lay in the uneven distribution of postjunctional alpha$_1$ and alpha$_2$ receptors. Their results indicate the presence of both receptors on venous smooth muscle, whereas arterial smooth muscle cells contain mainly postjunctional alpha$_1$ receptors.

Arterial or venous vasoconstriction (alpha$_1$ receptors) influences cardiac output in several ways that may be antagonistic (Fig. 14-23).[31] An acute increase in arteriolar adrenergic (alpha$_1$) tone increases peripheral vascular resistance, imposes additional afterload, and may reduce cardiac output. Arteriolar vasodilation produces opposite effects. Venous return can be increased by increasing volume or reducing venous capacitance. Therefore, acute venoconstriction, also an alpha$_1$ effect, increases preload and increases cardiac output within the limits of the contractile state of the myocardium, an effect opposite that of alpha$_1$ arteriolar constriction. Acute venodilation, a beta$_2$ effect, reduces venous return and may reduce cardiac output, as does venous pooling following alpha blockade.

The ratio of arteriolar resistance to venous resistance is important in adjusting cardiac output. Each catecholamine has a distinctive effect, qualitatively and quantitatively, on each vascular region.[43] Therefore, a knowledge of each drug's action in altering the ratio of arteriolar to venous resistance is of great importance in drug selection. A drug that increases preload, even though it possesses good inotropic properties, may not be appropriate in the treatment of cardiac failure with high filling pressures. It might be more appropriately used in a distributive shock syndrome such as sepsis. Venoconstriction and arteriolar constriction are both alpha$_1$ effects but have widely divergent effects on cardiac output. Proper drug selection, therefore, cannot be made solely on the basis of the net alpha and beta effect.

Table 14-14 is a summary of the available data on the relative potencies of the amines on the alpha$_1$ receptors of the resistance and capacitance vessels. Scant data permit inaccuracies, but the table is derived from sources that demonstrate remarkable consistency. It is offered as a clinical guide to drug selection. The peripheral receptors of both resistance and capacitance vessels subserve vasoconstriction, but with divergent effects on afterload and preload; therefore, the alpha$_1$ receptors have been subdivided into alpha$_1$ arterial (alpha$_{1a}$) and alpha$_1$ venous (alpha$_{1v}$). Note that methoxamine and phenylephrine, both pure alpha drugs, are equipotent arterial vasoconstrictors. Phenylephrine, however, is a potent venous constrictor, but methoxamine has virtually no effect on the capacitance vessels. Dopamine has potent venoconstrictor (alpha$_{1v}$) effect at doses at which few alpha$_{1a}$ or beta$_1$ effects are noted.

Drug Dosage and Adverse Effects. The major adverse effects of the sympathomimetic amines are related to excessive alpha or beta activity. The potential for harm can be understood in terms of receptor characteristics. Excessive beta$_1$ activity may increase contractility but increase heart rate and myocardial oxygen consumption beyond supply. Severe dysrhythmias are a frequent companion of excess beta$_1$ activity as a result of increased conduction velocity, automaticity, and ischemia. The beta$_2$ activity has the potential to increase cardiac output by reducing resistance (afterload) while reducing blood pressure. An excessive decrease in diastolic pressure, however, reduces obstructive coronary perfusion and may further aggravate myocardial ischemia. The beta$_1$ and beta$_2$ effects of adrenergic agonists are more useful clinically than alpha$_1$ effects and can be used for longer periods of time. Unfortunately, it is difficult to separate the inotropic, dromotropic, and chronotropic effects in the clinical setting. The characteristics of the ideal positive inotropic agent are listed in Table 14-15 for comparison with each drug as it is discussed.[31]

Drugs with prominent alpha$_1$ agonist effects may produce a desirable increase in blood pressure but reduce total flow due to increases in arteriolar resistance (afterload). A more

---

TABLE 14-14. Comparison of Relative Alpha$_1$ Catecholamine Responses on Peripheral Resistance and Capacitance Vessels*

Vasoconstriction			
Alpha$_1$ Arterial (alpha$_{1a}$)		**Alpha$_1$ Venous (alpha$_{1v}$)**	
Norepinephrine	+ + + + +	Norepinephrine	+ + + + +
Metaraminol	+ + + + +	Phenylephrine	+ + + + +
Phenylephrine	+ + + +	Metaraminol	+ + + +
Methoxamine	+ + + +	Dopamine	+ + +
Epinephrine	0 − + + + +†	Epinephrine	0 − + + + +†
Dopamine	0 − + + + +‡	Ephedrine	+ + +
Ephedrine	+ +	Mephentermine	+ ?
Mephentermine	+ +	Methoxamine	0 − + ?
Dobutamine	+ − 0	Dobutamine	?
Isoproterenol	0	Isoproterenol	0

*Drugs are listed in descending order of potency within each vascular region.

†Dose-dependent; beta effects of epinephrine predominate at low doses.

‡Dose-dependent; DA and beta effects predominate at low doses.

Reprinted with permission from Lawson NW, Wallfisch HK: Cardiovascular pharmacology: A new look at the "pressors." In Stoelting RK, Barash PG, Gallagher TJ (eds): Advances in Anesthesia, p 195. Chicago, Year Book Medical Publishers, 1986.

TABLE 14-15. Characteristics of the Ideal Positive Inotropic Agent

Enhances contractile state by increasing velocity and force of myocardial fiber shortening

Lacks tolerance

Does not produce vasoconstriction

No cardiac dysrhythmias

Does not affect heart rate

Controllability—immediate onset and termination of action

Elevates perfusion pressure by raising cardiac output rather than systemic vascular resistance

Redistributes blood flow to vital organs

Direct-acting—not dependent on release of endogenous amines

Compatible with other vasoactive drugs

Effective orally or parenterally

---

prominent alpha$_1$ venous constriction may improve cardiac output by increasing preload or precipitate failure if preload exceeds the contractile limits of the myocardium. An increase in afterload increases myocardial oxygen consumption, produces ischemia of other organs, reduces renal blood flow, and produces dangerous increases in coronary artery resistance.[201]

In general, the alpha effects of the sympathomimetics are of benefit only when used for specific indications and for the briefest possible time. Other measures are usually more effective in improving flow and are indicated before a pressor should be used. The only time an adrenergic amine should be used as a pressor or in a pressor dose range without consideration of flow is when arterial perfusion pressure must be increased immediately to prevent imminent death or morbidity.[202] Cardiopulmonary resuscitation is the primary example where a pressor effect is necessary to create diastolic coronary perfusion during closed or open heart massage. Any drug with strong alpha agonist properties seems equally effective in this regard. Epinephrine, with its added beta properties, is the first-line agent for this situation. Drugs that vasodilate, such as isoproterenol, have little use in this setting even if they possess inotropic properties.[7] Another situation in which a vasoconstrictor may be justified as a temporary measure is hypotension when cerebral, coronary, or extracorporeal bypass perfusion pressure is the prime consideration.

The prolonged use of adrenergic agonists with strong alpha properties commonly results in tachyphylaxis. This phenomenon is probably caused by increasing plasma volume loss through ischemic capillaries and down regulation of the adrenergic receptors. Precapillary sphincters are under local myogenic control and relax when hypoxic and acidotic, despite strong alpha stimulation. Postcapillary sphincters are more functional in a hypoxic and acidotic milieu but are under stronger central neurogenic control. Continued postcapillary tone in the face of precapillary relaxation increases hydrostatic pressure with a net loss of intravascular volume. These events are just a few of the explanations for the once mysterious so-called "levophed shock," in which patients were unable to be weaned from NE infusions.[51,55]

Dopamine is the only clinically available example of a DA agonist. This property has been put to effective clinical use in reducing resistance in the mesenteric and renal beds, mediating an improvement in perfusion of these regions in the low-flow state. Few complications have been ascribed to dopamine when used solely for this purpose.[85]

Low Output Syndrome. Cardiac output is dependent on the integration of synchrony, heart rate, contractility, afterload, and preload. Synchrony of atrioventricular contraction is an additional determinant when dysrhythmias develop (see Fig. 14-23).

Patients with the low cardiac output syndrome have abnormalities of the heart, blood volume, or blood flow distribution.[203] Those remaining in this state for more than 1 hour usually have dysfunction of all three components. Modern hemodynamic monitoring has pinpointed hypovolemia, relative or absolute, as the most common cause of the low-output syndrome, regardless of the etiology.[203,204] The use of a vasopressor or vasoconstrictor drug is rarely, if ever, warranted in absolute hypovolemia. Initial treatment with adrenergic amines in this setting is likely to delay volume repletion and potentiate the shock state. The proper hemodynamic management of septic shock, the most commonly seen distributive abnormality, remains controversial, but volume repletion is the primary consideration. Likewise, the initial treatment of cardiac dysfunction is optimum volume replacement, because hypovolemia is a frequent accompaniment of impaired myocardial performance. Ventricular performance may be improved solely on the basis of increased preload and the Frank-Starling mechanism.

The treatment of cardiogenic shock is an excellent example of the low-flow state that requires multiple autonomic interventions common to other forms of the low-output syndrome. An acute reduction of left ventricular contractility (inotropism) produces a cascade of events that worsen in cyclic fashion (Fig. 14-24).[205] One could draw this cascade beginning with any one of the five determinants of cardiac output. Loss of contractility produces a reduction in cardiac output, increased left ventricular end-diastolic pressure, and a host of compensatory reflexes, which are familiar. These compensatory mechanisms include the Frank-Starling law, increased sympathetic activity that augments contractility and rate. Chronic dysfunction produces a third compensatory mechanism, hypertrophy.

The attributes of the ideal inotropic drug are listed in Table 14-15. The inotropic agent needed for the patient illustrated in Figure 14-24 would be rapid-acting, short-lived, and would not increase heart rate, preload (unless hypovolemic), afterload, or infarct size. Since the ideal inotropic drug is not available, the peripheral side-effects of any inotropic agent become critical to selection because all are multireceptor agonists.

Myocardial failure exists when the heart cannot pump enough blood to meet metabolic needs. The clinical manifestations of heart failure result from peripheral circulatory derangements that are the result of the heart's forward output lagging behind the input. Venous pressure increases and produces congestion.

There are marked differences between chronic heart failure, from whatever the cause, and acute failure from infarction. These differences are not yet fully appreciated.[206] Patients with chronic heart failure have retention of sodium and water and are typically hypovolemic, whereas patients with acute heart failure are either normo- or commonly hypovolemic. Cardiomegaly is a common compensatory feature of chronic heart failure but is absent with acute heart failure. Circulating catecholamines and myocardial catecholamine content are decreased in chronic failure but markedly elevated in the acute infarct. Thus, the response to inotropic drugs in chronic heart failure is influenced not only by the lack of myocardial catecholamine stores but also by down regulation of beta receptors. The cardiac output in chronic failure is borderline to decreased, whereas it is

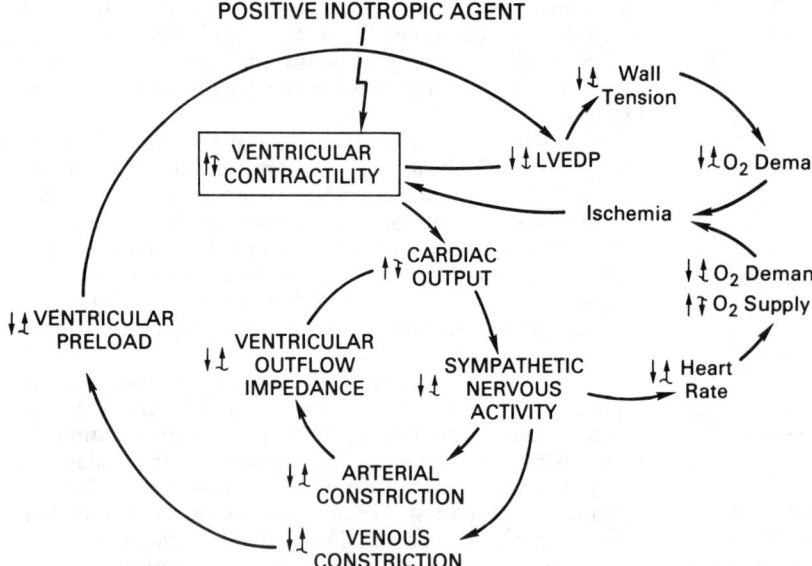

Figure 14-24. Reversal of heart failure by intervention ($\updownarrow$) with the ideal positive inotropic agent is depicted. (Reprinted with permission from Evans DB, Weishaar RE, Kaplan HR: Strategy for the discovery and development of a positive inotropic agent. Pharmacol Ther 16:303, 1982.)

usually normal or elevated with acute failure as a result of the compensatory mechanism.

Acute failure is the most common complication of infarction, occurring in 40–50% of patients, which reflects a 20–25% involvement of the myocardium. In contrast to the patient with chronic heart failure, this dysfunction is usually transient, lasting between 48–72 hours. Drugs with a predominant inotropic action are used alone or in combination to acutely improve cardiac contractility. Therefore, one has to be concerned that myocardial damage is not extended during this transient period by inappropriate inotropic or chronotropic support. This is not as major a concern in the patient with hypertrophy, in whom increased inotropism may actually reduce oxygen consumption by reducing ventricular mass.

Table 14-16 presents one approach to the management of

TABLE 14-16. Management of Low Output Syndrome Caused by Myocardial Dysfunction

1. Assure adequate ventilation and oxygenation
2. Relieve pain and symptoms of recurrent ischemia
3. Institute hemodynamic monitoring (pulmonary artery, pulmonary capillary wedge, and arterial pressures; urine output; cardiac output)
4. Optimize left ventricular filling pressure
5. Correct metabolic abnormalities
6. Control dysrhythmias (#2 priority if life-threatening)
7. Pharmacologic support
   a. Vasodilators
   b. Inotropic drugs
   c. Diuretics—chronic heart failure
8. Rule out "correctable" causes of shock (septal or left ventricle rupture, mitral regurgitation, acute aneurysm)
9. Mechanical support of circulation
10. Surgical correction if possible

Note: Hemodynamic monitoring is essential in confirming a diagnosis, optimizing filling pressures and cardiac output, selecting pharmacologic support, and avoiding complications. Adjustment of left ventricular filling pressure may require additional volume or a relative volume reduction with vasodilators. The diagnostic criteria for cardiogenic shock are not met until step 4 is accomplished.

---

cardiogenic shock listed in order of relative importance. The use of sympathomimetic support is placed in proper perspective. It emphasizes the essential role that invasive hemodynamic monitoring and volume management play in confirming a diagnosis of cardiogenic failure.[31] Although volume expansion and reduction of afterload may improve cardiac output, other pharmacologic interventions may still be necessary to optimize cardiac output and its distribution. Invasive monitoring is a prerequisite for the rational use of the vasoactive drugs to (1) establish that a sympathomimetic is necessary; (2) select drugs for the hemodynamic condition; (3) follow resultant hemodynamic changes, since many of the beneficial effects of the catecholamines are hidden to the clinical eye; and (4) avoid complications of pressor therapy that are visible to all. Drug selection for the low-output state remains the most enigmatic.

Table 14-17 is a summary of the hemodynamic effects of some of the currently popular and once popular sympathomimetic drugs.[31] Many of the hemodynamic effects are dose-related. The dose ranges are listed and a standard infusion rate cited. Standard rates of infusion are simply guidelines, and the actual dose administered should be determined by patient response. The doses are calculated assuming the use of calibrated infusors in which 60 drops equal 1 ml, or using a calibrated infusion pump.

Methoxamine and Phenylephrine. Methoxamine is the prototype pure vasoconstrictor. Phenylephrine produces similar actions, but there are important clinical differences. Table 14-11 demonstrates that methoxamine possesses only alpha$_1$ properties, and Table 14-14 demonstrates that it produces almost no venoconstriction (alpha$_{1v}$). Its only pharmacologic effects are to increase arterial resistance, increase afterload, and reduce flow, even though blood pressure is elevated. Few clinical uses for methoxamine remain. It has been useful for treating paroxysmal atrial tachycardias. A single intravenous dose of methoxamine can break a paroxysmal atrial tachycardia reflexly through baroreceptor stretch, obviating the need for use of digitalis or countershock (see Table 14-17). Carotid massage produces similar results by a similar mechanism. The calcium channel blockers will probably displace methoxamine even further in this regard.

TABLE 14-17. Dose Schedule and Hemodynamic Effects of the Adrenergic Agonists

Drug Listed from alpha to beta	Dosages IV Push Adults	IV Infusion*	Site of Activity Alpha$_{1a}$	Alpha$_{1v}$	Beta$_1$	Beta$_2$	DA	Hemodynamics ↑ = Increase; ↓ = Decrease; − = No change CO	Inotrop	HR	VR	TPR	RBF
Methoxamine	5–10 mg	N/R	+ + + +	0 − + ?	0	0	0	− ↓	−	Reflex ↓	−	↑ ↑	↓ ↓
Phenylephrine	50–100 µg	a. 10 mg/250 ml b. 40 µg·ml^{-1} c. 0.15–0.75 µg·kg^{-1}·min^{-1} d. 0.15 µg·kg^{-1}·min^{-1}	+ + + +	+ + + + +	0	0	0	− ↓	−	Reflex ↓	↑ ↑ ↑	↑ ↑	− ↓
Norepinephrine	N/R	a. 4 mg/250 ml b. 16 µg·ml^{-1} c. 0.01 − 0.1 µg·kg^{-1}·min^{-1} d. 0.1 µg·kg^{-1}·min^{-1}	+ +	+ + +	+ + + +	? +	0	↑ − ↓	↑	Reflex ↓	↑ ↑ ↑	↑ ↑ ↑	↓ ↓ ↓
Metaraminol	N/R	a. 100 mg/250 ml b. 400 µg·ml^{-1} c. 0.5–7 µg·kg^{-1}·min^{-1} d. 0.5 µg·kg^{-1}·min^{-1}	+ +	+ +	+ + +	0	0	− ↓	↑	Reflex ↓	↑	↑ ↑ ↑	↓ ↓ ↓
Epinephrine	0.3–0.5 ml 1 : 1000 (0.3–0.5 mg) sc—Asthma iv—Anaphylaxis	a. 1 mg/250 ml b. 4 µg·ml^{-1} 0.01–0.03 µg·kg^{-1}·min^{-1} c. 0.03–0.15 µg·kg^{-1}·min^{-1} 0.15–0.30 µg·kg^{-1}·min^{-1}	+ + + + + + + + +	+ + + + + + + + +	+ + + + + + + + + + + +	+ + + + + + + +	0	↑ ↑ ↑ − ↑ − ↓	↑ ↑ ↑ ↑ ↑ ↑	↑ ↑ ↑ ↑ ↑ ↑	↑ ↑ ↑	↑ ↑ ↑ ↑ ↑ ↑	↑ ↓ − ↓
	5 ml 1 : 10,000 (0.5 mg) cardiac arrest every 5 minutes	d. 0.015 µg·kg^{-1}·min^{-1}	+	+	+ + + +	+ + + +	0	↑ ↑	↑ ↑	↑ ↑	↑	↑	↑
Ephedrine	5–10 mg	N/R	+ +	+ + +	+ + +	+ +	0	↑	↑	↑	↑ ↑	↑	↑ − ↓
Mephentermine	15–30 mg	a. 500 mg/250 ml b. 2000 µg·ml^{-1} c. 4–8 µg·kg^{-1}·min^{-1} d. 4 µg·kg^{-1}·min^{-1}	0 − + +	+ ?	+ + + +	+ ?	0	↑	↑ ↑	↑	↑ ?	↑	↓ − ↑
Dopamine‡	N/R	a. 200 mg/250 ml b. 800 µg·ml^{-1} 0.05–5 µg·kg^{-1}·min^{-1} c. 2–10 µg·kg^{-1}·min^{-1} 10 µg·kg^{-1}·min^{-1}† d. 2 µg·kg^{-1}·min^{-1}	 + + + + + + 	+ + + + + + + + + + + + + + + +	 + + + + + + + + 	 + + + + + + + + + + 	+ + + + + + + + + +	↑ ↑ ↑ ↑ − ↓ −	— ↑ ↑ ↑ —	— − ↑ ↑ ↑ —	↑ ↑ ↑ ↑	− ↓ − ↑ ↑ ↑ − ↓	↑ ↑ ↓ ↑
Dobutamine‡	N/R	a. 250 mg/250 ml b. 1000 µg·ml^{-1} c. 2–30 µg·kg^{-1}·min^{-1} d. 5 µg·kg^{-1}·min^{-1}	0 − +	?	+ + + +	+ +	0	↑ ↑	↑ ↑	− ↑	?	−	− ↑
Isoproterenol	0.4 mg (0.2 ml of 2 µg·ml^{-1} solution) Third-degree heart block	a. 1 mg/250 ml b. 4 µg·ml^{-1} c. 0.15 µg·kg^{-1}·min^{-1} to desired effect d. 0.015 µg·kg^{-1}·min^{-1}			+ + + + + + + + + +	+ + + + + + + + + +		↑ − ↓	↑ ↑ ↑	↑ ↑ ↑	↓	↓ ↓	− ↑

*a. Mixture
 b. Concentration µg·ml^{-1}
 c. Dose range µg·kg^{-1}·min^{-1}
 d. Standard rate infusion
†"Rule of Six"
‡Dopamine and dobutamine employ the same doses. Dosage of either may quickly be calculated by multiplying patient's weight (kg) × 6 = mg added to 100 ml D5%W. The number of drops delivered through a calibrated infusor (60 drops = 1 ml) is the number of µg·kg^{-1}·min^{-1} infused into the patient. Example: 70 kg × 6 = 420; 420 mg/100 ml = 4200 µg·ml^{-1} or 70 µg/gtt; 5 µg·kg^{-1}·min^{-1} = 5 gtt/min.
N/R = not recommended; CO = cardiac output; Inotrop = contractility; HR = heart rate; VR = venous return (preload); TPR = peripheral resistance (afterload); RBF = renal blood flow.
Reprinted with permission from Lawson NW, Wallfisch HK: Cardiovascular pharmacology: A new look at the "pressors." In Stoelting RK, Barash PG, Gallagher TJ (eds): Advances in Anesthesia, p 195. Chicago, Year Book Medical Publishers, 1986.

Table 14-14 demonstrates that phenylephrine, considered a pure alpha drug, increases venous constriction more than arterial constriction.[196,197] Venous constriction may be its most redeeming feature when compared with the purely arteriolar effect of methoxamine. Acutely, venoconstriction favors venous return (preload), even though arterial resistance (afterload) also increases. The net effect may result in an increase in pressure and flow. Phenylephrine, like methoxamine, does not change cardiac output in normal individuals but can cause a decreased output in patients with ischemic heart disease.[55,207,208] It is rarely necessary to give a pure alpha pressor for extended periods, but phenylephrine has continued to be favored in operating rooms to sustain pressure during cardiopulmonary bypass as well as during cerebral and peripheral vascular procedures.[209] It

does not produce dysrhythmias as a direct effect. Phenylephrine is also useful in reversing right-to-left shunt in tetralogy of Fallot when patients are having "spells" during anesthesia.[31,43] A dose of 2 µg·kg^{-1} iv push may be used. The arterial vasoconstrictors may reduce the size of an ischemic injury when used in conjunction with intra-aortic balloon pumping or nitroglycerin.[210]

Norepinephrine and Metaraminol. NE and metaraminol produce similar hemodynamic effects. NE is the naturally occurring mediator of the SNS and the immediate precursor of epinephrine. It produces direct-acting hemodynamic effects on the alpha and beta receptors in a dose-related manner when given by infusion. Metaraminol possesses direct action but acts primarily by causing release of stored endogenous NE. Both drugs produce increases in cardiac output and blood pressure when given in low doses (see Table 14-17), primarily as a result of predominant beta action at this level.[211] Higher doses reduce flow because alpha arteriolar constriction supersedes the beta effects. Reflex bradycardias may occur, as with methoxamine and phenylephrine, despite active beta$_1$ stimulation.

Increased plasma levels of the endogenous catecholamines, NE and epinephrine, are the sympathetic milieu in which exogenous sympathomimetics are ordinarily given. NE is the catecholamine standard against which all other catecholamines are compared. It is the endogenous neurotransmitter of the sympathetic nervous system. NE administered intravenously has received an unseemly reputation over the years that is perhaps unmerited.[212] Current studies indicate that NE is being used in doses that are orders of magnitude greater than that necessary to obtain its best response. Complications such as renal failure and tissue necrosis are routine and can be expected when NE is used in this manner. Personal experience and the published experience of others also indicate that if an infusion of NE is used simply to titrate to blood pressure rather than measured flow, the amount of NE infused is five to ten times more than necessary to obtain the best oxygen delivery and oxygen consumption.[213,214] Most published dose infusion rates are based on blood pressure titration and as a result are too liberal. Although NE is less commonly used in the critically ill patient than other catecholamines, a resurgence of interest in this agent is noted in the literature. It has remained clinically useful because its effects are predictable, prompt, and potent.[215,216]

Objections to the use of NE (or metaraminol) for the treatment of cardiogenic shock are based on two considerations: (1) vasoconstriction increases the pressure work of the left ventricle, with an adverse effect on the oxygen economy of the already ischemic pump; and (2) these drugs cause further vasoconstriction and organ ischemia in a syndrome in which intense constriction may already have occurred.[55] The use of NE or metaraminol requires the use of invasive monitoring; otherwise, complications are to be expected. It is not usually necessary to elevate the systolic blood pressure above 90–100 mm Hg. At this level of infusion, the cardiac output will normally be increased as a beta effect without excessive peripheral vasoconstriction. Both NE and metaraminol are potent venoconstrictors, which should alter interpretation of venous filling pressures as a guide to adequate volume repletion.

Metaraminol is neither as prompt nor as potent as NE. Metaraminol can be given intramuscularly or intravenously without causing necrosis, which is commonly seen with the continued use of NE. Benefits of metaraminol are limited, however, because it is thought to depend on tissue NE levels for its efficacy. It loses its effectiveness during prolonged use because it displaces NE and replaces it as a false transmitter. It may also not be effective initially in patients who are receiving catechol depleters. Other undesirable effects associated with the use of NE and metaraminol include renal arteriolar constriction and aggravation of oliguria. In addition, prolonged therapy may produce a reduction in plasma volume as a result of fluid transudation at the capillary level. Indeed, in some instances, cardiogenic shock requiring continuous NE infusions has been reversed by fluid infusions.[55] The use of the minimal effective dose of these drugs in combination with careful invasive monitoring and attention to fluid management is the only way to avoid iatrogenic disasters.

Epinephrine. Epinephrine is the prototypical endogenous catecholamine. It is synthesized, stored, and released from the adrenal medulla and is the key hormonal element in the fight or flight response. It is the most widely used catecholamine in medicine. Epinephrine is used to treat asthma, anaphylaxis, cardiac arrest, and bleeding and to prolong regional anesthesia. The cardiovascular effects of epinephrine, when given systemically, result from its direct stimulation of both alpha and beta receptors. This is dose-dependent and is outlined in Table 14-17.

The effect of epinephrine on the peripheral vasculature is mixed.[217] It has predominantly alpha-stimulating effects in some beds (skin, mucosa, and kidney) and beta-stimulating actions in others (skeletal muscle). These effects are also dose-dependent. At therapeutic doses, beta-adrenergic effects predominate in the peripheral vessels, and total resistance may be reduced. Constriction, however, is maintained in the renal and cutaneous areas because of its dominant alpha effect in these areas. An increase in cardiac output with epinephrine may be due to a redistribution of blood to low resistance vessels in the muscle, but with further reduction in flow to vital organs. Cardiac dysrhythmias are a prominent hazard, and the strong chronotropic effects of epinephrine have limited its use or systematic investigation in the treatment of cardiogenic shock. In contrast, it is frequently used for cardiac failure after open heart surgery.

Some volatile anesthetics sensitize the myocardium to circulating catecholamines and induce cardiac dysrhythmias. This is especially true in the presence of hypoxia and hypercarbia. Halothane has the most pronounced cardiac-sensitizing action of the volatile anesthetics in use today. The mechanism has been thought to be related to the stimulation of alpha- and beta-adrenergic receptors, since blockade of these receptors consistently abolishes these cardiac dysrhythmias.[218,219] However, Kapur and Flacke demonstrated that calcium channel blockade is equally effective.[220] This is not surprising if the shared final pathway of beta and calcium-entry blockade proves to be correct (see Fig. 14-15).[221] The exact mechanism is further confused by studies showing that the myocardial depression produced by the volatile anesthetics is related to blockade of the slow calcium current.[222] These findings are compatible with the observations that beta blockade, calcium blockade, and general anesthetics produce myocardial depression.[223]

Intravenous and locally infiltrated adrenergic agents should be used cautiously during inhalation anesthesia, especially with halothane. The following schedule has been found to be relatively safe during halothane anesthesia.[218]

1. Epinephrine concentrations no greater than 1:100,000–1:200,000 (1:200,000 = 5 µg·ml^{-1}).
2. Adult dose should be no greater than 10 ml of 1:100,000 or 20 ml of 1:200,000 within 10 minutes.
3. Total should not exceed 30 ml of 1:100,000 (60 ml of 1:200,000) within 1 hour.

In another report, the dose of submucosally injected epinephrine necessary to produce ventricular cardiac dysrhythmias in 50% of patients anesthetized with a 1.25 MAC of a volatile anesthetic was 2.1, 3.4, and 6.7 µg·kg^{-1} during administration of halothane, enflurane, and isoflurane, respectively.[223] The incidence of cardiac dysrhythmias was eliminated when this dose was halved in patients anesthetized with halothane or isoflurane. In contrast with adults, children seem to tolerate higher doses of subcutaneous epinephrine without developing cardiac dysrhythmias.[224]

Ephedrine. Ephedrine is one of the most commonly used noncatecholamine sympathomimetic agents in the practice of anesthesia. It is used extensively for treating hypotension following spinal or epidural anesthesia. Ephedrine stimulates both alpha and beta receptors by direct and indirect actions. It is predominantly an indirect-acting pressor, producing its effects by causing NE release.[55] Tachyphylaxis develops rapidly and is probably related to the depletion of NE stores with repeated injection.[217] The cardiovascular effects of ephedrine (see Table 14-17) are nearly identical to those of epinephrine but less potent.[51,52] Its effects are sustained about ten times longer than those of epinephrine.

Ephedrine remains the pressor of choice in obstetrics because uterine blood flow improves linearly with blood pressure.[132,133] This effect is probably not related to its arteriolar vasoconstriction but rather to its venoconstrictive action. Ephedrine is a weak, indirect-acting sympathomimetic agent that produces venoconstriction to a greater degree than arteriolar constriction[187,189,225] (see Table 14-14). This may be its most important and unappreciated effect. It causes a redistribution of blood centrally, improves venous return (preload), increases cardiac output, and restores uterine perfusion. The mild beta action restores heart rate simultaneously with improved venous return. An increased blood pressure is noted as a result rather than a cause of these events. Mild alpha$_1$ arteriolar constriction does occur, but the net effect of improving venous return and heart rate is increased cardiac output (Fig. 14-25). Uterine blood flow is spared. This response, however, depends on the patient's state of hydration.

Dopamine is an attractive alternate vasopressor for obstetrics for similar reasons.[224] It produces strong alpha$_1$ venoconstriction and volume redistribution at infusion rates at which alpha$_{1a}$ or beta effects are minimal. The primary disadvantage of dopamine is its lack of immediate availability as an iv push drug. It requires more careful titration than ephedrine. The prophylactic administration of ephedrine before spinal blockade in obstetrics can produce misleading clinical estimates of volume status because of its effects on venous return and arterial pressure.

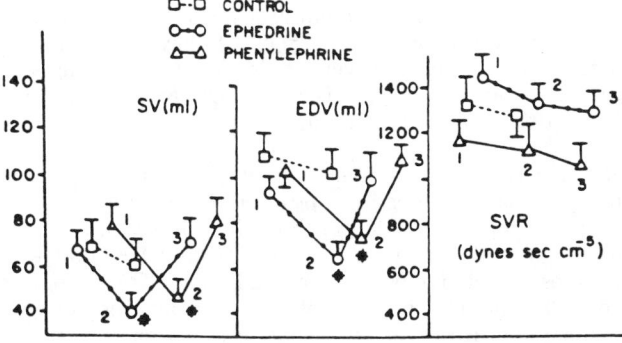

Figure 14-25. Stroke volume (SV), end-diastolic volume (EDV) and systemic vascular resistance (SVR) (1) before regional block; (2) during hypotension; and (3) after therapy with ephedrine or phenylephrine. The increase in stroke volume was related entirely to an increased venous return secondary to venoconstriction in these awake, healthy patients. The afterload effects of phenylephrine at higher doses predominate in patients with heart disease or myocardial depression and reduce cardiac output. (Reprinted with permission from Ramanathan S, Grant G: Vasopresser therapy for hypotension due to epidural anesthesia for cesarean section. Acta Anaesthesiol Scand 32:4, 1988.)

Mephentermine. Mephentermine is a rarely used direct- and indirect-acting sympathomimetic agent similar to metaraminol. Agonists with these properties are unpredictable and have largely been replaced by new and more selective agents.[55] Mephentermine has a direct, positive inotropic action on the heart with prolonged action (see Tables 14-11 and 14-17). The peripheral alpha effects of mephentermine appear to be the result of an indirect release of NE. Its peripheral effects are complex and unpredictable. Discrepancies between experimental and clinical observations are in part attributable to important differences in the physiologic status of experimental subjects and patients. Mephentermine increases cardiac output, heart rate, and peripheral vascular resistance in normal subjects; however, high doses result in decreases in peripheral resistance in patients in shock. This is presumably a direct vasodilating effect. A pronounced increase in venous return has been noted with mephentermine.[52] This is disputed by the studies of Zimmerman et al[195] and Schmid et al,[196] who indicate that mephentermine is a relatively weak venoconstrictor. Table 14-17 indicates its unknown status in this regard.

Dopamine. Dopamine is the immediate precursor of NE. The actions of dopamine as a neurotransmitter in the CNS have been well defined. It is also found in high concentrations of the postganglionic nerve terminals of the SNS and in the adrenal gland. Dopamine offers distinct advantages over many sympathomimetics in treating the low-output syndrome.[57] Dopamine is an agonist to all three types of adrenergic receptors, depending on the dosage used (see Table 14-17). This advantageous spectrum of activity is the reason it has become a drug of choice, after volume expanders, in managing shock in the surgical intensive care units.[83,180] The desired action can be selected by alteration of the infusion rate. Dopamine is primarily a direct-acting drug but causes some NE release in its beta dose range. Renal and mesenteric vascular dilation, mediated through the DA receptors, is produced at infusion rates of 0.5 to 5.0 $\mu g \cdot kg^{-1} \cdot min^{-1}$.[89,96] An increase in cardiac output may be noted at this dose level without a change in blood pressure or heart rate.[226] Improved perfusion is the result of a reduced afterload in the mesenteric vessels and an increased venous return (see Fig. 14-17; Fig. 14-26). Venoconstriction (alpha$_{1v}$) occurs at doses at which direct cardiac and peripheral arterial effects are minimal.[197] Increasing doses stimulate beta effects, which begin at about 2 $\mu g \cdot kg^{-1} \cdot min^{-1}$. The onset of alpha activity begins around 7 $\mu g \cdot kg^{-1} \cdot min^{-1}$. Infusion rates of 10 $\mu g \cdot kg^{-1} \cdot min^{-1}$ or higher produce more intense alpha vasoconstriction and may override any beneficial DA or beta effects. When vasoconstriction predominates, dopamine behaves like NE (Fig. 14-27).[202]

The distributive effects of dopamine are useful in the surgical patient, in whom sepsis is the most common distributive abnormality.[227] Dopamine can sustain cardiac output and renal and mesenteric function until definitive therapy is successful.[217] Dopamine is a proven cardiotonic drug after open heart surgery. It facilitates management of surgical patients with heart failure and helps avoid problems related to excessive infusion of intravenous fluids by support of cardiac output and urine excretion.[89,228] Dopamine increases mean pulmonary arterial pressure and is not recommended for patients in right-sided heart failure.[201,229,230,231] Although dopamine is frequently given to patients in cardiogenic shock, its positive inotropic, chronotropic, and vasoconstrictive effects may increase myocardial oxygen de-

Pulmonary Capillary Wedge Pressure (PCWP)

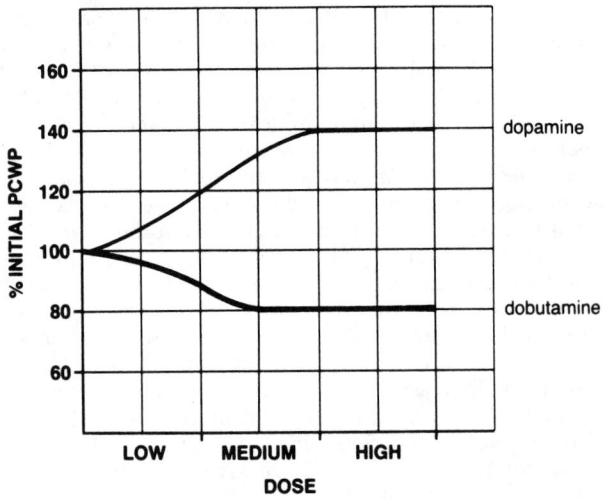

Figure 14-26. A decrease in venous capacitance has been demonstrated as an early effect of dopamine. An increase in pulmonary capillary wedge pressure may be noted. Dobutamine may decrease pulmonary capillary wedge pressure by increased inotropism as well as vasodilation with minimal effect on venous capacitance. (Redrawn with permission of Eli Lilly Co.)

mand. Increased venous return may not be desirable in this situation. Adverse effects of dopamine are tachycardia, nausea and vomiting, headache, and angina pectoris. Ventricular cardiac dysrhythmias may become troublesome, although the incidence is less than that with isoproterenol, epinephrine, or NE.[217] Excessive infusion can cause distant gangrene similar to that produced by NE. Dopamine inhibits insulin secretion and may contribute to hyperglycemia in the critically ill patient.[57] This drug's beneficial effects are best titrated by using invasive monitoring.

Systemic Vascular Resistance (SVR)

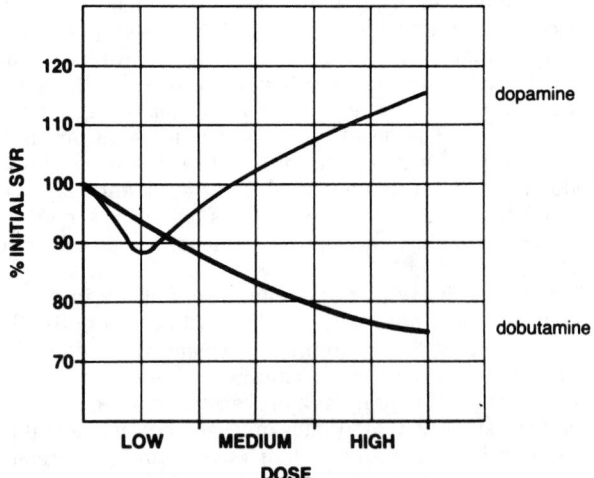

Figure 14-27. Dobutamine produces a net reduction in vascular resistance. Its weak alpha vasoconstrictive effects are balanced by a direct beta$_2$ vasodilation with little change in vascular tone. However, further reflex arterial vasodilation occurs with increased cardiac output. Low-dose dopamine dilates renal and mesentric arterial beds, which reduces afterload but increases resistance at increasing doses as a result of its predominant alpha effect.

Dobutamine. Dobutamine is a synthetic catecholamine, that is, a modification of isoproterenol, which is derived from dopamine.[55,232] It is an example of pharmacologic engineering in which modification of a basic molecular structure produced a useful drug. Variations in chemical structure among isoproterenol, dopamine, and dobutamine can be seen in Figure 14-8. Dobutamine has some clear advantages in certain clinical situations. It acts directly on beta$_1$-adrenergic receptors but exerts a much weaker beta$_2$-adrenergic action than isoproterenol.[209] It does not cause NE release or stimulate DA receptors. It produces a positive inotropic effect with minimal changes in heart rate or vascular resistance at standard rates of infusion (see Table 14-17).[56] A positive inotropic effect without a correspondingly strong chronotropic effect is an obvious advantage of dobutamine over isoproterenol. It is not totally devoid of chronotropic action. Dobutamine increases automaticity of the sinoatrial node and increases conduction through the atrioventricular node and ventricles. Troublesome tachycardias can occur in sensitive individuals, and caution should be exercised in giving dobutamine to patients with established atrial fibrillation and other tachydysrhythmias. Increases in heart rate may be seen at infusion rates exceeding $10-15$ $\mu g \cdot kg^{-1} \cdot min^{-1}$. Increases in cardiac output are primarily through its positive inotropic action and secondarily through reduction in afterload (see Figs. 14-17 and 14-27). Changes in arterial blood pressure may not occur. Dobutamine possesses very weak alpha properties, which can be unmasked by beta blockade. Administration of propranolol produces a prompt and dramatic increase in blood pressure. In the absence of adrenergic blockade, dobutamine increases coronary blood flow by reducing resistance.

With a half-life of 2 minutes, the controllability of dobutamine is superb. Tachyphylaxis is rare but may be noted if dobutamine is given for over 72 hours. This drug is to the cardiologist what dopamine is to the surgical intensivist. Dobutamine is of most value in patients with acute or chronic congestive failure from ischemic disease. It has proved to be as effective as dopamine and nitroprusside combined in the treatment of myocardial failure with infarction. Dobutamine is contraindicated in the patient with idiopathic hypertrophic subaortic stenosis.

Like isoproterenol, dobutamine seems to inhibit hypoxic pulmonary vasoconstriction.[57,229,233] It may, therefore, be useful in managing right ventricular failure following surgery for congenital heart disease or cor pulmonale. This observation requires confirmation.

Dopexamine. Dopexamine hydrochloride is a dopamine analogue that provides mild positive inotropism with systemic and renal vasodilation through stimulation of beta$_2$-adrenergic and dopamine receptors of both DA$_1$ and DA$_2$ subtypes. Its relative potency on the DA$_1$ and DA$_2$ receptors is only 0.3 and 0.17, respectively, that of an equipotent dose of dopamine. However, dopexamine has been reported to improve variables associated with renal function to a greater extent than could be attributed to an increased cardiac output alone.[234]

The relative effect of dopexamine on beta$_1$ receptors is only 0.1 that of dopamine but is 60 times more potent on beta$_2$ adrenoreceptors. This accounts for its weak inotropism but powerful vasodilator activity. Dopexamine is a more profound vasodilator than dobutamine. In addition, the dopamine receptor agonist properties of dopexamine should mediate additional, preferential renal vasodilation in contrast to dobutamine, which is inactive at dopamine receptors. The beta activity of dopexamine can be completely blocked with propranolol. Dopexamine has been found to be devoid of direct alpha-adrenoreceptor activity.[235] Despite its weak beta$_1$ agonist activity, it exerts prominent inotropic effects not only through stimulation of myocardial beta$_1$ receptors but with additional effect, like dobutamine, through inhibition of norepinephrine uptake.[236] Dopexamine inhibits hypoxic pulmonary vasoconstriction in animals primarily by stimulation of beta$_2$ adrenoreceptors.[237] This pharmacologic profile has proved to be beneficial in both the short- and long-term management of low-output left ventricular failure and perhaps right-sided heart failure.

Isoproterenol. Isoproterenol is a potent balanced beta$_1$ and beta$_2$ receptor agonist with no vasoconstrictor effects. It increases heart rate and contractility while decreasing systemic vascular resistance. Although it can increase cardiac output, it is not useful in shock because it redistributes blood to nonessential areas by its preferential effect on the cutaneous and muscular vessels.[203] As a result, it produces variable and unpredictable results on cardiac output and blood pressure in patients with cardiogenic shock. Isoproterenol is a potent dysrhythmogenic drug and extends myocardial ischemic areas. Deleterious effects on an evolving ischemic process include cardiac dysrhythmias, tachycardia, and reduced diastolic coronary perfusion pressure and time. Increased myocardial oxygen demand and only modest hemodynamic improvement make it an unattractive drug for patients in shock, especially after acute myocardial infarction.

Isoproterenol is helpful in managing cardiac failure associated with bradycardia, asthma, and cor pulmonale. It is also a useful chemical pacemaker in third-degree heart block until an artificial pacemaker can be inserted or the cause can be removed.[217] Chernow et al[57] and Zaritsky[55] suggest that isoproterenol might be useful in treating both idiopathic and secondary pulmonary hypertension. It has also been reported as useful in improving the forward flow in patients with regurgitant aortic valvular disease, but it should not be used if there is an accompanying stenosis.[210,226]

Clonidine—Alpha$_2$ Agonists. See the section on Antihypertensives.

Combination Therapy. Many combinations of vasoactive drugs are useful in making fine hemodynamic adjustments in the critically ill.[211,238] One of the first such combinations was used to prevent tissue necrosis caused by NE that could occur with or without extravasation.[52] Phentolamine, an alpha blocker (5–10 mg/4 mg of NE), was added to the infusion bottle to prevent the intense vasoconstriction of NE. No hemodynamic data are available describing possible benefits from the alpha blockade and afterload reduction of phentolamine.

The available sympathomimetic agents provide a wide range of hemodynamic effects. An even greater spectrum of activity can be achieved by combining different sympathomimetic drugs or sympathomimetics with vasodilators. For example, if a larger positive inotropic action and less vasoconstriction are desired, isoproterenol can be added to either dopamine or dobutamine. If an increase in afterload is desirable, the addition of NE to dopamine or dobutamine might be helpful.[239] Combinations are also useful in redistributing blood flow to vital organs despite adequate cardiac output. One of the advantages of dopamine in the surgical patient is its dose-related effect on vascular tone and cardiac contractility. Dopamine improves renal and mesenteric blood flow. Dobutamine may be used to increase global cardiac output, and dopamine can be added to the low-dose range to distribute a higher percentage of the increased cardiac output to the renal bed. Many combinations have been advocated.[193,239]

The existence of a finite number of adrenergic receptors implies that adrenergic agonists must compete for a limited number of receptor sites. Just as the net effect of a single drug is the algebraic sum of its receptor action, the combined effects of sympathomimetics also appear to be additive rather than synergistic. Many of the adrenergic combinations have been described as synergistic, but this may be a matter of clinical interpretation of a summated receptor effect that is simply more physiologically efficient. Summation can be used to advantage in selectively avoiding unwanted side-effects of one drug while supplementing its desired attributes with another.

The studied use of adrenergic combinations in patients with cardiac failure has been proposed because pathophysiology cannot be approached with the attitude that beta agonism is all good and alpha stimulation is all bad. The objective is to increase coronary perfusion and flow but decrease afterload. This is the effect achieved by the intra-aortic balloon pump. No single vasoactive agent can achieve this effect, but these conditions can be approached with combination therapy.[238]

Animal studies have shown that cardiac output and renal blood flow increase when dopamine-induced vasoconstriction is attenuated by alpha blockers. On this basis, vasodilators have been beneficially used in patients experiencing vasoconstriction who did not respond adequately to high-dose dopamine alone.[211] Recently, the short-acting vasodilators, sodium nitroprusside and nitroglycerin, have been successfully combined with dopamine or dobutamine. The use of nitroprusside or nitroglycerin improves these patients by reducing afterload. Nitroglycerin is a more potent venodilator than nitroprusside and appears more efficacious in reducing preload. Dobutamine and nitroprusside produce comparable increases in cardiac output in patients with congestive heart failure. When they are infused together, the increase in cardiac output is greater than when either drug is used alone.[193] In addition, there is a greater reduction in pulmonary wedge pressure and pulmonary vascular resistance. This combination improves both inotropism and afterload reduction. This action is similar to that produced by amrinone alone.

During combination therapy standard rates of infusion such as those outlined in Table 14-18 no longer apply, and invasive monitoring is mandatory for success. Obviously, it would be simpler to use one drug. Side-effects of combinations must be weighed in terms of the economy of myocar-

---

TABLE 14-18. Cardiovascular Effects of Ritodrine and Terbutaline[212-214,217]

Hemodynamics	% Change from Baseline	
	Ritodrine (%)	Terbutaline (%)
Systolic blood pressure	+12	+6
Diastolic blood pressure	−7	−7
Total peripheral resistance	−33	−23
Cardiac output	+50	52
Heart rate	+33	+28
Stroke volume	+20	+15

dial oxygen balance. A reduction of pressure work by the myocardium and better coronary perfusion may be offset by an increase in inotropic or chronotropic myocardial oxygen consumption.[240]

Tocolytics

The term *tocolytic* simply means to stop labor. Eighty-five percent of early neonatal deaths that are not related to lethal abnormalities are associated with premature labor.[241] Various pharmacologic agents have been used to (1) decrease stimulus to the myometrium (alcohol), or (2) prevent myometrial response to stimuli. Drugs belonging to the latter category include opioids, magnesium sulfate, prostaglandin inhibitors, and calcium channel inhibitors. Beta agonists have now become the focus of research in this area. The principal action of these drugs is to stimulate beta$_2$ receptors of the myometrium and produce relaxation (see Table 14-5).[242]

Metaproterenol and isoxsuprine were the first beta agonists to be used successfully. Unfortunately, these drugs are equipotent beta$_1$ and beta$_2$ agonists, and the side-effects of tachycardia and hypotension were unacceptable.[243] A second generation of beta-adrenergic drugs were applied in which the predominant action is beta$_2$. Ritodrine and terbutaline are receiving widespread use as tocolytic agents because of their predominant beta$_2$ agonism, which minimizes the undesirable beta$_1$ effects. Ritodrine is the only beta agonist tocolytic currently approved in the United States. It was specifically synthesized for this purpose and is structurally related to epinephrine.

All beta-agonist tocolytic agents have both beta$_1$ and beta$_2$ properties but in different proportions. The circulatory effects vary from one drug to another, depending on the degree of beta$_1$ stimulation. Table 14-18 compares the beta$_1$ cardiovascular effects of ritodrine and terbutaline while being used as tocolytics in humans. The side-effects of these drugs may result in serious consequences. Predictable complications in pregnant women include hyperglycemia with resultant hypokalemia (see Table 14-5).[50] All manner of cardiac dysrhythmias have been described, including ischemia and chest pain. The occurrence of pulmonary edema following the use of beta agonist tocolytics with and without corticosteroids has been described, although the mechanism is not clear.[244,245] Table 14-19 outlines contraindications for the use of beta agents for inhibiting labor.[246]

Nonadrenergic Sympathomimetic Agents. Table 14-4 classifies the drugs that mimic the SNS into two broad categories, adrenergic or nonadrenergic. Adrenergic agonists exert their action through adrenergic receptors by direct stimulation or indirectly *via* release of NE. Adrenergic agonists may

TABLE 14-19. Contraindications for Beta Tocolytic Therapy

Eclampsia or severe pre-eclampsia
Intrauterine infection
Maternal hyperthyroidism
Maternal cardiac disease
Uncontrolled maternal diabetes mellitus
Significant vaginal bleeding
Severe anemia or hypovolemia
Fetal anomaly incompatible with extrauterine life
Death *in utero*

be catecholamines or noncatecholamines by chemical configuration. Nonadrenergic sympathomimetic drugs also act indirectly by influencing the cAMP-calcium cascade, exclusive of the receptors (see Fig. 14-15). The function of the second messenger (cAMP) and the third messenger (Ca^{2+}) nearly always goes together.[120,121,247] This concept reinforces the recent appreciation of the homogeneity of action of a wide variety of drugs previously thought to be unrelated. Sympathomimetics have more pharmacologic similarities than differences.

Xanthines. The clinically important xanthine is theophylline-ethylenediamine (aminophylline).[210] Caffeine is a socially important xanthine. Aminophylline has been the mainstay in the treatment of asthma and bronchospasm since 1902 because of its strong beta$_2$ mimetic effect. Epinephrine, isoproterenol, and ephedrine are used to treat asthma for the same reason. Levels of cAMP in the cell are governed by a magnesium-dependent phosphodiesterase (see Fig. 14-15). This enzyme catalyzes the second messenger 3'5' cAMP to the less active 5' cAMP. Three major phosphodiesterase enzymes have been discovered that have been designated as PDE I, PDE II, and PDE III.[248] The xanthines are nonspecific phosphodiesterase inhibitors that interact with all three types. Inhibition of phosphodiesterase results in increased levels of cAMP and beta response (Fig. 14-15). Increases in cAMP by this mechanism are important when reviewing the many complicated interactions of the xanthines in the clinical setting.

Catecholamines influence the accumulation of cAMP by activating adenyl cyclase. Increased catecholamine levels, combined with the xanthines, may lead to synergistic adrenergic activity by increasing production and reducing breakdown of cAMP. Cardiac dysrhythmias are common in such circumstances and are further potentiated during general anesthesia with halothane.[249] Serious cardiac dysrhythmias and arrest have been produced with this combination when it has not been carefully controlled.

Intravenous aminophylline produces an increase in cardiac output as a result of its positive inotropic and chronotropic effects. It also reduces afterload by its beta$_2$ vasodilating effect.[217] The cardiac stimulating effects are still manifest in the presence of beta blockade because the xanthines are not receptor-dependent for their agonism. Thus, they may be temporarily useful in those situations where excessive beta blockade has been produced.[50] The inotropic effects are short-lived, lasting 20–30 minutes. Care must be taken during infusion, because common side-effects include hypotension and dysrhythmias. Seizures have also been reported.[249]

Phosphodiesterase Inhibitors. A new group of drugs has been developed that have pharmacologic properties approaching the characteristics of the ideal inotropic agent (see Table 14-15).[205] They do not rely on stimulation of beta and/or alpha receptors. They are the product of a search for a nonglycosidic, noncatecholamine inotropic agent. These drugs combine positive inotropism with vasodilator activity; like the xanthines, they are phosphodiesterase inhibitors but differ in that they selectively inhibit PDE III.[248] PDE I and II hydrolyze all cyclic nucleotides, whereas PDE III acts specifically on cAMP. The PDE III inhibitors apparently interact with PDE III at the cell membrane and impede the breakdown of cAMP.[250] cAMP levels increase and protein kinases are activated to promote phosphorylation of the sarcoplasmic reticulum in a cascade manner similar to the effects of adrenergic drugs. In cardiac muscle, phosphorylation increases the slow inward movement of calcium current, promoting increased intracellular calcium stores. Thus, inotropism increases. In vascular smooth muscle, increased cAMP activity accounts for the vasodilation, decreased peripheral vascular resistance, and lusitropism. Amrinone, like nitroprusside and nitroglycerin, promotes diastolic relaxation, which promotes ventricular filling.[185,251]

A variety of phosphodiesterase inhibitors are undergoing clinical trials.[251,252] The relative contribution of inotropism and vasodilation differs with each. Amrinone is the only phosphodiesterase inhibitor released for clinical use in the United States. It is the prototypical PDE III inhibitor. The degree of hemodynamic effect of these drugs depends on the dose, degree of inotropic reserve, and state of cAMP depletion.

AMRINONE. Amrinone is a bipyridine derivative that produces mild inotropic activity and strong vasodilatory effects. The characteristics of amrinone, compared with those of the ideal inotropic agent (see Fig. 14-24 and Table 14-15), rank it very near the ideal drug. It is the first oral inotrope available since the introduction of digitalis.[250,251] However, it is not currently prescribed in its oral form. Studies of single-dose and short-term oral and intravenous amrinone show dose-related improvements at rest in the cardiac index and the left ventricular stroke index (40–80% increase); left ventricular end-diastolic pressure (40% decrease); pulmonary capillary wedge pressure (16–44% decrease); pulmonary artery pressure (17–33% decrease); right atrial pressure (16–44% decrease); left ventricular ejection fraction (50% increase); and systemic vascular resistance (23–50% decrease). Significantly, heart rate and mean arterial pressure are not affected. Hemodynamic improvement is also noted when amrinone is used in combination with hydralazine. The improvement is greater than with either drug alone.[238] Peak response with an intravenous dose occurs after 5 minutes and reveals no evidence of tolerance over short-term trials (24 hours); it is compatible with other adrenergic agonists. It is an effective inotropic agent in patients receiving beta blockers. Its efficacy in the patient who has been digitalized has been demonstrated.

Intravenous amrinone therapy should be initiated with a 0.75 μg·kg^{-1} bolus given over 2–3 minutes. It is continued with a maintenance infusion of 5–10 μg·kg^{-1}·min^{-1}, adjusted by hemodynamic monitoring. An additional bolus dose of 0.75 μg·kg^{-1} may be given 30 minutes after initiation of therapy. Care must be taken not to give the bolus too quickly because sudden decreases in peripheral vascular resistance may occur and result in severe hypotension. Hypotension is not a major clinical problem with appropriate monitoring of ventricular filling pressures. The infusion should not exceed a total daily dose of 10 μg·kg^{-1}, including the bolus doses. Amrinone has the same range of infusion rates as dopamine and dobutamine, and dose calculation follows the "rule of six" described in Table 14-17.

Amrinone has two uncommon side-effects. Dose-related thrombocytopenia occurs in some patients taking long-term oral medication. This usually responds to dose reduction. Acute intravenous amrinone has not produced thrombocytopenia.[252–255] Centrilobular hepatic necrosis occurs in dogs given high doses of amrinone for periods exceeding 3 months. There is no evidence of such an effect in humans, but the implications of using halothane in a patient on amrinone are obvious. If the side-effects do not prove troublesome, this will be a valuable drug. It has a therapeutic index of approximately 100:1 as compared with 1.2:1 with the digitalis glycosides.

MILRINONE. Milrinone is an experimental bipyridine inotropic agent that is a derivative of amrinone.[256] It has nearly 20 times the inotropic potency of the parent compound. Milrinone is active both intravenously and orally and has beneficial short-term hemodynamic effects in patients with severe refractory congestive heart failure. Improvement of cardiac output appears to result from a combination of enhanced myocardial contractility and peripheral vasodilation. Treatment with oral milrinone for up to 11 months has been effective and well tolerated without evidence of fever, thrombocytopenia, or gastrointestinal effects. However, clinical efficacy in humans remains in question.

ENOXIMONE. Enoximone is a newer PDE III inhibitor that has proved beneficial in patients suffering from severely impaired myocardial function.[257] Enoximone is an imidazole derivative structurally unrelated to digitalis, catecholamines, or amrinone. It has not been implicated in platelet compromise. Its hemodynamic effects are similar to those produced by amrinone. It appears to be a more potent inotropic agent than amrinone, whose inotropic effect has been questioned. It produced pulmonary and systemic arteriolar vasodilation and can thus be classified as an inodilator. Heart rate has not been affected in the trial studies now under way. Any increase in myocardial oxygen consumption (MVo_2) by the increase in inotropism is countered by a decrease in afterload and reduced ventricular size.

Forskolin and BAY K 8644. Forskolin is an experimental drug with actions similar to those of the PDE inhibitors.[258,259] It produces marked positive inotropic and vasodilatory properties *in vitro* and *in vivo*. Forskolin acts directly on the catalytic unit of adenyl cyclase to cause stimulation of this enzyme. This results in increases in cardiac cAMP production, calcium influx into the myocardium, and increased contractility.

BAY K 8644 is an experimental drug that promotes calcium influx and increased myocardial contractility.[258,259] Unfortunately, it also promotes peripheral and coronary artery vasoconstriction. BAY K 8644, a calcium agonist, is structurally similar to nifedipine, a calcium-entry blocker.

Glucagon. Glucagon is a single-chain polypeptide of 29 amino acids that is secreted by pancreas alpha cells in response to hypoglycemia. The liver and kidney are responsible for its degradation. Known effects of this hormone in humans include[210,217,260]

1. Inhibition of gastric motility.
2. Enhanced urinary excretion of inorganic electrolytes.
3. Increased insulin secretion.
4. Hepatic glycogenolysis and gluconeogenesis.
5. Anorexia.
6. Inotropic and chronotropic cardiac effects.

Little attention was given to glucagon until 1968, when it was demonstrated to produce positive inotropic and chronotropic effects in the canine heart. Glucagon enhances the activation of adenyl cyclase in a manner similar to that of NE, epinephrine, and isoproterenol, but with an important difference. These cardiac actions of glucagon are not blocked by beta blockade or catecholamine depletion. Glucagon, in contrast to the xanthines, rarely causes dysrhythmias, even in the face of ischemic heart disease, hypokalemia, and digitalis toxicity. Glucagon may, in fact, possess antidysrhythmic activity in digitalis toxicity because it has been shown to enhance atrioventricular nodal conduction in patients with varying degrees of atrioventricular block. It should be used carefully in patients with atrial fibrillation. In humans, an intravenous dose of 1–5 mg of glucagon increases cardiac index, mean arterial pressure, and ventricular contractility, even in the presence of digitalis therapy.

Glucagon can be mixed in 5% dextrose in water and is stable for long periods. After a bolus dose, its action dissipates in approximately 30 minutes. A continuous infusion of 5 $\mu g \cdot kg^{-1} \cdot min^{-1}$ is augmented by an initial bolus of 50 $\mu g \cdot kg^{-1}$. Onset of action occurs in 1–3 minutes and peaks at 10–15 minutes.

Nausea and vomiting are common side-effects in the awake patient, especially following a bolus dose. Hypokalemia, hypoglycemia, and hyperglycemia are also seen. Despite the obvious benefits of glucagon in cardiac patients, its use has not become popular.[258] This may be related to its high cost and the multiple metabolic and physiologic effects that are common after its administration.

This pancreatic hormone may be of benefit when more conventional approaches have proved refractory in the following settings: (1) low cardiac output syndrome following cardiopulmonary bypass; (2) low cardiac output syndrome with myocardial infarction; (3) chronic congestive heart failure; and (4) excessive beta-adrenergic blockade.

Digitalis Glycosides. The most important actions of the digitalis glycosides are those affecting myocardial contractility, conduction, and rhythm. The glycoside most likely to be used by the anesthesiologist is digoxin.

The principal uses of digoxin are for the treatment of congestive heart failure and to control supraventricular cardiac dysrhythmias such as atrial fibrillation. Digoxin is one of the few positive inotropes that does not increase heart rate. Digoxin enhances myocardial inotropism and automaticity but slows impulse propagation through the conduction tissues.[261] Despite nearly two centuries of use, its mechanism of action is only modestly certain. Digitalis reciprocally facilitates calcium entry into the myocardial cell by blocking the $Na^+ K^+$ adenosine triphosphatese pump.[262] This calcium influx may account for its positive inotropic action because this inotropic response is not catecholamine– or beta receptor–dependent and is therefore effective in patients taking beta blocking drugs. The inhibition of this enzyme transport mechanism also results in a net K^+ loss from the myocardial cell. This contributes to digitalis toxicity with hypokalemia. Calcium potentiates the toxic effects of digitalis. Extreme caution should be observed when calcium is given to a patient taking digitalis or when digitalis administration is contemplated in the patient with hypercalcemia.

A common indication for the glycosides is in the chronic management of cardiac tachydysrhythmias. Cardiac dysrhythmias are, paradoxically, their most common side-effect. Synchrony of the cardiac beat is an important determinant of cardiac output, and digoxin can be beneficial when heart failure is caused by a tachydysrhythmia, even in ischemic myocardial disease. However, the use of beta or calcium channel blockers is increasing in this regard because they both reduce overall myocardial oxygen consumption.

The positive inotropic effects of digoxin are potentially beneficial in selected cases of the low cardiac output syndrome. Digoxin produces a dose-related increase in contractility in both normal and failing hearts. Limits are imposed on the upper reaches of inotropism by the development of serious dysrhythmias.

Confusion has arisen in the past about whether digitalis increases or decreases myocardial oxygen consumption. This was based on the observation that the increased ino-

tropism of digoxin increases MVo_2 in patients with normal hearts but decreases it in patients with heart failure. The tension developed within the ventricular wall is a prime determinant of oxygen consumption. By augmenting contractility, wall tension and MVo_2 at any given afterload will be decreased, with a reduction in ventricular radius and heart rate.[229,240] This may underlie the clinical observation that angina is often decreased by digoxin in patients with cardiomegaly, whereas angina may be markedly increased by digitalis in patients with ischemic disease without cardiomegaly.

Digitalis tends to increase the tone of the peripheral resistance vessels in normal subjects by a direct vasoconstrictor effect. Untreated congestive heart failure is accompanied by high peripheral vascular resistance owing to compensatory SNS activation. Successful treatment with digitalis usually reduces resistance as increased contractility improves cardiac output. This is the result of SNS release associated with improved cardiac function. Caution must be exercised, however, in giving intravenous digoxin or ouabain in a setting in which an increase in afterload would be deleterious. An immediate peripheral vasoconstrictor effect can occur, producing a transient worsening of congestive heart failure. Inconsistent hemodynamic benefit has occurred with digitalis in congestive heart failure following myocardial infarction. It has been of no benefit in cardiogenic shock and has proved potentially injurious in patients with uncomplicated myocardial infarction because of its vasoconstrictive properties and effects on myocardial oxygen consumption in the absence of cardiomegaly.

Digoxin is of potential value in patients with signs and symptoms of congestive heart failure caused by ischemic, valvular, hypertensive, and congenital heart disease.[230] Patients with cardiomyopathies and cor pulmonale may also benefit. Care must be taken to rule out conditions in which the use of digitalis is of no benefit and is potentially harmful. These include mitral stenosis with normal sinus rhythm and constrictive pericarditis with tamponade. Signs and symptoms of idiopathic hypertrophic subaortic stenosis are often exacerbated by digitalis. With increased strength of contraction, the muscular obstruction can be markedly increased. The same is true for the use of digitalis in patients with infundibular pulmonic stenosis, as occurs with tetralogy of Fallot. Any augmentation of contractility may further reduce an already diminished pulmonary blood flow. Beware of digitalis toxic reactions in the older age group and in patients suffering from arterial hypoxemia, acidosis, renal compromise, hypothyroidism, hypokalemia, or hypomagnesemia as well as in patients receiving quinidine or calcium channel blockers.

The issue of prophylactic digitalization of patients with diminished cardiac reserve who are about to undergo major surgical procedures remains controversial.[217,261] Indications for preoperative digitalis in which the prophylactic administration of digoxin should be considered include (1) previous heart failure, (2) increased heart size, (3) coronary flow disturbances according to electrocardiogram, (4) age over 60 years, (5) age over 50 years before lung surgery, (6) anticipated massive blood loss, (7) atrial flutter or fibrillation, (8) cardiovascular surgery, and (9) rheumatic valvular lesions.

When entertaining the possibility of perioperative digitalis administration, the following points must be considered:[31]

1. Myocardial oxygen balance is threatened in the nonfailing, nondilated heart.
2. The therapeutic-to-toxic ratio of digitalis is narrow.

3. Inotropic drugs that are less toxic and may be stopped immediately are readily available.
4. Verapamil or beta blockers are more efficacious for supraventricular tachydysrhythmias not initiated by heart failure.
5. Digitalis may cause serious dysrhythmias in the unstable patient.
6. Serum potassium concentrations may fluctuate in the surgical patient who is critically ill.
7. Any cardiac dysrhythmias that occur in the presence of digitalis must be considered a toxic phenomenon.
8. Digitalis-induced cardiac dysrhythmias are difficult to treat.
9. Renal compromise will result in toxic effects with standard maintenance doses.
10. Cardioversion may be dangerous after digitalis administration.
11. After initiation of digitalis therapy, the administration of alternative drugs becomes more complicated.

Digitalization is not an all or none state, and improved contractility is dose-related. Even a low dose will strengthen myocardial contractility. Within 10 minutes following an intravenous injection of 0.25–1.0 mg of digoxin, a marked improvement in presystolic ejection period can be seen. Once the desired effect has been gained, it is not necessary to continue administering the drug just because a digitalizing dose has not been reached. The goal, therefore, is to correct heart failure with the minimum effective dose necessary. The amount of digitalis should be guided by the clinical improvement of the patient. Control of the ventricular response provides a relatively straightforward end point in patients with atrial flutter or atrial fibrillation. Toxic symptoms should be searched for when digitalis is administered for control of heart rate. Toxic concentrations of digoxin that produce serious dysrhythmias are usually higher than doses required for a substantial inotropic effect. When evaluating a patient for digitalis toxic effects, the useful maneuver of carotid sinus pressure can give some clue to potential digitalis excess. Cardiac rhythm disorders such as second-degree atrioventricular block, accelerated atrioventricular junctional rhythm, or bradycardia may emerge in response to carotid sinus stimulation before they occur spontaneously. In recent years there has been an increased effort to use serum assays in an effort to define end points for digitalis administration. Serum levels, however, may not correlate with heart rate, tissue-bound levels, or toxicity.

Calcium Salts. Ringer established the importance of calcium in cardiac contraction more than 150 years ago. It is of great importance in the genesis of the cardiac action potential and is the key to controlling intracellular energy storage and utilization. Movement of extracellular calcium across membranes also governs the function of uterine smooth muscle as well as the smooth muscle of the blood vessels. Only recently have we begun to appreciate the critical role that calcium plays in a wide spectrum of biologic processes, from coagulation to neuromuscular transmission. The sympathomimetic drugs promote the transmembrane influx of calcium, whereas the beta blockers and calcium channel blockers inhibit such movement.

Despite its molecular simplicity, calcium is one of the least understood drugs.[263] Calcium chloride is often part of the treatment of ventricular fibrillation, even though the published data to support this indication are scarce. There are data confirming its capability to initiate ventricular fibrillation in a manner similar to that of epinephrine. Al-

though many of the effects of epinephrine are mediated by calcium, the two drugs are clearly not identical. The fact that epinephrine can improve debrillation success by strengthening the fibrillatory pattern is the apparent basis for the use of calcium salts in this setting. This assumption has not been experimentally or clinically documented.[264] The American Heart Association has recently recommended against the use of calcium during cardiac arrest except when hyperkalemia, hypocalcemia, or calcium-entry inhibitor toxicity is present.[265]

Traditionally, calcium gluconate has been preferred in pediatric patients and calcium chloride in adult patients. Previous data held that calcium chloride produced consistently higher and more predictable levels of ionized calcium than an equivalent dose of the other preparations.[266] Recent studies have shown, however, that ionization of any of the preparations is immediate and equally effective.[267,268] Intravenous calcium appears effective for the transient reversal of hypotension thought to be the result of myocardial depression from the potent volatile anesthetic drugs.[269] Some clinicians feel that recurrent intraoperative hypotension response to calcium chloride may be an indication for the administration of digoxin. Calcium chloride is also given at the termination of cardiopulmonary bypass to offset the myocardial depression associated with hypothermic potassium cardioplegia.[217] The use of calcium salts is clearly indicated during rapid or massive transfusions of citrated blood.[270] Citrate binds calcium, and rapid infusion rates of citrated blood result in myocardial depression that is reversible by calcium.

Three forms of calcium salts are available: calcium chloride, calcium gluconate, and calcium gluceptate. Calcium chloride produces only transient (10–20 minutes) increases in cardiac output.[261] If inotropic effects are needed for a longer period of time, other inotropic agents should be selected. Bolus doses of 2–10 $\mu g \cdot kg^{-1}$ (1.5 $\mu g \cdot kg^{-1} \cdot min^{-1}$) of calcium chloride can produce moderate improvement in contractility. The rapid administration of calcium salts, if the heart is beating, can produce bradycardia and must be used cautiously in the patient who is digitalized because of the hazard of producing toxic effects.

Calcium gluceptate can be given in a dose of 5–7 ml (4.5–6.3 mEq) and calcium gluconate in a dose of 10–15 ml (4.8–7.2 mEq). These doses are approximately equivalent to that suggested for calcium chloride. Calcium gluconate is unstable and is no longer in frequent use. All of the calcium salts will precipitate as calcium carbonate if mixed with sodium bicarbonate.

Antidepressant Drugs. *Monoamine Oxidase Inhibitors.* Monoamine oxidase inhibitors (MAOIs) and the tricyclic antidepressants are used to treat psychotic depression. These drugs are not used in the practice of anesthesia but are a source of potentially serious interactions in patients who are taking them chronically.

MAOIs (Table 14-20) block the oxidative deamination of endogenous catecholamines into inactive vanillylmandelic acid (see Fig. 14-12). They do not inhibit synthesis.[271] Thus, blockade of monoamine oxidase would produce an accumulation of NE, epinephrine, dopamine, and 5-hydroxylryptamine in adrenergically active tissues, including the brain. Alleviation of depression may be related to elevations of the endogenous catecholamines. Overdose with MAOIs is expressed as SNS hyperactivity. They may produce agitation, hallucinations, hyperpyrexia, convulsions, hypertension, and hypotension. Orthostatic hypotension is a common complaint in patients taking MAOIs.[272]

TABLE 14-20. Antidepressant Drugs	
Nonproprietary Name	**Trade Name**
Monoamine Oxidase Inhibitors	
Isocarboxazid	Marplan
Pargyline	Eutonyl
Phenelzine	Nardil
Tranylcypromine	Parnate
Tricyclic Antidepressants	
Imipramine	Imavate, Janimine, Presamine, SK-Pramine, Tofranil
Desipramine	Norpramin, Pertofrane
Amitriptyline	Amitril, Elavil, Endep
Nortriptyline	Aventyl, Pamelor
Doxepin	Adapin, Sinequan
Protriptyline	Vivactil
Amoxapine	Asendin
Maprotiline	Ludiomil
Nontricyclics	
Trazodone	Desyrel
Fluoxetine	Prozac
Bupropion	Wellbutrin

The action of sympathomimetic amines is potentiated in patients taking MAOIs. Indirect-acting sympathomimetics (ephedrine, tyramine) produce an exaggerated response as they trigger the release of accumulated catecholamines. Foods containing a high tyramine content such as cheese, red Italian wine, and pickled herring can also precipitate hypertensive crises.[272] SNS reflex stimulation is also intensified by tyramine. Meperidine has been reported to produce hypertensive crisis, convulsions, and coma with MAO inhibitors. Hepatotoxicity has been reported that does not seem to be related to dosage or duration of treatment. Its incidence is low but remains a factor in selecting anesthesia.

The MAOIs produce long-lasting, irreversible enzyme inhibition that is unrelated to duration of treatment. Regeneration of monoamine oxidase may, therefore, take weeks and has much the same effect on adrenergic metabolism as that of organophosphates on the cholinesterase system. MAOIs are known to intensify CNS depression caused by ethanol, analgesics, and general anesthesia. The depressive mechanism is not known.

The anesthetic management of patients taking MAOIs remains controversial, although recent data question the need to discontinue them preoperatively. Current recommendations for management include discontinuation of the drugs for at least 2 weeks before surgery; however, this recommendation is not based on controlled studies but rather is the result of limited case reports that suggest potent drug interactions.[271,273-275] A small number of studies found few adverse effects in humans taking MAOIs given analgesics, opioid anesthesia, or regional blocks. However, opioids that cause release of catecholamines (meperidine) or histamine (morphine) should be avoided in these patients.

Symptoms of SNS overdose or interactions due to MAOIs can be treated effectively with alpha blockers, ganglionic blockers, or direct-acting vasodilators.

Tricyclic antidepressants should not be substituted for the MAOIs in the perioperative period. Adverse CNS interactions similar to those encountered with the indirect sympathomiometic amines have been reported. A 2-week wash-out period is recommended before introducing tricyclic antidepressants to a patient taking an MAOI.

Tricyclic Antidepressants. This group of antidepressant drugs is referred to as tricyclic antidepressants because of their structure. The important tricyclic antidepressants are listed in Table 14-20. These drugs have almost replaced the MAOIs because they cause fewer side-effects.[271] The manner in which the tricyclic antidepressants relieve depression is not clear, but all of these agents block uptake of NE into adrenergic nerve endings. Just as with the MAOIs, high doses of the tricyclic antidepressants can induce seizure activity that is responsive to diazepam.

There is a tendency for patients taking tricyclic antidepressants to develop tachycardia and cardiac dysrhythmias. This may be related to high concentrations of NE in cardiac tissues. Other reported cardiovascular effects have included orthostatic hypotension, myocardial infarction, and precipitation of congestive heart failure.[276] Imipramine may cause hypotension and bradycardia as a result of direct cardiac depression. Death from overdose of tricyclic antidepressants is usually due to cardiac failure or the development of cardiac dysrhythmias that are refractory to treatment. Tricyclic antidepressants can also cause a central anticholinergic syndrome which is responsive to physostigmine.

Neuroleptic drugs may potentiate the effects of tricyclic antidepressants by competition with metabolism in the liver. Chronic barbiturate use increases metabolism of the tricyclic antidepressants by microsomal enzyme induction. Other sedatives, however, potentiate the tricyclic antidepressants in a manner similar to that occurring with the MAOIs. Atropine also has an exaggerated effect because of the anticholinergic effect of tricyclic antidepressants. Prolonged sedation from thiopental has been reported. Ketamine may also be dangerous in patients taking tricyclic antidepressants by producing acute hypertension and cardiac dysrhythmias. Likewise, muscle relaxants that produce tachycardia (pancuronium, gallamine) have been observed to produce serious ventricular cardiac dysrhythmias in humans and dogs pretreated with imipramine.

Despite these serious interactions, discontinuation of these drugs before surgery is probably not necessary. The latency of onset of these drugs is from 2–5 weeks; however, the excretion of tricyclic antidepressants is rapid, with approximately 70% of a dose appearing in the urine during the first 72 hours. One might consider a discontinuation of the drug for 72 hours, but the risk of recurrent depression may be greater than that of any untoward drug reaction. The long latency period for resumption of treatment militates against interrupted treatment. A thorough knowledge of the possible drug interactions and autonomic countermeasures obviates postponement.

Adrenergic Antagonists

Alpha Antagonists. Drugs that bind selectively to alpha-adrenergic receptors block the action of endogenous catecholamines at effector sites and alter the autonomic response. The resultant effects may be ascribed to unopposed beta-adrenergic receptors and are dependent upon the prevailing adrenergic tone. In the vasculature, for example, the response to the alpha blocker phenoxybenzamine may vary over a wide range in a single vascular bed, depending on its intrinsic state of constriction. Vessels with higher initial tone have a greater response to alpha blockade. Classically, alpha blockers are defined as drugs that convert the vascular

TABLE 14-21. Alpha-Adrenergic Blocking Drugs

	Type of Antagonism	Selectivity
Phenoxybenzamine	Noncompetitive	alpha$_1$ > α_2
Phentolamine	Competitive	α_1 = α_2
Tolazoline	Competitive	α_1 = α_2
Prazosin	Competitive	α_1 >> α_2
Yohimbine	Competitive	α_2 >> α_1

response to epinephrine from constriction to vasodilation.[277] Prominent clinical effects of alpha blockers include hypotension, tachycardia, and miosis. Nasal stuffiness, diarrhea, and inhibition of ejaculation are common side-effects.

The alpha blockers may be classified according to binding characteristics (Table 14-21). Phenoxybenzamine is a drug that binds covalently to the receptors and produces an irreversible blockade. It is relatively nonspecific and has antagonistic activity at several other receptor types as well.[278] Phentolamine, tolazoline, and prazosin are characterized by reversible binding and antagonism.

There are also important differences between the individual drugs with regard to relative receptor specificity. As with the beta blockers, some show greater affinity for one subset of alpha receptors than another. Phenoxybenzamine, for example, is 100 times more potent on alpha$_1$ than alpha$_2$ receptors. Prazosin is also markedly specific for alpha$_1$ receptors, whereas phentolamine has nearly equal blocking activity on both subsets. Phentolamine, therefore, by blocking presynaptic inhibitory alpha$_2$ receptors, causes greater NE release from the presynaptic terminal. The tachycardia as well as the reflex response to hypotension seen commonly with phentolamine is thought to be secondary to this enhanced NE release.

Phenoxybenzamine. Phenoxybenzamine is a haloalkylamine with predominantly alpha$_1$ antagonist activity. Because of the noncompetitive nature of the block, as discussed above, it has a relatively long duration of 24 hours. In the past it was the drug of choice for treating patients with pheochromocytoma in preparation for surgery. It has now been replaced with shorter-acting, more specific drugs such as phentolamine.

Phentolamine. Phentolamine is an imidazoline, which is a competitive antagonist at alpha$_1$ and alpha$_2$ receptors. The imidazolines also have some antihistaminic and cholinomimetic activity. The cholinomimetic activity may result in abdominal cramping and diarrhea, both of which are blocked by atropine. Tachycardia and hypotension are also common side-effects.[277] It also is commonly used in the diagnosis and treatment of pheochromocytoma. It is usually given in 2–5-mg iv boluses until adequate control of blood pressure is obtained.

Tolazoline. Tolazoline is also an imidazoline derivative and acts like phentolamine. It is less potent on peripheral alpha receptors, however, and some of its vasodilatory action has been ascribed to histamine-like activity. It effectively decreases pulmonary vascular resistance and has been used in neonates with respiratory distress syndrome to improve pulmonary blood flow. The effects, however, were detrimental and inconsistent.[279,280]

Prazosin. Prazosin is a piperazine derivative that has relative selectivity for alpha$_1$ receptors and, as a result, does not cause the tachycardia seen with phentolamine. Cardiovascular effects include decreased peripheral vascular resistance and venous return with little change in heart rate or cardiac output. When used alone, it is not remarkably effective in treatment of essential hypertension resulting from fluid retention. When combined with a diuretic, however, it is an effective antihypertensive drug. It should not be used with clonidine or alpha-methyldopa (discussed below), as it appears to decrease their effectiveness. Prazosin also may cause bronchodilation, and it decreases serum cholesterol and triglyceride levels.[281]

Yohimbine. Yohimbine is an alpha$_2$ antagonist (see Table 14-5). It blocks the action of clonidine on presynaptic receptors and increases NE release. It is mostly used as a research tool but has been used in the treatment of impotence and orthostatic hypotension.[282]

Beta Antagonists. The use of beta blocking drugs has markedly escalated in the last 10 years as more indications for their use have been found and more compounds have been developed.[283] They are among the most common drugs used in the treatment of cardiovascular disease, and frequently the anesthesiologist must deal with their effects and side-effects during anesthesia. There are now a variety of drugs available with beta blocking activity that may be distinguished by differing pharmacokinetic and pharmacodynamic characteristics.[284,285] Examples of drugs available for clinical use in the United States and their characteristics are listed in Table 14-22. Their structures are shown in Figure 14-28.

Several of these drugs are marketed on the basis of cardioselectivity, *i.e.*, antagonist activity is greater at beta$_1$ than beta$_2$ receptors in an isolated muscle preparation. Theoretically, this implies that these agents would be of greater benefit in treatment of patients with obstructive airway disease, diabetes mellitus, or peripheral vascular disease.[286] The practitioner must keep in mind, however, that this means *relative selectivity*, not *specificity*, and that beta blocking effects may be seen in all tissues if higher blood levels are reached (see Fig. 14-13). Clinical studies have not shown greater effectiveness of cardioselective beta blockers in treatment of hypertension[287] or diabetes mellitus,[288] and their relative effectiveness in the case of peripheral vascular disease is still controversial.[286]

The use of beta$_1$ selective blockers in patients with obstructive airway disease is also controversial. The degree of bronchoreactivity is an important consideration in their use. Patients with reactive airway disease may develop serious reductions in ventilatory function even with beta$_1$ selective drugs.[289] No beta blocker can be considered safe in patients with obstructive airway disease, and other types of drugs are available for treatment of supraventricular arrhythmias and hypertension.

Some beta antagonists have partial agonist activity at low doses. This is referred to as intrinsic sympathomimetic activity. Drugs with intrinsic sympathomimetic activity decrease resting heart rate less than those without it.[290] In the presence of similar degrees of beta blockade, however, all beta blockers blunt exercise-induced increases in heart rate to a similar extent.[288] The clinical relevance of this is unclear, but it has been implied that intrinsic sympathomimetic activity would be advantageous in patients treated with nonselective beta blockers who are troubled by brady-

TABLE 14-22. Beta-Adrenergic Blocking Drugs

Drug	Trade Name	Relative Beta₁ Selectivity	Membrane Stabilizing Activity	Intrinsic Sympatho-mimetic Activity	Plasma Half-life (H)	Oral Availability %	Lipid Solubility	Elimination	Preparations
Propranolol	Inderal	0	+	0	3–4	36	+ + +	Hepatic	Oral, iv
Nadolol	Cogard	0	0	0	14–24	34	0	Renal	Oral
Timolol	Blocadren	0	0	0	4–5	50	+	Hepatic and renal	Oral, eye drops
Pindolol	Visken	0	+	+ +	3–4	86	+	Hepatic and renal	Oral
Esmolol	Brevibloc	+ +	0	0	0–16	—	?	RBC esterase	iv
Acebutolol	Sectral	+	+	+	3–4	37*	0	Hepatic*	Oral
Atenolol	Tenormin	+ +	0	0	6–9	57	0	Renal	Oral
Metoprolol	Lopressor	+ +	0	0	3–4	38	+	Hepatic	Oral
Betaxolol	Kerlone	+ + +	+	0	14–22	89	0	Hepatic*	Oral
Penbutolol	Levatol	0	0	+	5	85	0	Hepatic*	Oral
Carteolol	Cartrol	0	0	+	6	85	0	Renal	Oral

* Primarily hepatic, but active metabolites are formed that must be renally excreted.

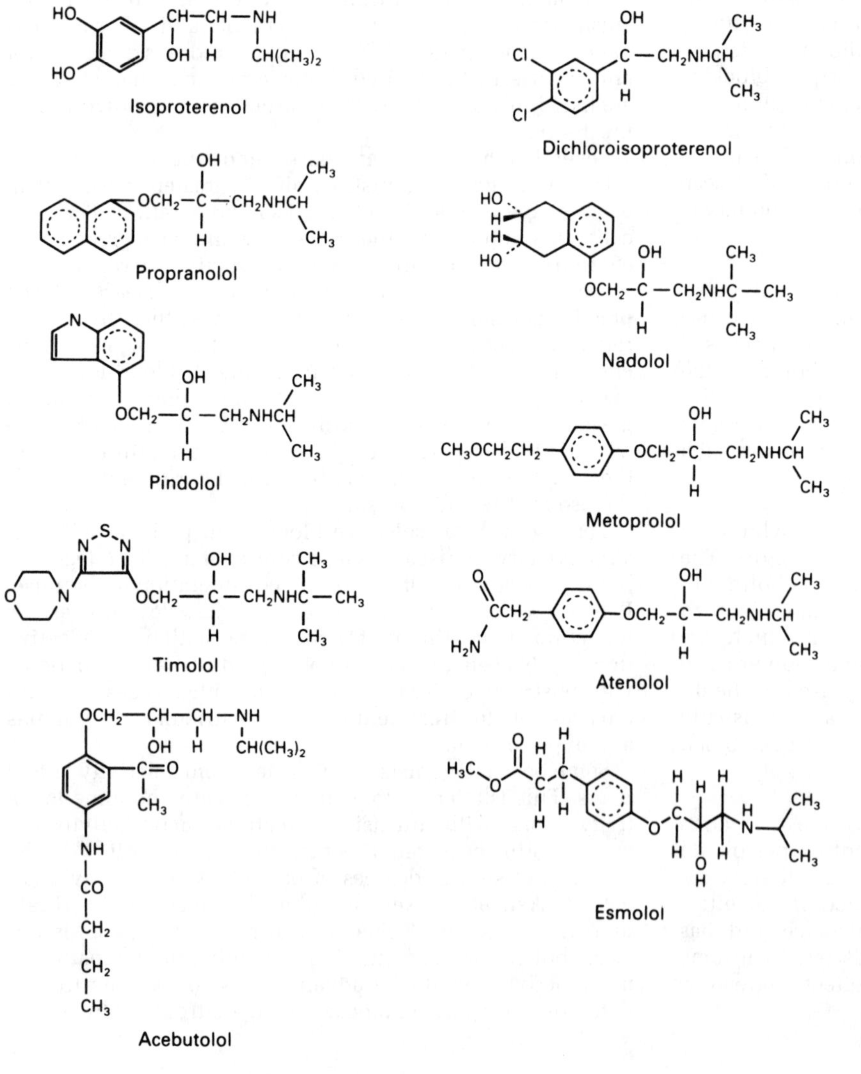

Figure 14-28. The structures of the commonly used beta blockers are compared with the pure beta agonist, isoproterenol, and the partial agonist, dichloroisoproterenol.

cardia or worsening ventricular failure.[291] A distinct advantage to intrinsic sympathomimetic activity in beta blockers has not been clearly shown in clinical studies.

Several of the beta blockers listed in Table 14-22 also have a local anesthetic-like effect on myocellular membranes at high doses. This effect is similar to that of quinidine in that phase 0 of the cardiac action potential is depressed, slowing conduction. This membrane-stabilizing activity is caused by the *d-isomer*, whereas the *l-isomer* is responsible for beta blocking activity. The clinical significance of membrane-stabilizing activity is also unclear.[285]

Propranolol. Propranolol is the prototype beta blocking drug against which all others are compared. It is nonselective and has no intrinsic sympathomimetic activity but does have membrane-stabilizing activity at higher doses. It is available in both iv and oral forms. It is highly lipophilic and is metabolized by the liver to more water-soluble metabolites, one of which, 17-OH propranolol, has weak beta blocking activity. There is a significant first-pass effect by the liver after oral administration of the drug. It is highly protein-bound, and the free drug level may be altered by other highly bound drugs. The elimination half-life is approximately 4 hours but the pharmacologic half-life is around 10 hours.

Hemodynamic effects include decreased heart rate and contractility. The major factors contributing to the decrease in blood pressure by propranolol are decreased cardiac output and renin release. Systemic vascular resistance may increase upon acute administration owing to blockade of beta$_2$-receptors in the peripheral vasculature. With chronic administration, however, peripheral vascular resistance decreases. This is thought to be secondary to decreased renin release and, possibly, decreased central SNS outflow.[282,292] Complications with the use of propranolol include bradycardia, heart block, worsening of congestive heart failure, bronchospasm, and sedation. During anesthesia with halothane, it may cause severe bradydysrhythmias.

Nadolol. Nadolol is a noncardioselective beta blocker with no membrane-stabilizing activity or intrinsic sympathomimetic activity. It is approximately equipotent to propranolol, but its effects are prolonged owing to slower elimination. It is relatively lipid-insoluble and is excreted 70% unchanged in urine and 20% in the feces. The elimination half-life is 24 hours. Because it is lipid-insoluble, it does not cross the blood-brain barrier, and sedation is less of a problem than with propranolol. Hemodynamic effects are the same as for propranolol. The main advantage of the drug is the capability for once per day dosing.

Timolol. Timolol is also noncardioselective with little intrinsic sympathomimetic activity and no membrane-stabilizing activity. It is the only beta blocker used as the *l*-isomer rather than the racemic mixture. It is five to ten times as potent as propranolol. Hepatic metabolism accounts for approximately 66% of its elimination, and another 20% is found unchanged in the urine. The elimination half-life is 5.6 hours, and the pharmacologic half-life is approximately 15 hours. It was first used topically for treatment of glaucoma but is now used in hypertension and has been shown to decrease the risk of reinfarction and death following myocardial infarction.[293] Its hemodynamic effects and side-effects are similar to those of other beta blockers. The anesthesiologist should also be aware that timolol eye drops may be absorbed systemically and cause bradycardia

and hypotension that are refractory to treatment with atropine.[294]

Pindolol. Pindolol is a nonselective beta blocker with membrane-stabilizing activity and intrinsic sympathomimetic activity. It is 10–40 times as potent as propranolol. It is lipid-soluble and metabolized by the liver but not as avidly extracted; therefore, its biologic availability after oral administration is more predictable. It is excreted 40% unchanged in the urine. The elimination half-life is 3.5 hours. It is useful in the treatment of angina pectoris, cardiac dysrhythmias, and hypertension. As discussed above, the clinical usefulness of the intrinsic sympathomimetic activity property is unclear.

Oxprenolol. Oxprenolol is similar to pindolol except for less intrinsic sympathomimetic activity and lower potency.

Metoprolol. Metoprolol is a relatively selective beta$_1$ blocking drug with beta$_2$ blocking effects at moderate and high doses. It has neither intrinsic sympathomimetic activity nor membrane-stabilizing activity. It has a possible advantage in patients with reactive airway disease at oral doses up to 100 mg·day^{-1}.[295] In this case, it should probably be used with a beta$_2$ mimetic drug. It is mostly metabolized in the liver, with only about 5% excreted unchanged in the urine. The elimination half-life is 3.5 hours. It has recently become available in iv as well as oral form; therefore it may be useful during anesthesia.

Atenolol. Atenolol is similar to metoprolol in that it is relatively cardioselective and has no intrinsic sympathomimetic activity or membrane-stabilizing activity. It is less lipophilic, however, and is eliminated primarily by renal excretion. The elimination half-life is 6–7 hours. The lack of first-pass metabolism results in more predictable blood levels after oral dosing.

Acebutolol. Acebutolol is a cardioselective beta blocker with intrinsic sympathomimetic activity and membrane-stabilizing activity.[296] It is metabolized in the liver and is subject to extensive first-pass metabolism. The primary metabolite is diacetolol (Fig. 14-29), which has a pharmacologic profile similar to that of the parent drug and is excreted renally.[297] The pharmacologic effects of the drug, therefore, are dependent on both hepatic transformation and renal excretion. The elimination half-life of acebutolol is 3–4 hours and of diacetolol 8–13 hours. Elimination is prolonged in the elderly and patients with renal disease. Acebutolol, like pindolol, has intrinsic sympathetic activity that makes it more advantageous than the other beta blockers in patients with bradydysrhythmias or myocardial failure.

Esmolol. Esmolol is a recently released beta blocker that has several uses in the perioperative period.[298-303] The most unique feature of the drug is the ester function incorporated into the phenoxypropanolamine structure. This allows for rapid degradation by esterases in the red blood cells and a resultant pharmacologic half-life of 10–20 minutes.[304]

Esmolol is cardioselective and appears to have little effect on bronchial or vascular tone at doses that decrease heart rate in humans. It has been used successfully in low doses in patients with asthma,[305] but caution is again advised when using beta blockers in these patients.[286]

Esmolol is metabolized rapidly in the blood by an esterase located in the red blood cell cytoplasm. It is different from

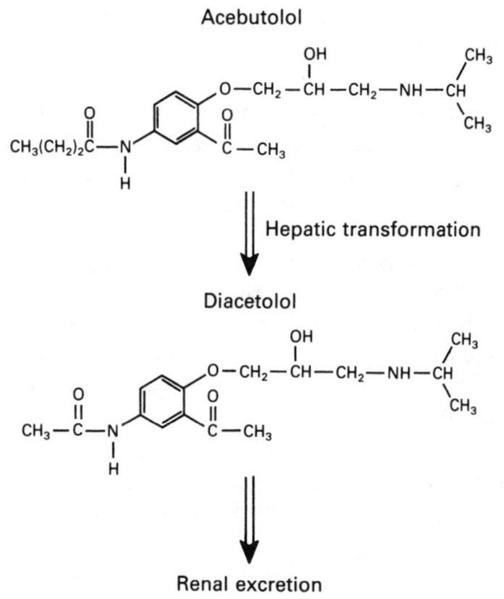

Acebutolol

Figure 14-29. Acebutolol is metabolized in the liver to diacetolol, which has a potency similar to that of the parent drug. Diacetolol is eliminated by renal excretion. The pharmacologic half-life of acebutolol, therefore, depends on both hepatic and renal function.

the plasma cholinesterase and is not inhibited to a significant degree by physostigmine or echothiophate but is markedly inhibited by sodium fluoride. There are no apparent important clinical interactions between esmolol and other ester-containing drugs. At the highest infusion rates (500 $\mu g \cdot kg \cdot min^{-1}$), esmolol does not prolong neuromuscular blockade by succinylcholine.[304]

Esmolol has proven to be quite useful in the perioperative period because of its capability to be administered intravenously and its short half-life.[306] This feature permits a trial of beta blockade in doubtful situations. Esmolol has been shown to blunt the response to intubation of the trachea[298,303] and is moderately effective in treating postoperative hypertension.[298,299] Most reported studies in humans have used doses of 50–500 $\mu g \cdot kg^{-1} \cdot min^{-1}$. The most beneficial approach seems to be a loading dose of 500 $\mu g \cdot kg \cdot min$, followed by continuous infusion of 50–300 $\mu g \cdot kg \cdot min$. Peak blockade appears to occur within 5 minutes. On discontinuation of the infusion, serum levels decline with an elimination half-life of 9 minutes. The heart rate response to isoproterenol returns to control in 20 minutes.

Betaxolol. Betaxolol hydrochloride is a $beta_1$ selective (cardioselective) adrenergic receptor antagonist and is freely soluble in water. It has weak membrane-stabilizing activity and no intrinsic sympathomimetic (partial agonist) activity. The preferential effect on $beta_1$ receptors is not absolute. Some $beta_2$ inhibitory activity can be expected in the bronchial and vascular musculature at higher doses. Absorption of an oral dose is complete, with an absolute bioavailability of 90% that is unaffected by ingestion of food or alcohol. The mean elimination half-life is from 14–22 hours. It is eliminated primarily by the liver but secondarily through the kidneys. Betaxolol is indicated in the management of hypertension. It may be used alone or concomitantly with other antihypertensive agents.

Penbutolol. Penbutolol is a synthetic beta receptor antagonist for oral administration. It is a nonselective beta receptor antagonist with some intrinsic sympathomimetic activity. Penbutolol does not appear to have any membrane-stabilizing properties, as does propranolol. Plasma elimina-

tion half-life is 5 hours in normal subjects. Ninety percent of radioactive penbutolol was found to be excreted in the urine. There is no change in the effective half-life of penbutolol in healthy patients versus those on renal dialysis. It is indicated primarily for the treatment of hypertension and may be used in combination with other antihypertensives.

Carteolol. Carteolol is a synthetic, nonselective, beta-adrenergic receptor blocking agent with intrinsic sympathetic activity. It possesses no significant membrane-stabilizing (local anesthetic) activity and is without value in treating intrinsic arrhythmias. Carteolol has equivocal effects on renin secretion because of its intrinsic sympathomimetic activity, in contrast to beta blockers without such activity, which inhibit renin. Carteolol is well absorbed with a half-life of approximately 6 hours. About 50–75% of the drug is eliminated by the kidneys; thus, renal impairment increases its half-life in proportion to the reduction in creatinine clearance. Carteolol is primarily indicated for the management of hypertension but may be used in combination with other potent drugs.

Mixed Antagonists. *Labetalol.* Labetalol is an antihypertensive drug with blocking activity at both alpha and beta receptors. The relative alpha/beta blocking effects are dependent upon the route of administration. After oral administration, the ratio of alpha/beta effectiveness is 1:3; however, when given intravenously, it is 1:7 (i.e., it is three and seven times more potent on beta than on alpha receptors, respectively). The alpha effects are primarily on $alpha_1$ receptors, whereas the beta effects are nonselective.

Hemodynamic effects consist primarily of decreased peripheral resistance and decreased or unchanged heart rate with little change in cardiac output.[306] Serum renin activity is decreased. Maintenance of lower heart rates in the presence of decreased systemic blood pressure is beneficial in controlling the myocardial oxygen supply/demand ratio and is a major benefit of labetalol in patients with coronary artery disease.[307]

Labetalol is eliminated by hepatic glucuronide conjugation. The elimination half-life after intravenous administration is 5.5 hours and 6–8 hours after oral use. Elimination is not markedly prolonged in patients with hepatic or renal failure. Another advantage of the drug is the ability to convert from iv to oral forms of the same drug after the patient is stable.[308,309,310]

For treatment of hypertension when used as a bolus, the initial dose is 0.25 $mg \cdot kg^{-1}$ intravenously over 2 minutes, then repeat every 10 minutes to a total of 300 mg. When used as a continuous infusion, it is usually started at 2 $mg \cdot min^{-1}$ and titrated to effect. Because there is an enhanced effect by inhalation anesthetics, these doses should be decreased when used intraoperatively.

Complications and contraindications are similar to those for the beta blockers. Labetalol should be used with caution in patients with compromised myocardial function because it may worsen heart failure. Also, owing to $beta_2$ blocking activity, the drug may induce bronchospasm in asthmatics. As with other beta blockers, abrupt withdrawal is not recommended.

Calcium Entry Blockers

Calcium is regarded as the universal messenger in cells and plays a critical role in a number of biologic processes.[120,121,247] It is involved in blood coagulation, a broad array of enzymatic reactions, the metabolism of bone, neuromuscular transmission, the electrical activation of various excitable membranes as well as endocrine secretion, and muscle contraction. Calcium initiates several physiologic events in the specialized automatic and conducting cells in the heart.[311] It is involved in the genesis of the cardiac action potential, and it links excitation to contraction and controls energy stores and utilization. Movement of extracellular calcium across membranes also governs the function of smooth muscle in bronchi and in coronary, pulmonary, and systemic arterioles. Its role in adrenergic effector response has been outlined in detail in the section on Molecular Pharmacology and Effector Response.

Membrane calcium channels are known to exist that provide a pathway for calcium influx across cell membranes that differs from calcium efflux movements associated with active pumps or exchange.[312] The inward calcium channel exhibits two distinguishing properties: (1) selectivity in that they have the ability to distinguish between ion species, and (2) excitability in that they have the property of responding to changes in membrane potential.[313]

Separate, ion-specific, channels for sodium and calcium influx are thought to exist. The status of these channels can vary to produce three kinetic states: resting, activated, and inactivated. Sodium channels are referred to as fast channels because the transition among resting, activated, and inactivated states is more rapid than among the calcium channels. Thus, calcium channels are often referred to as membrane "slow channels."[222]

Classification of calcium entry blockers has been difficult since their discovery. They were initially thought to be beta-adrenergic blocking drugs because of their sympatholytic action. Later they were called calcium antagonists. It is clear, however, that these drugs are not true pharmacologic antagonists of calcium. Instead, they interact with the cell membrane to control the intracellular concentration of calcium. The correct terminology for this group of drugs appears to be *calcium entry blockers*.[314] *Slow channel inhibitors* or *calcium channel blockers* are alternate terms.

The molecular structures of three clinically useful calcium entry blockers are seen in Figure 14-30. Calcium entry blockers are a heterogeneous group of drugs with dissimilar structures and electrophysiologic and pharmacologic properties.[221] Despite structural dissimilarities, this group shares some important actions that are consistent with the known importance of extracellular calcium and adrenergic function. Any drug that alters slow-channel kinetics could be expected to produce vasodilation, to depress cardiac conduction velocity (dromotropism), to depress contractility (inotropism), and to decrease heart rate (chronotropism). All calcium entry blockers do this, but with varying degrees of potency in the intact human and *in vitro* (Table 14-23).[315,316] Thus, despite their similarities, these drugs cannot be considered therapeutically interchangeable. Clinically, nifedipine is a potent coronary artery vasodilator

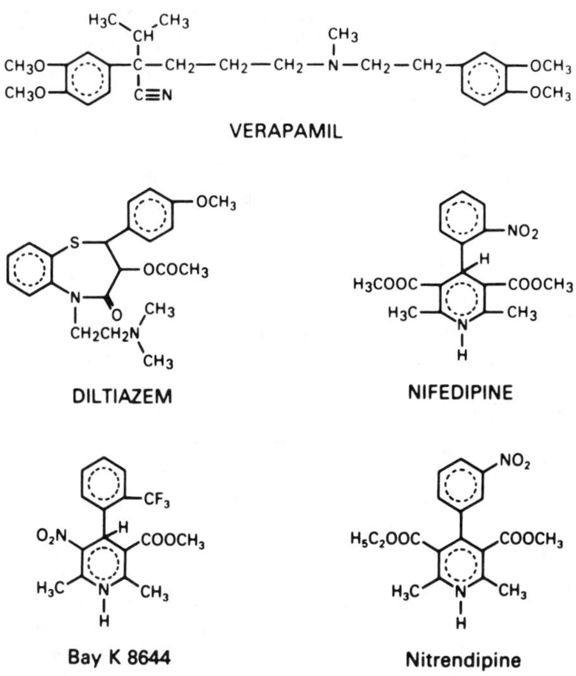

Figure 14-30. Structural formulas of the calcium entry blockers demonstrate dissimilar structures consistent with their dissimilar electrophysiologic and pharmacologic properties. They also share some similarities but cannot be considered therapeutically interchangeable. Nifedipine and nitrendipine are structurally similar and are both potent vasodilators; BAY K 8644 is also similar but is a calcium channel agonist.

with little direct effect on cardiac conduction. It may reduce dysrhythmias secondarily when increased coronary blood flow is of benefit. Verapamil is valued for its specific antidysrhythmic activity, but it is a myocardial depressant with little vasodilator activity. Verapamil also has slightly greater local anesthetic activity (fast-channel inhibition) than procaine on an equimolar basis.[317] The significance of this observation in humans has not been established.

The structural heterogenicity of this group of drugs also suggests more than one site and mechanism of action. Although the molecular basis of the action of these compounds is unknown, they are lipophilic, and it appears likely that they work by producing conformational changes in the cell membranes (see the section on Molecular Pharmacology and Effector Response).

The useful pharmacologic effects of the calcium entry blockers have been confirmed almost solely to the cardiovascular system, although the list of uses will likely grow.[222] Table 14-24 lists some of the areas of investigation in which they appear to be of clinical benefit.[318-321] Calcium entry

TABLE 14-23. Autonomic Effects of Calcium Entry Blockers in Intact Humans

	Verapamil	Diltiazem	Nifedipine	Lidoflazine
Negative inotropic	+	0/+	0	0
Negative chronotropic	+	0/+	0	0
Negative dromotropic	+ + + +	+ + +	0	0
Coronary vasodilation	+ +	+ + +	+ + + +	+ + + +
Systemic vasodilation	+ +	+ +	+ + + +	+ + +
Bronchodilation	0/+		0/+	

TABLE 14-24. Uses of Calcium Channel Blockers

Vascular Disorders	Nonvascular Disorders
Systemic hypertension	Bronchial asthma
Pulmonary hypertension	Esophageal spasm
Cerebral arterial spasm	Dysmenorrhea
Raynaud's phenomenon	Premature labor
Migraine	

blockers have been described, perhaps erroneously, as selective slow channel blockers. A review of the literature, however, suggests that these agents are not selective but rather that the slow channel effects on the cardiovascular system are just more apparent. Their lack of selectivity should not be surprising considering the critical role calcium plays in a wide variety of biologic processes. The sensitivity of a given tissue to the calcium entry blockers is related to that tissue's dependence on extracellular calcium for its function. This would explain the sensitivity of the calcium-dependent myocardium and smooth muscle to these blockers on the one hand and the apparent insensitivity of striated muscle on the other.[322] Extracellular calcium is relatively insignificant in the function of striated muscle, where the sarcoplasmic reticulum is the major storage organelle of calcium. Striated muscle can recycle intracellular calcium for prolonged periods, which is in keeping with its function of sustained contraction as opposed to the rhythmic or cyclic contraction of the myocardium and smooth muscle.

The drugs are all absorbed *via* the gastrointestinal tract, but the extensive first-pass hepatic extraction of verapamil limits its bioavailability orally (Table 14-25). Onset of action is equivalent for all three drugs and is consistent with rapid membrane transport. All three drugs are extensively protein-bound and subject to the effect of changes in plasma protein concentration and competition from other protein-bound drugs and metabolites, but final elimination of verapamil and nifedipine is primarily renal.

Verapamil

Verapamil is a calcium entry blocker that is administered intravenously for terminating supraventricular tachydysrhythmias.[323-326] Nearly all forms of supraventricular tachydysrhythmias are caused by re-entry using either the sinoatrial or the atrioventricular node as part of the circuit. Verapamil terminates these cardiac dysrhythmias by decreasing nodal conductivity, converting the unidirectional block of re-entry to a bidirectional block. In this regard, its action on supraventricular dysrhythmias is similar to that of quinidine on ventricular re-entry cardiac dysrhythmias.

TABLE 14-25. Comparative Pharmacology of Calcium Entry Blockers

	Verapamil	Diltiazem	Nifedipine
Dose			
Oral	80–160 mg tid	60–90 mg tid	10–20 mg tid
iv	75–150 $\mu g \cdot kg^{-1}$	75–150 $\mu g \cdot kg^{-1}$	5–15 $\mu g \cdot kg^{-1}$
Absorption			
Oral (%)	>90%	>90%	>90%
Bioavailability			
Oral (%)	<20%	? <20%	60–70%*
Onset			
Oral	15–20 minutes	20–30 minutes	15–20 minutes
iv	1 minute	?	1 minute
Sublingual	—	—	3 minutes
Peak Effect			
Oral	5 hours	30 minutes	1–2 hours
iv	5–30 minutes	?	1–3 hours
Elimination half-life	2–7 hours	4 hours	4–5 hours
Plasma protein binding	90%	80%	90%
Metabolism	70% First-pass hepatic	Deacetylated	80% to lactone
Elimination			
Renal	75%	35%	70%
Gastrointestinal (liver)	15%	75%	<15%
Side-Effects	Constipation, headache, vertigo, hypotension, atrioventricular conduction disturbances	Headache, dizziness, flushing, atrioventricular conduction disturbances, constipation	Headache, hypotension, flushing, digital dysesthesias, leg edema

* Light-sensitive.

Verapamil does not alter the action potential upstroke in fibers whose resting membrane potential is more negative than −60 mV, i.e., fast action potentials.[327] It does slow or prevent depolarization in cardiac tissue with a resting membrane potential that is less negative than −50 mV, i.e., calcium-dependent upstroke. Verapamil, therefore, has profound effects on pacemaker cells, which depend on the calcium current for depolarization.[328] It depresses the rate of sinus discharge, reduces conduction velocity, and increases refractoriness of the atrioventricular node. A dose-dependent increase in the PR interval and atrioventricular interval is produced on the electrocardiogram. This has been described as a quinidine-like effect similar to that produced by Class IA antidysrhythmic drugs (e.g., procainamide), which are also effective for supraventricular dysrhythmias. In contrast to the procainamide, verapamil does not increase the QRS or Q-T interval because it lacks activity on the sodium-dependent action potentials.

Verapamil is a first-line drug for treatment of supraventricular tachydysrhythmias (Table 14-26). The incidence of successful termination of paroxysmal atrial tachycardia (PAT) with verapamil in adults has approached 90%.[325] It is also effective in treating atrial fibrillation and atrial flutter by either converting to a sinus rhythm or slowing the ventricular response. The ventricular rate will slow as a result of decreased conduction velocity through the atrioventricular node even when conversion is not produced. Caution must be exercised in treating patients when the underlying cause of the atrial tachycardia, atrial fibrillation, or atrial flutter is the Wolff-Parkinson-White syndrome.[329] An accessory bypass tract lies near the atrioventricular node that participates in the re-entry of these tachydysrhythmias. Verapamil may terminate the tachydysrhythmia by its specific depressant effects on the atrioventricular node, which is one limb of the re-entrant pathway. It may also increase conduction velocity in the accessory tract, in which case the heart rate may actually increase.

Verapamil has no adverse effects on bronchial asthma or obstructive lung disease and may be selected over propranolol in patients with these conditions.[318] It should be avoided in patients with sick sinus syndrome, atrioventricular block, and the presence of heart failure, unless the heart failure is the result of a supraventricular tachycardia.

Studies further support the hypothesis that Ca^{2+} participates directly in the genesis of ventricular dysrhythmias (Fig. 14-31).[329,330] When sodium channels are inactivated by hypoxia, stretch, or hyperkalemia, the remaining Ca^{2+} currently can produce a depolarizing current in these abnormal cells, especially in the presence of catecholamines. The conversion of a fast response cell to a cell with slow response characteristics presents all the necessary ingredients for the re-entry phenomenon: slow depolarization and de-

TABLE 14-26. Actions of Calcium Entry Blockers

Verapamil

Vasodilator
  ↓ systemic vascular resistance → ↑ heart rate
  → ↑ ejection fraction and cardiac output
Small decrease in left ventricular dP/dt
Little or no change in coronary resistance
↓ conduction through atrioventricular node (↑ P-R interval)
Should not be given with digitalis or beta blockers

Diltiazem

More like verapamil than nifedipine
Dilates coronary more than systemic vessels and has less marked hemodynamic effects than nifedipine or verapamil
Little effect on cardiac output
Does not cause tachycardia
Effects on conduction system similar to those of verapamil
Less inotropic effect than verapamil

Nifedipine

Rapid onset of action, may be used sublingually
Potent peripheral vasodilator, may be useful in treatment of hypertension
Has little clinically important negative inotropic activity
Less tendency to produce cardiac decompensation than verapamil
Little effect on nodal activity and no antiarrhythmic activity; therefore causes no electrocardiographic changes
Increases coronary blood flow in normal and ischemic myocardium

layed conduction. The resulting ventricular dysrhythmias can usually be terminated with one of the Class I drugs as long as the resting membrane potential of the slow response is between −80 and −60 mV. Verapamil has been effective in terminating ventricular tachycardias and premature depolarizations in about two thirds of the treatment trials when other drugs have failed. The resting membrane potential of these abnormal "slow response" foci has been postulated to be less negative than −60 mV, a range in which lidocaine would be ineffective on the calcium current conduction and depolarization. More information is needed before recommendations can be made for verapamil in treating dysrhythmias other than supraventricular tachydysrhythmias. Other drugs are significantly more effective for the initial treatment of ventricular dysrhythmias.

The important side-effects of verapamil are directly related to its predominant pharmacologic action (see Table 14-26). It may produce unwanted atrioventricular conduction delays and bradycardia, resulting in cardiovascular collapse. Verapamil must be used very carefully, if at all, in the presence of propranolol. The combined effect has produced

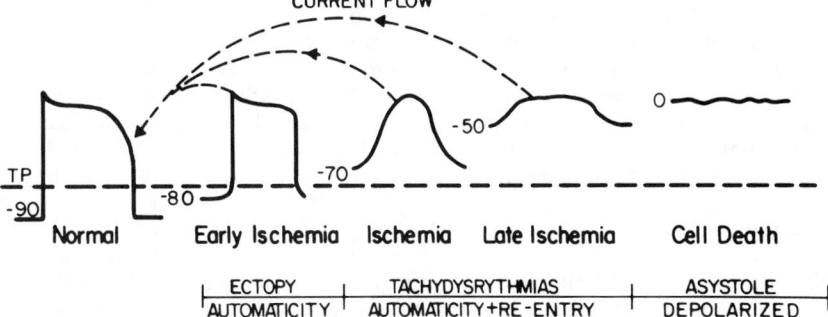

Figure 14-31. Verapamil may be useful in treating ventricular dysrhythmias when first-line drugs are ineffective. The source of the cardiac dysrhythmia has been speculated to have inoperative fast sodium channels and thus to be susceptible to a Calcium entry blocker in terminating re-entry.

complete heart block in animals and humans. It must be used carefully in digitalized patients for the same reason. No such interactions exist with nifedipine. The combination of beta blockade and nifedipine may be beneficial in patients with ischemic heart disease because the reflex tachycardia seen with nifedipine can be countered with beta blockade.

Nifedipine

Nifedipine is the most potent calcium entry blocker when tested in isolated tissue preparations. It is an equipotent cardiac depressant and vasodilator. Depression of inotropism and cardiac conduction, however, is not evident in the intact human. It does not effect baroreflex mechanisms and, as a result, the marked vasodilation is accompanied by increased SNS tone and afterload reduction (see Table 14-26).[222] A compensatory tachycardia may result, and cardiac output may actually increase as a result of the afterload reduction.

The most specific therapeutic application for nifedipine is coronary vasospasm (variant of Prinzmetal's angina).[221,316] It has been more successful than nitroglycerin for this purpose because it produces a more profound and predictable coronary vasodilation. It has also been extremely useful in other types of ischemic heart disease ranging from unstable angina to myocardial infarction. The decrease in myocardial oxygen demands that result from the reduced afterload and reduced left ventricular volume appears to be the mechanism for the relief of angina. Coronary vasodilation is another factor, but it is not known if this is the antianginal effect in patients with coronary artery disease. The dilating effect may last only 5 minutes, but the antianginal effect may last more than 1 hour.

Nifedipine is not available for intravenous use, but clinical practice has demonstrated that sublingual nifedipine is an effective therapeutic application with a nearly immediate onset of action.[221,223] One need only puncture the end of a nifedipine capsule and squirt it under the patient's tongue. Use of this technique is particularly applicable for the anesthesiologist in situations where oral medication cannot be given. We have also used sublingual nifedipine effectively in situations where perioperative hypertension and evidence of acute coronary ischemia coexist. In these circumstances, a reduction in afterload, coronary vasodilation, and reduced blood pressure are all achieved with the same drug.[331] Reflex tachycardia, if it occurs, can be managed with beta blockade without significant interaction with nifedipine.

Diltiazem

The hemodynamic effects of diltiazem lie somewhere between those of verapamil and nifedipine.[222] It is less potent than either of these two agents.[332] Diltiazem is a good coronary artery dilator but a poor peripheral vasodilator. It often produces bradycardia and delayed conduction, and reflex tachycardia is not a problem.[333] It appears to be an effective oral drug for the treatment of coronary disease in which cardiac dysrhythmias are troublesome. Cardiac dysrhythmias are noticeably a part of the clinical picture in patients suffering from coronary spasm.

Nicardipine

Nicardipine hydrochloride is a calcium channel blocker that can be administered orally and intravenously. It is the only calcium channel blocker that can be titrated intrave-

nously to achieve blood pressure response. Nicardipine is a smooth muscle relaxant producing vasodilation of peripheral and coronary arteries. It has a rapid onset of action, and the major effects last 10 to 15 minutes. Toxic metabolic products are not produced.[334] It has minimal cardiodepressant effects and does not decrease the rate of the sinus node pacemaker or slow conduction through the atrioventricular node. Renal failure does not affect the dosage, but the dosage should be reduced in the elderly and those with hepatic dysfunction. It is compatible with most crystalloid solutions.

Side-effects of nicardipine include headache, lightheadedness, flushing, and hypotension. Reflex tachycardia is not a frequent finding with nicardipine, as is the case with nitroprusside, hydralazine, or nifedipine.

Nimodipine

Nimodipine is highly lipophilic. It has a greater vasodilating affect on cerebral arteries than on vessels elsewhere because of its lipophilism, which promotes crossing the blood-brain barrier. Clinical studies demonstrate a favorable effect on the severity of neurologic deficits caused by cerebral vasospasm following subarachnoid hemorrhage. However, no radiographic evidence has been presented that nimodipine either prevents or relieves spasm of these arteries. The mechanism for clinical improvement is not known. It is primarily an oral drug that is rapidly absorbed, with a T-terminal half-life of approximately 8–9 hours. Earlier elimination rates are much more rapid, which results in a need to redose every 4 hours. The bioavailability of an oral dose is only 13%. Dosage should be reduced in patients with hepatic dysfunction. The primary indication for nimodipine is for the improvement of neurologic deficits caused by spasm following subarachnoid hemorrhage from a ruptured congenital aneurysm.

Felodipine

Felodipine is a second-generation calcium channel inhibitor that is currently under investigation by the Federal Drug Administration. Nimodipine and felodipine have demonstrated selectivity for vascular tissue beds. Whereas nimodipine preferentially dilates cerebral vessels, felodipine preferentially dilates peripheral resistance vessels. Neither has significant effects on cardiac muscle. This has important clinical implications in the treatment of hypertension. Early studies indicate that 10–20 mg of felodipine daily will reduce blood pressure without reducing cardiac output or heart rate. Coronary blood flow increases, but no effect on ventricular contraction or relaxation has been reported. This would make the drug appropriate for the active hypertensive patient.

Calcium Entry Blockers and Anesthesia

Evidence indicates that halothane depresses slow-channel kinetics. All of the potent inhalation anesthetics behave in a similar fashion in that they depress myocardial contractility and vascular tone in a dose-related manner.[335,336] Most studies indicate that the calcium entry blockers and inhalation anesthetics exert additive effects on the inward calcium current.[221,316] Opioid anesthetics do not appear to add anything to the effects of the calcium entry blockers.

Several recent studies indicate an interaction between the calcium entry blockers and the neuromuscular blocking drugs similar to that seen with the mycin antibiotics.[222] This interaction is not well defined, but in vitro and in vivo studies indicate a reduced margin of safety with these drug combinations. Calcium entry blockers appear to augment the effects of both depolarizing and nondepolarizing muscle relaxants.[337] These observations serve as a word of caution, since their clinical significance has not been defined. Prolonged apnea and relaxation have been reported when verapamil was used to treat a supraventricular tachycardia in a patient with Duchenne's muscular dystrophy.[338]

Calcium entry blockers should be continued until the time of surgery to maintain control of angina pectoris, hypertension, or cardiac dysrhythmias.[222] It could be anticipated that sudden discontinuation of these drugs theoretically could produce a rebound of symptoms, although this phenomenon has not been reported. Up regulation of calcium receptors would probably occur during periods of entry blockade.[339]

Verapamil may increase the toxicity of digoxin, the benzodiazepines, carbamazepine, oral hypoglycemics, and possibly quinidine and theophylline.[340] Cardiac failure, atrioventricular conduction disturbances, and sinus bradycardia may be more frequent with concurrent use of beta blockers, and severe hypotension and bradycardia may occur with bupivacaine. Decreased lithium effect and lithium neurotoxicity have both been reported with the concurrent use of verapamil.[341] The effects of verapamil may also be increased by cimetidine.[340]

Antihypertensives

Increased awareness and treatment of hypertension over the last 20 years has resulted in increasing numbers of patients presenting for anesthesia and surgery who are taking one or more antihypertensive medications (Table 14-27). These drugs are numerous, affect multiple organ systems, and have the potential for many deleterious interactions in the perioperative period. Most antihypertensive drugs blunt the ANS or its effector organs or cause reflex increases in ANS outflow. Most anesthetic agents also inhibit ANS tone to some degree[342] and may therefore have additive effects with antihypertensive drugs. In addition, patients with hypertension may exhibit greater lability in blood pressure intraoperatively and rebound hypertension in the postoperative period.[343-345] The anesthesiologist should therefore maintain a thorough understanding of the commonly used antihypertensive drugs. A rational approach to their perioperative use includes decisions as to holding or continuing them preoperatively, possible interactions with anesthetic drugs, and resumption of treatment postoperatively. The commonly used antihypertensive drugs are grouped below according to their primary mechanism of action and discussed briefly with emphasis on considerations for the anesthesiologist.

Diuretics

Diuretics are the most commonly prescribed drugs for hypertension. Their basic mechanisms of action are decreased plasma and extracellular volumes. Although the thiazides and furosemide have been shown to have vasodilating properties, the clinical significance of this effect is unclear. Chronic diuretic therapy results in decreased intravascular volume. The cardiovascular response to induction of anesthesia may therefore be accentuated, resulting in hypotension and tachycardia. Other problems associated with diuretic use include hypokalemia, hyponatremia, hypocalcemia, and hyperglycemia. Chronic hypokalemia is quite common with diuretic therapy and may predispose the patient to cardiac arrhythmias.[346] The clinical relevance of perioperative hypokalemia is unclear and has stirred considerable debate among anesthesiologists as to whether surgery should be postponed until plasma potassium levels are treated.[347,348]

TABLE 14-27. Antihypertensive Drugs for Perioperative Use

Drug	Dose	Latency	Duration	Side-Effects*
Diuretics				
Furosemide	20–40 mg iv	5–10 minutes	4 hours	Hypokalemia, hypovolemia
Sympatholytics				
Alpha-methyldopa	250–500 mg siv	20 minutes	24 hours	Sedation, hepatitis, hemolytic anemia
Clonidine	0.2 mg in 10 ml normal saline per rectum	20 minutes	12–24 hours	Sedation, dry mouth, withdrawal syndrome
Vasodilators				
Hydralazine	5–10 mg iv 10–40 mg im	15–20 minutes 20–40 minutes	4–6 hours	Lupus-like syndrome, drug fever, rash
Nifedipine	10 mg siv	5–10 minutes	7 hours	Headache, fluid retention
Verapamil	5 mg iv	2–5 minutes	4–6 hours	Heart block, myocardial failure
Diazoxide	300 mg siv	3–5 minutes	5–12 hours	Decreased cerebral blood flow, hyperuricemia
Sodium nitroprusside	0.25–0.5 $\mu g \cdot kg^{-1} \cdot min^{-1}$	1–2 minutes	2–5 minutes	Cyanide toxicity, increased cerebral blood flow
Nitroglycerin		2–5 minutes	3–5 minutes	Headache, fluid retention

Adrenergic Blocking Drugs

See Tables 14-21, 14-22, and 14-23

Doses shown are for 70-kg adult. iv = intravenous push, siv = slow intravenous infusion, im = intramuscular, sl = sublingual.

*All the drugs listed may also cause hypotension. All possible side-effects are not listed; the ones shown are the most common.

Adrenergic Receptor Antagonists

Beta Blockers. Beta-adrenergic receptor blockers are also commonly used now in the treatment of hypertension. They have been discussed in detail above, but certain comments about their perioperative use are pertinent here (see Table 14-22). Following the introduction of propranolol, several deleterious interactions (in particular, the enhanced negative inotropic and chronotropic effects of halothane) were noted with anesthetics. This resulted in a debate over whether or not the blocker should be discontinued preoperatively. Beta blocker therapy should be continued up to the time of operation. A withdrawal syndrome has been noted after acute discontinuation of chronic beta blocker therapy.[349,350] Also, the control of heart rate and blood pressure perioperatively is easier if chronic medications are continued and the anesthetic plan is altered rather than acutely stopping the chronic medications and administering a routine anesthetic plan.[351] Heart rate is a major determinant of myocardial oxygen demand. Tachycardia has recently been shown to increase the risk of poor outcome in patients with ischemic heart disease.[240,352] The control of heart rate therefore as well as of blood pressure is important perioperatively, and beta blocker therapy should be continued to maximize this control.

Alpha Blockers. The alpha blockers in use today include prazosin and phentolamine (see Table 14-21). Phentolamine is used almost exclusively in the diagnosis and treatment of pheochromocytoma. Prazosin is now commonly used to treat essential hypertension. When patients taking these drugs are to undergo anesthesia, it should be kept in mind that the normal ANS response to stress and inhalation anesthetic drugs may be completely blocked at the vascular effector site; therefore, elevations of catecholamines will not reflexly increase peripheral vascular resistance and may aciually decrease it if vascular beta receptors are left unopposed. In the presence of alpha blockade, we suggest preloading with intravenous fluids to ensure adequate central volume and careful titration of halogenated anesthetic drugs.

Sympatholytics

Sympatholytic drugs include those that block central SNS outflow or NE release from the presynaptic neuron at the effector site. Currently included in this group are alpha-methyldopa and clonidine.

Alpha-Methyldopa. Alpha-methyldopa is a catechol derivative that is enzymatically converted to active compounds by enzymes in the catecholamine synthesis chain (see Fig. 14-9). Alpha-methyldopamine and alpha-methylnorepinephrine are the primary metabolites. The precise mechanism responsible for decreased SNS tone is unclear, but it is thought that alpha-methylnorepinephrine, which is stored in presynaptic vesicles, is released and stimulates presynaptic alpha$_2$ receptors, thereby inhibiting NE release.[282] Because of the unique metabolism of alpha-methyldopa to the active compound and the storage of the metabolite in presynaptic vessicles, both the time to onset and duration of action are long. Even after intravenous administration, the peak effect may not be seen for several hours. Although the elimination half-life is 2 hours, the effect of an oral dose may last up to 24 hours.

Clonidine. Clonidine stimulates presynaptic alpha$_2$ receptors and inhibits NE release from both central and peripheral adrenergic terminals. It also has some alpha$_1$-agonist activity and in high oral doses may cause paradoxical hypertension by stimulating vascular alpha$_1$ receptors. Under normal circumstances, the alpha$_2$ effects predominate. The prominent antihypertensive effect is thought to be secondary to stimulation of alpha$_2$ receptors in the vasomotor centers of the medulla oblongata.[282] Whether these are presynaptic or postsynaptic receptors remains controversial;[277] however, the end result is decreased SNS and enhanced vagal tone. Peripherally, there is decreased plasma renin activity as well as decreased epinephrine and NE levels.[353]

Cardiovascular effects of clonidine include decreased peripheral vascular resistance and heart rate.[354] The cardiovascular response to exercise is usually maintained. Prominent side-effects include hypotension, sedation, and dry mouth.[355,356] One of the more worrisome complications of clonidine use is the occurrence of a withdrawal syndrome on acute discontinuation of the drug. This usually occurs about 18 hours after discontinuation and consists of hypertension, tachycardia, insomnia, flushing, headache, apprehension, sweating, and tremulousness. It lasts for 24–72 hours and is most likely to occur in patients taking more than 1.2 mg·day of clonidine. The withdrawal syndrome has been noted postoperatively in patients who were taken off clonidine for surgery.[357] It can be confused with anesthesia emergence symptoms, particularly in a patient with uncontrolled hypertension. Clonidine is not available for intravenous use, but symptoms of the withdrawal syndrome as well as routine postoperative hypertension can be treated with clonidine administered transdermally or rectally.[358] Withholding clonidine prior to surgery is not recommended.

Dexmedetomidine. Dexmedetomidine is a more selective alpha$_2$ agonist than clonidine.[359] It has a much shorter half-life (about 1.5 hours) and a more rapid onset of action (<5 minutes). The time to peak effect is 15 minutes. Intravenous dexmedetomidine provides excellent sedation, lowering of blood pressure and heart rate, and profound decreases in plasma catecholamines. Little respiratory depression is evident. Other studies have shown it to be an effective anxiolytic and sedative when used as premedication for anesthesia for minor gynecologic surgery. In an animal model, dexmedetomidine produces stereospecific and dose-dependent decreases in MAC.[360]

Clinical Possibilities

Flacke listed the potential uses of sympatholytic drugs in the future. In addition to the reducing effect of MAC and the absent respiratory depression, the following properties seem particularly valuable to the anesthesiologist:[360]

1. They are potent analgesics
2. They are sedatives and anxiolytics
3. They are antisialogogues
4. They may promote hemodynamic stability
5. Homeostatic reflexes remain intact
6. They attenuate opioid rigidity (in animals)
7. Their circulatory actions can be reversed.

Clonidine has also been used successfully as a substitute for opiates and nicotine during withdrawal. It reduces sympathetic hyperactivity with head injury and can be used as an analgesic in the subarachnoid and epidural spaces for the treatment of pain.

Converting Enzyme Inhibitors

The renin-angiotensin system is integrally related to the ANS in controlling blood pressure (see Fig. 14-18). The central role of the renin-angiotensin-aldosterone system in the regulation of fluid balance and hemodynamics was not fully appreciated until the discovery and clinical application of inhibitors of the angiotensin-converting enzyme.[151,152] Captopril, enalapril, and lisinopril inhibit converting enzyme and thereby prevent the conversion of angiotensin I to the active angiotensin II. These drugs have been highly effective in the treatment of all levels of essential hypertension as well as renovascular and malignant hypertension.[153-155] The cardiovascular effects normally involve only decreased peripheral vascular resistance. Cardiac output may remain normal or increase while the filling pressure remain unchanged. Thus, these drugs have been effective in the management of congestive heart failure as well.[361-363] There is usually no increase in SNS tone in response to the lowered blood pressure. ACE inhibition generally results in reductions in angiotensin-aldosterone, norepinephrine, and plasma antidiuretic hormone. This suppression is accompanied by a decrease in aldosterone and an improvement in cumulative plasma potassium levels, which are beneficial in both congestive heart failure and hypertension. It can be concluded that the major humoral responses to chronic congestive heart failure, even overlooking the effects of the diuretics, are affected by the release of angiotensin, aldosterone, and increased SNS tone.

Captopril, the first orally active compound, has proved highly effective in the treatment of all levels of hypertension and congestive heart failure. Enalapril is a second-generation (nonsulfhydryl) angiotensin-converting enzyme inhibitor. The omission of the sulfhydryl group possibly diminishes side-effects. Both captopril and enalapril combine a high degree of clinical efficacy with a low rate of side-effects. Both are eliminated *via* renal excretion and should be given in reduced doses in patients with renal dysfunction. Captopril has a shorter half-life and requires more frequent dosing than enalapril. Enalapril has to be converted by esterase in the liver and other tissues into the active compound, enalaprilat. Many new angiotensin-converting enzyme inhibitors are being developed that are eliminated *via* hepatic routes and may prove advantageous in renal failure. Lisinopril is one of these angiotensin-converting enzyme inhibitors that is absorbed as the active form and is very long-acting.

The angiotensin-converting enzyme inhibitors are associated with few side-effects and are increasingly popular in treating hypertension. Captopril may produce reversible neutropenia, dermatitis, and angioedema. Enalapril produces syncope, headache, and dizziness in about 1% of elderly patients. All angiotensin-converting enzyme inhibitors may cause hypotension in patients who are hypovolemic and taking diuretic therapy. Diuretic therapy should be discontinued 1 week before starting angiotensin-converting enzyme inhibitor therapy. The hypotensive effects are also enhanced by the concomitant use of calcium channel blockers. The angiotensin-converting enzyme inhibitors blunt the hypokalemic effects of thiazide diuretics and may magnify the potassium-sparing effects of spironolactone, triamterene, and amiloride. In addition, nonsteroidal anti-inflammatory drugs, including aspirin, may magnify the potassium-retaining effects of angiotensin-converting enzyme inhibitors.

Vasodilators

The drugs that directly relax smooth muscle to cause vasodilation reflexively increase ANS tone and are included here for the sake of a complete discussion of antihypertensive drugs.[159] These are discussed with emphasis on perioperative use.

Hydralazine. Hydralazine is the most commonly used vasodilator and can be given by the im, iv, and oral routes (Table 14-27). It relaxes smooth muscle tone directly, without interacting with adrenergic or cholinergic receptors. The mechanism of action is unknown. It is most potent in coronary, splanchnic, renal, and cerebral vessels, causing increased blood flow in each of these organs. The decrease in cardiac afterload is beneficial but, unfortunately, there is usually a concomitant reflex tachycardia that may be severe. It is commonly combined with a beta blocker such as propranolol. It may also cause fluid retention and is usually given chronically with a diuretic.[282]

Hydralazine is metabolized by hepatic acetylation, and oral bioavailability may be low owing to first-pass metabolism. The elimination half-life is about 4 hours, but the pharmacologic half-life is much longer as a result of avid binding of the drug to smooth muscle. The effective half-life is approximately 100 hours.[364] Side-effects include a lupus-like syndrome, drug fever, skin rash, pancytopenia, and peripheral neuropathy. The iv dose we recommend for perioperative use is 5–10 mg in an iv bolus every 15–20 minutes until blood pressure control is achieved. It may also be given 10–40 mg intramuscularly, but the response is slower.

Sodium Nitroprusside. Sodium nitroprusside is an extremely potent vasodilator that is available only for iv administration. It acts directly on smooth muscle, causing both arterial and venous dilation.[159,365] The mechanism of action is not entirely clear but appears to involve binding to a receptor on the surface of the myocyte, followed by activation of an intracellular vasodilator intermediate.

The action of sodium nitroprusside on both venous and arterial sides of the circulation causes decreases in cardiac preload as well as afterload. This results in decreased cardiac work; however, it has been suggested that sodium nitroprusside may further compromise ischemic myocardium in the presence of occlusive coronary artery disease by shunting blood away from the ischemic zone.[366]

Sodium nitroprusside is very useful during the perioperative period. It lowers blood pressure within 1–2 minutes, with the effect dissipating within 2 minutes after infusion is stopped. It is extremely potent and should be administered through a central venous line by infusion pump while continuously monitoring arterial pressure. The starting dose is $0.25-0.5$ $\mu g \cdot kg^{-1} \cdot min^{-1}$. It can be increased slowly as needed to control blood pressure, but chances for toxicity are greater if the dose of 10 $\mu g \cdot kg^{-1} \cdot min^{-1}$ is exceeded. The dose required for steady-state–induced hypotension is variable.

Chemically, sodium nitroprusside consists of a ferrous iron atom bound with five cyanide molecules and one nitric group. The ferrous iron reacts with sulfhydryl groups in red blood cells and releases cyanide.[367] Cyanide is reduced to thiocyanate in the liver and excreted in the urine. The half-life of thiocyanate is 4 days, and it accumulates in the presence of renal failure.[368] There is no evidence, however, that pre-existing hepatic or renal failure increases the likelihood of cyanide toxicity. Administration of high doses of sodium nitroprusside can result in cyanide toxicity. The cyanide molecule binds to cytochrome oxidase, interfering with electron transport and causing cellular hypoxia. This can be recognized by increasing tolerance to the drug, elevated mixed venous P_{O_2}, and metabolic acidosis. The treatment of cyanide toxicity consists of (1) administration of amyl nitrate (by inhalation or directly into the anesthesia circuit); (2) infusion of sodium nitrite 5 mg·kg^{-1} over 4–5 minutes; and (3) administration of sodium thiosulfate 150 mg·kg^{-1} in 50 ml water over 15 minutes.

The hypotensive effects of sodium nitroprusside may be potentiated by inhalation anesthetics and blood loss; therefore close perioperative monitoring is essential. It is commonly used to induce hypotension for decreasing blood loss in patients predisposed to major hemorrhage. Administration of sodium nitroprusside causes a reflex increase in sympathetic tone and renin release.[369] Drugs that blunt these reflexes markedly enhance its effects. Preoperative treatment with propranolol or captopril decreases the amount of sodium nitroprusside required for producing hypotension and thus decreases the potential for toxicity.[370,371]

Glyceril Trinitrate. Glyceril trinitrate, or nitroglycerin, is a venodilator used to treat myocardial ischemia (see Chapter 23). Its predominant action is on venules, causing increased venous capacitance and decreased cardiac preload. Effects on the arterial side are minimal except at very high doses. Upon iv administration effects can be seen within 2 minutes, and they usually resolve with 5 minutes of discontinuing the drug. Side-effects are minimal, and there is no potential for cyanide toxicity as with nitroprusside (NTP). Use of nitroglycerin for control of perioperative hypertension has been reported,[372] but because of its relatively weak arteriolar action it is not as useful as other drugs as an antihypertensive agent. In obstetric patients with pre-eclampsia, however, it may be chosen over nitroprusside to circumvent potential cyanide toxicity to the fetus.[373]

Diazoxide. Diazoxide is a direct-acting vasodilator that may be given intravenously and is useful in hypertensive emergencies. It has a greater effect on resistance than capacitance vessels, thus decreasing cardiac afterload with little effect on preload. It also causes fluid retention and induces a reflex sympathetic response.[282] The hypotensive effect is potentiated by diuretics, sympatholytics, and hypovolemia.

Diazoxide is usually administered as an iv bolus of 300 mg for a 70-kg adult. It is 90% bound to serum albumin; therefore a substantial portion of the initial bolus may not reach the site of action. Rapid boluses (less than 30 seconds) of 100 mg every 5 minutes are often recommended as an alternative to allow more free drug to reach the arterioles.[282] The hypotensive effect is usually obtained in 5–10 minutes and lasts 5–12 hours.

Calcium Entry Inhibitors

The calcium entry blockers verapamil, nifedipine, and nitrendipine may also be useful for treating hypertension in the perioperative period.[374,375] They are discussed in detail in the section on Adrenergic Antagonists—Calcium Channel Blockers.

Treatment of Postoperative Hypertension

The wide variety of antihypertensive agents discussed previously makes the treatment of hypertension in the recovery room easier because we can now choose from among multiple routes of administration and variable onsets and durations of action of the different agents.[376,377] However, treatment may become confusing unless the basic pharmacology of each drug is understood. Those drugs available for only oral administration are not routinely used because of unreliable gastrointestinal function during this period. The etiology of postoperative hypertension in each case should be considered. A determination should be made if this requires emergency therapy or is just urgent. Pain should be eliminated by assurance of adequate analgesia prior to therapy with antihypertensive agents. Also, because of the complex pathophysiology of hypertension, a thorough knowledge of each patient and his or her condition is mandatory in choosing a treatment regimen. The medications required for preoperative control may provide the most information in determining what will be necessary postoperatively. In particular, the use of drugs that may have an associated withdrawal syndrome such as clonidine or beta blockers should be noted as well if they were withheld prior to surgery. The volume status of the patient also is important. Fluid overload may require diuretic therapy. Volume depletion or hemorrhage may predispose to severe hypotension in response to routine doses of sympatholytics or vasodilators.

For severe elevations of blood pressure that require immediate treatment, we feel sodium nitroprusside is the drug of choice. Diazoxide and nifedipine (sublingual) are also useful but may take 5–10 minutes to work. In the presence of ischemic heart disease, sublingual nifedipine is very effective owing to its beneficial effects on coronary blood flow as well as blood pressure. Also, if nifedipine is readily available, it can usually be given and begin to work before a sodium nitroprusside infusion can be prepared. Central line placement may also be circumvented in choosing nifedipine over sodium nitroprusside. If control of blood pressure requires sodium nitroprusside, several of the slower acting agents may be used to wean the patient. Hydralazine, 5–10 mg intravenously, and propranolol 0.2–0.5 mg intravenously in repeated doses, are a commonly used approach. Propranolol can be titrated to maintain heart rate below 100 beats per minute and then hydralazine can be used to lower blood pressure to the desired level with boluses every 20–30 minutes. Labetalol, metoprolol, and esmolol may also be used intravenously. Esmolol has the advantage of being rapidly titratable.[301] Alpha-methyldopa may be used intravenously but takes much longer to work than clonidine. Clonidine can be given per rectum and begins to act in 10–20 minutes.[358] If conditions permit, it is helpful to use the drugs the patient was taking preoperatively to ease the transition in the postoperative period. Caution must be exercised if the hypertension is the result of excessive exogenous catecholamines, pheochromocytoma, or thyrotoxicosis. Alpha blockade should be started before beta blockade. The hypertension may, in fact, worsen if beta receptors are blocked first, leaving the alpha receptors unopposed.

REFERENCES

1. Axelrod J, Reisine TD: Stress hormones: Their interaction and regulation. Science 224:452, 1984
2. Pinsker MC: Anesthesia: A pragmatic construct. Anesthesiology 65:819, 1986
3. Weiner N, Taylor P: Neurohumoral transmission and the autonomic nervous system. In Gilman AG, Goodman LS, Rall TW et al (eds): The Pharmacological Basis of Therapeutics, p 66. New York, Macmillan, 1985
4. Koizumi K, Brooks CC: The autonomic nervous system and

its role in controlling visceral activities. In Mountcastle VB (ed): Medical Physiology, p 783. St. Louis, CV Mosby, 1974

5. Warwick R, Williams PL: The autonomic nervous system. In Warwick R, Williams PL (eds): Gray's Anatomy, 35th ed, p 1065. Philadelphia, WB Saunders, 1973

6. Guyton AC: The autonomic nervous system: The adrenal medulla. In Guyton AC (ed): Textbook of Medical Physiology, p 686. Philadelphia, WB Saunders, 1986

7. Bevan JA: Introduction. In Bevan JA (ed): Essentials of Pharmacology, p 108. New York, Harper & Row, 1976

8. Everett NB: The autonomic nervous system. In Everett NB (ed): Functional Neuroanatomy, p 242. Philadelphia, Lea & Febiger, 1971

9. Davson H, Eggleton MG: The autonomic nervous system. In Davson H, Eggleton MG (eds): Principles of Human Physiology, p 1131. Philadelphia, Lea & Febiger, 1962

10. White JC, Smithwick RH, Simeone FA: Physiology of visceral pain. In White JC, Smithwick RH, Simeone FA (eds): The Autonomic Nervous System, p 126. New York, Macmillan, 1952

11. Willis WD: The pain system: The neural basis of nociceptive transmission in the mammalian nervous system. In Gildenberg PL (ed): Pain and Headache, vol 8. New York, Karger, 1985

12. Lake CR, Chernow B, Feuerstein G: The sympathetic nervous system in man: Its evaluation and the measurement of plasma NE. In Ziegler MG, Lake CR (eds): Norepinephrine, p 1. Baltimore, Williams & Wilkins, 1984

13. Miller NE: Biofeedback and visceral learning. Ann Rev Psychol 29:373, 1972

14. Davies DS, Reid JL (eds): Central Action of Drugs in Blood Pressure Regulation. Baltimore, University Park Press, 1975

15. Lambert DH, Deane RS, Mazuzan JE: Anesthesia and the control of blood pressure in patients with spinal cord injury. Anesth Analg 61:344, 1982

16. Kewalramanii LS: Autonomic dysreflexia in traumatic myelopathy. Am J Phys Med 59:1, 1980

17. Axelrod J, Weinshilboum R: Catecholamines. N Engl J Med 287:237, 1972

18. Guyton AC: Rhythmic excitation of the heart. In Guyton AC (ed): Textbook of Medical Physiology, p 165. Philadelphia, WB Saunders, 1986

19. Flacke WE, Flacke JW: Cholinergic and anticholinergic agents. In Smith NT, Corbascio AN (eds): Drug Interaction in Anesthesia, p 160. Philadelphia, Lea & Febiger, 1986

20. Fujii AM, Vatner SF: Autonomic mechanisms regulating myocardial contractility in conscious animals. Pharmacol Ther 29:221, 1985

21. Yanowitz F, Preston JB, Abildskov JA: Functional distribution of right and left stellate innervation to the ventricles. Circ Res 18:416, 1966

22. Berne RM, Levy MN: Control of the heart. In Berne RM, Levy MN (eds): Cardiovascular Physiology, p 221. St. Louis, CV Mosby, 1977

23. Bexton RS, Milne JR, Cory-Pearce R et al: Effect of beta blockade on exercise response after cardiac transplantation. Br Heart J 49:584, 1983

24. Manger WM: Catecholamines in normal and abnormal cardiac function. In Kellerman JJ (ed): Advances in Cardiology, p 30. New York, Karger, 1982

25. Vatner SF: Regulation of coronary resistance vessels and large coronary arteries. Am J Cardiol 56:16E, 1985

26. Hillis LD, Braunwald E: Coronary-artery spasm. N Engl J Med 299:695, 1978

27. Shepard JT, Vanhoutte PM: Spasm of the coronary arteries: Causes and consequences (the scientist's viewpoint). Mayo Clin Proc 60:33, 1985

28. Kates RA, Stack RS, Hill RF et al: General anesthesia for patients undergoing percutaneous transluminal coronary angioplasty during acute myocardial infarction. Anesth Analg 65:815, 1986

29. Braunwald E: A symposium: Experimental and clinical aspects of coronary vasoconstriction. Am J Cardiol 56:672, 1985

30. Osswald W, Guimaraes S: Adrenergic mechanisms in blood vessels: Morphological and pharmacological aspects. Rev Physiol Biochem Pharmacol 96:54, 1983

31. Lawson NW, Wallfisch HK: Cardiovascular pharmacology: A new look at the "pressors." In Stoelting RK, Barash PG, Gallagher TJ (eds): Advances in Anesthesia, p 195. Chicago, Year Book Medical Publishers, 1986

32. Bevan JA: Some basis of differences in vascular response to sympathetic activity: Variations on a theme. Circ Res 45:161, 1979

33. Guyton AC: Local control of blood flow by the tissues, and nervous and humoral regulation. In Guyton AC (ed): Textbook of Medical Physiology, p 230. Philadelphia, WB Saunders, 1986

34. Nandiwada PA, Hyman AL, Kadowitz PJ: Pulmonary vasodilator responses to vagal stimulation and acetylcholine in the cat. Circ Res 53:86, 1983

35. Guyton AC: The pulmonary circulation. In Guyton AC (ed): Textbook of Medical Physiology, p 287. Philadelphia, WB Saunders, 1986

36. Benumof JL: The pulmonary circulation. In Kaplan JA (ed): Thoracic Anesthesia p 249. New York, Churchill-Livingstone, 1983

37. Benumof JL: One-lung ventilation and hypoxic pulmonary vasoconstriction: Implications for anesthetic management. Anesth Analg 64:821, 1985

38. Carlsson AJ, Bindslev L, Hedenstierna G: Hypoxia-induced pulmonary vasoconstriction in the human lung. Anesthesiology 66:312, 1987

39. Comroe JH: Reflexes from the lungs. In Comroe JH (ed): Physiology of Respiration, p 72. Chicago, Year Book Medical Publishers, 1979

40. Junod AF: Metabolism of vasoactive agents in lung. Am Rev Respir Dis 115:51, 1977

41. Youdim MBH, Bakhle YS, Ben-Harari RR: Inaction of monoamines by the lung. In Metabolic Activities of the Lung, p 105. Amsterdam, Ciba Foundation Symposium 78, Exerpta, Medica, 1980

42. Halter JB, Pflug AE, Tolas AG: Arterial-venous differences of plasma catecholamines in man. Metabolism 29:9, 1980

43. Pearl RG, Maze M, Rosenthal MH: Pulmonary and systemic hemodynamic effects of central nervous and left atrial sympathomimetic drug administration in the dog. J Cardiothorac Anesth 1:29, 1987

44. Bevan JA: Some basis of differences in vascular response to sympathetic activity. Circ Res 45:161, 1979

45. Miller R: Multiple calcium channels and neuronal function. Science 235:46, 1987

46. Carpenter RL, Mulroy MF: Edrophonium antagonizes combined lidocaine-pancuronium and verapamil-pancuronium neuro-muscular blockade in cats. Anesthesiology 65:506, 1986

47. Wood M: Cholinergic and parasympathomimetic drugs. Cholinesterases and anticholinesterases. In Wood M, Wood AJJ (eds): Drugs and Anesthesia, p 111. Baltimore, Williams & Wilkins, 1982

48. Thomas J, Fouad FM, Tarazi RC et al: Evaluation of plasma catecholamines in humans. Correlation of resting levels with cardiac responses to beta-blocking and sympatholytic drugs. Hypertension 5:858, 1983

49. Lake CR, Ziegler MG, Kopin IJ: Use of plasma norepinephrine for evaluation of sympathetic neuronal function in man. Life Sci 18:1315, 1976

50. Stoelting RK: Sympathomimetics. In Stoelting RK (ed): Pharmacology and Physiology in Anesthetic Practice, p 251. Philadelphia, JB Lippincott, 1987

51. Zaimis E: Vasopressor drugs and catecholamines. Anesthesiology 29:732, 1968

52. Smith NT, Corbascio AN: The use and misuse of pressor agents. Anesthesiology 8:58, 1970

53. Shepard JT, Vanhoutte PM: Neurohumoral Regulation. The Human Cardiovascular System, p 368. New York, Raven Press, 1984

54. Zsigmond EK: Catecholamines and anesthesia. In Oyama T (ed): Endocrinology and the Anaesthetist, p 225. New York, Elsevier, 1983

55. Zaritsky AL, Chernow B: Catecholamines, sympathomimetics. In Ziegler MG, Lake CR (eds): Frontiers of Clinical Neurosci-

ence, vol 2 (Norepinephrine), p 481. Baltimore, Williams & Wilkins, 1984

56. Kopin IJ: Catecholamine metabolism and the biochemical assessment of sympathetic activity. Clin Endocrinol Metab 6:525, 1977

57. Chernow B, Rainey TG, Lake CR: Catecholamines in critical care medicine. In Ziegler MG, Lake CR (eds): Frontiers of Clinical Neuroscience, vol 2 (Norepinephrine), p 368. Baltimore, Williams & Wilkins, 1984

58. Fuder H: Selected aspects of presynaptic modulation of noradrenaline release from the heart. J Cardiovasc Pharmacol 7 (suppl 5):S2, 1985

59. Kopin IJ: Metabolic degradation of catecholamines and relative importance of different pathways under physiological conditions and after the administration of drugs. In Blaschko H, Muscholl E (eds): Catecholamines: Handbook of Experimental Pharmacology, p 270. New York, Springer Verlag, 1972

60. Lefkowitz RJ: Beta-adrenergic receptors: Recognition and regulation. N Engl J Med 295:323, 1976

61. Maze M: Clinical implications of membrane receptor function in anesthesia. Anesthesiology 55:160, 1981

62. Wood M: Cholinergic and parasympathomimetic drugs. Cholinesterases and anticholinesterases. In Wood M, Wood AJJ (eds): Drugs and Anesthesia, p 111. Baltimore, Williams & Wilkins, 1982

63. Reardon DP, Bailey JC: Parasympathetic effects on electrophysiologic properties of cardiac ventricular tissue. J Am Coll Cardiol 2:1200, 1983

64. Von Euler US: A specific sympathomimetic ergone in adrenergic nerve fibers (sympathin) and its relation to adrenaline and noradrenaline. Acta Physiol Scand 12:73, 1946

65. Ahlquist RP: A study of the adrenotropic receptors. Am J Physiol 153:586, 1948

66. Exton JH: Mechanisms involved in α-adrenergic phenomena. Am J Physiol 248:E633, 1985

67. Lands AM, Arnold A, McAnliff JP et al: Differentiation of receptor systems activated by sympathomimetic amines. Nature 214:597, 1967

68. Ariens EJ, Simonis AM: Physiological and pharmacological aspects of adrenergic receptor classification. Biochem Pharmacol 32:1539, 1983

69. Kebabian JW, Calne DB: Multiple receptors for dopamine. Nature 277:93, 1979

70. Davey MJ: Alpha adrenoreceptors—an overview. J Mol Cell Cardiol 18:1, 1986

71. Dresel PE: Cardiac alpha receptors and arrhythmias. Anesthesiology 63:582, 1985

72. Maze M, Hayward E, Gaba DM: Alpha$_1$-adrenergic blockade raises epinephrine-arrhythmia threshold in halothane-anesthetized dogs in a dose-dependent fashion. Anesthesiology 63:611, 1985

73. Aubrey ML, Davey MJ, Petch B: Cardioprotective and antidysrhythmic effects of alpha-1 adrenoreceptor blockade during myocardial ischemia and reperfusion in the dog. J Cardiovasc Pharmacol 7:S93, 1985

74. Maze M, Segal IS, Bloor BC: Clonidine and other alpha$_2$ adrenergic agonists: Strategies for the rational use of these novel anesthetic agents. J Clin Anesth 2:146, 1988

75. Hoffman BB, Lefkowitz RJ: Alpha-adrenergic receptor subtypes. N Engl J Med 302:1390, 1980

76. Berthelesen S, Pettinger WA: A functional basis for classification of alpha adrenergic receptors. Life Sci 21:595, 1977

77. Langer SZ, Hicks PE: Alpha-adrenergic subtypes in blood vessels: Physiology and pharmacology. J Cardiovasc Pharmacol 6:S547, 1984

78. Ruffolo RR, De Marinas RM, Wise M et al: Structure-activity relations for alpha-2 adrenergic receptor agonists and antagonists. In Limbirt LE (ed): The α2-Adrenergic Receptors, p 115. Clifton NJ, Humana Press, 1988

79. Hyman AL, Kadowitz PJ: Evidence for existence of postjunctional α_1- and α_2-adrenoreceptors in cat pulmonary vascular bed. Am J Physiol 249:H891, 1985

80. Langer SZ: Presynaptic regulation of catecholamine release. Biochem Pharmacol 23:1793, 1974

81. Bryan LJ, Cole JJ, O'Donnell SR et al: A study designed to explore the hypothesis that the beta$_1$ adrenoceptors are "innervated" receptors and beta$_2$ adrenoceptors are "hormonal" receptors. J Pharmacol Exp Ther 216:395, 1981

82. Goldberg LI: Dopamine receptors and hypertension. Am J Med 77:37, 1984

83. Rajfer SI, Goldbert LI: Dopamine in the treatment of heart failure. Eur Heart J 3(suppl D):103, 1982

84. Peringer E, Jenner P, Donaldson IM et al: Metoclopramide and dopamine receptor blockade. Neuropharmacology 15:463, 1976

85. Yahr MD: Levodopa. Ann Intern Med 83:677, 1975

86. Goldberg LI, Volkman PH, Kohli JD: A comparison of the vascular receptor with other dopamine receptors. Ann Rev Pharmacol Toxicol 18:57, 1978

87. Solanki DR, Suresh M, Ethridge HC: The effects of intravenous cimetidine and metaclopramide on gastric volume and pH. Anesth Analg 63:599, 1984

88. Thorner MD: Dopamine is an important neurotransmitter in the autonomic nervous system. Lancet 1:662, 1975

89. Hilberman M, Maseda J, Stinson EB et al: The diuretic properties of dopamine in patients following open heart operations. Anesthesiology 61:489, 1984

90. Daly JW, Bruns RF, Snyder SH: Adenosine receptors in the central nervous system: Relationship to the central actions of methylxanthines. Life Sci 28:2083, 1981

91. Barrett JE, Tessel RE: Behavioral pharmacology of drugs affecting norepinephrine transmission. In Ziegler MG, Lake CR (eds): Frontiers of Clinical Neuroscience, vol 2 (Norepinephrine), p 160. Baltimore, Williams & Wilkins, 1984

92. Owall A, Gordon E, Lagerkranser M et al: Clinical experience with adenosine for controlled hypotension during cerebral aneurysm surgery. Anesth Analg 66:229, 1987

93. Engel G, Gothert M, Muller-Schweinitzer E et al: Evidence for common pharmacological properties of 5-hydroxy-tryptamine binding sites; presynaptic 5-hydroxytryptamine autoreceptors in CNS and inhibitory presynaptic 5-hydroxytryptamine receptors on sympathetic nerves. Naunyn Schmiedebergs Arch Pharmacol 324:116, 1983

94. Manchikanti L, Kraus JW, Fields SP: Cimetidine and related drugs in anesthesia. Anesth Analg 61:595, 1982

95. Lineberger AS, Sprague DH, Battaglini JW: Sinus arrest associated with cimetidine. Anesth Analg 64:554, 1985

96. Goldberg LI: The dopamine vascular receptor: New areas for biochemical pharmacologists. Biochem Pharmacol 24:651, 1975

97. Williams LT, Lefkowitz RJ: Receptor Binding Studies in Adrenergic Pharmacology. New York, Raven Press, 1979

98. Motulsky JH, Insel PA: Adrenergic receptors in man. N Engl J Med 302:18, 1982

99. Tell GP, Haour F, Saez JM: Hormone regulation of membrane receptors and cell responsiveness: A review. Metabolism 27:1566, 1978

100. Galant SP, Duriseti L, Underwood S et al: Decreased beta-adrenergic receptors on polymorphonuclear leukocytes after adrenergic therapy. N Engl J Med 299:933, 1978

101. Glaubiger G, Lefkowitz RJ: Elevated beta-adrenergic number after chronic propranolol treatment. Biochem Biophys Res Commun 78:720, 1977

102. Hoefke W: Clonidine: In Scriabine A (ed): Pharmacology of Antihypertensive Drugs, p 55. New York, Raven Press, 1980

103. Johnston RV, Nicholas DA, Lawson NW et al: The use of rectal clonidine in the perioperative period. Anesthesiology 64:288, 1986

104. Myers MG: Beta adrenoreceptor antagonism and pressor response to phenylephrine. Clin Pharmacol Ther 36:57, 1984

105. Williams LT, Lefkowitz RJ: Thyroid hormone regulation of β-adrenergic receptor number. J Biol Chem 252:2787, 1977

106. Sutherland EW, Robison GA: The role of cyclic-3'5' AMP in response to catecholamines and other hormones. Pharmacol Rev 18:145, 1966

107. Sutherland EW, Robison GA, Butcher RW: Some aspects of the biological role of adenosine 3'5' monophosphate. Circulation 37:279, 1968

108. Schramm M, Selinger Z: Message transmission: Receptor controlled adenylate cyclase system. Science 225:1350, 1984

109. Lefkowitz RJ, Cerione RA, Codina J et al: Reconstitution of the β-adrenergic receptor. J Membrane Biol 87:1, 1985

110. Gilman AG: Proteins and dual control of adenylate cyclase. Cell 36:577, 1984

111. Yatani A, Brown AM: Adrenergic modulation of cardiac calcium channel currents by a fast G protein pathway. Science 245:71, 1989

112. Sutherland EW, Oye I, Butcher RW: The action of epinephrine and the role of adenyl cyclase system in hormone action. Recent Prog Horm Res 21:623, 1965

113. Tomlinson S, MacNeil S, Brown BL: Calcium, cyclic AMP and hormone action. Clin Endocrinol 23:595, 1985

114. Lamers JM: Calcium transport systems in cardiac sarcolemma and their regulation by the second messenger cyclic AMP and calcium-calmodulin. Gen Physiol Biophys 4:143, 1985

115. Exton JH: Mechanisms involved in α-adrenergic phenomena. Am J Physiol 258:E633, 1985

116. Ignarro LJ, Kadowitz PJ: The pharmacological and physiological role of cyclic GMP in vascular smooth muscle relaxation. Annu Rev Pharmacol Toxicol 25:171, 1985

117. Berridge MJ: Inositol triphosphate and diaglycerol as second messengers. Biochem J 22:345, 1984

118. Marx JL: Polyphosphoinositide research updated. Science 235:974, 1987

119. Kariya T, Wille L, Dage R: Biochemical studies on the mechanism of cardiotonic activity of MDL 17,043. J Cardiovasc Pharmacol 4:509, 1982

120. Rasmussen H: The cycling of calcium as an intracellular messenger. Sci Am 261:73, 1989

121. Rasmussen H, Barret PO: Calcium messenger system: An integrated view. Pharmacol Rev 64:938, 1984

122. Levitzki P: From epinephrine to cyclic AMP. Science 241:800, 1988

123. Kreiger EM: Time course of baroreceptor resetting in acute hypertension. Am J Physiol 218:486, 1970

124. Flacke WE, Flacke JW: Cardiovascular physiology and circulatory control. Semin Anesth 1:185, 1982

125. Takeshima R, Dohi S: Circulatory responses to baroreflexes, Valsalva maneuver, coughing, swallowing, and nasal stimulation during acute cardiac sympathectomy by epidural blockade in awake humans. Anesthesiology 63:500, 1985

126. Berne RM, Levy MN: Coronary circulation and cardiac metabolism. In Berne RM, Levy MN (eds): Cardiovascular Physiology, p 221. St. Louis, CV Mosby Co, 1977

127. Guyton AC: Cardiac output, venous return, and their regulation. In Guyton AC (ed): Textbook of Medical Physiology, p 272. Philadelphia, WB Saunders, 1986

128. Sharpey-Schafer EP: Venous tone: Effects of reflex changes, humoral agents and exercise. Br Med Bull 19:115, 1963

129. Blinks JR: Positive chronotropic effect of increasing right atrial pressure in the isolated mammalian heart. Am J Physiol 196:299, 1956

130. Baron JF, Decauz-Jacolot A, Edouard A et al: Influence of venous return on baroreflex control of heart rate during lumbar epidural anesthesia in humans. Anesthesiology 64:188, 1986

131. Kotrly KT, Ebert TJ, Vucins E et al: Baroreceptor reflex control of heart rate during isoflurane anesthesia in humans. Anesthesiology 60:173, 1984

132. Greene NM: The cardiovascular system. In Greene NM (ed): Physiology of Spinal Anesthesia, p 43. New York, Kreiger Publishing, 1976

133. Greene NM: Perspectives in spinal anesthesia. Reg Anesth 7:55, 1982

134. Bailey PL, Stanley TH: Anesthesia for patients with a prior cardiac transplant. J Cardiothorac Anesth 4:38, 1990

135. Bexton RS, Milne JR, Cory-Pearce R et al: Effect of beta blockade on exercise response after cardiac transplantation. Br Heart J 49:584, 1983

136. Orlick AE, Ricci DR, Alderman EL et al: Effects of alpha adrenergic blockade upon coronary hemodynamics. J Clin Invest 62:459, 1978

137. Fowles RE, Reitz BA, Ream AK: Drug actions in a transplanted or artificial heart. In Kaplan JA (ed): Cardiac Anesthesia, vol 2 (Cardiovascular Pharmacology), p 641. New York, Grune & Stratton, 1983

138. Cannom DS, Rider AK, Stinson EB et al: Electrophysiologic studies in the denervated transplanted human heart: II. Response to norepinephrine, isoproterenol and propranolol. Am J Cardiol 36:859, 1975

139. Leachman RD, Cokkinos DVP, Cabrera R et al: Response of the transplanted, denervated human heart to cardiovascular drugs. Am J Cardiol 27:273, 1971

140. Bexton RS, Milne JR, Cory-Pearce R et al: Effect of beta blockade on exercise response after cardiac transplantation. Br Heart J 49:584, 1983

141. Shepard JT, Vanhoutte PM: Why nerves to coronary vessels? Symposium—Autonomic control of coronary tone: Facts, interpretations, and consequences. Fed Proc 43:2855, 1984

142. Moreland RS, Bohr DF: Adrenergic control of coronary arteries. Fed Proc 43:2858, 1984

143. Vanhoutte PM, Cohen RA: Effects of acetylcholine on the coronary artery. Fed Proc 43:2878, 1984

144. Feigl EO: Parasympathetic control of coronary blood flow. Fed Proc 43:2881, 1984

145. Loffelholz K, Muscholl E: Muscarinic inhibition of the noradrenaline release evoked by postganglionic sympathetic nerve stimulation. Naunyn Schmiedebergs Arch Pharmacol 265:1, 1969

146. Levy MN, Blattberg B: Effect of vagal stimulation on the overflow of norepinephrine into the coronary sinus during cardiac sympathetic nerve stimulation in the dog. Circ Res 107:508, 1976

147. Yasue H, Touyama M, Shimamoto M et al: The role of the autonomic nervous system in the pathogenesis of Prinzmetal's variant form of angina. Circulation 50:534, 1984

148. Schrier RW, Berl T, Anderson RJ: Osmotic and nonosmotic control of vasopressin release. Am J Physiol 236:F321, 1979

149. Coore HG, Randle PJ: Regulation of insulin secretion studied with pieces of rabbit pancreas incubated in vitro. Biochem J 93:66, 1964

150. Torretti J, Gerson J, Cates RP et al: β-adrenoreceptor blockade and tolerance to potassium. Anesthesiology 64:846, 1986

151. Todd PA, Heel RC: Enalapril: A review. Drugs 31:198, 1986

152. Frohlich E: Angiotensin converting enzyme inhibitors. Hypertension 13:I-125, 1989

153. Dzau VJ: Mechanism of action of angiotensin-converting enzymes (ACE) inhibitors in hypertension and heart failure. Drugs (suppl. 2):11, 1990

154. Weinberger MH: Angiotensin-converting enzyme inhibitors. Med Clin North Am 71:979, 1987

155. Stoelting RK: Antihypertensive drugs. In Stoelting RK (ed): Pharmacology and Physiology in Anesthetic Practice, p 294. Philadelphia, JB Lippincott, 1987

156. MacGregor GA, Dawes PM: Agonist and antagonist effects of Sar¹-Ala⁸-angiotensin II in salt-loaded and salt-depleted normal man. Br J Clin Pharmacol 3:483, 1976

157. Taylor P: Ganglionic stimulating and blocking agents. In Gilman AG, Goodman LS, Rall TW, Murad F (eds): The Pharmacological Basis of Therapeutics, 7th ed, p 315. New York, Macmillan, 1985

158. Vickers MD, Wood-Smith FG, Stewart HC: Cardiovascular drugs. In Vickers MD, Wood-Smith FG, Stewart HC (eds): Drugs in Anesthetic Practice, p 337. Boston, Butterworth, 1979

159. Stoelting RK: Peripheral vasodilators. In Stoelting RK (ed): Pharmacology and Physiology in Anesthetic Practice, p 307. Philadelphia, JB Lippincott, 1987

160. Taylor P: Cholinergic agonists. In Gilman AG, Goodman LS, Rall TW, Murad F (eds): The Pharmacological Basis of Therapeutics, p 100. New York, Macmillan, 1985

161. Stoelting RK: Anticholinesterase drugs and cholinergic agonists. In Stoelting RK (ed): Pharmacology and Physiology in Anesthetic Practice, p 217. Philadelphia, JB Lippincott, 1987

162. Vickers MD, Wood-Smith FG, Stewart HC: Parasympathomimetic and cholinergic agents: Anticholinesterases. In Vickers

MD, Wood-Smith FG, Stewart HC (eds): Drugs in Anesthetic Practice, p 306. Boston, Butterworth, 1979

163. Westfall TC: Muscarinic agents. In Bevan JA (ed): Essentials of Pharmacology, p 116. New York, Harper & Row, 1976

164. Westfall TC: Cholinesterase inhibitors. In Bevan JA (ed): Essentials of Pharmacology, p 120. New York, Harper & Row, 1976

165. Bell CMA, Lewis CB: Effect of neostigmine on integrity of ileorectal anastomoses. Br Med J 3:587, 1968

166. Wilkins JL, Hardcastle JD, Mann CV, Kaufman L: Effects of neostigmine and atropine on motor activity on ileum, colon, and rectum of anesthetized subjects. Br J Med 1:793, 1970

167. Brown EN, Daughety MJ, Petty WC: Integrity of intestinal anastomoses muscle relaxant reversal with neostigmine. Anesth Analg 1:117, 1973

168. Child CS: Prevention of neostigmine-induced colonic activity. Anesthesia 39:1083, 1984

169. Taylor P: Anticholinesterase agents. In Gilman AG, Goodman LS, Rall TW, Murad F (eds): The Pharmacological Basis of Therapeutics, p 110. New York, Macmillan, 1985

170. De Roetth A, Wong A, Dettbarn WD et al: Blood cholinesterase activity of glaucoma patients treated with phospholine iodide. Am J Ophthalmol 62:834, 1966

171. Milby TH: Prevention and management of organophosphate poisoning. JAMA 216:2131, 1971

172. Stoelting RK: Anticholinergic drugs. In Stoelting RK (ed): Pharmacology and Physiology in Anesthetic Practice, p 232. Philadelphia, JB Lippincott, 1987

173. Price NM, Schmitt LG, McGuire J et al: Transdermal scopolamine in the prevention of motion sickness at sea. Clin Pharmacol Ther 29:414, 1981

174. Wood M: Anticholinergic drugs: Anesthetic premedication. In Wood M, Wood AJJ (eds): Drugs and Anesthesia: Pharmacology for Anesthesiologists, p 141. Baltimore, Williams & Wilkins, 1982

175. Weiner N: Atropine, scopolamine, and related antimuscarinic drugs. In Gilman AG, Goodman LS, Rall TW, Murad F (eds): The Pharmacological Basis of Therapeutics, 7th ed, p 110. New York, Macmillan, 1985

176. Westfall TC: Antimuscarinic agents. In Bevan JA (ed): Essentials of Pharmacology, p 128. New York, Harper & Row, 1976

177. Duvoisin RC, Katz RL: Reversal of central anticholinergic syndrome in man by physostigmine. JAMA 206:1963, 1968

178. Spaulding BC, Choi SD, Gross JB et al: The effect of physostigmine on diazepam-induced ventilatory depression: a double-blind study. Anesthesiology 61:551, 1984

179. Snir-Mor I, Weinstock M, Davidson JT, Bahar M: Physostigmine antagonizes morphine-induced respiratory depression in human subjects. Anesthesiology 59:6, 1983

180. Ruiz CE, Weil MH, Carlson RW: Treatment of circulatory shock with dopamine: Studies on survival. JAMA 242:165, 1979

181. Resnekov L: University of Chicago Myocardial Infarction Research Unit: Comprehensive Clinical and Laboratory Research. Washington DC U.S. Public Health Service PH43-68-1334-A73, 1975

182. Resnekov L: Cardiogenic shock. Chest 83:893, 1983

183. Reinart K: Principles and Practice of SvO₂ Monitoring, pp 121–124. London, Intensive Care World, King and Worth, Publishers, vol 5, no 4, Dec 1988

184. Astiz ME, Rackow EC, Falk JL et al: Oxygen delivery and consumption in patients with hyperdynamic septic shock. Crit Care Med 15:26, 1987

185. Wynands JE: Amrinone: Is it the inotrope of choice? J Cardiothorac Anesth 3:45, 1989

186. Rothe CF: Physiology of venous return. Arch Intern Med 146:977, 1986

187. Stanton-Hicks M, Hock A, Stuhmeier K, Arndt JO: Venoconstrictor agents mobilize blood from different sources and increase intrathoracic filling during epidural anesthesia in supine humans. Anesthesiology 66:317, 1987

188. Lundberg J, Norgren L, Thomson D, Werner O: Hemodynamic effects of dopamine during thoracic epidural analgesia in man. Anesthesiology 66:641, 1987

189. Ramanathan S, Grant G, Turndorf H: Cardiac preload changes with ephedrine therapy for hypotension in obstetrical patients. Anesth Analg 65:S125, 1986

190. Butterworth JF, Austin JC, Johnson MD et al: Effect of total spinal anesthesia on arterial and venous responses to dopamine and dobutamine. Anesth Analg 66:209, 1987

191. Cubbold A, Folkow B, Kjellmer I et al: Nervous and local chemical control of pre-capillary sphincters in skeletal muscle as measured by changes in filtration coefficient. Acta Physiol Scand 57:180, 1963

192. Folkow B, Mellander S: Veins and venous tone. Am Heart J 68:309, 1964

193. Coffman JD, Lempert JA: Venous flow velocity, venous volume and arterial blood flow. Circulation 52:141, 1975

194. Sharpey-Schafer EP, Ginsburg J: Humoral agents and venous tone. Effects of catecholamines, 5-hydroxytryptamine, histamine and nitrites. Lancet 2:1337, 1962

195. Zimmerman BG, Abboud FM, Eckstein JW: Comparison of the effects of sympathomimetic amines upon venous and total vascular resistance in the foreleg of the dog. J Pharmacol Exp Ther 139:290, 1963

196. Schmid PG, Eckstein JW, Abboud FM: Comparison of the effects of several sympathomimetic amines on resistance and capacitance vessels in the forearm of man. Circulation 34:209, 1966

197. Marino RJ, Romagnoli A, Keats A: Selective venoconstriction by dopamine in comparison with isoproterenol and phenylephrine. Anesthesiology 43:570, 1975

198. Gurmaraes S, Osswald W: Adrenergic receptors in the veins of dogs. Eur J Pharmacol 5:133, 1969

199. McNay JL, McDonald RA, Goldberg LI: Direct renal vasodilatation produced by dopamine in the dog. Circ Res 16:510, 1965

200. DeMay J, Vanhoutte PM: Uneven distribution of postjunctional alpha₁ and alpha₂-like adrenoreceptors in canine arterial and venous smooth muscle. Circ Res 48:875, 1981

201. Rude RE: Pharmacologic support in cardiogenic shock. Adv Shock Res 10:35, 1983

202. Rajfer SI, Goldberg LI: Sympathetic amines in the treatment of shock. In Shoemaker WC, Thompson WL, Holbrook PR (eds): Textbook of Critical Care, p 490. Philadelphia: WB Saunders, 1984

203. Houston MC, Thompson WL, Robertson D: Shock diagnosis and management. Arch Intern Med 144:1433, 1984

204. Shoemaker WC: Fluid management. Semin Anesth 2:251, 1983

205. Makabali C, Weil MH, Henning RJ: Dobutamine and other sympathomimetic drugs for the treatment of low cardiac output failure. Semin Anesth 1:63, 1982

206. Roberts R: The role of diuretics and inotropic therapy in failure associated with myocardial infarction. Arch Int Physiol Biochem 92:S33–48, 1984

207. Rouke GA, Freund PR, Jacobsen AF et al: Effect of spinal anesthesia in geriatric patients with heart disease; choice of vasopressor therapy to reverse hemodynamic changes. Anesthesiology 73:A140, 1990

208. Schwinn DA, Reves JG: Time course and hemodynamic effects of alpha-1 adrenergic bolus administration in anesthetized patients with myocardial disease. Anesth Analg 68:571, 1989

209. Evans DB, Weishaar RE, Kaplan HR: Strategy for the discovery and development of a positive inotropic agent. Pharmacol Ther 16:303, 1982

210. Hug CC, Kaplan JA: Pharmacology—cardiac drugs. In Kaplan JA (ed): Cardiac Anesthesia, p 39. New York, Grune & Stratton, 1979

211. Bourdaris JP, Dubourg O, Gueret P et al: Inotropic agents in the treatment of cardiogenic shock. Pharmacol Ther 22:53, 1983

212. Mueller HS: Catecholamine support of the critically ill cardiac patient: Inotropic agents versus vasopressors α- or β-adrenergic agonists or both? Intensive Crit Care Digest 5:36, 1986

213. Desjars P, Pinaud M, Bugnon D et al: Norepinephrine therapy has no deleterious renal effects in human septic shock. Crit Care Med 17:426, 1989

214. Meadows D, Edwards JD, Wilkins RG *et al*: Reversal of intractable septic shock with norepinephrine therapy. Crit Care Med 16:663, 1988

215. Desjars P, Pinaud M, Potel G *et al*: A reappraisal of norepinephrine therapy in human septic shock. Crit Care Med 15:134, 1987

216. Stuart-Taylor ME, Crosse MM: A plea for noradrenaline. Anaesthesia 44:916, 1989

217. Waller JL: Inotropes and vasopressors. In Kaplan JA (ed): Cardiac Anesthesia, vol 2 (Cardiovascular Pharmacology), p 273. New York, Grune & Stratton, 1983

218. Wood M: Drugs and the sympathetic nervous system. In Wood M, Alistair JJ (eds): Drugs and Anesthesia. Baltimore, Williams & Wilkins, 1982

219. Maze M, Smith CM: Identification of receptor mechanism mediating epinephrine-induced arrhythmias during halothane anesthesia in the dog. Anesthesiology 59:322, 1983

220. Kapur PA, Flacke WE: Epinephrine-induced arrhythmias and cardiovascular function after verapamil during halothane anesthesia in the dog. Anesthesiology 55:218, 1981

221. Reves JG, Kissin I, Lell WA, Tosone S: Calcium entry blockers: Uses and implications for anesthesiologist. Anesthesiology 57:504, 1982

222. Stoelting RK: Calcium entry blockers. In Stoelting RK (ed): Pharmacology and Physiology in Anesthetic Practice, p 355. Philadelphia, JB Lippincott, 1987

223. Johnston RR, Eger EI, Wilson C: A comparative interaction of epinephrine with enflurane, isoflurane, and halothane in man. Anesth Analg 55:709, 1976

224. Karl HW, Swedlow DB, Lee KW *et al*: Epinephrine-halothane interactions in children. Anesthesiology 58:142, 1983

225. Ramanathan S, Grant GJ: Vasopressor therapy for hypotension due to epidural anesthesia for cesarean section. Acta Anaesthesiol Scand 32:1, 1988

226. Boudaris JP, Duborg O, Gueret P *et al*: Inotropic agents in the treatment of cardiogenic shock. Pharmacol Ther 22:53, 1983

227. Houston MC, Thompson WL, Robertson D: Shock diagnosis and management. Arch Intern Med 144:1433, 1984

228. Goldberg LI, Hsieh Y, Resnekov L: Newer catecholamines for treatment of heart failure and shock: An update on dopamine and a first look at dobutamine. Prog Cardiovasc Dis 19:327, 1977

229. Pank JR, Tinker JH: Cardioactive drugs and their monitorable effects. Semin Anesth 11:268, 1983

230. Lappas DG, Powell WMJ, Daggett WM: Cardiac dysfunction in the perioperative period, pathophysiological diagnosis and treatment. Anesthesiology 47:117, 1977

231. Murphy MB, Elliott WJ: Dopamine and dopamine receptor agonists in cardiovascular therapy. Crit Care Med 18:S14, 1990

232. Shoemaker WC, Appel PL, Kram HB: Hemodynamic and oxygen transport effects of dobutamine in critically ill general surgical patients. Crit Care Med 14:1032, 1986

233. Furman WR, Summer WR, Kennedy TP *et al*: Comparison of the effects of dobutamine, dopamine, and isoproterenol on hypoxic pulmonary vasoconstriction in the pig. Crit Care Med 10:371, 1982

234. Lokhandwala MF: Renal actions of dopexamine hydrochloride. Clin Intensive Care 1:163, 1990

235. Colardyn FC, Vandenbogaerde JF, Vogelaers DP *et al*: Use of dopexamine hydrochloride in patients with septic shock. Crit Care Med 17:999, 1990

236. McCormack DG, Barnes PJ, Evans TW: Effects of dopexamine hydrochloride on hypoxic pulmonary vasoconstriction in isolated rat lung. Crit Care Med 18:520, 1990

237. Baumann G, Felix SB, Filcek SAL: Usefulness of dopexamine hydrochloride versus dobutamine in chronic congestive heart failure and effects on hemodynamics and urine output. Am J Cardiol 65:748, 1990

238. Lawson N: Therapeutic combinations of vasopressors and inotropic agents. Semin Anesth 9:270, 1990

239. Lipman J, Plit M: A guide to the rational use of dopamine, dobutamine, and isoprenaline in patients who need inotropic support. S Afr Med J 65:506, 1984

240. Tinker JH: Perioperative myocardial infarction. Semin Anesth 1:253, 1982

241. Ferguson JE, Hensleigh PA, Kredenster D: Adjunctive use of magnesium sulfate with ritodrine for preterm labor tocolysis. Am J Obstet Gynecol 148:166, 1984

242. Schwarz R, Retzke U: Cardiovascular effects of terbutaline in pregnant women. Acta Obstet Gynecol Scand 62:419, 1983

243. Beneditti TJ: Maternal complications of parenteral β-sympathetic therapy for premature labor. Am J Obstet Gynecol 145:1, 1983

244. Pou-Martinez A, Kelly SH, Newell FD, Culbert CM: Postpartum pulmonary edema after ritodrine and betamethasone use. J Reprod Med 27:428, 1982

245. Semchyshyn S, Zuspan FP, O'Shaughnessy R: Pulmonary edema associated with the use of hydrocortisone and a tocolytic agent for the management of premature labor. J Reprod Med 28:47, 1983

246. Spielman RJ: Maternal effects and complications of beta-adrenergic therapy for premature labor. Resident Staff Phys 32:102, 1986

247. Rasmussen H: Cell communication, calcium ion and cyclic adenosine monophosphate. Science 170:404, 1970

248. Rutman HI, LeJemtel TH, Sonnenblick EH: Newer cardiotonic agents: Implications for patients with heart failure and ischemic heart disease. J Cardiothorac Anesth 1:59, 1987

249. Stirt JA, Sullivan SF: Aminophylline. Anesth Analg 60:587, 1981

250. Levy JH, Bailey JM: Amrinone: Pharmacokinetics and pharmacodynamics. J Cardiothorac Anesth 3:10, 1989

251. Hines R: Clinical applications of amrinone. J Cardiothorac Anesth 3:24, 1989

252. Braunwald E: A symposium: Amrinone. Am J Cardiol 56:1B, 1985

253. Braunwald E: Newer positive inotropic agents. Circulation 73(suppl): III 1–3, 1986

254. Benotti JR, Grossman W, Braunwald E *et al*: Effects of amrinone on myocardial energy metabolism and hemodynamics in patients with severe congestive heart failure due to coronary artery disease. Circulation 68:28, 1980

255. Ward A, Brogden RN, Heel RC *et al*: Amrinone—a preliminary review of its pharmacological properties and therapeutic use. Drugs 26:468, 1983

256. Baim DS, McDowell AV, Cherniles J *et al*: Evaluation of a new bipyridine inotropic agent—milrinone—in patients with severe congestive heart failure. N Engl J Med 309:748, 1983

257. Boldt J, Kling D, Moosdorf R, Hempelmann G: Enoximone treatment of impaired myocardial function during cardiac surgery; combined effects with epinephrine. J Cardiothorac Surg 4:462, 1990

258. Colucci WS, Wright RF, Braunwald E: New positive inotropic agents in the treatment of congestive heart failure. Part 1. N Engl J Med 314:290, 1986

259. Colucci WS, Wright RF, Braunwald E: New positive inotropic agents in the treatment of congestive heart failure. Part 2. New Engl J Med 314:349, 1986

260. Zaloga GP, Chernow B: Insulin, glucagon and growth hormone. In Chernow B, Lake CR (eds): The Pharmacologic Approach to the Critically Ill Patient, p 562. Baltimore, Williams & Wilkins, 1983

261. Stoelting RK: Digitalis and related drugs. In Stoelting RK (ed): Pharmacology and Physiology in Anesthetic Practice, p 269. Philadelphia, JB Lippincott, 1987

262. Haustein KO: Digitalis. Pharmacol Ther 18:1, 1983

263. Silverberg RA, Weil MH: Cardiopulmonary resuscitation. In Chernow B, Lake CR (eds): The Pharmacologic Approach to the Critically Ill Patient, p 140. Baltimore, Williams & Wilkins, 1983

264. Blecic S, De Backer D, Huynh CH *et al*: Calcium chloride in experimental electromechanical dissociation: A placebo-controlled trial in dogs. Crit Care Med 15:324, 1987

265. Montgomery WH, Donegan JD, McIntyre KM: Standards and guidelines for cardiopulmonary resuscitation (CPR) and emergency cardiac care (ECC). Part III: Adult advanced cardiac life support. JAMA 255:2933, 1986

266. White RD, Goldsmith RS, Rodriguez R et al: Plasma ionic calcium levels following injection of chloride, gluconate, and gluceptate salts of calcium. J Thorac Cardiovasc Surg 71:609, 1976

267. Bull J, Band DM: Calcium and cardiac arrest. Anesthesiology 35:1006, 1980

268. Cote CJ, Drop LJ, Daniels AL, Hoaglain DC: Calcium chloride versus calcium gluconate: Comparison of ionization and cardiovascular effects in children and dogs. Anesthesiology 66:465, 1987

269. Desai TK, Carlton RW, Thill-Baharozian M, Beheb MA: A direct relationship between ionized calcium and arterial pressure among patients in an intensive care unit. Crit Care Med 16:578, 1988

270. Marquez J, Martin D, Virji MA et al: Cardiovascular depression secondary to ionic hypocalcemia during hepatic transplantation in humans. Anesthesiology 64:457, 1986

271. Wong KC, Everett JD: Sympathomimetic drugs. In Smith NT, Corbascio AN (eds): Drug Interactions in Anesthesia, p 71. Philadelphia, Lea & Febiger, 1986

272. Stoelting RK: Drugs used in treatment of psychiatric disease. In Stoelting RK (ed): Pharmacology and Physiology in Anesthetic Practice, p 347. Philadelphia, JB Lippincott, 1987

273. Wong KC, Ashburn MA: Monamine oxidase inhibitors and anesthesia. Literature Scan: Anesthesiology Current Insights. Cedar Knoll, NJ, Word Medical Communication, April 1990

274. Hirshman CA, Lindeman K: MAO inhibitors: Must they be discontinued before anesthesia. JAMA 260:3507, 1988

275. Wells DG, Bjorksten AR: Monoamine oxidase inhibitors revisited. Can J Anaesth 36:1, 1989

276. Kosanin R: Anesthetic considerations in patients on chronic tricyclic antidepressant therapy. Anesth Rev 8:38, 1981

277. Weiner N: Drugs that inhibit adrenergic nerves and block adrenergic receptors. In Gilman AG, Goodman LS, Rall TW, Murad F (eds): The Pharmacological Basis of Therapeutics, p 181. New York, Macmillan, 1985

278. Nickerson M, Goodman LS: Pharmacological properties of a new adrenergic blocking agent: N, N-dibenzyl-b-chloroethylamine (dibenamine). J Pharmacol Exp Ther 89:167, 1947

279. Hickey PR, Hansen DD: Anesthesia and cardiac shunting in the neonate: Ductus arteriosus, transitional circulation, and congenital heart disease. Semin Anesth 3:106, 1984

280. Grover RF, Reeves JT, Blount SG: Tolazoline hydrochloride (priscoline) and effective pulmonary vasodilator. Am Heart J 61:5, 1961

281. Graham RM, Pettinger WA: Drug therapy: Prazosin. N Engl J Med 300:232, 1979

282. Ziegler MG: Antihypertensives. In Chernow B, Lake CR (eds): The Pharmacologic Approach to the Critically Ill Patient, p 303. Baltimore, Williams & Wilkins, 1983

283. Lowenthal DT, Saris SD, Packer J et al: Mechanisms of action and the clinical pharmacology of beta-adrenergic blocking drugs. Am J Med 77:119, 1984

284. Wood A: Pharmacologic differences between beta blockers. Am Heart J 108:1070, 1984

285. Shand DG: Comparative pharmacology of the β-adrenoreceptor blocking drugs. Drugs 25(suppl 2):92, 1983

286. McDevitt DG: Clinical significance of cardioselectivity. Prim Cardiol (suppl 1):165, 1983

287. Clausen N, Damsgaard T, Mellemgaard K: Antihypertensive effect of a nonselective and cardioselective (metoprolol) beta adrenergic blocking agent at rest and during exercise. Br J Clin Pharmacol 7:379, 1979

288. Woods LL, Wright AD, Kendall MJ, Black E: Lack of effect of propranolol and metoprolol on glucose tolerance in maturity-onset diabetes. Br Med J 281:1321, 1980

289. Chang LCT: Use of practolol in asthmatics: A plea for caution. Lancet 2:321, 1971

290. Silke B, Verma SP, Ahuja RC et al: Is the intrinsic sympathomimetic activity (ISA) of beta-blocking compounds relevant in acute myocardial infarction? Eur J Clin Pharmacol 27:509, 1984

291. Taylor SH, Silke MB, Lee PS: Intravenous beta-blockade in coronary heart disease. Is cardioselectivity or intrinsic sympathomimetic activity hemodynamically useful? N Engl J Med 306:631, 1982

292. Reid JL, Dean CR, Jones DH: Central actions of anti-hypertensive drugs. Cardiovasc Med Dec. 2:1185, 1977

293. Pratt CM, Young JB, Roberts R: The role of beta-blockers in the treatment of patients after infarction. Cardiol Clin 2:13, 1984

294. Frishman WH: Atenolol and timolol, two new systemic β-adrenoceptor antagonists. N Engl J Med 306:1456, 1982

295. Formgren H: The effects of metoprolol and practolol on lung function and blood pressure in hypertensive asthmatics. Br J Clin Pharmacol 3:1007, 1976

296. Wollman GL, Cody RJ, Tarazi RC, Bravo EL: Acute hemodynamic effects and cardioselectivity of acebutolol, practolol and propranolol. Clin Pharmacol Ther 25:813, 1979

297. Basil B, Jordan R: Pharmacological properties of diacetylol a major metabolite of acebutolol. Eur J Pharmacol 80:47, 1982

298. Gold MI, Sacks DJ, Grosnoff DB et al: Use of esmolol during anesthesia to treat tachycardia and hypertension. Anesth Analg 68:101, 1989

299. Gray RJ, Bateman TM, Czer LSC et al: Esmolol: A new ultrashort-acting beta-adrenergic blocking agent for rapid control of heart rate in postoperative supraventricular tachyarrhythmias. J Am Coll Cardiol 5:1451, 1985

300. Girard D, Shulman BJ, Thys DM, et al: The safety and efficacy of esmolol during myocardial revascularization. Anesthesiology 65:157, 1986

301. Reves J, Flezzani P: Perioperative use of esmolol. Am J Cardiol 56:57F, 1985

302. Gray R, Bateman TM, Czer LSC et al: Use of esmolol in hypertension after cardiac surgery. Am J Cardiol 46:49F, 1985

303. Menkhaus P, Reves JG, Kissin I et al: Cardiovascular effects of esmolol in anesthetized humans. Anesth Analg 64:327, 1985

304. Gorczynski R: Basic pharmacology of esmolol. Am J Cardiol 56:3F, 1985

305. Steck J, Sheppard D, Byrd R et al: Pulmonary effects of esmolol. Clin Res 33:472A, 1985

306. de Bruihn NP, Reves JG, Croughwell N et al: Pharmacokinetics of esmolol in anesthetized patients receiving chronic beta blocker therapy. Anesthesiology 66:323, 1987

307. Wilson DJ, Wallin JD, Vlachakis ND et al: Intravenous labetalol in the treatment of severe hypertension and hypertensive emergencies. Am J Med 75:95, 1983

308. Gagnon RM, Morissette M, Priesant S et al: Hemodynamic and coronary effects of intravenous labetalol in coronary artery disease. Am J Cardiol 49:1267, 1982

309. Weidmann P, De Chiatel R, Ziegler WH et al: Alpha and beta adrenergic blockade with orally administered labetalol in hypertension. Am J Cardiol 41:570, 1978

310. Berel M, Langlois S, Belleau LJ, Grose JH: Labetalol infusion in hypertensive emergencies. Clin Pharmacol Ther 37:615, 1985

311. Atlee JA: Normal electrical activity of the heart. In Atlee JA (ed): Perioperative Cardiac Dysrhythmias, p 16. Chicago, Year Book, 1985

312. Nayler WG, Poole-Wilson P: Calcium antagonists: Definition and mode of action. Basic Res Cardiol 76:926, 1981

313. Triggle DJ: Calcium antagonists: Basic chemical and pharmacological aspects. In Weiss GB (ed): New Perspectives on Calcium Antagonists, p 1. Baltimore, Williams & Wilkins, 1981

314. Henry PD: Comparative pharmacology of calcium antagonists: Nifedipine, verapamil, and diltiazem. Am J Cardiol 46:1047, 1980

315. Millard RW, Lathrop DA, Grupp G et al: Differential cardiovascular effects of calcium channel blocking agents: Potential mechanisms. Am J Cardiol 49:499, 1982

316. Reves JG: The relative hemodynamic effects of CA^{++} entry blockers: Uses and implications for anesthesiologists. Anesthesiology 61:3, 1982

317. Kraynack BJ, Lawson NW, Gintautas J: Local anesthetic effect of verapamil in vitro. Reg Anesth 7:114, 1982

318. So SY, Ip M, Lam WK: Calcium channel blockers and asthma. Lung 164:1, 1986

319. Schwartz ML, Rotmench HH, Vlasses PH, Ferguson RK: Cal-

cium blockers in smooth muscle disorders. Arch Intern Med 144:1425, 1984

320. Solomon GD, Steel JG, Spaccavento LJ: Verapamil prophylaxis of migraine. JAMA 250:2500, 1983

321. McLeod AA, Jewitt DE: Drug treatment of primary pulmonary hypertension. Drugs 31:177, 1986

322. Fleckenstein A: Specific pharmacology of calcium in myocardium, cardiac pacemakers, and vascular smooth muscle. Ann Rev Pharmacol Toxicol 17:149, 1977

323. Atlee JA: Drugs used for treatment of cardiac dysrhythmias. In Atlee JA (ed): Perioperative Cardiac Dysrhythmias, p 272. Chicago: Year Book, 1985

324. Hwang MH, Danoviz J, Pacold I et al: Double blind crossover randomized trial of intravenously administered verapamil. Arch Intern Med 144:491, 1984

325. Klein HO, Kaplinsky E: Digitalis and verapamil in atrial fibrillation and flutter. Is verapamil now the preferred agent? Drugs 31:185, 1986

326. Haft JI, Habbab MA: Treatment of atrial arrhythmias—effectiveness of verapamil when preceded by calcium infusion. Arch Intern Med 146:1085, 1986

327. Antman EM, Stone PH, Muller JE, Braunwald E: Calcium channel blocking agents in the treatment of cardiovascular disorders. Part I. Basic and clinical electrophysiologic effects. Ann Int Med 93:875, 1980

328. Morad M, Tung L: Ionic events responsible for the cardiac resting and action potential. Am J Cardiol 49:584, 1982

329. Atlee JA: Management of specific cardiac dysrhythmias. In Atlee JA (ed): Perioperative Cardiac Dysrhythmias, p 380. Chicago, Year Book, 1985

330. Clusin WT, Bristow MR, Karaguezian HS et al: Do calcium-dependent currents mediate ischemic ventricular fibrillation? Am J Cardiol 49:606, 1982

331. Given BD, Lee TH, Stone PH, Dzau VJ: Nifedipine in severely hypertensive patients with congestive heart failure and preserved ventricular systolic function. Arch Intern Med 145:281, 1985

332. Kraynack BJ: Calcium channel blocking agents: Side effects and drug interactions. Annual Refresher Course Lecture 238. American Society of Anesthesiology, 1983

333. Merin RG: Calcium (slow) channel blocking drugs. Annual Refresher Course Lecture 101. American Society of Anesthesiology, 1982

334. Halpern NA, Sladen RN, Goldberg JS et al: Nicardipine infusion for postoperative hypertension after surgery of the head and neck. Crit Care Med 18:950, 1990

335. Merin RG, Basch S: Are the myocardial functional and metabolic effects of isoflurane really different from those of halothane and enflurane? Anesthesiology 53:398, 1981

336. Hysing ES, Chelly JE, Doursout MF et al: Cardiovascular effects of and interaction between calcium blocking drugs and anesthetic in chronically instrumented dogs. III. Nicardipine and isoflurane. Anesthesiology 65:385, 1986

337. Carpenter RL, Mulroy MF: Edrophonium antagonizes combined lidocaine-pancuronium and verapamil-pancuronium neuromuscular blockade in cats. Anesthesiology 65:506, 1986

338. Zalman F, Perloff JK, Durant NN, Campion DS: Acute respiratory failure following intravenous verapamil in Duchenne's muscular dystrophy. Am Heart J 105:510, 1983

339. Snyder SH, Reynolds IJ: Calcium-antagonist drugs. N Engl J Med 313:995, 1985

340. Abramowicz M: Verapamil for hypertension. Med Lett Drugs Ther 29:37, 1987

341. Price WA, Giannini AJ: Neurotoxicity caused by lithium-verapamil synergism. J Clin Pharmacol 26:717, 1986

342. Roizen MF, Moss J, Muldoon SM: The effects of anesthesia, anesthetic adjuvant drugs, and surgery on plasma norepinephrine. In Ziegler MG, Lake CR (eds): Frontiers of Clinical Neuroscience, vol 2 (Norepinephrine), p 227. Baltimore, Williams & Wilkins, 1984

343. Goldman L, Caldera DL: Risks of general anesthesia and elective operation in the hypertensive patient. Anesthesiology 50:285, 1979

344. Prys-Roberts C: Hypertension, ischemic heart disease and anesthesia. Int Anesthesiol Clin 18:3, 1980

345. James TN: A cardiogenic hypertensive reflex. Anesth Analg 69:633, 1989

346. Holland DB: Diuretic-induced hypokalemia and ventricular arrhythmias. Drugs 28(suppl):86, 1984

347. Vitez T, Soper L, Wong KC, Soper P: Chronic hypokalemia and intraoperative dysrhythmias. Anesthesiology 63:130, 1986

348. McGovern B: Hypokalemia and cardiac arrhythmias. Anesthesiology 63:127, 1985

349. Boudoulas H, Lewis RP, Kates RE et al: Hypersensitivity to adrenergic stimulation after propranolol withdrawal in normal subjects. Ann Intern Med 86:433, 1977

350. Stoelting RK: Alpha- and beta-adrenergic receptor antagonists. In Stoelting RK (eds): Pharmacology and Physiology in Anesthetic Practice, p 280. Philadelphia, JB Lippincott, 1987

351. Avorn J, Everitt DE, Weiss S: Increased antidepressant use in patients prescribed β-blockers. JAMA 255:357, 1986

352. Slogoff S, Keats AS: Does perioperative myocardial ischemia lead to postoperative myocardial infarction? Anesthesiology 62:107, 1985

353. Maze M, Segal IS, Block BC: Clonidine and other alpha$_2$ adrenergic agonists. Strategies for the rational use of these novel anesthetic agents. J Clin Anesth 1:146, 1988

354. Flacke JW, Bloor BC, Flacke WE et al: Reduced narcotic requirement by clonidine with improved hemodynamic and adrenergic stability in patients undergoing coronary bypass surgery. Anesthesiology 67:11, 1987

355. Heideman SM, Sarnaik AP: Clonidine poisoning in children. Crit Care Med 18:618, 1990

356. Payen D, Quintin L, Plaisance P et al: Head injury: Clonidine decreases plasma catecholamines. Crit Care Med J 18:392, 1990

357. Brodsky JB, Brave JJ: Acute postoperative clonidine withdrawal syndrome. Anesthesiology 44:519, 1976

358. Johnston RV, Nicholas DA, Lawson NW et al: The use of rectal clonidine in the perioperative period. Anesthesiology 64:288, 1986

359. Aantaa R, Kanto J, Scheinin M et al: Dexmedetomidine, an α$_2$ adrenoreceptor agonist, reduces anesthesia requirements for patients undergoing minor gynecologic surgery. Anesthesiology 73:230, 1990

360. Flacke J: Opioid anesthesia and the alpha-2 agonists. Annual Refresher Course lectures. American Society of Anesthesiology lecture 235, 1990

361. Fyhrquist F: Clinical pharmacology of the ACE inhibitors. Drugs 32(suppl 5):33, 1986

362. Brunner HR, Nussberger J, Waeber B: Effects of angiotensin converting enzyme inhibition: A clinical point of view. J Cardiovasc Pharmacol (suppl 4):S73, 1985

363. Packer M: Converting-enzyme inhibition for severe chronic heart failure: Views from a skeptic. Int J Cardiol 7:111, 1985

364. O'Malley K, Segal JL, Israili ZH et al: Duration of hydralazine action in hypertension. Clin Pharmacol Ther 18:581, 1975

365. Cohn JN, Burke LP: Nitroprusside. Ann Intern Med 91:752, 1979

366. Chiarello M, Gold HK, Leinback RC: Comparison between the effects of nitroprusside and nitroglycerin on ischemic injury during acute myocardial infarction. Circulation 54:766, 1976

367. Tinker JH, Michenfelder JD: Sodium nitroprusside: Pharmacology, toxicology and therapeutics. Anesthesiology 45:340, 1976

368. Tinker JH, Michenfelder JD: Increased resistance to nitroprusside-induced cyanide toxicity in anuric dogs. Anesthesiology 50:40, 1980

369. Miller ED, Ackerly JA, Vaughn ED et al: The renin-angiotensin system during controlled hypotension with sodium nitroprusside. Anesthesiology 47:257, 1977

370. Khambatta HJ, Stone JG, Khan E: Propranolol alters renin release during nitroprusside-induced hypotension and prevents hypertension on discontinuation of nitroprusside. Anesth Analg 60:569, 1981

371. Woodside J, Garner L, Bedford RT et al: Captopril reduces the

dose requirement for sodium nitroprusside induced hypotension. Anesthesiology 60:413, 1984

372. Fremes SE, Weisel RD, Mickle D et al: A comparison of nitroglycerin and nitroprusside. I. Treatment of postoperative hypertension. Ann Thorac Surg 39:53, 1985

373. Hood D, Dewan D, James F et al: The use of nitroglycerin in preventing the hypertensive response to tracheal intubation in severe preeclampsia. Anesthesiology 63:399, 1985

374. Goa KL, Sorkin EM: Nitrendipine—A review of its pharmaco-dynamic and pharmacokinetic properties and therapeutic efficacy in the treatment of hypertension. Drugs 33:123, 1987

375. Guazzi M, Olivari MT, Polese A et al: Nifedipine, a new anti-hypertensive with rapid action. Clin Pharmacol Ther 22:528, 1977

376. Ferguson RK, Vlasses PH: Hypertensive emergencies and urgencies. JAMA 255:1607, 1986

377. Abramowicz M: Drugs for hypertension. Med Let Drugs Ther. Med Letter Inc 29(issue 730):1, 1987

15

Robert J. Fragen
Michael J. Avram

Nonopioid Intravenous Anesthetics

The dictionary defines *anesthesia* as a loss of sensation in a part of the body or in the body generally, induced by administration of a drug.[1] Anesthesiologists usually expand this definition in line with the concept of Woodbridge.[2] In 1957, he proposed four components of general anesthesia for drugs of limited or specific action comparable to Guedel's signs for general anesthesia with diethyl ether. His components are blockades of sensory, reflex, mental, and motor functions. Adequate sensory blockade results in minimal response to painful stimuli and is indicated by stability of the cardiovascular and respiratory systems. Troublesome cardiovascular, respiratory, and gastrointestinal reflexes are prevented by adequate reflex blockade. Sedation, amnesia, and unarousable deep sleep are produced by mental blockade. Motor blockade provides muscle relaxation and a quiet surgical field. No single intravenous anesthetic drug is yet available that can produce all the components of adequate anesthesia. Because the drugs available have relatively selective blocking actions, it is necessary to use a combination of drugs that together provide the desired effect.

Excluding ketamine, nonopioid intravenous (iv) anesthetics generally provide only the mental component of the anesthetic state, requiring the addition of analgesics, inhaled anesthetics, and/or muscle relaxants to provide the other components. Thus, the drugs discussed in this chapter are mainly amnestic, sedative (anxiolytic, ataraxic), and hypnotic. The terms *sleep*, *hypnosis*, and *unconsciousness* are used interchangeably in anesthesia literature to refer to the state of artificially induced (i.e., drug-induced) sleep.

Nonopioid iv drugs can be used initially as anesthetic induction drugs to produce the unconscious state, or they can be given by repeated injection or by infusion to maintain the mental component of the anesthetic state.

There has been an expanded research effort in recent years to discover more specific, controllable compounds that can be injected intravenously to provide selective hypnotic, analgesic, or muscle relaxant actions or that can be injected in combination to provide all the components of general anesthesia. Total iv anesthesia refers to general anesthesia administered only with injectable drugs, avoiding inhaled anesthetics entirely. The potential advantage of total iv anesthesia is its facility to provide each component of anesthesia with a dose of a specific drug sufficient to meet the particular needs of the patient and surgeon. When vola-tile inhalation anesthetics are administered, all the components of anesthesia are increased or decreased in intensity at the same time, as are their side-effects.

HISTORY

The iv route of drug administration became possible only after the careful descriptions of the vascular system by William Harvey in 1628 in *De Motu Cordis* and the introduction of the syringe by Rynd (1845) and Pravaz (1853) and of the hypodermic needle by Wood (1855). The first monograph on iv anesthesia was published by Ore, a Frenchman, at the University of Bordeaux in 1874. Unfortunately, he used chloral hydrate, which had a long duration of action and a very narrow margin of safety. At the end of the 19th century and early in the 20th century, hedonal, a derivate of urethane, was used for iv anesthesia, but it caused prolonged drowsiness, respiratory failure, tachycardia, and phlebitis. The use of procaine was reported by August Bier in 1909. All the early barbiturates were long-acting and unsatisfactory for anesthesia. In 1933, Hellmuth Weese described the first ultra–short-acting barbiturate, hexobarbital. The untoward effects he reported were respiratory depression, phlebitis, allergy, and convulsions.[3]

The most important barbiturate is thiopental, introduced in 1934. It was first described by Ralph Waters and coworkers at the University of Wisconsin, although some give credit for its introduction to John S. Lundy at the Mayo Clinic.[4] When thiopental was used as the sole anesthetic for battle casualties in World War II, it was termed the "ideal form of euthanasia" because of the many deaths associated with its administration to patients in shock.[5] Thiopental could have fallen into disuse as a result of this experience, but, instead, it became a major component of the concept of the narcosis-relaxant-analgesic anesthesia proposed by Reese and Gray in the United Kingdom.[6] They realized that drugs administered by the iv route bypassed the first-pass variability of absorption of drugs given orally or intramuscularly (im). Thus, modern iv anesthesia was born with the introduction of thiopental. However, it soon became apparent that this was not an ideal iv agent as a sole anesthetic, as an anesthetic induction agent, or as a maintenance anes-

TABLE 15-1. Intravenous Anesthetics and Their First Year of Clinical Administration

1934	Thiopental
1952	Thiamylal
1957	Methohexital
1957	Ketamine
1960	Gamma OH-butyric acid
1961	Propanidid
1964	Diazepam
1971	Althesin
1973	Etomidate
1977	Propofol
1978	Midazolam

thetic; it could not fulfill Reese and Gray's concept of the anesthetic triad.

It was not until 1952 that another successful iv anesthetic was discovered. Since that time, nine new agents have appeared (Table 15-1), all attempting to improve upon the major drawbacks of thiopental—slow recovery, respiratory depression, and cardiovascular depression. Of these drugs, gamma-hydroxybutric acid was never studied in the United States but is still used in some European countries. Both propanidid and althesin were withdrawn from the market because of an unacceptably high incidence of anaphylactoid reactions to their solvent, cremophor El (about 1:1000). Propofol was originally dissolved in cremophor El and caused anaphylactoid reactions,[7] but it is now produced with a safer solvent.

Before comparing the pharmacology of currently used iv anesthetic drugs, it is important to review the "ideal" properties of an iv anesthetic agent (Table 15-2).

For more than 50 years, anesthesiologists have circumvented thiopental's deficiencies, while investigators have continued to pursue the goal of finding a more ideal drug. Currently, there are no approved or investigational iv anesthetics that fulfill all the criteria for the ideal drug.

TABLE 15-2. Properties of an "Ideal" Intravenous Anesthetic Agent

Physicochemical and pharmacokinetic
  Water-soluble
  Long shelf life (>1 year)
  Stable on exposure to light (>1 day)
  Small volume (±10 ml) required for anesthetic induction
Pharmacodynamic
  Small interindividual variation
  Safe therapeutic ratio
  Onset in one arm–brain circulation time
  Short duration of effect
  Inactivated by rapid metabolism to nontoxic metabolites
  Rapid recovery
Hypersensitivity
  No anaphylaxis
  No histamine release
Side-effects
  No local toxicity
  No alterations in body organ function, except primary central
    nervous system effects
    Central nervous system
    Cardiovascular system
    Respiratory system
    Gastrointestinal system

CHEMISTRY AND FORMULATION

The thiobarbiturates, thiopental [5-ethyl-5-(1-methylbutyl)-2-thiobarbituric acid] and thiamylal [5-allyl-5-(1-methylbutyl)-2-thiobarbituric acid], and the methylated oxybarbiturate methohexital [α-dl-1-methyl-5-allyl-5-(1-methyl-2-pentynyl) barbituric acid] (Fig. 15-1), are the barbiturate induction drugs used in the practice of anesthesia. The sodium salts of these drugs, plus 6% by weight anhydrous sodium carbonate, must be reconstituted with either water or 0.09% sodium chloride, providing 2.5%, 2.0%, or 1.0% solutions of thiopental, thiamylal, or methohexital, respectively. The moderate alkalinity (pH 10 to 11) of the barbiturate solutions is maintained by the buffering action of the sodium carbonate in the presence of atmospheric carbon dioxide. Ringer's lactate solution should not be used to reconstitute any of the barbiturates, nor should the reconstituted barbiturates be mixed with acidic solutions of other drugs, because the decrease in alkalinity will result in the precipitation of the barbiturates as free acids. Properly reconstituted solutions of the thiobarbiturates are stable for up to 1 week if refrigerated; sterile water solutions of methohexital can be used up to 6 weeks after reconstitution.

The parenteral formulations of the benzodiazepine induction agents, diazepam (7-chloro-1,3-dihydro-1-methyl-5-phenyl-2H-1,4-benzodiazepin-2-one) and midazolam [8-chloro-6-(2'fluorophenyl)-1-methyl-4H-imidazo[1,5α][1,4] benzodiazepine] (Fig. 15-1), are quite different from each

Barbiturates

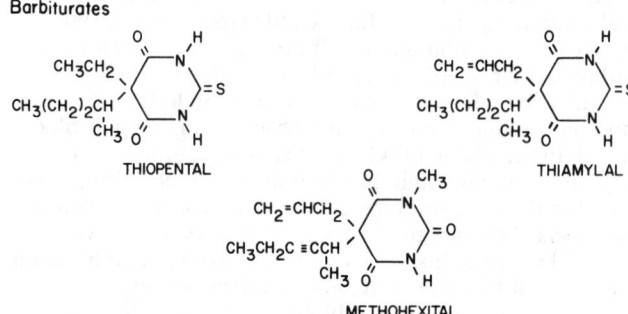

Benzodiazepines

Miscellaneous

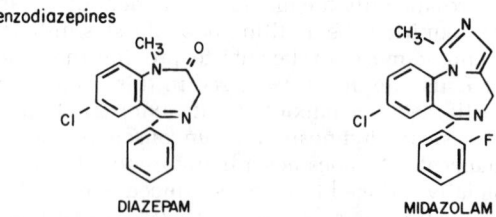

Figure 15-1. Agents used for the induction of general anesthesia. (Reprinted with permission from Fragen RJ, Avram MJ: Comparative pharmacology of drugs used for the induction of anesthesia. In Stoelting RK, Barash PG, Gallagher TJ [eds]: Advances in Anesthesia, p 103. Chicago, Year Book Medical Publishers, Inc, 1986.)

other owing to the availability of water-soluble salts of midazolam but not of diazepam. Diazepam is marketed as a 5 mg·ml^{-1} solution in a 50% organic (40% propylene glycol and 10% ethanol) vehicle that also contains a buffer and a preservative. Although diazepam is stable in solution, it cannot be mixed with solutions of other drugs; if it is, its solubility is reduced. The midazolam formulation, on the other hand, contains 1 or 5 mg·ml^{-1} of the hydrochloride salt in a buffered, pH 3.5, aqueous solution that is stable and compatible with saline, Ringer's lactate solution, and formulations of acidic salts of other drugs.

Although water-soluble salts and a 10% ethanolic formulation of etomidate [R-(+)-ethyl 1-(α-methylbenzyl)-1H-imidazole 5-carboxylate] (Fig. 15-1) exist, the only formulation available in the United States is a 2 mg·ml^{-1} solution in a 35% propylene glycol vehicle. While etomidate is stable in solution in this vehicle, it should not be diluted or mixed with other drug formulations.

Propofol (2,6-diisopropylphenol) (Fig. 15-1) is a hydrophobic liquid at room temperature. It is formulated as a 1% aqueous emulsion, containing 10% soybean oil, 2.25% glycerol, and 1.2% egg phosphatide[8] and is stable at room temperature. After shaking the ampule and opening it, propofol should be promptly drawn into a sterile syringe with aseptic technique because it can act as a culture medium if contaminated. Each ampule is meant for single patient use; the residual should be discarded at the end of each anesthetic. This formulation should not be mixed with other solutions.

The iv formulation of ketamine [(dl-2-(o-chlorophenyl)-2-(methyl-amino)-cyclohexanone] (Fig. 15-1) contains 10, 50, or 100 mg·ml^{-1} of the hydrochloride salt in a moderately acidic (pH 3.5 to 5.5) solution with a preservative. Ketamine is stable in solution but should not be mixed with solutions of the moderately alkaline barbiturates or with diazepam, with which it is commonly coadministered.

STRUCTURE–ACTIVITY RELATIONSHIPS

Structure–activity relationships are descriptions of the way in which modifications of the chemical structure of prototypical drugs affect their pharmacologic activities. The addition, modification, or removal of functional groups on the fundamental structure of a drug lends it physicochemical properties that affect the drug's ability to gain access to its site of action and to interact with its presumed receptor; they also determine the effect it will have on the receptor when interacting with it.[9] The structure–activity relationships for the anesthesia induction drugs are reasonably well described.

Modification of the structure of barbituric acid (Fig. 15-2A), 2, 4, 6-trioxohexahydropyrimidine, can convert the inactive compound into a hypnotic with a variety of pharmacologic activities.[10] The addition of aliphatic side chains in positions 5 and 5' introduces hypnotic activity to the molecule, particularly if at least one of the side chains is branched. The length of the side chains in the 5 and 5' positions can influence the duration of action of the barbituric acid derivatives as well as their potency; both pentobarbital and secobarbital contain relatively long (i.e., branched 5 carbon) side chains in position 5' and have a relatively short duration of action, whereas secobarbital is slightly more potent than pentobarbital because of the slightly longer (3 vs. 2 carbon) side chain in position 5. Replacement of the oxygen atom in position 2 of an active barbiturate

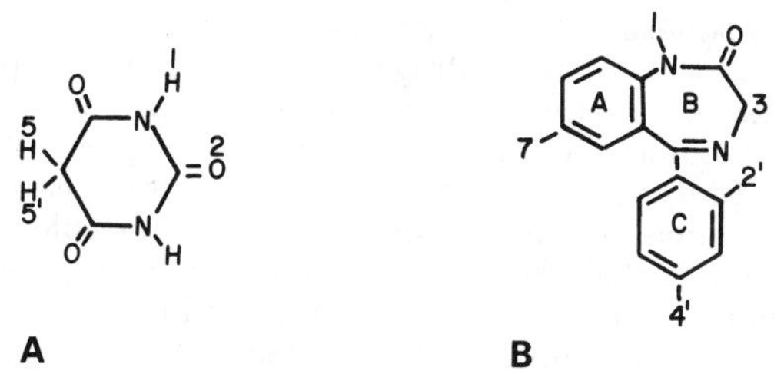

Figure 15-2. (A) Barbituric acid, (B) 5-phenyl-1,4 benzodiazepin-2-one ring system.

with a sulfur atom produces a drug with a faster onset and a shorter duration of action; the thiobarbiturates, thiopental and thiamylal (see Fig. 15-1), have a more rapid onset and shorter duration of action than their oxybarbiturate analogues, pentobarbital and secobarbital. Methylation of an active barbiturate in the 1 position produces a barbiturate such as methohexital (see Fig. 15-1), with a rapid onset and short duration of action at the expense of an increased incidence of excitatory side-effects. Thus, given basic hypnotic activity, any chemical modification of a barbiturate that increases its lipophilicity generally increases both its potency and rate of onset while shortening its duration of action.

The pharmacologic activity of the classic 5-phenyl-1,4 benzodiazepin-2-one ring system (Fig. 15-2B) can be affected by substitution in a number of positions.[11] The introduction of an electronegative group in position 7 on ring A, such as the chloro group in diazepam and midazolam (see Fig. 15-1), is nearly essential for typical benzodiazepine activity. A methyl group in position 1 on ring B, as in diazepam, increases biologic activity, whereas larger substituents in that position decrease it.

A halogen in position 2' of ring C, as in midazolam, increases pharmacologic activity, whereas any substituent in the 4' position very strongly decreases it. The fused imidazole ring contributes unique properties to midazolam (see Fig. 15-1).[12] The basicity of the imidazole nitrogen (pK$_a$ 6.15) allows the preparation of salts that are both soluble and stable in acidic aqueous solution (pH of approximately 3.5) yet lipophilic at physiologic pH. In addition, the methyl group in position 1 of the fused imidazole ring is metabolized rapidly by hepatic oxidation (hydroxylation), contributing, with redistribution, to its shorter duration of action; the methylene group in position 3 of the classic diazepine ring (Fig. 15-2B) is metabolized more slowly.

Imidazole derivatives have classically been used as antimycotic agents. Several 1-(1 aralkyl)-imidazole-5-carboxylic acid esters such as etomidate (see Fig. 15-1) are potent hypnotic drugs with good therapeutic indices.[13] Hypnotic activity in such a molecule requires the presence of both an alkyl branched carbon atom between the aryl moiety and the imidazole nitrogen and an ester moiety.

Propofol (see Fig. 15-1) is one of a series of di-ortho-substituted phenols with moderate to high hypnotic potencies and therapeutic ratios.[14] Sleeping time increases with increasing side chain length. Potency increases and induction time decreases with increasing length of the side chains up to a total of seven to eight carbon atoms. With side chains longer than this, potency is decreased, induction is slowed, and recovery is prolonged. The 2,6-di-sec-alkylphenols are generally more potent and have higher therapeutic ratios than the 2,6-di-n-alkylphenols, because potency and therapeutic ratios increase with increased steric compression of the phenolic hydroxyl group.

The cyclohexane ring geminally substituted with an aromatic ring and a basic nitrogen is essential to the phencyclindine-like activity of the arylcycloalkylamines, of which ketamine (see Fig. 15-1) is a member.[15] The potency of these compounds is influenced by substitutions on the nitrogen-containing side chain, but their pharmacologic activity is unaffected. An electron withdrawing group on the aromatic ring, such as the o-chloro group in ketamine, decreases the psychotropic activity of the molecule.

An important but often overlooked aspect of structure–activity relationships is the relationship of stereoisomerism to biologic activity. Many important molecules in biology and medicine contain one or more asymmetric carbon atoms. Except for the presence of the asymmetric centers, the stereoisomers of a given molecule are physically and chemically identical. Nonetheless, biologic activity is often predicated on the active stereoisomer of a given neurotransmitter, hormone, or drug interacting with the chiral active center of a receptor or enzyme.[16] Because side-effects are often due to the nonspecific action of drugs (i.e., they are often not receptor- or enzyme-mediated), the inactive stereoisomers can contribute significantly to the side-effects of the racemic mixture. Some isomers have been shown to have effects even at the receptor or enzyme opposite that of the active isomer. The "inactive" isomer, therefore, should be considered an impurity.[17]

Many barbiturates, including thiopental, thiamylal, and methohexital, have asymmetric carbon atoms in one of the side chains attached to carbon 5 of the barbiturate ring.[18] The (−) isomers of both thiopental and thiamylal are the most potent isomers in mice.[18,19] Methohexital, on the other hand, not only has an asymmetric carbon atom on one of the side chains attached to carbon 5 but also an asymmetric site at carbon 5 itself. It therefore has four stereoisomers, the most active of which, the β-1, is four to five times as potent as the least active, the α-1.[18,20] All the barbiturates are marketed as the racemic mixture.

The (+) isomer of etomidate is the only stereoisomer with hypnotic activity.[21] Etomidate is the only anesthetic induction drug with an asymmetric carbon atom that is marketed as the most active isomer.

The stereoisomers of ketamine have been tested in humans. The (+) isomer was reported to be 3.4 times as potent a hypnotic as the (−) isomer and, "at equianesthetic doses," to be an even more potent analgesic.[22] The (−) isomer, on the other hand, at an equally hypnotic dose, had more clinically important side-effects, including disturbing emergence reactions.[22] Nonetheless, ketamine is marketed as a racemic mixture.

Neither propofol nor the benzodiazepines contain asymmetric carbon atoms.

MECHANISMS OF ACTION

Given the enormous complexity of the central nervous system (CNS), it is hardly surprising that neither neurotransmission nor the mechanisms of anesthetic induction drugs are fully understood. There are many theories purporting to explain how various anesthetic agents work. Some of these theories suggest that anesthetics directly affect cell membranes (biophysical theories), whereas others suggest direct interaction with neurotransmitter systems (transmitter theories).[23-26] Although no drug has a single action and many drugs have a variety of actions, some of which are concentration-dependent, there is a substantial body of evidence suggesting that most of the anesthetic induction drugs

exert many of their effects by modulating GABAminergic transmission.[27-29] Such an action is consistent with the GABA (gamma-aminobutyric acid) transmitter theory of anesthetic action.[30]

GABA is the most common inhibitory neurotransmitter in the mammalian CNS. Activation of the postsynaptic GABA receptor increases chloride conductance through the ion channel, hyperpolarizing and, as a result, inhibiting the postsynaptic neuron. The GABA receptor is actually an oligomeric complex (Fig. 15-3) consisting of the GABA receptor and its associated chloride ion channel, the benzodiazepine receptor, the barbiturate receptor, and the picrotoxin binding site.[32] Both barbiturates and benzodiazepines, by activating distinct receptors on the GABA receptor complex, increase chloride ion flux initiated by the interaction of GABA with its receptor, thereby enhancing GABA-induced postsynaptic inhibition. Benzodiazepines bind to their receptor (possibly displacing an endogenous modulator of GABA function), producing an allosteric modification of the GABA receptor and increasing the efficiency of GABA receptor/effector (i.e., chloride ion channel) coupling. As a result, benzodiazepines increase the frequency of chloride ion channel openings produced by GABA.[26,27,29,33] Barbiturates, on the other hand, by binding to their receptor, decrease the rate of dissociation of GABA from its receptor and increase the duration of GABA-activated chloride ion channel openings.[24,28,29,33] There is evidence that the benzodiazepines and the barbiturates exert their anticonvulsant and anxiolytic actions through their interactions with the GABA receptor complex, but it is less certain that they produce their sedative/hypnotic effects by this mechanism.[31,34-36]

Like the barbiturates and benzodiazepines, propofol may enhance GABA-activated chloride ion channel function. However, it appears to do so through a separate recognition site on the GABA receptor complex or by a different mechanism than that described for the barbiturates and benzodiazepines.[37]

Etomidate may also modulate GABAminergic neurotransmission. In contrast to the increased affinity of the GABA receptor produced by barbiturates, etomidate appears to increase the number of GABA receptors, possibly by displacing endogenous inhibitors of GABA binding.[38]

Just as the dissociative anesthetic ketamine has actions that are significantly different from the other iv anesthetic induction drugs, it also has different effects on neurotransmission within the CNS. Although their effects on neuro-

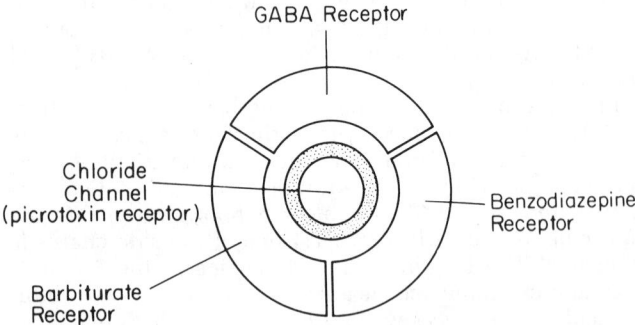

Figure 15-3. Representation of the hypothetical GABA_A receptor oligomeric complex. (Reprinted with permission from Olsen RW, Fischer JB, Dunwiddie TV: Barbiturate enhancement of γ-aminobutyric acid receptor binding and function as a mechanism of anesthesia. In Roth SH, Miller KW [eds]: Molecular and Cellular Mechanisms of Anesthetics, p 165. New York, Plenum, 1986.)

transmission are not as well described as the effects of barbiturates and benzodiazepines, arylcycloalkylamines have been reported to interact with CNS muscarinic acetylcholine receptors as antagonists and with opioid receptors as agonists.[39] The interaction of ketamine with the sigma opioid receptor may produce the dysphoric reactions to this drug.[40] Ketamine also blocks the N-methyl-D-aspartate receptor subclass of the putative neurotransmitter L-glutamate, possibly contributing to its anesthetic action.[41]

Until recently, there were no specific antagonists for the CNS effects of the iv anesthetic induction drugs. Physicians have attempted to antagonize their effects nonspecifically with drugs such as the anticholinesterase physostigmine because of its ability to produce relatively nonspecific cortical activation and arousal.[42] Flumazenil and Ro 15–3505 are specific benzodiazepine receptor antagonists. Flumazenil is a pure benzodiazepine receptor antagonist, whereas Ro 15–3505 is a more potent benzodiazepine receptor antagonist that may have very weak partial inverse agonist properties (i.e., it may behave slightly like the hypothetical endogenous modulator of GABA function at the benzodiazepine receptor).[43,44]

PHARMACOKINETICS

General

Selected pharmacokinetic parameters for the iv anesthetic induction drugs are listed in Table 15-3. (See also Chapter 13.)

Because the various studies may have different pharmacokinetic models and sampling times, it is difficult to compare the initial or central volumes of distribution (V_c) of these

drugs. However, the V_cs for all of them appear to exceed intravascular space. The rapid onsets of effects of most of these drugs suggest that the brain is part of their initial volume of distribution.

The action of these drugs is terminated through "dilution" in the body by redistribution from the relatively small V_c (including the brain) to the much larger total apparent volume of distribution Vd_{ss} (see below); this is taking place during the rapidly declining portions of the plasma concentration versus time relationship (Fig. 15-4). Vd_{ss} for benzodiazepines is approximately 1 l·kg^{-1}, suggesting relatively uniform distribution of the drugs throughout the body, whereas Vd_{ss}s for the other induction agents are 2 to 3 l·kg^{-1}, implying extensive uptake by some tissues of the body (Table 15-3).

Elimination clearance, the irreversible removal of drug from the body, begins the moment that a drug reaches the clearing organs (e.g., liver, kidneys) but becomes a dominant influence on the plasma drug concentration versus time relationship only after the end of the rapid decline in plasma drug concentrations characterizing the distribution phase (Fig. 15-4). The elimination clearances of these hepatically eliminated drugs range from very low to very high, whether expressed in ml·min^{-1} [53,62] or ml·min^{-1}·kg^{-1} (Table 15-3). The low, restrictive elimination clearances of diazepam and thiopental reflect their low hepatic extraction ratios. The fact that the extraction ratios of diazepam and thiopental are equal to the unbound fractions of these drugs suggests that their restrictive elimination is due to extensive protein binding (Table 15-3). The other induction drugs have much higher hepatic extraction ratios and elimination clearances despite the extensive protein binding of some. This implies that the rate of their dissociation from plasma proteins does

---

TABLE 15-3. The Pharmacokinetics of Intravenous Anesthesia Induction Drugs ($x \pm$ SD)*

Drug	V_c (l·kg^{-1})	Vd_{ss} (l·kg^{-1})	Vd_β (l·kg^{-1})	Cl_e (ml·min^{-1})	Cl_e (ml·min^{-1}·kg^{-1})	$T_{1/2\beta}$ (h)	Estimated Hepatic Extraction Ratio	Plasma Protein Binding (%)	Minimal Effective Plasma Concentration (µg·ml^{-1})
Thiopental[45]	0.53 ±0.18	2.34 ±0.75	3.46 ±1.54†	247†	3.4 ±0.4	12.0 ±5.5	0.15	83.4 ±1.4	19.2 ±6.3‡[46]
Methohexital[50]	0.35 ±0.10	2.2 ±0.7	3.68†	835†	10.9 ±3.0	3.9 ±2.1	0.50	73[51]	10[52]
Etomidate[53]	0.15 ±0.03	2.52 ±0.90	4.46 ±2.26	1210 ±303	17.9 ±5.6	2.9 ±1.1	0.90	76.9 ±1.0†[54]	0.307 ±0.076
Propofol[55]	0.35 ±0.16	2.3 ±0.8	5.02†	2090§ ±650	30§ ±8	1.9 ±0.6	Nearly 1.0?	96.8– 98[56]	1.07 ±0.13
Ketamine[57]	1.7†	3.1 ±0.9	5.1 ±0.7	1429†	19.1 ±2.5	3.1†	Nearly 1.0?	12[58]	0.640 ±0.213[59]
Diazepam[60]	0.31 ±0.12	1.13 ±0.28	1.53†	26.6 ±4.1	0.4†	46.6 ±14.2	0.03†	97.8 ±1.0	N.A.¶
Midazolam[62]	0.17 ±0.03	1.09 ±0.18	1.60 ±0.31	436 ±127	7.5 ±2.4	2.7 ±0.8	0.51†[62,63]	94 ±1.9[63]	0.157 ±0.079

*These data are not available for thiamylal.

†These values have been calculated by the present authors from data in the sources cited.

‡Pentobarbital is either an artifact encountered in the measurement of thiopental[48] or such a minor metabolite[49] that it cannot be considered to contribute to the CNS effects of thiopental.

§Whole blood clearance.

¶Not applicable because diazepam has several clinically important pharmacologically active metabolites, one of which has a half-life that is longer than that of diazepam.[61]

Modified with permission from Fragen RJ, Avram MJ: Comparative pharmacology of drugs used for the induction of anesthesia. In Stoelting RK, Barash PG, Gallagher TJ (eds): Advances in Anesthesia, p 103. Chicago, Year Book Medical Publishers, 1986.

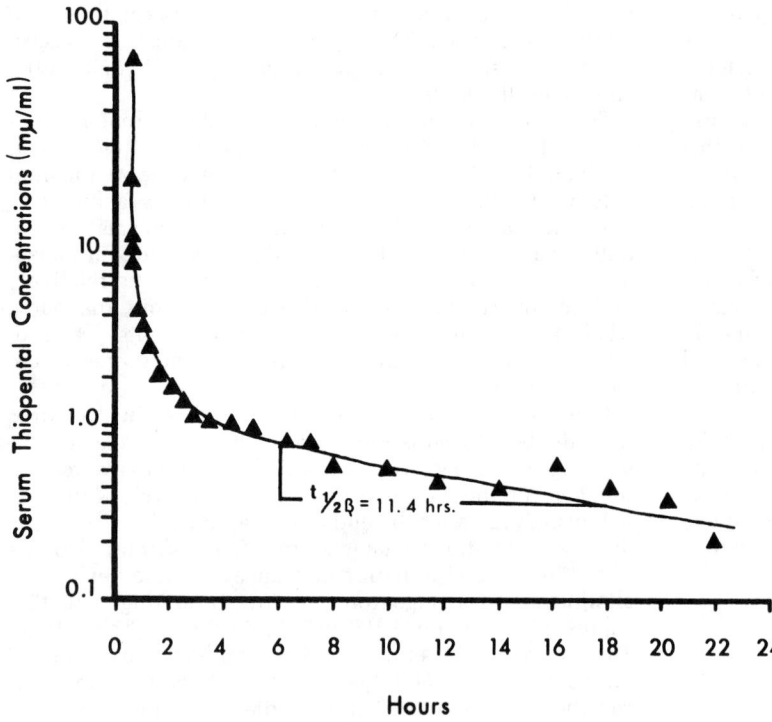

$t\frac{1}{2\beta} = 11.4$ hrs.

Figure 15-4. Serum thiopental concentrations versus time relationship after a rapid intravenous (bolus) administration of the drug. The triangles represent measured serum concentrations, and the line represents a computer-generated fit to a triexponential equation. (Modified with permission from Burch PG, Stanski DR: The role of metabolism and protein binding in thiopental anesthesia. Anesthesiology 58:146, 1983.)

not limit their rate of elimination. The extremely high elimination clearance of propofol suggests that there is a significant extrahepatic contribution to its clearance. Because of their high elimination clearances, etomidate and propofol are well suited pharmacokinetically for use by continuous iv infusion for sedation or hypnosis.

Elimination half-life ($T_{1/2\beta}$) is a pharmacokinetic variable depending directly on volume of distribution (Vd_β, which is useful only for calculating $T_{1/2\beta}$) and inversely on elimination clearance. The wide range of half-lives of these drugs, from less than 1 hour for propofol to over 40 hours for diazepam, is more a reflection of the large differences in the elimination clearances of the drugs than it is of the small differences in their volumes of distribution.

Pharmacodynamic modeling of the effects of the anesthetic induction drugs is extremely difficult, because there is no unequivocal measure of their effects. Stanski and colleagues are working in this complex area using changes in the processed EEG as measures of effect. They suggest that the number of waves per second from aperiodic electroencephalographic analysis be used as a measure of thiopental anesthetic depth; verbal responsiveness is lost at maximum electroencephalographic activation, whereas near burst suppression is necessary to prevent patient movement in response to noxious stimuli.[46] The voltage per second from aperiodic electroencephalographic analysis is proposed as a continuous electroencephalographic measure of the hypnotic effect of midazolam; midazolam increases the electroencephalographic voltage per second.[47]

Termination of Hypnotic Effect

The classic physiologic pharmacokinetic studies of the disposition of thiopental demonstrated that redistribution of drug from the brain to other less well-perfused tissues is the primary mechanism for the termination of the effects of

anesthetic induction drugs after rapid iv administration (Fig. 15-5).[65-67] Although never a principal factor, elimination clearance plays a more important role in terminating the effects of drugs with intermediate or high hepatic extraction ratios (e.g., methohexital; see Table 15-3)[50] than it does with drugs having low extraction ratios (e.g., thiopental; see Table 15-3).[45] When drugs such as the iv anesthetic induction drugs are administered in high doses, in multiple doses, or by continuous iv infusion, the importance of elimination clearance to the termination of drug effect increases as the size of the dose or duration of infusion increases. As an extreme example, the effect of thiopental administered for 42 to 89 hours by continuous iv infusion in cerebral

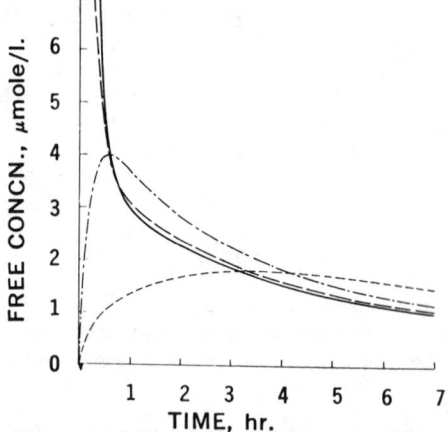

Figure 15-5. Free thiopental concentrations in blood (– – –), viscera (———), adipose (-----), and lean (—·—) body tissues after a rapid intravenous (bolus) administration of the drug. (Reprinted with permission from Bischoff KB, Dedrick RL: Thiopental pharmacokinetics. J Pharm Sci 57:1346, 1968.)

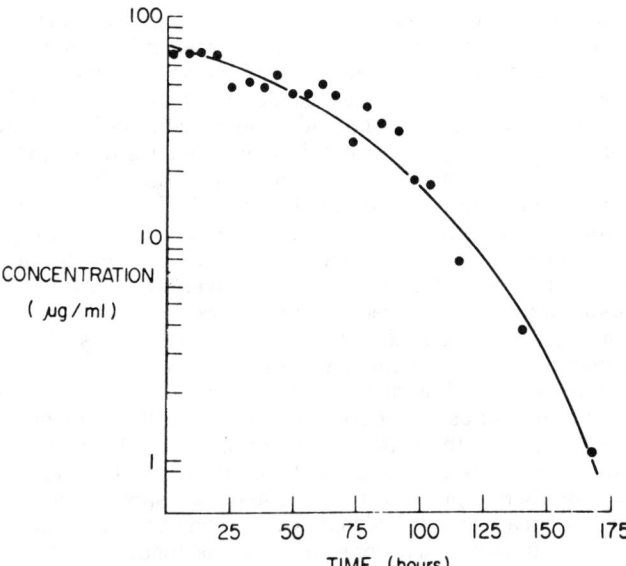

Figure 15-6. Plasma thiopental concentration versus time relationship after a 42-hour infusion of a total dose of 40,200 mg of the drug in cerebral resuscitation, illustrating nonlinear (Michaelis–Menten) elimination clearance. Note the difference between this postdrug administration relationship and that illustrated in Figure 15-4 for a standard dose of the same drug, which has typical distributional phases followed by linear elimination clearance. (Modified with permission from Stanski DR, Mihm FG, Rosenthal MH et al: Pharmacokinetics of high-dose thiopental used in cerebral resuscitation. Anesthesiology 53:169, 1980.)

resuscitation was terminated by nonlinear (i.e., Michaelis–Menten) elimination, with no contribution from redistribution (Fig. 15-6).[49]

Volatile Anesthetics and Pharmacokinetics

There is a growing body of literature on the effects of anesthetics, particularly volatile anesthetics, and on the absorption and disposition of drugs.[68] Most of these studies have examined the effects of volatile anesthetics on elimination clearance of drugs administered perioperatively.

Few studies have directly assessed the effects of volatile anesthetics on the elimination clearance of iv anesthetic induction drugs in humans. Nonetheless, there are suggestions that volatile anesthetic drugs decrease the elimination clearance of such high and intermediate extraction ratio drugs as etomidate,[53,69,70] ketamine,[71] and methohexital.[72] The elimination clearance of high extraction ratio drugs is usually reduced by a decrease in hepatic blood flow; the clearance of low extraction ratio drugs is reduced by a decreased hepatic extraction ratio, resulting from enzyme inhibition; the clearance of intermediate extraction ratio drugs is affected by changes in both hepatic blood flow and extraction ratio.[73] Most volatile anesthetics decrease hepatic blood flow.[74] There is also evidence from studies in rats,[75] dogs,[76] and sheep[77] that volatile drugs can affect a decrease in hepatic clearance by decreasing not only hepatic blood flow but also hepatic metabolism. Regardless of the mechanism, decreases in the clearances of induction agents by volatile anesthetics would prolong their elimination half-lives. Because the effects of standard doses of the induction drugs are largely terminated by redistribution, decreased elimination clearance and the resultant prolongation of elimination

half-life would result in a prolonged effect only after very high doses, multiple doses, or continuous iv infusions. The nonspecific stimulation of drug-metabolizing enzymes by volatile anesthetic drugs[78] is unlikely to be an acute effect and is, therefore, unlikely to affect the clearance of the anesthetic induction drugs.

The effects of the volatile anesthetics on the distribution of ketamine have been studied in the rat,[75] and on the distribution of propranolol in the dog.[79] Further studies on the effects of anesthetics on drug distribution, including studies in humans, must be conducted before it is possible to speculate on the implications of alterations in the distribution of induction drugs. Nonetheless, clinical experience suggests that any effect seldom has profound consequences.

Age and Pharmacokinetics

Elderly patients require significantly lower induction doses of the iv anesthetic drugs, including thiopental,[80-83] diazepam,[84] midazolam,[85,86] etomidate,[87] and propofol,[88] than do young patients. There are suggestions in the literature that the increased reactivity of elderly patients to the iv induction drugs has a pharmacokinetic rather than a pharmacodynamic basis.[80,83,87,89,90]

Anatomic and physiologic changes with aging could have important effects on the pharmacokinetics of the iv induction drugs. There is a decrease in the proportion of body weight represented by total body water and in lean body mass;[91] this could result in an increase in the total apparent volume of distribution of lipophilic drugs such as the induction drugs. An age-related decrease in cardiac output with a concomitant alteration in the distribution of systemic flow,[92] usually at the expense of drug-clearing organs, may decrease the elimination clearance of high-clearance drugs in the elderly. These changes could prolong the half-lives of drugs but cannot provide a pharmacokinetic explanation for the increased reactivity of the elderly to the iv induction drugs.

The change in the disposition of thiopental with aging has been the subject of several investigations. Since thiopental equilibrates very rapidly between plasma and the brain,[66] either a slower rate of drug transfer from the central to the fast compartment[89] or a decreased central volume of distribution[83] would explain the increased CNS and cardiovascular sensitivity of elderly patients to standard doses of thiopental. In addition to an age-related increase in both the volume of distribution and half-life of thiopental, Christensen and colleagues found a decrease in the rate at which the drug is transferred from the central to the fast compartment in the elderly.[89] Homer and Stanski found that the initial distribution volume of thiopental decreased with age,[83] resulting in less initial dilution of a dose of thiopental, but this observation could not be reproduced by others[93] and did not hold up on reanalysis.[94] Using a newly developed model that includes a description of late intravascular mixing, the only age-related early kinetic change Avram and coworkers found was a decrease in the fast intercompartmental clearance with age.[93] Stanski and Maitre found a similar kinetic change that provides the rationale for dose adjustment.[94]

Even when patient characteristics that vary with age and influence pharmacokinetics are included in a multiple linear regression model, age is still associated with decreased thiopental induction dose requirements.[95] Thus, age-related changes in thiopental dose requirements may be due to age-related changes in early intravascular mixing or pharmacodynamic changes not detectable with current techniques.

EFFECTS ON ORGAN SYSTEMS

Central Nervous System Effects

Intravenous anesthetics primarily modify activity within the CNS, alter consciousness, produce amnesia, and, in the case of ketamine, produce analgesia as well. These agents also affect the EEG, intracranial pressure, cerebral blood flow, cerebral metabolic rate for oxygen ($CMRo_2$), and intraocular pressure (IOP). Clinically, desirable effects include reductions in blood flow, metabolism, and pressures within the CNS as well as a sleep pattern on the EEG; these are especially important for patients with intracranial pathology and increased intracranial pressure.

Thiopental causes an increase in the amplitude and a slowing in the frequency of the EEG.[96] If the dose is high enough, burst suppression, and then a flat EEG will appear. Etomidate produces EEG effects similar to those exhibited after use of thiopental.[97] There is an initial increase in alpha amplitude followed by a progressive decrease in activity and, in some cases, periods of burst suppression. The myoclonic movements that occasionally occur during induction of anesthesia with etomidate are not associated with specific EEG changes of epileptiform activity, but convulsions have been reported following the use of etomidate.[98,99] Anesthetic induction doses of midazolam cause the awake alpha rhythm to change to a beta rhythm. After about 30 minutes, alpha activity returns, but some EEG effects are still seen an hour after drug administration.[100] This is not the classic sleep pattern but is similar to the EEG changes following the use of diazepam and other benzodiazepines. Ketamine anesthesia leads to increases in alpha, delta, and theta waves but results in no change in beta activity.[101] An induction dose of propofol caused an increase in alpha rhythm, then delta and theta activity. Propofol infusion rates greater than 9 $mg\cdot kg^{-1}\cdot h^{-1}$ can produce burst suppression lasting 15 or more seconds. The EEG returns to normal shortly after induction of anesthesia.[102]

Another index of CNS activity is evoked potential monitoring, commonly used since the mid-1980s. This monitoring is useful in detecting abnormalities of neural transmission in the spinal cord or intracranial structure. Anesthetics that could blunt the evoked response during the monitoring period would be detrimental, yet there is a scarcity of reports in the medical literature of well-controlled studies of the effects of iv anesthetics on the somatosensory-evoked potentials. Thiopental and propofol can be used safely for anesthetic induction and, in therapeutic doses, during anesthetic maintenance, because they elicit minimal alteration in somatosensory-evoked potentials. Etomidate, on the

other hand, increases the amplitude of somatosensory-evoked potentials transiently, sometimes mimicking the pattern at the onset of ischemia. It also alters the waveform, making the diagnosis of neurologic injury more difficult.[103]

Other CNS effects of etomidate, however, are beneficial for the neurosurgical patient. Cerebral blood flow, $CMRo_2$, and intracranial pressure are reduced in a dose-related fashion by etomidate,[104,105] the barbiturates,[106,107] the benzodiazepines,[108] and propofol.[109,110] An exception was described in a study in which intracranial pressure was unchanged after midazolam, 0.32 $mg\cdot kg^{-1}$, was given to patients with brain tumors, and intracranial pressure was over 20 mm Hg.[111] Because etomidate has the least effect on systemic blood pressure, it is more successful than other drugs in maintaining cerebral perfusion pressure. Some question the advisability of using propofol for patients with severe brain injury because the beneficial effect of a decrease in intracranial pressure may be more than offset by a decrease in cerebral perfusion pressure. This may be a special concern for the area of the brain that is in contact with a retractor during surgery.[113] The one drug that is inappropriate for patients with intracranial pathology is ketamine because it increases cerebral blood flow, intracranial pressure, and cerebrospinal fluid pressure.[101]

Many iv hypnotics have been used clinically and experimentally for brain protection against seizures caused by epilepsy[114-116] or by local anesthetic overdose.[117] Methohexital, however, would be an inadvisable choice for brain protection, as high doses (24 $mg\cdot kg^{-1}$), which suppress electroencephalographic activity, can cause refractory postoperative seizures.[118] There is also a report of ketamine inducing seizures in epileptics.[119]

Among the factors that may affect IOP are systemic arterial pressure, central venous pressure, patency of the drainage system for the aqueous humor, and diseases of the eyes themselves. All the nonopioid iv anesthetics except ketamine, by themselves, reduce IOP. This has been demonstrated with thiopental, diazepam, and midazolam (Table 15-4)[120] as well as with etomidate[121] and propofol.[122] If normal doses of these induction drugs are followed by administration of succinylcholine and tracheal intubation, however, IOP rises above control values. When a second dose of propofol, 1 $mg\cdot kg^{-1}$, was given just before succinylcholine administration, it offered protection against the usual rise in IOP in such circumstances; a second dose of thiopental offered no such protection.[121] Etomidate, 0.3 $mg\cdot kg^{-1}$,[123] and propofol, 2.1 $mg\cdot kg^{-1}$,[121] caused a sharper decrease in IOP than did thiopental, 4 to 5 $mg\cdot kg^{-1}$. Possible mechanisms for this decrease in IOP are an increase in the outflow of aqueous humor, relaxation of extraocular muscles, and pe-

---

TABLE 15-4. IOP Changes in mm Hg (Mean ± SEM)

Drug	Control	1 Minute	3 Minutes	After Succinylcholine	After Tube
Midazolam	16.3 ± 1.0	11.8 ± 0.9*	9.6 ± 1.0*	21.6 ± 1.0†	24.9 ± 1.9*
Diazepam	17.5 ± 0.8	12.1 ± 0.7*	11.5 ± 0.6*	23.7 ± 1.5*	26.6 ± 1.8*
Thiopental	17.8 ± 1.4	13.4 ± 1.4*	12.4 ± 1.7*	23.7 ± 2.3†	26.9 ± 2.6*

*$p < 0.001$ compared with control.

†$p < 0.01$ compared with control.

Reprinted with permission from Fragen RJ, Hauch T: The effects of midazolam maleate and diazepam in intraocular pressure in adults. In Aldrete JA, Stanley TH (eds): Trends in Intravenous Anesthesia, p 245. Chicago, Year Book Medical Publishers, 1980.

ripheral vasodilation. Thus, all the drugs except ketamine can be used safely to induce anesthesia for ophthalmologic surgery, even for the emergency patient with an open globe. Ketamine, however, can be safely administered to children for tonometry.[124] Although most of the reported studies concerning the effects of induction drugs on IOP used succinylcholine as the muscle relaxant, a nondepolarizing relaxant may be a more appropriate companion to iv induction agents for patients with open eye injuries.

The beneficial cerebral effects of the barbiturates, benzodiazepines, etomidate, or propofol are useless if the patient is allowed to cough, breath-hold, or strain or if hypercarbia is present. The cerebral vasculature is still capable of responding after induction doses of these hypnotic drugs. Because hypercarbia is the most important cerebral vasodilator, hypocarbia is the goal during intracranial surgery. Although benzodiazepines may be used to ameliorate the stimulatory effects of ketamine, midazolam does not protect against the rise in intracranial pressure caused by ketamine.[115]

Table 15-5 summarizes the relative CNS effects of these drugs. Other possible CNS effects are discussed under induction and recovery side-effects of these drugs.

Respiratory Effects

Nonopioid iv anesthetics are always given with other drugs such as opioids, volatile anesthetics, or skeletal muscle relaxants, all of which cause respiratory depression. Under general anesthesia, ventilation of the lungs can be assisted or controlled to maintain normocarbia, but if iv anesthetics are used as sedatives or hypnotics in spontaneously breathing patients, respiratory depression may occur. Thus, it is important to know the effects of these iv anesthetics on respiratory rate, tidal volume, bronchial smooth muscle, and respiratory reflexes. None of these drugs produce long-term respiratory depression or cause bronchoconstriction.

At one time, thiopental was blamed for causing airway spasm and increased sensitivity of airway reflexes, but it is more likely that these were due to the introduction of artificial airways or endotracheal tubes in inadequately anesthetized patients. Methohexital is associated with a higher incidence of hiccup and coughing than other iv anesthetics.

Intravenous induction drugs can reduce tidal volume and respiratory rate until apnea occurs. Respiratory depression is greater when opioid premedication is administered[125,126] or when the drug is injected rapidly. When propofol is given alone, the respiratory rate increases for the first 30 seconds, then rapidly decreases to apnea in most patients,[126] producing a more profound respiratory depression than does thiopental. Its main effect is on tidal volume rather than rate;[127] the rate returns to control values by 4 minutes after injection of 2.5 mg·kg^{-1}. When fentanyl is given before propofol induction, apnea occurs within 30 seconds after propofol is injected. When thiopental is used, tidal volume is depressed more than respiratory rate.[128] Etomidate causes a brief period of hyperventilation with a small increase in both tidal volume and respiratory rate toward the end of induction; this is followed by a period of short-lived respiratory depression or apnea.[129] Apnea following etomidate is less common than after barbiturate or propofol induction but more frequent than after midazolam, diazepam, or ketamine induction. It is also more frequent and of longer duration with opioid premedication and in older patients.

When midazolam was given to volunteers, tidal volume decreased about 40%, respiratory rate increased about 40%, but minute ventilation was unchanged. This effect was not dose-related over the dose range of 0.05 to 0.2 mg·kg^{-1} (Fig. 15-7). The highest dose, 0.2 mg·kg^{-1}, reduced oxygen saturation as a result of a longer duration of apnea.[130] Specific benzodiazepine antagonists reverse the respiratory depressant effects of the benzodiazepines; these effects are not reversed by the opioid antagonist, naloxone.[130]

Midazolam, given for anesthetic induction to patients with chronic obstructive pulmonary disease, produced a more profound and longer-lasting respiratory depression than it did in normal patients or than equivalent doses of thiopental produced in patients with pulmonary disease.[131]

Ketamine generates few respiratory effects. Its effect ranges from mild respiratory stimulation to mild depression,[132] depression being more common in spontaneously breathing elderly patients[133] or related to rapid administration of the drug.[134] Although all these induction drugs can be used safely for asthmatic patients, ketamine can be beneficial in relieving bronchospasm because of its sympathomimetic effect. After ketamine induction, cough and laryngospasm are rare and laryngeal reflexes are intact, but when a belladonna alkaloid is excluded from premedication, excess secretions can develop in the respiratory tract. The respiratory response to carbon dioxide continues during ketamine anesthesia.[135]

Table 15-6 summarizes the relative respiratory effects of equivalent doses of nonopioid iv drugs administered to induce general anesthesia. Slower injection times and lower doses, such as might be used for continuous infusion, result in less respiratory depression for each agent. For safety, one should be prepared to maintain the airway artificially and assist or control ventilation of the lungs when any of them are used.

Cardiovascular Effects

The effects of iv anesthetics on the cardiovascular system are more important than their effects on the respiratory system; there is no simple maneuver to counteract temporary cardiovascular depression in the way that artificial ventilation of the lungs is used to reverse temporary respiratory

TABLE 15-5. Cerebral Effects (Healthy Adults)*

	CBF	CPP	CMRo$_2$	ICP	IOP
Thiopental	– –	– –	– –	– –	–
Thiamylal	– –	– –	– –	– –	–
Methohexital	– –	– –	– –	– –	–
Etomidate	– –	0	– –	– –	–
Propofol	– –	– –	– –	– –	–
Ketamine	+ +	+	+	+	+
Diazepam	–	–	–	–	–
Midazolam	–	–	–	–	–

* + + to – – is a five-point scale qualitatively describing the relative increase (+, + +) or decrease (–, – –) or no effect (0) among the induction agents for each cerebral effect.

CBF = cerebral blood flow; CPP = cerebral perfusion pressure; CMRo$_2$ = cerebral metabolic rate of oxygen; ICP = intracranial pressure; and IOP = intraocular pressure.

Reprinted with permission from Fragen RJ, Avram MJ: Comparative pharmacology of drugs used for the induction of anesthesia. In Stoelting RK, Barash PG, Gallagher TJ (eds): Advances in Anesthesia, p 103. Chicago, Year Book Medical Publishers, 1986.

TABLE 15-6. Comparative Respiratory Effects

	Respiratory Depression	Bronchomotor Tone
Thiopental	+ +	0
Thiamylal	+ +	0
Methohexital	+ +	0
Etomidate	+	0
Propofol	+ +	0
Ketamine	0	+
Diazepam	+	0
Midazolam	+	0

Note: 0 to + + + represents a scale of increasing severity of respiratory depression or beneficial effect on bronchomotor tone; this is only a qualitative comparison of each drug.

depression. Unfortunately, all iv anesthetics are either cardiovascular depressants or stimulants. A number of factors that can influence the cardiovascular system of patients undergoing general anesthesia are listed in Table 15-7.

These factors can have multiple effects on hemodynamics. As a person goes from the awake to the unconscious state, blood pressure and heart rate decrease about 10%. This degree of change is expected after anesthetic induction. Resting sympathetic tone is high in nervous and hypertensive patients. Anesthetics causing vasodilation will, therefore, have a more profound effect in these patients. Hypercarbia causes vasodilation and stimulates release of catecholamines. The more rapid the injection, the greater the concentration of drug that reaches the heart and the more profound the cardiac effect of the induction drugs. Cardiovascular depression after anesthetic induction is greater in the hypovolemic patient. Restoration of blood vol-

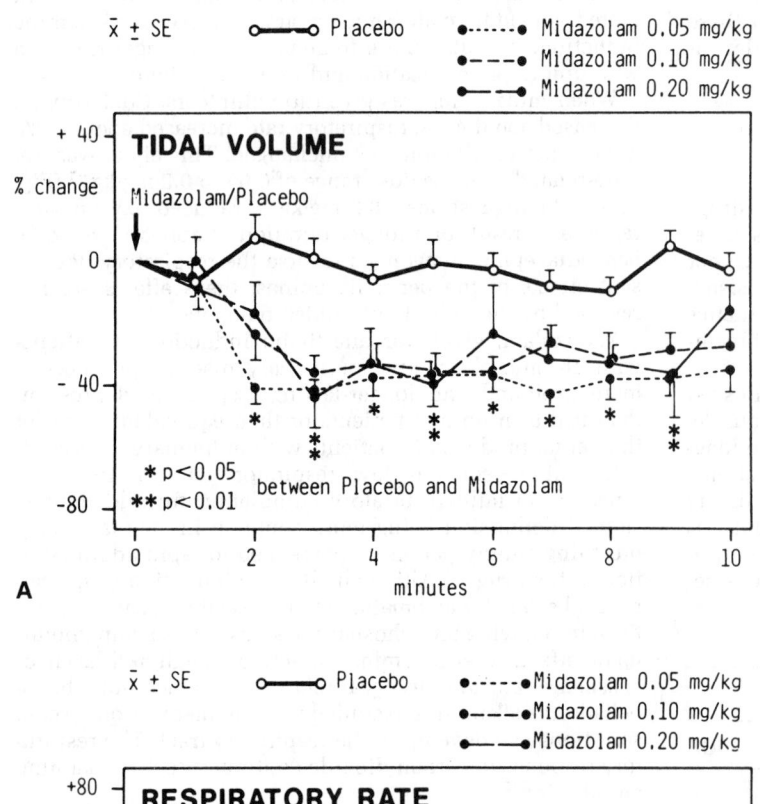

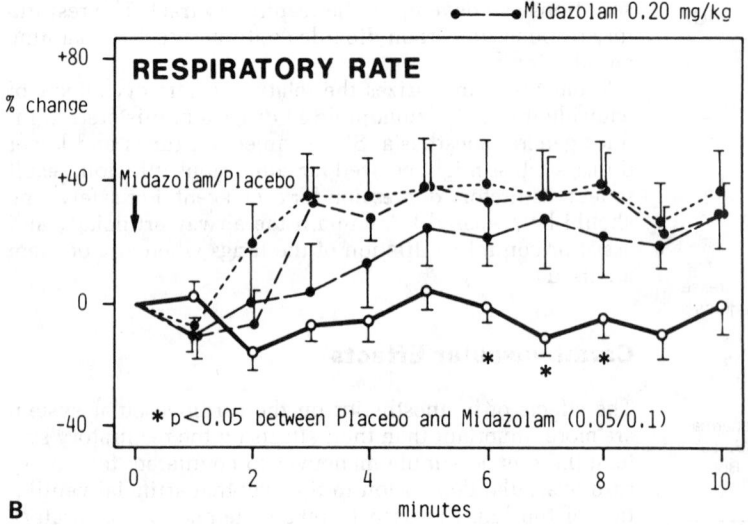

Figure 15-7. The *A* and *B* figures show the percentage changes in tidal volume and respiratory rate, respectively, for 10 minutes after the injection of three different doses of midazolam or a placebo. These doses of midazolam are within the therapeutic range for intravenous (iv) sedation to anesthetic induction. There were significant differences in respiratory effects between midazolam and placebo, but the effects were not different between the three midazolam doses. (Reprinted with permission from Forster A, Morel D, Bachmann M *et al:* Respiratory depressant effect of different doses of midazolam and lack of reversal with naloxone. A double-blind randomized study. Anesth Analg 62:920, 1983.)

TABLE 15-7. Factors Influencing the Cardiovascular System at the Time of Anesthetic Induction

1. Change from awake to unconscious state
2. Resting sympathetic tone
3. Ventilatory status
4. Speed of injection
5. Vascular volume
6. Pathophysiology of diseases affecting the autonomic nervous system or the cardiovascular system directly
7. Cardiovascular effects of ancillary drugs
8. Residual effects of cardiovascular drugs
9. Cardiovascular effects of premedicants

ume is the aim of good patient care prior to surgery, but when hypovolemia exists in the emergency patient, the barbiturates, benzodiazepines, and propofol must be used with extreme care, if at all.

Diseases of the cardiovascular system or autonomic nervous system may exaggerate the cardiovascular response to anesthetic drugs, or they may blunt the compensatory reflexes to drug-related cardiovascular changes. Premedicants and other drugs seldom produce cardiovascular effects except in the elderly and in patients with pre-existing cardiovascular disease; in such cases, changes in blood pressure or heart rate may occur. For example, morphine can cause bradycardia, and meperidine can cause tachycardia. Atropine increases heart rate. Slow heart rates are found in patients on digitalis, calcium channel blockers, and beta blockers. Because many of these factors may exist prior to iv induction of anesthesia, studies reporting different cardiovascular effects of the same iv induction drug may be misleading unless the modifying factors are considered.

The general effects of midazolam on circulation are shown schematically in Figure 15-8.[136] This pattern of drug action and body reaction pertains to most of the other induction drugs as well, except for etomidate and ketamine. Induction drugs may cause dilation of the capacitance or resistance vessels or may directly depress the myocardium,

blunt compensatory cardiovascular reflexes, affect the autonomic nervous system directly or centrally, or affect the conduction system. Other than sinus bradycardia or tachycardia, dysrhythmias are not produced by the induction drugs discussed here unless someone fails to counteract their respiratory depressant effects by ventilatory assistance.

Ketamine produces tachycardia by central sympathetic stimulation,[101] but concomitant administration of diazepam, droperidol,[101] thiopental,[137] midazolam,[138] volatile anesthetics,[137] or labetalol blunts this response. This chronotropic effect is partially responsible for the rise in blood pressure that occurs after ketamine administration. Tachycardia is exaggerated if pancuronium is given with ketamine. Other physiologic alterations that ketamine may produce include an adrenergic constriction of capacitance vessels with an increased venous return,[137] direct autonomic nervous system stimulation, and baroreceptor depression.[139] In another study, the baroreceptor mechanism remained intact after both ketamine and etomidate induction.[140] Ketamine actually has a direct vasodilating effect, but this is overcome by sympathetic stimulation[140] resulting in little change in systemic vascular resistance. In critically ill patients, the autonomic nervous system response may be absent, and the catecholamines may be depleted. In such patients, ketamine can be a cardiovascular depressant.[141] Ketamine is not recommended for patients with coronary artery disease because intraventricular pressures are elevated and contractility is increased,[139] resulting in increased myocardial oxygen demand.

Ketamine may be advantageous for some conditions. It is antidysrhythmogenic and counteracts both epinephrine-induced ventricular dysrhythmias and digitalis-induced dysrhythmias.[142] It is beneficial for patients in cardiogenic shock[101] or hypovolemic shock, as perfusion of the myocardial, renal, hepatic, and cerebral circulations improves with the rise in arterial pressure.[141] After ketamine induction in patients with pericardial effusion, either with or without constrictive pericarditis, the cardiac index remained stable; blood pressure, systemic vascular resistance, and right atrial pressure increased; and heart rate was unchanged from the

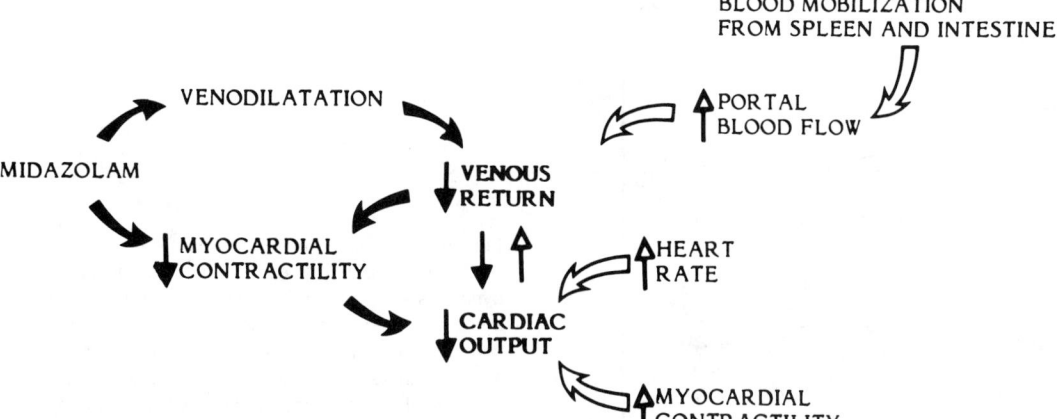

Figure 15-8. The hemodynamic changes that occur after midazolam are illustrated by the solid arrows on the left side of the figure. They evoke compensatory changes that attempt to return circulation toward normal and are depicted by the open arrows in the right side of the figure. This illustration is probably also correct for some of the other induction agents. (Reprinted with permission from Gelman S, Reves JG, Harris D: Circulatory responses to midazolam anesthesia: Emphasis on canine splanchnic circulation. Anesth Analg 62:135, 1983.)

usual tachycardia found in these patients.[138] Although ketamine is recommended for induction in such patients, it sometimes causes a decrease in cardiac output.[138] Children with congenital heart disease who were given ketamine, 2 mg·kg[−1], for anesthetic induction had preserved myocardial function. Although blood pressure and heart rate rose, there was no change in ejection fraction and no change in wall motion as determined by M-mode echocardiography.[143] Ketamine is the only iv induction drug that usually stimulates the cardiovascular system. It is thought to have a more pronounced effect on the right side of the heart and pulmonary circulation than on the left side of the heart and systemic vascular bed.[144]

In 1974, German investigators demonstrated minimal changes in cardiovascular and coronary hemodynamics associated with use of etomidate. Bruckner found that etomidate, 0.3 mg·kg[−1], produced a slight increase in cardiac index and a slight decrease in heart rate, arterial blood pressure, and systemic vascular resistance. The changes were maximal 3 minutes after injection, returned to control values over the next 5 minutes, and were of lesser magnitude than demonstrated by other iv hypnotics.[145] Kettler et al showed that the same dose of etomidate increased coronary blood flow 19% with no increase in myocardial oxygen consumption. Coronary vascular resistance decreased 19% with no change in coronary perfusion pressure (Fig.15-9).[146] This was interpreted as a mild nitroglycerin-like effect, suggesting that etomidate is a good anesthetic induction drug for patients with coronary artery disease who undergo either coronary artery bypass grafting or noncardiac procedures. Patients with valvular heart disease displayed a decrease of 10–20% in systemic arterial pressure, pulmonary artery pressure, and pulmonary capillary wedge pressure[138] without change in central venous pressure, heart rate, or electrocardiogram. Colvin et al demonstrated that etomidate caused less hypotension than did thiopental when each was given to patients with mild hypovolemia.[147] In one study of etomidate, an unchanged dP/dT with no change in preload or afterload implied unimpaired myocardial function. Of all

the rapidly acting iv hypnotics, etomidate produces the least detrimental cardiovascular changes;[148] this may be the main reason for its use.

Diazepam and midazolam rarely produce cardiovascular changes when used in low doses for premedication or iv sedation, provided that precautions are taken against ventilatory depression. In induction doses, these benzodiazepines usually cause mild cardiovascular changes but may cause significant cardiovascular effects.

In one study, both diazepam and midazolam transiently depressed baroreflex function and reduced norepinephrine plasma concentrations from awake levels. Epinephrine levels were only reduced by midazolam. None of these changes were as significant as those occurring after anesthetic maintenance concentrations of volatile anesthetic drugs.[149]

Results of a number of studies comparing diazepam with other hypnotic induction drugs illustrate its vascular and myocardial effects. Used for patients with coronary artery disease, diazepam, 0.1 to 0.5 mg·kg[−1], caused a decrease in mean arterial pressure of 7–18% but no change in heart rate, cardiac index, systemic vascular resistance, stroke index, or left ventricular stroke work index despite this fivefold difference in dose.[138] In another study, 5 to 8.5 mg of diazepam reduced left ventricular end-diastolic pressure (LVEDP), tension time index, and myocardial oxygen consumption for at least 20 minutes after injection.[150] There was no change in either coronary blood flow or coronary vascular resistance. The reduction in LVEDP could be due to a preload or afterload reduction; a nitroglycerin-like action on the circulation is unlikely. These changes resulted in improved cardiac function.

When diazepam, 5 mg, was given after morphine anesthesia, 2 mg·kg[−1], systolic blood pressure and heart rate decreased; cardiac output, stroke volume, and diastolic blood pressure decreased very slightly; and peripheral vascular resistance increased. A second dose of diazepam caused only a further decrease in systolic pressure and a further increase in peripheral resistance.[151]

Diazepam also caused more cardiovascular depression in

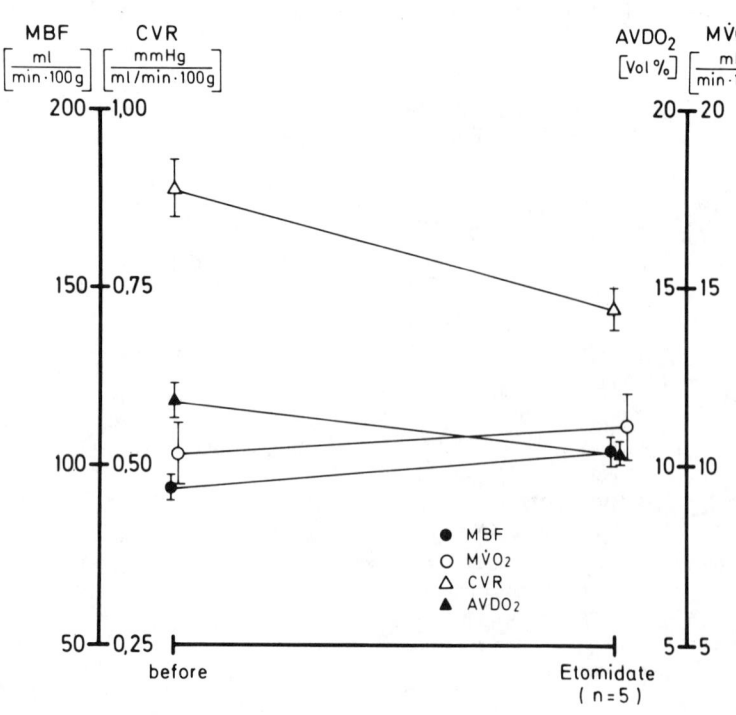

Figure 15-9. This figure illustrates the effect of 0.12 mg·kg[−1]·min[−1] of etomidate on coronary hemodynamics and myocardial oxygen consumption in a healthy patient. There was a mild decrease in coronary vascular resistance (CVR) and a corresponding increase in myocardial blood flow (MBF). Myocardial oxygen consumption (MV̇O₂) was unchanged because of a simultaneous decrease in the arteriocoronary venous oxygen difference (AVDO₂). (Reprinted with permission from Kettler D, Sonntag H, Donath V et al: Haemodynamics, myocardial function, oxygen requirements and oxygen supply to the human heart after administration of etomidate. Anaesthesist 23:116, 1974.)

patients with LVEDP more than 15 mm Hg and with mean ejection fractions less than 0.38 than in patients with LVEDP less than 15 mm Hg. Blood pressure decreased in both groups of patients. The pre-ejection period (PEP) lengthened, and the PEP/LVET (left ventricular ejection time) increased, suggesting that hypotension coincided with a reduction in myocardial performance.[152] Diazepam should be used with care in patients with coronary artery disease and elevated LVEDP.

Diazepam, 0.4 mg·kg^{-1}, caused a more profound decrease in peripheral resistance and arterial pressure than did thiopental, 3 mg·kg^{-1}, when either drug was given intravenously to healthy patients undergoing dental procedures in the semisupine position.[153] Thiopental usually has more depressant effects in supine patients. Tilting 12 volunteers before and after administering diazepam, 10 mg, caused no change in their measured hemodynamics.[154] Diazepam proved superior to thiopental as a hypnotic for cardioversion in an experiment in which premature ventricular contractions occurred in 11 of 18 patients who received thiopental but none who received diazepam. When cardioversion was performed in patients with mitral stenosis, cardiac output remained nearer to control values after diazepam.[154] When compared with methohexital for electroshock therapy anesthesia, diazepam was associated with more cardiac dysrhythmias.[155]

These studies show that diazepam has both peripheral vascular and direct myocardial effects, but the degree of these effects is mild compared with that of most hypnotic induction drugs.

Midazolam was originally considered twice as potent as diazepam on a milligram basis, but further experience suggested that it is probably even more potent. Differences in the cardiovascular effects produced by the two benzodiazepines in earlier studies may be attributed to the effects of nonequivalent doses as much as to real differences between them.

After midazolam induction, a small decrease in blood pressure and an increase in heart rate occur in patients with normal cardiovascular function. In premedicated patients with coronary artery disease, changes in these measurements are usually less than 20% of control values.[156] When midazolam was given for sedation to patients with coronary artery disease undergoing cardiac catheterization, no significant changes in hemodynamic measurements occurred.[157]

In another group of patients with stable coronary artery disease who were asleep after receiving iv midazolam, 0.2 mg·kg^{-1}, for cardiac catheterization, mean arterial pressure decreased 15% and LVEDP decreased 44%. Cardiac index, stroke index, and heart rate of these patients changed less than 15%, whereas systemic vascular resistance and V$_{max}$ were unchanged.[158] In the same study, effects of midazolam on coronary circulation were measured (Table 15-8). There were no electrocardiographic changes or changes in myocardial lactate extraction, nor was there an equivalent reduction in coronary blood flow and myocardial metabolism. When control pulmonary artery occlusion pressure (PAOP) exceeded 18 mm Hg and when the cardiac index was less than 2.2 l·min^{-1}·m^{-2}, induction of anesthesia with midazolam caused a significant reduction in PAOP toward normal; at the same time cardiac index and heart rate increased, whereas left ventricular stroke work index, systemic vascular resistance, and mean arterial pressure decreased. The 40% decrease in systemic vascular resistance in this group was about twice that which occurred in patients with PAOP less than 17 mm Hg.[159] It therefore can be

TABLE 15-8. Cardiovascular and Coronary Effects of Midazolam (x ± SD)

	Control	5 Minutes	15 Minutes
HR (beats·min^{-1})	81 ± 17	87 ± 16†	87 ± 15†
MAP (mm Hg)	109 ± 20	93 ± 15‡	92 ± 13‡
LVEDP (mm Hg)	7.7 ± 2.7	4.9 ± 2.4†	4.2 ± 2.6†
CSBF (ml·min^{-1})	134 ± 58	104 ± 38†	104 ± 30†
CVR (units)	0.84 ± 0.2	0.92 ± 0.2	0.91 ± 0.2
MVO$_2$ (ml·min^{-1})	16.8 ± 10.1	11.4 ± 4.4†	11.1 ± 3.6†
C(a-cs)O$_2$ (ml·dl^{-1})	12.1 ± 1.4	10.9 ± 1.5†	10.8 ± 1.3
Lact (a-cs)/lact a	0.45 ± 0.15	0.52 ± 0.15	0.44 ± 0.2
PcsO$_2$ (mm Hg)	22 ± 3	25 ± 0.4*	25 ± 4*

* = $p < 0.05$; † = $p < 0.01$; ‡ = $p < 0.001$.

HR = heart rate; MAP = mean arterial pressure; LVEDP = left ventricular end diastolic pressure; CSBF = coronary sinus blood; CVR = coronary vascular resistance; MVO$_2$ = myocardial oxygen consumption; C(a-cs)O$_2$ = aorta-coronary sinus oxygen-content difference; Lact(a-cs)/lact a = aorta-coronary sinus lactate concentration divided by aortic lactate concentration; PcsO$_2$ = oxygen tension in the coronary sinus. These measurements were made before and 5 and 15 minutes after midazolam, 0.2 mg·kg^{-1}, iv.

Adapted with permission from Marty J, Nitenberg A, Blanchet F et al: Effects of midazolam in the coronary circulation in patients with coronary artery disease. Anesthesiology 64:206, 1986.

concluded that midazolam can be used safely in patients with coronary artery disease.

However, midazolam, 0.075 or 0.15 mg·kg^{-1}, cannot be given safely to patients with coronary artery disease breathing oxygen after high-dose fentanyl, 75 μg·kg^{-1}. After high-dose fentanyl, there is significant venous pooling and both stroke index and systolic blood pressure decrease, the latter about 30%.[160] In contrast to diazepam, midazolam caused a decrease in cardiac index without a reduction in systemic vascular resistance. Midazolam also decreased coronary sinus blood flow and coronary perfusion pressure without altering coronary vascular resistance.

When midazolam was used to induce anesthesia for adults with valvular heart disease, pump function was maintained and there was a decrease in systemic vascular resistance.[161]

When flow was held constant during cardiopulmonary bypass, diazepam, 0.3 mg·kg^{-1}, caused a transient decrease in systemic vascular resistance, whereas systemic vascular resistance remained stable after midazolam, 0.2 mg·kg^{-1}. Venodilation was greater after midazolam, however.[162]

As suggested by Figure 15-8, midazolam would be a more cardiovascularly depressing drug without the compensatory mechanisms. It should, therefore, be used cautiously, if at all, in patients who are hypovolemic or beta blocked, have a blunted baroreflex, or have myocardial disease severe enough to prevent improvement in contractility. Tracheal intubation performed shortly after midazolam induction also returns blood pressure to control values; there is less tachycardia than when tracheal intubation follows shortly after thiopental induction.[156,163]

Barbiturates have more effects on the cardiovascular system than do benzodiazepines. Thiopental's main effects are to decrease cardiac output and increase heart rate. A decrease in cardiac output can be caused by (1) less ventricular filling (preload) owing to dilation of the capacitance vessels; (2) a direct negative inotropic effect; or (3) a decrease in central catecholamine outflow. The baroreceptor reflex is probably responsible for increased heart rate. Standard induction doses of thiopental usually produce an unchanged, or slightly decreased, mean arterial pressure and cardiac index in healthy patients as well as in patients with compensated heart disease.[138] However, cardiovascular depression is exaggerated if the patients have valvular heart disease, either left- or right-sided heart failure, cardiac tamponade, hypovolemia, or are elderly. Thiopental must be used cautiously, if at all, in these conditions. It is particularly dangerous for patients with "compensated shock"[164] and for those with a fixed cardiac output. (Digitalis reduces the depressant effect of thiopental on the heart.[165]) Methohexital, 1 mg·kg^{-1}, and thiopental, 3 mg·kg^{-1}, produce a similar decrease in myocardial contractility in healthy adults.[166] Induction doses of methohexital are associated with greater increases in heart rate than occurs with equivalent doses of thiopental. Although methohexital dilates capacitance vessels and has a direct myocardial effect, it may also cause some change in total peripheral resistance by either a central or a peripheral effect.[167] In most studies in healthy patients, thiopental had little effect on the resistance vessels. Regional blood flow is usually reduced. Thiopental decreases cerebral, hepatic, and renal blood flow and reduces central blood volume because blood pools in the splanchnic circulation. Although baroreceptor function is intact in healthy patients, thiopental may markedly decrease baroreceptor activity in hypersensitive patients.[168] Thiopental's myocardial depressant effects are more obvious when the baroreflex is blunted by volatile anesthetics, when there is beta-adrenergic blockade, or when insufficient myocardial reserve exists to sustain an increased heart rate.

High doses of thiopental or methohexital given to neurosurgical patients decreased blood pressure, stroke volume index, and systemic vascular resistance about 15%; heart rate increased.[118,169] The ventricular stroke work indices decreased, and other hemodynamic measurements remained stable. These were tolerable changes in patients with normal cardiovascular systems.[118,170] When thiopental, 6 mg·kg^{-1}, was given to patients with coronary artery disease, there was a parallel decrease in myocardial oxygen consumption and coronary blood flow.[171]

The most significant adverse cardiovascular effect of propofol is hypotension. Although the other induction agents may also cause hypotension, they concomitantly generate a greater degree of compensatory increase in heart rate. After propofol induction of anesthesia, blood pressure returns toward control values after a few minutes. Although not important for healthy patients, the temporary 15–20% decrease in systolic blood pressure is a slightly greater decrease than occurs after barbiturate induction in healthy patients, patients with coronary artery disease, or those with valvular heart disease.[172-176] However, when assessed by transesophageal echocardiography, propofol caused negative ionotropism but less pronounced and of shorter duration than that caused by thiopental.[177]

After receiving propofol, 2.5 mg·kg^{-1}, for coronary artery bypass grafting, patients who had no myocardial infarct for at least 3 months and an ejection fraction over 30% had a significant decrease in mean arterial pressure, systemic vascular resistance and left ventricular stroke work index; their heart rate increased. Table 15-9 shows the changes in hemodynamic variables after propofol induction of anesthesia as well as further changes that occurred when halothane was added. The changes were transient and without sequelae in these patients, but they probably represent both vasodilation and direct myocardial depression.[178] In an earlier study, propofol caused a 25% decrease in mean arterial pressure and a significant decrease in systemic vascular resistance; two of ten patients had a systolic blood pressure decrease of more than 70 mm Hg.[179] After intubation of the trachea, there was less cardiovascular stimulation than after thiopental induction, but propofol does not suppress the hemodynamic response to laryngoscopy and tracheal intubation.[179] It is the authors' opinion that propofol should be used with utmost caution, if at all, in patients who cannot tolerate temporary significant decreases in blood pressure.

The effects of propofol on coronary circulation were addressed in one study;[180] an induction dose of 2 mg·kg^{-1} was followed by a 200 μg·kg^{-1}·min^{-1} continuous infusion. Myocardial blood flow decreased 26%, myocardial oxygen consumption decreased 31%, and coronary vascular resis-

TABLE 15-9. Cardiovascular Effects of Propofol Versus Thiamylal in Patients with Coronary Artery Disease

		Control	T$_1$	T$_3$	T$_4$
MAP	(P)	97 ± 11	83 ± 18‡	75 ± 16*†	66 ± 9†
	(T)	95 ± 13	93 ± 10	95 ± 8	77 ± 11†
HR	(P)	60 ± 14	72 ± 19†	68 ± 12‡	71 ± 10†
	(T)	67 ± 12	75 ± 11‡	67 ± 8	71 ± 8
CI	(P)	2.4 ± 0.4	2.4 ± 0.4	2.4 ± 0.5	2.6 ± 0.6
	(T)	2.8 ± 1	2.8 ± 0.8	2.5 ± 0.6	2.4 ± 0.9
PAOP	(P)	16 ± 5	15 ± 5	14 ± 5	12 ± 4‡
	(T)	18 ± 3	18 ± 3	17 ± 3	15 ± 4
SVR	(P)	1565 ± 262	1246 ± 328‡	1146 ± 227*†	987 ± 291*†
	(T)	1426 ± 450	1379 ± 442	1522 ± 349	1307 ± 358
LVSWI	(P)	45 ± 10	28 ± 9†	30 ± 10†	28 ± 8†
	(T)	44 ± 15	37 ± 10‡	39 ± 9	29 ± 14

*$p < 0.01$ between groups; †$p < 0.01$ within groups; ‡$p < 0.05$ within groups; x̄ ± 1 SD.

T$_1$ = 1 minute after injection; T$_3$ = 3 minutes after injection; T$_4$ = 1 minute after halothane; P = propofol; T = thiamylal; MAP = mean arterial pressure; HR = heart rate; CI = cardiac index; PAOP = pulmonary artery occlusion pressure; SVR = systemic vascular resistance; LVSWI = left ventricular stroke work index.

Reprinted with permission from Profeta JP, Guffin A, Mikula S et al: The hemodynamic effects of propofol and thiamylal sodium for induction in coronary artery surgery. Anesth Analg 66:5142, 1987.

TABLE 15-10. Induction Characteristics of Propofol in Older Versus Younger Patients

Dose (mg·kg⁻¹)	% Induced		Systolic Blood Pressure Decreased >40 mm Hg		APNEA >1 min	
	<60	≥60	<60	≥60	<60	≥60
1.5	53	96	3	12	3	0
1.75	83	100	0	8	3	4
2	87	96	0	20	10	20
2.25	97	100	0	45	13	25

Reprinted with permission from Dundee JW, Robinson FP, McCollum JSC et al: Sensitivity to propofol in the elderly. Anaesthesia 41:482, 1986.

tance increased 19% without change in arterial–coronary sinus oxygen content difference.[180] A few patients had some myocardial lactate production, suggesting possible imbalance of regional myocardial oxygen demand and supply associated with propofol. In another study, there was no difference in the degree of hypotension between a rapid (5-second) injection and a slower (60-second) injection when propofol was given for anesthetic induction in young, healthy patients.[181] A slower injection time usually results in less hypotension. Elderly patients have more hypotension after propofol than younger patients; the degree of hypotension seems dose-related in the elderly (Table 15-10).[88]

The condition of patients when they enter a given study may influence their cardiovascular changes on induction of anesthesia. When propofol was used to induce anesthesia in patients with good ventricular function, right-sided pressures such as the central venous pressure, pulmonary artery pressure, and PAOP, as well as the systemic vascular resistance and pulmonary vascular resistance were unchanged.[182] When similar induction was performed on patients with impaired cardiac function, the reductions in cardiac index and mean arterial pressure were primarily related to a marked decrease in central venous pressure (16–29%) and PAOP (35–44%). Neither systemic vascular pressure nor pulmonary vascular resistance changed in these patients.[183]

Table 15-11 compares the relative hemodynamic effects of the various induction agents in healthy patients. All these agents can be used safely in healthy patients, but the data presented in this section should help the anesthesiologist make appropriate choices for patients with compromised cardiovascular function.

Hepatorenal Effects

None of these anesthetic induction drugs have adverse effects on the hepatic system,[136,184,185] even though those that cause hypotension can reduce hepatic blood flow. Most of the drugs decrease urine output because of an increase in antidiuretic hormone. Glomerular filtration and effective plasma flow decrease, and water and electrolyte reabsorption increase. Unlike opioids, the nonopioid induction drugs do not increase intrabiliary pressure. The barbiturates cause slight hyperglycemia and reduce carbohydrate metabolism.

Endocrine Effects

The suppression or release of central catecholamines by these drugs was discussed in the section concerning cardio-

TABLE 15-11. Cardiovascular Effects of IV Anesthetics (Healthy Adults)*

	MAP	HR	CO	SVR	Venodilation	dP/dT
Thiopental	−	+	−	0 to +	+	−
Thiamylal	−	+	−	NR	+	−
Methohexital	−	+ +	−	NR	+	−
Etomidate	0	0	0	0	0	0
Propofol	−	+	0	−	+	NR
Ketamine	+ +	+ +	+	+	0	0
Diazepam	0 to −	− to +	0	− to +	+	0
Midazolam	0 to −	− to +	0 to −	0 to −	+	0

* + + to − − is a five-point scale qualitatively describing the relative increase (+, + +) or decrease (−, − −) or virtually no effect (0) among the induction agents for each cardiovascular effect.

MAP = mean arterial pressure; HR = heart rate; CO = cardiac output; SVR = systemic vascular resistance; dP/dT = myocardial contractility; NR = not reported.

Reprinted with permission from Fragen RJ, Avram MJ: Comparative pharmacology of drugs used for the induction of anesthesia. In Stoelting RK, Barash PG, Gallagher TJ (eds): Advances in Anesthesia, p 103. Chicago, Year Book Medical Publishers, 1986.

vascular effects. None of these drugs appears to affect the anterior pituitary, thyroid, or adrenal medulla. Etomidate suppresses adrenal cortical function; its duration is dose-related. In anesthetic induction doses, it can suppress adrenocortical response to stress for 5 to 8 hours,[70] whereas an infusion produces a longer effect.[186] Etomidate causes a decrease in cortisol, 17-hydroxyprogesterone, aldosterone, and corticosterone production. It inhibits 17-α- and 11-β-hydroxylase and the cholesterol side chain cleavage enzyme.[186] Clinical doses of propofol and thiopental did not suppress the adrenocortical response to the stress of surgery or to adrenocorticotropic hormone stimulation (Fig. 15-10).[187] However, in high doses, *in vitro* thiopental acts on 11-β-hydroxylase, and propofol acts at the first stage of cholesterol synthesis.[188] Midazolam does not suppress adrenocortical function either; adrenocorticotropic hormone and β-endorphin levels increase at the end of surgery after etomidate or methohexital anesthesia[189] but are suppressed by midazolam. In this study, etomidate given by bolus and infusion to a mean dose of 63 mg suppressed the cortisol response to adrenocorticotropic hormone stimulation for 6 hours and the aldosterone response to adrenocorticotropic hormone stimulation for 20 hours, but without electrolyte changes.[189]

Allergic Effects

None of the recently introduced anesthetic induction drugs are associated with histamine release.[190] Histamine release has been reported after the use of barbiturates, and anaphylactoid reactions have been reported occasionally after the use of thiopental.[191-193] Histamine release is increased by high dosage and rapid injections.

Other Effects

None of these iv anesthetics have adverse effects on the reproductive system, but they can all cross the placenta to depress the fetus. Most drugs can be used safely for pregnant patients in normal induction doses. The benzodiazepines

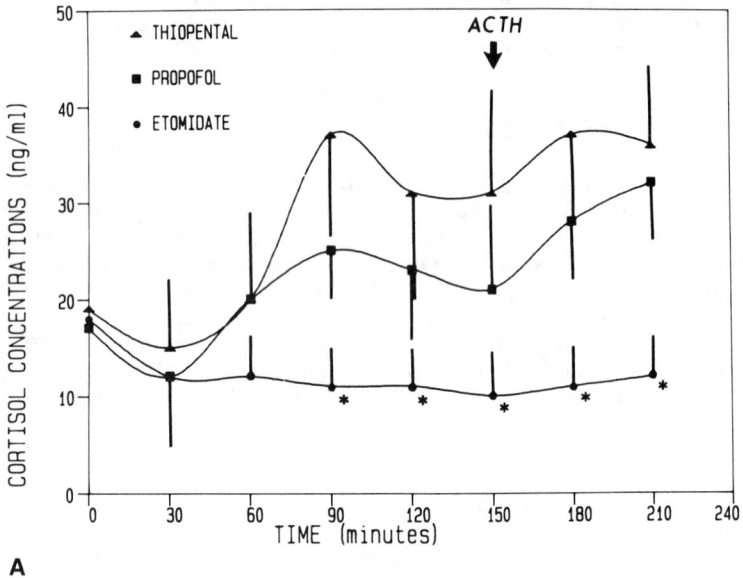

A

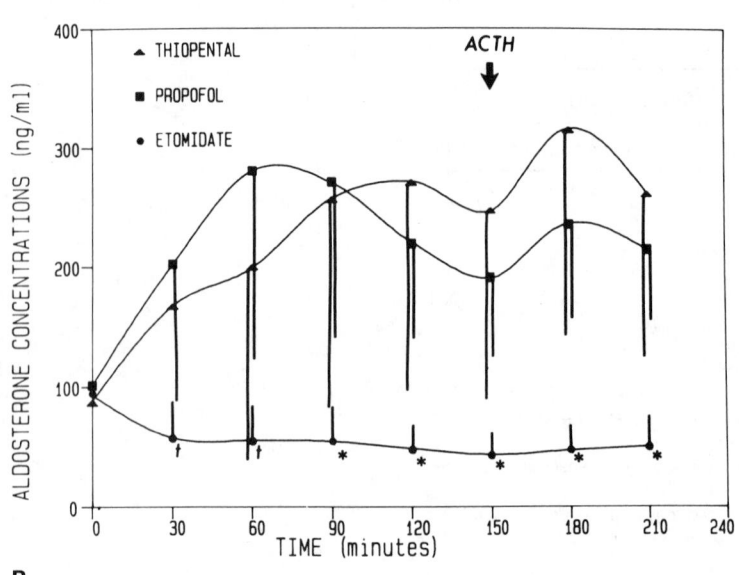

B

Figure 15-10. The *A* and *B* figures show the blood cortisol (*A*) and aldosterone (*B*) concentration before and after anesthetic induction with thiopental, propofol, and etomidate and after an ACTH stimulation test administered 150 minutes after injection of the hypnotic drug. Asterisks (*) show significant differences (*p* < 0.05) between blood concentrations of cortisol or aldosterone after etomidate and those after either thiopental or propofol at the same time. There were no significant differences between the hormone concentrations in patients receiving propofol or thiopental. (Reprinted with permission from Fragen RJ, Weiss HW, Molteni A: The effect of propofol on adrenocortical steroidogenesis: A comparative study with etomidate and thiopental. Anesthesiology 66:839, 1987.)

are discouraged for cesarean section anesthesia because diazepam in high doses is associated with hypotonic babies with low Apgar scores.[194] Midazolam is a poor choice for sedation with regional anesthesia because its amnestic effect may prevent the mother from remembering the birth of her baby.[195] The same may also be true of diazepam.

Propofol and the benzodiazepines can produce muscle relaxant effects in an *in vitro* model,[196,197] but neither propofol, thiopental, nor midazolam produced significant clinical effects on concomitantly administered muscle relaxants.[198,199] Propofol may affect muscles directly, and the benzodiazepines act through the spinal cord. Barbiturates, ketamine, and etomidate have no direct effects on skeletal muscles nor do they interact with the commonly used muscle relaxant drugs.[199]

USES DURING CLINICAL ANESTHESIA

Induction of Anesthesia

Intravenous induction drugs, with the exception of the benzodiazepines, are used primarily by anesthesiologists to induce general anesthesia. Table 15-12 lists the drugs and the ranges of commonly recommended induction doses. The pediatric dose is usually somewhat higher. This is illustrated by the recommended induction doses of 2.5–3.0 $mg \cdot kg^{-1}$ of propofol in unpremedicated children ages 3–12.[200] Although propofol is twice as potent as thiopental at its median effective dose (ED_{50}), the slope of the dose-response curve is less steep.[201]

To identify persons who might be particularly sensitive to these drugs, one can inject approximately 25% of the calculated dose initially and then observe the patient's level of consciousness, respiration, and cardiovascular response. If there is much effect from this low dose, the calculated dose based on population averages should be reduced. Differences in rapidity of the onset of effect for comparable induction doses depend upon the speed of injection, the central volume of distribution, and cardiac output. Most of these drugs act in one arm–brain circulation time. The exceptions are the benzodiazepines and ketamine. To reduce ketamine's side-effects, a 60-second injection time is recommended. Opioid premedication or opioids given intravenously shortly before the anesthetic induction drug also speed onset, especially with the benzodiazepines. When midazolam was titrated during early dose-ranging studies,[202] or given slowly over 20 to 30 seconds,[203] induction times were longer than after thiopental but shorter than after diazepam. Usually, when midazolam is administered over 5 seconds and preceded by iv fentanyl, 100 μg, for an adult, patients lose consciousness in about 1 minute. Normal induction doses of the barbiturates, etomidate, and propofol last 3 to 5 minutes when given alone and slightly

longer if other sedative drugs or opioids are given beforehand. Action of the benzodiazepines lasts 6 to 15 minutes, and ketamine lasts 10 to 15 minutes. The duration of effect can be prolonged by a higher initial dose, repeated fractional doses, or a continuous infusion.

Interactions can occur between two hypnotic drugs or between hypnotics and opioids at the time of anesthetic induction. Because midazolam and thiopental have a synergistic action, lower than normal doses of each can be combined for anesthetic induction (so-called coinduction).[204] If the normal dose of 0.2 $mg \cdot kg^{-1}$ of midazolam does not cause unconsciousness, a very low dose of thiopental, 50–100 mg, can be injected intravenously to successfully complete induction of anesthesia. Alfentanil decreases the induction dose requirement for midazolam. In mice and rats, benzodiazepines and opioids are synergistic for hypnotic effects but antagonistic for nociceptive effects.[205-207] Fentanyl administered intravenously a few minutes before induction did not change the single-dose pharmacokinetics,[208] or the propofol concentrations, or the time to recovery in patients who received a propofol infusion designed to maintain a plasma concentration of 3 $ng \cdot ml^{-1}$.[209]

Routes other than the intravenous one can be used to provide basal hypnosis or unconsciousness. Midazolam, thiamylal, and methohexital can induce unconsciousness with deep intramuscular (im) injection; midazolam is the least irritating. Any of these three drugs can be used to provide basal hypnosis in children. Ketamine, 4 to 6 $mg \cdot kg^{-1}$, has been used successfully by the im route for pediatric anesthesia. Thiopental and midazolam have also been administered rectally in children. Midazolam can be given intranasally in a dose of 0.1 $mg \cdot kg^{-1}$ to sedate children. By this route, the peak plasma concentration occurs 10 minutes after administration and is 57% of that achieved by the same dose of midazolam given intravenously.[211]

When sedative doses of midazolam or other hypnotic drugs are administered to patients, especially if concurrent opioids are given, oxygen saturation should be monitored by pulse oximetry to detect hypoxemia.

For all drugs, the anesthetic induction dose should be reduced for hypovolemic patients. Adequate time should be allowed for the initial dose to take effect when circulation time is slowed; otherwise, an overdose may be given. As previously mentioned, elderly patients normally have increased reactivity to standard doses of these drugs.

The incidence and severity of induction side-effects are usually related to dose, rate of injection, initial distribution volume, and the amount and type of premedication. A slower injection time may reduce side-effects but will also prolong induction. This is illustrated by a study in which propofol was infused at a rate of 300, 600, or 1200 $ml \cdot h^{-1}$ until loss of consciousness. Induction time was slowest with the lowest infusion rate, but the total dose used was less, resulting in less hypotension and apnea.[212] Opioids reduce the incidence and severity of side-effects caused by etomidate.

Pain on injection can occur whether the induction agents are dissolved in water or organic solvents, although patients who mention pain at the time of induction of anesthesia seldom remember or complain about it postoperatively. Its incidence is greater and more severe when the drug is injected into small hand veins rather than larger arm or antecubital veins. Opioid premedication given either intravenously or intramuscularly before the induction agent or lidocaine mixed with the induction drug can decrease both the incidence and severity of pain.[213] Midazolam, ketamine, and thiopental are the least irritating to the vein, whereas a

---

TABLE 15-12. Drug Doses (Healthy Adults)

Thiopental	3–5 $mg \cdot kg^{-1}$
Thiamylal	3–5 $mg \cdot kg^{-1}$
Methohexital	1–1.5 $mg \cdot kg^{-1}$
Etomidate	0.3 $mg \cdot kg^{-1}$
Propofol	1.5–2.5 $mg \cdot kg^{-1}$
Ketamine	0.5–1.5 $mg \cdot kg^{-1}$
Diazepam	0.3–0.6 $mg \cdot kg^{-1}$
Midazolam	0.15–0.4 $mg \cdot kg^{-1}$

disturbing incidence of pain on injection (up to 40%) accompanies use of methohexital, etomidate, propofol, and diazepam. When injected into the hand or wrist veins, propofol caused pain in all patients and methohexital caused pain in 80% of patients, whereas thiopental was injected without pain.[214] Because injectable diazepam is associated with a relatively high incidence of venous sequelae, it has been virtually replaced by midazolam for anesthetic use.

Excitement phenomena, which include fine skeletal muscle tremors, twitching, hiccup, or coughing, may accompany induction of anesthesia. They are low in incidence and severity following induction of anesthesia with midazolam, thiopental, ketamine, diazepam, and propofol. Myoclonus is reported after induction of anesthesia with etomidate, and any of these phenomena can be present when methohexital is used. Stark et al compared the incidence of excitatory effects after propofol with those following the barbiturates.[215] The data were published in tabular form by the manufacturer (Table 15-13). Propofol and thiopental were associated with fewer excitatory effects than was methohexital. The methyl group on the barbiturate molecule may be responsible for the higher incidence of excitement reactions to methohexital than to thiopental.[216] Mackenzie and Grant reported a 75% incidence of excitatory movements after methohexital induction compared with 20% following propofol induction.[217] When Doze et al compared propofol and methohexital in outpatient anesthesia, they, too, found a lower incidence of excitement after propofol induction.[218] Excitement phenomena occur after loss of consciousness, so they are not perceived by the patient. Usually, their duration of effect is less than 1 minute, and they are a mild annoyance.

Maintenance

Ketamine can be used by infusion to maintain both unconsciousness and analgesia, but the other drugs may only be suitable to maintain hypnosis (unconsciousness) in a balanced anesthesia technique or for sedation with regional or local anesthesia. This can be accomplished by using a continuous infusion or an intermittent bolus technique in which about 20–25% of the initial induction dose is given whenever further doses are necessary. Drugs with the highest elimination clearances are least likely to cause prolonged drowsiness when given by infusion, depending, of course, on the dose administered. Exponential infusion rates that follow the plasma decay curves are most likely to achieve and maintain a target blood concentration. They must be correlated with the clinical picture, and appropriate adjustments must be made in the infusion rate.

When propofol is used by infusion, rapid recovery of consciousness occurs after the infusion is terminated. When it was used in one study for iv sedation with regional anesthesia, the mean infusion rate was 3 mg·kg^{-1}·hr^{-1} in patients over age 65 years, and 4.1 mg·kg^{-1}·hr^{-1} in younger patients. Recovery occurred approximately 4 minutes from the end of the infusion when the mean infusion time was 98 minutes.[219] Propofol initially injected at 0.5 mg·kg^{-1} with an infusion that decreased in 10-minute increments from 5-4-3 mg·kg^{-1}·h^{-1} for sedation during subarachnoid block gave good sedation and quicker recovery than did midazolam when it was either reversed or allowed to wear off spontaneously.[220] For total iv anesthesia, Camu et al recommend an initial infusion of 6 to 9 mg·kg^{-1}·hr^{-1} for about 30 minutes following induction with propofol, 2 mg·kg^{-1}, followed by a maintenance infusion of 3 mg·kg^{-1}·hr^{-1}.[221] Willaert recommends an infusion rate of 9 mg·kg^{-1}·hr^{-1} for 30 minutes, then 4.5 mg·kg^{-1}·hr^{-1} when propofol is given with alfentanil, oxygen, and air.[222] Jenstrup et al used 9 mg·kg^{-1}·h^{-1} for 10 minutes, then 6 mg·kg^{-1}·h^{-1} after an induction dose of 1.5 mg·kg^{-1} with either alfentanil or fentanyl.[223] The blood concentrations of propofol were fairly steady even during cardiopulmonary bypass and hypothermia when propofol was infused during cardiac surgery under alfentanil anesthesia.[224] Methohexital was successfully administered by an infusion using a closed-loop feedback control as part of total intravenous anesthesia. The infusion rate was controlled by matching it to the median frequency of the EEG.[225]

Patients recovered more quickly from propofol than from methohexital when a maintenance dose of methohexital, 0.1 to 0.3 mg·kg^{-1}·min^{-1} after a 1.5-mg·kg^{-1} induction dose, was compared with a maintenance dose of 0.1 to 0.2 mg·kg^{-1}·min^{-1} of propofol after a 2-mg·kg^{-1} induction dose in patients breathing 67% nitrous oxide in oxygen.[226] Thiopental infusions must be used cautiously because they can be associated with prolonged recovery. Some authorities advocate using ketamine infusions for general surgical cases[227] or for thoracic surgery using one-lung ventilation.[228] Midazolam, used by intermittent bolus for hypnosis in a balanced anesthetic technique with fentanyl and nitrous oxide, proved superior to thiopental, because fewer supplemental drugs were needed to maintain an adequate depth of anesthesia.[229] Midazolam was associated with fewer emergency complications and more amnesia for early postoperative events.[229,230]

Etomidate is not approved for use as a maintenance hypnotic in the United States, but a 10% ethanolic form is available in other countries. It is not the recommended choice for prolonged infusion for critically ill patients in intensive care units unless supplemental steroids are administered, but after a 1- to 2-hour infusion, no serious harmful effects have been reported.[53] However, when compared with midazolam and methohexital infusions for sedation, short etomidate infusions caused less respiratory depression but more

TABLE 15-13. Incidence (% of Patients) of Excitatory Effects After Three Anesthetics

	N	Any Excitatory Effects	Spontaneous Movements	Twitching	Tremor	Hypertonus	Hiccup
Propofol	1459	13.9	8.7	3.0	0.8	1.9	2.3
Methohexital	86	41.9	10.5	17.4	2.3	1.2	26.7
Thiopental	123	7.3	4.1	1.6	0	0	1.6

Reprinted with permission of ICI Pharmaceuticals.

postoperative headache, nausea, and restlessness.[231] Diazepam is also not a good choice for infusions because of its long half-life, active metabolites, and venous irritation.

The side-effects during maintenance infusions are fewer than those seen during induction of anesthesia because a low dose is given per unit of time compared with that of an induction dose. However, an overdose can produce prolonged drowsiness.

A midazolam infusion can be successfully used to sedate children requiring artificial ventilation after cardiac surgery.[232,233] A blood level of 250 ng·ml^{-1} was necessary for adequate sedation, achieved with a 2 μg·kg^{-1}·min^{-1} infusion combined with morphine, 0.33 μg·kg^{-1}·min^{-1}. When controlled ventilation was changed to continuous positive airway pressure, morphine was discontinued and the rate of midazolam administration was increased to a mean of 4 μg·kg^{-1}·min^{-1} (range 2–5 μg·kg^{-1}·min^{-1}). When hepatic function was impaired, recovery was longer.[232] When midazolam or propofol was given by infusion to sedate patients after cardiac surgery, patients recovered consciousness more rapidly after propofol infusion.[234] Sedation following propofol infusion was easily controlled, and there was little cardiovascular depression.[234]

Midazolam is the most versatile of the nonopioid induction drugs. It can be used for children[235] as well as for adults for im premedication and iv sedation for surgical and diagnostic procedures[115] as well as for sedation in intensive care units and for induction of anesthesia. Midazolam has been given successfully by a patient-controlled analgesia apparatus both during epidural anesthesia[236] and in the intensive care unit.[237]

Benzodiazepines are also the only sedatives for which there is a specific antagonist. Flumazenil is a specific benzodiazepine antagonist that can reverse all the CNS effects of the benzodiazepines, including sedative-hypnotic, amnestic, muscle relaxant, and electroencephalographic effects. The antagonism of these benzodiazepine effects is not of equal magnitude or duration with a given dose of flumazenil. Titrating flumazenil to effect is a useful method of administration. It has been used in this way to reverse sedation produced by flunitrazepam,[238] diazepam,[239] and midazolam.[240] Effective sedation with rapid recovery can be provided by midazolam for trigeminal nerve thermocoagulation. After antagonizing midazolam with flumazenil to determine the correct radiofrequency probe placement, resedation can be established with lower doses of midazolam. When flumazenil was used to antagonize residual benzodiazepine effects at the end of the procedure, there was no resedation for 4 hours.[241] Flumazenil, 0.01 mg·kg^{-1}, antagonized both the sedative and amnestic effects of 2–5 mg of midazolam given intravenously to volunteers.[242] Flumazenil itself has no effect on memory.[243] However, when used to reverse higher doses of midazolam employed in the induction of general anesthesia in outpatient surgery, its duration of effect was too short.[243]

When flumazenil is used to reverse long-acting benzodiazepines, resedation is possible because the half-life of the antagonist is 0.7 to 1.8 hours owing to its high hepatic clearance.[244] In one study, some patients appeared to be asleep after receiving flumazenil but were wide awake when addressed.[240] An increase in delta activity on the EEG could explain this phenomenon. In another study in which flumazenil was used to reverse midazolam sedation when midazolam and fentanyl were used for total intravenous anesthesia, 95% of the patients became resedated.[245] No alteration in hemodynamics or respiration occurred when flumazenil was given to reverse diazepam sedation in patients with cardiac disease undergoing cardiac catheterization.[246]

Physostigmine, 2 mg, combined with glycopyrrolate, 0.2 mg, produces nonspecific reversal of hypnosis caused by benzodiazepines as well as other hypnotic drugs.[247] Aminophylline, 60 mg iv, can also counteract deep diazepam sedation, apparently by an adenosine blockade of GABA-receptors in the CNS. Aminophylline given to patients during benzodiazepine anesthesia could result in patient awareness.[248]

IMPACT OF PRE-EXISTING DISEASE

Ketamine is considered the preferred induction drug for children with tetralogy of Fallot or transposition of the great vessels. It should not be used in patients with Wolff-Parkinson-White syndrome.[249]

Acute intermittent porphyria and some other types of porphyria may be triggered by the barbiturates; they are contraindicated for patients with these diseases. There is some question about the safety of the benzodiazepines and ketamine for patients with porphyria, although ketamine has been used safely in such patients. Etomidate can be used for induction in the presence of this disease, but propofol has not undergone investigation in humans with porphyria.[249]

Although etomidate temporarily suppresses adrenocortical function, there is no contraindication to its use for any disease states. Patients with adrenocortical insufficiency, regardless of the etiology, are on maintenance cortisone therapy, usually with a boost in dose at the time that they come to surgery, which provides added protection against the stress of surgery and anesthesia.

Only the few disease states previously mentioned are currently known to contraindicate these induction drugs. None of these drugs trigger malignant hyperpyrexia.

RECOVERY

The time required for initial awakening, orientation to time and place, and return of normal psychomotor performance should be as short as possible after administration of the anesthetic drugs ceases. The quickest possible return of the patient's homeostatic mechanisms is the goal after any anesthetic. Early recovery is especially important in the expanding outpatient surgical population. Early discharge is not only desirable from the patient's viewpoint but may also be cost-saving. Adequate analgesia in the early postoperative period must also be provided. Because the anesthetic drug or maintenance hypnotic is usually only one of a number of drugs that constitute the anesthetic regimen, it is not the only drug that affects the duration of recovery. A number of studies have been performed in which short anesthetics differed from each other only in the induction drugs used.[98,176,219,226,250-254] In many of these studies, different induction drugs caused differences of only 5 to 10 minutes in time to awakening and orientation. Although some of the differences are statistically significant, they are not clinically important. Assuming that equivalent doses of the iv anesthetics are given to an ideal patient, time to recovery will increase in the following order, from most rapid to slowest: propofol, methohexital, etomidate, thiopental, midazolam, ketamine, and diazepam. Thus, propofol, having the fastest recovery, may become the induction drug of choice for healthy outpatients.

Mackenzie and Grant showed that psychomotor performance was impaired for 30 minutes following propofol administration, 60 to 90 minutes after methohexital administration, and up to 2 hours or longer after thiopental administration in outpatient anesthesia.[254] Patients undergoing ambulatory surgery who received propofol could walk 14 minutes sooner than those who received methohexital.[219] After propofol administration, awakening usually occurs at a blood concentration of about 1 μg·ml^{-1} and orientation at about 0.6 μg·ml^{-1}.[226]

Patients receiving midazolam became oriented 20 minutes later than those receiving thiopental. They also had a slower return of hand coordination, vigilance, spatial concepts, and short-term learning.[255] Return of these functions was slow enough for these authors to recommend that midazolam be avoided as an anesthetic induction drug for outpatients. Some investigators believe that midazolam induction is satisfactory for outpatients, even though some patients did not fully recover until 3 hours or more after surgery.[230,256] Patients should be eligible for discharge from an outpatient surgical facility by 2 hours after surgery or sooner. Recovery from midazolam usually takes twice as long as from thiopental. Its amnestic properties are another negative factor for its use as an induction drug for outpatients: Outpatients may seem quite alert but be unable to remember instructions given to them in the early postoperative period. After midazolam anesthesia, outpatient instructions should be in writing. Because the duration of amnesia is dose-related, amnesia is less prolonged with the lower doses of midazolam used for iv sedation. A 5-mg dose of midazolam produces amnestic effects in 1 to 2 minutes lasting for at least 32 minutes.[257]

Recovery after methohexital administration is perceived to be faster than after thiopental administration, but comparisons of the two do not always give consistent results.[200] Recovery after etomidate induction is similar to that after thiopental.[219] When ketamine is used in outpatients, they are usually ready for discharge by 2 hours, but occasionally recovery is prolonged.[134]

Recovery after continuous infusions may be prolonged when the redistribution sites are saturated, and recovery depends upon elimination clearance. Active metabolites, such as N-desmethyldiazepam, can prolong recovery. Drugs that have relatively low elimination clearances (hence, long elimination half-lives) can leave prolonged residual effects. Low doses of sedatives or opioids given postoperatively can have additive effects with the residual anesthetic drugs, causing resedation.

The early recovery period will be pleasant if the anesthetic drugs leave no emergence side-effects and if there is sufficient analgesia to obtund the pain of surgery.

Recovery side-effects are important because they may interfere with a patient's recovery and persist well into the postoperative period. Recovery side-effects are least common after administration of propofol and are compared with the effects of the barbiturates in Table 15-14.[215] Patients return to a clear-headed state sooner after propofol induction than after other induction agents. Because it also results in the lowest incidence of nausea and vomiting, propofol is well suited to induce anesthesia for outpatients. The apparent antiemetic effect of propofol is attributable to the drug itself and not to the intralipid-like emulsion.[258] Nausea and vomiting are also acceptably low in incidence following use of the benzodiazepines, barbiturates, and ketamine. After midazolam induction, the incidence of nausea and vomiting ranges from none to 15%; 15% is the incidence after other induction drugs. Of 1130 patients, the overall incidence of

TABLE 15-14. Incidence (% of Patients) of Recovery Side-Effects

	N	Headache	Nausea	Vomiting	Restlessness
Propofol	1223	2.2	2.0	2.5	1.6
Methohexital	86	9.3	12.8	10.5	3.5
Thiopental	79	1.3	10.1	10.1	2.5

Reprinted with permission of ICI Pharmaceuticals.

vomiting after midazolam was 3% during the investigational period.[115] Nausea and vomiting are frequent side-effects following induction of anesthesia with etomidate, especially when it is used for short anesthetics.[250]

Other factors in the perioperative period contribute to postoperative nausea, including the presence of pain, use of opioids, surgical site, and use of volatile anesthetics. Some authorities claim that nitrous oxide contributes because it dilates the bowel and increases middle ear pressure. However, one study claims that 60% nitrous oxide did not play a major role, but predisposing factors such as female gender, young adults, and a prior history of postoperative nausea are important.[259]

Emergence excitement occurs following etomidate and ketamine administration. When etomidate was used by bolus plus infusion as part of a total iv anesthetic technique, restlessness and disorientation occurred from early awakening until full orientation.[53] This has not been reported when etomidate was given only for induction of anesthesia. After ketamine induction, patients should recover in a quiet place without being disturbed. They may experience mood alterations, feelings of estrangement or isolation, negativism, hostility, apathy, drowsiness, and repetitive motor behavior. Diplopia or other visual disturbances sometimes occur on return of consciousness. Patients may have difficulty speaking or experience severe emergence delirium. These unpleasant emergence phenomena can be ameliorated or avoided by giving lorazepam, midazolam, diazepam, or thiopental before or with ketamine; or they can be used to treat the symptoms postoperatively. Because these drugs can prolong recovery from ketamine, midazolam, with its shorter duration of effect, may be the best of the benzodiazepines for this function. Droperidol may increase the incidence of vivid dreams when it is used to treat emergence reactions. Preoperative discussion with patients about the possibility of these symptoms occurring also reduces their incidence and severity.[134] If postoperative excitement occurs following administration of the other iv drugs, the anesthesiologist should consider other causes, such as pain or hypoxia.

Venous sequelae such as venous thrombosis, thrombophlebitis, or phlebitis may occur up to the 10th day after irritant iv drugs have been injected. There is less than a 5% incidence of these sequelae after most drugs, including midazolam, propofol, ketamine, and the barbiturates. Because both etomidate and diazepam are dissolved in propylene glycol, the incidence of venous sequelae is 10–20% following etomidate induction and up to 40% following diazepam induction.[184] Venous reactions usually involve a small segment of vein, are treated symptomatically, and rarely result in permanent damage.

If thiopental or thiamylal is extravasated, it is irritating, and tissue slough may occur. This is treated by heat to increase absorption of barbiturate. If the agent is injected intra-arterially, vascular spasm and gangrene can occur.[260] Local injection of vascular dilators or stellate ganglion blockade has been used to treat this unfortunate circumstance and should be carried out as soon as possible.

Other postoperative side-effects include a low incidence of headache after all the drugs, prolonged drowsiness (usually dose-related), and prolonged amnesia after midazolam is given in high doses or to the elderly.

If both induction and recovery side-effects are considered, midazolam appears to be the best induction drug because it is associated with the fewest side-effects. Methohexital causes a high incidence of induction side-effects, and the barbiturates are associated with a low incidence of recovery side-effects. Etomidate has both induction and recovery side-effects. Ketamine is pleasant for induction, but excitement on recovery can be troublesome. Propofol causes some induction side-effects, but recovery after its use is more rapid and pleasant than that following any of the other drugs described here.

DRUG INTERACTIONS

There is considerable potential for drug interactions during anesthesia and surgery for three reasons: (1) patients requiring anesthesia and surgery are often receiving other drugs; (2) the anesthetic frequently takes the form of polypharmacy; and (3) most drugs used during anesthesia acutely depress the CNS and inhibit protective reflexes.[261] Therefore, the possibility of drug interactions must always be on the mind of the vigilant anesthesiologist. However, the anesthesiologist need not memorize the long lists of drug interactions in books,[262] review articles, and compendia, because many of the drug interactions in those lists are either inaccurate or clinically unimportant and of purely academic interest.[261,263-265] Most clinically important adverse drug interactions can be avoided by understanding the pharmacology of the drugs being used and the mechanisms of interactions. Drug interactions can generally be classified as pharmaceutical, pharmacokinetic, or pharmacodynamic.[261,263-266]

Pharmaceutical interactions result from physicochemical incompatibilities of drug formulations with each other or with iv fluids. An acidic drug, such as a barbiturate, is dissolved in a basic medium and will precipitate as the free acid if the pH is lowered; a basic drug, such as ketamine, is dissolved in an acidic medium and will precipitate as the free base if the pH is raised. On the other hand, some drugs, such as diazepam, have limited solubility in aqueous media and will precipitate if there is an increase in the water:organic solvent ratio of their vehicle (see the section on Chemistry and Formulation). Additionally, some drugs are unstable in acidic or basic media; mixing a barbiturate with atracurium is likely to result not only in precipitation of the barbiturate but also in inactivation of atracurium by the Hofmann reaction, which occurs at basic pH. Pharmaceutical interactions are easily avoided by not mixing drugs or diluting them with iv fluids unless they are known to be compatible.

Pharmacokinetic drug interactions result from one drug interfering with the absorption or disposition of another. Since the anesthetic induction drugs are administered intravenously, the process of absorption is avoided. Because investigation into the interference of drugs with drug distribution is only beginning, the potential clinical implications of such interference remain speculative. Most research on pharmacokinetic drug interactions has focused on the effect of drugs on the elimination clearance of other drugs. Because the iv anesthetic induction drugs are eliminated almost exclusively by hepatic metabolism, potential pharmacokinetic interactions affecting hepatic drug clearance are the most relevant to this discussion.

One drug can affect the elimination clearance of another by altering the rate at which the other drug is delivered to the liver (i.e., hepatic blood flow) or the ability of hepatic enzymes to metabolize the drug (i.e., enzymatic induction or inhibition). The elimination clearance of high hepatic extraction ratio drugs (see Table 15-3) can be decreased by the lowered hepatic blood flow produced by drugs such as propranolol or the volatile anesthetics. Chronic treatment with drugs such as phenobarbital or rifampin induces hepatic microsomal enzyme activity, resulting in increased elimination clearance of drugs metabolized by these enzymes. Enzyme induction, however, is a slow process and is unlikely to occur after the acute administration of barbiturates during anesthesia. On the other hand, cimetidine therapy or the volatile anesthetics can inhibit enzymes, decreasing the hepatic elimination of drugs metabolized by various oxidative enzymes. Because the effects of single doses of the iv anesthetic induction drugs are terminated primarily by redistribution, drug interactions affecting the elimination clearance of these drugs are unlikely to alter their duration of action unless they are given in very large doses, in multiple doses, or by continuous infusion. In such cases, elimination clearance can play a significant role in the termination of drug effect.

Pharmacodynamic interactions occur when one drug increases or decreases the reactivity to another drug as a result of their action at the same receptor or in the same physiologic system. Pharmacodynamic interactions involving CNS depressant drugs such as the anesthetic induction drugs are the most common serious interactions reported. Nonetheless, the pharmacodynamic interactions of these drugs is quite predictable because of their well-defined pharmacologic actions and those of the drugs with which they interact. Thus, the induction dose requirement is decreased in the patient acutely intoxicated with alcohol but is increased in the sober chronic alcoholic. Chronic abusers of amphetamines or cocaine may be more sensitive to the depressant effects of the anesthetic induction drugs, whereas those acutely intoxicated with amphetamine or cocaine may require higher than standard doses for the induction of anesthesia. Caution in the administration of these powerful depressant drugs is always recommended when the potential for a pharmacodynamic drug interaction exists.

TOXICITY

One need look no further than the tragic consequences of administering thiopental to the hypovolemic casualties of the Japanese attack on Pearl Harbor[5] to realize the tremendous potential toxicity of the iv anesthetic induction drugs. New induction agents that will have less toxicity are constantly being sought; the failure of newly developed drugs, such as propanidid, althesin, and minaxolone, to achieve and maintain a position in the armamentarium of the anesthesiologist is often because of their unacceptable toxicity or "adverse effects."

The toxicity or "adverse effects" of the anesthetic induction drugs can be classified as (1) the effects of the drugs when administered in relative or absolute overdose, (2) side-effects of standard doses of the drugs, (3) abnormal or

TABLE 15-15. Summary of the Important Clinical Properties of the Intravenous Sedative/Hypnotics Used for Anesthetic Induction*

	Predictability of Induction	Induction Pain and Excitement	Cerebral Effects	Respiratory Effects	Cardiovascular Effects	Recovery Characteristics
Thiopental	+	0	+	−	−	+
Thiamylal	+	0	+	−	−	+
Methohexital	+	−	+	−	−	+
Etomidate	+	− −	+ +	0	+	−
Propofol	+	−	+	−	−	+ +
Ketamine	+	0	−	+	−	− −
Diazepam	−	− −	+	0	0	+
Midazolam	0	0	+	0	0	+

* + + to − − is a five-point qualitative scale describing the relative positive (+, + +), neutral (0), or negative (−, − −) effect of each agent in each category.

Reprinted with permission from Fragen RJ, Avram MJ: Comparative pharmacology of drugs used for the induction of anesthesia. In Stoelting RK, Barash PG, Gallagher TJ (eds): Advances in Anesthesia, p 103. Chicago, Year Book Medical Publishers, 1986.

unpredictable responses to standard doses, and (4) drug interactions.[267] Several reviews have been devoted exclusively to the subject.[268-270] The "adverse effects" of these agents can be minimized by administering doses appropriate for the patient's physiologic condition at the slowest rate practical for the clinical situation.

SUMMARY

Although thiopental is not the ideal iv anesthetic induction drug, the fact that it has no major disadvantages accounts for its long-standing position as the standard drug for this application. Few of the drugs developed to displace thiopental as the standard are used today. Those that have survived have properties that make their use in specific clinical situations advantageous, whereas other properties preclude their use as routine induction drugs. The important clinical properties of these drugs are summarized in Table 15-15.

The older induction drugs are not generally better than thiopental. Although not extensively studied, thiamylal appears to be similar to thiopental. Methohexital is associated with faster recovery after induction of anesthesia than is thiopental, but it also produces tachycardia and more excitatory effects on induction. Ketamine's advantages are its ability to produce somatic analgesia, bronchodilation, and cardiovascular stimulation, although in some situations the last may be a disadvantage. Disadvantages of ketamine are its adverse cerebral effects and psychotomimetic effects on recovery. When used for induction of anesthesia, diazepam produces less cardiovascular and respiratory depression than does thiopental, but induction of anesthesia is less predictable, recovery is slower, and venous complications are associated with its use.

The newer drugs, etomidate, midazolam, and propofol, are clearly superior to some of the older induction drugs for specific clinical applications but not to thiopental for routine induction of anesthesia. Etomidate causes less respiratory and cardiovascular depression than does thiopental and has more beneficial cerebral effects, but these advantages are often offset by induction and recovery side-effects. Midazolam has the advantages of diazepam, causes less cardiovascular and respiratory depression than thiopental, but results in a more prolonged recovery than that associated with thiopental induction. However, midazolam causes less frequent venous irritation than does diazepam and has a shorter elimination half-life. Propofol causes cardiovascular and respiratory depression equivalent to that produced by thiopental but has a shorter recovery time.

REFERENCES

1. Stedman's Medical Dictionary, p 73. Baltimore, Williams & Wilkins, 1953
2. Woodbridge PD: Changing concepts concerning depth of anesthesia. Anesthesiology 18:536, 1957
3. Frost EAM: Essays on the History of Anesthesia, p 31. Georgetown, McMahon Publishing, 1985
4. Pratt TW, Tatum AL, Hathaway HR et al: Sodium ethyl (1-methylbutyl) thiobarbiturate, preliminary experimental and clinical study. Am J Surg 31:464, 1935
5. Halford FJ: A critique of intravenous anesthesia in war surgery. Anesthesiology 4:67, 1943
6. Dundee JW: Historical vignettes and classification of intravenous anesthetics. In Aldrete JA, Stanley TH (eds): Trends in Intravenous Anesthesia, p 1. Chicago, Year Book Medical Publishers, 1980
7. Briggs LP, Clarke RSJ, Watkins J: An adverse reaction to the administration of disoprofol (Diprivan). Anaesthesia 37:1099, 1982
8. Glen JB, Hunter SC: Pharmacology of an emulsion formulation of ICI 35 868. Br J Anaesth 56:617, 1984
9. Albert A: Relations between molecular structure and biological activity: States in the evolution of current concepts. Ann Rev Pharmacol 21:13, 1971
10. Dundee JW: Molecular structure-activity relationships of barbiturates. In Halsey MJ, Millar RA, Sutton JA (eds): Molecular Mechanisms in General Anesthesia, p 16. New York, Churchill Livingstone, 1974
11. Sternbach LH: the benzodiazepine story. J Med Chem 22:1, 1979
12. Gerecke M: Chemical structure and properties of midazolam compared with other benzodiazepines. Br J Clin Pharmacol 16:11S, 1983
13. Godefroi EF, Janssen PAJ, Van der Eycken CAM et al: DL-1 (1-arylalkyl) imidazole-5-carboxylate esters. A novel type of hypnotic agent. J Med Chem 8:220, 1965
14. James R, Glen JB: Synthesis, biological evaluation, and preliminary structure–activity considerations of a series of alkylphenols as intravenous anesthetic agents. J Med Chem 23:1350, 1980

15. Cone EJ, McQuinn RL, Shannon HE: Structure–activity relationship studies of phencyclidine derivatives in rats. J Pharmacol Exp Ther 228:147, 1984

16. Simonyi M: On chiral drug action. Med Res Rev 4:359, 1984

17. Ariëns EJ: Stereochemistry, a basis for sophisticated nonsense in pharmacokinetics and clinical pharmacology. Eur J Clin Pharmacol 26:663, 1984

18. Andrews PR, Mark LC: Structural specificity of barbiturates and related drugs. Anesthesiology 57:314, 1982

19. Christensen HD, Lee IS: Anesthetic potency and acute toxicity of optically active disubstituted barbituric acids. Toxicol Appl Pharmacol 26:495, 1973

20. Gibson WR, Doran WJ, Wood WC et al: Pharmacology of stereoisomers of 1-methyl-5-(1-methyl-2-pentynyl)-5-allyl-barbituric acid. J Pharmacol Exp Ther 125:23, 1959

21. Heykants JJP, Meuldermans WEG, Michiels LJM et al: Distribution, metabolism and excretion of etomidate, a short-acting hypnotic drug, in the rat. Comparative study of $(R)-(+)$ and $(S)-(-)-$ etomidate. Arch Int Pharmacodyn Ther 216:113, 1975

22. White PF, Ham J, Way WL et al: Pharmacology of ketamine isomers in surgical patients. Anesthesiology 52:231, 1980

23. Ueda I, Kamaya H: Molecular mechanisms of anesthesia. Anesth Analg 63:929, 1984

24. Miller KW: General anesthetics. In Feldman SA, Scurr CF, Paton W (eds): Drugs in Anaesthesia: Mechanisms of Action, p 133. Baltimore, Edward Arnold, 1987

25. Nimmo WS: Hypnotics. In Feldman SA, Scurr CF, Paton W (eds): Drugs in Anaesthesia: Mechanisms of Action, p 125. Baltimore, Edward Arnold, 1987

26. Stone TW: Drugs interfering with synaptic transmission in the central nervous system. In Feldman SA, Scurr CF, Paton W (eds): Drugs in Anaesthesia: Mechanisms of Action, p 234. Baltimore, Edward Arnold, 1987

27. Costa E, Guidotti A: Molecular mechanisms in the receptor action of benzodiazepines. Ann Rev Pharmacol Toxicol 19:531, 1979

28. Ho IK, Harris RA: Mechanism of action of barbiturates. Ann Rev Phamacol Toxicol 21:83, 1981

29. Olsen RW: Drug interactions at the GABA receptor–ionophore complex. Ann Rev Pharmacol Toxicol 22:245, 1982

30. Cheng SC, Brunner EA: The effects of anesthetic agents on GABA metabolism in rat brain synaptosomes. In Hertz L, Kvamme E, McGeer EG et al (eds): Glutamine, Glutamate, and GABA in the Central Nervous System, p 653. New York, Alan R Liss, 1983

31. Olsen RW, Fischer JB, Dunwiddie TV: Barbiturate enhancement of γ-amino-butyric acid receptor binding and function as a mechanism of anesthesia. In Roth SH, Miller KW (eds): Molecular and Cellular Mechanisms of Anesthetics, p 165. New York, Plenum, 1986

32. Olsen RW: GABA-benzodiazepine-barbiturate receptor interactions. J Neurochem 37:1, 1981

33. Study RE: Barker JL: Diazepam and $(-)-$pentobarbital:Fluctuation analysis reveals different mechanisms for potentiation of γ-aminobutyric acid responses in cultured central neurons. Proc Natl Acad Sci 11:7180, 1981

34. Roth SH, Tan K-S, MacIver MB: Selective and differential effects of barbiturates on neuronal activity. In Roth SH, Miller KW (eds): Molecular and Cellular Mechanisms of Anesthetics, p 43. New York, Plenum, 1986

35. Macdonald RL, Skerritt JH, Werz MA: Barbiturate and benzodiazepine actions on mouse neurons in cell culture. In Roth SH, Miller KW (eds): Molecular and Cellular Mechanisms of Anesthetics, p 17. New York, Plenum, 1986

36. Ticku MK, Rastogi SK: Barbiturate-sensitive sites in the benzodiazepine-GABA receptor–ionophore complex. In Roth SH, Miller KW (eds): Molecular and Cellular Mechanisms of Anesthetics, p 179. New York, Plenum, 1986.

37. Concas A, Santoro G, Mascia MP et al: The general anesthetic propofol enhances the function of γ-aminobutyric acid-coupled chloride channel in the rat cerebral complex. J Neurochem 55:2135, 1990

38. Willow M: A comparison of the actions of pentobarbitone and

39. Vincent JP, Cavey D, Kamenka JM et al: Interaction of phencyclidines with the muscarinic and opiate receptors in the central nervous system. Brain Res 152:176, 1978

40. Sircar R, Zukin SR: Further evidence of phencyclidine/sigma opioid receptor commonality. In Clouet DH (ed): Phencyclidine: An Update, p 14. Rockville, Maryland, National Institute on Drug Abuse, 1986

41. Yamamura T, Harada K, Okamura A, Kammotsu O: Is the site of action of ketamine anesthesia the N-methyl-D-aspartate receptor? Anesthesiology 72:704, 1990

42. Friedman J: Physostigmine: The universal antagonist. In Aldrete JA, Stanley TH (eds): Trends in Intravenous Anesthesia, p 509. Chicago, Year Book Medical Publishers, 1980

43. Martin IL: The benzodiazepine receptor: Functional complexity. Trends Pharmacol Sci 5:343, 1984

44. Haefely W, Kyburz E, Gerecke M et al: Recent advances in the molecular pharmacology of benzodiazepine receptors and in the structure–activity relationships of their agonists and antagonists. In Testa B (ed): Advances in Drug Research, Vol 14, p 165. New York, Academic Press, 1985

45. Burch PG, Stanski DR: The role of metabolism and protein binding in thiopental anesthesia. Anesthesiology 58:146, 1983

46. Hung OR, Varvel JR, Shafer SL, Stanski DR: Use of EEG as a measure of thiopental anesthetic depth. Anesthesiology 73:A391, 1990

47. Bührer M, Maitre PO, Hung O, Stanski DR: Electroencephalographic effects of benzodiazepines. I. Choosing an electroencephalographic parameter to measure the effect of midazolam on the central nervous system. Clin Pharmacol Ther 48:544, 1990

48. Furano ES, Greene NM: Metabolic breakdown of thiopental in man determined by gas chromatographic analysis of serum barbiturate levels. Anesthesiology 24:796, 1963

49. Stanski DR, Mihm FG, Rosenthal MH et al: Pharmacokinetics of high-dose thiopental used in cerebral resuscitation. Anesthesiology 53:169, 1980

50. Hudson RJ, Stanski DR, Burch PG: Pharmacokinetics of methohexital and thiopental in surgical patients. Anesthesiology 59:215, 1983

51. Brand L, Mark LC, Snell MMcM et al: Physiologic disposition of methohexital in man. Anesthesiology 24:331, 1963

52. McMurray TJ, Robinson FP, Dundee JW et al: A method for producing constant plasma concentrations of drugs. Applications to methohexitone. Br J Anaesth 58:1085, 1986

53. Fragen RJ, Avram MJ, Henthorn TK et al: A pharmacokinetically designed etomidate infusion regimen for hypnosis. Anesth Analg 62:654, 1983

54. Meuldermans WEG, Heykants JJP: The plasma protein binding and distribution of etomidate in dog, rat and human blood. Arch Int Pharmacodyn Ther 221:150, 1976

55. Shafer A, Doze VA, Shafer S, White PF: Pharmacokinetics and pharmacodynamics of propofol infusions during general anesthesia. Anesthesiology 69:348, 1988

56. Major E, Verniquet AJW, Waddell TK et al: A study of three doses of ICI 35 868 for induction and maintenance of anaesthesia. Br J Anaesth 53:267, 1981

57. Clements JA, Nimmo WS: Pharmacokinetics and analgesic effect of ketamine in man. Br J Anaesth 53:27, 1981

58. Wieber J, Gugler R, Hengstmann JH et al: Pharmacokinetics of ketamine in man. Anaesthesist 24:260, 1975

59. Idvall J, Ahlgren I, Aronsen KF et al: Ketamine infusions: Pharmacokinetics and clinical effects. Br J Anaesth 51:1167, 1979

60. Klotz U, Avant GR, Hoyumpa A et al: The effect of age and liver disease on the disposition and elimination of diazepam in adult man. J Clin Invest 55:347, 1975

61. Greenblatt DJ, Shader RI, Divoll M et al: Benzodiazepines: A summary of pharmacokinetic properties. Br J Clin Pharmacol 11:11S, 1981

62. Avram MJ, Fragen RJ, Caldwell NJ: Midazolam kinetics in women of two age groups. Clin Pharmacol Ther 34:505, 1983

63. Allonen H, Ziegler G, Klotz U: Midazolam kinetics. Clin Pharmacol Ther 30:653, 1981
64. Fragen RJ, Avram MJ: Comparative pharmacology of drugs used for the induction of anesthesia. In Stoelting RK, Barash PG, Gallagher TJ (eds): Advances in Anesthesia, p 103. Chicago, Year Book Medical Publishers, 1986
65. Brodie BB, Bernstein E, Mark LC: The role of body fat in limiting the duration of action of thiopental. J Pharmacol Exp Ther 105:421, 1952
66. Price HL, Kovnat PJ, Safer JN et al: The uptake of thiopental by body tissues and its relation to the duration of narcosis. Clin Pharmacol Ther 1:16, 1960
67. Bischoff KB, Dedrick RL: Thiopental pharmacokinetics. J Pharm Sci 57:1346, 1968
68. Runciman WB, Mather LE: Effects of anaesthesia on drug disposition. In Feldman SA, Scurr CF, Paton W (eds): Drugs in Anaesthesia: Mechanisms of Action, p 87. Baltimore, Edward Arnold, 1987
69. Van Hamme MJ, Ghoneim MM, Ambre JJ: Pharmacokinetics of etomidate, a new intravenous anesthetic. Anesthesiology 49:274, 1978
70. Fragen RJ, Shanks CA, Molteni A et al: Effects of etomidate on hormonal response to surgical stress. Anesthesiology 61:652, 1984
71. Nimmo WS, Clements JA: Ketamine. In Prys-Roberts C, Hug CC, Jr (eds): Pharmacokinetics of Anaesthesia, p 235. Boston, Blackwell Scientific, 1984
72. Stanski DR: Pharmacokinetics of barbiturates. In Prys-Roberts C, Hugg CC, Jr (eds): Pharmacokinetics of Anaesthesia, p 112. Boston, Blackwell Scientific, 1984
73. Wilkinson GR, Shand DS: A physiological approach to hepatic drug clearance. Clin Pharmacol Ther 18:377, 1975
74. Larson CP, Mazze RI, Cooperman LH et al: Effects of anesthesia on cerebral, renal, and splanchnic circulation: Recent developments. Anesthesiology 41:169, 1974
75. White PF, Marietta MP, Pudwill CR et al: Effects of halothane anesthesia on the biodisposition of ketamine in rats. J Pharmacol Exp Ther 196:545, 1976
76. Reilly CS, Wood AJJ, Koshakji R et al: The effect of halothane on drug disposition: Contribution of changes in intrinsic drug metabolizing capacity and hepatic blood flow. Anesthesiology 63:70, 1985
77. Runciman WB, Mather LE, Ilsley AH et al: A sheep preparation for studying interaction between blood flow and drug disposition. II. Experimental applications. Br J Anaesth 56:1117, 1984
78. Linde HW, Berman ML: Nonspecific stimulation of drug-metabolizing enzymes by inhalation anesthetic agents. Anesth Analg 50:656, 1971
79. Gordon L, Wood AJJ, Koshakji RP et al: Acute effects of halothane on arterial and venous concentrations of propranolol in the dog. Anesthesiology 67:225, 1987
80. Dundee JW: The influence of body weight, sex and age on the dosage of thiopentone. Br J Anaesth 26:164, 1954
81. Christensen JH, Andreasen F: Individual variation in response to thiopental. Acta Anaesth Scand 22:303, 1978
82. Dundee JW, Hassard TH, McGowan WAW et al: The 'induction' dose of thiopentone: A method of study and preliminary illustrative results. Anaesthesia 37:1176, 1982
83. Homer TD, Stanski DR: The effect of increasing age on thiopental disposition and anesthetic requirement. Anesthesiology 62:714, 1985
84. Giles HG, MacLeod SM, Wright JR et al: Influence of age and previous use on diazepam dosage required for endoscopy. Can Med Assoc J 118:513, 1978
85. Gamble JAS, Kawar P, Dundee JW et al: Evaluation of midazolam as an intravenous anesthetic induction agent. Anaesthesia 36:868, 1981
86. Dundee JW, Halliday NJ, Loughran PG: Variation in response to midazolam. Br J Clin Pharmacol 17:645P, 1984
87. Arden JR, Holley FO, Stanski DR: Increased sensitivity to etomidate in the elderly: Initial distribution versus altered brain response. Anesthesiology 65:19, 1986
88. Dundee JW, Robinson FP, McCollum JSC et al: Sensitivity to propofol in the elderly. Anaesthesia 41:482, 1986
89. Christensen JH, Andreasen F, Jansen JA: Pharmacokinetics and pharmacodynamics of thiopentone: A comparison between young and elderly patients. Anaesthesia 37:398, 1982
90. Sear JW, Cooper GM, Kumar V: The effect of age on recovery: A comparison of the kinetics of thiopentone and althesin. Anaesthesia 38:1158, 1983
91. Bruce A, Andersson M, Arvidsson B et al: Body composition. Prediction of normal body potassium, body water and body fat in adults on the basis of body height, body weight and age. Scand J Clin Lab Invest 40:461, 1980
92. Bender AD: The effect of increasing age on the distribution of peripheral blood flow in man. J Am Geriatr Soc 13:192, 1965
93. Avram MJ, Krejcie TC, Henthorn TK: The relationship of age to the pharmacokinetics of early drug distribution: The concurrent disposition of thiopental and indocyanine green. Anesthesiology 72:403, 1990
94. Stanski DR, Maitre PO: Population pharmacokinetics and pharmacodynamics of thiopental: The effect of age revisited. Anesthesiology 72:412, 1990
95. Sanghvi R, Henthorn TK, Krejcie TC et al: Patient characteristics associated with the thiopental doses at clinical and EEG induction end points. Clin Pharmacol Ther 49:164, 1991
96. Kiersey DK, Bickford RG, Faulkner A: Electroencephalographic patterns produced by thiopental sodium during surgical operations: Description and classification. Br J Anaesth 23:141, 1951
97. Ghoneim MM, Yamada T: Etomidate: A clinical and electroencephalographic comparison with thiopental. Anesth Analg 56:479, 1977
98. Lees NW, Hendry JGB: Etomidate in urological outpatient anaesthesia. Anaesthesia 32:592, 1977
99. Gancher S, Laxer KD, Krieger W: Activation of epileptogenic activity by etomidate. Anesthesiology 61:616, 1984
100. Brown CR: Clinical electroencephalographic and pharmacokinetic studies of a water-soluble benzodiazepine, midazolam maleate. Anesthesiology 50:467, 1979
101. Silvay G: Ketamine. Mt Sinai J Med 50:300, 1983
102. Sebel PS, Lowdon JD: Propofol. A new intravenous anesthetic. Anesthesiology 71:260, 1989
103. McPherson RW, Sell B, Traystman RJ: Effects of thiopental, fentanyl, and etomidate on upper extremity somatosensory evoked potentials in humans. Anesthesiology 65:584, 1986
104. Moss E, Powell D, Gibson RM et al: Effect of etomidate on intracranial pressure and cerebral perfusion pressure. Br J Anaesth 51:347, 1979
105. Renou AM, Vernheit J, Macrez P et al: Cerebral blood flow and metabolism during etomidate anaesthesia in man. Br J Anaesth 50:1047, 1978
106. Astrup J, Rosenorn J, Cold GE et al: Minimum cerebral blood flow and metabolism during craniotomy. Effect of thiopental loading. Acta Anaesthesiol Scand 28:478, 1984
107. Bendtsen AO, Cold GE, Astrup J et al: Thiopental loading during controlled hypotension for intracranial aneurysm surgery. Acta Anaesthesiol Scand 28:473, 1984
108. Nugent M, Artru AA, Michenfelder JD: Cerebral effects of midazolam and diazepam. Anesthesiology 53:S8, 1980
109. Stephan H, Sonntag H, Schenk HD et al: Einfluss von Disoprivan (Propofol) auf die Durchblutung und den Sauerstoffverbrauch des Gehirns und die CO_2—Reactivität der Hirngefasse beim Menschen. Anaesthesist 36:60, 1987
110. Hartung HJ: Beeinflüssung des Intrakrahiellendrukes durch Propofol (Disoprivan). Anaesthesist 36:66, 1987
111. Dundee JW, Halliday NJ, Harper KW: Midazolam: A review of its pharmacological properties and therapeutic uses. Drugs 28:519, 1984
112. Pinaud M, Lelausque JN, Chetanneau A et al: Effects of propofol on cerebral hemodynamics and metabolism in patients with brain trauma. Anesthesiology 73:404, 1990
113. Moss E, Price DJ: Effect of propofol on brain retraction pressure and cerebral perfusion pressure. Br J Anaesth 65:823, 1990

114. Giese JL, Stanley TH: Etomidate: A new intravenous anesthetic induction agent. Pharmacotheraphy 3:251, 1983
115. Reves JG, Fragen RJ, Vinik MR et al: Midazolam: Pharmacology and uses. Anesthesiology 62:310, 1985
116. Helrich M, Papper EM, Rovenstine EA: Surital sodium: A new anesthetic for intravenous use. Preliminary clinical evaluation. Anesthesiology 11:33, 1950
117. deJong RH, Bonin JD: Benzodiazepines protect mice from local anesthetic convulsion and deaths. Anesth Analg 60:385, 1981
118. Todd MM, Drummond JC, U HS: The hemodynamic consequences of high-dose methohexital anesthesia in humans. Anesthesiology 61:495, 1984
119. Bennett DR, Madsen JA, Jordan WS et al: Ketamine anesthesia in brain-damaged epileptics: Encephalographic and clinical observations. Neurology 23:449, 1973
120. Fragen RJ, Hauch T: The effects of midazolam maleate and diazepam on intraocular pressure in adults. In Aldrete JA, Stanley TH (eds): Trends in Intravenous Anesthesia p 245. Chicago, Year Book Medical Publishers, 1980
121. Famewo CE, Adugbesian CO, Osuntakum OD: Effect of etomidate on intraocular pressure. Can Anaesth Soc J 24:712, 1977
122. Mirakhur RK, Shepherd WFI, Darrah WC: Propofol or thiopentone: Effects on intraocular pressure associated with induction of anaesthesia and tracheal intubation (facilitated with suxamethonium). Br J Anaesth 59:431, 1987
123. Calla S, Gupta A, Sen N et al: Comparison of the effects of etomidate and thiopentone on intraocular pressure. Br J Anaesth 59:437, 1987
124. Ausinsch B, Rayburn RL, Munson ES et al: Ketamine and intraocular pressure in children. Anesth Analg 55:773, 1976
125. Helrich M, Eckenhoff JE, Jones RE: Influence of opiates on the respiratory response of man to thiopental. Anesthesiology 17:459, 1956
126. Streisand JB, Nelson P, Bubbers S et al: The respiratory effect of propofol with and without fentanyl. Anesth Analg 66:S171, 1987
127. Taylor MB, Grounds RM, Mulrooney PD et al: Ventilatory effects of propofol during induction of anesthesia. Anaesthesia 41:816, 1986
128. Guerra F: Thiopental forever after. In Aldrete JA, Stanley TH (eds): Trends in Intravenous Anesthesia, p 143. Chicago, Year Book Medical Publishers, 1980
129. Kalenda K: Etomidate as an induction agent. Lancet 2:1143, 1976
130. Forster A, Morel D, Bachmann M et al: Respiratory depressant effect of different doses of midazolam and lack of reversal with naloxone. A double-blind randomized study. Anesth Analg 62:920, 1983
131. Gross JB, Zebrowski MB, Carel WD et al: Time course of ventilatory depression after thiopental and midazolam in normal subjects and in patients with chronic obstructive pulmonary disease. Anesthesiology 58:540, 1983
132. Corssen G, Gutierrez J, Reves JG: Ketamine in the anesthetic management of asthmatic patients. Anesth Analg 51:588, 1972
133. Stefanssen T, Wickerstrom I, Haljamae H: Haemodynamic and metabolic effects of ketamine anesthesia in the geriatric patient. Acta Anaesthesiol Scand 26:371, 1982
134. White PF, Way WL, Trevor AJ: Ketamine—Its pharmacology and therapeutic uses. Anesthesiology 56:119, 1982
135. Soliman MG, Brinale GF, Kuski G: Response to hypercapnia under ketamine anaesthesia. Can Anaesth Soc J 22:486, 1975
136. Gelman S, Reves JG, Harris D: Circulatory responses to midazolam anesthesia: Emphasis on canine splanchnic circulation. Anesth Analg 62:135, 1983
137. Johnstone M: The cardiovascular effects of ketamine in man. Anesthesia 31:873, 1976
138. Reves JG, Kissen I: Intravenous anesthetics. In Kaplan J (ed): Cardiac Anesthesia, p 3. New York, Grune & Stratton, 1983
139. Tweed WA, Minuckm, Mymin D: Circulatory responses to ketamine anesthesia. Anesthesiology 37:613, 1972
140. Altura BM, Altura BT, Carella A et al: Vascular smooth muscle and general anesthesia. Fed Proc 39:1584, 1981
141. Pedersen T, Engback J, Klausen NO et al: Effects of low-dose ketamine and thiopentone on cardiac performance and myocardial oxygen balance in high risk patients. Acta Anaesth Scand 26:235, 1982
142. Corssen G, Reves JG, Carter JR: Neuroleptanesthesia, dissociative anesthesia, and hemorrhage. Int Anesth Clin 12:145, 1974
143. Bini M, Reves JG, Berry D et al: Ejection fraction during ketamine anesthesia in congenital heart diseased patients. Anesth Analg 63:186, 1984
144. Gooding JM, Dimick AR, Tavakoli M: A physiologic analysis of cardiopulmonary response to ketamine anesthesia in noncardiac patients. Anesth Analg 56:813, 1977
145. Bruckner JB: Investigations in the effects of etomidate in the human circulation. Anaesthesist 23:322, 1974
146. Kettler D, Sonntag H, Donath V et al: Haemodynamics, myocardial function, oxygen requirements and oxygen supply to the human heart after administration of etomidate. Anaesthesist 23:116, 1974
147. Colvin MP, Savege TM, Newland PE et al: Cardiorespiratory changes following induction of anesthesia with etomidate in patients with cardiac disease. Br J Anaesth 51:551, 1979
148. Kettler D, Sonntag H, Donath V et al: Haemodynamics, myocardial function, oxygen requirements and oxygen supply of the human heart after administration of etomidate. In Doenicke AE (ed): Etomidate—An Intravenous Hypnotic Agent, p 81. New York, Springer, 1977
149. Marty J, Gauzit R, Lefebre P et al: Effects of diazepam and midazolam on baroreflex control of heart rate and on sympathetic activity in humans. Anesth Analg 65:113, 1986
150. Cote P, Guenet P, Bourossa M: Systemic and coronary hemodynamic effects of diazepam in patients with normal and diseased coronary arteries. Circulation 50:1210, 1974
151. Stanley TH, Bennett GM, Loeser EA et al: Cardiovascular effects of diazepam and droperidol during morphine anesthesia. Anesthesiology 44:255, 1976
152. Douchot PJ, Staub F, Berzina L et al: Hemodynamic response to diazepam-dependence on prior left ventricular and diastolic pressure. Anesthesiology 60:499, 1984
153. Rubin A, Allen GD, Everett GB: Induction of general anesthesia with diazepam or thiopental. A comparison of the cardiorespiratory effects. Anesthesia Progress 39, 1978
154. Dundee JW, Haslett WHK: The benzodiazepines. Br J Anaesth 42:217, 1970
155. Allen RE, Pitts FN Jr, Summers WK: Drug modification of ECT: Methohexital and diazepam II. Biol Psychiatry 15:257, 1980
156. Samuelson PN, Reves JG, Kouchoukos NT et al: Hemodynamic responses to anesthetic induction with midazolam or diazepam in patients in ischemic heart disease. Anesth Analg 60:802, 1981
157. Fragen RJ, Myers SN, Baressi V et al: Hemodynamic effects of midazolam in cardiac patients. Anesthesiology 51:S103, 1979
158. Marty J, Nitenberg A, Blanchet F et al: Effects of midazolam in the coronary circulation in patients with coronary artery disease. Anesthesiology 64:206, 1986
159. Reves JG, Samuelson PN, Lewis S: Midazolam maleate induction in patients with ischaemic heart disease. Haemodynamic observations. Can Anaesth Soc J 26:402, 1979
160. Heikkila M, Jalonen J, Arola M et al: Midazolam as adjunct to high-dose fentanyl anesthesia for coronary artery bypass grafting operation. Acta Anaesthesiol Scand 28:683, 1984
161. Schulte-Sasse U, Hess W, Tarnow J: Haemodynamic responses to induction of anaesthesia using midazolam in cardiac surgical patients. Br J Anaesth 54:1053, 1982
162. Samuelson PN, Reves JG, Smith LR et al: Midazolam versus diazepam. Different effects on systemic vascular resistance. Arzneimittelforschung 31:2268, 1981
163. Boralessa H, Senior DF, Whitwam JG: Cardiovascular response to intubation. Anaesthesia 38:623, 1983
164. Graves CL: Management of general anesthesia during hemorrhage. Int Anesth Clin 12(1):1, 1974
165. List WF: Digitalis—thiopentone effects on myocardial function. Anaesthesia 30:624, 1975

166. Blackburn JP, Conway CM, Leigh M et al: The effects of anaesthetic induction agents upon myocardial contractility. Anaesthesia 26:93, 1971

167. Bernhoff A, Eklund B, Kaijser L: Cardiovascular effects of short-term anaesthesia with methohexitone and propanidid in normal subjects. Br J Anaesth 44:2, 1972

168. Bristow JD, Prys-Roberts C, Fisher A et al: Effects of anesthesia on baroreflex control of heart rate in man. Anesthesiology 31:422, 1969

169. Filner BE, Karliner JS: Alteration of normal left ventricular performance by general anesthesia. Anesthesiology 45:610, 1976

170. Todd MM, Drummond JC, U HS: The hemodynamic consequences of high-dose thiopental anesthesia. Anesth Analg 64:681, 1985

171. Reiz S, Balfors E, Freedman A et al: Effects of thiopentone on cardiac performance, coronary haemodynamics and myocardial oxygen consumption in chronic ischemic heart disease. Acta Anaesthesiol Scand 25:103, 1981

172. Al-Khudairi D, Gordan G, Morgan M et al: Acute cardiovascular changes following disoprofol: Effects in heavily sedated patients with coronary artery disease. Anaesthesia 37:1007, 1982

173. Aun C, Major E: The cardiorespiratory effects of ICI 35 868 in patients with valvular heart disease. Anaesthesia 39:1006, 1984

174. Coates DP, Prys-Roberts C, Spelina RR et al: Propofol ('Diprivan') by intravenous infusion with nitrous oxide: Dose requirement and haemodynamic effects. Postgrad Med J 61 (Suppl 3):76, 1985

175. Fahy L, van Maurik GA, Utting JE: A comparison of the induction characteristics of thiopentone and propofol (2,6 di-isopropyl phenol). Anaesthesia 40:939, 1985

176. Rolly G, Versechelin L: Comparison of propofol and thiopentone for induction of anaesthesia in premedicated patients. Anaesthesia 40:945, 1985

177. Mulier JP, Wauters PF, VanAken H et al: Cardiodynamic effects of propofol in combination with thiopental: Assessment with transesophageal echocardiographic approach. Anesth Analg 72:28, 1991

178. Profeta JP, Guffin A, Mikula S et al: The hemodynamic effects of propofol and thiamylal sodium for induction in coronary artery surgery. Anesth Analg 66:S142, 1987

179. Patrick MR, Blair IJ, Feneck RO et al: A comparison of the hemodynamic effects of propofol ('Diprivan') and thiopental in patients with coronary artery disease. Postgrad Med J 61 (Suppl 3):23, 1985

180. Stephan H, Sonntag H, Schenk HD et al: Effects of propofol on cardiovascular dynamics, myocardial blood flow and myocardial metabolism in patients with coronary artery disease. Br J Anaesth 58:969, 1986

181. Rolly G, Versechelin L, Hughes L et al: Effects of speed of injection on induction of anaesthesia using propofol. Br J Anaesth 57:743, 1985

182. Lippman M, Paicius R, Gingerich S et al: A controlled study of hemodynamic effect of propofol vs. thiopental during anesthesia induction. Anesth Analg 65:S89, 1986

183. Williams JP, McArthur JD, Walker WE et al: The cardiovascular effects of propofol in patients with impaired cardiac functions. Anesth Analg 65:S166, 1986

184. Dundee JW: Intravenous Anesthetic Agents. Chicago, Year Book Medical Publishers, 1979

185. Kawar P, Briggs LP, Bahar M et al: Liver enzyme studies with disoprofol (ICI 35 868) and midazolam. Anaesthesia 37:305, 1982

186. Wagner RL, White PF: Etomidate inhibits adrenocortical function in surgical patients. Anesthesiology 61:647, 1984

187. Fragen RJ, Weiss HW, Molteni A: The effect of propofol on adrenocortical steroidogenesis: A comparative study with etomidate and thiopental. Anesthesiology 65:839, 1987

188. Robertson WR, Reader SCJ, Davidson B et al: On the biopotency and site of action of drugs affecting endocrine tissues with specific reference to the antisteroidogenic effect of anesthetic agents. Postgrad Med J 61(Suppl 3):145, 1985

189. Crozier TA, Beck D, Schlaeger M et al: Endocrinological changes following etomidate, midazolam or methohexital for minor surgery. Anesthesiology 66:628, 1987

190. Doenicke A, Lorenz W, Stenworth D et al: Effects of propofol 'Diprivan' on histamine release, immunoglobulin levels and activation of complement in healthy volunteers. Postgrad Med J 61(suppl 3):15, 1985

191. Doenicke A, Lorenz W, Beigl R: Histamine release after intravenous application of short-acting hynotics. Br J Anaesth 45:1097, 1973

192. Westacott P, Ramachandran PR, Jancelewicz Z: Anaphylactic reaction to thiopentone: A case report. Can Anaesth Soc J 31:434, 1984

193. Clarke RSJ: Hypersensitivity reactions. In Dundee JW (ed): Intravenous Anesthetic Agents, p 87. Chicago, Year Book Medical Publishers, 1979

194. Flowers CE, Rudolph AJ, Desmond MM: Diazepam (Valium) as an adjunct in obstetric analgesia. Obstet Gynecol 36:68, 1969

195. Camann W, Cohen MB, Ostheimer GW: Is midazolam desirable for sedation in parturients? Anesthesiology 65:441, 1986

196. Fragen RJ, Booij LHDJ, van der Pol F et al: Interactions of disopropyl phenol (ICI 35 868) with suxamethonium, vecuronium and pancuronium in vitro. Br J Anaesth 55:433, 1983

197. Driessen JJ, Vree TB, Booij LHDJ et al: Effect of some benzodiazepines on peripheral neuromuscular function in the rat in vitro hemidiaphragm preparation. J Pharm Pharmacol 36:244, 1984

198. Robertson EN, Fragen RJ, Booij LHDJ et al: Some effects of disopropyl phenol (ICI 35 868) on the pharmacodynamics of atracurium and vecuronium in anaesthetized man. Br J Anaesth 55:723, 1983

199. Nightingale P, Retts NV, Healy TN et al: Induction of anesthesia with propofol (Diprivan) or thiopentone and interaction with suxamethonium, atracurium and vecuronium. Postgrad Med J 61(suppl 3):31, 1985

200. Hannallah RS, Baker SB, Casey W et al: Propofol: Effective dose and induction characteristics in unpremedicated children. Anesthesiology 74:217, 1991

201. Leslie K, Crankshaw DP: Potency of propofol for loss of consciousness after single dose. Br J Anaesth 64:734, 1990

202. Fragen RJ, Gahl F, Caldwell N: A water-soluble benzodiazepine Ro 21-3981, for induction of anesthesia. Anesthesiology 47:41, 1978

203. Berggren L, Erickson I: Midazolam for induction of anesthesia in outpatients. A comparison with thiopentone. Acta Anaesth Scand 25:492, 1981

204. Tverskoy M, Fleyshman G, Bradley EL Jr et al: Midazolamthiopental anesthetic interaction in patients. Anesth Analg 67:342, 1988

205. Kissen I, Brown PT, Bradley EL Jr: Sedative and hynotic midazolam-morphine interactions in rats. Anesth Analg 71:137, 1990

206. Kissen I, Brown PT, Bradley EL Jr: Morphine and fentanyl anesthetic interactions with diazepam: Relative antagonism in rats. Anesth Analg 71:236, 1990

207. Rosland JH, Hole K: 1,4-Benzodiazepines antagonize opiate-induced antinociception in mice. Anesth Analg 71:242, 1990

208. Gill SS, Wright EM, Reilly CS; Pharmacokinetic interaction of propofol and fentanyl: Single bolus injection study. Br J Anaesth 65:760, 1990

209. Dixon J, Roberts FL, Tackley RM et al: Study of possible interactions between fentanyl and propofol using a computer-controlled infusion of propofol. Br J Anaesth 64:142, 1990

210. Wilton NCT, Leigh J, Rosen D et al: Preanesthetic sedation of preschool children using intranasal midazolam. Anesthesiology 69:972, 1988

211. Walbergh EJ, Willis RJ, Eckhert J: Plasma concentrations of midazolam in children following intranasal administration. Anesthesiology 74:233, 1991

212. Peacock JE, Lewis RP, Reilly CS et al: Effect of different rates of infusion of propofol for induction of anesthesia in elderly patients. Br J Anaesth 65:346, 1990

213. Redfern N, Stafford MA, Hull CJ: Incremental propofol for short procedures. Br J Anaesth 57:1178, 1985

214. Hynynen M, Kortilla K, Tammisto T: Pain on I.V. injection of propofol (ICI 35868) in emulsion formulation. Acta Anaesth Scand 29:651, 1985

215. Stark RD, Binks SM, Dutka VN et al: A review of the safety and tolerance of propofol ('Diprivan'). Postgrad Med J 61 (Suppl 3):152, 1985

216. Thornton JA: Methohexitone and its application in dental anaesthesia. Br J Anaesth 42:255, 1970

217. Mackenzie N, Grant IS: Comparison of propofol with methohexitone in the provision of anaesthesia for surgery under regional block. Br J Anaesth 57:1167, 1985

218. Doze VA, Westphal LM, White PF: Comparison of propofol with methohexital for outpatient anesthesia. Anesth Analg 65:1189, 1986

219. Mackenzie N, Grant IS: Propofol for intravenous sedation. Anaesthesia 42:3, 1987

220. Kestin IG, Harvey PB, Nixon C: Psychomotor recovery after three methods of sedation during spinal anaesthesia. Br J Anaesth 64:675, 1990

221. Camu F, Gepts E, Cockshott ID: Dose-response curves and elimination kinetics following infusions of 3, 6 and 9 mg/kg/hr Diprivan. Proceedings of the Industry Forum. Propofol (Diprivan) infusion techniques for intravenous sedation or maintenance of anaesthesia, p 14. VII European Congress of Anaesthesiology, Vienna, 1986

222. Willaert J: Diprivan: Infusion in total intravenous anaesthesia with oxygen-air. Proceedings of the Industry Forum. Propofol (Diprivan) infusion techniques for intravenous sedation or maintenance of anaesthesia, p 21. VII European Congress of Anaesthesiology, Vienna, 1986

223. Jenstrup M, Nielsen J, Fruergard K et al: Total I.V. anaesthesia with propofol-alfentanil or propofol-fentanil. Br J Anaesth 64:717, 1990

224. Massey NJA, Sherry KM, Oldroyd S et al: Pharmacokinetics of an infusion of propofol during cardiac surgery. Br J Anaesth 65:475, 1990

225. Schwilder H, Stoeckel H: Effective therapeutic infusions produced by closed-loop feedback control of methohexital administration during total intravenous anesthesia with fentanyl. Anesthesiology 73:225, 1990

226. Vinik HR, Shaw B, MacKrell T et al: A comparative evaluation of propofol for the induction and maintenance of general anesthesia. Anesth Analg 66:S189, 1987

227. Aldrete JA, McDonald JS: Low dose ketamine-diazepam prevents adverse reactions. In Aldrete JA, Stanley TH (eds): Trends in Intravenous Anesthesia, p 331. Chicago, Year Book Medical Publishers, 1980

228. Silvay G, Weinrich AI, Lumb P et al: Continuous infusion of ketamine for thoracic surgery using one-lung ventilation. In Aldrete JD, Stanley TH (eds): Trends in Intravenous Anesthesia, p 355. Chicago, Year Book Medical Publishers, 1980

229. Reves JG, Vinik R, Hirschfield AM et al: Midazolam compared with thiopentone as a hypnotic component in balanced anaesthesia: A randomized double-blind study. Can Anaesth Soc J 26:42, 1979

230. Crawford ME, Carl P, Andersen RS et al: Comparison between midazolam and thiopentone-based balanced anaesthesia for day care surgery. Br J Anaesth 56:165, 1984

231. Urquhart ML, White PF: Comparison of sedative infusions during regional anesthesia—methohexital etomidate and midazolam. Anesth Analg 68:249, 1989

232. Booker PD, Beechey A, Lloyd-Thomas AR: Sedation of children requiring artificial ventilation using an infusion of midazolam. Br J Anaesth 58:1104, 1986

233. Lloyd-Thomas AR, Booker PD: Infusions of midazolam in paediatric patients after cardiac surgery. Br J Anaesth 58:1109, 1986

234. Grounds RM, Lalor JM, Lumley J et al: Propofol infusion for sedation in the intensive care unit: Preliminary report. Br Med J 294:397, 1987

235. Rita L, Seleny FL, Mazurek A et al: Intramuscular midazolam for pediatric preanesthetic sedation: A double-blind controlled study with morphine. Anesthesiology 63:528, 1985

236. Park WY, Watkins PA: Patient-controlled sedation during epidural anesthesia. Anesth Analg 72:304, 1991

237. Loper KA, Ready LB, Brody M: Patient-controlled anxiolysis with midazolam. Anesth Analg 67:1118, 1988

238. Bello CN, Mathias L, Torres MA et al: Evaluation of the effects of Ro 15-1788 in clinical anesthesia. Anesth Analg 66:S11, 1987

239. Kirkegaard I, Knudsen I, Jensen S et al: Benzodiazepine antagonist Ro 15-1788. Antagonism of diazepam sedation in outpatients undergoing gastroscopy. Anaesthesia 41:1184, 1986

240. Freye E, Fournell A: The benzodiazepine antagonist Ro 15-1788 reverses midazolam-induced EEG changes postoperatively. Anesth Analg 66:S60, 1987

241. Harrop-Griffiths AW, Watson NA, Jewkes DA: Midazolam and flumazenil in the anaesthetic management of trigeminal nerve thermocoagulation. Br J Anaesth 64:586, 1990

242. McKay AC, McKinney MS, Clarke RSJ: Effect of flumazenil on midazolam induced amnesia. Br J Anaesth 65:190, 1990

243. Philip BK, Simpson TH, Hauch MA et al: Flumazenil reverses sedation after midazolam-induced general anesthesia in ambulatory surgical patients. Anesth Analg 71:371, 1990

244. Klotz U, Ziegler G, Ludwig L et al: Pharmacodynamic interaction between midazolam and a specific benzodiazepine antagonist in humans. J Clin Pharmacol 25:400, 1985

245. Klausen NO, Juhl O, Sorenson J et al: Flumazenil in total intravenous anaesthesia using midazolam and fentanyl. Acta Anaesthesiol Scand 32:409, 1988

246. Geller K, Halpern P, Chernilas J et al: Cardiorespiratory effects of antagonism of diazepam sedation with flumazenil in patients with cardiac disease. Anesth Analg 72:207, 1991

247. Caldwell CB, Gross JB: Physostigmine reversal of midazolam-induced sedation. Anesthesiology 57:125, 1982

248. Kanto J, Aaltonen L, Himberg JJ et al: Midazolam as an intravenous induction agent in the elderly: A clinical and pharmacokinetic study. Anesth Analg 65:15, 1986

249. Stoelting RK, Dierdorf SF (eds): Anesthesia and Co-existing Disease. New York, Churchill Livingstone, 1983

250. Fragen RJ, Caldwell NJ: Comparison of a new formulation of etomidate with thiopental—side effects and awakening times. Anesthesiology 50:242, 1979

251. Vinik R, Shaw B, Harris C et al: Randomized evaluation of induction and recovery from anesthesia with diprivan or thiopental sodium. Anesth Analg 65:S162, 1986

252. Jessup E, Grounds RM, Morgan M et al: Comparison of infusions of propofol and methohexitone to provide light general anaesthesia during surgery with regional block. Br J Anaesth 57:1173, 1985

253. Milligan KR, Howe JP, O'Toole DP et al: Outpatient anesthesia: Recovery after propofol, methohexital and thiopental. Anesth Analg 66:S118, 1987

254. Mackenzie N, Grant IS: Comparison of the new emulsion formulation of propofol with methohexitone and thiopentone for induction of anaesthesia in day cases. Br J Anaesth 57:725, 1985

255. Reitan JA, Porter W, Braunstein M: Comparison of psychomotor skills and amnesia after induction with midazolam or thiopental. Anesth Analg 65:933, 1986

256. Fragen RJ, Caldwell NJ: Awakening characteristics following anesthesia induction with midazolam for short surgical procedures. Arzneimittelforschung (Drug Res) 31:2261, 1981

257. Connor JT, Katz RL, Pagano RR et al: RO 21-3981 for intravenous surgical premedication and induction of anesthesia. Anesth Analg 57:1, 1978

258. McCollum JSC, Milligan KR, Dundee JW: The antiemetic action of propofol. Anaesthesia 43:239, 1988

259. Muir JJ, Warner MA, Offord KP et al: Role of nitrous oxide and other factors in postoperative nausea and vomiting. A randomized and blinded prospective study. Anesthesiology 66:513, 1987

260. Dohi S, Naito H: Intraarterial injection of 2.5% thiamylal does cause gangrene. Anesthesiology 59:154, 1983

261. Halsey MJ: Drug interactions in anaesthesia. Br J Anaesth 59:112, 1987

262. Smith NJ, Corbascio AN: Drug interactions in Anesthesia. Philadelphia, Lea & Febiger, 1986

263. Gibb D: Drug interactions in anaesthesia. Clin Anaesthesiology 2:485, 1984

264. Greenblatt DJ, Shader RI: Pharmacokinetics in Clinical Practice. Philadelphia, WB Saunders, 1985

265. Prescott LF: Clinically important drug interactions. In Avery GS (ed): Drug Treatment, Principles and Practice of Clinical Pharmacology and Therapeutics, p 236. New York, Adis Press, 1980

266. Soni N: Mechanisms of drug interactions. In Feldman SA, Scurr CF, Paton W (eds): Drugs in Anesthesia: Mechanisms of Action, p 408. Baltimore, Edward Arnold, 1987

267. Halsey MJ: Adverse effects of drugs used in anesthesia. Br J Anaesth 59:1, 1987

268. Clarke RSJ, Dundee JW: Adverse reactions to intravenous induction agents. In Thornton JE (ed): Adverse Reactions to Anaesthetic Drugs, p 29. New York, Excerpta Medica/Elsevier, 1981

269. Whitwam JG: Intravenous induction agents. Clin Anaesthesiology 2:515, 1984

270. Sear JW: Toxicity of I.V. anaesthetics. Br J Anaesth 59:24, 1987

16

Michael R. Murphy

Opioids

The term *opioids*, as it is used at present, is an all-inclusive term that distinguishes those drugs, natural or synthetic, that have morphine-like qualities as well as drugs that bind at morphine receptor sites.[1] The term is even applied to the sites themselves. Therefore, the term *opioid* may refer to drugs that are agonists (*e.g.*, morphine, fentanyl), agonist-antagonists (*e.g.*, butorphanol, nalorphine), antagonists (*e.g.*, naloxone), or the receptor sites for these drugs in the body (Fig. 16-1). The term *opiate* is often used interchangeably with *opioid*, but historically *opiate* designates drugs derived from opium (*e.g.*, morphine, codeine). The term *narcotic* often refers to opioids. However, this term is actually nonspecific, having been derived from the Greek word for stupor, and it describes any drug that produces sleep. Today *narcotics* may be used to describe any number of drugs that are used illegally, whether or not they possess true opioid characteristics.

HISTORY

Opium comes from the milky exudate of the unripe seed capsule of the poppy (*Papaver somniferum*), and the term is a derivative of the Greek word for juice. Although the psychological effects of opium apparently were known as far back as the ancient Sumerians, the first known recorded reference to poppy juice was Theophrastus in the 3rd century, B.C.[1] Opium is composed of more than 20 distinct alkaloids. It was not until 1806 that Surturner isolated one of these alkaloids, morphine, which he named for the Greek god of dreams, Morpheus. Further alkaloids, including codeine (Robiquet, 1832) and papaverine (Merck, 1848), were derived from opium over the next several years.

The syringe was invented by Rynd (1845) and Pravaz (1853), and the hollow needle by Wood (1855), opening the door for the use of parenteral morphine. Claude Bernard used morphine as a premedication in 1869. By 1900, morphine, 2 mg·kg^{-1}, plus scopolamine, 1–3 mg, was described by Schneiderlein for surgical anesthesia. Despite the patients' lack of recall of the surgical events, these episodes predated the use of muscle relaxants or controlled ventilation, necessitating the restraint of the patients during the procedure. Furthermore, a number of the patients died postoperatively, probably secondary to respiratory depres-

sion.[2-4] The use of opioids for surgical anesthesia fell into disfavor following these deaths.

In 1938, the first synthetic opioid, meperidine, was introduced by Eisleb and Schaumann.[1] In 1947, Neff *et al* reported that "Nitrous oxide and oxygen, plus intravenous (iv) Demerol, plus curarization, afford good anesthesia and excellent muscular relaxation."[5] Nitrous oxide plus various opioids became popular. In 1958, Bailey *et al* reported anesthesia for cardiac surgery with meperidine and oxygen alone following induction with thiopental.[6] High-dose morphine (0.5–1.0 mg·kg^{-1}) and 100% oxygen became popular following a report by Lowenstein and coworkers in 1969.[7] Despite the relative stability of the patients in this study, a number of patients in subsequent uses of this technique were deemed to have inadequate depth of anesthesia. Stanley *et al*, in an effort to overcome the problem of inadequate anesthesia, increased the morphine dose to 8–11 mg·kg^{-1} but encountered unacceptable side-effects, including increased fluid requirements and generalized edema.[8]

Whereas the continued search for more efficacious opioids for anesthesia has resulted in the introduction of a number of new synthetic agonists (the fentanyl family) in the last 30 years, the earlier search for a potent, nonaddicting analgesic produced an n-allyl derivative of morphine, nalorphine. Nalorphine antagonized the effects of morphine, precipitated acute abstinence in addicts, and, importantly, also had analgesic actions.[1,9] This discovery led to the development of other agonist-antagonist compounds (*e.g.*, pentazocine, butorphanol) and the relatively pure antagonist naloxone.

PHARMACOLOGY

Receptors and Endogenous Opioid Peptides

The importance of the mixed actions of nalorphine was not so much its clinical usefulness as the fact that it increased the evidence for and aided the search for opioid receptors in the body. It was known that morphine-like drugs were structurally similar and exhibited stereospecificity, which suggested opioid receptor sites on the surface of or within cells. When it was demonstrated that the opioid antagonist nalorphine also had analgesic (agonist) properties, the ho-

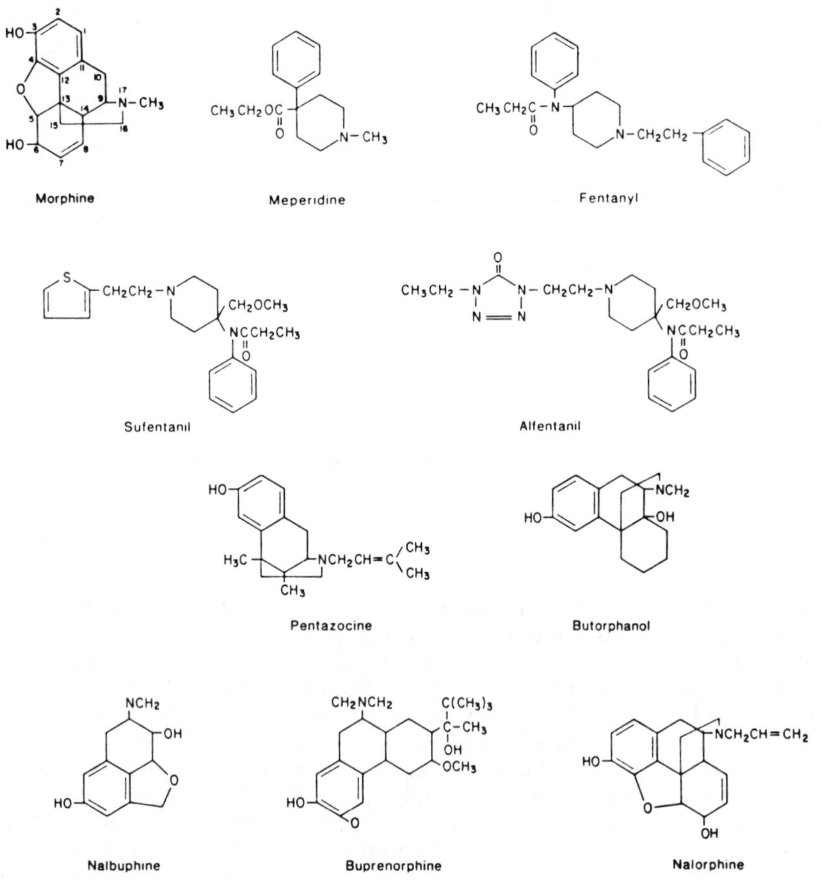

Figure 16-1. Chemical structures of opioid agonists (morphine, meperidine, fentanyl, sufentanil, alfentanil) and opioid agonist-antagonists (pentazocine, butorphanol, nalbuphine, buprenorphine and nalorphine).

mogeneous receptor theory was replaced by a heterogeneous receptor theory, originally proposing two receptors and eventually several.[10-12]

Martin *et al* identified three distinct opioid receptors.[1,10-12] Morphine and morphine-like drugs interact with the morphine or mu receptor to produce supraspinal analgesia, respiratory depression, indifference to environmental stimuli, bradycardia, miosis, hypothermia, physical dependence, and tolerance (Table 16-1). Ketocyclazocine is the prototype agonist for the kappa receptors, which are characterized by spinal analgesia, miosis, and sedation. The sigma receptors mediate dysphoric effects, hallucinations, tachypnea, tachycardia, and mydriasis; the typical agonist is N-allylnormetazocine (SKF–10,047). A delta and an epsilon receptor have been proposed to explain the relative potencies of opioid peptides and drugs to inhibit contraction of the isolated guinea pig ileum and mouse vas deferens. More recently, the mu receptor has been subdivided. Analgesia has been associated with the mu_1 but not with the mu_2 receptor, whereas respiratory depression is probably mediated by the mu_2 or delta receptors but not by mu_1.[1,11,12] The possibility of separating analgesia from respiratory depression apparently exists.

The realization of specific receptors in the mammalian central nervous system (CNS) and nerve plexuses of intestines for chemicals derived from plants started a search for endogenous opioid receptor ligands. A number of opioid peptides have been identified.[11-13] A review by Akil et al divides these into three opioid peptide families according to precursor.[13] The precursor for the first family is beta-endorphin/adrenocorticotropic hormone (also known as proopiomelanocortin). These peptides are primarily pro-

duced in the pituitary gland. The second group is from the enkephalin precursor (known as proenkephalin or proenkephalin A). These peptides include [Met]enkephalin and [Leu]enkephalin, and their opioid neuronal pathways include endocrine and CNS distributions. The enkephalins are also found in the adrenal medulla, gastrointestinal tract, and other structures; in the CNS, they are widely spread from cells in the cortex to cells in the spinal cord. The most recently described dynorphin/neoendorphin precursor (also known as prodynorphin or proenkephalin B) family is found primarily in gut, posterior pituitary, and brain.

The location of the opioid receptors and the endogenous ligands is related to their functions. For instance, those receptors and peptides involved in mediating analgesia are found in greater density in areas of the brain and spinal cord involved with pain sensation. The significance of a number of peptides, their locations, and the sites of the opioid receptors are not clearly understood. There is evidence that opioid peptides may be involved in numerous physiologic activities, including regulation of blood pressure, mood, appetite, thirst, sexual activity, memory, secretion of hormones, and interactions between the nervous and immune systems.[12] Continuing studies will provide answers to many questions and further explain the mechanism of actions of opioid drugs.

Central Nervous System Effects

Discussion of the CNS effects of opioids will focus on analgesia, drowsiness-consciousness, mood alteration, electroencephalographic changes, and emetic effects. Other effects

TABLE 16-1. Tentative Classification of Opiate Receptor Subtypes and Actions

Subtype	Prototypic Drugs	Proposed Actions
mu		
mu$_1$	Opioids and most opioid peptides	Supraspinal analgesia, including periaqueductal gray, nucleus raphe magnus, and locus coeruleus Prolactin release Free feeding and deprivation-induced feeding Acetylcholine turnover in the brain Catalepsy
mu$_2$	Morphine sulfate	Respiratory depression Growth hormone release (?) Dopamine turnover in the brain Gastrointestinal tract transit Guinea pig ileum bioassay Feeding Most cardiovascular effects
delta	Enkephalins	Spinal analgesia Dopamine turnover in the brain Mouse vas deferens bioassay Growth hormone release (?) Feeding
kappa	Ketocyclazocine and dynorphin	Spinal analgesia Inhibition of antidiuretic hormone release Sedation Feeding
epsilon	β-Endorphin	Rat vas deferens bioassay Hormone (?)
sigma	N-allylnormetazocine (SKF10,047)	Psychotomimetic effects Linked to N-methyl-d-aspartate

Reprinted with permission from Paseternak GW: Multiple morphine and enkephalin receptors and the relief of pain. JAMA 259:1362, 1988.

with a CNS component such as respiratory depression, cardiovascular responses, and endocrine responses are addressed later.

Analgesia is generally the primary reason that the opioids are given. The analgesia produced is a complex effect with components of suppression of transmission of noxious stimulation, reflex depression of afferent stimuli, and altered mental responses. There is minimal evidence of peripheral nervous system involvement in the analgesia produced by the opioids, but most of the effects are mediated by the receptors found in the spinal cord and brain.[14] The analgesia is unlike that produced by local anesthetic agents, which may block all sensation and motor ability by blocking neuronal transmission. The opioids are more selective for painful stimuli, leaving other sensory and motor modalities intact. A patient may be aware of the stimulus but may describe it as less or not painful at all.

Several areas (tracts/laminae) of the spinal cord are known to contain opioid receptors. The substantia gelatinosa, which serves as the main termination of the small afferent nerve fibers thought to be involved with pain, has the highest concentration of opioid receptors in the spinal cord.[14] The transmission of noxious stimuli is suppressed when the spinal cord opioid receptors are activated. Opioids applied locally by intrathecal or epidural techniques diminish pain.

Analgesia results when nociceptive stimuli to higher centers of the brain are depressed in the spinal cord. However, there are many supraspinal opioid receptor sites that act to modulate the sensory input from the spinal cord by descending neuronal pathways, and it has been suggested that the primary sites of analgesic actions of opioids are supraspinal. For instance, focal stimulation of the periaqueductal gray area of the midbrain will produce profound analgesia similar to that seen after the injection of high doses of morphine; naloxone will reverse both the focal stimulation or morphine-induced analgesia.[14] The actual mechanisms involved in opioid analgesia are complex and involve the modulation of painful stimuli by an intricate system of receptors in both afferent and efferent neuronal pathways.

Opioids are mood-altering drugs. Patients in distress report diminished pain, feelings of warmth and well-being, drowsiness, and, occasionally, euphoria. In normal, pain-free persons, the experience may not be pleasant but may produce feelings of lethargy and mental clouding. Alterations in mood and perception of surroundings are apparently mediated through the limbic system.[1,14]

Morphine-like drugs may produce drowsiness or sleep in some patients (especially the old or very ill), but even at very high doses unconsciousness is not assured. Occasionally, in patients in whom "anesthetic" doses of opioids have induced sleep, arousal may be elicited by noxious stimulation.[15] Morphine-like drugs do not produce amnesia without unconsciousness; the risk of awareness during surgery is present unless other CNS depressant drugs (e.g., nitrous oxide, scopolamine, barbiturates, benzodiazepines) are combined with the opioid as part of the anesthetic or preoperative medications.[16,17]

Constriction of the pupils (miosis) is produced by morphine and most mu and kappa opioid agonists in humans, presumably by an excitatory action on the autonomic segment of the nucleus of the oculomotor nerve.[1] The constriction is probably dose-related and considered pathognomonic of opioid toxicity but may be altered by other factors such as other drugs or asphyxia.

Opioids depress the cough reflex in part by a direct effect on the cough center in the medulla.[1] This suppression decreases the incidence and severity of cardiovascular stimulation with intubation of the trachea and improves tolerance of an endotracheal tube in ventilated patients.[18]

All the opioid analgesics in sufficient dosage will produce excitatory or convulsive activity in lower animals and probably in humans. There are considerable interspecies differences in the dosage required to produce seizures.[1,19,20] In humans, clinically useful, high doses of commonly used opioids producing profound analgesia ("anesthesia") do not produce seizures. Myoclonic and myotonic seizure–like movements reported in the literature are produced with no evidence of cortical seizure activity on the electroencephalogram (EEG).[21] The exception to this is meperidine. Very high doses of meperidine (>5 mg·kg^{-1}) may induce excitation and seizures. Meperidine is biotransformed to normeperidine, which is a potent CNS stimulant responsible for the excitatory symptoms.[1]

Opioids produce nausea and vomiting by stimulating the chemoreceptor trigger zone for emesis in the area postrema of the medulla.[1] The emetic effects are more common in ambulatory than in recumbent patients, suggesting a vestibular component. Morphine-like drugs have been shown to increase vestibular sensitivity. All clinically useful opioids produce nausea and vomiting, and, at equianalgesic doses, the incidence is not significantly lower than that of morphine. Opioids also depress the vomiting center, and higher plasma concentrations of opioids may overcome the chemoreceptor trigger zone stimulating effect. Nausea is less common with higher "anesthetic" doses or subsequent doses following an initial therapeutic dose.

Cardiovascular Effects

The relative stability of cardiovascular and myocardial responses found when high doses of morphine are used as the primary anesthetic led to the increased use of the opioids in patients in whom the cardiovascular depression produced by the potent inhalation agents is particularly detrimental.[7] However, there are cardiovascular changes produced by the opioids. Opioids produce a dose-dependent bradycardia, probably by stimulation of the vagal nucleus in the medulla.[22,23] Since the resultant bradycardia is mediated by the vagus nerve, it can be attenuated or blocked by atropine.[24] Experimentally, morphine has a direct effect on the sinoatrial node, but with clinically useful doses no effect on the sinoatrial node is seen.[25,26] Although bradycardia is the usual effect of opioids, large iv doses of meperidine and its congener alphaprodine have been associated with tachycardia, presumably related to their atropine-like structure.

Sufficiently high doses of all opioids produce direct depression of the myocardium.[18,27,28] However, the concentrations of opioids necessary to produce depression are hundreds to thousands of times greater than the peak plasma concentrations found clinically, even after very high "anesthetic" doses of opioid drugs. Except for meperidine, the opioids do not directly depress myocardial contractility at clinically useful doses. At doses as low as $2-2.5$ mg·kg^{-1}, meperidine may produce decreases in cardiac output and arterial pressure secondary to a significant negative ionotropic effect.[28,29] The use of meperidine as a primary anesthetic is limited.

The usual effect of morphine on the peripheral vasculature is arteriolar and venous dilation. Morphine is reported to have a direct action on vascular smooth muscle and to selectively block the venous vascular response to alpha-adrenergic stimulation; however, the primary mechanism for vasodilation is apparently histamine release (Fig. 16-2).[30-32] Meperidine and codeine also evoke the release of histamine, whereas fentanyl, sufentanil, and alfentanil do not.[32,33] Clinical and laboratory studies of the synthetic opioids fentanyl, sufentanil, and alfentanil on peripheral vascular resistance have been contradictory but tend to demonstrate a dose-related vasodilating effect.[34] The mechanism of action is controversial and may be the result of a direct action on the smooth muscle of the peripheral arterial system, neurogenic mechanisms, or both. In three animal species, fentanyl had no major effect on coronary arteriolar tone.[35]

Ventilatory Effects

All the agonist opioids produce a dose-dependent respiratory depression. It is likely that equianalgesic concentrations of the various available agonists produce equivalent respiratory depression. The differences occasionally noted by clinical observation generally have to do with the pharmacokinetics and pharmacodynamics of the different drugs as well as their relative potencies. The peak ventilatory effect of fentanyl injected intravenously is within $5-10$ minutes, whereas that of morphine may be as late as $30-60$ minutes and therefore not as obvious to someone who has

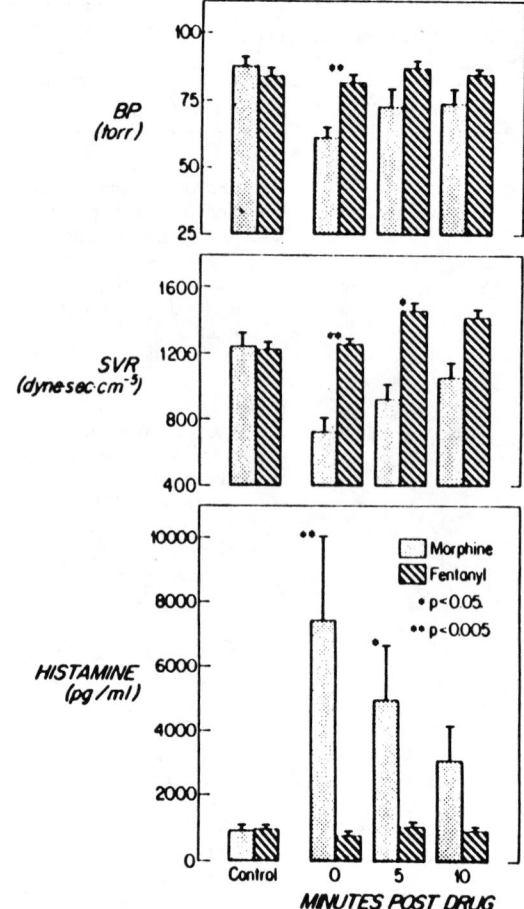

Figure 16-2. Intravenous administration of morphine, but not fentanyl, evokes declines in blood pressure (BP) and systemic vascular resistance (SVR) that parallel increases in the serum concentration of histamine (mean ± SE; *$p < 0.05$; **$p < 0.005$). (Reprinted with permission from Rosow CE, Moss I, Philbin DM et al: Histamine release during morphine and fentanyl anesthesia. Anesthesiology 56:93, 1982.)

injected the morphine but may no longer be observing the patient as carefully.[36-38] Furthermore, it is difficult to compare relative potencies of drugs that have radically different pharmacokinetic and pharmacodynamic timetables (Table 16-2).

Codeine is an opioid commonly used in place of morphine because it is alleged to produce less respiratory depression than morphine. Unfortunately, at the doses used, it also does not produce as much analgesia as morphine. In the same context, fentanyl is more acceptable as an intraoperative opioid because it does not produce as much (prolonged) respiratory depression postoperatively. Again, this is purely a kinetic-dynamic phenomenon related to the duration of action of fentanyl and morphine in the doses used.

It has been suggested that depression of ventilation may outlast the analgesic properties of some of the newer opioids or that respiratory depression may be greater with certain of these opioids at equianalgesic levels.[39] Although there is evidence to support these assumptions, they are by no means conclusive and may be related to the mechanisms of measurement as well as the effects of other CNS depressant drugs and sleep. Furthermore, a biphasic depression of ventilation has been proposed for fentanyl and possibly meperi-

TABLE 16-2. Estimated Relative Potencies and Dosages of Opioids

Drug (Trade Name)	Potency Ratio*	Analgesic Dose†	"Anesthetic" Dose‡
Morphine sulfate	1	10 mg	1–5 mg·kg^{-1}
Meperidine (Demerol)	0.1	100 mg	NA
Fentanyl (Sublimaze)	100	100 μg	50–150 μg·kg^{-1}
Sufentanil (Sufenta)	500–1000	10–20 μg	5–20 μg·kg^{-1}
Alfentanil (Alfenta)	10–20	500–1000 μg	100–200 μg·kg^{-1}
Pentazocine (Talwin)	0.3	30 mg	NA
Butorphanol (Stadol)	5	2 mg	NA
Nalbuphine (Nubain)	1	10 mg	NA
Buprenorphine (Buprenex)	30	0.3 mg	NA
Dezocine (Dalgan)	1	10 mg	NA

NA = not available, not applicable, or not advisable.

*Potency ratios are estimates relative to morphine sulfate as one and are purely guidelines.

†Dosages are variable, depending upon the patient's condition, other drugs administered, and pain levels.

‡High-dose opioids do not provide all of the requirements of general anesthesia. Supplemental drugs may be needed to guarantee amnesia/unconsciousness, relaxation, and sympathetic control.

dine (Fig. 16-3).[40,41] The biphasic response noted in the study by Becker and colleagues in surgical patients is most likely related to exogenous stimuli (or the lack thereof) in the postoperative period rather than to any inherent drug action or pharmacokinetic phenomenon.[36]

Opioids decrease the response of the respiratory centers in the brain stem to increases in CO_2. In normal subjects, when ventilatory response to increasing CO_2 is plotted with CO_2 on the abscissa of the graph, there is a relatively steep response (Fig. 16-4). When opioids are added in the awake subject, the response is shifted (displaced) to the right, but the slope of the line is not significantly changed.[42] The respiratory centers are reset for a higher CO_2 threshold, but the

sensitivity of the centers is not changed. If the subject goes to sleep, the line is shifted further to the right, and the slope of the response line is also depressed.[43] Much greater depression of ventilation is produced with loss of consciousness.

Lower doses of opioids tend to decrease breathing rate while maintaining tidal volume. As the dose is increased, tidal volume as well as breathing rate usually decreases. Irregular or periodic breathing may be induced as the pontine and medullary centers, which regulate rhythmicity of respiration, are depressed.[1] High enough doses may produce apnea even in an awake subject; however, the subject

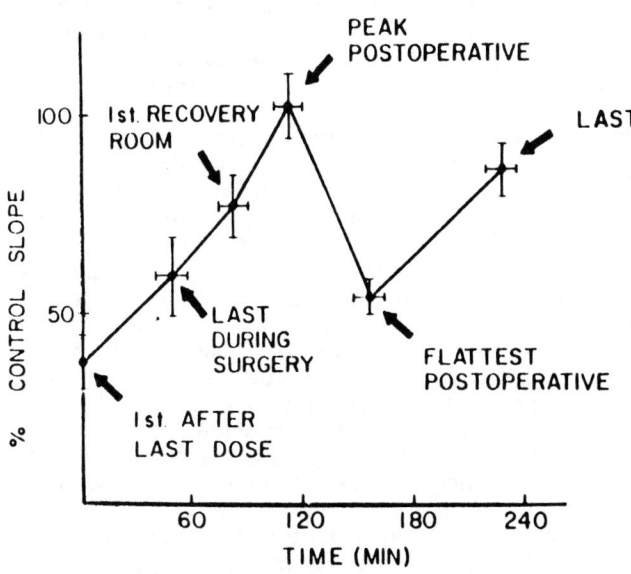

Figure 16-3. Carbon dioxide response slopes as percentages of control slope at the time of the last dose of fentanyl or Innovar (time = 0) and subsequently. Recurrence of depression of ventilation (flattest postoperative) corresponds to a time when external stimulation was reduced (mean ± SE). (Reprinted with permission from Becker L, Paulson B, Miller R et al: Biphasic respiratory depression after fentanyl-droperidol or fentanyl alone used to supplement nitrous oxide anesthesia. Anesthesiology 44:291, 1976.)

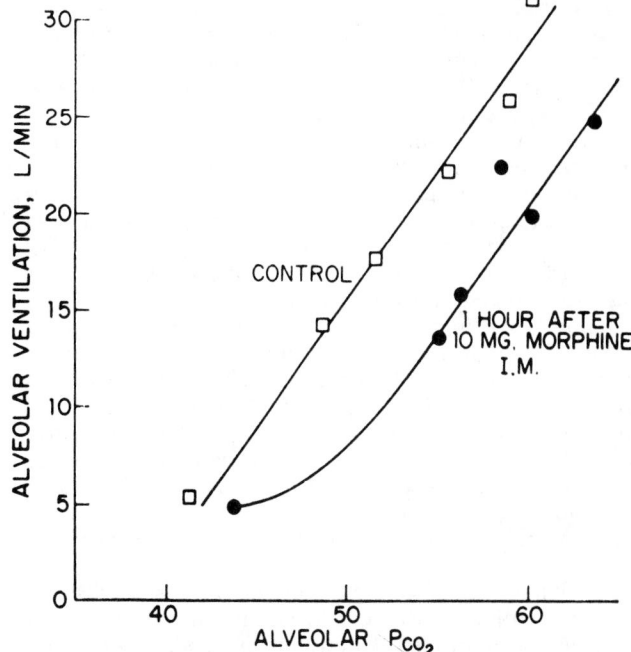

Figure 16-4. Respiratory response curves obtained before and 1 hour after 10 mg morphine sulfate was administered intramuscularly. The end-expiratory P_{CO_2} is plotted against the alveolar ventilation. (Reprinted with permission of Bellville JW, Seed JC: The effect of drugs on the respiratory response to carbon dioxide. Anesthesiology 21:727, 1960.)

can still breathe on command or if he or she makes a conscious effort.

Other CNS depressant drugs, such as the potent inhaled anesthetics, barbiturates, sedative-hypnotics, and alcohol, as well as sleep, increase the respiratory depressant action of the opioids. Pain, on the other hand, is a natural antagonist to the respiratory depressant action of opioids. Again, pain/analgesia and breathing are intertwined.

Older patients have lower dose requirements for depressants in general, and this includes the opioids. The increased sensitivity of older patients is probably related to pharmacokinetics.

Hepatorenal and Gastrointestinal Effects

The renal effects of opioids have been somewhat confusing because of the multitude of factors involved in urine formation.[44] Early animal experiments demonstrated a release of antidiuretic hormone by opioids. Studies in humans suggested that opioids do not release antidiuretic hormone but that surgical stimulation does. In fact, higher doses of opioids may tend to decrease the stress-related release of antidiuretic hormone.

A decrease in glomerular filtration rate with a subsequent decrease in urine output has been noted with opioids. However, if cardiovascular dynamics are unchanged, morphine does not decrease glomerular filtration rate, urine osmolarity, or urine output. When nitrous oxide is added as an anesthetic agent, significant decreases in glomerular filtration rate (40%–60%) and urine output are seen, even with minimal alterations in systolic and diastolic blood pressures.[44]

The diminution of urine output associated with opioids is probably not a result of direct opioid effects but rather surgical stresses that increase pituitary antidiuretic hormone secretion or altered renal hemodynamics as a result of sympathetic stimulation and vasoconstriction. It should also be noted that opioids increase ureteral and detrusor muscle tone, which may result in urinary retention requiring catheterization or reversal with naloxone.

There is no substantial evidence that the opioids themselves produce direct liver dysfunction in humans. However, morphine can produce symptoms of biliary colic owing to spasm of the sphincter of Oddi and the resulting rise of pressure in the biliary tract. Other agonist and agonist-antagonist opioids have also been implicated in sphincter pressure changes, and all probably obstruct flow through the ampulla.[45] Clinical manifestation of the spasm is inconsistent. In surgical patients requiring cholangiography, opioid-induced obstruction can result in unnecessary exploration of the common bile duct.[45] These situations may require reversal of the spasm. Reversal can be consistently accomplished with naloxone, but naloxone also reverses beneficial opioid effects. Other drugs that have been suggested to reverse the biliary spasm include nitroglycerin, glucagon, and atropine. The effect of these drugs is considerably less reliable.

Occasionally, in awake patients, the epigastric distress associated with biliary colic may mimic angina pectoris. In these patients, a differentiation must be made. If naloxone reverses the pain, it is probably biliary colic; if the pain increases or remains the same, it may be angina. Nitroglycerin can relieve both angina and colic and, therefore, may not be helpful in differentiation. Electrocardiographic changes usually indicate angina. The treatment of angina

may include repeated doses of opioids, whereas this approach would accentuate biliary colic.

The antidiarrheal effects of opium were used centuries before its analgesic effects were appreciated. Opioids decrease the motility of the gastrointestinal tract. Decreased gastric motility coupled with increased tone of the antrum may slow passage of gastric contents through the duodenum for up to 12 hours following morphine and retard absorption of orally administered drugs.[1] The danger of pulmonary aspiration in patients having general anesthesia who have eaten since or just prior to a dose of opioid is obvious. Throughout the rest of the intestine, there is an increase in resting tone, with periodic spasms, but a decrease in propulsive activity. The decrease in propulsive activity in the large intestine leads to desiccation of the feces and constipation. The effects of opioids on the intestine appear to be both peripherally (locally) and centrally mediated.[1] A number of opioid receptors have been identified in the gut and are a source for the study of opioids. Central actions on the intestines have been shown to be mediated by the vagus nerve.

Clinical observations suggest that meperidine, compared with other opioids, has a less intense spasmogenic effect on smooth muscle relative to its analgesic action. Meperidine tends to cause less constipation when given over prolonged periods of time. After equianalgesic doses, the increases in common bile duct pressures produced by meperidine are less than those produced by morphine but greater than those produced by codeine.[1]

Endocrine Effects

Opioids inhibit the release of the hypothalamic releasing factors, gonadotropin-releasing hormone and corticotropin-releasing factor, with the ultimate result of decreased plasma concentrations of luteinizing hormone, follicle-stimulating hormone, adrenocorticotropic hormone, beta-endorphin, testosterone, and cortisol. Concentrations of prolactin and growth hormone in plasma are increased by opioids, although they probably do not directly affect the release of antidiuretic hormone.[1,44]

The stress of surgery or trauma results in metabolic changes in the body designed to repair the damage. Generally, there are increases in the plasma concentrations of a number of substances, including cortisol, antidiuretic hormone, growth hormone, aldosterone, thyroid hormone, renin, glucose, and the catecholamines (epinephrine and norepinephrine).[46] In recent years, it has been noted that higher doses of opioids used for surgical anesthesia (especially the fentanyl drugs) modify or block the metabolic stress response to surgery ("stress-free anesthesia"). Generally, high-dose fentanyl family drugs plus oxygen either decrease or do not alter plasma concentrations of the catecholamines, cortisol, antidiuretic hormone, glucose, insulin, and growth hormone while increasing prolactin concentrations. If patients in whom these agents are administered are further stressed by cardiopulmonary bypass, the opioids are unable to block the release of antidiuretic hormone, growth hormone, glucose, and the catecholamines during or after bypass.[46,47] Preterm newborns and neonates, traditionally thought to be unable to perceive pain because of lack of myelination in the central nervous system, have also been shown to mount a substantial stress response to surgery that is altered by opioids in a manner similar to that seen in adults.[48]

Reproductive Effects

The opioid agonist analgesics are generally considered to be nonteratogenic and safe for use in women in early pregnancy. The placenta does not act as a barrier to opioid analgesics, and chronic or addictive use of opioids by the mother can addict her fetus/neonate. Neonates born of addicted mothers must be carefully observed and treated for signs of withdrawal.

Current methods for maternal pain relief are discussed in Chapter 46. Historically, several different opioid agonist analgesics have been used for the pain of labor. Morphine was originally popularized in combination with scopolamine as "twilight sleep." The sedation and amnesia produced by scopolamine are less popular today, and the technique has fallen into disuse.[49] Morphine produces more neonatal depression than does meperidine.[1] Part of this depression is related to the pharmacokinetics of morphine (a long-acting drug) versus meperidine (a short-acting drug). One study noted that babies delivered between 1 and 6 hours after the mother was given morphine showed signs of narcosis, with a peak incidence of depression at approximately 3.5 hours following maternal administration.[50] Neonates appear to be more sensitive to morphine than adults. This is probably related to increased permeability of the blood-brain barrier in the fetus/neonate. When directly administered morphine and meperidine are compared in the neonate, there is a greater shift of the ventilation–CO_2 response curve to the right with morphine than with meperidine.[49,50] Morphine has also been implicated in the prolongation of labor.[1]

Meperidine is more popular than morphine as an analgesic during labor. Therapeutic doses given once labor is well established do not appear to delay delivery, significantly alter rhythmic uterine contractions, or interfere with normal postpartum contraction or with involution of the uterus.[1,49]

Meperidine can obviously produce neonatal depression. The degree of depression is related to the total dose and time interval between maternal administration and delivery. Greater concentrations of meperidine are achieved in the fetus following iv rather than im administration to the mother owing to higher peak plasma concentrations in the mother with iv injection and the subsequent increased concentration gradient between the maternal and fetal blood. It has been suggested that meperidine doses of not more than 50–75 mg given intramuscularly more than 3 hours before delivery, or 25 to 50 mg given intravenously more than 2 hours before delivery, coupled with a regional block for delivery, ensure significant maternal pain relief with little or no detrimental neonatal effect.[49]

Some studies noting minor opioid depression of infants delivered within 1 hour of maternal administration of meperidine describe an increasing depression with time.[49,50] This apparent contradiction has been attributed to the accumulation of meperidine metabolites, particularly normeperidine, in the fetus. The higher pK_a of the metabolites makes them more likely to be trapped in the more acidotic fetus. Normeperidine has a longer half-life and is possibly a more potent respiratory depressant than meperidine in the fetus.

Alphaprodine (Nisentil) is less commonly used in obstetrics than in the past, when it was popular because of its good sedative properties and supposedly lower incidence of nausea and vomiting than meperidine.[49,50] The onset of analgesia with alphaprodine is rapid, within 5 minutes following subcutaneous administration or 1 to 2 minutes after iv administration, and its duration of action is short (approximately 2 hours). Its propensity to cause apnea, even at therapeutic doses, has made alphaprodine less popular. (Respiratory depression is a dose-related response—lower doses at more frequent intervals might be more useful.) Alphaprodine has also been associated with a decrease in fetal heart variability and a high incidence of sinusoidal fetal heart rate pattern.[50]

Neuromuscular Junction and Skeletal Muscle Effects

In clinical dosing, the opioids do not appear to have an effect on the neuromuscular junction of skeletal muscle or directly on skeletal muscle itself. However, all opioids given intravenously in high doses have the ability to produce rigidity of skeletal muscles, particularly in the chest and abdomen, but also in the extremities and jaw. Although rigidity is reported with morphine (2 mg·kg^{-1} plus nitrous oxide), it is more commonly seen with fentanyl and its analogues. Rigidity has been reported following iv doses of fentanyl as low as 80–200 µg (8% incidence) or with infusion rates as slow as 35 µg·min^{-1}.[20] The incidence of rigidity following 8 µg·kg^{-1} of fentanyl given intravenously was 100% in one study. In patients pretreated with low doses of nondepolarizing relaxants, rigidity is usually noted at approximately 15 µg·kg^{-1} of fentanyl.[20] Sufentanil and alfentanil in comparable doses act like fentanyl. There are reports of recurrence both intra- and postoperatively with fentanyl and sufentanil.[20,51]

The incidence and severity of rigidity may be increased by rapid infusion of the drug or the addition of nitrous oxide. Alternatively, the incidence and severity can be decreased by slower administration of opioids, deepening of anesthesia with potent inhalation agents or thiopental, or pretreatment with low doses of nondepolarizing muscle relaxants.[20] Jaffe and Ramsey reported a decreased incidence of rigidity in patients pretreated with metocurine (50 µg·kg^{-1}) but not those pretreated with pancuronium (12.5 µg·kg^{-1}) when compared with a nontreated group.[52] Other studies suggest that pancuronium is effective.

In severe cases, truncal rigidity may make ventilation of the patient's lungs difficult or impossible. Unconsciousness usually occurs before or with development of rigidity, but this is not always true. Severe rigidity may necessitate the use of a muscle relaxant to produce paralysis in an awake patient. Truncal rigidity can also create hemodynamic problems. If high airway pressures are used in an attempt to expand a rigid chest, the increased intrathoracic pressures may impede venous return and decrease cardiac output.

The mechanism of opioid-induced muscle rigidity is not clear. Even the site of the source of inability to ventilate the lungs has been called into question. Glottic rigidity and glottic closure as well as supraglottic airway obstruction have been described.[53,54] The mechanism is not at the neuromuscular junction and probably not at the spinal cord level but most likely is related to mu receptors in the caudate nucleus.[20,54]

TOXICOLOGY

In general, the opioid agonists are very safe drugs with high margins of safety. Coma, pinpoint pupils, and depression of ventilation suggest overdose. In most cases of overdose or poisoning with opioids, the common factors determining sequelae are depression of ventilation and hypoxia. If overdose is noted early and breathing is maintained before hypoxic damage, patients usually survive. Treatment is based on support of failing systems—ventilation, pulmonary edema, shock, tonic-clonic seizures. Initial treatment is support of respiration and iv doses of naloxone (0.2–0.4 mg, or 0.01 mg·kg^{-1} for children), repeated every 2 to 3 minutes until the patient is breathing and responsive or up to a total dose of about 10 mg. Doses of naloxone greater than 10 mg suggest an inaccurate diagnosis or a missed nonopioid drug overdose.[1]

Toxicologic studies in dogs using low to massive doses of different opioids have resulted in several conclusions. There is an inverse relationship between analgesic potency and toxic activity.[19] Weak opioids (meperidine, piritramide) may produce cardiac depression, seizures, and metabolic acidosis in doses that would be considered "anesthetic." Medium potency drugs (morphine, phenoperidine, and alfentanil) given in high doses, much greater than clinically used "anesthetic" doses, and high potency drugs (fentanyl and sufentanil) given in massive doses produce cardiovascular hyperactivity, seizures, and metabolic acidosis. The less potent the drug, the more severe the toxic manifestation. The higher the potency, the less severe the toxicity and the higher the dose at which it appears. For the more potent opioids, the toxic dose may be thousands of times greater than high therapeutic doses.[19]

ALLERGIC REACTIONS

Allergic reactions to opioid analgesics are uncommon and usually consist of urticaria or skin rashes. Anaphylactoid reactions to codeine and morphine have been reported and have been suggested as a mechanism for sudden death in iv heroin users.[1] At least one case of an apparent anaphylactoid allergic reaction to fentanyl has been reported.[55] It is not uncommon to see flushing, urticaria, or wheals at the site of injection in patients given morphine or codeine, which are known histamine releasers.[1,32] Meperidine, in a recent study, appears to be a more potent histamine releaser than morphine.[33] More potent opioids, fentanyl and sufentanil, do not appear to release systemically effective or measurable histamine levels, although a wheal and flare response may be elicited by intradermal testing.[32,33,56] In the same study of intradermally applied opioids in human volunteers, butorphanol produced a wheal but no flare, whereas alfentanil, nalbuphine, and naloxone did not produce either wheal or flare responses.[56]

PHARMACOKINETICS AND PHARMACODYNAMICS

Pharmacokinetics is the study of drug disposition in the body and includes the processes of absorption, distribution, biotransformation, and excretion (Table 16-3). Pharmacokinetic data are usually derived from measurement of concentrations of a drug in plasma. Opioids have no effect in plasma but have sites of action called receptors in certain specified tissues. It is the combination of the drug with its receptors that initiates an effect.

$$\text{drug} + \text{receptor} \leftrightharpoons \text{drug–receptor complex} \approx \text{effect}$$

The intensity of the effect is the result of the number of receptors occupied by the opioid. The drug–receptor interaction is reversible, and the effect may be increased or decreased by increasing or decreasing the receptor occupancy. The concentration of the drug at the receptor is more important than the concentration of the drug in plasma, but direct measurement of the concentration at the receptor is difficult or impossible in an intact patient or animal. Since plasma is the vehicle of transport of drugs to and from their sites of action, storage, biotransformation, and excretion, the concentration of drug in the plasma is generally proportional to (but not necessarily equal to) the concentration at these sites. Factors that influence the concentration of opioids in plasma affect their concentration at the receptors.

With iv administration of a drug, there is no delay from absorption. Peak concentrations in plasma occur almost immediately following bolus administration of opioids and then decrease rapidly as the drug is distributed to tissues of action, storage, biotransformation, or excretion. The onset and duration of action are related to the rise and fall of the number of receptors occupied. The uptake of the drug by a tissue is determined by its rate of delivery and the capacity of the tissue to accumulate the drug. Rate of delivery is primarily determined by blood flow, the concentration gradient between plasma and the tissue, and the permeability coefficient of the drug. For an opioid to reach a tissue, it must cross a biologic membrane, generally by dissolution and diffusion in the lipoprotein matrix of the membrane. For opioid drugs, the most important physiochemical properties that influence the rate of diffusion across biologic membranes (the permeability coefficient) are molecular size, ionization, and lipid solubility. Opioids are all relatively small molecules, and permeability is not significantly limited by size. Ionization is important, because nonionized drugs cross membranes more readily. The lower the pK$_a$ of the opioid, the greater the percentage of the drug that will be non-ionized at a particular pH (generally 7.4 in plasma) and the greater percentage of the drug available to cross membranes. Owing to the lipoprotein matrix of biologic membranes, the more lipid-soluble a drug, the faster it crosses.

The capacity of a tissue is determined by the affinity of the drug for the particular tissue (the tissue-plasma partition coefficient) and the mass of the tissue. Affinity is dependent upon drug binding, dissolution, active transport into the tissue, and pH-dependent partitioning of the drug between plasma and the tissue.

The concentration of the opioid in plasma is determined by its distribution and redistribution to its sites of action (receptors), storage (inactive sites), and tissues or organs of elimination. Elimination is the result of biotransformation and/or excretion. For the opioids, biotransformation is primarily in the liver. Biotransformation of the opioids is usually to an inactive metabolite or to a metabolite with considerably less activity than the parent drug. The most important exception to the rule is meperidine, which biotransforms in part to normeperidine, a drug with considerable activity. Biotransformation of the opioids usually facilitates excretion of the drug from the body at one or more sites—generally the kidneys.

Morphine

When morphine is administered intravenously, the decrease in the plasma concentration can be described by a biexponential or triexponential equation. Following an iv dose of 0.05–0.2 mg·kg^{-1}, there is an initial rapid distribution of the drug to tissues and organs. By 10 minutes,

TABLE 16-3. Pharmacokinetics of Opioid Agonists

	Rapid Distribution Half-Time (minutes)	Slow Distribution Half-Time (minutes)	Elimination Half-Time (hours)	Volume of Distribution (l·kg^{-1})	Clearance (ml·kg^{-1}·min^{-1})	Protein Binding (%)	pK_a
Morphine	1.2–2.5	9–13.3	1.7–2.2	3.2–3.4	15–23	26–36	7.93
Meperidine	4–17		3.2–7.9	2.8–4.2	5–17	58–82	8.5
Fentanyl	1.0–1.7	13–28	3.1–7.9	3.2–5.9	8–21	79–87	8.43
Sufentanil	1.4	17.7	2.7	1.7	13	92.5	8.01
Alfentanil	0.7–3.5	8.2–16.8	1.2–1.9	0.3–1	2.8–7.9	89–92	6.5

96–98% of the drug is cleared from plasma.[57] The initial rapid distribution phase has a half-time of 1.2–2.5 minutes in adults and children 1–15 years of age.[57-60] In those studies demonstrating triexponential curves, the slower distribution half-time is also relatively short (9–13.3 minutes). A morphine dose of approximately 1.0 mg·kg^{-1}, given at a rate of 5.0 mg·min^{-1} to elderly adult males, resulted in similar values of 1.3 and 19.8 minutes for the rapid and slow distribution phases.[58] The half-time of the terminal elimination phase for morphine using analytical methods specific for unchanged morphine is 1.7–2.2 hours.[57,59] Other studies have reported terminal elimination half-times as high as 2.9–4.5 hours.[58] The discrepancies among the studies are probably related to the employment of radioimmunoassay antibodies in the latter studies, which cross-react with morphine metabolites. This cross-reactivity will result in falsely high estimates of the concentration of morphine (especially at the later times when the concentration of metabolites is higher) and produce exaggerated elimination half-times.

Estimates of the volume of distribution for analgesic doses of morphine (0.05–0.2 mg·kg^{-1}) administered intravenously in adults are 3.2–3.4 l·kg^{-1}.[57,58,60] Whereas the volume of distribution for analgesic doses in children 1–15 years of age is 1.2 l·kg^{-1}, the estimated volume of distribution in elderly adults is 4.7 l·kg^{-1}.[58,59] The variabilities noted may be the result of many factors, including age, physical status, and anesthetic and surgical conditions. Nonetheless, the volume of distribution of morphine is relatively large, suggesting extensive tissue uptake. Since morphine is somewhat lipid-insoluble, the sequestration is most probably in nonfat tissues, with skeletal muscle containing the greater fraction because of its mass.

The clearance of morphine from the body is primarily the result of hepatic metabolism to morphine–glucuronide and other minor metabolites that are ultimately removed by the kidneys (Fig. 16-5). Less than 15% of a morphine dose is eliminated unchanged in the urine.[61,62] The clearance of morphine (15–23 ml·kg^{-1}·min^{-1}) is very high (approaching hepatic blood flow), indicating a high hepatic extraction ratio.[57,58] Because extraction of morphine from plasma is relatively complete, the elimination of morphine is dependent upon blood flow to the liver and the re-uptake of morphine from its sites of storage in the body. The large volume of distribution for morphine tends to keep the concentrations of morphine in plasma low, making re-uptake the rate-limiting step in elimination. The high hepatic extraction ratio also ensures that little orally administered morphine reaches the circulation owing to enterohepatic first-pass metabolism.

Stanski et al reported that 10 mg of morphine given intramuscularly had an absorption half-life of 7.7 (range 3–15) minutes with a 100% systemic availability.[58] Peak plasma concentrations were reached between 7.5–20 minutes after injection. Brunk and Delle found that 10 mg·kg^{-1} doses of morphine given intramuscularly or subcutaneously resulted in higher plasma concentrations than those seen after iv dosing in the period from 15 minutes to 3 hours after administration.[62] The iv doses are rapidly distributed out of the plasma, whereas the im or subcutaneous sites continue to release morphine into the plasma for distribution.

At physiologic pH (7.40), 23–36% of morphine is bound to plasma proteins—primarily albumin.[63,64] Only the unbound fraction (approximately 70%) would be available for distribution across membranes. Also, only non-ionized drugs readily distribute (cross) into the lipid phase of the membrane. The pK$_a$s for morphine (7.93/9.63 at 37°C) mean that only a small fraction (less than 10%) of morphine is normally non-ionized in plasma.[65,66] Furthermore, morphine is relatively lipid-insoluble with an octanol/water partition coefficient of 1.0.[66] The result is that only a small portion of the morphine found in plasma at any particular time readily crosses into the CNS. Acute changes in the concentration of morphine in plasma do not result in immediate changes in the levels in the CNS, and equilibrium between plasma and CNS levels of morphine is found only after prolonged steady-state levels of morphine in plasma.

It is interesting that morphine is considered to be a relatively long-acting opioid with analgesic effects lasting 4–5 hours although its elimination half-time is actually less than that for the reportedly shorter-acting drug fentanyl. And, although patients are aware of the effects of an iv dose of morphine within minutes of its injection, the peak effect of the dose may be delayed for over 15 minutes. A few reports in the literature have attempted to correlate plasma levels of morphine with analgesic intensity, but the studies show only crude and indirect comparisons. The studies have not been able to demonstrate a direct relationship between plasma concentrations of morphine and intensity of analgesia or respiratory depression.

Studies in animals also suggest that the blood–brain barrier is a significant impediment to the movement of morphine both into and away from its sites of analgesic and respiratory effects in the CNS. In dogs given an iv dose of 0.3 mg·kg^{-1} of morphine and allowed to breathe spontaneously, peak concentrations of morphine in the cerebrospinal fluid (CSF) did not occur until 15–30 minutes following injection (Fig. 16-6).[38] The delay probably reflects the low lipid solubility of morphine and the limitations imposed by biologic membranes on less lipid-soluble drugs. Diffusion of morphine from brain to CSF to plasma may occur and result in a concentration in CSF between that of plasma and brain. But once in the CSF, the elimination of morphine did not parallel its elimination from plasma.[38] These observations have been confirmed in other studies. One study that re-

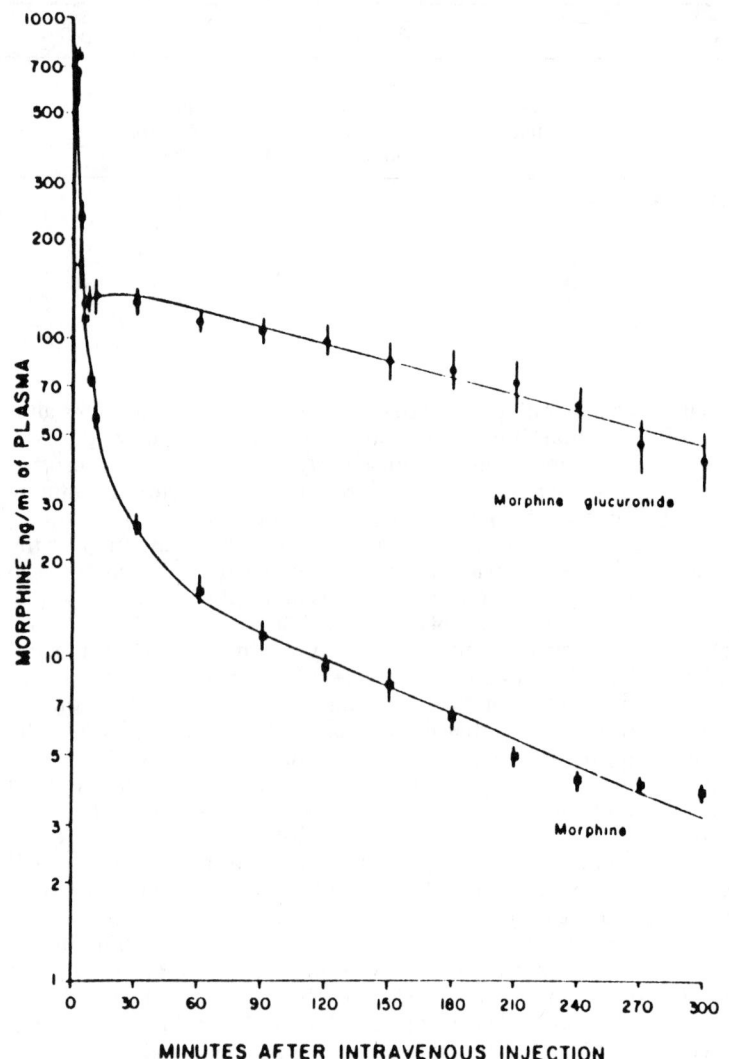

Figure 16-5. Plasma concentrations of morphine and its principal metabolite, morphine glucuronide, following intravenous administration of morphine (mean ± SE). (Reprinted with permission from Murphy MR, Hug CC Jr: Pharmacokinetics of intravenous morphine in patients anesthetized with enflurane-nitrous oxide. Anesthesiology 54:187, 1981.)

ported a delayed elimination of morphine from the brain in relation to that in plasma suggested that the slowed elimination was the result of a greater portion of the morphine existing in the ionized state in the relatively acid milieu of the brain.[67]

Ventilatory depression demonstrated by changes in the end-tidal CO_2 of spontaneously breathing dogs (Fig. 16-6) did not correlate with the concentration of morphine in either the plasma or the CSF.[38] Ventilatory depression is the pharmacodynamic effect of morphine measured in this study and probably most directly reflects the concentration of morphine at its receptors or sites of action. Plasma concentrations of morphine do not adequately reflect the intensity of effect of morphine, but the pharmacokinetic data do help explain the pharmacodynamics of the drug.

The literature suggests that a 10-mg dose of morphine is equivalent to approximately 20% nitrous oxide. Studies of the efficacy of a number of opioids to act as anesthetics or reduce the concentration of potent inhalation agents necessary to maintain minimal alveolar concentration (MAC) have been performed. In dogs given increasing iv doses of morphine, the end-tidal concentration of enflurane necessary to prevent movement to an applied tail-clamp can be reduced in a linear fashion up to a morphine dose of 5 mg·kg^{-1}.[15] A dose of 0.5 mg·kg^{-1} reduced the MAC of en-

flurane by 17%, 1.5 mg·kg^{-1} reduced MAC 32%, and 5 mg·kg^{-1} produced a 63% reduction in MAC. A fourfold increase in the dose of morphine to 20 mg·kg^{-1} reduced MAC to a maximum of 67%, which was not statistically different from the 63% reduction of the 5 mg·kg^{-1} dose. The effectiveness of morphine as an anesthetic appears to plateau at about 65% of a total MAC, suggesting that it does not provide complete anesthesia.

Similar studies in rats given subcutaneous doses of morphine found linear reductions of cyclopropane and halothane MAC up to a dose of 8 mg·kg^{-1}, in which the reductions were 55% and approximately 68%, respectively.[68] In the halothane study, further doses of 12 and 20 mg·kg^{-1} produced reductions of approximately 70% and 84%, demonstrating a response approaching plateau.

Meperidine

Intravenous injection of meperidine in normal subjects results in a biexponential decline of the concentration of meperidine in plasma. Meperidine has a relatively rapid tissue distribution half-time of 4–17 minutes.[69-72] The volume of distribution of meperidine is 2.8–4.2 l·kg^{-1}, indicating extensive tissue distribution similar to that seen with

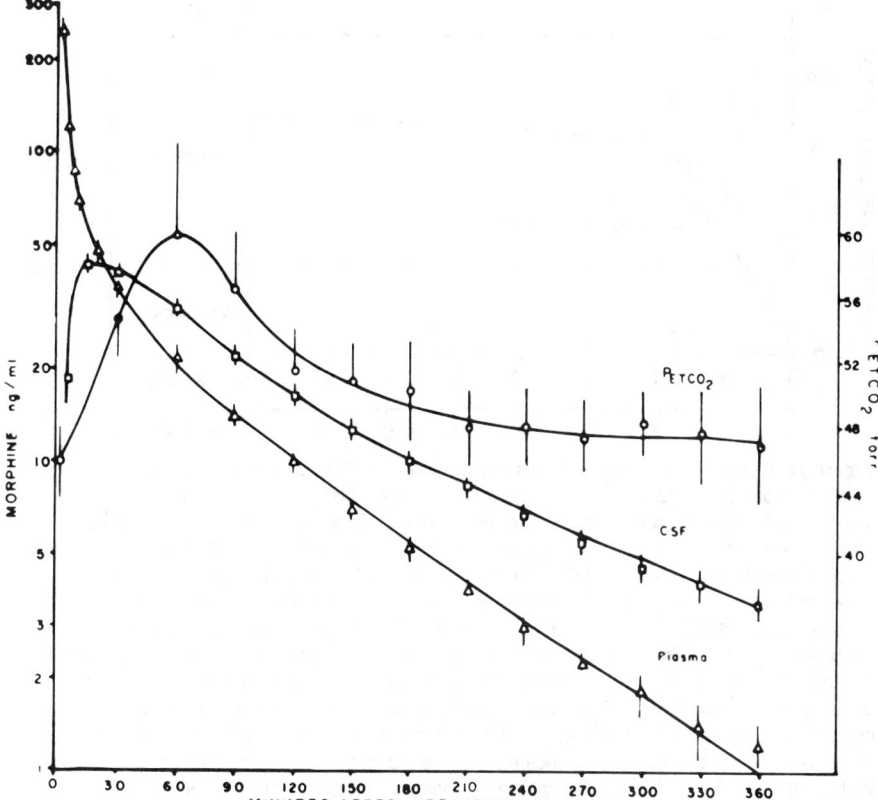

Figure 16-6. Cerebrospinal fluid (CSF) and plasma levels of morphine and end-tidal CO_2 (PET_{CO_2}) in six dogs given an 0.3 mg·kg^{-1} dose intravenously and allowed to ventilate spontaneously. Each point and vertical line represents the mean ± SEM. There is a lack of correlation between the concentrations of morphine in plasma, CSF, and the receptors for ventilatory depression as represented by the PET_{CO_2}. (Adapted with permission from Hug CC Jr, Murphy MR, Rigel EP et al: Pharmacokinetics of morphine injected intravenously into the anesthetized dog. Anesthesiology 54:38, 1981.)

morphine.[69-72] Meperidine also has a high clearance rate (10–17 ml·kg^{-1}·min^{-1}), which is slightly less than that of morphine.[69-73] The elimination half-time for meperidine is 3.2–4.1 hours, greater than that of morphine. After sampling for 24 hours, rather than the 6–7 hours sampled in the previous studies, even longer terminal half-lives (6–8 hours) and smaller clearances (4.9–7.6 ml·kg^{-1}·min^{-1}) were found.[74,75] Despite the longer elimination half-time for meperidine in relation to morphine, meperidine is a shorter-acting drug.

Meperidine's high clearance is indicative of a high hepatic extraction ratio. Meperidine is readily metabolized in the liver, and a number of metabolites are possible, the major ones being normeperidine, meperidinic acid, and normeperidinic acid. Normeperidine is found in plasma after repeat doses of meperidine and is eliminated much more slowly than is meperidine.[76] Normeperidine is an active metabolite, possessing twice the convulsive properties of meperidine with only half the analgesic effect.[76] Stambaugh et al found only 3.9% of an iv dose of meperidine excreted unchanged in the urine by 48 hours, whereas 4.2% was excreted as normeperidine.[70] The urinary excretion rates were 4.5% and 5.5% for meperidine and normeperidine, respectively, following im administration, and 3.3% and 6.2% after oral administration.

Absorption of an im dose of meperidine in postsurgical patients is extremely variable. Peak concentrations in plasma following 100-mg doses given at 4-hour intervals varied over a fivefold range among the patients. The peak concentrations were also associated with wide variations in the times to reach those peaks following im injection. The mean time to reach peak concentrations among the patients was 44 minutes but varied from 15 to 110 minutes.[77]

The free fraction of meperidine in plasma is 18–42%,

meaning that it is much more protein-bound than is morphine. Meperidine is primarily bound to alpha$_1$-acid glycoprotein (and, to a lesser extent, albumin). Meperidine protein binding can be affected by surgery and/or disease states that alter alpha$_1$-acid glycoprotein. Meperidine is also considerably more lipid-soluble than is morphine, with an octanol/water partition coefficient of 11.5 (morphine's is 1.0). The onset of action of meperidine is somewhat faster than that of morphine after both iv and im dosing. The duration of effect (2–3 hours) for analgesic doses is shorter than that of morphine, despite a longer elimination half-time for meperidine. The prolongation of morphine's pharmacodynamic effects has been examined.

Unlike morphine, there is a reasonable correlation between the plasma concentration of meperidine and the intensity of its effects. Austin et al found that the minimal effective analgesic concentration of meperidine in postsurgical patients was independent of the route of delivery (im vs iv) and ranged between 0.24 and 0.76 μg·ml^{-1}, with a mean of 0.46 μg·ml^{-1}.[78] The maximal blood concentration still associated with severe pain ranged from 0.10–0.98 μg·ml^{-1}, with a mean of 0.41 μg·ml^{-1}. These researchers concluded that concentrations of meperidine less than 0.10 μg·ml^{-1} did not alter the perception of pain. With gradual increases in blood concentrations, a critical point is reached, at which very small increases in concentration (0.05 μg·ml^{-1}) can produce complete analgesia. Although the variation of minimal analgesic concentrations was large among patients, the concentrations were stable and consistent for any individual. In practice, a meperidine concentration of 0.6 μg·ml^{-1} would produce suppression from severe pain 84% of the time, whereas 0.7 μg·ml^{-1} would produce relief from severe pain 95% of the time.[78] In another study,

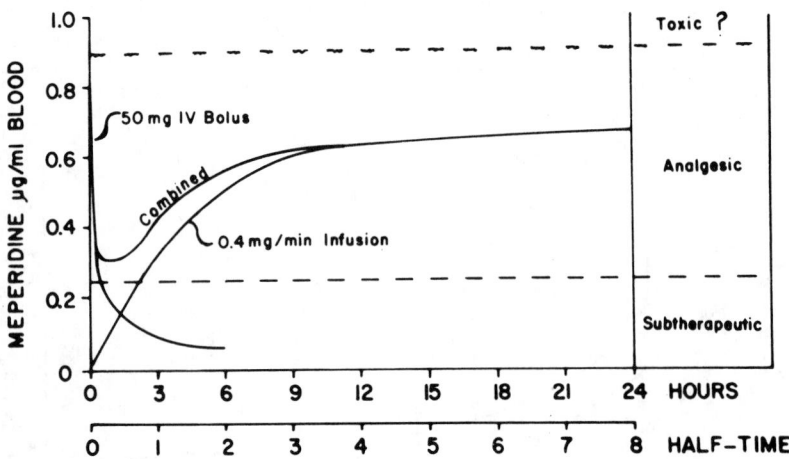

Figure 16-7. Simulation of blood levels of meperidine resulting from the combination of an intravenous bolus dose of 50 mg and a continuous infusion of 0.4 mg·min^{-1} begun at time zero. After the bolus dose alone, blood levels would initially be higher than necessary (near toxic?) and would fall into the subtherapeutic range after 20 to 40 minutes. With the continuous infusion of 0.4 mg·min^{-1}, it would take slightly more than 2 hours to reach the lowest analgesic concentrations. By combining the two methods of administration, blood levels of meperidine remain within the analgesic range; an additional bolus dose might be useful after about 20 minutes. An even better method would involve the use of a priming infusion to limit the peak concentration and to minimize the depth of the concentration trough. The toxic level of meperidine has not been defined; a concentration of 0.7 µg·ml^{-1} was estimated to provide relief of pain in 95% of cases and gave no evidence of clinically significant respiratory depression (or toxicity). (Reprinted with permission from Hug CC Jr: Improving analgesic therapy. Anesthesiology 53:441, 1980.)

healthy volunteers given 50 mg of meperidine intravenously had a maximal serum concentration of 0.52 µg·ml^{-1} observed in the first sample at 1 minute.[70] By 5 minutes, the concentration of meperidine in serum had decreased by one half to 0.25 µg·ml^{-1}. At 30 minutes, it was 0.14 µg·ml^{-1} and thereafter decreased more slowly. By 3 hours, the level was 0.11 µg·ml^{-1} and, at 8 hours, 0.07 µg·ml^{-1}. If the volunteers had been surgical patients, adequate analgesia would have been nonexistent or very short-lived following a single 50-mg bolus of meperidine.

The aforementioned data have added significance when it is noted that in patients given 100 mg of meperidine intramuscularly every 4 hours postoperatively, the concentration of meperidine in the blood of the patient was above the minimal analgesic concentration only about 35% of each 4-hour im dosing interval.[77] Variable pain control was the result of inadequate and unpredictable blood concentrations owing to unpredictable absorption from im sites of injection. The fact that there is a good correlation between blood concentration and pharmacodynamics (analgesia) allows the use of pharmacokinetic data to create a treatment regimen that produces satisfactory analgesia without significant toxicity. Just such a treatment plan was summarized in an editorial by Hug utilizing previously published data (Fig. 16-7) and was proved by Stapleton et al in patients.[79,80] An infusion of 0.4 mg·min^{-1}, preceded by a loading infusion of 1.0 mg·min^{-1} for 45 minutes followed by 0.53 mg·min^{-1} for 28 minutes, resulted in the abolition of severe pain after 3 hours and in continued analgesia for the 2-day study in postabdominal hysterectomy patients.[80]

Fentanyl

Much has been written about the variability of the pharmacokinetics of fentanyl in humans.[81,82] Excluding studies in which duration of sampling (less than 6 hours) was inadequate (too few samples were obtained at crucial times) or in which aortic cross-clamping or cardiopulmonary bypass intervened, the pharmacokinetic data are not quite so varied. Six studies, two in volunteers and four in surgical patients, appear to represent reasonable pharmacokinetic studies of fentanyl. The iv doses ranged from 5–10 µg·kg^{-1} and were given either as rapid bolus doses or as rapid infusions of up to 2.5 minutes, depending upon the study, except for the study by Scott and Stanski.[36,83-87] In this study, fentanyl was infused at 150 µg·min^{-1} until the appearance of delta wave activity in the raw EEG tracing (mean 717 µg).[87]

When fentanyl is injected intravenously, there is a very rapid decline in plasma concentration. In dogs given 10 or 100 µg·kg^{-1} of fentanyl intravenously, 98% of the dose was eliminated from plasma at 5 minutes and 99% by 30 minutes.[88] In volunteers, 98.6% of the injected dose has been eliminated from plasma by 60 minutes.[36] The concentration–time curve for fentanyl is described by either a biexponential or triexponential equation, depending upon the rate of injection or sampling times immediately following injection. In those studies in which fentanyl is given rapidly and sufficient numbers of samples are obtained early in the study, a triexponential decline in plasma concentrations is found.[36,83] In patients and volunteers, the rapid distribution half-time for fentanyl is 1.0–1.7 minutes, whereas the slower distribution phase is 13–28 minutes in the studies in which three phases are apparent.[36,83,87] Although there is no direct evidence in humans, animal studies suggest that the rapid distribution phase represents the equilibration of the vessel-rich group of tissues (e.g., brain, lung, heart) and plasma with skeletal muscle (Fig. 16-8).[89] The slower distribution (and redistribution) phase is the equilibration of the plasma/vessel-rich group of tissues and skeletal muscle with fat (Fig. 16-8).[89] The elimination half-time for fentanyl is 3.1–7.9 hours.[36,83–87] The 7.9 hour elimination half-time was found when plasma levels were sampled for 24 hours and is possibly more accurate than the 3.1–4.4 hour half-times obtained for the earlier studies in which levels were measured for 8 hours or less.

The pharmacokinetics and pharmacodynamics of fentanyl are very much influenced by its extreme lipid solubility, which allows it to cross biologic membranes very rapidly. Following iv injection in the rat, the uptake of fentanyl by the highly perfused (vessel-rich) group of tissues—heart, lung, and brain—reached a maximum at or before the first sampling at 1.5 minutes (Fig. 16-8).[89] The concentrations in these tissues paralleled the concentration of fentanyl in plasma and were therefore indistinguishable from plasma pharmacokinetically and are designated as part of the central compartment. The actual concentrations in these tissues were higher: two to three times greater in brain and heart than in plasma, and ten times greater in lung. Studies in humans have found that between 43 and 87% of an iv fentanyl dose may be sequestered in pulmonary tissue on the first pass through the lungs.[90] The uptake of fentanyl by skeletal muscle was somewhat slower than that for the central group of tissues and reached a maximum at about 5 minutes—the actual concentrations being two to four times greater than those in plasma. Maximal concentrations were found at 30 minutes in fat and were 35 times greater than those in plasma. Both skeletal muscle, because of its mass in relation to body size, and fat, because of its high partition coefficient for highly lipid-soluble drugs, act as storage sites for fentanyl. As the concentration of fentanyl in plasma decreases following its initial equilibration with adipose tissues, the fat, acting as a reservoir to maintain plasma concentrations, slowly releases the fentanyl back into the plasma for transport to the liver for biotransformation to excretable metabolites. This slow release maintains plasma concentrations and produces the relatively prolonged elimination half-time of 3.1–7.9 hours.[36,83-87]

Very little of a dose of fentanyl is eliminated by renal excretion as fentanyl. Only about 6.5% is eliminated as unchanged drug in the urine.[36] Fentanyl's high lipid solubility

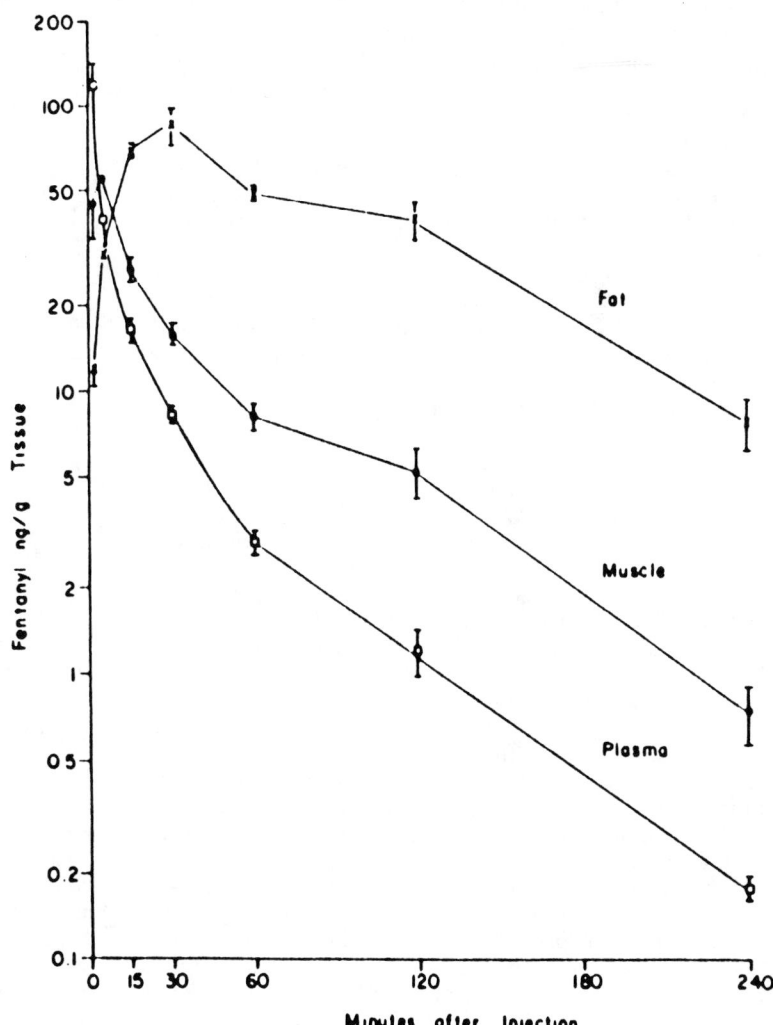

Figure 16-8. The short duration of a single dose of fentanyl reflects its rapid redistribution to inactive tissue sites such as fat and skeletal muscle with an associated decline in the serum concentration of drug. (Reprinted with permission from Hug CC, Murphy RR: Tissue redistribution of fentanyl and termination of its effects in rats. Anesthesiology 55:369, 1981.)

allows it to be readily reabsorbed from the renal tubules. Most of the fentanyl excreted by the kidneys is excreted as metabolites. Fentanyl metabolism is rapid and extensive in the liver. (Undefined extrahepatic sites appear to contribute to fentanyl metabolism in anhepatic dogs but are of little significance in the presence of a functioning liver.[91]) By 30 minutes after iv injection, the concentration of metabolites of fentanyl in plasma exceed the concentration of fentanyl, and the metabolites are eliminated at a much slower rate.[36] The primary route of metabolism is by N-dealkylation to norfentanyl and by hydroxylation of both fentanyl and nor-fentanyl to hydroxypropionyl fentanyl and hydroxypropionyl norfentanyl.[82,89] The pharmacologic activity, if any, of the fentanyl metabolites is not known.

The clearance of fentanyl is high, between 8 and 21 $ml\cdot kg^{-1}\cdot min^{-1}$.[1,36,83-87] These rates approach hepatic blood flow and indicate a high hepatic extraction ratio approaching 100%. With this high extraction ratio, hepatic metabolism is perfusion-dependent. The large volume of distribution, 3.2 to 5.9 $l\cdot kg^{-1}$, reflects the great tissue affinity of fentanyl. The slow release of fentanyl from muscle and fat keeps the plasma concentration relatively low and is the rate-limiting step in the elimination of fentanyl from the body.

The pK_a of fentanyl is 8.43. At pH 7.4, 91% of fentanyl is ionized.[82] Protein binding is approximately 79–87% at pH 7.4 and is consistent over large ranges of drug concentrations (100-fold or more).[36,82,86] The free fraction of fentanyl is therefore 13–21%. Changes in pH affect protein binding; pHs as low as 6.2 were associated with 38% bound drug, whereas increasing the pH increased binding to 90% at pH 7.6.

The pharmacodynamics of fentanyl, especially as related to ventilation, have been fairly well studied. Unlike morphine, there appears to be a fair correlation between the concentration of fentanyl in plasma and its pharmacologic effects on ventilation and probably analgesia. The onset of the effects of fentanyl is rapid. There is marked depression of ventilation within 2 minutes following iv injection of analgesic doses. In 7 volunteers injected over 90 seconds with iv doses of 3.2 or 6.4 $\mu g\cdot kg^{-1}$ of fentanyl base (equivalent to 5 or 10 $\mu g\cdot kg^{-1}$ of fentanyl citrate, which is the commercially available form), decreases in the sense of awareness and concern occurred during the injection of fentanyl.[36] By 2 minutes, the subjects were relaxed. These feelings were maximal between 5 and 10 minutes. Onset of ventilatory depression was as rapid, and apnea occurred in four subjects. A previous study in healthy subjects also noted the greatest ventilatory depression between 2 and 5 minutes following 6 $\mu g\cdot kg^{-1}$ of fentanyl administered intravenously.[92] Comparison of the pharmacokinetic study with the ventilatory study revealed a close relation between plasma levels of fentanyl and ventilatory depression as measured by increases in end-tidal CO_2 (Fig. 16-9).[36,92]

The same correlation has been demonstrated in dogs lightly anesthetized with enflurane/oxygen and breathing spontaneously. A 10-$\mu g\cdot kg^{-1}$ dose of fentanyl administered intravenously over 30 seconds produced an immediate onset of ventilatory depression; apnea occurred within 1.5 minutes.[37] Concentrations of fentanyl in CSF increased rapidly, with near maximal concentrations in the earliest sample taken at 2–3 minutes after injection. Following equilibration between plasma and CSF, there was a linear relationship between the log concentration of fentanyl in plasma and CSF and its effect (ventilatory depression) as measured by changes in end-tidal CO_2. This contrasts with the lack of correlation noted earlier with morphine (see Fig.

16-6). Ventilatory depression is an indirect measure of the concentration of the drug at its sites of action in the CNS.

The concentration of fentanyl in plasma and brain is proportional to dose.[88,89] When low doses are used, the concentration of drug in plasma and at its receptors rapidly falls below a threshold for effect. Increasingly higher doses will produce increasingly prolonged effects. Repetition of the same dose of fentanyl at set intervals produces accumulation of fentanyl in the body. Not only are there higher peak plasma concentrations following each injection but there are also proportional increases in end-tidal CO_2 and a more prolonged effect.[37]

When the pharmacodynamics of fentanyl were measured by EEG spectral edge analysis in patients, there was a measurable lag between fluctuations in plasma concentrations of fentanyl and its EEG slowing effects.[93] A time lag exists between the peak plasma concentration of fentanyl and its peak spectral edge effect; thereafter, the spectral edge changes and plasma concentrations parallel each other, but with a time lag of approximately 6 minutes. It is suggested

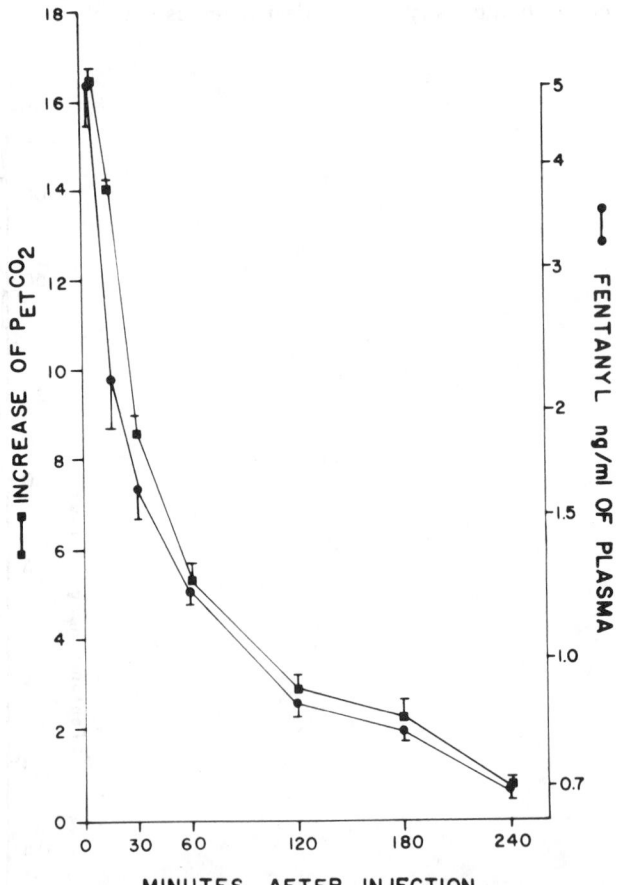

Figure 16-9. Comparison of the decline in log of ^{3}H-fentanyl plasma level in five subjects given 6.4 $\mu g\cdot kg^{-1}$ with the recovery from ventilatory depression (PET_{CO_2}) in ten subjects given 6 $\mu g\cdot kg^{-1}$ intravenously. A very close correlation between the plasma concentration and the ventilatory depression produced by fentanyl is evident. Ventilatory depression is an indirect measure of the concentration of fentanyl at its receptors. (Adapted with permission from McClain DA, Hug CC Jr: Intravenous fentanyl kinetics. Clin Pharmacol Ther 28:106, 1980.)

that the onset of the peak effect of fentanyl in patients is not quite as rapid as previously thought and that dosing should be 5–10 minutes before intense stimulation is anticipated. Clinically, this lag may not be as noticeable, since relatively higher than needed doses of fentanyl may raise the receptor levels of fentanyl beyond the threshold for pain or unconsciousness at some time earlier than the peak effect is seen. The lag between peak serum concentrations and peak effect (dynamics) has been attributed to the partitioning of fentanyl between serum and brain.[93] Because of fentanyl's great lipid solubility, it moves rapidly across the blood-brain barrier into the brain but then must fill a great number of nonreceptor storage sites. The suggestion is that fentanyl must fill a large depot before the concentration of drug at the receptor sites is adequate to produce the opioid effect.

Fentanyl has also been reported to produce a biphasic respiratory response noted as an increasing ventilatory depression in the recovery room following an apparent recovery from fentanyl and nitrous oxide anesthesia (see Fig. 16-4).[40] A number of pharmacokinetic studies have noted secondary increases in plasma concentrations of fentanyl in volunteers and patients.[36] These bumps in the concentration curves have been attributed to mobilization of fentanyl away from tissue storage areas back into the plasma secondary to increased perfusion of the storage areas. The most likely explanation is increased perfusion of skeletal muscles associated with movement in volunteers or during awakening from anesthesia in patients. In the report noted previously, the biphasic ventilatory depression is probably a result of the increased intensity of noxious stimulation and its antagonism of ventilatory effects immediately after surgery when the patients were awakened and transported to the recovery room. Later, when the patients were unstimulated, the residual respiratory depression produced by the remaining fentanyl was not antagonized by the stimulation and became more obvious.[36,40] Again, this report simply demonstrates that noxious stimulation is a natural antagonist to the effects of opioids and that unstimulated patients may become severely depressed postoperatively if the intensity of the stimulation is much less than it is intraoperatively.

Studies similar to those described for morphine to determine the ability of opioids to reduce the MAC of potent inhalation agents have been performed with fentanyl. In dogs, infusion of fentanyl produced stable plasma concentrations at which MAC determinations could be made. There is a dose-plasma concentration-related reduction in enflurane MAC with increasing concentrations of fentanyl up to a maximal reduction of approximately 66% at a plasma concentration of 30 ng·ml^{-1} (Fig. 16-10).[94] The maximal reduction of isoflurane MAC in dogs is the same at 67%.[95] These reductions are similar to those seen with high doses of morphine (63%) and suggest saturation of opioid receptors.

In another study using awake dogs, fentanyl was injected in increasing doses from 2.5 up to 100 μg·kg^{-1} at 5-minute intervals.[96] Plasma concentrations were then compared with the effects on pain responses, ventilation, and circulation. It is of interest that the analgesic effects could not be separated from the ventilatory or circulatory effects and that all these receptor-mediated effects were maximal at the same plasma concentration of fentanyl, 30 ng·ml^{-1}—the same maximal concentration noted in the enflurane MAC reduction study previously cited.

Although these studies were performed in dogs, and there certainly are species differences from humans, the differ-

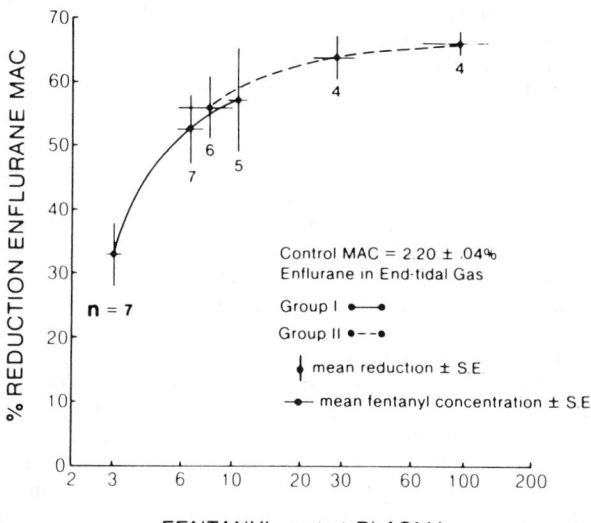

Figure 16-10. Percent reduction of enflurane MAC as a function of the logarithm of the plasma fentanyl concentration. Each point represents the mean concentration (±SEM) of fentanyl in plasma and the average percent (±SEM) reduction of enflurane MAC in the number of dogs indicated below the vertical standard error bar. Similar curves are produced by morphine, sufentanil, and alfentanil in the dog and may represent saturation of opioid receptors. (Adapted with permission from Murphy MR, Hug CC Jr: The anesthetic potency of fentanyl in terms of its reduction of enflurane MAC. Anesthesiology 57:485, 1982.)

ences may not be that great. In patients having cardiac surgery, plasma fentanyl levels of 15 ng·ml^{-1} were necessary for suppression of hemodynamic responses to noxious stimuli in 50% of subjects (EC$_{50}$).[97] Extrapolation of the data in this study suggests that the EC$_{90}$ (the effective concentration in 90% of the patients) would be approximately 30 ng·ml^{-1}. The 15 ng·ml^{-1} concentration in plasma was achieved by the administration of 50 μg·kg^{-1} fentanyl as a loading dose followed by an infusion of 0.5 μg·kg^{-1}·min^{-1}. It is probably not rational to give patients increasing doses of fentanyl once all opioid-effect receptors are occupied, because this will prolong the effect but not increase its intensity.

Sufentanil

Plasma levels of sufentanil for pharmacokinetic studies (and most opioid studies) are determined by radioimmunoassay. The sufentanil radioimmunoassay is accurate to a plasma concentration of 0.1 to 0.5 ng·ml^{-1}. Owing to the extreme potency of sufentanil (about ten times greater than fentanyl), smaller amounts of drug are given to attain the same clinical response as equally effective doses of fentanyl. Since fewer molecules are given, the plasma concentrations are low and may become undetectable before sufficient time has elapsed after administration to obtain enough concentration-time points for pharmacokinetic analysis.

The pharmacokinetics of sufentanil in animals are similar to that of fentanyl, and most pharmacokinetic properties of fentanyl can be applied to sufentanil. The earliest clinical study of merit on the pharmacokinetics of sufentanil was by Bovill *et al* in ten surgical patients not scheduled for cardiac surgery or bypass who had plasma levels of sufentanil determined for 8 hours following a 5 μg·kg^{-1} dose.[98]

The sufentanil concentration–time curve was best described by a triexponential equation in which 98% of the drug was cleared from plasma by 30 minutes. The rapid distribution half-time was 1.4 minutes, whereas the slower distribution phase was 17.7 minutes. These times are similar to those seen with fentanyl. The elimination half-time for sufentanil was 2.7 hours (164 minutes), which is somewhat less than that for fentanyl (3.1–7.9 hours).

The volume of distribution for sufentanil was 1.7 $l \cdot kg^{-1}$, which is somewhat less than that for fentanyl. This smaller volume of distribution coupled with a clearance of 13 $ml \cdot kg^{-1} \cdot min^{-1}$ for sufentanil (similar to that of fentanyl) accounted for the shorter elimination half-time of sufentanil compared with that of fentanyl.

No absolutely comparable studies exist; however, two studies are of particular interest. A study by Hudson et al described the pharmacokinetics of sufentanil in ten patients (ages 53–81 years) undergoing abdominal aortic surgery.[99] These patients were induced with 7.5 $\mu g \cdot kg^{-1}$ of sufentanil at 2.5 $\mu g \cdot kg^{-1} \cdot min^{-1}$ and given 5 $\mu g \cdot kg^{-1}$ at the same rate just prior to skin incision. Plasma levels of sufentanil were measured for 14–24 hours. Greeley et al studied five adolescent patients (ages 13–18 years) who received 10–16 $\mu g \cdot kg^{-1}$ of sufentanil as a bolus and underwent cardiovascular procedures.[100] Sufentanil concentrations in plasma were measured for 5 or 20 hours (no samples were obtained during or after extracorporeal circulation in those patients requiring cardiopulmonary bypass). No consistent differences in the pharmacokinetic parameters were noted whether measured for 5 or 20 hours.

The total sufentanil clearances in the Hudson et al and Greeley et al studies were 15 and 13 $ml \cdot min^{-1} \cdot kg^{-1}$, respectively, which is consistent with the 13 $ml \cdot min^{-1} \cdot kg^{-1}$ found by Bovill et al.[98-100] The rapid distribution and slower distribution half-times were 1.6 and 24.3 minutes in the Hudson et al study and 2.6 and 20.4 minutes in the Greeley study. However, there were large differences in the elimination half-times. Hudson et al reported an elimination half-time of 12.1 hours, whereas Greeley et al reported only 3.5 hours. These differences are owing to and a reflection of the large differences in the volumes of distribution from the two studies; Hudson et al reported 8.7 $l \cdot kg^{-1}$, whereas Greeley et al reported 2.8 $l \cdot kg^{-1}$. The differences in pharmacokinetic parameters for these two studies are very significant and are not readily explained. Differences in study design, surgical procedures, and patient population all contribute. The Greeley et al study tends to support the earlier Bovill et al study.

Sufentanil is highly protein-bound. At pH 7.40, 92.5% is protein-bound.[82] This large protein binding and sufentanil's volume of distribution suggest that sufentanil is highly lipophilic and extensively bound to tissues. As with fentanyl, the rate-limiting step for elimination from the body is re-uptake from peripheral tissues. The pK_a for sufentanil is 8.01 and 80% of sufentanil is ionized at pH 7.4.[82]

The pharmacodynamics of sufentanil has not been as well studied as that of fentanyl. However, the assumed similarities of the pharmacokinetics would suggest that the dynamics of fentanyl and sufentanil are similar. This assumption has generally held true, with sufentanil having a slightly more rapid onset of effect and a slightly shorter duration of action.

Sufentanil is the most potent opioid available for clinical use, being approximately five to ten times more potent than fentanyl. Studies in rats showed a reduction of halothane MAC of 90% with an infusion of $1 \cdot 10^{-3}$ $mg \cdot kg^{-1} \cdot min^{-1}$, suggesting the possibility of complete anesthesia with sufentanil as opposed to what has been observed with fentanyl.[101] Even though 90% MAC was achieved to tail-clamp response, the rats still opened their eyes or lifted their heads in response to loud noises or jarring, suggesting that complete anesthesia was not achieved.

In dogs, the reduction of enflurane MAC by sufentanil is essentially the same as that for fentanyl. At a sufentanil concentration in plasma of 48 $ng \cdot ml^{-1}$, produced by an infusion of 1.2 $\mu g \cdot kg^{-1} \cdot min^{-1}$, the MAC of enflurane was maximally depressed by 70%.[102] Despite its increased potency, sufentanil is probably not more efficacious as a complete anesthetic and requires adjuvant drugs (N_2O, benzodiazepines, other depressants) to produce complete anesthesia.

Alfentanil

Alfentanil has pharmacokinetic and pharmacodynamic properties that permit newer, more refined methods of administration. In pharmacokinetic studies when alfentanil is administered intravenously in patients as a bolus or rapid infusion (20–200 $\mu g \cdot kg^{-1}$), the decline in plasma concentration is described by either a bi- or triexponential equation. Where found, the initial rapid distribution half-time is 0.7–3.5 minutes.[87,103,104] The slower distribution half-time is 8.2–16.8 minutes.[103-107] In one study, 90% of the dose had disappeared from plasma by 30 minutes, whereas in another study, 96.4% was gone by 60 minutes.[103,104] The terminal elimination half-time for alfentanil is very short in these surgical patients. It varies between 70 and 111 minutes (1.2–1.9 hours).[103-107] In volunteers, the elimination half-time is very similar at 97 minutes.[86] The terminal elimination half-time for alfentanil is considerably shorter than those for fentanyl (3.1–7.9 hours).[36,83-87]

The volume of distribution is 0.3–1.0 $l \cdot kg^{-1}$ in surgical patients, and 0.4 $l \cdot kg^{-1}$ in volunteers.[86,87,103-107] The volume of distribution for fentanyl is considerably larger at 3.2–5.9 $l \cdot kg^{-1}$.[36,83-86] The clearance for alfentanil is 2.8–7.9 $ml \cdot kg^{-1} \cdot min^{-1}$ in surgical patients and 3.4 $ml \cdot kg^{-1} \cdot min^{-1}$ in volunteers.[86,87,103-107] The clearance for fentanyl is 11–21 $ml \cdot kg^{-1} \cdot min^{-1}$.[36,83-86]

The pharmacokinetics of alfentanil and fentanyl were compared in an editorial by Stanski and Hug (Figs. 16-11 and 16-12).[108] The following points were made:

1. Fentanyl (like most opioids) has a high clearance, approaching that of hepatic blood flow.
2. The elimination half-time of a drug is directly proportional to the volume of distribution and inversely proportional to clearance. Fentanyl's large volume of distribution limits the amount of drug available in plasma for elimination by the liver. Release of drug by the tissues (the rate-limiting step) keeps the plasma concentration low; thus, fentanyl has a relatively long terminal elimination half-time.
3. Fentanyl's short duration of action after a single dose results from redistribution rather than elimination. After very large or multiple smaller doses, accumulation of fentanyl occurs as a result of its long half-time, and redistribution is less effective in removing fentanyl from its sites of action in the brain.
4. The smaller volume of distribution of alfentanil (about one fourth to one sixth of fentanyl's) means that there is more alfentanil in the plasma for elimination by the liver (as opposed to being stored in tissues).
5. The clearance of alfentanil is approximately one half that of fentanyl. However, "the greater decrease of alfentanil's distribution volume relative to the decrease

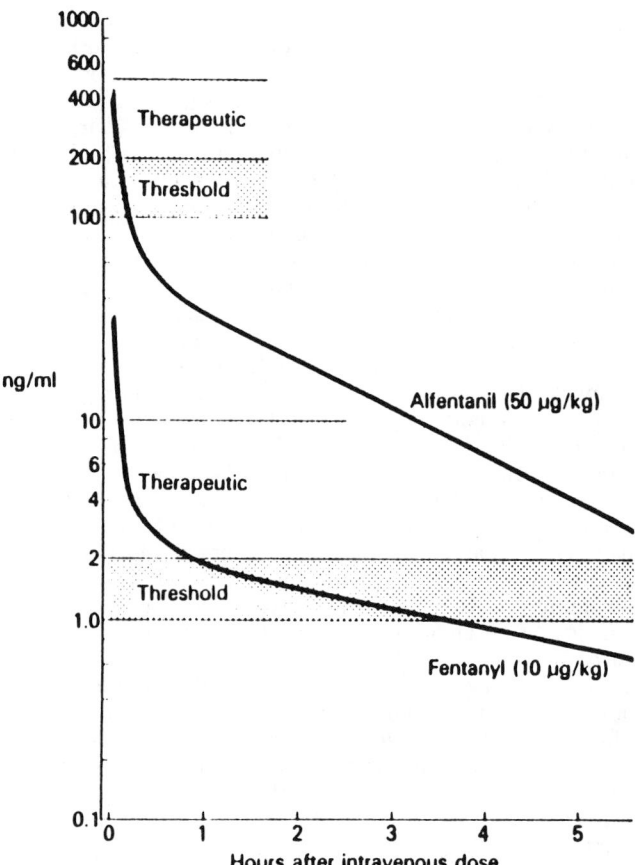

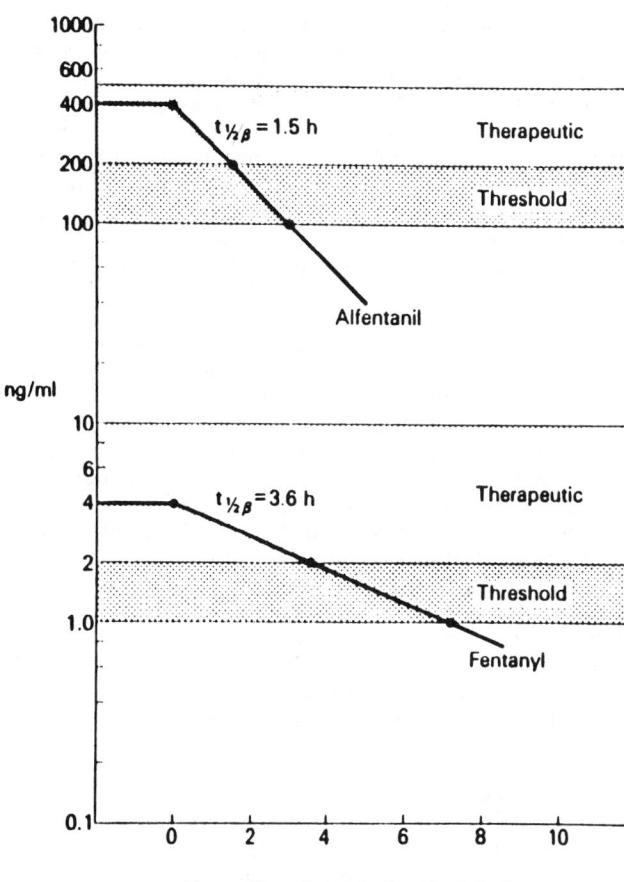

Figure 16-11. A comparison of serum decay curves following intravenous administration of fentanyl or alfentanil. Despite equivalent doses, the serum concentration of alfentanil greatly exceeds that of fentanyl owing in part to the small volume of distribution of alfentanil. (Reprinted with permission from Stanski DR, Hug CC Jr: Alfentanil—a kinetically predictable narcotic analgesic. Anesthesiology 57:435, 1982.)

Figure 16-12. The rate of decline in serum concentrations is such that concentrations compatible with spontaneous ventilation will be reached in about 3 hours after discontinuation of alfentanil and about 7.2 hours after discontinuation of fentanyl. (Reprinted with permission from Stanski DR, Hug CC Jr: Alfentanil—a kinetically predictable narcotic analgesic. Anesthesiology 57:435, 1982.)

in its clearance results in a significantly shorter terminal elimination half-time."[108]

Alfentanil is relatively lipid-soluble but considerably less so than fentanyl. The heptane:water coefficients at pH 7.4 and 37°C for alfentanil and fentanyl are 2.5 and 9.0, respectively.[86] The lower lipid solubility probably accounts for alfentanil's small volume of distribution. Alfentanil has a higher percentage of protein binding than does fentanyl. Approximately 89–92% of alfentanil is protein-bound.[86,105,107,109] However, with a pK_a of 6.5, 89% of alfentanil is non-ionized at pH 7.4. Since the non-ionized molecule moves more rapidly across biologic membranes, alfentanil's pK_a, coupled with its moderate lipid solubility, accounts for its rapid onset of action.[108,109]

Only about 0.4% of alfentanil is excreted unchanged in the urine at 24 hours following an iv bolus injection.[105] The high degree of protein binding of alfentanil decreases its glomerular filtration, whereas its prevalent non-ionized form favors reabsorption from the renal tubules.[110]

Alfentanil's small volume of distribution and short elimination half-time preclude significant accumulation of the drug in the body and render it a useful drug for continuous infusion. The rapid onset (1–2 minutes) and rapid equilibra-

tion between the plasma concentration of alfentanil and its CNS receptors also make alfentanil an excellent drug for titration to response.[93] There is a good correlation between plasma concentration and effect. Furthermore, plasma concentrations can be rapidly altered—either increased with boluses or increasing infusion doses or decreased by decreasing infusion rates—because of alfentanil's lack of accumulation and short elimination time.

Excellent data have been collected that demonstrate the plasma concentrations necessary to suppress responses to varying surgical stimuli. Although there is a 1.6 to 3.3-fold variability of concentration to suppress responses among patients anesthetized with alfentanil and 66% nitrous oxide, the response curves for individual patients is steep.[111] The plasma concentration of alfentanil that is necessary (along with 66% nitrous oxide) to obtund response to tracheal intubation in 50% of surgical patients studied (Cp_{50}) was 475 ng·ml^{-1}. The concentration necessary for skin closure was much less at 150 ng·ml^{-1}. The intensity of surgical stimulation varied considerably between these extremes. The important point is that stimulation does vary, and the amount of drug necessary to produce adequate analgesia needs to be altered frequently to meet this variation.

Alfentanil given by infusion with small bolus doses for

rapid increases in plasma levels can be used as effectively as an inhalation agent and actually probably more efficiently. High iv doses for induction (150 $\mu g \cdot kg^{-1}$) in combination with nitrous oxide rapidly establish levels sufficient for intubation of the trachea. Infusions of alfentanil can then maintain the plasma level. If the patient demonstrates no signs of light anesthesia (e.g., increases in blood pressure, heart rate, skeletal muscle movement), the infusion can progressively be decreased. If light anesthesia is noted, increases in the infusion rate and small bolus doses of alfentanil quickly restore adequate levels of analgesia. Because alfentanil does not accumulate to any significant degree in the body, the infusion can be turned off 15–20 minutes before the end of the procedure, with the likely expectation of recovery adequate for the patient to be safely taken to the postanesthesia care unit. This whole procedure is analogous to the use of a potent inhalation agent such as isoflurane.

Just as is seen with other agonist opioids, alfentanil produces a concentration-dependent reduction in the MAC of enflurane. Again, the effect plateaus at 70% reduction in enflurane MAC.[112] It is of interest that the concentration of alfentanil that produced the maximal reduction of MAC in response to tail-clamp (223 $ng \cdot ml^{-1}$) is similar to that required in combination with nitrous oxide to provide adequate anesthesia for skin incision in patients (279 $ng \cdot ml^{-1}$).[111,112] This fact suggests that the anesthetic efficacy of alfentanil in humans and dogs is similar.

DRUG INTERACTIONS

Since opioids are not complete anesthetics, they are often used in combination with other drugs (e.g., hypnotics, inhalation agents, muscle relaxants) to achieve the required anesthetic effects (unconsciousness, analgesia, skeletal muscle relaxation, and suppression of stress responses). It is known that increasing concentrations of opioids will produce a progressive decrease in the concentration of inhalation agents necessary to maintain anesthesia.[94,95,101,102] The potent inhalation agents (halothane, enflurane, isoflurane) are known dose-dependent cardiovascular depressants. Exaggerated cardiovascular depressive effects may be expected when they are added to a primarily opioid anesthetic or when opioids are added to a primarily inhalation anesthetic.[113,114] Doses of both agents may have to be significantly decreased when used in combination.

More commonly, nitrous oxide has been used in combination with the opioids to produce unconsciousness and amnesia and to potentiate analgesia in the so-called balanced anesthesia technique. In volunteers, nitrous oxide appears to produce a small negative inotropic and chronotropic cardiac effect combined with alpha stimulation of the peripheral vasculature.[115] Nitrous oxide in combination with opioids in patients has been associated with decreases in cardiac output, stroke volume, and heart rate, with variable effects on systemic vascular resistance.[116,117] These effects are measurable when nitrous oxide is added to opioids but may not be pronounced in patients with good left ventricular function. However, these myocardial depressant effects can be very significant in patients with poor left ventricular function and appear not to be the result of the opioid but primarily the nitrous oxide.[117,118] At least part of the depressant effects of nitrous oxide in the impaired heart may be related to the reduction of the inspired oxygen concentration with the high concentrations of nitrous oxide generally needed.[119]

Just as nitrous oxide is often used in combination with opioids to produce anesthesia, other hypnotics, primarily benzodiazepines and barbiturates, have been used to increase depth of anesthesia (unconsciousness) and amnesia. These combinations appear to be additive in their anesthetic-related effects.[120-122] Lower doses of both the opioid and hypnotic are needed to produce the desired state of anesthesia. Furthermore, the combination of even low to moderate doses of benzodiazepines and opioids may create a high risk for hypoxemia and apnea.[123] Thiopental in combination with morphine or fentanyl appears to antagonize some of the analgesic effect of the opioids.[121]

When benzodiazepines (e.g., diazepam, midazolam) are given alone in hypnotic (sleep-producing) doses, little or no changes in hemodynamics are seen. The same is true for high doses of fentanyl. However, the addition of low doses of a hypnotic to high doses of opioids may result in falls in blood pressure.[124] Occasionally, the effect may be profound and is characterized by decreases in blood pressure, systemic vascular resistance, and cardiac output. The hemodynamic effects are accompanied by decreases in circulating epinephrine and norepinephrine levels but no change in histamine levels with the fentanyl drugs. The mechanism appears to be an indirect centrally mediated decrease in vasoregulatory (mainly sympathetic) outflow from the CNS.[125] The reverse is also true. The addition of low doses of opioids to a benzodiazepine may result in hypotension. More frequently, the hemodynamic changes are not great when benzodiazepines and opioids are combined, and the changes produced are readily treatable. This combination is still clinically useful and commonly used to ensure amnesia.

Droperidol and scopolamine have been used as adjuvants to opioid anesthesia with insignificant hemodynamic changes. However, both have the potential for hemodynamic changes of their own, which are apparent when they are given in higher doses. Droperidol used alone occasionally produces unpleasant feelings of anxiety or excitement, even though the individual may appear very calm. These feelings are not noted when droperidol is used in combination with an opioid.

It has been suggested that the choice of muscle relaxant in combination with high-dose opioids may be important. The actions observed are an extension of the pharmacologic effects of the drugs. Opioids have a vagotonic effect and produce bradycardia. Pancuronium has a vagolytic effect and produces tachycardia. The combination may minimize or prevent changes in heart rate. The bradycardia produced by opioids may be beneficial to patients with ischemic heart disease, whereas tachycardia may increase ischemia. Vecuronium and metocurine either do not alter or may even potentiate the vagotonic effects of the opioids; lower heart rates are seen when these muscle relaxants are used.[126,127]

Drugs that affect metabolism of opioids, either directly or indirectly by decreasing liver blood flow, decrease the clearance of the opioid. Cimetidine, for instance, was shown to alter the elimination of fentanyl in dogs. Even acute administration of cimetidine, 10 $mg \cdot kg^{-1}$ intramuscularly the night before and 5 $mg \cdot kg^{-1}$ intramuscularly 90 minutes prior to 100 $\mu g \cdot kg^{-1}$ of fentanyl, resulted in an increase in the terminal elimination half-time of fentanyl from 155 to 340 minutes in these animals (Borel et al, personal communication). Propranolol has been shown to significantly decrease the first-pass uptake of fentanyl by the lungs; the potential pharmacodynamic effects have not been determined.[128] Patients who regularly consume alcohol appear to have a pharmacodynamic tolerance to alfentanil when compared with abstainers.[129]

Phenothiazines, monoamine oxidase inhibitors, and tricyclic antidepressants may exaggerate and prolong the depressant effects of opioids.[1] Severe reactions of excitation, delirium, hyperpyrexia, convulsions, and severe respiratory depression have been reported in patients on monoamine oxidase inhibitors given meperidine. Clonidine, a centrally acting preferential alpha₂-adrenergic agonist primarily used as an antihypertensive agent, has been shown to decrease opioid requirements for surgery.[130] Nifedipine, a calcium channel blocker, reportedly increased the analgesic effect of morphine postoperatively, independently of any effect on the metabolism of morphine.[131] Amphetamines enhance the analgesic effects of opioids.[1]

IMPACT OF PRE-EXISTING DISEASES

Age

Pre-existing diseases may alter responses to any drug. Choice of anesthesia-related drugs is generally determined following an evaluation of the patient's medical status and history. Many of the alterations in response (pharmacodynamics) are the result of pharmacokinetic changes produced by the disease.

Old age technically is not a disease but does produce changes in physiology and organ function that affect pharmacokinetics and pharmacodynamics. Furthermore, the elderly patient tends to have more ailments requiring drug intervention, thereby increasing the likelihood for drug interactions.

In general, increasing age is associated with decreasing ability of the kidneys and liver to clear drugs. Plasma concentrations of drugs, dependent upon clearance by these routes, may be increased in the elderly. This results in higher concentrations of the drug at sites of action. This increased action may be viewed as an increased sensitivity, because the intensity of the effect of a dose of drug seems to be greater than normal. In reality this is simply a concentration effect phenomenon. Generally, opioids are dependent on liver blood flow for clearance. Liver blood flow may be reduced by as much as 40–45% in the elderly.[132] Furthermore, enzyme function may be reduced; thus, lower doses and less frequent doses of opioids are needed in the elderly.

The elderly also tend to undergo changes in body composition. There is an increased proportion of adipose tissue in relation to body weight. Lean body mass is reduced. Lipid-soluble drugs tend to be more widely distributed with an increase in the volume of distribution.[132] There is also a decline of plasma albumin in the elderly, which may increase the free fraction for highly protein-bound drugs. Furthermore, it is possible that the blood-brain barrier is not as efficient in the elderly as in younger people, allowing more of a drug to cross from plasma to its sites of action in the CNS. This is apparently true in the fetus and newborn, in whom an immature blood-brain barrier is blamed for the apparent increased sensitivity of the neonates to certain drugs.

Although studies of the pharmacokinetics and pharmacodynamics of opioids in children are similar to those found in adults, both the elderly and neonates tend to demonstrate decreases in clearance of the opioids and increased intensity and prolongation of effects of these drugs.[83,100,133] However, variability is great, and dosages are not predictable based on age alone. It is suggested that cautious titration to the desired opioid effect, beginning with lowered initial doses, is appropriate.

Renal Disease

Only a small percentage of most opioids is excreted unchanged by the kidneys. Most of the opioids are first metabolized in the liver to metabolites that are readily excretable. Renal failure should not alter the dosage requirements tremendously. Renal failure does not appear to significantly affect the clearance of fentanyl or the fentanyl derivatives. Renal failure will result in increased concentrations of fentanyl metabolites in the plasma, but none is known to produce pharmacologic effects.

In contrast, both morphine and meperidine are metabolized to active metabolites. The major metabolite of meperidine, normeperidine, may readily accumulate to significant levels and result in prolonged respiratory depression and convulsions.[76] Meperidine is not a good choice for patients with renal failure.

The morphine-glucuronide metabolites are generally much less active than morphine, primarily because of their severely decreased ability to cross the blood-brain barrier; however, they are known to have opioid effects when injected directly into the CNS. It is possible that continued high plasma concentrations of these metabolites would result in some of the morphine-glucuronide crossing into the CNS, with resultant opioid effects. Naloxone reversible opioid toxicity has been reported as much as 1 week following the last dose of morphine in renal failure patients.[134]

Liver Disease

Because clearance of the opioids is heavily dependent on the liver, it would be anticipated that decreases in liver function or liver failure would significantly decrease the clearance of opioids. This is, in fact, the case. Pharmacokinetic studies in patients with liver failure, cirrhosis, and viral hepatitis who are given morphine, meperidine, or alfentanil usually demonstrate a tremendously smaller clearance than in normal subjects, and a prolonged elimination half-time with a relatively normal initial distribution. In these patients the volume of distribution is not significantly different from that of normal subjects.[71,135,136] Initial doses of opioids usually produce the expected intensity of effect, but it may be somewhat prolonged. Subsequent doses should be considerably lowered or delayed, since clearance of the drug is delayed and significant accumulation will result.

It is interesting that in patients with cirrhosis who were given fentanyl, 5 μg·kg^{-1} iv, no significant changes in clearance, volumes of distribution, or elimination half-time were seen. However, none of the patients in this study had severe liver disease; thus, some liver function was present. Fentanyl, unlike alfentanil, has a very large volume of distribution. Fentanyl's ultimate clearance is its reuptake from these peripheral compartments to the liver, where it is metabolized. In this instance, the amount of drug taken up from these storage areas was not great enough to saturate the liver's metabolizing systems, and no significant pharmacokinetic changes were noted. If, however, high or repeated doses of fentanyl are given, or if the patient has negligible liver function, more rapid accumulation of fentanyl will occur and a prolonged duration of effects will be found. The same reasoning is apparently true for sufentanil.[137]

Obesity

Because of the excessive adipose tissue of obese patients, it might be expected that highly lipophilic drugs such as fentanyl would have an increased volume of distribution and prolonged elimination half-time, whereas less lipophilic drugs, such as morphine, would be less affected. There are no studies to confirm the effect of obesity on morphine, but it is suggested that the dose be given according to ideal rather than actual body weight.

Fentanyl, in the only study available, was not affected by obesity. There were no significant differences of clearance, volume of distribution, or elimination half-time between normal controls and obese patients given fentanyl 10 $\mu g \cdot kg^{-1}$ intravenously.[138] It might still be assumed that accumulation of high or multiple doses will occur and prolong anesthesia, whereas responses to initial doses will be normal.

In a similar study of alfentanil (100 $\mu g \cdot kg^{-1}$ of lean body weight) in obese versus nonobese patients, it was found that the elimination half-time was double but the clearance was approximately one half the normal in the obese patients, and the volume of distribution was similar.[139] The reason for this reversal of expected results is not clear.

Neurologic Problems

It is a commonly held belief that opioids are inappropriate in patients with head trauma. The rationale is that respiratory depression and concomitant increases in CO_2 may further increase an already high intracranial pressure. Opioids may aggravate the effects of cerebral and spinal ischemia. The opioid effects of miosis, vomiting, and mental clouding may mask the important clinical signs of increasing CNS pathology.[1] In clinically useful doses, the direct effects of the synthetic opioids appear to be a parallel decrease in both cerebral blood flow and oxygen consumption with the induction of unconsciousness. These direct opioid effects are small, somewhat controversial, and probably more dependent on the combination of other anesthetic drugs.[140] In those patients in whom increased intracranial pressure is not a problem or in whom ventilation is mechanically supported, opioids are not specifically contraindicated.

CLINICAL USES OF OPIOIDS

Opioids have a number of clinical uses for the anesthesiologist. They are commonly used for premedication for surgical procedures. The feelings of well-being, warmth, and drowsiness, as well as the analgesia, make opioids a good choice for preoperative medications. They are frequently used in combination with sedatives or tranquilizers. The choice, dose, and route of administration of the opioid are dependent upon several factors, including whether the drug is given to the patient on the ward, in a preoperative holding area, or in the operating room itself. In general, longer-acting opioids such as morphine or meperidine, given intramuscularly, are used when the patient is medicated on the ward. These drugs may be given 1–3 hours prior to coming to the operating room with the expectation of a continuous, significant effect on arrival. Shorter-acting drugs such as fentanyl or sufentanil are less useful as ward premedicants because much of their activity has dissipated by the time the patient reaches the surgical suite. These shorter-acting drugs are very useful in the holding area or operating room, where they can easily be titrated to effect by incremental iv dosing. Alfentanil is probably not useful as a premedicant because of its extremely short action.

Opioids are also useful to aid induction of anesthesia. Lower doses reduce the amount of other induction agents necessary to induce anesthesia, whereas high doses may be used as the primary induction agent. The more rapid-acting fentanyl drugs are especially useful because they decrease the time necessary for induction when compared with morphine. Morphine must be given more slowly (5 $mg \cdot min^{-1}$ to avoid histamine release) and has a much slower onset of action. Meperidine has a relatively fast onset of action but cannot be used in high doses because of detrimental cardiac side-effects.

Maintenance of anesthesia is aided by opioid drugs. Again, they may be used as the primary anesthetic or in combination with the potent inhalation agents and/or nitrous oxide. The higher the dose of opioid, the less of the other anesthetic agents needed. Because of the significant myocardial depressant effects of the potent inhalation agents, opioids are frequently used in higher doses in patients with severe myocardial disease.

Most of the opioids used for clinical anesthesia have been given by infusion. Pharmacokinetic and pharmacodynamic considerations suggest that of the opioids commonly used in anesthesia, morphine is the least useful by infusion, whereas alfentanil would be the most useful, especially in shorter procedures. Fentanyl and sufentanil are often given by infusion and can be titrated so that they are fairly predictable. Alfentanil, because of its even more rapid onset and short duration, is more predictable and can be administered in a manner comparable to that in which the inhalation agents are administered.

Opioid analgesics are especially useful postoperatively for the relief of surgical pain. The choice of drugs and routes of administration are varied. For immediate control of severe pain, iv administration of rapid-acting drugs (fentanyl, sufentanil) is practical but probably will have to be repeated. Meperidine has a fairly rapid effect that will persist longer. Morphine is also excellent for postoperative pain, because it lasts longer but its onset is slower.

When patients return to the ward, most opioids are no longer given by iv route but rather intramuscularly because of the fear of respiratory depression from the high initial concentrations seen after iv injection. As discussed earlier, postoperative analgesia is frequently intermittent and inadequate. Other routes or techniques for analgesia are being increasingly used, including patient controlled analgesia pumps and epidural or intraspinal opioids. Spinally administered opioids are also used intraoperatively alone or in combination with general anesthesia. Spinal opioids have been beneficial for the relief of chronic pain syndromes.

Opioid analgesics have a role in the critical care unit, where they are used not only for relief of pain but also to help maintain patient comfort while on mechanical ventilation. The pharmacologic effects of the opioids make them excellent drugs for the mechanically ventilated patient. Depression of the cough reflex increases tolerance of the endotracheal tube; depression of ventilation helps prevent the patient from "fighting the ventilator"; sedation decreases anxiety; and analgesia increases patient comfort. No other single class of drugs will produce all these benefits for the mechanically ventilated patient.

OPIOID AGONIST-ANTAGONISTS AND PARTIAL AGONISTS

The agonist-antagonists and partial agonist drugs are characterized by their binding to opioid receptors, and the various effects produced reflect this binding (Table 16-4). The morphine-like drugs (agonists) are noted for their mu receptor activity—supraspinal analgesia, dose-dependent respiratory depression, and euphoria. Agonists–antagonists are thought to bind to mu receptors and can compete with the agonist for these sites. At mu receptors, either they may exert no action (competitive antagonist) or they may exert limited actions (partial agonists).[1] Buprenorphine (and the investigational drugs meptazinol, profadol, and propiram) have a high affinity for mu receptors but a low intrinsic activity (partial agonists). Nalorphine, pentazocine, nalbuphine, and butorphanol are competitive antagonists at mu receptors (and block the effects of morphine-like drugs) but have agonistic activity at other receptors (kappa and sigma). These drugs are classified as agonist-antagonists. It is believed that these drugs produce their analgesic and respiratory depressant effects by interaction with kappa receptors and that their psychomimetic and dysphoric effects are mediated by actions at the sigma receptors (Table 16-4). Agonist–antagonist opioid drugs are useful for the study of the opioid receptors and have stimulated the search for opioids with high analgesic potency, absent or limited respiratory depression, and low abuse potential.

Pentazocine

Pentazocine appears to produce its analgesic effects primarily by its agonistic activity at the kappa receptors. Parenterally, pentazocine is approximately one fourth as potent as morphine but exhibits a ceiling to both its respiratory depressant and analgesic effects. Doses beyond 30–50 mg do not produce proportionate increases in respiratory depression or analgesia. However, as the dose is increased, there is a high incidence of dysphoric, psychomimetic, and hallucinatory effects.

Pentazocine-related cardiovascular changes may be particularly significant to patients with reduced myocardial reserve. Pentazocine produces increases in systemic and pulmonary artery pressures, left ventricular end-diastolic pressure, and cardiac work.[141] It increases plasma epinephrine and norepinephrine concentrations unrelated to respiratory depression or carbon dioxide accumulation.[1]

Pentazocine has limited use for the anesthesiologist because of its dysphoric and cardiovascular effects as well as its limited analgesic effects. It also has significant abuse potential and can produce physical dependency. If given in sufficient doses to subjects dependent upon agonist analgesics, pentazocine produces withdrawal symptoms as a result of its mu antagonistic actions.[1]

Butorphanol

Butorphanol is a moderately potent analgesic that appears to have weak antagonistic effects at the mu receptors. It can be used before or after morphine-like drugs without tremendously altering their analgesic or anesthetic properties. However, butorphanol has been demonstrated to improve ventilation and the response to carbon dioxide following fentanyl, nitrous oxide, isoflurane anesthesia.[142]

Butorphanol is approximately five times more potent than morphine. A parenteral dose of 2–3 mg produces respiratory depression and analgesia equivalent to approximately 10 mg of morphine with an onset, peak, and duration of action similar to those of morphine.[1] Like pentazocine, its ventilatory depressant, analgesic, and anesthetic sparing effects do not increase proportional to dose and are limited. In dogs, butorphanol decreases the MAC for enflurane by 11% at a dose of 0.1 mg·kg^{-1}.[15] Doses 40 times larger do not further decrease MAC. Patients given 0.15 or 0.3 mg·kg^{-1} are easily aroused and follow commands appropriately (Moldenhauer CC et al, personal communication). Although butorphanol is limited as a primary anesthetic, it has been successfully used in conjunction with nitrous oxide or the potent inhalation agents in a balanced technique. Its cardiovascular effects are similar to those of pentazocine. The adjuvant agents used to produce balanced anesthesia in combination with butorphanol increase myocardial depression, which could be significant in cardiovascularly impaired patients but is probably not significant in healthy patients.

TABLE 16-4. Interactions of Morphine and Morphine-like Drugs with Opioid Receptors

	Receptor Types		
	μ	κ	σ
Effects	Supraspinal analgesia	Spinal analgesia	Dysphoria
	Respiratory depression	Respiratory depression	Hallucinations
	Euphoria	Sedation	Vasomotor stimulation
	Physical dependence	Miosis	
Drugs			
Morphine	Ag	Ag	0
Buprenorphine	pAg	—	0
Nalorphine	Ant	pAg	Ag
Pentazocine	Ant	Ag	Ag
Butorphanol	0	Ag	Ag
Nalbuphine	pAg/Ant	Ag	Ag
Naloxone	Ant	Ant	Ant

Abbreviations: Ag, agonist; pAg, partial agonist; Ant, antagonist; 0, no interaction.

Used with permission from Hug CC Jr: Semin Anesth 1:14, 1982.

The psychomimetic effects of butorphanol are similar to those of pentazocine at equianalgesic doses, but the incidence is somewhat less.[1] Since butorphanol has minimal mu receptor actions, it does not suppress or produce a withdrawal syndrome in patients dependent upon morphine-like drugs. Its abuse potential is considered minimal.

Nalbuphine

Nalbuphine is structurally related to the mu agonist oxymorphone and the antagonist naloxone.[1] It produces its analgesic effects at kappa receptors and is a moderately potent antagonist at mu receptors. It is considered equipotent to morphine at analgesic doses; 10 mg of im nalbuphine is approximately equivalent to 10 mg of im morphine. Nalbuphine has an onset, peak, and duration of effect similar to morphine. However, like other agonist-antagonist opioids, nalbuphine is limited in its effects. A dose of 0.5 mg·kg^{-1} of nalbuphine given intravenously in dogs reduced enflurane MAC by 8%.[15] Doses as high as 20 mg·kg^{-1} did not further decrease MAC. A ceiling effect for analgesia and ventilatory depression by nalbuphine has also been demonstrated in volunteers given nalbuphine or morphine in successive 0.15 mg·kg^{-1} doses.[143] Successive doses of morphine produced increasing ventilatory depression and analgesia in response to experimental pain. The initial dose of nalbuphine resulted in similar pain reduction and ventilatory depression as seen with morphine. However, further doses did not increase analgesia or ventilatory depression, and the authors concluded that the ceiling effect for respiratory depression of nalbuphine is paralleled by its limited analgesic effects. This study confirmed an earlier study that demonstrated a ceiling effect for respiratory depression by nalbuphine at 30 mg·70 kg^{-1}, which was equivalent to a morphine dose of 20 mg·70 kg^{-1}.[144] In surgical patients, nalbuphine doses as high as 3 mg·kg^{-1} were not sufficient to produce anesthesia and required the addition of diazepam, nitrous oxide, or halothane.[145] The Pco$_2$ remained at 45 mm Hg or less. Unlike pentazocine or butorphanol, nalbuphine does not appear to produce deleterious hemodynamic effects when given to patients with stable coronary artery disease or acute myocardial infarction.[1,145]

Nalbuphine produces fewer psychic side-effects than other agonist-antagonists at analgesic doses. It may produce an abstinence syndrome in subjects dependent upon morphine-like drugs.[1] The abuse potential is similar to that of pentazocine.

Because of the lower incidence of psychic side-effects and the hemodynamic stability noted with even high doses of nalbuphine, it has proved to be an effective drug to reverse the ventilatory depression of mu agonist-type drugs while maintaining reasonable analgesia. Nalbuphine has been shown to antagonize ventilatory depression produced by moderate and high doses of fentanyl.[146,147] High doses 0.1 to 0.3 mg·kg^{-1} iv) of nalbuphine have been used to antagonize opioid-induced ventilatory depression in noncardiac patients without adverse sequelae. In post–cardiac surgery patients, incremental doses (15 μg·kg^{-1}) of nalbuphine up to a total of 1–10 mg effectively decreased Pco$_2$ below 50 mm Hg, allowing extubation of the trachea of patients in the intensive care unit following fentanyl doses as high as 120 μg·kg^{-1}.[147] Adequate analgesia was maintained. Although the hemodynamic effects produced by nalbuphine are minimal, the rapid, partial reversal of the analgesia produced by mu agonists could result in significant catecholamine release. Titration to response is therefore recommended, es-

pecially in patients with limited cardiac reserve. Furthermore, respiratory depression will be produced by the nalbuphine itself. There is a ceiling to the depression, but nonetheless it is significant. The analgesia also has a ceiling, and in cases of severe pain, nalbuphine may not be adequate for pain control. Finally, renarcotization is a possibility, especially when lower doses of nalbuphine are titrated to minimal reversal of ventilatory depression.

Buprenorphine

Buprenorphine is a partial mu agonist that is highly lipophilic and can be administered sublingually, intramuscularly, or intravenously. Buprenorphine is 25 to 50 times more potent than morphine and produces analgesia and other CNS effects that are qualitatively similar to those of morphine.[1] Intramuscular doses of 0.4 mg, equivalent to about 10 mg of morphine, have a slower onset of effect and a prolonged duration of action. Peak respiratory depression may not occur for 3 hours. There is little relationship between the plasma concentration and duration of effect.

Depression of ventilation and other effects of buprenorphine can be prevented by prior administration of naloxone. However, because buprenorphine dissociates very slowly from mu receptors, even high doses of naloxone will not readily reverse the effects of buprenorphine once they have been produced.[1,148] Antagonism of ventilatory depression has been elicited by the stimulant effects of doxapram, but an infusion may be necessary because of the prolonged effect of buprenorphine.[148] Although there is probably a ceiling effect to the ventilatory depression produced by buprenorphine (it has been used to reverse fentanyl and sufentanil depression), significant clinical ventilatory depression has been reported.[148,149]

Buprenorphine is not useful as a sole anesthetic but is a satisfactory supplement for balanced anesthesia and is useful for postoperative pain management.[148-150] Because it is only a partial mu agonist but dissociates slowly from the receptor, buprenorphine may limit the effect of morphine-like drugs when given in conjunction with them. Buprenorphine may not be a good premedicant drug if mu agonists are to be used for anesthesia. It will also decrease the ability of mu agonists to relieve severe pain.

Hemodynamic effects are mild, even in cardiovascularly impaired patients. Usually, decreases in heart rate are seen, along with slight decreases in blood pressure.[148] The incidence of psychomimetic effects is low. A withdrawal syndrome, similar to that produced by morphine abstinence, can be seen when chronically administered buprenorphine is discontinued, with a delayed onset of up to 15 days. Buprenorphine can block or attenuate the subjective and physiologic effects of subcutaneous morphine (in doses of up to 120 mg) and has been suggested as a methadone substitute for the treatment of opioid addiction.[1] Buprenorphine has also been used as an epidural analgesic with effects similar to those of morphine.

Dezocine

Dezocine is an agonist-antagonist opioid that is as potent as or slightly more potent than morphine on a milligram per milligram basis. It has a more rapid onset and slightly shorter duration of action than morphine. Side-effects are similar, although dezocine does not appear to release histamine, at least in lower doses.[1,151] Studies in dogs suggest that dezocine may be more efficacious as an anesthetic supplement than other agonist-antagonists. A 58% reduction of enflurane MAC was produced in dogs with an iv dose of 20 mg·kg^{-1} of dezocine. This reduction is almost equal to the maximal reduction produced by the opioid agonists morphine and fentanyl (65%) studied under the same experimental conditions.[15,94,152] The upward slope of the dose-response curve at the 20 mg·kg^{-1} dose of dezocine suggested that greater reductions might be achieved at higher doses; however, this and higher doses were accompanied by severe hypotension or death in the enflurane anesthetized dog, primarily as a result of myocardial depression.[152] Dezocine is considerably more effective than other opioid agonist–antagonists as an anesthetic supplement, but further clinical studies are needed to determine its safety in high clinical doses.

ANTAGONISTS

Naloxone and naltrexone are oxymorphone derivatives that are generally considered to be "pure" antagonist opioids. Both drugs are competitive antagonists at mu, delta, kappa, and sigma opioid receptors. In moderate doses, they demonstrate no discernible activity except in the presence of stimulation of the opioid agonist receptors, either by drugs with agonist opioid effects or when the endogenous opioid systems are stimulated.[1] At very high doses, special effects of little clinical importance have been reported. Naloxone, at doses in excess of 0.3 mg·kg^{-1}, produces increases in systolic blood pressure and decreases performance on tests of memory.[1] Naltrexone, at high doses, may have produced mild dysphoria in one study, but no subjective effects were found in several other studies.[1]

Naloxone is used clinically to reverse unwanted opioid agonist effects (generally ventilatory depression and sedation). Remember that all opioid effects are reversed in parallel, including analgesia. The initial injection of high doses of naloxone postoperatively to patients given opioids for surgical procedures not only rapidly reverses respiratory depression but also suddenly unmasks pain, which may result in significant sympathetic and cardiovascular stimulation that may be detrimental to the patient. Intravenous bolus injections of naloxone, 0.1–0.4 mg, have resulted in reports of hypertension, atrial and ventricular dysrhythmias, pulmonary edema, and cardiac arrest.[153] It is suggested that, where possible, ventilation should be supported and naloxone titrated in incremental iv doses of 20–40 µg until the patient is appropriately ventilating but still comfortable.

Naloxone is readily titrated to response because it has a very rapid onset of effect. Peak effects are seen within 1–2 minutes after iv injection, since naloxone rapidly enters the brain.[154] The pharmacologic duration of effect is dose-dependent, but at appropriate doses it can be expected to be approximately 1–4 hours.[1] The plasma half-time of naloxone is 60–90 minutes.[154,155] The concentration of naloxone in the brain parallels that in the plasma. Naloxone is primarily cleared by metabolism in the liver.[1,155] The major metabolite is naloxone-3-glucuronide.

Because of naloxone's short half-time, there is a chance that renarcotization of patients may occur when naloxone has been used to reverse longer-acting opioids. Patients should be closely monitored for renarcotization. In one study, it was found that 5–10 µg·kg^{-1} of naloxone would readily reverse the ventilatory depression of 1.25–1.5 mg·kg^{-1} of morphine, but all the patients became renarco-

tized.[156] Satisfactory and prolonged reversal of morphine's ventilatory depression was achieved by a single 5 µg·kg^{-1} iv dose of naloxone followed 15 minutes later by a 10 µg·kg^{-1} im dose.

A more efficient method for titrating reversal is the use of a naloxone infusion. Intravenous infusions of naloxone in the range of 3–10 µg·kg^{-1}·hr^{-1}, following initial loading doses of 1.5–3.5 µg·kg^{-1}, have successfully been used to reverse the ventilatory depression of high doses of morphine (2 mg·kg^{-1}) and fentanyl (>100 µg·kg^{-1}).[157,158] These infusion rates are also useful to suppress the side-effects of spinal opioids, especially ventilatory depression and pruritus.[159] Infusion rates should be increased or decreased according to patient response.

Naloxone has been reported to be useful in the treatment of overdoses of alcohol, benzodiazepines, barbiturates, and clonidine; diagnosing physical dependency; and treating opioid addicts. Naloxone can be used to reverse the effects of agonist-antagonist opioids, but generally higher doses of naloxone are necessary because it has a greater affinity for mu receptors than for kappa and sigma receptors. Animal studies indicate that naloxone may be beneficial in the treatment of endotoxic and hypovolemic shock.

Naltrexone is a longer-acting competitive mu receptor antagonist, which is available for oral administration. Naloxone is not used orally, because most is rapidly metabolized in its first passage through the liver.[1] Naltrexone is used in oral doses of 100 mg or greater to prevent the euphoric effects of opioids in addicted patients.[1] Peak plasma concentrations are found within 1–2 hours, and the plasma half-time is 10 hours. Naltrexone has also been used to counteract the side-effects of spinal opioids used for chronic pain therapy or cesarean section. Oral naltrexone in doses of 3–12.5 mg has been shown to decrease the incidence of pruritus, nausea, and somnolence when administered prophylactically to cesarean section patients given intrathecal or epidural morphine. However, the incidence of pruritus was still high, and analgesia tended to be reversed at the higher doses.[160]

REFERENCES

1. Jaffe JH, Martin WR: Opioid analgesics and antagonists. In Gilman AG, Goodman LS, Rall TW et al (eds): The Pharmacological Basis of Therapeutics, 7th ed, p 491. New York, Macmillan, 1985
2. Foldes FF, Swerdlow M, Siker ES: Narcotics and Narcotic Antagonists, p 3. Springfield, Illinois, Charles C Thomas, 1964
3. Smith RR: Scopolamine-morphine anesthesia, with report of two hundred and twenty-nine cases. Surg Gynecol Obstet 7:414, 1908
4. Sexton JC: Death following scopolamine-morphine injection. Lancet 55:582, 1905
5. Neff W, Mayer EC, Perales M: Nitrous oxide and oxygen anesthesia with curare relaxation. Calif Med 66:67, 1947
6. Bailey P, Gerbode F, Garlington L: An anesthetic technique for cardiac surgery which utilizes 100% oxygen as the only inhalant. Arch Surg 76:437, 1958
7. Lowenstein E, Hallowell P, Levine FH et al: Cardiovascular response to large doses of intravenous morphine in man. N Engl J Med 281:1389, 1969
8. Stanley TH, Gray NG, Stanford W et al: The effects of high-dose morphine on fluid and blood requirements in open-heart operations. Anesthesiology 38:536, 1973
9. Lasagna L, Beecher HK: The analgesic effectiveness of nalorphine and nalorphine–morphine combinations in man. J Pharmacol Exp Ther 122:356, 1965
10. Martin WR: Opioid antagonists. Pharmacol Rev 10:452, 1967

11. Pasternak GW: Multiple morphine and enkephalin receptors and the relief of pain. JAMA 259:1362, 1988

12. Simon EJ: Opioid peptides and their receptors. In Estafanous FG (ed): Opioids in anesthesia II, p 20. Boston, Butterworth-Heinemann, 1991

13. Akil H, Watson SJ, Young E et al: Endogenous opioids: Biology and function. Ann Rev Neurosci 7:223, 1984

14. Kitahata LM, Collins JG, Robinson CJ: Narcotic effects on the nervous system. In Kitahata LM, Collins JG (eds): Narcotic Analgesics in Anesthesiology, p 57. Baltimore, Williams & Wilkins, 1982

15. Murphy MR, Hug CC Jr: The enflurane sparing effect of morphine, butorphanol, and nalbuphine. Anesthesiology 57:489, 1982

16. Lowenstein E: Morphine "anesthesia"—A perspective. Anesthesiology 35:563, 1971

17. Mummaneni N, Rao TLK, Montoya A: Awareness and recall with high-dose fentanyl–oxygen anesthesia. Anesth Analg 59:948, 1980

18. Barash P, Kopriva C, Giles R et al: Global ventricular function and intubation: Radionuclear profiles. Anesthesiology 53:S109, 1980

19. de Castro J, van de Walter A, Wouters L et al: Comparative study of cardiovascular, neurological and metabolic side-effects of eight narcotics in dogs. Acta Anaesthesiol Belg 30:5, 1979

20. Moldenhauer CC, Hug CC Jr: Use of narcotic analgesics as anaesthetics. Clin Anaesthesiology 2(1):107, 1984

21. Smith NT, Benthuysen JL, Bickford RG et al: Seizures during opioid anesthetic induction—are they opioid induced rigidity? Anesthesiology 71:852, 1989

22. Reitan JA, Stengert KB, Wymore MC et al: Central vagal control of fentanyl induced bradycardia during halothane anesthesia. Anesth Analg 57:31, 1978

23. Laubie M, Schmitt H, Vincent M: Vagal bradycardia produced by microinjections of morphine-like drugs into the nucleus ambiguus in anesthetized dogs. Eur J Pharmacol 59:287, 1979

24. Liu WS, Bidwai AV, Stanley TH et al: Cardiovascular dynamics after large doses of fentanyl and fentanyl plus N_2O in the dog. Anesth Analg 55:168, 1976

25. Urthaler F, Isobe JH, Gilmour KE et al: Morphine and autonomic control of the sinus node. Chest 64:203, 1973

26. Urthaler F, Isobe JH, James TN: Direct and vagally mediated chronotropic effects of morphine studied by selective perfusion of the sinus node of awake dogs. Chest 68:222, 1975

27. Goldberg AH, Padget CH: Comparative effects of morphine and fentanyl on isolated heart muscle. Anesth Analg 48:978, 1969

28. Strauer BE: Contractile responses to morphine, piritramide, meperidine and fentanyl: A comparative study of effects on the isolated ventricular myocardium. Anesthesiology 37:304, 1972

29. Freye E: Cardiovascular effects of high doses of fentanyl, meperidine and naloxone in dogs. Anesth Analg 53:40, 1974

30. Lowenstein E, Whiting RB, Bittar DA: Local and neurally mediated effects of morphine on skeletal muscle vascular resistance. J Pharmacol Exp Ther 180:359, 1972

31. Ward JW, McGrath RL, Weil JV: Effects of morphine on the peripheral vascular response to sympathetic stimulation. Am J Cardiol 29:656, 1972

32. Rosow CE, Moss I, Philbin DM et al: Histamine release during morphine and fentanyl anesthesia. Anesthesiology 56:93, 1982

33. Flacke JW, Flacke WE, Bloor BC et al: Histamine release by four narcotics: A double-blind study in humans. Anesth Analg 66:723, 1987

34. White DA, Reitan JA, Kien ND et al: Decrease in vascular resistance in the isolated canine hindlimb after graded doses of alfentanil, fentanyl, and sufentanil. Anesth Analg 71:29, 1990

35. Blaise GA, Witzeling TM, Sill JC et al: Fentanyl is devoid of major effects on coronary vasoreactivity and myocardial metabolism in experimental animals. Anesthesiology 72:535, 1990

36. McClain DA, Hug CC Jr: Intravenous fentanyl kinetics. Clin Pharmacol Ther 28:106, 1980

37. Hug CC Jr, Murphy MR: Fentanyl disposition in cerebrospinal fluid and plasma and its relationship to ventilatory depression in the dog. Anesthesiology 50:342, 1979

38. Hug CC Jr, Murphy MR, Rigel EP et al: Pharmacokinetics of morphine injected intravenously into the anesthetized dog. Anesthesiology 54:38, 1981

39. Epstein BS, Wurm SB: Opioids for monitored anesthesia care. In Estafanous FG (ed): Opioids in anesthesia II, p 179. Boston, Butterworth-Heinemann, 1991

40. Becker L, Paulson B, Miller R et al: Biphasic respiratory depression after fentanyl-droperidol or fentanyl alone used to supplement nitrous oxide anesthesia. Anesthesiology 44:291, 1976

41. Kaufman RD, Agleh KA, Bellville JW: Relative potencies and duration of action with respect to respiratory depression of intravenous meperidine, fentanyl and alphaprodine in man. J Pharmacol Exp Ther 208:73, 1979

42. Bellville JW, Seed JC: The effect of drugs on the respiratory response to carbon dioxide. Anesthesiology 21:727, 1960

43. Forrest WH, Bellville JW: The effect of sleep plus morphine on the respiratory response to carbon dioxide. Anesthesiology 25:137, 1964

44. Ruskis AF: Effects of narcotics on the gastrointestinal tract, liver, and kidneys. In Kitahata LM, Collins JG (eds): Narcotic Analgesics in Anesthesiology, p 143. Baltimore, Williams & Wilkins, 1982

45. Radnay PA, Brodman E, Mankikar D et al: The effect of equi-analgesic doses of fentanyl, morphine, meperidine and pentazocine on common bile duct pressure. Anaesthetist 29:26, 1980

46. de Lange S, Stanley TH, Boscoe JM et al: Catecholamine and cortisol responses to sufentanil-O_2 and alfentanil-O_2 anaesthesia during coronary artery surgery. Can Anaesth Soc J 30:248, 1983

47. Bovill JG, Sebel PS, Fiolet JWT et al: The influence of sufentanil on endocrine and metabolic responses to cardiac surgery. Anesth Analg 62:391, 1983

48. Anand KJS, Sippell WG, Aynsley-Green A: Randomized trial of fentanyl anaesthesia in preterm babies undergoing surgery: Effects on the stress response. Lancet 1:243, 1987

49. Clark RB, Seifen AB: Systemic medication during labor and delivery. In Wynn RM (ed): Obstetrics and Gynecology Annual, vol 12, p 165. Norwalk, Connecticut, Appleton-Century-Crofts, 1983

50. Brooks GZ, Ngeow YF: Narcotics: mother, fetus, and neonate. In Kitahata LM, Collins JG (eds): Narcotic Analgesics in Anesthesiology, p 157. Baltimore, Williams & Wilkins, 1982

51. Goldberg M, Ishak S, Garcia C et al: Postoperative rigidity following sufentanil administration. Anesthesiology 63:199, 1985

52. Jaffe TB, Ramsey FM: Attenuation of fentanyl-induced truncal rigidity. Anesthesiology 58:562, 1983

53. Scamman FL: Fentanyl-O_2-N_2O rigidity and pulmonary compliance. Anesth Analg 63:332, 1983

54. Benthuysen JL, Smith NT, Sanford TT et al: Physiology of alfentanil-induced rigidity. Anesthesiology 64:440, 1986

55. Bennett MJ, Anderson LK, McMillan JC et al: Anaphylactic reaction during anaesthesia associated with positive intradermal skin test to fentanyl. Can Anaesth Soc J 33:75, 1986

56. Levy JH, Brister NW, Shearin A et al: Wheal and flare responses to opioids in humans. Anesthesiology 70:756, 1989

57. Murphy MR, Hug CC Jr: Pharmacokinetics of intravenous morphine in patients anesthetized with enflurane-nitrous oxide. Anesthesiology 54:187, 1981

58. Stanski DR, Greenblatt DJ, Lowenstein E: Kinetics of intravenous and intramuscular morphine. Clin Pharmacol Ther 24:52, 1978

59. Dahlström B, Bolme P, Feychting J et al: Morphine kinetics in children. Clin Pharmacol Ther 26:354, 1979

60. Stanski DR, Paalzow L, Edlund PO: Morphine pharmacokinetics: GLC assay versus radioimmunoassay. J Pharm Sci 71:314, 1982

61. Yeh SY: Urinary excretion of morphine and its metabolites in morphine-dependent subjects. J Pharmacol Exp Ther 192:201, 1975

62. Brunk SF, Delle M: Morphine metabolism in man. Clin Pharmacol Ther 16:51, 1974

63. Olsen GD: Morphine binding to human plasma proteins. Clin Pharmacol Ther 17:31, 1975

64. Höllt V, Teschemacher H-J: Hydrophobic interactions responsible for unspecific binding of morphine-like drugs. Naunyn Schmiedebergs Arch Pharmacol 288:163, 1975

65. Kaufmann JJ, Semo NM, Koski WS: Microelectrometric titration measurement of the pK$_a$'s and partition and drug distribution coefficients of narcotics and narcotic antagonists and their pH and temperature dependence. J Med Chem 18:647, 1975

66. Herz A, Teschemacher H-J: Activities and sites of antinociceptive action of morphine-like analgesics. In Harper NJ, Simmonds AB (eds): Advances in Drug Research, p 79. New York, Academic Press, 1971

67. Nishitateno K, Ngai SH, Finck AD et al: Pharmacokinetics of morphine: Concentrations in the serum and brain of the dog during hyperventilation. Anesthesiology 50:520, 1979

68. Lake CL, DiFazio CA, Moscicki JC et al: Reduction in halothane MAC: Comparison of morphine and alfentanil. Anesth Analg 64:807, 1985

69. Mather LE, Tucker GT, Pflug AE et al: Meperidine kinetics in man: Intravenous injections in surgical patients and volunteers. Clin Pharmacol Ther 17:21, 1975

70. Stambaugh JE, Wainer IW, Sanstead JK: The clinical pharmacology of meperidine—Comparison of routes of administration. J Clin Pharmacol 16:245, 1976

71. Klotz U, McHorse TS, Wilkinson GR et al: The effect of cirrhosis on the disposition and elimination of meperidine in man. Clin Pharmacol Ther 16:667, 1974

72. Fung DL, Asling JH, Eisele JH et al: A comparison of alphaprodine and meperidine pharmacokinetics. J Clin Pharmacol 20:37, 1980

73. Dunkerley R, Johnson R, Schenker S et al: Gastric and biliary excretion of meperidine in man. Clin Pharmacol Ther 20:546, 1976

74. Verbeeck RK, Branch RA, Wilkinson GR: Meperidine disposition in man: Influence of urinary pH and route of administration. Clin Pharmacol Ther 30:619, 1981

75. Chan K, Tse J, Jennings F et al: Pharmacokinetics of low-dose intravenous pethidine in patients with renal dysfunction. J Clin Pharmacol 27:516, 1987

76. Szeto HH, Inturrisi CE, Houde R et al: Accumulation of normeperidine, an active metabolite of meperidine, in patients with renal failure or cancer. Ann Intern Med 86:738, 1977

77. Austin KL, Stapleton JV, Mather LE: Multiple intramuscular injections: A major source of variability in analgesic response to meperidine. Pain 8:47, 1980

78. Austin KL, Stapleton JV, Mather LE: Relationship between blood meperidine concentrations and analgesic response: A preliminary report. Anesthesiology 53:460, 1980

79. Hug CC Jr: Improving analgesic therapy. Anesthesiology 53:441, 1980

80. Stapleton JV, Austin KL, Mather LE: A pharmacokinetic approach to postoperative pain: Continuous infusion of pethidine. Anaesth Intensive Care 7:25, 1979

81. Reilly CS, Wood AJJ, Wood M: Variability of fentanyl pharmacokinetics in man. Computer predicted plasma concentrations for three intravenous dosage regimens. Anaesthesia 40:837, 1984

82. Mather LE: Clinical pharmacokinetics of fentanyl and its newer derivatives. Clin Pharmacokinet 8:422, 1983

83. Bentley JB, Borel JD, Nenad RE et al: Age and fentanyl pharmacokinetics. Anesth Analg 61:968, 1982

84. Koska AJ, Romagnoli A, Kramer WG: Effect of cardiopulmonary bypass on fentanyl distribution and elimination. Clin Pharmacol Ther 29:100, 1981

85. Haberer JP, Schoeffler P, Couderc E et al: Fentanyl pharmacokinetics in anaesthetized patients with cirrhosis. Br J Anaesth 54:1267, 1982

86. Bower S, Hull CJ: Comparative pharmacokinetics of fentanyl and alfentanil. Br J Anaesth 54:871, 1982

87. Scott JC, Stanski DR: Decreased fentanyl and alfentanil dose requirements with age. A simultaneous pharmacokinetic and pharmacodynamic evaluation. J Pharmacol Exp Ther 240:159, 1987

88. Murphy MR, Olson WA, Hug CC Jr: Pharmacokinetics of ^{3}H-fentanyl in the dog anesthetized with enflurane. Anesthesiology 50:13, 1979

89. Hug CC Jr, Murphy MR: Tissue redistribution of fentanyl and termination of effect in rats. Anesthesiology 55:369, 1981

90. Taeger K, Weninger E, Schmelzer F et al: Pulmonary kinetics of fentanyl and alfentanil in surgical patients. Br J Anaesth 61:425, 1988

91. Hug CC Jr, Murphy MR, Sampson JF et al: Biotransformation of morphine and fentanyl in anhepatic dogs. Anesthesiology 55:A261, 1981

92. Harper MH, Hickey RF, Cromwell TH et al: The magnitude and duration of respiratory depression produced by fentanyl and fentanyl plus droperidol in man. J Pharmacol Exp Ther 199:464, 1976

93. Scott JC, Ponganis KV, Stanski DR: EEG quantitation of narcotic effect: The comparative pharmacodynamics of fentanyl and alfentanil. Anesthesiology 62:234, 1985

94. Murphy MR, Hug CC Jr: The anesthetic potency of fentanyl in terms of its reduction of enflurane MAC. Anesthesiology 57:485, 1982

95. Murphy MR, Hug CC Jr: Efficacy of fentanyl in reducing isoflurane MAC; antagonism by naloxone and nalbuphine. Anesthesiology 59:A338, 1983

96. Arndt JO, Mikat M, Parasher C: Fentanyl's analgesic, respiratory, and cardiovascular actions in relation to dose and plasma concentration in unanesthetized dogs. Anesthesiology 61:355, 1984

97. Sprigge JS, Wynands JE, Whalley DG et al: Fentanyl infusion anesthesia for aortocoronary bypass surgery: Plasma levels and hemodynamic response. Anesth Analg 61:972, 1982

98. Bovill JG, Sebel PS, Blackburn CL et al: The pharmacokinetics of sufentanil in surgical patients. Anesthesiology 61:502, 1984

99. Hudson RJ, Bergstrom RG, Thomson IR et al: Pharmacokinetics of sufentanil in patients undergoing abdominal aortic surgery. Anesthesiology 70:426, 1989

100. Greeley WJ, Bruijn NP, Davis DP: Sufentanil pharmacokinetics in pediatric cardiovascular patients. Anesth Analg 66:1067, 1987

101. Hecker BR, Lake CL, DeFazio CA et al: The decrease of the minimum alveolar anesthetic concentration produced by sufentanil in rats. Anesth Analg 62:987, 1983

102. Hall RI, Murphy MR, Hug CC Jr: The enflurane sparing effect of sufentanil in dogs. Anesthesiology 67:518, 1987

103. Camu F, Gepts E, Rucquoi M et al: Pharmacokinetics of alfentanil in man. Anesth Analg 61:657, 1982

104. Bovill JG, Sebel PS, Blackburn CL et al: The pharmacokinetics of alfentanil (R39209). A new opioid analgesic. Anesthesiology 57:439, 1982

105. Schüttler J, Stoeckel H: Alfentanil (R39209) a new, short-action opiate: Pharmacokinetics and preliminary clinical experience. Anaesthesist 31:10, 1982

106. McDonnell TE, Bartkowski RR, Bonilla FA et al: Nonuniformity of alfentanil pharmacokinetics in healthy adults. Anesthesiology 57:A236, 1982

107. Meistelman C, Saint-Maurice C, Lepaul M et al: A comparison of alfentanil pharmacokinetics in children and adults. Anesthesiology 66:13, 1987

108. Stanski DR, Hug CC Jr: Alfentanil—A kinetically predictable narcotic analgesic. Anesthesiology 57:435, 1982

109. Meuldermans WEG, Hurkmans RMA, Heykants JJP: Plasma protein binding and distribution of fentanyl, sufentanil, alfentanil and lofentanil in blood. Arch Int Pharmacodyn Ther 257:4, 1982

110. Hug CC Jr, Chaffman M: Alfentanil: Pharmacology and Uses in Anesthesia, p 1. Auckland, New Zealand, ADIS Press, 1984

111. Ausems ME, Hug CC Jr, Stanski DR et al: Plasma concentra-

tions of alfentanil required to supplement nitrous oxide anesthesia for general surgery. Anesthesiology 65:362, 1986

112. Hall RI, Szlam F, Hug CC Jr: The enflurane-sparing effect of alfentanil in dogs. Anesth Analg 66:1287, 1987

113. Stoelting RK, Creasser CW, Gibbs PS: Circulatory effects of halothane added to morphine anesthesia in patients with coronary-artery disease. Anesth Analg 53:449, 1974

114. Bennett GM, Stanley TH: Cardiovascular effects of fentanyl during enflurane anesthesia in man. Anesth Analg 58:179, 1979

115. Eisele JH, Smith NT: Cardiovascular effects of 40 percent nitrous oxide in man. Anesth Analg 51:956, 1972

116. Stoelting RK, Gibbs PS: Hemodynamic effects of morphine and morphine–nitrous oxide in valvular heart disease and coronary-artery disease. Anesthesiology 38:45, 1973

117. Moffitt EA, Scovil JE, Barker RA et al: The effects of nitrous oxide on myocardial metabolism and hemodynamics during fentanyl or enflurane anesthesia in patients with coronary disease. Anesth Analg 63:1071, 1984

118. Eisele JH, Reitan JA, Massumi RA et al: Myocardial performance and N_2O analgesia in coronary-artery disease. Anesthesiology 44:16, 1976

119. Michaels I, Kay H, Barash P: Does nitrous oxide or a reduced FIO_2 alter hemodynamic function during high-dose fentanyl anesthesia? Anesthesiology 57:A44, 1982

120. Hall RI, Hug CC Jr: A quantitative description of the interaction of fentanyl and midazolam in reducing enflurane MAC in dogs. Can J Anaesth 35:S134, 1988

121. Kissin I, Mason JO, Bradley EL Jr: Morphine and fentanyl hypnotic interactions with thiopental. Anesthesiology 67:331, 1987

122. Kissin I, Vinik HR, Castillo R et al: Alfentanil potentiates midazolam-induced unconsciousness in subanalgesic doses. Anesth Analg 71:65, 1990

123. Bailey PL, Pace NL, Ashburn MA et al: Frequent hypoxemia and apnea after sedation with midazolam and fentanyl. Anesthesiology 73:826, 1990

124. Tomicheck RC, Rosow CE, Philbin DM et al: Diazepam–fentanyl interaction—Hemodynamic and hormonal effects in coronary artery surgery. Anesth Analg 62:881, 1983

125. Flacke JW, Davis LJ, Flacke WE et al: Effects of fentanyl and diazepam in dogs deprived of autonomic tone. Anesth Analg 64:1053, 1985

126. Salmenpera M, Peltola K, Takkunen O et al: Cardiovascular effects of pancuronium and vecuronium during high-dose fentanyl anesthesia. Anesth Analg 62:1059, 1983

127. Starr NJ, Sethna DH, Estafanous FG: Bradycardia and asystole following the rapid administration of sufentanil with vecuronium. Anesthesiology 64:521, 1986

128. Roerig DL, Kotrly KJ, Ahlf SB et al: Effect of propranolol on the first pass uptake of fentanyl in the human and rat lung. Anesthesiology 71:62, 1989

129. Lemmens HJM, Bovill JG, Hennis PJ et al: Alcohol consumption alters the pharmacodynamics of alfentanil. Anesthesiology 71:669, 1989

130. Flacke JW, Bloor BC, Flacke WE et al: Reduced narcotic requirements by clonidine with improved hemodynamic and adrenergic stability in patients undergoing coronary artery bypass. Anesthesiology 67:11, 1987

131. Carta F, Bianchi M, Argenton S et al: Effect of nifedipine on morphine-induced analgesia. Anesth Analg 70:493, 1990

132. Greenblatt DJ, Sellers EM, Shader RI: Drug disposition in old age. N Engl J Med 306:1081, 1982

133. Lynn AM, Slattery JT: Morphine pharmacokinetics in early infancy. Anesthesiology 66:136, 1987

134. Don HF, Dieppa RA, Taylor P: Narcotic analgesics in anuric patients. Anesthesiology 42:745, 1975

135. Ferrier C, Marty J, Bouffard Y et al: Alfentanil pharmacokinetics in patients with cirrhosis. Anesthesiology 62:480, 1985

136. Hasselström I, Eriksson S, Persson A et al: The metabolism and bioavailability of morphine in patients with severe liver cirrhosis. Br J Clin Pharmacol 29:289, 1990

137. Chauvin M, Ferrier C, Haberer JP et al: Sufentanil pharmacokinetics in patients with cirrhosis. Anasth Analg 68:1, 1989

138. Bentley JB, Borel JD, Gillespie TJ et al: Fentanyl pharmacokinetics in obese and nonobese patients. Anesthesiology 55:A117, 1981

139. Bentley JB, Finley JH, Humphrey LR et al: Obesity and alfentanil pharmacokinetics. Anesth Analg 62:251, 1983

140. McPherson RW, Feldman MA: Narcotics in neuroanesthesia. In Estafanous FG (ed): Opioids in anesthesia II, p 116. Boston, Butterworth-Heinemann, 1991

141. Alderman EL, Barry WH, Graham AF et al: Hemodynamic effects of morphine and pentazocine differ in cardiac patients. N Engl J Med 287:623, 1972

142. Bowdle TA, Greichen SL, Bjurstrom RL et al: Butorphanol improves CO_2 response and ventilation after fentanyl anesthesia. Anesth Analg 66:517, 1987

143. Gal TJ, DiFazio CA, Moscicki J: Analgesic and respiratory depressant activity of nalbuphine: A comparison with morphine. Anesthesiology 57:367, 1982

144. Romagnoli A, Keats AS: Ceiling effect for respiratory depression by nalbuphine. Clin Pharmacol Ther 27:478, 1980

145. Lake CL, Duckworth EN, DiFazio CA et al: Cardiovascular effects of nalbuphine in patients with coronary or valvular heart disease. Anesthesiology 57:478, 1982

146. Latasch L, Probst S, Dudziak R: Reversal by nalbuphine of respiratory depression caused by fentanyl. Anesth Analg 63:814, 1984

147. Moldenhauer CC, Roach GW, Finlayson CD et al: Nalbuphine antagonism of ventilatory depression following high-dose fentanyl anesthesia. Anesthesiology 62:647, 1985

148. Heel RC, Brogden RN, Speight TM et al: Buprenorphine: A review of its pharmacological properties and therapeutic efficacy. Drugs 17:81, 1979

149. Cook PJ, James IM, Hobbs KEF et al: Controlled comparison of i.m. morphine and buprenorphine for analgesia after abdominal surgery. Br J Anaesth 54:285, 1982

150. Kay B: A double-blind comparison between fentanyl and buprenorphine in analgesic-supplemented anesthesia. Br J Anaesth 52:453, 1980

151. Pandit SK, Kothary SP, Pandit UA et al: Double-blind placebo-controlled comparison of dezocine and morphine for postoperative pain relief. Can Anaesth Soc J 32:583, 1985

152. Hall RI, Murphy MR, Szlam F et al: Dezocine MAC reduction and evidence for myocardial depression in the presence of enflurane. Anesth Analg 66:1169, 1987

153. Smith G, Pinnock C: Naloxone—Paradox or panacea? Br J Anaesth 57:547, 1985

154. Ngai SH, Berkowitz BA, Yang JC et al: Pharmacokinetics of naloxone in rats and in man. Anesthesiology 44:398, 1976

155. Fishman J, Roffwarg H, Hellman L: Disposition of naloxone-7,-8,-^{3}H in normal and narcotic-dependent men. J Pharmacol Exp Ther 187:575, 1973

156. Longnecker DE, Grazis PA, Eggers GNN: Naloxone for antagonism of morphine-induced respiratory depression. Anesth Analg 52:447, 1973

157. Johnston RE, Jobes DR, Kennell EM et al: Reversal of morphine anesthesia with naloxone. Anesthesiology 41:361, 1974

158. Shupak RD, Harp JR: Reversible narcotic coma for neuroanesthesia. Anesthesiology 55:A230, 1981

159. Rawal N, Schött U, Dahlström B et al: Influence of naloxone infusion on analgesia and respiratory depression following epidural morphine. Anesthesiology 64:194, 1986

160. Abboud TK, Lee K, Zhu J et al: Prophylactic oral naltrexone with intrathecal morphine for cesarean section: Effects on adverse reactions and analgesia. Anesth Analg 71:367, 1990

17

Wendell C. Stevens
Harry G. G. Kingston

Inhalation Anesthesia

The role of the inhalation drugs in general anesthesia is changing. The number of patients who receive only inhalation drugs following induction of general anesthesia with an intravenous drug is decreasing and the use of intravenous drugs as adjuvants is increasing. The combination of intravenous and potent inhaled drugs might be called the new *balanced anesthesia*. A variety of drugs are chosen in order to derive the specific benefits of each. Thus, tachycardia occurring during isoflurane anesthesia may lead the anesthesiologist to administer an opioid to take advantage of the specific vagal actions of the opioid and to reduce the dose of isoflurane. Many anesthesiologists now prefer to decrease the total dose of a potent inhaled drug that a patient receives with any one of a number of intravenous drugs.

The inhaled anesthetics of greatest importance today are enflurane, halothane, and isoflurane, which are potent drugs, and nitrous oxide, which is a weaker drug. Potent drugs may be distinguished from nonpotent ones by their ability to produce respiratory paralysis in the presence of an adequate amount of oxygen. Discussion of these four drugs provides the major emphasis of this chapter. Although methoxyflurane is still available commercially, it is used infrequently. New compounds, desflurane and sevoflurane, are under clinical trial but as yet are not commercially available in the United States. Some of the physical characteristics of these compounds are given in Table 17-1. Their chemical structures are shown in Figure 17-1.

HISTORY

The recent introduction of desflurane and sevoflurane as inhaled anesthetic drugs represents the latest of the group of drugs whose lineage goes back to nitrous oxide, diethyl ether, and chloroform, all of which were introduced into clinical practice almost simultaneously. The search for new inhaled drugs continues because such drugs offer at least two general advantages over drugs administered by routes other than ventilatory: the ability to increase and decrease drug levels in the body at will and easy estimation of the concentration of anesthetic at the sites of action once the alveolar concentration is known. Since instruments of reasonable cost are now available to measure the alveolar concentration of anesthetic gases accurately and promptly, con-

trol of anesthetic dose can be done with great precision. Of course, we do not imply that anesthetics should be administered "by number" without close attention to the patient's requirements and the drugs' pharmacologic effects.

Advances in fluorine chemistry associated with nuclear research in the 1940s that allowed cost-effective incorporation of fluorine into molecules was pivotal to the development of modern anesthetics.[1] Prior to that time, the mainstays of inhalation anesthesia, cyclopropane, diethyl ether, and divinyl ether, were flammable. The nonflammable halogenated compounds chloroform and trichlorethylene were associated with hepatotoxicity or neurotoxicity and also were highly soluble in tissue.

In 1946, Robbins[2] reported studies of a series of fluorinated hydrocarbons. He showed that agents of a lower boiling point were more likely to produce convulsions than anesthesia. One of the fluorinated hydrocarbons, flurothyl, was actually used clinically as a convulsant in shock therapy. Halogenated aliphatic hydrocarbons and short-chain ethers with boiling points in the range of 50–100°C and containing a large proportion of fluorine as the halogen proved to be the best anesthetics. Some compounds with these components either have not withstood the test of practice or have been replaced by better drugs.

Fluroxene, the first of the new fluorinated anesthetics to be widely used clinically, was synthesized by Shukys in 1951 and evaluated by Krantz et al[3] and Sadove et al.[4] The requirements for testing drugs at that time were minimal, and rapid introduction of a new drug into clinical practice was common. Because fluroxene maintained cardiorespiratory function at near awake values, it maintained some popularity for nearly two decades, but several features limited its popularity.[5] These included flammability, some danger of ventricular arrhythmias, a high incidence of nausea and vomiting, and the threat of hepatotoxicity.[6]

Halothane was synthesized by Suckling in England in 1951,[7] tested in animals shortly thereafter, and introduced into clinical practice by 1956.[8,9] Halothane was readily accepted by the anesthesia community. Its nonflammability, favorable solubility characteristics, tolerance by patients at high inspired concentrations (overpressure), rapid induction, capacity to provide muscle relaxation, and an acceptably low incidence of nausea and vomiting as side-effects made it a drug far superior to other available anesthetics.

Methoxyflurane, synthesized before either fluroxene or

TABLE 17-1. Physical Characteristics of Anesthetics

Agent	Molecular Weight (g)	Boiling Point (760 mm Hg °C)	Vapor Pressure (mm Hg @ 20°C)	Liquid Density	Vapor/ Liquid (ml)	Chemical Stabilizer Necessary	Flammability Limits
Enflurane	184.5	56.5	175	1.517 (25°C)	198	No	None
Halothane	197.4	50.2	241	1.86 (20°C)	227	Yes	None
Isoflurane	184.5	48.5	238	1.496 (25°C)	196	No	None
Methoxyflurane	165	104.7	22.5	1.43 (20°C)	208	Yes	7% in air 5.4% in O_2
Nitrous oxide	44	−88.0	39,000	—	—	—	None in air
Sevoflurane	200	58.5	160	1.505 (20°C)	181	—	11% in O_2 10% in N_2O
Desflurane	168	23.5	664	1.45 (25°C)	211	No	20.8% in O_2 27.8% in N_2O 29.8% in N_2O/O_2

Physical data are from manufacturer's literature and from Wallin WF, Regan BM, Napoli MD *et al:* Sevoflurane: A new inhalational anesthetic agent. Anesth Analg 54:758, 1975; Vitcha JF: A history of Forane. Anesthesiology 35:4, 1971; and Halsey JM: Physiochemical properties of inhalational anesthetics. In Gray TC, Nunn JF, Utting JE (eds): General Anaesthesia, p 45. London, Butterworths, 1980.

halothane, was evaluated in humans by Artusio et al[10] in 1960. Perhaps it was tested because certain drawbacks in the use of halothane became apparent. These drawbacks included sensitization of the heart to the arrhythmic effects of epinephrine, cardiorespiratory depression, and the suspicion that halothane shared, along with other halogenated compounds such as chloroform, the danger of being a hepatotoxin. Methoxyflurane's favorable characteristics proved to be nonflammability, adequate muscle relaxation, and effective analgesia at low concentrations. Its high blood and tissue solubility, however, led to slow induction of anesthesia and exceedingly prolonged recovery. The greatest drawback to its use was nephrotoxicity.

The disadvantages of halothane, including hepatotoxicity,[11] encouraged the search for better inhaled anesthetics.[12] Out of hundreds of compounds tested by Terrell et al,[13,14] the two compounds enflurane and isoflurane have become important drugs in current clinical practice. Terrell centered his developmental work on the methyl-ethyl series of compounds because they tended to be stable, nonflammable, and excellent anesthetics.[14] The clinical trials of these two compounds proceeded nearly in parallel[15] involving patients[16,17] and human volunteers.[18,19] The extent of studies completed with each drug was far reaching compared to requirements for earlier compounds.[15,20-22]

A number of other drugs either have had only a brief trial clinically or are still in the evaluation process.[22] Among the former, halopropane ($CHF_2CF_2CH_2\ Br$) required prolonged time for induction of anesthesia and was excessively arrhythmogenic.[23] Teflurane (CF_3CHBrF) was associated with a high incidence of cardiac arrhythmias even in low concentrations.[24] Sevoflurane continues in the evaluative process and shows promise, particularly because of its low solubility in blood,[25] a property that may make it an excellent drug for use in outpatients. Desflurane ($CF_2HOCFHCF_3$) is the focus of intensive laboratory and clinical investigations. Its attractive properties are molecular stability and low blood solubility. Finally, aliflurane has been administered to a few patients[26] but it is not yet commercially available.

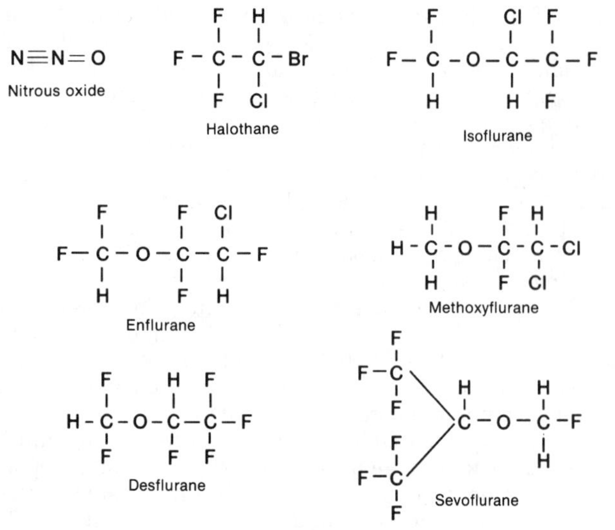

PHARMACOKINETICS OF INHALED ANESTHETICS

Uptake, Distribution, and Elimination

The inhaled drugs are distributed in the body according to the same principles that apply to other drugs (see Chapter 13). The gas anesthetics differ from most other drugs in that they enter the body through the lungs *via* ventilation. Thereafter, their absorption by blood and distribution to other tissues are determined by the solubility of the drug in blood (blood:gas partition coefficient), blood flow through the lungs, the subsequent distribution of blood to individual organs, solubility of anesthetics in the tissue (tissue:blood partition coefficient), and mass of the tissue.[27] Table 17-2 lists solubility characteristics of the inhaled anesthetics described in this chapter.

The goal of inhalation anesthesia is to develop and maintain a satisfactory partial pressure or tension of anesthetic at the site of anesthetic action, the brain. Tension refers to

Figure 17-1. Molecular structures of inhaled anesthetics.

TABLE 17-2. Partition Coefficients at 37°C

Agent	Blood: Gas	Brain: Blood	Liver: Blood	Muscle: Blood	Fat: Blood	Oil:Gas	Rubber: Gas		Other
Enflurane	1.91	1.4	2.1	1.7	36	98.5	74	(25°C)	Polyvinyl:gas 120 (25°C)
Halothane	2.3	2.9	2.6	3.5	60	224	120	(23°C)	Polyethylene:gas 26.3
									Soda lime:gas 1
Isoflurane	1.4	2.6	2.5	4.0	45	90.8	62	(25°C)	Polyethylene:gas 2 (25°C)
									Polyvinyl:gas 110 (25°C)
Methoxyflurane	12	2.0	1.9	1.3	49	970	630	(23°C)	
Nitrous oxide	0.47	1.1	0.8	1.2	2.3	1.4	1.2	(23°C)	
Sevoflurane	0.60	1.7	1.85	3.13	47.5	53.4	29.1		
Desflurane	0.42	1.29	1.31	2.02	27.2	18.7	19.3		

Physical data are from manufacturer's literature and from Eger EI II, Larson CP Jr, Severinghaus JW: The solubility of halothane in rubber, soda lime and various plastics. Anesthesiology 23:356, 1962; Wallin WF, Regan BM, Napoli MD *et al:* Sevoflurane: A new inhalational anesthetic agent. Anesth Analg 54:758, 1975; Eger RR, Eger EI II: Effects of temperature and age on the solubility of enflurane, halothane, isoflurane, and methoxyflurane in human blood. Anesth Analg 57:224, 1978; Yasuda N, Targ AG, Eger EI II: Solubility of I-653, sevoflurane, isoflurane, and halothane in human tissues. Anesth Analg 69:370, 1989; and Targ AG, Yasuda N, Eger EI II: Solubility of I-653, sevoflurane, isoflurane, and halothane in plastics and rubber composing a conventional anesthetic circuit. Anesth Analg 69:218, 1989.

the partial pressure of the gas with which the liquid is in equilibrium. Partial pressure, or tension, is related to concentration (percent) of anesthetic in the gas phase by the following formula:

Concentration
= (partial pressure ÷ barometric pressure) × 100

Induction of anesthesia is achieved, in a pharmacodynamic sense, when an anesthetizing partial pressure of anesthetic has been achieved in the brain. The brain or any individual tissue under consideration can be considered as the final site for a series of gradients in anesthetic partial pressure, which begins at the delivery hose exiting from the anesthetic machine. The gradients in gas tension may be arranged as follows: delivered > inspired > alveolar > arterial > tissue. In a purely pharmacokinetic interpretation, induction of anesthesia is complete when gas tensions in all tissues equal the alveolar tension. Until equilibrium is achieved, the gradients noted above continue to exist. This discussion of uptake and distribution of the inhaled drugs considers each gradient in succession.

First, a difference between delivered and inspired tension exists as long as uptake of anesthetic continues unless a nonrebreathing delivery system is being used. By definition, with a nonrebreathing system there is no difference between delivered and inspired tension. Use of high inflow rates to a circle system approximates a nonrebreathing system.[28] Anesthetic-system components can be arranged to favor preferential loss of anesthetic-poor gases during induction,[29] and the components of the anesthetic system can absorb anesthetics to widen a delivered-to-inspired tension difference.[30]

An inspired-to-alveolar tension difference can exist at the circuit-patient interface (Fig. 17-2). During induction of anesthesia, blood returning to the lung from tissues has an anesthetic tension lower than that in the alveoli. As a result, uptake of anesthetic drugs occurs from alveoli and causes an inspired-to-alveolar tension difference. The alveolar anesthetic concentration is of great importance during anesthesia with an inhaled drug because the arterial blood quickly equilibrates with the alveolar tension of the anesthetic[31] and, in turn, there is quick equilibration with the brain; therefore, the ability to measure or control the alveo-

lar tension of an anesthetic provides an indirect but reliable method to measure and control the brain tension (partial pressure) of an anesthetic.

The factors that govern the alveolar anesthetic tension are summarized in detail by Eger.[27] Achievement of an alveolar tension results from a balance between delivery of anesthetic to the lung by ventilation and uptake of anesthetic from the lung by blood and tissues. The inspired concentration and alveolar ventilation control delivery of anesthetic to the lung. The higher the inspired concentration, the more rapid the increase in alveolar concentration (concentration effect).[32] As alveolar (but not necessarily total) ventilation increases, more anesthetic molecules are delivered to the lung. Increasing alveolar ventilation makes alveolar gas more like the inspired gas, that is, lessens the inspired-to-alveolar concentration difference.

Administration of high concentrations of one gas (e.g., nitrous oxide) facilitates the rise in alveolar concentration of another gas (e.g., halothane), a phenomenon called the second gas effect (Fig. 17-3). The two components of the

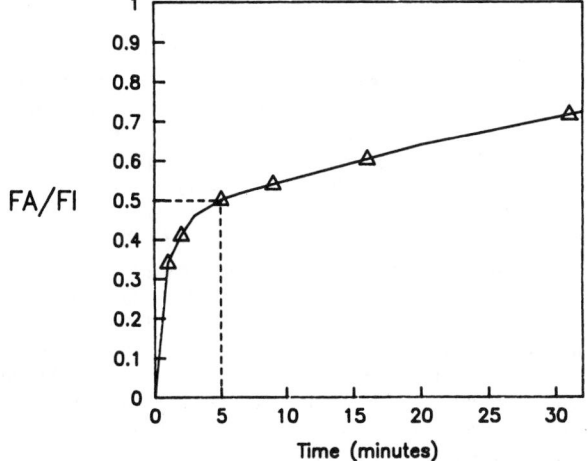

Figure 17-2. Depiction of the manner in which the alveolar concentration (FA) of an inhaled anesthetic approaches the inspired concentration (FI) over time. Assumptions include normal ventilation and cardiac output and blood:gas partition coefficient ~2.

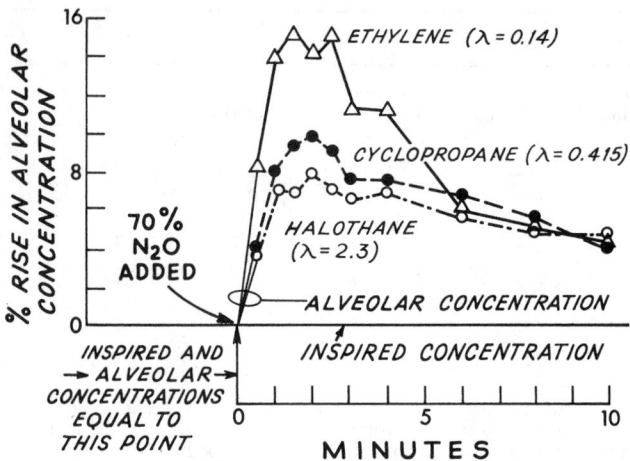

Figure 17-3. Average percent rise of the alveolar concentration of a second gas with the addition of 70% nitrous oxide. (Reprinted with permission from Stoelting RK, Eger EI II: An additional explanation for the second gas effect. Anesthesiology 30:273, 1969.)

second gas effect, increased ventilation (increased tracheal inflow) and the concentrating effect,[33] are operative at the alveolar level. Although a second gas effect exists for nearly any combination of inhaled drugs given simultaneously, it is most pronounced when nitrous oxide is used with a more potent drug such as halothane (the second gas). Despite nitrous oxide's relatively low blood solubility, the volume taken up early in anesthesia is high, as much as 1500 ml·min^{-1} or more, because it is delivered in high concentrations.[34]

The increase in alveolar concentration caused by delivery of anesthetic to the lung is opposed by uptake of anesthetic by the pulmonary capillary blood. Pulmonary capillary blood and alveolar anesthetic tensions are equal for any one alveolus–capillary unit; therefore, the next step in the tension gradient chain, the alveolar-to-arterial difference, ordinarily is small. This is particularly true when only minor ventilation-perfusion abnormalities exist.[31,34] Factors governing uptake include the anesthetic blood:gas partition coefficient, pulmonary blood flow, and the alveolar-to-mixed-venous tension difference. The higher the blood solubility of the anesthetic, the greater the uptake. Anesthetics act as ideal gases; therefore the quantity dissolved in blood per unit of pressure is the same for all partial pressures.[35] Their solubilities in blood and other tissues increase as temperature decreases but are not influenced by the patient's age.[36] Blood solubility of anesthetics increases soon after a meal,[37] and the blood:gas solubility of enflurane is lower in obese than nonobese patients.[38]

The last link in the chain of gradients, the blood-to-tissue tension difference, leads to uptake of anesthetic by tissues. Factors governing tissue uptake include the anesthetic tissue:blood partition coefficient, tissue blood flow, and the arterial-to-venous tension difference. Except for adipose tissue, the tissue:blood coefficients are generally quite similar to the blood:gas coefficients (see Table 17-2). Blood flow in relation to tissue mass is therefore of crucial importance in determining the capacity of the tissue for the anesthetic. A pertinent example of the importance of these factors in determining the rate of tissue anesthetic uptake is the rapid rise of alveolar and, therefore, myocardial concentration of anesthetics in infants.[39] A small amount of anesthetic is lost

via the skin and must, of course, be replaced by further uptake at the lung.[40]

When administration of an inhaled anesthetic is discontinued, removal of anesthetic from the body proceeds in a fashion that is nearly the reverse of induction. Emergence from anesthesia is more rapid with low blood or tissue anesthetic solubility, increased ventilation,[41] and replacement of nitrous oxide with nitrogen. The higher the concentration of nitrous oxide when elimination begins, the greater the effect on the rate of elimination of halothane.[42]

Recovery from anesthesia differs from induction in that anesthetic metabolism affects the rate of decrease of the alveolar anesthetic concentration. Although anesthetics are quite stable compounds, they are metabolized, usually to more polar compounds.[43] The amount of anesthetic removed from the body by metabolism is small compared with the amount exhaled. The amount metabolized is governed primarily by hepatic enzyme activity plus the amount and duration of availability of the anesthetic drug to the liver. The alveolar concentration of an anesthetic during induction and maintenance of anesthesia is influenced little by anesthetic metabolism because the amount of anesthetic administered or supplied to the patient far exceeds its uptake. During recovery however, as the alveolar concentration falls below the Km for metabolism of the drug (the partial pressure of anesthetic at which the rate of metabolism is one half the maximum rate of metabolism), a large fraction of the anesthetic presented to the liver is metabolized. As a result, the venous and alveolar concentrations decrease.[44,45] During the first few minutes of recovery, when the alveolar concentration is relatively high, drugs of lowest solubility exhibit the most rapid decline of alveolar concentration. Once the alveolar concentration decreases to the range of 0.01 minimum alveolar concentration (MAC), drugs that undergo considerable metabolism may be removed more rapidly than those resistant to metabolism, even though the former possess greater blood solubility. This factor accounts at least in part for the failure of the alveolar concentration of anesthetics to fall in strict accordance with their blood solubilities.

The Requirement for Anesthetics—Minimum Alveolar Concentration (MAC)

The pharmacokinetics of anesthetics (uptake and distribution) can be linked to pharmacodynamics (effect of the drug on the body) by consideration of anesthetic potency. The linkage exists because the desired alveolar concentration is what one strives to achieve and maintain during anesthesia. For the inhaled drugs, potency is commonly expressed as the MAC of the anesthetic. This is the alveolar concentration of anesthetic at 1 atm, which prevents movement in 50% of subjects in response to a painful stimulus (Table 17-3).[46-49] Various noxious stimuli have been used to provoke the response, including skin incision or electrical current.[47,49] Endpoints of response other than skeletal muscle movement have been proposed.[50] The 95% confidence limits for MAC are approximately 25% of the MAC value. A suggestion has been made that the dose of anesthetic preventing response to noxious stimuli in 95% of subjects, AD$_{95}$, more nearly approximates clinical anesthetic requirement.[51] In practice, the conventional MAC must be exceeded by a factor of 1.25–1.3 to assure surgical anesthesia in most patients.

Minimum alveolar concentration has been used when comparing the effects of equipotent doses of anesthetics on

TABLE 17-3. Minimum Alveolar Concentrations (MACs) in Humans as Percent of 1 Atmosphere

	MAC			MAC			
	With Oxygen	Reference Number	Age in Years	With N$_2$O	Reference Number	% N$_2$O	Age in Years
Enflurane	1.7	340	39 ± 3 SE	0.60	341	70	38 ± 2 SE
Halothane	0.77	47	42 ± 7 SD	0.29	55	66	
Isoflurane	1.15	342	44.2 ± 1.3 SE	0.50	342	70	46.3 ± 1.2 SE
Methoxyflurane	0.16	47	38 ± 9 SD	0.07	343	56	30–55
Nitrous oxide	104	50	21–35				
Sevoflurane	1.71	315	30–59	0.66	315	64	30–59
Desflurane	6.0	324	31–65	2.83	324	60	31–65

SE = standard error; SD = standard deviation.

TABLE 17-4. Physiologic or Pharmacologic Factors That Increase MAC

Increased central neurotransmitter levels (monoamine oxidase inhibitors, acute dextroamphetamine administration, cocaine, ephedrine, levodopa)
Hyperthermia
Chronic ethanol abuse*
Hypernatremia

*Determined in humans.

TABLE 17-5. Physiologic or Pharmacologic Factors That Decrease MAC

Metabolic acidosis
Hypoxia (Pao$_2$ < 38 mm Hg)
Induced hypotension ($\overline{AP}$ < 50 mm Hg)
Decreased central neurotransmitter levels (alpha-methyldopa, reserpine, chronic dextroamphetamine administration, levodopa)
Clonidine
Hypothermia
Hyponatremia
Lithium
Hypo-osmolality
Pregnancy
Acute ethanol administration*
Ketamine
Pancuronium*
Physostigmine (10 times clinical doses)
Neostigmine (10 times clinical doses)
Lidocaine
Opioids
Opioid agonist–antagonist analgesics
Barbiturates*
Chlorpromazine*
Diazepam*
Hydroxyzine*
Δ-9-Tetrahydrocannabinol
Verapamil

*Determined in humans.

various organ functions. The relative effects for anesthetics can be defined by calculating anesthetic or therapeutic indices, the dose producing a given effect divided by the MAC. For example, the dose of an anesthetic producing apnea when divided by the MAC defines its respiratory anesthetic index,[52] an index of the anesthetic's margin of safety.[53] The MAC has also been useful in quantifying the effect of other drugs or pathophysiologic states on anesthetic requirement. Factors increasing, decreasing, or not changing anesthetic requirement are summarized in Tables 17-4–17-6. A single explanation for the effect of these factors on MAC has not been found. Many seem to act through influences on central nervous system (CNS) catecholamine levels[54] or by direct CNS depression such as by opioids[55] or hypoxia.[56,57] Some drugs both increase and decrease the MAC, depending on dose or duration of administration. The acute administration of dextroamphetamines may increase the MAC, but chronic administration may decrease it.[58] Levodopa may initially increase and then decrease the MAC when high doses are used, but lower doses may decrease the MAC.[59] Some opioids exhibit a ceiling effect—an effect more promi-

TABLE 17-6. Physiologic or Pharmacologic Factors That Do Not Alter MAC

Duration of anesthesia*
Type of stimulation*
Gender*
Hypocarbia (Paco$_2$ to 21 mm Hg)*
Hypercarbia (Paco$_2$ to 95 mm Hg)
Metabolic alkalosis
Hyperoxia
Isovolemic anemia (hematocrit to 10%)
Systemic arterial hypertension *per se*
Thyroid function
Magnesium
Hyperkalemia
Hyperosmolality
Propranolol
Isoproterenol
Promethazine
Naloxone
Aminophylline

*Determined in humans.

nent for agonist-antagonist compounds than for agonists alone.[60,61] The inhaled drugs are considered to be nearly additive in their effects on MAC.[62,63] The most common interaction, that of nitrous oxide with a potent inhaled drug, provides a predictable reduction in requirement for the potent drug. The reduction is approximately equal to 1% of the MAC value for each volume-% alveolar nitrous oxide concentration. For example, 66% nitrous oxide will decrease the halothane requirement in middle-aged adults from 0.77% (MAC of halothane + oxygen) to 0.26% [0.77 − (0.77 × 0.66)]. Recent evidence indicates that the summation is not linear over the entire range of nitrous oxide concentrations.[64]

Pregnancy decreases the MAC when a sheep model is used,[65] but a decrease[48] or no change in the MAC is seen in the rat.[66] MAC is also influenced by age. In humans the MAC is lower in preterm neonates than in those at term. It is higher in term infants than in subjects at any other age.[67] Anesthetic requirement decreases with age; therefore an 80-year-old patient requires only three fourths the alveolar concentration for anesthesia of a young adult.[68]

At least two additional MAC values have been determined. One is MAC-awake, the dose at which response to the command "open your eyes" occurs.[69] The alveolar concentration at this point is approximately one half the standard MAC value. MAC-BAR is the alveolar concentration required to block the adrenergic response to noxious stimuli.[70] This value is approximately 1.5 times the standard MAC value.

EFFECTS OF INHALED ANESTHETICS ON ORGANS AND SYSTEMS

Central Nervous System

Inhaled anesthetics produce significant changes in mental function, cerebral oxygen consumption, cerebral blood flow (CBF), cerebrospinal fluid (CSF) dynamics, and CNS electrophysiology.

The changes in mental function, which are a necessary part of anesthesia, persist beyond the period of anesthetic administration and the immediate postoperative period. Following prolonged anesthesia, volunteers exhibit decreased intellectual function and an increased incidence of subjective symptoms. In one study, the effects of halothane exceeded those of isoflurane; the effect was greatest at 2 days following anesthesia and returned to near normal by 8 days.[71] Anesthesia with halothane or enflurane, when combined with nitrous oxide, led to altered psychomotor performance and driving skills.[72] The persistent mental effects of halothane may be caused in part by its biodegradation to bromide,[73] a CNS depressant. Some studies have also shown that trace concentrations of anesthetics can significantly impair perceptual, cognitive, and motor skills[74] or learning.[75] Other studies examining trace concentrations have failed to confirm impairment of psychomotor function.[76] It is probably safe to assume that concentrations of anesthetics in the brain several hours after surgery or present in the ambient air of an operating room are too low to impair most tests of mental function.

Each of the potent inhaled anesthetics decreases cerebral metabolic rate ($CMRo_2$), with the order of effect from greatest to least being isoflurane > enflurane ≥ halothane. The decrease in $CMRo_2$ is closely linked to cerebral electrical activity. With isoflurane it has been shown that once an

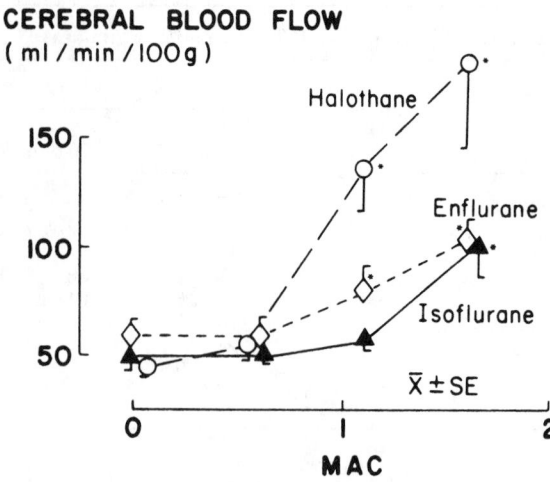

Figure 17-4. Cerebral blood flow measured in volunteers when awake and when anesthetized at varying MAC levels during controlled ventilation and normocapnea. (Reprinted with permission from Eger EI II: Isoflurane: A review. Anesthesiology 55:559, 1981.)

isoelectric electroencephalogram (EEG) is achieved, further increases in isoflurane concentration do not lead to further decreases in $CMRo_2$.[77] Enflurane results in decreased $CMRo_2$ at a time when the EEG demonstrates a spike-suppression pattern.[78] If seizure activity occurs, however, $CMRo_2$ may increase.[79] Brain hypoxia does not result from enflurane-induced seizures despite increased $CMRo_2$, most likely because CBF increases proportionately. The greatest decrease in $CMRo_2$ occurs during the transition from wakefulness to loss of consciousness.[80] The decrease in $CMRo_2$ produced by isoflurane may provide some cerebral protection during periods of oxygen deprivation if the oxygen deprivation itself has not abolished electrical activity.[81] Other workers have not reached the same conclusion.[82] Isoflurane-induced hypotension may produce sufficient cerebral vasodilation to maintain CBF at the prehypotensive levels, but during this time $CMRo_2$ decreases. Thus, cerebral oxygen supply-demand relationships may be somewhat better preserved by isoflurane than by halothane.[83]

Each of the inhaled agents, including nitrous oxide, produces cerebral vasodilation and an increase in CSF pressure. The order of potency for this effect is halothane > enflurane > isoflurane.[84] This cerebral vasodilation causes increased CBF and cerebral blood volume (Fig. 17-4). Nitrous oxide, either by itself or when added to one of the more potent drugs, can also produce cerebral vasodilation, but only to a modest degree. In the awake state, CBF is closely linked to $CMRo_2$; if $CMRo_2$ decreases, CBF decreases. Isoflurane may preserve this relationship better than the other anesthetics and may explain the smaller increase in CBF produced by isoflurane. The increase in CBF with anesthetics tends to attenuate with time. With halothane, Albrecht et al[85] demonstrated the normalization of CBF within 2 hours after induction of anesthesia.

Cerebrovascular responses to carbon dioxide are preserved when low concentrations of volatile anesthetics are used. Differences in the pattern of response exist, however. Hypocapnia will lead to a greater reduction in CBF during isoflurane than during halothane inhalation;[86] that is, the effect of isoflurane on regional CBF appears to be highly CO_2-dependent. In humans, critical regional CBF, the blood flow at which electroencephalographic evidence of cerebral ischemia occurs, is significantly lower with isoflurane than with halothane, approximately 10 ml·100 g^{-1}·min^{-1} and 18–20 ml·g^{-1}·min^{-1}, respectively.[87]

Studies in laboratory animals show that each of the potent inhaled drugs has important effects on CSF volume as well as on brain and cerebral blood volume. Anesthetics can affect both the production and reabsorption of CSF. Enflurane increases CSF production and increases the resistance to reabsorption of CSF.[88,89] Isoflurane does not result in any significant change in CSF production or reabsorption.[89,90] Halothane decreases the rate of CSF production but increases resistance to reabsorption.[91,92] As with the effects of anesthetics on CBF, these effects on CSF dynamics tend to return toward normal values with time, except with enflurane. Both the cerebrovascular and CSF dynamic effects of the anesthetics contribute to an effect on CSF pressure. In the presence of modest hypocapnia, isoflurane appears less likely to produce potentially dangerous increases in CSF pressure than enflurane or halothane.[84,93] Isoflurane may not be totally benign in this regard, however, because significant increases in CSF pressure have been reported in patients with brain tumors.[94] All evidence seems to indicate that enflurane is the least favorable drug with respect to control of CSF pressure.

The pattern of electroencephalographic changes with the various inhaled anesthetics is quite similar in that increased anesthetic concentration decreases EEG wave frequency and increases voltage. At high concentrations, the anesthetics may produce electrical silence, sometimes passing through a burst-suppression pattern.[95,96] The pattern of EEG dominance shifts from a posterior to an anterior location as anesthetic depth increases.[97] Unlike the other drugs, enflurane can produce high-voltage, repetitive spiking activity.[98] This activity can be attenuated or abolished by decreasing the enflurane dose or increasing the arterial carbon dioxide partial pressure (Paco$_2$).[98,99] Enflurane does not increase the risk of seizures in patients with epileptic foci.

Anesthetics also produce significant changes in sensory-evoked potentials and must be considered along with many other factors in interpreting these responses.[100-102] The magnitude of the effect differs depending on the type of evoked responses being recorded. Cortical responses are more affected than are subcortical responses. Enflurane, halothane, and isoflurane produce a dose-related decrease in the amplitude and an increase in the latency of cortical components of somatosensory-evoked potentials.[103] Nitrous oxide decreases somatosensory responses[104] and may produce greater attenuation of these responses than low concentrations of enflurane or isoflurane.[105,106] With respect to brain stem auditory-evoked potentials, enflurane,[107] halothane,[108,109] and isoflurane[110] each increase the latencies of certain peaks. Nitrous oxide does not increase latency but can decrease the amplitude of both visual- and auditory-evoked potentials.[101]

Respiratory System

Inhaled anesthetics, including nitrous oxide, have similar effects on breathing. Although these properties are similar, they need to be clearly understood in order to prepare safely for and manage the patient's ventilation in the perianesthetic period. Although this section emphasizes the effects of the drugs on breathing, the anesthetic state, per se, also alters other aspects of the respiratory system. Examples of the latter effects include the decrease of lung volume associated with induction of anesthesia and the change in the way gravitational factors affect diaphragm function.[111,112]

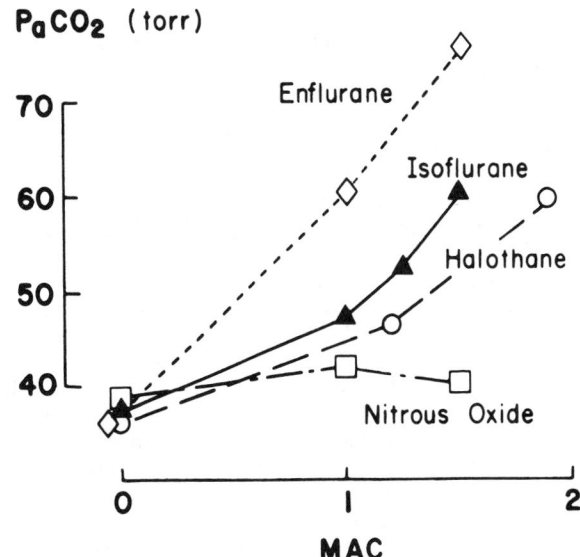

Figure 17-5. Paco$_2$ in spontaneous breathing volunteers when awake and anesthetized with enflurane, halothane, isoflurane, or nitrous oxide in oxygen. (Reprinted with permission from Eger EI II: Isoflurane: A review. Anesthesiology 55:559, 1981.)

Ventilatory Volumes and Frequency of Breathing

All inhaled anesthetics cause respiratory depression, with an elevation of Paco$_2$, in a dose-related manner (Fig. 17-5). Most inhaled anesthetics increase frequency of breathing and decrease tidal volume as anesthetic concentration increases.[19,113-115] These two changes counteract each other so that minute volume decreases less than might be expected from the decrease in tidal volume alone.[116] The increase in frequency as anesthetic depth increases is not a general property of all anesthetics because isoflurane tends not to increase frequency.[115] Nitrous oxide tends to increase respiratory frequency when added to isoflurane.[117] Adding 60% N$_2$O to 1 MAC halothane increases frequency to the same degree as an increase in the alveolar concentration of halothane alone from 0.8%–1.5%.[118] If minute volume is changed minimally, Paco$_2$ would be expected to change minimally unless other factors occur. Other factors do occur, however, including significant increases in wasted ventilation and small but consistent decreases in oxygen consumption and carbon dioxide production.

Effects on the Intercostal Muscle and Diaphragm

It is estimated that approximately 40% of normal tidal exchange is contributed by intercostal activity and 60% by the diaphragm.[119] In children and adolescents, halothane anesthesia decreases thoracic excursions but awake state abdominal excursions persist, presumably because the phrenic motor neuron pool is more resistant to depression than the intercostal motor neuron pool. The clinical result is a loss of intercostal function as depth of anesthesia increases. Recruitment of intercostals does not occur in response to increased chemical drive. Also, especially in children, active stabilization of the rib cage cannot occur to resist any inward motion that might take place in response to negative intrathoracic pressure. Diaphragm function is also depressed by anesthetics.[120] The effect is most prominent at high phrenic nerve stimulus frequencies, suggesting a direct muscle depressant effect of the anesthetics.[121]

Chemical Control of Breathing

The effects of anesthetics on the chemical control of breathing have probably received more emphasis than other respiratory effects. These effects certainly are important, because it is the loss of normal responses to chemical stimuli such as hypercarbia and hypoxia that so jeopardizes the patient in the perianesthetic period. The ventilatory response to carbon dioxide is depressed more or less proportionately to anesthetic dose,[19,113-115] except for diethyl ether,[114] but the hypoxic ventilatory response is blocked nearly completely by low concentrations of anesthesia.[122] Accordingly, during spontaneous breathing, as anesthetic concentration is increased, $Paco_2$ also increases. Duration of anesthesia does not affect the response, except with enflurane, with which $Paco_2$ returns toward normal values as anesthesia is prolonged.[19]

Apnea results if the anesthetic dose is high enough. The margin between the anesthetizing concentrations (MAC) and the concentration producing apnea (the respiratory anesthetic index) is least for enflurane. If apnea occurs, the apneic threshold is approximately 4 or 5 mm Hg below the $Paco_2$ maintained during spontaneous breathing, regardless of depth of anesthesia.[123] There are several clinical implications from these data. First, $Paco_2$ will be increased somewhat above normal during anesthesia if spontaneous breathing is allowed. The magnitude of the increase depends on the anesthetic dose. Second, one is limited in how low the $Paco_2$ can be maintained and still preserve spontaneous breathing as a guide to depth of anesthesia. It should be anticipated that the $Paco_2$ will be 50–55 mm Hg at surgical planes of anesthesia when the most potent inhaled anesthetics are used. Surgical stimuli will decrease this level by 4–5 mm Hg at an equivalent level of anesthesia.[124] Assisting ventilation just to the apneic threshold will only decrease the $Paco_2$ an additional 4 or 5 mm Hg. Nitrous oxide, when studied under hyperbaric conditions at 1–1.25 times MAC, does not increase the $Paco_2$ during spontaneous breathing.[125] Nitrous oxide is less depressant than the potent inhaled drugs but is not free of a significant effect.[126]

If the respiratory system is challenged by imposed increases of CO_2 during anesthesia, tidal volume increases but changes in frequency of breathing are relatively minor. All of the anesthetics produce an anesthetic dose-related depression of the ventilatory response to carbon dioxide (Fig. 17-6).[19,113-116] High doses can obliterate the response.

Anesthetic depression of the ventilatory response to hypoxia is potentially more harmful than depression of the hypercapnic ventilatory response. Knill et al[127-129] performed a number of elegant studies to show that anesthetics depress the hypoxic ventilatory drive in humans. Unlike the situation with anesthetic depression of the ventilatory CO_2 response, even subanesthetic concentrations of halothane, enflurane, and isoflurane markedly depress the hypoxic responses in humans, with the depression maximal at anesthetizing concentrations. Nitrous oxide significantly depresses the hypoxic response.[122] The normal augmentation of breathing produced by adding hypercarbia to hypoxia in the awake state is not observed during anesthesia.[129] The ventilatory response to metabolic acidemia is also depressed by anesthesia.[129] The absence of hyperpnea during hypoxemia means that a useful clinical sign of hy-

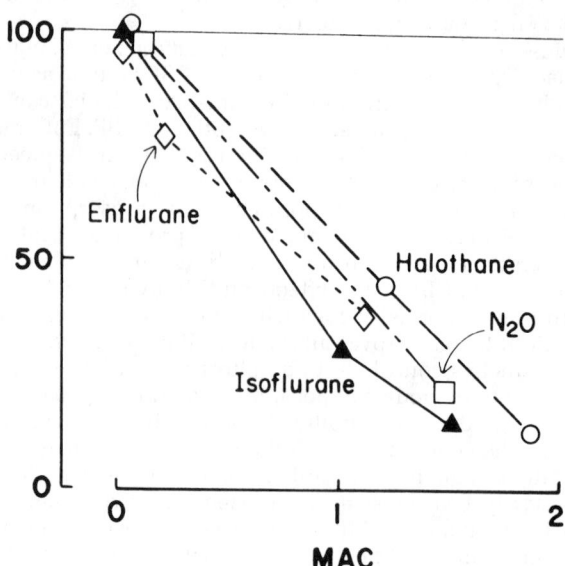

Figure 17-6. Percent change from awake values in the slope of the curve relating an increase in ventilation to imposed increases in $Paco_2$ in anesthetized volunteers. (Reprinted with permission from Eger EI II: Isoflurane: A review. Anesthesiology 55:559, 1981.)

poxia cannot be relied on during anesthesia. Another clinical implication of loss of the hypoxic ventilatory drive is the need for close observation during recovery from anesthesia.

Responses to Mechanical Loading

External. Another important aspect of ventilatory function is the response to mechanical loading, such as might be seen with partial occlusion of an endotracheal tube or the presence of a weight on the chest or abdomen.[130] In general, the ability of the anesthetized patient to respond to external (extrinsic) loads is better than the ability to respond to internal (intrinsic) ones. Anesthetized, spontaneously breathing adults can maintain normal ventilation despite increased resistance to breathing, such as might occur with small endotracheal tubes or an improperly attached humidifier in the anesthetic circuit,[131] but a number of workers have shown that the anesthetized patient is less able to compensate for an increase in resistive loads than the awake patient. Behrakis et al[132] found that the anesthetized patient is better able than the awake patient to compensate for a first loaded breath (the first breath after a resistance is placed in the airway). Thereafter the compensation is less complete in the anesthetized subject. Even subanesthetic concentrations of nitrous oxide may inhibit the normal response to resistive loads.[133] Moote et al[134] demonstrated in adults anesthetized with halothane at 1.1% that both resistive and elastic loads can be compensated for to a point but, if the loads are large enough, they may exceed the compensatory ability. Enflurane significantly alters the normal rib and abdominal wall synchrony when expiratory resistance is imposed. Lindahl et al[135] imposed resistive loads in children during N_2O/halothane anesthesia. They found a negligible effect on frequency of breathing and an initial decrease in tidal volume that returned to control levels in a fairly short time. In their study, the larger the child, the poorer the compensation, presumably because of the larger tidal volume and flow rates prior to the addition of resistance.

What happens when weights (such as a surgeon's elbow) are placed on the chest or abdomen? Recall that with anesthesia, the intercostal component of inspiration is decreased to a greater extent than the diaphragmatic component.[119] As a result, abdominal weights have a more profound effect than chest weights on breathing.[130] No compensation occurs with time, nor does an overshoot occur when the weights are removed.

Internal. An example of a major internal load is the increased expiratory resistance encountered in a patient with chronic obstructive pulmonary disease. Pietak et al[136] found a rough correlation between the degree of abnormality of forced expiratory volume in 1 second and the increase in $Paco_2$ during anesthesia. If spontaneous ventilation is allowed, inordinate hypoventilation may occur in such patients.

Responses to Surgery

Surgery and presumably the attendant pain stimulate breathing so that average $Paco_2$ values are lower than those without surgery.[124] The effect of surgery in lowering $Paco_2$ is about the same over a modest range of anesthetic concentrations. The decrease in $Paco_2$ is less than might have been expected from the increase in minute ventilation because CO_2 production increases. Rosenberg et al[137] measured 2-point ventilatory responses to CO_2 in patients receiving N_2O-enflurane anesthesia and found that ventilation was increased at each CO_2 level. The slopes of the ventilatory-response curves were roughly parallel so that no change in sensitivity occurred. Lam et al[138] also showed that surgery increased ventilation but did not alter the sensitivity to CO_2 or improve the hypoxic ventilatory response.

Airway Caliber

The potent inhaled agents do not differ markedly in their effects on bronchomotor tone. They all increase airway resistance to some degree because of loss of lung volume.[111] On the other hand, the potent inhaled drugs decrease airway resistance by causing bronchodilation[139,140] and by an effect on lung tissue pressure-volume hysteresis.[141] Heneghan et al[142] showed in humans that halothane decreases airway resistance to a greater extent than isoflurane. Halothane and isoflurane both attenuate increased airway resistance caused by hypocapnia.[143] Hirshman et al[143,144] studied the effects of anesthetics on both antigen-induced bronchoconstriction and bronchoconstriction resulting from topical stimulation and methylcholine. The potent agents blocked bronchoconstriction to a similar extent. The anesthetics did not block histamine release but rather blocked the bronchoconstrictor response to the mediator. All the potent inhaled anesthetics are effective for the patient with asthma, although halothane may be somewhat preferable to isoflurane because the latter has a pungent odor that can cause airway irritation.

Hypoxic Pulmonary Vasoconstriction

The phenomenon of diversion of blood away from atelectatic lung has been known for many years, but the relation of this diversion to hypoxia-induced pulmonary arterial constriction and the effect of anesthetic drugs on the response are more recent findings.[145-148] There is general agreement that the inhaled anesthetics depress the response in animals in a dose-related manner, but results with laboratory models may not apply under clinical conditions. Rees and Gaines[149] compared shunt fraction in patients undergoing one-lung anesthesia with ketamine or enflurane, drugs with differing effects on hypoxic pulmonary vasoconstriction in laboratory models, and found no differences in gas exchange in the patients. Neither halothane nor isoflurane decreased arterial oxygen tension (Pao_2) during one-lung ventilation of patients receiving opioid anesthesia,[150] and Carlsson et al[151] demonstrated no important clinical effect of isoflurane anesthesia on pulmonary vessel responses to hypoxia. These findings do not mean that selection of anesthetics is unimportant with regard to their effects on hypoxic pulmonary vasoconstriction. Rather, they mean that under clinical conditions with relatively low doses of inhaled drugs, the disease status of the lung and other effects of the anesthetics are of relatively greater importance.

Tracheal Ciliary Activity

Tracheal mucociliary flow[152,153] is inhibited by the inhaled anesthetics. This effect, when combined with a similar inhibition found with endotracheal intubation, inhalation of dry gases, and others, may contribute to postoperative pulmonary infections.

Circulatory System

Hemodynamics

Halothane, Enflurane, and Isoflurane. The circulatory effects of halothane,[154] enflurane,[155] isoflurane,[18] and nitrous oxide[156] have been determined in human volunteers not undergoing operations. Results from these studies are important starting points in the consideration of the circulatory effects of these drugs because the study methods were similar for all agents, the general physical status of the volunteers was similar and normal, and no surgical events affected the results. Knowing how the drugs affect healthy humans provides a basis for understanding how diseases or other events change the effects. To a large degree, the findings from the studies in volunteers have been substantiated by studies in patients.

All of the potent drugs decrease arterial pressure in a dose-related manner (Fig. 17-7). The mechanism of the decrease in blood pressure includes vasodilation, decreased cardiac output due to myocardial depression, and decreased sympathetic nervous system tone. With halothane, decreased cardiac output is the predominant cause (Fig. 17-8).[154] Halothane also increases venous compliance, and in patients who have high sympathetic tone, such as those with heart failure, halothane decreases systemic vascular resistance.[157] Enflurane causes both vasodilation and decreased myocardial contractility.[155] With isoflurane, a low peripheral resistance is the major cause of hypotension. Evidence of the relatively greater myocardial depression with halothane and enflurane is the greater increase in right atrial pressure seen with these drugs than with isoflurane. Nevertheless, isoflurane also fits the criteria for a myocardial depressant in that cardiac output may not decrease despite increased left ventricular filling pressure and decreased systemic vascular resistance.[158,159]

The inhaled anesthetics differ in their effects on heart rate.[160] The heart rate changes least with halothane and increases most with isoflurane. Because arterial pressure decreases and cardiac output is either stable or decreased,

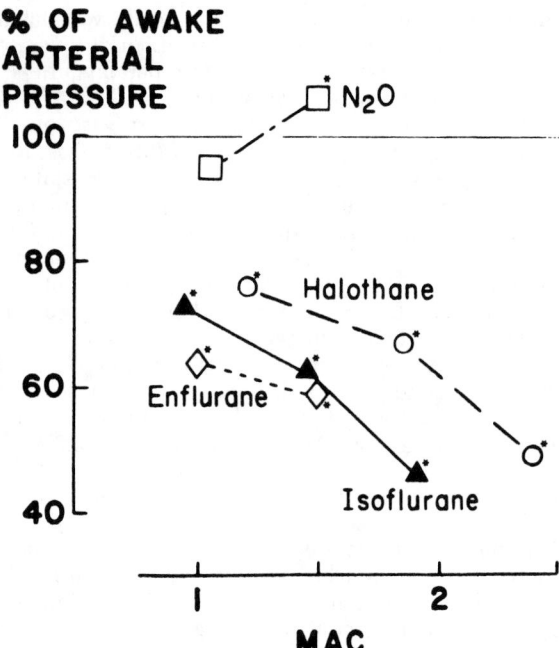

Figure 17-7. Percent change from awake values of mean arterial blood pressure in anesthetized, normocapnic volunteers. (Reprinted with permission from Eger EI II: Isoflurane: A review. Anesthesiology 55:559, 1981.)

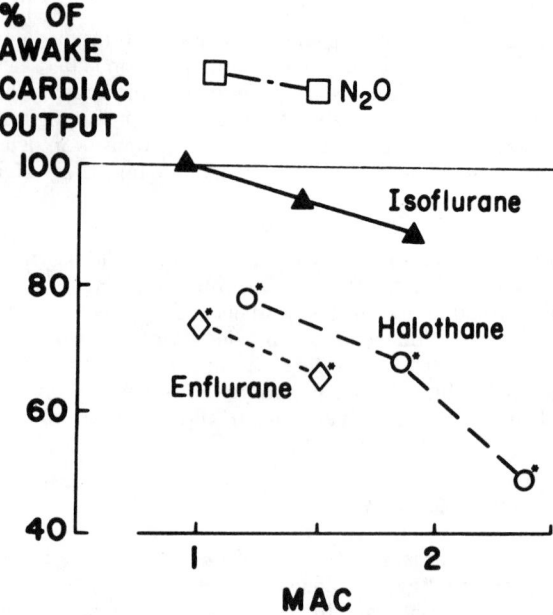

Figure 17-8. Percent change from awake values of cardiac output in anesthetized, normocapnic volunteers. (Reprinted with permission from Eger EI II: Isoflurane: A review. Anesthesiology 55:559, 1981.)

myocardial work is decreased with all the inhaled anesthetics.

Oxygen consumption is decreased approximately 10–15% below awake values in the anesthetized subject. As anesthetic dose is increased, the main reason for further decreases in oxygen consumption is decreased myocardial oxygen consumption.[161]

Anesthetics alter the distribution of cardiac output. Blood flow to the liver, kidneys, and gut is decreased, whereas blood flow to the brain, muscle, and skin is increased. Increases in muscle blood flow are most prominent with isoflurane.[18] Both isoflurane and halothane antagonize alpha-adrenergic–mediated vasoconstriction.[162]

The findings in human volunteers obtained during controlled ventilation and normocarbia are altered when breathing is spontaneous. The resultant increase in $Paco_2$ and decrease in mean airway pressure cause heart rate and cardiac output to increase and systemic vascular resistance to decrease. Mean arterial pressure differs little from values obtained during controlled ventilation at comparable MAC levels.[163-165]

In the awake subject, when $Paco_2$ is increased by adding CO_2 to the breathing system and ventilation is held constant, cardiac output increases, systemic vascular resistance decreases, and blood pressure changes little. The potent inhaled anesthetics attenuate this response to CO_2 in a dose-related manner.[165] Circulatory changes therefore may not provide a reliable clue that hypercarbia or hypoxemia is occurring intraoperatively as might be provided by a nonfunctioning anesthetic system valve, for example.[166]

As duration of anesthesia increases, there is recovery from the circulatory depressant effects of the anesthetics. This is especially true with halothane, to a lesser degree with enflurane, and to a yet smaller degree with isoflurane. The mechanism may involve beta-adrenergic stimulation[167]

leading to increased cardiac output, stroke volume, and decreased systemic vascular resistance.[154,168]

Nitrous Oxide. Nitrous oxide does not have a consistent hemodynamic effect. When given alone in a 40% concentration, it can decrease cardiac output.[156] When nitrous oxide is added to halothane in healthy volunteers, it lowers cardiac output and appears to stimulate the sympathetic nervous system, leading to increased systemic vascular resistance and increased arterial pressure.[126,169] For enflurane, the addition of nitrous oxide produces no change or small decreases in arterial pressure and cardiac output. Reduction of the enflurane concentration and substitution of some of the enflurane with nitrous oxide lead to less depression of circulatory variables than seen with enflurane alone.[170] For isoflurane at equivalent MAC levels, a nitrous oxide–isoflurane combination yields higher blood pressure than isoflurane alone, mainly because of greater systemic vascular resistance.[171] When nitrous oxide is given to patients with heart disease,[172,173] particularly in combination with opioids,[174] it causes hypotension and a decrease in cardiac output.

The pulmonary vascular effects of nitrous oxide are also variable. Patients with elevated pulmonary artery pressure may have further increases when nitrous oxide is added.[175] There is a significant correlation between the initial level of pulmonary vascular resistance and the additional increases produced by nitrous oxide.[176] Whereas nitrous oxide can increase pulmonary vascular resistance in adults, a study in infants failed to show further increases of pulmonary vascular resistance with the addition of nitrous oxide.[177] It is of interest that the decrease in pulmonary vascular resistance with isoflurane is less than the decrease in systemic vascular resistance.[178]

Intestinal Circulation. Splanchnic blood flow usually is decreased by anesthetics, an effect that is produced in two ways.[179] One is a decrease in hepatic perfusion owing to decreases in arterial pressure or cardiac output. The other is an increase in splanchnic vascular resistance caused by sympathetic stimulation such as occurs with surgical stimulation or increased $Paco_2$. The anesthetics also may have a direct effect on the hepatic circulation. Laboratory studies show that halothane and isoflurane have differing effects on hepatic vascular resistance.[180,181] Isoflurane produces hepatic arterial vasodilation and halothane does not. With both drugs, total hepatic blood flow decreases but oxygen delivery to the liver is better preserved with isoflurane. The hepatic oxygen supply-consumption ratio is higher during exposures to hypoxia with subanesthetic isoflurane than with equivalent doses of enflurane or halothane.[182] When nitrous oxide is added to halothane anesthesia, splanchnic blood flow decreases further.[183] Isoflurane may protect against renal and splanchnic vasoconstriction from somatic and visceral nerve stimulation.[184]

Reflex Control of the Circulation. Several studies have quantified the effects of the various inhaled anesthetics on these responses. Although the magnitude of the effect differs among the studies, it is clear that all of the inhaled agents,[185-187] including nitrous oxide,[188] attenuate baroreflex responses. Halothane attenuates both the pressor and depressor baroreflex responses.[185] Kotrly et al[187] found that the depression is less pronounced with isoflurane than others had shown for halothane or enflurane. Isoflurane depresses baroreflex control of heart rate in neonates.

In addition to effects on reflex changes in heart rate, vasomotor reflex responses are also attenuated by the anesthetics. In humans, application of lower body negative pressure and the resulting decrease in central blood volume do not result in as great an increase in peripheral resistance during halothane anesthesia as in awake subjects.[189] Baroreflex control of heart rate returns to awake levels soon following anesthesia. The rate of return of vasomotor reflexes after anesthesia is not known.

The attenuation of cardiovascular reflexes by anesthetics is important in determining the anesthetized patient's response to hemorrhage. Dogs anesthetized with halothane, enflurane, or isoflurane and subjected to graded hemorrhage showed no change in heart rate despite gradual decreases in arterial pressure.[190] In another study, nitrous oxide and halothane given at equal multiples of their MAC had similar depressant effects on the circulation of hypovolemic swine.[191]

Cardiac Dysrhythmias, Conduction, and Drug Interactions. Cardiac dysrhythmias may occur in 60% or more of patients undergoing anesthesia and surgery.[192] There are many mechanisms by which these dysrhythmias may occur, including altered physiology, autonomic imbalance, anesthetic agents, and other drugs. Anesthetics may affect pacemaker automaticity, impulse conduction, and refractoriness, which, in turn, may trigger re-entry phenomena.[192] Susceptibility of the heart to the dysrhythmic effects of epinephrine differs among anesthetics. Both enflurane and isoflurane are significantly less sensitizing than halothane (Fig. 17-9).[193,194] Epinephrine sensitivity is not closely related to the anesthetic dose.[195] Cardiac dysrhythmias due to interactions of the anesthetics and other vasoactive drugs also are less likely to occur with isoflurane than with halothane.[196] There may be a relationship between responsiveness of the alpha-adrenergic system and epinephrine sensitivity,[197] but the mechanism of the effect is unclear. The greater the degree of alpha-adrenergic responsiveness, the greater the epi-

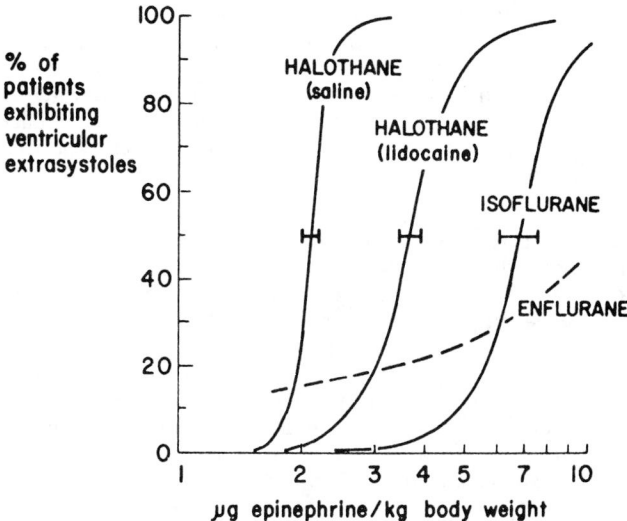

Figure 17-9. Percent of patients exhibiting three or more ventricular extrasystoles in response to a subcutaneous injection of epinephrine. (Reprinted with permission from the International Anesthesia Research Society from Johnston RR, Eger EI II, Wilson C: A comparative interaction of epinephrine with enflurane, isoflurane and halothane in man. Anesth Analg 55:709, 1976.)

nephrine sensitivity during halothane anesthesia. Children are less likely than adults to exhibit ventricular dysrhythmias from epinephrine during halothane anesthesia.[198]

Dysrhythmias may occur during halothane anesthesia in the presence of hypercarbia. The threshold for dysrhythmias is high, over 80 mm Hg.[199] During surgery the threshold decreases significantly. The tolerance for carbon dioxide is somewhat greater when nitrous oxide is added to halothane. Thiopental given prior to the potent inhaled drugs enhances epinephrine sensitivity, initially decreasing the dysrhythmic dose of epinephrine by approximately 50%.[200] Aminophylline is less likely to produce dysrhythmias during anesthesia with enflurane or isoflurane than with halothane.[201]

Enflurane, halothane, and isoflurane exert a direct negative chronotropic effect at the sinoatrial node.[192,202] Cardiac conduction is better preserved via normal pathways by isoflurane than by enflurane or halothane.[203] Conduction changes are believed to be a necessary part of the etiology of ventricular arrhythmias caused by re-entry of excitation. The volatile anesthetics do not appear to alter cardiac-pacing stimulation thresholds.[204] Atrioventricular junctional rhythms are common with all anesthetics, especially with enflurane and nitrous oxide.[192,205]

The cardiovascular effects of the inhaled anesthetics can be altered by other drugs. For example, the myocardial depression with isoflurane is enhanced by the calcium channel-blocking drug, verapamil, and is related to doses of each drug.[192,206-208] Some reversal of depression can be achieved by calcium administration. The data of Kapur et al[206] suggest that tolerance to verapamil is least with enflurane, next best with isoflurane, and best with halothane. In their study, the primary problem seen in halothane-treated animals was prolongation of the P-R interval; however, the interaction depends on both the halothane and verapamil doses. Anesthetics alter verapamil pharmacokinetics so that higher plasma levels of verapamil are achieved during anesthesia than in the awake state.[207] Diltiazem, another calcium channel blocker, has been used to treat premature ventricular contractions and tachyarrhythmias during halothane anesthesia.[209] It increases the threshold for epinephrine-induced dysrhythmias. Isoflurane interacts to prevent the reflex tachycardia that occurs with nicardipine.[210] Halothane and propranolol have similar cardiovascular-depressant effects and they appear to be additive.[211]

Coronary Circulation. Coronary autoregulation links coronary blood flow to myocardial oxygen demand. This relationship persists in the normal heart during anesthesia but may be perturbed by the inhaled anesthetics. In patients with normal coronary vessels, the effects of the drugs on coronary vessels are of minor importance compared with the influence of the major metabolic determinants of coronary blood flow and resistance. Differences in drug effects are more obvious and clinically relevant in the presence of coronary stenosis or occlusion.

Bollen et al[212] determined in isolated coronary vessels that halothane, more than isoflurane, relaxes coronary arteries that constrict in response to potassium or a prostaglandin compound. Using a dog model with coronary vessel stenosis or occlusion to produce a zone of myocardial blood flow deprivation, studies have shown that isoflurane is a potent coronary vasodilator and that it can steal blood away from ischemic zones of the myocardium.[213,214] It appears that isoflurane uncouples the generally close relationship between coronary blood flow and myocardial oxygen demand more than the other potent inhaled drugs. It produces greater dilation of intramyocardial arterioles than epicardial arteries.[215]

In patients with coronary artery disease receiving isoflurane, coronary blood flow is maintained despite decreased arterial pressure. At the same time, coronary sinus O_2 levels increase and, in some patients, lactate production occurs.[159] When hypotension is produced by isoflurane, animals with critical coronary stenosis may develop myocardial ischemia.[216] On the other hand, isoflurane has been shown to increase the tolerance to pacing-induced myocardial ischemia in humans,[217] and outcome studies have failed to associate use of isoflurane with a higher incidence of myocardial infarction or perioperative death when patients undergo coronary artery bypass operations.[218]

Enflurane also has prominent coronary vasodilating properties.[219] Nitrous oxide, when added to the potent inhaled agents, may have deleterious effects on the distribution of coronary blood flow.[172] When nitrous oxide is added to isoflurane, there is a further decrease in heart rate and arterial pressure.[173] Despite unchanged coronary flow, addition of nitrous oxide decreases myocardial oxygen extraction. Patients anesthetized with nitrous oxide and isoflurane may show large increases in coronary blood flow with only small decreases in oxygen consumption, suggesting autoregulation has been impaired. A similar effect occurs when nitrous oxide is added to enflurane anesthesia.

Renal Circulation. The primary effect of inhaled anesthetics on the kidney is mediated through their effects on the renal circulation. Renal blood flow generally does not decrease during anesthesia because autoregulation appears to be well preserved and a fall in systemic blood pressure is compensated for by a corresponding decrease in renal vascular resistance.[220] Glomerular filtration rates does decrease as a result of a fall in arterial pressure and, as a consequence of this, urine output decreases.[221] Since renal blood flow is preserved in a healthy patient, this reduction in urine output is not a cause for concern because urine flow is re-established when the blood pressure returns to normal levels.

Blood

Inhaled agents can have effects on hematopoiesis, individual cell elements, and coagulation. Anesthetics also can alter the function of elements of the immune response. This subject is covered in more detail in Chapters 52 and 53.

Hematopoiesis. Much of our concern about inhalation anesthetics and hematopoiesis involves a consideration of the potential toxic effects of nitrous oxide on the bone marrow and other tissues with rapidly dividing cells. Green and Eastwood noted dose-dependent depression of bone marrow in rats exposed to nitrous oxide.[222] Also, prolonged exposure to nitrous oxide will produce an anemia similar to pernicious anemia because of inhibition of the enzyme methionine synthetase, which is involved in the metabolism of vitamin B_{12}.[223] Although exposure of rats to 1% nitrous oxide for 1 week to 6 months has not been shown to be associated with bone marrow depression, sensitive tests of DNA biosynthesis such as deoxyuridine suppression[224] indicate that megaloblastic changes can occur in patients exposed to nitrous oxide for as little as 1 hour. Nunn et al[225] reported megaloblastic bone marrow changes in a seriously ill patient after 105 minutes of nitrous oxide anesthesia. Interestingly, the same patient required another anesthetic some 7 hours after the first, and on this occasion, 30 mg of folinic acid was given prior to the anesthetic. This anesthetic was not associated with bone marrow changes. Attempts have been made to use nitrous oxide to treat leukemia, but the effect of nitrous oxide on the bone marrow is apparently transitory, and the white blood cell count increases after withdrawal of the nitrous oxide.[226] At the concentrations in common clinical use, halogenated agents do not appear to adversely affect hematopoiesis.

White Blood Cells. Erskine and James[227] demonstrated that halothane has no effect on polymorphonuclear leukocyte chemotaxis in rabbits and that isoflurane, in fact, caused an increase in polymorphonuclear cell movement. Although inhaled agents have little or no effect on phagocytic engulfment of bacteria, both halothane and enflurane consistently cause transient inhibition of polymorphonuclear leukocytes. Metabolism function and killing activity were also reduced as demonstrated by changes in chemiluminescence during the phagocytosis of zymosan.[228] On the other hand, neither isoflurane nor nitrous oxide appears to inhibit polymorphonuclear cell function. The exact mechanism of this inhibition is unclear, but in some instances it may be due to the presence of serum factors.[229,230] Halothane also causes a reduction in the amount of interferon excreted by monocytes studied in vitro.[230] When halothane is administered in concentrations in common clinical use, there is no change in T-killer cell activity, although at concentrations greater than 4% T-cell inhibition can be demonstrated.[231] Halothane has also been shown to inhibit the formation of 5-lipoxygenase metabolites in leukocytes by inhibiting arachidonic acid release.[232] Thus, although it has been suggested that inhaled agents may unfavorably affect polymorphonuclear cell function in septic patients, it appears that this is a problem only in those patients who are not immunologically normal or in whom anesthesia has been protracted.[230,233] The clinical implications of leukocyte function modified by inhaled anesthetic agents are not clear, but lymphocytic immunologic activity can be altered for up to 24 hours after exposure to halothane 1%.[234]

Red Blood Cells. Since the shape and position of the oxygen dissociation curve are major factors influencing oxygen carriage, anesthesiologists have speculated about how this might be altered by inhaled drugs. Inhaled agents (including nitrous oxide) cause neither a shift in the oxygen dissociation curve nor a change in the affinity of hemoglobin for oxygen.[235] But, the measurement of blood gas tension by polarographic techniques *is* influenced by the presence of halothane, enflurane, and isoflurane but not by nitrous oxide or sevoflurane.[236]

Platelets. Volatile anesthetic drugs are imputed to cause increased bleeding during surgery, either by a direct effect on vascular smooth muscle or by altering platelet function. Halothane decreases the level of metabolic adenosine triphosphate within platelets and also decreases their ability to aggregate. The mild increase in bleeding time noted with halothane anesthesia is probably of little clinical significance and has not been demonstrated with either enflurane or isoflurane.[237]

More information about the toxic effects of inhaled agents on the bone marrow and cellular elements can be found in Chapters 4 and 18.

Neuromuscular System

The potent inhaled anesthetic agents not only potentiate the action of neuromuscular blocking drugs but also have muscle-relaxant properties of their own. Although the mechanism of this potentiation is not entirely clear, it appears that it is largely because of a postsynaptic effect at the neuromuscular junction.[238]

Although minor differences exist among them, all the potent inhaled anesthetics potentiate depolarizing relaxants. Isoflurane has a greater potentiating effect on succinylcholine block than does halothane and appears to accelerate the transition from Phase I to Phase II block when a succinylcholine infusion is used.[239] A similar effect is seen with enflurane.

Potent inhaled anesthetics have an even more profound potentiating effect on nondepolarizing muscle relaxants.[240] Isoflurane and enflurane potentiate neuromuscular blockade to a greater extent than either halothane or sevoflurane. Approximately three times as much *d*-tubocurarine is required to produce an equivalent level of neuromuscular blockade in patients receiving halothane than in those receiving isoflurane (Fig. 17-10).[241] A detailed description of individual muscle relaxants and how they are affected by potent inhaled agents can be found in Chapter 19.

Endocrine System

Islet Cell Function and Glucose Metabolism

During anesthesia, the blood glucose level is usually elevated both as a result of reduced insulin secretion and of tissue responsiveness to this hormone.[242] In the case of halothane and enflurane, the increase in blood glucose concen-

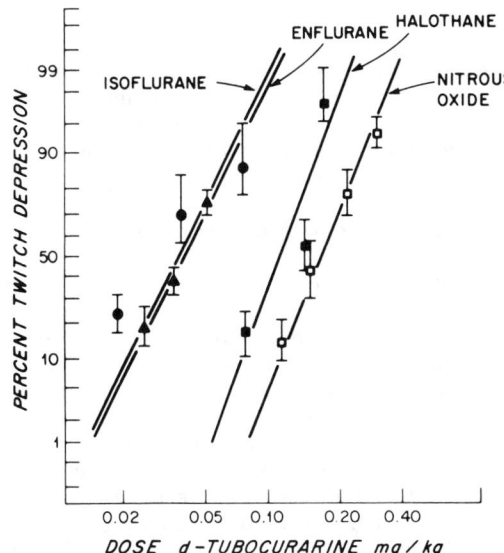

Figure 17-10. Interaction of 1.25 MAC isoflurane, enflurane, halothane, and 66% nitrous oxide with *d*-tubocurarine. (Reprinted with permission from Ali HH, Savarese JJ: Monitoring of neuromuscular function. Anesthesiology 45:216, 1976.)

tration during anesthesia is attributable mainly to a reduction in insulin release rather than to altered peripheral glucose utilization.[243] It has been speculated that the mechanism of action of anesthetic drugs on insulin secretion by the pancreas may be the result of an alteration in calcium availability, changes in microtubular or microfilament function, or even an effect of the agent on the plasma membrane itself. During surgery, sevoflurane appears to maintain plasma insulin at preanesthetic levels more consistently than other inhaled agents, which may be advantageous in patients with diabetes mellitus.

Antidiuretic Hormone

It has been suggested that all opioids and inhaled anesthetic drugs affect antidiuretic hormone release,[244] which may influence intraoperative renal function. With more accurate measurement of serum antidiuretic hormone, it has been demonstrated that neither opioid nor "light" halothane anesthesia, *per se*, stimulates release of antidiuretic hormone. Surgical stimulation, however, results in a massive release of antidiuretic hormone as part of the stress response.[245] Higher concentrations of anesthetics, *i.e.*, a "deeper" level of anesthesia, can modify this response.

Renin

Plasma renin activity varies very little as a result of anesthesia but is influenced by catecholamine release in the perioperative period and by the fluid status of the patient.

Serotonin

Inhaled anesthetic drugs, *per se*, do not protect against the effects of the carcinoid syndrome,[246] and although mechanical ventilation has been shown to be associated with more effective removal of serotonin by the lungs, halothane appears not to influence this process.

Testosterone

Halothane has been shown to significantly reduce the level of testosterone in the blood.[247] The level of testosterone falls intraoperatively and continues to decrease well into the postoperative period. The reason for this has not been established.

Surgical Stress and Endocrine Response

There is an increase in the activity of the hypothalamus and the pituitary and adrenal glands during surgical stress. The neuroendocrine aspects of this "stress response" are a result of both the anesthetic and the noxious stimuli caused by the surgical procedure. The extent of the stress can be quantified by measurement of serum levels of adrenocorticotropic hormone, cortisol, and catecholamines.

In a comparison of inhaled versus intravenous induction of anesthesia, inhaled induction of anesthesia was found to be more stressful than intravenous induction. Mask induction with halothane-oxygen anesthesia causes plasma norepinephrine levels to increase 15 minutes after the induction of anesthesia but they return to control levels some 45–60 minutes later.[248] This is attributed to increased norepinephrine release rather than to a decrease in the rate of removal from the tissues. Thus, anesthesia alone may be associated with hormonal changes that are independent of the response to surgery. Adrenocorticotropic hormone, beta-lipoprotein, cortisol, aldosterone, and dehydroepiandrosterone levels are all elevated in patients who are anesthetized for elective orthopedic procedures. The rise of aldosterone may be the result of elevated adrenocorticotropic hormone and serum renin levels. In a study of patients undergoing hysterectomy, Lacoumenta et al[249] noted that hormonal changes were similar in two groups of patients who received either 1.2 or 2.1 MAC of halothane. This suggests that higher concentrations of inhaled agent do not reliably suppress the endocrine response to surgical stimulation. Similar findings have been reported during isoflurane anesthesia.[250] This contradicts earlier work that suggested that the endocrine response could be attenuated with deeper levels of anesthesia. Comparing the stress response to surgery during either halothane or balanced anesthesia using fentanyl, it was found that halothane was less effective than fentanyl in preventing an increase in the concentration of plasma norepinephrine.[251] Yet enflurane is reported to be more effective than neurolept anesthesia in blocking sympathoadrenal responses to surgical stress and appears to inhibit the secretion of both epinephrine and norepinephrine from the adrenal medulla by a direct effect on the cell membrane. This is further substantiated by the fact that in a direct comparison between halothane and enflurane used to anesthetize children for adenoidectomy, the catecholamine levels increased with both drugs, but the increase was greater with halothane than with enflurane.[252]

Adrenal Medulla

In addition to information learned from the studies quoted above, our knowledge of the effect of anesthetic drugs on the hormones of the adrenal medulla has been enhanced by experience gained in the management of pheochromocytoma.[253] Since halothane is known to sensitize the myocardium to the dysrhythmic effects of epinephrine, enflurane, isoflurane, and now sevoflurane offer a theoretical advantage for the anesthetic management of a patient requiring resection of a pheochromocytoma.[254,255]

Thyroid Gland

Anesthetic agents can exert an effect on thyroid function by influencing secretion of thyroid-stimulating hormone (TSH) by the anterior pituitary gland, by a direct effect on the thyroid gland, or by attenuating the peripheral activity of the thyroid hormone. By measuring TSH and serum thyroxine levels simultaneously, Oyama et al[256] were able to show that neither the stress of surgery nor anesthesia with halothane or methoxyflurane influenced the release of TSH. Therefore, since patients anesthetized with halothane demonstrate a significant rise in serum thyroxine levels, it seems that TSH does not play an important role in the modulation of serum thyroxine either during anesthesia or during surgery.

Halothane-induced hepatotoxicity has been shown to occur in hyperthyroid rats, the explanation being that a new balance is created between glutathione and cytochrome P-450 activation. It has been demonstrated that the metabolism of halothane and enflurane is increased in hyperthyroid patients compared with euthyroid patients.[257] There is also a clinical impression that the anesthetic requirements of hypothyroid patients are less than those of patients without thyroid abnormality.[258]

Uterine and Fetal Effects

The inhaled anesthetics affect both the myometrium and the fetus.

Uterine Muscle

Volatile anesthetic drugs cause myometrial relaxation and can contribute to perinatal blood loss. Enflurane, isoflurane, and halothane are equally depressant to uterine smooth muscle at similar MAC values. This relaxation is clinically significant and results in greater blood loss when termination of pregnancy is performed under halothane anesthesia than when a nitrous oxide–opioid technique is used. Although MAC values in pregnancy are reduced, using 70% nitrous oxide in oxygen as the sole anesthetic is associated with a high incidence of intraoperative maternal awareness; therefore, low doses of inhaled halogenated drugs are commonly added. Although this practice could result in increased blood loss at the time of cesarean section as a result of myometrial relaxation, it has been shown that 0.5% halothane, 1.0% enflurane, or 0.75% isoflurane can be used safely to supplement an oxygen–nitrous oxide technique. In a study of 60 parturients at the time of cesarean section, it was shown that the use of isoflurane 1.0% or halothane 0.5% was not associated with increased maternal blood loss and that Apgar scores in infants delivered by this technique were good irrespective of the agent used.[259]

Fetal Effects

Inhaled drugs delivered to the mother cross the placenta and potentially affect the fetus. Halothane (1 MAC) has been shown to cause fetal hypotension even when this level of anesthesia results in little change in maternal blood pressure or pulse rate. Yet, although anesthesia with halothane (1 MAC) is associated with fetal hypotension owing to a decrease in fetal peripheral vascular resistance, fetal regional blood flow does not appear to be adversely affected. In an animal model in which fetal hypoxia was induced by occlusion of uterine blood flow, Baker et al showed that during asphyxia, regional and total brain, heart, and adrenal flow increased.[260] A similar response was seen when the animals were anesthetized, suggesting that during isoflurane-oxygen anesthesia, the balance of cerebral blood flow measured as supply-demand is maintained even during hypoxia.[260]

Enflurane and isoflurane have favorable cardiovascular and metabolic effects on the fetus during anesthesia for cesarean section. But because enflurane is partially metabolized to inorganic fluoride, there is a potential for the fetus to develop toxic reactions as a result of this. The total dose is small, however, and follow-up studies of infants delivered by cesarean section under enflurane anesthesia have not demonstrated any impairment of renal function.[261]

Because nitrous oxide can interfere with methionine synthetase and cell division, there is concern that its use during pregnancy may be associated with an increased incidence of fetal abnormalities. There is currently no evidence to suggest that this is the case.

SIGNS OF ANESTHESIA

When diethyl ether was a commonly used anesthetic, assessment of anesthetic depth was relatively easy. With anesthetic induction, the patient passed through stages of anesthesia that could be monitored by observation of pupils, muscle activity, tearing, respiratory patterns, and muscle relaxation.[262] With the onset of the modern era of anesthesia, however, the era that began when fluorinated inhaled drugs and muscle relaxants appeared, a problem began in determining what constitutes adequate anesthesia.[263] For example, in an effort to provide adequate conditions for surgery, muscle relaxants were given and one important sign of anesthesia, lack of movement, was removed.[264] The problem of assessing adequately the depth of anesthesia has persisted to the present time, especially when nitrous oxide is used as the primary anesthetic and is supplemented by other drugs to provide complete anesthesia.[265-267] Guedel's[262] description of reproducible physical signs for ether anesthesia no longer applies when anesthesiologists use a barbiturate for induction, inhaled drugs with low blood solubility for maintenance, and muscle relaxants. In addition, misinterpretation of respiratory signs can result in confusion of deep anesthesia with airway obstruction because the pattern of chest movement can be similar in both instances. Finally, pupillary dilation can reflect not only deep anesthesia but also sympathetic stimulation from hypercarbia or surgical stimulation.

Woodbridge[268] described well the concepts or components that constitute "general anesthesia." Although somewhat different terms are used in more recent literature, e.g., attenuation of the stress response rather than Woodbridge's depression of reflexes, the ideas are quite similar if not identical. The elements of the nervous system that are depressed during anesthesia include sensory (afferent), motor (efferent), reflex, and mental components. How does depression of each of these components contribute to clinical signs as a patient is anesthetized? What follows is a description of phenomena that occur as a patient is anesthetized with nitrous oxide combined with one of the potent inhaled drugs or with a potent drug used with oxygen alone.

Although it applied to diethyl ether, Artusio[269] was the first to describe the "lightest" or first stage of anesthesia, a stage of sensory and gentle mental depression virtually not used today except when providing analgesia with nitrous oxide or sedation with a more potent drug in an intensive care setting. Patients in this state open their eyes on command, breathe normally, and tolerate mild painful stimuli such as suturing of skin and superficial debridement. In general, airway and other reflexes remain intact.

Increasing the dose of anesthetic further may cause the patient to enter a stage of excitement. This stage is marked by muscle movement, retching, heightened laryngeal reflexes, disconjugate pupils, tachycardia, hypertension, and hyperventilation. Because many of these signs are unwanted, the goal should be to pass through this stage quickly by increasing the inspired concentration of the inhaled drug or by eliminating excitement altogether by use of an intravenous barbiturate. An excitement stage is quite likely to occur when nitrous oxide is used in concentrations exceeding 50% (vol/vol) because that closely approaches the estimated MAC awake for this drug.[270,271] MAC awake, although described as the anesthetic dose at which subjects begin to respond to commands, also defines a dose of anesthetic at which most patients lose consciousness and recall.[69]

The next deeper level of anesthesia, the level associated with the MAC, is notable by the absence of movement in response to a surgical incision. The MAC is that concentration at which 50% of patients do not move when a skin incision is made,[46] and when the MAC is exceeded by a factor of 1.25–1.3, the vast majority of patients will not move in response to an incision.[51] This level of anesthesia is associated with depression of each of the four elements of nervous system function. Sensory loss allows surgery to proceed without the patient's experiencing pain. There is loss of recall, although there are a few reports of recall occurring even at the deeper levels of anesthesia.[272] The incidence of recall is greatest when only low concentrations of anesthetics are used and neuromuscular blocking drugs are relied on to provide relaxation.[273] Evidence of reflex depression at this level of anesthesia is the absence of an increase of blood pressure or heart rate with surgical stimulation. A very pronounced autonomic response is indicative of a light level of surgical anesthesia. Finally, although the patient may not move when the incision is made, there may be insufficient motor relaxation for operations in the abdomen or thorax.

As anesthesia with the inhaled drugs deepens beyond the MAC, further respiratory, cardiovascular, and CNS depression occurs. It may be difficult or impossible to predict accurately the alveolar concentration of the anesthetic from assessment of clinical signs. This is because a given clinical sign, such as a change in blood pressure, is not affected by all anesthetics in the same way.[274,275] Furthermore, the impact of other drugs, age, debility, and surgical stimulation on clinical signs is unpredictable. Another mitigating factor is the alteration of circulatory effects of some anesthetics with time. For example, with halothane, the dose-response relationship between halothane and blood pressure that exists during the first hour of anesthesia is eliminated when anesthesia is prolonged.[274] Some recovery from the respiratory depression of enflurane occurs as anesthesia continues.[19] Monitoring the depth of anesthesia requires familiarity with the properties of each anesthetic and evaluation of the response of each patient to the anesthetic drug alone and to surgical stimulation.[275]

With further increases in alveolar concentration, a level of anesthesia can be achieved at which the autonomic response to noxious stimuli is totally blocked. This conforms to MAC-BAR, the MAC required to block the adrenergic and cardiovascular response to incision.[70] At this dose, one would not expect to see tachycardia or hypertension in response to surgical stimulation or other interventions such as endotracheal intubation.

As the concentration of potent inhaled anesthetics is deepened still further, the clinical picture is one of increasing depression of circulation and respiration. Although precise dose-response relationships may not exist,[274] arterial pressure and cardiac output are progressively reduced as the anesthetic dose is increased. Hypotension can be profound.

Changes in breathing are the most sensitive indices of depth of anesthesia, probably because breathing is less intimately under autonomic control than are circulatory functions. Movement of the diaphragm persists at levels of anesthesia that block intercostal muscle function.[118] For most drugs ventilatory frequency increases as anesthetic dose increases over a clinically useful range.[115] This change is accompanied by loss of active intercostal activity, leading to loss of thoracic expansion and persistence of only diaphragmatic descent.[276] A rocking breathing pattern results, often with a lower rib cage flaring, leading to an out-of-phase pattern of chest wall movement.[276] Unfortunately, liberal use of muscle relaxants, opioids, and controlled ventilation has prevented respiration from being a common monitor of anesthetic depth.

Pupillary and other eye signs of anesthetic depth do not follow a reliable dose-response relationship.[274,275] Eye movement is a somewhat better guide to depth than is pupillary diameter, and the presence of eye movement ordinarily is a sign of light anesthesia. Change of the eyes from conjugate to disconjugate positions with onset of surgery can usually be relied on as an indicator of the lightening level of anesthesia. Although lacrimation occurs even with deep levels of cyclopropane and ether, it is not apparent during deep enflurane, halothane, and isoflurane anesthesia. Conversely, the occurrence of lacrimation when it did not previously exist suggests a lightening level of anesthesia. Of the eye signs, pupillary diameter changes may be the least reliable indicator of anesthetic depth. This is because pupillary caliber is under sympathetic control.[274] A variety of variables can influence sympathetic activity, including drugs and $Paco_2$. As with newly appearing eye movement, acute pupillary enlargement with onset of surgery may be a sign of relatively light anesthesia, but it must be remembered that dilated pupils may also be a sign of cerebral hypoxia.

Some consideration of motor or efferent blockade is warranted. Muscle tone decreases as anesthetic depth increases.[277] The active abdominal expiratory effort that occurs as anesthesia is induced gradually becomes less intense and the abdomen becomes soft as a surgical plane of anesthesia is achieved.[276] Expiratory contraction of the rectus abdominis and other abdominal muscles gradually decreases as depth of anesthesia increases. The prominence of the recti is enhanced by contraction of the oblique and transverse abdominal muscles because their contraction makes the semilunar line more prominent. Stout patients with diastasis of the recti abdominus or with thin, incompetent recti often show paradoxical abdominal motion as consciousness is lost. This results from oblique and transverse muscle contraction during expiration that increases the intra-abdominal pressure during expiration, leading to protrusion of abdominal contents under or between the recti. Even profound levels of anesthesia will not obliterate muscle contraction from an electrocautery stimulus.

Although misjudgments about the level of anesthesia can occur, with practice and experience the adequacy of anesthesia ordinarily can be estimated from clinical signs.[265,276]

Accurate assessment is most difficult in the period after induction of anesthesia and before surgical stimulation begins. Tolerance of anesthesia may be poor, so that even very lightly anesthetized patients may be hypotensive at this time. If the concentration of anesthetic is reduced too much, these patients may move and exhibit hypertension, tachycardia, pupillary dilation, and salivation when surgery begins. Anesthetic depth should be viewed as a continuum, with patients maintained at various levels of the continuum depending on surgical requirements.[276] It is somewhat gratuitous, although true, to state that constant vigilance is necessary and that, when in doubt about the level of anesthesia, one should decrease the delivered concentration and closely observe the patient for changes in clinical signs. This will permit determination of whether this initial safest change in concentration, a decrease, was also the most appropriate change. We especially support the concept of tailoring the administered dose to the needs of the patient. This often includes light, deep, and intermediate levels in the same patient at various stages of the anesthetic.

CLINICAL USES AND TECHNIQUES

Several features about the clinical use of inhaled anesthetics lead to continued enthusiasm for these drugs by many anesthesiologists. Not all of the features are unique to the inhaled drugs; nonetheless, when taken in combination, they make these drugs versatile mainstays of the practice of anesthesia. The features include the ability to induce and maintain anesthesia regardless of age or habitus of the patient; presence of clinical signs that give an indication of depth of anesthesia; ability to increase or decrease depth of anesthesia at will; a predictable pattern of recovery from anesthesia; provision of all of the components of the anesthetic state in many patients without the use of adjuvants; knowledge of the concentration of the drug at the site of action; and the ability to deliver a broad range of oxygen concentrations. In the absence of enough outcome studies that allow us to know whether one technique of anesthesia is better than another, we believe the inhaled drugs will continue to be an important part of our armamentarium.

Induction of Anesthesia

Patient comfort and speed of induction lead many anesthesiologists to begin anesthesia with intravenous drugs and then to add inhaled agents. In these instances, consideration must be given to the safety and smoothness of the transition from anesthesia provided by the intravenous drugs to the maintenance state provided by the inhaled agents. Anesthesia provided by a single dose of a thiobarbiturate and depolarizing relaxant is brief because of their redistribution from brain and metabolism, respectively. There are four methods for quickly introducing an inhaled anesthetic in a concentration sufficient for the patient to tolerate the endotracheal tube and not to move when an incision is made. One is for the anesthesiologist to provide both high inspired anesthetic concentrations (overpressure) and controlled alveolar hyperventilation. Reference to the rate of rise of alveolar concentration toward the inspired concentration of an inhaled anesthetic is appropriate at this point. A typical pattern of the rate of rise of alveolar concentration toward the inspired concentration for a drug of intermediate blood solubility, such as isoflurane, is shown in Figure 17-2. In this example, it is assumed that alveolar ventilation maintains eucapnia. In order for a surgical level of anesthesia to be achieved within 5 minutes, the inspired concentration must be twice the desired alveolar concentration. For instance, when using isoflurane in a young adult, the inspired concentration required for induction to occur in 5 minutes or less with normal alveolar ventilation would be approximately 3%. It should also be recalled that the small influence of the second gas effect accompanying the use of nitrous oxide may further aid induction.[32,33]

A second approach to achieving an anesthetizing concentration of the inhaled drug during an intravenous induction is to administer supplemental doses of the sedative and relaxing drugs or to select intravenous drugs with more than ultrashort duration of action. This approach allows more time for inhaled induction to occur.

A third approach is to rely on a mixture of intravenous and inhaled drugs not only for induction but also for maintenance of anesthesia. Only a portion of the anesthetizing conditions are provided by the inhaled drugs. For example, one might combine intravenous opioids with a drug of low potency such as nitrous oxide, or subanesthetic concentrations of a potent agent such as enflurane. Because in the one instance a drug of low solubility is chosen and in the other only a low alveolar concentration of the anesthetic is needed, induction should be rapid.

A fourth approach is to use a potent drug of low blood solubility such as sevoflurane. This allows achievement of inhaled induction before loss of effect from the intravenous induction drugs occurs.

An inhaled induction with spontaneous breathing can be achieved with any of the potent drugs in oxygen alone or with nitrous oxide and oxygen. This can be done with or without a dose of thiobarbiturate or other injected drug. When thiobarbiturates are used, they cause some decrease in ventilation, thereby decreasing the speed of induction. The principles governing appropriate delivered and inspired anesthetic concentrations are similar to those noted above. Nitrous oxide speeds induction with potent drugs slightly (second gas effect). A novel approach to rapid induction is the inspiration of a single breath of a high concentration of potent drug followed by a brief period of breath-holding to allow redistribution of the gas molecules taken up by pulmonary capillary blood.[278]

It is tempting to perform an inhaled induction by controlled ventilation once the patient has received a thiobarbiturate and neuromuscular blocking drugs for an endotracheal intubation. A danger exists in attempting to achieve a rapid rise of alveolar concentration of the potent drugs by this method. A very rapid increase of brain and cardiac anesthetic concentrations can occur. Profound depression of both organs may occur rapidly even with drugs of high blood solubility that are ordinarily associated with slow induction of anesthesia. Reversal of the profound depression may be impeded by slow removal of drug from tissues owing to low organ blood flow, low flow abetted further by zealous hyperventilation, and resultant additional decreases in cardiac output. If spontaneous ventilation is preserved until surgical levels of anesthesia are achieved, less dependence is placed on circulatory parameters as the only signs of depth of anesthesia. Also, the respiratory depression of the anesthetic inhibits further uptake of the drug.[279] Ordinarily, apnea, the most profound respiratory depression, occurs before cardiac failure, the most profound circulatory depression.[280] A margin of safety is preserved when one avoids "pumping potent drugs into paralyzed patients."

The ease of induction with the inhaled drugs is influenced by features other than potency and tissue solubility. Patient acceptance depends in part on pungency of the drug and the airway irritability that accompanies its use.[281,282] Although experience and familiarity with a drug lead one to accommodate to or even overlook its drawbacks, it appears that isoflurane is accompanied by a greater incidence of breath-holding and coughing on induction than is halothane.[281-283] Each of the three commonly used potent drugs can produce hypotension and slow heart rates on induction in children.[284]

Maintenance of Anesthesia

Maintenance anesthesia can be provided with inhaled anesthetics alone without the use of adjuvants. On the other hand, some anesthesiologists prefer to add adjuvants to a primary inhaled technique. The weights given to factors governing this choice depend on personal experience, the significance attached to dangers of one drug compared with another, individual interpretation of results of experiments, and degree of concern about maintaining simplicity as opposed to polypharmacy in anesthesia care.

Unfortunately, relatively few results are available about outcome from anesthesia and surgery in relation to choice of anesthesia.[285] This represents an area of investigation in which pioneering studies such as those of Beecher et al[286] and Shnider et al[287] were followed by a significant hiatus until workers including Gold et al[288] and Warren et al[289] stimulated new interest in outcome studies.[218,290] The simplicity accompanying the use of only an inhaled drug to provide all the anesthetic components required for an intra-abdominal or intrathoracic procedure is attractive, but this approach may require deep levels of anesthesia, levels accompanied by systemic hypotension. This hypotension may be tolerated well by some patients and not by others. In such a situation, some anesthesiologists prefer to use lower concentrations of the inhaled drugs and to provide the needed relaxation with neuromuscular blocking drugs. This preference carries with it a decision to cope with the side-effects and complications of muscle relaxants. Similarly, one might elect to supplement inhaled drugs with opioids, but these, too, are not devoid of problems. One must be guided by the needs of the individual patient and apply knowledge of the specific pharmacology of the drugs.

There are a number of situations in which selection of an inhaled drug for maintenance of anesthesia is particularly indicated. The prominent vasodilating effects of enflurane and isoflurane or the myocardial effects of halothane may be advantageous in providing deliberate hypotension.[291,292] They are also effective for reversal of hypertension in the circumstance of cardiac surgery prior to and during cardiopulmonary bypass.[293] Finally, the potent inhaled anesthetics are excellent for patients with bronchospastic disorders. Unfortunately, one cannot prove the safety of one approach over another but only the absence of complications.

Surgery in outpatients requires prompt induction of and emergence from anesthesia. It may also require complete suppression of airway reflexes or profound muscle relaxation. The inhaled drugs provide these conditions. Rapid induction is limited by the pungency of isoflurane and desflurane, a limitation that is overcome by an intravenously administered drug. The rapid increase in alveolar concentration may produce profound circulatory depression. After brief operations recovery from anesthesia is rapid with all of the inhaled drugs, but especially so with nitrous oxide, sevoflurane, and desflurane. All the drugs tested thus far have detrimental effects on mental functions that persist beyond the time of overt wakefulness.[294]

Although outcome studies are not available, there is a body of experimental evidence that supports the idea that anesthesia for neurosurgery can be provided safely with inhaled drugs, among which isoflurane appears to produce more favorable conditions than the other drugs, including nitrous oxide. Isoflurane preserves well the dependence of cerebral vessel caliber on $Paco_2$,[86] decreases cerebral oxygen requirement, and has favorable effects on CSF dynamics.[90] It provides the advantage of precise control of anesthetic dose of an inhaled anesthetic and still preserves cerebral welfare. These comments do not mean that CSF pressure will not increase in any circumstances during isoflurane anesthesia.[94]

The inhaled drugs produce muscle relaxation by themselves and potentiate the effects of neuromuscular blocking drugs administered intravenously.[241] In some patients the muscle relaxation provided by the inhaled drug is sufficient. When neuromuscular blocking drugs are used with inhaled drugs, several issues need to be considered. The degree of potentiation of neuromuscular block depends on the anesthetic and the relaxant being used. Enflurane and isoflurane produce a similar degree of potentiation of d-tubocurarine blockade,[295] but enflurane produces greater potentiation of vecuronium blockade than does isoflurane or halothane.[296] The potent inhaled drugs produce greater potentiation of neuromuscular blockers than do combinations of nitrous oxide and intravenous drugs. Therefore the doses of relaxant drugs should be adjusted downward when using the potent inhaled agents. Decreasing the concentration of inhaled drug effectively decreases the effect of the neuromuscular blocking drug.[297] There is the potential for detrimental cardiac dysrhythmias when combining inhaled anesthetics with drugs that inhibit norepinephrine reuptake.[298] The relaxants by themselves do not necessarily affect the epinephrine sensitization produced by inhaled drugs.[299]

Inhaled Drugs as Part of Balanced Anesthesia Techniques

Little has been written about the popular current practice of balanced anesthesia, that is, the practice of combining inhaled drugs with sedatives, opioids, and other drugs that have effects on the CNS. The term balanced anesthesia when first coined by Lundy in 1925[300] referred to the use of a mixture of drugs, a "diet" of compounds, to provide the anesthetic state. A mixture was used with an eye to utilizing the advantages of small amounts of each drug, it was hoped without having to contend with the disadvantages of higher doses of any one drug. The term balanced anesthesia took on a different connotation when muscle relaxants were developed. The emphasis shifted to augmenting the effects of nitrous oxide. Nitrous oxide was the basic anesthetic, and its deficiencies as a complete anesthetic were overcome by adjuvants: sedation and amnesia by barbiturates or scopolamine; reflex suppression by belladonna drugs or opioids; analgesia by opioids; and muscle relaxation by neuromuscular blocking drugs. Deficiencies in a particular response were detected by clinical signs and the appropriate adjuvant was given.

In our opinion, the new era and scope of balanced anesthesia began when the cardiovascular benefits of morphine were described by Lowenstein et al.[301] Opioids became the favorite drugs of many to provide anesthesia for patients with advanced cardiovascular disease. But, as inadequate

suppression by opioids of reflex and motor responses (or even wakefulness) became apparent, the potent inhaled drugs were added to the anesthetic regimen. The concept of the new (or revival of the old) balanced anesthesia has matured further as the potential disadvantages of nitrous oxide have come more clearly into focus.[302] These include not only its cellular toxic effects but also its effects on breathing and on the circulation. We have returned more nearly to the original concept of balanced anesthesia described by Lundy.[300] Thus, sedation and amnesia are provided by barbiturates, benzodiazepines, or butyrophenones; reflex suppression and some portion of the anesthetic requirement are provided by an opioid, barbiturate, benzodiazepine, or butyrophenone; rapid induction of unconsciousness and relaxation for intubation are offered by the barbiturate-relaxant combination; and the remainder of the anesthetic requirement and reflex suppression are achieved by an inhaled anesthetic. Muscle relaxation is provided by a neuromuscular blocking drug given intravenously. Even when high doses of opioids are used to provide anesthesia, supplemental inhaled drugs often are given to attenuate hypertension, the dose being governed by the amount of drug needed to achieve the desired arterial pressure.[293] When the major component of the anesthetic is one of the inhaled drugs, an opioid may be used to decrease heart rate[303] or a benzodiazepine to ensure amnesia. These patterns of use of the inhaled agents reflect the variety of new drugs that are now available and the increased acceptance of polypharmacy. In addition, greater knowledge of pharmacokinetics and pharmacodynamics allows us to tailor several anesthetic drugs to clinical needs.

Recovery

Rate of recovery from anesthesia with an inhaled drug is quite predictable. The decrease in alveolar concentration is related to blood solubility of the anesthetic, alveolar ventilation, and duration of anesthesia.[304] The speed of recovery after short operations is not greatly dependent on solubility of the anesthetic. As anesthesia is prolonged, however, drugs of greater blood solubility are associated with significantly slower recovery. The more rapid the recovery from anesthesia, the earlier the need for analgesic drugs because the commonly used inhaled agents provide little anesthesia in low, subanesthetic concentrations. Despite this drawback, there may be an advantage to early return of protective airway and circulatory reflexes.

METHOXYFLURANE

As recently as 1983, one writer stated that "methoxyflurane is virtually no longer used in clinical anesthesia."[305] Rather, methoxyflurane now serves as a drug model of fluoride-related nephrotoxicity, one with which new and older drugs are compared because methoxyflurane provides such predictable effects. Introduced into clinical practice by Artusio et al[10] in 1960, methoxyflurane was used and acclaimed because one of its greatest drawbacks, high blood solubility, was also a strength. The drug persisted in the body to provide ongoing sedation and pain relief following surgery. Another advantage of the drug was its prominent analgesic property, leading to a role in its providing analgesia for labor via self-administration devices.[306] The clinical impression was that methoxyflurane was an excellent muscle-relaxing drug.

The report of putative methoxyflurane nephrotoxicity by Crandell et al[307] in 1966, however, set in motion a series of elegant studies by Mazze et al,[308,309] studies that in our view provided standards for assessment of the toxic effects of anesthetics on the kidney for the subsequent two decades. Although methoxyflurane could be administered safely if rigid limits to the total administered dose, e.g., MAC hours of anesthesia, were followed,[309] advantages of methoxyflurane over the other drugs did not warrant its continued use. Furthermore, reports of possible hepatotoxicity related to the use of methoxyflurane appeared.[310] For all of these reasons, although it is still available, methoxyflurane appears to be used rarely if at all in the United States.

SEVOFLURANE

The use of sevoflurane (fluoromethyl-1,1,1,3,3,3-hexa-fluoro-isopropyl ether) was first reported by Wallin et al in 1971.[311] This agent has a boiling point of 58.5°C and a very low solubility in blood (blood:gas partition coefficient = 0.6), a value very similar to that of nitrous oxide. This is associated with both a rapid induction of anesthesia and a rapid emergence from anesthesia. Sevoflurane is second only to desflurane (blood:gas solubility coefficient 0.4) in the speed at which induction of anesthesia can be accomplished.[316] Unlike halothane and isoflurane, for which the blood:gas solubility coefficient is significantly less in the very young, in the case of sevoflurane, it is the same in both pediatric and adult patients.[312] It is second only to desflurane in having a very low solubility in plastics and rubber.

Sevoflurane is bound and degraded by soda lime to a much greater extent than are halothane, isoflurane, or desflurane.[313] When sevoflurane was administered to rats it did not appear to be any more toxic than isoflurane in spite of these products of degradation, and it is in fact less toxic than halothane.[314] The MAC of sevoflurane in humans is 1.71 ± 0.07% which is reduced to 0.66% by the addition of 63% nitrous oxide.[315] As with other anesthetic agents, some loss occurs through the skin, although this is seen less with sevoflurane than with isoflurane.[40]

Two to three percent of the administered sevoflurane is metabolized, and after 1 MAC hour of exposure, the level of plasma inorganic fluoride is 22.1 $\mu mol \cdot l^{-1}$ as compared with 0.79 $\mu mol \cdot l^{-1}$ for desflurane.[317] This is similar to the levels seen with enflurane and is well below the generally accepted toxic limit of 50 $\mu mol \cdot l^{-1}$. These levels were short-lived, probably because of the rapid removal of sevoflurane from the body. Interestingly, the defluorinase-specific activity of sevoflurane is nearly identical to that of methoxyflurane; therefore, it is not the susceptibility to metabolism but other factors, in this instance the rapid pulmonary excretion, that account for much lower and more transient increases in serum fluoride with sevoflurane than methoxyflurane. In animal studies conducted thus far, there have been no reports of nephrogenicity or mutagenicity.

Preliminary reports based on animal studies suggest that sevoflurane decreased the synthesis of all serum proteins produced by the liver.[318] The precise mechanism by which this occurs is not clear at this time, since reduced hepatic blood flow, a potential cause of altered liver function, is not a consequence of sevoflurane.[319] Like the other halogenated agents, sevoflurane is also capable of triggering malignant hyperthermia.

Sevoflurane causes respiratory frequency and $Paco_2$ to increase in a manner similar to that of other potent inhaled drugs. Sevoflurane appears to cause less depression of diaphragmatic function than enflurane, although the reason for this has not been clearly established.[320] As with other potent inhaled agents, sevoflurane causes a decrease in systemic arterial pressure. It appears to cause a dose-dependent decrease in cardiac contractility and does not sensitize the myocardium to catecholamines.[319] Studies in rabbits indicate that although sevoflurane does not appear to cause an increase in cerebral blood flow, at 0.5–1.0 MAC it does cause a small but significant increase in intracranial pressure and a fall in cerebral oxygen uptake similar to that of isoflurane.[321] At this time sevoflurane has not yet received approval by the United States Food and Drug Administration, but it is available for use elsewhere in the world.

DESFLURANE

During the past 4 years the evaluation of a new inhalational anesthetic, desflurane, has proceeded rapidly. The first of a series of reports on its properties appeared in 1987.[322] Since that time an intense and thorough laboratory and clinical analysis of the compound has been carried out. Because it is not yet approved for routine clinical use, it was not included in the comparison of commonly available anesthetics in this chapter. It is likely to become available to clinicians in the near future.

Jones et al[319,323] in 1988 were the first to administer desflurane to humans. The first administrations followed several years of work by Eger and others in defining many of the properties of desflurane. The advantages that desflurane appeared to offer were low blood and tissue solubilities and molecular stability that resisted biodegradation. The last, in turn, may reduce the likelihood of toxicity from desflurane compared with other anesthetics.

The molecular formula of desflurane is $CF_2H-O-CFH-CF_3$ (Fig. 17-1). The presence of fluorine as the only halogen lends stability to the molecule. The stability is reflected in resistance to metabolism in the body or on exposure to soda lime. Its vapor pressure at 20°C is 664 mm Hg (see Tables 17-1 and 17-2). Thus, the compound is very near its boiling point at room temperature. Accurate delivery of desired amounts of the drug is accomplished by use of a vaporizer, which maintains near-constant temperature of the liquid anesthetic and supra-atmospheric pressure within the vaporizer. Other physical characteristics of importance are low blood:gas and blood:fat partition coefficients. Except for fat, its tissue and blood partition coefficients are similar to those of other agents (see Table 17-3).

The MAC of desflurane is 7.25% in healthy 18–30-year-old patients.[324] MAC decreased to 6.0% in 31–65-year-old patients. The reduction in MAC produced by concomitant use of nitrous oxide is similar to the effect of nitrous oxide on the MAC of other anesthetics. The relatively great potency of desflurane means it provides the advantage of simultaneously providing adequate anesthesia and high inspired oxygen concentrations. Thus, induction of and emergence from anesthetizing concentrations of desflurane can be accomplished nearly as rapidly as with nitrous oxide, even though the latter drug is not a complete anesthetic.

Desflurane's effects on many physiologic variables have been determined in humans. In some instances the studies include relatively small numbers of subjects at this early stage of the drug's evaluation. However, the range of the studies is remarkably large, and in many instances comparisons were made with currently used agents. Our analysis of the data available at this time leads us to conclude that desflurane and isoflurane have quite similar properties with the exception of blood and tissue solubilities and molecular stability.

Cerebral Effects. Desflurane produces cerebrovasodilation and decreases the cerebral oxygen requirement (CMRo$_2$).[325] If profound hypotension is induced, cerebral blood flow decreases but the reduction in CMRo$_2$ maintains the oxygen supply-demand balance.[326] The cerebrovascular CO$_2$ responsiveness is preserved during desflurane anesthesia. Desflurane's electroencephalographic effects are nearly identical to those of isoflurane, namely, decreased frequency and increased amplitude with increasing alveolar desflurane concentration.[327] Burst suppression begins to appear at about 1 MAC. An isoelectric pattern develops at slightly over 1.5 MAC. Studies in dogs have shown that the EEG becomes more active, that is, indicative of a lighter level of anesthesia, with time.[325] This onset of apparent tolerance is unique to desflurane. Mental function returns to normal more quickly following anesthesia with desflurane than with isoflurane.[328]

Cardiovascular Effects. Systemic arterial pressure decreases, systolic relatively more than diastolic pressure, and heart rate is maintained near control values.[319,329] Cardiac output remains near awake values at lighter planes of anesthesia. Regional hemodynamic effects include little dose-related change in renal blood flow, no change in hepatic arterial flow, and decrease in portal blood flow at 1.75 and 2.0 MAC levels.[330] Desflurane does not sensitize the myocardium to the dysrhythmic effects of epinephrine.[331] The effects just described are quite similar to those of isoflurane. Some differences between the drugs exist, however. In the presence of autonomic blockade, isoflurane is a more potent coronary artery dilator than desflurane.[332]

Respiratory Effects. Desflurane is a ventilatory depressant in humans.[333] Increases in respiratory frequency do not compensate for decreases in tidal volume that occur as alveolar desflurane is increased. Desflurane or the desflurane–nitrous oxide combination depresses the ventilatory response to CO$_2$. Increases in the Paco$_2$ with desflurane are equivalent to those produced by enflurane when each anesthetic is given at doses equivalent to about 1.66 MAC. Desflurane's effects on bronchomotor tone have not been reported.

Molecular Stability and Biotransformation. Desflurane is more resistant to breakdown by soda lime than are halothane, isoflurane and sevoflurane.[334] It also is more resistant to hepatic metabolism than the other potent halogenated anesthetics.[335,336] Its low blood and tissue solubility and molecular stability contribute to the minimal susceptibility to metabolism. These findings suggest desflurane has little toxic potential, a prediction borne out thus far in studies in laboratory animals[337] and humans.[319]

Neuromuscular Effects. Desflurane depresses neuromuscular function and also augments the actions of pancuronium and succinylcholine.[338] The magnitude of this augmentation produced by desflurane is similar to that of isoflurane. Alveolar desflurane equivalent to nearly 2 MAC was required to produce a decrement in the first response in a train-of-four sequence, but tetanic fade occurs at lower desflurane doses.

Kinetics. Desflurane's low solubility in blood and tissues results in a rapid approach of the partial pressures in blood

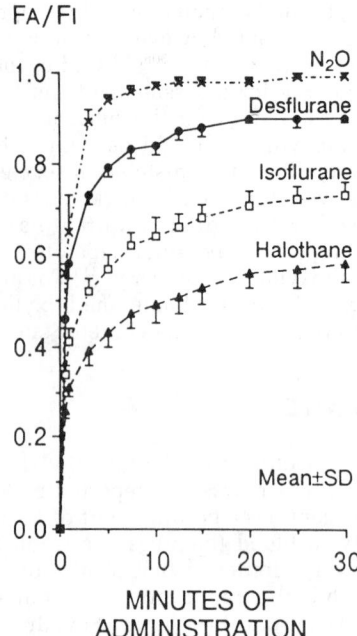

Figure 17-11. The ratios of end-tidal anesthetic concentrations (Fa) to inspired anesthetic concentrations (Fi) at constant Fi. (Reprinted with permission from Yasuda N, Lockhart SH, Eger EI II *et al.* Kinetics of desflurane, isoflurane, and halothane in humans. Anesthesiology 74:489, 1991.)

and tissue toward the inspired partial pressures[336] (Fig. 17-11). Hence, induction of anesthesia is rapid, limited only by the adequacy of alveolar ventilation and the rate at which the anesthesiologist can increase the inspired concentration. The latter is a factor in view of desflurane's pungency.[319] One should be able to change alveolar desflurane concentration rapidly in response to changing surgical requirement. Elimination of desflurane is rapid, so that recovery is prompt. Virtually all elimination of desflurane occurs *via* the lungs.

Overview

Desflurane's low blood and tissue solubility combined with adequate potency make it a very promising inhalation anesthetic. If further experience with desflurane establishes a putative low toxic potential, it will probably be used widely. Although the rapid recovery from brief anesthesia may not significantly shorten the time from the end of anesthesia to discharge from the hospital,[328] prompt return of mental function and normal control of the circulation and breathing seem satisfactory. Furthermore, the smaller influence of duration of anesthesia on recovery time[339] should be a significant advantage for desflurane in that awakening can occur quickly even after very long operations.

CONCLUSION

The list of characteristics of an ideal anesthetic is long.[15] A drug should provide rapid onset of action with predictable and, in most instances, rapid recovery from its effects. It should not have an effect on the brain or other organs that appears or persists after the time of anesthesia. It should be easy to administer, and its administration should be guided by clear signs of depth of anesthesia. The drug should possess a high safety margin in patients of all ages and physiognomies.

The search continues for drugs that approach these ideals. It appears that various anesthetic drugs may provide one or more of these ideal properties to a greater extent than other anesthetic agents but offer no benefit in other areas. For example, sevoflurane's solubility characteristics are of great advantage in terms of onset of action of anesthesia, alteration of depth of anesthesia, and recovery from anesthesia. Its respiratory effects, however, are not superior to those of other drugs, and the significance of its interactions with soda lime needs further clarification. We anticipate that future research for anesthetic drugs will be directed at the development of drugs with a high degree of specificity of action. As this research continues, anesthesia will likely be provided by a combination of drugs that the anesthesiologist believes will offer the patient as ideal anesthetic care as can be administered.

REFERENCES

1. Vitcha J: A history of Forane. Anesthesiology 35:4, 1971
2. Robbins J: Preliminary studies of the activity of fluorinated hydrocarbons. J Pharmacol Exp Ther 86:197, 1946
3. Krantz JC Jr, Carr J, Lu G et al: Anesthesia: Anesthetic action of trifluoroethyl vinyl ether. J Pharmacol Exp Ther 108:488, 1953
4. Sadove M, Balagot R, Linde H: Trifluoroethyl vinyl ether (Fluoromar): Preliminary clinical and laboratory studies. Anesthesiology 17:591, 1956
5. Cullen B, Eger EI II et al: Cardiovascular effects of fluroxene in man. Anesthesiology 32:218, 1970
6. Tucker W, Munson E, Holaday D et al: Hepatorenal toxicity following fluroxene anesthesia. Anesthesiology 39:104, 1973
7. Suckling C: Some chemical and physical factors in development of fluothane. Br J Anaesth 29:466, 1957
8. Johnstone M: Human cardiovascular response to fluothane anaesthesia. Br J Anaesth 28:392, 1954
9. Raventos J: Action of fluothane—new volatile anaesthetic. Br J Pharmacol 11:394, 1956
10. Artusio JF, Van Poznak A, Hunt R et al: Clinical evaluation of methoxyflurane. Anesthesiology 21:512, 1960
11. Subcommittee on the National Halothane Study: Summary of the National Halothane Study. JAMA 197:775, 1978
12. Burns T, Hall J, Bracken A et al: Fluorine compounds in anaesthesia. Anaesthesia 19:167, 1964
13. Terrell R, Speers L, Szur A et al: General anesthetics. I. Halogenated methylethyl ethers as anesthetic agents. J Med Chem 14:517, 1971
14. Terrell R: Physical and chemical properties of anaesthetic agents. Br J Anaesth 56:38, 1984
15. Stevens W, Eger EI II: Comparative evaluation of new inhalation anesthetics. Anesthesiology 35:125, 1971
16. Virtue R, Lund L, Phelps MJ et al: Difluoromethyl 1,1,2-trifluoro-2-chlorethyl ether as an anaesthetic agent: Results with dogs and a preliminary note on observations with man. Can Anaesth Soc J 13:233, 1966
17. Dobkin A, Nishioka K, Gengaje D et al: Ethrane (compound 347) anesthesia: A clinical and laboratory review of 700 cases. Anesth Analg 48:477, 1969
18. Stevens W, Cromwell T, Halsey M et al: The cardiovascular effects of a new inhalation anesthetic, Forane, in human volunteers at constant arterial carbon dioxide tension. Anesthesiology 35:3, 1971
19. Calverley R, Smith N, Jones C et al: Ventilatory and cardiovascular effects of enflurane during spontaneous ventilation in man. Anesth Analg 57:610, 1978
20. Raventos J, Spinks A: Methods of screening volatile anesthetics. Manchester Med Gaz 37:55, 1958
21. Burn J: Pharmacological screening of anaesthetics. Proc R Soc Med 52:95, 1959
22. Halsey M: Investigations on isoflurane, sevoflurane and other experimental anaesthetics. Br J Anaesth 53:43S, 1981
23. Fabian L, Gee H, Dowdy E et al: Laboratory and clinical investigations of a new fluorinated anesthetic compound, halopropane ($CHF_2CF_2CH_2Br$). Anesth Analg 41:707, 1962
24. Artusio JF, Van Poznak A: Laboratory and clinical investigations of teflurane, 1,1,1,2-tetrafluoro-2-bromethane (DA-708). Fed Proc 20:312, 1961
25. Kikuchi H, Morio M, Fujii K et al: Clinical evaluation and metabolism of sevoflurane in patients. Hiroshima J Med Sci 36:93, 1987
26. Holaday D, Jardines M, Greenwood W: Uptake and biotransformation of aliflurane (1-chloro-2-methoxy-1,2,3,3-tetrafluorocyclopropane, compound 26-P) in man. Anesthesiology 51:548, 1979
27. Eger EI II: Anesthetic Uptake and Action, pp 77–94. Baltimore, Williams & Wilkins, 1974
28. Hamilton W, Eastwood D: A study of denitrogenation with some inhalation anesthetic systems. Anesthesiology 16:861, 1955
29. Eger EI II, Ethans C: The effects of inflow, overflow and valve placement on economy of the circle system. Anesthesiology 29:93, 1968
30. Eger EI II, Larson CP Jr, Severinghaus J: The solubility of halothane in rubber, soda lime and various plastics. Anesthesiology 23:356, 1962
31. Eger EI II, Bahlman S: Is end-tidal anesthetic partial pressure an accurate measure of the arterial anesthetic partial pressure? Anesthesiology 35:301, 1971
32. Epstein R, Rackow H, Salanitre E et al: Influence of the concentration effect on the uptake of anesthetic mixtures: The second gas effect. Anesthesiology 25:364, 1964
33. Stoelting R, Eger EI II: An additional explanation for the second gas effect. Anesthesiology 30:273, 1969
34. Severinghaus JW: Role of lung factors. In Papper EM, Kitz RJ (eds): Uptake and Distribution of Anesthetic Agents, p 59. New York, McGraw Hill, 1963
35. Coburn CM, Eger EI II: The partial pressure of isoflurane or halothane does not affect their solubility in blood: Inhaled anesthetics obey Henry's law. Anesth Analg 65:672, 1986
36. Eger R, Eger EI II: Effect of temperature and age on the solubility of enflurane, halothane, isoflurane, and methoxyflurane in human blood. Anesth Analg 64:640, 1985
37. Munson E, Eger EI II, Tham M et al: Increase in anesthetic uptake, excretion, and blood solubility in man after eating. Anesth Analg 57:224, 1978
38. Miller M, Gandolfi A, Vaughan R et al: Disposition of enflurane in obese patients. J Pharmacol Exp Ther 215:292, 1980
39. Brandom B, Brandom R, Cook D: Uptake and distribution of halothane in infants: In vivo measurements and computer simulations. Anesth Analg 62:404, 1983
40. Lockhart S, Yasuda N, Peterson N et al: Comparison of percutaneous losses of sevoflurane and isoflurane in humans. Anesth Analg 72:212, 1991
41. Stoelting R, Eger EI II: The effects of ventilation and anesthetic solubility on recovery from anesthesia: An in vivo and analog analysis before and after equilibrium. Anesthesiology 30:290, 1969
42. Masuda T, Ikeda K: Effect of inspired nitrous oxide concentrations on the rate of fall of alveolar concentrations: Reversed concentration effect. Acta Anaesthesiol Scand 30:164, 1986
43. Cohen E, Van Dyke R: Biochemical aspects. In Cohen EN, Van Dyke RA (eds): Metabolism of Volatile Anesthetics, p 8. Reading, Massachusetts: Addison-Wesley, 1977
44. Cahalan M, Johnson B, Eger EI II: Relationship of concentrations of halothane and enflurane to their metabolism and elimination in man. Anesthesiology 54:3, 1981
45. Carpenter R, Eger EI, Johnson B et al: Pharmacokinetics of inhaled anesthetics in humans: Measurements during and after the simultaneous administration of enflurane, halothane, isoflurane, methoxyflurane and nitrous oxide. Anesth Analg 65:575, 1986

46. Merkel G, Eger EI II: A comparative study of halothane and halopropane anesthesia. Anesthesiology 24:346, 1963
47. Saidman L, Eger EI II, Munson E et al: Minimum alveolar concentrations of methoxyflurane, halothane, ether and cyclopropane in man: Correlation with theories of anesthesia. Anesthesiology 28:994, 1967
48. Quasha A, Eger EI II, Tinker J: Determination and application of MAC. Anesthesiology 53:315, 1980
49. Hornbein T, Eger EI II, Winter P et al: The minimum alveolar concentration of nitrous oxide in man. Anesth Analg 61:553, 1982
50. Kissin I, Morgan P, Smith L: Anesthetic potencies of isoflurane, halothane and diethyl ether for various end points of anesthesia. Anesthesiology 58:88, 1983
51. de Jong R, Eger EI II: MAC expanded: AD_{50} and AD_{95} values of common inhalation anesthetics in man. Anesthesiology 42:384, 1975
52. Regan M, Eger EI II: Effect of hypothermia in dogs on anesthetizing and apneic doses of inhalation agents. Determination of the anesthetic index (apnea/MAC). Anesthesiology 28:689, 1967
53. Wolfson B, Kielar C, Lake C et al: Anesthetic index—a new approach. Anesthesiology 38:583, 1978
54. Miller R, Way W, Eger EI II: The effects of alpha-methyldopa, reserpine, guanethidine, and iproniazid on minimum alveolar anesthetic requirement (MAC). Anesthesiology 29:1153, 1968
55. Saidman L, Eger EI II: Effect of nitrous oxide and of narcotic premedication on the alveolar concentration of halothane required for anesthesia. Anesthesiology 25:302, 1964
56. Cullen D, Eger EI II: The effects of hypoxia and isovolemic anemia on the halothane requirement (MAC) of dogs. 1. The effects of hypoxia. Anesthesiology 32:28, 1970
57. Cullen D, Cotev S, Severinghaus J et al: The effects of hypoxia and isovolemic anemia on the halothane requirement (MAC) of dogs. II. The effects of acute hypoxia on halothane requirement and cerebral surface Po_2, Pco_2, pH, and HCO_3. Anesthesiology 32:35, 1970
58. Johnston R, Way W, Miller R: Alteration of anesthetic requirement by amphetamines. Anesthesiology 36:357, 1972
59. Johnston R, White P, Way W et al: The effect of levodopa on halothane anesthetic requirements. Anesth Analg 54:178, 1975
60. Murphy M, Hug CC Jr: The enflurane sparing effect of morphine, butorphanol and nalbuphine. Anesthesiology 57:489, 1982
61. Lake C, DiFazio C, Moscicki J et al: Reduction in halothane MAC: Comparison of morphine and alfentanil. Anesth Analg 64:807, 1985
62. Miller R, Wahrenbrock E, Schroeder C et al: Ethylene—halothane anesthesia: Addition or synergism? Anesthesiology 31:301, 1969
63. Cullen S, Eger EI II, Cullen B et al: Observations on the anesthetic effect of the combination of xenon and halothane. Anesthesiology 31:305, 1969
64. Cole D, Kalichman M, Shapiro H et al: The non-linear potency of sub-MAC concentrations of nitrous oxide in decreasing the anesthetic requirement of enflurane, halothane, and isoflurane in rats. Anesthesiology 73:93, 1990
65. Palahniuk R, Shnider S, Eger EI II: Pregnancy decreases the requirement for inhaled anesthetic agents. Anesthesiology 41:82, 1974
66. Mazze R, Rice S, Baden J: Halothane, isoflurane, and enflurane MAC in pregnant and nonpregnant female and male mice and rats. Anesthesiology 62:339, 1985
67. Le Dez K, Lerman J: The minimum alveolar concentration (MAC) of isoflurane in preterm neonates. Anesthesiology 67:301, 1987
68. Gregory G, Eger EI II, Munson E: The relationship between age and halothane requirement in man. Anesthesiology 30:488, 1969
69. Stoelting R, Longnecker D, Eger EI II: Minimum alveolar concentrations in man on awakening from methoxyflurane, halothane, ether and fluroxene anesthesia: MAC awake. Anesthesiology 33:5, 1970
70. Roizen M, Horrigan R, Frazer B: Anesthetic doses blocking adrenergic (stress) and cardiovascular responses to incision—MAC BAR. Anesthesiology 54:390, 1981
71. Davison L, Steinhelber J, Eger EI II et al: Psychological effects of halothane and isoflurane anesthesia. Anesthesiology 43:313, 1975
72. Korttila K, Tammisto T, Ertama P et al: Recovery, psychomotor skills, and simulated driving after brief inhalational anesthesia with halothane or enflurane combined with nitrous oxide and oxygen. Anesthesiology 46:20, 1977
73. Tinker J, Gandolfi A, Van Dyke R: Elevation of plasma levels in patients following halothane anesthesia: Time correlations with total halothane dosage. Anesthesiology 44:194, 1976
74. Bruce D, Bach M, Arbit J: Trace anesthetic effects on perceptual, cognitive and motor skills. Anesthesiology 40:453, 1974
75. Cook T, Smith M, Winter P et al: Effect of subanesthetic concentrations of enflurane and halothane on human behavior. Anesth Analg 57:434, 1978
76. Ghoneim M, Mewaldt S, Petersen R: Memory effects of subanesthetic concentrations of nitrous oxide. Anesth Analg 59:540, 1980
77. Newberg L, Milde J, Michenfelder J: The cerebral metabolic effects of isoflurane at and above concentrations that suppress cortical electrical activity. Anesthesiology 59:23, 1983
78. Sakabe T, Maekawa T, Fujii S et al: Cerebral circulation and metabolism during enflurane anesthesia in humans. Anesthesiology 59:532, 1983
79. Wollman H, Smith A, Neigh J et al: Cerebral blood flow and oxygen consumption in man during electroencephalographic seizure patterns associated with enflurane anesthesia. In Brock M, Fieschi C, Ingvar D et al (eds): Cerebral Blood Flow, p 246. Berlin, Springer-Verlag, 1969
80. Stullken E, Milde J, Michenfelder J et al: The non-linear responses of cerebral metabolism to low concentrations of halothane, enflurane, isoflurane and thiopental. Anesthesiology 46:28, 1977
81. Newberg L, Michenfelder J: Cerebral protection by isoflurane during hypoxemia or ischemia. Anesthesiology 59:29, 1983
82. Nehis D, Todd M, Spetzler R et al: A comparison of the cerebral protective effects of isoflurane and barbiturates during temporary focal ischemia in primates. Anesthesiology 66:453, 1987
83. Newman B, Gelb A, Lam A: The effect of isoflurane-induced hypotension on cerebral blood flow and cerebral metabolic rate for oxygen in humans. Anesthesiology 64:307, 1986
84. Adams R, Cucchiara R, Gronert G et al: Isoflurane and cerebrospinal fluid pressure in neurosurgical patients. Anesthesiology 54:97, 1981
85. Albrecht R, Miletich D, Madala L: Normalization of cerebral blood flow during prolonged halothane anesthesia. Anesthesiology 58:26, 1983
86. Scheller M, Todd M, Drummond J: Isoflurane, halothane, and regional cerebral blood flow at various levels of $Paco_2$ in rabbits. Anesthesiology 64:598, 1986
87. Messick J, Casemen B, Milde L et al: Correlation of regional cerebral blood flow (rCBF) with EEG changes during isoflurane anesthesia for carotid endarterectomy: Critical rCBF. Anesthesiology 66:344, 1987
88. Artru A, Nugent M, Michenfelder J: Enflurane causes a prolonged and reversible increase in the rate of CSF production in the dog. Anesthesiology 57:255, 1982
89. Artru A: Effects of enflurane and isoflurane as resistance to reabsorption of cerebrospinal fluid in dogs. Anesthesiology 61:529, 1984
90. Artru A: Isoflurane does not increase the rate of CSF production in the dog. Anesthesiology 60:193, 1984
91. Artru A: Effects of halothane and fentanyl on resistance to reabsorption of CSF. J Neurosurg 60:252, 1984
92. Artru A: Effects of halothane and fentanyl on the rate of CSF production in dogs. Anesth Analg 62:581, 1983
93. Campkin T: Isoflurane and cranial extradural pressure: A study in neurosurgical patients. Br J Anaesth 56:1083, 1984
94. Grosslight K, Foster R, Colohan A et al: Isoflurane for neu-

roanesthesia: Risk factors for increases in intracranial pressure. Anesthesiology 63:533, 1985

95. Stockard J, Bickford R: The neurophysiology of anaesthesia. In Gordon EA (ed): Basis and Practice of Neuroanaesthesia, p 3. Amsterdam, Excerpta Medica, 1975

96. Eger EI II, Stevens W, Cromwell J: The electroencephalogram in man anesthetized with Forane. Anesthesiology 35:504, 1971

97. Tinker J, Sharbrough F, Michenfelder J: Anterior shift of the dominant EEG rhythm during anesthesia in a Java monkey. Anesthesiology 46:252, 1977

98. Neigh J, Garman J, Harp J: The electroencephalographic pattern during anesthesia with enflurane: Effects of depth of anesthesia, PaCO₂ and nitrous oxide. Anesthesiology 35:482, 1971

99. Lebowitz M, Blitt C, Dillon J: Enflurane-induced central nervous system excitation and its relation to carbon dioxide tension. Anesth Analg 51:355, 1972

100. Clark D, Rosner B: Neurophysiologic effects of general anesthetics. I. The electroencephalogram and sensory evoked responses in man. Anesthesiology 38:564, 1973

101. Lam AM: Monitoring neurologic evoked responses. ASA Refresher Courses in Anesthesiology 17:175, 1989

102. Grundy B: Intraoperative monitoring of sensory-evoked potentials. Anesthesiology 58:72, 1983

103. Peterson D, Drummond J, Todd M: Effects of halothane, enflurane, isoflurane, and nitrous oxide on somatosensory evoked potentials in humans. Anesthesiology 65:35, 1986

104. Sloan T, Koht A: Depression of cortical somatosensory evoked potentials by nitrous oxide. Br J Anaesth 57:849, 1985

105. McPherson R, Mahla M, Johnson R et al: Effects of enflurane, isoflurane, and nitrous oxide on somatosensory evoked potentials during fentanyl anesthesia. Anesthesiology 62:626, 1985

106. Sebel P, Flynn P, Ingram D: Effect of nitrous oxide on visual auditory and somatosensory evoked potentials. Br J Anaesth 56:1403, 1984

107. Dubois M, Sato S, Chassy J et al: Effects of enflurane on brainstem auditory evoked responses in humans. Anesth Analg 61:898, 1982

108. Uhl R, Squires K, Bruce D et al: Effect of halothane anesthesia on the human cortical visual evoked response. Anesthesiology 53:273, 1980

109. James F, Thornton C, Jones J: Halothane anaesthesia changes the early components of the auditory evoked responses in man. Br J Anaesth 54:787, 1982

110. Manninen P, Lam A, Nicholas J: The effects of isoflurane and isoflurane-nitrous anesthesia on brainstem auditory evoked potentials in humans. Anesth Analg 64:43, 1985

111. Rehder K, Mallow J, Fibuch E et al: Effects of isoflurane anesthesia and muscle paralysis on respiratory mechanics in normal man. Anesthesiology 41:477, 1974

112. Froese A, Bryan AC: Effects of anesthesia and paralysis on diaphragmatic mechanics in man. Anesthesiology 41:242, 1974

113. Munson E, Larson CP Jr, Babad A et al: The effect of halothane, fluroxene and cyclopropane on ventilation. Anesthesiology 27:716, 1966

114. Larson CP Jr, Eger EI II, Muallem M et al: The effects of diethyl ether and methoxyflurane on ventilation. II. A comparative study in man. Anesthesiology 30:174, 1969

115. Fourcade H, Stevens W, Larson CP Jr et al: The ventilatory effects of Forane, a new inhaled anesthetic. Anesthesiology 35:26, 1971

116. Devine J, Hamilton W, Pittinger C: Respiratory studies in man during fluothane anesthesia. Anesthesiology 19:11, 1958

117. Murat J, Saint-Maurice JP, Beydon L et al: Respiratory effects of nitrous oxide during isoflurane anesthesia in children. Br J Anaesth 58:1122, 1986

118. Wren W, Meeke R, Davenport J et al: Effects of nitrous oxide on the respiratory pattern of spontaneously breathing children during anaesthesia. Br J Anaesth 56:881, 1984

119. Tusiewicz K, Bryan A, Froese A: Contributions of changing rib cage-diaphragm interactions to the ventilatory depression of halothane anesthesia. Anesthesiology 47:327, 1977

120. Clergue F, Viires N, Lemesle P et al: Effect of halothane on diaphragmatic muscle function in pentobarbital-anesthetized dogs. Anesthesiology 64:181, 1986

121. Kochi T, Ide T, Ismo S et al: Different effects of halothane and isoflurane on diaphragmatic contractility in vivo. Anesth Analg 70:362, 1990

122. Knill R, Clement J: Variable effects of anaesthetics on the ventilatory response to hypoxaemia in man. Can Anaesth Soc J 29:93, 1982

123. Hickey R, Fourcade H, Eger EI II et al: The effects of ether, halothane and Forane on apneic thresholds in man. Anesthesiology 35:32, 1971

124. Eger EI II, Dolan W, Stevens W et al: Surgical stimulation antagonizes the respiratory depression produced by Forane. Anesthesiology 36:544, 1972

125. Eger EI II: Respiratory effects of nitrous oxide. In Eger EI II (ed): Nitrous oxide, p 109. New York, Elsevier, 1985

126. Hornbein T, Martin W, Bonica J et al: Nitrous oxide effects on the circulatory and ventilatory responses to halothane. Anesthesiology 31:250, 1969

127. Knill R, Manninen P, Clement J: Ventilation and chemoreflexes during enflurane sedation and anaesthesia in man. Can Anaesth Soc J 26:353, 1979

128. Knill R, Kieraszewicz H, Dodgson B et al: Chemical regulation of ventilation during isoflurane sedation and anaesthesia in humans. Can Anaesth Soc J 30:607, 1983

129. Knill R, Clement J: Ventilatory responses to acute metabolic acidemia in humans awake, sedated, and anesthetized with halothane. Anesthesiology 62:745, 1985

130. Nunn J, Ezi-Ashi T: The respiratory effects of resistance to breathing in anesthetized man. Anesthesiology 22:174, 1961

131. Slee TA, Sharar SR, Pavlin EG et al: The effects of airway impedance on work of breathing during halothane anesthesia. Anesth Analg 69:374, 1989

132. Behrakis P, Higgs B, Baydur A et al: Active inspiratory impedance in halothane-anesthetized humans. J Appl Physiol 54:1477, 1983

133. Royston D, Jordan C, Jones J: Effect of subanaesthetic concentrations of nitrous oxide on the regulation of ventilation in man. Br J Anaesth 55:449, 1983

134. Moote C, Knill R, Clement J: Ventilatory compensation for continuous inspiratory resistive and elastic loads during halothane anesthesia in humans. Anesthesiology 64:582, 1986

135. Lindahl S, Charlton H, Hatch D et al: Ventilatory responses to inspiratory mechanical loads in spontaneously breathing children during halothane anaesthesia. Acta Anaesthesiol Scand 30:122, 1986

136. Pietak S, Weenig C, Hickey R et al: Anesthetic effects on ventilation in patients with chronic obstructive pulmonary disease. Anesthesiology 42:160, 1975

137. Rosenberg M, Tobias R, Bourke D et al: Respiratory responses to surgical stimulation during enflurane anesthesia. Anesthesiology 52:163, 1980

138. Lam A, Clement J, Knill R: Surgical stimulation does not enhance ventilatory chemoreflexes during enflurane anaesthesia in man. Can Anaesth Soc J 27:22, 1980

139. Coon R, Kampine J: Hypocapnic bronchoconstriction and inhalation anesthetics. Anesthesiology 43:635, 1975

140. Kingston H, Hirshman C: Perioperative management of the patient with asthma. Anesth Analg 63:844, 1984

141. Warner D, Vetterman J, Brusasco V et al: Pulmonary resistance during halothane anesthesia is not determined only by airway calibre. Anesthesiology 70:453, 1989

142. Heneghan C, Bergman N, Jordan C et al: Effect of isoflurane on bronchomotor tone in man. Br J Anaesth 58:24, 1986

143. Hirshman C, Edelstein G, Peetz S et al: Mechanism of action of inhalational anesthesia on airways. Anesthesiology 56:107, 1982

144. Hirshman C, Bergman N: Halothane and enflurane protect against bronchospasm in an asthma dog model. Anesth Analg 57:629, 1978

145. Marshall BE: Hypoxic pulmonary vasoconstriction. Acta Anaesthesiol Scand Suppl 94:37, 1990

146. Bjertnaes L, Mundal R, Honje A et al: Vascular resistance in

atelectatic lungs: Effects of inhalation anaesthetics. Acta Anaesthiol Scand 24:109, 1980

147. Marshall C, Lindgren L, Marshall B: Effects of halothane, enflurane and isoflurane on hypoxic pulmonary vasoconstriction in rat lungs in vitro. Anesthesiology 60:304, 1984

148. Domino K, Borowec L, Alexander C et al: Influence of isoflurane on hypoxic pulmonary vasoconstriction in dogs. Anesthesiology 64:423, 1986

149. Rees D, Gaines GY III: One-lung anesthesia—a comparison of pulmonary gas exchange during anesthesia with ketamine or enflurane. Anesth Analg 63:521, 1984

150. Rogers S, Benumof J: Halothane and isoflurane do not decrease Pao₂ during one-lung ventilation in intravenously anesthetized patients. Anesth Analg 64:946, 1985

151. Carlsson A, Bindslev L, Hedenstierna G: Hypoxia-induced pulmonary vasoconstriction in the human lung. Anesthesiology 66:312, 1987

152. Forbes A, Horrigan R: Mucociliary flow in the trachea during anesthesia with enflurane, ether, nitrous oxide, and morphine. Anesthesiology 46:319, 1977

153. Lee K, Park S: Effect of halothane, enflurane, and nitrous oxide on tracheal ciliary activity in vitro. Anesth Analg 59:426, 1980

154. Eger EI II, Smith N, Stoelting R: Cardiovascular effects of halothane in man. Anesthesiology 32:396, 1970

155. Calverley R, Smith N, Prys-Roberts C et al: Cardiovascular effects of enflurane anesthesia during controlled ventilation in man. Anesth Analg 57:619, 1978

156. Eisele J, Smith N: Cardiovascular effects of 40 percent nitrous oxide in man. Anesth Analg 51:956, 1972

157. Reiz S, Bälfors E, Gustavsson B et al: Effects of halothane on coronary haemodynamics and myocardial metabolism in patients with ischaemic heart disease and heart failure. Acta Anaesthiol Scand 26:133, 1981

158. Merin R, Basch S: Are the myocardial functional and metabolic effects of isoflurane really different from those of halothane and enflurane? Anesthesiology 55:398, 1981

159. Moffitt E, Barker R, Glenn J et al: Myocardial metabolic and hemodynamic responses with isoflurane anesthesia for coronary arterial surgery. Anesth Analg 65:53, 1986

160. Eger EI II: The pharmacology of isoflurane. Br J Anaesth 56:71S, 1984

161. Theye R, Michenfelder J: Whole body and organ Vo₂ changes with enflurane, isoflurane and halothane. Br J Anaesth 47:813, 1975

162. Kenny D, Pelc LR, Brooks HL et al: Alteration of alpha 1 and alpha 2 adrenoreceptor mediated pressor responses by halothane and isoflurane anesthesia. Anesthesiology 71:224, 1989

163. Bahlman S, Eger EI, Halsey M et al: The cardiovascular effects of halothane in man during spontaneous ventilation. Anesthesiology 36:494, 1972

164. Cromwell T, Stevens W, Eger EI II et al: The cardiovascular effects of compound 469 (Forane) during spontaneous ventilation and CO₂ challenge in man. Anesthesiology 35:17, 1971

165. Cullen D, Eger EI II: Cardiovascular effects of carbon dioxide in man. Anesthesiology 41:345, 1974

166. Manninen P, Knill R: Cardiovascular signs of acute hypoxaemia and hypercarbia during enflurane and halothane anaesthesia in man. Can Anaesth Soc J 26:282, 1979

167. Price H, Skovsted P, Pauca A et al: Evidence for B-receptor activation produced by halothane in normal man. Anesthesiology 32:389, 1970

168. Ritter J, Shigezawa G, Roe S et al: Increasing myocardial oxygen demand during prolonged halothane anesthesia in dogs. Anesth Analg 62:788, 1983

169. Smith N, Eger EI II, Stoelting R et al: The cardiovascular and sympathomimetic responses to the addition of nitrous oxide to halothane in man. Anesthesiology 32:410, 1970

170. Smith N, Calverley R, Prys-Roberts C et al: Impact of nitrous oxide on the circulation during enflurane anesthesia. Anesthesiology 48:345, 1978

171. Dolan W, Stevens W, Eger EI II et al: The cardiovascular and respiratory effects of isoflurane–nitrous oxide anaesthesia. Can Anaesth Soc J 21:557, 1974

172. Moffitt E, Sethna D, Gary R et al: Nitrous oxide added to halothane reduces coronary flow and myocardial oxygen consumption in patients with coronary disease. Can Anaesth Soc J 30:5, 1983

173. Reiz S: Nitrous oxide augments the systemic and coronary haemodynamic effects of isoflurane in patients with ischaemic heart disease. Acta Anaesthesiol Scand 77:464, 1983

174. Lappas D, Buckley M, Laver M et al: Left ventricular performance and pulmonary circulation following addition of nitrous oxide to morphine during coronary-artery surgery. Anesthesiology 43:61, 1975

175. Hilgenberg J, McCammon R, Stoelting R: Pulmonary and systemic vascular responses to nitrous oxide in patients with mitral stenosis and pulmonary hypertension. Anesth Analg 59:323, 1980

176. Schulte-Sasse U, Hess W, Tarnow J: Pulmonary vascular responses to nitrous oxide in patients with normal and high pulmonary vascular resistance. Anesthesiology 57:9, 1982

177. Hickey P, Hansen D, Stratford M et al: Pulmonary and systemic hemodynamic effects of nitrous oxide in infants with normal and elevated pulmonary vascular resistance. Anesthesiology 65:374, 1986

178. Priebe H: Differential effects of isoflurane on regional right and left ventricular performances, and on coronary, systemic and pulmonary hemodynamics. Anesthesiology 66:262, 1987

179. Epstein R, Deutsch S, Cooperman L et al: Splanchnic circulation during halothane anesthesia and hypercapnia in normal man. Anesthesiology 27:654, 1966

180. Gelman S, Fowler K, Smith L: Regional blood flow during isoflurane and halothane anesthesia. Anesth Analg 63:557, 1984

181. Gelman S, Fowler K, Smith L: Liver circulation and function during isoflurane and halothane anesthesia. Anesthesiology 61:726, 1984

182. Matsumoto N, Rorie D, VanDyke R: Hepatic oxygen supply and consumption in rats exposed to thiopental, halothane, enflurane, and isoflurane in the presence of hypoxia. Anesthesiology 66:337, 1987

183. Seyde W, Ellis J, Longnecker D: The addition of nitrous oxide to halothane decreases renal and splanchnic flow and increases cerebral flow in rats. Br J Anaesth 58:63, 1986

184. Ostman M, Biber B, Martner J et al: Influence of isoflurane on renal and intestinal vascular responses to stress. Br J Anaesth 58:630, 1986

185. Duke P, Fownes D, Wade J: Halothane depresses baroreflex control of heart rate in man. Anesthesiology 46:184, 1977

186. Morton M, Duke P, Ong B: Baroreflex control of heart rate in man awake and during enflurane and enflurane–nitrous oxide anesthesia. Anesthesiology 52:221, 1980

187. Kotrly K, Ebert T, Vucins E et al: Baroreceptor reflex control of heart rate during isoflurane anesthesia in humans. Anesthesiology 60:173, 1984

188. Bagshaw R, Cox R: Nitrous oxide and the baroreceptor reflexes in the dog. Acta Anaesthesiol Scand 26:31, 1982

189. Ebert T, Kotrly K, Vucins E et al: Halothane anesthesia attenuates cardiopulmonary baroreflex control of peripheral resistance in humans. Anesthesiology 63:668, 1985

190. Weiskopf R, Townsley M, Riordan K et al: Comparison of cardiopulmonary responses to graded hemorrhage during enflurane, halothane, isoflurane, and ketamine anesthesia. Anesth Analg 60:481, 1981

191. Weiskopf R, Bogetz M: Cardiovascular actions of nitrous oxide or halothane in hypovolemic swine. Anesthesiology 63:509, 1985

192. Atlee JL, Bosnjak ZJ: Mechanisms for cardiac dysrhythmias during anesthesia. Anesthesiology 72:347, 1990

193. Johnston R, Eger EI II, Wilson C: A comparative interaction of epinephrine with enflurane, isoflurane, and halothane in man. Anesth Analg 55:709, 1976

194. Horrigan R, Eger EI II, Wilson C: Arrhythmias under enflurane anesthesia in man: A non-linear dose-response relationship and dose-dependent protection from lidocaine. Anesth Analg 57:547, 1978

195. Metz S, Maze M: Halothane concentration does not alter the threshold for epinephrine-induced arrhythmias in dogs. Anesthesiology 62:470, 1985

196. Tucker W, Rackstein A, Munson E: Comparison of arrhythmic doses of adrenaline, metaraminol, ephedrine and phenylephrine during isoflurane and halothane anaesthesia in dogs. Br J Anaesth 46:392, 1974

197. Spiss C, Maze M, Smith C: Alpha-adrenergic responsiveness correlates with epinephrine dose for arrhythmias during halothane anesthesia in dogs. Anesth Analg 63:297, 1984

198. Karl H, Swedlow DB, Lee KW et al: Epinephrine-halothane interactions in children. Anesthesiology 58:142, 1983

199. Robertson B, Clement J, Knill R: Enhancement of the arrhythmogenic effect of hypercarbia by surgical stimulation during halothane anaesthesia in man. Can Anaesth Soc J 28:342, 1981

200. Atlee JL III, Roberts F: Thiopental and epinephrine-induced dysrhythmias in dogs anesthetized with enflurane or isoflurane. Anesth Analg 65:437, 1986

201. Stirt J, Berger J, Sullivan S: Lack of arrhythmogenicity of isoflurane following administration of aminophylline in dogs. Anesth Analg 62:568, 1983

202. Bosnjak Z, Kampine J: Effects of halothane, enflurane and isoflurane on the SA node. Anesthesiology 58:314, 1983

203. Atlee JL III, Brownlee S, Burstrom R: Conscious-state comparisons of the effects of inhalation anesthetics on specialized atrioventricular conduction times in dogs. Anesthesiology 64:703, 1986

204. Zaidan J, Curling P, Craver JM Jr: Effect of enflurane, isoflurane, and halothane on pacing stimulation thresholds. PACE 8:32, 1985

205. Roizen M, Plummer G, Lichtor J: Nitrous oxide and dysrhythmias. Anesthesiology 66:427, 1987

206. Kapur P, Bloor B, Flacke W et al: Comparison of cardiovascular responses to verapamil during enflurane, isoflurane or halothane anesthesia in dogs. Anesthesiology 61:156, 1984

207. Rogers K, Hysing E, Merin R et al: Cardiovascular effects of and interaction between calcium blocking drugs and anesthetics in chronically instrumented dogs. II. Verapamil, enflurane, and isoflurane. Anesthesiology 64:568, 1986

208. Kates R, Kaplan J, Guyton R et al: Hemodynamic interaction of verapamil and isoflurane. Anesthesiology 59:132, 1983

209. Iwatsuki N, Katoh M, Ono K et al: Antiarrhythmic effect of diltiazem during halothane anesthesia in dogs and in humans. Anesth Analg 64:964, 1985

210. Hysing E, Chelly J, Doursout M et al: Cardiovascular effects of and interaction between calcium blocking drugs and anesthetics in chronically instrumented dogs. III. Nicardipine and isoflurane. Anesthesiology 65:385, 1986

211. Slogoff S, Keats A, Hibbs C et al: Failure of general anesthesia to potentiate propranolol activity. Anesthesiology 47:504, 1977

212. Bollen B, Tinker J, Hermsmeyer K: Halothane relaxes previously constricted porcine coronary artery segments more than isoflurane. Anesthesiology 66:748, 1987

213. Buffington C, Ranson J, Levine H et al: Isoflurane induces coronary steal in a canine model of chronic coronary occlusion. Anesthesiology 66:280, 1987

214. Reiz S, Balfors E, Sorensen M et al: Isoflurane—a powerful coronary vasodilator in patients with coronary artery disease. Anesthesiology 59:91, 1983

215. Sill J, Bove A, Nugent M et al: Effects of isoflurane on coronary arteries and coronary arterioles in the intact dog. Anesthesiology 66:273, 1987

216. Priebe H, Föex P: Isoflurane causes regional myocardial dysfunction in dogs with critical coronary artery stenoses. Anesthesiology 66:293, 1987

217. Tarnow J, Markschies-Hornung A, Schulte-Sasse U: Isoflurane improves the tolerance to pacing-induced myocardial ischemia. Anesthesiology 64:147, 1986

218. Slogoff S, Keats AS: Randomized trial of primary anesthetic agents on outcome of coronary artery bypass operations. Anesthesiology 70:179, 1989

219. Rydvall A, Häggmark S, Nyhmon H et al: Effects of enflurane on coronary haemodynamics in patients with ischaemic heart disease. Acta Anaesthesiol Scand 28:690, 1984

220. Bernard J-M, Doursout M-F, Wouters P et al: Effects of enflurane and isoflurane in hepatic and renal circulations in chronically instrumented dogs. Anesthesiology 74:298, 1991

221. Jarnberg P-O, Marrone B, Priano LL: Enflurane preserves renal blood flow. Anesthesiology 73:A572, 1990

222. Green C, Eastwood D: Effects of nitrous oxide inhalation on hemopoiesis in rats. Anesthesiology 24:341, 1963

223. Nunn J: Clinical aspects of the interaction between nitrous oxide and vitamin B_{12}. Br J Anaesth 59:3, 1987

224. Skacel P, Hewlett A, Lewis J et al: Studies of the haemopoietic toxicity of nitrous oxide in man. Br J Haematol 53:189, 1983

225. Nunn J, Chanarin I, Tanner A et al: Megaloblastic bone marrow changes after repeated nitrous oxide anaesthesia. Br J Anaesth 58:1469, 1986

226. Koblin DD: Nitrous oxide: A cause of cancer or chemotherapeutic adjuvant? Semin Surg Oncol 6:141, 1990

227. Erskine R, James M: Isoflurane but not halothane stimulates neutrophil chemotaxis. Br J Anaesth 64:723, 1990

228. Busoni P, Sarti A, De Martino M et al: The effect of general and regional anesthesia on oxygen-dependent microbicidal mechanisms of polymorphonuclear leukocytes in children. Anesth Analg 67:453, 1988

229. Mealy K, O'Farrelly C, Stephens R et al: Impaired neutrophil function during anesthesia and surgery is due to serum factors. J Surg Res 43:393, 1987

230. Stevenson GW, Hall SC, Rudnick S et al: The effect of anesthetic agents on the human immune response. Anesthesiology 72:542, 1990

231. Griffith C, Kamath M: Effect of halothane and nitrous oxide anaesthesia on natural killer lymphocytes from patients with benign and malignant breast disease. Br J Anaesth 58:540, 1986

232. Yamaoka A, Sumimoto H, Takeshige K et al: Inhibition of leukotriene formation in human leukocytes by halothane. Biochim Biophys Acta 918:284, 1987

233. Lieners C, Redl H, Schlag G et al: Inhibition by halothane, but not by isoflurane, of oxidative response to opsonized zymosan in whole blood. Inflammation 13:621, 1989

234. Ferrero E, Ferrero M, Marni A et al: In vitro effects of halothane on lymphocytes. Eur J Anaesthesiol 3:321, 1986

235. Lanza V, Mercadante S, Pignataro A: Effects of halothane, enflurane, and nitrous oxide on oxyhemoglobin affinity. Anesthesiology 68:591, 1988

236. Kambam J, Horton B, Parris W et al: Effect of sevoflurane on P50 and on measurement of oxygen tension. J Clin Monit 4:261, 1988

237. Hofmann J, Seidel U, Till U: Effect of halothane on metabolic ATP and induced aggregation of human blood platelets. Biomed Biochim Acta 48:337, 1989

238. Kobayashi O, Ohta Y, Kosaka F: Interaction of sevoflurane, isoflurane, enflurane and halothane with non-depolarizing muscle relaxants and their prejunctional effects at the neuromuscular junction. Acta Med Okayama 44:209, 1990

239. Donati F, Bevan D: Long-term succinylcholine infusion during isoflurane anesthesia. Anesthesiology 58:6, 1983

240. Keens S, Hunter J, Snowdon S et al: Potentiation of the neuromuscular blockade produced by alcuronium with halothane, enflurane and isoflurane. Br J Anaesth 59:1011, 1987

241. Miller R, Eger EI II, Way W et al: Comparative neuromuscular effects of Forane and halothane alone and in combination with d-tubocurarine in man. Anesthesiology 35:38, 1971

242. Hirsch I, McGill J, Cryer P et al: Perioperative management of surgical patients with diabetes mellitus. Anesthesiology 74:346, 1991

243. Ewart R, Rusy B, Bradford M: Effects of enflurane on release of insulin by pancreatic islets in vitro. Anesth Analg 60:878, 1981

244. Oyama T, Sato K, Kimura K: Plasma levels of antidiuretic hormone in man during halothane anaesthesia and surgery. Can Anaesth Soc J 18:614, 1971

245. Philbin D, Coggins C: Plasma antidiuretic hormone levels in

cardiac surgical patients during morphine and halothane anesthesia. Anesthesiology 49:95, 1978

246. Miller R, Boulukos P, Warner R: Failure of halothane and ketamine to alleviate carcinoid syndrome-induced bronchospasm during anesthesia. Anesth Analg 59:621, 1980

247. Oyama T, Aoki N, Kudo T: Effect of halothane anesthesia and of surgery on plasma testosterone levels in man. Anesth Analg 51:130, 1971

248. Joyce JT, Roizen MF, Gerson JI et al: Induction of anesthesia with halothane increases plasma norepinephrine concentrations. Anesthesiology 56:286, 1982

249. Lacoumenta S, Paterson J, Burrin J et al: Effects of two differing halothane concentrations on the metabolic and endocrine responses to surgery. Br J Anaesth 58:844, 1986

250. Gelman S, Rivas J, Erdemir H et al: Hormonal and haemodynamic responses to upper abdominal surgery during isoflurane and balanced anaesthesia. Can Anaesth Soc J 31:509, 1984

251. Campbell B, Parikh R, Naismith A et al: Comparison of fentanyl and halothane supplementation to general anaesthesia on the stress response to upper abdominal surgery. Br J Anaesth 56:257, 1984

252. Sigurdsson G, Lindahl S, Norden N: Catecholamine and endocrine response in children during halothane and enflurane anaesthesia for adrenoidectomy. Acta Anaesthiol Scand 28:47, 1984

253. Desmonts J, LeHouelleur J, Remond P et al: Anaesthetic management of patients with phaeochromocytoma: A review of 102 cases. Br J Anaesth 49:991, 1977

254. Suzukawa M, Michaels IAL, Ruzbarsky J et al: Use of isoflurane during resection of pheochromocytoma. Anesth Analg 62:100, 1983

255. Doi M, Ikeda K: Sevoflurane anesthesia with adenosine triphosphate for resection of pheochromocytoma. Anesthesiology 70:360, 1989

256. Oyama T, Matsuki A, Kudo T: Effect of halothane, methoxyflurane anaesthesia and surgery on plasma thyroid-stimulating hormone (TSH) levels in man. Anaesthesia 27:2, 1972

257. Servin F, Nivoche Y, Desmonts J et al: Biotransformation of halothane and enflurane in patients with hyperthyroidism. Anesthesiology 64:387, 1986

258. Murkin J: Anesthesia and hypothyroidism: A review of thyroxine physiology, pharmacology and anesthetic implications. Anesth Analg 61:371, 1982

259. Abboud T, D'Onofrio L, Reyes A et al: Isoflurane or halothane for cesarean section: Comparative maternal and neonatal effects. Acta Anaesthesiol Scand 33:578, 1989

260. Baker B, Hughes S, Shnider S et al: Maternal anesthesia and the stressed fetus: Effects of isoflurane on the asphyxiated lamb. Anesthesiology 72:65, 1990

261. Khristianson B, Magno R, Wickstrom I: Anesthesia for cesarean section. VI. Late effects on the infant of enflurane anesthesia for cesarean section. Acta Anaesthiol Scand 24:187, 1980

262. Guedel A: Inhalation Anesthesia: A Fundamental Guide, p 16. New York, Macmillan, 1951

263. Winterbottom E: Insufficient anesthesia. Br Med J 1:247, 1950

264. Neff W, Mayer E, Perales M: Nitrous oxide and oxygen anesthesia with curare relaxation. Calif Med 66:67, 1947

265. Mushin W: Analgesics as supplements during anaesthesia. Proc R Soc Med 44:840, 1951

266. Siker E: Analgesic supplements to nitrous oxide anesthesia. A review. Br Med J 2:1326, 1956

267. Utting J: Awareness in anaesthesia. Anaesth Intensive Care 3:334, 1975

268. Woodbridge P: Changing concepts concerning depth of anesthesia. Anesthesiology 18:536, 1957

269. Artusio JJ: Diethyl ether analgesia: A detailed description of the first stage of ether anesthesia in man. J Pharmacol Exp Ther 111:343, 1954

270. Wise R: Pain clinic and operative nerve blocks. In Churchill-Davidson HC (ed): A Practice of Anaesthesia, p 893. Chicago, Year Book Medical Publishers, 1984

271. Baskett P: The use of Entonox in the ambulance service. Proc R Soc Med 65:7, 1972

272. Bahl C, Wadwa S: Consciousness during apparent surgical anaesthesia. Br J Anaesth 40:289, 1968

273. Manizar J: Awareness, muscle relaxants and balanced anaesthesia. Can Anaesth Soc J 26:386, 1979

274. Cullen D, Eger EI II, Stevens W et al: Clinical signs of anesthesia. Anesthesiology 36:21, 1972

275. Eger EI II: Monitoring the depth of anesthesia. In Saidman LJ, Smith NT (eds): Monitoring in Anesthesia, p 1. Boston, Butterworths, 1978

276. Cullen SC, Larson CP Jr: Evaluation of anesthetic depth. In Cullen SC, Larson CP Jr (eds): Essentials of Anesthetic Practice, p 77. Chicago, Year Book Medical Publishers, 1974

277. Miller R: Monitoring of neuromuscular blockade. In Saidman LJ, Smith NT (eds): Monitoring in Anesthesia, p 193. Boston, Butterworths, 1978

278. Ruffle J, Snider M, Rosenberger J et al: Rapid induction of halothane anaesthesia in man. Br J Anaesth 57:607, 1985

279. Munson E, Eger EI II, Bowers D: Effects of anesthetic-depressed ventilation and cardiac output on anesthetic uptake: A computer nonlinear simulation. Anesthesiology 38:251, 1973

280. Wolfson B, Hetrick W, Lake C et al: Anesthetic indices—further data. Anesthesiology 48:187, 1978

281. Fisher D, Robinson S, Brett C et al: Comparison of enflurane, halothane, and isoflurane for diagnostic and therapeutic procedures in children with malignancies. Anesthesiology 63:647, 1985

282. Kingston H: Halothane and isoflurane anesthesia in pediatric outpatients. Anesth Analg 65:181, 1986

283. Buffington C: Reflex action during isoflurane anaesthesia. Can Anaesth Soc J 29:S35, 1982

284. Friesen R, Lichtor J: Cardiovascular effects of inhalation induction with isoflurane in infants. Anesth Analg 62:411, 1983

285. Keats AS: What do we know about anesthetic mortality? Anesthesiology 50:387, 1970

286. Beecher H, Todd D: A study of the deaths associated with anesthesia and surgery. Ann Surg 140:2, 1954

287. Shnider S, Papper E: Anesthesia for the asthmatic patient. Anesthesiology 22:886, 1961

288. Gold M, Schwam S, Goldberg M: Chronic obstructive pulmonary disease and respiratory complications. Anesth Analg 62:975, 1983

289. Warren T, Datta S, Ostheimer G et al: Comparison of the maternal and neonatal effects of halothane, enflurane, and isoflurane for cesarean delivery. Anesth Analg 62:516, 1983

290. Forrest JB, Cahalan MK, Rehder K et al: Multicenter study of general anesthesia. II. Results. Anesthesiology 72:262, 1990

291. Lam A, Gelb A: Cardiovascular effects of isoflurane-induced hypotension for cerebral aneurysm surgery. Anesth Analg 62:742, 1983

292. Fairbairn M, Eltringham R, Young P et al: Hypotensive anaesthesia for microsurgery of the middle ear. A comparison between isoflurane and halothane. Anaesthesia 41:637, 1986

293. Hess W, Arnold B, Shulte-Sasse U et al: Comparison of isoflurane and halothane when used to control intraoperative hypertension in patients undergoing coronary artery bypass surgery. Anesth Analg 62:15, 1983

294. Herbert M, Healy T, Bourke J et al: Profile of recovery after general anaesthesia. Br Med J 286:1539, 1983

295. Ali H, Savarese J: Monitoring neuromuscular function. Anesthesiology 45:216, 1976

296. Rupp SM, McChristian JW, Miller RD et al: Neostigmine and edrophonium antagonism of varying intensity neuromuscular blockade induced by atracurium, pancuronium, or vecuronium. Anesthesiology 64:711, 1986

297. Gencarelli P, Miller R, Eger EI II et al: Decreasing enflurane concentrations and d-tubocurarine neuromuscular blockade. Anesthesiology 56:192, 1982

298. Edwards R, Miller R, Roizen M et al: Cardiac responses to imipramine and pancuronium during anesthesia with halothane or enflurane. Anesthesiology 50:421, 1979

299. Schick L, Chapin J, Munson E et al: Pancuronium, d-tubocurarine, and epinephrine-induced arrhythmias during halothane anesthesia in dogs. Anesthesiology 52:207, 1980

300. Lundy J: Balanced anesthesia. Minn Med 8:399, 1925

301. Lowenstein E, Hallowell P, Levine F et al: Cardiovascular response to large doses of intravenous morphine in man. N Engl J Med 281:1389, 1969

302. Eger EI II: Should we not use nitrous oxide? In Eger EI II (ed): Nitrous Oxide/N₂O, p 339. New York, Elsevier, 1985

303. Cahalan M, Lurz F, Beaupre P et al: Narcotics alter the heart rate and blood pressure response to inhalation anesthesia. Anesthesiology 59:A26, 1983

304. Eger EI II: Recovery from anesthesia. In Eger EI II (ed): Anesthetic Uptake and Action, p 228. Baltimore, Williams & Wilkins, 1974

305. Rice S, Dooley J, Mazze R: Metabolism by rat hepatic microsomes of fluorinated ether anesthetics following ethanol consumption. Anesthesiology 58:237, 1983

306. Major V, Rosen M, Mushin W: Methoxyflurane as an obstetric analgesic: A comparison with trichloroethylene. Br Med J 2:1554, 1966

307. Crandell W, Pappas S, Macdonald A: Nephrotoxicity associated with methoxyflurane anesthesia. Anesthesiology 27:591, 1966

308. Mazze R, Trudell J, Cousins M: Methoxyflurane metabolism and renal dysfunction: Clinical correlations in man. Anesthesiology 35:247, 1971

309. Cousins M, Mazze R: Methoxyflurane nephrotoxicity. A study of dose-response in man. JAMA 225:1611, 1973

310. Lischner M: Fatal hepatic necrosis following surgery. Possible relation to methoxyflurane anesthesia. Arch Intern Med 120:225, 1967

311. Wallin R, Napoli MD: Sevoflurane (fluoromethyl-1,1, 1,3,3,3-hexafluoro-2-propyl ether): A new inhalational anesthetic agent. Fed Proc 30:442, 1971

312. Malviya S, Lerman J: The blood/gas solubilities of sevoflurane, isoflurane, halothane, and serum constituent concentrations in neonates and adults. Anesthesiology 72:793, 1990

313. Targ A, Yasuda N, Eger EI II: Solubility of I-653, sevoflurane, isoflurane, and halothane in plastics and rubber composing a conventional anesthetic circuit. Anesth Analg 69:218, 1989

314. Strum D, Eger EI II, Johnson B et al: Toxicity of sevoflurane in rats. Anesth Analg 66:769, 1987

315. Katoh T, Ikeda K: The minimum alveolar concentration (MAC) of sevoflurane in humans. Anesthesiology 66:301, 1987

316. Yasuda N, Targ A, Eger EI II et al: Pharmacokinetics of desflurane, sevoflurane, isoflurane, and halothane in pigs. Anesth Analg 71:340, 1990

317. Shiraishi Y, Ikeda K: Uptake and biotransformation of sevoflurane in humans: A comparative study of sevoflurane with halothane, enflurane, and isoflurane [see comments]. J Clin Anesth 2:381, 1990

318. Franks J, Kruskal J, Holaday D: Immediate depression of fibrinogen, albumin and transferrin synthesis by halothane, isoflurane, sevoflurane and enflurane. Anesthesiology 71:A238, 1989

319. Jones R: Desflurane and sevoflurane: Inhalation anaesthetics for this decade? Br J Anaesth 65:527, 1990

320. Ide T, Kochi T, Isono S et al: Diaphragmatic function during sevoflurane anaesthesia in dogs. Can J Anaesth 38:116, 1991

321. Scheller M, Tateishi A, Drummond J et al: The effects of sevoflurane on cerebral blood flow, cerebral metabolic rate for oxygen, intracranial pressure, and the electroencephalogram are similar to those of isoflurane in the rabbit. Anesthesiology 68:548, 1988

322. Eger EI II: Partition coefficients of I-653 in human blood, saline, and olive oil. Anesth Analg 66:971, 1987

323. Jones R, Cashman J, Mant T: Clinical impressions and cardiorespiratory effects of a new fluorinated inhalational anesthetic, desflurane (I-653), in volunteers. Br J Anaesth 64:11, 1990

324. Rampil I, Lockhart S, Zwass M et al: Clinical characteristics of desflurane in surgical patients: Minimum alveolar concentration. Anesthesiology 74:429, 1991

325. Lutz L, Milde J, Milde L: The cerebral functional, metabolic and hemodynamic effects of desflurane in dogs. Anesthesiology 73:125, 1990

326. Milde L, Milde J: The cerebral and systemic hemodynamics and metabolic effects of desflurane-induced hypotension in dogs. Anesthesiology 74:513, 1991

327. Rampil I, Lockhart S, Eger EI II et al: The electroencephalographic effects of desflurane in humans. Anesthesiology 74:434, 1991

328. Ghouri A, Bodner M, White P et al: Recovery profile after desflurane-nitrous oxide versus isoflurane-nitrous oxide in outpatients. Anesthesiology 74:419, 1991

329. Weiskopf R, Holmes M, Eger EI II et al: Cardiovascular effects of I-653 in swine. Anesthesiology 69:303, 1988

330. Merin R, Bernard J, Doursout M et al: Comparison of the effects of isoflurane and desflurane on cardiovascular dynamics and regional blood flow in the chronically instrumented dog. Anesthesiology 74:568, 1991

331. Weiskopf R, Eger EI II, Holmes M et al: Epinephrine induced premature ventricular contractions and changes in arterial blood pressure and heart rate during I-653, isoflurane, and halothane anesthesia in swine. Anesthesiology 70:293, 1989

332. Pagel PS, Kampine JP, Schmeling WT et al: Comparison of the systemic and coronary hemodynamic actions of desflurane, isoflurane, halothane, and enflurane. Anesthesiology 74:539, 1991

333. Lockart S, Rampil I, Yasuda N et al: Depression of ventilation by desflurane in humans. Anesthesiology 74:484, 1991

334. Eger EI II: Stability of I-653 in soda lime. Anesth Analg 66:983, 1987

335. Koblin D, Weiskopf R, Holmes M et al: Metabolism of I-653 and isoflurane in swine. Anesth Analg 68:147, 1989

336. Yasuda N, Lockhart S, Eger EI II et al: Kinetics of desflurane, isoflurane, and halothane in humans. Anesthesiology 74:489, 1991

337. Eger EI II, Johnson B, Strum D et al: Studies of the toxicity of I-653, halothane, and isoflurane in enzyme induced, hypoxic rats. Anesth Analg 66:1227, 1987

338. Caldwell J, Laster M, Magorian T et al: The neuromuscular effects of desflurane, alone and combined with pancuronium or succinylcholine in humans. Anesthesiology 74:412, 1991

339. Eger EI II, Johnson B: Rates of awakening from anesthesia with I-653, halothane, isoflurane, and sevoflurane: A test of the effect of anesthetic concentration and duration in rats. Anesth Analg 66:977, 1987

340. Gion H, Saidman LJ: The minimum alveolar concentration of enflurane in man. Anesthesiology 35:361, 1971

341. Torri G, Damia G, Fabian ML: Effects of nitrous oxide on the anaesthetic requirement of enflurane. Br J Anaesth 46:468, 1974

342. Stevens WC, Dolan WM, Gibbons RT et al: Minimum alveolar concentrations (MAC) of isoflurane with and without nitrous oxide in patients of various ages. Anesthesiology 42:197, 1975

343. Stoelting RK: The effects of nitrous oxide on the minimum alveolar concentration of methoxyflurane needed for anesthesia. Anesthesiology 34:353, 1971

18

Max T. Baker
Russell A. Van Dyke

Biochemical and Toxicological Aspects of the Volatile Anesthetics

In the past 25 years the metabolism, toxicity, and pharmacodynamics of the volatile anesthetics have come under careful study in an effort to understand the mechanisms of adverse effects sometimes seen following anesthesia with these agents. In the process, major strides have been made in understanding how these drugs interact with biologic systems; concomitantly there has been a decrease in the frequency of adverse reactions associated with their use. Information gained from research has led to the discontinued use of some anesthetics, such as fluroxene and methoxyflurane; the more selective use of others, such as halothane; and the development of newer ones, isoflurane and desflurane, that exhibit less of the properties thought to be involved in toxic processes.

Although anesthesia with the volatile anesthetics is safer than in the past, it is not as safe as possible, nor are all toxicological mechanisms known. Cellular processes are constantly being further elucidated, and many questions can be raised regarding the effects of anesthetics on newly discovered processes that may exist in both the normal state and in the altered physiologic states of patients needing anesthesia. Current thought in several areas of anesthetic research is shifting from the idea that the volatile agents influence cellular processes via nonspecific, poorly defined physical characteristics of the drugs themselves to the concept of anesthetic effect achieved through specific interactions with enzymes, receptors, or other cellular constituents.

In addition to contributing to decreased morbidity and mortality, research into anesthetic agents has increased our understanding of biologic systems. Examples include the use of halothane and methoxyflurane as substrates for cytochrome P-450, where knowledge of the mechanisms of oxidative and reductive dehalogenation has been expanded. Valuable information relating to the processes of chemically induced hepatotoxicity and role of oxygen tension in liver injury has similarly accrued through the study of anesthetic-induced hepatic necrosis in rats and guinea pigs.

ANESTHETIC METABOLISM

The biotransformation of anesthetic agents has been a major area of research. Many compounds appear to become toxic or to exhibit detrimental effects in the course of their metabolism to reactive metabolites.[1] It was initially believed that the halogenated anesthetics were biochemically inert, and the discovery that they were metabolized was a milestone in anesthetic toxicity research.[2] How the volatile anesthetics are metabolized, to what extent, and the biochemical consequences of their metabolism were major questions addressed. It was demonstrated early that initial anesthetic metabolism is performed by the important cytochrome P-450 enzymes,[3] the catalysts for most drug-metabolizing reactions. These enzymes are highly membrane bound and are located chiefly on the smooth endoplasmic reticulum of hepatocytes, but these are also found in low levels in other organs.[4] They can oxidize a multitude of lipophilic compounds by such processes as hydroxylation, n- or o-dealkylation, and epoxidation; moreover, certain substrates like halothane can be reduced.

The basic components of the cytochrome P-450 enzyme system include cytochome P-450, a hemoprotein with molecular weights ranging from 48,000 to 56,000, cytochrome P-450 reductase, a flavoprotein that supplies reducing equivalents to cytochrome P-450, and a lipid component that facilitates the interaction of the two proteins.[5] Oxidative metabolism by cytochrome P-450 entails the sequential transfer of two electrons from the reductase, which receives electrons from the reduced form of nicotinamide-adenine dinucleotide phosphate (NADPH), to the heme iron of P-450 and ultimately to molecular oxygen. The "active oxygen" generated on cytochrome P-450 then attacks a substrate bound to the active site of P-450 to add one atom of molecular oxygen to the substrate and generate one molecule of water.[5,6] Cytochrome b_5, which utilizes the reduced form of nicotinamide-adenine dinucleotide (NADH), has been implicated as a possible source for the second electron in some cytochrome P-450 reactions and therefore plays a role in drug metabolism.

Features of the cytochrome P-450 enzymes that are major determinants of metabolic rates and pathways are (1) the P-450 enzymes comprise multiple isozymes,[7,8] and (2) they are inducible.[9] Induction can be caused by exposure to one of hundreds of compounds and involves de novo synthesis, since both transcriptional and translational processes are stimulated to produce cytochrome P-450. A list of inducers includes many drugs, among them phenobarbital, cimetidine, phenytoin, isoniazid, some volatile anesthetics, and a number of environmental and industrial contaminants, including dioxin, 3-methylcholanthrene, DDT, acetone, and benzene. The cytochrome P-450 enzymes exhibit overlapping and selective substrate specificities and can be individually or broadly induced with select inducers.[10,11] For example, phenobarbital, a classic cytochrome P-450 inducer, can induce a spectrum of major forms in the rat; each of these forms tends to metabolize a wide range of large and small molecular weight substrates. Ethanol or isoniazid induce one form that metabolizes ethanol and other small compounds, including the volatile anesthetics. 3-Methylcholanthrene or β-naphthoflavone (β-NF) can induce several other forms (cytochromes P-448, or aryl hydrocarbon hydroxylases) that play lesser roles in the metabolism of drugs but are important in the metbolism of the planar carcinogenic polycyclic aromatic hydrocarbons.

There is now ample evidence for the multiple gene composition of cytochrome P-450 synthesis. Only a single decade separates the first report of a cytochome P-450 cDNA probe from the identification of least 71 complete cytochrome P-450 cDNAs or protein sequences in eight eukaryotic species and one prokaryote.[12] Fourteen families, based on sequence similarities, are currently recognized.[12,13] Each cytochrome P-450 is identified by its gene designation; in the nomenclature, Roman numerals indicate gene families, capital letters indicate subfamilies, and arabic numerals are used for individual genes.[8] Family I includes the two isozymes (IA1 and IA2) induced by 3-methylcholanthrene. Family II, with eight subfamilies, is the largest and includes a number of isozymes induced by phenobarbital. Subfamily

IIE includes the isozyme induced by ethanol, important in anesthetic metabolism. The enzymes in family III are selectively induced by pregnenolone 16α-carbonitrile and dexamethasone and are involved in the metabolism of steroid hormones.[13] Expression of the cytochrome P-450 isozymes depends not only on induction but also on such factors as the sex and physiologic state of the individual—obesity, fasting, diabetes, and the like. For example, P450IIE can be increased severalfold by fasting or diabetes. Streptozotocin-induced diabetes in rats can enhance enflurane and isoflurane metabolism, and this increased activity can be blocked by insulin.[14]

In addition to primary metabolism performed by cytochrome P-450, synthetic metabolism, or phase II metabolism,[1] is relevant for some anesthetics such as sevoflurane and fluroxene. Synthetic reactions are performed by the microsomal and cytosolic conjugating enzymes. Sulfotransferase, glucuronyltransferase, and glutathione-S-transferase can add sulfate, glucuronic acid, and glutathione, respectively, to polar functions of a drug or its metabolite prior to excretion.

Metabolic Pathways

Even though most halogenated anesthetics are similar in chemical composition (Fig. 18-1), they vary greatly in their rates and pathways of metabolism. Minor alterations in configuration, including the site, type, and number of halogen

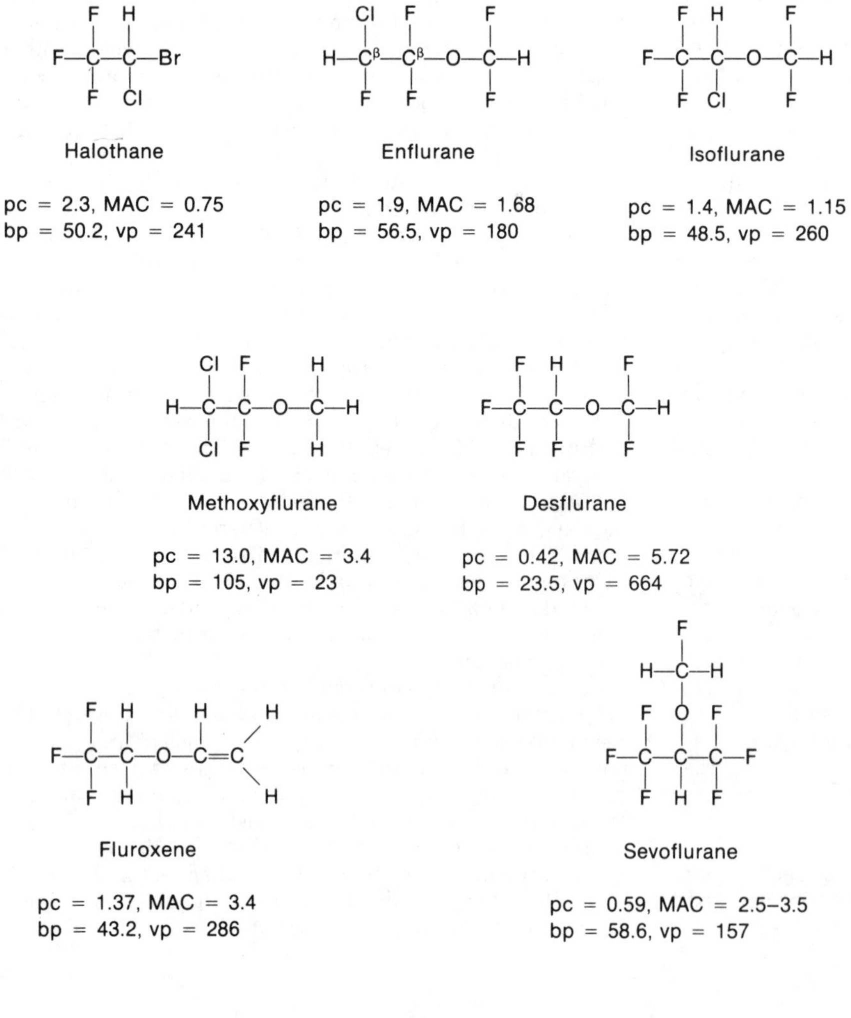

Figure 18-1. Chemical structures and properties of the volatile anesthetics. pc = blood : gas partition coefficient at 37°C, MAC = minimum alveolar concentration, bp = boiling point in Celsius degrees at 7600 mm Hg, vp = vapor pressure in mm Hg at 20°C.

substituents, can have major effects on the ability of cytochrome P-450 to degrade these compounds. Additionally, their solubility in biologic tissues is a factor governing their access to the metabolizing enzymes and their duration at the enzyme level. Cumulative studies in whole animals and microsomal systems (isolated endoplasmic reticulum) have shown that the rates of anesthetic metabolism follow the order: methoxyflurane > halothane > enflurane-sevoflurane > isoflurane > desflurane. In general, halogenation hinders metabolism, and the susceptibility of a halogen-substituted carbon to cytochrome P-450 oxidation is inversely related to the bond energy of the carbon-halogen bond. Bond energies follow the order: C–F > C–Cl > C–Br.[15] The solubility of the halogenated anesthetics in blood tends to follow the same order. Thus, the blood:gas partition coefficients of methoxyflurane, isoflurane, and desflurane are 13.0, 1.4, and 0.42, respectively (see Fig. 18-1).

Halothane

The mechanisms of oxidative anesthetic metabolism by cytochrome P-450 are thought to proceed in a manner analogous to hydroxylation. This involves attack by the activated oxgyen species generated by cytochome P-450 on a susceptible carbon atom of the anesthetic. The site of attack can lead to o-dealkylation of the ether anesthetics or direct oxidation of a carbon without ether cleavage.

The early finding that halothane ($CF_3CHBrCl$) forms bromide ion[16] and trifluoroacetic acid (TFA)[17] in animals and man indicated that halothane oxidation occurs on the chloro-bromo carbon (Fig. 18-2).[18,19] This was confirmed in microsomes and shown to be a cytochrome P-450–dependent reaction. TFA, however, is not a direct cytochrome P-450 product. Hydroxylation of the bromo-chloro carbon by cytochrome P-450 produces an unstable species that spontaneously dehydrobrominates, producing trifluoroacetyl acyl chloride. The trifluoroacetyl acyl chloride formed is a reactive intermediate that either binds to cellular macromolecules, primarily protein, or reacts with water to hydrolyze, eliminating chloride and forming TFA.[20,21]

Subsequent to the discovery that halothane is oxidized, it was demonstrated that 1,1,1-trifluoro-2-chloroethane (CTE) and 2-chloro-1,1-difluoroethene (CDE) were in vivo metabolites of halothane.[22] These metabolites are reductive products of halothane whose formation is also catalyzed by cytochrome P-450.[23,24] When reductive metabolism occurs, halothane serves as the electron acceptor from cytochrome P-450. This process is inhibited by molecular oxygen. As a

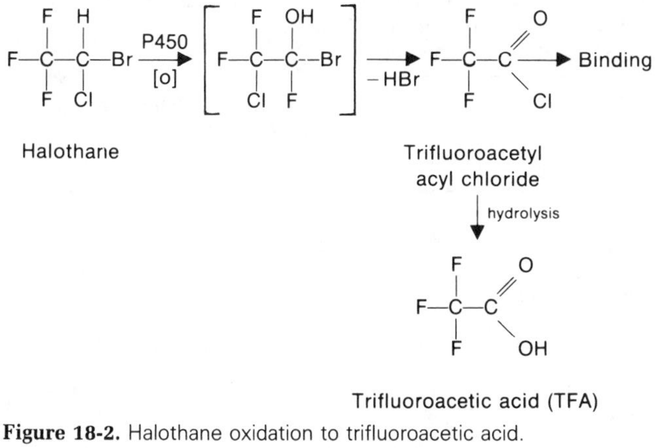

consequence, halothane reduction is facilitated in hypoxic or anoxic conditions. The ability of animals and man to produce CTE and CDE while breathing normal oxygen levels confirms that the distribution of oxygen in the liver is not uniform, with tissue oxygen in some areas being as low as 2–5%, the oxygen tensions at which reductive halothane metabolism occurs in vitro.[25] Oxidation is the major pathway of halothane metabolism, but, as shown in rats, reductive metabolism can be further enhanced, up to threefold or fourfold, if low oxygen is inhaled with halothane.[26]

The mechanism for halothane reduction by cytochrome P-450 has been extensively studied because of its link to halothane-induced liver necrosis in the hypoxic rat model.[20,24,27,28] Halothane reduction is a two-step process whereby a one-electron transfer to halothane results in CTE and a two-electron transfer produces CDE (Fig. 18-3). Apparently each cytochrome P-450 form that reduces halothane can produce both metabolites, and therefore CTE formation can be thought of as incomplete halothane reduction (see Fig. 18-2). CTE production by cytochrome P-450 entails the release of a halothane free radical that can bind to cellular macromolecules, particularly lipids, or can abstract a hydrogen atom from lipids to produce CTE. The binding and interaction of the free radical with lipids have been thought to be important in the halothane toxic mechanism because of the possibility of the reaction disrupting the normal lipid function in the cellular membranes.[29,30] Carbon-centered free radicals such as those formed from halothane attack the methylene bridge of an unsaturated fatty acid, potentially resulting in the formation of conjugated dienes during hypoxia and lipid peroxidation when oxygen tensions are restored.

CDE formation is a continuation of the reductive process in which a second electron is transferred to the halothane radical bound to cytochrome P-450 (see Fig. 18-3).[28] The halothane intermediate then undergoes beta elimination of fluoride to release CDE and inorganic fluoride. Reduced heme or other hemoproteins, like hemoglobin, can reduce halothane,[31] but CDE formation is specific to cytochrome P-450. To date, only the cytochrome P-450 hemoproteins have been shown to form CDE.

Investigations into the mechanisms of CDE formation have focused on the complex formed between halothane and cytochrome P-450, which is observable by spectral analysis during the two-electron reduction of halothane. The complex absorbs light maximally at 470 nm and has been shown to decay, without additional electron transfer, to release CDE.[28,32] The spectral entity was demonstrated to be a halothane-carbanion ferric iron–heme complex ($CF_3CClH^- \cdots Fe^{3+}$),[33] and has been proposed to be a steady-state intermediate in CDE formation. Nevertheless, the complex is a relatively stable entity that does not decay at a rate sufficient to account for the quantity of CDE formed in microsomes.[34] It therefore is not an obligatory intermediate in CDE formation, and the cytochrome P-450 forms not bound as complex more readily release CDE.

CDE and CTE are thought to be exhaled unchanged, yet examination of their potential metabolism showed that while CTE is largely inert to metabolism, CDE is readily defluorinated by cytochrome P-450. CDE oxidation occurs even under the low-oxygen conditions in which it is formed.[35] The products of CDE metabolism include inorganic fluoride and the non-halogen-containing compounds, glycolic acid and glyoxylic acid (see Fig. 18-3).[36] These two acids can be metabolized to carbon dioxide, possibly accounting for the carbon dioxide detected from halothane metabolism in vivo, as reported in early studies.[2] Ironically,

Figure 18-2. Halothane oxidation to trifluoroacetic acid.

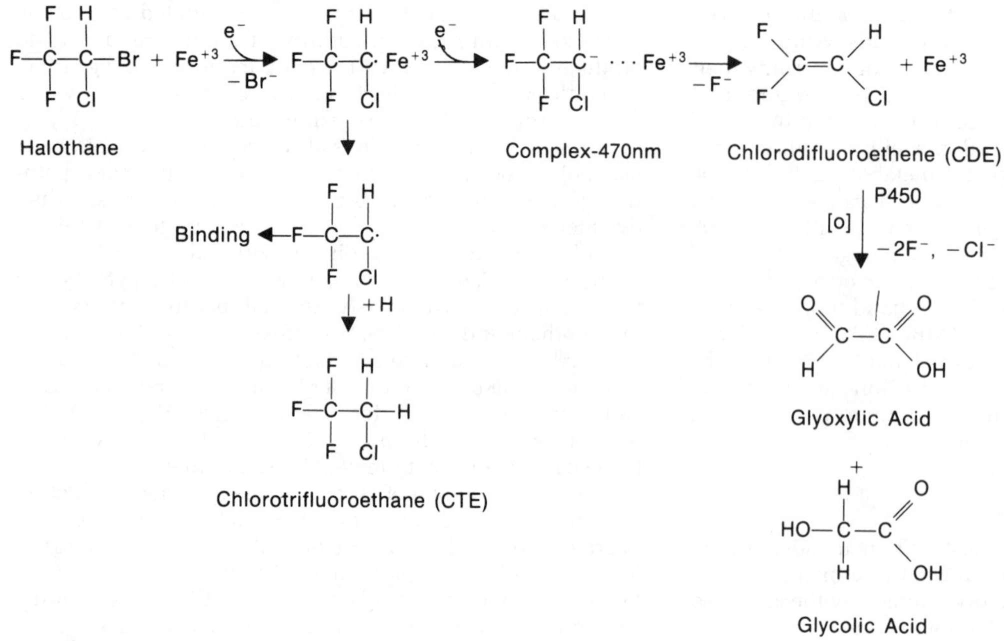

Figure 18-3. Mechanisms of halothane reduction and pathway of CDE oxidation.

CDE metabolism is stimulated by halothane itself, and results in covalent CDE-protein binding.[37] Although CDE is formed in low quantities, this evidence suggests that CDE biotransformation may also be of consequence in halothane exposures.

The extent of halothane metabolism has been reported to be 17–20% of the administered dose.[16] Assessment of metabolism by mass balance techniques, which are based on recovery of the parent anesthetic from exhaled gases, suggest that up to 46% of a subanesthetic dose of halothane may be metabolized (Table 18-1).[38] Metabolism varies greatly among individuals, however.[23,39] Although only a few patient factors have been identified as contributing to this variability, obesity apparently is one, as increased serum fluoride was observed in obese individuals following halothane inhalation.[40] The increased serum fluoride may be due to poorer oxygen delivery to the abdominal organs, thereby enhancing reductive metabolism, or it may represent a shift in the type of metabolism, from oxidative to reductive, independent of oxygen.

The cytochrome P-450 isozymes that metabolize halothane reduction to the greatest degree are one or more of the forms induced by phenobarbital and pregnenolone-16α-carbonitrile.[28,34] Halothane oxidation, on the other hand, is induced by phenobarbital and ethanol or isoniazid. The isozyme induced by ethanol, P450IIE1, is distinct from those induced by phenobarbital. This isozyme also oxidizes halothane to TFA at a greater rate than the phenobarbital-inducible forms.[41] It should be noted that the major route of halothane metabolism, oxidation to TFA, does not release fluoride, so that fluoride-induced renal toxicity is not a concern with halothane.

Enflurane

The metabolism of enflurane (CHF_2OCF_2CHClF), while considerably less than that of halothane, liberates fluoride and proceeds fast enough that there is some concern of it releasing sufficient fluoride to cause renal damage.[42,43] Analysis

of fluoride in early studies of enflurane by Chase et al[44] showed that urinary metabolites accounted for 2.4% of a dose of enflurane, but that figure was based on an average recovery of 82.7%, which suggests that the urinary metabolite value may have been underestimated. Mass balance studies indicate that metabolism may account for as much as 8% of a dose of administered enflurane.[38] In rat liver microsomes and in human urine, difluoromethoxydifluoroacetic acid (CHF_2OCF_2COOH) has been identified as the major enflurane metabolite.[45] Therefore cytochrome P-450 attacks the beta-ethyl carbon containing the chloride and fluorine substituents, and not the difluoromethyl carbon. This is consistent with fluorination conferring on carbon a greater resistance to oxidation. The proposed steps leading from hydroxylation to carboxylic acid formation are shown in Figure 18-4 and include a possible reactive intermediate, difluoromethoxydifluoroacetyl acyl fluoride. The ability of enflurane to bind covalently to macromolecules on metabolism is not clear, insofar as binding studies have not been

TABLE 18-1. Metabolism of Volatile Anesthetics as Assessed by Metabolite Recovery and Mass Balance Studies

	Magnitude of Metabolism (%)	
	Metabolite Recovery	Mass Balance
Isoflurane	0.2	0*
Enflurane	2.4	8.5
Halothane	11–25	46.1
Methoxyflurane	48	75.3

*Metabolism of isoflurane assumed to be zero for this calculation.

Data adapted with permission from Carpenter RL, Eger EL, Johnson BH et al: The extent of metabolism of inhaled anesthetics in humans. Anesthesiology 65:201, 1986.

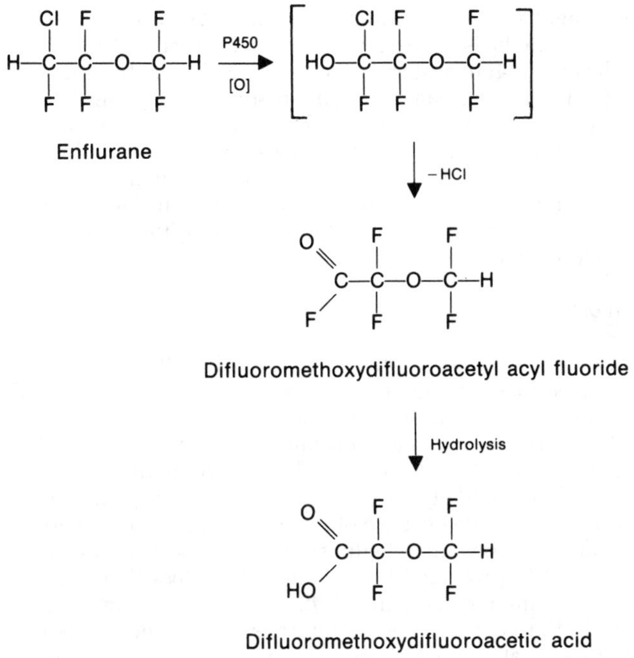

Enflurane

Difluoromethoxydifluoroacetyl acyl fluoride

Difluoromethoxydifluoroacetic acid

Figure 18-4. Pathway for the metabolism of enflurane by cytochrome P-450.

carried out with ^{14}C-labeled enflurane. However, there is indirect evidence (enflurane–microsomal adduct detection by anti-TFA IgG hapten antibodies in the liver) that binding does occur.[46]

Cousins et al[47] examined the serum and urinary inorganic fluoride concentrations in patients administered enflurane. Serum inorganic fluoride peaked at approximately 22 μM, a subtoxic level, 3 hours after anesthesia, and urinary fluoride peaked at 17 μM 5 hours after anesthesia. Both levels were maintained until 10 hours after anesthesia induction and then dropped steadily until reaching preanesthesia levels 4 days later. Despite these findings, several surgical patients have developed nephrotoxicity following enflurane anesthesia.[43] This led to the discovery by Rice et al[48,49] that isoniazid, when administered prior to enflurane anesthesia, led to enhanced enflurane defluorination, which accounted for the high levels of inorganic fluoride in individuals who developed nephrotoxicity following enflurane anesthesia. This paralleled the discovery that the metabolism of the volatile anesthetics, including enflurane, was enhanced by ethanol pretreatment.[50] It is now well recognized that this is due to the ability of ethanol and isoniazid to induce the same isozyme of cytochrome P-450, P450IIE1.[51]

Isoflurane

Isoflurane (CHF$_2$OCH$_2$ClCF$_3$) is an isomer of enflurane that has a slightly lower blood:gas partition coefficient than enflurane—1.4 vs. 1.9.[52,53] As with enflurane, the effect of the release of inorganic fluoride on metabolism was of early interest. Early work with isoflurane indicated a very low degree of defluorination.[54,55] In humans, the level of serum inorganic fluoride was found to transiently reach 4.4 μM 6 hours after anesthesia before returning to normal 2 days after the anesthetic episode. This represents only a modest rise above basal serum fluoride levels.

Studies of isoflurane biotransformation in microsomal preparations demonstrated that isoflurane could undergo

metabolism only in the presence of oxygen. Even though isoflurane, like halothane, possesses a trifluorinated carbon, the molecule as a whole does not have a configuration susceptible to reduction. In microsomes isoflurane has been shown to be oxidized to TFA and trifluoroacetaldehyde.[56] This suggests that cytochrome P-450 attacks the difluoromethyl carbon (o-dealkylation) and the alpha-ethyl carbon (o-insertion). o-Dealkylation can lead to trifluoroacetaldehyde and o-insertion to TFA (Fig. 18-5). However, trifluoroacetaldehyde can undergo non-cytochrome P-450 oxidation to TFA. Both mechanisms of metabolism may occur. Indirect evidence indicates that isoflurane binds to microsomal protein during metabolism, which could originate from the reactive acyl chloride or trifluoroacetaldehyde.[46,56] The form of the single-carbon products liberated from isoflurane and the other methyl ether anesthetics is not clear. Formaldehyde, formic acid, and carbon dioxide are possible initial products. The former two metabolites could enter the single-carbon pool to be metabolized to carbon dioxide.

Methoxyflurane

Studies of the metabolism of methoxyflurane (CH$_3$OCF$_2$ CCl$_2$H) have continued even as the clinical use of this drug in humans has ceased. Methoxyflurane is highly lipid soluble (blood:gas partition coefficient of 13)[57] and is readily metabolized.[58,59] It has been estimated by metabolite quanti-

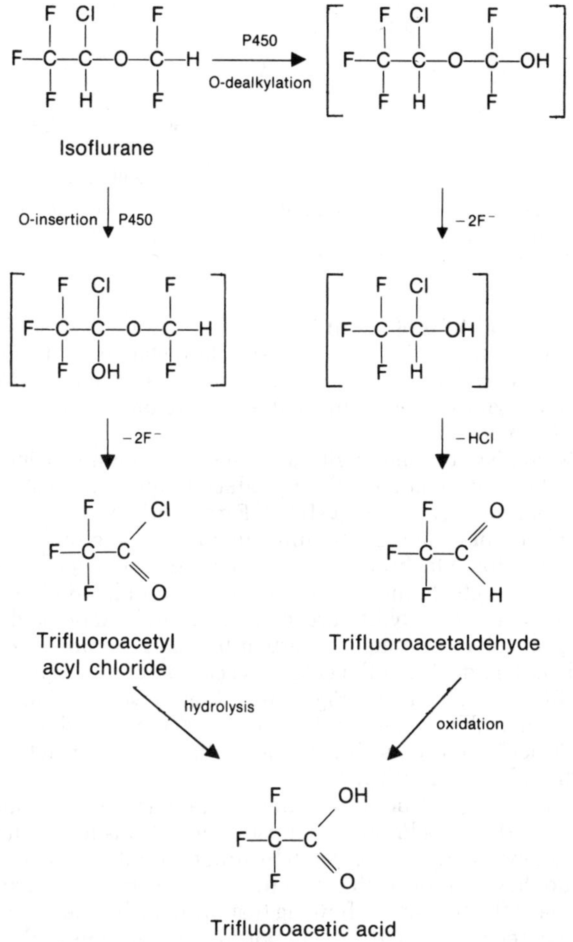

Isoflurane

Trifluoroacetyl acyl chloride

Trifluoroacetaldehyde

Trifluoroacetic acid

Figure 18-5. Pathways of isoflurane metabolism to trifluoroacetaldehyde and trifluoroacetic acid.

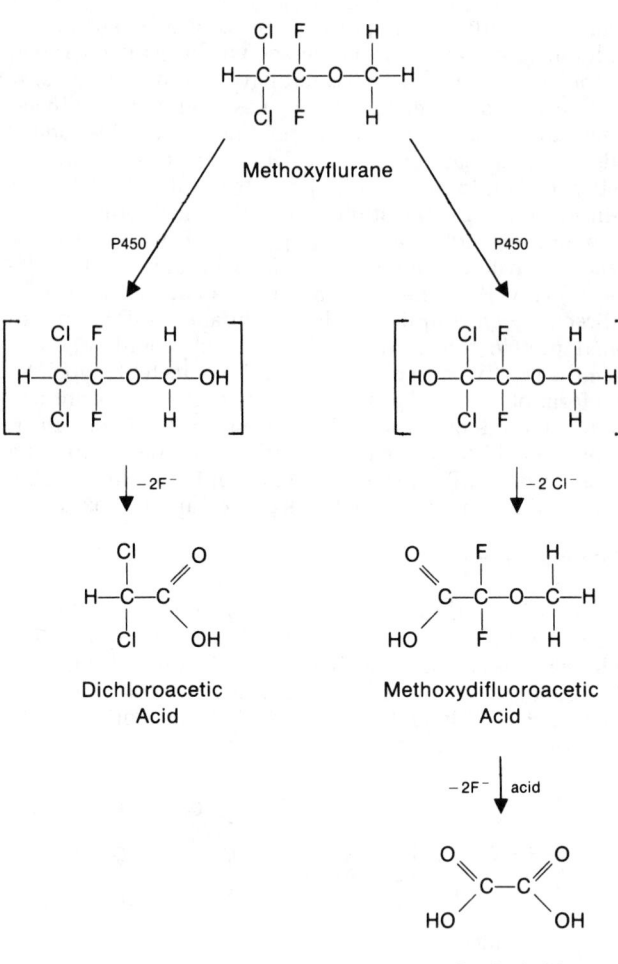

Figure 18-6. Metabolic pathways of methoxyflurane metabolism by cytochrome P-450.

quirement for P-450 oxidation of the ether function. That cytochrome b_5 is necessary was shown in reconstituted cytochrome P-450 systems, where cytochrome b_5 must be added for metabolism, and in microsomes, where antibodies to cytochrome b_5 inhibit methoxyflurane ether cleavage. Other substrates for cytochrome P-450 do not exhibit the cytochrome b_5 requirement. A possible explanation for this phenomenon is that methoxyflurane may induce a cytochrome b_5 dependence in P-450 LM2 (IIB4) through an unknown mechanism.[66]

Sevoflurane

Sevoflurane (fluoromethyl-1,1,1,3,3,3-hexafluoro-2-propyl ether) is an experimental anesthetic that has a blood:gas partition coefficient of 0.59.[67] Because of its low solubility it has a relatively high minimum alveolar concentration (MAC) value of 2.5–3.5% in rats.[68] This compound was originally thought likely to yield relatively large quantities of inorganic fluoride because of its high degree of fluorination. Sevoflurane does liberate fluoride on metabolism; however, the quantity produced is equivalent to or less than that released by the metabolism of enflurane. The amount of fluoride found in rats after sevoflurane anesthesia peaked at approximately 2.5 µM in untreated rats, and was higher in dogs (18–20 µM), although in both species levels decreased rapidly after anesthesia, returning to normal in 24 hours.[69] The relatively quick decline in plasma fluoride levels after cessation of anesthesia is likely due to the more rapid expiration of sevoflurane.

The metabolism of sevoflurane occurs by cytochrome P-450 attack on the fluoromethyl carbon to produce inorganic fluoride, 1,1,1,3,3,3-hexafluoroisopropanol, and a single-carbon product that has not been conclusively identified but is proposed to be carbon dioxide (Fig. 18-7).[69] Metabolism does not take place at the trifluorinated carbons because of the high degree of stability of the trifluorocarbons to direct enzymatic attack, thus accounting for the relatively low level of fluoride released from this anesthetic. Indeed, the hexafluoroisopropanol formed is a stable metabolite that does not undergo further cytochrome P-450 metabolism. It is, however, a relatively acidic alcohol that is subject to conjugation with glucuronic acid by glucuronyltransferase.[69] The sevoflurane molecule is not reduced by cytochrome P-450.

A major concern in the use of sevoflurane is its instability in soda lime. Halogenated hydrocarbons of appropriate structure tend to be unstable in base. Halothane is largely stable but can form small quantities of difluorochlorobromoethylene and trifluorochloroethane in soda lime.[70] For sevoflurane, the proton on the 2-propyl carbon is easily removed by base, forming a carbanion. The carbanion can rearrange, owing to the electron-withdrawing effects of the adjacent trifluorinated carbons, to release fluoride and produce an unsaturated carbon-carbon bond. Fluoromethyl 2,2-difluoro-1-(trifluoromethyl) vinyl ether $(CF_2C(CF_3)OCH_2F)$ is the major volatile product detected when sevoflurane is passed through soda lime.[71] A lesser product is fluoromethyl 2-methoxy-2,2-difluoro-1-(trifluoromethyl)ethyl ether $(CH_3OCF_2CH(CF_3)OCH_2F)$, whose formation may involve the reaction of the vinyl degradation product with methanol. The methanol is thought to originate from sevoflurane itself on soda lime. Thus it appears that sevoflurane is further broken down to single-carbon products. Indeed, vinyl fluorides are also unstable to base and hydrolyze to carboxylic acids.[72] The nonvolatile products of sevoflurane degradation, other than fluoride, have

fication that 46% of the inhaled methoxyflurane dose, almost three times that of halothane, is metabolized in humans.[60] Mass balance analysis shows that as much as 75% of methoxyflurane taken up at an exposure level of 0.0469% may be metabolized.[38]

Metabolism of methoxyflurane releases amounts of inorganic fluoride great enough to produce polyuria in rats and man (plasma levels > 50 µM).[61,62] Early work indicated that the ether moiety and the terminal dichloroethyl group were both sites for cytochrome P-450 oxidation. The major metabolic products found were inorganic fluoride, dichloroacetic acid, methoxydifluoroacetic acid, and oxalic acid.[63] Thus, attack on the methyl carbon liberates dichloroacetic acid, and oxidation of the beta-ethyl carbon produces methoxydifluoroacetic acid (Fig. 18-6). Methoxydifluoroacetic acid is unstable under acidic conditions, breaking down to oxalic acid and accounting for the oxalic acid obtained from methoxyflurane in vivo.[58]

Because of its structure, methoxyflurane is a unique substrate for the cytochrome P-450 isozymes. It was found that induction of cytochrome P-450 by different inducing agents did not have uniform effects on the metabolism of methoxyflurane at the two sites, showing that the cytochromes P-450 can be selective for different portions of the molecule.[59] Recently, Waskell et al[64,65] examined the metabolism of methoxyflurane and found an unusual cytochrome b_5 re-

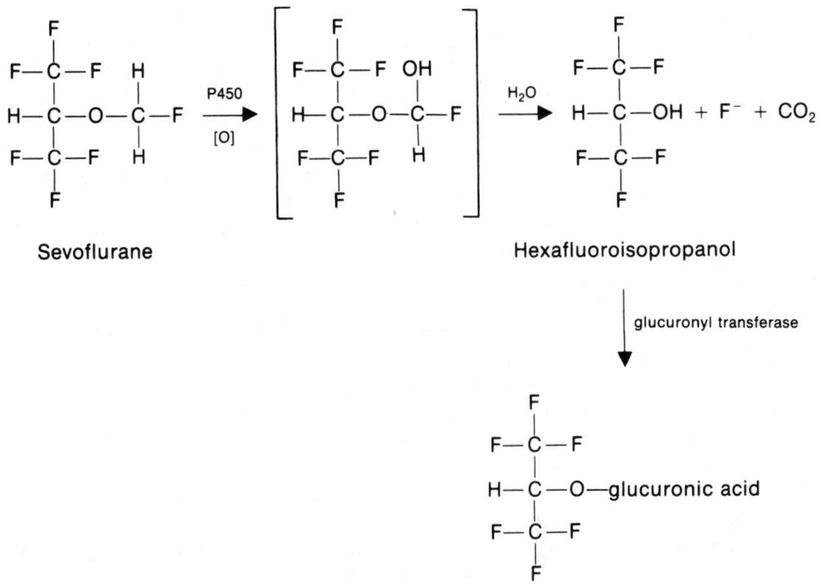

Figure 18-7. Metabolic pathway of sevoflurane.

not been identified. To date, no adverse reactions have been reported as a result of its instability; however, halogenated vinyl compounds are known to be metabolized to reactive intermediates.[73] It is important that as much as possible be known about this chemistry and the products involved.

Desflurane

Desflurane ($CHF_2OCHFCF_3$) is a newer agent with a low blood:gas partition coefficient (0.42) and high MAC value, 5.7% in rats.[74] It differs structurally from isoflurane only in that the alpha-ethyl carbon is fluorinated rather than chlorinated. Desflurane is highly resistant to metabolism.[75] Two major factors predict this. Its low solubility makes it difficult to maintain high intracellular levels, and substitution with fluorine instead of chlorine confers a greater resistance on the alpha-ethyl carbon to oxidation. In addition to its high resistance to metabolism, desflurane is very resistant to degradation in soda lime.[76]

Diethyl Ether

Although diethyl ether is not used in humans, it is still used extensively in animal research. It has been estimated that it is metabolized to as much as 5%.[2] Ether, like the halogenated anesthetics, is metabolized by cytochrome P-450. Its metabolites are ethanol and acetaldehyde, which are further metabolized by the alcohol-metabolizing system to acetic acid.[77] While phenobarbital induction increases microsomal ether metabolism, P450IIE1, induced by ethanol or acetone, metabolizes diethyl ether at more than twice the rate as the cytochromes P-450 induced by phenobarbital.[78] A concern with diethyl ether in research is its ability to strongly induce as well as inhibit P450IIE1, an important catalyst for the activation of the potent carcinogenic nitrosamines.[79,80]

Fluroxene

Fluroxene (2,2,2-trifluoroethyl vinyl ether) is no longer used, but it is an anesthetic whose metabolism is highly relevant to hepatotoxicity. Fluroxene is particularly suscep-

tible to metabolism because of its vinyl moiety. Unsaturated bonds are readily oxidized by cytochrome P-450 to initially form reactive epoxides.[73] Fluroxene in vivo is metabolized to trifluoroethanol glucuronide, TFA, and carbon dioxide; the carbon dioxide arises from the vinyl portion of the molecule.[81] Unlike all other fluorinated anesthetics, fluroxene does not release fluoride on metabolism.[82]

TOXICITY OF THE VOLATILE ANESTHETICS

The study of anesthetic organ toxicity initially focused on the development of hepatotoxicity and nephrotoxicity following the introduction of halothane and methoxyflurane. Shortly after these agents came into use, it was found that they were susceptible to metabolism,[2] which destroyed the concept that fluorinated anesthetics were inert materials that were quickly exhaled unchanged. This observation led to investigations into the relationships between metabolism and toxicity.

For methoxyflurane-induced renal injury, such a relationship was readily established. Renal dysfunction correlated with high plasma inorganic fluoride levels, which were determined to be the cause of the polyuria.[62] Roughly, plasma levels above 50 μM are thought to put individuals at high risk for kidney damage. The importance of enzyme induction was demonstrated in experiments in which untreated and phenobarbital-treated rats were exposed to methoxyflurane and examined for renal insufficiency. Those animals treated with phenobarbital had increased plasma fluoride levels and expressed renal injury, whereas low constitutive cytochrome P-450 levels in untreated rats were insufficient to generate enough fluoride for renal toxic effects to occur.[62] A similar phenomenon exists with fluroxene and liver necrosis. In rats, induction with phenobarbital and exposure to fluroxene for 3 hours resulted in a 100% lethal fulminant hepatic necrosis caused by fluroxene.[83] When rats were not induced or were administered a cytochrome P-450 inhibitor prior to fluroxene, toxicity was greatly reduced.[84] Although the toxic product of fluroxene has not been conclusively identified, the liver necrosis is likely due to oxidation of the vinyl portion of fluroxene to form a reactive metabolite.

Halothane Hepatotoxicity

In humans, halothane anesthesia is associated with mild and severe forms of hepatotoxicity, to which females are more susceptible than males.[85] The relationship of liver toxicity to halothane metabolism, while suspect, is not firm. The prevalence of severe halothane hepatitis in patient populations was determined to be approximately 1 in 30,000 of the individuals who were administered halothane.[86] This is an impressively low figure when one considers the diversity of such patients in terms of sex, nutritional status, physiologic condition, disease, stress, and the like. Interest in reductive halothane metabolism as a cause of hepatotoxicity followed the development of the hypoxic rat model of halothane-induced liver necrosis.[87] In this model, centrilobular necrosis could be produced in the male rat when animals were pretreated with phenobarbital and exposed to halothane (0.5–1.0%) for 2 hours under low-oxygen conditions (8–14%). Generally, lesions were observed 24 hours after exposure. These conditions—low oxygen and phenobarbital induction—are those that cause the greatest degree of halothane reduction to the free radical, the greatest binding of halothane to lipids, and the greatest conjugated diene formation in the liver. This model therefore appeared to confirm a role for reductive metabolism in the toxicity of halothane.

Further investigations into halothane hepatotoxicity shed doubt on the appropriateness of this model for representing the liver injury associated with halothane use in humans. Isoflurane and enflurane can produce toxicity under low-oxygen conditions,[88] yet these anesthetics are metabolized to low degrees by comparison with halothane, and undergo no reduction. Studies of the effects of low oxygen (10%) in phenobarbital-treated rats showed that liver toxicity occurred under low-oxygen conditions alone, without halothane.[89] Guinea pigs developed hepatotoxicity when exposed to halothane without cytochrome P-450 enzyme induction and under normoxic conditions.[90,91] Additional lines of evidence that argue against the hypoxic model include the observation that mice can be induced to metabolize halothane reductively to about the same extent as rats, but do not exhibit halothane hepatotoxicity.[92] Other halogenated compounds, such as DDT, readily form a reductive carbon-centered free radical that binds to lipids,[93] yet DDT has not been shown to be hepatotoxic in any species.

The influence of hyperthyroidism on anesthetic-induced centrilobular necrosis in rats was examined as a possible interactive factor. Exposure of triiodothyronine (T_3)-treated rats to 1% halothane in air for 2 hours resulted in hepatic necrosis.[94] Hepatic necrosis also occurred with enflurane (1.8%) and isoflurane (1.3%), but the incidence of necrosis with halothane was approximately three times that with isoflurane and enflurane.[95] Further investigations with the hyperthyroid model demonstrated that halothane liver toxicity developed regardless of whether the rats were hypoxic, normoxic, or hyperoxic, indicating that reductive metabolism is not related to this toxicity.[94] Oxidative metabolism of halothane also appears not to be involved.[96] The authors suggested that in the hyperthyroid model, toxicity is produced by the parent compound without metabolism. It is likely that the reserves of glycogen and other energy stores are exhausted by the thyroxin treatment, rendering the cell unable to cope with the insult of the xenobiotic.

An alternative hypothesis for the genesis of halothane liver necrosis, and one that is gaining favor, is that the necrosis results from a toxic immune response or hypersensitivity reaction. The basic elements of this mechanism are as follows. First, halothane in sufficient quantity binds to cellular constituents which in some manner are expressed on the surface of the hepatocyte. Upon recognition by the immune system, an antibody-antigen response occurs, eliciting cell damage.[97] Evidence for the possible involvement of the immune system came first from patients with halothane-induced liver necrosis. Their serum was found to contain antibodies that reacted specifically with halothane-altered hepatocytes.[98] The halothane-altered hepatocytes were believed to result from a covalently bound halothane-cellular constituent resulting from halothane metabolism. Neuberger et al[99] presented evidence that the expression of the antigen in rabbits is associated with the oxidative metabolism of halothane rather than with the reductive pathway. Further studies showed that the halothane antigens contain an adduct arising from a reaction with the trifluoroacetyl acyl chloride metabolite of halothane. That is, antigens formed in the liver reacted with a hapten-specific anti-TFA antibody, and generation of the antigen in rat was reduced when rats were treated with deuterated halothane.[100] Deuteration of halothane inhibits halothane oxidative metabolism but does not affect the reductive pathway.[18] The identity of the halothane antigens has been investigated and a cytochrome P-450 isozyme[101] and carboxylesterase[102] have been implicated as the halothane-adducted proteins.

The guinea pig model of halothane toxicity has been investigated in regard to both reductive halothane metabolism and an immune response as causes. It is thought that this model more closely resembles the toxicity in humans.[103] In addition to the facts that cytochrome P-450 induction is not required and that liver injury occurs under normoxia, both sexes are susceptible, and necrosis is delayed in onset and not seen until 48 hours after exposure.[91] Hypoxia does not exacerbate the halothane-induced liver toxicity. This appears to exclude a role for halothane reduction in halothane-induced liver necrosis in the guinea pig. In several strains of guinea pigs exposed to halothane, animals developed anti-TFA antibodies under conditions of oxidative halothane metabolism,[104] which suggests that the immunotoxic theory may be applicable to the guinea pig model.

Other Mechanisms of Anesthetic Toxicity

In addition to the above mechanisms, there is recent interest in the possibility that altered Ca^{2+} homeostasis in the hepatocyte is involved in halocarbon-induced liver injury.[105,106] Calcium plays a vital role in the regulation of many essential biochemical reactions and is held constant in the cytoplasm by an elaborate system. With extracellular calcium approximately 10^{-3} M and intracellular calcium approximately 10^{-7} M, gradients are maintained by regulatory sites located primarily on the membranes. Calcium enters the cell through either membrane voltage–sensitive channels, receptor-activated channels, or by nonspecific plasma membrane permeation.[107,108] Calcium is removed from the cell by an ATP-dependent calcium pump and an Na^+-Ca^{2+} exchange mechanism. Within the cell, calcium is pumped into the mitochondria and sequestered by endoplasmic reticulum and proteins on the plasma membrane.

Pathologic conditions will increase intracellular calcium outside the normal range.[109] The question remains as to whether increased intracellular calcium is a cause or the result of cell damage. However, our work has firmly established that the volatile anesthetics, halothane, enflurane, isoflurane, and sevoflurane, in clinical concentrations cause the release of calcium from intracellular stores in hepatocytes within seconds of their administration.[110,111] This has been studied with fura-2, aequorin, and $^{45}Ca^{2+}$, with similar results from each. A recent report offers the possibility that for the anesthetics, the initial response may lead to greater and more sustained calcium release. Farrell et al[112] found increases in calcium in the livers of guinea pigs 24 hours after exposure to halothane, and the increases were proportional to the severity of the liver necrosis. Evidence was presented that the increased calcium was due to impaired hepatic microsomal calcium uptake. New data indicate that intracellular calcium sequestration may be a mediator of toxic events and lead to cell death on exposure to other halocarbons,[113-115] including carbon tetrachloride, chloroform, and 1,1-dichloroethylene. The consequences of raising the intracellular Ca^{2+} are many. Ca^{2+} is a second messenger capable of turning on many other enzymes; as a result, normal hepatocyte function is altered, and presumably remains altered for the duration of the anesthetic.

Altered calcium flux may also play a role in ischemic damage to hepatocytes resulting from anesthetic exposure. Ischemic injury is associated with an increased cytoplasmic calcium concentration.[116] It is assumed by some that decreases in adenosine triphosphate (ATP) stores are responsible for the increased intracellular calcium; however, other mechanisms, such as an influx of Ca^{2+} from intracellular organelles, may also be possible.

EFFECTS OF VOLATILE ANESTHETICS ON DRUG METABOLISM

Like most compounds that interact with the cytochrome P-450 enzyme system, the volatile anesthetics can influence the activities of the drug-metabolizing enzymes. Such effects are important because they have the potential to influence the pharmacology and toxicology of other foreign compounds in the body. Volatile anesthetic agents can inhibit metabolism, which is their predominant effect; or, in certain situations, they facilitate the biotransformation of other drugs. These effects can be exerted in several fashions: by various direct interactions of the anesthetic agent with the cytochrome P-450 isozymes, by (in longer exposures) cytochrome P-450 enzyme induction, or possibly by altering the supply of drug that reaches the liver for metabolism. These several possibilities are discussed below.

Acute Inhibitory Anesthetic Effects

The ability of anesthetics to modify drug metabolism was initially demonstrated with diethyl ether. In early studies in rats, administration of ether concurrently with pentobarbital resulted in greater plasma levels of pentobarbital than in rats not given ether.[117] The authors concluded that ether was inhibitory to pentobarbital metabolism. This action of ether has since been confirmed with other drugs. Ether in whole rats has been shown to inhibit the metabolism of diphenylhydantoin,[118] antipyrine,[119] and aminopyrine.[120] In addition, it has been found to impair the metabolism of antipyrine in hepatocytes,[121] as well as the metabolism of ethanol,[122] which is partially metabolized by cytochrome P-450.[77] Ether is also a strong inhibitor of the biotransformation of the potent carcinogen, n-nitrosodimethylamine, in rat microsomes.[80,123]

Halothane is similarly an effective inhibitor of cytochrome P-450 activities, as has been demonstrated in vivo and in vitro with a number of substrates. In the whole rat, for example, halothane reduces the metabolism of ketamine,[124] propranolol,[125] diazepam,[126,127] and enflurane.[128] Inhibition of enflurane metabolism by halothane was also observed in surgical patients.[129] In rat liver microsomes, halothane was found to impair n-nitrosodimethylamine metabolism,[80] and in rat hepatocytes it inhibited antipyrine metabolism.[130] Additional substrates shown to be inhibited by halothane include the barbiturates amobarbital, hexobarbital, and pentobarbital, as was demonstrated in microsomes from phenobarbital-treated rats.[131]

Enflurane appears to be less potent than ether or halothane in inhibiting metabolism. However, in rats it has been shown to decrease aminopyrine demethylase without modifying aniline hydroxylase.[132] Enflurane, along with ether, halothane, and methoxyflurane, has been reported to impair the metabolism of mestranol in vivo in the rat.[133] In rat hepatocytes, enflurane inhibited antipyrine metabolism.[130] In contrast to ether and halothane, enflurane is not a particularly effective inhibitor of n-dimethylnitrosamine metabolism in microsomes. Similarly, in liver slices it was less effective than halothane in reducing the rate of elimination of diazepam.[126]

Studies of the effect of isoflurane on drug metabolism have been limited. It has been shown, however, that isoflurane in rats inhibits the oxidative metabolism of halothane,[134] and inhibits the demethylation of dimethylnitrosamine to about the same extent as do halothane and ether.[80] Comparisons of the effects of halothane, isoflurane, and enflurane on in vivo aminopyrine metabolism in the rat showed that enflurane anesthesia had no effect, while halothane and to a much lesser degree isoflurane increased the half-life of aminopyrine.[135]

Inhibitory Mechanisms

The mechanisms by which anesthetics inhibit drug metabolism are important, as the inhibition may be reversible or irreversible and may result from interactions with specific cytochrome P-450 isozymes. Ether's ability to inhibit metabolism is thought to be due to direct reversible interactions of the anesthetic with cytochrome P-450. Of the volatile anesthetics, ether is the broadest inhibitor of drug metabolism. This is attributed to its high lipid solubility,[136] which is a factor for compounds that interact with the lipophilic active sites of cytochrome P-450. Although the situation is not clear, ether as well as the other volatile anesthetics may inhibit cytochrome P-450 activity by competitively interacting with the lipophilic active sites of cytochrome P-450 or by nonspecifically interacting with the membrane-bound cytochrome P-450 complex. Although ether undergoes biotransformation,[77] it is not metabolized to reactive metabolites which inactivate cytochrome P-450 as occurs with halothane and fluroxene.

Halothane likely exerts effects in a similar manner as ether; however, more than one mechanism is involved. Halothane has a pronounced ability to rapidly and irreversibly inactivate cytochrome P-450 on metabolism. Several groups have shown a loss of cytochrome P-450 on halothane metabolism in vitro,[137,138] and this destruction, termed mechanism-based inactivation, was greater when halothane was metabolized at low oxygen levels, and with microsomes from phenobarbital-treated rats. These findings indicate that reductive metabolism is a more effective mechanism in destroying cytochrome P-450 and that the phenobarbital-induced forms are more susceptible to inactivation. The mechanism for the reductive cytochrome P-450 destruction is the formation of the halothane free radical, which attacks vital components of the cytochrome P-450 molecule, possibly the heme moiety.

In addition to this mechanism, other inhibitory processes may be at work as a consequence of halothane metabolism. On reduction, halothane forms a stable but reversible spectral complex with certain cytochrome P-450 forms, which can inhibit the cytochrome P-450 activity of the isozyme bound as complex.[34] Also, a reductive metabolite of halothane, 2-chloro-1,1-difluoroethene (CDE), is a strong mechanism-based inactivator of cytochrome P-450.[35,36] Although CDE is formed in low quantities *in vivo*, it is produced at the cytochrome P-450 active site, and its metabolism is not inhibited but enhanced by halothane.

A mechanism-based inactivation of cytochrome P-450 also occurs with fluroxene.[139] Fluroxene, like CDE, contains an ethenic moiety, a functional group that on oxidative attack by cytochrome P-450 destroys the enzyme.[140,141] In-depth studies of fluroxene and related ethylenic compounds show that on metabolism, the heme moiety of cytochrome P-450 is chemically altered and becomes nonfunctional.[140,142] In the case of fluroxene, a fluroxene metabolite–heme adduct is formed that can be detected by its fluorescence. Chloroform is similar to these agents in that its oxidative metabolism inactivates cytochrome P-450. The biochemical mechanisms differ, however. It is believed that chloroform inactivates cytochrome P-450 when it is metabolized to phosgene, a reactive and toxic metabolite that reacts with protein.[143,144]

The mechanisms by which isoflurane and enflurane inhibit metabolism involve direct interactions with the cytochrome P-450 enzymes. Isoflurane and enflurane, like diethyl ether, are not sufficiently metabolized to reactive intermediates to inactivate cytochrome P-450. The weaker inhibitory effect of these agents as compared with ether may relate to their lower lipid solubilities,[135] which is a function of their greater degrees of fluorination.

There are no reports of the effects of sevoflurane and desflurane on drug metabolism.

Direct Stimulatory Effects

Although inhibition of metabolism is the most prominent effect of the anesthetics, they can also enhance the metabolism of select substrates by direct interactions. For example, aniline but not aminopyrene metabolism in rat hepatic microsomes has been reported to be stimulated to various degrees by halothane and methoxyflurane.[131,145,146] K_{ms} and V_{ms} for aniline hydroxylase were both increased by the anesthetics in microsomes.[146]

A particularly strong enhancement (up to 3.5-fold) of the metabolism of CDE, the halothane metabolite, has been shown to be produced by halothane and isoflurane but not fluroxene.[35] The increased metabolism was greatest in microsomes from rats treated with phenobarbital and was not seen in microsomes from isoniazid-treated rats. In addition to greater fluoride production, halothane caused a greater degree of covalent CDE-macromolecular binding and cytochrome P-450 destruction due to CDE metabolism.[35,37] Enhanced metabolism by isoflurane is not restricted to CDE but has been determined to occur for the metabolism of the carcinogen vinylchloride (chloroethene) and for the metabolism of various gaseous fluorinated plastic monomers, including trifluorochloroethene and 1,1-difluoroethene.

The mechanism for acute stimulation of metabolism is not known, but several mechanisms are possible and may relate to the manner in which the select substrates interact with cytochrome P-450. The anesthetics may exert solvation effects to enhance access of the particular substrates to the active sites, or they may interact with the enzymes to increase the affinity of the substrates for cytochrome P-450. The anesthetics do not stimulate metabolism by enhancing the cytochrome P-450 electron transport system.[147]

Selective Anesthetic–Cytochrome P-450 Interactions

An important consideration in these effects is the ability of the anesthetics to interact with specific cytochrome P-450 forms. The cytochrome P-450 isozymes do not interact with all compounds in a similar manner; therefore it is unreasonable to expect anesthetic effects to be uniform for all substrates. For example, although isoflurane is not widely effective in inhibiting drug metabolism, recent data show that when it is present in microsomes from animals treated with a P450IIE1 inducer such as ethanol, dimethylnitrosamine metabolism is strongly inhibited.[80]

Investigations into the manner in which halothane interacts reductively with microsomal cytochrome P-450 show that these interactions are also selective for cytochrome P-450.[34] Halothane reduction is greatest in microsomes from phenobarbital-treated rats, and there is evidence that the phenobarbital-inducible form, PB-C (IIC6), is the isozyme preferentially inactivated by halothane reduction. Another phenobarbital-inducible isozyme, PB-B (IIB1), is the P-450 isozyme predominantly bound as complex which is protected from irreversible destruction by virtue of existing in complex. In microsomes from β-NF–treated rats, halothane destruction was much less extensive. Chloroform is different from halothane in that it has been shown to effectively destroy the cytochromes P-450 induced by both phenobarbital and β-NF.[144]

Interestingly, studies of halothane's effects on the disposition of propranolol, a chiral compound administered in racemic form, showed that halothane inhibition can have stereochemical consequences. Halothane impaired the intrinsic clearance of (−) – propranolol to greater degrees than it impaired the clearance of (+) – propranolol in dogs.[148] It is becoming evident that cytochrome P-450 can preferentially metabolize compounds based on their stereochemical configurations.[149] A possibility for this effect is that halothane may inhibit to a greater degree a cytochrome P-450 isozyme that preferentially metabolizes (−) – propranolol, or it may selectively impair the binding of one isomer of propranolol to cytochrome P-450 for metabolism.

Induction of Cytochrome P-450 by Anesthetics

Because of the impact that cytochrome P-450 induction can have on drug metabolism, the anesthetic agents have been tested for their ability to increase *in vivo* cytochrome P-450 synthesis and drug metabolism activities. Exposure to subanesthetic concentrations of diethyl ether (0.5% MAC) for 5 days (7 hours per day) in the rat increased liver cytochrome P-450 levels by 40%, whereas methoxyflurane was ineffective as an inducer.[150] Others have confirmed the cytochrome P-450–inducing effect of ether by a single exposure of ether at 1 MAC for 2 hours.[151]

The ability of halothane to induce cytochrome P-450 is less clear. A study of patients following surgery with halothane anesthesia revealed a small but significant increase in the clearance of antipyrine.[152] A comparative study of ether and halothane showed that while ether increased total cytochrome P-450, halothane did not.[151] Other studies of surgical patients showed that enflurane did not affect antipyrine metabolism,[153] and various chronic treatments of rats with enflurane did not modify aniline hyroxylase and decreased aminopyrine demethylase.[132] More recent studies considered the ethanol-inducible form of cytochrome P-450 (P450EII1), which is induced without altering cytochrome P-450 levels. Exposure of rats to diethyl ether or isoflurane induced the metabolism of n-nitrosodimethylamine demethylase.[78] Although halothane and enflurane have not been examined for their induction of P450EII1, because of the activity of isoflurane it may be expected that these agents would also induce as well as inhibit this isozyme of cytochrome P-450.

Other Mechanisms

In addition to direct effects on cytochrome P-450 and enzyme induction, anesthetics may indirectly alter drug metabolism. The indirect processes involved include decreased blood flow to the liver, which occurs with halothane anesthesia,[154] and alterations in drug–plasma protein binding. The former effect would decrease the supply of the drug to the liver for metabolism. Interference with drug–plasma protein binding would increase the free fraction of the drug in the bloodstream, making more available for metabolism. Enflurane and halothane are capable of inhibiting the binding of diazepam to human serum and albumin.[155] Stress, a factor in anesthetic situations, could also come into play. Chronic stress in rats has been found to impair the in vivo metabolism and excretion of antipyrine.[156]

SUMMARY

The volatile anesthetics can interact with cellular macromolecules and influence cellular processes in many ways. As exemplified by anesthetic metabolism and anesthetic effects on drug metabolism, the interactions and consequences of the interactions are highly dependent on the particular molecule. Therefore, for any particular adverse effect or mechanism, the anesthetics must be evaluated on an individual basis.

From the search for toxic anesthetic metabolites, it should be noted that only one product, inorganic fluoride, has been conclusively identified as a direct organ toxin. Fluoride is toxic to the kidney only after sufficiently high plasma fluoride levels have been achieved and maintained for a sufficiently prolonged time. Other metabolites, such as trifluoroacetyl acyl chloride or the halothane free radical, are highly suspect as toxins to liver not by themselves, but as adducts with cellular macromolecules.

It should also be recognized that apart from metabolism, the parent molecules can have profound effects on the function of the cell. Parent compound effects have not been excluded from involvement in toxic effects and may be a major reason why the newer agents, such as isoflurane, sevoflurane, and desflurane, appear to be less toxic. These agents are less soluble in biologic tissues and are present for only a brief period after anesthesia. Consequently, disruption of normal cell function is limited in duration.

Complicating the studies of anesthetic toxicity are the low occurrence of toxic effects in humans and the fact that the volatile anesthetics are commonly administered to individuals with altered physiologic states, such as obesity, enzyme induction, and organ manipulation. These states add enormously to the complexity of the toxic process and raise appropriate questions as to the validity of animal models for the study of liver toxicity in humans. Nevertheless, much progress has been made in understanding how anesthetics interact with the cell. It is remarkable that the volatile anesthetics can be safely administered to a large population with diverse medical problems. It attests to the skills of the anesthesiologists and the input of the research community regarding the use of these potent drugs.

REFERENCES

1. Sipes IG, Gandolfi AJ: Biotransformation of toxicants. In Klassen CD, Amdur MO, Doull J (eds): Casarett and Doull's Toxicology. New York, Macmillan, 1986
2. Van Dyke R, Chenowith M, Poznak AV: Metabolism of volatile anesthetics: I. Conversion in vivo of several anesthetics to $^{14}CO_2$ and chloride. Biochem Pharmacol 13:1239, 1964
3. Van Dyke RA: Metabolism of volatile anesthetics: III. Induction of microsomal dechlorinating and ether-cleaving enzymes. J Pharmacol Exp Ther 154:364, 1966
4. Schenkman JB, Kupfer D (eds): Hepatic Cytochrome P-450 Monooxygenase System. New York, Pergamon Press, 1982
5. Coon MJ, Persson AV: Microsomal cytochrome P-450: A central catalysis in detoxification reactions. In Jacoby WB (ed): Enzymatic Basis of Detoxification, vol 1, p 117. New York, Academic Press, 1980
6. Estabrook RW, Werringloer J: Cytochrome P-450: Its role in oxygen activation for drug metabolism. In Jerina DM (ed): Drug Metabolism Concepts. ACS Symposium Series. Washington, DC, American Chemical Society, 1977
7. Lu AYH, West SB: Multiplicity of mammalian microsomal cytochromes P-450. Pharmacol Rev 31:277, 1980
8. Nebert DW, Adesnik M, Coon MJ et al: The P450 gene superfamily: Recommended nomenclature. DNA 6:1, 1987
9. Conney AH: Pharmacological implications of microsomal enzyme induction. Pharmacol Rev 19:317, 1967
10. Waxman DJ: Interactions of hepatic cytochromes P-450 with steroid hormones: Regioselectively and stereospecificity of steroid metabolism and hormonal regulation of rat P-450 enzyme expression. Biochem Pharmacol 37:71, 1988
11. Guengerich FP, Dannan GA, Wright ST et al: Purification and characterization of liver microsomal cytochromes P-450: Electrophoretic, spectral, catalytic, and immunochemical properties and inducibility of eight isozymes isolated from rats treated with phenobarbital or B-naphthoflavone. Biochemistry 21:6019, 1982
12. Gonzales FJ: Molecular genetics of the P-450 superfamily. Pharmacol Ther 45:1, 1990
13. Juchau MR: Substrate specificities and functions of the P450 cytochromes. Life Sci 47:2385, 1990
14. Pantuck EJ, Pantuck CB, Conney AH: Effect of streptozotocin-induced diabetes in the rat on the metabolism of fluorinated volatile anesthetics. Anesthesiology 66:24, 1987
15. Anders MW, Pohl LR: Halogenated alkanes. In Anders MW (ed): Bioactivation of Foreign Compounds. Orlando, Florida, Academic Press, 1985
16. Rehder K, Forbes J, Alter H et al: Halothane biotransformation in man: A quantitative study. Anesthesiology 28:711, 1967
17. Cohen EN, Trudell JR, Edmunds HN, Watson E: Urinary metabolites of halothane in man. Anesthesiology 43:392, 1975
18. Sipes IG, Gandolfi AJ, Pohl LR et al: Comparison of the biotransformation and hepatotoxicity of halothane and deuterated halothane. J Pharmacol Exp Ther 214:716, 1980
19. Stier A: Trifluoroacetic acid as a metabolite of halothane. Biochem Pharmacol 13:154, 1964

20. Gandolfi AJ, White RD, Sipes IG, Pohl LR: Bioactivation and covalent binding of halothane in vitro: Studies with [3H]- and [14C]halothane. J Pharmacol Exp Ther 214:721, 1980
21. Satoh H, Gillette JR, Davies HW et al: Immunochemical evidence of trifluoroacetylated cytochrome P-450 in the liver of halothane-treated rats. Mol Pharmacol 28:468, 1985
22. Mukai S, Morio M, Fujii K, Hanaki C: Volatile metabolites of halothane in the rabbit. Anesthesiology 47:248, 1977
23. Gourlay GK, Adams JF, Cousins MJ, Sharp JH: Time-course of formation of volatile reductive metabolites of halothane in humans and an animal model. Br J Anaesth 52:331, 1980
24. Maiorino RM, Sipes IG, Gandolfi AJ et al: Factors affecting the formation of chlorotrifluoroethane and chlorodifluoroethylene from halothane. Anesthesiology 54:383, 1981
25. Lind RC, Gandolfi AJ, Sipes IG et al: Oxygen concentrations required for reductive defluorination of halothane by rat hepatic microsomes. Anesth Analg 65:835, 1986
26. Gourlay GK, Adams JF, Cousins MJ, Hall P: Genetic differences in reductive metabolism and hepatotoxicity of halothane in three strains of rats. Anesthesiology 55:96, 1981
27. Van Dyke RA, Gandolfi AJ: Anaerobic release of fluoride from halothane. Drug Metab Dispos 4:40, 1976
28. Ahr HJ, King LJ, Nastainczyk W, Ullrich V: The mechanism of reductive dehalogenation of halothane by liver cytochrome P-450. Biochem Pharmacol 31:383, 1982
29. Wood CL, Gandolfi AJ, Van Dyke RA: Lipid binding of a halothane metabolite: Relationship to lipid peroxidation in vitro. Drug Metab Dispos 4:305, 1976
30. Trudell JR, Bosterling B, Trevor AJ: Reductive metabolism of halothane by human and rabbit cytochrome P-450. Binding of 1-chloro-2,2,2-trifluoroethyl radical to phospholipids. Mol Pharmacol 21:710, 1982
31. Baker MT, Nelson RM, Van Dyke AR: The release of inorganic fluoride from halothane and halothane metabolites by cytochrome P-450, hemin, and hemoglobin. Drug Metab Dispos 11:308, 1983
32. Baker MT, Bates JN, Van Dyke RA: Stabilization of the reduced halocarbon-cytochrome P-450 complex of halothane by n-alkanes. Biochem Pharmacol 36:1029, 1987
33. Ruf HH, Ahr H, Nastainczyk W et al: Formation of a ferric carbanion complex from halothane and cytochrome P-450: Electron spin resonance, electron spectra, and model complexes. Biochemistry 23:5300, 1984
34. Baker MT, Vasquez MT, Chiang C-K: Evidence for the stability and cytochrome P450 specificity of the phenobarbital-induced reductive halothane-cytochrome P450 complex formed in rat hepatic microsomes. Biochem Pharmacol 41:1691, 1991
35. Baker MT, Bates JN, Leff SV: Stimulatory effects of halothane and isoflurane on fluoride release and cytochrome P-450 loss caused by the metabolism of 2-chloro-1,1-difluoroethene, a halothane metabolite. Anesth Analg 66:1141, 1987
36. Baker MT, Vasquez MT, Bates JN, and Chiang C-K: Metabolism of 2-chloro-1,1-difluoroethene to glyoxylic and glycolic acid in rat hepatic microsomes. Drug Metab Dispos 18:753, 1990
37. Baker MT, Bates JN: Metabolic activation of the halothane metabolite, [14C]2-chloro-1,1-difluoroethene, in hepatic microsomes. Drug Metab Dispos 16:169, 1988
38. Carpenter RL, Eger EI II, Johnson BH et al: The extent of metabolism of inhaled anesthetics in humans. Anesthesiology 65:201, 1986
39. Plummer JL, Van Der Walt JH, Cousins MJ: Reductive metabolism of halothane in children. Anaesth Intens Care 12:293, 1984
40. Young SR, Stoelting RK, Peterson C, Madura JA: Anesthetic biotransformation and renal function in obese patients during and after methoxyflurane or halothane anesthesia. Anesthesiology 42:451, 1975
41. Gruenke LD, Konopka K, Koop DR, Waskell LA: Characterization of halothane oxidation by hepatic microsomes and purified cytochromes P-450 using a gas chromatographic mass spectrometric assay. J Pharmacol Exp Ther 246:454, 1988
42. Loehning RW, Mazze RI: Possible nephrotoxicity from enflu-rane in a patient with severe renal disease. Anesthesiology 40:203, 1974
43. Eichhorn JH, Hedley-Whyte J, Steinman TI et al: Renal failure following enflurane anesthesia. Anesthesiology 45:557, 1976
44. Chase RE, Holaday DA, Fiserova-Bergerova V et al: The biotransformation of ethrane in man. Anesthesiology 35:262, 1971
45. Burke TR Jr, Branchflower RV, Lees DE, Pohl LR: Mechanisms of defluorination of enflurane: Identification of an organic metabolite in rat and man. Drug Metab Dispos 9:19, 1981
46. Christ DD, Satoh H, Kenna JG, Pohl LR: Potential metabolic basis for enflurane hepatitis and the apparent cross-sensitization between enflurane and halothane. Drug Metab Dispos 16:135, 1988
47. Cousins MJ, Greenstein LR, Hitt BA, Mazze RI: Metabolism and renal effects of enflurane in man. Anesthesiology 44:44, 1976
48. Rice SA, Talcott RE: Effects of isoniazid treatment on selected hepatic mixed-function oxidases. Drug Metab Dispos 7:260, 1979
49. Rice SA, Sbordone L, Mazze RI: Metabolism by rat hepatic microsomes of fluorinated ether anesthetics following isoniazid administration. Anesthesiology 53:489, 1980
50. Van Dyke RA: Enflurane, isoflurane, and methoxyflurane metabolism in rat hepatic microsomes from ethanol-treated animals. Anesthesiology 58:221, 1983
51. Koop DR, Crump BL, Nordblom GD, Coon MJ: Immunochemical evidence for induction of the alcohol-oxidizing cytochrome P-450 of rabbit liver microsomes by diverse agents: Ethanol, imidazole, trichloroethylene, acetone, pyrazole, and isoniazid. Proc Natl Acad Sci 82:4065, 1985
52. Knill RL, Lok PYK, Strupat JP, Lam AM: Blood solubility of isoflurane measured by a multiple gas phase equilibration technique. Can Anaesth Soc J 30:155, 1983
53. Lerman J, Gregory GA, Willis MM, Eger EI: Hematocrit and the solubility of volatile anesthetics in blood. Anesth Analg 63:911, 1984
54. Mazze RI, Hitt BA, Cousins MJ: Effect of enzyme induction with phenobarbital on the in vivo and in vitro defluorination of isoflurane and methoxyflurane. J Pharmacol Exp Ther 190:523, 1974
55. Holaday DA, Fiserova-Bergerova V, Latto IP, Zumbiel MA: Resistance of isoflurane to biotransformation in man. Anesthesiology 43:325, 1975
56. Bradshaw JJ, Ivanetich KM: Isoflurane: A comparison of its metabolism by humans and rat hepatic cytochrome P-450. Anesth Analg 63:805, 1984
57. Stoelting RK, Longshore RE: The effects of temperature on fluroxene, halothane, and methoxyflurane blood-gas and cerebrospinal fluid-gas partition coefficients. Anesthesiology 36:503, 1972
58. Van Dyke RA, Wood CL: Metabolism of methoxyflurane: Release of inorganic fluoride in human and rat hepatic microsomes. Anesthesiology 39:613, 1973
59. Ivanetich KM, Lucas SA, Marsh JA: Enflurane and methoxyflurane: Their interaction with hepatic cytochrome P-450 in vitro. Biochem Pharmacol 28:785, 1979
60. Sakai T, Takaori M: Biodegradation of halothane, enflurane, and methoxyflurane. Br J Anaesth 50:785, 1978
61. Cook TL, Beppu WJ, Hitt BA et al: A comparison of renal effects and metabolism of sevoflurane and methoxyflurane in enzyme-induced rats. Anesth Analg Curr Res 54:829, 1975
62. Mazze RI, Trudell JR, Cousins MJ: Methoxyflurane metabolism and renal dysfunction: Clinical correlation in man. Anesthesiology 35:247, 1971
63. Holaday DA, Rudofsky S, Treuhaft PS: The metabolic degradation of methoxyflurane in man. Anesthesiology 33:579, 1970
64. Canova-Davis E, Chiang JYL, Waskell L: Obligatory role of cytochrome b5 in the microsomal metabolism of methoxyflurane. Biochem Pharmacol 34:1907, 1985
65. Waskell L, Canova-Davis E, Philpot R et al: Identification of the enzymes catalyzing metabolism of methoxyflurane. Drug Metab Dispos 14:643, 1986

66. Lipka JJ, Waskell LA: Methoxyflurane acts at the substrate binding site of cytochrome P-450 LM2 to induce a dependence on cytochrome b_5. Arch Biochem Biophys 268:152, 1989

67. Wallin RF, Napoli MD: Sevoflurane, a new inhalational anesthetic agent. Anesth Analg 54:758, 1975

68. Cook TL, Beppu WJ, Hitt BA et al: Renal effects and metabolism of sevoflurane in fisher 344 rats: An in-vivo and in-vitro comparison with methoxyflurane. Anesthesiology 43:70, 1975

69. Martis L, Lynch S, Napoli MD, Woods EF: Biotransformation of sevoflurane in dogs and rats. Anesth Analg 60:186, 1981

70. Morio M, Fujii K, Mukai S, Kodama G: Decomposition of halothane by sodalime and the metabolites of halothane in expired gases. Excerpta Medica/International Congress Series (Abstracts of the 6th World Congress of Anaesthesiology), vol 387, pp 214–215, 1976

71. Hanaki C, Fujii K, Morio M, Tashima T: Decomposition of sevoflurane by sodalime. Hiroshima J Med Sci 36:61, 1987

72. Hudlicky M: Organic Fluorine Chemistry. New York, Plenum Press, 1971

73. Macdonald TL: Chemical mechanisms of halocarbon metabolism CRC Crit Rev Toxicol 11:85, 1983

74. Eger EI II, Johnson BH: MAC of I-653 in rats, including a test of the effect of body temperature and anesthetic duration. Anesth Analg 66:974, 1987

75. Koblin DD, Eger EI II, Johnson BH et al: I-653 resists degradation in rats. Anesth Analg 67:534, 1988

76. Eger EI II: Stability of I-653 in soda lime. Anesth Analg 66:983, 1987

77. Chengelis CP, Neal RA: Microsomal metabolism of diethyl ether. Biochem Pharmacol 29:247, 1980

78. Brady JF, Lee MJ, Li M et al: Diethyl ether as a substrate for acetone/ethanol-inducible cytochrome P-450 and as an inducer for cytochrome(s) P-450. Mol Pharmacol 33:48, 1987

79. Yang CS, Yoo J-SH, Ishizaki H, Hong J: Cytochrome P-450IIE1: Roles in nitrosamine metabolism and mechanisms of regulation. Drug Metab Rev 22:147, 1990

80. Tan Y, Keefer LK, Yang CS: Inhibition of microsomal N-nitrosodimethylamine demethylase by diethyl ether and other anesthetics. Biochem Pharmacol 36:1973, 1987

81. Blake DA, Rozman RS, Cascorbi HF, Krantz JC: Anesthesia LXXIV: Biotransformation of fluroxene. I. Metabolism in mice and dogs in vivo. Biochem Pharmacol 16:1237, 1967

82. Gion H, Yoshimura N, Holaday DA et al: Biotransformation of fluroxene in man. Anesthesiology 40:553, 1974

83. Harrison GG, Smith JS: Massive lethal hepatic necrosis in rats anesthetized with fluroxene, after microsomal enzyme induction. Anesthesiology 39:619, 1973

84. Ivanetich KM, Bradshaw JJ, Marsh JA et al: The role of cytochrome P-450 in the toxicity of fluroxene (2,2,2-trifluoroethyl vinyl ether) anaesthesia in vivo. Biochem Pharmacol 25:773, 1976

85. Touloukian J, Kaplowitz N: Halothane-induced hepatic disease. Semin Liver Dis 1:134, 1981

86. Summary of the National Halothane Study. JAMA 197:775, 1966

87. McLain GE, Sipes IG, Brown BR Jr: An animal model of halothane hepatotoxicity: Role of enzyme induction and hypoxia. Anesthesiology 51:321, 1979

88. Van Dyke RA: Effect of fasting on anesthetic-associated liver toxicity. Anesthesiology 44:A181, 1981

89. Shingu K, Eger EI II, Johnson BH: Hypoxia may be more important than reductive metabolism in halothane-induced hepatic injury. Anesth Analg 61:824, 1982

90. Lunam C, Cousins MJ, de la M Hall P: A guinea pig model of halothane associated hepatotoxicity in the absence of enzyme induction and hypoxia. J Pharmacol Exp Ther 232:801, 1985

91. Lunam CA, Cousins MJ, de la M Hall P: Guinea-pig model of halothane-associated hepatotoxicity in the absence of enzyme induction and hypoxia. J Pharmacol Exp Ther 232:802, 1985

92. Gorsky BH, Cascorbi HF: Halothane hepatotoxicity and fluoride production in mice and rats. Anesthesiology 50:123, 1979

93. Baker MT, Van Dyke RA: Metabolism-dependent binding of the chlorinated insecticide DDT and its metabolite, DDD, to microsomal protein and lipids. Biochem Pharmacol 33:255, 1984

94. Uetrecht J, Wood AJJ, Phythyon JM, Wood M: Contrasting effects on halothane hepatotoxicity in the phenobarbital-hypoxic and triiodothyronine model: Mechanistic implications. Anesthesiology 59:196, 1983

95. Berman ML, Kuhnert L, Phythyon JM, Holaday DA: Isoflurane and enflurane-induced hepatic necrosis in triiodothyronine-pretreated rats. Anesthesiology 58:1, 1983

96. Smith AC, Roberts SM, Berman LM et al: Effects of piperonyl butoxide on halothane hepatotoxicity and metabolism in the hyperthyroid rat. Toxicology 50:95, 1988

97. Pohl LR, Kenna JG, Satoh H, Christ D: Neoantigens associated with halothane hepatitis. Drug Metab Rev 20:203, 1989

98. Vergani D, Mieli-Vergani G, Alberti A et al: Antibodies to the surface of halothane-altered hepatocytes rabbit hepatocytes in patients with severe halothane-associated hepatitis. N Engl J Med 303:66, 1980

99. Neuberger J, Mieli-Vergani G, Tredger JM et al: Oxidative metabolism of halothane in the production of altered hepatocyte membrane antigens in acute halothane-induced hepatic necrosis. Gut 22:669, 1981

100. Kenna JG, Satoh H, Christ DD et al: Metabolic basis for a drug hypersensitivity: Antibodies in sera from patients with halothane hepatitis recognize liver neoantigens that contain the trifluoroacetyl group derived from halothane. J Pharmacol Exp Ther 245:1103, 1988

101. Satoh H, Gillette JR, Davies HW et al: Immunochemical evidence of trifluoroacetylated cytochrome P-450 in the liver of halothane-treated rats. Mol Pharmacol 28:468, 1985

102. Satoh H, Martin BM, Schulick AH et al: Human anti-endoplasmic reticulum antibodies in sera of patients with halothane-induced hepatitis are directed against a trifluoroacetylated carboxylesterase. Proc Natl Acad Sci USA 86:322, 1989

103. Lind RC, Gandolfi AJ, Brown BR, de la M Hall P: Halothane hepatotoxicity in guinea pigs. Anesth Analg 66:222, 1987

104. Siadat-Pajouh M, Hubbard AK, Roth TP, Gandolfi AJ: Generation of halothane-induced immune response in a guinea pig model of halothane hepatitis: Anesth Analg 66:1209, 1987

105. Recknagel RO: A new direction in the study of CC14 hepatoxicity. Life Sci 33:401, 1983

106. Farber JL: Calcium and the mechanisms of liver necrosis. Liver Dis 7:347, 1982

107. Gill DL: Sodium channel, sodium pump, and sodium-calcium exchange activities in synaptosomal plasma membrane vesicles. J Biol Chem 257:10986, 1982

108. Gill DL, Grollman EF, Kohn LD: Calcium transport mechanisms in membrane vesicles from guinea pig brain synaptosomes. J Biol Chem 256:184, 1981

109. Glende EA, Jr, Pushpendran CK: Activation of phospholipase A_2 by carbon tetrachloride in isolated rat hepatocytes. Biochem Pharmacol 35:3301, 1986

110. Iaizzo PA, Seewald MJ, Powis G et al: The effects of volatile anesthetics on Ca^{++} mobilization in rat hepatocytes. Anesthesiology 72:504, 1990

111. Iaizzo PA, Olsen RA, Seewald MJ et al: Transient increases of intracellular Ca^{++} induced by volatile anesthetics in rat hepatocytes. Cell Calcium 11:515, 1990

112. Farrell GC, Mahoney J, Bilous M, Frost L: Altered hepatic calcium homeostasis in guinea pigs with halothane-induced hepatotoxicity. J Pharmacol Exp Ther 247:751, 1988

113. Moore L: Inhibition of liver microsome calcium pump by in vivo administration of CCl_4, $CHCl_3$ and 1,1-dichloroethylene (vinylidene chloride). Biochem Pharmacol 29:2505, 1980

114. Brattin WO, Pencil SD, Waller RL et al: Assessment of the role of calcium ion in halocarbon hepatotoxicity. Environ Health Perspect 57:321, 1984

115. Agarwal AK, Mehendale HM: Perturbation of calcium homeostasis by CCl_4 in rats pretreated with chlordecone and phenobarbital. Environ Health Perspect 57:289, 1984

116. Chein KR, Abrams J, Serroni A et al: Accelerated phospholipid degradation and associated membrane dysfunction in irreversible ischemia liver cell injury. J Biol Chem 253:4809, 1978

117. Baedeland F, Greene NM: Effect of diethyl ether on tissue distribution and metabolism of pentobarbital in rats. Anesthesiology 19:724, 1958

118. Umdea T, Inaba T: Effects of anesthetics on diphenylhydantoin metabolism in the rat: Possible inhibition by diethyl ether. Can J Physiol Pharmacol 56:241, 1978

119. Johannessen W, Gadeholtt G, Aarbakke J: Effects of diethyl ether anaesthesia on the pharmacokinetics of antipyrine and paracetamol in the rat. J Pharm Pharmacol 33:365, 1981

120. Hanew T, Schenker S, Meredith CG, Henderson GI: The pharmacokinetic interaction of diethyl ether with aminopyrine in the rat. Proc Soc Exp Biol Med 175:64, 1984

121. Aune H, Olsen H, Morland J: Diethyl ether influence on the metabolism of antipyrine, paracetamol and sulphanilamide in isolated rat hepatocytes. Br J Anaesth 53:621, 1981

122. Aune H, Stowell AR, Morland J: Ether inhibition of ethanol metabolism in isolated rat liver parenchymal cells. Alcoholism Clin Exp Res 5:550, 1981

123. Keefer LK, Garland WA, Oldfield NF et al: Inhibition of n-nitrosodimethylamine metabolism in rats by ether anesthesia. Cancer Res 45:5457, 1985

124. White PF, Marietta MP, Pudwill CR et al: Effects of halothane anesthesia on the biodisposition of ketamine in rats. J Pharmacol Exp Ther 196:545, 1976

125. Reilly CS, Wood AJJ, Koshakji RP, Wood M: The effect of halothane on drug disposition: Contribution of changes in intrinsic drug metabolizing capacity and hepatic blood flow. Anesthesiology 63:70, 1985

126. Dale O, Gandolfi AJ, Brendel K, Schuman S: Rat liver slices and diazepam metabolism: In vitro interactions with volatile anaesthetic drugs and albumin. Br J Anaesth 60:692, 1988

127. Bell LE, Slattery JT, Calkins DF: Effect of halothane-oxygen anesthesia on the pharmacokinetics of diazepam and its metabolites in rats. J Pharm Exp Ther 233:94, 1985

128. Fish KJ, Rice SA: Halothane inhibits metabolism of enflurane in fisher 334 rats. Anesthesiology 59:417, 1983

129. Fish KJ, Rice SA, Weissman DB: Halothane inhibits metabolism of enflurane in surgical patients. Anesthesiology 61:A268, 1984

130. Aune H, Bessesen A, Olsen H, Morland J: Acute effects of halothane and enflurane on drug metabolism and protein synthesis in isolated rat hepatocytes. Acta Pharmacol Toxicol 53:363, 1983

131. Brown BR Jr: The diphasic action of halothane on the oxidative metabolism of drugs by the liver. Anesthesiology 35:241, 1971

132. Da Rocha-Reis MGF, Hipolito-Reis C: Effects of the inhalation of enflurane on hepatic microsomal enzymatic activities in the rat. Br J Anaesth 54:97, 1982

133. Hempel V, van Kugelgen C, Remmer H: Der Einfluß Narkosemittel auf den Fremdostaffabbau in der Leber. Anaesthesist 24:400, 1975

134. Fiserova-Bergerova V: Inhibitory effect of isoflurane upon oxidative metabolism of halothane. Anesth Analg 63:399, 1984

135. Wood M, Wood AJJ: Contrasting effects of halothane, isoflurane, and enflurane on in vivo drug metabolism in the rat. Anesth Analg 63:709, 1984

136. Allott PR, Steward A, Flook V, Mapleson WW: Variation with temperature of the solubilities of inhaled anaesthetics in water, oil, and biological media. Br J Anaesth 45:294, 1973

137. Krieter PA, Van Dyke RA: Cytochrome P-450 and halothane metabolism: Decrease in rat liver microsomal P-450 in vitro. Chem Biol Interact 44:219, 1983

138. De Groot H, Harnisch U, Noll T: Suicidal inactivation of microsomal cytochrome P-450 by halothane under hypoxic conditions. Biochem Biophys Res Commun 107:885, 1991

139. Murphy MJ, Guengerich FP, Kaminsky LS: Metabolism of fluroxene and analogous fluorinated ether anesthetics by highly purified cytochromes P-450 and the associated enzyme destruction. In: Coon MJ, Conney AH, Estabrook RW et al: Microsomes, Drug Oxidations, and Chemical Carcinogenesis, p 865. New York, Academic Press, 1980

140. Marsh JA, Bradshaw JJ, Sapeika GA et al: Further investigations of the metabolism of fluroxene and the degradation of cytochrome P-450 in vitro. Biochem Pharmacol 26:1601, 1977

141. Ortiz de Montellano PR, Kunze KL: Inactivation of hepatic cytochrome P-450 by allenic substrates. Biochem Biophys Res Commun 94:443, 1980

142. Ortiz de Montellano PR, Kunze KL, Beilan HS, Wheeler C: Destruction of cytochrome P-450 by vinyl fluoride, fluroxene, and acetylene: Evidence for a radical intermediate in olefin oxidation. Biochemistry 21:1331, 1982

143. Pohl LR, Martin JL, George JW: Mechanism of metabolic activation of chloroform by rat liver microsomes. Biochem Pharmacol 29:3271, 1980

144. Enosawa S, Nakazawa Y: Changes in cytochrome P-450 molecular species in rat liver in chloroform intoxication. Biochem Pharmacol 35:1555, 1986

145. Van Dyke RA, Rikans LE: Effect of the volatile anesthetics on aniline hydroxylase and aminopyrine demethylase. Biochem Pharmacol 19:1501, 1970

146. Korten K, Van Dyke RA: Acute interaction of drugs: I. The effect of volatile anesthetics on the kinetics of aniline hydroxylase and aminopyrine demethylase in rat hepatic microsomes. Biochem Pharmacol 22:2105, 1973

147. Hallen B, Johansson G: Inhalation anesthetics and cytochrome P-450-dependent reactions in rat liver microsomes. Anesthesiology 43:34, 1975

148. Whelan E, Wood AJJ, Koshakji R et al: Halothane inhibition of propranolol metabolism is stereoselective. Anesthesiology 71:561, 1989

149. Testa B: Substrate and product stereoselectivity in monooxygenase-mediated drug activation and inactivation. Biochem Pharmacol 37:85, 1988

150. Brown BR Jr, Sagalyn AM: Hepatic microsomal enzyme induction by inhalation anesthetics: Mechanism in the rat. Anesthesiology 40:152, 1974

151. Ross WT Jr, Cardell RR Jr: Proliferation of smooth endoplasmic reticulum and induction of microsomal drug-metabolizing enzymes after ether or halothane. Anesthesiology 48:325, 1978

152. Duvaldestin P, Mazze RI, Nivoche Y, Desmonts J-M: Enzyme induction following surgery with halothane and neurolept anesthesia. Anesth Analg 60:319, 1981

153. Duvaldestin P, Mauge F, Desmonts J-M: Enflurane anesthesia and antipyrine metabolism. Clin Pharmacol Ther 29:61, 1981

154. Gelman SI: Disturbance in hepatic blood flow during anesthesia and surgery. Arch Surg 111:881, 1976

155. Dale O, Nilsen OG: Displacement of some basic drugs from human serum proteins by enflurane, halothane, and their major metabolites: An in vitro study. Br J Anaesth 56:535, 1984

156. Pollack GM, Browne JL, Marton J, Haberer LJ: Chronic stress impairs oxidative metabolism and hepatic excretion of model xenobiotic substrates in the rat. Drug Metab Dispos 19:130, 1991

19

David R. Bevan
François Donati

Muscle Relaxants

PHYSIOLOGY AND PHARMACOLOGY

Structure

The cell bodies of neurons supplying skeletal muscle lie in the spinal cord. They receive and integrate information from several appendages, called dendrites, and from other nerve cells synapsing with the cell body. This information is carried *via* an elongated structure, the axon, to distant parts of the body.

Each nerve cell supplies many muscle cells (or fibers) a short distance after branching into as many nerve terminals. The nerve cell, together with the muscle fibers it innervates, is called the motor unit. The terminal portion of the axon is a specialized structure, the synapse, designed for the production and release of acetylcholine (ACh). The synapse is separated from the end-plate of the muscle fiber by a narrow gap, called the synaptic cleft, which is 20–50 nm in width (0.02–0.05 μm).[1]

The end-plate is a specialized portion of the membrane of the muscle fiber, characterized by folds and designed to respond to ACh. Most human muscle cells have only one end-plate, located near the midportion of the cell. Muscle cells have been classified according to their biochemical, morphologic, and functional characteristics. Slow twitch fibers tend to have a large aerobic capacity, slow contraction and relaxation times, and resistance to fatigue. The adductor pollicis, for example, contains mostly slow twitch fibers. Fast twitch fibers typically exhibit limited aerobic metabolism, have fast contraction and relaxation times, and are not resistant to fatigue. However, intermediate types exist. Furthermore, the biochemical, morphologic, and functional characteristics do not always coincide completely. As a result, much confusion has arisen in the literature.[2]

Nerve Stimulation

Nerve tissue is excitable; that is, it can carry electrical impulses generated when the cell membrane is depolarized, in response to either a chemical or an electrical stimulus. Under resting conditions, the electrical potential of the inside of a nerve cell is negative with respect to the outside (typically −90 mV). If this potential is made less negative (depolarization), sodium channels open and make the po-

tential positive for a short time (approximately 1 msec). This in turn depolarizes the next area of membrane, sodium channels open, and an electrical impulse, the action potential, propagates. In humans, conduction velocities in motor neurons are typically 40–70 m·sec^{-1}.

Under physiologic conditions, the source of action potentials in a nerve axon is the cell body, which is depolarized by neurotransmitters released by adjoining synapses. During anesthesia and surgery, a nerve may be stimulated electrically for the purpose of monitoring the neuromuscular junction. An action potential is generated provided that the current applied depolarizes the axon sufficiently to reach a certain threshold. The magnitude of the depolarization depends both on the current applied and on the duration of the stimulus.

A peripheral nerve is made up of a large number of axons of different thresholds, different sizes, and different distances from the stimulating electrode. Although each axon responds in an all-or-none fashion to the stimulus applied, not all axons respond to a given stimulus. Thus, in the absence of neuromuscular blockers, the relationship between the amplitude of the muscle contraction and current applied is sigmoidal.[3] At low currents, the depolarization is insufficient in all axons. As current increases, more and more axons are depolarized to threshold and the size of the muscle contraction increases. When the stimulating current reaches a certain level, all axons are depolarized to threshold and propagate an action potential. Increasing the current beyond this point does not increase muscle contraction; the stimulation is supramaximal (Fig. 19-1).

After firing once, a nerve axon cannot respond to further stimulation for a short time (usually 0.5–1 msec) called the refractory period. If the duration of stimulation is longer than the refractory period, repetitive stimulation of the axon may result.[1] For this reason, the current pulse applied must be short, less than 0.5 msec. Most commercially available stimulators deliver impulses lasting 0.1–0.2 msec.

Release of Acetylcholine

Acetylcholine is synthesized from choline and acetate and stored in the nerve ending. Electron micrographs of the synaptic area reveal a large number of vesicles concentrated near the cell membrane opposite the crests of the junctional

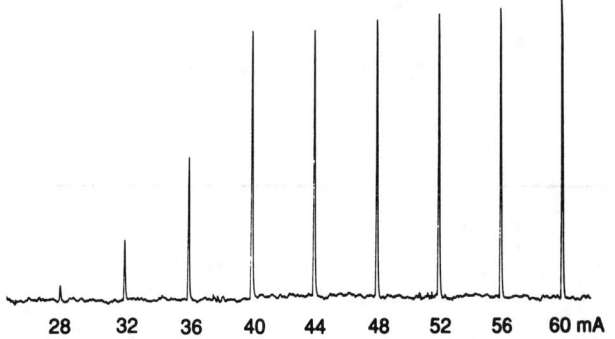

Figure 19-1. Example of increasing stimulating current in one patient. Current pulses, 0.2 msec duration, were delivered to the ulnar nerve at the wrist every 10 seconds. The force of contraction of the adductor pollicis was measured and appears as spikes. No twitch was seen if the current was 28 mA or less. At current strengths of 40 mA or greater, the current became supramaximal; increasing the current produced little change in force.

folds of the end-plate (Fig. 19-2).[4] These vesicles contain a high concentration of ACh, but some ACh is extravesicular.

Acetylcholine is released in packets or quanta, each containing about 5,000 to 10,000 molecules. In the absence of nerve stimulation, quanta are released spontaneously, at random, and this is seen as small depolarizations of the end-plate (miniature end-plate potential, or MEPP). When an action potential invades the nerve terminal, some 200–400 quanta are released spontaneously, unloading some 1 to 4 million ACh molecules into the synaptic cleft.[1] One quantum probably represents the contents of one vesicle, which discharges by fusing with the synaptic membrane. The short distance between the location of the vesicles and the receptor adds credence to this hypothesis. However, some observations suggest that extravesicular ACh is released preferentially, perhaps through pores in the synaptic membrane.[5] Knowledge of the exact release mechanism is not critical to the understanding of the action of neuromuscular blocking drugs.

Postsynaptic Events

The end-plate has 1 to 10 million receptors that are sensitive to ACh.[1] Structurally, these receptors consist of five glycoprotein subunits arranged in the form of a rosette and lying across the whole cell membrane (Fig. 19-3). Two of these noncontiguous subunits, called alpha subunits, are similar and each must bind simultaneously to an ACh molecule to induce a conformational change in the receptor structure. Thus an opening is made in the center of the rosette, allowing small ions to pass through the channel.[2,6] Sodium ions move inside along their concentration and electrical gradients, depolarizing the cell membrane. Potassium ions tend to move out, along their concentration gradient. If a large number of receptors open simultaneously, as occurs following release triggered by a nerve action potential, the depolarization attains or exceeds threshold, and an action potential is generated in muscle. This action potential propagates in the same way as a nerve action potential, and this electrical activity triggers the contraction process.

Thus, depolarization above threshold in a muscle fiber is followed by two distinct but related phenomena: an electrical event, the action potential, and a mechanical event, muscle contraction. The activity of a whole muscle is the sum of the response of the individual units, and can be measured either in terms of its electrical activity (by electromyography, or EMG) or its contractile force (by mechanomyography, or MMG). The EMG response of the muscles of the hand is 5–10 msec in duration, but the MMG response lasts approximately 150 msec (Fig. 19-4). Thus, for frequencies up to 100 Hz, the EMG response can be distinguished for each stimulus. However, summation of individual twitch responses occurs for frequencies greater than 7–10 Hz, and a tetanic response, greater in intensity than a muscle twitch, can be observed.

Nondepolarizing neuromuscular blocking drugs block the postsynaptic ACh receptor by binding to at least one of the two alpha subunits, thus preventing access by ACh. They may also enter and block the ion channel when it is open, but this "channel block" is of minor importance.[7] In the absence of neuromuscular blocking drugs there is a large proportion of spare receptors, i.e., a wide "margin of

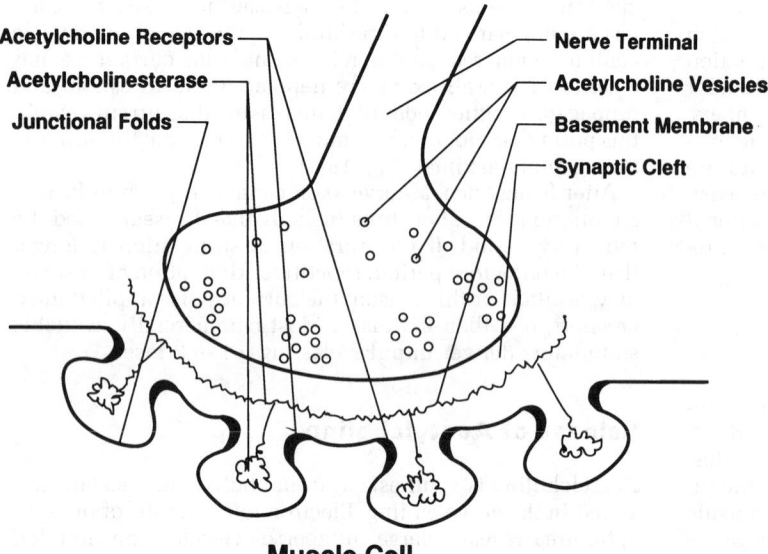

Acetylcholine Receptors

Acetylcholinesterase

Junctional Folds

Nerve Terminal

Acetylcholine Vesicles

Basement Membrane

Synaptic Cleft

Muscle Cell

Figure 19-2. Diagram of neuromuscular junction.

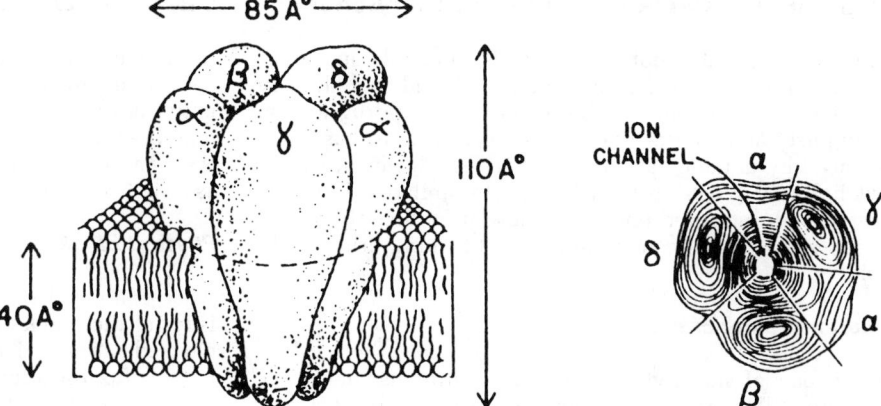

Figure 19-3. The nicotinic acetylcholine receptor consists of five glycoprotein subunits arranged to form an ion channel. The alpha subunits carry a recognition site for agonists and antagonists. (Reproduced with permission from Taylor P: Are neuromuscular blocking agents more efficacious in pairs? Anesthesiology 63:1, 1985.)

safety." In other words, only a small fraction of receptors need to bind to ACh in order to produce depolarization. This implies that neuromuscular blocking drugs must be bound to a large number of receptors before any blockade is detectable. Animal studies suggest that 75% of receptors must be occupied before twitch height decreases in the presence of d-tubocurarine, and that blockade is complete when 92% of receptors are occupied.[8] The actual number might vary depending on the type of muscle and the species studied,[9] but the general concept is applicable to humans. The point is that clinically detectable blockade occurs over a narrow range of receptor occupancy.

Acetylcholine is hydrolyzed very rapidly by the enzyme acetylcholinesterase, which is present in the folds of the end-plate as well as embedded in the basement membrane of the synaptic cleft. The presence of the enzyme in the synaptic cleft suggests that not all the ACh released reaches the end-plate; some is hydrolyzed en route.[2]

Some receptors are found on the muscle cell membrane outside the end-plate. Normally, the density of these extrajunctional receptors is low, but denervation leads to their proliferation. There is also a large number of extrajunctional receptors in fetal muscle, but they have disappeared by the time of birth in humans.

Presynaptic Events

There is growing evidence that presynaptic receptors have a regulatory role in the release of ACh. In the presence of neuromuscular blocking drugs, the EMG response decreases with stimulation frequencies greater than 0.15–0.1 Hz.[10] This "fade" probably reflects the decrease in ACh release that occurs with rapid stimulation. Under normal circumstances, a decrease in ACh release does not result in a decrease in muscle response because of the presence of a wide margin of safety. However, it would become apparent if this margin were reduced, such as in the presence of neuromuscular blocking drugs.

There are good reasons to believe that ACh release is maintained during high-frequency stimulation under physiologic conditions through presynaptic ACh receptors that regulate transmitter release.[2] These positive feedback receptors are blocked by small doses of nondepolarizing relaxants.[11] Although no direct evidence has been provided for this theory and no mechanism has been elucidated for the link between receptor activation and ACh output, several observations from various sources are highly suggestive of such a mechanism:

1. The relationship between twitch depression and fade is drug dependent and time dependent.[12]
2. Facilitatory drugs such as succinylcholine and neostigmine have clearly identifiable presynaptic effects.[13]
3. These effects can be blocked by nondepolarizing neuromuscular blocking drugs.[13]
4. Application of ACh through an electrode located near the neuromuscular junction does not produce fade in the presence of d-tubocurarine, whereas nerve stimulation does.[14]

Whatever the exact mechanism, fade can be regarded as a key property of nondepolarizing neuromuscular blocking drugs that is extremely useful for monitoring purposes.

NEUROMUSCULAR PHARMACOLOGY

Neuromuscular blocking drugs interact with the ACh receptor either by depolarizing the end-plate or by competing with ACh for binding sites. The former mechanism is characteristic of depolarizing drugs and the latter of nondepolarizing agents.

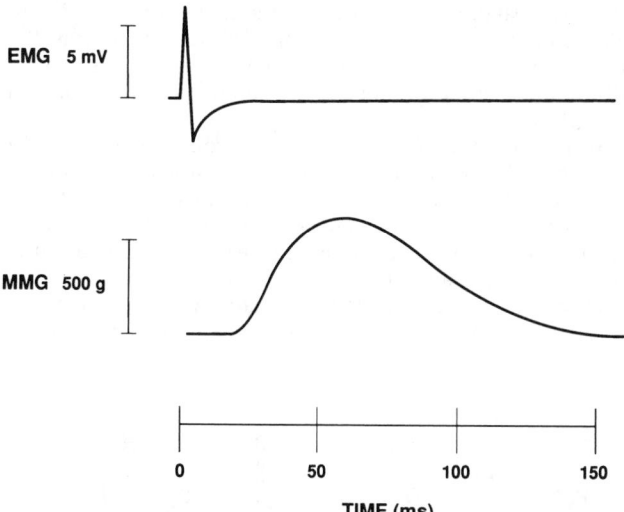

Figure 19-4. Typical electromyographic (EMG) and mechanomyographic (MMG) tracings of the adductor pollicis after single stimulation of the ulnar nerve. Note the longer duration and latency of the MMG response.

Depolarizing Blocking Drugs: Succinylcholine

Among drugs that depolarize the end-plate, only succinylcholine and decamethonium were introduced into clinical practice in North America. Decamethonium, a drug with a slow onset and intermediate duration of action, has been replaced by nondepolarizing alternatives. However, succinylcholine (Fig. 19-5) still enjoys great popularity despite a long list of undesired effects, because it is the only rapid-onset, short-duration neuromuscular blocking drug available.

Neuromuscular Effects

The effects of succinylcholine at the neuromuscular junction are still poorly understood. When it first reaches the postsynaptic receptor, succinylcholine exhibits ACh-like activity.[15] The membrane becomes depolarized and muscle activity follows. Succinylcholine also binds to extrajunctional receptors located on the muscle fiber and presynaptic receptors at the nerve terminal. The net effect is uncoordinated muscle activity that manifests clinically as fasciculations. Hyperkalemia is probably the result of the same phenomenon, that is, the large number of open ACh receptors allows potassium to flow from the inside to the outside of the muscle cells.

Although all ACh receptors might respond to succinylcholine, perhaps only presynaptic receptors are responsible for the fasciculations. The injection of succinylcholine is followed by intense nerve activity that can be blocked with small doses of nondepolarizing drugs. This suggests that presynaptic receptors are involved in the production of fasciculations and that they are blocked by defasciculating drugs. Following nerve stimulation, the twitch response may be greater than normal. This is due to repetitive stimulation, and the phenomenon is abolished by small doses of nondepolarizing drugs.[16]

The blocking effect of succinylcholine at the neuromuscular junction is probably due to desensitization. Prolonged exposure to an agonist leads to a state characterized by a lack of responsiveness of the receptor.[15] The time course required for this effect is milliseconds or seconds. Desensitization is also a property of ACh, but under physiologic conditions, breakdown of the transmitter is too rapid for desensitization to occur. Although brief by clinical standards, the duration of action of succinylcholine is many orders of magnitude longer than that of ACh, so that desensitization can take place.

Succinylcholine has yet another neuromuscular effect. In some muscles, like the masseter and to a lesser extent the adductor pollicis, a sustained increase in tension that may last for several minutes can be observed.[17,18] The mechanism of action of this tension change is uncertain, but it is blocked by large amounts of nondepolarizing drugs.[19] Masseter spasm, which has been associated with malignant hyperthermia, may be an exaggerated form of this response.

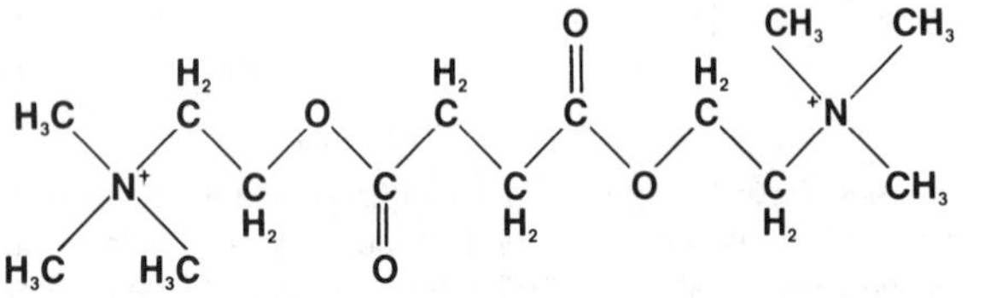

Figure 19-5. Structure of succinylcholine.

Characteristics of Depolarizing Blockade

After injection of succinylcholine, single twitch height is decreased. However, the response to high-frequency stimulation is sustained: train-of-four fade and tetanic fade are not observed. The block is antagonized by nondepolarizing agents and is potentiated by inhibitors of acetylcholinesterase, such as neostigmine and edrophonium.[20]

Phase II Block

After prolonged exposure to succinylcholine, the characteristics of the block change, and features of nondepolarizing blockade appear. Train-of-four and tetanic fade become apparent after the administration of 7–10 mg·kg^{-1}, which corresponds to 30–60 minutes of paralysis. Neostigmine or edrophonium can antagonize the block, which has been termed "nondepolarizing," "dual," or "phase II block." The last term is preferable because it does not imply any specific mechanism of action. The onset of phase II block coincides with tachyphylaxis, as more succinylcholine is required for the same effect.[21]

Pharmacology of Succinylcholine

Succinylcholine is rapidly hydrolyzed by plasma cholinesterase to choline and succinylmonocholine.[22] The latter has a weak neuromuscular blocking effect. Because of the rapid disappearance of succinylcholine from plasma, the maximum effect is reached rapidly. Subparalyzing doses (up to 0.3–0.5 mg·kg^{-1}) reach their maximal effect within approximately 1.5–2 minutes at the adductor pollicis,[23] and within 1 minute at more central muscles such as the masseter and the larynx. With larger doses (1–2 mg·kg^{-1}), abolition of twitch response can be reached even more rapidly.

The mean dose producing 50% blockade (ED$_{50}$) at the adductor pollicis is 0.15–0.2 mg·kg^{-1} with opioid–nitrous oxide anesthesia[24] and the ED$_{95}$ is in the range of 0.30–0.35 mg·kg^{-1}. In the absence of nitrous oxide, the ED$_{50}$ and ED$_{95}$ are increased to 0.3 and 0.5 mg·kg^{-1}, respectively.[23] These values are doubled if d-tubocurarine, 0.05 mg·kg^{-1}, is given as a precurarizing dose.[23] The time until full recovery of the MMG response is 10–12 minutes after a dose of 1 mg·kg^{-1} (Fig. 19-6).[25] No pharmacokinetic studies of succinylcholine have been performed, but the elimination half-life ($T_{1/2\beta}$) has been estimated, from the duration of action of various doses, at 2–4 minutes.[26]

Side Effects

Cardiovascular. Because of its structural similarity to ACh, succinylcholine is expected to have some parasympathetic activity. Sinus bradycardia with nodal or ventricular escape beats (or both) may occur, especially in children, and asystole has been described after a second dose of succinylcholine in adults. However, parasympathetic effects are infrequent and can be attenuated with atropine or glycopyrrolate.[27] Succinylcholine increases catecholamine release, and this effect may explain in part the low incidence of bradycardia. The exact nature of the interaction of succinylcholine with muscarinic receptors is, however, poorly understood, and the mechanism for the enhanced bradycardic effect of a second dose is not known.

Allergic Reactions. Succinylcholine has been incriminated as the trigger of allergic reactions more often than any other intravenous (iv) drug used in anesthesia. However, the prev-

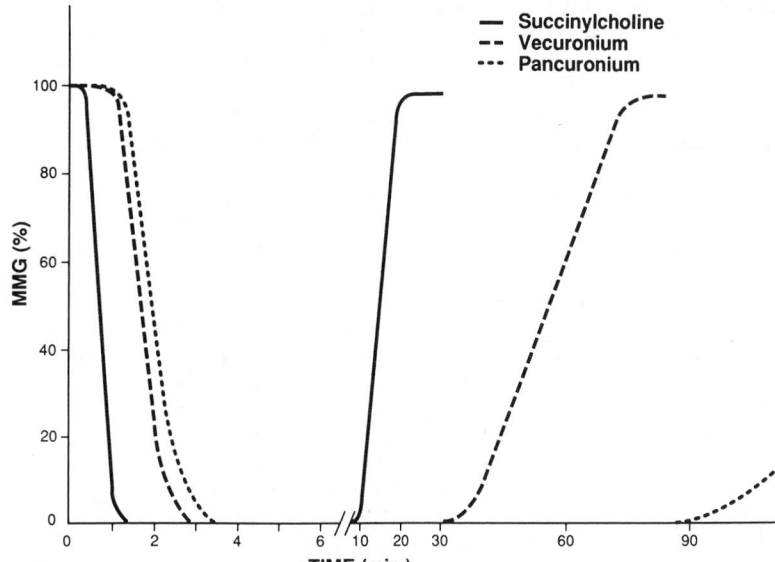

Figure 19-6. Approximate onset and recovery profiles for a short-acting drug, succinylcholine, 1.0 mg·kg^{-1}; an intermediate-acting drug, vecuronium, 0.1 mg·kg^{-1}; and a long-acting drug, pancuronium, 0.15 mg·kg^{-1}. Doses given are 2–2.5 × ED$_{95}$ for all three drugs.

alence is uncertain and the number of reported cases is low, in light of the widespread use of the drug.[1] Anaphylactic reactions that occur following the first exposure to a neuromuscular blocking drug may reflect sensitization that occurs from prior contact with cosmetics and soaps that also contain antigenic quaternary ammonium groups.

Fasciculations. The prevalence of fasciculations is high after the rapid injection of succinylcholine, especially in muscular adults. Although this is a benign side-effect of the drug, most clinicians prefer to prevent fasciculations. In this respect, a small dose of a nondepolarizing neuromuscular blocking drug given 3–5 minutes before succinylcholine is effective. d-Tubocurarine, 0.05 mg·kg^{-1}, gallamine, 0.2 mg·kg^{-1}, or atracurium, 0.03 mg·kg^{-1}, may be given for this purpose. Pancuronium, 0.01 mg·kg^{-1}, or vecuronium, 0.007 mg·kg^{-1}, are probably less effective as defasciculants. After administration of these nondepolarizing drugs, the dose of succinylcholine must be increased from 1 mg·kg^{-1} to 1.5–2 mg·kg^{-1} because of the antagonism between depolarizing and nondepolarizing drugs.[23] Care must be taken not to exceed these doses of nondepolarizing agents to avoid partial neuromuscular blockade in awake patients. The most common symptoms are blurred vision, heavy eyelids, and, occasionally, difficulty in swallowing or breathing. Other drugs such as diazepam, lidocaine, fentanyl, calcium, vitamin C, magnesium, and dantrolene have all been used to prevent fasciculations.[1] The results are no better than with nondepolarizing relaxants, and they may have undesirable effects of their own. "Self-taming," the administration of small (10 mg) doses of succinylcholine 1 minute before the intubating dose, is an effective tactic but has been largely abandoned because of the considerable blockade that may be produced by the "taming" dose.[1]

Muscle Pains. Generalized aches and pains, similar to the myalgias that follow violent exercise, are common 24–48 hours after succinylcholine administration. The relationship between muscle pains and fasciculations is not firmly established. Although many studies have failed to confirm that precurarization with a nondepolarizing neuromuscular blocking drug is of any value in the prevention of myalgias, the available evidence suggests there is a protective effect.[28]

Intragastric Pressure. Succinylcholine increases intragastric pressure, and this effect is blocked by precurarization. However, succinylcholine causes even greater increases in lower esophageal sphincter pressure.[29] Thus, succinylcholine does not appear to increase the risk of aspiration of gastric contents unless the esophageal sphincter is incompetent.

Intraocular Pressure. Intraocular pressure increases by 5–10 mm Hg after injection of succinylcholine, and precurarization with a nondepolarizing blocker has little or no effect on this increase.[30] For this reason, large doses of nondepolarizing neuromuscular blocking drugs are recommended for open eye injuries. However, it must be appreciated that other factors, such as inadequate anesthesia, elevated systemic blood pressure, and insufficient neuromuscular blockade during laryngoscopy and tracheal intubation, might increase intraocular pressure more than succinylcholine.[31]

Intracranial Pressure. Succinylcholine may increase intracranial pressure, and this response is probably diminished by precurarization.[32] Some of this change may be due to an increase in the partial pressure of carbon dioxide (P$_{CO_2}$) produced by fasciculations.[33] Again, laryngoscopy and tracheal intubation with inadequate anesthesia or muscle relaxation are likely to increase intracranial pressure even more than succinylcholine.

Hyperkalemia. Serum potassium increases by 0.5–1.0 mEq·l^{-1} after injection of succinylcholine. This increase is not prevented completely by precurarization. In fact, only large doses of nondepolarizing blockers abolish this effect.[34] Subjects with pre-existing hyperkalemia, such as patients in renal failure, do not have a greater increase in potassium levels, but the absolute level might reach the toxic range. However, severe hyperkalemia, occasionally leading to cardiac arrest, has been described in patients after major denervation injuries, spinal cord transection, peripheral denervation, stroke, trauma, extensive burns, and prolonged immobility with disease[1] and may be related to potassium loss *via* a proliferation of extrajunctional receptors.

Abnormal Plasma Cholinesterase. Plasma cholinesterase activity can be reduced by a number of endogenous and exogenous causes such as pregnancy, liver disease, uremia, malnutrition, burns, plasmapheresis, and oral contraceptives. These conditions usually lead to a slight, clinically unimportant increase in the duration of action of succinylcholine.[1,35]

A small proportion of patients (1:1500 to 1:3000 in the general population) have a genetically determined inability to metabolize succinylcholine. Plasma cholinesterase is either absent or an abnormal form of the enzyme is present. Only patients homozygous for the condition have prolonged paralysis (3–6 hours) after usual doses of succinylcholine (1–1.5 mg·kg[−1]). In heterozygous patients, the duration of action is only slightly prolonged.[35] Although whole blood or fresh frozen plasma can be given to accelerate succinylcholine metabolism in patients with low or absent plasma cholinesterase, the best course of action is probably mechanical ventilation of the lungs until full recovery of neuromuscular function can be demonstrated. Neostigmine and edrophonium are unpredictable in the reversal of abnormally prolonged succinylcholine blockade[36] and are best avoided.

Clinical Uses

The main indication for succinylcholine is to facilitate tracheal intubation. The dose required is approximately 1.0 mg·kg[−1], and must be increased to 1.5–2.0 mg·kg[−1] if a precurarizing dose of a nondepolarizing blocker has been used. Intubating conditions are optimal within 1–1.5 minutes.

Succinylcholine has also been used for maintenance of relaxation for up to 3 hours. However, because of the availability of nondepolarizing drugs for this purpose, succinylcholine infusions are indicated mainly for cases of less than 30 minutes' duration. Infusion rates for 90–95% blockade are approximately 50–100 μg·kg[−1]·min[−1] and need to be adjusted upward after 30–60 minutes because of tachyphylaxis.[21]

Children are slightly more resistant to succinylcholine than adults,[18] and doses of 1–2 mg·kg[−1] are required to facilitate intubation. In infants, 2–3 mg·kg[−1] may be required. Precurarization is not necessary in patients under 10 years of age because fasciculations are uncommon in this age group. Bradycardia is common in children unless atropine or glycopyrrolate is given.[27]

Nondepolarizing Drugs

Effects at the Neuromuscular Junction

Nondepolarizing neuromuscular blocking drugs bind to the postsynaptic receptor in a competitive fashion. An excess of ACh can tilt the balance in favor of neuromuscular transmission. To exert their effect, the nondepolarizing neuromuscular blocking drugs must bind to one of the alpha subunits of the receptor.[2] Blocking of the open channel is another possible mechanism of action, but current evidence suggests that its quantitative importance is small.[7] The concentrations of the drug are too low to produce important open channel blockade; and, more convincingly, an increase in ACh concentration, as occurs with the administration of anticholinesterase agents, should open more channels and offer the opportunity for more, not less, blockade.

As mentioned previously, the number of receptors that need to be bound to ACh to produce depolarization of the end-plate is only a small fraction of the total number of receptors. Thus, neuromuscular blockade in a given muscle is not apparent until a certain fixed proportion of receptors is occupied. Animal studies suggest that this fraction is approximately 75%.[8] However, not all end-plates within a muscle are similar. Some fail to transmit at 75% receptor occupancy, most require 80–90%, and the most resistant end-plates are blocked only when 92% receptor occupancy is reached.[8] Thus, partial neuromuscular blockade (>0% and <100%) occurs over a narrow range of receptor occupancy. Furthermore, it is not due to partial neurotransmission in all the end-plates, but to total blockade, which occurs only at some end-plates.

The *margin of safety* is reduced when high-frequency stimulation is used, because of a decrease in ACh release. Thus, fade following either train-of-four or tetanic stimulation will be detected at lower levels of receptor occupancy than depression of single twitch response. This critical receptor occupancy is greater for 100 Hz than for train-of-four stimulation and less for 30 Hz than for train-of-four stimulation.[37] However, although the principle of a decreased margin of safety for high-frequency stimulation should be retained, it is futile to attach too much importance to the actual receptor occupancy figures. The data are based on animal experiments, and the actual numbers vary with species and for different muscles within the same species.[9] Moreover, the correlation between certain clinical tests, such as hand grip and head lift, with receptor occupancy, is based more on conjecture than fact. It is possible to grade clinical tests in order of sensitivity and to assume that each test corresponds to a certain degree of receptor occupancy, but it is pointless to attach much importance to the figures.

Characteristics of Nondepolarizing Blockade

The fade observed in response to high-frequency stimulation is characteristic of nondepolarizing blockade. This fade can be observed if the stimulation rate exceeds 0.1–0.15 Hz. When EMG recordings are made in humans, fade reaches a maximum at 2 Hz and stays constant for frequencies up to 50 Hz.[10] With mechanical recordings, fusion of several individual responses occurs when the stimulation frequency exceeds the duration of the twitch. Thus, the initial peak is made up of the first few responses, the first being the strongest, and fade follows.

Tetanic stimulation is followed by post-tetanic facilitation, which is due to an increase in ACh release when the stimulation occurs soon after the tetanus. Thus, the response to nerve stimulation is increased. The intensity and duration of this effect depend on the frequency and duration of the tetanic stimulation. With a 50-Hz tetanus of 5 seconds' duration, post-tetanic facilitation lasts for less time than was previously thought, and twitch responses have been found to fall within 10% of their pretetanic values in less than 2 minutes, and in most cases in less than 1 minute (Fig. 19-7).[38]

Finally, nondepolarizing blockade can be antagonized with anticholinesterase agents such as edrophonium, neostigmine, or pyridostigmine. It is also antagonized by depolarizing agents such as succinylcholine, provided that the nondepolarizing blockade is intense and the succinylcholine dose is too small to produce a block of its own.

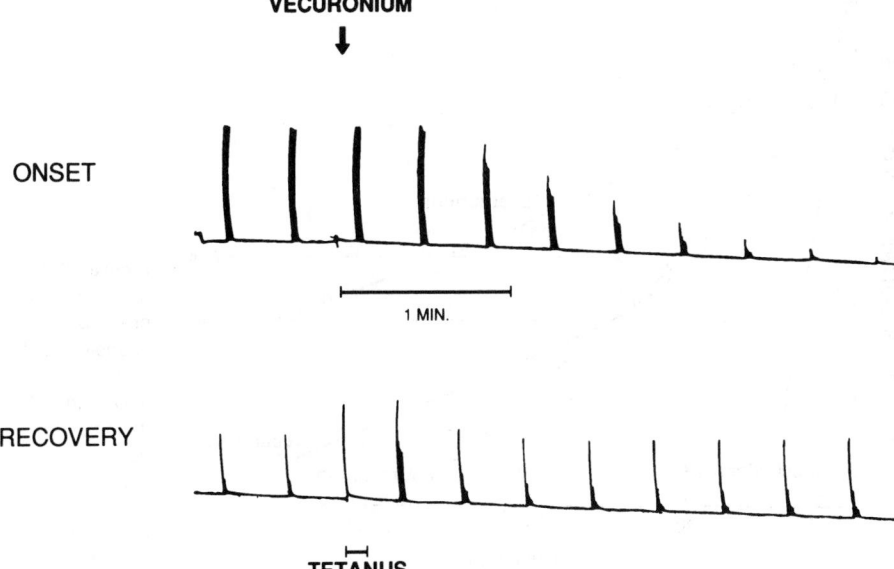

Figure 19-7. Characteristics of nondepolarizing blockade. Train-of-four responses are equal before the administration of vecuronium (*arrow*). For a given first twitch depression, fade is less during onset (*top*) than during recovery (*bottom*). Fade also occurs with a 5-second, 50-Hz tetanus (*bar*). Facilitation is apparent after the tetanus—*i.e.*, first twitch height and train-of-four ratio are increased, but only for the first two trains.

Pharmacokinetics

Plasma concentrations have been measured for all the nondepolarizing agents used clinically. The pharmacokinetic variables derived from these experiments depend on the dose given, the sampling schedule used, the accuracy of the assay, and the model chosen.[1] Thus, it is better to rely on the shape of the plasma concentration–time curve and relate duration of action to the concentration required for the desired effect, instead of basing decisions only on pharmacokinetic variables such as the elimination half-life.

With the exception of mivacurium, the pharmacokinetics of which are not well known as yet, all nondepolarizing drugs can be classified initially into three broad classes (Table 19-1):

1. long-acting drugs with long elimination half-lives (>1 hour) including *d*-tubocurarine, pancuronium, metocurine, gallamine, pipecuronium and doxacurium;
2. intermediate-acting drugs with intermediate elimination half-lives (atracurium); and
3. intermediate-acting drugs with long elimination half-lives. The drugs in this class, vecuronium and rocuronium (ORG 9426), depend on redistribution rather than elimination for termination of effect (Fig. 19-8).[39]

Nevertheless, pharmacokinetic analysis illustrates some of the common properties of these drugs. They all have a volume of distribution that is approximately equal to extracellular fluid volume (ECF) (0.2–0.4 l·kg^{-1}). In infants, in whom the ECF volume as a proportion of body weight is increased, the volume of distribution of *d*-tubocurarine parallels ECF volume quite closely.[40]

Onset and Duration of Action

Although the duration of action of nondepolarizing drugs is determined by the time required for plasma concentrations to decrease below a critical level, onset does not follow plasma concentrations. Whereas plasma concentrations reach a peak within 1–2 minutes after injection of the drug, the maximum blockade with most nondepolarizing agents is reached only after 5–7 minutes if subparalyzing doses are given. This discrepancy between concentration and block has been modeled mathematically by introducing the concept of a compartment, according to which the drug concentration is directly related to its effect. The access to this "effect compartment" is controlled by a rate constant (k_{eo}).[41,42] This rate constant corresponds to half-times of 5–10 minutes for most nondepolarizing drugs.[1]

The delay between peak plasma concentrations and blockade, represented by k_{eo}, is determined by all the factors that modify access of the drug to, and removal from, the neuromuscular junction. These factors include cardiac output, distance of the muscle from the heart, and muscle blood flow.[42] Thus, onset times are not the same in all muscles, because of different blood flows. If metabolism or redistribu-

TABLE 19-1. Typical Pharmacokinetic Data for Nondepolarizing Blockers in Adults, Except Where Stated

Drug	V_D (l·kg^{-1})	Cl (ml·kg^{-1}·min^{-1})	$T_{1/2\beta}$(min)
d-Tubocurarine			
Adults, 30–60 years	0.3–0.6	1–3	90–350
Elderly, 70–87 years	0.3	0.8	270
Neonates, <1 month	0.5	1.1	310
Infants, <1 year	0.5	1.0	305
Children, 1–4 years	0.3	1.5	170
Atracurium	0.2	5.5	20
Doxacurium	0.2	2.5	95
Gallamine	0.2	1.2	135
Metocurine	0.4	1.3	220
Mivacurium	NA	NA	NA
Pancuronium	0.3	1–2	100–130
Pipecuronium	0.3	2.4	140
Rocuronium	0.3	4.0	130
Vecuronium	0.4	4.5	110

V_D = volume of distribution, Cl = plasma clearance, $T_{1/2\beta}$ = elimination half-life.

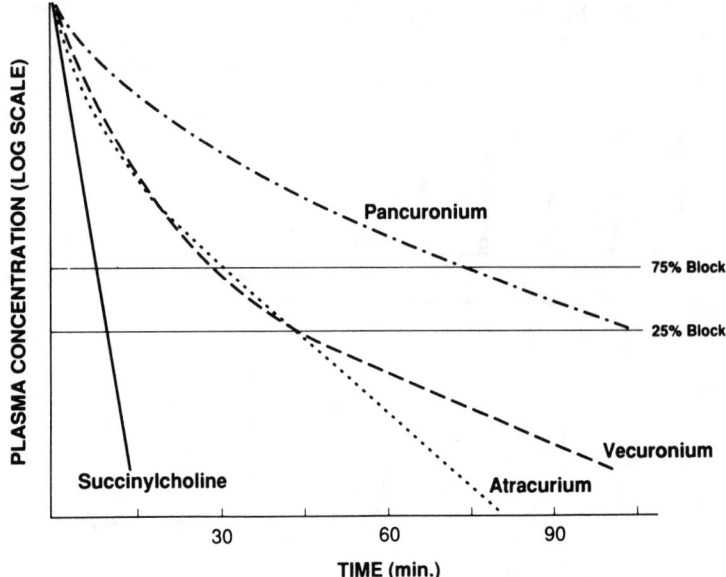

Figure 19-8. Plasma concentrations *vs.* time for four representative muscle relaxants. Concentrations are expressed as a function of each drug's concentration corresponding to 25% and 75% block. Succinylcholine is broken down very rapidly in the plasma; it is a short-acting drug. Pancuronium is a long-acting drug because of its long elimination time. Atracurium is an intermediate-duration drug and has an intermediate half-life. Vecuronium has an elimination half-life comparable with that of pancuronium. However, redistribution of the drug is very important and the duration of action is comparable with that of atracurium.

tion is very rapid the onset time is accelerated. This probably plays a role only for succinylcholine and mivacurium. Finally, there is growing evidence that potent drugs have a slower onset of action than less potent agents (Fig. 19-9).[43,44] This is because spare receptors must be occupied before blockade can be observed, and this requirement is independent of the potency of the drug. Thus, blockade of these spare receptors will occur faster, and onset will be more rapid, if more drug molecules are available—i.e., if potency is low.[42]

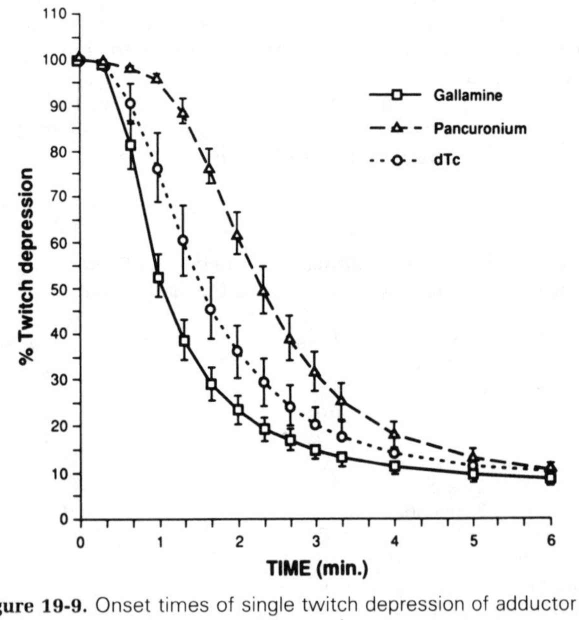

Time to maximal blockade is independent of dose if less than 100% block is attained. For most drugs, this value is 5–7 minutes.[42] For doxacurium, the most potent drug tested in humans, 10–15 minutes are required.[45] Once 100% block has been achieved, the time to disappearance of the twitch decreases with increasing dose. Onset and recovery times for nondepolarizing relaxants are shown in Table 19-2.

Individual Nondepolarizing Relaxants

Since 1942 nearly 50 nondepolarizing relaxants have been introduced into clinical anesthesia. This section discusses only those drugs currently available in North America and Europe. The first relaxant to undergo clinical investigation was Intocostrin,[1] the purified and standardized product of curare obtained from the plant *Chondodendrum tomentosum.* The pharmacologic action of *d*-tubocurarine is discussed first as the prototypical muscle relaxant.

***d*-Tubocurarine.** *d*-Tubocurarine is a monoquaternary ammonium compound. However, at body pH, the second nitrogen atom becomes protonated so that it possesses two positively charged centers (Fig. 19-10). The molecule undergoes minimal metabolism, so that 24 hours after its administra-

Figure 19-9. Onset times of single twitch depression of adductor pollicis after pancuronium (0.07 mg·kg⁻¹), *d*-tubocurarine (0.45 mg·kg⁻¹), and gallamine (2.4 mg·kg⁻¹). Although the maximum effect was identical in all three groups, the onset of blockade was fastest after gallamine. The mean time to 50% depression was 141 seconds for pancuronium, 99 seconds for *d*-tubocurarine, and 66 seconds for gallamine. (Reproduced with permission from Kopman AF: Pancuronium, gallamine, and *d*-tubocurarine compared: Is speed of onset inversely related to drug potency? Anesthesiology 70:915, 1989.)

TABLE 19-2. Typical Neuromuscular Activity of Nondepolarizing Blocking Drugs: Dose (ED₉₅), Onset to Maximum Effect, 25–75% Recovery Index (RI), and Time to 90% T1 recovery (T₉₀) After an ED₉₅ Dose in Adults

	ED$_{95}$ (mg·kg⁻¹)	Onset (min)	RI (min)	T$_{90}$ (min)
d-Tubocurarine	0.51	6	25–35	70–90
Atracurium	0.2	5–6	10–15	30
Doxacurium	0.025	10–14	NA	80–100
Gallamine	2.5	4–5	25–40	70–80
Metocurine	0.28	5	30–40	80–90
Mivacurium	0.08	3–6	6–8	25
Pancuronium	0.07	5–7	25	60
Pipecuronium	0.05–0.06	5–6	30–40	80–90
Rocuronium	0.3	3–4	10–15	30
Vecuronium	0.05	5–6	10–15	30

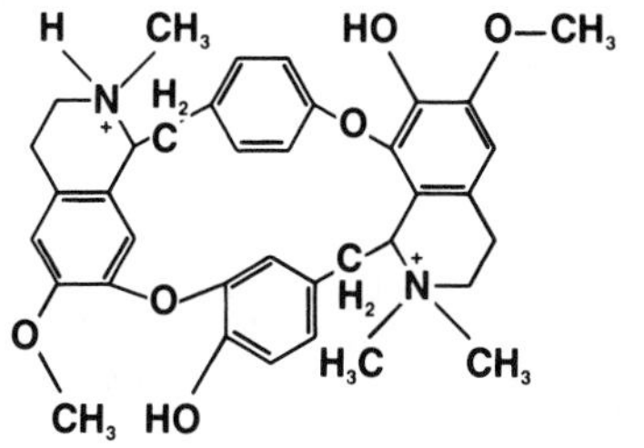

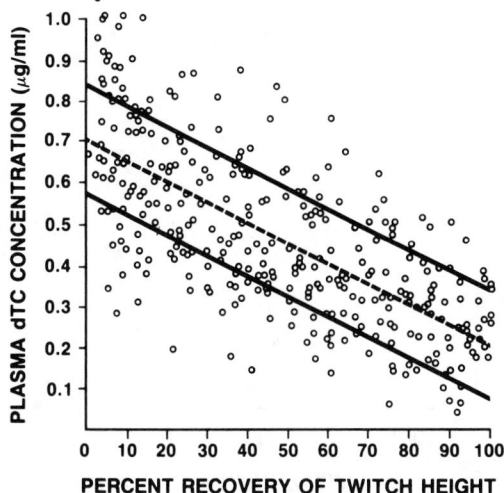

Figure 19-10. Structure of *d*-tubocurarine.

tion about 10% of the compound is found in the urine and 45% in the bile. It is 30–50% protein bound, but altered plasma protein does not appear to modify the pharmacokinetic or pharmacodynamic behavior.[46]

The development of a sensitive radioimmunoassay allowed the relationship between plasma concentration of *d*-tubocurarine and recovery from neuromuscular block to be demonstrated (Fig. 19-11).[47] As for most nondepolarizing relaxants, excretion is impaired in renal failure, with an increase in $T_{1/2\beta}$.[48]

Cardiovascular Effects. Hypotension frequently accompanies the administration of *d*-tubocurarine. In cats, autonomic ganglionic blockade occurs at similar doses as those that produce neuromuscular blockade.[49] In addition, *d*-tubocurarine causes vagal and sympathetic blockade, although clinically, bradycardia is more common than tachycardia.

In humans, *d*-tubocurarine causes dose-related histamine release,[50] and skin flushing is observed frequently. The hypotension can be reduced by pretreatment with the antihistamine promethazine or by administering *d*-tubocurarine slowly over 3 minutes. Thus, in humans, histamine release is probably more important than ganglionic blockade in the production of hypotension. Alternatively, a bolus injection of *d*-tubocurarine may induce the release of prostacyclin, which acts via H_1 receptors to produce hypotension.[51]

Age. The potency of *d*-tubocurarine on a mg·kg^{-1} basis is similar at all ages. However, the increased sensitivity of the neuromuscular junction in infants is concealed by the increased volume of distribution (see Table 19-1).[40,52] The onset of action is more rapid in the young as a result of a more rapid circulation time. However, the decreased glomerular filtration rate (GFR) in the very young and the very old results in an increase in $T_{1/2\beta}$ and prolonged duration of action.[53]

Burns. Patients with massive burns demonstrate resistance to *d*-tubocurarine and other nondepolarizing drugs that is dependent on the size of the burn and the time since injury.[54] The pharmacokinetic behavior of atracurium is unaltered in burn patients. Resistance is associated with higher concentrations of the free drug to produce a given degree of twitch suppression compared with nonthermally injured patients.[55] In contrast to denervation injury and an associated increase in extrajunctional cholinergic receptors that respond to ACh, the resistance to effects of nondepolarizing neuromuscular blocking drugs in patients with thermal injury is not associated with an increase in density of these receptors.[56] Thus, an altered affinity of the cholinergic receptors for ACh or nondepolarizing neuromuscular blocking drugs may be the basis for thermal injury–induced resistance to these drugs.

Clinical Use. The slow onset and long duration of action of *d*-tubocurarine have restricted its use, in doses of 15–30 mg·70 kg^{-1}, to the maintenance of relaxation during surgery. However, the dose-related cardiovascular effects were a stimulus for the production of alternative agents. Initially, this led to the introduction of pancuronium, which replaced the hypotension of *d*-tubocurarine with hypertension and tachycardia. More recently, drugs of intermediate duration—atracurium and vecuronium—have almost eliminated the use of *d*-tubocurarine because they have minimal cardiovascular activity. Some clinicians continue to use small doses of *d*-tubocurarine (3 mg·70 kg^{-1}) before succinylcholine ("precurarization") to reduce the incidence of fasciculations and muscle pains.

Atracurium. Atracurium is a bisquaternary ammonium benzylisoquinoline compound (Fig. 19-12) that was developed in an attempt to produce a short-acting muscle relaxant that would be independent of the liver and the kidney for termination of its action.[57] In humans, atracurium is metabolized both by the Hofmann reaction (nonenzymatic degradation at body temperature and pH) and by ester hydrolysis to several compounds (see Fig. 19-12). It has been estimated that two thirds of atracurium is degraded by ester hydrolysis and one third by Hofmann reaction.[58]

The metabolites of atracurium may be toxic. The quaternary monoacrylate, quaternary alcohol, and monoquaternary analogues produce neuromuscular blockade in high doses. Also, the quaternary monoacrylate, laudanosine, the quaternary alcohol, metholaudanosine, and the monoquaternary analogue decrease blood pressure, but at concentrations higher than those used in clinical practice.[59]

Laudanosine has been suspected of causing cerebral excitation. It has been shown to increase the MAC of halothane in rabbits.[60] At doses of 2–8 mg·kg^{-1} it produced wakening from halothane anesthesia, and at doses of 14–22 mg·kg^{-1} seizure activity was observed in dogs.[61] However, such doses are not used in humans. The clinical effects of laudanosine have been sought extensively but unsuccessfully.

PERCENT RECOVERY OF TWITCH HEIGHT

Figure 19-11. Relationship between twitch height and plasma *d*-tubocurarine concentration. (Reproduced with permission from Matteo RS, Spector S, Horowitz PE: Relation of serum *d*-tubocurarine concentration to neuromuscular blockade. Anesthesiology 41:441, 1974.)

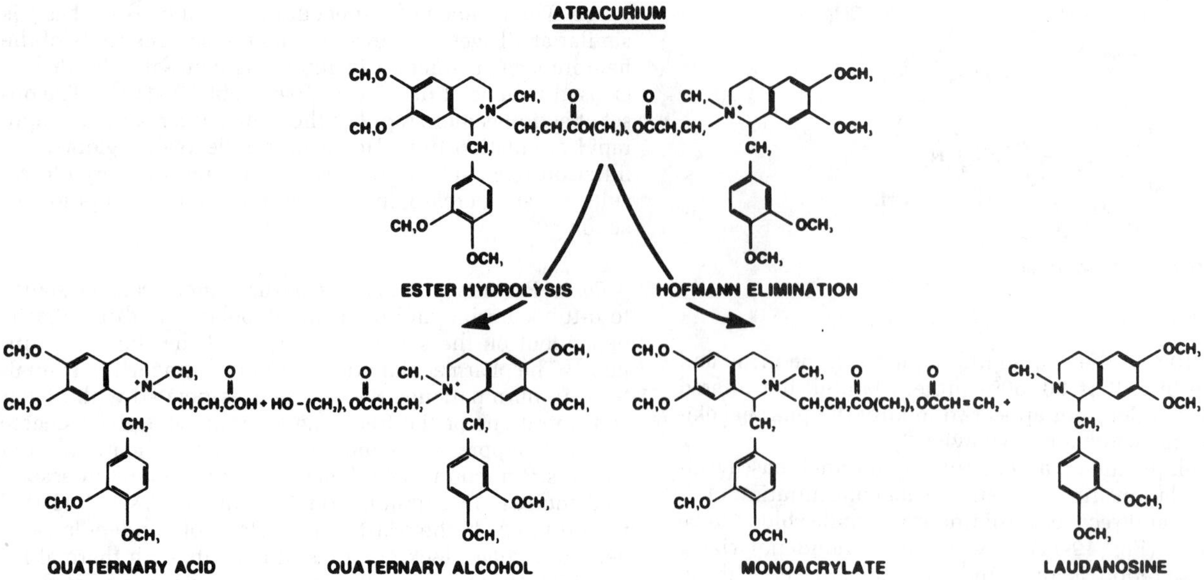

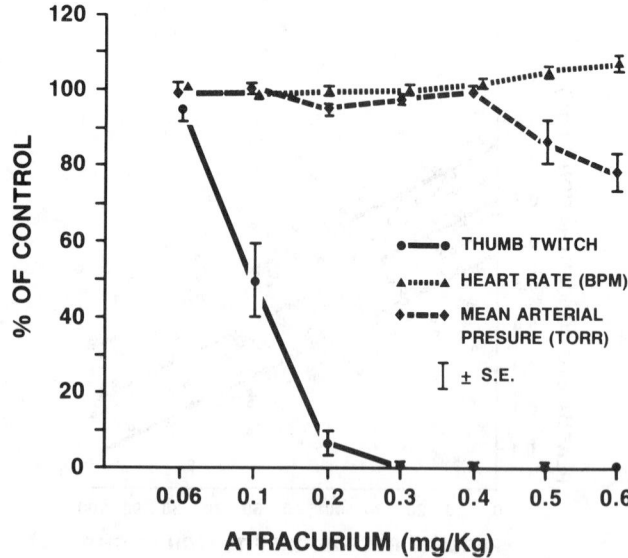

Figure 19-12. Structure of atracurium and its major metabolites.

There is also interest in the potential toxic effects of the highly reactive acrylates.[62]

Pharmacokinetics. The plasma concentration of atracurium decreases rapidly following iv administration (see Fig. 19-8). The conventional pharmacokinetic model that is used for other nondepolarizing relaxants may not be suitable for atracurium because it undergoes nonenzymatic degradation in the tissues as well as in plasma.

The onset of action of equipotent doses is similar for atracurium, pancuronium, d-tubocurarine, and vecuronium.[63] It is slower than succinylcholine but can be reduced if the dose is increased.[64] However, such acceleration is limited by hypotension and histamine release after large doses. The duration of action is also dose related. The time to 90% recovery of T1 after 0.4 mg·kg^{-1} is approximately 30 minutes, and this is prolonged by about 10% during halothane anesthesia.[64] The 25–75% recovery rate is rapid, on the order of 10–15 minutes (see Table 19-2).

Cardiovascular Effects. Atracurium is associated with few cardiovascular effects unless large doses (>2 × ED$_{95}$) are administered. The most common cardiovascular abnormality following smaller doses is the bradycardia that is most likely due to concomitant administration of opioids[65] or to vagal traction. Hypotension and tachycardia may accompany doses exceeding 0.4 mg·kg^{-1} (Fig. 19-13); these effects occur as a result of dose-related histamine release.[66] Similar changes occur after the use of d-tubocurarine or metocurine but at much lower doses (Table 19-3). The most obvious clinical manifestation of histamine release is skin flushing, but this is seldom associated with hypotension or bronchospasm. These responses can be avoided by slow injection over 1–3 minutes or by pretreatment with H$_1$ and H$_2$ receptor blockers.[67,68] Anaphylactoid reactions to atracurium have been described, but no more frequently than after other neuromuscular blocking drugs.[69]

Age. The potency of atracurium is similar in adults and children. When atracurium is given by infusion to the elderly, the reduction in dose requirement and the slower recovery time observed with vecuronium are not seen,[70]

presumably reflecting the organ independence of atracurium's elimination.

Clinical Uses. The short duration of action, rapid recovery, and absence of significant cardiovascular and cumulative drug effects have encouraged the use of atracurium as a continuous infusion (10 µg·kg^{-1}·min^{-1}) or as intermittent injections in several situations, including ambulatory surgery, cardiopulmonary bypass surgery, pheochromocytoma resection, and renal and hepatic disease. Large doses (0.5–0.6 mg·kg^{-1}) must be given if atracurium is used to produce rapid paralysis to facilitate tracheal intubation,[71] when conditions will also be influenced by the depth of anesthesia, airway reactivity, and the strength of the patient.

Figure 19-13. Neuromuscular, heart rate, and blood pressure responses to atracurium at various doses. (Reproduced with permission from Savarese JJ, Basta SJ, Ali HH *et al*: Neuromuscular and cardiovascular effects of BW 33A (atracurium) in patients under halothane anesthesia. Anesthesiology 57:A262, 1982.)

TABLE 19-3. Doses of Drugs Associated with Cardiovascular Changes

Drug	Dose (mg·kg^{-1})	Equivalent ED$_{95}$	Percentage of Control		
			BP	HR	Histamine
d-Tubocurarine	0.5	1	78	116	410
Metocurine	0.5	2	79	119	212
Atracurium	0.6	3	80	108	192

BP = blood pressure, HR = heart rate.
Adapted with permission from Basta SJ, Savarese JJ, Ali HH et al: Histamine releasing potencies of atracurium, dimethyl tubocurarine, and tubocurarine. Br J Anaesth 55:105S, 1983.

Doxacurium. Doxacurium is a long-acting nondepolarizing bisquaternary ammonium compound that is devoid of histamine-releasing or cardiovascular side-effects (Fig. 19-14). The pharmacokinetic behavior of doxacurium resembles that of pancuronium with respect to $T_{1/2\beta}$ and dependence on renal clearance for elimination from the circulation (see Table 19-1).[45,72,73] Doxacurium is also a weak substrate for plasma cholinesterase. The ED$_{95}$ for doxacurium is 30–40 µg·kg^{-1} (see Table 19-2).[74] Volatile anesthetics decrease doxacurium dose requirements by 20–40% compared with doses needed during N$_2$O-fentanyl anesthesia.[75] Although the place of doxacurium has yet to be clearly defined, it may be most useful in patients with ischemic heart disease who are undergoing prolonged anesthesia or long-term mechanical ventilation of the lungs. The slow onset time and prolonged duration of action make doxacurium inappropriate for facilitating tracheal intubation or for providing skeletal muscle relaxation during brief surgical procedures.

Gallamine. Gallamine was the first widely used synthetic neuromuscular blocking drug (Fig. 19-15) but has now been largely discarded as a result of the associated tachycardia. It is not metabolized but is excreted unchanged only *via* the kidney. Clearance is reduced by 80% in renal failure, and the $T_{1/2\beta}$ is prolonged fivefold.[76]

Cardiovascular Effects. In humans, gallamine is associated with a dose-dependent tachycardia and with increases in cardiac output and systemic vascular resistance. The vagal blocking action occurs predominantly at the postganglionic nerve terminal,[77] which is supplemented by some sympathetic nervous system stimulation.[78]

Clinical Use. Because of the associated tachycardia, gallamine is seldom used. When it was used to maintain relaxation it was usually given in doses of 1–2 mg·kg^{-1} following recovery from succinylcholine. It retains some popularity as a precurarizing agent in small doses, 10–20 mg, before succinylcholine administration.

Metocurine. Metocurine, produced by methylation of two hydroxy groups of d-tubocurarine (Fig. 19-16), is twice as potent as the parent compound and produces less histamine release. Like d-tubocurarine, it undergoes minimal metabolism. Within 48 hours of administration approximately half appears in the urine and another 2% appears in the bile.[79] Because metocurine is more dependent on renal function for excretion than is d-tubocurarine, clearance is disturbed to a greater degree in renal failure and in the elderly.

Cardiovascular Effects. In animals the separation between autonomic and neuromuscular effects of metocurine is greater than for d-tubocurarine,[49] and metocurine causes less histamine release than d-tubocurarine.[80] Consequently, changes in blood pressure and heart rate are not seen until doses greater than the ED$_{95}$ are administered.

Burns. Patients with burn injuries are resistant to all nondepolarizing relaxants, and the resistance to metocurine may be extensive. For example, an 8-year-old boy with a 35% surface burn required 12 times the normal dose of metocurine and 8 times the plasma concentration during the acute phase of the burn to produce complete neuromuscular blockade.[81]

Clinical Use. Because of its lack of cardiovascular effects, metocurine enjoyed a brief period of popularity before the introduction of atracurium and vecuronium. The combination of metocurine and pancuronium augmented neuromuscular block with opposing cardiovascular effects and was recommended for use in patients with severe cardiovascular disease.[82]

Mivacurium. Mivacurium is a short-acting nondepolarizing neuromuscular blocking drug that is hydrolyzed by plasma cholinesterase (Fig. 19-17).[83] The ED$_{95}$ of mivacurium is 0.08 mg·kg^{-1}; the time to onset of action is 3.3 minutes, and spontaneous recovery to 95% twitch height occurs in about 25 minutes (see Table 19-2). At 2 × ED$_{95}$ the onset time is 2.5 minutes and recovery to 95% twitch height occurs in about 31 minutes. The recovery time after discontinuing an infusion of mivacurium is about half that for atracurium or vecuronium infusions and is similar to that for succinylcholine.[84,85] The effect of anticholinester-

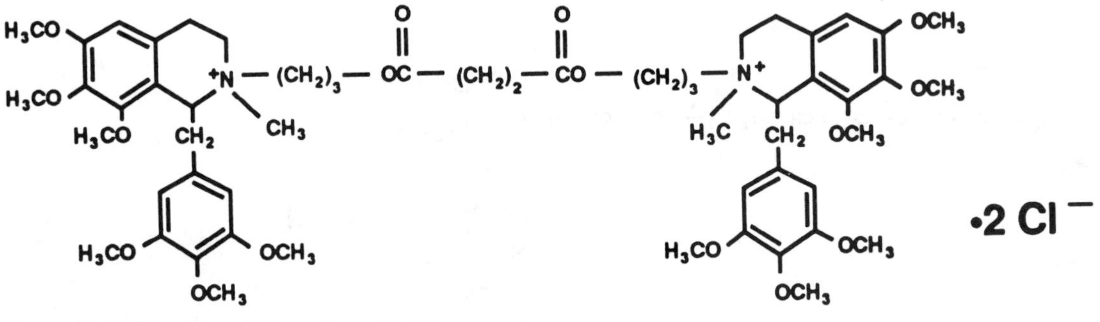

Figure 19-14. Structure of doxacurium chloride.

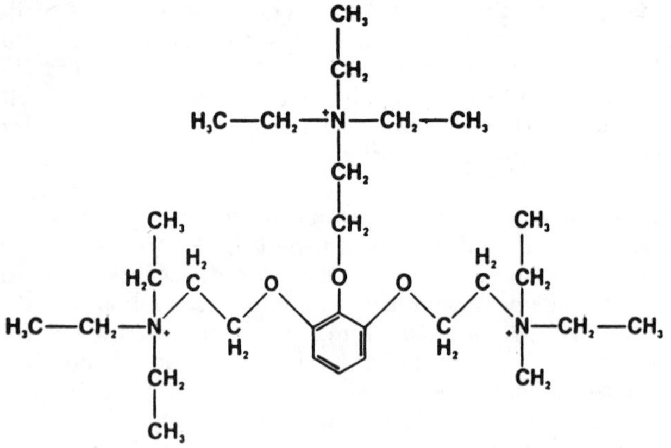

Figure 19-15. Structure of gallamine.

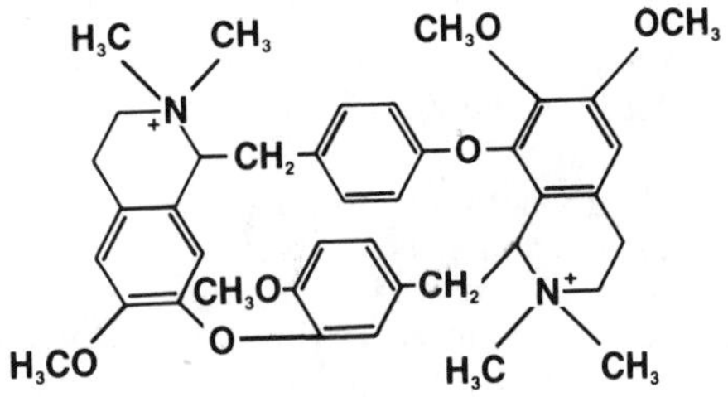

Figure 19-16. Structure of metocurine.

Pancuronium. Pancuronium (Fig. 19-18) is a long-acting, synthetic, nondepolarizing neuromuscular blocking drug developed from a series of bis-quaternary aminosteroid compounds.[87] The two quaternary groups were attached to a rigid steroid structure to maintain a constant interonium distance. Pancuronium is metabolized to a 3-OH compound that has one-half the neuromuscular blocking activity of the parent compound. Although values for protein binding varying from 20% and 87% have been described for pancuronium, the extent of binding does not appear to be important for its clinical activity. Clearance is decreased in renal and hepatic failure, demonstrating that excretion is dependent on both organs. The onset of action is more rapid in infants and children than in adults, and recovery is slower in the elderly.

Cardiovascular Effects. Pancuronium is associated with increases in heart rate, blood pressure and cardiac output, particularly after large doses (2 × ED_{95}). The cause is uncertain but includes a vagolytic effect at the postganglionic nerve terminal, a sympathomimetic effect as a result of blocking of muscarinic receptors that normally exert some braking on ganglionic transmission, and an increase in catecholamine release.[2] Pancuronium does not release histamine.

Clinical Use. The slow onset of action of pancuronium limits its usefulness in facilitating tracheal intubation. Administration in divided doses (priming principle) produces a small but measurable acceleration,[88] but the intermediate-acting compounds are more suitable when succinylcholine is contraindicated prior to tracheal intubation. In patients with myocardial ischemia, tachycardia should be avoided. Because these patients are often anesthetized with high doses of opioids, the use of pancuronium to provide muscle relaxation may offer some advantage over the use of cardiovascularly neutral relaxants.

Pipecuronium. Pipecuronium (Fig. 19-19) is a long-acting aminosteroid nondepolarizing neuromuscular blocking drug that is devoid of histamine-releasing or cardiovascular side-effects. It resembles pancuronium with respect to its potency, $T_{1/2\beta}$, and dependence on renal clearance for elimination from the circulation (see Table 19-1).[89-92] The ED_{95} is 50–60 $\mu g \cdot kg^{-1}$ iv, with 2 × ED_{95} producing adequate conditions for intubation of the trachea in about 3 minutes and a clinical duration of action of 80–120 minutes (see Table 19-2). Although the place of pipecuronium has yet to be clearly defined, it may be most useful in patients with ischemic heart disease who are undergoing prolonged anesthesia or long-term mechanical ventilation of the lungs. The slow onset time and the prolonged duration of action make pipecuronium of limited usefulness for facilitating tracheal

ase drugs is additive to the rapid rate of spontaneous recovery from mivacurium-induced neuromuscular blockade. Therefore, mivacurium is more rapidly reversed than are the longer acting nondepolarizing neuromuscular blocking drugs.

The cardiovascular response to mivacurium is minimal at doses up to 2 × ED_{95}, whereas administration of 3 × ED_{95} over 10–15 seconds evokes sufficient histamine release to lower mean arterial pressure transiently by about 15%.[83,86] Therefore, the cardiovascular effects of mivacurium are similar to those of atracurium.

Clinical Use. Although the place of mivacurium in clinical practice has not been clearly established, the rapid recovery makes it a useful drug for administration by continuous infusion. In some situations reversal may not be necessary and if this is shown to be safe, it will be a considerable benefit in outpatient anesthesia, where the administration of neostigmine or edrophonium may be accompanied by nausea and vomiting.

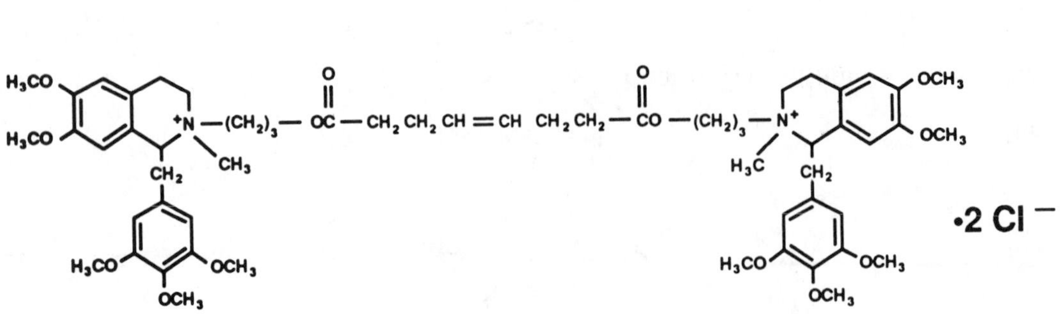

Figure 19-17. Structure of mivacurium chloride.

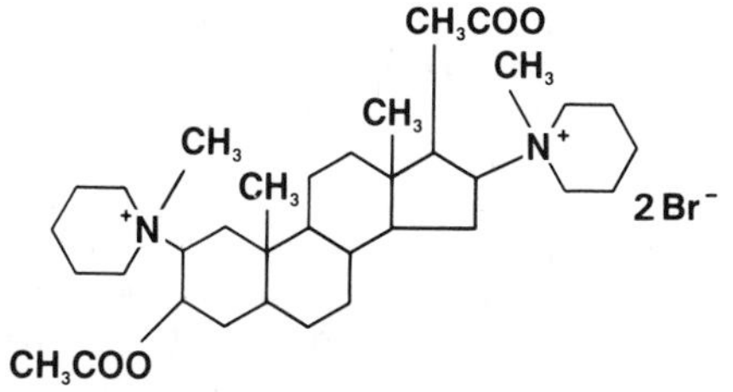

Figure 19-18. Structure of pancuronium.

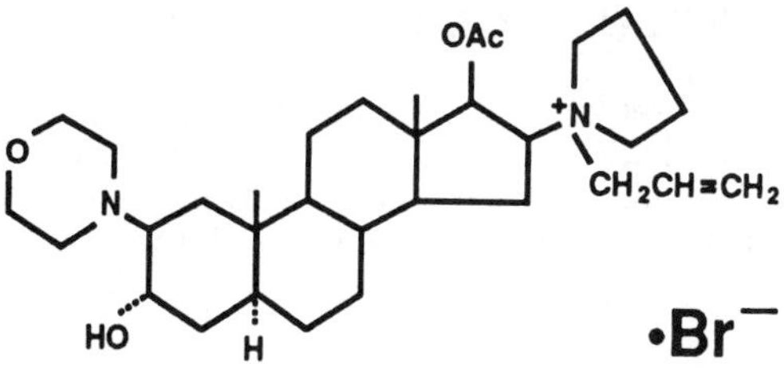

Figure 19-20. Structure of rocuronium (ORG 9426).

intubation or for providing skeletal muscle relaxation during brief surgical procedures.

Rocuronium. Rocuronium (Fig. 19-20) is a new aminosteroid neuromuscular relaxant currently undergoing clinical trials. Rocuronium has approximately one-seventh the potency of vecuronium. It has a more rapid onset but a similar duration of action[93] and similar pharmacokinetic behavior[94] as vecuronium. In animals it is devoid of cardiovascular effects.[95]

Cardiovascular Effects. In clinical doses no changes in heart rate or blood pressure have been observed. Rocuronium does not release histamine.

Clinical Use. The rapid onset and intermediate duration of action make rocuronium a potential replacement for succinylcholine in conditions in which rapid tracheal intubation is indicated. However, no studies have compared rocuronium with equipotent doses of succinylcholine.

Vecuronium. Vecuronium (Fig. 19-21) is an intermediate-acting aminosteroid neuromuscular relaxant without cardiovascular effects. It is a monoquaternary ammonium compound produced by demethylation of the pancuronium molecule at the 2-piperidino position.[96] The demethylation reduces the ACh-like characteristics of the molecule and increases its lipophilicity, which encourages hepatic uptake. Vecuronium undergoes spontaneous deacetylation to produce 3-OH, 17-OH, and 3,17-(OH)$_2$ metabolites. The most potent, 3-OH vecuronium, has about 60% of the activity of vecuronium, is excreted by the kidney, and has been found to be responsible for prolonged paralysis in intensive care patients.[97]

The pharmacokinetic variables of vecuronium are very similar to those of pancuronium, and the reason for vecuronium's shorter duration of action is that the plasma concentration decreases through the effective range far more rapidly, so that duration and recovery depend more on distribution than on elimination (see Fig. 19-8).[98] Recovery after long infusions of vecuronium (in excess of 6 hours) is slower than after a bolus dose[99] because the peripheral storage sites have become saturated, and a decrease in plasma concentration is then dependent on metabolism and excretion and not on redistribution.

Attempts have been made to reduce the time to onset of action of vecuronium and other nondepolarizing neuromuscular blocking drugs by using the priming principle.[100] This refers to the administration of a small, subparalyzing dose several minutes before the principal dose is given. For vecuronium, the best results have been obtained with a priming dose of 0.01 mg·kg^{-1}, followed 3–4 minutes later by 0.1 mg·kg^{-1}. The time to onset of maximal blockade is reduced by about 25%, but intubating conditions 2 minutes later are not as good as after succinylcholine.[101]

Cardiovascular Effects. Vecuronium usually produces no cardiovascular effects with clinical doses. It does not induce histamine release, although it may interfere with histamine metabolism.[102] Allergic reactions have been described, but no more frequently than after the use of other neuromuscular blocking drugs.

Clinical Use. The cardiovascular neutrality and intermediate duration of action make vecuronium a suitable agent for use in patients with ischemic heart disease or those undergoing short ambulatory surgery.

Large doses, with or without the priming principle, may be used to facilitate tracheal intubation when succinylcholine is contraindicated. For maintenance of relaxation, vecuronium may be given in intermittent boluses, 0.01–0.02 mg·kg^{-1}, or by continuous infusion. Infusion rates to maintain constant neuromuscular block vary considerably, and doses of 1–2 μg·kg·min^{-1} have been necessary to maintain 90% blockade. The wide individual variation suggests that dosing should be titrated with the help of neuromuscular monitoring. The likelihood of a lower incidence of residual skeletal muscle weakness postoperatively is an advantage of the use of intermediate-acting neuromuscular blocking drugs.

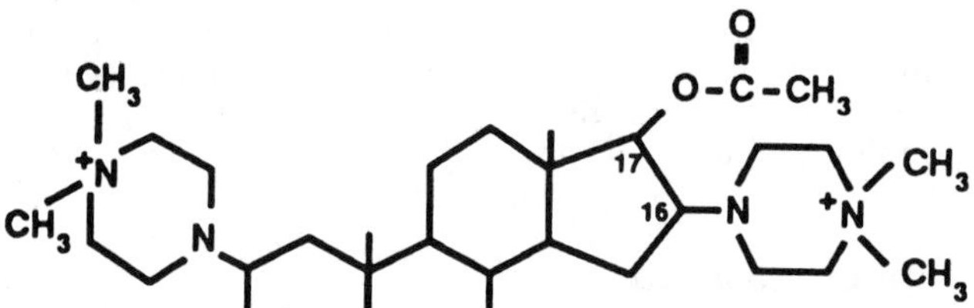

Figure 19-19. Structure of pipecuronium bromide.

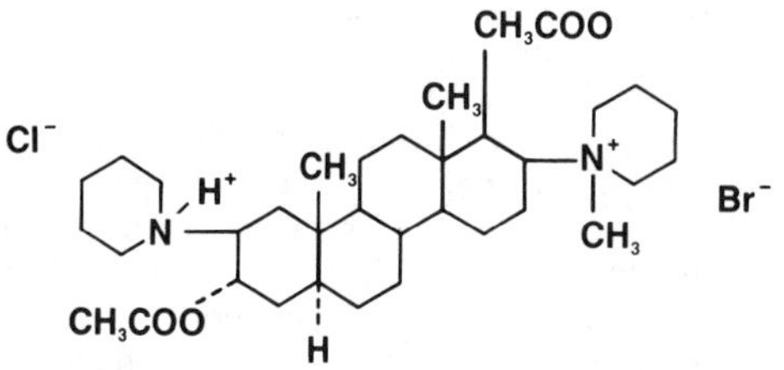

Figure 19-21. Structure of vecuronium.

DRUG INTERACTIONS

Interactions between neuromuscular blocking drugs and several anesthetic and nonanesthetic drugs have been suggested. Although some interactions have been confirmed, many remain as isolated case reports or theoretical possibilities.

Interactions with Anesthetic Agents

Inhalational Agents

The anesthetic vapors potentiate neuromuscular blockade when administered in high concentration. At clinical doses, shifts in the dose-response curves of d-tubocurarine, gallamine, pancuronium, metocurine-pancuronium combinations, atracurium, and vecuronium have been demonstrated.[103-108] Enflurane and isoflurane are more potent than halothane in potentiating the effect of d-tubocurarine and pancuronium, but enflurane produces greater potentiation of vecuronium than of halothane or isoflurane.[107] When atracurium was given by continuous infusion to children, the dose required to maintain constant blockade was reduced by about 30% during halothane (0.8%) or isoflurane (1.0%) administration.[109] Also, isoflurane[103] and nitrous oxide[110] have been shown to potentiate the effect of succinylcholine.

The cause of the potentiation is unknown, but the greater effect on tetanic and train-of-four responses than on single twitch responses suggests that prejunctional mechanisms are involved.[111] Also, the increased muscle blood flow caused by isoflurane may augment blockade by increasing the delivery of relaxant.

Intravenous Anesthetics

Potentiation of the action of nondepolarizing neuromuscular blocking drugs has been demonstrated with most iv induction agents in animals,[112] but this is of limited clinical importance.

Local Anesthetics

Lidocaine, procaine, and other local anesthetic agents produce neuromuscular blockade in their own right as well as by potentiating the effects of the depolarizing and nondepolarizing neuromuscular blocking drugs.[113] Gentamicin and lidocaine have additive effects, and profound neuromuscular blockade has been observed after their combined use in a patient given d-tubocurarine.[114]

Neuromuscular Blocking Drugs

Nondepolarizing-Nondepolarizing Interactions

Combinations of similar drugs, such as pancuronium-vecuronium and d-tubocurarine–metocurine, have additive effects. Other combinations tend to show potentiation. The first such synergism was demonstrated for pancuronium-metocurine combinations, and it was suggested that the combination may be used to reduce unwanted hemodynamic effects without prejudicing neuromuscular blockade.[82] Other combinations have also been shown to be synergistic (atracurium with d-tubocurarine, metocurine, or

pancuronium; vecuronium with atracurium or d-tubocurarine; d-tubocurarine with gallamine, alcuronium, or vecuronium). However, the synergism of these combinations is of little clinical importance.

Administration of a combination of relaxants does not affect the degree of protein binding of either drug, so the potentiation is not the result of an increase in unbound drug. An alternative is that one drug of the pair has predominantly presynaptic activity and the other acts postsynaptically.[115] Finally, the potentiation may be entirely of postsynaptic origin as a result of asymmetric binding of different relaxants to the alpha subunits of the ACh receptor.[116]

Nondepolarizing-Depolarizing Interactions

Depolarizing and nondepolarizing drugs are mutually antagonistic. When d-tubocurarine or other nondepolarizing agents are given before succinylcholine to prevent fasciculations and skeletal muscle pain, the succinylcholine is less potent and has a shorter duration of action[117] except after pancuronium administration, when the duration of action is prolonged because pancuronium inhibits plasma cholinesterase.[118] Conversely, the potency of the nondepolarizing drugs is enhanced when they are administered after succinylcholine.[119] Finally, the response to a small dose of succinylcholine at the end of an anesthetic in which a nondepolarizing drug has been used is difficult to predict. It may either antagonize or potentiate the blockade, depending on the degree of the nondepolarizing blockade.[120] If anticholinesterase has been given the effect of the succinylcholine is potentiated because of inhibition of succinylcholine antagonism.

Antibiotics

Neomycin and streptomycin are the most potent of the aminoglycosides in depressing neuromuscular function.[121] They augment both depolarizing and nondepolarizing block and their effects are potentiated by magnesium and antagonized by calcium but only partly by anticholinesterases.

The polymixins are the most potent of all antibiotics in their action at the neuromuscular junction. Their effect appears to be predominantly postjunctional. Reversal of the blockade is difficult: calcium and anticholinesterases are both inconsistent.

The lincosamines, clindamycin and lincomycin, have pre- and postjunctional effects and the blockade cannot be reversed with calcium or anticholinesterases.

Management of a prolonged blockade that is suspected to have arisen from a combination of antibiotics and neuromuscular blocking drugs is difficult. Only that portion of the blockade due to the neuromuscular blocking drug can be reversed with anticholinesterases. Management includes mechanical support of ventilation until spontaneous breathing resumes. It is better to avoid the syndrome by administering small doses of the most potent antibiotics, particularly when they are given by the iv, intraperitoneal, or intrapleural routes.

Anticonvulsants

Resistance to pancuronium, metocurine, and vecuronium but not to atracurium has been demonstrated in patients receiving the anticonvulsant phenytoin.[122,123]

Miscellaneous

Altered reactions to several other agents have been described.[1] These include potentiation of depolarizing and nondepolarizing blockade with beta-agonist and calcium channel blockers, and abnormal reactions in the presence of diuretics, corticosteroids, immunosuppressants, hypotensive agents, and several psychotropic drugs. Management of neuromuscular blockade in patients receiving other drugs is by titration of the dose with the help of a nerve stimulator.

DISEASES THAT ALTER THE RESPONSE TO MUSCLE RELAXANTS

Myasthenia Gravis

Myasthenia gravis is an autoimmune disease in which circulating antibodies produce a functional reduction in the number of ACh receptors.[124,125] The lesion is postsynaptic; the number of ACh quanta is normal and their content is either normal or increased.[126]

Diagnosis

The characteristic EMG finding in myasthenia gravis is a voltage decrement in response to repeated stimulation. Stimuli at 3 Hz show a fade in response to the second stimulus, and myasthenia gravis is diagnosed if the response to the fifth stimulus is reduced by more than 10%.[127] Latent myasthenia gravis may be revealed by testing after exercise. The diagnosis can be confirmed with the regional curare test.[128] A forearm tourniquet is applied, 0.5 mg d-tubocurarine is given iv, and the tourniquet is released after 4–5 minutes. Myasthenia is characterized by a pronounced fade in response to train-of-nine stimulation.

Edrophonium, 2–8 mg, produces brief recovery from myasthenia gravis. Finally, the diagnosis can be made by recognizing circulating ACh antibody.[129]

Response to Muscle Relaxants

Patients with myasthenia gravis are usually slightly resistant to succinylcholine,[130] but during recovery, phase II block develops rapidly and recovery is slow.[131]

Sensitivity to nondepolarizing neuromuscular blocking drugs led to the avoidance of d-tubocurarine or pancuronium except for diagnosis. The dose required to produce neuromuscular blockade is reduced by about 75%. Dose-response curves for atracurium and vecuronium have characterized the response more clearly.[132,133]

Anesthesia in Myasthenia Gravis

Traditionally, neuromuscular blocking drugs have been avoided in the patient with myasthenia gravis by the use of inhalational vapors with or without local anesthesia. More recently, there have been several reports of the successful use of atracurium or vecuronium[134,135] when these drugs are administered under neuromuscular monitoring. The use of atracurium and the avoidance of anticholinesterases seem to be particularly appropriate.

Two problems remain after thymectomy: postoperative anticholinesterase therapy and predicting the need for mechanical support of ventilation. In most patients, the dose of anticholinesterases is reduced for 1–2 days after surgery. The need for mechanical ventilation of the lungs is more likely in patients with long-standing disease (in excess of 6 years) or respiratory disease, those who are taking high doses of pyridostigmine (>750 mg·day^{-1}), and those with a vital capacity of less than 2.9 l.[136]

Myotonia

Myotonia is characterized by an abnormal delay in muscle relaxation after contraction. It exists in three forms—myotonic dystrophy (dystrophia myotonica, myotonia atrophica, Steinert's disease), myotonia congenita (Thomsen's disease), and paramyotonia congenita.

Diagnosis

Repeated nerve stimulation leads to a gradual but persistent increase in muscle tension. The EMG is pathognomonic; myotonic afterdischarges are seen in peripheral muscle and consist of rapid bursts of potential produced by tapping the muscle or moving the needle. They produce typical "dive-bomber" sounds on the loudspeaker.

Response to Muscle Relaxants

The characteristic abnormality in myotonia is a sustained, dose-related contracture after succinylcholine administration that makes ventilation difficult for 2–5 minutes.[137] The response to nondepolarizing drugs is normal, although myotonic responses have been observed after reversal with neostigmine.[138]

Anesthesia

Succinylcholine should be avoided and respiratory depressants used with care. Atracurium, without reversal, is an appropriate choice for relaxation.

Muscular Dystrophy

An increased incidence of morbidity and mortality has been described after anesthesia in the patient with Duchenne-type muscular dystrophy. In particular, there are several reports of cardiac arrest after administration of succinylcholine.[139,140]

Response to Muscle Relaxants

The response to depolarizing and nondepolarizing relaxants seems to be normal, although the regional curare test demonstrates a normal blockade that lasts longer than normal.[141] Patients with the rare syndrome, ocular muscular dystrophy, exhibited extreme sensitivity to d-tubocurarine but showed little response to anticholinesterases.[142]

There is considerable controversy of whether patients with Duchenne's muscular dystrophy are susceptible to malignant hyperthermia.[143,144]

Anesthesia

Succinylcholine should be avoided in patients with Duchenne's muscular dystrophy.

Upper Motor Neuron Lesions

Response to Muscle Relaxants

Patients with hemiplegia or quadriplegia as a result of central nervous system lesions have an abnormal response to depolarizing and nondepolarizing relaxants. Hyperkalemia and cardiac arrest have been described after succinylcholine administration, probably as a result of extrajunctional receptor spread. Hyperkalemia is usually seen from 1 week to 6 months after the lesion, so that recommendations for the avoidance of succinylcholine[145] may not be indicated in the patient with chronic weakness.[146]

Hemiplegic patients are resistant to nondepolarizing neuromuscular blocking drugs. Monitoring of the affected side shows that the blockade is less intense and recovery time is more rapid than on the unaffected side. However, the apparently normal side also demonstrates some weakness.[147]

Miscellaneous

Denervated skeletal muscle releases potassium after succinylcholine administration and is resistant to nondepolarizing neuromuscular blocking drugs. Contractures in response to succinylcholine have also been observed in amyotrophic lateral sclerosis, myotonia, and multiple sclerosis.[131] Succinylcholine is usually avoided in several neurologic diseases, including Friedreich's ataxia, polyneuritis, and Parkinson's disease, because of isolated reports of hyperkalemia.

MONITORING NEUROMUSCULAR BLOCKADE

Why Monitor?

The potential toxicity of neuromuscular blocking drugs is high because they interfere with the adequacy of alveolar ventilation. Ventilatory depression is an important cause of anesthesia-related mortality and morbidity, and the presence of residual neuromuscular blockade in this setting is undoubtedly an important factor.[148,149] In addition, the margin of safety is narrow because blockade occurs over a narrow range of receptor occupancy.[8,37] Moreover, there is considerable interindividual variability in response to the same dose of neuromuscular blocking drug.[150] Thus, it is important for the clinician to assess the effect of neuromuscular blocking drugs without the confounding influence of volatile agents, iv anesthetics, and opioids. To test the function of the neuromuscular junction, a peripheral nerve is stimulated electrically, and the response of the muscle is assessed.

Stimulator Characteristics

The response of the nerve to electrical stimulation depends on three factors: the current applied, the duration of the current, and the position of the electrodes. Stimulators should be able to deliver a maximum current in the range of 60–80 mA.[3] If the stimulator used delivers a constant voltage, the current delivered will depend on the impedance of the electrodes and of the tissues in between. Thus, most stimulators available for clinical use are designed to provide constant current, irrespective of impedance changes due to drying of the electrode gel, cooling, decreased sweat gland function, and so forth. However, this constant current feature does not hold for high impedances (>5 kOhm). Thus, electrodes should be firmly applied to the skin. A current display monitor on the stimulator is an asset, because accidental disconnection can be easily identified by a current approaching 0 mA. The duration of the current pulse should be long enough for all axons in the nerve to depolarize but short enough to avoid the possibility of exceeding the refractory period of the nerve. In practice, pulse durations of 0.1–0.2 msec are acceptable. At least one electrode should be on the skin overlying the nerve to be stimulated. If the negative electrode is used for this purpose, the threshold to supramaximal stimulation is less than for the positive electrode.[151,152] However, the difference is not large in practice. The position of the other electrode is not critical but it should not be placed in the vicinity of other nerves. There is no need to use needle electrodes. Silver–silver chloride surface electrodes, used to monitor the electrocardiogram, are adequate for peripheral nerve stimulation, without the risk of bleeding and infection. In practice, applying these electrodes along the course of a nerve gives the best results.

Monitoring Modalities

The reason why different stimulation modalities were introduced into clinical practice is that nondepolarizing neuromuscular blockade has characteristic features. When high-frequency stimulation is used, fade and post-tetanic facilitation can be observed. Thus, the following discussion refers mostly to nondepolarizing blockade.

Single Twitch

The simplest way to stimulate a nerve is to apply a single stimulus at intervals greater than 10 seconds. The amplitude of response is compared with a control, prerelaxant twitch height. However, because a control is required, the clinical usefulness of this mode of stimulation is limited.

Tetanus

When stimulation is applied at a frequency of 30 Hz or greater, the mechanical response of the muscle is fusion of individual twitch responses. Individual EMG responses can be discerned during nondepolarizing blockade and the mechanical response appears as a peak, followed by a fade (see Fig. 19-7). In the absence of neuromuscular blocking drugs, no fade is present and the response is sustained. The sensitivity of tetanic stimulation in the detection of residual neuromuscular blockade is greater than that of the single twitch test, and this sensitivity increases with frequency.[37] However, at frequencies greater than 100 Hz, some fade may be seen even in the absence of neuromuscular blocking drugs.[105] Thus, 50 Hz is used most commonly in practice. No control, prerelaxant response is required, as the degree of skeletal muscle paralysis can be assessed by the degree of fade following tetanic stimulation. However, the main disadvantage of this mode of stimulation is the post-tetanic facilitation (see Fig. 19-7), the extent of which depends on the frequency and duration of the tetanic stimulation. For a 50-Hz tetanus applied for 5 seconds, the duration of this interval appears to be only 1–2 minutes.[38] If a single twitch

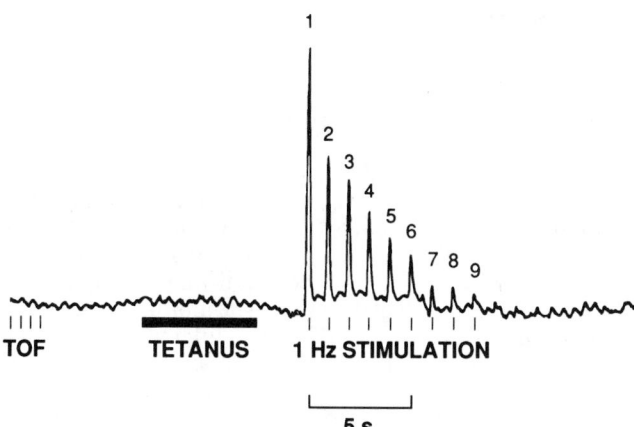

Figure 19-22. Post-tetanic count. During profound blockade, no response can be seen after train-of-four or tetanic stimulation. However if 1-Hz stimulation is applied after the tetanus, some twitches can be seen.

stimulation is performed during that time, the response is spuriously exaggerated.

Train-of-Four

With 2 Hz stimulation, the mechanical or electrical response decreases very little after the fourth stimulus, and the degree of fade is approximately equal to that found at 50 Hz.[10] Thus, applying train-of-four stimulation at 2 Hz provides approximately the same sensitivity as tetanic stimulation at 50 Hz. In addition, this relatively low frequency allows the response to be evaluated manually or visually. Moreover, the presence of a small number of impulses eliminates the problem of post-tetanic facilitation. Train-of-four stimulation can be repeated after a pause of 10 seconds. There is a fairly close relationship between single twitch depression and train-of-four response, and no control is re-

quired for the latter.[153] With single twitch blockade greater than 70–75%, not all four responses are visible. With blockade greater than 85–90%, only the first twitch is visible. In the range of 85–70% blockade, two to four twitches are visible. The train-of-four ratio, the height of the fourth twitch to that of the first twitch, is linearly related to first twitch height when blockade is less than 70%. When single twitch height has recovered to 100%, the train-of-four ratio is approximately 70%. Thus, train-of-four stimulation is a more sensitive indicator of neuromuscular blockade than single twitch stimulation.

Post-Tetanic Count

During profound neuromuscular blockade, there is no response to single twitch, tetanic, or train-of-four stimulation. To estimate the time required before the return of a response, one may use a technique that depends on the principle of post-tetanic facilitation. A 50-Hz tetanus is applied for 5 seconds, followed by a 3-second pause, and by stimulation at 1 Hz. The train-of-four and tetanic responses are undetectable, but facilitation produces a certain number of visible post-tetanic twitches (Fig. 19-22). For a given drug, the number of visible twitches correlates inversely with the time required for the return of single twitch or train-of-four responses.[154]

Double-Burst Stimulation

Train-of-four fade may be difficult to evaluate by visual or tactile means during recovery from neuromuscular blockade.[155] This can be overcome, to a certain extent, by applying two short tetanic stimulations and evaluating the ratio of the second to the first response. Many patterns have been suggested, but the most promising consists of two trains of three impulses at 50 Hz, separated by 750 msec.[156] The double-burst stimulation ratio correlates very closely with the train-of-four ratio (Fig. 19-23)[156,157] but is easier to detect manually.[157,158] At least 12–15 seconds must elapse between two consecutive double-burst stimulations.[156,157]

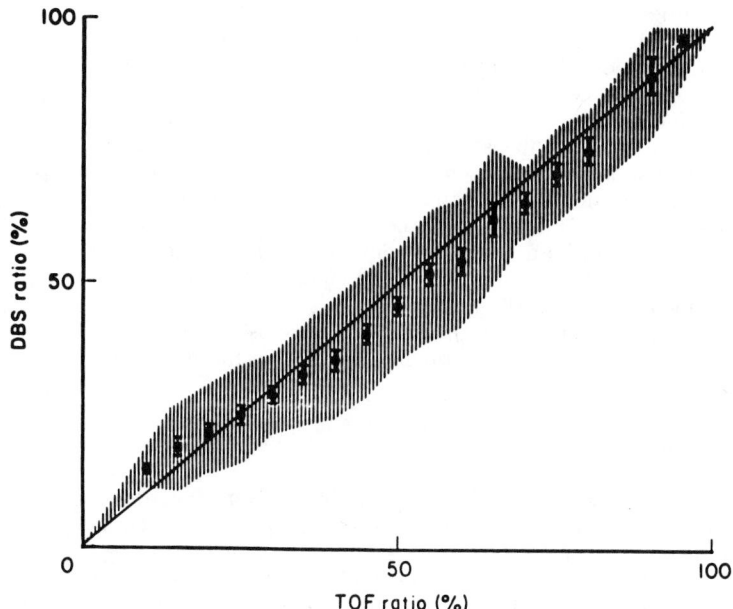

Figure 19-23. Relationship between double-burst stimulation (DBS) and train-of-four stimulation (TOF). The *shaded zone* shows 95% confidence limits and the line is the line of identity. (Reproduced with permission from Gill S, Donati F, Bevan DR: Clinical evaluation of double burst stimulation: Its relationship to train-of-four stimulation. Anaesthesia 45:543, 1989.)

Recording the Response

Visual and Tactile Evaluation

When electrical stimulation is applied to a nerve, the easiest and least expensive way to assess the response is to observe or feel the response of the muscle. This method is easily adaptable to any superficial muscle. However, serious errors in assessment can be made. In the case of evaluating the response of the adductor pollicis to ulnar nerve stimulation, the train-of-four count can be made reliably during a surgical procedure,[159] but the quantitative assessment of the train-of-four ratio is very difficult during recovery. Several studies suggest that train-of-four ratios as low as 0.3[155,157,158] can remain undetected. The detection rate for tetanic fade is no better.[160] With double-burst stimulation, fade can be detected reliably up to train-of-four ratios in the range of 0.5–0.6.[157,158]

Measurement of Force

A force transducer can overcome the shortcomings of one's senses. If applied correctly, the device provides accurate and reliable responses, displayed either as numbers or as an analog signal on a monitor such as an electrocardiogram screen. Unfortunately, transducers are applicable to only one muscle, usually the adductor pollicis. Force measurement can be used with single twitch, tetanus, train-of-four, double-burst, and post-tetanic stimulations. However, the availability of tetanus and double-burst stimulations is superfluous if accurate recording of the train-of-four response can be made.

Electromyography

It is possible to measure the electrical instead of the mechanical response of the skeletal muscle (see Fig. 19-4). One electrode should be positioned over the neuromuscular junction, which is usually close to the midportion of the muscle, and the other near the insertion of the muscle. A third, neutral electrode can be located anywhere else. Theoretically, any superficial muscle can be used for EMG recordings. In practice, such recordings are limited to the hypothenar eminence, the first dorsal interosseous, and the adductor pollicis muscles, which are supplied by the ulnar nerve. Most EMG recording devices compute the area under the EMG curve during a specified time window (usually 3–18 msec) after the stimulus is applied. This integrated EMG response is considered a better representation of the overall muscular activity than the measurement of peak response. There is usually good correlation between the EMG response and the force of the adductor pollicis if the EMG signal is taken from the thenar eminence.[161] The signal obtained from the hypothenar eminence is larger and less subject to movement artifacts, but it can underestimate the degree of paralysis when compared with the signal from the adductor pollicis.[162]

Accelerometry

Accelerometers respond to acceleration, which, according to Newton's law, should be proportional to force if mass remains unchanged. The device is usually attached to the tip of the thumb and a digital readout is obtained. The setup is very sensitive to inadvertent displacement of the thumb and, in the absence of neuromuscular blocking drugs, train-of-four ratios greater than 100% can be obtained.[163]

Choice of Muscle

It is impossible, for practical reasons, to monitor the skeletal muscles, which must be relaxed during surgery (e.g., the abdominal muscles), or the important muscles that must return to complete function postoperatively (e.g., the respiratory muscles). Thus, correlations must be made between monitored and other skeletal muscles. Unfortunately, different skeletal muscles in the body have different sensitivities to neuromuscular blocking drugs, and onset times are also different.

Adductor Pollicis

The adductor pollicis, supplied by the ulnar nerve, is accessible during most surgical procedures. Its force of contraction can be measured easily, and this measurement has become a standard in research. After injection of a dose of a neuromuscular blocking drug the time to maximal blockade is longer than in centrally located muscles.[164,165] The adductor pollicis is relatively sensitive to nondepolarizing neuromuscular blocking drugs, and during recovery it is blocked more than some respiratory muscles such as the diaphragm[164,165] and laryngeal adductors.[166]

Muscles of the Hypothenar Eminence

Ulnar nerve stimulation also produces flexion and abduction of the fifth finger. The hypothenar muscles are slightly more resistant to neuromuscular blocking drugs than is the adductor pollicis, the discrepancy being of the order of 15–20%.[162] Thus, a train-of-four ratio of 70% of the adductor pollicis corresponds to a train-of-four ratio of approximately 90% at the hypothenar eminence. The hypothenar eminence is particularly well suited for EMG recordings.

First Dorsal Interosseous Muscle

The EMG of the first dorsal interosseous muscle, also supplied by the ulnar nerve, can be obtained relatively easily and correlates well with adductor pollicis force.[167]

Orbicularis Oculi

Stimulation of the facial nerve produces contraction of the orbicularis oculi muscle. Onset of blockade is more rapid and recovery occurs sooner than at the adductor pollicis.[165] The time course of blockade correlates well with that of other resistant muscles such as the diaphragm.[165] Monitoring of the orbicularis oculi is probably indicated when profound blockade is desired. The facial nerve can be stimulated 2–3 cm posterior to the lateral border of the orbit.

Muscles of the Foot

The posterior tibial nerve, which can be stimulated behind the external malleolus, produces flexion of the big toe by contraction of the flexor hallucis. The response of this muscle is comparable to that of the adductor pollicis.[168] Stimulation of the external peroneal nerve produces dorsiflexion,[152] but the sensitivity of the muscles involved has not been measured.

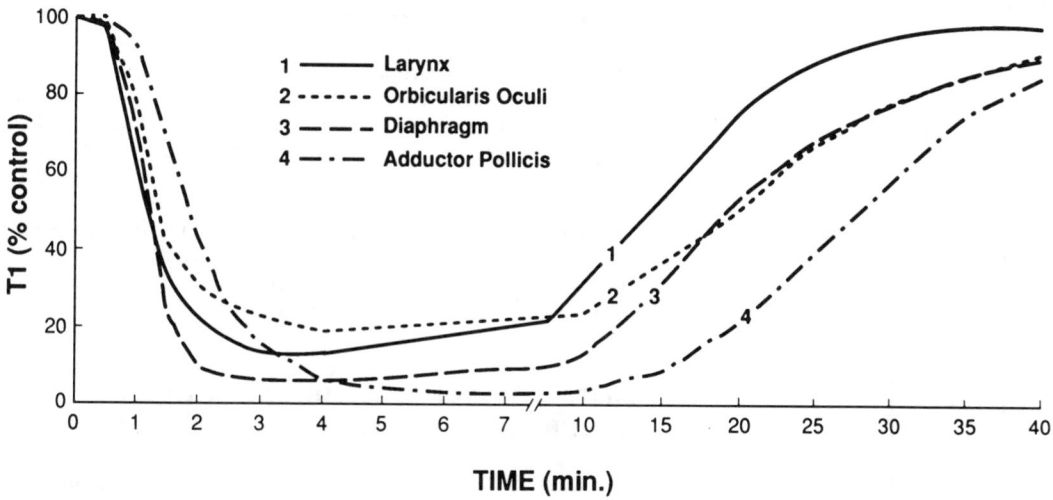

Figure 19-24. Onset and recovery after vecuronium, 0.07 mg·kg^{-1}, at various muscles, *vs.* time. Onset of action is more rapid at the larynx, orbicularis oculi, and diaphragm than at the adductor pollicis. Recovery occurs first at the larynx and last at the adductor pollicis. (Reproduced with permission from Donati F, Meistelman C, Plaud B: Vecuronium neuromuscular blockade at the diaphragm, the orbicularis oculi, and adductor pollicis muscles. Anesthesiology 73:870, 1990.)

Clinical Applications

Monitoring Onset

After induction of anesthesia, the intensity of the neuromuscular blockade must be assessed to determine the optimum time for tracheal intubation. In this setting, excellent conditions depend on relaxation of laryngeal and respiratory muscles. Onset is much quicker in these muscles than in the adductor pollicis,[164-166] and they are less sensitive to the action of muscle relaxants. Thus, blockade of the adductor pollicis is a very poor guide to adequate intubating conditions. The orbicularis oculi, which follows the profile of diaphragmatic[165] and possibly laryngeal blockade, appears to be a more appropriate choice (Fig. 19-24). Train-of-four fade takes longer to develop than single twitch depression (see Fig. 19-7),[12] and the train-of-four ratio should be of little importance during onset. Thus, single twitch stimulation at 0.1 Hz is preferred during onset of blockade. Although intubating conditions can be affected markedly by the depth of anesthesia, ideal intubating conditions might not be obtained unless blockade is observed at a resistant muscle, such as the orbicularis oculi.

Surgical Relaxation

Adequate surgical relaxation is usually obtained when fewer than two or three visible twitches are observed at the adductor pollicis. However, this criterion might prove inadequate in certain circumstances, when profound relaxation is required, because of the discrepancy between the adductor pollicis and other muscles. In this case, the post-tetanic count can be used at the adductor pollicis[154] provided that this type of stimulation is not repeated more often than every 2 to 3 minutes. A suitable alternative is the monitoring of the orbicularis oculi muscle,[165] which is more resistant to the effect of nondepolarizing muscle relaxants.

Monitoring Recovery

Complete return of neuromuscular function is desirable at the conclusion of surgery unless mechanical ventilation is planned. Thus, monitoring is useful in determining whether spontaneous recovery has progressed to a degree that allows reversal agents to be given, and to assess the effect of these agents.

The effectiveness of anticholinesterases depends directly on the degree of recovery present when they are administered. Preferably, reversal agents should be given only when four twitches are visible. The dose of anticholinesterase can also be adjusted according to the extent of recovery. For this assessment, using the adductor pollicis is preferable. This muscle is more sensitive and recovers later than those of the hypothenar eminence[169] or the orbicularis oculi.[165] If these skeletal muscles are used for monitoring purposes during recovery, allowance should be made for their greater resistance to skeletal muscle relaxants.

Finally, the adequacy of recovery should be assessed. Traditionally, a train-of-four ratio of 70% was considered to be the threshold below which residual weakness of the respiratory muscles could be present. Recent investigation suggests that, although some patients might have no clinical signs of weaknesses at train-of-four ratios of the adductor pollicis less than 70%, others might have demonstrable weakness at train-of-four ratios up to 80–90%.[170,171]

On the other hand, it has become apparent that human senses fail to detect either a train-of-four or tetanic fade when the train-of-four ratio is as low as 30%.[155,157,158] With double-burst stimulation, detection failures may occur at train-of-four ratios of 50–60%.[157,158] This indicates that clinical weakness can remain undetected. In this setting, the presence of force, EMG, or accelerometric equipment that provides an accurate response is a definite advantage. In any event, the evaluation should be completed by clinical tests, with the clinician bearing in mind that some of these tests can be affected by pain, depth of anesthesia, and patient cooperation.

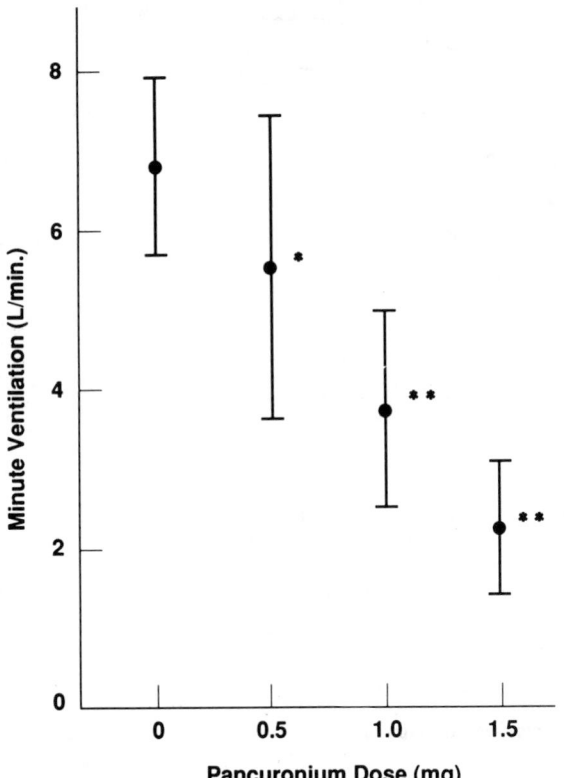

Figure 19-25. Minute ventilation in adults anesthetized with enflurane and given the cumulative dose of pancuronium indicated. (Reproduced with permission from Nishino T, Yokokawa N, Hiraga K et al: Breathing pattern of anesthetized humans during pancuronium-induced partial paralysis. J Appl Physiol 64:78, 1988.)

Anesthetized patients appear considerably more sensitive to the ventilatory effects of neuromuscular blocking drugs than awake patients.[172] Whereas tidal volume is preserved in awake patients receiving relatively high doses of neuromuscular blocking drugs, anesthetized patients have a decreased tidal volume and increased Pco_2 with doses of pancuronium as small as 0.5 mg (Fig. 19-25). The mechanism of this effect is uncertain, but the clinical implication is obvious.

Factors Affecting the Monitoring of Neuromuscular Blockade

Many drugs interfere with neuromuscular function, and these are dealt with elsewhere. However, certain situations make the interpretation of data on neuromuscular function different. For example, hypothermia decreases the response when neuromuscular blocking drugs are given. Thus, if the monitored hand is cold, the degree of paralysis will appear to be increased.[173] On the other hand, resistance to neuromuscular blocking drugs occurs with nerve damage, including peripheral nerve trauma, cord transection, and stroke. In this case, monitoring the involved limb would tend to underestimate the degree of muscle paralysis.[174,175] A noninvolved extremity should be used. The level of paralysis should also be adjusted for the type of patient and the type of surgery. For example, it is not necessary to paralyze frail individuals or patients at the extremes of age to the same extent as young muscular adults. The same applies to patients with debilitating muscular diseases.

It may be argued that neuromuscular monitoring has limited usefulness because the response of one skeletal muscle cannot be taken as representative of the whole body, because major errors in assessment can be made, and because monitoring does not seem to influence the amount of relaxant given or the incidence of postoperative residual block.[176] However, one must recognize that the effect of the neuromuscular blocking drug is the same whether or not monitoring is used. Neuromuscular monitoring can help in the diagnosis of inadequate skeletal muscle relaxation during surgery or insufficient recovery after surgery but does not, in itself, treat these conditions.

ANTAGONISM OF NEUROMUSCULAR BLOCKADE

The aim in the reversal of neuromuscular blockade is to ensure that the patient leaves the operating room with unimpaired skeletal muscle strength. There are some circumstances in which this is not desirable—for example, if it has been decided to continue mechanical support of ventilation into the postoperative period. Occasionally, complete recovery is unattainable.

Assessment of Neuromuscular Blockade

The principal goal of reversal is the re-establishment of spontaneous respiration and the ability to protect the airway from aspiration. Sensitive tests of pulmonary function such as vital capacity, maximum voluntary ventilation, and forced expiratory flow rate are difficult to perform in everyday practice, particularly when the patient is recovering from general anesthesia. Consequently, several indirect indices that are easier to measure have been correlated with the more specific tests of ventilatory function. Spontaneous ventilation adequate to prevent hypercapnia can be maintained despite considerable measurable skeletal muscle weakness if a patent airway is ensured.

Clinical Evaluation

Several crude tests have been suggested, including head lift for 5 seconds, tongue protrusion, arm lift for 45 seconds, and the ability to lift the legs off the bed. The maximum inspiratory pressure (MIP) has been correlated with tests of skeletal muscle strength (vital capacity, head lift, handgrip, leg raising) and of airway musculature (ability to swallow, approximate the vocal cords, maintain a patent airway, and elevate the mandible) in conscious volunteers receiving subparalyzing doses of d-tubocurarine.[177] The MIP was reduced successively. Head lift and leg raising were affected first, typically at an MIP of −53, and −50 cm H_2O, respectively. At an MIP of −25 cm H_2O or less, none of the subjects could swallow or maintain a patent airway, and handgrip was abolished. Nevertheless, as long as the mandible was elevated by an observer, the vital capacity was 40% of control and $P_{ET}CO_2$ was normal. Thus, the ability to maintain head lift for 5 seconds usually indicates sufficient strength to protect the airway and support ventilation.[177] Grip strength is more sensitive, but its assessment requires a dynamometer and preoperative control values, so that it is a less useful clinical tool. In infants and neonates, the ability to lift both legs off the table as a reflex response[178] appears to be as sensitive as the head lift in adults.

Evoked Responses to Nerve Stimulation

Clinical tests may be unobtainable in the patient recovering from anesthesia. Also, head lift may be impaired as a result of pain. Evoked responses to nerve stimulation are then appropriate. When the mechanical train-of-four ratio at the adductor pollicis is greater than 0.7, most clinical tests of neuromuscular function have returned to normal,[169,179-181] although, in some patients head lift may be impaired unless the train-of-four ratio is above 0.9.[170] This assumes that such a level of train-of-four recovery can be recognized, but subjective assessment of train-of-four fade is unreliable and is usually undetected until values are below 0.4–0.5.[155,157]

Detection of residual neuromuscular blockade is difficult unless the patient is awake and cooperative. Small degrees of paralysis will not be detected by train-of-four monitoring. However, this should not be interpreted as an excuse to avoid neuromuscular monitoring. Rather, train-of-four monitoring should be done to ensure that there is no detectable fade when the patient leaves the operating room. This will not guarantee full recovery, which awaits confirmation in the postanesthesia care unit when the patient is awake.

Residual Paralysis

Several studies have demonstrated that residual neuromuscular blockade is frequent in patients in the recovery room after surgery. Viby-Mogensen et al found, in 72 adult patients given d-tubocurarine, gallamine, or pancuronium, that the train-of-four ratio was less than 0.7 in 30 (42%) patients, and 16 of the 68 patients who were awake were unable to sustain head lift for 5 seconds.[182] Similar results have been obtained in Sweden,[183] Australia,[184] Canada,[170] and the United States.[185] The incidence of a train-of-four ratio below 0.7 is about 30% following the use of the longer acting agents—d-tubocurarine, pancuronium, alcuronium, and gallamine—but is reduced to less than 10% after using atracurium or vecuronium for operations lasting more than 2 hours.[170,185,186]

It is difficult to determine the importance of residual neuromuscular blockade. However, in a report on deaths occurring within 6 days of surgery, 11 of the 32 deaths due entirely to anesthesia were caused by postoperative ventilatory failure.[187] The presence of neuromuscular blockade was considered to be contributory in 6 of these deaths.[187]

Anticholinesterase Pharmacology

The pharmacologic principle involved in the reversal of muscle relaxants is the reduction of the effect of competitive blocking drugs by increasing the concentration of ACh at the neuromuscular junction.

Mechanism of Action

Neostigmine, edrophonium, and pyridostigmine inhibit acetylcholinesterase, but this may not be the only mechanism by which blockade is antagonized.

Neostigmine and pyridostigmine are attached to the anionic and esteratic sites of the acetylcholinesterase molecule and produce longer lasting inhibition than edrophonium. Neostigmine and pyridostigmine are inactivated by the interaction with the enzyme, whereas edrophonium is unaffected.[188]

Inhibition of acetylcholinesterase results in an increase

in the amount of ACh that reaches the receptor and in the time that ACh remains in the synaptic cleft. This causes an increase in the size and duration of the end-plate potentials.[189,190] Anticholinesterases also have presynaptic effects. In the absence of neuromuscular blocking drugs they potentiate the normal twitch response, in a way similar to succinylcholine, probably as a result of the generation of action potentials that spread antidromically.[2,13]

Anticholinesterases have other effects at the junction than inhibition of acetylcholinesterase. For example, the relationship between the train-of-four ratio and T1 depression is not the same for all agents.[191] Also, anticholinesterases react with single ACh receptors in vitro to decrease channel open time.[192]

The three anticholinesterases have a ceiling effect, at least in vitro.[193] Also, the effect of neostigmine may be modified by atropine[194] and by epinephrine;[2] both augment the ability of neostigmine to reverse the blockade.

Neostigmine Blockade

Large doses of anticholinesterases, greater than those used clinically, may produce neuromuscular blockade. Fade of both EMG and MMG responses has been observed during tetanic stimulation after clinical doses of neostigmine[195] but not edrophonium[196] were given to reverse neuromuscular blockade. Paradoxically, this neostigmine effect is antagonized with small doses of nondepolarizing neuromuscular blocking drugs. The mechanism involved is uncertain but appears to be of little clinical importance.

Potency

Dose-response curves have been constructed for edrophonium, neostigmine, and pyridostigmine. During a constant infusion of neuromuscular blocking drugs the curves are obtained by plotting the peak effect versus the dose of reversal agent. In this situation, neostigmine was found to be approximately 12 times as potent as edrophonium.[197] A similar relationship has been found during spontaneous recovery when the reversal agent was given at 10% T1 recovery and the values obtained at 10 minutes were used to construct the curves.[198] Potency ratios are difficult to determine because the slopes of the edrophonium and neostigmine curves are not parallel. In addition, the slope for edrophonium is flatter for train-of-four recovery than for T1 recovery,[199] and the curves shifted to the right when reversal of a more intense (99%) block was attempted (Fig. 19-26).[200] There is no difference in the dose-response relationship of anticholinesterases if vecuronium is infused instead of pancuronium.[201] However, there is a marked shift to the left for the curves obtained during vecuronium blockade if the reversal agent is given during spontaneous recovery.[202]

Pharmacokinetics

Following bolus iv injection, the plasma concentration of the anticholinesterases decreases rapidly during the first 5–10 minutes and then more slowly. Two-compartmental analysis has demonstrated similar values for the three drugs (Table 19-4).[203-206] Volumes of distribution are in the range of $0.7–1.4 \; l \cdot kg^{-1}$, and the $T_{1/2\beta}$ is 60–120 minutes. The drugs are water-soluble, ionized compounds so that their principal route of excretion is the kidney. Their clearances are in the range of $8–16 \; ml \cdot kg^{-1} \cdot min^{-1}$, which is much greater than the GFR because they are actively secreted into the

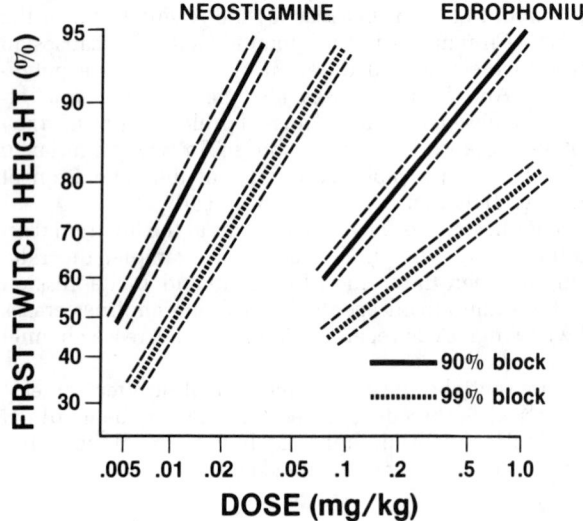

Figure 19-26. Dose-response curves for edrophonium and neostigmine in reversing 90%·and 99% atracurium block. (Reproduced with permission from Donati F, Smith CE, Bevan DR: Dose-response relationships for edrophonium and neostigmine as antagonists of moderate and profound atracurium blockade. Anesth Analg 68:13, 1989.)

tubular lumen.[207] Their clearance time is markedly reduced in patients in renal failure.

Pharmacodynamics

The onset of action of edrophonium (1–2 minutes) to peak effect is much more rapid than neostigmine (7–11 minutes) or pyridostigmine (15–20 minutes) (Fig. 19-27).[197,208-210] The reason for the differences is uncertain but may be related to the different rates of binding to the enzyme.

The duration of action corresponds to their pharmacokinetic behavior. In practice, the recovery of neuromuscular activity after reversal has two components: slow recovery from the relaxant and rapid, augmented recovery induced by the reversal agent. No recurarization should be expected after reversal unless the duration of action of the relaxants exceeds that of the reversal agents.

Factors Affecting Reversal

Several factors modify the rate of recovery of neuromuscular activity after reversal.

Block Intensity

The more intense the block at the time of reversal, the longer the recovery of neuromuscular activity (Fig. 19-28).[147,211,212] In addition, neostigmine is more effective than edrophonium or pyridostigmine in antagonizing intense (>90%) blockade.[199]

Anticholinesterase Dose

With more intense blockade a certain degree of recovery (train-of-four ratio > 0.7) can be obtained within a reasonable time (10 minutes) by increasing the dose of the reversal agent. However, because of the ceiling effect, there is little benefit in administering more than 0.07 mg·kg^{-1} neostigmine.

Attempts have been made to accelerate reversal by administering the anticholinesterase in divided doses—the priming principle. Although some acceleration can be demonstrated, the effect is small and of limited clinical importance.[213,214]

Choice of Relaxant

Recovery of neuromuscular activity after reversal is dependent on the rate of spontaneous recovery as well as the acceleration induced by the reversal agent. Consequently, the overall recovery of neuromuscular activity after administration of shorter-acting agents (atracurium, vecuronium) following the same dose of anticholinesterase is more rapid than after pancuronium, d-tubocurarine, or gallamine.[199,202] However, after prolonged infusions of vecuronium, spontaneous recovery becomes dependent on elimination and metabolism rather than redistribution. Thus the difference between vecuronium and pancuronium will be diminished because of their similar $T_{1/2\beta}$.[97] In addition, it appears that gallamine blockade is reversed more slowly than pancuronium blockade when neostigmine is given at the same degree of spontaneous recovery.[215]

Age

Recovery of neuromuscular activity occurs more rapidly[216] with smaller doses[217] of anticholinesterases in infants and children than in adults (Fig. 19-29). Thus, residual weakness in the postanesthesia care unit is found less frequently in children than in adults.[218]

Although the clearance of nondepolarizing relaxants is decreased in the elderly, the speed and extent of recovery after reversal are not affected,[51] probably because the elimination of anticholinesterases is also reduced.

TABLE 19-4. Mean Pharmacokinetic Variables for Anticholinesterases

Antagonist	Patient Status	V$_D$ (l·kg^{-1})	Cl (ml·kg^{-1}·min^{-1})	$T_{1/2\beta}$ (min)
Neostigmine	Normal	0.7	9.2	77
	Renal failure	1.6	7.8	181
Edrophonium	Normal	1.1	9.6	110
	Renal failure	0.7	2.7	206
Pyridostigmine	Normal	1.1	8.6	112
	Renal failure	1.0	2.1	379

V$_D$ = volume of distribution, Cl = plasma clearance, $T_{1/2\beta}$ = elimination half-life.

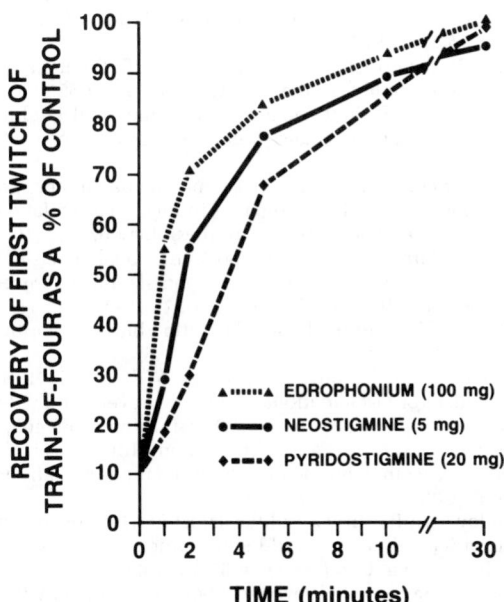

Figure 19-27. Onset of action of edrophonium, neostigmine, and pyridostigmine in the reversal of 90% pancuronium block. (From data of Ferguson A, Egerszegi P, Bevan DR: Neostigmine, pyridostigmine, and edrophonium as antagonists of pancuronium. Anesthesiology 53:390, 1980.)

Drug Interaction

Several drugs potentiate the action of neuromuscular blocking drugs, but there are few reports of impaired reversal. In the presence of enflurane and isoflurane, the reversal of pancuronium or vecuronium blockade is impaired, but only if administration of the vapor is continued during reversal.[219]

Renal Failure

Anticholinesterases are actively secreted into the tubular lumen,[207] so that their clearance is reduced in failure.[203-205] The rate and extent of recovery of pancuronium in renal failure after neostigmine are not impaired in renal failure, and "recurarization" does not occur.[220]

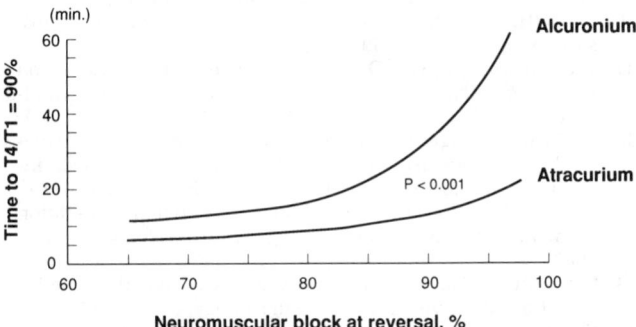

Figure 19-28. Relationship between time to recovery and prereversal twitch height after reversal of alcuronium, a long-acting relaxant, or atracurium blockade with edrophonium in children. (Reproduced with permission from Meretoja OA, Gebert R: Postoperative neuromuscular block following atracurium in children. Can J Anaesth 37:743, 1990.)

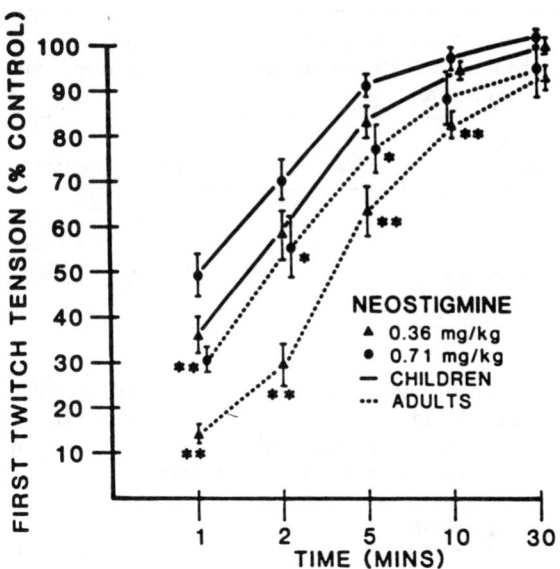

Figure 19-29. Comparison of recovery after reversal of 90% pancuronium blockade with neostigmine in adults and children. (Reproduced with permission from Meakin G, Sweet PT, Bevan JC et al: Neostigmine and edrophonium as antagonists of pancuronium in infants and children. Anesthesiology 59:316, 1983.)

Acid-Base Balance

The influence of acid-base disturbances on the reversal of neuromuscular blockade is poorly understood. Although it has been suggested that reversal is impaired in the ill, cachectic patient (neostigmine-resistant curarization) as a result of acidosis, this has been difficult to confirm in the laboratory.[221]

Other Effects

Cardiovascular Effects

Anticholinesterases provoke profound vagal stimulation. The time course of the vagal effects parallels the reversal of the block—rapid for edrophonium and slower for neostigmine. However, the bradycardia and bradyarrhythmias can be prevented with anticholinergic agents. Atropine has a rapid onset of action (1 minute), a duration of action of 30–60 minutes, and crosses the blood-brain barrier. Its time course makes it appropriate for use in combination with edrophonium,[197] whereas glycopyrrolate (onset, 2–3 minutes) is more suitable for use with neostigmine or pyridostigmine. As glycopyrrolate does not cross the blood-brain barrier, the incidence of memory deficits after anesthesia is less than after atropine.[209] If atropine is given with neostigmine, the dose is approximately half that of neostigmine (atropine, 20 $\mu g \cdot kg^{-1}$; neostigmine, 40 $\mu g \cdot kg^{-1}$). Such a combination leads to an initial tachycardia followed by a slight bradycardia. Atropine requirements are less with edrophonium (atropine, 7–10 $\mu g \cdot kg^{-1}$; edrophonium, 0.5 $mg \cdot kg^{-1}$).

Other Cholinergic Effects

Anticholinesterases produce increased salivation and bowel motility. Although atropine blocks the former, it appears to have little effect on peristalsis. Some reports claim an in-

TABLE 19-5. Recommended Doses of Neostigmine and Edrophonium, Based on Response to Train-of-Four (TOF) Stimulation

TOF Visible Twitches	Fade	Agent, Dose (mg·kg^{-1})
≤ 2	+ + + +	Neostigmine, 0.07
3–4	+ + +	Neostigmine, 0.04
4	+ +	Edrophonium, 0.5
4	±	Edrophonium, 0.25

crease in bowel anastomotic leakage after the reversal of neuromuscular blockade.[222] Others have held the use of anticholinesterases to be responsible for an increased incidence of vomiting after ambulatory surgery.[223]

Respiratory Effects

Anticholinesterases may cause an increase in airway resistance but anticholinergics reduce this effect. Several other factors, such as pain, the presence of an endotracheal tube, or light anesthesia, may predispose to bronchoconstriction at the end of surgery so that it is difficult to incriminate the reversal agents.

Clinical Use

Several reversal regimens have been proposed and are effective. In general, the more intense the blockade, the greater the dose of anticholinesterase that is required. However, there does not seem to be any advantage to giving more than the equivalent of neostigmine, 0.07 mg·kg^{-1}. Neostigmine is preferred to edrophonium for reversal of intense blockade, but the rapid action of edrophonium has the advantage of allowing the extent of reversal to be assessed in the operating room (Table 19-5).

REFERENCES

1. Bevan DR, Bevan JC, Donati F: Muscle Relaxants in Clinical Anesthesia. Chicago, Year Book Medical Publishers, 1988
2. Bowman WC: Pharmacology of Neuromuscular Function, 2nd ed. London, Wright, 1990
3. Kopman AF, Lawson D: Milliamperage requirements for supramaximal stimulation of the ulnar nerve with surface electrodes. Anesthesiology 61:83, 1984
4. Ellisman MH, Rash JE, Staehelin A, Porter KR: Studies of excitable membranes: II. A comparison of specialization at neuromuscular junctions and nonjunctional sarcolemmas of mammalian fast and slow twitch muscle fibers. J Cell Biol 68:752, 1976
5. Dunant Y, Israel M: The release of acetylcholine. Sci Am 252(4):58, 1985
6. Goudsouzian NG, Standaert FG: The infant and the myoneural junction. Anesth Analg 65:1208, 1986
7. Durant NN: The physiology of neuromuscular transmission. In Katz RL (ed): Muscle Relaxants: Basic and Clinical Aspects. Orlando, Florida, Grune & Stratton, 1984
8. Paton WDM, Waud DR: The margin of safety of neuromuscular transmission. J Physiol 191:59, 1967
9. Waud BE, Waud DR: The margin of safety of neuromuscular transmission in the muscle of the diaphragm. Anesthesiology 37:417, 1972
10. Lee C, Katz RL: Fade of neurally evoked compound electromyogram during neuromuscular block by d-tubocurarine. Anesth Analg 56:271, 1977
11. Baker T, Aguero A, Stanec A, Lowndes HE: Prejunctional effects of vecuronium in the cat. Anesthesiology 65:480, 1986
12. Bowman WC: Prejunctional and postjunctional cholinoceptors at the neuromuscular junction. Anesth Analg 59:935, 1980
13. Baker T, Stanec A: Drug actions at mammalian motor endings: The suppression of neostigmine-induced fasciculations by vecuronium and isoflurane. Anesthesiology 67:942, 1987
14. Gibb AJ, Marshall IG: Pre- and post-junctional effects of tubocurarine and other nicotinic antagonists during repetitive stimulation in the rat. J Physiol 351:275, 1984
15. Waud DR: The nature of "depolarization block." Anesthesiology 29:1014, 1968
16. Hartman GS, Flamengo SA, Riker WF: Succinylcholine: Mechanism of fasciculations and their prevention by d-tubocurarine or diphenylhydantoin. Anesthesiology 65:405, 1986
17. Van der Spek AFL, Fang WB, Ashton-Miller JA et al: The effects of succinylcholine on mouth opening. Anesthesiology 67:459, 1987
18. Plumley MH, Bevan JC, Saddler JM et al: Dose-related effects of succinylcholine on the adductor pollicis and masseter muscles in children. Can J Anaesth 37:15, 1990
19. Smith CE, Saddler JM, Bevan JC et al: Pretreatment with nondepolarizing neuromuscular blocking agents and suxamethonium-induced increases in resting jaw tension in children. Br J Anaesth 64:577, 1990
20. Lee C: Train-of-four fade and edrophonium antagonism of neuromuscular block by succinylcholine in man. Anesth Analg 55:663, 1976
21. Donati F, Bevan DR: Long-term succinylcholine infusion during isoflurane anesthesia. Anesthesiology 58:6, 1983
22. Litwiller RW: Succinylcholine hydrolysis. Anesthesiology 31:356, 1969
23. Szalados JE, Donati F, Bevan DR: Effect of d-tubocurarine pretreatment on succinylcholine twitch augmentation and neuromuscular blockade. Anesth Analg 71:55, 1990
24. Smith CE, Donati F, Bevan DR: Dose-response curves for succinylcholine: Single versus cumulative techniques. Anesthesiology 69:338, 1988
25. Walts LF, Dillon JB: Clinical studies on succinylcholine chloride. Anesthesiology 28:372, 1967
26. Cook DR, Wingard LB, Taylor FH: Pharmacokinetics of succinylcholine in infants, children, and adults. Clin Pharmacol Ther 20:493, 1976
27. Lerman J, Chinyanga HM: The heart rate response to succinylcholine in children: A comparison of atropine and glycopyrrolate. Can Anaesth Soc J 30:377, 1983
28. Pace NL: Prevention of succinylcholine myalgias: A meta-analysis. Anesth Analg 70:77, 1990
29. Smith G, Dalling R, Williams TIR: Gastro-oesophageal pressure gradient changes produced by induction of anaesthesia and suxamethonium. Br J Anaesth 50:1137, 1978
30. Cook JH: The effect of suxamethonium on intraocular pressure. Anaesthesia 36:359, 1981
31. Wynands JE, Crowell DE: Intraocular tension in association with succinylcholine and endotracheal intubation: A preliminary report. Can Anaesth Soc J 7:39, 1960
32. Stirt JA, Grosslight KR, Bedford RF, Vollmer D: "Defasciculation" with metocurine prevents succinylcholine-induced increases in intracranial pressure. Anesthesiology 67:50, 1987
33. Lanier WL, Milde JH, Michenfelder JD: Cerebral stimulation following succinylcholine in dogs. Anesthesiology 64:551, 1986
34. Gronert GA, Theye RA: Pathophysiology of hyperkalemia induced by succinylcholine. Anesthesiology 43:89, 1975
35. Whittaker M: Plasma cholinesterase variants and the anaesthetist. Anaesthesia 35:174, 1980
36. Viby-Mogensen J: Succinylcholine neuromuscular blockade in subjects homozygous for atypical plasma cholinesterase. Anesthesiology 55:429, 1981
37. Waud BE, Waud DR: The relation between the response to "train-of-four" stimulation and receptor occlusion during

competitive neuromuscular block. Anesthesiology 37:413, 1972

38. Brull SJ, Connelly NR, O'Connor TZ, Silverman DG: Effect of tetanus on subsequent neuromuscular monitoring in patients receiving vecuronium. Anesthesiology 74:64, 1991

39. Shanks CA: Pharmacokinetics of the nondepolarizing neuromuscular relaxants applied to calculation for bolus and infusion dosage regimens. Anesthesiology 64:72, 1986

40. Fisher DM, O'Keefe C, Stanski DR et al: Pharmacokinetics and pharmacodynamics of d-tubocurarine in infants, children, and adults. Anesthesiology 57:203, 1982

41. Sheiner LB, Stanski DR, Vozeh S et al: Simultaneous modeling of pharmacokinetics and pharmacodynamics: Application of d-tubocurarine. Clin Pharmacol Ther 25:358, 1979

42. Donati F: Onset of action of relaxants. Can J Anaesth 35:S52, 1988

43. Bowman WC, Rodger IW, Houston J et al: Structure:action relationships among some desacetoxy analogues of pancuronium and vecuronium in the anesthetized cat. Anesthesiology 69:57, 1988

44. Kopman AF: Pancuronium, gallamine, and d-tubocurarine compared: Is speed of onset inversely related to drug potency? Anesthesiology 70:915, 1989

45. Basta SJ, Savarese JJ, Ali HH et al: Clinical pharmacology of doxacurium chloride: A new long-acting nondepolarizing relaxant. Anesthesiology 69:478, 1988

46. Ghoneim MM, Kramer E, Barrow R et al: Binding of d-tubocurarine to plasma protein in health and disease. Anesth Analg 62:870, 1983

47. Matteo RS, Spector S, Horowitz PE: Relation of serum d-tubocurarine concentration to neuromuscular blockade. Anesthesiology 41:441, 1974

48. Miller RD, Matteo RS, Benet LZ et al: The pharmacokinetics of d-tubocurarine in man with and without renal failure. J Pharmacol Exp Ther 202:1, 1977

49. Hughes R, Chapple DJ: Effect of non-depolarizing neuromuscular blocking agents on peripheral autonomic mechanisms in cats. Br J Anaesth 48:59, 1976

50. Moss J, Roscow CE, Savarese JJ et al: Role of histamine in the hypotensive action of d-tubocurarine in humans. Anesthesiology 55:19, 1981

51. Hatano Y, Arai T, Noda J et al: Contribution of prostacyclin to d-tubocurarine-induced hypotension in humans. Anesthesiology 72:28, 1990

52. Matteo RS, Lieberman IG, Salanitre E et al: Distribution, elimination and action of d-tubocurarine in neonates, infants, children, and adults. Anesth Analg 63:799, 1984

53. Matteo RS, Backus WW, McDaniel DD et al: Pharmacokinetics and pharmacodynamics of d-tubocurarine and metocurine in the elderly. Anesth Analg 64:23, 1985

54. Martyn JAJ, Szyfelbein SK, Ali HH et al: Increased d-tubocurarine requirement following major thermal injury. Anesthesiology 52:352, 1980

55. Marathe PH, Dwersteg JF, Pavlin EG et al: Effect of thermal injury on the pharmacokinetics and pharmacodynamics of atracurium in humans. Anesthesiology 70:752, 1989

56. Marathe PH, Haschke RH, Slattery JT et al: Acetylcholine receptor density and acetylcholinesterase activity in skeletal muscle of rats following thermal injury. Anesthesiology 70:654, 1989

57. Stenlake JB, Waigh RB, Urwin J et al: Atracurium: conception and inception. Br J Anaesth 55:3S, 1983

58. Stiller RL, Cook DR, Chakravorti S: In vitro degradation of atracurium in human plasma. Br J Anaesth 57:1085, 1985

59. Chapple DJ, Clark JS: Pharmacological action of breakdown products of atracurium and related substances. Br J Anaesth 55:11S, 1983

60. Shi WZ, Fahey MR, Fisher DM et al: Laudanosine (a metabolite of atracurium) increases the minimal alveolar concentration of halothane in rabbits. Anesthesiology 63:584, 1985

61. Hennis PJ, Fahey MR, Canfell PC et al: Pharmacology of atracurium during isoflurane anesthesia in normal and anephric patients. Anesth Analg 65:743, 1986

62. Nigrovic V, Pandya JB, Klaunig JE, Fry K: Reactivity and toxicity of atracurium and its metabolites in vitro. Can J Anaesth 36:262, 1989

63. Miller RD, Rupp SM, Fisher DM et al: Clinical pharmacology of vecuronium and atracurium. Anesthesiology 61:444, 1984

64. Mirakhur RK, Lavery GG, Clarke RSJ et al: Atracurium in clinical anaesthesia: Effect of dosage on onset, duration and conditions for tracheal intubation. Anaesthesia 40:801, 1985

65. Hunter JM: Bradycardia after the use of atracurium. Br Med J 287:759, 1983

66. Savarese JJ, Basta SJ, Ali HH et al: Neuromuscular and cardiovascular effects of BW 33A (atracurium) in patients under halothane anesthesia. Anesthesiology 57:A262, 1982

67. Basta SJ, Savarese JJ, Ali HH et al: Histamine releasing potencies of atracurium, dimethyl tubocurarine, and tubocurarine. Br J Anaesth 55:105S, 1983

68. Scott RPF, Savarese JJ, Basta SJ et al: Atracurium: Clinical strategies for preventing histamine release and attenuating the haemodynamic response. Br J Anaesth 57:550, 1985

69. Jick H, Andrews EB, Tilson HH et al: Atracurium: A postmarketing surveillance study. Methods and US experience. Br J Anaesth 62:590, 1989

70. d'Hollander AA, Luyckx C, Barvais L et al: Clinical evaluation of atracurium besylate requirement for stable muscle relaxation during surgery: Lack of age-related effects. Anesthesiology 59:237, 1983

71. Schiller DJ, Feldman SA: Comparison of intubating conditions with atracurium, vecuronium and pancuronium. Anaesthesia 39:1188, 1984

72. Dressner DL, Basta SJ, Ali HH et al: Pharmacokinetics and pharmacodynamics of doxacurium in young and elderly patients during isoflurane anesthesia. Anesth Analg 71:498, 1990

73. Scott RPF, Norman J: Doxacurium chloride: A preliminary clinical trial. Br J Anaesth 62:375, 1989

74. Lennon RL, Hosking MP, Houck PC et al: Doxacurium chloride for neuromuscular blockade before tracheal intubation and surgery during nitrous oxide-oxygen-narcotic-enflurane anesthesia. Anesth Analg 68:255, 1989

75. Katz JA, Fragen RJ, Shanks CA et al: Dose-response relationships of doxacurium chloride in humans during anesthesia with nitrous oxide and fentanyl, enflurane, isoflurane, or halothane. Anesthesiology 70:432, 1989

76. Ramzan MI, Shanks CA, Triggs EJ: Gallamine disposition in surgical patients with chronic renal failure. Br J Clin Pharmacol 12:141, 1981

77. Lee Son S, Waud DR: Effects of non-depolarizing neuromuscular blocking agents on the cardiac vagus nerve in the guinea pig. Br J Anaesth 52:981, 1980

78. Brown BR, Crout JR: The sympathetic effect of gallamine on the heart. J Pharmacol Exp Ther 172:266, 1970

79. Meijer DKF, Weitering JG, Vermeer GA et al: Comparative pharmacokinetics of d-tubocurarine and metocurine in man. Anesthesiology 51:402, 1979

80. McCullogh LS, Stone WA, Delaunis AL et al: The effects of dimethyl tubocurarine iodide on cardiovascular parameters, postganglionic sympathetic activity and histamine release. Anesth Analg 51:554, 1972

81. Martyn JAJ, Matteo RS, Szyfellelbein SK et al: Unprecedented resistance to neuromuscular blocking effects of metocurine with persistence after complete recovery in a burned patient. Anesth Analg 61:614, 1982

82. Lebowitz PW, Ramsey FM, Savarese JJ et al: Combination of pancuronium and metocurine: Neuromuscular and hemodynamic advantages over pancuronium alone. Anesth Analg 60:12, 1981

83. Savarese JJ, Ali HH, Basta SJ et al: The clinical neuromuscular pharmacology of mivacurium chloride (BW 1090U): A short acting nondepolarizing ester neuromuscular blocking drug. Anesthesiology 68:723, 1988

84. Ali HH, Savarese JJ, Embree PT et al: Clinical pharmacology of mivacurium chloride (BW 1090U) infusion: Comparison with vecuronium and atracurium. Br J Anaesth 61:541, 1988

85. Brandom BW, Woelfel SK, Cook DR et al: Comparison of mi-

vacurium and suxamethonium administered by bolus and infusion. Br J Anaesth 62:488, 1989

86. Stoops CM, Curtis CA, Kovach DA et al: Hemodynamic effects of mivacurium chloride administered to patients during oxygen-sufentanil anesthesia for coronary artery bypass grafting or valve replacement. Anesth Analg 68:333, 1989

87. Buckett WR, Hewitt CL, Savage DS: Pancuronium bromide and other steroidal neuromuscular blocking agents containing acetylcholine fragments. J Med Chem 16:1116, 1973

88. Doherty WG, Breen PJ, Donati F et al: Accelerated onset of pancuronium with divided doses. Can Anaesth Soc J 32:1, 1985

89. Larijani GE, Bartkowski RR, Azad SS et al: Clinical pharmacology of pipecuronium bromide. Anesth Analg 68:734, 1989

90. Wierda JMKH, Richardson FJ, Agoston S: Dose-response relation and time course of action of pipecuronium bromide in humans anesthetized with nitrous oxide and isoflurane, halothane, or droperidol and fentanyl. Anesth Analg 68:208, 1989

91. Caldwell JE, Castagnoli KP, Canfell PC et al: Pipecuronium and pancuronium: Comparison of pharmacokinetics and duration of action. Br J Anaesth 61:693, 1988

92. Pittet J-F, Tassonyi E, Morel DR et al: Pipecuronium-induced neuromuscular blockade during nitrous oxide–fentanyl, isoflurane, and halothane anesthesia in adults and children. Anesthesiology 71:210, 1989

93. Wierda JMKH, de Wit APM, Kuizenga K, Agoston S: Clinical observations on the neuromuscular blocking action of ORG 9426, a new steroidal nondepolarizing agent. Br J Anaesth 64:521, 1990

94. Wierda JMHK, Kleef UW, Lambalk LM et al: The pharmacodynamics and pharmacokinetics of ORG 9426: A new nondepolarizing neuromuscular blocking agent in patients anaesthetized with nitrous oxide, halothane and fentanyl. Can J Anaesth 38:430, 1991

95. Muir AW, Houston J, Green KL et al: Effects of a new neuromuscular blocking agent (ORG 9426) in anaesthetized cats and pigs and in isolated nerve-muscle preparations. Br J Anaesth 63:400, 1989

96. Savage DS, Sleigh T, Carlyle I: The emergence of ORG NC 45, 1-[(2 beta, 3 alpha, 5, 16 beta, 17 beta)-3,17-bis(acetoxy)-2-(piperidinyl)-androstan-16-yl]-1-methyl-piperidinium bromide, from the pancuronium series. Br J Anaesth 52:3S, 1980

97. Segredo V, Malthay MA, Sharma ML et al: Prolonged neuromuscular blockade after long-term administration of vecuronium in two critically ill patients. Anesthesiology 72:566, 1990

98. Sohn YJ, Bencini AF, Scaf AHJ et al: Comparative pharmacokinetics and dynamics of vecuronium and pancuronium in anesthetized patients. Anesth Analg 65:233, 1986

99. Noeldge G, Hinsken H, Buzello W: Comparison between the continuous infusion of vecuronium and the intermittent administration of pancuronium and vecuronium. Br J Anaesth 56:473, 1984

100. Schwartz S, Ilias W, Lackner F et al: Rapid tracheal intubation with vecuronium: The priming principle. Anesthesiology 62:388, 1985

101. Mirakhur RK, Ferres CJ, Clarke RSJ et al: Clinical evaluation of ORG NC45. Br J Anaesth 55:119, 1983

102. Futo J, Kupferberg JP, Moss J et al: Vecuronium inhibits histamine N-methyltransferase. Anesthesiology 69:92, 1988

103. Miller RD, Way WL, Dolan WM et al: Comparative neuromuscular effects of pancuronium, gallamine, and succinylcholine during Forane and halothane anesthesia in man. Anesthesiology 35:509, 1971

104. Vitez TS, Miller RD, Eger EI et al: Comparison in vitro of isoflurane and halothane potentiation of d-tubocurarine and succinylcholine neuromuscular blocks. Anesthesiology 41:53, 1974

105. Fogdall RP, Miller RD: Neuromuscular blocking effects of enflurane, alone and combined with d-tubocurarine, pancuronium, and succinylcholine in man. Anesthesiology 42:173, 1975

106. Bennett MJ, Hahn JF: Potentiation of the combination of pancuronium and metocurine by halothane and isoflurane in humans with and without renal failure. Anesthesiology 62:759, 1985

107. Rupp SM, Miller RD, Gencarelli PJ: Vecuronium-induced neuromuscular blockade during enflurane, isoflurane, and halothane anesthesia in humans. Anesthesiology 60:102, 1984

108. Chapple DJ, Clark JS, Hughes R: Interaction between atracurium and drugs used in anaesthesia. Br J Anaesth 55:17S, 1983

109. Brandom BW, Rudd GD, Cook DR: Clinical pharmacology of atracurium in paediatric patients. Br J Anaesth 55:117S, 1983

110. Szalados JE, Donati F, Bevan DR: Nitrous oxide potentiates succinylcholine neuromuscular blockade in humans. Anesth Analg 72:18, 1991

111. Waud BE, Waud DR: Effects of volatile anesthetics on directly and indirectly stimulated skeletal muscle. Anesthesiology 50:103, 1979

112. McIndewar IC, Marshall RJ: Interaction between the neuromuscular block of ORG NC45 and some anaesthetic, analgesic and antimicrobial agents. Br J Anaesth 53:785, 1981

113. Matsuo S, Rao DBS, Chaudry I et al: Interaction of muscle relaxants and local anesthetics at the neuromuscular junction. Anesth Analg 57:580, 1978

114. Usubiaga JF, Wikinski JA, Morales RL: Interaction of intravenously administered procaine, lidocaine and succinylcholine in anesthetized subjects. Anesth Analg 46:39, 1967

115. Su PC, Su WL, Rosen AD: Pre- and post-synaptic effects of pancuronium at the neuromuscular junction of the mouse. Anesthesiology 50:199, 1979

116. Waud BE, Waud DR: Interaction among agents that block endplate depolarization competitively. Anesthesiology 61:420, 1984

117. Ferguson A, Bevan DR: Mixed neuromuscular block: The effect of precurarization. Anaesthesia 36:661, 1981

118. Stovner J, Oftedal N, Holmboe J: The inhibition of cholinesterase by pancuronium. Br J Anaesth 47:949, 1975

119. Krieg N, Hendrickx HHL, Crul JF: Influence of suxamethonium on the potency of ORG NC45 in anaesthetized patients. Br J Anaesth 53:259, 1981

120. Rouse JM, Bevan DR: Mixed neuromuscular block. Anaesthesia 34:608, 1979

121. Argov Z, Mastaglia FL: Disorders of neuromuscular transmission caused by drugs. N Engl J Med 301:409, 1979

122. Ornstein E, Matteo RS, Silverberg PA et al: Dose-response relationships for vecuronium in the presence of chronic phenytoin therapy. Anesth Analg 65:S116, 1986

123. Ornstein E, Schwartz AE, Matteo RS et al: Predictability of atracurium effect in phenytoin exposed patients. Anesthesiology 65:A112, 1986

124. Bender AN, Engel WK, Reingel SP et al: Myasthenia gravis: A serum factor blocking acetylcholine receptors of the human neuromuscular junction. Lancet 1:607, 1975

125. Drachman DB, Kao I, Pestronk A et al: Myasthenia gravis as a receptor disorder. Ann NY Acad Sci 274:226, 1976

126. Cull-Candy SG, Miledi R, Trautmann A et al: On the release of transmitter at normal, myasthenis gravis, and myasthenic syndrome affected human end-plates. J Physiol (London) 299:621, 1980

127. Ozdemiv C, Young RR: The results to be expected from electrical testing in the diagnosis of myasthenia gravis. Ann NY Acad Sci 274:203, 1976

128. Brown JC, Charlton JE: A study of sensitivity to curare in myasthenic disorders using a regional technique. J Neurol Neurosurg Psychiatry 38:27, 1975

129. Wojciechowski ARJ, Hanning CD, Pohl JEF: Postoperative apnoea and latent myasthenia gravis. Anaesthesia 40:882, 1985

130. Eisenkraft JB, Book WJ, Mann SM et al: Resistance to succinylcholine in myasthenia gravis: A dose-response study. Anesthesiology 69:760, 1988

131. Azar I: The response of patients with neuromuscular disorders to muscle relaxants: A review. Anesthesiology 61:173, 1984

132. Smith CE, Donati F, Bevan DR: Cumulative dose-response curves for atracurium in patients with myasthenia gravis. Can J Anaesth 36:402, 1989

133. Nilsson E, Meretoja OA: Vecuronium dose-response and

maintenance requirements in patients with myasthenia gravis. Anesthesiology 73:28, 1990

134. Green SJ, Shanks CA, Ronai AK et al: Atracurium-induced neuromuscular blockade in five myasthenic patients. Anesth Analg 64:221, 1985

135. Buzello W, Noeldge G, Krieg N et al: Vecuronium for muscle relaxation in patients with myasthenia gravis. Anesthesiology 64:507, 1986

136. Leventhal S, Orkin FK, Hirsh RA: Prediction of the need for postoperative mechanical ventilation in myasthenia gravis. Anesthesiology 53:26, 1980

137. Paterson IS: Generalized myotonia following suxamethonium. Br J Anaesth 34:340, 1962

138. Buzello W, Krieg N, Schlickewei A: Hazards of neostigmine in patients with neuromuscular disorders. Br J Anaesth 54:529, 1982

139. Smith CL, Bush GH: Anaesthesia and progressive muscular dystrophy. Br J Anaesth 57:1113, 1985

140. Larsen UT, Juhl B, Hein-Sørensen O et al: Complications during anaesthesia in patients with Duchenne's muscular dystrophy. Can J Anaesth 36:418, 1989

141. Brown JC, Charlton JE: Study of sensitivity to curare in certain neurological disorders using a regional technique. J Neurol Neurosurg Psychiatry 38:34, 1975

142. Robertson JA: Ocular muscular dystrophy: A cause of curare sensitivity. Anaesthesia 39:251, 1984

143. Gronert GA: Controversies in malignant hyperthermia. Anesthesiology 59:273, 1983

144. Rosenberg H, Heiman-Patterson T: Duchenne's muscular dystrophy and malignant hyperthermia: Another warning. Anesthesiology 59:362, 1983

145. Ginsberg H, Varejes L: The use of a relaxant in myasthenia gravis. Anaesthesia 10:177, 1955

146. Kardash K, Abou-Madi M, Trop D, Delorme M: Succinylcholine, motor dysfunction and potassium in brain tumor patients. Anesthesiology 71:A1139, 1989

147. Graham DH: Monitoring neuromuscular block may be unreliable in patients with upper motor-neuron lesions. Anesthesiology 52:74, 1980

148. Cooper AL, Leigh JM, Tring IC: Admissions to the intensive care unit after complication of anaesthetic techniques over 10 years: 1. The first 5 years. Anaesthesia 44:953, 1989

149. Tiret L, Desmonts JM, Hatton F et al: Complications associated with anaesthesia: A prospective study in France. Can Anaesth Soc J 33:336, 1986

150. Katz RL: Neuromuscular effects of d-tubocurarine, edrophonium and neostigmine in man. Anesthesiology 28:327, 1967

151. Rosenberg H, Greenhow DE: Peripheral nerve stimulator performance: The influence of output polarity and electrode placement. Can Anaesth Soc J 25:424, 1978

152. Hudes E, Lee KC: Clinical use of nerve stimulators in anaesthesia. Can J Anaesth 34:525, 1987

153. Ali HH, Utting JE, Gray TC: Quantitative assessment of residual antidepolarizing block: Part I. Br J Anaesth 43:473, 1971

154. Viby-Mogensen J: Clinical assessment of neuromuscular transmission. Br J Anaesth 54:209, 1982

155. Viby-Mogensen J, Jensen NH, Engbaek J et al: Tactile and visual evaluation of the response to train-of-four nerve stimulation. Anesthesiology 63:440, 1985

156. Engbaek J, Ostergaard D, Viby-Mogensen J: Double burst stimulation (DBS): A new pattern of nerve stimulation to identify residual neuromuscular block. Br J Anaesth 62:274, 1989

157. Gill S, Donati F, Bevan DR: Clinical evaluation of double burst stimulation: Its relationship to train-of-four stimulation. Anaesthesia 45:543, 1989

158. Drenck DE, Ueda N, Olsen NV et al: Manual evaluation of residual curarization using double burst stimulation: A comparison with train-of-four. Anesthesiology 70:578, 1989

159. Lee C: Train-of-4 quantitation of competitive neuromuscular block. Anesth Analg 54:649, 1975

160. Dupuis JY, Martin R, Tessonier JM, Tétrault JP: Clinical assessment of the muscular response to tetanic nerve stimulation. Can J Anaesth 37:397, 1990

161. Kopman AF: The effect of resting muscle tension on the dose-effect relationship of d-tubocurarine: Does preload influence the evoked EMG? Anesthesiology 69:1003, 1988

162. Kopman AF: The relationship of evoked electromyographic and mechanical responses following atracurium in humans. Anesthesiology 63:208, 1985

163. Viby-Mogensen J, Jensen E, Werner M et al: Measurement of acceleration: A new method of monitoring neuromuscular function. Acta Anaesthesiol Scand 32:45, 1988

164. Chauvin M, Lebrault C, Duvaldestin P: The neuromuscular blocking effect of vecuronium on the human diaphragm. Anesth Analg 66:117, 1987

165. Donati F, Meistelman C, Plaud B: Vecuronium neuromuscular blockade at the diaphragm, the orbicularis oculi, and adductor pollicis muscles. Anesthesiology 73:870, 1990

166. Donati F, Meistelman C, Plaud B: Vecuronium neuromuscular blockade at the adductor muscles of the larynx and adductor pollicis. Anesthesiology 74:833, 1991

167. Kopman AF: The dose-effect relationship of metocurine: The integrated electromyogram of the first dorsal interosseous muscle and the mechanomyogram of the adductor pollicis compared. Anesthesiology 68:604, 1988

168. Sopher MJ, Sears DH, Walts LF: Neuromuscular monitoring comparing the flexor hallucis brevis and adductor pollicis muscles. Anesthesiology 69:129, 1988

169. Dupuis JY, Martin R, Tétrault JP: Clinical, electrical and mechanical correlations during recovery from neuromuscular blockade with vecuronium. Can J Anaesth 37:192, 1990

170. Bevan DR, Smith CE, Donati F: Postoperative neuromuscular blockade: A comparison between atracurium, vecuronium, and pancuronium. Anesthesiology 69:272, 1988

171. Engbaek J, Ostergaard D, Viby-Mogensen J, Skovgaard LT: Clinical recovery and train-of-four ratio measured mechanically and electromyographically following atracurium. Anesthesiology 71:391, 1989

172. Nishino T, Yokokawa N, Hiraga K et al: Breathing pattern of anesthetized humans during pancuronium-induced partial paralysis. J Appl Physiol 64:78, 1988

173. Thornberry EA, Mazumdar D: The effect of changes in temperature on neuromuscular monitoring in the presence of atracurium blockade. Anaesthesia 43:447, 1988

174. Moorthy SS, Hildenberg JC: Resistance to non-depolarizing muscle relaxants in paretic upper extremities of patients with residual hemiplegia. Anesth Analg 59:624, 1980

175. Laycock JRD, Smith CE, Donati F, Bevan DR: Sensitivity of the adductor pollicis and diaphragm muscles to atracurium in a hemiplegic patient. Anesthesiology 67:851, 1987

176. Pedersen T, Viby-Mogensen J, Bang U et al: Does perioperative tactile evaluation of the train-of-four response influence the frequency of postoperative residual neuromuscular blockade? Anesthesiology 73:835, 1990

177. Pavlin EG, Holle RH, Schoene RB: Recovery of airway protection compared with ventilation in humans after paralysis with curare. Anesthesiology 70:381, 1989

178. Mason LJ, Betts EK: Leg lift and maximum inspiratory force, clinical signs of neuromuscular blockade reversal in infants and children. Anesthesiology 52:441, 1980

179. Ali HH, Kitz RJ: Evaluation of recovery from non-depolarizing neuromuscular blockade using a digital neuromuscular analyser: Preliminary report. Anesth Analg 52:740, 1973

180. Ali HH, Wilson RS, Savarese JJ, Kitz RJ: The effect of tubocurarine on indirectly elicited train-of-four muscle response and respiratory measurements in humans. Br J Anaesth 47:570, 1975

181. Brand JB, Cullen DJ, Wilson NE, Ali HH: Spontaneous recovery from nondepolarizing neuromuscular blockade: Correlation between clinical and evoked responses. Anesth Analg 56:55, 1977

182. Viby-Mogensen J, Jørgensen BC, Ørding H: Residual curarization in the recovery room. Anesthesiology 50:539, 1979

183. Lennmarken C, Löfström JB: Partial curarization in the postoperative period. Acta Anaesthesiol Scand 28:260, 1984

184. Beemer GH, Rozental P: Postoperative neuromuscular function. Anaesth Intens Care 14:41, 1986

185. Brull SJ, Silverman DG, Ehrenwerth J: Problems of recovery

and residual neuromuscular blockade: Pancuronium vs. vecuronium. Anesthesiology 69:A473, 1988

186. Jensen E, Engbaek J, Andersen BN et al: The frequency of residual neuromuscular blockade following atracurium (A), vecuronium (V) and pancuronium (P): A multicenter randomized study. Anesthesiology 73:A914, 1990

187. Lunn JN, Hunter AR, Scott DB: Anaesthesia-related surgical mortality. Anaesthesia 38:1090, 1983

188. Kitz RJ: The chemistry of anticholinesterase activity. Acta Anaesthesiol Scand 8:197, 1964

189. Fiekers JF: Interactions of edrophonium, physostigmine and methanesulfonyl fluoride with the snake end-plate acetylcholine receptor-channel complex. J Pharmacol Exp Ther 234:539, 1985

190. Kordas M, Brzin M, Majcen Z: A comparison of the effect of cholinesterase inhibitors on end-plate current and on cholinesterase activity in frog muscle. Neuropharmacology 14:791, 1975

191. Donati F, Ferguson A, Bevan DR: Twitch depression and train-of-four ratio after antagonism of pancuronium with edrophonium, neostigmine, or pyridostigmine. Anesth Analg 62:314, 1983

192. Wachtel RE: Comparison of anticholinesterases and their effects on acetylcholine-activated ion channels. Anesthesiology 72:496, 1990

193. Bartkowski RR: Incomplete reversal of pancuronium neuromuscular blockade by neostigmine, pyridostigmine, and edrophonium. Anesth Analg 66:594, 1987

194. Alves-do-Prado W, Corrado AP, Prado WA: Reversal by atropine of tetanic fade induced in cats by antinicotinic and anticholinesterase agents. Anesth Analg 66:492, 1987

195. Goldhill DR, Wainwright AP, Stuart CS, Flynn PJ: Neostigmine after spontaneous recovery from neuromuscular blockade: Effect on depth of blockade monitored with train-of-four and tetanic stimuli. Anaesthesia 44:293, 1989

196. Astley BA, Katz RL, Payne JP: Electrical and mechanical responses after neuromuscular blockade with vecuronium, and subsequent antagonism with neostigmine or edrophonium. Br J Anaesth 59:983, 1987

197. Cronelly R, Morris RB, Miller RD: Edrophonium: Duration of action and atropine requirement in humans during halothane anesthesia. Anesthesiology 57:261, 1982

198. Breen PJ, Doherty WG, Donati F et al: The potencies of edrophonium and neostigmine as antagonists of pancuronium. Anaesthesia 40:844, 1985

199. Donati F, McCarroll SM, Antzaca C et al: Dose-response curves for edrophonium, neostigmine, and pyridostigmine after pancuronium and d-tubocurarine. Anesthesiology 66:471, 1987

200. Donati F, Smith CE, Bevan DR: Dose-response relationships for edrophonium and neostigmine as antagonists of moderate and profound atracurium blockade. Anesth Analg 68:13, 1989

201. Gencarelli PJ, Miller RD: Antagonism of ORG NC45 (vecuronium) and pancuronium neuromuscular blockade by neostigmine. Br J Anaesth 54:53, 1982

202. Smith CE, Donati F, Bevan DR: Dose-response relationships for edrophonium and neostigmine as antagonists of atracurium and vecuronium neuromuscular blockade. Anesthesiology 71:37, 1989

203. Cronelly R, Stanski DR, Miller RD et al: Renal function and the pharmacokinetics of neostigmine in anesthetized man. Anesthesiology 51:222, 1979

204. Cronelly R, Stanski DR, Miller RD, Sheiner LB: Pyridostigmine kinetics with and without renal function. Clin Pharmacol Ther 28:78, 1980

205. Morris RB, Cronelly R, Miller RD et al: Pharmacokinetics of edrophonium in anephric and renal transplant patients. Br J Anaesth 53:1311, 1981

206. Morris RB, Cronelly R, Miller RD et al: Pharmacokinetics of edrophonium and neostigmine when antagonizing d-tubocurarine neuromuscular blockade in man. Anesthesiology 54:399, 1981

207. Rennick BR: Renal tubule transport of organic cations. Am J Physiol 9:F83, 1981

208. Miller RD, Van Nyhuis LS, Eger EI et al: Comparative times to peak affect and durations of action of neostigmine and pyridostigmine. Anesthesiology 41:27, 1974

209. Mirakhur RK: Antagonism of neuromuscular block in the elderly: A comparison of atropine and glycopyrrolate in a mixture with neostigmine. Anaesthesia 40:254, 1985

210. Ferguson A, Egerszegi P, Bevan DR: Neostigmine, pyridostigmine, and edrophonium as antagonists of pancuronium. Anesthesiology 53:390, 1980

211. Rupp SM, McChristian JW, Miller RD et al: Neostigmine and edrophonium antagonism of varying intensity neuromuscular blockade induced by atracurium, pancuronium, or vecuronium. Anesthesiology 64:711, 1986

212. Meretoja OA, Gebert R: Postoperative neuromuscular block following atracurium in children. Can J Anaesth 37:743, 1990

213. Abdulatif M, Naguib M: Accelerated reversal of atracurium blockade with divided doses of neostigmine. Can Anaesth Soc J 33:723, 1986

214. Szalados JE, Donati F, Bevan DR: Edrophonium priming for antagonism of atracurium neuromuscular blockade. Can J Anaesth 37:197, 1990

215. Miller RD, Lawson CP, Way WL: Comparative antagonism of d-tubocurarine, gallamine, and pancuronium-induced neuromuscular blockades by neostigmine. Anesthesiology 37:503, 1972

216. Meakin G, Sweet PT, Bevan JC, Bevan DR: Neostigmine and edrophonium as antagonists of pancuronium in infants and children. Anesthesiology 59:316, 1983

217. Fisher DM, Cronelly R, Miller RD, Sharma M: The neuromuscular pharmacology of neostigmine in infants and children. Anesthesiology 59:220, 1983

218. Baxter MM, Bevan JC, Samuel J et al: Postoperative neuromuscular function in pediatric day-care patients. Anesth Analg 72:504, 1991

219. Gill SS, Bevan DR, Donati F: Edrophonium antagonism of atracurium during enflurane anaesthesia. Br J Anaesth 64:300, 1990

220. Bevan DR, Archer DP, Donati F et al: Antagonism of pancuronium in renal failure: No recurarization. Br J Anaesth 54:63, 1982

221. Wirtavouri K, Salmenperä M, Tammisto T: Effect of hypocarbia and hypercarbia on the antagonism of pancuronium-induced neuromuscular blockade with neostigmine in man. Br J Anaesth 54:57, 1982

222. Aitkenhead AR: Anaesthesia and bowel surgery. Br J Anaesth 56:95, 1984

223. King MJ, Milazkiewicz R, Carli F, Deacock AR: Influence of neostigmine on postoperative vomiting. Br J Anaesth 61:403, 1988

20

Randall L. Carpenter
David C. Mackey

Local Anesthetics

Local anesthetics may be defined as drugs that block the generation and propagation of impulses in excitable tissues. Although the anesthesiologist is primarily concerned with the blocking effects of local anesthetic solutions on the spinal cord, spinal nerve roots, and peripheral nerves, these compounds also affect other excitable tissues, such as cardiac muscle,[1-4,22] skeletal muscle,[5,6] smooth muscle,[7] and brain.[8-10] This is an important consideration in local anesthetic toxicity. Local anesthetics are usually administered topically or by local infiltration, although they may also be delivered intravenously for regional anesthesia or for their systemic effects. A wide variety of substances, such as certain alpha and beta receptor blocking agents, volatile general anesthetics, alcohols, opioids, barbiturates and other anticonvulsants, tranquilizers, and plant and animal toxins may exhibit local anesthetic activity.[11-18] This discussion is limited to those local anesthetics utilized in clinical anesthesia, principally, the aminoesters and the aminoamides.

Acupuncture, hypnotism, refrigeration, and nerve compression are known to have been used for many years to alleviate surgical pain prior to the development and utilization of local anesthetic drugs, and the anesthetic and central nervous system stimulant effect derived from the leaves of the *Erythroxylon coca* bush had been recognized by Peruvian natives. In 1860, the alkaloid cocaine was isolated from the coca leaf by Niemann. In 1884, Koller reported the first use of a local anesthetic for surgery when he described the topical application of cocaine for ophthalmologic surgery. However, cocaine was found to be extremely toxic and addictive, and the search for a suitable substitute culminated in the synthesis of procaine, in 1904, by Einhorn. Procaine, the prototype aminoester local anesthetic, was first used clinically in 1905. Numerous other aminoester local anesthetics have been introduced subsequently, including tetracaine in 1932 and 2-chloroprocaine in 1955. In 1943, lidocaine was synthesized by Lofgren, and its clinical introduction 1 year later marked the first use of a new class of local anesthetics, the aminoamides. Several additional amide local anesthetics have been developed, including mepivacaine (1956), bupivacaine (1957), prilocaine (1959), and etidocaine (1971), and they have subsequently been placed into clinical use where they remain today. Ropivacaine, a new, long-acting aminoamide local anesthetic that may have reduced cardiovascular toxicity, is currently undergoing laboratory and clinical investigation.[19-23] There are several excellent reviews of the development of local anesthetics and local anesthesia for those who desire greater detail.[24-30]

CHEMISTRY OF LOCAL ANESTHETICS

The Local Anesthetic Molecule

In order to understand and predict the differences in biologic activity of local anesthetic agents, it is necessary to appreciate both the general structure of the local anesthetic molecule and the properties of each of its subunits. The typical, clinically employed, local anesthetic molecule is weakly basic in nature, containing an amine residue that contributes water solubility in its quaternary form and that is separated from a lipophilic domain by an intermediate alkyl chain (Fig. 20-1). The intermediate chain connecting the lipophilic head and the hydrophilic tail contains either an ester or an amide linkage, thus subdividing the clinically useful local anesthetics into two main groups: the aminoesters, which are metabolized by plasma cholinesterase, and the aminoamides, which are metabolized in the liver. The lipophilic portion of the molecule is usually an aromatic residue, contributed by a derivative of benzoic acid in the case of the aminoester anesthetics, or by a derivative of aniline in the case of the aminoamides.

Structure-Activity Relationships

In its tertiary form, the local anesthetic molecule is poorly soluble in water, but, because of its basic nature, it combines readily with acids to form water-soluble salts. Thus, for clinical utility, local anesthetics are usually prepared as their salt form, most often as hydrochlorides. In aqueous solution, the hydrochloride salt ionizes to yield a positively charged quaternary amine and a chloride anion. The charged, quaternary amine exists in solution in equilibrium with its uncharged, free-base, tertiary amine form (Fig. 20-2). The exact percentage of local anesthetic molecules in each of the two forms depends on the pK_a, or dissociation constant, of the local anesthetic and the pH of the sur-

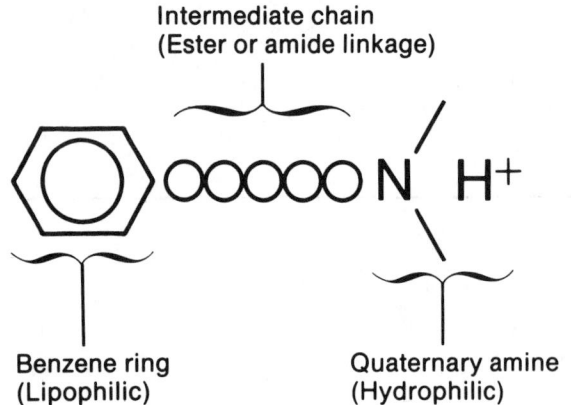

Figure 20-1. General structure of a local anesthetic molecule.

TABLE 20-1. Effect of pH on Local Anesthetic Base Dissociation

Agent	pK_a	Percentage of Total Drug in Base Form		
		$pH = 7.0$	$pH = 7.4$	$pH = 7.8$
Benzocaine	3.5	100	100	100
Mepivacaine	7.6	20	39	61
Lidocaine	7.9	11	24	44
Etidocaine	7.7	17	33	56
Bupivacaine	8.1	7	17	33
Tetracaine	8.6	6	14	28
Procaine	8.9	1	3	7
2-Chloroprocaine	9.1	0.8	2	5

Adapted with permission from the publisher from Tucker GT, Mather LE: Absorption and disposition of local anesthetics: Pharmacokinetics. In Cousins MJ, Bridenbaugh PO (eds): Neural Blockade in Clinical Anesthesia and Management of Pain, pp 48–49. Philadelphia, JB Lippincott, 1980.

rounding medium (Table 20-1). For example, as the pH is decreased, the equilibrium is shifted to favor the protonated form, and thus a relatively larger percentage of the local anesthetic will exist as positively charged, cationic molecules.

The degree of ionization is important, as it is the uncharged, free-base form that is most lipid-soluble and thus most able to traverse the lipid milieu of the axon membrane, its myelin sheath (if present), and the surrounding connective tissue coverings of the nerve fiber bundles and nerve.[31,32] As will be seen, both the lipophilic, neutral (free-base) form and the hydrophilic, charged (cationic) form of the local anesthetic molecule are involved in the blockade of the nerve impulse. Charged molecules probably gain access to specific receptors on the interior of the neuronal sodium channel *via* the aqueous pathway of the sodium channel pore, whereas neutral, uncharged forms interact with sodium channels through the lipid environment of the axon membrane (Fig. 20-3).[31,33-38]

The basic properties of a local anesthetic can be manipulated through alterations in its molecular structure.[39-42] For example, increasing the degree of alkyl substitution on the aromatic ring or on the tertiary amine increases lipid solubility and produces greater local anesthetic potency. Lengthening the intermediate chain increases anesthetic potency, but at the expense of increasing toxicity. Compounds containing ethyl esters, such as procaine and chloroprocaine, are more easily metabolized and produce less systemic toxicity. Molecular changes that lead to increased protein binding result in prolongation of the duration of local anesthetic action. Finally, when local anesthetic molecules contain asymmetric carbon atoms and thus can be resolved into optical isomers, an enantiomeric preparation of the local anesthetic may possess differing therapeutic and/or toxic qualities when compared with the racemic mixture.[19]

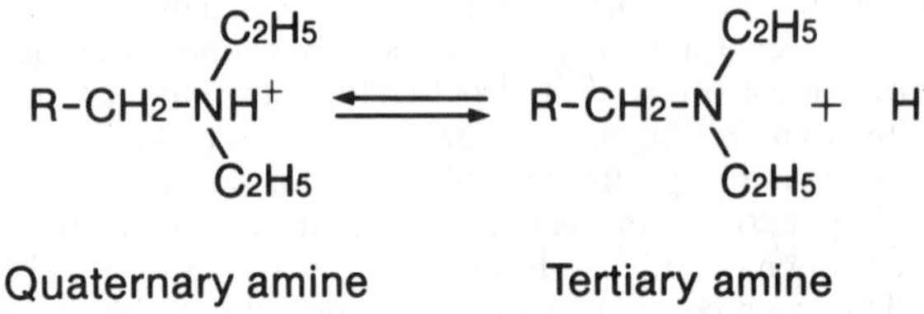

Commercial Preparations

Because the free-base form of most local anesthetics is poorly soluble in aqueous solution, they are prepared as hydrochloride salts dissolved in sterile water or normal saline. The solution is acidified to a pH of 4.40–6.40 to favor existence of the water-soluble, cationic, quaternary amine form of the local anesthetic molecule.[43,44] Unfortunately, this decreases the local anesthetic potency, and although it has been suggested that increasing the pH of the local anesthetic solution may shorten the onset and increase the duration of the blockade,[45,46] this also increases the risk of precipitation of the local anesthetic out of solution. The action of local anesthetics may also be potentiated by carbonation, with the suggested mechanism of action being a direct depressant effect of carbon dioxide on the axon, an increased conversion of the local anesthetic to the active cation form at the site of action inside the axon, or diffusion trapping of the local anesthetic inside the axon.[47-50]

Commercially prepared epinephrine-containing solutions must also be acidified, because alkaline solutions promote

$$R-CH_2-\overset{\overset{\displaystyle C_2H_5}{|}}{\underset{\underset{\displaystyle C_2H_5}{|}}{N}}H^+ \rightleftharpoons R-CH_2-\overset{\overset{\displaystyle C_2H_5}{|}}{\underset{\underset{\displaystyle C_2H_5}{|}}{N}} + H^+$$

Quaternary amine   Tertiary amine

Figure 20-2. The dissociation equilibrium of charged quaternary amine and uncharged tertiary amine local anesthetic molecules in an aqueous solution.

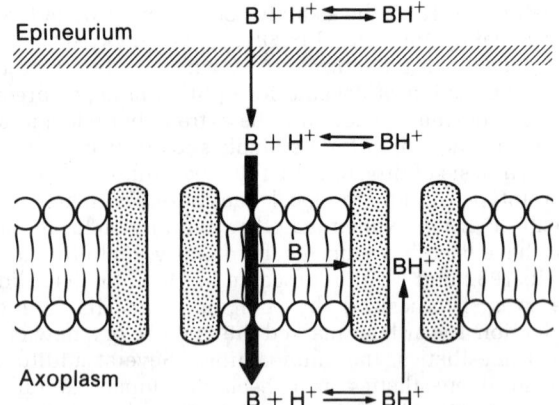

Figure 20-3. Local anesthetic access to the sodium channel. The uncharged molecule diffuses most easily across lipid barriers and interacts with the channel through the axolemma interior. The charged species formed in the axoplasm gains access to a specific receptor *via* the sodium channel pore.

oxidation of catecholamines.[51] However, recent evidence suggests that epinephrine-containing solutions can be alkalinized to a pH range of 7.0–8.0 for a time period of at least 2–6 hours without significant oxidation.[52,53] Antioxidants have also been added to epinephrine-containing solutions as well as to some local anesthetic solutions to retard their breakdown. The antioxidant sodium metabisulfite has been implicated in the reported neurotoxicity of 2-chloroprocaine, although this antioxidant has now been replaced by sodium ethylenediaminetetraacetic acid in 2-chloroprocaine solutions.

Because of their antibacterial and antifungal activity, antimicrobial preservatives are added to local anesthetic solutions contained in multidose vials. Preservative-containing local anesthetic solutions should not be used in spinal, epidural, or caudal anesthesia because of their potentially cytotoxic effects. The most frequently used antimicrobials are the paraben derivatives of para-hydroxybenzoate, such as methylparaben, ethylparaben, and propylparaben. The paraben derivatives are potent allergens and have been implicated in allergic reactions initially attributed to the local anesthetic.[54,55] Because of this, preservative-containing local anesthetics are not recommended for intravenous use.

Proper handling and storage of local anesthetics are important. Because of the possibility of small pieces of glass falling into single-dose ampules when they are opened, some manufacturers prefer to prepare their single-dose local anesthetic solutions in rubber-stoppered vials. However, it must be remembered that these containers do not contain antimicrobial preservatives and should not be used to disperse multiple doses of local anesthetic. Local anesthetic solutions that contain glucose may caramelize with prolonged heat. These solutions should be autoclaved only one time, and they should not remain in the autoclave any longer than necessary. Ampules of local anesthetic should never be sterilized by soaking in an antiseptic solution because of the potential for contamination through unnoticed cracks in the ampule.[56] Any local anesthetic solution containing a free aromatic amino group, such as 2-chloroprocaine and procaine, may be discolored by prolonged exposure to light. Similarly, epinephrine oxidizes with prolonged exposure to light.

MECHANISM OF ACTION OF LOCAL ANESTHETICS

Anatomy of the Peripheral Nerve

The basic unit of the peripheral nerve is the nerve fiber, composed of an axon that is enclosed almost its entire length by a sheath of Schwann cells. The axolemma of the axon is the continuation of the neuronal cell membrane, and it surrounds the axoplasm, the contents of the axon. Schwann cells, like neurons, are ectodermally derived and are vitally important in supporting the life and function of the axons they envelop.[57] The Schwann sheath of the larger peripheral axons contains concentric layers of myelin, a lipoid material that is composed of spiral wraps of the Schwann cell membrane itself.[58] Because of this, nerve fibers are often designated as myelinated or unmyelinated (Fig. 20-4; Table 20-2). Between successive Schwann cells along the length of the axon, there are small, nonmyelinated junctional regions, the nodes of Ranvier. Although the nodal regions of the nerve axon were originally thought to be entirely uncovered and uninsulated, in these areas investigators have more recently noted an array of microvillous interdigitations between the adjacent Schwann cells (Fig. 20-4).[59] A polyanionic ground substance matrix is found between the microvilli, and this organization of microvilli and negatively-charged ground substance may serve as a barrier to limit the access of local anesthetic molecules to the nodal axolemma.[60-63]

The nerve fibers of the peripheral nerve vary in thickness from less than 1 μm to greater than 20 μm. Delicate connective tissue layers around each fiber form the endoneurium. Groups of nerve fibers are bundled together by concentric layers of connective tissue, the perineurium, to form fascicles, and an additional outer layer of connective tissue cells and fibers, the epineurium, holds the fascicles together to form the peripheral nerve (Fig. 20-5).[64] These concentric coverings may be important in limiting the diffusion of local anesthetic into the nerve fibers.[65]

Physiology of the Nerve Fiber

The purpose of the peripheral nerves and their constituent nerve fibers is to carry information, and this is accomplished through electrical signals generated and conducted by neurons.[66] Although electrical potentials exist across the membranes of essentially all cells of the body, nerve cells possess the property of excitability, that is, they respond to stimuli by undergoing transient physiochemical changes that may alter the resting electrical potential of the cell and initiate a nerve impulse. Through the property of conductivity, the action potential, which is a rapid change in membrane potential, is propagated along the axolemma to its end. At the neuron terminal, a neurotransmitter is released, causing excitation of succeeding neurons or of effector cells, such as skeletal muscle.

The axolemma is typical of other cell membranes in that it is a fluid or dynamic mosaic structure of alternating oligosaccharides, globular proteins, and phospholipid bilayers

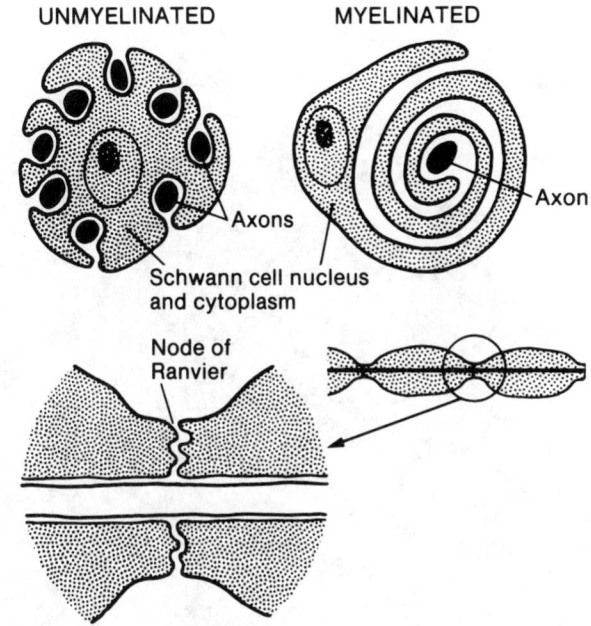

Figure 20-4. Unmyelinated and myelinated nerve fibers, with the microvillous interdigitations of two adjacent Schwann cells at a node of Ranvier.

TABLE 20-2. Classification of Nerve Fibers

Conduction/ Biophysical Classification	Anatomic Location	Myelin	Diameter (μ)	Rate (m·sec^{-1})	Function
A fibers					
A alpha	Afferent to and efferent	Yes	6–22	30–85	Motor and pro-
A beta	from muscles and joints				prioception
A gamma	Efferent to muscle spindles	Yes	3–6	15–35	Muscle tone
A delta	Sensory roots and afferent peripheral nerves	Yes	1–4	5–25	Pain Temperature Touch
B fibers					
	Preganglionic sympathetic	Yes	<3	3–15	Vasomotor Visceromotor Sudomotor Pilomotor
C fibers					
sC	Postganglionic sympathetic	No	0.3–1.3	0.7–1.3	Vasomotor Visceromotor Sudomotor Pilomotor
drC	Sensory roots and afferent peripheral nerves	No	0.4–1.2	0.1–2.0	Pain Temperature Touch

(Fig. 20-6).[67,68] The molecular constituents of the membrane are amphipathic, or structurally asymmetric, with one polar, or hydrophilic, end and one nonpolar, or hydrophobic, end. Since the membrane is in an aqueous environment, the polar groups of the lipids, proteins, and oligosaccharides are oriented so that they are in contact with water, and the nonpolar regions are sequestered within the membrane, away from the aqueous phase.

The axolemma is metabolically active, controlling transmembrane electrochemical potential by active transport in either direction and by controlling its own relative permeability to various ions. Adenosine triphosphate–dependent active transport results in the intracellular fluids containing a high concentration of potassium ions and a low concentration of sodium ions relative to the extracellular fluid. In addition to active transport, the membrane is specifically

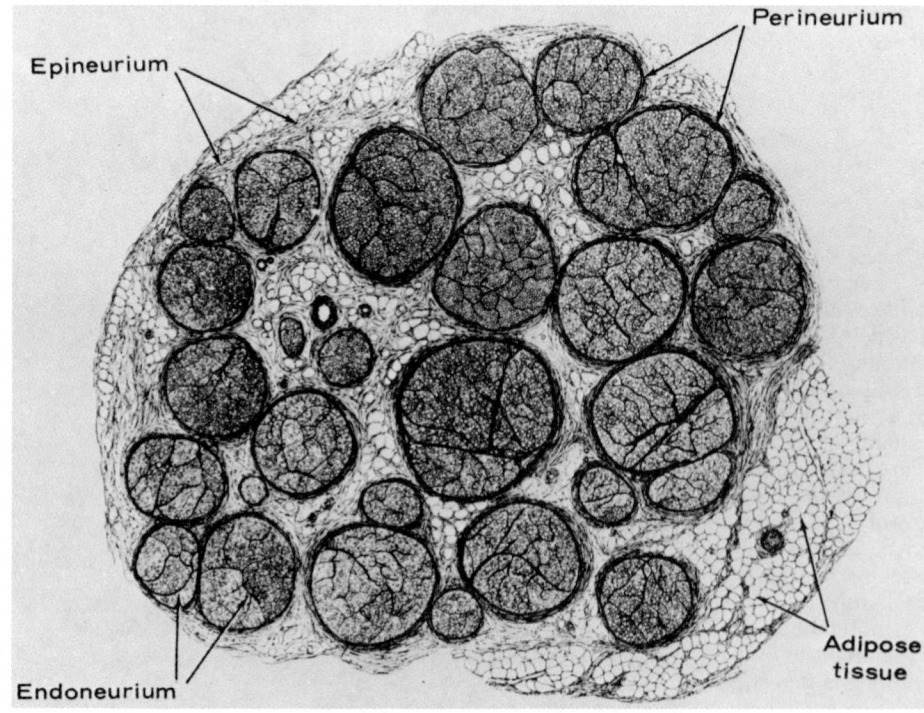

Figure 20-5. Drawing of a cross-section of a human ulnar nerve at very low magnification, illustrating the endoneurium, perineurium, and epineurium as well as the perineural vascular and adipose tissue. (Reprinted with permission from Angevine JB: The nervous tissue. In Fawcett DW (ed): A Textbook of Histology, p 336. Philadelphia, WB Saunders, 1986.)

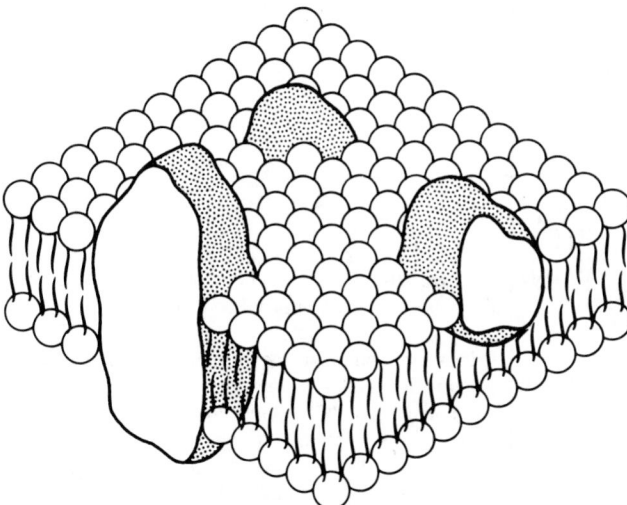

Figure 20-6. The fluid mosaic model of the structure of a typical cell membrane. Globular proteins are partially embedded in a fluid bilayer of phospholipid molecules. The polar groups of the protein molecules protrude from the membrane into the aqueous phase, and their nonpolar groups are buried in the hydrophobic membrane interior. Certain proteins extend entirely through the membrane, and these include those functioning as the ionic channels responsible for the electrical properties of cell membranes. (Redrawn with permission from Singer SJ, Nicolson GL: The fluid mosaic model of the structure of cell membranes. Science 175:723, 1972. Copyright 1972 by the AAAS.)

permeable to potassium ions and allows them to leak out of the cell faster than sodium ions can leak in. The difference in ionic concentration across the membrane results in an electrical potential, or charge, with the interior negative to the exterior in the resting state. The magnitude of the potential inside the membrane relative to the outside is determined by the ratio of the tendency for the ions to diffuse in one direction or the other, and the contribution of a particular ion is quantitated by the Nernst equation:

Membrane potential (millivolts)

$$= -61 \log \frac{\text{intracellular ion concentration}}{\text{extracellular ion concentration}}$$

The degree of importance of each of the ions in determining the voltage is proportional to the membrane permeability for that particular ion. Since, in the resting state, the neuronal membrane is very permeable to potassium and only slightly permeable to sodium, it is potassium, with its Nernst potential of -94 mV, that contributes the most to the membrane potential. However, because there is some contribution to the resting membrane potential by sodium and chloride ions, the membrane resting potential is more accurately calculated from the more complicated Goldman-Hodgkin-Katz equation, and averages -60 to -70 mV, with the cell interior negative relative to the exterior.[69]

Although electrical potentials exist across the cell membranes of most of the cells of the body, it is the development and propagation of rapid changes in membrane potential, the action potential, which allows nerve fibers to carry signals. This electrical excitability is possible because of the presence in the axolemma of voltage-sensitive ion channels that are specific for sodium, potassium, or calcium ions.[70-76] In response to voltage fluctuation, these channels sequentially open and close in gate-like fashion to allow the rapid diffusion of specific ions down their concentration gradients across the axolemma, so that the resultant ionic flux across the cell membrane depolarizes and repolarizes it (Fig. 20-7).

Although the sodium, potassium, and calcium ion channels are each important for initiation and propagation of the action potential in neurons, the properties of the sodium channel and its contribution to the action potential are the most important and best understood. Sodium channels exist in one of three states: closed (or resting), open, and inactivated (Fig. 20-8). When the membrane transiently becomes less negative relative to the resting potential (i.e., increases from the resting voltage of -70 mV toward zero) and the magnitude of the change is sufficient to reach a triggering value or initial threshold potential that is approximately -55 mV, a voltage-dependent conformational change in the closed or resting sodium channel is induced, so that the sodium permeability of the membrane is increased 500- to 5000-fold and the sodium ions are free to move down their electrochemical gradient into the cell. The sodium channel then closes to an inactivated state by voltage- and time-dependent mechanisms, resulting in the membrane's once again becoming impermeable to sodium ions.[77-83] Once inactivated, the sodium channel cannot reopen again until the membrane potential returns to a value near that of the original resting membrane potential, which allows the channel to first return to its closed, or resting, state. The voltage-dependent permeability changes, or gatings, of ion channels result from intrinsic electrical properties of the macromolecules that compose the channel.[84]

Sequential opening and closing of the ion-specific channels allows passive ion fluxes down electrochemical gradients. These ion fluxes change the transmembrane electrical potential and produce an action potential. Because the sodium channels open at the beginning of the action potential, a far greater amount of sodium ions enter the axon than potassium ions exit it. This results in the membrane potential becoming positive. Shortly after the onset of the action potential, the sodium channels close and voltage gating of the potassium channels occurs, resulting in greatly increased transmembrane permeability to potassium ions. At that point, the membrane potential returns to its baseline negative resting potential of approximately -70 mV after first undergoing a transient hyperpolarization (positive after potential) because some of the potassium channels remain open after the repolarization process is completed (Fig. 20-9).

For a signal to be transmitted by a nerve, it is necessary for an action potential to be conducted along a nerve fiber. If a local membrane depolarization is of sufficient magnitude to reach the critical threshold potential and trigger an action potential, the resultant voltage changes are usually of adequate strength to reach the initial threshold of the adjacent membrane segments and result in propagation of the action potential along the nerve fiber. This is called an "all-or-none phenomenon" because either the local depolarization reaches the initial threshold potential of adjacent membrane segments and propagates itself over the entire axolemma or it does not reach the necessary initial threshold voltage potential and the spread of depolarization stops.[85]

Once an action potential is initiated in an unmyelinated nerve fiber, it is propagated as a wave of depolarization that spreads at a constant speed, activating the sodium channels of each successive membrane segment as it travels along the axon. The larger the diameter of the fiber, the greater the speed of this impulse traveling along it.[85,86] Myelinization of nerve fibers is an adaptation that greatly increases the

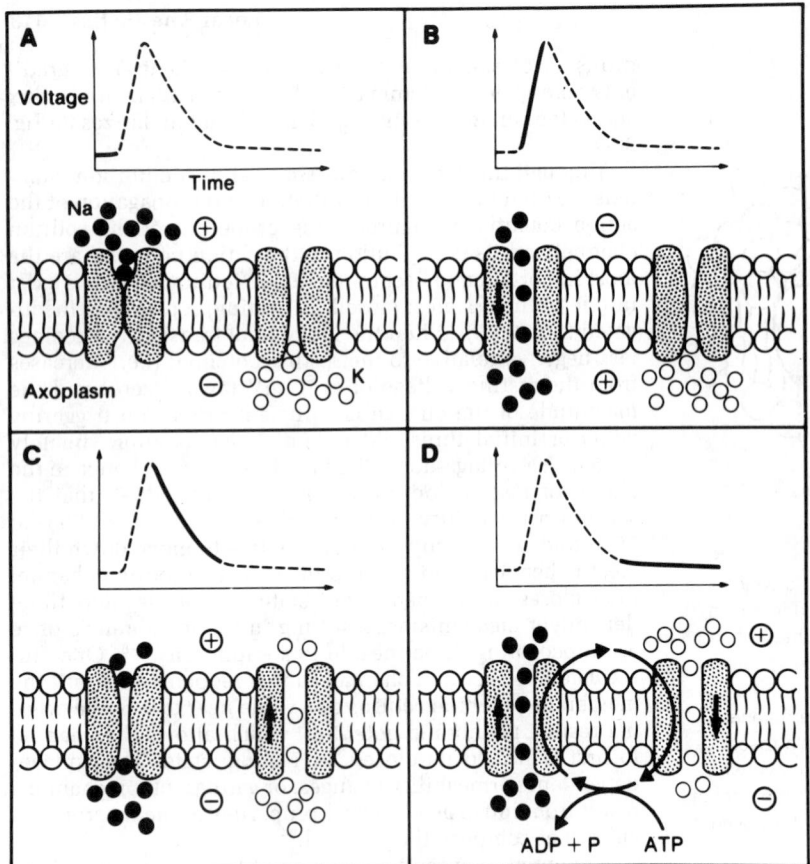

Figure 20-7. Sodium and potassium ion flux across the axolemma *via* specific channels and the resultant nerve action potential. At rest (*A*) an ATP-dependent pumping mechanism creates ionic gradients across the axolemma, with a relative excess of sodium ions (●) exterior to the cell and a relative excess of potassium ions (○) in the cell interior. During depolarization of the neuron (*B*), sodium channel pores open and sodium ions flow freely down their electrochemical gradient into the cell. During repolarization (*C*), sodium channels close and the axolemma is no longer permeable to sodium ions, but potassium ion channels open and potassium ions flow down their electrochemical gradient out of the cell. Upon completion of the action potential (*D*), sodium and potassium ions are actively transported back to the cell exterior and interior, respectively. (Redrawn with permission from Covino BG, Scott DB: Handbook of Epidural Anaesthesia and Analgesia, p 58. Orlando, Grune & Stratton, 1985.)

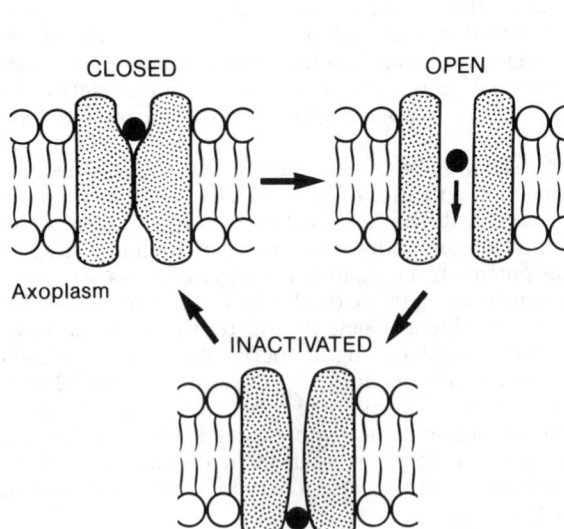

Figure 20-8. The three sodium channel states: closed or resting, open, and inactivated. Once inactivated, a sodium channel cannot reopen until the original resting membrane potential is reestablished, allowing the channel to first return to its closed, or resting, state.

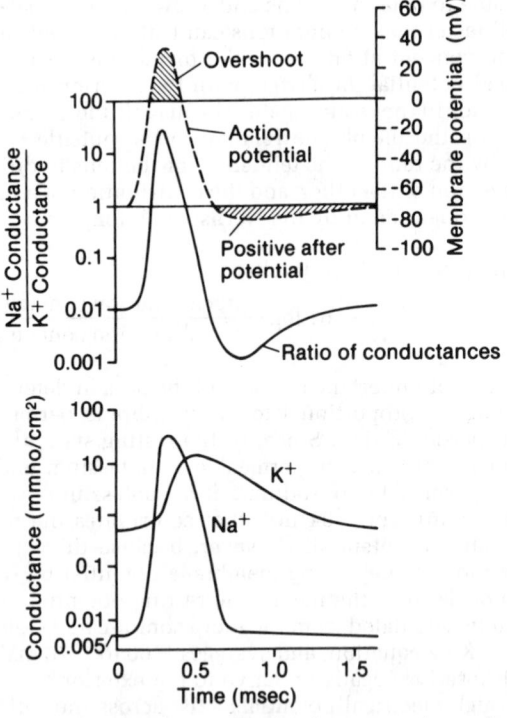

Figure 20-9. Sodium and potassium ion flux across the axolemma during an action potential. Note that sodium conductance increases several thousand-fold during the early stages of the action potential, yet potassium conductance increases only approximately 30-fold during the latter phase of the action potential. (Redrawn with permission from Guyton AC: Textbook of Medical Physiology, p 109. Philadelphia, WB Saunders, 1986.)

speed and efficiency of impulse transmission when compared with impulse transmission of unmyelinated nerve fibers of equal diameter.[87] Myelin is an excellent insulator, increasing the resistance to ion flow through the axolemma approximately 5000-fold. However, between successive Schwann cells along the length of the axon are the small, unmyelinated, junctional regions, the nodes of Ranvier, where ions can flow in relatively unimpeded fashion between the axoplasm and the extracellular fluid during an action potential. In addition, the nodal regions of the axolemma contain dense concentrations of sodium channels, which is in contrast to the internodal and perinodal regions, where few, if any, sodium channels exist.[88,89] Because of these factors, in myelinated nerve fibers, the action potential can occur only at the nodes of Ranvier; therefore the nerve impulse is forced to jump from node to node. This process, called saltatory conduction, contributes to increased speed and efficiency of neural transmission through several mechanisms. Because the nerve impulse jumps from node to node instead of spreading directly to adjacent axolemma segments, the velocity of conduction is increased an average of five to seven times. Since only the nodal regions of the axons depolarize, the total ion flux across the entire neural membrane is greatly decreased, and the energy expenditure needed to re-establish cationic gradients across the membrane after a series of depolarizations is less. Last, because conduction of the nerve impulse is an all-or-none phenomenon, propagation of the action potential may be more likely in myelinated fibers because the higher density of sodium channels in the nodal regions reduces the threshold for excitation by allowing generation of an action potential when a smaller percentage of the channels are activated.[79]

Electrophysiologic Effects of Local Anesthetics

Although local anesthetics alter potassium and calcium ion conductance across excitable membranes, inhibition of sodium ion influx across the neuronal cell membrane is the common mechanism of action through which all local anesthetic agents produce blockade of the nerve impulse.[4,7,91,92] To block the generation and conduction of the action potentials, local anesthetics must interfere with the function of the ion channels that specifically conduct sodium ions across the membrane.[90-96] The ionic gradients and resting membrane potential of the nerve are unchanged, but the increase in sodium permeability associated with the nerve impulse is inhibited. Since a wide variety of chemical compounds exhibit local anesthetic activity, it is unlikely that they all block sodium conductance in the same manner. Several theories regarding the mechanism of action of local anesthetics include calcium-mediated local anesthetic inhibition of sodium flux; interference with membrane permeability by expansion of membrane volume; local anesthetic-induced changes in the surface charge of the axolemma; and local anesthetic interaction with a specific receptor in the neuronal membrane.

Displacement of calcium from a membrane site that controls sodium permeability has been advanced as a mechanism of local anesthetic activity.[97] A low calcium ion concentration outside the neuron enhances local anesthetic activity, and an increasing external calcium concentration antagonizes the blocking action of local anesthetics. However, the direct actions of calcium and local anesthetics appear to be independent of each other.[98,99] Thus, it is unlikely

that calcium directly mediates the activity of local anesthetic agents.

A second theory regarding the mechanism of local anesthetic activity involves an application of the Meyer-Overton rule of anesthesia. It postulates that diffusion of the relatively lipophilic anesthetic molecules into the lipid component of the neuronal membrane expands the membrane to a critical volume and interferes with sodium conductance. Decreased sodium permeability could occur either through an increase in the lateral pressure in the membrane, which would directly compress the sodium channels, or through a conformational change in the proteins of the sodium channels brought about by an increase in the degree of the disorder of the membrane lipid molecules.[100-102] Local anesthetic agents have been shown both to increase the volume of lipid membranes and to increase their degree of disorder and, thus, fluidity.[103-107] High-pressure antagonism of the anesthetic activity of certain uncharged local anesthetic molecules, such as benzyl alcohol and benzocaine, has been shown to occur by some investigators and may be evidence for the applicability of the membrane expansion theory to the mechanism of action of these compounds.[108,109] However, pressure reversal has not been shown to occur in the case of charged local anesthetics, and there is no direct evidence that membrane expansion is important in their activity. These findings, as well as others, indicate that charged and uncharged local anesthetic molecules may have separate sites of action and that membrane expansion may be more important for the action of only the uncharged local anesthetics.[110]

A third proposal for the mechanism of action of local anesthetics involves the induction of alterations in the membrane surface charge. Because some of the neuronal membrane molecules contain hydrophilic, anionic tails that are arrayed so that they protrude outward from the membrane lipid to both the external (extracellular) and internal (axoplasmic) surfaces of the membrane, both surfaces of the axolemma are negatively charged relative to the membrane interior.[111,112] These fixed negative charges attract cations such as sodium and calcium, and these charge interactions add to the electrochemical resting potential to yield the net transmembrane potential.[113] The fixed negative charges of the membrane's two surfaces may also attract cationic local anesthetic molecules, aligning the charged local anesthetic molecule at the membrane-water interface with its nonpolar, aromatic domain in the membrane lipid and its hydrophilic, charged portion in the adjacent aqueous phase.[114] The cationic local anesthetic molecule thus neutralizes the fixed negative charges on the membrane surface to a variable degree and alters the transmembrane potential (Fig. 20-10).[115] If the local anesthetic molecule is absorbed to the extracellular side of the axonal membrane, the extra positive charges there could add to the already relatively positive extracellular charge and hyperpolarize the membrane, resulting in it being more difficult for an approaching nerve impulse to raise the transmembrane potential to depolarization threshold. On the other hand, if the local anesthetic molecule is absorbed into the intracellular side of the axonal membrane, the increase in positive charge could prevent sufficient repolarization of the membrane interior to allow for reactivation of sodium channels inactivated by a previous action potential. If sufficient sodium channels remain in the inactivated state, a subsequent action potential could not occur. Either mechanism could produce neural blockade.

The surface charge theory has the support of several investigators and also accounts for the antagonism between

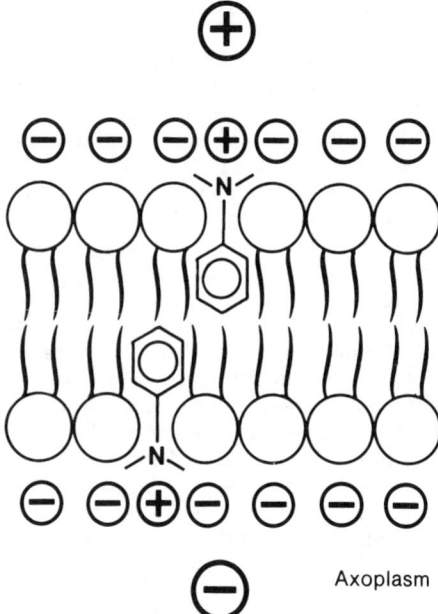

Axoplasm

Figure 20-10. Neutralization of membrane surface fixed negative charges by cationic local anesthetic molecules, according to the surface charge theory. The additional positive charges on the relatively positive-charged extracellular surface of the axolemma may hyperpolarize the membrane. The additional positive charges on the relatively negative-charged intracellular surface of the axolemma may prevent sufficient membrane repolarization for reactivation of sodium channels. Thus, additional positive charges provided by local anesthetic molecules at either axolemma surface could interfere with the development of action potentials. (Redrawn with permission from Scurlock JE: The mechanism of action of local anesthetics. Reg Anesth 2:5, 1977.)

divalent cations, such as calcium, and local anesthetic compounds.[114-117] Although the surface charge hypothesis may account for the action of charged local anesthetics, it does not explain the ability of uncharged local anesthetics, such as benzyl alcohol and benzocaine, to block nerve impulses. However, the failure of a single theory to satisfactorily explain the actions of all local anesthetic types does not necessarily invalidate it. Different local anesthetic molecules may have different mechanisms of action.

The fourth and most popular theory regarding the mechanism of action of local anesthetics proposes that they interact directly with specific receptors in the neuronal membrane.[118,119] These receptors, in turn, affect specific ion channels of the neuronal membrane in such a fashion that the ionic flux needed for initiation and propagation of the action potential is inhibited.

The structure of the sodium channel is apparently that of a lipoglycoprotein that spans the neuronal membrane and contains an aqueous pore that is able to discriminate between sodium and other ions, being selectively more permeable to sodium.[120-123] Intrinsic electrical properties of the macromolecules that compose the channel allow it to change configuration in response to changes in membrane potential, thus determining conductance of sodium ions across the axolemma. The distribution of the population of sodium channels between the resting and inactivated states, as previously described, is an important determinant of the refractory behavior of neurons. Immediately following an

action potential, many of the sodium channels are in the inactivated state and cannot be reopened by a subsequent voltage change.[123] Therefore, once an excitable membrane has been depolarized by an action potential, it cannot conduct a second impulse until it has first repolarized and thereby allowed inactivated sodium channels to return to the resting state. If an adequate number of sodium channels are not present in the resting state, sodium current sufficient for a second action potential cannot be generated.

The property of use- or frequency-dependent blockade, in which neuronal blockade by charged local anesthetic molecules increases with repetitive, brief membrane depolarizations, is one phenomenon that suggests direct interaction between sodium channel receptors and the charged local anesthetic molecule.[124,125] It is postulated that frequency dependence develops because charged, hydrophilic anesthetic molecules inhibit sodium ion conductance through the sodium channel by gaining access to a channel receptor, located within the channel itself, while the sodium channel pore is in the open state. Reversal of the local anesthetic inhibitory effect would also require an open channel pore to facilitate the dissociation of the local anesthetic molecule, and, thus, a closed channel containing a local anesthetic molecule would be slow to return to its uninhibited state. In contrast to charged anesthetics, neutral anesthetic compounds exhibit much less frequency-dependent blockade, and this may be the result of these molecules not being restricted to the aqueous phase, gaining access to a channel binding site through the lipid milieu of the membrane interior.[126,127] Local anesthetics may also shift the sodium channel population to a nonconducting state by binding preferentially to channels that have already been inactivated, preventing their return to the resting, depolarization-susceptible configuration.

In addition to interacting with sodium channels that are in the open and in the inactivated state, it appears that local anesthetics can also produce a tonic, or resting, block by binding with the channels in the resting state to prevent their voltage-induced activation.[123] This third type of local anesthetic sodium channel association appears to be much weaker. The discovery that the blocking potency of local anesthetic molecules is much greater when the interaction is with receptors of open or inactivated channels, as compared to those of resting channels, has led to the modulated receptor hypothesis of local anesthetic-receptor binding.[126,128-131] The variable state of the local anesthetic receptor determines the strength of its interaction with the local anesthetic molecule, and an excitable membrane with a higher depolarization frequency is more sensitive to the blocking effects of local anesthetics. The charged local anesthetics interact with all three sodium channel states, and the resultant variable drug potency is manifested as frequency-dependent blockade. Use or frequency dependence may be a mechanism by which a local anesthetic solution causes a differential blockade of the fibers within a given nerve.

At this time, it is uncertain as to where exactly the local anesthetic receptors of the sodium channel are located, and there may be at least three sites of local anesthetic binding (Fig. 20-11). One is located near the interior opening of the sodium pore and has a higher affinity for the more charged local anesthetic molecules, and one is located at the interface between the sodium channel structure and the surrounding membrane lipid, being more easily accessed by uncharged, lipophilic local anesthetic molecules.[123,132,133] In addition, there are a variety of other sodium channel sites where certain pharmacologic compounds and toxins spe-

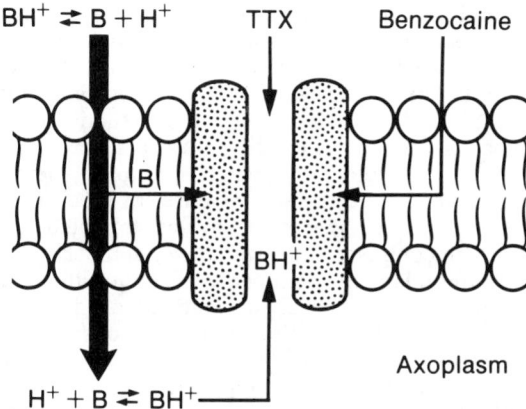

Figure 20-11. Sites of action of different types of local anesthetics. Aminoesters and aminoamides act at the axoplasmic surface of the sodium channels in their charged form (BH^+), or, to a lesser extent, at the intramembrane portion of the sodium channels in their base form (B). Uncharged local anesthetics, such as benzocaine, also act from within the membrane interior. Tetrodotoxin (TTX) and other biotoxins have sites of action at the external aspect of the sodium channels. (Redrawn with permission from Covino BG, Scott DB: Handbook of Epidural Anaesthesia and Analgesia, p. 64. Orlando, Grune & Stratton, 1985.)

cifically combine.[122] Tetrodotoxin, produced by several species of puffer fish, frogs, and newts; and saxitotoxin, produced by a marine dinoflagellate, are examples of other molecules that specifically bind to sodium channels. They directly interact with the outer aspect of the sodium channel to block sodium conductance.[134,135] A large number of sodium channel toxins exist, with differing modalities of sodium channel interaction.[136,137] Veratridine, a steroidal alkaloid, has been shown to preferentially inhibit C fibers in a frequency-dependent manner. Although toxins such as veratridine are not clinically important at present as local anesthetics, further investigation of these substances may produce new classes of local anesthetics that preferentially block nociceptive traffic.[138,139]

Minimum Blocking Concentration (C_m)

The minimum blocking concentration, or C_m, of a local anesthetic is the lowest concentration of anesthetic that blocks impulse conduction along a given nerve fiber or nerve within a specified time. The concept of C_m is analogous to the minimum alveolar concentration (MAC) of inhalational anesthetics and is a direct indication of the relative potency of a given anesthetic.[140] However, this value is determined *in vitro* and is extremely influenced by minor variations in experimental conditions.[141] For example, minor variations in the temperature, pH, or calcium ion concentration of the solution bathing the nerve will alter the value of C_m.[141-143] Similarly, the frequency of nerve stimulation also affects the apparent potency of the local anesthetic.

Despite the determination of differential potencies of local anesthetics *in vitro* (different C_ms), these relationships may not be directly applicable to clinical practice. Differences in diffusion, local tissue binding, systemic absorption, and nerve penetration affect the concentration of local anesthetic that ultimately develops in a nerve after injection of a given dose. Because intraneural concentrations of local anesthetics are rarely measured, clinical use is based on a dose-response relationship.

Dose-response relationships, in humans, suggest that pregnancy reduces the anesthetic requirement necessary to achieve a given level of epidural anesthesia.[144] *In vitro* comparison of nerve fibers from pregnant and nonpregnant rabbits suggests that pregnancy may increase the sensitivity of nerve membranes to local anesthetics.[145,146]

Differential Block

It has long been a clinical observation that all neuronal functions are not affected by local anesthetics in equal fashion. For example, blockade of the components of a peripheral nerve may proceed at different rates, with loss of sympathetic function first, followed by pin-prick sensation, touch, and temperature, and last motor function, or there may be relative sparing of one neuronal function over another, as in the low-dose bupivacaine labor epidural anesthesia that leaves motor tone relatively intact. Clinical findings such as these have given rise to the concept of differential blockade of the various nerve fiber types, and currently there are several potential explanations for the existence of this phenomenon. No uniformly accepted theory exists at present because of conflicting data generated by investigations performed under differing laboratory conditions and because of the difficulty of designing a suitable laboratory model. Also, there may very well be several independent mechanisms for differential blockade.

Peripheral nerve fibers have been classified according to size and function (see Table 20-2).[147,148] Myelinated somatic nerve fibers, or A fibers, are largest in diameter and conduct impulses the most rapidly. These are further divided according to progressively decreasing size into alpha, beta, gamma, and delta fibers. The alpha and beta fibers convey motor and proprioception information, the gamma fibers control muscle spindle tone, and the delta fibers, which are the smallest in diameter of the A fibers, transmit messages concerning pain, temperature, and touch. In contrast to the A fibers, which, as a group, are quite variable in diameter, ranging from 6 to 22 µm, the B and C fibers are much more uniform in size. The thinly myelinated B fibers are smaller in diameter than A fibers and have a preganglionic autonomic function. The unmyelinated C fibers are the smallest diameter nerve fibers, have the lowest rate of impulse conduction velocity, and contain postganglionic autonomic axons as well as axons conveying pain, temperature, and touch information.[149]

For many years, it was felt that differential blockade could be explained on the basis of the relative vulnerability of various neuronal fiber types to the blocking activity of local anesthetic solutions, with fiber diameter inversely proportional to susceptibility to local anesthetic blockade. Thus, the larger A fibers were thought to be less susceptible to blockade, whereas the small C fibers were thought to be the most easily blocked.[150] This inverse relationship between fiber size and susceptibility to local anesthetic blockade was drawn from *in vitro* data obtained using differently sized myelinated fibers only,[148] and it was subsequently shown that its application to the small C fibers did not hold true once C fibers were actually studied.[151-158] A delta and B fibers were found to be more susceptible to local anesthetic blockade than the relatively smaller C fibers, and later the largest A fibers were noted by some investigators to actually be the most susceptible of all to local anesthetic block. Thus, nerve fiber vulnerability to local anesthetic action varies directly with fiber size, the largest A fibers being the most sensitive and the small C fibers being the least sensitive.[159-161]

One explanation for the relative susceptibilities of different nerve fiber types to local anesthetic block involves the concept of conduction safety. A voltage change substantially greater than the action potential threshold of the adjacent membrane provides a margin of safety for continued conduction of the action potential. This ratio of the values of the nerve impulse voltage change to the adjacent membrane action potential threshold is termed the safety factor, and impulse propagation will fail if this value falls below 1, such as in local anesthetic blockade.[150,162,163] The conduction safety factor of smaller myelinated fibers may be less than that of larger myelinated fibers, making the smaller fibers more vulnerable to the effects of local anesthetics. Since local anesthetics must block at least three adjacent nodes of Ranvier to halt impulse propagation,[164] and since internodal distance is directly proportional to fiber size,[165] a relatively small distribution of local anesthetic solution may be sufficient to differentially block the smaller fibers (Fig. 20-12).[153,154] The conduction safety factor may be greater for nonmyelinated fibers, since only the immediately adjacent area of the axonal membrane must reach depolarization threshold for propagation of the action potential, whereas in myelinated fibers, the current generated at one node must be sufficient to depolarize the membrane of the next node some distance away. This may explain the relative *in vitro* resistance of nonmyelinated fibers to local anesthetic blockade.[63,166-168] An additional finding is that the safety factor of an individual nerve fiber is variable, depending on the location along the fiber itself, the degree of impulse activity, the CO_2 tension, and the local ionic gradients.[169-172] Because of the interaction of these factors, the relative effects of a local anesthetic upon different nerve fibers may be a dynamic phenomenon.

Although the large, fast-conducting A fibers have been found by some to be intrinsically the most sensitive to blockade by local anesthetics and the small, slow-conducting C fibers the least sensitive, this fact is not always immediately apparent in clinical situations involving nerve blocks. This may be a reflection of the relative rate of onset of block in different fiber types in contrast to the relative susceptibility of different fibers to local anesthetic blockade in the setting of a steady-state local anesthetic concentration. Because of the decreased ability of local anesthetic molecules to cross the multilayered lipoprotein membranes of the myelin sheath, the rate of onset of block is slower in A fibers when compared to the unmyelinated C fibers. Therefore, in contrast to the rapid onset of block in C fibers owing to the relatively unimpeded local anesthetic access to the axon, the slower local anesthetic blockade of A fibers depends on the pK_a and lipid partition coefficient of the local anesthetic molecule.[160,161,168,173] The lower the pK_a (and thus the greater the percentage of lipophilic, uncharged molecules at physiologic pH) and the greater the lipid partition coefficient of the local anesthetic molecule, the more rapid the onset of block in the A fibers. However, in high concentrations, even a relatively hydrophilic local anesthetic will produce a rapid block of A fibers because the greater diffusion gradient will cause a more rapid transit across the myelin sheath. Thus, the use of a lower concentration of a less lipid-soluble local anesthetic would be most likely to result in a differential blockade of A delta and C fibers at the onset of the nerve block.

The exact mechanism of differential blockade has not been conclusively demonstrated, and there may very well be more than one factor involved. Despite the general agreement that the unmyelinated C fibers are less sensitive to local anesthetics than the larger A and B fibers, the concepts of size-related differential susceptibility of myelinated nerve fibers to local anesthetic blockade, as well as of the myelin sheath as a barrier to local anesthetic diffusion, are not universally accepted.[174-180] The difference in the length of myelinated axon exposed to local anesthetic (i.e., the difference in the number of nodes of Ranvier bathed by anesthetic) may be the major clinical determinant in differential block.[181] It has been suggested that differential blockade may be the manifestation of a frequency-dependent process, with more rapidly firing fibers, such as those conveying sensory information, being more susceptible to blockade than slower firing fibers, such as somatic motor efferents.[170,182-185] Differential block may also be a reflection of the geographic arrangement of the nerve fibers within the peripheral nerve, with the outermost fibers blocked preferentially if the local anesthetic solution bathing the nerve is dilute enough so that there is a concentration gradient of local anesthetic extending from the outermost layers of the nerve to its center.[186,187]

PHARMACOKINETICS

Pharmacokinetics describes the movement of a drug through the body: movement into the bloodstream, movement from blood into tissues, and movement out of the body by metabolism and excretion. Pharmacodynamics describes the drug's effect on the body (usually expressed as a concentration-effect relationship). An understanding of pharmacokinetics enables anesthesiologists to predict the concentration of drug that will develop at the desired organ and thus to predict the effect that will be produced.

For regional anesthesia, local anesthetic is injected in close proximity to the site of desired effect so that local, physical factors become much more important than systemic pharmacokinetic factors for predicting the desired pharmacodynamic effect (e.g., neural blockade) (Fig. 20-13).

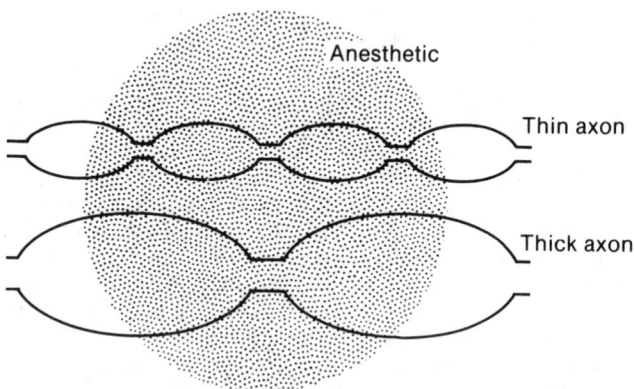

Figure 20-12. Differential blockade of myelinated nerve fibers of differing diameters. Internodal distance is proportional to axon diameter, and conduction blockade occurs when at least three adjacent nodes of a nerve fiber are exposed to blocking concentrations of the local anesthetic agent. Thus, equivalent spread of local anesthetic may produce conduction blockade of a thin axon but not the adjacent thick axon. (Redrawn with permission from Franz DN, Perry RS: Mechanisms for differential block among single myelinated and non-myelinated axons by procaine. J Physiol 236:207, 1974.)

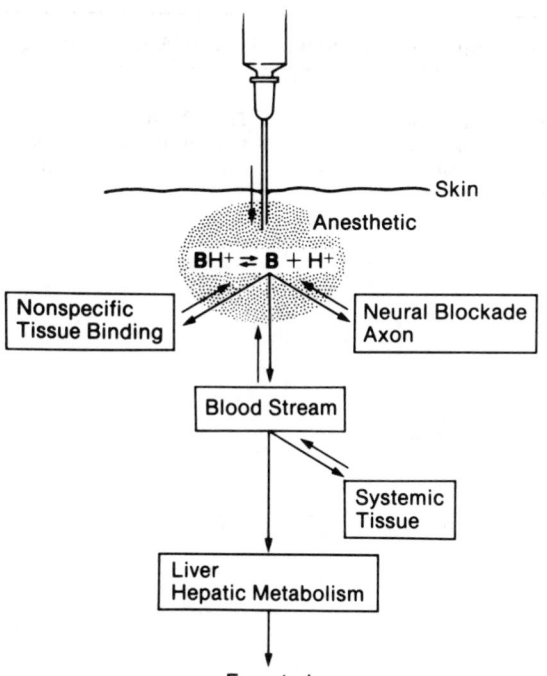

Figure 20-13. This figure depicts the factors determining the distribution of local anesthetic near the site of injection and within the body. A relatively high concentration of local anesthetic is injected in close proximity to a nerve bundle. Non-ionized anesthetic (**B**) diffuses into the axon and provides neural blockade. Nonspecific tissue binding (*e.g.*, to fat, muscle, or connective tissue) and absorption into the bloodstream reduce the mass of drug available to diffuse into neural tissue. Once absorbed into the bloodstream, the local anesthetics are distributed to systemic tissues and are metabolized in the liver to compounds that are primarily excreted by the kidney.

The goal in regional anesthesia is to use just enough local anesthetic to provide adequate anesthesia but less than the amount that will produce toxicity. Ideally, the minimum dose required would be determined by the minimum concentration of local anesthetic in the nerve necessary to produce the desired degree of neural blockade. However, the concentration that develops in neural tissue is difficult to predict because of the complex interaction of multiple factors, including (1) the proximity of the injected anesthetic to the nerve tissue, (2) the flow of anesthetic around the neural tissue, (3) diffusion across the tissue barriers and into neural tissue, (4) binding of anesthetic to local non-neural tissues, and (5) absorption into the vascular and lymph systems.

Thus, identical doses of local anesthetic used for the same block may result in markedly different concentrations of local anesthetic in the nerves, and dose-response relationships are extremely variable. Appreciation of this variability of effect, combined with the fact that many regional anesthetic techniques are performed with a single injection of drug, with no titration to effect, causes most anesthesiologists to use maximal doses of local anesthetic for regional blockade in an attempt to reduce the incidence of inadequate blocks. An understanding of pharmacokinetics allows us to predict peak blood levels resulting from a given dose of drug, and, it is hoped, define the maximum dose that can be administered and still avoid systemic toxicity.

In the following section, we will address local disposition of anesthetic, which is determined by bulk flow, diffusion, and systemic absorption. Then we will examine systemic distribution and elimination of absorbed anesthetic, interactions with other commonly used drugs, and the effects of coexistent disease.

Local Disposition

Bulk Flow

Because intraneural injection is painful and may result in nerve damage, local anesthetic should always be injected near the nerve.[188,189] The amount of anesthetic that reaches the nerve depends, to a large extent, on the proximity of injection to the nerve. The drug then needs to diffuse through connective tissue and past fat to reach the nerve (Fig. 20-13). The barriers to diffusion and the amount of adipose tissue vary considerably among different nerves in the body. For example, spinal nerve roots are floating free in cerebrospinal fluid, and the application of small amounts of local anesthetic produces profound blockade. In contrast, brachial plexus and sciatic nerves are surrounded by fascial sheaths and adipose tissue, and the application of large amounts of drug is necessary to provide reliable anesthesia.

It seems obvious that a larger volume of local anesthetic solution will spread by bulk flow to a greater extent, and should therefore produce a greater spread of nerve block. However, bulk flow and spread of anesthesia are not synonymous. For example, physical spread of local anesthetic solution in the epidural space is not directly correlated with the resulting clinical spread of anesthesia.[190,191] Concentration, or total mass of drug, also affects the spread, probably by influencing diffusion gradients. Separating the effects of volume, concentration, and mass is difficult.[192,193] It is likely that both factors are important: a minimum volume is necessary to provide adequate spread of local anesthetic around the nerves, and a minimum concentration is necessary to provide an adequate diffusion gradient for penetrance into the nerve. Furthermore, once above these minimum values, the total mass of drug becomes most important.[193]

Diffusion

After the local anesthetic is injected near the nerve, it must then move to the nerve, into the nerve, and within the nerve. These movements occur through the process of diffusion. During this process, the anesthetic is diluted by absorption into tissues, blood, and lymph. Although smaller compounds diffuse faster, the small range of differences in molecular weights of local anesthetics should not produce clinically significant differences in diffusion rates. Therefore, the rapidity and extent of diffusion depend to the largest extent upon the pK_a of the local anesthetic, the concentration of anesthetic injected, and possibly the lipid solubility.

Because the pK_a of all local anesthetics is higher than physiologic pH and higher than the pH of all commercially available local anesthetic solutions, most of the injected anesthetic is in the ionized, less lipid-soluble, form (see Table 20-1; Table 20-3). The ionized form of the drug diffuses poorly, whereas the non-ionized (free-base) form is thought to be freely diffusible (see Fig. 20-2). Consequently, the relatively high pK_a of tetracaine and procaine may, in part, explain these agents' relatively poor ability to spread and penetrate tissues. However, tetracaine is very effective when

TABLE 20-3. Chemical Structure, Physiochemical Properties, and Maximum Dose of Selected Local Anesthetic Agents

	Chemical Structure			Relative Lipid Solubility	Protein Binding (%)	pK$_a$	Equieffective Concentration (%)	Maximum Dose (mg)
	Aromatic End	Intermediate Chain	Amine End					
Aminoesters								
Procaine	H$_2$N-◯---	COOCH$_2$CH$_2$	-N(C$_2$H$_5$)(C$_2$H$_5$)	1	5	8.9	2	1000
2-Chloroprocaine	H$_2$N-◯(Cl)---	COOCH$_2$CH$_2$	-N(C$_2$H$_5$)(C$_2$H$_5$)	1	—	9.1	2	1000
Tetracaine	H$_9$C$_4$-N(H)-◯---	COOCH$_2$CH$_2$	-N(CH$_3$)(CH$_3$)	80	85	8.6	0.25	200
Aminoamides								
Lidocaine	◯(CH$_3$)(CH$_3$)---	NHCOCH$_2$	-N(C$_2$H$_5$)(C$_2$H$_5$)	4	65	7.9	1	500
Prilocaine	◯(CH$_3$)---	NHCOCH(CH$_3$)	-N(C$_3$H$_7$)(H)	1.5	55	7.7	1	900
Mepivacaine	◯(CH$_3$)(CH$_3$)---	NHCO	piperidine N-CH$_3$	1	75	7.6	1	500
Bupivacaine	◯(CH$_3$)(CH$_3$)---	NHCO	piperidine N-C$_4$H$_9$	30	95	8.1	0.25	200
Etidocaine	◯(CH$_3$)(CH$_3$)---	NHCOCH(C$_2$H$_5$)	-N(C$_2$H$_5$)(C$_3$H$_7$)	140	95	7.7	0.25	300

Adapted with permission from the publisher from Bonica JJ: Principles and Practice of Obstetric Analgesia and Anesthesia, p 476. Philadelphia, FA Davis, 1967.

injected into the subarachnoid space, where diffusion barriers are minimal.

Alkalinization of the injected solution increases the proportion of non-ionized drug and should facilitate diffusion.[46] In contrast, ampules of local anesthetic with epinephrine added have lower pH values than plain local anesthetic solutions and might, therefore, diffuse less readily.[44] Similarly, any factor that lowers extracellular pH, such as acidosis from local infection, will retard diffusion of local anesthetics because of increased ionization.

Higher concentrations, or greater total mass, of local anesthetic penetrate thicker nerve fibers, intensify the blockade, and may speed onset.[194,195] Presumably, this occurs because of increased diffusion gradients.

Local anesthetics with high lipid solubility would be expected to penetrate membranes more readily and have higher potency and longer duration. However, the ability to spread is offset by increased penetration into and nonspecific binding with fat, muscle, and other tissues. Thus, high lipid solubility might impede diffusion to the nerve receptor sites through nonspecific binding and delay the onset of anesthesia. Finally, local tissue binding may serve as a depot, slowly releasing local anesthetic to the nerve and prolonging duration. In conclusion, diffusion is affected by multiple factors whose ultimate interaction must often be observed and explained rather than predicted.

Kinetics of Nerve Block

In isolated nerve preparations, the sensitivity to local anesthetics is found by some authors to vary, depending on nerve diameter. Thus, in a clinical situation, the order of neural blockade might be expected to be analgesia, anesthesia, paresis, and finally paralysis. However, when the onset of neural blockade is critically examined for the brachial plexus, paresis occurs prior to analgesia.[186] Although these results appear to be inconsistent at first, this discrepancy can easily be explained by anatomic factors.

When local anesthetic is deposited near the brachial plexus, it must diffuse to the nerves before blockade results. Because the local anesthetic concentration at the outside of the nerve trunk is initially higher than in the center, the nerve bundles at the outside (mantle bundles) of the nerve trunk are blocked first, and onset of anesthesia is proximal to distal (Fig. 20-14). Motor nerve fibers are usually at the periphery of the nerve trunk and sensory fibers in the center (or core). Consequently, if the concentration of local anesthetic injected is sufficient to produce motor blockade, the onset of motor blockade precedes the onset of sensory blockade.[186] Similar results would not be expected for regional anesthetic techniques where diffusion barriers are minimal, such as spinal anesthesia.

Systemic Absorption

The rate of systemic absorption is an important factor in determining the peak blood level (Cmax) that results from injection of local anesthetic, the amount of local anesthetic remaining at the site of injection, and thus the duration of anesthesia. The most important factors affecting Cmax are (1) the total dose of local anesthetic, (2) the site of injection, (3) the physiochemical properties of the local anesthetic, and (4) the addition of vasoconstrictors.

The higher the total dose of local anesthetic administered, the higher the peak blood level that results (Fig. 20-15). This relationship between dose and maximum blood level is al-

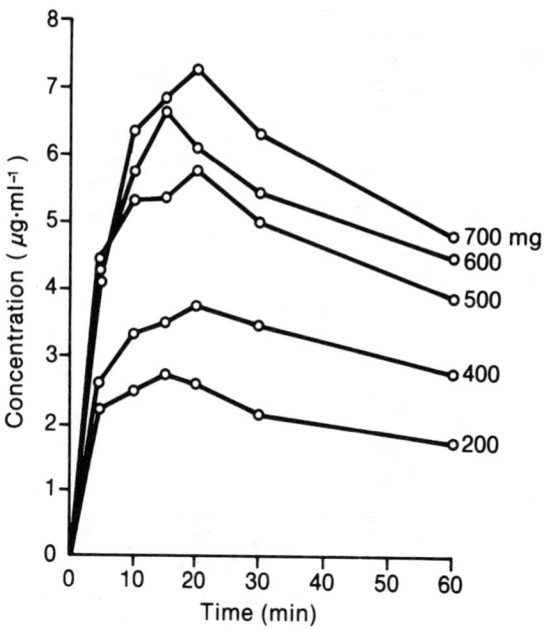

Figure 20-15. Mean plasma concentrations of lidocaine, resulting from epidural injection, increase with increasing doses. (From Braid DP, Scott DB: Dosage of lignocaine in epidural block in relation to toxicity. Br J Anaesth 38:596, 1966, with permission.)

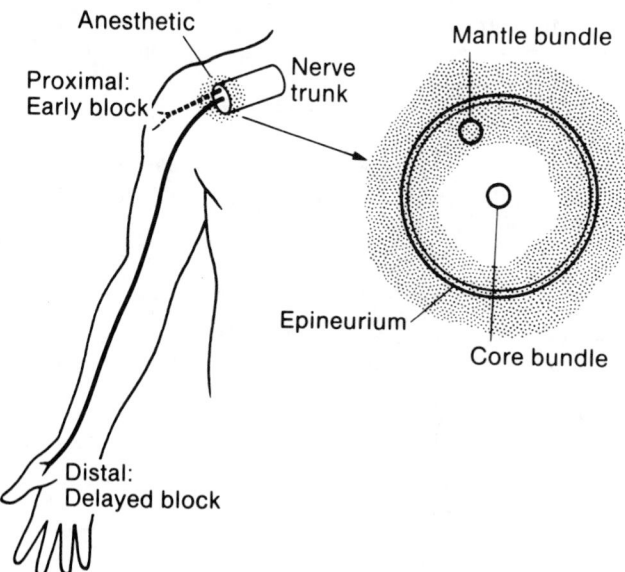

Figure 20-14. Representation of the somatotopic arrangement of fibers in the trunks of the brachial plexus. Nerve fibers in the mantle (or peripheral) bundles innervate the distal arm. The concentration gradient that develops during initial diffusion of local anesthetic into the nerve trunk causes onset of anesthesia to proceed from proximal to distal. (Modified with permission from de Jong RH: Physiology and Pharmacology of Local Anesthesia, p 66. Springfield, Charles C Thomas, 1977.)

most linear.[196,197] The effects of anesthetic concentration and the speed of injection on absorption rates are small.[196-198] Consequently, once the maximum safe total dose is identified, the concentration and volume used should be determined by anesthetic needs rather than by pharmacokinetic concerns.

Different sites of anesthetic injection have considerable variability in local blood flow and tissue binding. Absorption will be rapid from highly vascular sites and slower from sites with large amounts of fat and tissue that will bind the local anesthetic. In general, these effects are independent of the agent used.[199] Consequently, the rates of absorption differ between sites of injection to a greater extent than between anesthetic agents (Fig. 20-16).

The rate of absorption of local anesthetic from various sites decreases in the order intercostal > caudal > epidural > brachial plexus > sciatic/femoral. Rapid absorption is evidenced by high maximal blood levels and a relatively shorter time to reach maximum levels.[198] Absorption is also rapid after paracervical, pudendal, and subcutaneous infiltration of the vagina, whereas subcutaneous infiltration of the abdomen results in low levels.[196,199] Similarly, lidocaine sprayed on various parts of the respiratory tract results in concentrations similar to or lower than those expected for epidural injection.[199,200]

The interaction of local blood flow and tissue binding is apparent when looking at the above order. Although the epidural space is highly vascular compared to the intercostal space, peak blood levels are lower following epidural blockade than after intercostal blockade, probably as a result of greater fat binding in the epidural space. Similarly, although the epidural space has much greater vascularity than the subarachnoid space, the maximum blood levels seen after epidural or subarachnoid injection are not significantly different, probably as a result of greater nonspecific binding in the epidural space to fat and tissue.[201]

Physiochemical differences between local anesthetics

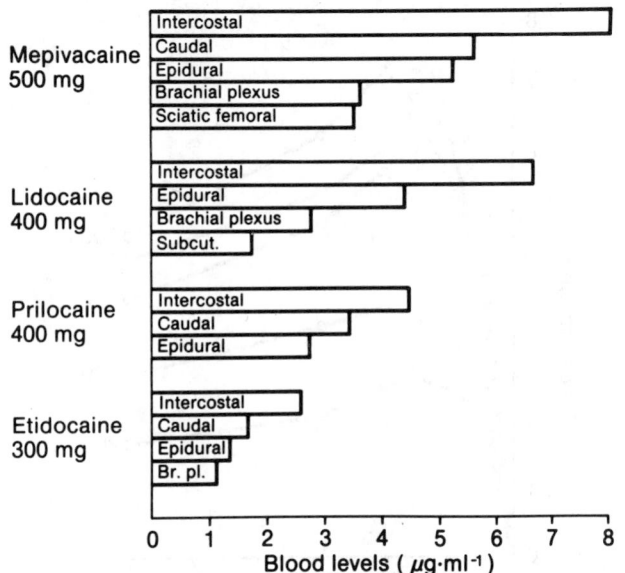

Figure 20-16. Peak serum levels of several local anesthetics resulting from various types of regional anesthetic procedures. (Reprinted with permission from Covino BG, Vassallo HG: Local Anesthetics: Mechanisms of Action and Clinical Use, p 97. New York: Grune & Stratton, 1976.)

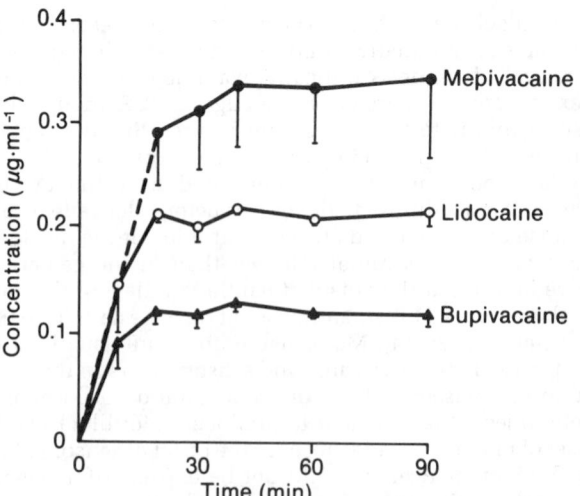

Figure 20-17. Blood concentrations of local anesthetic resulting from epidural injection of a mixture of equal milligram dosages of the three anesthetics (mean ± SE). (Reprinted with permission from Reynolds F: A comparison of the potential toxicity of bupivacaine, lignocaine, and mepivacaine during epidural blockade for surgery. Br J Anaesth 43:567, 1971.)

also significantly affect Cmax. For example, bupivacaine and etidocaine appear to produce greater vasodilation than lidocaine or mepivacaine.[202] Greater vasodilation should increase the rate of absorption of local anesthetic. However, the increment in Cmax for each 100 mg of bupivacaine or etidocaine injected into the epidural space is about half that observed for lidocaine and mepivacaine.[199] Furthermore, when equal doses of lidocaine, mepivacaine, and bupivacaine are injected together into the epidural space, the systemic blood levels that result are significantly different (Fig. 20-17).[203] Because local blood flow has to be the same when these drugs are injected together into the same space, the

difference in systemic absorption must reflect differences in local tissue binding, and, indeed, parallels the differences in lipid solubility (see Table 20-3).

Vasoconstrictors may be added to local anesthetic solutions to reduce systemic absorption and prolong duration.[204] These agents have variable effects but seem to be the most effective for reducing peak blood levels when administered with the shorter acting local anesthetics (lidocaine, mepivacaine, and prilocaine). From the above data, it appears that local tissue and nerve binding are more important than tissue blood flow in determining systemic absorption of edidocaine and bupivacaine. Perhaps this helps to explain why epinephrine is more effective at reducing Cmax and at prolonging the duration of lidocaine and mepivacaine than of bupivacaine or etidocaine (Table 20-4).

TABLE 20-4. Comparative Onset Times and Analgesic Durations of Various Local Anesthetic Agents and Effects of Addition of Epinephrine (5 μg·ml⁻¹) on Duration and Peak Plasma Levels (Cmax)

Anesthetic Technique	Anesthetic Agent	Usual Concentration (%)	Average Onset Time (min ± SE)	Average Analgesic Duration (min ± SE)	Addition of Epinephrine % Change Duration	Addition of Epinephrine % Change Cmax
Brachial plexus block (40–50 ml)	Lidocaine	1.0	14 ± 4	195 ± 26	+50	−20–30
	Mepivacaine	1.0	15 ± 6	245 ± 27	—	−20–30
	Bupivacaine	0.25–0.5	10 − 25	575	—	−10–20
	Etidocaine	0.5	9	572	—	−10–20
Epidural anesthesia (20–30 ml)	Lidocaine	2.0	15	100 ± 20	+50	−20–30
	Mepivacaine	2.0	15	115 ± 15	+50	−20–30
	Bupivacaine	0.5	17	195 ± 30	+0–30	−10–20
	Etidocaine	1.0	11	170 ± 57	+0–30	−10–20
Local infiltration	Lidocaine	0.5		75 (35–340)	+200	−50
	Mepivacaine	0.5		108 (15–240)	+120	—
	Bupivacaine	0.25		200 ± 33	+115	—

Adapted with permission from Covino BG, Vassallo HG: Local Anesthetics: Mechanism of Action and Clinical Use, pp 63, 81. New York, Grune & Stratton, 1976; and Tucker GT, Mather LE: Absorption and disposition of local anesthetics. In Cousins MJ, Bridenbaugh PO (eds): Neural Blockade in Clinical Anesthesia and Management of Pain, p 45. Philadelphia, JB Lippincott, 1980.

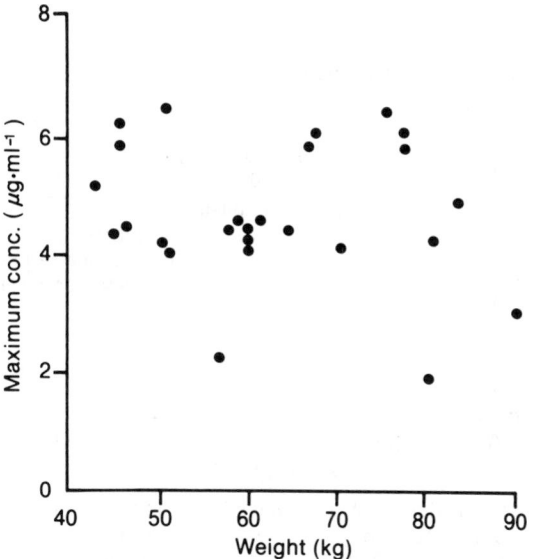

Figure 20-18. This scattergram illustrates the lack of correlation between body weight and the peak plasma concentration of lidocaine that results from epidural injection of 400 mg of lidocaine. (Reprinted with permission from Braid DP, Scott DB: Dosage of lignocaine in epidural block in relation to toxicity. Br J Anaesth 38:596, 1966.)

Physical and Pathophysiologic Factors

Although the maximum safe dose of a local anesthetic is frequently stated in terms of mg·kg^{-1}, there is no correlation between weight and peak plasma levels in adult patients (Fig. 20-18).[196,197] Acute hypovolemia slows the absorption of lidocaine after peridural injection, probably by decreasing cardiac output.[205] In contrast, increasing the cardiac output appears to increase absorption of local anesthetic.[206,207] Surprisingly, age and pregnancy do not appear to affect the rate of systemic absorption.[196,197,208-210]

Distribution and Elimination

Once local anesthetic is absorbed into the blood, it is usually distributed first to the lung. Local anesthetics have high solubilities in the lung, leading to a large uptake in lung tissue (Fig. 20-19).[211,212] This uptake of local anesthetic reduces the amount of drug that reaches the systemic circulation during accidental intravascular injection and thus could be considered protective.

Upon the anesthetic's reaching the systemic circulation, distribution is determined by tissue blood flow and the relative blood and tissue solubilities of the local anesthetic. Most of the local anesthetic is initially delivered to tissue groups with a high relative perfusion, the so-called vessel rich group (e.g., heart, brain, kidneys) (Fig. 20-19). Redistribution then occurs into tissues with lower relative perfusion, such as muscle and fat. Finally, local anesthetic is eliminated by metabolism and excretion.

Several factors have an important effect on distribution and elimination, including (1) protein binding, (2) clearance and metabolism, (3) physiologic effects of absorbed local anesthetic or peripheral blockade, and (4) other physical and pathophysiologic factors.

Protein Binding

Pharmacologic activity is generally related to unbound or free drug levels. The extent of protein binding, therefore, determines the amount of drug in the blood that is free, or available, to produce a pharmacologic effect.[213] The extent of protein binding varies considerably among the local anesthetics (see Table 20-3). Furthermore, as the concentration of local anesthetic increases, the percentage that is bound to protein decreases, probably as a result of saturation of binding sites (Fig. 20-20).[214]

Amide local anesthetics are primarily bound to alpha$_1$-acid glycoprotein and, to a lesser extent, to albumin.[211] The extent of protein binding varies considerably among patients. For example, the unbound lidocaine fraction may vary up to eightfold, being relatively low in patients with cancer and relatively high in neonates (Fig. 20-21).[215] Thus, differences in protein binding would lead to differences in the unbound drug fraction and could result in differences in the effects produced by the same total blood level of local anesthetic.

Another situation in which protein binding is important is in the understanding of placental transfer of drugs. The relatively low fetal:maternal plasma concentration ratio of bupivacaine compared with that of the shorter acting amides is assumed to imply that bupivacaine is safer for the infant. However, maternal plasma proteins bind approximately twice as much bupivacaine as fetal proteins.[216] Thus, the principal reason for differences in cord:maternal total

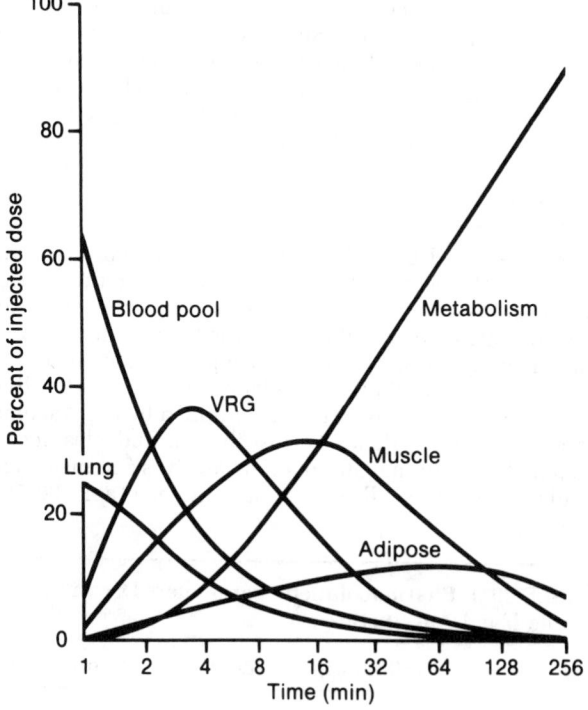

Figure 20-19. A perfusion model of the distribution of lidocaine in various tissues and its elimination from humans following an intravenous infusion for 1 minute (VRG = vessel rich group: different tissues grouped together because of relatively similar high tissue blood flows). Note the use of a logarithmic scale for time. (Reprinted with permission from Benowitz N, Forsyth RP, Melmon KL et al: Lidocaine disposition kinetics in monkey and man. I. Prediction by a perfusion model. Clin Pharmacol Ther 16:87, 1974.)

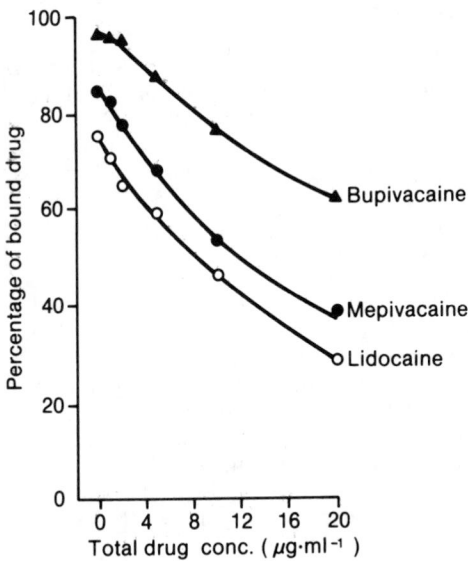

Figure 20-20. As the plasma concentration of local anesthetic increases, the percentage that is bound to plasma proteins decreases, and the percentage that is unbound, or free, increases. (Reprinted with permission from Tucker GT, Boyes RN, Bridenbaugh PO *et al:* Binding of anilide-type local anesthetics in human plasma: I. Relationships between binding, physiochemical properties, and anesthetic activity. Anesthesiology 33:287, 1970.)

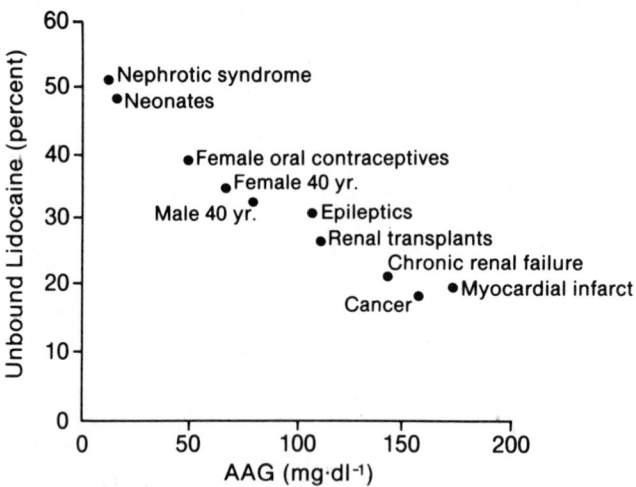

Figure 20-21. Relationship between the mean percentage of unbound, or free, lidocaine in plasma and the mean alpha$_1$-acid glycoprotein (AAG) concentration in various groups of patients. (Modified with permission from Routledge PA, Stargel WW, Barchowsky A *et al:* Control of lidocaine therapy: New perspectives. Ther Drug Monit 4:265, 1982.)

anesthetic concentrations is this difference in protein binding.[216,217] The concentration of unbound, pharmacologically active drug should equilibrate across the placenta and thus be similar in fetal and maternal blood. Indeed, intersubject variations in the fetal:maternal ratio are related, in large part, to individual variations in the extent of protein binding in maternal and fetal blood.[218]

Clearance

Clearance of a drug is defined as the volume of blood that is completely cleared of drug during a specific time period. Aminoamide local anesthetics are primarily cleared from the bloodstream by metabolism in the liver, with only prilocaine having any significant extrahepatic metabolism.[219,220] Because local anesthetics are highly extracted by the liver, the rate of clearance is largely determined by hepatic blood flow.[221] The net balance of distribution and clearance is such that the terminal elimination half-lives and mean body residence times of all amides are similar (Table 20-5).[211]

Mean body residence time represents the average time that drug molecules are present in the body.

Since the rate of clearance is similar for all amides but the duration of anesthesia is much different, lidocaine and mepivacaine tend to accumulate during continuous techniques, whereas bupivacaine accumulates only minimally.[222]

Aminoester local anesthetics are primarily cleared from the blood by plasma and liver cholinesterases. The pharmacokinetic parameters for 2-chloroprocaine have not been well defined because of its relatively rapid degradation in plasma. The *in vitro* blood half-life ranges from 7 to 20 seconds.[223] However, after epidural analgesia, the apparent half-life ranges from 1.5 to 6.4 minutes. This discrepancy probably results from the continuous uptake of anesthetic from the epidural space, even while chloroprocaine is being metabolized in the blood. This continued uptake makes it appear that chloroprocaine is being cleared from the blood more slowly. In this situation, in which absorption is slower than elimination, as it is after epidural anesthesia, the half-life reflects the absorption rate rather than the clearance rate. Thus, usual pharmacokinetic formulas, which are designed to describe intravenous administration of drugs, may not be entirely accurate for describing the pharmacokinetics of local anesthetics used for regional anesthesia.[211]

TABLE 20-5. Pharmacokinetic Parameters Describing the Disposition Kinetics of Amide Local Anesthetics

	Prilocaine	Lidocaine	Mepivacaine	Bupivacaine	Etidocaine
Vd_{ss} (liters)	191	91	84	73	134
$T_{1/2}$ (hours)	1.6	1.6	1.9	2.7	2.7
Cl (l·min^{-1})	2.37	0.95	0.78	0.58	1.11
MBRT (hours)	1.3	1.6	1.8	2.1	2.0

Vd_{ss} = volume of distribution (steady state); $T_{1/2}$ = terminal elimination half-life; Cl = systemic clearance; MBRT = mean body residence time.
Modified from Tucker GT: Pharmacokinetics of local anaesthetics. Br J Anaesth 58:717, 1986.

Although the aminoester local anesthetics are rapidly metabolized in normal patients, patients with abnormal or deficient plasma cholinesterases can exhibit signs of toxicity from usual dosages of 2-chloroprocaine.[224]

Finally, some metabolites of local anesthetics have been shown to be pharmacologically active. Monoethylglycinexylidide (MEGX), the metabolite that arises from N-deethylation of lidocaine, is near equipotent with lidocaine and can contribute to the occurrence of central nervous system toxicity.[225,226] Fortunately, MEGX levels are usually one-sixth to one-fourth of lidocaine levels, and the half-life of MEGX is comparable to that of lidocaine. However, MEGX accumulates in blood of patients in congestive heart failure and could contribute to toxicity even when plasma levels of lidocaine are in the therapeutic range.[225] Other metabolites may also have important pharmacologic effects; however, none have been identified to date.

Effects of Absorbed Local Anesthetic or Neural Blockade

The systemic effects of neural blockade, or of the absorbed local anesthetic itself, can alter the pharmacokinetics of the local anesthetics. Peripheral regional block techniques and local anesthetic blood levels commonly associated with regional anesthesia have minimal effects on blood flow.[226-228] In contrast, high thoracic levels of spinal or epidural anesthesia or high local anesthetic blood levels may significantly alter blood flow.[229-231]

Although these interactions initially seem to be straightforward and obvious, the effects are often surprising. For example, intravenous administration of lidocaine or bupivacaine decreases splanchnic resistance and increases hepatic blood flow.[227] One might expect that systemic absorption of local anesthetic during epidural blockade would produce the same effect. However, epidural blockade reduces hepatic blood flow, largely as a result of increased splanchnic vascular resistance.[232] Similarly, epidural anesthesia may produce significantly different systemic effects than spinal anesthesia, despite similar levels of sympathetic block, as a result of the higher blood levels of local anesthetic that occur with epidural anesthesia.[229-232]

Local anesthetics can directly reduce placental blood flow by vasoconstricting placental vascular beds and by stimulating myometrial contractility.[233,234] This effect is usually insignificant during routine peridural analgesia but can become significant after paracervical blockade or intravascular injection.

Physical and Pathophysiologic Factors

A reduction in cardiac output reduces the volume of distribution and plasma clearance of local anesthetics.[235,236] Reductions in clearance most likely result from a reduction in total hepatic blood flow.[237,238] As a result, a relatively low rate of lidocaine infusion can produce potentially toxic blood levels in some patients with cardiac failure.[235] However, plasma levels after peridural anesthesia are lower in the presence of decreased cardiac output, probably because of decreased absorption.[205] The ultimate result depends on the physiologic response of the patient to the particular regional technique and local anesthetic and is difficult to predict. To be safe, the total dose should be reduced when regional anesthesia is used in patients with cardiac failure.

Liver disease reduces plasma clearance and prolongs the half-life of lidocaine (Table 20-6) and probably of all local

TABLE 20-6. Effect of Disease on Lidocaine Pharmacokinetics

	$T_{1/2}$ (hours)	Vd_{ss} (l·kg^{-1})	Cl (ml·kg^{-1}·min^{-1})
Normal	1.8	1.32	10.0
Renal disease	1.3	1.2	13.7
Heart failure	1.9	0.88	6.3
Liver disease	4.9	2.31	6.0

$T_{1/2}$ = terminal elimination half-life; Vd_{ss} = volume of distribution (steady state); Cl = systemic clearance.

From Thomson PD, Melmon KL, Richardson JA et al: Lidocaine pharmacokinetics in advanced heart failure, liver disease, and renal failure in humans. Ann Intern Med 78:499, 1973.

anesthetics.[236,239] In contrast, renal disease has minimal effect.[236,240] Cholinesterase activity is reduced in newborns, pregnancy, renal or liver disease, and in patients who are debilitated or produce abnormal or insufficient amounts of enzymes.[241] Usually, enough cholinesterase activity remains, and the rate of absorption from the site of injection is slow enough that minimal accumulation of drug results. However, for patients with severely abnormal cholinesterase activity or in situations of accidental intravascular injection, these impairments of cholinesterase activity may lead to toxicity.[224]

Physiologic changes associated with old age would be expected to reduce the volume of distribution, the degree of protein binding, and the rate of elimination of local anesthetics, each contributing to increased plasma levels. Although some studies support this expectation,[198,242] numerous others do not.[196,208,209] However, the aged patient may accumulate higher plasma levels of local anesthetic with repeated dosages. Thus, the initial dose of local anesthetic need not necessarily be reduced in the elderly, but subsequent doses should be.[208,209] Pharmacologic changes at the other end of the age spectrum are much more dramatic. The elimination half-life of a local anesthetic may be prolonged two to three times in neonates.[243,244] Yet, children over 6 months of age distribute and eliminate intravenous lidocaine in a manner similar to that of adults.[245,246]

The effect of acid-base changes is complicated. Lactic acid produced in tissue could increase the total concentration of local anesthetic in that tissue. The non-ionized form of the drug crosses the cell membrane and becomes ionized to a greater extent in the acidic intracellular medium than it was in extracellular fluid, and the ionized local anesthetic is trapped (i.e., ion trapping), producing a higher total concentration within the cell. The effect that this higher concentration of ionized local anesthetic would have is purely speculative. However, the ionized form of the local anesthetic is thought to be active intracellularly. If so, there should be an increased pharmacologic effect that may be quite prolonged.

Similarly, fetal acidosis appears to result in greater transfer of local anesthetic from the mother to the fetus.[247] However, peak blood levels are not higher than for the nonacidotic fetus, perhaps because the local anesthetic is taken up and trapped in the acidotic fetal tissues.[248] In any case, there is no evidence that the acidotic fetus is more susceptible to local anesthetic-induced toxicity.

Acidosis of the plasma decreases protein binding, so that the free fraction of local anesthetic increases with decreasing pH.[249] Since there is less bound drug at a given total concentration of anesthetic, acidosis should increase the systemic effects of absorbed local anesthetics.

Drug Actions and Interactions

Concomitant administration of vasoactive drugs can affect cardiac output and modify the pharmacokinetics of local anesthetics through mechanisms previously discussed.[207,250] Halothane, cimetidine, and propranolol lower the clearance of lidocaine through inhibition of mixed function oxidases and/or decreased hepatic blood flow.[220,251,252] Most of the general anesthetics, except nitrous oxide, probably also lower clearance.[252] However, the mechanisms of action and relative effects may vary significantly among general anesthetics and patients.[220] These interactions suggest that toxic concentrations of local anesthetics could occur if any of these drugs are used concomitantly.

Because bupivacaine and diazepam are both highly protein-bound, it is possible that one might displace the other. Thus, diazepam has been suggested to have the potential to increase bupivacaine toxicity.[253] However, diazepam does not appear to be able to displace bupivacaine from serum binding sites.[254] Consequently, the use of diazepam to treat a toxic reaction will not increase the unbound fraction of bupivacaine.

Addition of epinephrine or phenylephrine to local anesthetics for regional blockade can decrease absorption, alter distribution, and increase the elimination rate of local anesthetics (see the section on Adjuvants and Combinations).[250,255,256] Similarly, beta-adrenergic agents increase clearance and volume of distribution of lidocaine.[207,257]

Combinations of Local Anesthetics

Mixtures of aminoester and aminoamide local anesthetics have been reported to combine the best characteristics of the individual agents.[258] For example, mixing chloroprocaine and bupivacaine is reported to produce a block with rapid onset and long duration.[259] In theory, combinations of local anesthetics may result in synergistic toxicity through competition for binding sites or metabolic enzymes or through inhibition of metabolic enzymes.[260,261] However, the systemic toxicity of local anesthetics appears to be merely additive, indicating that a mixture of bupivacaine and chloroprocaine might be less cardiotoxic than an equivalent dose of bupivacaine alone.[262] Despite the potential benefits of combining local anesthetics, clinical and laboratory evidence suggests that neural blockade produced by mixtures of local anesthetics is unpredictable and may not be any different than blockade produced by the individual agents.[263,264] Furthermore, prior administration of chloroprocaine reduces the ability of bupivacaine to produce neural blockade.[265] Thus, the clinical utility of anesthetic combinations remains to be clarified.

TOXICITY OF LOCAL ANESTHETICS

Allergic Reactions

True allergic reactions to local anesthetics are rare.[266] However, adverse reactions (e.g., local anesthetic overdose, fainting) appear to be common.[267-269] Differentiating between allergic and adverse reactions is often difficult because of the similarity of symptoms that may be produced.[268] Unlike most adverse reactions, however, allergic reactions are potentially fatal. Thus, many physicians are conservative and label patients as "allergic" to all "-caine" drugs, even when the signs and symptoms are consistent with an adverse reaction. This label can prove to be a problem in patients in whom the use of local anesthetics would be desirable.

Provocative skin testing has been advocated as a safe and effective procedure to differentiate between adverse and true allergic reactions to local anesthetics.[267,268,270] If the local anesthetic skin test and progressive challenge are negative, these authors maintain that it is safe to use the local anesthetic. However, the concept of skin testing with local anesthetics may not be scientifically sound, and the reliability of skin testing is questionable.[268,271] For example, local anesthetic compounds are too small to directly evoke an allergic response without prior conjugation to a carrier molecule. The immunologic response is initiated by, and directed against, this local anesthetic-carrier conjugate. Because appropriate local anesthetic-carrier conjugates are not available for skin testing, the reliability of skin testing is questionable. Finally, provocative testing engenders the risk of producing severe and potentially fatal reactions in patients who are truly allergic.[269,272]

Paraben derivatives have excellent bacteriostatic and fungistatic properties and are widely used in multidose local anesthetic preparations, other drugs, cosmetics, and foods. Despite the fact that a large percentage of the population has been exposed to parabens, the incidence of immediate toxicity to parenterally administered parabens is rare.[55] However, some patients thought to be allergic to local anesthetics were found to be allergic to the preservative methylparaben after more careful examination.[54,55,267] Finally, the potential for cross-sensitivity with some of the aminoester local anesthetics and p-aminobenzoic acid exists.[55] True allergy to aminoamide local anesthetics is exceedingly rare.

It is hoped that patients will not be denied the use of local anesthetics because of a wrong diagnosis of local anesthetic drug allergy. Cautious testing with local anesthetic drugs may be useful prior to surgery. If skin testing is negative, it should probably be followed by provocative challenge with an alternate local anesthetic, based on the history. Resuscitation equipment and trained individuals must be available when performing these tests, since severe systemic toxicity can be provoked by small quantities of local anesthetic.[269] The mechanism and treatment of allergic reactions to drugs are discussed in greater detail in Chapter 52.

Local Tissue Toxicity

When careful technique is utilized and when proper concentrations of local anesthetics are used, tissue toxicity is rare. However, serious neurotoxicity may result from the unintentional injection of large volumes or high concentrations of local anesthetic, from chemical contamination of the local anesthetic solution, or from neural ischemia produced by local pressure or hypotension.[273-277] Similarly, intraneural injection and direct trauma from the injection needle may produce neural deficit.[189]

Accidental subarachnoid injection of high doses of 2-chloroprocaine during the performance of epidural anesthesia has been reported to produce persistent and possibly permanent neurologic deficit.[273,276] Although animal models have produced conflicting results, it appears that both sodium bisulfite (the preservative) and a low pH are necessary to produce neurotoxicity.[276,278-280] 2-Chloroprocaine itself does not appear to be neurotoxic at clinical concentrations.[279,281] A new formulation of 2-chloroprocaine

(Nesacaine-MPF) which does not contain bisulfite does not appear to possess neurotoxic properties.

Systemic Toxicity

Systemic blood levels of local anesthetic produce a concentration-dependent continuum of effects ranging from therapeutic to toxic (Fig. 20-22). The appropriate use of local anesthetics for regional nerve blockade may occasionally result in minor signs of systemic toxicity but should rarely result in overt toxicity. Systemic toxicity most frequently results from one of two causes: (1) accidental intravascular injection, or (2) administration of an excessive dose of local anesthetic. The toxic effects of local anesthetics are primarily directed at the central nervous system and cardiovascular system, with the cardiovascular system being considerably more resistant. For example, four to seven times the dose of local anesthetic necessary to produce convulsions is required to produce cardiovascular collapse.[9]

Central Nervous System Toxicity

The toxic effects of local anesthetics on the central nervous system (CNS) are concentration-dependent (Fig. 20-22). Low concentrations produce sedation, whereas higher concentrations produce seizures.[9,282] The convulsant activity of local anesthetics probably results from selective depression of inhibitory fibers or centers in the CNS, allowing excessive excitatory input.[283] Seizures appear to originate in the subcortical brain structures, probably in the amygdala, with subsequent spread leading to grand mal seizures.[282,284] In general, CNS toxicity parallels anesthetic potency (Table 20-7).[9,285] Thus, the toxic:therapeutic ratios of local anesthetics are quite similar after intravenous administration.

Central nervous system toxicity is increased by raising the P_{CO_2}, decreasing the pH, or prior administration of a drug such as cimetidine that will slow elimination.[286-289] Ranitidine does not appear to increase CNS toxicity of local anesthetics, perhaps because it does not decrease hepatic blood flow.[289] Increasing arterial P_{CO_2} could increase CNS toxicity by increasing cerebral blood flow and increasing local anesthetic delivery to the brain, by increasing the concentration of ionized drug in the brain, or by a direct excit-

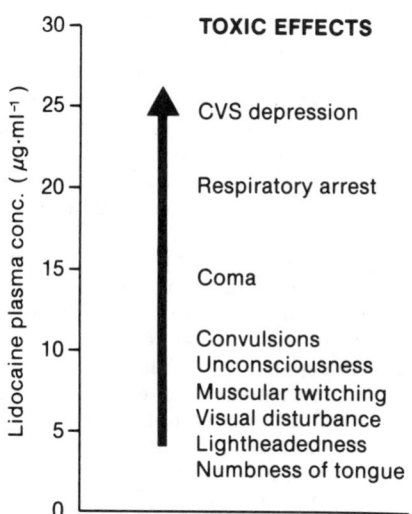

Figure 20-22. Continuum of toxic effects produced by increasing lidocaine plasma concentrations. CVS = cardiovascular system.

atory effect on subcortical structures.[286] Similarly, a decrease in pH may increase the concentration of ionized drug in the brain or may increase systemic distribution of local anesthetic to the brain.

Increasing the rate of intravenous drug administration produces systemic toxicity at a lower total dose of local anesthetic.[290] Similarly, electroencephalographic changes occur within one circulation after intravenous injection, indicating that the concentration of local anesthetic may also be an important determinant of the toxic effect.[282]

Central nervous system toxicity of local anesthetics is decreased by barbiturates, benzodiazepines, and inhalation anesthetics.[286,291-294] The effect of barbiturates and benzodiazepines is not surprising, as both are clinically useful for treating and preventing seizures. Inhalational anesthetics depress the central nervous system and probably raise the seizure threshold in a nonspecific manner.

Decreasing CNS toxicity of local anesthetics could be viewed as either beneficial or detrimental. If the peak blood levels obtained are relatively low, minor signs of local anesthetic toxicity would be masked, and this might be consid-

TABLE 20-7. Threshold for Production of CNS Toxicity by Local Anesthetics in Humans and Monkeys

| Agent | Relative Anesthetic Potency | Convulsive Threshold in Monkey | | Threshold for CNS Symptoms in Humans: Dose (mg·kg⁻¹) |
		Dose (mg·kg⁻¹)	Arterial Blood Level (μg·ml⁻¹)	
Procaine	1	—	—	19.2
Chloroprocaine	1	—	—	22.8
Lidocaine	2	14–22	18–26	6.4
Mepivacaine	2	18	22	9.8
Prilocaine	2	18	20	>6
Bupivacaine	8	4.3	4.5–5.5	1.6
Etidocaine	8	5.4	4.3	3.4
Tetracaine	8	—	—	2.5

Modified with permission from Covino BG, Vassallo HG: Local Anesthetics: Mechanism of Action and Clinical Use, p 126. New York, Grune & Stratton, 1976.

ered a beneficial effect. In the event that peak blood levels eventually become toxic, masking the early signs of toxicity may interfere with recognition of impending seizures or cardiovascular collapse. In this scenario, raising the CNS threshold would delay recognition and treatment and thus might be considered detrimental.[291,295]

Although toxic:therapeutic ratios for most local anesthetics are comparable after intravenous administration, these ratios are not necessarily indicative of the potential for toxicity when regional blockade is properly performed. For example, etidocaine is four times as toxic as lidocaine when both drugs are administered intravenously and only two times as toxic when the drugs are administered subcutaneously.[296] This discrepancy is probably explained by the observation that the more potent, more lipid-soluble anesthetics (e.g., bupivacaine, etidocaine) are absorbed into the systemic circulation much more slowly than the less potent agents (e.g., lidocaine, mepivacaine) (see Fig. 20-17). Thus, the toxic:therapeutic ratios for etidocaine or bupivacaine after properly performed regional anesthesia may be much greater than for lidocaine or mepivacaine.

Intra-arterial Injection

Accidental injection of a very low dose of local anesthetic into an artery can result in central nervous system toxicity. For example, grand mal seizures can occur after the injection of only 2.5 mg of bupivacaine into the vertebral artery during the performance of stellate ganglion block.[297] More worrisome, though, is the finding that low doses of local anesthetic injected into peripheral arteries, such as the brachial or femoral artery, can produce retrograde flow in the arterial system. This retrograde flow could allow direct access of local anesthetic to the cerebral circulation.[298] Thus, direct arterial injection may account for reports of systemic toxicity after the injection of low doses of local anesthetic.

Cardiovascular System Toxicity

Local anesthetics produce dose-related decreases in myocardial contractility and the rate of conduction of cardiac electrical impulses, and either contract or dilate vascular smooth muscle. Low concentrations may produce beneficial effects, such as prevention or treatment of arrhythmias.[299,300] In contrast, higher concentrations may produce refractory arrhythmias and cardiovascular collapse. Although the cardiovascular system (CVS) is more resistant to local anesthetic toxicity than is the CNS, CVS toxicity can be severe and difficult, if not impossible, to treat.[301]

Initially, the ratio of cardiac toxicity of local anesthetics was thought to parallel anesthetic potency.[302] More recent reports, however, suggest that bupivacaine and etidocaine may be relatively more cardiotoxic than would be predicted by their potency.[303,304] This relative increase in cardiotoxicity appears to result from more potent electrophysiologic effects.

Local anesthetics produce a dose-dependent delay in the transmission of impulses through the cardiac conduction system by their action on the cardiac sodium channels.[305,306] Sodium channel blockade develops during systole and dissipates during diastole. Both bupivacaine and lidocaine can block sodium channels rapidly during systole; however, bupivacaine dissociates from the sodium channel much more slowly during diastole.[305] Bupivacaine dissociates so slowly that the duration of diastole at physiologic heart rates (60–150 beats·min⁻¹) is insufficient for complete recovery of all sodium channels, and sodium channel block

accumulates (Fig. 20-23). In contrast, diastolic time during physiologic heart rates is sufficient for lidocaine to dissociate from the sodium channel before the next heart beat, and little accumulation of block results. Because sodium channel block accumulates with bupivacaine, it is much more potent in depressing traffic through the cardiac conduction system than would be predicted on the basis of local anesthetic potency. Thus, bupivacaine is approximately 70 times more potent than lidocaine in blocking cardiac conduction, at heart rates of 60–150 beats·min⁻¹; yet it is only four times more potent in blocking conduction in nerve tissues.[305] Although most research has focused on sodium channel blockade, bupivacaine and etidocaine also impair myocardial performance by producing a frequency-dependent block of sodium channels in myocardial muscle cells, and bupivacaine can effectively block potassium channels.[307,308] The interaction of these effects appears to further compound myocardial depression.

Cardiac arrhythmias and hypotension can also result from local anesthetic effects on the CNS.[309,310] Furthermore, bupivacaine and etidocaine are also relatively more cardiotoxic than lidocaine or mepivacaine through this indirect mechanism of action. Thus, the increased cardiac toxicity of etidocaine and bupivacaine most likely results from both direct actions on the heart and indirect actions on the CNS.[306,311,312]

Cardiovascular toxicity of local anesthetics is increased by hypoxia, acidosis, pregnancy, hyperkalemia, and the addition of epinephrine or phenylephrine to the local anesthetic solution and is possibly increased in neonates.[313–321]

Local anesthetics produce direct vasoconstriction or vasodilation of vascular smooth muscle and indirect effects through central stimulation of the autonomic nervous system and endocrine system.[312,322–324] The typical response at low concentrations is a minimal increase in mean arterial pressure due to increased total peripheral resistance.[227] At high concentrations, local anesthetics can either vasodilate or cause vasoconstriction.[234,322–324]

Appreciation of the potential for cardiac toxicity with bupivacaine and etidocaine has led to the search for a less

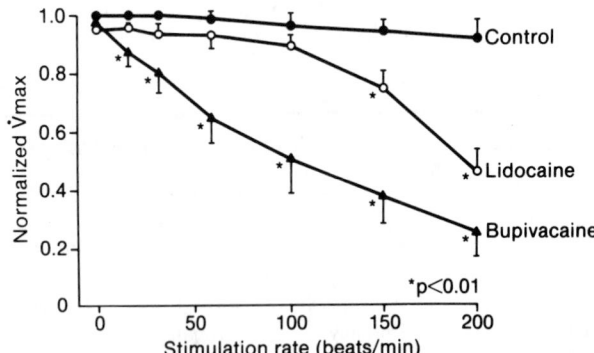

Figure 20-23. The effect of lidocaine (10 μg·ml⁻¹) and bupivacaine (1 μg·ml⁻¹) on maximum upstroke velocity (V̇max) of the action potential at different rates of stimulation (values are mean ± SD,* values significantly different from control, $p < 0.01$). Bupivacaine produced a progressive decrease in V̇max at stimulation rates above 3 beats·min⁻¹. Lidocaine did not significantly reduce V̇max until the stimulation rate increased to 150 beats·min⁻¹. (Reprinted with permission from Clarkson CW, Hondeghem LM: Mechanism for bupivacaine depression of cardiac conduction: Fast block of sodium channels during the action potential with slow recovery from block during diastole. Anesthesiology 62:396, 1985.)

toxic alternative. The most promising new agent, ropivacaine, is currently in clinical trials. Ropivacaine is structurally similar to bupivacaine and mepivacaine and like them is synthesized as a racemic mixture of L- and D-isomers. However, unlike the other local anesthetics, the commercial preparation of ropivacaine contains only the L-isomer. This preparation is based on the observation that the L-isomer has equal anesthetic potency to the D-isomer but is less cardiotoxic.[325] Indeed, evaluation in several animal species indicates that ropivacaine dissociates from sodium channels more rapidly than bupivacaine, produces less accumulation of sodium channel blockade at physiologic heart rates, and is less cardiotoxic than bupivacaine.[326-329] Initial studies in humans indicate that the potency and duration of action of ropivacaine are similar to those of bupivacaine.[325,330] Thus, even though the risk of cardiovascular toxicity has not been completely eliminated, it appears that ropivacaine offers clear advantages over bupivacaine and will likely replace bupivacaine in clinical practice once it is released for clinical use.[331]

Treatment of Systemic Toxicity

When local anesthetic-induced seizures occur, hypoxia, hypercarbia, and acidosis develop rapidly.[285,332] Furthermore, these metabolic changes greatly increase the toxicity of local anesthetics.[314] At the first signs of toxicity, oxygen must be delivered immediately. Administration of oxygen alone, by bag and mask, is often all that is necessary to treat seizures.[333] However, if seizure activity interferes with ventilation or is prolonged, anticonvulsant drug therapy is indicated.

The optimal drug for the initial treatment of local anesthetic-induced seizures is controversial. Because local anesthetic-induced seizures are usually of short duration, succinylcholine has been advocated as the treatment of choice.[333] Succinylcholine is rapid in onset and effectively facilitates ventilation. It also abolishes muscular activity, which decreases the severity of metabolic acidosis. However, neuronal seizure activity is not inhibited, and thus cerebral metabolism and oxygen requirements remain increased. Although muscle relaxation and ventilation with oxygen can prevent global cerebral ischemia, focal cerebral ischemia may not be prevented.[334,335] Consequently, succinylcholine may not be sufficient as a sole treatment.

Diazepam has been reported to be an effective anticonvulsant, with minimal side effects.[336] However, diazepam is relatively slow acting and may not stop seizures for 2–3 minutes after administration.[337] Thiopental acts more rapidly but may produce greater cardiorespiratory depression than that produced with benzodiazepines.[292,337] Furthermore, administration of barbiturates may decrease cardiac output and blood pressure to a greater extent than usual owing to a synergistic interaction with local anesthetics.[338]

Our suggestion would be to administer oxygen at the first sign of systemic toxicity, then use succinylcholine to facilitate ventilation. Finally, administer either a barbiturate or a benzodiazepine, as tolerated by the cardiovascular system, to reduce CNS metabolic demands. The need for oxygen, resuscitation equipment, and airway management skills when using local anesthetics should be obvious.

There is little information regarding the treatment of cardiovascular toxicity of local anesthetics in humans.[339,340] Animal data suggest that (1) high doses of epinephrine may be necessary to support the heart rate and blood pressure; (2) atropine may be useful for bradycardia; (3) DC cardioversion is often successful; and (4) ventricular arrhythmias are probably better treated with bretylium than with lidocaine.[341-345]

The best treatment for toxic reactions is prevention. Do not administer excessive doses of local anesthetic. Use meticulous technique, and utilize test doses whenever possible. It is also necessary to have knowledge of those doses of local anesthetic that should not be exceeded (Table 20-3). If toxic reactions occur, early detection and prompt support of ventilation and circulation are necessary.

Inhibition of Catecholamine Uptake by Cocaine

In addition to the CNS and CVS toxicities described above, cocaine causes norepinephrine and dopamine to accumulate at neuronal synapses by blocking the normal reuptake of these neurotransmitters. This explains the local vasoconstriction observed with this drug and why it is often preferred for use in vascular areas. Excess neurotransmitter acts on postsynaptic terminals in the CNS to produce myriad effects, ranging from euphoria and alertness to delirium, dysphoric agitation, and seizures. Excess neurotransmitters act through the sympathetic nervous system to cause hypertension, tachycardia, ventricular arrhythmias, myocardial infarction, and death.[345-349] Because cocaine is detoxified by plasma and liver cholinesterases, persons with cholinesterase deficiencies may be at increased risk for sudden death if they use cocaine.

Methemoglobinemia

Regional blockade performed with more than 500 mg of prilocaine is associated with methemoglobinemia.[350] It appears that prilocaine does not directly cause methemoglobinemia; rather, one of its metabolites is responsible. Thus, peak methemoglobin levels may not occur until 4–8 hours after administration and are directly related to the total dose of prilocaine administered.[350,351] Despite the finding that methemoglobinemia rarely reaches dangerous levels, the potential for cyanosis has surely limited the use of this drug. Prilocaine should probably not be used in obstetrics because fetal cyanosis interferes with newborn assessment and fetal blood is deficient in enzymes necessary to reduce methemoglobin.[350]

Methemoglobinemia is easily treated and rapidly reduced to hemoglobin by the administration of methylene blue (1–5 $mg \cdot kg^{-1}$) or, less successfully, of ascorbic acid (2 $mg \cdot kg^{-1}$).[351,352]

CLINICAL USES OF LOCAL ANESTHETICS

Features of an Ideal Local Anesthetic

Because anesthetic requirements vary considerably, no single set of local anesthetic properties can be considered ideal in all situations. For example, the ideal local anesthetic for laboring parturients would provide analgesia with no motor blockade. In contrast, many orthopedic surgeries require intense motor blockade.

In contrast to the clinical needs, the pharmacokinetic characteristics of an ideal anesthetic should be fairly uniform and would include slow systemic absorption (hence, low peak concentrations in the blood) and a high clearance from the blood leading to a short half-life. Additionally, the local anesthetic and any metabolites should be systemically inactive and nontoxic.[211]

It should be obvious that a local anesthetic with ideal properties for all clinical uses does not exist. Thus, the choice of local anesthetic must be individualized to each specific situation, and compromises, in terms of the ideal goal, are often necessary.

Choice of Local Anesthetic

Choice of a local anesthetic must take into consideration the duration of surgery, regional anesthetic technique employed, surgical requirements, the anesthesiologist's skills, the potential for local or systemic toxicity, and any metabolic constraints (see Table 20-4).

Usually, a local anesthetic is chosen that will, at least minimally, outlast the duration of surgery. For operations of brief duration, a short-acting local anesthetic will usually suffice. For prolonged operations, either a long-acting local anesthetic or a continuous anesthetic technique is chosen. Long-acting aminoamide local anesthetics, such as bupivacaine or etidocaine, have safety margins as good as if not better than short-acting drugs such as lidocaine and mepivacaine when injected properly because they have slower systemic absorption and they are more potent and can be injected in lower dosages.[199,203] Continuous techniques using a short-acting local anesthetic have many advantages, including the ability to closely match the duration of anesthesia and surgery. However, this technique results in greater systemic accumulation of local anesthetic or metabolites than occurs with long-acting aminoamide local anesthetics and may predispose to the development of tachyphylaxis.[203,221,353,354]

The concentration of local anesthetic necessary to provide neural blockade varies among block techniques. Larger nerves are more difficult to anesthetize and require higher concentrations of local anesthetic than smaller nerve fibers.[195] Thus, a higher concentration of local anesthetic is necessary for central neural blockade (e.g., epidural) than for peripheral blockade (e.g., posterior tibial nerve) (see Table 20-4). Even lower concentrations are necessary for subcutaneous infiltration. Similarly, when higher concentrations are used for a given technique, such as using 0.75% rather than 0.5% bupivacaine for epidural anesthesia, the intensity, duration, and speed of onset of neural blockade may be increased.[194]

The quality of sensory and motor blockade produced by the various anesthetics differs considerably. For example, intrathecal administration of tetracaine appears to provide greater motor blockade than does bupivacaine, whereas bupivacaine provides a longer duration of sensory analgesia.[355] Similarly, mepivacaine provides a greater degree of motor blockade than lidocaine for brachial plexus blockade, yet also provides a longer duration of sensory anesthesia.[186] When profound muscle relaxation is needed during surgery, mepivacaine and etidocaine may be the agents of choice for peripheral and epidural blockade (although high concentrations of bupivacaine provide excellent muscle relaxation), whereas tetracaine (or possibly lidocaine) may be preferred for spinal anesthesia.[356,357]

The potential for systemic toxicity should also be considered when choosing a local anesthetic. Rapid clearance of ester-type local anesthetics should greatly reduce the potential for systemic toxicity and provide a distinct advantage.[211] Indeed, chloroprocaine is so rapidly hydrolyzed that the risk of systemic toxicity is very low. However, its short duration of action limits its clinical utility. Tetracaine has a longer duration of action; however, it diffuses and spreads poorly through bodily tissues and is surprisingly toxic when administered intravenously.[9] Prilocaine has an extremely high clearance, which helps to minimize Cmax after a given dose and thus increases the margin of safety compared with the other aminoamide local anesthetics.[196,219]

Regional Anesthesia

Bupivacaine and lidocaine can be used for all regional blocks and are currently the most widely utilized local anesthetics. Mepivacaine is used extensively for peridural anesthesia and peripheral nerve blockade but not for spinal anesthesia. Etidocaine is relatively comparable to bupivacaine except that it produces more profound motor block. Consequently, its use is limited to surgical anesthesia. Prilocaine is rarely used because of its propensity to produce methemoglobinemia. Procaine is largely used for local infiltration. Tetracaine, cocaine, and benzocaine are useful for topical anesthesia, and tetracaine is widely used for spinal anesthesia. Chloroprocaine produces peridural blockade of short duration that is particularly useful for cesarean section because of the low potential for toxicity to mother and fetus.

Topical Anesthesia

Local anesthetics may be applied topically to provide anesthesia to such diverse sites as the eye, skin, tympanic membrane, oral mucosa, tracheobronchial tree, and rectum. To be effective topically, however, relatively high concentrations of local anesthetics are required (Table 20-8). Although increasing the concentration increases penetration of the tissues, the onset of anesthesia usually occurs in 5–10 minutes when applied to mucous membranes and in 30–60 minutes when applied to the skin. Systemic absorption is also greater from mucous membranes, as is the risk of toxicity if large volumes of local anesthetic are used.

Maximum Dose

Maximum doses of local anesthetic are frequently quoted for the safe administration of local anesthesia (i.e., avoidance of toxicity) (see Table 20-3). Unfortunately, these recommendations are general in nature and do not consider known pharmacokinetic variables. For example, different peak blood levels will result from the injection of the same dose of local anesthetic into different sites, yet maximum doses are quoted without consideration of the site of injection (see Fig. 20-16). Furthermore, the maximum recommended dose of local anesthetic may not be rational in terms of known systemic blood levels. For example, the maximum recommended dose of bupivacaine is often quoted as 200 mg. However, when intercostal nerve blocks were performed with 400 mg of bupivacaine, only one in ten patients had a peak blood level that approached the seizure threshold.[358] Because intercostal injection produces the highest local anesthetic blood level of any regional technique, other techniques should produce even lower blood levels and provide a greater margin of safety.[211] These data imply that the maximum recommended dose of bupivacaine is quite conservative. Finally, maximum doses are frequently quoted in terms of $mg \cdot kg^{-1}$, yet there is no evidence that weight significantly affects the peak blood level (see Fig. 20-18). The maximum doses given in Table 20-3 are

TABLE 20-8. Preparations of Local Anesthetics Intended for Topical Anesthesia

Anesthetic	Concentration (%)	Pharmaceutical Application Form	Intended Area of Use
Benzocaine	1–5	Cream	Skin and mucous membrane
	20	Ointment	Skin and mucous membrane
	20	Aerosol	Skin and mucous membrane
Cocaine	4	Solution	Ear, nose, throat
Cyclonine	0.5–1	Solution	Skin, oropharynx, tracheobronchial tree, urethra, rectum
Dibucaine	0.25–1	Cream	Skin
	0.25–1	Ointment	Skin
	0.25–1	Aerosol	Skin
	0.25	Solution	Ear
	2.5	Suppositories	Rectum
Lidocaine	2–4	Solution	Oropharynx, tracheobronchial tree, nose
	2	Jelly	Urethra
	2.5–5	Ointment	Skin, mucous membrane, rectum
	2	Viscous	Oropharynx
	10	Suppositories	Rectum
	10	Aerosol	Gingival mucosa
Tetracaine	0.5–1	Ointment	Skin, mucous membrane, rectum
	0.5–1	Cream	Skin, mucous membrane, rectum
	0.25–1	Solution	Nose, tracheobronchial tree

Reprinted with permission from Covino BG, Vassallo HG: Local Anesthetics: Mechanism of Action and Clinical Use, p 93. New York, Grune & Stratton 1976.

expressed in milligrams. Simple arithmetic indicates that a 1% solution of local anesthetic equals 10 mg·ml^{-1}.

A final consideration for determining the safe dose of local anesthetic is the skill of the anesthesiologist. Although proper injection of 200 mg of bupivacaine into the epidural space is very safe, as little as 50 mg injected intravenously or 2.5 mg injected intraarterially may be extremely toxic.[235,301] Thus, the skill of the anesthesiologist may be *the* major factor determining the toxic dose of a local anesthetic.

Antiarrhythmic Effects

Lidocaine has an antiarrhythmic effect that develops rapidly after intravenous infusion and dissipates quickly when the infusion is discontinued. Thus, it is easily titratable and extremely useful in situations where rapid control of ventricular arrhythmias is necessary. Bupivacaine, etidocaine, and mepivacaine have also been found to be effective antiarrhythmics.[299,300]

Blunting the Response to Tracheal Stimulation

Lidocaine, injected intravenously or topically applied to the larynx and trachea, is variably effective at blunting the hemodynamic response to intubation.[359-362] Intravenous lido-caine may also prevent the rise in intraocular pressure seen with tracheal intubation and the rise in intracranial pressure associated with tracheal suctioning.[363,364] Intravenous lidocaine also has been shown to suppress coughing and prevent reflex bronchoconstriction.[365,366]

Other Therapeutic Effects

Local anesthetics are anticonvulsants in low dosages and surprisingly have been promoted as effective treatment for status epilepticus.[367,368] Lidocaine blood levels of 1–2 μg·ml^{-1} provide systemic analgesia, reduce the minimum alveolar concentration for inhalational anesthetics, and have been used to treat both acute and chronic pain.[369,370] Lidocaine rapidly reduces raised intracranial pressure.[371] Intravenous infusions of local anesthetics can augment neuromuscular blockade.[372] Finally, infusions of local anesthetics can be used for general anesthesia.

ADJUVANTS AND COMBINATIONS

Epinephrine

Epinephrine has been reported to produce beneficial effects when added to virtually every available local anesthetic for nearly every regional anesthetic technique. These beneficial effects include the ability to (1) prolong the duration of anesthesia, (2) minimize the peak level of local anesthetic in the blood, (3) increase the intensity of the blockade, (4) reduce surgical bleeding, and (5) serve as a component of the test dose for regional anesthesia.

Prolonging the Duration of Anesthesia

In the concentrations typically used for regional anesthesia, local anesthetics universally cause local vasodilation. Epinephrine is added in an attempt to counteract this vasodilation, reduce absorption, and therefore prolong duration.[204] The ability of epinephrine to prolong duration is determined by the type of regional block, concentration of epinephrine, and type and concentration of local anesthetic utilized (see Table 20-4).[196,373,374]

The addition of epinephrine to tetracaine consistently prolongs the duration of spinal anesthesia.[357] When added to bupivacaine or lidocaine, the results are less certain; some authors find a prolonged duration of spinal anesthesia, whereas others are unable to detect any significant effect.[355,375-377] Epinephrine also prolongs the duration of most other regional anesthetic techniques (see Table 20-4). However, epinephrine is less effective when added to bupivacaine and etidocaine, probably because the long duration of action of bupivacaine and etidocaine does not appear to be a function of local blood flow.

Minimizing Peak Blood Levels of Local Anesthetic

Peak blood levels of local anesthetics can approach the toxic range when used for regional blockade, especially for intercostal and peridural techniques.[198] Epinephrine can decrease peak blood levels, presumably by producing local vasoconstriction and decreasing the rate of local anesthetic absorption. However, epinephrine is less effective in reducing peak blood levels when administered with bupivacaine and etidocaine (see Table 20-4).

Increasing the Intensity of Neural Blockade

Epinephrine has been considered for years to increase the intensity and quality of neural blockade. Hypalgesia or analgesia has been reported after the injection of epinephrine alone into the subarachnoid or epidural space.[378,379] Similarly, the intensity of motor and sensory blockade has been reported to be improved for spinal analgesia and for epidural anesthesia for labor and delivery.[373,380,381]

The increased intensity of analgesia may result from direct action of epinephrine on antinociceptive receptors in the spinal cord.[382] Epinephrine and other alpha-adrenergic agonists augment the ability of local anesthetics to block transmission of noxious stimuli in the spinal cord. Furthermore, the intensity and duration of these effects appear to depend on the dose of epinephrine.

Reducing Surgical Blood Loss

Subcutaneous, local infiltration of epinephrine-containing solutions can facilitate surgery by decreasing bleeding. The optimum concentration of epinephrine remains controversial.[383] Definite conclusions are difficult to make because the site of injection, the concentration of local anesthetic, and the concentration of epinephrine all seem to be important. However, most clinical evidence suggests that near-

maximal vasoconstriction occurs at epinephrine concentrations of 5 μg·ml^{-1} (1:200,000).

Optimal Concentration of Epinephrine

The optimal concentration of epinephrine for regional blockade is controversial. Since the degree of vasodilation is affected by the choice of local anesthetic, its concentration, and the site of injection, it is unlikely that one concentration of epinephrine is optimal for all regional techniques.[202,322] However, most authors agree that 5 μg·ml^{-1} of epinephrine is optimal. Although lower concentrations were initially thought to be ineffective, recent evidence suggests that concentrations as low as 1–2 μg·ml^{-1} may be sufficient.[383,384] In contrast, higher concentrations are more likely to produce toxicity from the absorbed epinephrine.[196,223,385] The maximum dose of epinephrine probably should not exceed 200–250 μg.[386] Reduced quantities should be used in patients who may be placed at risk if they develop hypertension or tachycardia, such as those with coronary artery disease.

Component of a Test Dose

A test dose is frequently used for peridural anesthetic techniques in an attempt to minimize the chance of accidental subarachnoid or intravascular injection. Subarachnoid injection is detected by the rapid onset of spinal anesthesia. Intravascular injection is more difficult but just as important to detect. If the test dose contains 15 μg of epinephrine, intravascular injection can be detected by an increase in the heart rate that begins in approximately 25 seconds, increases by at least 20%, and remains elevated for about 30 seconds.[387] These heart rate responses do not occur reliably in patients who are receiving beta-adrenergic blocking therapy.

Use in Obstetrics

The alpha-adrenergic effects of epinephrine may be dangerous to the fetus by decreasing uterine artery blood flow, and the beta-adrenergic effects may slow labor and increase the need for oxytocic supplementation.[388,389] Although some clinical studies have found epinephrine to be safe and free of these potential adverse effects, considerable controversy and uncertainty remain.[390-393] Some experts recommend the use of epinephrine in obstetrics, and others suggest that it should never be used.[394,395]

Systemic Effects

Administration of epinephrine with local anesthetics results in significantly higher systemic levels of epinephrine than when epinephrine is injected alone.[396] The absorbed epinephrine produces predominantly beta-adrenergic effects, with little evidence of alpha-adrenergic effects at doses up to 400 μg.[385] Thus, heart rate, contractility, and cardiac output are all increased, whereas peripheral vascular resistance and blood pressure usually decrease. Systemic absorption or accidental intravascular injection of epinephrine may produce a variety of undesirable side effects, including tachycardia, arrhythmias, tremor, hypertension, and possibly decreased uterine blood flow. In contrast to all other regional techniques, injection of epinephrine into the subarachnoid space does not appear to produce systemic effects.

Potential Contraindications to the Use of Epinephrine

Epinephrine should not be used in situations where its undesirable side effects would be particularly dangerous, such as patients with (1) severe or unstable angina; (2) malignant arrhythmias; (3) uncontrolled hypertension; or (4) uteroplacental insufficiency or fetal distress. Similarly, epinephrine should be avoided in patients with hyperthyroidism and patients on medications that modify the effects of catecholamines (e.g., tricyclic antidepressants or monoamine oxidase inhibitors). Finally, epinephrine should not be added to local anesthetics for peripheral nerve blocks in areas where there is not adequate collateral blood flow (e.g., digits, penis, wrist, ankle) or when performing intravenous regional anesthesia.

Phenylephrine

Phenylephrine is an alpha-adrenergic sympathomimetic that is effective for prolonging the duration of spinal and epidural anesthesia. However, phenylephrine does not appear to reduce peak blood levels of local anesthetic that result after epidural anesthesia, even when administered in doses that have vasoconstrictor effects equipotent with epinephrine.[256] Phenylephrine does not produce systemic effects when injected into the subarachnoid space, yet prominent alpha-adrenergic effects result when it is used for other regional techniques. The usual dose of phenylephrine used for prolongation of spinal anesthesia is 2–5 mg.

Vasopressin Analogues

Felypressin (octapressin) and ornipressin are synthetic drugs similar in structure to vasopressin but without the antidiuretic or coronary vasoconstrictor effects. These drugs increase the intensity and duration of local anesthesia, decrease systemic absorption, and decrease bleeding while producing minimal cardiovascular side-effects.[397-400] Octapressin and other catecholamines appear to have synergistic vasoconstrictor effects.[401] Finally, intravascular injection of octapressin-containing local anesthetic solutions appears to be less toxic than solutions that contain epinephrine.[399] Although these drugs enjoy considerable popularity in other countries, they are not currently available for use in the United States.

Carbonated Local Anesthetics

Carbonation of local anesthetics was first reported to hasten the onset and increase the intensity of local anesthesia over 20 years ago.[402] To this day, the clinical significance of this effect remains controversial, and commercially prepared solutions are not available in the United States for routine clinical use. The proponents of carbonated solutions speculate that the increased rate of onset of neural blockade results from more rapid intraneural diffusion and more rapid penetration of connective tissue sheaths around the nerve trunk.[47-50,403] The increased intensity of neural blockade is thought to result from the diffusion of carbon dioxide into the nerve, which reduces intraneural pH. This decrease in pH promotes ion trapping of the local anesthetic, increasing the intraneural concentration. Furthermore, carbon dioxide may have a direct anesthetic effect on the nerve membrane.[402] Several clinical studies report that carbonated local anesthetic solutions have advantages over typical solutions (prepared as the hydrochloride salt).[402-404]

In contrast, several studies report no clinical advantage of carbonated solutions.[405,406] Furthermore, carbonated solutions may have some disadvantages. For example, peak blood levels of local anesthetics are higher after regional blockade with carbonated local anesthetic solutions.[407] Similarly, a faster rate of onset of epidural blockade could result in a greater magnitude and rate of decline of blood pressure.[408] This effect could be especially detrimental in obstetric patients.

Sodium Bicarbonate

Addition of sodium bicarbonate to local anesthetic solutions will raise the pH and increase the concentration of non-ionized free base. For example, increasing the pH of a solution of lidocaine from 6 to 7 increases the percentage of non-ionized free base from less than 1% to 11% (see Table 20-2). The increased percentage of free base will theoretically increase the rate of diffusion and speed the onset of neural blockade.

Clinically, the addition of 1 mEq of sodium bicarbonate to each 10 ml of commercially prepared 1.5% lidocaine solution raises the pH to 7.15 and produces significantly faster onset of anesthesia and more rapid spread of sensory blockade.[46] Systemic blood levels were higher but not statistically different. Like carbonated solutions, the faster onset of these solutions may contribute to a greater magnitude and rate of decline in blood pressure.[408]

Dextran

The addition of dextran to local anesthetic solutions has been found to increase the duration of anesthesia.[409] Dextran also slows the rate of absorption of local anesthetic and epinephrine, when used, so that the peak blood levels are decreased.[396,410] However, the effect in individual patients is unpredictable, and dextran can provoke anaphylaxis.[411] Consequently, dextran is rarely added to local anesthetics for regional anesthesia.

Hyaluronidase

Hyaluronic acid is a viscous polysaccharide that inhibits diffusion of foreign substances within interstitial spaces of tissues. Hyaluronidase hydrolyzes hyaluronic acid, facilitating the spread of local anesthetics. Proponents of hyaluronidase suggest that it improves the success rate of some regional techniques and prevents hematoma formation if an artery is punctured.[412] However, the addition of hyaluronidase can increase Cmax, may provoke allergic reactions, may shorten the duration of anesthesia, and is technically awkward, since it cannot be heat sterilized (it is a protein).[412] Finally, most modern local anesthetic drugs diffuse rapidly; thus, the benefits of adding hyaluronidase are limited.

REFERENCES

1. Bean BP, Cohen CJ, Tsien RW: Lidocaine block of cardiac sodium channels. J Gen Physiol 81:613, 1983
2. Gintant GA, Hoffman BF: The role of local anesthetic effects

in the actions of antiarrhythmic drugs. In Strichartz GR (ed): Local Anesthetics p 213. Berlin, Springer-Verlag, 1987

3. Covino BG: Cardiovascular effects of regional anesthesia. In Covino BG, Fozzard HA, Rehder K et al (eds): Effects of Anesthesia, p 207. Bethesda, American Physiological Society, 1985

4. Courtney KR, Kendig JJ: Bupivacaine is an effective potassium channel blocker in heart. Biochim Biophys Acta 939:163, 1988

5. Steinback AB: Alteration of Xylocaine (lidocaine) and its derivatives of the time course of the end plate potential. J Gen Physiol 52:144, 1986

6. Sine SM, Taylor P: Local anesthetics and histrionicotoxin are allosteric inhibitors of the acetylcholine receptor. J Biol Chem 257:8106, 1982

7. Wali FA, Suer AH, Greenidge E et al: Local anaesthetics inhibit influx of calcium, sodium, and potassium into rat ileum, diaphragm, and human isolated saphenous vein. Gen Pharmacol 18:351, 1987

8. Garfield GM, Guigino L: Central effects of local anesthetic agents. In Strichartz GR (ed): Local Anesthetics, p 253. Berlin, Springer-Verlag, 1987

9. Liu PL, Feldman HS, Giasi R et al: Comparative CNS toxicity of lidocaine, etidocaine, bupivacaine, and tetracaine in awake dogs following rapid IV administration. Anesth Analg 62:375, 1983

10. Modica, PA, Tempelhoff R, White PF: Pro- and anticonvulsant effects of anesthetics (Part II). Anesth Analg 70:433, 1990

11. Zipf HF, Dittman ECH: General pharmacological effects of local anesthetics. In Lechat P (ed): Local Anesthetics, p 191. Oxford, Pergamon Press, 1971

12. Strichartz G: Use-dependent conduction block produced by volatile general anesthetic agents. Acta Anaesthesiol Scand 24:402, 1980

13. Haydon DA, Urban BW: The action of alcohols and other nonionic surface active substances on the sodium current of the squid giant axon. J Physiol 341:411, 1983

14. Sangarlangkarn S, Klaewtanong V, Jonglerttrakool P et al: Meperidine as a spinal anesthetic agent: A comparison with lidocaine-glucose. Anesth Analg 66:235, 1987

15. Kendig JJ: Barbiturates: Active form and site of action at node of Ranvier sodium channels. J Pharmacol Exp Ther 218:175, 1981

16. Courtney KR, Etter EF: Modulated anticonvulsant block of sodium channels in nerve and muscle. Eur J Pharmacol 88:1, 1983

17. Seeman P: The membrane actions of anesthetics and tranquilizers. Pharmacol Rev 24:583, 1972

18. Catterall WA: Neurotoxins that act on voltage-sensitive sodium channels in excitable membranes. Ann Rev Pharmacol Toxicol 20:15, 1980

19. Akerman B, Hellberg I-B, Trossvik C: Primary evaluation of the local anaesthetic properties of the amino amide agent ropivacaine (LEA 103). Acta Anaesthesiol Scand 32:571, 1988

20. Bader AM, Datta S, Flanagan H, Covino BG: Comparison of bupivacaine- and ropivacaine-induced conduction blockade in the isolated rabbit vagus nerve. Anesth Analg 68:724, 1989

21. Kopacz DJ, Carpenter RL, Mackey DC: Effect of ropivacaine on cutaneous capillary blood flow in pigs. Anesthesiology 71:69, 1989

22. Moller R, Covino BG: Cardiac electrophysiologic properties of bupivacaine and lidocaine compared with those of ropivacaine, a new amide local anesthetic. Anesthesiology 72:322, 1990

23. Scott DB, Lee A, Fagan D, Bowler GM et al: Acute toxicity of ropivacaine compared with that of bupivacaine. Anesth Analg 69:563, 1989

24. Fink BR: History of local anesthesia. In Cousins MJ, Bridenbaugh PO (eds): Neural Blockade in Clinical Anesthesia and Management of Pain, p 3. Philadelphia, JB Lippincott, 1980

25. Covino B: One hundred years plus two of regional anesthesia. Reg Anesth 11:105, 1986

26. Fink BR: Leaves and needles: The introduction of surgical local anesthesia. Anesthesiology 63:77, 1985

27. Lee JA: Some foundations on which we have built. Reg Anesth 10:99, 1985

28. Vandam LD: Some aspects of the history of local anesthesia. In Strichartz BR (ed): Local Anesthetics, p 1. Berlin, Springer-Verlag, 1987

29. Liljestrand G: The historical development of local anesthesia. In Lechat P (ed): International Encyclopedia of Pharmacology and Therapeutics, p 1. Oxford, Pergamon Press, 1971

30. Moore DC: Regional block: Its history in the United States since World War II. In Rupreht J, van Lieburg M, Lee JA et al (eds): Anaesthesia—Essays on Its History, p 128. Berlin, Springer-Verlag, 1985

31. Narahashi T, Frazier DT, Yamada M: The site of action and active form of local anesthetics. I. Theory and pH experiments with tertiary compounds. J Pharm Exp Ther 171:32, 1970

32. Ritchie JM, Ritchie B, Greengard P: The effect of the nerve sheath on the action of local anesthetics. J Pharm Exp Ther 150:160, 1965

33. Frazier DT, Narahashi T, Yamada M: The site of action and active form of local anesthetics. II. Experiments with quaternary compounds. J Pharm Exp Ther 171:45, 1970

34. Hille B: The pH-dependent rate of action of local anesthetics on the node of Ranvier. J Gen Physiol 69:475, 1977

35. Hille B: Local anesthetics: Hydrophilic and hydrophobic pathways for the drug-receptor reaction. J Gen Physiol 69:497, 1977

36. Hille B, Courtney K, Dum R: Rate and site of action of local anesthetics in myelinated nerve fibers. In Fink BR (ed): Molecular Mechanisms of Anesthesia. Progress in Anesthesiology, vol 1, p 13. New York, Raven Press, 1975

37. Ritchie JM: Mechanism of action of local anaesthetic agents and biotoxins. Br J Anaesth 47:191, 1975

38. Strichartz G: Interactions of local anesthetics with neuronal sodium channels. In Covino BG, Fozzard HA, Rehder K et al (eds): Effects of Anesthesia, p 39. Bethesda, American Physiological Society, 1985

39. de Jong RH: Local anesthetics, p 41. Springfield, Charles C Thomas, 1977

40. Eckenstam BA: The effect of the structural variation on the local analgetic properties of the most commonly used groups of substances. Acta Anaesthesiol Scand 25(Suppl):10, 1966

41. Buchi J, Perlia X: Structure-activity relations and physicochemical properties of local anesthetics. In Lechat P (ed): Local Anesthetics, p 39. Oxford, Pergamon Press, 1971

42. Courtney KR, Strichartz GR: Structural elements which determine local anesthetic activity. In Strichartz GR (ed): Local Anesthetics, p 53. Berlin, Springer-Verlag, 1987

43. Setnikar I: Ionization of bases with limited solubility. Investigation of substances with local anesthetic activity. J Pharm Sci 55:1190, 1966

44. Moore DC: The pH of local anesthetic solutions. Anesth Anal 60:833, 1981

45. Hilgier M: Alkalinization of bupivacaine for brachial plexus block. Reg Anesth 8:59, 1985

46. Di Fazio CA, Carron HO, Grosslight KR et al: Comparison of pH adjusted lidocaine solutions for epidural anesthesia. Anesth Analg 65:760, 1986

47. Catchlove RFH: The influence of CO_2 and pH on local anesthetic action. J Pharmacol Exp Ther 181A:298, 1972

48. Gissen AJ, Covino BG, Gregus J: Differential sensitivity of fast and slow fibers in mammalian nerve. IV. Effect of carbonation of local anesthetics (LA). Reg Anesth 10:68, 1985

49. Park WY, Hagins FM: Comparison of lidocaine hydrocarbonate with lidocaine hydrochloride for epidural anesthesia. Reg Anesth 11:128, 1986

50. Bokesch PM, Raymond SA, Strichartz GR: Dependence of lidocaine potency on pH and P_{CO_2}. Anesth Analg 66:9, 1987

51. Weiner N: Norepinephrine, epinephrine, and the sympathomimetic amines. In Gilman AG, Goodman LS, Rall TW et al (eds): Goodman and Gilman's The Pharmacological Basis of Therapeutics, 7th ed, p 158. New York, Macmillan, 1985

52. Parnass SM, Baughman VL, Miletich DJ et al: The effects of pH on the oxidation rate of epinephrine. Anesthesiology 67:A280, 1987

53. Bonhomme L, Benhamou, D, Martre BS et al: Chemical stability of bupivacaine epinephrine in pH-adjusted solutions. Anesthesiology 67:A279, 1987

54. Aldrete AJ, Johnson DA: Allergy to local anesthetics. JAMA 207:356, 1969

55. Nagel JE, Fuscaldo JT, Fireman P: Paraben allergy. JAMA 237:1594, 1977

56. Hutter CD: The Woolley and Roe case: A reassessment. Anaesthesia 45:859, 1990

57. Bray GM, Rasminsky M, Aguayo AJ: Interactions between axons and their sheath cells. Ann Rev Neurosci 4:127, 1981

58. Coggeshall RE: A fine structured analysis of the myelin sheath in rat spinal roots. Anat Rec 194:201, 1979

59. Landon N, Williams PL: Ultrastructure of the node of Ranvier. Nature 199:575, 1963

60. Langley OK, London DN: A light and electron histochemical approach to the nodes of Ranvier and myelin of peripheral nerve fibers. J Histochem Cytochem 15:722, 1967

61. London DN, Langley OK: The local chemical environment of nodes of Ranvier: A study of cation binding. J Anat 108:419, 1971

62. Langley OK: Local anesthetics and nodal polyanions in peripheral nerve. Histochem J 5:79, 1973

63. Gissen AJ, Covino BC, Gregus J: Differential sensitivity of fast and slow fibers in mammalian nerve: II. Margin of safety for nerve transmission. Anesth Analg 61:561, 1982

64. Angevine JB: The nervous tissue. In Fawcett DW (ed): A Textbook of Histology, p 311. Philadelphia, WB Saunders, 1986

65. Feng TP, Liu YM: The connective tissue sheath of the nerve as effective diffusion barrier. J Cell Comp Physiol 34:1, 1949

66. Stevens CF: The neuron. Sci Am 241:55, 1979

67. Singer SJ, Nicolson GL: The fluid mosaic model of the structure of cell membranes. Science 175:720, 1972

68. Pfenninger KH: Organization of neuronal membranes. Ann Rev Neurosci 1:445, 1978

69. Hille B: Ionic basis of resting and action potentials. In Hille B (ed): Handbook of the Nervous System. Handbook of Physiology, p 99. Baltimore, Williams & Wilkins, 1976

70. Hille B: Ionic channels in nerve membranes. Prog Biophys Mol Biol 21:1, 1970

71. Armstrong CM: Sodium channels and gating currents. Physiol Rev 61:644, 1981

72. Latorre R, Coronado R, Vergara C: K^+ channels gated by voltage and ions. Ann Rev Physiol 46:485, 1984

73. Schwarz W, Passow H: CA^{2+}-activated K^+ channels in erythrocytes and excitable cells. Ann Rev Physiol 45:359, 1983

74. Chiu SY, Ritchie JM: Potassium channels in nodal and internodal axonal membrane of mammalian myelinated fibres. Nature 284:170, 1980

75. Tsien RW: Calcium channels in excitable cell membranes. Ann Rev Physiol 45:341, 1983

76. DiPolo R, Beauge L: The calcium pump and sodium-calcium exchange in squid axons. Ann Rev Physiol 45:313, 1983

77. Catterall WA: The molecular basis of neuronal excitability. Science 223:653, 1984

78. Keynes RD: Ion channels in the nerve-cell membrane. Sci Am 240:126, 1979

79. Sigworth FJ: Sodium channels in nerve apparently have two conductance states. Nature 270:265, 1977

80. Aldrich RW, Corey DP, Stevens CF: A reinterpretation of mammalian sodium channel gating based on single channel recording. Nature 306:436, 1983

81. Goldman L, Schauf CL: Inactivation of the sodium current in myxicola giant axons. J Gen Physiol 59:659, 1972

82. Bezanilla F, Armstrong CM: Inactivation of the sodium channel: I. Sodium current experiments. J Gen Physiol 70:549, 1977

83. Aldrich RW, Corey DP, Stevens CF: A reinterpretation of mammalian sodium channel gating based on single recording. Nature 306:436, 1983

84. Agnew WS: Voltage-regulated sodium channel molecules. Ann Rev Physiol 46:517, 1984

85. Fozzard HA: Conduction of the action potential. In Berne RM *et al* (eds): Handbook of Physiology, sect 2, vol 1, p 335. Baltimore, Williams & Wilkins, 1979

86. Rall W: Core conductor theory and cable properties of neurons. In Brookhart JM, Mountcastle VB (eds): Handbook of Physiology, sect 1, vol 1, p 39. Baltimore, Williams & Wilkins, 1977

87. Ritchie JM: Physiological basis of conduction of myelinated nerve fibers. In Morell P (ed): Myelin, p 117. New York, Plenum, 1984

88. Ritchie JM, Chiu SY: Distribution of sodium and potassium channels in mammalian myelinated nerve. Adv Neurol 31:329, 1981

89. Waxman SG, Ritchie JM: Organization of ion channels in the myelinated nerve fiber. Science 228:1502, 1985

90. Taylor RE: Effect of procaine on electrical properties of squid axon membrane. Am J Physiol 196:1071, 1959

91. Courtney KR: Local anesthetics. Int Anesth Clin 26:239, 1988

92. Butterworth JF, Strichartz GR: Molecular mechanisms of local anesthesia: A review. Anesthesiology 72:711, 1990

93. Hille B: The common mode of action of three agents that decrease the transient change in sodium permeability in nerves. Nature 210:1220, 1966

94. Strichartz GR, Ritchie JM: The action of local anesthetics on ion channels of excitable tissues. In Strichartz GR (ed): Local Anesthetics. Handbook of Experimental Pharmacology, p 21. Berlin, Springer-Verlag, 1987

95. Strichartz G: Interactions of local anesthetics with neuronal sodium channels. In Covino BG, Fozzard HA, Rehder K *et al* (eds): Effects of Anesthetics, p 39. Bethesda, American Physiological Society, 1985

96. Strichartz GR, Ritchie JM: The action of local anesthetics on ion channels of excitable tissues. In Strichartz GR (ed): Local Anesthetics, p 21. Berlin, Springer-Verlag, 1987

97. Blaustein MP, Goldman DE: Competitive action of calcium and procaine on lobster axon. J Gen Physiol 49:1043, 1966

98. Arhem P, Frankenhaeuser B: Local anesthetics: Effects on permeability properties of nodal membrane in myelinated nerve fibres from xenopus. Potential clamp experiments. Acta Physiol Scand 91:11, 1974

99. Strichartz G: Molecular mechanisms of nerve block by local anesthetics. Anesthesiology 45:421, 1976

100. Shanes AM: Electrochemical aspects of physiological and pharmacological action in excitable cells. Part II: The action potential and excitation. Pharmacology 10:165, 1958

101. Johnson SM, Miller K: Antagonism of pressure and anaesthesia. Nature 228:75, 1970

102. Seeman P: The membrane expansion theory of anesthesia. In Fink BR (ed): Molecular Mechanisms of Anesthesia. Progress in Anesthesiology, vol 1, p 243. New York, Raven Press, 1975

103. Seeman P: The membrane actions of anesthetics and tranquilizers. Pharmacol Rev 24:583, 1972

104. Boulanger Y, Schreier S, Smith ICP: Molecular details of anesthetic-lipid interaction as seen by deuterium and phosphorus-31 nuclear magnetic resonance. Biochemistry 20:6824, 1981

105. Trudell JR, Cohen EN: Anesthetic-induced nerve membrane fluidity as a mechanism of anesthesia. In Fink BR (ed): Molecular Mechanisms of Anesthesia. Progress in Anesthesiology, vol 1, p 315. New York, Raven Press, 1975

106. Kelusky EC, Smith ICP: The influence of local anesthetics on molecular organization of phosphatidylethanolamine membranes. Mol Pharmacol 26:314, 1984

107. Smith ICP, Butler KW: Location and dynamics of anesthetics in membranes: A magnetic resonance view. In Covino BG, Fozzard HA, Rehder K *et al* (eds): Effects of Anesthesia, p 1. Bethesda, American Physiological Society, 1985

108. Kendig JJ, Cohen EN: Pressure antagonism to nerve conduction block by anesthetic agents. Anesthesiology 47:6, 1977

109. Seeman P: Anesthetics and pressure reversal of anesthesia (editorial). Anesthesiology 47:1, 1977

110. Mrose HE, Ritchie JM: Local anesthetics: Do benzocaine and lidocaine act at the same single site? J Gen Physiol 71:223, 1978

111. Hille B: Charges and potentials at the nerve surface, divalent ions and pH. J Gen Physiol 51:221, 1968

112. McLaughlin S, Harary H: Phospholipid flip-flop and the distribution of surface charges in excitable membranes. Biophys J 14:200, 1974

113. Wei LY: Role of surface dipoles on axon membrane. Science 163:280, 1969

114. Blaustein MP, Goldman DE: Action of anionic and cationic nerve-blocking agents: Experiment and interpretation. Science 153:429, 1966

115. McLaughlin S: Local anesthetics and the electrical properties of phospholipid bilayer membranes. In Fink BR (ed): Molecular Mechanisms of Anesthesia. Progress in Anesthesiology, vol 1, p 193. New York, Raven Press, 1975

116. Singer M: Effects of local anesthetics on phospholipid bilayer membranes. In Fink BR (ed): Molecular Mechanisms of Anesthesia. Progress in Anesthesiology, vol 1, p 223. New York, Raven Press, 1975

117. Aceves J, Machne X: The action of calcium and of local anesthetics on nerve cells, and their interaction during excitation. J Pharmacol Exp Ther 140:138, 1963

118. Strichartz GR: The inhibition of sodium currents in myelinated nerve by quaternary derivatives of lidocaine. J Gen Physiol 62:37, 1973

119. Hille B: Theories of anesthesia: General perturbations versus specific receptors. In Fink BR (ed): Molecular Mechanisms of Anesthesia. Progress in Anesthesiology, vol 2, p 1. New York, Raven Press, 1980

120. Hille B: Ionic channels in nerve membranes. Prog Biophys Mol Biol 21:1, 1970

121. Hille B: The permeability of the sodium channel to metal cations in myelinated nerve. J Gen Physiol 59:637, 1972

122. Ritchie JM: A pharmacological approach to the structure of sodium channels in myelinated axons. Ann Rev Neurosci 2:341, 1979

123. Strichartz GR, Ritchie JM: The action of local anesthetics on ion channels of excitable tissues. In Strichartz GR (ed): Local Anesthetics, Handbook of Experimental Pharmacology, p 21. Berlin, Springer-Verlag, 1987

124. Courtney KR: Mechanism of frequency-dependent inhibition of sodium currents in frog myelinated nerve by the lidocaine derivative GEA 968. J Pharmacol Exp Ther 195:225, 1975

125. Cahalan M, Shapiro BI, Almers W: Relationship between inactivation of sodium channels and block by quaternary derivatives of local anesthetics and other compounds. In Fink BR (ed): Molecular Mechanisms of Anesthesia. Progress in Anesthesiology, vol 2, p 17. New York, Raven Press, 1980

126. Hille B: Local anesthetics: Hydrophilic and hydrophobic pathways for the drug-receptor interaction. J Gen Physiol 69:497, 1977

127. Schwartz W, Palade PT, Hille B: Local anesthetics: Effect of pH on use-dependent block of sodium channels in frog muscle. Biophys J 20:343, 1977

128. Hondeghem LM, Katzung BG: Time- and voltage-dependent interactions of antiarrhythmic drugs with cardiac sodium channels. Biochim Biophys Acta 472:373, 1977

129. Courtney KR: Structure-activity relations for frequency-dependent sodium channel block in nerve by local anesthetics. J Pharmacol Exp Ther 213:114, 1980

130. Bean BP, Cohen CJ, Tsien RW: Lidocaine block of cardiac sodium channels. J Gen Physiol 81:613, 1983

131. Hondeghem LM, Katzung BG: Antiarrhythmic agents: The modulated receptor mechanism of action of sodium and calcium channel-blocking drugs. Ann Rev Pharmacol Toxicol 24:387, 1984

132. Khodorov B, Shishkova L, Peganov E et al: Inhibition of sodium currents in frog Ranvier node treated with local anesthetics: Role of slow sodium inactivation. Biochim Biophys Acta 433:409, 1976

133. Yeh JZ: Blockage of sodium channels by stereoisomers of local anesthetics. In Fink BR (ed): Molecular Mechanisms of Anesthesia, Progress in Anesthesiology, vol 2, p 35. New York, Raven Press, 1980

134. Ritchie JM, Rogart RB: The binding of saxitoxin and tetrodotoxin to excitable tissue. Rev Physiol Biochem Pharmacol 79:1, 1977

135. Cohen CJ, Bean BP, Colatsky TJ et al: Tetrodotoxin block of sodium channels in rabbit Purkinje fibers. Interactions between toxin binding and channel gating. J Gen Physiol 78:383, 1981

136. Honerjäger P: Cardioactive substances that prolong the open state of sodium channels. Rev Physiol Biochem Pharmacol 92:1, 1982

137. Strichartz G, Rando T, Wang GK: An integrated view of the molecular toxicology of sodium channel gating in excitable cells. Ann Rev Neurosci 10:237, 1987

138. Schneider M, Datta S, Strichartz G: A preferential inhibition of impulses in C-fibers of the rabbit vagus nerve by veratridine, an activator of sodium channels. Anesthesiology 74:270, 1991

139. Kendig JJ, Courtney KR: New modes of nerve block. Anesthesiology 74:207, 1991

140. de Jong RH: Clinical physiology of local anesthetic action. In Cousins MJ, Bridenbaugh PO (eds): Neural Blockade in Clinical Anesthesia and Management of Pain, p 27. Philadelphia, JB Lippincott, 1980

141. de Jong RH: Local Anesthesia, p 51. Springfield, Illinois, Charles C Thomas, 1977

142. Franz DN, Perry RS: Mechanisms for differential block among single myelinated and non-myelinated axons by procaine. J Physiol (Lond) 236:193, 1973

143. Rosenberg PH, Heavner JE: Temperature-dependent nerve-blocking action of lidocaine and halothane. Acta Anaesthesiol Scand 24:324, 1980

144. Bromage PR: Epidural Anesthesia, p 525. Philadelphia, WB Saunders, 1978

145. Datta S, Lambert DH, Gregus J et al: Differential sensitivities of mammalian nerve fibers during pregnancy. Anesth Analg 62:1070, 1983

146. Flanagan HL, Datta S, Lambert DH et al: Effect of pregnancy on bupivacaine-induced conduction blockade in the isolated rabbit vagus nerve. Anesth Analg 66:123, 1987

147. Gasser HS, Erlanger J: The role played by the sizes of the constituent fibers of a nerve trunk in determining the form of its action potential wave. Am J Physiol 80:522, 1927

148. Gasser HS, Erlanger J: The role of fiber size in the establishment of a nerve block by pressure or cocaine. Am J Physiol 88:581, 1929

149. de Jong R: Local Anesthetics, 2nd ed, p 56. Springfield, Illinois, Charles C Thomas, 1977

150. Raymond SA, Gissen AJ: Mechanisms of differential nerve block. In Strichartz GR (ed): Local Anesthetics, p 95. Berlin, Springer-Verlag, 1987

151. Everett GM, Goodsell JS: The greater resistance to procaine of slow fiber groups in some peripheral nerves. J Pharmacol Exp Ther 106:385, 1952

152. Everett GM, Toman JEP: Procaine block of fiber groups in various nerves. Fed Proc 13:352, 1954

153. Franz DN, Perry RS: Mechanisms for differential block among single myelinated and non-myelinated axons by procaine. J Physiol (Lond) 236:193, 1974

154. Ford DJ, Raj PP, Singh P et al: Differential peripheral nerve block by local anesthetics in the cat. Anesthesiology 60:28, 1984

155. Heavner JE, de Jong RH: Lidocaine blocking concentrations for B- and C-nerve fibers. Anesthesiology 40:228, 1974

156. Scurlock JE, Heavner JE, de Jong RH: Differential B and C fibre block by an amide- and an ester-linked local anaesthetic. Br J Anaesth 47:1135, 1975

157. Rosenberg PH, Heinonen E: Differential sensitivity of A and C nerve fibres to long-acting amide local anaesthetics. Br J Anaesth 55:163, 1983

158. Rosenberg PH, Heinonen E, Jansson SE et al: Differential nerve block by bupivacaine and 2-chloroprocaine. Br J Anaesth 52:1183, 1980

159. Gissen AJ, Covino BG, Gregus J: Differential sensitivities of mammalian nerve fibers to local anesthetic agents. Anesthesiology 53:467, 1980

160. Wildsmith JAW, Gissen AJ, Gregus J et al: Differential nerve blocking activity of amino-ester local anaesthetics. Br J Anaesth 57:612, 1985

161. Wildsmith JAW, Gissen AJ, Takman B et al: Differential nerve blockade: Ester v. amides and the influence of pK_a. Br J Anaesth 59:379, 1987

162. Tasaki I: Conduction of the nerve impulse. In Magoun HW

(ed): Handbook of Physiology, vol 1, Neurophysiology, p 108. Washington DC, American Physiological Society, 1959

163. Stampfli R: Overview of studies on the physiology of conduction in myelinated nerve fibers. In Waxman SG, Ritchie JM (eds): Demyelinating Diseases: Basic and Clinical Electrophysiology, p 11. New York, Raven Press, 1981

164. Tasaki I: Nervous Transmission, p 164. Springfield, Illinois, Charles C Thomas, 1953

165. Hiscoe NB: Distribution of nodes and incisures in normal and regenerated nerve fibers. Anat Rec 99:447, 1947

166. Nathan PW, Sears TA: Some factors concerned in differential nerve block by local anaesthetics. J Physiol (Lond) 157:565, 1961

167. Nathan PW, Sears TA: Differential nerve block by sodium-free and sodium-deficient solutions. J Physiol (Lond) 164:375, 1962

168. Gissen AJ, Covino BG, Gregus J: Differential sensitivity of fast and slow fibers in mammalian nerve: VI. Effect of pH on blocking action of local anesthetics. Reg Anesth 11:132, 1986

169. Grossman Y, Parnas I, Spira ME: Differential conduction block in branches of a bifurcating axon. J Physiol (Lond) 295:282, 1979

170. Raymond SA: Effects of nerve impulses on threshold of frog sciatic nerve fibres. J Physiol (Lond) 290:273, 1979

171. Raymond SA, Roscoe RF: After-effects of nerve impulses on threshold of frog sciatic fibers depends upon pH (pCO2). Soc Neurosci Abstracts 9:513, 1983

172. Malenka RC et al: Modulation of parallel fiber excitability by postsynaptically mediated changes in extracellular potassium. Science 214:339, 1981

173. Gissen AJ, Covino BG, Gregus J: Differential sensitivity of fast and slow fibers in mammalian nerve: III. Effect of etidocaine and bupivacaine on fast/slow fibers. Anesth Analg 61:570, 1982

174. Fink BR, Cairns AM: Differential peripheral axon block with lidocaine: Unit studies in the cervical vagus nerve. Anesthesiology 59:182, 1983

175. Fink BR, Cairns AM: Differential slowing and block of conduction by lidocaine in individual afferent myelinated and unmyelinated axons. Anesthesiology 60:111, 1984

176. Fink BR, Cairns AM: Diffusional delay in local anesthetic block in vitro. Anesthesiology 61:555, 1984

177. Fink BR, Cairns AM: Differential margin of safety of conduction in individual peripheral axons. Anesthesiology 63:65, 1985

178. Fink BR, Cairns AM: Differential effect of nerve fiber structure on block by local anesthetic. Anesthesiology 63:157, 1985

179. Fink BR: Mechanisms of differential epidural block. Anesth Analg 65:325, 1986

180. Fink BR, Cairns AM: Lack of size-related differential sensitivity to equilibrium conduction block among mammalian myelinated axons exposed to lidocaine. Anesth Analg 66:948, 1987

181. Fink BR: Mechanisms of differential axial blockade in epidural and subarachnoid anesthesia. Anesthesiology 70:851, 1989

182. Strichartz GR: The inhibition of sodium currents in myelinated nerve by quaternary derivatives of lidocaine. J Gen Physiol 62:37, 1973

183. Courtney KR, Kendig JJ, Cohen EN: Frequency-dependent conduction block: The role of nerve impulse pattern in local anesthetic potency. Anesthesiology 48:111, 1978

184. Scurlock JE, Meymaris E, Gregus J: The clinical character of local anesthetics: A function of frequency-dependent conduction block. Acta Anaesth Scand 22:601, 1978

185. Courtney KR: Structure-activity relations for frequency-dependent sodium channel block in nerve by local anesthetics. J Pharmacol Exp Ther 213:114, 1980

186. Winnie AP, LaVallee DA, DeSosa B et al: Clinical Pharmacokinetics of local anaesthetics. Canad Anaesth Soc J 24:252, 1977

187. Wildsmith JAW: Peripheral nerve and local anaesthetic drugs. Br J Anaesth 58:692, 1986

188. Kane RE: Neurologic deficits following epidural or spinal anesthesia. Anesth Analg 60:150, 1981

189. Selander D, Brattsand R, Lundborg G et al: Local anesthetics: Importance of mode of application, concentration and adrenaline for the appearance of nerve lesions. Acta Anaesthesiol Scand 23:127, 1979

190. Bromage PR: Spread of analgesic solutions in the epidermal space and their site of action: A statistical study. Br J Anaesth 34:161, 1962

191. Burn JM, Guyer PB, Langdon L: The spread of solutions injected into the epidural space. Br J Anaesth 45:338, 1973

192. Erdemir HA, Soper LE, Sweet RB: Studies of factors affecting peridural anesthesia. Anesth Analg 44:400, 1965

193. Bromage PR: Mechanism of action of extradural analgesia. Br J Anaesth 47(Suppl):199, 1975

194. Scott DB, McClure JH, Giasi RM et al: Effects of concentration of local anaesthetic drugs in extradural block. Br J Anaesth 52:1033, 1980

195. Galindo A, Hernandez J, Benavides O et al: Quality of spinal extradural anaesthesia: The influence of spinal nerve root diameter. Br J Anaesth 47:41, 1975

196. Scott DB, Jebson PJ, Braid DP et al: Factors affecting plasma levels of lignocaine and prilocaine. Br J Anaesth 44:1040, 1972

197. Braid DP, Scott DB: Dosage of lignocaine in epidural block in relation to toxicity. Br J Anaesth 38:596, 1966

198. Tucker GT, Moore DC, Bridenbaugh PO et al: Systemic absorption of mepivacaine in commonly used regional block procedures. Anesthesiology 37:277, 1972

199. Tucker GT, Mather LE: Clinical pharmacokinetics of local anaesthetics. Clin Pharmacokinet 4:241, 1979

200. Rosenberg PH, Heinonen J, Takasaki M: Lidocaine concentration in blood after topical anaesthesia of the upper respiratory tract. Acta Anaesthesiol Scand 24:125, 1980

201. Giasi RM, D'Agostino E, Covino BG: Absorption of lidocaine following subarachnoid and epidural administration. Anesth Analg 58:360, 1979

202. Blair MR: Cardiovascular pharmacology of local anaesthetics. Br J Anaesth 47S:247, 1975

203. Reynolds F: A comparison of the potential toxicity of bupivacaine, lignocaine and mepivacaine during epidural blockade for surgery. Br J Anaesth 43:567, 1971

204. Fink BR, Aasheim GM, Levy BA: Neural pharmacokinetics of epinephrine. Anesthesiology 48:263, 1978

205. Morikawa K-I, Bonica JJ, Tucker GT et al: Effect of acute hypovolaemia on lignocaine absorption and cardiovascular response following epidural block in dogs. Br J Anaesth 46:631, 1974

206. Bromage PR, Gertel M: Brachial plexus anesthesia in chronic renal failure. Anesthesiology 36:488, 1972

207. Mather LE, Tucker GT, Murphy TM et al: Hemodynamic drug interaction: Peridural lidocaine and intravenous ephedrine. Acta Anaesthesiol Scand 20:207, 1976

208. Bowdle TA, Freund PR, Slattery JT: Age-dependent lidocaine pharmacokinetics during lumbar peridural anesthesia with lidocaine hydrocarbonate or lidocaine hydrochloride. Reg Anesth 11:123, 1986

209. Veering BTH, Burm AG, van Kleef JW et al: Epidural anesthesia with bupivacaine: Effects of age on neural blockade and pharmacokinetics. Anesth Analg 66:589, 1987

210. Freund PR, Bowdle TA, Slattery JT et al: Caudal anesthesia with lidocaine or bupivacaine: Plasma local anesthetic concentration and extent of sensory spread in old and young patients. Anesth Analg 63:1017, 1984

211. Tucker GT: Pharmacokinetics of local anaesthetics. Br J Anaesth 58:717, 1986

212. Benowitz N, Forsyth RP, Melmon KL et al: Lidocaine disposition kinetics in monkey and man. I. Prediction by a perfusion model. Clin Pharmacol Ther 16:87, 1974

213. Tucker GT, Pharm B: Is plasma binding of local anesthetics important? Acta Anaesthesiol Scand 39:147, 1988

214. Tucker GT, Boyes RN, Bridenbaugh PO et al: Binding of anilide-type local anesthetics in human plasma: I. Relationships between binding, physicochemical properties, and anesthetic activity. Anesthesiology 33:287, 1970

215. Routledge PA, Stargel WW, Barchowsky A et al: Control of lidocaine therapy: New perspectives. Ther Drug Monit 4:265, 1982

216. Mather LE, Long GJ, Thomas J: The binding of bupivacaine to

maternal and foetal plasma proteins. J Pharm Pharmacol 23:359, 1971

217. Kennedy RL, Miller RP, Bell JU et al: Uptake and distribution of bupivacaine in fetal lambs. Anesthesiology 65:247, 1986

218. Thomas J, Long G, Moore G et al: Plasma protein binding and placental transfer of bupivacaine. Clin Pharmacol Ther 19:426, 1976

219. Arthur GR, Scott DH, Boyes RN et al: Pharmacokinetic and clinical pharmacological studies with mepivacaine and prilocaine. Br J Anaesth 51:481, 1979

220. Mather LE, Runciman WB, Carapetis RJ et al: Hepatic and renal clearances of lidocaine in conscious and anesthetized sheep. Anesth Analg 65:943, 1986

221. Tucker GT: Plasma binding and disposition of local anesthetics. Int Anesthesiol Clin 13:33, 1975

222. Van Zundert A, Burm A, Van Kleef J et al: Plasma concentrations of epidural bupivacaine in mother and newborn. Anesth Analg 66:435, 1987

223. Kuhnert BR, Kuhnert PM, Philipson EH et al: The half-life of 2-chloroprocaine. Anesth Analg 65:273, 1986

224. Smith AR, Hur D, Resano F: Grand mal seizures after 2-chloroprocaine epidural anesthesia in a patient with plasma cholinesterase deficiency. Anesth Analg 66:677, 1987

225. Halkin H, Meffin P, Melmon KL et al: Influence of congestive heart failure on blood levels of lidocaine and its active monodeethylated metabolite. Clin Pharmacol Ther 17:669, 1975

226. Lescanic ML, Miller ED, DiFazio CA: The effects of lidocaine on the whole body distribution of radioactivity labeled microspheres in the conscious rat. Anesthesiology 55:269, 1981

227. Klein SW, Sutherland RI, Morch JE: Hemodynamic effects of intravenous lidocaine in man. Can Med Assoc J 99:472, 1968

228. Wiklund L: Human hepatic blood flow and its relation to systemic circulation during intravenous infusion of bupivacaine or etidocaine. Acta Anaesthesiol Scand 21:189, 1977

229. Sivarajan M, Amory DW, Lindbloom LE: Systemic and regional blood flow during epidural anesthesia without epinephrine in the rhesus monkey. Anesthesiology 45:300, 1976

230. Sivarajan M, Amory DW, Lindbloom LE et al: Systemic and regional blood-flow changes during spinal anesthesia in the rhesus monkey. Anesthesiology 43:78, 1975

231. Bonica JJ, Berges PU, Morikawa K-I: Circulatory effects of peridural block: I. Effects of level of analgesia and dose of lidocaine. Anesthesiology 33:619, 1970

232. Kennedy WF, Everett GB, Cobb LA et al: Simultaneous systemic and hepatic hemodynamic measurements during high peridural anesthesia in normal man. Anesth Analg 50:1069, 1971

233. Greiss FC, Still JG, Anderson SG: Effects of local anesthetic agents on the uterine vasculatures and myometrium. Am J Obstet Gynecol 124:889, 1976

234. Gibbs CP, Noel SC: Response of arterial segments from gravid human uterus to multiple concentrations of lignocaine. Br J Anaesth 49:409, 1977

235. Prescott LF, Adjepon-Yamoah KK, Talbot RG: Impaired lignocaine metabolism in patients with myocardial infarction and cardiac failure. Br Med J 1:939, 1976

236. Thomson PD, Melmon KL, Richardson JA et al: Lidocaine pharmacokinetics in advanced heart failure, liver disease, and renal failure in humans. Ann Intern Med 78:499, 1973

237. Roth RA, Rubin RJ: Role of blood flow in carbon monoxide- and hypoxic hypoxia-induced alterations in hexobarbital metabolism in rats. Drug Metab Dis 4:460, 1976

238. Branch RA, Shand DG, Wilkinson GR et al: The reduction of lidocaine clearance by dl-propranolol: An example of hemodynamic drug interaction. J Pharmacol Exp Ther 184:515, 1973

239. Adjepon-Yamoah KK, Nimmo J, Prescott LF: Gross impairment of hepatic drug metabolism in a patient with chronic liver disease. Br Med J 4:387, 1974

240. Collinsworth KA, Strong JM, Atkinson AJ et al: Pharmacokinetics and metabolism of lidocaine in patients with renal failure. Clin Pharmacol Ther 18:59, 1975

241. Reidenberg MM, James M, Dring LG: The rate of procaine hydrolysis in serum of normal subjects and diseased patients. Clin Pharmacol Ther 13:279, 1971

242. Finucane BT, Hammonds WD, Welch MB: Influence of age on vascular absorption of lidocaine from the epidural space. Anesth Analg 66:843, 1987

243. Moore RG, Thomas J, Triggs EJ et al: The pharmacokinetics and metabolism of the anilide local anaesthetics in neonates. III: Mepivacaine. Eur J Clin Pharmacol 14:203, 1978

244. Mihaly GW, Moore RG, Thomas J et al: The pharmacokinetics of the anilide local anesthetics in neonates. I: Lignocaine. Eur J Clin Pharmacol 13:143, 1978

245. Ecoffey C, Desparmet J, Maury M et al: Bupivacaine in children: Pharmacokinetics following caudal anesthesia. Anesthesiology 63:447, 1985

246. Finholt DA, Stirt JA, DiFazio CA et al: Lidocaine pharmacokinetics in children during general anesthesia. Anesth Analg 65:279, 1986

247. Kennedy RL, Erenberg A, Robillard JE et al: Effects of changes in maternal-fetal pH on the transplacental equilibrium of bupivacaine. Anesthesiology 51:50, 1979

248. Friesen C, Yarnell R, Bachman C et al: The effect of lidocaine on regional blood flows and cardiac output in the non-stressed and the stressed foetal lamb. Can Anaesth Soc J 33:130, 1986

249. Denson D, Coyle D, Thompson G et al: Alpha₁-acid glycoprotein and albumin in human serum bupivacaine binding. Clin Pharmacol Ther 35:409, 1984

250. Bearn AG, Billing B, Sherlock S: The effect of adrenaline and noradrenaline on hepatic blood flow and splanchnic carbohydrate metabolism in man. J Physiol 115:430, 1951

251. Bowdle TA, Freund PR, Slattery JT: Propranolol reduces bupivacaine clearance. Anesthesiology 66:36, 1987

252. Burney RG, DiFazio CA: Hepatic clearance of lidocaine during N₂O anesthesia in dogs. Anesth Analg 55:322, 1976

253. Giasi RM, D'Agostino E, Covino BG: Interaction of diazepam and epidurally administered local anesthetic agents. Reg Anesth 5:8, 1980

254. Denson DD, Myers JA, Thompson GA et al: The influence of diazepam on the serum protein binding of bupivacaine at normal and acidic pH. Anesth Analg 63:980, 1984

255. Bonica JJ, Akamatsu TJ, Berges PU et al: Circulatory effects of peridural block. II. Effects of epinephrine. Anesthesiology 34:514, 1971

256. Stanton-Hicks M, Berges PU, Bonica JJ: Circulatory effects of peridural block: IV. Comparison of the effects of epinephrine and phenylephrine. Anesthesiology 39:308, 1973

257. Benowitz N, Forsyth RP, Melmon KL et al: Lidocaine disposition kinetics in monkey and man. II. Effects of hemorrhage and sympathomimetic drug administration. Clin Pharmacol Ther 16:99, 1974

258. Moore DC, Bridenbaugh LD, Bridenbaugh PO et al: Does compounding of local anesthetic agents increase their toxicity in humans? Anesth Analg 51:579, 1972

259. Cunningham NL, Major MC, Kaplan JA et al: A rapid-onset, long-acting regional anesthetic technique. Anesthesiology 41:509, 1974

260. Lalka D, Vicuna N, Burrow SR et al: Bupivacaine and other amide local anesthetics inhibit the hydrolysis of chloroprocaine by human serum. Anesth Analg 57:534, 1978

261. Raj PP, Ohlweiler D, Hitt BA et al: Kinetics of local anesthetic esters and the effects of adjuvant drugs on 2-chloroprocaine hydrolysis. Anesthesiology 53:307, 1980

262. de Jong RH, Bonin JD: Mixtures of local anesthetics are no more toxic than the parent drugs. Anesthesiology 54:177, 1981

263. Cohen SE, Thurlow A: Comparison of a chloroprocaine-bupivacaine mixture with chloroprocaine and bupivacaine used individually for obstetric epidural analgesia. Anesthesiology 51:288, 1979

264. Galindo A, Witcher T: Mixtures of local anesthetics: Bupivacaine-chloroprocaine. Anesth Analg 59:683, 1980

265. Corke BC, Carlson CG, Dettbarn W-D: The influence of 2-chloroprocaine on the subsequent analgesic potency of bupivacaine. Anesthesiology 60:25, 1984

266. Adriani J: Reactions to local anesthetics. JAMA 196:119, 1966

267. Aldrete JA, Johnson DA: Evaluation of intracutaneous testing for investigation of allergy to local anesthetic agents. Anesth Analg 49:173, 1970

268. Incaudo G, Schatz M, Patterson R et al: Administration of

local anesthetics to patients with a history of prior adverse reaction. J Allergy Clin Immunol 61:339, 1978

269. Brown DT, Beamish D, Wildsmith JAW: Allergic reaction to an amide local anaesthetic. Br J Anaesth 53:435, 1981

270. De Shazo RD, Nelson HS: An approach to the patient with a history of local anaesthetic hypersensitivity: Experience with 90 patients. J Allergy Clin Immunol 63:387, 1979

271. Fisher M McD: Intradermal testing in the diagnosis of acute anaphylaxis during anaesthesia—results of five years experience. Anaesth Intensive Care 7:58, 1979

272. Adriani T: Etiology and management of adverse reactions to local anesthetics. Int Anesthesiol Clin 10:127, 1972

273. Reisner LS, Hochman BN, Plumer MH: Persistent neurologic deficit and adhesive arachnoiditis following intrathecal 2-chloroprocaine injection. Anesth Analg 59:452, 1980

274. Ravindran RS, Bond VK, Tasch MD et al: Prolonged neural blockade following regional analgesia with 2-chloroprocaine. Anesth Analg 59:447, 1980

275. Gibbons RB: Chemical meningitis following spinal anesthesia. JAMA 3:900, 1969

276. Ready LB, Plumer MH, Haschke RH et al: Neurotoxicity of intrathecal local anesthetics in rabbits. Anesthesiology 63:364, 1985

277. Kane RE: Neurologic deficits following epidural or spinal anesthesia. Anesth Analg 60:150, 1981

278. Gissen AJ, Datta S, Lambert D: The chloroprocaine controversy. II. Is chloroprocaine neurotoxic? Reg Anesth 9:135, 1984

279. Wang BC, Hillman DE, Spielholz NI et al: Chronic neurological deficits and nesacaine-CE—an effect of the anesthetic, 2-chloroprocaine, or the antioxidant, sodium bisulfite? Anesth Analg 63:445, 1984

280. Ravindran RS, Turner MS, Muller J: Neurologic effects of subarachnoid administration of 2-chloroprocaine-CE, bupivacaine, and low pH normal saline in dogs. Anesth Analg 61:279, 1982

281. Ford DJ, Raj PP: Peripheral neurotoxicity of 2-chloroprocaine and bisulfite in the cat. Anesth Analg 66:719, 1987

282. Wagman IH, de Jong RH, Price DA: Effects of lidocaine on the central nervous system. Anesthesiology 28:155, 1967

283. de Jong RH, Robles R, Corbin RW: Central actions of lidocaine-synaptic transmission. Anesthesiology 30:19, 1969

284. de Jong RH, Walts LF: Lidocaine-induced psychomotor seizures in man. Acta Anaesthesiol Scand 23:598, 1966

285. Munson ES, Tucker WK, Ausinsch B et al: Etidocaine, bupivacaine, and lidocaine seizure thresholds in monkeys. Anesthesiology 42:471, 1975

286. de Jong RH, Wagman IH, Prince DA: Effect of carbon dioxide on the cortical seizure threshold to lidocaine. Exp Neurol 17:221, 1967

287. Alexander CH, Berko RS, Gross JB et al: The effect of changes in arterial CO_2 tension on plasma lidocaine concentration. Can J Anaesth 34:343, 1987

288. Englesson S: The influence of acid-base changes on central nervous system toxicity of local anaesthetic agents. Acta Anaesthesiol Scand 18:79, 1974

289. Kim KC, Tasch MD: Effects of cimetidine and ranitidine on local anesthetic central nervous system toxicity in mice. Anesth Analg 65:840, 1986

290. Scott DB: Evaluation of the toxicity of local anaesthetic agents in man. Br J Anaesth 47:56, 1975

291. Ausinsch B, Malagodi MH, Munson ES: Diazepam in the prophylaxis of lignocaine seizures. Br J Anaesth 48:309, 1976

292. de Jong RH, Heavner JE: Local anesthetic seizure prevention: Diazepam vs. pentobarbital. Anesthesiology 36:449, 1972

293. Feinstein MB, Lenard W, Mathias J: The antagonism of local anesthetic induced convulsions by the benzodiazepine derivative diazepam. Arch Int Pharmacodyn Ther 187:144, 1970

294. de Jong RH, Heavner JE, de Oliveira LF: Effects of nitrous oxide on the lidocaine seizure threshold and diazepam protection. Anesthesiology 37:299, 1972

295. Bernards CM, Carpenter RL, Rupp SM et al: Effect of midazolam and diazepam premedication on central nervous system and cardiovascular toxicity of bupivacaine. Anesthesiology 70:318, 1989

296. Adams HJ, Kronberg GH, Takman BH: Local anesthetic activity and acute toxicity. (±)-2-(ethylpropylamino)-2′,6′-butyroxylidide: A new long-acting agent. J Pharm Sci 61:1820, 1972

297. Kozody R, Ready LB, Barsa JE et al: Dose requirements of local anaesthetic to produce grand mal seizure during stellate ganglion block. Can Anaesth Soc J 29:489, 1982

298. Aldrete JA, Romo-Salas F, Arora S et al: Reverse arterial blood flow as a pathway for central nervous system toxic responses following injection of local anesthetics. Anesth Analg 57:428, 1978

299. Dunbar RW, Boettner RB, Gatz RN et al: The effect of mepivacaine, bupivacaine, and lidocaine on digitalis-induced ventricular arrhythmias. Anesth Analg 49:761, 1970

300. Chapin JC, Kushins LG, Munson ES et al: Lidocaine, bupivacaine, etidocaine, and epinephrine-induced arrhythmias during halothane anesthesia in dogs. Anesthesiology 52:23, 1980

301. Albright GA: Cardiac arrest following regional anesthesia with etidocaine or bupivacaine. Anesthesiology 51:285, 1979

302. Block A, Covino B: Effect of local agents on cardiac conduction and contractility. Reg Anesth 6:55, 1981

303. de Jong RH, Ronfeld RA, DeRosa R: Cardiovascular effects of convulsant and supraconvulsant doses of amide local anesthetics. Anesth Analg 61:3, 1982

304. Kotelko DM, Shnider SM, Dailey PA et al: Bupivacaine-induced cardiac arrhythmias in sheep. Anesthesiology 60:10, 1984

305. Clarkson CW, Hondeghem LM: Mechanism for bupivacaine depression of cardiac conduction: Fast block of sodium channels during the action potential with slow recovery from block during diastole. Anesthesiology 62:396, 1985

306. Nath S, Haggmark S, Johansson G et al: Differential depressant and electrophysiologic cardiotoxicity of local anesthetics: An experimental study with special reference to lidocaine and bupivacaine. Anesth Analg 65:1263, 1986

307. Lynch C: Depression of myocardial contractility in vitro by bupivacaine, etidocaine, and lidocaine. Anesth Analg 65:551, 1986

308. Courtney KR, Kendig JJ: Bupivacaine is an effective potassium channel blocker in heart. Biochim Biophys Acta 939:163, 1988

309. Thomas RD, Behbehani MM, Coyle DE et al: Cardiovascular toxicity of local anesthetics: An alternative hypothesis. Anesth Analg 65:444, 1986

310. Heavner JE: Cardiac dysrhythmias induced by infusion of local anesthetics into the lateral cerebral ventricle of cats. Anesth Analg 65:133, 1986

311. Kasten GW: Amide local anesthetic alterations of effective refractory period temporal dispersion: Relationship to ventricular arrhythmias. Anesthesiology 65:61, 1986

312. Edouard A, Berdeaux A, Langloys J et al: Effects of lidocaine on myocardial contractility and baroreflex control of heart rate in conscious dogs. Anesthesiology 64:316, 1986

313. Bosnjak ZJ, Stowe DF, Kampine JP: Comparison of lidocaine and bupivacaine depression of sinoatrial nodal activity during hypoxia and acidosis in adult and neonatal guinea pigs. Anesth Analg 65:911, 1986

314. Morishima HO, Covino BG: Toxicity and distribution of lidocaine in nonasphyxiated and asphyxiated baboon fetuses. Anesthesiology 54:182, 1981

315. Morishima HO, Pedersen H, Finster M et al: Bupivacaine toxicity in pregnant and nonpregnant ewes. Anesthesiology 63:134, 1985

316. Rosen MA, Thigpen JW, Shnider SM et al: Bupivacaine-induced cardiotoxicity in hypoxic and acidotic sheep. Anesth Analg 64:1089, 1985

317. Komai H, Rusy BF: Effects of bupivacaine and lidocaine on AV conduction in the isolated rat heart: Modification by hyperkalemia. Anesthesiology 55:281, 1981

318. Avery P, Redon D, Schaenzer G et al: The influence of serum potassium on the cerebral and cardiac toxicity of bupivacaine and lidocaine. Anesthesiology 61:134, 1984

319. Kambam JR, Kinney WW, Matsuda F et al: Epinephrine and phenylephrine increase cardiorespiratory toxicity of intravenously administered bupivacaine in rats. Anesth Analg 70:543, 1990

320. Torbiner ML, Yagiela JA, Mito RS: Effect of midazolam pre-

treatment on the intravenous toxicity of lidocaine with and without epinephrine in rats. Anesth Analg 68:744, 1989

321. Bernards CM, Carpenter RL, Kenter ME et al: Effect of epinephrine on central nervous system and cardiovascular system toxicity of bupivacaine in pigs. Anesthesiology 71:711, 1989

322. Johns RA, DeFazio CA, Longnecker DE: Lidocaine constricts or dilates rat arterioles in a dose-dependent manner. Anesthesiology 62:141, 1985

323. Johns RA, Seyde WC, DiFazio CA et al: Dose-dependent effects of bupivacaine on rat muscle arterioles. Anesthesiology 65:186, 1986

324. Fleisch JH, Titus E: Effect of local anesthetics on pharmacologic receptor systems of smooth muscle. J Pharmacol Exp Ther 186:44, 1973

325. Akerman B, Hellenberg I, Trossvik C: Primary evaluation of the local anesthetic properties of the amino amide agent ropivacaine (LEA 103). Acta Anaesthesiol Scand 32:571, 1988

326. Reiz S, Haggmark S, Johansson G, Nath S: Cardiotoxicity of ropivacaine—a new amide local anaesthetic agent. Acta Anaesthesiol Scand 33:93, 1989

327. Moller R, Covino BG: Cardiac electrophysiologic properties of bupivacaine and lidocaine compared with those of ropivacaine, a new amide local anesthetic. Anesthesiology 72:322, 1990

328. Feldman HS, Arthur GR, Covino BG: Comparative systemic toxicity of convulsant and supraconvulsant doses of intravenous ropivacaine, bupivacaine, and lidocaine in the conscious dog. Anesth Analg 69:794, 1989

329. Arlock P: Actions of three local anaesthetics: Lidocaine, bupivacaine and ropivacaine on guinea pig papillary muscle sodium channels (Vmax). Pharmacol Toxicol 63:96, 1988

330. Brown DL, Carpenter RL, Thompson GE: Comparison of 0.5% ropivacaine and 0.5% bupivacaine for epidural anesthesia in patients undergoing lower extremity surgery. Anesthesiology 72:633, 1990

331. Finucane BT: Ropivacaine—a worthy replacement for bupivacaine? Can J Anaesth 37:722, 1990

332. Moore DC, Crawford RD, Scurlock JE: Severe hypoxia and acidosis following local anesthetic-induced convulsions. Anesthesiology 53:259, 1980

333. Moore DC, Bridenbaugh LD: Oxygen: The antidote for systemic toxic reactions from local anesthetic drugs. JAMA 174:842, 1960

334. Posner JB, Plum F, Van Poznak A: Cerebral metabolism during electrically induced seizures in man. Arch Neurol 20:388, 1969

335. Tommasino C, Maekawa T, Shapiro HM: Local cerebral blood flow during lidocaine-induced seizures in rats. Anesthesiology 64:771, 1986

336. Munson ES, Wagman IH: Diazepam treatment of local anesthetic-induced seizures. Anesthesiology 37:523, 1972

337. Moore DC, Balfour RI, Fitzgibbons D: Convulsive arterial plasma levels of bupivacaine and the response to diazepam therapy. Anesthesiology 50:454, 1979

338. Richards RK, Smith NT, Katz J: The effects of interaction between lidocaine and pentobarbital on toxicity in mice and guinea pig atria. Anesthesiology 29:493, 1968

339. Davis NL, de Jong RH: Successful resuscitation following massive bupivacaine overdose. Anesth Analg 61:62, 1982

340. Mallampati SR, Liu PL, Knapp RM: Convulsions and ventricular tachycardia from bupivacaine with epinephrine: Successful resuscitation. Anesth Analg 63:856, 1984

341. Kendig JJ: Clinical implications of the modulated receptor hypothesis: Local anesthetics and the heart. Anesthesiology 62:382, 1985

342. Kasten GW, Martin ST: Bupivacaine cardiovascular toxicity: Comparison of treatment with bretylium and lidocaine. Anesth Analg 64:911, 1985

343. Kasten GW, Martin ST: Comparison of resuscitation of sheep and dogs after bupivacaine-induced cardiovascular collapse. Anesth Analg 65:1029, 1986

344. Kasten GW, Martin ST: Successful cardiovascular resuscitation after massive intravenous bupivacaine overdosage in anesthetized dogs. Anesth Analg 64:491, 1985

345. Chadwick HS: Toxicity and resuscitation in lidocaine- or bupivacaine-infused cats. Anesthesiology 63:385, 1985

346. Cregler LL, Mark H: Medical complications of cocaine abuse. N Engl J Med 315:1495, 1986

347. Wetli CV, Wright RK: Death caused by recreational cocaine use. JAMA 241:2519, 1979

348. Isner JM, Estes M, Thompson PD et al: Acute cardiac events temporally related to cocaine abuse. N Engl J Med 315:1438, 1986

349. Van Dyke C, Byck R: Cocaine. Sci Am March:128, 1982

350. Climie CR, McLean S, Starmer GA et al: Methaemoglobinaemia in mother and foetus following continuous epidural analgesia with prilocaine. Br J Anaesth 39:155, 1967

351. Lund PC, Cwik JC: Propitocaine (Citanest) and methemoglobinemia. Anesthesiology 26:569, 1965

352. Arens JF, Carrera AE: Methemoglobin levels following peridural anesthesia with prilocaine for vaginal deliveries. Anesth Analg 49:219, 1970

353. Inoue R, Suganuma T, Echizen H et al: Plasma concentrations of lidocaine and its principal metabolites during intermittent epidural anesthesia. Anesthesiology 63:304, 1985

354. Bromage PR, Pettigrew RT, Crowell DE: Tachyphylaxis in epidural analgesia: I. Augmentation and decay of local anesthesia. J Clin Pharmacol 9:30, 1969

355. Moore DC: Spinal anesthesia: Bupivacaine compared with tetracaine. Anesth Analg 59:743, 1980

356. Stanton-Hicks M, Murphy TM, Bonica JJ et al: Effects of extradural block: Comparison of the properties, circulatory effects and pharmacokinetics of etidocaine and bupivacaine. Br J Anaesth 48:575, 1976

357. Carpenter RL: How to optimize the success rate of spinal anesthesia. In Kirby RR, Brown DL (eds): Problems in Anesthesia, p 539. Philadelphia, JB Lippincott, 1987

358. Moore DC, Mather LE, Bridenbaugh PO et al: Arterial and venous plasma levels of bupivacaine following epidural and intercostal nerve blocks. Anesthesiology 45:39, 1976

359. Stoelting RK: Circulatory changes during direct laryngoscopy and tracheal intubation. Anesthesiology 47:381, 1977

360. Stoelting RK: Blood pressure and heart rate changes during short-duration laryngoscopy for tracheal intubation: Influences of viscous or intravenous lidocaine. Anesth Analg 57:197, 1978

361. Chraemmer-Jorgensen B, Hoilund-Carlsen PF, Marving J et al: Lack of effect of intravenous lidocaine on hemodynamic responses to rapid sequence induction of general anesthesia: A double-blind controlled clinical trial. Anesth Analg 65:1037, 1986

362. Laurito CE, Baughman VL, Polek WV et al: Aerosolized and intravenous lidocaine are no more effective than placebo for the control of hemodynamic responses to intubation. Anesthesiology 67:A29, 1987

363. Drenger B, Pe'er J, BenEzra D et al: The effect of intravenous lidocaine on the increase in intraocular pressure induced by tracheal intubation. Anesth Analg 64:1211, 1985

364. Yano M, Nishiyama H, Yokota H et al: Effect of lidocaine on ICP response to endotracheal suctioning. Anesthesiology 64:651, 1986

365. Yukioka H, Yoshimoto N, Nishimura K et al: Intravenous lidocaine as a suppressant of coughing during tracheal intubation. Anesth Analg 64:1189, 1985

366. Downes H, Gerber N, Hirshman CA: I.V. lignocaine in reflex and allergic bronchoconstriction. Br J Anaesth 52:873, 1980

367. Berry CA, Sanner JH, Keasling HH: A comparison of the anticonvulsant activity of mepivacaine and lidocaine. J Pharmacol Exp Ther 133:357, 1961

368. Bernhard CG, Bohm E, Hojeberg S: A new treatment of status epilepticus. Arch Neurol Psychiatr 74:208, 1955

369. Cassuto J, Wallin G, Hogstrom S et al: Inhibition of postoperative pain by continuous low-dose intravenous infusion of lidocaine. Anesth Analg 64:971, 1985

370. Fenning WR: The use of local anesthetics for "beneficial" systemic effects. In Kirby RR, Brown DL (eds): Problems in Anesthesia, p 539. Philadelphia, JB Lippincott, 1987

371. Bedford RF, Persing JA, Pobereskin L et al: Lidocaine or thio-

pental for rapid control of intracranial hypertension? Anesth Analg 59:435, 1980

372. Carpenter RL, Mulroy MF: Edrophonium antagonizes combined lidocaine-pancuronium and verapamil-pancuronium neuromuscular blockade in cats. Anesthesiology 65:506, 1986

373. Littlewood DG, Buckley P, Covino BG et al: Comparative study of various local anesthetic solutions in extradural block in labor. Br J Anaesth 51:47S, 1979

374. Tucker GT, Mather LE: Absorption and Disposition of Local Anesthetics. Pharmacokinetics, Neural Blockade in Clinical Anesthesia and Management of Pain, p 61. Philadelphia, JB Lippincott, 1980

375. Leicht CH, Carlson SA: Prolongation of lidocaine spinal anesthesia with epinephrine and phenylephrine. Anesth Analg 65:365, 1986

376. Chambers WA, Littlewood DG, Scott DB: Spinal anesthesia with hyperbaric bupivacaine. Effect of added vasoconstrictors. Anesth Analg 61:49, 1982

377. Chambers WA, Littlewood DG, Logan MR et al: Effect of added epinephrine on spinal anesthesia with lidocaine. Anesth Analg 60:417, 1981

378. Priddle HD, Andros GJ: Primary spinal anesthetic effects of epinephrine. Curr Res Anesth Analg 29:156, 1950

379. Bromage PR, Camporesi EM, Durant PA et al: Influence of epinephrine as an adjuvant to epidural morphine. Anesthesiology 58:257, 1983

380. Smith HS, Carpenter RL, Bridenbaugh LD: Failure rate of tetracaine spinal anesthesia with and without epinephrine. Anesthesiology 65:A193, 1986

381. Abouleish EI: Epinephrine improves the quality of spinal hyperbaric bupivacaine for cesarean section. Anesth Analg 66:395, 1987

382. Collins JG, Kitahata LM, Matsumoto M et al: Spinally administered epinephrine suppresses noxiously evoked activity of WDR neurons in the dorsal horn of the spinal cord. Anesthesiology 60:269, 1984

383. Siegel RJ, Vistnes LM, Iverson RE: Effective hemostasis with less epinephrine: An experimental and clinical study. Plast Reconstr Surg 51:129, 1973

384. Ohno H, Watanabe M, Saitoh J et al: Effect of epinephrine concentration on lidocaine disposition during epidural anesthesia. Anesthesiology 68:625, 1988

385. Kennedy WF Jr, Bonica JJ, Ward RJ et al: Cardiorespiratory effects of epinephrine when used in regional anesthesia. Acta Anaesthesiol Scand (Suppl) 22:320, 1966

386. Katz RL, Epstein RA: The interaction of anesthetic agents and adrenergic drugs to produce cardiac arrhythmias. Anesthesiology 29:763, 1968

387. Moore DC, Batra MS: The components of an effective test dose prior to epidural block. Anesthesiology 55:693, 1981

388. Hood DD, Dewan DM, Rose JC et al: Maternal and fetal effects of intravenous epinephrine containing solutions in gravid ewes. Anesthesiology 59:A393, 1983

389. Gunther RE, Bellville JW: Obstetrical caudal anesthesia: II. A randomized study comparing 1 per cent mepivacaine with 1 per cent mepivacaine plus epinephrine. Anesthesiology 37:288, 1972

390. Abboud TK, Sheik-ol-Eslam A, Yanagi T et al: Safety and efficacy of epinephrine added to bupivacaine for lumbar epidural analgesia in obstetrics. Anesth Analg 64:585, 1985

391. Jouppila R, Jouppila P, Hollmen A et al: Effect of segmental extradural analgesia on placental blood flow during normal labor. Br J Anaesth 50:563, 1978

392. Albright GA, Jouppila R, Hollmen A et al: Epinephrine does not alter human intervillous blood flow during epidural anesthesia. Anesthesiology 54:131, 1981

393. Jouppila R, Jouppila P, Kuikka J et al: Placental blood flow during caesarean section under lumbar extradural analgesia. Br J Anaesth 50:275, 1978

394. Albright GA: Epinephrine should be used with the therapeutic dose of bupivacaine in obstetrics. Anesthesiology 61:217, 1984

395. Marx GF: In reply to Ref. 394. Anesthesiology 61:218, 1984

396. Ueda W, Hirakawa M, Mori K: Acceleration of epinephrine absorption by lidocaine. Anesthesiology 63:717, 1985

397. Klingstrom P, Nylen B, Westermark L: A clinical comparison between adrenaline and octapressin as vasoconstrictors in local anesthesia. Acta Anaesthesiol Scand 11:35, 1967

398. Katz RL: Epinephrine and PLV-2: Cardiac rhythm and local vasoconstrictor effects. Anesthesiology 26:619, 1965

399. Akerman B: Effects of felypressin (Octopressin) on the acute toxicity of local anaesthetics. Acta Pharmacol Toxicol 27:318, 1969

400. Prokopiou AA, Pateromichelakis S, Rood JP: The effects of ornipressin and adrenaline on lignocaine nerve blocks. Acta Anaesthesiol Scand 30:647, 1986

401. Gerke DC, Frewin DB, Frost BR: The synergistic vasoconstrictor effect of octapressin and catecholamines on the isolated rabbit ear artery. Aust J Exp Biol Med Sci 55:737, 1977

402. Bromage PR, Burfoot MF, Crowell DE et al: Quality of epidural blockade. III. Carbonated local anaesthetic solutions. J Anaesth 39:197, 1967

403. Sukhani R, Winnie AP: Clinical pharmacokinetics of carbonated local anesthetics. I. Subclavian perivascular brachial block model. Anesth Analg 66:739, 1987

404. McClure JH, Scott DB: Comparison of bupivacaine hydrochloride and carbonated bupivacaine in brachial plexus block by the interscalene technique. Br J Anaesth 53:523, 1981

405. Martin R, Lamarche Y, Tetreault L: Comparison of the clinical effectiveness of lidocaine hydrocarbonate and lidocaine hydrochloride with and without epinephrine in epidural anaesthesia. Can Anaesth Soc J 28:217, 1981

406. Brown DT, Morison DH, Covino BG et al: Comparison of carbonated bupivacaine and bupivacaine hydrochloride for extradural anaesthesia. Br J Anaesth 52:419, 1980

407. Martin R, Lamarche Y, Tetreault L: Effects of carbon dioxide and epinephrine on serum levels of lidocaine after epidural anaesthesia. Can Anaesth Soc J 28:224, 1981

408. Parnass SM, Curran MA, Becker GL: Comparative hypotensive responses of the carbonated and hydrochloride salts of lidocaine in epidural blocks. Anesth Analg 66:S134, 1987

409. Navaratnarajah M, Davenport HT: The prolongation of local anaesthetic action with dextran. Anaesthesia 40:259, 1985

410. Adams H-A, Biscoping J, Kafurke H et al: Influence of dextran on the absorption of adrenaline-containing lignocaine solutions: A protective mechanism in local anaesthesia. Br J Anaesth 60:645, 1988

411. Bridenbaugh LD: Does the addition of low molecular weight dextran prolong the duration of action of bupivacaine? Reg Anesth 3:6, 1978

412. Moore DC: The use of hyaluronidase in local and nerve block analgesia other than spinal block: 1520 cases. Anesthesiology 12:611, 1951

IV

PREPARING FOR ANESTHESIA

21

C. Philip Larson Jr.

Evaluation of the Patient and Preoperative Preparation

Implementation of an anesthetic always begins with preoperative evaluation of the patient and development of an anesthetic plan. The purposes of the preoperative visit are (1) to learn as much about the patient as possible before administration of an anesthetic, (2) to plan the anesthetic and obtain the patient's agreement, (3) to answer the patient's questions and allay his or her fears and apprehensions as much as possible, (4) to reassure the patient that the anesthesiologist will do everything in his or her power to take the very best possible care of the patient during and after the operation, and (5) to order premedication or other patient care items. The time expended and the level of detail of the evaluation vary with many factors, including the nature and severity of the patient's illness and the complexity, urgency, and expected duration of the operation being proposed. Except in extreme emergencies such as acute uncontrolled bleeding into the head, chest, or abdomen, or acute fetal distress, sufficient time should be taken to garner all the information that is essential for planning an anesthetic that will be both safe and effective for the patient.

Whenever possible, it is desirable to perform the preoperative evaluation and development of an anesthetic plan well in advance of the operation and at a site that is away from the operating suite. The reasons for this are threefold: (1) it permits careful consideration of the history, physical examination, and laboratory data contained in the patient's chart in an unhurried manner; (2) it allows time if needed for procurement of additional laboratory data and/or consultations by other specialists; and (3) it allows time for quiet reflection and reconsideration of the data gathered and plans made, and perhaps consultation with colleagues regarding the anesthetic plan. Unfortunately, anesthetic evaluation and planning done at the operating room door immediately prior to the start of anesthesia and surgery sometimes result in inadequate data gathering, poor anesthetic planning, and resultant unnecessary anesthetic complications intraoperatively or postoperatively.

Today, many operations are performed in outpatient or ambulatory surgical facilities that are either special units in hospitals or free-standing facilities. In addition, many patients who are scheduled to undergo surgery in a hospital operating suite are not admitted to the hospital until the day of operation. As a result, most patients have their preoperative evaluation and planning done in a presurgical screening clinic or ambulatory surgical facility one or more days in advance of their scheduled operation. Because of the logistic problems that this kind of practice presents, the preoperative evaluation itself is generally done by a nurse practitioner trained in this field or by an available anesthesiologist, usually not the one who will be responsible for administering the anesthetic. Today, only when patients are seriously ill, need extensive preoperative evaluations or special preoperative treatments such as intravenous antibiotic therapy, or are already in the hospital for other reasons does the anesthesiologist have the luxury of making the preoperative visit in the traditional manner in the patient's hospital room the day before surgery. The prevailing practice is that most of the time anesthesiologists must rely on the anesthetic evaluations and plans made by a nurse practitioner or anesthesiologist colleagues when they see the patient for the first time the day of the operation. Ideal anesthetic practice in this modern climate dictates that the anesthesiologist at least review the records of the patients whom he or she will be anesthetizing the next day. Even better, some anesthesiologists have taken to telephoning their patients at home the evening before surgery and confirming the relevant findings and anesthetic plan with them. Regardless of what practice pattern is used, the anesthesiologist is responsible for gathering all the relevant information, developing an anesthetic plan, and confirming that plan with the patient prior to the start of administration of the anesthetic. The use of a detailed or automated health questionnaire that is completed by the patient in advance of seeing the anesthesiologist or nurse practitioner is extremely helpful both as a time saver and as a mechanism for capturing all important information.

CHART REVIEW

Preoperative evaluation of a patient begins with a review of the patient's chart. The relevant history, physical examination findings, and laboratory studies should be recorded in the chart and available for review. Commonly, patients will have had prior operations and received anesthetics in the same hospital or outpatient facility. If so, the anesthesiologist should review the records of the prior admission(s), placing special emphasis on the preoperative evaluation;

laboratory studies such as hematocrit reading and electrolyte panel, chest roentgenogram, and electrocardiogram; anesthetic and operative records; and the postoperative recovery. Much helpful information about how to manage a patient anesthetically can be obtained by reviewing records of earlier anesthetics used. Anesthesiologists should never discover after the fact that readily available records documented a prior myocardial infarction, a difficult tracheal intubation, poor venous access, or unexplained postoperative jaundice during administration of anesthesia, just to mention a few such problems.

Generally, anesthetic and operative records from other hospitals are hard to obtain, particularly on one day's notice or less; therefore the anesthesiologist must rely on the patient to provide details of significant past anesthetic or operative complications. However, if it is suspected on the basis of the preoperative experience that the patient has an unusual disorder that will affect delivery of the anesthesia, such as malignant hyperthermia, muscular dystrophy, or porphyria—and time permits—it is prudent to contact the medical records librarian of that hospital and request copies of the relevant records.

HISTORY AND PHYSICAL EXAMINATION

The extent of the history and physical examination which the anesthesiologist must do depends in large measure on what is available from the chart review. If a thorough report is in the patient's chart, the evaluation by the anesthesiologist will focus on confirmation of the major findings, followed by a supplemental history and examination that is specifically relevant to anesthesia. If a complete history and physical examination findings are not yet in the patient's chart, the anesthesiologist is obligated to complete a more detailed history and examination to ensure that at the conclusion of his or her visit all the essential information is in the patient's hospital record.

Before meeting the patient for the first time, the anesthesiologist should make certain that he or she appears professional. Whether in the outpatient or inpatient setting, most patients are accompanied by family and/or friends. At the outset of the interview, the anesthesiologist should greet and identify who the companions are, and determine from the patient if he or she would like them to stay during the history and physical examination. Confidentiality with respect to some bodily functions, prior operations, or drug use is important to some patients and should be respected. The anesthesiologist should also eliminate distractions, such as an operational television set, and maximize privacy by closing the patient's door or pulling a curtain around the patient's bed before beginning the interview.

Although history taking can be performed in many different ways, there are key elements in sequence and style that should be observed in order to establish rapport rapidly with the patient and maximize its efficiency. For example, when the anesthesiologist first introduces him- or herself, it is not uncommon for patients to immediately ask, "What kind of anesthetic are you going to give me?" or to state "I don't care what you do so long as I'm asleep," or "I don't want a spinal." At this juncture, the anesthesiologist should indicate that he or she is there to plan the best possible anesthetic with the patient but that this cannot be done until more information is known about the patient.

The best approach to the interview incorporates a standard format so that nothing is forgotten (Table 21-1) but tailors it to meet the circumstances of the individual patient. A good way to start the interview process is to ask patients

---

TABLE 21-1. General Outline of a Preoperative Patient Interview

1. Are you aware of the planned surgery? Do you know what operation is to be performed?
2. What problems caused you to go to the doctor? Details?
3. Treatments/medicines for the problems: dose, duration, effectiveness?
4. Current drug(s) use: reason, dose, duration, effectiveness, side-effects?
5. Tobacco or alcohol use: quantity?
6. Recreational drug use: quantity?
7. Drug allergies?
8. Prior anesthetic exposure(s): type, adverse effects?
9. General health and organ system review
   Circulatory system (hypertension, heart disease, angina, activity level)
   Respiratory system (cough, cold, sputum, pneumonia, asthma, stridor)
   Central nervous system (headache, dizziness, visual disturbances, stroke, seizure)
   Hepatic system (jaundice, hepatitis)
   Renal system (abnormal function)
   Gastrointestinal system (nausea, vomiting, reflux, diarrhea, weight change)
   Endocrine system (diabetes, thyroid condition, pheochromocytoma)
   Hematologic system (excessive bleeding, anemia)
   Musculoskeletal system (back or joint pains, arthritis)
   Dental system (loose teeth, caps)
   Reproductive system where appropriate (pregnant, preeclampsia)
   Obesity

---

if they are aware that their physician has scheduled them for surgery, and if they understand what surgery is to be performed. This is a valuable way to start because sometimes the contemplated surgery is contingent upon a particular laboratory study, and the surgeon may not have communicated the findings to the patient and affirmed the need for surgery in advance of the anesthesiologist's visit. The next logical line of questioning involves inquiring into what caused the patient to visit the physician or come to hospital. Patients who are contemplating surgery want to talk about why they need the operation, and some are put off if the anesthesiologist starts the interview with questions relating to what drugs they are taking or whether they have any trouble with their heart or lungs. How detailed this part of the interview will be depends on what is contained in the chart. If there is a thorough medical history available, the anesthesiologist need only review the highlights of the problem necessitating surgery. To complete the questioning about the problem requiring surgery, the anesthesiologist needs to know what treatments and/or drugs have been used, and in the case of the latter their dose, duration, and effectiveness.

Drug Evaluation and Interactions

Since the interview has been directed toward treatments and drug use, at this point it is timely to inquire about current drug use for whatever purpose. The spectrum of therapeutic drugs that patients may be taking and their anesthetic implications are myriad (Table 21-2). The inquiry should include questions about reason(s) for use, dose, duration of use, effectiveness, and any untoward effects from

(Text continues on page 549)

TABLE 21-2. Management of Drug Therapy in Relation to Anesthesia

Drug	Anesthetic Implication	Modification of Therapy
Analgesics		
Aspirin	Bleeding tendency due to functional impairment of platelets.	Stop aspirin therapy at least 10–14 days before elective surgery. Platelet transfusions as required in emergency surgery.

Opioids
  Morphine
  Meperidine
	Addiction	Use as needed.

Antibiotics		

Aminoglycosides
  Clindamycin
  Gentamicin
  Kanamycin
  Neomycin
  Streptomycin
	Can cause nondepolarizing neuromuscular block, potentiated by curare-like muscle relaxants; may be reversible with Ca^{2+} and/or neostigmine.	Avoid muscle relaxants or control their dosage carefully. Monitor neuromuscular blockade.

Cephalosporins
  Cefazolin
  Cefotaxime
  Cefotetan
	Allergic reaction	Avoid use

Vancomycin	Hypotension with rapid administration.	Administer at 10 mg·min^{-1} or less.
Anticholinesterases		
Echothiophate eye drops Organophosphate insect sprays	May prolong apnea following use of depolarizing muscle relaxants.	Avoidance or cautious use of muscle relaxants. Monitor neuromuscular blockade.
Anticoagulants		

Coumarin derivatives
  Dicumarol
  Warfarin
  Heparin
	Excessive bleeding with surgery. Occult bleeding, especially of GI tract, causing anemia and hypovolemia.	Stop therapy. Obtain coagulation screen. Avoid regional anesthesia if coagulation is abnormal. Reverse coumarin derivatives with vitamin K_1 oxide or heparin with protamine sulfate in emergency surgery.

Antidepressants		

Lithium preparations
  Eskalith
  Lithane
	Side-effects can include nausea and vomiting, diuresis with sodium loss, muscle weakness.	Continue until day of surgery. Anesthetic risk is probably less if disease is controlled. Use muscle relaxants carefully. Monitor neuromuscular blockade.

Monoamine oxidase inhibitors
  Isocarboxazid (Marplan)
  Pargyline
  Phenelzine (Nardil)
  Tranylcypromine (Parnate)
	Increased catecholamine stores. Alarming hypertensive response to directly and indirectly acting pressor amines. Prolonged effect of other drugs owing to decreased metabolism resulting from enzyme inhibition. Interaction between monoamine oxidase inhibitors and many other drugs may result in hypertension, hypotension, tachycardia, diaphoresis, convulsions, coma, respiratory depression, or hyperpyrexia. Alleged fatal interactions with opioids, especially meperidine, are poorly documented.	Replace with tricyclic antidepressants 2 weeks before surgery or use primarily volatile anesthetics. Avoid potent analgesics and use vasopressors cautiously. Local or conduction anesthesia without vasopressors is preferred. Be prepared to treat hypertension or hypotension.

Tricyclic antidepressants
  Amitriptyline (Elavil)
  Doxepin (Sinequan)
  Imipramine (Tofranil)
  Nortriptyline (Aventyl)
	Therapeutic doses may cause prolonged sleeping time and minor electrocardiographic changes. Cardiac or aged patients may show myocardial depression. Response to vasopressors may be exaggerated.	Continue until day of surgery. Anesthetic risk is probably less if depression is controlled.

Antidiabetic Agents		
Insulin	Hypoglycemia if long-acting agents are used.	Administer half of the regular dose of long-acting insulin on A.M. of surgery. Change from long-acting to short-acting injectable insulin if necessary. Ensure adequate glucose intake. Start fluid infusion in A.M.

Oral agents
  Chlorpropamide
  Phenformin
  Tolbutamide
		Omit oral agents prior to surgery.

(continued)

TABLE 21-2 (continued)

Drug	Anesthetic Implication	Modification of Therapy
Antihypertensives		
Clonidine (Catapres) Guanethidine Hydralazine (Apresoline) Methyldopa (Aldomet) Minoxidil (Loniten) Prazosin (Minipress) Reserpine	May potentiate hypotensive effects of anesthetic agents. Impairment of normal circulatory homeostasis with altered responses to endogenous catecholamines and pressor agents.	Continue therapy until day of surgery. Less risk from anesthesia if hypertension is controlled. Give myocardial depressant drugs cautiously.
Anti-inflammatory Drugs		
Indomethacin (Indocin) Naproxen (Naprosyn)	GI ulceration and bleeding. Decreased platelet aggregation and prolonged bleeding time.	Discontinue 2 weeks before surgery. Give platelet transfusions if necessary.
Antimetabolites		
Cyclophosphamide (Cytoxan) Doxorubicin (Adriamycin) Fluorouracil 6-Mercaptopurine Methotrexate	Thrombocytopenia and anemia.	Blood or platelet transfusions may be necessary.
Barbiturates and Other Sedative Hypnotics		

Barbiturates
   Pentobarbital
   Phenobarbital
   Secobarbital
	Barbiturates may cause hepatic microsomal enzyme induction, with increase of toxic metabolites of anesthetic agents.	Continue during hospitalization. Recognize increased or possibly decreased drug requirements for therapeutic effect.

Benzodiazepines
   Diazepam
   Flurazepam (Dalmane)
   Triazolam (Halcion)
	Tolerance: May need higher dose of anesthetic drugs.
	Dependence: Withdrawal may lead to abstinence syndrome.
		Treat abstinence syndrome as necessary. Doses of anesthetics may be greater (tolerance) or less from central nervous system depression.

Beta-Adrenergic Blockers		
Atenolol (Tenormin) Metoprolol (Lopressor) Propranolol (Inderal)	Bradycardia and myocardial depression. Summation with myocardial depressant action or vagotonic effect of anesthetic agents. Inability to compensate for blood loss with tachycardia. Decreased tolerance for cardiovascular stresses of anesthesia and surgery.	Continue drug but be prepared to treat hypotension with atropine, calcium, dopamine, etc.
Alpha- and Beta-Adrenergic Blockers		
Labetolol (Normodyne Trandate)	Bradycardia and myocardial depression augmented by anesthetic drugs. Nonallergic bronchospasm.	Continue drug, but be prepared to treat hypotension with atropine, calcium, dopamine, etc.
Calcium Channel Blockers		
Diltiazem (Cardizem) Nifedipine (Procardia) Verapamil (Calan, Isoptin)	Hypotension from myocardial depression or peripheral vasodilation.	Administer myocardial depressant anesthetics slowly.
Cardiac Glycosides		
Digitalis Digitoxin Digoxin	Danger of digitalis toxicity and cardiac arrhythmias, especially if K^+ is low. Vagotonic effect may summate with that of halothane or neostigmine.	If toxicity suggested, decrease digitalis or supplement K^+. Measure plasma digitalis levels if possible.
Diuretics		

Potassium losing agents
   Furosemide (Lasix)
   Mercurials
   Thiazides
	Hypokalemia. Hypochloremic metabolic alkalosis. Chronic dilutional hyponatremia may result.	Check serum electrolytes. May require supplemental potassium therapy before anesthesia. Evaluate blood and fluid volume.

Aldosterone antagonists Spironolactone	Hyperkalemia. Electrocardiographic changes, cardiac arrhythmias.	Check serum electrolytes. Careful monitoring of serum K^+. Evaluate blood and fluid volume.

Potassium-sparing agents
   Amiloridine
   Triamterine
   Triamterine with hydrochlorothiazide (Dyazide)
	Usually little change in electrolyte or acid-base status.	Check serum electrolytes. Evaluate blood and fluid volume.

(continued)

TABLE 21-2 (*continued*)

Drug	Anesthetic Implication	Modification of Therapy
Steroids		
Dexamethasone Hydrocortisone Prednisone Prednisolone	Hypotension from stress of anesthesia and surgery if regular doses of steroids were taken within 2 months preceding surgery.	Dexamethasone, 4–8 mg daily, or hydrocortisone 100 mg im every 6 hours commencing with premedication (1) for 3 days if major surgery; (2) for 24 hours if minor surgery; or (3) one dose if very brief procedure. Then taper to normal therapy.

the medication. Occasionally, patients or physicians will inquire as to whether a particular medication should be discontinued prior to anesthesia. Under most circumstances it is highly desirable for patients to continue their regular medications up to the time of anesthesia and operation. This is particularly true for drugs used to control hypertension, angina, arrhythmias, congestive heart failure, diabetes mellitus or other endocrine disorders, allergic reactions, or increased intracranial pressure. Rarely is discontinuance of a prescribed medication necessary to ensure safe anesthesia. The only exception would be for patients taking aspirin, nonsteroidal anti-inflammatory drugs, or other anticoagulants regularly. Regular ingestion of aspirin causes a prolongation of bleeding time that may[1] or may not[2] be associated with a predictable increase in blood loss. The cautious approach would be to check bleeding time preoperatively in any patient taking drugs that are thought to affect platelet function[3] and, if bleeding time is prolonged, to postpone surgery for several weeks until it has returned to normal.

It was believed for many years that patients taking monoamine oxidase inhibitors should stop taking these drugs at least 2 weeks before receiving an anesthetic because of the concern about hypertensive responses to anesthetic drugs, especially meperidine.[4,5] Recent reports, however, demonstrate that general anesthesia can be administered safely to patients taking monoamine oxidase inhibitors.[6-8]

Two drugs that are commonly used and abused are tobacco and alcohol. Each may have adverse effects on anesthetic management; therefore inquiry into their use and some quantitation of how much are necessary. Regular use of tobacco has several adverse effects that have implications for anesthesia. Its use makes the upper airway much more irritable to any foreign body, such as an endotracheal tube or suction apparatus. As a consequence, the combination of inadequate anesthesia (topical or general) and introduction of an endotracheal tube into the airway or its late removal at the conclusion of an anesthetic may cause excessive coughing and bucking, with attendant loss of lung volume, which in turn causes wheezing from marked decrease in airway size (often misdiagnosed as bronchospasm) and oxygen desaturation from ventilation–blood flow mismatching. There may also be a mobilization of thick secretions, causing partial or total obstruction of the airway or endotracheal tube. Continued use of tobacco usually causes patients to develop chronic bronchitis and pulmonary emphysema. Quantitation of tobacco use is usually recorded in pack-years or packs per week times number of years of smoking. Whether there is any benefit to the patient's stopping smoking the night before surgery is problematic. The only likely benefit would be a decrease in the content of carbon monoxide bound to hemoglobin, but documentation of improved outcome because of this is lacking.

Unlike tobacco, the effects of alcohol abuse are more subtle and involve the development of tolerance to drugs, including anesthetic drugs, nutritional deficiencies, and in its severest form cirrhosis of the liver causing esophageal varices, coagulopathies, and impairment of drug metabolism. Quantitation of alcohol use is usually expressed in the history as what is ingested, how often, and for how long.

An unfortunate circumstance is that many patients try street drugs such as marijuana, cocaine, or PCP, and a few are habituated to them. If patients are addicted to them, these drugs may increase the tolerance of patients for anesthetic drugs, necessitating use of higher doses of barbiturates, narcotics, or inhalation anesthetics than would otherwise be the case. Although it is rare, severe adverse reaction to anesthetic drugs has been reported in a patient addicted to amphetamines.[9] Therefore a complete interview must include questioning about the use of recreational drugs. An appropriate way to introduce this subject would be to say, "I need to know what types of drugs you are currently taking or have taken in the past. It is important for me to know about each one whether it's prescription, over-the-counter like aspirin, allergy medicine, or anything else or drugs for recreation because no matter how insignificant they may seem to you, drugs may have an adverse interaction with the anesthetic agents that I might need to use." While inquiring about drug use, it is timely to question the patient about any allergic responses to drugs, particularly antibiotics. If an allergy is claimed, as is commonly the case, it is necessary to inquire about its manifestations and target organs.[10] The reason for this is that many patients claim an allergy to narcotic drugs, particularly morphine or meperidine. When questioned, the allergy is usually "nausea and vomiting," which are common side-effects, not necessarily an allergic response to the opiates. The reason for making this distinction is that use of known allergic drugs is contraindicated, whereas drugs producing unpleasant side-effects may be administered if they are clearly needed and the side-effects are controllable. Rarely, patients may claim an anaphylactic reaction to a drug, with the target organ being the skin or mucus membranes (pruritus, erythema, urticaria, edema), the lungs (wheezing, tight chest, shortness of breath), the circulation (peripheral vasodilatation, shock) or the gastrointestinal tract (nausea, vomiting, abdominal pain, diarrhea).[11] There is no easy way to test preoperatively for a drug allergy; if it is suspected, the offending drug must be avoided.

Before concluding the drug evaluation section of the interview, the anesthesiologist must inquire about prior exposure to anesthetic drugs. This is easily accomplished by asking patients what prior operations they have had, and for each whether they went to sleep for the operation or had a nerve block. Patients rarely know what anesthetic drugs were used, except for thiopental, but if serious reactions occurred, most patients will know that and at least be able to give a general description of what happened. It is also necessary to inquire whether the patient knows if any other member of his or her family has had adverse responses to anesthetic drugs. The major thrust of this inquiry is to determine if the patient has one of the rare genetic disorders that may alter the elimination of anesthetic drugs.

The next step in history taking involves evaluation of the patient's general state of health followed by an in-depth, systematic review of the various organ system functions. One way to start is to ask the patient if he or she has any major problems other than the one that brought the patient to the physician. If the answer is yes, that area should be explored further. If the answer is no, a review of organ systems is appropriate (see Table 21-1).

Circulatory System

Most anesthesiologists begin with the circulatory system because cardiovascular problems are so common in surgical patients. The two major determinations to be made are whether the patient has hypertension and/or ischemic heart disease, with or without heart failure.

Hypertension can occur at any age but is more common with advancing age. The incidence of hypertension varies, depending upon the criteria used to define it. The most widely accepted definition of hypertension is a systolic blood pressure greater than 160 mm Hg and/or a diastolic blood pressure greater than 95 mm Hg. Using this definition, the Joint National Committee on Hypertension reported that about 45% of patients above the age of 65 years have hypertension.[12] The causes of hypertension are many (Table 21-3) but in most cases the etiology is unknown. In the preoperative evaluation of hypertension, the anesthesiologist must make every attempt to determine whether the hypertension is of primary or secondary origin.

The major organs at risk in the hypertensive patient are the heart, brain, and kidneys (Table 21-4). As the blood pressure increases, so do the risks for other cardiovascular complications such as stroke or coronary artery disease with attendant myocardial infarction or congestive heart failure.[13] The preoperative history should include questioning about whether the patient has hypertension, for how long and at what blood pressure, what the patient's activity level is and whether it has been affected by the hypertension, whether the patient has had angina, dizziness, or syncopal episodes, and whether the hypertension has been treated and if the treatment has made the patient feel better. Despite

TABLE 21-3. Etiology of Hypertension

Primary (idiopathic or essential) hypertension
Secondary hypertension
  Renal (end-stage renal disease or renovascular origin)
  Endocrine
    Pheochromocytoma
    Cushing's syndrome
    Primary aldosteronism
  Toxemia of pregnancy
  Mechanical (coarctation of the aorta)
  Neurogenic (increased intracranial pressure)

TABLE 21-4. Consequences of Untreated Hypertension

Heart

Myocardial hypertrophy secondary to increased peripheral resistance
Decreased intravascular volume
Coronary artery disease (ischemic heart disease)

Brain

Shift to right in autoregulation curve
Intracerebral occlusion or hemorrhage (stroke)

Kidneys

Decreased renal blood flow and glomerular filtration rate
Impaired sodium-conserving ability

numerous studies of hypertension, what should be done preoperatively for the patient with untreated hypertension remains controversial. In general, the prevailing view has been that except in emergencies, an untreated hypertensive patient should undergo complete medical evaluation and treatment for the hypertension before elective anesthesia and operation are carried out. Most authorities agree that if the hypertension is moderate or severe (systolic blood pressure greater than 195 mm Hg and/or diastolic blood pressure greater than 110 mm Hg), it should be treated before elective anesthesia and surgery are undertaken. However, if the untreated hypertension is mild (systolic less than 165 and diastolic less than 100), the need for treatment may rest with the presence of other adverse risk factors such as age, weight, history of smoking, history of angina, myocardial infarction or transient ischemic attacks, presence of hypercholesterolemia, or impaired glucose tolerance.[14] One study showed that in patients with mild hypertension and few risk factors, the incidence of intraoperative hypertension or hypotension, or perioperative cardiac arrhythmias or ischemia, or postoperative renal insufficiency was not different from in those patients who were normotensive or whose hypertension had been effectively treated.[14] Others have found that patients with untreated[15] and treated[16] hypertension are at increased risk for postoperative myocardial ischemia and infarction. If the decision is to proceed with the anesthetic and operation, the anesthesiologist must anticipate greater absolute intraoperative blood pressure decreases in such patients[17] and must manage the situation accordingly.

Like hypertension, coronary artery disease (ischemic heart disease) is common in the surgical population and requires careful preoperative evaluation. The objective of the preoperative evaluation is to determine the type, severity, and functional limitations of the heart disease. Potential risk factors for heart disease include age (over 45 years), obesity, hypertension, history of smoking, family history of coronary artery disease, diabetes, angina pectoris, prior myocardial infarction, and history of dysrhythmias or treatment for congestive heart failure. In one recent study, a history of dysrhythmias and preoperative use of digoxin for treatment of congestive heart failure were associated with a significantly increased incidence of adverse cardiac events postoperatively.[18] Whether patients who evidence myocardial ischemia preoperatively are at increased risk for postoperative cardiac complications remains controversial. In a study of 1023 patients undergoing coronary artery bypass grafting, Slogoff and Keats found that postoperative infarction was three times more likely to occur if perioperative ischemia was present.[19] Although others have found a similar correlation,[20] some investigators have not found any correlation between preoperative ischemia and postoperative cardiac complications either in patients undergoing coronary artery bypass grafting[21] or in those undergoing noncardiac surgery.[16,22] In addition to the obvious queries about these risk factors, specific questions about exercise tolerance and whether it is limited by angina or dyspnea should be asked. The usual assessment guideline is stair climbing. If a patient can climb two or more flights of stairs without stopping because of angina or dyspnea, cardiac reserve is probably good. Stable angina is not a contraindication to anesthesia and surgery.[23] In contrast, unstable angina as evidenced by chest pain at rest or with mild exercise or chest pain that varies in frequency or duration is a prodrome of ischemic heart disease and perhaps impending myocardial infarction. Symptoms suggestive of congestive heart failure that should be elicited include night coughing, insomnia because of diaphoresis or palpitations, and orthopnea. If these symptoms are present, anesthesia should not proceed until the heart disease has been evaluated fully except in emergencies.

Management of the patient with a history of prior myocardial infarction is relatively straightforward. It is well documented that the incidence of repeat myocardial infarction in the perioperative period is related to the time elapsed from the prior infarction. Operations performed within the first 3 months after a myocardial infarction are associated with a 30% incidence of perioperative reinfarction, whereas those performed between 3 and 6 months have a 15% incidence of perioperative reinfarction.[24-25] After 6 months, the incidence decreases to about 5%. One study indicates that if aggressive hemodynamic monitoring and prompt treatment of adverse cardiovascular events are used, the incidence of perioperative reinfarction decreases to 6% at less than 3 months, 2% at 3 to 6 months, and 1% thereafter.[26] If a repeat myocardial infarction does occur in these patients, the mortality is high (50–70%).[24-25] These studies indicate that all elective surgery should be postponed for 6 months after a myocardial infarction, and only emergency or urgent noncardiac surgery should be considered. This recommendation would be advisable regardless of whether the planned anesthetic is general, regional, or local. Patients who have undergone prior coronary artery bypass grafting do not appear to be at increased risk for perioperative infarction.[27-28]

Patients with other forms of cardiac disease, especially aortic stenosis or congestive heart failure, are at increased risk to develop cardiac complications postoperatively.[29,30,31] Evidence of these conditions on history or physical examination deserves careful evaluation before proceeding with anesthesia and surgery.

Physical examination of the cardiovascular system includes the items listed in Table 21-5.

Respiratory System

Detailed preoperative evaluation of the respiratory system is important for two reasons: (1) acute and chronic pulmonary diseases are common and second only to coronary artery disease as causes of mortality; and (2) respiratory malfunc-

TABLE 21-5. Physical Examination by the Anesthesiologist

1. Auscultation of the heart to determine rate, rhythm, and presence of aberrant sounds suggestive of valvular disease.
2. Auscultation of the lungs for rales suggestive of incipient heart failure.
3. Palpation of radial arteries for quality and rate.
4. Measurement of blood pressure in one or both arms if arteriosclerosis is suspected; effect of posture if hypovolemia is suspected (orthostatic hypotension).
5. Evaluation of venous filling in the arms, legs, and neck to assess fluid status.
6. Examination of skin for color (cyanosis, jaundice) and dependent parts for pitting edema.
7. Signs of increased intracranial pressure or cerebral ischemia from vasospasm, thrombosis, or embolism.
8. Signs of hepatic failure (ascites, tremor, confusion).
9. Signs of renal failure (hypertension, dysrhythmias, bleeding disorder).

tion is common in the postoperative period and is a major cause of postoperative mortality. Postoperative pulmonary complications are particularly common in the elderly, the obese, patients with a history of smoking, and those patients undergoing operations in the upper abdomen or thorax.[32] The evaluation should include a determination of the type, duration, and severity of the pre-existing lung disease and its reversibility by therapy. Specific questions include inquiry into the presence of dyspnea, a chronic night or morning cough, sputum production and color, sneezing, runny nose, sore throat, and prior episodes of colds or pneumonia. Patients usually know if they have hay fever or asthma, and the type and frequency of bronchodilator therapy used. Dyspnea is a particularly telling symptom; if it is absent on moderate exertion, the anesthesiologist can be confident that pre-existing lung disease is nonexistent or so minor that it will not present any anesthetic problems. If dyspnea is present, its severity should be quantitated in terms of occurrence at rest or with graded exercise. Stridor is also a symptom of importance and suggests partial upper airway obstruction. This symptom must be evaluated thoroughly before proceeding with anesthesia, because general anesthesia may convert partial obstruction into total, uncorrectable airway obstruction.

Except in its more advanced forms, it is difficult to distinguish chronic obstructive lung disease from chronic bronchitis by history and physical examination. In both diseases, patients generally have a history of smoking for many years and complain of dyspnea on exertion, morning cough, and moderate sputum production. With both diseases the patient may have prolonged exhalation with diffuse wheezing. As the chronic obstructive lung disease advances, the patient develops a barrel chest, breath sounds become distant, and use of accessory muscles of respiration is evident when the patient breathes. Severity of the disease can be quantitated by pulmonary function studies, which should be done before elective surgery is contemplated. Several measures can be taken to improve the patient's pulmonary status before anesthesia and operation. These include administering antibiotic therapy to resolve any existing pulmonary infection, chest physiotherapy, bronchodilator therapy, advising the patient to discontinue smoking, and teaching the patient to use incentive spirometry. Although discontinuing smoking will not improve lung function in a few weeks, it will decrease carboxyhemoglobin levels and improve mucociliary transport.[33-34] Preoperative education in the use of incentive spirometry will aid in correcting existing atelectasis and minimize its occurrence postoperatively.[35]

Patients with asthma that is in remission need no special preoperative therapy. Those who use a bronchodilator inhaler regularly should receive treatments the night before and the morning of operation at least 30 minutes before induction of anesthesia.

The patient with a cough or coryza suggestive of an impending cold presents a special dilemma to the anesthesiologist. If the operation is urgent or emergency in nature, the only decision is to proceed with the anesthetic. If the operation is elective, but because of other circumstances the patient or surgeon wants to proceed with the operation, the anesthesiologist must make a value judgment about the cost-benefit ratio of proceeding *versus* delaying the operation until the patient has recovered from the cold. The cost is that with endotracheal intubation and operative or postoperative atelectasis that are almost unavoidable, the patient may develop a postoperative pneumonia. The benefit is that the operation is completed as originally planned. Unfortunately, there are few data upon which to base a decision as to how to proceed. In a retrospective study in 3585 patients aged newborn to 20 years, Tait and Knight[36] found that those who had an uncomplicated upper respiratory tract infection were not at greater risk for intraoperative or postoperative complications than asymptomatic patients, even when endotracheal intubation was used. In contrast, Cohen and Cameron[37] found that children with upper respiratory tract infections were two to seven times more likely to experience respiratory-related adverse events during the perioperative period. If an endotracheal tube was inserted, the risk of respiratory complications increased 11-fold. The conservative approach would be to delay the operation if the patient has a fever or increased leukocyte count, or the operation is to be in the thorax or abdomen, or is contemplated to last longer than 1 hour.

Central Nervous System

Preoperative evaluation of the central nervous system involves assessment of central and peripheral nerve functions. Patients with symptomatic central nervous system diseases present with one or more of a variety of symptoms, including headache, nausea and vomiting, dizziness, visual disturbances, sensory abnormalities and/or motor weakness in one or more extremities, a sudden onset of seizures, or a history of a prior stroke. Unfortunately, some of these symptoms are not specific for central nervous system disease; therefore intracranial tumors may become quite large or intracranial aneurysms may rupture before the diagnosis is localized to the brain. The symptoms may be caused by ischemia from (1) stenosis or thrombosis of intracranial or extracranial cerebral vessels or emboli from the carotid arteries (transient ischemic attacks); (2) a mass effect compressing specific neurons in the motor, sensory, or visual cortex; (3) an increase in intracranial pressure causing distortion of brain tissue; or (4) an intracerebral hemorrhage that may increase intracranial pressure or cause vasospasm from the toxic effects of extravasated blood. Physical signs of increased intracranial pressure may include hyperten-

sion, bradycardia, arrhythmias, focal sensory or motor deficits, papilledema, slurred speech, generalized confusion or disorientation, or coma.

Patients with central nervous system tumors are treated with steroids, which generally lessen the edema formation and decrease or abolish the symptoms and signs of intracranial pressure (ICP) temporarily. Patients evidencing vasospasm from an intracranial hemorrhage may be treated with hypervolemic hemodilution, vasoactive drugs to control hypertension and/or tachycardia, or calcium channel blocking drugs (nimodipine). No treatment has been consistently successful in preventing or abolishing vasospasm. Current neurosurgical practice is shifting toward early operation following an intracerebral bleed provided that the patient is not obtunded.

Patients may evidence symptoms and signs of a peripheral neuropathy that may be attributable to one of many causes, including autonomic nervous system dysfunction, diabetes mellitus, or drug-induced neuropathy. Symptoms may include pain in one or more extremities, hypesthesia or diminished sensation, cold intolerance, and weakness or diminished function. Signs of a peripheral neuropathy may include pale, cold extremities with dry, atrophic skin, diminished peripheral pulses with slow capillary refill after blanching, sensory deficits, and decreased reflexes. When evaluating a patient with a peripheral neuropathy for appropriateness of an anesthetic, the anesthesiologist should focus on the type and extent of the neuropathy and whether it has changed in nature over time. If recent change has occurred, regional anesthesia is inadvisable. However, regardless of whether a regional or general anesthetic is planned, documentation of the neuropathy, preferably by a neurologist, is preferred before proceeding with the anesthetic.

Hepatic System

Disorders of the hepatic system have important implications for the anesthesiologist because

1. Many anesthetic drugs depend in part for their removal from the body by hepatic metabolism, and diminished hepatic function may prolong the anesthetic effect;
2. Coagulopathies may occur as a result of hepatic disease;
3. Hepatic insufficiency may occur postoperatively and be attributed rightly or wrongly to the anesthetic drugs used;
4. The hepatitis virus is virulent and easily transmitted from patient to anesthesiologist through contaminated blood or sputum. Knowledge of this possibility allows the anesthesiologist to take maximum precautions during care of the infected patient.

Most patients know if they have had jaundice or hepatitis in the past, although acute and chronic viral hepatitis do not always produce symptoms. Those symptoms that are present are usually nonspecific, such as fatigue, general malaise, or vague abdominal discomfort or pain. Additional findings on preoperative evaluation that might suggest hepatic disease include marked obesity with fatty infiltration of the liver, long-standing history of alcohol abuse resulting in alcoholic hepatitis, history of multiple blood transfusions, or use of drugs that are known to cause hepatitis. Except for jaundice, there are few physical findings of hepatitis until liver failure develops, as evidenced by spider nevi, ascites, generalized tremor, cyanosis, and confusion or disorientation. Definitive diagnosis of hepatic disease is made by laboratory analysis.

Renal System

Patients with disorders of the renal system generally present in one of two ways. Mild disorders include cystitis or incontinence in women and difficulty in voiding in men, usually due to prostatism. Discussion should be held with the patient regarding whether a bladder catheter will be used. At the other extreme are patients with a history of chronic renal disease often requiring dialysis. These patients may have symptoms and signs of hypertension and perhaps congestive heart failure. These result from release of renin from the kidney accompanied by the formation of angiotensin II, a potent vasopressor, along with fluid retention from decreased urinary output. They may also have findings of extreme fatigue, limited exercise tolerance, tachycardia from chronic anemia, dysrhythmias from hyperkalemia, easy bruising and bleeding from platelet dysfunction, and a history of infections resulting from suppression of the immune system by the chronic uremia. Appropriate laboratory studies will confirm the diagnosis of renal insufficiency. Patients evidencing hyperkalemia (serum potassium level greater than 5.5 $mEq \cdot l^{-1}$) or fluid overload should undergo dialysis before elective surgery is undertaken.

Gastrointestinal System

Preoperative evaluation of the gastrointestinal system includes questioning about the occurrence of nausea, vomiting, diarrhea, gastrointestinal bleeding, and gastric reflux, and a determination of current body weight and any recent weight change. A history of recurrent or persistent nausea, vomiting, bleeding, diarrhea, or weight loss should lead to a careful analysis of fluid and electrolyte status and the presence of anemia. Many patients state that prior anesthetics caused unpleasant postoperative nausea and vomiting. Whether that was attributable to the anesthetics or the use of opioid analgesics postoperatively cannot be determined; therefore the only recourse is to reassure the patient that everything will be done to try to minimize the occurrence of these effects after use of this anesthetic, including the use of antiemetics such as droperidol or metoclopramide.

A history of heartburn or gastric reflux should be taken seriously because it may signal the presence of an esopha-geal hiatus hernia, which may empty and cause pulmonary aspiration during induction of anesthesia. Any patient with evidence of a hiatus hernia may benefit from prophylactic drug therapy for acid aspiration as well as a rapid sequence induction with cricoid pressure until the airway is isolated by a sealed endotracheal tube. The same precautions should be taken for any patient with blood, food, or fluid in the stomach who requires an anesthetic.

Endocrine System

The endocrine diseases of concern in the preoperative period include diabetes mellitus, thyroid or parathyroid diseases, pheochromocytoma, carcinoid tumor, and adrenal cortical dysfunction.

Diabetes Mellitus

Diabetes mellitus is by far the most common endocrine disease, affecting an estimated 5–6 million people in the United States. Diabetes mellitus is a disorder of carbohydrate metabolism resulting in inappropriate hyperglycemia and glycosuria caused by impaired synthesis, secretion, or utilization of endogenous insulin. Diabetes is diagnosed when a standard, fasting blood glucose level is higher than 120 $mg \cdot dl^{-1}$, a 2-hour postprandial blood glucose level is greater than 140 $mg \cdot dl^{-1}$, or glycosuria is present. The majority of patients with diabetes (90%) are not dependent on insulin to maintain a normal blood glucose level, and they seldom develop acidosis or ketosis. Diet, weight control, and exercise are usually sufficient to maintain an acceptable blood glucose value in the Type II or noninsulin–dependent diabetic. The remaining 10% of diabetics are classified as having Type I or insulin-dependent diabetes, and they are highly susceptible to hyperglycemia, acidosis, ketosis, and the severe end-organ complications of diabetes, including hypertension and coronary artery disease, nephropathy, retinopathy, and neuropathy. Preoperative assessment of diabetes consists of determining which type of diabetes the patient has, and if it is Type I, whether secondary end-organ complications have developed. Generally, the history will distinguish between the two types of diabetes (Table 21-6). Age of the patient at onset of the diabetes is not an absolute distinguishing characteristic between Types I and II diabetes, since either type can occur at any age. Generally, patients with Type II diabetes can trace the onset of the disease to pregnancy, excessive weight gain, or following the use of a specific drug. Some patients do not know that they have diabetes until it is discovered during routine preoperative blood and urine examinations. Once diabetes is identified, it is essential, except in emergencies, to obtain a complete

TABLE 21-6. Clinical Types of Diabetes Mellitus

Event	Type I Insulin-Dependent	Type II Noninsulin-Dependent
Age at onset	Childhood	Middle age or elderly
Timing of onset	Abrupt	Gradual
Predisposing factors	Genetic	Obesity, pregnancy, drugs
Islet beta cell mass	90% loss	Mild to moderate decrease
Plasma insulin level	Absent or minimal	Normal, increased, or decreased
Control of diabetes	Insulin required	Diet, exercise may be enough
Acidosis, ketosis	Common	Rare

medical evaluation to determine whether the patient has any of the complications of the disease, and whether the diabetes and its complications are being optimally controlled. Since hypertension and coronary artery disease are common in diabetics, careful preoperative evaluation of the heart should be made. The presence of orthostatic hypotension or a decrease in blood pressure of more than 30 mm Hg upon the patient's moving from a supine to a standing position suggests the presence of cardiac autonomic neuropathy and impaired cardiac response to stress. The anesthesiologist should also be aware that autonomic dysfunction may cause the patient to have slow gastric emptying and predispose to pulmonary aspiration. Finally, the patients with Type I diabetes sometimes develop stiff joints including those in the neck and jaw, making endotracheal intubation more difficult.[38]

Maintaining "tight" control of the blood glucose concentration in the anesthetic period is inappropriate because of the extreme danger of hypoglycemia and the difficulty of its diagnosis, particularly during general anesthesia. The goals of anesthetic management of the diabetic patient are threefold:

1. To maintain the blood glucose level within the general range of 100–250 mg·dl^{-1} during anesthesia. This is best done by obtaining a blood glucose analysis the morning of operation and checking it every 1 to 2 hours during the operation.
2. To provide adequate fluid volume by starting an intravenous infusion the night before or the morning of operation. Generally, the fluid should contain dextrose, either 5 or 10%, and perhaps electrolytes, especially potassium, depending on the circumstances.
3. To individualize diabetic management for each patient rather than following a standard recipe.[39]

There are several satisfactory ways of accomplishing these goals. For the Type II diabetic who either takes no insulin or takes an oral hypoglycemic drug, no insulin is needed preoperatively. If the blood glucose level exceeds the acceptable range intraoperatively, it can be managed by the administration of regular insulin, 1–2 IU intravenously. As a rule of thumb, one unit of regular insulin given to the average adult generally decreases the blood glucose level about 25 mg·dl^{-1}. For the Type I diabetic, one satisfactory

approach is to give one half the dose of long-acting insulin that the patient usually takes the morning of operation and then give the other half after the patient has emerged from the anesthetic. Of course it is necessary to maintain a fluid infusion and monitor the blood glucose levels, in keeping with the goals noted above.

Thyroid and Parathyroid Diseases

Although diseases of the thyroid and parathyroid glands are uncommon, anesthesiologists occasionally encounter patients with malfunction of these glands manifested as hyperthyroidism, hypothyroidism, or hyperparathyroidism and hypercalcemia. Although most patients have received adequate medical therapy before the time of anesthesia administration and operation, it is important for the anesthesiologist to be aware of the clinical manifestations of these endocrine diseases (Table 21-7).[40] Hyperthyroidism is caused by excessive secretion of 3,5,3'-triiodothyronine (T_3) and thyroxine (T_4) from the thyroid gland owing to conditions such as Graves' disease, thyroiditis, or thyroid adenoma, or from a pituitary tumor secreting thyroid-stimulating hormone. The symptoms and signs of hyperthyroidism are those of hypermetabolism (Table 21-7), and the diagnosis is confirmed by finding increased levels of free and bound T_3 and T_4 in serum. Except in emergencies, preoperative preparation includes 2–6 weeks of therapy with propylthiouracil, which decreases the synthesis of thyroxine as well as decreasing the conversion of thyroxine into T_3, thus making the patient euthyroid. In addition, a beta-adrenergic blocking drug such as propranolol is often used to decrease heart rate, while watching carefully for any signs of congestive heart failure. In emergency circumstances or if a thyroid storm should develop (with hyperpyrexia, tachycardia, and disorientation), treatment with iodine and alpha- and beta-adrenergic blocking drugs may be necessary.

Hypothyroidism is more common than hyperthyroidism, affecting from 3–5% of the adult population. The lack of thyroid hormones results in the symptoms and signs of hypometabolism (see Table 21-7) and is confirmed by low serum levels of T_3 and T_4. Preoperative treatment consists of therapy with T_3 or T_4 as well as restoration of normal intravascular fluid volume and electrolyte status. Weinberg et al did not find any difference in many outcome variables

TABLE 21-7. Clinical Manifestations of Thyroid and Parathyroid Diseases

	Hyperthyroidism	Hypothyroidism	Hyperparathyroidism
General	Weight loss, heat intolerance, warm, moist skin	Cold intolerance	Weight loss, polydipsia
Cardiovascular	Tachycardia, atrial fibrillation, congestive heart failure	Bradycardia, congestive heart failure, cardiomegaly, pericardial or pleural effusions	Hypertension, heart block
Neurologic	Nervousness, tremor, hyperactive reflexes	Slow mental function, minimal reflexes	Weakness, lethargy, headache, insomnia, apathy, depression
Musculoskeletal	Muscle weakness, bone resorption	Large tongue, amyloidosis	Bone pains, arthritis, pathologic fractures
Gastrointestinal	Diarrhea	Delayed gastric emptying	Anorexia, nausea, vomiting, constipation, epigastric pain
Hematologic	Anemia, thrombocytopenia		
Renal		Impaired free water clearance	Polyuria, hematuria

Modified with permission from Roizen MF: Anesthesia for the patient with endocrine disease, Part I. Curr Rev Clin Anesth 6:43,1987.

as a result of anesthesia and surgery in 59 untreated hypothyroid patients compared with 59 euthyroid matched controls.[41] They concluded that there is not sufficient evidence to justify deferring needed surgery in patients until hypothyroidism has been corrected. Because patients with hypothyroidism may have excessively large tongues, the airway should be carefully evaluated for ease of tracheal intubation before induction of anesthesia.

Hyperparathyroidism causes excessive release of parathyroid hormone, which stimulates bone resorption and inhibits the renal excretion of calcium, in turn causing hypercalcemia. The clinical manifestations of hypercalcemia are nonspecific (see Table 21-7); therefore the diagnosis rests with laboratory confirmation of high serum calcium and parathyroid hormone levels. Preoperative management includes vigorous fluid therapy to correct hypovolemia and dilute the hypercalcemia and corticosteroid therapy to decrease calcium absorption from the gastrointestinal tract.

Pheochromocytoma

Pheochromocytomas are tumors of the chromaffin tissue of the sympathoadrenal system that cause symptoms and signs from the release of epinephrine and norepinephrine into the systemic circulation. Although pheochromocytomas are a rare cause of hypertension (less than 0.1% of all patients with hypertension),[42] they can cause severe morbidity and occasional mortality in the perioperative period if the disease is not diagnosed prior to anesthesia and surgery or if the disease is not managed carefully during and after surgery. The classic findings are intermittent hypertension, headache, sweating, and tachycardia (Table 21-8).[42] The hypertension and other signs and symptoms tend to be paroxysmal in nature because the release of catecholamines into the circulation is intermittent and because the half-life of circulating catecholamines is short (less than 1 minute) owing to their rapid enzymatic degradation by monoamine oxidase and catechol-o-methyl transferase and to reuptake. Years of excessive catecholamine production may cause hypovolemia, hyperglycemia, myocarditis, or cardiomyopathy, with myocardial infarction or congestive heart failure or intravascular hemorrhage into the brain or heart. The diagnosis is confirmed by the presence of increased plasma concentrations of epinephrine and/or norepinephrine, high levels of vanillylmandelic acid and metanephrine in the urine, and localization of the tumor by computed tomography or abdominal angiography.

Preoperative preparation of the patient with a pheochromocytoma includes administration of an alpha-adrenergic

TABLE 21-8. Clinical Manifestations of Pheochromocytoma*

Symptoms	Signs
Headache	Hypertension
Sweating	Orthostatic hypotension
Weight loss	Tachycardia
Nervousness	Dysrhythmias
Irritability	Myocarditis
Palpitations	Hypovolemia
	Hyperglycemia
	Polycythemia

*Most of the symptoms and signs are paroxysmal in nature.

blocking drug such as phenoxybenzamine, 20–250 mg·day^{-1}, or prazosin, 6–10 mg·day^{-1}, and a beta-adrenergic blocking drug such as propranolol, 120–480 mg·day^{-1}, several weeks prior to operation.[43] The beta-adrenergic blocking drug should never be started first, because used alone it may cause a sudden, severe hypertension. A relatively short-acting calcium channel blocking drug may also be useful by both attenuating the release of catecholamines and lessening their effects on target organs.[44] Once this pharmacologic therapy is begun, restoration of normal intravascular volume and management of the other manifestations of the disease can be accomplished with greater safety. Generally, it is appropriate to proceed with anesthesia and surgery when the symptoms have abated, the blood pressure is decreased and stable, dysrhythmias are absent or infrequent, and the hypovolemia has been corrected.

Carcinoid Syndrome

Carcinoid syndrome is a rare endocrine disorder caused by slow growing tumors, generally of the gastrointestinal tract, that release a variety of vasoactive amines and polypeptides into the circulation. The symptoms and signs depend upon the predominant substances being released from the tumor. If the primary substance is 5-hydroxytryptamine, the major findings are diarrhea, abdominal cramps, respiratory distress from bronchospasm, and hypertension. If the primary substances are histamine and bradykinin, the findings tend to be paroxysmal hypotension, cutaneous flushing, and bronchospasm. Removal of the primary tumor is usually not curative because 90% of patients have extensive metastases. However, primary tumor removal is necessary because of obstruction of the bowel, airway, or a major blood vessel. Medical treatment of this tumor involves administration of somatostatin or octreotide acetate in combination with ketanserin.[45] These drugs are thought to bind to specific receptors on the target cells for the amines and kinins, thereby preventing their normal actions. In addition to drug therapy, preoperative preparation includes fluid therapy to minimize hypovolemia and evaluation of the patient for carcinoid heart disease and congestive heart failure.

Adrenal Cortical Dysfunction

Dysfunction of the adrenal cortex may occur as a result of primary diseases of the adrenal cortex, from tumors of the pituitary gland, or most commonly from prolonged steroid therapy as treatment of connective tissue diseases such as rheumatoid arthritis or scleroderma. An excess of glucocorticoid (cortisol or its derivatives) causes Cushing's syndrome, which is characterized by truncal obesity, moon facies, skin striations, easy bruisability, hypertension, and hypovolemia. An excess of mineralocorticoid, primarily aldosterone, causes sodium retention, potassium depletion, polyuria, alkalosis, and clinical symptoms and signs associated with these electrolyte disturbances. Preoperative preparation consists of correction of fluid and electrolyte abnormalities, treatment of existing hypertension or diabetes, and steroid supplementation to cover the stress of anesthesia and surgery.

Hematologic System

The two major issues related to the hematologic system that are of concern preoperatively are the presence of an anemia and any disorder of hemostasis. Preoperative management of a patient with an anemia can be a vexing problem for the anesthesiologist. The principal reason for concern about an anemia is the fact that most of the oxygen delivered to tissues requires hemoglobin for its transport. Substantial decreases in hemoglobin result in substantial decreases in oxygen delivery to tissues, unless cardiac output is increased or body metabolism and oxygen consumption are decreased. Most anesthetics are associated with some decrease in cardiac output and some decrease in body metabolism as a result of the anesthetic effect itself as well as of a decrease of several degrees in body temperature that commonly occurs during anesthesia. The resultant effect may be an equivalent decrease in both oxygen demand and oxygen delivery. Unfortunately, there are no studies that document whether a decreasing hemoglobin concentration in blood is associated with increasing morbidity or mortality. Because of the high level of concern over transmission of the human immunodeficiency and hepatitis viruses, physicians are less willing to give patients transfusions just because an anemia is present and surgery is required. The long held but arbitrary values of a hemoglobin level of 10 $g \cdot dl^{-1}$ or a hematocrit value of 30% as a minimum below which elective surgery should not be performed are no longer considered valid. The risks of transfusion, although very small, are thought to be greater than the risks associated with performing anesthesia and surgery on patients with hemoglobin values of 8–10 $g \cdot dl^{-1}$ or hematocrit values of 25–30 $ml \cdot dl^{-1}$.

When faced preoperatively with a patient with anemia (arbitrarily defined as a hemoglobin value of less than 10 $g \cdot dl^{-1}$ or a hematocrit of less than 30 $ml \cdot dl^{-1}$), the anesthesiologist should ask three questions: what is the cause of the anemia; is the anemia acute or chronic; and will the patient benefit from delay of surgery and institution of medical therapy? Although there are many causes of anemia, the two of greatest concern to the anesthesiologist are anemias caused by blood loss and sickle cell anemia. Anemias resulting from acute blood loss generally require prompt surgical intervention; therefore the anesthesiologist usually must proceed with the anesthetic and plan to transfuse blood if the hemoglobin value decreases below 8 $g \cdot dl^{-1}$ during operation and additional blood loss is anticipated. Anemias owing to blood loss that is chronic, as evidenced by their long-standing nature and the lack of circulatory signs of anemia (e.g., tachycardia, orthostatic hypotension), might best be treated with medical therapy (including supplemental iron for several weeks) before proceeding with anesthesia and surgery. Patients with chronic anemia secondary to renal failure have adapted to their anemia and generally do not need preoperative transfusion. Sickle cell anemia is of special concern because its presence suggests the need to maintain full oxygen saturation of arterial blood and a normal cardiac output and blood pressure during anesthesia and surgery, although this is not always possible.

When anemia is present or substantial blood loss during surgery is anticipated, the trend today is toward the use of autologous blood donated by the patient a week or two before the anticipated surgery or the use of donor-directed blood. When the surgery is elective, the anesthesiologist should discuss with the patient and the surgeon what plans have been made for the availability of autologous or donor-directed blood, and if necessary should postpone surgery until such blood is available. Generally transfusion prior to surgery is only done when blood loss is acute or the patient is bleeding actively and signs of anemia and hypovolemia are present. With careful management, anesthesia and sur-

gery can be conducted safely even in the presence of severe anemia (hemoglobin 5 $g \cdot dl^{-1}$).[46] Although these are useful guidelines, the final decisions regarding management of the patient with anemia must be individualized according to his or her special needs and the anticipated effects of the anesthetic and operation.

Disorders of hemostasis may be of congenital origin, the classic example being hemophilia, or more commonly acquired owing to thrombocytopenia, which generally accompanies pre-eclampsia; platelet dysfunction, which commonly accompanies aspirin or other drug therapy; anticoagulant therapy; or liver disease. Patients generally know if they or members of their family bruise easily or bleed excessively when injured or cut. If patients do give a history of either of these problems, it is necessary to determine the onset, frequency, severity, site, and duration of the bleeding and what medications the patient is taking. This history usually reveals the etiology of the disorder, which can then be confirmed by laboratory tests. On physical examination, bleeding caused by platelet disorders generally occurs at mucocutaneous surfaces causing petechiae, superficial bruises, epistaxis, hematuria, or gastrointestinal bleeding, whereas bleeding caused by a deficiency in coagulation factors is deep bleeding into joints or muscles, often forming a palpable mass.[47] Except in emergency situations, anesthesia and operations should not proceed until the bleeding disorder has been characterized and treated. Regional anesthesia is almost invariably contraindicated in the presence of a bleeding disorder.

Musculoskeletal System

The most common musculoskeletal disorder is that of degenerative arthritis (osteoarthritis) or disk disease causing chronic back or joint pain. Generally, patients find some positions more comfortable than others, and when lying supine they prefer to have back or knee support. It is helpful to characterize what gives maximal support and then reassure the patient that you will attempt to provide that support while the operation is ongoing.

Less common but of greater concern is the presence of rheumatoid arthritis, which may have extensive systemic manifestations. These patients may give a history of chronic pain in joints of the neck, back, arms, legs, or hands relieved somewhat by taking aspirin, nonsteroidal anti-inflammatory drugs, or low doses of steroids. On physical examination one may find limited range of motion of the neck and temporomandibular joints and prominent nodes (Heberden's nodes) on the joints of the fingers. Rarely, patients may develop a change in voice or hoarseness owing to involvement of the cricoarytenoid joint in the disease process, thereby limiting vocal cord movement. Severe rheumatoid arthritis may cause symptoms and signs of myocarditis, pleuritis, or restrictive lung disease. The preoperative evaluation should include assessment of intravenous access, which may be difficult; what positioning will be needed to accomplish the operation; and if regional anesthesia is planned, whether positioning for it is possible.

If a regional anesthetic is planned, preoperative examination of the specific musculoskeletal site where the block is to be performed is useful. For example, if an epidural or spinal block is planned, examination of the spine for flexion and ease of identification of the spinous processes and interspaces is helpful in deciding whether to proceed with a block.

Dental System

The dental history includes questioning the patient about the presence of loose teeth, false teeth, or bridges that are removable and capped teeth that might be injured during endotracheal intubation. Some patients who have a full set of false teeth will ask if they can keep them in place during administration of the anesthetic or at least until they go to sleep. If the operation is expected to be short (less than 1 hour) and mask anesthesia is planned, I prefer to leave the false teeth in place because they make for a better mask fit. If endotracheal intubation is planned, the false teeth can be removed just prior to intubation. If the patient has had prior general anesthesia, it is vital to ask about any history of difficult intubation of the trachea. A negative history for difficult intubation does not preclude its possible occurrence.

A comprehensive physical examination of the dental system and airway should be performed in each patient even if endotracheal intubation is not planned (Table 21-9). Approximately 2 to 3% of patients have anatomic features that make tracheal intubation difficult. Findings that suggest that endotracheal intubation may be difficult include a small mouth, a narrow receding mandible or a protuberant maxilla (overbite), a large tongue or one whose mobility is limited, less than three fingerbreadths distance (less than 6 cm) between the mandible and the thyroid prominence, inability to place the head in the sniff position, and a short, full, or bull neck or the presence of a neck mass. Incorporating five variables (body weight, head and neck movement, jaw movement, receding mandible, and buck teeth) into a scoring system, Wilson and colleagues[48] tested them in 778 patients undergoing endotracheal intubation and found that the system correctly identified 95% of the difficult intubations. The scoring system falsely tagged 12% of the normal airways as being difficult.

Samsoon and Young,[49] using a scheme modified from Mallampati,[50] classified the airway into four classes based on the structures visible on direct examination of the oral cavity with the patient in the seated position, mouth open widely and tongue protruding to the maximum (Table 21-10). Of 15,360 patients evaluated, 13 had tracheas that were impossible to intubate under direct vision. On subsequent external examination, all but one were classified as having a Class IV airway, and all but the same one were graded as a Class III or IV at laryngoscopy. The one exception was a patient who had undiagnosed tracheal stenosis. Recently, Oates et al[51] compared the Mallampati and Wilson classifications in 675 patients and found that neither system predicted more than 50% of the difficult laryngoscopies. Of the patients who were predicted to be difficult,

only 3% proved to be difficult, thus giving a high rate of false-positive results.

TABLE 21-10. Airway Classification System of Samsoon and Young[49]

Class	Direct Visualization, Patient Seated	Laryngoscopic View
I	Soft palate, fauces, uvula, pillars	Entire glottis
II	Soft palate, fauces, uvula	Posterior commissure
III	Soft palate, uvular base	Tip of epiglottis
IV	Hard palate only	No glottal structures

Modified with permission from Mallampati RS, Gatt SP, Gugino LD et al: A clinical sign to predict difficult tracheal intubation: A prospective study. Can Anaesth Soc J 32:429, 1985.

Reproductive System

It is estimated that between 1 and 2% of pregnant women require anesthesia and surgery some time during the course of their pregnancy. Because most of the organogenesis occurs in the first trimester, there is concern that administration of anesthetic and other drugs during this period may result in fetal deformities (teratogenesis). Therefore it has generally been recommended that elective surgery be postponed until the second trimester. In the largest study to date involving 2565 pregnant women undergoing intercurrent surgery,[52] the incidence of congenital abnormalities in the fetus was no greater than that in a matched set of women with surgery-free pregnancies. However, the incidence of spontaneous abortion was greater in those undergoing surgery while pregnant than in the control group. Thus it is important to inquire about the menstrual history of all women of childbearing age and to advise those who are pregnant that they are at increased risk of having a spontaneous abortion if anesthesia and surgery are implemented but that the fetus is not at greater risk of developing congenital abnormalities.

Obesity

Many patients requiring anesthesia and surgery are overweight, but the major concern is with those who are morbidly obese. Morbid obesity is generally defined as being twice the ideal body weight. Ideal body weight in kilograms can be estimated by subtracting 100 from the patient's height in centimeters or calculated by determining the body mass index (BMI = weight [kg]/height [m^2]), assuming that a BMI of 30% above normal represents morbid obesity. The major preoperative concerns with the morbidly obese patient are the probable dysfunctions of the pulmonary and circulatory systems. Because of their greater body mass, such individuals have a higher oxygen demand and greater carbon dioxide production than normal patients and thus they must have a higher minute and alveolar ventilation. Their work of breathing is increased because of the mass of abdominal and chest wall fat that must be moved with each breath. The mass of fat also decreases lung volume, thereby decreasing pulmonary compliance and increasing the alveolar-arterial oxygen tension difference. Over time, this

TABLE 21-9. Preoperative Physical Examination of the Dental System and Airway

1. Ability to open mouth; size of oral cavity at lips
2. Presence of loose, false, or capped teeth; protruding incisors
3. Size and mobility of the tongue
4. Size and shape of mandible; maxillary overgrowth
5. Distance from the mandible to the prominence on the thyroid cartilage
6. Ability to place the head in the sniff position
7. Neck size and fullness; tracheal deviation
8. Ability to visualize the soft palate, fauces, uvula, and pillars

results in arterial hypoxemia, which in turn decreases oxygen supply to respiratory muscles, and morbidly obese patients hypoventilate rather than further increase the work of breathing. Some develop obstructive or central sleep apnea, which contributes further to the arterial hypoxemia and hypercarbia.

Morbidly obese patients must have an increased blood volume, red blood cell mass, and cardiac output in order to maintain blood flow to the muscles working to carry the weight. Ventricular enlargement ensues, and if arterial hypoxemia occurs, these patients develop congestive heart failure. Systemic and pulmonary hypertension are also common in morbidly obese patients because of the effects of the increased blood volume and arterial hypoxemia, and they also contribute to ventricular enlargement and congestive heart failure. Because of hypercholesterolemia, these patients may also have coronary artery disease. Other associated diseases include diabetes, hepatic insufficiency owing to fatty infiltration of the liver, and renal insufficiency.

Aside from evaluating the severity and treating the complications of morbid obesity, there is little that the anesthesiologist can do preoperatively to prepare the morbidly obese patient for anesthesia and surgery. Preoperative planning includes discussion with the surgeon regarding the patient's body position during surgery and any other special needs, and discussion with the patient regarding the need for direct arterial pressure monitoring, central venous pressure monitoring, and awake fiberoptic intubation of the trachea.

LABORATORY TESTS

Routine preoperative laboratory studies for all patients undergoing anesthesia and surgery include a determination of hemoglobin and hematocrit values, a differential blood cell count, and a urinalysis within 72 hours of surgery. The usefulness of these tests for all patients has been questioned, since abnormalities in blood cell count or urinalysis are seldom found in the absence of some indication of disease in the history or physical examination.[53] Furthermore, evidence suggests that when abnormalities are found in routine laboratory studies, they are rarely acted upon and they seldom affect the anesthetic or operative plan.[53,54] However, because these tests are a standard required for hospital accreditation by the JCAHO, they are routinely performed as part of the preoperative evaluation.

What laboratory tests are done beyond this minimum depends on many factors, including patient age, disease state, proposed operation, or preoperative drug therapy. The reason for ordering specific tests and how the results will influence the perioperative anesthetic plan should be clear when the tests are ordered. Obviously specific laboratory tests should be ordered when the history and physical examination suggest dysfunction of an organ system. For example, a chest roentgenogram, electrocardiogram, and blood chemistries (electrolytes, glucose and blood urea nitrogen levels) are indicated in any patient with symptoms or signs or pulmonary or cardiac disease or a history of diabetes or hepatic or renal disease. Patients with a history of a bleeding disorder should have tests for measurement of bleeding time, prothrombin time, and partial thromboplastin time. More sophisticated tests such as liver or pulmonary function tests, arterial blood gas analysis, echocardiography, angiography, computed tomography, or magnetic resonance imaging may be indicated by the history and physical examination.

What laboratory studies should be performed primarily because of the age of the patient? There is no clear consensus on this question, but in general it is customary for all patients over the age of 50 years to have an electrocardiogram, chest roentgenogram, and a blood chemistry panel, including electrolytes, creatinine/blood urea nitrogen, and glucose in addition to the routine tests, even if they are asymptomatic except for their surgical condition. Although it is recognized that the yield of these tests in terms of identification of an unsuspected disease is very small, they serve as useful baseline values for comparison should the patient develop unexpected complications in the perioperative period or for future surgical conditions that may arise.

Whether or not to proceed with anesthesia and surgery in the presence of an abnormal laboratory study finding depends on the severity of the abnormality, whether there is a reasonable likelihood that the abnormality will increase perioperative morbidity or mortality if uncorrected, and whether there is any reasonable chance that the abnormality can be corrected or improved preoperatively. For example, there is very little that the physician can do preoperatively to improve the condition of patients with chronic obstructive pulmonary disease if they are unresponsive to bronchodilator therapy and do not have a pulmonary infection. In contrast, there is much that might be done preoperatively for patients with coronary artery disease, including treating hypertension, decreasing heart rate, and treating arrhythmias and congestive heart failure. In most cases the decision about proceeding with anesthesia and surgery must be made after discussion with the surgeon, the patient, and the family.

CHOICE OF ANESTHETIC TECHNIQUE

Once the chart review, history, physical examination, and laboratory studies are completed and evaluated, it is time to discuss the choice of anesthetic technique with the patient. At the outset, it should be emphasized that the choice of anesthetic technique almost never matters, since outcome is determined by how that technique is implemented. Patients or surgeons may have a preference for general or regional anesthesia, and when they do, their wishes should be respected, unless there is a specific reason for selecting an alternative technique. There are a few circumstances in which a specific anesthetic technique is preferred or inappropriate. For example, regional anesthesia is preferred in patients with a full stomach if the block can be done safely and efficaciously. In contrast, regional anesthesia is usually difficult to implement and manage when the anesthesiologist cannot communicate with the patient because of a language barrier. Age is not a contraindication to regional anesthesia; caudal and axillary blocks can be effective and safe even in small children. Local anesthesia and monitored anesthesia care may be but are not always the safest forms of anesthesia for patients who are seriously ill and require surgical intervention. In one prospective study of 100,000 anesthetics administered for surgery, mortality within 7 days of operation was highest in those patients who received monitored anesthesia care.[55] Perhaps they were the most critically ill, but possibly the mortality in this group would have been lower if an anesthetic technique that allowed for greater intervention into patient variables had been used. Finally, it stands to reason that anesthesiologists will perform better using an anesthetic technique with which they are familiar rather than a less familiar technique.

Generally, when patients understand the surgical needs

and the anesthetic alternatives, they are willing to accept the recommended anesthetic technique. It is never appropriate to coerce a patient into accepting an anesthetic technique that he or she does not want. Ultimately, the patient must understand and consent to the technique to be used. Once this has been mutually agreed upon, the anesthesiologist should write a brief note in the patient's chart documenting the anesthetic findings, the American Society of Anesthesiologists' physical status classification (see below), the anesthetic technique to be used, and a statement indicating that the patient understands and agrees to the anesthetic plan with its attendant risks. The only remaining task is the writing of the preoperative orders (see Chapter 24).

THE RISKS OF ANESTHESIA

A final portion of the preoperative visit includes a discussion of the risks of anesthesia with the patient and/or the family. The desire to know about the risks of anesthesia varies among patients; some want to know all the potential risks in detail, whereas others prefer to know little or nothing about them, instead placing their faith and trust in the anesthesiologist to do his or her very best. In general, patients and their families recognize that anesthesia is not risk-free, and that as the patient's health deteriorates and his or her illness becomes more severe, the risks of anesthesia and surgery increase. This topic is best approached by asking the patient and/or family if they want to know about the risks of the proposed anesthetic procedure. If they reply "no," it is best to document their wishes in the chart and not discuss anesthetic risk further. There is nothing gained by instilling needless apprehension in a patient and family by citing serious risks that are generally ill-founded and undocumented.

If a patient or family wants more information about anesthetic risk, it is best to tailor the response in a graded manner, citing the more common and relatively innocuous risks first and then proceeding to the rarer and more serious ones if they seem to want more detail. Uncomfortable but not life-threatening risks of anesthesia include nausea and vomiting postoperatively; bruising or superficial thrombophlebitis at the site of the intravenous line; a sore throat or injury to the teeth if endotracheal intubation is planned; corneal abrasion; or a headache postoperatively if a spinal (or epidural) anesthetic is planned. Since it is impossible to give patients a statistical likelihood of any of these events, it is best to indicate that you will do all that you can to prevent them by using the appropriate medicines (e.g., antiemetics) or techniques (e.g., small endotracheal tube with careful insertion or small needle for spinal anesthesia) to minimize their occurrence, and if they occur, you will do everything you can to minimize the discomfort.

More serious complications from anesthesia and surgery that may occur in some patients because of predisposing conditions such as heart disease, chronic lung disease, renal or hepatic disease, or cerebrovascular insufficiency include arrhythmias, myocardial infarction, atelectasis and pneumonia, renal or hepatic insufficiency, or stroke. Patients who have had a prior myocardial infarction are at increased risk for repeat infarction from anesthesia and surgery, but the specific incidence varies depending on the interval since infarction and the intensity of cardiovascular monitoring and treatment (see section on Circulatory System). In discussing this issue with a patient with hypertension or myocardial ischemia, the anesthesiologist can only state that there may be an increased likelihood of myocardial infarction, depending on the type, complexity, and duration of the operation, and that careful monitoring and selective drug therapy will be used to try to prevent any cardiac complications.

Unfortunately, there are no data that the anesthesiologist can use to indicate the likelihood that a given patient will develop atelectasis and pneumonia or pulmonary embolism, renal or hepatic insufficiency, or stroke following anesthesia and operation. Although atelectasis is common postoperatively, pneumonia from aspiration or infection and pulmonary embolism are less so. In the absence of renal, hepatic, or cerebrovascular disease, postoperative complications involving these organ systems are rare and hence not to be expected. Even rarer are such complications as halothane hepatitis (estimated at 1 per 7000 exposures[56]), malignant hyperthermia (1 in 4500 general anesthetics with succinylcholine; 1 in 51,000 general anesthetics[57]), mismatched blood transfusion, patient awareness during operation, injury to the spinal cord or peripheral nerves, or burns.

In addition to patient disease, errors in anesthetic management may cause morbidity and mortality. Events such as anesthetic drug overdose; syringe swap and administration of the wrong drug; failure to provide adequate ventilation because of esophageal intubation, breathing circuit disconnects, hypoventilation, or airway mismanagement; equipment failure or misuse of equipment; and errors in judgment do occur and may cause disability or death in patients.[58] Keenan and Boyan[59] reported 27 cardiac arrests caused solely by anesthesia in 163,240 patients given anesthetics over a 15-year period (1969–1983) for an incidence of 1.7 per 10,000 anesthetics. The death rate was 0.9 per 10,000 anesthetics, which agrees with other studies that report an anesthetic death rate of about 1 per 10,000 anesthetics.[60,61] It has been suggested that the incidence of cardiac arrest and death from anesthesia may be less than the values cited above because of the recent widespread use of pulse oximetry and capnography during anesthesia and postanesthesia recovery. All of the studies cited above were performed before either of these modalities of monitoring were readily available. The only study that suggests that the incidence of death related to anesthesia is decreasing is that of Holland,[62] who reported an anesthetic mortality in New South Wales, Australia, of 1 per 10,250 anesthetics in 1970 and 1 per 26,000 anesthetics in 1984. Keats[63] questions the premise that better monitoring has caused a decrease in mortality due to anesthesia, believing that "new mechanisms of mortality are created at the same rate that we solve them." Although it is not zero, the incidence of cardiac arrest and death from anesthesia is extremely low, and this fact should be emphasized to those patients who ask about the possibility of this event. Comparison of the rarity of this event with the more common risk of death from an automobile accident is often cited to relieve anxiety and provide reassurance about the safety of anesthesia. Regardless of risk, every patient should be reassured that the anesthetic care and management will be done with utmost care, skill, and vigilance.

AMERICAN SOCIETY OF ANESTHESIOLOGISTS' PHYSICAL STATUS

In 1940, a committee of the American Society of Anesthetists, now known as the American Society of Anesthesiologists, was charged with developing a physical status classification for patients requiring anesthesia and surgery. The purpose of the classification was to standardize physical status categories for statistical studies and for hospital records so that more uniform interpretation of patient status would be possible. The committee developed six categories of physical status,[64] which were modified into five categories by Dripps et al in 1961.[65] The five category classification (Table 21-11) was adopted as a standard by the American Society of Anesthesiologists and remains the classification used by anesthesiologists and others to characterize physical status preoperatively.

The advantages of the physical status classification system of the American Society of Anesthesiologists are two-fold. First, it allows anesthesiologists and others to compare outcomes (complications or death) within their own institution or among institutions based on one standard criterion (physical status). In the final analysis, outcome is one important measure of how well the physicians are providing care. Second, and perhaps more important, it provides anesthesiologists with a quick summary of the physical status of a patient on a daily basis. Because patients are often not anesthetized by the same anesthesiologist who saw the patient preoperatively, a status of three or higher alerts the provider of the anesthetic that the patient has some serious physical problems and that extra care and vigilance are needed.

Although the physical status classification of the American Society of Anesthesiologists is a workable system, it has some drawbacks. First, the classifications are not sufficiently precise to ensure that all anesthesiologists will classify a given patient the same.[66] The greater the variations among anesthesiologists in their application of the classifications, the less meaningful are the comparisons based on the classification. Second, some anesthesiologists use the classification as a means of identifying "anesthetic risk." Although there are rough correlations between American Society of Anesthesiologists' physical status and mortality from anesthetics, it is not a precise risk classification. Patients who are in American Society of Anesthesiologists' categories 1 and 2 do have cardiac arrests and die from anesthesia because there are other causes of anesthetic deaths that have nothing to do with the physical status of the patient. Analyzing 645 postanesthetic deaths in 34,145 surgical patients, Marx et al[67] found a direct relationship between physical status and percentage of mortality. However, of the 27 deaths believed by the authors to be attributable primarily to anesthetic management, two were status 1 and one was status 2. Similar findings have been reported by Vacanti et al[68] in 68,388 anesthetic administrations and by Keenan and Boyan[59] in 163,240 anesthetic administrations.

Despite its shortcomings, the physical status classification

TABLE 21-11. Physical Status Classification of American Society of Anesthesiologists

Status*	Description
1	Healthy patient
2	Mild systemic disease
3	Severe systemic disease, not incapacitating
4	Severe systemic disease that is a constant threat to life
5	Moribund, not expected to live 24 hours irrespective of operation

* An E is added to the status number to designate an emergency operation.

TABLE 21-12. Preinduction Checklist

1. Check functional state of anesthesia machine, monitors, and suction
2. Prepare appropriate fluid infusion system
3. Prepare intravenous anesthetic drugs
4. Prepare equipment for general anesthesia (laryngoscope blade, endotracheal tube, stylet) or regional anesthesia (spinal or epidural kit)
5. Check room temperature, operating table function, special needs (e.g., warming/cooling blanket on table)
6. Identify and greet patient; transfer to operating table; inquire about night's sleep and current status
7. Examine chart for any changes or additional information since preoperative evaluation; verify premedication dose given and time
8. Start intravenous infusion
9. Apply monitors; obtain and chart baseline values
10. Discuss any changes in surgical plans or patient condition with surgeons

of the American Society of Anesthesiologists is sufficiently important that at the conclusion of the preoperative evaluation the anesthesiologist should assign each patient to one of the categories.

IMMEDIATE PREINDUCTION CHECKLIST

Prior to and after arrival of the patient in the operating room, the anesthesiologist must do several things to make delivery of the anesthetic as safe as possible (Table 21-12). Most of the items on this 10-point checklist are self-explanatory and need no elaboration. Item 3 is controversial and deserves greater consideration. Some in anesthesia practice believe that the anesthesiologist should prepare syringes containing emergency drugs such as atropine, ephedrine, and succinylcholine in advance of starting any anesthetic. I do not share that view for several reasons. First, I believe that anesthesiologists should be skilled enough in preoperative evaluation to know which patients might need one or more of these drugs and prepare it only for those patients. To prepare these drugs routinely before each day's anesthetic will result over time in tremendous waste of medications, supplies, and physician or technician time. Second, these drugs are rarely needed in minor emergencies and are ineffective (atropine and ephedrine) or dangerous (succinylcholine) in true emergencies. Third, when the drugs are drawn up and ready for use, there is a natural tendency to administer them at the first sign of changes in vital signs, without taking the time to evaluate the problem and its possible cause(s). Finally, the presence of additional loaded syringes increases the chances for syringe exchanges or switches and administration of the wrong drug. Emergency drugs should be prepared if the anesthesiologist has reasonable anticipation of their need but not as part of routine practice.

REFERENCES

1. Rubin RN: Aspirin and postsurgery bleeding. Ann Intern Med 89:1006, 1978
2. Amrein PC, Ellman L, Harris WH: Aspirin-induced prolongation of bleeding time and perioperative blood loss. JAMA 245:1825, 1981

3. George JN, Shatth SJ: The clinical importance of acquired abnormalities of platelet function. N Engl J Med 324:27, 1991

4. Shee JC: Dangerous potentiation of pethidine by iproniazid and its treatment. Br Med J 2:507, 1960

5. Taylor DC: Alarming reaction to pethidine in patients on phenelzine. Lancet 2:401, 1962

6. El-Ganzouri AR, Ivankovich AD, Braverman B, McCarthy R: Monoamine oxidase inhibitors: Should they be discontinued preoperatively? Anesth Analg 64:592, 1985

7. Wong KC: Preoperative discontinuation of monoamine oxidase inhibitor therapy: An old wives' tale? Semin Anesth 5:145, 1986

8. Wells DG: Monoamine oxidase inhibitors revisited. Can J Anaesth 36:64, 1989

9. Samuels SI, Maze A, Albright G: Cardiac arrest during cesarean section in a chronic amphetamine abuser. Anesth Analg 58:528, 1979

10. Stoelting RK: Allergic reactions during anesthesia. Anesth Analg 62:341, 1983

11. Bochner BS, Lichtenstein LM: Anaphylaxis. N Engl J Med 324:1785, 1991

12. Working Group on Hypertension in the Elderly: Statement on hypertension in the elderly. JAMA 256:70, 1986

13. Report of the Joint National Committee on Detection, Evaluation and Treatment of High Blood Pressure. Arch Intern Med 144:1045, 1984

14. Madhavan S, Alderman MH: The potential effect of blood pressure reduction on cardiovascular disease. Arch Intern Med 141:1583, 1981

15. Mangano DT: Perioperative cardiac morbidity. Anesthesiology 72:153, 1990

16. McHugh P, Gill NP, Wyld R et al: Continuous ambulatory ECG monitoring in the perioperative period; relationship of preoperative status and outcome. Br J Anaesth 66:285, 1991

17. Goldman L, Caldera DL: Risks of general anesthesia and elective operation in the hypertensive patient. Anesthesiology 50:285, 1979

18. Mangano DT, Browner WS, Hollenberg M et al: Association of perioperative myocardial ischemia with cardiac morbidity and mortality in men undergoing noncardiac surgery. N Engl J Med 323:1781, 1990

19. Slogoff S, Keats A: Does peri-operative myocardial ischemia lead to postoperative myocardial infarction? Anesthesiology 62:107, 1985

20. Raby K, Goldman L, Creager M et al: Correlation between preoperative ischemia and major cardiac events after peripheral vascular surgery. N Engl J Med 321:1296, 1989

21. Knight AA, Hollenberg M, London MJ et al: Perioperative myocardial ischemia: Importance of the preoperative ischemic pattern. Anesthesiology 68:681, 1988

22. Fegert G, Hollenberg M, Browner W et al: Perioperative myocardial ischemia in the non-cardiac surgical patient. Anesthesiology 69:A49, 1988

23. Elliot DL, Linz DH, Kane JA: Medical evaluation before operation. West J Med 137:351, 1982

24. Tarhan S, Moffitt EA, Taylor WF, Guiliani ER: Myocardial infarction after general anesthesia. JAMA 220:1451, 1972

25. Steen PA, Tinker JH, Tarhan S: Myocardial reinfarction after anesthesia and surgery. JAMA 239:2566, 1978

26. Rao TLK, Jacobs KH, El-Etr AA: Reinfarction following anesthesia in patients with myocardial infarction. Anesthesiology 59:499, 1983

27. Mahar LJ, Steen PA, Tinker JH et al: Perioperative myocardial infarction in patients with coronary artery disease with and without aorto-coronary artery bypass grafts. J Thorac Cardiovasc Surg 76:533, 1978

28. Akl BF, Talbot W, Neal JF, Havens D: Noncardiac operations after coronary revascularization. West J Med 136:91, 1982

29. Goldman L, Caldera DL, Nussbaum SR et al: Multifactorial index of cardiac risk in non-cardiac surgical procedures. N Engl J Med 297:845, 1977

30. Tinker JH, Noback CR, Vlietstra RE, Frye RL: Management of patients with heart disease for noncardiac surgery. JAMA 246:1348, 1981

31. Goldman L: Cardiac risks and complications of noncardiac surgery. Ann Intern Med 98:504, 1983

32. Tisi GM: Preoperative evaluation of pulmonary function. Am Rev Respir Dis 119:293, 1979

33. Krumholz RA, Chevalier RB, Ross JC: Changes in cardiopulmonary functions related to abstinence from smoking. Ann Intern Med 62:197, 1965

34. Stein M, Cassara EL: Preoperative pulmonary evaluation and therapy for surgery patients. JAMA 211:787, 1970

35. Bartlett RH, Gazzaniga AB, Geraghty TR: Respiratory maneuvers to prevent postoperative pulmonary complications—a critical review. JAMA 224:1017, 1973

36. Tait AR, Knight PR: Intraoperative respiratory complications in patients with upper respiratory tract infections. Can J Anaesth 34:300, 1987

37. Cohen MM, Cameron CB: Should you cancel the operation when a child has an upper respiratory tract infection? Anesth Analg 72:282, 1991

38. Salzarulo HH, Taylor LA: Diabetic "stiff joint syndrome" as a cause of difficult endotracheal intubation. Anesthesiology 64:366, 1986

39. Walts LF, Miller J, Davidson MB, Brown J: Perioperative management of diabetes mellitus. Anesthesiology 55:104, 1981

40. Roizen MF: Anesthesia for the patient with endocrine disease, Part I. Curr Rev Clin Anesth 6:43, 1987

41. Weinberg AD, Brennan MD, Gorman CA et al: Outcome of anesthesia and surgery in hypothyroid patients. Arch Intern Med 143:893, 1983

42. Manger WH, Gifford RW: Pheochromocytoma. New York, Springer-Verlag, 1977

43. Desmonts JM, Marty J: Anaesthetic management of patients with phaeochromocytoma. Br J Anaesth 56:781, 1984

44. Arai T, Hatano Y, Ishida H, Mori K: Use of nicardipine in the anesthetic management of pheochromocytoma. Anesth Analg 65:706, 1986

45. Creutzfeldt W, Stockman F: Carcinoids and carcinoid syndrome. Am J Med 82 (suppl 5B):4, 1987

46. Lichtenstein A, Eckhart WF, Swanson KJ et al: Unplanned intraoperative and postoperative hemodilution; Oxygen transport and consumption during severe anemia. Anesthesiology 69:119, 1988

47. Wallerstein RO: Laboratory evaluation of a bleeding patient. West J Med 150:51, 1989

48. Wilson ME, Spiegelhalter D, Robertson JA, Lesser P: Predicting difficult intubation. Br J Anaesth 61:211, 1988

49. Samsoon GLT, Young JRB: Difficult tracheal intubation; a retrospective study. Anaesthesia 42:487, 1987

50. Mallampati SR, Gatt SP, Gugino LD et al: A clinical sign to predict difficult tracheal intubation: A prospective study. Can Anaesth Soc J 32:429, 1985

51. Oates JDL, Macleod AD, Oates PD et al: Comparison of two methods for predicting difficult intubation. Br J Anaesth 66:305, 1991

52. Duncan PG, Pope WDB, Cohen MM, Greer N: Fetal risk of anesthesia and surgery during pregnancy. Anesthesiology 64:790, 1986

53. Kaplan EB, Sheiner LB, Boeckmann AJ et al: The usefulness of preoperative laboratory screening. JAMA 253:3576, 1985

54. Hubbell FA, Greenfield S, Tyler JL et al: The impact of routine admission chest x-ray films on patient care. N Engl J Med 312:209, 1985

55. Cohen MM, Duncan PG, Tate RB: Does anesthesia contribute to operative mortality? JAMA 260:2859, 1988

56. Touloukian J, Kaplowitz N: Halothane-induced hepatic disease. Semin Liver Dis 1:134, 1981

57. Ording H: Incidence of malignant hyperthermia in Denmark. Anesth Analg 64:700, 1985

58. Cooper JB, Newbower RS, Kitz RJ: An analysis of major errors and equipment failures in anesthesia management: Considerations for prevention and detection. Anesthesiology 60:34, 1984

59. Keenan RL, Boyan CP: Cardiac arrest due to anesthesia: a study of incidence and causes. JAMA 253:2373, 1985

60. Lunn JN: Anaesthetic mortality in Britain and France: methods and results of the British study. In Vickers MD, Lunn JN (eds):

562   Preparing for Anesthesia

Mortality in Anaesthesia, p 19. New York, Springer-Verlag, 1983

61. Derrington MC, Smith G: A review of studies of anaesthetic risk, morbidity and mortality. Br J Anaesth 59:815, 1987

62. Holland R: Anaesthetic mortality in New South Wales. Br J Anaesth 59:834, 1987

63. Keats AS: Anesthesia mortality in perspective. Anesth Analg 71:113, 1990

64. Saklad M: Grading of patients for surgical procedures. Anesthesiology 2:281, 1941

65. Dripps RD, Lamont A, Eckenhoff JE: The role of anesthesia in surgical mortality. JAMA 178:261, 1961

66. Owens WD, Felts JA, Spitznagel EL: ASA physical status classifications: A study of consistency of ratings. Anesthesiology 49:239, 1978

67. Marx GF, Mateo CV, Orkin LR: Computer analysis of postanesthetic deaths. Anesthesiology 39:54, 1973

68. Vacanti CJ, VanHouten RJ, Hill RC: A statistical analysis of the relationship of physical status to postoperative mortality in 68,388 cases. Anesth Analg 49:564, 1970

22

Stephen F. Dierdorf

Rare and Coexisting Diseases

Knowledge of the pathophysiologic characteristics of coexisting disease and an understanding of the implications of concomitant drug therapy are essential for the optimal management of anesthesia for an individual patient. In many instances, the nature of the coexisting disease has more impact on anesthesia than does the actual surgical procedure. A variety of rare disorders may influence the selection and management of anesthesia (Table 22-1). Economic constraints have increased the likelihood that patients with these diseases will present for outpatient surgery with incomplete preoperative evaluations. Consequently, the anesthesiologist must periodically update his or her diagnostic skills and clinical knowledge in order to recognize when additional evaluation may be required.

MUSCULOSKELETAL DISEASES

Muscular Dystrophy

There are several types of muscular dystrophy. Duchenne's muscular dystrophy, also known as pseudohypertrophic muscular dystrophy, is the most severe form. Duchenne's dystrophy is characterized by painless degeneration and atrophy of skeletal muscle. This disorder is a sex-linked recessive trait that is clinically evident in males. Typically, progressive skeletal muscle weakness develops that produces symptoms between the ages of 2 and 5 years. Progressive limitation of movement occurs, and these patients are usually confined to a wheelchair by the time they are 12 years of age. Axial skeletal muscle imbalance generally produces kyphoscoliosis, which often requires operative instrumentation for stabilization. Death occurs when patients are from 15–25 years of age and is secondary to congestive heart failure or pneumonia. Serum creatine kinase levels reflect the progression of skeletal muscle degeneration. Early in the patient's life the creatine kinase level is elevated. Later, as significant amounts of skeletal muscle have degenerated, the creatine kinase level decreases.

Cardiac muscle also degenerates in patients with this disease, as reflected by a progressive decrease in R wave amplitude on serial electrocardiograms (ECGs). Myocardial degeneration produces decreased myocardial contractility and in some cases mitral regurgitation secondary to papillary muscle dysfunction.[1] Nearly 60% of Duchenne patients between 6 and 10 years old have preclinical myocardial involvement.[2] Interestingly, myocardial abnormalities are usually confined to the lateral and posterobasal walls of the left ventricle.[3] However, obstruction of the right ventricular outflow tract can produce an insidious right-sided heart failure.[4] Degeneration of respiratory muscles is evidenced by the restrictive pattern of pulmonary function tests. Diminished muscle strength produces an ineffective cough and subsequent retention of secretions, which lead to pneumonia and, ultimately, death.

Becker's dystrophy is similar to Duchenne's dystrophy, but the onset is later and progression is slower. Other forms of muscular dystrophy include fascioscapulohumeral dystrophy and limb-girdle dystrophy. These types of dystrophies have clinical onset in adulthood and are not nearly as severe as Duchenne's muscular dystrophy.

Management of Anesthesia

Myocardial dysfunction in the patient with Duchenne's muscular dystrophy makes these patients potentially more sensitive to the myocardial depressant effects of potent inhaled anesthetics. There are numerous reports of cardiac arrest having occurred during induction of anesthesia.[5,6] Consequently, cardiac function must be monitored carefully during induction of anesthesia. Succinylcholine should not be used because massive rhabdomyolysis, hyperkalemia, and cardiac arrest can occur.[7-9] Some patients with Duchenne's muscular dystrophy are also susceptible to malignant hyperthermia, but this is unpredictable.[10] Nondepolarizing muscle relaxants can be used, although patients with Duchenne's muscular dystrophy may require a longer recovery time.[11]

Smooth muscle involvement results in hypomotility of the intestinal tract and delayed gastric emptying. The potential for aspiration of gastric contents is further enhanced by impaired swallowing mechanisms.[12] Precautions should be taken to prevent aspiration.

After operation, the patient with Duchenne's muscular dystrophy must be monitored closely for evidence of pulmonary dysfunction and retention of pulmonary secretions. Vigorous respiratory therapy and ventilatory support may be necessary.

TABLE 22-1. Coexisting Diseases That Influence Anesthesia Management

Musculoskeletal

Muscular dystrophy
Myotonic dystrophy
Myasthenia gravis
Eaton-Lambert (myasthenic)
  syndrome
Familial periodic paralysis
Guillain-Barré syndrome

Central Nervous System

Multiple sclerosis
Epilepsy
Parkinson's disease
Huntington's chorea
Alzheimer's disease
Amyotrophic lateral sclerosis
Creutzfeldt-Jakob disease

Anemias

Nutritional deficiency
Hemolytic
Hemoglobinopathies
Thalassemias

Collagen Vascular

Rheumatoid arthritis
Systemic lupus erythematosus
Scleroderma
Polymyositis

Skin

Epidermolysis bullosa
Pemphigus

Myotonic Dystrophy (Myotonia Dystrophica, Steinert's Disease)

Myotonic dystrophy is the most common form of a group of diseases known as the myotonias. Other forms of myotonia include congenital myotonia (Thomsen's disease) and paramyotonia. Myotonic dystrophy is transmitted as an autosomal dominant trait with symptoms occurring when patients are in the second or third decade of life. The hallmark of myotonic dystrophy is persistent contracture of skeletal muscle after stimulation. Myotonic contraction of affected muscle is not relieved by regional anesthesia, nondepolarizing muscle relaxants, or deep anesthesia. Relaxation may be induced by infiltration of the affected muscle with a local anesthetic. The administration of quinine, tocainide, or mexiletine may also alleviate myotonic muscle contracture. These drugs depress sodium influx into muscle cells and delay return of membrane excitability.[13,14] There is progressive involvement and deterioration of function in skeletal, cardiac, and smooth muscles. Although myocardial contractile tissue degenerates and affects ventricular systolic function, the cardiac conduction system, and in particular the His-Purkinje system, deteriorates more rapidly. Myocardial failure is rare, but cardiac dysrhythmias and atrioventricular block are common.[15,16] First-degree atrioventricular block may actually precede the onset of clinical symptoms. Sudden death may be a result of the abrupt onset of third-degree atrioventricular block. Although mitral valve prolapse occurs in 20% of patients with myotonic dystrophy, the prolapse is secondary to geometric changes of the heart caused by thoracic deformation. Systemic complications from mitral valve prolapse generally do not occur in patients with myotonic dystrophy.[17]

Pulmonary function studies demonstrate restrictive lung disease, mild arterial hypoxemia, and diminished ventilatory responses to hypoxia and hypercapnia.[18] Weakness of respiratory muscles diminishes the effectiveness of cough and may lead to pneumonia. Myotonia of respiratory muscles can produce intense dyspnea requiring therapy with antimyotonic medications such as procainamide.[19] Alteration of smooth muscle function produces gastric atony and intestinal hypomotility. Pharyngeal muscle weakness in conjunction with delayed gastric emptying increases the risk for aspiration of gastric contents.[20] Endocrine dysfunction also occurs in patients with myotonic dystrophy and produces diabetes mellitus, thyroid dysfunction, adrenal insufficiency, and gonadal atrophy. Other clinical features include cataract formation, frontal baldness, and mental deterioration.

Pregnancy often produces exacerbations of myotonic dystrophy. It has been suggested that the increased progesterone levels of pregnancy contribute to increased symptoms. Congestive heart failure is also more likely to occur during pregnancy.[21] Cesarean section must often be performed because of uterine smooth muscle dysfunction.[22]

Congenital myotonia (Thomsen's disease) develops during infancy or early childhood and usually manifests as a swallowing dysfunction because of an inability to relax the oropharyngeal muscles. The condition generally improves with age and does not affect a patient's life expectancy. Paramyotonia is the third and most rare of the myotonic syndromes. Myotonic contracture develops when the patient's environment is cold; warming will relax the contracted muscle. Hypokalemia has also been reported to produce muscle paralysis in patients with paramyotonia.[23]

Management of Anesthesia

Considerations for anesthesia in the patient with myotonic dystrophy include the presence of cardiac and respiratory muscle disease and the abnormal response to drugs used during anesthesia. Succinylcholine produces an exaggerated contracture, and its use should be avoided (Fig. 22-1). Succinylcholine-induced myotonia can make ventilation of the lungs and tracheal intubation difficult or impossible.[24] The patient's response to nondepolarizing muscle relaxants appears normal. Neostigmine, however, may precipitate myotonia when administered for reversal of neuromuscular blockade.[25] Consequently, when selecting a neuromuscular blocking drug, a shorter acting one such as atracurium or vecuronium would be useful.[26-28] The response to a peripheral nerve stimulator must be carefully interpreted because muscle stimulation may produce myotonia, which can be misinterpreted as sustained tetanus when significant neuromuscular blockade still exists. Patients with myotonia are quite sensitive to the respiratory depressant effects of opioids, barbiturates, benzodiazepines, and inhaled anesthetics. Depression of ventilation increases as the disease progresses and seems to result from depression of the central respiratory center and a peripheral muscle effect.[29] The response to propofol has been extremely varied. One report described intraoperative stability and rapid emergence.[30] Another reported exaggerated respiratory depression, hypotension, and ocular myotonia.[31] Because patients with myotonia have mitral valve prolapse and cardiac conduction abnormalities, cardiac dysrhythmias may occur. The preoperative ECG should be examined carefully for signs of atrioventricular conduction delay. Use of anesthetics known to delay conduction in the His-Purkinje system, specifically halothane, may be avoided for this reason.

Smooth muscle function is also affected by myotonia. Gastrointestinal motility is decreased and gastric emptying delayed. Precautions should be used to prevent pulmonary aspiration.[32]

Skeletal muscle weakness and myotonia are exacerbated during pregnancy. Labor is typically prolonged, and there is an increased incidence of postpartum hemorrhage from placenta accreta.[33] Anesthesia for cesarean section has been successful with general, spinal, and epidural anesthesia.[22,34] If general anesthesia is administered, it should be antici-

Succinylcholine (mg/kg)

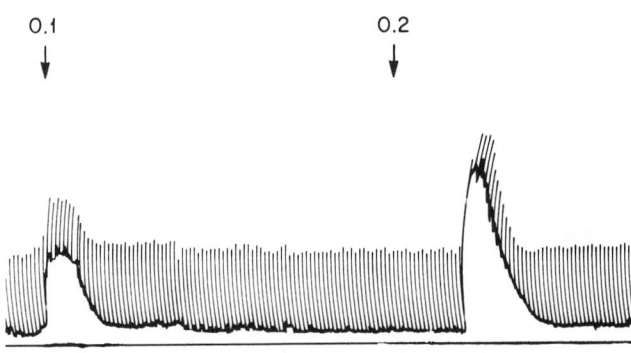

0.1

0.2

Figure 22-1. Administration of low doses of succinylcholine to a patient with myotonic dystrophy produces an exaggerated contraction of skeletal muscle. (Reprinted with permission from Mitchell MM, Ali HH, Savarese JJ: Myotonia and neuromuscular blocking drugs. Anesthesiology 49:44, 1978.)

pated that these patients will be sensitive to respiratory depressant drugs and will have a decreased ability to clear pulmonary secretions.[35]

Myasthenia Gravis

Myasthenia gravis is a disease of the neuromuscular junction caused by a decrease in the population of acetylcholine receptors. The incidence is one in 20,000, and female patients are affected twice as often as male patients. Myasthenia gravis is considered an autoimmune disease because circulating antibodies destroy or inactivate acetylcholine receptors. Seventy to ninety percent of myasthenic patients have antiacetylcholine receptor antibodies.[36] There is an apparent breakdown in tolerance of T and B cells to the acetylcholine receptor. This lack of tolerance activates T-helper cells, which produce antibodies specific for acetylcholine receptors.[37] This process initially occurs in the thymus. The central role of the thymus gland is certain, since 15–20% of patients with myasthenia have thymomas. In addition, myasthenics with thymic hyperplasia benefit from thymectomy.[38] Thymomas are more likely to occur in patients older than 30 years, whereas thymic hyperplasia frequently occurs in younger patients. Many myasthenic patients also have antinuclear, antithyroid, and antimuscle autoantibodies.[39]

The clinical hallmark of myasthenia gravis is skeletal muscle weakness. Typically there are periods of exacerbation alternating with remissions.

There are several types of myasthenia gravis. The classification is based on the skeletal muscle groups that are affected. Types of myasthenia gravis include generalized, ocular, bulbar, and shoulder-girdle. The course of the disease is frequently affected by environmental, physical, and emotional changes. Viral illness, pregnancy, and surgery may affect the patient with myasthenia gravis, but not predictably.[40] Patients with myasthenia gravis, especially those with thymoma, may have myasthenia gravis–related heart disease. Focal myocarditis is observed on histologic examination of cardiac muscle. Clinically this myocarditis produces dysrhythmias, particularly atrial fibrillation and atrioventricular block.[41]

Pregnancy may produce either exacerbation or remission of the disease. Forty percent of pregnant women have increased symptoms during gestation. Postpartum respiratory failure and death can occur. Fifteen to twenty percent of neonates born to myasthenic women have transient myasthenia resulting from the passive placental transfer of antiacetylcholine receptor antibodies. Neonatal myasthenia begins 12–48 hours after birth and may persist for several weeks. Neonatal skeletal muscle strength must be monitored carefully during the early neonatal period.[42]

Another interesting presentation of myasthenia gravis is isolated respiratory failure.[43,44] Consequently, undiagnosed myasthenia gravis should also be added to the differential diagnosis of respiratory failure.

Treatment modalities for myasthenia gravis may include the use of the following: cholinesterase inhibitors, thymectomy, corticosteroids, and immunosuppressants. Pyridostigmine is the most frequently used oral anticholinesterase for the treatment of myasthenia. Neostigmine, ambenonium, and distigmine (not yet available in the United States) are also used.[45] Consistent control of myasthenia with cholinesterase inhibitors can be quite challenging. Underdosage will result in increased skeletal muscle weakness, but an overdose will produce a "cholinergic crisis." Excessive doses of cholinesterase inhibitors produce abdominal cramping, diarrhea, vomiting, and skeletal muscle weakness that mimics the weakness of myasthenia. Corticosteroids produce remission in 80% of patients with myasthenia but also produce significant drug side-effects during long-term therapy.[46] Immunosuppressive therapy with azathioprine $(2.5 \text{ mg·kg}^{-1}\text{·day}^{-1})$ has been shown to reduce antiacetylcholine receptor antibody levels and produce clinical improvement.

Thymectomy has increased in popularity in recent years and can produce remission in nearly 80% of patients. The myasthenic patients that respond most dramatically to thymectomy are those with thymic hyperplasia and circulating receptor site antibodies.[47]

Management of Anesthesia

The primary concern in anesthesia for the patient with myasthenia gravis is the potential interaction between the disease, treatment of the disease, and neuromuscular blocking drugs. The uncontrolled or poorly controlled myasthenic patient is exquisitely sensitive to nondepolarizing muscle relaxants. Even low defasciculating doses of nondepolarizing muscle relaxants can produce significant respiratory muscle paralysis. Vecuronium and atracurium, because of their relatively rapid elimination, are useful nondepolarizing drugs for use in patients with myasthenia.[48-51] Myasthenic patients are clearly more sensitive to vecuronium, but clearance of the drug is normal in myasthenic patients.[52,53] The response of the myasthenic patient to succinylcholine is unpredictable. The untreated myasthenic demonstrates a resistance to succinylcholine. However, the myasthenic patient treated with cholinesterase inhibitors may exhibit a normal or prolonged response to succinylcholine.[54] Because of the patient's unpredictable response to succinylcholine, a nondepolarizing muscle relaxant is often preferred. Regardless of the muscle relaxant that is administered, careful monitoring with a peripheral nerve stimulator is highly recommended. Halothane and isoflurane have also been shown to depress neuromuscular transmission in myasthenic patients.[55,56] In addition, patients with myasthenia gravis are clinically more sensitive to the ventilatory depressant effects of barbiturates, inhaled anesthetics, and opioids.

TABLE 22-2. Comparison of Clinical Features Between Myasthenia Gravis and Eaton-Lambert (Myasthenic) Syndrome

	Myasthenia Gravis	Eaton-Lambert Syndrome
Sex distribution	Female > male	Male > female
Clinical features	Ocular and facial weakness	Proximal limb weakness
	Fatigue with activity	Improved strength with activity
	Normal reflexes	Reduced reflexes
	No myalgia	Myalgia common
Pharmacology	Sensitive to nondepolarizers	Sensitive to nondepolarizers and suc-cinylcholine
	Improved strength after anticholines-terases	No response to anticholinesterases
Pathology	Thymoma in 20–25%	Small-cell bronchogenic carcinoma

Modified with permission from Telford RJ, Hollway TE: The myasthenic syndrome: Anesthesia in a patient treated with 3,4 diamino pyridine. Br J Anaesth 64:363, 1990.

Ventilatory function must be carefully monitored in the postoperative period. The unpredictable interactions of the disease, treatment drugs, and anesthetic drugs can make postoperative mechanical ventilation of the lungs necessary. The need for postoperative mechanical ventilation is substantially increased when trans-sternal thymectomy is used as opposed to transcervical thymectomy.[57-59] The patient with myasthenia gravis requiring mechanical ventilation can be one of the most challenging to wean from ventilatory support. Skeletal muscle strength can vary significantly in a short period of time. It is imperative that sustained respiratory strength be confirmed before extubation of the trachea and resumption of independent, spontaneous ventilation.

Exacerbation of myasthenia gravis may occur in late pregnancy and the early postpartum period. Consequently, skeletal muscle relaxation produced by regional anesthesia in conjunction with inherent muscle weakness may lead to hypoventilation. Regional analgesia and anesthesia have been used successfully in myasthenic patients, but careful monitoring is necessary. Because 15–20% of infants born to myasthenic mothers may exhibit transient neonatal myasthenia within 1–21 days of birth, anticholinesterase therapy and mechanical ventilation of the lungs may be necessary.

Myasthenic Syndrome (Eaton-Lambert Syndrome)

The myasthenic syndrome is a disorder of neuromuscular transmission associated with carcinomas, particularly small-cell carcinoma of the lung. Myasthenic syndrome is considered to be an autoimmune disease in which IgG antibodies to presynaptic calcium channels are produced.[60] The result is a decreased release of acetylcholine in response to nerve stimulation.[61] Typically the patient is a 50- to 70-year-old man complaining of proximal extremity weakness. Unlike the patient with myasthenia gravis, the patient with myasthenic syndrome generally has increasing muscle strength with exercise and has no improvement in strength after anticholinesterase drugs are administered (Table 22-2).

Drugs from the aminopyridine group (4-aminopyridine and 3,4-diaminopyridine) promote calcium influx and calcium-dependent release of acetylcholine.[62,63] Reported experience with anesthesia in patients receiving aminopyri-

dines is limited, but it is recommended that their administration be continued up to the time of surgery.[64]

Patients with myasthenic syndrome are sensitive to the effects of both depolarizing and nondepolarizing muscle relaxants. Consequently, the doses of these drugs should be reduced, and neuromuscular function should be monitored carefully. Because this syndrome is difficult to diagnose, a high index of suspicion must be maintained in patients undergoing diagnostic procedures such as bronchoscopy and mediastinoscopy or exploratory thoracotomy for suspected carcinoma of the lung.

Familial Periodic Paralysis

Familial periodic paralysis is characterized by intermittent but acute episodes of skeletal muscle weakness or paralysis. Attacks begin when patients are in early childhood and may persist throughout their lives, although the frequency of episodes declines during middle age. There are three recognized forms of familial periodic paralysis: hypokalemic, normokalemic, and hyperkalemic (Table 22-3). It is believed that the defect involves abnormalities in the membrane transport of potassium and sodium.[65] The subsequent alterations in muscle membrane potentials may render the skeletal muscle inexcitable.

In the hypokalemic form, paralysis may be produced in the patient by his or her ingestion of carbohydrate loads, strenuous exercise, and infusion of glucose and insulin. Paralysis is generally incomplete and affects the limb and trunk muscles but spares the diaphragm. The low serum levels of potassium present during acute episodes often produce cardiac dysrhythmias. Treatment consists of potassium infusion and administration of acetazolamide or dichlorphenamide (carbonic anhydrase inhibitors).[66] Permanent skeletal muscle weakness can occur in some patients with hypokalemic familial periodic paralysis.[67] There are several anesthetic considerations for patients with familial periodic paralysis. If possible, any abnormalities should be corrected before surgery. During periods of hypokalemia, these patients may be sensitive to nondepolarizing muscle relaxants. Because they have unpredictable responses to neuromuscular blocking drugs, doses should be reduced and the response monitored with a peripheral nerve stimu-

TABLE 22-3. Clinical Features of Familial Periodic Paralysis

Type	Serum Potassium Concentration During Attack	Precipitating Factors	Other Features
Hypokalemic	<3 mEq·l⁻¹	Large meals Rest after strenuous exercise Glucose and insulin infusion	Changes of hypokalemia on ECG Cardiac dysrhythmias Sensitivity to nondepolarizing muscle relaxants
Normokalemic	3.0–5.5 mEq·l⁻¹	Alcohol Exercise Emotional stress	Muscle weakness persisting for as long as 14 days
Hyperkalemic	>5.5 mEq·l⁻¹	Exercise Potassium infusion Exposure to cold	Muscle weakness often localized to tongue and eyelids Sensitivity to succinylcholine

Reprinted with permission from Gibbs PS, Kim KC: Skin and musculoskeletal diseases. In Stoelting RK, Dierdorf SF, McCammon RL (eds): Anesthesia and Co-Existing Disease. New York, Churchill-Livingstone, 1988.

lator. Metabolic changes (alkalosis) or medications (glucose and insulin, diuretics) that reduce serum potassium levels may initiate an episode of paralysis.[68] It would be desirable to measure potassium levels during prolonged use of anesthetics. The ECG should be monitored continuously during anesthesia for evidence of cardiac dysrhythmias secondary to hypokalemia. After surgery, adequate skeletal muscle strength must be ascertained before mechanical ventilation of the lungs is discontinued. Monitoring of serum potassium levels in the postoperative period is also recommended after prolonged or complicated surgical procedures. A decrease in potassium levels may precede the onset of clinical muscle weakness.[69] Other recommendations include the avoidance of large carbohydrate loads and hypothermia. It should be remembered that any cause of severe potassium depletion, such as renal tubular acidosis or chronic diarrhea, can also produce skeletal muscle weakness.[70,71]

Hyperkalemic periodic paralysis is characterized by episodic muscle weakness that develops in association with increased levels of potassium. Attacks may be initiated by fasting, cold, rest after exercise, or potassium administration. Acute episodes of paralysis generally are treated with acetazolamide or diuretics. Epinephrine and metaproterenol are also effective.[65] This disorder may be confused with paramyotonia because cold may trigger skeletal muscle weakness in patients with either disease. The use of succinylcholine is best avoided because it may enhance potassium release from muscle cells and further increase serum potassium levels. Because of the potential for cardiac dysrhythmias, continuous ECG monitoring is recommended. If fasting is required, an intravenous infusion of glucose should be administered. Normothermia must also be maintained during anesthesia.

Normokalemic periodic paralysis can be triggered by a variety of stimuli, including alcohol ingestion, exercise, and emotional stress. Duration of skeletal muscle paralysis is quite variable but may exceed 14 days. Cardiac tachydysrhythmias are common during attacks. Recorded anesthesia experience with this form of periodic paralysis is extremely limited. Anesthetic considerations are similar to those for the hypokalemic form.[72]

Guillain-Barré Syndrome (Polyradiculoneuritis)

Guillain-Barré syndrome (polyradiculoneuritis, acute idiopathic polyneuritis) is characterized by the acute or subacute onset of skeletal muscle weakness or paralysis of the legs. Sensory disturbances such as paresthesias often precede the paralysis. Typically, the paralysis progresses cephalad within a few days to include the muscles of the trunk and arms. Difficulty in swallowing and impaired ventilation resulting from intercostal muscle paralysis often occur. Progression typically occurs over 10–12 days followed by gradual recovery. An acute course may develop from normal neurologic function to respiratory muscle paralysis within 48–72 hours. Other patients may have a subacute onset and relatively slow progression. Fifty to sixty-seven percent of patients with Guillain-Barré syndrome have a history of a respiratory tract or gastrointestinal tract viral illness within 4 weeks of the onset of neurologic symptoms. Cytomegalovirus, Epstein-Barr virus, and human immunodeficiency virus have all been implicated as causative agents of Guillain-Barré syndrome.[73] Other implicated etiologic agents include herpes virus, measles, vaccinations, and prior surgical procedures. Nerve demyelination that occurs is felt to be immunologically mediated, with a virus serving as an antigen. Although 85% of patients with this syndrome achieve a good or full recovery, chronic or recurrent neuropathy occurs in 3–5% of patients.[74]

The most serious immediate problem is ventilatory insufficiency. The vital capacity should be monitored frequently. If the vital capacity decreases to 15 or 20 ml·kg, mechanical ventilation of the lungs is indicated.[75] The more rapid the onset of quadriplegia, the more likely the need for prolonged mechanical ventilatory support.[76] Plasmapheresis has become the accepted therapy for Guillain-Barré syndrome. It has been demonstrated that plasmapheresis decreases the time to recovery and reduces the likelihood of residual neurologic effects.[77] The use of corticosteroids for the treatment of Guillain-Barré syndrome is controversial, and definitive studies have not been completed.

Autonomic nervous system dysfunction occurs in many

patients with Guillain-Barré syndrome. This dysfunction can produce wide fluctuations in blood pressure, tachycardia, cardiac dysrhythmias, and cardiac arrest.[78] Physical stimulation of the patient often precipitates hypertension, tachycardia, and cardiac dysrhythmias. Alpha- and beta-adrenergic blockade may be required for those patients.[79]

Management of Anesthesia

Autonomic nervous system dysfunction indicates that compensatory cardiovascular responses may be absent, resulting in significant hypotension secondary to postural changes, blood loss, or positive airway pressure. On the other hand, noxious stimuli such as laryngoscopic examination may produce exaggerated increases in heart rate and blood pressure. Direct-acting vasopressors or vasodilators may be required to control blood pressure. Cardiovascular function should be carefully monitored.

The use of succinylcholine should be avoided because of the danger of drug-induced potassium release and hyperkalemia. This risk may actually persist after clinical recovery from the disorder.[80] A nondepolarizing muscle relaxant with minimal cardiovascular effects, such as vecuronium, would be a useful choice for muscle relaxation. It is likely that mechanical ventilation will be required during the immediate postoperative period. Some patients with Guillain-Barré syndrome have pronounced sensory disturbances and benefit from the use of epidural opioids.[81,82]

It should be remembered that it can be very difficult to differentiate Guillain-Barré syndrome from other neurologic disorders such as anterior spinal artery syndrome or chronic inflammatory demyelinating polyneuropathy.[83]

CENTRAL NERVOUS SYSTEM DISEASES

Multiple Sclerosis

Multiple sclerosis is an acquired disease of the central nervous system characterized by multiple sites of demyelination in the brain and spinal cord. Plaques of demyelination are found most often in areas along spinal fluid pathways. The optic tracts and periventricular regions have a particular predilection for plaque formation.[84] Multiple sclerosis is primarily a disease of young adults, with the onset of symptoms occurring when patients are between the ages of 15 and 40 years.

The cause of multiple sclerosis appears to be multifactoral. The current theory is that multiple sclerosis is caused by a virus that either persists in the central nervous system or induces an autoimmune response.[85] The geographic correlation relative to susceptibility is impressive. The high-risk areas include the United States, Great Britain, Scandinavia, Europe, and New Zealand.

The symptoms of multiple sclerosis depend on the sites of demyelination in the brain and spinal cord. Demyelination of the optic tracts produces visual disturbances, whereas demyelination of oculomotor pathways usually produces nystagmus. Lesions of the spinal cord cause limb weakness and paresthesias. The legs are affected more frequently than the arms. Bowel retention and urinary incontinence are frequent complaints. Involvement of the brain stem can produce diplopia, trigeminal neuralgia, and at times alterations in ventilation that can lead to respiratory failure.[86-88] The course of multiple sclerosis is characterized by exacerbations of symptoms at unpredictable intervals over a period of several years. Residual symptoms eventu-

ally persist during remission and may lead to severe disability. In some patients the course is relatively benign, with infrequent periods of demyelination followed by prolonged remission. As is typical in many immune disorders, pregnancy is associated with an improvement in symptoms, but relapse frequently occurs in the postpartum period.[89]

The diagnosis of multiple sclerosis is initially made by clinical determination. Confirmation of the diagnosis can be made by chemical analysis of the cerebrospinal fluid and magnetic resonance imaging. Seventy percent of patients with multiple sclerosis have elevated levels of immunoglobulin G in the cerebrospinal fluid. Elevated levels of albumin in the cerebrospinal fluid are generally indicative of blood-brain barrier dysfunction.[90] Magnetic resonance imaging has been established as a sensitive diagnostic tool for multiple sclerosis and provides direct evidence of the location of demyelinated plaques in the central nervous system.[91]

There is no known cure for multiple sclerosis. Corticosteroids have been shown to promote remission and may do so by decreasing white matter edema and thereby enhancing nerve conduction through partially demyelinated nerve fibers.[92] Immunosuppressive therapy with azathioprine and cyclophosphamide has also been used, but with varying results.[93] Plasmapheresis has been employed with some benefit. Drugs used to treat skeletal muscle spasticity associated with multiple sclerosis include diazepam, dantrolene, and baclofen. Painful dysesthesias, tonic seizures, dysarthria, and ataxia are often treated with carbamazepine. Nonspecific therapeutic measures include the avoidance of excessive fatigue, emotional stress, and hyperthermia. Demyelinated nerve fibers are extremely sensitive to increases in temperature. A temperature increase of as little as 0.5°C may block conduction in demyelinated fibers.[94]

Management of Anesthesia

The effect of surgery and anesthesia on the course of multiple sclerosis is controversial. Some reports indicate that symptoms of multiple sclerosis are exacerbated by anesthesia, particularly regional anesthesia.[95,96] However, other studies report that anesthesia does not affect the course of multiple sclerosis.[86,97] A relatively high proportion of patients with multiple sclerosis who receive spinal anesthesia do have an exacerbation of symptoms after surgery.[98] It could be speculated that demyelinated areas of the spinal cord might be more sensitive to the effects of local anesthetics. This increased sensitivity could explain exacerbations after anesthesia. Intrathecal morphine in conjunction with spinal and general anesthesia has been used successfully in patients with multiple sclerosis.[99,100] Epidural anesthesia has been used for labor and delivery of female patients with multiple sclerosis. The neurologic relapse rate, however, was greater if bupivacaine in concentrations greater than 0.25% was used.[101] Certainly pyrexia and, most likely, metabolic changes induced by surgery and anesthesia could produce exacerbations of symptoms independent of the type of anesthesia. Despite the seeming confusion in the medical literature, certain conclusions seem warranted. Before surgery the patient with multiple sclerosis should be advised that surgery and anesthesia could produce a relapse of disease despite a well-managed anesthetic. The patient should have a thorough neurologic examination before operation to document coexisting neurologic deficits. After surgery the neurologic examination can be repeated so that findings can be compared. In view of the fact that spinal anesthesia can cause unpredictable exacerbations, use of this type of anesthesia should be reserved for special situations. The patient's temperature should be monitored closely during anesthesia, and even slight temperature elevations must be treated actively.

Selection of agents for general anesthesia should take into consideration potential interactions with medications the patient is receiving. For example, patients receiving corticosteroids may need corticosteroid supplementation during the perioperative period. Theoretically succinylcholine could produce an exaggerated release of potassium, although this has not been reported in patients with multiple sclerosis. Anticonvulsants such as carbamazepine and phenytoin can produce resistance to nondepolarizing muscle relaxants.[102]

Autonomic dysfunction caused by multiple sclerosis may produce exaggerated hypotensive effects of volatile anesthetics. Consequently, careful monitoring of cardiovascular function is indicated.

Epilepsy

A seizure disorder is a common manifestation of many types of central nervous system diseases. A seizure results from the excessive discharge of large numbers of neurons that become depolarized in a synchronous fashion. Idiopathic seizures generally begin when patients are children. The sudden onset of seizures in a young or middle-aged adult should arouse suspicion of focal brain disease, particularly a tumor. The onset of seizures after 60 years of age is usually secondary to cerebrovascular disease but can be a result of head injury, brain tumor, or metabolic disturbances.[103] The onset of seizures requires a thorough neurologic evaluation to determine the etiology.

There are several types of seizures and a number of classification techniques based on the International Classification of Epileptic Seizures (Table 22-4).[104,105] A description of the most frequently encountered types of seizures follows.

Grand Mal Seizure

A grand mal seizure is characterized by generalized tonic-clonic activity. All respiratory activity is arrested, and a period of arterial hypoxemia ensues. The tonic phase lasts for 20–40 seconds and is followed by the clonic phase. In the postictal phase the patient is lethargic and confused. Initial treatment is directed toward maintaining arterial oxygenation and stopping the seizure activity. Diazepam and thiopental are effective drugs for the treatment of acute seizures. Antiseizure drugs effective for seizure control and prevention are phenytoin, valproate, and carbamazepine.

Focal Cortical Seizure

Focal cortical seizures, also known as jacksonian epilepsy, may be sensory or motor, depending on the site of neuronal discharge. Usually there is no loss of consciousness, although the seizure activity may spread to produce a grand mal seizure.

Petit Mal Seizure

Petit mal seizures are characterized by a brief loss of awareness lasting about 30 seconds. Additional manifestations include staring, blinking, and rolling the eyes. There is an immediate resumption of consciousness. Petit mal seizures typically occur in children and young adults. Drugs used

TABLE 22-4. Classification of Seizures

Localization-Related Epilepsies and Syndromes

Idiopathic
  Benign childhood epilepsy
  Childhood epilepsy with occipital paroxysms

Generalized Epilepsies

Idiopathic
  Absence epilepsy
    Childhood
    Juvenile
  Benign neonatal convulsions
  Myoclonic epilepsy
    Neonatal
    Juvenile
  Grand mal seizures on awakening
Idiopathic and/or symptomatic
  West's syndrome
  Lennox-Gestaut syndrome
  Myoclonic-astatic seizures
  Myoclonic absences
Symptomatic
  Nonspecific etiology

Undetermined Epilepsies and Syndromes

With both generalized and focal seizures
  Neonatal seizures
  Severe myoclonic epilepsy of infancy
  Acquired epileptic aphasia

Special Syndromes

Febrile seizures
Alcohol-related seizures

Modified with permission from Riela AR: Management of seizures. Crit Care Clin 5:863, 1989.

for the treatment of petit mal seizures include valproate and ethosuximide.

Akinetic Seizure

Akinetic seizures are characterized by a sudden, brief loss of consciousness and loss of postural tone. These types of seizures generally occur in children and can produce severe head injury from a fall.

Myoclonic Seizure

Myoclonic seizures occur as isolated clonic jerks in response to a sensory stimulus. In most cases a single group of muscles is involved. Myoclonic seizures are often associated with degenerative and metabolic brain diseases.

Psychomotor Seizure

Psychomotor seizures are seen as an impairment of consciousness, inappropriate motor acts, hallucinations, amnesia, and unusual visceral symptoms. This type of seizure is usually preceded by an aura.

Status Epilepticus

Status epilepticus is a seizure disorder in which the seizure activity continues unabated for 30 minutes or longer. Status

TABLE 22-5. Anticonvulsant Drugs			
Drug Effects	Type of Seizure	Therapeutic Blood Level ($\mu g \cdot ml^{-1}$)	Side-Effects
Phenobarbital	Generalized	15–35	Sedation, increased drug metabolism
Valproate	Generalized; petit mal	50–100	Pancreatitis, hepatic dysfunction, thrombocytopenia
Phenytoin	Generalized; partial	10–20	Gingival hyperplasia, dermatitis, resistance to nondepolarizers
Carbamazepine	Generalized; partial	6–12	Cardiotoxic, hepatitis, resistance to nondepolarizers
Ethosuximide	Petit mal	40–100	Leukopenia, erythema multiforme
Primidone	Generalized; partial	6–12	Nausea, ataxia
Clonazepam	Petit mal	0.01–0.07	Ataxia

epilepticus can include all types of seizure activity. Grand mal status epilepticus is of the greatest concern because mortality can be as high as 20%. Typically grand mal status epilepticus lasts for 48 hours, with a seizure frequency of four to five per hour. As the seizure progresses, skeletal muscle activity diminishes and seizure activity may be evident only on the electroencephalogram (EEG). Respiratory effects of status epilepticus include inhibition of respiratory centers, uncoordinated skeletal muscle activity that impairs ventilation, and abnormal autonomic activity that produces bronchoconstriction. In addition to the danger of arterial hypoxemia from inadequate airway control, there is a high likelihood of permanent neuronal damage by continued seizures.[106] Diazepam is considered the drug of choice for the treatment of status epilepticus. Lorazepam has also been used for the initial treatment of status epilepticus. Because the effect of the benzodiazepines is transient, a longer acting anticonvulsant (e.g., phenytoin, phenobarbital) must also be administered.[107] Thiopental is also quite effective for the initial treatment of status epilepticus, but the effect is transient. Muscle relaxants may be required for tracheal intubation if a secured airway is necessary. Although muscle relaxants will terminate the skeletal muscle manifestations of a seizure, there is no effect on seizure activity in the brain. On rare occasions general anesthesia with halothane or isoflurane may be required for the treatment of status epilepticus.[108]

Management of Anesthesia

Patients receiving anticonvulsant medications should be maintained on their normal medication regimen until the time of surgery. After operation, medications should be given parenterally until oral intake can be resumed. In management of anesthesia for the patient with a seizure disorder, the potential influence of anticonvulsants on the response to anesthesia must be considered (see Table 22-5). Conversely, an anesthesia technique must be used that will not increase the likelihood of seizure activity. Because anticonvulsant drugs affect the liver and neuromuscular systems, the potential for significant drug interaction certainly exists. Stimulation of the hepatic microsomal enzymes by phenobarbital may accelerate and increase the magnitude of biotransformation of anesthetic drugs. Increased biotransformation of the volatile halogenated anesthetics may increase the risk of organ toxicity. Other known side-effects of anticonvulsants include leukopenia, anemia, and hepatitis

from phenytoin; pancreatitis, hepatic failure, and coagulopathy from valproate; and aplastic anemia, cardiotoxicity, and hypothyroidism from carbamazepine.[109,110]

Although most inhaled anesthetics, including nitrous oxide, have been reported to produce seizure activity, such activity during administration of halothane or isoflurane is extremely rare. Desflurane produces a dose-dependent depression of electroencephalographic activity similar to that of isoflurane.[111] Enflurane predictably produces spike and wave activity on the EEG, particularly when hypocarbia exists. Children seem to be particularly susceptible to enflurane-induced seizure activity.[112] It would appear that halothane, isoflurane, or desflurane is preferable to enflurane for anesthesia for patients with seizure disorders.

The use of ketamine is controversial. Ketamine has been shown to produce seizure activity in patients with known seizure disorders. However, there are also data indicating that ketamine is safe to use in patients with seizure disorders. It would seem reasonable to avoid the use of ketamine for patients with seizure disorders because alternative drugs such as barbiturates, benzodiazepines, and propofol are available.

Seizure-like activity has been reported to occur after the administration of fentanyl and sufentanil; however other studies have found no seizure activity after the use of these agents.[113-116] The reported seizure-like activity may represent myoclonic activity or some form of opioid-induced skeletal muscle rigidity. With the usual clinical doses, seizure activity after fentanyl or sufentanil is not likely.[117] In relatively high doses, fentanyl and sufentanil may produce seizures.[118,119] High-dose fentanyl (200–400 $\mu g \cdot kg^{-1}$) or sufentanil (40–160 $\mu g \cdot kg^{-1}$) should be used with caution in patients with seizure disorders. Anticonvulsant therapy does increase the fentanyl requirement for anesthesia. This increased fentanyl requirement could reflect enhanced metabolism by hepatic enzyme induction.[120]

Methohexital has also been reported to produce seizures in children.[121] Certainly methohexital has been used for many patients with seizure disorders without adverse effects. Although methohexital may not be contraindicated in patients with seizures, thiopental would be a useful alternative.

Propofol has not been extensively studied in humans with seizure disorders, although evidence from animal studies indicates that propofol is neither an anticonvulsant nor a convulsant drug.[122]

Another potential drug interaction in patients receiving

phenytoin and carbamazepine is the patient's resistance to nondepolarizing muscle relaxants.[102,123] The mechanism for this resistance appears to be pharmacodynamic rather than pharmacokinetic.

The patient with a seizure disorder should receive his or her normal therapeutic drug regimen up to and including the morning of surgery. After surgery, this regimen should be reinstituted as quickly as possible. A decline in blood levels of anticonvulsant drugs will only increase the likelihood of perioperative seizures.

Parkinson's Disease (Paralysis Agitans)

Parkinson's disease is a degenerative disease of the central nervous system caused by a loss of dopaminergic fibers in the basal ganglia of the brain. Subsequently dopamine is depleted in the basal ganglia. It has been conclusively demonstrated that Parkinson's disease is clearly secondary to dopamine deficiency.[124] Dopamine depletion produces diminished inhibition of the extrapyramidal motor system and unopposed action of acetylcholine. Parkinson's disease is one of the more common disabling neurologic diseases and affects 2.5% of the population older than 65 years.

The typical clinical features of Parkinson's disease include increases in spontaneous movements, cogwheel rigidity of the extremities, facial immobility, and a rhythmic tremor at rest. These features are all secondary to diminished inhibition of the extrapyramidal motor system as a result of depletion of dopamine from the basal ganglia. Other features that occur commonly in patients with Parkinson's disease include seborrhea, pupillary abnormalities, diaphragmatic spasm, and oculogyric crises. Mental depression can be severe enough to necessitate the use of antidepressant medications.

Parkinson's disease can be caused by a variety of disorders, including metabolic derangements, chemical agents, intracranial tumors, and arteriosclerotic changes. Other than in sporadic episodes of postencephalitic Parkinson's disease, there is no evidence that the disease is caused by a virus.[125]

The treatment of Parkinson's disease is directed toward increasing dopamine levels in the brain but preventing adverse peripheral effects of dopamine. Consequently, treatment protocols involve combinations of drugs used to achieve these goals. This approach does increase the likelihood of undesirable drug interactions, however. Levodopa, the immediate precursor of dopamine, is clearly the drug of choice for treatment of Parkinson's disease. Unlike dopamine, levodopa can cross the blood-brain barrier and is converted to dopamine. Because the decarboxylating enzyme responsible for converting levodopa to dopamine is also present outside the brain, the dose of levodopa must be increased to compensate for systemic degradation. The addition of a peripheral decarboxylase inhibitor such as carbidopa or benserazide reduces the levodopa requirement. Currently, the combination of levodopa and carbidopa is the most effective drug available for the treatment of Parkinson's disease.[126] Patients receiving prolonged levodopa therapy may become less sensitive to levodopa and require increased doses. Side-effects of levodopa administration include depletion of myocardial norepinephrine stores, peripheral vasoconstriction, and decreased intravascular volume with resultant orthostatic hypotension. In order to avoid some of the side-effects of prolonged levodopa therapy, a number of alternative drugs have been developed. Bromocriptine, pergolide, and lisuride are dopaminergic

agents that can relieve the tremor and rigidity of Parkinson's disease. Most studies with alternative drugs, however, indicate that levodopa is still the preferred treatment drug.[127] Side-effects of bromocriptine administration include hallucinations, nausea, orthostatic hypotension, angina pectoris, Raynaud-like digital vascular spasm, and cardiac dysrhythmias. Domperidone, a dopamine receptor antagonist, also prevents the peripheral side-effects of dopamine agonists. Domperidone does not cross the blood-brain barrier or interfere with the effective treatment of Parkinson's disease. Because decreased dopamine activity in the basal ganglia enhances the excitatory effects of acetylcholine, anticholinergic drugs such as trihexyphenidyl, benztropine, and diphenhydramine are often administered to patients with Parkinson's disease. Amantadine is an antiviral agent that also increases the release of dopamine in the brain, but its effects are short-lived.

Of other anti-Parkinson drugs, selegiline (Deprenyl) has proved to be the most useful. Selegiline is a selective monoamine oxidase-B inhibitor that prevents degradation of dopamine in the brain. Consequently, the central action of dopamine is enhanced. The primary role of selegiline in the treatment of Parkinson's disease is for patients in the very early stages of the disease when it has been shown that selegiline delays the onset of disability.[128] Selegiline can also be used in combination with low-dose levodopa during the early clinical phases of Parkinson's disease. Selegiline is metabolized to amphetamine and methamphetamine and could produce sympathomimetic activity. Selegiline does not produce hypertensive crises when administered with levodopa.[129]

Management of Anesthesia

Management of anesthesia is generally determined by potential interaction between anesthesia drugs and anti-Parkinson medications. The patient's therapeutic regimen should be administered on the morning of surgery. The half-life of levodopa is short, and interruption of therapy for more than 6 to 12 hours can result in severe skeletal muscle rigidity that interferes with ventilation. Phenothiazines and butyrophenones (droperidol) should be avoided because these drugs antagonize the effects of dopamine in the basal ganglia. The use of ketamine is controversial. Ketamine could potentially produce an exaggerated sympathetic nervous system response with resultant tachycardia and hypertension. Despite this concern, ketamine has been used without difficulty in patients treated with levodopa. Alfentanil has been reported to produce acute dystonic reactions in untreated patients with Parkinson's disease.[130] Theoretically halothane could cause cardiac dysrhythmias in patients receiving levodopa, but this has not been documented. The choice of muscle relaxant does not seem to be influenced by the presence of Parkinson's disease. Although there is one case report of hyperkalemia after administration of succinylcholine, further investigation has demonstrated that this was an isolated occurrence.[131]

The potential hazards of drug interactions in patients taking monoamine oxidase (MAO) inhibitors has been well publicized in the medical literature. The interaction between MAO inhibitors and meperidine appears to be the most significant. The success with the use of selegiline, a MAO B type inhibitor, for the treatment of Parkinson's disease increases the likelihood of having to anesthetize a patient who is receiving MAO inhibitors. Although there is little reported experience with anesthesia for patients receiving selegiline, anecdotal reports have indicated that anesthesia is generally uneventful. However, there have been reports of agitation, muscle rigidity, and hyperthermia in patients receiving meperidine and selegiline.[132] B-type MAO enzyme acts on phenylethylamine, benzylamine, tyramine, and dopamine, with little effect on epinephrine and norepinephrine.[133] Conceivably, this would explain why there is less risk of massive sympathetic discharge in patients receiving selective MAO type B inhibitors.

Autonomic dysfunction is common in patients with Parkinson's disease. Gastrointestinal dysfunction is very common and is manifested as excessive salivation, dysphagia, and esophageal dysfunction. Consequently, the patient with Parkinson's disease should be considered at risk for aspiration pneumonitis. The most consistent cardiovascular abnormality is orthostatic hypotension. The disease process undoubtedly produces hypotension, and this is further compounded by the tendency of anti-Parkinson drugs, such as bromocriptine and lisuride, to produce peripheral vasodilation.[134] Patients with Parkinson's disease would be more likely to develop exaggerated decreases in blood pressure in response to inhaled halogenated anesthetics.

In the postoperative period, patients with Parkinson's disease are more susceptible to developing confusion and even hallucinations. These alterations in mental function may not appear until the day after surgery.[135] The precise mechanism of this postoperative confusion is not known but could have significant impact on outpatient surgery in Parkinson patients.

Huntington's Chorea

Huntington's chorea is a premature degenerative disease of the central nervous system characterized by marked atrophy of the basal ganglia, particularly the caudate nucleus. Neurochemical analysis of the brain reveals reductions in gamma-aminobutyric acid and acetylcholine.[136] This disease is transmitted as an autosomal dominant trait, but appearance of significant clinical manifestations is delayed until a patient is 35 to 40 years old. The recent discovery of DNA markers for Huntington's chorea has made predictive testing available. Ethical and legal concerns, however, have significantly impacted on genetic screening programs.[137]

Disordered movement is the clinical hallmark of Huntington's chorea. In addition to the choreoathetosis, progressive dementia occurs. The disease progresses for several years, and accompanying mental depression makes suicide a frequent occurrence. Death usually results from malnutrition and aspiration pneumonitis. The duration of Huntington's chorea averages 17 years from the onset of symptoms to death.

There is no specific therapy for Huntington's chorea. Pharmacotherapy is directed at relief of mental depression and movement disorders. A number of drugs that affect central nervous system neurotransmitter function have been evaluated but have shown little promise. The most useful therapy for control of involuntary movements is with drugs such as the phenothiazines and butyrophenones that interfere with the neurotransmitter effects of dopamine.

Management of Anesthesia

As the disease progresses and the pharnygeal muscles become more involved, the risk of aspiration pneumonitis increases. Consequently, appropriate antiaspiration maneuvers must be employed. If preoperative and postoperative sedation are necessary, the butyrophenones or phenothi-

azines are logical choices. Reported anesthetic experience with patients with Huntington's chorea is too limited to allow the proposal of specific anesthetic techniques. Although there are no specific contraindications to the use of intravenous or inhaled anesthetics, delayed awakening and generalized tonic spasms have been reported after the administration of thiopental to one patient.[138] In contrast, after the administration of propofol a normal response with rapid recovery has been reported in a patient with Huntington's chorea.[139] Decreased plasma cholinesterase activity with a prolonged response to succinylcholine has also been reported.[140] It has also been suggested that these patients may be sensitive to the effects of nondepolarizing muscle relaxants.[141]

Alzheimer's Disease

Alzheimer's disease is the major cause of dementia in the United States. More than 2 million persons in the United States are afflicted with Alzheimer's disease, and it is the major reason that patients are admitted to nursing homes. As life expectancy for men and women increases, a larger proportion of the population will be susceptible to this disease. Although dementia can be caused by more than 60 disorders, Alzheimer's disease is responsible for 50–60% of the cases. Dementia is characterized by intellectual and cognitive deterioration that impairs social function. The clinical diagnosis of Alzheimer's disease can be made if a patient exhibits loss of memory and deficits in two or more areas of cognition. A mental status examination is central to the diagnosis of Alzheimer's disease. Any systemic cause of dementia, such as cerebral vascular disease, must be eliminated before the diagnosis of Alzheimer's disease is made. A cerebral computed tomographic scan and an EEG are helpful in diagnosis. Pathologic findings in the brain include a characteristic cortical atrophy and the presence of neurofibrillary tangles and neuritic plaques. Functionally there is a decrease in choline acetyltransferase and a subsequent cholinergic deficit. Interestingly, some studies have demonstrated an improvement in memory after the administration of physostigmine.[142] Unfortunately this effect is short-lived. Aluminum and aluminum silicate are found in the neurofibrillary tangles, but the significance of this finding is not clear. Many etiologies have been proposed for Alzheimer's disease. Viruses, neurotoxic metals and trace elements, biologic neurotoxins, and immune dysfunction have all been proposed as causative factors. Recently genetic factors have been demonstrated to be more important than previously thought. A genetic predisposition may render an individual more susceptible to environmental agents that produce Alzheimer's disease.[143,144]

Since the pathogenesis of Alzheimer's disease is not known, there can be no specific therapy. Proposed therapeutic regimens have included cholinesterase inhibitors, clonidine, cerebrovascular vasodilators, vitamins, and antidepressants.[145]

Management of Anesthesia

No specific complications have been reported with anesthesia for patients with Alzheimer's disease. However, a few speculations and suggestions seem warranted. Because of dementia, these patients may be disoriented and uncooperative. Sedative drugs, such as those used for preoperative medication, should be administered rarely because further mental confusion could result. There are no specific contraindications to the use of intravenous anesthesia, although an inhaled anesthetic would permit a more predictable return to the patient's preoperative level of mental function. It could be speculated that propofol would offer rapid recovery, but there has been no reported experience with propofol in patients with Alzheimer's disease. If an anticholinergic drug is required, glycopyrrolate, which does not cross the blood-brain barrier, would be preferable to scopolamine or atropine. Theoretically an anticholinergic drug that enters the brain could exacerbate the dementia. Finally, the patient's preoperative drug list should be reviewed for the possibility of interaction with anesthetics.

Amyotrophic Lateral Sclerosis

Amyotrophic lateral sclerosis (ALS) is a degenerative disease of motor cells throughout the central nervous system. Progression of the disease is relentless, and death generally follows within 3 years of diagnosis. Upper and lower motor neurons are involved almost exclusively. The cause of ALS is unknown, but proposed causes include a slow viral infection, toxins, immune dysfunction, impaired DNA repair, altered axonal transport, and trauma.[146] Although it has been speculated that previous infection with the polio virus might predispose a patient to the development of ALS in later life, data indicate that the incidence of ALS in postpoliomyelitis patients is actually decreased.[147]

The signs and symptoms reflect the upper and lower motor neuron dysfunction. Frequently reported initial manifestations are atrophy, weakness, and fasciculation of skeletal muscles, often beginning in the intrinsic muscles of the hand. Computed tomographic scanning of muscles demonstrates a symmetric atrophy of muscle and replacement of muscle tissue with fat.[148] As the disease progresses, the atrophy and weakness involve most skeletal muscles, including those of the tongue, pharynx, larynx, and chest. Pulmonary function studies demonstrate a decrease in vital capacity, forced expiration volume in 1 second, and maximal voluntary ventilation as the disease progresses.[149] Early symptoms of bulbar involvement include tongue fasciculations and dysphagia with pulmonary aspiration. The extraocular muscles usually are not involved. Although respiratory complications generally occur late in the course of the disease, some patients present initially with respiratory dysfunction.[150] Respiratory failure eventually results, and mechanical ventilation of the lungs is necessary. Prolonged ventilatory support presents legal and ethical dilemmas that may be compounded by the fact that these patients remain mentally competent and are clearly aware of the ultimate outcome.[151] Patients with ALS also have evidence of autonomic dysfunction manifested as an increased resting heart rate, orthostatic hypotension, and elevated resting levels of norepinephrine and epinephrine. There is usually decreased R-R interval variation on the ECG and a decreased heart rate response to the administration of atropine.[152]

Many therapeutic agents have been tried for patients with ALS, but with little success. Preliminary studies with the administration of thyrotropin-releasing hormone have produced transient improvement in some patients with ALS.[153]

Management of Anesthesia

Patients with lower motor neuron diseases such as ALS are vulnerable to hyperkalemia after the administration of succinylcholine. Patients with ALS may also have a prolonged response to nondepolarizing muscle relaxants. Bulbar involvement with dysfunction of pharyngeal muscles predisposes these patients to pulmonary aspiration. The need for postoperative ventilatory support is highly likely for the patient with ALS. There is no evidence that a specific anesthetic drug or combination of drugs is best for patients with ALS. Subclinical autonomic dysfunction undoubtedly produces exaggerated decreases in blood pressure in response to inhaled halogenated anesthetics.

Creutzfeldt-Jakob Disease

Creutzfeldt-Jakob disease is one of three disorders that constitute the class of diseases known as the human spongiform encephalopathies. The other two diseases in this group are kuru and Gerstmann-Staussler syndrome. Pathologically these disorders are also characterized by vacuolation of brain tissue and neuronal loss. They are most likely caused by an infectious agent, probably an atypical virus. Creutzfeldt-Jakob disease is a somewhat unique infectious disease in that the incubation time is long (years), and there is an absence of fever and inflammation. Creutzfeldt-Jakob disease is much less common than multiple sclerosis, but like multiple sclerosis, it is noted for its diverse presentations and varied neurologic signs.[154]

The typical clinical characteristics include subacute dementia, myoclonus, and electroencephalographic changes. The EEG pattern is relatively characteristic, with diffuse slow activity and periodic complexes. Because of the dementia and wide array of presenting symptoms, patients with Creutzfeldt-Jakob disease are often misdiagnosed as having psychiatric disorders. There is no specific therapeutic drug for the disease. Several antiviral drugs such as amantadine, idoxuridine, interferon, and vidarabine have been employed but with little success.

Management of Anesthesia

Creutzfeldt-Jakob disease is considered transmissible. There are reports of cases developing after accidental inoculation and surgery.[155-158] The transmission of Creutzfeldt-Jakob disease has been linked to contaminated dural graft material and pooled human growth hormone.[159,160] Consequently, appropriate precautions should be taken to protect other patients and medical staff. Three to ten percent formalin and 70% alcohol do not inactivate the Creutzfeldt-Jakob virus. Sodium hypochlorite 0.05% and sterilization with steam and ethylene oxide will destroy the virus.[161]

Although reported anesthetic experience with patients with Creutzfeldt-Jakob disease is limited, certain speculations and recommendations seem warranted. Patients with degenerative neurologic diseases are prone to aspirate gastric contents because they have impaired swallowing function and decreased activity of laryngeal reflexes. Therefore, appropriate antiaspiration maneuvers are indicated during anesthesia. Because lower motor neuron dysfunction also occurs in these patients, the use of succinylcholine should be avoided. The autonomic and peripheral nervous systems may also be involved.[162,163] This may produce abnormal cardiovascular responses to anesthesia and vasoactive drugs.

ANEMIAS

The causes of anemia are numerous (Table 22-6). Anemias can be conveniently classified as nutritional deficiency anemias, hemolytic anemias, hemoglobinopathies, and hemoglobin deficiency syndromes (thalassemias).

TABLE 22-6. Types of Anemias

Nutritional

Iron deficiency
Vitamin B_{12} deficiency
Folic acid deficiency

Hemoglobinopathies

Hemoglobin S

Hemolytic

Spherocytosis
Pyruvate kinase deficiency
Glucose-6-phosphate dehydrogenase deficiency
Immune-mediated
Drug-induced ABO incompatibility

Thalassemias

Thalassemia major (Cooley's anemia)
Thalassemia intermedia
Thalassemia minor

Irrespective of the cause of the anemia, compensatory physiologic mechanisms develop to offset the decreased oxygen-carrying capacity of the blood. Typically, in an otherwise healthy person symptoms do not develop from anemia until the hemoglobin level decreases below 7 g·dl^{-1}. Symptoms are highly variable and depend on other concurrent disease processes. Physiologic compensation includes increased plasma volume, increased cardiac output, and increased levels of red blood cell 2,3-diphosphoglycerate (2,3-DPG) (Table 22-7). Maximum levels of 2,3-DPG increase oxygen delivery by 30%.[164] Because elderly patients with chronic anemia have an increased plasma volume, transfusion of whole blood to these patients may result in congestive heart failure. Similarly, the myocardial depressant effects of anesthetics may be exaggerated in patients with increased cardiac output at rest as compensation for anemia.

The concern about transmission of the human immunodeficiency virus has clearly influenced the perioperative use of blood products and has radically altered recommendations for preoperative blood transfusion not only in normal patients but also in patients with chronic anemia. Traditional hematocrit levels that would have previously triggered the need for preoperative blood transfusion have been challenged.[165] Currently there is no universally accepted hematocrit level that demands that transfusion be carried out. The patient's physiologic status and coexisting diseases must be factored into a highly subjective decision.

TABLE 22-7. Compensatory Mechanisms to Increase Oxygen Delivery with Chronic Anemia

Increased cardiac output
Increased red blood cell 2,3-diphosphoglycerate levels
Increased P_{50}
Increased plasma volume
Decreased blood viscosity

Nutritional Deficiency Anemias

The three primary causes of nutritional deficiency anemias are iron deficiency, vitamin B_{12} deficiency, and folic acid deficiency.

Iron deficiency anemia produces the typical microcytic, hypochromic red blood cell. Iron deficiency anemia may be an absolute deficiency secondary to decreased oral intake or a relative deficiency caused by a rapid turnover of red blood cells (e.g., hemolysis). Measuring the hemoglobin and serum ferritin levels is a rapid and effective mechanism for differentiating true iron deficiency anemia from other causes.[166] Severe iron deficiency anemia can result in thrombocytopenia and neurologic abnormalities.[167,168]

Absorption of vitamin B_{12} by the gastrointestinal tract depends on production of intrinsic factor. Intrinsic factor is a glycoprotein produced by gastric parietal cells. Atrophy of the gastric mucosa causes a vitamin B_{12} deficiency and megaloblastic anemia. Vitamin B_{12} deficiency also may produce significant nervous system dysfunction. In adults this is usually manifest by a peripheral neuropathy secondary to degeneration of the lateral and posterior columns of the spinal cord. The neuropathy is evidenced by symmetric paresthesias with loss of proprioception and vibratory sensation, especially in the lower extremities. Parenteral vitamin B_{12} will reverse both the hematologic and neurologic changes. The neurologic abnormalities must be considered when regional anesthesia or peripheral nerve blocks might be used. Nitrous oxide inactivates the vitamin B_{12} component of methionine synthetase. Assessment of the impact on red blood cell production from exposure to clinical doses of nitrous oxide is controversial. Certainly, prolonged exposure to nitrous oxide results in megaloblastic anemia and neurologic changes similar to those seen in pernicious anemia.[169] It has also been reported that relatively short exposures to nitrous oxide may produce megaloblastic changes.[170-172] Congenital vitamin B_{12} deficiency produces severe neurologic impairment that can be only partially reversed with therapy.

Folic acid deficiency also produces megaloblastic anemia. Although peripheral neuropathy may occur, it is not as common as with vitamin B_{12} deficiency. Causes of folic acid deficiency include alcoholism, pregnancy, and malabsorption syndromes. Methotrexate, phenytoin, and ethanol are among the drugs known to interfere with folic acid absorption.

Hemolytic Anemias

Causes of hemolytic anemia include structural erythrocyte abnormalities, enzyme deficiencies, and immune hemolytic anemias.

Hereditary Spherocytosis

Hereditary spherocytosis is a disorder of red blood cell morphologic characteristics in which the red blood cell is rounded, more fragile, and more susceptible to hemolysis than the normal biconcave red blood cell. As a result of the increased fragility, the spleen destroys the abnormal red blood cells and a chronic anemia ensues. Although the exact cause of the osmotic fragility is not known, the red blood cell membrane does permit a greater influx of sodium into the cell.[173] Cholelithiasis from chronic hemolysis and elevation of the serum bilirubin concentration occur frequently in patients with hereditary spherocytosis. Patients with hereditary spherocytosis may have hemolytic crises develop accompanied by marked anemia, vomiting, and abdominal pain. These crises may be triggered by infection or folic acid deficiency.[174]

This disorder is treated by splenectomy, which is generally delayed until the patient is 6 years of age or older. Splenectomy before that age is associated with a high incidence of bacterial infections, especially those secondary to pneumococci. Before splenectomy, most patients require a folic acid supplement because there is excessive utilization of folic acid for red blood cell production. Transfusion is rarely necessary for patients with hereditary spherocytosis.

There are no special considerations during anesthesia for patients with hereditary spherocytosis. Preoperative transfusion is generally not necessary because adequate compensatory mechanisms for chronic anemia have developed in these patients.

Glucose-6-Phosphate Dehydrogenase Deficiency

Glucose-6-phosphate dehydrogenase (G-6-PD) deficiency is the most common of the inherited erythrocyte enzyme deficiencies. G-6-PD is one enzyme essential to the hexose monophosphate shunt. One percent of the black male population in the United States is afflicted by this disorder. Asian and Mediterranean populations are also susceptible to G-6-PD deficiency. Glucose-6-phosphate dehydrogenase initiates the hexose monophosphate shunt. This shunt produces nicotinamide-adenine dinucleotide phosphate, the major reducing compound of the red blood cell. Without nicotinamide-adenine dinucleotide phosphate the red blood cell is susceptible to damage by oxidation. A deficiency of G-6-PD results in decreased levels of reduced glutathione when the red blood cell is exposed to oxidant chemicals. This increases the rigidity of the red blood cell membrane and accentuates clearance of these stiff cells from the circulation. In severe forms of G-6-PD deficiency, oxidation produces denaturation of globin chains and causes intravascular hemolysis.[175] There are a number of drugs that accentuate the oxidative destruction of erythrocytes (Table 22-8), including analgesics, antibiotics, sulfonamides, and antimalarials. There is considerable variability in the hemolytic response to drugs; many drugs (e.g., aspirin) induce hemolysis only in very high doses.[176] These persons are unable to reduce methemoglobin produced by sodium nitrate, and therefore sodium nitroprusside and prilocaine should not be administered. Characteristically, the crisis begins 2 to 5 days following drug administration. Bacterial infections can also trigger hemolytic episodes. Presumably, oxidant compounds produced by active white blood cells may hemolyze susceptible red blood cells.

Anesthetic drugs have not been implicated as hemolytic agents; however, early postoperative evidence of hemolysis might indicate a G-6-PD deficiency syndrome.

TABLE 22-8. Drugs That Produce Hemolysis in Patients with Glucose-6-Phosphate Dehydrogenase Deficiency

Phenacetin	Nalidixic acid
Aspirin (high doses)	Isoniazid
Penicillin	Primaquine
Streptomycin	Quinine
Chloramphenicol	Quinidine
Sulfacetamide	Doxorubicin
Sulfanilamide	Methylene blue
Sulfapyridine	

Glutathione synthetase is another enzyme of the hexose monophosphate shunt, and deficiency of this enzyme may also produce anemia.

Pyruvate Kinase Deficiency

Pyruvate kinase is a glycolytic enzyme of the Embden-Meyerhof pathway. Clinically, these patients exhibit anemia, premature cholelithiasis, and splenomegaly. The degree of anemia varies from a very mild anemia that does not require transfusion to a severe transfusion-dependent anemia. The clinical features resemble those of patients with spherocytosis. There are no special considerations for anesthesia other than those for any patient with chronic anemia.

Other enzymes of the Embden-Meyerhof pathway include hexokinase, glucose phosphate isomerase, aldolase, triose phosphate isomerase, and phosphoglycerate kinase.[177]

Immune Hemolytic Anemias

The immune hemolytic anemias are characterized by immunologic alteration of the red blood cell membrane and are caused by drugs, disease, or erythrocyte sensitization.

By attaching to the erythrocyte membrane, drugs may form an immunologic complex that produces an antibody response. Levodopa, alpha-methyldopa, and penicillin can produce an immune hemolytic anemia. Collagen vascular diseases, neoplasms, and infections have been known to trigger an autoimmune hemolytic anemia. The classic example of erythrocyte sensitization is hemolytic disease of the newborn produced by Rh sensitization. An Rh-negative mother with Rh antibodies may produce hemolysis in an Rh-positive fetus. Differences in fetal and maternal ABO groups may also cause hemolysis. This is unusual because A and B antibodies are of the IgM class and do not readily cross the placenta.

Cold autoimmune hemolytic anemia is of special concern to the anesthesiologist because of the likelihood that the cold operating room environment and the hypothermia that are used during cardiopulmonary bypass may initiate a hemolytic crisis. Cold hemagglutinin disease is caused by IgM autoantibodies that react with the I antigen of red blood cells.[178] A hemolytic crisis can be triggered by exposure to cold. Maintaining a warm environment is essential for prevention of hemolysis.[179] Plasmapheresis to reduce the titer of the cold antibody is recommended prior to hypothermic procedures such as cardiopulmonary bypass.

Hemoglobinopathies

There are more than 300 different hemoglobinopathies described in the literature. Fortunately, most are quite rare and may never be encountered by an anesthesiologist during his or her career. Of the hemoglobinopathies, the most common in the United States are the sickle cell diseases. Eight to ten percent of black persons in the United States have the sickle cell trait, and 1 in 400 has sickle cell anemia.

Sickle Cell Disease

Hemoglobin S is a variant hemoglobin produced by substitution of valine for glutamic acid in the sixth position of the beta chain. When the hemoglobin deoxygenates, a gel structure is formed that produces structural changes in the red blood cell. The kinetics of gel formation by hemoglobin

TABLE 22-9. Hemoglobin S Variants

	Hemoglobin SS	Hemoglobin SC	Hemoglobin SA
Hemoglobin level (g·dl^{-1})	7–8	9–12	13–15
Life expectancy (years)	30	Slightly reduced	Normal
Propensity for sickling	+ + + +	+ +	+
Clinical features	Vaso-occlusive crises Pneumonia Papillary necrosis Splenic infarction Hepatomegaly Skin ulceration	Vaso-occlusive crises Retinal thrombosis Femoral head necrosis	Few under physio-logic conditions

S is complex, and factors such as rapidity of deoxygenation may determine how the hemoglobin gel polymerizes and deforms the red blood cell. Low oxygen tension and acidosis exaggerate sickle cell formation. Consequently, any condition that causes a decrease in oxygen tension (such as arterial hypoxemia) or decreased blood flow may produce sickling of red blood cells. Sickling begins at an oxygen tension less than 50 mm Hg and becomes most pronounced when the arterial oxygen tension decreases to 20 mm Hg. Local factors can also influence sickling. Systemic oxygenation may be adequate, but vascular occlusion may produce stasis with localized hypoxemia and initiate sickling. Similarly, if sickling occurs, increasing systemic oxygenation may not reverse the sickling if arteries supplying the area are occluded. It is better to prevent sickling than to treat it. The likelihood of sickling is directly related to the amount of hemoglobin S present in the blood.

The definitive diagnosis of sickle disease is made with hemoglobin electrophoresis. This test not only detects hemoglobin S but also reveals any other type of hemoglobin present. Although there are several variants of sickle cell disease, the most common are SS (sickle cell anemia), SA (sickle cell trait), SC, and S-thalassemia. In sickle cell anemia, 70–98% of the hemoglobin is S and the remainder is hemoglobin F (fetal). In patients with SA, 10–40% of the hemoglobin is hemoglobin S. Cells with hemoglobin S and C are less likely to sickle than those with SS but more likely to sickle than SA cells. The clinical severity of the disorder is also related to the amount of hemoglobin S (Table 22-9).

Clinical Manifestations. The patient with SA generally has a normal life expectancy and few complications with the hemoglobinopathy. Hemoglobin levels are usually normal. Sickling occurs only under extreme physiologic alterations; however, anesthesia and surgery may produce such alterations. Although the risk of anesthesia for patients with SA is considered small, there have been some reports of death from general anesthesia. Of the 514 patients with SA who received general anesthesia reported in the literature, there have been five deaths.[180,181] Not all of the deaths could be attributed totally to the sickle cell trait, however.

Patients with SS are the most severely affected of those with the sickle hemoglobinopathies. Clinical manifestations include chronic anemia and chronic hemolysis. Infarction of multiple organs is produced by occlusion of vessels with deformed erythrocytes. Generalized pulmonary fibrosis produces significant pulmonary dysfunction with an increased alveolar-to-arterial oxygen difference. Ultimately, cor pul-

monale is a significant cause of mortality in patients with SS.[182] Cardiac dysfunction characterized by decreased ventricular filling and reduced ejection fraction in conjunction with pulmonary dysfunction produces a reduced exercise tolerance.[183] Because of slow blood flow and decreased local oxygen tension, the renal medulla is particularly vulnerable to infarction and necrosis. Papillary necrosis secondary to medullary ischemia occurs frequently. There is often an inability to concentrate urine. Glomerular filtration declines with age, and nephrotic syndrome is relatively common.[184] Renal transplantation may ultimately be required.[185] By the time the patient is about 6 years of age, the spleen is virtually nonexistent because of repeated infarctions. The absence of splenic function increases the patient's vulnerability to bacterial infection. Chronic hemolysis of erythrocytes produces an elevated serum bilirubin level and results in a high incidence of cholelithiasis in patients with SS. Repeated cerebral infarction from large cerebral vessel occlusion and hemorrhage can produce neurologic dysfunction.[186] Priapism also occurs with increased frequency in patients with sickle cell disease. Most patients with SS die by 30 years of age.

The clinical manifestations of SC disease represent an intermediate severity between SA and SS hemoglobinopathies. Anemia is generally mild, with hemoglobin concentrations of 10–11 g·dl. Sickle cell crises are less common in patients with SC disease than in those with SS. Pulmonary dysfunction secondary to upper respiratory tract infections, pneumonia, and pulmonary embolization is relatively common in patients with SC disease. There are at least 40 other variants of the S hemoglobinopathy, some of which are quite rare. Hemoglobin SA, SS, and SC are the three most frequently encountered variants.

Treatment. Although the exact molecular nature of S hemoglobin has been known for over 40 years, no definitive treatment is available. The best treatment is prevention of sickling. Maintenance of good systemic oxygenation and hydration to maintain good tissue perfusion is essential. In some instances transfusion with normal adult hemoglobin (AA) to dilute the hemoglobin S erythrocytes and decrease blood viscosity is indicated. A variety of techniques aimed at reversing the sickling process, such as alkalinization, carbamylation, and acetylation, have been attempted but with little success. Because reversal of the sickling process is difficult, prevention becomes essential. Recently, long-term therapy with hydroxyurea has been demonstrated to increase levels of fetal hemoglobin in patients with sickle cell disease.[187] Fetal hemoglobin is composed of gamma globin chains rather than beta chains. The gamma globin chains are not affected by the genetic alteration that affects the beta chains of sickle cell disease. Increased levels of fetal hemoglobin inhibit polymerization of S hemoglobin and decrease the likelihood of sickling events.

Management of Anesthesia. Because arterial hypoxemia and vascular stasis are powerful stimuli for sickling, it is imperative that the risk of these be minimized during anesthesia and the postoperative period. Preoperative sedation should not depress ventilation. During surgery and the postoperative period, the inspired oxygen concentration should be increased to maintain or increase the arterial oxygen tension. Monitoring arterial hemoglobin saturation with a pulse oximeter is a useful noninvasive monitor for patients with sickle cell disorders. Although regional anesthesia is often used for these patients, administration of supplemental oxygen may still be indicated. Regional anesthesia may produce compensatory vasoconstriction and decreased oxygen delivery to nonblocked areas, making red blood cells in those areas vulnerable to sickling. Circulatory stasis can be prevented with adequate hydration and anticipation of intraoperative volume loss to avoid acute hypovolemia. The use of extremity tourniquets is controversial. There are no definitive studies documenting the safety or danger of tourniquet use. Some authors recommend that a tourniquet not be used for patients with hemoglobin S because of the potential dangers.[180] Other authors suggest that a tourniquet can be used if the tourniquet is critical to the success of the operation.[188] The environmental temperature should be controlled to maintain normothermia. Fever increases the rate of gel formation by S hemoglobin. Although hypothermia retards gel formation, the decreased temperature also produces peripheral vasoconstriction. Consequently, normothermia is desirable.

Although inhaled halogenated anesthetics accelerate precipitation of hemoglobin S *in vitro*, the clinical significance of this finding is not known. Maintenance of perfusion and oxygenation is more critical than the type of anesthesia. Because of low peripheral blood flow, hypothermia, and acidosis, cardiopulmonary bypass is especially dangerous for patients with sickle cell disease.[189] Intraoperative autotransfusion for patients with SS is controversial. There is evidence that autotransfusion can be used successfully if an exchange transfusion to dilute the number of hemoglobin S red blood cells is performed prior to anesthesia.[190]

The anesthesiologist should continue careful observation of the patient and monitoring of oxygenation into the postoperative period. Postoperative pain, analgesics, and transient pulmonary dysfunction may decrease arterial oxygen tension. Consequently, supplemental oxygen should be administered after surgery.

Although patients with SA are at less risk than patients with hemoglobin SS, the same precautions applied to patients with SS should be used for those with SA. The patient with SC hemoglobin is also at risk during anesthesia and should be treated accordingly.[191]

Thalassemia

Thalassemia represents a number of inherited disorders that result in production of abnormal globin chains of hemoglobin. There are alpha- and beta-thalassemias, depending on which globin chain is affected. Beta-thalassemia major, or Cooley's anemia, is the most severe of the thalassemias. Untreated Cooley's anemia usually results in death. Transfu-

sion therapy is essential but often produces iron toxicity. Iron toxicity can markedly reduce ventricular function, but chelation therapy with deferoxamine can reverse the myocardial dysfunction.[192] Splenectomy reduces transfusion requirements in some cases. Beta-thalassemia minor produces a mild hemolytic anemia and iron deficiency. Beta-thalassemia intermedia is an intermediate form of thalassemia but generally does not necessitate transfusion. Alpha-thalassemia produces a mild hemolytic anemia in most patients. Transfusion and splenectomy may be necessary in some patients with alpha-thalassemia.

Anesthetic considerations depend on the severity of the anemia. If the patient is transfusion-dependent, careful preoperative evaluation of hepatic and cardiac functions is warranted because of iron toxicity. When an anesthetic is selected, the likelihood of cardiomyopathy and hepatic dysfunction must be considered in addition to the effects of chronic anemia. Extramedullary hematopoiesis can produce hyperplasia of the facial bones and make direct laryngoscopic examination difficult.[193] Extramedullary hematopoiesis is also known to produce spinal cord compression and massive hemothorax in patients with thalassemia.[194,195]

COLLAGEN VASCULAR DISEASES

A number of diseases are classified as the collagen vascular or connective tissue diseases (Table 22-10). The four most common disorders of this group are rheumatoid arthritis, systemic lupus erythematosus, scleroderma, and polymyositis. Although many such patients can be categorized into discrete disease syndromes, many others with collagen vascular diseases are considered to have overlap syndromes with features of different disorders and cannot be conveniently classified. The origin of the collagen vascular diseases is unknown, but current theories implicate the immune system and its effects on the vascular bed. Although all these diseases have localized features involving the joints, each one also has diffuse systemic effects. Both the localized and systemic alterations in these patients are significant in the management of anesthesia.

Rheumatoid Arthritis

Rheumatoid arthritis is a chronic inflammatory disease characterized by a symmetric polyarthropathy and significant systemic involvement. Although genetics, immune responses, and inflammation are involved in the pathogenesis

---

TABLE 22-10. Collagen Vascular Diseases

Rheumatoid arthritis
Lupus
   Systemic lupus erythematosus
   Drug-induced lupus
   Discoid lupus
Scleroderma
   Progressive systemic sclerosis
   CREST syndrome (calcinosis cutis, Raynaud's phenomenon, esophageal dysfunction, sclerodactyly, telangiectasia)
   Focal scleroderma
Polymyositis
   Dermatomyositis
Overlap syndromes

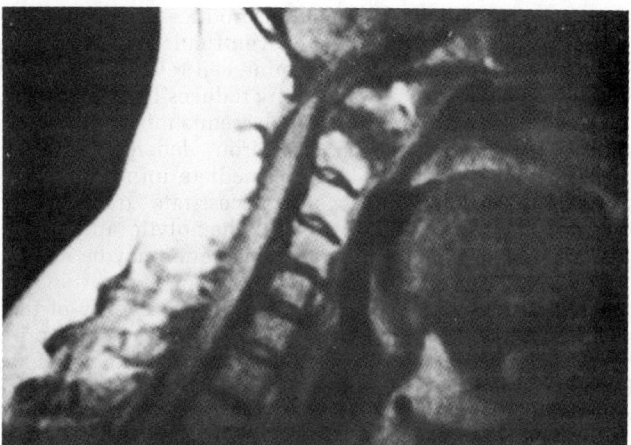

Figure 22-2. Magnetic resonance imaging scan of the cervical spine of a patient with rheumatoid arthritis. Note the significant degree of upper cervical cord compression. (Reprinted with permission from Johnston RA, Kelly IG: Surgery of the rheumatoid cervical spine. Ann Rheum Dis 49:847, 1990.)

TABLE 22-11. Extra-articular Manifestations of Rheumatoid Arthritis

Skin	***Peripheral Nervous System***
Raynaud's phenomenon	
Digital necrosis	Compression syndromes
	Mononeuritis
Eyes	
Scleritis	***Central Nervous System***
Corneal ulceration	Dural nodules
	Necrotizing vasculitis
Lung	
Pleural effusion	***Liver***
Pulmonary fibrosis	Hepatitis
Heart	***Blood***
Pericarditis	Anemia
Tamponade	
Coronary arteritis	
Aortic insufficiency	
Kidney	
Interstitial fibrosis	
Glomerulonephritis	
Amyloid deposition	

of rheumatoid arthritis, the cause is unknown. There are also infectious agents that produce rheumatoid arthritis-like diseases in animal models.[196] Irrespective of the etiologic agent, the synovial membrane undergoes change, beginning with cellular hyperplasia. The synovium is then invaded by lymphocytes, plasma cells, and fibroblasts. Ultimately, joint cartilage and bone are destroyed.

The hands and wrists are involved first, particularly the metacarpophalangeal and proximal interphalangeal joints. In the lower extremity the knee is involved most frequently. Compression of lower extremity peripheral nerves by the deformed knee can produce paresis and sensory loss over the lower leg. Cervical spine involvement is frequent and can produce odontoid erosion, atlantoaxial subluxation, apophyseal joint sclerosis, and diskovertebral joint narrowing.[197] Cervical spine changes can cause bony and ligamentous impingement on the spinal cord and produce a cervical myelopathy. The use of magnetic resonance imaging has demonstrated how frequently the cervical spine is affected by rheumatoid arthritis and how close even neurologically asymptomatic patients are to spinal cord compression[198] (Fig. 22-2). Synovitis of the temporomandibular joint may decrease jaw mobility. Cricoarytenoid arthritis is common and is evidenced by hoarseness, dysphagia, and stridor.

Extra-articular and systemic manifestations of rheumatoid arthritis are diverse (Table 22-11).[199] Pericardial thickening and/or effusion may lead to cardiac tamponade. Ventricular dysfunction may occur because of myocarditis and coronary arteritis. Formation of rheumatoid nodules in the cardiac conduction system can produce dysrhythmias. Aortitis with dilation of the aortic root can result in aortic insufficiency. Pleural effusions from pleural irritation frequently occur. Rheumatoid nodule deposition in the lung parenchyma in conjunction with costochondral arthritis produces restrictive pulmonary disease. Neurologic complications include peripheral nerve compression (carpal tunnel syndrome) and cervical nerve root compression. Mononeuritis multiplex is presumed to be caused by deposition of immune complexes in blood vessels supplying the affected nerves. Cerebral necrotizing vasculitis can also occur. Mild anemia is almost always present. The clinical complex of

rheumatoid arthritis, leukopenia (less than 2000/mm), and hepatosplenomegaly is termed Felty's syndrome.

Pharmacologic treatment of rheumatoid arthritis is directed at relief of pain and remission of the disease process. Nonsteroidal anti-inflammatory drugs include aspirin, phenylbutazone, indomethacin, ibuprofen, sulindac, and tolmetin. Aspirin is the standard against which all other drugs are compared. Unfortunately, significant side-effects occur with the chronic use of any of these drugs. Corticosteroids definitely reduce rheumatoid inflammation, but their deleterious side-effects are well known.

Although the parenteral administration of gold salts has been advocated for decades, gold is probably ineffective.[200] Other drugs recommended for remission include antimalarial drugs, penicillamine, and azathioprine. Many of these drugs cause anemia, thrombocytopenia, and hepatitis. Surgical procedures such as synovectomy, tenolysis, and joint replacement are performed to relieve pain and restore joint function.

Management of Anesthesia

Arthritic involvement of the temporomandibular joints, cricoarytenoid joints, and cervical spine can make tracheal intubation extremely difficult.[201] The mobility of these joints must be evaluated before operation so that the anesthesiologist can select an intubation technique. Fiberoptic laryngoscopic examination may be necessary. Since atlantoaxial instability is relatively common when the rheumatoid process involves the cervical spine, flexion of the neck could compress the spinal cord.[202] Neck pain with radiation to the occiput may be the first sign of cervical spine involvement.[203] Preoperative cervical radiographs or magnetic resonance imaging of the cervical spine may be necessary if the degree of cervical spine involvement is not known. Cricoarytenoid arthritis may be recognized by erythema and edema of the vocal cords. Involvement of the cricoarytenoid joints reduces the size of the glottic inlet and necessitates the use

TABLE 22-12. Adverse Effects of Drugs Used to Treat Collagen Vascular Diseases

Drug	Effects
Corticosteroids	Hypertension
	Osteoporosis
	Fluid retention
	Infection
Aspirin	Platelet dysfunction
	Peptic ulcer
	Hepatic dysfunction
	Hypersensitivity
Indomethacin	Peptic ulcer
	Hypertension
	Hyperglycemia
	Leukopenia
Gold	Aplastic anemia
	Dermatitis
	Nephritis
Antimalarials	Myopathy
	Retinopathy
Penicillamine	Glomerulonephritis
	Aplastic anemia
	Myasthenia
Azathioprine	Leukopenia
	Biliary stasis
Cyclophosphamide	Leukopenia
	Hemorrhagic cystitis

of a smaller than predicted tracheal tube. Exaggerated post-extubation edema and stridor may also occur.

The degree of cardiopulmonary involvement by the rheumatoid process influences the selection of the type of anesthesia. Functional evaluation of the lungs and heart is necessary if the clinical history suggests dysfunction. The need for postoperative ventilatory support should be anticipated if severe restrictive lung disease is present.

Medications the patient is receiving will influence the management of anesthesia (Table 22-12). Corticosteroid supplementation may be necessary during the operation, depending on the magnitude of the surgery. Aspirin will interfere with platelet function, and clotting may be abnormal. Many antirheumatoid drugs suppress red blood cell function, and anemia is common. The anti-inflammatory drugs also may alter hepatic function, which can influence the choice of anesthesia.

Restriction of joint mobility necessitates careful positioning during operation. The extremities should be positioned so as to minimize the risk of neurovascular compression and additional joint injury. Preoperative evaluation of joint motion helps determine how the extremities should be positioned.

There are many systemic effects of rheumatoid arthritis. The degree and type of systemic involvement must be considered when an anesthetic is selected for the patient with rheumatoid arthritis.[204]

Systemic Lupus Erythematosus

Systemic lupus erythematosus (SLE) is an autoimmune disease characterized by the production of antinuclear antibodies.[205] Anti-DNA antibodies are characteristic of SLE and

parallel the degree of organ involvement. It is unclear what the immunogen is; it could be a foreign DNA (e.g., bacterial DNA) or autologous DNA. There are also a number of drugs, including hydralazine, procainamide, alpha-methyldopa, phenytoin, carbamazepine, and isoniazid, that can produce characteristics of SLE in susceptible patients.

Although the clinical features of SLE are diverse, there are several areas of involvement common to most patients. Arthritis occurs in most patients and affects both large and small joints. Cutaneous manifestations include the characteristic erythematous butterfly rash over the nose and malar area, alopecia, and Raynaud's phenomenon. Glomerulonephritis from SLE is a significant cause of complications and death. Proteinuria, hypertension, and renal insufficiency frequently occur. During active phases of the disease, anemia, leukopenia, and thrombocytopenia are common.[206] Of special interest to the anesthesiologist is the effect of SLE on the central nervous system and the cardiopulmonary systems. The central nervous system manifestations of SLE include seizures, neuropathies, paralysis, and stroke.[207,208] Laryngeal involvement, including mucosal ulceration, cricoarytenoid arthritis, and recurrent laryngeal nerve palsy, has been reported in up to 30% of SLE patients.[209]

SLE produces a serositis that manifests as pleuritis and pericarditis in the cardiopulmonary systems. In addition to pleural effusions, pneumonitis and pulmonary hemorrhage occur. The pneumonitis may indicate primary pulmonary parenchymal involvement or be secondary to uremia or bacterial infection. Pericarditis is the most common cardiovascular manifestation of SLE. Despite the fact that more than 60% of patients with SLE have a pericardial effusion, tamponade is a relatively uncommon condition.[210] Cardiomyopathy may be secondary to direct involvement of cardiac muscle or secondary to hypertension, anemia, uremia, or coronary artery disease. A noninfectious endocarditis (Libman-Sacks endocarditis) often affects the mitral valve and can produce mitral insufficiency. Echocardiographic studies of SLE patients have demonstrated valvular lesions, decreased left ventricular compliance, and left ventricular dysfunction.[211-213]

There is no specific therapy for SLE. Therapy is based on specific symptoms and organ dysfunction. Nonsteroidal anti-inflammatory drugs are useful for treating arthritis. Glucocorticoids represent a mainstay of therapy because they are drugs with both anti-inflammatory and immunosuppressive effects. Immunosuppressive drugs such as cyclophosphamide and azathioprine have also been used. Interestingly, antimalarial drugs seem to have beneficial effects for patients with SLE. Despite nonspecific but beneficial effects of these drugs, their side-effects are not trivial and treatment produces significant morbidity in some patients.[214]

Despite the diverse nature of SLE and the potential for significant major organ dysfunction, careful evaluation and treatment of patients with a critical analysis of the risk-benefit ratio of different therapies have markedly improved survival.[215]

Management of Anesthesia

Because SLE is a multisystem disease with diverse clinical presentations and severity of organ dysfunction, careful preoperative evaluation is necessary. Anesthesia management is influenced not only by the degree of organ dysfunction but also by the drugs used to treat SLE.

Arthritic involvement of the cervical spine is unusual in patients with SLE. Consequently, tracheal intubation is generally not difficult. However, the potential for laryngeal involvement requires clinical evaluation of laryngeal function.

A preoperative echocardiogram may be useful for the detection of pericardial effusion and evaluation of ventricular function. Certainly cardiac dysfunction will influence the choice of drugs and monitors for anesthesia. Because renal dysfunction is so common in patients with SLE, renal function should be quantified before operation. Pulmonary function testing generally will reveal a restrictive type of disease. Although minor abnormalities in liver function are present in many patients with SLE, these generally are not clinically significant. However, a fatal lupoid hepatitis characterized by prolonged jaundice, hyperglobulinemia, and hepatomegaly develops in some patients.[216]

Because most patients with SLE receive corticosteroids, supplementation with steroids during the perioperative period is usually indicated. An initial intravenous dose of 1 mg·kg of hydrocortisone should be adequate, although the total steroid dose depends on the length and magnitude of the operation.

Although there are no specific contraindications to any particular type of anesthesia, it has been demonstrated that patients with SLE are at increased risk for postoperative infections and pulmonary complications.[217] In view of this increased risk, careful preoperative evaluation in conjunction with a prudent selection of monitors and anesthetic agents is critical to a successful outcome.

Scleroderma

Scleroderma (systemic sclerosis) is a collagen vascular disease that affects the skin, joints, and visceral organs. Microvascular changes produce tissue fibrosis and organ sclerosis. It appears that the vascular damage is produced by injury to vascular endothelial cells.[218] This injury results in vascular obliteration and leakage of serum proteins into the interstitial space. The proteins produce tissue edema, lymphatic obstruction, and ultimately fibrosis.[219] Another basic feature of scleroderma is excessive collagen synthesis. The entire pathologic sequence is most likely triggered by alterations in the humoral and cellular immune systems with activation of mast cells.[220]

The manifestations of scleroderma are observed most readily in the skin, which becomes thickened and swollen. Eventually the skin becomes atrophic, hair and sweat glands are lost, and small arteries become sclerotic. Raynaud's phenomenon occurs in 95% of patients with scleroderma and is often the initial manifestation of the disease. As the disease progresses, the skin becomes taut, resulting in immobility of underlying structures. Joint mobility may become severely restricted.

Renal involvement is extremely common and destruction of renal blood vessels leads to hypertension, anemia, chronic proteinuria, and progressive renal failure.

In the lung, scleroderma produces interstitial fibrosis and thickening of alveolar septa that impair oxygen diffusion. Sclerosis of the chest wall and diaphragm in conjunction with interstitial fibrosis produces a severe restrictive defect. Over 30% of scleroderma patients have some degree of pulmonary hypertension.[221] Ultimately, cor pulmonale can develop.

Myocardial fibrosis occurs in 60% of patients with scleroderma. Cardiac histologic findings include contraction band necrosis and replacement fibrosis. Coronary vascular reserve is diminished, as evidenced by abnormal cardiac per-

fusion scans. Administration of nifidepine has been shown to improve myocardial perfusion.[222] Despite the myocardial changes, a decreased resting ejection fraction is present in only 20% of patients with scleroderma.[223] Fibrous atrophy of the cardiac conduction system may explain the high incidence of delayed atrioventricular conduction and supraventricular dysrhythmias. Pericardial effusion is also a common finding.

In most patients with scleroderma, the esophagus is involved, which leads to gastroesophageal reflux and aspiration. In addition, small intestinal motility is decreased.

Many of the treatment modalities are directed at relieving the effects of scleroderma on various organs. Angiotensin-converting enzyme inhibitors such as captopril and enalapril are effective for the control of hypertension. Since scleroderma is an immune disorder, a number of cytotoxic immunosuppressive agents such as chlorambucil, azathioprine, and 5-fluorouracil have been used but with variable results. Administration of D-penicillamine has also produced some benefit, but significant side-effects of this drug are common.[224]

Management of Anesthesia

Much like SLE, scleroderma is a multiorgan disease with diverse manifestations. Consequently, the affected organ systems must be evaluated thoroughly so that a logical plan for anesthesia can be selected. There are no specific contraindications to the use of any type of anesthesia, although the selection is guided by the degree of organ dysfunction.

Tracheal intubation can be quite difficult. Lack of temporomandibular joint mobility may necessitate fiberoptic laryngoscopy with topical anesthesia. Orotracheal intubation may be preferable to nasotracheal intubation because of the fragility of the nasal mucosa and propensity for nasal hemorrhage. Tracheostomy may be necessary in severely affected patients.[225]

The patient with scleroderma is at risk for aspiration pneumonitis during the induction of anesthesia because of the high incidence of gastroesophageal reflux. Appropriate measures to prevent acid aspiration, such as the use of histamine-2 blocking agents and oral antacids, may be indicated.

Chronic arterial hypoxemia is often present because of restriction of lung expansion and impaired oxygen diffusion. Consequently, controlled mechanical ventilation of the lungs with an increased inspired oxygen concentration is generally necessary. Compromised myocardial function and decreased coronary vascular reserve often necessitate the use of invasive cardiovascular monitoring, as the response to inhaled anesthetics may be exaggerated. Venous access may be difficult to establish and a venous cutdown or central venous catheterization may be necessary. Muscle involvement may increase the sensitivity to muscle relaxants.[226]

The anesthesiologist is often consulted as to the efficacy of sympathetic blockade for the treatment of vasospasm secondary to Raynaud's phenomenon.

Polymyositis/Dermatomyositis

Polymyositis is an inflammatory myopathy affecting skeletal muscle. The diagnostic term dermatomyositis is used when characteristic skin lesions are associated with the myositis. Common presenting symptoms are proximal skeletal muscle weakness and the typical skin rash consisting of a violaceous rash over the patient's eyelids with an erythematous rash over the face, neck, and upper chest. The origin of polymyositis and dermatomyositis is unknown, but as with all of the collagen vascular diseases, altered cellular immunity is suspected. This concept is supported by the finding that 10–20% of dermatomyositis patients have neoplastic disease as well. It could be speculated that the same altered immunity that results in dermatomyositis also impairs the immune system's ability to eliminate neoplastic cells.[227] Serum creatine kinase levels are a sensitive indicator of muscle damage, although there is significant patient variability. Examination of skeletal muscle biopsy specimens reveals perivascular infiltrates, muscle degeneration, and interstitial infiltrates. Electromyography demonstrates short polyphasic motor units and muscle fibrillation.[228] Magnetic resonance imaging and P-31 spectroscopy may provide a unique opportunity to diagnose myositis and correlate dynamic changes with therapy.[229]

Thirty to seventy-five percent of patients with polymyositis have electrocardiographic abnormalities that are secondary to myocardial fibrosis or atrophy of the cardiac conduction system. Typical electrocardiographic findings include nonspecific ST-T wave changes, dysrhythmias, and bundle-branch block.[230] The magnitude of cardiac disease is an important prognostic factor.

Aspiration pneumonitis is one of the most common complications of polymyositis.[231] Pulmonary interstitial fibrosis with restrictive lung disease occurs in nearly 70% of patients. In addition to lung changes from aspiration, immunogenic dysfunction also contributes to histologic changes. Interstitial pneumonitis has a particularly poor prognosis.[232]

Most patients with myositis improve with corticosteroid therapy. The 25% of polymyositis patients who do not respond to corticosteroids are treated with immunosuppressive agents such as methotrexate, azathioprine, and cyclophosphamide.[233]

Management of Anesthesia

Although mobility of the temporomandibular joint is not as severely affected by polymyositis as by scleroderma, some patients with dermatomyositis present a real challenge for tracheal intubation. Adequate mandibular and cervical mobility must be ascertained before induction of anesthesia.

Although the typical electromyographic findings suggest the potential for hyperkalemia after administration of succinylcholine, this has not been documented. Atypical cholinesterase activity has also been reported in patients with dermatomyositis, but the significance of this finding is unclear.[234] Sensitivity to nondepolarizing muscle relaxants is also likely, although this has not been reported.[235] Adequate monitoring of neuromuscular function during anesthesia is certainly indicated.

Dysphagia usually occurs, and there is an increased likelihood of aspiration pneumonitis. Appropriate antiaspiration maneuvers should be used during induction of anesthesia. Gastrointestinal tract perforations are common in patients with dermatomyositis.[236]

The degree of cardiopulmonary dysfunction will influence the choice of anesthetic and selection of intraoperative monitors. Preoperative pulmonary and cardiac function studies provide useful information in patients with polymyositis. Because of the preoperative skeletal muscle weakness, postoperative ventilatory support of the lungs may be necessary.

SKIN DISORDERS

Epidermolysis Bullosa

Epidermolysis bullosa is a rare hereditary skin disorder. The basic defect is felt to be either increased collagenase production or an autoimmune disease in which antigens from the basement membrane stimulate an immune response.[237,238] The end result is loss of normal intercellular bridges and separation of skin layers. The separation of the skin layers results in intradermal fluid accumulation and bullae formation. Even minor skin trauma produces skin blisters. Lateral shearing forces applied to the skin are particularly damaging because of skin separation. Pressure applied perpendicular to the axis of the skin surface is not as hazardous.

Although there are over 25 different types of epidermolysis bullosa, they can be conveniently categorized into three groups, depending on where the actual skin separation occurs: epidermolytic (simplex), junctional, and dermolytic (dystrophic).[239] The simplex form is characterized by a benign course and normal development. In contrast, patients with the junctional form rarely survive beyond early childhood, usually dying from sepsis. The dystrophic form produces severe scarring of the fingers and toes, with pseudosyndactyly formation, esophageal stricture, and malnutrition (Fig. 22-3). Anemia and hypoalbuminemia are common and result from chronic infection and malnutrition. Severe anemia with repeated blood transfusion can result in iron toxicity and subsequent cardiomyopathy.[240] Most patients do not survive after the second decade of life. Mitral valve prolapse has also been reported in patients with epidermolysis bullosa.[241] Other diseases associated with epidermolysis bullosa include porphyria cutanea tarda, amyloidosis, multiple myeloma, diabetes mellitus, and hypercoagulable states. Secondary bacterial infection of the bullae with Staphylococcus aureus or beta-hemolytic streptococci is common. Glomerulonephritis may occur as a result of streptococcal infection. Albumin loss secondary to nephritis in addition to albumin loss into bullous lesions can produce significant hypovolemia that further impairs renal function.[242] Neoplastic degeneration of the epidermis is very common in patients with epidermolysis bullosa. Involvement of the esophageal mucosa usually causes esophageal stricture, which requires endoscopy and repeated esophageal dilatation.[243] Enamel hypoplasia of the teeth produces a high incidence of carious degeneration requiring extensive dental restoration.

Phenytoin, which inhibits collagenase activity, is used as therapy for epidermolysis, although only two thirds of patients have a favorable response to phenytoin. Corticosteroids have also been used but are probably not effective.

Management of Anesthesia

It is critical that trauma to the skin and mucous membranes be avoided or minimized in these patients. Trauma from tape, blood pressure cuffs, tourniquets, and adhesive electrocardiographic electrodes may cause bulla formation. The blood pressure cuff should be padded with a loose cotton dressing. Intravenous and intra-arterial catheters should be sutured or held in place with a gauze wrap rather than taped in place. Trauma from an anesthetic face mask must be reduced by gentle application against the skin. Lubrication of the mask and the patient's face can be quite helpful in reducing trauma. Use of upper airway instruments, including oropharyngeal and nasopharyngeal airways, should be kept

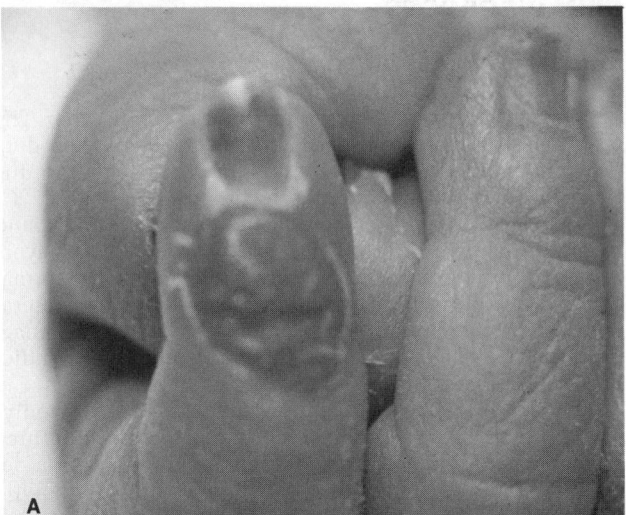

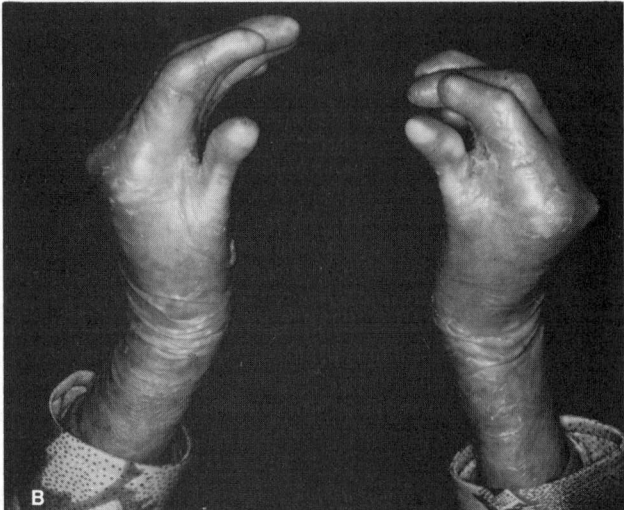

Figure 22-3. Epidermolysis bullosa. (*A*) Bullous lesion of the finger of a neonate with epidermolysis. (*B*) Hands of an older child with epidermolysis showing progression of the disease to produce severe scarring and pseudosyndactyly. (Courtesy of James E. Bennett, M.D., Division of Plastic Surgery, Indiana University School of Medicine.)

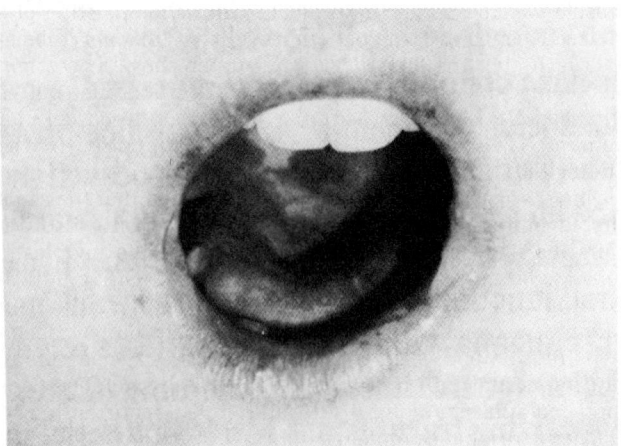

Figure 22-4. Severe microstomia in a child with epidermolysis bullosa. The inability to open the mouth can make tracheal intubation quite difficult. (Reprinted with permission from Wright JT: Comprehensive dental care and general anesthetic management of hereditary epidermolysis bullosa. Oral Surg Oral Med Oral Pathol 70:576, 1990.)

to a minimum because the squamous epithelium that lines the oropharynx and esophagus is more susceptible to trauma than is the columnar epithelium of the trachea. Laryngeal involvement is extremely rare, and tracheal bullae have not been reported. Frictional trauma to the oropharynx, as produced by an oral airway, may result in formation of large intraoral bullae and extensive hemorrhage from denuded mucosa.[244] Intraoral and oropharyngeal bullae are more likely to produce airway obstruction than is tracheal mucosal damage.[245] Hemorrhage from ruptured oral bullae has been successfully treated by application of epinephrine-soaked gauze to the bullae.[246] Tracheal intubation has been associated with only minimal complications and certainly should not be avoided if indicated.[247-249] When tracheal intubation is performed, the laryngoscope blade and tracheal tube should be well lubricated to avoid trauma to the oropharynx. Scarring of the oral cavity can result in a narrow oral aperture (microstomia) and immobility of the

tongue, which can increase the difficulty of laryngoscopy (Fig. 22-4). Use of an esophageal stethoscope should also be avoided because it may lead to formation of intraoral or esophageal bullae. Although the safety of tracheal intubation has been established for patients with the dystrophic form of epidermolysis bullosa, it has not been established in infants with the junctional form. The junctional form affects all mucosa including the respiratory epithelium.[250] However, the types of surgical procedures (intra-abdominal) required in infants with the junctional form usually mandate tracheal intubation.

Ketamine is a useful anesthetic for procedures that do not require skeletal muscle relaxation or intra-abdominal manipulation. Because patients with epidermolysis often require surgical procedures on the fingers and toes, use of ketamine is ideal. There are no known contraindications to the use of inhaled anesthetic drugs in these patients. Regional anesthesia, including spinal, epidural, and brachial plexus anesthesia, has been successfully used in patients with epidermolysis bullosa.[251,252]

Although porphyria has been reported to occur with increased frequency in patients with epidermolysis bullosa, this association is tenuous.[253] The type of porphyria with the alleged association is porphyria cutanea tarda, which does not have the same implications for anesthesia as acute intermittent porphyria.[254]

Pemphigus

Pemphigus is a vesiculobullous disease that may involve extensive areas of the skin and mucous membranes. It is an autoimmune disease in which there is a loss of cellular adhesiveness that leads to a separation of skin and mucous membrane epithelium. Most patients with pemphigus have IgG autoantibodies that bind to the surface of epidermal cells. These autoantibodies are highly specific and result in the excessive production of proteolytic enzymes that disrupt cell adhesion. There are several types of pemphigus, including pemphigus vulgaris, pemphigus vegetans, pemphigus foliaceus, and pemphigus erythematosus. Pemphigus vulgaris is the most common variant and is the most significant because of the high incidence of occurrence of oral lesions. Oral lesions occur in 50–70% of pemphigus patients and usually precede the onset of skin lesions. Involvement of the pharynx, larynx, esophagus, conjunctiva, urethra, cervix, and anus has also been reported.[255] Because extensive oropharyngeal involvement makes eating painful, patients may reduce oral intake to such an extent that malnutrition develops. Skin denudation and bullae formation can result in significant fluid and protein losses. The risk of secondary bacterial infection is great. As with epidermolysis bullosa, lateral shearing forces are more likely to produce bullae than is pressure exerted perpendicular to the skin surface. Treatment with systemic corticosteroids has reduced the mortality from 70% to as low as 5%.[256] The addition of immunosuppressants such as azathioprine, cyclophosphamide, methotrexate, and cyclosporine has further reduced mortality and decreased the incidence of corticosteroid-induced complications.

Pemphigus vegetans is most likely a subgroup of pemphigus vulgaris, as it is histologically similar to vulgaris. Common sites of involvement include the axilla, groin, flexural surfaces, and oral cavity. Pemphigus foliaceus (superficial pemphigus) is a less severe form of pemphigus in which acantholysis occurs high in the epidermis; the oral mucosa is not involved. Pemphigus erythematosus (Senear-Usher syndrome) is another form of superficial pemphigus. The lesions are characteristically erythematous, and hyperkeratotic patches are seen over the nose and malar area; the oral mucosa is not involved. Pemphigus can be induced by a number of drugs, including captopril, phenobarbital, piroxicam, and penicillamine.

Management of Anesthesia

Preoperative drug therapy and the extreme fragility of mucous membranes are of primary consideration for management of anesthesia in patients with pemphigus. Corticosteroid supplementation will undoubtedly be necessary during the perioperative period. Management of the upper airway and tracheal intubation should be performed as described for patients with epidermolysis bullosa. As in epidermolysis patients, ketamine has been used successfully in patients with pemphigus.[257] Regional anesthesia has also been used.[258]

There are no specific contraindications to the use of any inhaled or intravenous anesthetic; however, potential side-effects of treatment drugs and interactions with anesthetics must be considered. For example, methotrexate produces hepatorenal dysfunction and bone marrow suppression, and cyclophosphamide may prolong the effect of succinylcholine by inhibiting cholinesterase activity.

REFERENCES

1. Sanyal SK, Johnson WW, Dische WR et al: Dystrophic degeneration of papillary muscle and ventricular myocardium. Circulation 62:430, 1980
2. Nigro G, Comi LI, Politano L et al: The incidence and evolution of cardiomyopathy in Duchenne muscular dystrophy. Int J Cardiol 26:271, 1990
3. Perloff JK, Henze E, Schelbert HR: Alterations in regional myocardial metabolism, perfusion, and wall motion in Duchenne muscular dystrophy studied by radionuclide imaging. Circulation 69:33, 1984
4. Ellis FR: Inherited muscle disease. Br J Anaesth 52:153, 1980
5. Seay AR, Ziter FA, Thompson JA: Cardiac arrest during induction of anesthesia in Duchenne muscular dystrophy. J Pediatr 93:88, 1978
6. Chalkiadis GA, Branch KG: Cardiac arrest after isoflurane anaesthesia in a patient with Duchenne's muscular dystrophy. Anaesthesia 45:22, 1990
7. McKishnie JD, Muir JM, Girvan DP: Anaesthesia induced rhabdomyolysis—a case report. Can Anaesth Soc J 30:295, 1983
8. Rosenberg H: Neuromuscular blockade in the patient with neuromuscular disorders. Semin Anesth 4:9, 1985
9. Larsen UT, Juhl B, Hein-Sorensen O et al: Complications during anesthesia in patients with Duchenne's muscular dystrophy (a retrospective study). Can J Anaesth 36:418, 1989
10. Wang JM, Stanley TH: Duchenne muscular dystrophy and malignant hyperthermia—two case reports. Can Anaesth Soc J 33:492, 1986
11. Buzello W, Huttarsch H: Muscle relaxation in patients with Duchenne's muscular dystrophy. Br J Anaesth 60:228, 1988
12. Smith CL, Bush GH: Anaesthesia and progressive muscular dystrophy. Br J Anaesth 57:1113, 1985
13. Hook R, Anderson EF, Noto P: Anesthetic management of a parturient with myotonia atrophica. Anesthesiology 43:689, 1975
14. Streib EW: Successful treatment with tocainide of recessive generalized congenital myotonia. Ann Neurol 19:501, 1986
15. Perloff JK, Stevenson WG, Roberts NK et al: Cardiac involvement in myotonic muscular dystrophy (Steinert's disease): A prospective study of 25 patients. Am J Cardiol 54:1074, 1984
16. Forsberg H, Olofson B-O, Eriksson A et al: Cardiac involvement in congenital myotonic dystrophy. Br Heart J 63:119, 1990
17. Streib EW, Meyers DG, Sun SF: Mitral valve prolapse in myotonic dystrophy. Muscle Nerve 8:650, 1985
18. Jammes Y, Pouget J, Grimaud C et al: Pulmonary function and electromyographic study of respiratory muscles in myotonic dystrophy. Muscle Nerve 8:586, 1985
19. Fitting J-W, Leuenberger P: Procainamide for dyspnea in myotonic dystrophy. Am Rev Respir Dis 140:1442, 1989
20. Hannon VM, Cunningham AJ, Hutchinson M et al: Aspiration pneumonia and coma—an unusual presentation of dystrophica myotonia. Can Anaesth Soc J 33:803, 1986
21. Fall LH, Young WW, Power JA et al: Severe congestive heart failure and cardiomyopathy as a complication of myotonic dystrophy in pregnancy. Obstet Gynecol 76:481, 1990
22. Cope DK, Miller JN: Local and spinal anesthesia for cesarean section in a patient with myotonic dystrophy. Anesth Analg 65:687, 1986
23. Streib EW: Hypokalemic paralysis in two patients with paramyotonia congenita (PC) and known hyperkalemic/exercise-induced weakness. Muscle Nerve 12:936, 1989
24. Mitchell MM, Ali HH, Savarese JJ: Myotonia and neuromuscular blocking agents. Anesthesiology 49:44, 1978
25. Buzello W, Kreig N, Schlickewei A: Hazards of neostigmine in patients with neuromuscular disorders. Br J Anaesth 54:529, 1982
26. Nightengale P, Healy TEJ, McGuinness K: Dystrophica myotonia and atracurium. Br J Anaesth 57:1131, 1985
27. Stirt JA, Stone DJ, Weinberg G et al: Atracurium in a child with myotonic dystrophy. Anesth Analg 64:369, 1985
28. Boheimer N, Harris JW, Ward S: Neuromuscular blockade in dystrophia myotonica with atracurium besylate. Anaesthesia 40:872, 1985
29. Aldridge LM: Anaesthetic problems in myotonic dystrophy. Br J Anaesth 57:1119, 1985
30. White DA, Smyth DG: Continuous infusion of propofol in dystrophica myotonia. Can J Anaesth 36:200, 1989
31. Speedy H: Exaggerated physiological responses to propofol in myotonic dystrophy. Br J Anaesth 64:110, 1990
32. Ishizawa Y, Yamaguchi H, Dohi S et al: A serious complication due to gastrointestinal malfunction in a patient with myotonic dystrophy. Anesth Analg 65:1066, 1986
33. Jaffe R, Mock M, Abramowicz J et al: Myotonic dystrophy and pregnancy: A review. Obstet Gynecol Surv 41:272, 1986
34. Paterson RA, Tousignant M, Skene SD: Cesarean section for

twins in a patient with myotonic dystrophy. Can Anaesth Soc J 32:418, 1985

35. Blumgart CH, Hughes DG, Redfern N: Obstetric anaesthesia in dystrophica myotonica. Anaesthesia 45:26, 1990
36. Marchiori PE, dos Reis M, Quevedo ME et al: Acetylcholine receptor antibody in myasthenia gravis. Acta Neurol Scand 80:387, 1989
37. Steinman L, Mantegazza R: Prospects for specific immunotherapy in myasthenia gravis. FASEB J 4:2726, 1990
38. Fonseca V, Havard CWH: The natural course of myasthenia gravis. Br Med J 300:1409, 1990
39. Penn AS, Scotland DL, Lamme S: Antimuscle and antiacetylcholine receptor antibodies in myasthenia gravis. Muscle Nerve 9:407, 1986
40. Seybold ME: Myasthenia gravis. A clinical and basic science review. JAMA 250:2516, 1983
41. Hofstad H, Ohm O, Mork SJ et al: Heart disease in myasthenia gravis. Acta Neurol Scand 70:176, 1984
42. Plauche WC: Myasthenia gravis. Clin Obstet Gynecol 26:592, 1983
43. Mier A, Laroche C, Green M: Unsuspected myasthenia gravis presenting as respiratory failure. Thorax 45:422, 1990
44. Dushay KM, Zibrak JD, Jensen WA: Myasthenia gravis presenting as isolated respiratory failure. Chest 97:232, 1990
45. Havard CWH, Fonseca V: New treatment approaches to myasthenia gravis. Drugs 39:66, 1990
46. Donaldson DH, Ansher M, Horan S et al: The relationship of age to outcome in myasthenia gravis. Neurology 40:786, 1990
47. Mulder DG, Graves M, Herrmann C: Thymectomy for myasthenia gravis: Recent observations and comparisons with past experience. Ann Thorac Surg 48:551, 1989
48. Baraka A, Dajani A: Atracurium in myasthenics undergoing thymectomy. Anesth Analg 64:1127, 1984
49. Ramsey FM, Smith GD: Clinical use of atracurium in myasthenia gravis: A case report. Can Anaesth Soc J 32:642, 1985
50. Bell CF, Florence AM, Hunter JM et al: Atracurium in the myasthenic patient. Anaesthesia 39:961, 1984
51. Hunter JM, Bell CF, Florence AM et al: Vecuronium in the myasthenic patient. Anaesthesia 40:848, 1985
52. Nilsson E, Meretoja OA: Vecuronium dose-response and maintenance requirements in patients with myasthenia gravis. Anesthesiology 73:28, 1990
53. Eisenkraft JB, Book WJ, Papatestas AE: Sensitivity to vecuronium in myasthenia gravis: A dose-response study. Can J Anaesth 37:301, 1990
54. Abel M, Eisenkraft JB, Patel N: Response to suxamethonium in a myasthenic patient during remission. Anaesthesia 46:30, 1991
55. Nilsson E, Paloheimo M, Muller K et al: Halothane-induced variability in the neuromuscular transmission of patients with myasthenia gravis. Acta Anesthesiol Scand 33:395, 1989
56. Rowbottom SJ: Isoflurane for thymectomy in myasthenia gravis. Anaesth Intens Care 17:444, 1989
57. Sivak ED, Mehta A, Hanson M et al: Postoperative ventilatory dependence following thymectomy for myasthenia gravis. Cleve Clin Q 51:585, 1984
58. Leventhal SR, Orkin FK, Hirsch RA: Prediction of the need for postoperative mechanical ventilation in myasthenia gravis. Anesthesiology 53:26, 1980
59. Eisenkraft JB, Papatestas AE, Kahn CH et al: Predicting the need for postoperative mechanical ventilation in myasthenia gravis. Anesthesiology 65:79, 1986
60. Leys K, Lang B, Johnston I et al: Calcium channel autoantibodies in the Lambert-Eaton myasthenic syndrome. Ann Neurol 29:307, 1991
61. Azar I: The response of patients with neuromuscular disease to muscle relaxants: A review. Anesthesiology 61:173, 1984
62. McEvoy KM, Windebank AJ, Daube JR et al: 3,4-Diaminopyridine in the treatment of Lambert-Eaton myasthenic syndrome. N Engl J Med 321:1567, 1989
63. Agoston S, Van Weerden T, Westra P et al: Effects of 4-aminopyridine in Eaton-Lambert syndrome. Br J Anaesth 50:383, 1978
64. Telford RJ, Hollway TE: The myasthenic syndrome: Anesthesia in a patient treated with 3,4 diaminopyridine. Br J Anaesth 64:363, 1990
65. Bendheim PE, Reale EO, Berg BO: β-adrenergic treatment of hyperkalemic periodic paralysis. Neurology 35:746, 1985
66. Dalakas MC, Engel WK: Treatment of "permanent" muscle weakness in familial hypokalemic periodic paralysis. Muscle Nerve 6:182, 1983
67. Buruma OJS, Bots GTAM, Went LN: Familial hypokalemic periodic paralysis. Arch Neurol 42:28, 1985
68. Rollman JE, Dickson CM: Anesthetic management of a patient with hypokalemic familial periodic paralysis for coronary artery bypass surgery. Anesthesiology 63:526, 1985
69. Lema G, Urzua J, Moran S et al: Successful anesthetic management of a patient with hypokalemic familial periodic paralysis undergoing cardiac surgery. Anesthesiology 74:373, 1991
70. Christensen KS: Hypokalemic periodic paralysis secondary to renal tubular acidosis. Eur Neurol 24:303, 1985
71. Manary MJ, Keating JP, Hirshberg GE: Quadriparesis due to potassium depletion. Crit Care Med 14:750, 1986
72. Duncan PG: Neuromuscular diseases. In Katz J, Steward DJ (eds): Anesthesia and Uncommon Pediatric Diseases, p 509. Philadelphia, WB Saunders, 1987
73. England JD: Guillain-Barre syndrome. Annu Rev Med 41:1, 1990
74. Wijdicks EFM, Ropper AH: Acute relapsing Guillain-Barre syndrome after long asymptomatic intervals. Arch Neurol 47:82, 1990
75. Newton-John H: Prevention of pulmonary complications in severe Guillain-Barre syndrome by early assisted ventilation. Med J Aust 142:444, 1985
76. Ropper AH: Severe acute Guillain-Barre syndrome. Neurology 36:429, 1986
77. McKann GM: Guillain-Barre syndrome: Clinical and therapeutic observations. Ann Neurol 27(Suppl):S13-S16, 1990
78. Krone A, Reuther P, Fuhrmeister U: Autonomic dysfunction in polyneuropathies: A report of 106 cases. J Neurol 230:111, 1983
79. Moore P, James O: Guillain-Barre syndrome: Incidence, management, and outcome of major complications. Crit Care Med 9:549, 1981
80. Feldman JM: Cardiac arrest after succinylcholine administration in a pregnant patient recovered from Guillain-Barre syndrome. Anesthesiology 72:942, 1990
81. Rosenfeld B, Borel C, Hanley D: Epidural morphine treatment of pain in Guillain-Barre syndrome. Arch Neurol 43:1194, 1986
82. Connelly M, Shagrin J, Warfield C: Epidural opioids for the management of pain in a patient with Guillain-Barre syndrome. Anesthesiology 72:381, 1990
83. Covert CR, Brodie SB, Zimmerman JE: Weaning failure due to acute neuromuscular disease. Crit Care Med 14:307, 1986
84. Powell HC, Lampert PW: Pathology of multiple sclerosis. Neurol Clin 1:631, 1983
85. Ellison GW, Visscher BR, Graves MC et al: Multiple sclerosis. Ann Intern Med 101:514, 1984
86. Reder AT, Antel JP: Clinical spectrum of multiple sclerosis. Neurol Clin 1:573, 1983
87. Kuwahira I, Kondo T, Ohta Y et al: Acute respiratory failure in multiple sclerosis. Chest 97:246, 1990
88. Aisen M, Arlt G, Foster S: Diaphragmatic paralysis without bulbar or limb paralysis in multiple sclerosis. Chest 98:499, 1990
89. Birk K, Ford C, Smeltzer S et al: The clinical course of multiple sclerosis during pregnancy and the puerperium. Arch Neurol 47:738, 1990
90. Baum K, Nehring C, Girke W et al: Multiple sclerosis: Relations between MRI and CT findings, cerebrospinal fluid parameters and clinical features. Clin Neurol Neurosurg 92:49, 1990
91. Sola P, Scarpa M, Faglioni P et al: Diagnostic investigations in MS: Which is the most sensitive? Acta Neurol Scand 80:394, 1989
92. Compston DAS: The management of multiple sclerosis. Q J Med 70:93, 1989

93. Schapiro RT, Van den Noort S, Scheinberg L: The current management of multiple sclerosis. Ann NY Acad Sci 436:425, 1984

94. Eisen A: Neurophysiology in multiple sclerosis. Neurol Clin 1:615, 1983

95. Siemkowicz E: Multiple sclerosis and surgery. Anaesthesia 31:1211, 1976

96. Baskett PJF, Armstrong R: Anaesthetic problems in multiple sclerosis. Anaesthesia 25:397, 1970

97. Kytta J, Rosenberg PH: Anaesthesia for patients with multiple sclerosis. Ann Chir Gynaecol 73:299, 1984

98. Jones RM, Healy TEJ: Anaesthesia and demyelinating disease. Anaesthesia 35:879, 1980

99. Berger JM, Ontell R: Intrathecal morphine in conjunction with a combined spinal and general anesthetic in a patient with multiple sclerosis. Anesthesiology 66:400, 1987

100. Leigh J, Fearnley SJ, Lupprian KG: Intrathecal diamorphine during laparotomy in a patient with advanced multiple sclerosis. Anaesthesia 45:640, 1990

101. Bader AM, Hunt CO, Datta S et al: Anesthesia for the obstetric patient with multiple sclerosis. J Clin Anesth 1:21, 1988

102. Roth S, Ebrahim ZY: Resistance to pancuronium in patients receiving carbamazepine. Anesthesiology 66:691, 1987

103. Sung C-Y, Chu N-S: Epileptic seizures in elderly people: Aetiology and seizure type. Age Ageing 19:25, 1990

104. Gram L: Epileptic seizures and syndromes. Lancet 336:161, 1990

105. Thadani VM, Williamson PD: Classification of epileptic seizures and syndromes. Semin Neurol 10:328, 1990

106. Rawal K, D'Souza BJ: Status epilepticus. Crit Care Clin 1:339, 1985

107. Riela AR: Management of seizures. Crit Care Clin 5:863, 1989

108. Kofke WA, Young RSK, Davis P et al: Isoflurane for refractory status epilepticus: A clinical series. Anesthesiology 71:653, 1989

109. Tetzlaff JE: Intraoperative defect in haemostasis in a child receiving valproic acid. Can J Anaesth 38:222, 1991

110. Isojawi JIT, Pakarinen AJ, Myllyla VV: Thyroid function in epileptic patients treated with carbamazepine. Arch Neurol 46:1175, 1989

111. Rampil IJ, Lockhart SH, Eger EI et al: The electroencephalographic effects of desflurane in humans. Anesthesiology 74:434, 1991

112. Steen PA, Michenfelder JD: Neurotoxicity of anesthetics. Anesthesiology 50:437, 1979

113. Molbegott LP, Flashburg MH, Karasic HL et al: Probable seizures after sufentanil. Anesth Analg 66:91, 1987

114. Scott JC, Sarnquist FH: Seizure like movements during a fentanyl infusion with absence of seizure activity in a simultaneous EEG recording. Anesthesiology 62:812, 1985

115. Sebel PS, Bovill JG, Wauquier A et al: Effects of high-dose fentanyl anesthesia on the electroencephalogram. Anesthesiology 55:203, 1981

116. Bovill JG, Sebel PS, Wauquier A et al: Electroencephalographic effects of sufentanil anaesthesia in man. Br J Anaesth 54:45, 1982

117. Smith NT, Benthuysen JL, Bickford RG et al: Seizures during opioid anesthetic induction—are they opioid induced rigidity? Anesthesiology 71:852, 1989

118. Carlsson C, Smith DS, Keykhah MM et al: The effects of high dose fentanyl on cerebral circulation and metabolism in rats. Anesthesiology 57:375, 1982

119. Young ML, Smith DS, Greenberg J et al: Effects of sufentanil on regional cerebral glucose utilization in rats. Anesthesiology 61:564, 1984

120. Tempelhoff R, Modica PA, Spitznagel EL: Anticonvulsant therapy increases fentanyl requirements during anesthesia for craniotomy. Can J Anaesth 37:327, 1990

121. Rockoff MA, Gousdsouzian NG: Seizures induced by methohexital. Anesthesiology 54:333, 1981

122. Sebel PS, Lowdon JD: Propofol: A new intravenous anesthetic. Anesthesiology 71:260, 1989

123. Ornstein E, Matteo RS, Young WL et al: Resistance to metocurine-induced neuromuscular blockade in patients receiving phenytoin. Anesthesiology 63:294, 1985

124. Duvoisin RC: Etiology of Parkinson's disease: Current concepts. Clin Neuropharmacol 9 (suppl 1):S3, 1986

125. Lang AE, Blair RDG: Parkinson's disease in 1984: An update. Can Med Assoc J 131:1031, 1984

126. Drugs for parkinsonism. Med Lett Drug Ther 28:62, 1986

127. The Bromocriptine Multicentre Trial Group: Bromocriptine as initial therapy in elderly parkinsonian patients. Age Ageing 19:62, 1990

128. The Parkinson Study Group: Effect of deprenyl on the progression of disability in early Parkinson's disease. N Engl J Med 321:1364, 1989

129. DaPrada M, Keller HH, Pieri L et al: The pharmacology of Parkinson's disease: Basic aspects and recent advances. Experientia 40:1165, 1984

130. Mets B: Acute dystonia after alfentanil in untreated Parkinson's disease. Anesth Analg 72:557, 1991

131. Muzzi DA, Black S, Cucchiara RF: The lack of effect of succinylcholine on serum potassium in patients with Parkinson's disease. Anesthesiology 71:322, 1989

132. Zornberg GL, Bodkin JA, Cohen BM: Severe adverse interaction between pethidine and selegiline. Lancet 337:246, 1991

133. Golbe LI, Langston JW, Shoulson I: Selegiline and Parkinson's disease. Drugs 39:646, 1990

134. Korczyn AD: Autonomic nervous system disturbance in Parkinson's disease. Adv Neurol 53:463, 1990

135. Golden WE, Lavender RC, Metzer WS: Acute postoperative confusion and hallucinations in Parkinson disease. Ann Int Med 111:218, 1989

136. Shoulson I: Huntington's disease. Neurol Clin 2:515, 1984

137. Huggins M, Block M, Kanani SH et al: Ethical and legal dilemmas arising during predictive testing for adult-onset disease: The experience of Huntington disease. Am J Hum Genet 47:4, 1990

138. Davies DD: Abnormal response to anaesthesia in a case of Huntington's chorea. Br J Anaesth 38:490, 1966

139. Kaufman MA, Erb T: Propofol for patients with Huntington's chorea? Anaesthesia 45:889, 1990

140. Propert DN: Pseudocholinesterase activity and phenotypes in mentally ill patients. Br J Psychiatry 134:477, 1979

141. Lamont AMS: Brief report: Anaesthesia and Huntington's chorea. Anaesth Intens Care 7:189, 1979

142. Katzman R: Alzheimer's disease. N Engl J Med 314:964, 1986

143. Gautrin D, Gauthier S: Alzheimer's disease: Environmental factors and etiologic hypotheses. Can J Neurol Sci 16:375, 1989

144. Whitehouse PJ: Understanding the etiology of Alzheimer's disease. Neurol Clin 4:427, 1986

145. Mayeux R: Therapeutic strategies in Alzheimer's disease. Neurology 40:175, 1990

146. Tandan R, Bradley WG: Amyotrophic lateral sclerosis: Part 2. Etiopathogenesis. Ann Neurol 18:419, 1985

147. Armon C, Daube JR, Windebank AJ et al: How frequently does classic amyotrophic lateral sclerosis develop in survivors of poliomyelitis? Neurology 40:172, 1990

148. Kuther G, Rodiek SO, Struppler A: CT-scanning of skeletal muscles in amyotrophic lateral sclerosis. Adv Exp Med Biol 209:143, 1987

149. Ioli F, DiLorenzo G, Donner CF et al: Some remarks on lung function in amyotrophic lateral sclerosis. Adv Exp Med Biol 209:139, 1987

150. Carre PC, Didier AP, Tiberge YM et al: Amyotrophic lateral sclerosis presenting with sleep hypopnea syndrome. Chest 93:1309, 1988

151. Goldblatt D, Greenlaw J: Starting and stopping the ventilator for patients with amyotrophic lateral sclerosis. Neurol Clin 7:789, 1989

152. Chida K, Sakamaki S, Takasu T: Alteration in autonomic function and cardiovascular regulation in amyotrophic lateral sclerosis. J Neurol 236:127, 1989

153. Tandan R, Bradley WG: Amyotrophic lateral sclerosis: Part 1. Clinical features, pathology, and ethical issues in management. Ann Neurol 18:271, 1985

154. Bendheim PE: The human spongiform encephalopathies. Neurol Clin 2:281, 1984
155. Duffy P, Wolf J, Collins G et al: Possible person-to-person transmission of Creutzfeldt-Jakob disease. N Engl J Med 290:692, 1974
156. Bernoulli C, Siegfried J, Baumgartner G: Danger of accidental person-to-person transmission of Creutzfeldt-Jacob disease by surgery. Lancet 1:478, 1977
157. Gajdusek MD, Gibbs CJ, Asher DM et al: Precautions in medical care of, and in handling material from patients with transmissible virus dementia (Creutzfeldt-Jakob disease). N Engl J Med 297:1253, 1977
158. Brown P, Cathala F, Raubertas RF et al: The epidemiology of Creutzfeldt-Jakob disease. Neurology 37:895, 1987
159. Thadani V, Penar PL, Partington J et al: Creutzfeldt-Jakob disease probably acquired from a cadaveric dura mater graft. J Neurosurg 69:766, 1988
160. Marzewski DJ, Towfighi J, Harrington MG et al: Creutzfeldt-Jakob disease following pituitary-derived human growth hormone therapy. Neurology 38:1131, 1988
161. duMoulin GC, Hedley-Whyte J: Hospital-associated viral infection and the anesthesiologist. Anesthesiology 59:51, 1983
162. MacMurdo SD, Jakymec AJ, Bleyaert AL: Precautions in the anesthetic management of a patient with Creutzfeldt-Jakob disease. Anesthesiology 60:590, 1984
163. Sadeh M, Goldhammer Y, Chagnac Y: Creutzfeldt-Jakob disease associated with peripheral neuropathy. Isr J Med 26:220, 1990
164. Keith AS: Introduction to the anemias. In Wyngaarden JB, Smith LH (eds): Cecil's Textbook of Medicine, 17th ed, p 870. Philadelphia, WB Saunders, 1985
165. Levine E, Rosen A, Sehgal L et al: Physiologic effects of acute anemia: Implications for a reduced transfusion trigger. Transfusion 30:11, 1990
166. Cook JD, Skikne BS: Iron deficiency: Definition and diagnosis. J Int Med 226:349, 1989
167. Berger M, Brass LF: Severe thrombocytopenia in iron deficiency anemia. Am J Hematol 24:425, 1987
168. Bruggers CS, Ware R, Altman AJ et al: Reversible focal neurologic deficits in severe iron deficiency anemia. J Pediatr 117:430, 1990
169. Nunn JF, Chanarin J: Nitrous oxide inactivates methionine synthetase. In Eger EI (ed): Nitrous Oxide/N2O, p 211. New York, Elsevier-Dutton, 1985
170. Schilling RF: Is nitrous oxide a dangerous anesthetic for vitamin B-12 deficient subjects? JAMA 255:1605, 1986
171. Berger JJ, Modell JH, Sypert GW: Megaloblastic anemia and brief exposure to nitrous oxide—a causal relationship? Anesth Analg 67:197, 1988
172. Koblin DD, Tomerson BW, Waldman FM: Disruption of folate and vitamin B-12 metabolism in aged rats following exposure to nitrous oxide. Anesthesiology 73:506, 1990
173. Chang H, Miller DR: Hemolytic anemias: Membrane defects. In Miller DH (ed): Blood Diseases of Infancy and Childhood, 5th ed, p 262. St. Louis, CV Mosby, 1984
174. Hain WR: Diseases of blood. In Katz J, Steward DJ (eds): Anesthesia and Uncommon Pediatric Diseases, p 489. Philadelphia, WB Saunders, 1987
175. Morse EE: Toxic effects of drugs on erythrocytes. Ann Clin Lab Sci 18:13, 1988
176. Beutler E: Glucose-6-phosphate dehydrogenase deficiency. N Engl J Med 324:169, 1991
177. Hirono A, Forman L, Beutler E: Enzymatic diagnosis in nonspherocytic hemolytic anemia. Medicine 67:110, 1988
178. Park JV, Weiss CI: Cardiopulmonary bypass and myocardial protection: Management problems in cardiac surgical patients with cold autoimmune disease. Anesth Analg 67:75, 1988
179. Bedrosian CL, Simel DL: Cold hemagglutinin disease in the operating room. South Med J 80:466, 1987
180. Luban NLC, Epstein BS, Watson SP: Sickle cell disease and anesthesia. Adv Anesthesiol 1:289, 1984
181. The Anaesthesia Advisory Committee to the Chief Coroner of Ontario: Intraoperative death during cesarean section in a patient with sickle-cell trait. Can J Anaesth 34:67, 1987
182. Powars D, Weidman JA, Odom-Maryon T et al: Sickle cell chronic lung disease: Prior morbidity and the risk of pulmonary failure. Medicine 67:66, 1988
183. Balfour IC, Covitz W, Arensman FW et al: Left ventricular filling in sickle cell anemia. Am J Cardiol 61:395, 1988
184. Allon M: Renal abnormalities in sickle cell disease. Arch Intern Med 150:501, 1990
185. Gyasi HK, Zarroug AW, Matthew M et al: Anesthesia for renal transplantation in sickle cell disease. Can J Anaesth 37:778, 1990
186. Adams RJ, Nichols FT, McKie V et al: Cerebral infarction in sickle cell anemia: Mechanism based on CT and MRI. Neurology 38:1012, 1988
187. Rodgers GP, Dover GJ, Noguchi CT et al: Hematologic responses of patients with sickle cell disease to treatment with hydroxyurea. N Engl J Med 322:1037, 1990
188. Stein RE, Urbaniak J: Use of the tourniquet during surgery in patients with sickle cell hemoglobinopathies. Clin Orthop 151:231, 1980
189. Heiner M, Teasdale SJ, David T et al: Aortocoronary bypass in a patient with sickle cell trait. Can Anaesth Soc J 26:428, 1979
190. Cook A, Hanowell LH: Intraoperative autotransfusion for a patient with homozygous sickle cell disease. Anesthesiology 73:177, 1990
191. Rockoff AS, Christy D, Zeldis N et al: Myocardial necrosis following general anesthesia in hemoglobin SC disease. Pediatrics 61:73, 1978
192. Aldouri MA, Wonke B, Hoffbrand AV et al: High incidence of cardiomyopathy in beta-thalassemia patients receiving regular transfusion and chelation: Reversal by intensified chelation. Acta Haematol 84:113, 1990
193. Gibson JR: Anesthesia for sickle cell diseases and other hemoglobinopathies. Semin Anesth 6:27, 1987
194. Jackson DV, Randall ME, Richards F: Spinal cord compression due to extramedullary hematopoiesis in thalassemia: Long term follow-up after radiotherapy. Surg Neurol 29:389, 1988
195. Smith PR, Manjoney DL, Teitcher JB et al: Massive hemothorax due to intrathoracic extramedullary hematopoiesis in a patient with thalassemia intermedia. Chest 94:658, 1988
196. Phillips PE: Infectious agents in the pathogenesis of rheumatoid arthritis. Semin Arthritis Rheum 16:1, 1986
197. Wolfe BK, O'Keeffe D, Mitchell DM et al: Rheumatoid arthritis of the cervical spine: Early and progressive radiographic features. Radiology 165:145, 1987
198. Einig M, Higer HP, Meairs S et al: Magnetic resonance imaging of the craniocervical junction in rheumatoid arthritis: Value, limitation, indications. Skeletal Radiol 19:341, 1990
199. Krane SM, Simon LS: Rheumatoid arthritis: Clinical features and pathogenetic mechanisms. Med Clin North Am 70:263, 1986
200. Epstein WV, Henke CJ, Yelin EH et al: Effects of parenterally administered gold therapy on the course of adult rheumatoid arthritis. Ann Intern Med 114:437, 1991
201. Crosby ET, Lui A: The adult cervical spine: Implications for airway management. Can J Anaesth 37:77, 1990
202. Keenan MA, Stiles CM, Kaufman RL: Acquired laryngeal deviation associated with cervical spine disease in erosive polyarticular arthritis. Anesthesiology 58:441, 1983
203. White RH: Preoperative evaluation of patients with rheumatoid arthritis. Semin Arthritis Rheum 14:287, 1985
204. Reginster JY, Damas P, Franchimont P: Anaesthetic risks in osteoarticular disorders. Clin Rheumatol 4:30, 1985
205. Pisetsky DS, Grudier JP, Gilkeson GS: A role for immunogenic DNA in the pathogenesis of systemic lupus erythematosus. Arthritis Rheum 33:153, 1990
206. Pisetsky DS: Systemic lupus erythematosus. Med Clin North Am 70:337, 1986
207. Tsokos GC, Tsokos M, leRiche NGH et al: A clinical and pathologic study of cerebrovascular disease in patients with systemic lupus erythematosus. Semin Arthritis Rheum 16:70, 1986
208. Kitagawa Y, Goteh F, Koto A et al: Stroke in systemic lupus erythematosus. Stroke 21:1533, 1990

209. Espana A, Gutierrez JM, Soria C et al: Recurrent laryngeal nerve palsy in systemic lupus erythematosus. Neurology 40:1143, 1990
210. Doherty NE, Siegel RJ: Cardiovascular manifestations of systemic lupus erythematosus. Am Heart J 110:1257, 1985
211. Nihoyannopoulos P, Gomez PM, Joshi J et al: Cardiac abnormalities in systemic lupus erythematosus. Circulation 82:369, 1990
212. Crozier IG, Li E, Milne MJ et al: Cardiac involvement in systemic lupus erythematosus detected by echocardiography. Am J Cardiol 65:1145, 1990
213. Leung W-H, Wong K-I, Lau C-P et al: Doppler echocardiographic evaluation of left ventricular diastolic function in patients with systemic lupus erythematosus. Am Heart J 120:82, 1990
214. Klippel JH: Systemic lupus erythematosus. Treatment related complications superimposed on chronic disease. JAMA 263:1812, 1990
215. Jonsson H, Nived O, Sturfelt G: Outcome in systemic lupus erythematosus: A prospective study of patients from a defined population. Medicine 68:141, 1989
216. Mackay IR: Lupoid hepatitis and primary biliary cirrhosis: Autoimmune disease of the liver? Bull Rheum Dis 18:487, 1968
217. Papa MZ, Shiloni E, Vetto JT: Surgical morbidity in patients with systemic lupus erythematosus. Am J Surg 157:295, 1989
218. Kahaleh MB: Vascular disease in scleroderma. Rheum Dis Clin North Am 16:53, 1990
219. Rocco VK, Hurd ER: Scleroderma and scleroderma-like disorders. Semin Arthritis Rheum 16:22, 1986
220. Postlethwaite AE: Early immune events in scleroderma. Rheum Dis Clin North Am 16:125, 1990
221. Silver RM, Miller KS: Lung involvement in systemic sclerosis. Rheum Dis Clin North Am 16:199, 1990
222. Duboc D, Kahan A, Maziere B et al: The effect of nifedipine on myocardial perfusion and metabolism in systemic sclerosis. Arthritis Rheum 34:198, 1991
223. Owens GR, Follansbee WP: Cardiopulmonary manifestations of systemic sclerosis. Chest 91:118, 1987
224. Torres MA, Furst DE: Treatment of generalized systemic sclerosis. Rheum Dis Clin North Am 16:217, 1990
225. Thompson J, Conklin KA: Anesthetic management of a pregnant patient with scleroderma. Anesthesiology 59:69, 1983
226. Ringel RA, Brick JE, Brick JF et al: Muscle involvement in the scleroderma syndromes. Arch Intern Med 150:2550, 1990
227. Richardson JB, Callen JP: Dermatomyositis and malignancy. Med Clin North Am 73:1211, 1989
228. Hochberg MC, Feldman D, Stevens MB: Adult onset polymyositis/dermatomyositis: An analysis of clinical and laboratory features and survival in 76 patients with a review of the literature. Semin Arthritis Rheum 15:168, 1986
229. Park JH, Vansant JP, Kumar NG et al: Dermatomyositis: Correlative MR imaging and P-31MR spectroscopy for quantitative characterization of inflammatory disease. Radiology 177:473, 1990
230. Caro I: Dermatomyositis as a systemic disease. Med Clin North Am 73:1181, 1989
231. Dickey BF, Myers AR: Pulmonary disease in polymyositis/dermatomyositis. Semin Arthritis Rheum 14:60, 1984
232. Tazelaar HD, Viggiano RW, Pickersgill J et al: Interstitial lung disease in polymyositis and dermatomyositis. Am Rev Respir Dis 141:727, 1990
233. Oddis CV, Medsger TA: Current management of polymyositis and dermatomyositis. Drugs 37:382, 1989
234. Eielsen O, Stovner J: Dermatomyositis, suxamethonium action and atypical plasmacholinesterase. Can Anaesth Soc J 25:63, 1978
235. Ganta R, Campbell IT, Mostafa SM: Anaesthesia and acute dermatomyositis/polymyositis. Br J Anaesth 60:854, 1988
236. Downey EC, Woolley MM, Hanson V: Required surgical therapy in the pediatric patient with dermatomyositis. Arch Surg 123:1117, 1988
237. Fine JD: Epidermolysis bullosa. Int J Dermatol 25:143, 1986
238. Fine JD: Antigenic features and structural correlates of basement membranes. Arch Dermatol 124:713, 1988
239. Pearson RW: Clinicopathologic types of epidermolysis bullosa and their nondermatological complications. Arch Dermatol 124:718, 1988
240. Brook MM, Weinhouse E, Jarenwattananon M et al: Dilated cardiomyopathy complicating a case of epidermolysis bullosa dystrophica. Pediatr Dermatol 6:21, 1989
241. Banerjee AK: Mitral valve prolapse in a patient with epidermolysis bullosa. Br J Clin Pract 44:282, 1990
242. Mann JFE, Zeier M, Zilow E et al: The spectrum of renal involvement in epidermolysis bullosa dystrophica hereditaria: Report of two cases. Am J Kidney Dis 11:437, 1988
243. Kern IB, Eisenberg M, Willis S: Management of oesophageal stenosis in epidermolysis bullosa dystrophica. Arch Dis Child 64:551, 1989
244. Broster T, Placek R, Eggers GWN: Epidermolysis bullosa: Anesthetic management for cesarean section. Anesth Analg 66:341, 1987
245. Fisher GC, Ray DAA: Airway obstruction in epidemolysis bullosa. Anaesthesia 44:449, 1989
246. Pratilas V, Biezunski A: Epidermolysis bullosa manifested and treated during anesthesia. Anesthesiology 43:581, 1975
247. Boughton R, Crawford MR, Vonwiller JB: Epidermolysis bullosa—a review of 15 years' experience, including experience with combined general and regional anaesthetic techniques. Anaesth Intens Care 16:260, 1988
248. Wright JT: Comprehensive dental care and general anesthetic management of hereditary epidermolysis bullosa. Oral Surg Oral Med Oral Pathol 70:573, 1990
249. James I, Wark H: Airway management during anesthesia in patients with epidermolysis bullosa dystrophica. Anesthesiology 56:323, 1982
250. Holzman RS, Worthen HM, Johnson K: Anaesthesia for children with junctional epidermolysis bullosa (letalis). Can J Anaesth 34:395, 1987
251. Kaplan R, Strauch B: Regional anesthesia in a child with epidermolysis bullosa. Anesthesiology 67:262, 1987
252. Price T, Katz VT: Obstetrical concerns of epidermolysis bullosa. Obstet Gynecol Surv 43:445, 1988
253. Spargo PM, Smith GB: Epidermolysis bullosa and porphyria. Anaesthesia 44:79, 1989
254. Smith MF: Skin and connective tissue diseases. In Katz J, Steward DJ (eds): Anesthesia and Uncommon Pediatric Diseases, p 378. Philadelphia, WB Saunders, 1987
255. Korman NJ: Pemphigus. Dermatol Clin 8:689, 1989
256. Seidenbaum M, David M, Sandbank M: The course and prognosis of pemphigus. Int J Dermatol 27:580, 1988
257. Vatashsky E, Aronson HB: Pemphigus vulgaris: Anaesthesia in the traumatised patient. Anaesthesia 37:1195, 1982
258. Jeyaram C, Torda TA: Anesthetic management of cholecystectomy in a patient with buccal pemphigus. Anesthesiology 40:600, 1974

23

Henry Rosenberg   Jeffrey Fletcher
David Seitman

Pharmacogenetics

As a result of physiologic, metabolic, or anatomic changes, many inherited disorders have significant implications for anesthetic management. In this chapter we discuss the inherited disorders whose manifestations are enhanced or instigated by drugs usually used by anesthesiologists. In some cases, such as with the porphyrias, the manifestations may be induced by agents other than anesthetics. In contrast, in other enzymatic disorders, e.g., pseudocholinesterase deficiency, it would be extremely unlikely for a patient to have any problems until he or she were exposed to the depolarizing neuromuscular blocking agent succinylcholine. Malignant hyperthermia (MH) or malignant hyperpyrexia is perhaps the most significant inherited disorder that is triggered by exposure to anesthetic drugs.

MALIGNANT HYPERTHERMIA

Malignant hyperthermia was first formally described in 1960 in *Lancet* by Denborough and Lovell and subsequently in *The British Journal of Anaesthesia*.[1,2] That first case report laid the foundation for much of our understanding of the clinical presentations of MH. The patient was a young man who claimed that several of his relatives had died without apparent cause during anesthesia. He was anesthetized with halothane and developed tachycardia, hot sweaty skin, peripheral mottling, and cyanosis. Early recognition and symptomatic treatment saved the patient. It therefore became apparent that this new syndrome had the following elements: patients were otherwise healthy unless exposed to an anesthetic agent; temperature elevation was a hallmark; a heritable or genetic component was present; and a high mortality rate was found. In addition, with early recognition and treatment it was possible to abort the malignant effects of the syndrome.

In the 1960s other cases of MH were reported in increasing numbers, and a gene pool for MH was established in certain parts of the world. In addition, the association between porcine stress syndrome (PSS) or "pale soft exudative pork syndrome" and MH was described, thus providing an animal model for MH.[3] Porcine breeds such as the Landrace, Poland China, and Pietrain show the classic presentations of MH on induction of anesthesia with potent inhalation agents and succinylcholine.

In 1971 the first international symposium on MH was held in Toronto. During the 1970s many more clinical presentations of MH were reported. The development of an *in vitro* diagnostic test was suggested by Kalow *et al* based on exposure of a skeletal muscle biopsy specimen to caffeine and then halothane.[4] In 1975, at the Second International Symposium on Malignant Hyperhermia, Harrison's report showing that dantrolene could be effective in treating and preventing MH in pigs was brought to the attention of those interested in MH.[5] By 1979, a sufficient number of cases were described showing that intravenous dantrolene could successfully reverse the human form of MH, and the drug was approved for use by the Food and Drug Administration. During this decade studies of the pathophysiology of MH were also performed. By the late 1970s, it was apparent that MH most likely resulted from metabolic alterations in skeletal muscle. By the 1980s, regular workshops on MH were held every 2 to 4 years, with an increasing number of investigators becoming interested in this unusual syndrome. In the 1980s, lay organizations in the United States, Canada, and Great Britain were formed to disseminate information to patients affected by MH as well as to enhance awareness of the syndrome among physicians. A registry for MH was created in the United States in the late 1980s. Additional studies of the manifestations of MH and its association with other muscle disorders and the consolidation of our understanding and application of the muscle biopsy diagnostic halothane-caffeine contraction test have taken place in the 1980s. In addition, a variety of other tests for diagnosing MH were introduced, many of which subsequently were found to be of little or no validity.

A major step forward occurred in 1985, when the Lopez group directly demonstrated an increased intracellular concentration of calcium ion in muscle from MH-susceptible pigs and humans.[6] The intracellular calcium concentration dramatically increased during an MH crisis and was reversed by the administration of dantrolene. More widespread appreciation of MH and its clinical manifestations and greater preparedness for treating this potentially fatal but curable disorder occurred in this decade.

In the 1990s sophisticated molecular biologic techniques are being applied to identify the gene(s) for MH. In addition, we anticipate a further reduction in the mortality rate from this syndrome and a better understanding of its pathophysiologic characteristics, which we hope will lead to a less invasive diagnostic test than the one used at present.

Clinical Presentations

As our knowledge and understanding of MH have grown, the definition of MH has changed. At first MH was thought in all cases to be a heritable syndrome consisting of an extremely elevated body temperature, skeletal muscle rigidity, and acidosis associated with a high mortality rate. However, we have now begun to concentrate on the definition of MH in terms of its underlying pathophysiologic characteristics. MH is a hypermetabolic disorder of skeletal muscle with varied presentations, depending on species, breed, and triggering agents. An important pathophysiologic process in this disorder is intracellular hypercalcemia. Intracellular hypercalcemia activates metabolic pathways that if untreated result in adenosine triphosphate depletion, acidosis, membrane destruction, and cell death. Although a heritable component is present in many cases, it is not invariably apparent from patient family history. In addition, disorders that may have symptoms and signs similar to those of MH, such as neuroleptic malignant syndrome, may not have an inherited basis.

Classic Malignant Hyperthermia

Malignant hyperthermia may present in several ways. In almost all cases, the first manifestations of the syndrome occur in the operating room. However, MH also may occur in the recovery room or (rarely) even on return to the patient floor. In the classic case, the initial signs of tachycardia and tachypnea result from sympathetic nervous system stimulation secondary to underlying hypermetabolism and hypercarbia. Because most patients who receive general anesthesia are paralyzed, tachypnea usually is not recognized. Shortly after the increase in heart rate, an increase in blood pressure occurs, often associated with ventricular arrhythmias induced by sympathetic nervous system stimulation from hypercarbia or caused by hyperkalemia or catecholamine release. Thereafter, muscle rigidity or increase in muscle tone may become apparent. Desaturation of the blood in the operative field and then increase in body temperature, climbing at a rate of $1-2°C$ every 5 minutes, follow. With the increase in metabolism, the patient may "break through" the neuromuscular blockade. At the same time, the CO_2 absorbent becomes activated and warm to the touch (because the reaction with CO_2 is exothermic). The patient will display peripheral mottling and, on occasion, sweating and cyanosis. Blood gas analysis usually reveals hypercarbia and respiratory and metabolic acidosis without marked oxygen desaturation. A mixed venous sample will show even more dramatic evidence of CO_2 retention and metabolic acidosis.[7] Hyperkalemia, hypercalcemia, lactacidemia, and myoglobinuria are characteristic. Increase in creatinine phosphokinase levels is dramatic, often exceeding 20,000 units in the first 12–24 hours. Death results unless the syndrome is promptly treated. Even with treatment and survival, the patient is at risk for life-threatening myoglobinuric renal failure and disseminated intravascular coagulation. Another significant clinical problem is recrudescence of the syndrome within the first 24–36 hours.[8]

If succinylcholine is used during induction of anesthesia,

an acceleration of the manifestations of MH may occur such that tachycardia, hypertension, marked temperature elevation, and arrhythmias are seen over the course of 5–10 minutes. However, it is important to note that a completely normal response to succinylcholine may be present in some MH-susceptible patients. A potent inhalation agent apparently is necessary to trigger the syndrome in these cases.

Review of case reports of MH suggests that the syndrome becomes apparent most frequently shortly after anesthesia induction, particularly when succinylcholine is used, and at the end of the procedure as the patient is emerging from anesthesia.

Masseter Muscle Rigidity

Rigidity of the jaw muscles after administration of succinylcholine is referred to as masseter muscle rigidity (MMR). The association of this phenomenon with MH was underlined by many case reports of MMR preceding MH.[9,10] Although MMR probably occurs in patients of all ages, it is distinctly most common in children and young adults. Several studies have shown a peak age incidence at 8–12 years of age.[11] Characteristically, anesthesia is induced by inhalation with halothane, after which succinylcholine is administered. Snapping of the jaw or rigidity upon opening of the jaw is seen. However, this rigidity can be overcome with effort and usually abates within 2–3 minutes. A peripheral nerve stimulator usually reveals flaccid paralysis. However, increased tone of other muscles also may be noted. Repeat doses of succinylcholine do not relieve the problem. Tachycardia and arrhythmias are not infrequent. Only in rare cases does frank MH supervene immediately after MMR. More commonly (if the anesthetic is continued with a triggering agent) in 20 minutes or more the initial signs of MH appear. If the anesthetic is discontinued, the patient usually recovers uneventfully. However, within 4–12 hours, myoglobinuria occurs and creatinine phosphokinase elevation is detected.

Muscle biopsy testing by caffeine-halothane contracture test has shown that approximately 50% of patients who experience MMR are also susceptible to MH.[12] Therefore, most authorities recommend that anesthesia (if elective in nature) be discontinued and surgery postponed after an episode of MMR. With the introduction of end-tidal CO_2 monitoring, the availability of dantrolene, and enhanced understanding of MH, some have questioned the advice that all anesthetics must be discontinued after MMR. Instead, they recommend continuation with nontriggering anesthetics and the use of end-tidal CO_2 monitoring. If such a course is followed, it is nevertheless incumbent upon the anesthesiologist to discuss with the patient further diagnostic tests such as muscle biopsy for MH and to alert him or her to the possibility that MH may follow in subsequent procedures. The issue of whether to give dantrolene after an episode of MMR is also unresolved. It is our clinical impression that administration of dantrolene after MMR will prevent the characteristic myoglobinuria and marked elevation of creatinine phosphokinase. Recent reports indicate that when MMR is accompanied by rigidity of chest or limb, MH is more likely to follow than after isolated jaw rigidity.[13]

The differential diagnosis of MMR consists of (1) myotonic syndrome, (2) temporomandibular joint dysfunction, (3) underdosing with succinylcholine, or (4) not allowing sufficient time for succinylcholine to act before intubation. Signs of temporomandibular dysfunction as well as myotonia should be looked for in the postoperative period. Otherwise, patients need to be counseled regarding the need for a muscle biopsy and other diagnostic tests for MH.

If MMR were a rare phenomenon, it would be troublesome enough. However, based on several recent studies, this sign may occur in as many as 1 in 100 children anesthetized with halothane and given succinylcholine.[14] A third study based on the information supplied to the Danish Malignant Hyperthermia Registry showed that the incidence of MMR was 1 in 12,000 (including adults and children).[15] The discordance between the incidence of MH, which is felt to be in the range of 1 in 10,000–50,000 anesthetic administrations, and the higher incidence of MMR in children may relate to the following: (1) the retrospective nature of the studies, (2) a greater susceptibility to MH in the younger age groups, (3) a peculiarity of the innervation or muscle structure of children, (4) a peculiarity of the masseter muscle itself, and (5) false-positive results from the contracture test.

A variety of reports have shown that succinylcholine increases jaw muscle tone in all patients.[16] This normal agonistic effect of succinylcholine may account for some cases of MMR. The pathophysiology of jaw muscle tone increase is unknown.

Our advice regarding MMR is as follows:[17] (1) when it occurs, the anesthesiologist should, if at all possible, discontinue the anesthetic and postpone surgery. If end-tidal CO_2 monitoring and dantrolene are available and the anesthesiologist is experienced in managing MH, he or she may elect to continue with a nontriggering anesthetic. (2) After episodes of MMR, the patient should be observed carefully for a period of 12–24 hours. Administration of one to two $mg \cdot kg^{-1}$ of dantrolene should be considered. (3) The family should be informed of the episode of MMR and its implications. (4) Creatinine phosphokinase levels should be checked at 6, 12, and 24 hours after the episode. If the creatinine phosphokinase level is still grossly elevated at 12 hours, additional samples should be drawn until it begins to return to normal. Our recent studies have shown that if the creatinine phosphokinase level is greater than 20,000 IU in the perioperative period and a concomitant myopathy is not present, the diagnosis of MH can be made with virtual certainty.[18] (5) If muscle biopsy testing results are within normal limits after an episode of MMR, we currently do not recommend that other family members undergo testing but we advise that succinylcholine be avoided in future anesthetics for that patient.

A recent study by Littleford et al[11] has shown that acidosis and rhabdomyolysis occur after anesthesia is continued with an inhalation agent after MMR, although fulminant MH may not occur. To date, MMR has been documented only in association with succinylcholine, although it may occur after induction with any anesthetic agent, intravenous or inhalation, before succinylcholine administration. As such, many pediatric anesthesiologists avoid the use of succinylcholine except on specific indication. It is also of interest that a thiobarbiturate induction will greatly decrease the incidence of MMR.[19]

Other Presentations of Malignant Hyperthermia

Malignant hyperthermia may occur not only in the operating room but also in the early postoperative period, usually within the first few hours of recovery from anesthesia.

The characteristic tachycardia, tachypnea, hypertension, and arrhythmias indicate that an episode of MH may be about to follow. Isolated myoglobinuria in the postoperative period should also alert the anesthesiologist that a problem has occurred. Succinylcholine may cause rhabdomyolysis in patients who have other muscle disorders that may not be clinically obvious on cursory examination.[20] The presence of myoglobinuria mandates that the patient be referred to a neurologist for further investigation.

Neuroleptic Malignant Syndrome and Other Disorders Associated With Malignant Hyperthermia

The symptoms and signs of the neuroleptic malignant syndrome include fever, rhabdomyolysis, tachycardia, hypertension, agitation, muscle rigidity, and acidosis.[21] The mortality rate is about 20%. Dantrolene is an effective therapeutic modality in many cases of neuroleptic malignant syndrome. Therefore, it is not unusual for an anesthesiologist to be consulted in the management of patients with this disorder.

Although the resemblance of neuroleptic malignant syndrome to MH is striking, there are significant differences between the two. MH is acute, whereas neuroleptic malignant syndrome occurs after longer term drug exposure. Phenothiazines and haloperidol alone or in combination are usually triggering agents for neuroleptic malignant syndrome. Sudden withdrawal of drugs used to treat Parkinson's disease may also trigger neuroleptic malignant syndrome. Electroconvulsive therapy with succinylcholine does not appear to trigger the syndrome.[22] Also, neuroleptic malignant syndrome does not seem to be inherited, and there are no case reports of it in family members who have had an episode of MH.

Many believe that the changes in neuroleptic malignant syndrome are a reflection of dopamine depletion in the central nervous system by psychoactive agents. In support of this theory, therapy with bromocriptine, a dopamine agonist, is often useful in treatment of neuroleptic malignant syndrome.[23] Therefore, although there appear to be similarities between MH and neuroleptic malignant syndrome,[24] the common basis is not readily apparent. From an anesthesiologist's viewpoint, it is best to treat patients with neuroleptic malignant syndrome as though they were susceptible to MH until additional information is obtained, and to conduct electroconvulsive therapy without the use of succinylcholine or other triggering agents of MH.

Duchenne's muscular dystrophy and other muscular dystrophies have also been linked to MH. Some patients with Duchenne's muscular dystrophy who are anesthetized with MH-triggering agents (with or without succinylcholine) experience sudden cardiac arrest during surgery or in the very early postoperative period. Hyperkalemia, acidosis, and temperature elevation are usually seen.[25] In others, significant rhabdomyolysis occurs in the early postoperative period, which leads to muscle weakness and early death.[26] In a series of 10 muscle biopsy specimens from patients with Duchenne's muscular dystrophy and patients with a similar disorder, Becker's dystrophy, approximately 50% showed the typical halothane contractures in vitro that are observed in MH-susceptible patients.[27] Therefore, MH-triggering agents should not be used in patients with Duchenne's muscular dystrophy and related dystrophies. Dantrolene may worsen muscle weakness and should be given with caution.

Central core disease is an unusual myopathy characterized by muscle weakness. It is probably inherited in a recessive manner. Many cases of MH have been reported in patients with central core disease. Therefore, precautions regarding MH must be taken for all patients with central core disease.[28]

Another myopathy associated with MH is myotonia congenita. Only a few cases of MH have been reported in patients with myotonia congenita, far fewer than would be expected if there were a high coincidence of susceptibility to MH in such patients.

King or King-Denborough syndrome is a rare myopathy characterized by cryptorchidism, markedly slanted eyes, low-set ears, pectus deformity, scoliosis, small stature, and hypotonia. Several patients with this disorder have been diagnosed as MH-susceptible both clinically and by muscle biopsy.[29] Schwartz-Jampal syndrome, a myotonic-like condition, is also associated with MH.

One of the few metabolic disorders associated with MH is osteogenesis imperfecta.[30] Here again the association is sporadic. Despite a few well-documented cases of MH in patients with osteogenesis imperfecta, we have not confirmed MH susceptibility in three cases of osteogenesis imperfecta tested with the halothane-caffeine contracture test but have found typical contractures in one other biopsy.

Denborough et al have speculated that patients with MH are more likely to have offspring at risk for sudden infant death syndrome.[31] This observation needs further confirmation and investigation.

Pheochromocytoma may be mistaken for MH because of its presentation by tachycardia, hypertension, and fever during anesthesia. However, pheochromocytoma does not predispose to MH.[32]

Malignant Hyperthermia Outside the Operating Room

The concern that MH may occur outside the operating room without mediation of drugs in humans has been expressed repeatedly. This concern derives from the often repeated observation that an MH-like syndrome can occur in certain pig breeds in response to stressful situations. However, documented cases of fulminant MH occurring without drug intervention in humans have not been convincing. Gronert et al have described a patient who had episodic fevers and whose muscle biopsies tested positive for MH.[33] The fevers were controlled by dantrolene. Recently, Fishbein et al reported on two young patients who had apparent heat stroke and were also MH-susceptible.[34]

Some also believe that MH-susceptible patients are likely to die suddenly,[35] but the evidence is not convincing. Detailed information usually is not available regarding the medical history of young people who die suddenly and unexpectedly. Was there evidence of a recent infection? What were the results of previous medical examinations, drug levels, and other tests? Studies of sudden death in young people have found that infection and unrecognized cardiac disease account for more than half the causes of such death. Often the symptoms of such problems either are mild and not recognized or are ignored. About 10% of sudden unexpected deaths in healthy young adults result from a cerebral bleed, 25% from asthma and epilepsy, and about 15% from undetermined causes. Neuspiel and Kuller state that "both clinicians and coroners or medical examiners may have biased perceptions about sudden death in this age group."[36]

A great deal of debate and very few data characterize the discussions regarding sudden death and MH. A more widespread, easier to use diagnostic test and a better understanding of the pathophysiologic characteristics of MH are necessary to resolve this issue.

Drugs That Trigger Malignant Hyperthermia

It is clearly established that the potent inhalation agents, including methoxyflurane, cyclopropane, and ether, may trigger MH. Succinylcholine and decamethonium are also triggers. The status of many other drugs is less clear. Table 23-1 indicates the drugs we believe to be safe vs. those that are unsafe.

Local Anesthetics

Based on studies indicating that amide or ester local anesthetics do not trigger MH in susceptible swine and that amide local anesthetics do not trigger MH in susceptible humans, it seems clear that all local anesthetics are safe for MH-susceptible patients.[37,38] Preliminary studies of local anesthetics during an MH crisis (e.g., for arrhythmia control) do not show an exacerbation of MH by amide local anesthetics.

Catecholamines

Although plasma catecholamine concentration increases during an MH crisis, such an elevation is usually secondary to metabolic and cardiovascular changes. Sympathetic denervation by spinal anesthesia does not delay the onset of halothane-induced MH in susceptible pigs.[39] Other data also support the contention that vasopressors and other catecholamines are not involved in triggering MH.[40] Therefore, these drugs should be used as necessary but only with simultaneous treatment of the MH crisis.

Nondepolarizing Relaxants

Although curare is a suspected trigger of MH,[41] vecuronium, atracurium, pancuronium, and all other nondepolarizing drugs are considered safe to use in patients with MH.

TABLE 23-1. Safe Versus Unsafe Drugs in Malignant Hyperthermia

Unsafe Drugs	Safe Drugs
All inhalation agents (except nitrous oxide)	Althesin
Succinylcholine	Antibiotics
Potassium salts	Antihistamines
	Antipyretics
Insufficient Data/Controversial	Atracurium
	Barbiturates
Curare	Benzodiazepines
Phenothiazines	Droperidol
	Ketamine
	Local anesthetics
	Opioids
	Nitrous oxide
	Pancuronium
	Propofol
	Propranolol
	Vasoactive drugs
	Vecuronium

Anticholinesterases

Clinical studies have shown that anticholinesterase-anticholinergic combinations are safe for reversal of nondepolarizing relaxants in MH-susceptible patients.[42]

Phenothiazines

Phenothiazines increase intracellular calcium ion concentration and may cause contractures in vitro in muscle from MH-susceptible patients.[43] Phenothiazines also induce the related neuroleptic malignant syndrome. Therefore, although there have been several reports that phenothiazines are effective in managing temperature fluctuations during recovery from MH, these compounds should be used cautiously if at all in MH-susceptible patients.

Other Drugs

Digoxin, quinidine, and calcium salts do not induce MH in the swine caudal preparation.[44] Therefore, it is reasonable to assume that they are safe to use in clinical situations. However, potassium salts can trigger MH. This results from a depolarization of the muscle membrane, leading to muscle contracture. Neither ketamine nor propofol are MH triggers.[45]

Droperidol also seems to be safe, based on clinical experience and in vitro studies.[46]

Incidence and Epidemiology

Although the incidence of reported episodes of MH has increased, the mortality rate from MH has declined. In part these two trends reflect a greater awareness of the syndrome, earlier diagnosis, and better therapy. The incidence of MH varies from country to country, based on differences in gene pools. In the upper midwest of the United States, for example, there are many families containing large numbers of MH susceptibles. In contrast, other areas of the country and parts of the world have rarely reported MH. The overall incidence is said to be 1 in 50,000 anesthetics administered in adults and 1 in 15,000 anesthetics administered in children.[47] Results of large-scale studies of operative mortality are in general agreement with this figure. For example, a recent study in Great Britain revealed three cases of MH in 100,000 administered anesthetics. One of the better studies concerning the epidemiologic characteristics of MH is that of Ording.[15] Her study, based on information supplied to the Danish Malignant Hyperthermia Registry comprising the reported incidence of MH in the approximately 5,000,000 population in Denmark, revealed fulminant MH in approximately 1 in 250,000 administered anesthetics. However, if the definition of MH is expanded to include abortive cases of MH and is further refined to include only cases in which inhalation anesthetics and succinylcholine were used, the incidence was as high as 1 in 4000 anesthetic administrations!

Currently, the consensus is that the mortality from MH is approximately 10%. Indeed, the Malignant Hyperthermia Association of the United States is generally notified of two to four deaths from MH during the course of a year. However, the epidemiologic characteristics of MH are very difficult to define for the following reasons:

1. Widespread diagnostic testing for MH is difficult to apply.

2. The clinical diagnosis of MH is often questionable.
3. Triggering of MH even in susceptible patients may not occur upon an individual anesthetic exposure. In some cases susceptible patients have received triggering agents for up to 13 anesthetics without any problems, only to have MH triggered on the subsequent anesthetic.
4. A new central reporting agency for MH (the North American MH Registry) has only recently been established.
5. Triggering agent use varies among countries. Organizations such as the Malignant Hyperthermia Association (of Canada) as well as the Malignant Hyperthermia Association of the United States are in the process of creating central registries for the reporting of MH cases.

A better diagnostic test and better reporting of MH will certainly enhance our knowledge of the incidence of this syndrome.

Inheritance of Malignant Hyperthermia

Many of the reasons that limit our understanding of the epidemiologic characteristics of MH also limit our accurate assessment of its inheritance. It would seem that studies of the animal model would clarify the issue of inheritance, but this has not been the case. In certain reports the inheritance appears to be autosomal dominant,[48] whereas in others it is clearly autosomal recessive.[49] This difference may result from differences in breeds. In at least four breeds of swine, MH is quite common. Even in pigs, the breeding experiments may fail to clarify inheritance because the diagnosis of MH in swine is often based on the animal's exposure to 3–6% halothane by mask and observation of a clinical response. However, this test does not detect all those animals that are susceptible.[50] Variabilities in clinical presentation and the fact that MH is not regularly apparent on exposure to triggering agents, even in those that are susceptible, result in great difficulty in assessing the inheritance of MH in humans. The inheritance of MH in humans has been described as autosomal dominant, multifactorial, autosomal dominant with variable penetrance, and multigenetic.[51]

Our studies, as well as anecdotal reports from other diagnostic centers, have supported the concept of autosomal dominant inheritance by a single gene with variable penetrance. Representative examples of such clinical documentation of autosomal dominance are as follows.

1. A 34-year-old man died of the classic MH syndrome. Although his father had a history of ptosis, he had MH-negative results on muscle biopsy. His mother was too ill to have a biopsy performed. A maternal cousin was found to be MH-susceptible on the contracture test, as was his maternal uncle.
2. A 4-year-old child developed masseter rigidity during anesthesia with succinylcholine, with a postepisode level of creatinine phosphokinase of 8000 IU. Her two siblings had negative muscle biopsy results; however, her mother had MH-positive results. None of the children had had anesthesia previously.
3. An 8-year-old boy developed masseter rigidity with creatinine phosphokinase level elevation after receiving succinylcholine. His father stated that his own father had died of hyperthermia during surgery years

previously. The father was MH-susceptible on contracture testing.

Studies of large families have also documented an autosomal dominant pattern. McPherson and Taylor studied 93 families in whom MH occurred.[51] Although MH was often diagnosed by inference, based on creatinine phosphokinase elevations as well as clinical histories and in some cases contracture testing, various patterns of inheritance did emerge.

We therefore advise patients that 50% of siblings and 50% of children of the MH-susceptible patients are potentially at risk for this disorder. Although baseline creatinine phosphokinase determinations may be of no value in screening for MH, McPherson and Taylor reported that relatives of MH-susceptible patients with an elevated creatinine phosphokinase level (without recent trauma or muscle disorder) have a higher than 80% chance of being susceptible. However, relatives with a normal creatinine phosphokinase level may also be susceptible.

In cases of MH associated with a myopathy such as Duchenne's muscular dystrophy, it is not clear whether MH is a manifestation of the underlying myopathy—and therefore that those in a family who do not have evidence of a myopathy are not susceptible to MH—or whether the MH susceptibility is inherited apart from the myopathy—and therefore other family members may be at risk for MH.

Diagnostic Tests for Malignant Hyperthermia

In 1970, Kalow *et al* demonstrated that isolated muscle from MH-susceptible patients behaved abnormally in response to caffeine when tested *in vitro*.[4] Shortly thereafter, investigators demonstrated that muscle from MH-susceptible patients responded in an abnormal fashion to halothane. Although others have shown that potassium chloride, thymol, other inhalation anesthetic agents, and succinylcholine can induce greater contractures in muscle from MH-susceptible patients than from those who are nonsusceptible, treatment of muscle biopsy specimens with halothane, caffeine, and/or the combination has come to be the standard test for diagnosing MH susceptibility.[52]

Other tests have been proposed to differentiate patients with MH from those who are normal. Some tests use skeletal muscle biopsy specimens, such as the test that measures adenosine triphosphate concentration in isolated muscle after incubation with 4% halothane, whereas others employ blood elements such as platelets or white blood cells to determine susceptibility. Other less invasive tests also have been suggested to differentiate the MH-susceptible population, such as the twitch response to stimulation of the ulnar nerve during a period of tourniquet-induced ischemia. None of these tests are of value in determining MH status.

Tests That Have No Real Value in Diagnosis of Malignant Hyperthermia

Blood Tests. Hypotonic red blood cell lysis may help differentiate MH-susceptible swine from nonsusceptible swine. However, this test is not valid in humans.[53] Studies performed with red blood cells incubated with or without drugs have not shown any difference in hypotonic lysis between susceptible and nonsusceptible patients.

Creatinine Phosphokinase Tests. Creatinine phosphokinase determinations may be valuable in differentiating MH-susceptible swine populations.[54] However, this is not the case in humans. Creatinine phosphokinase is only useful in relatives of patients known to be susceptible to MH; in that instance, an elevated creatinine phosphokinase level predicts MH susceptibility with an approximate 70–80% accuracy rate. A normal creatinine phosphokinase level is not predictive.

Platelet Nucleotide Depletion Tests. Platelets from patients susceptible to MH were reported to have a greatly reduced energy concentration ratio (ATP + APD/hypoxanthine + AMP) compared with those from normal patients.[55] Several studies have failed to validate this test.[56]

Tests Using Skeletal Muscle Biopsy Specimens. Assay of the enzyme adenylate kinase was suggested as a possible marker for MH susceptibility. This has not been substantiated. Similarly, it was reported that myophosphorylase concentrations are elevated in susceptible patients, but this was not confirmed.[57]

Calcium Uptake and Calcium Adenosine Triphosphatase in Frozen Muscle. The advantage of this test was that samples could be frozen in liquid nitrogen and shipped to a laboratory that could perform this assay.[58] However, other studies have found that calcium uptake, as well as calcium adenosine triphosphatase, in frozen thin muscle sections does not differentiate MH-susceptible from nonsusceptible patients.[59] A double-blind study of 29 patients in whom the diagnosis of MH was made by halothane-contracture test versus the calcium uptake test showed a large number of false-positive results by the uptake test.

Skinned Fiber Tests. In this test isolated muscle cells are dissected, the membrane is disrupted either mechanically or chemically, and the response to caffeine is assessed in single fibers.[60] The advantage of the test is that muscle can be stored and shipped for analysis. However, the test is tedious and has technical difficulties. Testing with halothane cannot be performed either. At present, its results can only be considered supportive of the diagnosis by the standard halothane-caffeine contracture test.

Proteins in Malignant Hyperthermia. An abnormal protein in MH muscle was reported by one group.[61] However, subsequent studies have failed to confirm this finding.[62]

Less Invasive Tests. Enhanced response of the thenar muscles on stimulation of the ulnar nerve during a period of tourniquet ischemia was suggested to be a valid way of differentiating MH-susceptible from nonsusceptible patients. This finding also has not been substantiated by other investigators.[63]

Measurement of intracellular calcium release from white blood cells *in vitro* is also not a reliable test for MH.[64]

New Tests for Malignant Hyperthermia

We have recently reported that the ratio of inorganic phosphate to phosphocreatine is enhanced in MH-susceptible patients. Intracellular ratios of inorganic phosphate to phosphocreatine are measured easily by nuclear magnetic resonance spectrometry.[65] However, special equipment and personnel are necessary to perform this test. Other reports have suggested, based on nuclear magnetic resonance spectrometry, that recovery of adenosine triphosphate after exercise is delayed in MH-susceptible patients.

Although Lopez et al[6] have elegantly demonstrated that intracellular calcium concentration is elevated in muscle from MH-susceptible swine and further enhanced by exposure to halothane, this observation has not reached a practical level for introduction as a diagnostic test.

Halothane-Caffeine Contracture Test. This test is simple in concept and uncomplicated in operation.[66] Skeletal muscle is usually obtained from the vastus lateralis muscle by biopsy. Strips of muscle weighing approximately 100 mg and measuring 1–2 cm in length by 2–5 mm in width by 1–4 mm in thickness are cut and mounted in a standard muscle bath apparatus (Fig. 23-1). The tissue bath usually contains a modified Krebs solution at 37°C bubbled with O_2 and CO_2 (95%/5%), and the resting tension is adjusted to 2 g. The bundles are stimulated supramaximally with pulses of a frequency of 0.2 Hz for 2–10 milliseconds. After a 30-minute equilibration of CO_2/O_2, halothane is added to the mixture and the concentration is checked chromatographically.

Other strips are exposed to caffeine (see below). In our laboratory, patients are judged MH-susceptible when a contracture in one of the eight strips tested is greater than or equal to 0.7 g within a 5-minute exposure to 3% halothane[67] (Fig. 23-2) or greater than 0.5 g after exposure to 1–2% halothane. The European Malignant Hyperthermia Group has modified this halothane contracture test somewhat.[68] In this modification, the muscle is exposed to incremental doses of halothane and a contracture >0.2 g at a concentration of ≤2% halothane is considered abnormal. The halothane concentration is increased with each subsequent cycle.

The Caffeine Contracture Test. In the caffeine contracture test the muscle strips are mounted as already described. After a 30-minute equilibration period, strips are exposed to incremental concentrations of caffeine (0.125–16 mM) at twofold intervals. Two diagnostic criteria have been used in assessing the response to caffeine. The caffeine-specific concentration refers to that concentration that causes a 1-g contracture in the absence of halothane, based on a plot of the contracture response to incremental doses of caffeine. The second criterion is a contracture greater than or equal to 0.3 g to 2 mM caffeine. The latter is felt to be more accurate.

Halothane Plus Caffeine Contracture Test. This test is similar to the caffeine contracture test but is done in the presence of 1% halothane.

In our laboratory almost all MH-susceptible patients develop significant contractures on halothane exposure alone. Far fewer respond to caffeine alone. Indeed, false-negative results with a caffeine test only can be as high as 75%. Nevertheless, some patients display an abnormality on caffeine exposure but a normal response to halothane. Therefore, both tests should be used. The test combining halothane and caffeine has generated a great deal of controversy.[69] Patients whose muscle responds in a normal fashion to halothane and caffeine but in an enhanced fashion to the combination of halothane and caffeine have been termed as having "K" phenotypes. It has been hypothesized that patients with a K phenotype may respond to MH-triggering agents in a fashion similar to MH-susceptible patients but with a slower response. Through selective breeding, Nelson et al have identified pigs whose muscle responds in a manner that would correspond to a K phenotype. On exposure to halothane and after repeated doses of succinylcholine, serum lactate levels increase, pH levels decrease, and CO_2 excretion levels increase in these

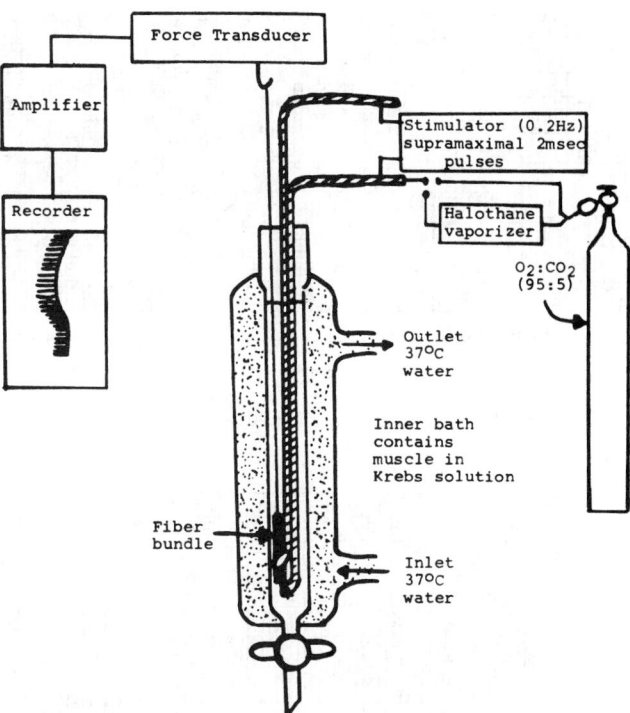

Figure 23-1. Diagram of the muscle bath apparatus used for contracture testing for diagnosing MH susceptibility.

animals.[70] However, gross fulminant MH is not observed. Studies using human tissue have shown that the contracture response of the K type can be found in up to 20% of the control population. Clearly this test variant will falsely diagnose many as MH-susceptible.

Pitfalls in the Contracture Test. Although at the present time more than 20 centers employ the caffeine-halothane contracture test for diagnosing MH, the criteria for differentiating susceptible from nonsusceptible patients are not always uniform among centers.

Incubation time, bath size, stimulation characteristics, and methods of introduction of halothane and caffeine are slightly different among centers. Most important, each laboratory needs to derive specimens from patients who are clearly and unequivocally normal and those who are clearly and unequivocally MH-susceptible. Unfortunately, it is not always possible to have complete agreement on the MH status of a patient. If an investigator determines the criteria for susceptibility in cases that are not unequivocally MH, a significant percentage of false-positive results can be reported. Recently North American Biopsy Centers and those in Europe have agreed upon a standard protocol and testing for MH and employ similar equipment and similar techniques.[71] This has facilitated the interchange of information and the creation of a larger pool of data for use in differentiating MH-susceptible from nonsusceptible patients. Within a short time, it is expected that well-defined criteria for differentiating MH will be established. A preliminary finding based on pooled data from many centers reveals a sensitivity of >96% and specificity of >80% for the contracture test. These are quite acceptable values.

One of the main problems in MH testing is that, rather than two separate groups being discernible on halothane-caffeine testing, instead there is a continuum of responses.[66] Susceptibility is determined by a response above or below

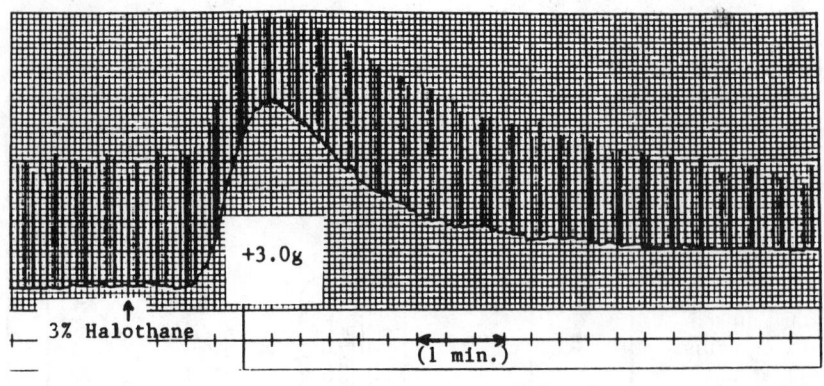

Abnormal Halothane Contracture

Figure 23-2. Muscle strips weighing approximately 150 mg and stimulated supramaximally are exposed to 3% halothane or incremental doses of caffeine. (*A*) A 3-g contracture is recorded from this strip from an MHS patient after exposure of the muscle to 3% halothane (*top*); a normal response to 3% halothane (*bottom*). (*B*) Contractures noted after exposure to 0.5, 1, and 2 mm caffeine in MHS muscle (*top*); no contracture response to the same caffeine concentrations. Twitch height augmentation is normal following caffeine addition (*bottom*).

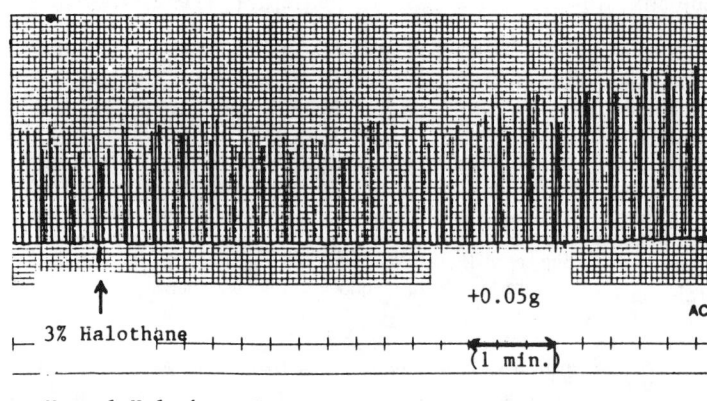

A   **Normal Halothane Contracture**

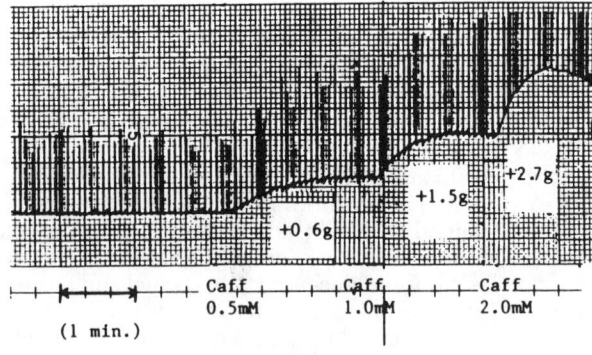

Abnormal Caffeine Dose Response

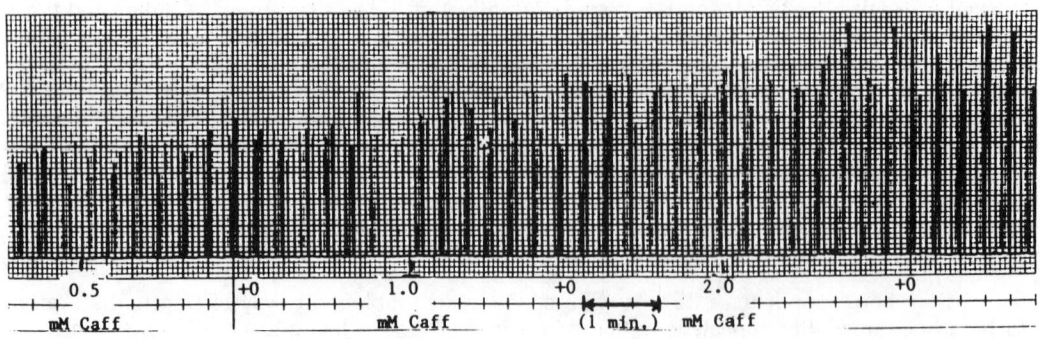

B   **Normal Caffeine Dose Response**

a certain threshold. In addition, there may be variability between individual strips from the same biopsy specimen. A recent estimate from our laboratory showed that only 52% of fiber bundles from patients diagnosed as MH-susceptible exhibited a positive response to halothane, whereas less than 25% of the strips tested positive for caffeine in biopsy specimens from 11 of 39 MH-susceptible patients. Therefore, to prevent sampling errors, it is best to test at least six strips for each patient. On the positive side, however, contracture response of 1 g to halothane alone is uniformly recognized as indicating MH susceptibility in all laboratories. Furthermore, there are no reported incidences of a patient who has been diagnosed as MH-negative by contracture testing who has subsequently experienced clinical episodes of MH. We have recently reported on 14 patients who were diagnosed as MH-negative by contracture testing and were exposed to halothane and succinylcholine without incident.[72]

Until such time as the basic biochemical defect of MH is uncovered, the halothane-caffeine contracture test will always be subject to differences in interpretation. However, the halothane-caffeine contracture test is currently the only diagnostic test for MH that has been confirmed in any manner by multiple centers throughout the world. We recommend that laboratories continue to do the halothane-caffeine contracture test but that they test with 3% halothane alone along with testing with caffeine alone. It is also necessary for each laboratory to establish its own controls and definitions of susceptibility, based on correlations with clinical events as well as standards of other laboratories.

Treatment of Malignant Hyperthermia

Malignant hyperthermia is a treatable disorder. If it is diagnosed early and treated promptly with proper continuing observation, the mortality rate should be close to zero. All institutions in which anesthetic agents are administered should have dantrolene available (36 ampules, i.e., 720 mg is recommended) and have a plan of management.

The Acute Episode

The following steps should be taken immediately when MH is diagnosed: (1) Administration of all inhalation agents and succinylcholine should be discontinued. (2) Hyperventilation with 100% oxygen should be instituted at high flow rates, and assistance should be secured. (It is usually helpful to have a cart available containing the agents for treatment of MH.) (3) Assistance should be obtained in mixing dantrolene. The present preparation of dantrolene is poorly soluble. Each ampule containing 20 mg should be mixed with 50 ml of sterile distilled water (not saline solution). Initial intravenous therapy should be started with a minimum dose of 2.5 mg·kg^{-1}, with repeat doses as needed.[73] Although it is often recommended that the maximum dose of dantrolene is 10 mg·kg^{-1}, more should be given as dictated by clinical circumstances. (4) Titration of dantrolene and bicarbonate to heart rate, body temperature, and Paco$_2$ is the best clinical guideline of therapy. (5) In fulminant cases in which significant metabolic acidosis is present, 2–4 mEq·kg^{-1} bicarbonate should be given. (6) If it is not already available, a capnometer should be obtained so that CO$_2$ excretion can be followed. (7) If at all possible, the anesthesia circuit and CO$_2$ absorbent should be changed because residual inhala-

tion anesthetics may contaminate the anesthesia circuit. If not, very high flows of oxygen should be used. (8) Dysrhythmia control usually follows hyperventilation, dantrolene therapy, and correction of acidosis. Calcium channel blocking agents should be avoided because they may induce hyperkalemia in the presence of dantrolene.[74] (9) Body temperature elevation should be managed by packing the patient with external ice packs and by use of gastric, wound, and rectal lavage. Gastric lavage is the quickest, most practical means for rapid temperature control. Some have recommended peritoneal dialysis and others cardiopulmonary bypass. Cooling should be stopped when body temperature reaches approximately 38°C to avoid hypothermia. (10) Although arterial blood gas determinations are useful for assessing acidosis, central mixed venous blood gas determinations (or, if not available, femoral venous blood gas readings) serve as a better guideline for therapy. Mixed venous CO$_2$ tension will be elevated and is a more appropriate measure of hypermetabolism. (11) Hyperkalemia should be managed in the usual fashion. The use of Ca^{2+} for acute treatment of hyperkalemia has not been investigated. During therapy of MH, hypokalemia frequently results. However, potassium replacement should be undertaken very cautiously, if at all, because potassium may retrigger an MH episode.

Ca^{2+} channel blockers should not be used in the acute treatment of MH, particularly when dantrolene is administered.[74] Several studies have shown that verapamil may interact with dantrolene to produce hyperkalemia and myocardial depression.

Management After the Acute Episode

After the acute episode, the clinician should be concerned about three complications of MH:

1. *Recrudescence of MH.* Although most cases of MH resolve promptly with therapy, some cases are difficult to control. Temperature fluctuations may occur for several days, and acute recrudescence may occur within hours of the first episode.[75]

2. *Disseminated intravascular coagulation.*[76] Disseminated intravascular coagulation has often been described in cases of MH, probably resulting from release of thromboplastins secondary to shock and/or release of cellular contents upon membrane destruction. The usual regimen for treatment of disseminated intravascular coagulation should be followed.

3. *Myoglobinuric renal failure.* Creatinine phosphokinase elevations may not occur for 6–12 hours after an MH episode and should be followed as a rough guide for therapy. However, myoglobinuria classically occurs within 4–8 hours of the episode; therefore, bladder catheterization is recommended. The guidelines for the dose and duration of dantrolene therapy after resolution of acute MH are empiric. It would seem prudent to continue dantrolene, 1–2 mg·kg^{-1} every 4 hours intravenously, for at least 24–36 hours. Some recommend conversion of dantrolene therapy from intravenous to oral form (4 mg·kg^{-1} per day or more) with continuation for several days.

Significant muscle weakness may follow MH, resulting from muscle destruction along with dantrolene administration; this should be managed symptomatically.

A variety of other electrolyte changes may occur, such as hypocalcemia and hyperphosphatemia. Sodium and chloride changes may occur secondary to fluid shifts during the acute episode. All these changes usually respond to control of the acute episode.

Dantrolene

In 1979 intravenous dantrolene was approved by the Food and Drug Administration for treatment of MH. Until that time, the primary use of dantrolene was in the management of spasticity. Dantrolene is a unique muscle relaxant. Unlike neuromuscular blocking agents (whose site of action is at the nicotinic receptor of the neuromuscular junction) or the nonspecific relaxants (which modulate spinal cord synaptic reflexes), dantrolene operates within the muscle cell itself by reducing intracellular levels of calcium. Most likely this results from a reduction of calcium release of sarcoplasmic reticulum or inhibition of excitation contracture coupling at the transverse tubular level. It has now been demonstrated that during an MH episode, dantrolene reduces intracellular calcium levels. Therefore, dantrolene is a specific and effective agent in the treatment of MH. In the usual clinical doses, dantrolene has little effect on myocardial contractility.[77]

Studies have also indicated that doses of neuromuscular blocking agents need not be changed significantly after dantrolene administration. However, the drug should be used cautiously in patients with neuromuscular disease.[78]

The serum level of dantrolene required for prophylaxis against MH is about 2.5 $\mu g \cdot ml^{-1}$. The half-life of intravenous dantrolene, which is the only form recommended, is approximately 12 hours. However, the therapeutic level of dantrolene usually persists for 4–6 hours after a usual intravenous dose of 2.5 $mg \cdot kg^{-1}$.[79] Therefore, dantrolene should be supplemented approximately every 4 hours after a clinical episode. Some muscle weakness may persist for 24 hours after dantrolene therapy is discontinued. Nausea and phlebitis are other complications of dantrolene administration. Hepatotoxicity has been demonstrated only with long-term use of oral dantrolene. Prophylaxis for MH should be carried out with intravenous or oral dantrolene (5 $mg \cdot kg^{-1}$ per 24 h).[80]

Management of the Patient Susceptible to Malignant Hyperthermia

Because of an increasing awareness of MH and more widespread use of diagnostic tests, it is not unusual for an anesthesiologist to be confronted with an MH-susceptible patient or a patient who has a family history of MH. The management of such patients should be carefully planned.

In the preoperative interview, the anesthesiologist should try to obtain sufficient information regarding previous episodes of MH and their documentation. The anesthesiologist should allow adequate time to reassure the patient and his or her family that he or she is familiar with MH and its implications and that appropriate prophylaxis and therapy will be instituted as necessary. It may be worth mentioning that there have been no deaths from MH in previously diagnosed MH-susceptible patients when the anesthesia team was aware of the problem. Some believe that anxiety may predispose a patient to MH and therefore recommend that anxiolytic agents be included in the premedication. Standard premedicant drugs such as opioids, benzodiazepines, ataractics, barbiturates, and antihistamines do not cause problems in MH-susceptible patients when administered in appropriate doses; however, we do not recommend phenothiazines for premedication. Anticholinergics are also used routinely.

Intravenous dantrolene sodium, 2.5 $mg \cdot kg^{-1}$, should be administered to those who have experienced an episode of MH. In others, dantrolene may be withheld provided that end-expired CO_2 is monitored and dantrolene is immediately available.[81] Although dantrolene may cause nausea and vomiting and, in some cases, complaints of pain at the injection site, patients should have no significant discomfort with the usual dose.

The anesthesia machine is prepared by draining or removing vaporizors, changing tubing and CO_2 absorbent, and flowing oxygen at 10 $l \cdot min^{-1}$ for 20 minutes.[82] Obviously, iced solutions and adequate supplies of dantrolene must be available in the vicinity of the operating room when MH-susceptible patients are anesthetized.

Exhaled CO_2 should be monitored because the earliest sign of MH is an increase in CO_2 production and excretion.[83] In the absence of capnography, arterial blood gas monitoring is recommended. Arterial and central venous monitoring is recommended for MH-susceptible patients, as dictated by the surgical procedure. Body temperature should be monitored by nasopharyngeal, rectal, or esophageal routes in all patients for all surgical procedures. Studies comparing skin temperature with core temperature during an MH crisis are lacking, but other studies have shown that forehead temperature may lag significantly behind core temperature.[84] Therefore, the value of peripheral temperature monitoring in detecting MH is not certain.

If possible, a regional, local, or major conduction anesthetic should be used with either amide or ester local anesthetics. If not possible, a barbiturate or narcotic induction followed by nitrous oxide, oxygen, and nondepolarizing relaxant with opioid supplementation is recommended. Other induction agents that have not been implicated in MH are midazolam, diazepam, droperidol, and propofol.

Neuromuscular blocking agents such as pancuronium, vecuronium, atracurium, and mivacurium are safe, according to animal and human studies. We routinely reverse nondepolarizing relaxants with anticholinesterase and anticholinergic agents.

At the worst, nitrous oxide is a weak triggering agent. Many thousands of safe anesthetics have been administered with nitrous oxide in MH-susceptible patients. Two cases have been reported in which early signs of MH have been documented despite the use of a safe anesthetic technique.[85] Therefore, even under the most controlled circumstances, the anesthesiologist should be alert to the early signs of MH.

We do not continue dantrolene after operation if there are no signs of MH. However, the patient must be observed closely for 4–6 hours. MH has not occurred after surgery when dantrolene pretreatment and safe anesthetic techniques were used. The patient may be discharged on the same day as surgery if indicated.

The same precautions should be taken for the obstetric patient as for the routine surgical patient. We are not convinced that the stress of labor may precipitate MH, and we recommend well-conducted epidural anesthesia for labor and delivery without dantrolene pretreatment but with careful monitoring of vital signs. If an emergency cesarean section with general anesthesia is necessary, dantrolene may be given intravenously along with nontriggering agents. In the very acute situation, anesthesia should be induced and dantrolene administration should be considered thereafter. The maternal/fetal partition ratio for dantrolene is probably 0.4.[86] Dantrolene has not been reported to produce significant problems for the fetus or newborn, but existing data are very scanty.

Malignant Hyperthermia in Species Other Than Pigs and People

Malignant hyperthermia has been reported sporadically in many species. Clinical episodes have been documented in cats, dogs (especially greyhound species), and horses. Capture myopathy is a syndrome characterized by temperature elevation, rhabdomyolysis, acidosis, and death in wild animals (e.g., zebra, elk) after prolonged chase.[87] This also has been suggested to be an MH variant.

Medicolegal Aspects

In this era of malpractice actions, it is not surprising that MH cases have been the subject of malpractice suits. Because MH may be considered an inborn genetic problem with a relatively fixed associated mortality that may go unrecognized before a patient's exposure to triggering agents, it may be used as a "cover" for other problems.

Fever, opisthotonic posturing, and neurologic abnormalities may accompany hypoxic brain injury, and because of their similarity to MH, MH may be incorrectly implicated in the differential diagnosis. Furthermore, after cardiac arrest from any cause, creatinine phosphokinase and potassium levels may be significantly elevated. We do not know of data concerning the incidence of litigation after the occurrence of MH.

Although some have stated that with the advent of dantrolene there should be no deaths from MH, this is probably unrealistic because in some cases the syndrome may be truly explosive and impossible to control with current therapy. Also, we are not completely familiar with all factors that lead to MH, including drugs that may trigger it, and the proper dose of dantrolene to employ in order to prevent recrudescence. Nevertheless, certain common themes underlie the basis for litigation in MH:

1. Failure to obtain a thorough personal history in regard to anesthetic problems and a family history of any unexplained perioperative problems.

2. Failure to monitor temperature continuously with an electronic temperature monitoring device. Several jury trial cases have been lost by the defense because the patient's temperature was not monitored. Intraoperative temperature monitoring is now considered a "standard of care" in the United States by the legal profession despite failure of the American Society of Anesthesiologists to recommend routine temperature monitoring during administration of all general anesthetics.

3. Failure to have adequate supplies of dantrolene on hand with a plan of management of MH.

4. Failure to investigate unexplained increases in body temperature and increased skeletal muscle tone (especially after succinylcholine administration) when associated with increased heart rate and arrhythmias.

Several examples of medicolegal cases involving these principles are described.

Increased heart rate developed in a 35-year-old man during a bowel resection for regional enteritis. His oral temperature by mercury thermometer was 37°C. The oral thermometer was left in place and the anesthesia continued with halothane and nitrous oxide. Toward the end of the procedure, there was a rapid increase in heart rate followed by an increase in body temperature. Despite cooling and administration of procainamide (this episode occurred in the predantrolene era) and other appropriate medical therapy, disseminated intravascular coagulopathy eventually developed and the patient died. The plaintiff won the case when it was tried by jury primarily because continuous electronic temperature monitoring was available and was not used.

Another case involved a young male patient who had shoulder surgery with halothane-nitrous oxide-oxygen. Again, temperature was not monitored continuously. Intraoperative tachycardia to about 150 beats·min^{-1} was treated with propranolol. At the end of the procedure, as the drapes were being removed, the patient felt warm. A temperature probe revealed a reading of nearly 40°C. Shortly thereafter cardiac arrest occurred, despite dantrolene administration, and the patient died. The case was settled out of court.

A man in his middle 30s had a dental procedure in a dental operatory (not in the hospital). Halothane anesthesia was administered by an anesthesiologist. Despite increasing heart rate and temperature elevation, the anesthetic was continued until the patient had a cardiac arrest. Dantrolene was not available. Access to the operatory was limited, and the patient died during transport to a nearby hospital. The case was settled out of court for an undisclosed sum. (Millions of anesthetics using MH-triggering agents are administered each year in dental operatories, outpatient surgical facilities, and, increasingly, physicians' offices. Standards and reviews operative at hospitals are not applied to these locations.)

Symptoms of bowel obstruction developed in a middle-aged man. He was taken to a local hospital, and anesthesia was administered with nitrous oxide-oxygen-halothane and succinylcholine. His temperature was not monitored, but an unexplained tachycardia (140–160 beats·min^{-1}) was present throughout the 2-hour procedure. On arrival in the intensive care unit after the operation, the patient was slightly hypotensive. Invasive monitoring was started. Despite marked metabolic and respiratory acidosis, a Pco_2 of 100 mm Hg, and a recorded temperature of nearly 42°C, MH was not diagnosed. A cooling blanket and antibiotics failed to arrest the decrease in the patient's blood pressure, which eventually led to cardiac arrest. A judgment against the physicians and hospital of $4.5 million dollars was reached.

Patient Support Services

To answer the needs of patients and families who wished to learn more about MH and of those families whose relatives have died from MH, two support groups were founded—the Malignant Hyperthermia Association (of Canada) and the Malignant Hyperthermia Association of the United States. Both groups serve as a repository of information about MH, provide names of physicians knowledgeable about MH and the location of MH diagnostic centers, and simply lend an ear to those with MH who have questions. Both organizations have an advisory committee of physicians but are run by volunteers who usually have a personal connection with MH. Both organize annual meetings for physicians and nonphysicians. The Malignant Hyperthermia Association of the United States publishes a quarterly newsletter, *The Communicator*, with excerpts from the medical literature, explanatory articles, questions and answers, and related information. In addition, a hotline has been organized so that a physician with an urgent question about MH can be placed in contact with a knowledgeable specialist. Approximately 30–40 calls a month are handled by this hotline.

The address of the Malignant Hyperthermia Association of the United States is P.O. Box 191, Westport, Connecticut

06881–0191. The hotline number is 209-634-4917. Ask for Index Zero.

The address of the Malignant Hyperthermia Association of Canada is Room 314, Elizabeth Wing, Toronto General Hospital, 101 College Street, Toronto, Ontario M5G1L7. The hotline number is 416-595-3000.

In 1989, the North American MH Registry was formed. Based in Hershey, Pennsylvania, the Registry will eventually be the repository for patient and family specific information for MH-susceptible patients. The address is Pennsylvania State University, Department of Anesthesia, College of Medicine, Hershey, Pennsylvania 17033–0850.

Physicians who want to provide patient services for MH must prepare for lengthy discussions about the disorder, because patients usually have only very limited information.

Pathophysiology and Etiology of Malignant Hyperthermia

Introduction

With the clinical implications of MH as a background, the pathophysiology and etiology can be more easily appreciated. Three major developments have contributed to the understanding of MH. The first was the recognition that the syndrome is genetically transmitted.[2] This finding is significant from a mechanistic standpoint because it suggests that a single inheritable anomaly might explain the abnormal response to anesthetics. A second finding was identification of a greater sensitivity of skeletal muscle from MH-susceptible patients to halothane and/or caffeine.[4] This was the basis for an in vitro system for patient diagnosis and study of the mechanisms underlying MH. The third was the recognition of similarities between human MH and porcine stress syndrome.[3] In addition to stress, the porcine stress syndrome could be triggered by halothane and succinylcholine, the two agents most often implicated in MH. Thus, an ideal animal model became available for studies of MH.

Pathogenesis and Etiology

Experimental Models for Malignant Hyperthermia

Although MH is rare in humans, breeding pigs for leaner meat and better musculature has resulted in the appearance of the MH gene (or genes) in relatively high frequency in a number of herds (e.g., Poland China, Landrace). This has been a major concern for breeders because the meat from pigs with MH is not marketable. This syndrome in pigs, which is similar to that in humans, can be elicited in the absence of anesthetics.[88] Although pigs administered MH-triggering anesthetics have provided a model for human MH, there is no evidence that a human stress syndrome exists in the majority of patients that is completely analogous to the porcine stress syndrome. Hence, there should be some caution in interpreting studies in swine because the gene(s) causing porcine MH may be different from those causing human MH. Certainly the mode of inheritance (autosomal recessive) in some breeds is different from that in humans (autosomal dominant). The occurrence of MH is rare in horses, dogs, and cats.[89] Of these, only the dog has been proposed as a model of human MH.[90]

Understanding the Malignant Hyperthermia Defect

A hypothesis explaining MH must account for the puzzling clinical observations surrounding this disorder. Most important, MH patients function normally in the absence of anesthetics. Therefore, the defect should not significantly interfere with normal muscle physiology. The defect, at least in humans, appears to be expressed only in skeletal muscle. Another common observation is that the expression of the syndrome shows a large variability among individuals. Patients do not respond to every exposure to anesthetics and the latency or severity of the MH syndrome can be highly variable, even in the same subject. Within the same biopsy specimen from an MH patient there can be considerable variability in the expression of the MH defect.[91] This is also true of cells from the same primary culture of skeletal muscle from these patients.[92] Therefore, the MH defect may not always be expressed in muscle, and up or down regulation of amount and/or activity, either regionally or throughout the muscle mass, is likely. The large interindividual variability may be explained by different genes causing MH in different families or by other predisposing factors being expressed differently in different patients or families. For example, swine age is clearly related to expression of porcine stress syndrome. In young swine (3–12 weeks) MH is not triggered by halothane or succinylcholine. Many different proteins have been reported to be altered in MH skeletal muscle. Thus it is reasonable to assume that a second messenger or modulating system may be altered in MH either as a primary defect or secondary to other abnormalities.

Skeletal Muscle—Site of the Malignant Hyperthermia Defect

Almost all evidence to date points to skeletal muscle as the site of the primary defect in MH.

Thermogenesis. The thermogenesis in MH is not initiated by the thermoregulatory centers in the central nervous system. Rather, the hypermetabolism is the result of a direct action of triggering agents on skeletal muscle. The in vitro contracture test for MH susceptibility is good evidence that skeletal muscle is the target tissue in MH.

Role of Calcium. Ultimately, the main problem in skeletal muscle is lack of control of myoplasmic Ca^{2+} concentration, which may be manifest clinically as muscle rigidity. Ca^{2+} levels are controlled by a complex interaction of Ca^{2+} release from the terminal cisternae, the adenosine triphosphate-driven Ca^{2+} pumps at the sarcoplasmic reticulum and sarcolemma, Na^+/Ca^{2+} exchange, several Ca^{2+} buffering proteins (calsequestrin, parvalbumin), and mitochondrial Ca^{2+} regulation. Although several of these systems may become involved as the MH syndrome progresses, the initial defect in Ca^{2+} regulation appears to be an increased sensitivity of the Ca^{2+} release mechanism in the terminal cisternae to halothane or other halogenated volatile anesthetics. The target of succinylcholine is not clear at this time. Dantrolene antagonizes Ca^{2+} release from the sarcoplasmic reticulum and can lower elevated Ca^{2+} levels and reverse an episode of MH.[94]

Organelles Within Skeletal Muscle That Exhibit a Malignant Hyperthermia-Associated Defect

Sarcolemma. Early studies suggesting involvement of the sarcolemma (muscle cell plasma membrane) in MH used indirect approaches or were not consistent in their findings. The most direct evidence for the manifestation of the MH defect at the sarcolemma has been the demonstration of a subtly altered Na^+ current in human primary cell cultures[92] and a defect in the sarcolemmal adenosine triphosphate–dependent Ca^{2+} transport in porcine muscle.[95]

Mitochondria. The uncoupling of Ca^{2+}-stimulated but not adenosine diphosphate-stimulated mitochondrial succinate oxidation has been demonstrated in pigs[96] and humans[97] susceptible to MH. These studies have been subjected to some undeserved criticism because they were not reproduced by other investigators.[98] However, it is essential that these studies be conducted at physiologic temperatures (37–40°C), since even the original studies did not find a similar defect at room temperature. Since contractures to halothane are only elicited at physiologic temperatures,[66] this temperature dependence of mitochondrial uncoupling appears to be an important observation.

Terminal Cisternae. The terminal cisternae of the sarcoplasmic reticulum are coupled to the t-tubules and are the sites of the Ca^{2+} release channel protein, or ryanodine receptor. Several investigators have found that the threshold of Ca^{2+} release from the terminal cisternae is low in *porcine* MH muscle.[99] However, this is not the case for human MH muscle.[100] The only report of altered Ca^{2+} release in human muscle was a slight (13%) increase in amount of release.[101] It is unclear how such a small difference relates to MH. No studies using isolated organelles have convincingly demonstrated a difference between normal and MH muscle in halothane-induced Ca^{2+} release.

Longitudinal Sarcoplasmic Reticulum. Whereas most early studies found no consistent manifestation of the MH defect in the longitudinal sarcoplasmic reticulum, a recent study has reported a structural defect in the major protein (Ca^{2+} adenosine triphosphatase) of this Ca^{2+} sequestering organelle in porcine muscle.[25] In addition, there was also a difference in MH compared to normal swine sarcoplasmic reticulum in thermal inactivation of the Ca^{2+} adenosine triphosphatase activity and a defect in polyadenylation of the enzyme.[102]

Proteins or Systems Reported Altered in Malignant Hyperthermia Muscle

Calcium Release Channel. Perhaps the most attractive hypothesis to explain MH is based on the observations that there is a low threshold of Ca^{2+}-induced Ca^{2+} release in porcine MH muscle[99] and that binding of the plant alkaloid ryanodine to the Ca^{2+} channel (often termed the ryanodine receptor) is abnormal in MH.[103] The hypothesis is attractive because it is simple to understand. However, it would be difficult to explain the intra- and interindividual variability in MH and the occurrence of nonrigid MH with such a hypothesis, especially since it would be expected that an altered calcium channel would lead to clinically apparent problems in the absence of anesthesia. Also, the threshold of Ca^{2+}-induced Ca^{2+} release is normal in human MH muscle,[100] and when the ryanodine binding studies are conducted using the same strain of swine for the MH– and MH+ groups and the influence of fatty acids is eliminated, there is no difference related to MH susceptibility.[104] In support of the ryanodine receptor as a defect in MH, however, some investigators have reported genetic linkage of the locus (chromosome 19q13.1) encoding the Ca^{2+} release channel with a positive contracture test.[105,106] However, many other genes, some with good potential for being the MH effect, are encoded in that region.[107] Also, recent studies have failed to show consistent linkage of contracture test results with the ryanodine receptor gene in humans (see below).

Sodium Channel. Recently Weiland et al[107a] have reported an alteration in the inactivation kinetics of the Na^+ currents in human MH muscle cultures. Although the sodium channel is not believed to be the primary defect in MH, this observation is important for several reasons: (1) it confirms the genetic component in human muscle, as all the cells are maintained in the same environment; (2) it is the only protein directly and specifically identified to have an altered function in human MH muscle; and (3) it demonstrates that cell culture systems can be used to study MH.

Elevated Fatty Acid Production. The observation of elevated fatty acid production was first reported in porcine muscle by Cheah and Cheah.[93] These findings were confirmed in human MH muscle[67] and, because of limitations in the techniques applied, were presumed to be due to elevated phospholipase A_2 activity. Subsequent studies have attributed the elevated fatty acid production to altered triglyceride-associated metabolism.[108]

Inositol 1,4,5-Trisphosphate Phosphatase. Inositol 1,4,5-trisphosphate is involved in Ca^{2+} mobilization in many cell types. The activity of an enzyme (inositol 1,4,5-trisphosphate phosphatase) regulating the inactivation of this second messenger has been shown to be deficient in porcine MH muscle.[109] The consequence of this deficiency is a tenfold elevated level of inositol 1,4,5-trisphosphate that could potentially raise Ca^{2+} levels.

Antioxidant Defense. The antioxidant defense system has been reported to be deficient in porcine MH muscle.[110] These interesting studies have suggested that vitamin E may be an antagonist of the MH episode.

Calcium-Adenosine Triphosphatase. A preliminary report has appeared that identifies a structural difference in the calcium-adenosine triphosphatase of porcine MH skeletal muscle.[102] Peptide maps of proteolytic digests of the enzyme differed from those of controls in that there was a deficiency in the polyadenylated mRNA for the protein and a greater resistance to thermal inactivation of the enzyme activity. Additionally, the sarcolemmal adenosine triphosphate–stimulated Ca^{2+} transport is deficient in porcine MH muscle.[95]

Acetylcholinesterase. Acetylcholinesterase activity is elevated in porcine MH muscle.[111] However, it is unlikely that this defect plays a role in the MH syndrome.

Phosphorylation Activity. Higher than normal levels of phosphorylation[112] and altered sensitivity to protein phosphatase inhibition[113] have been reported in porcine MH muscle. Altered phosphorylation could either be a primary or a secondary defect in MH.

Other Defects. The function of several other proteins has been reported to be altered in MH. However, these studies are unconvincing either because they use different strains of swine for the control and MH-susceptible groups or because they have not been verified over the years. For example, although fiber type was originally considered important in the response of MH skeletal muscle to triggering agents, these observations have not been substantiated.[114] Although catecholamines were proposed to trigger MH, this hypothesis has also not withstood testing. However, it is possible that catecholamines may worsen the episode.[115]

A Hypothesis to Explain Many Observations in Malignant Hyperthermia Muscle

Although the primary defect in MH is currently unknown, it is clear that the function or structure of several proteins is altered in MH skeletal muscle. We have identified one feature common to the majority of these proteins or systems. The Na^+ channel, acetylcholinesterase, and Ca^{2+}-adenosine triphosphatase are all proteins identified as acylated.[116] This means that these proteins bind fatty acids covalently on specific cysteine, serine, threonine, or glycine amino acid residues.[117] This is a dynamic process and is analogous to protein phosphorylation. In addition, the Ca^{2+} release channel protein has an N-terminal sequence[118] consistent with a myristoylation site (fatty acid amide bonded to glycine). Skeletal muscle from MH-susceptible patients has elevated fatty acid production.[67] Fatty acids modify the function of the Ca^{2+} release channel,[100] Na^+ channel,[119] and mitochondrial respiration.[96,97] Therefore, it appears that the effects of elevated fatty acid production in MH skeletal muscle must be accounted for when identifying proteins altered in MH. That is, some of the "defects" suggested to cause MH are merely artifacts occurring during organelle isolation secondary to failure to control fatty acid levels. The defect in the antioxidant system in MH muscle may be the result of excess fatty acids, since the double bonds of the unsaturated fatty acids are highly susceptible to oxidation. Conversely, the defect in the antioxidant defense system may be the cause of elevated fatty acid production.[120]

We believe, therefore, that the pathophysiologic change during MH results from protein function alteration secondary to elevated levels of certain fatty acids or their metabolic intermediates.

Using Molecular Biology to Understand Malignant Hyperthermia

Since MH is an inherited disorder, one or more gene defects will eventually be found to explain this syndrome.

Once the gene(s) have been identified, the protein abnormality may be identified and the pathophysiology understood. For example, based on the localization of the gene for Duchenne's dystrophy to the X chromosome, it was eventually determined that patients with this disorder did not manufacture a specific protein (terminal dystrophin), which is apparently needed for the maintenance of muscle cell integrity.

In the case of MH, chromosome 19 (in humans) and chromosome 6 (in pigs) have been identified as the site of the MH gene in a preliminary fashion. Using special techniques, it was determined that the inheritance of MH susceptibility (based on contracture test data) is inherited along with (or linked to) the inheritance of the gene that is responsible for encoding the proteins that make up the calcium release channel of skeletal muscle. This channel binds the plant alkaloid ryanodine and is termed the ryanodine receptor.

However, since those initial reports, other families have been identified in whom the inheritance of MH susceptibility was not linked to the gene encoding the ryanodine receptor.[121] One interpretation of these data is that MH is a heterogeneous disorder that may be caused in some families by defective proteins in the structure of the ryanodine receptor but in others by abnormalities in intermediate enzymes of fatty acid or triglyceride metabolism.

A practical explanation of these discordant findings has been offered recently. In MH pigs a specific base pair defect in the Ryanodine receptor gene has been found to be associated with MH susceptibility.[121a]

However, the same defect is found in only 1 of 60 human MH families screened by the same group. Therefore, in humans MH appears to be a heterogeneous disorder, but in pigs MH appears to be rather homogenous and perhaps different pathophysiologically.

Once the gene or genes for MH are determined, it will be possible to map them and to determine in what way the protein is abnormal.

In addition, since DNA may be found in white blood cells by harvesting white blood cells, the presence or absence of the abnormal gene will be determined and a "blood test" for MH will be possible.

The Future of Research in Malignant Hyperthermia

A greater understanding of the manner in which the Ca^{2+} release channel is regulated, especially by triggering agents and modifiers such as fatty acids, is needed. The fatty acid defect has to be distinguished as a primary or secondary defect in MH muscle. Alternate diagnostic tests that are more sensitive and specific than the contracture test also are crucial. In humans the defect appears to be expressed only in skeletal muscle, making a needle biopsy the approach most likely to succeed. DNA-based linkage studies, such as are currently being conducted,[105] have the power to identify the gene(s) causing MH without any knowledge of the function of the protein that the gene encodes. Also, molecular genetic approaches may be the only hope for a noninvasive diagnostic test. The defect in swine is not necessarily the same defect as that in most humans. Also, since more than one defect may cause MH in swine, the porcine studies may be important for identifying subpopulations of defects.

Summary

The MH gene or genes remain unidentified. The defect appears to be expressed only in skeletal muscle in humans, and MH-associated defects are manifest in virtually all organelles in skeletal muscle. Potential candidates for the defect are enzymes involved in triglyceride-fatty acid metabolism, inositol 1,4,5-trisphosphate phosphatase, or some aspect of phosphorylation or the antioxidant defense system. A disturbance in fatty acid metabolism, whether it is the primary defect in MH or a secondary effect, alters the function of several organelles and can lead to altered Ca^{2+} metabolism in skeletal muscle.

OTHER INHERITED DISORDERS

Inherited diseases affect every bodily organ and every physiologic and biochemical process. Some are mild and allow a relatively normal life span, whereas others are incompatible with extrauterine existence even for a few days. Adding to the complexity is a natural variability of genetic penetrance and expressivity even in a single family. All of these disorders have as a common feature an abnormality in one or more genes that affects the function of one or more enzymes. The metabolic basis of inherited diseases is the subject of several well-known books,[122,123] which may be consulted for an in-depth appreciation of our state of knowledge of many of these disorders (see also Chapter 22).

Disorders of Plasma Cholinesterase

Plasma cholinesterase, pseudocholinesterase, or nonspecific cholinesterase is an enzyme with a molecular weight of 320,000 and a tetrahedral structure. It is found in plasma and most tissue but not in red blood cells. Pseudocholinesterase degrades acetylcholine released at the neuromuscular junction.

The half-life of pseudocholinesterase has been estimated to be 8–16 hours. It is very stable in serum samples and can be stored for long periods of time at $-20°C$ with little or no activity loss. Cholinesterase is manufactured in the liver. Therefore, decreased plasma cholinesterase activity occurs in advanced cases of hepatocellular dysfunction.

Inherited variants of pseudocholinesterase are of interest to the anesthesiologist because the duration of action of succinylcholine, mivacurium, and, in some cases, ester-linked local anesthetics is a function of the activity of this enzyme system. Prolonged apnea after succinylcholine administration occurs in patients who have very low absolute activity of pseudocholinesterase or have enzyme variants.[124,125] These patients otherwise have no symptoms.

Many physiologic, pharmacologic, and pathologic factors can either increase or decrease the activity of this enzyme to a significant extent. However, it is only when there is a greater than approximately 75% decrease in the levels of the normal pseudocholinesterase that there is clinically evident prolongation of succinylcholine activity (see below). Table 23-2 lists some of the causes for variation in plasma cholinesterase activity.

Succinylcholine-Related Apnea

Succinylcholine is hydrolyzed by a two-step process, first to succinylmonocholine and then to succinic acid. It has been estimated that only about 5% of the injected drug reaches the end-plate region because of a combination of both hydrolysis and diffusion from the plasma. Urinary excretion and protein binding play unimportant roles in the disposition of the drug. The rate of metabolism determines the duration of action of succinylcholine.

There are a variety of assay procedures for pseudocholinesterase activity. However, most involve the reaction of a thiocholine (e.g., butyrylthiocholine) with serum or plasma containing cholinesterase. The reaction product is coupled with 5,5'-dithiobis-(2-nitrobenzoic acid) and forms a colored product that can be followed spectrophotometrically.

Kalow et al were the first to show that qualitative as well as quantitative differences in the pseudocholinesterase enzyme determine the duration of succinylcholine apnea.[126] Kalow found that in certain persons displaying succinylcholine sensitivity, the local anesthetic dibucaine (Nupercaine) inhibited the hydrolysis of a benzylcholine substrate less than it inhibited the reaction in those displaying a normal response to succinylcholine. The percentage inhibition of the reaction was termed the *dibucaine number*. It was found to be constant for a person and did not depend on the concentration of the enzyme. A report by Ravindran et al suggests that in patients with less than 10% of the normal pseudocholinesterase activity, the measurement of

TABLE 23-2. Some Causes of Changes in Cholinesterase Activity

Inherited

Cholinesterase variants that may lead to decreased or increased activity (*e.g.*, silent gene or C5 variant)

Physiologic

Decreases in last trimester of pregnancy
Reduced activity of the newborn

Acquired Decreases

Liver diseases
Carcinoma
Debilitating diseases
Collagen diseases
Uremia
Malnutrition
Myxedema

Acquired Increases

Obesity
Alcoholism
Thyrotoxicosis
Nephrosis
Psoriasis
Electroshock therapy[161]

Drugs Related to Diseases

Echothiophate iodide
Neostigmine
Pyridostigmine
Chlorpromazine
Cyclophosphamide
Monamine oxidase inhibitors
Pancuronium
Propanidid
Contraceptives
Organophosphorus insecticides
Hexafluorenium

Other Causes of Decreased Activity

Plasmapheresis
Extracorporeal circulation
Tetanus
Radiation therapy
Burns

The significance of these factors depends on the severity of disease, drug dosage, and individual variation.

Adapted from Whittaker M: Plasma cholinesterase variants and the anesthetist. Anaesthesia 35:174, 1980.

the dibucaine number (and the fluoride number) may be misleadingly low.[127]

A discontinuous distribution of dibucaine numbers suggested an inheritance pattern based on alteration at a single gene locus (Table 23-3). Those with dibucaine numbers in the range of 80 would be homozygous normal with a normal response to succinylcholine, those with dibucaine numbers of 20 would be homozygous atypical with a marked prolongation of succinylcholine activity, and those with dibucaine numbers in the 60 range would be heterozygotes and, in general, have a normal response to succinylcholine. This theory was substantiated by other workers.

Over the years, two other major allelic variants were discovered. In one case, the silent gene, the enzyme is not produced completely. In the other (fluoride-sensitive), there

TABLE 23-3. Biochemical Characteristics of Some Cholinesterase Variants

Genotype	Cholinesterase Activity (u/10)	Dibucaine Number	Fluoride Number	Chloride Number	Succinylcholine Number
EuEu	677–1860	78–86	55–65	1–12	89–98
EaEa	140–525	18–26	16–32	46–58	4–19
EuEa	285–1008	51–70	38–55	15–34	51–78
EuEf	579–900	74–80	47–48	14–30	87–91
EfEa	475–661	49–59	25–33	31–36	56–59
EfEs	351	63	26	25	81

Eu = normal enzyme gene; Ea = atypical enzyme gene; Ef = fluoride sensitive gene; Es = silent gene.
Reproduced with permission from Viby-Mogensen J: Succinylcholine neuromuscular blockade in subjects homozygous for atypical plasma cholinesterase. Anesthesiology 55:429, 1981.

is a differential inhibition of cholinesterase activity by fluoride.[128] In those with prolonged duration of succinylcholine activity with this genotype, fluoride ion inhibits the in vitro hydrolysis of substrate by the enzyme less than it does in normals. A fluoride number, similar to a dibucaine number, is thereby created. Other variants exist.

When there is a question of succinylcholine sensitivity, the absolute activity of the pseudocholinesterase should be determined as well as the dibucaine and fluoride numbers. In some cases, because of biologic variability or unusual combinations of genotype (e.g., combination of atypical and fluoride genes), it is helpful to use other inhibitors of the cholinesterase reaction in genotyping the patient. Bromide, urea, sodium chloride, and succinylcholine have been used to distinguish the various genotypes (Table 23-3).

Molecular genetic techniques have been successfully applied to pseudocholinesterase variants. La Du's laboratory has identified a point mutation in the gene for human serum cholinesterase in which a nucleotide change leads to an alteration of a single amino acid (adenine to guanine) in the protein. This change apparently alters the affinity of atypical cholinesterase for choline esters.[128a] Other base pair alterations account for other atypical variants, including the silent gene.

The identification of the genetic defect offers the prospect that more accurate and precise diagnostic tests for atypical pseudocholinesterase variants will be offered soon.

The frequencies of occurrence of the various genes vary to some extent with ethnic background. For example, South African blacks[129] and Eskimo populations have the silent gene much more frequently, patients with Huntington's chorea are more likely to have an Ef gene than are normal controls, and Israelis have a higher chance of having an atypical genotype than Americans. In European studies, the approximate percentages in the population of the genotypes are as follows: EuEu (96%), EuEa (2.5%), EuEf or EuEs (0.3%), EaEf (0.005%), EaEa (0.05%), and EfEf or EfEs* (0.006%).[130]

Atypical pseudocholinesterase may be associated with affective disorders.[131] Patients homozygous for atypical, fluoride, or silent genes as well as those with the combination of atypical with fluoride, atypical with silent genes, or fluoride with silent genes should wear Medic-Alert bracelets indicating that succinylcholine administration will lead to prolonged apnea. Relatives should be tested as well. There are only a few cholinesterase research units that investigate families and interpret results: Whittaker's in Great Britain,

Hanel and Viby-Mogensen's in Denmark, and Rosenberg's in the United States.

Clinical Implications of Pseudocholinesterase Abnormalities

Important questions for the anesthesiologist are: Which patients are at risk for development of an abnormal response to succinylcholine? What are the clinical characteristics of this response and treatment options?

Significant prolongation of succinylcholine's effects occurs in the following genotypes: EaEa, EfEf, EaEs, EfEa, and EsEs (Table 23-4). The more common situations in which homozygote normals and heterozygotes are at risk are as follows: patients who have been receiving echothiophate eye drops (up to 2 weeks after therapy is discontinued); patients who are undergoing plasmapheresis;[132] patients with severe liver disease; and patients (particularly heterozygotes) who have received succinylcholine after reversal of nondepolarizing blockade with neostigmine.

Viby-Mogensen has studied the question of plasma cholinesterase apnea in detail. His cholinesterase unit found that 6.2% of patients who displayed apnea for 50–250 minutes after a "usual" dose of succinylcholine had an acquired deficiency of plasma cholinesterase.[124] He then studied 70 patients who were genotypically normal for pseudocholinesterase and administered 1 mg·kg^{-1} of succinylcholine during a 50% nitrous oxide-oxygen-1% halothane anesthetic and followed the depression and return of thumb twitch. He found that there was indeed a relationship between the duration of apnea, the return of a full twitch response, and plasma cholinesterase activity.[133] However, only moderate prolongation of apnea was found when cholinesterase was depressed by as much as 70%. Apnea is only significantly prolonged with extreme depression of cholinesterase activity.

In a second study with a similar protocol, he found that heterozygotes having one normal gene (e.g., EuEa; EuEf) had a normal response to succinylcholine, including typical fasciculations and a depolarizing type of block with train-of-four stimulations.[134] However, heterozygotes without the usual gene (e.g., EaEf) had a prolonged response to succinylcholine, with apnea lasting as long as 24 minutes. Most showed typical fasciculations. Fade with train-of-four stimulations was the rule. It should be noted that others have found that heterozygotes with one normal gene display a prolonged response to succinylcholine under certain conditions. About one in 500 heterozygotes is prone to such a response.

Apnea develops in homozygous atypical patients (EaEa) when they are given succinylcholine, and it lasts from 120

*The abbreviations are defined as follows: Eu = normal enzyme gene; Ea = atypical enzyme gene; Ef = fluoride-sensitive gene; Es = silent gene.

TABLE 23-4. Hereditary Variants of Pseudocholinesterase Resulting from Four Allelic Genes

Genotype	Frequency in a British Population	Response to Succinylcholine	Typical Dibucaine Number	Typical Fluoride Number
N-N	96% normal	Normal	80	60
D-D	1 in 2000	Greatly prolonged	20	20
F-F	1 in 154,000	Moderately prolonged	70	30
S-S	1 in 100,000	Greatly prolonged	—	—
N-D	1 in 25	Slightly prolonged	60	45
N-F	1 in 200	Slightly prolonged	75	50
N-S	1 in 190	Slightly prolonged	80	60
D-F	1 in 20,000	Greatly prolonged	45	35
D-S	1 in 29,000	Greatly prolonged	20	20
F-S	1 in 150,000	Moderately prolonged	65	35

N = gene for normal pseudocholinesterase; D = gene for dibucaine-sensitive variant; F = gene for fluoride-sensitive variant; S = gene for absence of enzyme activity (silent gene).

Adapted from Lehmann H, Lidell J: Human cholinesterase (pseudocholinesterase): Genetic variants and their recognition. Br J Anaesth 41:243, 1969.

to more than 300 minutes.[125] The onset of neuromuscular block is similar to that in normals; however, there is fade in response to train-of-four stimulation. Contrary to Baraka's report, fasciculations do occur with succinylcholine in these patients.[135]

The other class of patients who regularly display prolonged apnea after succinylcholine administration are patients who are homozygous for the silent gene.

Treatment of Succinylcholine Apnea

The safest course of treatment after the patient fails to breathe within 10–15 minutes after succinylcholine administration is to continue mechanical ventilation until adequate muscle tone has returned. Two units of blood may contain adequate amounts of pseudocholinesterase to hydrolyze the succinylcholine.[136]

The use of cholinesterase inhibitors in treating succinylcholine apnea is controversial. When given along with blood or plasma, the improvement is rapid and lasting. If they are administered alone before there is evidence of fade with train-of-four stimulation, there may be a transient improvement followed by intensification of the neuromuscular block. The best chance for reversal of succinylcholine-related apnea in these situations occurs when no more than 0.03 mg·kg^{-1} of neostigmine is given 90–120 minutes after succinylcholine when a curare type of blockade is present.

C5 Variant

An isoenzyme of pseudocholinesterase has been demonstrated whereby the hydrolysis of succinylcholine is increased and, therefore, the duration of apnea is decreased after succinylcholine administration. The gene does not appear to be an allele of the Eu and Ea gene and is found infrequently in the population.[137]

Plasma Cholinesterase Abnormalities and the Metabolism of Local Anesthetics

Although the ester-linked local anesthetics (e.g., procaine, tetracaine, 2-chloroprocaine) are metabolized by pseudocholinesterase, prolongation of block and/or clinical toxic-

ity of these local anesthetics in homozygous atypical patients has rarely been documented.

Brodsky et al[138] have reported a normal caudal epidural anesthetic with the use of chloroprocaine in a patient with low plasma cholinesterase activity secondary to chronic echothiophate iodide therapy.

Raj et al reported that there were no clinical difficulties from prolonged elevation of the plasma concentration of chloroprocaine after epidural and brachial plexus block in homozygote atypicals.[139] On the other hand, Kuhnert et al have reported excessive somnolence and a prolonged chloroprocaine epidural block in a postpartum patient.[140] This patient also manifested sensitivity to succinylcholine during a postpartum anesthetic (prepregnancy response to succinylcholine was normal) and was believed to have either an EaEa or an EaEs genotype. Jatlow et al have shown delayed hydrolysis of cocaine in vitro with plasma from homozygote atypicals.[141] They theorized that such persons may be at risk for toxic reaction from normal doses of cocaine.

The Porphyrias

All the porphyrias result from a defect in heme synthesis. The heme pigments are tetrapyrroles that are the essential elements in hemoglobin, myoglobin, and the cytochromes, i.e., compounds that are involved in the transport of oxygen, activation of oxygen, and the electron transport chain. Cytochrome P-450 is a hemoprotein intimately involved in the conversion of lipid-soluble nonpolar drugs to soluble polar compounds that may be excreted in the urine.

A complete deficiency of enzymes that are involved in heme synthesis is incompatible with life. However, a partial deficiency may lead to the accumulation of one or more of the molecular intermediates in heme production. Such an accumulation of precursors is responsible for the clinical manifestations of the porphyrias (in as yet an unexplained manner).

The rate-limiting step in heme synthesis is the conjugation of succinyl-CoA with glycine to form delta aminolevulinic acid (the enzyme is aminolevulinic acid synthetase). In the porphyrias, there is a partial deficiency of enzymes subsequent to this initial step, which results in a stimula-

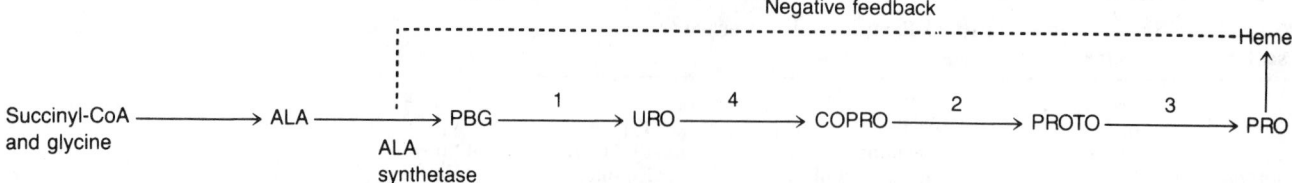

Figure 23-3. Biosynthesis of heme and sites of defects in certain porphyrias. (Abbreviations: ALA = aminolevulinic acid; PBG = porphobilinogen; URO = uroporphyrinogen; COPRO = copro-porphyrinogen; PROTO = protoporphyrinogen; PRO = protoporphyrin.) In intermittent acute porphyria, there is a partial deficiency of the enzyme at site 1. In hereditary coproporphyria, there is an enzyme deficiency at site 2. In variegate porphyria, the enzyme problem is at site 3. In porphyria cutanea tarda, there is a deficiency at site 4. (Reprinted with permission from Mees DL, Frederickson EL: Anesthesia and the porphyrias. South Med J 68:29, 1975.)

tion of this reaction to form aminolevulinic acid. The result is overproduction of intermediate products before the deficient step (Fig. 23-3).

The porphyrias generally manifest after puberty. Inheritance is through an autosomal dominant pattern, but congenital erythropoietic porphyria is inherited as an autosomal recessive pattern.

A functional classification for the anesthesiologist is based on a division of the porphyrias into inducible and noninducible forms. The inducible porphyrias are those in which the acute symptoms are precipitated upon drug exposure (Table 23-5).[142] These forms are acute intermittent porphyria, variegate porphyria, and hereditary coproporphyria. These porphyrias cause an acute neurologic syndrome and are therefore of interest to the anesthesiologist. Cutaneous manifestations, with particular sensitivity to ultraviolet light that is exhibited by skin fragility and bleeding, are the chief features of the other porphyrias. About 80% of patients with variegate porphyria are photosensitive. Some patients with hereditary coproporphyria also may have skin lesions. The porphyrias are very difficult to diagnose in the latent phase of the disorder. A variety of tests (e.g., the Watson-Schwartz test) or, more recently, direct assay of the intermediates themselves may be used in the acute state to measure the elevated levels of the heme intermediates. Variegate porphyria is common in South Africa, and acute intermittent porphyria is found with increasing frequency in Sweden. The inducible porphyrias are seen as a neurologic syndrome with a variety of presentations (Table 23-6).

The central, peripheral, and autonomic nervous systems may be involved in the porphyrias. A frequent manifestation is colicky abdominal pain, often with nausea and vomiting, which may suggest the diagnosis of acute abdomen, leading to exploratory laparotomy. Other symptoms are psychiatric disturbance, quadriplegia, hemiplegia, alterations of consciousness, and pain. Hyponatremia and hypokalemia may result from vomiting during the acute attack or may be related to hypothalamic disturbance. Death may result from paralysis of the respiratory muscles. The cause of these changes is unknown; they may be related to metabolites of the intermediates or result from deficiency of the heme pigment in the nerve cell itself.

An ever-increasing number of patients with concurrent human immunodeficiency virus and porphyria cutanea tarda are being recognized. The etiology of the association of these two disorders is unknown at this time.[143]

Because the porphyrias are unusual disorders, there is limited experience with the clinical use of many anesthetic drugs. In vitro studies suggest that certain anesthetics or anesthetic adjuvants may be contraindicated, but sufficient clinical experience is lacking (see below).[144]

Management of Patients with Porphyria

It is important to recognize porphyria in patients who are scheduled for surgery. It may become apparent through a careful family history and personal history related to anesthesia. A careful history in the patient with porphyria should concentrate on neurologic background and examination. Laboratory work should include electrolyte and blood urea nitrogen levels. Physical examination includes inspection of cutaneous lesions over the body.

In the anesthetic management of patients with porphyria, the chief concern is to avoid the administration of drugs that can induce a crisis; the drugs that induce cytochrome enzyme production can trigger the syndrome. Chief among those are the barbiturates; therefore, all barbiturates are con-

TABLE 23-5. Drugs Known to Precipitate Porphyria

Sedatives

Barbiturates
Hypnotics such as chlordiazepoxide, glutethimide, diazepam

Analgesics

Pentazocine, antipyrine, aminopyridine
Local anesthetics
Lidocaine

Anticonvulsants

Phenytoin, methsuximide

Antibiotics

Sulfonamides, chloramphenicol

Steroids

Estrogens, progesterones

Hypoglycemic sulfonylureas

Tolbutamide, chlorpropramide

Toxins

Lead, ethanol

Miscellaneous

Ergot preparations
Amphetamines
Methyldopa

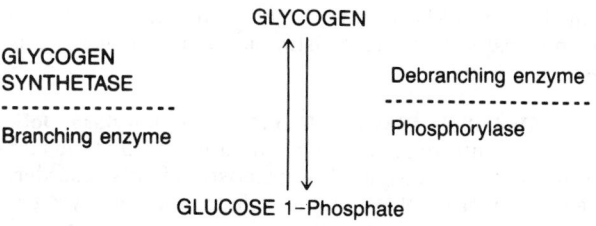

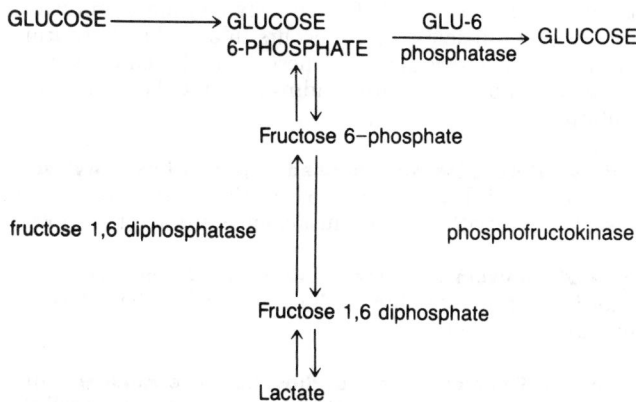

Figure 23-4. The glycogen-glucose-lactate pathway.

TABLE 23-6. Symptoms by Frequency in Variegate Porphyria

Abdominal pain	Pain in limbs
Vomiting	Confusion
Tachycardia	Abnormal behavior
Hypertension	Seizures
Neuropathy	Stupor
Pyrexia	

traindicated in porphyria. Ethyl alcohol, nonbarbiturate sedatives, hydantoin anticonvulsants, as well as a variety of other drugs also can induce a crisis (see Table 23-5). Endogenous factors, such as fasting, infection, and estrogens, may also precipitate porphyria. Diagnosis can be especially difficult because attacks may occur at a variable time period after drug administration or they may not occur at all despite administration of inducing drugs.

Propofol appears to be a safe induction agent.[145] Nitrous oxide, muscle relaxants, and opioids are unequivocally safe drugs. Experience with other inhalation agents and reversal agents has been favorable, but *in vitro* studies suggest that they might exacerbate a crisis.[146]

Most experts have advised that regional techniques be avoided to prevent confusion should neurologic signs develop after operation. However, recent reports of uneventful epidural anesthesia in the parturient with acute intermittent porphyria may indicate that this technique can be safely performed in these patients.[147] Blistered or fragile skin areas should be padded and given special attention. Glucose infusion should be started because starvation may induce an attack.

The acute attack should be treated with glucose infusion, and hyponatremia, hypokalemia, and hypomagnesemia should be treated. Pyridoxine and hematin also have been valuable in some cases. Supportive therapy for respiratory insufficiency and treatment of pain is also suggested.

Glycogen Storage Diseases

The metabolic pathways involving glucose degradation to lactate, glucose conversion to glycogen, and the breakdown of glycogen to glucose are important to the whole body biochemistry as well as to cellular physiology in general. The enzymatic steps involved in glucose metabolism have been studied intensively since the earliest days of modern biochemistry. The glycogen storage diseases are inherited and are characterized by dysfunction of one of the many enzymes involved in glucose metabolism. To date, several different glycogen storage disorders, each based on the deficiency of an enzyme involved in glucose metabolism, have been identified. Some of the glycogen storage diseases are incompatible with life past infancy, whereas others are not. Anesthetic experience with these diseases is limited, but several particular problems have been identified:[148]

> *Hypoglycemia.* This results from failure to metabolize stored glycogen to glucose; this is a constant risk of this disorder in these patients.
>
> *Acidosis.* This is related to fat and protein metabolism because glycogen stores are not metabolically available.
>
> *Cardiac and Hepatic Dysfunction.* This is secondary to destruction and displacement of normal tissue by the stored glycogen pools that accumulate.

Detailed descriptions of glucose metabolism are given elsewhere. Figure 23-4 outlines the glycogen-glucose-lactate pathway. There are, of course, multiple enzymatic steps to reach each of the end points.

Defects in Glucose Metabolism

Type I (Von Gierke's Disease; Glucose-6-Phosphate Deficiency). Inheritance is autosomal recessive. The prognosis is moderately good, with many patients surviving into adulthood. Short stature and liver enlargement are characteristic.

These patients tolerate fasting very poorly. Hypoglycemia, acidosis, and convulsions may be a problem. Prolonged bleeding has been described. Often, preoperative hyperalimentation is used to reduce liver glycogen stores. Portacaval shunt has been performed with limited success in these patients.[149]

Type II (Pompe's Disease). Inheritance of this disease is considered to be autosomal recessive. This is a devastating disease with a very poor prognosis. Death usually occurs in childhood. There is a deficiency of lysosomal acid maltase with an accumulation of glycogen in the lysosomes, especially in the heart, liver, muscle, and central nervous system. Cardiac compromise resulting from outflow obstruction of hypertrophied muscle occurs, as does congestive heart failure secondary to myocardial disruption by glycogen stores. A case report has been described in which halothane was used without incident.[150] In another case, halothane led to prompt hypotension and intractable cardiac failure.[151] A late-onset form with a better prognosis has been described as well.

Type III (Forbes' Disease; Debranching Enzyme Deficiency). Inheritance of this disease is autosomal recessive.

Type IV (Andersen's Disease; Branching Enzyme Deficiency). This is a very rare disorder, characterized by a defect in the synthesis of normal glycogen. Cirrhosis of the liver and death are characteristic before a patient reaches the age of 2 years.

Type V (McArdle's Disease; Muscle Phosphorylase Deficiency). An autosomal recessive inheritance pattern and cramping with exercise are characteristic of this disorder. There is an inability of skeletal muscle to mobilize glycogen stores with exercise, the usual fuel in muscle for sustained exercise. Myoglobinuria occurs with overexertion in these patients and may occur after succinylcholine administration as well. Muscle atrophy occurs in adulthood. Tourniquets should not be used in these patients, and frequent automated blood pressure readings should be done with caution.

Type VI (Hers' Disease; Reduced Hepatic Phosphorylase). A decreased ability to mobilize hepatic glycogen occurs in this disorder, with normal muscle and cardiac physiology.

Type VII (Muscle Phosphofructokinase Deficiency). This disorder is similar to McArdle's disease and is characterized by muscle cramping.

Type VIII (Deficient Hepatic Phosphorylase Kinase). This results from a deficiency in the regulatory enzyme controlling the phosphorylase enzyme. A case report has described fever and acidosis during succinylcholine, halothane, and ketamine anesthesia.[152] Liver transplantation has been used with success in the more severe forms of the glycogen storage diseases.

Defects of Fructose Metabolism

Fructose-6-phosphate is converted to fructose 1,6-diphosphate during glucose breakdown to lactate. Conversely, fructose 1,6-diphosphate is converted to fructose-6-phosphate by the enzyme fructose 1,6-diphosphatase during gluconeogenesis.

In fructose 1,6-diphosphatase deficiency, there is an inability to produce glycogen from lactate. Hypoglycemia may result. Acidosis has been reported because lactate is formed preferentially. In errors of fructose metabolism, like those of glucose metabolism, hypoglycemia and acidosis pose the greatest threats to the patient.[153]

The Mucopolysaccharidoses

The mucopolysaccharides are polysaccharides that yield mixtures of monosaccharides and derived products after hydrolysis. The mucopolysaccharides contain N-acetylated hexosamine in a characteristic repeating unit. For example, chondroitin sulfate A is a monosaccharide of d-glucuronic acid and N-acetyl d-galactosamine 4-sulfate. Monopolysaccharides are found in all cells.

The mucopolysaccharidoses are genetically determined diseases in which mucopolysaccharides are stored in tissues in abnormal quantities and excreted in large amounts in the urine. The disorders result from a deficiency of a specific lysosomal enzyme that is required to break down these compounds. As a result, mucopolysaccharides accumulate in tissues, producing specific clinical manifestations. There are seven basic forms of mucopolysaccharidoses and several subgroups. Most of the mucopolysaccharidoses are inherited as autosomal recessive traits. All the mucopolysaccharidoses are progressive, and

patients characteristically are marked by coarse facial features (gargoylism); associated skeletal abnormalities such as lumbar lordosis, stiff joints, chest deformity, dwarfing, and hypoplasia of the odontoid process (Morquio's syndrome); corneal opacities; limitation of joint motion; and heart, liver, and spleen enlargement resulting from mucopolysaccharide accumulation. Mental deterioration also occurs frequently.

The Hunter and Hurler syndromes are the best known variants of the mucopolysaccharidoses. The Hunter syndrome is an X-linked recessive disease.[154] Respiratory infection and heart disease, both valvular and ischemic, often lead to death when patients are young. Patients may commonly present for repair of inguinal hernia or ear, nose, and throat or orthopaedic procedures. The thick, soft tissues and the copious, thick secretions make perioperative and intraoperative airway management a particular problem. In Leroy's and Crocker's series, minor difficulties occurred with anesthesia in patients in more than one third of 60 operations.[154] Postoperative respiratory obstruction was noted in several cases. Because of the underlying heart disease, these patients should have electrocardiograms and echocardiographic tests performed before surgery.

Mucopolysaccharidosis IV (Morquio's syndrome) is associated with perhaps the most significant skeletal deformities. In addition to cardiovascular disorders and respiratory insufficiency from marked chest wall deformity, acute, subacute, or chronic myelopathy is extremely common. This is secondary to severe hypoplasia or absence of the odontoid process of the second cervical vertebra. In anesthesia care the head should be positioned carefully and precautions such as avoidance of succinylcholine should be taken with patients with spinal cord compromise.

These patients usually die of respiratory infection or cardiac failure resulting from valvular lesions or cardiomyopathy. Patients often require surgical correction of orthopaedic problems, corneal opacities, and carpal tunnel syndrome.

Other adverse reactions to anesthesia in patients with the mucopolysaccharidoses have been summarized recently.[155]

OTHER INHERITED DISORDERS

Osteogenesis Imperfecta

Osteogenesis imperfecta is seen in approximately 1 of 50,000 births. Most cases are autosomal dominant; some are autosomal recessive. The pathophysiologic characteristics include decreased collagen synthesis, which leads to osteoporosis; joint laxity; and tendon weakness. The manifestations of osteogenesis imperfecta are small bowed limbs, large head, short neck, blue sclerae, otosclerosis, joint laxity, brittle teeth, and a tendency to fractures. An increased bleeding tendency is also seen resulting from abnormal platelet function, and aortic and mitral valve dysfunction resulting from dilation of the valve ring.

The patient should be handled carefully because minor trauma may lead to fractures. Airway management may also be difficult because of cervical spine involvement with this disorder. Patients have short necks, and mandibular fractures frequently occur. The patient's cardiovascular status should be evaluated, especially mitral and aortic valve function. Kyphoscoliosis may also occur, with pulmonary compromise. Care should be taken to pad the pressure areas, particularly for long procedures. One should be prepared to obtain platelet transfusions. The patient's temperature should be monitored because hyperthermia (possibly resulting from central nervous system dysfunction) has been reported.[156] MH has also been associated with osteogenesis imperfecta.[30]

Neurofibromatosis (Von Recklinghausen's Disease)

Neurofibromatosis occurs in approximately one of 3000 births.[157] The inheritance pattern is autosomal dominant, but there is a varied expression. The pathophysiologic characteristics include localized fibromas of skin and nerve. Manifestations include café au lait spots and neuromas located along peripheral nerves inside and outside the central nervous system. Meningiomas, gliomas, and acoustic neuromas are not uncommon and are seen in two thirds of the cases. Laryngeal neurofibromas can lead to airway obstruction and dysphagia. Pheochromocytoma occurs in a small percentage of patients. Ten percent of patients with pheochromocytoma have neurofibromatosis. Scoliosis and kyphoscoliosis can also occur.

There are numerous anesthetic considerations for the patient with neurofibromatosis.[158,159] These include potential hypertensive crises resulting from pheochromocytomas or renal artery stenosis and hypersensitivity to nondepolarizing and depolarizing muscle relaxants. It is important to evaluate the airway because of the possibility of laryngeal tumors. Regional anesthesia may also be a problem in patients with fibromas involving the epidural space or peripheral nerves.

Marfan's Syndrome

Marfan's syndrome is caused by abnormal collagen production.[160] Its inheritance follows an autosomal dominant pattern. The classic clinical features of Marfan's syndrome include aortic regurgitation, joint laxity, spindly extremities, ectopia lentis, and weakened arterial walls. Death often occurs by the time the patient reaches the middle 30s. Aortic dissection is the most feared complication in the perioperative period. Consequently, hypertension should be aggressively controlled.

Ehlers-Danlos Syndrome

Ehlers-Danlos syndrome is inherited through an autosomal dominant pattern.[161] However, there are both X-linked recessive and X-linked dominant patterns of inheritance. The clinical features include hypermobile joints, bleeding tendency, hernias, and vascular dissection. The major problem relates to the bleeding tendency. The treatment plan for patients with Ehlers-Danlos syndrome is to evaluate their coagulation profile and to have large amounts of typed and crossed blood on hand.

Phenylketonuria

The inheritance of phenylketonuria follows an autosomal recessive pattern.[162] The inability to convert phenylalanine to tyrosine is the underlying defect. The clinical features include mental retardation and behavior abnormalities. These patients are prone to convulsions. Depression of the sympathoadrenal axis has also been seen. Hypoglycemia is common.

When anesthesia is administered, care should be taken to prevent hypoglycemia associated with preoperative fasting. The anesthesiologist should also remember that these patients can convulse. The precautions and appropriate plan for administering anesthesia include careful monitoring of blood glucose levels, avoidance of hypocarbia, avoidance of epileptogenic drugs, and continuation of all anticonvulsant therapy up to the time of surgery.

Prader-Willi Syndrome

The inheritance pattern of Prader-Willi syndrome is unknown.[163] Its clinical features include hypotonia, obesity, diabetes, hypogonadism, mental deficiency, and dental caries. The problems related to anesthesia are those that are secondary to the patient's hypoglycemia, obesity, and hypotonia. There are possible problems related to the neuromuscular blockade. The airway must be protected during surgery with an endotracheal tube, and during operation the blood glucose level should be monitored. Careful attention must also be paid to maintaining airway patency intraoperatively as well as postoperatively.

Riley-Day Syndrome (Familial Dysautonomia)

A deficiency of dopamine beta hydroxylase that leads to decreased norepinephrine at the nerve endings is thought to be the cause of Riley-Day syndrome.[164] This syndrome is inherited in an autosomal recessive fashion. Patients with Riley-Day syndrome exhibit copious pulmonary secretions, dysphagia, denervation supersensitivity, no sensitivity to pain, no response to histamine, and impairment of temperature control. The impairment of temperature control leads to intermittent fevers.

There are numerous problems related to anesthesia. These include corneal abrasions, excess secretions, pneumonia, labile blood pressure secondary to baroreceptor insensitivity and a decreased vascular volume, possible decreased response to hypoxia and hypercarbia, increased potential for aspiration because of swallowing problems, postural hypotension, and sensitivity to vasopressors.

Anesthesia management is well summarized by Axelrod et al.[165] Perioperative management should include diazepam (0.1–0.2 mg·kg^{-1} po) without an opioid. Cimetidine (5 mg·kg^{-1} iv) may be given on call. Intraoperative management should include temperature monitoring and careful blood pressure monitoring. Fresh gases should be humidified. Vasopressors need to be titrated carefully because of the hypersensitivity response. After operation secretions can be managed with chest percussion therapy. Postoperatively, narcotics should be avoided to minimize the risk of apnea.

REFERENCES

1. Denborough MA, Lovell RRH: Anaesthetic deaths in a family. Lancet 2:45, 1960
2. Denborough MA, Forster JFA, Lovell RRH et al: Anaesthesia deaths in a family. Br J Anaesth 34:395, 1962
3. Nelson TE: Porcine stress syndromes. In Gordon RA, Britt BA, Kalow W (eds): International Symposium on Malignant Hyperthermia, p 191. Springfield, Charles C Thomas, 1973
4. Kalow W, Britt BA, Terreau ME et al: Metabolic error of muscle metabolism after recovery from malignant hyperthermia. Lancet 2:895, 1970

5. Aldrete JA, Britt BA (eds): Second International Symposium on Malignant Hyperthermia. New York, Grune & Stratton, 1978

6. Lopez JR, Alamo L, Caputo C et al: Intracellular ionized calcium concentration in muscles from humans with malignant hyperthermia. Muscle Nerve 8:355, 1985

7. Gronert GA, Ahern CP, Milde JH: Treatment of porcine malignant hyperthermia: Lactate gradient from muscle to blood. Can Anaesth Soc J 33:729, 1986

8. Mathieu A, Bogosian AJ, Ryan JF et al: Recrudescence after survival of an initial episode of malignant hyperthermia. Anesthesiology 51:454, 1979

9. Donlon JV, Newfield P, Sreter I et al: Implications of masseter spasm after succinylcholine. Anesthesiology 49:298, 1978

10. Relton JES, Creighton RE, Conn AW et al: Generalized muscular hypertonicity associated with general anaesthesia. A suggested anaesthetic management. Can Anaesth Soc J 14:22, 1967

11. Littleford JA, Patel LR, Bose D et al: Masseter muscle spasm in children: Implications of continuing the triggering anesthetic. Anesth Analg 72:151, 1991

12. Ellis FR, Halsall PJ: Suxamethonium spasm. A differential diagnostic conundrum. Br J Anaesth 56:381, 1984

13. Hackl W, Mauritz W, Schemper M et al: Prediction of malignant hyperthermia susceptibility: Statistical evaluation of clinical signs. Br J Anaesth 64:425, 1990

14. Schwartz L, Rockoff MA, Koka BV: Masseter spasm with anesthesia: Incidence and implications. Anesthesiology 61:772, 1984

15. Ording H: Incidence of malignant hyperthermia in Denmark. Anesth Analg 64:700, 1985

16. Van Der Speck AFL, Fang WB, Ashton-Miller JA et al: The effects of succinylcholine on mouth opening. Anesthesiology 67:459, 1987

17. Rosenberg H: Trismus is not trivial. Anesthesiology 67:454, 1987

18. Rosenberg H, Fletcher JE: Masseter muscle rigidity and malignant hyperthermia susceptibility. Anesth Analg 65:161, 1986

19. Lazzell VA, Lerman J, Burrows FA, Creighton RE: Effect of thiopental on the incidence of masseter muscle rigidity after succinylcholine in infants and children. Anesthesiology 71:A1068, 1989

20. Miller ED, Sanders DB, Rowlingson JC et al: Anesthesia-induced rhabdomyolysis in a patient with Duchenne's muscular dystrophy. Anesthesiology 48:146, 1978

21. Caroff SN: The neuroleptic malignant syndrome. J Clin Psychiatry 41:679, 1980

22. Addonizio G, Susman VL: ECT as a treatment alternative for patients with symptoms of neuroleptic malignant syndrome. J Clin Psychiatry 48:102, 1987

23. Granato JR, Stern BJ, Ringel A et al: Neuroleptic malignant syndrome: Successful treatment with dantrolene and bromocriptine. Ann Neurol 14:89, 1983

24. Caroff SN, Rosenberg H, Fletcher JE et al: Malignant hyperthermia susceptibility in neuroleptic malignant hyperthermia syndrome. Anesthesiology 67:20, 1987

25. Kelfer H, Singer WN, Reynolds RN: Malignant hyperthermia in a child with Duchenne muscular dystrophy. Pediatrics 71:118, 1983

26. Smith CL, Bush GH: Anaesthesia and progressive muscular dystrophy. Br J Anaesth 57:1113, 1985

27. Heiman-Pattersohn TH, Natter H, Rosenberg H et al: Malignant hyperthermia susceptibility in X-linked muscle dystrophies. Pediatr Neurol 2:356, 1986

28. Frank JP, Harate Y, Butler JS et al: Central core disease and malignant hyperthermia syndrome. Ann Neurol 7:11, 1980

29. McPherson EW, Taylor CA: The King syndrome: Malignant hyperthermia, myopathy and multiple anomalies. Am J Med Genet 8:159, 1981

30. Rampton AJ, Kelly DA, Shanahan EC et al: Occurrence of malignant hyperpyrexia in a patient with osteogenesis imperfecta. Br J Anaesth 56:1443, 1984

31. Denborough MA, Galloway GJ, Hopkinson KC: Malignant hyperthermia and sudden infant death syndrome. Lancet 2:1068, 1982

32. Allen GC, Rosenberg H: Phaeochromocytoma presenting as acute malignant hyperthermia—a diagnostic challenge. Can J Anaesth 37:593, 1990

33. Gronert GA, Thompson RL, Onofrio BM: Human malignant hyperthermia: Awake episodes and correction by dantrolene. Anesth Analg 59:377, 1980

34. Fishbein WN, Muldoon SM, Deuster PA et al: Myoadenylate deaminase deficiency and malignant hyperthermia susceptibility: Is there a relationship? Biochem Med 34:344, 1985

35. Wingard DW: Malignant hyperthermia: A human stress syndrome? Lancet 2:1450, 1974

36. Neuspiel DR, Kuller DH: Sudden and unexpected death in childhood and adolescence. JAMA 264:1321, 1985

37. Wingard DW, Bobko S: Failure of lidocaine to trigger porcine malignant hyperthermia. Anesth Analg 58:855, 1979

38. Berkowitz A, Rosenberg H: Femoral block with mepivacaine for muscle biopsy in malignant hyperthermia patients. Anesthesiology 62:651, 1985

39. Gronert GA, Milde JH, Theye RA: Role of sympathetic activity in porcine malignant hyperthermia. Anesthesiology 47:411, 1977

40. Gronert GA, Milde JH, Taylor SR: Porcine muscle responses to carbachol, alpha and beta adrenoreceptor agonist, halothane or hyperthermia. J Physiol 307:319, 1980

41. Britt BA, Webb GE, LeDuc C: Malignant hyperthermia induced by curare. Can Anaesth Soc J 21:371, 1974

42. Ording H, Nielsen VG: Atracurium and its antagonism by neostigmine (plus glycopyrrolate) in patients susceptible to malignant hyperthermia. Br J Anaesth 58:1001, 1986

43. Hon CA, Landers DF, Platts AA: Effects of neuroleptic agents on rat skeletal muscle contracture in vitro. Anesth Analg 72:194, 1991

44. Gronert GA, Ahern CP, Milde J et al: Malignant hyperthermia not produced by CO_2, calcium or digoxin in porcine cardial or skeletal muscle: Triggering effects of potassium in skeletal muscle. Anesthesiology 64:24, 1986

45. Raff M, Harrison GG: The screening of propofol in MHS swine. Anesth Analg 68:750, 1989

46. Fletcher JE, Rosenberg H: *In vitro* studies of droperidol for use in human malignant hyperthermia. Anesthesiology 63:A302, 1985

47. Lunn JN, Farrow SC, Fowkes FGR et al: Epidemiology in anaesthesia. Br J Anaesth 59:803, 1982

48. Williams CH, Lasley JH: The mode of inheritance of the fulminant hyperthermia stress syndrome in swine. In Henschel EO (ed): Malignant Hyperthermia, Current Concepts, p 141. New York, Appleton-Century-Crofts, 1977

49. Seewald MJ, Eighinger HM, Lehmann-Horn F, Iaizzo PA: Characterization of swine susceptible to malignant hyperthermia by in vivo, in vitro and post-mortem techniques. Acta Anaesth Scand 35:345, 1991

50. Gallant EM, Rempel WE: Porcine malignant hyperthermia false negative in the halothane test. Am J Vet Res 48:488, 1987

51. McPherson EW, Taylor CA: The genetics of malignant hyperthermia: Evidence for heterogeneity. Am J Med Genet 11:273, 1982

52. Denborough MA: The pathopharmacology of malignant hyperpyrexia. Pharmacol Ther 9:357, 1980

53. Tolpin EI, Fletcher JE, Rosenberg H: Effects of anaesthetic agents on erythrocyte fragility: Comparison of normal and malignant hyperthermia susceptible patients. Can J Anaesth 34:366, 1987

54. Paasake RT, Brownell AKW: Serum creatine kinase level as a screening test for susceptibility to malignant hyperthermia. JAMA 255:769, 1986

55. Solomons CC, Masson NC: Platelet model for halothane-induced effects on nucleotide metabolism applied to malignant hyperthermia. Acta Anaesthesiol Scand 28:185, 1984

56. Lee MB, Adragna MHG, Edwards L: The use of a platelet nucleotide assay as a possible diagnostic test for malignant hyperthermia. Anesthesiology 63:311, 1985

57. Traynor CA, Van Dyke EA, Gronert GA: Phosphorylase ratio and susceptibility to malignant hyperthermia. Anesth Analg 62:324, 1983

58. Allen PD, Ryan JF, Jones DE et al: Correspondence: Sarcoplas-

mic reticulum calcium uptake in cryostat sections of skeletal muscle from malignant hyperthermia patients and controls. Muscle Nerve 9:474, 1986

59. Nagarajan K, Fishbein WN, Muldoon S: Calcium uptake in frozen muscle biopsy sections compared with other predictions of malignant hyperthermia susceptibility. Anesthesiology 66:680, 1987

60. Britt BA, Frodis W, Scott E et al: Comparison of the caffeine skinned fibre tension (CSFT) test with the caffeine-halothane contracture (CHC) test in the diagnosis of malignant hyperthermia. Can Anaesth Soc J 29:550, 1982

61. Blanck TJJ, Fisher YI, Thompson M et al: Low molecular weight proteins in human malignant hyperthermia muscle. Anesthesiology 61:589, 1984

62. Walsh MP, Brownell AKW, Littman V et al: Electrophoresis of muscle proteins is not a method for diagnosis of malignant hyperthermia susceptibility. Anesthesiology 64:473, 1986

63. Britt BA, Scott EA, Kleiman A et al: Failure of the tourniquet-twitch test as a diagnostic or screening test for malignant hyperthermia. Anesth Analg 66:1047, 1986

64. Ording H, Foder B, Scharff O: Cytosolic free calcium concentrations in lymphocytes from malignant hyperthermia. Br J Anaesth 64:341, 1990

65. Olgin J, Rosenberg H, Allen G et al: A blinded comparison of noninvasive, in vivo phosphorus nuclear magnetic resonance spectroscopy and the in vitro halothane/caffeine contracture test in the evaluation of malignant hyperthermia susceptibility. Anesth Analg 72:36, 1991

66. Fletcher JE, Rosenberg H: Laboratory methods for malignant hyperthermia. In Williams CH (ed): Experimental Malignant Hyperthermia, pp 121–140. New York, Springer-Verlag, 1988

67. Fletcher JE, Rosenberg H: In vitro muscle contractures induced by halothane and suxamethonium. 2. Human skeletal muscle from normal and malignant hyperthermia susceptible patients. Br J Anaesth 58:1433, 1986

68. Ellis FR, Halsall JP, Ording H et al: A protocol for the investigation of malignant hyperpyrexia (MH) susceptibility. Br J Anaesth 56:1267, 1984

69. Britt BA, Endrenyi L, Frodis W et al: Comparison of effects of several inhalation anaesthetics on caffeine-induced contractures of normal and malignant hyperthermic skeletal muscle. Can Anaesth Soc J 27:12, 1980

70. Nelson TE, Flewellen EH, Gloyna DF: Spectrum of susceptibility to malignant hyperthermia—diagnostic dilemma. Anesth Analg 62:545, 1983

71. Larach MG: Standardization of the caffeine halothane muscle contracture test. North American Malignant Hyperthermia Group. Anesth Analg 69:511, 1989

72. Allen GC, Rosenberg H, Fletcher JE: Safety of general anesthesia in patients previously tested negative for malignant hyperthermia susceptibility. Anesthesiology 72:619, 1990

73. Kolb ME, Horne ML, Martz R: Dantrolene in human malignant hyperthermia. Anesthesiology 56:254, 1982

74. Rubin AS, Zablocki AD: Hyperkalemia, verapamil and dantrolene. Anesthesiology 66:246, 1987

75. Fletcher R, Blennow G, Olsson AK et al: Malignant hyperthermia in a myopathic child. Prolonged postoperative course requiring dantrolene. Acta Anaesth Scand 26:431, 1982

76. Jensen AG, Bach V, Werner M et al: A fatal case of malignant hyperthermia following isoflurane anaesthesia. Acta Anaesth Scand 30:293, 1986

77. Britt BA: Dantrolene. Can Anaesth Soc J 31:61, 1984

78. Watson CB, Reierson N, Norfleet EA: Clinically significant muscle weakness induced by oral dantrolene. Sodium prophylaxis for malignant hyperthermia. Anesthesiology 65:312, 1986

79. Lerman J, McLeod ME, Strong HA: Pharmacokinetics of intravenous dantrolene in children. Anesthesiology 70:625, 1989

80. Allen GC, Cattran CB, Peterson RG, Lalande M: Plasma levels of dantrolene following oral administration in malignant hyperthermia-susceptible patients. Anesthesiology 69:900, 1988

81. Hackl W, Mauritz W, Schemper M et al: Prediction of malignant hyperthermia susceptibility: Statistical evaluation of clinical signs. Br J Anaesth 64:425, 1990

82. Beebe JJ, Sessler DI: Preparation of anesthesia machines for patients susceptible to malignant hyperthermia. Anesthesiology 69:395, 1988

83. Neubauer K, Kaufman RD: Another use for mass spectroscopy: Detection and monitoring of malignant hyperthermia. Anesth Analg 64:837, 1985

84. Vaughan MS, Cork RC, Vaughan RW: Inaccuracy of liquid crystal thermometry to identify cone temperature trends in postoperative adults. Anesth Analg 61:284, 1982

85. Ruhland G, Hinkle A: Malignant hyperthermia after oral and intravenous pretreatment with dantrolene in a patient susceptible to malignant hyperthermia. Anesthesiology 60:159, 1984

86. Shime J, Gare D, Andrews J, Britt B: Dantrolene in pregnancy: Lack of adverse effects on the fetus and newborn infant. Am J Obstet Gynecol 159:831, 1988

87. Harthorn AM, Young E: A relationship between acid base balance and capture myopathy in zebra (Equus burchelli) and apparent therapy. Vet Rec 95:337, 1974

88. Harrison GG: Porcine malignant hyperthermia—the saga of the "hot" pig. In Britt BA (ed): Malignant Hyperthermia, pp 103–136. Boston, Martinus Nijhoff Publishing, 1987

89. Klein L, Rosenberg H: Malignant hyperthermia in animals other than swine. In Britt BA (ed): Malignant Hyperthermia, pp 137–154. Boston, Martinus Nijhoff Publishing, 1987

90. Nelson TE: Malignant hyperthermia in dogs. J Am Vet Med Assoc 198:989, 1991

91. Allen GC, Fletcher JE, Huggins FJ, et al: Caffeine and halothane contracture testing in swine using the recommendations of the North American Malignant Hyperthermia Group. Anesthesiology 72:71, 1990

92. Wieland SJ, Fletcher JE, Rosenberg H, Gong QH: Malignant hyperthermia: Slow sodium current in cultured human muscle cells. Am J Physiol 257:C759, 1989

93. Cheah KS, Cheah AM, Waring JC: Phospholipase A2 activity, calmodulin, Ca^{2+} and meat quality in young and adult halothane-sensitive and halothane-insensitive British Landrace pigs. Meat Sci 17:37, 1986

94. Lopez JR, Allen PD, Alamo L et al: Myoplasmic free $[Ca^{2+}]$ during a malignant hyperthermia episode in swine. Muscle Nerve 11:82, 1988

95. Mickelson JR, Ross JA, Hyslop RJ et al: Skeletal muscle sarcolemma in malignant hyperthermia: Evidence for a defect in calcium regulation. Biochem Biophys Acta 897:364, 1987

96. Cheah KS, Cheah AM: Skeletal muscle mitochondrial phospholipase A2 and the interaction of mitochondria and sarcoplasmic reticulum in porcine malignant hyperthermia. Biochem Biophys Acta 638:40, 1981

97. Cheah KS, Cheah AM, Fletcher JE, Rosenberg H: Skeletal muscle mitochondrial respiration of malignant hyperthermia-susceptible patients. Ca^{2+}-induced uncoupling and free fatty acids. Int J Biochem 21:913, 1989

98. Heffron JJA: Mitochondrial and plasma membrane changes in skeletal muscle in the malignant hyperthermia syndrome. Biochem Soc Trans 12:360, 1984

99. Nelson TE: Abnormality in calcium release from skeletal sarcoplasmic reticulum of pigs susceptible to malignant hyperthermia. J Clin Invest 72:862, 1983

100. Fletcher JE, Tripolitis L, Erwin K et al: Fatty acids modulate calcium release from skeletal muscle heavy sarcoplasmic reticulum fractions: Implications for malignant hyperthermia. Biochem Cell Biol 68:1195, 1990

101. McSweeney DM, Heffron JJA: Uptake and release of calcium ions by heavy sarcoplasmic reticulum fraction of normal and malignant hyperthermia-susceptible human skeletal muscle. Int J Biochem 22:329, 1990

102. Mullikin-Kilpatrick D, Ekenbarger DM, Welch G et al: Microheterogeneity of the Ca^{2+} ATPase in skeletal muscle from pigs with malignant hyperthermia (MH). Anesthesiology 73:A696, 1990

103. Mickelson JR, Gallant EM, Litterer LA et al: Abnormal sarcoplasmic reticulum ryanodine receptor in malignant hyperthermia. J Biol Chem 263:9310, 1988

104. Vita GM, Fletcher JE, Tripolitis L et al: Altered [3H] ryanodine binding is not associated with malignant hyperthermia sus-

ceptibility in terminal cisternae preparations from swine. Biochem Int 23:563, 1991

105. McCarthy TV, Healy JMS, Heffron JJA et al: Localization of the malignant hyperthermia susceptibility locus to human chromosome 19q12-13.2. Nature 343:563, 1990

106. MacLennan DH, Duff C, Zorzato F et al: Ryanodine receptor gene is a candidate for predisposition to malignant hyperthermia. Nature 343:559, 1990

107. Levitt RC, McKusick VA, Fletcher JE, Rosenberg H: Gene candidate (letter). Nature 345:297, 1990

107a. Wieland SJ, Fletcher JE, Rosenberg M, Gong Q-H: Malignant hypothermia: Slow sodium current in cultured human muscle cells. Am J Physiol 257:C759, 1989

108. Fletcher JE, Rosenberg H, Michaux K et al: Fatty acids in muscle from patients susceptible to malignant hyperthermia. Eur J Anaesth 6:355, 1989

109. Foster PS, Gesini E, Claudianos C et al: Inositol 1,4,5,-trisphosphate phosphatase deficiency and malignant hyperpyrexia in swine. Lancet 1:124, 1989

110. Duthie GG, Arthur JR: The antioxidant abnormality in the stress-susceptible pig. Effect of vitamin E supplementation. Ann NY Acad Sci 570:322, 1989

111. Mickelson JR, Thatte HS, Beaudry TM et al: Increased skeletal muscle acetylcholinesterase activity in porcine malignant hyperthermia. Muscle Nerve 10:723, 1987

112. Joffe M, Salvage N, Sautoy CD et al: Kinase activity and protein phosphorylation in control and malignant hyperthermic skeletal muscle. Int J Biochem 23:443, 1991

113. Sim ATR, White MD, Denborough MA: Thiophosphorylation of skeletal muscle sarcoplasmic reticulum in porcine malignant hyperpyrexia. Int J Biochem 19:1217, 1987

114. Ording H, Hansen U, Theil Skovgaard L: Age, fiber type composition and in vitro contracture responses in human malignant hyperthermia. Acta Anaesthesiol Scand 32:121, 1988

115. Haggendal J, Jonsson L, Carlsten J: The role of sympathetic activity in initiating malignant hyperthermia. Acta Anaesthesiol Scand 34:677, 1990

116. Olson EN: Modification of proteins with covalent lipids. Prog Lipid Res 27:177, 1988

117. Grand RJA: Acylation of viral and eukaryotic proteins. Biochem J 258:625, 1989

118. Takeshima H, Nishimura S, Matsumoto T et al: Primary structure and expression from complementary DNA of skeletal muscle ryanodine receptor. Nature 339:439, 1989

119. Wieland SJ, Fletcher JE, Gong Q-H, Rosenberg H: Effects of lipid-soluble agents on sodium channel function in normal and MH-susceptible skeletal muscle cultures. In Blanck JJ, Wheeler DM (eds): Mechanisms of Anesthetic Action in Muscle, pp. 9–19. New York, Plenum Publishing Corporation, 1991

120. Van Kuijk FJGM, Sevanian A, Handelman GJ, Dratz EA: A new role for phospholipase A2: Protection of membranes from lipid peroxide damage. Trends in Bioch Sci 12:31, 1987

121. Levitt RC, Nouri N, Jedlicka AE et al: Evidence for molecular genetic heterogeneity in malignant hyperthermia susceptibility. Genomics, 11:543, 1991

121a. Fujii J, Otsu K, Zorzato F, DeLeon S, Khanna VK, Weiler JE, O'Brien PJ, MacLennan D: Identification of a mutation in porcine Ryanodine receptor associated with malignant hypothermia. Science 253:448, 1991

122. Nyhan WL, Sakata NO: Genetic and Malformation Syndromes in Clinical Medicine. Chicago, Year Book Medical Publishers, 1976

123. Stanbury JB, Wyngaarden JB, Frederickson DS: The Metabolic Basis of Inherited Disease. 6th ed. New York, McGraw-Hill, 1989

124. Viby-Mogensen J, Hanel HK: A Danish cholinesterase unit. Acta Anaesth Scand 21:405, 1977

125. Viby-Mogensen J: Succinylcholine neuromuscular blockade in subjects homozygous for atypical plasma cholinesterase. Anesthesiology 55:429, 1981

126. Kalow W, Genest K: A method for the detection of atypical forms of human serum cholinesterase. Determination of dibucaine numbers. Can J Biochem 35:339, 1957

127. Ravindran RS, Cummins DF, Pantazis KL et al: Unusual aspects of low levels of pseudocholinesterase in a pregnant patient. Anesth Analg 61:953, 1982

128. Harris H, Whittaker M: Differential inhibition of serum cholinesterase with fluoride. Recognition of two new phenotypes. Nature (London) 191:496, 1961

128a. McGuire M, Noguiera CG, Barttels CF, Lightstone H, Hayra A, Van Der Spek A, Lockridge O, La Du BN: Identification of the structured mutation responsible for the dibucaine-resistant (atypical) variant form of human cholinesterase. Proc Natl Acad Sciences USA 86:953, 1989

129. Krause A, Lane AB, Jenkins T: Pseudocholinesterase variation in southern Africa populations. South African Med J 71:298, 1987

130. Hanel HK, Viby-Mogensen J, Schaffalitzky de Muckadell OB: Serum cholinesterase variants in the Danish population. Acta Anaesthesiol Scand 22:505, 1978

131. Moorthy SS, Krishna G, Clark JH: Pseudocholinesterase and affective disorders. Anesth Analg 66:921, 1987

132. Patterson JL, Walsh ES, Hall GM: Progressive depletion of plasma cholinesterase during daily plasma exchange. Br Med J 2:580, 1979

133. Viby-Mogensen J: Correlation of succinylcholine duration of action with plasma cholinesterase activity in subjects with normal enzyme. Anesthesiology 53:517, 1980

134. Viby-Mogensen J: Succinylcholine neuromuscular blockade in subjects heterozygous for abnormal plasma cholinesterase. Anesthesiology 55:231, 1981

135. Baraka A: Absence of suxamethonium fasciculations in patients with atypical plasma cholinesterase. Br J Anaesth 47:419, 1975

136. Lovely MJ, Patteson SK, Beuerlein FJ, Chesney JT: Perioperative blood transfusion may conceal atypical pseudocholinesterase. Anesth Analg 70:326, 1990

137. Harris H, Hopkinson DA, Robson EB et al: Genetic studies on a new variant of serum cholinesterase detected by electrophoresis. Ann Hum Genet 26:359, 1963

138. Brodsky JB, Campos FA: Chloroprocaine analgesia in a patient receiving echothiophate iodide eye drops. Anesthesiology 48:288, 1978

139. Raj PP, Rosenblatt R, Miller J et al: Dynamics of local anesthetic compounds in regional anesthesia. Anesth Analg 56:110, 1977

140. Kuhnert BR, Philipson EA et al: A prolonged chloroprocaine epidural block in a postpartum patient with abnormal pseudocholinesterase. Anesthesiology 56:477, 1982

141. Jatlow P, Barash PG, Van Dyke C et al: Cocaine and succinylcholine sensitivity: A new caution. Anesth Analg 58:235, 1979

142. Murphy PC: Acute intermittent porphyria: The anaesthetic problem and its background. Br J Anaesth 36:801, 1964

143. Lafeuillade A, Dhiver C, Martin I et al: Porphyria cutanea tarda associated with HIV infection. AIDS 4:924, 1990

144. Mustajoki P, Heinonen J: General anesthesia in "inducible" porphyrias. Anesthesiology 53:12, 1980

145. McLoughlin C: Use of propofol in a patient with porphyria. Br J Anaesth 62:114, 1989

146. Parikh RK, Moore MR: Effect of certain anaesthetic agents on the activity of rat hepatic delta amino-levulinate synthetase. Br J Anaesth 50:1099, 1978

147. McNeill MJ, Bennet A: Use of regional anaesthesia in a patient with acute porphyria. Br J Anaesth 64:371, 1990

148. Cox JM: Anesthesia and glycogen storage disease. Anesthesiology 29:1221, 1963

149. Casson H: Anesthesia for portacaval bypass in patients with metabolic diseases. Br J Anaesth 47:969, 1975

150. Kaplan R: Pompe's disease presenting for anesthesia. Anesth Rev 7:21, 1980

151. Ellis FR: Inherited muscle disease. Br J Anaesth 52:153, 1980

152. Edelstein G, Hirshman CA: Hyperthermia and ketoacidosis during anesthesia in a child with glycogen-storage disease. Anesthesiology 52:90, 1980

153. Hashimoto Y, Watanabe H, Satou M: Anesthetic management of a patient with hereditary fructose 1,6 diphosphate deficiency. Anesth Analg 57:503, 1978

154. Leroy JG, Crocker AC: Clinical definition of the Hurler-Hunter phenotypes. Am J Dis Child 112:518, 1966

155. Sjogren P, Pedersen T, Steinmetz H: Mucopolysaccharidoses and anaesthetic risk. Acta Anaesth Scand 31:214, 1987

156. Oliverio RM: Anesthetic management of intramedullary nailing in osteogenesis imperfecta: Report of a case. Anesth Analg 52:232, 1973

157. Fisher MM: Anaesthetic difficulties in neurofibromatosis. Anaesthesia 30:648, 1975

158. Magbagbeola JA: Abnormal responses to muscle relaxants in patients with von Recklinghausen's disease. Br J Anaesth 42:710, 1970

159. Yamashita M, Matsuki A, Oyama T: Anaesthetic considerations in von Recklinghausen's disease (multiple neurofibromatosis). Anaesthetist 26:317, 1977

160. Pyevitz RE, McKusick VA: The Marfan syndrome: Diagnosis and management. N Engl J Med 300:172, 1979

161. Donlan P, Sisko F, Riley E: Anesthetic considerations for Ehlers-Danlos syndrome. Anesthesiology 52:266, 1980

162. Jackson SH: Inborn errors of metabolism. In Katz J, Benumof J, Kadis LB (eds): Anesthesia and Uncommon Diseases, 2nd ed, p 1. Philadelphia, WB Saunders, 1981

163. Palmer SK, Atlee JL: Anesthetic management of the Prader Willi syndrome. Anesthesiology 44:161, 1976

164. Brown BR, Watson PD, Taussig LM: Congenital metabolic diseases of pediatric patients. Anesthesiology 43:197, 1975

165. Axelrod FB, Donenfeld RF, Danzinger F, Turndorf M: Anesthesia in familial dysautonomia. Anesthesiology 68:631, 1988

24 John R. Moyers

Preoperative Medication

Anesthetic management for patients begins with preoperative psychological preparation and, if necessary, preoperative medication. Specific pharmacologic actions should be kept in mind when these drugs are administered before operation, and they should be tailored to the needs of each patient. The anesthesiologist should assess the patient's mental and physical condition during the preoperative visit. Because it is part of and the beginning of the anesthetic, choice of preoperative medication is based on the same considerations as the choice of anesthesia, for example, the patient's medical problems, requirements of the surgery, and the anesthesiologist's skills. Satisfactory preoperative preparation and medication facilitate an uneventful perioperative course. Poor preparation may begin a series of problems and misadventures.

No consensus exists on the choice of preoperative medications. Their use has been dominated in the past by tradition, which has been modified somewhat by the change in anesthetic agents and techniques over the years. Beecher stated that "empirical procedures firmly established in the habits of good doctors have a life, not to say, immortality of their own."[1] Similarly, "the emotional attachment of an anesthesiologist to his own regimen is often more obvious than his objective assessment of its effects."[2] Another reason for lack of consensus may be that several different drugs or combinations of drugs can accomplish the same goals. However, there is general agreement that most patients should enter the operating room after anxiety has been relieved and other specific goals have been met through preoperative preparation and medication. This should be accomplished without undue sedation's interfering with patient safety.

PSYCHOLOGICAL PREPARATION

Psychological preparation of the patient involves the preoperative visit and interview with the patient and family members. The anesthesiologist should explain anticipated events and the proposed anesthetic management in an effort to reduce anxiety and allay apprehension. Patients may perceive the day of surgery as the biggest day in their lives; they do not wish to be treated impersonally in the operating room.[3] Preoperative visits must be conducted efficiently but must be informative and reassuring and answer all questions. Most of the anesthesiologist's time is spent with an unconscious or sedated patient; therefore he or she must take time before the operation to earn the trust and confidence of that patient.

Most patients are anxious before surgery.[4-6] Studies show, depending on the intensity of inquiry, that from 40–85% of patients are apprehensive before surgery.[7,8] Preoperative anxiety states are at a high level, and patients expect apprehension to be relieved before they arrive in the operating room.[9,10] A study by Egbert et al showed that an average of 57.2% patients felt anxious before operation.[8] The highest levels of anxiety were noted in patients scheduled for major genitourologic surgery (79%) and for cancer surgery (85.7%). They found neither age nor sex differences in levels of apprehension among the study population. In a study of 500 adult patients scheduled for surgery, Norris and Baird found that female patients were more likely than male patients to be anxious before operation.[7] Also, they found an increased incidence of anxiety in female patients who weighed more than 70 kg and in patients previously or currently taking sedative drugs. They also documented a trend toward greater levels of anxiety in more ill patients. There was no difference in anxiety with regard to age, social status, nature of the operation, or previous hospital experience.

An informative and comforting preoperative visit may replace many milligrams of depressant medication. The study by Egbert and colleagues showed that more patients were adequately prepared for surgery after a preoperative interview than after 2 mg·kg^{-1} of pentobarbital given intramuscularly 1 hour before surgery (Table 24-1).[8] During unit rounds on the afternoon before surgery, the patients in their preoperative interview group were visited by the anesthesiologist, who discussed each patient's condition, the time of the operation, and the anesthetic. The patient was informed about perioperative events and asked about previous anesthetic experiences. The patients in this study who received pentobarbital for preoperative medication but had no interview appeared and felt drowsy but were not calm. Leigh et al investigated adult preoperative patients using objective tests of anxiety.[9] They found that the anesthesiologist's 10-minute preoperative visit produced lower anxiety levels before operation than no visit at all. Furthermore, they found that the preoperative visit was more effective than a booklet given to the patients the day before surgery, which

TABLE 24-1. Comparison of Preoperative Visit and Pentobarbital (2 mg·kg⁻¹ im) (Percentage of Patients)

	Felt Drowsy	Felt Nervous	Adequate Preparation
Control group	18	58	35
Pentobarbital only	30	61	48
Preoperative visit	26	40	65
Preoperative visit and pentobarbital	38	38	71

Data from Egbert LD, Battit GE, Turndorf H *et al:* The value of the preoperative visit by an anesthetist. JAMA 185:553, 1963.

TABLE 24-2. Various Goals for Preoperative Medication

1. Relief of anxiety
2. Sedation
3. Amnesia
4. Analgesia
5. Drying of airway secretions
6. Prevention of autonomic reflex responses
7. Reduction of gastric fluid volume and increased pH
8. Antiemetic effects
9. Reduction of anesthetic requirements
10. Facilitation of smooth induction of anesthesia
11. Prophylaxis against allergic reactions

Modified from Stoelting RK: Psychological preparation and preoperative medication. In Miller RD (ed): Anesthesia. New York, Churchill Livingstone, 1981.

was specifically designed to reassure them about anesthesia. The booklet was not a substitute for a proper preoperative visit and interview.

Psychological preparation cannot accomplish everything and will not relieve all anxiety. In addition to psychological preparation, there are other goals of preoperative medication. Control of pain and satisfactory levels of amnesia or sedation also cannot be achieved with consistent success at the preoperative visit alone. In addition, in emergency situations, there may be little or no time for a preoperative interview. Conversely, more seriously ill or elderly patients may not tolerate the physiologic effects of sedative medications. Always remember that the substitution of preoperative depressant drugs for a comforting and tactful preoperative visit may endanger patient safety.

PHARMACOLOGIC PREPARATION

The ideal drug or combination of drugs for preoperative pharmacologic preparation is as elusive as is the ideal anesthetic technique. Routine administration of the same drugs to all patients has fallen into disfavor as a selective approach has emerged. In selecting the appropriate drugs for preoperative medication, the patient's psychological condition and physical status must be considered. The patient's age also is important. Is the patient in the pediatric or the geriatric age group? The surgical procedure and its duration are important factors. Is this an outpatient procedure? Is it elective surgery or emergency surgery? The anesthesiologist must know the patient's weight; prior response to depressant drugs, including unwanted side-effects; and allergies. Finally, the anesthesiologist's experience and familiarity with certain preoperative medications more than others are determinants.

The goals to be achieved for each patient with preoperative medication are intimately involved in the selection process (Table 24-2). The desired goals may be multiple and should be tailored to the needs of each patient. Some of the goals, such as relief of anxiety and production of sedation, apply to almost every patient, whereas others are important only occasionally. Prophylaxis against allergic reactions applies in only a few instances. Prevention of autonomic reflexes mediated through the vagus nerve or an antiemetic effect may be better attempted immediately before the anticipated need rather than achieved at the time of preoperative medication. Administration of clonidine with diazepam 90–120 minutes before the induction of anesthesia blunts heart rate responses to laryngoscopic examination and reduces anesthetic requirements for inhaled and injected

drugs.[11,12] Conversely, most preoperative medication regimens do not produce sufficient obtundation to be clinically significant in reducing anesthetic requirement. Preoperative medication prevents preoperative elevations of plasma concentrations of beta-endorphins that normally accompany the stress response (Fig. 24-1).[13]

Some patients should not receive depressant drugs before surgery. Patients with little physiologic reserve, at the extremes of age, or with a head injury with hypovolemia would probably be harmed more than helped by many of the medications normally used before operation. In contrast, the conditions of others demand that attempts be made pharmacologically to reduce anxiety, increase gastric fluid pH, reduce gastric fluid volume, provide analgesia, or dry secretions in the airway to produce a safer perioperative course. For elective surgery, in most instances the anesthesiologist will want the patient to enter the operating room free of anxiety and sedated but easily arousable and cooperative. The patient should not be overly obtunded or display

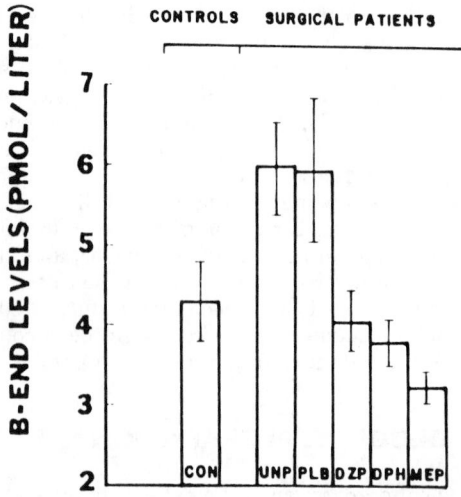

Figure 24-1. Plasma beta-endorphin (B-END) concentrations as measured in control (CON) patients or in presurgical patients receiving no premedication (UNP), intramuscular saline (PLB), oral diazepam 10 mg (DZP), intramuscular diphenhydramine 1 mg·kg⁻¹ (DPH), or intramuscular meperidine 1 mg·kg⁻¹ (MEP). Measurements were made 1 hour after treatment. Mean ± SEM. (Reprinted with permission from Walsh J, Puig MM, Lovitz MA *et al:* Premedication abolishes the increase in plasma beta-endorphin observed in the immediate preoperative period. Anesthesiology 66:402, 1987.)

other unwanted side-effects of the preoperative drugs. The patient who asks to be "asleep" before leaving the hospital room should be told that apprehension and sedation may be reduced but it would be unsafe to produce a comatose state. The time and route of administration of the preoperative medications are important. As a general rule, oral medications should be given to the patient in the hospital room 60–90 minutes before his or her arrival in the operating room. For full effect, intramuscular medications should be given at least 20 minutes and preferably 30–60 minutes before the patient's arrival in the operating room. Every attempt should be made to have the preoperative medications achieve their full effect before the patient's arrival in the operating room rather than after induction of anesthesia. The drug(s), doses, route of administration, and effects should be recorded on the anesthetic record. A list of common preoperative medications is presented in Table 24-3.

Finally, the choice of premedicant drugs is not based on a large body of scientific data that is either definitive or persuasive. The subject is difficult to study. Often the investigations involve only one dose of drug or one dose of a number of drugs given in combination. In some studies drugs are given parenterally, whereas in others they are administered orally or even rectally. Different investigations may study the effect of the drugs at different times after administration. The patients' responses and the investigators' observations of those responses are subjective and difficult to quantify. Also, the studies may involve heterogeneous groups of patients in whom the psychological preoperative preparation has not been standardized.

Sedative Hypnotics and Tranquilizers

Benzodiazepines

Benzodiazepines are among the most popular drugs used for preoperative medication (Table 24-4). They are used to produce anxiolysis, amnesia, and sedation. The anticonvulsant and muscle relaxant effects of the benzodiazepines are not usually important when preoperative medication is considered. Because the site of action of benzodiazepines is on specific receptors in the central nervous system, there is relatively little depression of ventilation or of the cardiovascular system with premedicant doses. Benzodiazepines have a wide therapeutic index and a low incidence of toxicity. Other than central nervous system depression, there are few side-effects of this group of drugs. Specifically, nausea and vomiting are not usually associated with administration of benzodiazepines for preoperative medication. These drugs are often used before operation to reduce the unpleas-

ant dreams and delirium that may occur after ketamine administration.[14]

There are some hazards and unwanted side-effects of the benzodiazepines. The central nervous system depression they cause is sometimes long and excessive, especially with use of lorazepam. There may be pain at the intramuscular or intravenous injection site with diazepam, as well as the possibility of phlebitis.[14] These drugs are not analgesic agents. Benzodiazepines may not always produce a calming effect but may cause agitation, as evidenced by restlessness and delirium in patients during labor and delivery.[15] However, in another study of patients during labor, a combination of benzodiazepines with an opioid produced satisfactory results.[16]

The proposed mechanisms of action of the benzodiazepines describe specific receptors and actions within the central nervous system (Fig. 24-2).[17,18] The sedative action is said to result from a facilitation or enhancement of inhibitory neurotransmission mediated by gamma-aminobutyric acid. The anxiolytic effect comes from the action of glycine-mediated inhibition of neuronal pathways in the brain stem and in the brain. The site of action of the benzodiazepines in producing amnesia is unknown.

Diazepam. The calming, amnesic, and sedative effects of diazepam make it a very popular choice for premedication.

TABLE 24-3. Common Preoperative Medications, Doses, and Administration Routes

Medication	Administration Route	Dose
Diazepam	Oral	5–20 mg
Lorazepam	Oral, im	1–4 mg
Midazolam	im	3–7 mg
	iv	Titration of 1.0–2.5-mg doses
Secobarbital	Oral, im	50–200 mg
Pentobarbital	Oral, im	50–200 mg
Morphine	im	5–15 mg
Meperidine	im	50–150 mg
Cimetidine	Oral, im, iv	150–300 mg
Ranitidine	Oral	50–200 mg
Metoclopramide	Oral, im, iv	5–20 mg
Atropine	im, iv	0.3–0.6 mg
Glycopyrrolate	im, iv	0.1–0.3 mg
Scopolamine	im, iv	0.3–0.6 mg

im = intramuscular; iv = intravenous.

Modified from Stoelting RK, Miller RD (eds): Basics of Anesthesia. New York, Churchill Livingstone, 1984.

TABLE 24-4. Comparison of Pharmacologic Variables of Benzodiazepines

	Diazepam	Lorazepam	Midazolam
Dose equivalent (mg)	10	1–2	3–5
Time to peak effect after oral dose (h)	1–1.5	2–4	0.5–1
Elimination half-time (h)	20–40	10–20	1–4
Clearance (ml·kg^{-1}·min^{-1})	0.2–0.5	0.7–1.0	6.4–11.1
Volume of distribution (l·kg^{-1})	0.7–1.7	0.8–1.3	1.1–1.7

Adapted from Reves JG, Fragen RJ, Vinick HR et al: Midazolam: Pharmacology and uses. Anesthesiology 62:310, 1985, and Stoelting RK: Pharmacology and Physiology in Anesthetic Practice. Philadelphia, JB Lippincott, 1987.

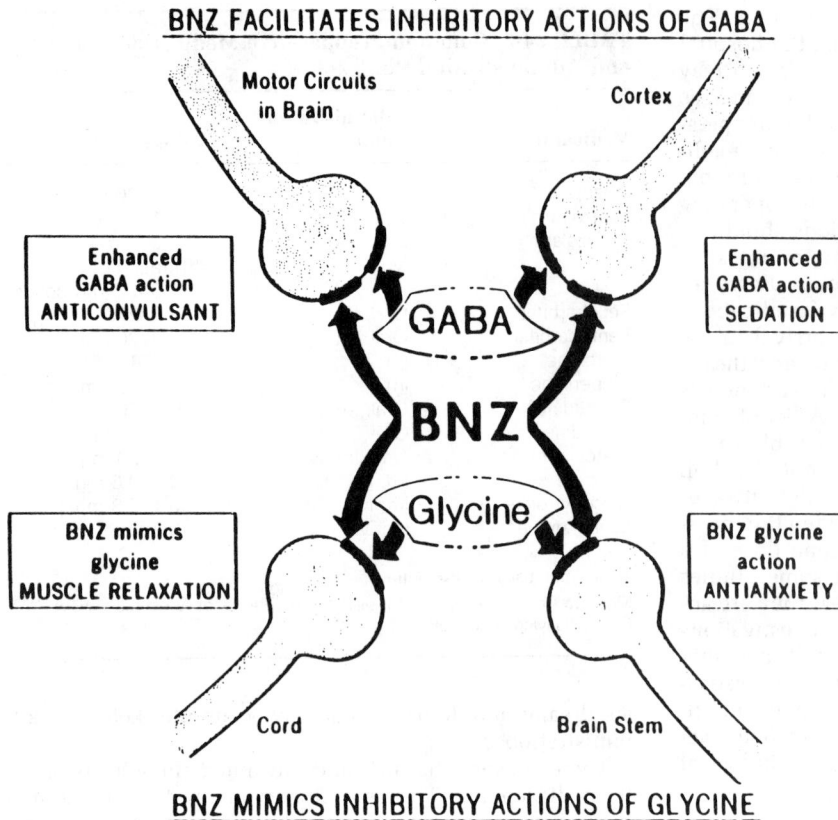

BNZ FACILITATES INHIBITORY ACTIONS OF GABA

Motor Circuits in Brain

Cortex

Enhanced GABA action **ANTICONVULSANT**

GABA

Enhanced GABA action **SEDATION**

BNZ

BNZ mimics glycine **MUSCLE RELAXATION**

Glycine

BNZ glycine action **ANTIANXIETY**

Cord

Brain Stem

BNZ MIMICS INHIBITORY ACTIONS OF GLYCINE

Figure 24-2. Schematic diagram of possible mechanisms for pharmacologic effects of benzodiazepines (BNZs). GABA = gamma aminobutyric acid. (Reprinted with permission from Richter JJ: Current theories about the mechanisms of benzodiazepines and neuroleptic drugs. Anesthesiology 54:66, 1981.)

It is the standard against which other benzodiazepines are usually compared. Because diazepam is insoluble in water and must be dissolved in organic solvents, pain may occur on intramuscular or intravenous injection. Phlebitis is often a sequela of intravenous injection. More than 90% of an oral dose of diazepam is rapidly absorbed. Peak effect after oral administration occurs within ½ to 1 hour and within 15–30 minutes in children (Fig. 24-3).[19] Diazepam does cross the placenta. Because the drug is highly protein-bound, patients with low serum albumin levels, such as those with cirrhosis

of the liver or chronic renal failure, may exhibit an increased effect of the drug.[17] Diazepam is metabolized by the hepatic microsomal enzymes to some metabolites that are active. Prolonged sedation resulting from active metabolites is usually seen after chronic use of diazepam rather than following the use of a single dose in the preoperative setting. The elimination half-time of diazepam is 21–37 hours in healthy volunteers. It may be prolonged in patients with cirrhosis or in elderly patients.[22] Because absorption is unpredictable after intramuscular injection and because of

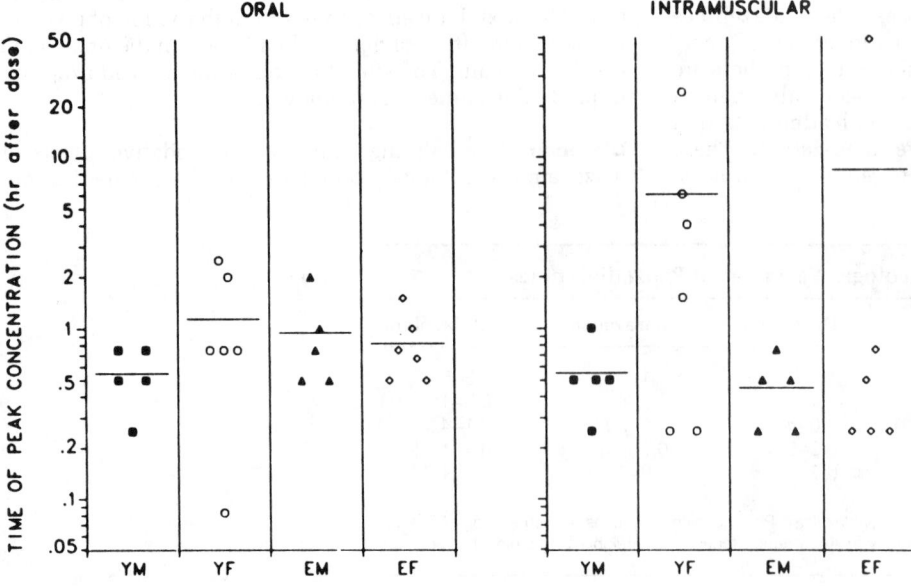

Figure 24-3. Individual and mean (*horizontal bar*) times of peak plasma concentrations after oral or intramuscular (deltoid) administration of diazepam, 5 mg, to adult patients (20–78 years old) categorized as young male (YM), young female (YF), elderly male (EM), and elderly female (EF) patients. (Reprinted with permission from Dwoll M, Greenblatt DJ, Ochs HR *et al*: Absolute bioavailability of oral and intramuscular diazepam: Effects of age and sex. Anesth Analg 62:1, 1983.)

pain with parenteral administration, many prefer to administer diazepam orally (Fig. 24-3).[19,23,24] Diazepam also may be given rectally.[25,26] It is not as reliable in preventing recall as lorazepam, but the antegrade amnesia effect may be enhanced by scopolamine.[27] There is no evidence for the production of retrograde amnesia after diazepam administration.[28]

There is little effect of diazepam outside the central nervous system. Minimal depression of ventilation, circulation, or hepatic or renal function occurs. Soroker *et al* demonstrated little or no effect on ventilation after diazepam administration.[29] Detectable $PaCO_2$ increases were demonstrable only after intravenous administration of 0.2 mg·kg^{-1} of diazepam in another study.[30] The increase in carbon dioxide results from a decrease in tidal volume. In another investigation, after intravenous doses of 0.4 mg·kg^{-1}, the slope of the carbon dioxide response curve decreased but it was not shifted to the right.[31] Despite the safety of relatively high intravenous doses of diazepam, respiratory arrest has been reported with as little as 2.5 mg.[32-34] Furthermore, ventilatory depression may be compounded by other depressant drugs, especially the opioids. There is little cardiovascular depression seen after the doses of diazepam used for preoperative medication. Indeed, higher intravenous doses produce little circulatory depression.[30,35] There is not much clinical effect on the neuromuscular junction after diazepam has been given for preoperative medication. There have been attempts to reduce myalgias and fasciculations produced by succinylcholine with diazepam.[36,37] The effect on fasciculations has been variable, but myalgias were reduced in one study.[36] Premedication with diazepam does not reliably prevent an increase in intraocular pressure after intubation of the trachea.[37-40] In animals, diazepam has reduced the seizure threshold for lidocaine, but this effect has not been proved in humans.[41]

Some controversy exists with regard to interaction of diazepam with other drugs. Cimetidine delays the hepatic clearance of diazepam.[42] The proposed mechanism is the inhibition of microsomal enzymes of cimetidine. There is

some question as to whether this is clinically significant when diazepam is used as a single dose before operation. Diazepam 0.2 mg·kg^{-1} has been shown to decrease the MAC for halothane.[43] The magnitude in reduction of anesthetic requirement from premedication doses may or may not be important to the anesthesiologist.

Lorazepam. Lorazepam resembles oxazepam and is five to ten times as potent as diazepam. Lorazepam can produce profound amnesia, relief of anxiety, and sedation (Fig. 24-4).[44-55] When lorazepam is compared with diazepam, their effects are very similar. However, unlike with administration of diazepam, pain on injection or phlebitis is not expected after lorazepam administration. Prolonged sedation is more likely after lorazepam administration. Even though the elimination half-life of diazepam is longer than that of lorazepam (20–40 hours vs. 10–15 hours), the effect of diazepam may be shorter because it more rapidly dissociates from the benzodiazepine receptor.[51]

Lorazepam is reliably absorbed both orally and intramuscularly. Maximal effect occurs 30–40 minutes after intravenous injection.[44] Bradshaw *et al* demonstrated clinical effects 30–60 minutes after oral administration of lorazepam.[52] A study by Blitt *et al* demonstrated that lack of recall was not produced until 2 hours after intramuscular injection.[53] Peak plasma concentrations may not occur until 2–4 hours after oral administration. Therefore, lorazepam must be ordered well before surgery so that the drug has time to be effective before the patient arrives in the operating room. Lorazepam also may be given sublingually.[54] As stated previously, the elimination half-life is 10–20 hours. The usual dose is about 25–50 µg·kg^{-1}. The dose for an adult should not exceed 4.0 mg.[44,45,55] With recommended doses, amnesia may be produced for as long as 4–6 hours without excessive sedation. Higher doses lead to prolonged and excessive sedation without more amnesia. Because of its length of action, lorazepam is not useful in instances in which rapid awakening is necessary, such as with outpatient anesthesia.[56] There are no active metabo-

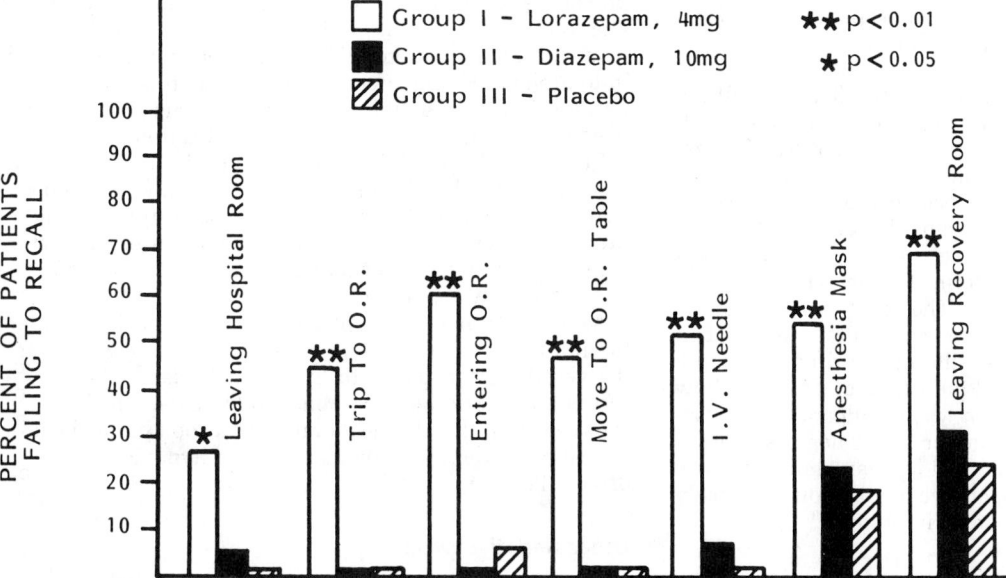

Figure 24-4. Percentage of patients in each group failing to recall specific events of the operative day. Medications were administered intramuscularly. (Reprinted with permission from Fragen RJ, Caldwell N: Lorazepam premedication: Lack of recall and relief of anxiety. Anesth Analg 55:792, 1976.)

lites of lorazepam, and because its metabolism is not dependent on microsomal enzymes, there is less influence on its effect from age or liver disease.[57] As with diazepam, little cardiorespiratory depression occurs with lorazepam.[58-63] However, there is the danger of unwanted respiratory depression in those with lung disease.[64]

Midazolam. The physicochemical properties of midazolam allow for its water solubility and rapid metabolism. As with other benzodiazepines, midazolam produces anxiolysis, sedation, and amnesia. It is two to three times as potent as diazepam because of its increased affinity for the benzodiazepine receptor. The usual intramuscular dose is 0.05–0.1 mg·kg^{-1} and titration of 1.0–2.5 mg at a time intravenously. There is no irritation or phlebitis with injection of midazolam. The incidence of side-effects after administration is low, although depression of ventilation and sedation may be greater than expected, especially in elderly patients or when the drug is combined with other central nervous system depressants.[65] There is more rapid onset of action and predictable absorption after intramuscular injection of midazolam than after diazepam. The time of onset after intramuscular injection is 5–10 minutes, with peak effect occurring after 30–60 minutes. The onset after intravenous administration of 5 mg would be expected to occur after 1–2 minutes. In addition to quicker onset, more rapid recovery occurs after midazolam administration when compared with diazepam. This probably results from the lipid solubility of midazolam and its rapid distribution in the peripheral tissues and metabolic biotransformation. For these reasons, midazolam usually should be given within an hour of induction.[66] Midazolam is metabolized by hepatic microsomal enzymes to essentially inactive hydroxylated metabolites.[66] H$_2$ receptor antagonists do not interfere with its metabolism.[67] The elimination half-life of midazolam is approximately 1–4 hours and may be extended in the elderly.[68] Tests show that mental function usually returns to normal within 4 hours of administration.[66] After administration of 5 mg, amnesia lasts from 20–32 minutes.[69,70] Intramuscular administration may produce longer periods of amnesia. The lack of recall may be augmented by concomitant administration of scopolamine.[71] The properties of midazolam make it ideal for shorter procedures.

Other Benzodiazepines. Oxazepam is another benzodiazepine that has been used for preoperative medication.[72,73] It is one of the pharmacologically active metabolites of diazepam. It is administered orally and is absorbed slowly after administration. Temazepam has been given in oral doses of 20–30 mg before surgery.[74-76] It must be given well before surgery because peak plasma levels do not occur until approximately 2½ hours after administration. Triazolam is a short-acting benzodiazepine.[77,78] The adult oral dose of the drug is 0.25–0.5 mg. Peak plasma concentrations occur in about 1 hour. Elimination half-life of the drug is 1.7–5.2 hours. However, a study by Pinnock et al did not show triazolam to be of short duration when compared with diazepam for premedication for minor gynecologic surgery.[78] Finally, because its effects may last for many hours, the use of chlordiazepoxide for preoperative medication has largely been replaced by the other benzodiazepines.[79]

Barbiturates

Use of barbiturates for preoperative medication is a time-tested practice with a long record of safety. These drugs are used primarily for their sedative effects. There is little cardiorespiratory depression associated with the usual preoperative doses.[80] The barbiturates may be given orally as well as parenterally, and the drugs are relatively inexpensive. Barbiturates are unlikely to produce sedation in the presence of pain. In fact, disorientation may result. Low doses of barbiturates have been said to be antianalgesic. The agents lack specificity of action on the central nervous system and have a lower therapeutic index than the benzodiazepines. Barbiturates should not be used in patients with certain kinds of porphyria. Barbiturate administration for pharmacologic preparation before surgery has been replaced in many instances by the use of benzodiazepines.

Secobarbital. Secobarbital usually is administered to adults in oral doses of 50–200 mg when used for preoperative medication. Onset usually occurs 60–90 minutes after administration, and sedative effects last 4 hours or longer. Indeed, even though secobarbital traditionally has been considered a "short-acting" barbiturate, it may impair performance for as long as 10–22 hours.[81]

Pentobarbital. Pentobarbital may be administered orally or parenterally. The oral dose used for adults is usually 50–200 mg. Pentobarbital has a biotransformation half-life of about 50 hours. Therefore, its use is not often suitable for shorter procedures. In an investigation by Dundee et al, 100 mg of pentobarbital given orally before surgery did not relieve anxiety or differ in effect from placebo.[82] These investigators postulated that higher doses may be necessary. In contrast, another study found pentobarbital equal to diazepam for the relief of preoperative anxiety.[83]

Butyrophenones

Intravenous or intramuscular doses of 2.5–7.5 mg of droperidol produce the appearance of sedation in patients before operation. Calmness and tranquility may be observed, but patients often state that they feel dysphoric and restless and even experience fear of death.[84] Patients' dysphoric feelings have led to refusal of surgery.[85,86] Because droperidol is a dopamine antagonist, extrapyramidal signs may appear after its administration.[87,88] This has been reported to occur in about 1% of patients. The butyrophenones also cause mild alpha-blocking effects. Another butyrophenone, haloperidol, is a long-acting antipsychotic drug that has been used infrequently for preoperative medication.

Currently, droperidol is usually administered for its antiemetic effect rather than its sedative properties (see the section on Antiemetics). Low clinical doses (up to 2.5 mg) of droperidol have been used before operation or just before emergence from anesthesia to prevent nausea and vomiting in the recovery room.

As a dopaminergic receptor blocker, droperidol counters the inhibitory effect of dopamine on the carotid body and the ventilatory response to hypoxia. Consequently, it preserves the carotid body response to hypoxia. For these reasons, it is said that droperidol may be a good premedication for patients who are dependent on the hypoxic ventilatory drive (Fig. 24-5).[89]

Other Sedative Drugs

Hydroxyzine. Hydroxyzine is a nonphenothiazine tranquilizer. It is often given for its proposed additive effects to opioids and does not cause an increase in side-effects.[90] Hydroxyzine has sedative action, anxiolytic properties, and limited analgesic properties. It does not produce amnesia.[47,91,92] It is an antihistamine and an antiemetic.[93]

Diphenhydramine. Diphenhydramine is a histamine receptor antagonist with sedative and anticholinergic activity. It is also an antiemetic. A dose of 50 mg will last 3–6 hours in an adult. Diphenhydramine has been used recently in combination with cimetidine, steroids, and other drugs for prophylaxis in patients with chronic atopy and for prophylaxis before chemonucleolysis and dye studies.[94] Diphenhydramine blocks the histamine receptor to prevent effects of histamine peripherally.

Phenothiazines. Promethazine, promazine, and perphenazine are often used in combination with opioids.[95,96] Phenothiazines have sedative, anticholinergic, and antiemetic properties. These effects, added to the analgesic effects of the opioids, have been used for preoperative medication.

Chloral Hydrate. Because of its anxiolytic and amnestic qualities, chloral hydrate was used in the past as a premedicant, often in the elderly. Since the advent of the benzodiazepines, chloral hydrate has played a much smaller role in preoperative medications.

Opioids

Morphine and meperidine are the most frequently used opioids for intramuscular preoperative medication. Recently the use of intravenous fentanyl just before surgery has become popular. Opioids are used when analgesia is needed before operation. It has been stated in the strict sense that "unless there is pain, there is no need for narcotic in preanesthetic medication."[97] For the patient experiencing pain before operation, the opioids can produce good analgesia and even euphoria. Opioids have been ordered for patients before operation to ameliorate the discomfort that may occur during regional anesthesia or the insertion of invasive monitoring catheters or large intravenous lines. The dose of opioid may need to be reduced in the debilitated or elderly patient.[98] The elderly patient often exhibits a reduced sensitivity to pain. Furthermore, elderly patients can have an increased analgesic response to opioids. Opioids also have been used before operation in the opioid-dependent patient.

Preoperative administration of opioids in other settings has been controversial. They have been given on the floor before surgery at the beginning of nitrous-opioid anesthetic. This is done in attempt to have a basal state of anesthesia on board when the patient arrives in the operating room and to get a preview of the patient's response to opioids. Opioids have been given to patients before operation to provide analgesia upon their awakening in the recovery room. The other approach is to titrate the opioid intravenously during emergence or upon the patient's arrival in the recovery room. Preoperative administration of opioids can lower anesthetic requirements.[99,100] This may or may not be clinically significant for a specific patient receiving a particular anesthetic technique. Some anesthesiologists use opioids in combination with other drugs before operation to facilitate anesthetic induction by mask. This is popular especially in patients in whom intravenous or rectal routes for induction agents cannot be used. It must be remembered that opioids will decrease ventilation during spontaneous breathing and therefore decrease uptake of inhalation drugs. If necessary, the anesthesiologist may want to use assisted or controlled ventilation of the lungs to overcome the respiratory depres-

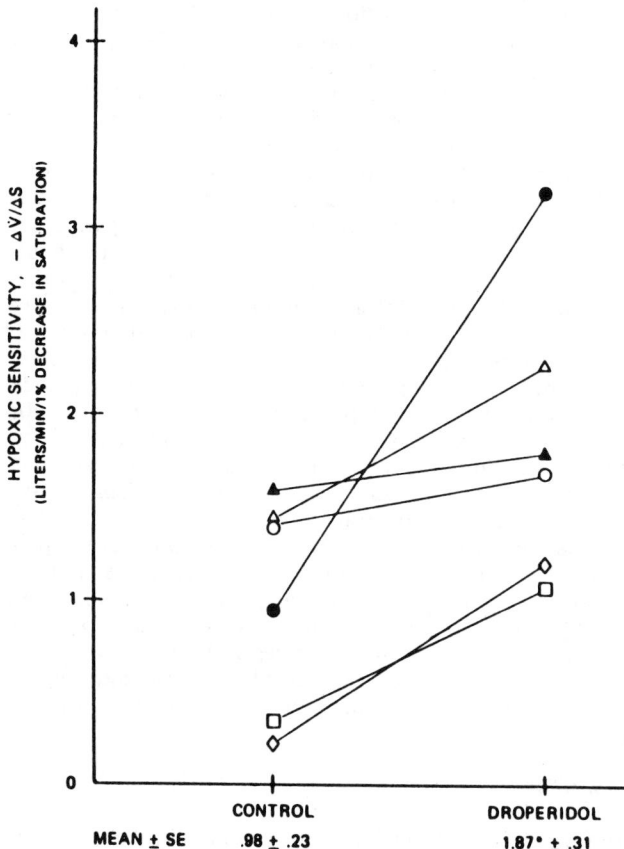

Figure 24-5. Hypoxic sensitivity (change in ventilation for each 1% decrease in oxygen saturation) is increased after intravenous administration of droperidol, 2.5 mg. Solid symbols represent repeated experiments on the same subjects as those represented by the open symbols. (Reprinted with permission from Ward DS: Stimulation of hypoxic ventilatory drive by droperidol. Anesth Analg 63:106, 1984.)

sant effects of the opioids. Finally, opioids are not the best drugs to relieve apprehension, produce sedation, or prevent recall.[101,102]

Administration of opioids has the potential for causing several side-effects. They usually exhibit no direct myocardial effects except in the case of very high doses of meperidine. However, opioids do interfere with the compensatory constriction of smooth muscles of the peripheral vasculature. This may lead to orthostatic hypotension. Histamine release after injection of morphine may compound these circulatory effects. As with most preoperative medications, it is probably safest to have the patient remain at bed rest after opioid premedication. The analgesic properties and respiratory depressant effects of opioids go hand in hand.[80] The decrease in the carbon dioxide drive at the medullary respiratory center may be prolonged. Furthermore, there is a decrease in the responsiveness to hypoxia at the carotid body after injection of only low doses of opioids.[103] In general, the opioid agonist-antagonists produce less respiratory depression, but they also produce less analgesia. Rather than euphoria, the opioids may produce dysphoria. When this side-effect does occur, it is most commonly seen in a patient who does not have pain before operation and has received the opioid premedication. Nausea and vomiting may result from opioid administration. Apomorphine is a profound emetic. The effect of opioids on the vestibular apparatus leading to motion sickness and/or stimulation of the medullary chemoreceptor trigger zone is a postulated reason for nausea and vomiting. Choledochoduodenal sphincter (sphincter of Oddi) spasm has been reported subsequent to injection of opioids.[104-105] The opioid produces smooth muscle constriction, which leads to right upper quadrant pain.[106] Pain relief may be achieved with naloxone or possibly glucagon.[107] Occasionally the pain from biliary tract spasm is difficult to differentiate from the pain of angina pectoris. The administration of nitroglycerin should relieve angina pectoris and pain resulting from biliary tract spasm; an opioid antagonist should relieve only pain resulting from biliary tract spasm. Some question the use of opioid premedication in patients with biliary tract disease. All opioids have the potential to induce choledochoduodenal sphincter spasm. Meperidine is less likely than morphine to produce this side-effect. Opioids may produce pruritus. Morphine, possibly through histamine release, often produces itching, especially around the nose. Opioids also may cause flushing, dizziness, and miosis.

Other drugs are often combined with opioids for their additive effects or to overcome the disadvantages of opioid side-effects. The sedative-hypnotics and scopolamine are often used with opioids to produce sedation, anxiolysis, and amnesia in addition to analgesia. Anesthesiologists often use the combination of morphine, a benzodiazepine, and/or scopolamine for pharmacologic preoperative preparation.

Morphine

Morphine is well absorbed after intramuscular injection. The onset of effect should occur within 15–30 minutes. The peak effect occurs in 45–90 minutes and lasts as long as 4 hours. After intravenous administration, the peak effect usually occurs within 20 minutes. Morphine is not reliably absorbed after oral administration. As with the other opioids, depression of ventilation and orthostatic hypotension may occur after injection of morphine. The effect of morphine on the chemoreceptive trigger zone may produce nausea and vomiting. Nausea and vomiting may also occur owing to a vestibular component. This has been postulated because the supine patient is less likely to complain of nausea and vomiting. After morphine administration, motility of the gastrointestinal tract is decreased. Also, gastrointestinal secretions may be increased. Inclusion of morphine in the preoperative medication reduces the likelihood that undesirable increases in heart rate will accompany surgical stimulation in the presence of volatile anesthetics.[108]

Meperidine

Meperidine is about one tenth as potent as morphine. It may be given orally or parenterally. A single dose of meperidine usually lasts 2–4 hours. The onset after intramuscular injection is unpredictable, and a great deal of variability in time to peak effect exists.[109] Meperidine is primarily metabolized in the liver. An increase in heart rate may be seen after meperidine administration, as may orthostatic hypotension.

Other Opioids

Codeine has been used orally in doses of 50–60 mg for adults for preoperative medication. An intramuscular dose of 120 mg is equal to about 10 mg of morphine. Codeine can be administered intravenously, but histamine release is very likely. There is an advantage with methadone in that it can

be given orally as well as intramuscularly. It is a long-acting opioid whose elimination half-life is approximately 35 hours.[110] Hydromorphone is another opioid that may be given orally as well as intramuscularly.

Opioid Agonist-Antagonists

Opioid agonist-antagonists have been chosen for preoperative medication in an attempt to reduce the ventilatory side-effects of pure opioid agonists.[111-115] However, there is a ceiling on the analgesia that can be produced by agonist-antagonist drugs. They are similar to the pure opioids with regard to side-effects. In addition, dysphoria may be even more likely to occur after their administration. Another issue to remember is that the agonist-antagonist drug can reduce the effectiveness of a pure opioid agonist needed to control postoperative pain. The most commonly used opioid agonist-antagonists are pentazocine, butorphanol, and nalbuphine.

Gastric Fluid pH and Volume

Many patients who come to the operating room are at risk for aspiration pneumonitis. The classic example is the patient with a "full stomach" who must have emergency surgery. The pregnant patient, the obese patient, the diabetic, and the patient with hiatus hernia or gastroesophageal reflux all may be at risk for aspiration of gastric contents and subsequent chemical pneumonitis (Fig. 24-6).[116] Although it is not certain, it is believed that in adults aspiration of a volume of gastric fluid greater than 25 ml with a pH lower than 2.5 will cause pulmonary sequelae. This has not and probably never will be proved in humans. However, using these guidelines, it has been estimated that 40–80% of patients scheduled for elective surgery may be at risk.[117-119] In addition, it has been shown that many outpatients exhibit an increase in gastric fluid volume (Fig. 24-7).[117] This raises the question of the necessity of prophylaxis for aspiration pneumonitis during induction of anesthesia and emergence and extubation of the trachea and during long mask cases in which silent regurgitation and aspiration may occur. However, clinically significant pulmonary aspiration of gastric contents is very rare in healthy patients having elective surgical procedures, and routine prophylaxis is questioned by many anesthesiologists.[119a,b]

The necessity of prolonged fasting (i.e., nothing by mouth after midnight) prior to induction of anesthesia for elective surgery has been challenged.[120,121,121a] Some institutions allow ingestion of clear liquids until 3 hours before surgery in selected patients. Indeed, gastric fluid volume immediately after induction of anesthesia is not increased by ingestion of 150 ml of water, coffee, or orange juice 2–3 hours earlier.[122] A similar study of Shevde and Trivedi described the administration of 240 ml of water, coffee, or pulp-free orange juice to healthy volunteers. All had gastric volumes of less than 25 ml with a slight decrease in pH within 2 hours of taking one of the three liquids.[123] There is concern about hypovolemia and hypoglycemia in the pediatric age group perioperatively after prolonged fasting. An investigation by Splinter and associates concluded that drinking clear fluid up to 3 hours before scheduled surgery does not have a measurable effect on gastric volume and pH of healthy children from the ages of 2–12 years.[124] Other studies in children and healthy adults scheduled for elective surgery have found similar results.[125-128a] Therefore, fears that ingestion of oral fluid on the morning of surgery will

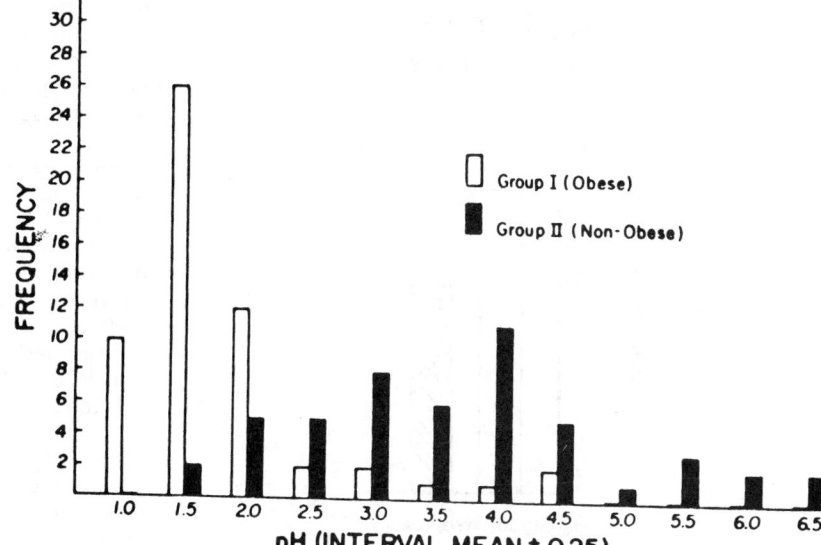

Figure 24-6. Frequency distribution of gastric fluid pHs in obese (45 kg more than predicted ideal weight) and nonobese patients. (Reprinted with permission from Vaughan RW, Bauer S, Wise L: Volume and pH of gastric juice in obese patients. Anesthesiology 43:686, 1975.)

invariably result in a predictable increase in gastric fluid volume are unfounded. It must be appreciated, however, that these data are from healthy patients not "at risk" for aspiration in the absence of opioid preoperative medication and apply only to ingestion of clear liquids.

Many different kinds of drugs have been used to alter gastric fluid volume and increase the pH of gastric fluid. Anticholinergics, H_2 receptor antagonists, antacids, and gastrokinetic agents have all been employed to reduce the possibility of aspiration pneumonitis.

Anticholinergics

Neither atropine nor glycopyrrolate has been shown to be very effective in increasing gastric fluid pH or reducing gastric fluid volume. A study by Stoelting demonstrated that when given intramuscularly 1–1½ hours before operation, neither atropine (0.4 mg) nor glycopyrrolate (0.2 mg) was successful in altering the gastric fluid pH or volume.[118] A similar study reported that glycopyrrolate ($4–5 \ \mu g \cdot kg^{-1}$) given before operation did not reduce the percentage of patients at risk for aspiration pneumonitis.[119] That is, in a

significant number of patients the gastric fluid pH remained below 2.5 and the gastric fluid volume was greater than 0.4 $ml \cdot kg^{-1}$. Giving higher doses of glycopyrrolate (0.3 mg) is not more effective. Furthermore, intravenous doses of anticholinergics may cause relaxation of the gastroesophageal junction (Fig. 24-8).[129] Theoretically, this may also occur after intramuscular doses. Therefore, the risk of aspiration pneumonitis may be increased, but this specific effect of intramuscular administration of anticholinergics for preoperative use has not been proved.

Histamine Receptor Antagonists

The H_2 receptor antagonists, cimetidine and ranitidine, reduce gastric acid secretion. They block the ability of histamine to induce secretion of gastric fluid with a high hydrogen ion concentration. Therefore, the H_2 receptor antagonists increase gastric fluid pH.[130] Their antagonism of the histamine receptor occurs in a selective and competitive manner. It is important to remember that these drugs cannot be expected to reliably affect gastric fluid volume or gastric-emptying time. Compared with other premedicants, cimeti-

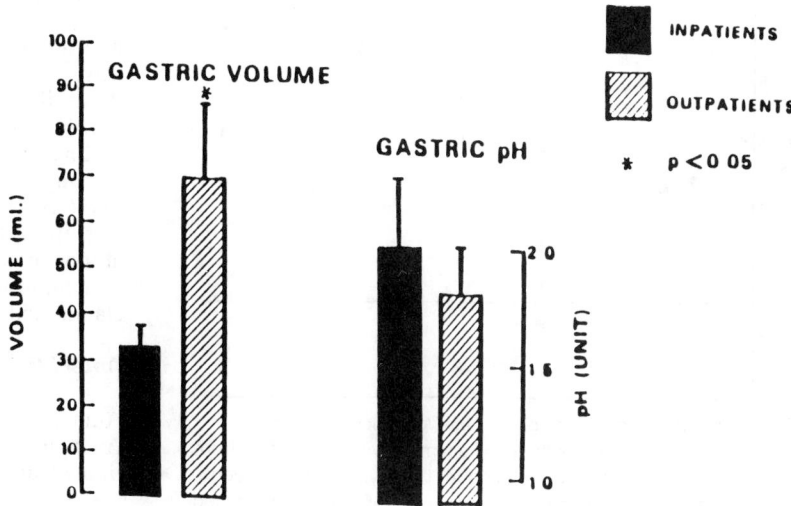

Figure 24-7. Gastric fluid volume and pH as measured for inpatients and outpatients. Mean ± SD. (Reprinted with permission from Ong BY, Palahniuk RJ, Cumming M: Gastric volume and pH in outpatients. Can Anaesth Soc J 25:36, 1978.)

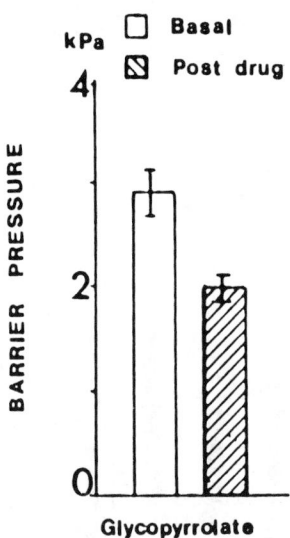

Figure 24-8. Barrier pressure (esophageal sphincter pressure minus gastric pressure) before and after intravenous administration of glycopyrrolate, 0.3 mg, to adult patients. Mean ± SE. (Reprinted with permission from Brock-Utne JG, Welman RS, Moshal MG *et al:* The effect of glycopyrrolate (Robinul) on the lower esophageal sphincter. Can Anaesth Soc J 25:144, 1978.)

dine and ranitidine have relatively few side-effects. Because there are few side-effects and because of the many elective patients at risk for aspiration pneumonitis, some anesthesiologists have advocated the preoperative use of H_2 receptor antagonists.[131] Multiple-dose regimens usually are more effective in consistently increasing gastric pH than a single dose before operation on the day of surgery (Fig. 24-9).[132] A multiple-dose regimen usually incorporates an oral dose of the H_2 receptor antagonist the night before surgery, followed by an intramuscular injection before operation on the day

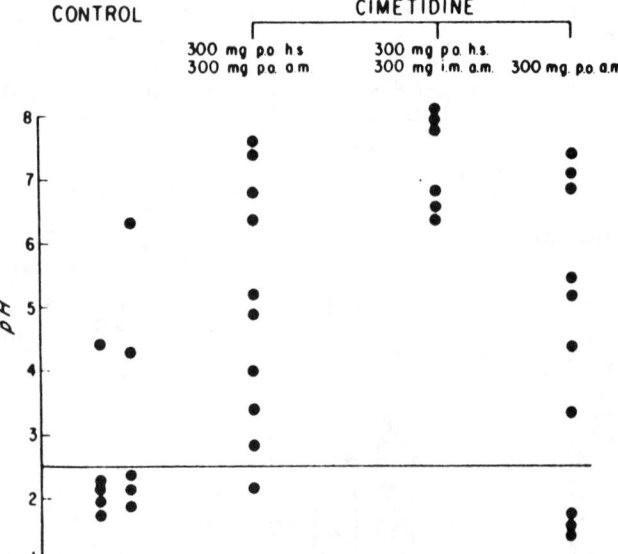

Figure 24-9. Distribution of gastric fluid pH in control and cimetidine-treated adult patients. (Reprinted with permission from Weber L, Hirshman CA: Cimetidine for prophylaxis of aspiration pneumonitis: Comparison of intramuscular and oral dosage schedules. Anesth Analg 58:426, 1979.)

of surgery. As with most other drugs, parenteral administration produces a more rapid onset than the oral route. Cimetidine or ranitidine also may be used for the allergic patient or in preparing a patient for exposure to a trigger of the allergic response, such as chymopapain or dye.

Cimetidine. Cimetidine usually is administered in 150–300 mg doses orally or parenterally.[132-136] Administration of 300 mg of cimetidine orally 1–1½ hours before surgery has been shown to increase the gastric fluid pH above 2.5 in 80% of patients.[133] There was no effect on gastric fluid volume. However, a study by Maliniak *et al* reported that cimetidine (300 mg) given intravenously 2 hours before operation increased gastric fluid pH and decreased gastric fluid volume.[136] Cimetidine can be given intravenously for those unable to take oral medications. It may be necessary to increase the dose for the very obese patient. Cimetidine can cross the placenta, but adverse fetal effects are unproved.[137,138] In one multicenter investigation, 126 patients were studied who were to have elective cesarean section with general anesthesia.[137] These patients received either 30 ml of an antacid 1–3 hours before operation or 300 mg of cimetidine orally at bedtime and again intramuscularly 1–3 hours before operation. There was an increase in gastric fluid pH and a reduction in gastric fluid volume in the cimetidine-treated group. Most important for this discussion, there were no differences in the neurobehavioral scores of the neonates between the two groups. The gastric effects of cimetidine last as long as 3 or 4 hours and therefore this drug is suitable for operations of that duration.[139]

Cimetidine has few side-effects, but there are some of note. It inhibits the hepatic mixed function oxidase enzyme system; therefore, it can prolong the half-life of many drugs, including diazepam, chlordiazepoxide, theophylline, propranolol, and lidocaine. The clinical significance of this after one or two preoperative doses of cimetidine is uncertain. There is also some question of hepatic blood flow reduction by cimetidine and a prolonged effect of the drug in patients with renal failure. Life-threatening cardiac dysrhythmias, hypotension, cardiac arrest, and central nervous system depression have been reported after cimetidine administration.[140,141] These side-effects may be especially likely to occur in critically ill patients after rapid intravenous administration. It has been postulated that airway resistance may increase in asthmatic patients because cimetidine could produce unopposed H_2 receptor-mediated bronchial constriction. As discussed previously, cimetidine does not affect gastric fluid already present.

Ranitidine. Ranitidine is more potent, specific, and longer acting than cimetidine. The usual oral dose is 50–200 mg. Ranitidine, 50–100 mg, given parenterally will decrease gastric fluid pH within 1 hour.[142,143] It is as effective in reducing the number of patients at risk for gastric aspiration as cimetidine and produces fewer cardiovascular or central nervous system side-effects.[144,145] The effects of ranitidine last up to 9 hours. Thus, it may be superior to cimetidine at the conclusion of lengthy procedures in reducing the risk of aspiration pneumonitis during emergence from anesthesia and extubation of the trachea.[134]

Antacids

Antacids are used to neutralize the acid in gastric contents. A single dose of antacid given 15–30 minutes before induction of anesthesia is almost 100% effective in increasing gastric fluid pH above 2.5.[118,146-148] The nonparticulate antacid, 0.3 M sodium citrate, is commonly given before operation when an increase in gastric fluid pH is desired. The nonparticulate antacids do not produce pulmonary damage themselves if aspiration of gastric fluid containing these antacids should occur.[149] Colloid antacid suspension may be more effective than the nonparticulate antacids in increasing gastric fluid pH.[150] However, aspiration of gastric fluid containing particulate antacids may cause significant and persistent pulmonary damage, despite the increase in gastric fluid pH.[151-154] The serious pulmonary sequelae have been manifested in the form of pulmonary edema and arterial hypoxemia.

Antacids work at the time given. There is no "lag time," as with the histamine receptor blockers. Antacids are effective on the fluid already present in the stomach. This makes them especially attractive in emergency situations for those patients who are able to take medications orally.

However, antacids do increase gastric fluid volume, unlike H₂ receptor blockers.[133,155-156] The risk of aspiration depends on both the pH and the volume of gastric content. The increase in gastric fluid volume from antacid administration may become readily apparent after repeated doses, such as during labor, during which opioid administration may also contribute to delayed gastric emptying.[157] Withholding antacids because of concern about increasing gastric volume is not warranted, considering animal evidence documenting increased mortality after aspiration of low volumes of acidic gastric fluid (0.3 ml·kg⁻¹, pH 1) compared with aspiration of large volumes of buffered gastric fluid (1–2 ml·kg⁻¹, pH ≥ 1.8).[158] Antacids may slow gastric emptying, and complete mixing with all gastric contents may be questionable in the immobile patient. The effect of antacids on food particles within the stomach is unknown.

Gastrokinetic Agents

Gastrokinetic agents are useful because of their effectiveness in reducing gastric fluid volume. Metoclopramide is an example of a gastrokinetic agent that may be administered before operation.

Metoclopramide. Metoclopramide is a dopamine antagonist that stimulates upper gastrointestinal motility, increases gastroesophageal sphincter tone, and relaxes the pylorus and duodenum.[159,160] It also has antiemetic properties. Metoclopramide speeds gastric emptying but has no known effect on acid secretion and gastric fluid pH. It may be administered orally or parenterally. A parenteral dose of 5–20 mg is usually given 15–30 minutes before induction. When the drug is administered intravenously over 3–5 minutes, it usually prevents the abdominal cramping that can occur from more rapid administration. An oral dose of 10 mg achieves onset within 30–60 minutes. The elimination half-life of metoclopramide is approximately 2–4 hours.

The clinical usefulness of the gastrokinetic agents is found in those patients who are likely to have large gastric fluid volumes, such as parturients, patients scheduled for emergency surgery who have just eaten, obese patients, patients with trauma, outpatients, and those with gastroparesis secondary to diabetes mellitus.

However, the administration of metoclopramide does not guarantee gastric emptying. Significant gastric fluid volume may still be present despite its administration.[129] The effect of metoclopramide on the upper gastrointestinal tract may be offset by concomitant atropine administration[160] or prior injection of opioids.[161] It will not further reduce gastric volume in patients undergoing elective surgery with already small gastric volumes.[162] It may not be effective after administration of sodium citrate.[163] In contrast, metoclopramide

may be especially effective in reducing the risk of aspiration pneumonitis when combined with an H₂ receptor antagonist (for example, ranitidine) before elective surgery.[164-166]

As mentioned previously, the drugs used to alter gastric fluid pH and volume are relatively free of side-effects. The risk-benefit ratio for these drugs in reducing the risk of pulmonary sequelae from aspiration is often very favorable. Indeed, the drugs do decrease the number of patients at risk. However, none of the drugs or combination of drugs is absolutely reliable in preventing the risk of aspiration pneumonitis in all patients all of the time. Therefore, they do not eliminate the need for careful anesthetic techniques to protect the airway during induction, maintenance, and emergence from anesthesia.

Antiemetics

There are several groups of patients in whom the antiemetic effects of drugs may be helpful in reducing nausea and vomiting. These are patients scheduled for ophthalmologic surgery, patients with a prior history of nausea and vomiting, patients scheduled for gynecologic procedures, and patients who are obese. Many anesthesiologists prefer not to administer antiemetics as part of a preoperative regimen but believe that antiemetics should be administered intravenously just before they are needed at the conclusion of surgery.

Droperidol

Droperidol has been administered, usually intravenously, in low clinical doses to prevent postoperative nausea and vomiting.[167-175] An investigation by Korttila et al showed that 1.25 mg of droperidol given intravenously 5 minutes before the conclusion of surgery reduced the incidence of nausea and vomiting after operation.[167] They found the antiemetic effect of droperidol to be better than that of either metoclopramide or domperidone. Another study by Santos and Datta demonstrated the effectiveness of droperidol as an antiemetic for patients having cesarean section with spinal anesthesia (Fig. 24-10).[168] However, low doses of droperidol may not always be effective in preventing nausea and vomiting.[169] Higher doses at the end of surgery may lead to excessive sedation in the recovery room.

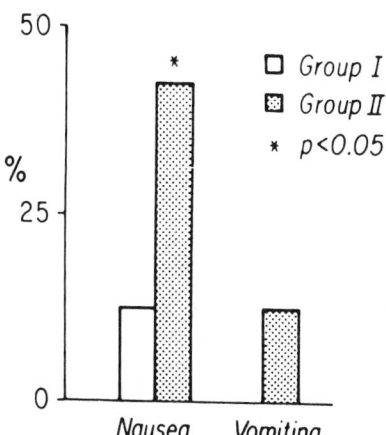

Figure 24-10. Incidence of nausea and vomiting after elective cesarean section after intravenous administration of droperidol, 2.5 mg (Group 1), or saline (Group 2). (Reprinted with permission from Santos A, Datta S: Prophylactic use of droperidol for control of nausea and vomiting during spinal anesthesia for cesarean section. Anesth Analg 63:85, 1984.)

TABLE 24-5. Comparison of Some of the Effects of Anticholinergic Drugs

	Atropine	Glycopyrrolate	Scopolamine
Increased heart rate	+ + +	+ +	+
Antisialagogue	+	+ +	+ + +
Sedation	+	0	+ + +

0 = no effect; + = small effect; + + = moderate effect; + + + = large effect.

Adapted from Stoelting RK: Pharmacology and Physiology in Anesthetic Practice. Philadelphia, JB Lippincott, 1991.

Metoclopramide

As mentioned in the previous section on gastrokinetic agents, metoclopramide does have antiemetic properties.[176-179] The effect is controversial and inconsistent, as demonstrated and discussed in the study by Cohen et al.[169] This may partially result from the brief duration of action of metoclopramide.

Other Antiemetics

Some of the phenothiazines, especially prochlorperazine, have antiemetic action. Hydroxyzine and diphenidol are two other drugs with antiemetic value.[93,175] Although it has antiemetic properties, domperidone has not been proved effective in reducing postoperative nausea and vomiting.[167]

Anticholinergics

Previously, anticholinergic drugs were widely used when inhalation anesthetics produced copious respiratory tract secretions and intraoperative bradycardia was a frequent danger.[180] The advent of newer inhalation agents has almost completely dispelled the routine use of anticholinergic drugs for preoperative medication. Their routine use has been questioned by several authors, who believe that the same care in selection of anticholinergics should be exhibited as in the choice of other drugs.[181-188] Specific indications for an anticholinergic before surgery are (1) antisialagogue effect, and (2) sedation and amnesia (Table 24-5). Uses that are less firmly established and not universally agreed upon include the preoperative prescription of anticholinergics for their vagolytic action or use in an attempt to decrease gastric acid secretion.

Antisialagogue Effect

Anticholinergics have been prescribed in a selective fashion when drying of the upper airway is desirable. For example, when endotracheal intubation is contemplated, an anesthesiologist may want to reduce secretions. In the study by Falick and Smiler, conditions were more often rated as satisfactory after endotracheal intubation when an anticholinergic drug had been administered.[189] The antisialagogue effect may be important for intraoral operations and instrumentations of the airway such as bronchoscopic examination. Administration of anticholinergics may be desirable before the use of topical anesthesia for the airway to prevent a dilutional effect of secretions and to allow contact of the local anesthetic with the mucosa.

Scopolamine is a more potent drying agent than atropine. It is less likely to increase heart rate and more likely to produce sedation and amnesia. Glycopyrrolate is a more potent and longer acting antisialagogue than atropine, with less likelihood of increasing heart rate.[190-192] Because glycopyrrolate is a quaternary amine, it does not easily cross the blood-brain barrier and does not produce sedation. Anticholinergics are not the only drugs that can dry secretions. As demonstrated by the study of Forrest et al, several other drugs and placebo (presumably a reflection of apprehension) can cause a patient to have a dry mouth before operation[193] (Table 24-6).

Sedation and Amnesia

When sedation and amnesia are desired before operation, scopolamine is frequently the anticholinergic chosen, especially in combination with morphine. Scopolamine and atropine both cross the blood-brain barrier. Scopolamine is a

TABLE 24-6. Incidence of Side-Effects One Hour After Preoperative Medication (Percentage of Patients)

Medication	Dry Mouth	Slurred Speech	Dizzy	Nauseated	Relaxed
Pentobarbital (50–150 mg)	29	27	10	7	2
Secobarbital (50–150 mg)	41	32	8	9	4
Diazepam (5–15 mg)	35	20	10	3	12
Hydroxyzine (50–150 mg)	45	31	6	2	9
Morphine (5–10 mg)	80	33	15	7	20
Meperidine (50–100 mg)	85	45	20	12	25
Placebo	34	21	7	12	4

Modified from Forrest WH, Brown CR, Brown BW et al: Subjective responses to six common preoperative medications. Anesthesiology 47:241, 1977.

much more potent sedative and amnestic drug than atropine. In a study of patient acceptance of preoperative medication, the combination of morphine and scopolamine was superior to that of morphine and atropine.[194] Scopolamine does not produce amnesia in all patients. It may not be as effective as lorazepam or diazepam in preventing recall. Scopolamine has an additive amnestic effect when combined with benzodiazepines. The study by Frumin et al showed that the combination of diazepam and scopolamine produced amnesia more often than did diazepam alone.[27]

Vagolytic Action

Vagolytic action of the anticholinergic drugs is produced through the blockade of effects of acetylcholine on the sinoatrial node. Atropine given intravenously is more potent than glycopyrrolate and scopolamine in increasing heart rate. The vagolytic action of the anticholinergic drugs is useful in the prevention of reflex bradycardia occurring during surgery. Bradycardia may result from traction on extraocular muscles or abdominal viscera, from carotid sinus stimulation, or after the administration of repeated doses of intravenous succinylcholine. The prevention of reflex bradycardia with intramuscular doses of the anticholinergics is unreliable, given the drug dosages and timing usually involved with preoperative medication administered on the unit. Many anesthesiologists prefer to give atropine or glycopyrrolate intravenously just before surgery and the anticipated bradycardic stimulus.[195] Atropine and glycopyrrolate given intravenously immediately before surgery have been equally effective in preventing bradycardia resulting from repeated doses of succinylcholine.[196]

Elevation of Gastric Fluid pH Level

High doses of anticholinergics often are needed to alter gastric fluid pH. Even then, when given in the preoperative setting, anticholinergics cannot be relied upon consistently to decrease gastric hydrogen ion secretion.[118,119] This function has largely been replaced by the use of histamine receptor antagonists (see the section on Gastric Fluid pH and Volume).

Side-Effects in Anticholinergic Drugs

Scopolamine and atropine may cause central nervous system toxicity, the so-called "central anticholinergic syndrome."[197] This is most likely to occur after the administration of scopolamine but can be seen after high doses of atropine. The symptoms of central nervous system toxicity resulting from anticholinergic drugs include delirium, restlessness, confusion, and obtundation. Elderly patients and patients with pain appear to be particularly susceptible.[198] The central nervous system toxic effect of anticholinergics has been reported to be potentiated by inhalation anesthetics.[199] Some clinicians have successfully treated the syndrome after it occurred with 1–2 mg of physostigmine intravenously.[199,200]

The anticholinergics relax the lower esophageal sphincter.[129] Theoretically, after parenteral administration of an anticholinergic drug, the risk of pulmonary aspiration of gastric contents is increased. This has yet to be proved as an important clinical issue.

Mydriasis and cycloplegia from anticholinergic drugs could be unwanted in patients with glaucoma because of resulting increased intraocular pressure. This seems un-

likely with the doses used for preoperative medication. Atropine and glycopyrrolate may be less likely to increase intraocular pressure than scopolamine.[201] In patients with glaucoma, most anesthesiologists feel safe in continuing medications for glaucoma up until the time of surgery and using atropine or glycopyrrolate when necessary (see Chapter 38).

Because anticholinergic drugs block vagal activity, relaxation of bronchial smooth muscle occurs and respiratory dead space increases.[202] The magnitude of the increase in dead space depends on prior bronchomotor tone, but increases as large as 25–33% have been reported. Anticholinergic drugs cause secretions to dry and thicken. Theoretically, a dose of anticholinergic drug given before operation could lead to inspissation of secretions and an increase in airway resistance. This may develop into more than a theoretical issue when patients with diseases such as cystic fibrosis are being considered.

Sweat glands of the body are innervated by the sympathetic nervous system and employ cholinergic transmission. Therefore, administration of anticholinergic agents interferes with the sweating mechanism, which may cause body temperature to increase. This side-effect of anticholinergic medication must be considered carefully in a child with a fever.

Atropine is more likely than glycopyrrolate or scopolamine to cause an increase in heart rate.[183] Unwanted increases in heart rate are much more likely after intravenous administration than after intramuscular administration. In fact, heart rate may transiently decrease after intramuscular administration as a result of a peripheral agonist effect of the anticholinergic agent.

Alpha₂ Adrenergic Agonists

Alpha₂ adrenergic agonists have been used as premedicants.[11,12,203-215] Clonidine in doses of 5 $\mu g \cdot kg^{-1}$ has been administered preoperatively to produce sedation, reduce maximum allowable concentration, and prevent hypertension and tachycardia from endotracheal intubation and surgical stimulation. It has even been used as part of anesthetic technique to produce induced hypotension.[215] After the administration of clonidine preoperatively, one is more likely to see episodes of hypotension and bradycardia during anesthesia when there are periods of little surgical stimulation. Furthermore, some anesthesiologists ask if preoperative alpha₂ adrenergic agonists are a substitute for a properly conducted anesthetic if appropriate attention is given to depth of anesthesia.

Other Drugs Given with Preoperative Medications

Although they are not preoperative medications in the strict sense, other drugs are often given at the time of preoperative medication. Examples of such drugs are insulin, steroids, antibiotics, and methadone for patients who are addicted to opioids. They may be prescribed by either the anesthesiologist or the surgeon to be given on the ward or in the operating room immediately before surgery. Regardless of these factors, their actions may affect the anesthetic, and the anesthesiologist must be knowledgeable about their administration and actions.

Antibiotics

Antibiotics are often administered immediately prior to operation for contaminated, potentially contaminated, or dirty surgical wounds. Prophylactic antibiotics may be warranted for "clean" surgical procedures when infection would be catastrophic. Other instances for the use of prophylactic antibiotics include in the immunosuppressed patient, in the aged or in patients taking steroids. Antibiotics given immediately before surgery are also used for the prevention of endocarditis. Patients with valvular heart disease, prosthetic valves, mitral valve prolapse, or other cardiac abnormalities may be endangered by bacteremia produced during surgery.[216] Antibiotic administration comes under the anesthesiologist's purview because of the desire to have such agents given immediately prior to exposure to pathogens, which is just before the beginning of surgery.

It has been estimated that 60–70% of surgical patients receive antibiotics just prior to surgery or intraoperatively. Cephalosporins are the most popular. However, no drug or combination of drugs may be relied on to protect against all potential pathogens in all patients for all types of surgery. As with any other medication, the anesthesiologist must know the side-effects and complications of the antibiotics to be administered. Some are associated with allergic reactions, hypotension, and bronchospasm, for example, penicillin and vancomycin. Allergic reactions from cephalosporin administration have been estimated to occur in about 5% of patients. A cross-reactivity of the cephalosporins in patients with a known penicillin allergy has been estimated at anywhere from 5–20%. The aminoglycosides, vancomycin, and the polymyxins have been implicated in nephrotoxicity. In addition, ototoxicity has resulted from aminoglycoside and vancomycin administration. Pseudomembranous colitis is a known complication of clindamycin administration. Finally, the aminoglycosides are known to extend the neuromuscular blocking effects of muscle relaxants.

Steroids

Steroid administration may be necessary immediately preoperatively in the patient treated for hypoadrenocorticism or in the patient with suppression of the pituitary-adrenal axis owing to present or previous administration of corticosteroids. It is impossible to identify the specific duration of therapy or dose of steroids that produces pituitary and adrenal suppression. Marked variability among patients exists. Certainly more suppression may be expected the higher the dose and the longer the duration of therapy. A conservative estimate is to consider treatment in any patient who has received corticosteroid therapy for at least 1 month in the past 6–12 months.

Because of disease states of the pituitary-adrenal axis or its suppression from steroid therapy, patients may not be able to respond to the stress of surgery. The dose and duration of supplemental steroid administration depend on an estimate of the stress of the surgical procedure in the perioperative period. One regimen is to administer 25 mg of cortisol preoperatively and then give an intravenous infusion of 100 mg of cortisol over the next 12–24 hours for adult patients.[217] Another method is to administer 100 mg of hydrocortisone intravenously before, during, and after surgery. This dose is meant to equal the estimated maximum amount of steroid that stress could produce in patients perioperatively. When considering whether to administer steroids or

a higher dose of steroids, the anesthesiologist should keep in mind that the risk-benefit ratio is usually very small.

Insulin

Anesthesia and surgery may interrupt the regular meal schedule and insulin administration of diabetics (see Chapters 21 and 45). Perioperative stress may increase serum glucose concentrations. A plan for perioperative insulin and glucose management must be agreed upon among the anesthesiologist, the surgeon, and the endocrinologist involved in the diabetic patient's care. There are several methods of doing this, none of which has proved superior to the others. One method is to administer one fourth to one half of the usual daily dose of intermediate-acting insulin preoperatively in the morning of surgery and begin an infusion of glucose-containing fluid. A second way is to administer no insulin or no glucose preoperatively and to measure serum glucose levels frequently during anesthesia. Regular insulin or glucose is then administered intra- and postoperatively as needed. A third method is to begin an infusion of insulin and glucose immediately preoperatively and to check serum glucose levels frequently.

Opioid Dependency

Withdrawal produced by drug cessation is a preoperative issue in the patient who is taking methadone or is dependent on other opioids. There should be an attempt to maintain opioid use at the usual level by continuing methadone or substituting other appropriate agents for methadone. The anesthesiologist should be cautioned about using agonist-antagonist drugs in these patients in the preoperative period for fear of producing withdrawal.

DIFFERENCES IN PREOPERATIVE MEDICATION BETWEEN PEDIATRIC AND ADULT PATIENTS

Differences between children and adults with regard to preoperative medication[218,219] include aspects of psychological preparation, the emphasis on oral medications when pharmacologic preparation is desired, and more frequent use of anticholinergics for their vagolytic activity. What remains the same is the need to assess the needs of each child individually and to tailor the psychological preparation and preoperative medication accordingly (see Chapter 48).

PSYCHOLOGICAL FACTORS IN PEDIATRIC PATIENTS

Hospital admission and major surgery can produce long-lasting psychological effects in some children.[220,221] The hospital stay is stressful and full of apprehension over the short term for almost all children. Psychological stress and anxiety are less likely to occur with minor procedures and brief hospitalizations.[222,223] Contrary to what one might believe, repeated hospitalizations have not been shown to increase the number of pediatric patients manifesting long-lasting psychological trauma.[221,224] The demeanor and communicative efforts of the anesthesiologist can make a difference to the child who is getting ready for a trip to the operating room, anesthesia, and surgery.

Age is probably the most important aspect when psychological preparation of the pediatric patient is considered.[219] A baby younger than 6 months of age is not emotionally upset when separated from his or her mother. Others in the health care team can substitute very easily. Preoperative preparation in this age group is often directed toward other goals, for example, obtundation of vagal reflex responses. However, preschool children are upset when separated from their mothers and fear the operating room. This is an age when hospitalization may be the most upsetting.[221,225,226] It is difficult to explain the forthcoming events to children in this age group. It is easier to communicate with patients from age 5 years to adolescence. The anesthesiologist can explain and offer reassurance about such issues as separation from parents and the home, operating room events, and any of the patient's perceived fears of surgery and anesthesia. Adolescent patients may already be anxious and apprehensive. They may also be worried about loss of consciousness, have a fear of death, or be apprehensive about what they will do or say after preoperative sedation or during anesthesia. The more fearful child may be difficult to identify.[219,227] This is usually the child who does not talk much during the preoperative interview and appears nonchalant or even detached. If these patients can be identified before operation, they are often candidates for heavy pharmacologic preparation.

Other important psychological aspects in preoperative preparation include the attitude and behavior of the parents, the socioeconomic status of the family, the magnitude of the planned surgery, and the hospital environment.[228,229]

Psychological Preparation

For the above reasons, a good preoperative visit and proper psychological preparation may be even more important in children than adults.[230-232] This is an art that is acquired by the anesthesiologist. The preoperative visit is a time of reassurance and explanation. It is an opportunity to gain the child's trust. Most anesthesiologists will want to involve the parents when possible. The child can then see the parents' acceptance of the anesthesiologist. Some hospitals have found motion pictures and slide shows to be helpful in preparing pediatric patients for the operating room.[228-234] The child may want to bring a personal belonging, such as a stuffed animal or blanket, to the operating room for security. Some children wish to take an active role by doing such things as holding the face mask during inhalation induction of anesthesia. It may be helpful in cases to have the parents accompany the child to the operating room suite.[235] In some hospitals parents may go into the operating room and stay until induction is complete.

Differences in Pharmacologic Preparation

The discussion of pharmacologic preparation for the pediatric patient presumes proper psychological preparation, a satisfactory operating room environment, and preparation for an efficient and timely induction of anesthesia.

Sedative-Hypnotics

As in adults, the sedative-hypnotic medications are used to reduce apprehension and produce sedation and amnesia. They are also used to facilitate smooth induction of anesthe-

sia when an inhalation method is to be used. The use of preoperative medication is controversial in pediatric patients. It has not been proved to reduce unwanted psychological outcome after surgery in anesthesia. It has been shown that the uneventful induction of anesthesia is less likely to produce long-lasting psychological problems in children.[221,225] After 6 months to 1 year of age, the child scheduled for a surgical procedure may benefit from a sedative hypnotic drug before surgery. There is some emphasis on avoiding intramuscular injections in children. The oral route is often used for preoperative medication in the older child, whereas in preschool children drugs may also be given rectally. Many sedative-hypnotic drugs have been prescribed for children before operation. The benzodiazepines and barbiturates have been chosen often, specifically diazepam and pentobarbital orally, which seem to be quite popular. Midazolam can be given intramuscularly or by the intranasal route (0.2 $mg \cdot kg^{-1}$). The most effective and acceptable route for midazolam is the oral route achieved by mixing 0.5–1.0 $mg \cdot kg^{-1}$ with a clear liquid (e.g., apple juice). It is effective in about 15 minutes and lasts for about an hour. Perhaps unique to the pharmacologic preparation of children is the rectal administration of methohexital (Fig. 24-11).[236] Methohexital (20–30 $mg \cdot kg^{-1}$) may be given immediately before operation, while the child is still in the parent's arms. The intramuscular route is also possible.

Opioids

There is the occasional need for opioid premedication in children. Methadone has the advantage of oral administration, usually prescribed in the 0.1–0.2 $mg \cdot kg^{-1}$ dose range.

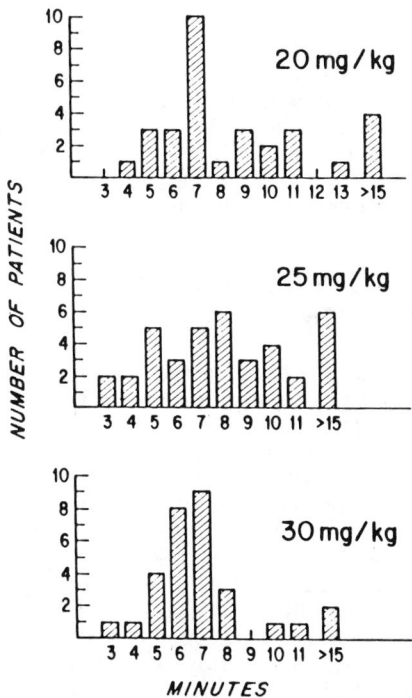

Figure 24-11. Frequency distribution of sleep induction times after rectal instillation of methohexital. Patients averaged 3.3 years in age and 15 kg in body weight. (Reprinted with permission from Liu LMP, Goudsouzian NG, Liu PL: Rectal methohexital premedication in children, a dose-comparison study. Anesthesiology 53:343, 1980.)

Intramuscular morphine and meperidine are used, often in combination with other premedications. Intramuscular morphine is often seen as part of the pharmacologic preparation for the child with congenital heart disease.[237-238] In many hospitals, opioids have been combined with sedative-hypnotic and anticholinergic drugs to make a "cocktail" that may be given orally for preoperative medication. Transmucosal administration of fentanyl in the form of a "fentanyl lollipop" (15–20 $\mu g \cdot kg^{-1}$) appears to be effective in producing sedation preoperatively. However, fentanyl lollipops significantly increase gastric volume and also increase the incidence of postoperative pruritus, nausea, and vomiting.[239-241] There are also ethical issues in delivering opioids in the form of candy. Sufentanil (3.0 $\mu g \cdot kg^{-1}$) given by the intranasal route has been shown to calm pediatric patients preoperatively. Again, postoperative nausea and vomiting and, in addition, respiratory complications have resulted in lack of enthusiasm for this technique.

Anticholinergics

Easily induced vagal reflexes make anticholinergics especially important in children.[238,242-244] Bradycardia may result from airway manipulation, surgical manipulation, or anesthetic drugs such as halothane or succinylcholine. Also, the child's cardiac output depends more on heart rate than does the adult's. If no contraindication exists, most pediatric patients receive atropine intravenously immediately after induction of anesthesia and placement of an intravenous catheter. If the intramuscular route has been used for atropine, it will often be administered immediately after the patient becomes unconscious during induction of anesthesia. Glycopyrrolate also has been used in children in this setting. Scopolamine has a place in premedication of the pediatric patient to produce sedation, amnesia, and drying of the airways. One must be aware of the hazards of administering an anticholinergic to a child with a fever or when inspissation of secretions is not wanted. Finally, it has been reported that patients with Down's syndrome appear to be sensitive to atropine.[245] This is especially evident with the effect on heart rate and mydriasis.

PREOPERATIVE MEDICATION FOR OUTPATIENTS

As with many aspects of preoperative medication, the pharmacologic preparation for outpatients is controversial (see Chapter 50).[51] Some anesthesiologists say premedication should be avoided. These patients are closer to their family and friends than inpatients, usually more minor surgery is scheduled, and postoperative obtundation and delayed discharge should be avoided.[246] Others believe a place exists for preoperative pharmacologic preparation for outpatients. In a study by Clark and Hurtig done in outpatients, intramuscular meperidine (1.0 $mg \cdot kg^{-1}$) and atropine (0.01 $mg \cdot kg^{-1}$) did not prolong recovery.[247] A retrospective analysis of 1553 patients by Meridy showed that preoperative medication with diazepam or hydroxyzine did not delay discharge after surgery in outpatients.[248] Oral diazepam 0.25 $mg \cdot kg^{-1}$ has been used successfully in adults to reduce anxiety before outpatient surgery,[249] as have low doses of intravenous midazolam. Horrigan et al reported that intravenous fentanyl (1–2 $\mu g \cdot kg^{-1}$) did not prolong recovery time in the outpatient setting in their study.[250] Some investigators have found a place for preoperative medication when

pediatric patients were scheduled for outpatient procedures.[251,252]

In some instances, antiemetic drugs may be desirable before operation for outpatients, for example, for patients scheduled for strabismus surgery, laparoscopic examination, and therapeutic abortions.[51] Nausea and vomiting are the most common reasons for delayed discharge in the ambulatory surgery setting. Low doses of droperidol have been used, with the consideration that higher doses can prolong recovery. Metoclopramide, hydroxyzine, transdermal scopolamine, and phenothiazines are other drugs that have been given before or during anesthesia to decrease the incidence of nausea and vomiting in the recovery room after outpatient surgery. One study has shown an increased gastric volume in outpatients.[117] Because of this and other factors, some authors recommend an H_2 receptor antagonist (cimetidine or ranitidine) combined with metoclopramide in selected outpatients.[253]

REFERENCES

1. Beecher HK: Preanesthetic medication. JAMA 157:242, 1955
2. Lyons SM, Clarke RSJ, Vulgaraki K: The premedication of cardiac surgical patients. Anaesthesia 30:459, 1975
3. Nicholson MJ: Preanesthetic preparation and premedication. In Hale DE (ed): Anesthesiology, p 202. Philadelphia, FA Davis, 1954
4. Baduer NH, Nielson W, Munk S et al: Preoperative anxiety: Detection and contributing factors. Can J Anaesth 37:414, 1990
5. Domar AD, Everett LL, Keller MG: Preoperative anxiety: Is it a predictable entity? Anesth Analg 69:763, 1986
6. Lichter JL, Johanson CE, Mhoon D et al: Preoperative anxiety—does anxiety level the afternoon before surgery predict anxiety level just before surgery? Anesthesiology 67:585, 1989
7. Norris W, Baird WLM: Pre-operative anxiety: A study of the incidence and aetiology. Br J Anaesth 39:503, 1967
8. Egbert LD, Battit GE, Turndorf H et al: The value of the preoperative visit by the anesthetist. JAMA 185:553, 1963
9. Leigh JM, Walker J, Janaganathan P: Effect of preoperative anesthetic visit on anxiety. Br Med J 2:987, 1977
10. Korttila K, Aromaa U, Tammisto T: Patient's expectations and acceptance of the effects of the drugs given before anaesthesia: Comparison of light and amnesic premedication. Acta Anaesth Scand 25:381, 1981
11. Ghignone M, Calvillo O, Quintin L: Anesthesia and hypertension. The effect of clonidine on perioperative hemodynamics and isoflurane requirements. Anesthesiology 67:3, 1987
12. Flacke JW, Bloor BC, Flacke WE et al: Reduced narcotic requirement by clonidine with improved hemodynamic and adrenergic stability in patients undergoing coronary bypass surgery. Anesthesiology 67:11, 1987
13. Walsh J, Puig MM, Lovitz MA et al: Premedication abolishes the increase in plasma beta-endorphin observed in the immediate preoperative period. Anesthesiology 66:402, 1987
14. Ong BY, Pickering BG, Palahniuk RJ et al: Lorazepam and diazepam as adjuncts to epidural anesthesia for cesarean section. Can Anaesth Soc J 29:31, 1982
15. Houghton DJ: Use of lorazepam as a premedicant for caesarean section. Br J Anaesth 55:767, 1983
16. McAuley DM, O'Neill MP, Moore J et al: Lorazepam premedication for labour. Br J Obstet Gynecol 89:149, 1982
17. Richter JJ: Current theories about the mechanisms of benzodiazepines and neurolytic drugs. Anesthesiology 54:66, 1981
18. Study RE, Barker JL: Cellular mechanisms of benzodiazepine action. JAMA 247:2147, 1982
19. Divoll M, Greenblatt DJ, Ochs HR et al: Absolute bioavailability of oral and intramuscular diazepam: Effect of age and sex. Anesth Analg 62:1, 1983

20. Greenblatt DJ, Koch-Weser J: Clinical toxicity of chlordiazepoxide and diazepam in relation to serum albumin concentration: A report from the Boston Collaborative Drug Surveillance Program. Eur J Clin Pharmacol 7:259, 1974

21. Kaplan SA, Jack ML, Alexander RJ et al: Pharmacokinetic profile of diazepam in man following single intravenous and chronic oral administration. J Pharm Sci 62:1289, 1973

22. Klotz I, Avant GR, Hoyumpa A et al: The effects of age and liver disease on the disposition and elimination of diazepam in adult man. J Clin Invest 55:347, 1975

23. Hillestad L, Hansen T, Melson H et al: Diazepam metabolism in normal man. Serum concentrations and clinical effects after intravenous intramuscular and oral administration. Clin Pharmacol Ther 16:479, 1974

24. Assaf RAD, Dundee JW, Gamble JAS: The influence of the route of administration on the clinical action of diazepam. Anaesthesia 30:152, 1975

25. Lundgren S: Comparison of rectal diazepam and subcutaneous morphine-scopolamine administration for outpatient sedation in minor oral surgery. Acta Anaesthesiol Scand 29:674, 1985

26. Ravnborg M, Hasselstrom L, Ostergard D: Premedication with oral and rectal diazepam. Acta Anaesthesiol Scand 30:132, 1986

27. Frumin MJ, Herekar VR, Jarvik ME: Amnesic actions of diazepam and scopolamine in man. Anesthesiology 45:406, 1976

28. Liu S, Miller N, Waye JD: Retrograde amnesia effects of intravenous diazepam in endoscopy patients. Gastrointest Endosc 30:340, 1984

29. Soroker D, Barzilay E, Konichezky S et al: Respiratory function following premedication with droperidol or diazepam. Anesth Analg 57:695, 1978

30. Rao S, Sherbaniuk RW, Prasad K et al: Cardiopulmonary effects of diazepam. Clin Pharmacol 14:182, 1973

31. Gross JB, Smith L, Smith TC: Time course of ventilatory response to carbon dioxide after intravenous diazepam. Anesthesiology 57:18, 1982

32. Braunstein MC: Apnea with maintenance of consciousness following intravenous diazepam. Anesth Analg 58:52, 1979

33. Wingard DW: Physostigmine reversal of diazepam-induced depression. Anesth Analg 56:348, 1977

34. Dalen JE, Evans GL, Banas JS et al: The hemodynamics and respiratory effects of diazepam (Valium). Anesthesiology 30:259, 1969

35. McCammon RL, Hilgenberg JC, Stoelting RK: Hemodynamic effects of diazepam and diazepam-nitrous oxide in patients with coronary artery disease. Anesth Analg 59:438, 1980

36. Davies AO: Oral diazepam premedication reduces the incidence of postsuccinylcholine muscle pains. Can Anaesth Soc J 30:603, 1983

37. Verma RS: Diazepam and suxamethonium muscle pain (a dose response study). Anaesthesia 37:688, 1982

38. Feneck RD, Cook JH: Failure of diazepam to prevent suxamethonium-induced rise in intra-ocular pressure. Anaesthesia 38:120, 1983

39. Kruger AE, Roelofse JA: Precautions against intra-ocular pressure changes during endotracheal intubation—a comparison of pretreatment with intravenous lignocaine and diazepam. S Afr Med J 63:887, 1983

40. Fjeldborg P, Hecht PS, Busted N et al: The effect of diazepam pretreatment on the succinylcholine-induced rise in intraocular pressure. Acta Anaesthesiol Scand 29:415, 1985

41. Moore DC, Balfour RI, Fitzgibbons D: Convulsive arterial plasma levels of bupivacaine and the response to diazepam therapy. Anesthesiology 50:454, 1979

42. Greenblatt DJ, Abernathy DR, Morse DS, et al: Clinical importance of the interaction of diazepam and cimetidine. N Engl J Med 310:1639, 1984

43. Perisho JA, Buechel DR, Miller RD: The effect of diazepam (Valium) in minimum alveolar anesthetic requirement (MAC) in man. Can Anaesth Soc J 18:563, 1971

44. Dundee JW, Lilburn JR, Nair SG et al: Studies of drugs given before anaesthesia. XXVI. Lorazepam. Br J Anaesth 49:1047, 1977

45. Heisterkamp DV, Cohen PT: The effect of intravenous premedication with lorazepam (Ativan), pentobarbital and diazepam on recall. Br J Anaesth 47:79, 1975

46. Pandit SK, Heisterkamp DV, Cohen PJ: Further studies of the antirecall effect of lorazepam: A dose-time-effect relationship. Anesthesiology 45:495, 1976

47. Wallace G, Mindlin LJ: A controlled double-blind comparison of intramuscular lorazepam and hydroxyzine as surgical premedicants. Anesth Analg 63:571, 1984

48. Aleniewski MI, Bulas BJ, Maderazo L et al: Intramuscular lorazepam versus pentobarbital premedication: A comparison of patient sedation, anxiolysis and recall. Anesth Analg 56:489, 1977

49. Russell WJ: Lorazepam as a premedicant for regional anaesthesia. Anaesthesia 38:1062, 1983

50. Pagano RR, Conner JT, Bellville JW et al: Lorazepam, hyoscine and atropine as IV surgical premedicants. Br J Anaesth 50:471, 1978

51. White PF: Pharmacologic and clinical aspects of preoperative medication. Anesth Analg 65:963, 1986

52. Bradshaw EG, Ali AA, Mulley BA et al: Plasma concentrations and clinical effects of lorazepam after oral administration. Br J Anaesth 53:517, 1981

53. Blitt CD, Petty WC, Wright WA et al: Clinical evaluation of injectable lorazepam as a premedicant: The effect on recall. Anesth Analg 55:522, 1976

54. Gale GD, Galloon S, Porter WR: Sublingual lorazepam: A better premedication? Br J Anaesth 55:761, 1983

55. Fragen RJ, Caldwell N: Lorazepam premedication: Lack of recall and relief of anxiety. Anesth Analg 55:792, 1976

56. George KA, Dundee JW: Relative amnesia actions of diazepam, flunitrazepam and lorazepam in man. Br J Clin Pharmacol 4:45, 1977

57. Kraus JW, Desmond PV, Marshall JP et al: Effects of aging and liver disease on disposition of lorazepam. Clin Pharmacol Ther 24:44, 1978

58. Gasser JC, Kaufman RD, Bellville JW: Respiratory effects of lorazepam, pentobarbital and pentazocine. Clin Pharmacol Ther 18:170, 1975

59. Comer WH, Elliott HW, Nomof W et al: Pharmacology of parenterally administered lorazepam in man. J Int Med Res 1:216, 1973

60. Conner JT, Katz RL, Bellville JW et al: Diazepam and lorazepam for intravenous surgical premedication. J Clin Pharmacol 18:285, 1978

61. Knapp RB, Fierro L: Evaluation of cardiopulmonary safety and effects of lorazepam as a premedicant. Anaesth Analg 53:122, 1974

62. Cormack RS, Milledge JS, Hanning CD: Respiration and amnesia after lorazepam or morphine premedication. Br J Anaesth 48:813, 1976

63. Dundee JW, Johnston HML, Gray RC: Lorazepam as a sedative—amnesia in an intensive care unit. Curr Med Res Opin 4:290, 1976

64. Denaut M, Yernault JC, DeCoster A: Double blind comparison of the respiratory effects of parenteral lorazepam and diazepam in patients with chronic obstructive lung disease. Curr Med Res Opin 2:611, 1975

65. Mohler H, Okada T: Benzodiazepine receptor: Demonstration in the central nervous system. Science 198:849, 1977

66. Reves JG, Fragen RJ, Vinick HR et al: Midazolam: Pharmacology and uses. Anesthesiology 62:310, 1985

67. Greenblatt DJ, Locniskar A, Scavone JM et al: Absence of interaction of cimetidine and ranitidine with intravenous and oral midazolam. Anesth Analg 65:176, 1986

68. Greenblatt DJ, Abernathy DR, Locniskar A et al: Effect of age, gender and obesity on midazolam kinetics. Anesthesiology 61:27, 1984

69. Dundee JW, Wilson DB: Amnesic action of midazolam. Anaesthesia 35:459, 1980

70. Connor JT, Katz RL, Pagano RR et al: R021-3981 for intravenous surgical premedication and induction of anesthesia. Anesth Analg 59:1, 1978

71. Fragen RJ, Funk DI, Avram MJ et al: Midazolam versus hy-

droxyzine as intramuscular premedicants. Can Anaesth Soc J 30:136, 1983

72. Barrett RF, James PD, McLeod KCA: Oxazepam premedication in neurosurgical patients. Anaesthesia 39:429, 1984
73. Greenwood BK, Bradshaw EG: Preoperative medication for day care surgery. A comparison between oxazepam and temazepam. Br J Anaesth 55:933, 1983
74. Amarasekera K: Temazepam as a premedicant in minor surgery. Anaesthesia 35:771, 1980
75. Beechy APG, Etringham RJ, Studd C: Temazepam as premedication in day surgery. Anaesthesia 36:10, 1981
76. Clark G, Ervin D, Yate P et al: Temazepam as premedication in elderly patients. Anaesthesia 37:421, 1982
77. Thomas D, Tipping T, Halifax R et al: Triazolam premedication. Anaesthesia 41:692, 1986
78. Pinnock CA, Fell D, Hunt PCW et al: A comparison of triazolam and diazepam as premedication for minor gynaecologic surgery. Anaesthesia 40:324, 1985
79. Greenblatt DJ, Shader RI: Benzodiazepines. N Engl J Med 291:1239, 1974
80. Smith TC, Stephen GW, Zeiger L et al: Effects of premedicant drugs on respiration and gas exchange in man. Anesthesiology 28:883, 1967
81. Koch-Weser J, Greenblatt DJ: The archaic barbiturate hypnotics. N Engl J Med 291:790, 1974
82. Dundee JW, Nair SG, Assof RAE et al: Pentobarbital premedication for anesthetic. Anaesthesia 31:1025, 1976
83. Hovi-Viander M, Kangas L, Kanto J: A comparative study of the clinical effects of pentobarbital and diazepam given orally as preoperative medication. J Oral Surg 38:188, 1980
84. Herr GP, Conner JT, Katz RL et al: Diazepam and droperidol as IV premedicants. Br J Anaesth 51:537, 1979
85. Lee CM, Yeakel AE: Patient refusal of surgery following Innovar premedication. Anesth Analg 54:224, 1975
86. Briggs RM, Ogg MJ: Patient's refusal of surgery following Innovar premedication. Plast Reconstr Surg 54:224, 1975
87. Rivera VM, Keichian AH, Oliver RE: Persistent parkinsonism following neurolept analgesia. Anesthesiology 42:635, 1975
88. Patton CM: Rapid induction of acute dyskinesis by droperidol. Anesthesiology 43:126, 1975
89. Ward DS: Stimulation of the hypoxic ventilatory drive by droperidol. Anesth Analg 63:106, 1984
90. Hupert C, Yacoub M, Turgeon LR: Effect of hydroxyzine on morphine analgesia for the treatment of postoperative pain. Anesth Analg 59:690, 1980
91. Wender RH, Conner JT, Bellville JW et al: Comparison of IV diazepam and hydroxyzine as surgical premedicants. Br J Anaesth 49:907, 1977
92. Belleville JW, Dorey F, Capparell D et al: Analgesic effects of hydroxyzine compared to morphine in man. J Clin Pharmacol 19:290, 1979
93. McKenzie R, Wadhewa RK, Uy NTL et al: Antiemetic effectiveness of intramuscular hydroxyzine compared with intramuscular droperidol. Anaesth Analg 60:783, 1981
94. Beaven MA: Anaphylactoid reactions to anesthetic drugs. Anesthesiology 55:3, 1981
95. Keats AS, Telford J, Kurosu Y: "Potentiation" of meperidine by promethazine. Anesthesiology 22:34, 1961
96. Conner JT, Bellville JW, Wender R et al: Morphine and promethazine as intravenous premedicants. Anesth Analg 56:801, 1977
97. Cohen EN, Beecher HK: Narcotics in preanesthetic medication—a controlled study. JAMA 147:1664, 1951
98. Belleville JA, Forrest WH, Miller E et al: Influence of age on pain relief from analgesics. JAMA 217:1835, 1971
99. Saidman LJ, Eger EI II: Effect of nitrous oxide and narcotic premedication on the alveolar concentration of halothane required for anesthesia. Anesthesiology 25:302, 1964
100. Tsunoda Y, Hattori Y, Takatsuko E et al: Effects of hydroxyzine, diazepam and pentazocine on halothane minimum alveolar anesthetic concentration. Anesth Analg 52:390, 1973
101. Conner JT, Bellville JW, Katz RL: Meperidine and morphine as intravenous surgical premedicants. Can Anaesth Soc J 24:559, 1977
102. Cormack RS, Milledge JS, Hanning CD: Respiratory effects and

amnesia after premedication with morphine or lorazepam. Br J Anaesth 49:351, 1977
103. Weil JV, McCullough RE, Kline JS: Diminished ventilatory response to hypoxia and hypercapnia after morphine in man. N Engl J Med 292:1103, 1975
104. Economou G, Ward-McQuaid JN: A cross-over comparison of the effect of morphine, pethidine and pentazine on biliary pressure. Gut 12:218, 1971
105. Greenstein AJ, Kaynan A, Singer A et al: A comparative study of pentazocine and meperidine on the biliary passage pressure. Am J Gastroenterol 58:417, 1972
106. Radnay PA, Brochman E, Mankikar D et al: The effect of equi-analgesic doses of fentanyl, morphine, meperidine, and pentazocine on common bile duct pressure. Anesthetist 29:26, 1980
107. Jones RM, Fiddian-Green R, Knight PR: Narcotic-induced choledochoduodenal sphincter spasm by glucagon. Anesth Analg 59:946, 1980
108. Cahalan MK, Lurz FW, Eger EI II et al: Narcotics decrease heart rate during inhalational anesthesia. Anesth Analg 66:166, 1987
109. Austin KL, Stapleton JV, Mather LE: Multiple intramuscular injections—a major source of variability in analgesic response to meperidine. Pain 8:47, 1980
110. Gourlay GK, Wilson PR, Glynn CJ: Pharmacodynamics and pharmacokinetics of methadone during the perioperative period. Anesthesiology 57:458, 1982
111. Laffey DA, Kay NH: Premedication with butorphanol: A comparison with morphine. Br J Anaesth 56:363, 1984
112. VanDam LD: Butorphanol. N Engl J Med 302:381, 1980
113. Hofmann RF, Weiler HH: Lorazepam and nalbuphine as local anesthetic ophthalmic surgery premedications. Ann Ophthalmol 15:64, 1983
114. Lake CL, Duckworth EN, DiFazio CA et al: Cardiorespiratory effects of nalbuphine and morphine premedication in adult cardiac surgical patients. Acta Anaesthesiol Scand 28:305, 1984
115. Pinnock CA, Bell A, Smith G: A comparison of nalbuphine and morphine as premedication agents for minor gynaecological surgery. Anaesthesia 40:1078, 1985
116. Vaughn RW, Bauer S, Wise L: Volume and pH of gastric juice in obese patients. Anesthesiology 43:686, 1975
117. Ong BY, Palahniuk RJ, Cumming M: Gastric volume and pH in outpatients. Can Anaesth Soc J 25:36, 1978
118. Stoelting RK: Responses to atropine, glycopyrrolate and Riopan on gastric fluid pH and volume in adult patients. Anesthesiology 48:367, 1978
119. Manchikanti L, Roush JR: The effect of preanesthetic glycopyrrolate and cimetidine in gastric fluid pH and volume in outpatients. Anesth Analg 63:40, 1984
119a. Olsson GL, Hallen B, Hambraeus-Jonzon K: Aspiration during anesthesia. A computer-aided study of 185,358 anaesthetics. Acta Anaesthesiol Scand 30:84, 1986
119b. Tiret L, Nwoche Y, Hatton F et al: Complications related to anaesthesia in infants and children: A prospective survey of 40,240 anaesthetics. Br J Anaesth 61:263, 1988
120. Goresky GV, Maltby JR: Fasting guidelines for elective surgical patients. Can J Anaesth 37:493, 1990
121. Miller M, Wishart HY, Nimmo WS: Gastric content of induction of anaesthesia: Is a 4 hour fast necessary? Br J Anaesth 55:1185, 1983
121a. Cote CJ: NPO after midnight for children—a reappraisal. Anesthesiology 72:589, 1990
122. Hutchinson A, Maltby JR, Reid CRG: Gastric fluid volume and pH in elective inpatients. Part I: Coffee or orange juice versus overnight fast. Can J Anaesth 35:125, 1988
123. Shevde K, Trivedi N: Effects of clear liquids on gastric volume and pH in healthy volunteers. Anesth Analg 72:528, 1991
124. Splinter WM, Schaefer SE, Zunder IH: Clear fluids three hours before surgery do not affect the gastric fluid contents of children. Can J Anaesth 37:498, 1990
125. Schreiner MS, Triebevassen A, Klon T: Ingestion of liquids compared with preoperative fasting in pediatric outpatients. Anesthesiology 72:593, 1990
126. Crawford M, Lerman J, Christensen S et al: Effects of duration

of fasting on gastric fluid pH and volume in healthy children. Anesth Analg 71:400, 1990

127. Splinter WM, Steward JR, Muir JG: The effect of preoperative apple juice on gastric contents, thirst, and hunger in children. Can J Anaesth 36:55, 1989

128. Splinter WM, Steward JR, Muir JG: Large volumes of apple juice preoperatively do not affect gastric pH and volume in children. Can J Anaesth 37:36, 1990

128a. Maltby JR, Lewis P, Martin A, Sutheriand LR: Gastric fluid volume and pH in elective patients following unrestricted oral fluid until three hours before surgery. Can J Anaesth 38:425, 1991

129. Brock-Utne JG, Rubin J, Welman S et al: The effect of glyco-pyrrolate (Robinul) on the lower esophageal sphincter. Can Anaesth Soc J 25:144, 1978

130. Black JW, Duncan WAM, Durant CJ et al: Definition and antag-onism of histamine H_2-receptors. Nature 236:385, 1972

131. Coombs DW: Aspiration pneumonia prophylaxis. Anesth An-alg 62:1055, 1983

132. Weber L, Hirshman CA: Cimetidine for prophylaxis of aspira-tion pneumonitis: Comparison of intramuscular and oral dose schedules. Anesth Analg 58:426, 1979

133. Stoelting RK: Gastric fluid pH in patients receiving cimeti-dine. Anesth Analg 57:675, 1978

134. Coombs DW, Hooper D, Colton T: Acid aspiration prophylaxis by use of preoperative oral administration of cimetidine. An-esthesiology 51:352, 1979

135. Manchikanti L, Kraus JW, Edds SP: Cimetidine and related drugs in anesthesia. Anesth Analg 61:595, 1982

136. Maliniak K, Vakil AH: Pre-anesthetic cimetidine and gastric pH. Anesth Analg 58:309, 1979

137. Hodgkinson R, Glassenberg R, Joyce TH et al: Comparison of cimetidine (Tagamet) with antacid for safety and effectiveness in reducing gastric acidity before elective cesarean section. Anesthesiology 59:86, 1983

138. Johnston JR, Moore J, McCaughey W et al: Use of cimetidine as an oral antacid obstetric anesthesia. Anesth Analg 62:720, 1983

139. Coombs DW, Hooper DW: Cimetidine as a prophylactic against acid aspiration at tracheal extubation. Can Anaesth Soc J 28:33, 1981

140. Cohen J, Weetman AP, Dargie HJ et al: Life threatening ar-rhythmias and intravenous injection of cimetidine. Br Med J 2:768, 1979

141. Shaw RG, Mashford ML, Desmond PV: Cardiac arrest after intravenous injection of cimetidine. Med J Aust 2:629, 1980

142. Durrant JM, Strunin L: Comparative trial of the effect of ra-nitidine and cimetidine on gastric secretion in fasting pa-tients at induction of anaesthesia. Can Anaesth Soc J 29:446, 1982

143. Harris PW, Morison DH, Dunn GL et al: Intramuscular cimeti-dine and ranitidine as prophylaxis against gastric aspiration syndrome. Can Anaesth Soc J 31:599, 1984

144. Zeldis JE, Friedman LS, Iselbacher KJ: Ranitidine: A new H_2-receptor antagonist. N Engl J Med 309:1368, 1983

145. Gillett GB, Watson JD, Langford RM: Ranitidine and single dose antacid therapy as prophylaxis against acid aspiration syndrome in obstetric practice. Anaesthesia 39:638, 1984

146. Viegas OJ, Ravindran RS, Shumacker CA: Gastric fluid pH in patients receiving sodium citrate. Anesth Analg 60:521, 1981

147. Gibbs CP, Spohr L, Schmidt D: The effectiveness of sodium citrate as an antacid. Anesthesiology 57:44, 1982

148. Manchikanti L, Grow JB, Collvier JA et al: Sodium citrate and metoclopramide in outpatient anesthesia for prophylaxis against aspiration pneumonitis. Anesthesiology 63:378, 1985

149. Gibbs CP, Hempling RE, Wynne JW et al: Antacid pulmonary aspiration. Anesthesiology 51:S290, 1979

150. Frank M, Evans M, Flynn P et al: Comparison of the prophy-lactic use of magnesium trisilicate, sodium citrate or cimeti-dine in obstetrics. Br J Anaesth 56:355, 1984

151. Bond VK, Stoelting RK, Gupta CD: Pulmonary aspiration syn-drome after inhalation of gastric fluid containing antacids. Anesthesiology 51:452, 1979

152. Gibbs CP, Schwartz DJ, Wynne JR et al: Antacid pulmonary aspiration in the dog. Anesthesiology 51:380, 1979

153. Heany GAH, Jones HD: Correspondence: Aspiration syndrome in pregnancy. Br J Anaesth 51:266, 1979

154. Schwartz J, Wynne JW, Gibbs CP et al: Pulmonary conse-quences of aspiration of gastric contents at pH values greater than 2.5. Am Rev Respir Dis 121:119, 1980

155. Foulkes E, Jenkins LC: A comparative evaluation of cimeti-dine and sodium citrate to decrease gastric acidity: Effective-ness at time of induction of anesthesia. Can Anaesth Soc J 23:29, 1981

156. Schmidt JF, Schierup L, Banning AM: The effect of sodium citrate on the pH and amount of gastric contents before general anesthesia. Acta Anaesthesiol Scand 28:263, 1984

157. O'Sullivan GM, Bullingham RE: Noninvasive assessment by radiotelemetry of antacid effect during labor. Anesth Analg 64:95, 1985

158. James CF, Modell JH, Gibbs CP et al: Pulmonary aspiration—effects of volume and pH in the rat. Anesth Analg 63:665, 1984

159. Murphy DF, Nally B, Gardiner J et al: Effect of metoclopra-mide on gastric emptying before elective and emergency cae-sarean section. Br J Anaesth 56:1113, 1984

160. Wyner J, Cohen SE: Gastric volume in early pregnancy: Effect of metoclopramide. Anesthesiology 57:209, 1982

161. Nimmo WS: Drugs, diseases and altered gastric emptying. Clin Pharmacokinet 1:189, 1976

162. Cohen SE, Jasson J, Talafre M-L et al: Does metoclopramide decrease the volume of gastric contents in patients undergoing cesarean section? Anesthesiology 61:604, 1984

163. Schmidt JF, Jorgensen BC: The effect of metoclopramide on gastric contents after preoperative ingestion of sodium citrate. Anesth Analg 63:841, 1984

164. Manchikanti L, Marrero TC, Roush JR: Preanesthetic cimeti-dine and metoclopramide for acid aspiration prophylaxis in elective surgery. Anesthesiology 61:48, 1984

165. Manchikanti L, Colliver JA, Marrero TC et al: Ranitidine and metoclopramide for prophylaxis of aspiration pneumonitis in elective surgery. Anesth Analg 63:903, 1984

166. O'Sullivan G, Sear JW, Bullingham RES et al: The effect of magnesium trisilicate, metoclopramide and ranitidine on gas-tric pH, volume and serum gastrin. Anaesthesia 40:246, 1985

167. Korttila K, Kauste A, Auvinen J: Comparison of domperidone, droperidol and metoclopramide in the prevention and treat-ment of nausea and vomiting after balanced general anesthe-sia. Anesth Analg 58:396, 1979

168. Santos A, Datta S: Prophylactic use of droperidol for control of nausea and vomiting during spinal anesthesia for cesarean section. Anesth Analg 63:85, 1984

169. Cohen SE, Woods WA, Wyner J: Antiemetic efficacy of droper-idol and metoclopramide. Anesthesiology 60:67, 1984

170. Tornetta FJ: A comparison of droperidol, diazepam and hy-droxyzine hydrochloride as premedication. Anesth Analg 56:496, 1977

171. Patton CM, Moon MR, Dannemiller JT: The prophylactic anti-emetic effect of droperidol. Anesth Analg 53:361, 1974

172. Iwamoto K, Schwartz H: Antiemetic effect of droperidol after ophthalmic surgery. Arch Ophthalmol 96:1378, 1978

173. Mortensen PT: Droperidol (dehydrobenzperidol): Postopera-tive antiemetic effect when given intravenously to gynaeco-logic patients. Acta Anaesth Scand 26:48, 1982

174. Karhunen U, Orko R: Nausea and vomiting after local anesthe-sia for cataract extraction in elderly female patients. Effect of droperidol premedication. Ophthalmic Surg 12:810, 1981

175. Winning TJ, Brock-Utne JG, Downing JW: Nausea and vom-iting after anesthesia and minor surgery. Anesth Analg 56:674, 1977

176. Clark MM, Stores JA: The prevention of postoperative vom-iting after abortion. Metoclopramide. Br J Anesth 41:890, 1969

177. Shah ZP, Wilson J: An evaluation of metoclopramide (Maxo-lon) as an antiemetic in anesthesia. Br J Anesth 44:865, 1972

178. Ellis FR, Spence AA: Clinical trials of metoclopramide (Maxo-lon) as an antiemetic in anaesthesia. Anaesthesia 25:368, 1970

179. Tornetta FJ: Clinical studies with the new antiemetic, met-oclopramide. Anesth Analg 48:198, 1969

180. Greenblatt DJ, Shader RI: Anticholinergics. N Engl J Med 288:1215, 1973

181. Clarke RSJ, Dundee JW, Moore J: Studies of drugs given before anesthesia. 4. Atropine and hyoscine. Br J Anaesth 36:648, 1964

182. Eger EI II: Atropine, scopolamine and related compounds. Anesthesiology 33:365, 1962

183. Mirakhur RK: Anticholinergic drugs. Br J Anaesth 51:671, 1979

184. Shutt LE, Bowes JB: Atropine and hyoscine. Anaesthesia 34:476, 1979

185. Holt AI: Premedication with atropine should not be routine. Lancet 2:984, 1961

186. Middleton JJ, Zitzer JM, Urbach KF: Is atropine always necessary before general anesthesia? Anesth Analg 46:51, 1967

187. Kessel J: Atropine premedication. Anaesth Intensive Care 2:77, 1974

188. Mirakhur RA, Clarke RSJ, Dundee JW et al: Anticholinergic drugs in anaesthesia. A survey of their present position. Anaesthesia 33:133, 1978

189. Falick YS, Smiler BG: Is anticholinergic premedication necessary? Anesthesiology 43:472, 1975

190. Wyant GM, Kao E: Glycopyrrolate methobromide. Effect on salivary secretion. Can Anaesth Soc J 21:230, 1974

191. Russell-Taylor WJ, Llewellyn-Thomas E, Seller EA: A comparative evaluation of intramuscular atropine, dicyclomine and glycopyrrolate using healthy medical students as volunteer subjects. Int J Clin Pharmacol 4:358, 1970

192. McCubbin TD, Brown JH, Dewar KMS et al: Glycopyrrolate as premedicant: Comparison with atropine. Br J Anaesth 51:885, 1979

193. Forrest WH, Brown CR, Brown BW: Subjective responses to six common preoperative medications. Anesthesiology 47:241, 1977

194. Conner JT, Bellville JW, Wender R et al: Morphine, scopolamine and atropine as intravenous surgical premedicants. Anesth Analg 56:606, 1977

195. Meyers EF, Tomeldan SA: Glycopyrrolate compared with atropine in prevention of the oculocardiac reflex during eye-muscle surgery. Anesthesiology 51:350, 1979

196. Sorensen O, Eriksen S, Hommegaard P et al: Thiopental-nitrous oxide-halothane anesthesia and repeated succinylcholine: Comparison of preoperative glycopyrrolate and atropine administration. Anesth Analg 59:686, 1980

197. Longo VG: Behavioral and electroencephalographic effects of atropine and related compounds. Pharmacol Rev 18:965, 1966

198. Smith DS, Orkin FK, Gardner SM et al: Prolonged sedation in the elderly after intraoperative atropine administration. Anesthesiology 51:348, 1979

199. Holzgrafe RE, Vondrell JJ, Mintz SM: Reversal of postoperative reactions to scopolamine with physostigmine. Anesth Analg 52:921, 1973

200. Duvoisin RC, Katz RL: Reversal of central anticholinergic syndrome in man by physostigmine. JAMA 206:1963, 1968

201. Garde JF, Aston R, Endler GC et al: Racial mydriatic response to belladonna premedication. Anaesth Analg 57:572, 1978

202. Severinghaus JW, Stupfel M: Respiratory dead space increase following atropine in man, and atropine, vagal or ganglionic blockade and hypothermia in dogs. J Appl Physiol 8:81, 1955

203. Maze M, Tranquilli W: Alpha-2 adrenoceptor agonists: Defining the role in clinical anesthesia. Anesthesiology 74:581, 1991

204. Kaukinen S, Pyykko K: The potentiation of halothane anesthesia by clonidine. Acta Anaesthesiol Scand 23:107, 1979

205. Bloor BC, Flacke WE: Reduction in halothane anesthetic requirement by clonidine, an alpha adrenergic agonist. Anesth Analg 61:741, 1982

206. Maze M, Birch B, Vickery RG: Clonidine reduces halothane MAC in rats. Anesthesiology 67:868, 1987

207. Flacke JW, Bloor BC, Flacke WE et al: Reduced narcotic requirement by clonidine with improved hemodynamic and adrenergic stability in patients undergoing coronary bypass surgery. Anesthesiology 67:11, 1987

208. Ghignone M, Quintin L, Duke PC et al: Effects of clonidine on narcotic requirements and hemodynamic response during induction of fentanyl anesthesia and endotracheal intubation. Anesthesiology 64:36, 1986

209. Ghignone M, Noe C, Calvillo O, Quintin L: Anesthesia for ophthalmic surgery in the elderly: The effects of clonidine on intraocular pressure, perioperative hemodynamics, and anesthetic requirement. Anesthesiology 68:707, 1988

210. Engelman E, Lipszyc M, Gilbart E et al: Effects of clonidine on anesthetic requirements and hemodynamic response during aortic surgery. Anesthesiology 71:178, 1989

211. Segal IS, Jarvis DA, Duncan SR et al: Clinical efficacy of oral-transdermal clonidine combinations during the perioperative period. Anesthesiology 74:220, 1991

212. Lieper DJ, Townsend GE: Improved hemodynamic and renal function with clonidine in coronary artery bypass grafting. Anesth Analg 70:s240, 1990

213. Orko R, Pouttu J, Ghignone M, Rosenberg PH: Effect of clonidine on hemodynamic responses to endotracheal intubation and on gastric acidity. Acta Anesthesiol Scand 31:325, 1987

214. Pouttu J, Scheinin B, Rosenberg PH et al: Oral premedication with clonidine: Effects on stress responses during general anesthesia. Acta Anaesthesiol Scand 31:730, 1987

215. Woodcock TE, Millar RK, Dixon F, Prys-Roberts C: Clonidine premedication for isoflurane induced hypotension. Br J Anaesth 60:388, 1988

216. Shulman ST, Amren DP, Bisno AL et al: Prevention of bacterial endocarditis. A statement for health professionals by the Committee on Rheumatic Fever and Infective Endocarditis of the Council on Cardiovascular Disease in the Young. Circulation 70:1123, 1984

217. Symreng T, Karlberg BE, Kågedal B et al: Physiological cortisol substitution on long-term steroid-treated patients undergoing major surgery. Br J Anaesth 53:949, 1981

218. Korsch BM: The child and the operating room. Anesthesiology 43:251, 1975

219. Steward DJ: Psychological preparation and premedication. In Gregory GA (ed): Pediatric Anesthesia, p 423. New York, Churchill Livingstone, 1983

220. Chapman AH, Loeb DG, Gibbons MJ: Psychiatric aspects of hospitalizing children. Archives of Pediatrics 73:77, 1956

221. Vernon DTA, Schulman JL, Foley JM: Changes in children's behavior after hospitalization. Am J Dis Child 111:581, 1966

222. Davenport HT, Werry JS: The effect of general anesthesia, surgery and hospitalization on the behavior of children. Am J Orthopsychiatry 40:806, 1970

223. Steward DJ: Experiences with an out-patient anesthesia service for children. Anesthesiology 52:877, 1973

224. Jessner L, Blom GE, Waldfogel S: Emotional implications of tonsillectomy and adenoidectomy on children. Psychoanal Study Child 7:126, 1952

225. Eckenhoff JE: Relationship of anesthesia to post-operative personality changes in children. Am J Dis Child 86:587, 1953

226. Beeby DG, Hughes JOM: Behaviour of unsedated children in the anaesthetic room. Br J Anaesth 52:279, 1980

227. Bothe A, Galdston R: A child's loss of consciousness: A psychiatric view of pediatric anesthesia. Pediatrics 50:252, 1972

228. Rothman PE: A note on hospitalism. Pediatrics 30:995, 1962

229. Tisza VB, Angoff K: A play program for hospitalized children: The role of the playroom teacher. Pediatrics 28:841, 1961

230. Booker PD, Chapman DH: Premedication in children undergoing day-care surgery. Br J Anaesth 51:1083, 1979

231. Jackson K: Psychological preparation as a method of reducing the emotional trauma of anesthesia in children. Anesthesiology 12:293, 1981

232. Visintainer MA, Wolfer JA: Psychological preparation for pediatric patients: The effect on children's and parents' stress responses and adjustment. Pediatrics 56:187, 1975

233. Vernon DTA, Bailey WC: The use of motion pictures in the psychological preparation of children for induction of anesthesia. Anesthesiology 40:68, 1974

234. Bevan JC, Johnston CJ, Haig MS et al: Preoperative parental anxiety predicts behavioural and emotional responses to induction of anaesthesia in children. Can J Anaesth 37:177, 1990

235. Melamed BG, Siegel LJ: Reduction of anxiety in children facing hospitalization and surgery by use of filmed modeling. J Consult Clin Psychol 43:511, 1975

236. Liu LMP, Goudsouzian NG, Liu PL: Rectal methohexital in

children, a dose-comparison study. Anesthesiology 53:343, 1980

237. McQuiston WO: Anesthetic problems in cardiac surgery in children. Anesthesiology 10:590, 1947

238. Moffitt EA, McGoon DC, Ritter DG: The diagnosis and correction of congenital cardiac defects. Anesthesiology 33:144, 1970

239. Feld LH, Champeau MW, van Steennis CA et al: Preanesthetic medication in children: A comparison of oral transmucosal fentanyl citrate versus placebo. Anesthesiology 71:374, 1989

240. Nicolson SC, Betts EK, Jobes DR et al: Comparison of oral and intramuscular preanesthetic medication for pediatric inpatient surgery. Anesthesiology 71:8, 1989

241. Goldstein-Dressner MC, Davis PJ, Kretchman E et al: Double-blind comparison of oral transmucosal fentanyl citrate with oral meperidine, diazepam, and atropine as preanesthetic medication in children with congenital heart disease. Anesthesiology 74:28, 1991

242. Gravenstein JS, Anton AH: Premedication and drug interaction. Clin Anesthesia 3:199, 1969

243. Rackow H, Salanitre E: Modern concepts in pediatric anesthesiology. Anesthesiology 30:208, 1969

244. Kessel J: Atropine premedication. Anaesth Intensive Care 2:77, 1974

245. Harris WS, Goodman RH: Hyper-reactivity to atropine in Down's syndrome. N Engl J Med 279:407, 1968

246. Korttila K, Linnoila M: Psychomotor skills related to driving after intramuscular administration of diazepam and meperidine. Anesthesiology 42:685, 1975

247. Clark AJM, Hurtig JB: Premedication with meperidine and atropine does not prolong recovery to the street fitness after out-patient surgery. Can Anaesth Soc J 28:390, 1981

248. Meridy HW: Criteria for selection of ambulatory surgical patients and guidelines for anesthetic management—a retrospective study of 1553 cases. Anesth Analg 61:921, 1982

249. Jakobsen H, Hertz JB, Johansen JR et al: Premedication before day surgery. Br J Anaesth 57:300, 1985

250. Horrigan RW, Moyers JR, Johnson BH et al: Etomidate vs. thiopental with and without fentanyl—a comparative study of awakening in man. Anesthesiology 52:362, 1980

251. Brustowicz RM, Nelson DA, Betts EK et al: Efficacy of oral premedication in pediatric outpatient surgery. Anesthesiology 60:475, 1984

252. Desjardins R, Ansara S, Charest J: Preanesthetic medication for paediatric day care surgery. Can Anaesth Soc J 28:141, 1981

253. Rao TLK, Suseela M, El-Etr AA: Metoclopramide and cimetidine to reduce gastric pH and volume. Anesth Analg 63:264, 1984

25

J. Jeff Andrews

Anesthesia Systems

INTRODUCTION

An anesthesia system consists of the various components that communicate with each other during the administration of inhalation anesthesia.[1] Delivery system components include the anesthesia machine, the vaporizers, the anesthetic circuit, and the ventilator. Removal of excess gas is accomplished by the scavenging system. A thorough understanding of these parts is essential to the safe practice of anesthesia. This chapter discusses the normal operation, function, and integration of major system components. More importantly, it illustrates some problems and hazards associated with each and describes appropriate preoperative checks.

ANESTHESIA MACHINES

Anesthesia machines have evolved from simple, pneumatic devices to sophisticated, computer-based, fully integrated anesthesia systems (Figs. 25-1 and 25-2). A few years ago, a rudimentary background in pneumatics sufficed for understanding these machines, but today an understanding of pneumatics, electronics, and even computer science is useful. Even though it is more difficult for the anesthesiologist to achieve a thorough understanding of modern anesthesia machines, it is essential to the safe practice of anesthesia. The anesthesiologist must be aware of design differences among various machines so that appropriate preoperative checks can be performed.

Anesthesia Machine Standards

The American National Standards Institute (ANSI) published the Z79.8-1979 machine standard in 1979.[2] This document was a landmark for the advancement of machine technology and patient safety because it provided guidelines for manufacturers regarding the minimum performance, design characteristics, and safety requirements for anesthesia machines. For almost a decade, the ANSI Z79.8-1979 standard was the guideline, but it has been superseded by the American Society for Testing and Materials (ASTM) F1161-88 standard.[3]

The two documents share many similarities, but a few major differences exist. The ANSI Z79.8-1979 standard addressed both flow meter controlled vaporizers and electrically heated vaporizers. The ASTM F1161-88 does not, since both these vaporizers are no longer manufactured in the United States. Several new requirements exist in the ASTM document that were not present in the ANSI 79.8-1979 standard. To meet the ASTM standard, newly manufactured anesthesia machines must have an oxygen analyzer, a breathing pressure monitor, and either an exhaled tidal volume monitor or a CO_2 monitor. These monitors must be in an enabled condition and functioning automatically when the machine is in use. The monitors must have a prioritized alarm system that groups alarms into three categories: high, medium, and low priority.[2,3]

Generic Anesthesia Machine

A generic two-gas anesthesia machine is shown in Figure 25-3. Both oxygen and nitrous oxide have two supply sources—a pipeline supply source and a cylinder supply source. The pipeline supply source is the primary gas source for the anesthesia machine. The hospital piping system provides gases to the machine at approximately 50 pounds per square inch gauge (psig), which is the normal working pressure of most machines. The cylinder supply source serves as a back-up if the pipeline fails. The oxygen cylinder source is regulated from 2200 to approximately 45 psig, and the nitrous oxide cylinder source is regulated from 745 to approximately 45 psig.[4-19]

A safety device traditionally referred to as the fail-safe system is located downstream from the nitrous oxide supply source. It serves as an interface between the oxygen and nitrous oxide supply sources. This device shuts off or proportionally decreases[4,5,15] the supply of nitrous oxide (and other gases) if the oxygen supply pressure decreases. Contemporary machines have an alarm device to monitor the oxygen supply pressure. An alarm is actuated at a predetermined oxygen pressure, such as 30 psig.[4,5,15]

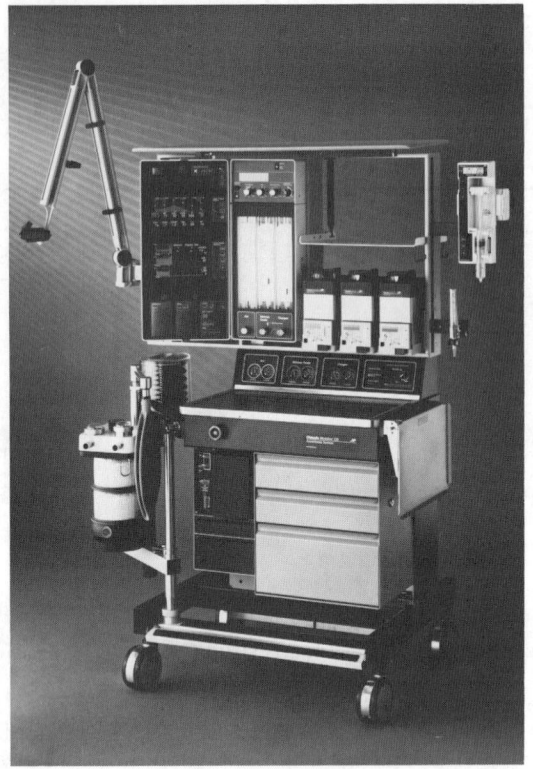

Figure 25-1. Ohmeda CD Anesthesia System. (Permission granted by Ohmeda, A Division of BOC Health Care, Inc, Madison, Wisconsin.)

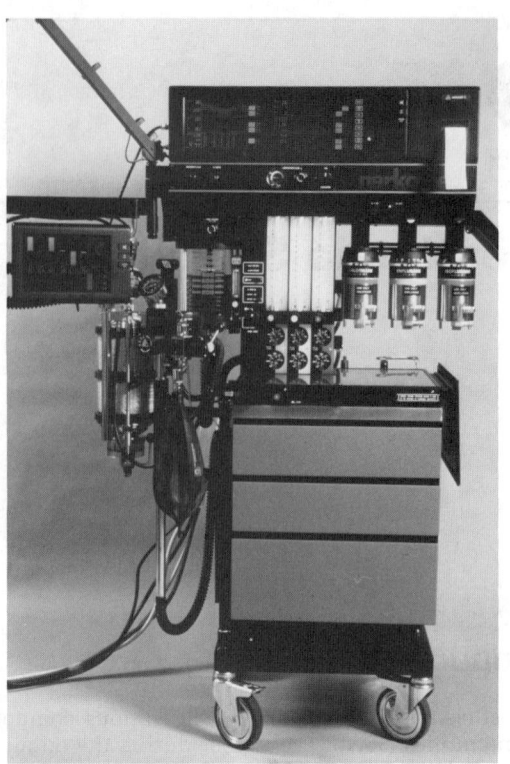

Figure 25-2. Narkomed 4 Anesthesia System. (Courtesy of North American Dräger, Telford, Pennsylvania.)

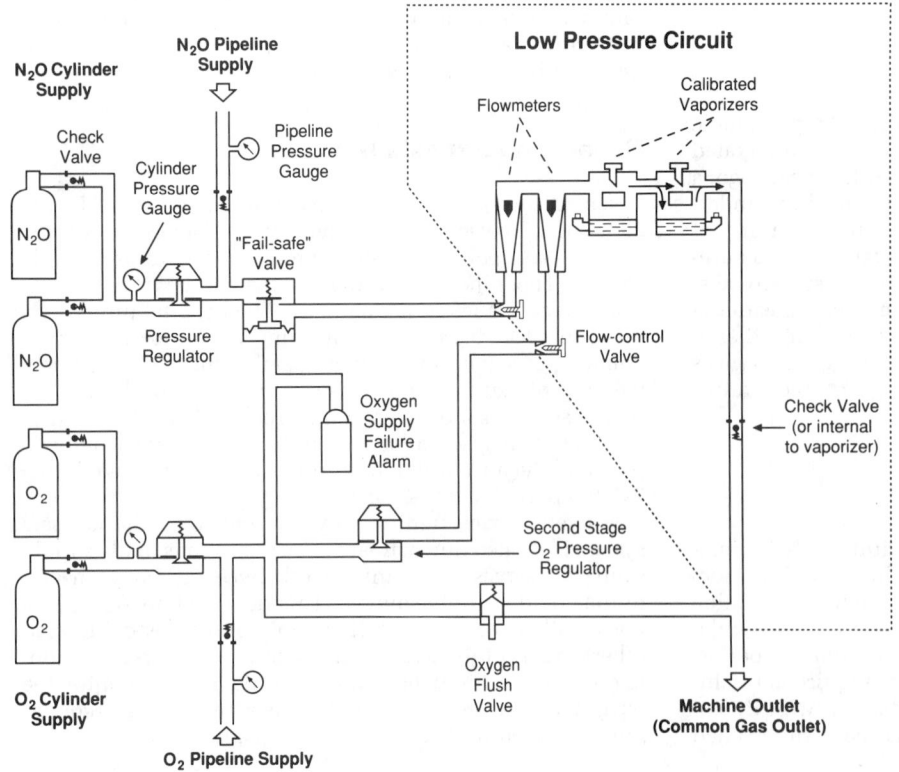

Figure 25-3. Diagram of a generic two-gas anesthesia machine. (Modified with permission from Check-Out, A Guide for Preoperative Inspection of an Anesthesia Machine. American Society of Anesthesiologists, Park Ridge, Illinois, 1987.)

Most Ohmeda machines have a second-stage oxygen regulator located downstream from the oxygen supply source. It is adjusted to a precise pressure level, such as 14 psig.[5,8-14] This regulator supplies a constant pressure to the oxygen flow control valve regardless of fluctuating oxygen pipeline pressures. For example, the flow from the oxygen flow control valve will be constant if the oxygen supply pressure is greater than 14 psig.

The flow control valves are an important anatomic landmark in the anesthesia machine because they separate the high-pressure circuit from the low-pressure circuit. The operator regulates flow entering the low-pressure circuit by adjusting the flow control valves. The flow travels through a common manifold, and it may be directed to a calibrated variable bypass vaporizer. Precise amounts of inhaled anesthetic can be added, depending on the vaporizer setting. The total fresh gas flow travels toward the common gas outlet.[4,5]

Many Ohmeda machines have a machine outlet check valve between the vaporizers and the common gas outlet.[5-12] Its purpose is to prevent back flow into the vaporizer, therefore minimizing the effects of downstream intermittent pressure fluctuations on agent concentration (see the section on Vaporizers, Intermittent Back Pressure). The presence or absence of a check valve *profoundly* influences the preoperative machine check (see the section on Checking Anesthesia Machines). The oxygen flush connection joins the mixed-gas pipeline between the one-way check valve and the common gas outlet. Thus the oxygen flush, when activated, has a "straight shot" to the common outlet.[4,5]

Pipeline Supply Source

The pipeline supply source is the primary gas source for the anesthesia machine. Most hospitals today have a central piping system to deliver medical gases such as oxygen, nitrous oxide, and air to the operating room. The central piping system must supply the anesthesia machine with the appropriate gas at the appropriate pressure for the machine to function properly. Unfortunately, this does not always occur.

In a survey of approximately 200 hospitals in 1976, 31% reported difficulties with the pipeline system.[20] The most common problem was inadequate oxygen pressure. This was followed by excessive pipeline pressures. The most devastating reported hazard, however, was accidental crossing of oxygen and nitrous oxide pipelines, which caused several deaths. This problem caused 23 deaths in a newly constructed wing of a general hospital in Sudbury, Ontario, during a 5-month period.[20,21]

The operator must take two actions if a pipeline crossover is suspected. First, the back-up oxygen cylinder should be turned on. Then, the pipeline supply must be disconnected. This second step is mandatory because the machine will preferentially use the 50 psig inappropriate pipeline supply source instead of the lower pressure (45 psig) oxygen cylinder source.[22]

Gas enters the anesthesia machine through the pipeline inlet connections (Fig. 25-3; see arrows). The pipeline inlet fittings are gas-specific Diameter Index Safety System (DISS) threaded body fittings. The DISS provides threaded noninterchangeable connections for medical gas lines, and this minimizes the risk of misconnection. A check valve is located downstream from the inlet. It prevents reverse flow of gases from the machine to the pipeline or to the atmosphere.[3]

A pipeline pressure gauge is mandated by the ASTM F1161-88 standard. It must be located on the pipeline side rather than on the machine side of the check valve (see Fig. 25-3).[3] Pressure measured in this location truly reflects pipeline pressure instead of pressure within the machine. For example, the gauge will read zero if the pipeline supply source is not connected to the anesthesia machine, irrespective of the on/off status of the cylinders. A value of 50 psig, however, does not guarantee that the pipeline is supplying the machine. The gauge will read 50 psig even when the check valve is stuck in the closed position. The operator should open the back-up cylinder if this problem is suspected.[22]

Some older anesthesia machines had a "pipeline" pressure gauge located on the machine side of the check valve. The gauge read approximately 50 psig when the machine was connected to the pipeline source. However, if the cylinders were turned on, the gauge read 45 psig even when the pipeline source was disconnected. If the operator did not recognize this subtle difference (45 versus 50 psig), cylinder depletion potentially resulted in a zero gas source status.[22]

Cylinder Supply Source

Anesthesia machines have reserve E cylinders if a pipeline supply source is not available or if the pipeline fails. Color-coded cylinders are attached to the anesthesia machine through the hanger yoke assembly. The hanger yoke assembly orients and supports the cylinder, provides a gas-tight seal, and ensures a unidirectional flow of gases into the machine.[4] Each hanger yoke is equipped with the Pin Index Safety System (PISS). The PISS is a safeguard introduced to eliminate cylinder interchanging and the possibility of accidentally placing the incorrect gas on a yoke designed to accommodate another gas. Two pins on the yoke are so arranged that they project into the cylinder valve. Each gas or combination of gases has a specific pin arrangement.[23]

Gas travels from the high-pressure cylinder source to the anesthesia machine when the cylinder is turned on (see Fig. 25-3). A check valve is located downstream from each cylinder if a double-yoke assembly is used. The check valve has several functions. First, it minimizes gas transfer from a cylinder at high pressure to one with low pressure. Second, it allows an empty cylinder to be exchanged for a full one while gas flow continues from the other cylinder into the machine with minimal loss of gas. Third, it minimizes leakage from an open cylinder to the atmosphere if one cylinder is absent.[4,5] A cylinder supply pressure gauge is located downstream from the check valves. The gauge will indicate the pressure in the cylinder having the higher pressure when two reserve cylinders of the same gas are opened at the same time.[17]

Each cylinder supply source has a pressure-reducing valve known as the cylinder pressure regulator. It reduces the high and variable storage pressure present in a cylinder to a lower, more constant pressure suitable for use in the anesthesia machine. The oxygen cylinder pressure regulator reduces the oxygen cylinder pressure from a high 2200 psig to approximately 45 psig. The nitrous oxide cylinder pressure regulator receives pressure of up to 745 psig and reduces it to approximately 45 psig.[4,5]

The cylinders should be turned off except during the preoperative machine checking period or when a pipeline source is unavailable. The reserve cylinder supply can be silently depleted if the cylinders are left on. This depletion occurs any time the pressure inside the machine decreases to a value lower than the regulated cylinder pressure. Oxygen pressure within the machine can decrease below 45 psig with oxygen flushing or with ventilator use, particularly at high peak flow rates. The pipeline supply pressures of all gases can be less than 45 psig if problems exist in the central piping system. If the cylinders are left on, they will eventually become depleted and no reserve supply will be available if there is a pipeline failure.[5,24]

Oxygen Supply Pressure Failure Safety Devices

Oxygen and nitrous oxide supply sources existed as independent entities in older models of anesthesia machines, and they were not pneumatically or mechanically interfaced. Therefore, abrupt or insidious oxygen pressure failure had the potential to lead to the delivery of a hypoxic mixture. The ASTM F1161-88 standard states that, "The anesthesia gas machine shall be designed so that whenever oxygen pressure is reduced from normal, and until flow ceases, the set oxygen concentration shall not decrease at the common outlet."[3] Contemporary anesthesia machines have a number of safety devices that act together in a cascade manner to minimize the risk of hypoxia as oxygen pressure decreases. Several of these devices are described below.

Pneumatic and Electronic Alarm Devices

Many older anesthesia machines have a pneumatic alarm device that sounds a warning when the oxygen supply pressure decreases to a predetermined threshold value such as 30 psig. The ASTM F1161-88 standard mandates that both an audible and a visual indication occur when the oxygen pressure falls below a manufacturer-specific pressure threshold.[3] Therefore, electronic alarm devices are now used to meet this guideline. The oxygen pressure threshold value for the Ohmeda Modulus II Plus and the Ohmeda CD is 27 psig.[13,14] It is 30 ± 3 for the North American Dräger Narkomed 2B, 3, and 4.[17-19]

Fail-Safe Systems

A fail-safe valve is present in the gas line supplying each of the flow meters except oxygen. This valve is controlled by oxygen pressure. It shuts off or proportionally decreases the supply of gases other than oxygen (nitrous oxide, air, carbon dioxide, helium, nitrogen) as the oxygen supply pressure decreases. Unfortunately, the term fail safe had led to the misconception that the device prevents administration of a hypoxic mixture. This is not the case. Machines that are not equipped with a proportioning system (see the section on Proportioning Systems) can deliver a hypoxic mixture under normal working conditions. The oxygen flow control valve can be closed intentionally or accidentally. Normal oxygen pressure will keep other gas lines open so that a hypoxic mixture can result.[4,5]

Ohmeda machines are equipped with a fail-safe valve known as the pressure-sensor shut-off valve. It is threshold in nature and is either open or closed. Figure 25-4 shows a nitrous oxide pressure-sensor shut-off valve with a threshold pressure of 20 psig.[9,10,12-14] An oxygen pressure greater than the threshold value is exerted on the mobile diaphragm in Figure 25-4A. This moves the piston, pin, and valve off the valve seat. Nitrous oxide flow passes freely to the nitrous oxide flow control valve. The oxygen supply pressure in

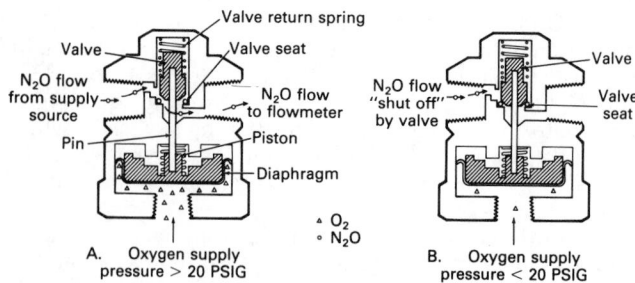

Figure 25-4. Pressure-sensor shut-off valve. The valve is open in *A* because the oxygen supply pressure is greater than the threshold value of 20 psig. The valve is closed in *B* because of inadequate oxygen pressure. (Redrawn with permission from Bowie E, Huffman LM: The Anesthesia Machine: Essentials for Understanding. Madison, Wisconsin, Ohmeda, A Division of BOC Health Care, Inc, 1985.)

Figure 25-4*B* is less than 20 psig, and the force of the valve return spring completely closes the valve.[5]

North American Dräger uses a fail-safe valve known as the Oxygen Failure Protection Device (OFPD) that interfaces the oxygen pressure with that of other gases, such as nitrous oxide, air, carbon dioxide, helium, and nitrogen.[15-19] It differs from Ohmeda's oxygen pressure-sensor shut-off valve because the OFPD is based on a proportioning principle rather than a threshold principle. The pressure of all gases controlled by the OFPD will decrease proportionally with the oxygen pressure. The OFPD consists of a seat-nozzle assembly that is connected to a spring-loaded piston (Fig. 25-5). The oxygen supply pressure in the left illustration is 50 psig. This pressure pushes the piston upward, forcing the nozzle away from the valve seat. Nitrous oxide or other gases advance toward the flow control valve at 50 psig. The oxygen pressure in the right illustration is zero psig. The spring is expanded and forces the nozzle against the seat, preventing flow through the device. Finally, the center illustration shows an intermediate oxygen pressure of 25 psig. The force of the spring partially closes the valve. The nitrous oxide pressure delivered to the flow control valve is 25 psig. There is a vast continuum of intermediate configurations between the extremes (0–50 psig) of oxygen supply pressure. These intermediate valve configurations are responsible for the proportional nature of the OFPD.[15]

Second-Stage Oxygen Pressure Regulator

Most contemporary Ohmeda machines have a second-stage oxygen pressure regulator set from 12–19 psig.[9-14] Oxygen flow meter output is constant when the oxygen supply pressure exceeds the set value. Ohmeda pressure-sensor shut-off valves are set at a higher threshold value (20–30 psig). This ensures that oxygen is the last gas flow to decrease if oxygen pressure fails.

Oxygen Ratio Monitor Controller

The Oxygen Ratio Monitor Controller (ORMC) is a complex safety device used on contemporary North American Dräger machines and is located downstream from the OFPD.[15-19] Both devices work together in a cascade manner when the oxygen supply pressure decreases. First, the OFPD proportionally decreases the pressure of the other gases, such as nitrous oxide.[15] Then, the spring-loaded ORMC shuts off the nitrous oxide slave control valve when the oxygen pressure

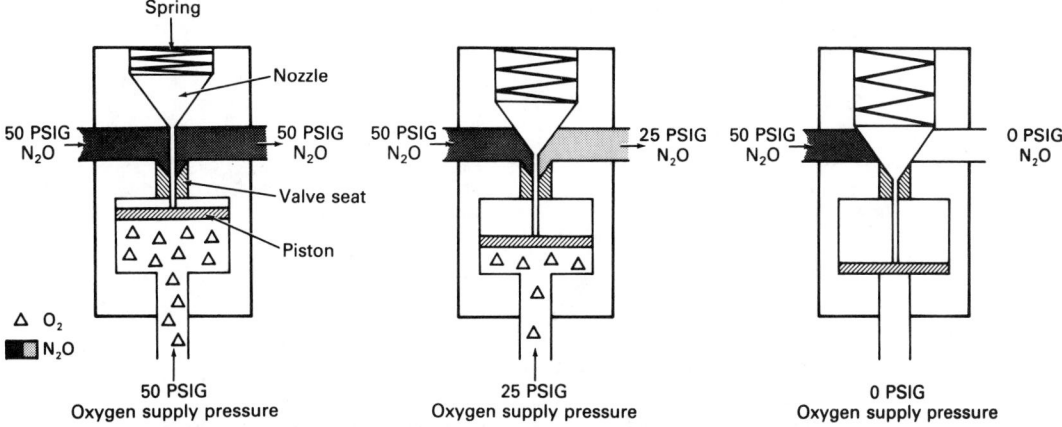

Figure 25-5. Oxygen Failure Protection Device—OFPD, which responds proportionally to changes in oxygen supply pressure. See text for details. (Redrawn with permission from Narkomed 2A Anesthesia System. Technical Service Manual, 6th ed. Telford, Pennsylvania, North American Dräger, June 1985.)

decreases below 10 psig. Thus, oxygen flow is the last to cease. This action represents only one function of the ORMC, which also serves as a proportioning device and an alarm system. The ORMC is discussed in detail in the section on Proportioning Systems.

Integration of Oxygen Pressure Failure Safety Devices

Different brands and models of anesthesia machines respond differently to an insidious decline in oxygen supply pressure.[25] Careful evaluation of a machine's response to a decline in oxygen supply pressure serves as a noninvasive "fingerprint" of the design of the internal anesthesia machine. Examples of such fingerprints are shown in Figure 25-6. They were generated in the following manner. All machine "E" cylinders were turned off, and a constant 50 psig nitrous oxide source was connected to the nitrous oxide pipeline inlet. With an initial oxygen pressure of 50 psig, the nitrous oxide and oxygen flow control valves were set to deliver 7 l·min^{-1} nitrous oxide and 3 l·min^{-1} oxygen. Total gas flow was calculated by adding the individual gas flows. An oxygen analyzer at the common outlet was used to determine the fresh gas oxygen concentration. The oxygen supply pressure was decreased in 5-psig decrements without changing the settings of the flow control valves. Gas flow and oxygen concentration were remeasured at each decrement, and the results were graphed.

Older Machines. Figure 25-6A represents the fingerprint of an older anesthesia machine that does not have a second-stage oxygen regulator. It does, however, have a threshold pressure-sensor shut-off valve set at 25 psig. A linear decline in oxygen flow occurs as the oxygen pressure decreases because of the absence of the second-stage regulator. Since the nitrous oxide supply pressure is adequate, the nitrous oxide flow remains constant at 7 l·min^{-1} until the 25 psig oxygen pressure threshold is reached. A vulnerable oxygen pressure zone exists from 50 to 26 psig because the fresh gas oxygen concentration decreases and total flow decreases. The oxygen concentration increases to 100% below 25 psig oxygen pressure because the nitrous oxide is shut off by the oxygen pressure-sensor shut-off valve.

Ohmeda Modulus II. Figure 25-6B is the fingerprint of an Ohmeda Modulus II. It has a pneumatic low oxygen supply

pressure alarm set at 30 psig, a pressure-sensor shut-off valve set at 20 psig, and a second-stage oxygen regulator set at 14 psig.[9,10] The oxygen flow remains constant as long as the oxygen pressure is greater than 14 psig. This is unlike older machines without the second-stage oxygen regulator. As the oxygen supply pressure decreases from 50 to 21 psig, the flow of oxygen and nitrous oxide remains constant at 3 l·min^{-1} and 7 l·min^{-1}, respectively. A pneumatic low oxygen pressure alarm sounds at 30 psig to alert the operator of a problem. It is important to note that when the alarm sounds, the oxygen concentration and the flows are identical to those noted at 50 psig. The nitrous oxide is shut off when the oxygen supply pressure decreases to 20 psig, which is the threshold pressure for the oxygen pressure-sensor shut-off valve. The oxygen concentration at that point increases to 100%. Oxygen flow remains constant at 3 l·min^{-1} from 20 to 15 psig because the second-stage oxygen regulator is set at 14 psig. Finally, there is a linear decrease in oxygen flow with decreasing oxygen supply pressure below 14 psig.

The Ohmeda Modulus II response to loss of oxygen supply pressure has several advantages over older machines. The oxygen concentration remains constant or increases, and the operator is alerted to a problem before flows decrease. Oxygen flow remains constant until the oxygen supply pressure is almost depleted because the value of the second-stage oxygen regulator is set at a low pressure.

North American Dräger Narkomed 2A ORMC. The North American Dräger Narkomed 2A ORMC response to decreasing oxygen supply pressure is unique and is shown in Figure 25-6C. Several safety devices are recruited as the oxygen supply pressure decreases. These include the OFPD, the electronic low oxygen pressure alarm set at 30 psig, and the ORMC. First, the OFPD proportionally decreases nitrous oxide pressure in response to reduced oxygen pressure.[15] Flow reductions are proportional, and the oxygen concentration of the fresh gas mixture remains constant at 30% from 50 psig to approximately 10 psig. The spring-loaded ORMC shuts off nitrous oxide flow entirely when the oxygen pressure is below 10 psig. The fresh gas oxygen concentration then increases to 100%.

An attractive feature of the Narkomed 2A response to decreasing oxygen pressure is that the oxygen concentration is maintained or increased. A vulnerable oxygen supply

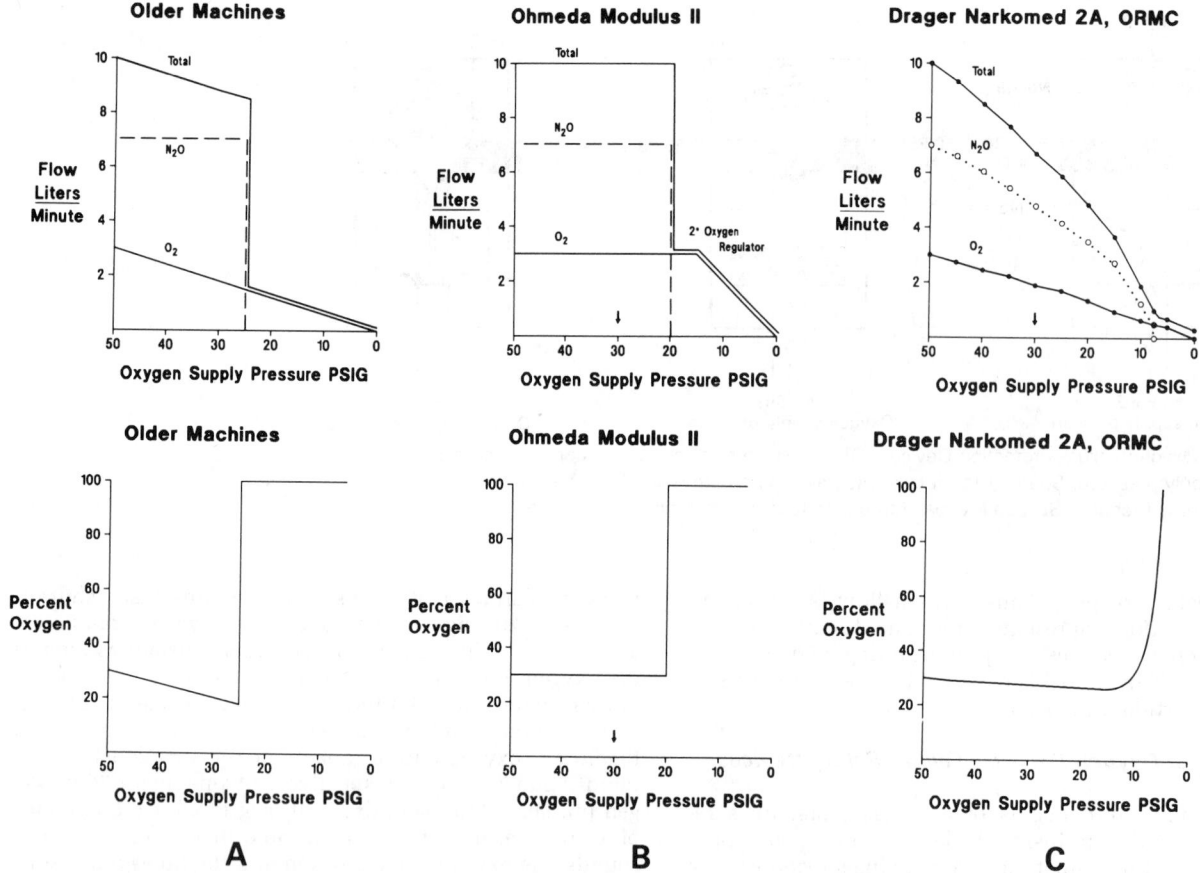

Figure 25-6. Response of three anesthesia machines to a gradual decline in oxygen supply pressure. The response of an older machine, an Ohmeda Modulus II, and a Dräger Narkomed 2A are shown in *A*, *B*, and *C*, respectively. *Vertical arrows* represent the oxygen supply pressure at which the low oxygen pressure alarm sounds. See text for details.

pressure zone theoretically exists from 50 to 31 psig because flows can decrease as much as 30% before the operator is alerted to an oxygen pressure problem. Clinically, however, this is probably insignificant because oxygen supply failure is usually complete and abrupt instead of gradual.

Flow Meter Assembly

The flow meter assembly (Fig. 25-7) precisely controls and measures gas flow to the common gas outlet. The flow control valve regulates the amount of flow that enters a tapered, transparent flow tube known as a Thorpe tube. A mobile indicator float inside the flow tube indicates the amount of flow passing through the flow control valve. The quantity of flow is indicated on a scale associated with the flow tube.[4,5]

Physical Principles of Flow Meters

Opening the flow control valve allows gas to travel through the space between the float and the flow tube. This space is known as the annular space (Fig. 25-8). The indicator float hovers freely in an equilibrium position where the upward force resulting from gas flow equals the downward force on the float resulting from gravity. The float moves to a new equilibrium position in the tube when flow is changed. These flow meters are commonly referred to as *constant*

pressure flow meters because the pressure decrease across the float remains constant for all positions in the tube.[4,23,26]

Flow tubes are tapered with the smallest diameter at the bottom of the tube and the largest diameter at the top. The term *variable orifice* designates this type of unit because the annular space between the float and the inner wall of the flow tube varies with the position of the float. The constriction created by the float can be tubular or orificial, depending upon the flow rate (Fig. 25-9). The characteristics of a gas that influence its flow rate through a given constriction are (1) its density and (2) its viscosity. Flow through the annular space is tubular at low flow rates. Poiseuille's law applies in this situation, and *viscosity* becomes dominant in determining gas flow rate. The annular space simulates an orifice at high flow rates, and gas flow rate then depends predominantly upon the *density* of the gas.[4,26]

Components of Flow Meter Assembly

Flow Control Valve Assembly. The flow control valve assembly is composed of a flow control knob, a needle valve, a valve seat, and a pair of valve stops.[4] The assembly can receive its pneumatic input either directly from the pipeline source (50 psig) or from a second-stage pressure regulator.[5] The flow control valves of contemporary North American Dräger machines are supplied by 50 psig.[15-19] In contrast, the flow control valves of contemporary Ohmeda products

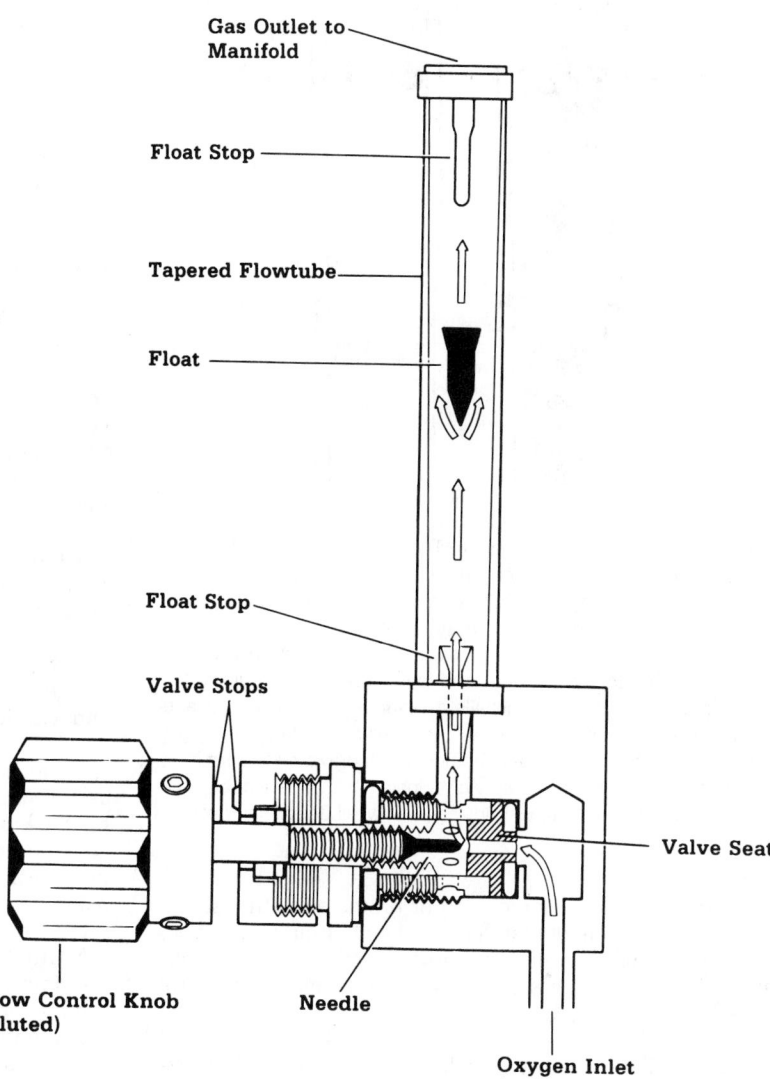

Gas Outlet to Manifold

Float Stop

Tapered Flowtube

Float

Float Stop

Valve Stops

Valve Seat

Flow Control Knob (Fluted)

Needle

Oxygen Inlet (16 PSIG)

Figure 25-7. Oxygen flow meter assembly. The oxygen flow meter assembly is composed of the flow control valve assembly plus the flow meter subassembly. (Reproduced with permission from Bowie E, Huffman LM: The Anesthesia Machine: Essentials for Understanding. Madison, Wisconsin, Ohmeda, A Division of BOC Health Care, Inc, 1985.)

are supplied by precision second-stage pressure regulators. On the Ohmeda Modulus II, the Modulus II Plus, and the CD, the oxygen flow control valve is supplied by 14 psig, and the nitrous oxide flow control valve is supplied by 26 psig.[9,10,13,14]

The location of the needle valve in the valve seat changes to establish different orifices when the flow control valve is

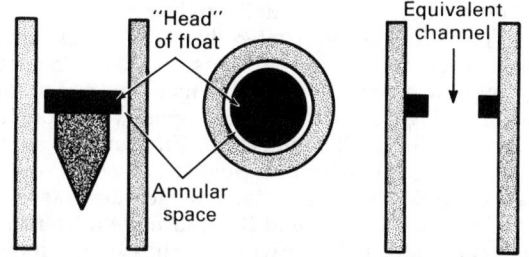

"Head" of float

Annular space

Equivalent channel

Figure 25-8. The annular space. The clearance between the head of the float and the flow tube is known as the annular space. It can be considered an equivalent to a circular channel of the same cross-sectioned area. (Redrawn with permission from Macintosh R, Mushin WW, Epstein HG: Physics for the Anaesthetist, 3rd ed. Oxford, England, Blackwell Scientific Publications, 1963.)

adjusted. Gas flow increases when the flow control valve is turned counterclockwise, and it decreases when the valve is turned clockwise. Extreme clockwise rotation results in damage to the needle valve and valve seat. Therefore, flow control valves are equipped with valve "stops" to prevent this occurrence.[5] The stops come into contact with each other at zero flow on most flow control valves. However, the oxygen flow control valve stops of the Ohmeda Modulus I, Modulus II, and the Modulus II Plus are set at an oxygen flow rate of approximately 200 ml·min^{-1}.[8-10,13] Thus, on contemporary Ohmeda machines, minimum oxygen flow results from incomplete closure of the oxygen flow control valve. On contemporary North American Dräger machines, the oxygen flow control valve does close completely. Minimum oxygen flow enters the oxygen flow tube just downstream from the flow control valve.[15-19]

Safety Features. Contemporary flow control valve assemblies have numerous safety features. The oxygen flow control knob is physically distinguishable from other gas knobs. It is distinctively fluted, projects beyond the control knobs of the other gases, and is larger in diameter. All knobs are color-coded for the appropriate gas, and the chemical formula or name of the gas is permanently marked on each.

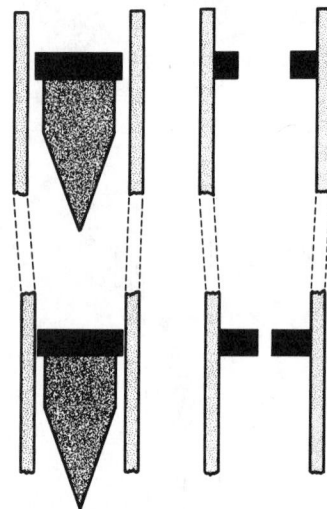

Figure 25-9. Flow tube constriction. The lower pair of illustrations represents the lower portion of a flow tube. The clearance between the head of the float and the flow tube is narrow. The equivalent channel is tubular because its diameter is less than its length. Viscosity is dominant in determining gas flow rate through this tubular constriction. The upper pair of illustrations represents the upper portion of a flow tube. The equivalent channel is orificial because its length is less than its width. Density is dominant in determining gas flow rate through this orificial constriction. (Redrawn with permission from Macintosh R, Mushin WW, Epstein HG: Physics for the Anaesthetist, 3rd ed. Oxford, England, Blackwell Scientific Publications, 1963.)

Flow control knobs are recessed or protected with a shield or barrier to minimize inadvertent change from a preset position. If a single gas has two flow tubes, the tubes are arranged in series and are controlled by a single flow control valve.[3]

Flow Meter Subassembly. The flow meter subassembly consists of the flow tube, the indicator float with float stops, and the indicator scale.[4]

Flow Tubes. Contemporary flow tubes are made of glass. Most have a single taper in which the inner diameter of the flow tube increases uniformly from bottom to top. Manufacturers provide double flow tubes for oxygen and nitrous oxide to provide better visual discrimination at low flow rates. A fine flow tube indicates flow from approximately 200 ml·min to 1 l·min^{-1}, and a coarse flow tube indicates flow from approximately 1 l·min^{-1} to 10–12 l·min^{-1}. The two tubes are connected in series and supplied by a single flow control valve. The total gas flow is that shown on the higher flow meter. Some older machines manufactured before the Z79.8 standard have two flow tubes for a single gas arranged in parallel. Each of the tubes has a flow control valve. The total flow is the sum of the individual flows.[4]

Indicator Floats and Float Stops. Several different types of bobbins or floats are used to indicate flow on contemporary anesthesia machines. Ohmeda employs a plumb-bob type float on the Modulus I, Modulus II, Modulus II Plus, and CD.[8-10,13,14] A rotating skirted float is used on the Ohmeda Excel Series.[12] North American Dräger machines are equipped with sapphire ball floats.[15-19] Flow is read at the top of the plumb-bob and skirted floats, but it is read at the center of the ball on the ball-type floats.[4]

Flow tubes are equipped with float stops at the top and bottom of the tube. The upper stop prevents the float from ascending to the top of the tube and plugging the outlet. It also ensures that the float will be visible at maximum flows instead of being hidden in the manifold. The bottom float stop provides a central foundation for the indicator when the flow control valve is turned off.[4,5]

Scale. The flow meter scale can be marked directly on the flow tube or located to the right of the tube.[3] Gradations corresponding to equal increments in flow rate are closer together at the top of the scale because the annular space increases more rapidly than does the internal diameter from the bottom to the top of the tube. Rib guides are used in some flow tubes with ball-type indicators to minimize this compression effect. They are tapered glass ridges that run the length of the tube. There are usually three rib guides that are equally spaced around the inner circumference of the tube. In the presence of rib guides, the annular space from the bottom to the top of the tube increases almost proportionally with the internal diameter. This results in a nearly linear scale.[4] Rib guides are employed on North American Dräger flow tubes.[15-17,19]

Safety Features. The flow meter subassembly for each gas on the Ohmeda Modulus I, Modulus II, and Modulus II Plus, and CD is housed in an independent, color-coded, pin-specific module. The flow tubes are adjacent to a gas-specific, color-coded backing. The flow scale and the chemical formula or name of the gas are permanently etched on the backing to the right of the flow tube. Flow meter scales are individually hand-calibrated using the specific float to provide a high degree of accuracy. The tube, float, and scale make an inseparable unit. The entire set must be replaced if any component is damaged.[8-10,13,14]

North American Dräger does not use a modular system for the flow meter subassembly. The flow scale, the chemical symbol, and the gas-specific color-coding are etched directly onto the flow tube.[15-19] The scale in use is obvious when two flow tubes for the same gas are used.

Problems with Flow Meters

Leaks. Flow meter leaks are a substantial hazard because the flow meters are located downstream from all machine safety devices except the oxygen analyzer.[1] Leaks can occur at the junction between the glass flow tube and the metal manifold because of problems associated with O-rings and gaskets. Glass flow tubes are the most fragile pneumatic component of the anesthesia machine. Gross damage is usually apparent, but subtle cracks and chips may be overlooked, resulting in errors of delivered flows.[27]

Eger et al in 1963 demonstrated that, in the presence of a flow meter leak, a hypoxic mixture is less likely to occur if the oxygen flow meter is located downstream from all other flow meters.[28] Figure 25-10 is a contemporary version of the figure in Eger's original publication. The unused air flow tube has a large leak. Nitrous oxide and oxygen flow rates are set at a ratio of 3:1. A potentially dangerous arrangement is shown in Figure 25-10A and B because the nitrous oxide flow meter is located in the downstream position. A hypoxic mixture can result because a substantial portion of oxygen flow passes through the leak, and all nitrous oxide is directed to the common gas outlet. A safer configuration that complies with the ASTM F1161-88 machine standard is shown in Figure 25-10C and D. The oxygen flow meter is located in the downstream position. A portion of the nitrous

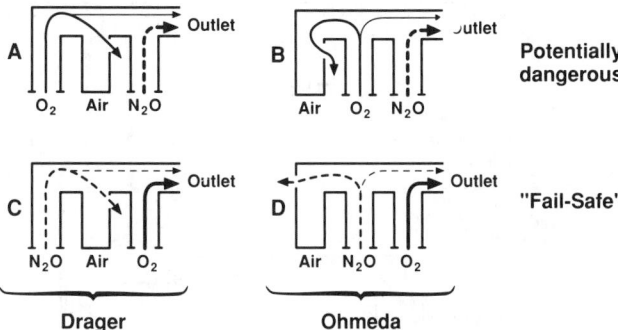

Figure 25-10. Flow meter sequence—a cause of hypoxia. In the event of a flow meter leak, a potentially dangerous arrangement exists when nitrous oxide is located in the downstream position (*A* and *B*). The safest configuration exists when oxygen is located in the downstream position (*C* and *D*). See text for details. (Modified with permission from Eger EI II, Hylton RR, Irwin RH *et al*: Anesthetic flow meter sequence—a cause for hypoxia. Anesthesiology 24:396, 1963.)

oxide flow escapes through the leak, and the remainder goes toward the common gas outlet. A hypoxic mixture is less likely to occur because all the oxygen flow is advanced by the nitrous oxide.[28] North American Dräger flow meters are arranged as in Figure 25-10C, and Ohmeda flow meters as in Figure 25-10D.

A leak in the oxygen flow tube can produce a hypoxic mixture even when oxygen is located in the downstream position (Fig. 25-11).[1,27] Oxygen escapes through the leak, and nitrous oxide flows toward the common outlet. This is particularly true at high nitrous oxide to oxygen flow ratios.

Inaccuracy. Flow error can occur even when flow meters are assembled properly with appropriate components. Dirt or static electricity can cause a float to stick, and the actual flow may be higher or lower than that indicated. Sticking is more common in the low flow range because the annular space is smaller. A damaged float can cause inaccurate readings because the precise relationship between the float and the flow tube is altered. Back pressure from the breathing circuit can cause a float to drop so that it reads less than the actual flow. Finally, if flow meters are not aligned properly in the vertical position, readings can be inaccurate because tilting distorts the annular space.[4,27,29]

Ambiguous Scale. Before the standardization of flow meter scales and the widespread use of oxygen analyzers, at least two deaths resulted from confusion created by ambiguous

scales.[27,29,30] The operator read the float position beside an adjacent but erroneous scale in both cases. Today this is less likely to occur because contemporary flow meter scales are marked either directly onto or to the right of the appropriate flow tube.[3] Confusion is minimized when the scale is etched directly onto the tube.

Proportioning Systems

Manufacturers have equipped their newer machines with proportioning systems in an attempt to prevent delivery of a hypoxic mixture. Nitrous oxide and oxygen are interfaced either mechanically or pneumatically so that the minimum oxygen concentration at the common outlet is 25%.

Ohmeda Link-25 Proportion Limiting Control System

Contemporary Ohmeda machines use the Link-25 System. The heart of the system is the mechanical integration of the nitrous oxide and oxygen flow control valves. It allows independent adjustment of either valve, yet automatically intercedes to maintain a minimum 25% oxygen concentration with a maximum nitrous oxide–oxygen flow ratio of 3:1. An increased nitrous oxide flow beyond this maximum ratio results in a proportional 3:1 increase in oxygen flow.[8-14]

Figure 25-12 shows the Ohmeda Modulus II Link-25 System. The nitrous oxide and oxygen flow control valves are identical. A 14-tooth sprocket is attached to the nitrous oxide flow control valve, and a 28-tooth sprocket is attached to the oxygen flow control valve. A chain physically links the sprockets. When the nitrous oxide flow control valve is turned two revolutions, or 28 teeth, the oxygen flow control valve will revolve once because of the 2:1 gear ratio. The final 3:1 flow ratio results because the nitrous oxide flow control valve is supplied by approximately 26 psig, whereas the oxygen flow control valve is supplied by 14 psig. Thus, the combination of the mechanical and pneumatic aspects of the system yields the final oxygen concentration.[9,10]

North American Dräger Oxygen Ratio Monitor Controller

North American Dräger's proportioning system, the Oxygen Ratio Monitor Controller (ORMC), is used on the North American Dräger Narkomed 2A, 2B, 3, and 4. It is a pneumatic oxygen–nitrous oxide interlock system designed to maintain a fresh gas oxygen concentration of at least 25 ± 3%. The device controls the fresh gas oxygen concentration to levels substantially higher than 25% at oxygen flow rates

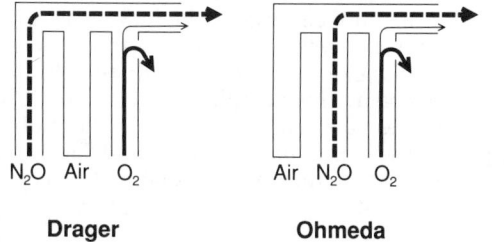

Figure 25-11. Oxygen flow tube leak. An oxygen flow tube leak can produce a hypoxic mixture regardless of flow tube arrangement. (Reprinted with permission from Andrews JJ: Inhaled anesthetic delivery. In Miller RD (ed): Anesthesia, 3rd ed, p 171. New York, Churchill Livingstone, 1990.)

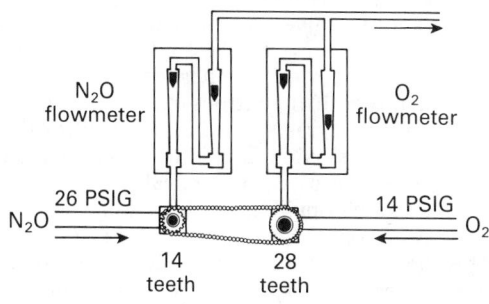

Figure 25-12. Ohmeda Link-25 Proportion Limiting Control System. See text for details.

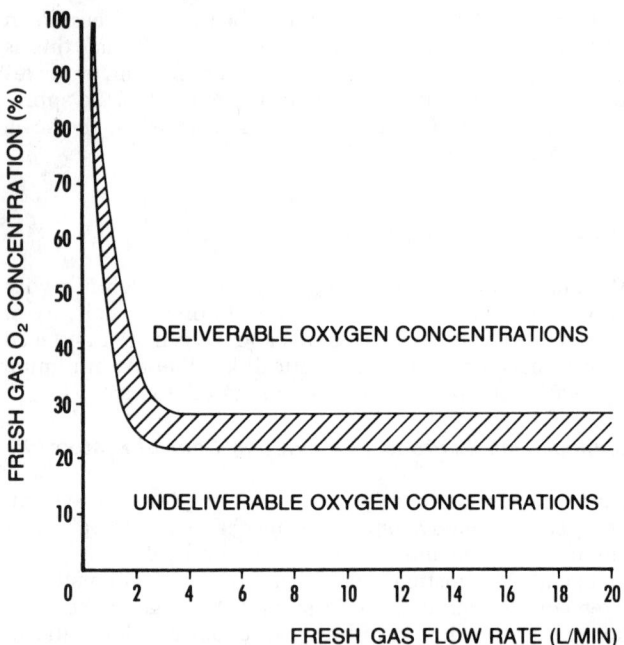

Figure 25-13. Oxygen concentration control curve for the North American Dräger Narkomed 2B, 3, and 4. The Oxygen Ratio Monitor Controller (ORMC) maintains a minimal fresh gas oxygen concentration of at least 25 ± 3% at flow rates greater than 1 l·min⁻¹. At flow rates less than 1 l·min⁻¹, the device controls the fresh gas oxygen concentration to levels substantially higher than 25%. (Redrawn with permission from Narkomed 3 Anesthesia System. Operator's Instruction Manual. Telford, Pennsylvania, North American Dräger, 1986.)

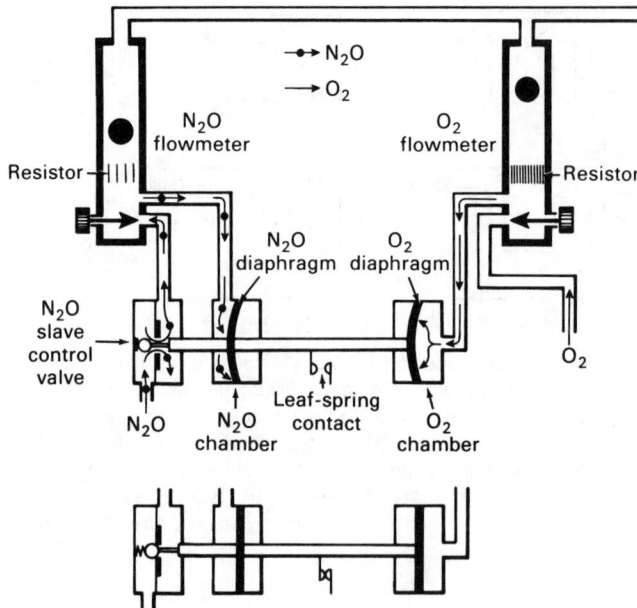

Figure 25-14. North American Dräger Oxygen Ratio Monitor Controller. See text for details. (Redrawn with permission from Schreiber P: Safety Guidelines for Anesthesia Systems. Telford, Pennsylvania, North American Dräger, 1984.)

less than 1 l·min⁻¹ (Fig. 25-13). The ORMC limits nitrous oxide flow to prevent delivery of a hypoxic mixture.[15-19] This is unlike the Ohmeda Link-25, which actively increases oxygen flow.

A schematic of the ORMC is shown in Figure 25-14. It is composed of an oxygen chamber, a nitrous oxide chamber, and a nitrous oxide slave control valve; all are interconnected by a mobile horizontal shaft. The pneumatic input into the device is from the oxygen and the nitrous oxide flow meters. These flow meters are unique because they have specific resistors located downstream from the flow control valves. These resistors create back pressures that are directed to the oxygen and nitrous oxide chambers. The relative value of these resistors ultimately dictates the value of the controlled fresh gas oxygen concentration. The back pressure in the oxygen and nitrous oxide chamber pushes against rubber diaphragms that are attached to the mobile horizontal shaft. Movement of the shaft regulates the nitrous oxide slave control valve that feeds the nitrous oxide flow control valve.[1,16]

If the oxygen pressure is proportionally higher than the nitrous oxide pressure, the nitrous oxide slave control valve opens to a larger degree, allowing more nitrous oxide to flow. As the nitrous oxide flow is increased manually, the nitrous oxide pressure forces the shaft toward the oxygen chamber. The valve opening becomes more restrictive and limits the nitrous oxide flow to the flow meter. Figure 25-14 illustrates the action of a single ORMC under different sets of circumstances. The back pressure exerted on the oxygen diaphragm, in the upper configuration, is greater than that exerted on the nitrous oxide diaphragm. This causes the

horizontal shaft to move to the left, opening the nitrous oxide slave control valve. Nitrous oxide is then able to proceed to its flow control valve and out through the flow meter. In the bottom configuration, the nitrous oxide slave control valve is closed because of inadequate oxygen back pressure.[1,16]

The ORMC has a dual role. It serves as a proportioning device and a monitor. An electrical contact attached to the mobile horizontal shaft activates an alarm when the ORMC is limiting the nitrous oxide flow to prevent a hypoxic fresh gas mixture. The alarm is functional only in the "O₂/N₂O" mode and not in the "All Gases" mode. However, the ORMC continues to control the oxygen–nitrous oxide ratio regardless of the alarm status.[15-19]

Limitations

Proportioning systems are not foolproof. Machines equipped with proportioning systems still can deliver a hypoxic mixture under the following conditions.

Wrong Supply Gas. Both the Link-25 and the ORMC will be fooled if a gas other than oxygen is present in the oxygen pipeline. In the Link-25 System, the nitrous oxide and oxygen flow control valves will continue to be mechanically linked, and a hypoxic mixture will proceed to the common outlet. The oxygen rubber diaphragm of the ORMC will recognize adequate "oxygen" pressure, and flow of both the wrong gas plus nitrous oxide will result. The oxygen analyzer is the only machine monitor that will detect this condition in both systems.

Defective Pneumatics or Mechanics. Normal operation of the Ohmeda Link-25 and the North American Dräger ORMC is contingent upon pneumatic and mechanical integrity. Pneumatic integrity in the Ohmeda System depends upon properly functioning second-stage regulators. A nitrous oxide–oxygen ratio other than 3:1 will result if the regulators are not precise. The chain connecting the two sprockets must be intact. A 97% nitrous oxide concentration can result if the chain is cut or broken.[31] In the North American Dräger System, a functional Oxygen Failure Protection Device (OFPD) is necessary to supply appropriate pressure to the ORMC. The mechanical aspects of the ORMC, such as the rubber diaphragms, the flow tube resistors, and the nitrous oxide slave control valve, must likewise be intact.

Leaks Downstream. The ORMC and the Link-25 function at the level of the flow control valves. A leak downstream from these devices, such as a broken oxygen flow tube (see Fig. 25-11), can result in the delivery of a hypoxic mixture. Oxygen escapes through the leak, and the predominant gas delivered at the common outlet is nitrous oxide. The oxygen analyzer is the only machine safety device that can detect the problem.[1] North American Dräger recommends a preoperative positive pressure leak test to detect such a leak.[15-19] Ohmeda recommends a preoperative negative pressure leak test because of the check valve located at the common outlet[6-10,12] (see the section on Checking Anesthesia Machines).

Inert Gas Administration. Administration of a third inert gas, such as helium, nitrogen, or carbon dioxide, can result in a hypoxic mixture because contemporary proportioning systems link only nitrous oxide and oxygen.[8-19] Use of an oxygen analyzer is especially mandatory if the operator uses a third inert gas.

Oxygen Flush Valve

The oxygen flush valve allows direct communication between the oxygen high-pressure circuit and the low-pressure circuit (see Fig. 25-3). Flow from the oxygen flush valve enters the low-pressure circuit downstream from the vaporizers and downstream from the Ohmeda machine outlet check valve. The spring-loaded oxygen flush valve stays closed until the operator opens it by depressing the oxygen flush button. Actuation of the valve delivers $35–75$ l·min^{-1} to the breathing circuit.[5]

The oxygen flush valve is associated with several hazards. A defective or damaged valve can stick in the fully open position, and this can cause barotrauma.[32] A valve sticking in a partially open position can cause patient awareness because the oxygen flow from the incompetent valve dilutes the inhaled anesthetic.[33] Normally functioning oxygen flush valves can cause problems. Overzealous intraoperative oxygen flushing can cause patient awareness. Oxygen flushing during the inspiratory phase of positive pressure ventilation can cause barotrauma. Excess volume cannot be vented from the breathing circuit because the ventilator relief valve is closed and the Adjustable Pressure Limiting (pop-off) Valve is either out of circuit or closed.[34] If a machine is equipped with a freestanding vaporizer downstream from the common gas outlet, oxygen flushing can deliver large quantities of inhaled anesthetic to the patient. Finally, inappropriate preoperative use of the oxygen flush to evaluate the low-pressure circuit for leaks can be misleading. This is particularly true on machines with a check valve at the common outlet.[35] Back pressure from the breathing circuit closes the check valve air-tight, and major low-pressure circuit leaks can go undetected (see the section on Checking Anesthesia Machines).

VAPORIZERS

Through the years, vaporizers have evolved from rudimentary ether inhalers to the present sophisticated variable bypass, temperature-compensated vaporizers. Bubble-through copper kettle vaporizers are no longer manufactured in the United States, and they are not addressed by the ASTM F1161-88 standard.[3] Therefore, this section is limited to newer variable bypass vaporizers. Certain physical principles are reviewed briefly before the discussion so that the design, construction, and operation of these vaporizers can be understood (see also Chapter 7).

Physics

Vapor Pressure

Inhaled volatile anesthetics exist in the liquid state at room temperature. When a volatile liquid is in a closed container, molecules escape from the liquid phase to the vapor phase until the number of molecules in the vapor phase is constant. These molecules bombard the wall of the container and create a pressure known as the saturated *vapor pressure*. More molecules enter the vapor phase, and the vapor pressure increases as the temperature increases (Fig. 25-15). Vapor pressure is independent of atmospheric pressure and is contingent only on the physical characteristics of the liquid and the temperature. The *boiling point* of a liquid is that temperature at which the vapor pressure equals atmospheric pressure.[36-38]

Latent Heat of Vaporization

Energy must be expended to convert a molecule from the liquid to the gaseous state because the molecules of a liquid tend to cohere. The *latent heat of vaporization* is defined as the number of calories required to change 1 g of liquid into vapor without a temperature change. The energy for vaporization must come from the liquid itself or from an outside source. The temperature of the liquid decreases during vaporization in the absence of an outside energy source.

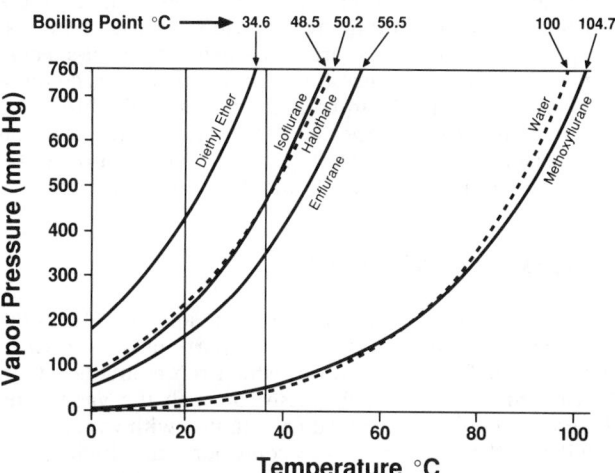

Figure 25-15. Vapor pressure versus temperature curves. (Modified with permission from Rodgers RC, Hill GE: Equations for vapour pressure versus temperature: Derivation and use of the Antoine equation on a hand-held programmable calculator. Br J Anaesth 50:420, 1978.)

Energy loss can lead to significant decreases in temperature of the remaining liquid. This temperature drop will greatly decrease vaporization.[36,38,39]

Specific Heat

The *specific heat* of a substance is the number of calories required to increase the temperature of 1 g of a substance by 1°C.[36,38,40] The substance can be solid, liquid, or gas. The concept of specific heat is important to the design, operation, and construction of vaporizers because it is applicable in two ways. First, the specific heat value for an inhaled anesthetic is important because it indicates how much heat must be supplied to the liquid to maintain a constant temperature when heat is lost during vaporization. Second, manufacturers select vaporizer metals that have a high specific heat to minimize temperature changes associated with vaporization.

Thermal Conductivity

Thermal conductivity is a measure of the speed with which heat flows through a substance. The higher the thermal conductivity, the better the substance conducts heat.[36] Vaporizers are constructed of metals that have relatively high thermal conductivity, which helps maintain a uniform temperature.

Vaporizer Classification

The Ohmeda Tec 4 and the North American Dräger Vapor 19.1 are classified as variable bypass, flow-over, temperature-compensated, agent-specific, out of circuit vaporizers. *Variable bypass* refers to the method for regulating output concentration. After the total gas flow enters the vaporizer's inlet, the concentration control dial adjusts the amount of gas that goes to the bypass chamber and to the vaporizing chamber. The gas channeled to the vaporizing chamber flows over the liquid agent and becomes saturated. Thus, *flow-over* refers to the method of vaporization. The Tec 4 and the Vapor 19.1 are classified as *temperature-compensated* because they are equipped with an automatic temperature-compensating device that helps maintain a constant vaporizer output over a wide range of temperatures. These vaporizers are classified as *agent-specific* and *out of circuit* because they are designed to accommodate a single agent and to be located outside the breathing circuit. Conversely, copper kettle vaporizers are classified as measured flow, bubble-through, non–temperature-compensated, multiple-agent, out of circuit vaporizers.[36]

Basic Design Principles

The total gas flow in a variable bypass vaporizer enters the vaporizer's inlet and splits into two portions, as shown in Figure 25-16. The first portion, which represents less than 20% of the total gas flow, passes through the vaporizing chamber, where it is enriched or saturated with vapor of the liquid anesthetic agent. The second portion, which represents more than 80% of the total gas flow, goes directly through the bypass chamber. Finally, both partial gas flows rejoin at the vaporizer outlet. The ratio of the two partial gas flows depends on the ratio of resistances in the two paths, that is, the resistance in the bypass chamber compared to the resistance in the vaporizing chamber. The con-

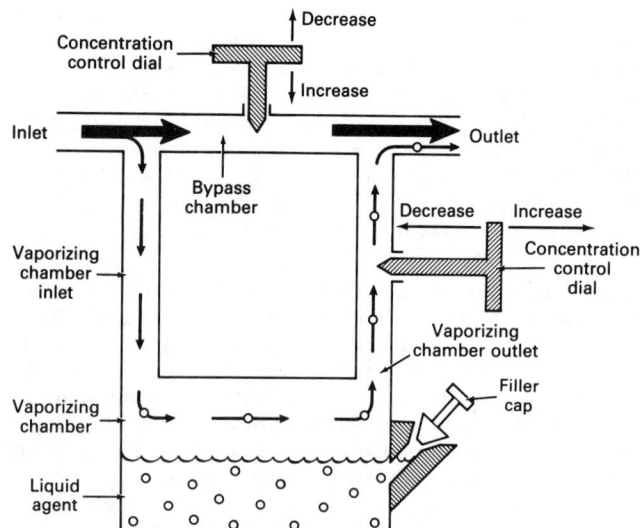

Figure 25-16. Generic variable bypass vaporizer. See text for details.

centration control dial can be located in the bypass chamber or in the vaporizing chamber outlet. A change in the dial setting causes a change in resistance, which alters the gas flow ratio.[41]

Factors That Influence Vaporizer Output

The output of an ideal vaporizer would be constant at varying conditions such as flow rates, temperatures, back pressures, and carrier gases. Designing such a vaporizer is difficult because, as ambient conditions change, the physical properties of gases and of vaporizers themselves can change.[41] Contemporary vaporizers approach being ideal but still have some limitations. Several factors are listed below that can influence vaporizer output.

Flow Rate

Variable bypass vaporizer output varies with the rate of gas flowing through them. This is particularly notable at extremes of flow rates. The output of all variable bypass vaporizers is less than the dial setting at low flow rates (less than 250 ml·min^{-1}). This results from the relatively high specific gravity of volatile anesthetic agents. Insufficient pressure is generated at low flow rates in the vaporizing chamber to upwardly advance the molecules. At extremely high flow rates such as 15 l·min^{-1}, the output of most variable bypass vaporizers is less than the dial setting. This is attributed to incomplete mixing and saturation in the vaporizing chamber. Also, the resistance characteristics of the bypass chamber and the vaporizing chamber can vary as flow increases. This can result in decreased output concentration.[41]

Figure 25-17 shows vaporizer output versus flow rate performance curves of three halothane vaporizers. These are the Fluotec Mark II, the Ohmeda Tec 4, and the North American Dräger Vapor 19.1. In contrast to the older Fluotec Mark II, the output of contemporary vaporizers is near linear over a wide range of flow rates because of design improvements. An extensive wick and baffle system is used in the Tec 4 and Vapor 19.1, which increases the effective surface area of the vaporizing chamber.[5,42,43] Also, both vaporizers have

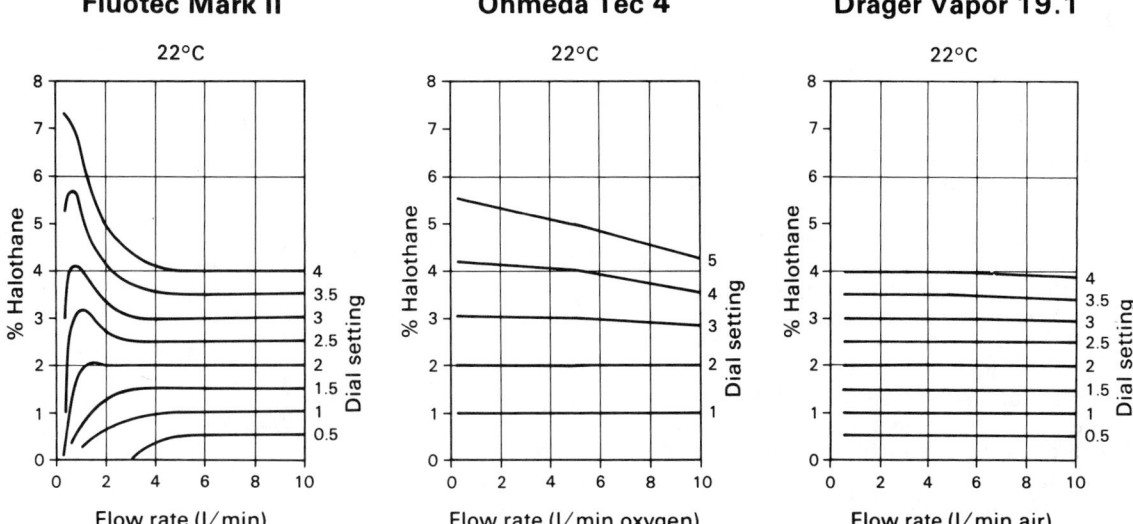

Figure 25-17. Output *versus* flow rate performance curves of the Fluotec Mark II, the Ohmeda Tec 4, and the North American Dräger Vapor 19.1. (Redrawn from data courtesy of Ohmeda, A Division of BOC Health Care, Inc, Madison, Wisconsin, and from data courtesy of North American Dräger, Telford, Pennsylvania.)

constant resistance characteristics over clinically useful flow rates.

Temperature

The output of older non–temperature-compensated vaporizers varies considerably with changes in temperature. This occurs because vapor pressure is a function of temperature. The output of contemporary temperature-compensated vaporizers, however, is almost linear over a wide range of temperatures. Several improvements in design are responsible for this linearity. Manufacturers have incorporated an automatic temperature-compensating mechanism in the bypass chamber to help maintain a constant vaporizer output with varying temperatures.[5,42,43] The valve can be a bimetallic strip or an expansion element. In either case, gas flow is apportioned in favor of the bypass chamber as temperature increases.[41] Wicks are placed in direct contact with the metal wall of the vaporizer to help replace heat that is used for vaporization. Vaporizers are constructed with metals

having relatively high specific heat and high thermal conductivity to minimize heat loss.

Figure 25-18 shows vaporizer output versus temperature performance curves for the Ohmeda Tec 4. Within the temperature range of 20–35°C, there is only a slight increase in vaporizer output associated with an increase in temperature.[43] Accuracy cannot be assured at temperatures outside this range because vapor pressure varies nonlinearly with temperature, whereas compensation varies linearly.

Intermittent Back Pressure

Intermittent back pressure associated with positive pressure ventilation or with oxygen flushing can result in higher vaporizer concentration than the dialed setting. This phenomenon is known as the *pumping effect*.[36,41,44-46] It is more pronounced at low flow rates, low dial settings, and low levels of liquid anesthetic in the vaporizing chamber. Additionally, the ventilator settings themselves are important because the pumping effect is exacerbated at rapid respiratory

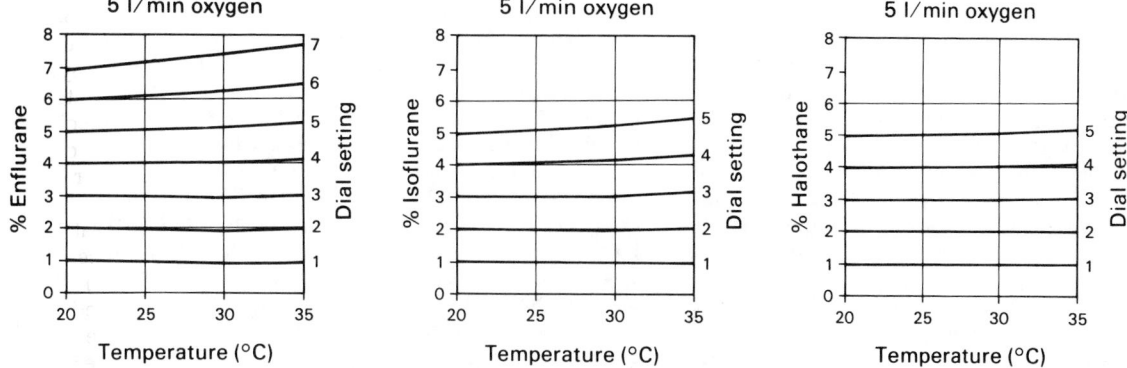

Figure 25-18. Output *versus* temperature performance curves of Ohmeda Tec 4 Vaporizers. (Redrawn with permission from Tec 4 Continuous Flow Vaporizer Operator's Manual. Steeton, England, Ohmeda, A Division of BOC Health Care, Inc, 1986.)

rates, high peak pressures, and rapid drops in pressure during expiration.[42-46] The Ohmeda Tec 4 and North American Dräger Vapor 19.1 are relatively immune from the pumping effect.[42,43] However, the pumping effect is clinically important to older variable bypass vaporizers such as the Fluotec Mark II.[44]

One proposed mechanism for the pumping effect is described as follows. Pressure is transmitted in a retrograde manner from the patient circuit to the vaporizer during the inspiratory phase of positive pressure ventilation. This produces a no-flow state within the vaporizer. Gas molecules are compressed in both the bypass chamber and the vaporizing chamber. Then, the back pressure is suddenly released during the expiratory phase of positive pressure ventilation. Vapor exits the vaporizing chamber via two routes. One portion leaves in the conventional manner through the vaporizing chamber outlet. However, another portion exists in a retrograde manner through the vaporizing chamber *inlet* and joins the bypass flow. This occurs because the output resistance of the bypass chamber is lower than that of the vaporizing chamber, particularly at low dial settings. The enhanced output concentration results from the increment of vapor that travels in the retrograde direction.[41,44-46]

Ohmeda and North American Dräger have addressed the pumping effect in the following manner. The vaporizing chambers of the Tec 4 and the Vapor 19.1 are smaller than those of older variable bypass vaporizers such as the Fluotec Mark II (750 ml).[42,43,45] Therefore, substantial volumes of vapor cannot be discharged from the vaporizing chamber into the bypass chamber during the expiratory phase. The North American Dräger 19.1 has a patented, long spiral tube that serves as the inlet to the vaporizing chamber.[42,45] When the pressure in the vaporizing chamber is released, some of the vapor enters this tube in a retrograde manner. The vapor does not enter the bypass chamber, however, because of tube length.[45] The Tec 4 has an extensive baffle system in the vaporizing chamber, and a one-way check valve has been inserted at the common outlet to minimize the pumping effect. This check valve may attenuate the pressure increase but does not prevent it, because gas still flows from the flow meters into the vaporizer during the inspiratory phase of mechanical ventilation.[36,47]

Carrier Gas Composition

Vaporizer output is influenced by the composition of the carrier gas that flows through the vaporizer (Fig. 25-19).[42,43,48-55] When the carrier gas is quickly switched from 100% oxygen to 100% nitrous oxide, there is a rapid transient decrease in vaporizer output, followed by a slow increase to a new steady-state value.[53,54] The transient decrease in vaporizer output is attributed to nitrous oxide's being more soluble than oxygen in halogenated liquid.[53] Therefore, the quantity of gas leaving the vaporizing chamber is transiently diminished until the inhaled anesthetic is totally saturated with nitrous oxide.

The explanation for the new steady-state output value is less well understood.[55] With contemporary vaporizers such as the North American Dräger 19.1 and the Ohmeda Tec 4, the steady-state output value is less when nitrous oxide is the carrier gas *versus* oxygen (Fig. 25-19B).[42,43] Conversely, the output of some older vaporizers is enhanced when nitrous oxide is the carrier gas instead of oxygen.[48,50] The steady-state plateau is achieved more rapidly with increased flow rates, regardless of the ultimate output value.[54] Factors that contribute to the steady-state response include the viscosity and density of the carrier gas, the relative solu-

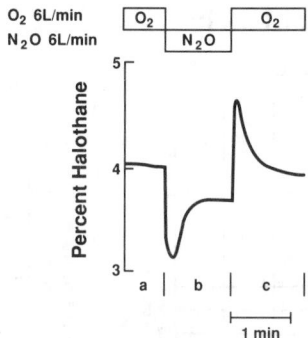

Figure 25-19. Halothane output of a North American Dräger Vapor 19.1 vaporizer with different carrier gases. The initial output concentration is approximately 4% halothane when oxygen is the carrier gas at flows of 6 l·min^{-1} (*a*). When the carrier gas is quickly switched to 100% nitrous oxide (*b*), the halothane concentration decreases to 3% within 8–10 seconds. Then, a new steady state concentration of approximately 3.5% is attained within 1 minute. See text for details. (Modified with permission from Gould DB, Lampert BA, MacKrell TN: Effect of nitrous oxide solubility on vaporizer aberrance. Anesth Analg 61:939, 1982.)

bilities of carrier gases in the liquid anesthetic, the flow splitting characteristics of the specific vaporizer, and the dial settings.[50,53-55]

Specific Vaporizers

Ohmeda Tec 4

The Ohmeda Tec 4 vaporizer system is used on most contemporary Ohmeda machines. As many as three Tec 4 vaporizers are attached to the Selectatec manifold that is located to the right of the flow meters. Vaporizer and manifold mechanisms combine to form an interlock system. The function of the interlock system is to (1) ensure that only one vaporizer can be turned on at a time; (2) ensure that gas flow enters only the vaporizer that is turned on; (3) minimize unwanted trace vapor after a vaporizer is turned off; and (4) lock the vaporizers into the gas circuit, ensuring that the vaporizer inlet and outlet ports seal correctly. Flow from the flow meters enters the vaporizer manifold and then moves only through the vaporizer, which is switched on, where it picks up a set concentration of anesthetic vapor. This gas mixture then flows out the vaporizer manifold to the common gas outlet.[13,43]

Each vaporizer has a single control dial with a concentration scale calibrated in percentage of anesthetic vapor per total volume. Turning on a vaporizer requires two simultaneous actions. The operator must depress the control dial release button, located to the left of the concentration control dial, and rotate the control dial counterclockwise. This prevents accidental displacement of the control dial from the off to the on position. A pair of mobile extension rods located behind the concentration control dial extend laterally when the vaporizer is turned on. If the lateral movement is transmitted either directly or indirectly to extension rods or another vaporizer on the manifold, that vaporizer cannot be turned on.[43]

Two different manifolds exist. An older version is present on the Ohmeda Modulus II and on the Ohmeda 8000.[9-11] If the center vaporizer is removed from this manifold, the lat-

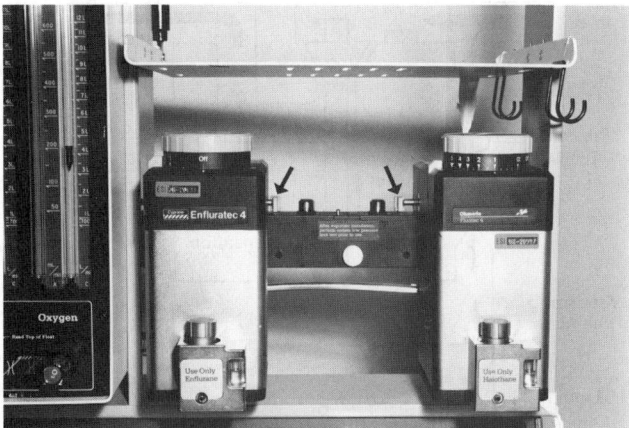

Figure 25-20. Improved interlock system of the Ohmeda Modulus II Plus with center vaporizer removed. The new manifold has a mobile bracket (see *arrows*), which allows communication between the extension rods of the two peripheral vaporizers. See text for details. (Reprinted with permission from Andrews JJ: Inhaled anesthetic delivery. In Miller RD (ed): Anesthesia, 3rd ed. New York, Churchill Livingstone, 1990.)

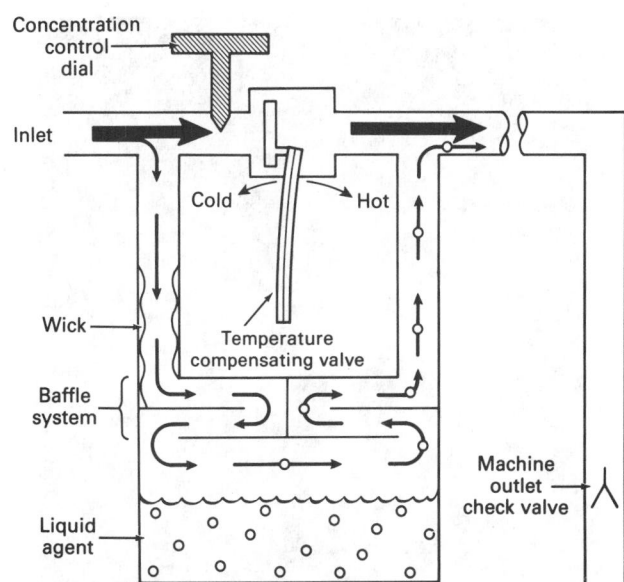

Figure 25-21. Simplified schematic of the Ohmeda Tec 4 Vaporizer. See text for details.

eral two vaporizers can be turned on simultaneously because their extension rods do not communicate. Either the left or the right vaporizer should be moved to the center position to correct the problem as indicated by the manifold warning label. Then, the interlock mechanism will function because the extension rods of the two vaporizers are in contact with each other.[9-11] The Ohmeda Modulus II Plus and the Ohmeda CD have an improved manifold (Fig. 25-20). Only a single inhaled anesthetic can be delivered even when the center vaporizer is removed. The new manifold has a mobile bracket (Fig. 25-20, arrows), which is free to move left or right. When a side vaporizer is turned on, the lateral movement of its extension rod is transmitted through the bracket to the other vaporizer. This prevents the second vaporizer from being turned on.[13,14]

Two filling mechanisms are available, including the screw-cap filler and the agent-specific keyed filler. The low location of the filler port minimizes overfilling in either case. The liquid capacity of the Tec 4 is 125 ml, and the amount retained by the wick system is 35 ml.[43]

A simplified diagram of the Ohmeda Tec 4 is shown in Figure 25-21. The total fresh gas flow enters the vaporizer's inlet and splits into two portions. The smaller first portion goes to the vaporizing chamber, which uses a wick and baffle system. The carrier gas becomes saturated with an anesthetic agent and rejoins the larger bypass flow at the vaporizer outlet. The concentration control valve determines the relative flows through the vaporizing and bypass chambers. Temperature compensation is automatically accomplished by the bimetallic strip, which influences flow through the bypass chamber. A one-way check valve is located at the common outlet of many Ohmeda machines to minimize the pumping effect.[5]

Ohmeda Tec 5

The Ohmeda Tec 5 vaporizer is an improved version of the Tec 4. The total liquid capacity of the Tec 5 is almost twice that of the Tec 4 (300 ml *versus* 160 ml). The operator uses only one hand instead of both to turn the Tec 5 on because of the newly designed control dial. The Tec 5 vaporizers

reside on the selectatec manifold with series arrangement. Both screw-cap and keyed fillers are available. Ohmeda recommends that the Tec 5 vaporizers be serviced every 3 years *versus* annually.[56]

North American Dräger Vapor 19.1

The North American Dräger Vapor Exclusion System is used on the Narkomed 2A, 2B, 3, and 4.[15-19] As many as three vaporizers are attached semipermanently to the vaporizer mounting bracket, which is located to the right of the flow meter bank (Fig. 25-22). A cam and lever interlock system is incorporated into the vaporizer bank, which prevents more than one vaporizer from being activated (Fig. 25-23). All unused vaporizers are locked in the zero position.[17,18] This external interlock system is different from the system used by Ohmeda in which the exclusion rods are an internal component of each vaporizer.[43,56] The North American Dräger interlock system continues to function when any of the three vaporizers are removed. However, a short-circuit block must be installed in place of the vaporizer, or a leak will occur.

The output of the North American Dräger 19.1 is regulated by a single concentration dial calibrated in percent and located on top of the vaporizer. When the control dial is set in the 0 position (off), fresh gas from the flow meter passes with almost no resistance through a bypass inside the vaporizer directly to the common outlet. Thus, the actual vaporizing portion of the 19.1 is completely separated from the fresh gas flow. Also, in the 0 position, the inlet and the outlet of the vaporizing chamber are interconnected and vented through a hole. This ensures that no pressure builds in the vaporizing chamber. The anesthetic loss caused by venting in the off position is less than 0.5 ml per 24 h at an ambient temperature of 22°C. Two types of filling mechanisms are available: the screw-cap filler or the safety, agent-specific, keyed filler. The liquid capacity of the 19.1 is 200 ml with a dry wick or 140 ml when the wick is wet.[42]

Figure 25-24 shows a simplified schematic of the North American Dräger Vapor 19.1 in the on position. Flow through the Vapor 19.1 is similar to that through the Tec 4,

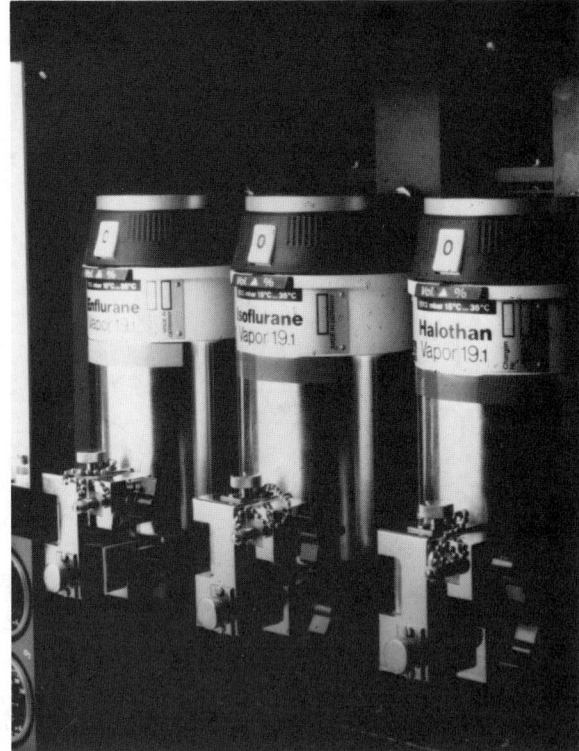

Figure 25-22. North American Dräger Vapor 19.1 Vaporizers with keyed filling devices. (Courtesy of North American Dräger, Telford, Pennsylvania.)

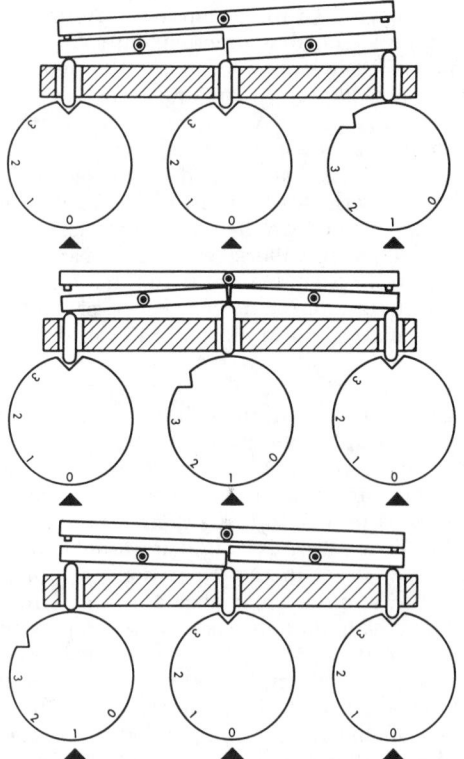

Figure 25-23. Three top views of North American Dräger's interlock system. A different vaporizer is turned on in each view. When one vaporizer is turned on, the other two are locked in the zero position. (Courtesy of North American Dräger, Telford, Pennsylvania.)

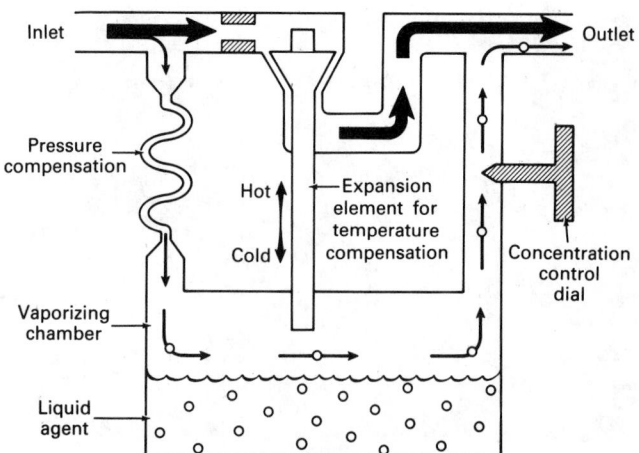

Figure 25-24. Simplified schematic of the North American Dräger 19.1 Vaporizer. See text for details.

but back pressure and temperature compensation are different. The Vapor 19.1 uses a patented, long, spiral tube as the inlet to the vaporizing chamber, which acts as a buffer against the pumping effect. Some inhaled anesthetic gas molecules do travel in a retrograde manner up this tube during the expiratory phase of the pumping effect. However, they do not reach the bypass chamber because of the tube length. North American Dräger does not employ a check valve at the common outlet because of this internal pressure compensation. Temperature compensation is achieved by an expansion element, which alters flow through the bypass chamber. The Vapor 19.1 has a wick and baffle system similar to that of the Tec 4.[42,43]

Desflurane Vaporizer

Contemporary variable bypass vaporizers such as the Ohmeda Tec 4 and Tec 5 and the North American Dräger 19.1 are unsuitable for controlled vaporization of desflurane because it has a vapor pressure near 1 atm (664 mm Hg) at room temperature.[57] The clinical trials with desflurane are conducted with pressurized vaporizers electrically heated to 23–25°C.[57-59] A back pressure regulator produces pressurization to 1550 mm Hg. This creates a condition in which the anesthetic has a relatively lower volatility. Pressurization eliminates the possibility of boiling at clinically useful temperatures. In a pressurized system, vapor pressure changes owing to temperature alterations are relatively small compared with the operating pressure. Therefore, temperature compensation is accomplished more easily. A supplemental heat source is necessary to overcome the high heat of vaporization requirements seen with desflurane. Compared with other halogenated anesthetics, more desflurane must be vaporized during a case because the minimum alveolar concentration (MAC) of desflurane is high (6–7%).[57] Without supplemental heat, cooling of the vaporizing chamber would be excessive.

Safety Features

The North American Dräger 19.1, the Ohmeda Tec 4, and the Ohmeda Tec 5 vaporizers have numerous safety features that have minimized or eliminated many hazards once associated with variable bypass vaporizers. Agent-specific, keyed filling devices help prevent filling a vaporizer with the wrong agent. Overfilling of these vaporizers is minimized because the filler port is located at the maximum safe liquid level. Today's vaporizers are soundly secured to the vaporizer manifold, and there is little need to move them. Thus, problems associated with tipping are minimized. Contemporary interlock systems prevent administration of more than one agent.[42,43,56]

Hazards

Contemporary Variable Bypass Vaporizers

Despite numerous safety features, some hazards are still associated with contemporary variable bypass vaporizers.

Misfilling. Vaporizers not equipped with keyed fillers have been commonly misfilled.[60] A potential for misfilling exists even on contemporary vaporizers equipped with keyed fillers.[61,62] Misfilling a contemporary variable bypass vaporizer with desflurane can theoretically cause desflurane overdose and hypoxemia. Safe delivery of desflurane requires unique safety features to prevent misfilling.

Tipping. Tipping can occur when vaporizers are incorrectly "switched out" or moved. However, tipping is unlikely when a vaporizer is attached to a manifold in the upright position. Excessive tipping can cause the liquid agent to enter the bypass chamber and can result in a high output concentration.[63] The Tec 4 is slightly more immune to tipping than the Vapor 19.1 because of the extensive baffle system of the former. However, if either vaporizer is tipped, it should not be used until it has been flushed for 20–30 minutes at high flow rates with the vaporizer set at a low concentration.[36]

Simultaneous Inhaled Anesthetic Administration. Two inhaled anesthetics can be administered simultaneously when the center Tec 4 vaporizer is removed from Ohmeda machines that have the older style vaporizer manifold. The left or right vaporizer should be moved to the central position if the central vaporizer is removed as indicated by the manifold label. The interlock system will then function properly because the two remaining vaporizers are adjacent.[9-11]

Leaks. Leaks often are associated with vaporizers.[36,64] A loose filler cap is the most common source of vaporizer leaks. They can occur at the O-ring junction between the vaporizer and its manifold. A vaporizer must be in the on position to detect a leak within it. Vaporizer leaks in the North American Dräger System can be detected with a conventional positive pressure leak test because of the absence of check valves. Ohmeda recommends a negative pressure leak testing device (suction bulb) to detect vaporizer leaks in the Modulus I, Modulus II, and the Excel because of the check valve at the machine outlet[8-10,12] (see the section on Checking Anesthesia Machines).

Freestanding (Add-On) Vaporizers

Freestanding, variable bypass vaporizers have been "added on" to many anesthesia machines between the common outlet and the patient circuit. This practice is fraught with hazards. Tipping is a substantial possibility because the vaporizer is not permanently affixed to the machine. Furthermore, multiple agents can be administered because at least one agent from the machine plus the agent from the freestanding vaporizer can be delivered. Oxygen flushing (35–75 l·min⁻¹) can deliver excess anesthetic agent from the freestanding vaporizer to the patient. Even though the inlet and outlet of freestanding vaporizers have different diameters, they can be connected in a reverse manner. Vaporizer output can be two times that indicated on the dial in this configuration.[65]

Many freestanding vaporizers have a check valve in the vaporizer outlet to minimize the pumping effect and to indicate reverse connection. This valve prevents detection of leaks in the low-pressure circuit when a traditional positive pressure leak test is performed. Also, an intraoperative disconnection between the machine outlet and the vaporizer inlet can go unnoticed if positive pressure ventilation is employed. The pressure from the breathing circuit closes the check valve during the inspiratory phase of mechanical ventilation, and the disconnection is not detectable by conventional means.[66]

ANESTHETIC CIRCUITS

Gas exits the anesthesia machine at the common gas outlet, and it then enters an anesthetic circuit. The function of an anesthetic circuit is not only to deliver oxygen and anesthetic gases to the patient but also to eliminate carbon dioxide. Carbon dioxide can be removed either by washout with adequate fresh gas inflow or by soda lime absorption. This discussion is limited to semiclosed rebreathing circuits and the circle system.

Mapleson Systems

Mapleson described and analyzed five different arrangements of fresh gas flow, tubing, mask, reservoir bag, and the expiratory valve to administer anesthetic gases.[67] They are now classically referred to as the Mapleson Systems, designated from A to E. Willis, Pender, and Mapleson added the F System to these original five.[68] The Mapleson circuits are shown in Figure 25-25. The amount of rebreathing associated with each type is highly dependent upon fresh gas flow rate. The performance of these circuits is best understood by studying the expiratory phase of the respiratory cycle.

Mapleson A

The Mapleson A is also known as Magill's circuit. It consists of a corrugated tube, a reservoir bag, a fresh gas inflow near the reservoir bag, and a spring-loaded expiratory valve near the patient (Fig. 25-25). Rebreathing during spontaneous ventilation in this circuit can be prevented with relatively low fresh gas flows. Upon exhalation, the patient end of the tubing is filled with dead space gas followed by the alveolar gas. This stream travels up the tubing and meets the fresh gas flowing into the circuit (Fig. 25-26 left). The pressure in the circuit increases and forces the expiratory valve to open, allowing the alveolar gas to escape. Most of the dead space gas is washed out if the fresh gas flow is adequate. During the inspiratory phase, the fresh gas flushes the dead space gas through the tubing toward the patient. Rebreathing of dead space gas poses no problem because it does not contain carbon dioxide. Several studies have confirmed Mapleson's original finding that rebreathing of alveolar gas can be prevented if the fresh gas flow is equal to or exceeds the patient's minute ventilation.[69,70] Rebreathing does not occur

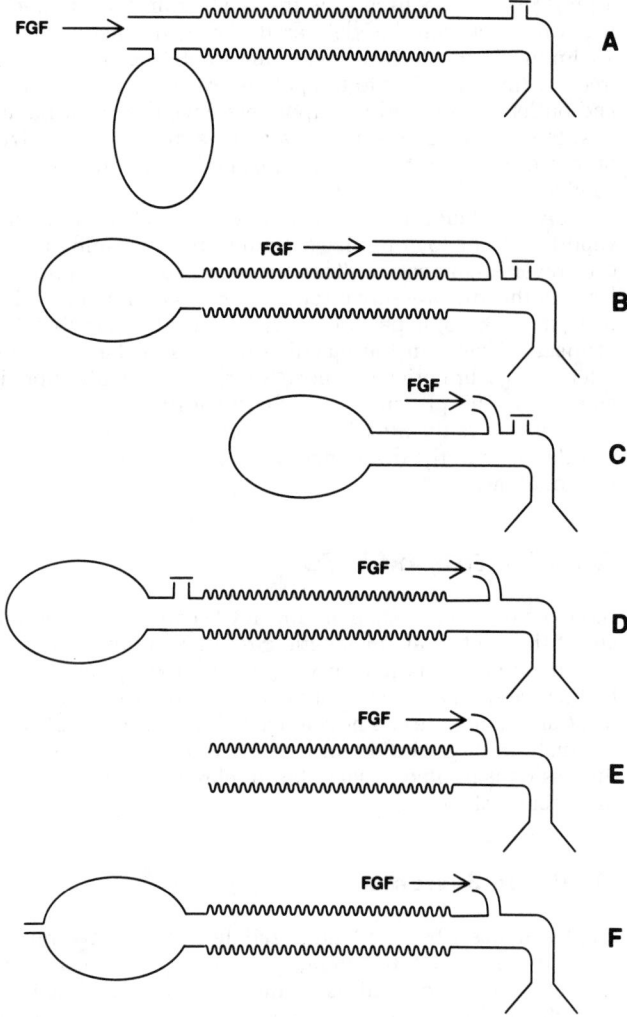

Figure 25-25. (A–F) Mapleson Breathing Systems. (Redrawn with permission from Willis BA, Pender JW, Mapleson WW: Rebreathing in a T-piece: Volunteer and theoretical studies of the Jackson-Rees modification of Ayre's T-piece during spontaneous respiration. Br J Anaesth 47:1239, 1975.)

until the fresh gas flow is below 70% of the patient's minute ventilation.

The Mapleson A Circuit is inefficient during controlled ventilation.[71] Expiratory valve resistance must be increased to ventilate the patient. Venting the gas in the circuit occurs during the inspiratory phase, and the alveolar gases are retained in the tubing during the expiratory phase (Fig. 25-26 right). Thus, alveolar gas is rebreathed with the ensuing breath before the pressure in the system increases enough to force the expiratory valve open. This can cause an increase in arterial carbon dioxide tension. Adequate carbon dioxide elimination using controlled ventilation with a Mapleson A System requires a fresh gas flow of greater than 20 l·min^{-1}. In practice, controlled ventilation should be avoided with this system.

Mapleson B

The Mapleson B System features the fresh gas inlet near the patient end just distal to the expiratory valve (see Fig. 25-25). This circuit functions similarly during both sponta-

neous and controlled ventilation, unlike the Mapleson A System. Location of the fresh gas inlet allows fresh gas to accumulate along with exhaled gases in the tubing (Fig. 25-26). The expiratory valve opens when pressure in the circuit increases, and a mixture of alveolar gas and fresh gas is discharged. During the next inspiration, the patient receives fresh gas flow from the machine and a mixture of retained fresh gas and alveolar gas from the tubing (Fig. 25-26). Composition of this inhaled mixture depends on fresh gas flow rate. Rebreathing can be prevented if the fresh gas flow rate is greater than twice the minute ventilation for both spontaneous and controlled ventilation.[71,72]

Mapleson C

The Mapleson C System is also known as the Water's Circuit without an absorber. Arrangement of its components is similar to that of the Mapleson B, but the large-bore tubing is shorter (see Fig. 25-25). This effectively reduces the reservoir volume and allows good mixing of fresh and exhaled gases. The inspired mixture contains more alveolar gas compared with the Mapleson B System. A fresh gas flow of twice the minute ventilation is required to prevent rebreathing.[72] Carbon dioxide will build up, although at a slower rate than with the Mapleson B Circuit, if rebreathing is allowed to occur.

Mapleson D

The Mapleson D Circuit can be described as a T-piece with an expiratory limb. The fresh gas inlet is located near the patient, and the expiratory valve is close to the reservoir bag (see Fig. 25-25). During the expiratory phase of spontaneous ventilation, fresh gas and alveolar gas flow down the expiratory limb (see Fig. 25-26). The expiratory valve opens as pressure increases in the circuit, and a portion of this mixture is expelled. The patient receives a combination of fresh gas and mixed gas from the tubing during the next inspiration. The content of this inspired mixture is determined by the rate of fresh gas flow, the patient's tidal volume, and the duration of the expiratory pause. A long expiratory pause (slow respiratory rate) allows the fresh gas to move down the tubing and flush the alveolar gas. A short expiratory pause (fast respiratory rate) provides inadequate time to flush the alveolar gas and allows rebreathing to occur. The amount of alveolar gas entering the tubing will increase if the patient's tidal volume is large. Rebreathing in this situation can be prevented by high fresh gas flows and a long expiratory pause. Mapleson determined that a fresh gas flow greater than two times the minute ventilation was enough to prevent rebreathing. Normocapnia can be maintained during spontaneous ventilation if the fresh gas flow is 100 ml·kg^{-1}·min^{-1} despite rebreathing.[73] Soliman and Laberge found that a flow rate of 206 ml·kg^{-1}·min^{-1} resulted in normocapnia in pediatric patients of ages 1–5 years.[74]

During the inspiratory phase of controlled ventilation, alveolar gas and dead space gas, instead of fresh gas, are forced out of the expiratory valve. Therefore, this system causes less rebreathing than the Mapleson B or C Systems. Bain and Spoerel have recommended the following fresh gas flow rates during controlled ventilation with the Mapleson D System:[73]

2 l·min^{-1} for infants weighing less than 10 kg
3.5 l·min^{-1} for patients weighing from 10–50 kg
70 ml·kg^{-1}·min^{-1} for patients weighing more than 60 kg

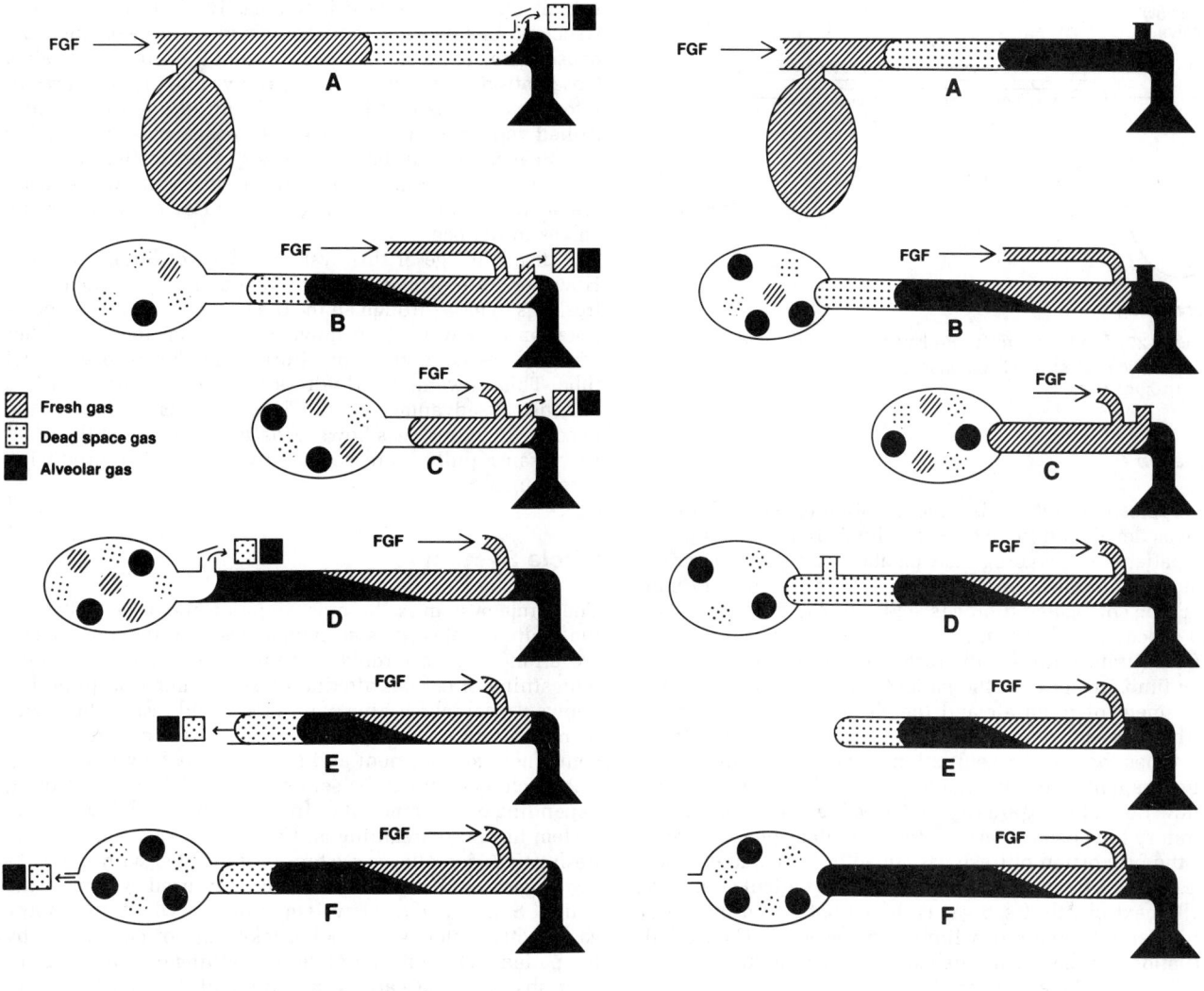

Spontaneous Ventilation   **Controlled Ventilation**

Figure 25-26. Gas disposition at end expiration during spontaneous (*left*) and controlled (*right*) ventilation in circuits *A–F*. (Modified with permission from Sykes MK: Rebreathing circuits: A review. Br J Anaesth 40:666, 1968.)

In each of these cases, the recommended tidal volume is 10 ml·kg^{-1} and the respiratory rate is 12–16 breaths per minute.

Bain Circuit

The Bain Circuit is a modification of the Mapleson D System. It is a coaxial circuit in which the fresh gas flows through a narrow inner tube within the outer corrugated tubing.[75] The central tube originates near the reservoir bag, but the fresh gas actually enters the circuit at the patient end (Fig. 25-27). Exhaled gases enter the corrugated tubing and are vented through the expiratory valve near the reservoir bag. The Bain Circuit may be used for both spontaneous and controlled ventilation. The fresh gas flows necessary to prevent rebreathing are similar to those of the Mapleson D System. Normocarbia during spontaneous ventilation requires a fresh gas flow of 200–300 ml·kg^{-1}, but a flow of only 70 ml·kg^{-1} will produce normocarbia during controlled ventilation.[73,76,77]

There are many advantages of this circuit. It is light weight, convenient, easily sterilized, and reusable. Scavenging of the gases from the expiratory valve is facilitated because it is located away from the patient. Exhaled gases in the outer reservoir tubing add warmth and humidity to inspired fresh gases. The hazards of the Bain Circuit include unrecognized disconnection or kinking of the inner fresh gas hose. These problems can cause hypercarbia from inadequate gas flow or increased respiratory resistance.

The outer tube should be transparent to allow inspection of the inner tube. The integrity of the inner tube can be assessed as described by Pethick.[78] High-flow oxygen is fed into the circuit while the patient end is occluded until the reservoir bag is filled. The patient end is opened, and oxygen is flushed into the circuit. If the inner tube is intact, the Venturi effect occurs at the patient end. This causes a decrease in pressure within the circuit, and the reservoir bag deflates. Conversely, a leak in the inner tube allows the fresh gas to escape into the expiratory limb, and the reservoir bag will remain inflated. This test is recommended as a part of the preanesthesia check if a Bain Circuit is used.

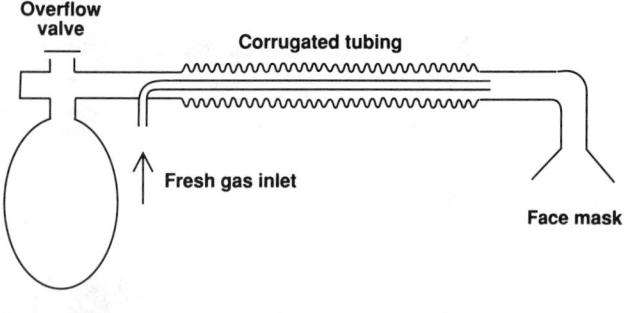

Figure 25-27. The Bain Circuit. (Redrawn with permission from Bain JA, Spoerel WE: A streamlined anaesthetic system. Can Anaesth Soc J 19:426, 1972.)

Mapleson E

The Mapleson E System is a modification of Ayre's T-piece that was developed in 1937 by Phillip Ayre for use in pediatric patients undergoing cleft palate repair or intracranial surgery.[79] It consists of a fresh gas inlet at the patient end and a long corrugated tubing (see Fig. 25-25). It has minimal dead space, no valves, and very little resistance.[80]

The expiratory limb is the reservoir. Volume of the expiratory limb greater than the patient's tidal volume prevents entrainment of room air and thereby prevents dilution of anesthetic gases and oxygen. A fresh gas flow greater than three times the minute ventilation prevents rebreathing.

During spontaneous ventilation, the fresh gas and exhaled gas flow down the expiratory limb (see Fig. 25-26 left). Peak expiratory flow occurs early in the expiratory phase. Therefore, the proportion of fresh gas added to the exhaled gases increases. The fresh gas accumulates at the patient end. During the next breath, fresh gas is drawn both from the fresh gas inlet and the expiratory limb or the reservoir. Controlled ventilation can be accomplished by intermittently occluding the end of the expiratory limb.

Mapleson F

The most commonly used T-piece system is the Jackson-Rees modification of Mapleson D.[81] This is a T-piece arrangement with a reservoir bag and incorporates a relief mechanism for venting exhaled gases. The relief mechanism is either an adjustable valve at the distal end of the reservoir bag or simply a hole in the side of the bag. During spontaneous ventilation when the patient exhales, the gases pass down the expiratory limb and mix with the fresh gas (see Fig. 25-26 left). The expiratory pause allows the fresh gas to push the exhaled gases down the expiratory limb. With the next inspiration, the inhaled gas mixture comes from the fresh gas flow and from the expiratory limb, including the reservoir bag. Considerations for fresh gas flow rates are similar to those for the Bain Circuit. Flow rates equivalent to three times the minute ventilation are recommended to prevent rebreathing.

The Jackson-Rees Circuit is commonly used for controlled ventilation during an anesthetic procedure and for transportation of the intubated patients. Fresh gas flow rates are similar to those in the Bain Circuit. The degree of rebreathing is affected by the management of venting and ventilation.

The Jackson-Rees System is popular for pediatric anesthesia, especially for head and neck surgery, because it is light

weight and can be positioned easily. It is simply constructed, inexpensive, and offers minimal resistance because there are no moving parts except the adjustable valve. Observation of the reservoir bag allows one to inspect respiratory excursions and judge the depth of anesthesia. Controlled ventilation can be instituted easily by squeezing the bag. Scavenging can be done either by enclosing the reservoir bag in a plastic chamber from which the waste gases are suctioned or by attaching various devices to the relief valves in the bag.

A disadvantage of this system is lack of humidification. However, this problem can be overcome by allowing the fresh gas to pass through an in-line heated humidifier. Incorporation of a water trap downstream from the humidifier accumulates condensed moisture from the fresh gas inlet tube. This prevents overhydration of the pediatric patient. Another disadvantage of the Jackson-Rees System is the need for high fresh gas flows. Finally, occlusion of the relief valve can rapidly increase the airway pressure, producing barotrauma.

Circle System

The circle system is the most popular breathing system in the United States. It is so named because its components are arranged in a circular manner. This system prevents rebreathing of carbon dioxide by soda lime absorption but allows partial rebreathing of other exhaled gases. The extent of rebreathing of the other exhaled gases depends upon component arrangement and the fresh gas flow rate.

A circle system can be semiopen, semiclosed, or closed, depending on the amount of fresh gas inflow.[82] A semiopen system has no rebreathing and requires a very high flow of fresh gas. A semiclosed system is associated with rebreathing of gases and is the most commonly used system in the United States. A closed system is one in which the inflow gas exactly matches that being taken up, or consumed, by the patient. There is complete rebreathing of exhaled gases after absorption of carbon dioxide, and the overflow (pop-off) valve is closed (see the section on Closed Circuit Anesthesia).

The circle system (Fig. 25-28) consists of seven components, including the following: (1) a fresh gas inflow source; (2) inspiratory and expiratory unidirectional valves; (3) inspiratory and expiratory corrugated tubes; (4) a Y-piece connector; (5) an Adjustable Pressure Limiting Valve or pop-off valve; (6) a reservoir bag; and (7) a canister containing a carbon dioxide absorbent. The unidirectional valves are placed in the system to ensure unidirectional flow through the corrugated hoses. The fresh gas inflow enters the circle by a connection from the common gas outlet of the anesthesia machine.

Numerous variations of the circle arrangement are possible, depending upon the relative positions of the unidirectional valves, the pop-off valve, the reservoir bag, the carbon dioxide absorber, and the site of fresh gas entry. However, to prevent rebreathing of carbon dioxide, three rules must be followed: (1) a unidirectional valve must be located between the patient and the reservoir bag on both the inspiratory and expiratory limbs of the circuit; (2) the fresh gas inflow cannot enter the circuit between the expiratory valve and the patient; and (3) the pop-off valve cannot be located between the patient and the inspiratory valve. If these rules are followed, any arrangement of the other components will prevent rebreathing of carbon dioxide.[83]

The most efficient circle system arrangement that allows

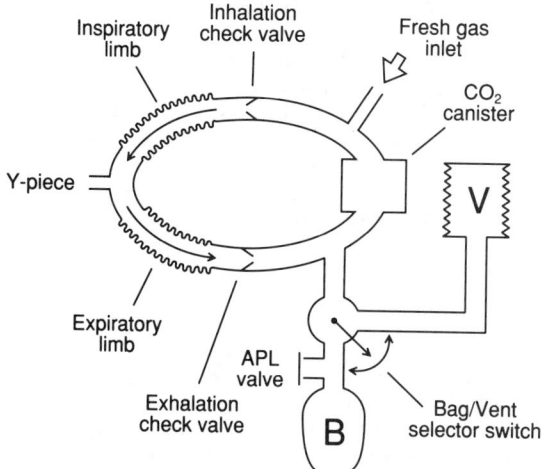

Figure 25-28. Components of the circle system. (Reprinted with permission from Andrews JJ: Inhaled anesthetic delivery systems. In Miller RD (ed): Anesthesia, 3rd ed, p 171. New York, Churchill Livingstone, 1990.)

the highest conservation of fresh gases is one with the unidirectional valves near the patient and the pop-off valve just downstream from the expiratory valve. This arrangement conserves dead space gas and preferentially eliminates alveolar gas. A more practical but less efficient arrangement is the one used on all contemporary anesthesia machines (Fig. 25-28). It is less efficient because it allows alveolar and dead space gas to mix before venting.[83,84]

The advantages of the circle system include a relative constancy of inspired concentration, conservation of respiratory moisture and heat, and minimization of operating room pollution. Additionally, it can be used for closed system anesthesia or with low oxygen flows. The major disadvantage of the circle system stems from its complex design. The circuit has approximately ten connections, all of which can disconnect and leak. Malfunctioning valves can cause serious problems. Rebreathing can occur if the valves stick in the open position. Total occlusion of the circuit can occur if the valves are stuck closed. Finally, the bulk of the circle system offers less convenience and portability than the Mapleson systems.

CARBON DIOXIDE ABSORPTION

Different anesthesia systems eliminate carbon dioxide with varying degrees of efficiency. This section is primarily concerned with the closed or semiclosed circle system, which requires carbon dioxide absorption in order to make rebreathing possible. Desirable features in the carbon dioxide absorption mechanism are lack of toxicity with common anesthetics, low resistance to air flow, low cost, ease of handling, and relative efficiency.

History

European scientists in the early 1900s were experimenting with the carbon dioxide absorptive properties of lime water and caustic sodas. However, the real impetus to develop efficient carbon dioxide absorptive techniques came from submarine and chemical warfare applications during World

War I.[85] In 1915, Wilson patented a new process to make soda lime, which greatly increased its efficiency.[86] Rebreathing techniques with carbon dioxide absorption were slow to gain in popularity until cyclopropane was introduced.[85] Cyclopropane was an expensive and explosive anesthetic agent. Many additions and refinements in soda lime have occurred since its invention, but the essential ingredients have remained unchanged.

Chemistry

Two formulations for carbon dioxide absorption are commonly used today. These are soda lime and baralyme. Soda lime consists of 94% calcium hydroxide, 5% sodium hydroxide, and 1% potassium hydroxide (an activator). Small amounts of silica are added to produce calcium and sodium silicate. This addition produces a hard compound and reduces dust formation. The efficiency of the soda lime absorption varies inversely with the hardness; therefore, little silicate is used in contemporary soda lime. Sodium hydroxide is the catalyst for the carbon dioxide absorptive properties of soda lime.[85,87]

Baralyme is composed of 80% calcium hydroxide and 20% barium hydroxide. Baralyme is more stable than soda lime and does not require a silica binder. Barium hydroxide is the catalyst. Baralyme is more dense than soda lime and is approximately 15% less efficient, based on weight in absorbing carbon dioxide. Water is required for both formulations, but baralyme contains water as the barium hydroxide octohydrate salt. Therefore, it may perform better in a dry climate.[85,87]

The soda lime used in the early days of carbon dioxide absorption was noted to regenerate its efficiency to absorb carbon dioxide after being exhausted.[88] The explanation for this regeneration is complex, but it is of little concern today. Regeneration is rarely seen today because of improved soda lime with less silica and the addition of potassium hydroxide. Baralyme has no regeneration capability.[85,87]

The size of the absorptive granules has been determined by trial and error, which represents a compromise between resistance to air flow and absorptive efficiency.[89] The smaller the granules, the more surface area is available for absorption. However, air flow resistance increases. The granular size of soda lime and baralyme in anesthesia practice is between 4 and 8 mesh. Resistance to air flow at this size is negligible. Mesh refers to the number of openings per linear inch in a sieve through which the granular particles can pass. A 4-mesh screen means that there are four quarter-inch openings per linear inch. An 8-mesh screen has eight eighth-inch openings per linear inch.[85]

The absorption of carbon dioxide by soda lime is a chemical and not a physical process.[88] Carbon dioxide combines with water to form carbonic acid. Carbonic acid reacts with the hydroxides to form sodium (or potassium) carbonate and water. Calcium hydroxide accepts the carbonate to form calcium carbonate and sodium (or potassium) hydroxide. The equations are as follows:

1. $CO_2 + H_2O \rightleftarrows H_2CO_3$
2. $H_2CO_3 + 2NaOH \ (KOH) \rightleftarrows Na_2CO_3 \ (K_2CO_3) + 2H_2O + Heat$
3. $Na_2CO_3 \ (K_2CO_3) + Ca(OH)_2 \rightleftarrows CaCO_3 + 2NaOH \ (KOH)$

Some carbon dioxide may react directly with $Ca(OH)_2$, but this reaction is much slower.

The reaction with baralyme differs from that of soda lime

because more water is liberated by a direct reaction of barium hydroxide and carbon dioxide.

1. $Ba(OH)_2 + 8H_2O + CO_2 \rightleftarrows BaCO_3 + 9H_2O + Heat$
2. $9H_2O + 9CO_2 \rightleftarrows 9H_2CO_3$

Then by direct reactions and by KOH and NaOH,

3. $9H_2CO_3 + 9Ca(OH)_2 \rightleftarrows CaCO_3 + 18H_2O + Heat$

Absorptive Capacity

The maximum amount of carbon dioxide that can be absorbed with the above equations is 26 l of CO_2 per 100 g of absorbent. However, channeling of gas through granules may substantially decrease this efficiency and allow only 10–20 l of carbon dioxide to actually be absorbed.[90]

Indicators

Ethyl violet is the pH indicator that is added to both soda lime and baralyme to help assess the functional integrity of the absorbent. It is a substituted triphenylmethane dye with a critical pH of 10.3.[87] Ethyl violet changes in color from colorless to violet when the pH of the absorbent decreases as a result of carbon dioxide absorption. The pH of fresh absorbent exceeds the critical pH, and the dye exists in its colorless form. As absorbent becomes exhausted, however, the pH decreases below 10.3, and ethyl violet changes to its violet form through alcohol dehydration.

Ethyl violet is not always a reliable indicator of the functional status of absorbent. Fluorescent lights can deactivate the dye so that the absorbent appears white even though it is exhausted.[91]

Historically, other pH indicators have been used to indicate absorbent exhaustion. All are acids or bases that change color when the hydrogen ion concentration changes. Other indicators and their respective colors are as follows: phenolphthalein (white → pink), clayton yellow (red → yellow), ethyl orange (orange → yellow), and mimosa z (red → white).[92]

Incompatibilities

It is an important and desirable feature to have carbon dioxide absorbents that are not intrinsically toxic and that are not toxic when exposed to common anesthetics. Soda lime fits this description, but it is important to note that when using an uncommon anesthetic, trichloroethylene, toxicity may result. In the presence of alkali and heat, trichloroethylene degrades into the cranial neurotoxin dichloroacetylene. Phosgene, a potent pulmonary irritant, is also produced. The resulting toxicities are manifested by cranial nerve lesions, encephalitis, and adult respiratory distress syndrome.[93]

A newer anesthetic, sevoflurane, is somewhat unstable in soda lime, but this apparently does not produce any toxic effects.[94] Soda lime and baralyme degrade sevoflurane, and the rate of degradation is a direct function of temperature. However, the degradation does not appear to be clinically relevant even in low-flow systems.[95]

ANESTHESIA VENTILATORS

The anesthesia ventilator can substitute for the breathing bag of the circle system, the Bain Circuit, and other breathing systems. A decade ago anesthesia ventilators were mere adjuncts to the anesthesia machine. Today, they have attained a prominent central role in newer anesthesia systems. This discussion focuses on the classification, operating, principles, and hazards of anesthesia ventilators.

Classification

Ventilators can be classified according to the power source, the drive mechanism, the cycling mechanism, and the bellows type.[96,97] The following section briefly reviews ventilator classification and terminology prior to the discussion of individual anesthesia machine ventilators.

Power Source

The power source required to operate a mechanical ventilator is provided by either compressed gas or electricity or both. Older pneumatic ventilators such as the Ohio Anesthesia Ventilator, the Ohio V5, and the Ohio V5A require only a pneumatic power source to function properly.[98-102] Contemporary electronic ventilators such as the North American Dräger AV-E, the Ohmeda 7000, and the Ohmeda 7810 require both an electronic and a pneumatic power source.[13,15-19,103,104]

Drive Mechanism

Most anesthesia machine ventilators are classified as double-circuit, pneumatically driven ventilators. In a double-circuit system, a driving force compresses a bag or bellows, which in turn delivers gas to the patient. Compressed gases provide the actual driving force. The ventilators are therefore pneumatically driven. The driving gas in the Ohmeda 7000 and the Ohmeda 7810 is composed of 100% oxygen.[13,103,104] In the North American Dräger AV-E, it is a mixture of oxygen and air because a Venturi device is employed.[15-19]

Cycling Mechanism

Most anesthesia machine ventilators are time cycled and provide ventilator support in the control mode. Initiation of inspiration is accomplished by a timing device. Older pneumatic ventilators use a fluidic timing device. Contemporary electronic ventilators use a solid-state timing device and are thus classified as time cycled and electronically controlled.

Bellows Classification

The direction of bellows movement during the expiratory phase determines the bellows classification. Ascending (standing) bellows ascend during the expiratory phase, whereas descending (hanging) bellows descend during the expiratory phase. Older pneumatic ventilators use weighted descending bellows, whereas most contemporary electronic ventilators have ascending bellows. Of the two configurations, the ascending bellows is safer. An ascending bellows will not fill if a disconnection occurs. The bellows of a descending bellows ventilator, however, will continue its upward and downward movement during a disconnection. The disconnection pressure monitor and the volume monitor may be "fooled" even if a disconnection is complete[1] (see the section on Breathing Circuit Problems).

Operating Principles

A generic ascending bellows ventilator is shown in Figure 25-29. It may be simplistically viewed as a breathing bag (bellows) located within a clear plastic box. The bellows physically separates the driving gas circuit from the patient gas circuit. The driving gas circuit is located outside the bellows, and the patient gas circuit is inside the bellows. During the inspiratory phase (Fig. 25-29 left), the driving gas enters the bellows chamber, causing the pressure within it to increase. This increase in pressure is responsible for two events. First, the ventilator relief valve closes. This prevents anesthetic gas from escaping into the scavenging system. Second, the bellows is compressed, and the anesthetic gas within the bellows is delivered to the patient's lungs. This compression action is analogous to the hand of the anesthesiologist squeezing the breathing bag.

During the expiratory phase (Fig. 25-29 right), the driving gas exits the bellows chamber. The pressure within the bellows chamber and within the pilot line declines to zero, causing the mushroom portion of the ventilator relief valve to open. Exhaled patient gas fills the bellows prior to any scavenging. This occurs because a weighted ball similar to that used in ball-type positive end–expiratory pressure valves is incorporated into the base of the ventilator relief valve. The ball produces 2–3 cm water of back pressure; therefore scavenging occurs only after the bellows fills completely and the pressure inside the bellows exceeds this pressure threshold. This design causes all ascending bellows ventilators to produce 2–3 cm water pressure of positive end–expiratory pressure within the breathing circuit. Scavenging occurs only during the expiratory phase, since the ventilator relief valve is open only during expiration.

Gas flow from the anesthesia machine into the breathing circuit is continuous, and it is independent of ventilator activity. During the inspiratory phase of mechanical ventilation, the ventilator relief valve is closed, and the breathing system Adjustable Pressure Limiting Valve (pop-off valve) is either closed or out of circuit. Therefore, the patient receives volume from the bellows and from the flow meters during the inspiratory phase. Factors that influence the correlation between set tidal volume and exhaled tidal volume include the flow meter settings, the inspiratory time, the compliance of the breathing circuit, external leakage, and the location of the tidal volume sensor.[13,14,103,104] Usually, the volume gained from the fresh gas flow during inspiration is counteracted by the volume lost to the breathing circuit compliance. The set tidal volume generally approximates the exhaled tidal volume. However, oxygen flushing during the inspiratory phase can result in barotrauma because excess volume cannot be vented.

Pneumatic Ventilators

Pneumatic ventilators performed the majority of mechanical ventilation in the operating room until recently. Although they have become less popular, many are still in use. Examples of pneumatic ventilators include the Ohio Anesthesia Ventilator, the Ohio V5, the Ohio V5A, and the North American Dräger AV. They are classified as pneumatically powered, double-circuit, pneumatically driven, descending bel-

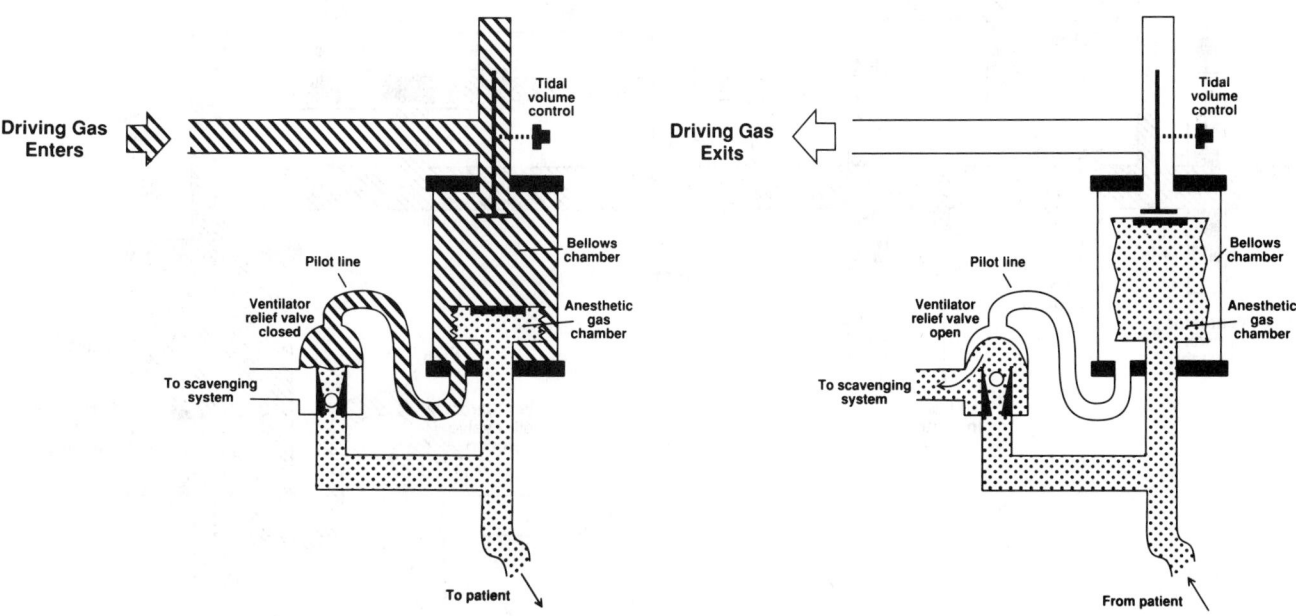

Inspiratory Phase Gas Flows   Expiratory Phase Gas Flows

Figure 25-29. Inspiratory and expiratory phase gas flows of a generic ascending bellows anesthesia ventilator. See text for details. (Reprinted with permission from Andrews JJ: Understanding your anesthesia machine and ventilator. In 1989 Review Course Lectures, p 59. Cleveland, International Anesthesia Research Society, 1989.)

lows, time cycled, fluidically controlled, tidal volume preset ventilators that are generally used in the control mode. All use a Venturi entrainment device drive-gas system. The entrained room air provides additional flow to the bellows chamber without substantially decreasing the oxygen supply pressure within the anesthesia machine.[98-102]

Pneumatic ventilators have several advantages. They require only a pneumatic power source. Therefore, they can be used effectively during an electrical power failure or in remote areas without electricity. The functional design of pneumatic ventilators is simple, and they are easy to operate. Most are mobile, freestanding units that can readily be moved from room to room. The fluidic control components have no moving parts and depend solely on gas flow and pressure to function. Maintenance is minimal, and an electrical background is not necessary to service the ventilators.

Disadvantages of pneumatic ventilators, however, outweigh the advantages. The major disadvantage is a possible unrecognized disconnection. This results from the descending bellows configuration coupled with a relatively low factory preset disconnection threshold pressure alarm limit such as 8–10 cm water pressure. Most pneumatic ventilators have only one alarm: the low-pressure disconnection alarm. This is in marked contrast to newer electronic ventilators, which may have multiple alarms. Finally, pneumatic

ventilators have a limited number of controls and lack versatility.

Electronic Ventilators

Contemporary electronic anesthesia machine ventilators, such as the North American Dräger AV-E, the Ohmeda 7000, and the Ohmeda 7810, are an integral portion of the global anesthesia system. Each is discussed below.

North American Dräger AV-E Anesthesia Ventilator

The North American Dräger AV-E is classified as a pneumatically and electronically powered, double-circuit, pneumatically driven, ascending bellows, time cycled, electronically controlled, tidal volume preset controller ventilator. The AV-E is standard equipment on contemporary North American Dräger anesthesia machines, and it is not available as a freestanding ventilator. It consists of two major components: the control assembly and the bellows assembly. The control assembly contains the electronic and pneumatic components of the ventilator. It is located above the flow meters and vaporizers, and it serves as a permanent shelf. The control assembly houses four controls. They include

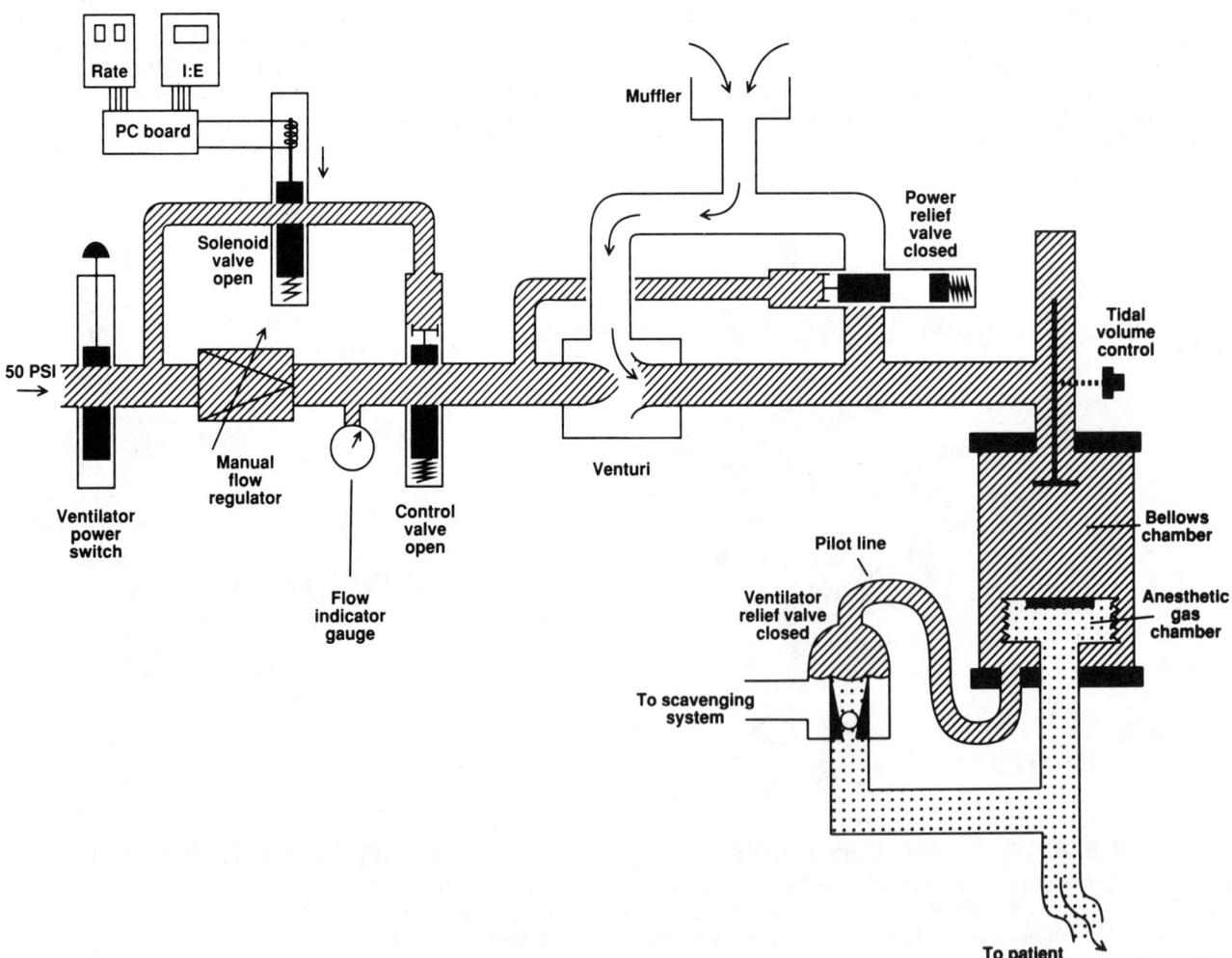

Figure 25-30. Inspiratory phase gas flows of the North American Dräger Av-E. See text for details.

the ventilator power switch, the frequency control, the I:E ratio control, and the inspiratory flow control. The bellows assembly is located to the left of the flow meters. The tidal volume scale on the plastic bellows housing ranges from 200 to 1400 ml, and it increases from bottom to top. The tidal volume adjustment knob is above the bellows chamber. Adjustment of the knob determines the location of the bellows stop, which limits the upward movement of the bellows within the bellows chamber to the desired tidal volume. The ventilator relief valve is behind the bellows chamber. The operator can observe the action of this valve because its dome is constructed of clear plastic.[15-19]

The operating principle of the AV-E is illustrated in Figures 25-30 and 25-31. Oxygen at 50 psig provides the pneumatic input to the driving gas circuit. Flow through this circuit is regulated by a solenoid valve that serves as an interface between the pneumatic and electric circuits of the ventilator. The electronic timing of the solenoid is determined by the settings of the frequency and I:E ratio controls. It is open during the inspiratory phase and closed during the expiratory phase.[15]

Inspiratory phase gas flows are illustrated in Figure 25-30. Oxygen at 50 psig passes through the solenoid valve and opens the control valve. This allows the preset gas flow from the flow regulator to proceed through the control valve to

the Venturi entrainment device. Back pressure from the Venturi device is directed to the power relief valve and closes it. Then oxygen from the flow regulator passes through the Venturi device, and a substantial volume of room air is entrained through the muffler. The flow of the driving gas increases considerably without depleting the oxygen pressure within the anesthesia machine because a Venturi device is used.[15]

The driving gas is forced into the bellows chamber, causing the pressure within it to increase. The pressure increases, resulting in two events. First, the ventilator relief valve closes. This prevents anesthetic gas from escaping into the scavenging system. Second, the bellows is compressed downward, and the anesthetic gas within the bellows is delivered to the patient's lungs. The ventilator relief valve remains closed as long as the bellows chamber contains pressure. The inspiratory pause time starts when the bellows is completely compressed, and it lasts until the bellows begins to ascend. The pressure in the bellows chamber, as preset by the flow regulator, cannot increase further. All excess pressure is released through the Venturi device entrainment port, and the Venturi device simultaneously ceases to entrain room air.[15] The volume of driving gas that enters and exits the bellows chamber during the inspiratory phase may be substantially greater than the tidal volume

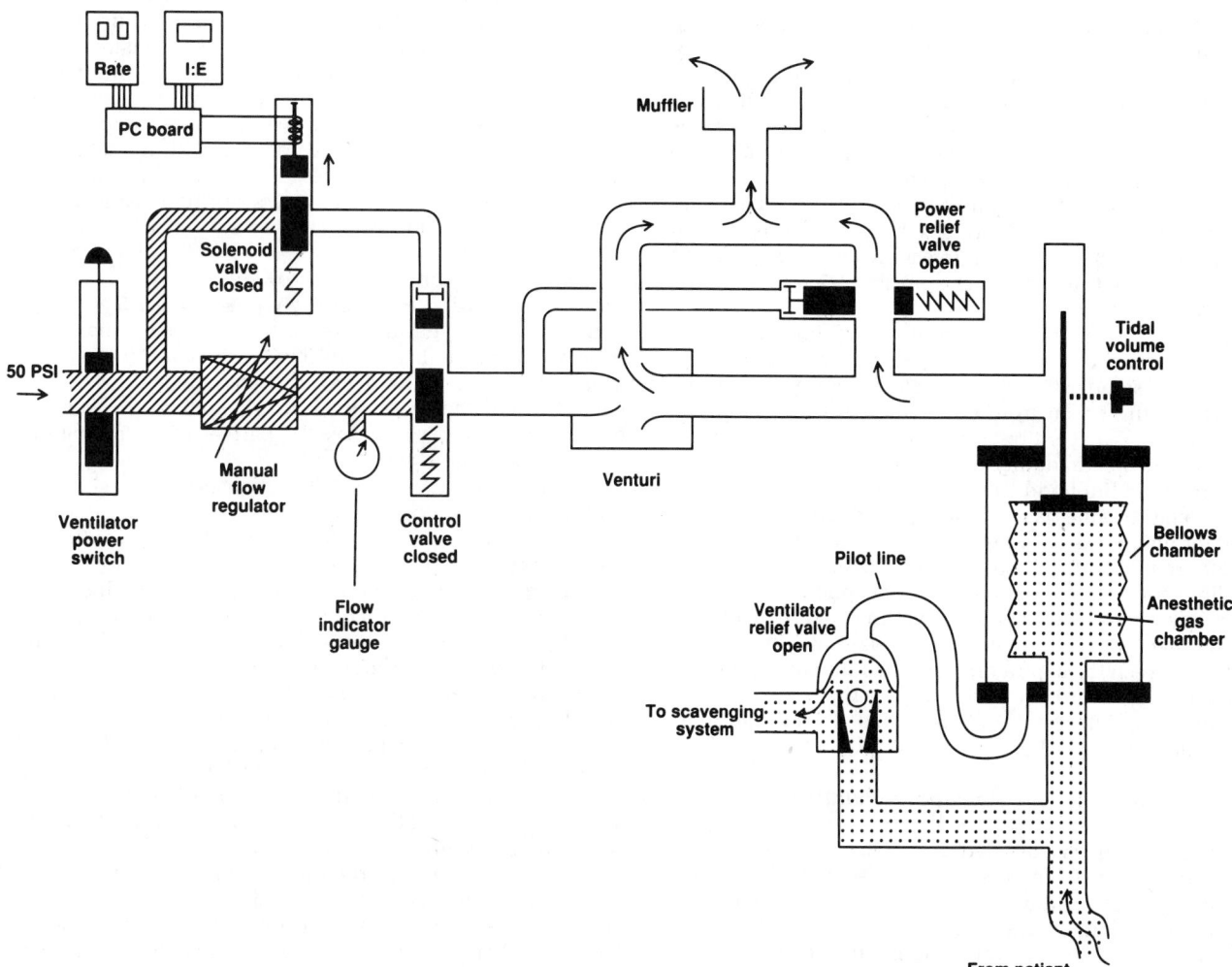

Figure 25-31. Expiratory phase gas flows of the North American Dräger AV-E. See text for details.

delivered. This is particularly true with slow rates and with prolonged inspiratory pause times.

The expiratory phase gas flows of the North American Dräger AV-E are shown in Figure 25-31. The expiratory phase begins when the electrical signal to the solenoid terminates. As soon as the electrical signal stops, the solenoid valve closes. This closure terminates the 50 psig gas supply to the control valve, which also closes. The preset gas flow from the flow regulator is interrupted by the control valve. This causes an immediate pressure decrease at the Venturi device, and no back pressure is supplied to the power relief valve, which opens. Then the driving gas within the bellows chamber can exit through the power relief valve and through the entrainment port of the Venturi device.[15] Regardless of the route taken, all driving gas is discharged through the ventilator muffler.

The pressure within the bellows chamber and in the pilot line declines to zero, causing the mushroom portion of the ventilator relief valve to open. To prevent premature outflow of anesthetic gas into the scavenging system, a weighted ball similar to those used in ball-type positive end–expiratory pressure valves is incorporated into the base of the ventilator relief valve. The ball produces 2 cm water back pressure. Thus the bellows extends fully, and 2 cm water pressure develops within the bellows chamber before anesthetic gas enters the scavenging system.[15]

Global examination of the inspiratory and expiratory gas flows of the North American Dräger AV-E reveals the importance of a clean, functional muffler. Much of the driving gas is entrained through the muffler during the inspiratory phase. All the driving gas exits through the muffler during the expiratory phase. Pressure within the bellows chamber and within the pilot line increases if the muffler becomes occluded. The ventilator relief valve remains closed if there is pressure within the bellows chamber. As a result, excess anesthetic gas cannot vent into the scavenging system, and patient airway pressure increases.[105] Two alarms should quickly alert the anesthesiologist when this scenario occurs—the continuing system pressure alarm and the high-pressure alarm.

Two ventilator monitors are available on the Narkomed 2B and Narkomed 3. The breathing pressure monitor, or Baromed, is standard equipment. Pressure input from the patient circuit can be from either the carbon dioxide absorber or the Y-piece. Pressure versus time waveforms are displayed on a cathode ray tube. The operator sets a high-pressure alarm limit and a threshold pressure alarm limit if preset default values are not acceptable. Alarms are provided for high pressure, pressure below the threshold for 15 and 30 seconds (apnea), continuing pressure above the set threshold for 15 seconds, and subatmospheric (≤ -10 cm water) pressure. The respiratory volume monitor, or Spiromed, is an optional monitor. The tidal volume sensor is located between the expiratory valve and the carbon dioxide absorber. Alarms are provided for low tidal volume (<70 ml), high respiratory rate (>99 breaths per minute), and reverse flow through the sensor (>20 ml).[17,18]

Ohmeda 7000 Electronic Anesthesia Ventilator

The Ohmeda 7000 is classified as a pneumatically and electronically powered, double-circuit, pneumatically driven, ascending bellows, time cycled, electronically controlled, and minute volume preset controller. It consists of two units: the control module and the bellows assembly. The control module is mounted above the flow meters on the

Ohmeda Modulus II. It has six controls, including the minute volume dial, the rate dial, the I:E ratio dial, the power switch, a sigh switch, and a manual cycle button. A tidal volume dial is not present on the Ohmeda 7000. The control module automatically calculates the tidal volume according to the setting of the minute volume and rate dials. The bellows assembly is mounted directly on the Ohmeda Gas Management System absorber using an interface manifold. The scale on the plastic bellows housing has a range of 100–1600 ml, and it increases from top to bottom. The ventilator relief valve cannot be seen during ventilator operation because it is inside the bellows assembly base.[103,104]

The operating principle of the Ohmeda 7000 is similar to that of the North American Dräger AV-E. Figure 25-32 is a schematic of the pneumatic circuitry of the Ohmeda 7000. The driving gas supply is 100% oxygen at 50 psig. A precision regulator reduces this pressure to 38 psig $\pm$ 0.5 psig. The regulated gas supply connects directly to a manifold of five solenoid valves. The control box electronically regulates the solenoid valves during the inspiratory time. Gas flow is directed through tuned orifices, which are calibrated for flows of 2, 4, 6, 8, 16, and 32 $l \cdot min^{-1}$. The range of flow selection is in 2 $l \cdot min^{-1}$ increments from 4 $l \cdot min^{-1}$ to 60 $l \cdot min^{-1}$. A precise volume of driving gas equal to the tidal volume is delivered to the bellows chamber at a specific rate, depending on the ventilator settings.[103,104]

During the inspiratory phase (Fig. 25-33 left), the control module delivers its computed driving gas flow into the bellows chamber. The bellows is compressed as the driving gas volume and pressure increase within the housing. Anesthetic gas is forced out of the bellows, through the patient circuit, and into the patient's lungs. Flow stops when the full volume of driving gas has been delivered into the bellows chamber. A relief valve located within the control module opens and vents excess driving gas into the atmosphere if excessive pressure occurs during the inspiratory phase. The threshold for this relief valve is 65 cm of water pressure.[103,104]

Anesthetic gas enters the bellows chamber from the patient circuit during the expiratory phase (Fig. 25-33 center and right). The ventilator relief valve, located inside the bellows chamber, has a threshold value of 2.5 cm water pressure. Therefore, it opens only when the bellows is fully extended and the pressure within the bellows exceeds 2.5 cm water pressure. Then, excess patient gas is popped off into the scavenging system.[103,104]

The operating principle of the Ohmeda 7000 is similar to that of the North American Dräger AV-E, but some differences exist. The Ohmeda 7000 does not use a Venturi device, and the driving gas is composed of 100% oxygen. Driving gas inflow rate is regulated by five solenoids instead of one. The Ohmeda 7000 control module delivers a precise driving gas volume to the bellows assembly, which displaces the bellows by the same amount. Therefore, the driving gas volume equals the tidal volume, and the bellows is only partially compressed during the inspiratory phase. North American Dräger's tidal volume, on the other hand, is derived from the position of a mechanical bellows stop. The driving gas volume may be substantially larger than the set tidal volume, and the bellows is fully compressed during inspiration. Because the two ventilators generate tidal volume by different means, the tidal volume scale on the plastic bellows housing differs on each one. On the Ohmeda 7000, the scale increases from top to bottom, whereas on the North American Dräger AV-E it increases from bottom to top.[15-19,103,104]

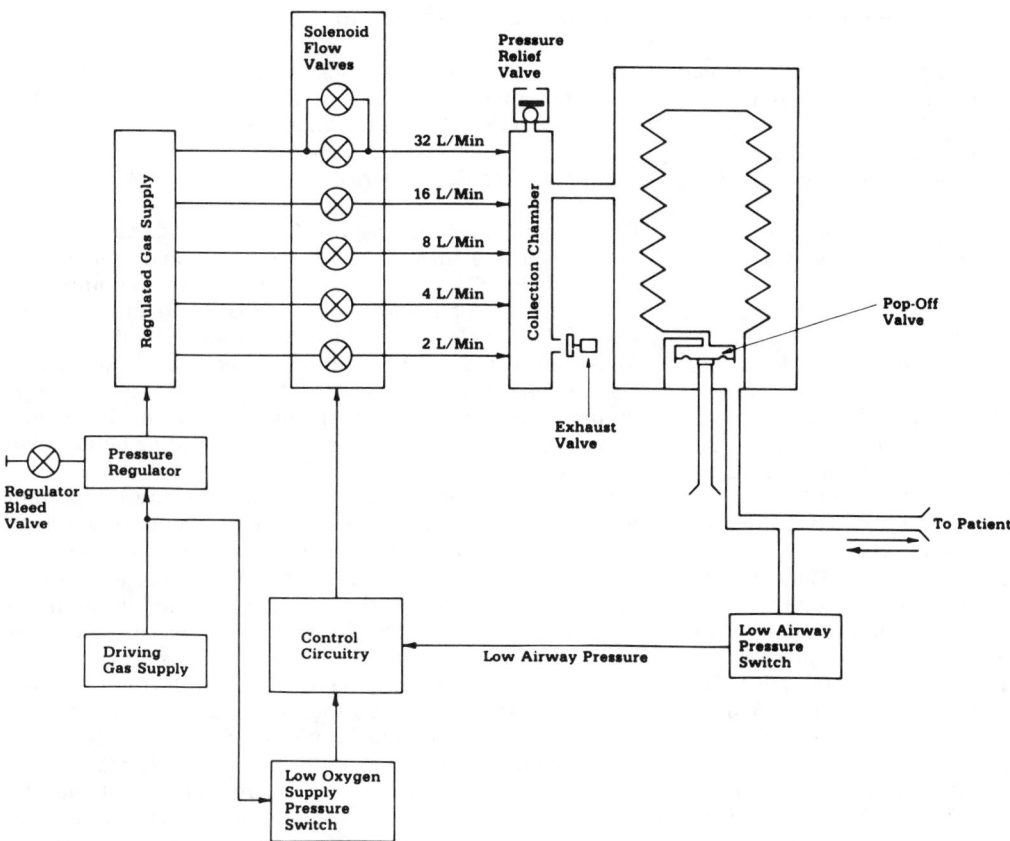

Figure 25-32. Diagram of the Ohmeda 7000 electronic anesthesia ventilator. See text for details. (Courtesy of Ohmeda, A Division of BOC Health Care, Inc, Madison, Wisconsin.)

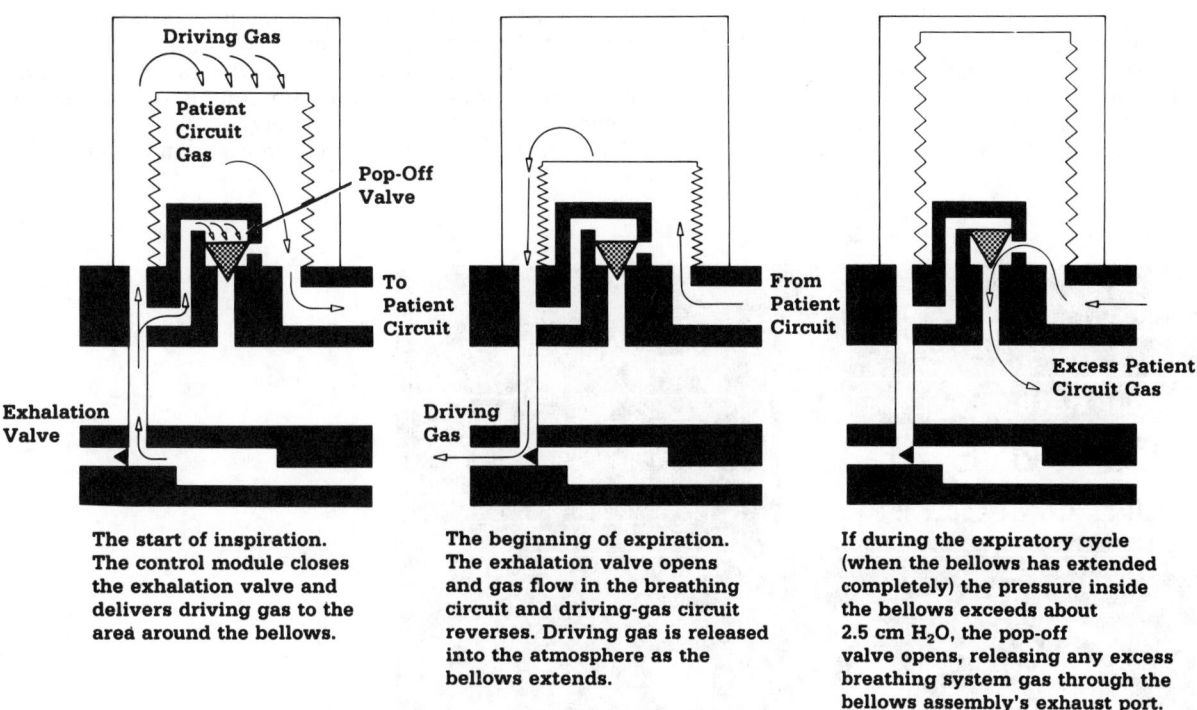

The start of inspiration. The control module closes the exhalation valve and delivers driving gas to the area around the bellows.

The beginning of expiration. The exhalation valve opens and gas flow in the breathing circuit and driving-gas circuit reverses. Driving gas is released into the atmosphere as the bellows extends.

If during the expiratory cycle (when the bellows has extended completely) the pressure inside the bellows exceeds about 2.5 cm H_2O, the pop-off valve opens, releasing any excess breathing system gas through the bellows assembly's exhaust port.

Figure 25-33. Inspiratory and expiratory phase gas flows of the Ohmeda 7000 and 7810 electronic anesthesia ventilator. See text for details. (Courtesy of Ohmeda, A Division of BOC Health Care, Inc, Madison, Wisconsin.)

Ohmeda 7810 Electronic Anesthesia Ventilator

The Ohmeda 7810 is standard equipment on the Ohmeda Modulus II Plus anesthesia system. It is classified as a pneumatically and electronically powered, double-circuit, pneumatically driven, ascending bellows, time cycled, electronically controlled, tidal volume preset, pressure limited controller. The 7810 serves not only as a ventilator but also as an oxygen analyzer, an airway pressure monitor, and a volume monitor. It combines these monitors and provides an integrated ventilator alarm system.[13]

The Ohmeda 7810 consists of two basic units: the control module and the bellows assembly. The bellows assembly of the 7810 is almost identical to that of the 7000, but the control module is substantially different. The control module of the 7810 (Fig. 25-34) has four dials, including the tidal volume dial, the rate dial, the inspiratory flow dial, and the inspiratory pressure limit dial. Other controls include the inspiratory pause button, the ventilator on/off switch, the alarm set pushwheels, the oxygen calibration thumbwheel, and the alarm silence button.[13]

The operating principle of the Ohmeda 7810 is very similar to that of the Ohmeda 7000, but the 7810 is more versatile. Many operators prefer the tidal volume preset feature of the 7810 compared with the minute volume preset of the 7000. The 7810 has more flexibility regarding I:E ratios. The 7000 is limited to I:E ratios of 1:1 through 1:3. The 7810, on the other hand, has a much broader continuum of I:E ratios that range from 1:0.33 (reverse I:E ratio) through 1:999. The 7810 has an inspiratory pause feature that increases the inspiration time by 25%. The 7000 does not have this feature. Probably the biggest advantage of the 7810 over the 7000 is the pressure limiting feature. The 7810 uses an operator adjustable, electronically controlled, automatic high-pressure relief system to manage excessive airway pressure. If the airway pressure exceeds the high-pressure threshold set by the operator, two events take place. The high-pressure alarm is activated, and the ventilator automatically releases the remaining driving gas into the atmosphere, terminating the inspiratory cycle. Active intervention is not required by the operator. If the high-pressure threshold is set appropriately, the possibility of barotrauma is minimized.[13,103,104]

Problems and Hazards

Numerous hazards are associated with anesthesia ventilators. They include problems with the breathing circuit, the bellows assembly, and the control assembly.

Breathing Circuit Problems

Breathing circuit disconnection is a leading cause of critical incidents in anesthesia.[106] The most common disconnection site is at the Y-piece. Disconnections can be complete or partial (leaks). A common source of leaks with older absorbers is failure to close the Adjustable Pressure Limiting Valve (or pop-off valve) upon initiation of mechanical ventilation. The bag/ventilator switch on contemporary absorbers helps minimize this problem. As mentioned above, disconnections manifest more readily with the ascending bellows because the bellows will not fill.[1]

Several disconnection monitors exist. The most important monitor is a vigilant anesthesiologist monitoring breath sounds, chest wall excursion, and mechanical monitors.

Pneumatic and electronic pressure monitors are helpful in diagnosing disconnections. Factors that influence monitor effectiveness include the disconnection site, the pressure sensor location, the threshold pressure alarm limit, the inspiratory flow rate, and the resistance of the disconnected breathing circuit.[107,108] Various anesthesia machines and ventilators have different locations for the pressure sensor and different values for the threshold pressure alarm limit (Table 25-1). The threshold pressure alarm limit may be factory preset or adjustable. An audible or visual alarm is actuated if the peak inspiratory pressure of the breathing circuit does not exceed the threshold pressure alarm limit. When an adjustable threshold pressure alarm limit is available, such as on the North American Dräger Narkomed 2A, 2B, 3, and 4, the operator should set the pressure alarm limit to within 5 cm water below the peak inspiratory pressure.[15-19] Figure 25-35 illustrates how a partial disconnection (leak) may be unrecognized by the low-pressure monitor if the threshold pressure alarm limit is set too low or if the factory preset value is relatively low.

Respiratory volume monitors are useful in detecting dis-

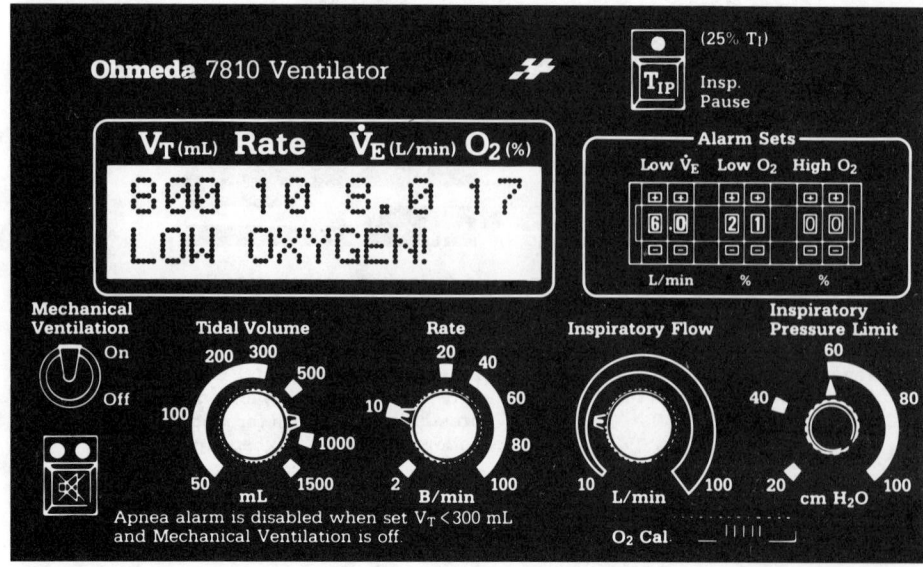

Figure 25-34. Ohmeda 7810 control assembly. (Courtesy of Ohmeda, A Division of BOC Health Care, Inc, Madison, Wisconsin.)

TABLE 25-1. Disconnection Pressure Monitors[8-10,13,15-18,98-104]

Machine/Ventilator	Location of Pressure Sensor	Threshold Pressure Alarm Limit (cm water)
Ohio Modulus I		
Model 21 Absorber	Patient side of expiratory valve	
Ohio Anesth Vent		10
Ohio V5 or V5A		8
Ohmeda Modulus II		
GMS Absorber	Patient side of expiratory valve	
Ohmeda 7000 Ventilator		6
Ohmeda Modulus II Plus		
GMS Absorber	Patient side of inspiratory valve	Δ4–9
Ohmeda 7810		PEEP* compensated
Dräger Narkomed 2A	CO₂ absorber or Y-piece	
Dräger AV-E		8, 12, 26
Dräger Narkomed 2B, 3	CO₂ absorber or Y-piece	5→30
Dräger AV-E		(12 default)

*PEEP = positive end–expiratory pressure.

connections. Volume monitors sense exhaled tidal volume, minute volume, or both. The user should bracket the high and low threshold volumes slightly above and below the exhaled volumes. For example, if the exhaled minute volume of a patient is $10 \ l \cdot min^{-1}$, reasonable alarm limits would be $8-12 \ l \cdot min^{-1}$.

Carbon dioxide monitors are probably the best devices to reveal patient disconnections. Carbon dioxide concentration is measured near the Y-piece either directly or by aspiration of a gas sample to the instrument. A drastic change in the difference between the inspiratory and end-tidal CO_2

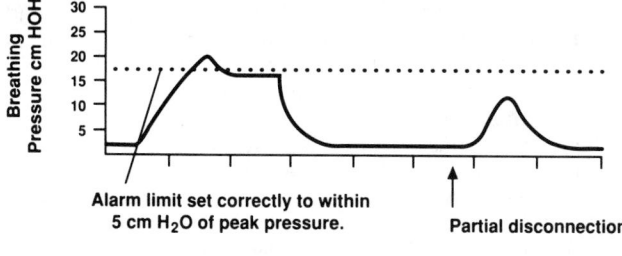

Alarm limit set correctly to within 5 cm H₂O of peak pressure.

Partial disconnection

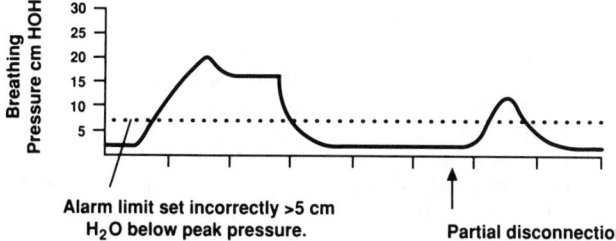

Alarm limit set incorrectly >5 cm H₂O below peak pressure.

Partial disconnection

Figure 25-35. Threshold pressure alarm limit. (*Top*) The threshold pressure alarm limit (*dotted line*) has been set appropriately. An alarm is actuated when a partial disconnection occurs (*arrow*) because the threshold pressure alarm limit is not exceeded by the breathing circuit pressure. (*Bottom*) A partial disconnection is unrecognized by the pressure monitor because the threshold pressure alarm limit has been set too low. (Redrawn with permission from Baromed Breathing Pressure Monitor. Operator's Instruction Manual. Telford, Pennsylvania, North American Dräger, August, 1986.)

concentration or the absence of CO_2 indicates a disconnection, a nonventilated patient, or other problems.[1]

Misconnections of the breathing system are not uncommon, despite efforts by standards committees to eliminate this problem by assigning different diameters to various hoses and terminals. Anesthesia machines, breathing systems, ventilators, and scavenging systems incorporate a multitude of hose terminals. Hoses have been connected to inappropriate terminals and even to various solid cylindrically shaped protrusions of the anesthesia machine.[1]

Occlusion (obstruction) of the breathing circuit may occur. Tracheal tubes can become kinked. Hoses throughout the breathing circuit are subject to occlusion by external mechanical forces that can impinge upon flow. Incorrect insertion of flow direction–sensitive components can result in a no-flow state.[1] Examples of these components include some positive end–expiratory pressure valves and cascade humidifiers. Depending on the location of the occlusion and the pressure sensor, a high-pressure alarm may alert the anesthesiologist to the problem.

Excess inflow to the breathing circuit from the anesthesia machine during the inspiratory phase can result in barotrauma. The best example of this phenomenon is oxygen flushing. Excess volume cannot be vented from the system during inspiration because the ventilator relief valve is closed and the Adjustable Pressure Limiting Valve is either out of circuit or closed.[34] A high-pressure alarm, if present, may be activated when the pressure becomes excessive. In the North American Dräger System, both audible and visual alarms are actuated when the high-pressure threshold is exceeded.[15-19] In the Modulus II Plus System, the Ohmeda 7810 ventilator automatically switches from the inspiratory to the expiratory phase when the adjustable peak pressure threshold is exceeded.[13] This minimizes the possibilities of barotrauma if the peak pressure threshold is set appropriately by the anesthesiologist.

Bellows Assembly Problems

Leaks can occur in the bellows assembly. Improper seating of the plastic bellows housing can result in inadequate ventilation because a portion of the driving gas is vented to the atmosphere. A hole in the bellows can lead to alveolar hyperinflation and possibly barotrauma in some ventilators because high-pressure driving gas can enter the patient circuit. The value on the oxygen analyzer may increase when the driving gas is 100% oxygen, or it may decrease if the driving gas is composed of an air-oxygen mixture.[109]

The ventilator relief valve can cause problems. Hypoventilation occurs if the valve is incompetent because anesthetic gas is delivered to the scavenging system during the inspiratory phase instead of to the patient. Gas molecules preferentially exit into the scavenging system because it represents the path of least resistance, and the pressure within the scavenging system can be subatmospheric. Ventilator relief valve incompetency can result from a disconnected pilot line, a ruptured valve, or a damaged flapper valve.[110,111] A ventilator relief valve stuck in the closed position can produce barotrauma. Excessive suction from the scavenging system can draw the ventilator relief valve to its seat and close the valve during both the inspiratory and expiratory phases.[1] Breathing circuit pressure escalates because excess anesthetic gas cannot be vented.

Control Assembly Problems

The control assembly can be the source of both electrical and mechanical problems. Electrical failure can be total or partial; the former is the more obvious. Some mechanical problems include leaks within the system, faulty regulators, and faulty valves. As mentioned previously, an occluded muffler can result in barotrauma (see the section on the North American Dräger AV-E). Obstruction of driving gas outflow closes the ventilator relief valve, and excess patient gas cannot be vented.[105]

SCAVENGING SYSTEMS

Scavenging is the collection and the subsequent removal of vented gases from the operating room.[113] Commonly, the amount of gas used to anesthetize a patient far exceeds the patient's needs. Therefore, scavenging minimizes operating room pollution. In 1982 the ANSI released the Z79.11-1982 guideline entitled "Scavenging Systems for Excess Anesthetic Gases." The document provided guidelines to manufacturers so that they could produce devices that safely and effectively scavenge excess anesthetic gas in order to reduce contamination in anesthetizing areas.[112]

Components

Scavenging systems have five components: (1) the gas collecting assembly, (2) the transfer tubing, (3) the scavenging interface, (4) the gas disposal tubing, and (5) an active or passive gas disposal assembly.[112] An active system uses a central vacuum to eliminate waste gases. The pressure of the waste gas itself produces flow through a passive system.

Gas Collection Assembly

The gas collection assembly captures excess anesthetic gas and delivers it to the transfer tubing.[112] Excess gas is vented from anesthesia systems through the Adjustable Pressure Limiting Valve and through the ventilator relief valve. All excess gas passes through these valves, accumulates in the

gas collection assembly, and is directed to the transfer tubing.

Transfer Tubing

The transfer tubing carries excess gas from the gas collecting assembly to the scavenging interface. The tubing must be either 19 mm or 30 mm, as specified by the ANSI Z79.11-1982 standard.[112] The tubing should be sufficiently rigid to prevent kinking, and it should be as short as possible to minimize the chance of occlusion. Some manufacturers color code the transfer tubing with yellow bands to distinguish it from 22-mm breathing system tubing. Many machines have separate transfer tubes for the Adjustable Pressure Limiting Valve and for the ventilator relief valve. The two are frequently "Y"ed together before they enter the scavenging interface.

Scavenging Interface

The scavenging interface is the most important component of the system because it protects the breathing circuit or ventilator from excessive positive or negative pressure.[113] The interface should limit the pressures immediately downstream from the gas collection assembly to between −0.5 and +10 cm water with normal working conditions.[112] Positive pressure relief is mandatory, irrespective of the type of disposal system used, to vent excess gas in case of occlusion downstream from the interface. If the disposal system is active (i.e., uses a vacuum), negative pressure relief is necessary to protect the breathing circuit or ventilator from excessive subatmospheric pressure. A reservoir is highly desirable with active systems, since it stores excess waste gas until the evacuation system can eliminate it. Interfaces can be open or closed, depending on the method used to provide positive and negative pressure relief.[113]

Open Interfaces. An open interface contains no valves and it is open to the atmosphere, allowing both positive and negative pressure relief. Open interfaces should be used only with active disposal systems that use a central vacuum system. Open interfaces require a reservoir because waste gases are intermittently discharged in surges, whereas flow to the active disposal system is continuous.[113]

Figure 25-36 shows four types of open interfaces used with active systems. The simplest is a T-tube shown in Figure 25-36A. Waste gas enters the top of the T-tube through the transfer tubing. Some of the gas is scavenged immediately to the active disposal system, whereas another portion collects in the reservoir tubing. The gas in the reservoir is subsequently removed between breaths. Positive relief and negative relief occur at the distal end of the reservoir tube. A safety hole in the reservoir provides positive and negative pressure relief if the distal end becomes occluded. Figure 25-36B is a coaxial system composed of a small inner tube and a large, corrugated outer tube. The proximal end of the small tube is open to the outer reservoir tube, and the distal end is connected to the active disposal system. Positive and negative relief occurs at the distal end of the corrugated hose, which is open to the atmosphere.[113]

Many contemporary anesthesia machines are equipped with open interfaces like those in Figure 25-36C and D.[114] An open canister provides reservoir capacity. The canister volume should be large enough to accommodate a variety of waste gas flow rates. Gas enters the system at the top of the canister and travels through a narrow inner tube to the

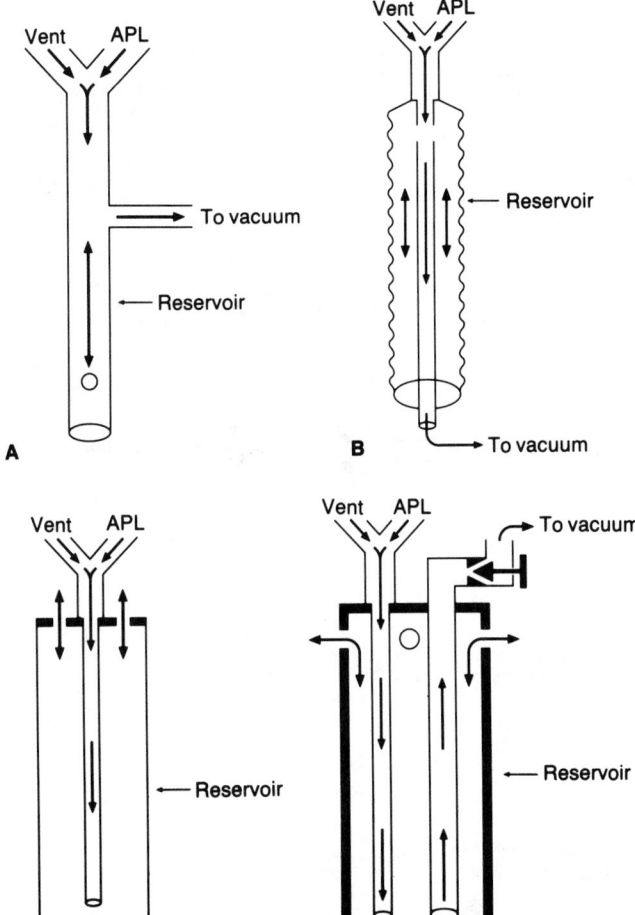

Figure 25-36. Open scavenging interfaces. Each requires an active disposal system. APL = Adjustable Pressure Limiting Valve. See text for details. (Modified with permission from Dorsch JA, Dorsch SE: Controlling trace gas levels. In Dorsch JA, Dorsch SE (eds): Understanding Anesthesia Equipment, 2nd ed, p 258. Baltimore, Williams & Wilkins, 1984.)

canister base. Gases are stored in the reservoir between breaths. Positive and negative relief is provided by holes in the top of the canister. The open interface shown in C differs somewhat from the one shown in D. The operator can regulate the vacuum by adjusting the vacuum control valve in D.[114]

The efficiency of an open interface depends upon several factors. The vacuum flow rate per minute must equal or exceed the minute volume of excess gases to prevent spillage. The volume of the reservoir and the flow characteristics within the interface are important. Spillage will occur if the volume of a single exhaled breath exceeds the capacity of the reservoir. Leakage can occur long before the volume of waste gas delivered to the reservoir equals the reservoir volume if large-scale turbulence occurs within the interface.[115]

Closed Interfaces. A closed interface communicates with the atmosphere through valves. All closed interfaces must have a positive pressure relief valve to vent excess system pressure if obstruction occurs downstream from the interface. A negative pressure relief valve is mandatory to protect

the breathing system from subatmospheric pressure if an active disposal system is used.[113] Two types of closed interfaces are commercially available. One has positive pressure relief only; the other has both positive and negative relief. Each type is discussed below.

Positive Pressure Relief Only. This interface (Fig. 25-37 left) has a single positive pressure relief valve and is designed to be used only with passive disposal systems. Waste gas enters the interface at the waste gas inlets. Transfer of the waste gas from the interface to the disposal system relies upon the pressure of the waste gas itself, since a vacuum is not used. The positive pressure relief valve opens at a preset value such as 5 cm water if an obstruction between the interface and the disposal system occurs.[116] A reservoir bag is not necessary.

Positive and Negative Pressure Relief. This interface has a positive pressure relief valve, at least one negative pressure relief valve, and a reservoir bag. It is used with active disposal systems. Figure 25-37 (right) is a schematic of North American Dräger's closed interface for suction systems. A variable volume of waste gas intermittently enters the interface through the waste gas inlets. The reservoir stores transient excess gas until the vacuum system eliminates it. The operator should adjust the vacuum control valve so that the reservoir bag is properly inflated (A) and not overdistended (B) or completely deflated (C). Gas is vented to the atmosphere through the positive pressure relief valve if the system pressure exceeds +5 cm H_2O. Room air is entrained through the negative pressure relief valve if the system pressure is more negative than −0.5 cm H_2O. A back-up negative pressure relief valve opens at −1.8 cm H_2O if the primary negative pressure relief valve becomes occluded.[15]

The effectiveness of a closed system in preventing spillage depends on the inflow rate of excess gas, the vacuum flow rate, and the volume of the reservoir. Leakage of waste gases into the atmosphere occurs only when the reservoir bag becomes fully inflated and the pressure increases sufficiently to open the positive pressure relief valve. In contrast, the effectiveness of an open system to prevent spillage depends not only on the volume of the reservoir but also on the flow characteristics within the interface.[115]

Gas Disposal Tubing

The gas disposal tubing conducts waste gas from the scavenging interface to the gas disposal assembly. It should be collapse-proof and should run overhead if possible to minimize the chance of occlusion.[112]

Gas Disposal Assembly

The gas disposal assembly ultimately eliminates excess waste gas. There are two types of disposal systems: active and passive.

The most common method for gas disposal is the active assembly, which uses a central vacuum. An interface with a negative pressure relief is mandatory because the pressure within the system is negative. A reservoir is very desirable, and the larger the reservoir, the lower the suction flow rate needed.[113,115]

A passive disposal system uses the pressure of the waste gas itself to produce flow through the system. Positive pressure relief is mandatory, but negative pressure relief and a reservoir are unnecessary. Excess waste gas can be elimi-

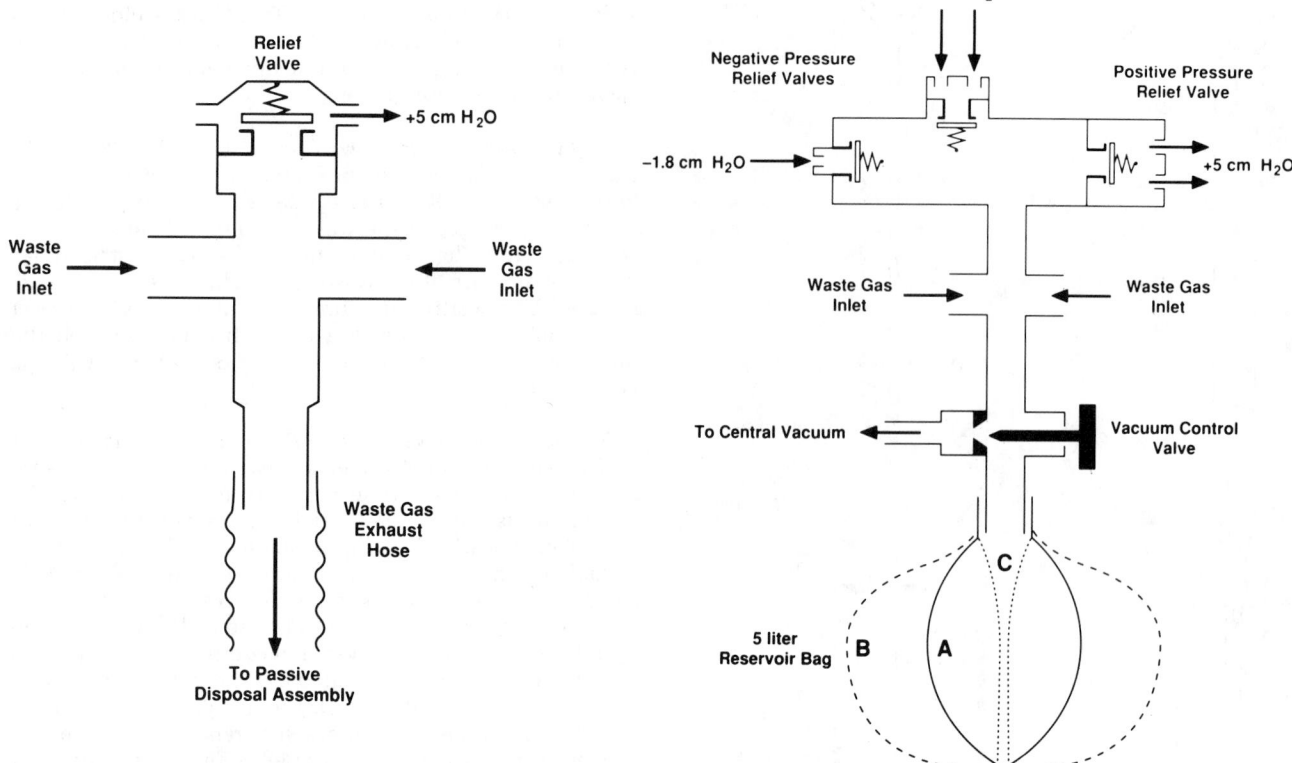

Figure 25-37. Closed scavenging interfaces. (*Left*) Interface used with a passive disposal system. (*Right*) Interface used with an active system. See text for details. (Modified with permission (*left*) from Scavenger Interface for Air Conditioning. Instruction Manual. Telford, Pennsylvania, North American Dräger, October 1984; (*right*) from Narkomed 2A Anesthesia System. Technical Service Manual. Telford, Pennsylvania. North American Dräger, 1985.)

nated in a number of ways, including venting through the wall, ceiling, or floor or to the room exhaust grill of a nonrecirculating air conditioning system.[113,115]

Hazards

Scavenging systems minimize operating room pollution, but they add complexity to the anesthesia system. A scavenging system extends the anesthesia circuit all the way from the anesthesia machine to the ultimate disposal site. This extension increases the potential for problems. Pressure alterations produced by obstruction or unopposed vacuum can be transferred to the anesthesia circuit and can potentially harm the patient.[115] Hazards associated with scavenging are discussed below.

Transmission of Excessive Positive Pressure to the Breathing System

Obstruction of scavenging pathways can cause excessive positive pressure to be transmitted to the breathing system. Some causes for obstruction include (1) compression of flexible tubing by wheels of the anesthesia machine,[117-119] (2) kinking of flexible tubing,[120] (3) plugging of a gas disposal tube with ice,[121] and (4) misassembling of the exhaust connector of a passive disposal system.[122] Obstruction can occur anywhere in the scavenging system, but it is particularly hazardous if an obstruction occurs upstream from the

scavenging interface because excess patient gas cannot be vented. Obstruction downstream from the interface is a smaller problem because excess gas will pop off through the positive pressure relief of the interface and not jeopardize the patient.[120]

Prior to the implementation of the ANSI Z79.11-1982 standard, a specific type of circle system misconnection was another cause of dangerously high pressure. The 22-mm expiratory hose of the circle system was incorrectly connected to the exhaust port of the Adjustable Pressure Limiting Valve rather than to the expiratory port of the carbon dioxide absorber.[118,123,124] This configuration prevented venting of excess gas, and therefore the pressure rapidly increased. This hazard was minimized when the ANSI Z79.11-1982 standard mandated either a 19-mm or 30-mm male fitting for the outlet of the gas collection assembly.[112]

Application of Excessive Negative Pressure to the Breathing System

Excessive negative pressure can be applied to the breathing system if an active disposal system is used.[113] This condition can occur if the negative pressure relief valve or port becomes obstructed or if the vacuum flow rate is excessive. Obstruction of the negative pressure relief valve or port can be caused by dust accumulation,[125] tape,[126] plastic bags,[127] or other objects. Mechanical problems can cause the valve to stick in the closed position.[128] Excessive vacuum can result from improper adjustment of the vacuum control knob on a closed scavenging interface or from misassembly of scavenging components.[129,130]

The ultimate consequences of applying excessive negative pressure to the breathing system depend on the design of the Adjustable Pressure Limiting Valve or the ventilator relief valve.[113,131] When a strong vacuum is applied to the exhaust side of some Adjustable Pressure Limiting Valves, gas flows across from the patient circuit to the vacuum. This causes the breathing bag to collapse, and excessive negative pressure can develop within the patient circuit.[125,128,129,131] Application of unopposed vacuum to the exhaust side of some diaphragm-type Adjustable Pressure Limiting Valves, on the other hand, can produce excessive positive pressure within the patient circuit. The subatmospheric pressure sucks the diaphragm against its seat, and flow across the valve ceases. Waste gas from the patient circuit cannot escape, and barotrauma can result.[1,16] A similar scenario can occur with some diaphragm-type ventilator relief valves. Excessive suction draws the ventilator relief diaphragm to its seat, and the valve closes. Excess gas cannot be scavenged, and barotrauma can result.[1,130]

Loss of Means of Monitoring

Ironically, scavenging systems have been blamed for being too effective. Inhaled anesthetic overdose was undetected in two cases because of the absence of smell of the anesthetic agent.[120,132] The efficient scavenging system concealed the strong odor of the inhaled anesthetic.

CHECKING ANESTHESIA MACHINES

A complete anesthesia apparatus checkout procedure should be performed each day before the first case. An abbreviated version should be performed before each subsequent case. Several checkout procedures exist, but the most popular one is the August 1986 Food and Drug Administration Anesthesia Apparatus Checkout Recommendations, reproduced in Appendix A.[133-136] The Food and Drug Administration checkout serves only as a generic guideline because the designs of different machines vary considerably. Also, many machines have been modified in the field. Therefore, specific checks must be performed on specific machines. The user must refer to the operator's manual for special procedures or precautions.

The three most important preoperative checks are (1) oxygen analyzer calibration, (2) the low-pressure circuit leak test, and (3) the circle system test. Each is discussed below.

Oxygen Analyzer Calibration

The oxygen analyzer is the most important machine monitor because it is the only machine safety device that evaluates the integrity of the low-pressure circuit. Other machine safety devices, such as the fail-safe system, the oxygen supply failure alarm, and the proportioning system, are all upstream from the flow control valves (see Fig. 25-3). The only machine monitor that detects problems downstream from the flow control valves is the oxygen analyzer. Calibration of this is described in the appendix of the Anesthesia Apparatus Checkout Recommendations, #13.

Low-Pressure Circuit Leak Test

The least well understood preoperative check is the low-pressure circuit leak test. (Appendix A, Anesthesia Apparatus Checkout Recommendations, #16). Several mishaps have resulted from application of the wrong leak test to the wrong machine.[29,64,137] Leaks in the low-pressure circuit can cause hypoxia or patient awareness under anesthesia.

The low-pressure leak test checks the integrity of the anesthesia machine from the flow control valves to the common outlet. It evaluates the portion of the machine that is downstream from all safety devices except the oxygen analyzer. The components located within this area are precisely the ones that are most subject to breakage and leaks. Flow tubes are the most delicate pneumatic components of the machine, and they can crack or break. A typical three-gas anesthesia machine has 16 O-rings in the low-pressure circuit. Leaks can occur at the interface between the glass flow tube and the manifold because of problems associated with O-rings and gaskets. Leaks can occur at the O-ring junction between the vaporizer and its manifold. Loose filler caps on vaporizers are a common source of leaks, and this can cause patient awareness.[138] Therefore, it is mandatory to perform the appropriate low-pressure leak test before every case. Many anesthesia machines have check valves located in the low-pressure circuit (Table 25-2). The presence or absence

TABLE 25-2. Check Valves and Recommended Leak Test[6-10,12-19]

Anesthesia Machine	Machine Outlet Check Valve	Vaporizer Outlet Check Valve	Leak Test Recommended by Manufacturer	
			Positive Pressure	Negative Pressure (Suction Bulb)
North American Dräger				
Narkomed 2A, 2B, 3, and 4	No	No	×	
Ohmeda Unitrol	Yes	Variable		×
Ohmeda 30/70	Yes	Variable		×
Ohmeda Modulus I	Yes	Variable		×
Ohmeda Modulus II	Yes	No		×
Ohmeda Excel Series	Yes	No		×
Ohmeda CD	No	No		×
Ohmeda Modulus II Plus	No	No		×

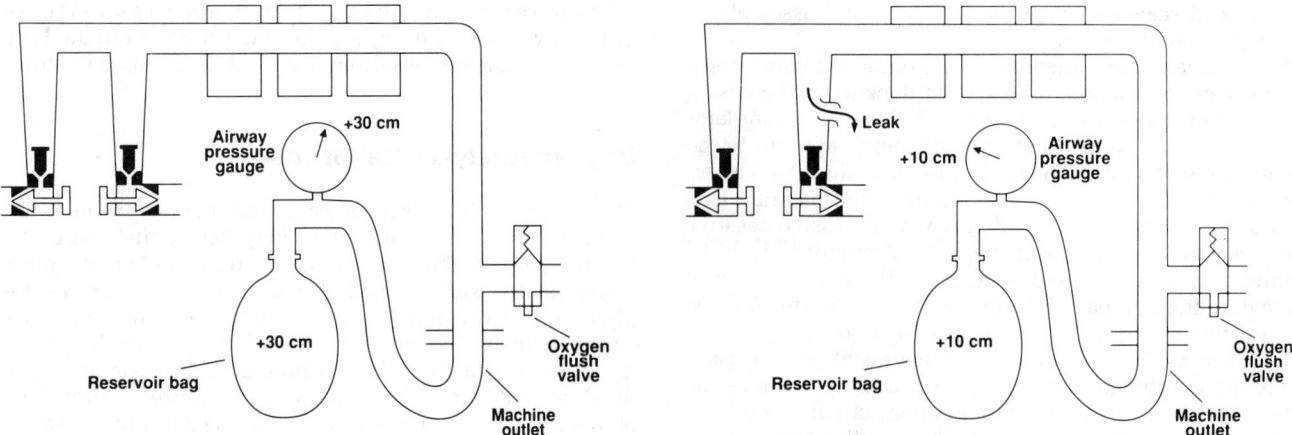

Figure 25-38. Traditional positive pressure leak test. (*Left*) An uninterrupted pipe is present from the flow control valves to the circle system airway pressure gauge. The value on the airway pressure gauge does not decline when the low-pressure circuit is leak-free. (*Right*) A leak in the low-pressure circuit is reflected by a decline in the value on the airway pressure gauge. (Reprinted with permission from Andrews JJ: Understanding anesthesia machines. In 1988 Review Course Lectures, p 78. Cleveland, International Anesthesia Research Society, 1988.)

of these check valves profoundly influences the type of leak test that should be used. Each is discussed as follows.

Machines Without Check Valves

A "traditional" positive pressure leak test using the circle system can be performed on machines that do not have check valves in the low-pressure circuitry (Table 25-2). The pop-off valve is closed, and the system is pressurized by use of the oxygen flush and flow from the oxygen flow control valve. The exact details of the test are outlined in Appendix A, Anesthesia Apparatus Checkout Recommendations, #16. An uninterrupted pipe is present from the flow control valves to the circle airway pressure gauge (Fig. 25-38). Therefore, a leak in the low-pressure circuit will be reflected by a decline in the value on the airway pressure gauge. This traditional test has two major advantages. First,

it does not require accessory test devices. Second, it can be performed quickly. The main disadvantage of the traditional test is its lack of sensitivity when compared with leak tests using special devices (see below). This lack of sensitivity occurs because the traditional test is volume-dependent. The pressurized volume in the breathing bag can mask leaks up to 250 ml·min^{-1}.

North American Dräger recommends a more sensitive positive pressure leak test for the Narkomed 2A, 2B, 3, and 4 (Fig. 25-39).[15-19] It is not volume-dependent because a positive pressure leak test device is substituted for the breathing bag. A no-flow state is created by turning the machine off. The pop-off valve is closed, and the inspiratory and expiratory valves are interconnected by a single breathing hose. The system is pressurized to 50 cm water by use of a squeeze bulb. The pressure decrease from 50 to 30 cm water should take 30 seconds or longer.

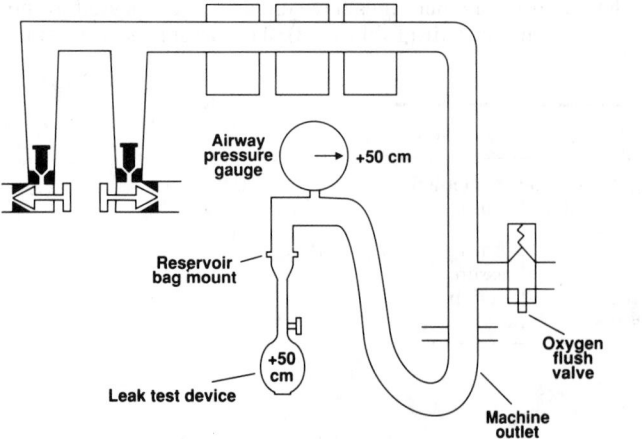
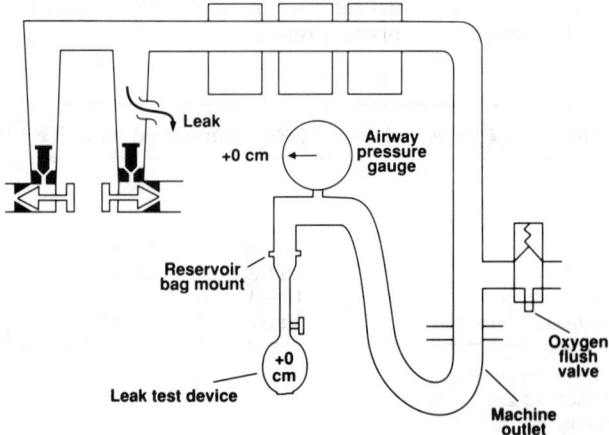

Figure 25-39. North American Dräger positive pressure leak test. (*Left*) A positive pressure leak test device is substituted for the reservoir bag. The low-pressure circuit is pressurized to 50 cm water using the squeeze bulb. (*Right*) A leak in the low-pressure circuit is reflected by a rapid decline in the value on the airway pressure gauge. (Reprinted with permission from Andrews JJ: Understanding anesthesia machines. In 1988 Review Course Lectures, p 78. Cleveland, International Anesthesia Research Society, 1988.)

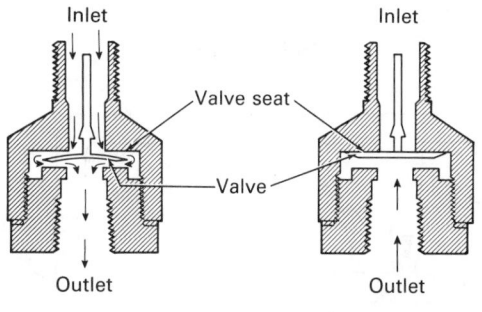

Figure 25-40. Machine outlet check valve. See text for details. (Reproduced with permission from Bowie E, Huffman LM: The Anesthesia Machine: Essentials for Understanding. Madison, Ohmeda, Inc, A Division of BOC Health Care, 1985.)

Machines With Check Valves

Most Ohmeda machines have a machine outlet check valve (see Table 25-2) to minimize the pumping effect. These include the Unitrol, the 30/70, the Modulus I and the Modulus II, and the Excel.[6-10,12] The check valve is located downstream from the vaporizers and upstream from the oxygen flush. It is open (Fig. 25-40 left) in the absence of back pressure. Gas flow from the manifold moves the rubber flapper valve off its seat and allows gas to proceed freely to the common outlet. The valve closes (Fig. 25-40 right) when back pressure is exerted on it.[5] Intermittent positive pressure and oxygen flushing close the valve.

Ohmeda recommends the use of a negative pressure leak test on the machines mentioned above (Fig. 25-41).[6-10,12] It is performed using a negative pressure leak testing device. This is a suction bulb device, and it is included with all Ohmeda machines requiring it. A no-flow state is established. (The flow control valves are turned off when the Unitrol is tested.[7] On the Modulus I and Modulus II, the master switch is turned off but the flow control valves are fully open.[8-10]) The leak testing device is attached to the common outlet. The bulb is compressed repeatedly until it remains collapsed. This action creates a vacuum in the low-pressure circuitry and opens the check valve. The machine is leak-free if the hand bulb remains collapsed for 30 seconds, but a leak is present if the bulb reinflates during this time period. The leak test must be repeated with each vaporizer in the on position to detect vaporizer leaks.

Ohmeda's rationale for the negative pressure leak test follows. First, the check valve separates the machine from the patient circuit. Pressurizing the circle system will only reveal leaks downstream from the check valve.[24] Second, the test is extremely sensitive because it is not volume-dependent. It can detect leaks as small as 30 ml·min⁻¹. Third, on the Modulus I and Modulus II, some components located *upstream* from the flow control valves are tested for leaks. These components include the oxygen flush, the pressure sensing system, and the pneumatics of the master on/off switch.

Inappropriate use of the oxygen flush valve to evaluate the low-pressure circuit for leaks can lead to a false sense of security despite the presence of huge leaks (Fig. 25-42).[29,35,64,137] Positive pressure from the patient circuit closes the check valve, and the value on the airway pressure gauge does not decline. The system appears to be tight, but in actuality, only the circuitry distal to the check valve is leak-free.[24] Thus, a vulnerable area exists from the check valve back to the flow control valves because this area is not checked by actuation of the oxygen flush. Addition of a freestanding vaporizer equipped with a check valve downstream from the common outlet creates an even larger vulnerable area.

Ohmeda Modulus II Plus and the Ohmeda CD

The Ohmeda Modulus II Plus and the Ohmeda CD Anesthesia Systems do not have a machine outlet check valve. Nevertheless, Ohmeda recommends the use of a negative pressure leak test because the test is extremely sensitive.[13,14] Also, a negative pressure leak test establishes a consistent method of checking all currently manufactured Ohmeda machines.

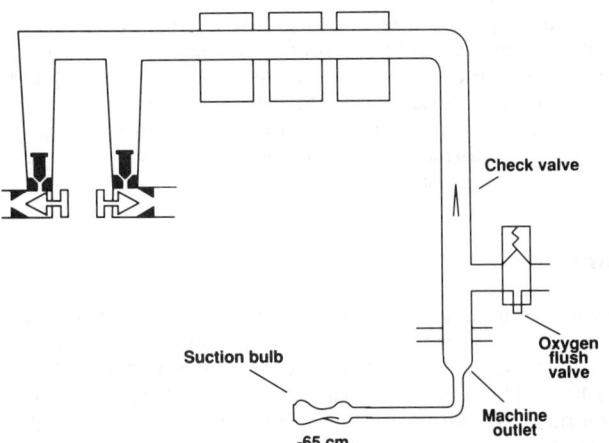
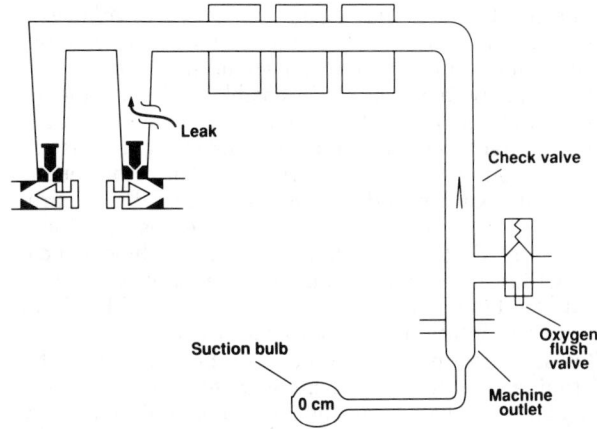

Figure 25-41. Ohmeda negative pressure leak test. (*Left*) A negative pressure leak testing device is attached directly to the machine outlet. Squeezing the bulb creates a vacuum in the low-pressure circuit and opens the check valve. (*Right*) When a leak is present in the low-pressure circuit, room air is entrained through the leak and the suction bulb inflates. (Reprinted with permission from Andrews JJ: Understanding anesthesia machines. In 1988 Review Course Lectures, p. 78. Cleveland, International Anesthesia Research Society, 1988.)

Circle System Test

The circle system test evaluates the integrity of the circle breathing system, which spans from the common gas outlet to the Y-piece. It has two parts—the *leak test* and the *flow test*. To thoroughly check the circle system for leaks and for valve integrity, both tests must be performed preoperatively.

The *leak test* is performed by closing the pop-off valve, occluding the Y-piece, and pressurizing the circuit to 30 cm water pressure using the oxygen flush. The value on the pressure gauge will not decline if the circle system is leak-free, but this does not assure valve integrity. The value on the gauge will read 30 cm water if the unidirectional valves are stuck shut or if the valves are incompetent. The *flow test* checks the integrity of the unidirectional valves. It is performed by removing the Y-piece from the circle system and breathing through the two corrugated hoses individually. The valves should be present, and they should move appropriately. The operator should be able to inhale but not be able to exhale through the inspiratory limb. The operator should be able to exhale but not inhale through the expiratory limb.

HUMIDIFICATION

Physiologic Considerations

The Mucus Blanket

The mucociliary blanket in the tracheobronchial tree provides a defense mechanism by which foreign particles and infectious debris are trapped and removed. Warm, humidified air is needed for this defense to function properly.[139,140] The upper airways warm and humidify the inspired air to 37°C and 95% humidity, despite wide variations in the external temperatures ranging from 0°C to 25°C and humidities of less than 45–55%. Air reaching the laryngeal opening varies only a degree centigrade under a wide range of conditions.[141] The large surface area and high vascularity of the mouth and nose warm and humidify 10,000 l of air every 24 hours. Nasal secretions amount to about 1 l·day^{-1}. Seventy-five percent of this moisture is used to humidify the inspired air. Most of this moisture is recaptured, limiting insensible water loss to only 25% or 250 ml·day^{-1}. However, fever, hyperventilation, endotracheal intubation, and inhalation of dry gases during an anesthetic procedure can dramatically increase this insensible loss in a patient.

Pseudostratified, ciliated, columnar epithelial cells of the respiratory tract keep the mucus blanket in a constant streaming motion toward the larynx.[142] Hence the mucus blanket is also known as the "mucus escalator."[141] The production and transport of the mucus as well as the ciliary movement is affected by various physical and biochemical factors. Ciliary activity is optimal between a pH of 6.8 and 7.2 and at a temperature of 28–33°C. Sodium chloride in 0.9% and 2% solution does not affect the ciliary activity. Opiates and nicotine directly depress the ciliary activity, but atropine inhibits it by increasing the viscosity of the mucus blanket. Inhaled anesthetics depress ciliary activity in concentrations required to produce general anesthesia.[140]

Precise administration of gases through the modern anesthesia machines depends on clean and dry anesthetic gases. These are supplied as anhydrous gases free of particulate matter because the presence of moisture can cause the valves to malfunction, orifices to distort, and flow meters to stray.[143] Inhalation of dry gases at room temperature or

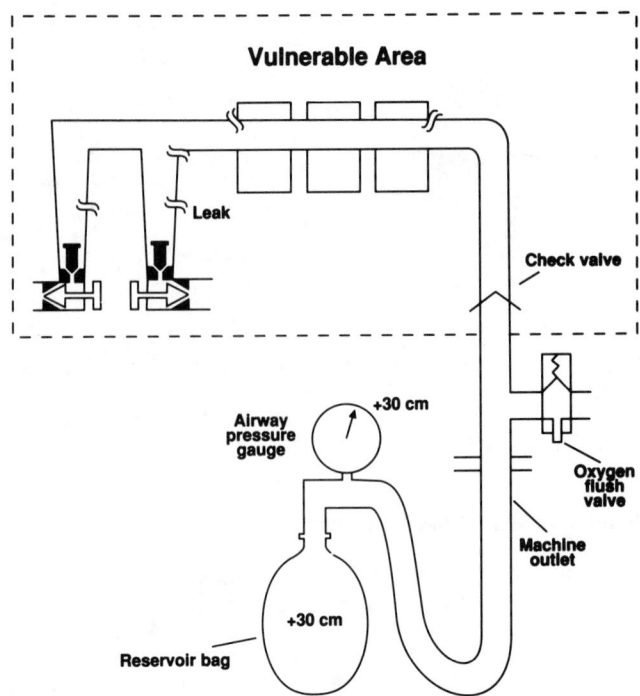

Figure 25-42. Schematic of an anesthesia machine with a machine outlet check valve. The area within the rectangle is not checked by the inappropriate use of the oxygen flush valve. The components located within this area are precisely the ones that are most subject to breakage and leaks. Positive pressure within the patient circuit closes the check valve, and the value on the airway pressure gauge does not decline despite leaks in the low-pressure circuit.

below requires that the lower respiratory passages humidify these gases.[144] In addition, endotracheal intubation bypasses nasopharyngeal air conditioning and compels the mucosa of the lower respiratory tract to perform the function of the nasopharynx.[141] Therefore, the water and heat losses from the respiratory tract become clinically significant in patients receiving unhumidified gases during a general anesthetic for any but the shortest surgical procedure. Breathing dry air can lead to desiccation of mucus, impairment of ciliary function and mucus escalator activity, retention of secretions, atelectasis, bacterial colonization, pneumonia, and heat loss. In order to minimize the postoperative pulmonary complications, warmth and humidity must be added from external sources to these dry gases as they enter the patient's airway.

Humidity

Vaporization is the conversion of a liquid into a gas. Humidity is not true gaseous water because atmospheric temperature exists below the critical temperature of water (374°C or 705°F).[142] The amount of water vapor a volume of gas can potentially contain depends on the temperature. The higher the temperature, the greater amount of water vapor a volume of gas can contain. The maximum amount of water that air can hold in the vapor state is called the saturated water content.[141] Figure 25-43 demonstrates that both the maximum water content of a gas and water vapor pressure increase exponentially with temperature.

Three terms are used to express water content of a gas:

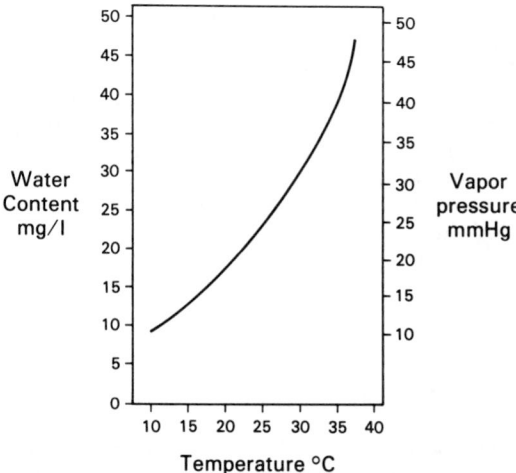

Figure 25-43. Maximum water content and water vapor pressure curve of a fully saturated gas. Both the maximum water content and the water vapor pressure increase exponentially with an increase in temperature.

Absolute humidity is the actual mass of water contained in a given volume of gas at a given temperature. Traditionally, this is measured as milligrams of water vapor per liter of gas ($mg \cdot l^{-1}$).

Maximum humidity is the maximum mass of water vapor that a given volume of gas can hold at a given temperature (saturated water content).

Relative humidity is a percentage expression of the actual water vapor content of a gas compared with its capacity to carry water at a given temperature.

The relative humidity can be computed if the temperature of the gas is known and either (1) the absolute humidity of the gas is known, or (2) the partial pressure of water vapor of the gas is known.[142] The percent relative humidity (% RH) can be calculated by any of the simple formulas listed below:

$$\% \, RH = \frac{\text{absolute humidity}}{\text{maximum humidity}} \times 100$$

$$\% \, RH = \frac{\text{actual water content}}{\text{maximum water content}} \times 100$$

$$\% \, RH = \frac{\text{actual water vapor pressure}}{\text{saturated water vapor pressure}} \times 100$$

Humidity deficit is the lack of sufficient water vapor for saturation. Room air is rarely saturated; therefore additional moisture must be added when air enters the respiratory tree. A primary humidity deficit exists when inspired room air is less than saturated at a given temperature. A secondary humidity deficit occurs when inhaled air is warmed from room temperature to body temperature. This is because the capacity of air to carry moisture increases when the inspired air is warmed.[142-144] Under normal conditions, the nasal mucosa and the upper airways pay this deficit by giving up heat and water.

The water content to correct the humidity deficit at standard room air conditions can be calculated. Inspired air at 21°C and 50% humidity contains only 9 $mg \cdot l^{-1}$ of water. Once inhaled, the water content must increase to 44 $mg \cdot l^{-1}$ at 37°C, and the humidity deficit is 35 $mg \cdot l^{-1}$:

Humidity deficit ($mg \cdot l^{-1}$) = maximum humidity (37°C)
                                  − absolute humidity (21°C)

Compressed oxygen is 100% dry even at room temperature. Forty-four milligrams of water vapor must be added to each liter of oxygen to achieve maximum humidity at 37°C. The relative humidity is zero in this instance. The humidity deficit is 44 $mg \cdot l^{-1}$ because the difference between maximum water content (44 $mg \cdot l^{-1}$) and absolute water content (0 $mg \cdot l^{-1}$) is 44 $mg \cdot l^{-1}$.

The loss of respiratory water can be calculated by the following formula:

Respiratory water loss $g \cdot h^{-1}$ = 60 VE (44-At)

Water loss is the product of the minute ventilation (VE) and the gradient of the inspired and exhaled water content. The water content of fully saturated exhaled air is 44 $mg \cdot l^{-1}$ at 37°C. The absolute water content of the inspired air at a given temperature is expressed as At. The hourly water loss for a 70-kg adult breathing a standard room air mixture (At = 9 $mg \cdot l^{-1}$) approximates 13 $g \cdot h^{-1}$. This value is near the estimated insensible daily respiratory water loss of 250 $ml \cdot day^{-1}$. Total body water loss through this mechanism would increase only to 16 $g \cdot h^{-1}$ if 100% anhydrous oxygen were administered. Thus, respiratory water loss resulting from humidity deficits has a negligible effect on body water balance and is replaced easily even in children. The importance of humidification of inspired gases is best understood in terms of the local preservation of the protective mucus blanket and thermal regulation.[145-148] Gases delivered at 37°C and those that are 50–75% saturated will maintain the integrity of the mucus blanket.

Heat Loss

Humidity deficits require energy in two ways. The first way is the simple necessity of warming the inspired gases to body temperature. The heat loss for this activity depends upon the minute ventilation, the temperature gradient between exhaled and inhaled gas, and the specific heat of the gas. It is expressed as follows:

Humidity heat loss/min = VE (37 − t) (specific heat)

The caloric requirements for this activity are estimated to be 40 $cal \cdot min^{-1}$ for modern breathing systems in which the gases are delivered at room temperature.[142] The cooler the gases, the higher the delivered energy cost will be.

The most significant loss of heat and caloric debt results from the cost of vaporizing water to cover the humidity deficit. Heat is expended to vaporize enough water to saturate the inspired air at body temperature. The caloric expenditure for this activity has been estimated to be about 550 $cal \cdot g^{-1}$ of water vaporized. Because anhydrous oxygen administration will require 16 $g \cdot hr^{-1}$ of water vapor, three times as many calories are expended per hour to humidify inhaled air. A depression of thermal regulation during general anesthesia compounds the heat loss and can produce a significant threat to anesthetized patients, particularly children. The administration of anesthetic gases at 37°C and 100% humidity can maintain body temperature in anesthetized patients and can even be used in some situations to rewarm patients who have been deliberately cooled. The temperature of inspired gases at the mouth or endotracheal tube as well as the humidifier's inspiratory temperature reading should be monitored. Temperatures in excess of 40°C at the endotracheal tube can produce hemorrhagic, bronchospastic tracheobronchitis. Temperatures of 40°C or

TABLE 25-3. Hazards of Nebulized Humidification

1. Overheating
2. Overhydration, pulmonary edema, water intoxication (especially in children)
3. Infection
4. Increase in airway resistance
5. Bronchopneumonia

less at the endotracheal tube connection are safe for rewarming and allow a margin of safety in temperature regulation.

Humidifiers

The rate of humidification (vaporization) is influenced by three factors: (1) the surface area for gas/water contact, (2) the duration of exposure, and (3) the temperature.[141]

There are two basic types of humidifying devices: vaporizers and nebulizers. Nebulizers deliver water in droplet form as an aerosol. Heated nebulizers can produce 100% humidity at body temperature. Despite their efficiency, they present certain hazards (Table 25-3). Nebulizers can transmit bacteria in the water droplets, but vaporizers cannot because there is no particulate matter.[149] Nebulizers also present the hazard of producing overhydration, water intoxication, and increased respiratory resistance, especially in children.[141,142] Vaporizers rarely add enough water to produce problems with water balance. The predominant humidifiers used on anesthesia machines are the vaporizer type because they are efficient enough and have a wider margin of safety than nebulizers.

Anesthesia Circuits and Humidity

The minimum recommended humidity for anesthesia is 60% or 12 mg·l^{-1}. Optimum values are between 14 and 30 mg·l^{-1} of water vapor. Simple moistening of the insides of corrugated hoses and of the reservoir bag has significantly increased the humidity in the circle system.[150] This achieves a water content of about 22 mg·l^{-1}. The humidity declines with time as evaporation within the circuit produces cooling. The adult or pediatric closed circle system can achieve a water content as high as 29 mg·l^{-1} when the gases are passed through a soda lime canister.[145,151,152] The relative humidity approaches 100% because of water production by neutralization during the process of carbon dioxide absorption by soda lime. Some of the water vapor also comes from the exhaled air. However, the temperature is still less than 37°C, and the pressure gradient for water vapor is from the lungs to air. A closed circuit provides ideal inspired humidity. Humidification probably is not necessary in units designed for total rebreathing (closed system) because water loss is of small magnitude. Humidification is required for systems that are open or semiopen and in which high gas flows are used for protracted periods of time.

Non-rebreathing circuits ordinarily deliver unhumidified gases. The Bain Circuit is an exception. It is a modification of the Mapleson D System (see the section on Anesthetic Circuits) and is conducive to the humidification of inspired gases.[142,153] The Bain Circuit is a coaxial circuit, and the inspiratory line is insulated by the warm exhaled gases in the outer expiratory tubing. This design minimizes decreases in temperature and humidity once the system is heated. An absolute humidity between 21–25 mg·l^{-1} can be achieved within 30 minutes of use. Relative humidity will increase to 100% in approximately 80 minutes.

Humidity does not affect oxygen analyzers unless excess condensation accumulates on the sensors.[154] This problem is minimized by the water-repelling membrane over the polymeric membrane. Condensation can occlude gas sampling lines for mass spectrometers and carbon dioxide monitors.

Humidifiers-Vaporizers

Vaporizers, in contrast to nebulizers, are derived from two basic prototypes: (1) the simple vaporizer, and (2) the heated vaporizer.[142] Simple vaporizers do not use heat and are designed to add only enough humidity to make the gas more comfortable. This type of humidifier is generally used only by mask or in an incubator. It allows the nasopharynx to provide the balance of humidification not provided by the humidifier. Although these devices may provide 100% humidity at room air temperature, they will supply only about a third of the humidity required for the lower respiratory tract at 37°C. Two types of simple vaporizers have been used: (1) the pass-over or blow-by humidifier, and (2) the bubble humidifier. Two other humidifiers have been classified as simple vaporizers but are actually nebulizers that do not utilize heat. These are called the jet and underwater jet humidifiers.

Three major types of heated vaporizers are commonly used: (1) the Hopkins, or pass-over, vaporizer, (2) the bubbler, and (3) the heated cascade humidifier.

1. The Hopkins, or pass-over, vaporizer is the simplest of the heated vaporizers. This type of humidifier is merely the heated version of the simple vaporizer. The large reservoir of the pass-over vaporizer is heated by an external hot plate element. It provides humidity by passing air over a relatively large surface area. This is the vaporizer used on the Emerson ventilator.[142]

2. Bubblers add vapor by evaporation of a stream of bubbles through a jar of water. A disadvantage of the bubbler is that the water in the jar is cooled as it evaporates. This lowers the temperature of the carrying gas and reduces its moisture-carrying capacity. The bubbler can only provide 20% relative humidity at body temperature unless it is heated. The deficit must be made up by the respiratory passages, and this may be poorly tolerated by a patient who already has lost mucociliary function. The addition of heat increases the performance of the bubbler, which is commonly used with nasal cannulas and oxygen masks.

3. Heated cascade humidifiers technically are bubblers. These devices deliver 100% humidity at body temperature. They break inspired gas into tiny bubbles and pass bubbles through heated water. These are the mainstream humidifiers used with anesthesia systems and are the most effective of all the evaporative humidifiers. These vaporizers are typified by the Bennett cascade vaporizer. A potential hazard associated with the Bennett is misconnection. It has a one-way check valve that retards the drift of humidity retrograde to the anesthesia machine.[142] Even though the inlet and outlet are labeled, they have the same diameter. Reverse hookup results in a no-flow state.

CLOSED CIRCUIT ANESTHESIA

During closed circuit anesthesia, the circle system Adjustable Pressure Limiting (pop-off) Valve is closed, and the gas delivery rate is adjusted to exactly match the uptake rate. The reservoir bag increases in size if delivery exceeds uptake, and the bag collapses if delivery is less than uptake. The composition of delivered gas must be appropriate to achieve the desired oxygen and anesthetic concentration while avoiding hypoxia, anesthetic overdose, or patient awareness. Delivering the perfect quantitative and qualitative blend of gases throughout the course of an anesthetic can be challenging because uptake kinetics is dynamic and physiologic variables may change.[155] Quantitative understanding of closed system anesthesia requires a thorough understanding of uptake and distribution of anesthetics (see Chapter 17).

History

In the 19th century Snow reported the use of a closed system.[155] Waters, in 1924, developed the to and fro closed circuit that delivered both oxygen–nitrous oxide and potent volatile liquid agents.[155] He described the successful use and advantages of a closed system in 1926.[156] Closed or very low-flow systems were used to advantage during the cyclopropane era, primarily because of the agent's high cost. With the clinical introduction of halothane, many anesthesiologists used halothane in closed systems.[155] The results were occasionally disastrous because of overdose.[157] Halothane's high potency, combined with increased use of controlled ventilation and muscle relaxants, may have contributed to this problem. Romagnoli used a modified Goldman ether drip feed to deliver liquid halothane into a closed system in 1960.[158] Hampton and Flickinger, in 1961, used intermittent injections of liquid halothane into the gas inlet of a rebreathing circuit.[159] Lowe developed the square root of time model in the mid-1970s to predict the rate of anesthetic tissue uptake over time.[155] His model is an invaluable guide to the anesthesiologist for administering volatile anesthetics during closed circuit anesthesia.

Advantages

Closed circuit anesthesia has several advantages. The use of oxygen, nitrous oxide, and inhaled anesthetic is minimal compared to an open system. Therefore, the cost is reduced.[160-164] Personnel exposure to trace gases in the operating room is minimized. Atmospheric pollution is also reduced. This is important because nitrous oxide and hydrochlorofluorocarbons (halothane, enflurane, and isoflurane) are known to destroy the earth's protective ozone layer.[161,165] Water losses are minimal during closed circuit anesthesia because all the exhaled carbon dioxide reacts with carbon dioxide absorbent, producing heat and water. The patient therefore rebreathes humidified gases. Tidal volume and expiratory flow rate can be accurately measured because the flow from the anesthesia machine is minimal. Expiratory volume and expiratory flow rate are completely patient-dependent.

Closed circuit anesthesia allows minute-to-minute direct monitoring of oxygen consumption. The flow rate indicated on the oxygen flow meter approximates the patient's oxygen consumption rate if the breathing bag volume remains constant. Hypermetabolic states, such as malignant hyperthermia, are easily detected by changes in steady-state oxygen consumption and carbon dioxide production. Quantitative assessment is possible for other physiologic parameters correlating with oxygen consumption. These include carbon dioxide production, alveolar ventilation, cardiac output, and fluid requirements.[155]

Changes in anesthetic concentration occur slowly in closed circuit anesthesia.[166] The approximate ventilatory system total capacity equals the volume of the circuit (7 l) plus the patient's functional residual capacity (3 l), or 10 l. Because flow rate into the system is typically small, the time constant is relatively long. (The time constant is defined as the capacity of a system divided by the flow rate into it.) The time constant for a "typical" closed circuit is 40 minutes (10,000 ml per 250 ml per minute), whereas the time constant for a "typical" open circuit is only 5 minutes (10,000 ml per 5000 ml per minute). Therefore, the concentration of anesthetics changes more gradually with closed circuits. These gradual concentration changes may sometimes be desirable in patients with hypertension, heart disease, diabetes, or similar diseases.

Disadvantages

Closed circuit anesthesia has several potential disadvantages. Administration of an anesthetic using a closed circuit is more complicated than using an open system with high fresh gas flows. The quantity of halogenated anesthetic introduced into the closed system must be exponentially tapered with time to maintain a constant arterial concentration. To maintain constant circuit volume, frequent flow meter adjustments may be necessary to maintain the delicate balance between delivery and uptake.[166] Also, adequate inspired oxygen concentration must be maintained throughout the case.

Dosage errors are possible with closed circuit anesthesia. The square root of time model predicts the quantity of anesthesia needed to achieve a specific level of anesthesia.[155] The model assumes (1) the appropriate dose is proportional to MAC, (2) the blood gas partition coefficient is "normal" and constant, (3) the cardiac output (or pulmonary blood flow) is normal, and it is proportional to the patient's weight (2 $kg^{3/4}$), and (4) pulmonary function is normal. The MAC of various anesthetics is constant under a wide variety of conditions, but it varies with age, metabolic factors, and administration of various drugs. Biologic variability exists in blood/gas partition coefficients between persons. Partition coefficients may vary within the same individual after a change in temperature, hematocrit, or diet.[155] Body size correlates with cardiac output in healthy patients, but it does not in patients with heart disease. Changes in cardiac output are common during the course of an anesthetic. Finally, many patients have pulmonary pathology with ventilation-perfusion mismatch.

A hypoxic mixture can potentially be delivered, particularly if nitrous oxide is used. Using a reliable oxygen analyzer, or using oxygen alone plus an inhaled anesthetic, minimizes this hazard. Without adequate pulmonary denitrogenation, the inspired nitrogen concentration can threaten adequate inspiratory oxygen concentration.[167] Morita, in 1985, demonstrated that after a short period of denitrogenation (6–8 minutes), average nitrogen concentration in the closed circuit increased from 6.4% to 16.2%. After long denitrogenation (33 minutes), the average nitrogen concentration increased from 1.0% to 5%.[168]

The long time constant of a closed circuit prevents rapid alteration of inspired gas concentrations. Opening the system allows fast alteration. An alternative to opening the system is using a charcoal filter to rapidly decrease the depth of anesthesia, maintaining the closed circuit.[169,170] The charcoal filter effectively adsorbs the halogenated anesthetic, but it does not remove nitrous oxide.[170]

Carbon dioxide absorbent is exhausted at a faster rate with closed circuit than with open circuit anesthesia. The Adjustable Pressure Limiting (pop-off) Valve of the circle system is located just downstream from the exhalation check valve (see Fig. 25-25), and this location optimizes absorbent use.[166] Most exhaled gas, rich in carbon dioxide, is vented through the relief valve during a high-flow open circuit anesthetic. Only a small portion of the total exhaled gas passes through the absorbent. Conversely, closed circuit absorbent handles 100% of the exhaled gas. Therefore, the utilization rate is increased, and there is a danger of rebreathing.[166]

Closed circuit anesthesia allows accumulation of waste products such as carbon monoxide. Endogenous carbon monoxide is a by-product of hemoglobin catabolism. Exogenous sources include cigarette smoke, automobile exhaust, and by-products of a wide variety of industrial processes.[171] Minor metabolic gases such as methane, acetone, and hydrogen or the common intoxicant ethanol can accumulate in the inspired gas.[168] Occasional flushing with fresh anesthetic gases reduces the concentrations of water-insoluble gases such as nitrogen, methane, and hydrogen. Highly soluble compounds, such as acetone and ethanol, are not readily removed by flushing.[168] Argon accumulates in closed circuit anesthesia when oxygen is supplied by an oxygen concentrator that uses a zeolitic molecular sieve.[172] Such oxygen contains 5% argon. Periodic opening of the circuit is necessary if it is totally closed. Volatile anesthetic metabolites can accumulate[173] but in clinically insignificant quantities.[174]

Equipment Needed

Anesthesia Machine

Contemporary Ohmeda and North American Dräger machines are suitable for closed circuit anesthesia. Ensuring that the machine and breathing circuit are leak-free requires extra care because of the low total gas flow. For example, a 100-ml leak in an open system is 2% of the total flow (100 ml per 5000 ml). The same leak in a closed circuit is 40% of the total flow (100 ml per 250 ml). Both manufacturers offer an optional low-flow kit. The flow meter scales in the low-flow range are expanded, and the flow rates are more accurate than those of standard flow meters. The minimum oxygen flow is reduced from 200 ml·min^{-1} to approximately 50 ml·min^{-1}. Flow values this low may be necessary for children, for adults with mild to moderate hypothermia, or for patients during deep inhalation volatile anesthesia.

Standard flow meters suffice if the minimum oxygen flow is equal to or lower than the patient's oxygen consumption. The Ohmeda CD has a minimum oxygen flow rate of 50 ml·min as a standard feature.[14] Contemporary North American Dräger machines have a minimum oxygen flow rate of 200 ml·min^{-1} when the gas selector switch reads O_2/N_2O. However, selecting the ''all gas'' mode decreases the minimum oxygen flow from 200 ml·min^{-1} to 0.[17-19]

Contemporary North American Dräger machines, such as the Narkomed 2B, 3, and 4, are incapable of delivering even a 50% nitrous oxide concentration at flow rates of less than 1 l·min^{-1} because of the ORMC safety device design (see Fig. 25-13).[17-19] Therefore, practitioners with North American Dräger machines commonly use oxygen alone plus inhaled anesthetic.

Circle System

As mentioned above, the circle system must be leak-free, and the endotracheal tube should be cuffed to avoid leaks between the trachea and the atmosphere.[166] The carbon dioxide absorbent must be functional because all exhaled gases pass through the canister. The rate of absorbent depletion is substantially higher in a closed than in an open circuit.

Ventilator

Contemporary ascending bellows ventilators such as the Ohmeda 7000, the Ohmeda 7800 series, and the North American Dräger AV-E are safe to use with closed circuit anesthesia. The ascending bellows configuration is safer than the descending configuration (see the section on Anesthesia Ventilators). Inadequate flow rates, increased oxygen consumption, and leaks all readily manifest with the ascending configuration because the bellows will not completely fill during the expiratory phase. With the descending configuration, the same problems are often unnoticed because the bellows will still fill during the expiratory phase. If the system has a leak, room air is entrained through the leak when the weighted bellows descends. Air entrainment causes an increase in the inspiratory nitrogen concentration and a decrease in the inspiratory oxygen concentration. If the system is tight, circuit volume decreases with inadequate flow rates or with increased oxygen consumption. During the expiratory phase, circuit pressures can become subatmospheric to levels as low as -10 to -30 cm water.

Vaporizer

Vapor can be added to the breathing circuit in three ways by the use of (1) out-of-circuit copper kettle or Vernitrol vaporizers, (2) out-of-circuit variable bypass vaporizers such as the Ohmeda Tec 4 and the North American Dräger Vapor 19.1, and (3) in-circuit liquid injection.[166] Copper kettles and Vernitrols are no longer manufactured in the United States. These vaporizers were used successfully in the past, but the ASTM F1161-88 standard does not address them.[3] Ohmeda no longer provides parts or service for Vernitrols. Variable bypass vaporizers, at low flow rates, are commonly incapable of delivering enough anesthetic early in the course of a closed circuit anesthetic because the patient's uptake is so high. Also, output of variable bypass vaporizers at flow rates less than 500 ml·min^{-1} is unpredictable.[52] Manufacturers do not publish vaporizer performance curves at flow rates of less than 250 ml·min^{-1}.

In-circuit liquid injection by syringe into the expiratory limb of the circle system achieves vaporization. This technique delivers the high concentrations of inhaled anesthetic necessary early in a case. The liquid is injected into the expiratory limb to allow adequate dilution by the circuit gas in order to avoid excessive inspired anesthetic concentrations of as high as 20–30%.[155] Direct contact between liquid anesthetic and the Ohmeda TVX flow cartridge, located on the expiratory limb, should be avoided. The polysulfone cartridge is degraded by halogenated hydrocarbons. Pooling of liquid halothane in the cartridge can create a hole in the cartridge, resulting in a circuit leak.[175]

Monitors

Closed circuit anesthesia is increasingly safer because improved monitors are available in many operating suites. An oxygen analyzer is mandatory to ensure adequate circuit oxygen concentration. An end-tidal CO_2 monitor detects rebreathing that occurs when the absorbent is depleted. Anesthetic agent monitors help ensure appropriate circuit anesthetic concentration, and this helps avoid over- or underdose.[166]

The high sampling rate of many side-stream gas analyzers sometimes causes problems during closed circuit anesthesia. The sampling rate can approach or exceed 300 ml·min^{-1}, and this value exceeds the total flow rate necessary for many closed circuit anesthetics. The patient may be deprived of necessary fresh gas if the sampling continues for extended periods.[176] This problem can be overcome by intermittent instead of continuous sampling.

A theoretical, ideal, multigas monitor for closed circuit anesthesia is the Ohmeda RASCAL II using Raman scattering technology. Inhaled anesthetic molecules are not destroyed during analysis by the RASCAL as they are by a mass spectrometer. After analysis, the unchanged gas molecules can be reintroduced into the breathing circuit, to maintain a constant volume. The monitor quantitates inspired and exhaled nitrogen concentration. Therefore, prior to induction, the degree of pulmonary denitrogenation can be assessed before closing the system. The monitor is also more accurate than infrared devices.

Technique: Square Root of Time Model

Several successful techniques have been used for closed system anesthesia. They range from basic liquid injection by syringe using routine circuit monitors to sophisticated, computer-based, servo-controlled, anesthesia delivery systems. As mentioned above, copper kettles and Vernitrols are no longer manufactured. Variable bypass vaporizers at low-flow rates are commonly incapable of delivering sufficient quantities of inhaled anesthetic early in the case. The use of nitrous oxide complicates the issue somewhat. The advantages of not using nitrous oxide include the ability to administer a higher inspiratory oxygen concentration and elimination of the possibility of delivering a hypoxic mixture due to nitrous oxide or nitrogen. Therefore, the following discussion is limited to liquid injection by syringe of volatile anesthetics using oxygen alone based upon Lowe's square root of time model.[155]

The square root of time model estimates the rate of anesthetic tissue uptake over time. Therefore, the model estimates the quantity of anesthetic needed to achieve a desired circuit anesthetic level, such as 1.3 MAC. The rate of anesthetic uptake is inversely proportional to the square root of time, and the cumulative anesthetic requirements are proportional to the square roots of time. The cumulative anesthetic dose necessary to achieve and maintain the desired arterial concentration for any given time period is equal to the area under the rate uptake curve.[155]

Figure 25-44 shows the predicted quantity of enflurane anesthetic necessary to anesthetize a 100-kg patient at 1.3 MAC. The *prime dose* is the amount of volatile anesthetic expressed in milliliters of vapor required to fill the ventilatory and arterial transport system with the desired anes-

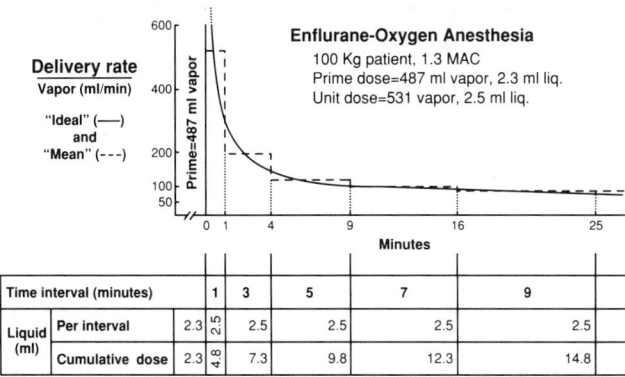

Time interval (minutes)		1	3	5	7	9
Liquid (ml)	Per interval	2.3 / 2.5	2.5	2.5	2.5	2.5
	Cumulative dose	2.3 / 4.8	7.3	9.8	12.3	14.8

Figure 25-44. Graphic representation of the first 25 minutes of a closed circuit anesthetic. *Upper graph:* The smooth curve indicates the ideal delivery rate to achieve and maintain a constant arterial concentration of 1.3 MAC enflurane in a 100-kg patient. The amount of anesthetic vapor absorbed between 0–1, 1–4, 4–9, and 9–16 minutes is equal. The area of each rectangle under the uptake curve is the same. *Lower table:* Time intervals, liquid injection dose schedules, and cumulative liquid dose are shown. The prime dose is given only once, and it can be introduced over any length of time. The unit dose is given during the first minute and repeated during subsequent time intervals. (Modified with permission from Lowe HJ, Ernst EA: The Quantitative Practice of Anesthesia: Use of the Closed Circuit. Baltimore, Williams & Wilkins, 1981.)

thetic concentration. The prime achieves a desired alveolar concentration in any desired time interval. Additional drug must be added during the anesthetic, as it is absorbed by the whole body tissues. The additional amount required is the same during the first minute, the next 3 minutes, the next 5 minutes, and subsequent intervals increasing by 2 minutes each. This *unit dose* is repeated at lengthening time intervals, and it maintains a desired alveolar concentration throughout anesthesia. Calculation of the unit dose requires a prediction of the MAC multiple needed for each individual patient and an estimate of the patient's cardiac output. Confirmation of an accurate unit dose prediction is determined by patient response within the first few minutes of an anesthetic. Shown below is the mathematical summary of the square root of time model.[155]

Rate of Tissue Uptake (milliliters of vapor/minute)

$$\dot{Q}an = \overbrace{\underbrace{\underbrace{\overbrace{f\,MAC \times \lambda\,B/G \times \dot{Q}}^{\text{minute arterial delivery}}}_{C_A}}_{Ca}}^{} \div \sqrt{t}$$

tissue uptake rate (ml·min^{-1})

$\dot{Q}an$ = rate of anesthetic tissue uptake (ml vapor·min^{-1})
  f = fraction or multiple
MAC = minimal alveolar concentration (ml vapor·dl^{-1})
λ B/G = blood/gas partition coefficient
  $\dot{Q}$ = cardiac output (dl·min^{-1})—equated with 2 kg$^{3/4}$
  C_A = alveolar anesthetic concentration (ml vapor·dl^{-1})
  Ca = arterial anesthetic concentration (ml vapor·dl^{-1})

TABLE 25-4.[155] Useful Values for Closed Circuit Anesthesia

Anesthetic	MAC 37°C	λ B/G 37°C	Molecular Weight	Specific Gravity g·ml^{-1} 20°C	ml vapor* ml liquid 37°C
Enflurane	1.7	1.9	184.5	1.52	210
Isoflurane	1.3	1.5	184.5	1.49	206
Halothane	0.75	2.4	197.4	1.86	240

* Milliliters vapor @ 37°C per ml liquid @ 20°C $= \dfrac{\text{Specific gravity} \times 22,400 \times (273 + °C)}{\text{Molecular weight} \times (273)}$

Modified with permission from Lowe HJ, Ernst EA: The Quantitative Practice of Anesthesia: Use of the Closed Circuit. Baltimore, Williams & Wilkins, 1981.

$\mathbf{Ca\dot{Q}}$ = amount anesthetic vapor delivered to tissues in 1 minute (ml·min^{-1})

t = time (minutes)—elapsed time of constant $\mathbf{Ca\dot{Q}}$

V_{vent} = volume of ventilatory delivery system (dl)

V_{vent} = $V_{circuit}$ + functional residual capacity

Prime Dose (milliliters of vapor)

Prime dose = amount needed to prime delivery system
= minute arterial delivery + amount to fill ventilatory system
= $\mathbf{Ca\dot{Q}}$ + (V_{vent} × CA)
≃ $\mathbf{Ca\dot{Q}}$ + 100 × f MAC in the "usual adult" patient

Cumulative Amount Absorbed (milliliters of vapor)

$$\int_0^t \dot{Q}\text{an dt} = \int_0^t f\,\text{MAC} \times \lambda\,\text{B/G} \times \dot{Q} \times t^{-1/2}\,dt$$
$$= 2f\,\text{MAC} \times \lambda\,\text{B/G} \times \dot{Q} \times t^{1/2}$$
$$= 2\mathbf{Ca\dot{Q}} \times t^{1/2}$$

Unit Dose (milliliters of vapor)

When t = 1 minute, unit dose is determined.

$$\text{Unit dose} = 2f\,\text{MAC} \times \lambda\,\text{B/G} \times \dot{Q} \times 1$$
$$= 2\mathbf{Ca\dot{Q}}$$

To clinically use the square root of time model with liquid injection, all the variables in the equations above must be known or estimated. Also, milliliters of vapor must be converted to milliliters of liquid anesthetic. Tables 25-4 through 25-6 provide data necessary to calculate both the prime and unit doses when using enflurane, isoflurane, or halothane.[155] The following example demonstrates the use of the square root of time model to calculate the prime and unit doses of liquid anesthetic needed to anesthetize a 100-kg patient with 1.3 MAC enflurane in oxygen (see Fig. 25-44):

TABLE 25-5.[155] Kg$^{3/4}$ Related to Physiologic Variables

Cardiac output or $\dot{Q}$ =	2 kg$^{3/4}$	dl·min^{-1}
O_2 consumption =	10 kg$^{3/4}$	ml·min^{-1}
CO_2 production =	8 kg$^{3/4}$	ml·min^{-1}
Fluids =	5 kg$^{3/4}$	ml·h^{-1}

Modified with permission from Lowe HJ, Ernst EA: The Quantitative Practice of Anesthesia: Use of the Closed Circuit. Baltimore, Williams & Wilkins, 1981.

Prime dose ≃ $\mathbf{Ca\dot{Q}}$ + 100 × f MAC
≃ f MAC × λ B/G × $\dot{Q}$ + 100 × f MAC
≃ (1.3)(1.7)(1.9)(2 kg$^{3/4}$) + 100 × (1.3)(1.7)
≃ (1.3)(1.7)(1.9)(2)(100$^{3/4}$) + (100)(1.3)(1.7)
≃ 266 + 221
≃ 487 ml vapor

≃ 487 ml vapor $\left(\dfrac{1\text{ ml liquid}}{210\text{ ml vapor}}\right)$ = 2.3 ml liquid

Unit dose = $2\mathbf{Ca\dot{Q}}$
= 2(266)
= 532 ml vapor

= 532 ml vapor $\left(\dfrac{1\text{ ml liquid}}{210\text{ ml vapor}}\right)$ = 2.5 ml liquid

After priming the circuit with 2.3 ml liquid enflurane, the 2.5-ml liquid unit dose could be injected at times 0, 1, and 4 minutes. However, to smooth induction, the total dose required for the first few minutes can be administered at an average rate. Many anesthesiologists, for example, use a 9-minute induction period. The total dose of liquid enflurane required for the first 9 minutes is 9.8 ml liquid (prime dose of 2.3 ml liquid + three unit doses of 2.5 ml). During the first 9 minutes, the average dose is 1.1 ml liquid per minute (9.8 ml liquid per 9 min). Therefore, 1.1 ml liquid are injected into the circuit at times 0, 1, 2, 3, 4, 5, 6, 7, and 8 minutes. During the subsequent 7-minute time interval (9–16 minutes), the 2.5-ml unit dose can be injected as a bolus, or if preferred introduced in smaller amounts throughout the interval. The dose must always be titrated to patient response.

TABLE 25-6. Kg Versus Kg$^{3/4}$

kg	kg$^{3/4}$	kg	kg$^{3/4}$
5	3.34	65	22.89
10	5.62	70	24.20
15	7.62	75	25.49
20	9.46	80	26.75
25	11.18	85	27.99
30	12.82	90	29.22
35	14.39	95	30.43
40	15.91	100	31.62
45	17.37	105	32.80
50	18.80	110	33.97
55	20.20	115	35.12
60	21.56	120	36.26

Computer-Controlled Closed Circuit Anesthesia

Computer-based, automatic control technology for administration of closed circuit anesthesia has been used clinically.[177-180] At least one system automatically controls oxygen delivery, nitrous oxide or air delivery, anesthetic delivery, and ventilation.[180] Servo controllers automatically regulate breathing circuit volume, oxygen concentration, end-tidal anesthetic concentration, and end-tidal P_{CO_2}. Automatic systems provide advantages of closed circuit anesthesia without encumbering the anesthesiologist with the more demanding control task.[180]

Acknowledgment. Selected portions of this chapter have appeared in Miller R (ed): Anesthesia, 3rd ed. New York, Churchill Livingstone, 1990. Reprinted with permission.

REFERENCES

1. Schreiber P: Safety guidelines for anesthesia systems. Telford, Pennsylvania, North American Dräger, 1984
2. American National Standards Institute: Minimum Performance and Safety Requirements for Components and Systems of Continuous Flow Anesthesia Machines for Human Use (ANSI Z79.8-1979). New York, American National Standards Institute, 1979
3. American Society for Testing and Materials: Minimum Performance and Safety Requirements for Components and Systems of Anesthesia Gas Machines (ASTM F1161-88). Philadelphia, American Society for Testing and Materials, 1988
4. Dorsch JA, Dorsch SE: The anesthesia machine. In Dorsch JA, Dorsch SE (eds): Understanding Anesthesia Equipment, 2nd ed, p 38. Baltimore, Williams & Wilkins, 1984
5. Bowie E, Huffman LM: The anesthesia machine: Essentials for understanding. Madison, Ohmeda, The BOC Group, Inc, 1985
6. 30/70 proportionate anesthesia machine. (Canadian version.) Madison, Ohio Medical Products, 1982
7. Ohmeda Unitrol Anesthesia System. Operation and Maintenance Manual. Madison, Ohmeda, The BOC Group, Inc, 1985
8. Modulus Anesthesia Gas Machine. Operation Maintenance. Madison, Ohio Medical Products, The BOC Group, 1981
9. Modulus II Anesthesia System. Operation and Maintenance Manual. Madison, Ohmeda, The BOC Group, Inc, 1985
10. Modulus II Anesthesia System. Service Manual. Madison, Ohmeda, The BOC Group, Inc, 1985
11. Ohmeda 8000 Anesthesia Machine. Operation and Maintenance Manual. Madison, Ohmeda, The BOC Group, Inc, 1985
12. Ohmeda Excel 110 and 210: Operation and Maintenance Manual. Madison, Ohmeda, The BOC Group, Inc, 1987
13. Modulus II Plus Anesthesia System: Operation and Maintenance Manual. Madison, Ohmeda, The BOC Group, Inc, 1988
14. Ohmeda CD Anesthesia System: Operation and Maintenance Manual. Madison, Ohmeda, The BOC Group, Inc, 1990
15. Narkomed 2A Anesthesia System: Technical Service Manual, 6th ed. Telford, Pennsylvania, North American Dräger, 1985
16. Narkomed 2A Anesthesia System: Instruction Manual, 7th ed. Telford, Pennsylvania, North American Dräger, 1985
17. Narkomed 2B Anesthesia System: Operator's Manual. Telford, Pennsylvania, North American Dräger, 1988
18. Narkomed 3 Anesthesia System: Operator's Instruction Manual. Telford, Pennsylvania, North American Dräger, 1986
19. Narkomed 4 Anesthesia System: Operations Instruction Manual. Telford, Pennsylvania, North American Dräger, 1990
20. Feeley TW, Hedley-Whyte J: Bulk oxygen and nitrous oxide delivery systems: Design and dangers. Anesthesiology 44:301, 1976
21. Pelton DA: Non-flammable medical gas pipeline systems. In Wyant GM (ed): Mechanical Misadventures in Anesthesia, p 8. Toronto, University of Toronto Press, 1978
22. Andrews JJ: Inhaled anesthetic delivery systems. In Miller RD (ed): Anesthesia, 3rd ed, p 171. New York, Churchill Livingstone, 1990
23. Adriani J: Clinical application of physical principles concerning gases and vapors to anesthesiology. In Adriani J (ed): The Chemistry and Physics of Anesthesia, 2nd ed, p 58. Springfield, Illinois, Charles C Thomas, 1962
24. Dorsch JA, Dorsch SE: Equipment checking and maintenance. In Dorsch JA, Dorsch SE (eds): Understanding Anesthesia Equipment, 2nd ed, p 401. Baltimore, Williams & Wilkins, 1984
25. Loeb RG, Ross WT, Lawson D: How modern anesthesia machines respond to a decrease in oxygen line pressure. Anesth Analg 66:S1, 1987
26. Macintosh R, Mushin WW, Epstein HG: Flowmeters. In Macintosh R, Mushin WW, Epstein HG (eds): Physics for the Anaesthetist, 3rd ed, p 196. Oxford, England, Blackwell Scientific Publications, 1963
27. Eger EI II, Epstein RM: Hazards of anesthetic equipment. Anesthesiology 24:490, 1964
28. Eger EI II, Hylton RR, Irwin RH et al: Anesthetic flowmeter sequence—a cause for hypoxia. Anesthesiology 24:396, 1963
29. Rendell-Baker L: Problems with anesthetic and respiratory therapy equipment. Int Anesthesiol Clin 20:1, 1982
30. Mazze RI: Therapeutic misadventures with oxygen delivery systems: The need for continuous in-line oxygen monitors. Anesth Analg 51:787, 1972
31. Abraham ZA, Basagoitia B: A potentially lethal anesthesia machine failure. Anesthesiology 66:589, 1987
32. Anderson CE, Rendell-Baker L: Exposed O_2 flush hazard. Anesthesiology 56:328, 1982
33. Anonymous: Internal leakage from anesthesia unit flush valves. Health Devices 10:172, 1981
34. Andrews JJ: Understanding your anesthesia machine and ventilator. In 1989 Review Course Lectures, p 59. Cleveland, International Anesthesia Research Society, 1989
35. Dodgson BG: Inappropriate use of the oxygen flush to check an anaesthetic machine. Can J Anaesth 35:336, 1988
36. Dorsch JA, Dorsch SE: Vaporizers. In Dorsch JA, Dorsch SE (eds): Understanding Anesthesia Equipment, 2nd ed, p 77. Baltimore, Williams & Wilkins, 1984
37. Macintosh R, Mushin WW, Epstein HG: Vapor pressure. In Macintosh R, Mushin WW, Epstein HG (eds): Physics for the Anaesthetist, 3rd ed, p 68. Oxford, England, Blackwell Scientific Publications, 1963
38. Adriani J: Principles of physics and chemistry of solids and fluids applicable to anesthesiology. In Adriani J (ed): The Chemistry and Physics of Anesthesia, 2nd ed, p 7. Springfield, Illinois, Charles C Thomas, 1962
39. Macintosh R, Mushin WW, Epstein HG: Vaporization. In Macintosh R, Mushin WW, Epstein HG (eds): Physics for the Anaesthetist, 3rd ed, p 26. Oxford, England, Blackwell Scientific Publications, 1963
40. Macintosh R, Mushin WW, Epstein HG: Specific heat. In Macintosh R, Mushin WW, Epstein HG (eds): Physics for the Anaesthetist, 3rd ed, p 17. Oxford, England, Blackwell Scientific Publications, 1963
41. Schreiber P: Anaesthetic Equipment: Performance, Classification, and Safety. New York, Springer-Verlag, 1972
42. Dräger Vapor 19.n Anaesthetic Vaporizer. Instructions for Use, 14th ed. Lubeck, Germany, Drägerwerk, 1990
43. Tec 4 Continuous Flow Vaporizer. Operator's Manual. Steeton, England, Ohmeda, The BOC Group, Inc, July, 1987
44. Hill DW, Lowe HJ: Comparison of concentration of halothane in closed and semi-closed circuits during controlled ventilation. Anesthesiology 23:291, 1962
45. Hill DW: The design and calibration of vaporizers for volatile anaesthetic agents. In Scurr C, Feldman S (eds): Scientific Foundations of Anaesthesia, 3rd ed, p 544. London, William Heineman Medical Books, 1982
46. Hill DW: The design and calibration of vaporizers for volatile anaesthetic agents. Br J Anaesth 40:648, 1968
47. Morris LE: Problems in the performance of anesthesia vaporizers. Int Anesthesiol Clin 12:199, 1974

48. Stoelting RK: The effects of nitrous oxide on halothane output from Fluotec Mark 2 vaporizers. Anesthesiology 35:215, 1971
49. Diaz PD: The influence of carrier gas on the output of automatic vaporizers. Br J Anaesth 48:387, 1976
50. Nawaf K, Stoelting RK: Nitrous oxide increases enflurane concentrations delivered by ethrane vaporizers. Anesth Analg 58:30, 1979
51. Prins L, Strupat J, Clement J: An evaluation of gas density dependence of anaesthetic vaporizers. Can Anaesth Soc J 27:106, 1980
52. Lin CY: Assessment of vaporizer performance in low-flow and closed-circuit anesthesia. Anesth Analg 59:359, 1980
53. Gould DB, Lampert BA, MacKrell TN: Effect of nitrous oxide solubility on vaporizer aberrance. Anesth Analg 61:938, 1982
54. Palayiwa E, Sanderson MH, Hahn CEW: Effects of carrier gas composition on the output of six anaesthetic vaporizers. Br J Anaesth 55:1025, 1983
55. Scheller MS, Drummond JC: Solubility of N_2O in volatile anesthetics contributes to vaporizer aberrancy when changing carrier gases. Anesth Analg 65:88, 1986
56. Tec 5 Continuous Flow Vaporizer. Operation and Maintenance Manual. Steeton, England, Ohmeda, The BOC Group, Inc, 1990
57. Jones RM: Desflurane and sevoflurane: Inhalation anaesthetics for this decade? Br J Anaesth 65:527, 1990
58. Jones RM, Cashman JN, Eger EI II et al: Kinetics and potency of desflurane (I-653) in volunteers. Anesth Analg 70:3, 1990
59. Miller ED, Greene NM: Waking up to desflurane: The anesthetic for the '90s? (editorial). Anesth Analg 70:1, 1990
60. Karis JH, Menzel DB: Inadvertent change of volatile anesthetics in anesthesia machines. Anesth Analg 61:53, 1982
61. Riegle EV, Desertspring D: Failure of the agent-specific filling device (letter to the editor). Anesthesiology 73:353, 1990
62. George TM: Failure of keyed agent-specific filling devices. Anesthesiology 61:228, 1984
63. Munson WM: Cardiac arrest: A hazard of tipping a vaporizer. Anesthesiology 26:235, 1965
64. Peters KR, Wingard DW: Anesthesia machine leakage due to misaligned vaporizers. Anesth Rev 14:36, 1987
65. Marks WE Jr, Bullard JR: Another hazard of free-standing vaporizers, increased anesthetic concentration with reversed flow of vaporizing gas. Anesthesiology 45:445, 1976
66. Capan L, Ramanathan S, Chalon J: A possible hazard with use of the Ohio ethrane vaporizer. Anesth Analg 59:65, 1980
67. Mapleson WW: The elimination of rebreathing in various semiclosed anaesthetic systems. Br J Anaesth 26:323, 1954
68. Willis BA, Pender JW, Mapleson WW: Rebreathing in a T-piece: Volunteer and theoretical studies of the Jackson-Rees modification of Ayre's T-piece during spontaneous respiration. Br J Anaesth 47:1239, 1975
69. Norman J, Adams AP, Sykes MK: Rebreathing with the Magill attachment. Anaesthesia 31:247, 1959
70. Kain ML, Nunn JF: Fresh gas economics of the Magill circuit. Anesthesiology 29:964, 1968
71. Sykes MK: Rebreathing during controlled respiration with the Magill attachment. Anaesthesia 31:247, 1959
72. Sykes MK: Rebreathing circuits: A review. Br J Anaesth 40:666, 1968
73. Bain JA, Spoerel WE: Flow requirements for a modified Mapleson D system during controlled ventilation. Can Anaesth Soc J 20:629, 1973
74. Soliman MG, Laberge R: The use of the Bain circuit in spontaneously breathing paediatric patients. Can Anaesth Soc J 25:276, 1978
75. Bain JA, Spoerel WE: A streamlined anaesthetic system. Can Anaesth Soc J 19:426, 1972
76. Ungerer MJ: A comparison between the Bain and Magill anesthetic systems during spontaneous breathing. Can Anaesth Soc J 25:122, 1978
77. Spoerel WE: Rebreathing and end tidal CO_2 during spontaneous breathing with the Bain circuit. Can Anaesth Soc J 30:148, 1983
78. Pethick SL: Letter to the editor. Can Anaesth Soc J 22:115, 1975
79. Ayre P: Endotracheal anesthesia for babies with special reference to hare-lip and cleft-palate operations. Anesth Analg 16:331, 1937
80. Ayre P: The T-piece technique. Br J Anaesth 28:520, 1956
81. Jackson-Rees G: Anaesthesia in the newborn. Br Med J 2:1419, 1950
82. Moyers J: A nomenclature for methods of inhalation anesthesia. Anesthesiology 14:609, 1953
83. Eger EI II: Anesthetic systems: Construction and function. In Eger EI II (ed): Anesthetic Uptake and Action, p 206. Baltimore, Williams & Wilkins, 1974
84. Eger EI II, Ethans CT: The effects of inflow, overflow and valve placement on economy of the circle system. Anesthesiology 29:93, 1968
85. Adriani J: Carbon dioxide absorption. In Adriani J (ed): The Chemistry and Physics of Anesthesia, 2nd ed, p 151. Springfield, Illinois, Charles C Thomas, 1962
86. Wilson RE: Soda lime: An absorbent for industrial purposes. J Ind Eng Chem 12:1000, 1920
87. Dewey & Almy Chemical Division: The sodasorb manual of CO_2 absorption. New York, W.R. Grace and Company, 1962
88. Foregger R: The regeneration of soda lime following absorption of CO_2. Anesthesiology 9:15, 1948
89. Hunt HE: Resistance in respiratory valves and canisters. Anesthesiology 16:190, 1955
90. Brown ES: Performance of absorbents: Continuous flow. Anesthesiology 20:41, 1959
91. Andrews JJ, Johnston RV Jr, Bee DE, Arens JF: Photodeactivation of ethyl violet: A potential hazard of sodasorb. Anesthesiology 72:59, 1990
92. Adriani J: Soda lime indicators. Anesthesiology 5:45, 1944
93. Case history 39. Accidental use of trichloroethylene (Trilene, Trimar) in a closed system. Anesth Analg 43:740, 1964
94. Strum D, Eger EI II, Johnson BH: Toxicity of sevoflurane in rats. Anesth Analg 66:769, 1987
95. Liu J, Laster MJ, Eger EI II et al: Absorption and degradation of sevoflurane and isoflurane in a conventional anesthetic circuit. Anesth Analg 72:785, 1991
96. Spearman CB, Sanders HG: Physical principles and functional designs of ventilators. In Kirby RR, Smith RA, Desautels DA (eds): Mechanical Ventilation, p 59. New York, Churchill Livingstone, 1985
97. McPherson SP, Spearman CB: Introduction to ventilators. In McPherson SP, Spearman CB (eds): Respiratory Therapy Equipment, 3rd ed, p 230. St. Louis, C.V. Mosby, 1985
98. Ohio Anesthesia Ventilator. Operation Maintenance. Madison, Ohio Medical Products, The BOC Group, Inc, 1982
99. Anesthesia Ventilator. Service Manual. Madison, Ohio Medical Products, The BOC Group, Inc, 1983
100. Ohio V5 Anesthesia Ventilator. Operation and Maintenance Manual. Madison, Ohmeda, The BOC Group, Inc, 1983
101. V5A Anesthesia Ventilator. Operation and Maintenance Manual. Madison, Ohmeda, The BOC Group, Inc, 1986
102. V5/V5A Anesthesia Ventilator. Service Manual. Madison, Ohio Medical Products, The BOC Group, Inc, 1983
103. 7000 Electronic Anesthesia Ventilator. Operation Maintenance. Madison, Ohmeda, The BOC Group, Inc, 1985
104. 7000 Electronic Anesthesia Ventilator. Service Manual. Madison, Ohmeda, The BOC Group, Inc, 1985
105. Roth S, Tweedie E, Sommer RM: Excessive airway pressure due to a malfunctioning anesthesia ventilator. Anesthesiology 65:532, 1986
106. Cooper JB, Newbower RS, Kitz RJ: An analysis of major errors and equipment failures in anesthesia management. Considerations for prevention and detection. Anesthesiology 60:34, 1984
107. Raphael DT, Weller RS, Doran DJ: A response algorithm for the low-pressure alarm condition. Anesth Analg 67:876, 1988
108. Slee TA, Pavlin EG: Failure of low pressure alarm associated with use of a humidifier. Anesthesiology 69:791, 1988
109. Feeley TW, Bancroft ML: Problems with mechanical ventilators. Int Anesthesiol Clin 20:83, 1982
110. Khalil SN, Gholston TK, Binderman J: Flapper valve malfunction in an Ohio closed scavenging system. Anesth Analg 66:1334, 1987

111. Sommer RM, Bhalla GS, Jackson JM: Hypoventilation caused by ventilator valve rupture. Anesth Analg 67:999, 1988

112. American National Standards Institute: American National Standard for Anesthetic Equipment—Scavenging Systems for Excess Anesthetic Gases (ANSI Z79.11-1982). New York, American National Standards Institute, 1982

113. Dorsch JA, Dorsch SE: Controlling trace gas levels. In Dorsch JA, Dorsch SE (eds): Understanding Anesthesia Equipment, 2nd ed, p 247. Baltimore, Williams & Wilkins, 1984

114. Open Reservoir Scavenger. Operator's Instruction Manual. Telford, Pennsylvania, North American Dräger, 1986

115. Gray WM: Scavenging equipment. Br J Anaesth 57:685, 1985

116. Scavenger Interface for Air Conditioning. Instruction Manual. Telford, Pennsylvania. North American Dräger, 1984

117. Davies G, Tarnawsky M: Letter to the editor. Can Anaesth Soc J 23:228, 1976

118. Tavakoli M, Habeeb A: Two hazards of gas scavenging. Anesth Analg 57:286, 1978

119. Mantia AM: Gas scavenging systems. Anesth Analg 61:162, 1982

120. O'Connor DE, Daniels BW, Pfitzner J: Hazards of anaesthetic scavenging: Case reports and brief review. Anaesth Intensive Care 10:15, 1982

121. Hagerdal M, Lecky JH: Anesthetic death of an experimental animal related to a scavenging system malfunction. Anesthesiology 47:522, 1977

122. Hamilton RC, Byrne J: Another cause of gas-scavenging-line obstruction. Anesthesiology 51:365, 1979

123. Flowerdew RM: A hazard of scavenger port design. Can Anaesth Soc J 28:481, 1981

124. Mann ES, Sprague DH: An easily overlooked malassembly. Anesthesiology 56:413, 1982

125. Seymour A: Possible hazards with an anaesthetic gas scavenging system. Anaesthesia 37:1218, 1987

126. Rendell-Baker L: Hazard of blocked scavenge valve. Can Anaesth Soc J 29:182, 1982

127. Patel KD, Dalal FY: A potential hazard of the Dräger scavenging interface system for wall suction. Anesth Analg 58:327, 1979

128. Mor ZF, Stein ED, Orkin LR: A possible hazard in the use of a scavenging system. Anesthesiology 47:302, 1977

129. Abramowitz M, McGill WA: Hazard of an anesthetic scavenging device. Anesthesiology 51:276, 1979

130. Malloy WF, Wightman AE, O'Sullivan D et al: Bilateral pneumothorax from suction applied to a ventilator exhaust valve. Anesth Analg 58:147, 1979

131. Sharrock NE, Leith DE: Potential pulmonary barotrauma when venting anesthetic gases to suction. Anesthesiology 46:152, 1977

132. Sharrock NE, Gabel RA: Inadvertent anesthetic overdose obscured by scavenging. Anesthesiology 49:137, 1978

133. Cooper JB: Toward prevention of anesthetic mishaps. Int Anesthesiol Clin 22:167, 1984

134. Spooner RB, Kirby RR: Equipment related anesthetic incidents. Int Anesthesiol Clin 22:133, 1984

135. Emergency Care Research Institute: Avoiding anesthetic mishaps through pre-use checks. Health Devices 11:201, 1982

136. Food and Drug Administration: Anesthesia Apparatus Checkout Recommendations, FDA, 8th ed. Rockville, Maryland, Food and Drug Administration, 1986

137. Comm G, Rendell-Baker L: Back pressure check valves a hazard. Anesthesiology 56:327, 1982

138. Dorsch JA, Dorsch SE: Hazards of anesthesia machines and breathing systems. In Dorsch JA, Dorsch SE (eds): Understanding Anesthesia Equipment, 2nd ed, p 289. Baltimore, Williams & Wilkins, 1984

139. Toremalm NG: Airflow pattern and ciliary activity in the trachea after tracheostomy. Acta Otolaryngol 53:442, 1961

140. Burton JDK: Effects of dry anesthetic gases on the respiratory mucous membrane. Lancet 1:235, 1962

141. Shapiro BA, Harrison RA, Kacmarek RM: Humidity and aerosol therapy. In Shapiro BA, Harrison RA, Kacmarek RM (eds): Clinical Application of Respiratory Therapy, p 90. Chicago, Year Book Medical Publishers, 1985

142. McPherson SP, Spearman CB: Humidifiers and nebulizers. In McPherson SP, Spearman CB (eds): Respiratory Therapy Equipment, 3rd ed, p 119. St. Louis, C.V. Mosby, 1985

143. Petty C: Anesthesia circuits. In Petty C (ed): The Anesthesia Machine, p 81. New York, Churchill Livingstone, 1987

144. Forbes AR: Humidification and mucus flow in the intubated trachea. Br J Anaesth 45:874, 1973

145. Chalon J, Ali M, Turndorf H et al: Humidification of Anesthetic Gases. Springfield, Illinois, Charles C Thomas, 1981

146. Tausk HC, Miller R, Roberts RB: Maintenance of body temperature by heated humidification. Anesth Analg 55:719, 1976

147. Elder PT: Accidental hypothermia. In Shoemaker WC, Thompson WL, Holbrook PR (eds): Textbook of Critical Care, p 85. Philadelphia, W.B. Saunders, 1984

148. Bernard JM, Pinaud M, Souron R: Perioperative hypothermia prevention. Acta Anaesthesiol Scand 31:521, 1987

149. Spaepen MS, Bodman HA, Kundsin RB: Prevalence and survival of microbe contaminants in heated nebulizers. Anesth Analg 57:191, 1978

150. Chase HF, Trotta R, Kilmore MA: Simple methods for humidifying non-rebreathing anesthesia gas systems. Anesth Analg 41:249, 1962

151. Chalon J, Simon RS, Ramanathan S: A high-humidity circle system for infants and children. Anesthesiology 49:205, 1978

152. Weeks DB: Humidification of anesthetic gases using heat-and-moisture exchangers. Anesth Rev 12:22, 1985

153. Ramanathan S, Chalon J, Capan L: Rebreathing characteristics of the Bain anesthesia circuit. Anesth Analg 56:822, 1977

154. Westenskow DR, Jordan WS, Jordan R: Evaluation of oxygen monitors for use during anesthesia. Anesth Analg 60:53, 1981

155. Lowe HJ, Ernst EA: The Quantitative Practice of Anesthesia: Use of the Closed Circuit. Baltimore, Williams & Wilkins, 1981

156. Waters RM: Advantages and technique of carbon dioxide filtration with inhalation anesthesia. Anesth Analg 5:160, 1926

157. Foster CA: Fatal cardiac arrest with fluothane. Lancet 1:1144, 1957

158. Romagnoli A, Cohen M, Diamond MJ: A safe and economical method of administering fluothane in closed circuit anaesthesia. Can Anaesth Soc J 7:186, 1960

159. Hampton LJ, Flickinger H: Closed circuit anesthesia utilizing known increments of halothane. Anesthesiology 22:413, 1961

160. Herscher E, Yeakel AE: Nitrous oxide-oxygen based anesthesia: The waste and its cost. Anesth Rev 4:29, 1977

161. Virtue RW: Anesthetic gas flows, costs and pollution. Anesth Rev 5:14, 1978

162. Patel A, Milliken RA: Costs of delivery of anesthetic gases re-examined—I. Anesthesiology 55:710, 1981

163. Virtue RW, Aldrete JA: Costs of delivery of anesthetic gases re-examined—II. Anesthesiology 55:711, 1981

164. Spain JA: Cost of delivery of anesthetic gases re-examined—III. Anesthesiology 55:711, 1981

165. Logan M, Farmer JG: Anaesthesia and the ozone layer. Br J Anaesth 63:645, 1989

166. Dorsch JA, Dorsch SE: The breathing system IV. In Dorsch JA, Dorsch SE (eds): Understanding Anesthesia Equipment, 2nd ed, p 210. Baltimore, Williams & Wilkins, 1984

167. Barton F, Nunn JF: Use of refractometry to determine nitrogen accumulation in closed circuits. Br J Anaesth 47:346, 1975

168. Morita S, Latta W, Hambro K et al: Accumulation of methane, acetone, and nitrogen in the inspired gas during closed-circuit anesthesia. Anesth Analg 64:343, 1985

169. Ernst EA: Use of charcoal to rapidly decrease depth of anesthesia while maintaining a closed circuit. Anesthesiology 57:343, 1982

170. Larsen VH, Severinsen I, Waaben J: Removal of halogenated anaesthetics from a closed circle system with a charcoal filter. Acta Anaesthesiol Scand 33:374, 1989

171. Middleton V, Poznak AV, Artusio JF et al: Carbon monoxide accumulation in closed circle anesthesia systems. Anesthesiology 26:715, 1965

172. Parker CJ, Snowdon SL: Predicted and measured oxygen concentrations in the circle system using low fresh gas flows with oxygen supplied by an oxygen concentrator. Br J Anaesth 61:397, 1988

173. Sharp JH, Trudell JR: Volatile metabolites and decomposition products of halothane in man. Anesthesiology 50:2, 1979

174. Eger ET II: Dragons and other scientific hazards. Anesthesiology 50:1, 1979
175. Ferderbar PJ, Hettler RE, Jablonski J et al: A case of breathing system leak during closed circuit anesthesia. Anesthesiology 65:661, 1986
176. Huffman LM, Riddle RT: Mass spectrometer and/or capnograph use during low-flow, closed circuit anesthesia administration. Anesthesiology 66:439, 1987
177. Ross JA, Wloch RT, White DC et al: Servo-controlled closed-circuit anaesthesia: A method for the automatic control of anaesthesia produced by a volatile agent in oxygen. Br J Anaesth 55:1053, 1983
178. O'Callaghan AC, Hawes DW, Ross JA et al: Uptake of isoflurane during clinical anaesthesia: Servo-control of liquid anaesthetic injection into a closed-circuit breathing system. Br J Anaesth 55:1061, 1983
179. Westenskow DR, Jordan WS, Hayes JK: Uptake of enflurane: A study of variability between patients. Anaesthesia 55:595, 1983
180. Ritchie RG, Ernst EA, Pate BL et al: Closed-loop control of an anesthesia delivery system: Development and animal testing. IEEE Transactions on Biomedical Engineering BME-34:437, 1987

APPENDIX
ANESTHESIA APPARATUS CHECKOUT RECOMMENDATIONS

This checkout, or a reasonable equivalent, should be conducted before administering anesthesia. This is a guideline which users are encouraged to modify to accommodate differences in equipment design and variations in local clinical practice. Such local modifications should have appropriate peer review. Users should refer to the operator's manual for special procedures or precautions.

* 1. *Inspect anesthesia machine for:*
     Machine identification number
     Valid inspection sticker
     Undamaged flow meters, vaporizers, gauges, supply hoses
     Complete, undamaged breathing system with adequate CO_2 absorbent
     Correct mounting of cylinders in yokes
     Presence of cylinder wrench
* 2. *Inspect and turn on:*
     Electrical equipment requiring warm-up (ECG/pressure monitor, oxygen monitor, etc.)
* 3. *Connect waste gas scavenging system:*
     Adjust vacuum as required
* 4. *Check that:*
     Flow-control valves are off
     Vaporizers are off
     Vaporizers are filled (not overfilled)
     Filler caps are sealed tightly
     CO_2 absorber bypass (if any) is off

Reproduced with permission from Food and Drug Administration: Anesthesia Apparatus Checkout Recommendations, FDA, 8th ed. Rockville, Maryland, Food and Drug Administration, 1986.

If an anesthetist uses the same machine in successive cases, the steps marked with an asterisk (*) need not be repeated or may be abbreviated after the initial checkout.

* 5. *Check oxygen (O_2) cylinder supplies:*
     a. Disconnect pipeline supply (if connected) and return cylinder and pipeline pressure gauge to zero with O_2 flush valve.
     b. Open O_2 cylinder, check pressure; close cylinder and observe gauge for evidence of high pressure leak.
     c. With the O_2 flush valve, flush to empty piping.
     d. Repeat as in b. and c. above for second O_2 cylinder, if present.
     e. Replace any cylinder less than about 600 psig. At least one should be nearly full.
     f. Open less full cylinder.
* 6. *Turn on master switch (if present):*
* 7. *Check nitrous oxide (N_2O) and other gas cylinder supplies:*
     Use same procedure as described in 5a. and b. above, but OPEN and CLOSE flow-control valve to empty piping.
     NOTE: N_2O pressure below 745 psig indicates that the cylinder is less than 1/4 full.
* 8. *Test flowmeters:*
     a. Check that float is at bottom of tube with flow-control valves closed (or at min. O_2 flow if so equipped).
     b. Adjust flow of all gases through their full range and check for erratic movements of floats.
* 9. *Test ratio protection/warning system (if present):*
     Attempt to create hypoxic O_2/N_2O mixture and verify correct change in gas flow and/or alarm.
*10. *Test O_2 pressure failure system:*
     a. Set O_2 and other gas flows to mid-range.
     b. Close O_2 cylinder and flush to release O_2 pressure.
     c. Verify that all flows fall to zero. Open O_2 cylinder.
     d. Close all other cylinders and bleed piping pressure.
     e. Close O_2 cylinder and bleed piping pressure.
     f. CLOSE FLOW CONTROL VALVES.
*11. *Test central pipeline gas supplies:*
     a. Inspect supply hoses (should not be cracked or worn).
     b. Connect supply hoses, verifying correct color coding.
     c. Adjust all flows to at least mid-range.
     d. Verify that supply pressures hold (45–55 psig).
     e. Shut off flow control valves.
*12. *Add any accessory equipment to the breathing system:*
     Add PEEP valve, humidifier, etc., if they might be used (if necessary remove after step 18 until needed).
13. *Calibrate O_2 monitor:*
     *a. Calibrate O_2 monitor to read 21% in room air.
     *b. Test low alarm.
     c. Occlude breathing system at patient end; fill and empty system several times with 100% O_2.
     d. Check that monitor reading is nearly 100%.
14. *Sniff inspiratory gas:*
     There should be no odor.
*15. *Check unidirectional valves:*
     a. Inhale and exhale through a surgical mask into the breathing system (each limb individually, if possible).
     b. Verify unidirectional flow in each limb.
     c. Reconnect tubing firmly.

##16. *Test for leaks in machine and breathing system:*
  a. Close APL (pop-off) valve and occlude system at patient end.
  b. Fill system via O_2 flush until bag just full, but negligible pressure in system. Set O_2 flow to 5 l/min.
  c. Slowly decrease O_2 flow until pressure *no longer rises* above about 20 cm H_2O. This approximates total leak rate, which should be no greater than a few hundred ml/min (less for closed circuit techniques).
  CAUTION: Check valves in some machines make it imperative to measure flow in step c. above when pressure *just stops rising.*
  d. Squeeze bag to pressure about 50 cm H_2O and verify that system is tight.

  17. *Exhaust valve and scavenger system:*
  a. Open APL valve and observe release of pressure.
  b. Occlude breathing system at patient end and ver-ify that negligible positive or negative pressure appears with either zero or 5 l/min flow and exhaust relief valve (if present) open with flush flow.

18. *Test ventilator:*
  a. If switching valve is present, test function in both bag and ventilator mode.
  b. Close APL valve if necessary and occlude system at patient end.
  c. Test for leaks and pressure relief by appropriate cycling (exact procedure will vary with type of ventilator).
  d. Attach reservoir bag at mask fitting, fill system, and cycle ventilator. Assure filling/emptying of bag.

19. *Check for appropriate level of patient suction.*
20. *Check, connect, and calibrate other electronic monitors.*
21. *Check final position of all controls.*
22. *Turn on and set other appropriate alarms for equipment to be used.*
    (Perform next two steps as soon as is practical)
23. *Set O_2 monitor alarm limits.*
24. *Set airway pressure and/or volume monitor alarm limits (if adjustable).*

A vaporizer leak can only be detected if the vaporizer is turned on during this test. Even then, a relatively small but clinically significant leak may still be obscured.

26
Linda C. Stehling

Management of the Airway

Airway management involves more than proficiency with tracheal intubation techniques. The anesthesiologist must understand the physiologic consequences and complications of endotracheal intubation and have knowledge of the anatomy, innervation, and pathologic conditions of the airway as well as of methods of assessment. He or she must be able to recognize patients in whom airway management may be difficult and be able to formulate and implement alternative plans in various clinical situations.

THE LARYNX

Anatomy

Located at the level of the fourth to sixth cervical vertebrae in the adult, the larynx is composed of cartilage, ligaments, and muscle. It is lined by mucous membrane, which is continuous with that of the pharynx and trachea. The laryngeal cavity extends from the laryngeal inlet to the caudal border of the cricoid cartilage. The larynx is bounded anteriorly by the epiglottis, posteriorly by the mucous membrane that extends between the arytenoid cartilages, and laterally by the aryepiglottic folds. The vocal folds (vocal cords, true cords) extend from the thyroid cartilage to the arytenoid cartilages. The rima glottidis is the triangular opening between the vocal cords. The portion of the laryngeal cavity above the vocal cords is the vestibule, which contains the ventricular folds (false vocal cords) (Fig. 26-1). In the adult, the area between the vocal cords is the narrowest part of the laryngeal cavity.

The infant's larynx differs from that of the adult in more than absolute size (Fig. 26-2). At birth, the epiglottis is at the midlevel of the first cervical vertebra (C1), the glottis is at the midlevel of C3, and the inferior margin of the cricoid is at the superior portion of C4. Descent of the laryngeal structures occurs, and by 3 years the epiglottis is at the level of C3, the glottis is at the intervertebral disk between C4 and C5, and the cricoid is at mid-C5. Little change occurs until puberty, when there is further descent of the glottis and cricoid owing to growth of the thyroid cartilage.[1] The infant's vocal cords are angled, whereas those of the adult are more perpendicular to the axis of the trachea. The epiglottis is less rigid, longer, and narrower. The angle between the glottis and epiglottis is more acute, and the aryepiglottic folds are redundant or closer to the midline. The infant's airway is narrowest at the cricoid.[1,2]

Innervation

Sensory and motor innervation of the larynx is provided by the vagus nerves. The internal branch of the superior laryngeal nerve is responsible for sensation down to the vocal cords and the recurrent laryngeal nerves are responsible for the area below the vocal cords. The cricothyroid muscle is innervated by the external branch of the superior laryngeal nerve, and the other laryngeal muscles are innervated by the recurrent laryngeal nerves.

Although the recurrent laryngeal nerves innervate the muscles responsible for both abduction and adduction, the abductor muscles appear to be more vulnerable to injury. Abductor paralysis occurs with mild to moderate nerve trauma, whereas severe trauma or sectioning of the nerves causes both abductor and adductor palsy. Following partial bilateral recurrent laryngeal nerve damage, the vocal cords lie near the midline, the airway aperture is small, and signs of airway obstruction quickly become apparent. With bilateral transection or severe nerve damage, the vocal cords remain in the midposition, and the airway is often adequate for normal respiration.

Function

The larynx primarily protects the lower airway by preventing foreign matter from entering it. Phonation is an important, but secondary, function.

AIRWAY ASSESSMENT

Although the same principles apply to patients outside the operating room, where decisions regarding emergency airway management must be based on less extensive evaluation, primary emphasis is placed here on management of patients having surgery. The patient's diagnosis and the proposed surgical procedure are often the first clues to potential difficulties with airway management as well as to the airway

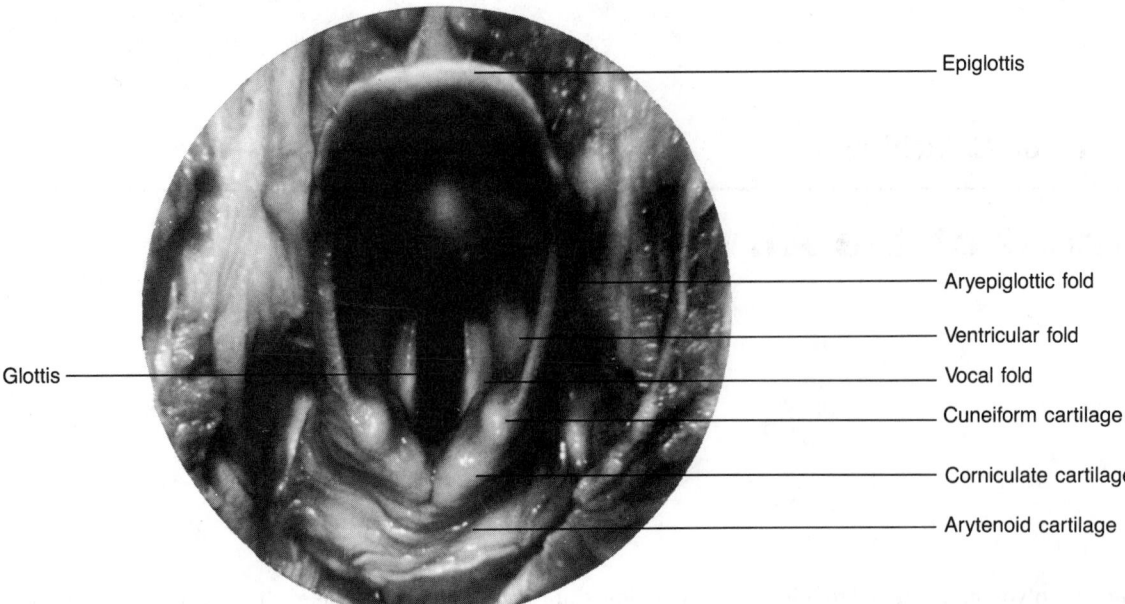

Epiglottis

Aryepiglottic fold

Ventricular fold

Vocal fold

Cuneiform cartilage

Corniculate cartilage

Arytenoid cartilage

Glottis

Figure 26-1. Anatomic specimen of adult human larynx.

equipment required. A thorough preoperative history and physical examination are essential.

History

The patient should be questioned about signs and symptoms suggestive of airway abnormalities, such as shortness of breath or hoarseness. Hoarseness in the patient with rheumatoid arthritis may indicate involvement of the cricoarytenoid cartilages and narrowing of the laryngeal opening.[3] Information should also be sought regarding previous surgery, trauma, or neoplasia involving the airway and prior anesthetic experiences. Whenever possible, previous anesthesia records should be reviewed, particularly if there is evidence suggesting that airway management may be difficult.

Physical Examination

The patient's head should be viewed in profile so that micrognathia, the most common feature associated with difficult laryngoscopy and intubation, can be detected. If the patient is seen only in the frontal plane, the degree of mandibular hypoplasia is frequently underestimated.

The presence of protruding or "buck" teeth, also best appreciated from the lateral aspect, may complicate endotracheal intubation. Conversely, it is often difficult to secure a tight seal with a face mask in edentulous patients. Loose, capped, and prosthetic teeth should be carefully noted. Occasionally it is preferable to extract loose teeth before airway manipulation to prevent them from being dislodged and possibly aspirated or swallowed. Nonfixed dental prostheses should be removed before anesthesia induction.

A cleft or long, high-arched palate, often associated with difficult tracheal intubation, may be an isolated finding or a component of a malformation syndrome. A relatively large, fixed tongue is more often found in patients with trisomy 21, the mucopolysaccharidoses, and the Beckwith-Weidemann syndrome. Although some conditions such as Treacher Collins and Goldenhar syndromes should be fa-

miliar to all anesthesiologists, the anesthetic implications of less common syndromes may not be as apparent, necessitating reference to texts dealing specifically with congenital anomalies.[4-6]

The ease of tracheal intubation can be predicted by having the seated patient open his or her mouth and protrude the tongue maximally. When the faucial pillars, soft palate, and uvula are easily visualized, direct laryngoscopic examination should be easy. Laryngoscopic examination may be easy or difficult if only the faucial pillars and soft palate are visible but the uvula is obscured by the tongue. When only the soft palate is visualized, exposure of the glottis is almost invariably difficult.[7,8]

Temporomandibular joint mobility is assessed by asking the patient to open the mouth. In the adult, the distance between the upper and lower central incisors is normally 4–6 cm. Joint function can be further evaluated if the anesthesiologist places a middle finger of each hand just inferior and posterior to the patient's ear lobes and the index fingers anterior to the tragus of the ears. When the patient opens

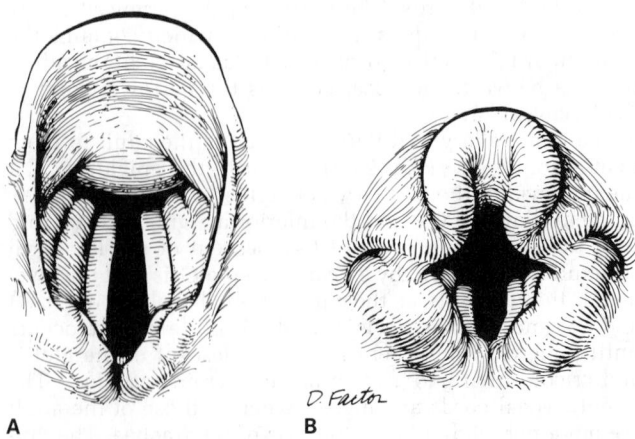

A   B

Figure 26-2. (A) Adult larynx. (B) Infant larynx. The infant's epiglottis is relatively long, stiff, and U-shaped.

the mouth maximally, the examiner should feel both rotation and forward gliding of the condylar heads bilaterally. If only the first phase of opening is palpated, limited opening of the mouth can be expected.[9] Occasionally, forward pressure on the angles of the mandible or grasping the mandible anteriorly and pulling it forward allows wider opening.[10]

Ankylosis of the temporomandibular joints is seen most frequently in patients with rheumatoid arthritis. However, it is also prevalent in patients with long-term Type I diabetes mellitus.[11] In patients who have sustained trauma or have an infection involving the mouth or neck, mobility may be restricted by pain rather than by deformity. The cause of the joint dysfunction must be determined because voluntary limitation of motion will disappear once anesthesia is induced and a muscle relaxant is administered. However, the use of general anesthesia and muscle relaxants may be contraindicated in patients with decreased temporomandibular joint mobility until an endotracheal tube has been positioned or a tracheostomy performed.

The patient's cervical spine mobility must be evaluated because endotracheal intubation usually involves extension of the neck. It is best to have the patient sit or stand during this examination, since the degree of restricted movement will be obscured if the patient's head is on a pillow. The normal range of flexion-extension of the neck varies from 165–90 degrees, with the range decreasing approximately 20% by the time the patient is 75 years old.[12] The patient with rheumatoid arthritis or ankylosing spondylitis may have virtually no neck mobility.[3,13] Although radiographic evidence of cervical spine involvement is present in 25–90% of patients with rheumatoid arthritis, approximately half have no symptoms.[14] Occult cervical spine fractures have been reported in approximately one third of patients with severe ankylosing spondylitis.[15] Long-standing diabetes mellitus is also associated with decreased cervical spine mobility.[11,16] Any type of movement that produces paresthesias or sensory or motor deficits must be noted and avoided during intubation of the trachea.

The probable ease of tracheal intubation also can be assessed by measurement of the distance, normally 6.5 cm or more in adults, between the lower border of the mandible and the thyroid notch when the patient's neck is fully extended. If the measurement is less than 6 cm, it will be impossible to visualize the larynx. If the distance is 6.5 cm

and the patient has prominent teeth, a thick neck, or decreased neck mobility, difficulty in visualizing the larynx should be anticipated.[17] The distance can be measured with a ruler or an intubation gauge (Fig. 26-3). The anesthesiologist can also use his or her fingers to assess the distance, but obviously this measurement varies with the examiner.

The neck should be palpated to detect masses and tracheal deviation. If the patient has a tracheostomy scar, the reason for the surgery must be determined. In patients with a tracheostomy in situ, it may be necessary to change the tube or use an adapter because some tubes are not compatible with anesthesia circuits.

A simple bedside test that is said to predict the difficulty of laryngoscopic examination and intubation in patients with the limited joint mobility syndrome associated with long-standing diabetes mellitus involves having the patient place the hands in the "prayer" position. Inability to oppose the interphalangeal joints is correlated with the degree of difficulty with intubation.[11]

Radiographic Studies

Standard anteroposterior and lateral view radiographs of the neck and chest may be indicated to evaluate the cervical spine and ascertain the diameter and position of the trachea in patients with known or suspected airway abnormalities. Odontoid hypoplasia is associated with a number of congenital disorders, including trisomy 21,[18] Morquio's and Klippel-Feil syndromes, osteogenesis imperfecta, certain types of dwarfism,[19] and congenital scoliosis. Atlantoaxial subluxation is the most common radiographic finding in rheumatoid arthritis, occurring in 25% of patients.[20] Rheumatoid patients at high risk of cervical spine involvement are the elderly and those with long-standing disease and neck symptoms. Computed tomography and magnetic resonance imaging may be useful in localizing and quantitating both intrinsic and extrinsic airway abnormalities.[21,22]

Laryngoscopy

A flexible fiberoptic nasopharyngoscope can be used by the anesthesiologist or otorhinolaryngologist to evaluate the pharynx and larynx. This examination can be performed with minimal discomfort in the awake patient and is especially useful in those with neoplasia involving the airway. However, visualization of the vocal cords, even if the laryngeal inlet appears adequate, does not guarantee that direct laryngoscopic examination and endotracheal intubation will be possible. A less reliable method of evaluating the glottis in the awake patient is indirect laryngoscopic examination with a laryngeal mirror.

Miscellaneous Studies

A variety of other measurements[23] and radiographic studies[24-26] have been employed to predict the likelihood of difficulty with laryngoscopic examination and intubation. Many are not practical for routine application. The five risk factors that are most consistently associated with difficulty are obesity, decreased head and neck movement, receding mandible, reduced jaw movement, and buck teeth.[27] A prospective study comparing the predictive value of a scoring system using these five factors (the Wilson risk-sum) and the classification of difficulty based on the view of pharyn-

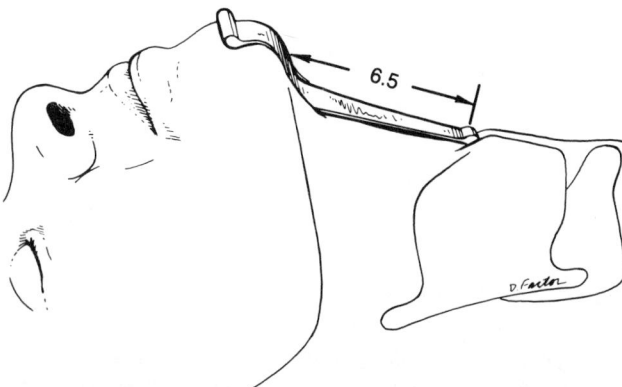

Figure 26-3. An intubation gauge can be used to estimate the degree of difficulty with endotracheal intubation. The distance between the lower border of the mandible and the thyroid notch is normally greater than 6.5 cm in the adult.

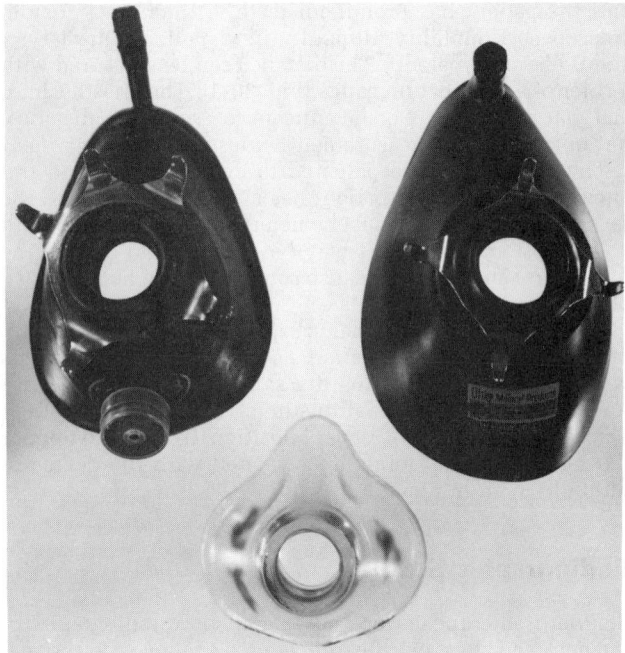

Figure 26-4. The Connell anatomic mask (*right*) is most often used for adults, whereas the Rendell-Baker-Soucek mask (*center*) is designed specifically for children. The Patil-Syracuse endoscopic mask (*left*) (Anesthesia Associates, San Marcos, California) has an endoscopic port for insertion of a fiberoptic endoscope and endotracheal tube.

geal structures obtained with the patient's mouth fully open and the tongue protruded[7] (the Mallampati test) was conducted in 675 patients. Both tests identified only 5 of 12 difficult laryngoscopic examinations and were much less sensitive and specific than originally described.[28]

No single test or classification can identify all patients in whom airway management will be difficult. Each anesthesiologist should formulate his or her own system for predicting the difficulty of laryngoscopy and endotracheal intubation and apply it to all patients preoperatively.

AIRWAY EQUIPMENT

Certain items of equipment such as masks, airways, laryngoscopes, and endotracheal tubes are essential for management of any patient, regardless of the anesthetic technique employed. The nature of the patient's pathologic condition or the surgical procedure may dictate that additional equipment, such as a fiberoptic endoscope, also be available.

Masks

The Connell anatomic mask (Fig. 26-4) is used most frequently for adults. It is available in a variety of sizes, and its malleable body allows it to be shaped to fit the patient's face. Rendell-Baker-Soucek masks (Fig. 26-4) are designed especially for children. Endoscopic masks (Fig. 26-4) may be employed during fiberoptic intubation of the trachea. Because flammable anesthetics are rarely used, it is no longer necessary to use carbon-containing black masks. Clear masks permit visualization of the mouth for secretions, emesis, and pinched lips.

Airways

Most oropharyngeal airways, available in several sizes and types, are made of plastic. Some are metal, including one specially designed for use during fiberoptic endotracheal intubation (Fig. 26-5). Nasopharyngeal airways are available in plastic and rubber. The binasal airway (Fig. 26-6) has an adapter for connection to the anesthesia circuit.

A new device, the laryngeal mask airway, consists of a tube to which is attached an elliptically shaped cuff that resembles a miniature face mask (Fig. 26-7). Four sizes are available for use in infants, children, and adults. General anesthesia is required for placement of the device. Once an adequate depth of anesthesia is achieved, the lubricated laryngeal mask, with the cuff deflated, is inserted blindly into the pharynx and guided digitally until resistance is felt as it enters the hypopharynx. Properly inserted, the airway lies with the mask tip resting against the upper esophageal sphincter, the sides toward the piriform fossae, and the upper border under the base of the tongue. Unlike other cuffed pharyngeal airways, it forms a seal around the laryngeal,

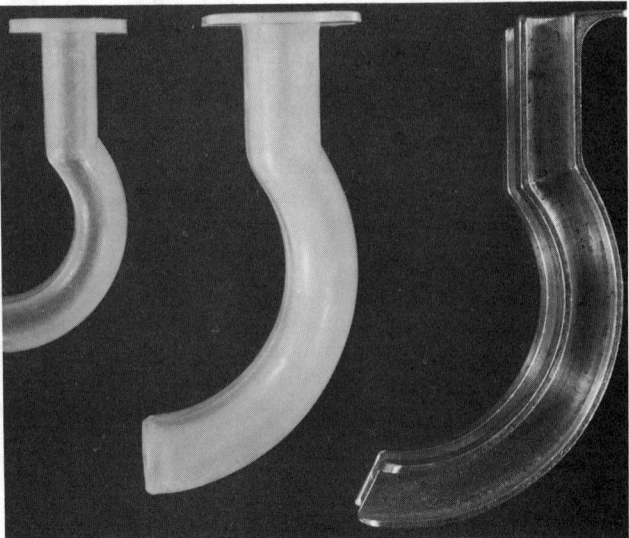

Figure 26-5. Oropharyngeal airways are available in sizes suitable for children (*left*) and adults (*center*). The Patil-Syracuse endoscopic airway (*right*) (Anesthesia Associates, San Marcos, California) has a central groove to keep the insertion tube of a fiberoptic endoscope in the midline and a slit at the distal end to direct the instrument into the larynx. Lateral channels are provided for suctioning.

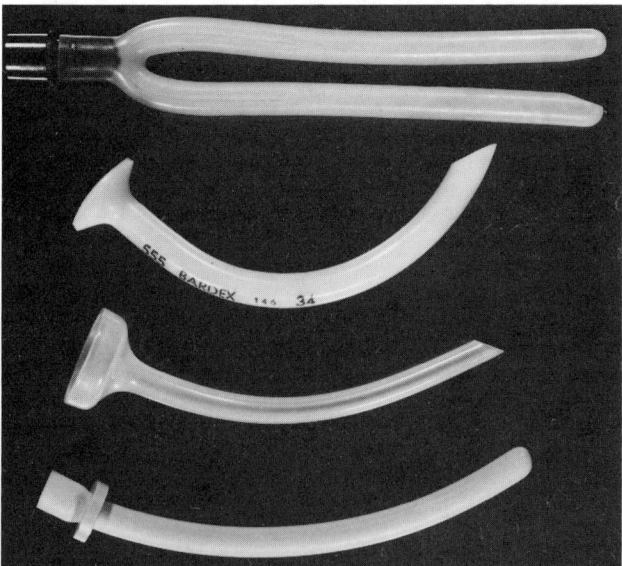

Figure 26-6. Nasal airways are shown.

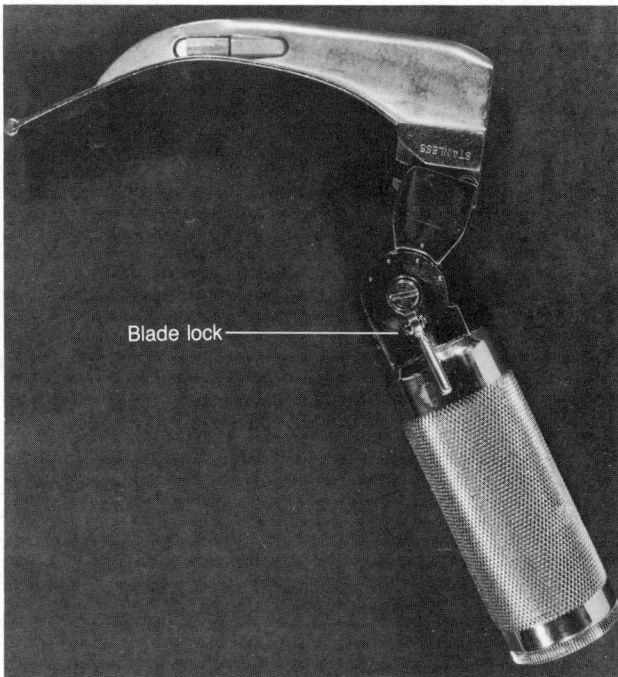

Figure 26-8. Short, adjustable laryngoscope handle (Anesthesia Associates, San Marcos, California) with blade lock to allow the blade to be positioned at different angles.

not the pharyngeal, perimeter. Two to thirty-five milliliters of air are used to inflate the cuff, depending on the size of the mask. The device is intended primarily for use in spontaneously breathing patients who are not at risk of aspiration of gastric contents. However, positive pressure ventilation can be employed. Potential complications include laryngospasm, most often the result of inadequate anesthesia, and airway obstruction due to improper insertion or positioning of the device. Favorable experience with the laryngeal mask airway has been reported in children[29,30] and adults.[31,32] In addition to being used in patients having elective surgery, the device has been employed in emergency situations when endotracheal intubation was impossible.[33] However, it must be remembered that its use does not preclude the aspiration of gastric contents.[34]

Laryngoscopes

Laryngoscopes are composed of a battery-containing handle and blade to which a bulb or fiberoptic light bundle is attached. Short handles are especially useful when patients who are obese or have short necks are intubated. One modification has a blade lock that allows the blade to be positioned at an angle of 180, 135, 90, or 45 degrees to the handle (Fig. 26-8).[35]

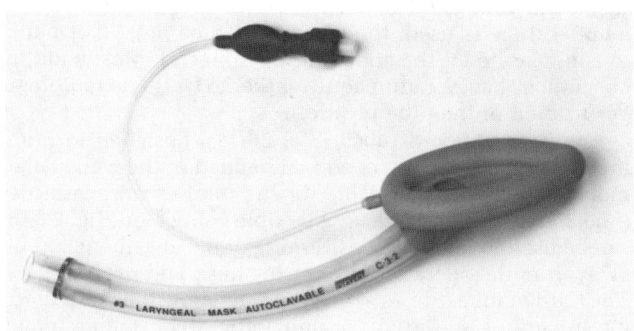

Figure 26-7. The laryngeal mask airway. (Courtesy of Dr. A.I.J. Brain.)

Curved and straight blades are the two general types available. The most commonly used are the Macintosh and Miller blades, which are manufactured in several sizes (Fig. 26-9). The tip of the curved blade is placed in the vallecula, superior to the epiglottis, whereas the tip of the straight blade is placed under the epiglottis to elevate it. Personal preference primarily determines the type of blade used for intubating adults. Alleged advantages of the curved blade include less potential for damage to the teeth and more space availability in the oropharynx for the endotracheal tube. Straight blades are usually used for children because it is easier to lift the base of the tongue and fix the epiglottis, thereby facilitating visualization of the glottis.

Proponents of the Macintosh blade claim that the incidence of laryngospasm and the magnitude of alterations in cardiac rate and rhythm are reduced because it does not contact the inferior surface of the epiglottis, which is innervated by the superior laryngeal nerve, a branch of the vagus. Rather, it is placed in the vallecula, which is innervated by the glossopharyngeal nerve. However, when studied, it was found that the incidence of changes in heart rate and rhythm was comparable with both curved and straight blades.[36] Because most patients receive a muscle relaxant before laryngoscopic examination, the theoretic advantage of decreased laryngospasm with a curved blade has assumed less significance.

The Bullard intubating laryngoscope (Circon ACMI, Stamford, CT) was designed for the difficult to intubate patient but can be used for direct laryngoscopic examination and intubation of patients with normal airways. Available in both pediatric[37] and adult styles (Fig. 26-10), the instrument combines an anatomically shaped rigid blade with a fiberoptic light source that permits laryngoscopy without the necessity for aligning the oral, pharyngeal, and tracheal axes as is required with conventional laryngoscopy. The clinical applications are similar to those for fiberoptic endoscopy and the time required to acquire skill in use of the instrument is similar.[38] Once the larynx is visualized

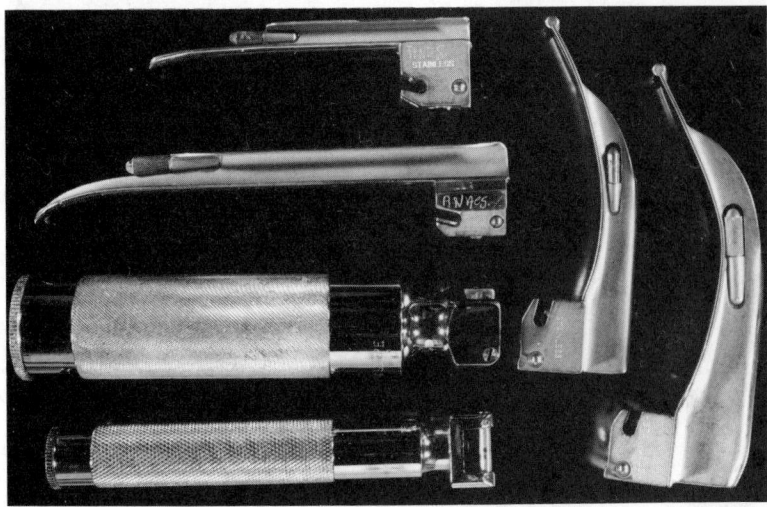

Figure 26-9. Laryngoscope handles and Miller (*above*) and Macintosh (*right*) blades.

through the eyepiece of the instrument, the endotracheal tube is guided into the glottis with an intubating forceps system or special introducing stylet.

Endotracheal Tubes

Endotracheal tubes are numbered according to the internal diameter. The approximate size and length of tubes for children are determined by the patient's age and size (see Table 48-3). However, there is significant variability, and tubes larger or smaller than the predicted size must be available. In general, a 7.0–8.5-mm internal diameter tube is appropriate for women and an 8.0–9.5-mm internal diameter tube is appropriate for men. In women, the length from the alveolar ridge to the tip of the tube should be approximately 21 cm, and in men, 23 cm.[39] Although some anesthesiologists select an endotracheal tube for children that is approximately the same size as the child's little finger, others rely on formulas based on age. A useful guideline for children older than 1 year is as follows:

$$\text{Endotracheal tube size (mm)} = 4 + \frac{\text{age (yr)}}{4}$$

$$= \frac{\text{age (yr)} + 16}{4}$$

The length of the tube can also be calculated:

$$\text{Length (cm)} = 12 + \frac{\text{age (yr)}}{2}$$

Nasotracheal tubes should be approximately 3 cm longer than orotracheal tubes.

Endotracheal tube resistance varies inversely with the tube size. Each millimeter decrease in tube size is associated with an increase in resistance of 25–100%. The work of breathing parallels changes in resistance. A 1-mm decrease in tube size increases the work of breathing by 34–154%, depending upon the ventilatory pattern.[40]

Most endotracheal tubes are made of semirigid plastic and are disposable. The label IT (implant tested) or Z-79 (for the Z-79 Committee on Anesthesia Equipment of the American National Standards Institute) signifies that the tube material is nontoxic to tissue.

Tubes used in older children and adults have cuffs that are inflated to seal the airway. Uncuffed tubes are usually employed in children younger than 8–10 years to decrease the risk of subglottic edema. In addition, the narrow subglottic area in young children provides an anatomic seal. When a cuffed tube is used, the size of the tube must be smaller to compensate for the added bulk of the cuff. Most endotracheal tubes have a radiopaque marker to facilitate radiologic verification of the tube position.

Anode or armored tubes (Fig. 26-11), designed to minimize kinking, have a wire coil embedded in the wall. Tubes molded with angles suitable for intraoral or intranasal use (Fig. 26-12) are available, or a flexible connector (Fig. 26-13) can be used to facilitate positioning of the anesthetic circuit away from the operative site during head and neck surgery. The Carden tube (Fig. 26-14) is placed below the vocal cords for surgery of the larynx or subglottic area. Double-lumen endobronchial or "split" tubes (Fig. 26-15) permit one or both lungs to be ventilated and are used primarily during thoracic surgery (see Chapter 34).

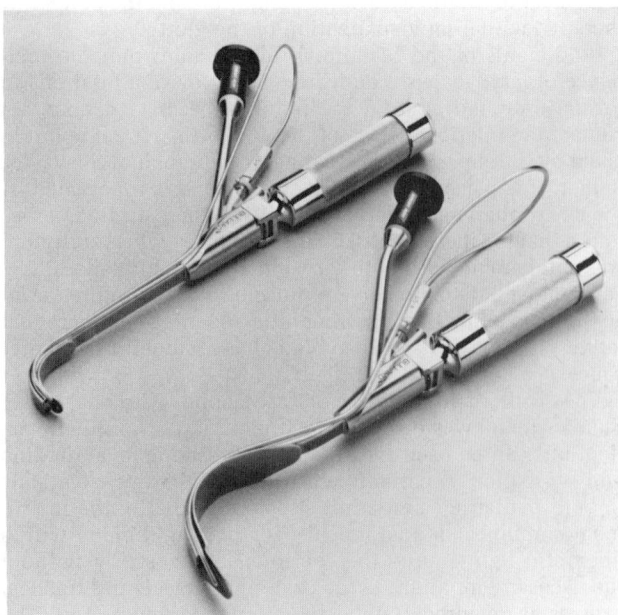

Figure 26.10. Bullard pediatric (*top*) and adult laryngoscopes with introducing stylets. (Courtesy of Circon ACMI, Stamford, Connecticut.)

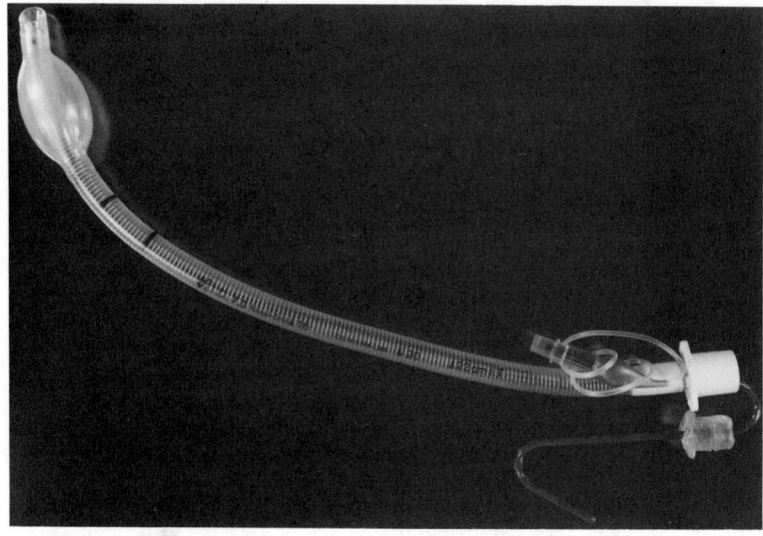

Figure 26-11. A flexible armored (anode) tube. A metal stylet is inserted into the tube to facilitate placement.

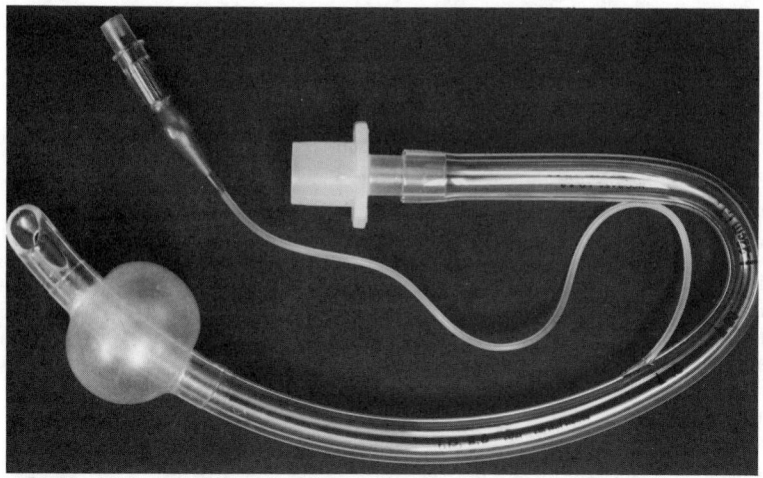

Figure 26-12. Preformed RAE tube for orotracheal intubation.

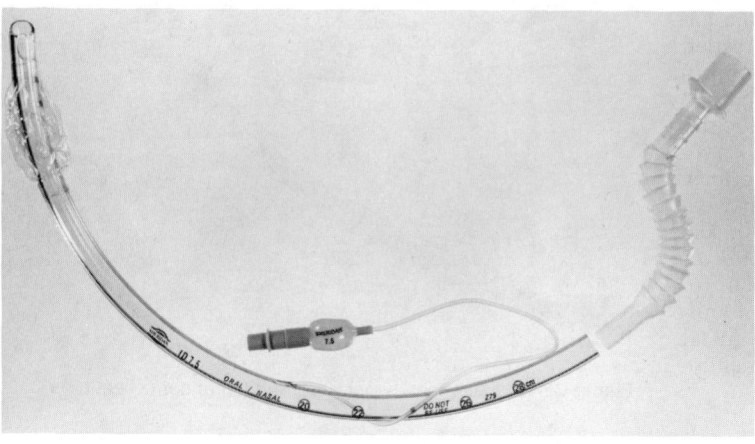

Figure 26-13. A flexible connector.

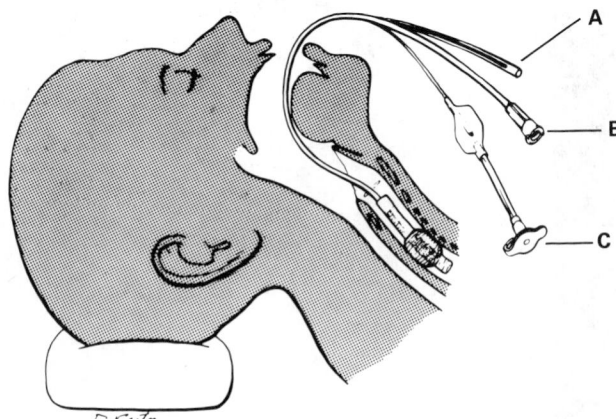

Figure 26-14. The Carden tube is positioned below the vocal cords for surgical procedures involving the larynx. It has a stylet (*A*) to facilitate placement, an adapter (*B*) for attachment to a jet ventilator, and a pilot tube (*C*) for cuff inflation.

Stylets

Malleable metal or firm rubber stylets are used to maintain the desired curve of the endotracheal tube during intubation. Although most are coated with a nonfriction covering to facilitate easy removal, they should be lubricated before insertion into the tubes. A modified stylet, the Flexguide (Scientific Sales International, Kalamazoo, MI), has a proximal thumb ring that is used to flex and guide the distal tip of the stylet into the laryngeal inlet.

A lighted stylet (Flexi-lum, Concept, Clearwater, FL) or lightwand is also available; this is a malleable stylet with a light bulb at the leading end and a battery in the handle. Laryngoscopy is not usually performed when the lighted stylet is employed. The operating room lights are dimmed, the patient's tongue is grasped with a gauze sponge and gently pulled forward, and the endotracheal tube containing the lighted stylet is inserted into the oropharynx and advanced. When the tip is correctly positioned in the midline just superior to the larynx, a glow is evident in the anterior neck. The tube is slid off the lightwand and advanced into the trachea. If the tip of the stylet enters the esophagus, the light is markedly diminished. The technique is useful in children[41] and adults.[42-44] General anesthesia can be employed; however, topical anesthesia and sedation are recommended when the technique is used in patients with known or suspected airway difficulty.[45]

Popular in Europe for many years, the Eschmann Introducer (Sims Surgical, Inc., Keene, NH) is a 60-cm gum elastic bougie that is angled 40 degrees approximately 3.5 cm from the distal end (Fig. 26-16). The introducer is threaded into the endotracheal tube and advanced until the tip protrudes from the tube. The tip of the introducer is guided into the larynx and the tube advanced over it. If difficulty is encountered in advancing the tube, counterclockwise rotation of the tube, so that the bevel is facing posteriorly rather than to the left, is often helpful.[46] Signs of appropriate placement, in addition to direct visualization, are "clicks" produced as the bougie slides over the tracheal cartilages and "hold up" as it reaches the small bronchi.[47] The introducer can also be modified to permit measurement of end-tidal carbon dioxide by drilling holes through the distal wall into the central hollow lumen and attaching an endotracheal tube adapter to the proximal end.[48]

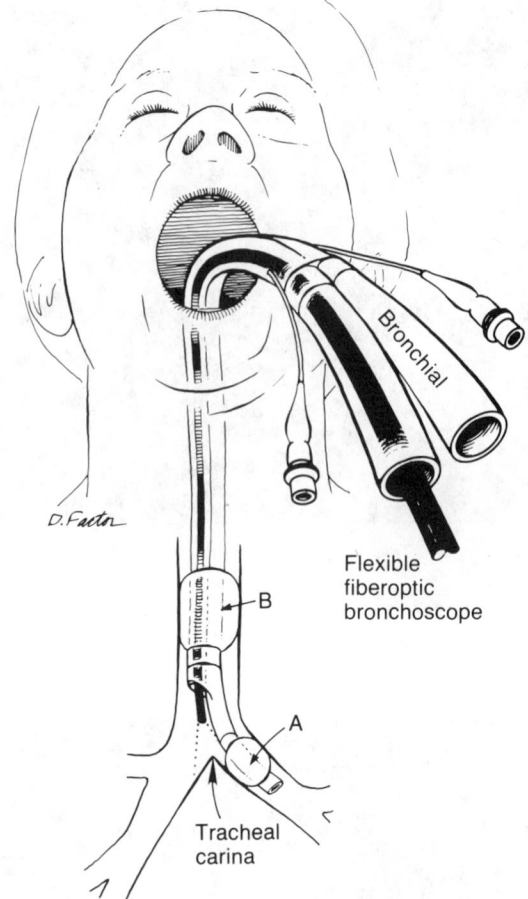

Figure 26-15. Double-lumen endobronchial tubes permit one or both lungs to be ventilated. The left endobronchial tube is positioned with the distal cuff (*A*) in the left bronchus and the proximal cuff (*B*) in the trachea. A fiberoptic bronchoscope can be used to confirm proper tube placement.

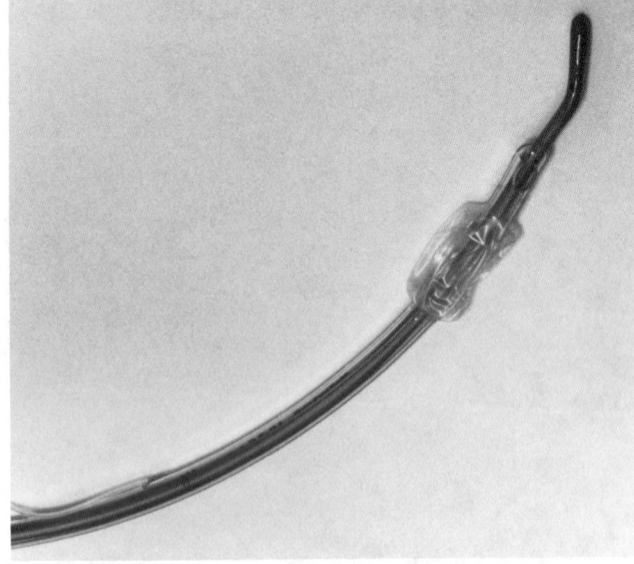

Figure 26-16. Eschmann stylet positioned in endotracheal tube.

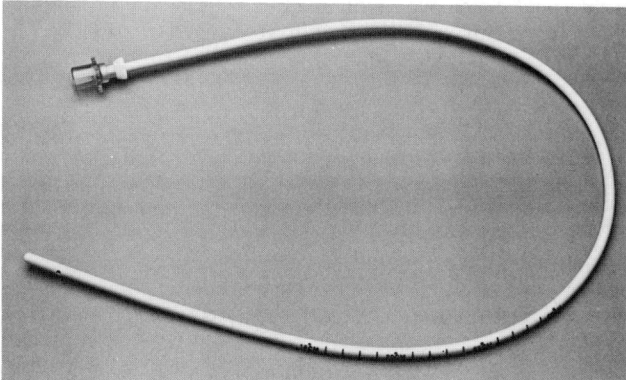

Figure 26-18. Endotracheal tube changer with adapter for attachment to anesthetic circuit or resuscitation bag if ventilation is necessary during tube changing procedure. (Courtesy of Cook Inc., Bloomington, Indiana.)

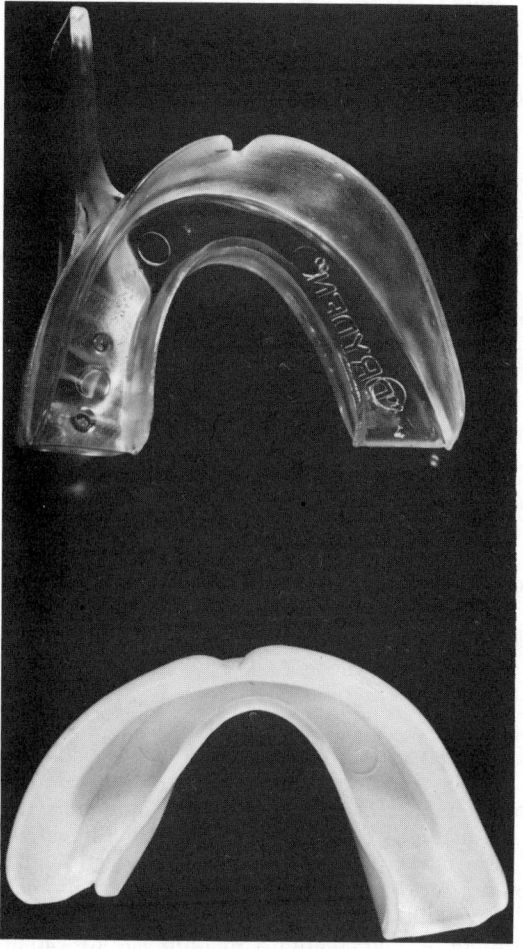

Figure 26-17. Dental guards used to protect the teeth from damage during laryngoscopic examination.

Ancillary Equipment

Soft plastic or rubber tooth protectors (Fig. 26-17) can lessen the chance of damage to the teeth. They are especially useful for protecting the upper teeth when the patient has caps or a fixed bridge. An alternative approach to protecting the teeth is affixing polyurethane sheeting with an adhesive backing (Success Polymers, Paramount, CA) to the flange of the laryngoscope blade.[49]

Although nasogastric tubes or ureteral catheters can be used to facilitate changing endotracheal tubes, airway exchange catheters are available (Fig. 26-18). The catheter is inserted into the existing endotracheal tube, the tube is withdrawn, the new endotracheal tube is threaded over the catheter, and the catheter is removed. If necessary, the patient can be ventilated through the catheter when the specially designed adapter is attached to the catheter and connected to the breathing circuit of an anesthesia machine, to a resuscitation bag, or to a jet injection ventilating device.

Mask Ventilation

The administration of oxygen by mask is an integral part of any general anesthetic unless the patient has a tracheostomy or endotracheal tube *in situ*. Although some anesthesiologists use a head strap to secure the mask prior to induction

of anesthesia, many patients are frightened by the mask and complain of a feeling of suffocation. One alternative is to allow the patient to hold the mask. Another is to apply the mask only after the patient has lost consciousness.

It is always advisable to have more than one size mask available because it is difficult to predict the most appropriate size. The mask is usually held in the anesthesiologist's left hand. Pressure exerted by the thumb and first finger opposes the mask to the patient's face. The other three fingers are placed on the patient's mandible, not the soft tissue of the neck. Many anesthesiologists find that hooking the small finger around the angle of the mandible is helpful in securing a tight mask fit. It may be necessary for the anesthesiologist to hold the mask with both hands, mandating the presence of another individual to assist with ventilation. The patient should be manually ventilated prior to administration of a muscle relaxant to ensure that ventilation is indeed possible. An exception is the patient at risk of aspiration of gastric contents, in whom positive pressure ventilation is usually avoided. If mask ventilation is not possible, it must be assumed that the airway is obstructed.

AIRWAY OBSTRUCTION

The most frequent site for airway obstruction is the oropharynx. With induction of anesthesia, there is relaxation of the jaw and tongue such that the base of the tongue falls back in contact with the posterior pharynx. To relieve this obstruction, the anesthesiologist should place his or her hands behind the angle of the patient's mandible and move it forward. Care must be taken to avoid putting pressure on the anterior structures of the neck, which can accentuate the obstruction. Other measures useful in opening the upper airway include slight extension of the neck, turning the head to the side, application of positive airway pressure to "distend" the soft tissue, and insertion of an oral or nasal airway. The oropharynx should be examined to ensure that the obstruction is not from a foreign body.

Airway obstruction can also be caused by reflex closure of the vocal cords, a condition known as laryngospasm. This typically occurs during "light" levels of anesthesia, when the larynx is irritated by contact with secretions, or when the patient experiences a painful stimulus. Partial laryngospasm is characterized by high-pitched phonation or "crowing." Total occlusion is characterized by no sounds but signs of airway obstruction such as retraction of the trachea or flaring of the nostrils.

The incidence of laryngospasm can be reduced by keeping the airway clear of foreign material, avoiding abrupt inhalation of high concentrations of volatile anesthetics, and establishing a "deep" level of surgical anesthesia before instrumentation of the airway or before allowing surgery to proceed. If laryngospasm occurs, it is usually brief and easily treated. Depending on the cause, treatment should include suctioning foreign material from the oropharynx, decreasing the inspired concentration of anesthetic, removing any painful stimulus, administering 100% oxygen, applying positive pressure to the airway, and placing the fingers behind the angles of the mandible to thrust the jaw forward. If these measures do not resolve the laryngospasm quickly, a rapidly acting muscle relaxant is usually administered.

ENDOTRACHEAL INTUBATION

General anesthesia is not, by itself, an indication for endotracheal intubation. In many cases endotracheal intubation is unnecessary, and occasionally it is contraindicated. Similarly, endotracheal intubation is not always required to treat airway obstruction. However, once it is determined that endotracheal intubation is necessary, the anesthesiologist must decide whether nasotracheal or orotracheal intubation is most appropriate, choose the type and size of laryngoscope and tube to use, decide whether the patient is to be intubated while awake or after induction of anesthesia, and decide whether a muscle relaxant can be used safely.

Indications for Endotracheal Intubation

Placement of an endotracheal tube is indicated when a patient is at risk for pulmonary aspiration of gastric contents. Endotracheal intubation is also necessary during operative procedures involving the head and neck, when a face mask would encroach on the surgical field. Patient position during surgery may dictate the need for placement of an endotracheal tube. It is essential for patients receiving general anesthesia in the prone and sitting positions and is usually necessary for those positioned laterally. Provision of a patent airway in patients with airway abnormalities and the need for prolonged positive pressure ventilation or repetitive tracheal suction are additional indications for endotracheal intubation. Intracranial, intrathoracic, and most intra-abdominal operations mandate endotracheal intubation.

Nasotracheal Versus Orotracheal Intubation

Orotracheal intubation is performed much more frequently than nasotracheal intubation. Indications for the latter include intraoral operative procedures during which the endotracheal tube could easily be displaced or obscure the operative site, and inability to open the patient's mouth. Nasotracheal intubation is contraindicated in the presence of intranasal abnormalities, extensive facial fractures, basilar skull fracture, and systemic coagulopathy. Bleeding is not unusual after nasotracheal intubation and can be excessive if the patient has a disorder of hemostasis. When nasotracheal intubation is planned, the patient should be asked if it is easier to breathe through one nostril than the other. If there is a difference, the nasotracheal tube should be passed through the presumably larger nasal passage after a topical vasoconstrictor such as phenylephrine or cocaine is applied. Endotracheal tubes used for nasotracheal intubation are usually smaller and longer than those used for orotracheal intubation.

Anesthesia for Intubation of the Trachea

Although most patients' tracheae are intubated after thiopental and succinylcholine administration, other anesthetic agents and muscle relaxants are frequently employed prior to intubation. "Fixed" agents such as thiopental, ketamine, opioids, sedatives, and muscle relaxants, which cannot be retrieved once given, must be administered judiciously. They may be contraindicated in patients with airway compromise or in those in whom it is anticipated that endotracheal intubation may be difficult. Muscle relaxants are particularly hazardous because they remove the patient's ability to protect the airway, and the loss of spontaneous ventilation precludes the anesthesiologist from guiding the endotracheal tube into the larynx by listening to breath sounds. If the anesthesiologist cannot *guarantee* that the patient's lungs can be ventilated by mask or that tracheal intubation may be accomplished with relative ease, administration of neuromuscular blocking agents is contraindicated.

Rapid Sequence Induction

A rapid sequence or so-called "crash" induction, the most common method of securing the airway in the patient with a full stomach, minimizes the chances of regurgitation and aspiration. Strict adherence to all details of the technique and the availability of an assistant are mandatory. All equipment, including the suction apparatus with a Yankauer or "tonsil" tip, must be checked before induction of anesthesia. Arguments can be advanced to justify placing the operating table in a head-up, head-down, or neutral (flat) position.[50] A 40-degree head-up tilt may be preferable because gravity will minimize the risk of passive regurgitation of gastric contents. Although many anesthesiologists remove an indwelling nasogastric tube because it may increase the risk of aspiration by making the esophageal sphincter less competent or interfere with obliteration of the esophagus during application of cricoid pressure, studies indicate that it is safe to leave the tube *in situ*.[51]

The patient is usually preoxygenated for 3–5 minutes; however, 2–3 minutes are adequate if the mask fits tightly.[52] Four maximally deep breaths within 30 seconds or three vital capacity breaths of 100% oxygen are alternate approaches[53] but probably offer a smaller margin of protection.[54] Respiration is not assisted until the airway is isolated in order to prevent air from being forced into the stomach. A nondepolarizing muscle relaxant may be administered before induction of anesthesia to minimize any increase in intragastric pressure from succinylcholine-induced muscle fasciculations. An assistant administers medications and applies cricoid pressure (Sellick's maneuver).[55] As soon as the drugs are injected, the assistant must apply cricoid pressure by placing his or her thumb and index finger on the cricoid cartilage and exerting pressure in an anteroposterior direction, occluding the esophagus (Fig. 26-19). The patient's trachea is intubated once muscle relaxation is evident, and the cuff of the endotracheal tube is inflated by the assistant. Cricoid pressure is maintained until proper placement of the endotracheal tube is assured.

Several modifications of the technique have been sug-

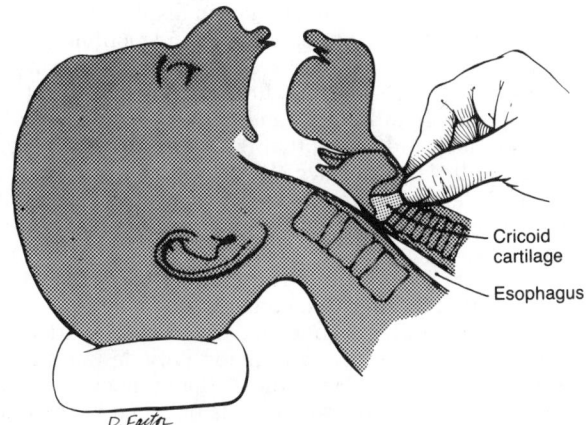

Figure 26-19. Cricoid pressure (Sellick's maneuver) is applied to occlude the esophagus and prevent aspiration of gastric contents.

gested. The necessity for avoiding manual ventilation has been questioned by investigators who did not demonstrate air entry into the stomach when cricoid pressure was applied as long as the airway remained patent.[56] Some anesthesiologists prefer to have the assistant apply gentle cricoid pressure until the patient loses consciousness and then increase the pressure. If active vomiting should occur, cricoid pressure must be released immediately or there is danger of esophageal rupture.[57] Proponents of the bimanual technique have the assistant place one hand behind the patient's neck, flexing it into the "sniffing" position, while applying conventional cricoid pressure with the other hand.[58] The cricoid yoke, a device that is purported to ensure consistent and adequate cricoid pressure, has also been advocated.[59]

INTUBATION OF THE TRACHEA IN THE AWAKE PATIENT

There are no absolute guidelines regarding indications for intubation of the trachea while the patient is awake. It is necessary in some patients with congenital or acquired airway lesions, a full stomach, intestinal obstruction, upper gastrointestinal bleeding, cervical spine abnormalities, and facial trauma. Topical anesthesia can be applied to the patient's tongue to decrease gagging during orotracheal intubation. Although they are only indicated under exceptional circumstances in patients at risk of aspiration of gastric con-

tents, superior laryngeal nerve blocks and translaryngeal injection of a local anesthetic significantly decrease the discomfort associated with intubation of the trachea while the patient is awake. Glossopharyngeal nerve blocks can also be performed to lessen the gag reflex.[60]

Local Anesthesia

Local anesthetic agents may be applied topically, infiltrated, or instilled. It must be remembered that local anesthetics are absorbed rapidly from mucous membranes, and recommended doses must not be exceeded.[61,62]

Topical anesthesia of the lips, tongue, and oropharynx can be provided by direct application of pledgets soaked with a local anesthetic. In edentulous patients, the anesthetic also should be applied to the gums. After the tip of the tongue has been anesthetized, it is grasped with a gauze sponge and pulled forward to facilitate access to the oral cavity. The tongue can be held by the patient or an assistant, so that the anesthesiologist has both hands available to continue application of the anesthetic. This is best achieved with cotton pledgets soaked in the local anesthetic (usually cocaine) and held with curved Krause forceps (Fig. 26-20). The superior surface of the tongue is anesthetized as the forceps are slowly advanced posteriorly. The pledgets then should be held in the piriform fossae for at least 2 minutes to anesthetize the internal laryngeal nerves.

Lidocaine aerosol is an effective, simple, and inexpensive method of topical anesthesia.[63] It can be employed alone or as an adjunct to other local anesthetic techniques. Ideally the patient is placed in a sitting position. A disposable nebulizer and face mask are used with an oxygen flow of approximately 8 l·min^{-1}. Phenylephrine (1 ml of 1% solution) can be added to the lidocaine (4 ml of 4% solution) as a vasoconstrictor. During the 5–7 minutes the patient breathes the mixture, the smaller nebulized particles are dispersed as far distally as the terminal bronchioles, whereas the larger particles remain in contact with the nasal and pharyngeal mucosa.

Another satisfactory technique that has the advantage of allowing the anesthesiologist to direct the local anesthetic into the nose and pharynx employs an atomizer containing local anesthetic attached by tubing to an oxygen tank (Fig. 26-21). A hole is made in the oxygen tubing near the connection to the atomizer. The anesthesiologist controls the particle size and velocity of mist emanating from the atomizer by occluding the hole in the tubing. Rest periods of approximately 15 seconds should be alternated with equal periods

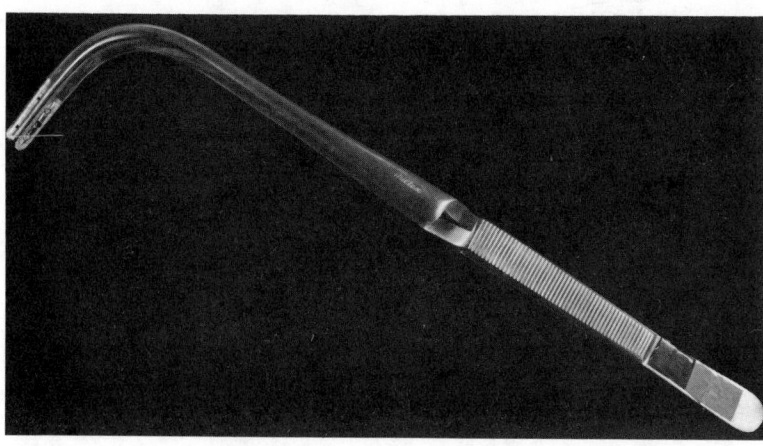

Figure 26-20. Krause forceps for grasping cotton swabs used to anesthetize the tongue and pharynx. The design facilitates application of local anesthetic to the piriform fossae.

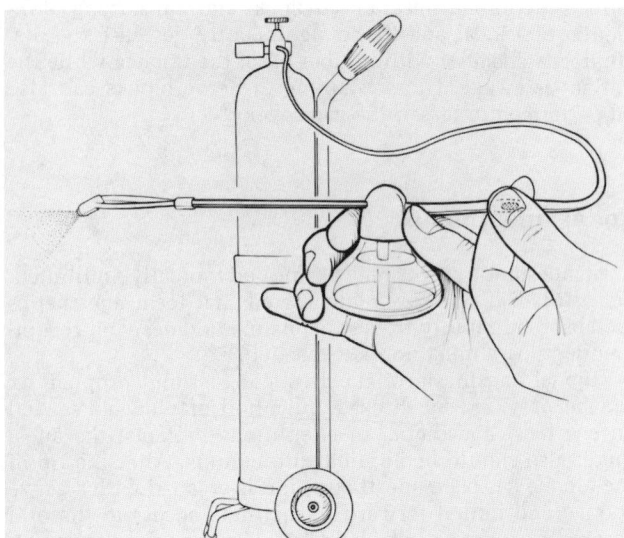

Figure 26-21. System for nebulizing local anesthetic prior to orotracheal or nasotracheal intubation. Digital occlusion of the hole in the oxygen tubing near the atomizer causes a fine mist of local anesthetic to be emitted from the atomizer when oxygen is flowing from the tank.

of nebulization. The total time required to achieve adequate topical anesthesia is approximately 10 minutes. Administration of an antisialagogue approximately an hour prior to initiating topical anesthesia may enhance the degree of anesthesia because secretions can impair local anesthetic contact with the mucosa.

Bilateral superior laryngeal nerve blocks can be performed to anesthetize the internal laryngeal nerves (Fig. 26-22). The nerves pierce the thyrohyoid membrane just inferior to the greater cornu of the hyoid bone. Application

of pressure to the opposite greater cornu displaces the laryngeal structures to the side to be blocked and facilitates identification of anatomic landmarks. After the skin is cleansed, the local anesthetic (3 ml of 2% lidocaine) is injected at the level of the thyrohyoid membrane with a 25-gauge needle. If air is aspirated, indicating that the pharynx has been entered, the needle is withdrawn slightly before the anesthetic is injected. Bilateral nerve blocks produce anesthesia of the inferior aspect of the epiglottis and the laryngeal outlet down to the vocal cords. The block should not be performed when there is local infection or tumor or when patients are at risk of aspiration of gastric contents.

Translaryngeal (often erroneously referred to as transtracheal) instillation of a local anesthetic provides anesthesia below the vocal cords. With the patient's neck fully extended, the cricothyroid membrane is palpated in the midline as a slight depression between the inferior border of the thyroid cartilage and the superior edge of the cricoid cartilage. The skin is cleansed and a 22-gauge needle is introduced perpendicular to the skin (Fig. 26-22). After air is aspirated, the local anesthetic (3–5 ml of 2–4% lidocaine) is injected. The needle should be removed immediately because the patient will cough vigorously. Alternatively, a small-gauge intravenous catheter can be inserted and, when air is aspirated, the inner stylet withdrawn. Local anesthetic can then be injected through the soft catheter without the risk of tracheal injury when the patient coughs.

Glossopharyngeal nerve blocks, in addition to producing anesthesia of the posterior third of the tongue, uvula, soft palate, and oropharynx, also abolish the gag reflex.[60] To perform the block, the patient's tongue is retracted to the contralateral side with a tongue depressor or the tongue is grasped with gauze and drawn forward to place the tonsillar pillar under tension (Fig. 26-23). Ideally, an angled tonsillar needle is used for injecting the local anesthetic, usually 3 ml of 1% lidocaine. The needle is inserted to a depth of 1 cm just behind the midpoint of the palatopharyngeal arch (posterior tonsillar pillar), aspiration is attempted, and the

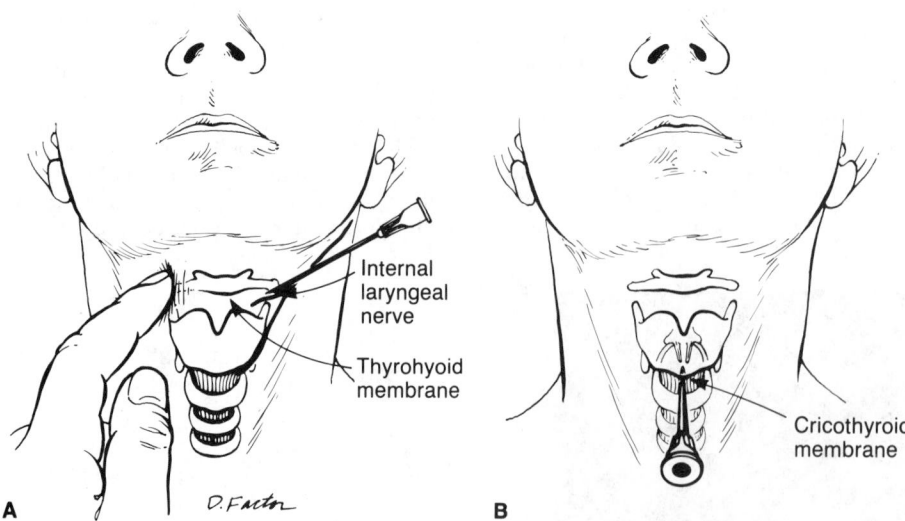

Figure 26-22. (A) When a superior laryngeal nerve block is performed, pressure is applied to the contralateral greater cornu of the hyoid to facilitate identification of anatomic landmarks. The needle is inserted at the level of the thyrohyoid membrane just inferior to the greater cornu of the thyroid cartilage. (B) Translaryngeal instillation of local anesthetic is performed to anesthetize the larynx below the vocal cords and the upper trachea. The needle is introduced through the cricothyroid membrane perpendicular to the skin.

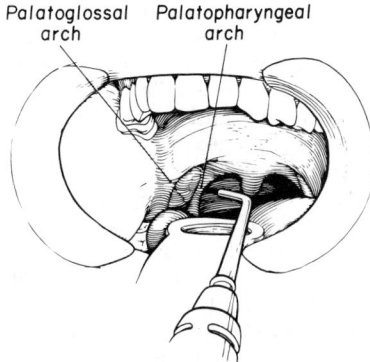

Figure 26-23. Glossopharyngeal nerve block is performed by injecting local anesthetic with a tonsillar needle behind the midpoint of the palatopharyngeal arch (posterior tonsillar pillar) into the lateral pharyngeal mucosa. A tongue depressor is used to retract the tongue and stretch the tonsillar pillars.

local anesthetic is injected. The block is repeated on the contralateral side. Preliminary results in a small number of patients indicate satisfactory results when a half-inch, 27-gauge needle is used to pierce the palatoglossal arch approximately 0.5 cm from the lateral margin of the root of the tongue at the point where it joins the floor of the mouth and 2 ml of 2% lidocaine is injected following aspiration.[64] The block should be used with caution, if at all, in patients at risk of aspiration of gastric contents. Not only does it abolish the gag reflex but soft-tissue relaxation can lead to airway obstruction. In patients with very active gag reflexes, the necessity for blocking the response must be weighed against the potential risk of aspiration.

When nasotracheal intubation is to be performed, the nasal passage should be anesthetized. Use of cocaine is preferable because it is a potent vasoconstrictor as well as topical anesthetic. Although the drug can be sprayed into the nose, best results are achieved when pledgets or cotton-tipped applicators soaked with the local anesthetic are placed in the nostrils and remain there for 3–5 minutes.

Orotracheal Intubation

The operating table should be positioned so that the patient's head is approximately at the level of the anesthesiologist's xiphoid process. In the adult, a pillow or pad is usually placed under the occiput to elevate the patient's head approximately 10 cm and thereby align the oral, pharyngeal, and laryngeal structures. Although this "sniffing" position should provide the most direct line of vision, some anesthesiologists find it easier to perform intubation when the patient's head is not elevated. Because children have relatively large heads, it is not necessary to use a pillow. Axial alignment is completed by extension of the atlanto-occipital joint, and the patient's mouth is opened as wide as possible. The laryngoscope blade is inserted in the right side of the mouth, and the tongue is moved toward the left as the blade is advanced. When a curved blade is used, the tip is advanced into the vallecula, the space between the base of the tongue and the pharyngeal surface of the epiglottis (Fig. 26-24). The epiglottis is elevated and the glottis exposed as

the handle of the laryngoscope is lifted forward and upward. In contrast, the tip of a straight blade is advanced beneath the laryngeal surface of the epiglottis to expose the glottic opening (Fig. 26-25). The most common errors made by the novice are levering on the upper incisors and trapping the lips between the laryngoscope blade and the teeth. The endotracheal tube should be observed until it passes through the vocal cords so that it can be ascertained that it is entering the larynx and the depth of insertion can be gauged. An assistant can apply external pressure to the thyroid cartilage to facilitate intubation of the trachea in the patient with an "anterior" larynx. In neonates and small children, the anesthesiologist can use the little finger of the left hand to apply pressure to the anterior neck.

If the endotracheal tube is too long, endobronchial intubation will occur. Right endobronchial intubation is far more likely to occur in adults because of the relative angles of the right and left bronchi. In children younger than 3 years of age, it has been claimed that the right and left tracheobronchial angles are approximately equal, making intubation of either bronchus equally likely.[65] Other studies refute this statement and confirm that even in premature infants, acci-

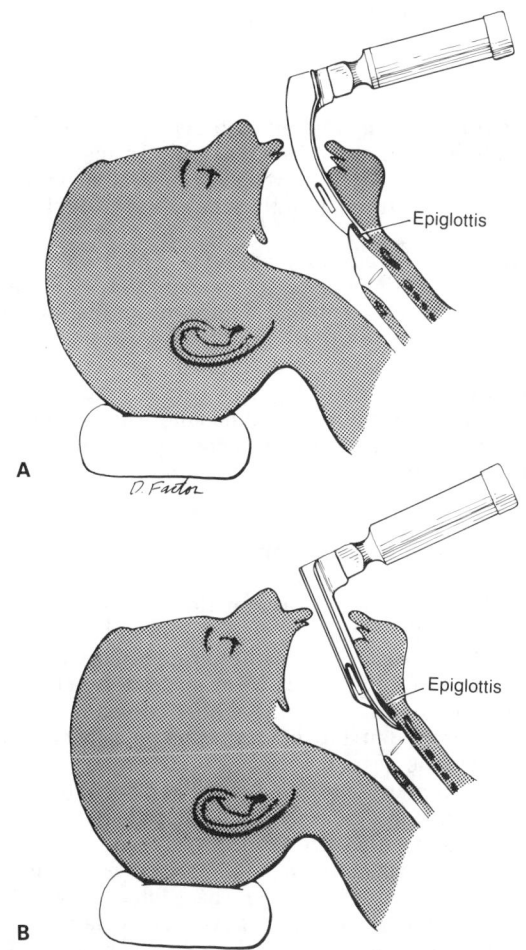

Figure 26-24. (A) When a curved laryngoscope blade is used, the tip of the blade is placed in the vallecula, the space between the base of the tongue and the pharyngeal surface of the epiglottis. (B) The tip of a straight blade is advanced beneath the epiglottis.

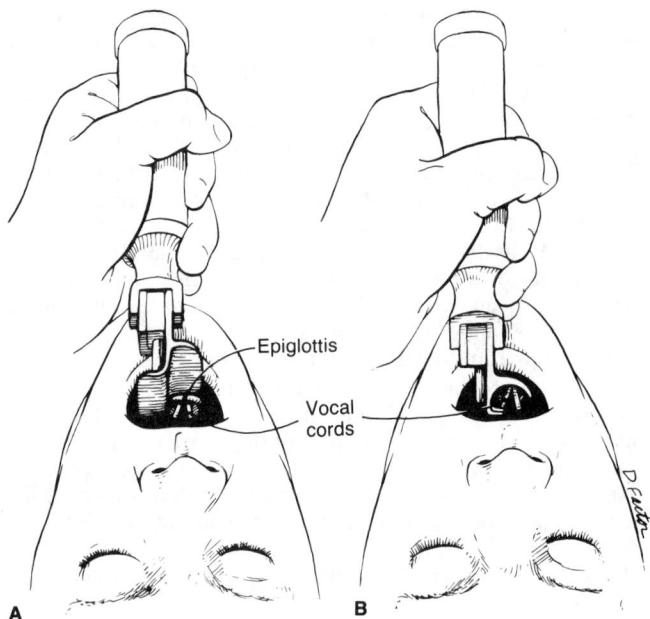

Figure 26-25. (A) The curved laryngoscope blade is placed in the vallecula, and the vocal cords are exposed as the handle is lifted upward and forward. (B) A straight blade is advanced beneath the laryngeal surface of the epiglottis to expose the glottic opening.

dental right endobronchial intubation is more probable than left endobronchial intubation.[66,67] However, the bevel of the endotracheal tube, not the tracheobronchial angle, may be the principal determinant of the side of endobronchial intubation.[68]

Once accurate tracheal placement is verified, the tube must be anchored securely to prevent later displacement into a bronchus or accidental extubation of the trachea. In patients with moist skin, tincture of benzoin should be applied before the tube is taped. In hirsute patients, cloth ties ("umbilical" or "hernia" tape) or Velcro straps should be used instead of adhesive tape. When these are not available, a surgical mask can be placed beneath the patient's head and the ties of the mask used to secure the tube.

Nasotracheal Intubation

Nasotracheal intubation can be performed under direct vision or a "blind" technique can be employed. If the patient states that it is easier to breathe through one nostril, that side should be used. A topical vasoconstrictor such as phenylephrine or cocaine should be applied. A soft nasal airway should be inserted first to determine the patency of the naris and to dilate the nasal passage.

If a general anesthetic is administered for intubation of the trachea, the nasal airway can be placed after the patient is anesthetized. Unless contraindicated, general anesthesia and a muscle relaxant are administered before laryngoscopic examination. The endotracheal tube is inserted into the nose until the tip is in the pharynx. Direct laryngoscopic examination is performed, the tip of the tube is visualized, and it is guided into the glottis. The direction of the tube is altered by rotating it to the right or left, as necessary. Occasionally, it is useful to rotate the patient's head (rather than the tube), especially in the patient with a deviated

septum. Flexion of the neck is necessary when the tip of the tube impinges on the anterior commissure of the glottis. Extension of the neck may facilitate intubation when the tube persistently enters the esophagus. If necessary, forceps are used to grasp and direct the tip of the tube (Fig. 26-26).

When "blind" nasotracheal intubation is employed, direct laryngoscopic examination is not performed. The technique is similar whether the patient is anesthetized or awake. Breath sounds are used to guide the tube into the glottis in the spontaneously breathing patient. The simplest technique is for the anesthesiologist to keep an ear close to the endotracheal tube in order to detect increased breath sounds as the tube nears the glottis. The major disadvantage of this technique is the potential for contamination of the anesthesiologist by patient secretions, particularly if coughing occurs as the tube enters the trachea. A whistle or amplifier can be placed in the tube to magnify the breath sounds[69] or a piece of tubing can be positioned in the endotracheal tube and attached to the anesthesiologist's stethoscope.[70] The endotracheal tube can also be connected to the anesthesia circuit initially and the end-tidal carbon dioxide waveform used to guide the tube into the trachea instead of relying on breath sounds.[71] An audio-capnometry intubation device that couples a carbon dioxide monitor and a voltage-controlled oscillator with a speaker has also been described.[72] The device yields an audible tone with a pitch that varies linearly with the carbon dioxide concentration.

Confirmation of Endotracheal Tube Placement

Visualization of the endotracheal tube entering the larynx, auscultation of the chest for breath sounds and of the epigastrium for absence of air entry into the stomach, and observation of chest motion during ventilation are common methods of ascertaining proper endotracheal tube placement. However, the position of the tube can be altered with changes in patient position, particularly flexion or extension of the neck, which can move the tube as much as 5 cm.[73]

Auscultation and observation of chest movement are notoriously inaccurate, particularly in obese patients and

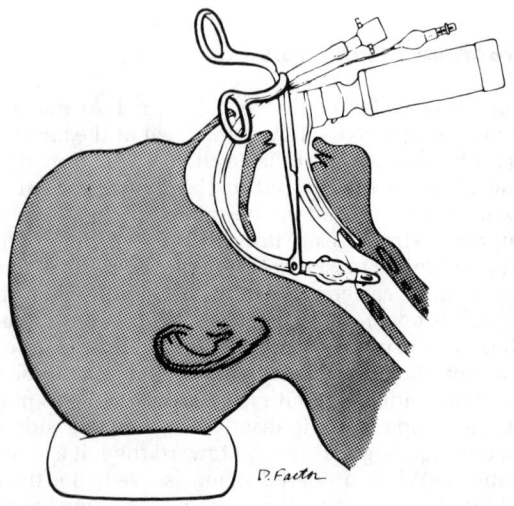

Figure 26-26. McGill forceps are used to grasp and direct the endotracheal tube during nasotracheal intubation.

those with lung disease. The presence of condensed water vapor in the tube lumen and movement of the reservoir bag usually but not always signify proper tube placement. Less practical methods are tactile examination via the oropharynx,[74] fiberoptic bronchoscopy, and chest radiography.

Detection of expired carbon dioxide with a capnograph or mass spectrometer provides the most reliable evidence of tracheal rather than esophageal intubation.[73] Although carbon dioxide can be detected initially with esophageal intubation if expired carbon dioxide entered the stomach during mask ventilation, the concentration is low and diminishes rapidly over three or four "breaths."

A single use device, the FEF end-tidal carbon dioxide detector (Fenem, New York, NY) can be used in the operating room as well as other areas where endotracheal intubations are performed (Fig. 26-27). It is interposed between the endotracheal tube and the anesthetic circuit and indicates the presence of carbon dioxide by a colorimetric change. Unlike infrared and mass spectrometers, the device is disposable, relatively inexpensive, weighs less than one ounce, has no moving parts, and requires no electrical power, calibration, or maintenance. Its reliability has been proved in several studies in surgical patients[75-78] as well as in the prehospital environment and emergency department.[79] The device is most useful for confirmation of endotracheal intubation in areas of the hospital other than the operating room where capnographs are not available and for use during out-of-hospital resuscitation. However, lack of a color change must be interpreted cautiously in the patient with cardiopulmonary arrest. It may indicate improper tube placement, inadequate cardiopulmonary resuscitation, or absence of cellular metabolism.[79]

PHYSIOLOGIC RESPONSES TO ENDOTRACHEAL INTUBATION

Hypertension, tachycardia, and increases in intracranial and intraocular pressure can occur in response to laryngoscopic examination and intubation.

Cardiovascular Responses

Laryngoscopic examination, with or without endotracheal intubation, provokes cardiovascular and sympathoadrenal responses.[80] The magnitude of the hypertensive response has been shown to correlate with the blood pressure changes associated with stressful events such as hospital admission.[81] It is impossible to compare the results of various clinical studies evaluating methods of attenuating the circulatory responses to laryngoscopy and intubation because of differences in patient populations, intervals between drug administration and laryngoscopy/intubation, duration of laryngoscopy, methods of drug administration, type and dosage of adjuvant drugs, and physiologic parameters measured. Most studies include only a few patients, and it is unknown whether the observed hemodynamic alterations influence morbidity and mortality.

Fentanyl (6–8 μg·kg⁻¹) is effective in attenuating or abolishing the tachycardia and hypertension associated with laryngoscopy and intubation.[82-84] In geriatric patients, administration of lower doses of fentanyl (1.5–3 μg·kg⁻¹) attenuates the hemodynamic effects of intubation but is often associated with hypotension in the period following intubation.[85]

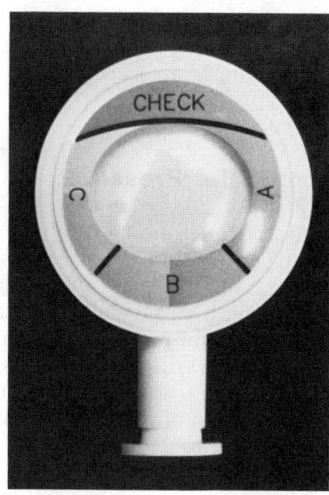

Figure 26-27. The FEF end-tidal carbon dioxide detector. The color ranges (A-C) indicate the approximate level of expired carbon dioxide.

Intravenous lidocaine (1.5 mg·kg⁻¹) also attenuates the hemodynamic responses to laryngoscopy and intubation.[85] For optimal effect, the lidocaine should be administered 3 minutes prior to intubation.[86] Inhalation of aerosolized lidocaine, gargling with viscous lidocaine, and translaryngeal administration of lidocaine are all inferior in effect to intravenous administration of the drug.[87]

Other drugs that appear to be effective are esmolol, by bolus injection[88] or infusion,[84] rapid infusion of sodium nitroprusside,[89] and intranasal nitroglycerin.[90] Although sublingual captopril reduces the pressor response to intubation, it is associated with a significant incidence of hypotension.[91]

The optimal means of attenuating the cardiovascular changes associated with laryngoscopic examination and intubation depend on the overall clinical situation. The approach to the patient with a full stomach, coronary artery disease, or known airway abnormalities differs from the approach to the healthy patient with normal airway anatomy scheduled for elective surgery. A combination of techniques may be employed, including achieving an adequate depth of anesthesia before laryngoscopic examination, administration of fentanyl (6–8 μg·kg⁻¹) or its equivalent, and intravenous administration of lidocaine (1.5 mg·kg⁻¹) approximately 3 minutes prior to laryngoscopy.

Intracranial Pressure Alteration

Although transient increases in intracranial pressure associated with laryngoscopic examination and intubation of the trachea are of no consequence in patients without intracranial abnormalities, they may be significant in patients with increased intracranial pressure. Although the exact mechanism for the increase is uncertain, possible explanations include light anesthesia, hypercarbia, inadequate relaxation during intubation, a direct cerebral vasodilating effect of the succinylcholine, skeletal muscle fasciculations, and cerebral stimulation caused by afferent muscle spindle activity during depolarization.[92-95] Induction of adequate anesthesia, plus use of techniques normally used to control increased intracranial pressure such as thiopental administration and hyperventilation before intubation of the trachea, will minimize this adverse effect of laryngoscopic examination and intubation. Intravenous but not translaryngeal administration of lidocaine is also useful in attenuating the response.[87]

Effects on Intraocular Pressure

The increase in arterial pressure associated with laryngoscopy and intubation can also induce an increase in intraocular pressure.[96] At least in children, this response is attenuated by pretreatment with intravenous lidocaine (1.5 mg·kg^{-1}).[97] Nebulized lidocaine is also effective but may obtund pharyngeal reflexes.[98] Although transient increases in intraocular pressure are of no consequence in most patients, prophylactic administration of lidocaine is advisable in patients with open eye injuries.

EXTUBATION OF THE TRACHEA

The trachea can be extubated while patients are deeply anesthetized or awake. Patients who are lightly anesthetized have active laryngeal reflexes and are prone to develop laryngospasm upon extubation of the trachea. Patients at risk of aspiration of gastric contents and those in whom reintubation would be difficult are best extubated while awake. Small children are usually extubated while awake because they have a high incidence of laryngospasm.

The consequences of coughing or "bucking" on the endotracheal tube are negligible in most patients. However, the associated hemodynamic alterations may harm those with increased intracranial or intraocular pressure or myocardial ischemia. In addition, undue tension on sutures can lead to bleeding or wound dehiscence. Administration of lidocaine (1.5 mg·kg^{-1}) approximately 3 minutes prior to extubation attenuates both the cardiovascular responses and coughing.

The pharynx is suctioned before extubation to remove secretions that can drain into the trachea or irritate the vocal cords and produce laryngospasm after the tube is withdrawn. Pressure on the breathing bag during tube removal may induce coughing and expulsion of any aspirated material.

COMPLICATIONS OF ENDOTRACHEAL INTUBATION

Complications can occur during intubation of the trachea or while the tube is *in situ* (Table 26-1).[99-106] Some are evident when they occur; others are recognized immediately following extubation of the trachea or in the days to weeks after the endotracheal tube is removed. The incidence of complications varies with the patient population, skill of the laryngoscopist, and conditions under which tracheal intubation is performed. The size, design, and composition of the endotracheal tube as well as the duration of tracheal intubation are also important.

Predisposing Factors

The patient's age influences the type of complications. The consequences of even slight edema of the airway are much more significant in children. In the infant, 1 mm of edema

TABLE 26-1. Complications of Endotracheal Intubation

During Intubation

Laryngospasm
Laceration, bruising of lips, tongue, and pharynx
Fracture, chipping, dislodgement of teeth or dental appliances
Perforation of trachea or esophagus[99]
Retropharyngeal dissection[100]
Fracture or dislocation of cervical spine[20]
Trauma to eyes
Hemorrhage
Bacteremia[101]
Aspiration of gastric contents or foreign bodies
Endobronchial or esophageal intubation
Dislocation of arytenoid cartilages[102] or mandible
Hypoxemia, hypercarbia
Bradycardia, tachycardia
Hypertension
Increased intracranial or intraocular pressure

With Tube in Situ

Accidental extubation
Endobronchial intubation
Obstruction or kinking
Bronchospasm
Ignition of tube by laser device
Aspiration
Sinusitis[103]
Excoriation of nose or mouth

Evident After Extubation

Laryngospasm
Aspiration of secretions, gastric contents, blood, or foreign bodies
Glottic, subglottic, or uvular edema[104]
Dysphonia, aphonia
Paralysis of vocal cords or hypoglossal, lingual nerves
Sore throat
Noncardiogenic pulmonary edema[105]
Laryngeal incompetence[106]
Soreness, dislocation of jaw
Tracheomalacia
Glottic, subglottic, or tracheal stenosis
Vocal cord granulomata or synechiae

decreases the cross-sectional area of the glottic opening approximately 70% and increases flow resistance at the cricoid approximately 16 times. The same degree of laryngeal edema is associated with no symptoms or mild hoarseness in the adult.

Some complications vary with the patient's sex. Granulomas of the larynx, although relatively rare, occur much more frequently in female patients, as does sore throat.[107] The duration of tracheal intubation correlates with the incidence and severity of some complications but not others. Postextubation glottic edema, aspiration, laryngeal stenosis, and vocal dysfunction are well-documented complications occurring in patients who have been intubated for a week or longer. However, the duration of translaryngeal intubation does not correlate with the incidence of granuloma formation.[108]

The type of endotracheal tube influences the incidence of both minor and major complications. Sore throat is a common complaint in patients who have had tracheal intubation. The reported incidence varies markedly and is as high as 90%. Also of interest is that approximately 15% of patients who receive general anesthesia by mask also complain of sore throat.[109] Lubrication of the tube does not appear to decrease and may actually increase the incidence of sore throat.[109,110] The use of a gauze bite block instead of a hard oropharyngeal airway has not been shown to decrease the incidence of sore throat. However, pharyngeal trauma correlates with the occurrence of sore throat, such as that caused by vigorous suctioning with stiff catheters.[111] The incidence of sore throat and hoarseness is reduced by using smaller endotracheal tubes.[112] Although low-volume cuffs appear to be associated with a lower incidence of sore throat, the consequence of prolonged contact of these cuffs with tracheal mucosa indicates that high-volume, low-pressure cuffs should be used for all but brief tracheal intubations.[107]

The inhalation anesthetic agent employed is also important. Nitrous oxide diffuses into the endotracheal tube cuff and increases the volume and pressure of the cuff.[113] These changes can be eliminated by inflation of the cuff with the same gas as that inspired, or with saline, or by periodic deflation of the cuff. Measurement of cuff pressures also has been recommended during prolonged operative procedures.[114]

Prevention of Complications

Endotracheal intubation obviously has hazards. Tubes should be placed only when indicated. Attention to detail during intubation of the trachea is essential and can prevent most minor complications. Adequate fixation prevents migration of the tube into a bronchus, accidental extubation of the trachea, and unnecessary tube motion, which may increase the incidence of airway irritation. When prolonged intubation of the trachea is indicated, the risks must be weighed against those of tracheostomy. For periods of a week or less, translaryngeal intubation generally is preferred to tracheostomy. However, the relative merits of endotracheal intubation and tracheostomy are less clear when an artificial airway is required for a longer period of time.[108] Laryngoscopic examination immediately after extubation of the trachea is useful in evaluating the airway for abnormalities.

THE DIFFICULT AIRWAY

The true incidence of difficulty with endotracheal intubation is unknown but has been reported to range between 1 and 3%.[115] Several studies have indicated that it is higher in obstetric than in surgical patients[8,116] and that the incidence of failed intubation in parturients may approach 1 in 500.[117] In the majority of patients the difficulty can and should be predicted. However, in a small percentage of cases there is no indication that exposure of the glottis will be difficult or impossible. Rarely, visualization of the larynx is possible when the patient is awake, but not after general anesthesia and muscle paralysis are induced. It is suggested that the larynx is shifted anteriorly when the normal tonic muscular activity associated with the conscious state is lost.[118]

The degree of difficulty with intubation that can be expected has been classified on the basis of the view obtained at laryngoscopy[119] (Fig. 26-28):

Grade 1. All or most of glottis visible; no difficulty anticipated.
Grade 2. Only posterior aspect of glottis visible; slight

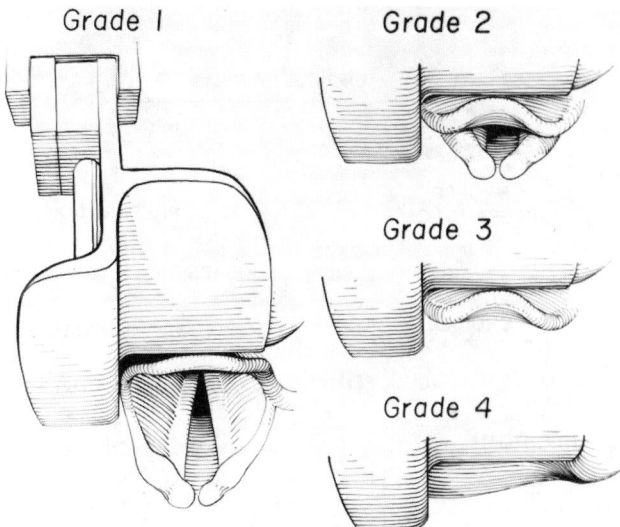

Figure 26-28. The grades of difficulty of endotracheal intubation based on the best view obtained at laryngoscopy.

difficulty anticipated. Pressure on larynx usually brings at least the arytenoid cartilages into view.
Grade 3. Only epiglottis, no part of glottis, visible; fairly severe difficulty anticipated.
Grade 4. Not even epiglottis visible; intubation impossible except by special methods.

A technique of simulating difficult intubation based upon this grading system has been proposed for improving the skills of anesthesia personnel, particularly students and residents, in dealing with unexpected difficult intubations.[119] After initial laryngoscopy, the blade is lowered so that the epiglottis descends and the view is converted from Grade 1 to Grade 3. Intubation is then attempted with an endotracheal tube containing an Eschmann (see Fig. 26-16) or other flexible introducer protruding from the tip of the tube. The introducer is advanced beneath the epiglottis in the midline, and the tube is advanced over it into the trachea. Proper placement of the endotracheal tube should be confirmed immediately by capnography. A high incidence of esophageal intubation has been reported when this teaching technique is employed.[120] Therefore, it should not be used in patients at risk of aspiration of gastric contents or when a delay in securing the airway might jeopardize the patient.

The optimal method of managing the patient in whom laryngoscopy and endotracheal intubation cannot be easily accomplished depends on the cause of the difficulty, whether it is anticipated, the nature and urgency of the surgical procedure, the patient's condition, and the personnel and equipment available. Having an organized approach to alternative methods of securing the airway[121] provides a basis for determining the types of equipment required and minimizes time lost in emergency situations (Fig. 26-29).

It is strongly recommended that every operating suite be equipped with an intubation cart containing adult and pediatric fiberoptic endoscopes, a light source, an assortment of laryngoscope blades, airways, endotracheal tubes and stylets, a cricothyrotomy set and means of transtracheal jet ventilation, and equipment for retrograde intubation. It is also advisable to have a copy of the algorithm for managing the difficult airway (Fig. 26-29) readily available in each operating room.

DIFFICULT AIRWAY ALGORITHM

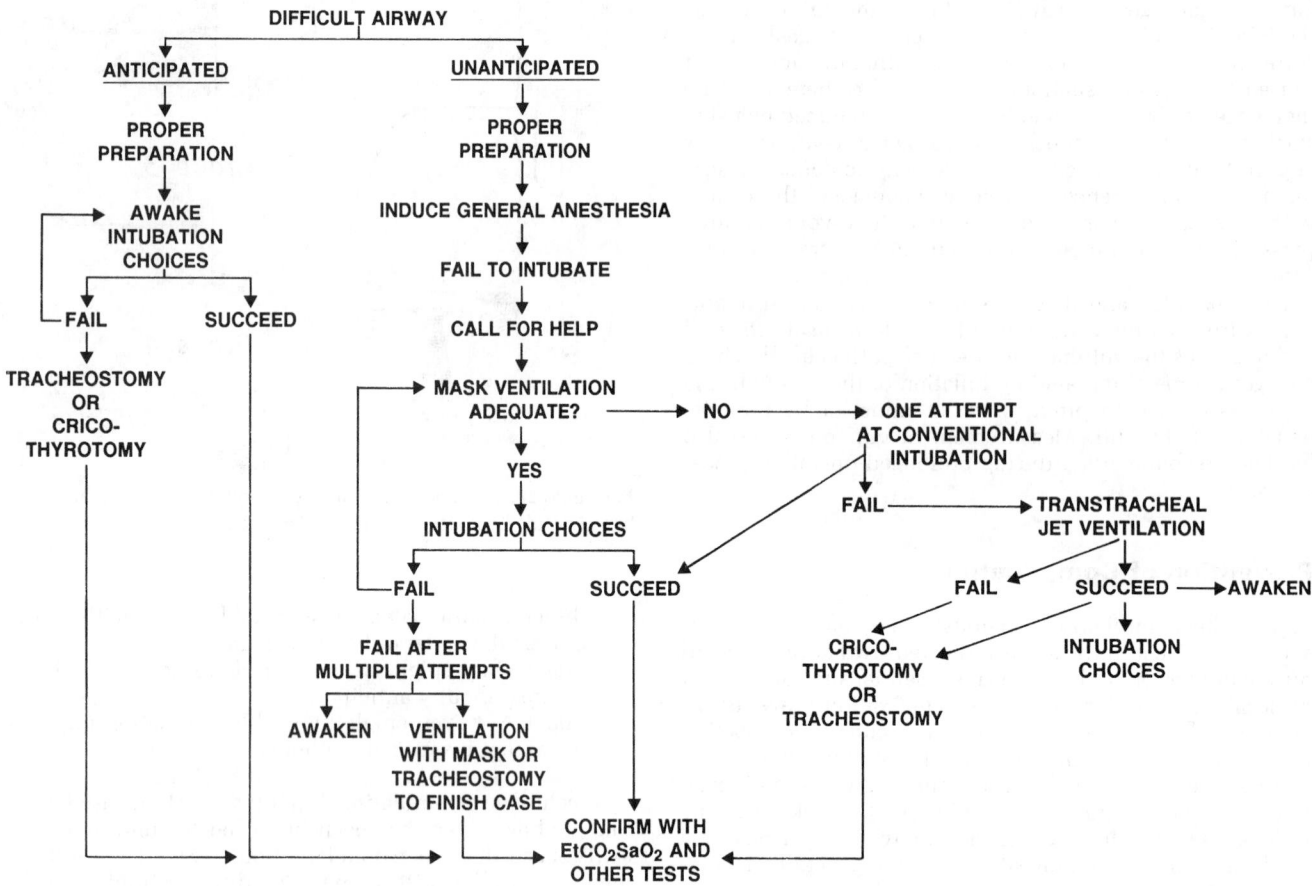

Figure 26-29. Algorithm for managing the patient with a difficult airway. (Modified from preliminary draft prepared by the American Society of Anesthesiologists' Task Force on Airway Management.)

Anticipated Airway Difficulty

The techniques to be employed should be decided upon in advance and all equipment thoroughly checked prior to the patient's arrival in the operating room. In addition to informing the patient of the potential problems, the anesthesiologist should notify the surgeon and operating room nurses that difficulty may be encountered and indicate whether special equipment is required. For example, rigid bronchoscopes and a light source as well as a tracheostomy set and appropriately sized tracheostomy tubes must be readily available in some circumstances. It may be necessary to request that an otolaryngologist be present in the operating room if the patient's surgeon is not experienced in performing tracheostomy. Eliciting the assistance of another anesthesiologist, particularly if he or she is more skilled in fiberoptic endoscopy or other specialized airway techniques, is also advisable.

Intubation performed while the patient is awake employing conventional laryngoscopy, a "blind" technique, or fiberoptic endoscopy is usually indicated in adults. The type of sedation and topical anesthesia administered must be individualized. In children, inhalation anesthesia with maintenance of spontaneous ventilation is often employed or, in some circumstances, ketamine is administered. The Bullard intubating laryngoscope or a lightwand can be used

in pediatric patients as well as in adults. Elective tracheostomy is appropriate for some surgical procedures involving the head and neck, such as laryngectomy, which entail tracheostomy during the course of the procedure. It is far better to perform a tracheostomy under controlled conditions than to resort to this technique once other measures have failed and the patient is *in extremis*.

Unanticipated Airway Difficulty

When the larynx cannot be visualized and an endotracheal tube cannot be placed, the anesthesiologist must consider the alternatives to airway management and formulate a plan based on the cause of the difficulty, the patient's condition, and the type and urgency of surgery. If the patient can be ventilated by mask, additional attempts at intubation may be justified or, in some situations, mask ventilation can be continued throughout the surgical procedure.

If the procedure is elective and multiple intubation attempts have resulted in airway trauma, the surgery is best cancelled and the patient allowed to emerge from anesthesia. If the difficulty is recognized before airway trauma occurs, the patient is stable, and an experienced fiberoptic endoscopist and appropriate equipment are available, consideration should be given to employing this technique. The patient whose condition is deteriorating because of cardiovascular instability or respiratory obstruction is rarely a candidate for fiberoptic endoscopy. If airway bleeding has been induced, fiberoptic visualization may be impossible. In such circumstances, cricothyrotomy with transtracheal ventilation or tracheostomy is preferable.

FIBEROPTIC ENDOSCOPY

Although the experienced endoscopist makes the procedure appear simple, fiberoptic laryngoscopic examination requires skill and practice.[17,122] Fiberoptic endoscopes are expensive, fragile instruments, and all individuals who use them should be trained by practitioners skilled in their use. Practice on a tracheobronchial model and intubation mannequin affords students the opportunity to develop skill in orienting and maneuvering the instrument and familiarity with the visual fields. Attendance at practical hands-on workshops,[123] practice on anesthetized, spontaneously breathing animals,[124] exposure of the epiglottis and vocal cords in patients recovering from general anesthesia,[125] intubation of awake, sedated patients, and finally intubation of patients with normal airways receiving general anesthesia[126] are ways of gaining facility with the instrument.

Fiberoptic intubation in conscious, sedated patients is not associated with significant hemodynamic alterations if adequate topical anesthesia is employed.[127,128] However, when fiberoptic orotracheal[129] or nasotracheal[130] intubation is compared with conventional laryngoscopic examination and intubation in patients receiving general anesthesia, the cardiovascular responses are greater with fiberoptic endoscopy.

Elective Fiberoptic Laryngoscopy

Fiberoptic endoscopic examination requires more time than conventional laryngoscopic examination, even when performed by an expert. It is imperative that the anesthetic technique be planned in advance, allowing sufficient time for induction of general anesthesia or for topical anesthesia and intravenous sedation to become effective. An assistant is useful when the procedure is performed with local anesthesia and mandatory if general anesthesia is administered. One person cannot monitor the patient, administer general anesthesia, and perform fiberoptic endoscopic examination.

Local anesthesia is often preferable, particularly in the patient with a precarious airway or if the endoscopist is not facile with the technique. Disadvantages of general anesthesia include relaxation of the tongue and pharyngeal tissues, which may make the technique more difficult, and time limitations imposed if the patient is apneic. When general anesthesia is chosen, use of an endoscopic mask with a port through which the fiberscope is passed permits uninterrupted anesthesia and ventilation during the procedure (Fig. 26-30). As an alternative, adequate anesthesia and ventilation of the lungs can be maintained in most patients with a binasal airway attached to the anesthetic circuit. In order to maintain the midline position of the fiberscope as it is advanced through the pharynx into the trachea, an endoscopic airway should be used. The Patil-Syracuse endoscopic airway (see Fig. 26-5), the Ovassapian fiberoptic intubating airway, or the Williams airway intubator is suitable. With the latter, the endotracheal tube is passed through the lumen of the airway.[131]

The largest fiberscope that will fit easily into the endotracheal tube should be used because visualization is improved and it is more difficult to thread a large endotracheal tube over a small, flexible endoscope. Orotracheal intubation permits use of a larger endotracheal tube and is associated with less tissue trauma and bleeding. However, it may be difficult to thread the endotracheal tube once the fiberscope is positioned in the trachea because of the acute angle formed between the oropharynx and the trachea. Retraction of the tongue and anterior displacement of the mandible usually effectively overcome this problem. Nasotracheal intubation is often easier to perform because the natural curve of the nasopharynx guides the tube into the larynx (Fig. 26-31).

A step-by-step procedure should always be followed when fiberoptic endoscopic examination is performed. The endoscopist initially must determine that the working elements of the endoscope and light source are functional. The sheath of the fiberscope must be lubricated thoroughly with a water-soluble jelly, beginning at the distal end and moving

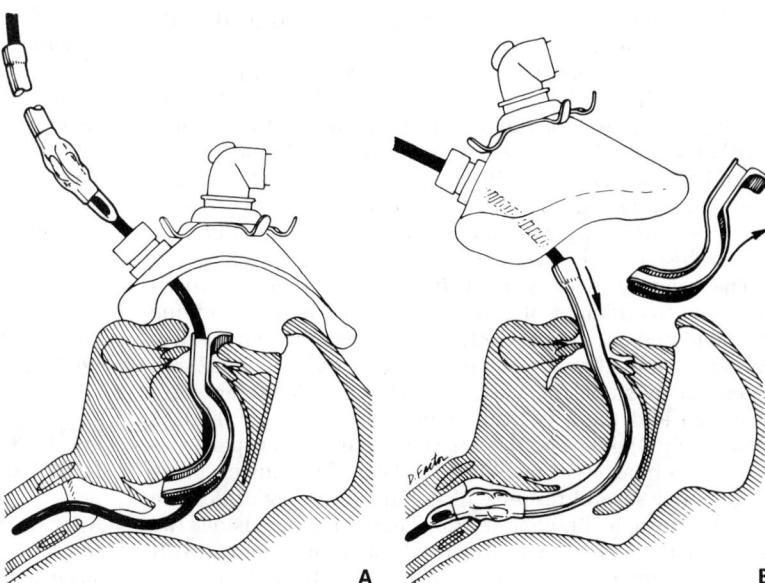

Figure 26-30. (A) The insertion tube of the fiberoptic endoscope and the endotracheal tube are introduced through the port of the endoscopic mask. (B) The endoscopic airway is removed and the endotracheal tube advanced into the trachea.

A **B**

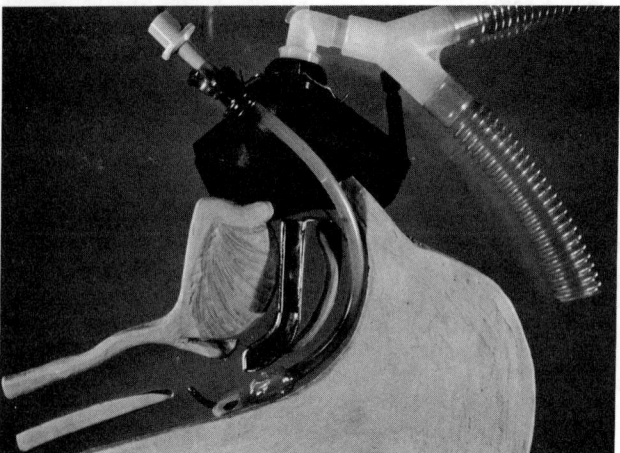

Figure 26-31. Model demonstrating use of endoscopic mask and airway during fiberoptic nasotracheal intubation.

proximally to avoid the lens. Products containing oil or petroleum jelly should not be used. The lens should be focused before use, not after the instrument is inserted. An antifog agent should be applied to the lens, or the tip of the fiberscope can be immersed in warm water immediately prior to use to minimize fogging of the lens. Visibility is enhanced if a constant oxygen flow is maintained through the operating channel of the instrument. In addition to providing a higher inspired oxygen concentration, the oxygen forces mucus, blood, and secretions away from the lens. Incorporation of a three-way stopcock in the suction tube allows alternating suction and oxygen flow.

The control section of the instrument is held in one hand, with the thumb positioned on the angle control and the index finger on the suction port. The fiberscope is threaded into the endotracheal tube and held fully extended with the other hand, and the angle knob is manipulated to ensure that the end of the fiberscope moves up and down rather than sideways. When orotracheal intubation is performed in the adult, the fiberscope is advanced 8–10 cm into the pharynx. If the fiberscope is in the midline and has been advanced the proper distance, the vocal cords will come into view as the tip is flexed upward. A local anesthetic agent can be instilled through the suction port directly onto the vocal cords if laryngeal anesthesia is inadequate. Slight rotation of the fiberscope may be necessary to bring the tip into the midline. The first view after it is advanced through the vocal cords will be the thyroid cartilage, not the tracheal cartilages. The tip of the fiberscope is straightened or returned to the neutral position and advanced until the tracheal cartilages and finally the carina are seen. The fiberscope is held firmly, the endotracheal tube is threaded into the trachea, and the endoscope is removed.

The primary reasons for technique failure are inexperience and insufficient planning. All too often the technique is considered only after multiple unsuccessful tracheal intubation attempts have resulted in tissue trauma, edema, and bleeding. In such circumstances anatomic landmarks are obscured and there is little chance of success. If there is insufficient light or if the instrument is not properly focused, the image will be blurred or hazy. The lens becomes fogged after several minutes of use. If suctioning or flowing oxygen through the channel does not improve vision, the instrument must be withdrawn, cleaned, and defogged. If the fiberscope easily advances more than 10 or 12 cm be-

yond the pharynx and no definable structures are evident, it can be assumed that it is in the esophagus. In this case the fiberscope should be withdrawn and the procedure repeated.

Emergency Fiberoptic Endoscopy

An antisialagogue should be administered as soon as the decision is made to proceed with fiberoptic endoscopy. If the esophagus was intubated or positive pressure ventilation resulted in stomach distention, a nasogastric tube should be inserted and the stomach decompressed. When mask ventilation is adequate, the patient is not at risk of aspiration of gastric contents, secretions and blood are not obscuring the airway, and an assistant is available, general anesthesia can often be continued and an endoscopic mask used. No additional muscle relaxants are administered, and it may be necessary to reverse a nondepolarizing relaxant to allow resumption of spontaneous ventilation. Cricoid pressure is applied in the patient at risk of aspiration of gastric contents, general anesthesia is discontinued, the muscle relaxant is reversed if necessary, the patient is allowed to awaken, and the endoscopic examination and intubation are performed with the patient awake.

The use of topical anesthesia and nerve blocks is controversial. The most conservative approach is to avoid use of all local anesthetics because it is impossible to ensure that topical anesthesia will be confined to the area above the vocal cords. Translaryngeal and superior laryngeal blocks are generally contraindicated. In the patient with a very active gag reflex, glossopharyngeal blocks can be considered in addition to topical anesthesia of the tongue. When motion of the vocal cords prevents passage of the endotracheal tube, spraying local anesthetic directly on the vocal cords through the working channel of the endoscope often allows passage of the tube into the glottis. Although favorable experience with translaryngeal and topical anesthesia in patients at high risk for aspiration has been described,[132] the risks of decreasing the patient's ability to protect his or her airway must be weighed against the difficulty of accomplishing intubation in the absence of adequate anesthesia.

Clinical Applications

The primary indication for fiberoptic endoscopy is endotracheal intubation. However, there are other diagnostic and therapeutic applications. The position of endotracheal, endobronchial,[133] and tracheostomy tubes[134] can be verified and the airway examined for abnormalities such as excessive secretions and smoke inhalation. In patients with mediastinal tumors, the functional anatomy of the airway can be evaluated and precise placement of endobronchial tubes relative to obstructive lesions can be confirmed.[135] The fiberoptic bronchoscope is also useful for placing segmental bronchial blockers and nasogastric tubes, changing endotracheal tubes,[136] facilitating retrograde intubation,[137] and performing tracheobronchial toilet.

OTHER SPECIALIZED TECHNIQUES OF AIRWAY MANAGEMENT

Altering the position of the patient's head and using a smaller endotracheal tube, different stylet, introducer, or laryngoscope blade are all that are necessary in most cases when endotracheal intubation is initially difficult. However, specialized equipment and techniques are necessary when these maneuvers fail. It is essential that the equipment be readily available and that the anesthesiologist be familiar with its use. Preassembled kits can be purchased or sets can be made from equipment available in the hospital. Some apparatus, e.g., equipment for transtracheal jet ventilation, should be immediately available in every anesthetizing location. Other devices should be kept in a consistent, designated, clearly marked place in the operating suite, preferably on a mobile intubation cart.

Retrograde Intubation

The retrograde technique is suitable for use in elective surgery when direct laryngoscopy is known or suspected to be difficult, or manipulation of the neck is contraindicated, and in some emergency situations. The skin over the cricothyroid membrane is cleansed and anesthetized and then punctured with an 18-gauge needle with the bevel directed cephalad at an angle of approximately 45 degrees. Once entry into the trachea has been confirmed by aspiration of air, a flexible 0.025–0.035-cm guidewire, 110–150 cm long, preferably with a J-tip, is introduced into the needle and threaded through the vocal cords into the pharynx and out the mouth. The needle is removed and the guidewire clamped at the level of the skin to prevent movement. With the guidewire held taut, the endotracheal tube is threaded over the guidewire into the trachea. Once proper placement of the endotracheal tube is verified, the guidewire is withdrawn through the mouth and the tube is connected to the anesthetic circuit.

Not infrequently, the endotracheal tube will "ricochet" around the guidewire because of the small diameter of the guidewire. Passing a catheter, endotracheal tube changer, or nasogastric tube antegrade over the guidewire effectively enlarges the diameter of the stylet and facilitates passage of the endotracheal tube. Rotating the tube 90 degrees counterclockwise is often helpful. An even better technique is threading the guidewire retrograde through the suction channel of a fiberoptic bronchoscope that is placed in the lumen of an appropriately sized endotracheal tube. The endotracheal tube is then positioned under direct vision and the guidewire removed via the proximal port of the suction channel.[137,138] If a retrograde intubation set is not used, it is essential that all components be tested in advance of their use in a patient to ascertain that they are compatible. If one is not available in the operating room, the J-wire can often be obtained from the radiology department.

Transtracheal Ventilation

A lifesaving measure when neither ventilation by mask nor endotracheal intubation is possible, transtracheal ventilation is accomplished by placing a 14- or 16-gauge over-the-needle catheter through the cricothyroid membrane. The catheter is directed caudally at an angle of 45 degrees to the skin. Once air is aspirated, indicating that the catheter is in the trachea, the stylet is removed, the catheter advanced, air again aspirated, and the catheter connected to an oxygen source. Inserting a 3-mm endotracheal tube adapter into the catheter hub permits attachment of the anesthesia circuit or a resuscitation bag. An alternate method of adapting to the circuit is to insert the adapter from a 7-mm endotracheal tube into the barrel of a 3-ml syringe from which the plunger

has been removed. However, ventilation with these systems will invariably be inadequate, and jet ventilation is preferable.[139]

A jet injector powered by regulated tank or wall oxygen is the preferred method of ventilation. Less desirable is a jet injector powered by unregulated oxygen pressure. The anesthesia machine flush valve can be used if a jet ventilator is not readily available. Noncompliant tubing is attached to the common outlet of the machine via a 4-mm endotracheal tube adapter. A one-quarter inch hose barb with a male Luer-Lok fitting is inserted in the other end of the tubing for connection to the transtracheal catheter.[139] (Fig. 26-32). Noncompliant oxygen tubing is used in order to bypass the compliant reservoir bag and corrugated tubing of the circle system.

It must be remembered that the only way the jetted inspired oxygen can be expired is through the upper airway. In the case of total upper airway obstruction, percutaneous transtracheal ventilation must be converted to a surgical cricothyroidotomy or tracheostomy and an endotracheal or tracheostomy tube inserted so that conventional intermittent positive pressure ventilation can be initiated as soon as possible. A commercially available cricothyrotomy catheter set (Cook Critical Care, Bloomington, IN) with a 6-mm inner diameter airway can also be used. The major complications of transtracheal jet ventilation are tissue emphysema and barotrauma with resultant pneumothorax.

Modifications of the transtracheal ventilation technique have been described, including use of a vessel dilator from a 7- or 9-gauge introducer kit. The vessel dilator is longer than a conventional intravenous catheter, firm, and resistant to kinking.[140] "Prophylactic" transtracheal ventilation can be employed while intubation is performed using a conventional or fiberoptic technique in patients who are known

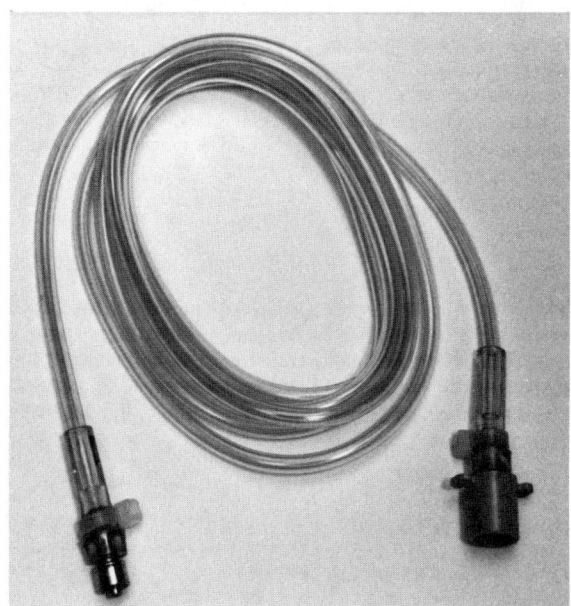

Figure 26-32. System for emergency transtracheal ventilation using the anesthesia machine flush valve. A 4-mm endotracheal tube adapter (*right*) connects to the common outlet of the anesthesia machine and a hose barb with a male Luer-lok fitting (*left*) is inserted into the other end of a piece of oxygen tubing for connection to the translaryngeal catheter. (Note that the adapters are bonded with plastic ties.)

to be difficult to intubate. While the patient is ventilated transtracheally, sedation or general anesthesia and a muscle relaxant can be safely administered without compromise of oxygenation.[141,142]

Fluoroscopic Techniques

The availability of fluoroscopy in most operating rooms has prompted some investigators to employ x-ray-guided endotracheal intubation in situations where movement of the neck is contraindicated or intubation is known to be difficult.[143,144]

Surgical Intervention

Although it has been performed much less frequently for airway management since the introduction of fiberoptic endoscopy, tracheostomy is indicated in some patients. However, surgical cricothyrotomy is preferred to tracheostomy in cases of acute airway obstruction because it is technically easier and can be performed more quickly. In addition, the cricothyroid membrane is less vascular than the area in which a standard tracheostomy incision is made, making bleeding less likely.[145]

REFERENCES

1. Westhorpe RN: The position of the larynx in children and its relation to the ease of intubation. Anaesth Intensive Care 15:384, 1987
2. Eckenhoff JE: Some anatomic considerations of the infant larynx influencing endotracheal intubation. Anesthesiology 12:401, 1951
3. Jenkins CL, McGraw RW: Anaesthetic management of the patient with rheumatoid arthritis. Can Anaesth Soc J 16:407, 1969
4. Katz J, Steward DJ: Anesthesia in Uncommon Pediatric Diseases. Philadelphia, WB Saunders, 1987
5. Jones KL: Smith's Recognizable Patterns of Human Malformation, 4th ed. Philadelphia, WB Saunders, 1988
6. Goldberg MJ: The Dysmorphic Child: An Orthopedic Perspective. New York, Raven Press, 1987
7. Mallampati SR, Gatt SP, Gugino LD et al: A clinical sign to predict difficult tracheal intubation: A prospective study. Can Anaesth Soc J 32:429, 1985
8. Sampson GLT, Young JRB: Difficult tracheal intubation. Anaesthesia 42:429, 1985
9. Block C, Brechner VL: Unusual problems in airway management. II. The influence of the temporomandibular joint, the mandible and associated structures on endotracheal intubation. Anesth Analg 50:114, 1971
10. Redick LF: The temporomandibular joint and tracheal intubation. Anesth Analg 66:675, 1987
11. Reisell E, Orko R, Maunuksela E-L, Lindgren L: Predictability of difficult laryngoscopy in patients with long-term diabetes mellitus. Anaesthesia 45:1024, 1990
12. Brechner VL: Unusual problems in the management of airways. I. Flexion-extension mobility of the cervical vertebrae. Anesth Analg 47:462, 1968
13. Sinclair JR, Mason RA: Ankylosing spondylitis. The case for awake intubation. Anaesthesia 39:3, 1984
14. Pellicci PM, Ranawat CS, Tsairis P et al: A prospective study of the progression of rheumatoid arthritis of the cervical spine. J Bone Joint Surg [Am] 63:342, 1981
15. Salathe M, Johr M: Unsuspected cervical fractures: A common problem in ankylosing spondylitis. Anesthesiology 70:869, 1989
16. Hogan K, Rusy D, Springman SR: Difficult laryngoscopy and diabetes mellitus. Anesth Analg 67:1162, 1988

17. Patil VU, Stehling L, Zauder HL: Fiberoptic Endoscopy in Anesthesiology. Chicago, Year Book Medical Publishers, 1983
18. Powell JF, Woodcock T, Luscombe FE: Atlanto-axial subluxation in Down's syndrome. Anaesthesia 45:1049, 1990
19. Berkowitz ID, Raja SN, Bender KS, Kopits SE: Dwarfs: Pathophysiology and anesthetic implications. Anesthesiology 73:739, 1990
20. Crosby DT, Lui A: The adult cervical spine: Implications for airway management. Can J Anaesth 37:77, 1990
21. Hotchkiss RS, Hall JR, Braun IF, Schisler JQ: An abnormal epiglottis as a cause of difficult intubation-airway assessment using magnetic resonance imaging. Anesthesiology 68:140, 1988
22. Schneider J, Probst R, Wey W: Magnetic resonance imaging—a useful tool for airway assessment. Acta Anaesthesiol Scand 33:429, 1989
23. Roberts JT: Functional anatomy of the larynx. Int Anesthesiol Clin 28:101, 1990
24. White A, Kander PL: Anatomical factors in difficult direct laryngoscopy. Br J Anaesth 47:468, 1975
25. Bellhouse CP, Dore C: Criteria for estimating likelihood of difficulty of endotracheal intubation with the Macintosh laryngoscope. Anaesth Intens Care 16:329, 1988
26. Horton WA, Fahy L, Charters P: Factor analysis in difficult tracheal intubation: Laryngoscopy-induced airway obstruction. Br J Anaesth 65:801, 1990
27. Wilson ME, Spiegelhalter D, Robertson JA, Lesser PL: Predicting difficult intubation. Br J Anaesth 61:211, 1988
28. Oates JDL, Macleod AD, Oates PD, et al: Comparison of two methods for predicting difficult intubation. Br J Anaesth 66:305, 1991
29. Grebenik CR, Ferguson C, White A: The laryngeal mask airway in pediatric radiotherapy. Anesthesiology 72:474, 1990
30. Johnston DF, Wrigley SR, Robb PJ, Jones HE: The laryngeal mask airway in paediatric anaesthesia. Anaesthesia 45:924, 1990
31. Brodrick PM, Webster NR, Nunn JF: The laryngeal mask airway: A study of 100 patients during spontaneous breathing. Anaesthesia 44:238, 1989
32. Maltby JR, Loken RG, Watson NC: The laryngeal mask airway: Clinical appraisal in 250 patients. Can J Anaesth 37:509, 1990
33. McClune S, Regan M, Moore J: Laryngeal mask airway for caesarean section. Anaesthesia 45:227, 1990
34. Griffin RM, Hatcher IS: Aspiration pneumonia and the laryngeal mask airway. Anaesthesia 45:1039, 1990
35. Patil VU, Stehling LC, Zauder HL: An adjustable laryngoscope handle for difficult intubations. Anesthesiology 60:609, 1984
36. Cozanitis DA, Nuuttila K, Merrett JD et al: Influence of laryngoscope design on heart rate and rhythm changes during intubation. Can Anaesth Soc J 31:155, 1984
37. Borland LM, Casselbrant M: The Bullard laryngoscope: A new indirect oral laryngoscope (pediatric version). Anesth Analg 70:105, 1990
38. Dyson A, Harris J, Bhatia K: Rapidity and accuracy of tracheal intubation in a mannequin: Comparison of the fiberoptic with the Bullard laryngoscope. Br J Anaesth 65:268, 1990
39. Owen RL, Cheney FW: Endobronchial intubation: A preventable complication. Anesthesiology 67:255, 1987
40. Bolder PM, Healy TEJ, Bolder AR: The extra work of breathing through adult endotracheal tubes. Anesth Analg 65:853, 1986
41. Holzman RS, Nargozian CD, Florence F; Lightwand intubation in children with abnormal upper airways. Anesthesiology 69:784, 1988
42. Ellis DG, Jakymec A, Kaplan RM, et al: Guided orotracheal intubation in the operating room using a lighted stylet: A comparison with direct laryngoscopic technique. Anesthesiology 64:823, 1986
43. Fox DJ, Castro T, Rastrelli AJ: Comparison of intubation techniques in the awake patient: The Flexi-lum surgical light (lightwand) versus blind nasal approach. Anesthesiology 66:69, 1987
44. Mehta S: Transtracheal illumination for optimal tracheal tube placement: A clinical study. Anaesthesia 44:970, 1989
45. Graham DH, Doll WA, Robinson AD, Warriner CB: Intubation with lighted stylet. Can J Anaesth 38:261, 1991

46. Dogra S, Flaconer R, Latto IP: Successful difficult intubation: Tracheal tube placement over a gum-elastic bougie. Anaesthesia 45:774, 1990

47. Kidd JF, Dyson A, Latto IP: Successful difficult intubation: Use of the gum elastic bougie. Anaesthesia 43:437, 1988

48. Artru AA, Schultz AB, Bonneu JJ: Modification of an Eschmann introducer to permit measurement of end-tidal carbon dioxide. Anesth Analg 68:129, 1989

49. Haddy S: Protecting teeth during endotracheal intubation. Anesthesiology 71:810, 1989

50. Salem MR: Anesthetic management of patients with "a full stomach." A critical review. Anesth Analg 49:47, 1970

51. Salem MR, Joseph NJ, Heyman HJ et al: Cricoid pressure is effective in obliterating the esophageal lumen in the presence of a nasogastric tube. Anesthesiology 63:443, 1985

52. Bertholid M, Read DH, Norman J: Preoxygenation—how long? Anaesthesia 38:96, 1983

53. Drummond GB, Park GR: Arterial oxygen saturation before intubation of the trachea. Br J Anaesth 56:987, 1984

54. Gambee AM, Hertzka RE, Fisher DM: Preoxygenation techniques: Comparisons of three minutes and four breaths. Anesth Analg 66:468, 1987

55. Sellick BA: Cricoid pressure to control regurgitation of stomach contents during induction of anaesthesia. Lancet 2:404, 1961

56. Lawes EG, Campbell I, Mercer D: Inflation pressure, gastric insufflation and rapid sequence induction. Br J Anaesth 59:315, 1987

57. Ralph SJ, Wareham CA: Rupture of the esophagus during cricoid pressure. Anaesthesia 46:40, 1991

58. Crowley DS, Giesecke AH: Bimanual cricoid pressure. Anaesthesia 45:588, 1990

59. Lawes EG: Cricoid pressure with or without the "cricoid yoke." Br J Anaesth 58:1376, 1986

60. Cooper M, Watson RL: An improved regional anesthetic technique for peroral endoscopy. Anesthesiology 43:372, 1973

61. Sutherland AD, William SRT: Cardiovascular responses and lidocaine absorption in fiberoptic-assisted awake intubation. Anesth Analg 65:389, 1986

62. Bromley L, Hayward A: Cocaine absorption from the nasal mucosa. Anaesthesia 43:356, 1988

63. Bourke DL, Katz J, Tonneson A: Nebulized anesthesia for awake endotracheal intubation. Anesthesiology 63:690, 1985

64. Woods AM, Lander CJ: Abolition of gagging and the hemodynamic response to awake laryngoscopy (Abstract). Anesthesiology 67:A220, 1987

65. Adriani J, Griggs TS: An improved endotracheal tube for pediatric use. Anesthesiology 15:466, 1954

66. Kubota Y, Toyoda Y, Nagata N et al: Tracheo-bronchial angles in infants and children. Anesthesiology 64:374, 1986

67. Tsuneto S, Yamashita M, Miyamoto Y: Tracheo-bronchial angles in neonates. Anesthesiology 67:151, 1987

68. Baraka A, Akel S, Muallem M et al: Bronchial intubation in children: Does the tube bevel determine the side of intubation? Anesthesiology 67:869, 1987

69. Patil VU, Stehling L, Zauder HL: An aid to blind endotracheal intubation. Anesth Analg 63:882, 1984

70. Shapiro H, Unger R: Blind, but not deaf or dirty, intubations. Anesthesiology 64:297, 1986

71. King H-K, Wooten DJ: Blind nasal intubation by monitoring end-tidal carbon dioxide. Anesth Analg 69:407, 1989

72. Omoigui S, Glass P, Martel DLJ et al: Blind nasal intubation with audio-capnometry. Anesth Analg 72:392, 1991

73. Birmingham PK, Cheney FW, Ward RJ: Esophageal intubation: A review of detection techniques. Anesth Analg 65:886, 1986

74. Chartes P, Wilkinson K: Tactile orotracheal tube placement test: Manual tactile examination of the positioned orotracheal tube to confirm laryngeal placement. Anaesthesia 42:801, 1987

75. Strunin L, Williams T: The FEF end-tidal carbon dioxide detector. Anesthesiology 71:621, 1989

76. Denman WT, Hayes M, Higgins D, Wilkinson DJ: The Fenem CO_2 detector device: An apparatus to prevent unnoticed oesophageal intubation. Anaesthesia 45:465, 1990

77. O'Flaherty DO, Adams AP: The end-tidal carbon dioxide detector: Assessment of a new method to distinguish oesophageal from tracheal intubation. Anaesthesia 45:653, 1990

78. Goldberg JS, Rawle PR, Zehnder JL, Sladen RN: Colorimetric end-tidal carbon dioxide monitoring for tracheal intubation. Anesth Analg 70:191, 1990

79. MacLeod BA, Heller MB, Yearly DM, Menegazzi JJ: Verification of endotracheal tube placement with colorimetric end-tidal CO_2 detection. Ann Emerg Med 20:267, 1991

80. Shibman AJ, Smith G, Achola KJ: Cardiovascular and catecholamine responses to laryngoscopy with and without tracheal intubation. Br J Anaesth 59:295, 1987

81. Bedford RF, Feinstein B: Hospital admission blood pressure: A predictor for hypertension following endotracheal intubation. Anesth Analg 59:367, 1980

82. Kautto UM: Attenuation of the circulatory response to laryngoscopy and intubation by fentanyl. Acta Anaesth Scand 26:217, 1982

83. Martin DE, Rosenberg H, Aukburg SJ et al: Low dose fentanyl blunts circulatory responses to tracheal intubation. Anesth Analg 61:680, 1982

84. Ebert JP, Pearson JD, Gelman S et al: Circulatory responses to laryngoscopy: The comparative effects of placebo, fentanyl and esmolol. Can J Anaesth 36:301, 1989

85. Splinter WM, Cervenko F: Haemodynamic responses to laryngoscopy and tracheal intubation in geriatric patients: Effects of fentanyl, lidocaine and thiopentone. Can J Anaesth 36:370, 1989

86. Tam S, Chung F, Campbell M: Intravenous lidocaine: Optimal time of injection before tracheal intubation. Anesth Analg 66:1036, 1987

87. Hamill JF, Bedford RF, Weaver DC et al: Lidocaine before endotracheal intubation: Intravenous or laryngotracheal? Anesthesiology 55:578, 1981

88. Sheppard S, Eagle CJ, Strunin L: A bolus dose of esmolol attenuates tachycardia and hypertension after tracheal intubation. Can J Anaesth 37:202, 1990

89. Stoelting RK: Attenuation of blood pressure response to laryngoscopy and tracheal intubation with sodium nitroprusside. Anesth Analg 58:116, 1979

90. Grover VK, Sharma S, Mahajan RP: Low-dose intranasal nitroglycerine attenuates pressor response. Anesthesiology 66:722, 1987

91. McCarthy GJ, Hainsworth M, Lindsay K et al: Pressor responses to tracheal intubation after sublingual captopril: A pilot study. Anaesthesia 45:243, 1990

92. Cottrell JE, Hartung J, Giffin JP et al: Intracranial and hemodynamic changes after succinylcholine administration in cats. Anesth Analg 62:1006, 1983

93. McLeskey CH, Cullen BF, Kennedy RD et al: Control of cerebral perfusion pressure during induction of anesthesia in high-risk neurosurgical patients. Anesth Analg 53:985, 1974

94. Burney RG, Winn R: Increased cerebrospinal fluid pressure during laryngoscopy and intubation for induction of anesthesia. Anesth Analg 54:687, 1975

95. Lanier WL, Milde JH, Michenfelder JD: Cerebral stimulation following succinylcholine in dogs. Anesthesiology 64:551, 1986

96. Murphy DF: Anesthesia and intraocular pressure. Anesth Analg 64:520, 1985

97. Lerman J, Kiskis AA: Effects of intravenous lidocaine and high-dose pancuronium on intraocular pressure in children (Abstract). Anesth Analg 64:185, 1985

98. Mostafa SM, Wiles JR, Dowd T et al: Effects of nebulized lignocaine on the intraocular pressure responses to tracheal intubation. Br J Anaesth 64:515, 1990

99. Johnson KG, Hood DD: Esophageal perforation associated with endotracheal intubation. Anesthesiology 64:281, 1986

100. O'Neill JE, Giffin JP, Cottrell JE: Pharyngeal and esophageal perforation following endotracheal intubation. Anesthesiology 60:487, 1984

101. Dinner M, Tjeuw M, Artusio JF: Bacteremia as a complication of nasotracheal intubation. Anesth Analg 66:460, 1987

102. Castella X, Gilabert J, Perez C: Arytenoid dislocation after tracheal intubation: An unusual cause of acute respiratory failure? Anesthesiology 74:613, 1991

103. Fassoulaki A, Pamouktsoglou P: Prolonged nasotracheal intubation and its association with inflammation of paranasal sinuses. Anesth Analg 69:50, 1989

104. Bogetz MS, Tupper BJ, Vigil AC: Too much of a good thing: Uvular trauma caused by overzealous suctioning. Anesth Analg 72:125, 1991

105. Lang SA, Duncan PG, Shephard AE, Ha HC: Pulmonary oedema associated with airway obstruction. Can Anaesth Soc J 37:210, 1990

106. Burgess GE, Cooper JR, Marino RJ et al: Laryngeal competence after tracheal extubation. Anesthesiology 51:73, 1979

107. Jensen PJ, Hommelgaard P, Sondergaard P et al: Sore throat after operation: Influence of tracheal intubation, intracuff pressure and type of cuff. Br J Anaesth 54:453, 1982

108. Bishop MJ, Weymuller EA, Fink BR: Laryngeal effects of prolonged intubation. Anesth Analg 63:335, 1984

109. Loeser EA, Stanley TH, Jordan W et al: Postoperative sore throat: Influence of tracheal tube lubrication versus cuff design. Can Anaesth Soc J 27:156, 1980

110. Stock MC, Downs JB: Lubrication of tracheal tubes to prevent sore throat from intubation. Anesthesiology 57:418, 1982

111. Monroe MC, Gravenstein N, Saga-Rumley S: Postoperative sore throat: Effect of oropharyngeal airway in orotracheally intubated patients. Anesth Analg 70:512, 1990

112. Stout DM, Bishop MJ, Dwersteg JF et al: Correlation of endotracheal tube size with sore throat and hoarseness following general anesthesia. Anesthesiology 67:419, 1987

113. Bernhard WN, Yost LC, Turndorf H et al: Physical characteristics of and rates of nitrous oxide diffusion into tracheal tube cuffs. Anesthesiology 48:413, 1978

114. Diaz JH: Continuous monitoring of intracuff pressures in endotracheal tubes. Anesthesiology 68:813, 1988

115. Williams KN, Carli F, Cormack RS: Unexpected, difficult laryngoscopy: A prospective survey in routine general surgery. Br J Anaesth 66:38, 1991

116. King TA, Adams AP: Failed tracheal intubation. Br J Anaesth 65:400, 1990

117. Davies JM, Weeks S, Crone LA, Pavlin E: Difficult intubation in the parturient. Can J Anaesth 36:668, 1989

118. Sivarajan M, Fink BR: The position and the state of the larynx during general anesthesia and muscle paralysis. Anesthesiology 72:439, 1990

119. Cormack RS, Lehane J: Difficult tracheal intubation in obstetrics. Anaesthesia 39:1105, 1984

120. Goldberg JS, Bernard AC, Marks RJ, Sladen RN: Simulation technique for difficult intubation: Teaching tool or new hazard? J Clin Anesth 2:21, 1990

121. McIntyre JWR: The difficult tracheal intubation. Can J Anaesth 34:204, 1987

122. Ovassapian A: Fiberoptic Airway Endoscopy in Anesthesia and Critical Care. New York, Raven Press, 1990

123. Dykes MHM, Ovassapian A: Dissemination of fibreoptic airway endoscopy skills by means of a workshop utilizing models. Br J Anaesth 63:595, 1989

124. Forbes RB, Murray DJ, Albanese MA: Evaluation of an animal model for teaching fibreoptic tracheal intubation. Can J Anaesth 36:141, 1989

125. Ovassapian A, Yelich SJ, Dykes MHM, Golman ME: Learning fibreoptic intubation: Use of simulators v. traditional teaching. Br J Anaesth 61:217, 1988

126. Coe PA, King TA, Towey RM: Teaching guided fibreoptic nasotracheal intubation: An assessment of an anesthetic technique to aid training. Anaesthesia 43:410, 1988

127. Ovassapian A, Yelich SJ, Dykes MHM, Brunner ER: Blood pressure and heart rate changes during awake fiberoptic nasotracheal intubation. Anesth Analg 62:951, 1983

128. Sutherland AD, Williams RT: Cardiovascular responses and lidocaine absorption in fiberoptic-assisted awake intubation. Anesth Analg 65:389, 1986

129. Smith JE: Heart rate and arterial pressure changes during fibreoptic tracheal intubation under general anaesthesia. Anaesthesia 43:629, 1988

130. Smith JE, Mackenzie AA, Sanghera SS, Scott-Knight VCE: Cardiovascular effects of fibrescope-guided nasotracheal intubation. Anaesthesia 44:907, 1989

131. Rogers SN, Benumof JL: New and easy techniques for fiberoptic endoscopy-aided tracheal intubation. Anesthesiology 59:569, 1983

132. Ovassapian A, Krejcie TC, Yelich SJ, Dykes MHM: Awake fibreoptic intubation in the patient at high risk of aspiration. Br J Anaesth 62:13, 1989

133. Benumof JL, Partridge BL, Salvatierra C, Keating J: Margin of safety in positioning modern double-lumen endotracheal tubes. Anesthesiology 67:729, 1987

134. Patil VU, Stehling LC, Zauder HL: Another use for the fiberoptic bronchoscope. Anesthesiology 55:484, 1981

135. Younker D, Clark R, Coveler L: Fiberoptic endobronchial intubation for resection of an anterior mediastinal mass. Anesthesiology 70:144, 1989

136. Rosenbaum SH, Rosenbaum LM, Cole RP et al: Use of the flexible fiberoptic bronchoscope to change endotracheal tubes in critically ill patients. Anesthesiology 54:169, 1981

137. Gupta B, McDonald JD, Brooks JHJ, Mendenhall J: Oral fiberoptic intubation over a retrograde guidewire. Anesth Analg 68:517, 1989

138. Lechman MJ, Donahoo JS, MacVaugh H: Endotracheal intubation using percutaneous retrograde guidewire insertion followed by antegrade fiberoptic bronchoscopy. Crit Care Med 14:589, 1986

139. Benumof JL, Scheller MS: The importance of transtracheal jet ventilation in the management of the difficult airway. Anesthesiology 71:769, 1989

140. Boyce JR, Peters G: Vessel dilator cricothyrotomy for transtracheal jet ventilation. Can J Anaesth 36:350, 1989

141. McLellan I, Gordon P, Khawaja S, Thomas A: Percutaneous transtracheal high frequency jet ventilation as an aid to difficult intubation. Can J Anaesth 35:404, 1988

142. Boucek CD, Gunnerson HB, Tullock WC: Percutaneous transtracheal high-frequency jet ventilation as an aid to fiberoptic intubation. Anesthesiology 67:247, 1987

143. Innocente F, Ori C, Giron GP: Tracheal intubation under fluoroscopic control: X-ray-guided orotracheal intubation in three cases of impossible direct laryngoscopy. Anaesthesia 45:675, 1990

144. Davidson, AJ, Reynolds AC, Stewart ET: Use of a flexible radiopaque directable catheter for difficult tracheal intubations. Anesthesiology 55:605, 1981

145. Miller RL: Invasive methods for securing an airway. Int Anesthesiol Clin 28:115, 1990

27

John T. Martin

Patient Positioning

Positioning a patient for a surgical procedure is frequently a compromise between what the anesthetized patient can tolerate, both structurally and physiologically, and what the surgical team requires for access to their anatomic targets.[1,2] Physiologic instability resulting from disease or injury may be magnified by rapidly moving a seriously ill patient from bed to transport cart, through corridors and elevators, and onto the operating table. Induction of anesthesia and positioning may need to be delayed until that patient is hemodynamically stable, or establishment of the intended surgical posture may need to be modified to match the patient's tolerance. This chapter presents the physiologic significance of various positions in which a patient may be placed during an operation, briefly describes the techniques of establishing the positions, and discusses the potential complications of each posture.

Careful attention should be paid to accurate terminology when discussing positioning. *Decubitus* is a loosely defined term[3] that is used in this chapter to indicate the part of the patient that is in contact with the supporting surface of the operating table. With suitable descriptors, the term *recumbent* can have the same meaning. Thus, the term *left lateral decubitus position* describes a patient whose left shoulder and hip rest on the operating table and whose right side is accessible to the surgeon. A dangerous jargonistic synonym, *right chest position,* is sometimes used, but it should be scrupulously avoided; it could lead to the patient's being turned onto the right chest and hip, with a resulting incorrect and potentially catastrophic incision on the exposed left side.

Statistics concerning the consequences of improper patient positioning are sparse. Based on records of settled claims, Cheney et al[4] presented valuable information about nerve damage subsequent to anesthesia, but they emphasized that their statistics did not relate to the population as a whole. Much of our information still comes from problems with single cases. Not infrequently, attempts to determine the etiology of complications alleged to be caused by patient positioning are unconscionably biased; on some occasions medicolegal conclusions have been shaped by assumptions and assertions made by persons having no familiarity with that particular case or with proceedings in an operating room in general. *Careful descriptive, but laconic, notations about positions employed during anesthesia and surgery,* *as well as brief comments about special protective measures such as eye care and pressure point padding, should be an obligatory part of every anesthesia record.* Only in this manner can subsequent inquiries be properly answered on behalf of the patient and the care team.

DORSAL DECUBITUS POSITIONS

Physiology

Circulation

In the horizontal supine position (Fig. 27-1A), the influence of gravity on the vascular system is minimal and intravascular pressures from head to foot vary little from mean pressures at the level of the heart; therefore, almost no perfusion gradient exists between the heart and arteries in either the head or the lower extremities. Similarly, venous gradients from the periphery to the right atrium consist principally of the cyclic intrathoracic pressure changes that occur with respiration.

If the patient in the dorsal decubitus position is tilted head high or head low, the effects of gravity on blood flow in the head or the feet can become quite significant as the gradient to or from the heart increases. Pressures have been shown to change by 2 mm Hg for each 2.5 cm that a given point varies in vertical height above or below the reference point at the heart.[5]

When the lower extremities are below the level of the heart, blood pools in the distensible dependent vessels, causing a reduction in effective circulating volume, cardiac output, and systemic perfusion. If the head is high and blood pressure measured at the level of the heart is low, the blood pressure in the brain is decreased further according to the magnitude of the head elevation.

The cardiovascular response to a head-up tilt of 75 degrees maintained for 3 minutes can be a useful indicator of the magnitude of acute blood loss.[6] If sustained tilt causes an increase in heart rate of more than 25 beats·min^{-1} but does not produce hypotension or syncope, the blood volume deficit is 9–14 ml·kg^{-1}. If syncope occurs on tilting, the deficit is likely to be as much as 20 ml·kg^{-1}. Hypo-

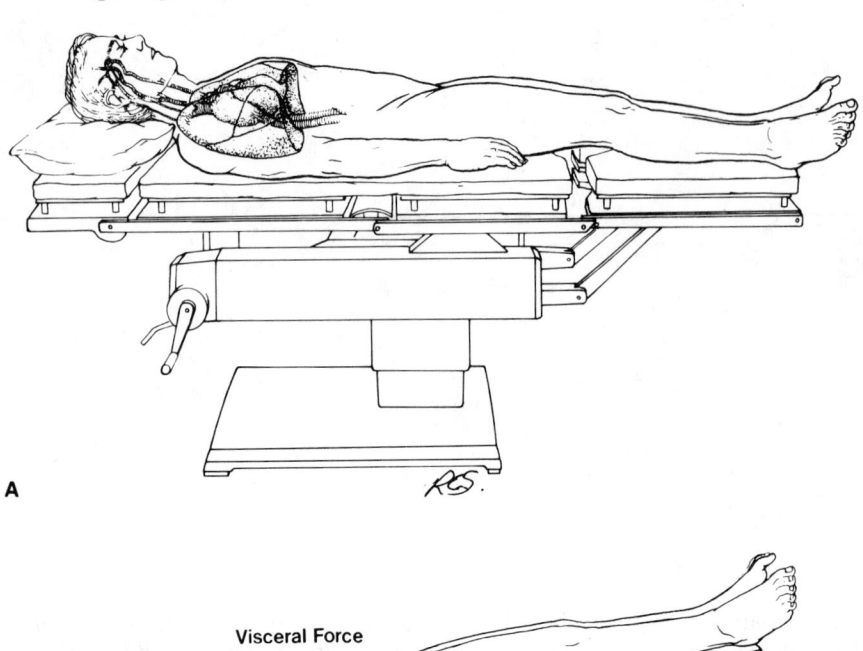

A

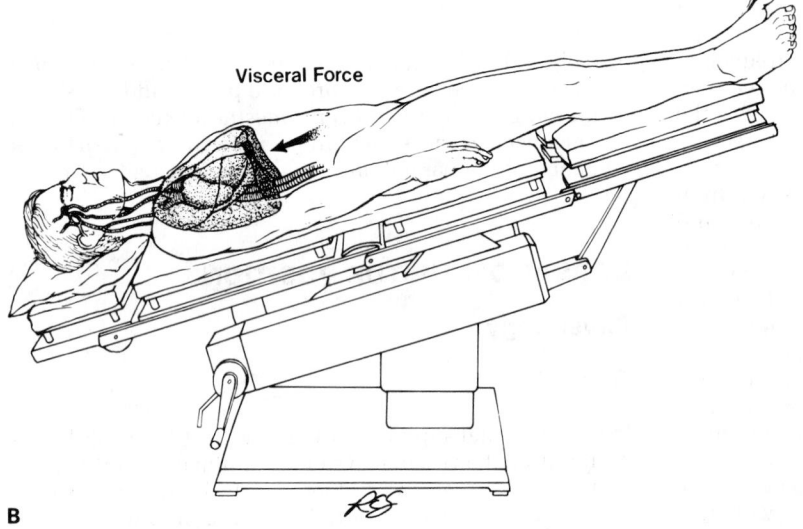

Visceral Force

B

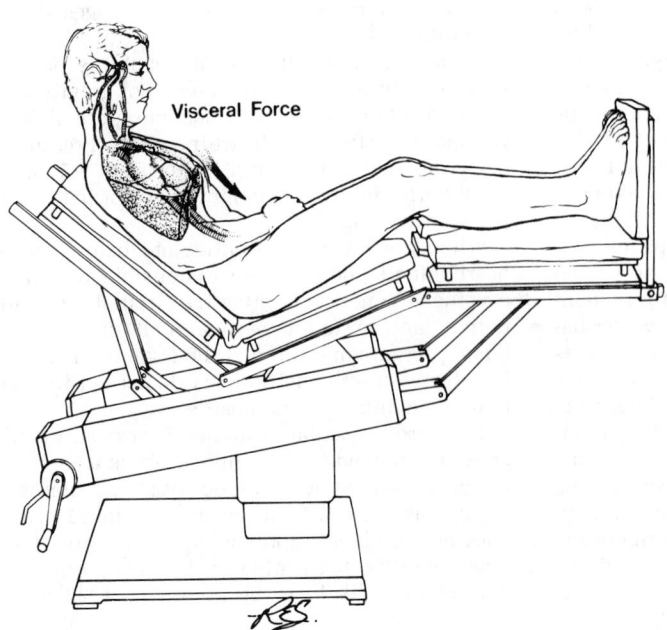

Visceral Force

C

Figure 27-1. (*A*) Supine adult with minimal gradients in the horizontal vascular axis. Pulmonary blood volume is greatest dorsally. Viscera displace the dorsal diaphragm cephalad. Cerebral circulation is slightly above heart level if the head is on a small pillow. (*B*) Head-down tilt aids blood return from lower extremities but encourages reflex vasodilation, congests vessels in the poorly ventilated lung apices, and increases intracranial blood volume. (*C*) Elevation of the head shifts abdominal viscera away from the diaphragm and improves ventilation of the lung bases.
According to the gradient above the heart, pressure in arteries of the head and neck decreases; pressure in accompanying veins may become subatmospheric.

tension without tilting indicates a deficit in excess of 20 ml·kg^{-1}.

If the head is tilted down (Fig. 27-1B), pressure in the cerebral veins increases in proportion to the gradient upward to the heart. Many alert patients so positioned complain of a rapidly occurring, pounding vascular headache. In the presence of intracranial pathology, a head injury, or a stroke, elevations of cerebral venous pressure resulting from head-down tilt may provoke or intensify cerebral edema and dangerously raise intracranial pressure. Head-down tilt also increases cerebrospinal fluid pressure within the cranial vault, adding its effect to the total intracranial pressure elevation.

Kubal et al[7] have shown that myocardial oxygen consumption can increase in awake patients scheduled for coronary artery bypass grafting when they are placed in mild degrees of head-down tilt as a means of distending jugular vessels and facilitating the percutaneous introduction of pulmonary artery catheters. Measurements suggested that an acute volume loading of the heart had occurred with the onset of the head-down tilt. Angina recurred in some patients, and one developed electrocardiographic changes indicative of myocardial ischemia.

Head-down tilt has been used to treat hypotension. A well-entrenched practice that was based on the suggestions of physiologist Walter Cannon during World War I,[8] this maneuver has been shown to be counterproductive.[9] Although it does increase central blood volume by recovering pooled blood from caudad portions of the body, and although cardiac output is increased transiently, the enlarged central blood mass activates baroreceptors on the great vessels of the chest and neck.[10] The result is rapid peripheral vasodilation, unchanged or reduced cardiac output, and decreased organ perfusion. In a study of patients in intensive care units, Sibbald and associates found that head-down tilt caused an unpredictable further decrease in mean arterial pressure in a significant number of patients who were already hypotensive.[9]

In the microcirculation, natural and spontaneous fluctuations in blood flow exist to serve the nutritive requirements of the tissues.[11] When an awake human is supine and motionless, the spontaneous fluctuations weaken progressively until they disappear in approximately 1 hour. The subject then becomes uncomfortable, and tissue blood flow continues to decrease if immobility is enforced.[12] A normal flow pattern returns if the subject becomes restless and moves about.

In the absence of hypocarbia, hypovolemia, or hypothermia, a similar impairment of changes in microcirculatory distribution of blood flow occurs after the induction of anesthesia, despite early augmentation of tissue flow owing to the vasodilative properties of the anesthetic agents. Normal tissue perfusion is re-established by awakening movements of the patient at the end of anesthesia.[12]

West et al[13] have identified three separate perfusion zones in the pulmonary circulation, based on the interrelationship among pressures in the alveoli, arterioles, and venules.

In Zone 1, alveolar pressure exceeds either arterial or venous pressure and perfusion of the lung unit is prevented. Although it is rarely present in a normal lung, Zone 1 can be produced by pulmonary hypotension, excessive positive end-expiratory pressure, or overdistention of alveolar units from large tidal volumes during intermittent positive pressure ventilation.

In Zone 2, arterial pressure exceeds alveolar pressure, whereas alveolar pressure remains higher than venous pressure. This relationship is found in nondependent portions of the lung, and perfusion is the result of a fluctuating balance between arterial and alveolar pressures.

In Zone 3, hydrostatic forces in the dependent portion of the lung have produced venous congestion, and perfusion is determined by the difference between arterial pressure and venous pressure.

In the dorsal recumbent positions, the pulmonary circulation tends to be most congested along the dorsal body wall and least congested substernally. When the patient is tilted head high, Zone 3 moves toward the lung bases and optimum ventilatory mechanics. If the tilt is head-down, Zone 3 shifts cephalad into the poorly ventilated lung apices and can be expected to intensify abnormal ventilation-perfusion ratios.

Respiration

In the supine position, mobile abdominal viscera gravitate toward the dorsal body wall and press the dorsal parts of the diaphragm cephalad. The displacement lengthens muscle fibers in that portion of the diaphragm and increases the strength and effectiveness of its contractions during spontaneous ventilation. The benefit is improved aeration of the congested, compacted, and less compliant lung bases. With head-up tilt (see Fig. 27-1C), the visceral weight shifts away from the diaphragm and ventilation is enhanced. In the head-down position, the visceral mass, its weight potentially increased by the presence of abdominal fat, fluid, or tumors, can cause significant respiratory embarrassment by impeding caudad excursions of the contracting diaphragm and preventing adequate expansion of the lung bases.

In the supine position, gravity-induced vascular congestion forces the dorsal portions of the lung to function as a Zone 3.[13] Consequently, the compliance of the area is reduced, and passive ventilation tends to distribute gas preferentially to substernal units where pulmonary blood volume is less. To prevent development of a clinically significant ventilation-perfusion imbalance during use of controlled ventilation, tidal volumes must be used that are greater than the average amount that is sufficient for the spontaneously breathing conscious patient.[14]

Variations of the Dorsal Decubitus Position

Supine

Horizontal. In the traditional horizontal supine position, the patient lies on the back with a small pillow beneath the head (see Fig. 27-1A). The arms are either comfortably padded and restrained alongside the trunk or abducted on well-padded arm boards. Either arm (or both) may be extended ventrally and the flexed forearm secured to an elevated frame in such a way that perfusion of the hand is not compromised, no skin to metal contact exists that might cause electrical burns if a cautery is used, and the brachial neurovascular bundle is neither stretched nor compressed at the axilla. (See the left arm arrangement in Fig. 27-15.) The lumbar spine may need padded support to prevent a postoperative backache (see the section on Dorsal Decubitus Complications). Bony contact points at the occiput, elbows, and heels should be padded.

Although the horizontal supine posture has a long history of widespread use, it does not place hip and knee joints in neutral positions and is poorly tolerated for any length of time by an immobilized, awake patient.

Contoured. A contoured supine posture (Fig. 27-2C) has been termed the *lawn chair position*.[15] It is established by arranging the surface of the operating table so that the trunk-thigh hinge is angulated about 15 degrees and the thigh-knee hinge is angulated a similar amount in the opposite direction. The patient then lies comfortably with hips and knees each flexed gently. Quite often a person who has been required to lie motionless on a rigid horizontal table and then is changed to the contoured supine position will offer an almost involuntary expression of relief and appreciation.

As in the horizontal supine position, the patient should have a pad or pillow beneath the occiput, elbows, and heels. Arms can be positioned as described for the horizontal supine posture.

Frog-Leg. On occasion a gynecologist or a pelvic surgeon may wish to place a supportive hand in the patient's vagina at some point during a laparotomy. Placing the patient supine with the knees bent and the soles of the feet together (the *frog-leg* position, Fig. 27-3) separates the thighs sufficiently to permit access to the perineum and vagina for the surgeon standing at the side of the patient's abdomen. If the patient's skeleton is stiff, lateral spread of the knees may seriously stress the hips; a pad of sufficient size should be used to support each knee (1) to minimize the opportunity for postoperative hip and back pain and (2) to prevent a dislocated hip or fracture of an osteoporotic femur during the operation.

With a patient in the supine position, a mobile abdominal mass, such as a very large tumor or a pregnant uterus, can rest on the great vessels of the abdomen and compromise cardiac output. This is known as the aortocaval syndrome or the supine hypotensive syndrome. A significant degree of perfusion can be restored if the compressive mass is rolled toward the left hemiabdomen by manual compression, a mechanical device producing leftward displacement, leftward tilt of the table top, or a wedge under the right hip.[16] In some quarters this modification of the dorsal decubitus position is referred to as semisupine.

Lithotomy

Standard. In the standard lithotomy position (Fig. 27-4), the patient lies supine with arms crossed on the trunk or extended laterally to less than 90 degrees on arm boards. Each lower extremity is flexed at the hip and knee, and both limbs are simultaneously elevated and separated so that the perineum becomes accessible to the surgeon. For most gynecologic procedures, the patient's thighs are flexed about 90 degrees on the trunk and the knees are bent sufficiently to maintain the lower legs nearly parallel to the floor. More acute flexion of either knees or hips can threaten to angulate and compress major vessels at either joint.

Numerous devices are available to hold legs that are elevated during delivery or operation. Each should be fitted to the stature of the individual patient.

When the legs are to be lowered to the original supine position at the end of the procedure, they should first be brought together at the knees and ankles in the sagittal plane and then lowered slowly together to the table top. This minimizes torsion stress on the lumbar spine that would occur if each leg were lowered independently. It also permits gradual accommodation to the increase in the circulatory capacitance, thereby avoiding sudden hypotension.[17]

Low. For most urologic procedures and for many procedures that require simultaneous access to the abdomen and

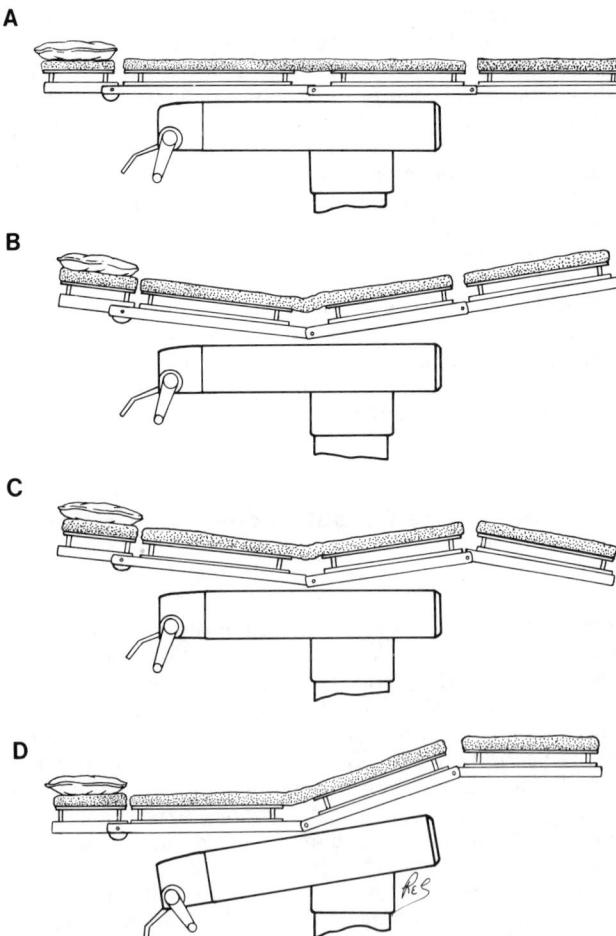

Figure 27-2. Establishment of the contoured supine ("lawnchair") position. (*A*) Traditional flat supine table top. (*B*) Thighs flexed on trunk. (*C*) Knees gently flexed in final body position. (*D*) Trunk section leveled to stabilize floor-supported arm board. (Reproduced with permission from Martin JT [ed]: Positioning in Anesthesia and Surgery, 2nd ed. Philadelphia, WB Saunders, 1987.)

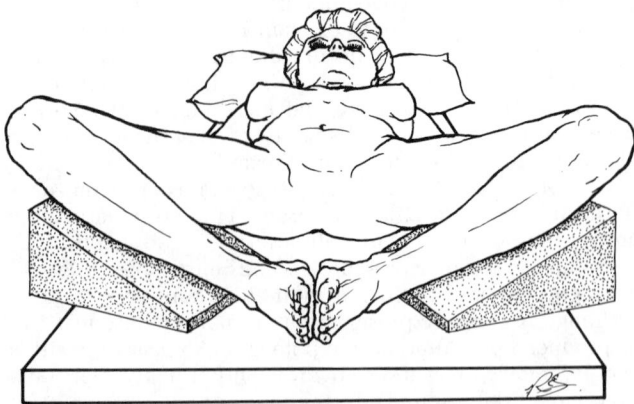

Figure 27-3. The frog-leg position for simultaneous access to the abdomen and vagina. See text. (Reproduced with permission from McLeskey CH [ed]: Geriatric Anesthesiology. Baltimore, Williams & Wilkins, in press.)

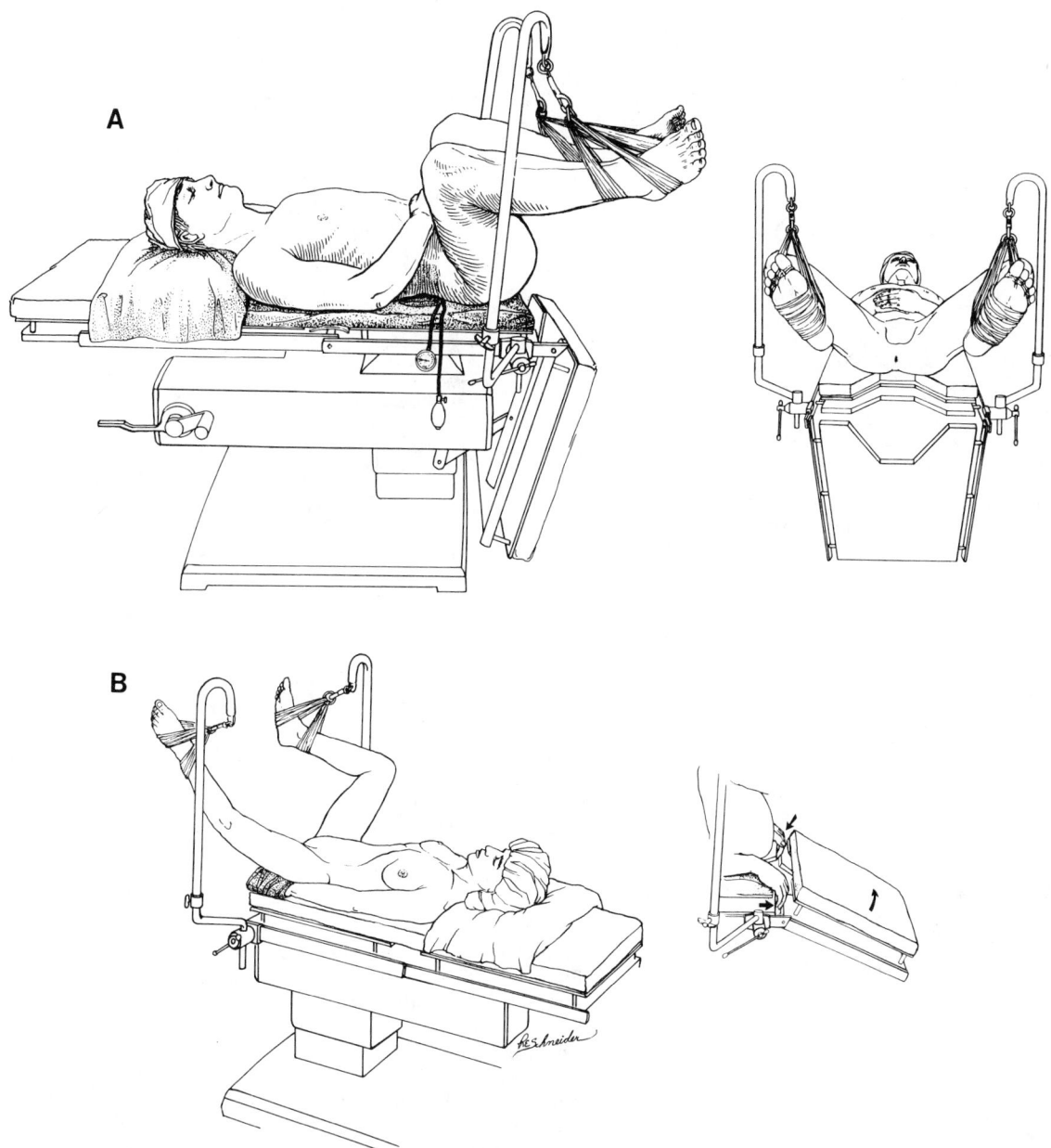

Figure 27-4. Standard lithotomy position. (*A*) Thighs are flexed slightly more than 90 degrees on abdomen; knees are flexed enough to bring lower legs roughly parallel to the table top. Arms are retained on boards, across the abdomen, or at sides of patient. (*B*) Note the possibility for a scissoring injury to fingers as the leg section of the table top is returned to horizontal. Towel-wrapping the hands helps keep the digits out of the hinge. (Modified with permission from Figures 7-1 and 8-1 of Martin JT [ed]: Positioning in Anesthesia and Surgery, 2nd ed. Philadelphia, WB Saunders, 1987.)

perineum, the degree of thigh elevation in the lithotomy position is only about 30–45 degrees (Fig. 27-5). This reduces perfusion gradients to and from the lower extremities and improves access to a perineal surgical site for members of the operating team, who are placed on the lateral aspect of either leg.

High. Some surgeons prefer to improve access to the perineum by suspending the patient's feet from high poles. The effect is to have the patient's legs almost fully extended on the thighs (Fig. 27-6) and the thighs flexed 90 degrees or more on the trunk. The posture produces a significant uphill gradient for arterial perfusion into the feet, requiring careful avoidance of hypotension. Less mobile patients may tolerate this posture poorly because of angulation and compression of the contents of the femoral canal by the inguinal ligament (Fig. 27-6*A*), or stretch of the sciatic nerve (Fig. 27-6*B*), or both.

Exaggerated. Transperineal access to the retropubic area requires that the patient's pelvis be flexed ventrally on the spine, the thighs be almost forcibly flexed on the trunk, and

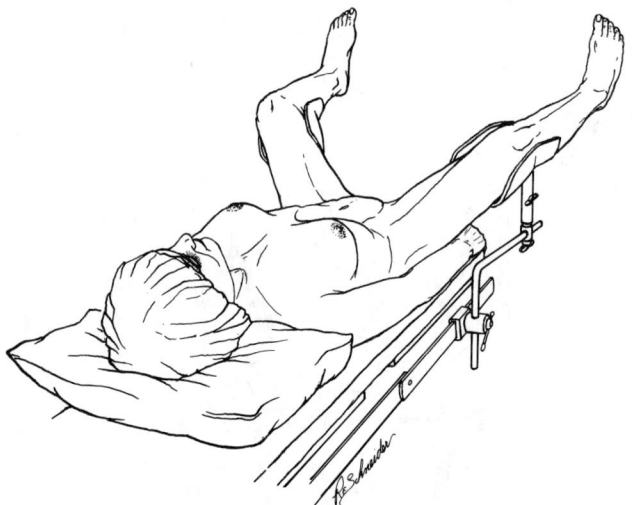

Figure 27-5. Low lithotomy position for perineal access, transurethral instrumentation, or combined abdominoperineal procedures.

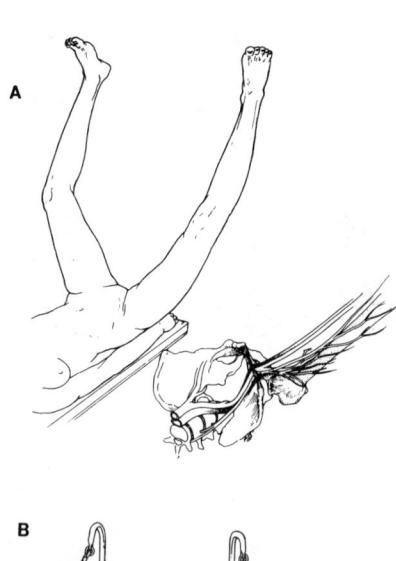

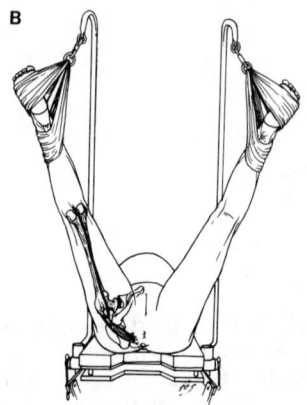

Figure 27-6. High lithotomy position. Note potential for angulation and compression/obstruction of contents of femoral canal (*A insert*) and/or stretch of sciatic nerve (*B*). (*A* reproduced with permission from McLeskey CH [ed]: Geriatric Anesthesiology. Baltimore, Williams & Wilkins, in press. *B* reproduced with permission from Martin JT [ed]: Positioning in Anesthesia and Surgery, 2nd ed. Philadelphia, WB Saunders, 1987.)

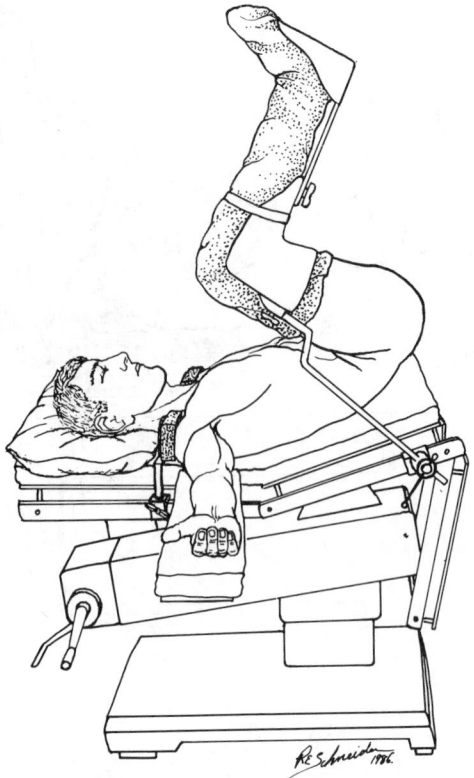

Figure 27-7. The exaggerated lithotomy position of Young. Shoulder braces, usually needed to stabilize the torso, are placed over the acromioclavicular area to minimize compression of the brachial plexus and adjacent vessels. (Reprinted with permission from Martin JT [ed]: Positioning in Anesthesia and Surgery, 2nd ed. Philadelphia, WB Saunders, 1987.)

the lower legs be aimed skyward so as to be out of the way (Fig. 27-7). The result places the long axis of the symphysis pubis almost parallel to the floor. This exaggerated lithotomy position stresses the lumbar spine, produces a significant uphill gradient for perfusion of the feet, and may restrict ventilation because of abdominal compression by bulky thighs. It can be tolerated under anesthesia but can rarely be assumed by an awake patient. Control of ventilation is usually necessary. If painful lumbar spine disease exists, an alternative surgical position may need to be chosen beforehand in order to avoid severely accentuating the lumbar distress postoperatively.

Lithotomy Plus Trendelenburg

Frequently some degree of head-down tilt is added to one of the lithotomy positions. If the tilt is great enough, and particularly in the instance of the exaggerated lithotomy position, the patient may slide cephalad unless protected by well-padded shoulder braces that are properly located over the acromioclavicular joints.

Depending on the degree of head depression, the addition of tilt to the lithotomy position combines the worst features of both the lithotomy and the Trendelenburg postures. The weight of abdominal viscera on the diaphragm adds to whatever abdominal compression is produced by the flexed thighs of an obese patient or of one placed in an exaggerated lithotomy position. Ventilation should be assisted or controlled.

Trendelenburg

Some time during the 1860s, Bardenhauer, an innovative German surgeon in Cologne, began to elevate the hips of patients to gravitate the viscera cephalad and help expose pathology deep within the pelvis.[18] That novel practice, tilting a patient 30–45 degrees head down (Fig. 27-8), was adopted and popularized by Friedrich Trendelenburg of Leipzig prior to 1870. However, its publication apparently awaited an article by Meyer, an American pupil of Trendelenburg, in 1885.[19]

During World War I, Walter Cannon, the eminent physiologist, espoused the notion that the Trendelenburg position was advantageous in the treatment of shock. He believed that it improved circulatory return from the lower extremities and improved cerebral circulation.[8] Although he repudiated that opinion in 1923,[20] the use of the "Trendelenburg" position to treat shock remained a common practice until recently. Reports of Cole in 1952,[21] Weil in 1957,[22] Guntheroth *et al* in 1964,[23] Taylor and Weil in 1976,[24] and Sibbald's group[9] in 1979 have carefully detailed the disadvantages of the Trendelenburg position as a means of treating shock. Nevertheless, the tenacious persistence of the practice has been astonishing, particularly among older physicians.

An alternate position that is useful for treating supine patients with perfusion deficits, such as moderate hypovolemia from blood loss or vasodilation from spinal anesthesia, is mild elevation of the lower extremities with the trunk remaining horizontal (see Fig. 27-2D). The blood volume in the legs is thought to be "autotransfused" into the central circulation by the maneuver. With the thorax level and a small pillow placed under the patient's head, changes in pulmonary function should be minimal and cerebral blood volume should be relatively unchanged.

Because of vasocompensation, whatever increase in mean arterial pressure accompanies elevation of the legs may be transient. In most instances, however, the rational therapy for the perfusion deficits described above is volume infusion rather than postural adjustment.

Reich and associates,[25] studying well-instrumented, anesthetized patients, have compared circulatory variables in the level supine position with those recorded after 3 minutes of marked (60-degree) elevation of the lower extremities or after 3 minutes of 20 degrees of head-down tilt. They found that head-down tilt only minimally increased cardiac output and mean arterial pressure, whereas leg raising slightly increased mean arterial pressure without affecting cardiac output. In each posture there was evidence of deteriorating pulmonary function and right ventricular stress. They urged caution in the use of either maneuver in patients with pulmonary disease or right ventricular compromise.

Cephalad displacement of the diaphragm and obstruction of its caudad inspiratory stroke accompany the Trendelenburg position because of gravity-shifted abdominal viscera. Consequently, the work of spontaneous ventilation is increased for an anesthetized patient in a posture that already worsens the ventilation-perfusion ratio by gravitational accumulation of blood in the poorly ventilated lung apices. During controlled ventilation, higher inspiratory pressures are needed to expand the lung.

Intracranial vascular congestion and increased intracranial pressure can be expected to result from head-down tilt. The position should be used for patients with intracranial pathology only in the rare instances in which a surgically useful alternate posture cannot be found. The operation should then be as brief as possible, and the need for postoperative neurologic intensive care should be anticipated.

The classic Trendelenburg position employed 30–45 degrees of head-down tilt and required some means of preventing the patient from sliding cephalad out of position. Hewer developed a contoured mattress with raised areas that supported the Achilles tendons, lumbar spine, and neck.[26] This English device has not been widely used in the United States. Wristlets attached to the rail at the operating table edge have been used, but they have the potential of stretching the brachial plexuses as the weight of the patient hangs from the fixed wrists. Ischemia of the hands also is a possibility if the wristlets are too tight.

Shoulder braces are best tolerated if placed over the

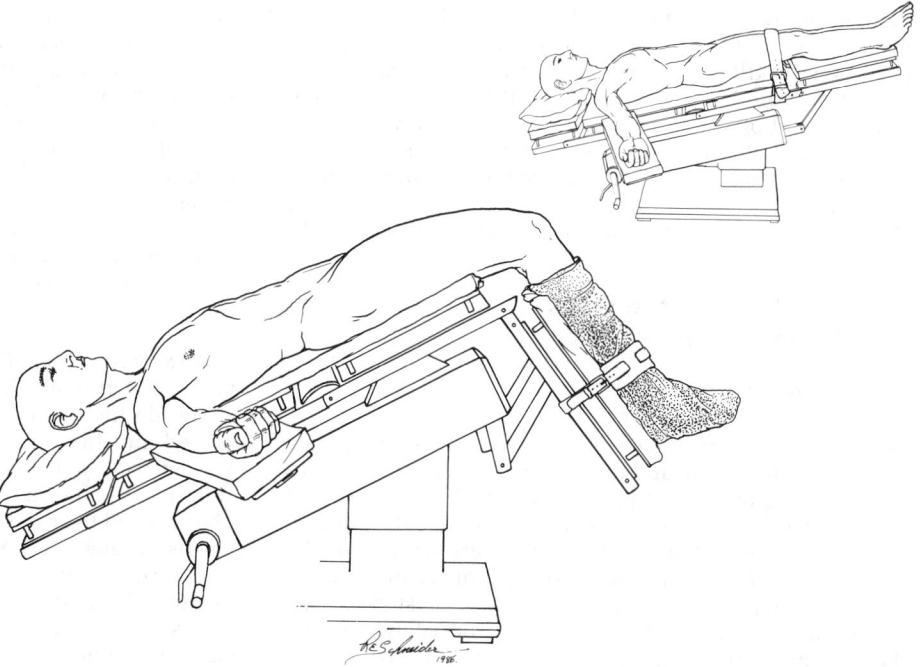

Figure 27-8. Head-down tilt. *Foreground* figure shows traditional steep (30- to 45-degree) tilt described by Trendelenburg. Leg restraints and knee flexion stabilize the patient, avoiding the need for wristlets or shoulder braces that threaten the brachial plexus. *Upper* figure shows 10 to 15 degrees of head-down tilt (the Scultetus position), which is more common in modern surgical procedures. (Reprinted with permission from Martin JT [ed]: Positioning in Anesthesia and Surgery, 2nd ed. Philadelphia, WB Saunders, 1987.)

acromioclavicular joints, but care must be taken to see that the shoulder is not forced sufficiently caudad to trap and compress the brachial neurovascular bundle between the clavicle and the first rib. If the braces are placed medially against the root of the neck, they may easily compress neurovascular structures that emerge from the area of the scalene musculature.

Anklets and bent knees are a satisfactory method of retaining the tilted patient in position (see Fig. 27-8) if the anklets are not excessively tight and if the flexed knee joint is placed sufficiently caudad of the leg-thigh hinge of the table top so that the adjacent firm edge of the depressed leg section of the table cannot indent the patient's proximal calf. Should it be allowed to do so, compressive ischemia and phlebitis are likely to result.

Scultetus

The usual amount of head-down tilt now employed in most surgical suites is probably about 10–15 degrees (Fig. 27-8 insert). This corresponds not to the position of Trendelenburg (Fig. 27-8) but to one referred to as the *scultetus position*.[3,27] The name appears to be derived from that of the German surgeon, Johann Schultes (1595–1645), who was known as Scultetus and for whom the bandage is named.

Although the scultetus position does not threaten to dislodge the patient, its minimal head-down tilt has been shown to cause an increase in myocardial oxygen consumption in spontaneously ventilating patients.[7] The use of head-down tilt as a method of increasing the caliber of veins in the superior caval circuit in order to assist in the insertion of central catheters should be seriously questioned in patients with impaired myocardial perfusion. It should be avoided in the presence of increased intracranial pressure.

In a study of 34 premedicated adults whose hearts were initially in sinus rhythm, Keusch and associates[28] compared the electrocardiographic effects of introducing a pulmonary artery catheter with a self-sealing diaphragm via the right internal jugular vein with each patient first in 5–10 degrees of head-down tilt (posture A) and then in 5 degrees of head-up tilt with right tilt (posture B, semisupine). Access to the pulmonary artery was equally swift in either position. Although the overall incidence of dysrhythmias was similar in both groups (A: 29 out of 34, B: 26 out of 34), during head-up right tilt the patients had only half as many malignant dysrhythmias (8 out of 26) as they did when head-down (17 out of 29). In most instances, head-down tilt malignant dysrhythmias changed to benign ones when the patient was placed in the head-up right tilt position, further confirming the head-down position as an unnecessary choice to facilitate pulmonary artery catheter insertion.

Complications of the Dorsal Decubitus Positions

Postural Hypotension

Depending on the resilience of the patient's vasocompensatory mechanisms, postural hypotension may be seen when a head-elevated position is being established. On a statistical basis, it can be presumed to be the most frequent complication of a head-elevated posture. If mean arterial pressure at the circle of Willis remains above 60 mm Hg in a patient who is not hypertensive, the postural hypotension may require little treatment other than to appropriately decrease the concentration of anesthetic drugs in order to preserve compensatory reflexes. If the degree of hypotension encountered is more severe, further head elevation should be delayed until decreasing the level of anesthetic; in addition, judicious use of fluids and vasopressors can re-establish effective perfusion.

Postural hypotension may also appear in the presence of inadequately replaced blood loss when the intravascular space has been functionally increased either by lowering the legs to horizontal at the termination of the lithotomy position or by returning a head-down tilt to horizontal. Volume repletion is the indicated therapy.

Pressure Alopecia

Prolonged compression of hair follicles can produce hair loss. Abel and Lewis[29] described patients who had pain, swelling, and exudation where the occiput had been supporting the weight of the head for long periods of time in the Trendelenburg position. Alopecia occurred between the 3rd and 28th postoperative day; regrowth was complete within 3 months. Use of tight head straps to hold anesthetic face masks and prolonged hypotension and hypothermia have also been associated with compression alopecia.[30] Frequently turning the patient's head during long operations[31] and use of padded, soft head supports are recommended to reduce the risks of this complication.

Pressure-Point Reactions

Weight-bearing bony prominences can develop ischemic necrosis of overlying tissue unless proper padding is applied. Hypothermia and vasoconstrictive hypotension may enhance the process. The heels, the elbows, and the sacrum are particularly vulnerable and should be carefully padded as a prophylactic routine. This is particularly important when patients are thin or when the operation will be prolonged.

Brachial Plexus Injuries

Root Injuries. Shoulder braces placed tight against the base of the neck can compress and injure the roots of the brachial plexus. Braces, if needed at all, are less harmful when placed more laterally over the acromioclavicular joint.

The dorsal decubitus positions do not usually threaten structures within the patient's neck unless considerable lateral displacement of the head occurs. In that position the roots of the brachial plexus on the side of the obtuse head-shoulder angle can be stretched and damaged. If the upper extremity is fixed at the wrist, the stretch injury of the plexus can be accentuated as the head moves laterally away from the anchoring point of the wrist. Similarly, exaggerated rotation of the head away from an extended arm can be associated with a brachial plexus injury.

Sternal Retraction. Frequently, the patient undergoing a median sternotomy has both arms padded and secured alongside the torso. An alternative is to have one arm abducted and the other arm restrained alongside the trunk. Vander Salm et al[32,33] described first rib fractures and brachial plexus injuries associated with median sternotomies. They related the extent of the injury to the amount of retractor displacement of the rib, with the most severe injury being caused by displacement sufficient to produce a first rib fracture. Roy and associates,[34] in a study of 200 consecutive adults scheduled for cardiac surgery *via* a median sternotomy, positioned the left arm either abducted and padded on an arm board with the palm supinated or secured by a draw sheet alongside the trunk; the right arm was always placed alongside the trunk. They found a 10% incidence of upper extremity nerve injury that was not influenced by internal mammary artery harvest, internal jugular vein catheterization, or left arm position. Surgical manipulation was more contributory than extremity positioning in producing trauma to the brachial plexus.

Compression Between Clavicle and First Rib. If the shoulder is allowed to move dorsally, or if the supine patient shifts cephalad while the upper extremity is anchored by wristlets at the level of the hip, the clavicle may be pressed forcibly against the underlying first rib. In the process, the subclavian neurovascular bundle can be compressed and its structures injured. Occasionally, a dampened pulse at the wrist will identify this situation in the sitting position; support under the elbow is required to lift the shoulder and relieve the obstruction.

Long Thoracic Nerve Dysfunction. Several lawsuits have centered on postoperative serratus anterior muscle dysfunction and winging of the scapula (Fig. 27-9) alleged to be the result of position-related injuries to the long thoracic nerve of Bell, which arises from nerve roots C5, C6, and C7. Because C5 and C6 fibers of the nerve course through the middle scalene muscle and emerge from its lateral border to join the fibers from C7, it has been proposed that neuropathies of the long thoracic nerve are traumatic in origin.[35] Johnson and Kendall[36] described the widely variable etiology of serratus anterior muscle paralysis in a review of 111 cases and found only 13% occurring after either a surgical procedure or an obstetric delivery. Because the nerve is not routinely involved in a stretch injury of the brachial plexus and because the plexus is not routinely involved when long thoracic nerve dysfunction occurs, the relationship between

postoperative long thoracic nerve palsy and patient positioning remains speculative. Based on evidence of Foo and Swann[37] plus data from recent litigations, Martin[38] concluded that in the absence of demonstrable trauma, postoperative dysfunctions of the long thoracic nerve were quite likely the result of coincidental neuropathies, possibly of viral origin.

Axillary Trauma from the Humeral Head. Excessive abduction of the arm on an arm board may thrust the head of the humerus into the axillary neurovascular bundle. The bundle is stretched at that point and its neural structures may be damaged. In the same manner, vessels can be compressed or occluded and perfusion of the extremity can be jeopardized.

Radial Nerve Compression. The radial (musculospiral) nerve, arising from roots C6–8 and T1, passes dorsally and laterally around the middle and lower portions of the humerus in the musculospiral groove. At a point on the lateral aspect of the arm about three finger breadths proximal to the lateral epicondyle of the humerus, the nerve can be compressed against the underlying bone and injured. Pressure from the vertical bar of an anesthesia screen or a similar device against the lateral aspect of the arm[39] and excessive cycling of an automatic blood pressure cuff[40] have been implicated in causing damage to the radial nerve. Postoperative radial nerve dysfunction is a relatively rare reason for malpractice litigation.[41]

Clinical manifestations of a radial nerve lesion include wrist drop, weakness of abduction of the thumb, inability to extend the metacarpophalangeal joints, and loss of sensation in the web space between the thumb and index finger.[42] Radial nerve function can be rapidly assessed by noting the patient's ability to actively extend the distal phalanx of the thumb.[43]

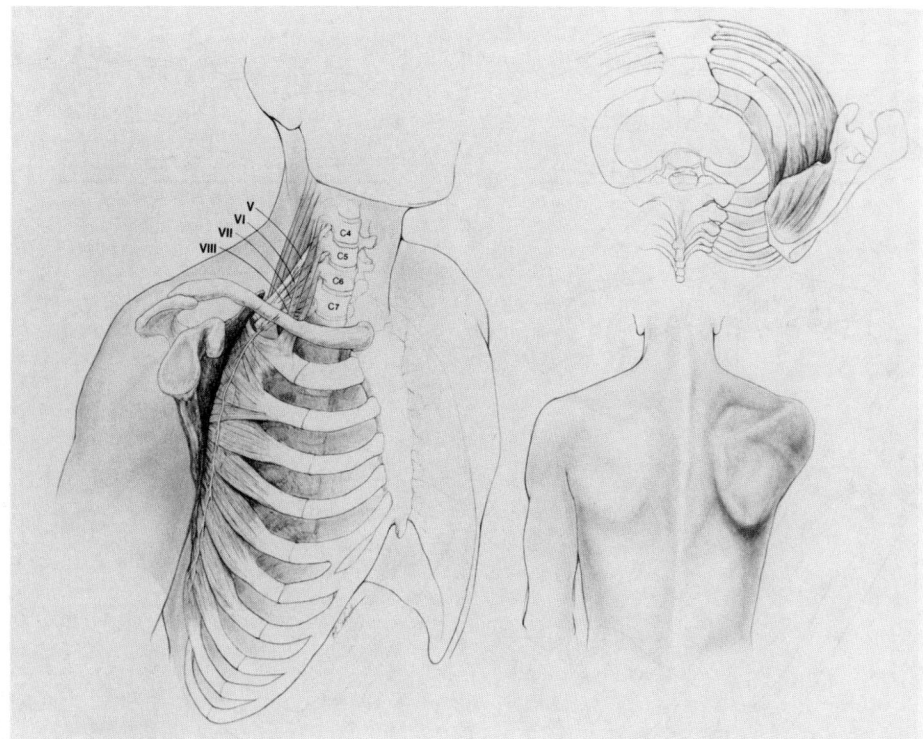

Figure 27-9. Scapular winging. The serratus anterior muscle (*upper right*) is supplied solely by the long thoracic nerve that branches immediately from C5, C6, C7, and sometimes C8 (*left figure*). Arising on the lateral ribs and inserting on the deep surface of the scapula, the muscle keeps the shoulder girdle approximated to the dorsal rib cage. Long thoracic nerve palsy allows dorsal protrusion of the scapula (*lower right*). See text. (Reproduced with permission from Martin JT: Postoperative isolated dysfunction of the long thoracic nerve: A rare entity of uncertain etiology. Anesth Analg 69:614, 1989.)

Median Nerve. Isolated injuries to the median nerve allegedly owing to positioning are extemely uncommon and the mechanism is obscure.[41] A more likely source of injury is iatrogenic manipulation of the vessels adjacent to the nerve in the antecubital fossa as might occur during venipuncture. A quick check of sensation over the dorsal and palmar surfaces of the distal phalanges of the first and second fingers will identify an acute injury.

Ulnar Nerve at the Elbow. The ulnar nerve passes dorsal to the medial epicondyle of the humerus through the cubital tunnel, the groove between the medial epicondyle and the olecranon process of the ulna, and continues into the forearm. Direct trauma to the nerve at the level of the elbow is not uncommon and is a frequent cause of litigation.[41] It can occur during sleep or anesthesia if the arm of a supine person rests on the flexed elbow with the forearm across the trunk. The nerve can also be compressed in some patients as the arm lies abducted on an arm board with the hand pronated and the contents of the cubital tunnel trapped between bone and the relatively firm surface of the board. Supination of the hand will almost always shift the weight of the elbow onto the olecranon process (Fig. 27-10) and offer the nerve a high degree of protection. As an additional precaution, soft padding should be added routinely to the pressure point of each elbow whether the arm is placed on

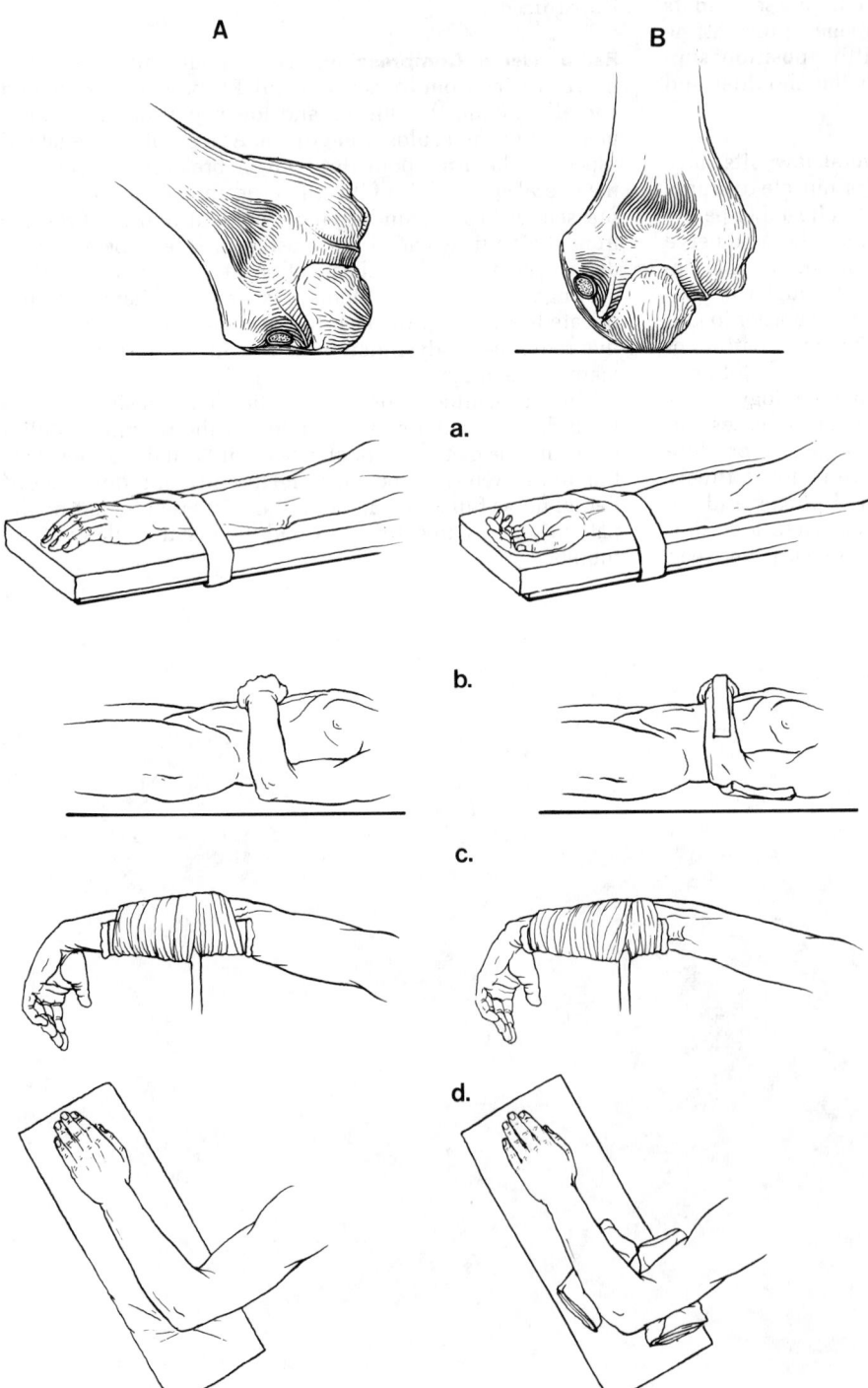

A B

a.

b.

c.

d.

Figure 27-10. The ulnar nerve at the cubital tunnel. Column A shows postures that threaten the nerve with compression between supporting surface and overlying bone. Column B indicates safer posture (as in supination) or protective padding to lessen the risks. (Modified from Wadsworth TG: The cubital tunnel and the external compression syndrome. Anesth Analg 53:303, 1974. Reproduced with permission from Martin JT [ed]: Positioning in Anesthesia and Surgery, 2nd ed. Philadelphia, WB Saunders, 1987.)

an arm board, retained at the side of the patient, or arranged in some other manner that risks pressure on the cubital tunnel. Automatically cycled blood pressure cuffs have also been proposed as a cause of ulnar nerve injuries.[44]

Clinical manifestations of ulnar nerve dysfunction vary with the location and the extent of the lesion.[45] However, rapid assessment can identify an acute injury if a pin prick cannot be felt in the fifth finger.[43]

Because ulnar nerve injury is relatively common, a wise precaution during the preanesthetic interview is to inquire about a history of ulnar neuropathies ("crazy bone" problems) or previous surgery at the elbow. If such a history is indicated, the finding must be recorded and a discussion with the patient or family should present the possibility of a postoperative recurrence despite special precautions of padding and positioning.

The time of recognition of digital anesthesia associated with ulnar nerve dysfunction may be quite important in establishing the origin of the postoperative syndrome. If ulnar hypesthesia or anesthesia is noted promptly after the end of anesthesia, as in the recovery facility, the condition is likely to be associated with events that occurred during anesthesia or surgery. If the recognition is delayed for many hours, the likelihood of cause shifts from the intraanesthetic period to postoperative events. In a review of closed claims, Kroll and associates[41] commented that postoperative ulnar dysfunction can occur as a result of events in the postanesthetic period and that certain susceptible patients may develop nerve injury "despite conventionally accepted methods of positioning and padding."

Opioids may mask dysesthesias and pain postoperatively, but even strong analgesics cannot mask a loss of sensation due to nerve dysfunction. Ulnar nerve function should be routinely assessed in the recovery room and the resultant observations recorded on the patient's record.

Arm Complications

An arm board that is hyperabducted, whether intentionally or by inadvertent pressure from the hip of a surgical assistant, is dangerous. It can force the head of the humerus into the axillary neurovascular bundle and damage nerves and vessels to the arm. Abduction of the arm to more than 90 degrees from the trunk should be avoided. An arm board should be securely attached to the operating table to prevent its accidental release.

An arm that is not properly secured can slip over the edge of the table or arm board, resulting in injury to the capsule of the shoulder joint by excessive dorsal extension of the humerus, fracture of the neck of an osteoporotic humerus, or injury to the ulnar nerve at the elbow. Conversely, in the unlikely event that the retaining strap is excessively tight across the supinated forearm (Fig. 27-11), the potential exists for pressure to compress the anterior interosseous nerve, a branch of the median nerve in the upper forearm that courses with its artery along the volar surface of the tough interosseous membrane. The result is an ischemic injury to the distribution of the nerve and artery that resembles a compartment syndrome in the lower extremity (see following discussion) and may require prompt surgical decompression.[46]

Backache

Lumbar backache can be worsened by the ligamentous relaxation that occurs with anesthesia. Loss of normal lumbar curvature in the supine position is apparently the issue. Several folded towels, or an inflatable bladder of a blood

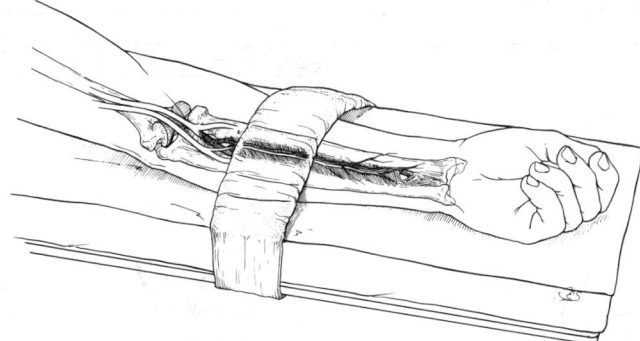

Figure 27-11. Arm restraint, if excessively tight, can compress the anterior interosseous nerve and vessel against the interosseous membrane in the volar forearm to produce an ischemic neuropathy. (Reproduced with permission from McLeskey CH [ed]: Geriatric Anesthesiology. Baltimore, Williams & Wilkins, in press.)

pressure cuff, if placed under the lumbar spine before the induction of anesthesia, may help retain lordosis and make a patient with known lumbar distress more comfortable. An exception to this is the patient with palpable tender points in the lumbar area; the pressure of the pad may create enough distress for the patient to object strongly to its presence.

Elevation of the legs can worsen the pain of a herniated nucleus pulposis. When the lithotomy position is contemplated for a patient with a history of low back pain or a lumbar disk, gentle passive attempts to have the patient assume the posture prior to anesthesia may be helpful in determining whether the position can be tolerated.

Perineal Crush Injury

The supine patient who is placed on a fracture table for repair of a fractured femur usually has the pelvis retained in place by a perineal pole (Fig. 27-12), while the foot of the injured extremity is fixed to a mobile rest. A worm gear on the rest lengthens the distance between the foot and the pelvis so the bone fragments can be distracted and realigned. Unless the pole is well padded, severe pressure can be exerted on the pelvis, and damage can occur to the genitalia and the pudendal nerves. Complete loss of penile sensation has been reported following use of the fracture table.[47,48] The correct position for the pole is against the pelvis between the genitalia and the uninjured limb.[47]

Compartment Syndrome

If, for whatever reason, perfusion to a lower extremity is inadequate, a compartment syndrome may develop. Characterized by ischemia, hypoxic edema, elevated tissue pressure within fascial compartments of the leg, and extensive rhabdomyolysis, the syndrome produces extensive and potentially lasting damage to the muscles and nerves within the compartment. Because the pathology is at tissue level, distal pulses and capillary refill may remain intact while a compartment syndrome is developing in an extremity; thus they are not useful indicators of the ongoing process. Ferrihemate, resulting from myoglobin destruction, exerts a direct toxic effect on renal tubular epithelium, and renal failure is likely.[49] Circulating debris from infections in the involved extremities is apt to be filtered by pulmonary microvasculature.

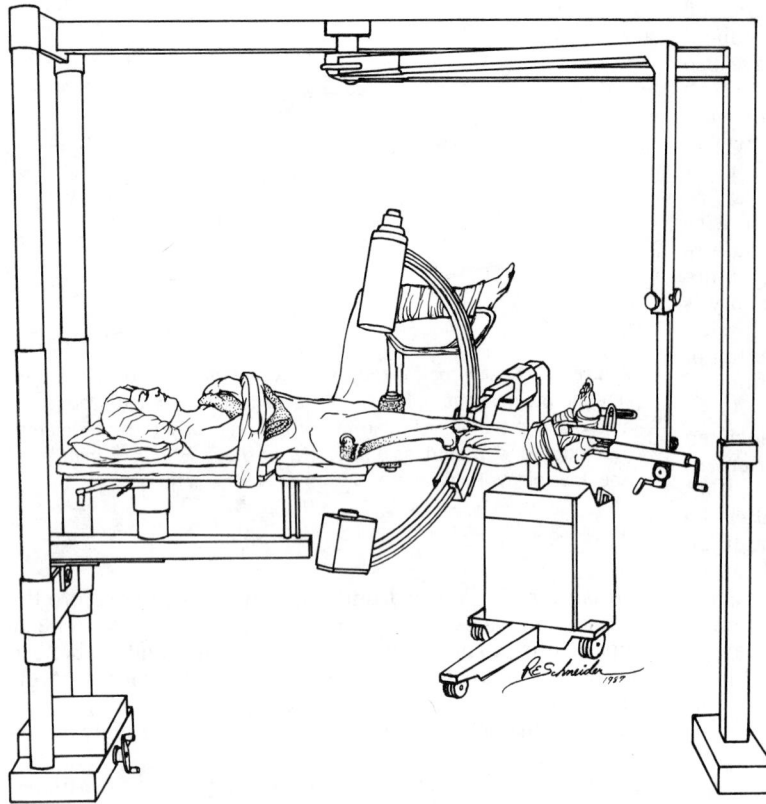

Figure 27-12. Traction table with perineal post stabilizing patient while leg is elongated to reposition bone ends. Elevated leg risks hypoperfusion; pelvic post threatens genitalia. (Reproduced with permission from Martin JT [ed]: Positioning in Anesthesia and Surgery, 2nd ed. Philadelphia, WB Saunders, 1987.)

Causes of a compartment syndrome while a patient is in any of the dorsal decubitus positions include (1) systemic hypotension and loss of driving pressure to the extremity (augmented by elevation of the extremity); (2) vascular obstruction of major leg vessels by intrapelvic retractors, by excessive flexion of knees or hips, or by undue popliteal pressure from a knee crutch; and (3) external compression of the elevated extremity by straps or leg wrappings that are too tight, by the inadvertent pressure of the arm of a surgical assistant, or by the weight of the extremity against a poorly supportive leg holder.[50] A tight strap on an arm board has been alleged to have compressed the anterior interosseous neurovascular bundle and created a forearm compartment syndrome. Posture times in excess of 5 hours have been a common factor in literature anecdotes of postlithotomy compartment syndromes. For lengthy procedures in the lithotomy position, well-padded holders that immobilize the limb by supporting the foot without compressing the calf or popliteal fossa seem to be the least threatening choices.

Usually, decompressive fasciotomies are the only means of terminating the cycle of ischemia and compartment edema. Alkalinizing the urine and promoting diuresis may reduce the degree of renal damage.

Finger Injury

In 1968, Courington and Little[51] described the amputation of a young woman's fingers that were caught between the leg and thigh sections of the operating table as the leg section was returned to the horizontal position at the termination of an operation, during which the patient was in the lithotomy position (see Fig. 27-4B). Welborn has advocated using a towel to create a boxing glove–like wrap on the hands of lithotomized patients in order to prevent such a

tragic misadventure.[52] Carefully removing the patient's hands from the risky position prior to raising the foot of the table is less troublesome and probably as safe.

LATERAL DECUBITUS POSITIONS

Physiology

Circulatory

In the lateral decubitus position the patient is turned onto one side of the trunk and stabilized to prevent accidental rolling toward either the supine or the prone posture. It is of practical and legal importance to repeat the statement made earlier in the Introduction, namely, that the side of the body that rests on the table is the side that determines the name of the position (left side down = left lateral decubitus position).

If the legs are maintained in the long axis of the body, almost no pressure gradients exist along the great vessels from head to foot. Small hydrostatic differences will be detected between the values recorded simultaneously by blood pressure cuffs placed on the two arms.

If the lower extremities are flexed laterally at the hips and allowed to remain below the level of the heart, blood will pool in the distensible vessels of the dangling legs because of gravity-induced increases in venous pressure and resultant venous stasis. Wrapping the legs and thighs in compressive bandages is a common method to combat venous pooling. Lateral flexion of the lower extremities can also partially or completely obstruct venous return to the inferior vena cava. A small support should be placed just caudad of the down-side axilla to lift the thorax enough to relieve pressure on the axillary neurovascular bundle and prevent disturbed blood flow to the hand.

In the low-pressure pulmonary circuit, hydrostatic gradients occur between the two hemithoraces. Although the degree of gravity-induced lateral displacement of the heart is different in the two lateral decubitus positions, it is generally true that most of the down-side lung lies below the level of the atrium and that the up-side lung lies above it. Vascular congestion of the down-side lung resembles a Zone 3 of West et al,[13] whereas the relative hypoperfusion of the up-side lung resembles a Zone 2. Kaneko et al[53] found that the transition between Zone 3 and Zone 2 occurred at approximately 18 cm above the most dependent part of the lung.

If the cervical spine of the patient who is placed in a lateral decubitus position is carefully maintained in alignment with the thoracolumbar spine, almost no gradient will occur between pressures in the mediastinum and those in the head. However, if the head is improperly supported and sufficient lateral angulation of the neck occurs in either direction, obstruction of jugular flow may be produced.

Respiratory

In the presence of a supple chest, the lateral decubitus position can decrease the volume of the down-side hemithorax. The weight of the chest may force the down-side rib cage into a less expanded conformation. Gravity-induced shifts of mediastinal structures toward the down-side chest wall tend to further reduce the volume of the dependent lung. Abdominal viscera force the down-side diaphragm cephalad if the long axis of the trunk is horizontal or head-down.

Spontaneous ventilation can partially compensate for the diaphragmatic stretching in the dependent hemithorax because the contractile efficiency of the elongated diaphragmatic muscle fibers is increased. The compacted lung base and Zone 3 vascular congestion decrease compliance and interfere with the distribution of gas during intermittent positive pressure ventilation. An elevated kidney rest that is placed against either the down-side rib margin or flank, or that migrates into that position as the patient shifts on it, further interferes with movement of the down-side hemidiaphragm and passive ventilation of the dependent lung.

The up-side hemithorax is much less compressed than the dependent side, and because the lung lies above the level of the atria, it has less vascular congestion than the down-side lung. As a result, unless contralateral flexion has stretched the up-side flank muscles to the point of rigidity and limited excursions of the costal margin, intermittent positive pressure ventilation is directed preferentially to the more compliant up-side lung. The result can easily be excessive ventilation of the underperfused up-side lung and hypoventilation of the congested down-side lung. The potential for a clinically significant ventilation-perfusion mismatch is obvious, particularly in the presence of pulmonary disease.

Variations of the Lateral Decubitus Positions

Standard (Horizontal) Lateral Position

In the horizontal lateral decubitus position (Fig. 27-13), the patient is rolled onto one side on a flat table surface and stabilized in that posture by flexing the down-side thigh to almost 90 degrees on the trunk. The down-side knee is bent to retain the leg on the table and improve stabilization of

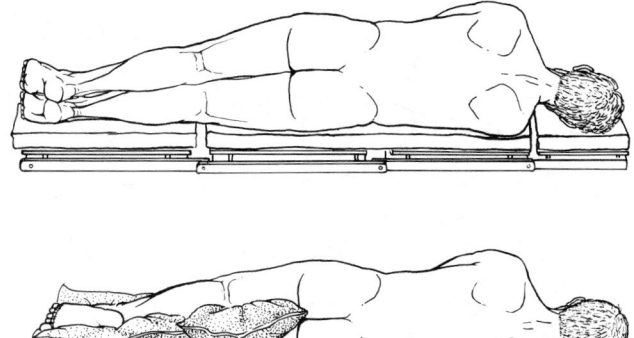

Figure 27-13. The standard lateral decubitus position. Proper head support, axillary roll, and leg pillow arrangement are shown on lower figure. Down-side leg is flexed at hip and knee to stabilize torso. Retaining straps and pad for down-side peroneal nerve are not shown. (Reproduced with permission from Martin JT [ed]: Positioning in Anesthesia and Surgery, 2nd ed. Philadelphia, WB Saunders, 1987.)

the trunk. The peroneal nerve of that side is padded to minimize compression damage caused by the weight of the legs. The up-side thigh and leg are extended comfortably, and pillows are placed between the lower extremities. The head is supported by pillows or a head rest so that the cervical and thoracic spines are properly aligned. A small pad (commonly but incorrectly referred to as an axillary roll), thick enough to raise the thorax and prevent excessive compression of the shoulder, is placed just caudad to and out of the down-side axilla. It should ensure adequate perfusion of the down-side hand and minimize circumduction of the dependent shoulder, which might stretch its suprascapular nerve.

Arms may be extended ventrally and retained on a single arm board with suitable padding between them, or they may be individually retained on a padded two-level arm support that can also help to stabilize the thorax (Fig. 27-14A). An alternate method of arm arrangement is to flex each elbow and place the arms on suitable padding on the table in front of the patient's face (Fig. 27-14B).

The patient is stabilized in the lateral position by the use of one or more retaining tapes stretched across the hip and fixed to the underside of the table top. Care must be taken to see that the hip tapes lie safely between the iliac crest and the head of the femur rather than over the head of the femur in a compressive manner that could result in its aseptic necrosis (Fig. 27-14B lower insert). An additional restraining tape may be used across the thorax if needed; it is functional and safe if placed just caudad of the axilla, where it has little effect on thoracic expansion, but it can be dangerous if placed across the costal margins, where it inevitably restricts ventilation.

Semisupine and Semiprone

The semilateral postures are designed to allow the surgeon to reach anterolateral (semisupine) and posterolateral (semiprone) structures of the trunk. The semiprone position is commonly used in the postoperative management of patients who have had surgical procedures within the upper airway and in the recovery room care of children.

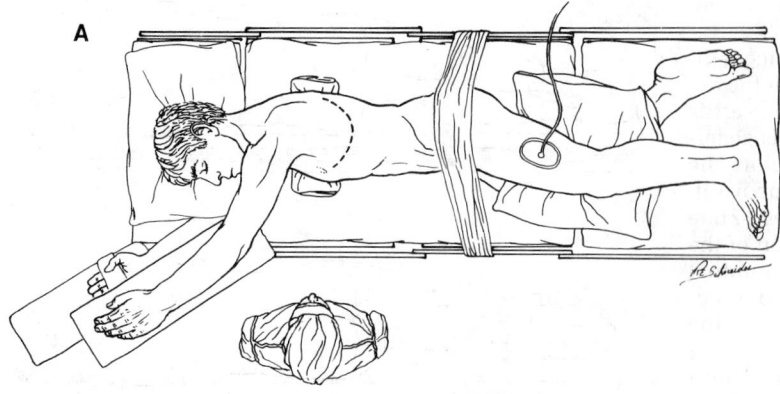

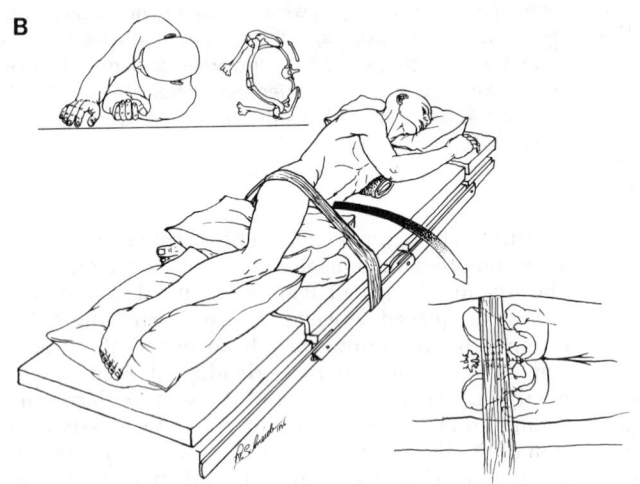

Figure 27-14. Lateral position with arms (*A*) arranged on two-tiered arm supports or (*B*) positioned in front of the patient's head either on pillows or on the table surface. Note the location of the stabilizing strap(s) between the iliac crest and the head of the up-side femur (*B, lower right*) rather than on the head of the femur. Potential ventral relocation of the torso can threaten the down-side axillary neurovascular bundle (*B, upper left*). (Reproduced with permission from Martin JT [ed]: Positioning in Anesthesia and Surgery, 2nd ed. Philadelphia, WB Saunders, 1987.)

In the semisupine position the up-side arm must be carefully supported so that it is not hyperextended and so that no traction or compression is applied to the brachial and axillary neurovascular bundles (Fig. 27-15). The supporting bar should be well wrapped to prevent electrical grounding contact (Fig. 27-15A). Sufficient noncompressible padding should be placed under the dorsal torso (Fig. 27-15, large figure) and hip to prevent the patient from rolling supine and stretching the anchored extremity. The pulse of the restrained wrist should be checked to ensure adequate circulation in the elevated arm and hand (Fig. 27-15B).

If the patient in the semiprone position is rolled more than about halfway between lateral and prone positions, the down-side arm is usually placed dorsal to the torso to avoid stress on that shoulder (Fig. 27-16). The down-side lower extremity is straight, whereas the up-side lower extremity is flexed at the hip and knee in order to prevent further pronation.

Sims' Position

In 1857 the prominent New York City gynecologist, J. Marion Sims, began to use a modification of the lateral position for operations on the perineum, rectum, vagina, and bladder[54] (Fig. 27-17). Subsequently, it became widely used as a birthing posture. It resembles the semiprone position in that the down-side lower extremity is extended, the up-side is flexed at the hip and knee to expose the perineum, and the patient rolls slightly ventrad.

Flexed Lateral Positions

Lateral Jackknife. The lateral jackknife position places the down-side iliac crest over the hinge between the back and thigh sections of the table (Fig. 27-18). The table top is angulated at that point to flex the thighs on the trunk laterally. After the patient has been suitably positioned and restrained, the chassis of the table is tipped so that the uppermost surface of the patient's flank and thorax becomes essentially horizontal. As a result, the feet are below the level of the atria, and significant amounts of blood may pool in distensible vessels in each leg.

The lateral jackknife position is usually intended to stretch the up-side flank and widen intercostal spaces as an asset to a thoracotomy incision. However, in terms of lumbar stress, restriction by the taut flank of upside costal margin motion, and pooling of blood in depressed lower extremities, its physiologic price is high. Actually, its usefulness to the surgeon is brief and it is rarely used. Once the rib-spreading retractor is placed in the incision, the position is of no value for the rest of the operation.[55]

Kidney. The kidney position (Fig. 27-19) resembles the lateral jackknife position, but it adds the use of an elevated rest (the "kidney rest") under the down-side iliac crest in order to increase the amount of lateral flexion and improve access to the up-side kidney under the overhanging costal margin. Unlike the lateral jackknife position, the kidney position does not have a useful alternative for a flank approach

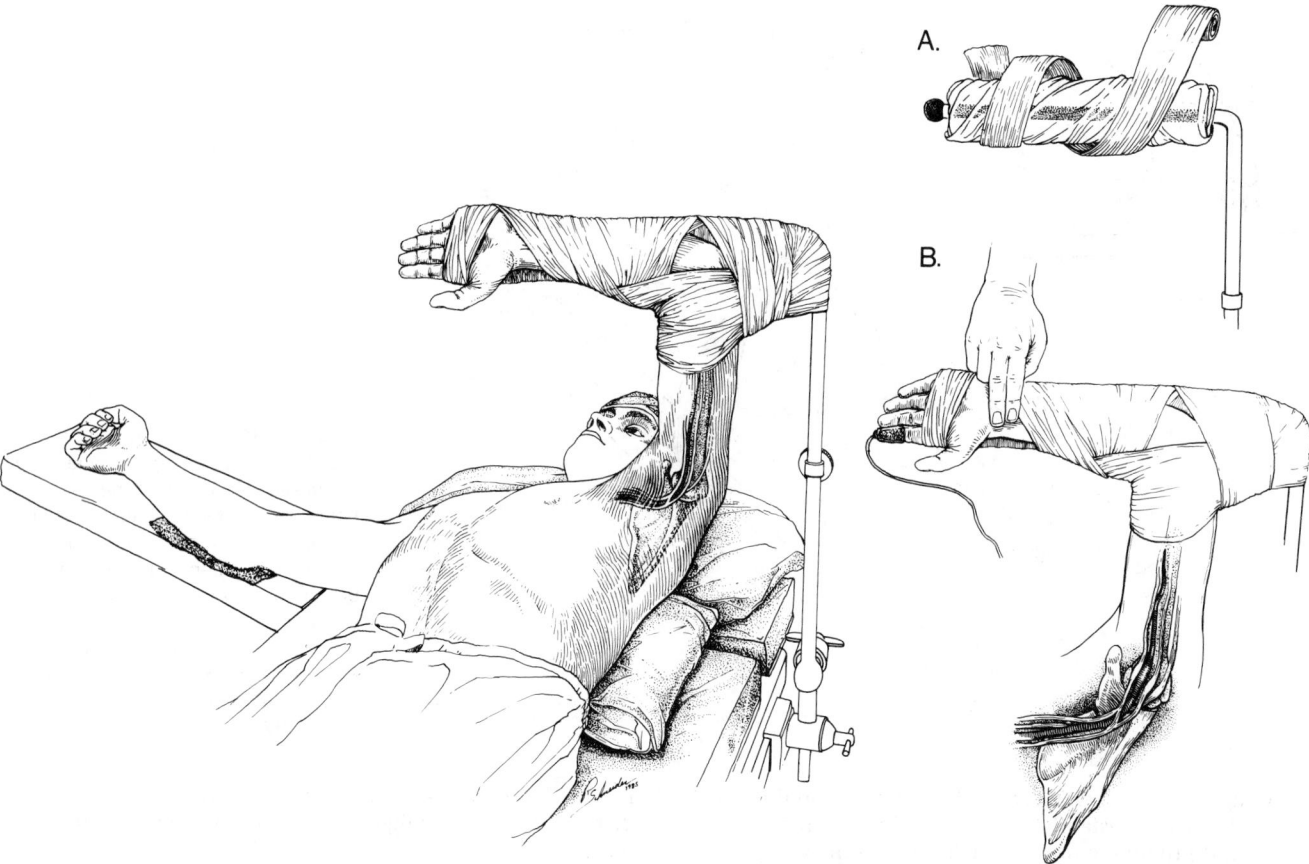

Figure 27-15. The semisupine position with dorsal pads supporting the torso, the extended arm padded at the elbow, and the elevated arm restrained on a well-cushioned adjustable overhead bar (*A*). Axillary contents (*B*) are not under tension and are not compressed by the head of the humerus, and a pulse oximeter ensures that the digital circulation is not compromised. The position is safe only if the arm does not become a hanging mechanism to support the torso. (Reproduced with permission from Collins VJ [ed]: Principles of Anesthesiology, 3rd ed. Philadelphia, Lea & Febiger, in press.)

to the kidney. Thus, the physiologic insults associated with the posture need to be limited by vigilant anesthesia and rapid surgery. Strict stabilizing precautions should be taken to prevent the patient from shifting on the table in such a manner that the elevated rest relocates into the down-side flank and becomes a severe impediment to ventilation of the dependent lung.

Complications of the Lateral Decubitus Positions

Eyes and Ears

Injuries to the dependent eye are unlikely if the head is properly supported during and after the turn from the supine to the lateral position. If the patient's face turns toward the mattress, however, and the lids are not closed, preventable abrasions of the surface of the eye can occur. Direct pressure on the globe can displace the crystalline lens or, particularly if systemic hypotension is present, can cause retinal ischemia.

In the lateral position, the weight of the head can press the down-side ear against a rough or wrinkled supporting surface. Careful padding with a pillow or a foam sponge is

usually sufficient protection against contusion of the ear. The external ear should also be palpated to assure that it has not been folded over in the process of placing support beneath the head.

Neck

Lateral flexion of the neck is possible when the head of a patient in the lateral position is inadequately supported. If the cervical spine is arthritic, postoperative neck pain can be troublesome. Pain from a symptomatic protrusion of a cervical disk can be intensified unless the head is carefully positioned so that flexion, extension, or rotation is avoided. Patients with unstable cervical spines can be intubated while awake and turned gently into the operative position while repeated neurologic checks, with which the patient cooperates and responds, are accomplished to detect the development of a positioning injury.[56]

Suprascapular Nerve Injury

Ventral circumduction of the dependent shoulder can rotate the suprascapular notch away from the root of the neck (Fig. 27-20). Since the suprascapular nerve is fixed both paravertebrally and at the notch, circumduction can stretch the

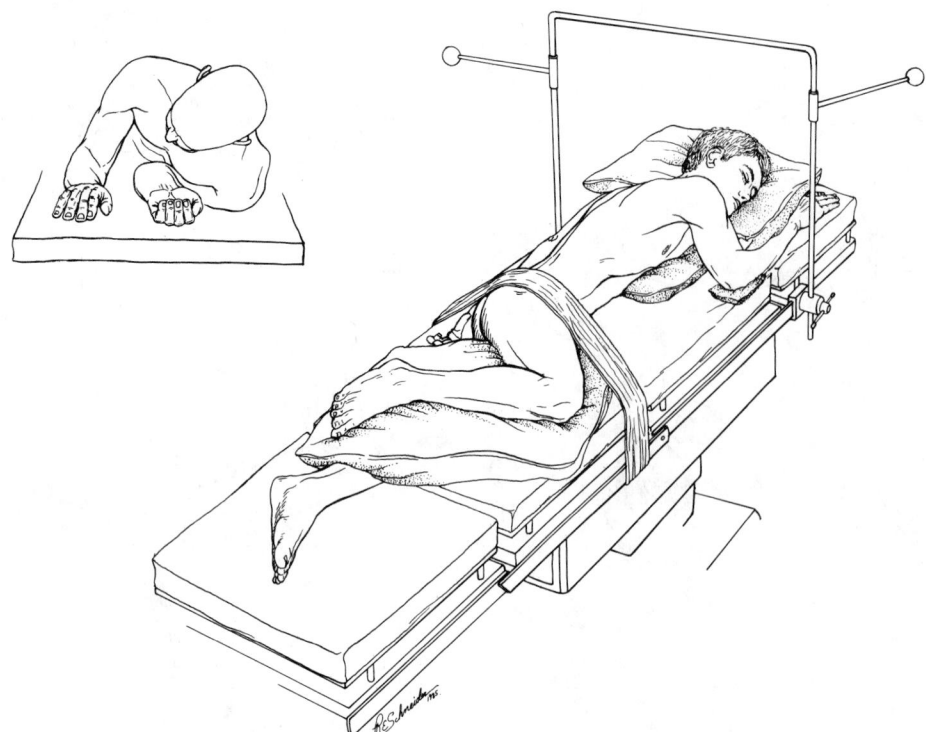

Figure 27-16. The semiprone position with the down-side leg extended and the up-side leg flexed at the knee, permitting moderate ventral rotation of the trunk. The down-side arm should be just behind the trunk to prevent axillary compression as shown in the insert. (Reproduced with permission from Martin JT [ed]: Positioning in Anesthesia and Surgery, 2nd ed. Philadelphia, WB Saunders, 1987.)

nerve and produce troublesome diffuse, dull shoulder pain. The diagnosis is established by blocking the nerve at the notch and producing pain relief. Treatment may require resecting the ligament over the notch to decompress the nerve. A supporting pad placed under the thorax just caudad of the axilla and thick enough to raise the chest off the shoulder should prevent a circumduction stretch injury to the nerve.

Long Thoracic Nerve

Instances of postoperative winging of the scapula (see Fig. 27-9) have followed use of the lateral decubitus position.[38] Although coincidental viral neuropathies of the long thoracic nerve may play a major etiologic role in postoperative appearances of scapular winging in patients for whom only a dorsal decubitus position was used, the possibility of trauma to the nerve while establishing the lateral position is difficult to refute.

Unstable Thorax

When the rib cage is unstable following an injury, turning the patient onto the injured side should be avoided if there

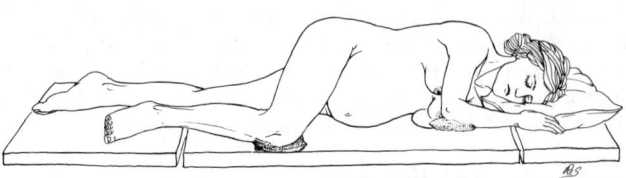

Figure 27-17. The Sims position, used as a means of access to the structures of the perineum. (Reproduced with permission from Martin JT [ed]: Positioning in Anesthesia and Surgery, 2nd ed. Philadelphia, WB Saunders, 1987.)

is a useful alternate position. Sharp ends of fractured ribs, displaced by the weight of the thorax, can puncture the down-side lung.

Atelectasis

Atelectasis of an imprisoned and poorly expanding dependent lung can occur in the lateral decubitus positions, particularly in the flexed lateral positions, if the flexion point is in the flank or on the costal margin instead of at the down-side iliac crest. Careful positioning and adequate passive intermittent positive pressure ventilation should reduce the risk. Application of 10 cm H_2O positive end-expiratory pressure has also proved effective.[57]

Aseptic Necrosis of the Up-Side Femoral Head

Compression of the head of the femur into the acetabulum by pressure from a misplaced restraining tape in the lateral decubitus position can result in aseptic necrosis of the hip. Obstruction of the nutrient artery to the femoral head is the assumed cause, and the incidence of the complication is not known. Nevertheless, the tapes that stabilize the patient should be carefully placed across the up-side hip on the soft tissue in the space between the head of the femur and the crest of the ilium in order to avoid direct pressure on the femoral head (see Fig. 27-18).

Unstable Spine

Turning a patient with an unstable vertebral column into the lateral position requires careful teamwork and a sufficient number of personnel to ensure gentle handling. Bivalve frames such as the Foster and Stryker are rarely used. If the trachea is intubated while the patient is awake, neurologic evaluations can be accomplished while the slow turn is in progress as well as after the final position is estab-

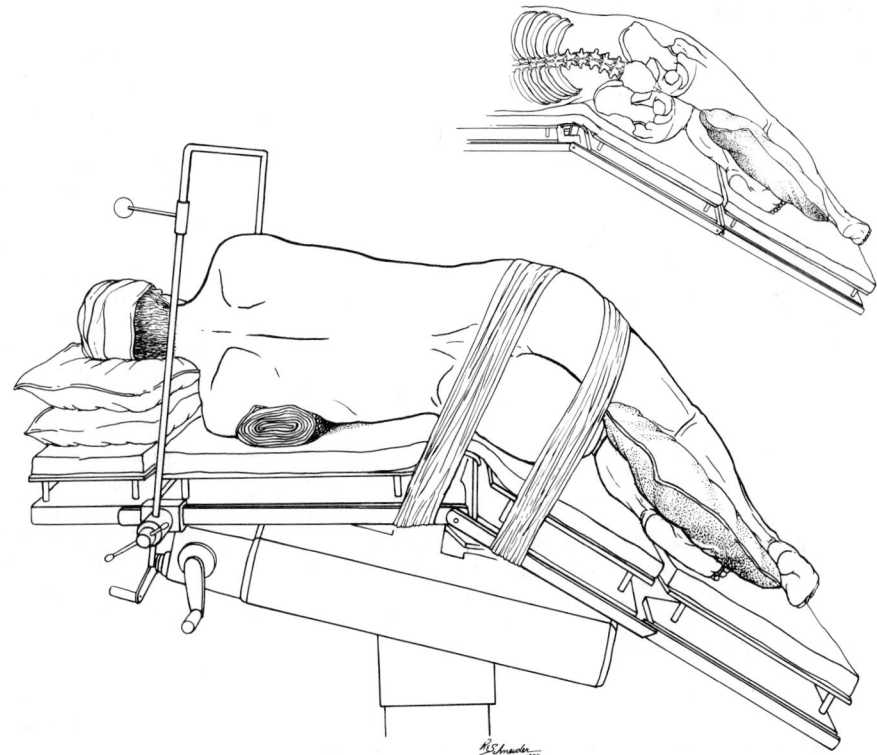

Figure 27-18. The lateral jackknife position, intended to open intercostal spaces. Note the properly placed restraining tapes (*large figure*) thrusting cephalad to retain the iliac crest at the flexion point of the table and prevent caudad slippage, which compresses the down-side flank (*insert*). (Reproduced with permission from Martin JT [ed]: Positioning in Anesthesia and Surgery, 2nd ed. Philadelphia, WB Saunders, 1987.)

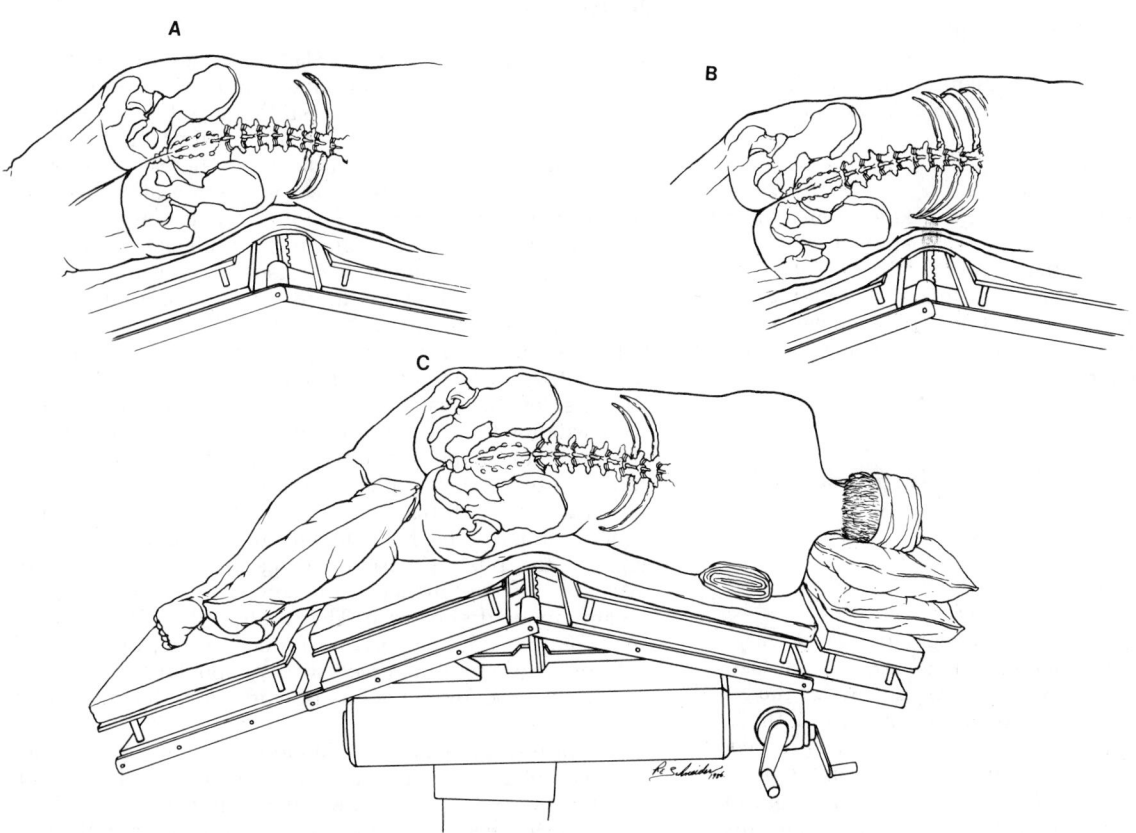

Figure 27-19. The flexed lateral (kidney) position. Upper panels show improper locations of the elevated transverse rest, the flexion point of the table, in the flank (*A*) or at the lower costal margin (*B*) to impede ventilation of the down-side lung. (*C*) The iliac crest at the proper flexion point, allowing the best possible expansion of the down-side lung. Restraining tapes deleted for clarity. (Reproduced with permission from Martin JT [ed]: Positioning in Anesthesia and Surgery, 2nd ed. Philadelphia, WB Saunders, 1987.)

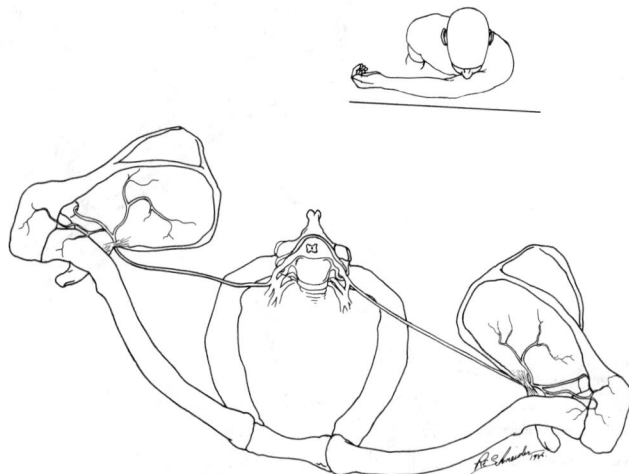

Figure 27-20. Circumduction of the arm displacing the scapula and stretching the suprascapular nerve between its anchoring points at the cervical spine and the suprascapular notch. (Reproduced with permission from Martin JT [ed]: Positioning in Anesthesia and Surgery, 2nd ed. Philadelphia, WB Saunders, 1987.)

lished.[56] Use of somatosensory-evoked potential recordings before and after the turn may also be helpful. Having the responsible surgeon present and involved in establishing the desired position is prudent. Final support of the head and extremities should be accomplished prior to release of the patient by members of the turning team. Resumption of the supine position and movement of the patient to a bed or a transport cart require equally meticulous attention.

Peroneal Nerve Injury

Pressure from weight of the down-side knee against the mattress may compress the common peroneal nerve as it courses laterally around the neck of the fibula. The patient's inability to dorsiflex the foot and loss of sensation over the dorsum of the foot indicate dysfunction of the nerve.[58] Padding the area of the head of the fibula is usually a sufficient precautionary measure.

VENTRAL DECUBITUS (PRONE) POSITIONS

Physiology

Circulatory

In the prone position, the circulatory dynamics vary according to the postural modification in use. If the legs remain essentially horizontal, pressure gradients in the blood vessels are minimal. If the patient is kneeling, or if the table chassis is rotated head high, significant pooling of venous blood in distensible dependent vessels is likely to occur.

With the patient lying on the soft abdominal wall, pressure of compressed viscera is transmitted to the dorsal surface of the abdominal cavity. Mesenteric and paravertebral vessels are compressed, causing engorgement of veins within the spinal canal. Obstruction of the inferior vena cava can produce immediate, visible distention of vertebral veins.[59] Because bleeding from incised vessels about the spine is increased under these circumstances, numerous

modifications of the prone position have been created to free the abdomen from pressure, reduce the congestion of intraspinal veins, and facilitate surgical hemostasis.[60,61]

If the head of a prone patient is below the level of the heart, venous congestion of the face and neck becomes evident. Turning the patient's head can alter arterial perfusion and venous drainage in both extracranial and intracranial vessels. Conjunctival edema, most abundant in the downside eye, is usual and reflects the influence of gravity on accumulation of extravascular fluid. If the head is above the level of the heart, mean vascular pressures are decreased according to the distance above the heart, air entrainment in open veins is possible, and conjunctival edema is less evident or absent.

Kaneko et al[53] described the perfusion of the entire lung of prone subjects in terms that subsequently fit the Zone 3 of West.[13] Backofen and Schauble[62] found that even the carefully established and supported prone position caused a significant fall in stroke volume and cardiac index, despite the development of increased vascular resistance in both the systemic and pulmonary circuits. No significant changes were detected in mean arterial pressure, right atrial pressure, or pulmonary artery occlusion pressure. On the basis of these observations, they recommend that in patients whose cardiovascular status is precarious, invasive hemodynamic monitors be introduced to detect otherwise unrecognizable deterioration of cardiac function caused by positioning.[62]

Respiratory

Using computed tomography, Gattinoni's group at the University of Milan[63] found a dramatic redistribution of computed tomographic densities from the dorsal (paravertebral supine) to the ventral (substernal) portions of the lungs when subjects were turned from the supine to the prone position. The original areas of compression atelectasis reopened when those parts of the lung became nondependent, whereas fresh areas of compression atelectasis formed rather promptly in newly dependent areas of the lung. In their study group, they found no change in oxygenation or shunting when pronation occurred.

If the thorax is supple or compliant, the body weight of an anesthetized prone patient compresses the anteroposterior diameter of the relaxed chest to a degree that is real but poorly defined. If the particular prone posture in use allows the pressure of the abdominal viscera to be sufficient to force the diaphragm cephalad, the lung is shortened along its long axis. With both the dorsoventral and the cephalocaudad dimensions of the lung decreased, and in the presence of the relative vascular congestion of a Zone 3 of West,[13,53] the compliance of the compacted prone lung can be anticipated to decrease. The result of decreased pulmonary compliance in a poorly positioned, prone, anesthetized patient is either an increased work of spontaneous ventilation or the need for higher inflation pressures during passive inspiration.

Proper positioning can retain more nearly normal pulmonary compliance by minimizing the cephalad shift of the diaphragm caused by compressed abdominal viscera. If the patient is arranged so that the abdomen hangs free, the loss of functional residual capacity is less in the prone position than in either the supine or the lateral position.[64] Rehder et al[65] noted that the weight of the freed abdominal contents had an "inspiratory effect on the diaphragm" when the pronated patient was properly supported by pads under the shoulder girdle and pelvis.

Variations of the Ventral Decubitus Position

Full (Horizontal) Prone

In the so-called "full" or "horizontal" prone position (Fig. 27-21), the requirement to elevate the trunk off the supporting surface so that the ventral abdominal wall is freed of compression almost always results in the head and lower extremities being below the level of the spine. If the table top is angulated at the trunk-thigh hinge in order to remove the lumbar lordosis and separate the lumbar spinous processes, and if the chassis is then rotated head-up sufficiently to level the patient's back, a significant perfusion gradient may develop between the legs and the heart. Wrapping the legs in compressive bandages minimizes pooling of blood in distensible vessels and supports venous return.

Various ventral supports, including parallel rolls of tightly packed sheets, padded and adjustable metal frames, and four-pillar frames, have been devised to free the abdomen from compression.[60,61] Each has merit, and no specific unit is unquestionably superior to all others. The choice is based on the physique of the patient, the requirements of the surgical procedure, and the available equipment.

Pronated patients with limited mobility of the neck, a history of postural neck pain, or a history suggesting a symptomatic cervical disk should have their heads retained in the sagittal plane, either with a skull-pin head clamp[66] or with a device similar to the rocker-based face rest being developed by Ray.[67] If the neck is pain-free and its mobility is satisfactory, the head can be turned laterally and supported on one of several soft sponge devices that prevents pressure on the down-side eye and ear.[68,69] However, forced rotation of the pronated head should be carefully avoided lest it induce postoperative neck pain.[69]

When a patient is scheduled to be pronated after induction of anesthesia, the preanesthetic interview should obtain and record information about any limitations that may exist in his or her ability to raise the arms overhead during work or sleep.[67] If the patient is symptomatic, the arms should be retained alongside the torso after pronation. (See the discussion of the Thoracic Outlet Syndrome.) If the arms are placed alongside the head (*i.e.*, extended ventrally at the shoulder, flexed at the elbow, and abducted onto arm boards), the musculature about the shoulders should be under no tension, neither humeral head should stretch or compress its axillary neurovascular bundle, ulnar nerves at the elbow should be padded, and the pulses at the wrists should remain full.

Prone Jackknife

The prone jackknife posture is used to provide access to the sacral, perianal, and perineal areas as well as to the lower alimentary canal (Fig. 27-22). The thighs are flexed on the trunk more than is usual in the full prone position, and management of the table surface hinges determines the degree of flexion available.[70]

Kneeling

Kneeling positions have been used to improve operative conditions in the lumbar and cervico-occipital areas (Fig. 27-23). Numerous frames have been constructed to support the weight of a kneeling patient, and their usefulness again depends on local use and the physique of the patient. If the vertebral column is unstable, kneeling frames are not as useful as parallel longitudinal supports, because kneeling risks application of shearing forces at the fracture site with the potential for damage of the contents of the spinal canal. In massively obese patients who must be operated on in the prone position, kneeling frames tend to prevent pressure on the abdomen more successfully than longitudinal frames.

Complications of the Ventral Decubitus Positions

Eyes and Ears

The eyes and ears are at risk in the prone position even when the head is turned to one side. The eyes should be lubricated, the lids closed, and each eye should be protected in some manner so that the lids cannot be accidentally separated and the cornea scratched. The eyes should also be protected against the head turning medially after positioning as well as against pressure being exerted on the globe.

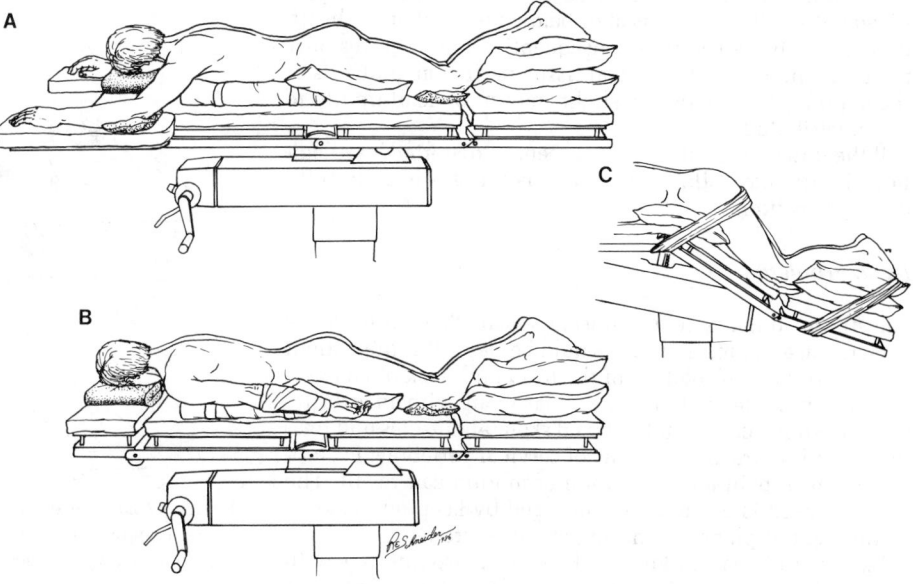

Figure 27-21. The classic prone position. (*A*) Flat table with relaxed arms extended alongside patient's head. Parallel chest rolls extend from just caudad of clavicle to just beyond inguinal area, with pillow over pelvic end. Elbows and knees are padded, and legs are bent at the knees. Head is turned onto a C-shaped foam sponge that frees the down-side eye and ear from compression. (*B*) Same posture with arms snugly retained alongside torso. (*C*) Table flexed to reduce lumbar lordosis; subgluteal are straps placed after the legs are lowered to provide cephalad thrust and prevent caudad slippage. (Reproduced with permission from Martin JT [ed]: Positioning in Anesthesia and Surgery, 2nd ed. Philadelphia, WB Saunders, 1987.)

A

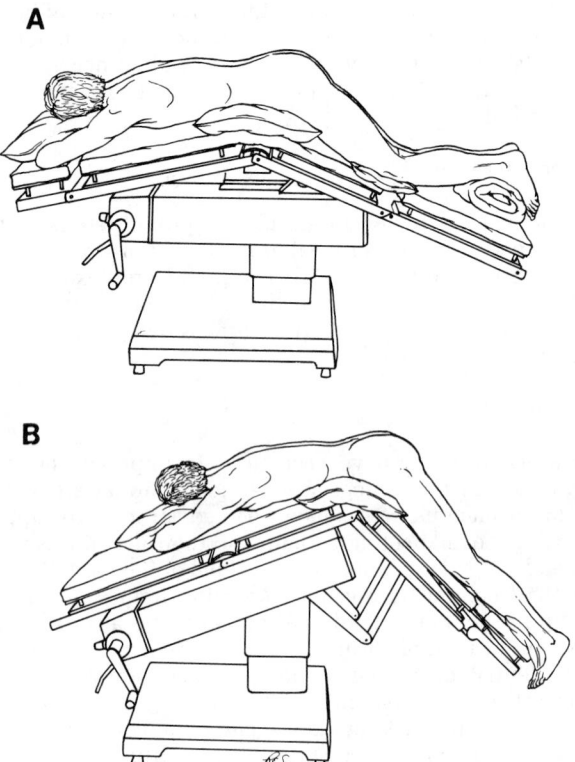

B

Figure 27-22. The prone jackknife positions. (*A*) Low jackknife position with the trunk-thigh hinge of the table used as the flexion point and augmented by a pillow under the pelvis. (*B*) Full jackknife position with the thigh-leg hinge of the table used as the flexion point to achieve more acute angulation of the hips on the torso. (Reproduced with permission from Martin JT [ed]: Positioning in Anesthesia and Surgery, 2nd ed. Philadelphia, WB Saunders, 1987.)

Monitoring wires and intravenous tubing should be checked after pronation to see that none has migrated underneath the head. If the head is retained in the sagittal plane, the eyes should be checked after positioning to assure that they are safe from compression by the head rest.

Conjunctival edema usually occurs in the eyes of the pronated patient if the head is at or below the level of the heart. It is generally transient, inconsequential, and requires only re-establishment of the normal tissue perfusion gradients of the supine position, or of a slight amount of head-up tilt, to be redistributed.

If the down-side external ear is bent or distorted, cartilaginous injury may follow. Soft foam padding is usually sufficient protection.

Neck Problems

Anesthesia impairs reflex muscle spasm that protects the skeleton against motion that would be painful if the patient were alert. Lateral rotation of the head and neck of an anesthetized, pronated patient, particularly one with an arthritic cervical spine, can stretch relaxed skeletal muscles and ligaments and injure articulations of cervical vertebrae. Postoperative neck pain and limitation of motion can result. The arthritic neck is usually best managed by keeping the head in the sagittal plane when the patient is prone.

Extremes of head and neck rotation can also interfere with flow in either the ipsilateral or contralateral vessels to and from the head. Excessive head rotation can reduce flow in both the carotid[71] and vertebral systems.[72] Impaired cerebral perfusion is the obvious consequence.

Brachial Plexus Injuries

Stretch injuries to the roots of the brachial plexus (Fig. 27-24A) on the side contralateral to the turned face are possible if the contralateral shoulder is held firmly caudad by a wrist restraint. If an arm is placed on an arm board alongside the head, care must be taken to ensure that the head of the humerus is not stretching and compressing the axillary neurovascular bundle (Fig. 27-24B,C).

When an arm is placed on an arm board alongside the head, the forearm naturally pronates. As a result, the ulnar nerve, lying in the cubital tunnel (the groove between the olecranon process and the medial epicondyle of the humerus), is vulnerable to being compressed by the weight of the elbow (Fig. 27-24D). Consequently, the medial aspect of the elbow must be well padded and its weight borne principally on the medial epicondyle.

Repetitious and prolonged inflations of automated blood pressure cuffs may result in injurious compression of either the radial nerve in the musculospiral groove above the elbow or the ulnar nerve prior to its entering the cubital tunnel[41,44] (Fig. 27-24E).

Thoracic Outlet Syndrome

Some patients complain of paresthesias in their arms after working with items on an overhead shelf, changing an overhead light bulb, or sleeping with one or both arms elevated alongside the head. The most likely explanation for the distress is the presence of a thoracic outlet syndrome with compression of the brachial plexus and subclavian vessels near the first rib.

As noted previously, all patients scheduled to be pronated should be questioned in the preanesthetic interview about their ability to function with arms elevated overhead, and their responses should be recorded on the charts.[61] A useful technique of inquiry if the history is in question is to have the patient clasp hands behind the occiput during the interview (Fig. 27-25). If the patient describes dysesthesias caused by having the arms overhead, or if dysesthesias

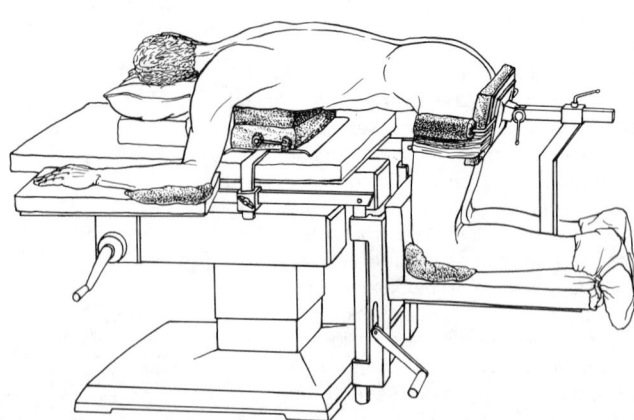

Figure 27-23. The Andrews kneeling frame with Wiltse's thoracic jack in use. (Reproduced with permission from Martin JT [ed]: Positioning in Anesthesia and Surgery, 2nd ed. Philadelphia, WB Saunders, 1987.)

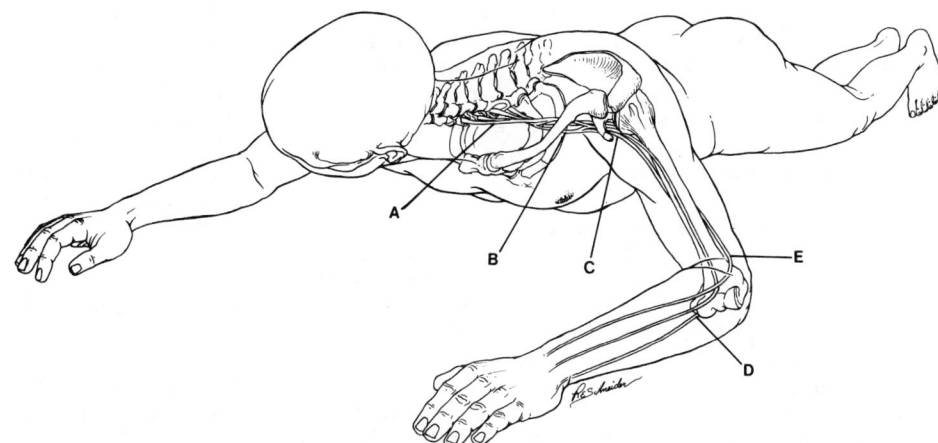

Figure 27-24. Sources of potential injury to the brachial plexus and its peripheral components when the patient is in the prone position. (*A*) Neck rotation stretching roots of the plexus. (*B*) Compression of the plexus and vessels between the clavicle and first rib. (*C*) Injury to the axillary neurovascular bundle from the head of the humerus. (*D*) Compression of the ulnar nerve before, beyond, and within the cubital tunnel. (*E*) Area of vulnerability of the radial nerve to lateral compression proximal to the elbow. (Reproduced with permission from Martin JT [ed]: Positioning in Anesthesia and Surgery, 2nd ed. Philadelphia, WB Saunders, 1987.)

occur while the patient is in the clasped hands on occiput position during the interview, during the operation the upper extremities should be retained alongside the trunk in the prone position. Agonizing, debilitating, and unremitting postoperative pain has been known to follow overhead arm placement in pronated patients who have had prior discomfort in their arms in that position.[61]

Unstable Chest Wall

If they are pronated and the weight of the thorax rests on the sternum and rib cage, patients with an unstable chest wall are apt to dislodge jagged ends of ribs into adjacent lung tissue. In most instances alternate surgical postures are possible and should be chosen despite the surgical inconve-

nience that may result. If the prone position must be used following a destabilizing injury to the thorax, serious consideration should be given to the prophylactic introduction of chest tubes situated so as to allow removal of intrapleural air during surgery.

Breast Injuries

Female breasts of average size can be stretched and injured if forced laterally by ventral chest supports when a patient is pronated. Medial and cephalad displacement seems better tolerated. Massive breasts of a very large patient, if forced laterally, may not cause distress to the patient; however, if the arms are retained alongside of the torso, the huge breasts may force each arm far enough laterally to cause the surgical

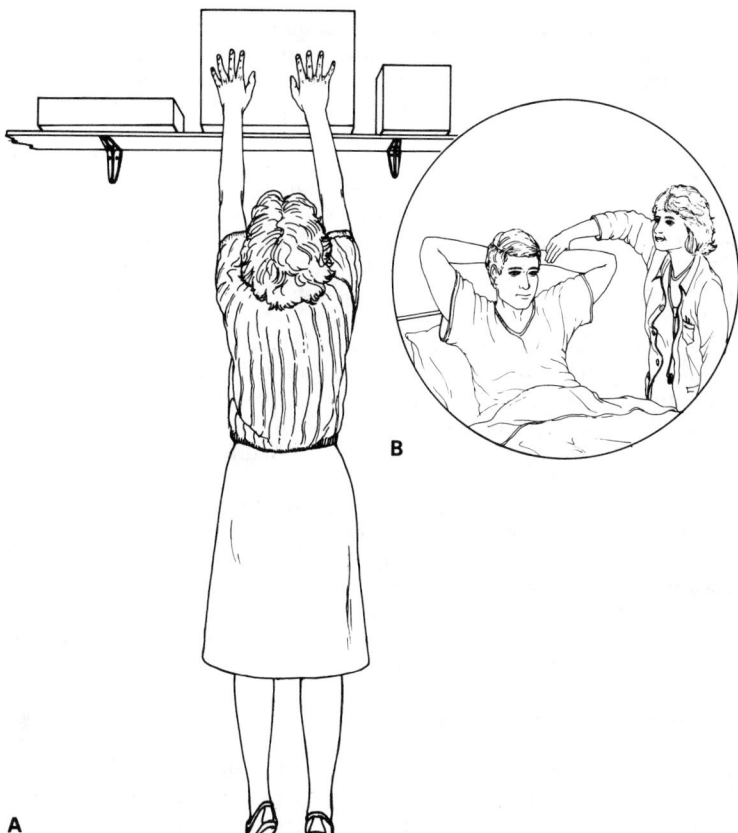

Figure 27-25. Assessment of a potential thoracic outlet syndrome. (*A*) The patient has a history of distress when trying to work or sleep with arms over head. (*B*) Interview was carried out with patient's hands clasped on occiput and radial pulses checked for damping. (Reproduced with permission from McCleskey CH [ed]: Geriatric Anesthesiology. Baltimore, Williams & Wilkins, in press.)

team difficulty in reaching the depths of an incision in the dorsal midline. Direct pressure on breasts containing enhancement prostheses can rupture the prosthesis. Tense skin grafts over mastectomy sites require considerable soft padding to prevent pressure necrosis and loss of the graft during a lengthy procedure in the prone position.

Coronary Artery Grafts

Mediastinal contents shift somewhat ventrad when a patient assumes the prone position. Apparently, the degree to which the ventrodorsal dimension of a stable chest is compressed by pronation can vary with the patient and the type of ventral supporting system used. Weinlander et al[73] have reported an occurrence with a patient who had received a coronary artery bypass graft 8 years previously and who had, in the interim, been successfully anesthetized for a lumbar laminectomy done in the prone position on longitudinal chest rolls. The patient subsequently needed a repeat laminectomy, and he was anesthetized and placed on a kneeling frame. The sternum was elevated by a pad to relieve venous congestion of the head and neck. Electrocardiographic evidence of myocardial ischemia followed placement of the sternal pad, was not relieved by drug therapy, and necessitated intra-aortic balloon pump support for emergency coronary artery revascularization following the laminectomy. Although a number of questions remain unanswerable, Weinlander's group felt that sternal compression resulting from the pad adversely affected the previously functional coronary artery grafts and probably caused the ischemia.[73] The implication that a sternal pad compresses the chest more than does a longitudinal frame is interesting but further proof is needed.

The Unstable Spine

Pronating the patient whose spine is unstable requires skillful teamwork. (See also the previous discussion of Lateral Decubitus Positions.) Enough people should be part of the turning team to control the weight being lifted without allowing sudden shifts of the patient's posture. Participation of the principal surgeon should be a requirement if stabilizing traction must be removed during positioning. Keeping the patient sedated but awake during tracheal intubation in the supine position permits multiple neurologic evaluations during pronation and final positioning to ensure that the maneuvers caused no new deficits.[56]

Use of bivalve nursing frames, such as the Foster or Stryker, allows anesthesia and intubation to be accomplished with the patient on the dorsal shell of the frame while traction is unchanged. Depending on the position of the neck in traction and the mobility of the mandible, fiberoptic or "blind" techniques may be needed for tracheal intubation. Addition of the ventral shell to the frame provides firm fixation of the patient during pronation. Removal of the dorsal shell after the turn permits the operation to be carried out on the remaining ventral shell without further risk from positioning torsion and without removing the corrective traction. Once the patient is pronated, care must be taken to assure the stability of transoral anesthesia devices and the safety of the eyes and face.

Abdominal Compression

Compression of the abdomen by the weight of the trunk of the prone patient can cause viscera to force the diaphragm cephalad enough to impair ventilation. If intra-abdominal

pressure approaches or exceeds venous pressure, return of blood from the pelvis and lower extremities is reduced or obstructed. Because the vertebral venous plexuses communicate directly with the abdominal veins, increased intra-abdominal pressure is transmitted to the perivertebral and intraspinal surgical field in the form of venous distention and increased difficulty with hemostasis. All of the various supportive pads and frames, when properly used, are designed to remove pressure from the abdomen and avoid these problems.[59-61]

Viscerocutaneous Stomata

Stomata that drain visceral contents into containers affixed to the abdominal wall are at risk in the prone position if they lie against a part of the ventral supporting frame or pad (Fig. 27-26). Compressive ischemia of the stomal orifice can cause it to slough. Surgical repair may be needed.

Knee Injuries

Extremely heavy patients, or those who have a pathologic condition of the knees, can have their knee joints injured in the kneeling position if the supportive ledges are not heavily padded (see Figure 27-23). Often there is no suitable alternative position for these patients, and the possibility of postoperative knee problems caused by the kneeling prone position should be carefully discussed in the preanesthetic interview.

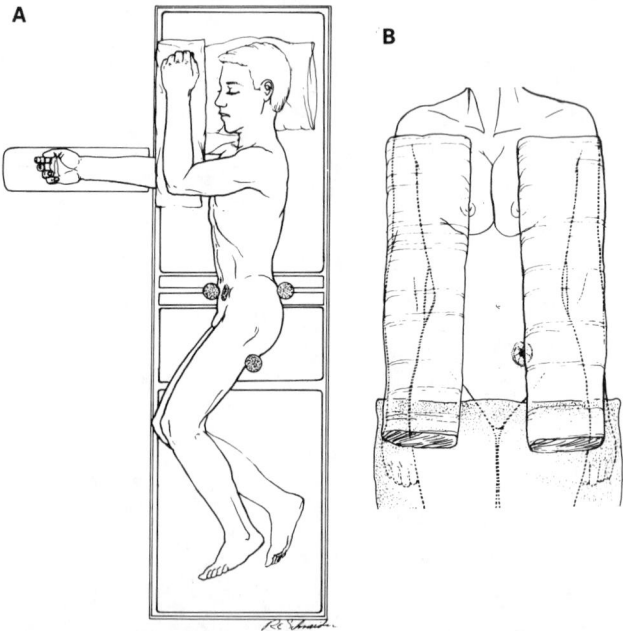

Figure 27-26. Postural supports compromising visceral stoma. Both (*A*), the vertical abdominal support of a device designed to maintain a patient in the lateral position, and (*B*), the longitudinal chest rolls supporting a pronated patient, can cause ischemic compression of a viscerocutaneous anastomosis and subsequent necrosis. Surgical repair of the stoma may be needed. (Reproduced with permission from McLeskey CH [ed]: Geriatric Anesthesiology. Baltimore, Williams & Wilkins, in press.)

HEAD-ELEVATED POSITIONS

Physiology

Circulatory

Coonan and Hope have reviewed circulatory changes that occur in alert humans with the change from the supine to the erect position.[74] As the head is raised above the level of the heart, pressure gradients develop and increase with the degree of elevation. Blood shifts from the upper body toward the feet. Atrial filling pressures decrease, sympathetic tone increases, parasympathetic tone decreases, the renin-angiotensin-aldosterone system is activated, and fluid and electrolytes are retained by the kidneys.[75,76] Intrathoracic blood volume decreases as much as 500 ml, pulmonary vascular resistance can double, and left atrial pressure falls more than right atrial pressure.[77] Cardiac output decreases 20–40%, and stroke volume falls by as much as 50%. Heart rate can increase by 30%. The arterial tree constricts, and systemic vascular resistance increases 30–60% to maintain a steady or increased mean arterial pressure, but the venous capacitance system is essentially unaffected.[78,79] Oxygen consumption by the tissues is unchanged; therefore the reduced oxygen supply (reduced cardiac output) causes an increased arteriovenous oxygen content difference.[80]

Cerebral blood flow decreases by approximately 20% with high head elevation.[78] Renal blood flow decreases as much as 30% (as much as 76% in massively obese patients in the sitting position), glomerular filtration decreases, and reduced secretion of antidiuretic hormone and aldosterone results in retention of water and sodium.[81]

Albin et al[82,83] and Dalrymple[84] noted similar alterations in cardiovascular parameters when the head-elevated position was established after patients were anesthetized. Although significant changes were not encountered with less than 60 degrees of head-up tilt, the magnitude of changes was often greater than the awake patient values presented above. The alterations increased progressively for more than 1 hour after the final posture was achieved. The question arose as to whether an impaired circulatory system could or should adjust to these stresses.

It can be inferred that the presence of intracranial pathology may exacerbate potentially harmful reductions in cerebral blood flow associated with head elevation.[85] In the anesthetized, seated patient, mean arterial pressure should be measured at the level of the circle of Willis, since that site is more reliable as an indicator of cerebral perfusion pressure in the head-elevated posture than is measurement at the level of the arm or wrist.[74]

Respiratory

As the patient becomes more upright in the head-elevated dorsal decubitus position, the inspiratory stroke of the diaphragm becomes less impeded by the bulk of abdominal viscera. Spontaneous chest wall motion requires less effort, and less pressure is needed to inflate the lungs during passive inspiration. Functional residual capacity increases in the head-elevated positions.[86] Age-related increases in shunting are less in the head-elevated position than in the supine position.[86] Gurtner[87] found that the diffusing capacity for oxygen was reduced in the sitting position as a result of the gravity-related decreases in perfusion of the upper portions of the lungs. Slutsky et al, however, found no difference between the supine position and the sitting position when measuring the ventilatory responses to hypoxia in volunteers.[88]

Variations of the Head-Elevated Positions

Sitting

The full sitting position, characterized by the patient sitting upright in a chair, is uncommon in current practice. It was used frequently for instillation of air prior to pneumoencephalography but was rarely chosen as a surgical position. It has disappeared as well in modern dental offices.

The classic sitting position for surgery places the patient in a semi-reclining posture on an operating table, with the legs elevated to about the level of the heart and the head flexed ventrally on the neck (Fig. 27-27). Head flexion should not be sufficient to force the chin into the suprasternal notch. (See the section on Midcervical Tetraplegia.) Compressive wraps around the legs reduce pooling of blood in the lower extremities. The head is held in place by some type of a face rest or by a three-pin skull fixation frame.

Supine, Head Elevated

A dorsal recumbent position with the head of the patient elevated somewhat is used for many operations involving the ventral and lateral aspects of the head (Fig. 27-28) and neck and occasionally, with the neck flexed, for transcranial access to the top of the brain. Its purpose is to improve access to the surgical target for the operating team as well as to drain blood and irrigation solutions away from the wound. The back section of the surgical table can be elevated as needed to produce a low sitting position (Fig. 27-28A), or the entire table can be rotated head-high with the patient's extended legs supported by a foot rest (Fig. 27-28B). Although the degree of tilt involved is not great, small pressure gradients are created along the vascular axis that can pool blood in the lower extremities or entrain air in patulous vessels that are incised above the level of the heart.

Vidabaek has described a position (Fig. 27-29) that uses a modest degree of head elevation along with a carefully arched thoracolumbar spine to improve access to the organs of the upper abdomen.[89] In a small series, he noted its usefulness to the surgeon as well as its associated difficulties for patients with precarious cardiovascular systems. For a similar purpose, a posture once widely used but long since discredited because of its trauma to the thoracolumbar spine placed the anesthetized patient in the horizontal supine position and then elevated the "kidney rest" [also known at that time as the "gallbladder rest"] against the T12–L1 vertebrae to violently arch the back and improve access to the gallbladder beneath the right costal margin. Happily, the posture did not permit intraoperative cholangiography and its use was abandoned.

For operations around the shoulder joint, the patient is often placed in a head-elevated semisupine position, with the upper torso rotated slightly toward the nonsurgical shoulder and supported by a firm roll or pad (Fig. 27-30). The upper trunk is moved laterally until the surgical shoulder extends beyond the edge of the operating table. The torso is supported so that the hips are on the table, the surgical shoulder is off and above the table edge, and the head rests on either a pillow (Fig. 27-30A) or a horseshoe head rest (Fig. 27-30B). Access is thereby provided to both

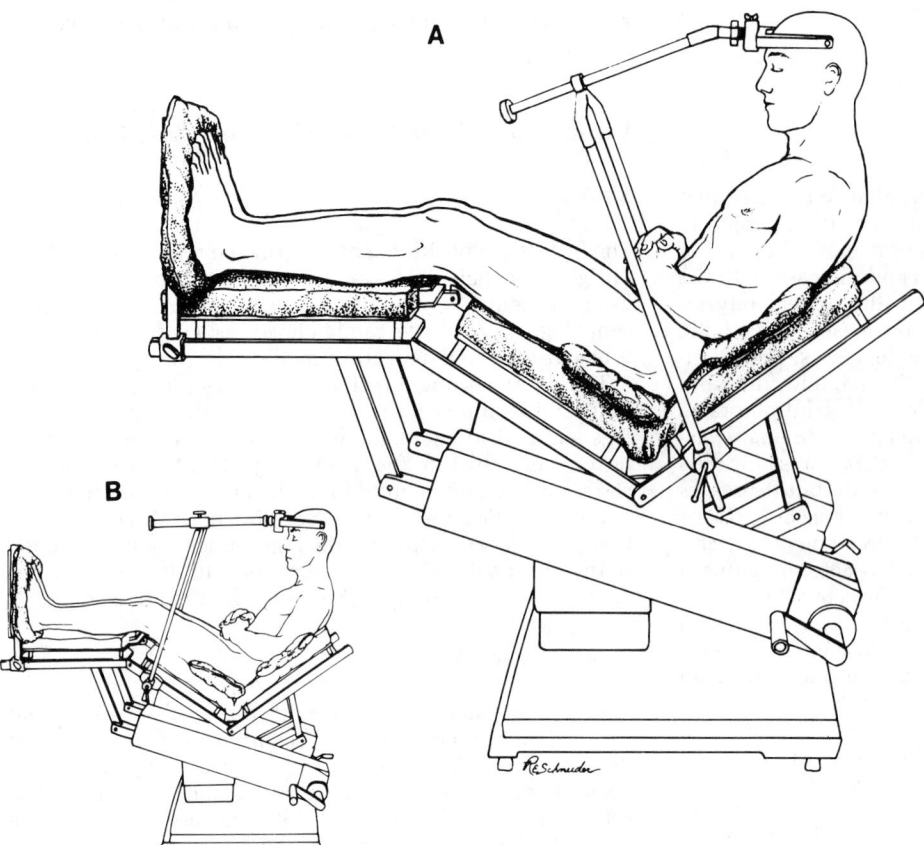

Figure 27-27. The conventional neurosurgical sitting position, with legs approximately at the level of the heart. (A) The frame of the headholder is properly clamped to the side rails of the trunk section of the table so that the patient's torso can be leveled in the event of a venous air embolus at the cervico-occipital operative site. (B) The frame is clamped to the side rails of the thigh section of the table, making it difficult or impossible to level the back section in an emergency. (Reproduced with permission from Martin JT [ed]: Positioning in Anesthesia and Surgery, 2nd ed. Philadelphia, WB Saunders, 1987.)

the dorsal and ventral aspects of the shoulder girdle. The surgical arm remains on the ventral torso and is prepared and draped to be mobile in the surgical field. This posture has been called the *barber chair position*.[90]

Lateral, Head Elevated

The lateral decubitus position with the head somewhat elevated, a means of access to occipitocervical pathology, has also been referred to as the *park bench position*.[91] All the stabilizing requirements needed for the usual lateral decubitus position apply. The head is held firmly in a three-pin skull fixation holder, which can be readjusted as needed during surgery. Although the degree of head elevation used is mild, the position does not completely remove the threat of air embolization. The anesthesiologist has good access to the patient's face and ventral thorax for purposes of monitoring, manipulation, and resuscitation.

Prone, Head-Elevated

The ventral decubitus posture with the table rotated head-high (Fig. 27-31) has become a widely used replacement for the sitting position as a means of access to dorsal structures of the head and neck. Usually the perceived advantage of the position is the avoidance of air embolization. Although the pressure gradients for air entrainment into patulous veins are less than in the full sitting position, the hazard is not eliminated. As a result of the positive pressure inflation cycle of passive ventilation, a bothersome recurrent flux of cerebrospinal fluid into and out of the exposed wound may be encountered. The posture also severely restricts resuscitative access to the ventral thorax.

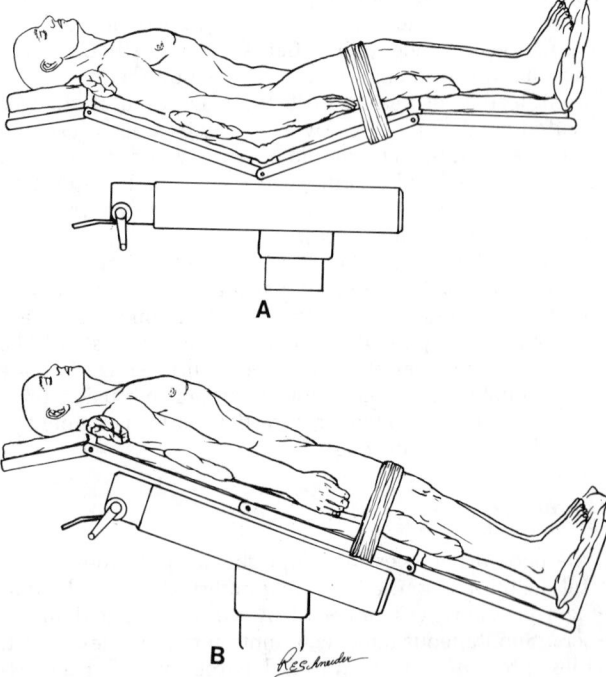

Figure 27-28. Head-elevated positions often used for operations about the ventral and ventrolateral aspects of the head, face, neck, and cervical spine. (A) The legs are at approximately heart level and the gradient into the head is appreciable but slight. (B) The flat table and foot rest are useful when a thyroidectomy is planned under regional anesthesia. (Reproduced with permission from Martin JT [ed]: Positioning in Anesthesia and Surgery, 2nd ed. Philadelphia, WB Saunders, 1987.)

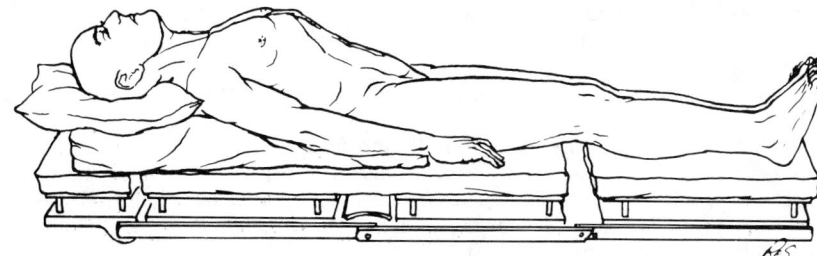

Figure 27-29. The xiphoid-high posture of Vidabaek used to gain access to the upper abdomen. (Reproduced with permission from Martin JT [ed]: Positioning in Anesthesia and Surgery, 2nd ed. Philadelphia, WB Saunders, 1987.)

Complications of the Head-Elevated Positions

Postural Hypotension

In the anesthetized patient, establishing any of the head-elevated positions is frequently accompanied by some degree of reduction in systemic blood pressure. The normal protective reflexes are inhibited by drugs used during anesthesia. Measuring mean arterial pressures at the level of the circle of Willis is recommended to assess cerebral perfusion pressures more accurately. Treatment of hypotension consists of temporarily delaying the elevation of the head as the patient is positioned; reducing the concentration of an-

esthetic drugs; infusing crystalloids or colloids to increase effective circulating volume; and using appropriately small amounts of a vasopressor as a temporary expedient.

Air Embolus

Air embolization is potentially lethal. In the bloodstream, air migrates to the heart, where it creates a compressible foam that destroys the propulsive efficiency of ventricular contraction and irritates the conduction system. Air can also move into the pulmonary vasculature, where bubbles obstruct small vessels and compromise gas exchange, or it can cross through a patent foramen ovale to the left side of the heart and the systemic circulation (see Chapter 32).

Opportunities for venous air embolization via an incised vein in a surgical wound located above the heart increase with the degree of elevation of the operative site. Although the occurrence of air emboli is a relatively frequent phenomenon in head-elevated positions, most of the emboli are small in volume, clinically silent, and recognizable only by sophisticated detection techniques. Nevertheless, the potential for continuing and dangerous accumulations of entrained air requires immediate detection of the embolization, a careful search for its portal of entry, and prompt treatment of its clinical effects.

Air embolism may be diagnosed by the presence of one or several of the following, in any order: a change in heart

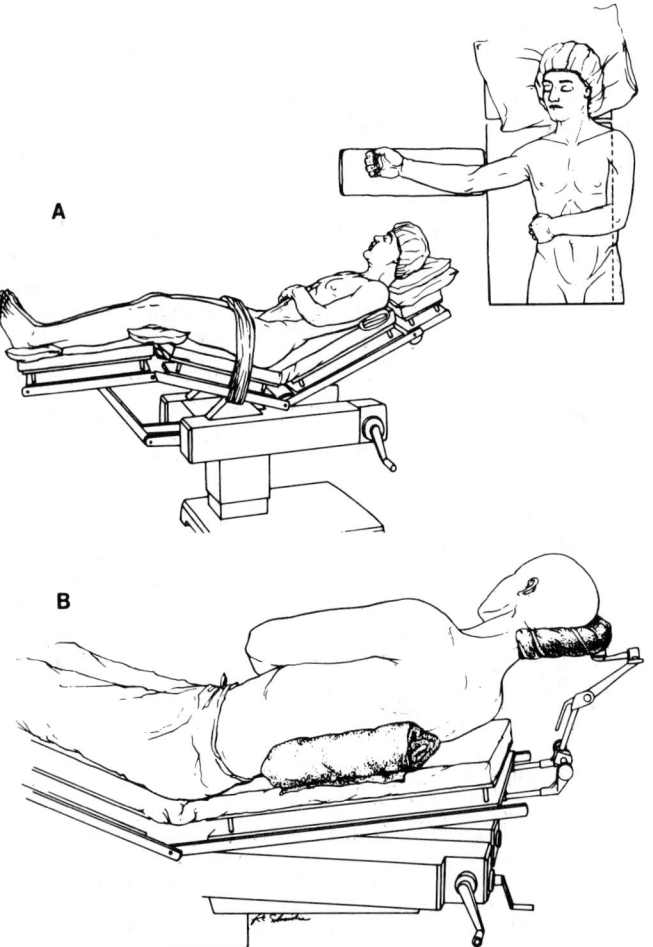

Figure 27-30. The barber chair position for surgery around the shoulder joint. See text. (A reprinted with permission from Martin JT [ed]: Positioning in Anesthesia and Surgery, 2nd ed. Philadelphia, WB Saunders, 1987.)

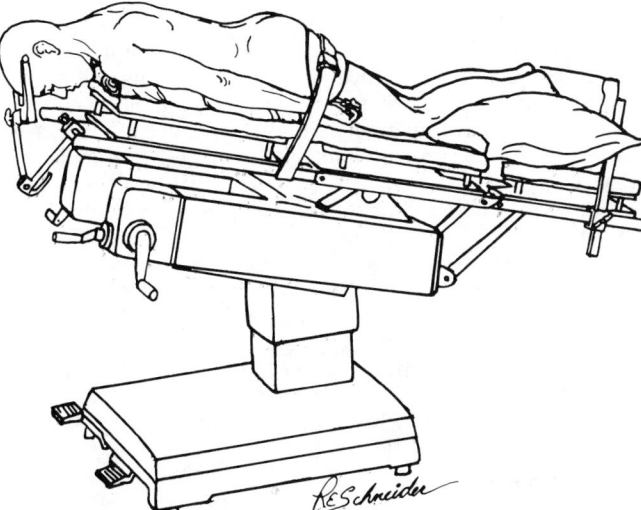

Figure 27-31. The skull-pin head rest used to stabilize a patient in the head-elevated prone position. Note the chest rolls used to free the abdomen from compression and the gluteal strap to minimize caudad slippage after head-up tilt. (Reproduced with permission from Martin JT [ed]: Positioning in Anesthesia and Surgery, 2nd ed. Philadelphia, WB Saunders, 1987.)

sounds noted by a parasternal Doppler probe; a cardiac murmur; cardiac dysrhythmias; hypotension; a decrease in expired carbon dioxide; and the sudden appearance of vigorous spontaneous ventilation despite continuing mechanical ventilation.

Approximately 20–35% of the population[92] have a residual foramen ovale that is functionally closed as long as pressure in the left atrium exceeds that in the right. However, in the sitting position, right atrial pressure can be higher than left. That gradient, augmented by the presence of air in the right side of the heart, intermittent positive pressure ventilation and positive end-expiratory pressure, may be sufficient to reopen an existing probe-patent but functionally closed foramen ovale. Air in the right atrium thereby gains paradoxical access to the coronary, cerebral, and systemic circulations.[93] In anesthetized and newly positioned patients, Perkins-Pearson et al[94] suggest that if pulmonary artery occlusion pressures are lower than right atrial pressures, this is an indication that the head-elevated posture should be abandoned in favor of a position in which the head is level with the heart.

Cucchiara and associates[95] have injected agitated saline through a right-sided heart catheter and used transesophageal echocardiography to detect paradoxical passage of fluid across the atrial septum. Positive airway pressure aided in determining paradoxical flow in 3 of their 20 patients.

Pneumocephalus

In the usual craniotomy procedure, most of the brain lies subjacent to the incision. After the dura is incised, cerebrospinal fluid is removed to improve working conditions, and the surgical field is open to the air. During the subsequent closure of the craniotomy, most of the air escapes from the wound and any residual pneumocephalus is of little consequence. When an incision is made through the dura in the posterior fossa or cervical spine of a seated patient, however, the bulk of the brain lies above the incision. Cerebrospinal fluid drains downward out of the wound, and tissue retraction can allow air to bubble up over the surfaces of the brain to become trapped in the upper reaches of the cranium.[96] When brain mass is decreased by ventricular drainage, steroids, and diuresis, the space available to a pneumocephalus is enlarged. Diffusion of nitrous oxide into the accumulated air, or the warming of trapped gas, can produce a tension pneumocephalus with signs of increased intracranial pressure and delayed awakening from anesthesia.

Toung et al[97] found postoperative pneumocephalus in all of a group of seated patients and in most of those who had been in the prone or the park bench position. Intraventricular air was present in most of the seated patients and was rare in those in the other positions. None of their group of 100 patients had neurologic changes attributable to the trapped intracranial air. Standefer et al[98] reported a 3% incidence of symptomatic (tension) pneumocephalus in seated, anesthetized patients whose duras were opened.

Ocular Compression

Pressure from a padded head rest on the eyes of a patient who has been placed in a head-elevated position can dislocate a crystalline lens or render the globe ischemic. Unilateral blindness has been reported as a result.[99] Modern skull-pin head clamps that grip firmly when properly applied have made ocular compression in the sitting position a rarity. In the head-elevated lateral decubitus or prone position, the threats to the eyes are those described in the preceding discussions of those nonelevated postures.

Edema of the Face, Tongue, and Neck

McAllister[100] has encountered severe postoperative macroglossia, apparently due to venous and lymphatic obstruction caused by prolonged, marked neck flexion. The patient's chin was firmly against the chest and an oral airway was in place to protect the endotracheal tube. Ellis et al[101] reported a similar patient who needed a tracheostomy because of massive swelling of the tongue, lips, pharynx, and epiglottis occurring shortly after extubation at the end of administration of a lengthy anesthetic in the sitting position that involved deliberate hypotension. Extremes of neck flexion, with or without head rotation, have been widely used to gain access to structures in the posterior fossa and cervical spine, but their potential for damage should be understood and the degree of flexion modified accordingly.

Midcervical Tetraplegia

This devastating injury occurs following marked flexion of the neck, with or without rotation of the head, and is attributed to stretching of the spinal cord with resulting compromise of its vasculature in the midcervical area. An element of spondylosis or a spondylotic bar may be involved.[102,103] The result is paralysis below the general level of the fifth cervical vertebra. Although the reports in the literature have generally described the condition as occurring after the use of the sitting position, midcervical tetraplegia has also occurred after prolonged, nonforced head flexion for intracranial surgery in the supine position. The role of a tethered cord in the production of the syndrome has not been established. No useful preoperative evaluation can as yet establish the potential for this complication.

Reversible changes in somatosensory evoked protentials elicited by stimulation of the median nerve have been found to occur after neck flexion.[104,105] However, in studies with monkeys, Cottrell et al[106] have shown that somatosensory evoked potentials may not be sensitive enough to detect midcervical tetraplegia, and Levy and associates[107] have suggested using motor-evoked potentials for this purpose.

Sciatic Nerve Injury

Stretch injuries of the sciatic nerve can occur in some seated patients if the hips are markedly flexed without bending the knees. Prolonged compression of the sciatic nerve as it emerges from the pelvis is possible in a thin, seated patient if the buttocks are not suitably padded. Foot drop may be the result of injuries to either the sciatic nerve or the common peroneal nerve and can be bilateral.

REFERENCES

1. Martin JT (ed): Positioning in Anesthesia and Surgery, 2nd ed. Philadelphia, WB Saunders, 1987
2. Anderton JM, Keen RI, Neave R (eds): Positioning the Surgical Patient. London, Butterworths, 1988
3. Dorland's Illustrated Medical Dictionary, 27th ed. Philadelphia, WB Saunders, 1988
4. Cheney FW, Posner K, Caplan RA et al: Standard of care and anesthesia liability. JAMA 261:1599, 1989
5. Enderby GEH: Postural ischemia and blood pressure. Lancet 1:185, 1954
6. Green DM, Metheny D: Estimation of acute blood loss by tilt test. Surg Gynecol Obst 84:1045, 1947

7. Kubal K, Komatsu T, Sanchala V et al: Trendelenburg position used during venous cannulation increases myocardial oxygen demands. Anesth Analg 63:239, 1984

8. Porter WT: Shock at the front. Boston Med Surg J 175:874, 1916

9. Sibbald WJ, Patterson NAM, Holliday RL et al: The Trendelenburg position: Hemodynamic effects in hypotensive and normotensive patients. Crit Care Med 7:218, 1979

10. Dripps RD, Comroe JH Jr: Circulatory physiology: The adjustments to blood loss and postural changes. Surg Clin North Am 26:1368, 1946

11. Burch GE: Method for recording simultaneously the time course of digital rate and of digital volume of inflow and outflow during a single pulse cycle in man. J Appl Physiol 7:99, 1954

12. Hope CE: Personal observations quoted in Coonan TJ, Hope CE: Cardiorespiratory effects of changes of body position. Can Anaesth Soc J 30:424, 1983

13. West JB, Dollery CT, Naimark A: Distribution of blood flow in isolated lung: Relations to vascular and alveolar pressures. J Appl Physiol 19:713, 1964

14. Froese AB, Bryan AC: Effects of anesthesia and paralysis on diaphragmatic mechanics in man. Anesthesiology 41:242, 1974

15. Martin JT: The lawn chair (contoured supine) position. In Martin JT (ed): Positioning in Anesthesia and Surgery, 2nd ed, p 37. Philadelphia, WB Saunders, 1987

16. Smith BE: Unusual patients: Obstetrics. In Martin JT (ed): Positioning in Anesthesia and Surgery, 2nd ed, p 266. Philadelphia, WB Saunders, 1987

17. Little DM: Posture and anesthesia. Can Anaesth Soc J 7:2, 1960

18. Wilcox S, Vandam LD: Alas, poor Trendelenburg and his position! A critique of its uses and effectiveness. Anesth Analg 67:574, 1988

19. Meyer W: Ueber die Nachbehandlung des hohen Steinschnittes sowie ueber Verwenbarkeit desselben zur Operation von Blasenscheidenfisteln. Arch Klin Chir 31:494, 1885

20. Cannon WB: Traumatic Shock. New York, Appleton and Co, 1923

21. Cole F: Head lowering in the treatment of hypotension. JAMA 150:273, 1952

22. Weil MH: Current concepts in the management of shock. Circulation 16:1097, 1957

23. Guntheroth WG, Abel FL, Mullins GL: The effect of Trendelenburg's position on blood pressure and carotid flow. Surg Gynecol Obstet 119:354, 1964

24. Taylor J, Weil MH: Failure of the Trendelenburg position to improve circulation during clinical shock. Surg Gynecol Obstet 124:1005, 1976

25. Reich DL, Konstadt SN, Hubbard M, Thys DM: Do Trendelenburg and passive leg raising improve cardiac performance? Anesth Analg 67:S184, 1988

26. Hewer CL: Latest pattern of non-slip mattress. Anaesthesia 8:198, 1953

27. Collins VJ: Principles of Anesthesiology, p 163. Philadelphia, Lea & Febiger, 1976

28. Keusch DJ, Winters S, Thys DM: The patient's position influences the incidence of dysrhythmias during pulmonary artery catheterization. Anesthesiology 70:582, 1989

29. Abel RR, Lewis GM: Postoperative alopecia. Arch Dermatol 81:72, 1960

30. Gormley T, Sokoll MD: Permanent alopecia from pressure of a headstrap. JAMA 199:157, 1967

31. Lawson NW, Mills NL, Ochsner JL: Occipital alopecia following cardiopulmonary bypass. J Thorac Cardiovasc Surg 71:342, 1976

32. Vander Salm TJ, Cereda J-M, Cutler BS: Brachial plexus injury following median sternotomy. J Thorac Cardiovasc Surg 80:447, 1980

33. Vander Salm TJ, Cutler BS, Okike ON: Brachial plexus injury following median sternotomy. Part II. J Thorac Cardiovasc Surg 83:914, 1982

34. Roy RC, Stafford MA, Charlton JE: Nerve injury and musculoskeletal complaints after cardiac surgery: Influence of internal mammary artery dissection and left arm position. Anesth Analg 67:277, 1988

35. Gregg JR, Labosky D, Harty M et al: Serratus anterior paralysis in the young athlete. J Bone Joint Surg 61A:825, 1979

36. Johnson JTH, Kendall HO: Isolated paralysis of the serratus anterior muscle. J Bone Joint Surg 37A:567, 1955

37. Foo CL, Swann M: Isolated paralysis of the serratus anterior. J Bone Joint Surg 65B:552, 1983

38. Martin JT: Postoperative isolated dysfunction of the long thoracic nerve: A rare entity of uncertain etiology. Anesth Analg 69:614, 1989

39. Britt BA, Gordon RA: Peripheral nerve injuries associated with anesthesia. Can Anaesth Soc J 11:514, 1964

40. Bickler PE, Schapera A, Bainton CR: Acute radial nerve injury from use of an automatic blood pressure monitor. Anesthesiology 73:186, 1990

41. Kroll DA, Caplan RA, Posner K et al: Nerve injury associated with anesthesia. Anesthesiology 73:202, 1990

42. Chusid JG: Correlative Neuroanatomy and Functional Neurology, p 145. Los Altos: Lange Medical Publications, 1985

43. McAlpine FS, Seckel BR: Peripheral nervous system complications. In Martin JT (ed): Positioning in Anesthesia and Surgery, 2nd ed, p 303. Philadelphia, WB Saunders, 1987

44. Sy WP: Ulnar nerve palsy possibly related to the use of automatically cycled blood pressure cuff. Anesth Analg 60:687, 1981

45. Chusid JG: Correlative Neuroanatomy and Functional Neurology, p 149. Los Altos: Lange Medical Publications, 1985

46. Hill NA, Howard FM, Huffer BR: The incomplete anterior interosseous nerve syndrome. J Hand Surg 10A:4, 1985

47. Hofmann A, Jones RE, Schoenvogel R: Pudendal nerve neuropraxia as a result of traction on the fracture table. J Bone Joint Surg 64A:136, 1982

48. Lindenbaum SD, Fleming LL, Smith DW: Pudendal nerve palsies associated with closed intramedullary femoral fixation. J Bone Joint Surg 64A:934, 1982

49. Orken DE: Modern concepts of the role of nephrotoxic agents in the pathogenesis of acute renal failure. In Edwards: Drugs affecting kidney function and metabolism. Progr Biochem Pharmacol 7:219, 1972

50. Matsen FA III: Compartmental syndrome. A unified concept. Clin Orthop Rel Res 113:8, 1975

51. Courington FW, Little DM Jr: The role of posture in anesthesia. Clin Anesth 3:24, 1968

52. Welborn SG: The lithotomy position: Anesthesiologic considerations. In Martin JT (ed): Positioning in Anesthesia and Surgery, 2nd ed, p 57. Philadelphia, WB Saunders, 1987

53. Kaneko K, Milic-Emily J, Dolovich MB et al: Regional distribution of ventilation and perfusion as a function of body position. J Appl Physiol 21:767, 1966

54. Sims JM: In Silver Suture in Surgery. The Anniversary Discourse Before the New York Academy of Medicine. Nov. 18, 1857. New York, Samuel S. and William Wood, 1858

55. Lawson NW: The lateral decubitus position: Anesthesiologic considerations. In Martin JT (ed): Positioning in Anesthesia and Surgery, 2nd ed, p 156. Philadelphia, WB Saunders, 1987

56. Lee C, Barnes A, Nagel EL: Neuroleptanalgesia for awake pronation of surgical patients. Anesth Analg 56:276, 1977

57. Brismar B, Hedenstierna G, Lundquist H et al: Pulmonary densities during anesthesia with muscular relaxation—a proposal of atelectasis. Anesthesiology 62:422, 1985

58. Chusid JG: Correlative Neuroanatomy and Functional Neurology, p 157. Los Altos, Lange Medical Publications, 1985

59. Smith RH: The prone position. In Martin JT (ed): Positioning in Anesthesia and Surgery, 2nd ed, p 79. Philadelphia, WB Saunders, 1978

60. Singh I: The prone position: Surgical aspects. In Martin JT (ed): Positioning in Anesthesia and Surgery, 2nd ed, p 181. Philadelphia, WB Saunders, 1987

61. Martin JT: The prone position: Anesthesiologic considerations. In Martin JT (ed): Positioning in Anesthesia and Surgery, 2nd ed, p 191. Philadelphia, WB Saunders, 1987

62. Backofen JE, Schauble JR: Hemodynamic changes with prone positioning during general anesthesia. Anesth Analg 64:194, 1985

63. Gattinoni L, Pelosi P, Vitale G et al: Body position changes redistribute lung computed-tomographic density in patients with acute respiratory failure. Anesthesiology 74:15, 1991

64. Douglas WW, Rehder K, Beynen FM et al: Improved oxygenation in patients with acute respiratory failure: The prone position. Am Rev Respir Dis 115:559, 1977

65. Rehder K, Knopp TJ, Sessler AD: Regional intrapulmonary gas distribution in awake and anesthetized-paralysed prone man. J Appl Physiol 45:528, 1978

66. Reid SA, Grundy BL: The head-elevated positions: Surgical aspects: The neurosurgical skull clamp. In Martin JT (ed): Positioning in Anesthesia and Surgery, 2nd ed, p 71. Philadelphia, WB Saunders, 1987

67. Martin JT: The prone position: Anesthesiologic considerations. In Martin JT (ed): Positioning in Anesthesia and Surgery, 2nd ed, p 201. Philadelphia, WB Saunders, 1987

68. Martin JT: Positioning the aged surgical patient. In McLeskey CH (ed): Geriatric Anesthesiology. Baltimore, Williams & Wilkins, in press.

69. Gravenstein N, Grundy BL, Reid SA: Complications of positioning: The central nervous system. In Martin JT (ed): Positioning in Anesthesia and Surgery, 2nd ed, p 291. Philadelphia, WB Saunders, 1987

70. Martin JT: The prone position: Anesthesiologic considerations. In Martin JT (ed): Positioning in Anesthesia and Surgery, 2nd ed, p 196. Philadelphia, WB Saunders, 1987

71. Sherman DD, Hart RG, Easton JD: Abrupt change in head position and cerebral infarction. Stroke 12:2, 1981

72. Toole JF: Effects of change of head, limb and body position on cephalic circulation. N Engl J Med 279:307, 1968

73. Weinlander CM, Coombs DW, Plume SK: Myocardial ischemia due to obstruction of an aortocoronary bypass graft by intraoperative positioning. Anesth Analg 64:933, 1985

74. Coonan TJ, Hope CE: Cardio-respiratory effects of change of body position. Can Anaesth Soc J 30:424, 1983

75. Sonkodi S, Agabiti-Rosei E, Fraser R et al: Response of the renin-angiotensin-aldosterone system to upright tilting and to intravenous frusemide: Effect of prior metoprolol and propranolol. Br J Clin Pharmacol 13:341, 1982

76. Williams GH, Cain JP, Dluly RG et al: Studies on the control of plasma aldosterone concentration in normal man. 1. Response to posture, acute and chronic volume depletion and sodium loading. J Clin Invest 51:1731, 1972

77. Fournier P, Mensch-Dechene J, Ranson-Bitker B et al: Effect of sitting up on pulmonary blood pressure, flow and volume in man. J Appl Physiol 46:36, 1979

78. Gauer OH, Thron HL: Postural changes in the circulation. In Hamilton WF, Dow P (eds): Handbook of Physiology, Section 2, Vol 3, p 2409. Washington DC, American Physiological Society, 1965

79. Ward RJ, Danziger F, Bonica JJ et al: Cardiovascular effects of change of posture. Aerospace Med 37:257, 1966

80. Bevegard S, Holmgren A, Jonsson B: The effect of body position on the circulation at rest and during exercise, with special reference to the influence on the stroke volume. Acta Physiol Scand 49:279, 1960

81. Rhodes JM, Graham-Brown RAC, Sarkany I: Reversible renal failure in an obese patient: Hazard of sitting with feet continuously elevated. Lancet 2:96, 1979

82. Albin MS, Janetta PJ, Maroon JC et al: Anaesthesia in the sitting position. In Recent Progress in Anesthesiology and Resuscitation. Amsterdam, Excerpta Medica International Congress Series No. 347, 1974

83. Albin MS, Babinski M, Wolf S: Cardiovascular response to the sitting position (letter). Br J Anaesth 52:961, 1980

84. Dalrymple DG: Cardiorespiratory effects of the sitting position in neurosurgery. Br J Anaesth 51:1079, 1979

85. Shenkin HA, Scheuerman EB, Spitz EB et al: Effect of change of posture upon cerebral circulation of man. J Appl Physiol 2:317, 1949

86. Don HF: The measurement of trapped gas in the lungs at functional residual capacity and the effects of posture. Anesthesiology 35:582, 1971

87. Gurtner GH: Interrelationships of factors affecting pulmonary diffusing capacity. J Appl Physiol 30:619, 1979

88. Slutsky AS, Goldstein RG, Rebuck AS: The effect of posture on ventilatory response to hypoxia. Can Anaesth Soc J 27:445, 1980

89. Vidabaek F: Posture with elevated and extended thorax. Acta Anaesth Scand 24:458, 1980

90. Day LJ: Unusual Positions: Orthopedics: Surgical aspects. In Martin JT (ed): Positioning in Anesthesia and Surgery, 2nd ed, p 223. Philadelphia, WB Saunders, 1987

91. Gilbert RGB, Brindle F, Galindo A: Anesthesia for Neurosurgery, p 126. Boston, Little, Brown, 1966

92. Hagen PT, Scholz DG, Edwards WD: Incidence and size of patent foramen ovale during the first ten decades: A necropsy study of 965 normal hearts. Mayo Clin Proc 59:17, 1984

93. Gronert GA, Messick JM, Cucchiara RF et al: Paradoxical air embolism from a patent foramen ovale. Anesthesiology 50:548, 1979

94. Perkins-Pearson NAK, Marshall WK, Bedford RF: Atrial pressures in the seated position: Implications for paradoxical air embolism. Anesthesiology 57:493, 1982

95. Cucchiara RF, Seward JB, Nishimura RA et al: Identification of patent foramen ovale during sitting position craniotomy by transesophageal echocardiography with positive airway pressure. Anesthesiology 63:107, 1985

96. Kitahata LM, Katz JD: Tension pneumocephalus after posterior fossa craniotomy, a complication of the sitting position. Anesthesiology 44:448, 1976

97. Toung TKJ, McPherson RW, Ahn H: Pneumocephalus: Effects of patient position on incidence of aerocele after posterior fossa and upper cervical cord surgery. Anesth Analg 65:65, 1986

98. Standefer M, Bay JW, Trusso R: The sitting position in neurosurgery: A retrospective analysis of 488 cases. Neurosurgery 14:649, 1984

99. Hollenhorst RW, Svein HJ, Benoit CF: Unilateral blindness occurring during anesthesia for neurosurgical operations. Arch Ophthalmol 52:819, 1954

100. McAllister RG: Macroglossia—a positional complication. Anesthesiology 40:199, 1974

101. Ellis SC, Bryan-Brown CW, Hyderally H: Massive swelling of the head and neck. Anesthesiology 42:102, 1975

102. Hitselberger WE, House WF: A warning regarding the sitting position for acoustic tumor surgery. Arch Otolaryngol 106:69, 1980

103. Wilder BL: Hypothesis: The etiology of midcervical quadriplegia after operation with the patient in the sitting position. Neurosurgery 11:530, 1982

104. McCallum JE, Bennett MH: Electrophysiologic monitoring of spinal cord function during intraspinal surgery. Surg Forum 26:469, 1975

105. McPherson RW, Szymanski J, Rogers MC: Somatosensory evoked potential changes in position-related brain stem ischemia. Anesthesiology 61:88, 1984

106. Cottrell JE, Hassan NF, Hartung J et al: Hyperflexion and quadriplegia in the seated position. Anesthesiol Rev 5:34, 1985

107. Levy WJ, York OH, McCaffrey M et al: Motor evoked potentials from transcranial stimulation of the motor cortex in humans. Neurosurgery 15:287, 1984

28 Hugh C. Gilbert
Jeffery S. Vender

Monitoring the Anesthetized Patient

Monitoring represents the process by which anesthesiologists recognize and evaluate potential physiologic problems in patients in a timely manner. The term is derived from *monere*, which in Latin means to remind or admonish. In perioperative care, monitoring implies that anesthesiologists will

1. Be observant and vigilant (clinical monitoring),
2. Employ appropriate monitors during and after anesthesia (instrumentation and/or electronic monitoring),
3. Interpret information from all monitoring modes, including those incorporated into the anesthetic delivery system (clinical judgment), and
4. Initiate corrective therapy when indicated (clinical safety).

The goal of monitoring is to enhance patient safety during anesthesia by identifying prognostic trends. Effective monitoring of both the patient and the equipment used for administering anesthesia should, in theory, diminish preventable mishaps as well as reduce poor outcomes that may follow surgical procedures, disease processes, or adverse effects related to the administration of anesthesia. Monitoring devices improve the capability for adequate warning because they can make repetitive measurements at higher frequencies than humans, they increase the specificity of clinical judgments (e.g., human observation of the color of blood *versus* oximetric measurement), and they do not fatigue. The value of a given monitor depends on several factors, including the clinical expertise of the anesthesiologist, the clinical setting, the anesthetic technique, and the specific equipment in use. It is important to recognize that "all morbidity or mortality associated with anesthesia care is not preventable or due to human error or equipment failure. Some of it, as in all specialties, occurs as a result of the patient's disease, and associated factors beyond anyone's control."[1]

Monitoring has become an essential aspect of anesthesia, and a plethora of medical devices are available that can be utilized. In this chapter, we focus attention on many different monitoring modalities that have been incorporated into standards of care or have been recommended as equipment that enhances the potential safety of anesthesia delivery. This chapter is not meant to be a comprehensive text on

clinical monitoring, nor is it our intent to discuss monitoring organ function. Many important monitors, such as electrocardiographs, and technologic advances such as intraoperative ST segment analysis are discussed elsewhere. Likewise, the descriptions of the technologic and scientific principles incorporated into monitoring devices have been simplified for clarity.

Eliminating preventable mishaps and injuries is an important reason for monitoring in anesthesia. Monitoring equipment should not be denied on the basis of its expense. Judge Learned Hand suggests that one must spend as much money to prevent an accident as the cost of that accident multiplied by the probability of the occurrence.[2] This legal ruling drives the quest for the designing, testing, and marketing of myriad "user-friendly" monitoring devices. The question of choice of monitors and their usefulness is a matter of convention, technology, politics, litigation, and personal taste. Standards for intraoperative monitoring have been adopted by The American Society of Anesthesiologists (adopted 1988, revised 1990)[3] (see Chapter 5, Appendix). Their application in the United States has become almost universal as a result of their incorporation into state regulations on standards of medical practice and at the insistence of insurance carriers.[4] These standards define in the most general way the minimum requirements for patient monitoring during anesthesia care.

Standard I requires qualified personnel to be present in the operating room for the continuous monitoring of the patient throughout the conduct of all general or regional anesthetics and during monitored anesthesia care. Standard II focuses attention on continually evaluating the patient's oxygenation, ventilation, circulation, and temperature. The following are specifically mandated: (1) using an oxygen analyzer that has a low oxygen concentration limit alarm; (2) a quantitative assessment of blood oxygenation (pulse oximetry); (3) determining the adequacy of ventilation by clinical signs; (4) verifying the correct placement of endotracheal tubes by clinical assessment and identification of carbon dioxide in the expired gas; (5) using disconnect alarms (low-pressure monitors) when a mechanical ventilator is in use; (6) continuously displaying the electrocardiogram; determining the heart rate and arterial blood pressure at least every 5 minutes; continually evaluating either heart tones, pulse trace or pulse character; and having a means to continuously measure changes in body temperature as clinically indicated. Quantitative monitoring of expired CO_2 (end-tidal CO_2 analysis) from the time of endotracheal intubation is strongly encouraged. Pulse oximetry is specifically suggested to satisfy the monitoring of blood oxygenation during anesthesia care.

The ASA standards emphasize the importance of melding physical signs (clinical monitoring) with instrumentation to promote safety. Electronic monitoring, no matter how sophisticated or comprehensive, does not necessarily reduce the need for clinical skills such as inspection, palpation, and auscultation. While the authors believe that, in general, electronic monitors are powerful tools that augment clinical judgments when properly utilized, there is very little evidence that "high tech" monitoring, by itself, reduces morbidity or mortality. Moreover, there is considerable controversy over the importance of specific monitors in unique clinical situations.

Monitoring can be classified as invasive, minimally invasive, or noninvasive. Invasive monitors place patients at risk for complications related to their application and use. Anesthesiologists must contemplate the vulnerability of patients to complications when assessing monitoring needs.

Consider the question of cardiac output and its distribution during anesthesia. If the patient is conscious, circulatory adequacy might be assessed using clinical monitoring by appraising the quality of the pulse and changes in blood pressure. Restlessness, mental clouding, or confusion may suggest a detrimental change in cerebral blood flow, or an acute drug toxicity, or perhaps hypoxemia unrelated to blood flow.

If a general anesthetic were administered instead of regional anesthesia, clinical signs relating to cerebral function would not be apparent. Our ability to judge the adequacy of cardiac output under general anesthesia can be severely limited. Although it may be possible to estimate the adequacy of perfusion by measuring urine output or assessing skin color, many factors associated with surgery and anesthesia often limit the reliability of these clinical signs. In this example, assessment of the central venous pressure or even measuring the cardiac output may be of importance in determining the conduct of the anesthetic or intraoperative medical therapy.

During anesthesia, therapeutic judgments are made from information obtained from instrumentation. The accuracy, reliability, and precision of clinical measurements constitute fertile areas of anesthesia research. Although statistical methods such as linear regression and the calculation of correlation coefficients are often used to evaluate the accuracy of new monitoring devices, they do not necessarily provide clinicians with information regarding applicability or usefulness.[5] The correlation coefficient (r) is not a measure of agreement but of association (see Chapter 3).

Clinicians expect monitoring devices to be engineered for accuracy, reproducibility, appropriate response times, and ease of use and maintenance. The performance of instruments such as medical gas analyzers is easily quantified by standard criteria of performance and calibration. Other monitoring systems such as continuous noninvasive cardiac output monitors or continuous arterial pressure measuring devices are more difficult to quantify because their reference standards exhibit bias (defined as the mean difference between measurements), and the study populations (surgery patients) are often skewed. Today, studies comparing two methods of monitoring often use method-comparison analysis to test accuracy (between technique variability). Method-comparison studies measure the precision and

trends of bias.[6] Mean differences between the two measurements (bias) estimate the systematic error. The standard deviation of the differences determines the precision of the measurement and is an estimate of the random error. Bias plots display the percentage difference of the measurement in question compared with the mean of the reference measurement and the measurement obtained by the test device.

Patient monitoring is rapidly changing, and the appearance of new devices is inevitable as advances in biomedical engineering find their way into the marketplace. National and international standards for patient safety and design are already commonplace. The Association for the Advancement of Medical Instrumentation has published guidelines to promote patient and operator safety and reduce the stress and distractions associated with medical monitoring.[7]

The proliferation of alarm tones during anesthesia care can be disturbing and may paradoxically reduce clinical vigilance. Monitoring systems may be insufficiently sensitive to reject errors and can create a cacophony of distracting signals. During routine anesthesia care, a minimum of five alarms (inspired oxygen, airway pressure, oximetry, blood pressure, and heart rate) are usually present. Unfortunately, a high frequency of spurious alarms occurs during routine anesthesia monitoring.[8] Integration of alarm signals is an important area of continuing evaluation.

There is great interest in standardizing the characteristics of alarm tones in order to prioritize messages and enhance their specificity. Audible alarms are designed to permit silencing and have user-adjusted set points. High-priority alarms should automatically reset after 120 seconds.

At no time in the history of anesthesia have practitioners had the capability to routinely monitor diverse physiologic variables in real time, often noninvasively, as they do today. Our understanding of the physiologic effects of anesthesia and its inherent risks is enhanced by utilizing appropriate intraoperative physiologic monitoring.

INSPIRATORY AND EXPIRED GAS MONITORING

Inspired Oxygen Monitoring

The concentration of oxygen in the anesthetic circuit must be measured. Although sensors are sometimes placed on the expired limb, they are usually on the inspired limb. This ensures that a hypoxic oxygen concentration is not delivered but does not guarantee the adequacy of arterial oxygenation. Three types of oxygen analyzers have been introduced for clinical use: paramagnetic, polarographic, and galvanic cell analyzers. (Other methods for monitoring inspired oxygen important to anesthesia care are described in the section on Multiple Expired Gas Analysis.) Specifications for clinical instruments include a fast response time (2–10 seconds), accuracy (±2%), and stability when exposed to humidity and inhalation agents.

Gases that are attracted to a magnetic pole are termed paramagnetic. Oxygen is a highly paramagnetic gas. Traditional paramagnetic oxygen analyzers, although very accurate, are fragile, have long response times, and are sensitive to weakly paramagnetic gases, e.g., nitrous oxide and water vapor, and therefore they do not meet the criteria for anesthesia oxygen monitoring.[9] Recently, a fast paramagnetic oxygen sensor has been developed for use in anesthesia. Using an alternating magnetic field, this device measures the pressure difference between two gas conduits (air and expired gas) when the gases are exposed to the magnetic field. The amplitude of the signal from a differential pressure transducer is proportional to the difference in the P_{O_2} between the two gas streams.[10] Differential paramagnetic oximetry has been incorporated into a variety of operating room monitors that display breath-by-breath oxygen waveforms (Datex Medical Instruments, Inc, Tewksbury, MA).

Galvanic cell analyzers meet the criteria for operative monitoring. These analyzers measure the flow of current produced when oxygen diffuses across a membrane and is reduced to molecular oxygen at the anode of an electrical circuit. The electron flow (current) is proportional to the partial pressure of oxygen (oxygen fuel cell). Galvanic cell analyzers require regular replacement of the galvanic sensor capsules.

Polarographic oxygen analyzers are based on the principle of the Clark electrode, which consists of a platinum or gold cathode and a silver anode. The electrodes are immersed in a potassium chloride electrolyte solution and connected to a battery and current meter. Oxygen diffuses through a gas-permeable polymeric membrane and then participates in the following reaction at the platinum cathode: $O_2 + 2H_2O + 4e^- \rightarrow 4\ OH^-$. The current change is proportional to the area of the platinum electrode, the diffusion characteristics of the electrolyte, and the number of oxygen molecules surrounding the electrode.[11] The response time is approximately 10–60 seconds. Polarographic oxygen electrodes are very versatile and are important components of gas machine inspired O_2 analyzers, blood gas analyzers, and transcutaneous and transconjunctival oxygen analyzers. Regular preventive maintenance (electrodes, membrane, electrolyte gel, and battery) is necessary. Comparisons of failure rate and life spans of galvanic cell analyzers and polarographic devices have been reported.[12]

Oxygen analyzers are equipped with visual and auditory alarms. When the sensor is placed in the inspiratory limb, oxygen analyzers are helpful in detecting a disconnection in the fresh gas flow. If the sensor is placed in the expiratory limb, endotracheal tube disconnects may also be identified.[13]

Monitoring of Expired Gases

Monitoring of expired gases has become increasingly common. Expiratory CO_2 monitoring has evolved as an important physiologic and safety monitor for assessing variables such as ventilation, cardiac output, distribution of blood flow, and metabolic activity. Respiratory gas and anesthetic agent analysis aids in the diagnosis of air embolism or airway leaks (CO_2 and N_2), quantifies vaporizer function, and complements the physiologic and safety features of measuring end-expired CO_2.

Infrared Capnography

Capnometry is the measurement and numeric representation of the CO_2 concentration (PKa) or partial pressure (mm Hg) during inspiration and expiration. A capnogram is a continuous concentration-time display of the CO_2 concentration sampled at a patient's airway during ventilation. Capnography is the continuous monitoring of a patient's capnogram.

The capnogram is divided into four distinct phases (Fig. 28-1). The first phase (A-B) represents the initial stage of expiration. Gas sampled during the initial phase of expiration occupies the anatomic dead space and is normally devoid of CO_2.

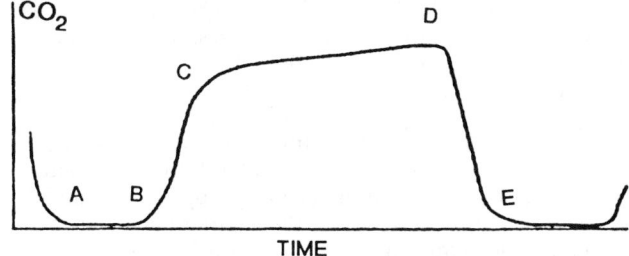

Figure 28-1. The normal capnogram. Point D delineates the end-tidal CO_2. $ETCO_2$ is the best reflection of the alveolar CO_2 tension.

void of CO_2. At point B, CO_2-containing gas presents itself at the sampling site, and a sharp upstroke (B-C) is seen in the capnogram. The slope of this upstroke is determined by the evenness of ventilation and alveolar emptying. Phase C-D represents the alveolar or expiratory plateau. During phase C-D, alveolar gas is being sampled. Normally, this part of the waveform is almost horizontal and delineates the ventilation-weighted average concentration of CO_2 in alveolar gas. Point D is the highest value and is called the end-tidal CO_2 ($ETCO_2$). $ETCO_2$ is the best reflection of the alveolar CO_2 tension ($PaCO_2$). As the patient begins to inspire, fresh gas (CO_2 free) is entrained, and there is a steep downstroke (D-E) back to baseline. Normally, unless rebreathing of CO_2 occurs, the baseline approaches zero.

Several methods for the quantification of CO_2 have been applied to patient monitoring systems. One of the most commonly used methods is based on infrared absorption. Asymmetric, polyatomic molecules like CO_2 absorb infrared light at specific wavelengths. A beam of infrared light is split and passes through the gas sample and a reference standard. The amount of infrared energy absorbed in the gas sample is cross-referenced against the control, and the concentration of CO_2 is calculated and displayed.

Modern capnometers compensate for interference from nitrous oxide, which absorbs some infrared at the same wavelength (4.3 μm) as CO_2 molecules. Instrument calibration is performed by zeroing the monitor to room air (0.05% CO_2) and then introducing a gas sample containing a known percentage of CO_2. Exhaling into the sampling tube should create a capnogram with an end-tidal CO_2 reading of 38–42 mm Hg.

Two basic systems of gas sampling are currently available. Sidestream sampling is the most commonly employed technique. Airway gas is aspirated and pumped through small-bore tubes to a distant measuring device. Although simple to use, sidestream sampling has some limitations. Secretions may obstruct air flow and influence the character of the capnogram. Condensate (water vapor) can potentially contaminate the system and produce falsely elevated CO_2 readings. Sidestream machines have a variable but unavoidable lag time between sample aspiration and detection. The rate of gas aspiration affects the accuracy of the CO_2 reading as well as the character of the capnogram. Typically, sampling flow rates range from 50–250 ml·min^{-1}. High sampling rates tend to produce good quality capnograms owing to axial mixing along the tube. If the sampling flow rate exceeds airway gas flow, entrainment of fresh gas contaminates the specimen and reduces the estimate of $PaCO_2$. This is of particular concern in the pediatric population or when using low-flow anesthesia in children or adults.

"Mainstream" or "flow-through" devices reduce or eliminate the problems associated with condensate errors, lag time, and sampling flow rates. Unfortunately, these devices are cumbersome, bulky, and heavy. They increase dead space and may produce additional stress on the endotracheal tube unless carefully supported.

The use of capnography is dependent on an understanding of the relationship between arterial, alveolar, and end-tidal CO_2. $ETCO_2$ provides a clinical estimate of the arterial CO_2 ($PaCO_2$). This concept assumes the following: ventilation and perfusion in the lungs are appropriately matched; CO_2 is easily diffusible across the capillary-alveolar membrane; and no sampling errors occur during measurement. If the above conditions are met, changes in $ETCO_2$ reflect changes in $PaCO_2$ even if it is assumed that all alveoli do not empty at the same time, e.g., $ETCO_2 \approx PaCO_2$ (alveolar) $\approx PaCO_2$ (arterial).

Using an idealized mathematic model of ventilation:perfusion, the $PaCO_2$ to $PaCO_2$ (hence $ETCO_2$) difference is zero. If the gradient between $PaCO_2$ and $ETCO_2$ is constant and small, capnography provides a noninvasive, continuous, real-time reflection of ventilation. The typical gradient during general anesthesia is about 5–10 mm Hg. Unfortunately, a maldistribution of ventilation and perfusion (increased $\dot{V}/\dot{Q}$) or gas sampling problems result in a widening of this gradient. A widening of the $PaCO_2$-$ETCO_2$ gradient makes an indirect assessment of $PaCO_2$ more problematic, especially if the change is dynamic.

Gas sampling errors also affect the $PaCO_2$-$ETCO_2$ gradient. As discussed earlier, sidestream analyzers can dilute the patient's tidal breath with fresh gas, producing a falsely low $ETCO_2$. This problem can be significant in neonates, infants, and small children with small tidal volumes.[14] The site of sampling can also affect accuracy.[15] The least error appears when the sampling site is on the endotracheal tube connector. Loose connections and system leaks are an additional source of sampling error.

The respiratory rate and pattern can also alter accuracy. Shallow tidal breaths, a prolongation of the expiratory phase of ventilation, uneven alveolar emptying, and small airway obstruction tend to increase the gradient between $PaCO_2$ and $ETCO_2$.

$\dot{V}/\dot{Q}$ maldistribution is a common cause of an increased $PaCO_2$-$PaCO_2$ gradient, which increases the $PaCO_2$-$ETCO_2$ gradient. Dead space ventilation is the extreme example of $\dot{V}/\dot{Q}$ mismatch in which there is a complete absence of perfusion in the presence of adequate alveolar ventilation. Since only perfused alveoli can participate in gas exchange, the nonperfused alveoli have a $PaCO_2$ of zero. The ventilation-weighted average of the perfused and nonperfused alveoli will determine the $ETCO_2$. The greater the dead space ventilation, the lower the $ETCO_2$ and the greater the $PaCO_2$-$ETCO_2$ gradient.

Conditions that increase $\dot{V}/\dot{Q}$ mismatch (dead space) reduce the usefulness of $ETCO_2$ monitoring. The common clinical causes associated with a widened $PaCO_2$-$ETCO_2$ gradient include embolic phenomena (thrombus, fat, air, amniotic fluid); hypoperfusion states; and chronic obstructive pulmonary disease. In contrast, shunt producing pathology (perfusion without ventilation) causes minimal changes in the $PaCO_2$-$ETCO_2$ gradient.

Capnography has been employed to identify appropriate placement of endotracheal tubes, indirectly assess the $PaCO_2$, monitor potential changes in perfusion and dead space, and detect added CO_2 in anesthesia circuits.

Anesthesiologists are fully aware of the importance of verifying that an endotracheal tube is properly placed in the trachea. Auscultation of the lungs has long been the primary method of identifying endotracheal tube placement, but capnography appears to have further decreased the potential for accidental esophageal intubations. Since the esophageal or gastric gas concentration is primarily composed of inspired gas, it should contain exceedingly small amounts of CO_2. Following an esophageal intubation, the first one or two "breaths" may contain some CO_2, but the concentration should approach zero after four or five "breaths." The CO_2 waveform should be observed beyond the sixth breath before an opinion is reached regarding the sampling of alveolar gas.[16] A continuous, stable CO_2 waveform ensures the presence of alveolar ventilation but does not necessarily indicate that the endotracheal tube is properly positioned within the trachea (e.g., above the carina).

The reliability of $ETCO_2$ as a quantitative estimate of ventilation depends on the stability of the $\dot{V}/\dot{Q}$ relationships. Any process that increases dead space widens the $PaCO_2$-$PECO_2$ gradient (Table 28-1). In most situations, the $PaCO_2$ should exceed the $PECO_2$.

Increases in $ETCO_2$ can be expected when CO_2 production exceeds ventilation, e.g., as in hyperthermia, or when an exogenous source of CO_2 is present, e.g., during CO_2 insufflation, bicarbonate infusion, or rebreathing (Table 28-1).

A sudden drop of the $ETCO_2$ to near zero followed by the absence of a CO_2 waveform is a potentially life-threatening problem that could indicate malposition of an endotracheal tube in the pharynx or esophagus, disruption of airway integrity (disconnection or obstruction), disruption of sampling lines, or a sudden cardiac arrest. When a *sudden drop* of the $ETCO_2$ occurs, it is essential to quickly verify the integrity of ventilation and identify physiologic and mechanical factors that might account for a zero line capnogram. The adequacy of cardiopulmonary resuscitation can be assessed by capnography. Restoration of pulmonary blood flow is associated with an increase in $ETCO_2$.

Abrupt decreases in the $ETCO_2$ are often associated with an altered cardiopulmonary status, e.g., embolism or hypoperfusion. *Gradual reductions* in $ETCO_2$ often reflect decreases in $PaCO_2$ that occur following increases in minute ventilation or a reduction of the metabolic rate.

The size and shape of the capnogram waveform can be quite informative. A slow rate of rise of the second phase (B-C) is suggestive of either chronic obstructive pulmonary disease or acute airway obstruction. A normally shaped capnogram with an increase in $ETCO_2$ suggests alveolar hypoventilation or an increase in CO_2 production. Transient increases in $ETCO_2$ are often seen during tourniquet release, aortic unclamping, or the administration of bicarbonate.

Multiple Expired Gas Analysis

Three techniques are available that permit monitoring of the entire spectrum of respiratory and anesthetic gases. The most commonly employed technique for multiple gas monitoring is similar to infrared capnography. Asymmetric molecules such as CO_2, N_2O, water vapor, and the potent inhalation agents absorb infrared light at specific wavelengths.[17] Single-room multifiltered instruments designed to detect and display respiratory gases and inhalation vapors of interest have been clinically available since 1989. Since O_2 and N_2 do not absorb infrared light, multiple gas analyzers must incorporate several detection technologies to measure and display all the gases of interest.

Intraoperative breath-by-breath analysis of respiratory and anesthetic gases requires either monitoring devices in every anesthetizing location (dedicated mass spectrometry,

TABLE 28-1. Changing ETCO$_2$: Common Etiologies

Increases in ETCO$_2$	Decreases in ETCO$_2$
Changes in CO$_2$ Production	
Hyperthermia	Hypothermia
Sepsis	Hypometabolism
Malignant hyperthermia	
Muscular activity	
Changes in CO$_2$ Elimination	
Hypoventilation	Hyperventilation
Rebreathing	Hypoperfusion
	Embolism

infrared absorption, or Raman scattering) or a single instrument (mass spectrometer) with a fast response that can be multiplexed to sample, measure, and display the results in 15–30 different anesthetizing locations.

Multiroom mass spectrometer systems collect respiratory samples using long nylon or Teflon tubes that end at a rotating valve that permits room-to-room time-shared sampling. Gas samples enter the mass spectrometer, where they are bombarded by an electron beam that fragments the gas molecules. Each gas has characteristic ion fragments, which then are transported from the ionization chamber to a detection chamber. In the detection chamber, the ion fragments pass through a magnetic field. In the magnetic field, the fragments spin in a circle of a specific diameter based on their respective mass/charge ratio. In magnetic sector instruments, detector plates are positioned precisely in the trajectory of the ion fragments of interest. Impacts between the detector plate and the ion fragments create electric currents.

The current generated from each detection plate is proportional to the fraction of gas in the original sample. The current is analyzed using a sophisticated computer program that identifies the mass spectrum of the ion fragments and calculates the percentage of each gas or vapor in the sample. Concentration-time profiles with reports of inspired and expired end-tidal values can be generated or stored by the network's computer system.

Quadrapole instruments use varying magnetic fields induced between an electrode array (quadrapole lens), which separates the ions by mass/charge ratios and directs them to a single detector for analysis.

A major defect of multiplexed mass spectrometry systems is their inability to continuously sample and display ETCO$_2$. This problem has been solved by including dedicated in-line infrared CO$_2$ scanners that interact with the sensitive and accurate mass spectrometer and its computer system to display an accurate breath-by-breath capnogram. The secondary CO$_2$ scanner serves as a back-up qualitative capnograph when the mass spectrometer's detector function needs repair.

The initial capital investment for multiplexed mass spectrometry systems is high. Single room mass spectrometry is also available (Ohmeda 6000 Multigas Monitor, Madison, WI). Whereas the benefit of mass spectrometry in reducing critical incidents has been difficult to quantify, the concept of respiratory gas and agent monitoring has gained acceptance, and alternative instrumentation for single location gas analysis is currently available.

A unique approach to multiple gas analysis is based on Raman scattering. Raman scattering results when photons generated by a high-intensity argon laser collide with gas molecules. Following impact, gas molecules are momentarily excited to unstable vibrational and rotatory states. As they return to their normal state, photons of a characteristic frequency are emitted. The scattered photons are measured as peaks in a spectrum that determines the concentration and composition of respiratory gases and inhalation vapors.

Raman spectroscopy offers the following advantages when compared with operating room mass spectrometry: each gas is analyzed independently, calibration is simple, and response time is fast.[18] Unlike what occurs in mass spectrometers, the gas molecules are unaltered during the detection process and can be returned to the anesthesia circuit. Raman spectroscopy can distinguish the concentration of all volatile anesthetic agents, CO$_2$, N$_2$O, O$_2$, and N$_2$, and it accurately estimates gas concentrations in the presence of nonmeasured gases such as helium. An instrument using Raman technology (RASCAL, Ohmeda, Salt Lake City, UT) is commercially available and has undergone clinical trials.[18] Comparisons with mass spectrometry reveal a similar degree of accuracy.

The clinical indications for routine CO$_2$ and O$_2$ gas monitoring are well documented. Instrumentation that provides measurement of nitrogen and all the anesthetic vapors provides clinically relevant information that, although not mandated, is desirable. Nitrogen (N$_2$) monitoring provides quantification of washout during preoxygenation. A sudden rise in N$_2$ in the exhaled gas indicates either introduction of air from leaks in the anesthesia delivery system or venous air embolism.[19,20] Critical events that can be detected by analysis of respiratory gases and anesthesia vapors are listed in Table 28-2.[21]

Oxygen Monitoring

The assessment of oxygenation is an integral part of anesthesia practice. Hypoxemia is a common etiologic cause of morbidity and mortality. Early detection and prompt intervention may limit the sequelae of hypoxemia. The clinical signs associated with hypoxemia, e.g., tachycardia, tachypnea, altered mental status, and/or cyanosis, are often masked or difficult to appreciate when the patient is under anesthesia.

TABLE 28-2. Gas Analysis and the Detection of Critical Events

Event	Monitoring Modality
Error in gas delivery system	O$_2$, N$_2$, agent, CO$_2$
Anesthesia machine malfunction	O$_2$, N$_2$, agent, CO$_2$
Vaporizer malfunction or contamination	Agent
Anesthesia circuit leaks	N$_2$, CO$_2$
Endotracheal cuff leaks	N$_2$, CO$_2$
Poor mask fit	N$_2$, CO$_2$
Hypoventilation	CO$_2$
Airway obstruction	CO$_2$
Air embolism	N$_2$, CO$_2$
Disconnection	CO$_2$
Malignant hyperthermia	CO$_2$
Circuit hypoxia	O$_2$
Vaporizer overdose	Agent

Modified with permission from Knopes KD, Hecker BR: Monitoring anesthetic gases. In Lake CL (ed): Clinical monitoring. Philadelphia, WB Saunders, 1990.

The mechanisms of hypoxemia are multifactorial. Oxygen analyzers (previously discussed) assess oxygen delivery (FIO_2) to the patient. Other noninvasive technologies are available to detect the presence of arterial hypoxemia. Arterial oxygen monitors do not ensure adequacy of oxygen delivery or utilization to or by the tissues. These monitors are not a replacement for arterial blood gas measurements when they are indicated.

Pulse Oximetry

Pulse oximetry has rapidly become the standard of care for monitoring oxygenation during anesthesia. Extensive reviews of pulse oximetry are available in the literature.[22-26]

Pulse oximeters measure pulse rate and oxygen saturation of hemoglobin (SpO_2) on a noninvasive, continuous basis. A relationship exists between hemoglobin saturation and oxygen tension—the oxyhemoglobin dissociation curve (Fig. 28-2). On the steep part of the curve, a predictable correlation exists between SaO_2 and PO_2. In this range, the SaO_2 is a good reflection of the extent of hypoxemia and the changing status of arterial oxygenation. This relationship is altered by shifts in the curve to the right (increased O_2 affinity) or to the left. At a PO_2 of 75 mm Hg or greater, the SaO_2 plateaus and loses its ability to reflect changes in PaO_2. Factors that shift the oxyhemoglobin dissociation curve are discussed in Chapter 10.

Pulse oximetry is based on several premises:

1. The color of blood is a function of oxygen saturation.
2. The change in color results from the optical properties of the hemoglobin molecule and its interaction with oxygen.
3. The instrument measures the absorption of specific wavelengths of light relative to the ratio of oxygenated (O_2Hb) and reduced hemoglobin (Hb).

Pulse oximeters combine the use of plethysmography and spectrophotometric analysis to measure hemoglobin saturation (see also Chapter 7). The spectrophotometric principle

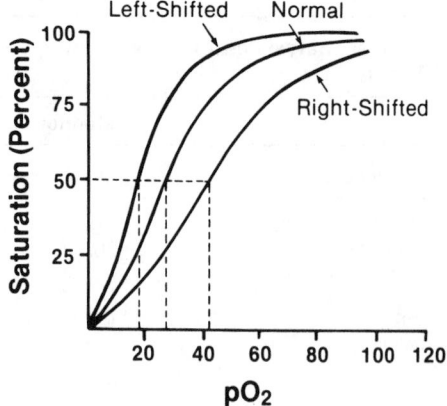

Figure 28-2. The oxyhemoglobin dissociation curve. The relationship between arterial saturation of hemoglobin and oxygen tension is represented by the sigmoid-shaped oxyhemoglobin dissociation curve. When the curve is left-shifted, the hemoglobin molecule binds oxygen more tightly. (Reproduced with permission from Brown M, Vender JS: Non-invasive oxygen monitoring. Crit Care Clin 4:493, 1988.)

for determining oxygen saturation is based on the Beer-Lambert Law. At a constant light intensity and hemoglobin concentration, the intensity of light transmitted through the sample is a logarithmic function of the oxygen saturation of hemoglobin.[27] Two wavelengths of light are required to distinguish between O_2Hb and reduced Hb. Typically, the wavelengths employed are red (660 nm) and near infrared (940 nm). These wavelengths produce maximal differences in light absorption of O_2Hb and reduced Hb. Light-emitting diodes function as the light source. The two wavelengths are passed through an arterial bed. The percentage of O_2Hb and reduced Hb is determined by measuring the ratio of infrared and red light transmitted to a photodetector.

The oxygen saturation measured by a pulse oximeter is not the same as the SaO_2 measured by a laboratory co-oximeter. The pulse oximeter measures the "functional" saturation of hemoglobin. Functional saturation represents the amount of O_2Hb reported as a percentage of the total of reduced Hb and O_2Hb. (Functional SaO_2 = O_2Hb/ O_2Hb + reduced Hb × 100.) Laboratory co-oximeters use multiple wavelengths that distinguish other types of Hb, e.g., carboxy (COHb) and methemoglobin (MetHb). These instruments measure the "fractional" saturation, which is determined by the following: fractional SaO_2 = O_2Hb/(O_2Hb + reduced Hb + COHb + MetHb) × 100.

This feature explains why an SpO_2 measurement can exceed the SaO_2 reading reported by a laboratory co-oximeter. MetHb and COHb are typically in low concentrations, except in certain pathologic conditions.

In addition to spectrophotometric analysis, the pulse oximeter utilizes a plethysmographic waveform to differentiate the pulsatile "arterial" Hb saturation from the nonpulsatile "venous" blood and absorption from other tissues such as skin, muscle, and bone.[28] The pulsatile arterial bed (e.g., a finger) is positioned between the light-emitting diodes and the photodetector. The amount of light detected is altered by the pulsatile waveform, creating a change in the length of the light path. The amplitude of the detected light depends on the changing arterial pulse, the wavelength of light used, and the oxygen saturation of the arterial blood. The absence of a pulsatile waveform, e.g., extreme hypothermia or hypoperfusion, limits the ability of a pulse oximeter to calculate the SpO_2.

The clinical application of pulse oximetry is quite extensive. The monitoring of SpO_2 has been utilized in all patient age groups to detect and prevent hypoxemia. The clinical benefits of pulse oximetry are enhanced because the instrument is noninvasive, continuous, autocalibrating, has a quick response time, and is easy to use.

Clinical accuracy is typically reported to be ±2–3% for a wide range of SpO_2 values (70–100%).[29] Accuracy and response time vary, depending on the manufacturer, patient characteristics, study methodology, and sensor placement.[30] The appropriate use of pulse oximetry necessitates an appreciation of both physiologic and technical limitations. Despite the numerous clinical benefits of pulse oximetry, other factors can greatly impact on its accuracy and reliability.

Since pulse oximetry measures functional hemoglobin saturation, a factitiously high SpO_2 results when carboxyhemoglobin or methemoglobin levels are above normal. SpO_2 should not be regarded as an early warning device except when conditions exist in which oxygenation is impaired and the hemoglobin saturation has already encroached upon the steep portion of the oxyhemoglobin dissociation curve. Shifts in the oxyhemoglobin dissociation curve also influence the relationship between PaO_2 and SpO_2.

Poorly perfused (low-flow) conditions caused by hypothermia, hypotension, altered vascular resistance, or the use of vasoactive drugs can reduce the pulsatile signal, limiting the instrument's ability to calculate an accurate estimate of SaO_2. It is often necessary to change sensor sites to obtain an optimal signal.

Motion may interfere with the pulse oximeter. Motion artifacts occur commonly in awake, agitated, or shivering patients. Neonates and pediatric patients are prone to create artifacts caused by motion. Signal averaging reduces the impact of motion but also lengthens the response time. Software algorithms for artifact rejection and signal identification have been incorporated into clinical instruments. The presence of a heart rate discrepancy between the electrocardiogram and the pulse oximeter should alert the user to the potential for motion artifact.

Ambient light can contaminate a light-emitting diode signal[31] as can other light sources such as xenon, radiant warmers, fluorescent lights, or phototherapy devices. The oximeter sensor should be covered to reduce light contamination. Light-emitting diode sensors may lose their specificity to emit the proper wavelength when exposed to cold environments.

The presence of any substance in the blood that absorbs light in the red or infrared spectrum may produce spurious SpO_2 readings. Methylene blue absorbs light in the red range (668 nm), causing a reduction in the calculated SpO_2.[32] Indigo carmine and indocyanine green have lesser effects on the SpO_2. Nail polish can alter the spectra of emitted light, depending on the color and number of coats applied. Blue, black, and green produce the most significant reductions of SpO_2.[33]

The presence of dysfunctional hemoglobins can alter the ability of the SpO_2 to reflect the true SaO_2. COHb is read as O_2Hb by pulse oximeters, producing a falsely high SpO_2. COHb causes a leftward shift in the oxyhemoglobin dissociation curve. In patients with suspected increases in COHb, the SaO_2 should be checked using a laboratory co-oximeter.

MetHb also influences the accuracy of pulse oximetry. MetHb absorbs both red and infrared light. At a high level of MetHb, the SpO_2 tends to be 85%, irrespective of the actual PaO_2 or SaO_2. Fetal Hb has limited influence on the accuracy of the SpO_2.

In general, pulse oximeters are simple to use and provide excellent information for monitoring the adequacy of arterial oxygenation. Complications from the use of pulse oximetry are most commonly caused by errors in data interpretation. Reports of burns and pressure necrosis in infants exist but are quite infrequent.[34]

The scope of pulse oximetry is increasing. Today, most clinical devices have sensors that utilize transmittance technology. Reflectance instruments have also been developed that permit the application of oximetric sensors to alternative sites, including the chest and forehead. Tracking the plethysmographic signal over flat surfaces is technically difficult. Further development is still needed to ensure accuracy and clinical efficacy.

Transcutaneous Oxygen Monitoring

Although pulse oximetry and capnography have become the most commonly employed devices in anesthesiology, other modalities have been successfully utilized for oxygen and carbon dioxide monitoring. In the 1970s, transcutaneous oxygen monitoring was popular when caring for neonates and premature infants having cardiorespiratory difficulties.[35]

The transcutaneous oxygen sensor utilizes a polaro-

TABLE 28-3. Clinical Utility of $Ptco_2$

Cardiac Output	PaO_2	$Ptco_2$ Trends
Normal	Normal	PaO_2
Normal	Decreased	PaO_2
Decreased	Normal	Flow
Decreased	Decreased	Oxygen delivery

graphic oxygen electrode to measure oxygen that diffuses to the skin's surface from the dermal capillary bed. The electrode is a miniaturized modification of the standard Clark electrode (see Chapter 7).

Transcutaneous oxygen tension ($Ptco_2$) is not identical to the PaO_2 (Table 28-3). Under normal circumstances, oxygen flow through the skin is very low and the $Ptco_2$ is considerably lower than the PaO_2. Heating the cutaneous electrode to 43°C allows oxygen to diffuse more rapidly through the stratum corneum; shifts the oxyhemoglobin dissociation curve to the left, thereby increasing the local oxygen tension; and arterializes the dermal capillary bed (except in severely compromised low-flow states).[36] Heating compensates for the low diffusion of oxygen across the skin. In neonates and young infants, there is a good correlation between $Ptco_2$ and PaO_2. In adults, heating the skin is only partially successful in enhancing cutaneous oxygen flow, thus reducing the usefulness of $Ptco_2$.

The correlation between $Ptco_2$ and PaO_2 is directional.[36] However, the correlation is lessened if skin perfusion is compromised. $Ptco_2$ is flow-dependent. During shock states, the $Ptco_2$ tends to correlate with changes in cardiac output. If hypoxemia and hypoperfusion coexist, the $Ptco_2$ trend indicates changes in oxygen delivery, which is defined as the product of cardiac output and arterial oxygen content. Therefore, decreasing $Ptco_2$ could be utilized as a continuous, noninvasive, early warning monitor of tissue perfusion (hypoperfusion). An arterial blood gas determination is essential to determine whether a reduction in $Ptco_2$ is the result of changes in gas exchange or perfusion.

Several additional limitations and risks have been associated with $Ptco_2$ monitoring. Hypothermia reduces cutaneous blood flow; edema or obesity may interfere with oxygen diffusion. Nitrous oxide and halothane can react with the $Ptco_2$ electrode, causing an upward drift of the $Ptco_2$.[37] The site of application can produce variability in the measured $Ptco_2$. The preferred sites are the chest and abdomen. Use of peripheral sites tends to underestimate PaO_2, even when perfusion is normal.

Proper sensor application is crucial for accuracy of transcutaneous gas monitoring. A loose or dislodged sensor will be influenced by room air oxygen. Excessive external pressure tends to compress the dermal capillaries, producing a falsely low $Ptco_2$ reading. Other limitations include a 10–20 minute warm-up time, calibration requirements, a slow response time, and electrode drift.[38]

Skin burns are the most common complication associated with $Ptco_2$ monitoring. The incidence of burns appears to be a function of the cutaneous electrode temperature and the duration of monitoring at the same location. In neonates, changing the sensor site every 2 hours reduces the likelihood of thermal injury. Adults can tolerate a 44°C sensor for up to 6 hours without thermal injury. Under normal use, the underlying skin appears hyperemic and erythematous. This usually resolves within 24 hours following removal of the electrode.

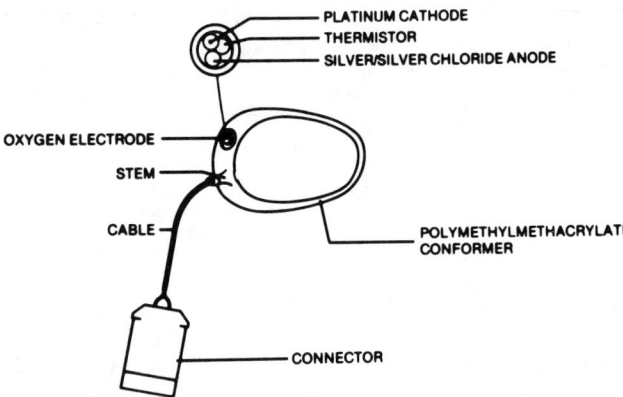

Figure 28-3. The conjunctival oxygen monitoring probe. (Reproduced with permission from Brown M, Vender JS: Non-invasive oxygen monitoring. Crit Care Clin 4:493, 1988.)

Transconjunctival Oxygen Monitoring

Transconjunctival oxygen monitoring ($Pcjo_2$) provides an additional method with which to assess arterial oxygenation.[24] Similar to $Ptco_2$, the $Pcjo_2$ monitor utilizes a miniaturized Clark electrode. The electrode is fitted into a polymethyl methacrylate ophthalmic conformer and rests against the palpebral conjunctiva. The device requires a two-point calibration prior to placement over the eye. Figure 28-3 diagrams the scleral conformer and electrode assembly.

In contrast to $Ptco_2$, $Pcjo_2$ electrodes are unheated. The capillary vessels of the palpebral conjunctiva are close to the surface and are not covered by a "thick" layer of oxygen-consuming tissue.[39] $Pcjo_2$ electrodes have a faster response time (60 seconds) compared with transcutaneous electrodes. The $Pcjo_2$ value is always less than the measured Pao_2. Analogous to the $Ptco_2$ value, accuracy is greatest when hemodynamic stability exists. Since population studies demonstrate a wide individual variation in $Pcjo_2$ measurements, the monitor is best used as an indicator of changes in Pao_2 within a given individual. In general, $Pcjo_2$ reflects changes in Pao_2, cardiac output, and oxygen delivery, as described for $Ptco_2$.

$Pcjo_2$ monitors oxygenation of a tissue bed vascularized by a branch of the ophthalmic artery, making $Pcjo_2$ a potentially important monitor during carotid endarterectomy.[40] $Pcjo_2$ reflects changes produced by cross-clamping, manipulation, or arterial obstruction. $Pcjo_2$ is least affected by global low flow states, since both the cerebral and ophthalmic circulations are preferentially preserved compared with peripheral arterial flow. Complications of $Pcjo_2$ monitoring are rare.[41] Mild irritation or corneal abrasions may occur. Chemosis of the conjunctiva and allergic reactions to the polymers of the ophthalmic conformer have been recognized.

Transcutaneous and Transconjunctival Carbon Dioxide Monitoring

Surface electrodes for CO_2 monitoring have also been developed. The fundamental concepts for $Ptcco_2$ and $Pcjco_2$ monitoring are similar to those described for O_2 monitoring.

The $Ptcco_2$ electrode is based on the Stowe-Severinghaus CO_2 electrode (see Chapter 7). Although CO_2 diffuses through the skin more readily than O_2, heating the $Ptcco_2$ electrode is still necessary. Heat shortens the response time and improves the correlation with $Paco_2$ measurements. Since heating the skin increases the local metabolic rate, $Ptcco_2$ tends to exceed the $Paco_2$ by a multiple of 1.3, and many devices incorporate a correction factor to improve the correlation with $Paco_2$.[38] Unlike the $Ptco_2$, a decrease in perfusion causes an increase in the $Ptcco_2$ as a result of locally augmented CO_2 production. $Ptcco_2$ instruments require calibration and maintenance, and there is a tendency for them to drift over time. When the limitations of the instrument are understood, $Ptcco_2$ is a reasonable noninvasive method for monitoring the prevailing tendency of the $Paco_2$. The clinical applications of $Ptcco_2$ and $Pcjco_2$ during anesthesia have been quite limited. Utilization of $Ptcco_2$ has gained greater acceptance in neonatal and pediatric patients.

BLOOD PRESSURE MONITORING

Intraoperative measurement and recording of arterial blood pressure has been an essential aspect of anesthesia care and is mandated as an important indicator of the adequacy of circulation during anesthesia.[3] Systemic blood pressure monitoring is commonly performed indirectly using encircling cuffs or directly by inserting an arterial line and transducing the arterial pressure trace. The means and methods for the estimation of arterial blood pressure are not stipulated, and today anesthesiologists have at their disposal a variety of techniques for measuring changes in systolic, diastolic, mean arterial, and pulse pressures.

Traditionally, anesthesiologists routinely measure and record the systolic and diastolic pressures at 5-minute intervals. Changes in systolic blood pressure have been correlated with changes in myocardial oxygen requirements.[42] Diastolic pressure is an important determinant of the adequacy of coronary perfusion.[43] Mean arterial pressure (the integrated mean of the pressure wave) represents the "hydrostatic force" that powers diffusion and filtration functions. Mean arterial pressure (P) is often used in conjunction with resistance (R) when estimating organ perfusion (Q) or cardiac output ($Q \approx P/R$).

Arterial Pressure Wave

The size, shape, and transmission of the pressure wave throughout the arterial circulation are complex and are related to the dynamics of pulsatile flow, the acceleration and deceleration of blood, the elasticity of the large conducting arteries, and a modulated impedance that controls regional blood flow. Factors that contribute to the propagation and character of the pressure pulse include the energy content imparted by ventricular systole (1–600 watts); contour transformation by the vascular tree; and reflective waves that are produced at the periphery. Arterial pressure is created by the interaction of myocardial and vascular factors imparting potential and kinetic energy to a dynamic arterial blood volume.

Estimates of pressure recorded in the ascending aorta are expected to be fundamentally different from those measured in a peripheral artery. Figure 28-4 demonstrates the paradox that as blood pressure is examined from the aorta to the distal arteries, the pressure appears to increase.[44] The tapering of peripheral arteries confines the pressure trace energy, producing an increase in systolic pressure. Measurements

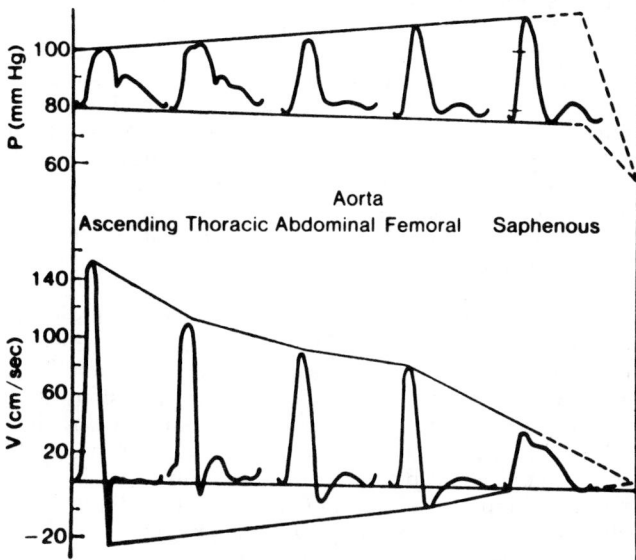

Figure 28-4. Blood pressure and velocity measurements in normal arteries of dogs. As measurements are made further away from the ascending aorta, estimates of systolic pressure increase while the blood velocity decreases. The apparent increases in blood pressure occur as a result of reflected waves. (Reproduced with permission from Milnor WR: Hemodynamics. Baltimore, Williams & Wilkins, 1989.)

from sites where impedance differences exist demonstrate interference from reflected waves. Therefore, the character of the pressure wave as well as of the values measured are different at various locations in the arterial tree. In peripheral arteries, intra-arterial measurements demonstrate that although systolic pressure is higher, mean pressure is lower than in the aorta, resulting from forward wave propagation and wave reflection.[45] Reflection is an inherent characteristic of the arterial tree and produces resonant waves that are directed back toward the proximal aorta.

Arterial blood pressure represents the lateral pressure exerted on arteries by blood as it flows. During the cardiac cycle, an arterial pulse wave results as the left ventricular stroke volume is ejected into the blood-filled arterial vascular tree. The elasticity of the aorta and conducting arteries (arterial tree compliance) and physiologic factors such as blood volume, stroke volume, cardiac output, and peripheral vascular resistance determine the beat-to-beat arterial blood pressure.

Direct and indirect measurements of arterial blood pressure are, to a great extent, dependent on our ability to evaluate the quality and character of the arterial pulse wave. Many factors influence the accuracy of blood pressure monitoring. Monitoring techniques, no matter how simple or sophisticated, are often constrained by the natural properties of fluid motion and physiologic alterations that may influence accuracy and precision. Since blood is relatively incompressible, blood pressure measurements rely on devices (transducers) that convert pressure (force/unit area) into another form of energy (see Chapter 7). The traditional Riva-Rocci auscultatory method utilizes sound waves produced when blood flow is restored in the brachial artery following its occlusion.

Maintaining an adequate blood pressure is important for preserving organ function, and intraoperative management

of blood pressure is an inherent part of anesthesia. Blood pressure is presumed to serve as an indicator of the adequacy of tissue perfusion or of cardiac function. Although the relationship between blood flow, pressure, and peripheral resistance is well known ($\dot{Q} = P/R$), pressure by itself cannot be considered a reliable index of the adequacy of perfusion.[46]

Discrepancies between indirect methods of estimating systemic blood pressure and intra-arterial pressure measurements occur frequently. Indirect measurements of the arterial blood pressure are dependent on changes in flow or volume, and indirect estimates of diastolic and systolic blood pressures frequently are lower than simultaneously recorded intra-arterial measurements. Although some of the differences are related to the constraints of hydraulically coupled transducing systems, it is probable that real differences exist based on differing methodology, since intra-arterial blood pressure monitoring is based on force displacement rather than transformations in flow or volume.

Indirect Measurement of Arterial Blood Pressure

The simplest method of blood pressure determination estimates systolic blood pressure by palpating the return of the arterial pulse while an occluding cuff is deflated. Modifications of this technique include the observance of the return of Doppler sounds, the transduced arterial pressure trace, or a photoplethysmographic pulse wave.[47]

Auscultation of the Korotkoff sounds permits estimation of both systolic (SP) and diastolic (DP) blood pressures. Mean arterial blood pressure (MAP) can be calculated using an estimating equation (MAP = DP + 1/3SP-DP). Comparisons of direct intra-arterial pressure recordings with auscultation can show considerable divergence. Korotkoff sounds result from turbulent flow within an artery in response to the mechanical deformation from the blood pressure cuff. Systolic blood pressure is signaled by the appearance of the first Korotkoff sound. Disappearance of the sounds or a muffled tone signals the diastolic blood pressure.

The detection of sound changes is subjective and prone to errors based on deficiencies in sound transmission or hearing. Cuff deflation rate also influences accuracy. Quick deflations (>3 mm Hg per second) underestimate blood pressure. Palpation and auscultatory techniques require pulsatile blood flow and are unreliable during conditions of low flow.[48] These techniques are reasonably accurate when aneroid gauges are within calibration, the encircling cuff is appropriately sized and positioned, the inflation is above the true systolic pressure, and the Korotkoff sounds or pulse is properly identified.

Blood Pressure Cuffs

All cuff-based blood pressure measurements require the application of encircling blood pressure cuffs that contain inflatable bladders. Estimates of arterial blood pressure are related to either the equilibration of the pressure within the bladder (palpatory, auscultatory, and Doppler) or the changes of pressure and motion of the bladder during deflation (oscillometry). The American Heart Association recommends that the bladder width should approximate 40% of the circumference of the extremity. Bladder length should be sufficient to encircle at least 60% of the extremity.[49] Falsely high estimates result when blood pressure cuffs are too small, when they are applied too loosely, when the extremity is below heart level, or when uneven compression is transmitted to the underlying artery. Falsely low estimates result when cuffs are too large, when the extremity is above heart level, or following quick deflations.

Doppler sphygmomanometry is based on the detection of the Doppler-shift signal following the restoration of blood flow upon deflation of a blood pressure cuff (see Chapter 7). Studies have demonstrated good correlation of Doppler sphygmomanometry with direct arterial measurements of systolic arterial blood pressure.[50] Compact battery-operated Doppler devices are helpful in clinical situations, in which it is difficult to determine systolic arterial blood pressure indirectly because of low flow.[51] The Doppler-shift signal is best identified over the compressed arterial wall using a coupling gel to enhance the transmittance of the sound waves.

Since 1976, microprocessor-controlled oscillotonometers have replaced auscultatory and palpatory techniques for routine intraoperative blood pressure monitoring. Oscillometry accurately and directly measures mean blood pressure by sensing the point of maximal fluctuations in cuff pressure produced while deflating a blood pressure cuff.

Modern microprocessor-controlled oscillotonometers (e.g., Dinamap, Critikon Inc, Tampa, FL) measure systolic and diastolic blood pressures and mean arterial pressure by sampling oscillations in the cuff and determining parameter identification points for each respective measurement.[52,53] Substantial differences exist among the many microprocessor-controlled oscillotonometers with respect to their proprietary parameter identification points and method of operation. In a generic microprocessor-controlled oscillotonometer, cuff pressure is sensed by a pressure transducer whose output is digitized for processing. After the cuff is inflated by an air pump, cuff pressure is held constant while oscillations are sampled. If no oscillations are sampled, the computer opens a deflation valve, and the next level is sampled for oscillations. Artifact-rejection algorithms are implemented by the step-wise deflation–parameter identification points cycle. Microprocessor-controlled oscillotonometers compare the amplitude of oscillation pairs and numerically display their estimates. Figure 28-5 graphically depicts the responses of a Dinamap. During this inflation cycle, the ef-

fect of respiratory variation, a premature ventricular complex, and cuff movement are demonstrated.

Automated oscillometry has been demonstrated to correlate well with direct intra-arterial measurement of mean arterial and diastolic blood pressures.[54] Microprocessor-controlled oscillotonometers may underestimate systolic blood pressure, with mean errors reported from −6.9 to −8.6 mm Hg when compared with direct radial artery pressures.[55] The Association for the Advancement of Medical Instrumentation states that microprocessor-controlled oscillotonometers have a mean error of less than 5 mm Hg when compared with a centrally placed arterial line.[52]

Oscillometry requires the careful evaluation of several cardiac cycles at each increment of deflation in order to smooth out pronounced respiratory variations or motion artifacts. Cuff movement or erratic pulse transmission influences the accuracy of all microprocessor-controlled oscillotonometers. The time necessary to display the measured mean arterial blood pressure and the estimates of systolic and diastolic pressures vary, depending on the proprietary software that integrates the inflation/deflation cycle and the analysis of the amplitude of oscillations. In the anesthetized patient, automated oscillometry is usually accurate and versatile. A variety of cuff sizes make it possible to utilize oscillometry in all age groups. Although upper arm cuffs are most commonly employed, other locations may be acceptable for cuff placement, including the thigh, calf, ankle, or lower arm. Modern instruments incorporate faster access modes that are useful in situations in which rapid changes in arterial blood pressure are anticipated.

Indirect Continuous Noninvasive Techniques

Peñaz has described a method that holds the size of the digital arteries of a finger constant and alters the pressure within a finger cuff.[56] The device uses infrared light and detects oscillations within the finger cuff. Using a very fast servomechanism and pump, the Finapres adjusts the pressure in the finger cuff during each cardiac cycle, preventing the digital arteries from expanding (loading) during systole and vice versa (unloading) during diastole. The device modulates cuff pressure so that the plethysmographic excur-

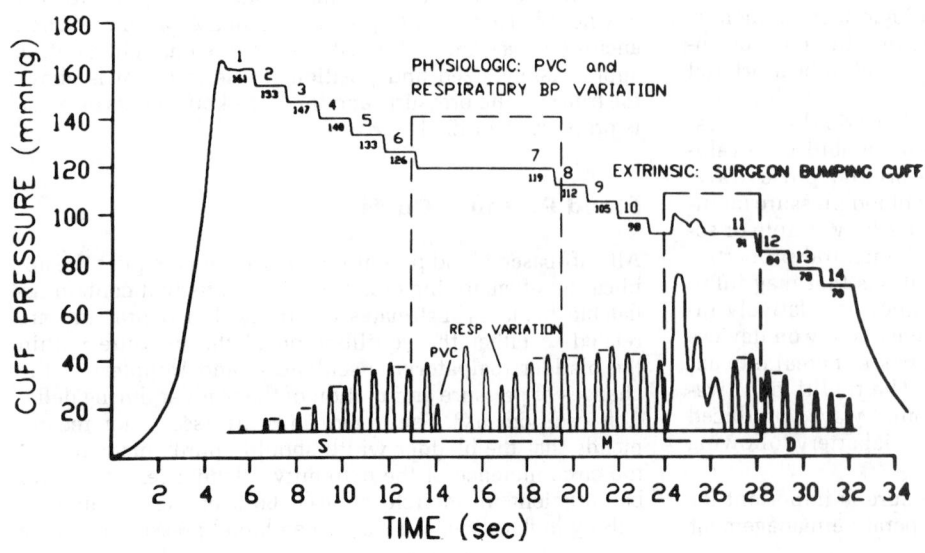

Figure 28-5. Diagram illustrating motion artifact, a premature ventricular contraction, and respiratory artifact as sensed by a Dinamap noninvasive blood pressure monitor. (Reproduced with permission from Ramsey M: Blood pressure monitoring: Automated oscillometric devices. J Clin Monit 7:56, 1991.)

sions are kept to a minimum. Transmural arterial pressure is constrained so that the variations in cuff pressure are identical to the finger arterial pressure pulsations. Photoplethysmography creates a calibrated arterial pressure trace.

Arterial spasm following cardiopulmonary bypass or following administration of phenylephrine has been demonstrated to affect the reliability of early prototypes of the Finapres.[57] The device is susceptible to hydrostatic errors resulting from changing the position of the transducer-servomechanism.

Another unique approach to providing continuous, noninvasive blood pressure monitoring is based on measuring the pulse wave velocity. Studies have identified a linear relationship between the pulse wave velocity and changes in mean arterial blood pressure.[58] ARTRAC estimates systolic and diastolic blood pressures by measuring the pulse wave velocity and changes in blood volume using two photometric sensors placed on the forehead and a digit. The technique requires calibration from a cuff-based or invasive arterial blood pressure reading. Since the technology utilizes the alternating portion of two reflectance oximeter probes, the instrument also calculates oxygen saturation. Clinical trials have demonstrated that ARTRAC can detect beat-to-beat changes in arterial blood pressure and compares favorably with intra-arterial pressure estimates.

Arterial tonometry is another promising technology for noninvasive, continuous blood pressure monitoring. Tonometry can be performed using any superficial artery that is in close proximity to an underlying bone, e.g., the radial, dorsalis pedis, or temporal artery. Accurate tonometric measurements require flattening of the artery so that a force displacement transducer located in the tonometer senses the force due to blood pressure. A computer controls a pneumatic bladder that maintains the "hold-down pressure" to create the correct geometry for the transducer to track arterial pressure. Currently available instruments incorporate multiple sensors in the tonomoter housing, which greatly simplifies the task of positioning and increases the precision of estimates of the measurements.

After placement, the instrument automatically performs a calibration using oscillometry. Periodic cuff measurements adjust the continuous estimate derived from tonometry. Clinical studies suggest that arterial tonometry can provide accurate, reliable, real-time blood pressure values and pressure waveforms that compare favorably with invasive blood pressure measurements.[59] Although tonometry is a promising technology, its performance during low-flow states or when peripheral vascular resistance is increased has not been studied. Motion artifacts are another potential concern.

Problems Associated With Noninvasive Monitoring

Cuff-based pressure monitoring systems are inherently safer than invasive monitoring. When clinical circumstances require frequent blood pressure readings, it is advisable to periodically move the cuff to alternative sites in order to reduce the possibility of nerve injury, extremity edema, or petechiae formation. Failure to deflate the cuff increases venous pressure and, if the cuff is left unattended, could reduce tissue perfusion. Ulnar neuropathy has been described following the use of automated cycled blood pressure cuffs. Compression of the ulnar nerve can be avoided by applying the encircling cuff proximal to the ulnar groove.

Automated sequencing may alter the timing of intravenous drug administration when the intravenous access site is located in the same extremity. Difficulty occurs with automated cuff cycling instruments in determining appropriate deflation cycles in patients with tremors or shivering. Aside from the errors related to movement, a compartment syndrome attributed to a prolonged inflation cycle has been described.[60]

Hydrostatic errors occur when blood pressure cuffs are placed on extremities that are above or below the level of the right atrium. The hydrostatic offset can be mathematically corrected by adding (above) or subtracting (below) 0.7 mm Hg for each centimeter that the cuff is off the horizontal plane of the heart.

Invasive Measurement of Arterial Blood Pressure

Indwelling arterial cannulation not only offers anesthesiologists the opportunity to monitor beat-to-beat changes in arterial blood pressure but also provides vascular access for arterial blood sampling. Although thought of as the gold standard, intra-arterial techniques are subject to many sources of error based on the physical properties of fluid motion and the performance of the catheter-transducer-amplification system used to sense, process, and display the pressure pulse wave. Ideally, a transduced intra-arterial pressure trace faithfully emulates the beat-to-beat changes that occur in the arterial vascular tree during systolic ejection.

Direct arterial blood pressure monitoring utilizes saline-filled tubings that transmit the force of the pressure pulse wave to a transducer that converts the beat-to-beat pressure changes into voltage changes (see Chapter 7). These voltage changes are amplified, filtered, and displayed as the arterial pressure trace. High fidelity recordings of the arterial pressure trace and their analysis (Fourier series or power spectrum analysis) indicate that the arterial pressure wave (input) contains frequencies from 1–30 Hz (1 Hz = 60 cycles per second). Most of the frequency components contained in the arterial pressure wave are below 10 Hz.

The behavior of transducers, fluid couplings, signal amplification, and displays can be described by a second-order differential equation in which the mass, elasticity, and resistance of the transducing system are related to input. Solving the equation predicts the output (transduced arterial pressure trace) and characterizes the system's performance.

The fidelity of any fluid-coupled transducing system is constrained by two properties: damping (ζ) and natural frequency (Fo). Zeta (ζ) describes the tendency for "fluid" in the measuring system to extinguish motion. Fo describes the tendency for the measuring system to resonate.

The fidelity of the transduced pressure depends on optimizing ζ and Fo, thus permitting the to-and-fro movement of the coupling tubing and transducer to faithfully reproduce the range of frequencies contained in the arterial pressure wave. This can be described as the system's band width. The band width is represented by the frequency response beginning at 0 (no perturbations) to the frequency at which the system begins to resonate (ring) and amplify and distort the arterial wave signal. Resonance occurs at the Fo. Conventional disposable transducers coupled with 60 inches of pressure tubing have a Fo of approximately 20–30 Hz.

Damping lowers the effective band width. If the system is underdamped ($\zeta = 0.2$), the effective band width is reduced by 20%. Optimally damped systems have a band width of approximately two thirds of the Fo. If Fo ap-

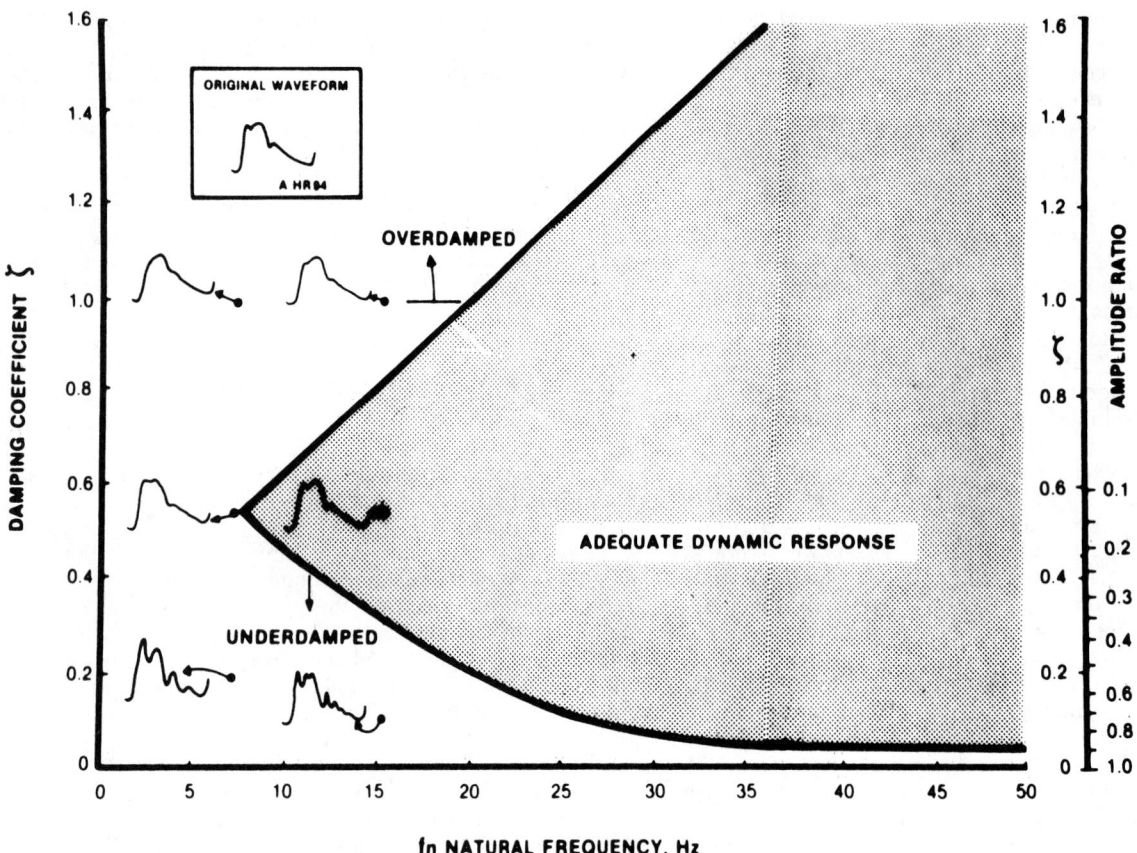

Figure 28-6. The relationship between the frequency of fluid-filled transducing systems and damping. The shaded area represents the appropriate range of damping for a given natural frequency (F_n). The size of the wedge is also dependent on the steepness of the arterial pressure trace and heart rate. (Reproduced with permission from Gardner RM: Direct blood pressure measurement-dynamic response requirements. Anesthesiology 54:231, 1981.)

proaches the frequencies found in the arterial pressure wave (<10 Hz), estimates of the systolic blood pressure will increase because the fluid-filled coupling system resonates. Figure 28-6 demonstrates the effect of damping on the character of an arterial pressure trace.

Studies have demonstrated that fidelity is optimized when catheters and tubings are very stiff, the mass of the fluid is small, the number of stopcocks is limited, and the connecting tubing is not excessive. Air bubbles lower the natural frequency of catheter-transducer systems.[61,62]

In clinical practice, underdamped catheter-transducer systems tend to overestimate systolic pressure by 15–30 mm Hg and amplify artifact (catheter whip). Excessive increases in ζ reduce fidelity and underestimate systolic pressure. Overdamping reduces the fidelity of the system and underestimates the systolic blood pressure. Dynamic calibration can determine the fidelity of the pressure recording system. In clinical practice, it is sufficient to place the transducer at the level of the right atrium, open the stopcock to the atmosphere, and balance the electronic amplifying system to display "zero"; attaching a calibrated mercury manometer to the stopcock will permit a stepwise calibration (static calibration). Periodic checks of the reference point zero are necessary to detect and eliminate transducer drift.

Since many therapeutic decisions are based on changes in arterial blood pressure, it is imperative that anesthesiologists understand the physical limitations imposed by fluid-filled pressure transducer systems. Significant exaggeration of pressure measurements should be expected when a fluid-filled pressure transducer system has a resonant frequency in the range of the pressure wave frequencies occurring in the circulation. Systolic pressure is underestimated when measured with overdamping systems and overestimated by underdamped or resonating systems. Similar errors occur for the estimation of diastolic pressure. Mean pressure estimates are accurately monitored even when conditions of damping and resonance are not optimal.

Monitor manufacturers filter the transducer signal, removing the higher frequencies carried in the electrical signal and thereby reducing the fidelity of the monitoring system. Filtering (electrical damping) is beneficial in reducing noise from electrocautery and improving overall performance.

Today's modern monitors digitize the electrical signal, which permits software-specific analysis of time-weighted averages or the graphic display of the pressures of interest over time. Numeric displays of pressure values are based on proprietary algorithms requiring interpretation before initiating therapy. During anesthesia, the character of the displayed arterial waveform may vary greatly from central aortic pressure. This is particularly true during the harvesting of internal mammary arteries and following cardiopulmonary bypass, when significantly lower systolic and mean radial artery pressures are frequently observed.[63,64]

Arterial Cannulation

The radial artery remains the most popular site for cannulation because of its accessibility and the presence of a collateral blood supply. In the past, assessment of the patency of the ulnar circulation by performance of an Allen's test has been recommended prior to radial artery cannulation. Allen's test is performed by compressing both radial and ulnar arteries while the patient tightens his or her fist. Releasing pressure on each respective artery determines the dominant vessel supplying blood to the hand. The prognostic value of the Allen's test in assessing the adequacy of the ulnar collateral circulation may have been overestimated.[65,66]

Abnormal radial artery blood flow following the removal of arterial lines occurs frequently. Studies suggest that blood flow normalizes in 3–70 days.[66,67] Radial artery thrombosis can be minimized by using nontapered 20–22 gauge catheters constructed of Teflon, avoiding polypropylene-tapered catheters, and reducing the duration of arterial cannulation.[67-69] During cannula removal, the potential for thromboembolism may be diminished by compressing the proximal and distal arteries while aspirating the cannula during withdrawal.[70]

Many cannulation sites have been used for direct arterial blood pressure monitoring (Table 28-4). Three techniques for cannulation are common: direct arterial puncture, guidewire-assisted cannulation (Seldinger's technique), and the transfixion-withdrawal method. When assessing an appropriate upper extremity location for arterial cannulation, it is important to check the cuff blood pressure in each arm prior to selection and avoid using arterial access distal to angiography.[71]

A necessary condition for percutaneous placement is identification of the arterial pulse. Doppler flow probes are helpful in clinical situations in which the location of the arterial pressure pulse is difficult to palpate.

Complications of Invasive Monitoring

Arterial cannulation is regarded as an invasive procedure with a documented morbidity. Ischemia following radial artery cannulation resulting from thrombosis, proximal emboli, or prolonged shock has been described.[71,72] Contributing factors include severe atherosclerosis, diabetes, low cardiac output, and intense peripheral vasoconstriction. Ischemia, hemorrhage, thrombosis, embolism, cerebral air embolism, aneurysm formation, arteriovenous fistula formation, and infection have occurred as the direct result of arterial cannulation, arterial blood sampling, or high pressure flushing.

Continuous flush devices are incorporated into disposable transducer kits and infuse at $3–6$ ml·h^{-1}. In neonates, the infusion volume may contribute to fluid overload. Continuous flush devices have little effect on the blood pressure measurement. However, pressurized flush devices may serve as a source of an air embolism. Removing air from the pressure bag, stopcocks, and tubings minimizes the potential for air embolism.

Special Problems of Invasive Monitoring

Invasive monitoring is indicated if known or suspected cardiovascular instability is anticipated during the administration of anesthesia. Invasive monitoring is necessary when noninvasive techniques do not afford accurate or convenient measurements of blood pressure or when frequent arterial blood gases or blood sampling is required.

Arterial catheter systems increase the risk of infection. Aseptic technique for catheter placement, although prudent and necessary, does not eliminate the potential for bacterial contamination during blood sampling. Shinozaki and colleagues[73] found that 16.2% of arterial catheter system stopcocks became contaminated, suggesting that arterial blood sampling is an important source of bacterial contamination of transducer systems.

Direct arterial pressure monitoring requires constant vigilance. The data displayed need to be correlated before therapeutic interventions are initiated. Sudden increases in blood pressure may represent a hydrostatic error because the position of the transducer was not adjusted following the elevation of the operating room table. Sudden decreases often result when blood pressure tracings become damped because the arterial catheter is partially kinked. Before initiating therapy, the transducer system should be "rezeroed" and the patency of the arterial cannula verified. This will ensure the accuracy of the measurement and avoid a potentially dangerous medication error.

TABLE 28-4. Arterial Cannulation

Arterial Cannulation Site	Clinical Points of Interest
Ulnar	Complications similar to those for radial artery Primary source of hand blood flow
Brachial	Insertion site medial to biceps tendon Median nerve damage is potential hazard Can accommodate 18-gauge cannula
Axillary	Insertion site at junction of pectoralis major and deltoid muscles Specialized catheter kit available
Femoral	Easy access in low-flow states Potential for local and retroperitoneal hemorrhage Longer catheters preferred
Dorsalis pedis	Posterior tibial artery collateral circulation Higher systolic pressure estimates Adequate collateral flow needs verification

CENTRAL VENOUS AND PULMONARY ARTERY MONITORING

Central venous pressure cannulas are important portals for intraoperative vascular access and the assessment of changes in cardiac function. For surgical procedures in which the risk of air embolization is high, a properly placed central venous pressure catheter can assist in the diagnosis and treatment of this potentially lethal occurrence. Monitoring central venous pressure by observing changes in a fluid-filled manometer continues to be an option for appraising the fluid volume status of patients. Today, it is common to continuously measure central venous pressure using a saline-filled catheter-transducer system identical to those described for arterial pressure monitoring.

Percutaneous insertion of central venous pressure catheters is a skill that every anesthesiologist needs to acquire. The right internal jugular vein is the preferred site for cannulation by anesthesiologists because it is accessible from the head of the operating table, has a predictable anatomy, and has a high success rate of use in both adults and children.[74] Left-sided internal jugular cannulation can also be utilized but is less desirable because of the potential for damaging the thoracic duct or difficulty in maneuvering catheters through the jugular-subclavian junction. Additionally, the potential for accidental puncture of the left carotid artery and embolization to the left dominant cerebral hemisphere are often cited as reasons to avoid left-sided internal jugular cannulation.

Three techniques for right internal jugular vein insertion (posterior, central, and anterior) have been described based on their relationship with the two heads of the sternocleidomastoid muscle.[75] Many excellent descriptions of the anatomic landmarks are available for study. The following key points will aid in successful and safe internal jugular vein cannulation:

- Position patients carefully to adequately assess landmarks;
- Whenever possible, use a head-down position (Trendelenburg) to distend the vessel and avoid air embolization;

- The course of the internal jugular vein is variable but customarily follows a line from the mastoid process along the clavicular head of the sternocleidomastoid muscle;
- Use 22-gauge "seeker" needles before placing large-bore catheters or sheaths.
- Verification of venous access is essential before passing large-bore catheters or sheaths (e.g., by assessment of blood oxygen saturation, oxygen tension, color, pressure, or waveform). Failure to do so may lead to accidental cannulation of the carotid artery.

Alternatives to the internal jugular vein include the external jugular vein, subclavian vein, antecubital vein, and femoral vein. Table 28-5 lists problems or risks associated with various access sites.

Central Venous Pressure Monitoring

Whereas the value of central venous access (for administration of drugs and fluids) cannot be argued, the benefit of central venous pressure monitoring has been the subject of much debate. Central venous pressure is essentially equivalent to right atrial pressure. Conditions that affect right atrial pressure are reflected by changes in the central venous pressure. The normal central venous pressure waveform consists of three peaks (a, c, and v waves) and two descents (x, y), each resulting from the ebb and flow of blood in the right atrium. Corresponding events occur in the left atrium (Fig. 28-7).[84]

The character of the central venous pressure tracing is dependent on many factors, including heart rate, heart rhythm (conduction disturbances), tricuspid valve function, normal and abnormal intrathoracic pressure changes, and changes in right ventricular compliance.

When tachycardia is present, the central venous pressure waves fuse, limiting their diagnostic value. In patients with atrial fibrillation, a waves are absent. In patients in whom "resistance" to the emptying of the right atrium is present, large a waves are observed. Examples include impaired right atrial emptying owing to tricuspid stenosis, right ven-

TABLE 28-5. Central Venous Cannulation Sites

Location	Advantages	Disadvantages	Reference
Right internal jugular	Accessible Good landmarks	Carotid artery puncture Trauma to brachial plexus Pneumothorax	Shah[76] Belani[77]
External jugular	Superficial location Safety	Lower success rate Sheath placement Kinks at subclavian vein Subclavian trauma Two sets of valves	Jobes[78]
Subclavian	Accessible Good landmarks	Pneumothorax Hemothorax Chylothorax Pleural effusion	Borja[79]
Antecubital	Limited complications	Lowest success rate Thrombosis Thrombophlebitis Catheter shearing	Webre[80]
Femoral	High success rate	Catheter sepsis Thrombophlebitis	Bansmer[81] Burri[82]

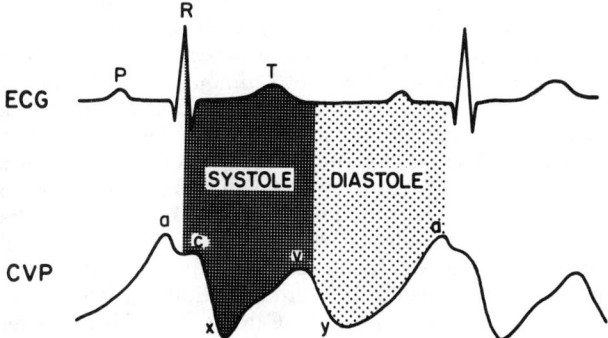

Figure 28-7. The normal central venous pressure trace. (Redrawn with permission from Mark JB: Central venous pressure monitoring: Clinical insights beyond the numbers. J Cardiothorac Vasc Anesth 5:163, 1991.)

tricular hypertrophy due to pulmonic stenosis, or acute or chronic lung disease associated with pulmonary hypertension. Conditions in which right ventricular compliance is abnormal often demonstrate large a waves.

Venous wave changes are also of diagnostic significance. Tricuspid regurgitation (valvular or functional) typically produces giant v waves (regurgitant c-v waves) that begin immediately following the QRS complex. Large v waves may suggest right ventricular ischemia and failure, constrictive pericarditis, or cardiac tamponade. In these conditions, the compliance of the right ventricle is frequently compromised. Diagnosis of right ventricular ischemia is often difficult. A prominent v wave in the central venous pressure tracing is suggestive of right ventricular papillary muscle ischemia and tricuspid regurgitation.[83] The central venous pressure waveform in patients with diminished right ventricular compliance often demonstrates elevated pressures with prominent a and v waves, which together may form an m or w configuration.[84]

Central venous pressure monitoring is helpful in the diagnosis and treatment of pericardial tamponade, in which equalization of diastolic filling pressures typically occurs. As the central venous pressure tracing becomes monophasic, the y descent is lost. Equalization of diastolic filling pressures (central venous pressure, right ventricular diastolic pressure, pulmonary diastolic pressure (PDP), pulmonary wedge pressure) is a characteristic of hemodynamically significant pericardial constriction and cardiac tamponade (see section on Pulmonary Artery Monitoring).[85]

TABLE 28-6. Complications Common to All Central Venous Pressure Catheter Placement Techniques

Accidental arterial puncture
  Hematoma
  False aneurysm
  Arteriovenous fistula
Poor positioning of catheter during placement
  Wall perforation
  Dysrhythmias
Injury to surrounding structures
Clot and fibrinous sleeve formation
Thrombosis of the vein
  Embolus
Catheter-related infections
Guidewire embolus
Bleeding

Following treatment, a dramatic drop in filling pressures, restoration of systemic blood pressure, and a normalization of the central venous pressure waveform should occur.

In patients with left-sided (or combined) heart disease, central venous pressure monitoring is often unreliable in estimating left ventricular filling pressures. Reliable estimates of left atrial pressure are indispensable in patients with hemodynamically significant mitral or aortic disease and in patients with poor ventricular function (often defined by an ejection fraction <0.4). Since central venous pressure monitoring is less invasive and less costly than pulmonary artery monitoring, and offers unique understanding of right-sided hemodynamic events, it is appropriate to utilize it whenever its benefits outweigh the risk of its placement.

Complications of Central Venous Catheters

Significant complications resulting from central line placement occur infrequently. Potentially serious complications have been described for virtually every vascular access location, suggesting that experience and supervision are important considerations when contemplating central venous pressure catheter placement. Table 28-6 lists complications of central venous pressure catheter placement that are common to all venipuncture sites. Table 28-7 focuses attention on the specific complications that have been described for internal jugular and subclavian access. The following sections highlight several complications of central venous catheterization that are of particular interest to anesthesiologists.

Venous Air Embolism

The possibility of venous air embolism during central venous pressure catheter placement or following its removal is a potentially serious occurrence that can be avoided by eliminating the conditions necessary for air entrainment. Venous air embolism may result when a syringe, iv cap, stopcock, or iv connector is removed from a needle, catheter, or sheath that is placed in a vein with a subatmospheric pressure. Since the iv access device maintains the patency of the vein, air can enter the venous circulation through the device. This can be avoided by using the Trendelenburg position to increase venous pressure and by limiting the time the catheter is open to air.

Catheter Shearing, Catheter and Guidewire Emboli

Catheter shearing may result when central venous catheters inserted through a metal needle are pulled back so that the needle bevel shears the catheter. This complication has di-

---

TABLE 28-7. Complications Common to Subclavian and Internal Jugular Central Venous Pressure Catheters

Puncture of pleura or lung
  Pneumothorax
Hemothorax and or hemomediastinum
Puncture of the lymphatic ducts
  Chylothorax or chylomediastinum
Intravenous fluid infusion errors
  Pleural effusion
Injury to surrounding structures

minished in frequency with the introduction of guidewire (Seldinger) techniques. However, there is the potential for migration of the sheared distal fragment or the entire guidewire.

Infection

Central venous catheters have been identified as important sources of nosocomial infections and sepsis. Catheter contamination may occur at the time of insertion (poor technique) or result from colonization from a distant infected site (hematogenous spread) or occur as the consequence of skin contamination at the insertion site. Both local and systemic infections have been reported. The risk of central venous catheter infections is approximately 4%.[86] Maintaining sterility and preventing catheter-related infections require appropriate dressing and tubing changes based on institutional guidelines.

Pulmonary Artery Monitoring

The development of the flow-directed, balloon flotation pulmonary artery catheter was a major advance in hemodynamic monitoring and it has become an important tool in the quantitative assessment of cardiopulmonary function. Right-sided heart pressures as estimated by the central venous pressure are often unreliable determinants of left ventricular filling pressures. This is particularly true of patients who are elderly or have pre-existing cardiopulmonary disease.[87-89]

The original indication for pulmonary artery monitoring was for the management of complicated myocardial infarctions.[90] Numerous articles have since reviewed the various applications and benefits of pulmonary artery monitoring.[91,92] Indications for pulmonary artery monitoring are broadly defined. Typically, the indications for pulmonary artery monitoring have been predicated on specific patient pathology, e.g., cardiac pathology, pulmonary diseases, shock, and renal failure. Alternatively, if the pulmonary artery catheter is viewed as a physiologic monitor, insertion should be guided by the information needed for diagnosis and therapy. If the following information is deemed necessary, a pulmonary artery catheter is indicated for measuring (1) intracardiac pressures, (2) thermodilution cardiac output, (3) mixed venous oxygen saturation, and (4) derived hemodynamic indices, e.g., systemic vascular resistance and left ventricular stroke work index. This information can help define the clinical problem, monitor the progression of hemodynamic dysfunctions, and guide the response to therapy.

The measurement of intracardiac pressures can be used to indirectly assess left ventricular preload, diagnose the existence of pulmonary hypertension, or differentiate cardiac and noncardiac causes of pulmonary edema. Equalization of all intracardiac diastolic pressures is highly suggestive of a constrictive cardiac process such as cardiac tamponade. Analysis of the central venous pressure and pulmonary artery port pressure waveforms provide diagnostic insights into the functional characteristics of both the right and left ventricles.

Pulmonary artery catheters allow for the rapid and reproducible measurements of thermodilution cardiac output (see the section on Monitoring Cardiac Function). Cardiac output measurements are helpful for assessing cardiac function, calculating oxygen delivery (CO × arterial O_2 content), and assessing cardiac performance.

Access to mixed venous blood from the pulmonary artery port (discussed later) provides an indirect assessment of the balance between O_2 delivery and O_2 utilization. Additionally, the mixed venous oxygen saturation ($S\bar{v}o_2$) is needed to calculate the mixed venous oxygen content ($C\bar{v}o_2$). $C\bar{v}o_2$ is necessary for the calculation of intrapulmonary (Equation 28-1) or intracardiac shunts (Equation 28-2):

$$\frac{Cco_2 - Caco_2}{Cco_2 - C\bar{v}o_2} = \frac{\dot{Q}s}{\dot{Q}t} \tag{28-1}$$

$$\frac{Sao_2 - SRAo_2}{Sao_2 - S\bar{v}o_2} = \frac{\dot{Q}p}{\dot{Q}s} \tag{28-2}$$

where Cco_2 = capillary O_2 content, Cao_2 = arterial O_2 content, $C\bar{v}o_2$ = mixed venous O_2 content, $\dot{Q}s/\dot{Q}t$ = shunt fraction, Sao_2 = arterial O_2 saturation, $SRAo_2$ = right atrial O_2 saturation, $S\bar{v}o_2$ = mixed venous O_2 saturation, $\dot{Q}p/\dot{Q}s$ = pulmonary-to-systemic shunt.

Hemodynamic measurement is often predicated on the manipulation of preload, afterload, and contractility. Several of the derived indices of hemodynamic function necessitate the measurement of a cardiac output (Table 28-8).

The proper clinical use of pulmonary artery catheters depends on the interpretation and validity of the information obtained,[91,93] which in turn are dependent on (1) a properly functioning pressure monitoring system, (2) correctly identifying the "true" pulmonary capillary wedge pressure (PCWP), and (3) an understanding of the various factors that affect the relationship of PCWP and other cardiac pressures and volumes and ventricular function.

The technical concerns of pressure monitoring are addressed in the section on Invasive Measurement of Arterial Blood Pressure. Measurement errors caused by equipment

TABLE 28-8. Derived Hemodynamic Variables

Name	Abbreviation	Calculation	Units
Cardiac index	CI	CO/BSA	$1 \cdot min^{-1} \cdot m^{-2}$
Systemic vascular resistance	SVR	(MAP-CVP/CO) × 80	$dynes \cdot cm \cdot sec^{-5}$
Pulmonary vascular resistance	PVR	(MPAP-PCWP/CO) × 80	$dynes \cdot cm \cdot sec^{-5}$
Stroke index	SI	CI/Heart Rate	$cc \cdot beat^{-1} \cdot m^{-2}$
Left ventricular stroke work index	LVSWI	SI × (MAP-PCWP) × 0.0136	$g \cdot m \cdot beat^{-1} \cdot m^{-2}$
Right ventricular stroke work index	RVSWI	SI × (MPAP-CVP) × 0.0136	$g \cdot m \cdot beat^{-1} \cdot m^{-2}$

BSA = body surface area; MAP = mean arterial pressure; CVP = central venous pressure; MPAP = mean pulmonary arterial pressure; PCWP = pulmonary capillary wedge pressure.

misuse or malfunction may invalidate the clinical use-fulness of pulmonary artery catheter measurements. The various techniques for intravascular cannulation, pulmonary artery catheter insertion, and equipment set-up are well described elsewhere.[90] Catheter placement can be achieved by using changes in vascular waveforms or by direct observation under fluoroscopy. The greatest source of error in pulmonary artery monitoring appears to be related to the inappropriate interpretation or utilization of the transduced pressure wave. Figure 28-8 depicts the transduced pressure waves as a pulmonary artery catheter is floated to the wedged position.

Hemodynamic monitoring necessitates an appreciation of the various physiologic determinants of cardiac output and oxygen delivery. The pulmonary artery catheter is used to measure intracardiac pressure, in particular the PCWP. PCWP is used to indirectly assess left ventricular preload (left ventricular end-diastolic volume or LVEDV) by reflecting changes in left ventricular end-diastolic pressure (LVEDP).

It has been well demonstrated that right-sided pressures often are poor indicators of left ventricular filling, either as absolute numbers or in terms of direction of change in response to therapy.[88] Figure 28-9 depicts the relationship between the various pressures in the cardiopulmonary system.[94] The correlation of these pressures as estimates of LVEDP or LVEDV is directly related to their proximity to the left ventricle. Assuming an open conduit from the catheter tip to the left ventricle, when the pulmonary artery catheter is in the "wedged" position, the right-sided heart chambers and valves are bypassed. During end diastole, there is cessation of forward blood flow, and a static fluid column is presumed to exist from the left ventricle to the pulmonary artery catheter tip. Ideally, changes in LVEDP are reflected by all proximal pressures (pulmonary artery end-diastolic pressure (PAEDP), PCWP, pulmonary venous pressure, left atrial pressure). Alterations in internal or external forces applied to the open conduit during wedge measurements may invalidate this relationship.

Factors Affecting the Interpretation of Pulmonary Artery Catheter Data

Normally, pulmonary vascular resistance and the impedance to pulmonary blood flow are minimal. Any significant increase in pulmonary vascular resistance alters the relationship between PCWP and PAEDP. Acute or chronic parenchymal pulmonary diseases, emboli, alveolar hypoxia, acidosis, hypoxemia, and many vasoactive drugs increase pulmonary vascular resistance, thereby altering the relationship between PCWP and PAEDP. Tachycardia shortens ventricular diastole, reducing distal runoff of pulmonary blood flow and thereby increasing pulmonary vascular resistance.[93] When the above situations exist, the PAEDP cannot be assumed to reflect distal diastolic pressures, including the PCWP.

The accurate measurement of the PCWP can be grossly affected by the position of the catheter tip in the pulmonary artery and by changes in intrathoracic pressure. West described a gravity-dependent difference between ventilation and perfusion in the lung.[95] The variability in pulmonary blood flow is a result of differences in pulmonary artery (PA), alveolar (Palv), and venous pressures (PV) and is categorized into three distinct zones (see Chapters 33 and 34). In Zone I, Palv is greater than PA or PV. In Zone II, Palv is greater than PV but less than PA. Only in Zone III do PA

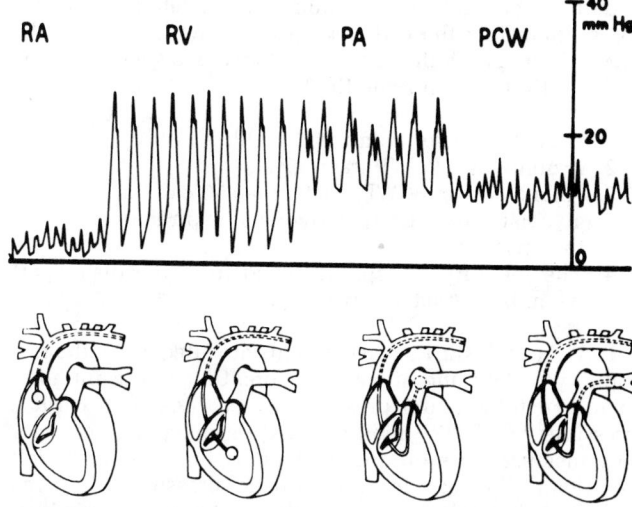

Figure 28-8. Pressure tracing observed during the flotation of a pulmonary artery catheter. (Reproduced with permission from Dizon CT, Barash PG: The value of monitoring pulmonary artery pressure in clinical practice. Conn Med 41:622, 1979.)

and PV exceed Palv, allowing for uninterrupted blood flow and a continuous communication with distal intracardiac pressures. Increases in alveolar pressure, decreases in perfusion (e.g., hypovolemia, decreased cardiac output), or changes in position can convert areas of Zone III into either Zone I or Zone II. Accurate measurement necessitates a pulmonary artery catheter tip to be placed in Zone III. Since pulmonary artery catheters are flow-directed, they usually advance to areas of highest flow. The effect of alveolar pressure is also dependent on pulmonary compliance. The less compliant the lung, the less alveolar pressure is transmitted to the vascular bed.

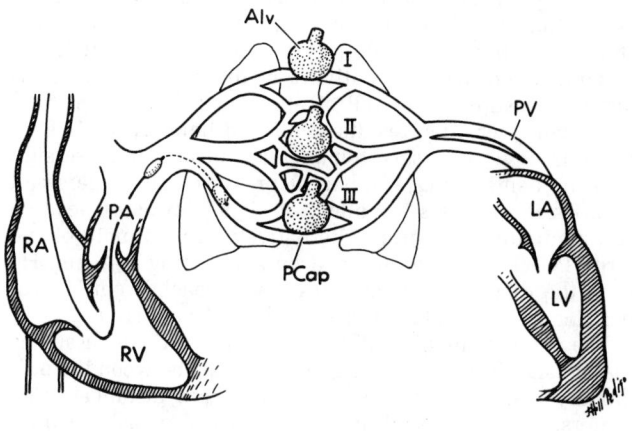

Figure 28-9. The anatomical position of a pulmonary artery catheter in the pulmonary artery. The dashed line positions the inflated balloon in the "wedged" position. (RA = right atrium; RV = right ventrical; PA = pulmonary artery; ALV = alveolus; Pcap = pulmonary capillary; PV = pulmonary vein; LA = left atrium; LV = left ventrical.) I, II, and III characterize the relationship of $P_{alveolar}$, $P_{arterial}$, P_{venous} as described by West. The bottom of the figure shows a progressive correlation of vascular pressures. (Reproduced with permission from Vender JS: Invasive cardiac monitoring. Crit Care Clin 4:455, 1988.)

Catheter position can be confirmed by a lateral chest film to ascertain that the catheter tip is below the level of the left atrium. The following characteristics suggest that the catheter tip is not in Zone III:[96]

1. A PCWP greater than the PAEDP,
2. A nonphasic PCWP tracing,
3. An increase in PCWP greater than 50% of the increased alveolar pressure (positive end-expiratory pressure therapy), and
4. The inability to aspirate blood from the distal port when the catheter is wedged.

PCWP and PAEDP measurements are affected by the respiratory pattern and airway pressure. Changes in intrathoracic and intrapleural pressures affect transmural cardiac pressures.[97,98] PCWP monitoring does not reflect changes in transmural pressure (net distending pressure of the left ventricle). Changes in intrathoracic pressure affect the PCWP-LVEDP relationship. With spontaneous or positive pressure ventilation, intrathoracic pressure is closest to atmospheric pressure at end expiration. Therefore, PCWP measurements should be estimated at end expiration.

Positive end-expiratory pressure therapy can induce changes in both intravascular and intrapleural pressure.[99] During positive end-expiratory pressure, alveolar pressure is increased, potentially converting Zone III areas to Zone II. If positive end-expiratory pressure is transmitted across the alveoli, intrapleural pressure also increases. The amount of pressure transmitted is dependent on the intrapulmonary compliance. Positive end-expiratory pressure also can alter ventricular distensibility and decrease venous return. This causes a disproportionate increase in PCWP (and LVEDP) when compared with changes in LVEDV.

The effect of positive end-expiratory pressure (at less than 10 cm H_2O) on the PCWP is minimal if the pulmonary artery catheter is located in Zone III.[91] Higher levels of positive end-expiratory pressure can influence the PCWP-LVEDV relationship. When this situation arises, trends in the PCWP rather than absolute numbers are used to guide therapy. During positive end-expiratory pressure therapy, it is not recommended that the ventilator be disconnected in an effort to measure the PCWP at atmospheric pressure.[88,93,98] This maneuver often results in marked hemodynamic fluctuations or unnecessary hypoxemia. Intrapleural pressure measurements using esophageal pressure transducers can be utilized to assess the effect of higher levels of positive end-expiratory pressure. Alternatively, an estimate of the "true PCWP" can be obtained by subtracting 1–2 mm Hg from the displayed wedge pressure for each 5 cm H_2O of positive end-expiratory pressure above 10 cm H_2O.

The relationship of PCWP and left atrial pressure assumes that no significant pressure gradient exists between the pulmonary veins and the left atrium. In rare instances (e.g., tumors, fibrosis, vasculitis, and atrial myxomas), obstruction of the pulmonary veins may cause the pulmonary venous pressure to exceed the left atrial pressure.[98] In patients with endotoxemia, localized pulmonary venoconstriction has been described.[100]

Left atrial pressure is assumed to reflect the LVEDP. Pathologic obstruction at the mitral orifice (mitral stenosis, myxoma, or clot) can interfere with this relationship. The presence of large v waves secondary to mitral regurgitation, noncompliant left atrium, or left-to-right intracardiac shunting can be misinterpreted as an unwedged pulmonary artery tracing. As with central venous pressure tracings, v

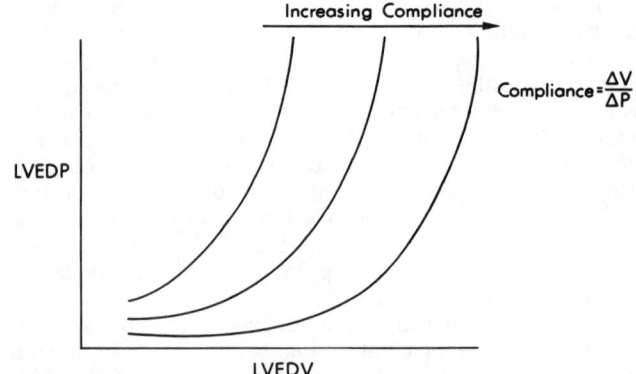

Figure 28-10. Typical ventricular compliance curve. (Reproduced with permission from Vender JS. Invasive cardiac monitoring. Crit Care Clin 4:455, 1988.)

waves occur at the end of ventricular systole when the left atrium is maximally filled. The size of the pulmonary artery v wave is mostly related to changes in left atrial compliance rather than regurgitant volume. When large v waves are present, the best estimate of LVEDP is the difference between the a and v wave pressures rather than the PCWP.[93]

Decreases in left ventricular compliance, aortic regurgitation, and premature closure of the mitral valve may reverse the normal pressure gradient when the LVEDP is greater than the left atrial pressure.[101,102] Therefore, the accuracy of the measured pulmonary pressures and their correlation with LVEDP do not ensure a valid reflection of preload. Preload (length of the myocardial fibers at end diastole) is best determined by measuring the LVEDV. The relationship between LVEDP and LVEDV is not linear.

Figure 28-10 graphically depicts the relationship between left ventricular pressure and volume.[91] Note that a series of curves are shown representing several of a family of curves, each demonstrating that the curvilinear relationship between LVEDP and LVEDV is dependent on ventricular compliance. Therefore, the relationship between left atrial preload and LVEDV is complex and dependent upon both ventricular compliance and transmural cardiac pressures.

Patients often have varying ventricular compliance resulting from inherent alterations in ventricular stiffness.[101-103] Ventricular compliance is a dynamic factor that can be influenced by many physiologic and pathologic variables. The compliance curves suggest that at low preloads, larger increases in LVEDV produce smaller changes in LVEDP. Conversely, at higher preloads, a similar change in LVEDV produces a greater pressure change. For a given LVEDV, any decrease in ventricular compliance results in an increase in LVEDP. This explains the development of hydrostatic pulmonary edema at normal LVEDV.

Some of the commonly recognized factors that decrease ventricular compliance are shown in Table 28-9. Increases

---

TABLE 28-9. Decreased Left Ventricular Compliance: Common Etiologies

Myocardial ischemia	Cardiac tamponade
Restrictive myopathies	Myocardial fibrosis
Right-to-left intraventricular shunts	Inotropic drugs
Aortic stenosis	Hypertension

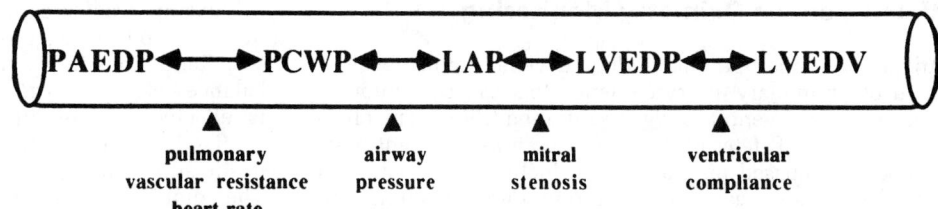

Figure 28-11. The pulmonary artery monitoring cascade. The factors listed below the figure can have a profound effect on the correlation between the listed pressures and on LVEDV.

in ventricular compliance are associated with the use of vasodilators, with congestive myopathies, and with regurgitant mitral or aortic valves.

The data provided by pulmonary artery catheter pressure monitoring must be interpreted in view of the pathophysiologic and respiratory effects that influence the relationship between the available pressures (PAEDP and PCWP) and the physiologic variables that we wish to discern (LVEDP and LVEDV). Even when the PCWP accurately reflects changes in LVEDP, changes in ventricular compliance mitigate the correlation with LVEDV (preload). Appropriate utilization of pulmonary artery catheters necessitates an appreciation and understanding of these pitfalls and limitations.[93,100,103] Figure 28-11 depicts the pressure cascade and factors that commonly affect the PCWP-LVEDV relationship.

The use of pulmonary artery catheters is also associated with numerous complications.[104] The frequency of any particular complication varies among published reports. Factors that appear to reduce complications include experience, supervision, and attention to details. One large study suggests a low incidence of morbidity and mortality.[76] The majority of complications can be categorized into three groups: (1) insertion risks (see Tables 28-6 and 28-7), (2) catheter passage risks (advancement and removal), and (3) risk associated with use (maintenance).

Insertion risks are identical to those described for placement of central venous catheters. Complications of advancement and removal are related to problems associated with cardiac performance or structure. Dysrhythmias are the most common complication of catheter passage.[105] Right bundle-branch blocks and even complete heart block have been reported during catheter advancement.[106] Intravenous lidocaine can be administered either therapeutically or prophylactically during advancement.[107] If heart block is a concern, a catheter with pacing capabilities should be employed. Table 28-10 lists the complications that have been associated with catheter advancement and removal.

Coiling, looping, and/or knotting are more common in low-flow states, with large intracardiac cavities, when smaller diameter catheters are utilized, or when an excessively long catheter is inserted.[107,108]

Knotting of a pulmonary arterial catheter around other structures, e.g., pacing wires, papillary muscles, or chordae tendineae, can be a serious complication. If the knot cannot

be withdrawn through the introducer or venotomy site, fluoroscopic disentanglement or surgical removal may be required. Proper placement of pulmonary artery catheters must be confirmed by a chest radiograph after insertion.

Difficult insertions can be anticipated in patients with right ventricular enlargement, low-flow states, or tricuspid valvular disease. In these situations, special patient positioning (head-up, left side down), deep breathing, or fluoroscopic guidance may be necessary.

Numerous complications have been associated with the continued use of pulmonary artery catheters.[91,109,110] Table 28-11 lists many of these but is not all-inclusive.

The most dramatic and potentially catastrophic complication is pulmonary artery perforation and hemorrhage.[111] Predisposing risk factors for perforation and hemorrhage include hypothermia, the presence of pulmonary hypertension, and poor insertion technique. The mortality rate from this complication is high if patients have a coagulopathy or are on anticoagulation medication. Perforations and subsequent hemorrhage can be avoided by restricting "overwedging," continuously monitoring the pulmonary arterial pressure trace to recognize spontaneous "wedging," minimizing the number of balloon inflations, and using proper technique during balloon inflations. Serious pulmonary hemorrhage may require single lung ventilation and surgical intervention.

Catheter-related infections (sepsis or endocarditis) are well-recognized causes of morbidity that can be minimized when infection control protocols are implemented.[109,112]

New Modalities of Pulmonary Artery Catheter Monitoring

Since the advent of pulmonary artery catheters, several modifications have been developed to enhance their monitoring capabilities. The first significant change in pulmonary artery catheters was the incorporation of a thermistor at their tip, permitting the measurement of cardiac output. Other features have been introduced for clinical use or evaluation. These include mixed venous oximetry, capability to monitor right ventricular ejection fraction, and continuous cardiac output capabilities. Additionally, pulmonary artery catheters have been manufactured with pacing capabilities.

TABLE 28-10. Complications of Pulmonary Artery Catheter Passage

Dysrhythmias	Heart block
Knotting	Kinking or coiling
Valvular damage	
Perforation of the pulmonary artery, right atrium or right ventricle	

TABLE 28-11. Complications of Pulmonary Artery Catheter Presence

Thrombosis	Pulmonary infarction
Pulmonary artery rupture	Thrombocytopenia
Sepsis	Valvular damage
Endocarditis	Thromboembolism
Balloon rupture (right-to-left shunt)	Dysrhythmias

Mixed Venous Oximetry Monitoring

Advances in fiberoptic technology have led to the development of pulmonary artery catheters that can continuously measure mixed venous oxygen saturation ($S\overline{v}o_2$). The clinical relevance of determining $S\overline{v}o_2$ on an intermittent basis has been discussed previously and includes calculation of mixed venous oxygen content, intrapulmonary shunt, and oxygen consumption. Continuous $S\overline{v}o_2$ monitoring provides information on the minute-to-minute assessment of total tissue oxygen balance, e.g., the relationship between oxygen delivery and oxygen consumption.

Oxygen delivery ($\dot{D}o_2$) equals the arterial oxygen content times the cardiac output ($\dot{D}o_2 = [Hb \times 13.8] \times CO$). The constant 13.8 represents the volume of oxygen carried by hemoglobin converted to unit of grams per liter. This equation does not include the dissolved oxygen content, which in most cases is insignificant. Oxygen consumption ($\dot{V}o_2$) is determined by the difference between arterial and venous oxygen delivery (venous $\dot{D}o_2$). The relationship between $S\overline{v}o_2$, $\dot{V}o_2$, and $\dot{D}o_2$ is demonstrated in the following equation, which is derived from the Fick relationship:

$$S\overline{v}o_2 = Sao_2 - (\dot{V}o_2/(Hb \times 13.8) \times CO)$$

$S\overline{v}o_2$ varies directly with cardiac output (CO), Hb, and Sao_2 and inversely with $\dot{V}o_2$. The normal $S\overline{v}o_2$ is 75%, which indicates that under normal conditions, tissues extract 25% of the oxygen delivered. An increase in $\dot{V}o_2$ or a decrease in arterial oxygen content ($Sao_2 \times Hb$) is compensated by increasing CO or tissue oxygen extraction. Increases in oxygen extraction are reflected by a decrease in $S\overline{v}o_2$. At critical levels of oxygen delivery, $S\overline{v}o_2$ plateaus because oxygen consumption is maximal.[113] When the $S\overline{v}o_2$ is less than 30%, tissue oxygen balance is compromised, and anaerobic metabolism ensues.[113] It is imperative to recognize that $S\overline{v}o_2$ is determined by the variables mentioned above and therefore is not a direct reflection of changes in CO exclusively. A normal $S\overline{v}o_2$ does not ensure a normal metabolic state but suggests that oxygen kinetics are either normal or compensated. Figure 28-12 demonstrates an $S\overline{v}o_2$ recording in a patient recovering from cardiac surgery. In this example, a decrease in $S\overline{v}o_2$ is found in spite of marked increases in CO, suggesting an imbalance between $\dot{D}o_2$ and $\dot{V}o_2$. Reductions in $\dot{V}o_2$, e.g., reducing shivering, restore the balance between oxygen consumption and delivery, which is reflected by a step-up of the $S\overline{v}o_2$.

Mixed venous oximetry is a powerful tool for both diagnostic and therapeutic assessments in critically ill patients. The combination of continuous Sao_2 and $S\overline{v}o_2$ monitoring (termed dual oximetry) provides continuous information regarding the cardiopulmonary effects of positive end-expiratory pressure.[114]

As with all monitoring, there are technologic and physiologic limitations associated with mixed venous oximetry.[91,93] Although a low $S\overline{v}o_2$ is considered ominous, a normal or high $S\overline{v}o_2$ does not necessarily indicate adequate tissue oxygen balance. $S\overline{v}o_2$ is a global measurement and does not ensure the adequacy of regional (specific vital organs) tissue oxygen balance. The following pathophysiologic conditions may be associated with normal or high $S\overline{v}o_2$ levels: sepsis, arteriovenous fistulae, peripheral shunts, cirrhosis, left-to-right intracardiac shunts, cyanide poisoning, hemoglobinopathies, and unintentioned pulmonary artery catheter wedging.

MONITORING CARDIAC FUNCTION

Cardiac output and hemodynamic variables derived from estimates of blood pressure and flow are important indices of myocardial performance and the status of the circulatory system. Estimates of the rate of blood flow pumped by the heart (cardiac output), although not performed as a routine measurement during anesthesia, are of great importance when managing critically ill patients or patients with documented or newly acquired cardiac dysfunction.

Fick Cardiac Output

The earliest technique for CO measurement was first proposed by Adolph Fick in 1870. Modern invasive techniques are all based on adaptations of Fick's principle, which states that the size of a fluid stream can be calculated by instilling an indicator into the stream and measuring the concentration difference over time between the inflow and outflow. Traditionally, oxygen has been used as the indicator substance where CO is determined by measuring the oxygen consumption ($\dot{V}o_2$) and dividing it by the arteriovenous content difference ($Cao_2 - C\overline{v}o_2$). The direct Fick method is invasive because of the need to sample arterial and mixed venous blood from the pulmonary artery or right ventricle.

The direct Fick CO technique is considered to be the standard for comparing other methods of CO determination. The technique assumes that a steady state exists with respect to oxygen saturation, oxygen consumption, and CO during the period of data collection. Values are inaccurate if cardiac, pulmonary, or hepatic shunts are present.[115] Fick CO has been superseded by the thermodilution technique, which was introduced into clinical practice in 1971.[116]

Adaptations of the direct Fick CO technique have been described. With the advent of continuous mixed venous oximetry, Davies and coworkers have described a method for the continuous measurement of cardiac output by the Fick technique using the Westenskow system for continuous $\dot{V}o_2$ and pulse oximetry.[117,118] Recently, Morton described a non-

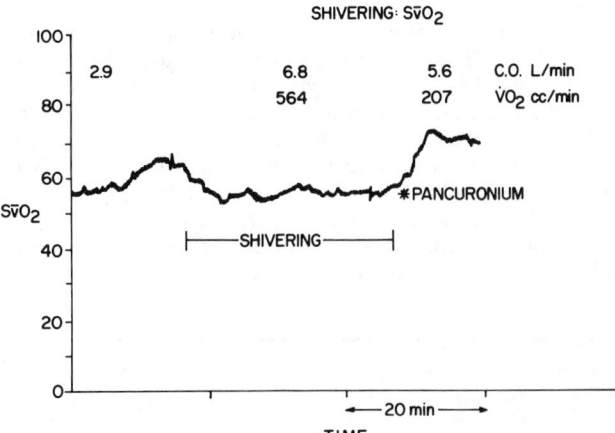

Figure 28-12. This $S\overline{v}o_2$ recording in a postcoronary artery bypass patient demonstrates the effects of shivering and its treatment, and the relationship between $S\overline{v}o_2$, cardiac output (CO), and metabolic rate $\dot{V}o_2$. (Reproduced with permission from Vender JS: Invasive cardiac monitoring. Crit Care Clin 4:455, 1988.)

invasive method to calculate CO using CO_2 as the indicator.[119]

Indicator Dilution Techniques

Indicator dilution determinations of CO are based on a concept proposed by Stewart and tested by Hamilton and colleagues.[120,121] A known amount of indicator (usually indocyanine green dye) is injected into a central venous pressure catheter, and arterial blood is withdrawn at a constant rate and assayed by an in-line photodensitometer. The output of the photodensitometer is graphed as a concentration-time curve. Today, computers calculate the average concentration over time (area under the curve). Since the area appears in the denominator of the equation, a smaller area produces a larger CO.

Thermodilution CO determination is the most widely utilized adaptation of the indicator dilution principle. This technique was first described by Fegler in 1952.[122] Today, cooled 5% dextrose or 0.9% saline is injected into the central venous pressure port of a thermodilution pulmonary artery catheter. A thermistor in the pulmonary artery records the decrease in temperature as the "cooled blood" passes through the pulmonary artery. Computers contend with the complexity of the thermodilution CO equation which, while similar to that for dye dilution, includes the following factors: specific heat of blood and indicator, specific gravity of blood and indicator, the volume of the injectate, catheter size, and the area of the blood temperature curve. (The numerator contains the volume of injectate, the temperature difference between injectate and blood, and the computational constant. The denominator is the integral of the temperature change over time.) Unlike what occurs in dye dilution, the small amount of cold solution does not recirculate. Comparison studies suggest that either room temperature or an iced injectate can be used for clinical measurements of thermodilution CO.[123] Iced injectate produces a more exacting curve with a better signal-to-noise ratio.

When properly performed, thermodilution CO determination correlates very well with both direct Fick and dye dilution determinations.[124,125] In clinical practice, triplicate determinations are averaged to increase precision. Differences in values of 12–15% are not of clinical significance.[131]

Alterations in right-sided cardiac output vary during the respiratory cycle.[126] Thermodilution CO measurements at peak inspiration or end expiration have less variability.[127] Precision is enhanced by maintaining consistency of the injection rate (2–4 seconds), the injection volume (10 ml), and measurement of injectate temperature as it enters the circulation.[128,129] Repetition of injections should be delayed for at least 90 seconds to allow for a steady thermal environment.

There are numerous sources of inaccuracies when determining CO by thermodilution. Observation of the thermal curve is helpful in assessing the accuracy of thermodilution CO determinations. Low amplitude curves result when injectate volume is too small, the temperature differential between injectate and patient is small, or the thermistor is improperly positioned.[125] Tricuspid or pulmonic regurgitation and intracardiac shunts may produce recirculation errors.[124] A diminished height of the concentration-time curve can occur from incomplete filling of the syringe, loss of injectate through leaks, or a thrombus insulating the pulmonary artery thermistor. Each of these results in a falsely high CO reading. Intravenous infusions can influence CO determinations. It has been recommended that rapid infusions be maintained either at a constant rate or discontinued prior to CO determination.[130] Irregularities in the thermal curve should be evaluated prior to initiation of therapy based on determination of cardiac output.

Continuous Cardiac Output Pulmonary Artery Catheters

Several different technologies have been assessed for the determination of continuous cardiac output from pulmonary artery catheters. Pulsed thermodilution uses a filament that intermittently heats blood proximal to a thermistor. The change in the thermistor output is proportional to the blood flow. Clinical validation of this unique methodology is under investigation.

Doppler ultrasound is an important method for evaluating blood flow (see below). Incorporation of Doppler flow probes on pulmonary artery catheters offers the potential to continuously monitor CO. Doppler pulmonary artery CO has been evaluated with variable results. Other pulmonary artery catheter systems using intracardiac impedance and injectionless cold thermodilution are under investigation. At present these methodologies are not available for clinical use.

Right Ventricular Ejection Fraction

Calculation of right ventricular ejection fraction and end-diastolic volume may be performed using a special pulmonary artery catheter that employs a rapid response thermistor and a computer system that analyzes the exponential decay of the pulmonary artery temperature over several cardiac cycles. Injectate is administered in the right atrium, and the ejection fraction is determined by subtracting the mean residual fraction from the cardiac output.[132]

Application of this technology includes any clinical condition in which impairment of right ventricular function is suspect (e.g., sepsis, adult respiratory distress syndrome, pulmonary hypertension, right coronary artery disease). The accuracy of right ventricular ejection fraction has been questioned when dysrhythmias, tricuspid regurgitation, or improper catheter positioning is present. Further clinical studies are needed to confirm the clinical utility of right ventricular ejection fraction catheters.

Noninvasive Techniques for Cardiac Output Determination

The quest for technically simple, nontraumatic methods for accurately estimating CO has a long history. Two methods are currently available for clinical use.

Impedance plethysmography is based on measuring the pulsatile change in resistance during the cardiac cycle. Four electrodes are applied to the neck and thorax. Impedance measurements are made in two pairs while a continuous small electric current is applied across the thorax. Stroke volume is proportional to the ventricular ejection time and the maximum rate of impedance change during systole (max dZ/dT).[133] Electrode placement is an important source of error.[134] Other factors that influence bioimpedance include intrathoracic fluid shifts and changes in hematocrit. Although impedance plethysmography has not gained wide use, the technique offers clinicians a quick method for determining CO with minimal direct patient risk.

Continuous wave or pulsed wave Doppler ultrasonography can measure the velocity of blood in the ascending or descending aorta. CO is calculated by multiplying the time-weighted average velocity of blood flow by an estimate of aortic cross-sectional area that can be directly measured or predicted from a nomogram. Accuracy and precision are dependent on the reliability of the estimate of aortic diameter and the alignment of the Doppler probe to the blood flow jet (laminar flow). Velocity measurements are most accurate when the Doppler beam and flow are parallel (angle or incidence = 0). In clinical practice, velocity measurements are not considered accurate when the angle exceeds 25 degrees. Suprasternal, transtracheal, and transesophageal probes have been designed for determining CO using continuous wave Doppler ultrasonography. Incorporating the Doppler probe in an endotracheal tube decreases the difficulty in positioning and maintaining probe alignment during surgery. Comparison studies question the precision and accuracy of CO determinations using suprasternal, transesophageal, and transtracheal Doppler techniques.[135-137]

Intraoperative Echocardiography

Intraoperative cardiac imaging utilizing two-dimensional transesophageal echocardiography (TEE) has added a new dimension to monitoring cardiac function during anesthesia and surgery.

Intraoperative echocardiography can assess the functional integrity of heart valves,[138] determine intracardiac blood flow relationships, estimate intracardiac volumes, and quantify ventricular contractility. Transesophageal echocardiography is superior to precordial Doppler in the early recognition of venous air embolism.[139] Since most tissues interfere with sound wave penetration, the mounting of multiple Doppler probes on gastroscopic instruments permits the precise alignment of structures of interest.

Transesophageal echocardiography uses sound waves to penetrate tissues. When ultrasound strikes the interface of tissues of different densities, a portion of the energy is reflected back. The greater the difference in density, the greater the reflection. The time required for the reflected sound to return to the piezoelectric crystals is related to the distance from the transducer. Therefore, transesophageal echocardiography can define anatomic structures by the "brightness" of the reflected energy and the time interval from transmission to reception of signal. If the transesophageal echocardiography monitoring system permits Doppler echocardiography, it is possible to display the two-dimensional image and also quantify flow. Today, color-coded Doppler flow imaging is incorporated into transesophageal echocardiography monitoring systems providing real-time images of intracardiac blood flow as well as two-dimensional structural analysis.

Transesophageal echocardiography is contraindicated in patients with esophageal strictures, esophagitis, esophageal varices, or previous esophageal surgery. TEE offers anesthesiologists the opportunity for monitoring global ventricular function, assessing intraoperative embolic events, assessing regional myocardial contractility or ischemia, and visualizing intraoperative valvular function and blood flow. The clinical applications of transesophageal echocardiography are evolving as anesthesiologists begin to gain experience in operating the system or as cardiologists skilled in this technique perform intraoperative transesophageal echocardiography examinations during surgery (Table 28-12).

MONITORING NEUROLOGIC FUNCTION

The best assessment of neurologic function is a thorough clinical neurologic examination that permits the evaluation of the integration of brain and spinal cord. Anesthesia, sedation, the use of muscle relaxants as well as the extent of neuropathology or trauma may significantly impair the sensitivity of or even the ability to perform a clinical neurologic examination in the operating room. For this reason, monitoring of neurologic function has become an important aspect of neuroanesthesia care. Intraoperative neurologic

TABLE 28-12. Clinical Application of Intraoperative Transesophageal Echocardiography

Application	Mode	View	Reference
Global Cardiac Function			
Ejection fraction	2-D	Short axis	Konstadt et al[140]
Cardiac output	2-D	Short axis	Thys et al[141]
Effects of anesthesia and surgery	2-D	Short axis	Roizen et al[142]
Regional Wall Motion			
Segmental wall ischemia	M-mode	Short axis	Elliott et al[143]
	2-D	Short axis	Smith et al[144]
Anatomic Assessment			
Mitral valve function	Contrast 2-D	Long axis	Goldman et al[145]
	Color flow	Long axis	Czer et al[146]
Aortic valve cusps	2-D	Short axis	
Aortic valve mobility	2-D	Long axis	
Aortic valve function	Contrast 2-D	Long axis	Equaras et al[147]
Aortic aneurysms and dissections	Color flow	Long axis	Hashimoto et al[148]
Congenital heart disease	Color flow	Short and long axis	Cyran et al[149]
Intracardiac air	2-D	Long axis	Cucchiara et al[139]

monitoring can guide anesthesia and surgical decision making.

Preservation of optimal neuronal environment through monitoring spontaneous or evoked neural activity has become the mainstay of monitoring neurologic function. Anesthesia can influence synaptic transmission and/or electrical activity directly or by altering physiologic factors such as ventilation, blood flow, or blood pressure. Anesthetic agents, the means and methods utilized to administer them, and alterations in autoregulation all have clinically important effects on the systems used to monitor neurologic function. The effects of anesthetic management on cerebral blood flow, metabolism, and brain monitoring are discussed in Chapter 32.

Intracranial Pressure Monitoring

Intracranial pressure monitoring was initially utilized in the management of trauma, where the relationship between uncontrolled intracranial pressure elevation and fatality has been firmly established.[150,154] Intracranial pressure can be monitored by insertion of an intracranial bolt, insertion of a ventricular catheter, insertion of an epidural transducer, or placing a fiberoptic sensor in the epidural space. Each of these techniques is invasive, requiring a burr hole for intracranial access.

The cerebrospinal fluid pressure wave is pulsatile, having variations in amplitude that correlate with the cardiac and ventilatory cycles. Normal intracranial pressure is less than 15 mm Hg.

Two abnormal cerebrospinal fluid waveforms have been described. A waves or plateau waves exhibit 50–100 mm Hg increases in intracranial pressure for several minutes and are associated with acute increases in cerebral blood volume. B waves are defined by their lower amplitude and shorter duration.[151]

Subarachnoid Devices

The subarachnoid bolt (Richmond bolt) is a hollow stainless steel device that is screwed into a burr hole and fluid coupled to a transducer system or fluid-filled manometer that is "zeroed" at the level of the ear. The tip of the bolt is extradural, and a small dural opening allows subdural pressures to be measured. Withdrawal of cerebrospinal fluid is not possible, and the bolt may become occluded. The transducing system should not contain a continuous infusing or flush device. Subarachnoid bolts are easy to place, produce accurate pressure measurements, and reduce the potential for infection. Pressure/volume determinations can sometimes be performed by adding a small volume of fluid to the transducing system and determining the change in pressure; however, intracranial compliance testing is best done with an intraventricular catheter.

Intraventricular catheters permit the monitoring of intracranial pressure as well as the withdrawal of cerebrospinal fluid. Compliance estimates can also be determined by noting the pressure response to the injection of a small volume of saline. Catheters may clot or kink, and occasionally it is necessary to flush the system. Flushing of the tubing or catheter can be hazardous because of the disturbed pressure-volume relationships found in many neurosurgical patients. Bacterial contamination of intraventricular catheters and tubings is a serious complication and limits their utility as a routine technique for intracranial pressure monitoring.[152]

Epidural Devices

Epidural sensors reduce the potential for infection because the dura is not opened. A self-contained electronically coupled epidural transducer has been designed for the continuous monitoring of intracranial pressure. The transducer is housed in a bolt that screws directly into a small burr hole. The epidural transducer's accuracy depends on intimate contact with the dura, which transmits the cerebrospinal pressure waves.[153] Cerebrospinal fluid sampling and compliance estimates cannot be determined by this method.

A fiberoptic monitoring system has been designed to continuously monitor intracranial pressure. The system is microprocessor-controlled and requires the placing of a specialized, disposable sensor between the inner table of the skull and the dura. The sensor contains an optically linked membrane that deforms as the dura transmits the intracranial pressure wave. The deformation reduces the optical transmission in a fiberoptic bundle. A microprocessor-controlled pneumatic pump adds air into the sensor, equalizing the light transmission between two transmission fiberoptic bundles. The pressure that equalizes the light transmission is directly proportional to the intracranial pressure. Other fiberoptic probes have been developed that can be placed in the lateral ventricles or cerebral cortex.

Assessment of Intracranial Pressure Monitoring

Epidural techniques do not permit sampling of cerebrospinal fluid, nor can they be used to monitor compliance. The nonfluid coupled systems cannot be "rezeroed" after placement, and baseline drift can be a problem during prolonged intracranial pressure monitoring. Intracranial pressure–guided therapy assumes that cerebral perfusion pressure (CPP = MAP − ICP) is uniformly distributed and that intracranial hypertension will result in either ischemia or displacement or compression of brain tissue. Intracranial pressure monitoring does not measure neural function or neural recovery.

The Electroencephalogram

The electroencephalogram (EEG) represents the spontaneous electrical activity of the cerebral cortex as recorded from either the scalp or surface electrodes. The EEG signal originates from postsynaptic excitatory and inhibitory potentials of the pyramidal cells located in the outer cerebral cortex.

The EEG signal has several characteristics that make it particularly difficult to measure and evaluate accurately in the operating room. Signal processing is difficult because of the small voltages, 10–100 μV (1000 times smaller than electrocardiogram signals) and the variation in frequencies recorded, 1–30 Hz. Conventional EEG analysis utilizes scalp electrodes positioned at standardized points in relation to cranial dimensions, which allows correlation of EEG findings from one patient to another.

The voltage difference between a pair of EEG electrodes is amplified and compared to the voltage of a reference electrode (ground) using a process called differential amplification. Differential amplification removes artifacts that are common to the EEG electrodes and the reference electrode. The resulting signal is then passed through electronic filters, which reduce or remove unwanted frequencies. The amplified and filtered signals (8–16 channels) are then displayed as a graph of amplitude (voltage) over time.

In unanesthetized patients, the EEG is a composite of two factors: background rhythms regulated by "pacemaker neurons" of the brain stem and local electrical activity resulting from the cortical neurons underlying the active electrode. During periods of ischemia, "neuronal illness," or while the patient is under anesthesia, EEG activity generally decreases in both amplitude and frequency. Generation of EEG activity consumes approximately 50% of the total oxygen of the cerebral cortex.

EEG monitoring has been advocated for the intraoperative detection of cerebral ischemia during deliberate hypotension or during carotid endarterectomy; for the intraoperative or perioperative assessment of pharmacologic interventions; for the identification of epileptic foci; or for the assessment of coma or brain death.[155,156]

Deep anesthesia, cerebral ischemia, or other pathologic states abolish or reduce normal neural EEG activity (alpha and beta rhythms), and slower frequencies (delta and theta) predominate. Alterations in EEG amplitude can result from synchronization or desynchronization of EEG activity or cortical depression. Sleep or surgical anesthesia typically increases amplitude (synchronization), whereas arousal characteristically decreases amplitude (desynchronization). Deep levels of anesthesia may decrease amplitude of the EEG by direct depression of cortical activity or by depressing "pacemaker" regulation. High concentrations of isoflurane and desflurane can cause periods of electrical silence interspersed with brief episodes of high-frequency activity (burst suppression).

The benefit of intraoperative EEG monitoring depends on the specificity of on-line analysis of the EEG output (voltage versus time tracings) and correlation with the identifiable changes that relate to reversible surgical insults. Unfortunately, many intraoperative events of interest (e.g., regional ischemia) are not associated with specific alterations in the EEG patterns. EEG interpretation requires experienced observers and the ability to integrate the changes with anesthetic, physiologic, and surgical events.

Several signal processing techniques have been utilized to produce displays of EEG information to improve the ability to interpret changes or evaluate trends. Usually the raw EEG is amplified, filtered, and digitized and then processed to create topographic or graphic displays of the processed EEG signal. Real-time analysis using Fourier transformations to identify amplitudes and frequencies of interest or using aperiodic analysis permits the display of amplitude (voltage) and frequency that can be graphically shown so that novices can identify the changes of interest present in the EEG.

A variety of EEG processing monitors are available for clinical use. All EEG processing monitors quantify and display changes in frequency when the EEG slows, and display changes in amplitude when it flattens. In the operating room, comparison of right- and left-sided EEG activity is of great interest, and several monitors process and display two EEG channels simultaneously. Instruments using Fourier transformations create power spectrum plots that graph the EEG amplitude (power) over the frequency range of interest during a specified sampling period or epoch. These plots of power (y axis) versus frequency (x axis) can be displayed as a series that places the plots one in front of the other (z axis) to produce the compressed spectral array that allows observation over time. The spectral edge frequency has been utilized by investigators as a descriptor summarizing the behavior of the power spectrum during anesthesia.[157]

This spectral edge is the frequency that is just above 95% of the power contained in the raw EEG. The spectral array can be density-modulated using color or gray scale to denote power while displaying time (x axis) and frequency (y axis). Density modulation eliminates the hidden valleys that occur when using a compressed spectral array of epochs. Monitors using aperiodic analysis of the EEG display output as vertical spikes on an xyz plot. The size of the spike indicates amplitude, whereas the horizontal position and color are determined by the frequency. Time is displayed on the z axis, with new data advancing in front of the previous display.

Today, instrumentation and software exist to map the frequency spectrum of the entire standard EEG. This is done by using EEG information at discrete electrode positions and interpolating to estimate the EEG between the electrodes. This allows a continual map to be graphically displayed across the entire head when multiple electrodes are used. Brain mapping transfers an immense amount of EEG data into a pictorial image of brain function. This quantitative EEG technique is currently an investigational tool that may provide insight into the distribution of electrical activity associated with the administration of anesthetics.[158] Intraoperative multichannel EEG mapping is technically feasible and could identify and monitor the potentially deleterious effects of cerebral hypoxia during anesthesia.

Evoked Potentials

Evoked potentials are useful because they monitor the functional integrity of specific brain stem, visual, or peripheral neural pathways. Evoked potentials represent a small electrical signal generated in neural pathways following periodic neural stimulation. In the cortex and subcortex, the evoked potential signals are much smaller than the background EEG, such that computer signal averaging and filtering are used to remove the random background electrical activity. The averaged evoked response is then displayed as a plot of voltage over time. Three sensory pathways are commonly utilized intraoperatively to monitor neural function (see Chapter 32).

Brain stem auditory evoked responses are produced by stimulation of the cochlea using pulsed sound. Five to seven waves are displayed following processing from recording electrodes placed near the ear and cortex. Brain stem auditory evoked responses provide functional assessment of the auditory pathway (ear and brain stem) and are useful in assessing function in comatose patients and in the intraoperative monitoring of neural function during surgical procedures of the cerebellopontine angle, floor of the 4th ventricle, or 5th, 7th, or 8th cranial nerves. Brain stem auditory evoked responses monitor subcortical neural pathways and may remain normal in the face of severe cortical dysfunction and deep anesthesia.

Visual evoked potentials are produced by flashing light to stimulate the retina and recording the response using electrodes placed over the occipital cortex. Visual evoked potentials allow assessment of the integrity of the visual pathway. Visual evoked potentials are very sensitive to anesthetic effects and are technically difficult to monitor intraoperatively. Visual evoked potentials may be helpful in procedures on the visual system, during resection of pituitary tumors and craniopharyngiomas, and during procedures in the vicinity of the optic tracts (e.g., anterior cerebral artery aneurysms).

Somatosensory evoked potentials are produced by stimulating either the median or the ulnar nerves of the upper extremity, or the common peroneal or posterior tibial nerves of the lower extremity, using small electrical impulses similar to those produced by a neuromuscular blockade monitor. Recording electrodes are traditionally placed over the peripheral nerve stimulated, the lumbar spine, the brachial plexus, the cervical spine, and the scalp. The responses observed at the cervical spine and scalp represent peaks produced by multiple generators in the brain stem, thalamus, and sensory cortex. The somatosensory evoked potentials traverse the long tracts in the central nervous system, giving them the broadest potential for intraoperative monitoring.

Somatosensory evoked potentials have been utilized to monitor cerebral function and ischemia associated with cerebral procedures or subarachnoid hemorrhage; spinal cord function during instrumentation of the spine; and spinal cord function during thoracoabdominal surgery.[159,160] In the spinal cord, ischemia or injury to the posterior or lateral columns produces a deterioration characterized by a decreasing amplitude and increasing latency of the somatosensory evoked potentials tracing. The presence of somatosensory evoked potentials responses and their normalization are thought to be sensitive indicators of a favorable prognosis. Monitoring of somatosensory evoked potentials is an extension of the sensory neurologic examination and does not specifically evaluate the function of the motor pathways.

Motor evoked potentials are currently investigational monitors. They are recorded from peripheral nerves or from electromyographic activity of muscle after stimulation of the motor cortex, using electrical or magnetic impulses or by electrical stimulation of motor pathways of the spinal cord. Motor evoked potentials have significant implications for anesthesiologists because they are sensitive to inhalation anesthesia and may require a controlled neuromuscular blockade when the electromyogram is recorded. In addition, transcranial magnetic stimulation of the motor strip has been associated with hypertension.[161,162] Nevertheless, motor evoked potentials are of importance because they allow assessment of spinal motor tracts, which are missed with somatosensory evoked potentials monitoring.

Facial nerve monitoring is a specialized form of motor evoked potential that is in common use during surgery of the posterior fossa. Here, intentional stimulation or surgical irritation of the facial nerve causes muscular contraction of the face. Responses can be visually evaluated (obicularis oculi or obicularis oris muscle). Additionally, electrodes can be placed in the muscle and the electromyogram recorded or amplified to produce an audible feedback signal. Like the motor evoked potential, pharmacologic muscle relaxation must be carefully titrated. The facial nerve is rather insensitive to anesthetic influence.

As with the EEG, assessment of evoked potential changes

is often difficult because alterations may result from ischemia, neural path disruption, and pressure or distortion of neural structures as well as from anesthesia, blood pressure, temperature, or technical variables. During anesthesia, it is preferable to monitor the contralateral area not at risk as well as the area at risk in order to differentiate changes resulting from surgery or other global variables. Guidelines for personnel, equipment, and documentation of evoked potentials monitoring have been published by the American Electroencephalographic Society.[163]

Noninvasive Monitoring of Cerebral Hemodynamics, and Oxygen Delivery: Future Considerations

Transcranial ultrasonography is a noninvasive method that has been used to assess the status of the intracranial circulation.[164,165] The technique is based on using a 2-MHz Doppler probe that permits estimation of velocity of blood flow by detecting the Doppler shift following the ultrasonic penetration of the temporal bone. Transcranial ultrasonography has the potential to assess intracranial arterial occlusions irrespective of etiology and to monitor ipsilateral internal carotid artery blood velocity.

Transcranial ultrasonography has been utilized to diagnose cerebral emboli and to monitor the blood flow velocity following recanalization. Its potential clinical utility for intraoperative management requires further evaluation. Difficulties attributable to insufficient penetration through the temporal bone can be expected in up to 30% of patients.[166] Recent interest in using transcranial ultrasonography as an early warning of critical reductions in cerebral perfusion during anesthesia has been reported.[167]

Near infrared spectroscopy NIS has been heralded as a technology that not only can monitor cerebral oxygen delivery but also can assess cerebral hemodynamics.[168] This methodology is possible because infrared light (650–1100 nm) penetrates the scalp and skull, permitting assessment of light-absorbing molecules such as O_2Hb and reduced Hb. Other light-absorbing molecules exist for evaluation by near infrared spectroscopy, including many cytochromes and the vascular marker, indocyanine green.

Preliminary studies suggest that near infrared spectroscopy can be adapted to measure brain oxygen saturation using infrared technology similar to that used in pulse oximetry.[169-171] In the brain, venous oximetry signals (reduced Hb) predominate over arterial signals (O_2Hb), and therefore near infrared spectroscopy oximetry represents a composite of the two compartments, which is referred to as regional cerebral Hb oxygen saturation. Regional cerebral Hb oxygen saturation correlates best with cerebral $S\bar{v}o_2$. Cerebral $S\bar{v}o_2$ and the regional cerebral Hb oxygen saturation are sensitive indicators of changing regional cerebral oxygen extraction resulting from systemic hypoxia, regional cerebral oligemia, or anemia.

NEUROMUSCULAR MONITORING

Clinical criteria for assessing intraoperative relaxation and subsequent reversal are imprecise and subjective when compared with evoked motor testing.[178,179] (Table 28-13). For this reason, it is desirable to monitor the status of the neuromuscular junction with a nerve stimulator when using neuromuscular blocking agents during anesthesia (see also Chapter 19).

TABLE 28-13. Clinical Criteria for Normalization of Neuromuscular Transmission

Test	Reference
Head lift >5 seconds	Gal[172]
Sustained hand grip	Russell[173]
Sustained arm lift >45 seconds	Stanec[174]
Sustained leg lift (infants)	Mason[175]
Negative inspiratory force ≥ −20	Ali[176]
Vital capacity of 15 ml·kg^{-1}	Brand[177]

Nerve stimulators permit precise, individualized dosing of neuromuscular blocking agents. During induction, nerve stimulation can identify the onset time of the neuromuscular block and serve as a guide for the titration of neuromuscular blocking agents. Since the sensitivity of patients to neuromuscular blocking agents varies, nerve stimulators permit adjustment of the degree of blockade to match clinical needs. During emergence from anesthesia, nerve stimulators are of great help in assessing the optimal time to initiate reversal or in diagnosing and treating potential impairments in neuromuscular transmission in the early postoperative period.

Stimulation of a motor nerve and evaluation of the resultant motor response are the foundations upon which neuromuscular junction monitoring is based. Motor responses to electrical stimulation, although intended to assess the neuromuscular junction, also depend on the functional status of the muscle and the electrical characteristics of the stimuli. Three features constitute neuromuscular junction monitoring: the stimulating electrodes, the nerve stimulator, and the recording technique. For clinical assessment, surface stimulation using detached metal electrodes or pregelled electrocardiographic electrodes is favored. Skin resistance is an important variable in determining the adequacy of the stimulation current. Preparing the electrode site with a degreasing agent ensures that the stimulus current is adequate. Needle electrodes offer the lowest impedance and can be placed subcutaneously following the induction of anesthesia.

The responses of stimulated motor units are not uniform with respect to the onset or resolution of neuromuscular blocking agents, and the diaphragm is particularly resistant to blockade by both nondepolarizing and depolarizing neuromuscular blocking agents.[180,181] Since the evoked tension of muscles varies with the current applied, the electrical characteristics of the output of nerve stimulators are clinically relevant.[182] Clinically useful instruments should deliver a monophasic square wave having a pulse width of 200–300 μsec and an output current 20–25% greater than the current necessary to stimulate all the muscle fibers supplied by the stimulated nerve.[182] Stimulators may have adjustable outputs from 0–60 mA or deliver a fixed output.

Various stimulus patterns have been described for the clinical assessment of neuromuscular function, and the stimulation modes of clinical instruments may be switched to support any of the following patterns: 0.5–1 second twitch (0.5–1 Hz), train-of-four, tetanic stimulation, and double-burst stimulation. Monitoring the onset and depth of neuromuscular blockade may require using several stimulation modes.

Single-twitch stimulation is very valuable in assessing the effect of depolarizing blockade. The degree of relaxation is determined by dividing the response following relaxation by the control response, and the duration of blockade is defined as the time for the twitch response to recover to the control response. Responses are depicted in Figure 28-13. Single-twitch responses are not always reliable in monitoring the depth of nondepolarizing blocks because the response to single-twitch stimulation is dependent on stimulus frequency.[183,184]

Today, train-of-four has become the most popular method of stimulation.[183] Train-of-four is more sensitive than single twitch in estimating the degree of blockade following administration of nondepolarizing muscle relaxants.[185] Train-of-four is performed by delivering four supramaximal stimuli (>30 mA) every 0.5 seconds (2 Hz). The degree of nondepolarizing blockade is determined by estimating the ratio of the fourth response to the first response, expressed as a percent of the first "twitch height." The extent of a nondepolarizing block is proportional to the degree of fade. Fade is the clinical response resulting from the reduced postsynaptic (end plate) function following nondepolarizing neuromuscular blockade.

Depolarizing blockade can also be evaluated using train-of-four stimulation. During a depolarizing block, all four responses are smaller than the initial response. Fade is not present unless a phase II block is developing (see Chapter 19).

Criteria for the adequacy of the reversal of neuromuscular blocking agents based on comparison studies in human volunteers using thumb twitch, train-of-four ratio, and effort-dependent pulmonary function tests demonstrate that pulmonary function is adequate with train-of-four ratios of ≥0.70[172,177] Healthy patients may tolerate train-of-four ratios of ≤0.40.[186]

Traditionally, the response to tetanic stimulation has been advocated as an important tool in assessing neuromuscular transmission following intense nondepolarizing blockade. Tetanic stimulation utilizes a 5-second volley of supramaximal stimuli at a frequency of 50 Hz, followed by single twitches of 1 Hz. When neuromuscular transmission is normal or during a pure depolarizing block, the response observed following tetanic stimulation is a sustained twitch height. During a nondepolarizing blockade (or Phase II blockade following administration of succinylcholine), the response observed following tetanic stimulation demonstrates an increase in the twitch height (post-tetanic facilitation) and fades. The degree and duration of post-tetanic facilitation are dependent on the extent of neuromuscular blockade. The degree of fade is dependent not only on the extent of blockade present but also on the stimulation characteristics (frequency, duration) and on how often the tetanic stimulus has been applied.

Tetanic stimulation is very painful and should be performed only in anesthetized patients. During intense neuromuscular blockade, muscle responses following train-of-four and single-twitch stimulation may not be present. Post-tetanic responses appear before train-of-four, permitting quantification from the time of the appearance of post-tetanic facilitation. Counting the number of post-tetanic responses (post-tetanic count) reflects on the depth of relaxation. As the block dissipates, the number of post-tetanic responses increases until the train-of-four response can be quantified.

In clinical practice, responses to nerve stimulation are quantified either by observation or by feeling the strength of response. Visual and tactile assessments are often insensitive to residual blockade when compared with transduced recordings of the evoked responses to stimulation. During recovery, there is a need for a sensitive and reliable method to evaluate residual nondepolarizing blockade. Double-burst stimulation was designed to enhance the ability to detect residual blockade in recovering patients who might have or develop residual weakness.[187] The thumb response is observed following ulnar nerve stimulation. Double-burst stimulation utilizes short tetanic bursts separated by a pause of 750 μsec. Various double-burst stimulation patterns have been studied. The most widely reported stimulation patterns use three 0.2 msec volleys of tetany followed by a 750 μsec pause and a repeat volley of either two or three tetanic stimulations (double-burst stimulation 3.2 and 3.3, respectively). If weakness or fade is felt or observed following double-burst stimulation, then the corresponding train-of-four is expected to be equal or less than 0.7. The absence of

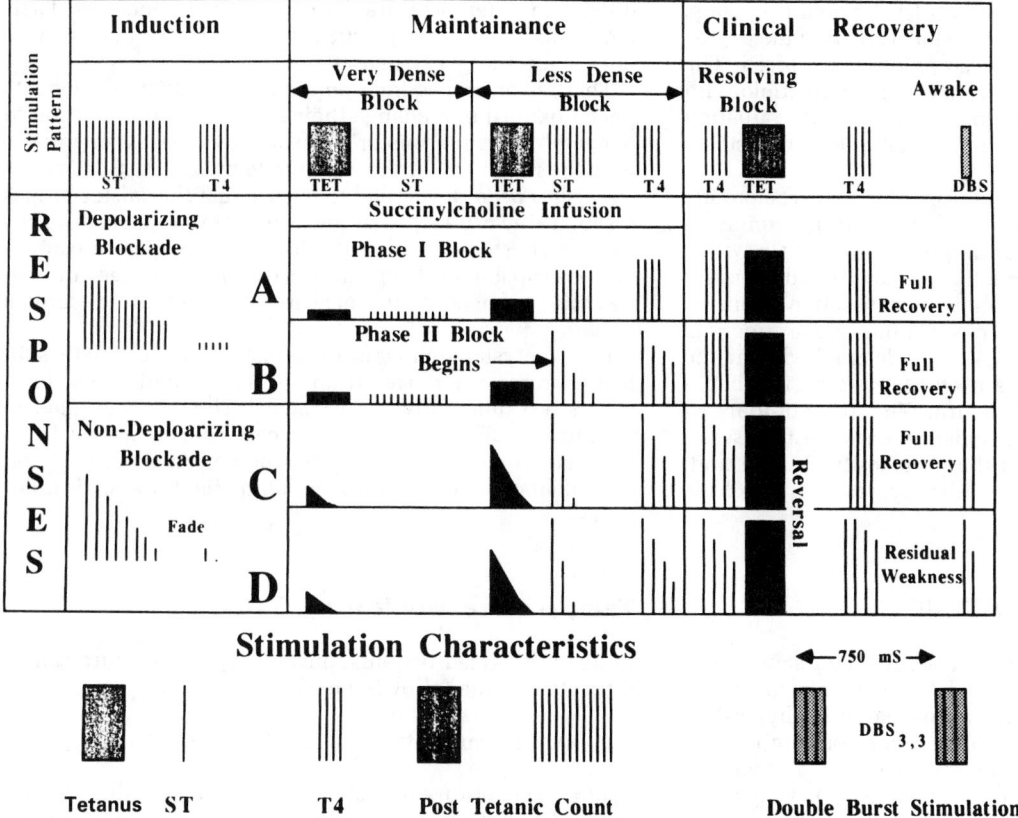

Figure 28-13. Assessing neuromuscular function. This diagram simulates the clinical responses observed following neuromuscular stimulation. Stimulation patterns are depicted in the upper panel. (ST = single twitch; T4 = train of four; TET = tetanus; DBS = double burst stimulation.) The following four situations are demonstrated by the letters: A, the normal use of a succinylcholine infusion; B, the development of a phase II block; C, a nondepolarizing blockade that is reversed with full recovery; and D, a nondepolarizing blockade that demonstrates residual weakness.

fade following a double-burst stimulation of 3:3 indicates that clinically significant residual neuromuscular blockade is not present.[188] Double-burst stimulation correlates well with train-of-four ratios measured during electromyography.[187] Double-burst stimulation offers clinicians a simple visual or tactile method for assessing neuromuscular function in patients recovering from general anesthesia.

A variety of stimulation sites are available for observing or recording the motor response to nerve stimulation. In clinical practice, the ulnar nerve at the wrist or elbow, the facial nerve at the stylomastoid or at the lateral canthal fold, and the mandibular nerve at the mandibular condyle are favorite stimulation sites.[189] When the face or arms are not available, stimulation of the peroneal nerve at the neck of the fibula or the posterior tibial nerve posterior to the medial malleolus can be used to monitor motor responses. Clinical judgments based on responses of the adductor pollicis or facial muscles overestimate the degree of blockade of the diaphragm, which is particularly resistant to neuromuscular block.[190]

Evoked responses of muscles following nerve stimulation may be quantified by displaying a processed electromyograph or by measuring acceleration or force developed during muscle contraction. The electromyograph measures the compound action potential of the muscle that results following nerve stimulation. Electrodes are placed over a muscle innervated by the stimulated nerve, and the electrical signal resulting from the excitation of the muscle is electronically processed to create a graphic display of the muscle's response, expressed as a percentage of control or as a train-of-four ratio. The response is proportional to the number of muscle fibers activated during supramaximal nerve stimulation. Electromyographic monitoring does not require special arm boards and can be performed on any muscle in any size patient; it will predict the neuromuscular refractory period with precision. Monitoring the compound electromyogram is principally a research technique that can be adapted to the clinical setting.[191]

Mechanomyography measures the force of the muscle contraction following nerve stimulation. A force displacement transducer is applied to the thumb (adductor pollicis muscle), and the twitch tension resulting from adduction of the thumb in response to ulnar stimulation is measured and electronically processed and shown on a display unit. Accuracy depends on maintaining a constant thumb angle and appropriate resting tension. Mechanomyography is principally a research and teaching tool. However, the output of force displacement transducers can be displayed in the operating room using the pressure ports.[192]

Recently, it has become possible to simplify the quantification of neuromuscular transmission by monitoring acceleration rather than force displacement. A small acceleration transducer is applied to the thumb, and the ulnar nerve is stimulated. When this electrode is exposed to force, a voltage change proportional to the force developed during muscle contraction is processed, and data evaluating the degree of neuromuscular blockade are graphically displayed. The output of acceleration transducers can be compatible with operating room display units to permit a visual evaluation of the train-of-four ratio, twitch height, or post-tetanic count.

Electromyography, mechanomyography, and accelerometry permit accurate evaluation of the status of neuromuscular blockade and recovery. During induction, single-twitch stimulation is helpful in identifying ideal conditions for intubation of the trachea. Following intubation, train-of-four stimulation effectively tracks neuromuscular function. If a dense neuromuscular blockade is desirable during the surgery, post-tetanic count is useful to determine when a train-of-four response will return. The train-of-four response is ideal in monitoring moderate blockade and assessing the extent of reversal. In the postanesthesia care unit, double-burst stimulation may identify residual blockade without pain.

MONITORING TEMPERATURE

The ability to monitor body temperature is a standard of care in anesthesia. The potential for accidental heat loss (hypothermia) or the risk of triggering malignant hyperthermia requires the continual observation of temperature changes. Although an intact thermoregulatory system normally maintains central body temperature, perioperative hypothermia commonly results from anesthetic-induced inhibition of thermoregulation. Inhibition of thermoregulation occurs during both general and regional anesthesia.[193-195] Additionally, the operating room environment and surgical exposure contribute to heat losses resulting from evaporation, convection, and conduction (see Chapter 7).

Hypothermia develops when thermoregulation fails to control the balance between metabolic heat production and environmental heat loss. The anticipated response to hypothermia, including increases in heat production (nonshivering thermogenesis and shivering) and decreases in heat losses (decreased sweating and vasoconstriction), are impaired during anesthesia. Therefore, anesthetized patients often behave like poikilotherms until core temperature approaches a new set point for thermoregulation. All patients are at risk for developing hypothermia. Those at greatest risk include the elderly, burn patients, neonates, and patients with spinal cord injuries.

Hyperthermia occurs rarely and may develop in anesthetized patients who have a genetic predisposition and have been exposed to anesthetic agents that trigger malignant hyperthermia (see Chapter 23). Other causes of intraoperative hyperthermia include exposure to endogenous pyrogens, increases in metabolic rate secondary to thyrotoxicosis or pheochromocytoma, anticholinergic blockade of sweating, or excessive environmental warming.

Thermometry

Clinical thermometry requires an accuracy of ±0.1°C. Several techniques can be utilized to continuously monitor temperature in anesthetized patients. Thermocouple temperature probes contain a circuit made of two dissimilar metals. One junction is used to measure body temperature and the other is placed in a thermally neutral reference. An electromotive force (Seebeck effect) is proportional to the difference in temperature between the two junctions. Thermocouple systems may drift if the reference junction does not remain thermally neutral.

Thermistor probes incorporate semiconducting elements (metal oxides) that change their resistance in proportion to temperature. A thermistor's resistance varies exponentially with the reciprocal of the absolute temperature. Special circuitry has been developed to ensure that thermistor probes respond linearly to physiologic temperature changes, thus reducing hysteresis and drift. Thermistor temperature monitors are capable of determining very small changes in temperature as needed to measure thermodilution cardiac output.

Liquid-crystal temperature detectors can estimate skin temperature over ranges from 34–40°C. Liquid-crystal detectors are inherently inaccurate.[196] They are designed to monitor the temperature underneath their adhesive back. Accuracy, to a large degree, depends on maintaining good skin contact and minimizing nonpatient thermal influences.[197]

Temperature Monitoring Sites

In unanesthetized patients, mean body temperature can be estimated by the following equation:

$$\text{Mean temperature} = 0.85\ T_{central} + 0.15\ T_{skin}.$$

Central temperature is customarily measured using temperature probes placed in the external auditory canal (tympanic probe), nasopharynx, esophagus (esophageal stethoscope), bladder (Foley catheter), rectum, or blood (pulmonary artery catheter). During routine noncardiac surgery, temperature differences between these sites are very small.[198] During and following cardiopulmonary bypass or deliberate hypothermia, gradients between these sites are to be anticipated. When cooling anesthetized patients, changes in rectal temperature often lag behind changes in central temperature. Likewise, during rewarming, probe locations residing in regions of high blood flow often reflect blood temperature rather than central temperature. Therefore, the adequacy of rewarming is best judged by measuring temperature at several locations.

Complications of thermometry are rare. Electrical burns have been reported to occur if current leakage is present.[199] Tympanic probes must be utilized with care because perforation of the tympanic membrane is possible.

COMPUTERS AND MONITORING

Computers are an integral part of intraoperative monitoring. Most of the devices and instruments used during anesthesia have microprocessors to control their operation. Computers are used routinely in dedicated monitoring units for data acquisition, signal processing, and display of specific physiologic variables. Computerization of the anesthesia workplace has occurred insidiously because of the ubiquity of computer chips in electrical engineering. Unfortunately, microprocessor-based monitoring devices function independently, and the anesthesiologist's workplace has become cluttered with displays, controls, and alarms. Today, computerization has the potential to centralize and coordinate the monitoring of physiologic parameters, display specific advisories and warnings, and automatically generate the anesthesia record.

Although computer engineering has created many "smart" monitors, e.g., intraoperative ST segment electrocardiographic analysis, human interaction is an important aspect of the integration and use of computers for the monitoring of intraoperative physiologic parameters and anesthesia delivery systems. Anesthesia information management and data collection are evolving areas of interest.

Since most modern monitors contain their own microprocessors, it is possible to transfer both processed and raw data to other computer systems for information management. Special types of interfaces have been developed for transferring information between processors. Today, electrical cables are used for this purpose. A standard for medical information, the medical information bus, reduces the difficulty in connecting monitors for centralized information processing and data collection. Electrical links require rigid adherence to standards of electrical safety. Data transfer incorporates checks to identify that the communication network between the computers is sending and receiving information according to a configured pattern.

Most of the signals from medical monitoring equipment, e.g., transduced arterial pressure, are contained in varying DC voltages. Conversion of voltages to binary output must occur before the signal can be either transmitted or processed. Analog-to-digital converters digitize analog signals for computer processing. Analog-to-digital converters use sampling algorithms to digitize complex analog signals. For high fidelity data sampling, the sampling rate must be twice the rate of the highest frequency contained in the analog signal (Nyquist's theorem). Sampling of analog waveforms at an incorrect rate will result in a digitized wave that differs markedly from the original information. Many analog-to-digital converters are required for real-time, on-line data transfers in anesthesia information processing. On-line digital data acquisition and data transfer are not discernible to the anesthesiologist, and errors or artifacts can be difficult to detect.

Figure 28-14 graphically depicts the interrelationships associated with data acquisition and information processing.

Output devices such as printers, plotters, and video displays can assist the anesthesiologist in assessing multiple physiologic variables and implementing and coordinating "smart" alarms. Computer programs are available to automate anesthesia recordkeeping. Whereas physiologic data are easily transmitted for automated recordkeeping through the medical information bus, drug and fluid administration information and annotations of care or events require input by the anesthesiologist. Input devices such as keyboards, keypads, touch screens, and track-balls (mice) can be adapted for data entry or control of video output.

Proponents of automated anesthesia records believe that they will enhance clinical care, render historical data more meaningful, and make quality assurance issues easily identifiable.[200] Opponents of automation cite issues of confidentiality and artifact detection and recognition.[201] Anesthesia records are important documents when physicians defend their clinical judgments in a court of law. Accuracy, legibility, and completeness of documentation enhance the credibility of the defendant as a competent practitioner. Computerization of the anesthetic record offers advantages to practicing anesthesiologists. Comparison studies suggest that automated recordkeeping is more accurate and complete than hand charting.[202]

FUTURE TRENDS IN MONITORING THE ANESTHETIZED PATIENT

Diagnostic and therapeutic advances in medicine have had a great impact on the strategies and techniques available for intraoperative monitoring. This chapter has focused attention on the monitoring environment of the operating suite, the importance of understanding the practical limitations of specific monitoring devices, and the integration of monitoring and vigilance to enhance the safety of anesthesia practice.

Unfortunately, technologically advanced and "essential"

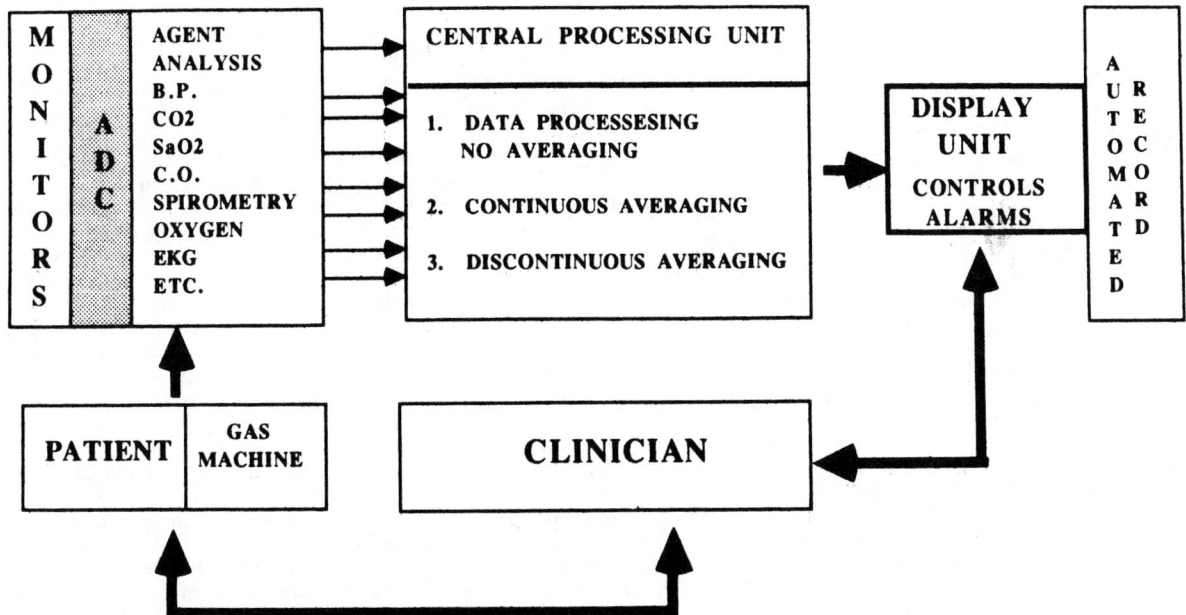

Figure 28-14. The computerization of monitoring functions. The diagram represents the integration of monitoring devices. The bold arrows represent the feedback loops between the patient, the anesthesiologist, the gas machine, and all monitoring devices.

monitoring may not be appropriate or even feasible in some locations or situations. The best example is the vexing problem of monitoring anesthetized patients during magnetic resonance imaging. Many of our "essential" monitors do not perform well or seriously diminish the quality of magnetic resonance imaging scans when they are utilized. Mandates for essential monitoring by themselves may not solve all of our problems regarding safety, nor do they guarantee vigilance.

Today's anesthesia practice has narrowed the distinction between laboratory medicine and patient monitoring. Technologic advances in instrument design have made it possible to have ready access to serum chemistries, hematologic profiles, assessment of anticoagulation function, and arterial blood gas levels. Stat laboratories adjacent to operating rooms and intensive care areas have enhanced the opportunity to monitor the physiologic milieu of the patient perioperatively.

Miniaturization of ion-specific electrodes and similar devices (chemical field effect transistors) may provide clinicians with instrumentation that conveniently and continuously monitors in vivo physiologic parameters of interest.[203] In situ catheter-tip chemical transducers can be engineered using ion-specific electrode concepts. Catheter-tip transducers to analyze pH, CO_2, and O_2 are technically feasible, and periodically reports of their application appear. However, problems relating to membrane stability, anticoagulation, and drift limit the potential for in vivo ion-specific electrode monitoring.

The quest for the continuous measurement of arterial blood gases underscores how technology has narrowed the distinction between laboratory medicine and patient monitoring. The current clinical practice of intermittent sampling of arterial blood will undoubtedly be revised as new technologies are adapted to provide clinicians with monitoring instruments that perform better, reduce costs, or provide information in real time. Continuous measurement of arterial oxygen tension is now technically feasible.[204,205]

REFERENCES

1. Pierce EC: Historical prospectives. Int Anesthesiol Clin 22:1, 1984
2. Schwartz WB, Komesar NK: Doctors, damages, and deterrence. An economic view of medical malpractice. N Engl J Med 298:1282, 1978
3. The Standards for Intraoperative Monitoring, pp. 670–671. Directory of Members, Park Ridge IL, American Society of Anesthesiologists, 1991
4. Whitcher C, Ream AK, Parsons D et al: Anesthetic mishaps and the cost of monitoring. A proposed standard for monitoring. J Clin Monit 4:5, 1988
5. LaMantia KR, O'Connor T, Barash PG: Comparing methods of measurement: An alternative approach. Anesthesiology 72:781, 1990
6. Bland JM, Altman DG: Statistical methods for assessing agreement between two methods of clinical measurement. Lancet 1:307, 1986
7. Association for the Advancement of Medical Instrumentation: Human Factors, Engineering Guidelines and Preferred Practices for the Design of Medical Devices. Arlington, VA, 1988
8. Kestin IG, Miller BR, Lockhart CH: Auditory alarms during anesthesia monitoring. Anesthesiology 69:106, 1988
9. Ellis FR, Nunn JF: The measurement of gaseous oxygen tension utilizing paramagnetism: An evaluation of the "Servomex" OA.150 analyzer. Br J Anaesth 40:569, 1968
10. Meriläinen PT: A differential paramagnetic sensor for breath-by-breath oximetry. J Clin Monit 6:65, 1990
11. Crampton Smith A, Hahn CEW: Electrodes for the measurement of oxygen and carbon dioxide tensions. Br J Anaesth 41:431, 1969
12. Mayer RM: Oxygen analyzers: Failure rates and life spans of galvanic cells. J Clin Monit 6:196, 1990
13. McGarrigle R, White S: Oxygen analyzers can detect disconnections. Anesth Analg 63:464, 1985
14. Schieber RA, Nomnoum A, Sugden A et al: Accuracy of expiratory carbon dioxide measurements using the coaxial and circle breathing circuits in small subjects. J Clin Monit 1:149, 1985
15. Badgwell JM, McLeod ME, Lerman J, Creighton RE: End tidal PCO_2 measurements sampled at the distal and proximal end of the endotracheal tube in infants and children. Anesth Analg 66:959, 1987
16. Linko K, Paloheimo M, Tammisto T: Capnography for detection of accidental esophageal intubation. Acta Anesthesiol Scand 27:199, 1983
17. Mogue LR, Rantala B: Capnometers. J Clin Monit 4:115, 1988
18. Westenskow DR, Smith KW, Coleman DL et al: Clinical evaluation of a Raman scattering multiple gas analyzer for the operating room. Anesthesiology 70:350, 1989
19. Matjasko J, Gunselman J, Delaney J, Mackenzie CF: Sources of nitrogen in the anesthesia circuit. Anesthesiology 65:229, 1986
20. Matjesko J, Petrozza P, Mackenzie CF: Sensitivity of end-tidal nitrogen in venous air embolism in dogs. Anesthesiology 65:418, 1985
21. Knopes KD, Hecker BR: Monitoring anesthetic gases, p 485. In Lake CL (ed): Clinical Monitoring. Philadelphia, WB Saunders, 1990
22. Barker SJ, Tremper KK: Pulse oximetry: Application and limitations. Int Anesth Clin 25:155, 1987
23. Kelloher JF: Pulse oximetry. J Clin Monit 5:37, 1989
24. Brown M, Vender JS: Non-invasive oxygen monitoring. Crit Care Clin 4:493, 1988
25. Craig KC: Clinical application of pulse oximetry. Probl Resp Care 2:255, 1989
26. Lamiell JM: Pulse oximetry. Probl Crit Care 5:44, 1991
27. Severinghaus JW, Astrup PB: History of blood gas analysis. VI Oximetry. J Clin Monit 2:270, 1986
28. Wukitsch MW, Petterson MT, Tobler DR et al: Pulse oximetry: Analysis of theory, technology and practice. J Clin Monit 4:290, 1988
29. Chapman KR, Lio FLW, Watson RM et al: Range of accuracy of two wavelength oximetry. Chest 89:540, 1986
30. Tremper KK, Barker SJ: Pulse oximetry. Anesthesiology 70:98, 1989
31. Eisele JH, Downs D: Ambient light affects pulse oximeters. Anesthesiology 67:864, 1987
32. Scheller MS, Unger RJ, Kelner MJ: Effects of intravenously administered dyes on pulse oximetry. Anesthesiology 65:550, 1986
33. Cote CJ, Goldstein A, Fuchman WH et al: The effect of nail polish on pulse oximetry. Anesth Analg 67:683, 1988
34. Miyaska K, Ohata J: Burns, erosion and sun tan with the use of pulse oximetry in infants. Anesthesiology 67:1008, 1987
35. Huch R, Huch A, Albani M et al: Transcutaneous PO_2 monitoring in the routine management of infants and children with cardiorespiratory problems. Pediatrics 57:681, 1976
36. Tremper KK, Shoemaker WC: Transcutaneous oxygen monitoring of critically ill adults, with and without low flow shock. Crit Care Med 9:706, 1981
37. Tremper KK, Barker SJ, Blatt DH et al: Effects of anesthetic agents on the drift of a transcutaneous oxygen tension sensor. J Clin Monit 2:234, 1986
38. Blanton HM: Transcutaneous gas monitoring. Probl Crit Care 5:69, 1991
39. Kwan M, Fatt I: A noninvasive method of continuous arterial oxygen tension estimation from measured palpebral conjunctival oxygen tension. Anesthesiology 35:309, 1971
40. Shoemaker WC, Lawner P: Method for continuous conjunctival oxygen monitoring during carotid artery surgery. Crit Care Med 11:946, 1983
41. Abraham E: Conjunctival oxygen tension monitoring. Int Anesth Clin 25:97, 1987

42. Braunwald E: Control of myocardial oxygen consumption: Physiologic and clinical considerations. Am J Cardiol 27:416, 1971

43. Hoffman JIE, Buckberg GD: The myocardial supply:demand ratio. A critical review. Am J Cardiol 41:327, 1978

44. MacDonald DA: Blood Flow in Arteries. London, Edward Arnold, 1974

45. O'Rourke MF, Yainuma T: Wave reflections and the arterial pulse. Arch Intern Med 144:366, 1984

46. Milnor WR: Hemodynamics. Baltimore, Williams & Wilkins, 1982

47. Wallace CT, Baker JD, Alpert CC et al: Comparison of blood pressure measurement by Doppler and by pulse oximetry techniques. Anesth Analg 66:1018, 1987

48. Cohn JN: Blood pressure measurement in shock. JAMA 199:118, 1967

49. Kirkendall WM, Feinleib M, Freis ED et al: Recommendation for human blood pressure determination by sphygmomanometers. Subcommittee of the AHA postgraduate education committee. News from the American Heart Association 1146A, 1981

50. Stegall HF, Kardon MB, Kemmerer WT: Indirect measurement of arterial blood pressure by Doppler ultrasonic sphygmomanometry. J Appl Physiol 25:793, 1968

51. Poppers PJ, Epstein RM, Donham RT: Automatic ultrasound monitoring of blood pressure during induced hypotension. Anesthesiology 35:431, 1972

52. Ramsey M: Blood pressure monitoring: Automated oscillometric devices. J Clin Monit 7:56, 1991

53. Nystrom E, Reid KH, Bennett R et al: A comparison of two automated indirect arterial blood pressure meters: with recordings from a radial arterial catheter in anesthetized surgical patients. Anesthesiology 62:526, 1985

54. Ramsey M III: Noninvasive automatic determination of mean arterial pressure. Med Biol Eng Comput 17:11, 1979

55. Epstein RH, Huffnagle S, Barkowski RR: Comparative accuracies of a finger blood pressure monitor and an oscillometric blood pressure monitor. J Clin Monit 7:161, 1991

56. Peñaz J: Photoelectric measurement of blood pressure volume and flow in the finger. Digest, 10th International Conference of Medical Biological Engineers, Dresden 104, 1973

57. Kurki T, Smith NT, Head N et al: Noninvasive continuous blood pressure measurement from the finger: Optimal measurement conditions and factors affecting reliability. J Clin Monit 3:6, 1987

58. Bramwell JC, Hill AV: The velocity of the pulse wave in man. Proc R Soc Lond 93:298, 1922

59. Kammotsu O, Ueda M, Otsuka H et al: Arterial tonometry for noninvasive, continuous blood pressure monitoring during anesthesia. Anesthesiology 75:333, 1991

60. Celoria G, Dawson JA, Teres D: Compartment syndrome in a patient monitored with an automated blood pressure cuff. J Clin Monit 3:139, 1987

61. Gardner RM: Blood pressure—dynamic response needs. Anesthesiology 54:227, 1981

62. Hipkins SF, Rutten AJ, Runciman WB: Experimental analysis of catheter-manometer systems in vitro and in vivo. Anesthesiology 71:893, 1989

63. Stern DH, Gerson JI, Allen FB et al: Can we trust the direct radial artery pressure immediately after cardiopulmonary bypass? Anesthesiology 62:557, 1985

64. Kinzer JB, Lichtenthal PR, Wade LD: Loss of radial artery pressure trace during internal mammary artery dissection for coronary artery bypass graft surgery. Anesth Analg 64:1134, 1985

65. McGregor AD: The Allen test—an investigation of its accuracy by fluorescein angiography dye. J Hand Surg 12:82, 1987

66. Slogoff S, Keats AS, Arlund C: On the safety of radial artery cannulation. Anesthesiology 59:42, 1983

67. Bedford RF, Wollman H: Complications of percutaneous radial artery cannulation: An objective prospective study in man. Anesthesiology 38:228, 1973

68. Davis FM, Steward JM: Radial artery cannulation. Br J Anesth 52:674, 1980

69. Downs JB, Rackstein AD, Klein EF, Hawkins IF: Hazards of radial artery catheterization. Anesthesiology 38:283, 1973

70. Bedford RF: Removal of radial artery thrombi following percutaneous cannulation for monitoring. Anesthesiology 46:430, 1977

71. Vender JS, Watts RD: Differential diagnosis of hand ischemia in the presence of an arterial cannula. Anesth Analg 61:465, 1982

72. Wilkins RG: Radial artery cannulation and ischaemic damage: A review. Anaesthesia 40:896, 1985

73. Shinozaki T, Dean RS, Mazuzan JE et al: Bacterial contamination of arterial lines: A prospective study. JAMA 249:233, 1983

74. Sanford TJ: Internal jugular vein cannulation versus subclavian cannulation: An anesthesiologist's view: The right internal jugular vein. J Clin Monit 1:58, 1985

75. Blitt CD: Catheterization Techniques for Invasive Cardiovascular Monitoring. Springfield, Ill, Charles C Thomas, 1981

76. Shah KB, Rao TLK, Laughlin S et al: A review of pulmonary artery catheterization in 6,245 patients. Anesthesiology 61:271, 1984

77. Belani KG, Buckley JJ, Gordon JR, Castenada W: Percutaneous cervical venous line placement: A comparison of the internal and external jugular routes. Anesth Analg 59:40, 1980

78. Jobes DR, Schwartz AJ, Greenhow DE et al: Safer jugular vein cannulation: Recognition of arterial puncture and preferential use of the external jugular route. Anesthesiology 59:353, 1987

79. Borja AR, Hinshaw JR: A safe way to perform infraclavicular subclavian catheterization. Surg Gynecol Obstet 130:673, 1970

80. Webre DR, Arens JF: Use of cephalic and basilic veins for introduction of central venous catheters. Anesthesiology 38:389, 1973

81. Bansmer G, Keith D, Tesluk H: Complications following use of catheters of inferior vena cava. JAMA 167:1606, 1958

82. Burri C, Ahnefeld FW: The Caval Catheter. Berlin, Springer-Verlag, 1978

83. Trager MA, Feinberg BI, Kaplan JA: Right ventricular ischemia diagnosed by an esophageal electrocardiogram and right atrial pressure tracing. J Cardiothorac Anesth 1:123, 1987

84. Mark JB: Central venous pressure monitoring: Clinical insights beyond the numbers. J Cardiothorac Anesth 5:163, 1991

85. Sharkey SW: Beyond the wedge: Clinical physiology and the Swan-Ganz catheter. Am J Med 83:111, 1987

86. Maki DG: Infections associated with intravascular lines. In Swartz M, Remington J (eds): Current Topics in Clinical Infectious Disease, pp 309–363. New York, McGraw-Hill, 1982

87. Civetta JM, Gabel JC: Flow directed pulmonary artery catheterization. Indications and modification of technique. Ann Surg 176:753, 1972

88. Civetta JM, Gabel JC: Flow directed pulmonary artery catheterization. Indications and modifications of technique. Ann Surg 176:753, 1972

89. Samii K, Counseiller C, Viars P: Central venous pressure and pulmonary wedge pressure. Arch Surg 111:1122, 1976

90. Swan HJC, Ganz W, Forrester JS et al: Catheterization of the heart in man with the use of flow directed balloon tipped catheters. N Engl J Med 283:447, 1970

91. Vender J: Pulmonary artery catheter monitoring. Anesth Clin North Am 6:743, 1988

92. Amin DK, Shah PK, Swan JHC: The Swan-Ganz catheter: Indications for insertion. J Crit Ill 1:54, 1986

93. Tuman KJ, Carroll GC, Ivankovich AD: Pitfalls of interpretations of pulmonary artery catheter data. J Cardiovasc Anesth 3:625, 1989

94. Matthay MA: Invasive hemodynamic monitoring in critically ill patients. Clin Chest Med 4:234, 1983

95. West JB, Dollery CT, Naimark A: Distribution of blood flow in isolated lung: Relation to vascular and alveolar pressures. J Appl Physiol 19:713, 1984

96. Marini JJ: Obtaining meaningful data from the Swan-Ganz catheter. Crit Care Clin 2:572, 1988

97. Marini JJ, O'Quin R, Culver BH et al: Estimation of transmural cardiac pressure during ventilation with PEEP. J Appl Physiol 53:384, 1982

98. O'Quin R, Marini JJ: Pulmonary artery occlusion pressure.

Clinical physiology, measurement, and interpretation. Am Rev Respir Dis 128:319, 1983

99. Pepe PE, Marin JJ: Occult positive end-expiratory pressure in mechanically ventilated patients with airflow obstruction. Ann Rev Respir Dis 126:166, 1982

100. Marini JJ: Hemodynamic monitoring with the pulmonary artery catheter. Crit Care Clin 2:551, 1986

101. Carlile PV: Pitfalls in the interpretation of hemodynamic data. Prog Crit Care Med 2:69, 1985

102. Jardin F, Farcot JC, Boisante L et al: Influence of positive end-expiratory pressure on left ventricular performance. N Engl J Med 304:387, 1981

103. Weber KT, Janiold JS, Shroff S et al: Contractile mechanics and interaction of the right and left ventricles. Am J Cardiol 47:686, 1981

104. Puri VK, Carlson RW, Bander JT et al: Complications of vascular catheterization in the critically ill. Crit Care Med 8:495, 1980

105. Voukydis PC, Cohen SI: Catheter-induced arrhythmias. Am Heart J 88:588, 1974

106. Murray IP: Complications of invasive monitoring. Med Instrum 15:85, 1981

107. Salmenpera M, Peltola K, Rosenberg P: Does prophylactic lidocaine control cardiac arrhythmias associated with pulmonary artery catheterization? Anesthesiology 56:210, 1982

108. Amin DK, Shah PK, Swan JHC: The Swan-Ganz catheter: Insertion technique. J Crit Ill 1:38, 1986

109. Davies MJ, Cronin KD, Damainque E: Pulmonary artery catheterization. An assessment of risks and benefits in 220 surgical patients. Anesth Intens Care 10:9, 1982

110. Band JD, Mahi DG: Infections caused by arterial catheters used for hemodynamic monitoring. Am J Med 67:735, 1979

111. Barash PG, Nardi D, Hammond G et al: Catheter-induced pulmonary artery perforation, mechanisms, management and modifications. J Thorac Cardiovasc Surg 82:5, 1981

112. Heard SO, Davis LF, Shevertz RJ et al: Influence of sterile protective sleeves on the sterility of pulmonary artery catheters. Crit Care Med 15:499, 1987

113. Mohsinifar Z, Goldbach P, Tachkin DP et al: Relationship between O_2 delivery and O_2 consumption in the adult respiratory distress syndrome. Chest 84:267, 1983

114. Räsänen J, Downs JB: Titration of continuous positive airway pressure by real-time dual oximetry. Crit Care Med 15(a):395, 1987

115. Taylar SH, Silke B: Is the measurement of cardiac output useful in clinical practice? Br J Anaesth 60:90S, 1988

116. Ganz W, Donoso R, Marcus HS et al: A new technique for measurement of cardiac output by thermodilution in man. Am J Cardiol 27:392, 1971

117. Davies GG, Jebson PJR, Glasgow BM, Hess DR: Continuous Fick cardiac output compared to thermodilution cardiac output. Crit Care Med 14:881, 1986

118. Westenskow DR, Culter CA, Wallace WD: Instrumentation for monitoring gas exchange and metabolic rate in critically ill patients. Crit Care Med 12:183, 1984

119. Morton WD: The non-invasive determination of cardiac output in children. Anesthesiology 69:223, 1988

120. Hamilton WF, Moore JW, Kinsman JM et al: Studies on circulation IV: Further analysis of the injection method, and of changes in hemodynamics under physiologic and pathologic conditions. Am J Physiol 99:534, 1932

121. Truccone NJ, Spontnitz HM, Gersony WM et al: Cardiac output in infants and children after open-heart surgery. J Thorac Cardiovasc Surg 71:410, 1976

122. Fegler G: Measurement of cardiac output in anesthetized animals by thermodilution method. Q J Exp Physiol 39:153, 1954

123. Shellock FG, Riedinger MS, Bateman TM, Gray RJ: Thermodilution cardiac output determination in hypothermic postcardiac surgery patients: Room vs ice temperature injectate. Crit Care Med 668, 1983

124. Fischer AP, Benis AM, Jurado RA et al: Analysis of errors in measurement of cardiac output by simultaneous dye and thermal dilution in cardiothoracic surgical patients. Cardiovasc Res 12:190, 1978

125. Levett JM, Replogle RL: Thermodilution cardiac output: A critical analysis and review of the literature. J Surg Res 27:392, 1979

126. Jansen JRC, Schreuder JJ, Bogaard JM et al: Thermodilution technique for measurement of cardiac output during artificial ventilation. J Appl Physiol 51:584, 1981

127. Stevens JH, Raffin TA, Mihm FG et al: Thermodilution cardiac output measurement. JAMA 253:2240, 1985

128. Pearl RG, Rosenthal MH, Nelson L et al: Effect of injectate volume and temperature on thermodilution cardiac output determination. Anesthesiology 64:798, 1986

129. Meissner H, Glanert G, Stackmeir B et al: Indicator loss during injection in the thermodilution system. Res Exp Med 159:183, 1973

130. Wetzel RC, Latson TW: Major errors in thermodilution cardiac output measurement during rapid volume infusion. Anesthesiology 62:684, 1985

131. Stetz CW, Miller RG, Kelly CE, Raffin TA: Reliability of the thermodilution method in the determination of cardiac output in clinical practice. Am Rev Respir Dis 126:1002, 1982

132. Kay H, Afshari M, Barash PG et al: Measurement of ejection fraction by thermal dilution techniques. J Surg Res 34:337, 1983

133. Kubicek WG, Karnegis JN, Patterson RP et al: Development and evaluation of an impedance cardiac output system. Aerospace Med 37:1208, 1966

134. Bernstein DP: A new stroke volume equation for thoracic electrical bioimpedance: Theory and rationale. Crit Care Med 14:902, 1986

135. Kamal GD, Symreng T, Starr J: Inconsistent esophageal Doppler cardiac output during acute blood loss. Anesthesiology 72:95, 1990

136. Siegel LC, Shafer SL, Martinez GM et al: Simultaneous measurements of cardiac output by thermodilution, esophageal Doppler, and electrical impedance in anesthetized patients. J Cardiothorac Anesth 2:590, 1988

137. Abrams JH, Weber RE, Holman KD: Continuous cardiac output determination using transtracheal Doppler: Initial results in humans. Anesthesiology 71:11, 1989

138. Goldman ME, Mindich BP, Stavile K et al: Intraoperative contrast two-dimensional echocardiography to assess mitral valve operations. J Am Coll Cardiol 4:1035, 1984

139. Cucchiara RF, Nugent M, Seward JB et al: Air embolism in upright neurosurgical patients: Detection and localization by two-dimensional transesophageal echocardiography. Anesthesiology 60:353, 1984

140. Konstadt SN, Thys D, Mindich BP et al: Validation of quantitative intraoperative transesophageal echocardiography. Anesthesiology 65:418, 1986

141. Thys DM, Hillel Z, Goldman ME et al: A comparison of hemodynamic indices derived by invasive monitoring and two-dimensional echocardiography. Anesthesiology 67:630, 1987

142. Roizen M, Beaupre P, Alpert R et al: Monitoring with two-dimensional transesophageal echocardiography. Comparison of myocardial function in patients undergoing supraceliac, suprarenal-infraceliac, or infrarenal aortic occlusion. J Vasc Surg 1:300, 1984

143. Elliott PL, Schauble JF, Weiss J et al: Echocardiography and LV function during anesthesia. Anesthesiology 53:S105, 1980

144. Smith J, Cahalan M, Benefield D et al: Intraoperative detection of myocardial ischemia in high risk patients: Echocardiography versus two-dimensional transesophageal echocardiography. Circulation 72:1015, 1985

145. Goldman ME, Mindich BP, Stavile K et al: Intraoperative contrast two-dimensional echocardiography to assess mitral valve operations. J Am Coll Cardiol 4:1035, 1984

146. Czer LSC, Maurer G, Bolger AF et al: Intraoperative evaluation of mitral regurgitation by Doppler color flow mapping. Circulation 76(suppl 3):III108, 1987

147. Equaras BG, Pasalodos J, Gonzalez V et al: Intraoperative contrast two-dimensional echocardiography: Evaluation of the presence and severity of aortic and mitral regurgitation during cardiac operations. J Thorac Cardiovasc Surg 89:573, 1985

148. Hashimoto S, Kumada T, Osakada G et al: Detection of the

entry by color Doppler in dissection aortic aneurysm. Clinical significance of the transesophageal color Doppler. Circulation 76(suppl 4): IV 37, 1987

149. Cyran SE, Meyer RA, Bailey WW et al: Intraoperative transesophageal echocardiographic assessment of congenital heart disease in children. Circulation 76(suppl 4): IV 172, 1987

150. Miller JD, Becker DP, Wand JD et al: Significance of intracranial hypertension in severe head injury. J Neurosurg 47:501, 1977

151. Risberg J, Lundberg N, Ingvar DH: Regional cerebral blood volume during acute transient rises of the intracranial pressure (plateau waves). J Neurosurg 31:303, 1969

152. Rosner MJ, Becker DP: ICP monitoring: Complications and associated factors. Clin Neurosurg 23:494, 1976

153. Koster WG, Kupers MH: Intracranial pressure and its epidural measurement. Med Prog Technol 7:21, 1980

154. Saul TG, Druker TB: Effect of intracranial pressure monitoring and aggressive treatment on mortality in severe head injury. J Neurosurg 56:498, 1982

155. Manheimer WH, Keats AS, Chamberlin JA: Safety in hypotension anesthesia. Surgery 54:883, 1963

156. Sundt TM Jr: The ischemic tolerance of neural tissue and the need for monitoring and selective shunting during carotid endarterectomy. Stroke 14:93, 1983

157. Scott JC, Ponganis KV, Stanski DR: EEG quantification of narcotic effect. The comparative pharmacodynamics of fentanyl and alfentanil. Anesthesiology 62:234, 1985

158. Engelhardt W, Carl G, Maurer K: Electroencephalographic mapping during isoflurane anesthesia for treatment of mental depression. J Clin Monit 7:23, 1991

159. Symon L, Haragadine J, Zawirski M et al: Cerebral conduction time as an index of ischemia in subarachnoid haemorrhage. J Neurol Sci 44:95, 1979

160. Kaplan BJ, Friedman WA, Alexander JA, Hampson SR: Somatosensory evoked potential monitoring of spinal cord ischemia during aortic surgery. Neurosurgery 19:82, 1986

161. Hallett M, Cohen LG: Magnetism: A new method for stimulation of nerve and brain. JAMA 262:538, 1989

162. Levy WJ, York DH, McCaffrey M, Tanzer F: Motor evoked potential from transcranial stimulation of the motor cortex in humans. Neurosurgery 15:287, 1984

163. American Electroencephalographic Society: Guidelines for intraoperative monitoring of evoked potentials. J Clin Neurophysiol 4:397, 1987

164. Bishop CCR, Powell S, Rutt D, Browse NL: Transcranial Doppler measurement of middle cerebral flow velocity: A validation study. Stroke 17:913, 1986

165. Arnolds B, von Reutern G-M: Transcranial Doppler sonography: Examination, technique, and normal reference values. Ultrasound Med Biol 12:115, 1986

166. Kaps M, Damian MD, Teschendorf U, Dorndorf W: Transcranial Doppler ultrasound finding in middle cerebral artery occlusion. Arch Neurol 47:960, 1990

167. Benichou H, Bergeron P, Ferdani M et al: Pre- and intraoperative transcranial Doppler: Prediction and surveillance of tolerance to carotid clamping. Ann Vasc Surg 5:21, 1991

168. McCormick PW, Stewart M, Goetting MG et al: Noninvasive cerebral optical spectroscopy for monitoring oxygen delivery and hemodynamics. Crit Care Med 19:89, 1991

169. Takatani S, Cheung PW, Ernst EA: A noninvasive tissue reflectance oximeter. Ann Biomed Eng 8:1, 1980

170. Kuikka J, Ahonen A, Koivula A et al: An intravenous isotope method for measuring regional cerebral blood flow (rCBF) and blood volume (rCBV). Phys Med Biol 22:958, 1977

171. Chance B, Leigh JS, Miyake, H et al: Comparison of time-resolved and unresolved measurements of deoxyhemoglobin in brain. Proc Natl Acad Sci USA 85:4971, 1988

172. Gal TJ, Goldberg SK: Relationship between respiratory muscle strength and vital capacity during partial curarization in awake subjects. Anesthesiology 54:141, 1981

173. Russell WJ, Serle DG: Hand grip force as an assessment of recovery from neuromuscular blocking. J Clin Monit 3:87, 1987

174. Stanec A, Heyduk J, Stanec G, Orkin LR: Tetanic fade and post-tetanic tension in the absence of neuromuscular blocking agents in anesthetized man. Anesth Analg 57:102, 1978

175. Mason LJ, Betts E: Leglift and maximum inspiratory force, clinical signs of neuromuscular blockade reversal in neonates and infants. Anesthesiology 52:441, 1980

176. Ali HH, Wilson RS, Savarese JJ, Kitz RJ: The effect of tubocurarine on indirectly elicited train-of-four muscle response and respiratory measurements in humans. Br J Anaesth 47:570, 1975

177. Brand JB, Cullen DJ, Wilson NE, Ali HHH: Spontaneous recovery from non-depolarizing neuromuscular blockade: Correlation between clinical and evoked responses. Anesth Analg 56:55, 1977

178. Viby-Mogensen J, Jorgenson BC, Ording H: Residual curarization in the recovery room. Anesthesiology 50:390, 1979

179. Lennmarken C, Lofstrom JB: Partial curarization in the postoperative period. Acta Anesthesiol Scand 28:260, 1984

180. Caffrey RR, Warren ML, Backer KE: Neuromuscular blockade monitoring comparing the orbicularis oculi and adductor pollicis muscles. Anesthesiology 65:95, 1986

181. Pansard J-L, Chauvin M, Lebrault C et al: Effect of an intubating dose of succinylcholine and atracurium on the diaphragm and the adductor pollicis muscle in humans. Anesthesiology 67:326, 1987

182. Kopman AF, Lawson D: Milliamperage requirements for supramaximal stimulation of the ulnar nerve with surface electrodes. Anesthesiology 61:83, 1984

183. Ali HH, Utting JE, Gray C: Stimulus frequency in the detection of neuromuscular blockade in humans. Br J Anesth 42:967, 1970

184. Ali HH, Savarese JJ: Stimulus frequency and dose-response curve to d-tubocurarine in man. Anesthesiology 52:36, 1980

185. Lee CM: Train of 4 quantification of competitive neuromuscular block. Anesth Analg 54:649, 1975

186. Beemer GH, Rozenthal P: Postoperative neuromuscular function. Anesth Intensive Care 14:41, 1986

187. Engbaek J, Ostergaard D, Viby-Mogensen J: Double burst stimulation (DBS): A new pattern of nerve stimulation to identify residual neuromuscular block. Br J Anaesth 62:274, 1989

188. Drenck NE, Ueda N, Olsen NV et al: Manual evaluation of residual curarization using double burst stimulation: A comparison with train-of-four. Anesthesiology 70:578, 1989

189. Nakatsuka M, Franks P, Keenan R: A method of rapid sequence induction using high dose narcotics with vecuronium or vecuronium and pancuronium in patients with coronary artery disease. J Cardiothorac Anesth 2:177, 1988

190. Donati F, Antzaka C, Bevan DR: Potency of pancuronium at the diaphragm and the adductor pollicis muscle in humans. Anesthesiology 65:1, 1986

191. Lee C, Katz RL, Arnold SJL, Glaser B: A new instrument for continuous recording of the evoked compound electromyogram in the clinical setting. Anesth Analg 56:260, 1977

192. Stanec A: Adductor pollicis monitor. Anesth Analg 63:1139, 1984

193. Sessler DI, Olofsson CI et al: The thermoregulatory threshold in humans during halothane anesthesia. Anesthesiology 68:836, 1988

194. Sessler DI, Olofsson CI, Rubinstein EH: The thromoregulatory threshold in humans during nitrous oxide-fentanyl anesthesia. Anesthesiology 69:337, 1988

195. Stjernstrom H, Hennberg S et al: Oxygen consumption and heat balance during TURP. Anesthesiology 61:A258, 1984

196. Vaughan MS, Cork RC, Vaughan RW: Inaccuracy of liquid-crystal thermometry to identify core temperature trends in postoperative adults. Anesth Analg 61:284, 1984

197. Lees DE, Schuette W, Bull J et al: An evaluation of liquid-crystal thermometry as a screening device for intraoperative hyperthermia. Anesth Analg 57:669, 1978

198. Cork RC, Vaughan RW, Humphrey LS: Precision and accuracy of intraoperative temperature monitoring. Anesth Analg 62:211, 1983

199. Parker EO: Electrosurgical burn at the site of an esophageal temperature probe. Anesthesiology 61:93, 1984

200. Eichhorn JH, Edsall DW: Computerization of anesthesia information management. J Clin Monit 7:71, 1991
201. Ream AK: Automating the recording and improving the presentation of the anesthesia record. J Clin Monit 5:270, 1989
202. Lerou JGC, Dirksen R, van Daele M et al: Automated charting of physiological variables in anesthesia: A quantitative comparison of automated versus handwritten anesthesia records. J Clin Monit 4:37, 1988
203. Berman JH, Hebert NC: Ion selective microelectrode. In *Advances in Experimental Medicine and Biology*, vol 50. New York, Plenum Press, 1974
204. Barker SJ, Tremper KK, Hyatt J et al: Continuous fiberoptic arterial oxygen tension measurements in dogs. J Clin Monit 3:48, 1987
205. Shapiro BA, Cane RD, Chomka CM, et al: Evaluation of a new intraarterial blood gas system in dogs. Crit Care Med 15:361A, 1987

29

James R. Zaidan

Electrocardiography

Cardiac dysrhythmias occur at any time in the perioperative period. Although Levy and Lewis reported the development of dysrhythmias and sudden death during chloroform administration as early as 1911,[1,2] it was not until 1968 that Vanik and Davis reported the incidence of perioperative dysrhythmias in a large series of patients:[3] 34% of the patients with heart disease in their study developed dysrhythmias. Interestingly, dysrhythmias occurred in 16.3% of the otherwise healthy patients. Administering regional anesthesia did not improve the incidence of dysrhythmias in the healthy patients. Kuner et al, in a study of Holter monitoring of 154 operative patients, reported that 62% of the patients had dysrhythmias.[4] As in the Vanik and Davis study, Kuner et al suggested that regional anesthesia did not reduce the incidence of perioperative dysrhythmias.

These perioperative studies must be compared with the occurrence of cardiac dysrhythmias in the normal population. In 92 healthy children aged 7–11 years,[5] heart rate varied between 37 and 197 beats·min^{-1}. Junctional rhythms appeared in 45% of the children. Premature atrial and ventricular contractions occurred in 21%. Another study of healthy medical students[6] revealed heart rates ranging from 37–180 beats·min^{-1}. Minimal heart rates during sleep ranged from 33–55 beats·min^{-1}. Twenty-eight percent had sinus arrests persisting longer than 1.75 seconds. Premature ventricular contractions occurred in 50% of the subjects, and 6% developed Wenckebach second-degree atrioventricular (AV) block. With these studies of unanesthetized subjects in mind, dysrhythmias occurring during anesthesia do not appear quite so ominous.

The decision to treat perioperative dysrhythmias depends on the overall cardiac status of the patient. For instance, a healthy patient undergoing uncomplicated surgery should not necessarily receive treatment for a junctional rhythm that does not significantly change blood pressure and clinical signs of perfusion. Conversely, this same dysrhythmia occurring in a patient with tight aortic stenosis might cause profound hemodynamic changes that require rapid treatment to prevent cardiovascular collapse.

This chapter aims to acquaint the reader with the electrocardiographic monitoring required to facilitate rapid diagnosis of intraoperative dysrhythmias. It will include lead placement and the surface electrocardiogram (ECG), methods of obtaining intracavitary ECGs, vector analysis, electro-physiology, and mechanisms of dysrhythmias. Discussions of specific dysrhythmias encompass supraventricular nodal, and ventricular dysrhythmias, bundle-branch and AV nodal blocks, ischemic patterns, drug and electrolyte effects, and pacemakers.

THE NORMAL ELECTROCARDIOGRAM

The electrocardiographic deflections separate into waves, complexes, intervals, and segments. Multiple waves form complexes, whereas intervals include waves and segments. Table 29-1 describes each of these deflections and their electrophysiologic significance. Sinoatrial (SA) nodal activity and atrial repolarization are invisible on the surface ECG.

Figure 29-1 reveals a normal surface ECG. Note that the P wave and T wave are upright in every lead except AVR and that the ST segment is isoelectric with the PR segment. With a standard paper speed of 25 mm·sec^{-1}, each millimeter represents 0.04 sec. Figure 29-1 therefore represents a

TABLE 29-1. Electrophysiologic Significance of Electrocardiogram Deflections

Deflection	Significance
P wave	Impulse spreads through atrium and AV node
P–R internal	1. Conduction from AV node to Purkinje fibers
	2. Atrial repolarization
QRS complex	Ventricular activation
Q wave	Any negative wave occurring before the R wave
R wave	Any positive wave
S wave	Any negative wave occurring after the R wave
ST segment	Occurs when the majority of myocardial cells are in phase 2 (plateau phase)
	Elevation or depression indicates ischemia
Q–T interval	Indicator of total ventricular depolarization and repolarization time; inversely proportional to heart rate
T wave	Represents ventricular repolarization
U wave	Related to ventricular repolarization

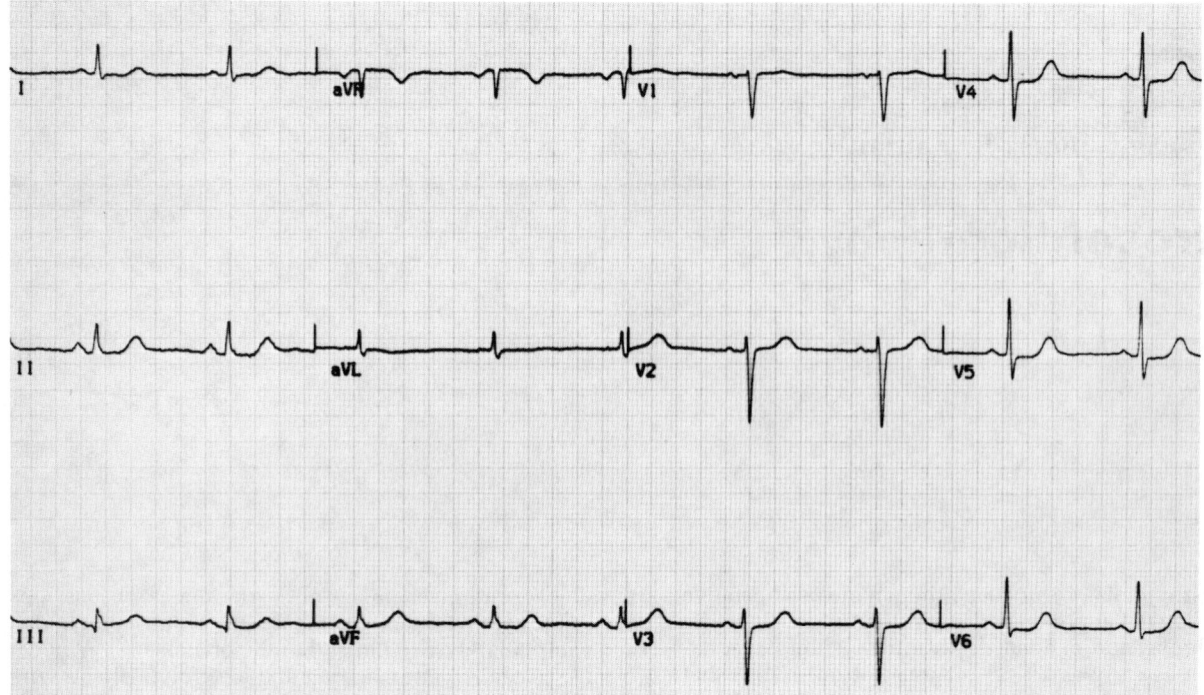

Figure 29-1. Normal ECG with sinus bradycardia.

P-R interval of 0.152 sec (normal range 0.12–0.20), a QRS duration of 0.088 sec (normal <0.10 sec), and a rate-corrected Q-T interval of 0.421 sec. Figures 29-2 through 29-5 show different types of intraoperative interference that the anesthesiologist can encounter.

Figure 29-6 reveals the importance of calibrating and appropriately filtering the electrocardiographic signal. The first line, an ECG that was incorrectly calibrated, has almost 9 mm of ST segment elevation. Correctly calibrated to 1 mV·cm^{-1} in the second line, the same patient had only 1.5 mm ST segment elevation. Changes in low-frequency filtering create the difference in ST segment elevation noted be-

tween the second and third tracings in Figure 29-6. The middle trace is filtered between 0.5 and 50 Hz, and the bottom trace is filtered from 0.05 to 100 Hz. Greater filtering of the ECG signal at the lower end of the signal (0.5 Hz vs. 0.05 Hz) distorts the ST segment change associated with ischemia. Generally accepted electrical filtering extends from 0.05 Hz high pass and 100 Hz low pass. Therefore, the third trace in Figure 29-6 is correctly filtered and reveals that the patient had a 4-mm ST segment change. Although intraoperative lead placement tends to be haphazard, in fact, standardized placement helps interpret the ECG. Table 29-2 describes correct lead placement.

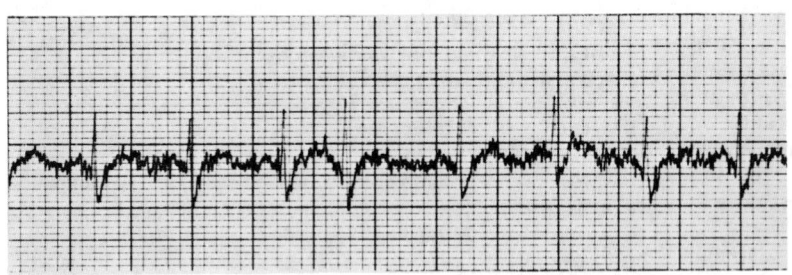

Figure 29-2. Muscle artifact in the baseline makes it impossible to differentiate a premature atrial contraction from a junctional escape. Note the fourth R wave.

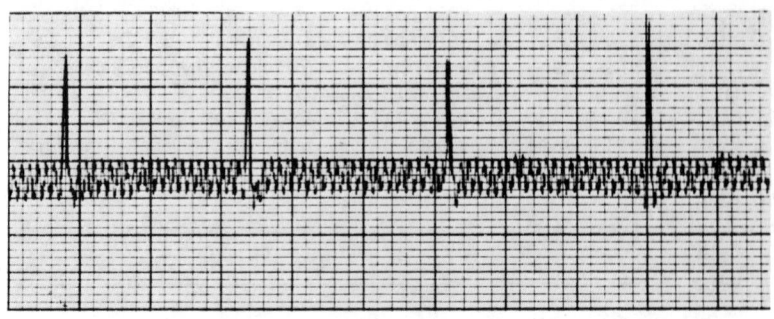

Figure 29-3. A 60-cycle interference affects the baseline.

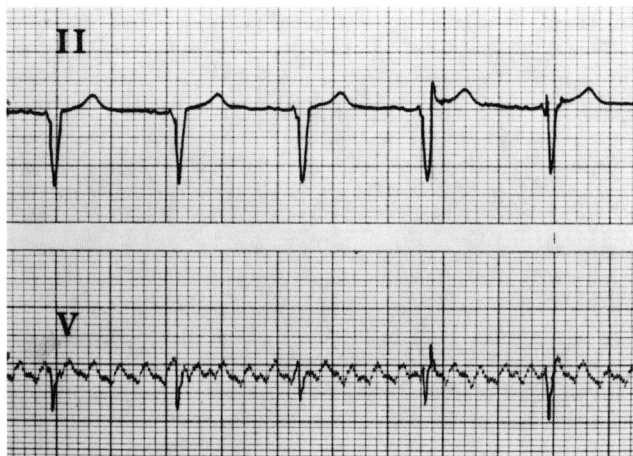

Figure 29-4. The arterial pump head in the cardiopulmonary bypass machine distorts the ECG so that it appears like atrial flutter. This problem is created by the motor revolving within the column of blood in the arterial tubing.

Impulses detected by the surface electrodes combine to cause deflections on the recorder in such a way that positive deflections have forces directed toward the electrode and negative deflections have forces directed away from the electrode. Electrical forces traveling perpendicular to the electrode do not cause a deflection on the ECG recorder and are therefore "invisible."

Three standard electrodes (right arm, left arm, and left leg) form a triangle, first described by Einthoven, in which the R wave voltage in lead II should normally equal the combined voltages of leads I plus III. In the standard bipolar limb leads I, II, and III, each electrode equally influences the recorded ECG from locations on the extremities distant from the heart. Placing an exploring electrode close to the heart on the precordium and an indifferent electrode distant from the heart on an extremity lessens the influence of the indifferent electrode on the final ECG pattern. The "C" leads perform this task. The C leads are named according to the location of their indifferent electrode: C_F, left leg indifferent; C_R, right arm indifferent; and C_L, left arm indifferent. As an example, locating the left arm electrode (indifferent) over the left upper chest and the left leg electrode (exploring) over the V_1 position and selecting lead III on the ECG monitor modify the C_L lead so that it is called the MC_{L1} lead.[7]

Connecting the combined left leg, left arm, and right arm electrodes through 5000 ohm resistances to a common terminal eliminates the indifferent electrode's influence on the precordial lead. Leads V_1–V_6, therefore, are considered unipolar and describe the impulse occurring under the surface electrode. Another type of unipolar lead is the limb lead. These leads are the commonly used V_R, V_L, and V_F leads that are augmented in height by disconnecting the right arm (V_R), left arm (V_L), or left leg (V_F) electrodes from the common terminal. Augmentation performed by the ECG machine renames these leads aV_R, aV_L, and aV_F, respectively.

One can also record impulses from inside the heart if the monitor is appropriately electrically isolated. These intracavitary ECGs, which are called the *atrial electrogram* (AEG) and the *ventricular electrogram* (VEG), help to characterize complex atrial dysrhythmias. Figure 29-7 shows a typical AEG, and Figure 29-8 describes the intracavitary electrograms associated with placing an electrode into the ventricle. It is best when diagnosing a dysrhythmia simultaneously to record the AEG and a surface lead II ECG. The VEG is not as clinically useful as the AEG. An esophageal ECG also can help to diagnose arrhythmias.[8] The esophageal probe, which contains large surface area electrodes, records impulses from the atrium or the ventricle.[9-11]

A special type of intracavitary electrogram, called the His bundle recording, requires multiple electrodes, special filtering, and fluoroscopy. After the impulse travels through the AV node, it enters the bundle of His. As shown in Figure 29-9, the very small His bundle deflection is located approximately midway between the atrial and ventricular deflections. Measuring the time between the P wave or R wave and His deflection estimates the time required for an impulse to travel from the atrium, through the AV node and bundle of His, to the ventricular conducting system. Normal conduction time intervals in the His bundle electrogram have wide variations. To ensure an accurate His bundle recording, the AEG and VEG recordings must be approximately equal in height (mV). Also, pacing from the electrode that is recording the His bundle deflection might produce a QRS complex identical to the surface lead's QRS complex. Once the catheter achieves good position, one can measure the PA (10–50 msec), SA (60–125 msec), and HV (35–55 msec) intervals.[12-16] The PA interval, measuring the time from the beginning of the surface P wave to the beginning of the intra-atrial recording, estimates atrial activation time. The AH interval indicates the time for the impulse to proceed through the AV node, whereas the HV interval records the time necessary for the impulse to conduct through the His–Purkinje system. These intervals can be used to determine the effects of anesthetic drugs on conduction.[17]

Three methods exist for determining heart rate. The first method notes the number of 0.04 sec units (1 mm) between R waves, multiplies 0.04 sec times this number of units, and divides this number into 60. The second method quickly estimates heart rate. If two R waves have 5 mm between them (0.2 sec), the heart rate is 300. Each 0.2-sec increase in the RR interval indicates a decrease in the heart rate to 150, 100, 75, 60, 50, 43, 37, 35, and finally 30 beats·min^{-1}

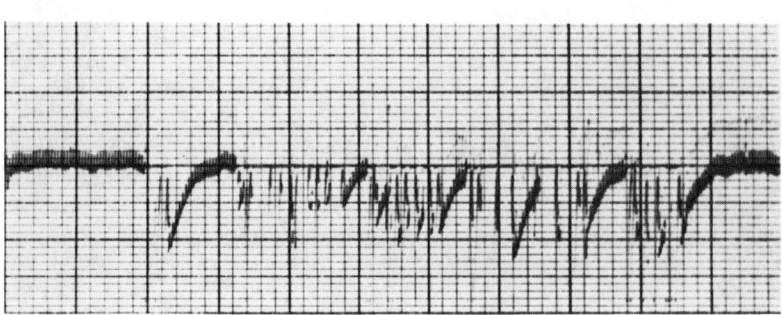

Figure 29-5. The electrocautery totally distorts the electrogram.

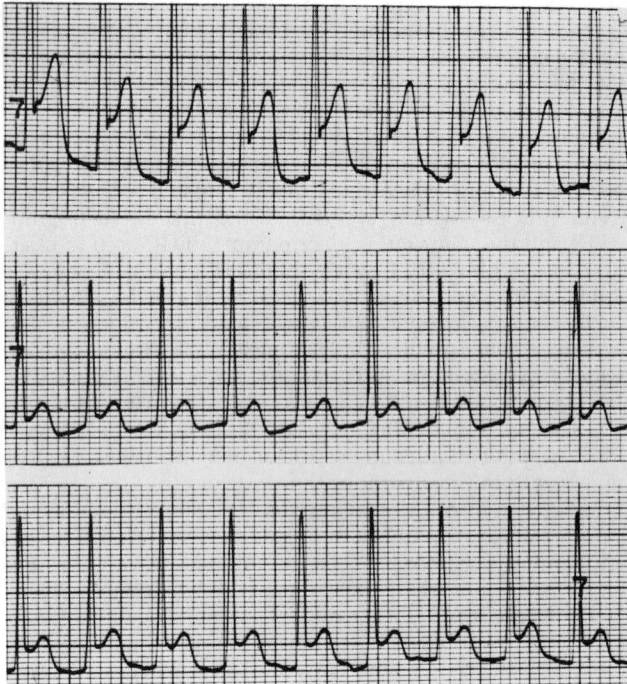

Figure 29-6. A noncalibrated ECG (*top*) artifactually depicts 9-mm ST segment elevation. The calibrated *middle* and *bottom* traces are filtered from 0.5–50 Hz and 0.05–100 Hz, respectively. The *bottom* trace is correctly filtered for ECG diagnosis of ST segment change and reveals a 4-mm elevation.

if there were 10 0.2-sec units between R waves. The third method of determining heart rate involves knowing the number of seconds in the sweep speed of the ECG monitor. If the ECG monitor's sweep speed is 5 sec, the heart rate is 12 times the number of R waves in one sweep.

VECTORS AND ELECTRICAL AXIS

The sum of all of the impulses describes the electrical axis of the heart. One can determine an axis for the QRS complex, the P wave, and the T wave, and deviations from each normal axis have clinical significance. To determine an axis, one must first know the hexaxial reference system shown in Figure 29-10. Note that the standard limb leads are at

TABLE 29-2. Correct Electrocardiogram Lead Placement

Lead	Location
R_A	Right wrist
R_L	Right ankle
L_A	Left wrist
L_L	Left ankle
V_1	4th intercostal space, right of sternum
V_2	4th intercostal space, left of sternum
V_3	Between V_2 and V_4
V_4	5th intercostal space, left midclavicular line
V_5	5th intercostal space, left anterior axillary line
V_6	5th intercostal space, left midaxillary line

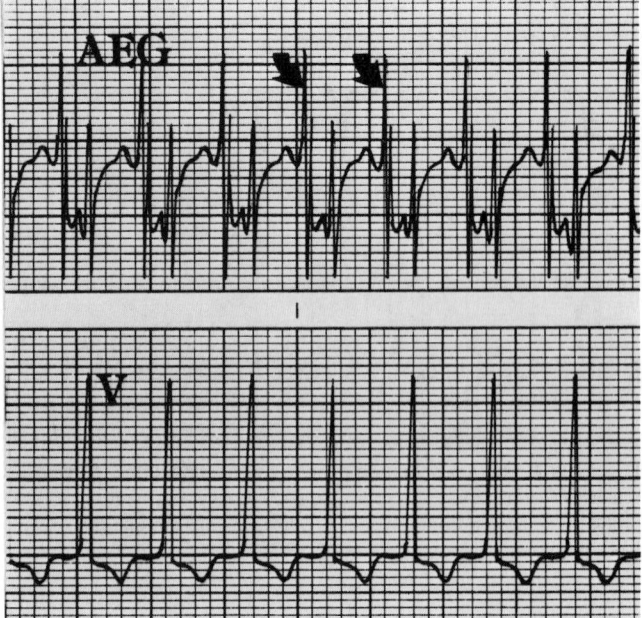

Figure 29-7. The AEG (*top*) clearly reveals atrial depolarizations compared to the V_5 lead (*bottom*). The *arrows* point out P waves on the AEG.

60-degree angles to each other, and that the augmented limb leads are oriented at 120-degree angles. Lead I, located at 0 degrees, points directly to the right and aV_F points directly downward. The directions of the other leads are easily placed by remembering the 60/120 degree rule. The heart is

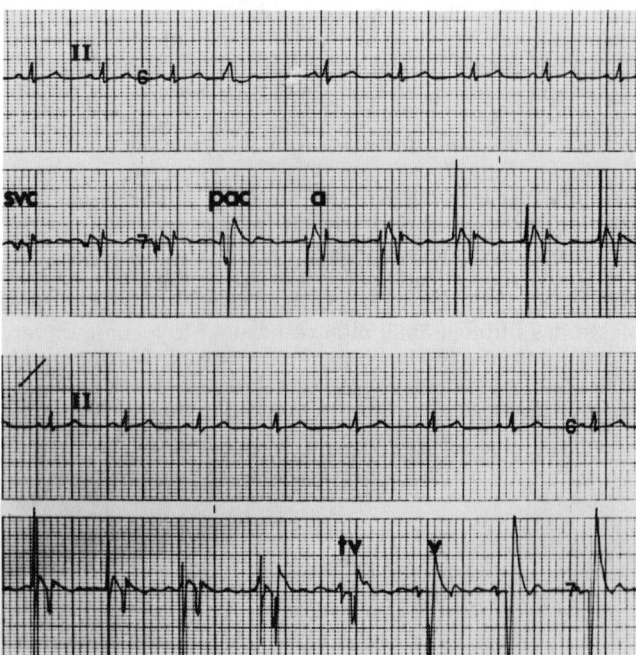

Figure 29-8. Determine the exact location of an intracardiac electrode by observing the electrogram. In this example, the electrogram clearly shows the electrode as it enters the superior vena cava (SVC), atrium (A), tricuspid valve (TV), and ventricle (V). One premature atrial contraction (PAC) occurs.

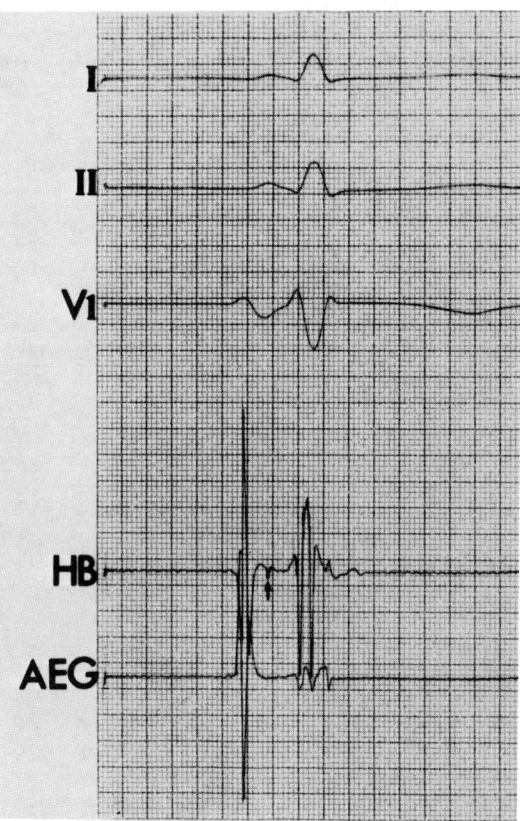

Figure 29-9. The His bundle recording requires special catheters and electrical filtering. Leads I, II, and V₁ are surface ECG leads. HB is the His recording showing the His deflection at the *arrow*. The atrial and ventricular depolarizations are approximately equal in height compared to the atrial electrogram (AEG). (Courtesy of Paul Walter, M.D.)

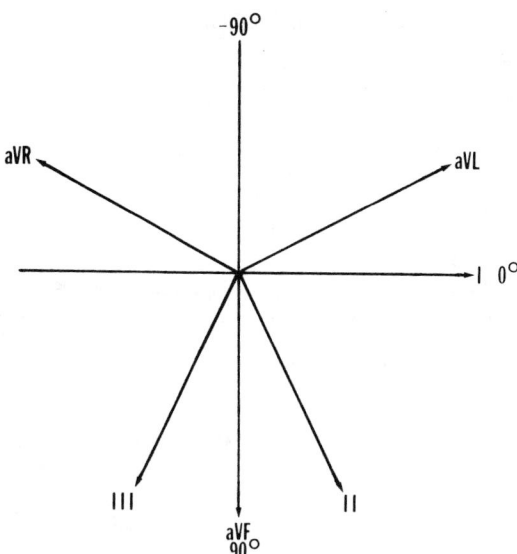

Figure 29-10. The hexaxial reference system shows that leads I, II, and III are at 60-degree angles to each other, and leads aV_R, aV_L, and aV_F are at 120-degree angles.

theoretically placed on the hexaxial reference system so that the septum lies on lead I, the left ventricle lies in the quadrant described by lead I and −90 degrees, and the right ventricle lies in the quadrant between lead I and +90 degrees. The first method of determining the QRS axis looks at the QRS complex with the highest voltage. The axis would point toward that lead on the hexaxial reference system if the voltage were positive and away from that lead if the voltage were negative. In Figure 29-1, leads I and II have approximately the same height R wave (6 mm). This configuration would place the R wave axis equidistant between leads I and II. Since lead I is 0 degrees and lead II is +60 degrees, the estimated R wave axis by this method is +30 degrees. The second system first finds the ECG lead with equiphasic voltage (equal positive and negative voltage) and then looks at the voltage in lead II. The axis will be perpendicular to the equiphasic lead and toward lead II if lead II is predominantly positive but away from lead II if lead II is predominantly negative. Using Figure 29-1, lead III is slightly positive but approximately equiphasic. A positive lead II places the R wave axis perpendicular to lead III and toward lead II, or in the vicinity of +40 to +50 degrees. The final system of determining the QRS axis specifically measures the voltage in two of the standard limb leads and plots them on the hexaxial system. This last method, although it is simple in concept and can be performed by hand, is usually calculated by computer systems. The nor-

mal QRS axis is −30 +90 degrees. Minus 30 degrees to −90 degrees indicates a left axis deviation and +90 − 180 degrees indicates a right axis deviation. Left and right axis deviations can be normal variations. Right axis deviations, however, should alert one to left posterior hemiblock, right ventricular hypertrophy, emphysema, or pulmonary embolus. Left anterior hemiblock and abdominal tumors or fluid that rotate the heart to the left are possibilities for left axis deviation.[18] One may use the same methods to determine P wave and T wave axes. The T wave axis generally points in the same direction as the QRS axis and should be within 50 degrees of the QRS axis. The P wave axis should point between leads I and II but slightly closer to lead II. Because the sum of all electrical forces in the atria points toward lead II, monitor this lead to see the most easily discernible P wave. A leftward shift of the P wave axis indicates left atrial enlargement, and a rightward shift indicates right atrial enlargement. A right P wave axis deviation greater than +60 degrees is strong evidence of chronic lung disease.[19]

ELECTROPHYSIOLOGY

A rapid influx of sodium ions through the cellular membrane creates phase 0 of the action potential and determines its maximal amplitude, overshoot, and rate of rise (Vmax).[20] Hodgkin and Huxley later found that although sodium influx depolarizes, potassium extrusion repolarizes the membrane.[21] Hagiwara and Nakajina described two inward currents in cardiac conduction tissue.[22] One current, the fast channel responsible for phase 0 of the action potential, was due to the influx of sodium ions, and a second, slower current found later in the action potential was due to the influx of calcium ions.

The action potential encompasses five different phases (Figure 29-11A). Phase 0 occurs when an impulse of sufficient amplitude opens an activation "gate" or channel located in the external surface of the membrane that initiates

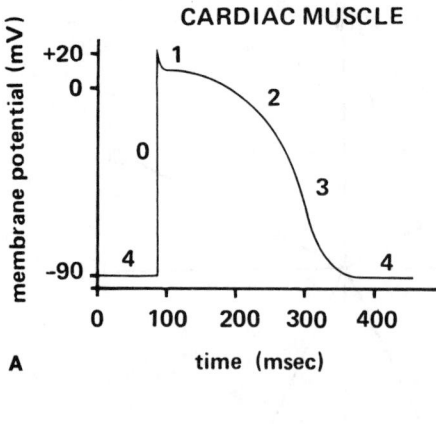

A

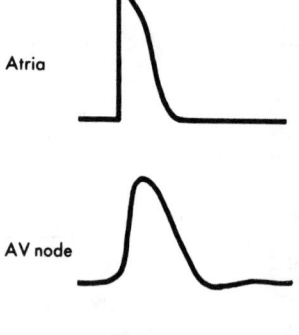

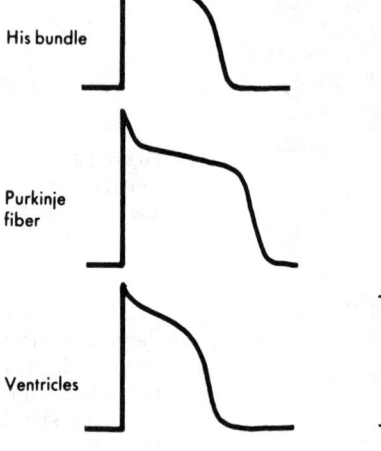

B

Figure 29-11. (*A*) Five phases (phase 0–4) constitute the cardiac action potential. These phases are described in the text. (*B*) Relationships of typical action potentials throughout the conduction system. Note the progressive lengthening of phase 2 from the atrium to the Purkinje fiber and then the shortening of phase 2 in ventricular muscle. (Reproduced with permission from Marriott HJL, Conover MHB: Advanced Concepts in Arrhythmias. St Louis, CV Mosby, 1983.)

entrance of sodium ions. Almost at the same instant, inactivation gates located in the internal surface of the membrane begin closing to impede the inward flow of sodium ions. The inactivation gates close slightly slower than the activation gates open. This slight delay is the period in which sodium enters the cell. Phase 1, extending from the peak of phase 0 to the beginning of the plateau phase, is thought to occur secondary to the beginning of an outward potassium current and an inward chloride current.[23,24] During phase 2 the slow calcium channel that opened during phase 0 remains open because of its prolonged inactivation time constant of up to 500 msec. Calcium entrance counterbalances potassium extrusion, so that for up to 200 msec the transmembrane potential does not change. Phase 2, therefore, is called the plateau phase of the action potential. Phase 3 occurs when the slow inward flow of calcium ions diminishes and the outward potassium current continues.[25] The flow of potassium ions increases as the transmembrane voltage becomes more negative.

After reaching the maximal negative membrane potential, called the *maximal diastolic potential*, SA nodal cells begin spontaneously depolarizing during phase 4. Spontaneous depolarization in SA nodal cells is caused by the movement of calcium ions into the cell. When the SA nodal cell reaches the threshold potential, sodium quickly flows into the cell to create another phase 0. Automaticity in Purkinje fibers, unlike in SA cells, is not secondary to calcium influx but either to a slow decrease in an outward potassium current[26] or to an increasing diastolic inward sodium current.[27]

Ventricular muscle normally does not have a phase 4 or a maximal depolarization potential but rather has a constant resting membrane potential.

Figure 29-11*B* describes the appearance of action potentials in different areas of the heart. One notable fact is the lengthening of the action potential duration in the distal Purkinje system and its shortening in ventricular muscle.[28] This lengthening of the action potential duration in distal conducting fibers compared with ventricular muscle protects the ventricular muscle from receiving impulses in their relative refractory period.[29] Impulses entering ventricular muscle during the repolarizing phase could potentially fibrillate the heart.

Action Potentials and the Electrocardiogram

The relationship between multiple action potentials and the ECG is easy to visualize when it is remembered that myocardial cells depolarize in sequence over a period of time.[30] It is this time delay in the onset of phase 0 of the first action potential to the onset of phase 0 of the last action potential that inscribes the electrocardiographic pattern. The peak of the R wave occurs when the membrane potentials among the myocardial cells beneath the electrode are at their greatest differences. Phase 2, occurring simultaneously in most cells, creates a short period of time in which there are minimal voltage differences among the action potentials. Because the ECG electrode records no voltage difference, the

ECG pattern becomes isoelectric and forms the ST segment. Phase 3 action potential delays create the T wave.

MECHANISMS OF DYSRHYTHMIAS

Several cellular mechanisms create dysrhythmias. These mechanisms either spontaneously initiate an impulse or require ongoing impulse formation with a circuit.

Automatic Mechanisms

Changes in Normal Automaticity

Cells in various areas of the heart display automaticity. These areas include the SA and distal AV nodes, bundle of His, bundle branches, Purkinje cells, and even cells in tricuspid and mitral valves.[31-33] Normally, only SA nodal cells display sufficiently rapid automaticity and a less negative maximal diastolic potential to reach threshold before the other potential pacemaker cells.[34,35] Changes in automaticity imply that slow depolarization during phase 4 of the action potential reaches threshold at a rate different than normal and is simply an enhancement of normal physiology. The slope of phase 4 could increase or decrease, causing an increase or decrease in heart rate or the ectopic rate.

Abnormal Automaticity

Normal atrial and ventricular myocardial cells do not display phase 4 depolarization. Changing the resting membrane potential to -60 mV, however, creates abnormal automaticity through slow-response action potentials.[36-38] A less negative transmembrane potential not only initiates spontaneous depolarization in cells that normally do not have this type of activity[39,40] but also permits spontaneously depolarizing cells to reach threshold before a pacemaker cell with a more negative transmembrane potential. In this instance, even ventricular or atrial muscle can initiate ectopic beats or tachycardias. Table 29-3 lists the effects of changes in maximal diastolic potential, threshold potential, and slope of phase 4 on heart rate.

Oscillatory Currents

Spontaneous oscillations can occur in transmembrane potentials. These oscillations in resting transmembrane potentials do not require a previous action potential to initiate them and are thought by some to cause spontaneous impulses.[41] According to Lin et al, oscillatory currents that develop in response to repolarization are caused by calcium-initiated release of intracellular calcium that triggers a Na^+-Ca^{2+} exchange.[42]

Triggered Activity

Another mechanism responsible for cardiac dysrhythmias is the presence of early and delayed afterdepolarizations.[43] Described by Bozler in atrial muscle[44] and by Cranefield and Aronson in Purkinje fibers,[45] delayed afterdepolarizations occur after the cell has fully repolarized. Early afterdepolarizations occur before completion of membrane repolarization. Both types of afterdepolarizations can trigger another action potential of sufficient magnitude to reach the thresh-

TABLE 29-3. Effect of Changes in Action Potential on Heart Rate

Change	Effect
Increase slope of phase 4	Higher heart rate if in SA nodal cell
	Escape beats or ectopic focus
Decrease slope of phase 4	Slower heart rate if in SA nodal cell
	Less chance of escape beats or irritable focus
Less negative threshold	Slower heart rate if in SA nodal cell
	Less chance of escape beats or ectopic focus
More negative threshold	Faster heart rate if in SA nodal cell
	Escape beats or irritable focus
Less negative maximal diastolic potential	Higher heart rate if in SA nodal cell
	Escape beats or ectopic focus
More negative maximal diastolic potential	Slower heart rate if in SA nodal cell
	Less chance of escape beats or irritable focus

old potential. The dysrhythmias thereby created are called *triggered dysrhythmias*.

It is unclear how oscillatory currents described above relate to early afterdepolarizations. They may represent the same phenomenon,[46] although Lin et al state that oscillatory currents are self-initiating,[42] whereas afterdepolarizations require a preceding depolarization.

The molecular mechanism responsible for creating afterdepolarization remains unclear. Because cardiac glycosides are known to cause these depolarizations, the mechanism of afterdepolarization is likely related to calcium.[46] The magnitude of afterdepolarizations is increased by catecholamines and high levels of extracellular calcium.[47]

Re-entry

Re-entry, another dysrhythmogenic mechanism, can be ordered or random.

Ordered Re-entry

Schmitt and Erlanger described the requirements for re-entry in 1929.[48] These requirements are a complete circuit by which an impulse can return to the beginning of the pathway, unequal conduction velocities in each limb of the circuit, and a unidirectional block.[46] Re-entrant circuits that follow definite anatomic pathways are called *ordered re-entry*. Re-entrant circuits can be found in loops of Purkinje fibers;[49] in unbranched collections of Purkinje fibers;[50] in the AV node;[51] at the junction of the atrium with the SA or at AV nodes;[52,53] and at the junction of the Purkinje fibers with myocardial cells.[54] They give rise to many types of supraventricular dysrhythmias. Wolff-Parkinson-White syndrome and AV nodal re-entrant tachycardia are examples of ordered re-entry.

Random Re-entry

In 1940, Wiggers noted that rapid rates of pacing fibrillated dog hearts.[55] Fibrillation requires a certain volume of myocardial cells for its initiation and persistence and represents fragmented wavefronts that are randomly conducted and blocked throughout the atrium or ventricle. The fragmented impulses block whenever they meet refractory tissue and retrogradely conduct to reactivate other limbs of the small circuits. Individual cells not receiving impulses in an orderly fashion respond by randomly contracting whenever they receive an impulse. Allessie et al suggest that the block does not necessarily require anatomically defined areas such as ischemia or infarction.[56] The blocks, however, can be the propagating impulse itself, creating a functionally inactive area of tissue. Atrial fibrillation is one example of random re-entry.

Reflection

It is possible for a quite small section of tissue, such as a group of myocardial cells, to have depressed conduction. Part of this section of tissue also could have total unidirectional blockade, while the remainder could continue transmitting impulses (Fig. 29-12). The transmitted impulse can reverse its direction, retrogradely proceed through the unidirectionally blocked area, and re-enter the proximal segment. This type of re-entry is called *reflection*. Reflection develops in longitudinally conducting fibers when a zone of depressed conduction separates two segments of normally conducting tissue.[57] Rozanski et al subdivided reflection into two types.[58] In their experiments, Rozanski et al characterized the action potentials of proximal (P) and distal (D) segments of ventricular muscle fibers separated by a nonelectrolytic sucrose gap (G) that represented the zone of depressed conduction. Normally conducting tissue would not retrogradely conduct to the proximal segment. A secondary depolarization that prolonged the action potential duration in the proximal segment of the ventricular fiber characterizes Type I reflection (Fig. 29-13). Type II reflection (Fig. 29-14) occurs when the impulse returns to the segment proximal to the block after the proximal segment has fully repolarized. In Type II reflection, the proximal segment actually develops two action potentials, the second of which can re-enter normal areas. Reflection potentially causes premature beats.

Parasystole

Parasystole is the simultaneous existence of two totally independent pacemaker sites. As an example, one site could be in the sinus node that conducts normally, with a second site located in the distal Purkinje fibers. The second pacemaker site is protected from overdrive suppression by entrance block. If exit block does not exist, the secondary pacemaker continues discharging into the myocardium and causes an ectopic ventricular beat. This mechanism causes ventricular bigeminy, trigeminy, and so forth, depending on the discharge rate of the parasystolic site. It is very much like a patient having an asynchronous pacemaker that does not sense intrinsic electrical activity. This patient's ECG would reveal at least three different QRS morphologies: the sinus beat, the parasystolic ventricular beat, and fusion beats or a combination of the sinus and parasystolic beats.

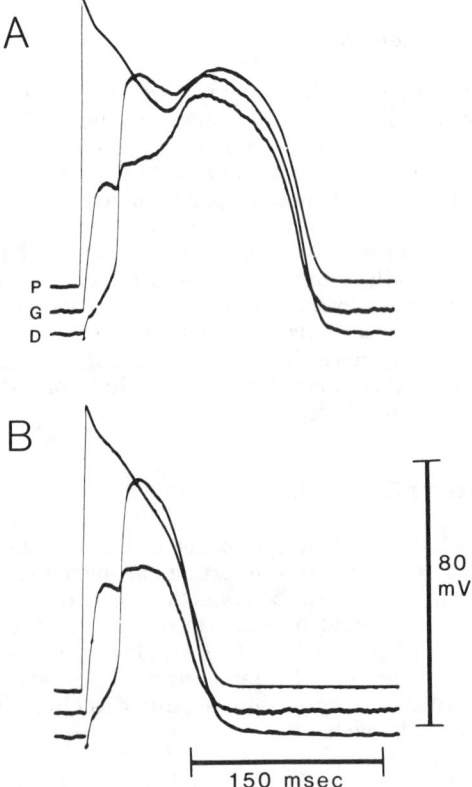

Figure 29-13. (*A*) Type I reflection appears as a prolongation of phase 2 of depolarization in a proximal segment of a small section of ventricular muscle that was electrically divided into proximal (P) and distal (D) segments by a sucrose bath (G). (*B*) Conduction in the three segments when reflection does not occur. (From Rozanski GJ, Jalife J, Moe GK: Reflected reentry in nonhomogeneous ventricular muscle as a mechanism of cardiac arrhythmias. Circulation 69:163, 1984. Reprinted by permission of the American Heart Association, Inc.)

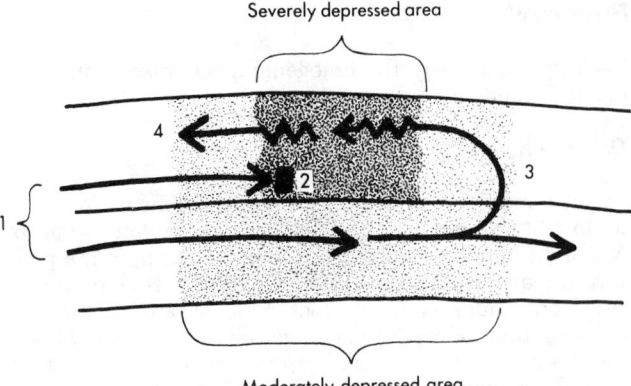

Figure 29-12. Illustration of reflection, in which the impulse (1) blocks in an ischemic area (2). The original impulse reflects at (3) and returns through the severely depressed area to its origin (4). (Reproduced with permission from Marriott HJL, Conover MHB: Advanced Concepts in Arrhythmias. St Louis, CV Mosby, 1983.)

ANTIDYSRHYTHMIC DRUG CLASSIFICATION

Anesthesiologists use many antidysrhythmic drugs. It is important to know the pharmacologic properties of these drugs to avoid their potentially serious side-effects. Antidysrhythmic drugs are classified according to the drug's effect on a single myocardial cell's action potentials (Tables 29-4 and 29-5).[59]

Class I

These membrane-stabilizing drugs block rapid sodium channels. Because of this effect, they reduce conduction velocity (reduce slope of phase 0 and decrease overshoot) and prolong the effective refractory period. Their ability to change conduction velocity and the refractory period makes them useful in treating re-entrant dysrhythmias. Automatic arrhythmias are terminated because Class I drugs also slow phase 4 of depolarization. Investigators have further subdivided the Class I drugs according to the degree of effect on the cell's action potential. Class IA drugs moderately reduce the slope of phase 0 and prolong the action potential duration. Class IB agents have little effect on phase 0, but they increase the potassium repolarization current and therefore decrease the refractory period. Class IC drugs markedly slow phase 0 and conduction but only minimally affect repolarization.

Class II

These agents, the beta blocking drugs, terminate dysrhythmias solely by their action on the beta-1 and beta-2 receptors.[60]

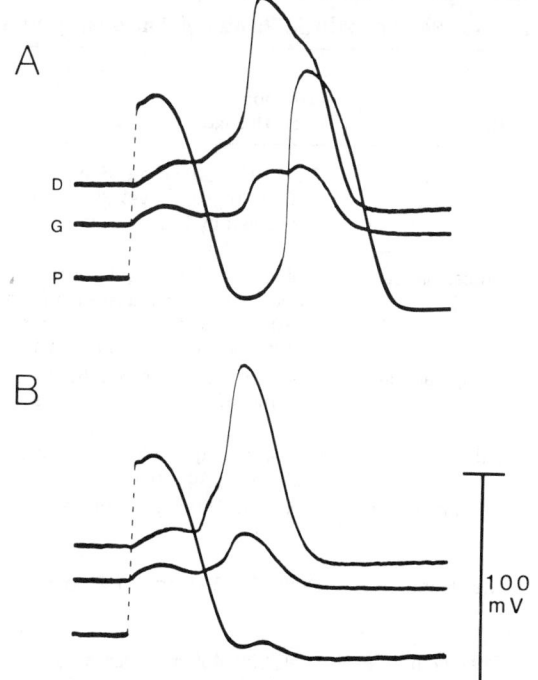

Figure 29-14. (A) Type II reflection appears as a second action potential occurring in the proximal segment of a small section of ventricular muscle that was electrically divided by a sucrose gap. P = proximal segment; D = distal segment; G = sucrose gap. (B) Conduction in the three segments when reflection does not occur. (From Rozanski GJ, Jalife J, Moe GK: Reflected reentry in nonhomogeneous ventricular muscle as a mechanism of cardiac arrhythmias. Circulation 69:163, 1984. Reprinted by permission of the American Heart Association, Inc.)

TABLE 29-4. Classification of Antidysrhythmic Drugs

Class	Electrophysiologic action	Drugs
I. Membrane-stabilizing agents		
A	Depress phase 0 (dV/dt)	Quinidine
	Slow conduction moderately	Procainamide
	Prolong repolarization	Disopyramide
B	Minimal effect on phase 0 of the action potential	Lidocaine
		Mexiletine
	Shorten repolarization	Tocainide
		Phenytoin
C	Markedly depress phase 0 of the action potential	Encainide
		Flecainide
	Marked slowing of conduction	Lorcainide
	Minimal effect on repolarization	
II. Beta-adrenergic blocking agents		Propranolol
		Atenolol
		Metoprolol
III. Prolong repolarization	No effect on phase 0 of the action potential	Amiodarone
		Bretylium
IV. Calcium channel blockers		Verapamil
		Diltiazem

Reprinted with permission from Platia EV: Management of Cardiac Arrhythmias, p 134. Philadelphia, JB Lippincott, 1987.

TABLE 29-5. Pharmacologic Profile of Antidysrhythmic Drugs

Class	Drug	Commonly Used Dosage	Elimination Half-Life	Therapeutic Plasma Level ($\mu g \cdot ml^{-1}$)	Side-Effects
IA	Quinidine	Oral: 200–600 mg q 6–8 hours iv: 6–10 mg·kg^{-1} over 30 minutes followed by 2–3 mg·min^{-1}	6 hours	2–6	Quinidine syncope, conduction disturbances, nausea, vomiting, diarrhea, thrombocytopenia, hypotension
	Procainamide	Oral: 250–1000 mg q 4 hours (q 6 hours for sustained-release form) iv: 10–20 mg·kg^{-1} over 20–40 minutes followed by 2–6 mg·min^{-1}	2–4 hours	4–12 (8–15, N-acetyl procainamide)	Conduction disturbances, nausea, diarrhea, fever, lupus syndrome, hypotension
	Disopyramide	Oral: 150–300 mg q 6–8 hours iv: 2 mg·kg^{-1} over 3–5 minutes	6–8 hours	5–7	Cardiac depression, conduction disturbances, anticholinergic symptoms
IB	Lidocaine	iv: 1–2 mg·kg^{-1} bolus followed by 20–40 μg·kg^{-1}·min^{-1}	1–2 hours	2–5	Drowsiness, hallucination, seizures, paranoid ideation
	Tocainide	Oral: 400–600 mg q 8 hours	13–15 hours	4–10	Tremor, dizziness, ataxia, paresthesia, rash, hepatitis, nausea, vomiting
	Mexiletine	Oral: 150–300 mg q 6–8 hours	10–20 hours	0.75–2.0	Tremor, convulsions, dizziness, photosensitivity, dermatitis, hypotension, nausea, vomiting
	Phenytoin	Oral: 200–400 mg once daily iv: 50–100 mg every 5 minutes to maximum 1 g	24 hours	10–18	Hypotension, vertigo, lethargy, dysarthria, gingivitis, macrocytic anemia, lupus, pulmonary infiltrates
	Moricizine (ethmozine)	Oral: 75–200 mg q 8 hours	4–10 hours		Dizziness, headache, pruritus
IC	Encainide	Oral: 25–75 mg q 6–8 hours iv: 0.5–1 mg·kg^{-1} over 15 minutes	3–4 hours	0.01–0.02	Conduction disturbances, blurred vision, nystagmus, dizziness, ataxia, vertigo, paresthesia, nausea, proarrhythmic
	Flecainide	Oral: 100–200 mg q 12 hours iv: 2 mg·kg^{-1} over 10 minutes	18–20 hours	0.2–1.0	Blurred vision, headache, lightheadedness, ataxia, proarrhythmic
	Lorcainide	Oral: 100–200 mg q 12 hours iv: 1–2 mg·kg^{-1} over 30 minutes	7–13 hours (norlorcainide, 24 hours)	0.05–0.3 0.08–0.3	Sleep disturbances, nightmares, tremor, hyponatremia, nausea, diarrhea
Unclassified					
	Propafenone	Oral: 100–300 mg q 8 hours iv: 2 mg·kg^{-1} over 15 minutes	4–8 hours	0.5–2.0	Dizziness, metallic taste, conduction disturbances, nausea
II	Propranolol (beta$_1$/beta$_2$)*	Oral: 20–80 mg q 6 hours iv: 0.5–1 mg q 2 minutes to maximum 6–10 mg	3–6 hours	0.05–0.1	Depression, fatigue, AV block, bradycardia, myocardial depression
	Acebutolol (beta$_1$/beta$_2$)	Oral: 600–1200 mg once daily	24 hours		As above
	Atenolol (beta$_1$)*	Oral: 50–200 mg once daily	24 hours		As above
	Nadolol (beta$_1$/beta$_2$)	Oral: 40–240 mg once daily	24 hours		As above
	Timolol (beta$_1$/beta$_2$)	Oral: 20–60 mg	15 hours		As above
III	Amiodarone	Oral: 800–1600 mg·day^{-1} for 2 weeks, then 200–600 mg·day^{-1} maintenance iv: 5–10 mg·kg^{-1} bolus over 5–15 minutes; then 800–1600 mg·day^{-1} as a continuous infusion or in divided doses	13–60 days		Corneal deposits, gastrointestinal disturbances, altered thyroid function, interstitial pulmonary disease, peripheral neuropathy, bradycardia, conduction block, hepatic dysfunction
	Bretylium	iv: 5–10 mg·kg^{-1} bolus over 10–30 minutes, then 1–4 mg·min^{-1}	6–8 hours	0.8–2.0	Transient hypertension, sinus tachycardia, postural hypotension, proarrhythmic

(continued)

TABLE 29-5 *(continued)*

Class	Drug	Commonly Used Dosage	Elimination Half-Life	Therapeutic Plasma Level ($\mu g \cdot ml^{-1}$)	Side-Effects
IV	Verapamil	Oral: 80–160 mg q 6–8 hours iv: 5–10 mg bolus, repeated after 10 minutes to a maximum of 20 mg Continuous infusion: 1–5 $\mu g \cdot kg^{-1} \cdot min^{-1}$	4–8 hours	0.1	Cardiac depression, hypotension, AV block, asystole, edema, head-ache, constipation
	Diltiazem	Oral: 60–90 mg q 6 hours	3–5 hours		Edema, postural hypotension
V	Digoxin	Oral: 1–1.5 mg in divided doses over 24 hours for digitalization; 0.125–0.25 mg once daily for maintenance iv: 0.75–1 mg in divided doses over 24 hours for digitalization	1.5 days	1–2	Anorexia, nausea, vomiting, diar-rhea, malaise, fatigue, confusion, headache, colored vision, arrhyth-mias, aggravation of heart failure

* Beta$_1$/beta$_2$, noncardioselective beta blockers; beta$_1$, cardioselective beta blockers.
Reprinted with permission from Platia EV: Management of Cardiac Arrhythmias, p 135. Philadelphia, JB Lippincott, 1987.

Class III

Drugs in the third category of antidysrhythmics prolong the action potential duration and therefore lengthen the refractory period. Bretylium, which initially releases norepinephrine and then later inhibits its release, extends the refractory period in His–Purkinje fibers and ventricular muscle cells.[61] By lengthening the refractory period in the His–Purkinje and ventricular cells and therefore decreasing the dispersion of refractoriness, bretylium decreases the chance of microre-entry. A totally different drug, amiodarone, functions similarly to bretylium but is not limited to Purkinje and ventricular muscle cells.[62]

Class IV

These drugs exert their influence primarily in the AV and SA nodes by blocking calcium channels. They have little if any effect on the fast sodium channels. Despite the fact that nifedipine is a calcium channel blocking agent, it is not considered an antidysrhythmic drug but rather a coronary vasodilator.

Class V

This group, the cardiac glycosides, exerts its antidysrhythmic effect through the parasympathetic system.[63] It creates supraventricular and ventricular dysrhythmias by initiating triggered activity and increasing the slope of phase 4 of depolarization. Treatment of digitalis-induced dysrhythmias includes withholding the drug, administering potassium if the serum concentration is low, and possibly administering phenytoin, a drug known to terminate triggered activity.

SUPRAVENTRICULAR TACHYCARDIAS

Any tachycardia originating above the bundle of His is considered a supraventricular tachycardia. Included in this group of dysrhythmias are sinus arrhythmia and sinus tachycardia, atrial fibrillation and flutter, re-entrant dysrhythmias, atrial tachycardia, multifocal atrial tachycardia, and AV junctional tachycardia. This section presents a brief discussion of each category of supraventricular tachycardia.

Sinus Dysrhythmia

Sinus dysrhythmia is a normally occurring variation in heart rate that occurs with respiration. In older patients, however, the phenomenon can be symptomatic in the presence of hypothyroidism, digitalis, and calcium channel blocking drugs (Fig. 29-15).

Sinus Tachycardia

One of the most common dysrhythmias observed by the anesthesiologist is sinus tachycardia (Fig. 29-16). Causes include arterial hypoxemia, hypoventilation, light anesthesia, hypovolemia, hyperthermia, and antimuscarinic drugs. Treatment, directed toward correcting the underlying cause, includes evaluation of oxygenation and ventilation, deepening anesthesia, appropriate volume replacement, and possibly administration of beta blocking drugs. Pacing and cardioversion do not assume a role in controlling sinus tachycardia.

AV block generally does not occur in the presence of sinus tachycardia. Because impulses conduct through the AV node with gradual slowing, however, it is possible for AV nodal block to occur at a rate of 180–200 beats·min^{-1}. AV nodal block rarely occurs in hearts free of disease but can potentially occur at lower rates in patients with coro-

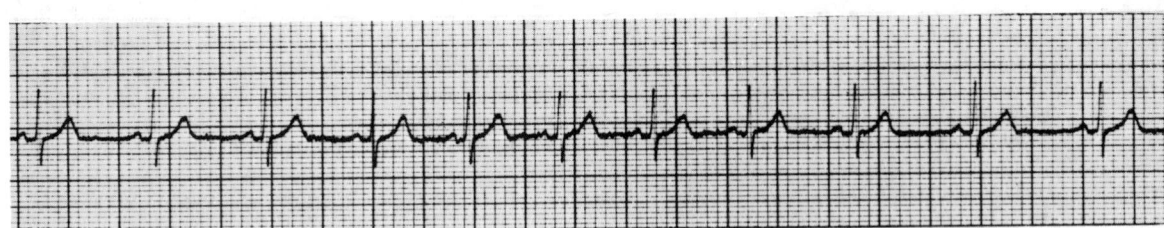

Figure 29-15. Sinus dysrhythmia.

nary artery or valvular heart disease. If tachycardia-induced AV block occurs in patients with heart disease, consider a beta₁ blocking agent such as metoprolol in intravenous doses of 0.5 mg titrated to effect with a maximum dose of 5 mg. As atrial rate slows, 1:1 AV nodal conduction should resume.

Atrial Fibrillation

Atrial fibrillation produces an irregularly irregular QRS pattern and a fibrillatory baseline (Fig. 29-17). If the diagnosis is not obvious, recording the AEG will confirm the presence of the fibrillatory baseline (Fig. 29-18).

Atrial fibrillation is associated with higher mortality in some patients.[64] Patients with chronic atrial fibrillation without associated cardiovascular disease have a higher mortality rate than patients in sinus rhythm. Patients with paroxysmal atrial fibrillation were found to suffer a higher mortality rate only in the presence of cardiac disease such as mitral stenosis and coronary artery disease. The Framingham study shed light on antecedent factors for developing atrial fibrillation.[65,66] There is a 2% risk of developing atrial fibrillation over a 20-year period. This risk increases in the presence of congestive heart failure, rheumatic heart disease, and hypertensive cardiovascular disease. The average time to death after developing atrial fibrillation was 6 years. Investigators have demonstrated an increased risk of developing atrial fibrillation with increasing left atrial size, especially if the left atrial size is greater than 4.5 cm.[67]

Patients with atrial fibrillation persisting longer than approximately 1 week can develop an atrial thrombus and,

eventually, an arterial embolus. Many patients experiencing chronic atrial fibrillation therefore take warfarin.

Patients with chronic atrial fibrillation without other significant cardiac disease generally are hemodynamically stable without major beat-to-beat changes in blood pressure if the ventricular response is 70–100 beats·min⁻¹ (Fig. 29-19). Acute onset of atrial fibrillation, however, can create extreme hemodynamic instability. Initially, the very high ventricular rate substantially reduces ventricular filling. The end result is a high rate and low cardiac output and blood pressure.

Treatment focuses on controlling heart rate by cardioversion and drug administration. Atrial pacing assumes no role in the treatment of atrial fibrillation. If the ventricular response is at bradycardic levels, therapy is to increase heart rate using ventricular inhibited pacing. Cardioversion remains the mainstay of therapy in hemodynamically unstable patients. Beginning with 50 watts (joules), incrementally increase the energy output to a maximum of 300 joules. Assure synchronization of the defibrillator to avoid initiating ventricular fibrillation. Drug therapy consists of cardiac glycosides, verapamil, and beta-adrenergic blocking agents.[68-71] Do not use verapamil or digitalis if the atrial fibrillation occurs in the presence of Wolff-Parkinson-White syndrome because these drugs could increase the ventricular rate.[72,73]

The blood pressure should respond to acute control of the heart rate. Although it will not convert atrial fibrillation to sinus rhythm, propranolol will lower the ventricular rate, allow for ventricular filling, and eventually increase the blood pressure. If blood pressure does not sufficiently increase after rate control, consider using an alpha-adrenergic

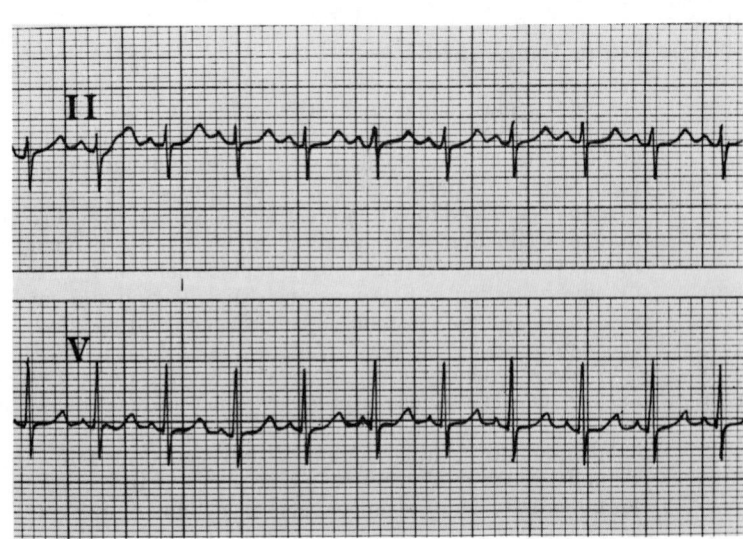

Figure 29-16. At a rate of 125 beats·min⁻¹ and P waves occurring on a 1:1 basis with the R waves, this ECG shows sinus tachycardia.

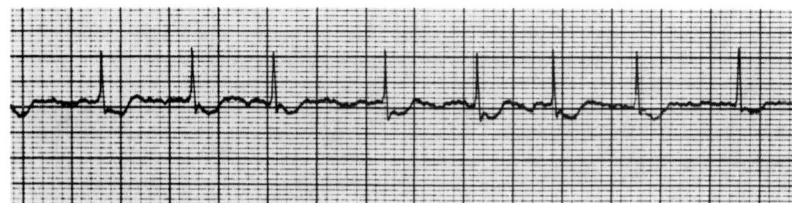

Figure 29-17. This ECG demonstrates atrial fibrillation. It has a fibrillatory baseline and irregularly irregular R waves.

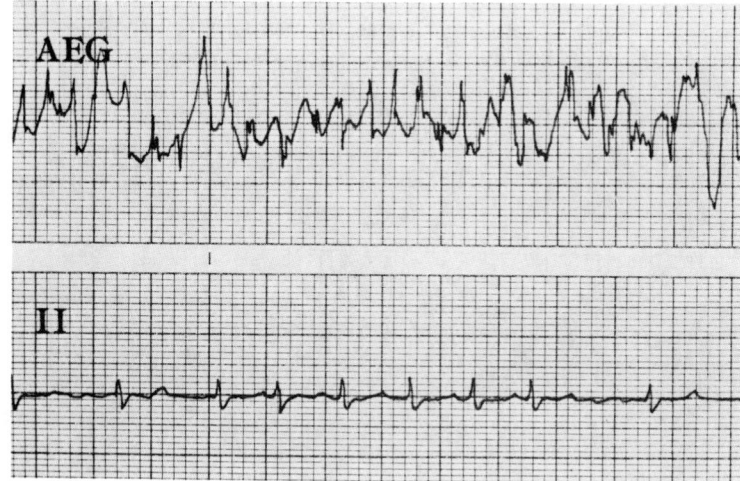

Figure 29-18. The atrial electrogram (*top*) clearly reveals a fibrillatory pattern and is consistent with atrial fibrillation. The simultaneous surface ECG is shown in the *bottom* tracing.

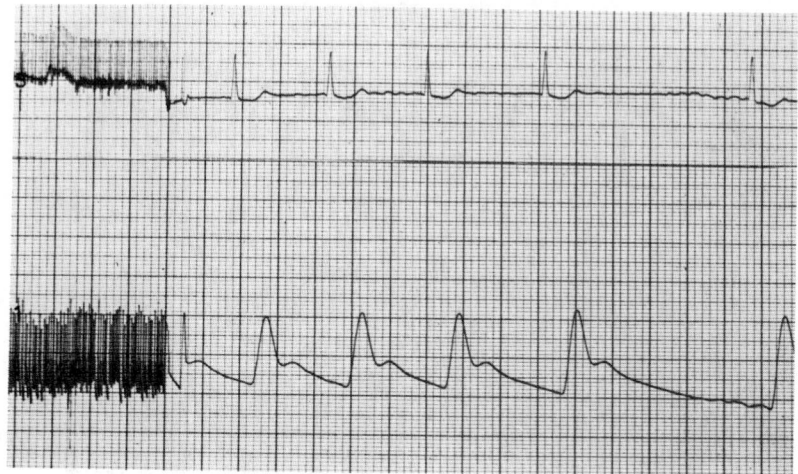

Figure 29-19. Atrial fibrillation has a characteristic tracing in the aterial pressure line. Like the ECG, the pressure tracing is irregularly irregular occasionally with long pauses, but if the heart rate remains between 70 and 100 beats·min^{-1}, the blood pressure should remain stable.

agent such as phenylephrine. Varapamil will convert atrial fibrillation to sinus rhythm more effectively than beta blocking agents. Because acute hypokalemia could cause atrial fibrillation, judicious potassium replacement through a central intravenous catheter potentially can revert fibrillation to sinus rhythm without other therapy.

Atrial Flutter

Atrial flutter occurs less commonly than atrial fibrillation. This dysrhythmia is diagnosed by noting a saw-toothed baseline with inverted P waves on the surface ECG (Fig. 29-20). The AEG unquestionably diagnoses atrial flutter (Fig. 29-21). Occasionally, the AEG will show a combination of fibrillation and flutter, as noted in Figure 29-22. Two types of atrial flutter occur.[74,75] Type I flutter has an atrial rate of 250–350 beats·min^{-1}, whereas Type II flutter has higher atrial rates of 340–430 beats·min^{-1}. Because of failure of AV conduction at high atrial rates, the ventricular response to Type I and Type II atrial flutter is approximately 150 beats·min^{-1}.

Automaticity and re-entry cause atrial flutter; however, re-entry is the more common cause.[76,77]

The treatment of atrial flutter includes rapid atrial pacing, vagal maneuvers, cardioversion, and drug administration. Exact placement of an electrical impulse within the atrial cycle terminates re-entrant Type I atrial flutter. Clinically, it is almost impossible to place a stimulus in the precise location in the atrial electrical cycle to block the circuit

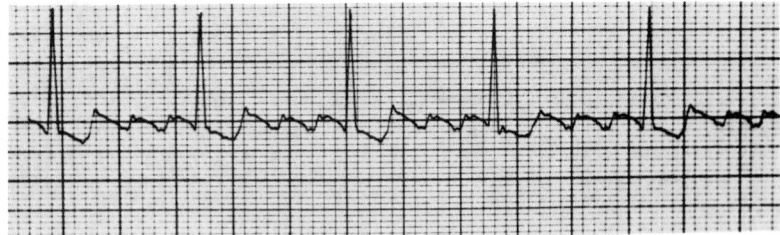

Figure 29-20. A saw-toothed baseline composed of inverted P waves helps to diagnose atrial flutter. In this ECG, the atrial rate is 250, characteristic of type I flutter, and the ventricular rate is 57.

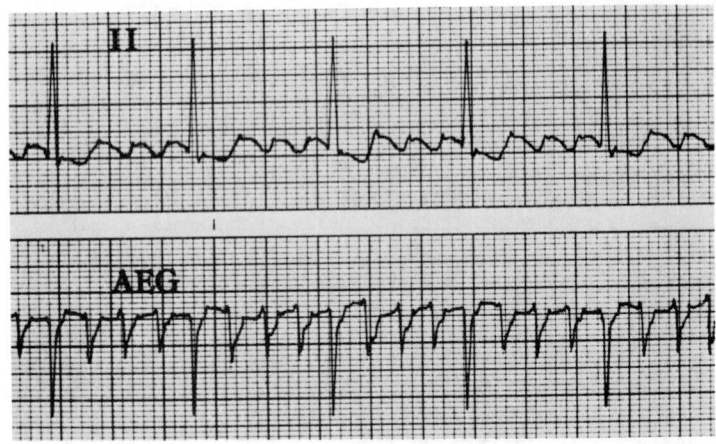

Figure 29-21. The atrial electrogram (*bottom*) clearly reveals atrial flutter waves. The *top* trace is lead II.

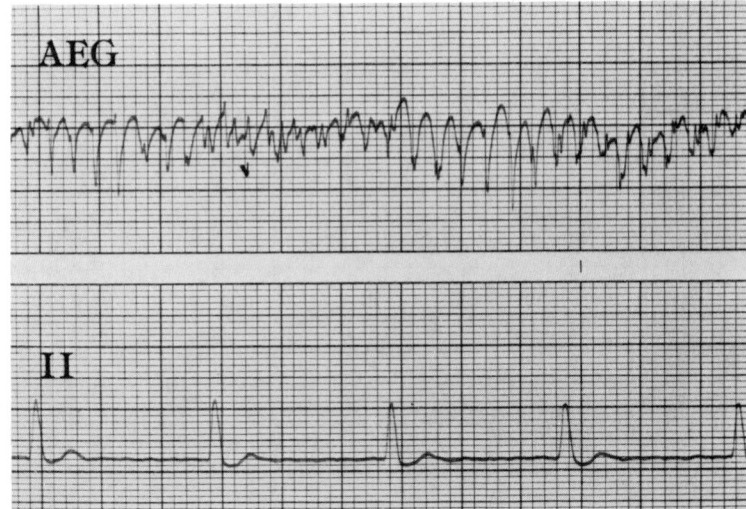

Figure 29-22. The atrial electrogram (*top*) is a fibrillation-flutter pattern reminiscent of ventricular torsades de pointes.

and terminate the dysrhythmia. Rapid atrial pacing, which delivers up to 800 stimuli per minute, performs this task. Waldo *et al* have shown that atrial pacing at the flutter rate will entrain the atrium but not break the re-entry.[78] One must pace higher than the flutter rate and create a morphologic change in the flutter wave in order to terminate this dysrhythmia. Type II atrial flutter generally will not terminate with rapid atrial pacing techniques.

Vagal maneuvers, such as carotid massage, do not always convert atrial flutter to sinus rhythm. Conversion occurs with increased vagal tone only if the re-entrant circuit includes the AV node. If the re-entrant circuit is located en-

tirely within atrial tissue, carotid massage could slow the ventricular response and reveal previously undiagnosed atrial flutter waves without terminating the dysrhythmia.

Cardioversion is another form of treatment. Atrial flutter responds to energy levels as low as 25 joules.[79]

As in atrial fibrillation, the goal of drug therapy is control of ventricular rate. AV nodal blocking drugs such as verapamil, glycosides, and beta-adrenergic blockers represent primary drug therapy. Class IA antidysrhythmics may convert atrial flutter to sinus rhythm. By slowing the atrial flutter rate, thereby decreasing concealed conduction, and by their vagolytic action, Class IA agents can increase the ventricular rate.[80] Class IA agents commonly are used in conjunction with beta-adrenergic blocking drugs to control the ventricular rate.

Atrioventricular Nodal Re-entrant Tachycardia

Another supraventricular tachycardia involves re-entry in the AV node. The AV node is a highly complex structure that can dissociate into two conducting pathways that join proximally and distally into common pathways.[81-83] The AV node, therefore, represents a location for a re-entrant dysrhythmia. In fact, it is possible to have two forms of AV nodal re-entrant tachycardia.[84] The more common form (slow-fast) conducts slowly through the anterograde limb and rapidly through the retrograde limb, whereas the less common form (fast-slow) conducts rapidly through the anterograde limb and slowly through the retrograde limb. The slow-fast type of this dysrhythmia begins with a premature atrial beat and has its inverted P wave inscribed within the QRS complex because retrograde conduction is very rapid. The fast-slow form of this dysrhythmia begins with either a ventricular or an atrial premature complex, or sinus tachycardia. The P wave occurs after the QRS complex because atrial activation takes place by way of the slow retrograde pathway.

Treatment focuses on vagal maneuvers, cardioversions, rapid atrial pacing, and drugs. Because of re-entrant circuit includes the AV node, stimulating the parasympathetic system with a Valsalva maneuver or very careful carotid artery massage should terminate this dysrhythmia. Rapid atrial pacing and DC cardioversion starting with 25 joules also should readily convert the dysrhythmia to sinus rhythm. Verapamil is the drug of choice;[85] however, glycosides, beta-adrenergic blockers, and edrophonium can also terminate the dysrhythmia. Class IA agents are less effective than the other antiarrhythmic drugs. Adenosine recently has been used to treat this dysrhythmia. Adenosine's vasodilating effects reduce systemic blood pressure by as much as 50%. The hypotension, easily missed without an arterial catheter, persists only for a short period of time, because adenosine's half-life is approximately one second. Adenosine is not considered first-line therapy for an AV nodal re-entrant tachycardia.

Atrioventricular Reciprocating Tachycardia

This dysrhythmia is one of several supraventricular tachycardias that occur in patients with *pre-excitation syndrome* or *Wolff-Parkinson-White syndrome* (Fig. 29-23). These patients have two AV nodal conducting pathways: one pathway is the normal AV node, bundle of His, and Purkinje system, and the second pathway is the anomalous AV nodal bypass tract or Kent's bundle. The atrial impulse normally conducts over both of these pathways, leading to a short P-R interval (<0.12 sec) and a widened QRS complex with a delta wave or initial slurring of the P-R interval into the QRS complex.[86] The re-entrant circuit in Wolff-Parkinson-White syndrome includes an atrium and a ventricle, the normal AV conducting pathway, and the anomalous tract.

Wolff-Parkinson-White syndrome includes two subgroups, depending on the direction of the major deflection within the V_1 QRS complex. The QRS complex in Type A has an R wave visible in V_1, whereas the QRS complex in Type B contains an S wave in V_1. An R wave in V_1 indicates that the impulse arrives in the left ventricle and travels toward the V_1 electrode, and an S wave in V_1 describes an impulse that begins in the right ventricle and spreads toward the left ventricle away from the V_1 electrode. The QRS duration depends on several factors.[87] If the impulse traveling through the accessory pathway arrives at the ventricle many milliseconds before the impulse traveling through the AV node, the QRS complex will be very wide and bizarre. If, however, the two impulses arrive at approximately the same time, the QRS complex will be of normal duration. Abnormal repolarization leads to ST–T wave abnormalities.

Concealed Wolff-Parkinson-White syndrome occurs when the accessory pathway conducts only in a retrograde direction. Absence of anterograde conduction in the accessory pathways masks all of the electrocardiographic findings of Wolff-Parkinson-White syndrome (short PR interval, delta wave, widened QRS complex), but these patients still develop supraventricular tachycardias.[88]

Patients with Wolff-Parkinson-White syndrome can develop atrial fibrillation, atrial flutter, or the reciprocating tachycardia. Treatment focuses on controlling ventricular rate and reducing the dispersion of the refractory periods and conduction velocities of the two conducting pathways. Vagal maneuvers are a reasonable first-line therapy. Intraoperative onset of a supraventricular tachycardia could require

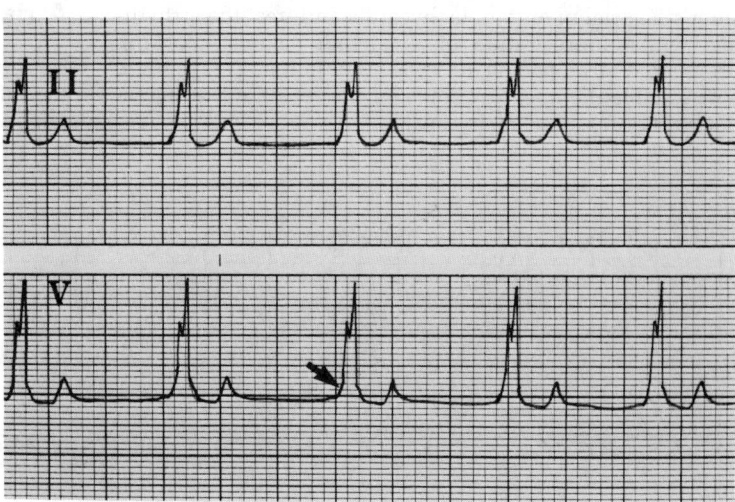

Figure 29-23. Wolff-Parkinson-White syndrome includes a short P-R interval (approximately 0.08 sec), a delta wave (*arrow*), and an intraventricular conduction delay.

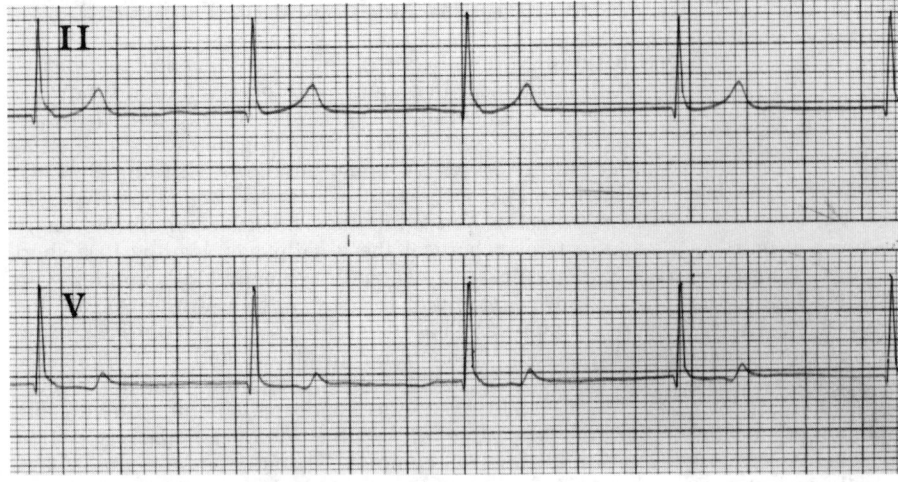

Figure 29-24. Idiojunctional rhythms (rate = 40 beat-sec·min^{-1}) commonly have visible P waves in the QRS complex. The P waves are noted here in the terminal phase of the R wave and cause the slurring effect.

cardioversion if hypotension occurs. The Class IA antidysrhythmics, quinidine, procainamide, and disopyramide, increase refractoriness in the accessory pathway and should help to terminate the reciprocating dysrhythmia and maintain sinus rhythm. Beta blockade is also a reasonable therapeutic choice. Avoid administering digoxin, however, because it decreases the refractory period of the accessory pathway. If the patient develops atrial fibrillation, digoxin will allow conduction of an excessive number of impulses into the ventricle and increase the likelihood that ventricular fibrillation will occur. The decision to use digoxin or verapamil should be based on electrophysiologic studies performed by the cardiologist. Occasionally, however, a patient will benefit from the effects of digoxin.

Sinoatrial Re-entrant Tachycardia

Occasionally, the SA node forms part of a re-entrant circuit that includes the atrium.[89] Premature atrial beats are an initiating event of this dysrhythmia. During the tachycardia, the P waves appear similar to the normal P wave, and the patient can have a rate similar to that in sinus tachycardia. A distinguishing feature is its abrupt onset. If the patient's heart rate suddenly increases to 150–180 beats·min^{-1}, consider sinoatrial re-entrant tachycardia and treat the arrhythmia with administration of a calcium channel blocking drug, rapid atrial pacing, or vagal stimulation. Verapamil is a reasonable therapeutic choice for the re-entrant tachycardia but not for sinus tachycardia.

Accelerated Atrioventricular Junctional Tachycardia

AV nodal cells normally have a phase 4 of depolarization that permits a rate of 40–60 beats·min^{-1} (Figs. 29-24 and 29-25). Although it is normally suppressed by SA nodal activity, the AV node occasionally increases its rate through enhanced automaticity. The factors causing enhanced automaticity in the AV node include hypokalemia, digitalis intoxication, and ischemia.[90] When the junctional rate increases to 70–100 beats·min^{-1}, the dysrhythmia is called an accelerated AV junctional rhythm (Fig. 29-26). An accelerated junctional tachycardia occurs when the heart rate surpasses 100 beats·min^{-1}. The hemodynamic effect of a junctional rhythm reflects independent atrial and ventricular contractions with atrial cannon waves and hypotension alternating with a normal central venous pressure tracing and normal blood pressure (Fig. 29-27).

These dysrhythmias are secondary to enhanced automaticity; therefore, rapid atrial pacing is not a therapeutic option. In the presence of intact AV conduction, atrial pacing restores atrial kick. Consider using AV sequential pacing if the patient has AV nodal block with the junctional rhythm.

Atrial Tachycardia

The final group of supraventricular tachydysrhythmias is the atrial tachycardias. These dysrhythmias, entirely contained within the atrium, have re-entry and enhanced nor-

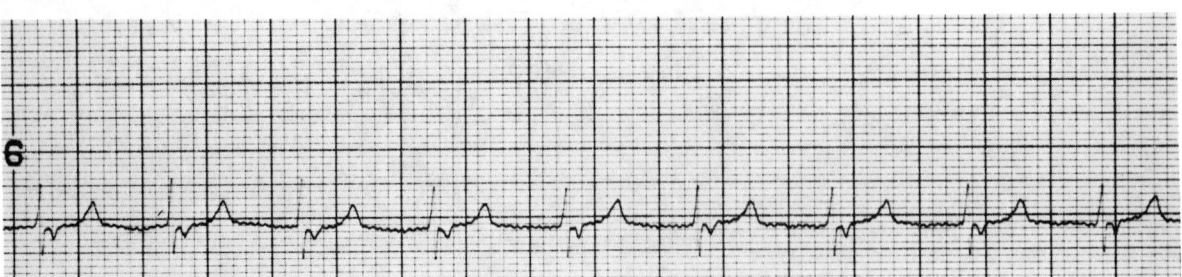

Figure 29-25. This ECG demonstrates retrogradely conducted and therefore inverted P waves.

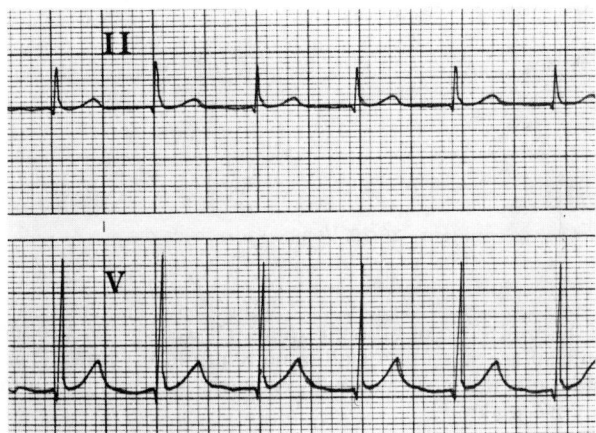

Figure 29-26. An accelerated idiojunctional rhythm occurs when the junctional escape mechanism increases to more than 70 beats·min^{-1}. In this case, the rate is 77 beats·min^{-1}, and the P waves slur the terminal phase of the R waves.

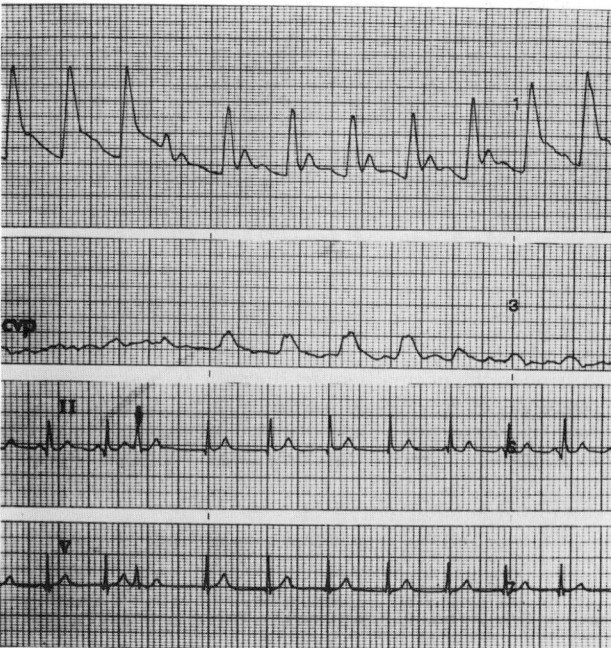

Figure 29-27. The sudden onset of an idiojunctional rhythm occurs with an aberrantly conducted junctional beat (*arrow*). The loss of atrial kick causes a loss of blood pressure (*top*) and the appearance of cannon waves on the central venous pressure monitor (*second trace*). The reappearance of the sinus mechanism restores arterial pressure, and the atrial cannon waves disappear.

mal or abnormal automaticity as their pathophysiologic mechanisms. Because the re-entrant atrial tachycardias do not include the SA or AV nodes in their circuit, vagal maneuvers will not terminate the dysrhythmia. Class IA drugs can successfully convert atrial tachycardia to sinus rhythm. Chronic lung disease and digitalis intoxication are common antecedents. It is nearly impossible to differentiate between an automatic atrial tachycardia and a re-entrant atrial tachycardia without using specialized electrophysiologic testing.

Multifocal atrial tachycardia occurs in patients with chronic lung disease, coronary artery disease, and hypokalemia. This type of atrial tachycardia has varying P-P, P-R, and R-R intervals and at least three different P wave morphologies.[91] Cardiac glycosides do not convert multifocal atrial tachycardia to sinus rhythm. Restoring potassium and magnesium levels, or administering procainamide or quinidine, however, can stop the dysrhythmia.[92,93] Unfortunately, this dysrhythmia commonly recurs.

VENTRICULAR DYSRHYTHMIAS

Ventricular irritability presents as unifocal and multifocal premature contractions, ventricular tachycardia, and ventricular fibrillation (Figs. 29-28 through 29-30). The differ-

ential diagnosis of ventricular irritability during anesthesia should include myocardial ischemia with all of its possible antecedent factors; hypercarbia; direct stimulation from surgery and central monitoring catheters; reflex enhancement of parasympathetic tone; and drug interactions. Ventricular premature contractions associated with increased pulmonary artery pressures are caused by hypoventilation and arterial hypoxemia until proved otherwise.

Ventricular irritability occurring during myocardial ischemia probably originates through a re-entrant mechanism because programmed stimulation initiates and terminates ventricular tachycardia.[94] More recently, clinical studies in patients with ventricular aneurysms and ventricular dysrhythmias revealed that resection of areas of the ventricle that had continuous electrical activity during diastole re-

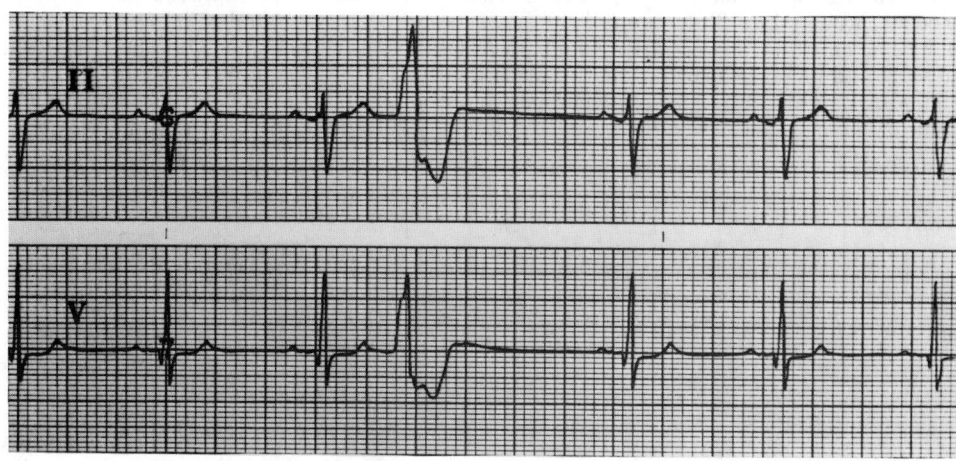

Figure 29-28. It is difficult to distinguish an aberrantly conducted beat from a premature ventricular contraction, which is itself aberrantly conducted. This ECG likely reveals a premature ventricular contraction because it is unrelated to atrial activity, is fully compensated (see text), and has an increased QRS duration. The normal P wave occurs in the T wave of the premature ventricular contraction.

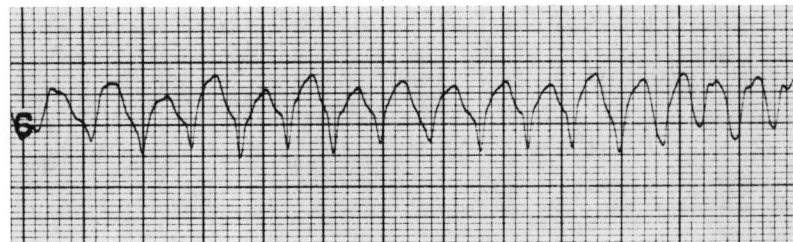

Figure 29-29. Ventricular tachycardia.

sulted in ablation of the arrhythmia.[95-97] Animal studies in infarcted dog heart models revealed that electrical activity occurring in the normally quiet diastolic period was related to ingrowth of scar tissue into myocardial tissue. This ingrowth of scar separated and disoriented myocardial muscle cells so that activation of this area was prolonged.[98] Investigators believe also that ventricular dysrhythmias occur as a result of triggered activity.[43,99]

The clinical impression is that for a premature ventricular contraction to cause ventricular tachycardia, the premature ventricular contraction must fall on the T wave.[100] In fact, a premature ventricular beat located any place in the cardiac cycle can initiate ventricular tachycardia.[101-103] A depolarization traversing any repolarizing area can initiate re-entry and ventricular tachycardia. The surface ECG reflects the electrical events not in one cell but rather in all of the myocardial cells. For this reason, small areas of myocardium repolarize at various times around the T wave, not just during the peak of the T wave; therefore, a premature ventricular contraction occurring late in the ST segment or after the T wave could cause ventricular tachycardia.

Hypercarbia with its associated hypertension and tachycardia potentially causes ventricular irritability. Also, reflex bradycardia secondary to surgical manipulation or laryngoscopy can result in idioventricular escape complexes. More direct causes of ventricular irritability include direct manipulation from pulmonary and esophageal surgical procedures and right ventricular stimulation from a pulmonary artery catheter.

Combinations of drugs may also cause ventricular dysrhythmias. Chronic administration of imipramine followed by pancuronium and halothane is associated with increased serum norepinephrine levels and ventricular dysrhythmias.[104] Aminophylline plus halothane but not enflurane creates ventricular irritability if the serum concentration of aminophylline is greater than the therapeutic range.[105]

Epinephrine combines with the volatile anesthetics to cause ventricular irritability.[106-108] The irritability appears to occur through the alpha receptor;[109,110] however, the beta$_1$ and beta$_2$ effects at lower doses could decrease diastolic pressure and increase heart rate and secondarily cause ventricular irritability in patients with coronary artery disease. Johnson et al[106] determined in dogs that enflurane required

the highest dose of epinephrine, 10.9 μg·kg^{-1}, to produce ventricular irritability. Isoflurane required 6.7 μg·kg^{-1} and halothane, the most sensitizing volatile anesthetic, required only 2.1 μg·kg^{-1}.

Treatment of ventricular irritability focuses on terminating the premature beats as quickly as possible while determining and correcting the cause. Ensure oxygenation and ventilation, remove the surgical stimulus that may have caused parasympathetic effects, and quickly treat hypertension and tachycardia. Consider the possibility that a pulmonary artery catheter might be coiled within the ventricle. It is seldom necessary to insert a pulmonary artery catheter farther than 25% of the patient's height in centimeters. Bradycardia may result in ventricular escape beats. If the bradycardia has a sinus or an idiojunctional mechanism, increase heart rate by administering an antimuscarinic agent or by atrial pacing if atrial electrodes are available. Drug therapy consists of lidocaine, 1 mg·kg^{-1}, followed by an infusion at a rate of 2–4 mg·min^{-1}. Also useful is bretylium, 5 mg·kg^{-1}, with a 1–4 mg·min^{-1} infusion. Procainamide is occasionally useful. Administer 30 mg·kg^{-1} of procainamide up to a maximal dose of 1 g until the dysrhythmia terminates, then maintain the serum level with an infusion of 1–4 mg·min^{-1}. Stop the infusion of procainamide if the QRS complex widens by 50%.

It is important but very difficult to distinguish ventricular complexes from aberrant supraventricular complexes.[111] Unfortunately, lead II, the most commonly used ECG lead, cannot adequately distinguish ventricular contractions from aberrantly conducted beats (Figs. 29-31 through 29-33). Problems arise because ventricular tachycardias and bundle-branch blocks have deep Q waves (QS pattern) in lead II. Another problem is that dissociated atrial activity, usually thought to imply ventricular tachycardia, occurs also during junctional tachycardia. If retrograde AV conduction remains intact, ventricular tachycardia can create retrograde P waves.[112] Finally, although we think of a fusion beat as a supraventricular complex combining with a ventricular complex, it is possible, as shown by Kistin, that a supraventricular complex and an aberrantly conducted junctional complex can join to form a fusion beat.[113] Despite all of the pitfalls in differentiating supraventricular from ventricular complexes, clinicians generally accept the following criteria

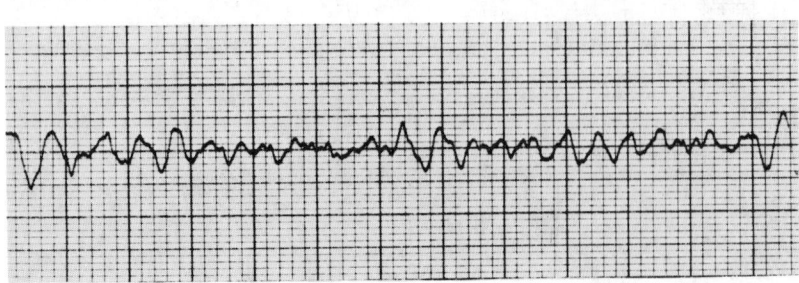

Figure 29-30. Ventricular fibrillation.

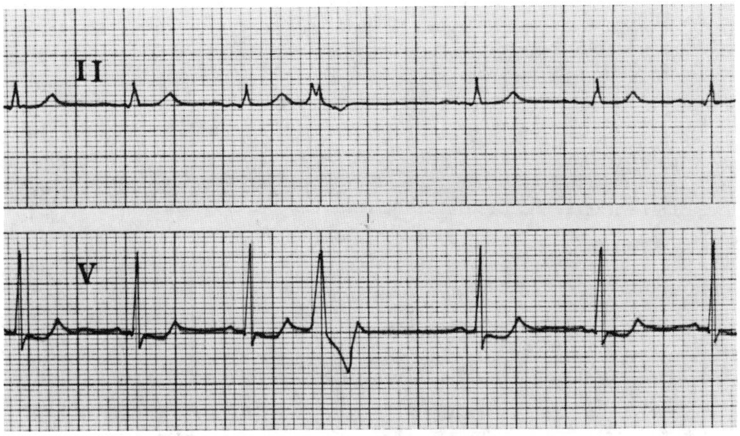

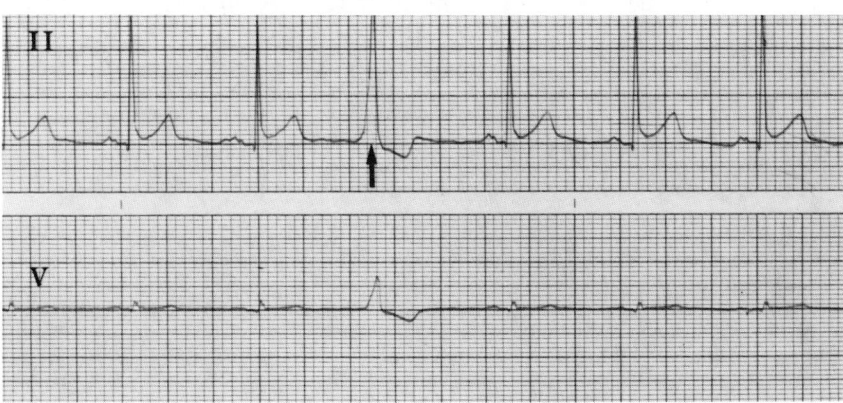

Figure 29-31. Full compensation indicates a ventricular origin; however, QRS duration (0.14 sec) and similar initial forces (upward) imply aberrant conduction.

as indicative of ventricular activity:

1. QRS complex >0.12 sec
2. Full compensation (two normal R-R intervals equals the R-R interval circumscribing the premature beat)
3. Dissociated from atrial activity
4. Premature in relation to the sinus beats
5. R or qR in V_1 with taller left "rabbit ear"
6. Deep QS (>15 mm) in V_6

Wellens *et al* characterized the criteria for diagnosing ventricular ectopy.[114] When in doubt, treat a wide QRS complex as though it were ventricular in origin.

Torsades de Pointes

An unusual variety of ventricular tachycardia, torsades de pointes (Fig. 29-34), occurs in patients with prolonged Q-T intervals. The various causes of the Q-T interval prolongation include congenital prolongation; antidysrhythmic drugs such as procainamide, quinidine, and disopyramide; subarachnoid hemorrhage; and electrolyte disturbances.[115-118] It commonly occurs just after aortic unclamping during cardiac surgery. It is associated with variant angina and occurs in the presence of bradycardia.[119] The electrocardiographic pattern is one of ventricular tachycardia twisting around a central axis.

The importance of torsades de pointes is that one must avoid administering the usual antidysrhythmic drugs. Treatment includes correcting the underlying electrolyte problem, pacing for bradycardia, and cardioversion.

BUNDLE-BRANCH BLOCK

Ventricular activation proceeds in parallel, not in series. If one of the bundle branches slows or blocks conduction, the impulses quickly travel to the normal ventricle. The impulse then slowly conducts through the intraventricular septum and blocked ventricle. The electrocardiographic pattern reflects this concept.

Right Bundle-Branch Block

The septum depolarizes from left to right, as is normal, before the left ventricular muscle mass depolarizes from the septum toward the free wall (right to left). Finally, the right ventricular electrical forces depolarize from the septum toward the right ventricular free wall (left to right). Overall, the ECG in V_1 initially shows an upward deflection (septal activation toward V_1); second, a downward deflection (left ventricular activation away from V_1); and third, another upward deflection (unopposed right ventricular forces toward V_1) (Fig. 29-35). This pattern in V_1 is an rSR' deflection.

Left Bundle-Branch Block

Abnormal right to left septal activation simultaneously occurs with right ventricular activation. The septal forces overwhelm the right ventricular forces. The left ventricle activates from the septum toward the free wall. Overall, the ECG in V_6 contains an initial upward deflection (right ventricular and septal forces combined), followed by a minimal

Figure 29-32. This QRS complex (*arrow*) is probably a premature junctional with aberrant conduction.

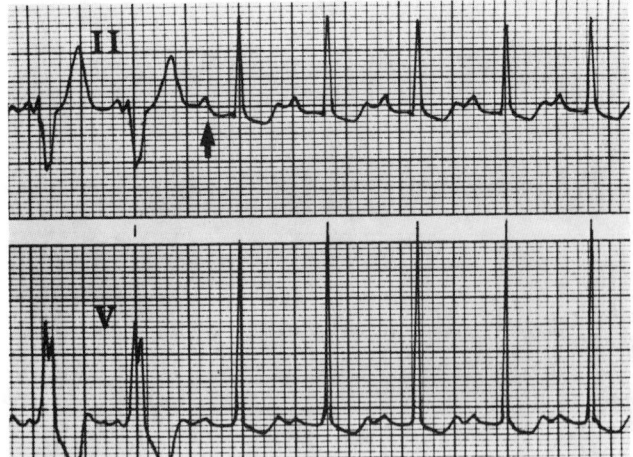

Figure 29-33. A short P-R interval finds the bundle branches somewhat refractory, leading to bundle-branch block (first two QRS complexes). An increased time for the impulse to conduct through the AV node (first-degree block starting at *arrow*) finds the bundle branches fully repolarized and capable of normally conducting the impulse. The first two QRS complexes, therefore, represent aberrant conduction and not ventricular contractions.

downward deflection (septal activation finishing), quickly followed by another upward deflection (left ventricular activation). The pattern in V_6, therefore, is an R wave with a notch at the peak (Fig. 29-36). Leads I and aV_L can have the same general ECG patterns as V_6. Figure 29-37 compares leads I, V_1, and V_6 in right and left bundle-branch block.

Abnormal repolarization would be expected in the presence of abnormal depolarization. T waves should travel secondarily in a direction opposite to the terminal forces of the QRS complex. It is abnormal for T waves to move in the same direction as the terminal force of the QRS complex.[120]

Bundle-branch blocks occasionally associate with abnormal left or right axis deviation. Combined complete left bundle-branch block and left axis deviation are associated with a higher mortality rate.[121,122] Bundle-branch patterns can occur either as a single complex or as runs of complexes related to heart rate. Premature atrial beats that are very early in the cardiac cycle can meet a refractory bundle branch that has not fully repolarized. Also, a very late premature atrial beat can meet a bundle branch that has already slightly depolarized during phase 4. In this instance, conduction could be slow enough to create an electrocardiographic picture of bundle-branch block. In some patients with heart disease, a bundle-branch block can occur during episodes of tachycardia.

The Hemiblocks

It is possible for the left bundle-branch to have a block distal to its division into the anterior and posterior fascicles. A block occurring in one of the fascicles is called a *hemiblock*. It is difficult to relate a specific anatomic lesion in the left bundle-branch to the electrocardiographic patterns associated with the hemiblocks.[123,124] In posterior hemiblock (Fig. 29-38), look for a right axis deviation and sometimes a Q wave in leads II, III, and aV_F, and in anterior hemiblock (Fig. 29-39), look for a left axis deviation.[125]

Problems arise when trying to determine which patient with a bifascicular block would require perioperative temporary pacing. In a study of 544 patients with chronic bifascicular block and trifascicular disease, McAnulty et al reported that only 19 patients suffered from heart block. Of 160 deaths, 42% were attributable to tachycardia and acute myocardial infarction rather than bradycardia associated with heart block.[126] Predictors of sudden death were coro-

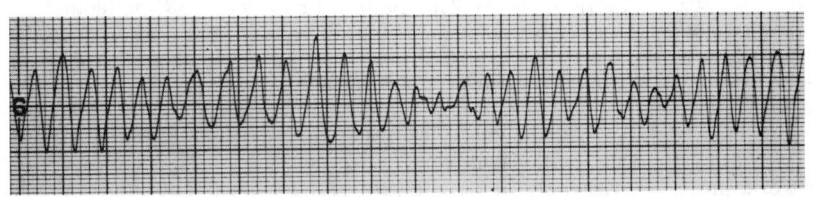

Figure 29-34. A torsades de pointes pattern of ventricular tachycardia occurs when the depolarization waves twist around a central axis. Altered concentrations of myocardial potassium, calcium, or magnesium and prolonged Q-T interval syndrome, either drug-induced or congenital, accompany this ECG pattern.

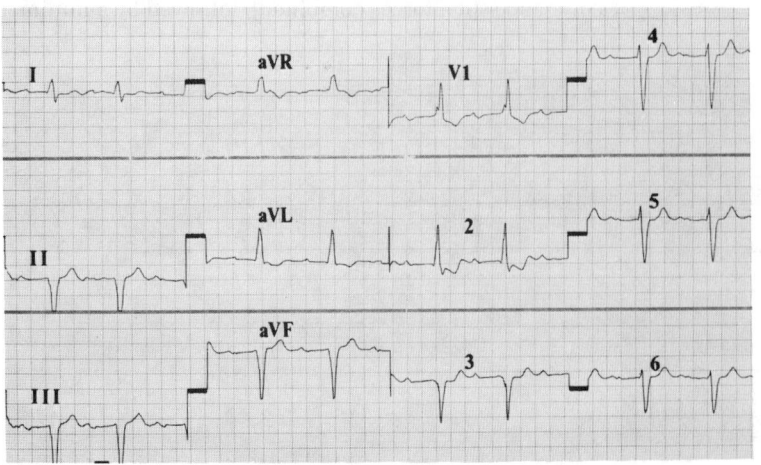

Figure 29-35. Diagnose right bundle-branch block by noting the QRS configuration in lead V_1. This patient also had a first-degree AV block. (Reprinted with permission from Zaidan JR, Curling PE: Cardiac dysrhythmias: Recognition and management. In Stoelting RK, Barash PG, Gallagher TH [eds]: Advances in Anesthesia, vol 2, p 232. Chicago, Year Book Medical Publishers, 1985.)

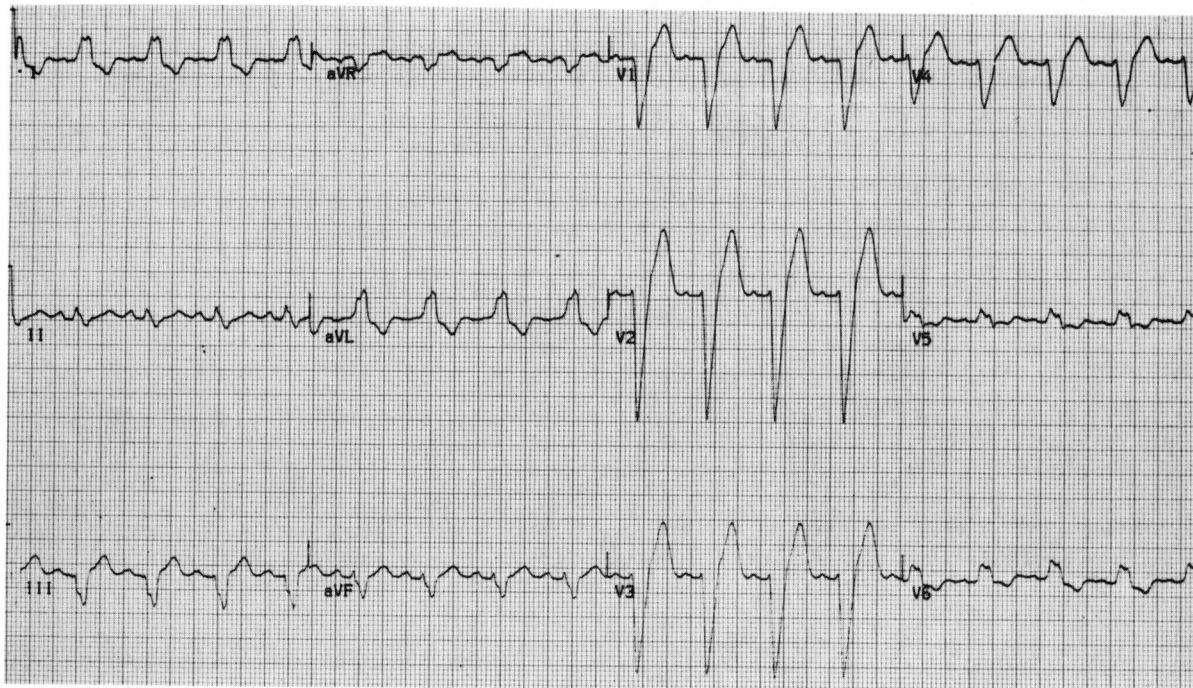

Figure 29-36. The pattern in lead V_6 is consistent with left bundle-branch block.

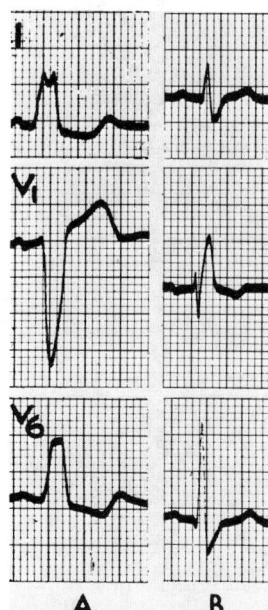

Figure 29-37. Comparison of left (*A*) and right (*B*) bundle-branch blocks in leads I, V_1, and V_6. (Reprinted with permission from Marriott HJL: Practical Electrocardiography, 7th ed, p 64. Baltimore, Williams & Wilkins, 1983.)

nary artery disease and increasing age. Denes *et al* investigated sudden cardiac deaths in 30 patients of 277 who had chronic bifascicular block. Death was associated with coronary artery disease and ventricular arrhythmias rather than heart block.[127] Two Framingham studies of newly acquired right and left bundle-branch block also imply that sudden death is related to cardiovascular abnormalities other than complete heart block.[128,129] Investigations of anesthetized patients reveal the almost nonexistent chance of developing a perioperative complete heart block from bifascicular block.[130,131] What the studies in anesthetized subjects do not address is the incidence of developing a third-degree block when the patient has either chronic bifascicular block plus first-degree block or evidence of trifascicular disease. In these latter two situations, if the patient is scheduled for major surgery associated with rapid fluid and electrolyte shifts and potentially major blood loss, one should at least have pacing capabilities immediately available. Pacing can take the form of a typical ventricular electrode, a pulmonary artery catheter, or a transcutaneous system.[132]

HEART BLOCK

First-degree block occurs when the impulse requires a prolonged period to traverse the AV node. All the impulses reaching the AV node from the atrium successfully cross the node and enter the ventricle. The ECG reflects first-degree block as a P-R interval longer than 0.21 sec (Fig. 29-40). The incidence of first-degree block in the normal population is approximately 1%.[133]

Second-degree block, indicating that some but not all of the impulses cross the AV node, occurs in two forms. Type I second-degree block is diagnosed by noting a progressively lengthening P-R interval until a P wave is not followed by a QRS complex (Fig. 29-41). The problem is progressive slowing of conduction within the AV node.[134] Although Type I second-degree block can be associated with cardiac disease such as ischemic heart disease, aortic valve disease, mitral valve prolapse, and atrial septal defects; it is also found in athletes who have no cardiac symptoms.[135,136]

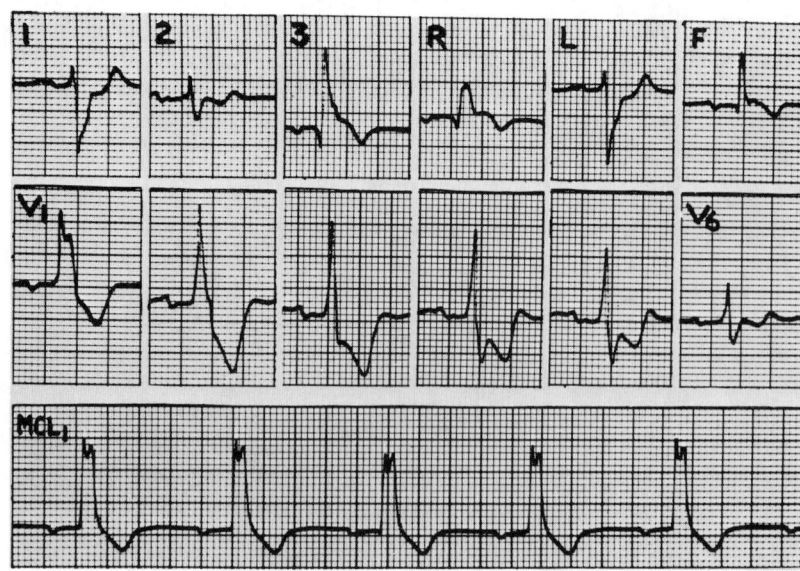

Figure 29-38. Right axis deviation indicating left posterior hemiblock is diagnosed in this case by noting an R wave axis of approximately 120 degrees. (Reprinted with permission from Marriott HJL: Practical Electrocardiography, 7th ed, p 91. Baltimore, Williams & Wilkins, 1983.)

Twenty-three percent of the 35 athletes experienced second-degree block compared with only 6% of the control group. As the P-R interval progressively lengthens, the R-P interval must progressively shorten. If Type I second-degree block occurs after an acute inferior myocardial infarction, it generally does not proceed to a third-degree block.[137]

Type II second-degree block, the more serious of the two types of second-degree block, occurs in the bundle branches. For this reason, bundle-branch block frequently accompanies Type II block. To diagnose this dysrhythmia, one must see unvarying P-R intervals in the conducted beats, and if two consecutive P waves conduct, the consecutive P-R intervals must be equal (Figs. 29-42 and 29-43).

Third-degree or complete AV block occurs when no impulses cross the AV node. The ventricles will respond either by developing asystole or an idioventricular or idiojunc-

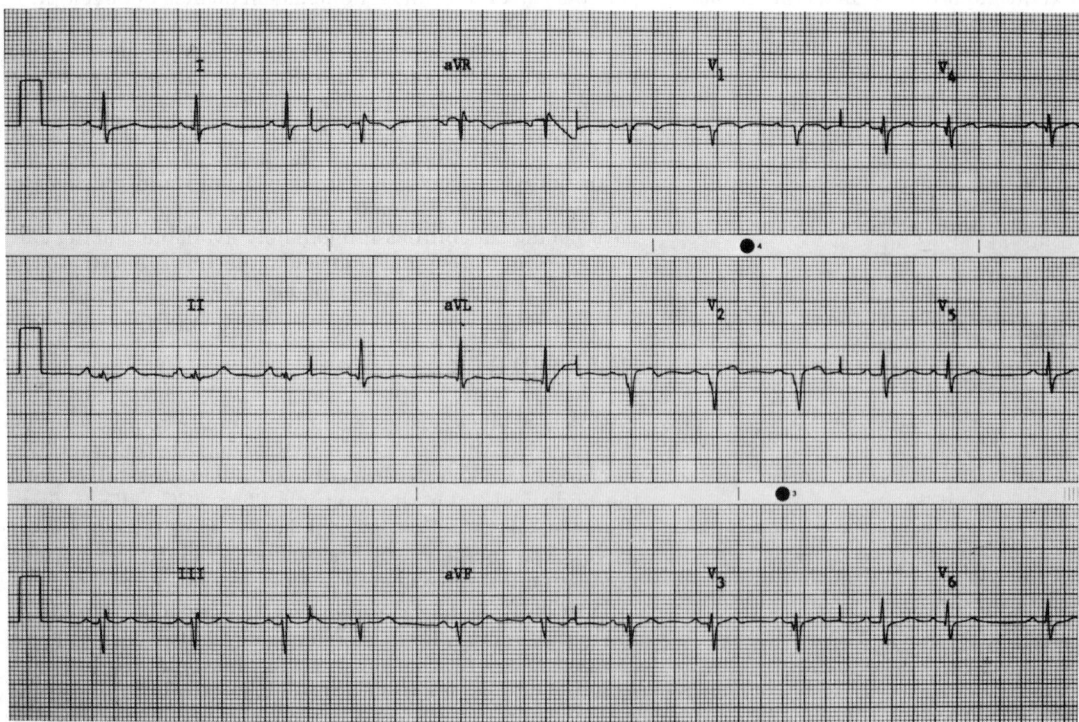

Figure 29-39. Noting the R and S wave deflections in leads I, II, and III will indicate the R wave axis. As a rough estimate, note the lead in which the R and S waves add to zero (lead II). The R wave axis will be perpendicular to lead II. Since lead III is negative, the axis points away from lead III and would be in the quadrant between 0 degrees and −90 degrees. The exact axis is −30 degrees, a left axis deviation consistent with left anterior hemiblock.

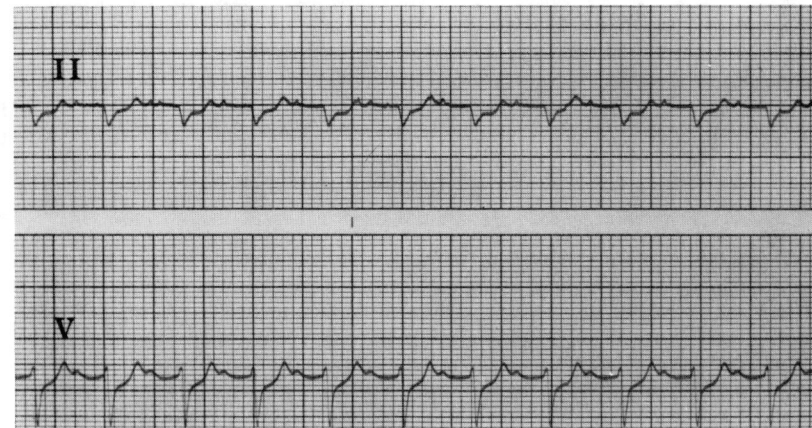

Figure 29-40. First-degree block carries a prolonged P-R interval >0.21 sec. All of the impulses proceed through the AV node. This ECG also contains ST segment depression.

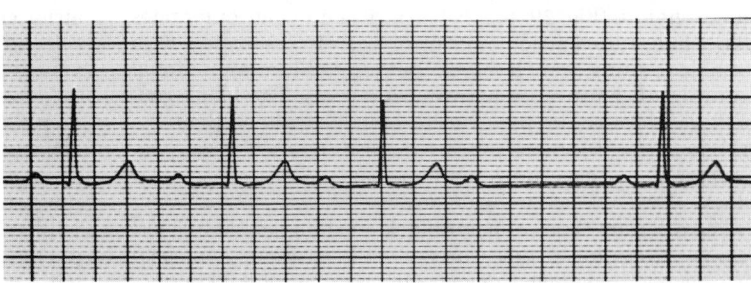

Figure 29-41. Diagnose Type I second-degree AV block by noting progressively lengthening P-R intervals until complete block occurs. This cycle repeats with identical P-R intervals. (Reprinted with permission from Zaidan JR, Curling PE: Cardiac dysrhythmias: Recognition and management. In Stoelting RK, Barash PG, Gallagher TH [eds]: Advances in Anesthesia, vol 2, p 235. Chicago, Year Book Medical Publishers, 1985.)

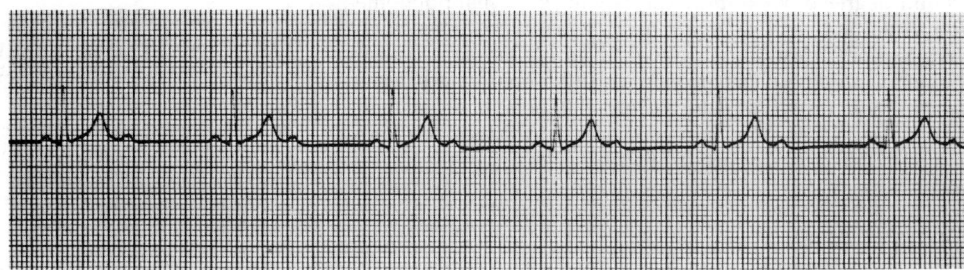

Figure 29-42. Diagnose Type II second-degree AV block by noting identical P-R intervals in the conducted beats. In this case, the block is 2:1, indicating two P waves for each QRS complex.

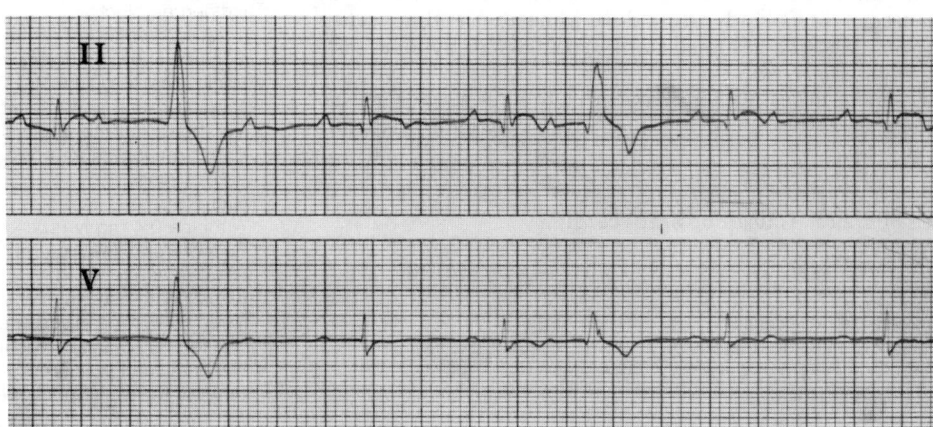

Figure 29-43. Type II 2:1 second-degree block with either premature junctional or ventricular contractions.

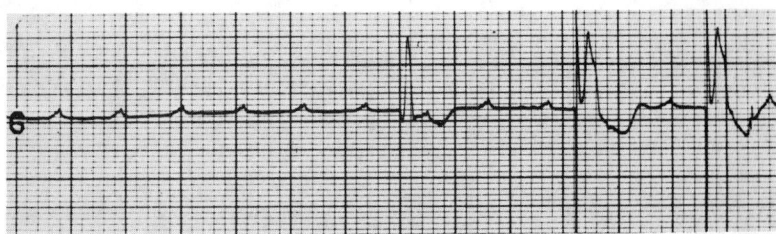

Figure 29-44. Third-degree block with one junctional escape beat and initiation of ventricular pacing occurred in this patient. Occurrence of P waves without some escape beats is correctly called asystole.

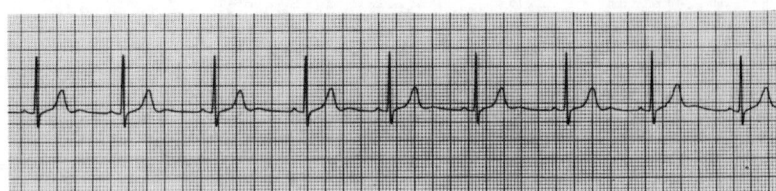

Figure 29-45. Sinus bradycardia is defined as a heart rate below 60 beats·min^{-1}.

tional rhythm (Fig. 29-44).[135] The atrial and ventricular rates dissociate. Idioventricular control will be associated with a wide bundle-branch block pattern and idiojunctional control will have more narrow complexes. The block generally is located in the bundle branches rather than the AV node.[138-140] Ischemic heart disease, Lev's disease, and Lenegre's disease are common causes of trifascicular block.[141,142]

The different types of heart block must be related to heart rate to determine if disease is actually present. A normal heart generally shows signs of fatigue of AV nodal conduction at approximately 180–200 beats·min^{-1}. If this person were atrially paced at 250 beats·min^{-1}, probably a second-degree AV block would occur, even if the AV node were perfectly normal. This person does not actually have a second-degree block but is experiencing a normal phenomenon. A patient with ischemic heart disease, however, might have normal AV conduction until atrial pacing increases the heart rate to 90 beats·min^{-1}. At this rate, second-degree heart block might develop. Both subjects have second-degree heart block by electrocardiographic criteria, but only one has clinically important disease.

BRADYCARDIA

Sinus rates below 60 beats·min^{-1} classically fall into the category of sinus bradycardia (Fig. 29-45). Both well-trained athletes and critically ill patients with heart disease experience sinus bradycardia. Table 29-6 outlines several of the causes of sinus bradycardia during anesthesia. Bradycardia must always be assumed to be secondary to hypoxia until proved otherwise.

It is not necessary for bradycardia to have a sinus mechanism. Causes of nonsinus bradycardia include premature atrial complexes with nonconducted premature P waves, SA nodal block, third-degree block associated with an idioventricular rhythm, and atrial fibrillation or flutter.

Treatment of bradycardia (outlined in Table 29-7) depends on the hemodynamic and electrocardiographic responses. Maintenance of the sinus mechanism without ventricular or junctional escape beats and no loss of blood pressure in an otherwise healthy patient dictates vigilance with no specific treatment. In fact, uncontrolled treatment of bradycardia sometimes creates more problems. A patient with a "tight" left main coronary artery lesion can be asymptomatic at a heart rate of 40 beats·min^{-1}. Increasing the patient's rate to 90 beats·min^{-1} likely will cause myocardial ischemia. Before treating bradycardia, consider the pos-

TABLE 29-6. Causes of Bradycardia

Vagal reflexes
Hypoxia
Intracranial hypertension
Anticholinesterase drugs
Beta blocking drugs
Digitalis preparations

TABLE 29-7. Treatment of Bradycardia

Ensure oxygenation
Sinus, no escape beats, otherwise healthy:
　No treatment, unless hypotensive
Sinus or idiojunctional, vagally induced, with hypotension and possibly escape beats:
　Removal of vagal influence
　Atropine 0.4 mg iv repeated
　Ephedrine 5 mg iv repeated, if necessary
　Possible atrial pacing
Sinus, with hypertension:
　Treat hypertension
　Do not increase rate until hypertension is controlled
Third-degree block:
　Treat ischemia
　Sequential pacing if atrial activity intact
Chronic atrial fibrillation:
　Stop digoxin if serum concentration is high
　Ventricular pacing to physiologic rate
　Cardioversion might not be successful
Beta blockade:
　Stop drug
　Atropine 0.4 mg iv repeated
　Isoproterenol (4–8 μg·ml^{-1}) 0.5–2 μg·min^{-1}
　Atrial or sequential pacing
Anticholinesterase-induced (muscle relaxant reversal):
　Atropine 0.4 mg iv repeated
Increased intracranial pressure:
　Hyperventilation, diuretics
　Surgery to relieve pressure

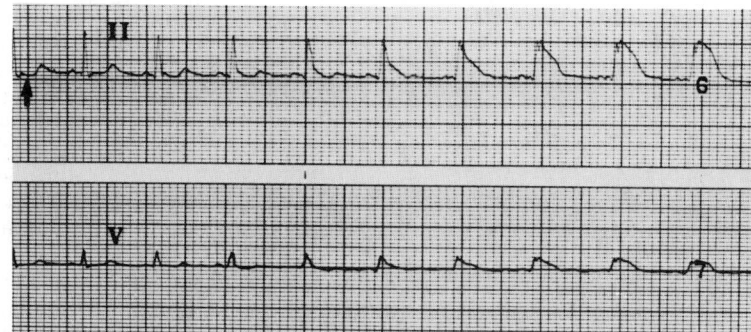

Figure 29-46. Aortic cross-clamping (*arrow*) after initiation of cardiopulmonary bypass resulted in an intraventricular conduction delay and ST segment change within three beats.

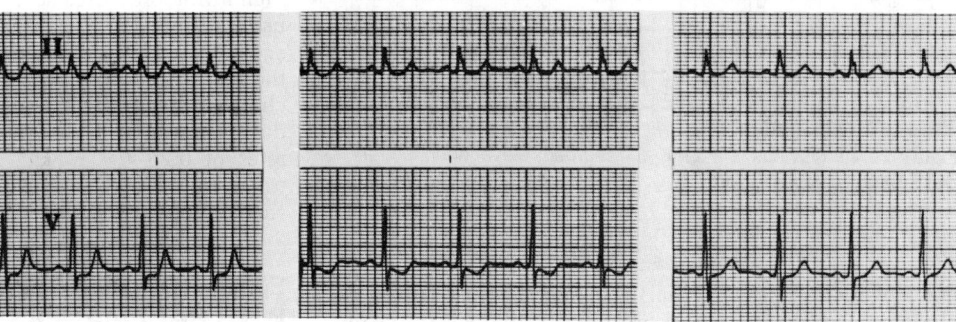

Figure 29-47. ST segment depression is evident in leads II and V₅ (*left*). This patient had chest pain. Metoprolol decreased the heart rate from 96 to 80 beats·min⁻¹ (*middle*) with an obvious improvement in the ST segment changes. Pain resolved within a few minutes after decreasing the heart rate, and the ST segments became isoelectric.

sibility that a tachycardia is potentially worse than bradycardia. Do not administer an antimuscarinic agent to a patient who has a reflex sinus bradycardia secondary to hypertension. Treating the hypertension will return the heart rate to more physiologic levels. Atrial pacing, when available, allows precise control of heart rate.

MYOCARDIAL ISCHEMIA AND INFARCTION

One of the initial electrocardiographic events in the presence of decreased oxygen delivery to the myocardium is T wave inversion. If coronary flow does not return, the ST segment elevates and takes with it the inverted T wave. At this point, re-establishment of coronary flow will allow the ST-T wave changes to revert to normal. Continued insufficient oxygen delivery, however, eventually changes the QRS complex into a persistent QS complex or Q wave (Figs. 29-46 through 29-52). This pattern of necrosis develops because the impulse no longer enters the area of the necrotic tissue. The electrical forces that formerly approached the ECG electrode do not exist; therefore, the electrode records activity directed toward the opposite side of the heart and away from the electrode. The overall electrocardiographic picture is a negative deflection recorded in the area of the necrosis and an unopposed, enhanced, positive deflection recorded from the other side of the heart.

An infarct has an area of necrosis associated with Q waves, an area of injury associated with ST segment changes, and a larger area of ischemia that creates T wave changes. Electrodes placed directly on the heart can record each of these separate areas. An electrode located on the body's surface, however, simultaneously records all three of these areas. The result is probably T wave changes, ST segment elevation, and Q waves recorded from one surface electrode. Characteristically, the Q wave must be 0.03 sec in duration, the ST segments are convex upward (dome-shaped), and the T wave is pointed with two equal limbs.

Locating the exact position of an infarct is not well defined.[143] We can predict the general area of the heart affected by the infarct by observing specific electrocardiographic leads. Table 29-8 indicates these areas. If limb and precordial leads reveal persistent ST-T wave changes, the patient experienced a subendocardial infarct.[144]

Other subtle electrocardiographic changes suggest but are

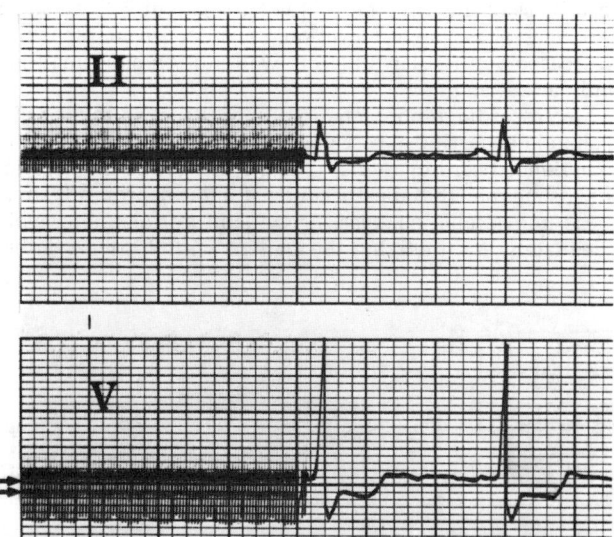

Figure 29-48. The ECG recorder can reveal ST segment depression even at very slow speeds. Note the lighter colored ink between the arrows and this area's corresponding location when the recorder was increased to 25 mm·sec⁻¹. This lighter colored area disappeared when the ST segments returned to the baseline.

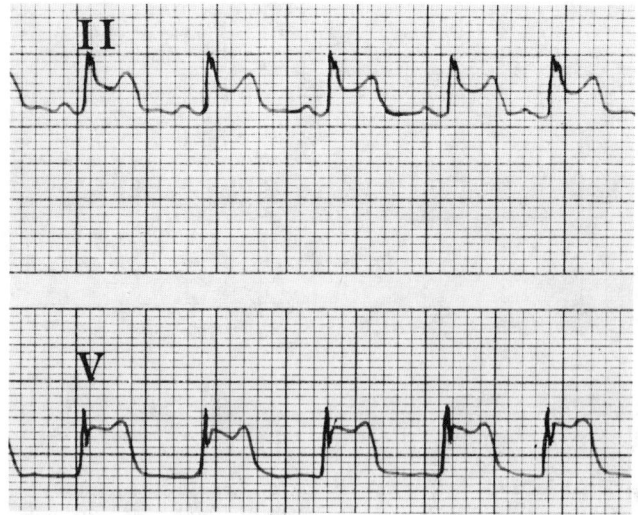

Figure 29-49. Obvious is a 3-mm ST segment elevation in lead II and a 6-mm elevation in V_5.

disease. In fact, it is the light anesthesia that causes hypertension and tachycardia. A lightly anesthetized patient must receive supplemental anesthetic drugs. Occasionally, the anesthesiologist will find it necessary to use beta-adrenergic blocking drugs such as propranolol, esmolol, or metoprolol, alpha-adrenergic blocking drugs such as phentolamine, the alpha-beta blocking drug labetalol, and directly acting vasodilators such as nitroprusside and nitroglycerin to control hypertension and tachycardia. Hypotension presents more difficult therapeutic problems. Although one might think that a hypotensive patient should not receive a vasodilator, reducing preload with nitroglycerin can restore the myocardial oxygen balance, increase contractility and secondarily increase cardiac output and blood pressure; therefore, if high filling pressures accompany the hypotension, consider using nitroglycerin as a first-line drug, followed by a $beta_1$ agonist such as dobutamine. If low filling pressures led to the hypotension, then volume replacement becomes the choice therapy. Patients experiencing ST segment elevation during anesthesia can receive a nitroglycerin infusion at rates of $0.25-0.5$ $\mu g \cdot kg^{-1} \cdot min^{-1}$ or 10 mg of sublingual nifedipine. Volatile anesthetic agents plus nifedipine can cause hypotension.

not diagnostic of myocardial ischemia. These changes include a perfectly horizontal ST segment that abruptly converts into the T wave, inverted U waves, and postextrasystolic T wave changes.[145-147]

An atrial infarct is more difficult to diagnose than a ventricular infarct. Suspect an atrial infarct when a patient experiencing a ventricular infarct develops an atrial dysrhythmia.[148] Electrocardiographic signs of an atrial infarct include a change in the contour of the P wave and significant P-R interval elevation in lead I associated with P-R interval depression in lead III.[149]

The ST segment change during exercise is significant if it undergoes 1-2 mm of depression 0.08 sec after the J point regardless of the direction of the ST segment.[150-152] If stress produces ST segment elevation, consider severe ischemia, decreased ventricular function, wall motion abnormalities, and variant angina.[153-157]

Electrocardiographic changes indicative of myocardial ischemia occurring at rest portend infarction. If the patient experienced cardiovascular changes that led to the myocardial ischemia, the anesthesiologist should promptly treat these undesirable changes. A common mistake is to avoid adequately anesthetizing the patient with coronary artery

ELECTROCARDIOGRAMS ASSOCIATED WITH PACEMAKERS

Increased use and sophistication of pacemakers create the possibility of misinterpretation of their ECG. The location of the electrodes and the type of generator determine the appearance of the ECG. The generator can stimulate the atrium, ventricle, or both chambers sequentially. Electrodes located in the atrium will create P waves, and ventricular electrodes will cause a left bundle-branch block if they are on the right ventricle or a right bundle-branch block if they are on the left ventricle.

At this time, almost all implanted pacemakers are programmable. Programmability implies that one can easily change the rate, voltage output, sensitivity, and other parameters. Two common generators have the three-letter designation, VVI and DDD. VVI indicates that stimulation (first letter) and sensing (second letter) take place in the ventricle (V). "I" indicates that if the pacemaker's sensing circuit detects sufficient R wave voltage (usually about ±2 mV), the generator turns off (the sensing circuit inhibits the pacing circuit). With a VVI generator, one would expect to see ventricular pacing or no pacing, depending on the patient's

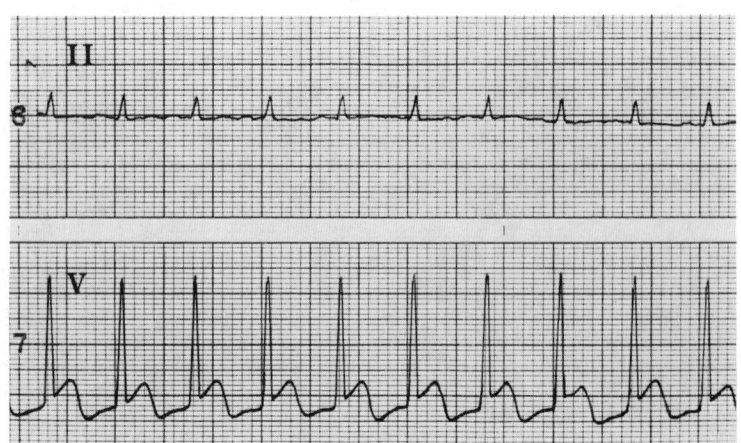

Figure 29-50. Lead II does not always reveal ST segment changes simultaneously with lead V_5.

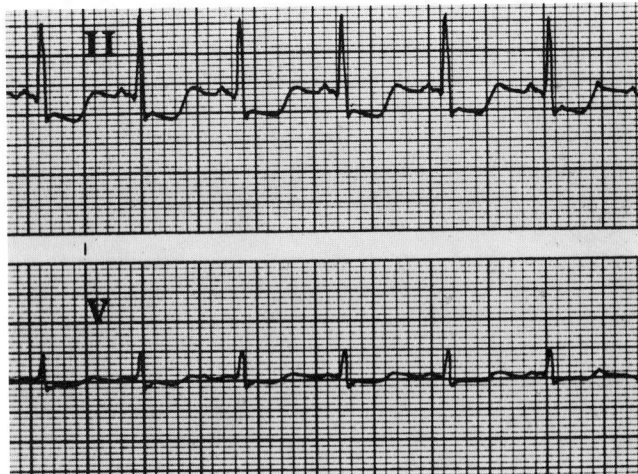

Figure 29-51. In this example, lead II showed signs of ischemia not evident in V_5. This patient had right coronary artery disease.

TABLE 29-8. Locating the Myocardial Infarct

Area of Infarct	Affected ECG Leads
Anterior	I, aV_L, V_3, V_4
Inferior	II, III, aV_F
Lateral	I, aV_L, V_5, V_6
Posterior	Reciprocal changes in V_1, V_2
Anterolateral[172]	V_{1-6}
Anteroseptal[173]	V_{1-4}
Inferolateral[174]	Inferior + V_5, V_6
Right ventricle[175,176]	V_{4R}–V_{6R}

intrinsic heart rate. A DDD pacemaker stimulates the atrium and ventrical (dual) and senses P waves from the atrium and R waves from the ventricle (dual). If it senses a P wave, the generator waits the programmed period of time (the P-R interval) and then either triggers an impulse into the ventricle if an R wave does not occur or continues pacing in the inhibited mode if the R wave does occur. The "fully automatic" DDD pacemaker can have four levels of pacing that depend on the patient's heart rate and P-R interval: (1) total AV sequential pacing; (2) atrial pacing without ventricular pacing; (3) ventricular pacing without atrial pacing; and (4) no pacing.

The pacemaker with a VVIR generator responds to motion of the patient. It is programmable for the incremental increase in pacing rate and the sensitivity to movement. A patient could experience a 5 beat·min^{-1} rate increase with maximal motion, or a 10 beat·min^{-1} rate increase with minimal motion, depending on the program. The implication for the anesthesiologist is that shivering or muscle fasciculation from a depolarizing relaxant could increase the pacing rate.

Pacemakers must receive at least a simple evaluation before the patient can proceed to surgery. If the generator is less than 2 years old, does not produce pacing impulses

when the patient's heart rate is above 72 beats·min^{-1}, and does produce pacing impulses associated with a peripheral pulse when the heart rate slows, probably the pacemaker system is properly functioning. The pacemaker should continue to function throughout the operative period unless one of several events occurs. Table 29-9 outlines the events that can cause intraoperative failure. One of the more important factors associated with pacemaker failure is the electrocautery. A magnet used to convert a programmable VVI, VVIR, DDD, or DDDR pacemaker to VOO (asynchronous) activity does not prevent reprogramming but rather increases the likelihood that the generator will reprogram. The clinician will be unaware of this change as long as the magnet remains over the generator. If the magnet is not used, reprogramming is less likely, but a change in the program could be immediately evident. Place the magnet on the generator if it changes to a program that causes loss of pacing. Remove the magnet only when the patient is fully monitored, and be prepared to use the programming device if the patient's heart no longer paces. Once the device is plugged in and turned on, place the magnetic coil over the generator and push the red button. This red button, found on all the programming devices, will convert the pacemaker to the VVI mode, a rate of 70 beats·min^{-1}, and an output of 5 volts. Call the patient's cardiologist to determine what other type of program the patient might require.

A special type of pacemaker, the automatic implantable cardioverter defibrillator (AICD), automatically cardioverts or defibrillates patients experiencing ventricular tachydysrhythmias. The earliest design permitted only defibrillation;[158,159] however, electrophysiologic studies revealed that patients develop ventricular tachycardia before fibrillation and that tachycardia requires less conversion energy than fibrillation.[160,161] The latest models of the AICD are therefore designed to test for and treat both tachycardia and fibrillation. The AICD analyzes two parameters to help it decide when to discharge. One of these parameters is the heart rate, and the second is the probability density function. The probability density function analyzes the amount of time that the ECG tracing is away from the baseline. As an example, a normal ECG remains on the baseline for a large part of the cardiac cycle. Ventricular tachycardia, however, crosses but does not remain on the baseline as it moves toward a negative deflection. When the AICD senses a rate greater than 155 beats·min^{-1} and a probability density function suggesting extensive time away from the baseline, it releases an impulse of 25 joules through the ventricular lead system. The generator recycles three more times and releases 30 joules of energy if sensing suggests that the tachydysrhythmia was not terminated. The clinical implication for the anesthesiologist is the patient's ischemic heart disease and nonischemic cardiomyopathy, the leading indica-

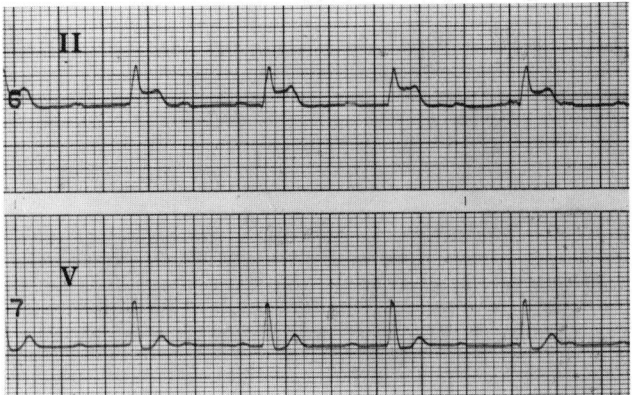

Figure 29-52. ST segment elevation, seen here in lead II, implies variant angina. The patient had AV dissociation and probably also third-degree AV block.

TABLE 29-9. Causes and Treatment of Pacemaker Failure

Change	Causes	Result	Considerations
Acute K+ changes			
Extracellular K+ decrease	Hyperventilation Acute diuretic therapy	Pacing loss	Increase output external generator
Extracellular K+ increase	Myocardial ischemia Depolarizing muscle relaxants Rapid K+ replacement	Pacing-related ventricular fibrillation	Treat ischemia Lidocaine $CaCl_2$
Electromagnetic interference	Electrocautery	Pacing loss Reprogramming	The pacemaker generator must not be between the ground plate and the active electrode of the electrocautery
Myocardial infarction	Increase in size of electrode (dead tissue) and therefore decreased charge at the electrode-tissue interface	Pacing loss	Increase output of external generator; possible cardiopulmonary resuscitation

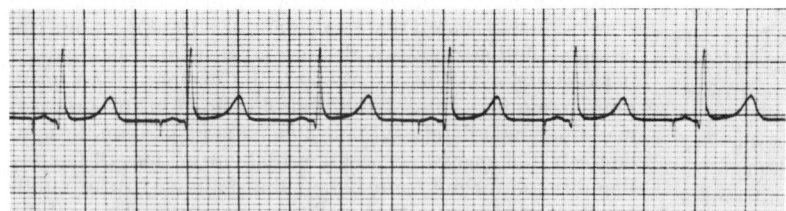

Figure 29-53. Normal atrial pacing. A P wave follows each pacing impulse, and each P wave travels to the ventricle.

tions for insertion of the AICD in a vast majority of these patients.[162] It is important to determine the preoperative cardiac status of the patient before developing an anesthetic management plan.

It is also important to know how to manage the generator during the operative procedure. It is possible that the electrocautery could trigger the charging-discharging cycle. For this reason, the AICD should be deactivated before the start of surgery. Turning the generator off and on is performed by placing the magnet over the pacemaker and listening for a high-pitched tone. The continuous tone reveals that the generator is inactive, whereas the R wave synchronous beep indicates that the generator is active. When the patient is in the operating room and fully monitored for surgery, place the magnet over the pacemaker for 30 seconds and wait for the synchronous beeping tone to become a continuous tone before removing the magnet. Reactivate the generator before transporting the patient to the postanesthesia care unit. Immediately stop the electrocautery if the tone sounds during surgery.

The remainder of this section presents commonly used normally and abnormally functioning pacemakers (Figs. 29-53 through 29-61).

OTHER CONDITIONS AFFECTING THE ELECTROCARDIOGRAM

Several other conditions that acutely affect the ECG could involve a patient scheduled for emergency surgery.

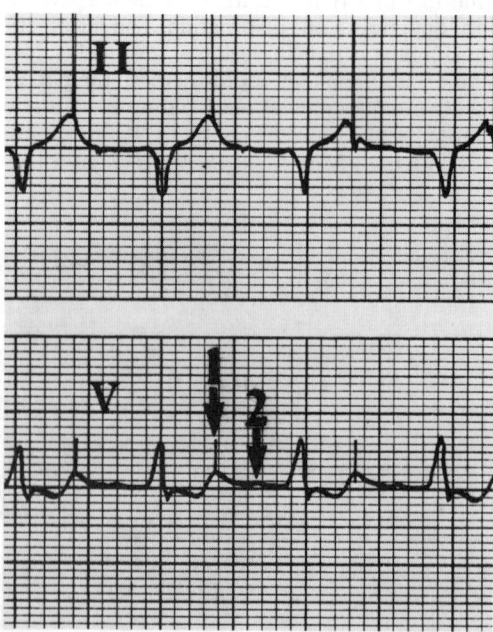

Figure 29-54. This patient had a long delay between the atrial pacing impulse (*arrow 1*) and the P wave (*arrow 2*). This situation can occur after cardiopulmonary bypass and cardioplegia.

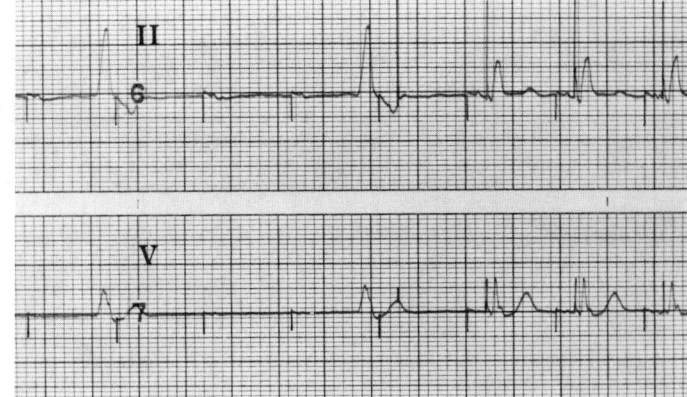

Figure 29-55. Atrial pacing created an atrial depolarization that was not conducted to the ventricle. The first two QRS complexes are ventricular escapes, whereas the last three are associated with sequential pacing.

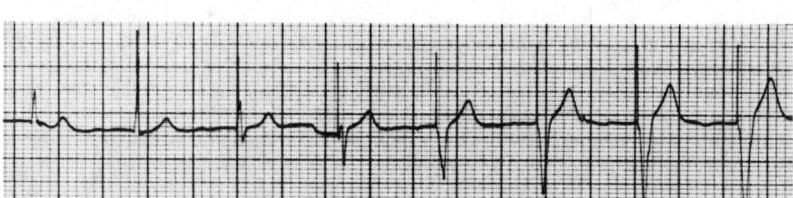

Figure 29-56. Normal ventricular inhibited pacing showing, in sequence, a junctional escape, two pseudofusion beats, three fusion beats, and two ventricularly paced beats.

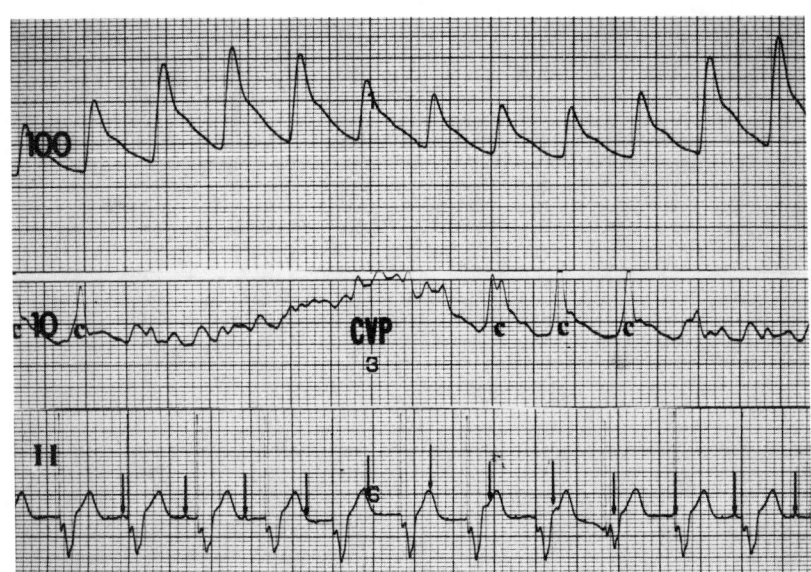

Figure 29-57. Ventricular pacing with continued atrial activity (*arrows*) results in hemodynamic effects much like a junctional rhythm. The arterial blood pressure (*top* trace) decreases, and cannon waves (c) appear on the CVP tracing (*middle* trace). The third trace is lead II (100 = 100 mm Hg; 10 = 10 mm Hg).

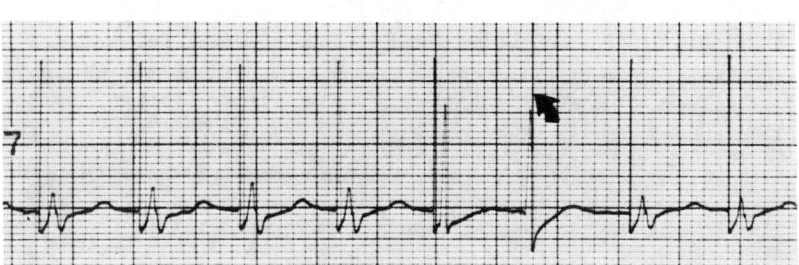

Figure 29-58. The pacing spike at the *arrow* occurs after the peak of the R wave, showing abnormal sensing. The fifth complex is a fusion beat.

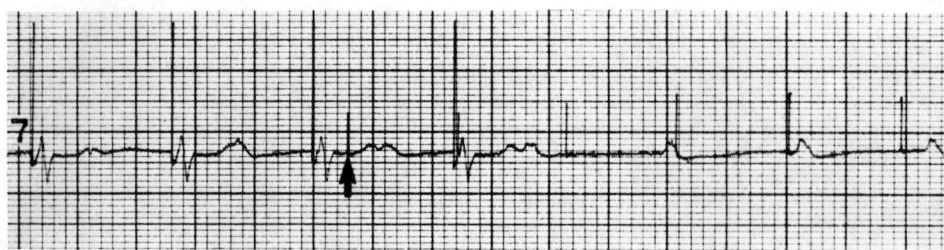

Figure 29-59. A second, temporary pacemaker, turned on at the *arrow,* inhibited the patient's implanted pacemaker. The temporary pacemaker was not functioning and did not take over ventricular pacing. Only unrelated P waves occur.

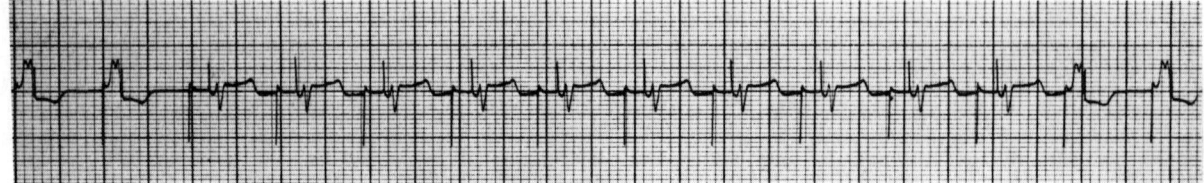

Figure 29-60. AV sequential pacing reversed accidentally when the atrial pacing electrode touched the ventricle (first three and last two QRS complexes). Ventricular pacing occurred with the atrial impulse, and the ventricular impulse therefore found a refractory ventricle. Had the P-R interval been set to approximately 300 msec, the ventricular impulse could have initiated ventricular tachycardia or fibrillation by stimulating the ventricle in the repolarization period.

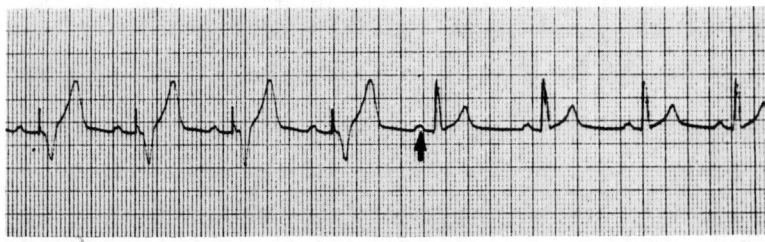

Figure 29-61. Illustration of one aspect of totally automatic, or DDD pacing. P wave sensing occurs (no impulse found before the P wave). The P wave took longer than the pacemaker's P-R interval to cross the AV node; therefore, the ventricular circuit activated, and ventricular pacing occurred (first four complexes). The P wave crossed the AV node in a sufficiently short time period to inhibit the ventricular circuit at the *arrow.* An intraventricular conduction delay is evident.

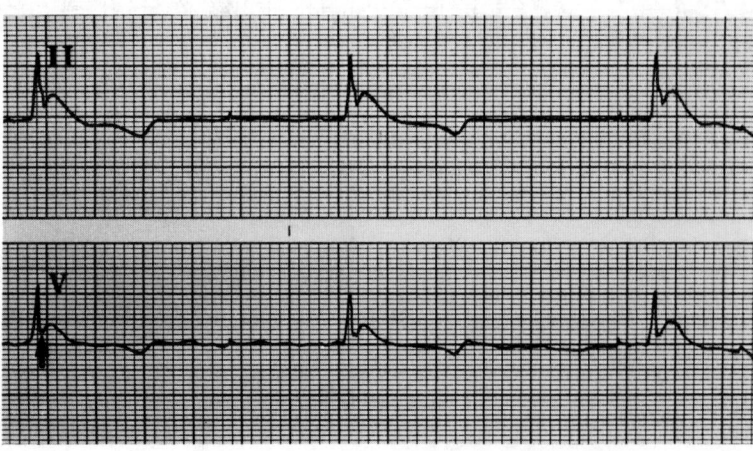

Figure 29-62. Osborne waves (*arrow*) occur during hypothermia. Note that the Osborne wave is not an elevation of the ST segment.

TABLE 29-10. Electrocardiogram Associated with Electrolyte Abnormalities

Electrolyte Change	ECG Response
Hypokalemia	ST segment depression
	T wave flattening and inversion
	Tall U wave
Hyperkalemia	Tall T wave
	P-R interval prolongation
	ST segment depression
	QRS widening
	Ventricular fibrillation
Hypocalcemia	Prolonged Q-T interval
Hypercalcemia	Short Q-T interval
	ST segment may disappear

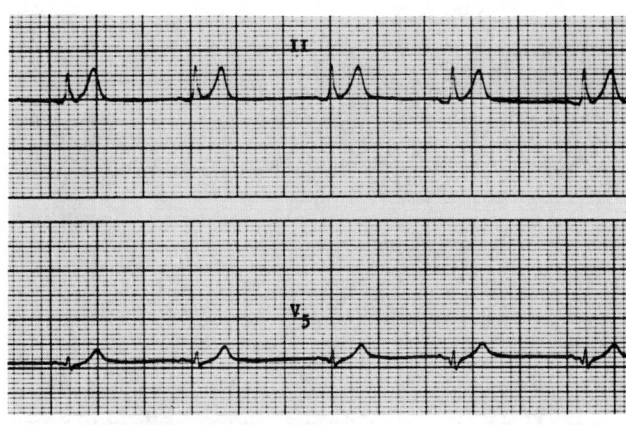

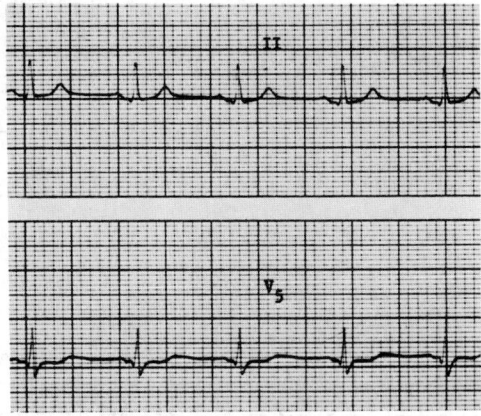

Figure 29-63. Elevated myocardial potassium creates peaked T waves in relation to the R wave (*top* tracings). The *bottom* tracings show the ECG a short while after the patient received glucose and insulin.

Acute Pericarditis

The ST stage develops first in acute pericarditis. It is characterized by elevated ST segments in many leads. The PR segment commonly undergoes depression.[163,164]

The T wave stage composing the second phase of acute pericarditis persists for 10 days to 2 weeks. Widespread T wave inversion is the characteristic finding.

Pericardial Effusion

Electrocardiographic findings characteristic of pericardial effusion include low QRS voltage, ST segment elevation, and electrical alternans. A patient experiencing electrical alternans of the P waves as well as the QRS complexes likely will have a malignant pericardial effusion.[165-167]

Intracranial Hemorrhage

Intracranial hemorrhage produces bradycardia and wide inverted T waves many times coupled with an inverted U wave.[168,169] Conversely, intracranial hemorrhage can mask myocardial ischemia by changing an inverted T wave to the upright position.[170]

Hypothermia

Moderate hypothermia above approximately 32°C does not change the ECG. Below 30°C, bradycardia and an elevation of the J point develop (Fig. 29-62). Atrial fibrillation occurs below 29°C.[171]

Electrolytes

Electrocardiographic changes associated with electrolyte abnormalities are listed in Table 29-10 (Figs. 29-63 and 29-64). These electrocardiographic changes may exist in the presence of normal serum electrolytes. Conversely, the ECG can be normal in the presence of abnormal serum electrolytes. Myocardial concentrations and transmembrane gradients, not serum electrolyte concentrations, create the electrocardiographic changes.

Monitoring Catheters

Atrial and ventricular dysrhythmias and right bundle-branch block can occur when a pulmonary arterial catheter floats through the heart and into the pulmonary artery (Fig.

Figure 29-64. Transient T wave enhancement and R wave changes were evident after the patient received 2 mEq of potassium through a central catheter. The *broad arrows* follow the T wave changes, whereas the *narrow arrows* trace the R wave changes. The heart rate also decreased. One can diagnose these changes even when the recorder speed is slow (25 mm·min⁻¹).

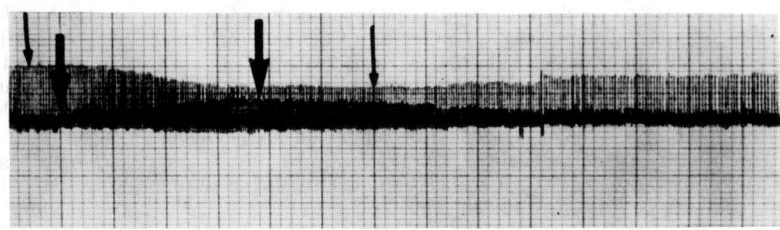

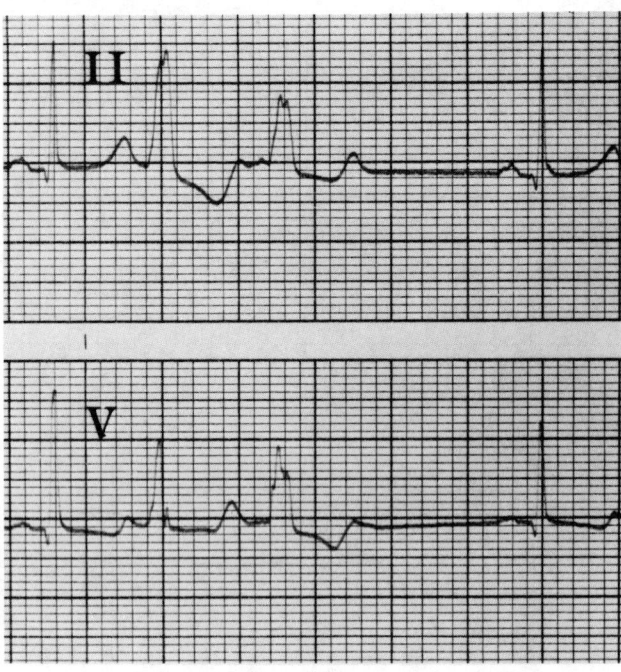

Figure 29-65. The pulmonary arterial catheter created these electrocardiographic changes as it floated through the right ventricular outflow tract. It is difficult to distinguish between atrial and ventricular catheter-related dysrhythmias; however, these changes are most likely ventricular in origin.

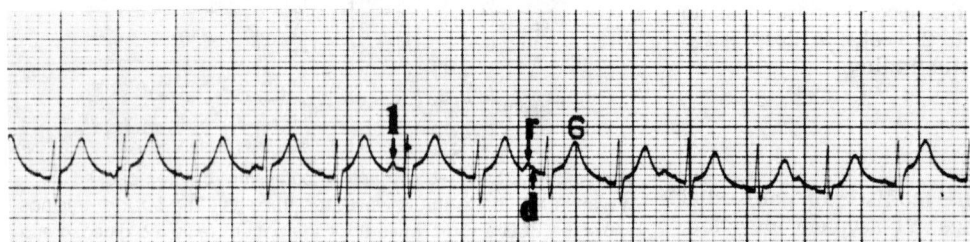

Figure 29-66. The heart transplant patient has recipient P waves (*arrow* r) and donor P waves (*arrow* d). They occasionally superimpose (*arrow* 1).

29-65). Advancing a pulmonary artery catheter introduced through the right internal jugular vein no more than 25% of the patient's height in centimeters measured from the skin entry point should avoid dysrhythmias caused by coiling within the atrium or ventricle.

Heart Transplantation

Heart transplantation creates an unusual ECG with P waves originating from the donor's heart and from the recipient's SA node and remaining atrial tissue. The donor's P wave will remain associated with the QRS complexes, and the recipient's atrial activity will dissociate from the QRS complexes (Fig. 29-66).

REFERENCES

1. Levy AG, Lewis T: Heart irregularities resulting from the inhalation of low percentages of chloroform vapor and their relationship to ventricular fibrillation. Heart 3:99, 1911
2. Levy AG: Sudden death under light chloroform anesthesia. J Physiol 42:3, 1911
3. Vanik PE, Davis HS: Cardiac arrhythmias during halothane anesthesia. Anesth Analg 47:299, 1968
4. Kuner J, Enescu V, Utsu F et al: Cardiac arrhythmias during anesthesia. Dis Chest 52:580, 1967
5. Southall DP, Johnston F, Shinebourne EA et al: A 24-hour electrocardiographic study of heart rate and rhythm patterns in populations of healthy children. Br Heart J 45:281, 1981
6. Brodsky M, Wu D, Denes P et al: Arrhythmias documented by 24 hour continuous electrocardiographic monitoring in 50 male medical students without apparent heart disease. Am J Cardiol 39:390, 1977
7. Marriott HJL, Fogg E: Constant monitoring for cardiac dysrhythmias and blocks. Mod Concepts Cardiovasc Dis 39:103, 1970
8. Kates RA, Zaidan JR, Kaplan JA: Esophageal lead for intraoperative electrocardiographic monitoring. Anesth Analg 61: 781, 1982
9. Copeland GD: Clinical evaluation of a new esophageal electrode, with particular reference to the bipolar esophageal electrocardiogram. Am Heart J 57:862, 1959
10. Enselberg CD: The esophageal electrocardiogram in the study of atrial activity and cardiac arrhythmias. Am Heart J 41:382, 1951
11. Prystowsky EN, Pritchett EL, Gallagher JJ: Origin of the atrial electrogram recorded from the esophagus. Circulation 61: 1017, 1980
12. Narula OS, Scherlag BJ, Samet P et al: Atrioventricular block: Localization and classification by His bundle recordings. Am J Med 50:146, 1971
13. Damato A, Schnitzler RN, Lay SH: Recent advances in the bundle of His electrograms. In Yu PN, Goodwin JF (eds): Progress in Cardiology, p 181. Philadelphia, Lea & Febiger, 1973
14. Gallagher JJ, Damato AN: Technique of recording His bundle activity in man. In Grossman W (ed): Cardiac Catheterization and Angiography, p 213. Philadelphia, Lea & Febiger, 1974

15. Castellanos A Jr, Castillo C, Agha A: Contribution of His bundle recording to the understanding of clinical arrhythmias. Am J Cardiol 28:499, 1971

16. Rosen KM: Evaluation of cardiac conduction in the cardiac catheterization laboratory. Am J Cardiol 30:701, 1972

17. Atlee JL, Brownlee SW, Burstrom RE: Conscious-state comparisons of the effects of inhalation anesthetics on specialized atrioventricular conduction times in dogs. Anesthesiology 64:703, 1986

18. Marriott HJL: Electrical axis. In Marriott HJL (ed): Practical Electrocardiography, p 32. Baltimore, Williams & Wilkins, 1983

19. Fowler NO, Daniels C, Scott RC et al: The electrocardiogram in cor pulmonale with and without emphysema. Am J Cardiol 16:500, 1965

20. Hodgkin AL, Katz B: Ionic currents underlying activity in the giant axon of the squid. J Physiol 108:37, 1949

21. Hodgkin AL, Huxley AF: A quantitative description of membrane current and its application to conduction and excitation in nerve. J Physiol 117:500, 1952

22. Hagiwara S, Nakajina S: Differences in Na and Ca spikes as examined by application of tetrodotoxin, procaine, and manganese ions. J Gen Physiol 49:793, 1966

23. Katz AM: Cardiac action potential. In Katz AM: Physiology of the Heart, p 229. New York, Raven Press, 1977

24. Kenyon JL, Gibbons WR: Effects of low-chloride solutions on action potentials of sheep cardiac Purkinje fibers. J Gen Physiol 70:63, 1977

25. Trautwein W: Membrane currents in cardiac muscle fibers. Physiol Rev 59:973, 1973

26. Bigger JT: Mechanisms and diagnosis of arrhythmias. In Braunwald E (ed): Heart Disease: A Textbook of Cardiovascular Medicine, p 630. Philadelphia, WB Saunders, 1980

27. DiFrancesco D: A new interpretation of the pacemaker current in calf Purkinje fibers. J Physiol 314:359, 1981

28. Myerburg RJ, Stewart JW, Hoffman BF: Electrophysiological properties of the canine peripheral AV conducting system. Circ Res 26:361, 1970

29. Myerburg RJ: The gating mechanism in the distal AV conducting system. Circulation 43:955, 1971

30. Surawicz B, Saito S: Exercise testing for detection of myocardial ischemia in patients with abnormal electrocardiograms at rest. Am J Cardiol 41:943, 1978

31. Wit AL, Fenoglio JJ, Wagner BM et al: Electrophysiological properties of cardiac muscle in the anterior mitral valve leaflet and the adjacent atrium in dog. Possible implications for the genesis of atrial dysrhythmias. Circ Res 32:731, 1973

32. Bassett AL, Wit AL: Ectopic impulses originating in the tricuspid valve and contiguous atrium. Fed Proc 33:445, 1974

33. Fenoglio JJ: Canine mitral complex, ultrastructure and electromechanical properties. Circ Res 31:417, 1972

34. Hoffman BF, Cranefield PF: Electrophysiology of the Heart. New York, McGraw Hill, 1960

35. Norma A, Irisawa H: A time and voltage-dependent potassium current in the rabbit sinoatrial node cell. Pfluegers Arch 366:251, 1976

36. Katzing B: Effects of extracellular calcium and sodium on depolarization-induced automaticity in guinea pig papillary muscle. Circ Res 37:118, 1975

37. Brown HF, Noble ST: Membrane currents underlying delayed rectification and pacemaker activity in frog atrial muscle. J Physiol (London) 204:717, 1969

38. Imaniski S, Surawicz B: Automatic activity in depolarized guinea pig ventricular myocardium: Characteristics and mechanisms. Circ Res 39:751, 1976

39. Lazzara R, El-Sherif M, Sherlag BJ: Electrophysiological properties of canine Purkinje cells in one day old myocardial infarction. Circ Res 33:722, 1973

40. Hordof AJ, Edie R, Malm JR et al: Electrophysiological properties and response to pharmacologic agents of fibers from diseased human atria. Circulation 54:774, 1976

41. DeHaan RL, DeFelice LJ: Electrical noise and rhythmic properties of embryonic heart cell aggregates. Fed Proc 37:2132, 1978

42. Lin CI, Kotake H, Vassalle M: On the mechanism underlying the oscillatory current in cardiac Purkinje fibers. J Cardiovasc Pharm 8:906, 1986

43. Cranefield PF: Action potentials, afterpotentials, and arrhythmias. Circ Res 41:415, 1977

44. Bozler E: The initiation of impulses in cardiac muscle. Am J Physiol 138:273, 1943

45. Cranefield PF, Aronson RS: Initiation of sustained rhythmic activity by single propagated action potentials in canine Purkinje fibers exposed to sodium-free solution or to ouabain. Circ Res 34:477, 1974

46. Hoffman BF, Rosen MR: Cellular mechanisms for cardiac arrythmias. Circ Res 49:1, 1981

47. Ferrier GR: Digitalis arrhythmias: Role of oscillatory afterpotentials. Prog Cardiovasc Dis 19:459, 1977

48. Schmitt FO, Erlanger J: Directional differences in the conduction of the impulse through heart muscle and their possible relation to extrasystolic and fibrillary contractions. Am J Physiol 87:326, 1929

49. Wit AL, Cranefield PF, Hoffman BF: Slow conduction and reentry in the ventricular conducting system. II. Single and sustained circuit movement in networks of canine and bovine Purkinje fibers. Circ Res 30:11, 1972

50. Wit AL, Hoffman BF, Cranefield PF: Slow conduction and reentry in the ventricular conducting system. I. Return extrasystole in canine Purkinje fibers. Circ Res 30:1, 1972

51. Mendez C, Moe GK: Demonstration of a dual AV nodal conduction system in the isolated rabbit heart. Circ Res 23:378, 1966

52. Han J, Malozzi AM: Sinoatrial reciprocation in the isolated rabbit heart. Circ Res 22:355, 1965

53. Bigger JT Jr, Goldreyer BN: The mechanism of paroxysmal supraventricular tachycardia in man. Circulation 42:673, 1970

54. Sasyniuk BI, Mendec C: A mechanism for reentry in canine ventricular tissue. Circ Res 28:3, 1971

55. Wiggers CS: The mechanism and nature of ventricular fibrillation. Am Heart J 20:399, 1940

56. Allessie MA, Bouke FIM, Schopman FJG: Circus movements in rabbit atrial muscle as a mechanism of tachycardia. III. The "leading circle" concept: A new model of circus movement in cardiac tissue without the involvement of an anatomical obstacle. Circ Res 41:8, 1977

57. Antzelevitch C, Moe GK: Electronically mediated delayed conduction and reentry in relation to "slow responses" in mammalian ventricular conducting tissue. Circ Res 49:1129, 1981

58. Rozanski GJ, Jalife J, Moe GK: Reflected reentry in nonhomogeneous ventricular muscle as a mechanism of cardiac arrhythmias. Circulation 69:163, 1984

59. Harrison DC: Antiarrhythmic drug classification: New science and practical application. Am J Cardiol 56:185, 1985

60. Single BN, Jewitt DE: Beta-adrenergic receptor blocking drugs in cardiac arrhythmias. Drugs 7:426, 1974

61. Heissenbuttel RH, Bigger JT: Bretylium tosylate: A newly available antiarrhythmic drug for ventricular arrhythmias. Ann Intern Med 91:229, 1979

62. Singh BN, Nademanee K, Josephson MA et al: The electrophysiology and pharmacology of verapamil, flecainide, and amiodarone: Correlations with clinical effects and antiarrhythmic actions. Ann NY Acad Sci 432:210, 1984

63. Gillis RA, Onset JA: The role of the nervous system in the cardiovascular effects of digitalis. Pharmacol Rev 31:19, 1980

64. Gajowski J, Singer RB: Mortality in an insured population with atrial fibrillation. JAMA 245:1540, 1981

65. Kannel WB, Abbott RD, Savage DD et al: Epidemiologic features of chronic atrial fibrillation: The Framingham study. N Engl J Med 306:1018, 1982

66. Kannel WB, Abbott RD, Savage DD et al: Coronary heart disease and atrial fibrillation: The Framingham study. Am Heart J 106:389, 1983

67. Henry WL, Morganroth J, Pearlman AS et al: Relation between echocardiography determined left atrial size and atrial fibrillation. Circulation 53:273, 1976

68. Hartel G, Louhija A, Konttinen A et al: Value of quinidine in

maintenance of sinus rhythm after electric conversion of atrial fibrillation. Br Heart J 32:57, 1970

69. Hartel G, Louhija A, Konttinen A: Disopyramide in the prevention of recurrence of atrial fibrillation after electroconversion. Clin Pharmacol Ther 15:551, 1974

70. Waxman HL, Myerburg RJ, Appel R et al: Verapamil for control of ventricular rate in paroxysmal supraventricular tachycardia and atrial fibrillation or flutter. Ann Intern Med 94:1, 1981

71. Weiner P, Bassan MM, Jarchovsky J et al: Clinical course of acute atrial fibrillation treated with rapid digitalization. Am Heart J 105:223, 1983

72. Sellers TD, Bashmore TM, Gallagher JJ: Digitalis in the preexcitation syndrome: Analysis during atrial fibrillation. Circulation 56:260, 1977

73. Gulamhusein S, Ko P, Carruthers SG et al: Acceleration of the ventricular response during atrial fibrillation in the Wolff-Parkinson-White syndrome after verapamil. Circulation 65:348, 1982

74. Waldo AL, MacLean WAH: Diagnosis and Treatment of Cardiac Arrhythmias Following Open Heart Surgery, p 115. Mt Kisco, NY, Futura, 1980

75. Wells JL, MacLean WAH, James TN et al: Characterization of atrial flutter. Studies in man after open heart surgery using fixed atrial electrodes. Circulation 60:66, 1979

76. Boineau JP: Atrial flutter: A synthesis of concepts. Circulation 72:249, 1985

77. Guiney TE, Lown B: Electrical conversion of atrial flutter to atrial fibrillation: Flutter mechanism in man. Br Heart J 34:1215, 1972

78. Waldo AL, MacLean WAH, Karp RB et al: Entrainment and interruption of atrial flutter with atrial pacing: Studies in man following open heart surgery. Circulation 56:737, 1977

79. Treatment of cardiac arrhythmias. Med Lett Drugs Ther 25:21, 1983

80. Sung RJ, Myerburg RJ, Castellanos A: Electrophysiological demonstration of concealed conduction in the human atrium. Circulation 58:940, 1978

81. Anderson RH, Becker AE, Brechenmacker C et al: Ventricular preexcitation: A proposed nomenclature for its substrates. Eur J Cardiol 3:27, 1975

82. Mendez C, Moe GK: Demonstration of a dual AV nodal conduction system in the isolated rabbit heart. Circ Res 19:378, 1966

83. Moe GR, Preston JB, Burlington H: Physiological evidence for a dual AV transmission system. Circ Res 4:357, 1956

84. Sung RJ, Styperek JL, Myerburg RJ et al: Initiation of two distinct forms of atrioventricular nodal reentrant tachycardia during programmed ventricular stimulation in man. Am J Cardiol 42:404, 1978

85. Waxman HL, Myerburg RJ, Appel R et al: Verapamil for control of ventricular rate in paroxysmal supraventricular tachycardia and atrial fibrillation or flutter: A doubleblind randomized cross-over study. Ann Intern Med 94:1, 1981

86. Wolff L, Parkinson J, White PD: Bundle branch block with short PR interval in healthy young people prone to paroxysmal tachyarrhythmia. Am Heart J 5:685, 1930

87. Wellens HJJ: The Wolff-Parkinson-White syndrome. In Mandel WJ (ed): Cardiac Arrhythmias: Their Mechanisms, Diagnosis, and Management, p 342. Philadelphia, JB Lippincott, 1980

88. Gillette PC: Concealed anomalous cardiac conduction pathways: A frequent cause of supraventricular tachycardia. Am J Cardiol 40:848, 1977

89. Narula OS: Sinus node reentry: A mechanism for supraventricular tachycardia. Circulation 50:1114, 1974

90. Sung RJ, Change MS, Chiang BN: Clinical electrophysiology of supraventricular tachycardia. Cardiol Clin 1:225, 1983

91. Shine KI, Kastor J, Yurchak PM: Multifocal atrial tachycardia: Clinical and electrocardiographic features in 32 patients. N Engl J Med 279:344, 1968

92. Iseri LT, Fairshter RD, Hardemann JL et al: Magnesium and potassium therapy in multifocal atrial tachycardia. Am Heart J 110:789, 1985

93. Levine JH, Michael JR, Guarnieri T: Treatment of multifocal atrial tachycardia with verapamil. N Engl J Med 312:21, 1985

94. Wellens HJJ, Duren D, Lie KI: Observations on mechanisms of ventricular tachycardia in man. Circulation 54:237, 1976

95. Josephson ME, Horowitz LN, Farshidi A: Continuous local electrical activity: A mechanism of recurrent ventricular tachycardia. Circulation 57:659, 1978

96. Marcus NH, Falcone RA, Harken AH et al: Body surface late potentials: Effects of endocardial resection in patients with ventricular tachycardia. Circulation 70:632, 1984

97. Wiener I, Mindich B, Pitchon R: Fragmented endocardial electrical activity in patients with ventricular tachycardia: A new guide to surgical therapy. Am Heart J 107:86, 1984

98. Gardner PI, Ursell PK, Fenoglio JJ et al: Electrophysiologic and anatomic basis for fractionated electrograms recorded from healed myocardial infarcts. Circulation 72:596, 1985

99. Kieval RS, Johnson NJ, Rosen MR: Triggered activity as a cause of bigeminy. J Am Coll Cardiol 8:644, 1986

100. Lown B, Temte JV, Arter WJ: Ventricular tachyarrhythmias: Clinical aspects. Circulation 47:1364, 1973

101. Thanavaro S, Kleiger RE, Miller JP et al: Coupling interval and types of ventricular ectopic activity associated with ventricular runs. Am Heart J 106:484, 1983

102. Bleifer SB, Karpman HL, Sheppard JJ et al: Relation between premature ventricular complexes and development of ventricular tachycardia. Am J Cardiol 31:400, 1973

103. Chou TC, Wenzke F: The importance of R on T phenomenon. Am Heart J 96:191, 1978

104. Edwards RP, Miller RD, Roizen MF et al: Cardiac response to imipramine and pancuronium during anesthesia with halothane or enflurane. Anesthesiology 50:421, 1979

105. Stirt JA, Berger JM, Riker SM et al: Arrhythmogenic effects of aminophylline during halothane anesthesia in experimental animals. Anesth Analg 59:410, 1980

106. Johnson RR, Eger EI, Wilson C: A comparative interaction of epinephrine with enflurane, isoflurane, and holothane in man. Anesth Analg 55:709, 1976

107. Zahed B, Miletick DJ, Ivankovich AD et al: Arrhythmic doses of epinephrine and dopamine during halothane, enflurane, methoxyflurane, and fluroxene in goats. Anesth Analg 56:207, 1977

108. Sumikawa K, Ishizaka N, Suzaki M: Arrhythmogenic plasma levels of epinephrine during halothane, enflurane, and pentobarbital anesthesia in the dog. Anesthesiology 58:322, 1983

109. Maze M, Smith CM: Identification of receptor mechanism mediating epinephrine-induced arrhythmias during halothane anesthesia in the dog. Anesthesiology 59:322, 1983

110. Spiss CK, Maxe M, Smith CM: Alpha-adrenergic responsiveness correlates with epinephrine dose for arrhythmias during halothane anesthesia in dogs. Anesth Analg 63:297, 1984

111. Marriott HJL: Aberrant ventricular conduction and the diagnosis of tachycardia. In Marriott HJL (ed): Practical Electrocardiography, p 211. Baltimore, Williams & Wilkins, 1983

112. Marriott HJL: Differential diagnosis of supraventricular and ventricular tachycardia. Geriatrics 25:9, 1970

113. Kistin AD: Problems in the differentiation of ventricular arrhythmia with abnormal QRS. Prog Cardiovasc Dis 8:1, 1966

114. Wellens HJJ, Bar FW, Lie KI: The value of the electrocardiogram in the differential diagnosis of a tachycardia with a widened QRS complex. Am J Med 64:27, 1978

115. Strasberg B, Sclarovsky S, Endberg A et al: Procainamide-induced polymorphous ventricular tachycardia. Am J Cardiol 47:1309, 1981

116. Reynolds EW, Vanderark CR: Quinidine syncope and the delayed repolarization syndromes. Mod Concepts Cardiovasc Dis 45:117, 1976

117. Nicholson WJ, Martin CE, Gracey JG et al: Disopyramide-induced ventricular fibrillation. Am J Cardiol 43:1053, 1979

118. Carruth JE, Silverman ME: Torsade de pointes: Atypical ventricular tachycardia complicating subarachnoid hemorrhage. Chest 78:886, 1980

119. Krikler DM, Curry PVL: Torsade de pointes, an atypical ventricular tachycardia. Br Heart J 38:117, 1976

120. Henry EI: Significance of the relation of QRS and T-waves in bundle branch block: A useful electrocardiographic sign. Am Heart J 54:407, 1957

121. Dhingra RC, Amat-Y-Leon F, Wyndham C et al: Significance of left axis deviation in patients with chronic left bundle branch block. Am J Cardiol 42:551, 1978
122. Rabkin SW, Mathewson FA, Tate RB: Natural history of left bundle branch block. Br Heart J 43:164, 1980
123. Rizzon P, Rossi L, Baissus C et al: Left posterior hemiblock in acute myocardial infarction. Br Heart J 35:711, 1975
124. Rossi L: Histopathology of conducting system in left anterior hemiblock. Br Heart J 38:1304, 1976
125. Marriott HJL: The hemiblocks and trifascicular block. In Marriott HJL (ed): Practical Electrocardiography, p 84. Baltimore, Williams & Wilkins, 1983
126. McAnulty JH, Rahimtoola SH, Murphy E et al: Natural history of "high-risk" bundle-branch block: Final report of a prospective study. N Engl J Med 307:137, 1982
127. Denes P, Dhingra RC, Wu D et al: Sudden death in patients with chronic bifascicular block. Arch Intern Med 137:1005, 1977
128. Schneider JF, Thomas E, Kreger BE et al: Newly acquired right bundle-branch block. Ann Intern Med 92:37, 1980
129. Schneider JF, Thomas E, Kreger BE: Newly acquired left bundle-branch block: The Framingham study. Ann Intern Med 90:303, 1979
130. Pastore JO, Yurchak PM, Janis KM et al: The risk of advanced heart block in surgical patients with right bundle branch block and left axis deviation. Circulation 57:677, 1978
131. Rooney SM, Goldiner PL, Muss E: Relationship of right bundle-branch block and marked left axis deviation to complete heart block during general anesthesia. Anesthesiology 44:64, 1976
132. Zoll PM, Zoll RH, Falk RH et al: External noninvasive temporary cardiac pacing: Clinical trials. Circulation 71:937, 1985
133. Johnson RL: Electrocardiographic findings in 67,375 asymptomatic individuals. VII. A-V block. Am J Cardiol 6:153, 1960
134. Narula OS: Wenckebach type I and type II atrioventricular block (revisited). Cardiovasc Clin 6:138, 1974
135. Marriott HJL: Atrioventricular block: Conventional approach. In Marriott HJL (ed): Practical Electrocardiography, p 322. Baltimore, Williams & Wilkins, 1983
136. Viitasalo MT, Kala R, Eisalo A: Ambulatory electrocardiographic recording in endurance athletes. Br Heart J 47:213, 1982
137. Lown B, Losowsky BD: Artificial cardiac pacemakers. II. N Engl J Med 283:971, 1970
138. Lepeschkin E: The electrocardiographic diagnosis of bilateral bundle branch block in relation to heart block. Prog Cardiovasc Dis 6:445, 1964
139. Steiner C, Lau SH, Stein E et al: Electrophysiological documentation of trifascicular block as the common cause of complete heart block. Am J Cardiol 28:436, 1971
140. Rosenbaum MB, Elizari MV, Kretz A et al: Anatomical basis of A-V conduction disturbances. Geriatrics 25:132, 1970
141. Lev M: Anatomic basis for atrioventricular block. Am J Med 37:742, 1964
142. Lenegre J: Etiology and pathology of bilateral bundle branch block in relation to complete heart block. Prog Cardiovasc Dis 6:409, 1964
143. Roberts WC, Cardin JM: Locations of myocardial infarcts: A confusion of terms and definitions. Am J Cardiol 42:868, 1978
144. Yu PNG, Stewart JM: Subendocardial myocardial infarction with special reference to the electrocardiographic change. Am Heart J 39:862, 1950
145. Evans W, McRae C: The lesser electrocardiographic signs of cardiac pain. Br Heart J 14:429, 1952
146. Gerson MC, Phillips JF, Morris SN et al: Exercise-induced U wave inversion as a marker of stenosis of the left anterior descending coronary artery. Circulation 60:1014, 1979
147. Mann RH, Burchell HB: The sign of T wave inversion in sinus beats following ventricular extrasystoles. Am Heart J 47:504, 1954
148. Marriott HJL: Myocardial infarction. In Marriott HJL (ed): Practical Electrocardiography, p 373. Baltimore, Williams & Wilkins, 1983
149. Liu CK: Atrial infarction of the heart. Circulation 23:331, 1961
150. Kurita A, Chaitman BR, Bourassa MG: Significance of exercise-induced junction S-T depression in evaluation of coronary artery disease. Am J Cardiol 40:492, 1977
151. Rijneke RD, Ascoop CA, Talmon JL: Clinical significance of upsloping ST segments in exercise electrocardiography. Circulation 61:671, 1980
152. Stuart RJ, Ellestad MH: Upsloping S-T segments in exercise stress testing. Am J Cardiol 37:19, 1976
153. Yasui H: Comparison of coronary arteriography findings during angina pectoris associated with ST elevation or depression. Am J Cardiol 47:539, 1981
154. Stiles GL, Rosati RA, Wallace AG: Clinical relevance of exercise-induced ST segment elevation. Am J Cardiol 46:931, 1980
155. Sriwattanakomen S, Ticzon AR, Zubritsky SA et al: ST segment elevation during exercise: Electrocardiographic and arteriographic correlation in 38 patients. Am J Cardiol 45:762, 1980
156. Specchia G, deServi S, Falcone C et al: Coronary arterial spasm as a cause of exercise-induced ST segment elevation in patients with variant angina. Circulation 59:948, 1979
157. Specchia G, deServi S, Falcone C et al: Significance of exercise-induced ST segment elevation in patients without myocardial infarction. Circulation 63:46, 1981
158. Mirowski M, Mower MM, Staewen WS et al: Standby automatic defibrillator: An approach to prevention of sudden coronary death. Arch Intern Med 126:158, 1970
159. Mirowski M, Reid PR, Mower MM et al: Termination of malignant ventricular arrhythmias with an implanted automatic defibrillator in human beings. N Engl J Med 303:322, 1980
160. Livelli FD Jr, Bigger JT Jr, Reiffel JA et al: Response to programmed ventricular stimulation: Sensitivity, specificity and relation to heart disease. Am J Cardiol 50:452, 1982
161. Reid PR, Mirowski M, Mower MM et al: Clinical evaluation of the internal automatic cardioverter-defibrillator in survivors of sudden cardiac death. Am J Cardiol 51:1608, 1983
162. Reid PR, Griffith SC, Mower MM et al: Implantable cardioverter-defibrillator: Patient selection and implantation protocol. PACE 7 (Part II):1331, 1984
163. Bruce MA, Spodick DH: Atypical electrocardiogram in acute pericarditis: Characteristics and prevalence. J Electrocardiol 13:61, 1980
164. Spodick DH: Electrocardiogram in acute pericarditis. Distributions of morphologic and axial changes by stages. Am J Cardiol 33:470, 1974
165. Bashour FA, Cochran PW: The association of electrical alternans with pericardial effusion. Dis Chest 44:146, 1963
166. McGregor M, Baskind E: Electrical alternans in pericardial effusion. Circulation 11:837, 1955
167. Nizet PM, Marriott HJL: The electrocardiogram and pericardial effusion. JAMA 198:169, 1966
168. Hersh C: Electrocardiographic changes in subarachnoid hemorrhage, meningitis, and intracranial space occupying lesions. Br Heart J 26:785, 1964
169. Surawicz B: Electrocardiographic pattern of cerebrovascular accident. JAMA 197:913, 1966
170. Gould L, Reddy RC, Kollali M et al: Electrocardiographic normalization after cerebral vascular accident. J Electrocardiol 14:191, 1981
171. Emslie-Smith D: The significance of changes in the electrocardiogram in hypothermia. Br Heart J 21:343, 1959
172. Myers GB: Correlation of electrocardiographic and pathologic function in large anterolateral infarcts. Am Heart J 36:838, 1948
173. Myers GB: Correlation of electrocardiographic and pathologic findings in anteroseptal infarction. Am Heart J 36:535, 1948
174. Myers GB. Correlation of electrocardiographic and pathologic findings in posterolateral infarction. Am Heart J 38:837, 1949
175. Erhardt LR, Sjögren A, Wahlberg I: Single right-sided precordial lead in the diagnosis of right ventricular involvement in myocardial infarction. Am Heart J 91:571, 1976
176. Croft CH, Nicod P, Corbett JR et al: Detection of acute right ventricular infarction by right precordial electrocardiography. Am J Cardiol 50:421, 1982

V

MANAGEMENT OF ANESTHESIA

30

Benjamin G. Covino*
Donald H. Lambert

Epidural and Spinal Anesthesia

The introduction of regional anesthesia into clinical practice is attributed to Carl Koller,[1] a young Viennese ophthalmologist, who employed cocaine in 1884 for topical anesthesia of the cornea in patients scheduled for eye surgery. In 1885, Corning[2] accidentally performed the first spinal anesthetic while performing experiments on the action of cocaine on the spinal nerves of dogs. Corning coined the term spinal anesthesia in 1888. In 1898, Sicard described the toxic effects of subarachnoid cocaine.[3] August Bier is considered the father of spinal anesthesia. In 1899, he reported that he and his assistant had performed spinal anesthesia on each other and then employed this technique to provide anesthesia for surgical procedures.[4] In 1899, Tait and Caglieri[5] performed the first spinal anesthesia for surgery in the United States. However, Matas[6] provided the first description of spinal anesthesia in the United States.

Cathelin,[7] in France, is believed to have performed the first caudal epidural anesthetic in surgical patients in 1901. In 1921, Pages[8] described the lumbar approach to the epidural space for surgical patients. However, Dogliotti[9] is usually given credit for describing a more practical approach to the lumbar epidural space and for popularizing the use of segmental epidural analgesia for surgery. Epidural and spinal anesthesia continue to be two of the most popular regional anesthetic procedures employed for surgery, obstetrics, and postoperative analgesia. Today, spinal anesthesia is probably the most widely employed regional anesthetic technique for surgical patients. The introduction of continuous epidural techniques has helped to popularize the use of this procedure, particularly for analgesia during labor and for postoperative analgesia.

*Shortly after the completion of this chapter, the anesthesia community was shocked and saddened to learn of the untimely death of Dr. Benjamin G. Covino. Ben Covino's career was synonymous with revelations concerning local anesthesia and the application of regional anesthesia. We shall all miss this kindhearted and authoritative mentor.—D.H.L.

RATIONALE FOR THE USE OF EPIDURAL AND SPINAL ANESTHESIA

Anesthesia can clearly influence the physiologic state of patients during the intraoperative and postoperative periods. In some patients, regional anesthesia may be preferable to general anesthesia for certain surgical procedures in which either form of anesthesia may be employed. Prospective studies have elucidated the influence of various anesthetic techniques on the endocrine-metabolic responses to surgery, perioperative blood loss, frequency of thromboembolic complications, cardiopulmonary complications, postoperative recovery phase, and morbidity and mortality.[10]

Metabolic and Endocrine Alterations

Regional anesthesia itself appears to have little influence on endocrine function and metabolic activity. A decrease in plasma epinephrine and norepinephrine levels has been reported following epidural and spinal anesthesia that extends to the upper thoracic dermatomes.[11]

With regard to metabolic products, epidural anesthesia extending to the midthoracic level does not produce any significant changes in blood glucose, lactate, alanine, free fatty acids, glycerol, or ketones.[12,13] Spinal anesthesia extending to the upper thoracic dermatomal levels inhibits the release of insulin, which usually occurs in response to hyperglycemia.[12]

Surgical stimulation results in an increase in plasma concentrations of cortisol, aldosterone, renin, vasopressin, growth hormone, epinephrine, norepinephrine, glucose, and lactate. Most of these surgically induced endocrine and metabolic changes can be inhibited by adequate afferent blockade (Tables 30-1 and 30-2).

Epidural anesthesia can block the increase in plasma prolactin, growth hormone, adrenocorticotropic hormone, and

TABLE 30-1. Effect of Epidural Anesthesia on Surgically Induced Endocrine Functions

Endocrine Parameters	Surgery	Epidural Blockade
Pituitary Hormones		
Prolactin	Increase	Inhibit
Growth hormone	Increase	Inhibit
ACTH	Increase	Inhibit
ADH	Increase	Inhibit
Adrenal and Renal Hormones		
Cortisol	Increase	Inhibit
Aldosterone	Increase	Inhibit
Renin	Increase	Inhibit
Epinephrine	Increase	Inhibit
Norepinephrine	Increase	Inhibit
Pancreatic Hormones		
Insulin	No effect	Decrease
Glucagon	No effect	No effect
Thyroid Hormones		
Thyroxine	No effect	No effect
Triiodothyronine	Decrease	No effect

ACTH = adrenocorticotropic hormone; ADH = antidiuretic hormone.

antidiuretic hormone associated with surgery. Epidural anesthesia also inhibits the surgically induced increase in plasma cortisol, aldosterone, renin, epinephrine, and norepinephrine.[14] The extent of the epidural blockade and the site of surgery influence the degree of inhibition of these various hormones.

A decrease in plasma insulin levels has been observed following surgery performed under epidural anesthesia, whereas there was little or no change in plasma glucagon.[12,15] Glucose tolerance is much less affected by surgery if epidural rather than general anesthesia is employed.[16] Epidural anesthesia does not appear to exert a significant influence on changes in plasma thyroxine or plasma triiodothyronine levels during surgery.[17]

Increases in plasma glucose, lactate, and 3-hydroxybutyrate, which usually occur following the start of surgery, can be effectively inhibited by epidural anesthesia.[13,15] Surgical

TABLE 30-2. Effect of Epidural Anesthesia on Surgically Induced Changes in Metabolic Functions

Metabolic Parameters	Surgery	Epidural Blockade
Glucose	Increase	Inhibit
Lactate	Increase	Inhibit
3-Hydroxybutyrate	Increase	Inhibit
Glycerol	Increase	Inhibit
Free fatty acids	Increase	Inhibit
Alanine	Decrease	No effect
Cyclic adenosine monophosphate	Increase	Inhibit

procedures involving the lower abdomen performed under epidural anesthesia are associated with decreased levels of plasma glycerol and free fatty acids.[13] Upper abdominal surgical procedures or analgesia extending to only the lower thoracic dermatomes has not been associated with similar changes in free fatty acids.[18]

The ability of epidural or spinal anesthesia to inhibit the release of pituitary hormones is probably attributable to the blockade of afferent nociceptive pathways. On the other hand, the inhibition of the release of adrenal cortical hormones, such as cortisol, may result from an inhibition of efferent pathways or, more likely, from the inhibition of the release of adrenocorticotropic hormone from the pituitary gland during afferent blockade. Inhibition of the release of catecholamines from the adrenal medulla is probably related to the blockade of efferent autonomic pathways. Similarly, the decrease in the release of insulin from the pancreas is probably owing to the blockade of efferent sympathetic fibers to the pancreas.

The inability of epidural and spinal anesthesia to block the endocrine-metabolic stress response for upper abdominal surgical procedures may be due to a failure to block afferent pathways conducted through the vagus nerve. However, vagus nerve blockade by local infiltration failed to inhibit the increase in cortisol blood levels observed during surgery in the upper abdominal area carried out under epidural anesthesia. The stress associated with an upper abdominal surgical procedure may be sufficiently great that it is difficult for an epidurally or intrathecally administered local anesthetic to inhibit completely all nociceptive afferent pathways.

Blood Loss

A number of studies have evaluated intraoperative blood loss during various surgical procedures performed under either general or regional anesthesia. The average intraoperative blood loss was 22–50% lower during total hip replacements performed under epidural or spinal anesthesia compared with similar procedures performed under general anesthesia.[19,20] Blood loss was reduced by 37% during retropubic prostatectomy and 18% during transurethral prostatectomy performed under regional anesthesia compared with general anesthesia.[22] Spinal anesthesia has been associated with a reduction in intraoperative blood loss of 45% during abdominal hysterectomies.[23] However, other studies involving abdominal surgery failed to demonstrate any difference in blood loss between general and regional anesthesia.[24,25]

The diminished bleeding during regional anesthesia may be related to the hypotension caused by the sympathetic block. Hypotensive anesthesia with halothane and nitroprusside also results in a similar reduction in intraoperative blood loss during hip replacement. Some studies have shown that the decreased blood loss during epidural blockade was not associated with a significant reduction in blood pressure. It has been postulated that epidural or spinal anesthesia may lead to a redistribution of blood flow away from the operative site, resulting in a reduced blood loss.[21]

Thromboembolic Complications

Thromboembolic complications have been reported to be reduced 50–60% when hip surgery is performed under lumbar epidural anesthesia.[20,21,26] A similar reduction was observed during prostatectomy.[22] Epidural anesthesia did not significantly reduce thromboembolic complications following abdominal surgical procedures.[25,27]

The mechanism responsible for the reduction in thromboembolism is probably an increased blood flow to the lower extremities following sympathetic blockade by regional anesthesia. An additional factor may be an increase in fibrinolytic activity during regional anesthesia.[28,29]

Cardiopulmonary Complications

Continuous epidural analgesia for postoperative pain relief may ameliorate the usual postoperative deterioration of pulmonary function. A comparison of intramuscular morphine, continuous intravenous morphine, or continuous epidural bupivacaine for postoperative pain relief following cholecystectomy revealed that patients given epidural analgesia had better analgesia than patients receiving morphine, had significantly higher arterial oxygen tensions during the first 3 postoperative days, and had a lower incidence of pulmonary complications and chest infections.[30] In a review of multiple studies in which regional or general anesthesia had been employed for various surgical procedures, 25 of 198 patients (13%) who received regional anesthesia developed postoperative pulmonary complications in contrast to 43 of 203 patients (21%) in the general anesthesia group.[14] This suggests that regional anesthesia may alter the rate of postoperative pulmonary complications.

The cardiovascular effects of general or regional anesthesia in healthy patients do not differ markedly. Both general anesthesia and epidural or spinal anesthesia may cause a decrease in blood pressure. The hypotension related to general anesthesia is usually due to a decrease in cardiac output, whereas spinal or epidural blockade decreases systemic vascular resistance secondary to sympathetic blockade. However, a comparison of neuroleptic anesthesia and epidural anesthesia combined with light general anesthesia in patients with a recent history of myocardial infarction scheduled for major abdominal surgery revealed significant differences in the two groups with regard to various hemodynamic parameters.[31] A mean pulmonary artery occlusion pressure of greater than 18 mm Hg was observed in 75% of the neuroleptic anesthesia patients compared with in 17% of the epidural group. A decrease in coronary vascular resistance of greater than 25% occurred in 57% of the neuroleptic anesthesia patients compared with 13% of the epidural patients. All the neuroleptic anesthesia patients demonstrated an increase in myocardial oxygen consumption of more than 25% compared with only one patient in the epidural group with such an increase. Fifty percent of the neuroleptic anesthesia patients showed ST-T segment depression of greater than 1 mm compared with 13% in the epidural group. Finally, ventricular arrhythmias developed intraoperatively in 36% of the neuroleptic anesthesia patients, whereas only 8% of the epidural patients showed signs of ventricular arrhythmias. No difference in the frequency of perioperative myocardial infarction or 1-month postoperative mortality existed between the two groups. Two patients in the neuroleptic anesthesia group and one patient in the epidural group suffered an intraoperative myocardial infarction. In addition, three patients in the neuroleptic anesthesia group developed a myocardial infarction during the first postoperative week. Two patients in the neuroleptic anesthesia group and one patient in the epidural group died within the first postoperative month. The results of this study suggest that patients with diagnosed cardiac disease who undergo major noncardiac surgery may develop more serious alterations in coronary hemodynamics and may be at greater risk in terms of myocardial ischemia and ventricular arrhythmias when a general anesthetic, rather than a regional anesthetic technique, is employed.

Additional data have been forthcoming suggesting that epidural anesthesia may actually be beneficial in patients with coronary artery disease, presumably because of the blockade of sympathetic innervation of the heart. For example, lumbar or thoracic epidural anesthesia with 0.5% bupivacaine resulted in a decrease in left ventricular loading and improvement in global and regional ventricular functions in patients with coronary artery disease.[32,33] It was also suggested that volume loading should be limited prior to the induction of epidural anesthesia in such patients.[32] In addition, thoracic epidural anesthesia was reported to increase the diameter of stenotic coronary artery segments without a dilation of coronary arterioles, leading to a reduction in ischemic chest pain in patients at rest.[34]

Morbidity and Mortality

Little difference in perioperative mortality exists between various anesthetic techniques in relatively healthy patients scheduled for elective surgery. In elderly patients admitted for emergency repair of hip fractures, contradictory results have been reported.[35,36] A lower mortality within the 1-month postoperative period was observed in several studies in patients in whom spinal anesthesia had been employed compared with those in whom general anesthesia had been used. However, no difference in the number of deaths during a 1–2 year postoperative period was observed in patients in whom an emergency repair of a hip fracture was carried out under either spinal or general anesthesia.[36,37] Therefore, emergency surgery performed under spinal anesthesia in elderly patients who presumably have a certain degree of cardiac disease may be associated with a lower morbidity and mortality, but only during the immediate, i.e., 1–2 weeks, postoperative period. Epidural anesthesia and postoperative epidural analgesia may improve the outcome in high-risk patients in whom major surgical procedures are performed.[38] When compared with a control group of patients in whom general anesthesia and parenteral opiates for postoperative analgesia were employed, patients who received epidural anesthesia and analgesia had a significant reduction in the overall postoperative complications rate, incidence of cardiovascular failure, and major infectious complications. In summary, data exist that suggest that regional anesthesia may be beneficial in high-risk surgical patients.

ANATOMY

Bony Structures

The spinal canal extends from the foramen magnum to the sacral hiatus. The bony arches of the vertebra posterior to the vertebral bodies form a continuum that makes up the spinal canal (Fig. 30-1). The spaces between the vertebrae are occupied by the spinal ligaments. The vertebral column consists of seven cervical, 12 thoracic, and five lumbar vertebrae. The sacrum and coccyx are caudad extensions of the vertebral column. The shape and size of the vertebrae differ in the cervical, thoracic, and lumbar areas (Fig. 30-2). The

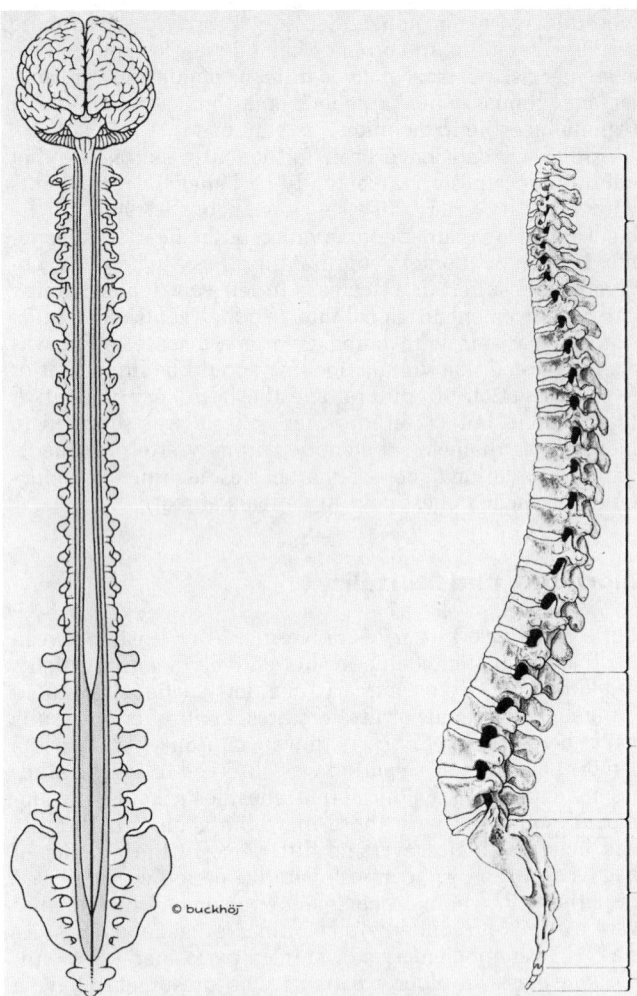

Figure 30-1. (*Left*) The spinal canal runs from the foramen magnum to the sacral hiatus. (*Right*) The vertebral column is composed of 7 cervical, 12 thoracic, and 5 lumbar vertebrae, with the sacrum and coccyx inferiorly. The vertebrae vary in size and shape according to their position and function. (Reproduced with permission from Covino BG, Scott DB: Handbook of Epidural Anaesthesia and Analgesia, p 10. Orlando, Grune & Stratton, 1985.)

vertebrae increase in size from the cervical to the lumbar areas, which is related to the function of the vertebrae in the various locations. Cervical vertebrae are smallest and have the least weight-bearing function. The lumbar vertebrae are largest in size and support the greatest amount of weight.

The vertebrae consist of a vertebral body behind which is a bony arch. The arch consists of two pedicles anteriorly and two laminae posteriorly. The transverse processes are formed by the junction of the pedicles and laminae, whereas the spinal process is formed from the union of opposing laminae.

The spinal processes vary in their angulation in the cervical, thoracic, and lumbar regions. The degree of angulation influences the direction of a needle to be placed in the epidural or subarachnoid space. In the cervical, lower thoracic, and lumbar regions, the spinal processes are almost horizontal, and the needle may be directed at right angles to the sagittal plane. However, in the midthoracic region, the

spinal processes have a marked caudad angulation that is maximal between the T3 and T7 vertebrae. Thus, an epidural or spinal needle must be inserted at varying degrees from the horizontal plane in order to enter the epidural or subarachnoid space. The sacrum is formed by the fusion of the five sacral vertebrae, and the coccyx is attached to the caudad end of the sacrum.

Ligaments

The vertebrae are joined together posteriorly by a series of short ligaments. The laminae of the vertebrae are connected by the ligamentum flavum, whereas the posterior spinous processes are connected by the interspinous ligaments. The supraspinous ligaments run superficial to the tips of the spinal processes. The vertebral bodies are separated anteriorly by the intervertebral disks, and the anterior longitudinal ligament runs from the base of the skull to the sacrum, with an attachment to the disks and the adjacent margins of the vertebral bodies. The posterior longitudinal ligament connects the posterior surface of the vertebral bodies and forms the anterior wall of the vertebral canal. The interverte-

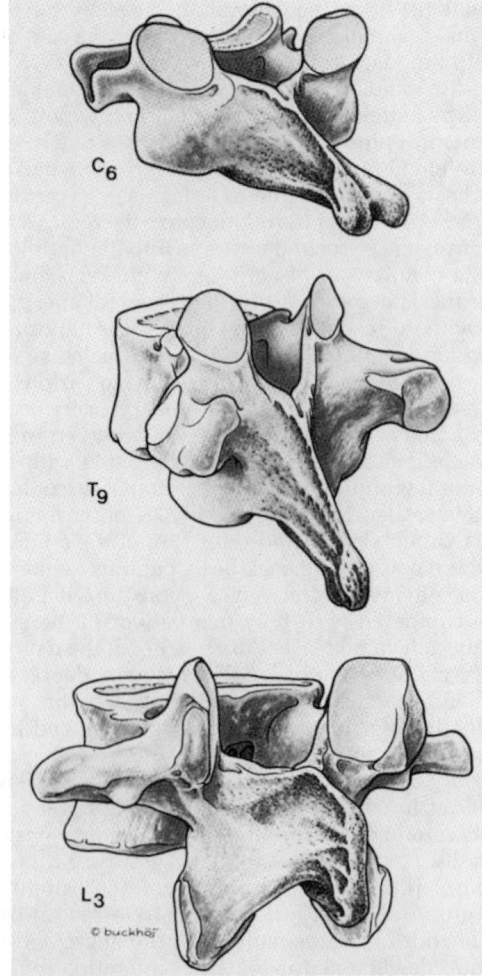

Figure 30-2. Oblique views of a cervical, a thoracic, and a lumbar vertebra. (Reproduced with permission from Covino BG, Scott DB: Handbook of Epidural Anaesthesia and Analgesia, p 11. Orlando, Grune & Stratton, 1985.)

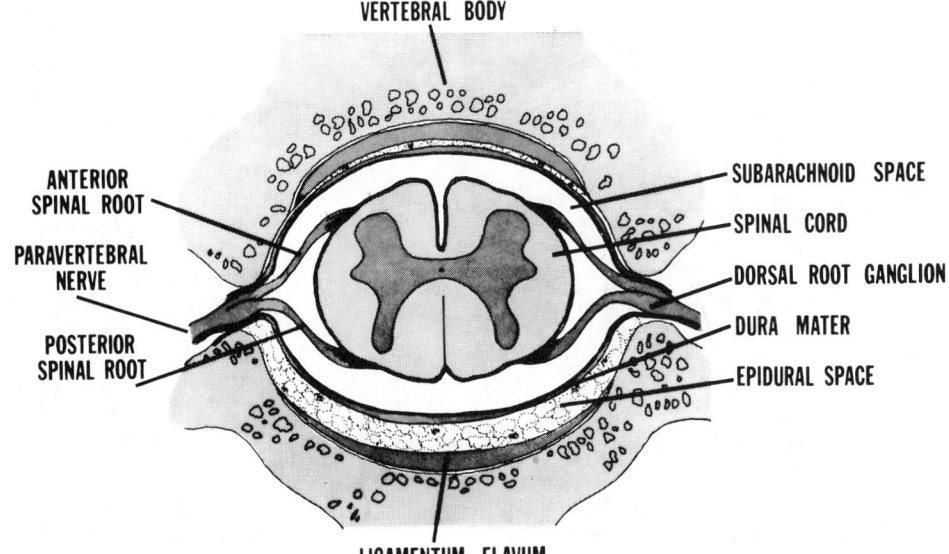

Figure 30-3. Cross-sectional diagram of the vertebral column and spinal cord. (Reproduced with permission from Covino BG, Vassallo HG: Local Anesthetics: Mechanism of Action and Clinical Use, p 76. New York, Grune & Stratton, 1976.)

bral foramina exist as openings between the vertebral pedicles through which the spinal nerves pass.

Epidural Space

The spinal canal contains the spinal cord and its coverings, the pia mater, arachnoid mater, and dura mater. The epidural space (Fig. 30-3) is located between the dura mater and the connective tissue covering the vertebrae and the ligamentum flavum. The epidural space has been described as a potential space, since normally it is completely filled with a loose type of connective tissue, fatty tissue, and blood vessels. It is particularly rich in venous plexuses. No free fluid exists in the epidural space. However, solutions injected into the epidural space spread in all directions among the loose tissue structures that occupy this area.

The subdural space is the area between the arachnoid mater and the dura mater. It is also a potential space, since it contains lymph. The pia mater is closely attached to the spinal cord and the spinal nerves. The area between the arachnoid mater and the pia mater is the subarachnoid space, which contains cerebrospinal fluid (Fig. 30-3).

The space within the spinal canal is primarily occupied by the spinal cord that extends from the foramen magnum to the first or second lumbar vertebra. The spinal cord has a longitudinal cylindric shape that is somewhat flattened anteroposteriorly, particularly in the lumbar region. The cord is characterized by cervical and lumbar enlargements. Below the lumbar area, the cord tapers into the conus medullaris, from which the filum terminale continues down to attach to the coccyx.

The anterior and posterior (dorsal) spinal nerve roots exit from the spinal cord and then join to form the spinal nerves at each intervertebral space. The spinal nerves leave the spinal canal via the intervertebral foramina (Fig. 30-3). The dorsal root ganglia are located on the dorsal spinal roots just prior to the junction at which the ventral and dorsal roots unite. In the cervical and thoracic regions, the spinal nerves immediately leave the spinal canal by way of intervertebral foramina shortly after their formation. However, because the spinal cord ends at the level of L1–2, the lower lumbar and sacral nerve roots extend for some distance within the spinal canal as the cauda equina before leaving the spinal canal to enter the sacral epidural space (Fig. 30-4).

As the spinal nerves leave the spinal canal through the intervertebral foramina, they divide into anterior and posterior primary rami. The posterior rami supply the skin and muscles of the back, whereas the anterior rami supply the rest of the body. Each spinal segment supplies a specific region of the skin and a specific number of muscles. In the cervical, brachial, and lumbosacral regions, the anterior rami join to form the various nerve plexuses. The cutaneous distribution of the spinal nerves is shown in Figure 30-5.

Autonomic Nervous System

Sympathetic and parasympathetic nerves are important considerations in epidural and spinal anesthesia, since blockade of these nerves can lead to profound physiologic changes. The preganglionic nerves of the sympathetic nervous system originate in nerve cells in the lateral column of the gray matter of the spinal cord. These preganglionic fibers pass from the spinal cord through the spinal nerves from the T1 to the L2 level. After the spinal nerves exit through the intervertebral foramina, the preganglionic sympathetic nerve fibers leave the spinal nerves to become part of the white rami communicantes, which run to the sympathetic chain. The preganglionic fibers then run up or down the sympathetic chain to synapse within specific sympathetic ganglia. The sympathetic chain extends the length of the spinal column along the anterolateral aspect of the vertebral bodies. In the cervical region, the sympathetic ganglia make up the superior cervical, middle cervical, and stellate ganglia. In the thoracic region, the sympathetic chain gives rise to the splanchnic nerves, which pass through the diaphragm and terminate in the celiac plexus. In the abdominal area, these nerves connect with the celiac, aortic, and hypogastric plexuses. The sympathetic chain ends in the pelvis on the anterior surface of the sacrum.

Postganglionic sympathetic nerves originate in the various ganglia and are widely distributed to various organs. Postganglionic sympathetic nerves play an important role in controlling cardiac function, vascular tone, gastrointestinal tone, and motility.

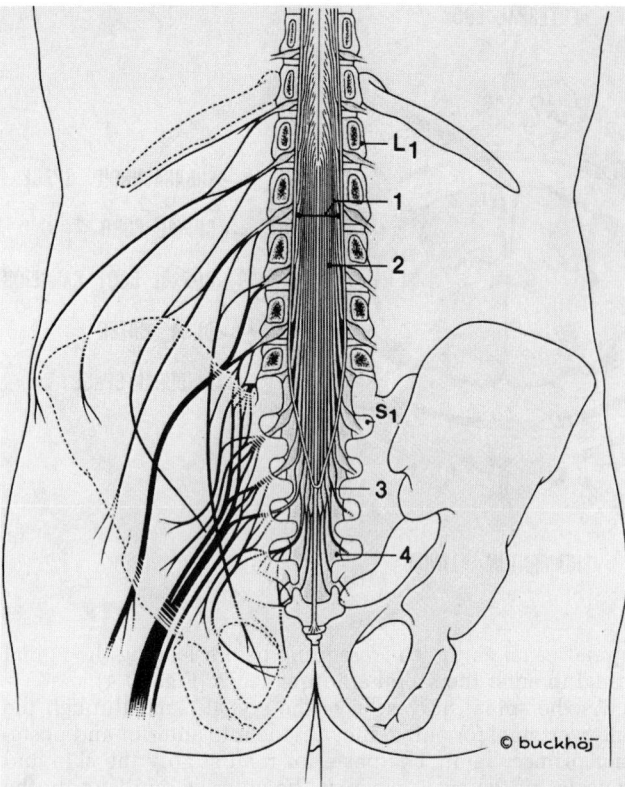

Figure 30-4. Schematic diagram of the cauda equina and the formation of the lumbosacral plexus. (1) Cauda equina. (2) Subarachnoid space. (3) Dorsal root ganglion. (4) Sacral epidural space. (Reproduced with permission from Covino BG, Scott DB: Handbook of Epidural Anaesthesia and Analgesia, p 24. Orlando, Grune & Stratton, 1985.)

Preganglionic parasympathetic nerve fibers are contained within the cranial nerves, or in the second, third, or fourth sacral nerves. The preganglionic parasympathetic fibers extend to the various organs that they innervate and synapse within the walls of these organs with the short postganglionic parasympathetic fibers. The parasympathetic nervous system is also of importance in terms of regulating cardiovascular and gastrointestinal function.

Blood Supply of the Spinal Canal

The anterior spinal artery and posterior spinal arteries and their branches supply blood to the spinal cord, spinal roots, and meninges (Fig. 30-6). The anterior spinal artery is formed by the union of two branches of the terminal portion of the vertebral artery at the level of the foramen magnum. The anterior spinal artery then descends along the median sulcus on the anterior surface of the cord to the conus medullaris and then terminates as an arteriole on the filum terminale. The anterior spinal artery supplies the anterior two thirds of the spinal cord. Two posterior spinal arteries are located on each side of the posterior surface of the cord. They arise from the posterior inferior cerebellar arteries and descend on the dorsal surface of the cord medial to the dorsal nerve roots. The posterior spinal arteries supply the posterior one third of the spinal cord.

Branches of the vertebral, deep cervical, intercostal, and lumbar arteries enter the vertebral canal through the intervertebral foramina. These spinal branches divide into anterior and posterior radicular arteries that travel along the nerve roots to reach the cord, where they anastomose with the anterior and posterior spinal arteries. One of the radicular arteries is considerably larger than the rest and represents the major blood supply to the lower two thirds of the cord. This particular branch is known as the arteria radicularis magna, or the artery of Adamkiewicz. It is located in the lower thoracic or upper lumbar area and is more common on the left side.

Blood from the contents of the spinal canal drains into a tortuous venous plexus in the pia mater, which contain six longitudinal veins. These connect with the internal vertebral plexus in the epidural space, from which blood flows by way of the intervertebral veins into the azygos and hemiazygos systems.

PATIENT EVALUATION AND PREPARATION FOR EPIDURAL AND SPINAL ANESTHESIA

The preanesthetic evaluation and examination of patients scheduled for epidural or spinal anesthesia should be no less vigorous than for patients scheduled for general anesthesia. The anesthesiologist should explain to patients the reasons for suggesting an epidural or spinal anesthetic technique and the potential advantages of these techniques. Patients should be made aware of what they might hear or see in an operating room if the decision is made to have them remain awake during a surgical procedure. Although a complete medical history should be obtained on any patient scheduled for surgery, a careful evaluation of the patient's cardiovascular and neurologic status should be made if epidural or spinal anesthesia is selected. A presurgical physical examination should have been performed by the surgical staff and reviewed by the anesthesiologist. The patient's drug history should be taken, since many agents that affect the cardiovascular system, such as adrenergic blocking agents or antihypertensive agents, may influence the patient's physiologic response to epidural or spinal blockade.

Physical examination of the patient's back should be made to determine the appropriate site of entry of the epidural or spinal needle. Any spinal deformities or excessive calcification that may make epidural or spinal anesthesia difficult, or, in fact, impossible should be noted. Any history of back problems or trauma to the spinal canal should be elicited from the patient, which again may determine the feasibility of performing a central neural block in a particular patient.

Laboratory data required preoperatively for patients scheduled for epidural or spinal anesthesia are similar to those required for general anesthetic patients. However, particular attention should be paid to the coagulation profile to determine the possibility of any coagulation defects and any laboratory data that might be indicative of abnormal bleeding tendency. Coagulation profiles and, possibly, bleeding times should be obtained on any patient who has been on anticoagulants preoperatively, even if the anticoagulants have been discontinued prior to surgery. Similar studies should be available on patients who have been taking medications that are known to influence platelet adhesiveness and that may result in prolonged bleeding times.

The technique of epidural or spinal anesthesia should be described to the patient. The advantages relative to general anesthesia and the possible complications of epidural or spinal anesthesia intraoperatively and postoperatively

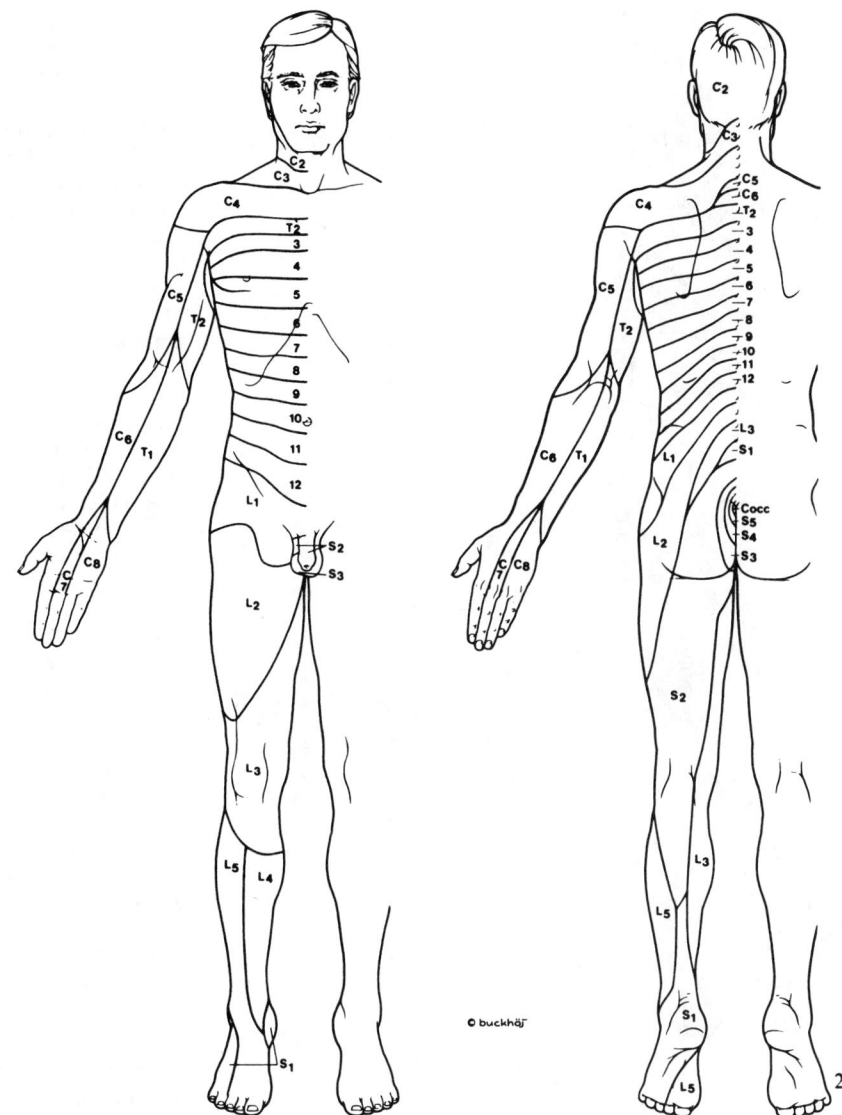

Figure 30-5. Cutaneous distribution of the spinal nerves. (Reproduced with permission from Covino BG, Scott DB: Handbook of Epidural Anaesthesia and Analgesia, p 25. Orlando, Grune & Stratton, 1985.)

should also be explained. Patient concerns regarding remaining in an awake state intraoperatively should not be an automatic contraindication to the use of an epidural or spinal anesthetic technique. Various forms of sedation may be employed intraoperatively. The use of earphones for listening to music or other forms of entertainment can provide a distraction for patients during the procedure. Alternatively, general anesthetic agents in sufficiently low concentrations to allow patients to sleep but not be fully anesthetized may also be utilized. If a combined general and regional anesthetic technique is suggested for a particular patient, the primary anesthetic procedure is the epidural or spinal, and the general anesthetic should be merely sufficient to allow a state of somnolence rather than a state of full general anesthesia. Patients in whom a combined general and regional anesthetic procedure is anticipated may or may not require intubation of the trachea. The choice of intubation of the trachea will depend on the ability to maintain a patent airway with a mask and the position of the patient intraoperatively.

Preoperative medication for patients scheduled for epi-

dural or spinal anesthesia is dependent on the level of anxiety of the patient, the ability of the anesthesiologist to allay fear and anxiety, and the ability of the patient to tolerate some pain associated with insertion of the epidural or spinal needle. Anticholinergic agents are probably not indicated in patients scheduled for regional anesthesia.

INDICATIONS AND CONTRAINDICATIONS FOR EPIDURAL AND SPINAL ANESTHESIA

Table 30-3 includes a list of those surgical procedures that can be performed under epidural or spinal anesthesia. Surgical procedures in the upper abdomen have been performed under high spinal anesthesia, but today, lumbar or thoracic epidural techniques are usually employed. There are relatively few absolute contraindications to epidural and spinal anesthesia. These include localized infection at the puncture site, patients who refuse regional anesthesia, severe uncorrected hypovolemia, uncorrected coagulation defects, or pathologic situations resulting in excessive bleed-

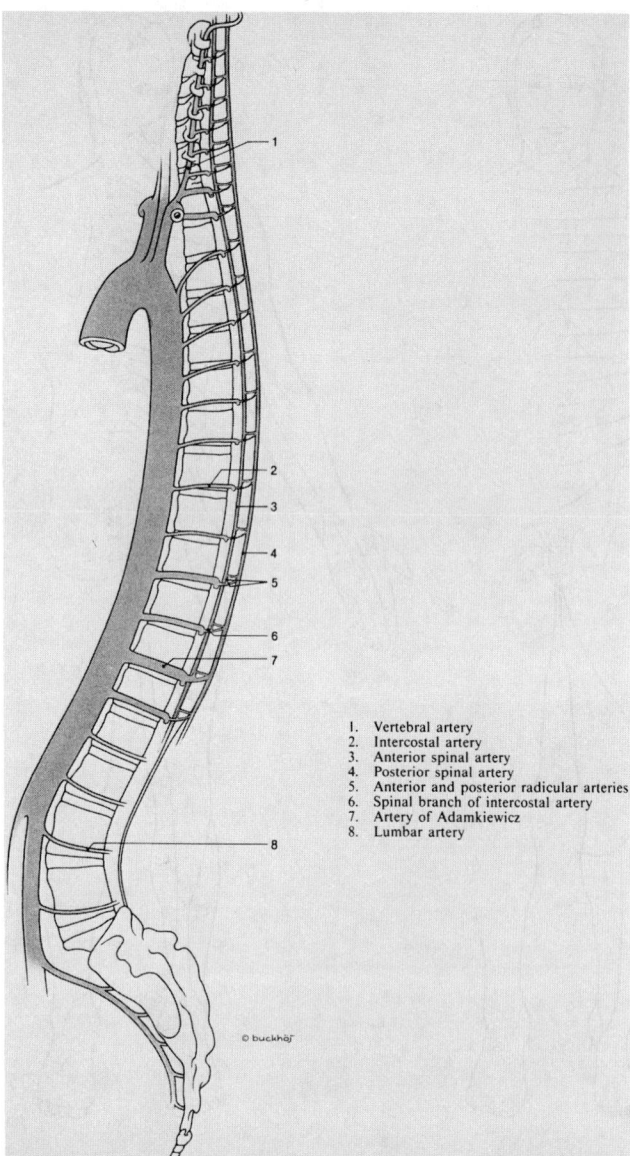

1. Vertebral artery
2. Intercostal artery
3. Anterior spinal artery
4. Posterior spinal artery
5. Anterior and posterior radicular arteries
6. Spinal branch of intercostal artery
7. Artery of Adamkiewicz
8. Lumbar artery

© buckhoj

Figure 30-6. Blood supply of the spinal cord. Radicular arteries, which run in the anterior and posterior nerve roots to the cord, are derived from the vertebral artery in the neck, the intercostal arteries in the thorax, and the lumbar arteries in the abdomen. The artery of Adamkiewicz is the main supply of the lower two thirds of the cord. (Reproduced with permission from Covino BG, Scott DB: Handbook of Epidural Anaesthesia and Analgesia, p 21. Orlando, Grune & Stratton, 1985.)

ing times and anatomic abnormalities that make epidural or spinal techniques difficult or impossible. Relative contraindications include generalized infection, such as bacteremia, neurologic disorders such as multiple sclerosis, and minidose heparin therapy. In these cases, the benefits of employing epidural or spinal anesthesia may sometimes outweigh the risks.

TECHNICAL ASPECTS

The most important landmarks for performance of a lumbar epidural or spinal block are the vertebral spinal processes and the iliac crests (Fig. 30-7). The spinous processes clearly

define the midline. A line drawn between the iliac crests crosses the fourth lumbar vertebra. Thus, the interspace above this line represents the L3–4 interspace, and the space below the line is the L4–5 interspace. These spaces are usually chosen for insertion of the epidural or spinal needle, since the spinal cord ends at the L1–2 level. For thoracic epidural blocks, a line passing between the inferior angle of the scapulae crosses the seventh thoracic vertebra. The T7–8 interspace is usually the site of needle entry for a midthoracic epidural block.

Epidural Blockade

The epidural space is most easily entered in the lumbar region, since the spinous processes are not angulated in relation to the vertebral body, and the space between adjacent laminae, covered by the ligamentum flavum, is wide. The patient should be positioned with the lumbar spine in maximal flexion so that the intervertebral spaces are maximally opened. This can be done in the lateral or the sitting position. In the lateral position, the patient's knees are flexed as high as possible in front of the abdomen, and the head is bent onto the chest. In the sitting position, the patient's body should be flexed with the elbows resting on the knees or on a table, and the head bent with the chin on the chest.

Numerous prepackaged and sterile kits are available for epidural blocks. A 17- or 18-gauge Tuohy needle is most commonly employed. The curved Huber point is designed to decrease the possibility of accidental dural puncture and facilitate the passage of a plastic catheter into the epidural space. Various types of epidural needles are available, such as the Crawford needle, which has a short blunt bevel, and the Weiss needle, with wings attached to the needle hub. The latter is particularly useful if a hanging drop technique is employed.

TABLE 30-3. Surgical Procedures Often Performed Under Spinal or Epidural Anesthesia

1. Any intra-abdominal procedure
2. Gynecologic procedures
     Hysterectomy
     Cone biopsy
     D & C
     Ovarian cystectomy
3. Obstetric procedures
     Cesarean section
     Circlage
     Vaginal delivery
4. Herniorraphies
5. Lower limb procedures
     Orthopedic
     Vascular
     Amputations
6. Urologic procedures
     Transurethral resections
     Cystoscopy
     Open prostatectomies
     Penile implant
     Orchiectomy
7. Perineal and rectal surgery
     Bartholin's cyst
     Rectal fissures
     Hemorrhoids
8. Others

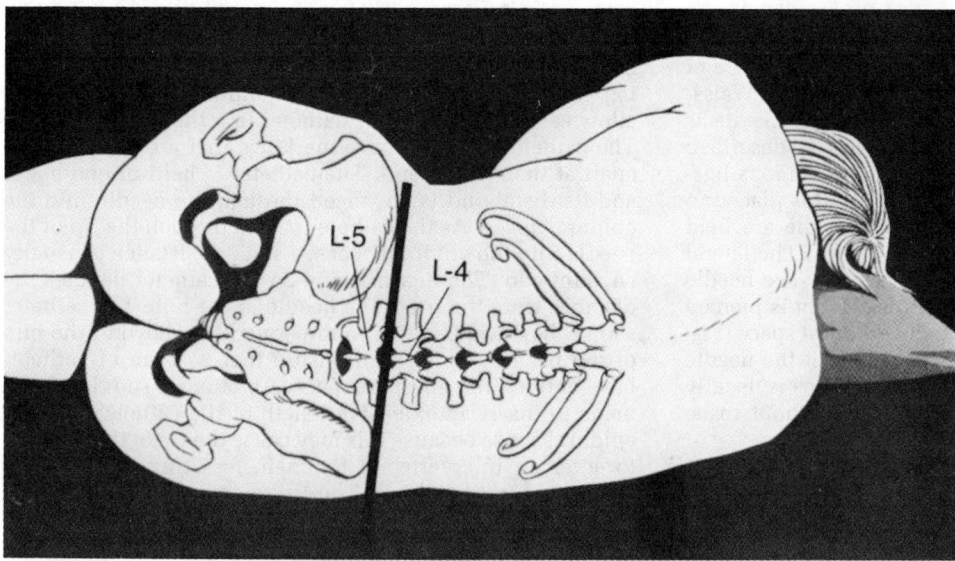

Figure 30-7. Patient position for epidural and/or spinal anesthesia. Anatomic landmarks are illustrated.

Epidural blocks should only be attempted in a location where complete anesthetic equipment is readily available, including an anesthetic machine and resuscitative equipment and drugs. An intravenous infusion should be initiated prior to the performance of an epidural block. In addition, blood pressure, heart rate, and an electrocardiogram should be recorded prior to and during the epidural procedure.

Epidural anesthesia must be performed utilizing an aseptic technique. The patient's back should be sterilized with an antiseptic solution. The decision to employ sterile drapes is at the discretion of the anesthesiologist, but it is useful to ensure a sterile field. The anesthesiologist should wear a mask and sterile surgical gloves.

The iliac crest is observed or palpated, and the L3–4 interspace identified. The L2–3 and L4–5 spaces should also be identified, and the space that appears to offer the easiest access to the epidural space is chosen for needle insertion (see Fig. 30-7). An intradermal wheal is raised with a local anesthetic over the chosen interspace. Subcutaneous infiltration may also be employed to decrease the pain associated with insertion of the epidural needle and to identify the appropriate direction for the epidural needle. A 16- or 18-gauge needle is used to perforate the skin in order to facilitate penetration with the epidural needle. The skin should be held firmly over the spinous process above the chosen interspace with the index and middle finger of one hand while the epidural needle is inserted in the middle of the chosen interspace at right angles to the skin with the opposite hand.

The most common method to identify the epidural space is the loss of resistance technique. There are many variations of this technique. Usually, a syringe containing saline or air is attached to the needle lying in the interspinous ligament (Fig. 30-8). If the needle is properly positioned, it will be difficult to inject at this point. At this time, the direction of the tip of the needle should be slightly cephalad.

The dorsum of the noninjecting hand is placed on the patient's back, and the thumb and index or middle finger are used to grasp the hub of the needle. This hand is used to advance the needle. The opposite hand is placed on the

plunger of the syringe, and gentle but continuous pressure is applied. Resistance to advancement of the plunger is noted as the needle is advanced toward the ligamentum flavum. As the needle passes through the ligamentum flavum and enters the epidural space, a sudden loss of resistance occurs. The saline or air can be injected with ease into

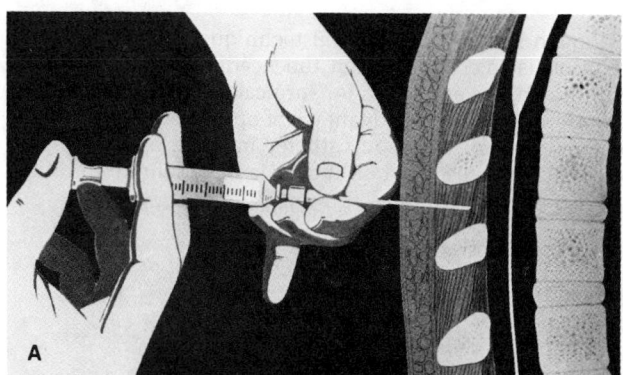

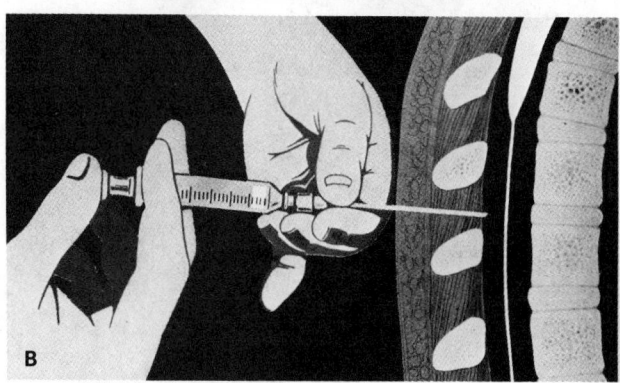

Figure 30-8. Correct hand positions for the loss of resistance method of identifying the epidural space. The needle should be advanced slowly and firmly (A), until loss of resistance is encountered, signifying entry of the needle into the epidural space (B).

the epidural space. The advancement of the needle should cease once the epidural space has been identified.

The hanging drop technique is based on the presence of negative pressure in the epidural space. A winged, Weiss-type epidural needle is usually employed. The needle is inserted percutaneously in the same fashion as described above. Once the needle is engaged in the interspinous ligament, the stylet is removed and a drop of fluid is placed in the hub of the needle. The wings of the needle are held with the thumb and index finger of both hands. The lateral surface of the hands rest on the patient's back. The needle is slowly advanced until the ligamentum flavum is pierced and the hanging drop is sucked into the epidural space (Fig. 30-9). At this point, no further advancement of the needle should occur. Identification of the epidural space is usually confirmed by the injection of saline or air without resistance.

A midline approach is most commonly employed for insertion of the epidural needle. However, for thoracic epidural anesthesia in the midthoracic region, where the spinous processes are markedly angulated, or in patients who cannot flex their spines adequately, or where there is excessive vertebral calcification, a paramedian or lateral approach to the epidural space may prove useful. The needle is inserted 1.0–1.5 cm lateral to the midline on a level with the upper border of the spinous process below the selected interspace. Following cutaneous penetration, the needle is directed in a cephalad and mediad direction in order to perforate the ligamentum flavum and enter the epidural space in the midline. Identification of the epidural space is accomplished by a loss of resistance or by the hanging drop technique.

Catheter Placement

Although single-shot epidural techniques (local anesthetic solution is injected through the needle and the needle is withdrawn) are employed for surgical procedures of limited duration, the primary advantage of epidural blockade is the ability to insert a plastic catheter into the epidural space and provide anesthesia or analgesia of indefinite duration.

A variety of commercial epidural catheters are available. Some have a single terminal opening, whereas others may have several lateral holes with or without a terminal opening. Most but not all catheters are supplied with a stylet to allow easier passage of the catheter into the epidural space. The catheters usually have markings that are spaced 1 cm apart at their distal end. The catheter is held in one hand, and its distal end is advanced through the needle into the epidural space. As the catheter passes through the tip of the needle into the epidural space, a slight resistance is usually encountered. The first marking on the catheter denotes the distance from the tip of the needle to the hub. The catheter should be advanced two to three markings beyond the hub of the needle, which will ensure that 2–3 cm of catheter have entered the epidural space. An attempt should not be made to insert an extensive length of the catheter into the epidural space because this may cause the tip of the catheter to enter an intervertebral foramen, resulting in an inadequate epidural blockade. The tip of the epidural needle is usually directed in a cephalad or caudad direction in the hope of advancing the catheter in a cephalad or caudad direction. However, radiologic studies indicate that the direction of the needle tip does not guarantee the direction of the catheter in the epidural space.

Once the catheter has been inserted into the epidural space, the needle is slowly withdrawn. The needle should be withdrawn over the catheter with one hand while the other hand applies gentle inward pressure on the catheter to ensure that it is not withdrawn with the needle (Fig. 30-10). No attempt should ever be made to withdraw a catheter back through the needle, since this may result in shearing of a portion of the catheter in the epidural space.

Once the needle and stylet have been withdrawn, the catheter is taped to the patient's back, usually with a loop formed as the catheter exits from the back to prevent kinking of the catheter. The catheter is taped to the patient's back from the point of cutaneous exit up to the shoulder, so that injections can be made at the head of the table. A syringe adapter is fastened to the proximal end of the catheter, to which a syringe may then be attached. A bacterial filter may also be employed between the catheter and the syringe.

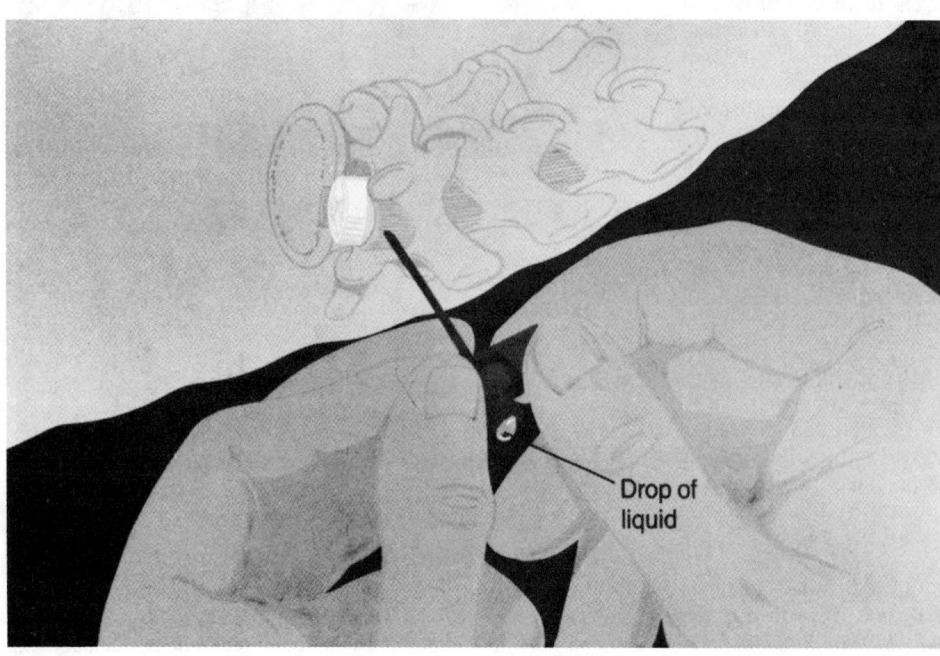

Drop of liquid

Figure 30-9. Correct hand position for using the hanging drop method of locating the epidural space. The needle should be moved slowly until the drop is sucked into the needle, signifying entry of the needle tip into the epidural space.

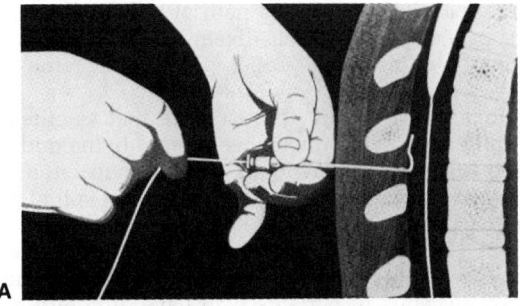

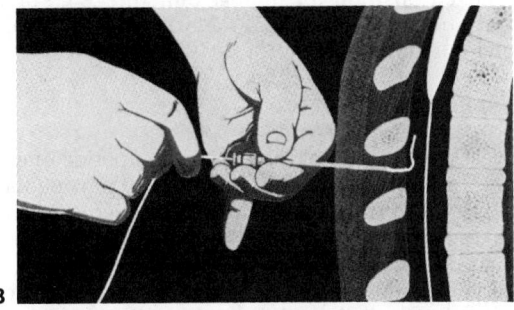

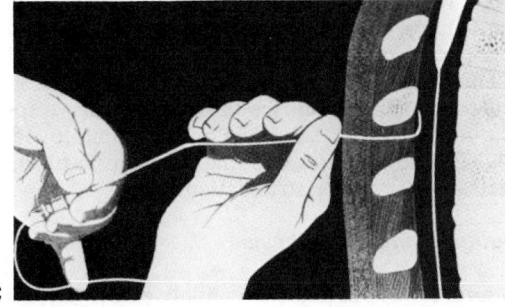

Figure 30-10. Removing the needle following insertion of the catheter. With one hand holding the catheter, the other hand should pull the needle (*A*) until both hands meet (*B*). When the needle is free, it should be removed by holding the catheter and gently easing the needle off with the other hand (*C*).

Test Dose

A local anesthetic test dose is recommended to detect an accidental intravascular or subarachnoid placement of the needle or catheter. Three to four milliliters of a local anesthetic solution with epinephrine, e.g., 3–4 ml of 1.5% lidocaine with 1:200,000 epinephrine, should be used as a test dose. Heart rate and blood pressure should be monitored. An intravascular injection is usually detected by the increase in heart rate and blood pressure that occurs following the intravascular injection of epinephrine. Failure to elicit an increase in heart rate or blood pressure is often but not always indicative of a nonintravascular injection. For example, patients on chronic beta-adrenergic receptor blockers do not demonstrate an increase in heart rate following the intravenous injection of epinephrine.[39]

Following the administration of the test dose, sensory and motor function in the lower limbs should be assessed in order to detect the possibility of an accidental subarachnoid injection. If any signs of an intravascular injection are noted, no further injections should be made, the epidural needle or catheter should be withdrawn, and the entire placement

procedure should be reinstituted at another interspace. If signs of an intrathecal injection are observed, spinal anesthesia may be considered as an alternative to epidural anesthesia.

Because of the relatively rapid absorption of drugs from the epidural space and the relatively high doses required for epidural blockade, the main portion of injectate should be given slowly and, preferably, in a fractionated dose regimen. In the latter instance, volumes of 3–5 ml of anesthetic solution are administered intermittently at 3- to 4-minute intervals. The patient should be continually evaluated for signs of an accidental intravascular or intrathecal injection. The total dose of drug administered depends on the physical status of the patient and the location of the surgical procedure. The dermatomal analgesic level can be evaluated by pin-prick or use of an alcohol swab at approximately 1-minute intervals during and following the intermittent injection of the anesthetic solution.

Spinal Anesthesia

Spinal anesthesia is usually induced with the patient in the lateral decubitus or the sitting position. The lateral decubitus position has the advantage that it is more comfortable for the patient and the patient is not as likely to experience a faint. The disadvantage is that it is often difficult to communicate the posture that the anesthesiologist would like the patient to assume. Furthermore, it is easy for patients to make their backs lordotic at the precise moment when an arched-out back is more desirable. Last, if the patient is obese, it is more difficult to locate the midline with the patient in the lateral decubitus position.

The advantage of the sitting position is that the proper curvature of the back for lumbar puncture is easier to obtain. The correct posture is easily communicated to the patient by asking him or her to merely lean forward. Another advantage is that it is more difficult for the patient to move away from the needle when in this position. The sitting position is also helpful for patients with certain injuries. For example, it is often less painful for patients with hip fractures to achieve a sitting position than to lie on either side. The major disadvantage to this position is the increased incidence of fainting. Preparation of the patient's back for spinal anesthesia is the same as previously described for epidural anesthesia.

Midline Approach

The L4–5 interspace is the site most commonly used for spinal anesthesia. The spinal cord ends at the L1–2 interspace in adults (it ends at L2 in small children). However, even at this level, the spinal cord has tapered, becoming the filum terminale, and the possibility of damaging the cord with the spinal needle is remote. Therefore, lumbar puncture performed at L2 and below is virtually free of risk of injuring the spinal cord itself. Nerve injury involving the cauda equina is, on the other hand, possible, although extremely rare, since these structures are free to move away from the advancing needle.

The anesthesiologist should choose the interspace below L2, which appears to afford the easiest access to the subarachnoid space. A skin wheal is raised with local anesthetic in the midline of the chosen interspace. The spinal needle, with the bevel parallel to the dural fibers, is inserted through the skin wheal in the midline and parallel to the spinous processes. Some prefer a two-handed method of advancing the needle. However, advancement of the needle with thumb and index finger of one hand while identifying the appropriate space with the fingers of the opposite hand appears to afford greater opportunity for successful lumbar puncture. The needle is angled slightly cephalad and is advanced slowly and gently until it lodges in the supraspinous ligament. Once lodged in the supraspinous ligament, the direction that the tip of the needle will take is "fixed by the ligament" and is no longer under the control of the anesthesiologist. Any attempts to guide or change the direction of the needle tip by bending its shaft will not be successful. The needle is slowly advanced without bending it through the ligaments toward the dura. A "firming up" is often noticed as the needle enters the ligamentum flavum and a distinct "pop or click" is heard as it leaves this ligament and enters the dura. If cerebrospinal fluid is not obtained, or if blood, paresthesia, or bone is encountered, the needle is withdrawn to the subcutaneous tissue and redirected, and the process of advancing the needle is repeated. If, after one or two attempts, cerebrospinal fluid is not obtained, it is best to move to another interspace. Usually, unless there is some anatomic problem, lumbar puncture is successful after one or two attempts. Time should not be wasted at an interspace where problems are encountered.

Some anesthesiologists prefer to use an introducer to guide the spinal needle in the proper direction. If an introducer needle is used, it is inserted in the center of the skin wheal and directed along the intended path of the spinal needle, stopping short of the ligamentum flavum. The spinal needle is then inserted via the introducer through the ligamentum flavum and the dura and into the subarachnoid space. If resistance is encountered, the introducer and the needle are withdrawn to the subcutaneous plane and redirected.

The incidence of postdural puncture headache is related to needle gauge and patient age.[40,41] A 25- or 26-gauge needle should be employed in young patients. However, 22-gauge needles may be used in elderly patients. Skill with lumbar puncture can be improved by using larger (22-gauge) needles in patients 60 years of age and older. These larger needles facilitate lumbar puncture and help to build confidence with the technique without increasing the incidence of postlumbar puncture headache in this age group. Once the spinal needle has entered the subarachnoid space and flow has been achieved, it is not necessary to rotate it. The volar surface of the nondominant hand is placed on the patient's back, and the hub of the needle is grasped between the thumb and index finger. The syringe containing the spinal anesthetic solution is securely attached to the needle, a small amount of cerebrospinal fluid is gently aspirated to verify that the needle has not been dislodged, and the spinal anesthetic solution is injected. Once the solution has been injected, the needle is removed and the patient is positioned for surgery.

Paramedian or Lateral Approach

This technique is performed at a distance of 1.5–2.0 cm lateral to the midline opposite the center of the selected interspace. The needle is directed medially at an angle of approximately 25 degrees with the midline and at right angles to the vertebral column. If bone is encountered, the needle is withdrawn slightly and then readvanced in a slightly cephalad or caudad direction. Often, the needle can be "walked" off the bone into the ligamentum flavum and, thence, into the subarachnoid space. Minimal resistance is encountered as the needle is advanced until the ligamentum

flavum is reached because the path of the needle is lateral to the supra- and interspinous ligaments. Free flow of cerebrospinal fluid indicates proper placement of the spinal needle.

The advantages of this approach are that calcified ligaments and osteophytes, often encountered in the midline in the aged patient, are avoided. Furthermore, the opening between the vertebrae through which the spinal needle passes en route to the cerebrospinal fluid is larger when approached from this direction as compared with the midline approach. This is especially true and may be particularly advantageous in patients who have difficulty assuming the flexed position for lumbar puncture, e.g., pregnant patients, patients with rheumatoid arthritis, and patients in the prone position.

Taylor Approach

The lowest prominence of the posterior superior iliac spine is located, and a skin wheal is raised 1.0 cm medial and 1.0 cm caudad to this point. The spinal needle is directed through the skin wheal, medially and cephalad, in such a manner as to enter the spinal canal in the midline at the lumbosacral (L5–S1) interspace. As with the lateral or paramedian approach, if the needle contacts the bony sacrum, it may be "walked off" into the lumbosacral foramen.

The advantages of this technique are the same as for the lateral or paramedian approach. In addition, the Taylor approach employs the largest interspace in the vertebral column and, therefore, should be the easiest place to perform lumbar puncture. This technique has been employed to ensure low segmental levels of spinal anesthesia for urologic and rectal surgery in geriatric patients.

Continuous Spinal Anesthesia

This technique, which had been widely employed, declined in popularity because of the increased use of continuous epidural anesthesia and the high incidence of postdural puncture headache. In recent years various microcatheters have become available for continuous spinal anesthesia. A 32-gauge catheter is available that can pass through a 26-gauge needle, whereas 27- and 28-gauge catheters have been introduced for use with 22-gauge needles.[42] The technique of continuous spinal anesthesia is quite simple. The subarachnoid space is located with a 22- or 26-gauge needle in the fashion described above. The 27-, 28-, or 32-gauge catheter is then threaded 2–3 cm beyond the tip of the needle. The needle is withdrawn and the catheter taped to the patient's back. Occasionally, the catheter fails to thread easily most likely because of encountering a nerve root or the posterior dural boundary of the subarachnoid space.[42] The 32-gauge catheter has a stylet embedded in its wall and requires careful lateral support at the needle hub during advancement to avoid kinking.

MECHANISM OF SPINAL AND EPIDURAL ANESTHESIA

Spinal Blockade

Nerve fibers are classified on the basis of size and degree of myelination. Size and degree of myelination, in turn, determine the conduction velocity. Fiber size is also related to function and sensitivity to local anesthetics. Table 30-4

TABLE 30-4. Classification of Nerve Fibers on the Basis of Fiber Size, Relating Size to Fiber Function and Sensitivity to Local Anesthetics

Fiber Group	Diameter (µm)	Conduction Velocity (m · s⁻¹)	Modality Subserved	Sensitivity to Local Anesthetics (Subarachnoid Procaine-%)
A (Myelinated)				
Alpha	20	100	Large motor Proprioception	1
Beta	↑	↑	Small motor Touch Pressure	1
Gamma	↓	↓	Muscle Spindle	1
Delta	4	5	Temperature Sharp pain	0.5
B (Myelinated)	3	3–14	Preganglionic Autonomic	0.25
C (Unmyelinated)	0.5–1	1.2	Dull pain Temperature Touch	0.5

Reproduced with permission from Winnie AP: Differential diagnosis of pain mechanisms. In Hershey SG (ed): ASA Refresher Courses in Anesthesiology 6:171, 1978. Copyright 1978, The American Society of Anesthesiologists.

shows the sensitivity of the various fiber types to the subarachnoid injection of procaine and the classic concept relating local anesthetic blockade to fiber size, as described by Gasser and Erlanger in 1929.[43]

Recent studies in isolated nerves have suggested that the classic concept may be incorrect.[44] These studies have shown that the large myelinated fibers are more sensitive to local anesthetic blockade than the smaller unmyelinated fibers. However, *in vivo* diffusion of local anesthetics to the membrane receptor site and interaction with those receptors are both involved in determining the apparent sensitivity of the various nerve fibers to local anesthetic blockade. Thus, in spinal anesthesia, the anatomy of the dorsal roots brings small-diameter nerve fibers close to the nerve root surface, thereby shortening the diffusion path of a drug instilled into the spinal subarachnoid space. The diffusion path to the large-diameter fibers, which are situated deep to the nerve bundle, is longer. This makes it appear that the small-diameter fibers are more susceptible to drug action than the large-diameter fibers.

The amount of local anesthetic employed during spinal anesthesia represents an overdose in relation to the minimum concentration required to block the various nerve fiber types. Furthermore, the distribution of the local anesthetic in the spinal subarachnoid space results in a relatively rapid blockade of all fiber types during clinical spinal anesthesia.

Spinal anesthesia is induced with the express purpose of interrupting the nociceptive A delta and C fiber afferents (dorsal roots) that subserve the pain modality. At the same time, the proprioceptive and sympathetic afferent fibers (dorsal root) and motor and sympathetic (both ventral root) nerve fibers are also blocked. Blockade of motor and proprioceptive fibers is also desirable because it improves the surgical operative conditions and patient comfort. Nociceptive viscerosensory afferent sympathetic fiber impulses trav-

eling *via* the sympathetic trunk must also be interrupted for the patient to remain comfortable during the surgical procedure. Since these fibers enter the spinal cord *via* the dorsal root, they are blocked along with the other fibers in this structure.

Epidural Blockade

The dorsal and the ventral spinal roots appear to be the primary sites of action of epidurally administered local anesthetic agents because of the unique anatomy of the membranous structures around the spinal roots. In this area, the dura mater is relatively thin and arachnoid granulations are believed to be present; these granulations increase the surface area available for diffusion of anesthetic agents from the epidural space into the subarachnoid space.[45] Local anesthetics administered epidurally are concentrated in spinal roots to a greater extent than in either the dorsal root ganglion or the spinal cord itself.[46] Additional evidence favoring the spinal roots as the initial site of action of epidurally administered local anesthetics is obtained from clinical studies evaluating the onset pattern of epidural blockade. A significant delay in onset of anesthesia at the S1 and S2 dermatomal levels is usually observed following the epidural administration of various local anesthetics.[47] In some cases, little or no anesthesia is present at the S1 and S2 levels, although adequate anesthesia is obtained above and below those dermatomes. This delay of or failure to achieve anesthesia in the S1–2 region is believed to be related to the large size of the nerve roots in this area. The increased fiber size of the nerve roots, which is owing to a greater density of connective tissue, impedes the rate of diffusion of local anesthetic agents to the nerve membrane receptor sites. The spinal cord may also represent a site of action of epidurally injected local anesthetic drugs. Tissue distribution studies following the epidural administration of labeled local anesthetics have shown that these agents can cross the dura and penetrate the spinal cord. However, the concentration of local anesthetics in the spinal cord following epidural administration was less than that found in the spinal roots.[46] During the recovery phase from epidural blockade, analgesia regresses from the highest to the lower dermatomes in a caudad direction, similar to the regression observed following subarachnoid blockade. This suggests that spinal cord blockade does occur following epidural administration of local anesthetic agents, but the initial onset of anesthesia is probably related to inhibition of conduction in spinal roots.

PHYSIOLOGIC EFFECTS OF SPINAL AND EPIDURAL BLOCKADE

Spinal Blockade

Spinal anesthesia profoundly affects the cardiovascular system and, to a lesser degree, the pulmonary, hepatic, renal, and endocrine systems. Sympathetic nerve fiber blockade is unavoidable during spinal anesthesia. The preganglionic sympathetic nerve fibers originate in the lateral horn of the spinal cord and exit via the ventral roots. Because of the distribution of local anesthetic solution during the conduct of spinal anesthesia, these fibers are blocked along with the other fibers in the ventral roots.

The degree of sympathetic efferent denervation is often unpredictable and may be quite extensive during spinal anesthesia. Since the sympathetic B fibers are among the smallest in the body, it is generally assumed that the level of sympathetic blockade during spinal anesthesia exceeds the level of sensory anesthesia because the B fibers are more sensitive to the action of local anesthetics. Gissen et al[44] have shown that B fibers are blocked at intermediate concentrations and that C fibers are the most resistant to block. As mentioned above, the sympathetic fibers may be blocked to a greater extent than somatic sensory fibers because they are more peripherally located in the nerve roots.

An alternative explanation lies in the anatomy of the distribution of the sympathetic nerve fibers. Sympathetic preganglionic fibers leaving the spinal cord travel up or down segments before entering the sympathetic ganglia. Therefore, sensory blockade, for example, to the fourth thoracic dermatome, may be associated with interruption of sympathetic activity as high as the first thoracic level. It has, in general, been assumed that sympathetic blockade exceeds somatic blockade by two dermatomes.[48] However, Chamberlain and Chamberlain,[49] utilizing thermographic measurements of skin temperature during lidocaine or tetracaine spinal anesthesia, have recently shown that skin temperature increases (assumed to represent sympathetic blockade) occurred as much as six dermatomal levels higher than the somatic sensory block. These findings may explain the profound hypotension sometimes associated with relatively low sensory levels of spinal anesthesia.

The Cardiovascular System

Numerous studies have been conducted on the cardiovascular effects of spinal anesthesia. For example, Ward et al reported that a level of spinal anesthesia to T5 resulted in an increase in pulse rate of 3.7%.[50] Generally, spinal anes-

thesia is associated with a slowing of the pulse rate, depending on the level of block, premedication, the patient's age, and the patient's position. Bradycardia is caused by blockade of the cardioaccelerator fibers and diminished venous return. The cardioaccelerator fibers arise from the T1–4 dermatomes. Levels of spinal anesthesia that include these dermatomes not only inhibit the cardiac accelerator nerves but also result in total preganglionic sympathetic blockade that produces venodilation and decreased venous return. The decreased venous return activates great vein and right atrial cardiac receptors that reflexly slow the heart.[51]

Ward et al also showed a decrease in mean arterial blood pressure of 21.3%, whereas the decline in total peripheral resistance was only 5.0%. The hypotension seen with spinal anesthesia is clearly the result of a decrease in cardiac output (17.7%). The decline in cardiac output results from venodilation and decreased stroke volume (25.4%). It should be appreciated that all of these cardiovascular effects associated with spinal anesthesia are the direct result of preganglionic sympathetic blockade by the local anesthetic.

The Respiratory System

Many studies have shown that even high levels of spinal anesthesia have little, if any, effect on resting ventilatory mechanics.[52] Furthermore, it has also been shown that blood gas tensions are only slightly affected under these conditions.[53] On the other hand, intercostal muscle paralysis resulting from high levels of spinal anesthesia does interfere with the ability to cough and clear secretions.[54]

The Renal System

The preganglionic sympathetic innervation of the kidney arises from the T11–L1 dermatomes. Despite levels of spinal anesthesia above these dermatomes, autoregulation maintains renal blood flow as long as the mean arterial blood pressure remains higher than 80 mm Hg. Spinal anesthesia resulting in hypotension, sufficient to cause renal hypoperfusion, is accompanied by transient decreases in glomerular filtration and urinary output. Restoration of the blood pressure results in recovery of renal function.[55]

The Gastrointestinal System

The effect of spinal anesthesia on hepatic blood flow and function is minimal. Hepatic blood flow is diminished in direct proportion to any reduction in arterial blood pressure. There are no major changes in hepatic function following spinal anesthesia, even in situations in which there are dramatic decreases in blood pressure, such as when deliberate hypotension has been produced to minimize surgical blood loss.[56,57]

The innervation of the bowel is both sympathetic and parasympathetic. The parasympathetic innervation arises from the vagus nerve and the hypogastric nerves (S2–4). The sympathetic innervation comes from the T5–L1 dermatomes. Spinal anesthesia is capable of blocking all the sympathetic fibers innervating the bowel and the hypogastric nerves. The vagus nerve, of course, remains unblocked. The result of spinal anesthesia to the T5 dermatome is to contract the intestines, increase peristalsis and secretion, and relax sphincters. The contracted state of the bowel during spinal anesthesia may improve the surgical field.

The etiology of nausea during spinal anesthesia is poorly understood. Possible causes include the unopposed vagal activity, increased peristalsis, hypotension, cerebral hypoxia, and adjuvant medications used for sedation. If nausea is persistent, the operative conditions obviously will be poor. The combination of nausea and a high spinal blockade may increase the risk of aspiration because the ability to clear secretions and protect the larynx is diminished with high spinal anesthesia.[54]

Epidural Blockade

Administration of local anesthetics in sufficient dosage into the epidural space inhibits conduction of sensory, motor, and autonomic fibers. The small unmyelinated sensory fibers are usually affected initially following epidural injection because of the lack of diffusion barriers. The larger, heavily myelinated motor fibers of the A type are usually much more resistant to blockade because of the thick myelin sheath surrounding them, which serves as a barrier to the diffusion of local anesthetics. The rate of blockade of preganglionic autonomic B fibers varies according to the dosage of local anesthetic and the specific drug administered into the epidural space. Sympathetic blockade sufficient to cause systemic hypotension rarely occurs before sensory anesthesia is well established. Thus, sensory analgesia is usually the first indication of successful epidural blockade.

Hemodynamic Effects

Interruption of sympathetic impulses can lead to cardiovascular alterations following the establishment of epidural anesthesia. In most patients, cardiovascular changes are not very marked. On the other hand, profound hypotension may be observed in some patients following the onset of epidural anesthesia. The changes in blood pressure, heart rate, and cardiac output are related to the level of blockade, the amount of drug administered, the specific local anesthetic employed, the inclusion of a vasoconstrictor in the anesthetic solution, and the cardiovascular status of the patient (Fig. 30-11).

The dermatomal level of sympathetic blockade determines the degree of hypotension following the epidural administration of local anesthetics. Blocks below T5 are seldom associated with marked hypotension because of compensatory vasoconstriction in unblocked segments. Higher blocks not only prevent compensatory vasoconstriction but also affect the cardiac sympathetic nerves that arise in the T1–4 segments. At these dermatomal levels of block, a fall in heart rate and cardiac output may occur. The blockade of sympathetic fibers to the heart and the failure to block the vagus nerves can cause vasovagal attacks, which are associated with profound bradycardia and, in some patients, with transient cardiac arrest. This may represent the most common cause of profound hypotension following high levels of epidural anesthesia. The venous capacitance vessels are also affected by the sympathetic blockade. Pooling can occur if the venous return is obstructed by gravity or a pregnant uterus. Thus, patients are very susceptible to the head-up posture, which causes expansion of the capacitance vessels and can lead to a marked decrease in venous return and cardiac output.

Relatively large amounts of local anesthetic drugs are required to achieve a satisfactory degree of epidural blockade. The local anesthetic agents are absorbed rather rapidly and may produce systemic effects involving the cardiovascular

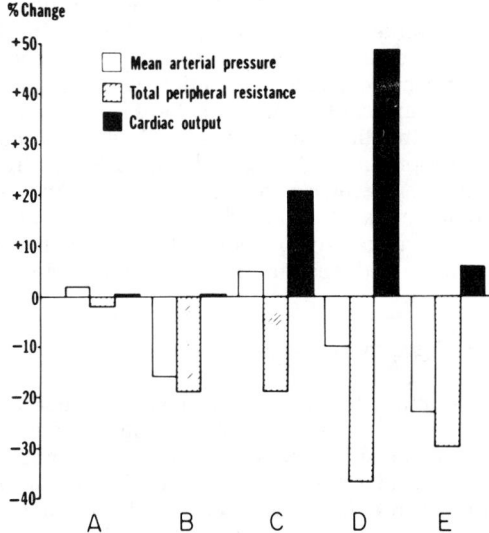

Figure 30-11. Cardiovascular effects of epidural anesthesia as influenced by analgesic dermatomal level, epinephrine, and presence of hypovolemia. The sensory level of anesthesia was T5 at A, D, and E; T1 at B; and T2–3 at C. Epinephrine was present at D and E. Hypovolemia was present at E. (Modified and reproduced with permission from Covino BG, Vassallo HG: Local Anesthetics: Mechanism of Action and Clinical Use, p 137. New York, Grune & Stratton, 1976.)

system. Most local anesthetic agents produce a biphasic effect on the cardiovascular system. For example, it has been shown that blood levels of lidocaine of less than 4 $\mu g \cdot ml^{-1}$ following epidural blockade resulted in a slight increase in blood pressure owing mainly to an increase in cardiac output. Doses of epidural lidocaine that produce blood levels in excess of 4 $\mu g \cdot ml^{-1}$ caused hypotension owing in part to the negative inotropic action of lidocaine and the peripheral vasodilator effect of this agent.[58]

Differences in the onset of epidural anesthesia occur as a function of the specific agent employed. The more rapidly acting agents, such as chloroprocaine and etidocaine, tend to produce a more profound degree of hypotension because of the more rapid blockade of sympathetic fibers. In addition, certain agents, such as etidocaine, can penetrate myelinated fibers more readily and, again, may be associated with a more profound degree of sympathetic blockade and hypotension.

A more profound degree of hypotension may occur following the use of epinephrine-containing local anesthetics for epidural blockade. The absorbed epinephrine is believed to stimulate beta$_2$-adrenergic receptors in peripheral vascular beds, leading to an enhanced state of vasodilation and a fall in diastolic pressure.[59] The beta$_1$-adrenergic receptor stimulating effect of epinephrine results in an increase in heart rate and cardiac output that counteracts the peripheral vasodilator state to some extent. Although absorbed epinephrine may be responsible for the early cardiovascular changes observed following epidural block, the more prolonged hypotension seen with local anesthetics containing epinephrine is probably related to the achievement of a more profound degree of sympathetic blockade.

Cardiovascular depression is more severe and more dangerous following the production of epidural anesthesia in hypovolemic subjects.[60] Epidural anesthesia in mildly hypovolemic volunteers was associated with profound hypotension and bradycardia. Hypovolemia is usually accompanied by compensatory vasoconstriction, which is abolished by the block, and cardiovascular collapse may ensue. The addition of epinephrine to the anesthetic solution may result in a less profound degree of hypotension in hypovolemic subjects. However, even the positive inotropic and chronotropic action of absorbed epinephrine cannot completely counteract the hypotensive effect of epidural blockade owing to the reduced circulating blood volume in these patients.

Effects on Regional Blood Flow

The sympathetic nervous system plays an important part in regulating regional blood flow. Blockade of sympathetic nerve fibers and resulting loss of vasomotor tone will, therefore, cause considerable change in the distribution of cardiac output, and epidural anesthesia will produce significant changes in blood flow to various organs, depending on the level of blockade achieved. Investigations in monkeys have shown that a T10 dermatomal level of anesthesia resulted in an increase in lower limb blood flow but no significant change in coronary, cerebral, renal, or hepatic blood flow.[61] High levels (T1) of epidural blockade caused a 55% decrease in coronary blood flow. This decrease in coronary blood flow occurred concomitantly with a 47% decrease in mean arterial blood pressure. The decrease in myocardial work was greater than the decrease in coronary flow. The low coronary flows may be related, in part, to extensive sympathetic blockade or to the peripheral vasodilator effect of lidocaine, both of which cause systemic hypotension and decreased coronary perfusion.

A significant decrease in cerebral blood flow of approximately 35% was also observed following achievement of a T1 dermatomal level of epidural anesthesia. Normally, cerebral blood flow is kept constant owing to autoregulation, but below a critical arterial pressure the blood flow decreases and is compensated for by increased oxygen extraction from the arterial blood.

Renal blood flow also decreased significantly following attainment of a T1 level of epidural anesthesia in the studies in monkeys. A 31–37% decrease in renal blood flow occurred at the time when mean arterial blood pressure and cardiac output were markedly reduced, suggesting that renal autoregulation may also be affected by hypotension.

Significant decreases in total hepatic blood flow of 20–40% were observed following achievement of a T1 level of anesthesia. These changes in hepatic blood flow followed a 14–47% decrease in mean arterial pressure.

Limited studies have been conducted in humans with regard to regional blood flow during epidural anesthesia. A 14% decrease in renal blood flow was observed in volunteers when a T5 level of epidural blockade was produced.[62] This change in renal blood flow occurred despite the lack of a significant decrease in mean arterial pressure and cardiac output. On the other hand, hepatic blood flow changes during epidural anesthesia in humans parallel changes in mean arterial pressure.

The effect of epidural blockade on blood flow in the lower limbs below the level of blockade is predictable. A marked increase in blood flow in the lower limbs below the level of block is accompanied by a compensatory decrease in blood flow in the upper limbs above the level of blockade.[63] As a result, blood pressure may not change very much with a low level of epidural anesthesia. However, high levels of epidural blockade cause inhibition of sympathetic outflow to both upper and lower limbs, resulting in extensive vasodilation and a marked decrease in peripheral vascular resistance. Under these conditions, limb blood flow is directly related to the patient's blood pressure.

PHARMACOLOGIC CONSIDERATIONS

Spinal Anesthesia

The selection of a specific local anesthetic for spinal anesthesia is related to a number of factors, such as

1. The desired segmental level of sensory anesthesia.
2. The duration of the surgical procedure.
3. The intensity of the motor blockade desired.

Greene[64] has reviewed the factors that are believed to influence the distribution of local anesthetics in the cerebrospinal fluid (Table 30-5). The density of the local anesthetic solution, the shape of the spinal canal, and the position of the patient are probably the most important factors involved.[65]

Density, Specific Gravity, and Baricity

Local anesthetics used for spinal anesthesia are described as hypobaric, isobaric, or hyperbaric. Hypobaric solutions are less dense than cerebrospinal fluid, whereas isobaric and hyperbaric solutions are equally dense and more dense than cerebrospinal fluid, respectively.

Density is the weight in grams of 1 ml of a solution $(g \cdot ml^{-1})$ at a specific temperature.

Specific gravity is the ratio of the density of a solution at a specific temperature to the density of water at that same temperature.

Baricity is the ratio of the density of a (local anesthetic) solution at a specific temperature to the density of cerebrospinal fluid at that same temperature.[64] Some authors have used specific gravity to determine the baricity of local anesthetic solutions. Baricity, in this case, is the ratio of the specific gravity of a local anesthetic solution at a specific temperature to the specific gravity of cerebrospinal fluid at the same temperature. This is less accurate than determining baricity from density.

An isobaric local anesthetic solution has a baricity of unity, whereas hypobaric and hyperbaric solutions have baricities less than and greater than unity, respectively. It is important to note that density varies inversely with temperature. Therefore, a local anesthetic that has the same density as cerebrospinal fluid at 37°C[66] will be more dense (hyperbaric) at room temperature than cerebrospinal fluid at 37°C. However, the clinically important density of local anesthetic solutions is that which is measured at 37°C because during spinal anesthesia, local anesthetic solutions rapidly equilibrate with the temperature of cerebrospinal fluid.[67]

The density of normal human cerebrospinal fluid with 95% confidence limits at 37°C is 1.0001 to 1.0005. Therefore, local anesthetic solutions with baricity less than 0.9998 (99.9% confidence limits) at 37°C will be hypobaric in all patients. Similarly, local anesthetic solutions at 37°C with baricity greater than 1.0008 (99.9% confidence limits) will be reliably hyperbaric in all patients. Because of the

TABLE 30-5. Factors Influencing Distribution of Local Anesthetics in Cerebrospinal Fluid*

Patient Characteristics

Age
Height
Weight
Gender
Intra-abdominal pressure
Anatomic configuration of spinal column
Position

Technique of Injection

Site of injection
Direction of injection
 Direction of needle
 Direction of bevel
Turbulence
 Rate of injection
 Barbotage

Diffusion

Characteristics of Spinal Fluid

Composition
Circulation
Volume
Pressure
Density

Characteristics of Anesthetic Solution

Density
Hypobaric solutions
Isobaric solutions
Hyperbaric solutions
Amount of anesthetic
Concentration of anesthetic
Volume injected
 Isobaric solutions
 Hypobaric solutions
 Hyperbaric solutions
Vasoconstrictors

*Hypothetical or demonstrable.

Reproduced with permission from Greene NM: Distribution of local anesthetic solutions within the spinal subarachnoid space. Anesth Analg 64:715, 1985.

normal variability in the density of cerebrospinal fluid, it is difficult to know precisely that a local anesthetic solution will, in fact, be isobaric in all patients. Nevertheless, local anesthetic solutions with densities between 0.9998 and 1.0008 behave functionally as if they have the same density as cerebrospinal fluid.[64]

The local anesthetics most commonly used for spinal anesthesia in the United States are lidocaine, bupivacaine, and tetracaine (Table 30-6). Procaine is also available for spinal anesthesia but is not widely used.

Dibucaine is a popular spinal anesthesia agent outside of the United States. However, it is no longer available in the United States.

Local anesthetic solutions used for spinal anesthesia are generally formulated with sodium chloride to make them isotonic. Solutions without added glucose either are isobaric (e.g., lidocaine, tetracaine, and dibucaine) or are very close to isobaric (bupivacaine is very slightly hypobaric). Procaine that is formulated as a 10% solution for spinal anesthesia is hyperbaric. Hyperbaric solutions of lidocaine, tetracaine, bupivacaine, and dibucaine are prepared by adding glucose in sufficient quantity to increase their density to greater than 1.0008. Other agents may be used to make a local anesthetic solution hyperbaric. For example, 1% tetracaine is sometimes made hyperbaric by mixing it in a 1:1 ratio with 10% procaine. Hypobaric solutions of procaine, tetracaine, and dibucaine are prepared by diluting them with distilled water to a density of less than 0.9998. Dilution of lidocaine with distilled water to make it hypobaric results in concentrations of lidocaine too low to provide adequate spinal anesthesia. The adequacy of spinal anesthesia with a hypobaric solution of bupivacaine is not well documented at this time. Table 30-6 summarizes the density and baricity of the commonly used spinal anesthetic solutions.

Effect of Baricity and Patient Position on Spinal Anesthesia

Utilizing an *in vitro* model of the spinal canal and injecting into it local anesthetic solutions colored with methylene blue dye, the effect of baricity, gravity (patient position), and shape of the spinal canal on the distribution of local anesthetics can be observed within the spinal subarachnoid space. Isobaric solutions remain in the vicinity of the injection site, hyperbaric solutions gravitate to dependent areas, and hypobaric solutions "float" to the least dependent areas. The shape of the average human spinal canal with the patient in the supine position is such that there is a lumbar lordosis (high point) at the L3–4 interspace and a thoracic kyphosis (low point) at the T5–6 interspace (Fig. 30-12). These curves influence the distribution of hyperbaric and hypobaric solutions within the spinal subarachnoid space. The distribution of isobaric solutions is unaffected by the shape of the spinal canal.

For surgical procedures performed with the patient in other than the supine position, the baricity of the local anesthetic solution and gravity have been employed to "direct" the local anesthetic toward the spinal nerves innervating the surgical site. For example, hemorrhoidectomy with the patient in the lithotomy position is often performed under saddle block spinal anesthesia. This is accomplished by administering a hyperbaric local anesthetic solution with the patient in the sitting position and allowing the solution to gravitate to the sacral nerves. Alternatively, hemorrhoidectomy in the prone jackknife position and hip surgery in the lateral recumbent position are often performed under hypobaric spinal anesthesia. In these cases, the spinal anesthesia is performed with the patient positioned for the surgical procedure that results in an uppermost position of the

TABLE 30-6. Density and Baricity of Local Anesthetics Commonly Used for Spinal Anesthesia

Agent	Usual Concentration (%)	Glucose Concentration (%)	Density (37°C)	Baricity (37°C)
CSF			1.0003	1.0000
Procaine	2.5	DW	0.9986	0.9983 (HO)
Procaine	10.0		1.0107	1.0104 (H)
Lidocaine	2.0	S	1.0007	1.0004 (I)
Lidocaine	5.0	7.5	1.0265	1.0262 (H)
Bupivacaine	0.5	S	0.9993	0.9990 (HO*)
Bupivacaine	0.75	8.25	1.0230 (CAL)	1.0227 (H)
Tetracaine	<0.33	DW	<0.9980	<0.9977 (HO)
Tetracaine	0.5	S	1.0000	0.9997 (HO*)
Tetracaine	0.5	5.0	1.0136	1.0133 (H)
Dibucaine	0.66	S	0.9967	0.9964 (HO)
Dibucaine	0.5	S	0.9992	0.9990 (HO*)
Dibucaine	0.25	5.0	1.0111	1.0108 (H)

CSF = cerebrospinal fluid; CSF density (37°C) 99.9% confidence limits = 0.9998–1.0008. Dibucaine is no longer manufactured. DW = distilled water; S = saline; HO = hypobaric; I = isobaric; H = hyperbaric; HO* = solution considered to be clinically isobaric; CAL = approximate value calculated from specific gravity.
Reproduced with permission from Lambert DH, Covino BG: Hyperbaric, hypobaric and isobaric spinal anesthesia. Res Staff Phys 33:79, 1987.

surgical site and the spinal nerves to be anesthetized. After injection, the hypobaric solution "floats" up to the nerves innervating the surgical site. These relationships are illustrated in Figure 30-13. It is important to note that surgery performed on areas innervated by nerves below the L1 dermatome may be easily performed with an isobaric solution. Since these solutions are unaffected by patient position, the spinal anesthesia can be induced in the most convenient position for the patient and the anesthesiologist. The patient can then be turned to the position dictated by the surgical procedure. Because spinal nerves L1–S5 pass through the cerebrospinal fluid into which the isobaric solution is injected, anesthesia in all of these dermatomes will result (Fig. 30-14).

Hyperbaric solutions of lidocaine and tetracaine are probably the most common solutions employed for spinal anesthesia. Hyperbaric solutions achieved their popularity because of the belief that it is easier to control the spread of these solutions.

Guidelines for Use of Hyperbaric and Isobaric Solutions

The following is a practical guide to the use of anesthetic solutions of varying baricity, depending on the surgical site.[68]

Surgery Above the L1 Dermatome

1. Hernias
2. Any intra-abdominal surgery
3. Radical orchiectomy (groin incision)
4. Gynecologic surgery requiring T10 dermatomal level of anesthesia (e.g., D&C, circlage, cone biopsy)
5. Cesarean section
6. Vaginal delivery

A hyperbaric solution is used for the surgical or obstetric procedures listed above. Hyperbaric solutions gravitate to the thoracic kyphosis in the supine patient, assuring an adequate level of spinal anesthesia. The thoracic kyphosis is at T6 in the average patient.

Hyperbaric Solutions

1. Lidocaine 5%, dextrose 7.5% (manufactured premixed)
2. Bupivacaine 0.75%, dextrose 8.25% (manufactured premixed)
3. Bupivacaine 0.375%, dextrose 5% (mix equal volumes of 0.75% bupivacaine and 10% dextrose)
4. Tetracaine 0.5%, dextrose 5% (mix equal volumes of 1% tetracaine and 10% dextrose)

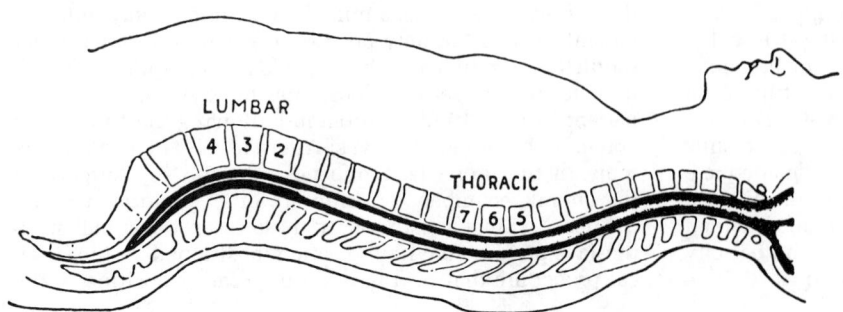

Figure 30-12. The shape of the spinal canal with the patient in the supine horizontal position. The lumbar lordosis produces a high point at L3, whereas the thoracic kyphosis produces a low point at T6. (Reproduced with permission from Lee JA, Atkinson RS: Sir Robert MacIntosh's Lumbar Puncture and Spinal Analgesia: Intradural and Extradural, p 138. Endinburgh, Churchill Livingstone, 1978.)

For the preceding surgical procedures, an isobaric solution is ideal. As indicated above, these solutions tend to remain in the lower dermatomes, providing intense anesthesia of prolonged duration.

Isobaric Solutions

1. Lidocaine 2% (epidural solution)
2. Bupivacaine 0.5% (epidural solution)
3. Bupivacaine 0.75% (epidural solution)
4. Tetracaine 0.5% (mix equal volumes of 1% tetracaine and preservative-free saline)

Any procedure performed below the L1 dermatome that is usually done with a hypobaric solution can be carried out equally well with an isobaric solution. Therefore, hypobaric solutions are rarely required, except for the occasional patient in whom anesthesia is induced in the jackknife posi-

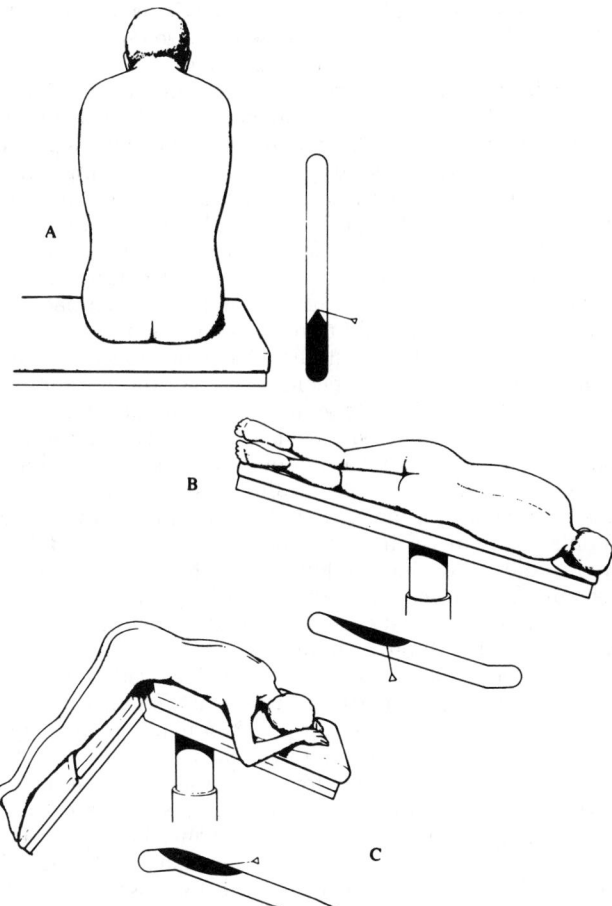

Figure 30-13. The effect of position and baricity on the distribution of a local anesthetic in the spinal subarachnoid space. The tubular figures to the right are meant to represent the dural sac, which contains the cerebrospinal fluid. The darkened areas indicate the disposition of the local anesthetic solution. (*A*) The patient is in the seated position undergoing "saddle block." A hyperbaric solution, which gravitates to the most dependent area, is used. (*B*) The patient is in the right lateral recumbent position with head-down tilt for left hip surgery. A hypobaric solution that "floats" to the uppermost area is employed. (*C*) The patient is in the prone jackknife position for rectal surgery. Again, a hypobaric solution is used. All three procedures could be done equally well with an isobaric solution. Isobaric solutions are unaffected by position and remain localized to the site of injection. (Reproduced with permission from Lambert DH, Covino BG: Hyperbaric, hypobaric, and isobaric spinal anesthesia. Res Staff Phys 33:79, 1987. Copyright 1987, Romaine Pierson Publishers.)

Surgery Below the L1 Dermatome

1. All lower limb orthopedic surgery (includes hip surgery)
2. Genitourinary surgery (transurethral resection of the prostate, transurethral resection of bladder tumor, cystoscopy, penile implant, scrotal orchiectomy)
3. Perineal surgery (Bartholin's cyst)
4. Lower limb vascular surgery (femoral-popliteal bypass graft)
5. Amputations of the lower limbs
6. Rectal surgery

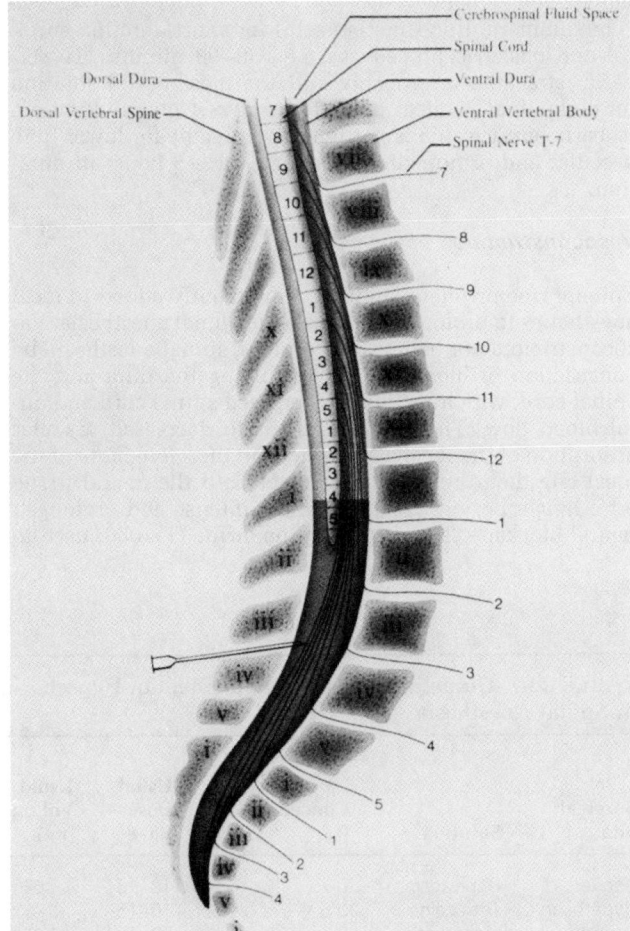

Figure 30-14. Longitudinal section through the distal portion of the vertebral column and spinal cord. Notice that the spinal cord terminates at the L1 vertebral body and that the spinal nerves extend downward for considerable distances before exiting beneath their respective vertebral bodies. Isobaric local anesthetics injected into the spinal subarachnoid space at the L3–4 interspace clinically occupy the darkened area and block all spinal nerves distal to L1. Furthermore, isobaric solutions tend to remain localized and are unaffected by patient position. (Reproduced with permission from Lambert DH, Covino BG: Hyperbaric, hypobaric, and isobaric spinal anesthesia. Res Staff Phys 33:79, 1987. Copyright 1987, Romaine Pierson Publishers.)

tion. Table 30-7 summarizes the agents used for spinal anesthesia, the dosages employed, and the usual durations for surgery performed at sites above or below the L1 dermatomes. Hyperbaric and isobaric lidocaine provide surgical anesthesia of approximately 1–2 hours, respectively. Tetracaine and bupivacaine are similar in terms of anesthetic duration. The hyperbaric solutions provide approximately 2 hours of surgical anesthesia above the L1 level, whereas the isobaric solutions provide 3–4 hours' duration below the L1 level. Differences do exist between tetracaine and bupivacaine. Compared with bupivacaine, epinephrine appears to prolong the anesthetic duration of tetracaine to a greater extent above the L1 dermatome.[69,70] Sensory analgesia below the L1 level appears more pronounced with bupivacaine. For example, the frequency of tourniquet pain is significantly lower in bupivacaine-treated patients compared with tetracaine-treated patients.[71,72] On the other hand, the intensity of motor blockade appears to be more profound when tetracaine is employed for spinal anesthesia.

In summary, lidocaine is useful for short-duration surgical and obstetric procedures, *i.e.*, 30–90 minutes. Hyperbaric tetracaine is probably still the most useful solution for abdominal surgical procedures of 2–4 hours' duration. Isobaric bupivacaine is particularly valuable for lower limb vascular and orthopedic procedures of 2–5 hours in duration.

Vasoconstrictors

Epinephrine or phenylephrine is frequently added to local anesthetics to prolong the duration of spinal anesthesia. Vasoconstrictors are believed to prolong spinal anesthesia by constriction of blood vessels supplying the dura and the spinal cord, which results in decreased spinal cord and dural blood flow. This, in turn, leads to decreased vascular absorption of the local anesthetic, and therefore more of the local anesthetic remains in contact with the neural tissue for a longer period, creating a more intense and prolonged neural blockade. The dose of epinephrine (1:1000) used to extend the duration of spinal anesthesia is usually 0.2–0.3 ml (200–300 μg). The recommended dosage for phenylephrine (1% solution) is 0.2–0.5 ml (2–5 mg).

The ability of vasoconstrictors to prolong the duration of spinal anesthesia may vary, depending on the specific local anesthetic employed. Epinephrine and phenylephrine have been shown to prolong the duration of spinal anesthesia induced with tetracaine.[69] It has been reported that epinephrine did not significantly prolong two- and four-segment (lower thoracic) regression of spinal anesthesia with lidocaine and bupivacaine.[70,73] Nevertheless, the duration of anesthesia in the lumbar and sacral dermatomes was prolonged by the addition of epinephrine to lidocaine and bupivacaine. Other studies have demonstrated that vasoconstrictors can significantly prolong the duration of lidocaine- and bupivacaine-induced spinal anesthesia.[74-77]

Kozody et al[78-80] have shown that lidocaine and tetracaine increased whereas bupivacaine decreased spinal cord and dural blood flow in dogs. Tetracaine was responsible for the greatest increase in blood flow. Epinephrine was found to inhibit the increase in spinal cord and dural blood flow produced by lidocaine and tetracaine. These results suggest that epinephrine should markedly prolong the action of tetracaine and moderately increase the duration of lidocaine but not alter the duration of bupivacaine.

Epinephrine and phenylephrine are believed to prolong spinal anesthesia primarily by vasoconstriction. However, a direct antinociceptive effect in the spinal cord may also be operative.[81] In this regard, the alpha$_2$ adrenergic receptor agonist, clonidine, has been found to produce analgesia following intrathecal administration and to enhance the efficacy of central neural blocks with local anesthesics.[82,83] The most profound effect of adding a vasoconstrictor to the spinal anesthetic solution occurs in the lumbosacral region. This is most likely due to the fact that the concentrations of the local anesthetic and the vasoconstrictor are greatest here because this is the customary site of injection.

In general, vasoconstrictors appear useful in prolonging the duration of spinal anesthesia below L1 with all local anesthetic agents. Thus, the duration of spinal anesthesia

---

TABLE 30-7. Guidelines for the Employment of Hyperbaric and Isobaric Solutions in Spinal Anesthesia

Surgical Site	Solution	Concentration (%)	Usual Dose (mg)	Usual Volume (ml)	Usual Duration No EPI* (hours)	Usual Duration 0.2 mg EPI (hours)
Above L1: Hyperbaric	Bupivacaine	0.75	10–15	1.5–2	2	2
	Tetracaine	0.5	10–15	2–3	3	3
	Lidocaine	5.0	50–75	1–1.5	1	1
Below L1: Isobaric	Bupivacaine	0.5	15	3	3–4	4–6
	Tetracaine	0.5	15	3	3–4	4–6
	Lidocaine	2.0	60	3	1–2	2–4

*EPI = Epinephrine.

Isobaric solutions of bupivacaine and lidocaine are not yet approved by the Federal Drug Administration for spinal anesthesia. However, this use has been reported in numerous publications. Solutions intended for spinal anesthesia should NOT contain any preservatives or antioxidants, such as methylparaben, sodium bisulfite, or sodium metabisulfite.

Reproduced with permission from Lambert DH, Covino BG: Hyperbaric, hypobaric, and isobaric spinal anesthesia. Res Staff Phys 33:79, 1987.

TABLE 30-8. Agents for Epidural Blockade

Agent	Usual Concentration (%)	Usual Onset (minutes)	Usual Duration of Surgical Anesthesia	Main Clinical Use
Chloroprocaine	2–3	5–15	30–90	Obstetrics
Lidocaine	1–2	5–15	60–120	Obstetrics Surgery
Mepivacaine	1–2	5–15	60–150	Surgery
Prilocaine	1–3	5–15	60–150	Surgery
Bupivacaine	0.25–0.75	10–20	120–140	Obstetrics Surgery
Etidocaine	1–1.5	5–15	120–240	Surgery

for orthopedic or vascular procedures in the lower extremities may be prolonged by the addition of a vasoconstrictor to lidocaine, bupivacaine, or tetracaine. However, for abdominal surgical procedures, vasoconstrictors added to lidocaine or bupivacaine may not be as efficacious as they are with tetracaine in terms of prolonging anesthetic duration.

Epidural Anesthesia

Local anesthetic agents intended for epidural (Table 30-8) use may be classified as follows:

1. Agents of low anesthetic potency and short duration of action (e.g., chloroprocaine),
2. Agents of intermediate anesthetic potency and duration of action (e.g., lidocaine, mepivacaine, and prilocaine), and
3. Agents of high anesthetic potency and prolonged duration of action (e.g., bupivacaine and etidocaine).[84]

In terms of latency, chloroprocaine, lidocaine, mepivacaine, prilocaine, and etidocaine possess a relatively rapid onset of action. Bupivacaine has a relatively slow onset of anesthesia. Procaine and tetracaine are rarely used for epidural blockade because of their slow onset of action.

Chloroprocaine has enjoyed popularity as an epidural anesthetic agent for obstetric use. This local anesthetic is characterized by a rapid onset time and a wide therapeutic ratio in terms of systemic toxicity for mother and fetus. The very short duration of chloroprocaine limits its usefulness for surgical epidural anesthesia except for short ambulatory procedures or unless a catheter technique is employed.

Lidocaine, mepivacaine, and prilocaine are similar in terms of their anesthetic profile when used for epidural blockade. Lidocaine may possess a slightly shorter onset time, whereas mepivacaine and prilocaine produce a longer duration of anesthesia than lidocaine when these drugs are used without a vasoconstrictor. Prilocaine is systemically the least toxic of the various amide local anesthetics. Unfortunately, doses above 600 mg are associated with the occurrence of methemoglobinemia, which has limited the use of this drug. Nevertheless, it is an excellent local anesthetic if such doses are not exceeded.

Bupivacaine and etidocaine are employed as epidural drugs of relatively long duration. They differ considerably in their anesthetic profile, although they are both potent,

long-acting local anesthetics. Bupivacaine is widely used for both surgical and obstetric epidural anesthesia. It is of particular value for continuous epidural blockade during labor. When used as a 0.25% solution, it provides satisfactory sensory analgesia with minimal motor blockade. The 0.5% solution is also used during labor, but at the expense of greater motor blockade. Thus, the patient in labor can be rendered pain-free and still be able to move her legs. In addition, bupivacaine usually provides 1–3 hours of adequate analgesia, although this depends greatly on the dosage. The onset of anesthesia is relatively slow, frequently requiring 15–20 minutes for development of an adequate epidural blockade. For surgical procedures, the 0.75% concentration of bupivacaine appears more useful than the 0.25% or 0.5% solution. The latency is shortened, the depth of analgesia is more profound, and skeletal muscle relaxation is improved. However, 0.75% bupivacaine is no longer recommended for obstetric anesthesia because of reports of severe cardiotoxic reactions.

Etidocaine is especially useful for surgical procedures. When used as a 1.5% solution, this drug provides the most rapid onset of any local anesthetic administered epidurally. Initial signs of analgesia appear in 3–5 minutes and may be complete in 10 minutes. Etidocaine shows little sensory-motor discrimination. Thus, dosages of this drug that provide satisfactory analgesia invariably produce profound motor blockade. In surgical situations in which optimal skeletal muscle relaxation is desirable, etidocaine has proved a valuable local anesthetic for epidural use, since it combines a rapid onset, duration of 3–4 hours, and a satisfactory quality of analgesia combined with profound skeletal muscle relaxation. However, this marked effect on motor function renders etidocaine of limited value for obstetric analgesia.

Recently, a new amide local anesthetic agent, ropivacaine, has been employed for epidural anesthesia.[85] This agent, which is a propyl derivative of mepivacaine but is prepared as the pure S-isomer, has an epidural clinical profile similar to that of bupivacaine. Ropivacaine has been compared with bupivacaine at 0.5 and 0.75% concentrations.[86,87] The two agents appear similar in terms of onset, potency, spread, and differential sensory-motor blockade. The duration of motor blockade is reported to be significantly shorter for ropivacaine compared with bupivacaine.

The quality of epidural blockade is influenced primarily by the local anesthetic employed. Other factors that may influence the adequacy of epidural blockade include

(1) dose, volume, and concentration of the local anesthetic agent; (2) addition of a vasoconstrictor to the local anesthetic solution; (3) site and speed of injection; (4) patient position; and (5) patient age, height, and clinical status.

Dose, Volume, and Concentration of the Local Anesthetic Agent

The volume of the anesthetic solution administered into the epidural space may influence the vertical spread of anesthesia. For example, 30 ml of 1% lidocaine produced a level of analgesia following lumbar epidural administration that was 4.3 dermatomes higher than that achieved by 10 ml of 3% lidocaine.[88] However, the relationship between spread and volume of local anesthetic solution is neither linear nor predictable. The essential qualities of epidural anesthesia, that is, onset, depth, and duration of sensory analgesia and motor blockade, are related to the mass of drug rather than to variations in volume or concentration of solution. For example, a comparison of 600 mg of prilocaine administered epidurally either as 30 ml of a 2% solution or as 20 ml of a 3% solution failed to show any difference in onset, adequacy, or duration of anesthesia and onset, depth, and duration of motor blockade.[89] An increase in the dosage of local anesthetic administered epidurally will tend to decrease the onset time, increase the frequency of satisfactory anesthesia, and significantly prolong the duration of anesthesia (Fig. 30-15). Studies with bupivacaine administered epidurally in obstetrics have shown that increasing the concentration from 0.125% to 0.5% while maintaining the same volume of injection shortened the latency time, improved the incidence of satisfactory analgesia, and increased the duration of sensory anesthesia. In addition, the degree and duration of motor blockade were enhanced by an increase in the concentration and dosage of bupivacaine.[90]

Addition of a Vasoconstrictor

Epinephrine is frequently added to local anesthetic solutions intended for epidural administration in order to increase the depth of blockade and significantly prolong the duration of anesthesia. The effect of epinephrine is believed to be related primarily to its effects on the local vasculature, which cause a decrease in absorption of the local anesthetic. Thus, more of the drug remains in the epidural space and is available for diffusion to the spinal roots and cord to produce a more profound degree and longer duration of anesthesia. A 1:200,000 (5 $\mu g \cdot ml^{-1}$) concentration of epinephrine is usually employed when used in conjunction with a drug such as lidocaine. Although other vasoconstrictor drugs, such as phenylephrine, have also been used as additives to solutions of local anesthetics intended for epidural anesthesia, the available evidence suggests that epinephrine is the most effective vasoconstrictor.[91]

Prilocaine, bupivacaine, and etidocaine administered epidurally do not appear to benefit from the addition of epinephrine as much as lidocaine or mepivacaine. In the case of bupivacaine, the effect of epinephrine on the frequency and duration of adequate anesthesia depends on the concentration of bupivacaine employed for epidural blockade. The frequency of adequate anesthesia and/or the duration of sensory analgesia is improved when epinephrine 1:200,000 is added to 0.125% and 0.25% bupivacaine for epidural blockade in obstetric patients.[90] However, the addition of epinephrine to 0.5% and 0.75% bupivacaine intended for epidural use in either obstetric or surgical patients is not

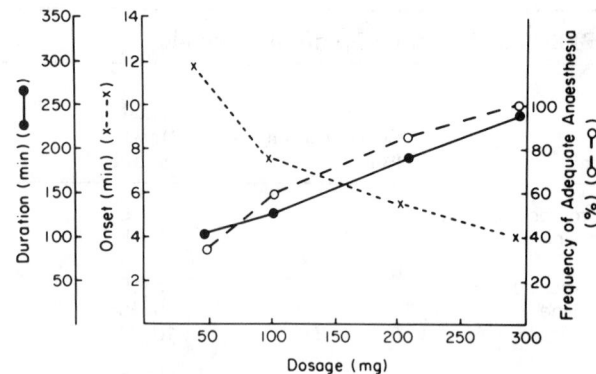

Figure 30-15. The effect of increasing dosage of local anesthetic agent on the onset, duration, and frequency of adequate anesthesia during epidural anesthesia. Increasing the dose decreases the onset time while increasing the duration and frequency of adequate anesthesia.

associated with a significant improvement in the frequency of adequate anesthesia.[90,92] The duration was prolonged in some studies but not in others.[92,93] The addition of epinephrine to either bupivacaine or etidocaine does appear to increase the profoundness of motor blockade.[92]

Site and Speed of Injection

Injection of local anesthetics into different epidural sites produces marked differences in the spread of anesthesia. For example, injections of small volumes, i.e., 3–5 ml, into the relatively narrow midthoracic epidural space results in a discrete but wide segmental blockade. Lumbar epidural administration usually requires the use of volumes of 15–25 ml to achieve surgical anesthesia. Cephalad spread occurs more easily than caudad spread following lumbar epidural injections, in part because of the negative intrathoracic pressure and the resistance afforded by the narrowing of the epidural space at the lumbosacral junction. A significant delay or absence of analgesia or both at the first and second sacral segments are frequently observed following lumbar epidural injections. This has been attributed in part to the narrowing of the epidural space at the lumbosacral junction and to the thickness of the spinal roots in this area.[47] Caudal anesthesia usually requires greater amounts of drug owing to loss of solution through the anterior sacral foramina and the rapid vascular absorption from this site. Little cephalad spread beyond the lumbosacral junction occurs following caudal injections because of the peculiar anatomy of the epidural space in this region.

Rate of injection appears to have little effect on the profile of epidural anesthesia. Twenty milliliters of 2% lidocaine injected into the lumbar epidural space at a rate of 1 ml·sec^{-1} and 1 ml·3 sec^{-1} did not influence the duration of anesthesia or motor block or the level of anesthesia in a clinically significant manner.[79] Greater patient discomfort may be associated with the rapid injection of local anesthetics into the epidural space.

Patient Position

Posture was originally thought to influence the spread of epidural analgesia.[94] However, studies involving the use of radioisotopes administered in the epidural space failed to demonstrate any effect of posture on the spread of these materials in the epidural space.[95] Controversy exists concerning the onset of sensory anesthesia following the epidural administration of local anesthetics to patients in the sitting or lateral decubitus position. Some studies have suggested a greater spread in patients in the lateral decubitus position.[94] Other investigators have failed to confirm these findings.[96] In general, patient position *per se* does not appear to predictably influence the spread or duration of epidural anesthesia in a fashion similar to that following the administration of local anesthetics into the subarachnoid space.

Age, Height, and Pregnancy

Discrepancies exist between studies that evaluated the influence of age and height of patients on the spread of anesthetics in the epidural space.[96,97] Originally, the level of epidural blockade was reported to be related to height and age. Other investigators have failed to demonstrate any correlation between age, height, and spread of epidurally administered local anesthetics. More recent studies comparing the spread of anesthetic solution in patients of varying age have shown little correlation between the maximal dermatomal analgesic level obtained and the age of patients up to the age of 40 years.[98] Patients 40 years and older did show a greater spread of epidural anesthesia compared with patients less than 40 years of age when the volume and dose of local anesthetic solution were the same in both groups. However, the mean difference between the various age groups was only two to three segments. The enhanced spread of epidural anesthesia in older patients may be related to the compliance of the epidural space. Epidural compliance has been reported to increase with advancing age, and the spread of epidural anesthesia was directly related to compliance of the epidural space.[99]

Pregnancy is believed to affect the level of epidural anesthesia. For example, similar levels of anesthesia were obtained following the use of 6–10 ml of 2% lidocaine in obstetric patients and 15–30 ml of 2% lidocaine in nonpregnant patients.[100] This difference is believed to be related to inferior vena caval compression in pregnancy, which results in a marked distention of the epidural venous plexi. Recent studies suggest that the greater sensitivity and spread of epidural anesthetics in pregnant patients may be related to hormonal rather than mechanical factors. The dose per segment requirements of epidurally administered local anesthetics was decreased in patients during their first trimester of pregnancy compared with a similar group of nonpregnant patients.[101] Since distention of venous plexi by inferior vena caval occlusion is not a factor at this early stage of pregnancy, the increased sensitivity to local anesthetics is believed to be related to hormonal influences. Moreover, isolated nerve studies have confirmed a more rapid onset of conduction blockade and a greater sensitivity to local anesthetics in nerves from pregnant rabbits compared with nerves from nonpregnant animals.[102,103]

COMPLICATIONS OF SPINAL AND EPIDURAL ANESTHESIA

Spinal Blockade

Complications associated with spinal anesthesia may be classified as minor or major. Minor complications consist of limited, transient alterations in physiologic function. Hypotension, the high spinal block with depression of ventilation, postdural puncture headache, and back pain fall into the minor complications category. The major complications category consists largely of neurologic injuries—isolated nerve injuries, meningitis, and cauda equina syndrome. Fortunately, the major complications of spinal anesthesia occur infrequently. Although the minor complications occur with greater frequency, they are, in general, easy to manage.

Hypotension

Hypotension during spinal anesthesia is the result of decreased cardiac output, which in turn is the result of decreased venous return. The amount of venous pooling and, therefore, decreased venous return are directly related to the degree of sympathectomy, which in turn is related to the level of the spinal blockade. The degree of hypotension that can be tolerated depends on the age and physical status of the patient. Elderly patients with cardiac and cerebrovascular disease may be at risk, if the blood pressure is allowed to decline to low levels during spinal anesthesia. Although the absolute level of hypotension that can be tolerated by these patients is not known, it is probably best not to allow the mean blood pressure to decline more than 20% in these individuals.

In pregnancy, placental perfusion is dependent upon maternal blood pressure. Maintaining maternal mean blood pressure above 100 mm Hg ensures placental perfusion and improves fetal outcome. On the other hand, young, healthy, nonpregnant individuals may experience greater falls in blood pressure without ill effects.

Attention to a few details will minimize the occurrence of hypotension. These include adequate hydration prior to the induction of spinal anesthesia and proper positioning of the patient once spinal anesthesia is induced. Both of these maneuvers improve venous return, cardiac output, and blood pressure. All patients should have fluid deficits replaced prior to spinal anesthesia. An additional 500 ml of balanced salt solution usually mitigates the response to venodilation due to sympathectomy. Patients with congestive heart failure should receive less fluid because their vascular systems are already at or above capacity. Once the spinal anesthetic drug has been injected, positioning the patient so as to ensure adequate venous return is paramount. Usually the horizontal supine position is all that is required. If, however, after adequate fluid loading and after the patient is in the supine horizontal position the blood pressure cannot be maintained in the desired range, moving to a slight head-down position, so that the right atrium is below the great veins, often improves the situation. The head-down tilt need not be steep. A modest Trendelenburg position of 5–10 degrees will improve venous return without greatly exaggerating the cephalad spread of the spinal anesthetic. Occasionally, despite both of these maneuvers, the blood pressure needs to be supported with vasoactive agents. Patients should not be placed in the head-up position so as to prevent an exaggerated cephalad spread of the local anesthetic; this will tend to cause a more profound degree of hypotension.[104]

During spinal anesthesia, systemic vascular resistance (arteriolar dilation) is only minimally decreased. The major decline in mean arterial pressure is decreased cardiac output resulting from decreased venous return. Therefore, vasopressors that constrict veins in preference to arterioles provide a more rational method for treating the hypotension that results from spinal anesthesia. Drugs commonly used are ephedrine, mephentermine, and phenylephrine. Ephedrine and mephentermine have mixed alpha and beta receptor activity and are potent venoconstrictors, whereas phenylephrine is an alpha receptor agonist and a more potent arteriolar constrictor. While improving venous return, ephedrine and mephentermine also increase heart rate. Phenylephrine increases blood pressure by arteriolar constriction, with little or no change or a decline in heart rate.[105-107]

One approach to treating hypotension during spinal anesthesia is to administer boluses of ephedrine (5–10 mg) intravenously. Usually, one or two boluses are all that is required. Occasionally, however, it is necessary to administer a vasoconstrictor for more prolonged periods. Under these conditions, an intramuscular injection of ephedrine (25–50 mg) or an infusion of phenylephrine (10 mg in 250 ml of D5W or balanced salt solution) is indicated because tachyphylaxis precludes the intravenous administration of ephedrine or mephentermine for prolonged intervals.[108]

Postdural Puncture Headache

Postdural puncture (spinal) headache is believed to be owing to decreased cerebrospinal fluid pressure resulting from the leakage of cerebrospinal fluid through the opening in the dural sheath created by the lumbar puncture needle. Postdural puncture headache is probably the most common complication of spinal anesthesia. The incidence of spinal headache is believed to be related to age, sex, pregnancy, size of the dural puncture needle, direction of the needle bevel, and the angle at which the needle penetrates the dura.[40,41,109-111] The headache is classically described as frontal or occipital, is made worse by erect posture, is improved in the recumbent position, and may be accompanied by tinnitus and/or photophobia. A true postdural puncture headache must have a postural component, i.e., be made worse by the sitting or standing position. It is important to remember that many patients may have a headache postoperatively that is not related to the dural puncture.

Table 30-9 shows the effect of sex, age, and needle size on the incidence of postdural puncture headache. Women appear to be more prone to develop a postdural puncture headache than men.[40] This may be related to the influence of hormones, e.g., progesterone and estrogen. Age is inversely related and needle diameter is directly related to the incidence of postdural headache. Midline approaches to the subarachnoid space result in greater leakage of cerebrospinal fluid than paramedian approaches.[111] Midline approaches may, therefore, result in a higher incidence of postdural puncture headache. Inserting the spinal needle with the bevel parallel to the orientation of the dural fibers, as opposed to cutting across them with the bevel inserted at right angles to the fibers, has been reported to decrease the incidence of postdural puncture headache.[110] The incidence of postdural puncture headache is higher in pregnant patients than in nonpregnant females. At the Brigham and Women's Hospital, the incidence of postspinal headache in obstetric patients averages approximately 7%, despite the use of 26-gauge needles. Once again, hormonal factors may be involved. However, an interesting alternative explanation is the increased incidence of postdural puncture headache associated with the concentration of glucose injected with the local anesthetic.[112] Figure 30-16 shows a direct relationship between the incidence of spinal headache and the amount of glucose contained in the local anesthetic solution. Some controversy exists concerning the incidence of postdural puncture headache following the use of epidural catheters for continuous spinal anesthesia. The frequency of postdural puncture headache has been reported to vary from less than 1% to 60% with the use of large needles and catheters.[113-115] The use of the 32-gauge microcatheter resulted in a postdural puncture headache incidence of 4% in a relatively young age population.[42] In order to minimize the frequency of postdural puncture headache, the following guidelines have been suggested in terms of catheter size for continuous spinal anesthesia:

1. Up to age 50: 32-gauge catheter and 27-gauge needle
2. 50–65 years: 27- or 28-gauge catheter and 22-gauge needle
3. More than 65 years: 19- or 20-gauge catheter and 18-gauge needle

Once the diagnosis of postdural puncture headache is confirmed, three methods of therapy are available: (1) analgesics, bed rest, and hydration; (2) epidural blood patch; and (3) intravenous caffeine.

Nearly all postdural puncture headaches resolve without therapy in time. Bed rest, analgesics, and hydration are often satisfactory for the patient who has had extensive surgery and who is unlikely to be ambulatory postoperatively.

TABLE 30-9. Relation of Sex, Age, and Needle Gauge Used for Lumbar Puncture to Incidence of "Spinal" Headache

	Number of Spinal Anesthetics	Number of "Spinal" Headaches	Percent
Sex			
Male	4063	302	7
Female	5214	709	14
Vaginal delivery	938	220	22
Other procedures	4276	489	12
Totals	9277	1011	21
Age (Years)			
10–19	537	51	10
20–29	1994	321	16
30–39	1833	261	14
40–49	1759	192	11
50–59	1736	133	8
60–69	1094	45	4
70–79	297	7	2
80–89	27	1	3
Totals	9277	1011	11
Needle Gauge			
16	839	151	18
19	154	16	10
20	2698	377	14
22	4952	430	9
24	634	37	6

Reproduced with permission from Vandam LD, Dripps RD: Long-term follow up of patients who received 10,098 spinal anesthetics: III. Syndrome of decreased intracranial pressure (headache and occular and auditory difficulties). JAMA 161:586, 1956. Copyright 1956, American Medical Association.

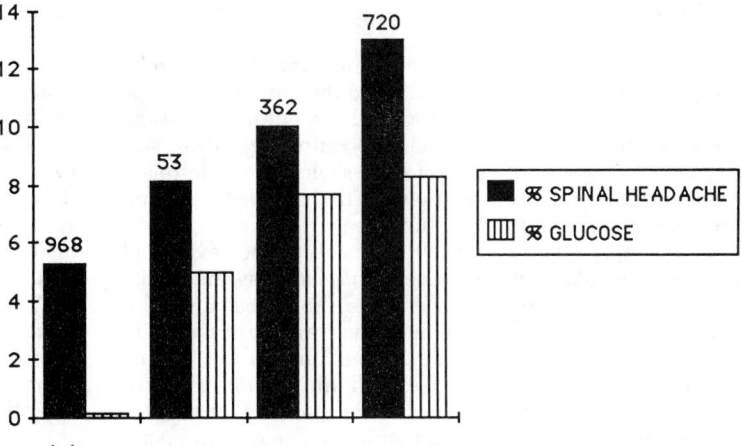

Figure 30-16. The relationship between glucose concentration of the spinal anesthetic and the incidence of spinal headache. As the glucose concentration increases, the incidence of spinal headache also increases. Tet-proc = tetracaine 0.5%-procaine 5% (no dextrose); lido = lidocaine (5%); bupiv = bupivacaine (0.75%); and dex = dextrose (concentration as indicated by the open bars). The numbers above the solid bars indicate the number of spinal anesthetics. (Reproduced with permission of the author: Naulty JS: Unpublished, 1985.)

Hydration in the form of "forcing fluids" is done with the intent of increasing the production of cerebrospinal fluid so that cerebrospinal fluid production exceeds loss through the dural puncture site, thus restoring the cerebrospinal fluid pressure to normal. Some authors have recommended the use of pitressin to augment the process by preventing diuresis.[116]

If a postdural puncture headache persists following 24 hours of rest, fluid, and analgesic therapy, the patient should be offered an epidural blood patch. This is accomplished by placing a needle in the epidural space in the vicinity of the dural puncture and injecting 10–20 ml of autologous blood aseptically. The optimum amount of blood injected has been determined to be 15 ml in the average patient.[117] This procedure is very effective. If relief of the headache is not observed, the procedure may be repeated. If two epidural blood patches are not effective in curing the headache, the diagnosis of postdural puncture headache is suspect. Complications associated with epidural blood patch are minimal. Low back pain and nuchal discomfort are the most common complaints, and these usually resolve in 24–48 hours with analgesics. Epidural saline has been recommended for postdural puncture headache[118] but does not appear to be as efficacious as an epidural blood patch.[119]

Recently, the use of caffeine infusions for the treatment of postdural puncture headache has been reinvestigated. The initial studies involving caffeine were conducted by Sechzer and Abel.[120,121] The mechanism by which caffeine infusion reverses spinal headache is not clear, although it may be related to its vasoconstrictor action. Jarvis et al[122] have shown that 80% of patients with postdural puncture headache, infused with D5-Ringer's lactate solution (1) containing caffeine sodium benzoate (500 mg), followed by an additional infusion of 1000 ml of D5-Ringer's lactate solution, resulted in significant improvement in symptoms. Oral caffeine has also been reported to decrease the severity of postdural puncture headache.[123]

Extensive Spread of Spinal Blockade

High spinal anesthesia with respiratory and vascular embarrassment can occur in any patient. However, the patients most susceptible to high spinal anesthesia are parturients. This may result from a number of factors—e.g., decreased cerebrospinal fluid volume, the use of hyperbaric solutions in the presence of an exaggerated lumbar lordosis, increased neuronal sensitivity to local anesthetics, or ventilatory insufficiency due to the enlarged uterus. High spinal anesthesia is most likely to occur shortly after the induction of spinal anesthesia. Nevertheless, late occurring respiratory distress has been reported. It is important, therefore, to closely monitor the patient during and following the induction of spinal anesthesia until the level has significantly regressed.

Most patients become agitated with a high spinal, and nausea and hypotension are frequently seen. These symptoms should alert the anesthesiologist to the possibility that the spinal anesthesia is higher than desired. The diagnosis should be made as quickly as possible and can be made in combination with the treatment. The patient should be given oxygen, preferably by mask attached to the anesthesia circuit. Ask the patient to take a deep breath and observe intercostal muscle function and the movement of the reservoir bag. Good intercostal muscle function and exchange of large volumes of oxygen from the reservoir bag are inconsistent with high spinal anesthesia. Agitation, nausea, and hypotension most likely represent exaggerated sympathectomy. Treatment consists of restoring the blood pressure with positioning, fluids and/or vasopressors, and reassurance. Lack of intercostal muscle function and minimal movement of the reservoir bag indicate very high spinal anesthesia. Again, the treatment consists of supporting the blood pressure and reassurance while assisting ventilation. Usually, the phrenic nerves are spared and diaphragmatic breathing will produce adequate ventilation. This may not be the case in the parturient, in whom the enlarged uterus interferes with diaphragmatic excursions. Inadequate ventilation may require induction of general anesthesia and assisted ventilation of the lungs following endotracheal intubation. Intubation of the trachea is especially indicated for the patient at risk for aspiration.

When spinal anesthetics spread to the cervical region, the concentration of the local anesthetic in the upper regions is not great. Therefore, the exaggerated spread is usually short-lived, and respiratory function can be expected to return relatively quickly. It is usually advisable, however, to keep the patient unconscious until the surgical procedure is complete once intubation of the trachea has been accomplished.

Backache

Surprisingly, backache following spinal anesthesia is relatively infrequent. It may be related to the spinal anesthetic procedure itself. Small hematomas, ligamentous irritation, reflex skeletal muscle spasm, and positioning during surgery are also possibilities. Profound skeletal muscle relaxation occurs with spinal anesthesia. This, coupled for example with the lithotomy position, may result in ligament strain postoperatively. Backache does occur, however, and it sometimes takes on the same significance as the spinal headache. Serious neurologic damage should be ruled out. Otherwise, reassurance, rest, heat, and analgesics usually rectify the problem. Physical examination and the "laying on of hands" is often beneficial and should be done if practical. Occasionally, paraspinous muscle spasm is the culprit, and skeletal muscle relaxant medication, e.g., diazepam, can help.

Nausea

Nausea during spinal anesthesia can be a vexing problem. Because nausea can be a symptom of cerebral ischemia, it is imperative that the anesthesiologist think first of providing oxygen and determining if severe hypotension is the cause when nausea appears. Treatment involves restoration of the arterial blood pressure while providing oxygen therapy. Datta et al[124] have shown that immediate treatment of arterial hypotension in parturients minimizes the incidence of nausea during cesarean section.

Another cause of nausea during spinal anesthesia is an imbalance between the parasympathetic and sympathetic nervous systems resulting from chemical sympathectomy or from parasympathetic-mediated traction reflexes from surgical manipulation. Atropine (0.4 mg) may help, but not invariably. Adjuvant medications, especially opioids, may cause nausea in some cases. In this instance, small amounts of droperidol (0.625 mg) may be beneficial.[125]

Major Neurologic Injuries

Major neurologic injuries are extremely rare following spinal anesthesia. This is due, in part, to the use of disposable spinal kits and the relative safety and low doses of the local anesthetics employed. The prepackaged sterile spinal kits have virtually eliminated meningitis as a complication of spinal anesthesia. A review[126] of 11 spinal anesthetic studies involving approximately 65,000 patients with various agents lists 31 cases of neurologic sequelae (an incidence of 1:2000). Many of these 31 sequelae were exacerbations of previous neurologic diseases.[127]

The possible causes of neurologic injury include (1) spinal cord ischemia, (2) needle trauma, (3) chemical contamination of local anesthetic solutions, and (4) toxicity of the local anesthetic solutions themselves. Spinal cord ischemia is believed to be associated with prolonged arterial hypotension in combination with a precarious anterior spinal arterial blood supply. Neurologic injury resulting from needle trauma is extremely rare. It usually results from multiple attempts during difficult lumbar puncture.[128] Contamination of local anesthetic solutions with detergents or other chemicals has been responsible, in some cases, for the production of neurologic sequelae following spinal anesthesia. For example, cases of aseptic meningitis have been attributed to soaking syringes with disinfectants.[129] The use of disposable equipment has virtually eliminated this complication and bacterial meningitis. The incidence of neurologic complications owing to spinal anesthesia has decreased since the 1940s, probably because of the use of disposable equipment and elimination of solutions containing substances such as alcohol, acacia, and strychnine.[130] Recently several cases of sensory-motor deficits have been reported following continuous spinal anesthesia, particularly with the use of a 28-gauge catheter.[131] The cause may be related to the caudal location of the catheter such that the anesthetic solution fails to spread in a cephalad direction. This may lead to the administration of excessive doses of local anesthetic, which may result in neural damage.

When a major neurologic complication occurs following spinal anesthesia, a neurologist should be consulted and every effort should be made to determine the etiology of the neurologic injury. Neurologic injury can be caused by an errantly placed needle or injection of the wrong substance into the subarachnoid space. However, nerve injury can also result from other causes, e.g., pre-existing neurologic lesion, retractors, the birth process, or pressure on nerves resulting from faulty positioning during surgery.

Unfortunately, there is often little that can be done once neurologic injury has occurred. With the exception of evacuation of a hematoma or drainage of an abscess, treatment is usually symptomatic. The best therapy, however, is attention to details and avoidance of injury.

Epidural Anesthesia

Toxicity Caused by Local Anesthetics

Relatively high doses of local anesthetic agents are required in order to achieve adequate sensory anesthesia for surgery following epidural administration. In addition, the epidural space contains numerous venous plexuses, which may be penetrated by an epidural needle or catheter, leading to the accidental intravascular administration of local anesthetic agents. As a result, toxicity may occur either because of the administration of an excessive amount of drug extravascularly or because of accidental intravascular injection. The blood and tissue levels of local anesthetic agents associated with systemic toxic reactions are determined by the rate of absorption, tissue redistribution, metabolism, and excretion of the anesthetic compound.

The systemic absorption and potential toxicity of epidurally administered local anesthetics are related to the site of injection, addition and dosage of a vasoconstrictor, and the pharmacologic profile of the local anesthetic itself. Little difference in the rate of absorption is seen following cervical, thoracic, or lumbar epidural injections.[132] However, with caudal injections, mean peak venous blood levels are significantly higher than those following lumbar epidural injections.[84] This may reflect the greater lateral spread of the injected solution and exposure to a larger vascular surface area in the caudal canal.

Blood levels of local anesthetics are related to the total dose of drug administered. For most local anesthetics, a linear relationship exists between the amount of drug administered and the resultant peak blood level (Fig. 30-17). For example, the mean venous blood level of lidocaine increased from approximately 1.5 $\mu g \cdot ml^{-1}$ to 4 $\mu g \cdot ml^{-1}$ as the total dose administered into the lumbar epidural space was increased from 200 to 600 mg.[84] For certain local anesthetics, such as bupivacaine and etidocaine, a nonlinear relationship has been observed between the total dose administered and the peak venous blood level. This may be attributable to the high lipid solubility of bupivacaine and

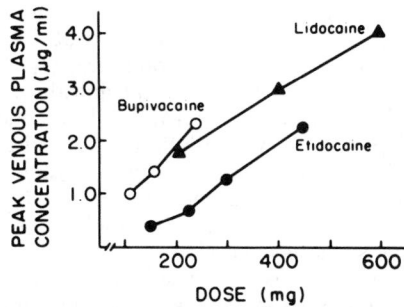

Figure 30-17. Relationship between the amount of drug administered epidurally and the resultant peak blood levels. For lidocaine, a linear relationship is observed. Bupivacaine and etidocaine demonstrate a nonlinear relationship.

etidocaine, which results in sequestration of these drugs in epidural fat such that the rate of systemic absorption is less when relatively low doses are used. However, when high doses are administered, lipid depots may be saturated so that more free drug is available for absorption. The peak blood level achieved following epidural blockade is a function of the dose in milligrams and does not appear to be related to either the concentration or the volume of the local anesthetic solution employed. No significant difference in the venous plasma levels of different local anesthetics has been observed following the lumbar epidural administration of these drugs at varying volumes and concentrations if the total dose was the same.[84]

Many local anesthetic solutions contain a vasoconstrictor agent, usually epinephrine, in a concentration of 5 μg·ml^{-1} (1:200,000). A concentration of 5 μg·ml^{-1} of epinephrine appears to be optimal in terms of reducing the rate of absorption of local anesthetic agents, such as lidocaine and mepivacaine, from the lumbar epidural space.[133] The vascular uptake from the epidural space of local anesthetics such as prilocaine, bupivacaine, and etidocaine appears to be less influenced by the addition of a vasoconstrictor than is the vascular uptake of lidocaine and mepivacaine.[133-135]

Differences exist in the rate of absorption of various local anesthetics from the epidural space. For example, prilocaine blood levels are significantly lower than those of lidocaine following lumbar epidural administration of equal doses of both drugs. This difference may reflect the greater vasodilator activity of lidocaine, but more important is the larger distribution volume and the rapid rate of elimination of prilocaine.[136] Among the more potent drugs, etidocaine blood levels are significantly lower than those of bupivacaine if equal doses of both local anesthetics are administered epidurally.[136] This may be related, in part, to the greater lipid solubility, the larger distribution volume, and more rapid rate of elimination of etidocaine.[120] The lower blood level of etidocaine has practical clinical implications. Although 1.0–1.5% etidocaine is required to provide a similar degree of sensory analgesia as 0.5–0.75% bupivacaine, no difference in blood levels or potential toxicity exists between the two drugs following lumbar epidural administration.

Systemic Toxicity of Local Anesthetic Agents

When properly performed, epidural anesthesia does not usually result in blood levels of local anesthetics that are sufficient to cause systemic effects. However, accidental intravascular injection or the administration of an excessive amount of local anesthetic into the epidural space can result in high blood and tissue levels that will cause profound systemic effects.

The central nervous system is particularly susceptible to the systemic actions of local anesthetics.[137] The signs and symptoms of central nervous system toxicity are as follows: initially, feelings of numbness of the legs and tongue, lightheadedness, and dizziness are usually reported, followed frequently by visual and auditory disturbances, such as difficulty in focusing and tinnitus. Other subjective central nervous system symptoms include disorientation and occasional feelings of drowsiness. Objective signs of an excitatory central nervous system effect include shivering, skeletal muscular twitching, and tremors, involving at first muscles of the face and distal parts of the extremities. This may progress to generalized convulsions of a tonic-clonic nature. If a sufficiently high dose of a local anesthetic agent is administered systemically, these initial signs of central nervous system excitation are rapidly followed by a state of generalized central nervous system depression. Seizure activity ceases and depression of ventilation and, ultimately, apnea occur.

In general, the cardiovascular system appears to be more resistant to the effects of local anesthetics than the central nervous system. However, local anesthetics can cause profound cardiovascular toxicity.[137]

The sequence of cardiovascular events that usually occurs following the accidental intravascular administration of local anesthetics is as follows. At relatively nontoxic blood levels of these drugs, either no change in blood pressure or a slight increase in blood pressure may be observed. The slight increase in blood pressure may be related to an increase in cardiac output and heart rate that has been seen in some animal preparations and is believed to be caused by an enhancement of sympathetic activity by these drugs. In addition, the direct vasoconstrictor action of local anesthetics on certain peripheral vascular beds at low concentrations may be responsible, in part, for a slight increase in systemic blood pressure. As the blood level of local anesthetic agents approaches toxic concentrations, a fall in blood pressure is usually the first sign of a systemic effect. The hypotension appears to be related to the negative inotropic action of these agents, which results in a decrease in cardiac output and stroke volume. The initial reduction in blood pressure is transient in nature and is spontaneously reversible in most patients. However, if the amount of local anesthetic administered is excessive, a profound and irreversible state of cardiovascular depression occurs. This is the result not only of the negative inotropic action of the local anesthetics but also of massive peripheral vasodilation. Local anesthetic toxicity is best avoided by administering these agents slowly into the epidural space or by the use of a fractionated dose technique, as described previously.

Treatment of central nervous system toxicity consists initially of maintaining a patent airway and assisting ventilation of the lungs with oxygen. Most convulsive reactions are of brief duration and terminate spontaneously. If convulsive activity persists for more than 1–2 minutes, therapy should be instituted. Central nervous system depressants, such as iv thiopental or diazepam, are most frequently employed to terminate convulsive activity. Succinylcholine has also been advocated as a means of controlling the muscular activity associated with convulsions. In addition, succinylcholine will facilitate endotracheal intubation in a convulsing patient in whom ventilation of the lungs cannot be adequately supported.

Hypotension caused by local anesthetic–induced toxicity is probably best treated with a drug like ephedrine that has positive inotropic activity and a peripheral vasoconstrictor action.

Local Tissue Toxicity

The potential of epidurally administered local anesthetics to cause localized nerve damage is very low. The accidental subarachnoid injection of high doses of local anesthetics may be of concern, since the spinal cord and spinal roots lack a connective tissue sheath. Most local anesthetics are free of local neural irritation in the concentrations employed for epidural anesthesia. Some concern has existed with regard to the local irritant properties of chloroprocaine owing to reports of prolonged sensory-motor deficits in patients following the accidental subarachnoid injection of large amounts of this local anesthetic.[138,139] Experimental studies have indicated that the combination of the low pH and sodium bisulfite in solutions of chloroprocaine may be responsible for the neurotoxic effects rather than the chloroprocaine itself.[140] It is obvious that epidural blockade should be performed with great care to avoid the accidental intrathecal injection of large amounts of local anesthetics. Again, a fractionated dose technique should preclude the intrathecal administration of large amounts of local anesthetics.

The sensory-motor deficits related to the use of chloroprocaine solutions containing sodium bisulfite have resulted in a change in the formulation of this anesthetic solution. The antioxidant, sodium bisulfite, has been replaced by ethylenediaminetetra-acetic acid (EDTA). This has led to reports of intense back pain following the epidural administration of relatively large volumes of chloroprocaine solution containing EDTA.[141] This phenomenon has been reported to occur primarily in ambulatory surgical patients and not in obstetric cases. The back pain may be related to the calcium binding properties of EDTA in the paraspinal muscles, resulting in severe muscle spasm and back pain. The pain is responsive to parenteral or epidural opiates. The intravenous administration of calcium was reported to decrease the incidence and severity of back pain.[142]

Technique-Related Complications

Hypotension. This is the most common cardiovascular complication of epidural anesthesia and results primarily from widespread sympathetic blockade. The hemodynamic effects of epidural blockade are similar to those previously described for spinal blockade. However, because of the slower onset of sympathetic blockade following epidurally administered local anesthetics, an excessive fall in arterial pressure is usually not seen in normovolemic patients. Epidural blockade to the T10 level seldom causes any decrease in arterial pressure. Blocks extending into the upper thoracic segments frequently result in a decrease in mean arterial pressure of no more than 10–20 mm Hg. The vasodilation below the level of sympathetic blockade is usually compensated for by vasoconstriction above the level of blockade, such that the decrease in blood pressure is relatively mild. On the other hand, an extremely high level of sympathetic blockade resulting in a reduction in cardiac output can lead to a profound fall in blood pressure. In addition, in hypovolemic patients or patients in whom inferior vena caval occlusion is present, epidural blockade can result in a severe degree of hypotension. As is the case with spinal blockade, patients should be kept supine or in a slightly head-down position in order to increase venous return and ensure an adequate cardiac output that will tend to prevent a marked fall in blood pressure.

The combined use of light general anesthesia and epidural blockade will generate a greater fall in blood pressure owing to the peripheral vasodilation produced by the epidural blockade and the negative inotropic action of the general anesthetic. However, in healthy patients, the decrease in blood pressure is usually well tolerated, unless the depth of general anesthesia is excessive.

Treatment of hypotension caused by sympathetic blockade is dependent on the degree of hypotension and the physical status of the patient. In most healthy patients, a fall of approximately 20 mm Hg in mean arterial pressure is usually well tolerated and may be beneficial in terms of decreasing blood loss. If the fall in blood pressure is excessive or occurs in patients with cardiovascular disease in whom it is important to maintain blood pressure, positioning of patients in a head-down position and administration of fluids are frequently adequate to reverse the hypotensive state. A marked fall in blood pressure owing to extensive sympathetic blockade may require pharmacologic intervention. If the extent of the sympathetic blockade is sufficiently great to cause a fall in heart rate, atropine should be administered to treat the bradycardia. In addition, the use of vasopressor agents may be required to reverse the profound state of hypotension. An intravenous infusion of an alpha-adrenergic receptor stimulant, such as phenylephrine, may be employed. Drugs such as ephedrine or mephentermine, which possess both alpha- and beta-receptor stimulating activity, may be of value. Some authors have advocated the intramuscular use of ephedrine prophylactically in order to prevent a decrease in blood pressure following the induction of epidural anesthesia. However, this is rarely necessary in healthy patients or if the dose of epidurally administered local anesthetic is controlled in order to avoid an excessive level of sympathetic blockade.

Ventilatory Complications. Epidural blockade rarely has any profound effect on ventilation. Even epidural blockade extending to the upper thoracic dermatome is usually not associated with a significant degree of ventilatory depression. Although high epidural blocks may result in paralysis of intercostal muscles, the diaphragm is usually able to function normally and achieve adequate ventilation of the lungs. In certain patients, such as the grossly obese, diaphragmatic activity may be inadequate, and assisted ventilation of the lungs is required.

Accidental Subdural or Subarachnoid Injections. Profound depression of ventilation following the performance of an epidural block is usually indicative of an accidental subdural or subarachnoid injection. The inadvertent administration of local anesthetics subdurally or intrathecally always represents a potential complication of epidural blockade. The hemodynamic and respiratory consequences of a high spinal blockade have been discussed previously. An accidental subdural injection would result in hemodynamic and ventilatory changes similar to those seen following an accidental high spinal blockade. However, the onset of hypotension and ventilatory depression following a subdural injection is usually slower than that observed following an accidental intrathecal injection. Treatment of hypotension or ventilatory depression caused by high accidental spinal blockade is the same as that described previously. The accidental intrathecal or subdural administration of local anesthetics is best prevented by the use of a fractional dose technique when performing an epidural blockade. Early signs of motor weakness, extensive spread of sensory anesthesia, and hypotension following the administration of 3–4 ml of local anesthetic solution are usually indicative of an inadvertent subarachnoid injection.

Dural Puncture and Postspinal Headache. Accidental puncture of the dura is always a potential risk when performing an epidural blockade. Spinal headache does not always occur following dural puncture with a 17- or 18-gauge epidural needle. In older patients in whom epidural anesthesia is performed, dural puncture is frequently not associated with the occurrence of a spinal headache. However, in younger patients and, in particular, pregnant patients, dural puncture during an attempted epidural block results in a high incidence of postspinal headache. Some authorities have advocated the immediate use of an epidural blood patch in such patients in whom dural puncture has occurred during an attempted epidural blockade. However, since the extent to which the dura has been punctured is unknown, and since not all patients develop a classic spinal headache, it is probably prudent to wait 12–24 hours postoperatively to determine if a spinal headache develops and then offer the patient the option of an epidural blood patch.

Neural Damage. Neurologic deficits may occur following epidural blockade, although the incidence of this problem is low. A review of seven epidural studies involving approximately 45,000 patients listed 40 cases of neurologic sequelae, 22 of which were simply identified as paresthesias.[126] Neurologic deficits are usually due to trauma, anterior spinal artery syndrome, or space-occupying lesions, such as a hematoma. The etiology and management of these neural injuries are similar to those described previously for spinal anesthesia. The concurrent use of epidural anesthesia and anticoagulants is a concern with regard to the possible dangers associated with the puncture of an epidural vein and the development of an epidural hematoma.[143] Epidural anesthesia should not be attempted in a patient who is fully anticoagulated or in patients in whom an abnormal coagulation profile or bleeding time is present. Anticoagulation of a patient following the placement of an epidural catheter does appear justified. Studies involving several thousand patients have been reported in which patients have been anticoagulated with heparin primarily for vascular surgical procedures following the placement of an epidural catheter and no epidural hematomas occurred.[144,145] Concern is frequently expressed with regard to patients in whom an epidural vein is punctured during an attempted epidural block and in whom heparinization is planned for the surgical procedure. Puncture of an epidural blood vessel should not be an automatic cause for cancellation of surgery or abandonment of the epidural technique. If heparinization is not accomplished until 30–60 minutes following the puncture of the epidural blood vessel, this should allow sufficient time for clot formation to occur at the site of the venous puncture. The use of minidose heparin or oral anticoagulants to prevent postoperative deep venous thrombosis may restrict the use of epidural anesthesia. However, reports exist in which epidural anesthesia has been employed in patients on oral anticoagulants without adverse complications.[144]

Nevertheless, the potential risk of an epidural hematoma should be fully explained to any patient in whom an epidural anesthetic is employed and in whom anticoagulant therapy is anticipated. In addition, these patients should be carefully monitored preoperatively to evaluate their coagulation profile and examined postoperatively to determine whether any signs of neurologic deficits related to a space-occupying lesion are present.

Catheter Complications. Insertion of plastic catheters into the epidural space is usually a simple and safe procedure. Complications related to catheter insertion may occur, although the incidence is very low. Catheters may be inserted directly into a blood vessel or, more rarely, may be placed into the subarachnoid space. Negative aspiration of blood is not a guarantee that a catheter has not been placed into an epidural vein. Thus, the use of an epidural test dose or a fractionated dose regimen is advocated in order to avoid the intravascular injection of an excessive dose of local anesthetic.

The most common concern associated with the use of an epidural catheter involves the breaking off of a segment of the catheter in the epidural space.[146] This usually occurs if an attempt is made to withdraw a catheter through the epidural needle. A catheter must never be withdrawn backward through the epidural needle. If it is not possible to advance the catheter into the epidural space, the needle and catheter should be withdrawn together and the procedure repeated at another interspace. If an epidural catheter is sheared, most authorities believe that it is best to inform the patient of this occurrence but indicate that no attempt should be made to retrieve the catheter segment. Catheter segments remaining in the epidural space are rarely associated with clinically significant problems. It has also been reported that epidural catheters can curl and turn on themselves in the epidural space and can actually form a knot, such that it may be difficult to remove them from the epidural space. This is an extremely rare occurrence and is usually due to attempts to advance an excessive length of catheter into the epidural space.[146] For this reason, catheters should never be advanced more than 2–3 cm into the epidural space.

The introduction of microcatheters for continuous spinal anesthesia has resulted in reports of sheared spinal catheters.[42] The tensile strength of the microcatheters varies considerably. In addition, these catheters may stretch and break if care is not taken during the removal process. The patient should be placed in the lateral decubitus position if any resistance or catheter stretching is noted during removal. In the case of a sheared spinal catheter, the same procedure is recommended as for a sheared epidural catheter.

CAUDAL ANESTHESIA

Caudal anesthesia is produced by placement of local anesthetic solution in the epidural space *via* a needle or catheter introduced through the sacral hiatus into the sacral canal. The patient may be positioned in either the lateral or the prone position, with the latter position preferred for palpating bony landmarks. The sacral hiatus and the adjacent sacral cornu are identified (usually about 5 cm from the tip of the coccyx in the midline), and an 18-gauge, 7-cm needle is inserted at a 45-degree angle into the sacral hiatus between the two cornua. The needle is advanced through the sacrococcygeal membrane until the sacrum is contacted. At this point, the needle is withdrawn a small distance and the angle is changed to 5–15 degrees before advancing the needle in the sacral canal for a distance of about 2 cm. Further advancement of the needle increases the risk of dural puncture because the dural sac typically extends to the level of S2. Aspiration tests are necessary to confirm the absence of cerebrospinal fluid or blood. A test dose of local anesthetic solution containing epinephrine is then injected. Approximately twice the dose of local anesthetic solution (3 ml of drug per spinal segment) is needed for caudal compared with lumbar epidural anesthesia because of the relatively large sacral canal and free leakage of solution through sacral foramina. Although infection is rare, the nearness of this approach to the rectum requires strict aseptic technique. In adults, most anesthesiologists prefer the lumbar rather than the caudal (sacral) approach to the epidural space because the former is a more predictable and easier technique to use.

Caudal anesthesia is becoming a popular technique for provision of anesthesia and postoperative analgesia in pediatric patients.[147] In contrast to in adults, the sacral hiatus is usually easy to locate in children (especially neonates), and local anesthetic dose requirements seem more predictable. The needle should not be advanced more than 1 cm into the sacral canal because the dural sac may extend more caudal in children compared with in adults.

REFERENCES

1. Koller K: Über die Verwendung des Cocain zur Anasthesirung am Auge. Wien Med Blatter 7:1352, 1884
2. Corning JL: Spinal anesthesia and local medication of the cord. NY J Med 42:483, 1885
3. Sicard A: Essais d'injections microbiennes toxiques et therapeutiques, par voie cephalo-racidenne. CR Soc Biol (Paris) 50:472, 1898
4. Bier A: Versüche über Cocainisirung des Ruckensmarkes. Deutsch Z Chir 51:361, 1899
5. Tait D, Caglieri G: Experimental and clinical notes on the subarachnoid space. Trans Med Soc Calif 35:6, 1900
6. Matas R: Report of successful spinal anesthesia. Medical news. JAMA 33:1650, 1899
7. Cathelin MF: Une novelle voie d'injection rachidienne. Methode des injections epidurales par le procede du canal sacre. Applications a l'homme. CR Soc Biol (Paris) 53:452, 1901
8. Pages F: Anesthesia metamerica. Rev Sanid Mil Madr 11:351, 1921
9. Dogliotti AM: Anesthesia. Chicago, SB Dubour, 1939
10. Carron H, Covino BG: Influence of anaesthetic procedures on surgical sequelae. Reg Anesth 7(suppl), 1982
11. Enqquist A, Brandt MR, Fernandes A et al: The blocking effect of epidural analgesia on the adrenocortical and hyperglycemic response to surgery. Acta Anaesthesiol Scand 21:330, 1977
12. Halter JB, Pflug AE: Relationship of impaired insulin secretion during surgical stress to anesthesia and catecholamine release. J Clin Endocrinol 51:1093, 1980
13. Kehlet H, Brandt MR, Prange Hanson A et al: Effect of epidural analgesia on metabolic profiles during and after surgery. Br J Surg 66:543, 1979
14. Kehlet H: Influence of regional anesthesia on postoperative morbidity. Ann Chir Gynaecol 73:171, 1984
15. Brandt MR, Kehlet H, Binder C et al: Effect of epidural analgesia on the glycoregulatory endocrine response to surgery. Clin Endocrinol 5:107, 1976
16. Brandt MR, Kehlet H, Faber O et al: C-peptide and insulin during blockade of the hyperglycemic response to surgery by epidural analgesia. Clin Endocrinol 6:167, 1977
17. Brandt MR, Kehlet H, Skovsted L et al: Rapid decrease in plasma-triiodothyronine during surgery and epidural analgesia independent of afferent neurogenic stimuli and of cortisol. Lancet 2:1333, 1976
18. Hallberg D, Oro L: Free fatty acids of plasma during spinal anaesthesia in man. Acta Med Scand 178:281, 1965
19. Keith I: Anaesthesia and blood loss in total hip replacement. Anaesthesia 32:444, 1977
20. Modig J, Hjelmstedt A, Sahlstedt B et al: Comparative influences of epidural and general anaesthesia on deep vein thrombosis and pulmonary embolism after total hip replacement. Acta Chir Scand 147:125, 1981
21. Modig J, Borg T, Karlstrom G et al: Thromboembolism after total hip replacement: Role of epidural and general anesthesia. Anesth Analg 62:174, 1983
22. Hendolin H, Mattila MAK, Poikolainen E: The effect of lumbar epidural analgesia on the development of deep vein thrombosis of the legs after open prostatectomy. Acta Chir Scand 147:425, 1981
23. McKenzie PJ, Wishart HY, Dewar MS et al: Comparison of the effects of spinal anaesthesia and general anaesthesia on postoperative oxygenation and perioperative mortality. Br J Anaesth 52:49, 1980
24. Hendolin H, Tuppurainen T, Lahtinen J: Thoracic epidural analgesia and deep vein thrombosis in cholecystectomized patients. Acta Chir Scand 148:405, 1982
25. Mellbring G, Dahlgren S, Reiz S et al: Thromboembolic complications after major abdominal surgery: Effect of thoracic epidural analgesia. Acta Chir Scand 149:263, 1983
26. Davis FM, Laurenson VG: Spinal anaesthesia or general anaesthesia for emergency hip surgery in elderly patients. Anaesth Intensive Care 9:352, 1981
27. Hjortso NC, Andersen T, Froosig F et al: A controlled study of the effect of epidural analgesia with local anaesthetics and morphine on morbidity after abdominal surgery. Acta Anaesthesiol Scand 29:790, 1985
28. Modig J, Borg T, Bagge L et al: Role of extradural and of general anaesthesia in fibrinolysis and coagulation after total hip replacement. Br J Anaesth 55:625, 1983
29. Simpson PJ, Radford SG, Forster SJ et al: The fibrinolytic effects of anaesthesia. Anaesthesia 37:3, 1982
30. Cuschieri RJ, Morran CG, Howie JC et al: Postoperative pain and pulmonary complications: Comparison of three analgesic regimens. Br J Surg 72:495, 1985
31. Reiz S, Balfors E, Sorenson MB et al: Coronary hemodynamic effects of general anesthesia and surgery: Modification by epidural analgesia in patients with ischemic heart disease. Reg Anesth 7(suppl):S8, 1982
32. Baron JF, Coriat P, Mundler O et al: Left ventricular global and regional function during lumbar epidural anesthesia in patients with and without angina pectoris. Influence of volume loading. Anesthesiology 66:621, 1987
33. Blomberg S, Emanuelsson H, Ricksten SE: Thoracic epidural anesthesia and central hemodynamics in patients with unstable angina pectoris. Anesth Analg 69:558, 1989
34. Blomberg S, Emanuelsson H, Kvist H et al: Effects of thoracic epidural anesthesia on coronary arteries and arterioles in patients with coronary artery disease. Anesthesiology 73:840, 1990
35. McLaren AD: Mortality studies. A review. Reg Anaesth 7(suppl):S192, 1982
36. McKenzie PJ, Wishart HY, Dewer MS et al: Long-term outcome after repair of the fractured neck of the femur. Br J Anaesth 56:581, 1984
37. Valentin N, Lomholt B, Jensen JS et al: Spinal or general anaesthesia for surgery of the fractured hip? A prospective study of mortality in 578 patients. Br J Anaesth 58:284, 1986
38. Yeager MP, Glass DD, Neff RH et al: Epidural anesthesia and analgesia in high-risk surgical patients. Anesthesiology 66:729, 1987
39. Soni V, Peeters C, Covino B: Value and limitations of test dose prior to epidural anesthesia. Reg Anesth 6:23, 1981
40. Vandam LD, Dripps RD: Long term follow up of patients who received 10,098 spinal anesthetics: III. Syndrome of decreased intracranial pressure (headache and occular and auditory difficulties). JAMA 161:586, 1956
41. Bromage PR: Neurologic complications of regional anesthesia for obstetrics. In Shnider SM, Levinson G (eds): Anesthesia for Obstetrics, 2nd ed, p 317. Baltimore, Williams and Wilkins, 1987
42. Hurley RJ, Lambert DH: Continuous spinal anesthesia with a microcatheter technique: Preliminary experience. Anesth Analg 70:97, 1990

43. Gasser HS, Erlanger J: The role of fiber size in establishment of a nerve block by pressure or cocaine. Am J Physiol 88:581, 1929

44. Gissen AJ, Covino BG, Gregus J: Differential sensitivities of mammalian nerve fibers to local anesthetic agents. Anesthesiology 53:467, 1980

45. Shantha TR, Evans JA: The relationship of epidural anesthesia to neural membranes and arachnoid villi. Anesthesiology 37:543, 1972

46. Bromage PR, Joyal AC, Binney JC: Local anesthetic drugs. Penetration from the spinal extradural space into the neuraxis. Science 140:392, 1963

47. Galindo A, Hernandez J, Benavides O et al: Quality of spinal extradural anesthesia: The influence of spinal nerve root diameter. Br J Anaesth 47:41, 1975

48. Greene NM: The area of differential block during spinal anesthesia with hyperbaric tetracaine. Anesthesiology 19:45, 1958

49. Chamberlain DP, Chamberlain BDL: Changes in skin temperature of the trunk and their relationship to sympathetic blockade during spinal anesthesia. Anesthesiology 65:139, 1986

50. Ward RJ, Bonica JJ, Freund FG et al: Epidural and subarachnoid anesthesia: Cardiovascular and respiratory effects: JAMA 191:275, 1965

51. Greene NM: Physiology of Spinal Anesthesia, 3rd ed, p 95. Baltimore, Williams & Wilkins, 1981

52. Askrog VF, Smith TC, Eckenhoff JE: Changes in pulmonary ventilation during spinal anesthesia. Surg Gynecol Obstet 119:563, 1964

53. DeJong RH: Arterial carbon dioxide and oxygen tensions during spinal block. JAMA 191:608, 1965

54. Egbert LD, Tamersoy K, Deas TC: Pulmonary function during spinal anesthesia: The mechanism of cough depression. Anesthesiology 22:882, 1961

55. Kennedy WF Jr, Sawyer TK, Gerbenshagen HJ et al: Simultaneous systemic cardiovascular and renal hemodynamic measurements during high spinal anesthesia in man. Acta Anaesthesiol Scand (suppl) 37:163, 1970

56. Greene NM, Bunker JP, Kerr WS et al: Hypotensive spinal anesthesia: Respiratory, metabolic, hepatic, renal and cerebral effects. Ann Surg 140:641, 1954

57. Kennedy WF Jr, Everett GB, Cobb LA et al: Simultaneous systemic and hepatic hemodynamic measurements during high spinal anesthesia in normal man. Anesth Analg 49:1016, 1970

58. Bonica JJ, Berges PU, Morikawa K: Circulatory effects of peridural block: I. Effect of level of analgesia and dose of lidocaine. Anesthesiology 33:619, 1971

59. Bonica JJ, Akamatsu TJ, Berges PU et al: Circulatory effects of peridural block: II. Effect of epinephrine. Anesthesiology 34:514, 1972

60. Bonica JJ, Kennedy WF, Akamatsu TJ et al: Circulatory effects of peridural block: III. Effects of acute blood loss. Anesthesiology 36:219, 1972

61. Sivarajan M, Amory DW, Lindbloom LE: Systemic and regional blood flow during epidural anesthesia without epinephrine in the rhesus monkey. Anesthesiology 45:300, 1976

62. Kennedy WF, Sawyer TK, Gerbershagen HU et al: Systemic cardiovascular and renal hemodynamic alterations during peridural anesthesia in normal man. Anesthesiology 31:414, 1969

63. Stanton-Hicks M, Murphy TM, Bonica JJ et al: Effects of peridural block: V. Properties, circulatory effects, and blood levels of etidocaine and lidocaine. Anesthesiology 42:398, 1975

64. Greene NM: Distribution of local anesthetic solutions within the subarachnoid space. Anesth Analg 64:715, 1985

65. Wildsmith JAW, McLure JH, Brown WT et al: Effects of posture on the spread of isobaric and hyperbaric amethocaine. Br J Anaesth 53:273, 1981

66. Levin E, Muravchick S, Gold MI: Density of normal human cerebrospinal fluid and tetracaine solutions. Anesth Analg 60:814, 1981

67. Ernst EA: In-vitro changes of osmolality and density of spinal anesthetic solutions. Anesthesiology 29:104, 1968

68. Lambert DH, Covino BG: Hyperbaric, hypobaric and isobaric spinal anesthesia. Res Staff Phys 33:79, 1987

69. Armstrong IR, Littlewood DG, Chambers WA: Spinal anesthesia with tetracaine—effect of added vasoconstrictors. Anesth Analg 62:793, 1983

70. Chambers WA, Littlewood DG, Scott DB: Spinal anesthesia with hyperbaric bupivacaine: Effect of added vasoconstrictors. Anesth Analg 61:49, 1982

71. Concepcion M, Lambert DH, Welch KA et al: Tourniquet pain during spinal anesthesia: A comparison of plain solutions of tetracaine and bupivacaine. Anesth Analg 67:828, 1988

72. Stewart A, Lambert DH, Concepcion M et al: Decreased incidence of tourniquet pain during spinal anesthesia with bupivacaine: A possible explanation. Anesth Analg 67:833, 1988

73. Chambers WA, Littlewood DG, Logan MR et al: Effect of added epinephrine on spinal anesthesia with lidocaine. Anesth Analg 60:417, 1981

74. Lawrence VS, Rich CR, Magitsky L et al: Spinal anesthesia with isobaric lidocaine 2% and the effect of phenylephrine. Reg Anesth 9:17, 1984

75. Racle JP, Benkhadra A, Poy JY et al: Effect of increasing amounts of epinephrine during isobaric bupivacaine spinal anesthesia in elderly patients. Anesth Analg 66:882, 1987

76. Vaida GT, Moss P, Capan LM et al: Prolongation of lidocaine spinal anesthesia with phenylephrine. Anesth Analg 65:781, 1986

77. Moore DC, Chadwick HS, Ready LB: Epinephrine prolongs lidocaine spinal: Pain in the operative site the most accurate method of determining local anesthetic duration. Anesthesiology 67:416, 1987

78. Kozody R, Ong B, Palahniuk RJ et al: Subarachnoid bupivacaine decreases spinal cord blood flow in dogs. Can Anaesth Soc J 32:216, 1985

79. Kozody R, Palahniuk RJ, Biehl DR: Spinal cord blood flow following subarachnoid lidocaine. Can Anaesth Soc J 32:472, 1985

80. Kozody R, Palahniuk RJ, Cumming MO: Spinal cord blood flow following subarachnoid tetracaine. Can Anaesth Soc J 32:23, 1985

81. Collins JG, Kitahata LM, Matsumoto M et al: Spinally administered epinephrine suppresses noxiously evoked activity of WDR neurons in the dorsal horn of the spinal cord. Anesthesiology 60:269, 1984

82. Coombs DW, Saunders RL, Lachance D et al: Intrathecal morphine tolerance: Use of intrathecal clonidine, DADLE, and intraventricular morphine. Anesthesiology 62:358, 1985

83. Nishikawa T, Dohi S: Clinical evaluation of clonidine added to lidocaine solution for epidural anesthesia. Anesthesiology 73:853, 1990

84. Covino BG, Scott DB: Handbook of Epidural Anaesthesia and Analgesia, p 70. Orlando, Grune & Stratton, 1985

85. Concepcion M, Arthur GR, Steele SM et al: A new local anesthetic, ropivacaine. Its epidural effects in humans. Anesth Analg 70:80, 1990

86. Brown DL, Carpenter RL, Thompson GE: Comparison of 0.5% bupivacaine for epidural anesthesia in patients undergoing lower-extremity surgery. Anesthesiology 72:633, 1990

87. Concepcion M, Steele S, Bader A, Arthur R: Comparison of 0.75% ropivacaine and 0.75% bupivacaine for epidural anesthesia. Anesthesiology 73:A791, 1990

88. Erdermir HA, Soper LE, Sweet RB: Studies of the factors affecting peridural anesthesia. Anesth Analg 44:400, 1965

89. Covino BG, Bush DF: Clinical evaluation of local anaesthetic agents. Br J Anaesth (suppl) 47:289, 1975

90. Littlewood DG, Buckley P, Covino BG et al: Comparative study of various local anesthetic solutions in block in labour. Br J Anaesth 51:47S, 1979

91. Stanton-Hicks M, Berges PU, Bonica JJ: Circulatory effects of peridural block: IV. Comparison of the effects of epinephrine and phenylephrine. Anesthesiology 39:308, 1973

92. Sinclair CJ, Scott DB: Comparison of bupivacaine and etidocaine in extradural blockade. Br J Anaesth 56:147, 1984

93. Kier L: Continuous epidural analgesia in prostatectomy: Comparison of bupivacaine with and without epinephrine. Acta Anaesthesiol Scand 18:1, 1974

94. Bromage PR: Spread of analgesic solutions in the epidural

space and their site of action: A statistical study. Br J Anaesth 34:161, 1962

95. Nishimura N, Kitahara T, Kusakafe T: The spread of lidocaine and I131 solution in the epidural space. Anesthesiology 20: 785, 1959

96. Park MY, Hagins FM, Massengale MD et al: The sitting position and anesthetic spread in the epidural space. Anesth Analg 63:863, 1984

97. Bromage PR: Aging and epidural dose requirements. Br J Anaesth 41:1016, 1969

98. Park WY, Massengale M, Kim S-I et al: Age and the spread of local anesthetic solutions in the epidural space. Anesth Analg 59:768, 1980

99. Hirabayashi Y, Shimizu R, Matsuda I, Inoue S: Effect of extradural compliance and resistance on spread of extradural analgesia. Br J Anaesth 65:508, 1990

100. Hehre FW, Moyes AZ, Senfield RM et al: Continuous lumbar peridural anesthesia in obstetrics: II. Use of minimal amounts of local anesthetics during labor. Anesth Analg 44:89, 1965

101. Fagraeus L, Urban BJ, Bromage PR: Spread of epidural analgesia in early pregnancy. Anesthesiology 58:184, 1983

102. Datta S, Lambert DH, Gregus J et al: Differential sensitivities of mammalian nerve fibers during pregnancy. Anesth Analg 62:1070, 1983

103. Flanagan HL, Datta S, Lambert DH et al: Effect of pregnancy on bupivacaine-induced conduction blockade in the isolated rabbit vagus nerve. Anesth Analg 66:123, 1987

104. Greene NM: Present concepts of spinal anesthesia. ASA Refresher Courses in Anesthesiology 7:131, 1979

105. Butterworth JF IV, Austin JC, Johnson MD et al: Effect of total spinal anesthesia on arterial and venous responses to dopamine and dobutamine. Anesth Analg 66:209, 1987

106. Butterworth JF IV, Piccione W, Berrizbeitia LD et al: Augmentation of venous return by adrenergic agonist during spinal anesthesia. Anesth Analg 65:612, 1986

107. Greene NM: Abbott Lecture. Perspectives in spinal anesthesia. Reg Anesth 7:55, 1982

108. Gilman AG, Goodman LS, Gilman A: The Pharmacologic Basis of Therapeutics, 6th ed, p 163. New York, Macmillan, 1980

109. Gielen M: Post dural puncture headache (PDPH): A review. Reg Anesth 14:101, 1989

110. Mihic DN: Postspinal headache and relationship of needle bevel to longitudinal dural fibers. Reg Anesth 10:76, 1985

111. Ready LB, Cuplin S, Haschke RH, Nessly M: Spinal needle determinants of rate of transdural fluid leak. Anesth Analg 69:457, 1989

112. Naulty JS, Hertwig L, Hunt CO et al: Influence of local anesthetic solution on postdural puncture headache. Anesthesiology 72:450, 1990

113. Denny N, Masters RW, Pearson D et al: Postdural puncture headache after continuous spinal anesthesia. Anesth Analg 77:791, 1987

114. Guiffrida JG, Bizzari DV, Masi R et al: Continuous procaine spinal anesthesia for cesarean section. Anesth Analg 51:117, 1972

115. Norris MD, Leighton GL: Continuous spinal analgesia after accidental dural puncture in parturients. Society of Obstetric Anesthesia and Perinatology Annual Meeting, Madison, Wisconsin, 1990

116. Zuspan FP: Treatment of postpartum post spinal headache. Obstet Gynecol 16:1, 1960

117. Szeinfeld M, Ihmeidan IH, Moser MM et al: Epidural blood patch: Evaluation of the volume and spread of blood injected into the epidural space. Anesthesiology 64:820, 1986

118. Crawford JS: Prevention of headache consequent on dural puncture. Br J Anaesth 44:598, 1972

119. Shnider SM, Levinson G: Anesthesia for cesarean section. In Shnider SM, Levinson G (eds): Anesthesia for Obstetrics, p 165. Baltimore, Williams & Wilkins, 1987

120. Sechzer PH, Abel L: Post-spinal anesthesia headache treated

with caffeine. Evaluation with demand method. Part I. Curr Ther Res 24:307, 1978

121. Sechzer PH: Post-spinal anesthesia headache treated with caffeine. Part II: Intracranial vascular distention, a key factor. Curr Ther Res 26:440, 1979

122. Jarvis AP, Greenawalt JW, Fagraeus L: Intravenous caffeine for post-dural puncture headache. Reg Anesth 11:42, 1986

123. Camann WR, Murray RS, Mushlin PS et al: Effects of oral caffeine on postdural puncture headache: A double-blind placebo controlled trial. Anesth Analg 70:181, 1990

124. Datta S, Alper MH, Ostheimer GO et al: Method of ephedrine administration and nausea and hypotension during spinal anesthesia for cesarean section. Anesthesiology 56:68, 1982

125. Santos A, Datta S: Prophylactic use of droperidol for control of nausea and vomiting during spinal anesthesia for cesarean section. Anesth Analg 63:85, 1984

126. Kane RE: Neurologic deficits following epidural or spinal anesthesia. Anesth Analg 60:150, 1981

127. Vandam LD, Dripps RD: Exacerbation of pre-existing neurologic disease after spinal anesthesia. N Engl J Med 255:843, 1956

128. Dripps RD, Vandam LD: Hazards of lumbar puncture. JAMA 147:1118, 1951

129. Garfield JM, Andriole GL, Vetto JT et al: Prolonged diabetes insipidus subsequent to an episode of chemical meningitis. Anesthesiology 64:253, 1986

130. Greene NM: Neurological sequelae of spinal anesthesia. Anesthesiology 22:682, 1961

131. Rigler ML, Drasner K, Krejcie TC: Cauda equina syndrome after continuous spinal anesthesia. Anesth Analg 72:275, 1991

132. Mayumi T, Dohi S, Takahashi T: Plasma concentrations of lidocaine associated with cervical, thoracic and lumbar epidural anesthesia. Anesth Analg 62:578, 1983

133. Braid DP, Scott DB: The systemic absorption of local analgesic drugs. Br J Anaesth 37:394, 1965

134. Lund PC, Bush DF, Covino BG: Determinants of etidocaine concentration in the blood. Anesthesiology 42:497, 1975

135. Abdel-Salam AR, Vonwiller JB, Scott DB: Evaluation of etidocaine in extradural block. Br J Anaesth 47:1081, 1975

136. Tucker GT, Mather LE: Clinical pharmacokinetics of local anaesthetics. Clin Pharmacokinet 4:241, 1979

137. Covino BG: Toxicity of local anesthetics. Adv Anesth 3:37, 1986

138. Ravindran RS, Bond VK, Tasch MD et al: Prolonged neural blockade following regional analgesia with 2-chloroprocaine. Anesth Analg 58:447, 1980

139. Reisner LS, Hochman BN, Plumer MH: Persistent neurological deficit and adhesive arachnoiditis following intrathecal 2-chloroprocaine injection. Anesth Analg 58:452, 1980

140. Gissen AJ, Datta S, Lambert D: The chloroprocaine controversy: II. Is chloroprocaine neurotoxic? Reg Anesth 9:135, 1984

141. Hynson JM, Sessler DI, Glosten B: Back pain in volunteers after epidural anesthesia with chloroprocaine. Anesth Analg 72:253, 1991

142. Dirkes J: Treatment of Nesacaine-MPF-induced back pain with calcium chloride (letter). Anesth Analg 70:463, 1990

143. Varkey GP, Brindle GF: Peridural anaesthesia and anticoagulant therapy. Can Anaesth Soc J 21:106, 1974

144. Odoom JA, Sih IL: Epidural analgesia and anticoagulation therapy. Experience with one thousand cases of continuous epidurals. Anaesthesia 38:254, 1983

145. Rao TLK, El-Etr AA: Anticoagulation following placement of epidural and subarachnoid catheters: An evaluation of neurologic sequelae. Anesthesiology 55:618, 1981

146. Bromage PR: Epidural Analgesia, p 664. Philadelphia, WB Saunders, 1978

147. Broadman LM: Regional anesthesia for the pediatric outpatient. Anesth Clin NA 5:53, 1987

31

Michael F. Mulroy

Peripheral Nerve Blockade

GENERAL PRINCIPLES

Regional anesthesia of the extremities and of the trunk is a useful alternative to general anesthesia in many situations. Regional techniques have attracted renewed interest because of awareness of their salutary role in reducing the stress response to anesthesia and surgery,[1] in reducing postoperative complication rates,[2] and for their potential in improving outpatient anesthesia recovery.[3] Regional techniques are also the most favored choice of anesthesia by anesthesiologists,[4] but their application is often limited by inconsistent teaching in our residency training programs.[5] They are not applicable for every patient or procedure, but familiarity with the techniques described in this chapter and in Chapter 30 will broaden the alternatives we have to offer patients. The specific advantages of regional techniques are mentioned briefly as appropriate in this chapter but are discussed in greater detail in chapters relating to specific surgical situations. Some aspects of the selection of drugs and equipment and the preparation, sedation, and monitoring of patients must be modified when dealing with regional anesthesia and are discussed before the description of specific techniques.

Local Anesthetic Drug Selection and Doses

The pharmacology of local anesthetics is reviewed at length in Chapter 20. A few points deserve emphasis, particularly in regard to peripheral nerve blockade. Although high concentrations of drug are needed to produce anesthesia in the epidural space, lower concentrations (e.g., 1% lidocaine, 0.25% or 0.5% bupivacaine) are more appropriate on peripheral nerves because of concerns about local and systemic toxicity. Local toxicity of these anesthetics appears to be concentration-dependent[6,7] (unless injected directly intraneurally); thus, high concentrations are best avoided. Lower concentrations are also indicated because larger volumes are often required to anesthetize poorly localized peripheral nerves or to block a series of nerves (such as the intercostals). The use of a high-concentration solution presents the patient with a high total milligram dose of local anesthetic, which may produce toxic blood levels. In simplest terms, one can use twice as much 1% lidocaine as 2%

lidocaine before reaching the same level of concern about toxicity.[8] For both of these reasons, high concentrations are best avoided in peripheral nerve blockade.

The absorption of drug and the duration of anesthesia vary with the dose, drug, location injected, and presence of vasoconstrictors. The anesthesiologist must remain aware that the highest blood levels of local anesthetic occur after intercostal blockade, followed by epidural, caudal, and brachial plexus blockade. Similarly, the duration is dependent upon the blood supply of the area of injection. Equivalent doses of local anesthetic may produce only 3 to 4 hours of anesthesia in the epidural space but 24 to 36 hours on the sciatic nerve. Care should be taken in choosing drugs of appropriate concentration, duration, and total dose. Specific comments are made in conjunction with each of the techniques described, but familiarity with the material and tables in Chapter 20 is needed for appropriate choices. In general, the addition of epinephrine 1:200,000 is advantageous in prolonging the duration of blockade and in reducing the systemic blood levels of local anesthetic. Its use is not appropriate in the vicinity of "terminal" blood vessels, such as in the digits or penis, or when using an intravenous regional technique, but generally all the recommended doses and drugs in this chapter include the addition of epinephrine to the solution.

Nerve Localization

A few general principles apply to methods of nerve localization. The blockade techniques associated with reliable *proximity of nerves to bones or arteries* are the easiest technically to perform (e.g., epidural, intercostal, axillary). Less reliable landmarks, such as the psoas compartment or obturator foramen, require either large volumes of local anesthetic solution or the establishment of a distinct paresthesia of the desired nerve to provide adequate anesthesia. *Paresthesias* have been recommended as the ultimate sign of successful localization, and the older dictum of "no paresthesia, no anesthesia" has merit. Nevertheless, there are some potential problems associated with this technique. Of greatest concern is the potential for intraneural injection if paresthesias are obtained. This is usually signaled by a complaint from the patient of a "cramping" or "aching" pain during the initial injection. If this occurs, the needle should be immediately withdrawn by a few millimeters and a small test injection repeated. Even without intraneural injection, residual neuropathy of peripheral nerves appears more likely if paresthesias are obtained. Selander et al[9] have reported a 2.8% incidence of residual ulnar neuropathy when paresthesias were used to locate nerves compared with a 0.8% incidence with other techniques of axillary blockade. Although careful technique and attention to needle design (see below) and drugs (see Chapter 20) may reduce this, caution should be taken when using paresthesias for nerve localization. A third problem with this technique is the inevitable discomfort associated with it; patient education and sedation must be handled appropriately (see below).

One alternative method for nerve localization is the use of a *nerve stimulator*. This is based on the observation that a low-current electrical impulse applied to a peripheral nerve will produce stimulation of the motor fibers and, thus, will identify the proximity of the nerve without actual needle contact or patient discomfort (or cooperation). This technique is particularly suited to the patient who is uncooperative as a result of inebriation or heavy sedation. Since the nerve stimulator does not actually have to contact the nerve to produce a motor response, its use may reduce the chance for nerve injury. Its use does not improve the success rate of regional anesthesia in a training program,[10] since a familiarity with the anatomy and the techniques is necessary to bring the needle into proximity with the nerve. Nevertheless, this is a promising adjunct to regional anesthesia, and some comments about appropriate use of these devices are warranted.

The ideal stimulator should have a variable amperage output.[11] This allows a high current to be delivered in the exploration phase and then a progressively lower current to document proximity of the nerve. Whereas 10 mA can be used to produce the first motor twitch, actual injection of anesthetic should be delayed until stimulation is produced by as little as 0.1 mA. At that point, 2–3 ml of local anesthetic should be sufficient to abolish motor twitch and indicates that it is appropriate to inject the remainder of the proposed dose. The accuracy of the localization can be improved by the use of insulated needles. A plastic sheath along the shaft allows the current flow to be concentrated at the tip and is more likely to produce stimulation only when the tip is near the nerve fiber rather than after the tip has moved past its target.[12] Current flow can also be improved by using the positive (red) pole of the stimulator as the ground (or reference) electrode and the negative (black) lead as the connection to the needle itself. Despite these steps the stimulator is still only an adjunct to nerve localization and not a reliable substitute for good technique. Its potential advantages must be weighed against the small amount of extra time involved in its use and the usual requirement for an assistant to operate the machine while the anesthesiologist performs the actual blockade.

Equipment

In addition to the nerve stimulator, some other items of regional blockade equipment deserve general comment. The most frequent discussion in this regard is the debate over disposable *versus* reusable *trays*. This is a matter of personal preference and of economy. If a large volume of regional anesthetics is performed in an institution, the cost of maintenance of trays (technician time and sterilization) will be less than the use of disposable equipment.[13] Reusable

trays also allow the department to select high-quality needles and syringes to meet their specifications. Manufacturers usually do not produce disposable equipment to the same high tolerances that characterize reusable instruments. On the other hand, there are a large number of quality disposable kits available on the market today, and many of the major manufacturers will customize their packages at the request of large institutions willing to commit to purchasing a sufficient volume. The use of disposable trays also provides the advantage of placing the burden of sterilization on the manufacturer, although the liability for checking the sterility of contents always remains with the user. In the final analysis, cost is a major factor, but personal choice is usually the critical element.

For greater safety and efficacy, the *needles* used for regional techniques require some modifications from the standard injection needles (Fig. 31-1). First, for most cases of peripheral blockade, the "short bevel" or "B bevel" is used. This shorter angulation of the bevel (16–20 degrees vs conventional 12–13 degrees) was introduced by Selander et al[14] and has been shown to produce less injury to nerves, perhaps by pushing the nerve away rather than piercing it when contact is made. Other modifications, such as the "pencil point"–insulated needle, have also been introduced in attempts to reduce nerve injury. Another feature of regional blockade needles is the addition of a "security bead" to the shaft. This small bead is added approximately 6 mm from the juncture of the shaft and the hub and prevents the shaft of the needle from retracting below the skin in the event that it becomes separated from the hub. These two modifications are useful features for peripheral nerve blockade. In addition, the regional anesthesiologist should have an assortment of needle sizes and lengths available for various types of blockade.

Special *syringes* are also useful for performing peripheral nerve blockades. Although glass syringes are often preferred for epidural techniques, the loss of resistance is rarely needed in peripheral blockade. Plastic or glass may be equally useful. With respect to size, a 10-ml syringe is usually a good compromise. Large volumes are usually required for peripheral nerve blockade, so that 3-ml and 5-ml syr-

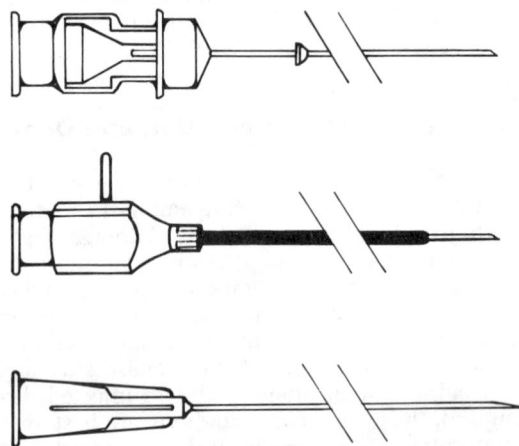

Figure 31-1. Regional anesthesia needles. Characteristic features of needles used for peripheral nerve blockade include the "security bead" on the shaft just below its juncture with the hub (*top*) and the shorter bevel angle compared with standard Quincke-type needle points (*bottom*). Further modifications to enhance the use of a nerve stimulator include the attachment prong for the electrode and the insulated shaft (*middle*).

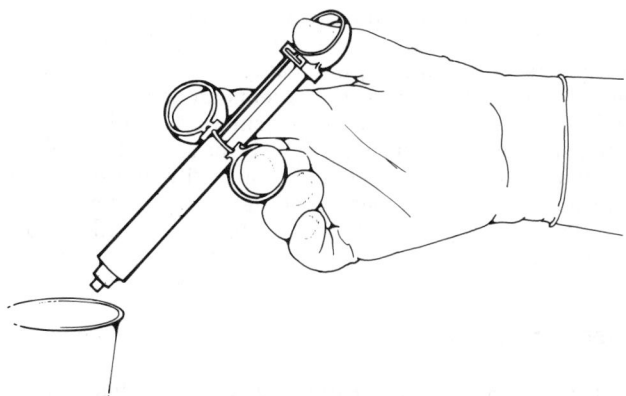

Figure 31-2. The three-ring ("control") syringe. Use of this adaptation to the plunger of a standard 10-ml syringe allows greater control of injection, easier aspiration, and the opportunity to refill the syringe with one hand. Plastic adapters are available for disposable syringes as demonstrated; glass syringes are supplied with a metal plunger and ring attached. (Reproduced with permission from Mulroy M: Handbook of Regional Anesthesia. Boston, Little, Brown, 1989.)

inges are rarely adequate. Larger than 10-ml volume often presents such bulk and weight that fine control is hampered. If a larger syringe is used, it is usually advisable to have an assistant manipulate the syringe and have it attached to the needle by a short length of extension tubing. The use of finger rings (the "control syringe") is helpful in controlling injection and allowing the operator to refill the syringe with one hand (Fig. 31-2). Luer-Lok adaptors for the syringe-hub connection are also advantageous. Although friction fittings produce tight seals, the amount of force required for attaching or removing the syringe may displace a needle that has been meticulously maneuvered into the appropriate close contact with a nerve.

The selection of *antiseptic solutions* is usually a local preference. Organic iodine preparations are the current standard for skin asepsis. They are usually nonirritating to tissues and carry the added advantage of a distinct color. Colorless preparation solutions are dangerous because of the possibility of confusion with (or contamination of) local anesthetic solutions. Colored alcohol solutions are acceptable skin cleansers for many of the simple infiltrations that do not require extensive preparation. For major deep blockade, a wide area of skin preparation is more desirable, and the borders of the clean area can be extended by draping on four sides with sterile towels. Regional anesthesia does not require the same degree of sterile preparation and gowning as indicated for surgery, but strict attention to asepsis is desirable to reduce the chance of infection.

Common Complications

Although specific complications of each of the individual techniques are discussed in the following sections, there are a few recurrent common problems of peripheral nerve blockade that merit mention. *Systemic toxicity of local anesthetics* is the most serious concern. This syndrome, as well as the problems of allergy and other unique toxicities, is addressed in Chapter 20. Central nervous system excitation and myocardial depression are the two most common hazards associated with high blood levels of local anesthetics. No peripheral nerve blockade using significant quanti-

ties of local anesthetic should be performed without appropriate resuscitation equipment immediately available. This includes blockades using small quantities of anesthetic but near cerebral vessels, such as stellate ganglion or cervical plexus blockade. With peripheral nerve blockade, careful use of a test dose and small incremental injections are needed if intravascular injection is a risk. Although attention is usually focused on this possibility, toxicity can also occur owing to slow absorption of high doses. Patients should be observed carefully for 20–30 minutes following injection, since peak levels occur at this time.

Peripheral *neuropathy* usually results from intraneural local anesthetic injection or needle trauma, although it should be kept in mind that there are other causes.[15] Careful attention should be paid to positioning the patient with numb extremities. Postoperative follow-up is important in confirming that neurologic function has returned to normal. If a deficit is detected, early neurologic assessment is critical in determining whether a pre-existent neuropathy was involved.[16] Fortunately, most of these syndromes resolve uneventfully, but full recovery of some peripheral injuries requires several months as a result of slow regeneration of injured peripheral nerves. Sympathetic concern and involvement of the anesthesiologist in arranging physical therapy during recovery help reduce patient dissatisfaction.

Other minor complications such as *pain at the site of injection* and local *hematoma* formation are not uncommon but are usually of short duration and respond to reassurance by the anesthesiologist. Hematoma around a peripheral nerve is not of the same significance as that in the epidural or subarachnoid space. Again, expressed concern and help with local therapy and analgesics alleviate patient dissatisfaction.

PATIENT PREPARATION

Patient Selection

In general, all patients scheduled for extremity, thoracic, abdominal, or perineal surgery should be considered candidates for a regional anesthetic technique. This can be used as the only anesthetic, as a supplement to provide analgesia and muscle relaxation along with general anesthesia, or as the initial step for provision of prolonged postoperative analgesia such as with intercostal blockade or continuous epidural anesthesia. *Patient refusal* can often be an impediment to regional anesthesia, although this is frequently a "relative" refusal. Often the patient's real objections to "being awake" or "being aware" can be managed by the use of sedatives and amnestic drugs. True unwavering refusal of "any needles" is a contraindication to regional anesthesia, although gentle attempts at patient education should be offered. Other contraindications include local *infection* and perhaps systemic *coagulopathy*. The presence of pre-existing *neurologic disease* is often discussed. Some data are available in the case of spinal anesthesia, but the use of peripheral nerve blockade in this situation is unclear. A classic example is whether an arm blockade should be used for a scheduled ulnar nerve transposition at the elbow. Although some physicians will avoid any procedure that may confuse the picture of postoperative neuropathy, others believe that if there is a clear difference in the potential injury and the pre-existent disease, regional techniques are appropriate. There are no clear answers in this regard, and full patient education and cooperation are most appropriate. Finally, the level of *patient anxiety* is an important consideration. Extreme apprehension regarding surgery will necessitate heavy sedation, and the advantages of regional anesthesia in providing rapid recovery, alertness, and protection of airway reflexes may be negated. The use of regional anesthesia in these situations is a matter of judgment and experience.

Premedication and Sedation

The best preparation for a regional technique is careful patient education. Calm, gentle explanation of the technique as it is performed will reduce most patient anxiety to a manageable level. In most cases, however, supplemental medication is also useful. In addition to the general comments about premedication discussed in earlier chapters, regional anesthesia techniques have some special requirements. First, sedation must be adjusted to the required level of patient cooperation. If paresthesias are to be sought, medication must be light enough to allow patient identification and reporting of nerve contact. Although a mild dose of opioid (50–100 μg of fentanyl or equivalent) will help ease the discomfort of nerve localization, patient awareness must be maintained. This does not preclude the use of an amnestic agent, and midazolam in 1–3 mg doses may provide excellent amnesia at levels of consciousness that still allow cooperation. This is also an excellent supplement in the outpatient setting, where short duration of effect is desired. If paresthesias are not needed, as in intercostal blockade, heavy sedation may allow greater patient tolerance of the injections. In such situations, longer-acting opioids such as 8–12 mg of morphine and more sedative-amnestics such as scopolamine may be useful. Although intramuscular premedication is common with hospitalized patients, careful titration of intravenous drugs at the time of the blockade is the most effective way to adjust the level of sedation to individual patient needs and sensitivities.

Monitoring

Along with the consideration of degree of sedation is the question of the appropriate degree of monitoring for patients receiving regional anesthetic techniques. Although current discussions of "monitoring" typically revolve around mechanical and electrical devices, repetitive assessment of the patient's *mental status* when receiving local anesthetics is of paramount importance. The anesthesiologist must maintain verbal contact with these patients on a frequent basis and ideally have an uninvolved assistant available to assess the level of consciousness at all times. There are no electrical or mechanical devices that detect rising blood levels of local anesthetic; close observation for peak levels owing to intravenous (within 2 minutes) and subcutaneous (about 20 minutes) absorption is essential. An *electrocardiogram* (ECG) is appropriate to detect the pulse rise seen with epinephrine when it is included in a test dose. It is also useful in case systemic toxicity occurs with bupivacaine, particularly whenever high doses of that drug are used. Other pulse counters such as mechanical meters and pulse oximeters are also useful when monitoring the pulse rate change with epinephrine. *Blood pressure* monitoring should be performed, as with use of any anesthetic. A baseline pressure should be obtained whenever any sympathetic blockade is performed and at frequent intervals thereafter. Other circumstances in which blood pressure measurement is important include following the injection of celiac plexus anes-

thesia or to detect intravascular epinephrine injection. Beyond these specific comments, the standards for monitoring and recordkeeping on any patient undergoing regional anesthesia are the same as for patients undergoing any general anesthetic. One must be particularly careful not to be lulled into a false sense of security because it is "just a regional anesthetic." Patients may still develop life-threatening cardiovascular or ventilatory depression owing to delayed absorption of local anesthetic or too liberal use of sedation.

Discharge Criteria

Concern is occasionally expressed about discharging patients from Postanesthesia Care Units when an extremity is still anesthetized. If regional anesthesia is administered to provide prolonged analgesia, numbness may be expected to persist for 10 (with intercostal anesthesia) to 24 (with sciatic blockade) hours after bupivacaine administration. It is clearly unreasonable to delay discharge in this situation, and patients have been successfully discharged to the floors as long as their mental alertness is adequate. Even outpatients may be discharged home with numb arms or legs as long as the patient is reliable and adequate instruction about care of the insensitive extremity is provided. The major problem arises with orthostatic hypotension following sympathetic blockade. Patients receiving celiac plexus blockade or spinal or epidural sympathectomies should be assessed for stable blood pressure and ambulated gradually before discharge from close supervision.

SPECIFIC TECHNIQUES

The remainder of this chapter is devoted to the details of the performance of specific types of blockade, arranged by sections of the body. No attempt has been made to describe every regional technique practiced but to focus on those of clinical usefulness to the anesthesiologist. The common methods are described, recognizing that several alternative approaches have been advocated in each case.

Head and Neck

Regional anesthesia of the head and neck has limited surgical application. Concern about control and maintenance of the airway makes many anesthesiologists uncomfortable with regional techniques when intraoperative airway intervention is awkward. Nevertheless, occasionally there are patients who may benefit from regional techniques in the head or neck. More commonly, the techniques of trigeminal nerve blockade and occipital nerve blockade are used for diagnostic or neurolytic blockade for chronic pain syndromes. Cervical plexus blockade is useful for some surgical procedures on the neck, and topical/regional airway anesthesia is effective in reducing the subjective discomfort and hemodynamic responses to intubation.

Trigeminal Nerve Blockade

Sensory and motor nerve function of the face is provided by the branches of the 5th cranial (trigeminal) nerve. The roots of this nerve arise from the base of the pons and send sensory branches to the large gasserian (or semilunar) ganglion, which lies on the superior margin of the petrous bone

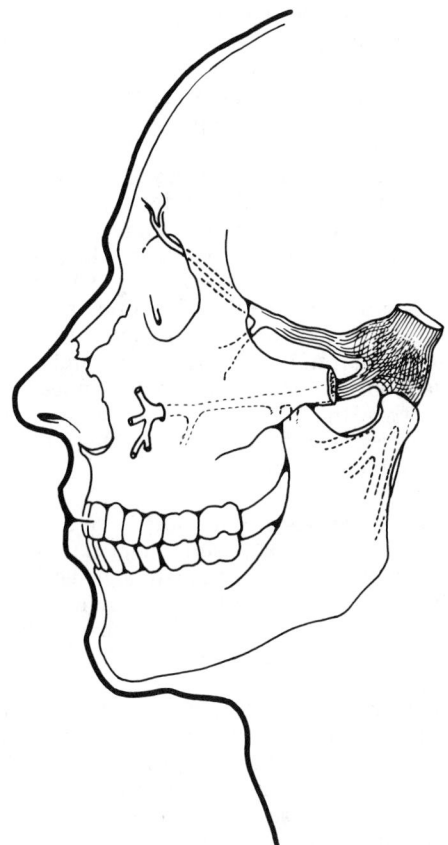

Figure 31-3. Lateral view of major branches of the trigeminal nerve. Each major branch exits the skull by a separate foramen. The ophthalmic branch travels in the orbit. The maxillary and mandibular branches emerge from the skull medial to the lateral pterygoid plate, which serves as the landmark for their identification. (Reproduced with permission from Mulroy M: Handbook of Regional Anesthesia. Boston, Little, Brown, 1989.)

just inside the skull above the foramen ovale. A smaller motor fiber nucleus lies behind it and sends motor branches to one terminal nerve, the mandibular. The three major branches of the trigeminal each have a separate exit from the skull (Fig. 31-3). The uppermost ophthalmic branch passes through the sphenoidal fissure into the orbit. The main terminal fibers of this nerve, the frontal nerve, bifurcate into the supratrochlear and supraorbital nerves. These two branches traverse the orbit along the superior border and exit on the front of the face in the easily palpated supraorbital notch for the former and along the medial border of the orbit for the latter.

The two major branches of the trigeminal nerve are the middle (maxillary) and lower (mandibular). The maxillary nerve contains only sensory fibers and exits the skull through the foramen rotundum. It passes beneath the skull anteriorly through the sphenomaxillary fossa. At this point, it lies medial to the lateral pterygoid plate on each side. At the anterior end of this channel, it again moves superiorly to re-enter the skull in the infraorbital canal in the floor of the orbit. Within the sphenomaxillary fossa, it branches to form the sphenopalatine nerves and to give off the posterior dental branches. The anterior dental nerves arise from the main trunk as it passes through the infraorbital canal. The terminal infraorbital nerve emerges from the foramen of the

same name just below the eye and lateral to the nose and gives off the terminal palpebral, nasal, and labial nerves. The mandibular nerve is the third and largest branch of the trigeminal, and the only one to receive motor fibers. It exits the skull posterior to the maxillary nerve through the foramen ovale. At this point, it is just posterior to the lateral pterygoid plate of the sphenoid bone. The motor nerves separate into an anterior branch immediately below the foramen ovale. The main branch continues as the inferior alveolar nerve medial to the ramus of the mandible. This nerve curves anteriorly to follow the mandible and exits as a terminal branch through the mental foramen. The mental nerve provides sensation to the lower lip and jaw.

Gasserian Ganglion Blockade. Ideally, the simplest blockade of the trigeminal nerve is performed in the central ganglion, which includes all three branches, and it is frequently recommended for treatment of disabling trigeminal neuralgia. In fact, this blockade is technically the most difficult and has the most undesirable potential for the complications of subarachnoid injection of anesthetic after neurolytic blockade. Residual numbness of the face is sometimes unpleasant, and a neuritis may be as unpleasant as the original condition. Protective corneal sensation may also be lost, and special care of the eye may be needed. Nevertheless, it is a technique useful in severe cases of trigeminal neuralgia that are unresponsive to more peripheral blockade. Alcohol injection has been performed in the past, although radiofrequency ablation by neurosurgeons has become more accepted recently. The procedure for blockade follows:

1. Three landmarks are needed to help locate the foramen ovale. First, a skin wheal is raised 3 cm lateral to the corner of the mouth on the involved side. A second mark is made on the skin 1 cm anterior to the midpoint of the zygoma (the midpoint lies just above the deepest part of the sigmoid notch of the mandible). The third landmark is the pupil of the eye on the ipsilateral side.
2. A 12.5-cm needle is introduced through the skin wheal on the cheek. The needle is advanced posteriorly in the sagittal plane formed by an imaginary line between the pupil and the point of insertion. As it moves posteriorly, it is angled superiorly toward the third point (anterior to the midpoint of the zygomatic arch). If advanced properly, the needle will pass through the muscles of the cheek without entering the oral cavity and will contact the base of the skull medial to the mandible and the zygoma. If it has remained in the plane of the pupil, it will be near the foramen ovale.
3. Once bone is contacted, the needle is withdrawn and reinserted to angle slightly more posteriorly until the foramen is entered. At this point, paresthesias of the maxillary branch are sought. The needle should not be advanced more than 1 cm beyond the opening of the foramen. If there is any question about localization, biplanar fluoroscopy is useful in confirming position.
4. After localization of the nerve, careful aspiration is performed to detect unwanted subarachnoid placement of the needle. Two milliliters of 1% lidocaine injected slowly usually produce anesthesia of all three sensory branches. If alcohol is used, the anesthesia is preceded by a severe burning sensation; this can be reduced by prior injection of a few drops of local anesthetic.

Superficial Trigeminal Nerve Branch Blockade. Fortunately, most anesthetic applications of trigeminal blockade

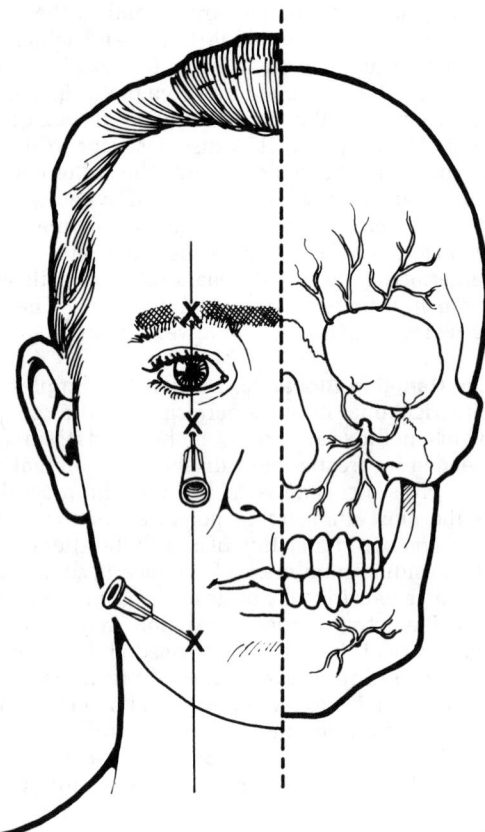

Figure 31-4. Terminal branches of the trigeminal nerve. Each of the three terminal branches (the supraorbital, infraorbital, and mental) exits its respective bony canal in the same sagittal plane, approximately 2.5 cm from the midline. The infraorbital canal is angled slightly cephalad, while the mental canal can be entered if the needle is directed medially and slightly caudad. (Reproduced with permission from Mulroy M: Handbook of Regional Anesthesia. Boston, Little, Brown, 1989.)

can be more easily performed by injection of the individual terminal superficial branches. This is relatively simple, since the three superficial branches and their associated foramen all lie in the same sagittal plane on each side of the face (Fig. 31-4). Each of these foramina are readily palpable, and these nerves can be easily blocked with superficial injections of small quantities of local anesthetic. Although the bony landmarks are usually sufficient themselves, paresthesias are desirable before alcohol injection. Each of these blocks can be performed with the patient in the supine position. The procedure for blockade follows:

1. The supraorbital notch is easily palpated along the medial superior rim of the orbit, usually 2.5 cm from the midline. Two to three milliliters of local anesthetic injected immediately in the vicinity of the notch produce anesthesia of the ipsilateral forehead. Anesthesia of the supratrochlear nerve by superficial infiltration of the medial aspect of the orbital rim is needed if the band of anesthesia is to cross the midline.
2. The infraorbital foramen lies below the inferior orbital rim in the same plane at approximately the same distance from the midline as the supraorbital notch (usually 2.5 cm). If the foramen cannot be palpated directly, it can be sought by gently probing with a small-gauge needle. This needle should be introduced

through a skin wheal approximately 0.5 cm below the expected opening, because the canal angles cephalad from this point toward the orbital floor. Again, injection of a small quantity of local anesthetic immediately in the vicinity of the foramen produces anesthesia of the middle third of the ipsilateral face.
3. The mental nerve also emerges approximately 2.5 cm from the midline, usually midway between the upper and lower borders of the mandible. The mental canal angles medially and inferiorly so that, in this case, needle insertion should start approximately 0.5 cm above and 0.5 cm lateral to the anticipated location of the orifice if it cannot be palpated directly. In older patients, resorption of the superior margin of the mandibular bone will make the foramen appear to lie more superiorly along the ramus. Again, 2 ml of local anesthesia injected into the canal produces anesthesia of the mandibular area.

Maxillary Nerve Blockade. If anesthesia in superior dental nerves is also required or if superficial infraorbital nerve blockade does not produce adequate anesthesia, proximal block of the maxillary nerve is required. This can be performed by a lateral approach to the sphenopalatine fossa (Fig. 31-5). The procedure for blockade follows:

1. The patient lies supine with a small towel under the occiput and the head turned slightly away from the side to be blocked. The zygomatic arch is marked along its course, and the patient is asked to open and close the mouth slowly so that the curved upper border of the mandible can be identified. The lowest point of the mandibular notch is palpated, and an "X" marked at this spot, which is usually at the midpoint of the zygoma. A skin wheal is raised at the "X" after the appropriate skin preparations.
2. With the patient's jaw in the open position, a 7.5-cm needle is introduced through the "X" and directed 45

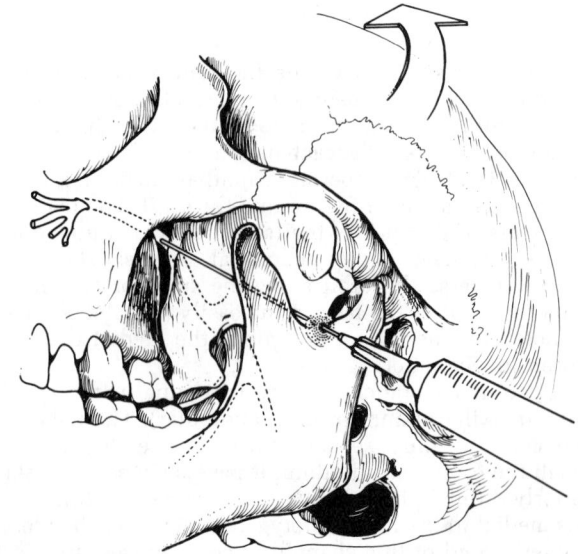

Figure 31-5. Lateral approach to the maxillary nerve. The needle is introduced through the skin just over the notch of the mandible and directed anteriorly and cephalad to identify the pterygoid plate. As the needle is advanced anteriorly off the plate, the maxillary nerve is encountered before it re-enters the skull in the infraorbital canal in the base of the orbit. (Reproduced with permission from Mulroy M: Handbook of Regional Anesthesia. Boston, Little, Brown, 1989.)

degrees cephalad and slightly anterior. This direction should be toward the imagined posterior border of the globe of the eye.

3. The needle should contact the pterygoid plate. It is then withdrawn and redirected slightly anterior until it succeeds in passing beyond the pterygoid plate. At this point, the nerve should lie approximately 1 cm deeper. A paresthesia in the nose or the upper teeth confirms the nerve localization.

4. Anesthesia can be achieved by injecting 5 ml into the fossa, either on obtaining the paresthesia or blindly by advancing 1 cm beyond the plate.

The major complication of concern is spread of the anesthetic to adjacent structures, especially to the nerves in the orbit.

Mandibular Nerve Blockade. This nerve can also be blocked for inferior dental pain. It is the only branch where anesthesia carries the risk of loss of motor (mastication) function (Fig. 31-6). The procedure for blockade follows:

1. Head position and landmarks are the same as those described for the maxillary nerve blockade.

2. A 2-inch needle is introduced through the skin wheal and directed medially but slightly posterior and without the cephalad angulation required for maxillary nerve anesthesia. This leaves the needle approximately perpendicular to the skin in all planes.

3. When the pterygoid plate is contacted, the needle is redirected posteriorly until it passes beyond the plate. It should contact the nerve 0.5 to 1 cm deep to this point.

4. Paresthesia of the jaw or cheek confirms identification

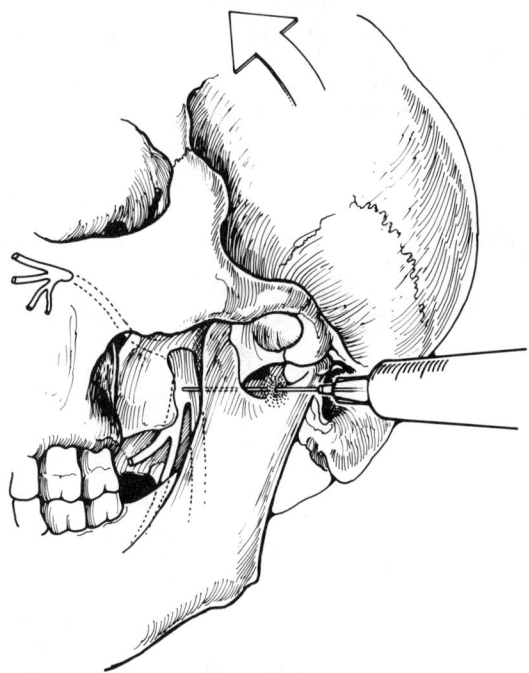

Figure 31-6. Lateral approach to the mandibular nerve. The needle is introduced in the same manner as for the maxillary nerve block but directed posteriorly. After contacting the pterygoid plate, it is directed farther posteriorly until it passes behind the plate, where it should encounter the nerve. (Reproduced with permission from Mulroy M: Handbook of Regional Anesthesia. Boston, Little, Brown, 1989.)

of the nerve. Five to ten milliliters of solution injected incrementally at this point should produce anesthesia of the terminal branches. If paresthesias are essential, exploration should be carried gently cephalad and caudad from the initial point where the needle passes posterior to the plate. As with maxillary blockade, paresthesias can be painful to the patient, and the use of an assistant to secure the head is occasionally necessary.

Facial nerve anesthesia can occasionally be seen when large volumes are injected to block the mandibular nerve. This is of little consequence unless neurolytic agents are used. A more serious complication is the possibility of intravascular injection in this highly vascularized area. Injection should be performed incrementally with small quantities, and constant observation for signs of central toxicity.

Cervical Plexus Blockade

Sensory and motor fibers of the neck and posterior scalp arise from the nerve roots of the 2nd, 3rd, and 4th cervical nerves. This cervical plexus is unique in that the sensory fibers separate from the motor fibers early in their course and can be blocked separately. Classic plexus anesthesia along the tubercles of the vertebral body produces both motor and sensory blockade. The transverse processes of the cervical vertebrae form peculiar elongated troughs for the emergence of their nerve roots. These troughs lie immediately lateral to a medial opening for the cephalad passage of the vertebral artery. The trough at the terminal end of the transverse process divides into an anterior and a posterior tubercle, which can often be easily palpated. These tubercles also serve as the attachments for the anterior and middle scalene muscles, which thus form a compartment for the cervical plexus as well as for the brachial plexus immediately below. The compartment at this level is less developed than the one formed around the brachial plexus. The motor branches (including the phrenic nerve) curl anteriorly around the lateral border of the anterior scalene and proceed caudad and medially toward the muscles of the neck. They give anterior branches to the sternocleidomastoid muscle as they pass behind it. The sensory fibers, as mentioned, also emerge behind the anterior scalene muscle but separate from the motor branches and continue laterally to emerge superficially under the posterior border of the sternocleidomastoid muscle. They provide sensory anesthesia to the anterior and posterior skin of the neck and shoulder.

Anesthesia of either the superficial cervical nerves or the cervical plexus itself can be used for operations on the lateral or anterior neck. Thyroidectomy and carotid endarterectomy fall into this category, although supplemental local infiltration of the thyroid gland may occasionally be necessary because of sensory innervation from cranial nerves. In carotid surgery, local infiltration of the carotid bifurcation may be necessary to block reflex hemodynamic changes associated with glossopharyngeal stimulation. Cervical plexus anesthesia alone is rarely adequate for shoulder surgery. It is preferable to perform interscalene anesthesia of the brachial plexus for these procedures, since the likelihood of adequate motor relaxation is greater and the cervical plexus is usually blocked incidentally. The procedure for cervical plexus blockade follows:

1. The patient is placed supine with a small towel under the head, with the head turned slightly to the side opposite the one to be blocked.

2. The mastoid process is identified and marked. The

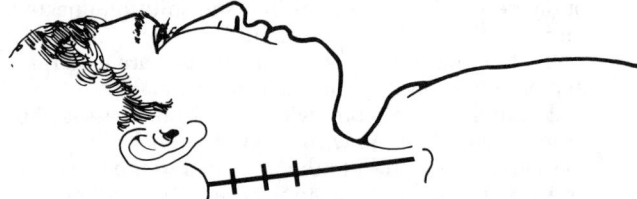

Figure 31-7. Superficial landmarks for cervical plexus blockade. A line is drawn from the mastoid process to the prominent tubercle of the 6th cervical vertebra. The transverse processes of the 2nd, 3rd, and 4th cervical vertebrae lie 0.5 cm posterior to this line and at 1.5-cm intervals below the mastoid. (Reproduced with permission from Mulroy M: Handbook of Regional Anesthesia. Boston, Little, Brown, 1989.)

transverse processes can often be palpated. If not, the most prominent tubercle, that of the 6th cervical vertebra, is marked, and a line is drawn between it and the mastoid process (Fig. 31-7).

3. The cervical processes should be felt approximately 0.5 cm posterior to the line drawn between the mastoid and the 6th cervical tubercle. The 2nd vertebral process should lie approximately 1.5 cm below the mastoid itself. (There is no process for the first vertebra.)

4. The 3rd and 4th processes lie approximately 1.5 cm below their respective superior neighbors.

5. Skin wheals are raised at the three "X" marks that have been placed over the transverse processes.

6. A 3.75-cm needle is introduced perpendicular to the skin and directed posterior and slightly caudad at each "X" until it rests on the transverse process. It is important to maintain a caudad direction in order to avoid entry directly into the intervertebral foramina. The needle is walked caudad. It should slip off the bone if it is truly on the process rather than continuing to contact bone if it is on the vertebral body. It is important to contact the transverse process as far laterally as possible in order to avoid any contact of the needle with the vertebral artery (Fig. 31-8).

7. Paresthesias are usually not necessary. A syringe is

connected to the needle, and 5 ml of local anesthetic solution is deposited along the transverse process. Anesthesia should follow within 5 minutes in the distribution of the nerve.

The major potential complication of this procedure is intravascular injection into the vertebral artery. Again, injection should be made in small increments, with frequent observation of the patient's mental status and frequent aspiration to detect intravascular placement. If the needle is advanced too far medially into the vertebral foramen, epidural or even subarachnoid anesthesia may be produced. This is more likely in the cervical region because of longer sleeves of dura that accompany these nerve branches. Again, frequent aspiration and careful lateral placement of the needle are important.

Phrenic nerve blockade occurs frequently with deep cervical plexus anesthesia. This blockade is not indicated in any patient who is dependent upon his or her diaphragm for tidal ventilation, nor is bilateral blockade desirable in most patients. Recurrent laryngeal nerve or vagal blockade can also occur because of diffusion of the local anesthetic. This is a troublesome but not serious complication. It may interfere with the ability to evaluate vocal cord function following thyroid surgery.

Superficial Cervical Plexus Blockade. This is performed in the same position as deep cervical plexus blockade and results in anesthesia only of the sensory fibers of the plexus. The procedure for blockade follows:

1. An "X" is made along the posterior border of the sternocleidomastoid muscle at the level of the 4th cervical vertebra. This usually corresponds with the junction of the external jugular vein as it crosses the posterior border of the muscle (Fig. 31-9).

2. A skin wheal is raised at this mark, and superficial local anesthetic infiltration is performed along the posterior border of the sternocleidomastoid muscle 4 cm above and below the level of the "X." Ten to 12 ml

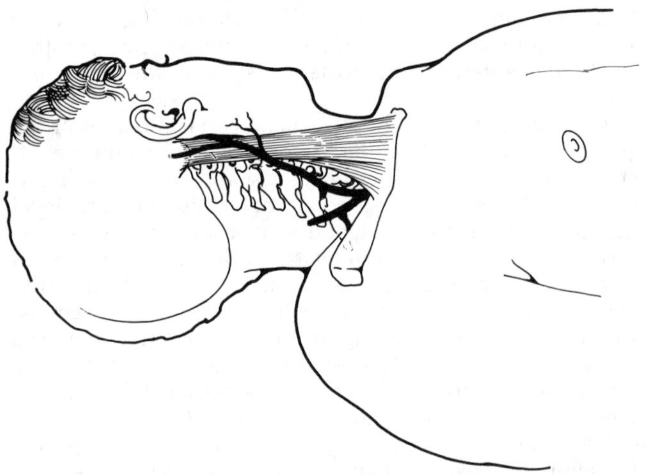

Figure 31-8. Anatomy of deep cervical plexus blockade. The transverse processes lie under the lateral border of the sternocleidomastoid muscle, each with a distal trough or sulcus that defines the path of nerve exit. (Reproduced with permission from Mulroy M: Handbook of Regional Anesthesia. Boston, Little, Brown, 1989.)

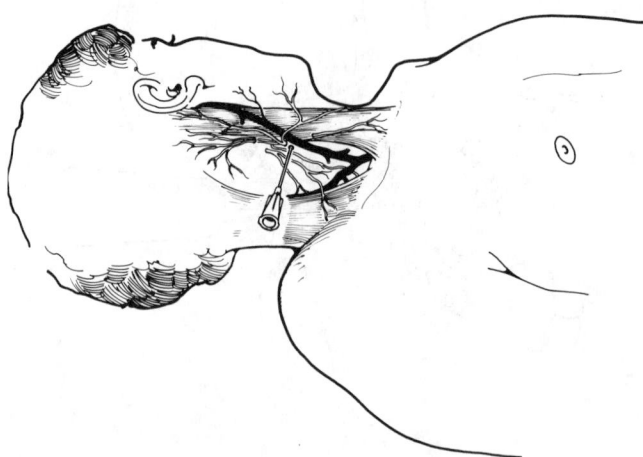

Figure 31-9. Superficial cervical plexus blockade. The sensory fibers of the plexus all emerge from behind the lateral border of the sternocleidomastoid muscle. A needle inserted at its midpoint, usually where the external jugular vein crosses the muscle, can be directed superiorly and inferiorly to block all these terminal branches. (Reproduced with permission from Mulroy M: Handbook of Regional Anesthesia. Boston, Little, Brown, 1989.)

of local anesthetic solution usually provide sensory anesthesia of the anterior neck and shoulder.

Occipital Nerve Blockade

The ophthalmic branch of the trigeminal nerve provides sensory innervation of the forehead and anterior scalp, but the remainder of the scalp is innervated by fibers of the greater and lesser occipital nerves, terminal branches of the cervical plexus. These nerves can be blocked by superficial injection at the point on the posterior skull where they emerge from below the muscles of the neck (Fig. 31-10). Anesthesia is rarely used for surgical procedures; it is more often applied as a diagnostic step in evaluating head and neck pain complaints. The procedure for blockade follows:

1. The block is performed in the sitting position, with the patient leaning the head forward to expose the prominent nuchal ridge of bone at the posterior base of the skull.
2. The external occipital protuberance is identified in the midline, and a mark is placed lateral to this prominence along the nuchal line at the lateral border of the insertion of the erector muscles of the neck, usually 2.5 cm from the midline. The branches of the greater occipital nerve usually pass laterally from behind the muscle to cross the nuchal line at this point.
3. After skin preparation, a small needle is introduced through the mark to the depth of the skull itself. A ridge of 1–4 ml of local anesthetic (1% lidocaine or equivalent) is then deposited across the path of the emerging nerves just above the level of the bone. Paresthesias are occasionally encountered but are not essential to obtaining simple skin anesthesia.
4. If more anterior anesthesia of the scalp is required, the lesser occipital nerve branches are also blocked by advancing the needle subcutaneously from this point in an anterior direction toward the mastoid process. A band of anesthetic solution is deposited along the line

between the skin entry and the mastoid. A larger volume (6–8 ml) is required.

Complications of this technique are rare. Care must be taken not to advance the needle anteriorly under the skull, as the foramen magnum might be entered unintentionally with a long needle. Local hematoma may be produced with the superficial injection, but this is only a temporary problem.

Airway Anesthesia

Manipulation of the airway either during laryngoscopy or during endotracheal intubation is often associated with laryngospasm, coughing, and undesirable cardiovascular reflexes. The anesthesiologist can abolish or blunt these reflexes by anesthetizing one or all of the sensory pathways involved. The nasal mucosa is innervated by fibers of the sphenopalatine ganglion, a branch of the middle division of the 5th cranial nerve. These branches lie on the lateral wall of the nasal passages on each side, under the mucosa just posterior to the middle turbinate (Fig. 31-11). The branches of these fibers continue caudad to provide sensory innervation to the superior portion of the pharynx, uvula, and tonsils. Anesthesia of the maxillary branch of the trigeminal nerve is possible but not a practical solution for airway anesthesia. Transmucosal topical application of local anesthetic is more appropriate. Below the sphenopalatine fiber distribution, sensory innervation of the oral pharynx and supraglottic regions is provided by branches of the glossopharyngeal nerve. These nerves lie laterally on each side of the pharynx submucosally in the region of the posterior tonsillar pillar. Direct submucosal injection can be performed but carries the risk of unintentional intravascular injection into several blood vessels in this area. Topical anesthesia of the terminal branches in the mouth and throat is again an easier approach. The larynx itself is innervated by the superior laryngeal branch of the vagus nerve in the area above the vocal cords. This branch leaves the main vagal trunk in the carotid sheath and passes anteriorly. Its internal branch penetrates the thyrohyoid membrane and

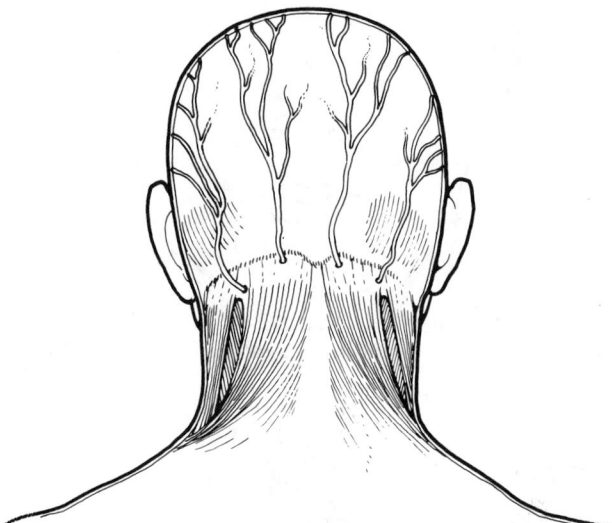

Figure 31-10. Occipital nerve blockade. The greater and lesser branches of the occipital nerve emerge from under the muscles at the level of the nuchal ridge on the posterior scalp. They can be easily blocked by a subcutaneous ridge of anesthetic solution. (Reproduced with permission from Mulroy M: Handbook of Regional Anesthesia. Boston, Little, Brown, 1989.)

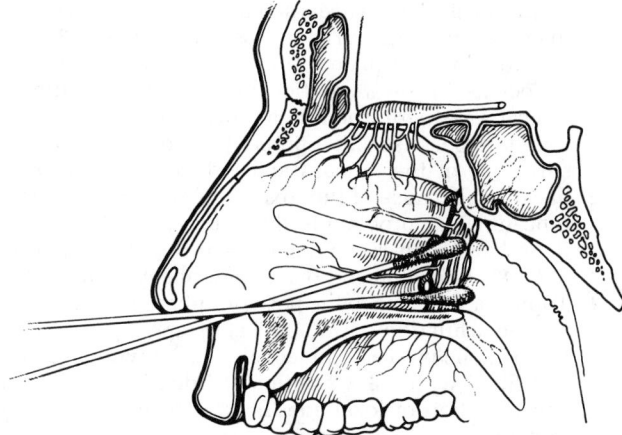

Figure 31-11. Nasal airway anesthesia. Cotton pledgets soaked with anesthetic are inserted along the inferior and middle turbinates to produce anesthesia of the underlying sphenopalatine ganglion by transmembrane diffusion of the solution. Wide pledgets also are needed to provide maximal topical anesthesia and vasoconstriction of the nasal mucosa. (Reproduced with permission from Mulroy M: Handbook of Regional Anesthesia. Boston, Little, Brown, 1989.)

divides to provide the sensory fibers to the cords, epiglottis, and arytenoids.

The recurrent laryngeal nerve provides innervation to the areas below the vocal cords, including motor innervation for all but one of the intrinsic laryngeal muscles. The trachea itself is also innervated by the recurrent laryngeal nerve. Topical anesthesia is again the simplest approach to this nerve.

Airway anesthesia can be performed by anesthetizing one or all of these sensory distributions. Full anesthesia will facilitate procedures such as nasal intubation or fiberoptic laryngoscopy. Airway anesthesia below the vocal cords might best be avoided if there is concern about potential aspiration, as this may blunt the reflex cough reaction to the presence of foreign bodies in the trachea. Topical postpharyngeal anesthesia may also ablate protective laryngeal reflexes.

In the performance of airway anesthesia, the patient can be anesthetized in the supine position, although many patients find it more comfortable to be semiupright or sitting when topical anesthesia is sprayed into the posterior pharynx. These positions allow them greater ease in swallowing excess solutions and may reduce gagging. In whatever position chosen, there should be a firm support behind the head to reduce the possibility of involuntary withdrawal motions by the patient, which might dislocate needles being used for injections. The procedure for airway anesthetic administration follows:

1. For nasal mucosal anesthesia, cotton pledgets soaked with anesthetic solution are introduced through the nares and passed along the turbinates all the way to the posterior end of the nasal passage (Fig. 31-11). A second set of pledgets is introduced with a cephalad angulation to follow the middle turbinate back to the mucosa overlying the sphenoid bone. This pledget is the more critical one, since anesthesia in this mucosal area is most likely to anesthetize the branches of the sphenopalatine ganglia as they pass along the lateral wall of the airway. Bilateral anesthesia is preferable, even if a nasal tube is to be inserted only on one side; bilateral blockade of the sphenopalatine fibers will also produce posterior pharyngeal anesthesia caudad to this level. The pledgets should be allowed to remain in contact with the nasal mucosa for at least 2–3 minutes to allow adequate diffusion of local anesthetic.

   Cocaine in a 4% solution has been the traditional topical anesthetic for this application because of its unique vasoconstrictive properties. Cocaine produces shrinkage of the mucosa and reduces the chance of bleeding. Because of the toxicity of cocaine and a significant abuse problem in this country, alternate solutions have been recommended—primarily a mixture of 3–4% lidocaine and 0.25–0.5% phenylephrine.[17,18]

2. Topical anesthesia to the posterior pharynx can be performed while the nasal applicators are in place. This can be done with a commercial spray or with an atomizer filled with a 4% solution of lidocaine. (A higher concentration of local anesthetic is required in order to penetrate mucosal membranes.) For effective anesthesia in the posterior pharyngeal wall, topical application is performed in two stages. First, the tongue itself is sprayed with a local anesthetic, and the patient is encouraged to gargle and swallow the residual liquid in the mouth. The numb tongue is then grasped with a gauze pad with one hand while the spray device is inserted into the mouth with the other. The patient is then encouraged to take rapid deep breaths ("pant like a puppy") while the spray is applied on inspiration. The inspiratory flow of gases should be enough to draw the lidocaine solution into the posterior pharynx and even to the vocal cords themselves. If superior laryngeal nerve blockade has been performed prior to this, it is likely that the aerosol will be carried into the trachea itself. Again, a few minutes are needed for adequate onset of topical anesthesia in the pharynx. Topical anesthesia is less effective if there are copious secretions. Premedication with an anticholinergic is frequently beneficial.

3. Superior laryngeal nerve blockade can also be performed while the nasal pledgets are in place (Fig. 31-12). This nerve is blocked bilaterally by identifying the superior ala of the thyroid cartilage, which usually lies just inferior to the posterior portion of the hyoid bone on each side. A 5-ml syringe with a 1% lidocaine solution with a 23-gauge 1.75-cm needle is used. The index finger of one hand retracts the skin of the neck caudad down over the thyroid cartilage; the needle is inserted until it rests on the superior margin of the cartilage. The tension on the skin is then released, and the needle is withdrawn slightly and allowed to walk superiorly off the cartilage. The needle is then reinserted and passed through the thyrohyoid membrane, which is perceived as a discernible resistance. After careful aspiration, 2.5 ml of solution is injected into the space below the membrane. This procedure is repeated on the opposite side. This blockade can be performed as part of total airway anesthesia or it can be used independently to provide increased acceptance of indwelling endotracheal tubes in the intensive care unit.[19]

4. Tracheal anesthesia can be performed by a direct transcrycoid ("transtracheal") injection. This is accomplished by raising a small skin wheal over the cricothyroid membrane. A 20-gauge intravenous catheter is then inserted gently through this skin wheal and

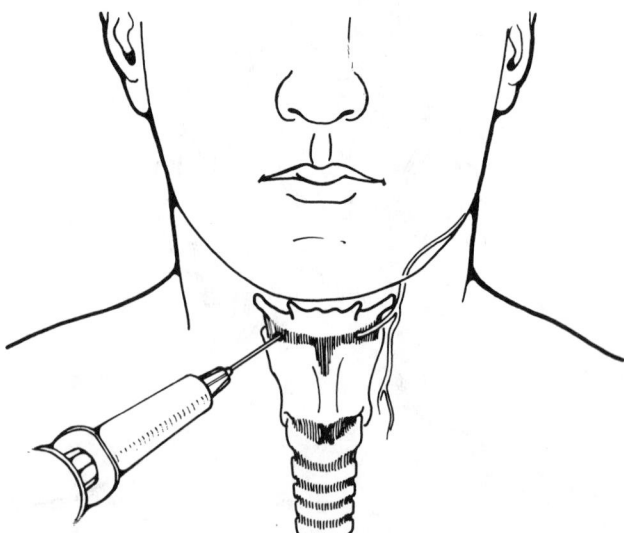

Figure 31-12. Superior laryngeal nerve blockade. The needle is advanced superiorly off the lateral wing of the thyroid cartilage to drop through the thyrohyoid membrane. (Reproduced with permission from Mulroy M: Handbook of Regional Anesthesia. Boston, Little, Brown, 1989.)

through the membrane. Entry into the trachea can be confirmed by the ability to aspirate air through the catheter. The steel stylet is then removed, and the plastic catheter is left in the trachea. A syringe with 4 ml of 4% lidocaine is attached to the catheter, and the local anesthetic is sprayed into the trachea during inspiration. The flow of air usually carries the local anesthetic distally; the resultant cough continues to spread the anesthetic more proximally up to the underside of the vocal cords and the larynx. Not uncommonly, if the local anesthetic is injected while the patient forcibly exhales, it is possible to obtain adequate anesthesia of the trachea, larynx, and posterior pharynx, without the need for either steps 2 or 3.

5. After each of these steps has been completed, the pledgets can be removed from the nasal passages and nasal intubation performed. If tracheal or laryngeal anesthesia has been omitted because of concern about aspiration, there should be some pharmacologic intervention to reduce the cardiovascular response to the passage of the tube into the trachea. This can be facilitated by pretreatment with intravenous beta-adrenergic blocking drugs, by administration of sedation, or by administration of rapid-acting thiobarbiturates immediately after the airway is secured.

Complications of these techniques are rare. Systemic toxicity from the local anesthetics is a distinct possibility because of the large quantities of drug required to produce sufficient mucosal anesthesia. If all four stages of airway anesthesia are undertaken, the total milligram doses applied usually exceed the maximal recommended dose for peripheral injection. Fortunately, the mucosal absorption is less than the peripheral absorption, but close attention to the patient's mental status and preparation for treatment of toxicity are necessary. As has been mentioned, aspiration of gastric contents is also a possibility when the protective reflexes of the airway are interrupted. Precautions should be taken in the form of the usual prophylaxis to reduce stomach acidity as well as provision for suction and adequate oxygenation if emesis or regurgitation occurs.

Upper Extremity

The innervation of the upper extremity is conveniently derived from five closely approximated nerve roots, extending from the 5th cervical to the 1st thoracic segment of the spinal cord. These roots undergo a series of mergers and divisions that produce the terminal nerves of the arm and hand. The plexus branches are close enough to each other to allow reliable anesthesia to be achieved at several points associated with consistent bony or vascular landmarks.

In their proximal course, the nerve roots all lie in a well-demarcated fascial envelope formed by the anterior fascia of the middle scalene muscle and the posterior fascia of the anterior scalene. These muscles attach to the posterior and anterior tubercles of the transverse processes of the cervical vertebrae from which the nerves emerge. The tubercle can be used as a faithful landmark to guide localization of the nerve, and the fascial planes serve to keep anesthetic solution injected between them in close proximity to the nerve bundle. The fascia extends outward for a variable distance from the lateral border of the muscles to enclose the nerves in a "sheath," which can extend into the axilla. This enclosed bundle passes over the 1st rib just behind the midpoint of the clavicle (and just posterior to the insertion of the anterior scalene on the rib), where it is joined by the subclavian artery, which rises from the mediastinum to cross the rib and pass into the axilla. At the midpoint of the rib, the plexus has consolidated into only three trunks; these rapidly subdivide into the terminal branches. The musculocutaneous nerve is the first branch to leave the companionship of its partners as it passes into the body of the coracobrachialis muscle high in the axilla. As the individual nerves form, separate compartments in the sheath are formed by developing septa, and reliable blockade of all the nerves with a single injection is not practical distal to the axilla.

Although many techniques of approach to the brachial plexus have been described, there are basically three anatomic locations where anesthetics are placed: (1) the interscalene groove near the transverse processes; (2) the subclavian sheath at the 1st rib; and (3) the axillary sheath surrounding the artery in the axilla. Because of the specific configuration of the nerves at each of these levels, the anesthesia produced is significantly different with each approach and applicable to different situations.[20] Interscalene injection at the level of the 6th cervical transverse process produces extension of the blockade to the lower fibers of the cervical plexus and, thus, is ideally suited for shoulder operations and upper arm procedures. It frequently spares the lowest branches of the plexus, the C8 and T1 fibers, which innervate the caudad (ulnar) border of the forearm. Blockade at the level of the 1st rib is most reliable in producing anesthesia of all four terminal nerves of the forearm and hand. The axillary technique is simpler but carries the risk of missing the musculocutaneous nerve that departs the sheath high in the axilla and, thus, might produce inadequate anesthesia of the forearm. The choice of the appropriate approach depends not only on the patient's anatomy but also on the site of surgery.

The terminal branches can also be anesthetized by local anesthetic injection along their peripheral courses as they cross the joint spaces, or by the injection of a dilute local anesthetic solution intravenously below a pneumatic tourniquet on the upper arm.

Interscalene Approach

This technique was first popularized by Winnie,[21] who stressed the advantages of the fascial sheath provided by the "envelope" of muscles that surround the origins of the brachial plexus in the neck. Localization of the nerves uses a combination of the muscular and bony landmarks surrounding the nerves. The procedure for blockade follows:

1. The patient is positioned supine, with the head turned to the side opposite that to be blocked. A small towel is placed under the occiput. The arm on the side to be blocked is held at the side, and the patient is asked to hold the shoulder down by pretending to reach for the hip or knee.
2. The lateral border of the sternocleidomastoid muscle is identified and marked, and the patient is then asked to raise the head slightly into a "sniffing" position. This tenses the scalene muscle behind the sternocleidomastoid muscle, and the groove between the anterior and middle scalene is palpated by rolling the fingers posteriorly off the lateral border of the sternocleidomastoid muscle. This groove is marked along its entire extent, as high up as possible. The patient then relaxes the muscles of the neck, and the level of the cricoid cartilage is marked. The index fin-

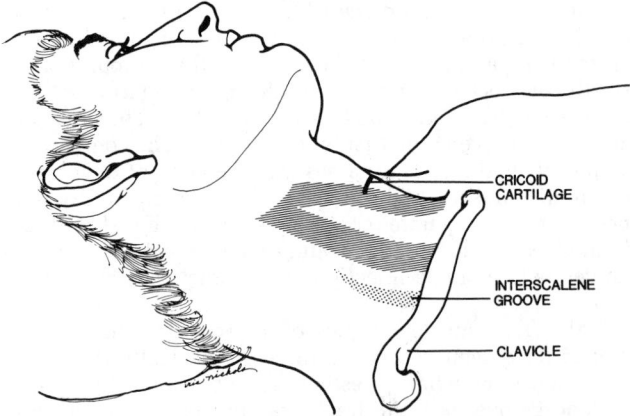

Figure 31-13. Superficial landmarks for interscalene brachial plexus blockade. The sternocleidomastoid muscle is identified, and the anterior scalene muscle is found by moving the fingertips over the lateral border of the larger muscle while it is slightly tensed. The groove between the anterior and middle scalene muscles can usually be felt easily, along with the tubercle of the 6th cervical vertebra, which lies at the level of the cricoid cartilage. (Reproduced with permission from Mulroy M: Handbook of Regional Anesthesia. Boston, Little, Brown, 1989.)

ger then gently palpates in the groove at the level of the cricoid (Fig. 31-13). The prominent transverse process of the 6th cervical vertebra can often be felt directly.

3. After aseptic skin preparation, a skin wheal is raised in the groove at the level of the cricoid. A 22-gauge 3.75-cm needle is introduced through the wheal *perpendicular to the skin in all planes* so that it is directed medially, caudad, and slightly posteriorly. Resting one hand on the clavicle allows better control of the syringe (Fig. 31-14).
4. The needle is advanced until the tubercle is contacted or a paresthesia is elicited (or a motor twitch is obtained with a nerve stimulator) (Fig. 31-15). If bone is contacted before nerve, the needle is withdrawn and

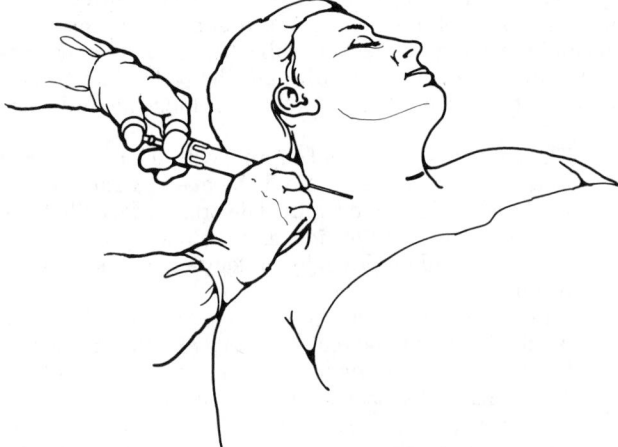

Figure 31-14. Hand position for interscalene blockade. The needle is directed medially and caudad into the interscalene groove while one hand exerts constant control of the depth by resting on the clavicle. (Reproduced with permission from Mulroy M: Handbook of Regional Anesthesia. Boston, Little, Brown, 1989.)

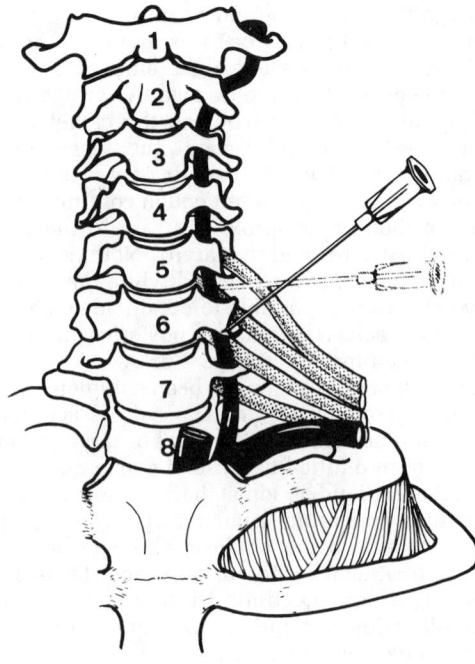

Figure 31-15. Needle direction for interscalene blockade. The needle is always kept in a caudad direction; medial insertion will allow the point to pass into the intervertebral foramen and produce epidural, spinal, or intra-arterial injection of anesthetic. Note the relation of the vertebral artery and the nerve roots to the transverse processes. (Reproduced with permission from Mulroy M: Handbook of Regional Anesthesia. Boston, Little, Brown, 1989.)

redirected in small steps in an anteroposterior (AP) plane until the nerves are identified.

5. Once the nerve is located (usually a paresthesia to the thumb or upper arm), the needle is fixed in this position with one hand while 25–30 ml of local anesthetic solution is injected. Careful aspiration is performed first, and the initial injection is performed in small increments to detect intraneural or intra-arterial placement of the needle. A larger volume (30–40 ml) is required if greater spread is desired, such as to the cervical plexus or inferiorly to the C8 to T1 fibers.
6. If arm surgery requiring a tourniquet is planned, a subcutaneous ring of anesthetic across the axilla is usually required to block the superficial intercostobrachial fibers crossing from the chest wall into the axilla.

Complications from this approach are related to the structures located in the vicinity of the tubercle. The cupola of the lung is close and can be contacted if the needle is directed too far inferior. Pneumothorax should be considered if cough or chest pain is produced while exploring for the nerve. If the needle is allowed to pass directly medially, it may enter the intervertebral foramina, and injection of local anesthetic may produce spinal or epidural anesthesia. The vertebral artery passes posteriorly at the level of the 6th vertebra to lie in its canal in the transverse process; direct injection into this vessel can rapidly produce central nervous system toxicity and convulsions. Careful aspiration and incremental injections are helpful in avoiding both of these potential problems.

Even with appropriate injection, the local anesthetic solution will spread to contiguous nerves. This may produce cervical plexus blockade with high volumes, which may be desirable if shoulder surgery is contemplated. The involvement of the motor fibers of the cervical roots also produces diaphragmatic paralysis,[22] which may be a problem in patients with respiratory insufficiency. The phrenic nerve may be blocked by lower volumes because of diffusion to the anterior side of the anterior scalene or because of inappropriate injection anterior to the muscle.

Neuropathy of the C6 root is a potential problem, because the needle may unintentionally pin the nerve root against the tubercle and predispose to intraneural injection. The needle should be withdrawn slightly if the first injection produces the characteristic "crampy" pain sensation.

Inadequate anesthesia is most likely to occur in the ulnar distribution. As mentioned previously, this can be reduced by the use of higher volumes. Supplemental local anesthesia of the ulnar nerve may also be helpful.

Supraclavicular Approach

The description of the approach to the brachial plexus at this level is originally attributed to Kulenkampff, but the current recommended technique is based on the modifications recommended by Moore[23] and Winnie and Collins.[24] The current technique avoids the originally described medial direction of the needle, which may contact the pleura. It uses the same anatomic consideration, however, in that it attempts to intercept the nerve trunks at their closest approximation to one another as they pass over the 1st rib. The procedure for blockade follows:

1. The patient lies in the same position as for interscalene blockade, with the ipsilateral arm held at the side and pulled downward to exaggerate the landmarks of the clavicle and the neck muscles.
2. The outline of the clavicle is drawn on the skin, as well as the interscalene groove (as described previously). The midpoint of the clavicle is marked. An "X" is placed posterior to this midpoint in the interscalene groove, usually 1 cm behind the clavicle. The groove ideally extends all the way to the 1st rib, where the muscles insert, but palpation of the rib is usually difficult. On the thin patient, the pulsation of the subclavian artery can be appreciated in the groove or just anterior to it.
3. After aseptic preparation, a skin wheal is raised at the mark, and a 3.75-cm 22-gauge needle attached to a 10-ml syringe is introduced in the sagittal plane and advanced caudad until the 1st rib is contacted (Figs. 31-16 to 31-18). It is important that the direction of the needle remain perpendicular to the rib, which usually requires that the syringe remain parallel to the axis of the head and neck. If the rib is not contacted, careful exploration should be carried out first laterally to the mark and, last of all, medially. The greatest danger of contacting the pleura occurs when probing medially.
4. If a paresthesia is produced during the course of exploration, the anesthetic solution is injected while the needle is fixed in position. Twenty-five to forty milliliters of 1% lidocaine or 0.25% bupivacaine may produce adequate analgesia; higher concentrations will produce anesthesia and profound motor blockade. Multiple paresthesias are not usually required, since there are only three trunks at this level and the sheath that encloses them is well defined.
5. If a paresthesia is not obtained on needle insertion, exploration is continued until the rib is identified. A 5-cm needle may be needed to reach the rib in the

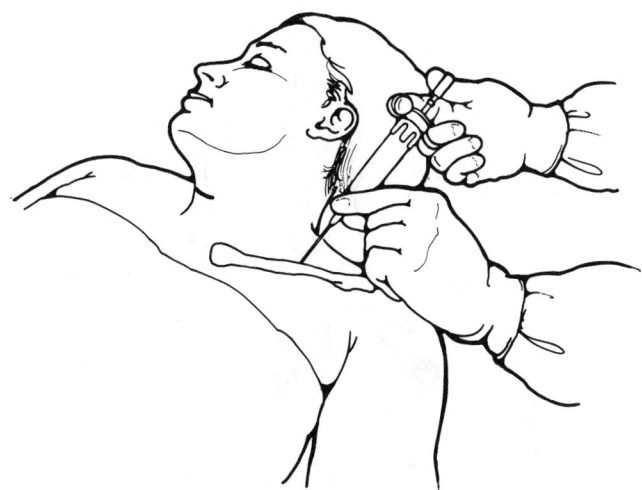

Figure 31-16. Hand position for supraclavicular blockade. The needle is directed caudad behind the midpoint of the clavicle in the interscalene groove. Again, control of depth is maintained by the hand resting on the clavicle. The syringe is kept in the sagittal plane parallel to the patient's head to prevent medial angulation, which would increase the chance of pneumothorax. (Reproduced with permission from Mulroy M: Handbook of Regional Anesthesia. Boston, Little, Brown, 1989.)

heavier patient. Once the rib is contacted, the needle is walked in an AP plane until a paresthesia is found. Again, the needle is kept in the safe sagittal plane on the dorsal surface of the rib during exploration. If the needle advances beyond the anterior or posterior border of the rib as it curves medially at these two points, it is simply redirected in the opposite direction until the rib is found again. Medial direction is avoided. While exploring along the direction of the rib, the nee-

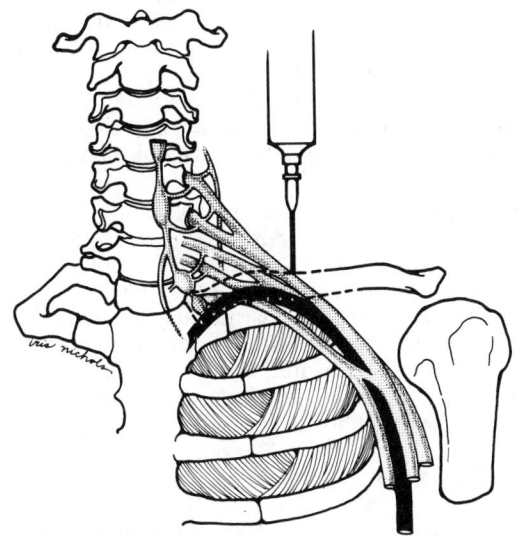

Figure 31-17. Needle direction for supraclavicular blockade (AP view). The needle is directed downward onto the first rib, where it can be expected to contact the three trunks of the brachial plexus as they cross over the rib. The rib at this point lies along the AP plane of the body. (Reproduced with permission from Mulroy M: Handbook of Regional Anesthesia. Boston, Little, Brown, 1989.)

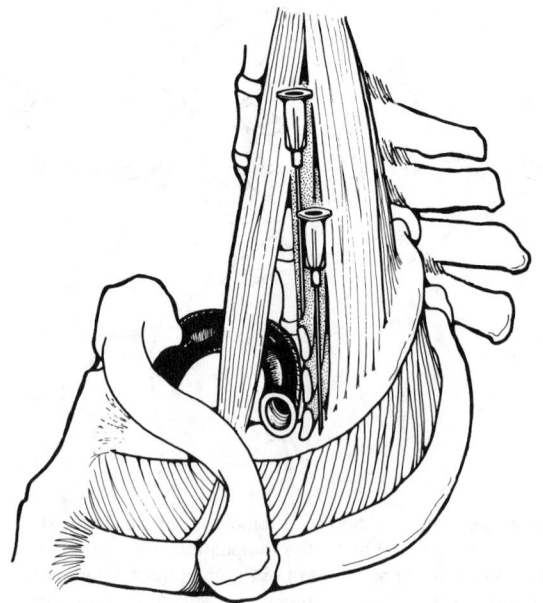

Figure 31-18. Needle direction for supraclavicular blockade (lateral view). The subclavian artery rises from the chest to join the three trunks of the brachial plexus in crossing over the first rib. The nerves usually lie posterior to the artery at this point, although they rapidly encircle it as it becomes the axillary artery. Note that once the needle contacts the rib, it should be withdrawn almost completely to the skin before redirection, since short steps along the bone may simply "push" the nerves ahead of the needle. (Reproduced with permission from Mulroy M: Handbook of Regional Anesthesia. Boston, Little, Brown, 1989.)

dle should be withdrawn almost to the skin before redirection for each pass. If it is lifted only a few millimeters from the rib, it may simply push the nerve bundle ahead of it without making contact.

6. If no paresthesia is obtained, the artery can be used as a landmark. Once it is entered with the needle, a series of injections posterior to it can be used to produce a "wall" of 40 ml of anesthetic solution in this area.

7. If a tourniquet is to be used, a ring of subcutaneous anesthesia should be infiltrated along the axilla to block the sensory fibers from the chest wall that cross here to innervate the inner aspect of the upper arm.

Pneumothorax is the most serious complication of this technique. Although it is rare in experienced hands,[25] it does occur more frequently with this approach to the brachial plexus than with any other approach. This may limit the use of this technique, particularly in outpatients, in whom the insertion of a chest tube would then require hospitalization. The other complications of peripheral blockade do not occur with any greater frequency with this blockade than with other methods of blockade.

Axillary Technique

Of the central approaches, the axillary technique carries the least chance of pneumothorax and thus may be ideal for the outpatient. The nerves are anesthetized around the axillary artery, where they have regrouped into their terminal branches. The technique does generate some controversy because of the observation that at this point the single sheath may be broken up into separate compartments by

fascial septa, which now surround the individual nerves. Although the septa do not limit diffusion of drug in every case,[26] Thompson and Rorie[27] have identified several patients in whom the development of these divisions has limited the spread of anesthetic to other nerves at this level. This has led to the recommendation that local anesthetic be injected at multiple sites with this technique in contrast to the single injections possible with the other approaches. Another obstacle to the single-injection technique at this level is the early departure of the musculocutaneous branch from the sheath high in the axilla. In light of these controversies, several variations of this technique are possible.

Classic Approach, Seeking Paresthesias. This is probably the most common practice. The procedure for blockade follows:

1. The patient lies supine with the arm extended 90 degrees from the side and flexed at the elbow. Extension beyond 90 degrees will potentially compress the axillary artery because of the pressure from the head of the humerus and may make identification of the landmarks more difficult. A pillow under the forearm also reduces rotation of the shoulder joint, which can obscure the pulse.

2. The axillary artery is marked as high in its course in the axilla as is practical. It is usually felt in the intramuscular groove between the coracobrachialis and the triceps muscles. It also passes between the insertions of the pectoralis major and the latissimus dorsi muscles on the humerus.

3. After aseptic preparation, a skin wheal is raised over the proximal portion of the artery. The index and middle fingers of the nondominant hand straddle the artery just below this point, both localizing the pulsation and compressing the sheath below the intended site of injection (Fig. 31-19).

4. A three-ring syringe with a 2.5-cm short bevel needle is held in the other hand, and the needle is introduced alongside the artery seeking a paresthesia. Ideally, the

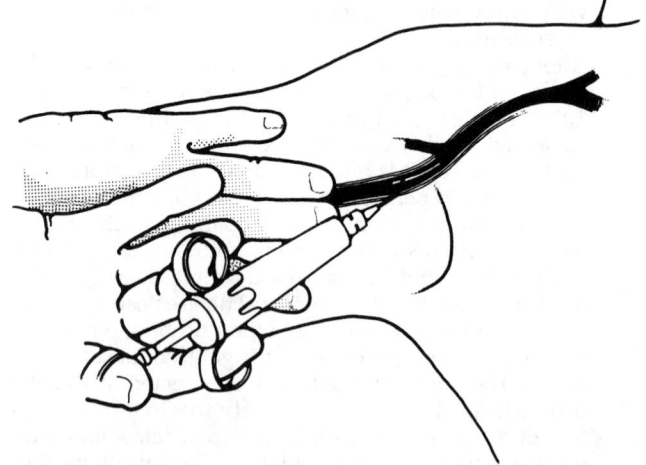

Figure 31-19. Hand position for axillary blockade. Two fingers of equal length straddle the artery while the needle is introduced along its long axis with a central angulation. The palpating fingers serve not only to identify the vessel but also to compress the perivascular sheath and encourage the spread of anesthetic solution centrally. (Reproduced with permission from Mulroy M: Handbook of Regional Anesthesia. Boston, Little, Brown, 1989.)

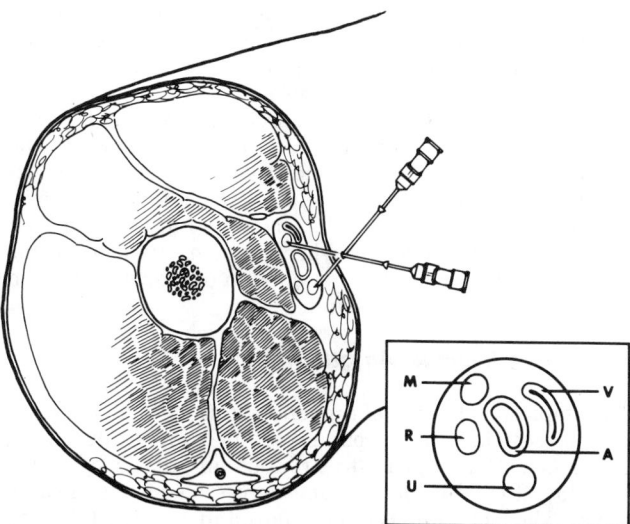

Figure 31-20. Needle position for axillary injection. The median and musculocutaneous nerves lie on the superior side of the artery, although the latter may have already departed the axillary sheath at the level of injection. The ulnar nerve lies inferior, and the radial nerve is inferior and posterior.

nerves serving the area of proposed surgery are sought first. The median and the musculocutaneous nerves lie on the superior aspect of the artery (as viewed by the operator), whereas the ulnar and radial nerves lie below and behind the vessel (Fig. 31-20).

5. When a paresthesia is obtained, the contents of the syringe are injected, taking precautions to avoid intraneural injection. Firm pressure is maintained on the distal sheath to encourage the solution to move centrally from the point of injection, hopefully to include the point of origin of the musculocutaneous nerve. At this point, the anesthesiologist may elect to fix the needle in position, refill the syringe, and inject a total dose of 25–40 ml of anesthetic solution near this single paresthesia. As an alternative, the larger bolus may be injected from a 50-ml syringe attached to the needle by an intravenous extension tube.

6. If other paresthesias are desired, they should be elicited within 5 minutes of the original injection. Beyond this time, spread of the solution may produce hypesthesia of the other nerves, which prevents their identification. A second paresthesia should be sought on the side of the artery opposite the original one. With this approach, 15–20 ml of solution is injected following elicitation of each paresthesia.

7. If separate supplementary anesthesia of the musculocutaneous nerve is sought, it can be obtained by injecting an additional 5–10 ml of anesthetic solution into the body of the coracobrachialis muscle. This muscle can be easily grasped between the thumb and forefinger, and the entry into its fascial compartment is readily identified. This step may be required even if 40 ml of solution is used in the perivascular injection, since the musculocutaneous nerve may be spared as often as 25% of the time even with this or larger volumes.[28]

Alternate Approach of Multiple Injections Without Paresthesias. As an alternative to the classic technique, anesthesia can be obtained without seeking paresthesias. This approach may reduce nerve injury.[29] The technique is identical to that just described except that no paresthesias are elicited and the anesthetic solution is simply injected on each side of the artery in multiple small increments covering the entire perivascular area and producing a "wall" of solution that intercepts the paths of each of the branches. This approach is potentially less reliable and requires meticulous attention to localization of the artery and the surrounding fascial compartment.

Transarterial Approach. This is another alternative that seeks to avoid paresthesias. Again, the preparation and landmarks are identical to those of the classic approach. Here the artery is deliberately entered directly with the needle. The needle is advanced through the vessel until aspiration confirms that it has passed just posterior; at this point, half the anesthetic solution is injected incrementally with careful attention to avoid intravascular placement. The needle is then withdrawn back through the vessel until aspiration confirms that it is just anterior to the artery. The other half of the solution is injected.

This technique is simple and effective and should be kept in mind as an alternative while the classic approach is being used. If paresthesias cannot be obtained with the former or (more commonly) if the vessel is unintentionally entered during the search, the transarterial approach should be used.

The complications of all these approaches are minimal compared with those of the other central approaches. The problem of neuropathy is the foremost consideration. Hematoma can occur if the vessel is punctured, but this is rarely a problem. The use of small-gauge needles may reduce this possibility.

Distal Upper Extremity Blockade

As in the leg, the nerves to the hand can be blocked at the point where they cross the two major joints, the elbow and the wrist (Fig. 31-21). At these two levels, the overlying muscles are thinned and the bony landmarks are more prominent, allowing easier identification of the nerves. Peripheral blockade is usually not quite as dense as central blockade but may be useful in anesthetizing one branch that was missed with a central blockade or in providing very localized anesthesia on the hand. Since the sensory branches to the forearm from the musculocutaneous nerve and the internal cutaneous nerve have already branched so extensively that adequate anesthesia of the forearm is not easily obtained, blockade at the elbow really produces no greater anesthesia than blockade at the wrist.

Blockade at the Elbow. Two nerves to the hand cross this joint on the inner aspect, whereas the ulnar travels posteriorly in its well-known superficial groove. The procedure for blockade follows:

1. The ulnar nerve is blocked by injection of 1–4 ml of local anesthetic proximal to the groove formed by the medial condyle of the humerus and the olecranon. This is easily done with the joint flexed at about 30 degrees. Further flexion may cause the nerve to roll medially and anterior to the condyle. Paresthesias can usually be readily obtained, but direct injection on a paresthesia or directly into the groove under pressure is not advised because of the risk of damage to the nerve. If the injection is made deep to the fascia, anesthesia should commence within 5 minutes.

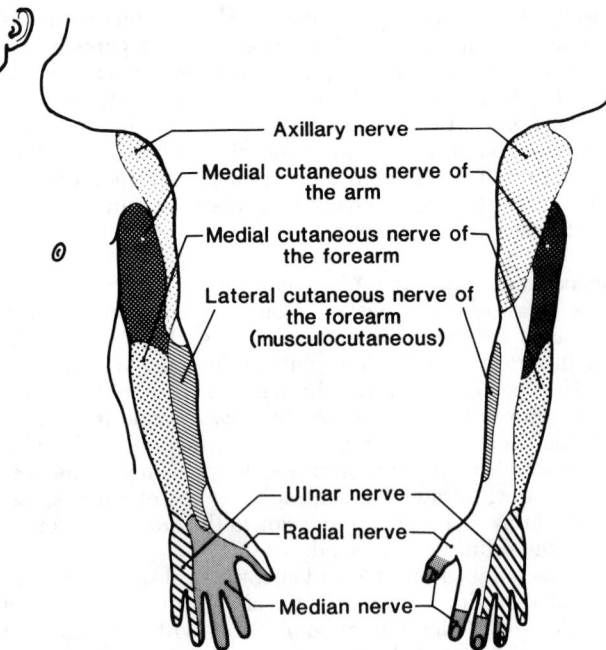

Figure 31-21. Sensory dermatomes of the arm. Sensation is provided by the terminal nerves, as identified. This pattern is different from the classic dermatomal distribution of the nerve roots. Different patterns of anesthesia develop if the blockade is performed at the root level (interscalene blockade) *versus* the terminal nerve level (axillary blockade). (Reproduced with permission from Mulroy M: Handbook of Regional Anesthesia. Boston, Little, Brown, 1989.)

2. The median nerve crosses the joint in the company of the brachial artery. A line is drawn between the two condyles on the inner aspect of the joint, and a skin wheal is raised at the point where this line crosses the pulsation of the brachial artery, usually 1 cm to the ulnar side of the biceps tendon. A needle is introduced perpendicularly at this point, and paresthesias are sought immediately adjacent to the artery. Five milliliters of solution are sufficient to produce anesthesia, and, again, intraneural injection is carefully avoided.

3. The radial nerve is identified along the same intracondylar line, approximately 2 cm lateral to the biceps tendon. Another skin wheal is raised here, and, again, a needle is inserted to search for paresthesias in a fan-shaped pattern. If paresthesias are not obtained, a "wall" of anesthetic solution can be deposited here but with less chance of reliable anesthesia.

Blockade at the Wrist. The nerves lie more superficially at this joint and are closely associated with easily identified landmarks (Fig. 31-22). For this reason, blockade at this level is usually preferred to other distal approaches. The procedure for blockade follows:

1. The ulnar nerve lies between the ulnar artery and the flexor carpi ulnaris. A skin wheal is raised at the level of the styloid process on the palmar side of the forearm between these two landmarks. A small-gauge needle is inserted, and 3 ml of solution is injected into the area, with or without paresthesias.

2. At the same level on the forearm, the median nerve lies between the tendons of the palmaris longus and the flexor carpi radialis. If only the palmaris longus

can be felt, the nerve is just to the radial side of this tendon. A skin wheal is raised, and a needle is inserted until it pierces the deep fascia. Three milliliters of solution will produce anesthesia.

3. The radial nerve requires a broader injection, as it has already started to ramify as it crosses the wrist. The anatomic "snuffbox" formed by the tendons of the extensor pollicus longus and extensor pollicus brevis tendons is located, and 3 ml of solution is injected here. A subcutaneous wheal is then raised from this point, extending over the dorsum of the wrist 3–4 cm onto the back of the hand.

Intravenous Regional Anesthesia

The simplest technique of arm anesthesia is the injection of local anesthetic into the venous system below an occluding tourniquet. This appears to produce anesthesia by direct diffusion of the anesthetic from the vessels into the nearby nerves. The technique is often referred to as a *Bier block*, in honor of August Bier who first described anesthesia produced in this manner. His technique required a cutdown and ligation of a vein; the modern adaptation is elegant in its simplicity. The procedure for blockade follows:

1. A small-gauge (20 or 22) intravenous plastic catheter is inserted in the arm to be blocked on the dorsum of the hand. It is taped firmly in place, and a heparin port or small syringe is attached and saline is injected to maintain patency. A pneumatic tourniquet is applied over the upper arm.

2. The arm is elevated to promote venous drainage. An elastic bandage may be applied to produce further exsanguination. After exsanguination, the touniquet is inflated to 300 mm Hg or 2.5 times the systolic blood

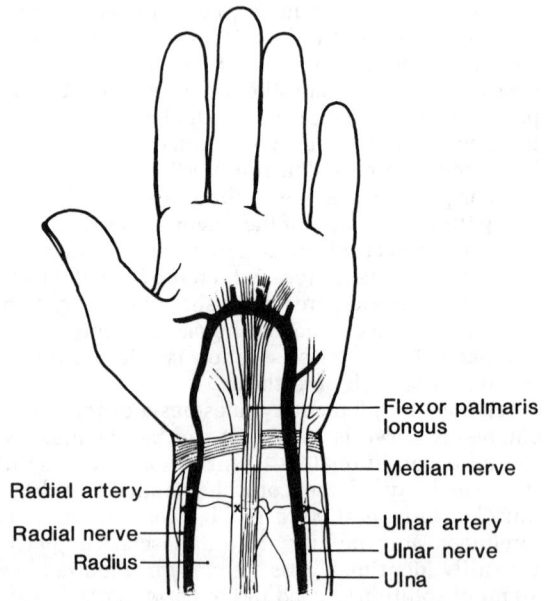

Figure 31-22. Terminal nerves at the wrist. The median nerve lies just to the radial side of the flexor palmaris longus. The ulnar and radial nerves lie just "outside" their respective arteries. The radial nerve has already begun branching at this level and must be blocked by a wide subcutaneous ridge of anesthetic. (Reproduced with permission from Mulroy M: Handbook of Regional Anesthesia. Boston, Little, Brown, 1989.)

pressure and is tested carefully for adequate occlusion of the radial pulse.

3. The arm is returned to the horizontal position, a 50-ml syringe with 0.5% lidocaine or prilocaine (or 0.25% bupivacaine) is attached to the previously inserted cannula, and the contents are injected. The forearm will discolor, and the patient will perceive a transient "pins and needles" sensation as anesthesia ensues over the following 5 minutes. Epinephrine should *not* be added to the local anesthetic solution.

4. For short procedures, the cannula can be removed at this point. If surgery may extend beyond 1 hour, the cannula can be left in place and reinjected after 90 minutes.

5. Beyond 45 minutes of surgery, many patients will experience discomfort at the level of the tourniquet. Special "double-cuff" tourniquets are available for this blockade to alleviate this problem. The proximal cuff is inflated first, allowing anesthesia to be induced in the area under the distal cuff. If discomfort ensues, the distal cuff is inflated over the anesthetized area of skin, and the uncomfortable proximal cuff is released. This step is critical, since the major risk of this procedure is premature release of solution into the circulation. If a double cuff is used, both cuffs should be tested before starting and the proper sequence for inflation and deflation meticulously followed. The potential for leakage of anesthetic into the circulation is greater with these narrower cuffs used in the double setup. Since the "shifting" process also increases the potential for unintentional release of anesthetic, the use of a single wider cuff may be better for short procedures.

6. If surgery is completed in less than 20 minutes, the tourniquet is left inflated for at least that total period of time. If 40 minutes have elapsed, the tourniquet can be deflated as a single maneuver. Between 20 and 40 minutes, the cuff can be deflated, reinflated immediately, and finally deflated after a minute to delay the sudden absorption of anesthetic into the systemic circulation.[30]

7. The duration of anesthesia is minimal beyond the time of tourniquet release. Although bupivacaine may produce a slight prolongation of analgesia, the advantage is short.

The simplicity of this technique is offset by the significant risk of systemic local anesthetic toxicity if the tourniquet fails or is released prematurely. Careful testing of the tourniquet and slow injection of solution into a peripheral (not antecubital) vein will reduce the chance of leakage under the tourniquet.[31] Systemic blood levels are time-dependent,[32] and careful attention should be paid to the sequence of tourniquet release and patient monitoring during this period. A separate intravenous site for injection of resuscitation drugs is needed as well as ready availability of all needed equipment. With careful attention to these details, this technique is one of the most effective and reliable available to the anesthesiologist.

Trunk

Anesthesia of the abdomen and chest is most simply obtained with spinal and epidural injections of local anesthetics, as discussed in Chapter 30. In some situations, a narrower band of intercostal or paravertebral anesthesia is preferable, or epidural injection may be hazardous because of infection or coagulopathy. In many clinical situations, it may also be desirable to separate the anesthesia of the somatic and sympathetic fibers that inevitably occurs in combination when these axial blockades are performed. The sympathetic nerves separate from their somatic counterparts early in their course, which makes independent somatic and sympathetic blockade a practical consideration. Sympathetic blockade is most commonly performed at the major ganglia, particularly the stellate, celiac, and lumbar plexus. These blockades often require multiple injections and are technically more difficult than axial anesthesia, but they do offer advantages in certain clinical situations.

The somatic nerves of the chest emerge from their respective intervertebral foramina and pass through the narrow triangular-shaped paravertebral space. In this triangle, they give off the sympathetic branch and also a small dorsal branch, which provides sensation to the midline of the back. The main trunks then pass into the intercostal groove along the ventral caudad surface of each rib. An artery and vein travel along with each of these nerves in the groove under the protection of the overhanging external edge of the rib. The fasciae of the internal and external intercostal muscles provide interior and external borders of this intercostal groove. As the nerves travel beyond the midaxillary line, they give off a lateral sensory branch while the main trunk continues on to the anterior abdominal wall to provide sensory and motor innervation for the trunk and abdomen down to the level of the pubis. The intercostal groove becomes much less well defined anterior to the midaxillary line, and the nerve begins to move away from its protected position. The lowermost intercostal nerve (the 12th) is much less closely applied to its accompanying rib and is less easy to identify and anesthetize using a classic intercostal blockade technique. The upper lumbar roots form the ilioinguinal nerves, which pass laterally within the muscles of the abdominal wall at the level of the iliac crest and eventually move anteriorly to provide innervation of the groin region as the ilioinguinal nerves.

The anatomic basis for separate sympathetic anesthesia is produced by the early separation of sympathetic fibers from their somatic roots in the form of the white rami communicantes, which separate from the somatic nerves shortly after their emergence from the intervertebral foramina and join the sympathetic ganglia, which lie anteriorly on each side of the vertebral bodies. These preganglionic fibers of the sympathetic system usually arise only from the 1st thoracic through the 2nd lumbar segments. The spinal ganglia formed by these fibers constitute the sympathetic trunks, which extend upward into the neck and caudad along the lumbar spine. They give terminal sympathetic branches to all the areas of the body. The sympathetic innervation of the head and the lower extremities is derived from fibers that originate from the spinal cord, join sympathetic trunks, and then pass cephalad or caudad along the chain of ganglia before reaching their target organs. Segmental sympathetic innervation of the body from the cervical to the sacral roots is provided by postganglionic nerves departing from the chains (the gray rami communicantes), which rejoin the somatic nerves early in their course. In the head (where motor and sensory innervation is by cranial nerves), the sympathetic fibers reach their end organs by traveling with the arterial vascular supply. The sympathetic ganglia in the neck lie along the lateral border of the relatively flat vertebral bodies. In the chest, the vertebral bodies become more rounded, and the chain of ganglia lies more posteriorly on the lateral side of the vertebral body near the head of each rib. In the abdomen and pelvis, the sympathetic chains begin to move anteriorly and lie on the ventral surface of the vertebral bodies and thus are more widely separated from their respective somatic nerves.

Intercostal Nerve Blockade

Anesthesia of the intercostal nerves provides both motor and sensory anesthesia of the entire abdominal wall from the xiphoid to the pubis. The 6th to 11th ribs are usually easily identified, and their accompanying nerves are reliably blocked by injections along the easily palpated sharp posterior angulation of the ribs, which occurs between 5–7 cm from the midline in the back.[33] Ribs above the 5th are difficult to palpate because of the overlying scapula and paraspinous muscles and are thus most easily blocked using the paravertebral technique. Establishing five or six levels of intercostal nerve blockade is a useful anesthetic procedure for providing analgesia and motor relaxation for upper abdominal procedures such as cholecystectomy and gastric surgery. This form of anesthesia usually requires supplementation with light general anesthesia or an additional sympathetic blockade, since much of the intraperitoneal and subdiaphragmatic sensation is carried by other nerve trunks. This form of anesthesia for upper abdominal surgery offers the advantages of muscle relaxation without the necessity of an accompanying sympathetic blockade (unless celiac plexus blockade is chosen as an optional supplement). Intercostal blockade with long-acting amide local anesthetics also provides postoperative analgesia for 8–12 hours, which may greatly facilitate patient satisfaction and immediate recovery.[34] Unilateral blockade of these nerves is a useful treatment for the pain of rib fracture and also serves to reduce postoperative analgesia requirements in patients with subcostal incisions. Several segments must be blocked in each of these applications because of the overlap of the intercostal nerves. This technique is also useful in reducing the pain associated with the insertion of chest tubes or percutaneous biliary drainage procedures. The procedure for blockade follows:

1. For the performance of intercostal blockade, the patient may be in the lateral, sitting, or prone position. For operative anesthesia, the prone position is most practical. A pillow is placed under the abdomen in order to provide slight flexion of the thoracic spine. The arms are draped over the edge of the stretcher or operating table so that the scapula falls away laterally from the midline. The anesthesiologist stands at the patient's side. Most anesthesiologists prefer to stand on the side that allows their dominant hand to hold the syringe at the caudad end of the patient.

2. The spinous processes in the midline from T6 through T12 are marked (Fig. 31-23). The ribs are then identified along the line of their most extreme posterior angulation. For the 12th rib, this is usually 7 cm from the midline. At the level of the 6th rib, this posterior angulation is best appreciated somewhat more medially, usually 5 cm from the midline. These two ribs are marked first at their inferior borders, and a line is drawn between these two points. The rest of the ribs between them are identified, and a mark is placed on the inferior border of each rib along the angled parasagittal plane identified by the first line between the 6th and 12th ribs.

3. After aseptic preparation, light sedation is provided for the patient, and a skin wheal is raised at each mark.

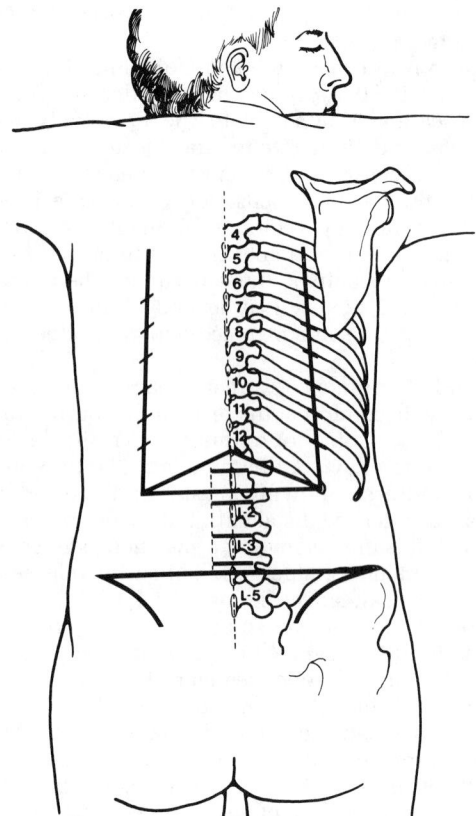

Figure 31-23. Landmarks for intercostal blockade. The inferior borders of the ribs are identified at their most prominent points on the back. The marks then usually lie along a line that angles slightly medially from the 12th to the 6th rib. The triangle drawn between the 12th ribs and their spinous processes is used for the celiac plexus blockade. (Reproduced with permission from Mulroy M: Handbook of Regional Anesthesia. Boston, Little, Brown, 1989.)

4. The ribs are usually blocked starting with the lowermost and moving upward. The 12th rib is not closely associated with its intercostal nerve, and a reliable blockade is not usually possible. For upper abdominal procedures, blockade of this nerve can be omitted without jeopardizing the anesthesia.

5. Starting with the lowest rib on the side closest to the anesthesiologist, the index finger of the cephalad hand is placed on the skin above the identifying mark; this finger should lie immediately over the midpoint of the rib. The skin is then retracted in a cephalad direction, so that the previous mark now lies over the rib itself, somewhat toward the inferior side. The anesthesiologist's other hand inserts a 22-gauge 3.75-cm needle directly onto the rib. This needle is attached to a 10-ml syringe filled with local anesthetic. The syringe and needle are held in such a way that they maintian a constant 10-degree cephalad angulation.

6. Once the needle is safely "parked" on the dorsal surface of the rib, the cephalad hand releases the tension on the skin and takes control of the needle and syringe (Fig. 31-24). This is done by placing the ulnar border of the hand firmly against the skin and grasping the hub of the needle firmly between the thumb and index finger. The middle finger of this hand rests

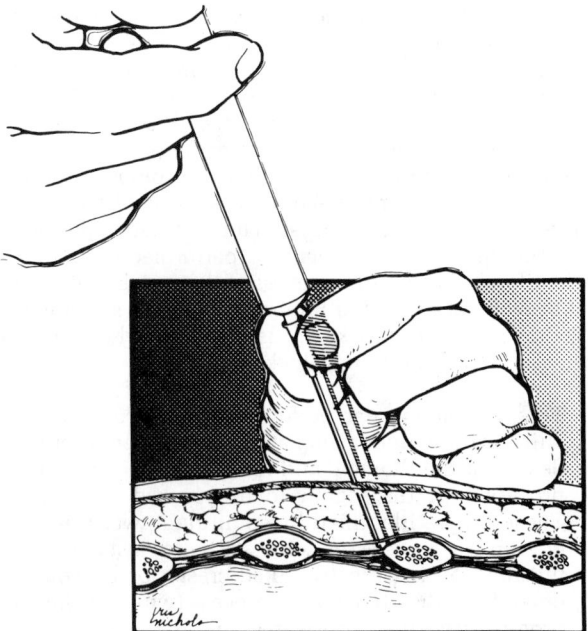

Figure 31-24. Hand and needle positions for intercostal blockade. The depth of the needle is controlled by the hand resting on the back. The other hand injects solution when the needle is under the rib, but that is the only function performed while the needle is near the pleura. (Reproduced with permission from Mulroy M: Handbook of Regional Anesthesia. Boston, Little, Brown, 1989.)

along the shaft of the needle to provide guidance. Once the syringe is firmly gripped by the cephalad hand, the fingers of the caudad hand are placed in an "injection" position, either in the rings of a three-ring syringe or on the plunger of a straight syringe.

7. The needle and syringe are then raised slightly off the bone and "walked" in a caudad direction until they pass below the inferior border of the rib. The entire needle and syringe unit is kept at a 10-degree cephalad angle to the rib at all times. As it passes the inferior border, the needle is advanced 4–6 mm under the rib, with the needle actually pointing slightly cephalad into the intercostal groove.

8. Once in the groove, aspiration is performed, and 3–5 ml of local anesthetic solution is injected. Generally, 0.25% bupivacaine produces good sensory anesthesia, whereas 0.5% bupivacaine is required for prolonged anesthesia with motor blockade. Aspiration is not reliable in preventing intravascular injection of the anesthetic; a slight "jiggling" motion of the needle during the injection will reduce this chance by ensuring that the needle is in a vessel only transiently if it does occur.

9. As soon as the injection is complete, the needle is withdrawn from the groove and moved cephalad and parked again on the safe dorsal surface of the rib. The fingers of the caudad hand are then removed from the injection position and assume control of the syringe again. The cephalad hand now relinquishes control and is moved up to the next rib to repeat this cyclic process.

10. The six or seven designated ribs on each side are blocked in this process by progressively moving up the back, with control of the syringe alternating between the cephalad and caudad hands at the time of

injection. The ribs on the opposite side are blocked in a similar manner. This can be done with the anesthesiologist standing on the same side and reaching across the back, or by moving to the opposite side of the patient. If the contralateral blockades are performed from the opposite side of the bed, an attempt should be made to "switch hands," so that the functions of the cephalad and caudad hands remain the same even though the right and left hands have changed roles. It is sometimes more difficult for operators to control the syringe with their nondominant hand. It is worth the effort, since attempting to hold the syringe in the cephalad hand often makes maintenance of the proper cephalad angulation difficult. The syringe often ends up being rotated along its long axis as it is moved to the caudad edge of the rib, with the result that by the time the needle moves off the rib, it is pointed in a caudad rather than a cephalad direction. This produces an injection of solution away from the nerve rather than into the groove.

11. If the intercostal nerve blockades are to be supplemented by a number of somatic paravertebral nerve blockades or sympathetic blockade of the celiac plexus, these are performed at the end of intercostal anesthesia. Care should be taken to adjust the total dose of drug in such combinations of techniques so that the maximal recommended amounts are not exceeded.

Despite frequent concern about the incidence of pneumothorax with intercostal blockade, this complication is rare in experienced hands.[35] This depends primarily upon maintaining strict safety features of the described technique. Primarily, emphasis should be placed on absolute control of the syringe and needle at all times, particularly during the injection. This control requires that the cephalad hand, which is securely resting on the back, is the one that controls the depth of needle insertion. The needle rests on the safe dorsal side surface of the rib at all other times except for the brief moment of injection.

A common complication is related to the sedation required to perform this blockade in the prone position. The 12 to 14 needle insertions are uncomfortable, and patients usually require some narcotic and amnesic sedation. Overdose can lead to airway obstruction and respiratory depression in the prone position. Ideally, the sedation should be administered by an assistant who will monitor the patient's airway and breathing closely while the anesthesiologist is performing the blockade. Care should be exercised in patients with reflux esophagitis to avoid regurgitation and aspiration during this procedure. Attention must also be paid to the patient's mental status, since this blockade produces the highest blood levels of local anesthetics when compared with any other regional anesthetic technique. Because this blockade is frequently supplemented by a light general anesthetic for surgery, signs of systemic toxicity are rarely seen because of the overlying general anesthetic. When the blockade is performed for postoperative pain relief, the dose should be reduced to 0.25% bupivacaine in order to minimize the chance for toxicity.

Although one of the advantages of this blockade is the avoidance of sympathetic blockade and its attendant cardiovascular changes, it is possible to produce partial spinal or epidural anesthesia if the injection is made close to the midline and the anesthetic tracks along a dural sleeve to the epidural or subarachnoid space.[36] This appears to be more likely if intrathoracic injection is performed intraoperatively by a surgeon. Hypotension may result in this situation. Hypotension has also been observed rarely when this blockade is used for postoperative pain relief in a patient who has received generous doses of opioids. Once the local anesthetic succeeds in relieving the pain, the patient's intrinsic sympathetic response is reduced, and the respiratory depressant effect of previously injected opioids is unmasked. Patients should be observed for at least 20–30 minutes following performance of intercostal blockade. Respiratory insufficiency can also be seen if the intercostal muscles are blocked in a patient who is dependent on them for ventilation. Patients with chronic obstructive disease with ineffective diaphragm motion are not good candidates for this technique.

Paravertebral Blockade

The upper five ribs are more difficult to palpate laterally, and blockade of their associated intercostal nerves is best performed with a paravertebral injection. This approach is technically more difficult and has slightly greater potential for complications because of the proximity of the lung and of the intervertebral foramina. Anatomically, the injection is made into the triangle formed by the intervertebral body, the pleura, and the plane of the transverse processes (Fig. 31-25). The intervertebral foramina at each level lie between the transverse processes and approximately 2 cm anterior to the plane formed by the transverse processes in their associated fasciae. At this point, the sympathetic ganglia lie very close to the somatic nerves, and coincidental sympathetic blockade is usually attained. This is also related to the injection of larger volumes of local anesthetic that is required because location of the nerve is less reliable with this technique. Nevertheless, it is a useful technique for segmental anesthesia, particularly of the upper thoracic segments. It is also useful if a more proximal blockade is needed, such as to relieve the pain of herpes zoster or of a proximal rib fracture.

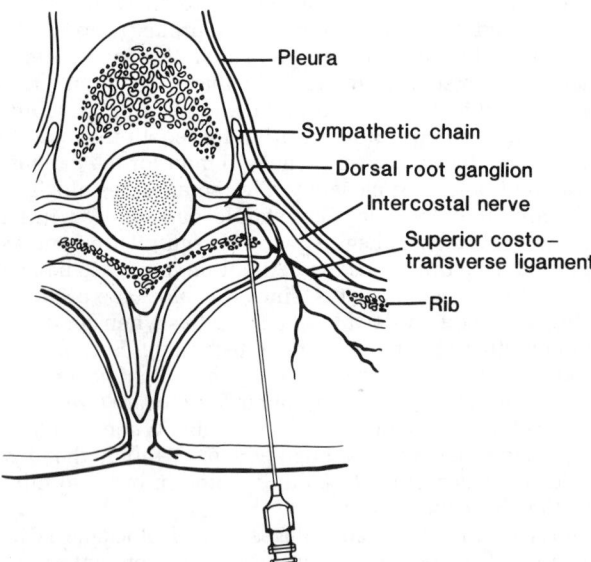

Figure 31-25. Paravertebral blockade. As it exits the intervertebral foramen, the thoracic somatic nerve enters a small triangular space formed by the vertebral body, the plane of the transverse process, and the pleura. Medial direction of the needle is obviously important in reducing the chance of a pneumothorax.

The paravertebral approach varies somewhat, depending upon the spinal level. In the upper thoracic spine, the transverse process is located lateral to the spinous process of the vertebral body above it. In the lower thoracic spine, the spinous processes are less steeply angled, so that the 11th and 12th spinous processes lie between the associated transverse processes. In the lumbar region, the spinous processes are straight, and the transverse processes lie opposite their own respective spinous process. Thus, paravertebral blockade in the upper thoracic region is performed at each level by identifying the spinous process of the vertebra *above* the level to be blocked; in the lumbar region, the spinous process of the level to be blocked is used to locate the transverse process. The procedure for blockade follows:

1. This blockade is also performed in the prone position, with a pillow under the patient's abdomen to produce flexion of the thoracic and lumbar spine. The spinous processes in the region to be blocked are marked. These can be identified by counting upward from the 4th lumbar process (which usually lies just at or above the line joining the two iliac crests) or by counting down from the 7th cervical process (which is the most prominent in the cervical region).

2. Transverse lines are drawn across the cephalad border of the spinous processes and extended laterally to overlie the transverse process (approximately 1–4 cm). In the lumbar region, the lines overlie the transverse process of the associated vertebra. In the thoracic region, they indicate the transverse process of the vertebral body immediately below the associated spinous process. Finally, a vertical line is drawn parallel to the spine 3–4 cm lateral to it joining the transverse lines from the spinous processes. For a diagnostic blockade, a single nerve may need to be anesthetized. For pain control, several levels must be identified. The injection of at least three segments (as in intercostal blockade) is required to produce reliable segmental blockade because of sensory overlap.

3. Following aseptic skin preparation, skin wheals are raised at the intersections of the vertical and transverse lines.

4. A 22-gauge needle is introduced through the skin wheal in the sagittal plane and directed slightly cephalad to contact the transverse process. A 7.5-cm needle is usually required in the average patient, and the transverse process will lie between 3 and 5 cm from the skin. Gentle cephalad or caudad exploration may be required to identify the bone. The depth of the transverse process is carefully noted on the needle shaft.

5. The needle is now withdrawn from the transverse process and "walked" inferiorly to pass below its caudad edge. This usually requires more perpendicular direction relative to the skin. The needle is advanced 2 cm below the transverse process and angled slightly medial to attempt to contact the vertebral body. Paresthesias are not sought unless a neurolytic injection is planned. When the needle has entered the paravertebral space, 5–10 ml of local anesthetic solution is injected after careful aspiration.

The complication of pneumothorax is more likely in the thoracic region with this technique than with intercostal blockade.[37] The needle should be directed medially as it passes below the transverse process and never more than 2 cm beyond the transverse process (see Fig. 31-25). If cough or chest pain occurs, a chest x-ray should be performed to rule out pneumothorax. Subarachnoid injection is also more likely in the thoracic area because of the extension of the dural sleeves to the level of the intervertebral foramina. Careful aspiration is important but may not prevent the unintentional injection of local anesthetic into a subdural pocket. Total spinal anesthesia can result with a 5- to 10-ml injection. Systemic toxicity is also a possibility because of the need for relatively large volumes of local anesthetic. Attention must be paid to the total milligram dosage injected. The volume required for each level obviously limits the concentrations that can be used and the total number of levels that can be blocked. If lumbar paravertebral injections are combined with intercostals, the concentration and total volume for both blockades may have to be reduced.

Intrapleural Anesthesia

Upper abdominal analgesia can also be obtained by inserting an epidural catheter into the intrapleural space for injection or infusion of local anesthetic. The anesthetic appears to diffuse through the parietal pleura onto the intercostal nerves and produce anesthesia similar to injection of multiple intercostal nerve blocks. It may also act upon the sympathetic nerves by diffusion to the ganglia lying along the anterior vertebral borders.

1. As with intercostal block, the technique can be performed with the patient in the prone, lateral, or sitting position.
2. The 7th or 8th intercostal space is identified 8–10 cm from the midline and marked at the upper border of the lower rib.
3. A skin wheal is made at this site, and a Tuohy epidural needle is inserted with the bevel directed cephalad and advanced over the inferior rib in a slightly medial and cephalad angle through the intercostal muscles. Once in the intercostal layers, the stylet is removed, and an air-filled 5-ml glass syringe is attached.
4. The needle is advanced farther until the parietal pleura is punctured, signaled by a negative pressure that moves the plunger of the syringe forward. The syringe is removed, and a standard epidural catheter is threaded 5–6 cm beyond the tip. Aspiration is performed to exclude perforation of the lung or a blood vessel.
5. Twenty milliliters of 0.5% bupivacaine with epinephrine is injected into the pleural space, and the catheter is carefully taped to the skin. Reinjection is required every 3–6 hours, or a constant infusion of 0.25% bupivacaine ($0.125 \text{ ml·kg}^{-1}\text{·h}^{-1}$) can be initiated.

There have been several enthusiastic reports of success with this technique,[38] but several limitations have been described. Pain relief is usually reliable, and respiratory depression is not a problem. However, the duration is short enough that large quantities of local anesthetic are required to maintain analgesia, and systemic toxicity has been reported in 1.3% of patients.[39] The incidence of pneumothorax (averaging 2%) is not inconsequential, especially with first attempts. Puncture of the lung also occurs, apparently with a higher incidence if a "loss of resistance" technique is used rather than the passive identification process described above. A major limitation is the unilateral analgesia, which limits this technique to procedures such as cholecystectomy and nephrectomy, rib fracture, and herpetic pain.

Loss of local anesthetic solution to thoracostomy drainage makes this technique less reliable for thoracotomy pain.

The technique is relatively new. Its ultimate utility, especially in comparison to that of epidural opioid infusion, remains unclear.

Sympathetic Blockade—Stellate Ganglion

Separate blockade of the sympathetic fibers of the upper extremity and head can be achieved by a single injection of a local anesthetic on the stellate ganglion. The ganglion is the large fusion of the first thoracic sympathetic ganglion with the lower cervical ganglion on each side, and it lies on the generally flat lateral border of the vertebral body of C7. All the fibers to the middle and superior cervical ganglia pass through this lowermost collection and thus can be anesthetized with a single injection. Although technically simple, the location of this ganglia in close proximity to the carotid artery, the vertebral artery, and the pleura makes this a challenging blockade. It is very useful in providing pain relief for sympathetic dystrophies of the upper arm. Stellate ganglion blockade may relieve the pain of acute herpes zoster infection of the head or neck region. It has also been advocated as a means of reducing post-thoracotomy pain by blocking the sympathetic sensory fibers to the pleural cavity. The procedure for blockade follows:

1. The patient is placed in a supine position with a small towel or pillow under the neck, and the arms are held at the side.
2. The medial border of the sternocleidomastoid muscle on the involved side is marked with a pen, as is the level of the cricoid cartilage. Gentle palpation approximately 2 cm lateral to the cartilage often reveals the anterior tubercle of the transverse process of the 6th cervical vertebra (Chassaignac's tubercle). A circle is marked over this tubercle, and an "X" is placed 1.5–2 cm caudad to this mark at the same distance from the midline. This "X" should overlie the tubercle of the 7th cervical vertebra and should fall at the medial border of the sternocleidomastoid muscle body and approximately two fingerbreadths above the clavicle itself.
3. A skin wheal is made at the "X" after aseptic skin preparation.
4. With the index and middle finger of one hand, the sternocleidomastoid muscle and the carotid sheath are retracted laterally (Fig. 31-26). A 22- or 25-gauge 3.75-cm needle is introduced through the "X" and passed directly posterior until it rests on bone. Paresthesia of the brachial plexus implies that the needle is too far laterally and has passed beyond the transverse process. It may have to be readjusted slightly more medially and perhaps more cephalad or caudad.
5. Once bone is contacted, the needle is withdrawn a few millimeters, and very careful aspiration is performed to rule out contact with the vertebral artery. A 2-ml test dose is injected to further evaluate an unrecognized intravascular position. The patient's mental status must be closely observed.
6. If no change occurs, a total of 10 ml of local anesthetic can be injected incrementally with frequent aspiration. One percent lidocaine or 0.25% bupivacaine or their equivalents are more than adequate to produce anesthesia of the sympathetic nerves.
7. Onset of sympathectomy is usually indicated by the appearance of a Horner's syndrome on the ipsilateral

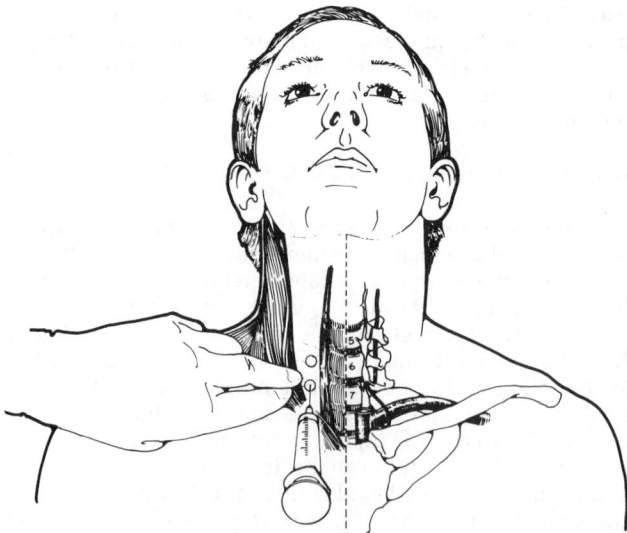

Figure 31-26. Stellate ganglion blockade. The sternocleidomastoid muscle and the carotid sheath are retracted laterally with one hand while the needle is introduced directly onto the lateral border of the 7th vertebral body, just medial to the transverse process. The vertebral artery is passing posteriorly at this level to enter its canal in the transverse processes, but here it lies near the level of intended injection. After contacting bone, the needle is withdrawn slightly and careful aspiration is performed before incremental injection. (Reproduced with permission from Mulroy M: Handbook of Regional Anesthesia. Boston, Little, Brown, 1989.)

side. Ptosis, miosis, and anhydrosis usually develop within 10 minutes as well as vasodilation in the arm. Nasal congestion is another common sign usually associated with Horner's syndrome.

As implied, there are several potential complications of stellate ganglion blockade related to the surrounding anatomy. The pleura can be punctured, with resulting pneumothorax. Intravascular injection is the most serious complication because of the close proximity of the vertebral artery to the site of injection. Careful aspiration and incremental injections are essential. Only a few milligrams of local anesthetic are required to produce cerebral symptoms when injected directly into the vertebral circulation. Cardiovascular changes are possible with the loss of the cardiac accelerator fibers from the cervical sympathetic ganglia. This is particularly a problem if bilateral blockade is performed—a procedure rarely indicated. Hoarseness from recurrent laryngeal nerve paralysis is a minor but troublesome side-effect. Somatic anesthesia of the brachial plexus nerves can be produced by injection behind the level of the tubercle, and phrenic nerve paralysis has also been reported. Subarachnoid injection is also a possibility if the needle is misplaced. The close association of so many vital structures has discouraged the use of neurolytic agents in the region of the stellate ganglion.

Sympathetic Blockade—Celiac Plexus

The thoracic sympathetic ganglia send branches anteriorly that merge as greater and lesser splanchnic nerves to pass below the diaphragm and around the aorta to coalesce in a diffuse periaortic supplementary sympathetic ganglion known as the *celiac plexus*. This extensive network is generally located at the level of the 1st lumbar vertebra in the retroperitoneal space along the aorta at the level of the origin of the celiac artery. Fibers from this ganglion send postganglionic innervation to all the intra-abdominal organs and appear to carry pain sensation from many of the intraperitoneal organs such as the pancreas and liver. Injection into this retroperitoneal space allows anesthetic solution to diffuse around the ganglia and the splanchnic nerves to provide blockade of these fibers.[40] This blockade produces supplementary intra-abdominal anesthesia when used in conjunction with intercostal blockade or general anesthesia. It is more commonly applied as a neurolytic sympathetic blockade for the relief of pain from malignancy of the pancreas, liver, or other upper abdominal organs.[41] The procedure for blockade follows:

1. As with intercostal blockade, the patient is placed in the prone position with the thoracic spine flexed by the use of a pillow under the abdomen.
2. The spinous processes of the 12th thoracic and the 1st lumbar vertebral bodies are identified and marked along their entire extent. The 12th rib is likewise identified and marked 7 cm from the midline. A line is drawn between the 12th ribs on each side, usually crossing the midline at the level of the spinous process of the 1st lumbar vertebra. Lines are also drawn from the spinous process of the 12th thoracic vertebra to the points on these ribs on both sides. The net result is a shallow triangle, with the spinous process of the 12th vertebra at its apex.
3. Skin wheals are raised bilaterally at the marks along the ribs after aseptic skin preparation. Deeper infiltration of local anesthetic with a 22-gauge needle is often helpful in improving patient tolerance of this procedure.
4. On each side, a 12.5-cm 22- or 20-gauge needle is introduced through the skin wheals and advanced anteriorly and medially and cephalad along the two lines of the triangle that was previously drawn (Fig. 31-27). The needle should be passed at approximately a 45-degree angle anteriorly so that it will contact the lateral body of the vertebral body of L1 at a depth of approximately 5 cm from the skin. (The 12th spinous process partially overlies the L1 vertebral body.)
5. When contact with a vertebral body is made, the needle is withdrawn several centimeters, and the angle of insertion is steepened so that it advances more anteriorly with subsequent passage, hoping to "walk off" the anterior border of the vertebral body. The periosteum may be encountered several times during this attempt and should always be palpated gently because of the associated discomfort. Intravenous sedation may be required for tolerance of this blockade, although it must be kept to a minimum if evaluation of a diagnostic pain blockade is desired.
6. Once the anterior border of the vertebral body is reached, the needle is advanced 2–3 cm beyond this, and careful aspiration is performed. On the left side, advancement should be halted whenever aortic pulsation is appreciated. If the artery is unintentionally punctured, the needle should be withdrawn slightly and cleared immediately of blood. On the right side, the needle can often be advanced a centimeter or two further than the needle on the left side.
7. If radiologic confirmation is desired, it is obtained at this point, before injection of the anesthetic. The bony landmarks themselves are usually sufficient to

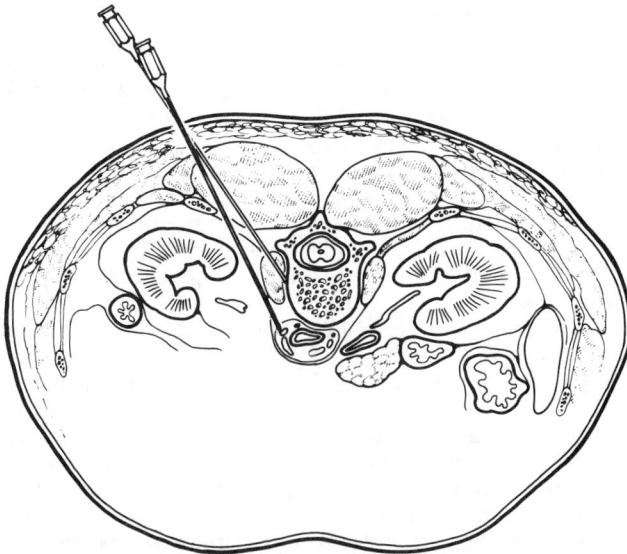

Figure 31-27. Celiac plexus blockade. The surface landmarks are described in Figure 31-23. The needles are advanced medially and superiorly to contact the lateral aspect of the vertebral body. They are then advanced more anteriorly to pass beyond the vertebra to the prevertebral space where the greater and lesser splanchnic nerves and their subsequent celiac plexus lie. No attempt is made to advance the needles to the anterior aspect of the vessels. (Reproduced with permission from Mulroy M: Handbook of Regional Anesthesia. Boston, Little, Brown, 1989.)

identify the retroperitoneal space anterior to the first lumbar vertebral body. If neurolytic agents are to be used or if the anatomy is difficult, x-ray confirmation may be desirable. Although simple flat-plate radiographs are usually sufficient, the use of fluoroscopy may be indicated in difficult cases. The use of a computed tomographic scan is not economically justified except in the most difficult of anatomic localizations.

8. Careful aspiration is performed, and a test dose is injected on each side to rule out subarachnoid or intravascular injection.
9. A large volume of local anesthetic solution is required. Twenty to 25 ml of 0.75% lidocaine or 0.25% bupivacaine are usually adequate, but a large volume is needed to diffuse in the retroperitoneal space to reach the ganglia.
10. The most reliable sign of successful anesthesia is the disappearance of pain in cancer patients or the appearance of hypotension in normal patients. Pain patients must remain supine for several hours and should have appropriate intravenous fluid supplementation to avoid orthostatic hypotension. Gradual ambulation is mandatory.

Hypotension is the most common complication of celiac plexus blockade. As mentioned previously, it can be reduced by the administration of a liter of balanced salt solution before performing the blockade. The most serious complication is the development of paralysis from unrecognized subarachnoid injection of a neurolytic drug.[42] Radiographic confirmation of needle location is advisable before injection of any neurolytic drug. Even with correct placement of neurolytic drugs, back pain is common and may require intravenous opioids. This pain can be reduced by diluting the alco-

hol solution with an equal volume of local anesthetic, such that a total volume of 50 ml is injected, consisting of 25 ml of alcohol and 25 ml of anesthetic. Even with this approach, diaphragmatic irritation (manifested as shoulder pain) is not uncommon. The duration of pain relief in the chronic pain patient is unpredictable but is often sufficient for 2–6 months. The blockade appears to be repeatable as often as necessary, although a trial diagnostic blockade with a local anesthetic agent is indicated before each use of neurolytic drugs. One minor side-effect of celiac plexus blockade is the increased peristalsis of the gut that is produced by the shift in the balance of the parasympathetic and sympathetic innervations. This may produce diarrhea within the first 12 hours after the blockade and may be a source of relief to patients on chronic opioid therapy for cancer pain.

Sympathetic Blockade—Lumbar

Lumbar sympathetic blockade combines some of the anatomic considerations for stellate ganglion blockade and paravertebral anesthesia. As with the sympathetic innervation of the head and arm, the sympathetic nerves to the lower extremities all exit the cord above the 2nd lumbar vertebra and all pass through a common "gateway" ganglia in the sympathetic chain at the L2 level. Thus, as in the neck, sympathetic blockade of the lower extremity can be achieved by a single injection of one ganglion. The approach to this ganglion is very similar to paravertebral anesthesia, as discussed previously, except that in the lumbar region, the sympathetic chain lies much more anterior from the somatic nerves, and thus a clean separation of sympathetic blockade from somatic blockade can be attained more easily.

As in the upper extremity, lumbar sympathectomy can be used in the treatment of sympathetic dystrophies or herpes zoster in an early stage. It is also occasionally used in the lower extremities in the presence of severe vascular disease to give some indication of whether a patient would profit from permanent chemical or surgical sympathectomy. The procedure for blockade follows:

1. The patient position is similar as that for celiac plexus blockade. The patient lies prone with a pillow under the lumbar spine.
2. The spinous processes of the 2nd and 3rd lumbar vertebrae are identified and marked over their entire course. A horizontal line is drawn through the midpoint of the 2nd lumbar spinous process and extended 5 cm to either side of the midline. An "X" is placed at this point, which should overlie the space between the transverse process of the 2nd and 3rd vertebrae or the caudad edge of the second transverse process.
3. A skin wheal is raised after aseptic skin preparation at each "X."
4. A 10-cm needle is introduced on each side through the "X," angled 30 to 45 degrees cephalad, and advanced until it contacts the transverse process (Fig. 31-28).
5. The depth of the needle insertion is marked, and the needle is then withdrawn slightly, angled caudad, and "walked" inferiorly off the transverse process (usually in a direction perpendicular to the skin). A slight medial angulation is used in the hope of contacting the vertebral body below the transverse process. The needle is advanced 5 cm below the depth of the transverse process. If it encounters a vertebral body, it is angled slightly more anteriorly to "walk off" that body at the desired depth.

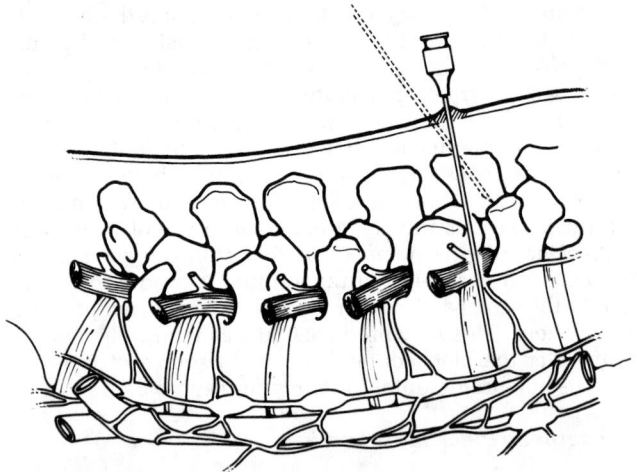

Figure 31-28. Lumbar sympathetic blockade. The needle is first placed on the transverse process of the 2nd lumbar vertebra and then advanced below it to pass 5 cm deeper. The needle can be angled slightly medially to contact the body of the vertebra; the sympathetic chain lies along the anterior margin of these bodies. (Reproduced with permission from Mulroy M: Handbook of Regional Anesthesia. Boston, Little, Brown, 1989.)

6. Once the needle is in position, careful aspiration is performed, and a test dose is injected on both sides. Ten milliliters of local anesthetic solution injected on each side should produce sympathetic blockade. Again, 1% lidocaine, 0.25% bupivacaine, or an equivalent concentration is more than sufficient to produce sympathetic nerve blockade. If a neurolytic drug such as phenol is used, confirmation of needle position by radiography should be obtained. A slightly more caudad site of injection may be more effective for neurolytic blockade;[43] injection of smaller quantities at several levels may be more appropriate for neurolytic drugs.
7. Care is taken not to inject anesthetic solution as the needle is withdrawn, because this may produce a somatic nerve blockade as the needle passes the course of the L2 nerve root.
8. Vasodilation and increase in skin temperature should be noted within the leg in 5–10 minutes. This can be quantitated objectively if a skin temperature probe is placed on the foot before the start of the blockade.

Complications with this technique are unusual, but, again, intravascular or subarachnoid injection can be a potential problem. The most troublesome and frequent complication is simultaneous blockade of the 2nd lumbar somatic nerve root. This produces a band of anesthesia across the lateral and anterior thigh. This may confuse the evaluation of a diagnostic sympathetic blockade.

Ilioinguinal Blockade

The L1 nerve root (occasionally joined by a branch of the T12 root) provides sensory anesthesia to the lowermost portion of the abdominal wall and the groin by means of its superior iliohypogastric branch and its inferior ilioinguinal branch. These nerves travel in a path very similar to that of the intercostal nerves, but without the convenient bony landmark of a rib to identify them. Nevertheless, they can be anesthetized relatively easily in the groin because of their

relationship to the anterosuperior iliac spine. Anesthesia of these two nerves is useful in providing lower abdominal wall anesthesia to supplement intercostal blockade. It is more commonly used to produce field anesthesia for hernia repair surgery. Anesthesia of these nerves alone is not sufficient for hernia repair, and subcutaneous infiltration is also necessary. The procedure for blockade follows:

1. The patient lies in a supine position, and the anterosuperior iliac spine is identified. An "X" is placed on the skin 2.5 cm medial to the spine and slightly cephalad.
2. After aseptic preparation, a skin wheal is raised at the "X."
3. A 2.5-cm 22-gauge needle is introduced through the "X" and directed perpendicular to the skin until it reaches the fascia of the external oblique muscle. A "wall" of local anesthetic solution is then laid down between this point and the iliac spine and also opposite the mark on an imaginary line extending toward the umbilicus. Injections are made at and below the level of the external oblique, with some solution injected at the level of the internal oblique. A total of 10–15 ml of anesthetic is usually required. A solution of 1% lidocaine, 0.25% bupivacaine, or an equivalent is adequate.
4. If field anesthesia for hernia repair is required, further subcutaneous infiltration of anesthetic is performed along the skin crease of the groin and along the imaginary line extending to the umbilicus. This produces a triangular-shaped area of skin anesthesia. For hernia operations, further anesthesia of the spermatic cord is required. This is usually performed by local injections in the area of the cord and the internal ring. Although epinephrine is useful in the subcutaneous and ilioinguinal blockade, it should be avoided in solutions used to anesthetize the base of the penis or the spermatic cord.

Further anesthesia of the groin area and below can be obtained by blockade of the femoral and lateral femoral cutaneous nerves (see next section), but this may result in unwanted weakness of the leg musculature, which may prevent ambulation.

Complications of this procedure are extremely rare. Hematoma formation and unwanted motor blockade of the femoral nerve are possible. These complications are rare. More commonly, anesthesia produced by this technique is inadequate for hernia repair because the patient is still able to perceive the discomfort of peritoneal traction. Administration of local anesthesia by the surgeon or systemic opioids may be required.

Penile Blockade

If surgery is confined to the penis (e.g., circumcision, urethral procedures), the organ should be blocked with simple local infiltration. Two skin wheals are raised at the dorsal base of the penis, one on each side just below and medial to the pubic spine. A 22-gauge 3.75-cm needle is introduced on each side, and 5 ml of anesthetic is deposited superficially and deep along the lower border of the pubic ramus to anesthetize the dorsal nerve. An additional 5 ml is infiltrated in the subcutaneous tissue around the underside of the shaft to produce a complete ring of anesthetic. A larger needle or a second injection site may be needed to complete the ring. Twenty to twenty-five milliliters of 0.75% lidocaine or 0.25% bupivacaine usually suffices. Epinephrine is strictly avoided.

Lower Extremity

The nerves to the lower extremity are most easily blocked by the spinal, caudal, or epidural techniques described in Chapter 30. There are occasions when anesthesia by these routes is contraindicated because of systemic sepsis or coagulopathy, or when selective anesthesia of one leg or foot is needed. Peripheral nerve blockade is possible because the motor and sensory fibers to the lower extremities are somewhat similar to those of the upper extremities in that they form a series of intertwined branching roots and divisions that are enclosed in a fascial sheath before they emerge as the terminal nerves to the extremity. They can also be successfully blocked by a single injection in one plane, although the anatomic landmarks identifying this fascial sheath are not as clearly defined as those in the upper extremity. Because of this, the majority of lower extremity blockades are performed more distally, where the nerves have already separated into terminal branches. Thus, in addition to the fascial compartment approach (psoas blockade), there are peripheral approaches described at the hip, at the knee, and at the ankle.

The nerves to the legs emerge from the roots of the 2nd lumbar though the 3rd sacral spinal segments (Fig. 31-29). The upper nerve roots from the 2nd to the 4th lumbar vertebrae form the lumbar plexus, which then ramifies to eventually form the lateral femoral cutaneous, femoral, and obturator nerves. These primarily provide sensory–motor innervation of the upper leg, although a branch of the femoral nerve commonly extends along the medial side of the knee as far down as the big toe. A branch of this lumbar plexus, the lumbosacral trunk of L4 and L5, joins the sacral fibers to form the major trunks of the large nerve of the posterior thigh and lower leg, the sciatic. The sciatic nerve is made up of two main trunks, the tibial and the common peroneal, which divide just above the knee. As in the brachial plexus, the upper nerve roots emerge from their foramina into a compartment lined by the fasciae of muscles anterior and posterior to it. In this case, the quadratus lumborum is posterior, whereas the posterior fascia of the psoas muscle provides the anterior border of the compartment. The sacral roots have a similar envelope except that the posterior border is the bone of the ilium, which prevents approach with a needle.

The lumbar plexus branches form their three terminal nerves early. Each of these pass anteriorly and laterally to circle around the pelvis and emerge anteriorly in the groin. The femoral nerve is the only one to continue in the fascial compartment formed by the psoas fascia as it passes into the groove between the psoas and the iliac muscles. The femoral nerve becomes associated with the femoral artery in the area of the groin and passes under the inguinal ligament just lateral to the artery. The lateral femoral cutaneous nerve migrates laterally early and passes under the inguinal ligament near the anterosuperior iliac spine. The third branch of the lumbar plexus, the obturator, remains somewhat medial and posterior in the pelvis and emerges under the superior ramus of the pubis through the obturator foramen to supply motor and sensory fibers to the medial thigh and medial border of the knee.

The branches of the sacral plexus also travel laterally within the pelvis before exiting posteriorly through the sciatic notch as the sciatic nerve. This largest nerve of the body

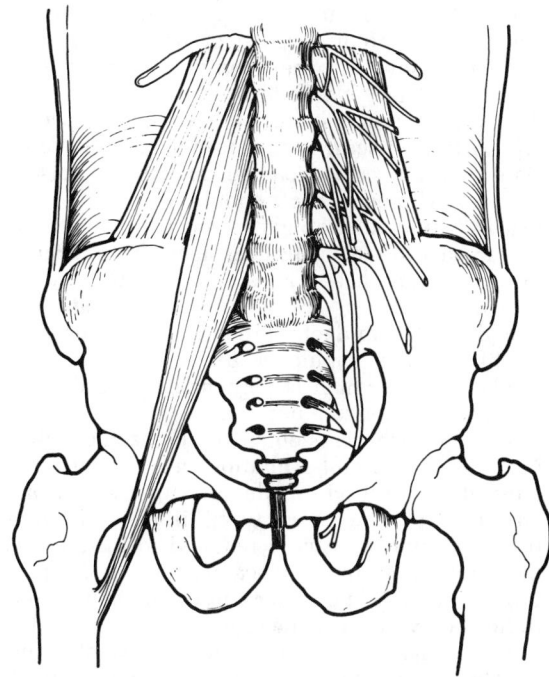

Figure 31-29. Psoas compartment anatomy. The roots of the lumbar plexus emerge from their foramina into a fascial plane between the quadratus lumborum muscle posteriorly and the psoas muscle anteriorly. The origin of the lumbosacral plexus is broader than the corresponding brachial plexus in the neck, and the lower sacral roots cannot be easily reached by a single injection. (Reproduced with permission from Mulroy M: Handbook of Regional Anesthesia. Boston, Little, Brown, 1989.)

is actually the conjunction of two trunks. The lateral trunk forms from the roots of L4 through S2 and eventually emerges as the common peroneal nerve. Other branches of L4 through S3 form the medial trunk, eventually becoming the tibial nerve. These combined nerves exit through the sciatic notch and pass anteriorly to the piriformis muscle between the ischial tuberosity and the greater trochanter of the femur. They curve caudad and descend the posterior thigh immediately behind the femur. After their bifurcation high in the popliteal fossa, the peroneal nerve provides the motor and sensory fibers to the anterior calf and dorsum of the foot, whereas the tibial nerve remains posterior and provides sensation to the calf and sole of the foot. Thus, there are three major branches that cross the knee—the femoral, tibial, and peroneal. By the time these nerves reach the ankle, there are five branches that cross this joint to provide innervation for the skin and muscles of the foot.

Psoas Compartment Blockade

As described previously, the roots of the lumbar plexus lie in an envelope similar to the interscalene fascial compartment in the neck (Fig. 31-29). Unfortunately, this fascial compartment is more difficult to identify in the lower than in the upper extremity and lies much deeper beneath the skin than its equivalent in the neck. Nevertheless, it is useful to attempt if single-injection anesthesia of the leg is desired.[44] The procedure for blockade follows:

1. The patient is placed in the prone or the lateral position. The spinous processes of the lumbar vertebrae

are identified, and an "X" is placed on the skin 5 cm lateral to the spinous process of the 3rd lumbar vertebra. This is similar to the technique described for lumbar paravertebral blockade.

2. After aseptic preparation, a skin wheal is raised at the "X." A 10-cm needle is advanced perpendicular to the skin in all planes and passed through the muscles of the back. The nerve roots should lie at a depth of between 7–10 cm. Although in some patients the well-demarcated fascial planes can identify the entry into the perineural sheath, anesthesia is much more reliable if paresthesias are obtained. If they are not obtained at a 10-cm depth, probing with the needle in a fan-like manner should be performed in a cephalad caudad plane (which is perpendicular to the known paths of the emerging nerves).

3. When a paresthesia is obtained, the needle is fixed in position, and careful aspiration and administration of a test dose are used to rule out intravascular or subarachnoid placement. Forty milliliters of local anesthetic solution is usually required to fill the sheath. Lidocaine, 1.5% or bupivacaine, 0.5%, is adequate to provide sensory and motor anesthesia. Lower concentrations provide adequate sensory anesthesia with less profound motor blockade. Fifteen to twenty minutes may be required for spread of the anesthetic to all the roots of the lumbosacral plexus. It may take longer to produce anesthesia of the caudad branches (the lower sacral fibers that form the tibial nerve).

Complications of this technique are rare, although hematoma in the muscle sheath and neuropathy of the nerves are possible. Inadequate anesthesia of some of the branches may occur more frequently than these rare complications.

Anesthesia at the Level of the Hip

Many anesthesiologists feel more confident when administering regional anesthesia in the hip region when paresthesias are sought for each of the major nerves. This technique is cumbersome and usually requires the patient to assume at least two separate positions for the injections. The anesthesia is more reliable but also requires a larger volume of anesthetic drug. Each of the four nerves may be blocked selectively on an individual basis. Anesthesia of the lateral femoral cutaneous nerve is occasionally used to provide sensory anesthesia for obtaining a skin graft from the lateral thigh. It can also be blocked as a diagnostic tool to identify cases of meralgia paresthetica. A sciatic nerve blockade alone provides adequate anesthesia for the sole of the foot and lower leg. Procedures on the knee require anesthesia of the femoral and the obturator nerves. Anesthesia of the lateral femoral cutaneous is also required if a tourniquet is to be placed on the thigh during foot surgery.

Sciatic Nerve Blockade, Classic Posterior Approach. This is the most commonly described approach to the sciatic nerve and requires that the patient be able to lie in the lateral position and flex the hip and the knee (Fig. 31-30). The procedure for blockade follows:

1. The patient lies with the side to be blocked uppermost and rolls slightly anterior, flexing the knee so that the ankle of the involved side rests on top of the knee of the opposite side. This position tends to rotate the femur so that the trochanter is more easily palpated and the muscles overlying the sciatic nerve become stretched.

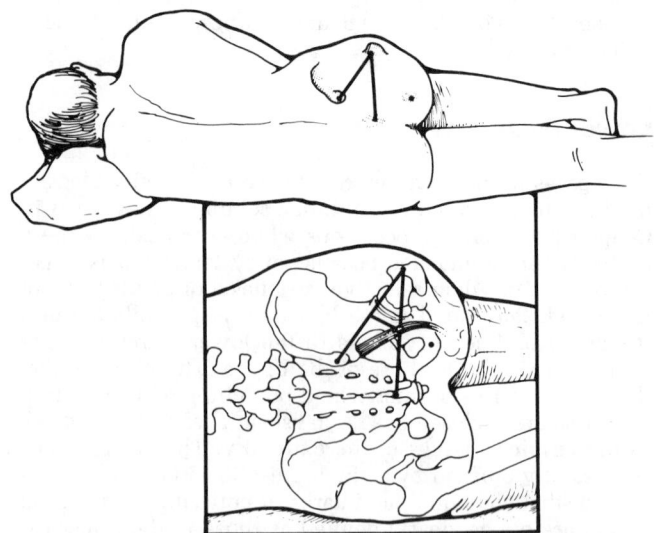

Figure 31-30. Sciatic nerve blockade, classic posterior approach. With the patient in the lateral position and the hip and knee flexed, the muscles overlying the sciatic nerve are stretched to allow easier identification. The nerve lies beneath a point 5 cm caudad along the perpendicular line that bisects the line joining the posterosuperior iliac spine and the greater trochanter of the femur. This is also usually the intersection of that perpendicular line with another line joining the greater trochanter and the sacral hiatus. (Reproduced with permission from Mulroy M: Handbook of Regional Anesthesia. Boston, Little, Brown, 1989.)

2. The superior aspect of the greater trochanter of the hip is marked with a circle. A similar circle is placed on the posterosuperior iliac spine, and a line is drawn between these two points.

3. A perpendicular line is drawn from the midpoint of this original line and extended 5 cm in the caudad direction. An "X" is marked at this point. A third line drawn between the greater trochanter and the sacral hiatus should intersect this "X." In the taller patient, the original perpendicular may need to be extended caudad to intersect with the third line, and the nerve may lie closer to the intersection of the second and third lines than to the original "X."

4. A skin wheal is raised at the "X" after aseptic skin preparation.

5. A 10-cm needle is introduced perpendicular to the skin in all planes, and paresthesias of the lower leg and foot are sought. If they are not obtained at the full depth of the needle, the needle is withdrawn to the skin and reintroduced in a fanwise fashion in a path perpendicular to the imagined course of the nerve in the hip. This path can usually be visualized by following the muscular groove on the back of the thigh up and into the imagined position of the sciatic notch. The bony edges of the sciatic notch itself may be encountered. These should be noted, and the search continued. The nerve should lie at approximately this depth as it emerges from inside the pelvis. Paresthesias are critical in this blockade, since the blind infiltration of a large quantity of local anesthetic rarely produces adequate anesthesia because of multiple muscle planes in this area. If a paresthesia cannot be obtained in the first 10 minutes, the landmarks should be reassessed. Alternatively, the blockade can be performed with a nerve stimulator, which will also reduce patient discomfort.

6. When a paresthesia to the foot is obtained, the needle is held immobile, and 25 ml of local anesthetic is injected. Again, 1.5% lidocaine, 0.5% bupivacaine, or the equivalent is adequate. A lower concentration may be needed if several nerves are to be blocked, which would then require a large total volume of anesthetic in several locations.

Sciatic Nerve Blockade, Supine Approach (Lithotomy). If a patient is uncomfortable in the lateral position or cannot be turned to the side because of a fracture or pain, the nerve can be blocked with the patient in the supine position. An assistant is required to elevate the leg into a lithotomy type position so that the posterior aspect can be reached. The procedure for blockade follows:

1. With the patient supine, the hip is flexed by an assistant so that the upper leg is at a 90-degree angle to the torso.
2. The greater trochanter is identified as well as the ischial tuberosity, and a line is drawn between these two. An "X" is marked on the midpoint of this line.
3. A skin wheal is raised at the "X" after aseptic skin preparation. A 10-cm needle is introduced, and paresthesias are sought in a direction along the length of this line (which is perpendicular to the course of the nerve).
4. When a paresthesia is obtained, 25 ml of local anesthetic is injected.

Lateral Femoral Cutaneous Nerve Blockade. The other three nerves of the leg can be blocked at the level of the hip with the patient in the supine position. If no paresthesias are sought, the patient can be sedated more heavily than was used for the sciatic nerve blockade. If the single-injection technique (see below) is used, paresthesias are needed and sedation should be lighter. The procedure for blockade follows:

1. In the supine position, the anterosuperior iliac spine is identified and marked. An "X" is placed on the skin 2.5 cm below and 2.5 cm medial to the spine.
2. A skin wheal is raised at the "X" after aseptic preparation.
3. A 3.75-cm 22-gauge needle is introduced through the wheal and directed laterally until a "pop" is felt as it pierces the fascia lata. Three to five milliliters of local anesthetic solution is injected as the needle is withdrawn slowly. The needle is then reinserted slightly medially, and the procedure is repeated until a "wall" of anesthesia has been spread over a 5-cm area above and below the fascia lata extending medially from the level of the anterosuperior spine. A total of 15–20 ml of local anesthetic may be required. No paresthesias are sought.

Femoral Nerve Blockade. This blockade can be performed blindly without eliciting paresthesias, or paresthesias can be sought for a "three-in-one" blockade (see below). The procedure for blockade follows:

1. In the supine position, a line is drawn from the antero-superior iliac spine to the pubic tubercle. The femoral artery is identified as it passes below this line, and an "X" is marked on the skin lateral to the artery 2.5 cm below the line.
2. After aseptic preparation, a skin wheal is raised at the mark.

3. A 5-cm 22-gauge needle is introduced through the "X" and passed perpendicular to the skin until it lies next to the artery and slightly deep to it (Fig. 31-31). Entry into the vessel is not sought, but the needle should be easily perceived to be moving with pulsation of the vessel if it is in sufficient proximity.
4. Five milliliters of local anesthetic are injected slowly as the needle is withdrawn. The needle is then reinserted slightly more laterally, and the process is repeated again until another "wall" of anesthesia has been laid down lateral to and slightly deep to the femoral artery.
5. Anesthesia of the medial thigh should ensue within 5–10 minutes.

Obturator Nerve Blockade. This nerve is more difficult to locate because of its depth, but anesthesia is essential for operations in the area of the knee. The procedure for blockade follows:

1. In the supine position, the pubic tubercle is identified, and an "X" is placed 1.5 cm below and 1.5 cm lateral to this structure. This should lie medial to the femoral artery, and a line drawn between the three "X's" used

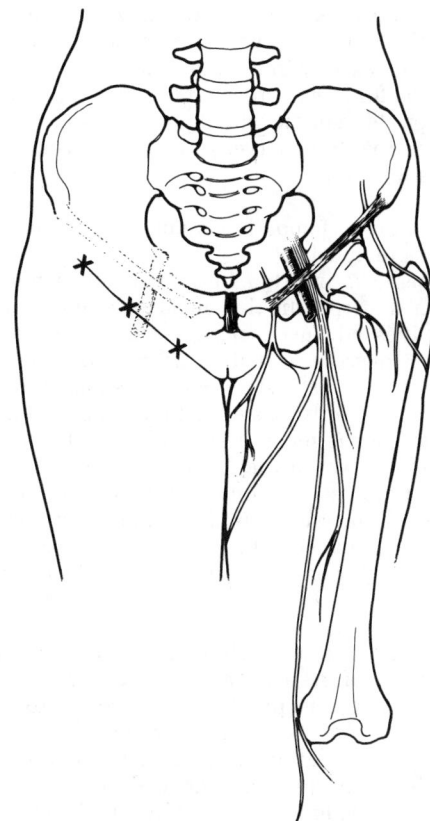

Figure 31-31. Blockade of the anterior lumbosacral branches in the groin. The lateral femoral cutaneous nerve emerges approximately 2.5 cm medial to the anterosuperior iliac spine and is best blocked 2.5 cm caudad to this point. The femoral nerve emerges alongside and slightly posterior to the femoral artery and is again easily approached approximately 2.5 cm below the inguinal ligament. On that same line, the obturator nerve emerges from the obturator canal but is deeper and less reliably located. (Reproduced with permission from Mulroy M: Handbook of Regional Anesthesia. Boston, Little, Brown, 1989.)

for these three nerve blockades should be parallel to the line between the superior spine and the pubic tubercle.

2. After aseptic skin preparation, a skin wheal is raised at the "X," and a 7.5-cm 22-gauge needle is introduced through the "X" perpendicular to the skin.

3. The needle is advanced until it contacts bone, which should be the inferior ramus of the pubis. The needle is withdrawn slightly and redirected laterally and slightly caudad to enter the obturator foramen. It is advanced another 2–3 cm, and 5 ml of anesthetic is injected as the needle is withdrawn through the presumed depth of the obturator foramen.

4. The needle is then reinserted slightly more laterally, and the process is repeated again until 20 ml of anesthetic solution has been injected to form another "wall" along the presumed path of the obturator nerve (see Fig. 31-31).

Lumbar Plexus ("Three-in-One") Blockade. Winnie et al[45] have popularized the concept of a single-injection blockade for the lumbar plexus, utilizing the fascial plane that the femoral nerve travels in as it crosses the pelvis. The object of this blockade is to inject a large quantity of local anesthetic solution in this plane so that it will spread upward into the pelvis and anesthetize the obturator and lateral femoral cutaneous nerves at the point where they still travel in conjunction with the femoral nerve. Because it is essential to have the needle exactly in the plane of the nerve, paresthesias are critical for this approach. Light sedation is therefore more appropriate than for the relatively "blind" traditional approaches to the three nerves of the groin. The procedure for blockade follows:

1. Preparation for femoral nerve blockade is made as described previously.

2. The needle is inserted in a cephalad manner rather than in a perpendicular angle recommended previously. It is advanced alongside the artery angled at about 45 degrees so that it passes under the inguinal ligament. A paresthesia is sought, recognizing that the nerve lies slightly posterior to and occasionally partially under the femoral artery. When the paresthesia is obtained, the needle is fixed and the fingers of an assistant are used to compress the femoral artery and the neural sheath below the inguinal ligament while the operator injects 40 ml of anesthetic solution. The injection is performed incrementally after careful aspiration.

Complications of these techniques are rare. Hematomas can occur in any of the areas of injection and are annoying but rarely serious. The problem of systemic toxicity is a major one because of the large volumes of anesthetic solution required. As mentioned previously, careful attention must be paid to the total milligram dose involved when these multiple injections are used. Neuropathy is a possibility. Interneural injection must be avoided by watching for signs of any discomfort at the time of actual injection.

Popliteal Fossa Blockade

The nerves of the lower leg can also be anesthetized by injections at the level of the knee.[46] The success of this technique depends upon locating the sciatic nerve near its bifurcation into the tibial and peroneal branches high in the popliteal fossa (Fig. 31-32). Supplemental anesthesia of the femoral nerve is needed in order to block its terminal saphenous branch, which serves the medial anterior calf and the dorsum of the foot. The procedure for blockade follows:

1. The patient is placed in a prone position. The triangular borders of the popliteal fossa are outlined by drawing the borders of the biceps femoris and the semitendinosus muscles. The base of the triangle is the skin crease behind the knee. The patient can help identify the muscles by slightly flexing the lower leg.

2. After the triangle is drawn, a perpendicular line is drawn from the midpoint of the base to the apex of the triangle. Five centimeters from the base, an "X" is drawn 1 cm lateral to this bisecting line.

3. After aseptic skin preparation, a skin wheal is raised at the "X."

4. A 7.5-cm or 10-cm needle is introduced through the "X" and directed 45 degrees cephalad along the middle of the triangle (Fig. 31-33). The nerves should be passing down the back of the leg parallel to the bisecting line of the triangle. A fanwise search is conducted perpendicular to this line until the nerve is contacted. If the femur is contacted by the needle, the depth is noted. The nerve should lie midway between the skin and the femur.

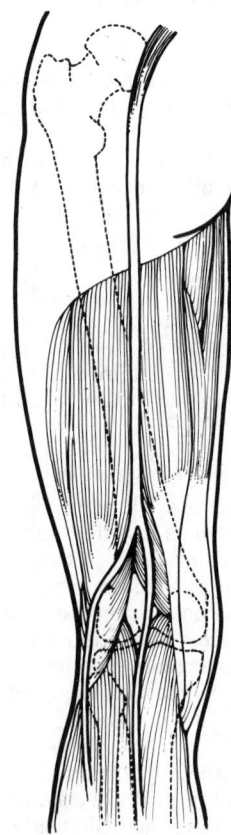

Figure 31-32. Popliteal fossa blockade. The two major trunks of the sciatic bifurcate in the popliteal fossa 7–10 cm above the knee. A triangle is drawn using the heads of the biceps femoris and the semitendinosus muscles and the skin crease of the knee; a long needle is inserted 1 cm lateral to a point 5 cm cephalad on the line from the skin crease that bisects this triangle. (Reproduced with permission from Mulroy M: Handbook of Regional Anesthesia. Boston, Little, Brown, 1989.)

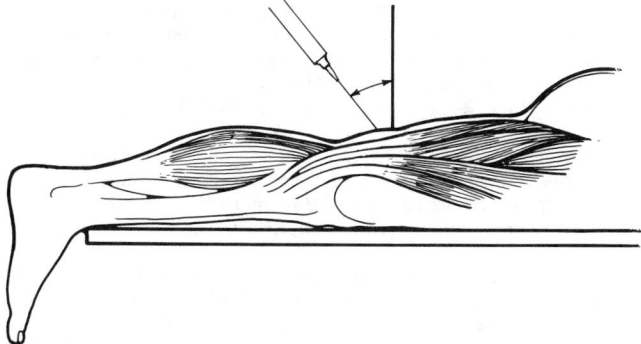

Figure 31-33. Popliteal fossa blockade, needle direction. The needle is inserted at the point described in Figure 31-32 and angled 45 degrees cephalad. The nerves usually are contacted halfway between the skin and the femur. (Reproduced with permission from Mulroy M: Handbook of Regional Anesthesia. Boston, Little, Brown, 1989.)

5. Once a paresthesia is obtained, the needle is fixed in position and 30–40 ml of local anesthetic solution is injected.
6. The femoral branches can be injected in the same position by raising a subcutaneous wheal of 5–10 ml of local anesthetic along the medial tibial head just below the knee.

Ankle Blockade

All the nerves of the foot can be blocked at the level of the ankle.[47] Although this approach is ideal in producing the least amount of immobility of the lower extremity, it is technically more difficult because at least five nerves must be anesthetized (Fig. 31-34). Several of these nerves can be blocked by simple infiltration of a "wall" of anesthesia, but increased reliability can be produced by seeking paresthesias of the major branches. If paresthesias are not sought, this blockade may actually be less time consuming than other techniques, even though five separate injections are required. The procedure for blockade follows:

1. The *posterior tibial nerve* is the major nerve to the sole of the foot. It can be approached with the patient either in the prone position or with the hip and knee flexed so that the foot rests on the bed. The medial malleolus is identified, along with the pulsation of the posterior tibial artery behind it. A needle is introduced through the skin just behind the posterior tibial artery and directed 45 degrees anteriorly, seeking a paresthesia in the sole of the foot. Five milliliters of a local anesthetic will produce anesthesia if a paresthesia is identified. If not, a fan-shaped injection of 10 ml can be performed in the triangle formed by the artery, the achilles tendon, and the tibia itself.
2. *Sural nerve.* With the foot in the same position, the other posterior nerve of the ankle can be blocked by injection on the lateral side. The subcutaneous injection of a ridge of anesthesia behind the lateral malleolus filling the groove between it and the calcaneus will produce anesthesia of the sural nerve. This will require another 5 ml of local anesthetic.
3. *Saphenous nerve.* The last three branches of the ankle lie anteriorly. The patient is either turned supine, or the leg can now be extended so that attention of the anesthesiologist is turned to the anterior surface. The

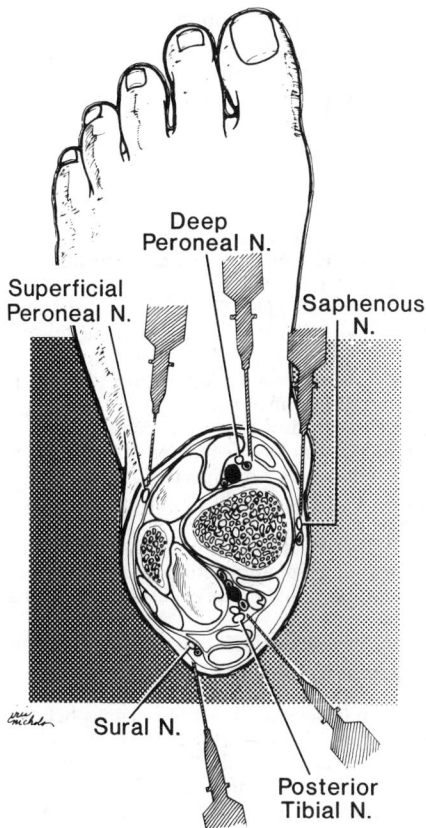

Figure 31-34. Ankle blockade. Injections are made at five separate nerve locations. The superficial peroneal nerve, sural nerve, and saphenous nerve are usually blocked simply by subcutaneous infiltration, since they may have already generated many superficial branches as they cross the ankle joint. Paresthesias can be sought in the posterior tibial or the deep peroneal nerve, but the bony landmarks usually suffice to provide adequate localization for the deeper injections. (Reproduced with permission from Mulroy M: Handbook of Regional Anesthesia. Boston, Little, Brown, 1989.)

saphenous nerve is anesthetized by infiltrating 5 ml of local anesthetic around the saphenous vein at the level where this vein passes anterior to the medial malleolus. A wall of anesthesia between the skin and the bone itself will suffice to block the nerve.
4. *Deep peroneal nerve.* This is the major nerve to the dorsum of the foot and lies in the deep plane of the anterior tibial artery. Pulsation of the artery is sought at the level of the skin crease on the anterior midline surface of the ankle. If it can be felt, 5 ml of local anesthetic is injected just lateral to this. If the artery is not palpable, the tendon of the extensor hallucus longus can be identified by asking the patient to extend the big toe. Injection can be made into the deep planes below the fascia using either one of these landmarks.
5. *Superficial peroneal branches.* Finally, a subcutaneous ridge of anesthetic solution is laid along the skin crease between the anterior tibial artery and the lateral malleolus. This subcutaneous ridge will overlie the previous subfascial injection for the deep peroneal nerve. Another 5–10 ml of local anesthetic may be required to cover this area.

Anesthesia of the foot should ensue within 10 minutes after the performance of these five injections. Complications of this blockade are rare, although neuropathy can be produced. Care should be taken not to pin any of the deep nerves against the bone at the time of injection, and intraneural injection should be avoided as usual.

REFERENCES

1. Kehlet H: The modifying effect of general and regional anesthesia on the endocrine-metabolic response to surgery. Reg Anesth (suppl) 7:S38, 1982
2. Yeager MP, Glass DD, Neff RK et al: Epidural anesthesia and analgesia in high-risk surgical patients. Anesthesiology 66:729, 1987
3. Wetchler BV: Anesthesia for Ambulatory Surgery, pp 225–269. Philadelphia, JB Lippincott, 1985
4. Buffington CW, Ready LB, Horton WG: Training and practice factors influence the use of regional anesthesia; implications for resident education. Reg Anesth 10:2, 1985
5. Bridenbaugh LD: Are anesthesia resident programs failing regional anesthesia? Reg Anesth 7:26, 1982
6. Selander D, Brattsand R, Lundborg G et al: Local anesthetics: Importance of mode of application, concentration, and adrenaline for the appearance of nerve lesions. Acta Anaesth Scand 23:127, 1979
7. Ready LB, Plummer MH, Haschke RH et al: Neurotoxicity of intrathecal local anesthetics in rabbits. Anesthesiology 63:364, 1985
8. Kelly DA, Henderson AM: Use of local anesthetic drugs in hospital practice. Br Med J 286:1784, 1983
9. Selander D, Edshage S, Wolff T: Paresthesiae or no paresthesiae? Acta Anesthesiol Scand 23:27, 1979
10. Smith BL: Efficacy of a nerve stimulator in regional anesthesia; experience in a resident training programme. Anaesthesia 31:778, 1976
11. Pither CE, Raj PP, Ford DJ: The use of peripheral nerve stimulators for regional anesthesia. Reg Anesth 10:49, 1985
12. Bashein G, Haschke RH, Ready LB: Electrical nerve location: Numerical and electrophoretic comparison of insulated vs uninsulated needles. Anesth Analg 63:919, 1984
13. McMahon DJ: Managing regional anesthesia equipment. In Brown DL: Problems in Anesthesia, vol 1, no 4, pp 592–596. Philadelphia, JB Lippincott, 1987
14. Selander D, Dhuner KG, Lundborg G: Peripheral nerve injury due to injection needles used for regional anesthesia. Acta Anaesthesiol Scand 21:182, 1977
15. Thompson GE: Perioperative nerve injuries. In Brown DL: Problems in Anesthesia, vol 1, no 4, pp 580–587. Philadelphia, JB Lippincott, 1987
16. Marinacci AA, Rand CW: Electromyogram in peripheral nerve complications following general surgical procedures. West J Surg 67:199, 1959
17. Gross JB, Hartigan ML, Schaffer DW: A suitable substitute for 4% cocaine before blind nasotracheal intubation: 3% lidocaine–0.25% phenylephrine nasal spray. Anesth Analg 63:915, 1984
18. Sessler CN, Vitaliti JC, Cooper KR et al: Comparison of 4% lidocaine/0.5% phenylephrine with 5% cocaine: Which dilates the nasal passages better? Anesthesiology 64:274, 1986
19. Gotta AW, Sullivan CA: Anesthesia of the upper airway using topical anesthesia and superior laryngeal nerve block. Br J Anaesth 53:1055, 1981
20. Lanz E, Theiss D, Jankovic D: The extent of blockade following various techniques of brachial plexus block. Anesth Analg 62:55, 1983
21. Winnie AP: Interscalene brachial plexus block. Anesth Analg 49:455, 1970
22. Urmey WF, Talts KH, Sharrock NE: One hundred percent incidence of hemidiaphragmatic paresis associated with interscalene brachial plexus anesthesia as diagnosed by ultrasonography. Anesth Analg 72:498, 1991
23. Moore DC: Regional Block. Springfield, Illinois, Charles C Thomas, 1954
24. Winnie AP, Collins VJ: The subclavian perivascular technique of brachial plexus anesthesia. Anesthesiology 25:353, 1964
25. Moore DC, Bridenbaugh LD: Pneumothorax: its incidence following brachial plexus block analgesia. Anesthesiology 15:475, 1954
26. Partridge BL, Katz J, Benirschke K: Functional anatomy of the brachial plexus sheath: Implications for anesthesia. Anesthesiology 66:743, 1987
27. Thompson GE, Rorie DK: Functional anatomy of the brachial plexus sheaths. Anesthesiology 59:117, 1983
28. Vester–Andersen T, Christiansen C, Sorensen M et al: Perivascular axillary block II: Influence of injected volume of local anesthetic on neural blockade. Acta Anaesthesiol Scand 27:95, 1983
29. Selander D: Axillary plexus block: Paresthetic or perivascular (editorial). Anesthesiology 66:726, 1987
30. Sukhani R, Garcia CJ, Munhall RJ et al: Lidocaine disposition following intravenous regional anesthesia with different tourniquet deflation techniques. Anesth Analg 68:633, 1989
31. Grice SC, Morell RC, Balestrieri FJ et al: Intravenous regional anesthesia: Evaluation and prevention of leakage under the tourniquet. Anesthesiology 65:316, 1986
32. Tucker GT, Boas RA: Pharmacokinetic aspects of intravenous regional anesthesia. Anesthesiology 34:538, 1971
33. Moore DC, Bush WH, Scurlock JE: Intercostal nerve block: A roentgenographic anatomic study of technique and absorption in humans. Anesth Analg 59:815, 1980
34. Bridenbaugh PO, DuPen SL, Moore DC et al: Postoperative intercostal nerve block analgesia versus narcotic analgesia. Anesth Analg 52:81, 1973
35. Moore DC, Bridenbaugh LD: Pneumothorax: Its incidence following intercostal nerve block. JAMA 182:1005, 1962
36. Sury MRJ, Bingham RM: Accidental spinal anesthesia following intrathoracic intercostal nerve blockade. Anaesthesia 41:401, 1986
37. Eason MJ, Wyatt R: Paravertebral thoracic block—a reappraisal. Anaesthesia 34:638, 1979
38. Reiestad F, Stromskag KE: Intrapleural catheter in the management of postoperative pain. Regional Anesth 11:89, 1986
39. Stromskag KE, Minor B, Steen PA: Side effects and complications related to intrapleural analgesia: An update. Acta Anaesthesiol Scand 34:473, 1990
40. Moore DC, Bush WH, Burnett LL: Celiac plexus block: A roentgenographic, anatomic study of technique and spread of solution in patients and corpses. Anesth Analg 60:369, 1981
41. Brown DL, Bulley K, Quiel EL: Neurolytic block for pancreatic cancer pain. Anesth Analg 66:869, 1987
42. Cherry DA, Lamberty J: Paraplegia following coeliac plexus block. Anesth Intensive Care 12:59, 1984
43. Umeda S, Arai T, Hatano Y et al: Cadaver anatomic analysis of the best site for chemical lumbar sympathectomy. Anesth Analg 66:643, 1987
44. Chayen D, Nathan H, Chayen M: The psoas compartment block. Anesthesiology 45:95, 1976
45. Winnie AP, Ramamurthy S, Durrani Z: The inguinal paravascular technique of lumbar plexus anesthesia. "The 3-in-1 block." Anesth Analg 52:989, 1973
46. Rorie DK, Byer DE, Nelson DO et al: Assessment of block of the sciatic nerve in the popliteal fossa. Anesth Analg 59:371, 1980
47. Schurman DJ: Ankle block anesthesia for foot surgery. Anesthesiology 44:342, 1976

32

Audrée A. Bendo   John Hartung

Ira S. Kass   James E. Cottrell

Neurophysiology and Neuroanesthesia

NEUROPHYSIOLOGY

To understand how anesthetics act on the nervous system and how these actions may affect the practice of neuroanesthesia, one first needs to understand the basic principles of neurophysiology. The following description of cellular neurophysiology provides background information only; greater detail may be sought elsewhere.[1-4]

Membrane Potentials

Neurons have an electrical potential across their cell membrane owing to different intra- and extracellular ion concentrations. These concentration differences lead to an opposing voltage called the equilibrium potential. The Nernst equation is a method for calculating the equilibrium potential for a single ion. The Nernst or equilibrium potential for potassium (E_K) at 37°C can be calculated as:

$$E_K = -61 \log (K_i/K_o)$$

where K_i is the potassium concentration inside the cell and K_o is its concentration outside the cell.[4] This value is approximately -90 mV, yet the membrane potential for most neurons at rest is usually closer to -70 mV. This is because both sodium and potassium ions contribute to the resting membrane potential. An ion's contribution to the membrane potential of a neuron is determined by its conductance, which is proportional to the membrane's permeability for that ion. Because the conductance to potassium (g_K) is much higher than the sodium conductance (g_{Na}) in an unexcited neuron, the resting membrane potential is nearer to the potassium equilibrium potential than the sodium equilibrium potential ($E_{Na} = +45$ mV). The following equation is useful for calculating a cell's membrane potential:

$$E_m = [g_K(E_K) + g_{Na}(E_{Na}) + g_x(E_x)]/(g_K + g_{Na} + g_x)$$

where x refers to other ions.[4]

The conductance of ions across the cell membrane is through channels, which are proteins that span the membrane and have a hydrophilic pore that allows the ions to pass through. Many channels predominantly let one species of ion pass. The sodium channel (Fig. 32-1) is highly selective for sodium and lets very little potassium pass through it; the potassium channel (Fig. 32-2) is likewise selective for potassium. These channels are controlled by gates that open and close. During rest, most of the sodium channels have their gates closed, while more of the potassium channels' gates are in the open position. The opening and closing of the gates for the ion channels control the conductance of the cell membrane for that ion.

Neurons signal over long distances by propagating action potentials, which are brief and rapid depolarizations of the membrane along their axons. The action potential is caused by a fast increase in the sodium conductance (because of the opening of the sodium activation gate) and a slower increase in the potassium conductance. These conductance changes are triggered by a depolarization of the cell membrane, and therefore the channels that open in response to the depolarization are described as voltage-sensitive channels. When the neuron depolarizes past a threshold voltage level, an action potential is generated. The peak voltage of the action potential is approximately $+20$ mV; this level is attained because at the peak the sodium conductance is much greater than the potassium conductance. The voltage during the action potential returns rapidly to resting levels (repolarizes) because of the following: (1) the sodium conductance shuts itself off by closing a second gate (inactivation gate) in the channel (Fig. 32-1), and (2) the potassium conductance increases, due to the opening of potassium channels. A detailed description of membrane potentials, ion channels, gating and action potentials can be found in Aidley,[1] Hille,[2] and Kandel and Schwartz.[4]

Synaptic Transmission

Neurons communicate using chemical synapses. The chemical, called a transmitter, is released from the presynaptic neuron, diffuses across the synaptic cleft and combines with a receptor molecule on the postsynaptic neuron. The release of the neurotransmitter is initiated by an action potential traveling down the axon of the presynaptic neuron, causing the depolarization of the presynaptic terminal. This depolarization leads to the opening of voltage-dependent calcium channels and the entry of calcium from the extra-

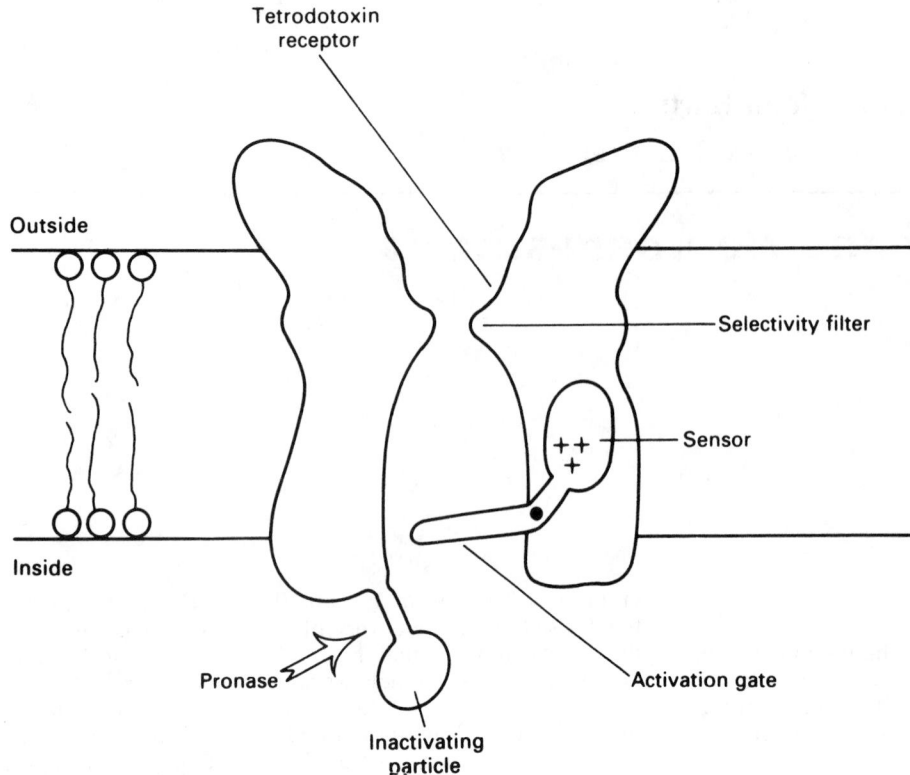

Tetrodotoxin
receptor

Outside

Selectivity filter

Sensor

++
+

Inside

Pronase

Activation gate

Inactivating
particle

Figure 32-1. Sodium channel. The selectivity filter allows sodium but not potassium to pass through. The channel is open and allows sodium through when both the activation gate and the inactivation gate, which is also called the inactivating particle, are in the open position. Closing either gate will block the passage of ions. (Reprinted with permission from Aidley DJ: The Physiology of Excitable Cells. New York, Cambridge University Press, 1989.)

cellular fluid into the terminal. Vesicles containing the neurotransmitter then fuse with the terminal membrane, releasing the neurotransmitter into the synaptic cleft. The combination of the neurotransmitter with its receptor located on the postsynaptic cell alters ion channels associated with the receptor. These channels are described as ligand gated channels. The opening of these ion channels leads to a change in the membrane potential of the postsynaptic neuron. If the transmitter is excitatory this postsynaptic neuron is depolarized and, therefore, more likely to generate an action potential. If the transmitter is inhibitory, the neuron is hyperpolarized and made less likely to generate an action potential.

There are numerous neurotransmitters in the brain; for purposes of discussion, we will examine two common neurotransmitters and their receptors.[3,5]

Gamma-amino-butyric acid (GABA) is a major inhibitory amino acid transmitter that is active throughout the brain and reduces the excitability of neurons by hyperpolarizing them. There are two major GABA receptors. Activation of the $GABA_a$ receptor opens chloride channels,[6] and its activity is enhanced by benzodiazepines and barbiturates. The $GABA_b$ receptor is thought to either open potassium channels or close calcium channels, it does not affect chloride channels.[7] The response to $GABA_b$ receptor activation has a slower onset and a more prolonged activation than the $GABA_a$ receptor. Both receptors may be present on the same neuron, providing a mechanism for rapid and prolonged action.

Glutamate is the major excitatory transmitter in the brain. Its activation depolarizes neurons, making it more likely that they will fire action potentials. There are three types of glutamate receptors that have been named for their preferen-

tial pharmacologic agonists. The AMPA and kainate receptors allow sodium and potassium but not calcium through their channels.[8,9] These channels are responsible for the normal excitatory responses seen with glutamate. The third glutamate receptor, the n-methyl-d-aspartate receptor (NMDA), is activated when neurons are depolarized; the channels associated with this receptor are not opened by glutamate at normal resting membrane potentials. These channels allow passage of calcium as well as sodium and potassium.[8,9] NMDA receptor activation is important in changing a neuron's excitability to last over a period of hours and days (long-term potentiation); this has been correlated with learning in animals.[9] Glutamate receptors have also been associated with neuronal injury after anoxia.[10]

The above is a simple description of how synapses operate to convey information from one neuron to another. This process is finely controlled; there are neurotransmitters that act on presynaptic terminals to regulate the amount of transmitter that the terminal releases.[3] Indeed some neurons have receptors on their presynaptic terminals, called autoreceptors, that reduce the amount of transmitter that terminal releases in response to the build up of that same transmitter in the synapse. This is a way of controlling the concentration of transmitter in the synaptic cleft. There are compounds called neuromodulators that, when applied to a neuron alone, have no observable effect on the excitability of that neuron but alter the effect of other excitatory or inhibitory inputs to that neuron. These neuromodulators are released in the same manner as neurotransmitters; indeed, it is possible for the same substance to be a neuromodulator at one synapse and a neurotransmitter at another. Furthermore, some synapses have been shown to release two neuroactive compounds from the same presynaptic terminal,

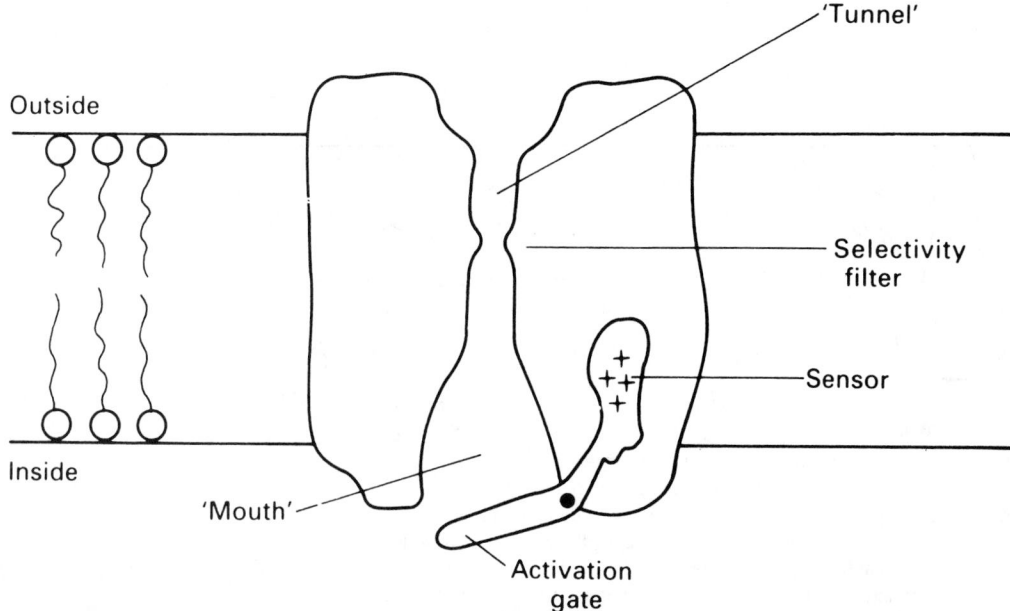

Figure 32-2. Potassium channel. The selectivity filter allows potassium but not sodium to pass through the channel. This channel is thought to have only an activation gate that opens to allow ions through the channel; the channel closes by closing this gate. (Reprinted with permission from Aidley DJ: The Physiology of Excitable Cells. New York, Cambridge University Press, 1989.)

these so-called cotransmitters can have synergistic actions on the postsynaptic terminal. Many of the peptide neurotransmitters are released as cotransmitters with a nonpeptide transmitter.

The binding of a transmitter to a receptor as described earlier can directly cause the opening of an ion channel, leading to a change in the neuron's membrane potential. Neurotransmitters also work through intracellular second messengers. One example of a second messenger is cyclic AMP, which activates protein kinases to phosphorylate proteins and change their activity. Ion channels may be phosphorylated as well as have many intracellular proteins. A group of proteins that bind guanosine triphosphate (GTP), called G proteins, are activated when a transmitter binds a specific receptor molecule. In some cases these G proteins activate ion channels directly, but in others they can either stimulate (G_s) or inhibit (G_i) adenylate cyclase, the enzyme that converts ATP into cyclic AMP[1] (Fig. 32-3). G proteins have also been implicated in the phosphatidylinositol second-messenger system; in this case, a transmitter binds to a receptor, which causes another G protein (G_p) to activate phospholipase C (Fig. 32-4). This membrane-bound enzyme breaks down a membrane phospholipid into diacylglycerol and inositol trisphosphate, both of which are second messengers. Diacylglycerol activates protein kinase C, which will then phosphorylate other proteins, whereas inositol trisphosphate increases cytosolic calcium by releasing calcium from intracellular stores (endoplasmic reticulum).[11]

Brain Metabolism

The main substance used for energy production in the brain is glucose.[12] When oxygen levels are sufficient, glucose is metabolized to pyruvate in the glycolytic pathway (Fig.

32-5). This biochemical process generates ATP from ADP and inorganic phosphate and produces NADH from NAD. Pyruvate from this reaction then enters the citric acid cycle which, with regard to energy production, primarily generates NADH from NAD. The mitochondria use oxygen to couple the conversion of NADH back to NAD with the production of ATP from ADP and inorganic phosphate. This process, called oxidative phosphorylation, yields three ATP molecules for each NADH converted. This pathway yields 38 ATP molecules for each glucose molecule metabolized.[13]

This pathway requires oxygen; if oxygen is not present the mitochondria can neither make ATP nor regenerate NAD from NADH. Glycolysis requires NAD as a cofactor

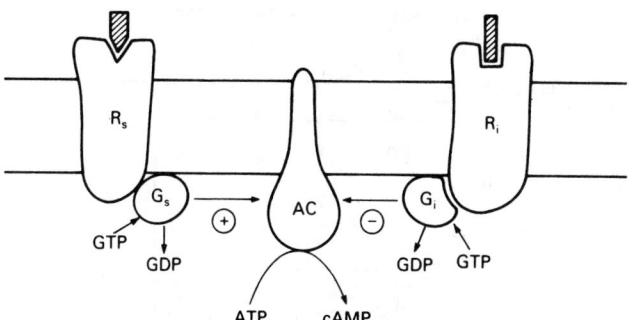

Figure 32-3. G proteins and adenylate cyclase. Different transmitters bind to either a stimulatory receptor (R_s) or an inhibitory receptor (R_i). Both are coupled to GTP-binding proteins (G proteins). G_s stimulates adenylate cyclase to increase cAMP levels; G_i inhibits adenylate cyclase and decreases cAMP levels. (Reprinted with permission from Aidley DJ: The Physiology of Excitable Cells. New York, Cambridge University Press, 1989.)

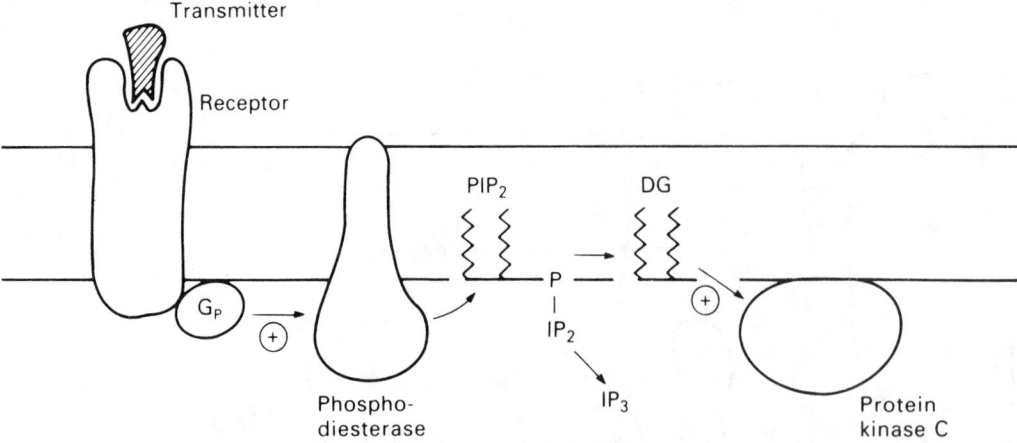

Figure 32-4. G proteins and phosphodiesterase. A transmitter binds to a receptor activating a G protein (G_p), which activates the membrane-bound enzyme phosphodiesterase.This enzyme converts phosphatidylinositol-4,5-bisphosphate (PIP_2) into inositol 1,4,5-triphosphate (IP_3), which is water soluble and causes the release of calcium from endoplasmic reticulum and diacylglycerol, which is lipid soluble and remains in the membrane to activate protein kinase C. Protein kinase C will in turn phosphorylate certain other proteins, altering their activity. (Reprinted with permission from Aidley DJ: The Physiology of Excitable Cells. New York, Cambridge University Press, 1989.)

and is blocked in its absence. Thus, in the absence of oxygen, glycolysis proceeds by a modified pathway termed "anaerobic glycolysis"; this modification involves the conversion of pyruvate to lactate-regenerating NAD. There is a net hydrogen ion production, which lowers the intracellular pH. A major problem with anaerobic glycolysis, in addition to lowering pH, is that only two molecules of ATP are formed for each molecule of glucose metabolized.[13] This level of ATP production is insufficient for meeting the brain's energy needs.

When the oxygen supply to a neuron is reduced, mechanisms that reduce and/or slow the fall in ATP levels include: (1) the utilization of phosphocreatine stores (a high-energy phosphate that can donate its energy to maintain ATP levels), (2) the production of ATP at low levels by anaerobic glycolysis, and (3) a rapid cessation of spontaneous electrophysiologic activity.[14]

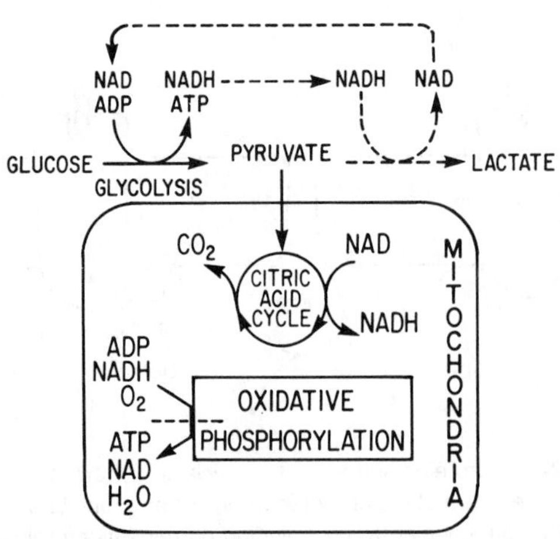

Pumping ions across the cell membrane is the largest energy requirement in the brain (Table 32-1). The sodium, potassium, and calcium concentrations of a neuron are maintained against large electrochemical differences with respect to the outside of the cell. When a neuron is not excited (firing action potentials), there is a slow leak of potassium out of the cells and of sodium into the cells. Neuronal activity markedly increases the flow of potassium, sodium, and calcium; this increases the rate of ion pumping required to maintain the neuron's ion concentration. Because ion pumping uses ATP as an energy source, the ATP requirement of active neurons is greater than that for "resting neurons." If energy production does not meet the demand of energy use in the brain, the neurons first become unexcitable and then may become irreversibly damaged.[14,15]

Neurons require energy to maintain their structure and internal function. The cell's membranes, internal organelles, and cytoplasm are made of carbohydrates, lipids, and proteins that require energy for their synthesis. Ion channels, enzymes, and cell structural components are important protein molecules that are continuously formed, modified, and broken down in the cell. If ATP is not available, protein synthesis can not continue and the neuron will die. Carbohydrates and lipids are also continuously synthesized and degraded in normally functioning neurons; their metabolism also requires energy. Most cellular synthesis takes place in the cell body, thus energy is required for transport

Figure 32-5. Energy metabolism in the brain. Dotted lines indicate reactions that occur during ischemia. The dotted line across the oxidative phosphorylation reaction indicates that this reaction is blocked during ischemia.

TABLE 32-1. Cellular Processes That Require Energy

1. Pumping ions across membranes
2. Metabolism of proteins, lipids, carbohydrates, and other molecules
3. Transporting of molecules within cells

of components down the axon to the nerve terminal. The importance of this transport is illustrated by the death of the distal end of an axon when it is severed from its cell body. Thus, energy is required to maintain the integrity of neurons even in the absence of electrophysiologic activity.

The overall metabolic rate for the brain of a young adult man (mean age, 21 years) is 3.5 ml $O_2 \cdot min^{-1} \cdot 100 \ g^{-1}$ brain tissue or 5.5 mg glucose$\cdot min^{-1} \cdot 100 \ g^{-1}$.[12] This rate is virtually the same in elderly men (mean age, 71 years). Children (mean age, 6 years) have a markedly higher metabolic rate of 5.2 ml $O_2 \cdot min^{-1} \cdot 100 \ g^{-1}$ brain tissue. While the reasons for this high metabolic rate are unknown, it may reflect extra energy requirements for the growth and development of the nervous system.[12]

Cerebral Blood Flow

The brain receives approximately 15% of the cardiac output, yet it has only 2% of total body weight.[12] The disproportionately large blood flow is owing to the high metabolic rate of the brain. Global blood flow and metabolic rate remain fairly stable. Regional blood flow and metabolic rate of the brain can change dramatically; when metabolic rate goes up in a region of the brain, the blood flow to that region also increases. The mechanism of this coupling of blood flow and metabolism is not known; however, an increase in either potassium or hydrogen ion concentrations in the extracellular fluid surrounding arterioles may lead to dilatation and increased flow. Other agents that may mediate the coupling are calcium, adenosine and the eicosinoids (e.g., prostaglandins, thromboxane).[14] None of these mechanisms need be exclusive, and more than one or all of them may contribute to this exquisite coupling of flow and metabolism.

Increasing carbon dioxide levels causes vasodilatation and increased blood flow (Fig. 32-6). Doubling the carbon dioxide from 40 to 80 mm Hg doubles the flow; reducing the carbon dioxide from 40 to 20 mm Hg halves the flow.[16,17] These changes are transient, and blood flow returns to normal in 6–8 hours, even if the altered carbon dioxide levels are maintained. These effects may be related to hydrogen ion concentration. High carbon dioxide levels increase the extracellular hydrogen ion concentration and blood flow, while low carbon dioxide levels decrease the extracellular hydrogen ion concentration and reduce blood flow. The bicarbonate concentration in the extracellular fluid of the brain adjusts, bringing the pH back to normal, even though the carbon dioxide levels remain altered.[18] This has important clinical implications to reduce cerebral blood flow for patients hyperventilated for prolonged periods. If normocarbia is rapidly reestablished, brain interstitial fluid pH will decrease and cerebral blood flow will increase dramatically, perhaps increasing intracranial pressure.

If a patient is hypoventilated, carbon dioxide increases, pH decreases, and blood flow increases throughout the brain. The arterioles could become maximally dilated throughout the brain, impeding the ability to direct flow to areas of high metabolic demand. Thus, this luxury flow caused by high carbon dioxide levels throughout the brain could "steal" blood flow from areas that require extra oxygen and produce metabolites. This is particularly important during focal ischemia with the blockage of an intracerebral artery. The vessels supplying collateral flow to the area of the blocked artery would already be maximally dilated due to the metabolic demands of the ischemic tissue, and high $Paco_2$ would cause blood flow to be shunted away to areas

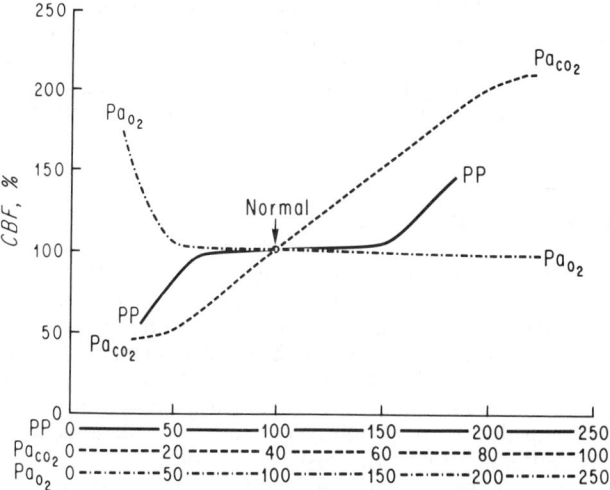

Figure 32-6. The effect of perfusion pressure (PP), arterial carbon dioxide pressure (Paco2), and arterial oxygen pressure (Pao2) on cerebral blood flow. Each parameter on the abscissa is varied independently while the other parameters are held at their normal levels. (Reprinted with permission from Michenfelder JD: Anesthesia and the Brain, pp 6, 94–113. New York, Churchill Livingstone, 1988.)

of less demand.[19] The blood flow to the brain can be manipulated to advantage during focal ischemia. Reducing carbon dioxide with hyperventilation or reducing metabolism with agents such as thiopental would reduce blood flow to most areas of the brain, while the vessels in the ischemic area would be maximally dilated because of low pH. These manipulations, which are sometimes called inverse steal or the "Robin Hood effect" (rob from the rich, give to the poor), could have the effect of maximizing blood flow to compromised areas.[20] The clinical relevance of flow redistribution due to hypocarbia has been questioned.[21]

The cerebral blood flow autoregulates with respect to pressure changes. In normotensive individuals, mean arterial blood pressure can vary from 50 to 150 mm Hg and cerebral blood flow will be maintained constant because of an adjustment of the cerebral vascular resistance (Fig. 32-6). This phenomenon is a myogenic response of the arterioles owing to their ability to constrict in response to an increased distending pressure. This response takes a few minutes to develop; therefore, after a rapid increase in mean arterial pressure, there is a short period (about 1–3 min) of increased blood flow.[22] If mean blood pressure falls below 50 mm Hg, then cerebral blood flow is reduced; at a pressure of 40 mm Hg, mild symptoms of cerebral ischemia occur.[23] Patients who are hypertensive demonstrate a shift of autoregulation to higher pressures.[24] Their lower limit of autoregulation could be well above 50 mm Hg; their upper limit for autoregulation is also increased. This shift, due to hypertrophy of the vessel wall, takes 1 or 2 months to become established.[23] Autoregulation can be abolished by trauma, hypoxia, and certain anesthetic and adjuvant anesthetic drugs. When blood pressure exceeds the autoregulated range, it usually causes a disruption of the blood–brain barrier and cerebral edema.

The cerebral vasculature is also regulated by neurogenic factors that seem to have their greatest influence on the larger cerebral vessels. They control flow to large areas of the brain and play less of a role in the regulation of local cerebral blood flow.[23] The innervation includes cholinergic, adrenergic, and serotonergic systems. Sympathetic activation leads to increased mean arterial blood pressure and shifts the autoregulatory curve to the right, increasing the pressure at which the breakthrough of autoregulation occurs.[24]

Cerebrospinal Fluid

The neurons in the brain are exquisitely sensitive to changes in their environment. Small alterations in extracellular ion levels can alter neuronal activity profoundly. Substances that circulate in the blood, such as catecholamines, if not sequestered from direct contact with the brain, might also disrupt brain function. Thus composition of the fluid surrounding the brain is tightly regulated and distinct from extracellular fluid in the rest of the body (Table 32-2).[25] There are two barriers, the blood–brain barrier and the blood–cerebrospinal fluid barrier, that maintain the difference between blood and cerebrospinal fluid (CSF) composition.

Brain capillary endothelial cells (the blood–brain barrier) have tight junctions that prevent extracellular passage of substances between the endothelial cells. They also have a low level of pinocytotic activity that reduces the transport of large molecules across the cells. In addition, processes of astrocyte glial cells are interposed between the neurons of the brain and the capillaries. The functional importance of the astrocytes to the blood–brain barrier is currently unknown; however, they are located wherever the blood–brain barrier is present and appear to be necessary for the development and perhaps the maintenance of the barrier. The blood–brain barrier impedes the flow of ions such as potassium, calcium, magnesium, and sodium; polar molecules such as glucose, amino acids, and mannitol; and macromolecules such as proteins.[25] Lipid soluble compounds, water, and gases such as carbon dioxide, oxygen, and volatile anesthetics pass rapidly through the blood–brain barrier. Many substances that do not cross the blood–brain barrier are required for brain function; these substances are transported across the capillary endothelial cell by carrier-mediated processes. These processes consist of either active transport, which requires the expenditure of energy, or passive transport, which does not. Passive transport, which is also referred to as facilitated diffusion, can only move molecules into the brain if their concentration in the blood is higher than their concentration in the brain. Glucose is an example of a molecule that enters the brain by passive transport. All of these transport processes have a limited capacity. The blood–brain barrier can become disrupted by acute hypertension, osmotic shock, disease, tumor, trauma, irradiation, and ischemia.

Cerebrospinal fluid is primarily formed in the choroid plexus of the cerebral ventricles. The capillaries of the choroid plexus have fenestrations and intercellular gaps that allow free movement of molecules across the endothelial cells; however, they are surrounded by choroid plexus epithelial cells, which have tight junctions and form the basis of the blood–cerebrospinal fluid barrier. It is these cells that secrete the CSF. The CSF volume in the brain is between 100 and 150 ml; it is formed and reabsorbed at a rate of 0.3–0.4 ml·min^{-1}. This allows a complete replacement of the CSF volume 3–4 times a day. The blood–CSF barrier is similar to the blood–brain barrier in that it allows the free movement of water, gases, and lipid-soluble compounds but

TABLE 32-2. Composition of Cerebrospinal Fluid (CSF) and Serum in Humans[25]

Component	CSF	Serum
Sodium (mEq·l^{-1})	138.0	140.0
Postassium (mEq·l^{-1})	2.8	4.0
Calcium (mEq·l^{-1})	2.4	4.6
Magnesium (mEq·l^{-1})	2.7	1.8
Chloride (mEq·l^{-1})	124.0	99.0
Glucose (mg·dl^{-1})	60.0	99.0
Protein (g·dl^{-1})	0.05	7.08

requires carrier-mediated active or passive transport processes for glucose, amino acids, and ions. Proteins are largely excluded from the CSF. The CSF is primarily formed by the transport of sodium, chloride, and bicarbonate with the osmotic movement of water. Two clinically used substances that reduce CSF formation are furosemide, which inhibits the sodium and chloride combined transport and acetazolamide, which reduces bicarbonate transport by inhibiting carbonic anhydrase.[26] The CSF flows from the lateral ventricles to the third and fourth ventricles and then to the cisterna magna. It then flows around the brain and spinal cord in the cerebral and spinal subarachnoid space. The fluid in the subarachnoid space provides cushioning for the brain, reducing the effect of head trauma. The CSF is absorbed into the venous system of the brain by the villi in the arachnoid membrane. These arachnoid villi allow one-way flow of CSF from the subarachnoid space into the venous sinuses when CSF pressure is greater than the pressure in these sinuses. Owing to the high rate of CSF formation and its absorption into the venous system, proteins and other matter released into the brain extracellular fluid are removed. If the foramina connecting the ventricles or the arachnoid villi are blocked, then pressure builds and hydrocephalus occurs.

Intracranial Pressure

The brain is enclosed in the cranium, which has a fixed volume; therefore, if any of the components located in the cranial vault increase in volume, the intracranial pressure will increase (Table 32-3). An increase in volume of one of these components can increase intracranial pressure (ICP) and result in two major deleterious effects on the organism. The first is to reduce blood flow to the brain. The cerebral perfusion pressure is determined by the mean arterial pressure minus the ICP. If ICP increases to a greater extent than mean arterial pressure, then cerebral perfusion pressure is reduced. If ICP rises sufficiently, then the brain can become ischemic. The second important effect of increased ICP is

TABLE 32-3. The Three Major Components Occupying Space in the Skull

1. The brain, which includes neurons and glia
2. The cerebrospinal fluid and extracellular fluid
3. The blood perfusing the brain

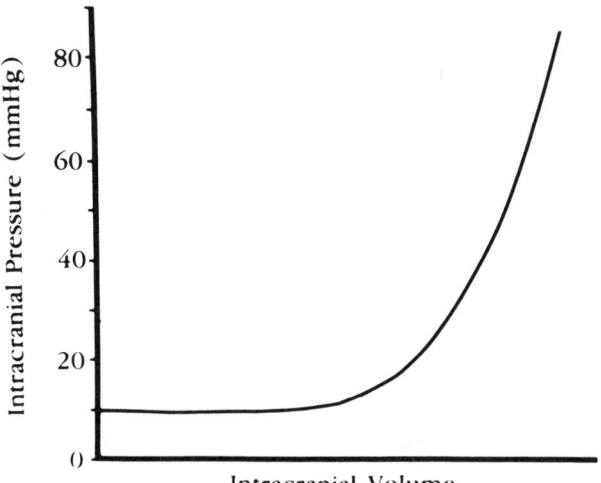

Figure 32-7. The effect of increasing volume on intracranial pressure. At first, as volume is increased, pressure does not increase, owing to the elastance of intracranial structures. This elastance is exceeded and then a small increase in volume can cause a large increase in intracranial pressure. (Modified from Miller JD, Garibi J, Pickard JD: The effects of induced changes of cerebrospinal fluid volume during continuous monitoring of ventricular pressure. Arch Neurol 28:265, 1973.)

its ability to induce brain herniation. This herniation could be across the meninges, down the spinal canal, or through an opening in the skull. Herniation can rapidly lead to neurologic degeneration and death.

The ICP in humans is normally less than 10 mm Hg.[27] Under normal circumstances, a small increase in intracranial volume will not greatly increase ICP because of the elastance of the components located in the cranium (Fig. 32-7). After a certain point, however, the capacity of the system to adjust to increased volume is exceeded and even a small increase in volume will increase ICP.[28] Increases in ICP can be caused by the following: (1) increased CSF volume owing to blockage of the circulation or absorption of the CSF as described above; (2) increased blood volume owing to vasodilatation or hematoma; and (3) increased brain tissue volume caused by a tumor or edema.

Brain edema is typically classified as cytotoxic or vasogenic.[29] The former is due to neuronal damage, which leads to increased sodium and water in the brain cells, and therefore an increase in intracellular volume. Vasogenic edema is caused by a breakdown of the blood–brain barrier and the movement of protein from the blood into the brain's extracellular space. Water moves osmotically with the protein increasing the extracellular fluid volume in the brain.

Pathophysiology

When the blood supply to the brain is limited, ischemic damage to neurons can occur—the brain is the most sensitive organ to ischemic damage.[14] To understand the rationale of the treatments used to protect the brain against ischemic damage, one needs an appreciation of the pathophysiologic mechanisms that may lead to this damage. The central event precipitating damage is reduced energy production due to blockage of oxidative phosphorylation. This causes ATP production per molecule of glucose to be re-

duced by 95%. At this rate of production ATP levels fall, leading to the loss of energy-dependent homeostatic mechanisms. The activity of ATP-dependent ion pumps is reduced and the intracellular levels of sodium and calcium increase, while intracellular potassium levels decrease (Fig. 32-8). These ion changes cause the neurons to depolarize and release excitatory amino acids such as glutamate. High levels of glutamate further depolarize the neurons and allow more calcium to enter through the NMDA receptor channel. The high intracellular calcium level is thought to trigger a number of events that could lead to the anoxic damage. These include increasing the activity of proteases and phospholipases.[30] The latter would increase the levels of free fatty acids and free radicals. Free radicals are known to damage proteins and lipids, while free fatty acids interfere with membrane function. In addition, there is a buildup of lactate and hydrogen ions. All of these processes, coupled with the reduced ability to synthesize proteins and lipids due to the reduced ATP levels, may lead to the irreversible damage with ischemia. In addition, phospholipase activation leads to the production of excess arachidonic acid which, upon reoxygenation, can form eicosanoids including thromboxane, prostaglandins, and leukotrienes. These substances can cause strong vasoconstriction and reduce blood flow in the postischemic period. Thus, procedures that may protect against ischemic damage should interfere with these mechanisms (Table 32-4). Specific agents that might accomplish these objectives will be detailed in the section on brain protection later in the chapter.

Ischemia can be either global or focal in nature; an example of the former would be cardiac arrest, the latter a localized stroke. While the mechanisms leading to neuronal damage are probably similar for both, there are important distinctions between the two. In focal ischemia there are three regions. The first receives no blood flow and responds the same as globally ischemic tissue; the second, called the penumbra, receives collateral flow and is partially ischemic; the third is normally perfused. If the insult is maintained for a prolonged period, the neurons in the penumbra will die. More neurons in the penumbra region will survive if collateral blood flow is increased. Mechanisms such as inverse steal (described in the Cerebral Blood Flow section of this chapter) will enhance collateral blood flow and, therefore, neuron survival in focal but not global ischemia.

Epileptic seizures are sudden, excessive, and synchronous discharges of large numbers of neurons. Aside from those patients with epilepsy, epileptic seizures are seen in patients with: ionic and electrolyte imbalances, disorders of brain metabolism, infection, brain tumor, brain trauma, or elevated body temperature.[31] The EEG record shows spikes, which are rapid changes in voltage corresponding to excess activity in many neurons. During the seizure, sodium and calcium ions enter the cells and potassium leaves. Thus the cells use more energy (ATP) for ion pumping even though they can not maintain normal ion levels. High extracellular potassium may be responsible for the large and progressive depolarization of the neurons that is seen with seizures. The mechanisms that lead to permanent neuronal damage with epilepsy may be similar to those that damage cells during ischemia. Intracellular calcium levels rise, which may precipitate the damage. It is clear that during seizures the energy demand and, therefore, the cerebral metabolic rate and blood flow increase greatly. Thus in conditions in which blood flow to the brain may be compromised, it is imperative to avoid seizures. Antiseizure medications increase neuronal inhibition or reduce excitatory processes in the

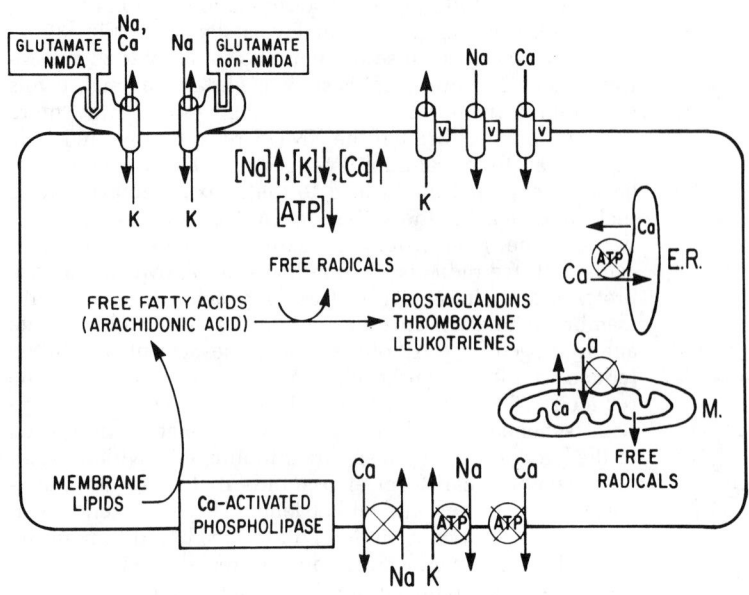

NEUROTRANSMITTER GATED CHANNELS

VOLTAGE SENSITIVE CHANNELS

EVENTS DURING ISCHEMIA

Figure 32-8. The effect of ischemia on ion and metabolite levels in neurons. For clarity, ion channels are shown on the top membrane and ion pumps on the bottom membrane; their actual location can be on any membrane surface. Circles indicate energy-driven pumps, × through the circle indicates that this pump is blocked or has reduced activity during ischemia. *V* indicates a voltage-dependent channel.

brain. Seizures may be accompanied by systemic lactic acidosis, reduced arterial oxygenation, and increased carbon dioxide; therefore it is important to maintain ventilation, oxygenation, and blood pressure. Prolonged or recurring seizures can lead to profound brain damage.

Brain trauma can directly lead to permanent physical neuronal damage. This primary damage can be caused by brain herniation or severing of blood vessels in the brain, resulting in direct ischemia. Reversal of the primary damage is not possible; however, much of the brain injury in trauma patients is secondary and occurs following the initial insult.[32] Calcium influx resulting from the trauma has been implicated as a trigger for the damage.[33] It is important to prevent the secondary ischemia that frequently follows brain trauma and is possibly due to the release of vasoconstrictive substances during reperfusion.[34] In addition hemorrhage may increase intracranial blood volume and ICP, reducing cerebral perfusion pressure. The intracranial blood can be damaging by directly promoting free-radical formation using the iron in hemoglobin. Secondary damage can be reduced with proper treatment such as monitoring and, if necessary, reducing ICP, maintaining blood flow, reducing vasospasm, and perhaps using pharmacologic agents that interfere with the cascade of events that lead to neuron damage.

TABLE 32-4. Procedures That May Protect Against Ischemic Damage

1. Maintaining ATP levels by reducing the metabolic rate
2. Blocking sodium or calcium influx
3. Scavenging free radicals
4. Blocking receptors for excitatory amino acids
5. Maintaining blood flow

Brain tumors are expanding, space-occupying lesions that may lead to significant increases in ICP, which could lead to reduced cerebral perfusion pressure or brain herniation. Frequently the blood vessels supplying the tumor have a leaky blood–brain barrier that may contribute to vasogenic brain edema and elevated ICP.

Thus for several pathophysiologic events in the brain, ionic imbalance (particularly, high intracellular calcium levels) has been implicated as a possible cause of the brain damage. A common mechanism of neuronal cell death for various pathophysiologic events may exist.

NEUROANESTHESIA

Effects of Anesthetics and Other Adjunctive Drugs on Brain Physiology

Volatile Anesthetics

Halothane, enflurane, and isoflurane have direct vasodilatory effects that increase cerebral blood flow (Table 32-5). Halothane with nitrous oxide (1.5 MAC) has been shown to increase blood flow almost 65%, while enflurane and isoflurane have a lesser effect at equal anesthetic potency.[35] Enflurane increased blood flow approximately 35% while isoflurane showed an even smaller increase. The increase in cerebral blood flow returns to baseline levels after approximately 3 hours of the initial exposure to 1.3 MAC of anesthetic.[36] The importance of increased cerebral blood flow is its influence on intracranial pressure. Increasing blood flow would tend to increase the amount of blood in the head, which under conditions of abnormal intracranial elastance could lead to large increases in ICP. A 1984 ani-

TABLE 32-5. Effects of Anesthetics on CBF/CMRO₂

Anesthetic	CBF	CMRO₂	CBF/ CMRO₂ Coupling	Direct Cerebral Vasodilatation
Halothane	↑ ↑ ↑	↓	No	Yes
Enflurane	↑ ↑	↓	No	Yes
Isoflurane	↑ or 0	↓ ↓	Yes	Yes
N₂O alone	↑	↑	Probably yes	Not known
N₂O with volatile anesthetics	↑	↑	Probably yes	—
N₂O with intravenous anesthetics	0	0	—	—
Thiopental	↓ ↓ ↓	↓ ↓ ↓	Yes	No
Etomidate	↓ ↓ ↓	↓ ↓ ↓	Yes	No
Propofol	↓ ↓	↓ ↓	Yes	No
Midazolam	↓ ↓	↓ ↓	Yes	No
Ketamine	↑ ↑	↑	Yes	Yes
Fentanyl	↓ or 0	↓ or 0	—	No
Sufentanil	Not known	0	—	
Alfentanil	Not known	Not known	—	

0 = no change; — = data inclusive or no data.

mal study surprisingly found that halothane and isoflurane increased ICP equally, even though halothane caused a greater increase in cerebral blood flow.[37] This may be explained by the finding that isoflurane and halothane increase cerebral plasma volume similarly.[38] These volatile anesthetics reduce the cerebral metabolic rate; isoflurane reduces the metabolic rate to a greater extent than halothane.[37] Indeed it is thought that isoflurane's metabolic effect, which reduces cerebral blood flow, competes with its direct vasodilatory action to limit the net increase in cerebral blood flow with this agent. Enflurane has been shown to induce seizure type discharges; this effect is potentiated by hypocapnia. Seizures induced with 1.5 MAC enflurane, hypocapnia, and an auditory stimulus increased cerebral metabolic rate and blood flow by 50%.[39] The above considerations have led to isoflurane becoming the choice volatile anesthetic for neuroanesthetic cases.

Sevoflurane, an anesthetic not yet available in the United States, is similar to isoflurane with respect to its effects on cerebral blood flow, cerebral metabolic rate, and intracranial pressure.[40] In rats, sevoflurane induces substantially smaller increases in ICP, single pial arteriole diameter, and flow than does isoflurane,[41] and most recently sevoflurane was proven protective during incomplete ischemia compared to fentanyl with N₂O.[42] Desflurane, another new anesthetic, increased cerebral blood flow and decreased the cerebral metabolic rate in an animal study.[43] One MAC desflurane has been shown to substantially increase ICP in neurosurgical patients with supratentorial mass lesions despite establishment of (13–33 mm Hg) hypocapnia,[44] though 0.5 MAC desflurane with N₂O may not alter ICP compared to 0.5 MAC isoflurane with N₂O.[45]

Nitrous oxide can increase cerebral blood flow and intracranial pressure.[46,47] Barbiturates and hypocapnia in combination may prevent these increases. There are indications that, even when given independently, barbiturates, benzodiazepines, and morphine are effective in blunting nitrous oxide's effect on cerebral blood flow and intracranial pressure.[48,49] In contrast, a volatile anesthetic may add to the increases in cerebral blood flow obtained with nitrous oxide.[50] Although the data on nitrous oxide's effect on brain metabolism are far from unequivocal, the evidence seems to indicate that there can be a substantial increase in cerebral metabolic rate if nitrous oxide is administered alone.[46] Although nitrous oxide is commonly used in neuroanesthesia, it seems unwise to use it when either intracranial pressure is high or elastance is abnormal, unless care is taken to counteract these effects.

Intravenous Anesthetics

Barbiturates decrease the cerebral metabolic rate and cerebral blood flow.[47-51] A major problem with barbiturates is that they can substantially reduce mean arterial blood pressure which, if not controlled, can reduce cerebral perfusion pressure. At high doses (10–55 mg·kg⁻¹), thiopental can produce an isoelectric EEG and decrease the cerebral metabolic rate by 50%.[52] This direct metabolic effect of thiopental leads to constriction of the cerebral vasculature and thereby reduces cerebral blood flow. Barbiturates are also effective in reducing elevated intracranial pressure and controlling epileptiform seizures.[53] Methohexital is an exception with regard to epileptiform activity; it can activate some seizure foci in patients with temporal lobe epilepsy.[54]

Etomidate, like the barbiturates, reduces cerebral metabolic rate and cerebral blood flow.[55-57] In addition to the indirect effect of reduced cerebral metabolism on blood flow, etomidate is also a direct vasoconstrictor even before metabolism is suppressed.[56] Its advantage over the barbiturates is that it does not produce clinically significant cardiovascular depression. A problem with etomidate and the reason why it is not commonly used is that it suppresses the adrenocortical response to stress.[58]

Propofol is a rapidly acting intravenous anesthetic that, like etomidate and the barbiturates, reduces the cerebral metabolic rate and cerebral blood flow.[59,60] It is able to reduce intracranial pressure; however, because it also reduces mean arterial blood pressure, its effect on cerebral perfusion pressure must be carefully monitored.[61] Because propofol is a newly released drug, there are relatively few studies examining its cerebral effects and the above results need further confirmation.

Benzodiazepines have been shown to reduce cerebral metabolic rate and cerebral blood flow[62,63]; however, this effect is not as pronounced as that with the barbiturates. As with the barbiturates, the blood flow reduction by benzodiazepines is thought to be secondary to a reduction in cerebral metabolic rate. Benzodiazepines may reduce intracranial pressure due to their effect on cerebral blood flow. Flumazenil is a benzodiazepine antagonist that has been shown to reverse the cerebral metabolic rate, cerebral blood flow, and intracranial-pressure lowering effects of the benzodiazepine, midazolam.[64] Thus flumazenil may cause problems in patients with high intracranial pressure or abnormal intracranial elastance.

The opioid anesthetics, morphine and fentanyl, cause either a minor reduction or no effect on cerebral blood flow and cerebral metabolic rate when compared with conditions in the unstimulated brain[65,66]; however, if the patient is aroused or in pain, they can cause a modest reduction in these parameters.[67] There is controversy concerning the effects of sufentanil: some studies demonstrate a reduction in cerebral blood flow and metabolism,[68,69] whereas others report an increase in blood flow and intracranial pressure.[70,71] The latter study found no increase in intracranial pressure with fentanyl.[71] The duration of the increased blood flow and intracranial pressure effects of sufentanil in the above studies was short and could be overcome by hypocapnia. In animal studies, alfentanil decreased cerebral blood flow and metabolism after 35 minutes and had no significant effect on ICP.[72] In patients with brain tumors, alfentanil increased cerebrospinal fluid pressure.[73] Its effect on cerebrospinal fluid pressure was less than that found with sufentanil but greater than that found with fentanyl. Alfentanil had the greatest effect on mean arterial blood pressure and cerebral perfusion pressure.[71]

Ketamine, a dissociative anesthetic, activates certain areas in the brain and can increase cerebral blood flow and cerebral metabolic rate.[74-76] It is therefore not commonly used in neuroanesthesia.

BRAIN PROTECTION

Procedures or drugs chosen to protect the brain during an ischemic event should augment, or at least not interfere with, the mechanisms listed in Table 32-4.

Techniques to Prevent Brain Damage

When ischemia reduces supply, maintenance of ATP by inducing hypothermia remains the *sine qua non* for reducing demand. Michenfelder has estimated a 50% reduction in $CMRO_2$ as temperature decreased from 37 to 27°C, followed by a decrease to less than 8% of normal oxygen consumption at 17°C.[16] The need for formal tests of the protective effect of profound hypothermia are obviated by the observation that human brains often recover after an hour of total cerebral ischemia during intentional circulatory arrest at 12–15°C. Although moderate hypothermia to 28°C is routinely used during noncirculatory-arrest cardiopulmonary bypass surgery, its protective efficacy has been presumed, probably accurately, but should be tested prospectively. A laboratory investigation indicates that protection afforded by intraischemic mild hypothermia accrues primarily from reduction of glutamate and dopamine release,[77] and other studies have shown that mild hypothermia (34–31°C) improves neurologic outcome even when induced subsequent to an ischemic insult.[78]

Unfortunately, with regard to neuronal membrane integrity and ionic leaks of Na, K, and Ca, the deleterious effects of hypothermia develop more slowly but are qualitatively similar to the effect of hypoxia.[79] Hypothermia is not, however, nearly as dangerous as normothermic hypoxia, because reduced metabolic rate reduces the production of toxic metabolites. Accordingly, patients subjected to deep hypothermia with circulatory arrest can often reestablish ionic gradients if reperfusion is accomplished—a reasonably reliable prospect for patients undergoing a cardiopulmonary bypass procedure, but unreliable when recirculation depends upon a heart that has its own imbalances to overcome. Much research has been directed toward enabling homeothermic mammals to gain the benefits of hypothermia without paying the costs, as do hibernators. If that research succeeds, we may eventually be able to provide brain protection during protracted periods of "ischemic" CBF and even induce circulatory arrest in neurosurgical patients more routinely.

Anesthetic and Adjuvant Drugs

Barbiturates

Maintenance of ATP by reduction of $CMRO_2$ is the mainstay of pharmacologic brain protection. Barbiturate administration is the only such intervention that has proven useful in humans.[80-91] In addition to lowering $CMRO_2$, pentobarbital often reduces elevated ICP that is refractory to hyperventilation and mannitol.[83,92,93] Experiments in primates indicate that some of the protective effect of barbiturates during focal ischemia can be attributed to vasoconstriction in areas of healthy brain that shunts CBF to injured areas.[94,95] Barbiturates have also been shown to reduce calcium influx,[96,97] inhibit free radical formation,[98-100] and reduce cerebral edema.[101,102] Among the most intriguing of the potentially protective mechanisms of barbiturates is their ability to block Na channels.[103,104]

While the ability of barbiturates to protect brains from global ischemia remains controversial,[16,19] the only large, randomized human study to date found only statistically insignificant trends in favor of barbiturate protection as a resuscitative measure subsequent to cardiac arrest.[105]

Midazolam

Midazolam is a benzodiazepine that reduces $CMRO_2$ in humans[106] and other mammals.[107] Consistent with *in vitro* results demonstrating that midazolam protects hippocampal neurons against anoxic damage by maintaining ATP levels and reducing calcium influx,[108] Baughman *et al* have found that midazolam protects rats after incomplete global ischemia.[109]

Etomidate

Etomidate also reduces $CMRO_2$ and has demonstrated protective effects in laboratory studies,[56] however, etomidate's usefulness may be limited by its propensity to constrict cerebral vasculature before it suppresses $CMRO_2$.

Propofol

Propofol is an induction drug that reduces $CMRO_2$ and has been shown to protect hippocampal neurons from seven minutes of anoxia.[110]

Channel Blockers

Specific ionic channel blockers may have a role to play in clinical brain protection. Only nimodipine has shown efficacy in humans,[111-114] with its beneficial effect probably resulting more from vascular relaxation than from direct neuronal effects.[115,116] Studies of humans after stroke from cerebral aneurysm rupture and cerebral ischemic disease have demonstrated positive effects even though nimodipine was given subsequent to the ischemic event.[111,112,114] Nimodipine administration following ventricular fibrillation has been shown to have a positive effect in a subgroup of patients who had delays (13 min) in initiation of life support techniques.[113] Other calcium channel blockers, particularly flunarizine,[117] have shown promise of direct neuronal protection in laboratory studies,[118,119] but replication of lidoflazine's initial laboratory success has failed in comatose humans after cardiac arrest.[120,121] Magnesium reduces Ca entry and is powerfully protective *in vitro* but has not shown promise *in vivo*.[122] Sodium channel blockers should contribute to stabilization of neuronal membranes during ischemia, and both lidocaine[123-125] and phenytoin[126] have shown promise in the laboratory.[127]

Much attention has also recently been focused on the excitotoxic hypothesis of cerebral damage.[128-130] As discussed, cerebral ischemia causes excessive release of the excitatory neurotransmitter glutamate. Both NMDA and non-NMDA glutamate receptor blockers may prove beneficial. Although NMDA antagonist MK-801 has given mixed results in this regard,[131-135] the non-NMDA glutamate receptor antagonist NBQX has shown promise in a laboratory model of global ischemia,[136] as has the competitive NMDA blocker CGS-19755.[137]

Free Radical Scavengers

Free radical scavengers are a likely candidate for inclusion in defense against ischemic brain damage. After disappointing results with glucocorticoid administration subsequent to cardiac arrest in humans,[138] a large, randomized, controlled trial has shown that methylprednisolone reduced spinal-cord deficits if administered within 8 hours of injury.[139] Vitamin E has proven protective *in vitro*,[140] with supportive evidence *in vivo*,[141] as has U74006F. This 21-aminosteroid has shown protection after complete cerebral ischemia in dogs,[142] after cerebral vasospasm in rabbits,[143] after middle cerebral artery occlusion in rats,[144] after traumatic injury in rats,[145] and for treatment of brain edema in rats.[146] Nevertheless, in a study of incomplete ischemia in the rat, U74006F did not markedly improve outcome.[147] Superoxide dismutase has demonstrated experimental promise as a free radical scavenger that protects during reperfusion,[148] and the hydroxyl scavenger dimethylthiourea has shown an ability to reduce infarct size and brain edema after middle cerebral artery occlusion in rats without affecting cerebral blood flow.[149]

Progress and Prospects

Several recent developments have improved our ability to protect the central nervous system from ischemic damage. Nimodipine, for example, has benefited victims of acute ischemic stroke,[111] poor-grade aneurysm patients,[112] and patients who received delayed resuscitation after ventricular fibrillation.[113] Methylprednisolone has been shown to improve outcome after spinal cord injury in humans,[139] and

other free radical scavengers are demonstrating protective effects in the laboratory.[140-149] New glutamate receptor antagonists have brought the excitotoxicity hypothesis to center stage.[131,133,136,137,150] Combined pharmacotherapies,[151] including the NMDA-receptor blocker MK-801 with nimodipine,[132] are showing protective effects in the laboratory. Platelet activating factor antagonism is continuing to demonstrate postischemic protection in a variety of rodents.[152-155] In addition, renewed success with neural implants,[156] laboratory success in neuronal regeneration,[157,158] and the ability to culture continuously a human cortical neuronal cell line[159] have advanced the prospects for recovery from permanent damage.

Nevertheless, improvements in our ability to prevent and treat perioperative neurologic injury have so expanded the range and severity of conditions amenable to surgical intervention that we are seeing more patients, a higher percentage of whom would have been considered too sick for surgery just 10 years ago. The magnitude of our challenge has kept pace with the effectiveness of our solutions. These events are exciting and offer hope that new and better drugs and techniques will be developed over the next decade.

MONITORING

Electroencephalogram

The electroencephalogram (EEG) can be used to monitor cerebral function during general anesthesia. Because of the size and complexity of most EEG equipment, the need for trained personnel, and the difficulty in obtaining, interpreting and storing the raw EEG, its use in the operating room has been limited. With recent advances in technology and computer processing, signal processed EEG monitors are becoming practical to use in the operating room.

The EEG waves recorded on the surface of the scalp are spontaneous electrical potentials generated by the pyramidal cells of the granular cortex. The EEG signal consists of graded summations of inhibitory and excitatory postsynaptic potentials (PSPs) that create dipole fields in the dendrites of the pyramidal cells.[160] When a number of dipoles develop at once, the summation creates electrical potentials that are large enough to produce detectable voltages on the scalp.

The EEG waveforms are interpreted by pattern recognition and quantification. Specific complexes are described in terms of morphology, spatial and temporal distribution, and reactivity of the waveforms. Quantification involves measuring frequency and amplitude. Frequency is measured in Hertz (Hz) and is defined as the number of times per second the wave crosses the zero voltage line. Amplitude, which is measured in microvolts (μV), is the electrical height of the wave. The frequency bands are divided into delta (0–3 Hz), theta (4–7 Hz), alpha (8–13 Hz), and beta (above 13 Hz) rhythms (Table 32-6).

The traditional EEG is a plot of voltage against time. Sixteen channels are usually recorded. EEG waveform changes associated with anesthetic drugs, Pao$_2$, Paco$_2$, and temperature are described in Table 32-7.

The EEG response to anesthetic agents can vary from cortical excitation through depression to isoelectricity. Usually, anesthetic induction produces a decrease in alpha and an increase in beta activity. As the depth of anesthesia increases, EEG frequency decreases until theta and delta activity predominate. By further increasing the dose of anesthesia, the EEG changes to a burst suppression pattern, which coincides with near maximal depression of cerebral meta-

TABLE 32-6. EEG Frequency Ranges

Delta rhythm (0–3 Hz)	Deep sleep, deep anesthesia, or pathologic states (*e.g.,* brain tumors, hypoxia, metabolic encephalopathy)
Theta rhythm (4–7 Hz)	Sleep and anesthesia in adults; hyperventilation in awake children and young adults
Alpha rhythm (8–13 Hz)	Resting, awake adult with eyes closed, predominantly seen in occipital leads
Beta rhythm (>13 Hz)	Mental activity, light anesthesia

bolic activity. Complete electrical silence or isoelectricity follows an additional increase in anesthesia.

Efforts to use the EEG as a monitor of depth of anesthesia have been unsuccessful because of the variety of agents used during an anesthetic and because some anesthetic agents do not follow the general pattern described above (Fig. 32-9).[161,162] EEG verification of burst suppression and electrical silence is valuable when determining the dose required to induce and maintain barbiturate coma.

Other physiologic parameters that affect EEG waveforms are $Paco_2$,[163] temperature[164] and sensory stimulation.[165] Hypocarbia causes EEG slowing. Mild hypercarbia causes increased frequency, and severe hypercarbia produces a decrease in frequency and amplitude. When body temperature

TABLE 32-7. EEG Changes Associated with Anesthetic Drugs, Pao₂, Paco₂ and Temperature

Increased Frequency

Barbiturates (low dose)
Benzodiazepines (low dose)
Etomidate (low dose)
N₂O (30–70%)
Inhalation agents (<1 MAC)
Ketamine
Hypoxia (initially)
Hypercarbia (mild)
Seizures

Decreased Frequency/Increased Amplitude

Barbiturates (moderate dose)
Etomidate (moderate dose)
Opioids
Inhalation agents (>1 MAC)
Hypoxia (mild)
Hypocarbia (moderate to extreme)
Hypothermia

Decreased Frequency/Decreased Amplitude

Barbiturates (high dose)
Hypoxia (mild)
Hypercarbia (severe)
Hypothermia (<35°C)

Electrical Silence

Barbiturates (coma dose)
Etomidate (high dose)
Isoflurane (2 MAC)
Hypoxia (severe)
Hypothermia (<15–20°C)
Brain death

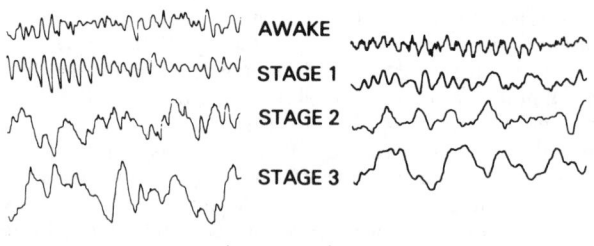

ALFENTANIL EEG   FENTANYL EEG

AWAKE
STAGE 1
STAGE 2
STAGE 3

50 µV   1 sec.

Figure 32-9. EEG changes with increasing doses of fentanyl and alfentanil: Awake, mixed alpha (8–13 Hz) and beta (>13 Hz) activity; Stage 1, slowing with alpha spindles; Stage 2, more slowing, theta activity present (4–7 Hz); Stage 3, maximal slowing, delta waves present (<4 Hz) with high amplitude. (Reprinted with permission from Scott JC, Ponaganis KV, Stanski DR: EEG quantification of narcotic effect: The comparative pharmacodynamics of fentanyl and alfentanil. Anesthesiology 62:234, 1985.)

falls below 35°C, hypothermia causes a progressive slowing of activity. Complete electrical silence occurs at 15–20°C. Sensory stimulation is associated with EEG activation.

The most significant contribution that EEG monitoring may make to patient care is the early detection of cerebral hypoxia and ischemia. Inadequate partial pressure of oxygen or insufficient cerebral blood flow is reflected within seconds in the EEG.[166,167,168] Hypoxia may initially produce EEG activation, which is followed by slowing and eventually electrical silence.[169] Cerebral ischemia causes progressive slowing of the EEG and voltage attenuation that proceeds to electrical silence.[167]

When monitoring an EEG during anesthesia, the changes resulting from hypoxia or ischemia must be distinguished from the variety of drug and physiologic effects that also may influence the EEG. Because of this, the EEG must always be interpreted within the clinical context in which it is observed.

A specific intraoperative application of the EEG is the localization of epileptic foci during surgery for intractable epilepsy. For these procedures, recording electrodes are applied on or in the brain, and a light general anesthetic is administered to avoid pharmacologic cortical depression, which would prevent provocative seizure activity. Provocative techniques and agents such as hyperventilation, low dose barbiturates, enflurane, and etomidate have been used to activate the foci.[170-172]

Computerized EEG Processing

The development of the computer-processed EEG has facilitated intraoperative EEG monitoring. The methods of analysis used to process the EEG include power-spectrum, zero-cross, and aperiodic analysis. The most widely used and best validated technique is power-spectrum analysis, which uses a computer to perform a Fourier transformation. A given epoch of EEG (usually 2–8 sec) is converted from a plot of voltage against time to a plot of power (amplitude squared) against frequency. With this technique, data are displayed in one of three formats: the compressed spectral array (CSA), the density spectral array (DSA), and the band spectral array (BSA) or power bands. For example, to generate the CSA format, the Fourier transformation converts the irregular EEG waves to equivalent sine waves of known frequency and power (Fig. 32-10).[166] This display shows time and power as one axis (vertical) and frequencies on the horizontal axis. The Fourier spectral data from successive segments are stacked one on top of the other creating a pseudo three-dimensional display, that is, the plot is shifted vertically with time and compressed. A major advantage of power-spectrum analysis is that it retains almost all the information in the original EEG. Power-spectrum analysis has documented value as a monitor of cerebral ischemia and possible value in the determination of anesthetic depth.[168,173,174] The main disadvantages of this analysis technique are lack of detection of spike activity, inclusion of artifact within frequency bands, and limited review of raw EEG data to determine reliability of the ongoing input.

An early method used for processing the EEG was the zero-cross analysis. The zero-cross frequency or mean frequency of the EEG is estimated by counting the number of times the EEG waveform crosses the zero-voltage axis.[175] Aperiodic analysis is a variant of the zero-cross method. With this technique, each waveform is analyzed in relation to its frequency, amplitude, and time of occurrence. Aperiodic analysis does not rely on averaging many waveforms over a given epoch. The signal is broken into the four component frequencies, with the amplitudes at each frequency in each hemisphere displayed. Aperiodic analysis of the EEG can be used quite effectively to detect the presence of intraoperative cerebral ischemia (Fig. 32-11).[176]

Several technical matters must be considered to effectively implement intraoperative electrophysiologic monitoring. Awake controls should be obtained prior to induction of general anesthesia. Monitoring should be continuous throughout anesthesia and continue until the patient is awake. Bilateral data must be obtained, especially during cerebrovascular procedures. For example, during a carotid endarterectomy, bilateral changes may indicate anesthetic or systemic effects, whereas ipsilateral changes on the operated side are more likely consistent with surgical trauma or ischemia. Marked changes in anesthetic depth, systemic blood pressure (BP), $Paco_2$, and brain temperature must be avoided in order to distinguish between anesthetic and physiologic effects on the EEG and those due to hypoxia or ischemia.

There is controversy concerning the number of EEG channels required for appropriate intraoperative monitoring. The traditional electrophysiologist recommends eight or more channels for ischemia monitoring. Many of the available computerized-processing devices analyze only two channels, although machines that analyze four, eight and 16 or more channels are currently available. In general, with the application, testing, and maintenance of eight or more electrodes, electrophysiologic monitoring becomes extremely time consuming for the anesthesiologist who is working alone, and usually requires technical support. Therefore, for routine intraoperative use, a minimum of two and perhaps four channels are recommended. As the computerized-processed EEG devices become more sophisticated and easier to use by the nonelectrophysiologist, the intraoperative application and analysis of four or more channels will become more practical.

Evoked Potentials

Evoked potentials (EPs) are used intraoperatively to monitor the integrity of specific sensory and motor pathways. Sensory evoked potentials (SEPs) evaluate the functional integ-

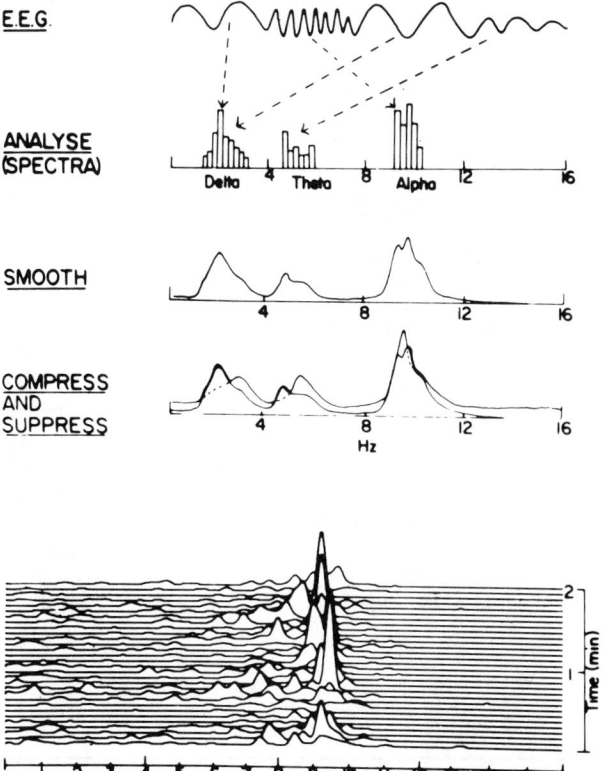

Figure 32-10. Schematic diagram of technique used to generate compressed spectral array. Below the diagram is an example of compressed spectra of the alpha rhythm from a normal subject. (Reprinted with permission from Stockard JJ, Bickford RG: The neurophysiology of anesthesia. In Gordon E (ed): A Basis and Practice of Neuroanesthesia, 2nd ed, p 20. Amsterdam, Elsevier Science Publishing, 1981.)

rity of ascending sensory pathways, whereas motor evoked potentials (MEPs) test the functional integrity of descending motor pathways.

There are major differences between EPs and the EEG. The EEG is a recording of spontaneous, random electrical activity, that has a nonspecific function and generates a relatively large signal, e.g., 50 μV or more. Evoked potentials are comparatively small amplitude responses (0.1–20 μV) to a specific stimulus that are pathway specific.

Sensory Evoked Potentials

The application of a sensory stimulus, e.g., a click, flash, or shock—results in an afferent nerve impulse that can be detected by appropriately placed surface electrodes as transient potential differences. The amplitude of these EPs is very small and obscured by normal background bioelectric activity from the EEG, EKG, muscle activity, and other extraneous electrical activity. Signal averaging is required to extract the evoked responses from this background noise. The background noise is random and is eliminated by the averaging process.

Three SEP modalities are employed clinically; somatosensory, auditory, and visual. The waves of the evoked po-

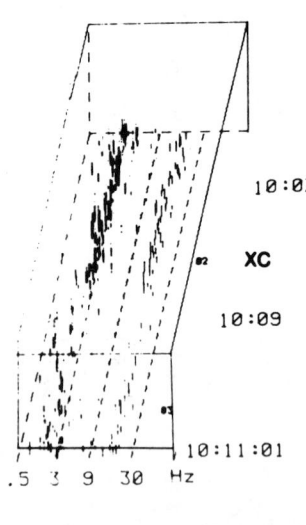

LEFT HEMI 5 MIN (Snap)

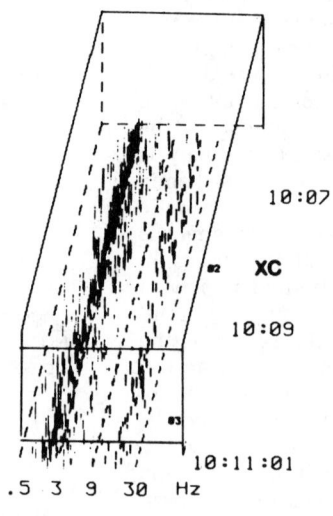

RIGHT HEMI 5 MIN (Snap)

Figure 32-11. EEG as displayed by a Lifescan Monitor using aperiodic analysis. This photograph was obtained approximately 3 minutes after occlusion (marked "XC") of the left carotid artery. Frequency is displayed on the *x* axis. The amplitude of each mapped EEG wave is a vertical "pole." Time is displayed on the diagonal axis, with the most recent time at the bottom front of the box. This display shows attenuation of activity on the left with occlusion that is more apparent in the higher frequency range. The regional cerebral blood flow with occlusion was 9 ml·100 g⁻¹·min⁻¹. (Reprinted with permission from Spackman TN, Faust RJ, Cucchiara FR *et al:* A comparison of aperiodic analysis of the EEG with Standard EEG and cerebral blood for detection of ischemia. Anesthesiology 66:229, 1987.)

TABLE 32-8. Effects of Intravenous and Inhaled Agents on Sensory Evoked Potentials

	BAEPs		cSSEPs		VEPs	
	Lat	Amp	Lat	Amp	Lat	Amp
Intravenous Agents						
Thiopental						
4–6 mg·kg⁻¹	0	0	0	0	—	—
20 mg·kg⁻¹	↑	0	↑	↓	↑	↓
75 mg·kg⁻¹	↑	↓	↑	↓	↑	↓
Pentobarbital						
9–18 mg·kg⁻¹	↑	↓	↑	↓	↑	↓
Droperidol						
0.1 mg·kg⁻¹	—	—	↑	↓	—	—
Diazepam						
0.1 mg·kg⁻¹	0	0	↑	↓	—	—
Midazolam	—	—	0	↓	—	—
Meperidine	—	—	↑	↑ / ↓	—	—
Morphine	—	—	↑	↓	—	—
Fentanyl	0	0	↑	↓	—	—
Sufentanil	0	0	0	↓	—	—
Alfentanil	0	0	0	↓	—	—
Etomidate						
0.05–0.3 mg·kg⁻¹·min⁻¹	0	0	↑	↑	—	—
Propofol						
2–6 mg·kg⁻¹	0	0	↑	↓	—	—
Inhalation Agents						
Enflurane	↑	0	↑	↑ *	↑	↓
Halothane	↑	0	↑	↓	↑	0
Isoflurane	↑	0	↑	↓ *	↑	↓
Nitrous oxide	0	0	0	↓	↑	↓

BAEPs = brain stem auditory evoked potentials, cSSEPs = cortical somatosensory evoked potentials, VEPs = visual evoked potentials, ↑ = increased, ↓ = decreased, Lat = latency, Amp = amplitude, 0 = no change, — = no data.
*1.5 MAC enflurane and isoflurane (but not halothane) will occasionally abolish the cortical evoked response to median nerve stimulation.

tential are thought to represent potentials from specific neural generators. The individual peaks in the waveform are described in terms of polarity (negative, positive), poststimulus latency (msec), and peak-to-peak amplitude (μV or nV). They are also described by the distance separating the neural generators and recording electrodes (near-field, far-field).

Anesthetic Considerations for Sensory Evoked Potential Recording

Compromise or injury of a neurologic pathway is manifested as an increase in the latency and/or a decrease in the amplitude of evoked potential waveforms. Accordingly, anesthetic, physiologic, and environmental factors capable of producing this pattern of alteration must be controlled when recording evoked potentials. All anesthetics that have been studied influence evoked potentials to some extent. Table 32-8 summarizes the known effects of intravenous and inhaled agents.[177-199] The sensitivity of evoked potentials to drug effects varies with the sensory modality being monitored. Evoked potentials of cortical origin (i.e., the cortical component of the SSEP and the VEP) are more vulnerable to anesthetic influences than brain stem potentials (e.g., BAEPs and the subcortical components of the SSEP). In general, to obtain satisfactory intraoperative SEP recordings, it is important to maintain constant anesthetic drug levels. Specifically, bolus administration of intravenous agents and step changes in inspired inhalation agent concentration must be avoided, especially at times when neurologic injury might occur. When recording cortical evoked potentials (SSEPs or VEPs), one should employ intravenous techniques. High concentrations of volatile agents essentially eliminate cortical evoked potentials. However, end-tidal concentrations of 0.5 MAC halothane, enflurane, and iso-

flurane are compatible with satisfactory recordings in patients who are neurologically normal.

In general, volatile agents cause a dose-dependent increase in latency and a decrease in amplitude of the cortical SSEP or VEP.[177-183] As exemplified in a study by Peterson et al (Fig. 32-12), reductions in SSEP amplitude greater than 50% were observed with 1 MAC halothane, 0.5 MAC enflurane, and 0.5 MAC isoflurane, all administered with 60% N_2O in oxygen.[177] The authors concluded that halothane disrupted the SSEP the least, and enflurane disrupted the most. In another study, halothane was found to be the most disruptive, and enflurane the least disruptive.[178] Although the results are inconsistent, these studies demonstrate that inhalation agents cause dose-dependent changes in SSEPs, producing marked attenuation in 1 MAC concentrations. The effects of inhalation agents on VEPs are similar to the effects on cortical SSEPs except that halothane has been shown to increase latency without changing amplitude.[180,182] Nitrous oxide alone has been shown to produce significant decreases in amplitude with minimal latency changes in the cortical SSEP, but it decreases both amplitude and latency in the VEP.[179,184,185]

Brain stem responses are considerably more resistant to anesthetic influences than are cortical responses. For example, clinically used concentrations of the inhaled agents tend to increase the latencies of the BAEP with minimal amplitude effects.[186-188] Most anesthetic regimens are compatible with recording of brain stem responses. However, as with the other evoked potential modalities, large step changes (greater than 0.5 MAC) in inspired inhalation agent concentration should be avoided during critical periods.

Studies on the effects of intravenous agents demonstrate that induction doses of thiopental, etomidate, and fentanyl preserve SSEP recordings.[189] Increasing doses of thiopental result in dose-dependent increases in latency and decreases in amplitude in cortical SSEPs and progressive increases in

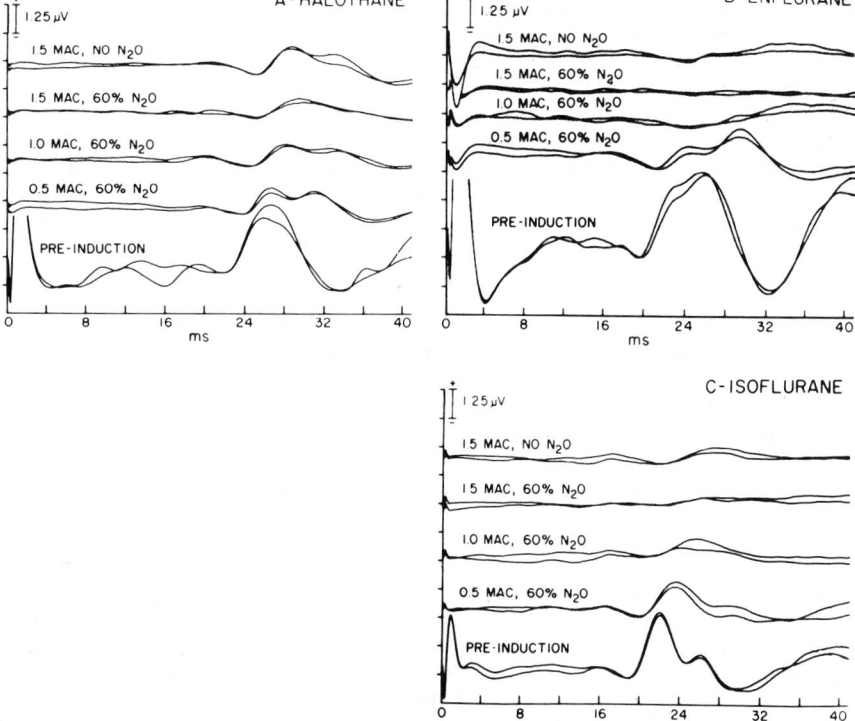

Figure 32-12. The responses of cortical somatosensory evoked potentials to various minimal alveolar concentrations (MACs) of halothane, enflurane, and isoflurane. A marked alteration of evoked potentials occurs at 1 MAC and higher levels of inhaled agents and a modest improvement of the response occurs when N_2O is withdrawn. (Reprinted with permission from Peterson DO, Drummond JC, Todd MM: Effects of halothane, enflurane, isoflurane and nitrous oxide on somatosensory evoked potentials in humans. Anesthesiology 65:35, 1986.)

latency in BAEPs.[190] Very high doses of thiopental, exceeding that which produces an isoelectric EEG, alter SSEPs and BAEPs predictably, but waveforms are preserved.[191] VEPs are more sensitive than the other sensory modalities to the effects of barbiturates, with only the early potentials persisting at low doses and increasing in latency at higher doses.[191] Either bolus administration or intravenous infusions of etomidate causes increases in latency and increases in amplitude of cortical SSEPs and slight decreases in amplitude of cervical potentials.[192] Etomidate produces minimal changes in the early or subcortical peaks of the BAEP, but causes a dose-dependent attenuation and prolongation of the middle latency cortical peaks.[193] The benzodiazepines also alter SEPs. Diazepam causes increases in latency and decreases in amplitude of SSEPs and no change in BAEPs.[194] Midazolam decreases the amplitude without changing the latency of SSEPs.[192] Propofol increases the latency and decreases the amplitude of cortical SSEPs.[195] The effects of propofol infusions on auditory BAEPs and middle latency peaks are similar to etomidate. Propofol causes no change in BAEPs and produces an increase in latency and decrease in amplitude of middle latency potentials in a dose-dependent manner.[196]

The opioids in general produce dose-dependent increases in latency and variable changes in amplitude of SSEPs. Fentanyl and morphine cause dose-dependent increases in latency of all waves and decreases in amplitude.[197,198] The administration of high-dose fentanyl (up to 60 $\mu g \cdot kg^{-1}$), has been shown to be compatible with reproducible recordings of SSEPs.[198] Narcotics produce minimal to no effect on BAEP recordings.[199] Because narcotics preserve SEP recordings even in relatively high doses, they are recommended for use as infusions during intraoperative monitoring. As with all intravenous agents used, bolus administration should be avoided during critical times when neurologic injury might occur.

Physiologic factors such as temperature, systemic blood pressure, and arterial tensions of oxygen and carbon dioxide can alter SEPs and must be controlled during intraoperative recording. Both hypothermia and hyperthermia alter all SEPs.[200-202] In addition, fluids used to irrigate the brain or spinal cord can cause marked changes in recordings despite normal core temperature measurement. Therefore, body temperature irrigating fluids should be used. Systemic hypotension below levels of cerebral autoregulation produces progressive decreases in amplitude of cortical SSEPs until the waveform is lost, with no change in latency.[203,204] It seems, however, that BAEPs may be resistant to profound levels of hypotension (e.g., a MAP of 20 mm Hg in dogs).[203] During scoliosis surgery, SSEP changes have been observed that resolved with increases in systemic blood pressure, suggesting that spinal cord manipulation during "safe" levels of hypotension may cause significant ischemia.[205] Changes in arterial tensions of oxygen and carbon dioxide also alter SEPs, probably reflecting changes in blood flow or oxygen delivery to neural structures.[206,207] Isovolemic hemodilution has been shown to alter SEPs; however, the changes in SSEPs and VEPs only became significant at hematocrits below 15%.[208]

Motor Evoked Potentials

A motor evoked potential (MEP) can be produced by direct (epidural) or indirect (transosseous) stimulation of the brain or spinal cord. Following transcranial stimulation, the signal descends through both the dorsolateral and ventral spinal cord. It is primarily localized in the pyramidal tracts, and can be recorded from spinal cord, peripheral nerve, and muscle using conventional electromyographic (EMG) and evoked potential averaging techniques. Stimulation of the motor cortex elicits contralateral peripheral nerve signals, EMG signals, or limb movements.

Transosseous activation of motor neurons can be accomplished by either electrical or magnetic stimulation. Transcranial electrical stimulation of the motor cortex is achieved by delivering brief electrical shocks through electrodes on the skin.[209] Percutaneous electrical stimulation can be uncomfortable. Elevations of arterial blood pressure and heart rate have been reported in awake and anesthetized patients.[209] If the rate of transcortical stimulation is slowed, these cardiovascular responses may return to normal.

Transcranial magnetic stimulation is produced by placing a magnetic coil over the motor cortex.[210] This technique is painless, noninvasive, and does not require direct contact with the scalp. Because high-resistance tissues such as bone and skin are transparent to magnetic fields, smaller voltages can be used to stimulate neural elements below the surface. With magnetic stimulation, there is concern about movement of metallic objects that lie within the magnetic field.

With either electrical or magnetic stimulation, there is theoretical concern that repetitive cortical stimulation can induce epileptic activity, neural damage, and cognitive or memory dysfunction. Current guidelines for transcranial MEP stimulation recommend intermittent rather than continuous stimulation over several hours and cautious use in patients with a history of seizures, possible skull fractures, or implanted metallic devices.[211] Disruptions of the calvarium, i.e., a skull fracture, could focus the current toward certain regions of the brain and potentially cause neural damage. Other situations of concern are patients with cardiac pacemakers and central venous and pulmonary artery catheterization. Transcranial MEP stimulation should probably be avoided in these patients until collaborative safety studies are performed.

There are several potential indications for intraoperative monitoring of MEPs. The ability to monitor conduction in both sensory and motor pathways during spinal cord surgery would be particularly informative. For example, during scoliosis surgery, a direct monitor of motor pathway function would obviate the need for the intraoperative wake-up test and provide continuous information about motor function throughout the surgical procedure. During intracranial procedures that involve large or complicated vascular lesions and potential compromise to the motor cortex or tracts, the ability to guide the surgical resection by monitoring motor function may prevent postoperative motor deficits. Paralysis is an unpredictable complication that can occur following aortic aneurysm surgery. Although SSEPs have been used to identify intraoperative spinal cord dysfunction during aortic cross-clamping, a monitor of motor function would provide more specific information.

The effects of anesthetic agents on MEPs are under investigation. Recent reports and observations show the MEP to be more sensitive than SEPs to anesthetics. For example, sedative doses of midazolam and fentanyl cause a decrease in the amplitude of the EMG response.[212] An induction dose of midazolam can produce profound and prolonged attenuation of MEPs.[213] Induction with thiopental or anesthesia with N_2O and isoflurane are reported to produce loss of potentials.[212] Increasing N_2O concentration gradually attenuates and abolishes MEPs at a concentration of 66% in rats, while SSEPs are minimally altered.[214] A concentration of 50% N_2O is reported to cause a minimal response alteration and appears to be compatible with monitoring.[215] In primates, anesthetic doses of ketamine and etomidate cause minimal MEP response alterations and are compatible with monitoring.[216,217] Muscle relaxants affect the recorded EMG response by depressing myoneural transmission. By using a continuous muscle relaxant induction technique and maintaining one to two twitches in a train of four, reliable MEP responses have been recorded. Although it appears that MEPs are more sensitive to the effects of anesthetic agents, reliable responses can be recorded with a nitrous oxide-narcotic technique and with agents such as ketamine or etomidate. It appears that agents with CNS inhibitory action (e.g., thiopental and midazolam) produce profound changes in MEP responses and should be avoided. As with SEPs, hypothermia, hypoxia, and hypotension can also alter MEPs under anesthesia.

Intracranial Pressure Monitoring

Since Lundberg's[218] report in 1960, continuous intracranial pressure (ICP) monitoring has been used to guide the perioperative management of patients with head injury, ruptured intracranial aneurysm, brain tumor, cerebrovascular occlusive disease, and hydrocephalus. For example, during intracranial procedures, knowledge of ICP and arterial blood pressure allows precise titration of pharmacologic agents during induction and establishment of anesthesia and guides positioning of the patient to avoid venous engorgement or bleeding.[219] Intracranial hypertension resulting from application of the bone flap or head dressing at the conclusion of surgery can also be observed and treated.[220] Postoperatively, ICP monitoring allows early detection and prompt treatment of brain swelling or hemorrhage. Another indication for intraoperative ICP monitoring is to detect intracranial hypertension in the multiple trauma patient during a non-neurosurgical procedure.[221]

There is no doubt that ICP monitoring can serve as an early warning system for impending disaster.[222,223] Whether or not outcome is improved by monitoring and controlling ICP is more difficult to prove.[224,225]

Techniques used to monitor ICP include: a ventricular catheter, a subarachnoid bolt, and a variety of epidural transducers (Fig. 32-13). The intraventricular catheter is the standard method of monitoring ICP. This technique requires a small scalp incision and a burr hole through the skull. A soft, nonreactive plastic catheter is introduced into the lateral ventricle and connected with sterile tubing filled with saline to an external transducer. The intraventricular catheter measures CSF pressures reliably. It allows therapeutic CSF drainage and can also be used for compliance testing. There are, however, several potential problems with this technique. In a patient with severe brain swelling or a large mass lesion and small ventricles, it may be technically difficult to locate the lateral ventricle. Besides not being able to pass the catheter into the CSF, there is a possibility of brain tissue damage, hematoma, and infection.[226] Infection is a common complication of ventriculostomy and appears to be related to the length of catheterization (5 days or more), older age, and steroid administration.[226,227] Furthermore, this device depends upon the transmission of ICP through fluid-filled tubes that can block, thus dampening or obliterating the recording.

The subarachnoid bolt is a currently used method for monitoring ICP.[228] It is usually fitted into a burr hole made 2–3 cm anterior to the frontoparietal suture line, with the tip of the bolt passing through incised dura. The advantages

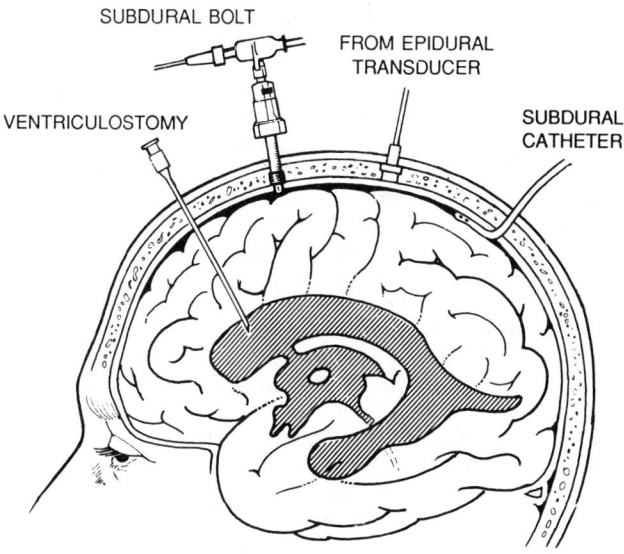

Figure 32-13. Techniques used to measure intracranial pressure.

of the bolt are that it does not require brain-tissue penetration or knowledge of ventricular position, and can be placed in any skull location that avoids major venous sinuses. There are several disadvantages with using this technique. The bolt cannot be used to lower ICP by CSF drainage or to test compliance reliably. As with the intraventricular catheter, the bolt is connected to a transducer with tubing filled with sterile saline. Not only can the tubing block, but also brain substance can obstruct the tip of the bolt; in either situation, the recording may become damped or lost. Drilling side holes just proximal to the tip of the bolt compensates for this problem to some extent. Subarachnoid devices are easily inserted, but can malfunction if they are not coplanar to the brain surface or if they become loose. The major complication of this procedure is infection, commonly meningitis, osteomyelitis, or a localized infection, which has been shown to be related to duration of monitoring, older age, and steroid administration.[226] Epidural bleeding and focal seizures, if the bolt is inserted too deeply, can also occur.

A variety of epidural transducers have been developed. The two primary types used are a device that has a pressure-sensitive membrane mounted close to or contacting the dura and the Ladd epidural transducer, based on the principle of the Numoto pressure switch.[229,230] The main advantage to using an epidural transducer is the extradural placement. If infection occurs, it is separated from the brain by the dura. The disadvantages of monitoring with an epidural transducer are technical problems in calibrating the transducer in situ, inability to perform compliance testing or to aspirate fluid to decrease ICP, and the high cost of the equipment.

A relatively new development in ICP monitoring has been that of a miniaturized fiberoptic device (Camino Laboratories, San Diego, CA). This sensing device is mounted at the end of a 4-French fiberoptic bundle and can be inserted through a 2-mm burr hole. This monitor senses changes in the amount of light reflected off a pressure-sensitive diaphragm located at the tip of a fiberoptic catheter. Mean pressure can be displayed digitally or as a pressure wave form. With this device, it is possible to insert the tip of the catheter into the subdural, intraparenchymal, or intraventricular compartments. Because it is a solid state monitor, the problems of infection, leaks, catheter occlusion, and drift that exist with fluid- or air-filled systems are minimized or avoided. Animal and human studies show that pressure recordings obtained with the fiberoptic catheter are accurate and reliable.[231,232] Another advantage is that it allows direct measurement of brain tissue pressure, which may be important in edema formation and regional capillary blood flow. The main disadvantage of this device is that it cannot be recalibrated *in situ*. In a recent study, cumulative drift was analyzed.[232] Because cumulative drift became significant by the fifth day, the authors suggested that the monitor be replaced after 5 days. Another limitation of the fiberoptic device is that it cannot be used for CSF drainage or compliance testing unless it is used in conjunction with a ventriculostomy.

Noninvasive transducers have been designed to measure anterior fontanelle pressure in newborns and infants.[233,234] These devices record relative changes in fontanelle pressure, which correlates closely with ICP. Accurate pressure recordings require coplanar application of the transducer.

All of the clinically available monitors have recognized advantages and disadvantages. Despite the problems associated with these devices, ICP monitoring provides useful information for evaluating the patient's condition, progress, and need for therapy. The primary cost to the patient is infection; therefore, the overall benefit to the patient far outweighs this cost.

NEURORADIOLOGY

The methods most commonly used are computed tomography (CT), magnetic resonance imaging (MRI), angiography, and myelography. These procedures require the patient's total immobility. Therefore, in uncooperative patients, specifically children and adults who are fearful, and those who are retarded or obtunded, general anesthesia will be required. All the standard equipment and monitors required for the administration of a general anesthetic and possible cardiopulmonary resuscitation must be present. (See also Chapter 54.)

Computed Tomography Scan

The CT scan produces a series of images by computerized processing of x-ray absorption measurements (photon attenuation data as measured by sodium iodide crystals rotating about the patient's head).[235] Performance of a brain scan requires that the patient lie on a table with his head inside a rotating gantry that makes a 180° arc producing one axial slice or cut. Depending on the generation of the scanner, the rotation may take from a few seconds to 4.5 minutes per cut. Eight cuts are usually required for a complete examination of the head. When contrast enhancement is indicated, the dye is infused intravenously and the scan is repeated. The patient must remain supine and immobile throughout the entire scan.

The radiation exposure during CT is similar to that of a conventional skull x-ray (1.0–2.5 rad).[236] Exposure values for personnel attending the patient are minimal (e.g., 1–2 mrad·h^{-1} for the anesthesiologist positioned next to the scan).[236] However, radiation monitoring badges and lead aprons should be worn by personnel who participate in CT scanning on a regular basis.

Magnetic Resonance Imaging

Magnetic resonance imaging is a noninvasive diagnostic technique that is superior to CT in many central nervous system disorders.[237] This technique employs a strong magnetic field and radio frequency (RF) pulses to generate images.[238] In the presence of a magnetic field and RF pulses, certain atomic nuclei (nuclei with an odd number of protons, for example ^{1}H nuclei) act like magnets and are aligned within the magnetic field. When the RF pulse is discontinued, the nuclei relax, emitting an electrical signal that is detected by a receiver coil and used to reconstruct the image. The magnet of the MRI system is in the form of a tube that can accommodate the human body. The patient must remain still during the investigation, which may last 1 hour, to prevent imaging artifacts.

The MRI is an extremely valuable diagnostic tool that provides excellent contrast between grey and white brain matter. Because there is no dental or bony artifact, it is superior to the CT scan in examining the posterior fossa.[239] Furthermore, MR images can be displayed in axial, coronal, or sagittal planes. Until recently, the MRI has been restricted to medically stable patients because of monitoring constraints. The high-static magnetic field (0.12–2.00 tesla [T]) and the RF energy transmitted during image acquisition may damage or cause malfunction of electrical, electronic, or mechanical life-support and monitoring equipment. Conversely, the RF energy generated by these devices can interfere with MR signal detection, producing artifacts that degrade the image. Another problem unique to MRI is that ferromagnetic substances placed within the magnetic field are propelled toward the scanner.

Laryngoscopes are not magnetic, but the batteries are. Therefore, to use a laryngoscope within the scanning room, plastic- or paper-coated batteries must be used.[240] A prebent RAE tube is recommended because of limited vertical space within the scanner. Very long breathing tubes are required, and either pipeline gases or a remotely placed anesthesia machine can be used. Aluminum cylinders can be used safely within the scanning room. An MRI-compatible ventilator (225/SIMV ventilator, Monaghan Medical Corp., Plattsburg, NY) has been designed and used successfully.[241] This ventilator is pneumatically driven, volume cycled, and has fluidic controls. The ventilator is completely powered by high-pressure oxygen delivered by a wall source or from large cylinders placed outside the imaging room, and electronic parts have been replaced with plastic, aluminum, or other nonmetallic alloys.

The need to avoid ferrous metal makes the implementation of monitoring during MRI challenging.[242,243] Monitoring of heart beat and respiration can be achieved using nonmetallic precordial or esophageal stethoscopes; however, the drum-like noise of the scanner may obscure auscultated heart and breath sounds. A standard vascular Doppler has also been used to monitor heart rate. Capnography is possible with long tubing and high-powered suction. Changes in respiratory rate can be observed, even though the end-tidal CO_2 reading may not reflect actual values. Blood pressure is easily measured with an ordinary cuff and long-pressure tubing without metal connections. The blood pressure dial must be kept away from the magnetic field. Automated blood pressure devices without metal connectors have also been used. Using nonmetallic components, intraarterial pressure and ICP monitoring have been described.[243] Transducers are affixed along the side of the magnet at its midpoint to minimize artifact. Shielded electric extension cables couple the transducers to the monitors located outside the scanning room. There have been reports of image degradation with the pulse oximeter, but using a long-probe lead and placing the oximeter a distance from the magnet may help. Monitoring of the ECG is a problem because the wires interfere with the image. Alternatively, finger plethysmography and ECG telemetry have been used.

Guidelines for using the MRI have been issued by the National Radiological Protection Board.[244] It is recommended that women in the first trimester of pregnancy not be scanned because of possible developmental consequences. Patients with demand pacemakers should not be scanned because the varying magnetic field can induce electric currents in the pacemaker wires, which may be mistaken for the natural electrical activity of the heart, inhibiting pacemaker output.[242] Intracranial clips used to treat aneurysms can move and become displaced when exposed to the magnetic field. Patients who have a large metallic implant or prosthesis can be scanned until the heat at the site of the implant or prosthesis becomes uncomfortable. There is a possibility that induced currents can affect myocardial contractility or produce arrhythmias. Full resuscitation facilities should be available.

Angiography

Angiography is used to delineate the vasculature of the brain or spinal cord. Catheters are usually introduced through the femoral, brachial, or axillary artery. With catheter techniques, contrast material is injected into the internal carotid artery, eliminating common carotid artery puncture and facial discomfort in the distribution of the external carotid artery. Spinal cord angiography involves selective studies and subtraction techniques. Because the injection of contrast can exacerbate the already damaged spinal cord, these procedures are usually performed without general anesthesia in order to monitor the patient's neurologic status.

There are several risks and problems associated with angiography. Arterial spasm, hematoma, and local infection can occur at the site of needle puncture. Subintimal dissection or occlusion of the vessel may result from injection into the vessel wall. Iodine-containing contrast media produce vasodilation and a burning sensation in the distribution of the injected vessel. Septicemia, cerebral embolism, anaphylactic reactions to the iodinated contrast material and, rarely, seizures or death are all potential complications of cerebral angiography.

The introduction of low-ionic and nonionic contrast material has reduced both the discomfort and toxicity associated with angiography. Because of this, patients usually do not require general anesthesia and are able to tolerate the procedure with minimal or no sedation. When general anesthesia is requested for children or uncooperative adults, the angiogram quality may be enhanced by hyperventilation.[245,246] Hypocarbia allows greater concentration of contrast material by slowing cerebral circulation and improves clarity by constricting cerebral vessels.[245,246]

Myelography

Myelography requires spinal lumbar puncture, the injection of contrast material, and the prone position. It is uncommon for the anesthesiologist to be involved in myelography except for studies in children or uncooperative adults. Metriz-

amide is a water-soluble contrast agent that has been used for myelograms. Because of its rapid absorption from the CSF, metrizamide does not require aspiration at the end of the procedure, but it is associated with allergic reactions and mental changes ranging from headache to confusion to convulsions. Any drug that lowers the epileptogenic threshold (e.g., phenothiazines or ketamine) should be avoided in patients who are receiving metrizamide. The newer, nonionic contrast media (iohexol and iopamidol) are associated with a reduced incidence of side effects and are replacing metrizamide in current practice.

Adverse Reactions from Contrast Media

Contrast media are radiopaque, iodine-containing salts that can be injected into arteries, veins, or CSF spaces. Both neurotoxic and allergic reactions have been reported following administration. Neurotoxic reactions are more likely to complicate angiographic investigations and include dizziness, convulsions, unconsciousness, hemiplegia, blindness, and aphasia.[247] These effects are related to the hyperosmolality of the contrast agent. Contrast media may temporarily impair the blood–brain barrier or cross it during disease,[248] causing CNS damage by a direct necrotizing effect that is associated with hypoxic microvascular damage.[249] A critical factor appears to be the concentration of the agent.[250] If slurring of speech or confusion is observed, the procedure should be terminated. The occurrence and persistence of more serious CNS problems may require therapy with steroids, low molecular weight dextran, or vasopressor-induced elevation of systemic blood pressure to improve blood flow to areas that may be ischemic. The introduction of hypoosmolar contrast agents should reduce the CNS toxicity associated with angiography.

Allergic reactions to contrast media vary from pruritus, burning on injection, and mild skin rashes to wheezing, dyspnea, syncope, and cardiovascular collapse (see Chapter 52). These reactions most likely result from nonimmunologic release of histamine and other vasoactive mediators from mast cells and basophils.[251] A prospective study conducted by the International Society of Radiologist's Committee on Contrast Media[252] reported in 1975 a 2.33% incidence of nonfatal reactions to contrast media in 27,628 vascular studies. Four fatal reactions were reported in this group. This incidence of adverse reactions in patients with a history of allergy were twice that of the general population, and in patients with a history of reaction to a previous investigation, adverse reactions were three times that of the general population.

Prophylaxis with steroids and antihistamines is recommended in patients with a history of allergies or specific reaction to contrast media. These patients should be evaluated by an allergist and medicated for 36–48 hours prior to the injection of contrast. Several regimens have been proposed, all including a corticosteroid (e.g., prednisone) and an antihistamine (diphenhydramine or hydroxyzine) in various combinations and doses before, during, and after the investigation.[253,254] A further reduction in the reaction rate has been reported with the addition of ephedrine sulfate (25 mg, po, 1 h prior to the investigation).

Mild allergic reactions require little more than reassurance and perhaps intravenous diphenhydramine. More severe reactions, e.g., respiratory distress, hypotension, or syncope can be treated initially with subcutaneous epinephrine. Be prepared, however, for all degrees of resuscitation, because emergent therapy for bronchospasm, laryngeal edema, hypotension, arrhythmias, and full cardiopulmonary arrest may be required.

ANESTHETIC MANAGEMENT OF NEUROSURGICAL PATIENTS

The administration of anesthesia to neurosurgical patients requires an understanding of the basic principles of neurophysiology and the effects of anesthetic agents on intracranial dynamics as reviewed in the previous sections of this chapter.

Preoperative Evaluation

During the preoperative evaluation, the patient's overall medical condition must be considered and integrated into the formulation of an anesthetic management plan. Neurosurgical procedures tend to be lengthy, requiring unusual positioning of the patient and the institution of special techniques such as hyperventilation, cerebral dehydration, and deliberate hypotension. Not all patients can tolerate the position desired by the surgeon; this must be addressed and, if possible, evaluated preoperatively. Further, in patients with cardiac disease, routine institution of osmotherapy or hyperventilation may compromise organ function. Such patients must be medically optimized and, when indicated, cardiac monitoring should be instituted. Except for neurosurgical emergencies (e.g., head trauma or impending herniation), most neurosurgical procedures can be delayed to treat medically unstable conditions.

The preoperative evaluation must include a complete neurologic examination with special attention to the patient's level of consciousness, presence or absence of increased ICP, and extent of focal neurologic deficits. The signs and symptoms frequently associated with intracranial hypertension are headache, nausea, papilledema, unilateral pupillary dilation, and oculomotor or abducens palsy. With advanced stages of intracranial hypertension, the patient exhibits a depressed level of consciousness and irregular respiration. The clinical signs do not reliably indicate the level of ICP. Only a direct CSF pressure measurement can be used to quantitate the pressure; however, indirect evidence of elevated ICP can be determined by evaluating the MRI or CT scan for a mass lesion accompanied by a midline shift of 0.5 cm or encroachment of expanding brain on CSF cisterns.[255]

The location of the lesion in the supratentorial or infratentorial compartment will determine the clinical presentation and anesthetic management. Supratentorial disease is usually associated with problems in the management of intracranial hypertension, whereas infratentorial lesions cause problems related to mass effects on vital brain stem structures and elevated ICP due to obstructive hydrocephalus.

Fluid and electrolyte abnormalities are common in patients with reduced levels of consciousness. Patients are usually dehydrated and develop electrolyte abnormalities because of decreased fluid intake, iatrogenic water restriction, neuroendocrine abnormalities and diuresis from diuretics, steroid-related hyperglycemia, and radiographic contrast agents. Fluid and electrolyte abnormalities must be corrected prior to induction of anesthesia to prevent cardiovascular instability.

COMMON INTRACRANIAL PATHOLOGY

I. Supratentorial-Intracranial Tumors

Supratentorial tumors (meningiomas, gliomas, and metastatic lesions) change intracranial dynamics predictably. Initially, when the lesion is small and slowly expanding, volume-spatial compensation occurs by compression of the CSF compartment and nearby cerebral veins, which prevents increases in ICP.[256] As the lesion grows, however, compensatory mechanisms are exhausted and further increases in tumor mass cause progressively greater increases in ICP. Primary or metastatic tumors or chronic subdural hematomas can present as chronic mass lesions. Because of the ability of the intracranial compartment to compensate up to a point, patients may exhibit minimal neurologic dysfunction despite the presence of a large mass, elevated ICP, and shifts in the position of brain structures.

Significant changes in ICP can occur with supratentorial tumors if they develop a central area of hemorrhagic necrotic tissue or a wide border of brain edema. As the tumor enlarges, it can outstrip its blood supply, developing a central hemorrhagic area that may expand rapidly, increasing ICP. Brain edema surrounding the tumor increases the effective bulk of the tumor and represents an additional portion of the brain that is not autoregulating. In such situations of compromised intracranial compliance, small increases in arterial pressure may produce large increases in cerebral blood flow, which can markedly increase intracranial volume and ICP with the attendant complications.

Anesthetic Techniques and Drugs

The goal of neuroanesthetic care for patients with supratentorial tumors is to maximize therapeutic modalities that reduce intracranial volume. Intracranial pressure must be controlled before the cranium is opened, and optimal operating conditions must be obtained by producing a slack brain that facilitates surgical dissection. Various maneuvers and pharmacologic agents have been used to reduce brain bulk. For example, fluid restriction, administration of diuretics or steroids, hyperventilation, and systemic blood pressure control may be implemented preoperatively to reduce cerebral edema and brain bulk, thereby reducing ICP. The application of these methods selectively or together, when necessary, is often accompanied by marked clinical improvement.

Clinical Control of Intracranial Hypertension

The traditional approach to fluid management in neurosurgical patients is to restrict fluid intake (Table 32-9).[257] Fluid restriction decreases brain water content, thereby reducing formation of cerebral edema and lowering ICP. When water intake is limited to about one-third to one-half of daily fluid requirements, the reduction in ICP occurs over a period of several days. Severe water restriction has been shown to be only modestly effective in reducing brain water content.[258] Following experimental water restriction in dogs, brain water content decreased 1% after 24 hours, with only an additional reduction of 1% over the next 72 hours, whereas muscle water content decreased by 5% and body weight by 11% after 4 days of water restriction.[258]

Severe fluid restriction over several days can cause hypovolemia, resulting in hypotension, inadequate renal perfusion, electrolyte and acid–base disturbances, hypoxemia, and reductions in cerebral blood flow. Fluid restriction may

TABLE 32-9. Clinical Control of Intracranial Hypertension

Fluid restriction
Diuretics: Osmotic, tubular
Corticosteroids
Hyperventilation
Blood pressure control
Position to improve cerebral venous return
Anesthetics agents: Thiopental, lidocaine, etomidate

be instituted preoperatively as well as postoperatively. When instituted preoperatively, the patient's volume must be restored before induction of anesthesia to prevent hypotension in response to anesthetic agents and positive pressure ventilation. Fluid resuscitation and maintenance fluids in the routine neurosurgical patient are provided with glucose-free isotonic crystalloid solutions to prevent increases in brain water content. The crystalloid solutions are given as necessary to maintain cardiac filling pressures and urine output. For the routine craniotomy, the patient receives hourly maintenance fluids and replacement of half the urine output and two to three times the blood loss.

Solutions containing glucose are avoided in all neurosurgical patients with normal glucose metabolism, since these solutions can exacerbate ischemic damage and cerebral edema.[259-262] Glucose administration augments ischemic damage by increasing anaerobic lactate production.[263] Lactate is thought to enhance postischemic brain injury. Intravenous fluids containing glucose and water (D5 0.45% saline or D5W) are particularly problematic, since the glucose is metabolized and the free water remains in the intracranial fluid compartment, resulting in brain edema. Brain edema can interfere with surgical exposure and, after closure of the skull, can compromise cerebral perfusion.

Rapid brain dehydration and ICP reduction are often obtained by administering diuretics. There are two diuretics that are employed: the osmotic diuretic, mannitol, and the loop diuretic, furosemide. Mannitol is given as an intravenous infusion in a dose of 0.25–1.0 $g \cdot kg^{-1}$. Its action begins within 10–15 minutes and is effective for approximately 2 hours. Larger doses produce a longer duration of action but do not necessarily reduce ICP more effectively.[264] Furthermore, larger doses and repeated administration can result in metabolic derangement. Mannitol is effective when the blood–brain barrier is intact. Mannitol decreases ICP by increasing plasma osmotic pressure, thereby reducing brain interstitial and intracellular volume.[265] When the blood–brain barrier is disrupted, mannitol may enter the brain and increase osmolality. Mannitol could pull water into the brain as the plasma concentration of the agent declines and cause a rebound increase in ICP. This rebound increase in ICP may be prevented by maintaining a mild fluid deficit.[266] Mannitol has been shown to cause vasodilation of vascular smooth muscle, which is dependent on dose and administration rate.[267-269] Mannitol-induced vasodilation affects intracranial and extracranial vessels and can transiently increase cerebral blood volume and ICP while simultaneously decreasing systemic blood pressure.[267,269] Because mannitol may initially increase ICP, it should be given cautiously and in conjunction with maneuvers that decrease intracranial volume (e.g., steroids or hyperventilation).

Hypertonic agents such as mannitol should also be administered cautiously in patients with congestive heart failure. In these patients, the transient increase in intravascular volume may cause pulmonary edema. Furosemide may be a better agent to reduce ICP in patients with impaired cardiac reserve. Prolonged use of mannitol may produce dehydration, electrolyte disturbances, hyperosmolality, and impaired renal function.

The loop diuretic, furosemide, reduces ICP by inducing a systemic diuresis, decreasing CSF production, and resolving cerebral edema by improving cellular water transport.[270-272] Furosemide lowers ICP without increasing cerebral blood volume or blood osmolality; however, it is not as effective as mannitol in reducing ICP.[271] Furosemide can be given alone as a large initial dose (0.5–1 $mg \cdot kg^{-1}$) or as a lower dose with mannitol (0.15–0.30 $mg \cdot kg^{-1}$). Combined mannitol and furosemide diuresis has been shown to be more effective than mannitol alone in reducing ICP and brain bulk but causes more severe dehydration and electrolyte imbalances.[273] With combined therapy, it is necessary to monitor electrolytes intraoperatively and replace potassium as indicated.

Corticosteroids reduce edema around brain tumors;[274,275] however, steroids require many hours or days before a reduction in ICP becomes apparent. The administration of steroids preoperatively frequently causes neurologic improvement that can precede the ICP reduction. One explanation for this is that the neurologic improvement is accompanied by partial restoration of the previously abnormal blood–brain barrier.[276] The mechanism of action of edema reduction by steroids is unknown. Postulated mechanisms of action for steroidal reduction in brain edema are brain dehydration, prevention of lysosomal activity, enhanced cerebral electrolyte transport, improved brain metabolism, promotion of water and electrolyte excretion, and inhibition of a vascular permeability factor.[276,277] The potential complications of continuous perioperative steroid administration are hyperglycemia, glucosuria, gastrointestinal bleeding, electrolyte disturbances, and increased incidence of infection. Therefore, the potential risks and benefits of continuous steroid administration need to be evaluated in these patients.

Hyperventilation to a $Paco_2$ of 25–30 mm Hg is the mainstay of acute and subacute management of intracranial hypertension. As discussed previously, hyperventilation reduces brain volume by decreasing cerebral blood flow through cerebral vasoconstriction. For every mm Hg change in $Paco_2$, CBF changes by 4%. Hyperventilation is only effective when the CO_2 reactivity of the cerebrovasculature is intact. Impaired responsiveness to changes in CO_2 tension occurs in areas of vasoparalysis, which are associated with extensive intracranial disease such as ischemia, trauma, tumor, and infection.

The autoregulation of cerebral blood flow has been discussed as has the relationship between blood pressure and ICP when autoregulation is disturbed. The therapeutic goals are to maintain cerebral perfusion pressure and to control intracranial dynamics so that cerebral ischemia, edema, hemorrhage, and herniation are avoided. Severe hypotension results in cerebral ischemia and should be treated with volume replacement, inotropes, or vasopressors as dictated by clinical need. Severe hypertension, conversely, can worsen cerebral edema and cause intracranial hemorrhage and herniation. The beta-adrenergic blockers, propranolol and esmolol, the alpha-adrenergic blocker, phentolamine, and combined alpha- and beta-adrenergic blocker, labetalol, are effective in reducing systemic blood pressure in patients with raised ICP with minimal or no effect on CBF or ICP.

For most neurosurgical patients, a neutral head position,

elevated 30°, is recommended to decrease ICP by improving venous drainage. Flexing or turning of the head may obstruct cerebral venous outflow, causing a dramatic ICP elevation that has been shown to resolve with resumption of a neutral head position.[278] Lowering the head impairs cerebral venous drainage, which can quickly result in an increase in brain bulk and ICP.

The application of positive end-expiratory pressure (PEEP) to mechanically ventilated patients can potentially increase ICP.[279] This effect can occur when PEEP increases central venous pressure, impairing cerebral venous outflow and cardiac output. When PEEP is required to maintain oxygenation, it should be applied cautiously and with appropriate monitoring to minimize decreases in cardiac output and increases in ICP. PEEP levels of 10 cm H_2O or less have been used without significant increases in ICP or decreases in cerebral perfusion pressure.[280] When higher levels of PEEP are required to optimize the PaO_2–PEEP–CPP relationship, both central venous pressure and ICP monitoring are indicated.

The administration of pharmacologic agents that increase cerebral vascular resistance can acutely reduce ICP. Thiopental, etomidate, and lidocaine are potent cerebral vasoconstrictors that can be used for this purpose. The effects of these agents on CBF, $CMRO_2$, ICP, and CPP are reviewed in this chapter. These agents are usually administered during induction of anesthesia but may also be administered in anticipation of noxious stimuli or to treat persistently elevated ICP in the intensive care unit.

Premedication

Lethargic patients do not receive premedication. Patients who are alert and anxious may receive an anxiolytic (e.g., diazepam 0.1 mg·kg^{-1}, po) before coming to the operating room. If there is any doubt about the patient's level of consciousness, the patient may be given sedation or analgesics in the operating room after an intravenous route is established. For the preinduction insertion of invasive monitoring devices in an awake, conversant patient, premedicants (e.g., small doses of opioids) should be considered to alleviate the discomfort from needle punctures.

Monitoring

In addition to the routine monitors, measurement of intraarterial blood pressure, arterial blood gases, central venous pressure, and urinary output is recommended for all major neurosurgical procedures. An arterial cannula is inserted before induction of anesthesia to continuously monitor blood pressure and to estimate cerebral perfusion pressure. When the arterial pressure transducer is at head level, cerebral perfusion pressure is calculated as the difference between mean arterial pressure and the CVP in patients without incracranial hypertension or the ICP in those with intracranial hypertension. With direct arterial pressure monitoring, the hemodynamic consequences of the pharmacologic agents administered during anesthesia are recognized instantly. In addition, the arterial catheter provides ready access for intraoperative measurement of arterial blood gases, hematocrit, serum electrolytes, and osmolality. Radial, femoral, or brachial arteries are suitable for short-term cannulation; however, after ulnar artery collateral blood flow is tested, cannulation of the radial artery is preferred.

Because most neurosurgical patients are dehydrated preoperatively and then subjected to intraoperative diuresis, the measurement of cardiac preload and urinary output is important. A right atrial catheter reflects cardiac preload and is used to determine the preoperative fluid deficit and rate of intraoperative fluid infusion. When possible, the CVP catheter should be inserted through an antecubital vein instead of the jugular or subclavian veins.[281] This avoids increased ICP from both the head down position and decreased cerebral venous outflow. The position of the antecubital CVP can be verified by chest x-ray, transducer pressure wave form, or p-wave configuration on the ECG.

Urinary output is also measured as an indicator of perioperative fluid balance. During craniotomy, a diuresis occurs initially following the administration of osmotic or loop diuretics. A reduced urine output may reflect either hypovolemia or release of antidiuretic hormone.

The insertion of an ICP monitor for supratentorial tumor operations is controversial. ICP monitoring is an invasive procedure that can cause bleeding or infection.[226] When performed with local anesthesia before induction, the procedure can be uncomfortable to the patient. The major benefits of perioperative ICP monitoring have been discussed in the section on ICP monitoring.

Muscle Relaxants

For many years, there has been a controversy (recently resolved) regarding the relationship of succinylcholine administration and ICP elevation. Intravenous administration of succinylcholine is reported to produce activation of the EEG and increases in cerebral blood flow and ICP in dogs with normal brains.[282,283] These cerebral effects have been attributed to succinylcholine-induced increases in muscle afferent activity that produce cerebral stimulation. In many, but not all patients with compromised intracranial compliance, succinylcholine has been shown to increase ICP.[284,285] This increase can be blocked with a full, paralyzing dose of vecuronium or a pretreatment (defasciculating) dose of metocurine.[284,285] The nondepolarizing agent apparently eliminates the massive afferent input to the brain after succinylcholine.

To achieve muscle relaxation for intubation of the trachea, succinylcholine is not recommended for elective neurosurgical cases; however, succinylcholine remains the best agent for achieving total paralysis for the rapid sequence intubation of the trachea. Therefore, in an emergency room or ICU setting, when there is a risk of aspiration or a need for immediate reassessment of neurologic status, succinylcholine should be used. Simultaneously, an effort should be made to control anesthetic depth to protect against the ICP elevating effects of such noxious stimuli as laryngoscopy, intubation, or tracheal suctioning. In the hemiplegic (or paraplegic) patient, succinylcholine is avoided because of the risk of hyperkalemia.[286] Succinylcholine-induced hyperkalemia has also been reported following closed head injury and ruptured cerebral aneurysms in patients who were not hemiplegic or paraplegic.[287-289]

Nondepolarizing muscle relaxants are used during induction and maintenance of anesthesia in neurosurgical patients. Those agents that release histamine are avoided, however. Histamine alone may lower blood pressure and increase ICP, thus lowering cerebral perfusion pressure.[290] When the blood–brain barrier is disrupted, histamine can produce cerebrovasodilation and increases in cerebral blood flow.[291] Because of d-tubocurare's potent histamine releasing property, it is not recommended for use in neurosurgical patients. Metocurine causes less histamine release than d-tubocurare but could also cause cerebrovasodilation and increases in cerebral blood volume and ICP by the same mechanism. Atracurium in intubating doses (0.5 mg·kg^{-1}) has been reported to have no significant effect on ICP, blood pressure, or cerebral perfusion pressure in neurosurgical patients.[292,293] The release of laudanosine by atracurium does not appear to have clinical significance in humans.[294] Laudanosine has been reported to produce seizure activity in animals.[295]

Pancuronium administration has no apparent effect on ICP, CBF, or $CMRO_2$.[296,297] When administered in intubating doses (0.1 mg·kg^{-1}), pancuronium's vagolytic effects can cause an increase in heart rate and blood pressure, which might have deleterious effects in some neurosurgical patients. In patients with elevated ICP, vecuronium is currently the agent of choice for intubation and surgical paralysis. Vecuronium has no effect on ICP, heart rate, or blood pressure in neurosurgical patients.[298] To achieve relatively rapid airway control (within 90 sec) a priming dose of vecuronium (0.01 mg·kg^{-1}) can be administered followed by a higher dose (0.10 mg·kg^{-1}), or high doses of vecuronium (to 0.4 mg·kg^{-1}) can be safely administered without hemodynamic consequence.[299,300]

Induction, Maintenance, and Emergence

When the patient is brought into the operating room, a gross neurologic examination should be repeated and documented because changes in the patient's neurologic status can occur overnight. In patients with elevated ICP by clinical exam, CT scan and/or ICP measurement, osmotherapy may be indicated prior to induction of anesthesia. Following the application of appropriate monitoring devices, the cooperative patient is asked to hyperventilate while preoxygenation is provided. Before laryngoscopy and intubation of the trachea, the patient is smoothly and deeply anesthetized with agents that reduce ICP. In the presence of elevated ICP, thiopental is commonly used to induce anesthesia; however, an alternative agent such as midazolam can be used depending on the patient's medical condition. The following induction sequence is suggested. The intravenous administration of thiopental (4–6 mg·kg^{-1}) is followed by an opioid (fentanyl, 3–5 μg·kg^{-1}), and muscle relaxant. If no airway difficulties are anticipated, vecuronium (0.1 mg·kg^{-1}) is administered while controlled hyperventilation with 100% oxygen is instituted. In patients who have been vomiting because of elevated ICP, cricoid pressure is applied during mask ventilation. To deepen the anesthetic, fentanyl is administered in 50 μg increments to a total dose of 10–15 μg·kg^{-1}, depending on the blood pressure response. Lidocaine (1.5 mg·kg^{-1}) is also administered intravenously 90 seconds before intubation to suppress laryngeal reflexes.[301] When the peripheral muscle twitch response disappears, an additional 2–3 mg·kg^{-1} bolus of thiopental is administered, and endotracheal intubation is performed as rapidly and smoothly as possible. An esmolol infusion or bolus may also be used to reduce the heart rate and blood pressure response to laryngoscopy and intubation.[302] After induction of anesthesia, ventilation of the lung is controlled mechanically and adjusted to maintain arterial carbon dioxide tension ($Paco_2$) between 25 and 30 mm Hg. An arterial blood gas is drawn after intubation to establish the arterial end-tidal CO_2 gradient.

The most commonly administered maintenance anesthetics for patients with supratentorial tumors are nitrous oxide-opioid and nitrous oxide-volatile inhalational agents. In practice, the opioid most frequently employed is fentanyl, and the volatile agent most frequently employed is isoflurane. In patients with elevated ICP or low compliance, some clinicians avoid the administration of either nitrous oxide or high concentrations of isoflurane (i.e., greater than 1.0%). Alternatively, an opioid-isoflurane (0.5–1.0% concentration) or a totally intravenous technique may be employed. The intravenous technique is especially useful when severe intracranial hypertension exists and the brain is tight despite adequate hyperventilation and the administration of steroids and diuretics. A thiopental infusion (1–6 mg·kg^{-1}·h^{-1}), fentanyl boluses or infusion (1–4 μg·kg^{-1}·h^{-1}), and/or a lidocaine infusion (1.5 mg·kg^{-1} bolus followed by 1–4 mg·min^{-1}) can be administered in cases of severe intracranial hypertension.

Emergence from anesthesia should be as smooth as possible, avoiding straining or bucking on the endotracheal tube. Bucking can cause arterial hypertension and elevated ICP during termination of anesthesia, which can lead to postoperative hemorrhage and cerebral edema.[303] To avoid bucking during emergence, muscle relaxants are not reversed until the head dressing is applied. Intravenous lidocaine (1.5 mg·kg^{-1}) can be administered 90 sec before suctioning and extubation to minimize cough, straining, and hypertension. Antihypertensive agents such as labetalol and esmolol are also administered during emergence to control systemic hypertension.

In the usual craniotomy for excision of a supratentorial tumor, the conduct of the anesthetic is aimed at awakening and extubating the patient at the end of the procedure. The removal of a large tumor improves the patient's intracranial compliance, and hypercarbia required to drive ventilation in the emerging patient is usually well tolerated. The patient is extubated only when fully reversed from paralysis, and when he is awake and following commands. If the patient is not responsive, the endotracheal tube remains in place until the patient is awake and following commands. A brief neurologic examination is performed before and after extubation of the trachea. The patient is positioned with his head elevated 30° and transferred to the recovery room with oxygen by mask and oxygen saturation monitoring. Close monitoring and care, including frequent neurologic evaluations, are continued in the recovery room.

II. Infratentorial Intracranial Tumors

The perioperative management of infratentorial tumors poses significant surgical and anesthetic challenges because of the relatively confined space within the posterior fossa. The posterior fossa contains the medulla, pons, cerebellum, major motor and sensory pathways, primary respiratory and cardiovascular centers, and lower cranial nerve nuclei. Because of the posterior fossa's small size, a localized tumor can significantly compromise these vital brain stem structures and cranial nerves. Consequently, when evaluating patients with infratentorial tumors, the anesthesiologist should be aware that these patients have the potential to develop profound neurologic damage. Patients may exhibit depressed levels of consciousness secondary to increased ICP from obstructive hydrocephalus and/or exhibit signs of brain stem compression with depressed respiration and cranial nerve palsies. Preoperative endotracheal intubation and respiratory support may be required.

Special Anesthetic Considerations

Surgical Position. A major challenge of infratentorial surgery is preventing further neurologic damage from surgical position and exploration. There is considerable controversy among neurosurgeons as to the best position for infratentorial surgery.

Exploration of the posterior fossa has been traditionally

performed in the sitting position because it provides excellent surgical exposure and facilitates venous and cerebrospinal fluid drainage. From the standpoint of the anesthesiologist, the sitting position provides better ventilation and easier access to the chest, airway, endotracheal tube, and extremities. Furthermore, facial and conjunctival edema are reduced; however, the sitting position is associated with significant risks. In older or debilitated patients, the sitting position can produce cardiovascular instability, resulting in hypotension with cerebral and cardiovascular compromise. A significant risk of venous air embolism occurs in patients operated on in the sitting position, and an attendant risk of paradoxical air embolism may also occur in patients with a probe patent foramen ovale or other right-to-left shunt.

Other problems associated with the sitting position are peripheral nerve injury, pneumocephalus, jugular venous obstruction and quadriplegia. Peripheral nerve injuries to the ulnar, sciatic, or lateral peroneal nerves can result if care is not taken in positioning and padding the respective pressure points. Pneumocephalus occurs frequently in patients who have surgery performed in the sitting position.[304] Pneumocephalus may develop into tension pneumocephalus postoperatively, producing serious neurologic dysfunction.[305] Nitrous oxide has been implicated in the genesis of tension pneumocephalus.[305] Because of this, when used, nitrous oxide should be discontinued after dural and cranial closure and avoided if surgery recurs within 7 days. Jugular venous obstruction causing swelling of the face and tongue may result from hyperflexion of the neck.[306] To avoid this, head flexion should be limited by placing two fingers between the mandible and sternum. Para-, tri- and quadriplegia have been reported following surgery in the sitting position. This complication has been attributed to mechanical compression of the cervical spinal cord or vertebrobasilar blood vessels and stretching of spinal cord blood vessels causing ischemia during head flexion.[307] If hypotension occurs, the brain stem and cervical spinal cord is rendered even more vulnerable to an ischemic insult. During surgical positioning for posterior fossa exploration, cases of position-related brain stem and cervical spinal cord ischemia have been reported.[308,309] Therefore, flexion of the head on the cervical spine may be hazardous in some patients with large posterior fossa tumors and in elderly or arthritic patients. A preoperative examination of the mobility of the cervical spine, including a review of radiologic studies to determine the width of the cervical canal, should be performed to establish whether the patient can tolerate the position required for surgery. In addition, the application of sensory evoked potential monitoring during positioning for surgery may be used to detect position-related ischemia.

Other positions used for posterior fossa exploration are the lateral, prone, and park bench or three-quarters prone, positions. These alternative positions have been advocated because of the lower incidence of air emboli and greater cardiovascular stability. Potential disadvantages of these positions are malignant cerebellar edema and venous hemorrhage. To date, there is no evidence that surgical position affects postoperative outcome. In a 1988 study that reviewed 579 posterior fossa craniectomies, patients in the sitting position had less blood loss and postoperative cranial nerve dysfunction than patients operated on in the horizontal position (supine, prone, lateral, and park bench), and there was no difference in the incidence of hypotension and postoperative cardiopulmonary complications between groups.[310] The incidence of venous air embolism in this series of patients was significantly greater in sitting versus horizontal patients (45% versus 12%), but it was not associated with a significantly increased morbidity or mortality.[310] The authors concluded that there are significant advantages and disadvantages to both sitting and horizontal positions and that these positions can be used safely.

As more surgeons are being trained to use lateral or prone positions, the number of cases performed in the sitting position is declining. No matter what position is chosen, the selection should be based on the location of the tumor, surgical exposure, the patient's medical condition, and consideration of the risks and benefits.

Monitoring. During posterior fossa exploration, surgical retraction or manipulation of the brain stem or cranial nerves can cause significant cardiac dysrhythmias or alterations in blood pressure. Adequate warning, and thus early notification of the surgeon, of brain stem compromise can be obtained by monitoring the electrocardiogram for alterations in cardiac rate and rhythm. In addition, direct arterial pressure monitoring provides continuous information on sudden changes in systemic blood pressure and an estimate of cerebral perfusion pressure. (To estimate cerebral pressure in the sitting position, the transducer should be zeroed to the highest point on the skull.) The hemodynamic consequences of dysrhythmias or air embolism are also instantly recognized with direct arterial pressure monitoring.

More recently, electrophysiologic monitoring of sensory evoked potentials has been used to detect ischemia and compromise of the brain stem or cranial nerves. For example, brain stem auditory evoked potentials are monitored during surgery for acoustic neuroma to help preserve function of the eighth cranial nerve or during posterior fossa procedures to monitor brain stem ischemia. Depending on the tumor's location, somatosensory evoked potentials may also be used to detect brain stem compromise. Position-related ischemia has been observed during monitoring with either brain stem auditory or somatosensory evoked potentials.[308,309] Electromyography is used during acoustic neuroma surgery to test seventh nerve function when the face is not accessible to palpation or visual assessment.

Venous Air Embolism. Venous air embolism may occur whenever the operative field is elevated 5 cm or more above the right atrial level. Whereas the incidence of air embolism is 25–35% among patients operated on in the sitting position, entrainment of air also occurs during operations performed in the lateral, supine, or prone positions. Air may also pass directly through the pulmonary circulation or through right-to-left intracardiac shunts (e.g., probe-patent foramen ovale) to the coronary and cerebral circulation when right atrial pressure exceeds left atrial pressure. A reported 51% of patients develop right atrial pressure greater than left atrial pressure in the sitting position, and of these, 7% may experience paradoxical air embolism.[311] The primary pathophysiologic event in venous air embolism is intense vasoconstriction of the pulmonary circulation, which results in ventilation–perfusion mismatch, interstitial pulmonary edema, and reduced cardiac output (CO) as pulmonary vascular resistance increases.

A precordial Doppler ultrasonic transducer is the most sensitive monitor of venous air embolism clinically available and it detects amounts of air as small as 0.25 ml. The transducer is placed over the right sternal border between the third and sixth intercostal spaces. Correct positioning is verified by injecting a 10-ml bolus of saline into the right atrial catheter. The resultant turbulent flow changes the Doppler sounds to a typical "mill-wheel" sound, which is similar to the sounds produced by intravascular air.

The capnograph is also useful for detecting the occurrence of venous air embolism. Small volumes of intravascular air produce a ventilation–perfusion mismatch, which is reflected in a reduced end-expired CO_2. The capnograph complements the capabilities of the Doppler by differentiating hemodynamically insignificant emboli that are heard with the Doppler from significant emboli. Doppler sounds without reduction in end-tidal CO_2 usually indicate insignificant amounts of air.

The use of mass spectrometry in the operating room provides measurement of exhaled concentrations of both CO_2 and N_2. The advantage of knowing the value of end-expired N_2 is the ability to calculate the volume of entrained air.[312]

Unlike the precordial Doppler, the 2-D transesophageal echocardiogram[313] has the advantage of monitoring air in the left and right cardiac chambers. It has been shown to be as sensitive as the precordial Doppler in detecting small amounts of entrained air. Therefore, this new monitor offers promise for better intraoperative detection of both venous and arterial air embolism. In addition, 2-D echocardiography during a valsalva maneuver can be used to determine the presence of a probe-patent foramen ovale preoperatively. If a patent foramen ovale is detected, another position should be chosen because the possibility of a paradoxical embolus exists.

Early diagnosis of air embolism is essential for successful treatment. The precordial Doppler unit is considered the basic monitoring device for detection of air embolism and is most effective when used in conjunction with at least one other monitoring modality (e.g., a capnograph or a pulmonary artery catheter). The clinical significance of air embolism detected by Doppler ultrasonography can be assessed by an increase in pulmonary artery pressure or a decrease in end-expired CO_2.[314] A Doppler in conjunction with either a capnograph or a pulmonary artery catheter usually detects air before physiologic alteration begins. Treatment is directed at preventing further influx of air.[315] The surgical field is flooded with saline and packed, and bone edges are waxed. Nitrous oxide, if present, is discontinued to prevent further expansion of embolized air. Neck veins are compressed as a means of increasing jugular venous pressure, which prevents further air entry and helps to localize the source of air. Aspiration of air from a right atrial (RA) catheter is attempted. The position of the RA catheter may be confirmed by a chest film, by using a saline-filled catheter as a unipolar lead and following the configuration of the P waves on the ECG, or by transducing a venous wave form. Evidence suggests that maximal retrieval of injected air can be obtained from a multiorificed catheter tip that is positioned at the junction of the superior vena cava and the right atrium.[316] If necessary, vasopressors and volume infusion can be used to treat hypotension. In patients with a probe-patent foramen ovale, administration of positive end-expiratory pressure should be avoided to prevent increases in right atrial pressure and a right-to-left shunt.

Pulmonary artery catheterization has been advocated for patients who undergo surgery in the sitting position. A change in pulmonary artery pressure (PAP) correlates with the hemodynamic significance of the embolus because PAP increases proportionally with the volume of air that enters the pulmonary arteries. In addition, the catheter identifies patients at risk for paradoxical air embolism, i.e., patients who develop a right atrial pressure greater than pulmonary capillary wedge pressure (PCWP). When this occurs, measures to elevate PCWP, such as volume loading or repositioning, are undertaken,[317] however, use of the pulmonary artery catheter for recovery of air has been disappointing.

Anesthetic Management. When selecting an anesthetic technique for patients in the sitting position, conditions of particular concern are cardiovascular stability and risk of air embolism. In changing an anesthetized patient from the supine to sitting position, a mild transient postural hypotension occurs in about one-third of cases and marked hypotension in about 2–5% of cases.[318,319] General anesthesia with positive-pressure ventilation is associated with a reduction in blood pressure mainly caused by a decrease in cardiac output. As patients are placed into the sitting position, venous return is impeded, causing further reductions in cardiac output and blood pressure.[318,319] Therefore, efforts are directed at promoting venous return and maintaining cardiac output during the anesthetic management of these patients. An opioid-nitrous oxide-oxygen technique has been shown to cause the least impairment of cardiovascular performance when patients are placed in the sitting position.[319] Measures to avoid hypotension are also instituted. These include adequate preoperative hydration, wrapping the legs with Ace bandages, and flexing the patient's hips and knees at heart level. The patient's position is slowly changed, titrating position against systemic blood pressure. Administration of fluids (balanced salt solutions) and small amounts of vasopressors may be necessary.

Because nitrous oxide expands embolized air, general anesthesia without nitrous oxide has been advocated by some for anesthetizing patients in the sitting position; however, this would necessitate the use of a volatile anesthetic agent. In some patients, the use of a volatile agent may increase the risk of focal or generalized ischemia from an increase in ICP and an anesthetic-induced reduction in blood pressure. Therefore, the risks and benefits of using nitrous oxide versus a volatile agent for neurosurgical procedures with an increased potential for air embolism should be discussed and individualized. In general, a balanced anesthetic technique (nitrous oxide-oxygen-opioid-muscle relaxant) combined with controlled hyperventilation is recommended for maximal cardiovascular stability and control of intracranial hypertension. If air embolism occurs, nitrous oxide is discontinued. Nitrous oxide may be reintroduced cautiously with concurrent Doppler monitoring to determine whether the embolized air remains a threat.

Postoperative Concerns. The potential for significant cardiorespiratory and neurologic deterioration exists in the immediate postoperative period following posterior fossa exploration. Therefore, direct arterial pressure and ECG monitoring should be continued for the first 24–48 hours postoperatively, and neurologic examinations should be performed frequently.

Central apnea requiring postoperative ventilatory support may result from extensive posterior fossa exploration causing damage to respiratory centers.[320] If respiratory centers have been manipulated but not destroyed, respiratory impairment is temporary. Postoperative impairment of swallowing and pharyngeal sensation may occur secondary to stretch or manipulation of cranial nerves IX, X, and XII. These patients are at increased risk for aspiration pneumonia or hypoxia and therefore should remain intubated until airway protective reflexes return.

Systemic hypertension frequently occurs following posterior fossa surgery and requires immediate treatment to prevent brain edema and hematoma formation. Postoperative hypertension usually resolves within the first 24 hours. Atrial and ventricular ectopic beats may also occur within the first 24 hours.

Because of the proximity of respiratory and cardiovascular centers, any edema, hematoma, or infarction of the brain stem and cerebellum can produce serious compromise. When a patient fails to awaken satisfactorily from anesthesia, bleeding or acute swelling of the structures in the posterior fossa must be suspected. In addition, patients who are awake and talking may become unresponsive secondary to obstructive hydrocephalus or brain stem compression. Level of consciousness is an early reliable sign of brain stem compression. More serious signs are systemic hypertension, bradycardia, and irregular or absent respirations. Reintubation and prompt surgical intervention to relieve pressure on the brain stem are necessary.

The preoperative level of consciousness and intraoperative conditions will determine whether the patient is extubated at the end of the procedure. A patient with a depressed level of consciousness preoperatively should not be expected to improve immediately following surgery. In general, patients who require preoperative mechanical ventilation usually require postoperative mechanical ventilation. Furthermore, if the surgical procedure is extensive, producing an engorged, swollen brain, postoperative mechanical ventilation is usually necessary.

III. Pituitary Tumors

The pituitary gland is located at the base of the skull in the sella turcica, a bony cavity within the sphenoid bone, and it is divided into anterior (adenohypophysis) and posterior (neurohypophysis) lobes. A fold of dura (the diaphragma sella) on the superior surface of the sella is pierced by the infundibular stalk, which connects the posterior lobe of the pituitary gland to the hypothalamus. The hypothalamus regulates hormone release from the anterior pituitary through regulatory peptides (hypothalamic releasing and inhibiting factors) that reach the anterior pituitary by a complex portal vascular system. Control of hypothalamic secretion is complex and occurs from neuronal and chemical influences including feedback from target organ hormones. The large glandular anterior pituitary secretes at least seven hormones. The smaller posterior pituitary stores and secretes two hormones, antidiuretic hormone (ADH) and oxytocin, which are synthesized in specialized hypothalamic neurons and transported as granules in axons down the pituitary stalk to the posterior pituitary gland. The anterior and posterior pituitary hormones are listed in Table 32-10.

Pituitary tumors can be divided into two general categories, nonfunctioning and hypersecreting.[321] Nonfunctioning pituitary tumors are usually diagnosed when they become large and produce symptoms related to mass effects by impinging on adjacent structures. Headache, impaired vision, cranial nerve palsies, increased ICP, and hypopituitarism may result. The most common nonfunctioning tumors are chromophobe adenomas, craniopharyngiomas, and meningiomas. As these tumors enlarge, they can cause selective or global impairment of pituitary function by compressing the normal gland. A sudden enlargement of the pituitary caused by spontaneous hemorrhage or infarction into the tumor produces a symptom complex known as pituitary apoplexy, a life-threatening condition characterized by acute neurologic deficits and a rapid decline in pituitary function. Therapy includes rapid administration of corticosteroids and emergency surgical decompression.

Functioning pituitary adenomas produce an excess of one or more of the hormones of the anterior pituitary and, therefore, are usually diagnosed when the tumors are small. The

TABLE 32-10. Pituitary Gland Hormones

Anterior Pituitary	Posterior Pituitary
Growth hormone	Antidiuretic hormone
Prolactin	Oxytocin
Gonadotropins: Follicle-stimulating hormone, luteinizing hormone	
Adrenocorticotropic hormone	
Beta-lipotropin	
Thyroid-stimulating hormone	

most frequently occurring are prolactinomas followed by growth hormone (GH) and adrenocorticotropic hormone (ACTH) secreting adenomas. Adenomas secreting thyrotropin (TSH) or follicle-stimulating hormone (FSH) and luteinizing hormone (LH) are rare. Adenomas secreting both GH and prolactin (PRL) are common, however. Prolactinomas may produce the amenorrhea–galactorrhea syndrome in females and decreased libido and impotence in males. Excessive production of GH prepuberty results in gigantism and postpuberty results in acromegaly. Cushing's disease develops from an ACTH-secreting adenoma that causes bilateral adrenal hyperplasia.

Special Anesthetic Considerations

Preoperative Evaluation. The preoperative evaluation of patients with pituitary tumors requires an assessment of endocrine function and associated medical disorders. Endocrine tests are performed in the basal state and are supplemented by appropriate provocative tests (Table 32-11). These tests diagnose hyper- or hypofunctioning tumors, the extent of endocrine disturbance, and the adequacy of treatment. A thorough discussion of endocrinologic testing can be found elsewhere.[322]

In Cushing's disease, the increased ACTH and cortisol can produce multiple systemic effects such as diabetes mellitus with insulin-resistant hyperglycemia, hyperaldosteronism with hypokalemia and metabolic alkalosis, hypertension, mild congestive heart failure, and obesity. These patients require preoperative evaluation and management of hypertension, diabetes, and electrolyte imbalances, and a cardiovascular evaluation for ischemic heart disease and congestive heart failure.

TABLE 32-11. Preoperative Endocrine Studies for Pituitary Tumors

Basal levels of pituitary hormones: GH, PRL, ACTH, TSH, FSH, LH
Serum levels: Cortisol (am and pm), thyroxine, testosterone, estradiol
Urinary levels: 17-ketosteroids, 17-hydroxycorticosteroids, free cortisol, estrogens
Provocative and suppression tests as indicated: GH reserve—glucagon stimulation; GH suppression—glucose suppression (acromegaly); prolactin reserve—chlorpromazine or thyrotropin-releasing hormone provocative testing; low- and high-dose dexamethasone suppression (Cushing's syndrome), metyrapone test (Cushing's syndrome)
Posterior pituitary function tests: ADH reserve—serum and urine osmolality before and after 8–12 hours of water deprivation

Patients with acromegaly exhibit a general overgrowth of skeletal, connective, and soft tissues. Hands and feet become markedly enlarged and facial features become coarse. All major organs increase in size, including the heart, lungs, liver, and kidneys. These patients also require an evaluation for systemic hypertension, diabetes, ischemic heart disease, cardiomegaly, and congestive heart failure, with appropriate medical management instituted before surgery. Significant anatomic airway changes can occur in acromegalics, making airway management difficult.[323,324] Facial bone hypertrophy, particularly of the mandible and nose, thick tongue and lips, and hypertrophy of nasal turbinates, soft palate, tonsils, epiglottis, and larynx create difficulties with mask fit and visualization of the larynx. Glottic stenosis caused by soft tissue overgrowth may cause preoperative hoarseness and dyspnea. These patients usually require a smaller endotracheal tube than anticipated based on the size of the patient's facial features, and may be predisposed to postextubation edema. Stretching or compression of the recurrent laryngeal nerves from laryngeal soft tissue or thyroid gland enlargement may result in vocal cord paralysis. Because of these anatomic changes, a thorough preoperative airway examination is required. Patients complaining of hoarseness, dyspnea, or inspiratory stridor should undergo indirect laryngoscopy and x-ray examination of the neck to analyze airway conformation and lumen diameter. Based on this evaluation, preparations for difficult airway management and intubation should be anticipated. For patients with difficult airways and glottic abnormalities, an awake intubation with a fiberoptic laryngoscope is recommended. This obviates the need for a tracheostomy in all but the most severe cases. Patients without upper airway or vocal cord involvement can be managed in the routine manner.

Pressure effects on the normal pituitary gland from parasellar tumors or other lesions can cause panhypopituitarism. Patients who have panhypopituitarism require replacement therapy with appropriate hormones. These patients should be euthyroid before surgery. Glucocorticoid replacement is required when thyroxine replacement is started to avoid stressing an insufficient adrenocortical axis. Because glucocorticoids are also necessary to facilitate renal excretion of a water load, diabetes insipidus is usually not observed in the patient with pituitary insufficiency until cortisol replacement therapy is instituted. Preoperatively, the patient with panhypopituitarism will be receiving oral steroid and thyroxine therapy and, when indicated, intranasal instillation of synthetic vasopressin.

During the preanesthetic evaluation, the size and location of the tumor and its effect on intracranial dynamics should be determined. Pituitary microadenomas do not produce mass effects. Pituitary tumors with suprasellar extension, craniopharyngiomas, and other suprasellar tumors may exert a mass effect. In these patients, the CT scan or MRI and the neurologic examination are evaluated for signs of increased ICP. All patients scheduled for pituitary surgery are given supplemental short-acting glucocorticoid therapy perioperatively.[325] Because the surgery involves manipulation or removal of the anterior pituitary, transient or permanent deficiency of ACTH and cortisol secretion may result. To assess function of the optic nerves and chiasm, a visual examination including examination of the visual fields is performed. When transsphenoidal surgery is planned, an otolaryngologic examination of the nasal passages and nasopharynx is also performed, and a nasal culture is obtained to guide antibiotic therapy in the event of postoperative infection.

Surgical Considerations. Since the introduction of the operating microscope, transsphenoidal excision has been recommended for all pituitary tumors that do not have marked suprasellar extension. Advantages of the transsphenoidal approach include the following: lower morbidity and mortality rates with decreased incidence and severity of diabetes insipidus, elimination of frontal lobe retraction and external scars, magnified visualization and removal of small tumors, which spares normal tissue, decreased frequency of blood transfusions, and shorter hospitalization. Relative disadvantages include: the possibility of cerebrospinal fluid leakage and meningitis (which is rare with the use of antibiotics), inability to visualize neural structures adjacent to a large tumor, inaccessibility of tumors extending into middle and anterior fossae, and the possibility of bleeding from cavernous sinuses or carotid arteries (which can lead to intracranial hemorrhage, brain stem compression, and significant blood loss). The transcranial approach to the sella permits direct visualization of suprasellar structures: the vascular sinus ring, optic chiasm, hypothalamus, and pituitary stalk. This approach is recommended for pituitary tumors of uncertain diagnosis and those that have significant suprasellar extension with optic nerve or hypothalamic involvement. With this approach, there is potential for damage to the olfactory nerves, frontal lobe vasculature, and optic nerves and chiasm. In addition, the incidence of permanent diabetes insipidus and anterior pituitary insufficiency is increased.

Anesthetic Considerations. The anesthetic management of patients undergoing pituitary surgery is not fundamentally different from those undergoing other craniotomies. Basic neuroanesthetic principles apply whether the transsphenoidal or transcranial approach is used. With the transcranial approach, however, intraoperative measures to control ICP are instituted since pressure effects, the necessity for brain retraction, and the potential for greater blood loss exist.

During transsphenoidal procedures, central venous pressure and urinary output are not routinely measured. When the patient is positioned with a significant head-up tilt, however, air embolism may occur during this procedure.[326] Therefore, precordial Doppler monitoring and right atrial catheterization are recommended for detection and treatment of air embolism when a significant surgical site–cardiac gradient (15° or more) exists.

Evoked potential monitoring of visual evoked potentials may be used during pituitary surgery to monitor direct compression or compromise of blood supply to optic nerves and chiasm. Technical difficulties that cause intraoperative recording problems include changes in pupil size, deviation of eyes, goggle size and bulkiness, and stimulus delivery (light flashes). Because visual evoked potentials are entirely cortical in origin, they are also more vulnerable to the effects of general anesthetics.

For transsphenoidal procedures, a sublabial incision and dissection through the nasal septum is performed; therefore, oral endotracheal intubation is required. The nasal septum is usually prepared with 4% cocaine pledgets placed in the nares, followed by injection of 2% lidocaine with epinephrine 1–200,000 to the submucosa. This combination develops a dissection plane, decreases bleeding, and buffers the hypertensive response to nasal dissection. Initially, the cocaine and epinephrine may cause hypertension, tachycardia, and dysrhythmias, and drugs to treat these responses should be available. Following oral endotracheal intubation, the oropharynx is packed with saline-soaked gauze to minimize blood pooling in the glottis, esophagus, and stomach.

Although lumbar cerebrospinal fluid drainage is commonly employed during transcranial procedures, it is usually not indicated during transsphenoidal procedures unless an intraoperative air study is planned. When the surgical lesion has suprasellar extension, delineation of the superior margin is facilitated by injection of air or N_2O–oxygen mixture into the subarachnoid space. When air is injected, N_2O must be discontinued from the anesthetic mixture because it rapidly diffuses into the air-filled closed space, increasing the volume of injected air. Injection of N_2O–oxygen mixture permits continuation of inhaled N_2O.

Potential intraoperative complications during transsphenoidal procedures relate to the anatomic landmarks surrounding the sella turcica. The cavernous sinuses occupy the lateral walls of the sella and contain venous structures, the internal carotid artery, and cranial nerves III, IV, V, and VI. The optic chiasm with its associated optic nerves and tracts lies directly above the diaphragma sella in front of the pituitary stalk. Surgical manipulation in the region surrounding the sella can result in the following: hemorrhage from the venous sinuses or internal carotid artery, arterial spasm or thrombotic occlusion secondary to arterial manipulation, venous air embolism if head-up tilt is excessive, cranial nerve weakness secondary to trauma or stretching, and visual complications secondary to damage of the optic nerve or chiasm.[327]

Following transsphenoidal surgery, the patient will awaken with nasal packing and be required to breathe through the mouth postoperatively. Therefore, these patients must be fully awake and following commands before extubation of the trachea.

Postoperative Concerns. In the immediate postoperative period following either transsphenoidal or transcranial procedures, the primary concerns are corticosteroid coverage and fluid balance. Dexamethasone followed by prednisone is given for 5 days after surgery or until postoperative testing shows an intact pituitary–adrenal axis. Fluid balance is assessed by strict attention to hourly fluid intake and output and urine specific gravity. Development of diabetes insipidus is uncommon during surgery but may occur early in the postoperative course. Diabetes insipidus is commonly seen during the first 12 hours postoperatively and usually lasts for 2–4 days. Diagnosis is based on the following: polyuria (2–15 l·day^{-1}); hypernatremia; high serum osmolality (≥ 300 mOsm·kg^{-1}); decreased urine osmolality (≤ 200 mOsm·kg^{-1}); and decreased urine specific gravity (1.005 or less). Therapy includes replacement of

urine losses with intravenous fluids. When urinary volumes are excessive, exogenous vasopressin is given. In patients who develop permanent diabetes insipidus, vasopressin tannate-in-oil is used until intranasal desmopressin can be prescribed.

Other complications of pituitary tumor surgery include cerebrospinal fluid rhinorrhea, hypothalamic injury or stroke, cerebral ischemia, and meningitis. Following transsphenoidal surgery, patients must be carefully monitored in the recovery room for airway obstruction caused by bleeding and secretions in the pharynx. Frequent neurologic examinations are performed to note any changes in mental status. Patients who have had an uncomplicated hospital course after transsphenoidal surgery are often discharged within 5–6 days.

CEREBROVASCULAR MALFORMATIONS

I. Intracranial Aneurysms

The incidence of cerebral aneurysms in North America is estimated to be 2,000 per 100,000 (1 in 50), with the incidence of subarachnoid hemorrhage (SAH) from a ruptured aneurysm 12 per 100,000 (1 in 8000).[328] Therefore, most aneurysms are small and asymptomatic, remaining undetected throughout life. The factors that cause aneurysms to enlarge and rupture are not well defined, and there are no known specific risk factors predisposing patients to aneurysmal rupture. The patients are usually young, with a peak age-related incidence for rupture in the fifth decade of life, and the incidence for females slightly higher than that for males.[329] Before age 40, aneurysms occur predominantly in men, while after age 40 more women are afflicted. The incidence of SAH varies according to country and racial group.[330]

Following a SAH from a ruptured intracranial aneurysm, patients are assigned a clinical grade based on the degree of cerebral dysfunction present. Two classifications are currently in use: Botterell's original classification and the modification proposed by Hunt and Hess.[331,332] These classifications are used by neurosurgeons to estimate surgical risk and outcome (Table 32-12). Higher grades, or patients who are clinically more impaired, are associated with the presence of cerebral vasospasm, intracranial hypertension, and increased surgical mortality.

The presence of blood in the subarachnoid space causes an abrupt, marked rise in ICP, which often results in systemic hypertension and dysrhythmias. The abrupt increase in ICP accounts for the acute onset of a sudden, severe headache. The classic presentation of aneurysmal SAH is that of

TABLE 32-12. Classification and Surgical Risk of Patients with Subarachnoid Hemorrhage

Grade	Criteria	Perioperative Mortality Rates (%)
I	Asymptomatic, or minimal headache and slight nuchal rigidity	0–5
II	Moderate to severe headache, nuchal rigidity, no neurologic deficit other than cranial nerve palsy	2–10
III	Drowsiness, confusion, or mild focal deficit	10–15
IV	Stupor, moderate to severe hemiparesis, possibly early decerebrate rigidity, and vegetative disturbance	60–70
V	Deep coma, decerebrate rigidity, moribund appearance	70–100

severe headache associated with stiff neck, photophobia, nausea, vomiting, and often transient loss of consciousness. With this presentation, the diagnosis of SAH is obvious. In about 50% of patients, a small bleed or "warning leak" precedes a major aneurysmal rupture.[333] Warning symptoms and signs tend to be mild and nonspecific (headache, dizziness, orbital pain, slight motor or sensory disturbance) and are generally ignored or misdiagnosed by both patient and physician. A greater awareness among the medical community of the warning signs of aneurysmal rupture would benefit this patient population. When patients are operated on electively before a major rupture, the overall morbidity and mortality is markedly reduced.[334,335]

The diagnosis of SAH is made by the combination of clinical findings and a CT scan. This is followed by angiography of both carotid and vertebral arteries to define the cause. Aneurysms are classified according to location and size. They arise at a branch or bifurcation, usually at a point where a major vessel makes a turn changing the axial flow of blood.

There are several potential complications of SAH and surgical treatment of aneurysms. The most important of these are intracranial hypertension, rebleeding, vasospasm, and hydrocephalus. Intracranial hypertension is present to some degree in most patients following a SAH. In the uncomplicated case, intracranial hypertension does not require specific treatment. Intracranial pressure gradually returns to normal by the end of the first week. If an intracerebral hemorrhage, intraventricular hemorrhage, vasospasm, or hydrocephalus develops, intracranial hypertension may be severe and require treatment. Patients may require emergency ventriculostomy, steroids, diuretics or intubation and hyperventilation. Intracranial pressure should be lowered gradually, especially in patients with unclipped aneurysms. Abrupt lowering of ICP by lumbar puncture, ventricular drainage, or rapid infusion of mannitol can induce rebleeding.

Rebleeding occurs most commonly during the first 24 hours following initial SAH. The chance of rebleeding is about 4% within the first day; after 48 hours, it is 1.5% per day with a cumulative rebleeding rate of 19% by the end of 2 weeks.[336] Recurrent aneurysmal hemorrhage is a devastating complication associated with increased morbidity and mortality.

Traditional medical treatment for a patient with a recent SAH is designed to prevent rebleeding. Patients are nursed in a quiet environment. Bed rest, sedation (benzodiazepines or barbiturates), and analgesics (codeine) are recommended to minimize stress. Anticonvulsants are prescribed for seizure prophylaxis. There is a 5% incidence of early seizures in patients after SAH.[335] Blood pressure is controlled and stabilized. Attention is paid to fluid balance, with volume expansion if signs of cerebral ischemia develop, and to proper nutrition.

In many centers, antifibrinolytic drugs (epsilon aminocaproic acid and tranexamic acid) are administered to patients following SAH. Because SAH stimulates an increase in CSF fibrinolytic activity, antifibrinolytic drugs are administered to retard lysis of the fibrin-platelet plug that seals the aneurysmal rent, thus preventing rebleeding; however, their use is controversial.[337-339] Although the frequency of rebleeding is reduced following the administration of antifibrinolytic agents, there is an increase in the frequency of ischemic complications, hydrocephalus and thromboembolism, and outcome is similar to those patients not receiving the drugs. Therefore, any benefit derived from the use of antifibrinolytics may be offset by the associated complications. The

only effective therapy to prevent rebleeding is clipping the aneurysm.

A major cause of morbidity and mortality in the patient who has recovered from SAH is cerebral vasospasm.[340] Angiographic evidence of vasospasm can be detected in up to 70% of these patients. However, clinical vasospasm with ischemic deficits is observed in approximately 30% of patients, most often between days 4 and 12, with a peak at 6–7 days following SAH.[340] The clinical syndrome of vasospasm is often heralded by worsening headache and increasing blood pressure. It is characterized by progressive symptoms of confusion and lethargy, followed by focal motor and speech impairments corresponding to the arterial territory involved. The syndrome may resolve gradually or progress to coma and death within a period of hours to days.

The mechanism responsible for vasospasm is unknown; however, structural and pathologic changes have been demonstrated in the vessel wall.[341,342] There is also evidence that vasospasm after SAH correlates with the amount of blood in the subarachnoid space, and removal of the clot may decrease the incidence and severity of ischemic deficits.[340,343,344] Several approaches to prevent cerebral vasospasm have been suggested, from removal of clotted blood around intracranial arteries within the basal subarachnoid cisterns to the use of agents that lyse clots (plasmin), neutralize spasmogenic substances (antithrombin III, haptoglobin, sodium nitrite), combat free radical reactions, or neutralize focal intracranial acidosis.[344] None of these approaches has proven conclusively effective in the prevention of vasospasm. More recently, the calcium antagonist nimodipine has been investigated. The use of a calcium antagonist is based on the assumption that contraction of cerebral arterial smooth muscle cells is a calcium-dependent phenomenon that should be inhibited by preventing influx of extracellular calcium. Nimodipine has not been shown to prevent or reverse narrowing of major cerebral arteries, but evidence suggests that it may prevent or reverse ischemic neurologic deficits.[345-347] These reported beneficial effects may arise from improvement in collateral blood flow produced by dilation of smaller vessels or by improvement of the brain's tolerance to ischemia. Patients who receive nimodipine prophylaxis prior to surgery may experience a transient lowering of systemic blood pressure during anesthesia, but they are not reported to be at increased risk for intraoperative hemodynamic instability.[348]

When symptomatic vasospasm develops, an effective treatment is increasing cerebral perfusion pressure. This is accomplished by intravascular volume expansion and induced hypertension and by reduction in ICP. Intracranial pressure is reduced by ventricular drainage if ventriculomegaly exists or with infusion of mannitol in the absence of enlarged ventricles. Intravascular volume expansion is accomplished with infusion of crystalloid, colloid, or blood to a pulmonary capillary wedge pressure of 15–18 mm Hg or a central venous pressure of 12 mm Hg. If this regimen does not reverse the deficit, a vasopressor (dopamine, dobutamine) is introduced to raise systemic blood pressure until the neurologic deficits subside or reverse. The major complications of this therapy are pulmonary edema and cardiac failure in patients at risk and rebleeding in patients with unclipped aneurysms. Hypervolemic hypertensive therapy has been shown to reverse at least 70% of the neurologic deficits caused by vasospasm when treatment is initiated prior to infarction.[340,349] Hemodilution has also been suggested as an adjunct to hypervolemic hypertensive therapy; however, its use is controversial. Hemodilution decreases blood viscosity and improves cerebral blood flow, but it also decreases blood oxygen content.[350] The optimal hematocrit thought to maximize the oxygen delivery to tissues has been estimated at 33%, but may be higher in ischemic brain.[350,351]

The timing of surgery for a patient with a ruptured intracranial aneurysm is controversial. The advantages of early surgery (within 72 hours of SAH) are the prevention of early rebleeding; the removal of cisternal clots, possibly reducing the incidence of vasospasm; and securing of the aneurysm, allowing relative safety in the treatment of vasospasm. There is also a reduction in medical complications because patients require less bed rest and fewer pharmacologic agents. A major disadvantage of early operation is that surgery is performed on a freshly injured brain with impaired autoregulation. Similar operative morbidity and mortality rates have been reported for early and delayed surgery.[352-354] The use of contemporary microsurgical techniques, spinal fluid drainage, and balanced anesthesia (e.g., barbiturate–opioid–relaxant) with mild hyperventilation and diuretics provide brain relaxation for surgical dissection in the acutely injured brain, making early surgery possible.

Proponents of delayed surgery (days 10–14) claim the following advantages: the brain has recovered from the SAH; vasospasm has resolved; and the incidence of severe postoperative vasospasm may be reduced. Another advantage to delaying surgery is that coexisting medical conditions can be diagnosed and treated prior to surgery. Similar operative results have been reported for early and delayed surgery, and in a recent report of the International Cooperative Study, the overall outcome at 6 months following initial SAH was equivalent between early and delayed surgical groups.[355] In this study, the postoperative risk of vasospasm following early surgery was equivalent to the risk of rebleeding and vasospasm in patients waiting for delayed surgery. The initiation of aggressive therapy for postoperative vasospasm (nimodipine prophylaxis and/or hypervolemic hypertensive therapy) may influence future outcome results following early surgery.

Special Anesthetic Considerations

Preoperative Evaluation. When the neurologic examination is performed, the patient's clinical grade is noted (Table 32-12). The patient's CT scan or MR image is evaluated for the presence of cerebral edema, midline shift, ventricular distortion, hydrocephalus, and hematoma to assess the presence and severity of intracranial hypertension. The severity, acuteness, and stage of the SAH, the presence of intracranial hypertension, and the timing of surgery will determine the anesthetic management. Because the circle of Willis is proximal to the hypothalamus, a SAH in this area can cause a variety of disturbances related to hypothalamic dysfunction, e.g., electrocardiographic (ECG) changes, temperature instability, various changes in endocrine (pituitary) function, and a variety of electrolyte disturbances.[335,356,357] Sympathetic overactivity and overstimulation of both adrenal cortex and medulla can contribute to hypertension and diabetes, requiring treatment with insulin.[335,358]

Electrolyte abnormalities frequently occur secondary to the syndrome of inappropriate antidiuretic hormone (SIADH) secretion or diabetes insipidus.[335,356,359] Hyponatremia is the most common electrolyte disturbance detected and is often associated with a high urinary sodium and osmolality, which is expected with SIADH. Unlike a patient with SIADH, however, the patient with SAH usually has a contracted intravascular volume despite hyponatremia. The events leading to volume depletion with hyponatremia are

unknown. The suggested treatment is water restriction and replenishment of intravascular volume with colloid or blood.[360] The factors contributing to intravascular volume contraction in these patients are supine diuresis secondary to increased thoracic blood volume, negative nitrogen balance, decreased erythropoiesis, increased catecholamine levels, and iatrogenic blood loss. The most severe form of electrolyte imbalance seen after SAH is hypernatremia and hyperosmolality, which carries a grave prognosis.[359] This can lead to the syndrome of hyperosmolar coma, which is associated with severe intracranial hypertension. Attempts to treat hypernatremia and hyperosmolality with hypotonic solutions can lead to an exacerbation of intracranial hypertension, resulting in an irreversible condition or death. Fluid restriction, diuretics, and steroids used in the management of SAH and intracranial hypertension may further aggravate dehydration and electrolyte abnormalities. Fluid balance and electrolyte abnormalities should be corrected prior to surgery.

Most aneurysm surgery requires significant intravascular volume shifts (diuresis followed by volume loading) and extensive systemic blood pressure manipulations (periods of deliberate hypotension). Therefore, patients with a history of hypertension, ischemic heart disease and/or congestive heart failure must be in optimal condition to tolerate the hemodynamic changes required for this surgery. Depending on the degree of cardiovascular disease, inadvertent or deliberate hypotension may be poorly tolerated. When patients have significant hypertension, the blood pressure should be lowered gradually to normotensive levels to avoid cerebral ischemia. Agents such as propranolol, labetalol, or methyldopa are used in neurosurgical patients because these agents do not affect cerebral blood volume or ICP. A more extensive review of drugs to treat hypertension and to induce hypotension is discussed elsewhere.[361] When the systemic blood pressure is lowered, a critical level below which neurologic deficits occur may be observed. Systemic blood pressure below this level should be avoided intraoperatively.

Electrocardiographic abnormalities are commonly associated with ruptured cerebral aneurysms.[362] The ECG changes include ST-segment depression or elevation, T-wave inversion or flattening, U-waves, prolonged Q–T intervals, and dysrhythmias. The clinical significance of the abnormalities is unknown. Subendocardial infarction following severe SAH in otherwise previously healthy patients has been reported.[363] These changes may be related to abnormal release of catecholamines induced by hypothalamic dysfunction and may result from an increased uptake of epinephrine by the myocardium.[335,357,358] Focal areas of necrosis in the myocardium have been observed in postmortem microscopic examination.[364] The ECG changes are not necessarily associated with increased operative morbidity and mortality or consistent increases in serum myoglobin or creatine kinase.[365] They usually resolve within 10 days following SAH and require no special treatment. When cardiac dysrhythmias and occasional frank subendocardial ischemia result in cardiac failure, appropriate treatment must be instituted.

Anesthetic Management. The anesthetic goals for intracranial aneurysm surgery are to avoid aneurysm rupture, maintain cerebral perfusion pressure and transmural aneurysm pressure, and provide a "slack" brain. Intraoperative aneurysm rupture occurs in approximately 20% of patients and is associated with high morbidity and mortality.[366] Cerebral perfusion pressure is maintained by using drugs in doses that avoid sudden or profound decreases in systemic blood pressure or increases in ICP. Similarly transmural pressure, which is defined as the difference between mean arterial pressure and ICP, must be maintained. (The pressure within an aneurysm is equal to the systemic blood pressure.) The relationship between transmural pressure and wall stress or tension of the aneurysm is linear. An increase in mean arterial pressure or fall in ICP will increase transmural pressure, wall stress, and risk of aneurysm rupture.[367] Methods to control brain volume and ICP, such as hyperventilation, diuretics, spinal drainage, and head position, facilitate surgical exposure and minimize the retraction pressure that can cause tissue injury.

Patients in Hunt's grade I or II who appear anxious should receive premedication as previously described. A pulmonary artery catheter is recommended in Hunt's grade III or higher to provide a more accurate measure of the patient's volume status and cardiac function intraoperatively and postoperatively in the prevention or management of cerebral vasospasm. Electrophysiologic monitoring with the EEG or SSEPs may be used to monitor brain function during induced hypotension.[368,369] When barbiturates are administered for brain protection, the EEG is used to guide the dose required to achieve a burst suppression pattern.

To minimize the risk of hypertension and aneurysmal rupture during induction of anesthesia, intravenous lidocaine and beta-blockers such as propranolol, labetalol, or esmolol have been recommended. During induction, esmolol is particularly effective because of its rapid onset and short duration of action. Following induction, ventilation is mechanically controlled to maintain the $Paco_2$ at 35 mm Hg if ICP is normal.[370] This $Paco_2$ is selected to maintain cerebral blood flow in the presence of vasospasm and deliberate hypotension and to prevent excessive lowering of ICP that can increase aneurysmal transmural pressure. If intracranial hypertension is present, the $Paco_2$ is lowered to 25–30 mm Hg. A deep plane of anesthesia must be established prior to insertion of head pins, scalp incision, turning the bone flap, and opening the dura in order to avoid a hypertensive response. When intracranial hypertension is present, anesthesia should be deepened with additional doses of thiopental and fentanyl until the skull is opened.

The drugs most frequently used to maintain anesthesia during aneurysm surgery are fentanyl and thiopental (bolus dosing or infusions) in conjunction with isoflurane in oxygen. In conditions of poor intracranial compliance, a continuous infusion of thiopental (2–3 $mg \cdot kg^{-1} \cdot h^{-1}$ following a bolus dose of 5 $mg \cdot kg^{-1}$) is recommended as the primary anesthetic for aneurysm surgery in conjunction with a fentanyl infusion (1–4 $\mu g \cdot kg^{-1} \cdot h^{-1}$) and one-half MAC concentration of isoflurane in oxygen. The total dose of fentanyl should not exceed 10–12 $\mu g \cdot kg^{-1}$, unless postoperative ventilation is planned. Potential disadvantages to using thiopental are blood pressure instability and prolonged recovery from anesthesia. With this technique, a pulmonary artery catheter should be inserted to monitor and optimize cardiovascular performance and intravascular volume. Following an uneventful aneurysm clip application, the thiopental infusion is discontinued to prevent a delay in recovery.

Several techniques are instituted during aneurysm surgery to provide a "slack" brain and facilitate dissection. These are hyperventilation of the lungs, osmotic diuresis, barbiturate administration, and CSF drainage. A lumbar subarachnoid catheter or spinal needle is inserted following induction to allow CSF drainage during the procedure. Excessive loss of CSF must be avoided during insertion of the lumbar drain because it can decrease ICP, thus increasing aneurysmal transmural pressure and the potential for rupture. Removal of CSF after opening of the dura is done cautiously with guidance by the surgeon.

Prior to aneurysm clipping, isotonic crystalloid solutions without glucose are administered to replace overnight fluid losses and provide hourly maintenance fluid requirements. When the aneurysm is secured, intraoperative fluid deficits are replaced and additional volume is administered. At the time of aneurysm dissection, blood is available for transfusion in case the aneurysm ruptures. A bolus of thiopental (3–5 $mg \cdot kg^{-1}$) is given before temporary occlusion of a major intracranial vessel and before aneurysm clipping. Induced hypotension, if planned, should begin when the surgeon begins his dissection of the aneurysm. Following aneurysm clipping, the central venous pressure and pulmonary capillary wedge pressure are raised to 10–12 mm Hg or 15–18 mm Hg, respectively, with crystalloid, colloid, or blood. A postoperative hematocrit between 30–35% is desirable. As discussed previously, intravascular volume expansion with hemodilution is recommended to reduce the risk of postoperative cerebral vasospasm.[351]

When considering the use of deliberate hypotension, the risk–benefit ratio must be assessed for each patient. The potential benefit of hypotension must be weighed against the risk of causing cerebral ischemia or ischemia to other organs. Patients with a history of cardiovascular disease, occlusive cerebrovascular disease, intracerebral hematoma, fever, anemia, and renal disease are not good candidates for induced hypotension. Such patients should only be subjected to moderate reductions in systemic blood pressure (20–30 mm Hg), if at all. The most commonly used agents to induce hypotension are sodium nitroprusside, nitroglycerine, trimethaphan, and isoflurane. Which agent is best for neurovascular procedures is the subject of much debate and is discussed in a following section of this chapter.

Low-grade hypothermia (32°C) is recommended during aneurysm surgery to enhance the brain's ability to tolerate ischemia. Hypothermia reduces the cerebral metabolic requirements for oxygen by 7–13% for each degree centigrade that the temperature is lowered, thereby prolonging safely tolerated periods of cerebral ischemia. More profound levels of hypothermia (30°C and below) are associated with complications such as cardiac dysrhythmias, hypotension, acidosis, coagulation defects, and rewarming shock and are not recommended for the routine cerebral aneurysm surgery. Profound hypothermia and circulatory arrest are used to resect otherwise inoperable giant basilar cerebral aneurysms.

The temporary occlusion of a feeding artery to produce an acute reduction in focal blood flow is common practice during aneurysm surgery.[371] The advantages of temporary clipping are that it produces a slack aneurysm and eliminates the need for induced hypotension and its systemic effects. Depending on the location of the aneurysm, either somatosensory evoked potentials or brain stem auditory evoked potentials can be used to monitor the safety of temporary occlusion.

The major intraoperative complication of aneurysm surgery is hemorrhage. When an aneurysm ruptures intraoperatively, there is potential for major ischemic damage from hypotension and the surgical efforts to control bleeding. Hemorrhagic death is also possible. The following management is recommended: rapid infusion of blood to maintain blood volume and reduction of mean arterial pressure to 40–50 mm Hg to decrease the rate of bleeding. If bleeding continues to be excessive, the mean arterial pressure is briefly lowered to 30 mm Hg. Finally, one or both of the carotid arteries can be compressed to produce a bloodless field.

The primary goals at the conclusion of surgery are to avoid coughing, straining, hypercarbia, and hypertension. For patients in grades I and II who have no intraoperative complications, the endotracheal tube should be removed in the operating room and a neurologic examination performed. Patients who have intraoperative complications or have depressed consciousness preoperatively (grades III–V) should remain intubated and receive mechanical ventilation until their neurologic status improves.

Postoperative Concerns. Variation in systemic blood pressure is common postoperatively and contributes significantly to morbidity and mor- tality in patients following aneurysm repair. Causes of hypertension include preexisting hypertension, pain, and CO_2 retention from residual anesthesia. The administration of sodium nitroprusside for induced hypotension may cause a significant rebound increase in systemic blood pressure from plasma renin activity, which can persist for some time into the postoperative period. The treatment of postoperative hypertension is critical to prevent the formation of cerebral edema or hematoma. Antihypertensive drugs should be administered after respiratory depression and pain are eliminated as causes. The hypertensive response usually subsides within 12 hours. When indicated, preoperative antihypertensive drugs are reinstituted and maintained.

After clipping of the aneurysm, cerebral vasospasm continues to pose a threat to neurologic integrity. Postoperative hypotension must be avoided, and the patient's intravascular volume must be accurately assessed with either a central venous pressure or pulmonary artery catheter. As previously discussed, a higher than normal intravascular fluid volume should be maintained.

II. Arteriovenous Malformations

An arteriovenous malformation (AVM) of the brain consists of a tangle of congenitally malformed blood vessels that form an abnormal communication between the arterial and venous systems. The arterial afferents flow directly into venous efferents without the usual resistance of an intervening capillary bed, and thus oxygenated blood is shunted directly into the venous system, leaving surrounding brain tissue transiently or permanently ischemic. These lesions predominate in males over females (2:1), with the onset of complaints between the ages of 10 and 30. The chief clinical features are parenchymal or subarachnoid hemorrhage, focal epilepsy, and progressive focal neurologic sensory-motor deficits occurring in a child or young adult. A vein of Galen AVM in infants may present with hydrocephalus and/or high output cardiac failure. The natural history of AVMs is not completely understood.[372-374] The risk of hemorrhage is 2–3% per year. The rate of rebleeding is 6% in the first year after a hemorrhage and about 2% per year thereafter.[373] Mortality from initial hemorrhage is high with reports between 10–30%. Recurrence of hemorrhage with a fatal outcome is a constant danger. There are several options for the management of AVMs that include: surgical excision, embolization, high-energy therapy (proton beam, gamma rays, or conventional x-rays), a combination of the above, and leaving AVMs alone. Arteriovenous malformations of suitable size and location can be managed success-

fully with surgical excision. In one report, elective surgery for excision of AVMs was associated with a mortality of 5% and only 3% for supratentorial lesions.[375] Morbidity also varies with the location of the mass. To avoid intraoperative or postoperative massive brain swelling or hemorrhage of large AVMs, operations may be staged or follow preoperative embolization.

Special Anesthetic Considerations

In addition to providing anesthesia for craniotomy and resection of the AVM, anesthesia may be required for radiologic embolization of the AVM. Closed embolization of cerebral AVMs is uncomfortable and invasive; however, general anesthesia is not mandatory. It has been performed successfully with various combinations of sedative drugs (fentanyl–droperidol or fentanyl–midazolam) that allow neurologic examinations during the procedure and permit immediate diagnoses of complications.[376] Children, uncooperative patients, and those with intracranial hypertension or airway problems usually require general anesthesia. General anesthesia does not allow direct neurologic assessment. Potential complications of embolization procedures are embolic or ischemic stroke and hemorrhage from the AVM, either acute or delayed.[376,377]

The anesthetic management of patients with AVMs is similar to the management of patients for aneurysm surgery. Depending on the presentation, the anesthetic approach is modified. For example, a large bleed may present with symptoms relating to mass effects and require maneuvers to reduce ICP. High flow through a large intact AVM may cause a "steal" with resulting cerebral ischemia and require different techniques to improve cerebral perfusion pressure. With more extensive lesions, hypothermia and high-dose barbiturates have been recommended for brain protection. Induced hypotension may also be required to reduce lesion size and blood flow.

After removal of the AVM, breakthrough cerebral edema or hemorrhage may result. This occurs when the blood flow from the surgically obliterated AVM is diverted to the surrounding brain. The smaller vessels in the brain surrounding the AVM are not accustomed to the higher pressure-flow state, and autoregulation is exceeded, resulting in severe brain swelling, edema, and hemorrhage. Immediate treatment should include the simultaneous application of high-dose barbiturates, osmotic diuretics, hyperventilation, and maintenance of a low-normal mean arterial blood pressure.[378] When marked brain swelling occurs intraoperatively, the patient should remain intubated, hyperventilated, and sedated postoperatively. Hypertension during emergence and postoperatively must be controlled, preferably with beta-blockers, to prevent bleeding into the bed of the AVM.

DELIBERATE HYPOTENSION

Intentional reduction of blood pressure to hypotensive levels during surgery gained popularity in Britain subsequent to its advocacy by Griffiths and Gillies in 1948.[379] Nicholas Greene brought the "hypotensive spinal" or "Gillies technique" to the United States in 1952,[380] and by the end of that decade, deliberate hypotension was in common practice. While the efficacy of inducing hypotension in order to reduce blood loss remains somewhat controversial,[381] the technique is widely used and recommended for that purpose.[382]

The use of deliberate hypotension for cerebral aneurysm clip ligation is also controversial, though it has many advocates and Michenfelder credits the technique as the preeminent contribution that anesthetic management has made to the reduction of mortality from aneurysm surgery over the last 15 years.[383] Decreasing aneurysm transmural pressure during manipulation of the aneurysmal sac will theoretically decrease the potential for rupture. Note that the thinner the wall, the greater the wall stress at any given pressure. Therefore, either an increase in mean arterial pressure (MAP), or a fall in cerebrospinal fluid (CSF) pressure or brain tissue pressure will increase transmural pressure, the wall stress, and the risk of rupture. Nevertheless, it is difficult to confirm the usefulness of deliberate hypotension in prevention of aneurysm rupture. The only published study directly comparing hypotension with normotension found no difference in the frequency of aneurysm rupture during surgery.[384] In addition, some argue that deliberate hypotension can increase the likelihood of vasospasm, seriously impair borderline ischemic brain tissue, and impair autoregulation.[385,386] While it is too early to determine the cost-benefit ratio of inducing hypotension during cerebral arteriovenous malfunction embolization, results thus far suggest that hypotension facilitates the embolization process.[387]

Most practitioners agree that reduction of mean arterial pressure to 50 mm Hg can be well tolerated by the normal, healthy brain.[388] However, patients with chronic hypertension usually lose cerebral blood flow autoregulation at 50 mm Hg, so their blood pressure should only be reduced by 50 mm Hg below their normal pressure.[382] Other contraindications to all but the most moderate reductions in blood pressure (20–30 mm Hg) include fever, anemia, occlusive cerebrovascular disease, and intracerebral hematoma. Although hyperventilation is a useful technique for reducing intramural pressure through cerebral vasoconstriction, its use in conjunction with hypotension may aggravate the risk of partial ischemia.[389] Accordingly, ventilation during hypotension should be adjusted to maintain normocarbia.

TABLE 32-13. Adverse Effects from SNP Infusion[390-397]

Cyanide and thiocyanate toxicity
Rebound hypertension
Intracranial hypertension
Blood coagulation abnormalities
Increased pulmonary shunting
Hypothyroidism
Decrease in myocardial, liver, and skeletal muscle oxygen reserves
Possible damage to mitochondria

Commonly Used Drugs

Sodium Nitroprusside

Sodium nitroprusside (SNP) continues to be the most widely used drug to induce hypotension because of its rapid onset, relatively consistent effect, and short half-life. Adequate blood flow to vital organs is maintained at perfusion pressures above 50 mm Hg. Sodium nitroprusside primarily dilates resistance vessels, either by interfering with sulfhydryl groups or by blocking intracellular calcium activation. In addition, SNP may increase cyclic GMP. Cardiac output is unaffected by SNP. Possible adverse effects are listed in Table 32-13.

Cyanide (CN) is produced when SNP is metabolized (see Figure 32-14). One milligram of SNP contains 0.44 mg of CN. Toxic blood levels (greater than 100 $\mu g \cdot dl^{-1}$) occur when greater than 1 $mg \cdot kg^{-1}$ SNP is administered within 2.5 hours or when greater than 0.5 $mg \cdot kg^{-1} \cdot h^{-1}$ is administered within 24 hours. Death from CN has occurred after 4–12 $mg \cdot kg^{-1}$ CN. Death following SNP secondary to CN has been reported in a pediatric patient when blood CN level was 400 $\mu g \cdot dl^{-1}$.[390] Greater risk of CN toxicity exists in patients who are nutritionally deficient in cobalamins (vitamin B_{12} compounds) or in dietary substances containing sulfur.

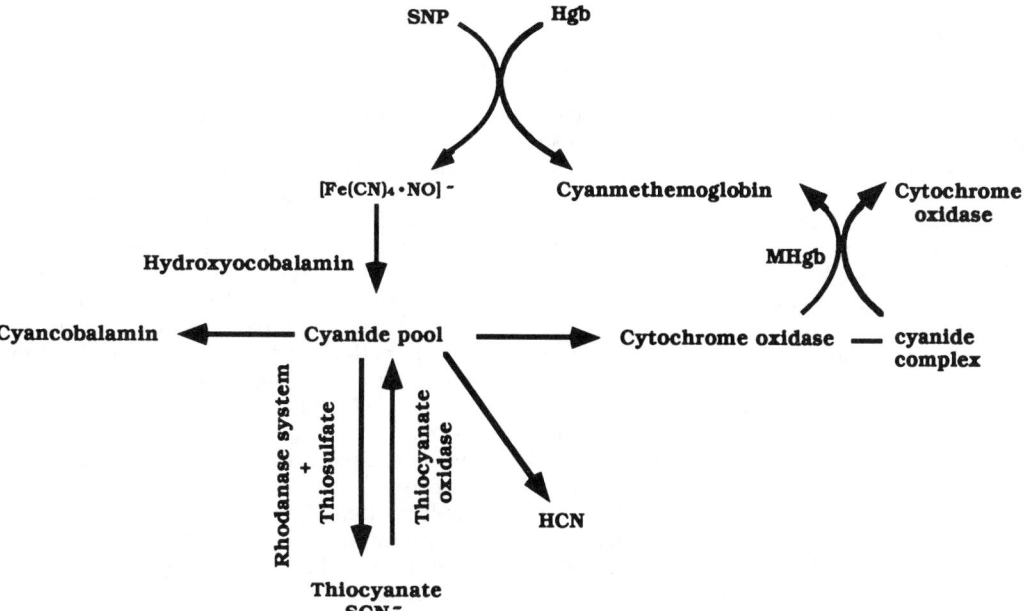

Figure 32-14. Red blood cell biotransformation of sodium nitroprusside. (SNP = sodium nitroprusside; Hgb = hemoglobin; mHgb = methemoglobin; SCN = thiocyanate; HCN = hydrogen cyanide.)

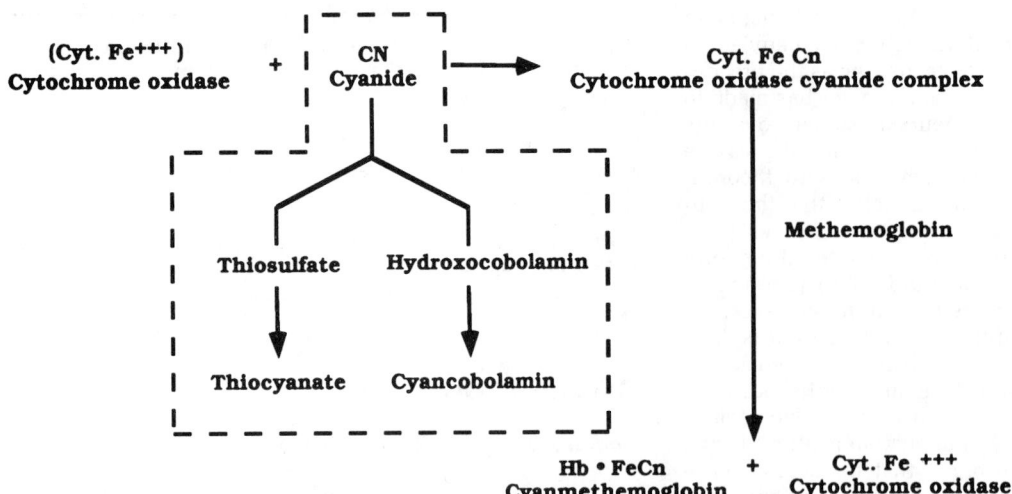

Figure 32-15. Tissue cytochrome oxidase combines with cyanide to form cytochrome oxidase-cyanide complex. Methemoglobin frees cyanide from complex, forming cyanmethemoglobin. Other potential pathways to prevent toxicity include the addition of thiosulfate or hydroxocobolamin. (The *dashed line* indicates treatment of cyanide toxicity.)

Measurement of blood CN and pH will enable detection of abnormalities in high-risk patients for whom larger than recommended amounts of SNP have been used. Treatment should consist of intravenous thiosulfate except in those patients with abnormal renal function, for whom hydroxocobalamin is recommended (see Figure 32-15). Circulating levels of thiocyanate increase when renal function is compromised, and central nervous system abnormalities result when thiocyanate levels reach $5-10$ mg·dl^{-1}. Fortunately, recent research indicates that captopril can be used to lower the dose requirement of SNP and thereby reduce the consequent build up of cyanide.[398]

Another strategy for reducing the potential for cyanide toxicity is to maintain SNP-like pharmacodynamics while greatly reducing SNP dosage in a 1:10 mixture with trimethaphan.[399]

Systemic and pulmonary hypertension occur after abrupt discontinuance of SNP.[391] This results from increased plasma renin activity (PRA) caused either by ischemic or dilated renal vessels. Gradual SNP discontinuance, preoperative propranolol, and converting enzyme inhibitors (captopril) will attenuate this response until increased PRA returns to normal (plasma half-life, 30 min).

Based on results obtained in dogs, Michenfelder and Milde have argued that SNP dilates cerebral capacitance vessels regardless of anesthetic background, and in addition, dilates cerebral resistance vessels when autoregulation is blunted by a volatile agent.[400] Under either circumstance, if venous return is impeded by a mass lesion, SNP will cause an increase in cerebral blood volume (CBV).[401] Accordingly, SNP causes increased intracranial pressure (ICP) in patients with low intracranial compliance.[401] In the closed cranium, an increase in ICP can cause hemispheric reductions in CBF due to regional reductions in CPP. In the open cranium with open dura, SNP-induced cerebral vasodilatation is not likely to affect regional CBF,[402] but may disturb local perfusion, especially in areas under retraction and areas that are distant from the site of small to moderate size craniotomies. Steroids and sedatives may improve intracranial compliance and allow SNP administration prior to opening of the dura. If this is to be done, ICP should be monitored continuously.

Sodium nitroprusside can cause platelet disintegration and inhibition of platelet aggregation,[393] and SNP-induced abnormalities in blood coagulation can exacerbate increased bleeding caused by vasodilation.[394]

Increased pulmonary shunting occurs in patients with normal pulmonary function after SNP-induced hypotension, but fibrosed pulmonary vessels of patients with chronic obstructive lung disease show little response to SNP, and shunting increases are not significant.[390] Recent work has demonstrated a significant relationship between age and SNP sensitivity, with lower doses capable of inducing equally profound hypotension in older patients.[403] It is possible that further elucidation of this age-dosage relationship will allow more appropriate age-specific administration of SNP with a consequent amelioration of SNP-related complications.

Nitroglycerin (NTG)

Nitroglycerin (NTG) directly dilates capacitance vessels,[404] has a short half-life, and no clinically significant toxic metabolites. Resistance to NTG has been reported in some patients receiving nonvolatile anesthetics.[405] As with SNP, low intracranial compliance contraindicates NTG use prior to dural opening unless steroids, diuretics, or sedatives have improved compliance. Even with the dura open, both nitrates entail some risk of increased CBV and significant brain swelling.[391,405] Also similar to SNP, pulmonary shunting increases in patients with normal pulmonary function in contrast to those with chronic obstructive pulmonary disease (COPD), after NTG-induced hypotension. Recent research indicates that NTG reduces cardiac index compared with SNP at a mean arterial pressure of 40 mm Hg.[406]

Effects of nitroprusside and nitroglycerin on microcirculation are markedly different. In animal experiments that have continuously monitored local tissue PO$_2$ in skeletal muscle, liver, and myocardium, tissue PO$_2$ is dramatically reduced while arterial PO$_2$ remains within normal range during sodium nitroprusside infusion. This clinically relevant finding has been confirmed by measurement in patients.[407] In support of these findings, Franke et al have shown by capillaroscopy that sodium nitroprusside predominantly dilates precapillaries, while nitroglycerin acts on all microvascular segments.[408] During hypotension using either drug, pressure is decreased to the same extent on the arteriolar side; however, on the venous side, there is only a decrease with nitroglycerin. Accordingly, the pressure difference between the arteriolar side and the venule side, which is of greater importance for capillary perfusion, remains unchanged with nitroglycerin but decreases significantly with sodium nitroprusside. Furthermore, Franke et al found that a significant volume of blood is diverted through arteriovenous shunts during sodium nitroprusside hypotension.

Trimethaphan

Trimethaphan blocks sympathetic ganglia, resulting in resistance and capacitance vessel relaxation, which usually decreases arterial pressure. Trimethaphan's short plasma half-life makes for easy control, but histamine release has been reported to cause bronchospasms[409] and potential ICP increases.[410] The speed of infusion and altered autoregulation may also influence trimethaphan's effect on ICP.[411] Myoneural blockade has been reported after administration of trimethaphan, probably due to its chemical resemblance to neuromuscular blocking agents.[412] Trimethaphan is recommended for mean arterial pressure (MAP) reductions above 50 mm Hg because electroencephalographic (EEG) slowing with high-voltage wave activity and increased brain lactate concentrations have been reported to accompany trimethaphan-induced reduction of MAP below 50 mm Hg.[395] These findings accord well with evidence that trimethaphan reduces blood flow at all levels of the spinal cord in dogs.[413]

Halothane, Enflurane, Isoflurane, and Desflurane

Halothane, enflurane, isoflurane, and desflurane[414] hypotension are produced by increasing their respective inspired concentrations. Decreased blood pressure results from varying degrees of myocardial depression and peripheral vascular dilatation. Potential adverse effects include autoregulatory loss of vital organ blood flow, reduction in cerebral perfusion pressure (CPP) as MAP decreases, ICP increase in patients with intracranial masses, increased cerebral edema, and accumulation of anaerobic metabolites.[412] In addition, enflurane alters CSF dynamics, which may cause further increases in ICP.[415] Enflurane may also induce seizure activity in certain patients, especially during hypocapnia.

Isoflurane has been recommended for deliberate hypotension because of its rapid onset of action, ease of control, and rapid reversal on discontinuance.[416] Macnab et al have determined that, relative to SNP, isoflurane blunts the stress response to induced hypotension.[417] The hypotension that results from isoflurane is primarily a consequence of peripheral vascular dilation, with maintenance of CO except at higher inspired concentrations. Reports of worsening of ST-segment changes and shunting of blood from collateral-dependent regions in the myocardium have caused concern about using isoflurane in patients with myocardial disease.[418] Pulmonary shunting and dead space are not increased during isoflurane-induced hypotension.

Because of isoflurane's ability to reduce $CMRO_2$ by 50% at 1.5–2 MAC while maintaining cerebral blood flow,[419] cerebral protection seemed likely. However, Bendo et al[420] have found that clinical doses of isoflurane are not as protective as thiopental in the in vitro hippocampal slice model, and Nehls et al[421] have demonstrated that isoflurane

does not afford protection following focal ischemia. In addition, Van Aken et al[422] have demonstrated loss of autoregulation for 60 minutes following discontinuance of isoflurane and increases in CBF, which could worsen edema and ischemia and increase neurologic deficits. Gelb et al have recently tested the hypothesis that isoflurane-induced hypotension provides a measure of protection relative to SNP-induced hypotension during middle cerebral artery occlusion in monkeys.[423] Unfortunately, they found no difference in neurologic scores or lesion size between the isoflurane and SNP groups. Bendo et al recently demonstrated that isoflurane-induced hypotension increased brain edema and neurologic deficits in dogs with cryolesions when compared with similar dogs that received labetalol-induced hypotension. Thus α and combined α and β drugs such as labetalol and esmolol, a short-acting beta-blocker, may be superior hypotensive drugs for use in neurosurgical patients.

Adenosine Triphosphate

Adenosine triphosphate (ATP) has been used to induce hypotension in humans.[424-426] Advantages include prompt onset and short duration. Adenosine triphosphate is metabolized to adenosine and PO_4 with adenosine being responsible for vasodilation. Adenosine is metabolized to uric acid and conflicting reports exist as to the amount that accumulates. Unfortunately, ATP and adenosine dilate cerebral vessels and impair a dog's autoregulation,[427] and appear to blunt autoregulation in humans.[428]

Esmolol and Labetalol

Esmolol, an ultra short-acting cardioselective beta-adrenergic blocker with an estimated half-life of approximately 9 minutes has been used to decrease blood pressure by itself[429] or in combination with other agents.[430,431] Esmolol's cardiac depressant properties indicate caution in attempting to use it as a primary hypotensive drug.

Labetalol, a combined alpha- and beta-blocker is likewise better used in combination therapies when inducing hypotension, not only because of bradycardia, but also because of its lack of potency.[432] Both esmolol and labetalol have properties advantageous to neurosurgical patients because they do not dilate cerebral vessels, increase heart rate, cause rebound hypotension, or have toxic metabolites.[433]

HEAD INJURY

The annual incidence of head injury in the United States is approximately 300 per 100,000 population.[434,435] Approximately 600,000 people each year sustain severe head injuries. Forty-five thousand people die, and significant residual disability remains in more than 20% of survivors.[436] Head injury occurs most frequently in young and otherwise healthy individuals. Males are affected two to three times more often than females in all age groups and are more likely to sustain severe head trauma. More than 50% of patients with severe head trauma have multiple injuries resulting in significant blood loss, systemic hypotension, and hypoxia.[435] Causes of head injury include motor vehicle accidents, falls, physical assault, firearm accidents, domestic accidents, birth trauma, and work-related and sports injuries. Motor vehicle accidents cause more than 50% of all head injuries and greater than 70% of all fatal head injuries.[434,437,438] In the pediatric population, greater than 90%

of all severe head injuries are related to motor vehicle accidents.[439]

Classification of severe head injury is based on the Glasgow Coma Scale (Table 32-14), which defines neurologic impairment in terms of eye opening, speech, and motor function.[440,441] The total score that can be obtained is 15, and severe head injury is determined by a score of 7 or less persisting for 6 hours or more. The Glasgow Coma and Glasgow Outcome Scales permit comparison of the severity of injury between patients and institutions and allow outcome prediction.[434,439-442] The prognosis after head injury depends on the type of lesion sustained, the age of the patient, as well as the severity of the injury as defined by the Glasgow Coma Scale.[434,439,443,444] In general, mortality is closely related to the initial score on the coma scale. For any given lesion and score, however, the elderly have a poorer outcome than do younger patients.[439,444,445]

Following head trauma, the primary injury results from the biomechanical effect of forces applied to the skull and brain at the time of the insult and is manifested within milliseconds. For those victims who survive long enough to be admitted to the hospital, the management goal is to initiate timely and appropriate therapy to prevent secondary brain injury. With early intervention by trained personnel at the scene of the injury and rapid referral to a center equipped to treat patients with severe head injuries, a significant decrease in mortality should be accomplished.[439] When the initial injury is not fatal, subsequent neurologic damage and systemic complications should be preventable in a large proportion of patients. Currently, there is no treatment for the primary injury. Secondary injury caused by hypoxia, anemia, hypotension, hypercarbia, or intracranial hypertension can be prevented, however.

Primary injury or biomechanical trauma to brain parenchyma includes concussion, contusion, laceration, and hematoma. Not all severely head-injured patients require surgery. Generalized brain injury with edema or contusion is a common finding in patients, whether or not a surgically correctable mass lesion is present. Diffuse cerebral swelling occurs because of sudden intracerebral congestion and hyperemia. Twenty-four hours or more after the initial insult, cerebral edema develops in the extracellular spaces of the white matter. Nonoperative treatment of diffuse cerebral swelling includes hyperventilation, diuresis with mannitol and furosemide, and barbiturates in conjunction with ICP monitoring.

Depressed skull fractures and acute epidural, subdural, and intracerebral hematomas usually require craniotomy. Chronic subdural hematomas are often evacuated through burr holes. Depressed skull fractures under lacerations should be elevated and debrided within 24 hours to minimize the risk of infection. Bony fragments and penetrating objects should not be manipulated in the emergency room, as they may be tamponading a lacerated vessel or dural sinus. Traumatic epidural hematoma is an infrequent complication of head injury, usually the result of an automobile accident. The initial injury tears middle meningeal vessels or dural sinuses and causes unconsciousness. When a spasm and clot occur in the vessel(s), the bleeding stops and the patient recovers, experiencing a lucid interval. Over the next several hours, the vessel bleeds and the patient rapidly deteriorates (especially with arterial bleeding). In rapidly deteriorating conditions, treatment should not be delayed pending radiologic evaluation. Emergency evacuation is necessary. Venous epidural hematomas develop more slowly, and there may be time for diagnostic testing. The clinical presentation of acute subdural hematomas ranges from minimal deficits to unconsciousness and signs of a mass lesion (hemiparesis, unilateral decerebration, and pupillary enlargement). A lucid interval may occur. The most common cause of subdural hematoma is trauma, but it may occur spontaneously and is associated with coagulopathies, aneurysms, and neoplasms. It is considered acute if the patient becomes symptomatic within 72 hours, subacute between 3–15 days, and chronic after 2 weeks. Subacute and chronic subdural hematoma are usually observed in patients over 50 years of age. A history of head trauma may be absent. The clinical presentation in these patients may vary from focal signs of brain dysfunction to a depressed level of consciousness or development of an organic brain syndrome. Intracranial hypertension is usually associated with acute subdural hematoma. Intensive medical therapy to correct elevated ICP and control brain edema and swelling may be required prior, during, and after hematoma evacuation. With intracerebral hematomas, the clinical picture may vary from minimal neurologic deficits to deep coma. Large, solitary intracerebral hematomas should be evacuated. Lesions causing delayed neurologic deterioration from fresh hemorrhage are also evacuated but carry a poor prognosis. Depending on the degree of cerebral injury, patients with intracerebral hematomas may require intensive medical therapy to control intracranial hypertension and cerebral edema. Coup and contracoup injuries usually cause cerebral contusion and intracerebral hemorrhage. In general, contused brain tissue is not removed; however, occasionally contused tissue over the frontal or temporal poles may be removed to control edema formation and prevent herniation.

Emergency Therapy

Before securing the airway in a head-injured patient, a quick assessment of the patient's neurologic status and concomitant injuries should be made. Fifteen percent of patients with severe head injury have an associated cervical spinal cord injury.[446] Therefore, unless a cervical spine fracture has been excluded by radiographic evaluation, cervical alignment by axial traction is necessary during emergent intubation. Facial fractures and soft tissue edema can pre-

TABLE 32-14. Glasgow Coma Scale[440,441]

Eye Opening

Spontaneous	4
To speech	3
To Pain	2
None	1

Best Verbal Response

Oriented	5
Confused	4
Inappropriate	3
Incomprehensible	2
None	1

Best Motor Response

Obeys commands	6
Localizes	5
Withdraws	4
Flexion	3
Extension	2
None	1

vent direct visualization of the larynx. In this situation, a fiberoptic intubation of the trachea or intubation with an illuminated stylet may be attempted. In the presence of severe facial or laryngeal injuries, a cricothyrotomy may be required. Nasal intubations are avoided in the presence of a suspected basal skull fracture, severe facial fractures, and bleeding diathesis. For patients without facial injuries, the simplest and most expeditious approach to intubation is preoxygenation followed by rapid sequence induction with cricoid pressure and maintenance of axial traction. All head-injured patients are assumed to have full stomachs. Awake, oral intubation without anesthetic agents may be possible in the severely injured patient, but this is difficult in the awake or uncooperative, combative patient. Depending on the patient's cardiovascular status, virtually any of the intravenous induction agents, except ketamine, can be used. The choice of muscle relaxants is controversial. Succinylcholine can increase ICP. In the setting of acute airway compromise, full stomach, and need to perform subsequent neurologic examinations, the benefits of rapid onset and termination of action of succinylcholine may outweigh the risk of transiently increasing ICP.

Following control of the airway in the head-injured patient, attention should focus on resuscitation of the cardiovascular system. Transient hypotension after head injury is not uncommon, but sustained hypotension usually results from hemorrhage secondary to other systemic injuries.[447] These injuries must be sought and aggressively treated. Traumatized brain is more vulnerable to secondary injury from hypotension and hypoxia than is normal brain.[448] Severe hypotension or shock is associated with an increase in morbidity and mortality.[447,449]

Circulating blood volume can be restored with either isotonic crystalloid or colloid solutions. Hypotonic solutions are more likely to increase brain water content than isotonic fluids such as 0.9% saline, 6% hydroxyethyl starch in 0.9% saline, and 5% albumin in 0.9% saline.[450,451] Since lactated Ringer's solution is slightly hypoosmolar, it may in large quantities contribute to edema formation.[450] In addition, large volumes (>500 ml) of 6% hydroxyethyl starch can cause coagulopathies. Substantial blood loss requires transfusion with crossmatched blood. A minimal hematocrit between 30–33% is recommended to maximize oxygen transport. The goal in the management of the hypotensive patient with head injury is to maintain the cerebral perfusion pressure between 60–120 mm Hg. When indicated, an ICP monitor is inserted to guide fluid resuscitation and prevent severe elevations in ICP.

Hypertension, tachycardia, and increased cardiac output often develop in patients with isolated head trauma, especially young adults.[452] Electrocardiographic abnormalities and fatal arrhythmias have been reported.[453] The hyperdynamic circulatory responses and ECG changes may result from a surge in epinephrine that accompanies head injury.[452,454] Both labetalol and esmolol can be used to control hypertension and tachycardia in this situation.

In some patients, severe intracranial hypertension precipitates reflex arterial hypertension and bradycardia (Cushing's triad). A reduction in systemic blood pressure in these patients can further aggravate cerebral ischemia by reducing cerebral perfusion pressure. Systemic blood pressure must be lowered cautiously when intracranial hypertension is severe. In such cases, a reduction of intracranial pressure may interrupt this reflex response.

Following stabilization of head-injured patients, including control of airway and systemic blood pressure, therapeutic interventions to control intracranial hypertension are

instituted. The head is elevated 15–20° and maintained in a neutral position without rotation or flexion. Hyperventilation to a $Paco_2$ of 25–30 mm Hg is a very rapid and effective intervention. Mannitol, 0.25–1 $g \cdot kg^{-1}$, may be given to lower ICP acutely, or a combination of furosemide and mannitol may be administered. Used together, furosemide and mannitol work synergistically, hastening the onset of ICP decrease and prolonging the effect of lower doses of mannitol.[455] Barbiturates are used to control ICP when other measures have failed.[456] Appropriate monitoring must be instituted and hypotension avoided.

Anesthetic Management

The patient is evaluated by CT scan and taken directly to the operating room. There is usually minimal time available for resuscitation and preanesthetic assessment. Information that should be obtained preoperatively is described in Table 32-15. The anesthetic management is a continuation of the initial resuscitation, including airway management, fluid and electrolyte balance, and ICP control. The routine monitors for major neurosurgical procedures are applied. Anesthetic management is directed at avoidance of secondary brain injury. Intraoperative hypotension secondary to blood loss or precipitated by anesthetic drugs should be avoided by appropriate volume expansion. Maintenance of ventilation ($Paco_2$ between 25 and 30 mm Hg) and oxygenation ($Pao_2 > 60$ mm Hg) is extremely important. Positive end-expiratory pressure may be used if necessary (5–10 cm H_2O does not adversely affect ICP).

Intraoperative brain swelling or herniation from the operative site may complicate hematoma decompression. Such causes as improper patient positioning, contralateral intracerebral hematoma, venous drainage obstruction from packing, and acute hydrocephalus from intraventricular hemorrhage must be eliminated. In this setting, the adequacy of hyperventilation must also be verified. A large alveolar-arterial CO_2 gradient may exist, so that end-tidal CO_2 may not reflect arterial CO_2. The respiratory system and equipment should be reviewed to ensure normal peak inspiratory and expiratory pressures. Hemopneumothorax, high intraabdominal pressures, a kinked endotracheal or expiratory tube, and a stuck expiratory valve can produce marked peak inspiratory or expiratory pressures as well as hypoxemia and hypercarbia. Fluid and electrolyte balance must be reevaluated in patients with cerebral swelling. Mannitol loses its effect after 1–3 hours, and it may be necessary to repeat the mannitol bolus to increase osmolarity. Volume overload and hyponatremia may also cause cerebral swelling and must be corrected. If cerebral swelling persists, the anesthetic should be converted to opioid and thiopental infusions with oxygen and air. Thiopental may be given in a

---

TABLE 32-15. Preanesthetic Assessment of the Head-Injured Patient

Airway (cervical spine)
Breathing: Ventilation and oxygenation
Circulatory status
Associated injuries
Neurologic status (Glasgow Coma Scale)
Preexisting chronic illness
Circumstances of the injury: time of injury, duration of unconsciousness, associated alcohol or drug use

---

series of boluses over 5–10 minutes to a total dose of 5–25 mg·kg^{-1}, followed by an infusion of 4–10 mg·kg^{-1}·h^{-1}. To avoid barbiturate-induced myocardial depression and hypotension, it may be necessary to increase preload and add a vasopressor such as dopamine. Malignant brain swelling may require removal of brain tissue and a temporary scalp closure with a loose dural patch to minimize ICP after closure.

Emergence from anesthesia usually involves transporting an intubated, ventilated, and anesthetized patient to the intensive care unit. Even in an uncomplicated craniotomy for evacuation of hematoma, a period of postoperative ventilation is recommended as brain swelling is maximal 12–72 hours after injury. Hypertension and coughing or bucking on the endotracheal tube should be avoided as this can lead to significant intracranial bleeding. Labetalol and esmolol can be used to treat hypertension, and supplemental barbiturates are given to sedate the patient.

Systemic Sequelae

The systemic effects of head injury are diverse and can complicate management.[457] These include cardiopulmonary problems (airway obstruction, hypoxemia, shock, adult respiratory distress syndrome, neurogenic pulmonary edema, electrocardiographic changes); hematologic problems (disseminated intravascular coagulation); endocrinologic problems (pituitary dysfunction, i.e., diabetes insipidus, syndrome of inappropriate ADH); metabolic problems (nonketotic hyperosmolar hyperglycemic coma); and gastrointestinal problems (stress ulcers, hemorrhage). Conditions not discussed elsewhere in this chapter will be reviewed.

Aspiration, pneumonia, fluid overload, and trauma-related adult respiratory distress syndrome are common causes of pulmonary dysfunction in head-injured patients. A fulminant pulmonary edema may also occur. Neurogenic pulmonary edema (NPE) is characterized by marked pulmonary vascular congestion, intraalveolar hemorrhage, and a protein-rich edema fluid. Specific features of this syndrome are its rapid onset, its relationship to hypothalamic lesions, and the ability to prevent or attenuate it by alpha-blockers and central nervous system depressants. Neurogenic pulmonary edema is thought to result from massive sympathetic discharge from injured brain secondary to intracranial hypertension. Traditional therapy for pulmonary edema of cardiac origin is ineffective, and the outcome is frequently fatal. Therapy is directed at reducing intracranial hypertension, providing supportive respiratory care, and blocking sympathetic hyperactivity.[458]

In head-injured patients, several clotting abnormalities may be present. Disseminated intravascular coagulation (DIC) has been reported after mild and severe brain trauma and anoxic brain damage, and it presumably develops following release of brain tissue thromboplastin into the systemic circulation.[459] Treatment of the underlying disease process usually results in spontaneous recovery of the coagulation defects. Occasionally, administration of cryoprecipitate, fresh frozen plasma, platelet concentrates, and blood may be required.

Anterior pituitary insufficiency following head injury is a rare occurrence. However, patients exhibiting posttraumatic diabetes insipidus may develop a delayed impairment of anterior pituitary hormones, requiring replacement therapy. Posterior pituitary dysfunction occurs more frequently following head trauma. Diabetes insipidus (DI) may occur following craniofacial trauma and basilar skull fractures. Its clinical presentation includes polyuria, polydipsia, hypernatremia, high-serum osmolality, and dilute urine. Frequently, posttraumatic DI is transient, and treatment is based on water replacement. If the patient cannot maintain fluid balance, exogenous vasopressin may be administered. The syndrome of inappropriate antidiuretic hormone (SIADH) secretion is associated with hyponatremia, serum and extracellular fluid hypoosmolality, and renal excretion of sodium, urine osmolality greater than serum osmolality, and normal renal and adrenal function. The patient develops symptoms and signs of water intoxication (anorexia, nausea, vomiting, irritability, personality changes, and neurologic abnormalities). SIADH secretion usually begins 3–15 days after trauma, lasting no more than 10–15 days with appropriate therapy. Treatment includes water restriction with or without hypertonic saline.

Many factors in neurosurgical patients predispose to nonketotic hyperosmolar hyperglycemic coma (NHHC) such as steroids, prolonged mannitol therapy, hyperosmolar tube feedings, phenytoin, and water restriction.[457] Diagnostic criteria for NHHC are hyperglycemia, glucosuria, absence of ketosis, plasma osmolality greater than 330 mOsm·kg^{-1}, dehydration, and central nervous system dysfunction. Hypovolemia and hypertonicity are the immediate threats to life. Serum sodium may be high, normal, or low, depending on the state of hydration. Serum potassium is low. Serial laboratory tests are essential. Once sodium deficits are replaced and blood pressure and urine output are stable, water deficits are replaced with 0.45% saline. Hyperglycemia usually responds to relatively small doses of insulin. Intermittent furosemide therapy may be given for cerebral edema prophylaxis in the elderly, the adult-onset diabetic, or the patient with compromised renal function.

REFERENCES

1. Aidley DJ: The Physiology of Excitable Cells. New York, Cambridge University Press, 1989
2. Hille B: Ionic Channels of Excitable Membranes. Sunderland, Massachusetts, Sinauer Associates, 1984
3. Cooper JR, Bloom FE, Roth RH: The Biochemical Basis of Neuropharmacology. New York, Oxford University Press, 1986
4. Kandel ER, Schwartz JH: Principles of Neural Science. New York, Elsevier, 1985
5. Siegel G, Agranoff B, Albers RW et al: Basic Neurochemistry. New York, Raven Press, 1989
6. Brunn-Meyer SE: The GABA/benzodiazepine receptor-chloride ionophore complex: Nature and modulation. Prog Neuropsychopharmacol Biol Psychiatry 11:365, 1987
7. Bormann J: Electrophysiology of GABAa and GABAb receptor subtypes. TINS 11:112, 1988
8. Watkins JC, Evans RH: Excitatory amino acid transmitters. Annu Rev Pharmacol Toxicol 21:165, 1981
9. Macdermott AB, Dale N: Receptors, ion channels and synaptic potentials underlying the integrative actions of excitatory amino acids. TINS 10:280, 1987
10. Kass IS, Chambers G, Cottrell JE: The n-methyl-d-aspartate antagonists aminophosphonovaleric acid and MK-801 reduce anoxic damage to dentate granule and CA 1 pyramidal cells in the rat hippocampal slice. Exp Neurol 103:116, 1989
11. Berridge MJ: Regulation of ion channels by inositol trisphosphate and diacylglycerol. J Exp Biol 124:323, 1986
12. Sokoloff L: Circulation and energy metabolism of the brain. In Basic Neurochemistry, p 565. New York, Raven Press, 1989
13. Lehninger AL: Principles of Biochemistry. New York, Worth Publishers, 1982
14. Siesjo BK: Cell damage in the brain: A speculative synthesis. J Cereb Blood Flow Metab 1:155, 1981

15. Hansen AJ: Effect of anoxia on ion distribution in the brain. Physiol Rev 65:101, 1985
16. Michenfelder JD: Anesthesia and the Brain, pp 23–55, 94–113. New York, Churchill Livingstone, 1988
17. Smith AL, Wollman H: Cerebral blood flow and metabolism: Effects of anesthetic drugs and techniques. Anesthesiology 36:378, 1972
18. Plum F, Siesjo BK: Recent advances in CSF physiology. Anesthesiology 42:708, 1975
19. Mihm FG, Cottrell JE, Hartung J et al: Cerebral damage and pharmacological intervention. In Newfield P, Cottrell JE (eds): Neuroanesthesia: Handbook of Clinical and Physiologic Essentials, p 59. Boston, Little, Brown and Co, 1991
20. Michenfelder JD: Cerebral blood flow and metabolism. In Cucchiara RF, Michenfelder JD (eds): Clinical Neuroanesthesia, p 1. New York, Churchill Livingstone, 1990
21. Greenfield, JC, Rembert JC, Tindall GT: Transient changes in cerebral vascular resistance during the Valsalva maneuver in man. Stroke 15:76, 1984
22. Lassen NA: Cerebral and spinal cord blood flow. In Cottrell JE, Turndorf H (eds): Anesthesia and Neurosurgery, p 1. St Louis, CV Mosby, 1986
23. Strandgaard S, Olesen J, Skinhoj E et al: Autoregulation of brain circulation in severe arterial hypertension. Br Med J 1:507, 1973
24. Bill A, Linden J, Linden M: Sympathetic effect on cerebral blood vessels in acute arteriole hypertension. Acta Physiol Scand 96:27A, 1976
25. Hochwald GM: Cerebrospinal fluid mechanisms. In Cottrell JE, Turndorf H (eds): Anesthesia and Neurosurgery, p 33. St Louis, CV Mosby, 1986
26. Artru AA: Cerebrospinal fluid dynamics. In Cucchiara RF, Michenfelder JD (eds). Clinical Neuroanesthesia, p 41. New York, Churchill Livingstone, 1990
27. Lundberg N: Monitoring of the intracranial pressure. In Critchley M, O'Leary JL, Jennett B (eds): Scientific Foundations of Neurology, p 356. Philadelphia, FA Davis, 1972
28. Miller JD, Garibi J, Pickard JD: The effects of induced changes of cerebrospinal fluid volume during continuous monitoring of ventricular pressure. Arch Neurol 28:265, 1973
29. Fishman RA: Brain edema. N Engl J Med 293:706, 1975
30. Siesjo BK: Cerebral circulation and metabolism. J Neurosurg 60:883, 1984
31. Wasterlain CG: Epileptic seizures. In Siegel G, Agranoff RW, Albers BW, et al (eds): Basic Neurochemistry, p 797. New York, Raven Press, 1989
32. Bruce DA: Management of severe head injury. In Cottrell JE, Turndorf H (eds): Anesthesia and Neurosurgery, p 150. St Louis, CV Mosby, 1986
33. Young W, Koreh I: Potassium and calcium changes in injured spinal cords. Brain Res 365:42, 1986
34. Hall ED, Wolf DL: A pharmacological analysis of the pathophysiologic mechanisms of posttraumatic spinal cord ischemia. J Neurosurg 64:951, 1986
35. Eintrei C, Leszniewski W, Carlson C: Local application of Xenon for measurement of regional cerebral blood flow during halothane enflurane and isoflurane anesthesia in humans. Anesthesiology 63:391, 1985
36. Boarini DJ, Kassel NF, Sprowell JA et al: Comparison of systemic and cerebrovascular effects of isoflurane and halothane. J Neurosurg 15:400, 1984
37. Todd MM, Drummond JC: A comparison of the cerebrovascular and metabolic effects of halothane and isoflurane in the cat. Anesthesiology 60:276, 1984
38. Weeks JB, Todd MM, Warner DS et al: The influence of halothane isoflurane and pentobarbital on cerebral plasma volume in hypocapnic and normocapnic rats. Anesthesiology 73:461, 1990
39. Michenfelder JD, Cucchiara RF: Canine cerebral oxygen consumption during enflurane anesthesia and its modification during induced seizures. Anesthesiology 40:575, 1974
40. Scheller MS, Tateishi A, Drummond JC et al: The effects of sevoflurane on cerebral blood flow, cerebral metabolic rate for oxygen, intracranial pressure, and the electroencephalogram

are similar to those of isoflurane in the rabbit. Anesthesiology 68:548, 1988
41. Lu GP, Gibson JA Jr, Frost EAM, et al: Cerebral vasodilating effect of sevoflurane vs isoflurane. Anesthesiology 73(3A): A625, 1990
42. Werner C, Kochs E, Hoffman WE et al: The effects of sevoflurane on neurological outcome from incomplete ischemia in rats. J Neurosurg Anesth 3(3):237, 1991
43. Lutz LJ, Milde JH, Milde LN: The cerebral functional, metabolic and hemodynamic effects of desflurane in dogs. Anesthesiology 73:125, 1990
44. Muzzi DA, Losasso TJ, Dietz NM et al: The effect of desflurane on cerebrospinal fluid pressure in neurosurgical patients. Anesthesiology 73(3A):A1215, 1990
45. Muzzi D, Daltner C, Losasso T et al: The effect of desflurane and isoflurane with N_2 on cerebrospinal fluid pressure in patients with supratentorial mass lesions. J Neurosurg Anesth 3(3):202, 1991
46. Pellegrino DA, Miletich DJ, Hoffman WE et al: Nitrous oxide markedly increases cerebral cortical metabolic rate and blood flow in the goat. Anesthesiology 60:405, 1984
47. Moss E, McDowall DG: ICP increases with 50 percent nitrous oxide in oxygen in severe head injuries during controlled ventilation. Br J Anaesth 51:757, 1979
48. Phirman JR, Shapiro HM: Modification of nitrous oxide induced intracranial hypertension by prior induction of anesthesia. Anesthesiology 46:150, 1977
49. Hoffman WE, Miletich DJ, Albrecht RF: The effects of midazolam on cerebral blood flow and oxygen consumption and its interaction with nitrous oxide. Anesth Analg 65:729, 1986
50. Sakabe T, Kuramoto T, Kumagae S et al: Cerebral responses to the addition of nitrous oxide to halothane in man. Br J Anaesth 48:957, 1976
51. Pierce EC, Lambertsen CJ, Deutsch S et al: Cerebral circulation and metabolism during thiopental anesthesia and hyperventilation in man. J Clin Invest 41:1664, 1964
52. Michenfelder JD: The interdependency of cerebral function and metabolic effects following massive doses of thiopental in the dog. Anesthesiology 41:231, 1974
53. Shapiro HM, Galindo A, Wyte SR et al: Rapid intraoperative reduction of intracranial pressure with thiopentone. Br J Anaesth 45:1057, 1973
54. Rockoff MA, Goudsouzian NG: Seizures induced by methohexital. Anesthesiology 54:333, 1981
55. Renou AM, Vernhiet J, Macrez P et al: Cerebral blood flow and metabolism during etomidate anesthesia in man. Br J Anaesth 50:1047, 1978
56. Milde LN, Milde JH, Michenfelder JD: Cerebral functional, metabolic, and hemodynamic effects of etomidate in dogs. Anesthesiology 63:371, 1985
57. Davis DW, Mans AM, Biebuyck JF et al: Regional brain glucose utilization in rats during etomidate anesthesia. Anesthesiology 64:751, 1986
58. Fragen KJ, Shanks CA, Molteni A et al: Effects of etomidate on hormonal responses to surgical stress. Anesthesiology 61:652, 1984
59. Dam M, Ori C, Pizzolato G et al: The effects of Propofol anesthesia on local cerebral glucose utilization in the rat. Anesthesiology 73:499, 1990
60. Van Hemelrijck J, Fitch W, Mattheussen M et al: Effect of propofol on cerebral circulation and autoregulation in the baboon. Anesth Analg 71:49, 1990
61. Pinaud M, Lelausque J-N, Chetanneau A et al: Effects of propofol on cerebral hemodynamics and metabolism in patients with brain trauma. Anesthesiology 73:404, 1990
62. Nugent M, Artru AA, Michenfelder JD: Cerebral metabolic, vascular, and protective effects of midazolam maleate: Comparison to diazepam. Anesthesiology 56:172, 1982
63. Forster A, Juge O, Morel D: Effects of midazolam on cerebral blood flow. Anesthesiology 56:453, 1982
64. Fleischer JE, Milde JH, Moyer TP et al: Cerebral effects of high-dose midazolam and subsequent reversal with RO-1788 in dogs. Anesthesiology 68:234, 1988
65. Jobes DR, Kennell EM, Bush GL et al: Cerebral blood flow

and metabolism during morphine-nitrous oxide anesthesia in man. Anesthesiology 47:16, 1977

66. Vernhiet J, Renou AM, Orgogozo JM et al: Effects of diazepam fentanyl mixture on cerebral blood flow and oxygen consumption in man. Br J Anaesth 50:165, 1978

67. Drummond JC, Shapiro HM: Cerebral Physiology. In Miller RD (ed). Anesthesia. New York, Churchill Livingstone, 1990

68. Murkin JM, Farrar JK, Tweed WA: Sufentanil anaesthesia reduces cerebral blood flow and cerebral oxygen consumption. Can J Anaesth 35:S131, 1988

69. Young WL, Prohovnik I, Correll JW et al: A comparison of the cerebral hemodynamic effects of sufentanil and isoflurane in humans undergoing carotid endarterectomy. Anesthesiology 71:863, 1989

70. Milde LN, Milde JH, Gallagher WJ: Effects of sufentanil on cerebral circulation and metabolism in dogs. Anesth Analg 70:138, 1990

71. Marx W, Shah N, Long C et al: Sufentanil, alfentanil, and fentanyl: Impact on cerebrospinal fluid pressure in patients with brain tumors. J Neurosurg Anesth 1:3, 1989

72. Lutz LJ, Milde JH, Milde LN: Cerebral effects of alfentanil in dogs with reduced intracranial compliance. J Neurosurg Anesth 1:169, 1989

73. Jung R, Free K, Shah N et al: Cerebrospinal fluid pressure in anesthetized patients with brain tumors: Impact of fentanyl vs alfentanil. J Neurosurg Anesth 1:136, 1989

74. Davis DW, Mans AM, Biebuyck JF et al: The influence of ketamine on regional brain glucose use. Anesthesiology 69:199, 1988

75. Takeshita H, Okuda Y, Sari A: The effects of ketamine on cerebral circulation and metabolism in man. Anesthesiology 36:69, 1972

76. Cavazutti M, Porro CA, Biral GP et al: Ketamine effects on local cerebral blood flow and metabolism in the rat. J Cereb Blood Flow Metab 7:806, 1987

77. Busto R, Globus M, Dietrich WD et al: Effect of mild hypothermia on ischemia-induced release of neurotransmitters and free fatty acids in rat brain. Stroke 26(7):904, 1989

78. Hoffman WE, Werner C, Baughman VL et al: Post-ischemic treatment with hypothermia improves outcome from incomplete cerebral ischemia in rats. J Neurosurg Anesth 3(1):34, 1990

79. Hochachka PW: Defense strategies against hypoxia and hypothermia. Science 231:234, 1986

80. Nussmeier NA, Arlund C, Slogoff S: Neuropsychiatric complications after cardiopulmonary bypass: Cerebral protection by a barbiturate. Anesthesiology 64:165, 1986

81. Spetzler RF, Martin N, Hadley MN et al: Microsurgical endarterectomy under barbiturate protection: A prospective study. J Neurosurg 65:63, 1986

82. Hicks RG, Kern DR, Horton DA: Thiopental and cerebral protection under EEG control during carotid endarterectomy. Anaesth Intensive Care 14(1):22, 1986

83. Levin AB, Duff TA, Javid MJ: Treatment of increased intracranial pressure. A comparison of different hypersomotic agents and the use of thiopental. J Neurosurg 5(5):570, 1979

84. Lawner PM, Simeone FA: Treatment of intraoperative middle cerebral artery occlusion with pentobarbital and extracranial-intracranial bypass. Case report. J Neurosurg 51(5):710, 1979

85. Spetzler RF, Selman WR, Roski RA et al: Cerebral revascularization during barbiturate coma in primates and humans. Surg Neurol 17(2):111, 1982

86. Sokoll MD, Kassell NF, Davies LR: Large dose thiopental anesthesia for intracranial aneurysm surgery. J Neurosurg 10(5):555, 1982

87. Markowitz IP, Adinolfi MF, Kerstein MD: Barbiturate therapy in the postoperative endarterectomy patient with a neurologic deficit. Am J Surg 148:221, 1984

88. McMeniman WJ, Fletcher JP, Little JM: Experience with barbiturate therapy for cerebral protection during carotid endarterectomy. Ann R Coll Surg Engl 66:361, 1984

89. Bendtson AO, Cold GE, Astrup J: Thiopental loading during controlled hypotension for intracranial aneurysm surgery. Acta Anaesthesiol Scand 28:473, 1984

90. Zaidan JR, Klochany A, Martin WM et al: Effect of thiopental on neurologic outcome following coronary artery bypass grafting. Anesthesiology 74:406, 1991

91. Todd MM, Hindman BJ, Warner DS: Barbiturate protection and cardiac surgery: A different result. Anesthesiology 74(3):402, 1991

92. Marshall LF, Smith RW, Shapiro HM: The outcome with aggressive treatment in severe head injuries. Part II: Acute and chronic barbiturate administration in the management of head injury. J Neurosurg 50(1):26, 1979

93. Marshall LF, Shapiro HM et al: Pentobarbital therapy for intracranial hypertension and metabolic coma in Reyes' syndrome. Crit Care Med 6(1):1, 1978

94. Branston NM, Hope T, Symon L: Barbiturates in focal ischemia of primate cortex: Effects on blood flow distribution, evoked potential, and extracellular potassium. Stroke 10(6):647, 1979

95. Kofke WA, Nemoto EM, Hossman KA: Brain blood flow and metabolism after global ischemia and post insult thiopental therapy in monkeys. Stroke 10(5):554, 1979

96. Blaustein MP, Ector AC: Barbiturate inhibition of calcium uptake by depolarized nerve terminals in vitro. Mol Pharmacol 11:369, 1975

97. Leslie SW, Friedman MB, Wilcox RE et al: Acute and chronic effects of barbiturates on depolarization-induced calcium influx into rat synaptosomes. Brain Res 185:409, 1980

98. Demopoulos HE, Flamm ES, Pietronigro DD et al: Free radical pathology and antioxidants in regional cerebral ischemia and central nervous system trauma. In Cottrell JE, Turndorf H (eds): Anesthesia and Neurosurgery, pp 246–279. St Louis, CV Mosby, 1986

99. Smith DS, Margue JJ: Inhibitory effects of different barbiturates on lipid peroxidation in brain tissue in vitro: Comparison with the effects of promethazine and chlorpromazine. Anesthesiology 53(3):186, 1980

100. Olson JJ: Cerebral radioprotection by pentobarbital: Dose-response characteristics and association with GABA agonist activity. J Neurosurg 72(5):749, 1990

101. Smith AL: Anesthetics and cerebral edema. Anesthesiology 45:64, 1976

102. Clasen RA, Pandolfii S, Casey D: Furosemide and pentobarbital in cryogenic cerebral injury and edema. Neurology 24:642, 1974

103. Frenkel C, Duch DS, Urban BW: Molecular actions of pentobarbital isomers on sodium channels from human brain cortex. Anesthesiology 72:640, 1990

104. Abramowicz AE, Kass IS, Cottrell JC: Thiopental attenuates anoxia-induced Na and K concentration changes in the rat hippocampal slice (abstract). Anesthesiology 73(3A), 1990

105. Brain Resuscitation Clinical Trial I Study Group: Randomized clinical study of thiopental loading in comatose survivors of cardiac arrest. N Engl J Med 314(7):397, 1986

106. Foster A, Juge O, Morel D: Effects of midazolam on cerebral blood flow in human volunteers. Anesthesiology 56:453, 1982

107. Hoffman WE: Benzodiazepines and antagonists: Effects on ischemia. J Neurosurg Anesthesiol 1(3):272, 1989

108. Abramowicz AE, Kass IS, Chambers G et al: Midazolam improves electrophysiologic recovery after anoxia and reduces changes in ATP levels and calcium influx during anoxia in the rat hippocampal slice. Anesthesiology 74:1121, 1991

109. Baughman VL, Hoffman WE, Miletich DJ et al: Cerebral metabolic depression and brain protection produced by midazolam and etomidate in the rat. J Neurosurg Anesthesiol 1(1):22, 1989

110. Rosenberg RB, Kass IS, Cottrell JC: Propofol improves electrophysiologic recovery after anoxia in the rat hippocampal slice (abstract). Anesthesiology 75(3A), 1991

111. Gelmers HJ, Gorter K, De Weerdt CJ: A controlled trial of nimodipine in acute ischemic stroke. N Engl J Med 318(4):203, 1988

112. Petruk K, West M, Mohr G: Nimodipine treatment in poor-grade aneurysm patients: Results of a multicenter double-blind placebo-controlled trial. J Neurosurg 68:505, 1988

113. Roine RO, Kaste M, Kinnunen A et al: Nimodipine after resus-

citation from out-of-hospital ventricular fibrillation: A placebo-controlled, double-blind, randomized trial. JAMA 264 (24):3171, 1990

114. Allen GS, Ahn HS, Preziosi TJ: Cerebral arterial spasm—A controlled trial of nimodipine in patients with subarachnoid hemorrhage. N Engl J Med 308(11):619, 1983

115. Kass IS, Cottrell JE, Chambers G: Magnesium and cobalt, not nimodipine, protect neurons against anoxic damage in the rat hippocampal slice. Anesthesiology 69:710, 1989

116. Heiss WD, Holthoff V, Pawlik G: Effect of nimodipine on regional cerebral glucose metabolism in patients with acute ischemic stroke as measured by positron emission tomography. J Cereb Blood Flow Metab 10(1):127, 1990

117. De Ryck M: Animal models of cerebral stroke: Pharmacological protection of function. Eur Neurol 30(Suppl 2):21, 1990

118. Borgers M: Effects of Ca2⁺-entry blockers on ischemic brain. J Neurosurg Anesthesiol 1(4):368, 1989

119. Sakabe T: Calcium entry blockers in cerebral resuscitation. Magnesium 8:238, 1989

120. Brain Resuscitation Clinical Trial II Study Group: A randomized clinical study of a calcium-entry blocker (lidoflazine) in the treatment of comatose survivors of cardiac arrest. N Engl J Med 324(18):1225, 1991

121. Plum F: Vulnerability of the brain and heart after cardiac arrest (editorial). N Engl J Med 324(18):1278, 1991

122. Warner DS: Magnesium and the injured brain. J Neurosur Anesthiol 1(4):360, 1989

123. Sustch G, Rubinstein EH: Minor effect of lidocaine on brain electrical recovery after 5 minutes of almost complete cerebral ischemia in the rabbit. J Neurosurg Anesthesiol 3(1):39, 1991

124. Rasool N, Faroqui F, Rubinstein EH: Lidocaine accelerates neuroelectrical recovery after incomplete global ischemia in rabbits. Stroke 21:929, 1990

125. Sutsch G, Rubinstein EH: Lidocaine accelerates recovery of brain electrical activity after 3 minutes of complete ischemia in the rabbit. J Neurosurg Anesthesiol 3(2):124, 1991

126. Artru AA, Michenfelder JD: Cerebral protective, metabolic, and vascular effects of phenytoin. Stroke 11:377, 1980

127. Gelb AW: Local anesthetics in cerebral ischemia. J Neurosurg Anesthesiol 1(4):383, 1989

128. Choi DW: NMDA antagonists and hypoxic neuronal injury. J Neurosurg Anesthesiol 1(4):357, 1989

129. Collins RC, Dobkin BH, Choi DW: Selective vulnerability of the brain. New insights into the pathophysiology of stroke. Ann Intern Med 110:992, 1989

130. Koh JY, Goldberg MP, Hartley DM et al: Non-NMDA receptor-medicated neurotoxicity in cortical culture. J Neurosci 10(2): 693, 1990

131. Papagapiou MP, Auer RN: Regional neuroprotective effects of the NMDA receptor antagonist MK-801 (Dizocilipine) in hypoglycemic brain damage. J Cereb Blood Flow Metab 10: 270, 1990

132. Uematsu D, Araki N, Greenberg JH et al: Combined therapy with MK-801 and nimodipine for protection of ischemic brain damage. Neurology 41:88, 1991

133. Kass IS, Chambers G, Cottrell JE: The N-methyl-D-aspartate antagonists aminophosphonovaleric acid and MK-801 reduce anoxic damage to dentate granule and CAI pyramidal cells in the rat hippocampal slice. Exper Neurol 103:116, 1989

134. Corbett D, Evans S, Thomas C: MK-801 reduced cerebral ischemic injury by inducing hypothermia. Brain Res 514:300, 1990

135. Gill R, Woodruff GN: The neuroprotective actions of kynurenic acid and MK-801 in gerbils are synergistic and not related to hypothermia. Eur J Pharm 176:143, 1990

136. Sheardown MJ, Nielsen EO, Hansen PJ et al: 2,3-Dihydroxy-6-nitro-7-sulfamoyl-benzo(F)quinoxaline: A neuroprotectant for cerebral ischemia. Science 247:571, 1990

137. Grotta JC, Picone CM, Ostrow PT: CGS-19755, a competitive NMDA receptor antagonist, reduces calcium-calmodulin binding and improves outcome after global cerebral ischemia. Ann Neurol 27(6):612, 1990

138. Jastremski M, Sutton-Tyrell K, Vaagenes P: Glucocorticoid treatment does not improve neurological recovery following cardiac arrest. JAMA 262(24):3427, 1989

139. Bracken MB, Shepard MJ, Collins WF: A randomized, controlled trial of methylprednisolone or naloxone in the treatment of acute spinal-cord injury. N Engl J Med 322(20):1405, 1990

140. Acosta D, Kass IS, Cottrell JE: Effect of a-Tocopherol and free radicals on anoxic damage in the rat hippocampal slice. Exp Neurol 97:607, 1987

141. Suzyki J, Fujimoto S, Mizoi K et al: The protective effect of combined administration of anti-oxidants and perflurochemicals on cerebral ischemia. Stroke 15:672, 1984

142. Natale JE, Schott RJ, Hall ED et al: The 21-aminosteroid U74006F reduces systemic lipid peroxidation, improves neurologic functions, and reduces mortality after cardiopulmonary arrest in dogs. Prog Clin Biol Res 308:391, 1989

143. Zuccarello M, Marsch JT, Schmitt G et al: Effect of the 21-aminosteroid U-74006F on cerebral vasospasm following subarachnoid hemorrhage. J Neurosurg 71:98, 1989

144. Young W, Wojak JC, DeCrescito V: 21-Aminosteroid reduces ion shifts and edema in the rat middle cerebral artery occlusion model of regional ischemia. Stroke 19:1013, 1988

145. Aoki N, Lefer AM: Protective effects of a novel nonglucocorticoid 21-Aminosteroid (U74006F) during traumatic shock in rats. J Cardiovasc Pharmacol 15:205, 1990

146. Hall ED, Travis MA: Inhibition of arachidonic acid-induced vasogenic brain edema by the non-glucocorticoid 21-aminosteroid U74006F. Brain Res 451:350, 1988

147. Hoffman WE, Prekezes C: The 21-aminosteroid does not markedly improve outcome from incomplete ischemia in the rat. J Neurosurg Anesthesiol 3(2):96, 1991

148. Pereira BM, Chan PH, Weinstein J et al: Cerebral protection during reperfusion with superoxide dismutase in focial cerebral ischemia. Adv Neurol 52:97, 1990

149. Martz D, Beer M, Betz L: Dimethylthiourea reduces ischemic brain edema without affecting cerebral blood flow. J Cereb Blood Flow Metab 10:352, 1990

150. Gotti B, Benavides J, Mackenzie ET et al: The pharmacotherapy of focal cortical ischemia in the mouse. Brain Res 522:290, 1990

151. Ginsberg M: The potential of combination pharmacotherapy in cerebral ischemia. In Kriegelstein K, Oberpichler H (eds): Pharmacology of Cerebral Ischemia, pp 499–510. Stuttgart, Wissenschaftliche Verlagsgesellschaft mbH, 1990

152. Spinnewyn B, Blavet N, Clostre F et al: Involvement of platelet activating factor (PAF) in cerebral post-ischemic phase on mongolian gerbils. Prostaglandins 34:337, 1987

153. Bielenberg GW, Wagener G: Infarct reduction by PAF-antagonists after MCA occlusion in the rat. J Cereb Blood Flow Metab 9(1):S274, 1989

154. Oberpichler H, Sauer Dirk, Robberg C et al: PAF-antagonist, gink golide B, reduces post-ischemic neuronal damage in rat brain hippocampus. J Cereb Blood Flow Metab 10:133, 1990

155. Duverger D, Spinnewyn B, Blavet N et al: Systemic administration of a PAF-antagonist, BN50739, protects against cerebral ischemia. In Kriegelstein J, Oberpichler H (eds): Pharmacology of Cerebral Ischemia, pp 409–413. Stuttgart: Wissenschaftliche Verlagsgesellschaft mbH, 1990

156. Lindvall O, Brudin P, Widner H et al: Grafts of fetal dopamine neurons survive and improve motor function in Parkinson's disease. Science 247:574, 1990

157. Skaper SD, Leon A, Toffanno G: Neuroplasticity and repair following injury to the central nervous system. J Neurosurg Anesth 1(4):377, 1989

158. Kuhlengel KR, Bunge MB, Burton H: Implantation of cultured sensory neurons and schwann cells into lesioned neonatal rat spinal cord: Implant characteristics and examination of corticospinal tract growth. Comp Neurol 293(1):74, 1990

159. Ronnett GV, Hester LD, Nye JS et al: Human cortical neuronal cell line: Establishment from a patient with unilateral megaloencephaly. Science 248:603, 1990

160. Kiloh LG, McComas AJ, Osselton JW et al: The neural basis of the EEG. In Kiloh LG, McComas AJ, and Osselton JW (eds):

Clinical Electroencephalography, 4th ed, p 24. London, Butterworth Publishers, 1981

161. Scott JC, Ponaganis KV, Stanski DR: EEG quantification of narcotic effect: The comparative pharmacodynamics of fentanyl and alfentanil. Anesthesiology 62:234, 1985

162. Michenfelder JD, Cucchiara RF: Canine cerebral oxygen consumption during enflurane anesthesia and its modification during induced seizures. Anesthesiology 40:575, 1974

163. Woodbury DM, Rollins LT, Gardner MD et al: Effects of carbon dioxide on brain excitability and electrolytes. Am J Physiol 192:79, 1958

164. Levy WJ: Quantitative analysis of EEG changes during hypothermia. Anesthesiology 60:291, 1984

165. Moruzzi G, Magoun HW: Brain stem reticular formation and activation of the EEG. Electroencephalogr Clin Neurophysiol 1:455, 1949

166. Stockard JJ, Bickford RG: The neurophysiology of anesthesia. In Gordon E (ed): A Basis and Practice of Neuroanesthesia, 2nd ed, pp 3–49. Amsterdam, Elsevier, 1981

167. Trojaborg W, Boysen G: Relation between EEG, regional cerebral blood flow and internal carotid artery pressure during carotid endarterectomy. Electroencephalogr Clin Neurophysiol 34:61, 1973

168. Rampil IJ, Holzer JA, Quest DO et al: Prognostic value of computerized EEG analysis during carotid endarterectomy. Anesth Analg 62:186, 1983

169. Hugelin A, Bonvallet M, Dell P: Activation reticulaire et corticule d'origine chemoceptive au cours de l'hypoxie. Electroencephalogr Clin Neurophysiol 11:325, 1959

170. Flemming DC, Fitzpatrick J, Fariello RG et al: Diagnostic activation of epileptogenic foci by enflurane. Anesthesiology 52:431, 1980

171. Gancher S, Laxer KD, Krieger W: Activation of epileptogenic activity by etomidate. Anesthesiology 61:616, 1984

172. Musella L, Wilder BJ, Schmidt RP: Electroencephalographic activation with intravenous methohexital in psychomotor epilepsy. Neurology 21:594, 1971

173. Chiappa KH, Burke SR, Young RR: Results of electroencephalographic monitoring during 376 endarterectomies: Use of a dedicated minicomputer. Stroke 10:381, 1979

174. Rampil IJ, Matteo RS: Changes in spectral edge frequency correlate with the hemodynamic response to laryngoscopy and intubation. Anesthesiology 67:139, 1987

175. Levy WJ, Shapiro HM, Maruchak G et al: Automated EEG processing for intraoperative monitoring: A comparison of techniques. Anesthesiology 53:223, 1980

176. Spackman TN, Faust RJ, Cucchiara RF et al: A comparison of a periodic analysis of the EEG with standard EEG and cerebral blood for detection of ischemia. Anesthesiology 66:229, 1987

177. Peterson DO, Drummond JC, Todd MM: Effects of halothane, enflurane, isoflurane and nitrous oxide on somatosensory evoked potentials in humans. Anesthesiology 65:35, 1986

178. Pathak KS, Amaddio BS, Scoles PV et al: Effects of halothane, enflurane, and isoflurane in nitrous oxide on multi-somatosensory evoked potentials. Anesthesiology 70:207, 1989

179. McPherson RW, Mahla M, Johnson R et al: Effects of enflurane, isoflurane, and nitrous oxide on somatosensory evoked potentials during fentanyl anesthesia. Anesthesiology 62:626, 1985

180. Domino EF, Corssen G, Sweet RB: Effects of various general anesthetics on the visually evoked response in man. Anesth Analg 42:735, 1963

181. Burchiel KG, Stockard JJ, Myers RR et al: Visual and auditory evoked responses during enflurane anesthesia in man and cats. Electroencephalogr Clin Neurophysiol 39:434P, 1973

182. Uhl RR, Squires KC, Bruce DL, Starr A: Effect of halothane anesthesia on the human cortical visual evoked response. Anesthesiology 53:273, 1980

183. Chi OZ, Field C: Effects of isoflurane on visual evoked potentials in humans. Anesthesiology 65:328, 1986

184. Sloan TB, Koht A: Depression of cortical somatosensory evoked potentials by nitrous oxide. Br J Anaesth 57:849, 1985

185. Sebel PS, Flynn PJ, Ingram DA: Effect of nitrous oxide on visual, auditory and somatosensory evoked potentials. Br J Anaesth 56:1403, 1984

186. Dubois MY, Sato S, Chassy T et al: Effects of enflurane on brainstem auditory evoked responses in humans. Anesth Analg 61:898, 1982

187. Manninen PH, Lam AM, Nicholas JP: The effects of isoflurane and isoflurane-nitrous oxide anesthesia on brainstem auditory evoked potentials in humans. Anesth Analg 64:43, 1985

188. Thornton C, Heneghan CPH, James MFM et al: Effects of halothane or enflurane with controlled ventilation on auditory evoked potentials. Br J Anaesth 56:315, 1984

189. McPherson RW, Sell B, Traystman RJ: Effects of thiopental, fentanyl and etomidate on upper extremity somatosensory evoked potentials in humans. Anesthesiology 65:584, 1986

190. Drummond JC, Todd MM, Sang H: The effect of high dose sodium thiopental on brainstem auditory and median nerve somatosensory evoked responses in humans. Anesthesiology 63:249, 1985

191. Sutton LN, Frewen T, Marsh R et al: The effects of deep barbiturate coma on multimodality evoked potentials. J Neurosurg 57:178, 1982

192. Koht A, Schütz W, Schmidt G et al: Effects of etomidate, midazolam, and thiopental on median nerve somatosensory evoked potentials and the additive effects of fentanyl and nitrous oxide. Anesth Analg 67:435, 1988

193. Thornton C, Heneghan CPH, Navaratnarajah M et al: Effect of etomidate on the auditory evoked response in man. Br J Anaesth 57:554, 1985

194. Grundy BL, Brown RH, Greenberg BA: Diazepam alters cortical potentials. Anesthesiology 51:538, 1979

195. Maurette P, Simeon F, Castagnera L et al: Propofol anaesthesia alters somatosensory evoked cortical potentials. Anaesthesia 43:44, 1988

196. Savoia G, Esposito C, Belfiore F et al: Propofol infusion and auditory evoked potentials. Anaesthesia 43:46, 1988

197. Pathak KS, Brown RH, Cascorbi HF et al: Effects of fentanyl and morphine on intraoperative somatosensory cortical-evoked potentials. Anesth Analg 63:833, 1984

198. Schubert A, Peterson DO, Drummond JC et al: The effect of high-dose fentanyl on human median nerve somatosensory evoked responses. Anesth Analg 65:S136, 1986

199. Samra SK, Lilly DJ, Rush NL et al: Fentanyl anesthesia and human brainstem auditory evoked potentials. Anesthesiology 61:261, 1984

200. Grundy BL, McPhail J, Bottoms C et al: Effect of hypothermia on somatosensory evoked potentials during cardiopulmonary bypass (abstract). Electroencephalogr Clin Neurophysiol 58:41P, 1984

201. Stockard JJ, Sharbrough FW, Tinker JA: Effects of hypothermia on the human brainstem auditory response. Ann Neurol 3:368, 1978

202. Dubois M, Coppola R, Buchsbaum MS et al: Somatosensory evoked potentials during whole body hyperthermia in humans. Electroencephalogr Clin Neurophysiol 52:157, 1981

203. Eng DY, Dong WK, Bledsoe SW et al: Electrical and pathologic correlates of brain hypoxia during hypotension. Anesthesiology 53:S92, 1980

204. Kobrine AI, Evans DE, Rizzoli AH: Relative vulnerability of the brain and spinal cord to ischemia. J Neurol Sci 45:65, 1980

205. Grundy BL, Nash CL, Brown RH: Arterial pressure manipulation alters spinal cord function during correction of scoliosis. Anesthesiology 54:249, 1981

206. Nakagawa Y, Ohtsuka T, Tsura M et al: Effects of mild hypercapnia on somatosensory evoked potentials in experimental cerebral ischemia. Stroke 25:275, 1984

207. Grundy BL, Heros RC, Tung AS et al: Interoperative hypoxia detected by evoked potential monitoring. Anesth Analg 60:437, 1981

208. Nagao S, Roccaforte P, Moody RA: The effects of isovolemic hemodilution and reinfusion of packed erythrocytes on somatosensory and visual evoked potentials. J Surg Res 25:530, 1978

209. Levy WJ, York DH, McCaffrey M et al: Motor evoked poten-

tials from transcranial stimulation of the motor cortex in humans. Neurosurgery 15:287, 1984

210. Maccabee PJ, Amassian VE, Cracco RQ et al: Stimulation of the human nervous system using the magnetic coil. J Clin Neurophysiol 8:38, 1991

211. Agnew WF, McCreery DB: Considerations for safety in the use of extracranial stimulation for motor evoked potentials. Neurosurgery 20:143, 1987

212. Tung HC, Drummond JC, Bickford RG: The effects of anesthetic and sedative agents on magnetic motor evoked responses (abstract). Anesthesiology 69:A313, 1988

213. Ghaly RF, Stone JL, Levy WJ et al: The effect of an anesthetic induction dose of midazolam on motor potentials evoked by transcranial magnetic stimulation in the monkey. J Neurosurg Anesthesiol 3:20, 1991

214. Zentner J, Ebner A: Nitrous oxide suppresses the electromyographic response evoked by electrical stimulation of the motor cortex. Neurosurgery 24:60, 1989

215. Ghaly RF, Stone JL, Levy WJ et al: The effect of nitrous oxide on transcranial magnetic-induced electromyographic responses in the monkey. J Neurosurg Anesthesiol 2:175, 1980

216. Ghaly RF, Stone JL, Aldrete A et al: Effects of incremental ketamine hydrochloride doses on motor evoked potentials (MEPs) following transcranial magnetic stimulation: A primate study. J Neurosurg Anesthesiol 2:79, 1990

217. Ghaly RF, Stone JL, Levy WJ et al: The effect of etomidate on motor evoked potentials induced by transcranial magnetic stimulation in the monkey. Neurosurgery 27:936, 1990

218. Lundberg N: Continuous recording and control of ventricular fluid pressure in neurosurgical practice. Acta Psychiatr Neurol Scand 36(Suppl 149):1, 1960

219. Shapiro HM, Wyte SR, Harris AB et al: Acute intraoperative intracranial hypertension in neurosurgical patients: Mechanical and pharmacologic factors. Anesthesiology 37:399, 1972

220. Leech P, Barker J, Fitch W: Changes in intracranial pressure and systemic arterial pressure during termination of anesthesia. Br J Anaesth 46:315, 1974

221. Palmer MA, Perry JF Jr, Fischer RP et al: Intracranial pressure monitoring in the acute neurologic assessment of multiinjured patients. J Trauma 19:497, 1979

222. Lobato RD, Rivas JJ, Portillo JM et al: Prognostic value of the intracranial pressure levels during the acute phase of severe head injuries. Acta Neurochir [Suppl] 28:70, 1979

223. Marshall LF, Smith RW, Shapiro HM: The outcome with aggressive treatment in severe head injuries. Part 1: The significance of intracranial pressure monitoring. J Neurosurg 50:20, 1979

224. Saul TG, Ducker TB: Effect of intracranial pressure monitoring and aggressive treatment on mortality in severe head injury. J Neurosurg 56:498, 1982

225. Uzzell BP, Obrist WD, Dolinskas CA et al: Relationship of acute CBF and ICP findings to neuropsychological outcome in severe head injury. J Neurosurg 65:630, 1986

226. Rosner MJ, Becker DP: ICP monitoring: Complications and associated factors. Clin Neurosurg 23:494, 1976

227. Narayan RK, Pulla RS, Kishore MD et al: Intracranial pressure: To monitor or not to monitor? J Neurosurg 56:650, 1982

228. Vries JK, Becker DP, Young HF: A subarachnoid screw for monitoring intracranial pressure. J Neurosurg 39:416, 1973

229. Koster WG, Kuypers MH: Intracranial pressure and its epidural measurement. Med Prog Technol 7:21, 1980

230. Numoto M, Slater JP, Donaghy RMP: An implantable switch for monitoring intracranial pressure. Lancet 1:578, 1966

231. Ostrup RC, Luersson TG, Marshall LF et al: Continuous monitoring of intracranial pressure with a miniaturized fiberoptic device. J Neurosurg 67:206, 1987

232. Crutchfield JS, Narayan RK, Robertson CS et al: Evaluation of a fiberoptic intracranial pressure monitor. J Neurosurg 72:482, 1990

233. Bunegin L, Albin MS, Rauschhuber R et al: Intracranial pressure measurement from the anterior fontanelle utilizing a pneumoelectronic switch. Neurosurgery 20:726, 1987

234. Rochefort MJ, Rolfe P, Wilkinson AR: New fontanometer for continuous estimation of intracranial pressure in the newborn. Arch Dis Child 62:152, 1987

235. Hounsfield GN: Computerized transverse axial scanning (tomography): Part I. Description of system. Br J Radiol 46:1016, 1973

236. Perry BJ, Bridges C: Computerized transverse axial scanning (tomography): Part III. Radiation dose considerations. Br J Radiol 46:1048, 1973

237. Stark DD, Bradley WG: Magnetic resonance imaging. St Louis, CV Mosby, 1988

238. McCullough EC, Baker HL Jr: Nuclear magnetic resonance imaging. Radiol Clin North Am 20:3, 1982

239. McGinnis BD, Brady TJ, New PFJ: Nuclear magnetic resonance imaging of tumors in the posterior fossa. J Comput Assist Tomogr 7:575, 1983

240. Geiger RS, Cascorbi HF: Anesthesia in an NMR scanner. Anesth Analg 63:622, 1984

241. Dunn V, Coffman CE, McGowan JE et al: Mechanical ventilation during magnetic resonance imaging. Magn Res Imaging 3:169, 1985

242. Roth JL, Nugent M, Gray JE: Patient monitoring during magnetic resonance imaging. Anesthesiology 62:80, 1985

243. Barnett GH, Ropper AH, Johnson KA: Physiologic support and monitoring of critically ill patients during magnetic resonance imaging. J Neurosurg 68:246, 1988

244. Saunders RD, Smith H: Safety aspects of NMR clinical imaging. Br Med Bull 40:148, 1984

245. Dallas SH, Moxen CP: Controlled ventilation for cerebral angiography. Br J Anaesth 41:597, 1969

246. Edmonds-Seal J, du Bonley G, Bostick T: The effect of intermittent positive pressure ventilation upon cerebral angiography with special reference to the quality of the films—A preliminary communication. Br J Radiol 40:957, 1967

247. Junck L, Marshall WH: Neurotoxicity of radiologic contrast agents. Ann Neurol 13:469, 1983

248. Numaguchi Y, Fleming MS, Hasao K et al: Blood brain barrier disruption due to cerebral arteriography: CT findings. J Comput Assist Tomogr 8:936, 1984

249. Margolis G, Tarazi AK, Grimson KS: Contrast medium injury to the spinal cord produced by aortography: Pathologic anatomy of the experimental lesion. J Neurosurg 13:349, 1956

250. Margolis G, Tindall GT, Phillips RL et al: Evaluation of roentgen contrast agents used in cerebral arteriography: I. A simple screening method. J Neurosurg 15:30, 1958

251. Olin T: Adverse reactions to intravascularly administered contrast media. Acta Radiol [Diagn] (Stockh) 27:257, 1986

252. Shehadi WH: Adverse reactions to intravascularly administered contrast media: A comprehensive study based on a prospective survey. Am J Roentgenol Radium Ther Nucl Med 124:145, 1975

253. Greenberger PA, Patterson R, Tapio CM: Prophylaxis against repeated radiocontrast media reactions in 857 cases. Arch Intern Med 145:2197, 1985

254. Lasser EC, Berry CC, Talner LB et al: Pretreatment with corticosteroids to alleviate reaction to intravenous contrast material. N Engl J Med 317:845, 1987

255. Tabaddor K, Danziger A, Whisoff HS: Estimation of intracranial pressure by CT scan in closed head trauma. Surg Neurol 18:212, 1982

256. Kullberg G, Sundberg G: ICP and CSF absorption impairment after subarachnoid hemorrhage, pp 224–227. Berlin, Springer-Verlag, 1980

257. Shenkin HA, Bezier HS, Bonzarth WF: Restricted fluid intake: Rational management of the neurosurgical patient. J Neurosurg 45:432, 1976

258. Jelsma LF, McQueen JD: Effect of experimental water restriction on brain water. J Neurosurg 26:35, 1967

259. Sieber FE, Smith DS, Traystman RJ et al: Glucose: A reevaluation of its intraoperative use. Anesthesiology 67:72, 1987

260. Pulsinelli WA, Waldman S, Rawlinson D et al: Moderate hyperglycemia augments ischemic brain damage: A neuropathologic study in the rat. Neurology 32:1239, 1982

261. Pulsinelli WA, Levy DE, Sigsbee B et al: Increased damage after ischemic stroke in patients with hyperglycemia with or without established diabetes mellitus. Am J Med 74:540, 1983

262. Lanier W, Strangland KJ, Scheithauer BW et al: The effects of dextrose infusion and head position on neurologic outcome after complete cerebral ischemia in primates: Examination of a model. Anesthesiology 66:39, 1987

263. Welsh FA, Ginsberg MD, Rieder W et al: Deleterious effect of glucose pretreatment on recovery from diffuse cerebral ischemia in the cat. II. Regional metabolite levels. Stroke 11:355, 1980

264. Marshall LF, Smith RW, Rauscher LA et al: Mannitol requirements in brain-injured patients. J Neurosurg 48:169, 1978

265. Muizelaar JP, Lutz HA III, Becker DP: Effect of mannitol on ICP and CBF and correlation with pressure autoregulation in severely head-injured patients. J Neurosurg 61:700, 1984

266. Hooshang H, Dove J, Houff S et al: Effects of diuretics and steroids on CSF pressure. Arch Neurol 21:499, 1969

267. Ravussin P, Abou-Madi M, Archer D et al: Changes in CSF pressure after mannitol in patients with and without elevated CSF pressure. J Neurosurg 69:869, 1988

268. Cote CJ, Greenhow DE, Marshall BE: The hypotensive response to rapid intravenous administration of hypertonic solutions in man and in the rabbit. Anesthesiology 50:30, 1979

269. Domaingue CM, Nye DH: Hypotensive effect of mannitol administered rapidly. Anaesth Intensive Care 13:134, 1985

270. Domer FR: Effects of diuretics on cerebrospinal fluid formation and potassium movement. Exp Neurol 24:54, 1969

271. Cottrell JE, Robustelli A, Post K et al: Furosemide- and mannitol-induced changes in intracranial pressure and serum osmolality and electrolytes. Anesthesiology 47:28, 1977

272. Clasen RA, Pandolfi S, Casey D: Furosemide and pentobarbital in cryogenic cerebral injury and edema. Neurology 24:642, 1974

273. Schettini A, Stahurski B, Young HF: Osmotic and osmotic loop diuresis in brain surgery: Effects on plasma and CSF electrolytes and ion excretion. J Neurosurg 56:679, 1982

274. Galicich JH, French LA: Use of dexamethasone in the treatment of brain tumors and brain surgery. Am Proc 12:169, 1961

275. Miller JD, Sakalas R, Ward JD et al: Methylprednisolone treatment in patients with brain tumors. Neurosurgery 1:114, 1977

276. Bouzarth WF, Shenkin HA: Possible mechanisms of action of dexamethasone in brain injury. J Trauma 14:134, 1974

277. Bruce JN, Criscuob GR, Merrill MJ et al: Vascular permeability induced by protein product of malignant brain tumors: Inhibition by dexamethasone. J Neurosurg 67:880, 1987

278. Shapiro HM: Intracranial hypertension. Anesthesiology 43:449, 1975

279. Shapiro HM, Marshall LF: Intracranial pressure responses to PEEP in head-injured patients. J Trauma 18:254, 1978

280. Cooper KR, Boswell PA, Choi SC: Safe use of PEEP in patients with severe head injury. J Neurosurg 63:552, 1985

281. Smith SL, Albin MS, Ritter RR et al: CVP catheter placement from the antecutibal veins using a J-wire catheter guide. Anesthesiology 60:238, 1984

282. Lanier WL, Milde JH, Michenfelder JD: Cerebral stimulation following succinylcholine in dogs. Anesthesiology 64:551, 1986

283. Lanier WL, Iaizzo PA, Milde JH: Cerebral function and muscle afferent activity following i.v. succinylcholine in dogs anesthetized with halothane: The effects of pretreatment with defasciculating doses of pancuronium. Anesthesiology 71:87, 1989

284. Minton MD, Grosslight KR, Stirt JA et al: Increases in intracranial pressure from succinylcholine: Prevention by prior nondepolarizing blockade. Anesthesiology 65:165, 1986

285. Stirt JA, Grosslight KR, Bedford RF et al: "Defasciculation" with metocurine prevents succinylcholine-induced increases in intracranial pressure. Anesthesiology 67:50, 1987

286. Cooperman LH, Strobel GE, Kennal EM: Massive hyperkalemia after administration of succinylcholine. Anesthesiology 32:161, 1970

287. Thomas ET: Circulatory collapse following succinylcholine: Report of a case. Anesth Analg 48:333, 1969

288. Stevenson PH, Birch AA: Succinylcholine-induced hyperkalemia in a patient with a closed head injury. Anesthesiology 51:89, 1979

289. Iwatsuki N, Kuroder H, Ameha K et al: Succinylcholine-induced hyperkalemia in patients with ruptured cerebral aneurysm. Anesthesiology 53:64, 1980

290. Edvinsson L, Mackenzie ET: Amine mechanisms in the cerebral circulation. Pharmacol Rev 28:275, 1977

291. Vesely R, Hoffman WE, Gil KS et al: The cerebrovascular effects of curare and histamine in the rat. Anesthesiology 66:519, 1987

292. Minton MD, Stirt JA, Bedford RF et al: Intracranial pressure after atracurium in neurosurgical patients. Anesth Analg 64:1113, 1985

293. Rosa G, Orfei P, Sanfilippo M et al: The effects of atracurium besylate (Tracrium®) on intracranial pressure and cerebral perfusion pressure. Anesth Analg 65:381, 1986

294. Standaert FG: Magic bullets, science, and medicine. Anesthesiology 63:577, 1985

295. Hennis PJ, Fahey MR, Canfell PC et al: Pharmacology of laudanosine in dogs. Anesthesiology 65:56, 1986

296. McLeskey CH, Cullen BF, Kennedy RD et al: Control of cerebral perfusion pressure during induction of anesthesia in high-risk neurosurgical patients. Anesth Analg 53:985, 1974

297. Lanier WL, Milde JH, Michenfelder JD: The cerebral effects of pancuronium and atracurium in halothane-anesthetized dogs. Anesthesiology 63:589, 1985

298. Stirt JA, Maggio W, Haworth C et al: Vecuronium: Effect on intracranial pressure and hemodynamics in neurosurgical patients. Anesthesiology 67:570, 1987

299. Ginsberg B, Glass PS, Quill T et al: Onset and duration of neuromuscular blockade following high-dose vecuronium administration. Anesthesiology 71:201, 1989

300. Toboada JA, Rupp SM, Miller RD: Refining the priming principle for vecuronium. Anesthesiology 64:243, 1986

301. Hammil JF, Bedford RF, Weaver DC et al: Lidocaine before endotracheal intubation: Intravenous or laryngotracheal. Anesthesiology 55:578, 1981

302. Cucchiara RF, Benefiel DJ, Matteo RS et al: Evaluation of esmolol in controlling increases in heart rate and blood pressure during tracheal intubation. Anesthesiology 65:528, 1986

303. Leech P, Barker J, Fitch W: Changes in intracranial pressure and systemic arterial pressure during termination of anesthesia. Br J Anaesth 46:315, 1974

304. Young TJK, McPherson RW, Ahn H: Pneumocephalus: Effect of patient position on the incidence of aerocele after posterior fossa surgery. Anesth Analg 65:65, 1986

305. Artru AA: Nitrous oxide plays a direct role in the development of tension pneumocephalus intraoperatively. Anesthesiology 57:59, 1982

306. Ellis SC, Bryan-Brown CW, Hyderally H: Massive swelling of the head and neck. Anesthesiology 42:102, 1975

307. Wilder BL: Hypothesis: The etiology of midcervical quadriplegia after operation with the patient in the sitting position. Neurosurgery 11:530, 1982

308. McPherson RW, Szymanski T, Rogers MC: Somatosensory evoked potential changes in position related brainstem ischemia. Anesthesiology 61:88, 1984

309. Grundy BL, Procopio PT, Janetta PJ: Evoked potential changes produced by positioning for retromastoid craniectomy. Neurosurgery 10:766, 1982

310. Black S, Ockert DB, Oliver WC et al: Outcome following posterior fossa craniectomy in patients in the sitting or horizontal positions. Anesthesiology 69:49, 1988

311. Perkins-Pearson NAK, Marshall WK, Bedford RF: Atrial pressures in the seated position: Implications for paradoxical air embolism. Anesthesiology 57:493, 1982

312. Matjasko J, Petrozza P, Mackenzie CF: Sensitivity of end-tidal nitrogen in venous air embolism detection in dogs. Anesthesiology 63:418, 1985

313. Cucchiara RF, Nugent M, Seward JB et al: Air embolism in

upright neurosurgical patients: Detection and localization by two-dimensional echocardiography. Anesthesiology 60:353, 1984

314. Drummond JC, Prutow RJ, Scheller MS: A comparison of the sensitivity of pulmonary artery pressure, end-tidal carbon dioxide, and end-tidal nitrogen in the detection of venous air embolism in the dog. Anesth Analg 64:688, 1985

315. Albin MS, Babinski M, Maroon JC et al: Anesthetic management of posterior fossa surgery in the sitting position. Acta Anaesthesiol Scand 20:117, 1976

316. Bunegin L, Albin MS, Helsel PE et al: Positioning the right atrial catheter: A model for reappraisal. Anesthesiology 55:343, 1981

317. Colohan ART, Perkins NAK, Bedford RF et al: Intravenous fluid loading as prophylaxis for paradoxical air embolism. J Neurosurg 62:839, 1985

318. Albin MS, Babinski M, Wolf S: Cardiovascular responses to the sitting position. Br J Anaesth 52:1961, 1980

319. Marshall WK, Bedford RF, Miller ED: Cardiovascular responses in the seated position—Impact of four anesthetic techniques. Anesth Analg 62:648, 1983

320. Artru AA, Cucchiara RF, Messick JM: Cardiorespiratory and cranial nerve sequelae of surgical procedures involving the posterior fossa. Anesthesiology 52:83, 1980

321. Randall RV: Clinical presentation of pituitary adenomas. In Laws ER, Randall RV, Kern EB et al (eds): Management of Pituitary Adenomas and Related Lesions with Emphasis on Transsphenoidal Surgery, p 15. New York, Appleton-Century-Crofts, 1982

322. Kohler J: Clinical Endocrinology. New York, John Wiley & Sons, 1986

323. Kitahata LM: Airway difficulties associated with anaesthesia in acromegaly. Br J Anaesth 43:1187, 1971

324. Hassan SZ, Matz GJ, Lawrence AM et al: Laryngeal stenosis in acromegaly: A possible cause of airway difficulties associated with anesthesia. Anesth Analg 55:57, 1976

325. Messick JM, Laws ER, Abbond CF: Anesthesia for transsphenoidal surgery of the hypophyseal region. Anesth Analg 57:206, 1978

326. Newfield P, Albin MS, Chestnut JS et al: Air embolism during transsphenoidal pituitary operations. Neurosurgery 2:39, 1978

327. Laws ER, Kern EB: Complications of transsphenoidal surgery. In Laws ER, Randall RV, Kern RB et al (eds): Management of Pituitary Adenomas and Related Lesions with Emphasis on Transsphenoidal Surgery, p 329. New York, Appleton-Century-Crofts, 1982

328. Kassell NF, Torner JC: Epidemiology of intracranial aneurysms, anesthetic considerations in the surgical repair of intracranial aneurysms. In Varkey GP (ed): International Anesthesiology Clinics. Boston, vol 20, p 89. Little, Brown and Co, 1982

329. Boarini DJ, Kassell NF: Cerebral aneurysm management: Neurologic aspects. In Cottrell JE, Turndorf H (eds): Anesthesia and Neurosurgery, 2nd ed, p 407. St Louis, CV Mosby, 1986

330. Suzuki J, Hori S, Sakurai Y: Intracranial aneurysms in the neurosurgical clinics in Japan. J Neurosurg 35:34, 1971

331. Botterell EH, Longhead WM, Scott JW et al: Hypothermia and interruption of the carotid or carotid and vertebral circulation in the surgical management of intracranial aneurysms. J Neurosurg 13:1, 1956

332. Hunt WE, Hess RM: Surgical risk as related to time of intervention in the repair of intracranial aneurysms. J Neurosurg 28:14, 1968

333. Sekkar LN, Heros RC: Origin, growth, and rupture of saccular aneurysms: A review. Neurosurgery 8:248, 1981

334. Leblanc R: The minor leak preceding subarachnoid hemorrhage. J Neurosurg 66:35, 1987

335. Heros RC, Kistler JP: Intracranial arterial aneurysm—An update. Stroke 14:628, 1983

336. Kassell NF, Torner JC: Aneurysmal rebleeding: A preliminary report from the Cooperative Aneurysm Study. J Neurosurg 13:479, 1983

337. Kassell NF, Torner JC, Adams HP: Antifibrinolytic therapy in the acute period following aneurysmal subarachnoid hemorrhage. J Neurosurg 61:225, 1984

338. Vermeulen M, Lindsay KW, Murray GD et al: Antifibrinolytic treatment in subarachnoid hemorrhage. N Engl J Med 311:432, 1984

339. Adams HP, Kassell NF, Torner JC et al: Predicting cerebral ischemia after aneurysmal subarachnoid hemorrhage: Influences of clinical condition, CT results and antifibrinolytic therapy. A report of the Cooperative Aneurysm Study. Neurology 37:1586, 1987

340. Kassell NF, Sasaki T, Colohan ART et al: Cerebral vasospasm following aneurysmal subarachnoid hemorrhage. Stroke 16:562, 1985

341. Hughes JT, Schianchi PM: Cerebral artery spasm: A histological study at necropsy of the blood vessels in cases of subarachnoid hemorrhage. J Neurosurg 48:515, 1981

342. Peerless SJ, Kassell NF, Kometsu K et al: Cerebral vasospasm: Acute proliferative vasculopathy? II. Morphology. In Wilkins RH (ed): Cerebral Arterial Spasm: Proceeding of the Second International Workshop, p 88. Baltimore, Williams & Wilkins, 1980

343. Kistler JP, Crowell RM, Davis KR et al: The relation of cerebral vasospasm to the extent and reaction of subarachnoid blood visualized by CT scan. A prospective study. Neurology (New York) 33:424, 1983

344. Wilkins RH: Attempts at prevention or treatment of intracranial arterial spasm: An update. Neurosurgery 18:808, 1986

345. Allen GS, Ahn HS, Preziosi TJ et al: Cerebral arterial spasm—A controlled trial of nimodipine in patients with subarachnoid hemorrhage. N Engl J Med 308:619, 1983

346. Zabramski J, Spetzler RF, Bonstelle C: Chronic cerebral vasospasm: Effect of calcium antagonists. Neurosurgery 19:129, 1986

347. Germano IM, Bartkowski HM, Cassel ME et al: The therapeutic value of nimodipine in experimental focal cerebral ischemia. J Neurosurg 67:81, 1987

348. Stullken EH, Balestrieri FJ, Prough DS et al: The hemodynamic effects of nimodipine in patients anesthetized for cerebral aneurysm clipping. Anesthesiology 62:346, 1985

349. Kassell NF, Peerless SJ, Durward QJ et al: Treatment of ischemic deficits from vasospasm with intravascular volume expansion and induced arterial hypertension. Neurosurgery 11:337, 1982

350. Kee DB, Wood JH: Rheology of the cerebral circulation. Neurosurgery 15:125, 1984

351. Awad IA, Carter P, Spetzler RF et al: Clinical vasospasm after subarachnoid hemorrhage: Response to hypervolemia, hemodilution and arterial hypertension. Stroke 18:365, 1987

352. Ljunggren B, Brandt L, Kagstrom E et al: Results of early operations for ruptured aneurysms. J Neurosurg 54:473, 1981

353. Suzuki J, Onuma T, Yoshimoto T: Results of early operation on cerebral aneurysms. Surg Neurol 11:407, 1979

354. Samson DS, Hodosh RM, Reid WR et al: Risk of intracranial aneurysm surgery in the good grade patient: Early versus late operation. Neurosurgery 5:522, 1979

355. Kassell NF, Torner JC, Jane JA et al: The International Cooperative Study on the timing of aneurysm surgery. J Neurosurg 73:37, 1990

356. Debros FM, Sundaram P: Preanesthetic evaluation. In Varkey, GP (ed): Anesthetic Considerations in the Surgical Repair of Intracranial Aneurysms. International Anesthesiology Clinics, vol 20(2), p 71. Boston, Little, Brown and Co, 1982

357. Wilkins RH: Hypothalamic dysfunction and intracranial arterial spasm. Surg Neurol 4:472, 1975

358. Benedict GR, Loach AB: Clinical significance of plasma adrenaline and nor-adrenaline in patients with subarachnoid hemorrhage. J Neurol Neurosurg Psychiatry 41:113, 1978

359. Takaku A, Shindo K, Tanaka S et al: Fluid and electrolyte disturbances in patients with intracranial aneurysms. Surg Neurol 11:349, 1979

360. Nelson PB, Seif SM, Maroon JC et al: Hyponatremia in intracranial disease: Perhaps not the syndrome of inappropriate

secretion of antidiuretic hormone (SIADH). J Neurosurg 55:938, 1981

361. Newman M, Reves JG, McKay RD: Cardiovascular therapy. In Newfield P, Cottrell JE (eds): Neuroanesthesia: Handbook of Clinical and Physiologic Essentials, 2nd ed, pp 129–160. Boston, Little, Brown and Co, 1991

362. Cruickshank JM, Neil-Dwyer G, Brice J: Electrocardiographic changes and their prognostic significance in subarachnoid hemorrhage. J Neurol Neurosurg Psychiatry 37:755, 1974

363. Offerhause L, van Gool J: Electrocardiographic changes and tissue catecholamines in experimental subarachnoid hemorrhage. Cardiovasc Res 3:433, 1969

364. Doshi R, Neil-Dwyer G: Hypothalamic and myocardial lesion after subarachnoid hemorrhage. J Neurol Neurosurg Psychiatry 40:821, 1977

365. Rudehill A, Gordon E, Sundquist K et al: A study of ECG abnormalities and myocardial specific enzymes in patients with subarachnoid hemorrhage. Acta Anaesthesiol Scand 26:344, 1982

366. Batjer H, Samson D: Intraoperative aneurysmal rupture: Incidence, outcome, and suggestions for surgical management. Neurosurgery 18:701, 1986

367. Ferguson G: Physical factors in the initiation, growth, and rupture of human intracranial aneurysms. J Neurosurg 3:666, 1972

368. Jones TH, Chiappa KH, Young RR et al: EEG monitoring for induced hypotension for surgery of intracranial aneurysms. Stroke 10:292, 1979

369. Friedman WA, Kaplan BL, Day AL et al: Evoked potential monitoring during aneurysm operation: Observations after fifty cases. Neurosurgery 20:678, 1987

370. Sullivan HG, Keenan RL, Isrow L et al: The critical importance of PaCO₂ during intracranial aneurysm surgery. J Neurosurg 52:426, 1980

371. Jabre A, Symon L: Temporary vascular occlusion during aneurysm surgery. Surg Neurol 27:47, 1987

372. Drake CG: Arteriovenous malformations of the brain: The options for management. N Engl J Med 309:308, 1983

373. Graf CJ, Perret GE, Torner JC: Bleeding from cerebral arteriovenous malformations as part of their natural history. J Neurosurg 58:331, 1983

374. Brown RD, Wiebers DO, Forbes G et al: The natural history of unruptured intracranial arteriovenous malformations. J Neurosurg 68:352, 1988

375. Drake CG: Cerebral arteriovenous malformations: Considerations for and experience with surgical treatment in 166 cases. Clin Neurosurg 26:145, 1979

376. O'Mahony BJ, Bolsin SNC: Anaesthesia for closed embolization of cerebral arteriovenous malformations. Anaesth Intensive Care 16:318, 1988

377. Brian JE, Eleff S, McPherson RW: Immediate hemodynamic management following subarachnoid hemorrhage during embolization of cerebral vascular abnormalities. J Neurosurg Anesth 1:63, 1989

378. Marshall LF, Hoi SU: Treatment of massive intraoperative brain swelling. Neurosurgery 13:412, 1983

379. Griffiths HWC, Gillies J: Thoracolumbar splanchnicectomy and sympathectomy: Anesthetic procedure. Anaesthesia 3:134, 1948

380. Greene NM: Hypotensive spinal anesthesia. Surg Gynecol Obstet 95:331, 1952

381. Donald JR: Induced hypotension and blood loss during surgery. J R Soc Med 75:149, 1982

382. Miller ED Jr: Deliberate hypotension. In Miller RD (ed): Anesthesia, 2nd ed, pp 1949–1970. New York, Churchill Livingstone, 1986

383. Michenfelder JD: Forward. In Varkey GP (ed): Anesthetic Considerations in the Surgical Repair of Intracranial Aneurysms, pp xiii–xiv. Boston, Little, Brown, and Co, 1982

384. Dahlgren BE, Gordon E, Steiner L: Evaluation of controlled hypotension during surgery for intracranial arterial aneurysms. Excerpta Medica Int Congress Series 200:1232, 1968

385. Adams JH, Brierley JB, Conner RCR: The effect of systemic

hypotension upon the human brain: Clinical and neuropathological observations in 11 cases. Brain 89:235, 1966

386. Eckenhoff JE, Lesch M: Deliberate hypotension—A devil's advocate analysis. In Eckenhoff JE (ed): Controversy in Anesthesia, pp 105–113. Philadelphia, WB Saunders, 1979

387. O'Mahony BJ, Bolsin SN: Anaesthesia for closed embolisation of cerebral arteriovenous malformations. Anaesth Intensive Care 16:318, 1988

388. Shapiro HM: Neurosurgical anesthesia and intracranial hypertension. In Miller RD (ed): Anesthesia, 2nd ed, pp 1563–1620. New York, Churchill Livingstone, 1986

389. Harp JR, Wollman H: Cerebral metabolic effects of hyperventilation and deliberate hypotension. Br J Anaesth 45:256, 1973

390. Casthely PA, Lear S, Cottrell JE et al: Intrapulmonary shunting during induced hypotension. Anesth Analg 61:231, 1982

391. Cottrell JE, Illner P, Kittay MJ et al: Rebound hypertension after sodium nitroprusside-induced hypotension. Clin Pharmacol Ther 27:32, 1980

392. Davies DW, Kadar D, Steward DJ et al: A sudden death associated with the use of sodium nitroprusside for induction of hypotension during anesthesia. Can Anaesth Soc J 22:547, 1975

393. Mehta P, Mehta J, Miale TD: Nitroprusside lowers platelet count. N Engl J Med 299:1134, 1978

394. Hines R, Barash PG: Infusion of sodium nitroprusside induces platelet dysfunction in vitro. Anesthesiology 70:611, 1989

395. Michenfelder JD, Theye RA: Canine systemic and cerebral effects of hypotension induced by hemorrhage, trimethaphan, halothane, or nitroprusside. Anesthesiology 46:188, 1977

396. Michenfelder JD, Tinker JH: Cyanide toxicity and thiosulfate protection during chronic administration of sodium nitroprusside in the dog. Anesthesiology 47:441, 1977

397. Endrich B, Franke N, Peter K et al: Induced hypotension: Action of sodium nitroprusside and nitroglycerin on the microcirculation. A micropuncture investigation. Anesthesiology 66:605, 1987

398. Woodside J Jr, Garner L, Bedford RJ: Captopril reduces the dose requirement for sodium nitroprusside induced hypotension. Anesthesiology 60:413, 1984

399. Miller R, Toth C, Silva DA: Nitroprusside versus a nitroprusside-trimethaphan mixture: A comparison of dosage requirements and hemodynamic effects during induced hypotension for neurosurgery. Mt Sinai J Med (NY) 54(4):308, 1987

400. Michenfelder JD, Milde JH: The interaction of sodium nitroprusside, hypotension, and isoflurane in determining cerebral vasculature effects. Anesthesiology 69:870, 1988

401. Cottrell JE, Patel KP, Ransohoff JR: Intracranial pressure changes induced by sodium nitroprusside in patients with intracranial mass lesions. J Neurosurg 48:329, 1978

402. Pinaud M, Souron R, Lelausque JN et al: Cerebral blood flow and cerebral oxygen consumption during nitroprusside-induced hypotension to less than 50 mm Hg. Anesthesiology 70:255, 1989

403. Wood M, Hyman S, Wood AJJ: A clinical study of sensitivity to sodium nitroprusside during controlled hypotensive anesthesia in young and elderly patients. Anesth Analg 66:132, 1987

404. Mason DT, Zelis R, Amsterdam EA: Actions of the nitrates on the peripheral circulation and myocardial oxygen consumption: Significance in the relief of angina pectoris. Chest 59:296, 1971

405. Cottrell JE, Gupta B, Rappaport H et al: Intracranial pressure during nitroglycerin-induced hypotension. J Neurosurg 53:309, 1980

406. Maktabi M, Warner D, Sokoll M: Comparison of nitroprusside, nitroglycerin, and deep isoflurane for induced hypotension. J Neurosurg 19:350, 1986

407. Hauss J, Schonleben K, Spiegel H et al: Nitroprusside- and nitroglycerin-induced hypotension: Effects on hemodynamics and on the microcirculation. World J Surg 6:241, 1982

408. Franke N, Endrich B, un Messmer K: Veranderungen der Mikrozirkulation bei Gabe von Natriumnitroprussid und Nitroglycerin. Schweiz Med Wochenschr 111:1017, 1981

409. Ivankovitch AD, Miletich DJ, Tinker JH: Nitroprusside and other short acting hypotensive agents. Int Anesthesiol Clin 16(2):132, 1978

410. Stoyka WW, Schutz H: The cerebral response to sodium nitroprusside and trimethaphan controlled hypotension. Can Anaesth Soc J 22:275, 1975

411. Karlin AD, Hartung J, Cottrell JE: Rate of induction of hypotension with trimethaphan modifies the intracranial pressure response in cats. Br J Anaesth 61:161, 1988

412. Cottrell JE, Van Aken H, Gupta B et al: Induced hypotension. In Cottrell JE, Turndoff H (eds): Anesthesia and Neurosurgery, 2nd ed, pp 418–443. St Louis, CV Mosby, 1986

413. Wilton NCT, Tait AR, Kling TF et al: The effect of trimethaphan-induced hypotension on canine spinal cord blood flow: Measurement at different cord levels using radiolabelled microspheres. Spine 13:490, 1988

414. Milde LN, Milde JH: Cerebral and systemic hemodynamic and metabolic effects of desflurane-induced hypotension in dogs. Anesthesiology 74:513, 1991

415. Artru AA: Enflurane causes a prolonged and reversible increase in the rate of CSF fluid in the dog. Anesthesiology 57:255, 1982

416. Lam AM, Gelb AW: Cardiovascular effects of isoflurane-induced hypotension for cerebral aneurysm surgery. Anesth Analg 62:742, 1983

417. Macnab MSP, Manninen PH, Lam AM et al: The stress response to induced hypotension for cerebral aneurysm surgery: A comparison of two hypotensive techniques. Can Anaesth Soc J 35(2):111, 1988

418. Reiz S, Balfors E, Bredgaard M: Coronary hemodynamic effects of general anesthesia and surgery. Regional Anesth [Suppl] 7:S8–S18, 1982

419. Madsen, JB, Cold GE, Hansen ES: Cerebral blood flow and metabolism during isoflurane-induced hypotension in patients subjected to surgery for cerebral aneurysms. Br J Anaesth 59:1204, 1987

420. Bendo AA, Kass IS, Cottrell JE: Comparison of the protective effect of thiopental and isoflurane against damage in the rat hippocampal slice. Brain Res 403:136, 1987

421. Nehls DG, Todd MM, Spetzler RF et al: A comparison of the cerebral protective effects of isoflurane and barbiturates during temporary focal ischemia in primates. Anesthesiology 66:453, 1987

422. Van Aken H, Fitch W, Graham DI: Cardiovascular and cerebrovascular effects of isoflurane-induced hypotension in the baboon. Anesth Analg 65:565, 1986

423. Gelb AW, Boisvert DP, Tang C et al: Primate brain tolerance to temporary focal cerebral ischemia during isoflurane- or sodium nitroprusside-induced hypotension. Anesthesiology 70:678, 1989

424. Numajiri Y, Mokuji T, Kagami K: ATP induced hypotensive anesthesia during prosthetic hip surgery (in Japanese). J Clin Anesthesiol 3:279, 1979

425. Owall A, Jarnberg PO, Brodin LA et al: Effects of adenosine-induced hypotension on myocardial hemodynamics and metabolism in fentanyl anesthetized patients with peripheral vascular disease. Anesthesiology 68:416, 1988

426. Owall A, Lagerkranser M, Sollevi A: Effects of adenosine-induced hypotension on myocardial hemodynamics and metabolism during cerebral aneurysm surgery. Anesth Analg 67:228, 1988

427. Van Aken H, Puchstein C, Anger C et al: Changes in intracranial pressure and compliance during adenosine triphosphage-induced hypotension in dogs. Anesth Analg 63:381, 1984

428. Lagerkranser M, Bergstrand G, Gordon E et al: Cerebral blood flow and metabolism during adenosine-induced hypotension in patients undergoing cerebral aneurysm surgery. Acta Anaesthiol Scand 33:15, 1989

429. Ornstein E, Matteo RS, Weinstein JA et al: A controlled trial of esmolol for the induction of deliberate hypotension. J Clin Anesth 1:31, 1988

430. Edmonson R, Del Valle O, Shah N et al: Esmolol for potentia-tion of nitroprusside-induced hypotension: Impact on the cardiovascular, adrenergic, and renin-angiotensin systems in man. Anesth Analg 69:202, 1989

431. Ornstein E, Young WL, Ostapkovich N et al: Deliberate hypotension in patients with intracranial arteriovenous malformations: Esmolol compared with isoflurane and sodium nitroprusside. Anesth Analg 72:639, 1991

432. Cope DHP, Crawford MC: Labetalol in controlled hypotension. Br J Anaesth 51:1, 1979

433. Van Aken H, Puchstein C, Schweppe ML et al: Effect of labetalol on intracranial pressure in dogs with and without intracranial hypertension. Acta Anesth Scand 26:615, 1982

434. Klauber MR, Barrett-Connor E, Marshall LF et al: The epidemiology of head injury: A prospective study of an entire community. San Diego County, California, 1978. Am J Epidemiol 5:500, 1981

435. Miller JD: Assessing patients with head injury. Br J Surg 77:241, 1990

436. Kurtzke JF: The current neurologic burden of illness and injury in the United States. Neurology 32:1207, 1982

437. Kalsbeek WD, McLaurin RL, Harris BSG III et al: The national head and spinal cord injury survey: Major findings. J Neurosurg 53:S19, 1980

438. Jennett B, McMillan R: Epidemiology of head injury. Br Med J 282:101, 1981

439. Alberico AM: Outcome after severe head injury. J Neurosurg 67:648, 1987

440. Teasdale G, Jennett B: Assessment of coma and impaired consciousness: A practical scale. Lancet 2:81, 1974

441. Jennett B: Assessment of the severity of head injury. J Neurol Neurosurg Psychiatry 39:647, 1976

442. Jennett B, Bend M: Assessment of outcome after severe brain damage: A practical scale. Lancet 1:480, 1975

443. Gennarelli TA, Spielman GM, Langfitt TW et al: Influence of the type of intracranial lesions on outcome from severe head injury—A multicenter study using a new classification system. J Neurosurg 56:26, 1982

444. Berger MS, Pitts LH, Lovely M et al: Outcome from severe head injury in children and adolescents. J Neurosurg 62:194, 1985

445. Luerssen T, Klauber M, Marshall LF: Outcome from head injury related to patient's age. J Neurosurg 68:409, 1988

446. Heiden JS, Weiss MH, Rosenberg AW et al: Management of cervical spinal cord trauma in Southern California. J Neurosurg 43:732, 1975

447. Miller JD: Head injury and brain ischemia: Implications for therapy. Br J Anaesth 57:120, 1985

448. Jenkins LW, Marmarou A, Lewett W et al: Increased vulnerability of the traumatized brain to early ischemia. In Baethmann A, Go GK, Unterberg A (eds): Mechanisms of Secondary Brain Damage, p 273. New York, Plenum Publishing, 1986

449. Newfield P, Pitts LH, Kaktis JV: The influence of shock on mortality after head trauma (abstract). Crit Care Med 8:254, 1980

450. Tommasino C, Moore S, Todd MM: Cerebral effects of isovolemic hemodilution with crystalloid or colloid solutions. Crit Care Med 16:862, 1988

451. Poole GV Jr, Prough DS, Johnson JC et al: Effects of resuscitation from hemorrhagic shock on cerebral hemodynamics in the presence of an intracranial mass. J Trauma 27:18, 1987

452. Clifton GL, Robertson CS, Kyper K et al: Cardiovascular response to severe head injury. J Neurosurg 59:447, 1983

453. McLeod AA, Neil-Dwyer G, Meyer CHA et al: Cardiac sequelae of acute head injury. Br Heart J 47:221, 1982

454. Clifton GL, Ziegler M, Grossman R: Circulating catecholamines and sympathetic activity after head injury. Neurosurgery 8:10, 1981

455. Wilkinson HA, Rosenfeld S: Furosemide and mannitol in the treatment of acute experimental intracranial hypertension. Neurosurgery 12:405, 1983

456. Eisenberg HM, Frankowski RF, Contant CF et al: High dosage barbiturate control of elevated intracranial pressure in patients with severe head injury. J Neurosurg 69:15, 1988

457. Matjasko MJ: Multisystem sequelae of severe head injury. In Cottrell JE, Turndorf H (eds): Anesthesia and Neurosurgery, 2nd ed, p 188. St Louis, CV Mosby, 1986

458. Colgan FS, Sawa T, Geneyk LG *et al*: Protective effects of beta blockade on pulmonary function when intracranial pressure is elevated. Crit Care Med 11:368, 1983

459. Miner ME, Kaufman HH, Graham SH *et al*: Disseminated intravascular coagulation fibrinolytic syndrome following head injury in children: Frequency and prognostic implications. J Pediatrics 100:687, 1982

33

M. Christine Stock
Ronald A. Harrison

Respiratory Function in Anesthesia

Anesthesiologists directly manipulate pulmonary function to a greater extent than any other organ system. Thus, a sound and thorough working knowledge of applied pulmonary physiology is essential to the safe conduct of anesthesia. This chapter discusses pulmonary anatomy, the control of ventilation, oxygen and carbon dioxide transport (ventilation-perfusion relationships), lung volumes and pulmonary function testing, and abnormal physiology and anesthesia.

FUNCTIONAL ANATOMY OF THE LUNGS

Volumes by Gray[1] and Netter[2] illustrate the basic anatomy of the lungs excellently and give a complete and fully detailed description of human lung anatomy. This chapter emphasizes functional lung anatomy, with structure described as it applies to the mechanical and physiologic function of the lungs.

Thorax

The human thorax is composed of 12 thoracic vertebral bodies, 12 pairs of ribs, and the sternum. It provides rigid protection of the organ systems that lie interior to it, and provides the superstructure for the bellows system, which moves gas in and out of the lungs. The thoracic cage is shaped like a truncated cone, with small superior and large inferior openings and diaphragms attached at the base. The thoracic vertebral column provides major vertical support for the thorax. Anteriorly, the sternum renders support and is so named because of its sword-like appearance. The sternum's individual components consist of a handle (the manubrium), a body (corpus sterni), and a tip (the xiphoid process). The upper border of the manubrium, positioned between the two sternoclavicular joints, forms the suprasternal notch. It lies in the same horizontal plane as the midportion of the second thoracic vertebral body. The sternal angle, an important anatomic landmark, is formed by the junction of the manubrium and the sternal body with the second rib. The sternal angle is located in the horizontal plane that passes through the vertebral column at the T4 or T5 level. This plane demarcates the superior from the inferior mediastinum.

Of the 12 pairs of ribs, five pairs are true ribs that have direct, cartilaginous connections to both the vertebral column and the sternum. The five pairs of "false ribs" are only indirectly cartilaginously joined to the sternum, and the last two ribs are free-floating ribs. All ribs articulate with thoracic vertebral bodies so that their anterior portion and the sternum can be raised and lowered with expiration and inspiration. Each rib has an artery, nerve, and vein that runs under the inferior lip of the rib. The predominant ventilatory changes in thoracic diameter occur in the anteroposterior direction in the upper thoracic region and in the lateral or transverse direction in the lower portion of the thorax.[3]

Muscles of Ventilation

The ventilatory musculature has been the focus of considerable scientific attention. The ventilatory muscles are endurance muscles that pump the thoracic bellows, thereby moving gas in and out of the lungs. Poor nutrition, chronic obstructive pulmonary disease with gas trapping, and increased airway resistance predispose to the development of ventilatory failure, owing to ventilatory muscle fatigue.[4]

The ventilatory muscles include the diaphragm, intercostal muscles, abdominal muscles, cervical strap muscles, sternocleidomastoid muscle, and the large back and intervertebral muscles of the shoulder girdle. The primary ventilatory muscle is the diaphragm, with minor contributions from the intercostal muscles. Normally, at rest, inspiration requires work and expiration is passive. As ventilatory effort increases, abdominal muscles assist with rib depression and increase intra-abdominal pressure to facilitate forced exhalation. With a further increase in effort, the cervical strap muscles help to elevate the sternum and upper portions of the chest. Finally, the large back and paravertebral muscles of the shoulder girdle become important during maximum ventilatory effort.

Generally, muscles that raise the ribs are functionally inspiratory, whereas muscles that lower the ribs are important primarily during expiration. In a person with normal lung parenchyma, both breathing and coughing can be performed exclusively by the diaphragm.

Ventilatory muscles must create sufficient force to lift the ribs to create subatmospheric pressure in the intrapleural space. Breathing is an endurance phenomenon, i.e., something that is done repetitively over a long period of time. The type of muscle fiber correlates with fatigability and oxidative capacity.[5] Fatigue-resistant fibers are characterized by a slow-twitch response to electrical stimulation. They comprise approximately 50% of the diaphragmatic fibers and, because of their high oxidative capacity, function mostly as endurance units.[6] Fast-twitch muscle fibers that are susceptible to fatigue have rapid responses to electrical stimulation. Fast-twitch fibers impart strength; they allow the muscle to produce greater force over a short period of time. Thus, fast-twitch fibers are useful during brief periods of maximal ventilatory effort, and slow-twitch fibers provide endurance.[7]

To perform work, a muscle must be firmly anchored at both its origin and insertion. The diaphragm is unique because its insertion is mobile: an untethered central tendon that originates from fibers directly attached to the vertebral bodies and the costal portions of the lower ribs and sternum. Diaphragmatic contraction results in descent of the diaphragmatic dome and expansion of the thoracic base. These changes result in decreased intrathoracic and intrapleural pressure, and a corresponding increase in intra-abdominal pressure.

The electrical activity of the ventilatory muscles is informative of the function of the muscles during different types of ventilatory effort.[8] During breathing at rest, there is a gradual and progressive rise in the electrical activity of the diaphragm during the early portion of inspiration; and the electrical activity gradually falls to zero by late inspiration.[9] However, during forced exhalation or expulsive efforts such as coughing, diaphragmatic electrical activity remains high even throughout expiration.[10] The intercostal muscles are active primarily during inspiration, and debate continues as to their significance during expiration. The muscles of the abdominal wall, the most powerful muscles of expiration, are important for expulsive efforts such as coughing.[11] These muscles increase intra-abdominal pressure by compressing the abdominal contents. In addition, some flexion of the trunk and depression of the lower ribs occurs.

The cervical strap muscles elevate and fix the first two ribs. They are active even during spontaneous ventilation at rest. The cervical strap muscles are the most important inspiratory accessory muscles. Their importance is magnified if diaphragmatic function is impaired, as in patients with cervical spinal cord transection. The primary function of the sternocleidomastoid muscle is to elevate the sternum, thus increasing the anteroposterior diameter of the chest wall. The large back muscles, such as the pectoralis major and minor, the latissimus dorsi, and the serratus anterior, are used to augment inspiration by enlarging the rib cage during very high levels of ventilatory activity.

Lung Structures

With an intact respiratory system, the expandable lung tissue completely fills the pleural cavity. The visceral and parietal pleurae are constantly in contact with each other, creating a potential intrapleural space in which pressure drops when the diaphragms descend and the rib cage expands. The resultant subatmospheric intrapleural pressure is a reflection of the opposing and equal forces between the lung tissue and chest wall structures at functional residual capacity (FRC). With inspiration, the intrapleural pressure becomes more negative as the chest wall expands. The intrapleural space normally has a slightly subambient pressure (-2 to -3 mm Hg) at FRC. When the thorax is opened, the

TABLE 33-1. Major Divisions of the Lung

Lung Side/Lobe	Bronchopulmonary Segment
Right	
Upper	Apical
	Anterior
	Posterior
Middle	Medial
	Lateral
Lower	Superior
	Medial basal
	Lateral basal
	Anterior basal
	Posterior basal
Left	
Upper	Apical posterior
	Anterior
Lingula	Superior
	Inferior
Lower	Superior
	Posterior basal
	Anteromedial basal
	Lateral basal

healthy lung retracts because pressures within both the alveolar spaces and along the visceral pleurae are ambient.

In both the right and left lungs are oblique fissures that separate the upper from the lower lobes. In addition, the right lung has a horizontal fissure separating the middle and lower lobes. Major divisions of the right and left lung are listed in Table 33-1. Working knowledge of the bronchopulmonary segments is important for localizing lung pathology, interpreting lung radiographs, identifying lung regions during bronchoscopy, and operating on the lung. Each bronchopulmonary segment is separated from its adjacent segments by well-defined connective tissue planes. Therefore, pulmonary pathology initially tends to remain segmental.

The lung parenchyma can be subdivided into three airway categories based on functional lung anatomy (Table 33-2). The conductive airways provide basic gas transport, but no gas exchange takes place in them. The next group of airways, which have smaller diameters, are transitional airways. They are conduits for gas movement, and additionally perform limited gas diffusion and exchange. Finally, the smallest respiratory airways' primary function is gas exchange. Ventilation-perfusion ($\dot{V}A/\dot{Q}$) relationships are defined by these respiratory airways and are the essence of true respiration.

Conventionally, airways with diameters of 2 mm or greater are considered large airways and create 90% of total airway resistance. By the seventh airway generation, the

TABLE 33-2. Functional Airway Divisions

Type	Function	Structures
Conductive	Bulk gas movement	Trachea to terminal bronchioles
Transitional	Bulk gas movement Limited gas exchange	Respiratory bronchioles Alveolar ducts
Respiratory	Gas exchange	Alveoli Alveolar sacs

internal diameter has decreased to approximately 2 mm and the cumulative cross-sectional area is more than 5.0 cm². The number of alveoli increases progressively with age, starting at approximately 24 million at birth and reaching the final adult count of 300 million by the age of 8–9 years. The alveoli are associated with about 250 million precapillaries and 280 billion capillary segments. Each capillary segment is minimally in contact with two adjacent alveoli. This arrangement results in approximately 70 m² surface area for gas exchange.

Conductive Airways

In the adult, the trachea is a fibromuscular tube approximately 10–12 cm long with an outside diameter of approximately 20 mm. Structural support is provided by 20 U-shaped hyaline cartilages, with the open part of the U facing posteriorly. The cricoid membrane tethers the trachea to the cricoid cartilage at the level of the sixth cervical vertebral body. The trachea enters the superior mediastinum and bifurcates at the sternal angle (the lower border of the fourth thoracic vertebral body). Normally, half of the trachea is intrathoracic and half is extrathoracic. Both ends of the trachea are attached to mobile structures. Thus, the carina can move superiorly as much as 5 cm from its normal resting position. Airway "motion" becomes important in the intubated patient. In the adult, the tip of an orotracheal tube moves an average of 3.8 cm with flexion and extension of the neck, but can travel as far as 6.4 cm.[12] In infants and children, tracheal tube movement with respect to the trachea is even more critical: movement of even 1 cm can move the tube out of the trachea or below the carina.

The tracheal wall includes several cellular structures that are important in removing mucus from the lungs.[13] The tracheal epithelial layer is composed primarily of pseudostratified columnar ciliated epithelium. Interspersed between the cells are goblet cells and brush cells. Chronic exposure to irritants such as tobacco smoke increases the number of mucus-producing goblet cells and decreases the number of ciliated cells,[14] resulting in an increased volume of secretions and reduced ability to remove them. The cilia beat in an organized and coordinated manner and create metachronal wave movement of the superficial "gel" mucus layer toward the mouth. Brush cells appear to be the source of low-viscosity fluid for the serous layer. The histologic structures of other larger airways are similar to those in the trachea.

The next airway generation is composed of the right and left main-stem bronchi. The diameter of the right bronchus is generally greater than that of the left. In the adult, the right bronchus leaves the trachea at approximately 25 degrees from the vertical tracheal axis, whereas the angle of the left bronchus is approximately 45 degrees. Thus, inadvertent endobronchial intubation or aspiration of foreign material is more likely to occur in the right lung than the left. Further, the right upper lobe bronchus dives almost directly posterior at approximately 90 degrees from the right main bronchus. Foreign bodies and fluid that are aspirated by a supine subject usually fall into the right upper lobe. In children less than 3 years old, the angles created by the right and left main-stem bronchi are approximately equal, with takeoff angles of about 55 degrees.

The right main bronchus is approximately 2.5 cm long prior to its initial branching into lobar bronchi. However, in somewhat less than 10% of adults, the right upper lobe bronchi depart from the right main-stem bronchus less than 2.5 cm from the carina. Further, in approximately 2–3% of adults, the right upper lobe bronchus opens into the trachea, above the carina. After the right upper and middle lobe bronchi divide from the right main bronchus, the main channel becomes the right lower lobe bronchus. The left main bronchus is approximately 5 cm long prior to its initial branching point to the left upper lobe and the lingula, and then continues on as the left lower lobe bronchus.

Eighteen segmental bronchi form the next generation of airways (see Table 33-1). Their anatomic positions are important for normal clearance of secretions and for postural drainage. Depending on the lung segment, successive bronchial generations (prior to the appearance of bronchioles) number between 8 and 13. Each successive generation beyond the segmental bronchi undergoes progressive and significant increases in total cross-sectional area (Table 33-3). Weibel's morphometric data, based on dichotomous airway division, result in the total cross-sectional area estimates that appear in Table 33-3.[15] Histologically, the ciliated epithelial cells gradually turn into an ever greater number of cuboidal epithelial cells similar to those in primary bronchioles. Bronchi, defined as airways containing some cartilaginous elements, become as small as 1 mm in diameter.

In general, the histologic structures of the larger bronchi are identical to those of the trachea. At the level of medium-sized bronchi, the eighth to tenth airway generations, the cartilage plates become less helical and less well developed and occur less regularly. The bronchial mucous glands and goblet cells progressively become fewer after the tracheal bifurcation but persist to the level of the smallest bronchi. The numbers of mucous glands and of serous acini also decrease. The venous plexus that surrounds the epithelial wall becomes more extensive in the peripheral bronchi. The fibromuscular cylindrical arrangement that creates elastic

TABLE 33-3. Dimensions and Numbers of Airways

Airway Generation	Airway Name	Diameter (cm)	Cumulative Cross-sectional Area (cm²)
0	Trachea	1.80	2.54
1	Main-stem bronchi	1.22	2.33
2	Lobar bronchi	0.83	2.13
3	Segmental bronchi	0.56	2.00
4	Subsegmental bronchi #1	0.45	2.48
8	Subsegmental bronchi #5	0.18	6.95
16	Terminal bronchiole	0.06	180
17	Respiratory bronchiole #1	0.05	300
20	Alveolar duct #1	0.045	1600
23	Alveolar sac	0.041	11,800

Based on data from Weibel.[15]

recoil in the airways is more prominent than in the peripheral bronchi. This muscular arrangement facilitates changes in both length and caliber of the airways during normal inspiration and expiration.

The bronchioles typically have diameters less than 1 mm. They are devoid of cartilaginous support and have the highest proportion of smooth muscle in the wall, in relation to intraluminal diameters. There are approximately three to four bronchiolar generations, the final generation being the terminal bronchiole. The terminal bronchiole is the last airway component that is not directly involved in gas exchange. Goblet cells are not found in bronchioles, and there is a continued gradual transition from ciliated epithelial cells to cuboidal epithelium.

Transitional Airways

The respiratory bronchiole, which follows the terminal bronchiole, is the first place in the tracheobronchial tree where gas exchange occurs. Respiratory bronchioles are characterized by intermittent alveolar outpockets and histologically by a gradual change from cuboidal epithelium to squamous cells. The respiratory bronchioles make up a small part of the total adult respiratory surface area. In adults, two or three generations of respiratory bronchioles eventually lead to alveolar ducts. There are usually four to five generations of alveolar ducts, each with multiple openings into alveolar sacs. The closely spaced multiple openings of the alveolar ducts are an integral part of the lung parenchyma. During the ventilatory cycle, traction forces tend to distort their structure. The normal architecture is maintained by a framework consisting of elastic collagenous reticular fibers and slender bundles of smooth muscle fibers. The final divisions of alveolar ducts terminate in alveolar sacs that open into alveolar clusters.

Respiratory Airways and the Alveolar-Capillary Membrane

Intact alveoli range between 100 and 300 μm in diameter. The configuration of an alveolus depends on its location in the lung.[16] The peripherally positioned alveoli, which lie just beneath the pleura or along the bronchopulmonary segmental planes, are dome-shaped and open widely into alveolar sacs. Deeper alveoli share straight flat walls with adjacent alveoli, and may have four to six sides. The intra-alveolar septa form the supportive latticework and are composed of elastic, collagenous, and reticular fibers. The pulmonary capillaries also are incorporated into and supported by this fibrous lattice.

The pulmonary capillary beds are the densest capillary networks in the body. The calculated diameter for pulmonary capillaries is between 10 and 14 μm. This extensive vascular branching system starts with pulmonary arterioles in the region of the respiratory bronchioles. Each alveolus is closely associated with approximately 1000 short capillary segments.

The alveolar-capillary interface is complicated but well designed to facilitate gas exchange. On electron microscopy, the alveolar wall consists of a thin capillary epithelial cell, a basement membrane, a pulmonary capillary endothelial cell, and a surfactant lining layer. The flattened, squamous Type I alveolar cells cover approximately 80% of the alveolar surface. Type I cells contain flattened nuclei and extremely thin cytoplasmic extensions that provide the surface for gas exchange. The volume of a Type I cell is twice that of a Type II alveolar cell (see below), but its surface is

50 times greater.[17] Type I cells are highly differentiated and metabolically limited, which makes them highly susceptible to injury. When Type I cells are damaged severely, Type II cells replicate and modify to form new Type I cells.[18]

Type II alveolar cells are interspersed among Type I cells, primarily at alveolar-septal junctions. These polygonal cells have vast metabolic and enzymatic activity and manufacture surfactant.[19] The enzymatic activity required to produce surfactant is only 50% of the total enzymatic activity present in Type II alveolar cells.[20] The remaining enzymatic activity modulates local electrolyte balance and endothelial and lymphatic cell functions.[21] Both Type I and Type II alveolar cells have tight intracellular junctions, thus providing a relatively impermeable barrier to fluids.

Type III alveolar cells, alveolar macrophages, are an important element of lung defense. Their migratory and phagocytic activities result in the ingestion of foreign materials within alveolar spaces.[22]

Finally, numerous finger-like projections of the capillary endothelial cells greatly increase their surface area. They also provide intimate contact between the capillary endothelial cell and the entire circulating blood volume. Capillary endothelial cells are ideally suited for metabolism of circulating substances. Thus, the alveolar-capillary membrane has two primary functions: transport of oxygen and carbon dioxide, and the widely varied metabolic activities of local and humoral substances.

Collateral Ventilation

Airways 1 mm or less in diameter are susceptible to blockage, resulting in accumulation of fluids and secretions and inhibition of gas exchange, especially oxygen transport. The pores of Kohn were the first structures described to provide collateral ventilation. They render intra-alveolar communication and are located in the interspaces between the alveolar-capillary networks.[23] Conduits that afford direct communication between small respiratory bronchioles and neighboring alveoli also create collateral ventilation and may be more important. These communications are of larger diameter than the pores of Kohn, 30 μm versus 8–10 μm, and their anatomic position allows access to a greater number of alveoli.[24]

Mediastinum

The space between the right and left mediastinal pleurae contains the thoracic components of the cardiovascular and gastrointestinal systems, the great vessels, nerves, nerve plexuses, lymphatics, and connective tissue. The mediastinum consists of superior and inferior compartments. The inferior compartment is subdivided further into anterior, middle, and posterior portions. The middle portion of the inferior mediastinum, which contains the pericardial sac and its contents, is the largest subcompartment. Because mediastinal structures are in intimate contact with the pleural surfaces, the viscera housed within the mediastinum are subject to the cyclic pressure changes generated in the intrapleural space.

Pulmonary Vascular Systems

Two major circulatory systems supply blood to the lungs—the pulmonary and bronchial vasculature networks. The pulmonary vascular system delivers mixed venous blood from the right ventricle to the pulmonary capillary bed by way of the pulmonary arteries. After gas exchange occurs in the pulmonary capillary bed, oxygen-rich and carbon dioxide-poor blood is returned to the left atrium *via* the pulmonary veins. The pulmonary veins run independently along the intralobar connective tissue planes. The pulmonary arteries contain a specialized connective tissue that maintains blood vessel patency despite changes in lung volume and intrathoracic pressure during breathing or a change in body position. The pulmonary capillary system adequately provides for the metabolic and oxygen needs of the alveolar parenchyma. However, the bronchial system must provide oxygen to the conductive airways and pulmonary vessels. Anatomic connections between the bronchial and pulmonary venous circulations create an absolute shunt of approximately 2% of the total cardiac output.

LUNG MECHANICS

Lung movement is entirely passive and responds to forces external to the lungs. During spontaneous ventilation, the external forces are produced by ventilatory muscles. The lungs' response is governed by the impedance of the chest wall and the airways. This impedance, or hindrance, falls mainly into two categories: (1) elastic work to overcome the elastic recoil of the lung and gas-liquid interface, and (2) resistance to gas flow.

Elastic Work

The lungs' natural tendency is to collapse; thus, expiration is normally passive as gas flows from the lungs when the elastic recoil produces smaller alveoli. The thoracic cage exerts an outwardly directed force and the lungs exert an inwardly directed force that together result in a subatmospheric intrapleural pressure. Because the outward force of the thoracic cage exceeds the inward force of the lung, the overall tendency of the lung is to remain inflated when it resides within the thoracic cage. At FRC, the outward and inward forces on the lung are equal. Thus, at passive end-exhalation, the respiratory muscles are relaxed so that the lung and chest wall always return toward FRC. Gravitational forces create a more subatmospheric pressure in nondependent areas of the lung than in dependent areas. In the upright adult, the difference in intrapleural pressure from the top to the bottom of the lung is approximately 7 cm H_2O.

Surface tension at an air-fluid interface produces forces that tend to further reduce the area of interface. The gas pressure within a bubble is always higher than the surrounding gas pressure because the surface of the bubble is in a state of tension. The alveoli resemble bubbles in this respect, although alveolar gas communicates with the atmosphere *via* the airways. The pressure inside a bubble is higher than the surrounding pressure by an amount depending on the surface tension of the bubble's liquid and the radius of curvature, according to the La Place equation: $P = 2T/R$, where P is the pressure within the bubble (dyn/cm^2), T is the surface tension of the liquid (dyn/cm), and R is the radius of the bubble (cm).

During expansion, the surface tension in the lung increases to 40 mN·m^{-1}, a value close to that of plasma. During contraction, the surface tension falls to 19 mN·m^{-1}, a lower value than that of any other known fluid. The alveoli experience hysteresis, that is, different pressure-volume re-

lationships, during expansion and contraction. In contrast to a bubble, the pressure within an alveolus decreases as the radius of curvature decreases. Thus, gas tends to flow from larger to smaller alveoli to maintain stability and prevent lung collapse.

The alveolar transmural pressure gradient is the difference between intrapleural and alveolar pressure and is directly proportional to lung volume. Intrapleural pressure can be safely measured with a percutaneously inserted catheter,[25] but this technique is rarely performed clinically. Esophageal pressure can be used as a reflection of intrapleural pressure, but measurement of esophageal pressure is fraught with technical difficulties and can only be performed in the upright, seated individual with the esophageal balloon in the midesophagus.

If the lungs are slowly inflated and deflated, the pressure-volume curve during inflation differs from that obtained during deflation. The two curves form a hysteresis loop that becomes progressively broader as the tidal volume is increased (Fig. 33-1). A greater pressure than anticipated is required during inflation, and recoil pressure is less than expected during deflation. Thus, the lung accepts deformation poorly under stress, and, once deformed, assumes its original shape slowly and with effort. This phenomenon, another example of elastic hysteresis, is important for the maintenance of normal lung compliance. However, for the purposes of this discussion, it will be ignored.

The sum of the pressure-volume relationships of the thorax and lung results in a sigmoidal curve (Fig. 33-2). The vertical line drawn at end-expiration coincides with FRC. Normally, humans breathe on the steepest part of the sigmoidal curve, where compliance is highest. The compliance of the curve is represented by the slope of the curve ($\Delta V/\Delta P$). In restrictive diseases the curve shifts to the right or the slope is depressed, or both. These changes result in smaller FRCs and lower lung compliance. When lung compliance is small, larger changes in intrapleural pressure are

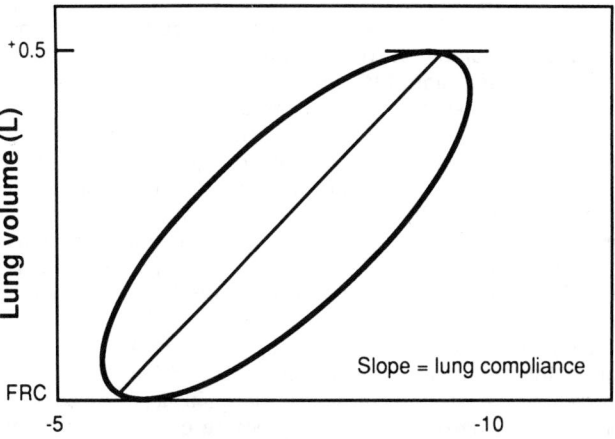

**Intrapleural pressure (cmH2O)
Relative to atmospheric pressure**

Figure 33-1. Dynamic pressure-volume loop of resting tidal volume. Quiet, normal breathing is characterized by hysteresis of the pressure-volume loop. The lung is more resistant to deformation than expected, and returns to its original configuration less easily than expected. The slope of the line connecting the zenith and nadir lung volumes is lung compliance, approximately 500 ml per 3 cm H_2O = 167 ml per cm H_2O.

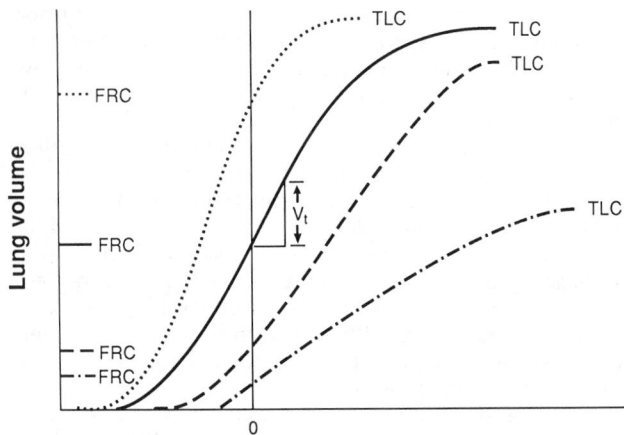

Transpulmonary pressure

Figure 33-2. Pulmonary pressure-volume relationships at different levels (total lung capacity). The solid line depicts the normal pulmonary pressure-volume relationships but ignores hysteresis. Humans normally breathe on the linear, steep part of this sigmoidal curve, where the slope, which is equal to compliance, is greatest. The *vertical line* at zero defines FRC, regardless of the position of the curve on the graph. Mild restrictive lung disease, indicated by the *dashed line,* shifts the curve to the right with little change in slope. However, with restrictive disease, the patient breathes on a lower FRC, at a point on the curve where the slope is less. Severe restrictive pulmonary disease profoundly depresses the FRC and diminishes the slope of the entire curve (*dashed-dotted line*). Obstructive disease (*dotted line*) elevates both FRC and compliance. (FRC = functional residual capacity; TLC = total lung capacity.)

needed to create the same tidal volume; typically, smaller tidal volumes are inspired more rapidly. Thus, patients with decreased lung compliance typically breathe with rapid, shallow ventilatory patterns. The ventilatory rate is one of the most sensitive indices of lung compliance. Continuous positive airway pressure (CPAP) will shift the vertical line to the right, thus allowing the patient to breathe on a steeper and more favorable portion of the volume-pressure curve.

On the other hand, in diseases that increase lung compliance, FRC increases and the pressure-volume curve shifts to the left and steepens. Less elastic work is required to inspire, but elastic recoil is reduced significantly. Chronic obstructive lung disease and acute asthma are the most common examples of this process. If lung compliance and FRC are sufficiently high, the patient must use ventilatory muscles to actively expire. The difficulty these patients experience in emptying the lungs is compounded by the increased airway resistance.

Both compliance and inspiratory elastic work can be measured for a single breath by measuring airway (Paw) and intrapleural (Ppl) pressures and tidal volume. Lung compliance, the slope of the volume-pressure curve, is given by the equation

$$C_L = \frac{\Delta V}{\Delta P_L} = \frac{V_T}{P_{L_i} - P_{L_e}} = \frac{V_T}{[(Paw_i - Ppl_i) - (Paw_e - Ppl_e)]}$$

where P_L is transpulmonary pressure, V_T is tidal volume, Paw_e and Paw_i are expiratory and inspiratory Paw, and Ppl_e and Ppl_i are expiratory and inspiratory Ppl.

Elastic work (Wel) is performed during inspiration only, expiration being passive during normal breathing. The area within the triangle in Figure 33-2 describes the work per-

formed to inspire. The equation that yields elastic work (and the area of the triangle) is

$$Wel = \frac{1}{2}(V_T)(P_{L_i} - P_{L_e})$$
$$= \frac{1}{2}(V_T)[(Paw_i - Ppl_i) - (Paw_e - Ppl_e)]$$

Resistance to Gas Flow

Both laminar and turbulent flow exist within the respiratory tract, usually in mixed patterns. The physics of each, however, is significantly different and worth consideration.

Laminar Flow

Below critical flows, gas proceeds through a straight tube as a series of concentric cylinders that slide over one another. Thus, fully developed flow has a parabolic profile with a velocity of zero at the cylinder wall and a maximum velocity at the center of the advancing "cone." Peripheral cylinders tend to be stationary and the central cylinder moves fastest. This type of streamlined flow is usually inaudible. The advancing conical front means that some fresh gas reaches the end of the tube before the tube has been completely filled with fresh gas. That is, significant alveolar ventilation can occur when the tidal volume (V_T) is less than anatomic dead space, a fact that was noted by Roher in 1915[26] and is very important in high-frequency ventilation. Gas flowing in a straight, unbranched tube meets resistance that can be calculated by the following equation:

$$R = \frac{8 \times \text{length} \times \text{viscosity}}{\pi r^4} = \frac{P_B - P_A}{\text{flow}}$$

where P_B and P_A are barometric and alveolar pressures. The inverse relationship between flow and the fourth power of the radius (r^4) explains the critical importance of narrowed air passages. Viscosity is the only physical gas property that is relevant under conditions of laminar flow. Helium has a low density, but its viscosity is close to that of air. Helium will not improve gas flow if the flow is laminar. For practical purposes this is not a problem because flow is usually turbulent when airway resistance is evaluated.

Turbulent Flow

High flow rates, particularly through branched or irregularly shaped tubes, disrupt the orderly flow of laminar gas. Turbulent flow is usually audible and almost invariably present when high resistance to gas flow is problematic. Turbulent flow usually presents with a square front so that no fresh gas will reach the end of the tube until the amount of gas entering the tube is almost equal to the volume of the tube. Thus, turbulent flow effectively purges the contents of a tube. Four conditions that will change laminar flow to turbulent flow are high gas flows, sharp angles within the tube, branching in the tube, and a change in the tube's diameter.

During turbulent flow, the driving pressure is:

1. proportional to the square of the required gas flow rate,
2. proportional to gas density and independent of viscosity, and
3. inversely proportional to the fifth power of the radius of the tube.

Resistance, defined for laminar flow as the pressure gradient divided by flow rate, is not constant, as it is with laminar flow, but increases in proportion to the flow rate. A detailed description of these phenomena is beyond the scope of this chapter, but the reader is referred to descriptions by Nunn.[27]

Increased Airway Resistance

Increased resistance can be due not only to bronchiolar hyperreactivity but also to mucosal edema, mucous plugging, epithelial desquamation, and foreign bodies. The normal response to increased inspiratory resistance is increased inspiratory muscle effort, with little change in FRC.[28] Accessory muscles are brought into play according to the degree of resistance. Emphysematous patients retain remarkable ability to preserve an adequate alveolar ventilation, even with gross airway obstruction. In patients with preoperative FEV_1 values <1 liter, there was no correlation between FEV_1 and the partial pressure of carbon dioxide in arterial blood ($Paco_2$), which was normal in most patients. Further, asthmatic patients compensate well for increased airway resistance, and also keep the mean $Paco_2$ in the lower end of normal range.[29] Thus, an increased $Paco_2$ in the setting of increased airway resistance deserves serious attention.

There are two principal compensatory mechanisms for high *inspiratory* resistance. The muscle spindles indicate that the inspiratory muscles have failed to shorten by the intended amount. Their afferent discharge augments the activity in the motor neuron pool of the anterior horn. The conscious subject can detect very small increases in inspiratory resistance.[30] The other compensatory mechanism is driven by an elevated $Paco_2$.[31]

Expiratory resistance against 10 cm H_2O does not result in activation of the expiratory muscles in conscious or anesthetized subjects. The initial work to overcome expiratory resistance initially is performed by the inspiratory muscles. The subject augments inspiratory force until a sufficiently high lung volume is achieved so that elastic recoil overcomes expiratory resistance.[32] This response is clearly unlike what might be expected from activation of the Breuer-Hering reflex; however, this reflex is very weak in man. The conscious subject normally uses expiratory muscles to overcome expiratory pressures that are 10 cm H_2O greater than inspiratory Paw. The immediate effects of excessive resistance are probably less important than the long-term response. The ventilatory muscles can fatigue, thus precipitating ventilatory failure.

CONTROL OF VENTILATION

Mechanisms that control ventilation are extremely complex, requiring integration with many parts of the central and peripheral nervous systems (see Fig. 33-4). The respiratory centers were first localized in the brain stem in 1812 by LeGallois, who demonstrated that breathing did not depend on an intact cerebrum but on a small region of the medulla near the origin of the vagus nerves.[33] Countless studies in the past two centuries have greatly increased our knowledge and understanding of the anatomic components of ventilatory control. However, experimental work performed in animals is difficult to apply to man because of interspecies variation.

Generation of Ventilatory Pattern

Before we describe the brain stem structures responsible for the generation of a ventilatory pattern, certain terms will be defined. The term *eupnea* (literally, "good breathing") refers to normal breathing: continuous rhythmic inspiratory and expiratory movement without undue interruption. *Apnea* ("no breathing") is the cessation of ventilatory *effort* with lung volume at FRC. On the other hand, *apneusis* is cessation of ventilation with the lungs filled to total lung capacity.[34] In *apneustic ventilation*, apneusis alternates with expiratory spasm.[35] Finally, *Biot's ventilation* is characterized by a series of ventilatory gasps interposed between periods of apnea, frequently referred to as agonal ventilation.[36]

A *respiratory center* is a specific area in the brain that integrates neural traffic to cause spontaneous ventilation. There are several discrete respiratory centers within the pontine and medullary reticular formations that function as the control system (Fig. 33-3).[37]

Initial descriptions of brain stem respiratory functions are based on classic ablation and electrical stimulation studies.[38-41] Another method for localizing respiratory centers entails recording action potentials from different areas of the brain stem with microelectrodes. This method is based on the assumption that local brain activity that occurs in phase with respiratory activity is evidence that the area under study has "respiratory neurons."[42] These techniques are imperfect for precisely localizing discrete respiratory centers.

Medullary Centers

The medulla oblongata contains the most basic ventilatory control areas in the brain. Specific areas are active primarily during inspiration or expiration, with many neural inspiratory or expiratory interconnections. The inspiratory centers that reside in the *dorsal respiratory group* (DRG) are located in the dorsal medullary reticular formation. The DRG is the source of elementary ventilatory rhythmicity[43,44] and functions as the "pacemaker" for the respiratory system.[45] Whereas resting lung volume occurs at end-expiration, the electrical activity of the ventilatory centers is at rest at end-inspiration. The rhythmic activity of the DRG persists even when all incoming peripheral and interconnecting nerves are sectioned or blocked completely. The result is ataxic, gasping ventilation with frequent maximum inspiratory efforts: apneustic breathing.

The *ventral respiratory group* (VRG) functions as the expiratory coordinating center and is located in the ventral medullary reticular formation. The inspiratory and expiratory neurons function by a system of reciprocal innervation, or negative feedback.[42] When the DRG creates an impulse to inspire, inspiration occurs, and then the DRG impulse is quenched by a reciprocating VRG impulse. This VRG transmission prohibits further use of the inspiratory muscles, thus allowing passive expiration to occur.

Pontine Centers

The pontine centers process information that originates in the medulla. The *apneustic center* is located in the middle or lower pons. With activation, this center sends impulses to inspiratory DRG neurons and is designed to sustain inspiration. Electrical stimulation results in inspiratory spasm.[46] The middle and lower pons contain specific areas for phase-spanning neurons.[47] These neurons assist with the transition between inspiration and expiration and do not exert direct control over ventilatory muscles.

The *pneumotaxic respiratory center* is in the rostral pons. A simple transection through the brain stem that isolates this portion of the pons from the upper brain stem reduces

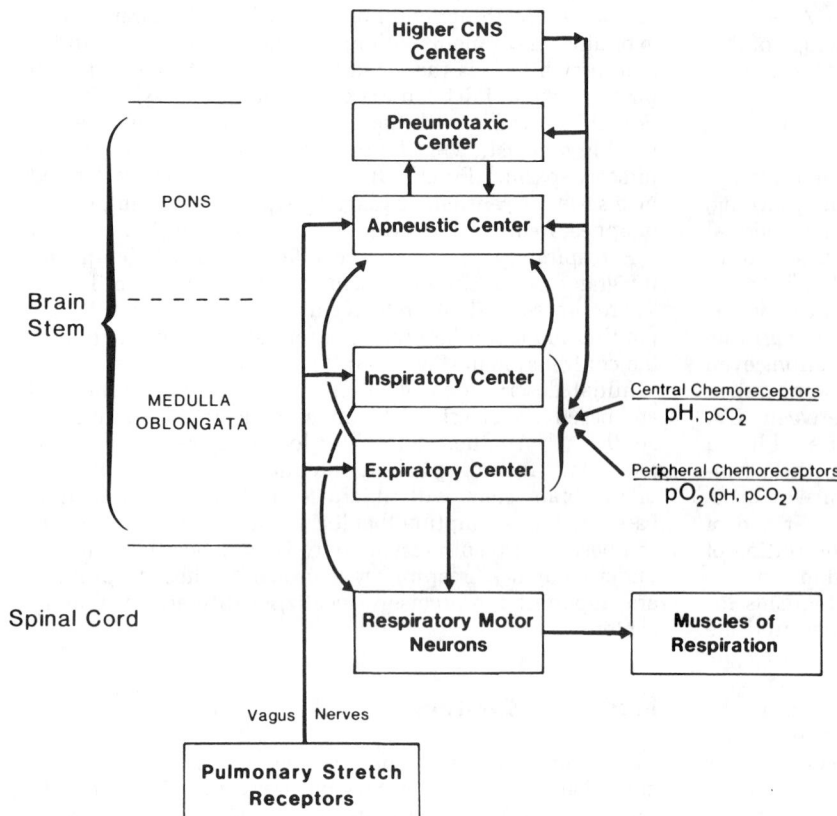

Figure 33-3. Classic CNS respiratory centers. Diagram illustrates major respiratory centers, neurofeedback circuits, primary neurohumoral sensory inputs, and mechanical outputs.

ventilatory rate and increases tidal volume. If both vagus nerves are additionally transected, apneusis results.[48] Thus, the primary function of the pneumotaxic center is to limit the depth of inspiration. When maximally activated, the pneumotaxic center secondarily increases ventilatory frequency. The pneumotaxic center performs no pacemaking function and has no intrinsic rhythmicity.

Higher Respiratory Centers

Many higher brain structures clearly affect ventilatory control processes. In the midbrain, stimulation of the reticular activating system increases the rate and amplitude of ventilation.[49] The cerebral cortex also affects breathing pattern, although precise neural pathways are not known.[50] Occasionally, the ventilatory control process becomes subservient to other regulatory centers. For example, the respiratory system plays an important role in the control of body temperature, because it supplies a large surface area for heat exchange. This is especially important in animals, in which panting is a primary means of dissipating heat. Then, ventilatory pattern is influenced by neural input from descending pathways from the anterior and posterior hypothalamus to the pneumotaxic center of the upper pons.

Vasomotor control and certain respiratory responses are closely linked. Stimulation of the carotid sinus not only decreases vasomotor tone but also inhibits ventilation. Alternatively, stimulation of the carotid body chemoreceptors (see Chemical Control of Breathing) results in an increase in both ventilatory activity and vasomotor tone.[51,52]

Reflex Control of Ventilation

Reflexes that directly influence ventilatory pattern usually do so to prevent airway obstruction (Fig. 33-4). *Deglutition,* or swallowing, involves the glossopharyngeal and vagus nerves. Stimulation of the anterior and posterior pharyngeal pillars of the posterior pharynx induces swallowing. During swallowing, inspiration ceases momentarily, usually is followed by a single large breath, and briefly increases ventilation. The ventilatory centers that coordinate breathing and deglutition have not been identified.[53]

Vomiting significantly modifies normal ventilatory activity.[54] Swallowing, salivation, gastrointestinal reflexes, rhythmic spasmodic ventilatory movements, and significant diaphragmatic and abdominal muscular activity must be coordinated over a very brief interval. Because of the obvious risk of aspirating gastric contents, it is advantageous to inhibit inspiration during vomiting. Input into the respiratory centers occurs from both cranial and spinal cord nerves.

Coughing results from stimulation of the tracheal subepithelium, especially along the posterior tracheal wall and carina.[55] Coughing also requires coordination of both airway and ventilatory muscle activity. An effective cough requires deep inspiration, then forced exhalation against a momentarily closed glottis to increase intrathoracic pressure, thus allowing an expulsive expiratory maneuver.

Proprioception in the pulmonary system, the qualitative knowledge of the gas volume within the lungs, probably arises from smooth muscle spindle receptors. These proprioceptors are sensitive to pressure changes and are located within the smooth muscle of all airways.[56] Airway stretch reflexes can be demonstrated during distention of isolated

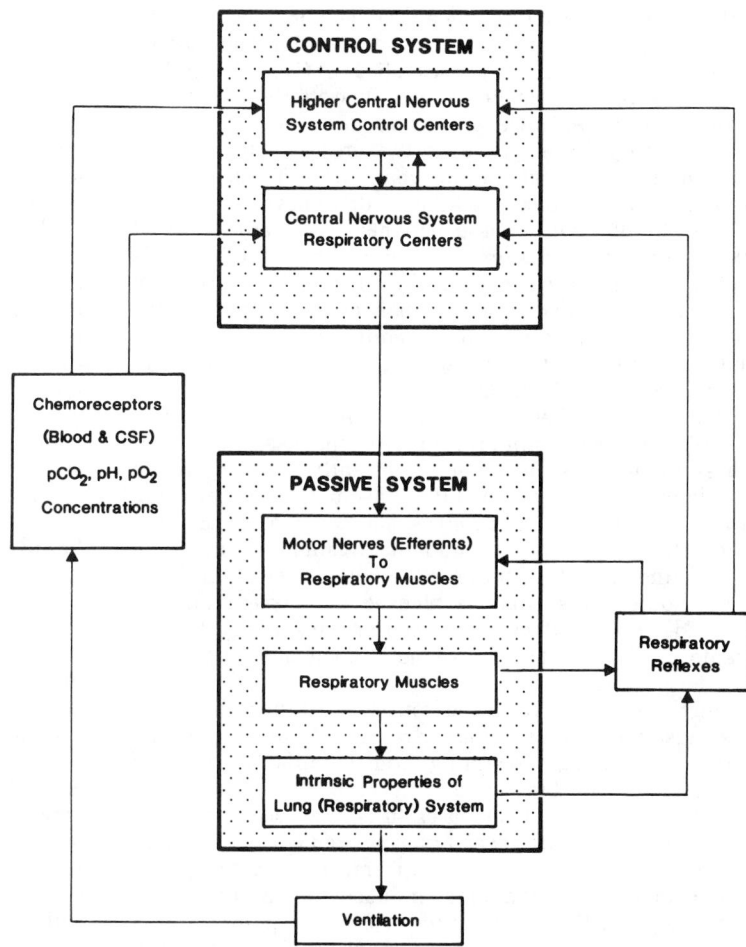

Figure 33-4. Model of the respiratory system. The two major subdivisions are (1) the ventilation control system component, which acts on (2) the passive respiratory system component.

airways, so that airway pressure, rather than volume distention, appears to be the primary stimulation.[57] Clinical conditions in which pulmonary airway stretch receptors are stimulated include pulmonary edema and atelectasis. Certain drugs, such as acetylcholine, pilocarpine, and histamine, that are administered in doses large enough to decrease lung compliance also enhance the stretch reflex.[58] In contrast, airway stretch receptors are inhibited by inhalation of vaporized water, intravenously administered antihistamines, and topically administered local anesthetics.

Golgi tendon organs (tendon spindles) occur in series arrangements within ventilatory muscles and facilitate proprioception. The intercostal muscles are rich in tendon spindles, whereas the diaphragm has a limited number. Thus, the pulmonary stretch reflex primarily involves the intercostal muscles but not the diaphragm.[59] When the lungs are full and the chest wall is stretched, these receptors send signals to the brain stem that inhibit further inspiration.

In 1868, Breuer and Hering reported that lightly anesthetized, spontaneously breathing animals would cease or decrease ventilatory effort during sustained lung distention.[60] This response was blocked by bilateral vagotomy. The *Breuer-Hering reflex* is prominent in lower order mammals such as rabbits but is only weakly present in man. The Breuer-Hering reflex is so active in lower mammals that even 5 cm H_2O CPAP will induce apnea. In man, however, the reflex is only weakly present, as evidenced by the fact that humans will continue to breathe spontaneously with

CPAP in excess of 40 cm H_2O. This inflation reflex is associated with inspiratory muscle inhibition as documented by marked reductions in electrical activity of both the phrenic nerve and the diaphragmatic muscle itself. The second component of the Breuer-Hering reflex, the deflation reflex, produces increased ventilatory muscle activity following sustained lung deflation. This reflex is not significant in man.

Both pulmonary and airway stretch reflexes operate secondary to the pacemaking and modulating effects of the brain stem ventilatory control centers.

Chemical Control of Ventilation

Peripheral Chemoreceptors

In a simplistic view of chemical ventilatory control, the peripheral chemoreceptors primarily respond to lack of oxygen, and the central nervous system (CNS) receptors primarily respond to changes in Pco_2, pH, and acid-base disturbances.

The peripheral chemoreceptors are composed of the carotid and aortic bodies.[61,62] The carotid bodies, located at the bifurcation of the common carotid artery, have predominantly ventilatory effects. The aortic bodies, which are scattered about the aortic arch and its branches, have predominantly circulatory effects. The neural output from the carotid body reaches the central respiratory centers by way of the afferent glossopharyngeal nerves. Output from the aortic bodies travels to the medullary centers *via* the vagus nerve. Both carotid and aortic bodies are stimulated by decreased Pa_{O_2}, but not by decreased Sa_{O_2} or Ca_{O_2}. When Pa_{O_2} falls below 100 mm Hg, neural activity from these receptors begins to increase. However, it is not until the Pa_{O_2} reaches 60–65 mm Hg that neural activity increases sufficiently to substantially augment minute ventilation. Thus, patients who depend on hypoxic ventilatory drive have Pa_{O_2} values in the mid-60s. Once these patients' Pa_{O_2} values exceed 60–65 mm Hg, ventilatory drive diminishes and Pa_{O_2} falls until ventilation is again stimulated by arterial hypoxemia. When mechanical ventilation is being discontinued for the patient dependent on hypoxic ventilatory drive, the Pa_{O_2} must fall below 65 mm Hg so that the patient will regain the hypoxic ventilatory drive.

The carotid bodies also are sensitive to decreased pH_a, but this response is minor. Similarly, changes in Pa_{CO_2} do not stimulate these receptors sufficiently to alter minute ventilation. Increases in blood temperature, hypoperfusion of the carotid bodies themselves, and some chemicals will stimulate these receptors. Sympathetic ganglion stimulation by nicotine or acetylcholine will stimulate the carotid and aortic bodies; this effect is blocked by hexamethonium. Blockade of the cytochrome electron transport system by cyanide will prevent oxidative metabolism, and thus stimulate these receptors also.

Ventilatory effects resulting from stimulation of the receptors cause increased ventilatory rate and tidal volume. Hemodynamic changes resulting from stimulation of these receptors include bradycardia, hypertension, increases in bronchiolar tone, and increases in adrenal secretion. The carotid body chemical receptors have been termed *ultimum moriens* ("last to die"). The peripheral receptor's response to hypoxemia is resistant to the influences of anesthesia and tissue hypoxia that may depress central responses. However, the peripheral receptor's response is not sufficiently robust to reliably increase ventilatory rate or minute ventilation to herald the onset of arterial hypoxemia during general anesthesia or recovery from anesthesia.

Central Chemoreceptors

Approximately 80% of the ventilatory response to inhaled carbon dioxide originates in the central medullary centers. Acid-base regulation involving carbon dioxide, H^+, and bicarbonate is related primarily to chemosensitive receptors located in the medulla close to or in contact with the cerebrospinal fluid (CSF). The chemosensitive areas of the brain stem are in the infralateral aspects of the medulla near the origin of cranial nerves IX and X. The exact location of the chemosensitive area, whether intracellular or extracellular, is still debated, although the area just beneath the surface of the ventral medulla is exquisitely sensitive to the extracellular fluid H^+ concentration.[63] Although the central response is the major factor in the regulation of breathing by carbon dioxide, carbon dioxide has little direct stimulating effect on these chemosensitive areas. These receptors are primarily sensitive to changes in H^+ concentration. Carbon dioxide has a potent but indirect effect by reacting with water to form carbonic acid, which disassociates into hydrogen and bicarbonate ions.[64]

Increased Pa_{CO_2} is a more potent ventilatory stimulus than increased arterial H^+ concentration from a metabolic source. Carbon dioxide, but not H^+, passes readily through the blood-brain and blood-CSF barriers. Local buffering systems immediately neutralize H^+ in arterial blood and body fluids. In contrast, the CSF has minimal buffering capacity.

Thus, once carbon dioxide crosses into the CSF, H^+ are created and trapped in the CSF, resulting in a CSF H^+ concentration considerably greater than that found in the blood. Because carbon dioxide crosses the blood-brain barrier readily, the P_{CO_2} values in the CSF, cerebral tissue, and jugular venous blood rise quickly and to the same degree as the Pa_{CO_2}, although the central values are approximately 10 mm Hg above those measured in arterial blood.

The ventilatory response to changes in Pa_{CO_2} (increased V_T, increased respiratory rate) is rapid and peaks within a minute or two after the change in Pa_{CO_2}. With the same level of carbon dioxide stimulation, the resultant increase in ventilation declines over a period of several hours, probably as a result of bicarbonate ions that are actively transported from the blood into the CSF through the arachnoid villi.[65] Central medullary chemoreceptors also respond to temperature change. Cold CSF (with normal pH) or local anesthetic applied to the medullary surface will depress ventilation.

Ventilatory Response to Altitude

Ventilatory response and adaptation to high altitude are good examples of the integration of peripheral and central chemoreceptor control of ventilation. The following mechanism of acclimatization was proposed by Severinghaus and coworkers in 1963 and has since been confirmed.[66]

Following ascent from sea level to 4000 m, acute exposure to high altitude and low P_{IO_2} would result in arterial hypoxemia. This decrease in Pa_{O_2} activates the peripheral hypoxemic ventilatory drive by stimulating the carotid and aortic bodies, and causes increased minute ventilation. As minute ventilate increases, Pa_{CO_2} and CSF P_{CO_2} decrease and cause concomitant increases in pH_a and CSF pH. The alkaline shift of the CSF decreases ventilatory drive *via* medullary chemoreceptors, partially offsetting hypoxemic drive. A temporary equilibrium is attained within minutes, with Pa_{CO_2} only 2–5 mm Hg below normal and Pa_{O_2} approximately 45 mm Hg. This initially profound hypoxemia probably causes the acute respiratory distress and other associated symptoms (headache, diarrhea) associated with rapid ascent. However, the CNS is able to restore CSF pH to normal (7.326) by pumping bicarbonate ions out of the CSF over 2–3 days. In 2–3 days, CSF bicarbonate concentration decreases approximately 5 $mEq \cdot l^{-1}$ and restores CSF pH to within 0.01 pH unit of values at sea level. Then, centrally mediated ventilatory drive returns to normal, and hypoxic drive and stimulation of peripheral receptors can proceed unopposed. Thus, after 3 days' exposure to 4000 m altitude, ventilatory adaptation would result in a new equilibrium, with Pa_{CO_2} approximately 30 mm Hg and Pa_{O_2} approximately 55 mm Hg. Following descent to sea level, the low CSF bicarbonate concentration persists for several days, and the climber "overbreathes" until CSF bicarbonate and pH values return to normal.

Breath-holding

Most adults with normal lungs and gas exchange can hold their breaths approximately 1 minute when breathing room air without previously hyperventilating. After 1 minute of breath-holding under these circumstances, Pa_{O_2} decreases to approximately 65–70 mm Hg and Pa_{CO_2} increases approximately 12 mm Hg. In the absence of supplemental oxygen and hyperventilation, the "breakpoint" is remarkably constant at a Pa_{CO_2} of 50 mm Hg.[67,68] However, if the individual breathes 100% oxygen prior to breath-holding, he should be able to hold his breath for 2–3 minutes, or until Pa_{CO_2} rises to 60 mm Hg. Hyperventilation sufficient to reduce Pa_{CO_2} to 20 mm Hg can lengthen the period of breath-holding to 3–4 minutes.[69] Hyperventilation with 100% oxygen prior to breath-holding should extend the apneic period to 6–10 minutes. The Pa_{CO_2} rate of rise in awake, preoxygenated adults with normal lungs who hold their breaths without previous hyperventilation is 7 mm Hg·min^{-1} in the first 10 seconds, 2 mm Hg·min^{-1} in the next 10 seconds, and 6 mm Hg·min^{-1} thereafter.[68]

The duration of voluntary breath-holding is directly proportional to lung volume at onset. This is probably related both to oxygen stores in the alveoli and to the rate at which Pa_{CO_2} rises. With smaller lung volumes, the same amount of carbon dioxide is emptied into a smaller volume during the apneic period, thus increasing the carbon dioxide concentration more rapidly than occurs with larger lung volumes. Of note, apneic patients during general anesthesia effectively "breath-hold" at FRC rather than at vital capacity, which would tend to accelerate the rate of rise of carbon dioxide. Despite this difference in lung volume, the rate of rise of Pa_{CO_2} in apneic anesthetized patients is 12 mm Hg during the first minute and 3.5 mm Hg·min^{-1} thereafter, significantly lower than in the awake state.[70,71] During anesthesia, metabolic rate and carbon dioxide production are significantly less than during ambulatory wakefulness, which probably accounts for the different rates of rise in carbon dioxide levels.

Hyperventilation with room air prior to prolonged breath-holding during exercise is inadvisable. During underwater swimming after poolside hyperventilation, the urge to breathe is first stimulated by a rising Pa_{CO_2}. Swimmers who hyperventilate with room air prior to swimming long distances underwater frequently lose consciousness from arterial hypoxemia before the Pa_{CO_2} is sufficiently increased to stimulate the "need" to breathe.

Hyperventilation rarely is followed by an apneic period in awake humans, despite a markedly depressed Pa_{CO_2}. However, minute ventilation may decrease significantly. Aggressive intermittent positive pressure breathing treatments for patients with chronic obstructive pulmonary disease (COPD) can depress minute ventilation sufficiently to create arterial hypoxemia if they breathe room air after cessation of therapy.[72] In contrast, even mild hyperventilation during general anesthesia will produce prolonged apneic periods.[73]

Quantitative Aspects of Chemical Control of Breathing

The ventilatory responses to oxygen and carbon dioxide can be assessed quantitatively. Unfortunately, the quantitative indices of hypoxemic sensitivity are not clinically useful because the normal range is very wide. The reader is referred to more comprehensive sources for a discussion of the quantitative indices of hypoxemic sensitivity.[74]

Ventilatory responses to Pa_{CO_2} changes are measured in several ways, provided that carbon dioxide production remains constant. When subjects voluntarily increase minute ventilation to a prescribed level, the Pa_{CO_2} decreases hyperbolically. The plot of minute ventilation (independent variable) and Pa_{CO_2} (dependent variable) is the *metabolic hyperbola* (Fig. 33-5). The metabolic hyperbola is cumbersome to evaluate and difficult to use clinically.

The curve more commonly used is the Pa_{CO_2} *ventilatory response curve* (see Fig. 33-5). It describes the effect of changing Pa_{CO_2} on the resultant minute ventilation. Usu-

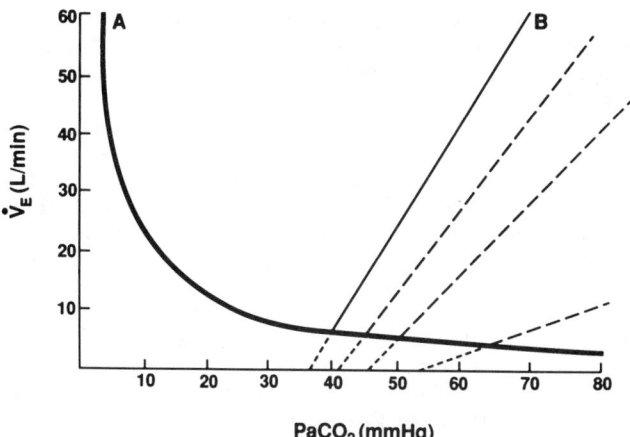

Figure 33-5. Carbon dioxide–ventilatory response curve. The metabolic hyperbola, curve *A*, is generated by varying $\dot{V}_E$ and measuring changes in carbon dioxide concentration. The hyperbolic configuration makes it cumbersome for clinical use. The carbon dioxide–ventilatory response curve, *B*, is linear between approximately 20 and 80 mm Hg. It is generated by varying Pa_{CO_2} (usually by controlling inspired carbon dioxide concentration) and measuring the resultant $\dot{V}_E$. This is the most commonly used test of ventilatory response. The slope defines "sensitivity"; the setpoint, or resting Pa_{CO_2}, occurs at the intersection of the metabolic hyperbola and the carbon dioxide–ventilatory response curve; and the apneic threshold can be obtained by extrapolating the carbon dioxide–ventilatory response curve to the x-intercept. In the absence of surgical stimulation, increasing doses of potent inhaled anesthesia or opioids will shift the curve to the right and eventually depress the slope (*dashed lines*). Painful stimulation will reverse these changes to varying and unpredictable degrees.

ally, subjects inspire carbon dioxide to raise Pa_{CO_2}, and the effect on minute ventilation is measured. Creating these curves and observing how they change in a variety of circumstances allows quantitative study of factors that affect the chemical carbon dioxide control of ventilation. The carbon dioxide response curve approaches linearity in the range most often encountered in life: at Pa_{CO_2} values between 20 and 80 mm Hg. Once the Pa_{CO_2} exceeds 80 mm Hg, the curve becomes parabolic, with its peak ventilatory response at a Pa_{CO_2} between 100 and 120 mm Hg. Increasing the Pa_{CO_2} above 100 mm Hg allows carbon dioxide to act as a ventilatory and CNS depressant, the origin of the term "carbon dioxide narcosis."

The slope of the carbon dioxide response curve is considered to represent carbon dioxide sensitivity. Normal carbon dioxide sensitivity ranges from 0.5 to 0.7 l·min^{-1}·mm Hg^{-1} CO_2. When Pa_{CO_2} reaches 100 mm Hg, carbon dioxide sensitivity is at its peak, and normally reaches as high as a 2.0 l·min^{-1}·mm Hg^{-1} CO_2. The setpoint, the point of intersection of the carbon dioxide response curve and the metabolic hyperbola, defines normal resting Pa_{CO_2}. Extrapolation of the carbon dioxide response curve to the x-intercept (where minute ventilation is 0) defines the *apneic threshold*, which normally occurs at a Pa_{CO_2} of approximately 32 mm Hg in awake adults. The slope of the curve is a measure of the response of the entire ventilatory mechanism to carbon dioxide stimulation.

Once Pa_{O_2} exceeds 100 mm Hg, it no longer influences the carbon dioxide response curve. When the Pa_{O_2} is between 65 and 100 mm Hg, its effect on the carbon dioxide response curve is small. However, when Pa_{O_2} falls below

65 mm Hg, the carbon dioxide response curve shifts to the left and its slope increases, probably as a result of increased ventilatory drive stimulated by the peripheral chemoreceptors. Thus, during measurements of carbon dioxide ventilatory response, the subject should breathe supplemental oxygen.

The carbon dioxide response curve can be generated rapidly by increasing the fraction of inspired carbon dioxide (F_{ICO_2}) by requiring the subject to rebreathe exhaled gas. The results obtained with this technique are less pure because the F_{ICO_2} is not controlled.

Three clinical states result in a left shift and/or a steepened slope of the carbon dioxide response curve. These same three situations are the only causes of true hyperventilation, *i.e.*, an increase in minute ventilation such that the decreased Pa_{CO_2} creates respiratory alkalemia (either primary or compensatory). Situations resulting in enhanced carbon dioxide response are (1) arterial hypoxemia, (2) metabolic acidemia, and (3) central etiologies. Examples of central etiologies that cause hyperventilation include drug administration, intracranial hypertension, hepatic cirrhosis, and nonspecific arousal states such as anxiety and fear. Aminophylline, salicylates, and norepinephrine stimulate ventilation independent of peripheral chemoreceptors. Opioid antagonists, given in the absence of opioids to presumably normal people, do not stimulate ventilation. However, when given after opiate administration, they do reverse the effects of opioids on the carbon dioxide response curve.

Ventilatory depressants displace the carbon dioxide response curve to the right or decrease its slope, or both. Changes in physiology that depress ventilation include metabolic alkalemia, denervation of peripheral chemoreceptors, normal sleep, and drugs. During normal sleep, the carbon dioxide response curve is displaced to the right, with the degree of displacement depending on the depth of sleep. Usually, Pa_{CO_2} increases up to 10 mm Hg during deep sleep. Hypoxemic responses are not impaired by sleep, which is convenient for continued survival at high altitude.

Opioids displace the carbon dioxide response curve to the right with little change in slope at sedative doses. With higher, "anesthetic" doses, the curve shifts farther to the right and its slope is depressed, simulating the effect of potent inhalation agents on the carbon dioxide response curve (see Fig. 33-5). Opioids induce pathognomonic changes in ventilatory patterns: a decreased ventilatory rate with an increased tidal volume. Not until opioids nearly induce apnea is tidal volume decreased. Large narcotic doses can result in apnea before consciousness is lost. Like sex, breathing requires both ability and desire.

Barbiturates in sedative or light hypnotic doses have little effect on the carbon dioxide response curve. In doses adequate to allow skin incision, barbiturates shift the carbon dioxide response curve to the right. The ventilatory pattern resulting from barbiturate administration is characterized by decreased tidal volume and increased ventilatory rate. Potent inhaled anesthetics displace the carbon dioxide response curve to the right and decrease the slope, the degree depending on the anesthetic dose and the level of surgical stimulation. As the inhaled anesthetic dose increases, the carbon dioxide response curve eventually becomes horizontal (slope = 0), resulting in essentially no ventilatory response to Pa_{CO_2} changes.

Potent inhaled anesthetics and opioids both displace the set point to the right, implying that the resting, steady-state Pa_{CO_2} is higher and minute ventilation lower. Further, when the carbon dioxide response curve shifts to the right, the apneic threshold also increases (see Fig. 33-5). Surgical

stimulation reverses the ventilatory response changes induced by inhaled anesthetics and opioids, but the degree of reversal is not predictable. Enflurane, halothane, and isoflurane all produce qualitatively similar carbon dioxide ventilatory responses. At equipotent doses, when administered with oxygen, the greatest to least ventilatory depression occurs with enflurane, halothane, and isoflurane.

OXYGEN AND CARBON DIOXIDE TRANSPORT

This chapter discusses only *external* respiration, in which oxygen moves from the ambient environment into the pulmonary capillaries and carbon dioxide leaves the pulmonary capillaries to enter the atmosphere. The movement of gas across the alveolar-capillary membrane depends on the integrity of the pulmonary and cardiac systems. Unless it is otherwise stated, the reader should assume that the ventilation and perfusion of alveolar-capillary units are normal. Abnormal distribution of ventilation or perfusion of the lungs is discussed later (see Ventilation-Perfusion Relationships).

Bulk Flow of Gas (Convection)

Convection, in which all gas molecules move in the same direction, is the primary mechanism responsible for gas flow in large and most small airways, down to the bronchi and bronchiolar airways of the 14th or 15th generation. Because the cross-sectional area of the airways progressively increases as gas moves toward the lung periphery, the average velocity of gas particles decreases as they travel toward the alveoli. As a result, the greatest part of airway resistance occurs in the larger airways, where gas molecules travel more quickly. During normal quiet ventilation, gas flow within convective airways is mainly laminar, thus reducing resistance to gas flow (see Resistance to Gas Flow).

Gas Diffusion

Diffusion is random molecular motion that results in the complete mixing of all gases. In the lung, diffusion gradually becomes the predominant mode of gas transport, beginning with the terminal bronchioles (16th airway generation). Once gas reaches the small alveolar ducts, alveolar sacs, and alveoli, both diffusion and regional V/Q relationships influence gas transport. Historically, clinicians assumed that defects in gas diffusion were responsible for arterial hypoxemia. However, the most frequent cause of arterial hypoxemia is physiologic shunt (see Ventilation-Perfusion Relationships).[75]

Carbon dioxide is 20 times as diffusible across membranes as oxygen molecules; therefore, carbon dioxide crosses membranes easily. As a result, hypercarbia is never the result of defective diffusion, but rather the result of inadequate alveolar ventilation with respect to carbon dioxide production.

True diffusion defects that create arterial hypoxemia are rare. When diffusing capacity is measured, the most common reason for a measured decrease in diffusing capacity (see Pulmonary Function Testing) is mismatched ventilation and perfusion that functionally results in a decreased surface area available for diffusion.

Distribution of Ventilation and Perfusion

The efficiency with which oxygen and carbon dioxide exchange at the alveolar-capillary level highly depends on the matching of capillary perfusion and alveolar ventilation. At this level, the marriage between the lung and the circulatory system must be well-matched and intimate.

Distribution of Blood Flow

Blood flow within the lung is mainly gravity dependent. Because the alveolar-capillary beds are not composed of rigid vessels, the pressure of the surrounding tissues can influence the resistance to flow through the individual capillaries. Thus, blood flow depends on the relationship between pulmonary artery pressure (Ppa), alveolar pressure (PA), and pulmonary venous pressure (Ppv̄) (Fig. 33-6). West created a lung model that divides the lung into three zones.[76,77] Zone I conditions occur in the highest part of the lung, independent of body position, above the level where pulmonary artery pressure is equal to alveolar pressure. Because alveolar pressure is approximately equal to atmospheric pressure, pulmonary artery pressure in Zone I is subatmospheric, but necessarily greater than pulmonary venous pressure (PA > Ppa > Ppv̄). Alveolar pressure that is transmitted to the pulmonary capillaries promotes their collapse, with a consequent theoretical blood flow of zero to this lung region. Thus, Zone I receives ventilation in the absence of perfusion, and creates alveolar dead space ventilation. Normally, Zone I areas exist only to a limited extent. However, in conditions of decreased pulmonary artery pressure, such as hypovolemic shock, Zone I enlarges.

Zone III occurs in the most gravity-dependent areas of the lung where Ppa > Ppv̄ > PA and blood flow is primarily governed by the pulmonary arterial to venous pressure difference. Because gravity also increases pulmonary venous pressure, the pulmonary capillaries become distended. Thus, perfusion in Zone III is lush, resulting in capillary perfusion in excess of ventilation, or physiologic shunt.

Finally, Zone II occurs from the lower limit of Zone I to the upper limit of Zone III, where Ppa > PA > Ppv̄. The pressure difference between pulmonary artery and alveolar pressure determines blood flow in Zone II. Pulmonary venous pressure has little influence. Well-matched ventilation and perfusion occur in Zone II, which contains the majority of alveoli.

Distribution of Ventilation

Alveolar pressure is the same throughout the lung; therefore, the more negative intrapleural pressure at the apex results in physically larger, more distended apical alveoli than in other areas of the lung. The transpulmonary pressure (Paw − Ppl), or distending pressure of the lung, is greater at the top and lower at the bottom, where intrapleural pressure is less negative. Despite the smaller alveolar size, more ventilation is delivered to dependent pulmonary areas. The decrease in intrapleural pressure at the base of the lungs during inspiration is greater than at the apex because of diaphragmatic proximity. Thus, more gas is sucked into dependent areas of the lung.

Ventilation-Perfusion Relationships

As discussed above, the majority of blood flow is distributed to the gravity-dependent part of the lung. During a spontaneous breath, the largest portion of the tidal volume also reaches gravity-dependent lung. Thus, the nondependent area of the lung receives a lower proportion of both ventilation and perfusion, and dependent lung receives greater proportions of ventilation and perfusion. Nevertheless, ventilation and perfusion are not matched perfectly, and a variety of V̇A/Q̇ ratios result throughout the lung. The ideal V̇A/Q̇ ratio of 1 is believed to occur at approximately the level of the third rib. Above this level, ventilation occurs slightly in excess of perfusion, while below the third rib the V̇A/Q̇ ratio becomes less than 1 (Fig. 33-7).

In a simplified model, gas exchange units can be divided into normal (V̇A/Q̇ = 1:1), dead space (V̇A/Q̇ = 1:0), shunt (V̇A/Q̇ = 0:1), or a silent unit (V̇A/Q̇ = 0:0) (Fig. 33-8). Although this model is helpful in understanding V̇A/Q̇ relationships and their influences on gas exchange,[78] V̇A/Q̇ really occurs as a continuum. In the lungs of a healthy, upright, spontaneously breathing individual, the majority of alveolar-capillary units are normal gas exchange units. The V̇A/Q̇ ratio varies between absolute shunt, in which V̇A/Q̇ equals 0, to absolute dead space, in which V̇A/Q̇ is infinity. Rather than absolute shunt, most units with low V̇A/Q̇ mismatch receive decreased ventilation relative to blood flow. Similarly, most dead space units are not absolute but are characterized by low blood flow relative to ventilation.

Hypoxic pulmonary vasoconstriction, stimulated by alve-

Figure 33-6. Distribution of blood flow in the isolated lung. In Zone 1, alveolar pressure (PA) exceeds pulmonary artery pressure (Ppa), and no flow occurs because the vessels are collapsed. In Zone 2, arterial pressure exceeds alveolar pressure, but alveolar pressure exceeds pulmonary venous pressure (Ppv̄). Flow in Zone 2 is determined by the arterial-alveolar pressure difference (Ppa − PA), which steadily increases down the zone. In Zone 3, pulmonary venous pressure exceeds alveolar pressure, and flow is determined by the arterial-venous pressure difference (Ppa − Ppv̄), which is constant down this pulmonary zone. However, the pressure across the vessel walls increases down the zone, so that their caliber increases, as does flow. (Reproduced with permission from West JB, Dollery CT, Naimark A: Distribution of blood flow in isolated lung: Relation to vascular and alveolar pressures. J Appl Physiol 19:713, 1964.)

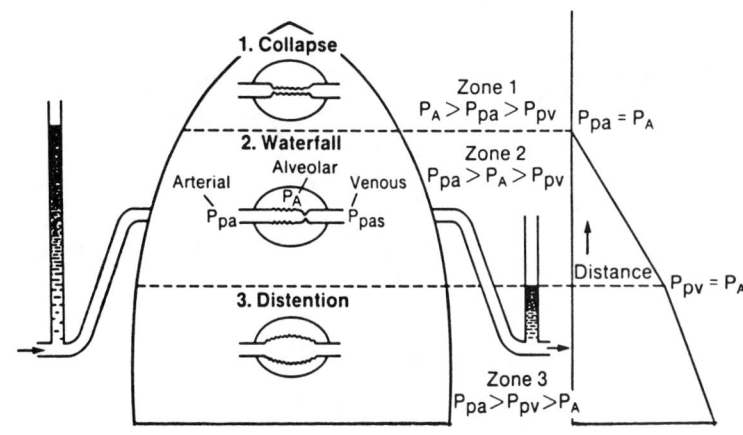

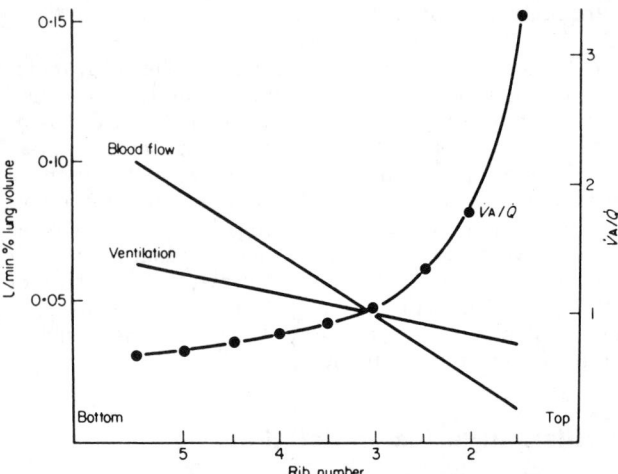

Figure 33-7. Distribution of ventilation, blood flow, and ventilation-perfusion ratio in the normal, upright lung. Straight lines have been drawn through the ventilation and blood flow data. Because blood flow falls more rapidly than ventilation with distance up the lung, ventilation-perfusion ratio rises, slowly at first, then rapidly. (Reproduced with permission from West JB: Ventilation/Blood Flow and Gas Exchange, 4th ed. Oxford, England, Blackwell Scientific Publications, 1985.)

olar hypoxia, severely decreases blood flow. Thus, poorly ventilated alveoli also receive minuscule blood flow. Further, decreased regional pulmonary blood flow results in bronchiolar constriction and diminishes the degree of dead space ventilation.[79,80] When either of these phenomena occurs, the shunt or dead space units effectively become silent units in which little ventilation or perfusion occurs.

Many pulmonary diseases result in both physiologic shunt and dead space abnormalities. However, most disease processes can be characterized as producing either primarily shunt or dead space in their early stages.

Physiologic Dead Space

Each inspired breath is composed of gas that contributes to alveolar ventilation (VA) and gas that becomes dead space ventilation (VD). Thus, tidal volume (VT) = VA + VD. In the normal, spontaneously breathing person, the ratio of alveolar to dead space ventilation for each breath is 2:1. Conveniently, the rule of "1, 2, 3" applies to normal, spontaneously breathing persons. For each breath, 1 ml·lb^{-1} (body weight) becomes VD, 2 ml·lb^{-1} becomes VA, and 3 ml·lb^{-1} constitutes the VT.

Physiologic dead space consists of anatomic and alveolar dead space. Anatomic dead space ventilation, approximately 2 ml·kg^{-1} ideal body weight, accounts for the majority of physiologic dead space.[81] It arises from ventilation of the oronasopharynx to the terminal and respiratory bronchioles, where little gas exchange occurs. Clinical conditions that modify anatomic dead space include tracheal intubation, tracheostomy, and large lengths of ventilator tubing between the tracheal tube and the ventilator Y-piece.

Alveolar dead space ventilation arises from ventilation of alveoli where there is little or no perfusion. Because disease changes anatomic dead space little, physiologic dead space is primarily influenced by changes in alveolar dead space.

The clinician's primary focus is on conditions that significantly increase alveolar dead space ventilation.[82] The most common etiology of acutely increased physiologic dead space is an abrupt decrease in cardiac output.[83] Rapid changes in physiologic dead space ventilation most often arise from changes in pulmonary blood flow, resulting in decreased perfusion to ventilated alveoli. Other pathologic conditions that interfere with pulmonary blood flow include pulmonary embolism, whether due to thrombus, fat,

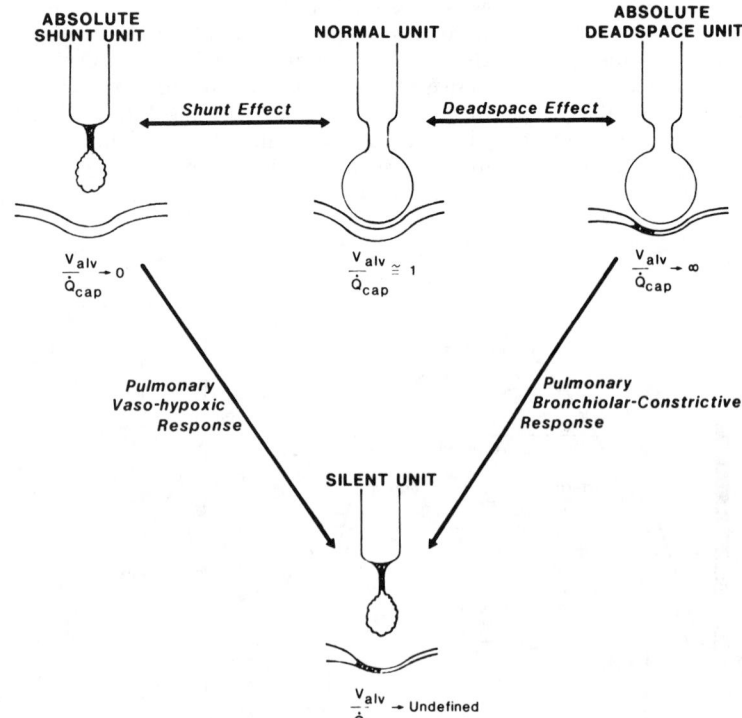

Figure 33-8. Continuum of ventilation/perfusion relationships. Gas exchange is maximally effective in normal lung units and only partially effective in shunt and deadspace effect units. It is totally absent in silent units, absolute shunt, and deadspace units.

air, or amniotic fluid. Chronic pulmonary diseases can create dead space ventilation by chronically changing the relationship between alveolar ventilation and blood flow; this alteration is especially prominent in patients with COPD. Further, acute diseases such as adult respiratory distress syndrome can cause an increase in dead space ventilation owing to intense pulmonary vasoconstriction. Finally, therapeutic or supportive manipulations such as positive pressure ventilation or positive airway pressure therapy can increase alveolar dead space because depressed venous return to the right heart will decrease cardiac output.[84] Intravenous fluid administration will usually overcome this problem.

Increases in dead space ventilation primarily affect carbon dioxide elimination and have little influence on arterial oxygenation until dead space ventilation exceeds 80–90% of minute ventilation ($\dot{V}E$).

Assessment of Physiologic Dead Space

Because the lung receives nearly 100% of the cardiac output, assessment of physiologic dead space ventilation in the acute setting yields valuable information about pulmonary blood flow and, ultimately, about cardiac output. If pulmonary blood flow decreases, the most likely cause is a decreased cardiac output. Thus, it is clinically useful to be able to readily assess the degree of physiologic dead space ventilation.

There are two easy and several difficult ways to assess dead space ventilation. A comparison of minute ventilation and Pa_{CO_2} allows a gross qualitative assessment of physiologic dead space ventilation. The Pa_{CO_2} is determined only by alveolar ventilation and $\dot{V}_{CO_2}$. If $\dot{V}_{CO_2}$ remains constant, Pa_{CO_2} also will remain constant as long as minute ventilation supplies the same degree of alveolar ventilation. If the spontaneously breathing individual must increase minute ventilation to maintain the same Pa_{CO_2}, he has experienced an increase in dead space ventilation because less of the minute ventilation is contributing to alveolar ventilation. Alternatively, a mechanically ventilated patient with a fixed minute ventilation and no increase in $\dot{V}_{CO_2}$ also experiences an increased dead space ventilation if the Pa_{CO_2} rises. Hence, when Pa_{CO_2} in a mechanically ventilated patient increases, it is necessary to determine if the cause is increased dead space ventilation or an increased $\dot{V}_{CO_2}$. A rule of thumb for mechanically ventilated patients is that doubling baseline minute ventilation decreases Pa_{CO_2} from 40 to 30 mm Hg, and quadrupling minute ventilation decreases Pa_{CO_2} from 40 to 20 mm Hg.

The mechanically ventilated patient with normal lungs has a dead space to alveolar ventilation ratio (V_D/V_A) of 1:1 rather than 1:2, as during spontaneous ventilation. If mechanical V_T is 1000 ml, 500 ml contributes to V_A and 500 ml contributes to V_D. At rest, the required $\dot{V}_A$ with normal $\dot{V}_{CO_2}$ is approximately 60 ml·kg^{-1}·min^{-1}. A 70-kg man would then require a $\dot{V}_A$ of 4200 ml·min^{-1}. During spontaneous breathing, the required $\dot{V}E$ would be 6300 ml, but during mechanical ventilation $\dot{V}E$ would have to be 8400 ml·min^{-1}. With this calculation made, if a 70-kg resting patient requires $\dot{V}E$ much in excess of 8400 ml·min^{-1}, either $\dot{V}_D$ or $\dot{V}_{CO_2}$ is increased.

With properly functioning equipment, the difference between Pa_{CO_2} and end-tidal P_{CO_2} ($P_{ET}CO_2$) is widened only by changes in dead space ventilation. Measurement of this difference is simple, readily obtainable, somewhat inexpensive and yields reliable information relative to the degree of dead space ventilation. Clinical situations that change

pulmonary blood flow sufficiently to increase dead space ventilation can be detected by comparing $P_{ET}CO_2$ with temperature-corrected Pa_{CO_2}. Yamanaka and Sue[85] found that the $Pa - P_{ET}CO_2$ in ventilated patients varied linearly with the dead space to tidal volume ratio (V_D/V_T), and that $P_{ET}CO_2$ correlated poorly with Pa_{CO_2}. Thus, in the critically ill, mechanically ventilated patient and in anesthetized patients, monitoring $P_{ET}CO_2$ gives far more information about ventilatory efficiency or dead space ventilation than it does about the absolute value of Pa_{CO_2}. The Pa_{CO_2} will be greater than or equal to $P_{ET}CO_2$ unless the patient inspires carbon dioxide.

Anesthesiologists commonly measure $P_{ET}CO_2$ to detect venous air embolism during anesthesia. A lowered cardiac output alone, in the absence of venous air embolism, may sufficiently decrease pulmonary perfusion so that dead space ventilation increases and $P_{ET}CO_2$ falls. Thus, a depressed $P_{ET}CO_2$ is a sensitive but nonspecific monitor. Air in the pulmonary arteries mechanically interferes with blood flow and also causes pulmonary arterial constriction, further decreasing pulmonary blood flow. A decreased $P_{ET}CO_2$ suggests that a physiologically significant air embolism has occurred. The same physiologic considerations apply to detecting pulmonary thromboembolism.

Depressed cardiac output is probably the most common cause of acutely decreased pulmonary blood flow and increased physiologic dead space ventilation in the operating room and intensive care unit. Weil et al[86] observed a linear correlation between $P_{ET}CO_2$ and cardiac output during resuscitation in pigs when Pa_{CO_2} was kept constant ($r = 0.79$). They concluded that the increase in $P\bar{v}CO_2$ and the concurrent decrease in $P_{ET}CO_2$ reflected a critical reduction in cardiac output, which diminished alveolar blood flow to the extent that carbon dioxide clearance by the lung failed to keep pace with systemic carbon dioxide production.

Some clinicians use the divergence of $P_{ET}CO_2$ from Pa_{CO_2} as a reflection of pulmonary blood flow for other applications. During intentional pharmacologic or surgical manipulation of pulmonary blood flow, the difference between Pa_{CO_2} and $P_{ET}CO_2$ serves as a useful physiologic monitor of the effectiveness of these interventions. Further, regarding $P_{ET}CO_2$ as a reflection of pulmonary perfusion is a useful tool for studying and monitoring the effectiveness of closed-heart massage during resuscitation efforts. Murray and coworkers[87] suggested that an appropriate positive end-expiratory pressure (PEEP) level could be chosen based on the difference between Pa_{CO_2} and $P_{ET}CO_2$. They hypothesized that this gradient should be smallest when there is maximal recruitment of perfused, functional gas units without alveolar overdistention that would create dead space ventilation. The study demonstrating the usefulness of this concept was performed in dogs; it has been difficult to apply this concept in humans. These applications take advantage of $Pa - P_{ET}CO_2$ as an estimate of physiologic dead space ventilation, which can be calculated more precisely if mixed-expiratory $P\bar{E}CO_2$ is known.

The most quantitative technique used to measure physiologic dead space utilizes a modification of the Bohr equation,

$$\frac{V_D}{V_T} = \frac{Pa_{CO_2} - P\bar{E}CO_2}{Pa_{CO_2}}$$

where $P\bar{E}CO_2$ is the P_{CO_2} from the mixture of all expired gases. In spontaneously breathing patients, normal V_D/V_T is between 0.2 and 0.4, or approximately 0.33. In patients receiving positive pressure ventilation, V_D/V_T becomes approximately 0.5. The major limitation of this measurement is the difficulty in collecting exhaled gas for $\bar{P}\text{E}\text{CO}_2$. Exhaled gases, collected in cumbersome 8-liter bags, can easily be contaminated with inspired air or supplemental oxygen. The measurement also will be inaccurate if the patient does not maintain a steady pattern of ventilation. Therefore, extreme care must be taken to ensure that all measurements are performed accurately. In practice, this measurement is rarely performed.

Physiologic Shunt

Whereas physiologic dead space ventilation applies to areas of the lung that are ventilated but poorly perfused, physiologic shunt occurs in lung that is perfused but poorly ventilated. Physiologic dead space primarily affects carbon dioxide elimination; physiologic shunt primarily inhibits arterial oxygenation. Defective to absent gas exchange can be the net effect of either abnormality in the extreme.[88] The physiologic shunt ($\dot{Q}\text{sp}$) is that portion of the total cardiac output ($\dot{Q}\text{t}$) that returns to the left heart and systemic circulation without receiving oxygen in the lung. When pulmonary blood is not exposed to alveoli or when those alveoli are devoid of ventilation, the result is *absolute shunt*, in which $\dot{V}\text{A}/\dot{Q} = 0$. *Shunt effect*, or *venous admixture*, is the more common clinical phenomenon and occurs in areas where alveolar ventilation is deficient compared to the degree of perfusion: $0 < \dot{V}\text{A}/\dot{Q} \ll 1$. Because blood passing through areas of absolute shunt receives *no* oxygen, arterial hypoxemia resulting from absolute shunt is not reversed with supplemental oxygen. Alternatively, supplemental oxygen supplied to patients with arterial hypoxemia due to venous admixture will increase the PaO_2. Although ventilation to these alveoli is deficient, they do carry a small amount of oxygen to the capillary bed.

A small percentage of venous blood normally bypasses the right ventricle and empties directly into the left atrium. This anatomic, absolute shunt arises from the venous return from the pleural, bronchiolar, and thebesian veins. This venous drainage accounts for 2–5% of total cardiac output and explains the small shunt that normally occurs. Anatomic shunts of greatest magnitude usually are associated with congenital heart disease that causes right-to-left shunt. Intrapulmonary anatomic shunts, such as arteriovenous malformations, can also cause anatomic shunt. Intrapulmonary arteriovenous malformations are observed in patients with advanced hepatic cirrhosis.[89] Examples of diseases causing absolute shunt include acute lobar atelectasis, extensive acute lung injury, advanced pulmonary edema, and consolidated pneumonia. Examples of disease entities that produce venous admixture include mild pulmonary edema, postoperative atelectasis, and chronic obstructive pulmonary disease.

Physiologic Shunt Calculation

The clinical reference standard for the calculation of physiologic shunt fraction is derived from a two-compartment pulmonary blood flow model where one compartment (gas exchange) represents the perfect alveolar-capillary marriage and the other compartment (shunt) receives pulmonary capillary blood flow with no ventilation. Using the Fick relationship, the following equation can be derived:

$$\frac{\dot{Q}\text{sp}}{\dot{Q}\text{t}} = \frac{\text{Cc}'\text{O}_2 - \text{CaO}_2}{\text{Cc}'\text{O}_2 - \text{C}\bar{\text{v}}\text{O}_2}$$

where $\text{Cc}'\text{O}_2$ and $\text{C}\bar{\text{v}}\text{O}_2$ are end-capillary and mixed venous oxygen contents respectively. Because this equation is based on an artificial two-compartment model, the absolute value is physically meaningless. A calculated $\dot{Q}\text{sp}/\dot{Q}\text{t}$ of 25% physically means that *if* the lung existed in two compartments, 25% of the cardiac output would travel through the shunt compartment. Because the lung does not exist in two compartments, this equation grossly estimates pulmonary gas exchange defects. Nevertheless, it remains our best tool for clinically evaluating the efficiency with which the lungs oxygenate arterial blood. Observing shunt fraction change with therapeutic intervention or on the progress of disease is more valuable than knowing the absolute value *per se*.

Because hemoglobin concentration is uniform throughout the vascular system, the oxygen contents in the shunt equation are determined primarily by oxyhemoglobin saturation. Thus, the shunt equation can be approximated by substituting saturation values for each term; the new value, called *ventilation-perfusion ratio* (VQI),[90] is determined as follows:

$$\text{VQI} = \frac{\text{Sc}'\text{O}_2 - \text{SaO}_2}{\text{Sc}'\text{O}_2 - \text{S}\bar{\text{v}}\text{O}_2} = \frac{1 - \text{SaO}_2}{1 - \text{S}\bar{\text{v}}\text{O}_2}$$

If the patient is neither breathing a hypoxic gas mixture nor has a methemoglobin or carboxyhemoglobin value in excess of 5–6%, $\text{Sc}'\text{O}_2$ must equal 1 because the model requires a perfect alveolar-capillary interface. This substitution results in the final expression in the equation above.

SaO_2 and $\text{S}\bar{\text{v}}\text{O}_2$ can be estimated continuously with pulse oximetry and by using a pulmonary artery catheter with oximetry capability. By interfacing the outputs of these two devices with a computer, VQI can be calculated continuously.

The greatest advantage of calculating $\dot{Q}\text{sp}/\dot{Q}\text{t}$ or VQI to assess arterial oxygenation is that these values include the contribution of mixed venous blood. Oxygen tension–based indices do not reflect mixed venous contribution to arterial oxygenation and can be misleading.[90] Even if venous admixture is small, mixed venous blood with very low oxygen content will magnify the effect of a small shunt. Oxygen tension–based indices, for example $\text{PaO}_2/\text{FIO}_2$, alveolar to arterial PO_2 difference ($\text{DA}-\text{aO}_2$), and $\text{PaO}_2/\text{PAO}_2$, do not take into account the influence of $\text{C}\bar{\text{v}}\text{O}_2$ on the arterial oxygenation process. Therefore, in critically ill patients who are hypoxemic, the insertion of a pulmonary artery catheter to assess shunt and to measure cardiac output may be essential to understanding the influence of cardiac function on arterial oxygenation.

$\text{DA}-\text{aO}_2$ is a useful quantitative assessment of arterial oxygenation mainly when arterial hemoglobin is well saturated. When PaO_2 is below 150 mm Hg (and certainly when it is below 100 mm Hg), the relationship between oxygen content and oxygen tension is nonlinear. Normal $\text{DA}-\text{aO}_2$ is less than 5 mm Hg when hemoglobin is well saturated with oxygen.

The assessment of arterial oxygenation requires knowledge at least of FIO_2 and either PaO_2 or SaO_2. Further assessment of the efficiency with which the lungs oxygenate the arterial blood can be estimated from oxygen tension–based indices, but these do not take into account the contribution of mixed venous blood to arterial oxygenation. Mixed venous blood can become extremely desaturated in the critically ill patient owing to inadequate cardiac output, anemia, arterial hypoxemia, or increased $\dot{V}\text{O}_2$. The best knowledge of the efficiency with which the lungs oxygenate the arterial blood can be obtained only by calculating shunt fraction or VQI.

PULMONARY FUNCTION TESTING

Anesthesiologists frequently care for patients with significant pulmonary dysfunction in the perioperative and intraoperative periods. Factors predisposing to an increased risk of pulmonary complications include the type of operation, smoking, obesity, and age. When pulmonary function tests are abnormal, the incidence of postoperative pulmonary complications is increased.[91,92] Therefore, it is imperative that the anesthesiologist be able to interpret tests of pulmonary function intelligently and know which tests to request if pulmonary dysfunction is suspected. This section discusses lung volumes, tests of pulmonary mechanics, and diffusing capacity.

Lung Volumes and Capacities

Known, reproducible pulmonary gas volumes and capacities provide a reliable basis for comparison between normal and abnormal measurements.[93] Because normal measurements vary with size, height is most frequently used to define "normal." Lung capacities are composed of two or more lung volumes. Lung volumes and capacities are schematically illustrated in Figure 33-9.

Tidal volume is the volume of gas that moves in and out of the lungs during quiet breathing and is approximately 6 to 8 ml·kg^{-1}. Tidal volume falls with decreased lung compliance or when the patient has reduced ventilatory muscle strength.

Vital capacity is usually approximately 60 ml·kg^{-1}, but

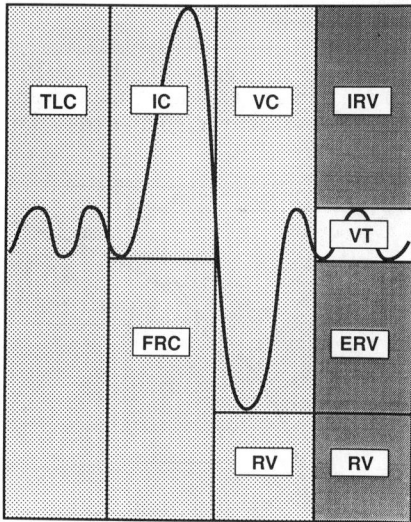

Figure 33-9. Lung volumes and capacities. The darkest bar on the far right depicts the four basic lung volumes that sum to create TLC. Other lung capacities are composed of two or more lung volumes. The overlying spirographic tracing orients the reader to the relationship between the lung volumes and capacities and the spirogram. (ERV = expiratory reserve volume; FRC = functional residual capacity; IC = inspiratory capacity; IRV = inspiratory reserve volume; RV = residual volume; VT = tidal volume; TLC = total lung capacity; VC = vital capacity.)

may vary as much as 20% from normal in healthy individuals. Vital capacity correlates well with the capability for deep breathing and effective coughing. It can be decreased by restrictive pulmonary disease such as pulmonary edema or atelectasis. It also may be reduced by mechanical factors such as pleural effusion, pneumothorax, pregnancy, large ascites, or ventilatory muscle weakness.

The *inspiratory capacity* is the largest volume of gas that can be inspired from the resting expiratory level and frequently is decreased in the presence of significant extrathoracic airway obstruction. This measurement is one of the few simple tests that can detect extrathoracic airway obstruction. Most routine pulmonary function tests measure only exhaled flows and volumes, which may be relatively unaffected by extrathoracic obstruction until it is severe. Changes in the absolute volume of inspiratory capacity usually parallel changes in vital capacity. *Expiratory reserve volume* is not of great diagnostic value.

Functional residual capacity is the volume of gas remaining in the lungs at passive end-expiration. *Residual volume* is that gas remaining within the lungs at the end of forced maximal expiration. The FRC serves two primary physiologic functions. It determines the point on the pulmonary volume-pressure curve for resting ventilation (see Fig. 33-2). The line tangential to the pulmonary volume-pressure curve at FRC defines lung compliance. Thus, FRC determines the elastic pressure-volume relationships within the lung. Further, FRC is the resting expiratory volume of the lung. As such, it greatly influences relationships within the lung. When FRC is reduced, venous admixture (low $\dot{V}_A/\dot{Q}$) increases and results in arterial hypoxemia. (See also the section on Lung Mechanics.)

The FRC also may be used to quantify the degree of pulmonary restriction. Disease processes that reduce FRC and lung compliance include acute lung injury, pulmonary edema, pulmonary fibrotic processes, and atelectasis. The FRC decreases 10% when a healthy subject lies down. Ventilatory muscle weakness or paralysis also will decrease FRC.

In contrast, patients with chronic obstructive pulmonary disease have excessively compliant lungs that recoil less forcibly. Their lungs retain an abnormally large volume at the end of passive expiration, a phenomenon called *gas trapping*.

FRC Measurement

The FRC and residual volume must be measured indirectly because residual volume cannot be removed from the lung. The alveolar nitrogen concentration (PAN$_2$) is assumed to be approximately 78% and to be in equilibrium with the atmosphere. In actuality, PAN$_2$ is slightly less than atmospheric PN$_2$ because of displacement by the respiratory gases, especially carbon dioxide and water vapor. The multiple breath nitrogen washout test is performed by having the subject breathe 100% oxygen for several minutes so that alveolar nitrogen is gradually "washed out." With each breath, the volume of gas and the concentration of nitrogen in the exhaled gas are measured. A rapid nitrogen analyzer coupled to a spirometer or pneumotachometer provides a breath-by-breath analysis of nitrogen washout. Electronic signals proportional to nitrogen concentrations and exhaled volumes (or flow, if a pneumotachometer is used) are integrated to derive the exhaled volume of nitrogen for each breath. Then the values for all breaths are summed to provide a total volume of nitrogen washed out of the lungs. The test is continued for 7 minutes or until the alveolar nitrogen concentration is reduced to less than 7%. FRC is calculated using the equation:

$$FRC = \frac{N_2 \text{ volume} \times [N_2]_f}{[N_2]_i}$$

where $[N_2]_i$ and $[N_2]_f$ are the fractional concentrations of alveolar nitrogen at the beginning and at the end of the test, respectively. These values can be obtained from the initial and final end-tidal nitrogen concentrations. For each minute of oxygen breathing, approximately 40 ml of nitrogen is removed from the blood and tissue. A factor of 0.04 $ml \cdot min^{-1}$ multiplied by the duration of the test in minutes must be subtracted from the calculated FRC value. Finally, the FRC must be corrected to BTPS.

Pulmonary Mechanics

Forced Vital Capacity

The FVC is the volume of gas that can be expired as forcefully and rapidly as possible after maximal inspiration. Normally, FVC is equal to vital capacity. Because forced expiration causes transpulmonary pressures that are greater than normal, bronchiolar collapse, obstructive lesions, and gas trapping are all exaggerated. Thus, FVC may be reduced in chronic obstructive diseases even when the vital capacity appears near normal. FVC nearly always is decreased by restrictive diseases. FVC values < 15 $ml \cdot kg^{-1}$ are associated with an increased incidence of postoperative pulmonary complications.[92] Finally, FVC is largely dependent on patient effort and cooperation.

Forced Expiratory Volume

FEV_T is the volume of gas expired over a given time interval during the FVC maneuver. The interval, described by the subscript T, is the time elapsed in seconds from the onset of expiration.

Because FEV_T records a volume of gas expired over time, it is actually a measure of flow. By assessment of expiratory flow at specific intervals, the severity of airway obstruction can be ascertained. Decreased FEV_T values are common in both obstructive and restrictive disease patterns. The validity of the test depends largely on the cooperation of the subject. The most important application of FEV_T is its correlation with the patient's FVC. Normal subjects can expire at least three quarters of FVC within the first second of the forced expiratory maneuver. The $FEV_{1.0}$, the most frequently employed value, is normally greater than or equal to 0.75.

Normally, an individual can expire 50–60% of FVC in 0.5 second, 75–85% in 1 second, 94% in 2 seconds, and 97% in 3 seconds. Cooperative patients with obstructive disease will exhibit a reduced FEV_T/FVC in most cases. On the other hand, patients with restrictive disease usually have normal FEV_T/FVC ratios. The validity of the evaluation of the FEV_T/FVC is highly dependent on patient cooperation and effort. It is possible to deliberately produce an artificially low FEV_T/FVC.

Forced Expiratory Flow

$FEF_{25-75\%}$ is the average flow rate during the middle half of the FEV maneuver. This test is also called maximum mid-expiratory flow rate (MMFR).

The length of time required for a subject to expire the middle half of the FVC is divided into 50% of the FVC. The spirogram in Figure 33-10 marks the place from 25% to 75%

of FVC, constituting the middle 50% of FVC. The straight line connecting the 25% and 75% volumes has a slope approximately equal to average flow. A normal value for a healthy 70-kg man is approximately 4.7 $l \cdot sec^{-1}$ (or 280 $ml \cdot min^{-1}$). Normally, both the absolute value and the percentage of predicted value for the individual being studied are recorded. A normal value is 100% ± 25% of predicted. Decreased flow rates indicate medium-sized airway obstruction. This value is typically normal in restrictive diseases. This test is fairly sensitive in the early stages of obstructive airway disease. Decreased $FEV_{25-75\%}$ frequently will be observed before other obstructive manifestations occur. Although somewhat effort dependent, the test is much more reliable and reproducible than $FEV_{1.0}/FVC$.

Maximum Voluntary Ventilation

Maximum voluntary ventilation (MVV) is the largest volume of gas that can be breathed in 1 minute by voluntary effort. The MVV is measured by having the subject breathe as deeply and as rapidly as possible for 10, 12, or 15 seconds. The results are extrapolated to 1 minute. The subject should set his own rate and move more than his tidal volume but less than his vital capacity in each breath.

MVV measures the endurance of the ventilatory muscles and indirectly reflects lung-thorax compliance and airway resistance. MVV is the best ventilatory endurance test that can be performed in the laboratory. Normal values may vary by as much as 30% from normal, so that only large reductions in MVV are significant. Healthy, young adults average approximately 170 $l \cdot min^{-1}$. Values are lower in women, and decrease with age in both sexes. Because this maneuver exaggerates air trapping and exerts the ventilatory muscles, MVV is decreased greatly in patients with moderate to severe obstructive disease. MVV is usually normal in patients with restrictive disease because limitation of pulmonary expansion usually does not impede the action of ventilatory muscles.

Flow-Volume Curves

The flow-volume curve graphically demonstrates the flow generated during a forced expiratory maneuver followed by a forced inspiratory maneuver, compared to the volume ex-

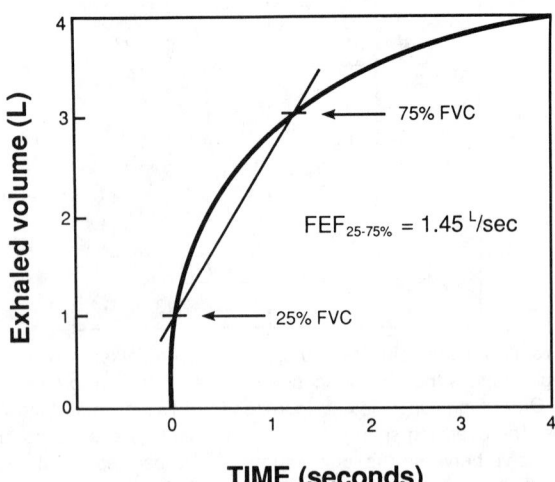

Figure 33-10. $FEF_{25-75\%}$. The spirogram depicts a 4-liter FVC on which the points representing 25% and 75% FVC are marked. The slope of the line connecting these points is the $FEF_{25-75\%}$.

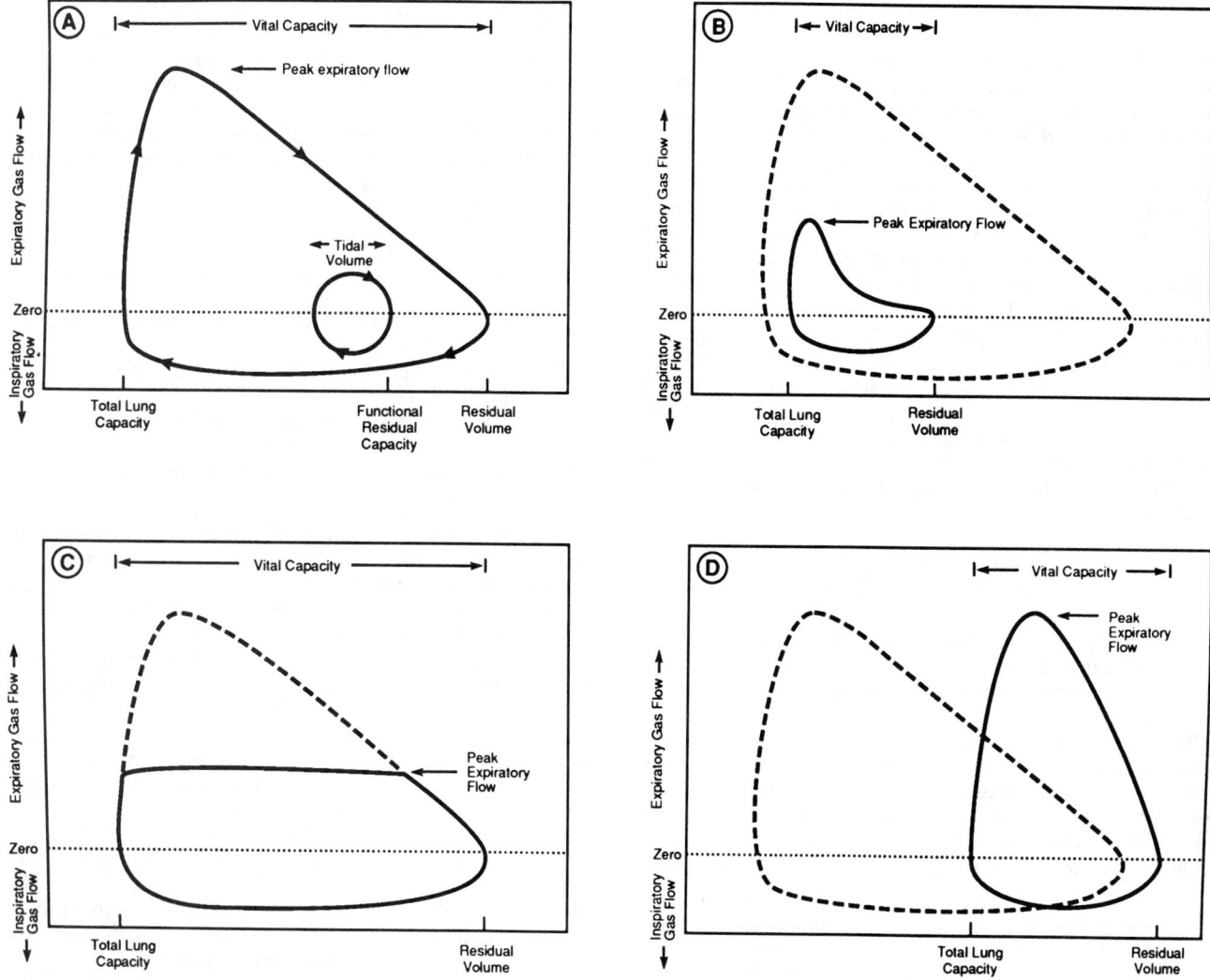

Figure 33-11. Flow-volume loops. Curve *A* is a normally configured adult flow-volume loop. The slope of the loop after the subject reaches peak expiratory flow is nearly linear. Obstructive pulmonary disease, caused by increased airway resistance in the bronchial tree, results in curve *B,* with markedly decreased peak expiratory flow and a "scooped out" appearance for the remainder of expiration. Residual volume is larger and vital capacity is smaller than normal. Curve *C* results from upper airway (extrathoracic) airway obstruction. A flattened expiratory curve with decreased peak expiratory flow is pathognomonic of upper airway obstruction. Curve *D* is found in restrictive lung disease that results in a miniature flow-volume loop with normal peak expiratory flows and a normal-shaped curve. However, residual volume, total lung capacity, and vital capacity are all proportionally reduced.

pired (Fig. 33-11). The subject forcibly exhales completely, then immediately and forcibly inhales to vital capacity. The expired and inspired volumes are plotted on the abscissa and flow is plotted on the ordinate. Although a variety of numbers can be generated from the flow-volume loop, the configuration of the loop itself is probably the most informative part of the test.

Significant decreases in flow or volume are evident in a single graphic display. Obstructive diseases are accompanied by decreased flows and restrictive processes by decreased volumes. The shape of the expiratory curve is largely independent of patient effort, with flow determined mainly by the elastic recoil properties of the lungs (from 75% of TLC down to residual volume). Normally, the flow decreases linearly with volume over most of the vital capac-

ity range, so that the expiratory curve is linear (see Fig. 33-11A). In those with obstructive lung disease, flow decreases particularly at lower lung volumes, and the flow-volume loop takes on a scooped-out appearance (see Fig. 33-11B). Obstruction of the upper airway and trachea is accompanied by characteristic limitations to expiratory and inspiratory flow that result in a flat, ovoid loop. Thus the flow-volume loop is useful in the diagnosis of large airway and extrathoracic airway obstruction (see Fig. 33-11C).

Restrictive disease usually results in relatively normal peak expiratory flows and a linear decrease in flow, but the lung volume itself is decreased (see Fig. 33-11D). Moderate to severe restriction results in equal flows at all lung volumes and appears as a miniature flow-volume loop.

Carbon Monoxide Diffusing Capacity

Because P_{O_2} in the pulmonary capillary blood varies with time as it moves through the pulmonary capillary bed, oxygen cannot be used to assess diffusion capacity. A gas mixture containing carbon monoxide is the traditional diagnostic gas used to measure diffusing capacity. Its partial pressure in the blood is nearly zero, and its affinity for hemoglobin is 200 times that of oxygen.[94] Carbon monoxide diffusing capacity (D_{LCO}) collectively measures all the factors that affect the diffusion of gas across the alveolar-capillary membrane. The D_{LCO} is recorded in ml of $CO \cdot min^{-1} \cdot mm\ Hg^{-1}$ at STPD.

In persons with normal hemoglobin concentrations and normal $\dot{V}_A/\dot{Q}$ matching, the main factor limiting diffusion is the alveolar-capillary membrane. Small amounts of carbon dioxide and inspired gas can produce measurable changes in the concentration of inspired gas compared to expired gas. There are several methods for determining D_{LCO}, but all methods measure diffusing capacity according to the equation

$$D_{LCO} = \frac{ml\ CO\ transferred \cdot min^{-1}}{mean\ P_{ACO} - mean\ capillary\ P_{CO}}.$$

The average value for resting subjects when the single-breath method is used is 25 ml $CO \cdot min^{-1} \cdot mm\ Hg^{-1}$. D_{LCO} values can increase to two or three times normal during exercise.

The D_{LO_2} may be estimated from the D_{LCO} by multiplying D_{LCO} by 1.23, although the D_{LCO} is usually the reported value. D_{LCO} can be divided by the lung volume at which the measurement was made to obtain an expression of diffusing capacity per unit lung volume.

Some of the other factors that can influence D_{LCO} are:

1. Hemoglobin concentration: decreased hemoglobin concentration decreases the D_{LCO};
2. Alveolar P_{CO_2}: an increased P_{ACO_2} raises D_{LCO};
3. Body position: the supine position increases D_{LCO}; and
4. Pulmonary capillary blood volume.

Diffusing capacity is decreased in alveolar fibrosis associated with sarcoidosis, asbestosis, berylliosis, oxygen toxicity, and pulmonary edema. These states are frequently categorized as diffusion defects, but low D_{LCO} probably is related more closely to loss of lung volume or capillary bed perfusion. D_{LCO} is decreased in obstructive disease because of the decreased alveolar surface area, loss of capillary bed, the increased distance from the terminal bronchiole to the alveolar-capillary membrane, and $\dot{V}_A/\dot{Q}$ mismatching. Diffusing capacity also is decreased by space-occupying lesions and lung resection. In short, most states that decrease the measured D_{LCO} actually cause abnormal $\dot{V}_A/\dot{Q}$ matching. Very few disease states truly inhibit oxygen diffusion across the alveolar-capillary membrane.

Preoperative Pulmonary Function Testing

Preoperative assessment of pulmonary function may alert the anesthesiologist to the special needs of a patient with respiratory disease and may allow improvement of pulmonary function before an elective operation. There are no accepted guidelines to determine which patients should undergo pulmonary function testing preoperatively. However, patients who may benefit from preoperative therapy (e.g., to reverse bronchospasm) or for whom quantitative baseline values would be helpful in subsequent postoperative management should undergo preoperative pulmonary function testing. Ideally, tests should be chosen to quantify specific pulmonary problems. Patients in whom the clinical suspicion of markedly impaired function should be high include the following:

1. Patients with any chronic disease that involves the lungs.
2. Heavy smokers with a history of persistent cough or wheezing.
3. Patients with chest wall and spinal deformities.
4. Morbidly obese patients.
5. Patients who will require single lung anesthesia or who will have lung resected.
6. Patients with severe neuromuscular disease.

These people usually can be identified from the preoperative history and physical examination. The object of testing is to predict the likelihood of pulmonary complications and to identify patients who may benefit from therapy to improve pulmonary function preoperatively.

Formal preoperative pulmonary evaluation includes a history and physical examination, chest radiograph, arterial blood gas analysis, and screening spirometry. A history of sputum production, of wheezing or dyspnea, of exercise tolerance, and of other phenomena that limit daily activities may yield more practical information than formal testing. Arterial blood analysis, which should be sampled while the patient breathes room air, adds information regarding gas exchange and acid-base balance. Screening spirometry yields FVC, $FEV_{1.0}$, and $FEV_{1.0}/FVC$ values and the forced midexpiratory flow rate. These results allow classification of lung disease into restrictive, obstructive, or mixed patterns. Further, they quantify the severity of disease.

Patients with obstructive airway disease and decreased expiratory flows may benefit from preoperative bronchodilator therapy and formal pulmonary toilet. High-risk patients with COPD who receive bronchodilation, chest physical therapy, deep breathing, forced oral fluids ($\geq 3\ l \cdot day^{-1}$), preoperative instruction in postoperative respiratory techniques, and who stop smoking experience postoperative pulmonary complications at a rate approximately equal to that observed in normal patients.[95-97] Interestingly, although a regimen like this significantly reduces the incidence of postoperative pulmonary complications,[98] airway obstruction and arterial hypoxemia are not measurably reversed during the 48–72 hours of preoperative therapy.[99] It is possible that the reduced complication rate results from the additional attention that these patients receive rather than from the specific regimen employed.

ANESTHESIA AND OBSTRUCTIVE PULMONARY DISEASE

Patients with marked obstructive pulmonary disease are at increased risk for both intraoperative and postoperative pulmonary complications. For example, patients with reduced $FEV_{1.0}/FVC$ or reduced midexpiratory flow not only suffer airway obstruction but usually exhibit increased airway reactivity. Because of the hazard of provoking reflex bronchoconstriction during laryngoscopy and tracheal intubation, patients with COPD or asthma should receive aggressive bronchodilator therapy preoperatively. High alveolar concentrations of potent inhalational anesthetics will blunt airway reflexes and reflex bronchoconstriction[100] but require a fairly robust cardiovascular system. Adjunctive intravenous administration of opioids and lidocaine prior to airway instrumentation will decrease airway reactivity.

Spontaneous ventilation during general anesthesia in patients with severe obstructive disease is more likely to result in hypercarbia than in patients with normal pulmonary function.[101] Preoperative $FEV_{1.0}$ reduction is related to the $Paco_2$ increase. Therefore, controlled mechanical ventilation with ventilatory rates less than 10 per minute should prevent hypercarbia, minimize $\dot{V}A/\dot{Q}$ mismatch, and allow time for exhalation. Low ventilatory rates necessitate larger tidal volumes, which may predispose the patient to pulmonary barotrauma because of high peak airway pressures. Inspiratory flows should be adjusted to keep peak airway pressure below 40 cm H_2O.[102,103] Higher inspiratory flows produce a shorter inspiratory time and a longer expiratory time. Thus, a balance that avoids high peak airway pressure yet allows the longest possible expiratory time should be sought.

Finally, depending on the procedure and the duration of anesthesia, one ideally would extubate the patient's trachea at the end of the operation. The irritating tracheal tube increases both airway resistance and reflex bronchoconstriction, limits the ability of the patient to clear secretions effectively, and increases the risk of iatrogenic infection. For some patients with obstructive disease (for example, the young asthmatic), many advocate tracheal extubation during deep anesthesia at the conclusion of the operation.

The Effect of Smoking on Pulmonary Function

Smoking affects pulmonary function in many ways. The irritant smoke decreases ciliary motility and increases sputum production. Thus, these patients have a high volume of sputum and decreased ability to clear it effectively. As smoking habits persist over months and years, airway reactivity and the development of obstructive disease become problematic. Early in the disease, mild $\dot{V}A/\dot{Q}$ mismatch, bronchitic disease, and airway hyperreactivity are primary problems. Later, these problems are accompanied by gas trapping, flattened diaphragmatic configuration (which decreases the efficiency with which the diaphragm functions), and barrel chest deformity. Lung compliance increases significantly, so that limited elastic recoil prevents complete passive emptying. As a result, many patients exhale forcibly to reduce gas trapping.

Smoking also affects gas exchange. With gas trapping, ventilation and perfusion become increasingly mismatched. Large areas of dead space ventilation and venous admixture occur. Carbon dioxide elimination is inefficient because of dead space ventilation. The typical minute ventilation for patients with advanced obstructive lung disease can be 1½ to 2 times normal. In addition, venous admixture produces arterial hypoxemia that is exquisitely sensitive to low concentrations of supplemental oxygen. Gas exchange is further impaired by the increased carboxyhemoglobin concentration that results from inspiring smoke. The carboxyhemoglobin concentration normally is less than 1%. However, in smokers, it can be as high as 8–10%.

Finally, smokers are at increased risk for developing head and neck cancers, which may influence airway management.

ANESTHESIA AND RESTRICTIVE DISEASE

Restrictive disease, characterized by proportional decreases in all lung volumes, results in low lung compliance. The decreased FRC not only produces low lung compliance, it also results in arterial hypoxemia because of low $\dot{V}A/\dot{Q}$ mismatching. These patients typically breathe rapidly and shallowly.

Positive pressure ventilation of patients with restrictive disease is fraught with high peak airway pressures because more pressure is required to expand stiff lungs. Lower mechanical tidal volumes at more rapid rates reduce the risk of barotrauma but augment ventilation-induced cardiovascular depression and increase the extent of atelectasis. Larger tidal volumes and lower rates result in less cardiovascular compromise, but the higher peak airway pressure increases the risk of barotrauma.[104] A variety of ventilatory schemes have been developed to ventilate patients with profound restrictive lung disease (see Chapter 59). The use of PEEP will increase FRC and reverse arterial hypoxemia, and by itself will not cause barotrauma.[105] During controlled mechanical ventilation, the cardiovascular effects of PEEP can be profound, although most cardiovascular changes can be reversed by allowing spontaneous ventilation or by intravenous fluid administration. Inotropes or pressors rarely are required when cardiovascular function is depressed as a consequence of increased mean airway pressure.

Because the FRC is small, a lower oxygen store is available during apneic periods. Even preoxygenation with an Fio_2 of 1.0 can result in arterial hypoxemia seconds after the cessation of breathing. Patients with severe restrictive diseases tolerate apnea poorly. Because arterial hypoxemia develops so rapidly, transportation of these patients within the hospital should be performed with a pulse oximeter or some other form of continuous evaluation of arterial oxygenation.

FRC decreases 10–15% in supine, healthy, spontaneously breathing individuals. Controlled ventilation further reduces FRC only slightly.[106] General anesthesia consistently decreases FRC by a further 5–10%,[107] which usually results in decreased lung compliance.[108] The FRC reaches its nadir within the first 10 minutes of anesthesia[107,109,110] and is independent of whether ventilation is spontaneous or controlled. The diminished FRC persists in the postoperative period,[111] but may be restored postoperatively by the use of PEEP or CPAP.[107,112,113] However, once positive airway pressure is removed, FRC plummets to previously diminished levels, which reach a new postoperative nadir 12 hours after operation.[114] After upper abdominal operations, which are associated with the highest incidence of postoperative pulmonary complications, FRC recovers over 3–7 days. With the use of intermittent CPAP by mask, FRC will recover within 72 hours.[115] Patients use incentive spirometers appropriately only 10% of the time unless therapy is supervised.[116] Stir-up regimens are as effective as incentive spirometry at preventing postoperative pulmonary complications,[115] are less expensive than supervised incentive spirometry, and thus are preferred over incentive spirometry therapy. After mediasternotomy for cardiac operations, FRC does not return to normal for several weeks, regardless of postoperative pulmonary therapy.[117] The persistently low FRC in this population probably is due to mechanical factors such as a widened mediastinum, intrapleural fluid, and altered chest wall compliance.

REFERENCES

1. Goss CM (ed): Gray's Anatomy of the Human Body, 29th ed. Philadelphia, Lea & Febiger, 1966
2. Netter FH: Respiratory System. In Divertic MB, Brass A (eds): Ciba Collection of Medical Illustrations, vol 7. Ciba, 1979
3. Wade OL: Movements of thoracic cage and diaphragm in respiration. J Physiol (Lond) 124:193, 1954
4. Gillespi DJ, Marsh HMM, Divertie MB et al: Clinical outcome of respiratory failure in patients requiring prolonged (> 24 hours) mechanical ventilation. Chest 90:364, 1986
5. Burke RE, Levine DN, Zojas FE et al: Mammalian motor units: Physiologic histochemical correlation in these types of cat gastrocnemius. Science 174:709, 1971
6. Lieberman DA, Falkner JA, Craig AB Jr et al: Performance and histochemical composition of guinea pig and human diaphragm. J Appl Physiol 34:233, 1973
7. Roussos C, Macklin PT: Diaphragmatic fatigue in man. J Appl Physiol 43:189, 1977
8. Murphy AJ, Koepec GH, Smith EM et al: Sequence of action of diaphragm and intercostal muscles during respiration: II. Expiration. Arch Phys Med 40:337, 1959
9. Petit JM, Milic-Emili G, Delhez L: Role of the diaphragm in breathing in conscious normal man: An electromyographic study. J Appl Physiol 15:1101, 1960
10. Coryllos PN: Action of the diaphragm in cough: Experimental and clinical study on the human. Am J Med Sci 194:523, 1937
11. Campbell EJM, Green JH: The behavior of the abdominal muscles and intra-abdominal pressure during quiet breathing and increased pulmonary ventilation: A study in man. J Physiol (Lond) 127:423, 1955
12. Conrardy PA, Goodman CR, Lainge F et al: Alteration of endotracheal tube position: Flexion and extension of the neck. Crit Care Med 4:8, 1976
13. Rhodin JAG: An Atlas of Ultrastructure. Philadelphia, WB Saunders, 1963
14. Auerbach O, Stout AP, Hammond EC et al: Changes in bronchial epithelium in relation to cigarette smoking and in relation to lung cancer. N Engl J Med 265:253, 1961
15. Weibel ER: Morphometrics of the lung. In Fenn WO, Rahn H (eds): Handbook of Physiology, Section 3, Vol 1, p 285. Washington DC, American Physiological Society, 1964
16. Krahl VE: Microstructure of the lung. Arch Environ Health 6:37, 1963
17. Gail DB, L'Enfant CJM: Cells of the lung: Biology and clinical implications. Am Rev Respir Dis 127:366, 1983
18. Bachoven M, Weibel ER: Basic pattern of tissue repair in human lungs following unspecific injury. Chest 65:145, 1974
19. Kikkawa Y, Yoneda K, Smith F: The type II epithelial cells of the lung: Chemical composition and phospholipid synthesis. Lab Invest 32:295, 1975
20. Fishman AP: Non-respiratory function of lung. Chest 72:84, 1977
21. Mason RJ, Williams MC, Widdicombe JH: Secretion and fluid transport by alveolar type II epithelial cells. Chest 81(suppl):61, 1982
22. Hocking WG, Golden DW: The pulmonary-alveolar macrophage. N Engl J Med 301:580, 1979
23. Macklin CC: Alveolar pores and their significance in the human lung. Arch Pathol 21:202, 1936
24. Lambert MW: Accessory bronchio-alveolar channels. Anat Rec 127:472, 1957
25. Downs JB: A technique for direct measurement of intrapleural pressure. Crit Care Med 4:207, 1976
26. Rohrer F: Der Strömungswiderstand in den menschlichen Atemwegen. Pflugers Arch [Ges Physiol] 162:225, 1915
27. Nunn JF: Resistance to gas flow and airway closure. In: Applied Respiratory Physiology, p 50. Boston, Butterworths, 1987
28. Fink BR, Ngai SH, Holiday DA: Effect of air flow resistance on ventilation and respiratory muscle activity. JAMA 168:2245, 1958
29. Palmer KNV, Diament ML: Effect of aerosol isoprenaline on blood-gas tensions in severe bronchial asthma. Lancet 2:1232, 1967
30. Campbell EJM, Freedman S, Smith PS, Taylor ME: The ability of man to detect added elastic loads to breathing. Clin Sci 20:223, 1961
31. Nunn JF, Ezi-Ashi TI: The respiratory effects of resistance to breathing in anesthetized man. Anesthesiology 22:174, 1961
32. Campbell EJM: The effects of increased resistance to expiration on the respiratory behavior of the abdominal muscles and intraabdominal pressure. J Physiol 136:556, 1957
33. LeGallois CJJ: Expériences sur le Principe de la Vie, p 325. Paris, D'Hautel, 1812
34. Lumsden TL: The regulation of respiration: Part I. J Physiol (Lond) 58:81, 1923
35. Hoff HE, Breckenridge CG: The medullary origin of respiratory periodicity in the dog. Am J Physiol 158:157, 1949
36. Hoff HE, Breckenridge CG: Intrinsic mechanisms in periodic breathing. AMA Arch Neurol Psychiatry 72:11, 1954
37. Brodie DA, Borison HL: Evidence for a medullary inspiratory pacemaker: Functional concept of central regulation of respiration. Am J Physiol 188:347, 1957
38. Comroe JH Jr: The effects of direct chemical and electrical stimulation of the respiratory center in the cat. Am J Physiol 139:490, 1943
39. Ngai SH, Wang SC: Organization of central respiratory mechanisms in the brainstem of the cats: Localization by stimulation and destruction. Am J Physiol 190:343, 1957
40. Pitts RF: The differentiation of respiratory centers. Am J Physiol 134:192, 1941
41. Pitts RF, Magoun HW, Ranson SW: Localization of the medullary respiratory centers in the cat. Am J Physiol 126:673, 1939
42. Salmoiraghi GC, Burns BD: Localization and patterns of discharge of respiratory neurons in the brainstem of a cat. J Neurophysiol 23:2, 1960
43. Cohen MI: Neurogenesis of respiratory rhythm in the mammal. Physiol Rev 51:1105, 1979
44. Guz A: Regulation of respiration in man. Ann Resp Physiol 37:303, 1975
45. Pitts RF, Magoun HW, Ranson SW: The origin of respiratory rhythmicity. Am J Physiol 127:654, 1939
46. Lumsden TL: Observations on the respiratory centers in the cat. J Physiol (Lond) 57:153, 1923
47. Cohen MI, Wang SC: Respiratory neuronal activity in the pons of the cat. J Neurophysiol 22:33, 1959
48. Stella G: On the mechanism of production and the physiologic significance of "apneusis." J Physiol (Lond) 93:10, 1938
49. Kabat H: Electrical stimulation of points in the forebrain and mid-brain: The resultant alterations in respiration. J Comp Neurol 64:187, 1936
50. Kaada BR: Somato-motor, autonomic and electrocorticographic responses to electrical stimulation of "rhinencephalic" and other structures in primates, cat and dog: A study of responses from the limbic, subcallosal, orbito-insular, piriform and temporal cortex, hippocampus-fornix and amygdala. Acta Physiol Scand 24(suppl 83):1, 1951
51. Chai CY, Wang SC: Localization of central cardiovascular control mechanism in lower brainstem of the cat. Am J Physiol 202:25, 1962
52. Uvnas B: Central cardiovascular control. In Handbook of Physiology, Section I, vol II: Neurophysiology, p 1131. Washington DC, American Physiological Society, 1960
53. Bosma JF: Deglutition: Pharyngeal stage. Physiol Rev 37:275, 1957
54. Wang SC, Borison HL: The vomiting center: A critical experimental analysis. AMA Arch Neurol Psychiatry 63:928, 1950
55. Gaylor JB: The intrinsic nervous mechanisms of the human lung. Brain 57:143, 1934
56. von Euler C: On the role of proprioceptors in perception and execution of motor acts with special reference to breathing. In Pengelly LD, Rebuck AS, Campbell JBL (eds): Loaded Breathing, p 139. Longman, Don Mills, 1974

57. Davis HL, Fowler WS, Lambert EH: Effect of volume and rate of inflation and deflation on transpulmonary pressure and response of pulmonary stretch receptors. Am J Physiol 187:558, 1956

58. Dawes GS, Comroe JH Jr: Chemoreflexes from the heart and lungs. Physiol Rev 34:167, 1954

59. Jung-Caillot MC, Duron B: Number of neuromuscular spindles and electrical activity of the respiratory muscles. In Durm B (ed): Respiratory Centers and Afferent Systems, p 165. Paris, INSERM, 1976

60. Hering E, Breuer J: Die Sebsteuerung der Atmung durch den Nervus vagus. Stizber Akad Wiss Wien 57(II):672, 1868

61. Biscoe TJ: Carotid body: Structure and function. Physiol Rev 58:604, 1978

62. Coleridge HM: Thoracic chemoreceptors in the dog: A histological and electrophysiologic study of the location, innervation and blood supply of the aortic bodies. Circ Res 26:235, 1970

63. Leusen I: Regulation of cerebrospinal fluid composition with reference to breathing. Physiol Rev 52:1, 1972

64. Cohen MI: Discharge patterns of brainstem respiratory neurons in relation to carbon dioxide tension. J Neurophysiol 31:142, 1968

65. Heinemann HO, Golaring RM: Bicarbonate and the regulation of ventilation. Am J Med 57:361, 1974

66. Severinghaus JW, Mitchell RA, Richardson BW et al: Respiratory control at high altitude suggesting active transport regulation of CSF pH. J Appl Physiol 18:1155, 1166, 1963

67. Ferris EB, Engel GL, Stevens CD, Webb J: Voluntary breath holding. J Clin Invest 25:734, 1946

68. Stock MC, Downs JB, McDonald JS et al: The carbon dioxide rate of rise in awake apneic man. J Clin Anesth 1:96, 1988

69. Engle GL, Ferris EB, Webb JP et al: Voluntary breatholding: II. The relation of the maximum time of breatholding to the oxygen tension of the inspired air. J Clin Invest 23:734, 1946

70. Eger EI, Severinghaus JW: The rate of rise of Pa_{CO_2} in the apneic anesthetized patient. Anesthesiology 22:419, 1961

71. Stock MC, Schisler JQ, McSweeney TD: The Pa_{CO_2} rate of rise in anesthetized patients with airway obstruction. J Clin Anesth 1:328, 1989

72. Wright FG, Foley MF, Downs JB et al: Hypoxemia and hypocarbia following intermittent positive-pressure breathing. Anesth Analg 55:555, 1976

73. Fink BR: The stimulant effect of wakefulness on respiration: Clinical aspects. Br J Anaesth 33:97, 1961

74. Berger AJ, Mitchell RA, Severinghaus JW: Regulation of respiration: Part III. N Engl J Med 297:194, 1977

75. West JB: Ventilation/Blood Flow and Gas Exchange, 4th ed. Oxford, England, Blackwell Scientific Publications, 1985

76. West JB, Dollery CT, Naimark A: Distribution of blood flow in isolated lung: Relation to vascular and alveolar pressures. J Appl Physiol 19:713, 1964

77. West JB, Dollery CT: Distribution of blood flow and the pressure-flow relations of the whole lung. J Appl Physiol 20:175, 1965

78. Bendixen HH, Egbert LD, Hedley-Whyte J et al: Respiratory Care. St Louis, CV Mosby, 1965

79. Benumof JL, Pirla AF, Johanson I et al: Interaction of $P\bar{v}_{O_2}$ with Pa_{O_2} on hypoxic pulmonary vasoconstriction. J Appl Physiol 51:871, 1981

80. Swenson EW, Finley TN, Guzman SV: Unilateral hypoventilation in man during temporary occlusion of one pulmonary artery. J Clin Invest 40:828, 1961

81. Fowler WS: Lung function studies: II. The respiratory deadspace. Am J Physiol 154:405, 1948

82. Fisher SR, Duranceau A, Floyd RD et al: Comparative changes in ventilatory deadspace following micro- and massive emboli. J Surg Res 20:195, 1976

83. Freeman J, Nunn JF: Ventilation-perfusion relationships after hemorrhage. Clin Sci 24:135, 1963

84. Bergman NA: Effect of varying respiratory waveforms on distribution of inspired gas during artificial ventilation. Am Rev Respir Dis 100:518, 1969

85. Yamanaka MK, Sue DY: Comparison of arterial-end-tidal P_{CO_2} difference and deadspace/tidal volume ratio in respiratory failure. Chest 92:832, 1987

86. Weil MH, Bisera J, Trevino RP et al: Cardiac output and end-tidal carbon dioxide. Crit Care Med 13:907, 1985

87. Murray IP, Modell JH: Early detection of endotracheal tube accidents by monitoring carbon dioxide concentration in respiratory gas. Anesthesiology 59:344, 1983

88. West JB: Ventilation-perfusion relationships. Am Rev Respir Dis 116:919, 1977

89. Meler C, Naeije R, Delchamps P et al: Pulmonary and extra-pulmonary contributions and hypoxia in liver cirrhosis. Am Rev Respir Dis 139:632, 1989

90. Räsänen J, Dows JB, Malec DJ, Oates K: Oxygen tensions and oxyhemoglobin saturations in the assessment of pulmonary gas exchange. Crit Care Med 15:1058, 1987

91. Block AJ, Olson GN: Preoperative pulmonary function testing. JAMA 235:257, 1976

92. Tisi GM: Preoperative evaluation of pulmonary function. Am Rev Respir Dis 119:293, 1979

93. Christi RV: Lung volume and its subdivisions. J Clin Invest 11:1099, 1932

94. Apthorp GH, Marshall R: Pulmonary diffusing capacity: A comparison of breath-holding and steady-state methods using carbon monoxide. J Clin Invest 40:1775, 1961

95. Stein M, Cassara EL: Preoperative pulmonary evaluation and therapy for surgery patients. JAMA 211:787, 1970

96. Milledge JS, Nunn JF: Criteria for fitness for anaesthesia in patients with chronic obstructive lung disease. Br Med J 3:670, 1975

97. Williams CD, Brenowitz JB: "Prohibitive" lung function and major surgical procedures. Am J Surg 132:703, 1976

98. Gracey DR, Divertie MB, Didier EP: Preoperative pulmonary preparation of patients with chronic obstructive pulmonary disease: A prospective study. Chest 76:123, 1979

99. Petty TL, Brink GA, Miller NW, Corsello PR: Objective functional improvement in chronic airway obstruction. Chest 57:216, 1970

100. Yakaitas RW, Blitt CP, Anguillo JP: End tidal halothane concentration for endotracheal intubation. Anesthesiology 47:386, 1977

101. Pietak W, Weenig CS, Hickey RF et al: Anesthetic effects on ventilation in patients with chronic obstructive pulmonary disease. Anesthesiology 42:160, 1975

102. Connors AF, McAferee D, Gray BA: Effect of inspiratory flow rate on gas exchange during mechanical ventilation. Am Rev Respir Dis 124:537, 1981

103. Tuxen DV, Lane S: The effects of ventilatory pattern on hyperinflation, airway pressures, and circulation in mechanical ventilation of patients with severe airflow obstruction. Am Rev Respir Dis 136:872, 1987

104. Petersen GW, Baier H: Incidence of pulmonary barotrauma in a medical ICU. Crit Care Med 11:67, 1983

105. Pepe PE, Hudson LD, Carrico CJ: Early application of positive end-expiratory pressure in patients at risk for the adult respiratory distress syndrome. N Engl J Med 311:281, 1984

106. Bergofsky EH: Ions and membrane permeability in the regulation of the pulmonary circulation. In Fishman AP, Hect H (eds): The Pulmonary Circulation and Interstitial Space, p 269. Chicago, University of Chicago Press, 1969

107. Brisner B, Hedenstierna G, Lundquist H et al: Pulmonary densities during anesthesia with muscular relaxation: A proposal of atelectasis. Anesthesiology 62:422, 1985

108. Don HF, Robson JG: The mechanics of the respiratory system during anesthesia. Anesthesiology 26:168, 1965

109. Don HF, Wahba M, Cuadrado L et al: The effects of anesthesia and 100 percent oxygen on the functional residual capacity of the lungs. Anesthesiology 32:251, 1970

110. Westbrook PR, Stubbs SE, Sessler AD et al: Effects of anesthesia and muscle paralysis on respiratory mechanics in normal man. J Appl Physiol 34:81, 1973

111. Alexander JI, Spence AA, Parikh RK et al: The role of airway closure in postoperative hypoxemia. Br J Anaesth 45:34, 1975

112. Wyche MQ, Teichner RL, Kallost T et al: Effects of continuous positive-pressure breathing on functional residual capacity

and arterial oxygenation during intra-abdominal operation. Anesthesiology 38:68, 1973

113. Rose DM, Downs JB, Heenen TJ: Temporal responses of functional residual capacity and oxygen tension to changes in positive end-expiratory pressure. Crit Care Med 9:79, 1981

114. Craig DB: Postoperative recovery of pulmonary function. Anesth Analg 60:46, 1981

115. Stock MC, Downs JB, Gauer PK et al: Prevention of postoperative pulmonary complications with CPAP, incentive spirometry and conservative therapy. Chest 87:151, 1985

116. Lyager S, Wernberg M, Rajani N et al: Can postoperative pulmonary complications be improved by treatment with Bartlett-Edwards incentive spirometer after upper abdominal surgery? Acta Anaesthesiol Scand 23:312, 1979

117. Stock MC, Downs JB, Cooper RB et al: Comparison of continuous positive airway pressure, incentive spirometry, and conservative therapy after cardiac operations. Crit Care Med 12:969, 1984

34
James B. Eisenkraft   Steven M. Neustein
Edmond Cohen

Anesthesia for Thoracic Surgery

The number of noncardiac thoracic surgical operations has dramatically increased in recent years and is expected to increase further in the future. A report using data from the National Center for Health Statistics in the USA showed that in 1979, approximately 53,000 procedures on the lung and bronchus were performed; this number had grown to 73,000 in 1983.[1] Mediastinoscopies increased from 33,000 in 1979 to 44,000 in 1983. The increase in this type of surgery has been associated with and sometimes made possible by advances in anesthesia care. Indeed, thoracic anesthesia is developing into a subspecialty in its own right, with a number of reference texts devoted exclusively to this subject.[2-4]

The physiologic, pharmacologic, and clinical considerations for the patient undergoing pulmonary surgery are reviewed, followed by sections on anesthesia for diagnostic and therapeutic procedures, high-frequency ventilation, and special situations, including bronchopleural fistula and tracheal reconstruction. A discussion of myasthenia gravis is included because of the relationship between the thymus gland and myasthenia, and because thymectomy is one of the most commonly performed thoracic surgical procedures in these patients. The chapter concludes with a review of the postoperative management of the thoracic surgical patient.

PREOPERATIVE EVALUATION

In addition to the routine assessment for major surgery, the preoperative evaluation of the patient for thoracic surgery should focus on the extent and severity of pulmonary disease and of cardiovascular involvement.

History

Dyspnea

Dyspnea occurs when the requirement for ventilation is greater than the patient's ability to respond appropriately. Dyspnea is quantitated as to the degree of physical activity required to produce it, the level of activity possible (e.g., ability to walk on level ground or climb stairs), and manage-

ment of daily activities. Severe exertional dyspnea usually implies a significantly diminished ventilatory reserve and a forced expiratory volume in 1 second (FEV_1) of less than 1500 ml, with possible need for postoperative ventilatory support.

Cough

Recurrent productive cough for 3 months of the year for 2 consecutive years is necessary to make the diagnosis of chronic bronchitis. Cough indirectly increases airway irritability. If the cough is productive, the volume, consistency, and color of the sputum should be assessed. Sputum should be cultured to rule out infection and to establish whether there is a need for preoperative antibiotic therapy. Blood-stained sputum or episodes of gross hemoptysis should alert the anesthesiologist to the possibility of a tumor invading the respiratory tract, e.g., the mainstem bronchus, which might interfere with endobronchial intubation.

Cigarette Smoking

Cigarette smoking increases the risk of chronic lung disease and malignancy as well as the incidence of postoperative pulmonary complications. The number of pack-years (packs smoked per day multiplied by the number of years) is directly related to measurable changes in respiratory air flow and closing capacity, making these patients prone to postoperative atelectasis and arterial hypoxemia.[5]

Physical Examination

The physical examination of the patient should address in particular the following aspects.

Respiratory Pattern

The presence of cyanosis and clubbing, the breathing pattern, and the type of breath sounds should be noted.

Cyanosis. The presence of peripheral cyanosis (in the fingers, toes, or ears) should be distinguished from causes of poor circulation (acrocyanosis). The presence of central cyanosis (in the buccal mucosa) is usually secondary to arterial hypoxemia. If cyanosis is present, the arterial saturation is 80% or less (Pao_2 less than 50–52 mm Hg), which indicates a limited margin of respiratory reserve.

Clubbing. Clubbing is often seen in patients with chronic lung disease, malignancies, or congenital heart disease associated with right-to-left shunt.

Respiratory Rate and Pattern. A patient's inability to complete a normal sentence without pausing for breath is an indication of severe dyspnea. Inspiratory paradox, the abdomen moving in while the chest moves out, suggests diaphragmatic fatigue and respiratory dysfunction. The patient should be assessed for paroxysmal retraction (Hoover's sign), limited diaphragmatic movement because of hyperinflation, asymmetry of chest movement secondary to phrenic nerve involvement, hemothorax, pleural effusion, and pneumothorax. The pattern and rate of breathing have important roles in distinguishing between obstructive and restrictive lung disease. For a constant minute ventilation, the work done against air flow resistance decreases when breathing is slow and deep. Work done against elastic resistance decreases when breathing is rapid and shallow (e.g., as in pulmonary infarct, pulmonary fibrosis).

Breath Sounds. Wet sounds (crackles) are usually caused by excessive fluid in the airways and indicate sputum retention or edema. Dry sounds (wheezes) are produced by high-velocity air flow through bronchi and are a sign of airway obstruction. Distant sounds are an indication of emphysema and possibly bullae. The trachea should be in the midline. Displacement of the trachea may be secondary to a number of causes, including mediastinal mass, and should alert the anesthesiologist to a potentially difficult intubation of the trachea and/or airway obstruction on induction of anesthesia.

Evaluation of the Cardiovascular System

One of the most important factors in the evaluation of patients scheduled for thoracic surgery is the presence of an increase in pulmonary vascular resistance (PVR) secondary to a fixed reduction in the cross-sectional area of the pulmonary vascular bed. The pulmonary circulation is a low-pressure, high-compliance system that is capable of handling an increase in blood flow by recruitment of normally underperfused vessels. This acts as a compensatory mechanism, which normally prevents an increase in pulmonary arterial pressure. In chronic obstructive pulmonary disease (COPD), there is distention of the pulmonary capillary bed with reduced ability to tolerate an increase in blood flow (reduced compliance). Such patients demonstrate an increase in PVR when cardiac output increases because of a reduced ability to compensate for an increase in pulmonary blood flow. This results in pulmonary hypertension, signs of which include a narrowly split second heart sound, increased intensity of the pulmonary component of the second heart sound, and right ventricular and atrial hypertrophy.

An increase in PVR is of significance in the management of the patient during anesthesia because several factors such as acidosis, sepsis, hypoxia, and application of positive end-expiratory pressure all further increase the PVR and increase the likelihood of right ventricular failure.

In patients with ischemic or valvular heart disease, the function of the left side of the heart should also be carefully evaluated. This is discussed elsewhere in this volume (Chapter 36).

Laboratory Studies

Electrocardiogram

A patient with COPD may present with electrocardiographic features of right atrial and ventricular hypertrophy and strain. These include a low-voltage QRS complex due to lung hyperinflation and poor R-wave progression across the precordial leads. An enlarged P wave ("P pulmonale") in standard lead II is diagnostic of right atrial hypertrophy. The electrocardiographic changes of right ventricular hypertrophy are an R/S ratio of greater than 1.0 in lead V_1 (i.e., R-wave voltage exceeds S-wave voltage).

Chest Radiography

Hyperinflation and increased vascular markings are usually present with COPD. Prominent lung markings often occur in bronchitis, whereas they are decreased in emphysema, particularly at the bases where actual bullae may be present in severe cases. Hyperinflation, with an increased anteroposterior chest diameter, may be present, together with an enlarged retrosternal air space of greater than 2 cm in diameter seen in a lateral chest radiograph.

The location of the lung lesion should be assessed by posteroanterior and lateral projections on chest radiography. In addition to tracheal or carinal shift, a mediastinal mass may indicate a difficult intubation, a difficult and bloody dissection, difficulty in using a double-lumen tube (because of deviation of the mainstem bronchus), or a collapsed lobe owing to bronchial obstruction with possible sepsis. Review of a computed tomographic study is also useful and will often provide more information about tumor size and location than the chest radiograph.

Arterial Blood Gas. A common finding in arterial blood gas analysis of COPD patients is hypoventilation and CO_2 retention. The "blue bloaters" (chronic bronchitics) are cyanotic, hypercarbic, hypoxemic, and usually overweight. They are in a state of chronic respiratory failure and have a reduced ventilatory response to CO_2. In these patients, the high $Paco_2$ increases cerebrospinal fluid bicarbonate concentration, the medullary chemoreceptors become reset to a higher level of CO_2, and sensitivity to CO_2 is decreased. These patients hypoventilate when given high oxygen concentrations because of a decreased hypoxic drive.

The "pink puffers" (patients with emphysema) typically are thin, dyspneic, and pink, with essentially normal blood gas values. They present with an increase in minute ventilation to maintain their normal $Paco_2$, which explains the increase in work of breathing and dyspnea.

Pulmonary Function Testing and Evaluation for Lung Resectability. There are three goals in performing pulmonary function tests in patients scheduled for lung resection. The first goal is to identify those patients at risk of increased morbidity and mortality postoperatively. In thoracic surgery for lung cancer, the specific question is: How much lung tissue may be safely removed without making the patient a pulmonary cripple? This should be weighed against the 1-year mean survival of the surgically untreated lung carcinoma. The second goal is to identify those patients who will need short- or long-term ventilatory support postoperatively. The third goal is to evaluate the beneficial effect and reversibility of airway obstruction with the use of bronchodilators.

Effects of Anesthesia and Surgery on Lung Volumes. Anesthesia and postoperative medications can cause changes in lung volumes and ventilatory pattern (see Chapter 33). Total lung capacity (TLC) decreases after abdominal surgery but not after surgery on an extremity.[6] Vital capacity (VC) is reduced by 25–50% within 1–2 days following surgery and generally returns to normal after 1–2 weeks. Residual volume (RV) increases by 13%, whereas expiratory reserve volume (ERV) decreases by 25% following lower abdominal surgery and 60% following upper abdominal and thoracic surgery. Tidal volume (VT) decreases by 20% within 24 hours following surgery and gradually returns to normal after 2 weeks. Pulmonary compliance decreases by 33%, with similar reductions in functional residual capacity (FRC) secondary to small airway closure. Most of the patients who undergo lung resection are smokers with a certain degree of COPD and are prone to postoperative complications in direct relation to the amount of lung to be resected (lobectomy or pneumonectomy) and to the severity of the preoperative lung disease.

Spirometry. Forced vital capacity (FVC), FEV_1, and peak expiratory flow rate (PEFR) can be measured at the patient's bedside using a spirometer. The measurement can be recorded as a volume-time trace or as a flow-volume loop.

A VC of at least three times the VT is necessary for an effective cough.[7] A VC of less than 50% of predicted or less than 2 l is an indicator of increased risk.[8] An abnormal preoperative VC can be identified in 30–40% of postoperative deaths. A patient with an abnormal VC has a 33% chance of complications and a 10% risk of postoperative mortality.

FEV_1 is a more direct indication of airway obstruction. An FEV_1 of less than 800 ml in a 70-kg male is probably incompatible with life and is an absolute contraindication to lung resection. Mortality in patients with an FEV_1 greater than 2 l is 10% and in patients below 1 l is between 20–45%.[9]

The ratio FEV_1/FVC is useful in differentiating between restrictive and obstructive disease. It is normal in restrictive disease, since both decrease, whereas in obstructive disease the ratio is generally low, since the FEV_1 is markedly reduced.

Maximum voluntary ventilation is a nonspecific test and is an indicator of both restriction and obstruction. Although maximum voluntary ventilation has not been systematically evaluated as a predictor of morbidity, it is generally accepted that a maximum voluntary ventilation below 50% of predicted value is an indication of high risk.

A ratio of residual volume-to-total lung capacity (RV/TLC) of greater than 50% is generally indicative of a high-risk patient for pulmonary resection. Mittman[10] found that a RV/TLC ratio of greater than 40% was associated with a 30% mortality compared with a 7% mortality when RV/TLC was less than 40% (normal range 20–25%).

Flow-Volume Loops. The flow-volume loop displays essentially the same information as a spirometer but is more convenient for measurement of specific flow rates (Fig. 34-1). The shape and peak air flow rates during expiration at high lung volumes are effort-dependent but indicate the patency of the larger airways. Effort-independent expiration occurs at low lung volumes and usually reflects small airways re-

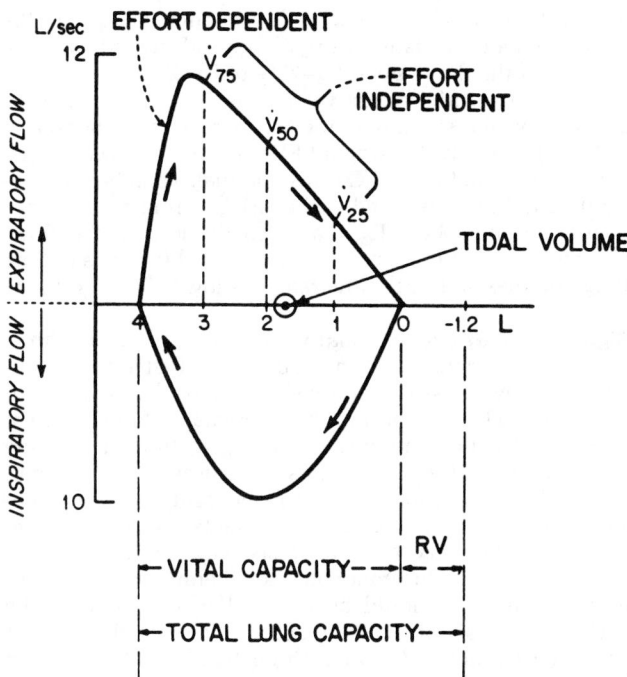

Figure 34-1. Flow volume loop in a normal subject. $\dot{V}_{75}$, $\dot{V}_{50}$, and $\dot{V}_{25}$ represents flow at 75, 50, and 25% of vital capacity, respectively. (RV = residual volume). (Reproduced with permission from Goudsouzian N, Karamanian A: Physiology for the Anesthesiologist, 2nd ed. Norwalk, Appleton-Century-Crofts, 1984.)

sistance, best measured by maximum mid-expiratory flow rate between 25 and 75% of vital capacity ($MMEFR_{25-75}$).

In general, patients with obstructive airways disease (Fig. 34-2), such as asthma, bronchitis, and emphysema, have grossly reduced FEV_1/FVC ratios because of increased airways resistance and a reduction in FEV_1. Peak expiratory flow rate and maximum voluntary ventilation are usually reduced, whereas TLC increases secondary to increases in

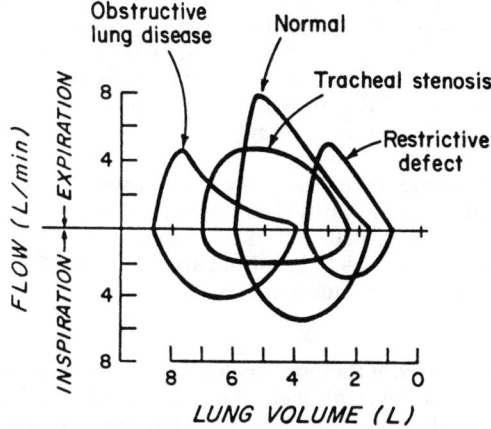

Figure 34-2. Flow volume loops relative to lung volumes (1) in a normal subject, (2) in a patient with COPD, (3) in a patient with fixed obstruction (tracheal stenosis), and (4) in a patient with pulmonary fibrosis (restrictive defect). Note the concave expiratory form in the patient with COPD and the flat inspiratory curve in the patient with a fixed obstruction. (Reproduced with permission from Goudsouzian N, Karamanian A: Physiology for the Anesthesiologist, 2nd ed. Norwalk, Appleton-Century-Crofts, 1984.)

RV. In these patients, the effort-independent portion of the flow-volume curve is markedly depressed inward, with reduction of the flow rate at 25–75% of FVC.

In patients with restrictive disease (Fig. 34-2), such as pulmonary fibrosis and scoliosis, there is a reduction in FVC with a relatively normal FEV_1. Since the airways resistance is normal, FEV_1/FVC is also normal. Total lung capacity is markedly reduced, whereas maximum voluntary ventilation and $MMEFR_{25-75}$ are usually normal. The flow-volume curves of these patients are normal in shape but the lung volumes and peak flow rates are lower (Fig. 34-2).

Significance of Bronchodilator Therapy. Pulmonary function tests are usually performed before and after bronchodilator therapy to assess the reversibility of the airways obstruction.[11] This is useful in the assessment of the degree of airway obstruction and the patient's effort ability. Following treatment with bronchodilators, increases in PEFR compared with a baseline indicate reversibility of airway obstruction (often seen in asthmatic patients). A 15% improvement in pulmonary function tests may be considered a positive response to bronchodilator therapy and indicates that this therapy should be initiated preoperatively. The overall prognosis of COPD is better related to the level of spirometric function following bronchodilator therapy than to a baseline function.

Split-Lung Function Tests. Regional lung function studies serve to predict the functioning of the lung tissue that would remain after lung resection. A whole (two) lung test may fail to estimate whether the amount of postresection lung tissue will allow the patient to function at a reasonable level of activity without disabling dyspnea or cor pulmonale.

Regional Perfusion Test. This involves the intravenous injection of insoluble radioactive xenon (^{133}Xe). The peak radioactivity of each lung is proportional to the degree of perfusion of each lung.

Regional Ventilation Test. Using an inhaled, insoluble radioactive gas, the peak radioactivity over each lung is proportional to the degree of ventilation. Combining radiospirometry with whole lung testing (FEV_1, FVC, maximal breathing capacity [MBC]) has resulted in a fair degree of correlation between predicted volumes and pulmonary function tests measured after pneumonectomy. It is generally held that a FEV_1 of 800 ml is the minimum accepted volume for postresection survival.

Regional Bronchial Balloon Occlusion Test. This test basically simulates the postresection condition preoperatively by using balloon occlusion of the bronchus to the segment of the lung to be resected. Spirometry and arterial blood gas analysis are then performed with the remaining functional lung.

Pulmonary Artery Balloon Occlusion Test. The postoperative stress on the right ventricle and remaining pulmonary vascular bed can be simulated by occluding the pulmonary artery of the lung to be resected using a specially designed balloon-tipped pulmonary artery catheter that has a pressure-sensing port just proximal to the balloon. This test may be done with or without exercise. If upon balloon occlusion of the pulmonary artery of the lung to be resected the mean pulmonary artery pressure increases above 40 mm Hg, PaO_2 is less than 60 mm Hg, or $PaCO_2$ is greater than 45 mm Hg, it is unlikely that the patient will be able to tolerate pneumonectomy without developing respiratory failure or cor pulmonale postoperatively.

The preoperative pulmonary evaluation of patients considered for lung resection is summarized as follows. First, a whole lung test with spirometry and arterial blood gases should be done. If any of the following values—$PaCO_2 > 40$ mm Hg, $FEV_1 < 50\%$, FVC < 2 l, MBC < 50%, or RV/TLC > 50%—is found to be outside these limits, a second level of split-lung function testing should be done to estimate the exact contribution of the resected portion of the lung to either ventilation or perfusion. Conventional spirometry should yield a predicted postresection FEV_1 greater than 800 ml. If these criteria cannot be met, surgery is usually contraindicated. A postoperative simulation of ventilation or perfusion by bronchial or pulmonary artery occlusion can produce additional information, and risk-benefit ratio must be considered for each individual patient.

PREOPERATIVE PREPARATION

The wide spectrum of physiologic changes occurring during thoracic surgery puts patients at great risk of developing postoperative complications. Morbidity and mortality increase when these changes are superimposed on an acutely or chronically compromised patient. Several conditions show particular correlations with postoperative complications. Such conditions include infection, dehydration, electrolyte imbalance, wheezing, obesity, cigarette smoking, cor pulmonale, and malnutrition. Proper vigorous preoperative preparation can improve the patient's ability to face the surgery with a reduced risk of morbidity and mortality. Stein et al[12] found that postoperative pulmonary complications developed in 4 of 17 well-prepared patients compared with 13 of 17 unprepared patients; therefore, it is important that conditions predisposing to postoperative complications be effectively treated preoperatively.

Smoking

Approximately 33% of adult patients presenting for surgery are smokers, and there is now extensive evidence that they are at increased risk for developing postoperative respiratory complications.[13,14] Smoking increases airway irritability, decreases mucociliary transport, and increases secretions. Smoking also decreases FVC and MMEFR, thereby increasing the incidence of postoperative pulmonary complications.[15] On the other hand, cessation of smoking for a period of longer than 4–6 weeks prior to surgery is associated with a decreased incidence of postoperative complications.[14,16,17] Furthermore, cessation of smoking for 48 hours prior to surgery has been shown to decrease the level of carboxyhemoglobin, to shift the oxyhemoglobin dissociation curve to the right, and to increase tissue oxygen availability. It should be emphasized that most of the beneficial effects of cessation of smoking, such as improvement in ciliary function, improvement in closing volume, increase in MMEFR, and reduction in sputum production, usually occur 2–3 months following the cessation of smoking.

Infection

Acute or chronic infection should be vigorously treated prior to surgery. Broad-spectrum antibiotics, such as ampicillin or tetracycline, are commonly used. Treatment of the acutely ill patient will depend upon the results of the Gram stain of the sputum and on blood culture findings. In one prospective study, the incidence of mortality was lower (9%) in the group treated with prophylactic antibiotics compared with 17% of the untreated patients, and a lower incidence of postoperative pulmonary infection was shown as well.[18] Although not all surgeons administer antibiotics prophylactically to their patients, infection, when present preoperatively, should be vigorously treated.

Hydration and Removal of Bronchial Secretions

Correction of hypovolemia and electrolyte imbalance should be accomplished prior to surgery, since hydrating the patient decreases the viscosity of the bronchial secretions and facilitates their removal from the bronchial tree. Humidification using a jet humidifier or ultrasonic mist system is extremely useful. The use of mucolytic drugs, such as acetylcysteine (Mucomyst), or of oral expectorants (potassium iodide), can be of benefit to patients with viscous secretions.[19,20] Commonly used methods for removing the secretions from the bronchial tree include postural drainage, vigorous coughing, chest percussion, deep breathing, and the use of an incentive spirometer. These often require patient cooperation and frequent verbal encouragement to maximize the beneficial effect.

Wheezing and Bronchodilation

The presence of acute wheezing represents a medical emergency, and elective surgery should be postponed until effective proper treatment has been instituted. Chronic wheezing is often seen in patients with COPD and is attributable to the presence of gas flow obstruction secondary to smooth muscle constriction, accumulation of secretions, and mucosal edema. Smooth muscle contraction may occur in small airways only (detectable by changes in forced expiratory flow [FEF] 25–75%) or may be widespread, with a large reduction of FEV_1 and FVC. The efficacy of bronchodilators in reversing the bronchospastic component is extremely important. A trial of bronchodilators and measurement of their effects on pulmonary function should be performed in any patient who shows evidence of air flow obstruction.[21] Several classes of bronchodilators are available.

Sympathomimetic Drugs

Sympathomimetic drugs increase the formation of 3'5'-cyclic adenosine monophosphate (cAMP). The balance between cAMP, which produces bronchodilation, and cyclic guanosine monophosphate (cGMP), which produces bronchoconstriction, determines the state of contraction of the bronchial smooth muscle.[22] Thus, increasing cAMP production causes relaxation of the bronchial tree. Sympathomimetic drugs, such as epinephrine, isoproterenol, isoetharine, and ephedrine, all have mixed $beta_1$ and $beta_2$ sympathetic agonist effects. The $beta_1$ (cardiac effects) of these drugs are often undesirable in treating patients with COPD. Selective $beta_2$ sympathomimetic drugs, such as albuterol, terbutaline, and metaproterenol, given as inhaled aerosols, are the preferred drugs in the treatment of bronchospasm, particularly in patients with cardiac disease.

Phosphodiesterase Inhibitors

Phosphodiesterase inhibitors inhibit the breakdown of cAMP by cytoplasmic phosphodiesterase. The methylxanthines, such as aminophylline, increase the level of cAMP, resulting in bronchodilation. In addition, aminophylline improves diaphragmatic contractility and increases the patient's resistance to fatigue.[23] Therapeutic blood levels of aminophylline are $5-20 \ \mu g \cdot ml^{-1}$ and can be achieved by giving a loading dose of $5-7 \ mg \cdot kg^{-1}$ infused over 20 minutes, followed by a continuous iv infusion of $0.5-0.7 \ mg \cdot kg^{-1} \cdot h^{-1}$. Aminophylline may cause ventricular arrhythmias, and this side-effect should be borne in mind when treating patients who have myocardial ischemia.

Steroids

Although they are not true bronchodilators, steroids are traditionally considered to decrease mucosal edema and may prevent the release of bronchoconstricting substances. They are of questionable benefit in an acute bronchospastic situation. Steroids may be given orally, parenterally, or in aerosol form, such as beclomethasone by inhaler.

Cromolyn Sodium

Cromolyn sodium stabilizes mast cells and inhibits degranulation and histamine release. It is useful in the prevention of bronchospastic attacks but is of little value in the treatment of the acute situation.

Parasympatholytics

Parasympatholytics include atropine and ipratropium. In the past, atropine has been avoided in patients with COPD and bronchitis because of the concern regarding increases in the viscosity of mucus produced by this agent. However, atropine blocks the formation of cGMP and, therefore, has a bronchodilator effect. Marini et al[24] found that inhaled atropine alone improved FEV_1 in 85% of patients with COPD. When atropine was given together with terbutaline, the FEV_1 improved in 93% of patients, whereas terbutaline alone improved FEV_1 in only 56% of patients. Therefore the antimuscarinic drugs such as atropine potentiate the bronchodilator effect of the sympathomimetic agents.

In conclusion, the preoperative preparation of the patient for thoracic surgery should focus on those conditions that are treatable prior to surgery so that the patient is in optimal condition at the time of surgery.

INTRAOPERATIVE MONITORING

All patients undergoing thoracic surgical procedures require monitoring with an electrocardiogram (lead II and/or V_5), chest and/or esophageal stethoscopes for heart and breath sound auscultation, and a temperature probe. A chest stethoscope should be placed over the dependent hemithorax to assess dependent lung ventilation. In addition, a noninvasive blood pressure monitoring system can be used during surgery. Pulse oximetry has become the standard of care during the administration of anesthesia and is especially valuable during thoracic surgery because hypoxemia is not uncommon during one-lung ventilation. The pulse oximeter analyzes the pulsatile component of absorbance of light at two wavelengths, 660 nm (red) and 940 nm (infrared). The ratio of the pulse added absorbances permits estimation of arterial oxygen saturation of hemoglobin via an empiric algorithm.[25,26] The pulse oximeter saturation reading is designated SpO$_2$.

Arrhythmias occur commonly both during and following thoracic surgery, making the usual need for continuous electrocardiographic monitoring even more important. Supraventricular tachyarrhythmias occurring intraoperatively may be caused by cardiac manipulation. Arrhythmias occurring during one-lung ventilation may be a sign of inadequate oxygenation or ventilation. Arrhythmias occurring postoperatively may be related to sympathetic nervous system stimulation from pain or to a reduced pulmonary vascular bed from the lung resection. Patients presenting for lung resection often have chronic obstructive pulmonary disease owing to cigarette smoking, have right-sided heart strain, and are prone to multifocal atrial tachyarrhythmias.

The axis of electrocardiogram (ECG) lead II parallels that of the P wave, making this lead useful for arrhythmia detection. The simultaneous monitoring of lead V_5 also allows for monitoring of anterolateral wall myocardial ischemia.[27] The use of multiple leads facilitates a greater sensitivity of ischemia detection.[28] The following types of invasive monitoring are also indicated and have led to markedly improved patient care.

Direct Arterial Catheterization

Peripheral arterial cannulation has become an essential tool for the anesthesiologist in the management of patients undergoing major thoracic surgical procedures. It allows for continuous beat-to-beat measurement of blood pressure as well as frequent sampling for the determination of arterial blood gases. The risk, when utilizing 20-gauge Teflon catheters in the radial artery, has been shown to be extremely low, and any risk can be further decreased by ensuring patency of the ulnar artery. This can be done by the use of a modified Allen test, digital plethysmography, or Doppler ultrasonography.[29] Although the Allen test is a commonly performed technique, its usefulness has recently been challenged. Permanent ischemic complications have been reported in patients with normal Allen test results,[30-32] and catheterization in patients with abnormal Allen test findings has not resulted in ischemic sequelae.[33] The incidence of ischemic complications following radial arterial catheterization has been reported to be 0.01%.[33]

Continuous blood pressure readings are critical during thoracic surgery, since surgical manipulations or intravascular volume shifts can cause sudden major changes in the blood pressure. Immediate recognition of the change allows time for proper identification of the etiology and the institution of appropriate treatment.[34] A recently introduced noninvasive method (Penaz finger blood pressure cuff) provides continuous blood pressure measurements, but it can be rendered inaccurate by arterial spasm and does not allow for the drawing of blood samples.[35]

Serial blood gas determinations are essential in the management of patients undergoing one-lung anesthesia or during cases in which part of the lung may be "packed away" for a period of time. Arterial hypoxemia is commonly seen owing to increased pulmonary shunting and inadequate hypoxic pulmonary vasoconstriction. Significant changes in acid-base status as well as hyper- or hypoventilation can also be determined. The arterial blood samples can be used to confirm the readings obtained by pulse oximetry as well as to aid in the interpretation of transcutaneous arterial oxygen tension values (i.e., respiratory versus cardiac abnor-malities) and end-tidal CO$_2$ concentrations (i.e., inadequate ventilation versus shunting).

A radial arterial catheter can be placed in either extremity during thoracic surgery. For a mediastinoscopic examination, it is useful to place the catheter in the right arm and to use it to monitor compression of the innominate artery by the mediastinoscope.[36] This can help to avoid central nervous system complications resulting from inadequate cerebral blood flow through the right carotid artery (see the section on Mediastinoscopy). During thoracotomy, the radial arterial catheter is often placed in the dependent arm to aid in stabilizing the catheter. However, a roll must be placed under the patient to protect the axilla and avoid compression of the axillary artery and brachial plexus in this arm. In rare cases, the arterial catheter can be placed in the brachial, femoral, or dorsalis pedis artery if the ulnar collateral circulation is thought to be inadequate.[37] The incidence of complications of these sites is similar to that for radial artery cannulation.[38,39]

Central Venous Pressure Monitoring

The central venous pressure (CVP) is usually measured as an indication of right atrial and right ventricular pressures. It is a useful monitor if the factors affecting it are realized and its limitations are understood. The CVP reflects the patient's blood volume, venous tone, and right ventricular performance; however, it is also affected by central venous obstructions and alterations of intrathoracic pressure (e.g., positive end-expiratory pressure).[29] Serial measurements are more useful than an individual number, and the response of the CVP to a volume infusion is a useful test of right ventricular function. The CVP reflects right-sided heart function and not left ventricular performance (Fig. 34-3). The combination of the CVP to monitor right atrial pressure and the esophageal stethoscope to "monitor" left atrial pressure (e.g., rales, S$_3$) is still a useful monitoring technique in patients with good left ventricular function. A CVP catheter is often used in patients with good left ventricular function during thoracic surgical procedures for either monitoring or infusion/insertion applications. CVP monitoring is needed when there may be large volume shifts (e.g., pneumonectomy) or the patient is hypovolemic. Uses of a CVP catheter include: (1) insertion of a transvenous pacemaker where necessary; (2) infusion of vasoactive drugs; and (3) insertion of a pulmonary arterial catheter, which may subsequently be required during surgery or in the postoperative period.

The CVP catheter can be placed centrally from either the external or the internal jugular vein, from the subclavian veins, or from one of the arm veins. The success rate is highest using the right internal jugular vein, and a pacemaker or pulmonary arterial catheter can be inserted most easily from this vein.[40] The major disadvantage of using the external jugular vein during thoracotomy is that the catheter often kinks when the patient is turned to the lateral decubitus position. The subclavian technique leads to a high incidence of pneumothorax that can be disastrous if it occurs in the dependent lung during one-lung ventilation.

Pulmonary Artery Catheterization

The use of the pulmonary artery catheter (PAC) allows measurements of left-sided filling pressures, the determination of cardiac output by thermodilution, calculation of derived hemodynamic and respiratory parameters (e.g., systemic vascular resistance and intrapulmonary shunt, respec-

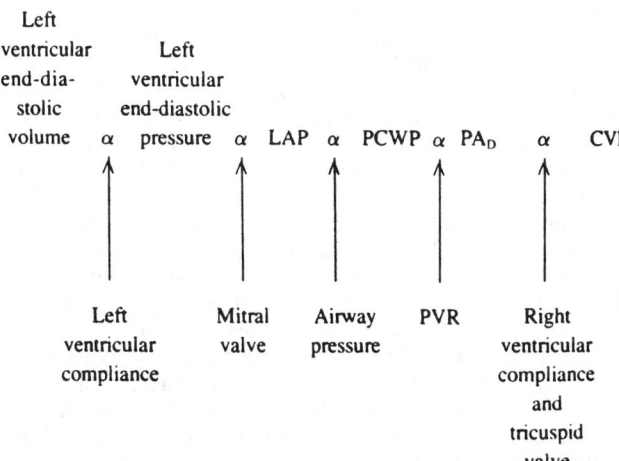

Left ventricular end-diastolic volume α Left ventricular end-diastolic pressure α LAP α PCWP α PA$_D$ α CVP

Left ventricular compliance | Mitral valve | Airway pressure | PVR | Right ventricular compliance and tricuspid valve

Figure 34-3. Directional changes in CVP may reflect alterations in left ventricular performance. However, in the presence of severe pulmonary disease or alteration in valve function, CVP is a poor monitor of left ventricular function. (LAP = left atrial pressure; PCWP = pulmonary capillary wedge pressure; PA$_D$ = pulmonary artery diastolic pressure.) (Reproduced with permission from Kaplan JA [ed]: Cardiac Anesthesia, p 192. New York, Grune & Stratton, 1979.)

tively), and clinical use of Starling function curves. In addition, advanced versions of the basic catheter allow measurement of mixed venous oxygen saturation or right ventricular ejection fraction as well as the application of atrial or ventricular pacing. The PAC is indicated during thoracic surgery in specific situations (Table 34-1).[34]

In the past, CVP catheters were used to monitor patients with left-sided heart disease or pulmonary disease; however, the CVP has been shown to have a poor correlation with the left atrial pressure in these types of patient. Many studies have shown the disparity between left- and right-sided pressures owing to the many factors separating the CVP reading from the true left ventricular preload (see Fig. 34-3).

TABLE 34-1. Indications for Pulmonary Artery Catheterization in Thoracic Surgery

1. Patients with known cardiovascular disease, with or without heart failure
2. Surgery in which cross-clamping of the thoracic aorta is anticipated
3. Patients with respiratory failure
4. Patients with suspected or diagnosed pulmonary emboli
5. Patients who have undergone previous cardiac surgery
6. When a pneumonectomy is anticipated
7. When significant shifts of intravascular volume are anticipated
8. When sepsis is present
9. Patients who receive continuous infusions of inotropes or vasodilators
10. Patients with pulmonary hypertension or elevated pulmonary vascular resistance
11. When cor pulmonale is present
12. Patients treated with bleomycin

Reproduced with permission from Kaplan JA (ed): Thoracic Anesthesia. New York, Churchill Livingstone, 1983.

The PAC is most reliably inserted via the right internal jugular vein using a modified Seldinger technique that has been extensively described.[29] Insertion of the PAC through either the external jugular vein or the subclavian vein often leads to obstruction of the catheter when the patient is placed in the lateral decubitus position. Complications of PAC insertion and use can be divided into immediate and long term.[41] Immediate complications include the development of supraventricular and ventricular arrhythmias during insertion, onset of a right bundle-branch block and/or complete heart block in patients with a pre-existing left bundle-branch block, and all the potential complications of inserting a needle into a central vein (e.g., arterial puncture, hematoma formation, pneumothorax, nerve damage, Horner's syndrome, air embolization, or thoracic duct injury).[42,43] The incidence of carotid artery cannulation with the 18-gauge "access" catheter has been reported to be 4%, and in this series the No. 8 French introducer was inserted into the carotid artery in five patients.[44] The incidence of arrhythmias is lowered by changing the position of the patient from Trendelenburg to a head-up right lateral tilt position prior to flotation of the pulmonary artery catheter.[45] Long-term complications of the PAC include balloon rupture and gas embolization, pulmonary infarction, pulmonary artery rupture, knotting of the catheter in the right ventricle, infection, vascular obstruction, and erroneous diagnosis from misinterpretation of data.[46,47]

Pulmonary artery rupture is the most serious complication associated with the use of the PAC and in a series of over 6000 patients was reported to occur in 0.6% of the cases.[48] Risk factors for this complication include hypothermia, pulmonary hypertension, anticoagulation, and being elderly or female.[39] Pulmonary artery perforation most commonly manifests as hemoptysis.

Management of pulmonary artery rupture and massive airway hemorrhage includes protecting the nonbleeding lung by placement of a double-lumen endotracheal tube. This allows suctioning and application of continuous positive airway pressure to the bleeding lung, which is not possible if the single-lumen tube is merely advanced into the bronchus of the nonbleeding lung. If a single-lumen tube is already in place, another alternative is the placement of a bronchial blocker alongside the tracheal tube after the site of bleeding is identified. The bleeding most often comes from the right side, since the pulmonary artery catheter floats to the right side in most cases. Bronchoscopy may allow identification of the bleeding site. Other treatment modalities include the use of positive end-expiratory pressure, inflation of the pulmonary artery catheter balloon to tamponade the bleeding, and the administration of protamine, if possible, if the patient has been anticoagulated with heparin.[39] Fluid resuscitation is essential, and if the bleeding continues surgical exploration and lung resection may be necessary.

Misinterpretation of data from a PAC is a real risk in a patient with cardiac and pulmonary disease undergoing thoracic surgery with one-lung ventilation. These errors can be produced by altered ventilatory modes, location of the PAC tip, ventricular compliance changes, or ventricular independence.[46,47] A major limitation of the PAC is the assumption that the pulmonary capillary wedge pressure (PCWP) is a good approximation of left ventricular end-diastolic volume. The use of the PCWP to directly assess preload assumes a linear relationship between ventricular end-diastolic volume and ventricular end-diastolic pressure. However, alterations in ventricular compliance affect

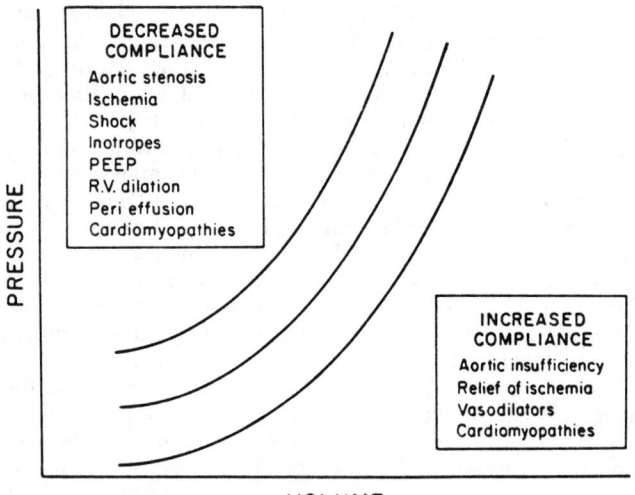

Figure 34-4. The left ventricular compliance is the relationship between the LVEDP and the LVEDV. An increased compliance shifts the curve down and to the right, whereas a decreased compliance shifts it up and to the left. Examples of increased and decreased compliance are shown in the boxes. Peri effusion = pericardial effusion. (Reproduced with permission from Kaplan JA [ed]: Cardiac Anesthesia, 2nd ed, p 207. Orlando, Grune & Stratton, 1987.)

this pressure-volume relationship during surgery. Reductions in ventricular compliance can be seen with myocardial ischemia, shock, right ventricular overload, or pericardial effusion (Fig. 34-4). Numerous investigators have demonstrated a poor correlation between PCWP and left ventricular end-diastolic volume in acutely ill patients.[46,47,49] This correlation is further worsened by the application of positive end-expiratory pressure.[50] Therefore, whenever the PCWP is used to estimate left ventricular preload, the number must be interpreted in light of the clinical situation. The interdependence of the right and left ventricles must also be remembered when interpreting PCWP.[51] Ventricular interdependence can cause misdiagnosis when the interventricular septum encroaches on the left ventricular cavity, leading to elevated values of PCWP. An elevated PCWP associated with a decreased cardiac output can be interpreted as left ventricular failure, when, in fact, there may not be an increased left ventricular end-diastolic volume but a decreased volume due to compression of the left ventricle by a distended right ventricle (Fig. 34-5). This situation can occur with acute respiratory failure and high levels of positive end-expiratory pressure.[52] Techniques such as echocardiography, which directly measure ventricular dimensions, are necessary to resolve this complex situation.

	PCWP	Cardiac Output	LVEDV
LV failure	↑	↓	↑
Ventricular interdependence	↑	↓	↓

Figure 34-5. Comparison of left ventricular failure and ventricular interdependence. (PCWP = pulmonary capillary wedge pressure; LVEDV = left ventricle end–diastolic volume.) (Reproduced with permission from Keefer JR, Barash PG: Pulmonary artery catheterization. In Blitt CD [ed]: Monitoring in Anesthesia and Critical Care Medicine. New York, Churchill Livingstone, 1985.)

Since the highest percentage of pulmonary blood flow is to the right lower lobe, the tip of a flow-directed PAC is usually located in the right lower lobe. During a left thoracotomy with one-lung ventilation, the catheter tip would then be in the dependent lung and should produce accurate hemodynamic measurements. However, during a right thoracotomy with one-lung ventilation, the catheter tip should be in the nondependent lung. Cohen et al reported that during right thoracotomies with the tip of the PAC catheter in a West Zone 1 or 2 region of the right lung, hemodynamic measurements may be inaccurate.[53] These authors found that cardiac output measurements were lower during right thoracotomies than left thoracotomies, and the derived parameters of stroke volume index and oxygen delivery were also inappropriately low (Fig. 34-6). It was thought that these results were attributable to the fact that the PAC tip located in the collapsed lung was affected by abnormalities in blood flow owing to hypoxic pulmonary vasoconstriction. This hypothesis is supported by the concurrent finding that the mixed venous oxygen saturation also decreased during right thoracotomies as compared with during left thoracotomies. This decrease in mixed venous oxygen saturation may have been caused by stagnation of blood flow through the partially collapsed lung. Therefore, hemodynamic data derived from a PAC in the nondependent collapsed lung must be carefully evaluated.

Assessment of right ventricular function is made difficult by the complex geometry and shape of the right ventricle. The thermodilution technique used to measure cardiac output with the PAC can also determine right ventricular ejection fraction if a fast-response thermistor is used. There are numerous situations during thoracic surgery when decreased right ventricular function precludes adequate right-sided heart output to a normal left ventricle. Since the right ventricle is very sensitive to increases in afterload, right ventricular function can be evaluated by comparing right ventricular ejection fraction with a measure of right ventricular afterload, such as pulmonary vascular resistance.[54] Right ventricular function curves may be even more useful than left ventricular function curves in patients with chronic pulmonary disease undergoing thoracic surgical procedures.

The multipurpose PAC, with five pacing electrodes, is now widely available. This catheter can be used for atrial, ventricular, or atrioventricular sequential pacing in patients who require a PAC for hemodynamic monitoring.[55] Indications for the pacing PAC are (1) intermittent third-degree heart block; (2) second-degree heart block; (3) left bundle-branch block; (4) digitalis toxicity; and (5) severe bradycardia.

A major development in the area of PAC monitoring has been the addition of fiberoptic bundles for light transmission, allowing continuous measurement of oxygen saturation of the mixed venous blood ($S\bar{v}O_2$) by an oximeter. Four mechanisms can account for a decreased $S\bar{v}O_2$: (1) decreased SaO_2; (2) decreased cardiac output; (3) increased oxygen consumption; and (4) decreased hemoglobin concentration. $S\bar{v}O_2$ represents a measure of global tissue oxygen extraction and consumption and is generally directly related to cardiac output via the Fick formula. The monitoring of $S\bar{v}O_2$ has been evaluated in patients undergoing one-lung anesthesia.[56] The change from two-lung to one-lung ventilation was accompanied by increases in heart rate, mean pulmonary artery pressure and cardiac index, and decreases in mixed venous oxygen saturation ($S\bar{v}O_2$) and arterial saturation (SaO_2). The changes in cardiac index did not correlate significantly with changes in $S\bar{v}O_2$. Changes in $S\bar{v}O_2$ were

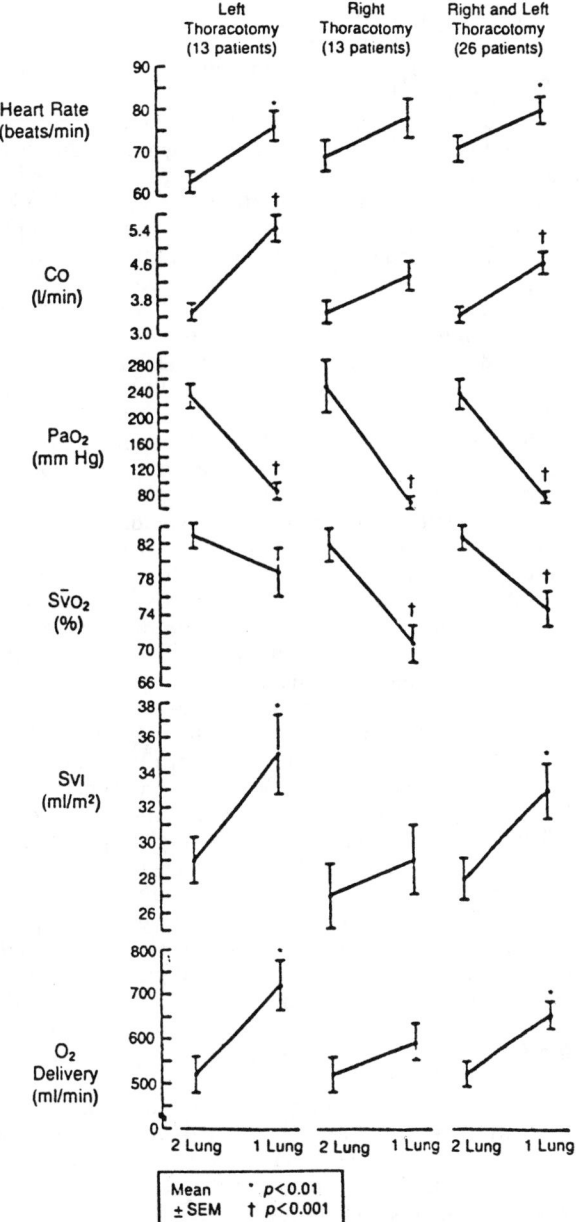

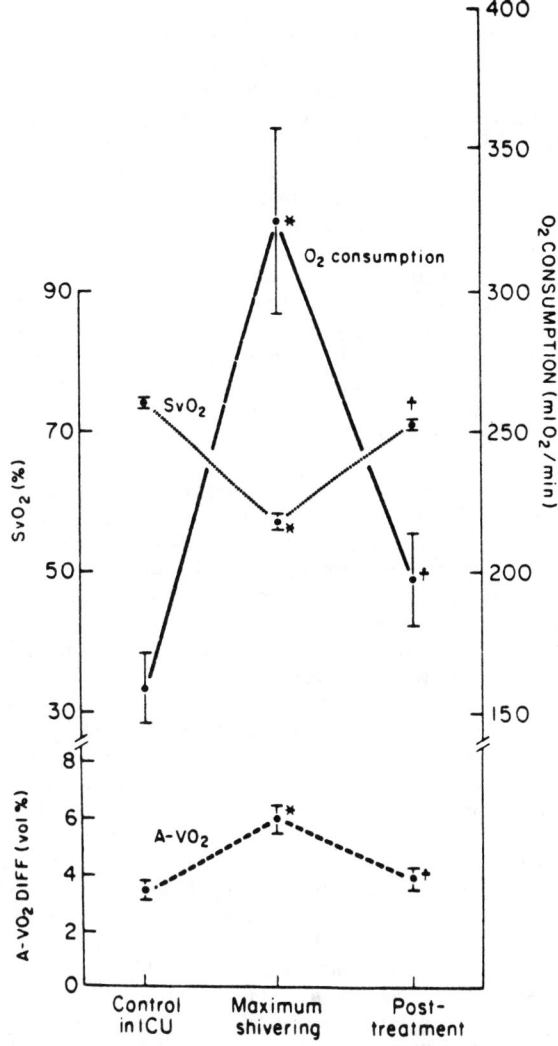

Figure 34-6. Oxygen delivery variables with left and right thoracotomies (see text for explanation). (CO = cardiac output; S$\bar{v}$o$_2$ = mixed venous O$_2$ saturation; SVI = stroke volume index.) (Reproduced with permission from Cohen E, Eisenkraft JB, Thys DM et al: Hemodynamics and Oxygenation During One Lung Anesthesia: Right Versus Left, p 126. Phoenix, Proceedings of the Society of Cardiovascular Anesthesiologists Meeting, April 1985.)

Figure 34-7. Postoperative shivering in a group of patients after coronary artery bypass graft operation produced a decrease in S$\bar{v}$o$_2$ due to a doubling of total body O$_2$ consumption. This was corrected after treatment with meperidine or pancuronium. (Reproduced with permission from Guffin A, Girard D, Kaplan JA: Shivering following cardiac surgery: Hemodynamic changes and reversal. J Cardiothorac Anesth 1:24, 1987.)

mainly dependent on changes in Sao$_2$. This type of monitoring may be of value, however, in the detection of patients who are unable to compensate for a decreased Pao$_2$ by increasing cardiac output and, therefore, have a compromised oxygen delivery system. For example, Guffin et al showed that shivering after intrathoracic surgery led to a marked decrease in S$\bar{v}$o$_2$ as a result of an increased oxygen consumption, which could not be compensated for by changes in cardiac output (Fig. 34-7).[57] Utilizing this type of catheter, many oxygen delivery parameters can be calculated during and after thoracic surgery.

The accuracy of the Shaw Opticath pulmonary artery catheter (Oximetrix Inc., Mountain View, CA) and the Swan-Ganz Oximetry TD Catheter (American Edwards Laboratories, Santa Ana, CA) was recently studied.[58] Both systems were accurate in assessment of S$\bar{v}$o$_2$, as they both correlated well with an in vitro reference S$\bar{v}$o$_2$, (r = 0.88). Comparison with in vitro S$\bar{v}$o$_2$ was recommended at 12-hour intervals because there was more than a 5% error in 20% of the Oximetrix system measurements and 13% of the Edwards system measurements.[58]

Monitoring of Oxygenation and Ventilation

Oxygenation

During the administration of all thoracic surgical anesthetics, the concentration of oxygen in the breathing system must be measured using an oxygen analyzer with a low oxygen concentration limit alarm. Such analyzers vary in sophistication from fuel cells, polarographic and paramagnetic analyzers, to mass and Raman spectrometers that can monitor all the gases used during anesthesia. Adequacy of blood oxygenation must also be ensured, and adequate illumination and exposure of the patient are necessary to assess the color of shed blood or the presence of cyanosis of the lips, nail beds, or mucous membranes. Most patients undergoing thoracic surgical or diagnostic procedures have an arterial catheter in place for continuous monitoring of blood pressure and sampling of arterial blood for arterial blood gas determinations. In such cases, baseline arterial blood gas values should be obtained with an $FIO_2 = 0.21$ (room air) prior to starting the procedure and repeated regularly and/or whenever indicated during surgery. Arterial blood is usually analyzed for oxygen tension (PaO_2), and saturation (SaO_2) is calculated from the oxygen-hemoglobin dissociation curve, correcting for temperature, pH, and $PaCO_2$.

The oxygen content of arterial blood can be assessed using a bench co-oximeter, such as the IL282 (Instrumentation Laboratory, Lexington, MA), which uses spectrophotometric principles to measure the total hemoglobin (Hb_{TOT}), which represents 100% ($g \cdot dl^{-1}$) and the percentages of oxyhemoglobin (HbO_2), methemoglobin (MetHb), and carboxyhemoglobin (COHb). Deoxygenated (reduced) hemoglobin (RHb) is the difference between 100% and the sum of COHb, MetHb, and HbO_2. The oxyhemoglobin percentage* (HbO_2, previously termed fractional concentration) is the more important index for assessing oxygen content. The oxygen saturation of available hemoglobin* (total amount of hemoglobin available to bind oxygen, or SaO_2%, and previously known as functional saturation) will differ from HbO_2%, depending upon the amount of dyshemoglobins (COHb, MetHb) present. Thus, if the hemoglobin concentration is 15 $g \cdot dl^{-1}$, and 1 g of hemoglobin combines with 1.34 ml O_2 when fully saturated, the formula (15 × HbO_2% × 1.34) provides the more accurate estimate of ml $O_2 \cdot dl^{-1}$ of blood than using (15 × SaO_2% × 1.34) or using the calculated saturation from a saturation nomogram based upon PaO_2.†

Pulse oximetry is now routinely employed (indeed in many locales it is a standard of care) for noninvasively obtaining a quantitative assessment of oxygenation. A sensor containing two light-emitting diodes and one photodetector is placed on a fingertip or earlobe. The light-emitting diodes emit light at 660 and 940 nm, and transmittance of light is measured by the photodetector. The ratio of the amplitude of the pulse-added absorbance signal at 660 nm to that at 940 nm is related, *via* an algorithm, to a previously empirically determined measure of oxygenation (SaO_2 or HbO_2%) and is displayed as the pulse oximeter's estimate of oxygen saturation, SpO_2).[59,60] Although subject to certain limitations (*i.e.*, presence of dyshemoglobins, dyes, hypothermia, low cardiac output states, heating lamps, and use of diathermy), pulse oximeters are fairly accurate in estimating oxygenation over the range of 60–100%. Their value has also been demonstrated during one-lung ventilation, when rapid assessment of oxygenation is extremely important, and when blood gas analysis may involve some delay (Fig. 34-8).[61] Pulse oximetry does not eliminate the need for arterial

blood gas analysis during thoracic surgery, however, and may be unreliable in certain circumstances.[62] Certainly a low SpO_2 reading provides the clinician with an indication for sampling and laboratory analysis of arterial blood, but an erroneously high SpO_2 reading may also occur.[63]

The monitoring of transcutaneous oxygen tension ($PtcO_2$) has also been used during thoracic surgery and one-lung anesthesia. Although these monitors are noninvasive and continuous, a warm-up time is required before use, and the skin underlying the sensor must be heated to 45°C to arterialize the blood. Generally, $PtcO_2$ is approximately 80% of actual arterial oxygen tension (PaO_2) and is accurate only when the patient is hemodynamically stable with a cardiac index in excess of 2.2 $l \cdot min^{-1} \cdot m^{-1}$. During periods of hypotension, $PtcO_2$ does not follow PaO_2 but decreases. Thus, a low $PtcO_2$ may be misleading in the presence of an adequate PaO_2 and poor tissue perfusion.[64] For these reasons, pulse oximetry is usually preferred over transcutaneous oxygen monitoring during thoracic surgery.

The most recent advance in continuous monitoring of oxygenation is the "optode," a fiberoptic probe for continuous intra-arterial measurement of PaO_2. The device consists of a single optical fiber with a luminescent dye coating at the tip. It is heparin-coated, less than 0.5 mm in diameter, and passes easily through a 20-gauge arterial cannula. It does not appear to interfere with the arterial pressure waveform, and blood samples can easily be withdrawn from the cannula with the optode in place. A flash lamp emits light that excites the molecules of the luminescent dye. The excited electrons of the dye can either decay to a lower energy level by emitting light or react with oxygen without light emission. Thus, the light emitted is inversely proportional to the amount of oxygen. This device has been evaluated, but further improvements in accuracy are required for use at a low PaO_2.[65,66] Nevertheless, once improved, *the optode holds great promise for use in thoracic surgical patients*, since it also permits simultaneous arterial pressure monitoring and arterial blood sampling.

Ventilation

All patients must be continually monitored to ensure adequate ventilation. Monitoring includes qualitative signs such as chest excursion (visual observation of the lungs when the chest is open), observation of the reservoir bag, and auscultation of breath sounds. An esophageal or precordial stethoscope should be used routinely. In addition, during one-lung ventilation, a stethoscope should be placed on the chest wall under the ventilated dependent lung. During controlled ventilation, circuit low- and high-pressure alarms with an audible signal must be utilized. The respiratory rate, VT, minute volume, and inflation pressures should be observed.

Adequacy of ventilation should be confirmed by monitoring arterial blood gases, $PaCO_2$ in particular. This may be estimated continuously and noninvasively by using a capnometer or some more sophisticated gas monitoring system. The end-tidal CO_2 concentration represents alveolar CO_2 ($PACO_2$), which approximates $PaCO_2$. There is normally a small arterial to alveolar CO_2 gradient (4–6 mm Hg), depending on alveolar dead space. The capnogram waveform is also helpful in diagnosing airway obstruction, incomplete relaxation, and even malposition of the double-lumen tube.[67] In the latter application, a capnograph is coupled with each port of the double-lumen tube (one or two capnographs may be used), and the correct position of the double-lumen tube is identified by simultaneous and synchronous

---

*National Committee for Clinical Laboratory Standards, Villanova, Pennsylvania. Vol 2, no 10, p 342, 1982.

$$†HbO_2\% \ (fractional \ saturation) = \frac{HbO_2}{Hb_{TOT}}$$

$$SaO_2\% \ (functional \ saturation) = \frac{HbO_2}{HbO_2 + RHb}$$

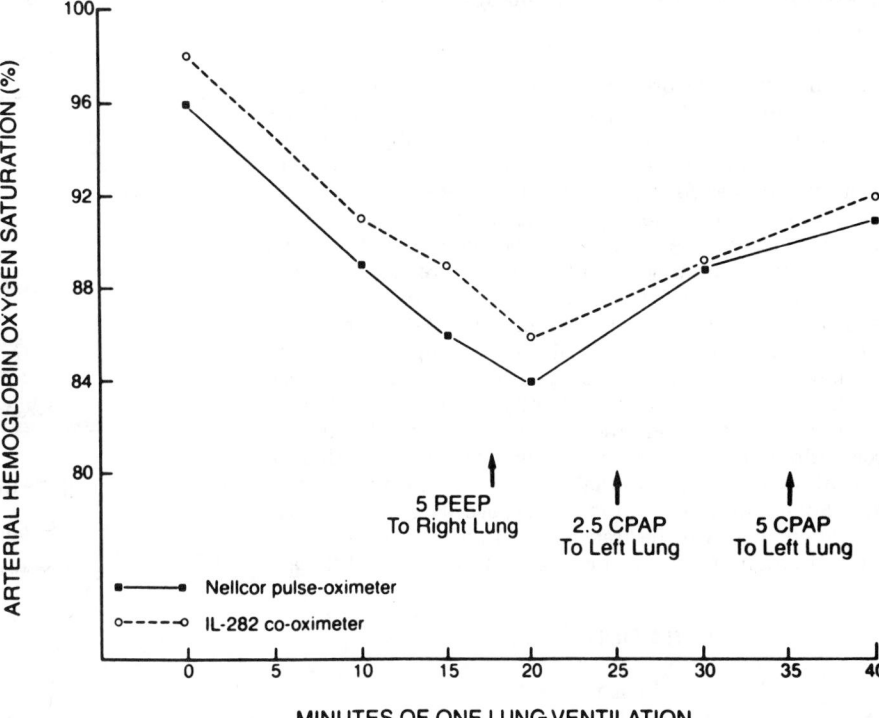

Figure 34-8. Changes in hemoglobin oxygen saturation during one-lung ventilation. Early detection of hypoxemia with pulse oximetry facilitates prompt treatment with positive end-expiratory pressure (5 cm H_2O) and incremental continuous positive airway pressure (2.5–5 cm H_2O) until arterial saturation is returned to an acceptable level. (PEEP = positive end-expiratory pressure; CPAP = continuous positive airway pressure.) (Reproduced with permission from Brodsky JB, Shulman MS, Swan M: Pulse oximetry during one-lung ventilation. Anesthesiology 65:213, 1985.)

CO_2 readings on each of the two analyzers. The waveforms from each lung are examined for shape, height, and rhythm, depending on the correct position of the tube as well as on the ventilation-perfusion ratio for each lung.[67] A decrease in end-tidal CO_2 in the gas from one lumen of the double-lumen tube suggests malposition of the tube. During one-lung ventilation, systemic hypoxemia is usually a greater problem than hypercarbia.[68] This is because CO_2 is some 20 times more diffusible than oxygen and $Paco_2$ is more dependent upon ventilation, as compared with Pao_2, which is more dependent upon perfusion.

Physiology of the Lateral Decubitus Position

Ventilation and blood flow in the upright position have been discussed in a previous chapter (see Chapter 33). These variables will now be considered as they pertain to the lateral decubitus position under five circumstances that are encountered during thoracic surgery.[69]

Lateral Position, Awake, Breathing Spontaneously, Chest Closed

In the lateral decubitus position, the distribution of blood flow and ventilation is similar to that in the upright position but turned by 90 degrees (Fig. 34-9). Blood flow and ventilation to the dependent lung are significantly greater than to the nondependent lung. Good $\dot{V}/\dot{Q}$ matching at the level of the dependent lung results in adequate oxygenation in the awake patient breathing spontaneously. There are two important concepts in this situation. First, since perfusion is gravity-dependent, the vertical hydrostatic gradient is smaller in the lateral as compared to the upright position; therefore, zone 1 is usually less extended. Second, in regard to ventilation, the dependent hemidiaphragm is pushed higher into the chest by the abdominal contents as com-

pared with the nondependent lung hemidiaphragm. During spontaneous ventilation, the conserved ability of the dependent diaphragm to contract will result in an adequate distribution of VT to the dependent lung. Since most of the perfusion is to the dependent lung, the $\dot{V}/\dot{Q}$ matching in this position is maintained similar to that in the upright position.

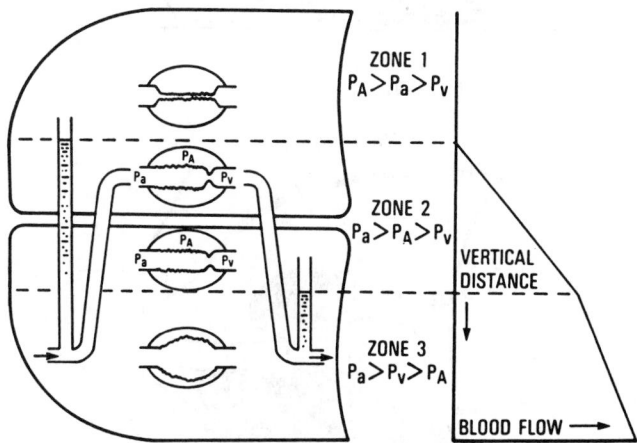

Figure 34-9. Schematic representation of the effects of gravity on the distribution of pulmonary blood flow in the lateral decubitus position. Vertical gradients in the lateral decubitus position are similar to those in the upright position, and cause the creation of zones 1, 2, and 3. Consequently, pulmonary blood flow increases with lung dependency and is largest in the dependent lung and least in the nondependent lung. (Pa = pulmonary artery pressure; PA = aveolar pressure; Pv = pulmonary venous pressure.) (Reproduced with permission from Benumof JL: Physiology of the open-chest and one lung ventilation. In Kaplan JA [ed]: Thoracic Anesthesia. New York, Churchill Livingstone, 1983.)

Lateral Position, Awake, Breathing Spontaneously, Chest Open

Controlled positive pressure ventilation is the most common way to provide adequate ventilation and ensure gas exchange in an open-chest situation. Frequently, thoracoscopy is performed using intercostal blocks with the patient breathing spontaneously in order to allow proper lung examination. The thoracoscope provides an adequate seal of the open chest to prevent a "free" open-chest situation. Two complications can arise from the patient breathing spontaneously with an open chest. The first is mediastinal shift, usually occurring during inspiration (Fig. 34-10). The negative pressure in the intact hemithorax, compared with the less negative pressure of the open hemithorax, can cause the mediastinum to move vertically downward and push into the dependent hemithorax. The mediastinal shift can create circulatory and reflex changes that may result in a clinical picture similar to that of shock and respiratory distress. Sometimes, depending on the severity of the distress, the patient needs to be tracheally intubated immediately, with initiation of positive pressure ventilation, and the an-

EXPIRATION

Pneumothorax

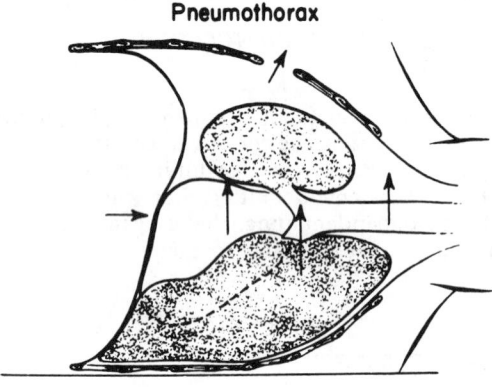

INSPIRATION

Pneumothorax

Figure 34-10. Schematic representation of mediastinal shift in the spontaneously breathing open-chested patient in the lateral decubitus position. During inspiration, negative pressure in the intact hemithorax causes the mediastinum to move downward. During expiration, relative positive pressure in the intact hemithorax causes the mediastinum to move upward. (Reproduced with permission from Tarhan S, Moffitt EA: Principles of thoracic anesthesia. Surg Clin North Am 53:813, 1973.)

EXPIRATION

Pneumothorax

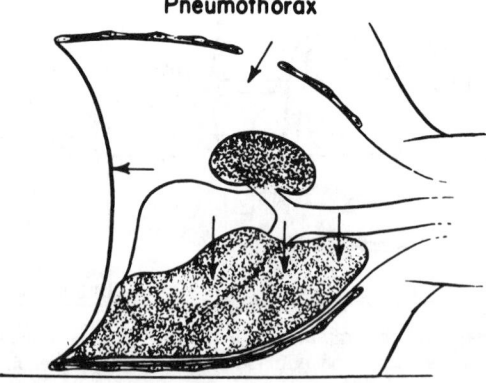

INSPIRATION

Pneumothorax

Figure 34-11. Schematic representation of paradoxical respiration in the spontaneously breathing open-chested patient in the lateral decubitus position. During inspiration, movement of gas from the exposed lung into the intact lung and movement of air from the environment into the open hemithorax cause collapse of the exposed lung. During expiration, the reverse occurs, and the exposed lung expands. (Reproduced with permission from Tarhan S, Moffitt EA: Principles of thoracic anesthesia. Surg Clin North Am 53:813, 1973.)

esthesiologist must be prepared to intubate the patient in this position without disturbing the surgical field. The second phenomenon is paradoxical breathing (Fig. 34-11). During inspiration, the relatively negative pressure in the intact hemithorax compared with atmospheric pressure in the open hemithorax can cause movement of air from the nondependent into the dependent lung. The opposite occurs during expiration. This gas movement reversal from one lung to the other represents wasted ventilation and can compromise the adequacy of gas exchange. Paradoxical breathing is increased by a large thoracotomy or by an increase in airways resistance in the dependent lung. Positive pressure ventilation or adequate sealing of the open chest will eliminate paradoxical breathing.

Lateral Position, Anesthetized, Breathing Spontaneously, Chest Closed

The induction of general anesthesia does not cause significant change in the distribution of blood flow but has an important impact on the distribution of ventilation. The majority of the VT enters the nondependent lung, and this

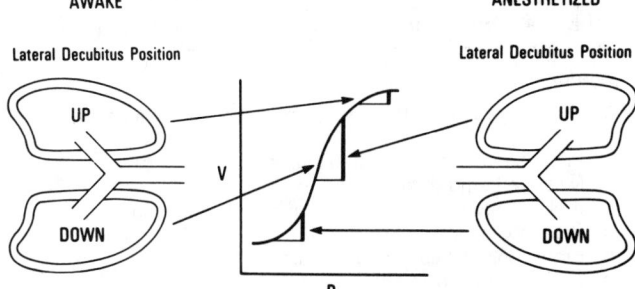

AWAKE   ANESTHETIZED

Lateral Decubitus Position   Lateral Decubitus Position

Figure 34-12. The left-hand side of the schematic shows the distribution of ventilation in the awake patient (closed chest) in the lateral decubitus position, and the right-hand side shows the distribution of ventilation in the anesthetized patient (closed chest) in the lateral decubitus position. The induction of anesthesia has caused a loss in lung volume in both lungs, with the nondependent (up) lung moving from a flat, noncompliant portion to a steep compliant portion of the pressure-volume curve, and the dependent (down) lung moving from a steep compliant part to a flat, noncompliant part of the pressure-volume curve. Thus, the anesthetized patient in the lateral decubitus position has the majority of tidal ventilation in the nondependent lung (where there is the least perfusion) and the minority of tidal ventilation in the dependent lung (where there is the most perfusion). (V = volume, P = pressure.) (Reproduced with permission from Benumof JL: Physiology of the open-chest and one lung ventilation. In Kaplan JA [ed]: Thoracic Anesthesia. New York, Churchill Livingstone, 1983.)

results in a significant $\dot{V}/\dot{Q}$ mismatch. Induction of general anesthesia causes a reduction in the volumes of both lungs secondary to a reduction in FRC. Any reduction in volume in the dependent lung is of a greater magnitude than that in the nondependent lung, for several reasons. First, the cephalad displacement of the dependent diaphragm by the abdominal contents is more pronounced and is increased by paralysis. Second, the mediastinal structures pressing on the dependent lung and/or poor positioning of the depen-

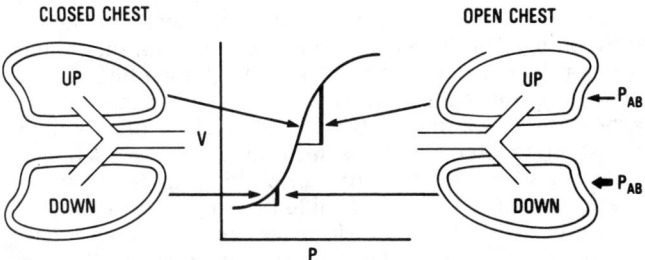

CLOSED CHEST   OPEN CHEST

Figure 34-13. This schematic of a patient in the lateral decubitus position compares the closed-chested anesthetized condition with the open-chested anesthetized and paralyzed condition. Opening the chest increases nondependent lung compliance and reinforces or maintains the larger part of the tidal ventilation going to the nondependent lung. Paralysis also reinforces or maintains the larger part of tidal ventilation going to the nondependent lung because the pressure of the abdominal contents (P_{AB}) pressing against the upper diaphragm is minimal, and it is, therefore, easier for positive pressure ventilation to displace this less resisting dome of the diaphragm. (V = volume, P = pressure.) (Reproduced with permission from Benumof JL: Physiology of the open-chest and one lung ventilation. In Kaplan JA [ed]: Thoracic Anesthesia. New York, Churchill Livingstone, 1983.)

dent side of the operating table prevent the lung from expanding properly. The above-mentioned factors will move lungs to a lower volume on the S-shaped volume-pressure curve (Fig. 34-12). The nondependent lung moves to a steeper position on the compliance curve and receives most of the VT, whereas the dependent lung will be on the flat noncompliant part of the curve.

Lateral Position, Anesthetized, Breathing Spontaneously, Chest Open

Opening the chest has little impact on the distribution of perfusion. However, the upper lung is now no longer restricted by the chest wall and is free to expand, resulting in a further increase in $\dot{V}/\dot{Q}$ mismatch as the nondependent lung is preferentially ventilated owing to a now increased compliance.

Lateral Position, Anesthetized, Paralyzed, Chest Open

During paralysis and positive pressure ventilation, diaphragmatic displacement is maximal over the nondependent lung, where there is the least amount of resistance to diaphragmatic movement caused by the abdominal contents (Fig. 34-13). This further compromises the ventilation to the dependent lung and increases the $\dot{V}/\dot{Q}$ mismatch.

One-Lung Ventilation, Anesthetized, Paralyzed, Chest Open

During two-lung ventilation in the lateral position, the mean blood flow to the nondependent lung is assumed to be 40% of cardiac output, and 60% of cardiac output goes to the dependent lung (Fig. 34-14). Normally, venous admixture (shunt) in the lateral position is 10% of cardiac output and is equally divided as 5% in each lung. Therefore, the average

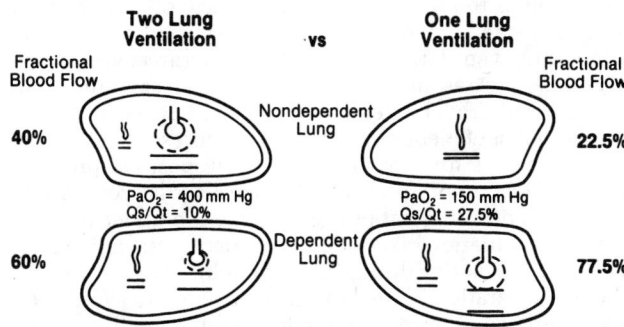

Figure 34-14. Schematic representation of two-lung ventilation *versus* one-lung ventilation. Typical values for fractional blood flow to the nondependent and dependent lungs, as well as Pao$_2$ and $\dot{Q}_s/\dot{Q}_t$ for the two conditions, are shown. The $\dot{Q}_s/\dot{Q}_t$ during two-lung ventilation is assumed to be distributed equally between the two lungs (5% to each lung.) The essential difference between two-lung and one-lung ventilation is that, during one-lung ventilation, the nonventilated lung has some blood flow and therefore an obligatory shunt, which is not present during two-lung ventilation. The 35% of total flow perfusing the nondependent lung, which was not shunt flow, was assumed to be able to reduce its blood flow by 50% by hypoxic pulmonary vasoconstriction. The increase in Q$_s$/Q$_t$ from two-lung to one-lung ventilation is assumed to be due solely to the increase in blood flow through the nonventilated, nondependent lung during one-lung ventilation. (Reproduced with permission from Benumof JL: Anesthesia for Thoracic Surgery. Philadelphia, WB Saunders, 1987.)

percentage of cardiac output participating in gas exchange is 35% in the nondependent lung and 55% in the dependent lung.

One-lung ventilation creates an obligatory right-to-left transpulmonary shunt through the nonventilated, nondependent lung, since the $\dot{V}/\dot{Q}$ ratio of that lung is zero. In theory, an additional 35% should be added to the total shunt during one-lung ventilation. However, assuming active hypoxic pulmonary vasoconstriction, blood flow to the nondependent hypoxic lung will be reduced by 50% and therefore will be (35/2) = 17.5%. To this must be added 5%, which is the obligatory shunt through the nondependent lung. The shunt through the nondependent lung will therefore be 22.5% (Fig. 34-14).[70] Together with the 5% shunt in the dependent lung, total shunt during one-lung ventilation is $22.5 + 5 = 27.5\%$. This results in a PaO_2 of approximately 150 mm Hg ($FIO_2 = 1.0$).

Since 72.5% of the perfusion is directed to the dependent lung during one-lung ventilation, the matching of ventilation in this lung is important for adequate gas exchange. The dependent lung is no longer on the steep, compliant portion of the volume-pressure curve because of reduced lung volume and FRC. There are several reasons for this reduction in FRC, including general anesthesia, paralysis, pressure of abdominal contents, compression by the weight of mediastinal structures, and suboptimal positioning on the operating table. Other considerations that impair optimal ventilation to the dependent lung include absorption atelectasis, accumulation of secretions, and the formation of a fluid transudate in the dependent lung. All of these create a low $\dot{V}/\dot{Q}$ ratio and a large $P(A-a)O_2$ gradient.

ONE-LUNG VENTILATION

Absolute Indications for One-Lung Ventilation

Separation of the lungs to prevent spillage of pus or blood from an infected or bleeding source is an absolute indication for one-lung ventilation (Table 34-2). Life-threatening complications, such as massive atelectasis, sepsis, and pneumonia, can result from bilateral contamination. Bronchopleural and bronchocutaneous fistulae both represent low-resistance pathways for the VT delivered by positive pressure ventilation, and both prevent adequate alveolar ventilation. Giant cysts or unilateral bullae may rupture under positive pressure ventilation. This can be avoided by selective lung ventilation. Finally, during bronchopulmonary lavage, an effective separation of the lungs is mandatory to avoid accidental spillage of fluid from the lavaged lung to the nondependent ventilated lung.

Relative Indications for One-Lung Ventilation

In clinical practice, a double-lumen tube is commonly used for a lobectomy or pneumonectomy; these represent relative indications for lung separation. Upper lobectomy, pneumonectomy, and thoracic aortic aneurysm repair are relatively high-priority indications. These procedures are technically difficult, and optimal surgical exposure and a quiet operative field are highly desirable. Lower or middle lobectomy and esophageal resection are of lower priority. Nevertheless, many surgeons are accustomed to operating with a collapsed lung, which minimizes lung trauma from retractors and manipulation, helps surgeons to better visualize lung anatomy, and facilitates identification and separation of an-

TABLE 34-2. Indications for One-Lung Ventilation

Absolute

1. Isolation of each lung to prevent contamination of a healthy lung:
   a. Infection (abscess, infected cyst)
   b. Massive hemorrhage
2. Control of distribution of ventilation to only one lung
   a. Bronchopleural fistula
   b. Bronchopleural cutaneous fistula
   c. Unilateral cyst or bullae
   d. Major bronchial disruption or trauma
3. Unilateral lung lavage

Relative

1. Surgical exposure—high priority
   a. Thoracic aortic aneurysm
   b. Pneumonectomy
   c. Upper lobectomy
2. Surgical exposure—low priority
   a. Esophageal surgery
   b. Middle and lower lobectomy
   c. Thoracoscopy under general anesthesia

Modified from Benumof JL: Physiology of the open chest and one-lung ventilation. In Kaplan JA (ed): Thoracic Anesthesia, p 299. New York, Churchill Livingstone, 1983.

atomic structures and lung fissures. Thoracoscopy, if not performed with an intercostal block in the spontaneously breathing patient, is greatly facilitated by collapse of the lung under examination.

Methods of Lung Separation

Bronchial Blockers

Bronchial Blocker. Lung separation can be achieved with a reusable bronchial blocker. Magill described an endobronchial blocker that is placed with the help of a bronchoscope and directed to the nonventilated lung. Inflation of the cuff at the distal end of the blocker serves to block ventilation to that lung. The lumen of the blocker permits suctioning of the airway distal to the catheter tip. Depending on the clinical circumstance, oxygen can be insufflated through the catheter lumen. A conventional endotracheal tube is then placed in the trachea. This technique can be useful in achieving selective ventilation in children under 12 years of age, since the smallest double-lumen tube available at present is a No. 28 French. However, since the blocker balloon requires a high distending pressure, it easily slips out of the bronchus into the trachea, obstructing ventilation and losing the seal between the two lungs. This displacement can be secondary to changes in position or to surgical manipulation. The loss of lung separation can be a life-threatening situation if it is performed to prevent spillage of pus, blood, or fluid from bronchopulmonary lavage. For this reason, bronchial blockers are rarely used in present-day practice.

Arterial Embolectomy Catheter. Selective airway occlusion can be achieved by the use of Fogarty catheters designed for embolectomy procedures.[71] Placement of the embolectomy catheter is best performed under direct vision with the aid of a fiberoptic bronchoscope. A conventional endotracheal tube is then placed alongside the catheter after withdrawing the bronchoscope.

Univent Tube. Introduced in 1982 by Fuji Systems Corporation, Tokyo, Japan, the Univent is a single-lumen endotracheal tube with a movable endobronchial blocker. In this tube, the bronchial blocker is housed in a small channel bored in the endotracheal tube wall. Following intubation of the trachea, the movable blocker is manipulated into the desired mainstem bronchus with the aid of a fiberoptic bronchoscope.[72-75] Disadvantages of the Univent tube are that correct positioning of the blocker may be difficult to achieve or maintain. The Univent tube may be ideal for cases in which changing tubes (e.g., from single- to double-lumen) may be difficult (such as mediastinoscopy followed by thoracotomy), or in cases of bilateral lung transplant.

Single-Lumen Endobronchial Tubes

Historically, a number of single-lumen tubes were designed for insertion into a mainstem bronchus in order to achieve lung separation.[2-4] However, these tubes are rarely, if ever, used today because of technical difficulties and less satisfactory performance.

Double-Lumen Endobronchial Tubes

These tubes are currently the most widely used means of achieving lung separation and one-lung ventilation. There are several different types of double-lumen tube, but all are essentially similar in design in that two catheters are bonded together. One lumen is long enough to reach a mainstem bronchus, and the second lumen ends with an opening in the distal trachea. Lung separation is achieved by inflation of two cuffs, the proximal tracheal cuff, and the distal bronchial cuff located in the mainstem bronchus (see the section on Positioning Double-Lumen Tubes). The endobronchial cuffs of right-sided tubes are slotted or otherwise designed to allow ventilation of the right upper lobe, since the right mainstem bronchus is too short to accommodate both the right lumen tip and a right bronchial cuff.

Carlens. A left-sided double-lumen tube with a carinal hook to aid in positioning and to minimize dislocation is shown in Figure 34-15. It is made of red rubber, and each catheter has a D-shaped cross-sectional lumen. Although the carinal hook may help in the correct placement of the tube, it can increase difficulty during insertion, cause vocal cord trauma, and can sometimes be amputated and lost during the insertion and manipulation of the tube.

White. This tube is essentially a right-sided Carlens tube (Fig. 34-16). It is used for right endobronchial intubations and left-sided surgical procedures. The distal endobronchial cuff is slotted to permit ventilation of the right upper lobe bronchus.

Robertshaw. This is a double-lumen tube available in left- and right-sided forms without a carinal hook, which makes insertion easier (Fig. 34-17). This tube has the advantages of having D-shaped large diameter lumina that allow easy suctioning and offer low resistance to gas flow and a fixed curvature to facilitate proper positioning and to reduce the possibility of kinking. The original red rubber tubes are available in three sizes: small, medium, and large. Clear, polyvinyl chloride (PVC) disposable Robertshaw design double-lumen tubes are now in wide use. These tubes are

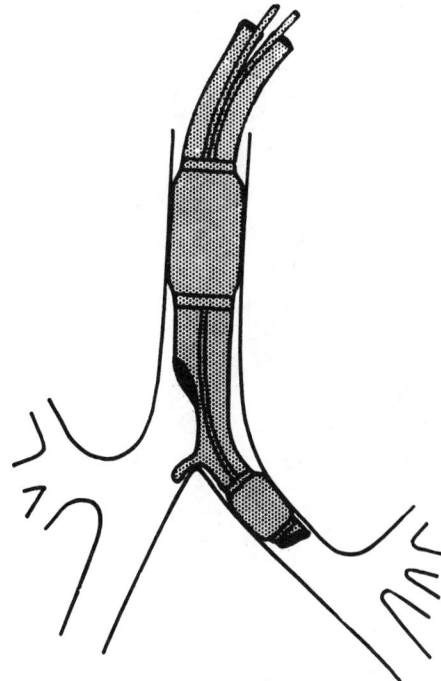

Figure 34-15. Left mainstem endobronchial intubation using a Carlens tube. Note carinal "hook" used for correct positioning. (Reproduced with permission from Hillard EK, Thompson PW: Instruments used in thoracic anaesthesia. In Mushin WW [ed]: Thoracic Anaesthesia, p 315. Oxford, Blackwell Scientific, 1963.)

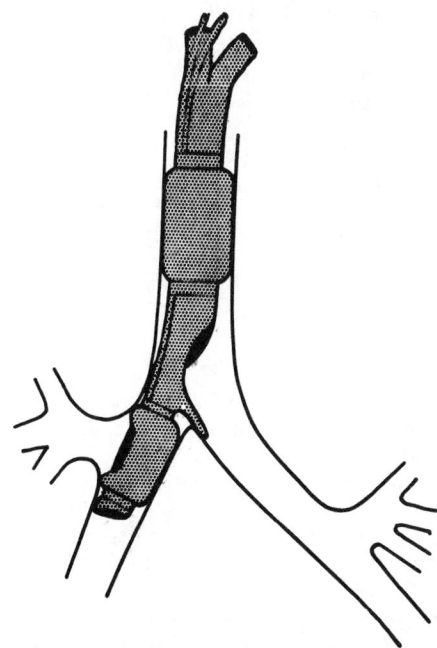

Figure 34-16. Right mainstem endobronchial intubation with a White tube. Note the slot in the endobronchial cuff to facilitate ventilation of the right upper lobe. (Reproduced with permission from Hillard EK, Thompson PW: Instruments used in thoracic anaesthesia. In Mushin WW [ed]: Thoracic Anaesthesia, p 309. Oxford, Blackwell Scientific, 1963.)

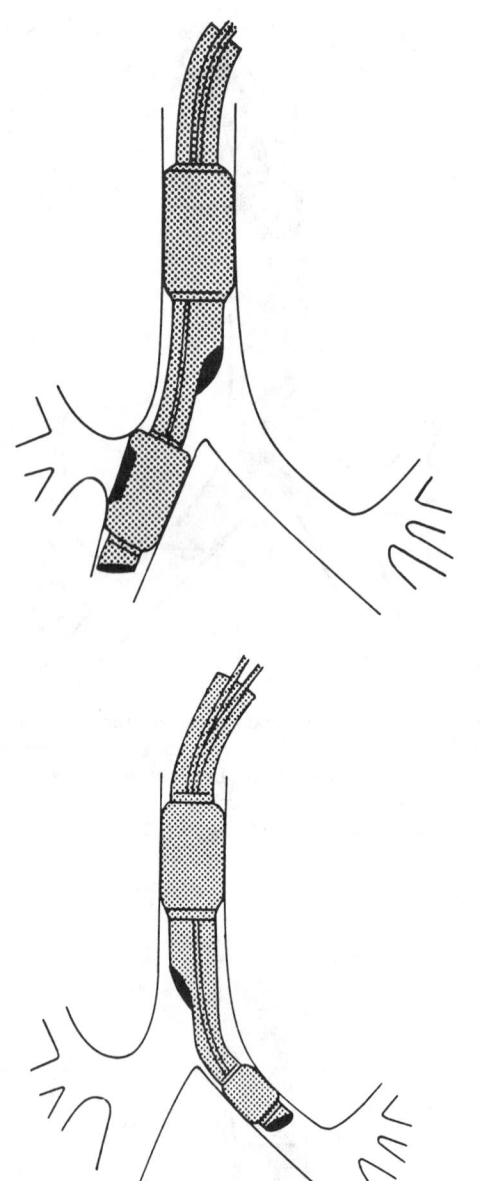

Figure 34-17. Right- and left-sided Robertshaw tubes. (Reproduced with permission from Wilson RS: Endobronchial intubation. In Kaplan JA [ed]: Thoracic Anesthesia. New York, Churchill Livingstone, 1983.)

available in a right or left design and in French sizes 35, 37, 39, and 41. A French size 28 has been made available for use in pediatric cases. The advantages of the disposable tubes include relative ease of insertion, proper positioning, easy recognition of the blue color of the endobronchial cuff when fiberoptic bronchoscopy is used, confirmation of position on a chest radiograph using the radio-opaque lines in the wall of the tube, and continuous observation of tidal gas exchange and of respiratory moisture through the clear plastic. The right-sided endobronchial tube is designed to minimize occlusion of the right upper lobe. The right endobronchial cuff is doughnut-shaped and allows the right upper lobe ventilation slot to ride over the right upper lobe orifice. The tube is also suitable for use in long-term ventilation in the intensive care unit because it has a high-volume low-pressure cuff. These are now considered the tubes of

choice for achieving lung separation and one-lung ventilation.

Despite the availability of disposable double-lumen tubes, many centers continue to use the red rubber Robertshaw tubes. There are several reasons for this. First, the cost of reusable tubes is significantly less than that of the disposable tubes. Second, some anesthesiologists believe that although the red rubber tubes may be more difficult to insert, they are less likely to dislocate during patient positioning and surgical manipulation. Third, during insertion of the double-lumen tube, the tracheal cuff often directly rubs against the patient's upper teeth. If these teeth are prominent and sharp, the thin-walled tracheal cuffs of the disposable tubes are much more likely to tear as compared with the thicker-walled cuffs of the red rubber tubes. Fourth, if the wrong size of disposable tube is selected and insertion is attempted, the tube cannot be reused because sterility is compromised. This does not apply to the red rubber tubes, which withstand repeated sterilization.

Positioning Double-Lumen Tubes. This section concentrates on the insertion of Robertshaw-type double-lumen tubes (both disposable and nondisposable), since they are the most widely used. Prior to insertion, the double-lumen tube should be prepared and checked. The tracheal cuff (low-pressure, high-volume) can accommodate up to 20 ml of air, and the bronchial cuff should be checked using a 3-ml syringe. The tube should be coated liberally with lubricating ointment and the stylet should be withdrawn, lubricated, and gently placed back into the bronchial lumen without disturbing the tube's preformed curvature. The Macintosh 3 blade is preferred for intubation of the trachea, since it provides the largest area through which to pass the tube. The insertion of the tube is performed with the distal concave curvature facing anteriorly. After the tip of the tube is past the vocal cords, the stylet is removed and the tube is rotated through 90 degrees. A left-sided tube is rotated 90 degrees to the left and a right-sided tube is rotated to the right. Advancement of the tube ceases when moderate resistance to further passage is encountered, indicating that the tube tip has been firmly seated in the mainstem bronchus. It is important to remove the stylet before rotating and advancing the tube in order to avoid tracheal or bronchial lacerations. Rotation and advancement of the tube should be performed gently and under continuous direct laryngoscopy to prevent hypopharyngeal structures from interfering with proper positioning. Once the tube is thought to be in the proper position, a sequence of steps should be performed to check its location.

First, the tracheal cuff should be inflated and equal ventilation of both lungs established. If breath sounds are not equal, the tube is probably too far down and the tracheal lumen opening is in a mainstem bronchus or is lying at the carina. Withdrawal of the tube by 2–3 cm usually restores equal breath sounds. The second step is to clamp the right side (in the case of the left-sided tube) and remove the right cap from the connector. Then the bronchial cuff is slowly inflated to prevent an air leak from the bronchial lumen around the bronchial cuff into the right tracheal lumen. This ensures that excessive pressure is not applied to the bronchus and helps avoid laceration. Inflation of the bronchial cuff rarely requires more than 2 ml of air. The third step is to remove the clamp and check that both lungs are ventilated with both cuffs inflated. This will ensure that the bronchial cuff is not obstructing the contralateral hemithorax, either totally or partially. The final step is to selectively clamp each side and watch for absence of movement and breath sounds on the ipsilateral side, while the ventilated side should have clear breath sounds, chest movement that feels compliant, respiratory gas moisture with each tidal ventilation, and no air leak. If peak airway pressure during two-lung ventilation is 20 cm H_2O, it should not exceed 40 cm H_2O for the same tidal volume during one-lung ventilation.

Other methods that have been used for ensuring the correct placement of a double-lumen tube include fluoroscopy, chest x-ray, selective capnography, and the use of an underwater seal. Determination of the presence of air leaks when positive pressure is applied to one lumen of double-lumen tube is easily done in the operating room. If the bronchial cuff is not inflated and positive pressure is applied to the bronchial lumen of the double-lumen tube, gas will leak past the bronchial cuff and return through the tracheal lumen. If the tracheal lumen is connected to an underwater seal system, gas will be seen to bubble up through the water. The bronchial cuff can then be gradually inflated until no gas bubbles are seen and the desired cuff seal pressure can be attained. This test is of extreme importance when absolute lung separation is needed, such as during bronchopulmonary lavage.

The most important advance in checking the proper position of a double-lumen tube is the introduction of the pediatric fiberoptic bronchoscope. Recently, Smith et al showed that when the disposable double-lumen tube was thought to be in correct position by auscultation and physical examination, subsequent fiberoptic bronchoscopy showed that 48% of tubes were, in fact, malpositioned.[76] When using a left-sided double-lumen tube, the bronchoscope is usually first introduced through the tracheal lumen. The carina is visualized and no bronchial cuff herniation should be seen. The upper surface of the blue endobronchial cuff should be just below the tracheal carina. The bronchial cuff of the disposable double-lumen tube is easily visualized because of its blue color. The bronchoscope should then be passed through the bronchial lumen and the left upper lobe orifice should be identified. When a right-sided double-lumen tube is used (Fig. 34-18), the carina should be visualized through the tracheal lumen, but more important, the orifice of the right upper lobe bronchus should be identified when the bronchoscope is passed through the right upper lobe ventilating slot of the double-lumen tube. Pediatric fiberoptic bronchoscopes are available in several sizes: 5.6, 4.9, and 3.6 mm in external diameter. The 4.9 mm-diameter bronchoscope can be passed through double-lumen tubes of French sizes 37 and larger. The 3.6 mm-diameter bronchoscope is easily passed through all sizes of double-lumen tube. In general, it is recommended that the largest size that can pass through the lumen of a double-lumen tube be used, since it provides better visualization and facilitates identification of the bronchial anatomy.

Problems of Malposition of the Double-Lumen Tube. The use of a double-lumen tube is associated with a number of potential problems, the most important of which is malposition. There are several possibilities for tube malposition. The double-lumen tube may be accidentally directed to the side opposite the desired mainstem bronchus. In this case, the lung opposite the side of the connector clamped will collapse. Generally inadequate separation, increased airway pressures, and instability of the double-lumen tube occur. In addition, because of the morphology of the double-lumen tube curvatures, tracheal or bronchial lacerations may result. If a left-sided double-lumen tube is inserted into the right mainstem bronchus, it will obstruct the ventilation to

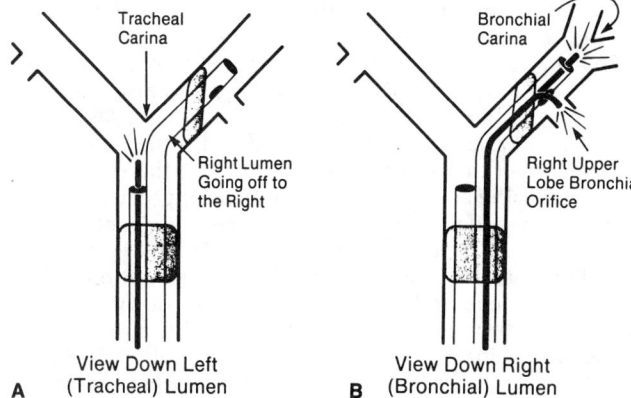

Figure 34-18. Use of fiberoptic bronchoscope to determine the position of a right-sided double-lumen tube. (*A*) When the bronchoscope is passed down the left (tracheal) lumen, the endoscopist should see a clear view of the tracheal carina and right lumen going off into the right mainstem bronchus. (*B*) When the bronchoscope is passed *via* the right (bronchial) lumen, the endoscopist should see the bronchial carina off in the distance; when the bronchoscope is flexed cephalad and passed through the right upper lobe ventilation slot, the right upper lobe bronchial orifice should be visualized. (Reproduced with permission from Benumof JL: Intraoperative considerations for all thoracic surgery. In Benumof JL: Anesthesia for Thoracic Surgery. Philadelphia, WB Saunders, 1987.)

the right upper lobe (Fig. 34-19 right). It is therefore essential to recognize and correct such a malposition as soon as possible.

Second, the double-lumen tube may be passed too far down into either the right or the left mainstem bronchus. In this case, breath sounds will be very diminished or not audible at all over the contralateral side. This situation is corrected when the tube is withdrawn until the opening of the tracheal lumen is above the carina.

Third, the double-lumen tube may not be inserted far enough with the bronchial lumen opening above the carina. In this position, good breath sounds will be heard bilaterally when ventilating through the bronchial lumen, but no breath sounds will be audible when ventilating through the tracheal lumen, since the inflated bronchial cuff obstructs gas flow arising from the tracheal lumen. The cuff should

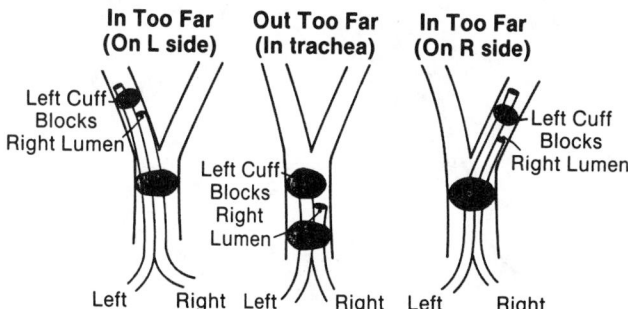

Figure 34-19. Diagram showing the three major malpositions of a left-sided double-lumen endotracheal tube. The tube can be in too far on the left (*left*), out too far (*center*), or down the right mainstem bronchus (*right*). In each case, the left cuff, when fully inflated, can completely block the right lumen. (Reproduced with permission from Benumof JL: Intraoperative considerations for all thoracic surgery. In Benumof JL: Anesthesia for Thoracic Surgery. Philadelphia, WB Saunders, 1987.)

be deflated and the double-lumen tube rotated and advanced into the desired mainstem bronchus.

Fourth, a right-sided double-lumen tube may occlude the right upper lobe orifice (Fig. 34-20). The mean distance from the carina to the right upper lobe orifice is 2.3 ± 0.7 cm in males, and 2.1 ± 0.7 cm in females.[77] With the right-sided double-lumen tubes, the ventilatory slot in the side of the bronchial catheter must overlie the right upper lobe orifice to permit ventilation of this lobe. The margin of safety, however, is extremely small, and varies from 1 to 8 mm.[77] It is, therefore, difficult to ensure proper ventilation to the right upper lobe and to avoid dislocation of the double-lumen tube during surgical manipulation. When right endobronchial intubation is required, a disposable right-sided double-lumen tube is perhaps the best choice because of the slanted doughnut shape of the bronchial cuff, which allows the ventilation slot to ride off the right upper lobe ventilation orifice and increases the margin of safety.

Fifth, the left upper lobe orifice may be obstructed by a left-sided double-lumen tube. Traditionally, it was believed that the take-off of the left upper lobe bronchus was at a safe distance from the carina and that it would not be obstructed by a left-sided double-lumen tube. However, the mean distance between the left upper lobe orifice and the carina is 5.4±0.7 cm in males and 5.0±0.7 cm in females.[77] The average distance between the openings of the right and left lumina on the left-sided disposable tubes is 6.9 cm.[4]

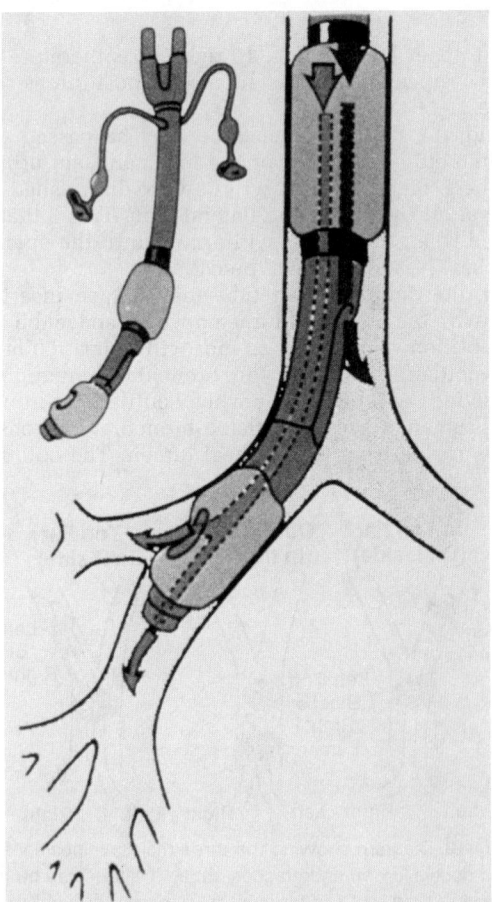

Figure 34-20. A right-sided Robertshaw design double-lumen tube showing the slotted endobronchial cuff overlying the origin of the right upper lobe bronchus. Malposition of the tube may cause the bronchial cuff to occlude the origin of the right upper lobe bronchus.

Therefore, an obstruction of the left upper lobe is possible while the tracheal lumen is still above the carina. There is also a 20% variation in the location of the blue endobronchial cuff on the disposable tubes, since this cuff is attached by hand at the end of the manufacturing process.

Finally, bronchial cuff herniation may occur and obstruct the bronchial lumen if excessive volumes are used to inflate the cuff. The bronchial cuff has also been known to herniate over the tracheal carina, and in the case of a left-sided double-lumen tube, to obstruct ventilation to the right mainstem bronchus.

Another rare complication with double-lumen tubes is tracheal rupture. Guernelli et al[78] reported 5 of 2700 patients with tracheobronchial rupture caused by intubation with Carlens tubes. Most of these ruptures were thought to be secondary to the carinal hook or use of an inappropriately sized tube. Overinflation of the bronchial cuff, inappropriate positioning, and trauma owing to intraoperative dislocation that resulted in bronchial rupture have also been described in association with the Robertshaw tube and the disposable double-lumen tube.[79] Therefore, the pressure in the bronchial cuff should be monitored and decreased if the cuff is found to be overinflated. If absolute separation of the lungs is not needed, the bronchial cuff should be deflated and then reinflated slowly to avoid excessive pressure on the bronchial walls. The bronchial cuff should also be deflated during any repositioning of the patient unless lung separation is absolutely required during this time.

Contraindications to Use of the Double-Lumen Tube. Use of a double-lumen tube to achieve lung separation is relatively contraindicated in situations where there is a lesion in the airway itself or a difficult upper airway that results in poor laryngeal visualization. It is also relatively contraindicated in some critically ill patients in whom short periods of apnea or hypoxemia, which may occur during insertion of a double-lumen tube, may be life-threatening. In patients requiring rapid intubation (e.g., with a full stomach), a double-lumen tube is not necessarily contraindicated, since the disposable tubes with stylets are as easily inserted as single-lumen tubes in most cases.

MANAGEMENT OF ONE-LUNG VENTILATION

This section discusses the management of one-lung ventilation in a paralyzed patient in the lateral decubitus position with an open chest. Inspired oxygen fraction (FIO$_2$), VT and respiratory rate, dependent lung, positive end-expiratory pressure, and nondependent lung continuous positive airway pressure are reviewed and an approach to the management of one-lung ventilation is presented.

Inspired Oxygen Fraction

Usually, an FIO$_2$ of 1.0 is used during one-lung ventilation. This high oxygen concentration serves to protect against hypoxemia during the procedure. In many studies, an FIO$_2$ of 1.0 has been used and resulted in a shunt of 25–30% and mean PaO$_2$ values between 150 and 210 mm Hg during one-lung ventilation.[80-83] In addition to a higher margin of safety, high inspired oxygen fractions cause vasodilatation of the vessels in the dependent lung, which increases the capability of this lung to accept blood flow redistribution due to nondependent lung hypoxic pulmonary vasoconstriction. A high FIO$_2$ may, however, cause absorption ate-

TABLE 34-3. Mean Pao_2 During One-Lung Ventilation Using $Fio_2 \leq 0.5$

Investigators	Ref. No.	No. of Patients	Fio_2	Two Lungs Pao_2 (mm Hg)	One Lung Pao_2 (mm Hg)
Lunding and Fernandes	85	6	0.50	163	77
Lunding and Fernandes	85	15	0.25	98	67
Khanam and Branthwaite	257	28	0.40	NR	73
Torda et al	86	9	0.50	116	64
Torda et al	86	10	0.35	126	62
Jenkins et al	87	10	0.50	165	87
Cohen et al	88	20	0.50	248	80

NR = not reported.

lectasis and potentially further increase the degree of shunt because of the collapsed alveoli.[84] The risk can be reduced by using a lower Fio_2, by the application of positive pressure ventilation, or by the use of a high VT and positive end-expiratory pressure. Theoretically, a high Fio_2 can also cause lung injury owing to oxygen toxicity, although this complication is unlikely to occur in the time frame of a surgical operation. Lower oxygen concentrations have been used in the past[85,86] and more recently[87,88] with resulting Pao_2 values as shown in Table 34-3.

The use of an Fio_2 less than 1.0 during one-lung ventilation offers the benefits of reducing the risk of absorption atelectasis and may permit use of lower concentrations of potent inhaled anesthetics, which in higher concentrations might be more depressant to the myocardium, particularly in high-risk patients. An Fio_2 of less than 1.0 may also be indicated in patients with bleomycin toxicity.[90] The combination of N_2O/O_2 with pulse oximetry monitoring may represent an optimal solution in such cases. However, the risk/benefit ratio for each patient should always be carefully considered.

Tidal Volume and Respiratory Rate

During one-lung ventilation, the dependent lung should be ventilated with a VT of 10–12 ml·kg^{-1}. Tidal volumes ranging between 8–15 ml·kg^{-1} produced no significant effect on transpulmonary shunt or Pao_2.[89] A VT of less than 8 ml·kg^{-1} can result in a decrease in FRC and enhanced formation of atelectasis in the dependent lung. A VT of greater than 15 ml·kg^{-1} can increase the pulmonary vascular resistance of the dependent lung (similar to the application of positive end-expiratory pressure) and divert blood flow into the nondependent lung. The value of 10–12 ml·kg^{-1} is a middle range between 8–15 ml·kg^{-1} and appears to have the least effect on Pao_2 and percent shunt ($\dot{Q}s/\dot{Q}t\%$).[82]

The respiratory rate should be adjusted to maintain a $Paco_2$ of 35 ± 3 mm Hg. Elimination of CO_2 is usually not a problem during one-lung ventilation if the double-lumen tube is positioned correctly. The shunt during one-lung ventilation has little influence on $Paco_2$ values, since the arterio-venous Pco_2 difference is normally only 6 mm Hg. Furthermore, CO_2 is 20 times more diffusible than O_2. It is also important not to hyperventilate the patient's lungs because hypocapnia will increase vascular resistance in the dependent lung, inhibit nondependent lung hypoxic pulmonary vasoconstriction, increase shunt, and decrease Pao_2. Hypocarbia is thought to inhibit hypoxic pulmonary vasoconstriction secondary to a vasodilator effect. Since hy-

pocarbia can only be achieved by hyperventilating the dependent lung, it will raise the mean intra-alveolar pressure and therefore the vascular resistance in that lung. Finally, one-lung ventilation decreases the VD/VT ratio and enhances CO_2 elimination.

Positive End-Expiratory Pressure to the Dependent Lung

The beneficial effect of selective positive end-expiratory pressure 10 cm H_2O ($PEEP_{10}$) to the dependent lung is caused by an increased lung volume at end-expiration (FRC), which improves the V/Q relationship in the dependent lung. The increase in FRC prevents airway and alveolar closure at end-expiration. Therefore, it is not surprising that attempts have been made to improve oxygenation during one-lung ventilation by the application of positive end-expiratory pressure to the dependent lung. However, the results were somewhat disappointing (Table 34-4). Most of the studies showed either no change in Pao_2, a decrease, or a slight increase in Pao_2,[83,88,89,91] probably owing to the positive end-expiratory pressure inducing an increase in lung volume that caused compression of the small interalveolar vessels and increased pulmonary vascular resistance. If this increase in resistance is limited to the dependent lung, blood flow can only be diverted to the nondependent lung, increasing $Qs/Qt\%$ and further decreasing Pao_2.

The studies of positive end-expiratory pressure cited above used an $Fio_2 = 1.0$ with a mean Pao_2 during one-lung ventilation of between 150–200 mm Hg, at which further improvement in Pao_2 is clinically unnecessary. The possibility that in a diseased dependent lung (low lung volume and low V/Q ratio) with a low Pao_2 (below 80 mm Hg) during one-lung ventilation the application of positive end-expiratory pressure can improve Pao_2 has been addressed by Cohen et al.[92] Using an $Fio_2 = 0.5$ in 18 patients, 11 patients had a Pao_2 below 80 mm Hg during one-lung ventilation. The application of 10 cm H_2O PEEP significantly increased Pao_2 in 10 out of 11 patients. In the other group of seven patients who had a Pao_2 greater than 80 mm Hg with one-lung ventilation, the application of 10 cm H_2O PEEP did not improve mean Pao_2. It was concluded from this study that the application of 10 cm H_2O PEEP during one-lung ventilation in patients with a low Pao_2 may increase FRC to normal values, resulting in a lower pulmonary vascular resistance and in an improved V/Q ratio and Pao_2. Presumably, patients with a higher Pao_2 had a dependent lung with an adequate FRC, and the application of positive end-expiratory pressure had the negative effect of redistrib-

TABLE 34-4. Effect of Positive End-Expiratory Pressure on PaO2 During One-Lung Ventilation in Humans

Investigators	Ref. No.	No. of Patients	FIO2	PEEP cm H2O	PaO2 (mm Hg) During One-Lung Ventilation With ZEEP	PaO2 (mm Hg) During One-Lung Ventilation With PEEP
Tarhan and Lundborg	80	14	1.0	10	170	120
Aalto-Setala et al	258	11	1.0	5	160	153 (NS)
Capan et al	83	11	1.0	10	155	85
Katz et al	89	17	1.0	10 ($V_T = 7$ ml·kg^{-1})	184	157 (NS)
Katz et al	89	17	1.0	10 ($V_T = 7$ ml·kg^{-1})	210	162
Cohen et al	92	17	0.5	10	80	105 (NS)

PEEP = positive end-expiratory pressure; ZEEP = zero end-expiratory pressure; NS = not statistically significant; VT = tidal volume.

uting blood flow away from the dependent ventilated lung (Fig. 34-21).

Continuous Positive Airway Pressure to the Nondependent Lung

The single most effective maneuver to increase PaO2 during one-lung ventilation is the application of continuous positive airway pressure to the nondependent lung. This has been clearly demonstrated in several studies.[83,88,93-95] A lower level of continuous positive airway pressure (5–10 cm H2O) maintains the patency of the nondependent alve-

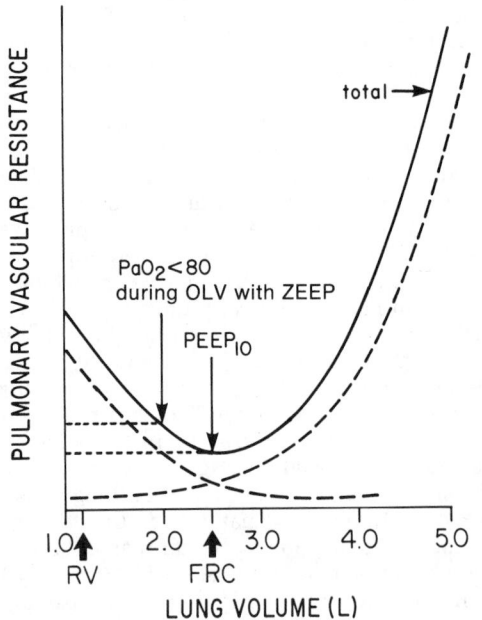

Figure 34-21. Effect of 10 cm H2O PEEP on FRC. It is postulated that, in patients having PaO2 < 80 mm Hg with ZEEP, FRC is low. PEEP10 increases FRC and thereby increases PaO2. (PEEP10 = positive end-expiratory pressure (10 cm H2O); OLV = one-lung ventilation; FRC = functional residual capacity; RV = residual volume; ZEEP = zero end-expiratory pressure.)

oli, allowing some oxygen uptake to occur in the distended alveoli. The continuous positive airway pressure should be applied after delivering a tidal volume to the nondependent lung to keep it slightly expanded. The continuous positive airway pressure, applied by insufflation of oxygen under positive pressure, will keep this lung "quiet" and prevent it from collapsing completely. Inflation of oxygen without maintaining a positive pressure failed to improve PaO2,[83,93] although some improvement in PaO2 occurred after 45 minutes of one-lung ventilation (from 140 ± 107 to 206 ± 76 mm Hg) with oxygen insufflation only.[96] Intermittent reinflation of the collapsed (nondependent) lung with oxygen also resulted in a significant improvement in PaO2.[97] The beneficial effects of continuous positive airway pressure 10 cm H2O (CPAP10) are not attributable solely to the effect of positive pressure in causing blood flow diversion away from the collapsed lung, since Alfery et al showed in dogs that the hyperinflation of nitrogen into the nondependent lung under 10 cm H2O failed to improve PaO2.[93]

The application of high-level continuous positive airway pressure (15 cm H2O) is not beneficial. At this pressure, the lung becomes overdistended, which interferes with surgical exposure. Also, this level of continuous positive airway pressure might have hemodynamic consequences, whereas CPAP10 has been shown to have no significant hemodynamic effects.[88,98]

Continuous positive airway pressure can be applied to the nondependent lung using a number of simple systems.[99-102] All of these systems have essentially the same features: an oxygen source, tubing to connect the oxygen source to the nonventilated lung, a pressure relief valve, and a pressure gauge. The catheter to the nondependent lung is usually insufflated with 5 l·min^{-1} of oxygen using a modified Ayre T-piece pediatric circuit, and the valve on the expiratory limb is adjusted to the desired pressure as read on the attached gauge (Fig. 34-22). Instead of a pressure gauge or manometer inserted into the circuit, Brown et al described the use of a weighted pop-off valve, such as a ball or spring-loaded positive end-expiratory pressure valve.[103]

High-frequency ventilation (HFV) with oxygen to the nondependent lung and conventional ventilation to the dependent lung has also been used to improve PaO2 during one-lung ventilation (see the section on High-frequency Ventilation).

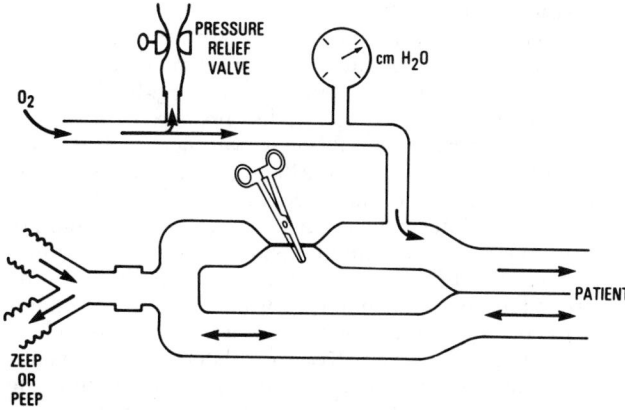

Figure 34-22. Schematic of a simple, selective up-lung continuous positive airway pressure system. The fresh inflow of oxygen is restricted or limited by a pressure release valve and, therefore, a constant distending airway pressure to the nonventilated lung occurs. The dependent lung can be ventilated with positive end-expiratory pressure (PEEP) or zero end-expiratory pressure (ZEEP). (Reproduced with permission from Benumof JL: Physiology of the open-chest and one lung ventilation. In Kaplan JA [ed]: Thoracic Anesthesia. New York, Churchill Livingstone, 1983.)

Clinical Approach to Management of One-Lung Ventilation

Once the patient is in the lateral position, the position of the double-lumen tube should be rechecked. Two-lung ventilation should be maintained for as long as possible, and when one-lung ventilation needs to be instituted, it is recommended that an $FiO_2 = 1.0$ be used. The lungs should be ventilated using a VT of 10–12 ml·kg^{-1} at a rate adjusted to maintain $PaCO_2$ at 35±3 mm Hg. This is usually monitored with the use of a capnometer or other multigas analyzer.

Following the initiation of one-lung ventilation, PaO_2 can continue to decrease for up to 45 minutes.[89] Close monitoring of arterial blood gases or use of a pulse oximeter should be available throughout the operative period. It is also essential to work closely with the surgeon. If there are any questions concerning the position of the double-lumen tube position and if fiberoptic bronchoscopy is not available, the surgeon can palpate the tube and help to manipulate it into the correct position with direct digital guidance.

If hypoxemia occurs during one-lung ventilation, the position of the double-lumen tube should be rechecked using a fiberoptic bronchoscope. If the dependent lung is not severely diseased, a satisfactory PaO_2 on two-lung ventilation should not decrease to dangerously hypoxic levels on one-lung ventilation. If a left thoracotomy is being performed using a right-sided double-lumen tube, the ventilation to the right upper lobe should be ensured. After the tube position has been confirmed as correct, CPAP$_{10}$ should be applied to the nondependent lung following a VT that expands the lung. In most cases, the PaO_2 will increase to a safe level. If a continuous positive airway pressure device is not readily available and the PaO_2 is below 80 mm Hg, PEEP$_{10}$ can be applied to the dependent lung. CPAP$_{5-10}$ with PEEP$_{5-10}$ can be applied in different combinations in search of optimal oxygenation.

In the very rare case in which the PaO_2 remains low despite all of these maneuvers, intermittent two-lung ventilation can be reinstituted with the surgeon's cooperation.

Also, depending on the stage of surgical dissection, if a pneumonectomy is being performed, ligation of the pulmonary artery will eliminate the shunt.

During one-lung ventilation, the peak airway pressure, the effective VT delivered (measured by a spirometer), and the shape of the capnogram should be checked continuously. A sudden increase in peak airway pressure may be secondary to tube dislocation because of surgical manipulation, resulting in impaired ventilation. In addition, continuous auscultation by a stethoscope over the dependent lung is extremely important.

If any questions arise about the stability of the patient, or if the patient becomes hypotensive, dusky, or tachycardic, two-lung ventilation should be resumed until the problem has been resolved. Because of pericardial manipulation (during left thoracotomy in particular) and pulling on the great vessels, cardiac arrhythmias and hypotension are not uncommon. Cardiotonic drugs should be prepared and kept available for use during any thoracic surgical procedure. It should be remembered that the majority of thoracic surgical procedures represent only relative indications for one-lung ventilation. The benefits of one-lung ventilation should always be weighed against the risks to the patient.

CHOICE OF ANESTHESIA FOR THORACIC SURGERY

The choice of anesthetic technique for a thoracic surgical procedure must take into account the patient's cardiovascular and respiratory status and the particular effects of anesthetic drugs on these and other organ systems.

Thoracic surgical patients are more likely than others to have increased airway reactivity and a propensity to develop bronchoconstriction. This is because many of these patients are cigarette smokers and have chronic bronchitis and/or COPD. In addition, surgical manipulation of the airways and bronchial tree by instruments, a double-lumen tube, or the surgeon makes bronchoconstriction more likely to occur. The potent inhalation anesthetics halothane, enflurane, and isoflurane have all been shown to decrease airways reactivity and bronchoconstriction provoked by hypocapnia or inhaled or irritant aerosols. Their mechanism of action is probably a direct one on the airway musculature itself, and these agents are, therefore, the drugs of choice in patients with reactive airways. For an inhalation induction, halothane might be preferable, since it is the least pungent of the three drugs, although once the patient is asleep isoflurane may be the preferred drug because it raises the cardiac arrhythmia threshold and provides greater cardiovascular stability. Fentanyl does not appear to influence bronchomotor tone, but morphine may increase tone by a central vagotonic effect and by releasing histamine.

In most patients, anesthesia is safely induced with a barbiturate—thiopental or thiamylal. In patients with reactive airways, ketamine may be the drug of choice for induction of anesthesia because it has a bronchodilator effect and has been successfully used in the treatment of asthma. Thiopental has been associated with bronchospasm in asthmatic patients, although the reactivity in such cases may be related to inadequate levels of anesthesia prior to instrumentation of the airway.

The muscle relaxants of choice for thoracic procedures are those that lack a histamine-releasing or vagotonic effect and that have some sympathomimetic effect. In this respect, pancuronium and vecuronium probably represent the drugs of choice. Succinylcholine is useful to provide rapid profound relaxation for intubation of the trachea and is not associated with an increase in airways reactivity.

Intravenous lidocaine ($1-2$ mg·kg^{-1}) can be used prior to manipulations of the airway to prevent reflex bronchospasm. It has also been given by infusion to depress airway reactivity in patients who have poor cardiovascular function and cannot tolerate normal doses of the potent inhaled agents. Intravenous lidocaine has also been used to treat bronchospasm occurring during anesthesia. Lidocaine nebulized and administered *via* the airways has a similar salutary effect on bronchial tone.

Atropine may be used to block the antimuscarinic effects of acetylcholine and thereby protect against cholinergically induced bronchoconstriction. It may be administered intravenously or in nebulized form (see the section on Bronchoscopy).

HYPOXIC PULMONARY VASOCONSTRICTION

General anesthesia may impair pulmonary gas exchange, and arterial hypoxemia may occur as a result. In patients undergoing halothane-oxygen anesthesia with spontaneous two-lung ventilation, Nunn found a calculated shunt of 14% of pulmonary blood flow as compared with a calculated shunt of 1% in normal conscious supine patients measured using the same techniques.[104] He suggested that the large shunt observed was probably due to perfusion of totally unventilated parts of the lung. Marshall et al confirmed this and concluded that postoperative hypoxemia may also be a result of the residual effects of the anesthetic on venous admixture.[105] With this background, many investigators have studied the regulation of the pulmonary circulation through a homeostatic mechanism called hypoxic pulmonary vasoconstriction, which normally diverts blood away from hypoxic regions of the lung and thereby optimizes the gas exchange function of the lung.

Hypoxic pulmonary vasoconstriction was first described by Von Euler and Liljestrand in 1946.[106] They were studying changes in the pulmonary circulation of the cat in response to changes in inspired gas mixtures and found that 10.5% inspired O_2 (in N_2) mixtures caused an increase in pulmonary arterial pressure. Breathing 100% O_2 caused a decrease in pulmonary arterial pressure. They concluded that the increased pressure during hypoxia was caused by a direct effect on the pulmonary vessels. Whereas they delivered hypoxic gas mixtures to both lungs, others have studied the effects of the size of the hypoxic segment and the size of the hypoxic stimulus on perfusion pressure and on flow diversion. Thus, Marshall et al studied the effects of changing FIO_2 in lung segments of seven different sizes in a dog model.[107] In each test, the rest of the lung received oxygen, whereas hypoxic pulmonary vasoconstriction in the test segment was demonstrated by both increased perfusion pressure and diversion of blood flow away from the hypoxic test segment. Marshall et al found that pulmonary perfusion pressure increased with the size of the hypoxic segment from zero (smallest hypoxic segment) to approximately 2.2 times baseline for the hypoxic whole lung. Flow diversion, as a percentage of flow to the test segment under normoxic conditions, decreased with increasing size of the hypoxic test segment from a maximum of 75% for very small segments to zero when the whole lung was made hypoxic. Flow diversion increased linearly as PaO_2 was decreased over the range of $128-28$ mm Hg. In both flow diversion and changes in perfusion pressure, the response to hypoxic pulmonary vasoconstriction was predictable, continuous, and maximal

at a predicted PaO_2 of 30 mm Hg (4% oxygen). Thus, hypoxic pulmonary vasoconstriction causes a rise in both perfusion (pulmonary arterial) pressure and flow diversion.

The choice of anesthetic technique for one-lung ventilation must take into consideration the effects on oxygenation and therefore on hypoxic pulmonary vasoconstriction. Normally, collapse of the nonventilated, nondependent lung results in activation of reflex hypoxic pulmonary vasoconstriction in this lung. This causes local increases in pulmonary vascular resistance and diversion of blood flow to other better oxygenated parts of the pulmonary vascular bed (i.e., the dependent oxygenated and ventilated lung). The stimulus to hypoxic pulmonary vasoconstriction appears to be a function of both PaO_2 and $P\bar{v}O_2$ in isolated rat lungs ventilated with hypoxic mixtures, but in the atelectatic lung the stimulus is the $P\bar{v}O_2$.[108] A decrease in cardiac output may potentiate hypoxic pulmonary vasoconstriction by lowering $S\bar{v}O_2$. The response is believed to be accounted for by each smooth muscle cell in the pulmonary arterial wall responding to the oxygen tension in its vicinity. Because hypoxic pulmonary vasoconstriction causes flow diversion, PaO_2 should be higher than if there were no hypoxic pulmonary vasoconstriction. The relationship between PaO_2 and the size of the hypoxic segment (Fig. 34-23) shows that, when little of the lung is hypoxic, hypoxic pulmonary vasoconstriction has little effect on PaO_2 because shunt will be small in this situation. When most of the lung is hypoxic, there is no significant normoxic region to which the hypoxic region can divert flow, and then it does not matter, in terms of PaO_2, whether the hypoxic region has active hypoxic pulmonary vasoconstriction or not. When the amount of lung made hypoxic is $30-70\%$, such as occurs during one-lung ventilation, there may be a large difference between the PaO_2 to be expected with normal hypoxic pulmonary vasoconstriction compared to that expected in its absence. Hypoxic pulmonary vasoconstriction can raise PaO_2 from potentially dangerous levels to higher and safer ones. Conversely, inhibition of hypoxic pulmonary vasoconstriction may cause or contribute to hypoxemia during anesthesia.

Effects of Anesthetics on Hypoxic Pulmonary Vasoconstriction

All of the inhalation and many of the intravenous drugs used in anesthesia have been studied for their effects on hypoxic pulmonary vasoconstriction. The results have not always been consistent. Benumof has classified the preparations used to study these effects as *in vitro, in vivo*, nonintact, *in vivo* intact, and human studies.[109] In the *in vitro* preparations, such as isolated rat lungs in which all variables could be controlled, it was found that hypoxic pulmonary vasoconstriction was depressed in a dose-related manner by all potent inhaled anesthetics[110] but not by intravenous agents.[111] In the *in vivo*, nonintact preparations, such as dogs in which the left lower lobe had been isolated for ventilation purposes, the inhaled agents had variable effects on hypoxic pulmonary vasoconstriction,[112,113] whereas intravenous agents had no effect.[114] In the *in vivo*, intact dog preparations, inhaled agents have been shown to depress hypoxic pulmonary vasoconstriction,[115] whereas intravenous drugs had no effect.[116] Based upon the results of the above three types of preparation, it is generally believed that inhaled agents inhibit hypoxic pulmonary vasoconstriction, whereas intravenous drugs do not have this effect.

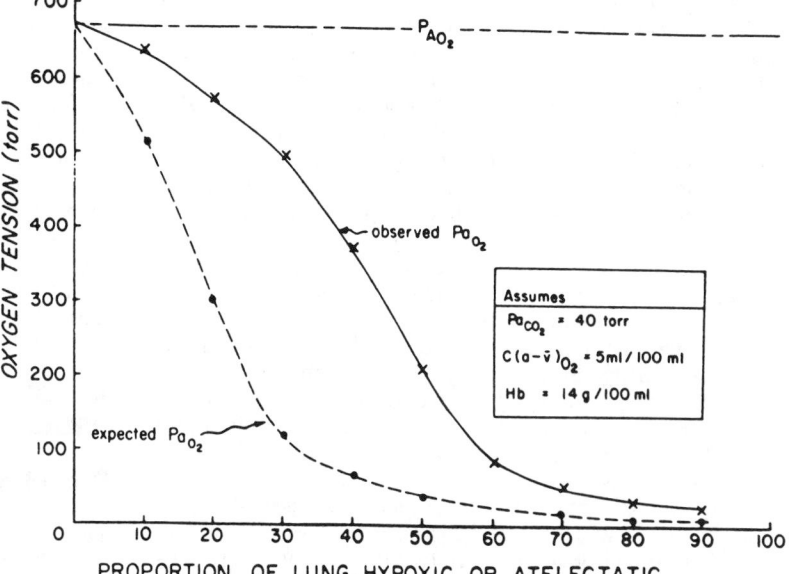

Figure 34-23. Role of hypoxic vasoconstriction in preserving Pa_{O_2} (in dogs). Assumptions are shown in insert. Lung is ventilated with $F_{IO_2} = 1.0$, while increasing portions of lung are subjected to hypoxia or atelectasis. In the absence of hypoxic pulmonary vasoconstriction, the expected Pa_{O_2} would follow the broken line, whereas in the presence of an active hypoxic pulmonary vasoconstriction response, observed Pa_{O_2} is maintained close to the solid line. (P_{AO_2} = aveloar P_{O_2}; Pa_{O_2} = arterial P_{O_2}.) (Adapted with permission from Marshall BE et al: HPV in dogs: Effects of lung segment size and oxygen tension. J Appl Physiol 51:1543, 1981.)

Human studies are perhaps the most significant because of their applicability to the clinical situation. Bjertnaes used perfusion scans (scintigraphy) to assess the effect of anesthetics on human hypoxic pulmonary vasoconstriction.[117] In his patients, lung separation was achieved using a double-lumen tube. One lung could then be ventilated with 100% O_2 and the other with 100% nitrogen. Hypoxic pulmonary vasoconstriction was assessed in the presence and absence of ether, halothane, and intravenous drugs (thiopental and fentanyl). Based upon his scintigraphic findings, Bjertnaes concluded that the inhaled agents, in clinically useful concentrations, inhibited hypoxic pulmonary vasoconstriction in humans.[117]

Jolin Carlsson et al used separate lung ventilation and a triple gas washout technique to study hypoxic pulmonary vasoconstriction in eight patients.[118] They demonstrated the presence of hypoxic pulmonary vasoconstriction in response to 8% O_2 in 92% nitrogen in the test lung but found no further change with the addition of 1.0 or 1.5% end-tidal isoflurane, and blood gas readings remained essentially unaltered. Attempts to use higher concentrations caused unacceptable hypotension. These authors concluded that isoflurane might be indicated for anesthesia in the presence of lung disease or during one-lung ventilation, since arterial oxygenation might be better preserved than would be the case with an anesthetic that more effectively inhibited hypoxic pulmonary vasoconstriction. Thus, although it is possible that higher concentrations of isoflurane might have caused a clear change in the differential blood flow distribution, at clinically used concentrations the effect of hypoxic pulmonary vasoconstriction in their subjects was all but unmeasurable.

Others have studied the effects on oxygenation of intravenous and inhalation anesthetic techniques during one-lung ventilation. Weinreich et al[119] used a ketamine infusion and found a lower incidence of hypoxemia (defined as $Pa_{O_2} < 70$ mm Hg) than other studies reporting the use of halothane for one-lung ventilation. Rees and Gaines[120] compared a ketamine-oxygen technique with an enflurane (1–3% inspired)-oxygen technique for one-lung ventilation and found no differences between the groups in Pa_{O_2} or shunt.

These findings suggested that ketamine afforded no advantage over enflurane during one-lung ventilation.

Rogers and Benumof[121] compared the effects of inhaled (isoflurane and halothane) with intravenous (methohexital and ketamine) anesthesia during one-lung ventilation and concluded that the inhalation drugs at about 1-minimum alveolar concentration (MAC) do not significantly affect hypoxic pulmonary vasoconstriction in humans, as evidenced by a lack of significant differences in Pa_{O_2} between use of the two techniques. The conclusions of this study have been questioned because the period of clinical exposure to the potent inhaled agents was very short. Thus clinically relevant tissue concentrations of anesthetic may not have been achieved.

In a subsequent study, Benumof et al investigated the changes in Pa_{O_2} and shunt that occurred following conversion from 1 MAC halothane or isoflurane anesthesia to intravenous anesthesia (fentanyl, diazepam, and sodium thiopental) during one-lung ventilation for thoracic surgery in 12 patients.[122] In this study, they found that during one-lung atelectasis, 1 MAC halothane anesthesia slightly but significantly increased shunt and decreased Pa_{O_2} (compared with intravenous anesthesia), whereas 1 MAC isoflurane anesthesia very slightly but nonsignificantly increased shunt and decreased Pa_{O_2} (compared with intravenous anesthesia). Fundamental differences between the two studies[121,122] were in the duration of the periods of one-lung ventilation with the potent inhaled agent and in the MAC multiples of the drugs used. In the earlier study,[121] end-tidal concentrations of halothane and isoflurane were kept constant for approximately 20 minutes at 1.45 and 1.15 MAC, respectively. In the later study,[122] patients were maintained on one-lung anesthesia with the potent inhaled agent (1 MAC) for 40 minutes before final measurements under these conditions were taken.[122] The authors also concluded that halothane and isoflurane had only a small inhibitory effect on the one-lung hypoxic pulmonary vasoconstriction response.[122]

The contrast between the results of the *in vitro* and *in vivo* studies is sufficiently striking to suggest that other variables are obscuring the effects of inhibition of hypoxic pulmonary vasoconstriction in the *in vivo* studies. One such variable is cardiac output, which is altered to a markedly different extent by different inhaled agents. Studying this relationship, Marshall found that the effectiveness of hypoxic pulmonary vasoconstriction varied inversely with cardiac output.[123] Thus, during the administration of halothane, a direct inhibition of hypoxic pulmonary vasoconstriction may be offset by the enhanced responsiveness accompanying decreased cardiac output, with the result that flow diversion and gas exchange (as assessed by PaO_2) and, by inference, hypoxic pulmonary vasoconstriction may also appear to be unaffected. This may explain the findings in some of the human studies.

Thus, overall, the potent inhaled anesthetics are the drugs of choice during thoracic surgery. The technique chosen should, however, always be dictated by the needs of the particular patient, so that, in the presence of cardiovascular instability or poor oxygenation when depression of hypoxic pulmonary vasoconstriction is a possibility, a balanced technique may be chosen. A recent study suggests that propofol in doses of 6 to 12 $mg \cdot kg^{-1} \cdot hr^{-1}$ does not abolish hypoxic pulmonary vasoconstriction during one-lung ventilation in humans.[124] The subject of anesthetics and hypoxic pulmonary vasoconstriction has been extensively reviewed by Eisenkraft.[125]

Other Determinants of Hypoxic Pulmonary Vasoconstriction

Aside from potent inhaled agents, other drugs and maneuvers used during anesthesia may also have an inhibitory effect on regional or whole-lung hypoxic pulmonary vasoconstriction. Factors associated with an increase in pulmonary arterial pressure antagonize the effect of increased resistance caused by hypoxic pulmonary vasoconstriction and result in increased flow to the hypoxic region. Such indirect inhibitors of hypoxic pulmonary vasoconstriction include mitral stenosis, volume overload, thromboembolism, hypothermia, vasoconstrictor drugs, and a large hypoxic lung segment. Direct inhibitors of hypoxic pulmonary vasoconstriction include infection; vasodilator drugs, such as nitroglycerin and nitroprusside; hypocarbia; and metabolic alkalemia. All of these potential inhibitors should be considered when evaluating a patient for hypoxemia during thoracic surgery.

Potentiators of Hypoxic Pulmonary Vasoconstriction

Whereas in the past most of the research effort has been directed to studying inhibition of hypoxic pulmonary vasoconstriction, more recent research has investigated substances that may potentiate it. Almitrine, a respiratory stimulant drug, has been found to improve PaO_2 in patients with COPD and to have this effect in the absence of ventilatory stimulation. Indirect evidence suggested that it may potentiate hypoxic pulmonary vasoconstriction in intact dogs, although a subsequent and more extensive study with dogs concluded that almitrine caused nonspecific pulmonary vasoconstriction that was greater in the 100% oxygen-ventilated lung than in the hypoxic lung regions, thus causing a reduction of the hypoxic pulmonary vasoconstriction response.[126]

It has been suggested that prostaglandins may play a role in hypoxic pulmonary vasoconstriction inhibition and therefore prostaglandin inhibitors have been investigated as potentiators of hypoxic pulmonary vasoconstriction. Ibuprofen, a cyclo-oxygenase inhibitor, has been found to potentiate hypoxic pulmonary vasoconstriction in hypoxic isolated rat lung preparations and to reverse the inhibition of hypoxic pulmonary vasoconstriction caused by halothane.[127] In an animal model, lidocaine has also been found to have salutary effects in terms of reversing depression of hypoxic pulmonary vasoconstriction.[128] The value, if any, of such potentiators in humans undergoing one-lung anesthesia has not yet been reported.

ANESTHESIA FOR DIAGNOSTIC PROCEDURES

Bronchoscopy

The translaryngeal approach to bronchoscopy was first described by Killian at the turn of the century, when he introduced an esophagoscope under topical anesthesia with cocaine to remove an aspirated pork bone from a patient's right bronchus. Early bronchoscopes were of the rigid type, but in 1966 the Machida and Olympus Companies introduced the first practical bronchofiberscopes. Since then, these have been improved dramatically and have simplified many otherwise complicated bronchoscopies. The indications for bronchoscopy are shown in Table 34-5 and the instruments of choice in Table 34-6. Operator preferences and experience may play a major role in the choice of instrument.

Prior to the performance of bronchoscopy, the patient must be evaluated preoperatively for chronic lung disease, respiratory obstruction, bronchospasm, coughing, hemoptysis, and infectivity of secretions. Medications should be reviewed, and the need for a more major procedure should always be anticipated. Thus, bronchoscopy may lead to thoracotomy or sternotomy. The planned technique for bronchoscopy should be discussed with the surgeon preopera-

---

TABLE 34-5. Indications for Bronchoscopy

Diagnostic	Therapeutic
Cough	Foreign bodies
Hemoptysis	Accumulated secretions
Wheeze	Atelectasis
Atelectasis	Aspiration
Unresolved pneumonia	Lung abscess
Diffuse lung disease	Reposition endotracheal tubes
Preoperative evaluation	Placement of endobronchial
Rule out metastases	tubes
Abnormal chest x-ray	Laser surgery of the airway
Assess local disease recurrence	
Recurrent laryngeal nerve palsy	
Diaphragm paralysis	
Acute inhalation injury	
Exclude tracheoesophageal fistula	
During mechanical ventilation	
Selective bronchography	

Adapted from Landa JF: Indications for bronchoscopy. Chest 73 (suppl): 686, 1978, with permission of author and publisher.

TABLE 34-6. Instruments of Choice for Bronchoscopy

Rigid

Foreign bodies
Massive hemoptysis
Vascular tumors
Small children
Endobronchial resections

Fiberoptic/Flexible

Mechanical problems of neck
Upper lobe and peripheral lesions
Limited hemoptysis
During mechanical ventilation
Pneumonia, for selective cultures
Positioning of double-lumen tubes
Difficult intubation
Checking position of endotracheal tube
Bronchial blockade

Combination

Positive cytologic findings with negative chest x-ray results

Adapted from Landa JF: Indications for bronchoscopy. Chest 73 (suppl): 686, 1978, with permission of author and publisher.

tively, and all equipment and connectors should be checked for compatibility. Monitoring during bronchoscopy should include an electrocardiogram, a blood pressure cuff, a precordial stethoscope, and a pulse oximeter. If thoracotomy is planned, an arterial cannula should also be placed as well as other monitors (e.g., pulmonary arterial or central venous pressure catheters) that may be indicated by the patient's condition. Many anesthetic techniques are useful for bronchoscopy.

Local Anesthesia

The patient should first be pretreated with a drying agent, such as atropine, glycopyrrolate, or scopolamine. The local anesthetics most commonly used are lidocaine and tetracaine. In all cases, the total dose of anesthetic must be considered and the potential for toxicity recognized. A nebulizer can be used to spray the oropharynx and base of the tongue, or the patient may gargle viscous lidocaine. The tongue is then held forward, and pledgets soaked in local anesthetic are held in each piriform fossa using Krause forceps to achieve block of the internal branch of the superior laryngeal nerve. Tracheal anesthesia is achieved by a transtracheal injection of local anesthetic, or by spraying the vocal cords and trachea under direct vision using a laryngoscope, or *via* the suction channel of the bronchofiberscope. Alternatively, a superior laryngeal nerve block can be performed by an external approach, and a glossopharyngeal block can be used to depress the gag reflex. These blocks cause depression of airway reflexes, so that patients must be kept on nothing by mouth for several hours following the examination. If a fiberoptic bronchoscopic examination is to be performed transnasally, the nasal mucosa should be pretreated topically with 4% cocaine, and/or viscous lidocaine may be administered through the nares. Local anesthesia for bronchoscopy has the advantage that the patient is awake, cooperative, and breathing spontaneously. Sedatives may be added to make the patient more comfortable. Disadvantages of local anesthesia include poor tolerance of any

bleeding by the patient and the occasional lack of patient cooperation.

General Anesthesia

General anesthesia for bronchoscopy is often combined with topical laryngeal anesthesia so that less general anesthesia is needed. A balanced technique uses N_2O/O_2, incremental doses of an intravenous drug such as thiopental, an opioid (e.g., fentanyl), and a muscle relaxant (e.g., succinylcholine, atracurium, or vecuronium). A potent inhaled anesthetic technique (e.g., O_2/halothane or N_2O/O_2/halothane) is also satisfactory, although the use of N_2O may cause some optical distortion for the surgeon because of changes in the refractive index of the gas mixture. Additionally, the use of N_2O and potent inhaled agents creates an operating room contamination problem for the waste anesthesia gases, but limited scavenging may be possible by placing a suction catheter in the patient's oropharynx. Unless there is some contraindication, ventilation of the lungs is generally controlled. In any patient undergoing a thoracic diagnostic procedure for a suspected malignancy, the possibility of the myasthenic syndrome with sensitivity to nondepolarizing muscle relaxants must always be considered. Muscle relaxant doses should be titrated to effect using a neuromuscular monitoring system.

Rigid Bronchoscopy

A modern rigid ventilating bronchoscope is essentially a hollow tube with a blunted, beveled tip. Various sizes and designs are available, but in all a side arm is provided for connection to an anesthesia source. A number of techniques have been described for maintaining ventilation and oxygenation during rigid bronchoscopic examination.

Apneic Oxygenation

Following preoxygenation and induction of general anesthesia and skeletal muscle paralysis, oxygen is insufflated at $10-15$ l·min^{-1} *via* a small catheter placed above the carina. If the patient has been adequately denitrogenated, this technique can provide adequate oxygenation for more than 30 minutes.[129] The apneic period should not be allowed to extend beyond 5 minutes, however, since the technique is limited by build-up of CO_2 (at a rate of 3 mm Hg·min^{-1}), respiratory acidosis, and cardiac arrhythmias. Fraoli et al[130] demonstrated that the FRC/body weight ratio is important in considering apneic oxygenation techniques and recommended that only patients with predicted FRC/body weight ratios of 50 ml·kg^{-1} or more have apneic oxygenation for longer than 5 minutes.

Apnea and Intermittent Ventilation

Oxygen and anesthesia gases are delivered to the bronchoscope *via* the anesthesia circuit. Ventilation is only possible when the eyepiece is in place, and this limits the period for instrumentation by the surgeon. Intermittent ventilation of the lungs is achieved by squeezing the reservoir bag. In this way, assuming a good bronchoscope fit in the airway, compliance is constantly monitored, the risk of barotrauma is reduced, and VT may be estimated. The disadvantage of this technique is that with prolonged bronchoscopies, poor levels of blood gases, and in particular hypercarbia, may result. This may lead to cardiac arrhythmias.

Sanders Injection System

Sanders applied the Venturi principle to provide ventilation of the lungs by attaching a jet ventilator to the bronchoscope.[131] Oxygen from a high-pressure source (50 psig) is delivered, *via* a controllable pressure-reducing valve and toggle switch, to a 2.5–3.5 cm 18- or 16-gauge needle inside and parallel to the long axis of the bronchoscope. When the toggle switch is depressed, the jet of oxygen entering the bronchoscope entrains air, and the air/oxygen mixture resulting at the distal tip of the bronchoscope emerges at a pressure to provide adequate ventilation and oxygenation. The intraluminal tracheal pressure is a function of the driving pressure from the reducing valve, the size of the needle jet, and the length, internal diameter, and design of the bronchoscope. Increasing the size of the needle jet increases the total gas flow for any given driving pressure. For each combination of gas driving pressure, jet orifice, and bronchoscope diameter, only one inflation pressure can be attained, regardless of the volume or compliance of the lung. As long as the proximal end of the bronchoscope is open, the system is strictly pressure-limited, and the pressure will not rise because of obstruction at the distal end. Pressure varies inversely with the cross-sectional area of the bronchoscope, so that insertion of a suction catheter or biopsy forceps into the lumen causes the intratracheal pressure to increase. Provided there is not a tight fit between the bronchoscope and the airway, the risk of barotrauma is unlikely. If the fit is tight, driving pressure should be reduced.

The advantages of the Sanders system are that because continuous ventilation is possible (since the presence of an eyepiece is not necessary for ventilation of the lungs), the duration of the bronchoscopy procedure is minimized but the efficiency also permits extended bronchoscopy. A disadvantage is that entrainment of air by the oxygen jet results in a variable FIO_2 at the distal end of the bronchoscope, ventilation of the lungs may be inadequate if compliance is poor, and adequacy of ventilation may be difficult to assess. Giesecke *et al* have compared the intermittent ventilation and the Sanders technique and found that PaO_2 was satisfactory with either method but it was higher in the intermittent ventilation group.[132] $PaCO_2$ was lower and arterial pH higher in the Sanders group, indicating superiority of this method, particularly for long procedures.

The basic Sanders technique has been modified to increase FIO_2 and to deliver N_2O and potent inhaled anesthetics. Carden[133] has replaced the 16-gauge oxygen jet with a longer jet (Carden side arm) that allows ventilation with 100% oxygen and the development of much higher pressures at the tracheal end of the bronchoscope, while using a driving pressure of 50 psig. The Sanders injector system may also be used with a ventilating bronchoscope, the side arm of which is connected to a supply of anesthesia gases, so that the injection jet will entrain the anesthesia gases.

Mechanical Ventilator

Ventilation of the lungs may be achieved by attaching a mechanical ventilator to an anesthesia circuit connected to the bronchoscope side arm.

High-Frequency Positive Pressure Ventilation

High-frequency positive pressure ventilation has been used in conjunction with rigid bronchoscopy and compared to the Sanders injector in patients with tracheobronchial stenosis. With high-frequency positive pressure ventilation of up to 150 breaths·min^{-1}, blood gases were identical with both techniques. At a frequency of 500 breaths·min^{-1}, oxygenation deteriorated and CO_2 was not removed effectively. High-frequency positive pressure ventilation has the advantage that the tracheobronchial wall remains perfectly immobilized during ventilation.[134]

Other Techniques

Cuirass ventilation, external chest compression, and a ventilating catheter or endotracheal tube placed alongside the bronchoscope have also been used to provide ventilation during bronchoscopy.

Fiberoptic Bronchoscopy

The new generations of fiberscope, with their improved optics and smaller diameters, have revolutionized bronchoscopy. Examination of the fifth order of bronchial branching is now possible, and the diagnostic potential of this instrument is thereby enhanced. The flexibility has also been applied in preoperative assessment of the airway, management of difficult tracheal intubations, endotracheal tube positioning and change, bronchial toilet, correct positioning of double-lumen tubes, bronchial blockade, and evaluation of the larynx and trachea.[3,135]

Nasal fiberoptic bronchoscopy under topical anesthesia is well tolerated by most awake patients. A suction catheter in the mouth is useful to remove oral secretions. Oral insertion is also possible in both awake and asleep patients and should be performed *via* a specially designed airway, which guides the fiberscope over the back of the tongue and prevents potential damage to it by the patient's teeth.

Physiologic Changes Associated with Fiberoptic Bronchoscopy. In all patients, insertion of the fiberoptic bronchoscope is associated with hypoxemia. The average decline in PaO_2 is 20 mm Hg and lasts for 1–4 hours after the procedure. By 24 hours the blood gas levels are usually back to normal. It is therefore recommended that if the initial PaO_2 is <70 mm Hg ($FIO_2 = 0.21$), bronchoscopy should be performed only with the administration of supplemental oxygen. This can be provided using mouth-held nasal prongs, using a special face mask with a diaphragm through which the fiberscope can be passed, or *via* an endotracheal tube with a T-piece diaphragm adapter.

During and after fiberoptic bronchoscopy, patients develop increased airway obstruction. Matsushima et al[136] studied alterations in pulmonary mechanics in 35 patients and found that insertion of the bronchoscope was associated with an increase in FRC (17–30%) and decreases in PaO_2, VC, FEV_1, and forced inspiratory flow. All had returned to baseline by 24 hours. These changes are thought to be secondary to direct mechanical activation of irritative reflexes in the airway and, possibly, also to mucosal edema. They may be avoided if atropine, either intramuscular or aerosolized into the airway, is administered preoperatively. Isoproterenol has a similar salutary effect on lung function but is associated with an increased incidence of cardiac arrhythmias. Overall, atropine is recommended as premedication for fiberoptic bronchoscopy. Concern that atropine may have an overall undesirable effect by increasing viscosity of secretions in patients with COPD is unsubstantiated.

The standard adult fiberoptic bronchoscope has an external diameter of 5.7 mm and a 2 mm-diameter suction channel. If suction at 1 atm is applied to the fiberscope, air is removed at a rate of 14 l·min^{-1}. If the fiberscope is in the airway, this will cause decreases in F_{IO_2}, P_{aO_2}, and FRC, leading to decreased P_{aO_2}. Suctioning should therefore be kept brief. The adult fiberscope will pass through endotracheal tubes of 7.0 mm or greater internal diameter. Clearly, passage through an endotracheal tube decreases the cross-sectional area available for ventilating the patient, so that if fiberscopy is planned, the largest possible diameter endotracheal tube should be used.

Insertion of the bronchoscope also causes a significant positive end-expiratory pressure (PEEP) effect, which may result in barotrauma in ventilated patients. If the patient is already being ventilated with positive end-expiratory pressure, the PEEP should be discontinued prior to the passage of the fiberscope. A postendoscopy chest x-ray film is advisable to exclude the presence of mediastinal emphysema or pneumothorax. In patients whose tracheae are intubated with endotracheal tubes of less than 8.0 mm internal diameter, use of pediatric fiberscopes, which have smaller diameters, would be more appropriate.

The suction channel of the adult fiberoptic bronchoscope has been used to oxygenate and ventilate the lungs of patients. By attaching a jet ventilation system (similar to that used to drive the Sanders injector for rigid bronchoscopy) to the suction connection at the head of a fiberoptic bronchoscope, Satyanarayana et al[137] were successful in ventilating lungs of patients undergoing gynecologic procedures. A driving pressure of 50 psig of oxygen was used with a ventilatory rate of 18–20 breaths per minute. Tracheal pressures of 6–8 mm Hg, tracheal oxygen concentrations of 88–93%, and P_{aO_2} values of 340–478 mm Hg were obtained. This technique permits adequate ventilation of patients with normally compliant lungs and chest walls but to date has not been attempted in patients with lung disease. Ventilation of the lungs should only be performed with the tip of the instrument in the trachea, as a more peripheral location may produce barotrauma.

Neodymium-yttrium-aluminum garnet (Nd-YAG) lasers have recently been used for the resection of obstructing and endobronchial lesions. This procedure is performed under general anesthesia. The lasers may be introduced into the bronchial tree through a fiberoptic bundle passed via the suction port of the fiberoptic bronchoscope. During laser resection, F_{IO_2} should be kept to a minimum and titrated against oxygen saturation (as continuously monitored by pulse oximeter) in order to make endotracheal fire less likely.[138] Laser therapy of bronchial tumors is also possible using a rigid bronchoscope.[139] Vourc'h et al found that high-frequency positive-pressure ventilation via a rigid bronchoscope provided satisfactory operating conditions for laser resection of tracheal tumors and had the advantage of producing airway immobility.[134] This subject is reviewed in more detail elsewhere.[140]

Complications of Bronchoscopy

Complications of rigid bronchoscopy include mechanical trauma to the teeth, hemorrhage, bronchospasm, loss of a sponge, bronchial or tracheal perforation, subglottic edema, and barotrauma. The incidence of complications is much lower with fiberoptic bronchoscopy. Nevertheless, complications may arise owing to overdose with topical anesthetic, insertion trauma, local trauma, hemorrhage, upper airway obstruction related to passage of the instrument through an area of tracheal stenosis, hypoxemia, and bronchospasm. In most cases, it is best to intubate the trachea with an endotracheal tube in patients following bronchoscopy under general anesthesia. This permits avoidance or treatment of

some of these problems, particularly the increased airway irritability. Intubation also facilitates effective suctioning of the trachea and bronchi and allows the patient to recover more gradually from general anesthesia. Overall, with careful evaluation of the patient and an understanding of the techniques employed, bronchoscopy is a relatively safe procedure.[141]

DIAGNOSTIC PROCEDURES FOR MEDIASTINAL MASSES

Patients with an anterior mediastinal mass present a special problem for the anesthesiologist. Although such masses may cause superior vena cava obstruction that is obvious, they may also cause obstruction of major airways and cardiac compression, which are less obvious and may become apparent only upon induction of anesthesia. Neuman et al[142] described three cases of anterior mediastinal mass, in two of which airway obstruction occurred following induction of anesthesia and onset of paralysis. In the first case, total occlusion of the trachea starting 2–3 cm above the carina and extending to both mainstem bronchi was observed, and a bronchoscope was passed through the obstruction. In the second case, extrinsic compression of the left mainstem bronchus occurred on inspiration during recovery from anesthesia. In the third case of anterior mediastinal mass, flow-volume studies were performed with the patient in the upright and supine positions and demonstrated marked reductions in FEV_1 and PEFR in the latter position. These findings suggested potential obstruction with onset of anesthesia, and radiotherapy to the mediastinum was commenced, after which the flow-volume studies showed improved function. The planned surgical procedure was then performed under local anesthesia.

One disadvantage of preoperative radiation therapy is that it may affect tissue histologic appearance, thereby preventing an accurate diagnosis. Furthermore, if the patient is a child, it may be difficult to obtain tissue samples under local anesthesia. Ferrari and Bedford reported a series of 44 patients ages 18 years or less with anterior mediastinal masses who underwent general anesthesia prior to radiation or chemotherapy, even in the presence of cardiorespiratory symptoms.[143] Although no fatalities occurred, seven patients developed airway compromise. These authors concluded that general anesthesia may be safely induced prior to radiation therapy and that the benefits of obtaining an accurate tissue diagnosis outweighed the risks.[143] Others have disagreed with these conclusions, stating that anesthesia is not safe when the reported rate of life-threatening complications is 16–20%.[144,145]

Airway obstruction caused by an anterior mediastinal mass has been attributed to changes in lung and chest wall mechanics associated with changes in position or to onset of paralysis in muscles that previously maintained airway patency. Neuman et al have proposed a flow chart (Fig. 34-24) describing the preoperative evaluation of a patient with an anterior mediastinal mass in order to avoid life-threatening total airway obstruction.[142] It is important to determine in the history if the patient has dyspnea in the supine position and to examine the computed tomographic (CT) scan to determine the extent of the tumor and its effect on surrounding structures. If such obstruction occurs, it may be relieved by passage of a rigid bronchoscope or anode tube past the obstruction, by direct laryngoscopy,[146] or by changing the position of the patient.

In a situation in which the biopsy procedure cannot be

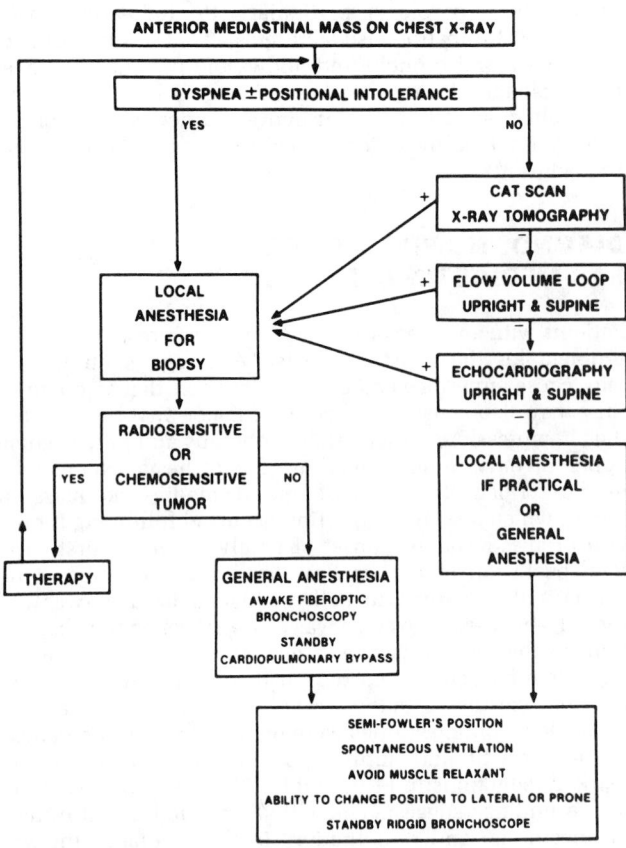

Figure 34-24. Flow chart describing the preoperative evaluation of the patient with an anterior mediastinal mass. + indicates positive finding; − indicates negative work-up. (Reproduced with permission from Neuman GG, Weingarten AE, Abramowitz RM et al: Anesthetic management of the patient with an anterior mediastinal mass. Anesthesiology 60:144, 1984.)

performed under local anesthesia and there is concern that muscle paralysis may result in airway compression, a fiberoptic intubation of the awake patient followed by general anesthesia with spontaneous ventilation has been described for thoracotomy.[147] Thus, during spontaneous inspiration, the normal transpulmonary pressure gradient distends the airways and helps to maintain their patency, even in the presence of extrinsic compression.

Mediastinoscopy

Mediastinoscopy was introduced by Carlens[148] as a means of assessing spread of carcinoma of the bronchus. The lymphatics of the lung drain first to the subcarinal and paratracheal areas and then to the sides of the trachea, the supraclavicular areas, and the thoracic duct. Examination of these nodes has provided a tissue diagnosis and greater selectivity of patients for thoracotomy. It is most useful in right-lung tumors, since left-lung cancers tend to spread to subaortic nodes that are more accessible by an anterior mediastinoscopy in the second or third interspace (Chamberlain procedure). Apart from diagnostic uses, mediastinoscopy has also been employed to place electrodes for atrial-triggered pacing.[149] The transcervical approach to the thymus is another adaptation of this technique.

The anesthetic considerations for mediastinoscopy follow naturally from an understanding of the anatomy of this pro-

cedure and its potential complications. For cervical mediastinoscopy, the patient is placed in a reverse Trendelenburg position, and the mediastinoscope is inserted into the superior mediastinum *via* a transverse incision just above the suprasternal notch. The instrument is advanced along the anterior aspect of the trachea and passes behind the innominate vessels and the aortic arch (see Fig. 34-25). The left recurrent nerve is vulnerable as it loops around the aortic arch, and any of these structures may be traumatized. Because of scarring, previous mediastinoscopy is a contraindication to a repeat examination. Relative contraindications include superior vena cava obstruction, tracheal deviation, and aneurysm of the thoracic aorta.

Preoperative evaluation should include a search for airway obstruction or distortion. Review of a computed tomographic scan is very helpful in this regard. Evidence of impaired cerebral circulation, history of stroke, or signs of the Eaton-Lambert syndrome resulting from oat cell carcinoma should be sought. Blood must be available for the procedure, because hemorrhage is a real risk and may be life-threatening.

Mediastinoscopy may be performed under local anesthesia, and this approach is claimed to offer greater simplicity and safety in patients with limited pulmonary reserve or in those with cerebrovascular disease.[150] However, most surgeons and anesthesiologists prefer general anesthesia using an endotracheal tube and continuous ventilation, as this offers a more controlled situation and greater flexibility in terms of surgical manipulation. The anesthetic technique should include a muscle relaxant to prevent the patient from coughing, since this may produce venous engorgement in the chest or trauma by the mediastinoscope to surrounding structures.

The morbidity of mediastinoscopy has been reported as 1.5–3.0%, and mortality as 0.09%.[151] The most common complication is hemorrhage (0.73%) because of the proximity of major vessels and the vascularity of certain tumors. Tamponade may be the only recourse, and thoracotomy or median sternotomy may be required to achieve hemostasis. Needle aspiration of any structure is essential prior to any biopsy's being taken. If severe bleeding occurs, induced arterial hypotension may be helpful in reducing the size of the tear in a vessel. If bleeding is venous, fluids given *via* an upper limb vein may enter the mediastinum, in which case a large-bore catheter should be placed in a lower limb vein.[152] A venous laceration may also result in air embolism, particularly if the patient is breathing spontaneously. Therefore some recommend the use of a precordial Doppler probe if the risk of air embolism is likely.

Pneumothorax is the second most common complication (0.66%). It is usually right-sided, often recognized at the time of the occurrence, and is treated according to size. A symptomatic pneumothorax should be treated by chest tube decompression.

Recurrent laryngeal nerve injury occurred in 0.34% of cases and was permanent in 50% of these cases.[151] The nerve may be damaged by the mediastinoscope or be involved in tumor. Such injury is not a problem unless both nerves are damaged, in which case upper airway obstruction may result. Autonomic reflexes may be initiated by manipulation of the trachea or of the aorta, the latter having pressor receptors located in the arch. Vagally mediated reflexes may be blocked by atropine.

"Apparent" cardiac arrest has been reported by Lee and Salvatore.[153] They monitored the right radial pulse using a plethysmograph, and the tracing suddenly disappeared in the presence of a normal electrocardiogram. A normal pulse returned after the mediastinoscope was removed, and the

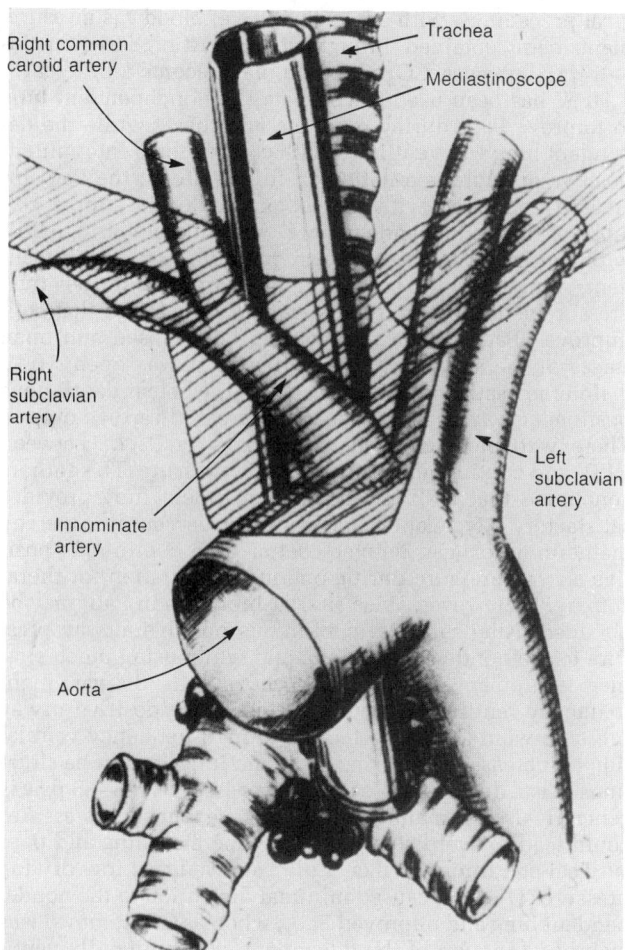

Right common carotid artery

Trachea

Mediastinoscope

Right subclavian artery

Innominate artery

Left subclavian artery

Aorta

Figure 34-25. Anatomic relationships during mediastinoscopy. Note the position of the mediastinoscope behind the right innominate artery and aortic arch and anterior to the trachea. (Reproduced with permission from Carlens E: Mediastinoscopy: A method for inspection and tissue biopsy in the superior mediastinum. Dis Chest 36: 343, 1959.)

cause of the apparent arrest was pressure on the innominate artery by the instrument (see Fig. 35-25). Decreases in right arm as compared to left arm blood pressure were found by Petty in four of seven cases undergoing mediastinoscopy.[36] Duration was 15–360 seconds. This is of particular significance if there is a history of impaired cerebral circulation or transient ischemic attacks or if a carotid bruit is present, since transient left hemiparesis has been reported following mediastinoscopy.[151] It is, therefore, recommended that blood pressure be monitored in the left arm and that the right radial pulse be measured continuously during mediastinoscopy. A decrease in the right radial pulse would be an indication for repositioning the mediastinoscope, especially in a patient with a history of cerebrovascular disease.

Other reported complications, which may require prompt intervention by the anesthesiologist, include acute tracheal collapse,[154] tension pneumomediastinum, mediastinitis, hemothorax, and chylothorax.[155] A chest radiograph taken in the immediate postoperative period is a useful precaution in all patients who have undergone mediastinoscopy.

Thoracoscopy

Thoracoscopy involves the insertion of an endoscope into the thoracic cavity and pleural space. It is used for the diagnosis of pleural disease, effusions, and infectious disease (especially in immunosuppressed and patients with acquired immunodeficiency syndrome) and for staging procedures, chemical pleurodesis, and lung biopsy. It is also used in therapeutic procedures such as CO_2 laser treatment of spontaneous pneumothorax or bullous emphysema and Nd-YAG laser vaporization of malignant pleural tumors.[155a] A small incision is made in the lateral chest wall, and with the insertion of the instrument fluid and biopsy specimens are easily obtained.

This procedure may be performed using local, regional, or general anesthesia, the choice depending upon the expected duration of the procedure and the physical status of the patient. The most common methods are local anesthetic infiltration or intercostal nerve blocks two spaces above and below the usual sixth intercostal space. Intercostal blocks also anesthetize the parietal pleura. The addition of a stellate ganglion block helps to suppress the cough reflex that is sometimes provoked during manipulation of the hilum of the lung.

When air enters the pleural cavity under inspection, a partial pneumothorax occurs, permitting good surgical visualization. Changes in PaO_2, $PaCO_2$, and electrocardiographic rhythm are usually minimal when the procedure is performed using local or regional anesthesia.[156] The physiology of this situation was discussed in the section on Lateral Position, Awake, Breathing Spontaneously, Chest Open.

With local anesthesia, the spontaneous pneumothorax is usually well tolerated because the skin and chest wall form a seal around the thoracoscope and limit the degree of lung collapse. Occasionally, however, the procedure is poorly tolerated, and general anesthesia must be induced. The insertion of a double-lumen tube with the patient in the lateral position may be difficult, in which case the patient may be temporarily placed in the supine position for the intubation.

If general anesthesia is required, either a single- or a double-lumen tube may be used. Positive pressure ventilation will interfere with visualization via the endoscope, however, and therefore a double-lumen tube is preferable. Additionally, if pleurodesis is being performed, general anesthesia via a double-lumen tube allows for complete re-expansion of the lung and avoids the pain associated with instillation of talc for recurrent pneumothorax. To overcome the pathophysiologic effects of the pneumothorax, although small, a high FIO_2 is recommended for either local or general anesthesia. Blood gas monitoring may not be essential, but pulse oximetry during this procedure is extremely useful.

ANESTHESIA FOR SPECIAL SITUATIONS

Management of patients with bronchopleural fistulas, empyema, cysts, bullae, and those requiring tracheal reconstruction is considered here. Many of these cases are appropriately managed using high-frequency ventilatory techniques; therefore, these techniques are described first.

High-Frequency Ventilation

With conventional positive pressure ventilation, VT and rates usually exceed or approach those in the normal spontaneously breathing patient. Gas transport to the alveoli occurs by convection in the larger airways and then by convection and molecular diffusion in the more distal airways and alveoli. High-frequency ventilation differs from conventional positive pressure ventilation in that smaller VT and more rapid rates are used. Gas transport may depend more on molecular diffusion, high-velocity flow, and coaxial gas flow in the airways, with gas in the center moving distally and that in the periphery moving proximally.

There are three different types of high-frequency ventilation. High-frequency positive pressure ventilation (HFPPV) uses small VT at rates of 60–120 breaths·min^{-1} (1–2 Hz). The ventilator used (e.g., Bronchovent) has a negligible internal compliance, so that the VT generated, which usually approximates the dead space volume, equals the volume set on the ventilator and represents all fresh gas. The high instantaneous gas flows generated facilitate gas exchange and movement in the conducting airways.

HFPPV may be delivered via an open or a closed system. An example of the former would be the percutaneous placement of a transtracheal catheter or placement of a catheter via the nose or mouth with its distal end above the carina. Inflow is intraluminal, and outflow is extraluminal. This technique has been used during bronchoscopy and tracheal resection and reconstructive surgery. When open systems are used, the gas outflow pathway is not established mechanically and depends upon natural airway patency. It is, therefore, subject to compromise. Also, aspiration is a potential complication with open systems.

The closed system is superior, since it integrates both airway patency and outflow protection. A closed system is represented by a catheter placed within a short segment of an endotracheal tube for delivery of the HFPPV, whereas the remainder of the tube lumen represents the exit pathway for gas. A quadruple-lumen endotracheal tube (Hi-Lo Jet Tracheal Tube, Mallinckrodt Inc, Argyle, NY) has been designed specifically for delivery of HFPPV. One lumen is for the HFPPV delivery, one for gas outflow, one for cuff inflation, and one for measuring airway pressures at the distal end of the tube. The use of a closed system also permits application of positive end-expiratory pressure, a situation not possible with an open arrangement.

High-frequency jet ventilation (HFJV) uses a pulse of a small jet of fresh gas introduced from a high-pressure source (50 psig) into the airway via a small catheter or additional lumen in an endotracheal tube. Rates used are usually 100–400 breaths·min^{-1}. The fresh gas jet entrains gas from an injection cannula side port reservoir. This system is somewhat analogous to the Sanders injector system described in the bronchoscopy section, and FIO_2 is similarly variable. The jet and entrained gas flows cause forward motion of the mass of gas in the airways. HFJV can be used with an open system or with a closed arrangement, as described above. In the latter, positive end-expiratory pressure may be added to enhance oxygenation. Also, using high fresh gas flows from an anesthesia circuit, inhaled anesthetics may be delivered as an entrained gas mixture.

High-frequency oscillation ventilation (HFOV) employs a mechanism that oscillates gas at rates of 400–2400 breaths·min^{-1}. It has not been described in association with thoracic surgical procedures. In this system, VT is small (50–80 ml), and gas exchange occurs via enhanced molecular diffusion and coaxial airway flow.

The potential advantages offered by HFPPV during thoracic anesthesia would be as follows: lower VT and inspiratory pressures result in a "quiet" lung field for the surgeon, with minimal movements of airway, lung tissue, and mediastinum. Thus, HFPPV has been used to ventilate both the nondependent and the dependent lung during thoracic sur-

gical procedures, with adequate arterial blood gas measurements being obtained throughout.[157,158] At high frequencies (>6 Hz), however, CO_2 retention may become a problem.

HFJV has been used to ventilate the nondependent lung to improve PaO_2 during one-lung anesthesia while the dependent lung was ventilated with conventional intermittent positive-pressure ventilation.[159] In this study, the PaO_2 increased compared with that obtained during simple collapse of the nondependent lung. A study comparing HFJV with continuous positive airway pressure to the nondependent lung during conventional intermittent positive-pressure ventilation to the dependent lung found that both improved PaO_2 significantly during both closed and open stages of the surgery.[160] When the chest was open, HFJV maintained satisfactory cardiac output, whereas continuous positive airway pressure usually decreased cardiac output. There were no significant differences in $PaCO_2$ between HFJV and continuous positive airway pressure. The authors concluded that HFJV to the nondependent lung provides satisfactory oxygenation and good cardiac output, thereby maintaining oxygen delivery better than continuous positive airway pressure during one-lung ventilation for thoracotomy.[160] However, since similar increases in PaO_2 may be obtained using selective continuous positive airway pressure to the nondependent lung and while using much simpler equipment than that necessary to deliver high-frequency ventilation, the use of continuous positive airway pressure would seem preferable to high-frequency ventilation to increase PaO_2 during most one-lung anesthesia situations. Also, during HFJV, a driving pressure of 25–35 psig is generally used to maintain normocapnia, but such pressures could lead to overdistention of the operated lung and poor surgical conditions. Wilks et al[159] showed that low driving pressures (15 psig) caused minimal distention to the nondependent lung and improved PaO_2, whereas CO_2 removal was mainly a function of the dependent, conventionally ventilated lung. In certain situations, however, HFJV to the nondependent lung may offer some advantage. Thus, Morgan et al[161] have described combined unilateral HFJV and contralateral intermittent positive-pressure ventilation in the management of a patient who required a right lower lobectomy for bronchial carcinoma associated with emphysema, pneumoconiosis, and a previous thoracoplasty for pulmonary tuberculosis. These authors and others recommend consideration of the use of this technique in any patient requiring partial lung resection in the presence of severe pulmonary impairment.[162,163]

The lower pressures and VT associated with high-frequency ventilation result in a small leak via bronchopleural fistulae, and HFJV is now generally considered the conservative treatment of choice in this condition. Another advantage of high-frequency ventilation is that the rapid rate small VT can be delivered via small tubes or catheters, so that if an airway has to be divided, the passage of a small tube across the surgical field will permit ventilation of the distal airway and lung tissue. This use has been applied during sleeve resection of the lung, tracheal reconstruction, and surgery for tracheal stenosis. In all three situations, the surgeon is able to work easily around the small catheter used to provide the high-frequency ventilation.

Conventional intermittent positive-pressure ventilation (650 ml × 14 breaths·min^{-1}) to the dependent lung has been compared to HFJV (150–200 breaths·min^{-1}; minute volume 10–15 l) to the dependent lung during one-lung ventilation in ten patients, using $FIO_2 = 0.5$.[87] There were no significant differences between the groups in PaO_2, $PaCO_2$, or hemodynamic indices, although shunt fraction was higher in the

HFJV group. A significant positive end-expiratory pressure effect was also noted in this group but not in the intermittent positive-pressure ventilation group. The unintentional generation of positive end-expiratory pressure during HFJV is well known and is thought to be due to expiratory flow limitation. The positive end-expiratory pressure to the dependent lung increases pulmonary vascular resistance in this lung and causes diversion of blood flow to the nondependent, nonventilated lung, thereby increasing shunt fraction (32.9% vs 42.4%). These authors concluded that the theoretical benefits of HFJV on the cardiovascular system are outweighed by the effects of mean airway pressure increasing shunt to the nonventilated lung during one-lung anesthesia.[87] Although adequate gas exchange was maintained with HFJV during one-lung anesthesia with $FIO_2 = 0.5$, these authors found that it was more difficult to assess the adequacy of ventilation during HFJV and, therefore, recommended against its routine use during one-lung anesthesia.[87]

Bronchopleural Fistula and Empyema

A bronchopleural fistula is an abnormal communication between the bronchial tree and the pleural cavity. Occasionally, there is an additional communication to the surface of the chest, a bronchopleural cutaneous fistula. A bronchopleural fistula occurs most commonly following pulmonary resection for carcinoma. Other causes include traumatic rupture of a bronchus or bulla (sometimes caused by barotrauma or positive end-expiratory pressure), penetrating chest wound, or spontaneous drainage into the bronchial tree of an empyema cavity or lung cyst. The incidence of fistula is higher following pneumonectomy than following other types of lung resection. The problems associated with bronchopleural fistula and empyema are that positive pressure ventilation may result in contamination of healthy lung, loss of air, decreased alveolar ventilation leading to CO_2 retention, and the development of a tension pneumothorax.

If an empyema is present, it should first be drained under local anesthesia prior to any surgery to close the bronchopleural fistula. Drainage is performed with the patient sitting up and leaning toward the affected side. It must be recognized that empyemas are often loculated and that complete drainage is not always possible. A drain to an underwater seal system is left in the cavity prior to administration of anesthesia for surgery of the bronchopleural fistula, and following the drainage of an empyema, a chest radiograph should be obtained to determine the efficacy of the procedure.

The priorities in the anesthetic management of bronchopleural fistula are the isolation of the affected side in terms of contamination and ventilation. The ideal approach is intubation of the trachea while the patient is awake using a double-lumen tube with the patient breathing spontaneously. Supplemental oxygen should be administered, and the patient should be constantly reassured. Neuroleptanalgesia is satisfactory in providing a suitably cooperative patient, and the airway is then pretreated with topical anesthesia. The endobronchial tube selected should be such that the bronchial lumen is on the side opposite the bronchopleural fistula. Section of the largest possible tube provides a close fit in the trachea, which helps to stabilize the tube. Once the tube is adequately positioned in the trachea, there may be a considerable outpouring of pus from the tracheal lumen if an empyema is present, and therefore this lumen should be immediately suctioned using a large-bore suction catheter. The healthy and, possibly, the affected lung may then be ventilated; adequacy of oxygenation and ventilation is assessed by pulse oximetry and arterial blood gas analysis.

An alternative technique is to insert the double-lumen tube under general anesthesia, with the patient breathing spontaneously to avoid a tension pneumothorax. With either technique, the chest drainage tube must be left unclamped to avoid any bouts of coughing and to prevent the build-up of a tension pneumothorax in the event that a predisposing valvular mechanism exists. In patients who do not have an empyema, use of a single-lumen tube has been described and may be satisfactory if the bronchopleural fistula and air leak are small. A rapid sequence induction with ketamine or thiopental followed by a relaxant has also been described but is associated with considerable risk of contamination and tension pneumothorax.

Bronchopleural fistula may also be treated conservatively using various ventilatory techniques. Thus, the bronchus of the normal lung may be intubated and ventilated, allowing the bronchopleural fistula to rest and heal. This approach may result in an intolerable shunt, however, and positive end-expiratory pressure may be necessary to maintain PaO_2. Differential lung ventilation via a double-lumen tube has also been described, the healthy lung being ventilated with normal VT, while the affected lung is exposed to a smaller VT[164] or to continuous positive airway pressure with oxygen at pressures just below the critical opening pressure of the fistula. The critical opening pressure of the bronchopleural fistula can be assessed by determining the lowest level of continuous positive airway pressure that must be applied to the bronchus on the affected side to produce continuous bubbling via the underwater seal chest drain.

For large bronchopleural fistulae, HFJV may be the nonsurgical treatment of choice. The use of small VT results in minimal gas loss through the fistula, which may heal more quickly. In addition, hemodynamic effects are usually minimal, and spontaneous efforts at ventilation are usually abolished, thereby decreasing the work of breathing and eliminating the need for relaxants or excessive sedation.

Bishop et al[165] demonstrated that HFJV may not always be superior to conventional ventilation in the conservative management of bronchopleural fistula. They showed that HFJV is less effective in reducing the ventilatory leak through a bronchopleural fistula when the peripheral leak is combined with severe injury and decreased compliance in the remainder of the lung than when only an airway is disrupted. In the seven patients they reported on, HFJV was compared with controlled ventilation of the lungs, and it was found that adequate gas exchange could not be achieved at comparable mean airway pressures with HFJV, although peak airway pressures decreased. Indeed, in some patients, flow through the bronchopleural fistula actually increased with HFJV. These authors concluded that HFJV should be used selectively in patients with bronchopleural fistula.[165]

Lung Cysts and Bullae

Air-filled cysts of the lung are usually bronchogenic, postinfective, infantile, or emphysematous. They may be associated with COPD or be an isolated finding. A bulla is a thin-walled space filled with air that results from the destruction of alveolar tissue. The walls are, therefore, composed of visceral pleura, connective tissue septa, or compressed lung tissue. In general, bullae represent an area of end-stage emphysematous destruction of the lung.

Patients may be considered for surgical bullectomy when dyspnea is incapacitating, when the bullae are expanding, when there are repeated pneumothoraces owing to rupture of bullae, or if the bullae compress a large area of normal lung. Most of these patients have severe COPD and CO_2 retention and little functional respiratory reserve. The first consideration in management is that a high FIO_2 should be maintained. If the bulla or cyst communicates with the bronchial tree, positive pressure ventilation may cause it to expand or even to rupture if it is compliant, producing a situation analogous to tension pneumothorax. If the bulla is very compliant, most of the applied VT may be wasted in this additional dead space. Nitrous oxide should be avoided, since it causes expansion of any air spaces within the body, including bullae. Once the chest is open, even more of the VT may enter the compliant bulla, which is no longer limited by chest wall integrity, and an increase in ventilation is needed until the bulla is controlled.

The anesthetic management of these patients is challenging, particularly if the disease is bilateral. A pulse oximeter is very helpful in the continuous assessment of oxygenation. Ideally, a double-lumen tube is inserted with the patient awake or under general anesthesia but breathing spontaneously. The avoidance of positive pressure ventilation (when possible) helps to decrease the likelihood of the potential problems described above, although it must be recognized that oxygenation may be precarious with spontaneous ventilation. Once the endotracheal tube is in place, each lung may be controlled separately, and adequate ventilation can be applied to the healthy lung if bilateral disease is not present. Gentle positive pressure ventilation with rapid, small VT and pressures not to exceed 10 cm H_2O may be used during the induction and maintenance of anesthesia, especially if the bullae have been shown to have no or only poor bronchial communication by preoperative ventilation scanning. While the surgery is being performed, as each bulla is resected, the operated lung can be separately ventilated to check for air leaks and the presence of additional bullae.

If positive pressure ventilation is to be applied prior to opening the chest, the possibility of a tension pneumothorax must be kept in mind, and treatment should be readily available. The diagnosis of pneumothorax may be made by a unilateral decrease in breath sounds (this may be difficult to distinguish in a patient with bullous disease), increase in ventilatory pressure, progressive tracheal deviation, wheezing, or cardiovascular changes. Treatment of a pneumothorax involves the rapid placement of a chest tube. An added risk of chest tube placement is the creation of a bronchopleural-cutaneous fistula, which causes problems for ventilation. Alternatively, general anesthesia is induced only after the surgeon has prepared the operative field and draped the patient. In the event of sudden deterioration in the patient's condition during induction, the surgeon may perform an immediate median sternotomy. In any event, the time from induction of anesthesia to sternotomy must be kept to a minimum.

In order to avoid these problems in a patient with known bullae, HFJV has been used in a patient with a large bulla undergoing coronary artery bypass graft[166] and in another patient undergoing bilateral bullectomy.[167] If bilateral bullectomy is to be performed, a median sternotomy is generally used. Benumof[168] has described the use of sequential one-lung ventilation using a double-lumen tube in the management of a patient needing bilateral bullectomy. The side with the largest bulla and least lung function, as assessed preoperatively by ventilation and perfusion scans, should be operated on first. In this way, the lung with the better function should support gas exchange first. If hypoxemia develops during this one-lung situation, application of continuous positive airway pressure to the nonventilated lung during the deflation phase of a tidal breath should increase PaO_2.

In an extreme situation in which no respiratory reserve exists, it may not be possible to maintain an adequate PaO_2 on one-lung ventilation, and in such a situation the use of an extracorporeal oxygenator and femorofemoral bypass may be needed. Heparinization is an additional surgical problem in such cases. Such a severe situation may also be well suited to surgery in a hyperbaric chamber. Oxygenation can be ensured, and the cyst or bulla will diminish in size under hyperbaric conditions.

Unlike most cases of pulmonary resection, patients following bullectomy are left with a greater amount of functional lung tissue than was previously available to them, and the mechanics of respiration are improved. At the end of the procedure, the double-lumen tube is replaced by a single-lumen tube, and the patients generally require several days to be weaned from the respirator. During this time, the positive airway pressure used should be minimized to avoid causing a pneumothorax owing to rupture of suture or staple lines or of residual bullae.

Anesthesia for Resection of the Trachea

Tracheal resection and reconstruction are technically difficult for the surgeon and challenging for the anesthesiologist.[169,170] Indications for this type of procedure include congenital lesions (agenesis, stenosis), neoplasia (primary or secondary), injuries (direct, indirect), infections, and postintubation injuries (caused by an endotracheal tube or tracheotomy). For the surgical team, the major problems are the maintenance of ventilation to the lungs while the airway is being operated on, and the integrity of the anastomoses postoperatively. In this respect, the presence of lung disease that is of sufficient severity to require postoperative ventilatory support is a relative contraindication to tracheal resection or reconstruction.

Monitoring of these patients should include an arterial cannula placed in the left radial artery to permit continuous measurement of blood pressure during periods of innominate artery compression. Steroids should be administered to help reduce any tracheal edema, and a high FIO_2 should be used throughout the procedure to ensure an adequate oxygen reserve at all times in the FRC, so that temporary interruptions of ventilation are less likely to produce hypoxemia.

Numerous methods have been reported to provide oxygenation and ventilation of the lungs during these procedures. A small-bore anode tube may be pushed through and distal to an upper lesion, so that resection may occur around the tube. This technique is useful only in mild stenoses. Alternatively, an endotracheal tube may be passed via the glottis to above the stenosis, and a sterile endotracheal or bronchial tube may later be inserted into the trachea opened distal to the site of stenosis, with the sterile anesthesia tubing being led across the surgical field. Following resection of the lesion, the sterile and distally placed endotracheal tube is withdrawn, and the upper tube (originally passed through the glottis) is advanced across the anastomosis. With low tracheal or bronchial lesions, resection and reconstruction may be performed around an endobronchial or double-lumen tube. During these procedures, the patient is kept in a head-down position to minimize aspiration of blood and debris into the alveoli, and ventilation must be carefully monitored throughout.

Clearly, the presence of large-bore tubes in the airway may make these resections technically difficult, and the use of high-frequency ventilation techniques may improve surgical access. Thus, a small-diameter catheter or catheters may be placed across or through the stenotic lesion or transected airway(s) and ventilation to the distal airways and lungs maintained using HFPPV or HFJV. Potential disadvantages of these high-frequency ventilation techniques are that, by necessity, the system is "open" (see the section on High-frequency Ventilation), and egress of gas during exhalation may be compromised if the stenosis is tight. Also, the catheter may become occluded by blood and become displaced, and distal aspiration of debris or blood may occur. With complex resections, two anesthesia teams with two machines and anesthesia circuits or sets of ventilating equipment may be necessary to ensure adequate ventilation of the two distal airway segments, although during carinal resections, HFPPV to the left lung alone generally provides adequate oxygenation and ventilation.

In very difficult cases, cardiopulmonary bypass has been used to provide oxygenation and carbon dioxide removal during the period of resection, while following resection, anesthesia can be maintained *via* a standard endotracheal tube. With the use of cardiopulmonary bypass comes an attendant risk of massive hemorrhage as a result of the necessary heparinization.

Following tracheal resection or reconstructive surgery, patients should be kept with their neck and head flexed in order to reduce tension on the anastomotic suture lines. In some cases, this is maintained by using sutures between the chin and the anterior chest wall. Extubation of the trachea is performed as early as possible, so as to minimize tracheal trauma due to the endotracheal tube and cuff.

Bronchopulmonary Lavage

This procedure involves irrigation of the lung and bronchial tree and is used as a treatment for alveolar proteinosis, radioactive dust inhalation, cystic fibrosis, bronchiectasis, and asthmatic bronchitis. Lung lavage is performed under general anesthesia using a double-lumen tube, so that one lung may be ventilated while the other is being treated with lavage fluid.[140,171]

The preoperative assessment of these patients should include ventilation-perfusion scans, so that lavage can be performed first on the more severely affected lung (i.e., the one with the least ventilation). If involvement is equal, the left lung is generally lavaged first, since gas exchange should be better through the larger right lung. Patients are premedicated and supplied with supplemental oxygen *en route* to the operating room.

Anesthesia is induced with an intravenous drug and maintained with an inhaled agent in oxygen to maintain the highest possible FIO_2. Muscle relaxation facilitates placement of the double-lumen tube, and the cuff seal should be checked to maintain perfect separation at a pressure of 50 cm H_2O to prevent leakage of lavage fluid around the cuff. A fiberoptic bronchoscope is useful to check the position of the bronchial cuff of the double-lumen tube. Other monitoring should include an arterial catheter, and oxygenation should be continuously monitored by pulse oximetry. A stethoscope should be placed over the ventilated lung to check for rales, the presence of which may indicate leakage of lavage fluid into this lung.

The patient is maintained on an $FIO_2 = 1.0$ throughout the procedure. Prior to lavage this serves to denitrogenate the lungs, so that only oxygen and carbon dioxide remain. Instillation of fluid then allows these gases to be absorbed, resulting in greater access by the fluid to the alveolar spaces than if the more insoluble nitrogen bubbles remained.

Once the trachea is intubated, the patient is turned so that the side to be lavaged is lowermost, and the double-lumen tube position and seal are checked once again. With the patient in a head-up position, warmed heparinized isotonic saline is infused by gravity from a reservoir 30 cm above the midaxillary line, into the catheter to the dependent lung, while the nondependent lung is ventilated. When fluid ceases to flow in (usually after 700–1000 ml in an adult), the patient is placed in a head-down position and fluid is allowed to drain out. The lavage is continued until the effluent is clear (as opposed to the milky fluid that drains initially when lavage is being performed for alveolar proteinosis), at which point the lung is suctioned and ventilation is re-established with large VT (and pressures), since compliance will be decreased owing to loss of surfactant. With each lavage, inflow and outflow volumes are monitored so that the patient is not "drowned" in fluid and there is no excessive absorption or leakage to the ventilated side. At least 90% of the saline volume should be recovered with each lavage. Two-lung ventilation is re-established and, as compliance improves, an air-oxygen mixture (addition of nitrogen) may be introduced to help maintain alveolar patency. After a further period of ventilation, most patients' tracheae can be extubated in the operating room. In the post-treatment period, patients are encouraged to cough and engage in breathing exercises to fully re-expand the treated lung. After 3 days to a week following lavage of the first lung, the patient may return to the operating room for lavage of the other lung.

Problems sometimes encountered with this procedure include spillage of lavage fluid from the treated to the ventilated lung. This must be managed by stopping the lavage and ensuring functional separation of the lungs before continuing. Double-lumen tube positioning is critical. Spillage may cause profound decreases in oxygenation, which may necessitate terminating the procedure and maintaining two-lung ventilation with oxygen and positive end-expiratory pressure.

During periods when lavage fluid is being instilled into the dependent lung, oxygenation usually improves because the increased intra-alveolar pressure caused by the fluid produces diversion of the pulmonary blood flow to the nondependent, ventilated lung (Fig. 34-26). Conversely, when the fluid is drained out of the dependent lung, hypoxemia may occur.[172,173] In some cases in which severe hypoxemia was anticipated during right lung lavage, the risk has been reduced by passing a balloon-tipped catheter into the right main pulmonary artery (checked by x-ray study) and inflating the balloon during periods of right lung drainage. In this way, blood flow to the dependent, right, nonventilated lung would be minimized during periods of drainage. This technique is not without risk (e.g., pulmonary artery rupture) and is reserved for those patients considered to be at greatest risk for hypoxemia during lavage.

If the patient has recently had a diagnostic open lung biopsy, a bronchopleural fistula may be present. If this is a possibility, a chest tube should be inserted on the side of

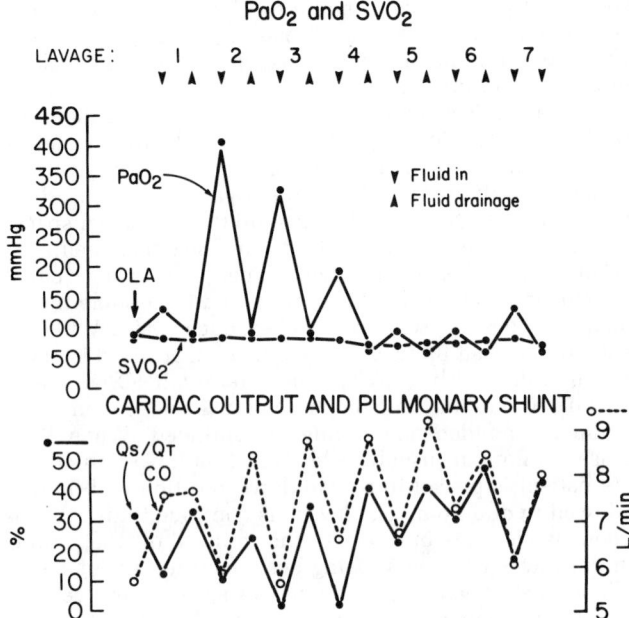

Figure 34-26. Changes in Pao$_2$, Sv̄o$_2$, CO, and Q̇$_s$/Q̇$_t$ during seven unilateral lung lavages. Instillation of fluid caused an increase in Pao$_2$, decreases in CO and in Q̇$_s$/Q̇$_t$, and no change in Sv̄o$_2$. (Sv̄o$_2$ should be read as % on the ordinate scale.) (Pao$_2$ = arterial oxygen tension; Sv̄o$_2$ = mixed venous oxygen saturation; CO = cardiac output; Q̇$_s$/Q̇$_t$ = intrapulmonary shunt; OLA = one-lung anesthesia.) (Reproduced with permission from Cohen E, Feinberg BI, Camunas JC: Unilateral Lung Lavage, p 112. Phoenix, Society of Cardiovascular Anesthesiologists Meeting, April 1985.)

the bronchopleural fistula, and this side should be lavaged first. The chest drain is removed several days later.

Limitations in the sizes of available double-lumen tubes preclude their use for lavage in patients weighing less than 40 kg. In such cases, cardiopulmonary bypass may be required to provide oxygenation during lavage.[174]

Myasthenia Gravis

The thoracic anesthesiologist will most likely have to manage myasthenia gravis (MG) patients for thymectomy, which is now considered the treatment of choice in most cases of MG. MG is a disorder of the neuromuscular junction, the function of which is altered routinely in the modern practice of anesthesia. The worldwide prevalence of the disease is 1 per 20,000 to 30,000 of the population; it is more common in females than males in a 6:4 ratio. People of any age may be affected, but peaks of incidence occur in the third decade for females and the fifth decade for males. MG is a chronic disorder characterized by weakness and fatigability of voluntary muscles with improvement following rest. Onset is frequently slow and insidious, any skeletal muscle or group of muscles may be affected, and the condition is associated with relapses and remissions. The most common onset is ocular, and, if the disease remains localized to the eyes for 2 years, the likelihood of progression to generalized MG is low. In some cases, the disease is generalized and may involve the bulbar musculature, causing problems with breathing and swallowing. Peripheral muscle involvement may cause weakness, clumsiness, and difficulty in holding up the head or in walking. The most commonly used clinical classification of MG is shown in Table 34-7.[175]

TABLE 34-7. Clinical Classification of Myasthenia Gravis[175]

I Ocular Myasthenia—Involvement of ocular muscles only. Mild with ptosis and diplopia. Electrophysiologic testing of other musculature is negative for MG.

IA Ocular Myasthenia with peripheral muscles showing no clinical symptoms but showing a positive electromyogram for MG.

II Generalized Myasthenia

IIA Mild—Slow onset, usually ocular, spreading to skeletal and bulbar muscles. No respiratory involvement. Good response to drug therapy. Low mortality rate.

IIB Moderate—As IIA but progressing to more severe involvement of skeletal and bulbar muscles. Dysarthria, dysphagia, difficulty chewing. No respiratory involvement. Patient's activities limited. Fair response to drug therapy.

III Acute Fulminating—Rapid onset of severe bulbar and skeletal weakness with involvement of muscles of respiration. Progression usually within 6 months. Poor response to therapy. Patient's activities limited. Low mortality rate.

IV Late Severe—Severe MG developing at least 2 years after onset of Group I or Group II symptoms. Progression of disease may be gradual or rapid. Poor response to therapy and poor prognosis.

The basic abnormality in MG is a decrease in the number of postsynaptic acetylcholine receptors at the end plates of affected muscles. This causes a decrease in the margin of safety of neuromuscular transmission. MG is an autoimmune disorder, and most of the affected patients have circulating antibodies to the acetylcholine receptors. These antibodies may cause complement-mediated lysis of the postsynaptic membrane, direct blockade of the receptors, or modulate the receptor turnover such that the degradation rate exceeds the resynthesis rate. Studies of the end-plate area show loss of synaptic folds and a widening of the synaptic cleft.[176]

The diagnosis of MG is suspected from the history and confirmed by pharmacologic, electrophysiologic, and/or immunologic testing. Patients cannot sustain or repeat muscular contraction. The electrical counterpart of this is a decrement in the muscle action potentials evoked by repetitive stimulation of a motor nerve. Mechanical and electrical (electromyography) decrements improve with 2–10 mg of intravenous edrophonium (Tensilon test). Myasthenic patients characteristically are sensitive to d-tubocurarine. When the routine electromyographic results are equivocal, a regional curare test may be performed using a tourniquet to isolate the limb and to limit the action of the drug. In the regional curare test, electromyograms are performed before and after the administration of 0.2 mg curare. In equivocal cases, a positive result of a test for antiacetylcholine receptor antibodies is considered diagnostic.

Medical Therapy

Anticholinesterases are used to prolong the action of acetylcholine at the postsynaptic membrane and may also exert their own agonist effect at the acetylcholine receptors. They are the most commonly used therapy in MG (Table 34-8). Myasthenic patients learn to regulate their medication and titrate dose against optimum effect. Overdosage causes the muscarinic effects of acetylcholine (Ach) and may cause a cholinergic crisis. Underdose causes weakness or a myasthenic crisis. In a patient with weakness, distinction be-

TABLE 34-8. Anticholinesterase Drugs Used to Treat Myasthenia Gravis

| Drug | Dosage (mg) | | | Efficacy |
	Oral	iv	im	
Pyridostigmine (Mestinon)	60	2.0	2.0–4.0	1
Neostigmine (Prostigmin)	15	0.5	0.7–1.0	1
Ambenonium (Mytelase)	6	Not available		2.5

tween the two types of crisis may be made by performing a Tensilon test or by examining pupillary size, which will be large (mydriatic) in a myasthenic but small (miotic) in a cholinergic crisis. Muscarinic side effects are treatable with atropine.

The immunologic basis of MG has led to the use of immunosuppressive drugs, such as steroids, azathioprine, cyclophosphamide, and, most recently, cyclosporine. Steroids often produce initial deterioration before an improvement. The usual regimen is prednisone 1 mg·kg^{-1} on alternative days. The other drugs mentioned represent third and fourth lines of treatment.

Plasma exchange or plasmapheresis may produce dramatic but transient improvements in muscle strength with decreases in antiacetylcholine receptor antibody titers. Usually reserved for severe MG, plasma exchange has been shown to improve respiratory function in both operated and nonoperated MG patients. Plasmapheresis causes a decrease in plasma cholinesterase levels that may prolong the effect of drugs, such as succinylcholine, which are normally broken down by this enzyme system.

Abnormalities are found in 75% of thymus glands removed from MG patients (85% show hyperplasia; 15% thymoma). Following thymectomy, some 75% of patients either go into remission or are improved. Thymectomy is now considered the treatment of choice in most patients with MG, exceptions being those in Osserman Class I.[177] A retrospective controlled study of 80 MG patients who were treated medically and matched (as regards age, sex and severity and duration of MG) with 80 treated by thymectomy showed that the group treated surgically lived longer and showed more clinical improvement than the group treated medically.[178] Thymectomy may be performed either *via* a classic sternum-splitting approach or transcervically using a technique similar to mediastinoscopy. Controversy exists over which is the best surgical approach to thymectomy. Although a more radical thymectomy can be performed by the trans-sternal route, the morbidity would appear to be greater than by the transcervical route. Furthermore, the results in terms of clinical improvement and remission rates following transcervical thymectomy are reported to be equally as good as those following trans-sternal thymectomy.[179]

Management of General Anesthesia

When possible, MG patients should be admitted for elective surgery while in remission. Upon admission, the patient's physical and emotional states should be optimized. Other diseases occasionally associated with MG should be excluded (Table 34-9). The patient's current drug therapy should be reviewed and possible drug interactions considered. Because patients are less active while in the hospital, their anticholinesterase dosage may need to be decreased. If the patient has a history of respiratory disease or bulbar

involvement, preoperative evaluation should include respiratory function studies. Breathing exercises and instruction in the use of incentive spirometers may be indicated. Patients should be told of the possible need for postoperative intubation of the trachea and ventilation of the lungs. Myasthenic patients should be scheduled to be the first case of the day in the operating room. Patients on steroid therapy should receive perioperative coverage.

Since the myasthenic patient's trachea is to be intubated and the lungs ventilated for the planned procedure, anticholinesterase therapy should be withheld on the morning of surgery so that the patient is weak on arrival at the operating room. This avoids interactions with other drugs used in the operating room. Anticholinesterase therapy may be continued if the patient is physically or psychologically dependent on it. Premedication is satisfactorily achieved with a benzodiazepine or barbiturate. Opioids are generally avoided because of the risk of producing respiratory depression.

Monitoring should be as dictated by the patient's state and planned surgical procedure but should include an assessment of neuromuscular transmission (mechanomyogram/twitch monitor or integrated electromyographic monitor) if agents affecting neuromuscular transmission are to be used.[180]

Induction of anesthesia is readily achieved with a short-acting barbiturate. In elective cases intubation of the trachea, maintenance, and relaxation are readily achieved using potent inhaled anesthetics. Anesthesia may be deepened using halothane, enflurane, or isoflurane and the trachea intubated under their effect. Myasthenic patients are more sensitive than normals to the neuromuscular depressant effects of the potent inhaled agents. Thus, while concentrations of 3.5% enflurane are needed to produce twitch depression in normals, as little as 1% enflurane or 0.4% isoflurane may produce profound depression in MG patients.[181] In MG patients isoflurane 1.9 MAC end-tidal concentration induced a neuromuscular block of 30–50%, whereas halothane 1.8 MAC induced a block of 10–20%. Both agents produced fade in the train of four ratio of 41% and 28%, respectively.[182] Because these drugs are easily administered and withdrawn, they are the most commonly used anesthetic drugs for MG patients. At the end of the procedure, the drug is discontinued and recovery of neuromuscular function begins.

Nondepolarizing Relaxants. In some cases, MG patients cannot tolerate the cardiovascular depressant effects of the potent inhaled anesthetics, in which case muscle relaxants

TABLE 34-9. Disorders Associated with Myasthenia Gravis

Thymoma	Multiple sclerosis
Thyroid disease	Ulcerative colitis
hyperthyroidism	Leukemia
hypothyroidism	Lymphoma
thyroiditis	Convulsive disorders
Idiopathic thrombocytopenic	Extrathymic neoplasia
purpura	Polymyositis
Rheumatoid arthritis	Sjögren's syndrome
Systemic lupus	Scleroderma
erythematosus	
Anemias	
pernicious	
hemolytic	

may be employed, titrating dose against monitored effect. MG patients are sensitive to the nondepolarizing relaxants. A usual defasciculating dose in a normal patient may represent an ED_{90} in an MG patient.[177] All the nondepolarizing relaxants have been successfully and uneventfully used, with careful monitoring, in MG patients. They should be titrated in $^1/_{10}$ to $^1/_{20}$ of the usual dose. At present atracurium is probably the preferred agent because of its short elimination half-life (20 minutes), small volume of distribution, lack of cumulative effect, and high clearance. The Hofmann elimination pathway results in atracurium having very reproducible pharmacodynamics and kinetics, and most patients do not require reversal if monitored carefully. A recent review suggests that the ED_{90} of atracurium in MG patients is approximately one fifth of that in normal patients.[183] Relaxation is readily maintained thereafter using an atracurium infusion, and recovery time is not prolonged with this drug. Although other nondepolarizing agents may be used, they do have cumulative effects, which may represent a potential disadvantage. If necessary, the nondepolarizers may be reversed by increments of anticholinesterase drugs while carefully monitoring neuromuscular transmission to obtain maximum antagonism yet avoid a cholinergic crisis. All anticholinesterases have been safely used. Edrophonium may be the drug of choice, since its onset of action is rapid and higher doses have a prolonged duration of action. Because of the risk of cholinergic crisis with anticholinesterase agents, the rapid, predictable, spontaneous recovery from atracurium may represent an additional advantage in that reversal may not be necessary.[180]

The sensitivity of MG patients to nondepolarizing relaxants is very variable, depending upon the individual patient, the severity of MG, and the treatment. There are conflicting reports as to the sensitivity of MG patients who are in remission. All such patients should be considered sensitive to nondepolarizers until proved otherwise.[177]

Succinylcholine. MG patients are resistant to the neuromuscular blocking effects of succinylcholine. The ED_{95} is 2.6 times normal in these patients.[184] Clinically, however, the use of succinylcholine has been without incident, with normal clinical doses producing adequate relaxation for endotracheal intubation and a normal recovery time, despite the occasionally reported early onset of phase II block. Doses of $0.2-1.0$ mg·kg^{-1} have been used in a number of MG patients, and most did not show fasciculation before becoming paralyzed.[177] Fade in response to train-of-four stimulation was observed in some patients during recovery, but recovery was not delayed. It should be noted that the prior administration of an anticholinesterase may complicate the response to succinylcholine by delaying its metabolism.

When a rapid sequence intubation of the trachea is required, rapid onset of muscle relaxation may be achieved with succinylcholine or with moderate doses of a nondepolarizer, in the latter case, with an associated prolongation of effect. A succinylcholine (1.5 mg·kg^{-1})-vecuronium (0.01 mg·kg^{-1}) sequence has been safely used in three MG patients for thymectomy. The authors suggested that this technique may be particularly advantageous when rapid sequence induction of anesthesia is indicated.[185]

Other Drug Interactions. Medications with neuromuscular blocking properties should be used with caution in patients with MG, particularly if relaxants are being used concurrently. Such drugs include antiarrhythmics (quinidine, procainamide, calcium channel blockers), diuretics (by causing hypokalemia), nitrogen mustards, quinine, and aminoglycoside antibiotics. Dantrolene has been used safely in a patient with MG.[186]

Recovery from Anesthesia. Recovery from anesthesia must be carefully monitored in these patients. Extubation of the trachea should be performed when the patients are responsive and able to generate negative inspiratory pressures of greater than -20 cm H_2O. Following extubation of the trachea, patients are carefully observed in the recovery area or the intensive care unit. As soon as possible, patients should resume their usual pyridostigmine regimen. Cases of mild respiratory depression may be treatable with parenteral anticholinesterase; more severe cases may require reintubation of the trachea and mechanical ventilation of the lungs. In the immediate postoperative period, postthymectomy patients often show a marked improvement in their condition and a decreased need for anticholinesterase therapy.

Postoperative Respiratory Failure. Myasthenic patients are at increased risk of developing respiratory failure postoperatively.[187] There have been several attempts at predicting preoperatively which MG patients will require prolonged postoperative ventilation of the lungs.[188] For patients who underwent trans-sternal thymectomy, Leventhal et al[189] found that positive predictors were a duration of MG greater than 6 years; history of chronic respiratory disease, other than that directly caused by MG; pyridostigmine dosage greater than 750 mg·day^{-1}; and a preoperative vital capacity of less than 2.9 l. This predictive system has not been found useful when applied in MG patients undergoing trans-sternal thymectomy at other centers and is of no value in MG patients undergoing other types of surgical procedure.[188] Each patient should, therefore, be treated on his or her own merits.

A more recent study of trans-sternal thymectomy patients suggested that the need for postoperative mechanical ventilation correlated best with preoperative maximum static expiratory pressure.[190] It was concluded that expiratory weakness, by reducing cough efficacy and ability to clear secretions, was the main predictive determinant. Adequate clearance of secretions is essential in these patients and may occasionally necessitate bronchoscopy.

In general, the postoperative morbidity in terms of respiratory failure is lower following transcervical than transsternal thymectomy.[179,188] Techniques described that may be useful in reducing postoperative ventilatory failure include preoperative plasma exchange and high-dose steroid therapy perioperatively.[180] If the anticipated duration of the surgical procedure is 1–2 hours, preoperative oral anticholinesterase therapy may be of value, since the peak effect of the drug will coincide with the conclusion of the surgical procedure and attempts at tracheal extubation.[177]

Postoperative Care

In the immediate postoperative period, pain relief for MG patients is usually provided by opioid analgesics, such as meperidine, but in reduced doses. The analgesic effect of morphine and other opioid analgesics has been reported as being increased by anticholinesterases, which has led to the recommendation that the dose of opioid analgesics be reduced by one third in patients receiving anticholinesterase therapy.[191] Combined regional and general anesthesia techniques have also been used to provide good surgical conditions and improved postoperative analgesia in MG patients undergoing thymectomy. Combined epidural-general anesthesia has been reported to provide excellent intra- and postoperative conditions for both surgeon and patient.[192,193]

Myasthenic Syndrome (Eaton-Lambert Syndrome)

The myasthenic syndrome is a very rare disorder of neuromuscular transmission, which is sometimes associated with small-cell carcinoma of the lung. Complaints of weakness may be mistaken for MG, but in Eaton-Lambert syndrome symptoms do not respond to administration of anticholinesterases or steroids, and activity *improves* strength. The defect in this condition is thought to be prejunctional, associated with diminished release of acetylcholine from nerve terminals, and improved by agents such as 4-aminopyridine, guanidine, and germine that increase repetitive firing. Affected patients are particularly sensitive to the effects of all muscle relaxants, which should be used with great caution or avoided entirely. The possibility of Eaton-Lambert syndrome should be considered in all patients with known malignant disease and those patients undergoing diagnostic procedures for suspected carcinoma of the lung. Anesthesia considerations in these patients are essentially the same as in those with MG.[180,194]

POSTOPERATIVE MANAGEMENT AND COMPLICATIONS

Atelectasis

Patients who require thoracotomy often have pre-existing pulmonary disease which, when combined with the operative procedure, is likely to result in significant pulmonary dysfunction and possibly pneumonia. Atelectasis, the most significant cause of postoperative morbidity, has been reported to occur in up to 100% of patients undergoing thoracotomy for pulmonary resection.[195] It occurs more frequently in the basal lobes than in the middle or upper lung regions. It may be secondary to reduction of normal respiratory effort due to splinting from pain, obesity, intrathoracic blood and fluid accumulation, and decreased compliance, all of which lead to rapid shallow constant VT. Such a respiratory pattern produces small airway closure and obstruction with inspissated secretions, resulting ultimately in alveolar air resorption and terminal airway collapse. A poor cough and limited clearance of secretions add to the problem. Other sources of atelectasis include mucus plugging, which can obstruct a lobe or even an entire lung, and incomplete re-expansion of the remaining lung tissue following one-lung anesthesia. The diagnosis of atelectasis can be made by clinical findings, chest x-ray film, or arterial blood gas analysis. This problem is best resolved by increasing resting lung volume or FRC. FRC can be increased by an increase in transpulmonary pressure (difference between airway and intrapleurál pressures: PL = [Paw − Ppl]) or in lung compliance.

The tracheae of many patients can be extubated shortly after brief thoracic surgical procedures using standard extubation criteria. However, most patients with COPD undergoing extensive thoracic surgical procedures require postoperative ventilation to avoid atelectasis and other pulmonary complications.[196] Mechanical ventilation raises airway pressure and, to a lesser extent, intrapleural pressure; therefore, transpulmonary pressure increases. Most postoperative thoracotomy patients are ventilated using intermittent mandatory ventilation and positive end-expiratory pressure. Ventilation settings include: VT = 12 ml·kg^{-1}, rate 8 breaths·min^{-1}, FiO$_2$ = 0.5 and positive end-expiratory pressure 5–20 cm H$_2$O. The goal is to keep the PaO$_2$ between 80–100 mm Hg and the PaCO$_2$ and pH normal. The intermittent mandatory ventilation rate is decreased as tolerated to two breaths per minute, and then the positive end-expiratory pressure level is reduced to 5 cm H$_2$O. When arterial blood gases are adequate at these settings and the VC is greater than 10 ml·kg^{-1}, inspiratory force is greater than −20 cm H$_2$O, and the level of consciousness is adequate, the patient's trachea is ready for extubation.[197]

In addition to the use of incentive spirometry and bronchodilators, coughing and clearance of secretions, and mobilizing the patient, adequate analgesia is essential to the prevention and treatment of atelectasis. Atelectasis caused by collapse of lung tissue distal to a mucus plug can be treated by positioning the patient in the lateral decubitus position with the fully expanded lung in the dependent position. This improves ventilation-perfusion matching and facilitates clearance of mucus from the nondependent obstructed lung.[198] However, the patient should not be placed with the operative side in the dependent position following a pneumonectomy because of the risk of cardiac herniation.[198]

Postoperative Pain Control

After extubation of the trachea, respiratory therapy and pain management become critical components of postoperative care. Adequate postoperative pain control is necessary to ensure a good respiratory effort. Administration of intravenous opioids has been the standard form of pain management for years. These drugs may improve pulmonary function slightly or allow respiratory therapy maneuvers; however, meperidine (50 mg) has been shown to be relatively ineffective at allowing patients to increase their ability to cough. Advantages of intravenous opioids are the ease of administration, relatively low toxicity, and the lack of a need for close medical supervision. The key disadvantage is the inadequate pain relief leading to postoperative atelectasis and great discomfort on the part of the patient. The administration of sufficient narcotic to treat pain adequately is likely to cause sedation and respiratory depression.

Patient-controlled analgesia is a newer method of administering intravenous narcotics. It consists of an infusion pump that delivers a programmed amount of drug when a patient presses a button. A minimum lockout time period from the previous dose is programmed, and a basal continuous infusion can also be provided. This method of treatment has been reported to reduce the amount of postoperative pain, drug use, sedation, and pulmonary complications.[199-201]

Patient-controlled analgesia also eliminates the time delays associated with personnel-administered medications and in general is very well accepted by patients.[199] Subcutaneous patient-controlled analgesia with hydromorphone has been reported to be as effective as intravenous patient-controlled analgesia.[202] Complications related to the use of patient-controlled analgesia are presented elsewhere in this volume (see Chapter 57).

Many clinicians have suggested the use of intercostal nerve blocks before, during, or after thoracic surgery to decrease pain and improve postoperative respiratory function.

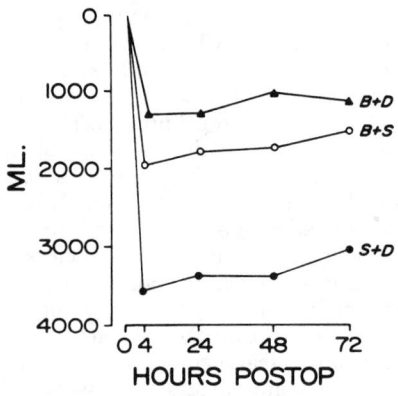

CHANGE IN VITAL CAPACITY FROM CONTROL

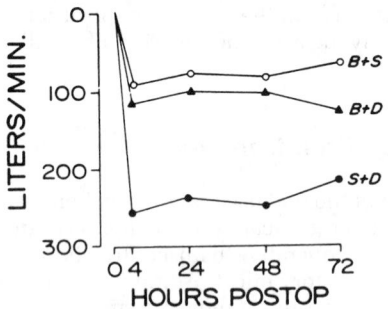

CHANGE IN FORCED EXPIRATORY FLOW
RATES FROM CONTROL

Figure 34-27. (*Top*) Mean decrease in vital capacity from control and after thoracotomy with intercostal nerve block; (*bottom*) mean decrease in forced expiratory flow rates from control and after thoracotomy with intercostal nerve block. Nerve block performed with the following solutions: bupivacaine-dextran (B + D); bupivacaine-saline (B + S); saline-dextran (S + D). (Reproduced with permission from Kaplan JA, Miller ED, Gallagher EG: Postoperative analgesia for thoracotomy patients. Anesth Analg 54:774, 1975.)

Studies have documented a decrease in requirements for postoperative opioids, improved respiratory function (Fig. 34-27), and some decrease in time of hospital stay.[203-206] The intercostal block can be performed externally before or after surgery using a standard technique. However, the easiest method during thoracic surgery is to have the surgeon perform the block under direct vision from inside the thorax while the chest is open. Bupivacaine, 0.5%, in doses of 2–3 ml, can be placed in the five intercostal spaces around the incision and in intercostal spaces where chest tubes will be placed. This provides for 6–24 hours of moderate pain relief, but patients still complain of diaphragmatic and shoulder discomfort caused by the chest tubes. Higher volumes of local anesthetic (e.g., 5–10 ml) should not be used in the intercostal space because of the high absorption rate and attendant systemic toxicity that can be produced as well as the possibility of pushing the drug centrally and producing a paravertebral sympathetic or epidural block with central sympatholysis and severe hypotension.[207] The placement of catheters in intercostal grooves intraoperatively allows for a continuous postoperative intercostal nerve block.[208] The

technique reduces pain and improves pulmonary function.[209,210] Although bupivacaine has been used in most reports, lidocaine has also been used.[211]

A prolonged duration intercostal nerve block may be obtained by cryoanalgesia, a technique of freezing the nerve under direct vision at the time of thoracotomy.[212] A cryoprobe is applied directly to the nerve to disrupt the axon but not the support structures. In this way, conduction is interrupted until the nerve regenerates over the next 1–6 months, by which time full structure and function are usually restored.[213] Hypoesthesia in the scar and adjacent skin is a common late finding.[214] During the postoperative period, the patients are numb in the segments thus treated. Ideally, any drains or chest tubes should be located within the area made analgesic with the cryoprobe so as to minimize immediate postoperative discomfort. Cryoanalgesia provides excellent analgesia when supplemented with other pain treatments.[215,216] Since cryoanalgesia is of prolonged duration, it is not used routinely following thoracotomy but rather in cases in which prolonged analgesia would be necessary, such as following surgery for chest trauma.

A recent approach to postoperative pain control after thoracic surgery is the use of epidural or intrathecal opioids. Epidural morphine has been shown to produce profound analgesia lasting from 16–24 hours after thoracotomy and not to cause a sympathetic block or sensory or motor loss.[217] These are significant advantages over other methods of administering opioids or local anesthetics. The opioids have been successfully used by both the thoracic and lumbar epidural routes. Morphine, in a dose of 5–7 mg diluted in 15–20 ml of fluid, has been used in the lumbar epidural technique. This technique has led to a 30% increase in postoperative expiratory flow rates without significant side-effects, even in patients with chronic lung disease.

Epidural morphine has recently been shown to reduce pain and improve respiratory function in post-thoracotomy patients.[218] The successful use of lumbar epidural sufentanil or fentanyl diluted to 20 ml has also been reported.[219-220] There has been one report of severe respiratory depression with epidural fentanyl and several reports with sufentanil.[220-222] The addition of epinephrine, 5 μg·ml^{-1}, to sufentanil administered in the thoracic epidural space decreases the plasma concentration of sufentanil and increases the duration of block.[223] Lumbar epidural hydromorphone (1.25–1.5 mg) has been reported to provide excellent analgesia, with fewer side-effects than epidural morphine.[224] Severe respiratory depression has been reported in one patient who received hydromorphone *via* a thoracic epidural catheter.[225] A prophylactic low-dose infusion of naloxone, or nalbuphine, an agonist-antagonist drug, can reduce the incidence of respiratory depression.[226,227]

Subarachnoid (intrathecal) morphine, in a dose of 10–15 μg·kg^{-1}, has also been successfully used after thoracic surgery. With this technique, the drug acts directly on the spinal cord, and analgesia can be produced with a lower dose than by the epidural or intravenous routes. Gray et al[228] showed the effectiveness of this technique in postthoracotomy pain management. When morphine is given intrathecally prior to the induction of anesthesia, a reduction in the dose of anesthetic drugs required may occur.[229,230] However, Wynands et al showed that intrathecal morphine (1.5 mg) did not reduce postoperative pain or improve respiratory parameters in a group of patients anesthetized with fentanyl undergoing intrathoracic surgery (Fig. 34-28).[231] The authors stated that this was because the opioid receptors were saturated by the intravenous fentanyl. All previous studies showing the benefits of epidural or intrathecal opioids have

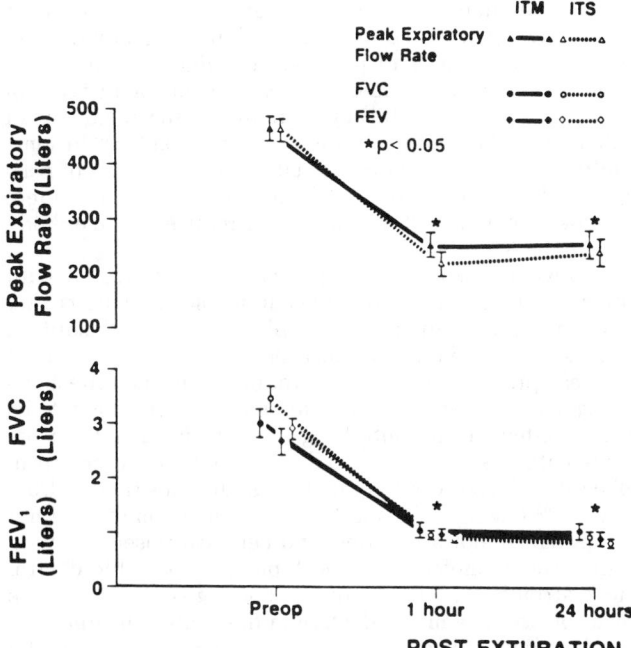

Figure 34-28. FVC, FEV$_1$, and PEFR measured preoperatively (Preop) and 1 and 24 hours after extubation. $p < 0.05$ when compared with baseline values. (ITM = intrathecal morphine; ITS = intrathecal saline.) (Reproduced with permission from Wynands JE, Casey WF, Ralley FF *et al:* The role of intrathecal morphine in the anesthetic management of patients undergoing coronary artery bypass surgery. J Cardiothoracic Anesth 1:510, 1988.)

been performed after anesthetic techniques that were not dependent on high doses of opioids. All patients who have received intrathecal or epidural opioids must be closely observed for potential side-effects. These include delayed respiratory depression, urinary retention, pruritus, nausea, and vomiting, and they appear to be dose-related. All these effects may be reversed with naloxone.

Interpleural analgesia is the most recently developed technique for postoperative pain treatment.[232] Although the mechanism has not been fully elucidated, the injection of local anesthetic between the pleural layers is thought to block multiple intercostal nerves or the pain fibers traveling with the thoracic sympathetic chain. The surgeon can place the catheter intraoperatively under direct vision while the chest is open. Catheter malposition has been documented following percutaneous placement, especially if the patient is not breathing spontaneously.[233] The chest tubes should not be suctioned for about 15 minutes following injection of local anesthetic to avoid loss of the anesthetic into the drainage. The efficacy of interpleural blockade for postthoracotomy pain relief has been reported to be both poor[234,235] and good.[216-236,237]

Respiratory Therapy Techniques

Physiotherapy is one of the oldest forms of therapy for the prevention and treatment of respiratory complications. Techniques include postural drainage, breathing exercises, vibration, deep breathing, coughing, and percussion. Many clinicians feel that chest physiotherapy is useful despite the sparse data to support its physiologic benefits. Decades ago, it was also felt that forced exhalation against resistance would create increased airway pressures and inflation of the lungs. Thus, water-filled blow bottles were designed for postoperative use. However, studies subsequently showed that a forced exhalation decreases the expiratory transpulmonary pressure and lung volumes and should be avoided in postoperative patients. Bartlett *et al* suggested that the blow bottles were only useful because of the large inspiration that preceded the forced exhalation.[238]

Intermittent positive-pressure breathing has also been used extensively in the postoperative period to prevent and treat respiratory insufficiency. However, most of the studies demonstrated little physiologic benefit. In fact, some authors showed that intermittent positive-pressure breathing could be harmful after thoracotomy because of the hypoventilation that subsequently occurred after the forced hyperventilation.[239] The hyperventilation led to a decreased FRC and Paco$_2$ secondary to the decreased expiratory transpulmonary pressure.

Incentive spirometry is the most widely used postoperative respiratory care device. This device, producing a long, deep breath, has been shown to cause less complications and atelectasis than intermittent positive-pressure breathing, blow bottles, or chest physiotherapy.[240] Patients with a decreased FRC and decreased Pao$_2$ experience a reduction of atelectasis on chest x-ray study and improved arterial oxygenation. Bartlett showed that the technique produces an increase in inspiratory transpulmonary pressure but not an increase in expiratory pressure.[238] Expiratory transpulmonary pressure can best be increased by the use of continuous positive airway pressure by mask. This technique was first described in the mid-1930s. Andersen *et al* compared mask continuous positive airway pressure to chest physiotherapy, postural drainage, and endotracheal suction in the treatment of postoperative atelectasis.[240] They found that 15 cm H$_2$O continuous positive airway pressure applied once an hour for 25–35 breaths led to a clinically significant improvement within 12 hours, whereas the other techniques produced little change. This technique appears to be very useful in the treatment of atelectasis in order to avoid reintubation of the trachea in patients after surgery. Gastric distention, regurgitation, and pulmonary aspiration are the potential dangers of mask continuous positive airway pressure.

Other Complications After Thoracic Surgery

The other major complications after thoracic surgery can be grouped into cardiovascular, pulmonary, and related problems (Table 34-10). The cardiovascular complications are often the most difficult to manage in patients with associated respiratory insufficiency. The low cardiac output syndrome and postoperative cardiac arrhythmias are the most common and life-threatening of these problems. In the postoperative period, advanced hemodynamic monitoring is used to make the differential diagnosis of left or right ventricular failure and the low output syndrome. The key monitor is the pulmonary arterial catheter that facilitates the construction of Starling function curves.[241] New diagnostic modalities, such as echocardiography, may be required to rule out the presence of pericardial effusions or tamponade after opening the pericardium during certain types of thoracic surgical procedure. The low cardiac output syndrome must be differentiated from hypovolemia resulting from intrathoracic hemorrhage, tamponade, pulmonary emboli, or the effects of mechanical ventilation with positive end-expiratory pressure. Postoperative fluid administration can

TABLE 34-10. Complications of Thoracic Surgery

I. Cardiovascular complications
  Hypotension
  Low-output syndrome
  Dysrhythmias
  Postoperative hypertension
  Myocardial ischemia and infarction
  Pacing problems
II. Pulmonary complications
  Pulmonary emboli
  Bronchopleural fistula
  Empyema and mediastinitis
  Pulmonary torsion
  Tracheostomy problems
  Diagnostic procedure complications
  Chest wall complications
  Pleural drainage
  Pulmonary hemorrhage
III. Related complications
  Monitoring equipment
  Neurologic—central and peripheral

lead to pulmonary edema resulting from the resection of lung tissue and the concomitant reduction of the pulmonary vascular bed. A postoperative pulmonary embolism can originate from the remaining pulmonary artery stump or tumor tissue. Therapeutic interventions for postoperative myocardial dysfunction include inotropic drugs, vasodilators, and combinations of these drugs, as needed, to improve ventricular function. The goal is to shift the Starling function curve up and to the left by reducing preload of either the left or the right side of the heart and increasing cardiac output. Vasodilators are very effective at decreasing right ventricular afterload and improving right ventricular function, since this side of the heart is especially afterload-dependent.[242] Combinations of inotropes and vasodilators, such as isoproterenol and nitroglycerin, or combined drugs, such as amrinone, can be especially useful in the treatment of right-sided heart failure.

Postoperative cardiac dysrhythmias are common after thoracic surgery. Patients undergoing pulmonary resection have postoperative supraventricular tachycardias with a frequency and severity proportional to both their age and the magnitude of the surgical procedure. Many factors contribute to these dysrhythmias, including underlying cardiac disease, degree of surgical trauma, intraoperative cardiac manipulation-stimulation of the sympathetic nervous system by pain, a reduced pulmonary vascular bed, effects of anesthetics and cardioactive drugs, and metabolic abnormalities.

Beck-Nielson reported on cardiac dysrhythmias in a series of 300 thoracotomies for lung resection and found that atrial fibrillation occurred in 20% of patients with malignant disease but in only 3% with benign disease.[243] A 22% incidence of dysrhythmias has been reported following pneumonectomies.[244] Multifocal atrial tachycardia often occurs in patients with chronic obstructive pulmonary disease and concomitant right-sided cardiac dysfunction. The right side of the heart may be further strained by the reduction in the size of the pulmonary vasculature from the lung resection, and especially following right pneumonectomy. The prophylactic use of digitalis in thoracic surgical patients is controversial, particularly in patients with signs of congestive heart failure. Factors against its use include the potential toxic effects of the drug and the difficulty in assessing adequacy of digitalization in the absence of heart failure. A prospective, placebo-controlled, randomized study demonstrated no advantage to prophylactic digitalization of patients undergoing thoracic surgery.[245] A factor in favor of its use is the drug's efficacy in reducing the incidence of potentially fatal complications in older patients.[246] In some studies it has been reported to reduce the incidence of perioperative dysrhythmias.[247,248] If digitalis is to be instituted, normokalemia should be ensured to reduce the likelihood of digitalis toxicity.

Supraventricular tachycardias can also be treated with either beta blocking or calcium channel blocking drugs after ruling out underlying reversible physiologic abnormalities, such as hypoxia. Verapamil has been the standard treatment for these problems until the introduction of the ultrashort-acting beta blocker, esmolol. Esmolol has been shown to be equally effective in controlling the ventricular rate in patients with postoperative atrial fibrillation or flutter and in increasing the conversion rate to regular sinus rhythm from 8–34%.[249] Owing to its short duration of action (beta elimination half-life of 9 minutes) and beta$_1$-cardioselectivity, it is the drug of choice in the postoperative period to control these arrhythmias. Doses of 50–200 $\mu g \cdot kg^{-1} \cdot min^{-1}$ have been shown to be most effective in the control of supraventricular tachycardias. A bolus of 1.5–2.0 $mg \cdot kg^{-1}$ of esmolol has been shown to effectively blunt the hemodynamic responses to both extubation[250] and intubation.[251]

Hemorrhage and pneumothorax are always major concerns after intrathoracic surgery. Because of these problems, interpleural thoracostomy tubes with an underwater seal system are routinely used after thoracic surgery. Slippage of a suture on any major vessel or airway in the chest can lead to the slow or rapid development of hypovolemic shock or a tension pneumothorax. Drainage of more than 200 ml·hr^{-1} of blood is an indication for surgical re-exploration for hemorrhage. Management of the pleural drainage system is fraught with confusion. The chest bottles must be kept below the level of the chest, and the tubes should not be clamped during patient transport. These tubes can be lifesaving, but errors in technique can lead to serious complications. The creation of a pneumothorax in the nonoperative chest by central venous catheter placement is very hazardous, since this lung is essential both intraoperatively during one-lung anesthesia and postoperatively following contralateral lung resection. Dehiscence of the bronchial stump may lead to the formation of a bronchopleural fistula, which carries a mortality rate of 20%.[252] Surgical treatment may be needed, in which case ventilation of the patient may be difficult because of loss of tidal volume through the fistula. A double-lumen endobronchial tube positioned in the contralateral mainstem bronchus or the use of HFJV may be required for safe management. HFJV allows ventilation with lowered peak airway pressures. However, there have been reports in which ventilation by HFJV was difficult.[165,253,254] If a double-lumen endobronchial tube is placed, the lung with the fistula can be ventilated independently with either continuous positive airway pressure or HFJV.[164,255]

Both central and peripheral neurologic injuries can occur during intrathoracic procedures. Such injuries often result in serious and disabling loss of function and are very distressing to the patient. Peripheral nerves can be injured, either in the chest or in other parts of the body, by pressure or stretching.[256] It has been recognized for years that the majority of these postoperative neuropathies are caused by malpositioning of the patient on the operating table, with subsequent stretching or compression of the nerves. The nerve injury may be apparent immediately after surgery or may not become obvious until several days later. These patients often complain of a variety of unpleasant sensations, including paresthesias, coldness, pain, or anesthesia in the area supplied by the affected nerves. The brachial plexus is especially vulnerable to trauma during thoracic surgery owing to its long superficial course in the axilla between two points of fixation, the vertebrae above and the axillary fascia below. Stretching is the chief cause of damage to the brachial plexus, with compression having only a secondary role.[256] Branches of the brachial plexus may also be injured lower in the arm by compression against objects such as an ether screen or other parts of the operating table. Intrathoracic nerves can be directly injured during a surgical procedure by being transected, crushed, stretched, or cauterized. The intercostal nerves are the ones most frequently injured during intrathoracic surgical procedures. The recurrent laryngeal nerve can become involved in lymph node tissue and injured at the time of a node biopsy, especially when the biopsy is performed through a mediastinoscope. This nerve can also be injured during tracheostomy or radical pulmonary dissections. The phrenic nerve is frequently injured during pericardiectomy, radical pulmonary hilar dissections, division of the diaphragm during esophageal surgery, or dissection of mediastinal tumors.

Prevention is the treatment of choice for all these intraoperative nerve injuries. Analgesics may be necessary to control postoperative pain in the distribution of the nerve injury and to aid in maintaining joint mobility during the healing phase. Subsequent surgical procedures may be necessary to move a swollen ulnar nerve at the elbow or to stent a partially paralyzed vocal cord.

REFERENCES

1. Rutkow IM: Thoracic and cardiovascular operations in the United States, 1979 to 1984. J Thorac Cardiovasc Surg 92:181, 1986
2. Kaplan JA (ed): Thoracic Anesthesia, 2nd ed. New York, Churchill Livingstone, 1991
3. Marshall BE, Longnecker DE, Fairly HB: Anesthesia for Thoracic Procedures. Oxford, Blackwell Scientific, 1987
4. Benumof JL: Anesthesia for Thoracic Surgery. Philadelphia, WB Saunders, 1987
5. Beck GJ, Doyle CA, Schacter FN: Smoking and lung function. Am Rev Respir Dis 155:149, 1981
6. Tisi GN: Preoperative evaluation of pulmonary function: Validity, indications, and benefits. Am Rev Respir Dis 119:293, 1979
7. O'Donoghue WJ, Baker JP, Bell GM et al: Respiratory failure in neuromuscular disease: Management in respiratory intensive care unit. JAMA 235:733, 1976
8. Gass GD, Olsen GN: Clinical significance of pulmonary function tests. Preoperative pulmonary function testing to predict postoperative morbidity and mortality. Chest 89:127, 1986
9. Lockwood P: Lung function test results and the risk of postthoracotomy complications. Respiration 30:529, 1973
10. Mittman C: Assessment of operative risk in thoracic surgery. Am Rev Respir Dis 84:197, 1961
11. Traver GA, Chine MG, Burrows B: Predictors of mortality in chronic obstructive pulmonary disease—a 15-year follow-up study. Am Rev Respir Dis 119:895, 1979
12. Stein M, Koota GM, Simon M et al: Pulmonary evaluation of surgical patients. JAMA 181:765, 1962
13. Jones RM, Rosen M, Seymour L: Smoking and anaesthesia (editorial). Anaesthesia 42:1, 1987
14. Jones RM: Smoking before surgery: The case for stopping smoking. Br Med J 290:1763, 1985
15. Buist AS, Sexton GV, Nagy JM et al: The effects of smoking cessation and modification of lung function. Am Rev Respir Dis 123:149, 1981
16. Pearce AC, Jones RM: Smoking and anesthesia: Preoperative abstinence and preoperative morbidity. Anesthesiology 61:576, 1984
17. Warner MA, Tinker JH, Divertie MB: Preoperative cessation of smoking and pulmonary complications in pulmonary dysfunction. Anesthesiology 59A:60, 1983
18. Cooper DKL: The incidence of postoperative infection and the role of antibiotic prophylaxis in pulmonary surgery: A review of 221 consecutive patients undergoing thoracotomy. Br J Dis Chest 75:154, 1981
19. Chopru SK, Tuplin GV, Simmons DH et al: Effects of hydration and physical therapy on tracheal transport velocity. Am Rev Respir Dis 115:1009, 1977
20. Scheffiner AC: The mucolytic activity and mechanism of action and metabolism of acetylcysteine. Pharmacol Ther 1:47, 1964
21. Lertzman MM, Chernich RM: Rehabilitation of patients with chronic obstructive disease. Chest 73 (suppl):927, 1978
22. Crabb-Johnson DC, Chir B, Andrew JL: Bronchodilator therapy. N Engl J Med 297:476, 1977
23. Aubier M, DeTroyer A, Sampson M et al: Aminophylline improves diaphragmatic contractility. N Engl J Med 249:305, 1981
24. Marini JJ, Lakshmimara Y, Kradyan WA: Atropine and terbutaline aerosols in chronic bronchitis. Chest 80:285, 1981
25. Tremper KK, Barker SJ: Pulse oximetry. Anesthesiology 70:98, 1989
26. Alexander CM, Teller LE, Gross JB: Principles of pulse oximetry: Theoretical and practical considerations. Anesth Analg 68:368, 1989
27. Kaplan JA, King SB: The precordial electrocardiographic lead (V5) in patients who have coronary artery disease. Anesthesiology 45:570, 1976
28. London MJ, Hollenberg M, Wong MG et al: Intraoperative myocardial ischemia. Localization by continuous 12-lead electrocardiography. Anesthesiology 69:232, 1988
29. Kaplan JA: Hemodynamic monitoring. In Kaplan JA (ed): Cardiac Anesthesia, 2nd ed, p 179. Orlando, Grune & Stratton, 1987
30. Baker RJ, Chunprapaph B, Nyhus LM: Severe ischaemia of the hand following radial artery catheterization. Surgery 80:449, 1976
31. Mangano DJ, Hickey RF: Ischemic injury following uncomplicated radial artery catheterization. Anesth Analg 58:55, 1979
32. Slogoff S, Keats AS, Arlund C: On the safety of radial artery cannulation. Anesthesiology 59:42, 1983
33. Bedford RF, Wollman H: Complications of percutaneous radial artery cannulation: An objective prospective study in man. Anesthesiology 38:228, 1973
34. Nobak CR: Intraoperative monitoring. In Kaplan JA (ed): Thoracic Anesthesia, p 197. New York, Churchill-Livingstone, 1983
35. Smith NT, Hesseling KH, deWit B: Evaluation of two prototype devices producing non-invasive, pulsatile, calibrated blood pressure measurement from a finger. J Clin Monit 1:17, 1985
36. Petty C: Right radial artery pressure during mediastinoscopy. Anesth Analg 58:428, 1979
37. Gurman GM, Kriemerman S: Cannulation of big arteries in critically ill patients. Crit Care Med 13:217, 1985
38. Russell JA, Joel M, Hudson RJ et al: Prospective evaluation of radial and femoral artery catheterization sites in critically ill adults. Crit Care Med 11:936, 1983
39. Ehrenwerth J, Urban MK: Monitoring during thoracic surgery. In Brodsky JB (ed): Problems in Anesthesia, p 306. Vol 4, no 2, Philadelphia, JB Lippincott, 1990
40. Verweis J, Kester A, Stroes W et al: Comparison of 3 methods for measuring central venous pressure. Crit Care Med 14:288, 1986
41. Sznajder JI, Zveibil FR, Bitterman H et al: Central vein catheterization: Failure and complication rates by 3 percutaneous approaches. Arch Intern Med 146:259, 1986

42. Shah KB, Rao TLK, Laughlin S et al: A review of pulmonary artery catheterization in 6245 patients. Anesthesiology 61:271, 1984

43. Patel C, Laboy V, Venus B et al: Acute complications of pulmonary artery catheter insertion in critically ill patients. Crit Care Med 14:195, 1986

44. Jobes DR, Schwartz AJ, Greenhow E et al: Safer jugular vein cannulation: Recognition of arterial pressure and preferential use of the external jugular route. Anesthesiology 59:351, 1983

45. Keusch DJ, Winters S, Thys DM: The patient's position influences the incidence of dysrhythmias during pulmonary artery catheterization. Anesthesiology 70:582, 1989

46. Nadeau S, Noble WH: Misinterpretation of pressure measurements from the pulmonary artery catheter. Can Anaesth Soc J 33:352, 1986

47. Schmitt EA, Brannigan CO: Common artifacts of pulmonary artery pressures: Recognition and interpretation. J Clin Monit 2:4, 1986

48. Shah KB, Rao TLK, Laughlin S et al: A review of pulmonary artery catheterization in 6,245 patients. Anesthesiology 61:271, 1984

49. Raper R, Sibbald WJ: Misled by the wedge. Chest 89:427, 1986

50. Tuman KJ, Carroll G, Ivankovich AD: Pitfalls in interpretation of the pulmonary artery catheter data. J Cardiothorac Anesth 3:625, 1989

51. Kaul S: The interventricular septum in health and disease. Am Heart J 112:568, 1986

52. Jardin F, Farcot JC, Boisante L et al: Influence of PEEP on left ventricular performance. N Engl J Med 304:387, 1981

53. Cohen E, Eisenkraft JB, Thys D et al: Hemodynamics and oxygenation during OLA. Right vs left. Anesthesiology 63:3A, A566, 1985

54. Hines R, Barash PG: Right ventricular failure. In Kaplan JA (ed): Cardiac Anesthesia, 2nd ed, p 995. Orlando, Grune & Stratton, 1987

55. Zaidan J, Freniere S: Use of a pacing pulmonary artery catheter during cardiac surgery. Ann Thorac Surg 35:633, 1983

56. Thys DM, Cohen E, Eisenkraft J: Mixed venous oxygen saturation during thoracic anesthesia. Anesthesiology 69:1005, 1988

57. Guffin A, Girard D, Kaplan JA: Shivering following cardiac surgery: Hemodynamic changes and reversal. J Cardiothorac Anesth 1:24, 1987

58. Reinhart K, Moser N, Rudolph T et al: Accuracy of two mixed venous saturation catheters during long term use in critically ill patients. Anesthesiology 69:769, 1988

59. Pologe JA: Pulse oximetry. Technical aspects of machine design. In Tremper KK, Barker SJ (eds): Int Anesthesiol Clin, Advances in Oxygen Monitoring, p 137. Boston, Little Brown & Co, 1987

60. Eisenkraft JB: Pulse oximeter desaturation due to methemoglobinemia. Anesthesiology 68:279, 1988

61. Brodsky JB, Shulman MS, Swan M et al: Pulse oximetry during one-lung ventilation. Anesthesiology 63:212, 1985

62. Desiderio DP, Wong G, Shah N et al: A clinical evaluation of pulse oximetry during thoracic surgery. J Cardiothorac Anesth 4:30, 1990

63. Van Norman G, Cheney FW: Falsely elevated oximeter reading dangerous on one lung. Park Ridge, Illinois, Anesthesia Patient Safety Foundation Newsletter 4:23, 1989

64. Tremper KK, Konchigeri HN, Cullen BF et al: Transcutaneous monitoring of oxygen tension during one-lung anesthesia. J Thorac Cardiovasc Surg 88:22, 1984

65. Barker SJ, Tremper KK, Heitzmann HA: Continuous fiberoptic arterial oxygen tension in dogs. Crit Care Med 15:403, 1987

66. Barker SJ, Tremper KK, Hyatt J, Heitzmann H: Comparison of three oxygen monitors in detecting endobronchial intubation. J Clin Monit 4:240, 1988

67. Shafieha MA, Sit J, Kartha R et al: End-tidal CO_2 analyzers in proper positioning of double-lumen tubes. Anesthesiology 64:844, 1986

68. Riley RH, Marcy JH: Unsuspected endobronchial intubation—detection by continuous mass spectrometry. Anesthesiology 63:203, 1985

69. West JB, Dollery CT, Naimark A: Distribution of blood flow in isolated lung. Relation to vascular and alveolar pressures. J Appl Physiol 19:713, 1964

70. Marshall BE, Marshall C, Benumof JL et al: Hypoxic pulmonary vasoconstriction in dogs: Effects of lung segment size and oxygen tension. J Appl Physiol 51:1543, 1981

71. Ginsberg RJ: New Techniques for one lung anesthesia using an endobronchial blocker. J Thorac Cardiovasc Surg 32:542, 1981

72. Inoue H, Shohtsu A, Ogawa J et al: New device for one-lung anesthesia: Endotracheal tube with movable blocker. J Thorac Cardiovasc Surg 83:940, 1982

73. Hultgren BL, Krishna PR, Kamaya H: A new tube for one lung ventilation: Experience with the Univent tube. Anesthesiology 65:3A, A481, 1986

74. Karwande SV: A new tube for single lung ventilation. Chest 92:761, 1987

75. MacGillivay RG: Evaluation of a new tracheal tube with a movable bronchus blocker. Anaesthesia 43:687, 1988

76. Smith G, Hirsch N, Ehrenwerth J: Sight and sound: Can double-lumen endotracheal tubes be placed accurately without fiberoptic bronchoscopy? Br J Anaesth 58:1317, 1987

77. Benumof JL, Partridge BL, Salvatierra C et al: Margin of safety in positioning modern double-lumen endotracheal tubes. Anesthesiology 67:729, 1987

78. Guernelli N, Bragaglia RB, Briccoli A et al: Tracheobronchial rupture due to cuffed Carlens tubes. Thorac Surg 28:66, 1979

79. Wagner DL, Gammage GW, Wong ML: Tracheal rupture following the insertion of a disposable double-lumen endotracheal tube. Anesthesiology 63:698, 1985

80. Tarhan S, Lundborg RO: Carlens endobronchial catheter versus regular endobronchial tube during thoracic surgery: A comparison of blood gas tensions and pulmonary shunting. Can Anaesth Soc J 18:594, 1971

81. Kerr JH, Crampton Smith A, Prys-Roberts C et al: Observations during endobronchial anesthesia II, oxygenation. Br J Anaesth 46:84, 1974

82. Flacke JW, Thompson DS, Read RC: Influence of tidal volume and pulmonary artery occlusion on arterial oxygenation during endobronchial anesthesia. South Med J 69:619, 1976

83. Capan LM, Turndorf H, Patel K et al: Optimization of arterial oxygenation during one-lung anesthesia. Anesth Analg 59:847, 1980

84. Dantzker DR, Wagner PD, West JB: Instability of lung units with low V/Q ratio during O_2 breathing. J Appl Physiol 38:886, 1975

85. Lunding M, Fernandes A: Arterial oxygen tensions and acid-base status during thoracic anaesthesia. Acta Anaesthesiol Scand 11:43, 1967

86. Torda TA, McCulloch CH, O'Brinh HD et al: Pulmonary venous admixture during one-lung anaesthesia: Effect of inhaled oxygen tension and respiration rate. Anaesthesia 29:272, 1974

87. Jenkins J, Cameron EWJ, Milne AC et al: One-lung anaesthesia. Cardiovascular and respiratory function compared during conventional ventilation and HFJV. Anaesthesia 42:938, 1987

88. Cohen E, Eisenkraft JB, Thys DM et al: Oxygenation and hemodynamic changes during one-lung ventilation. J Cardiothorac Anesth 2:34, 1988

89. Katz JA, Larlane RG, Rairby HB et al: Pulmonary oxygen exchange during endobronchial anesthesia: Effect of tidal volume and PEEP. Anesthesiology 56:164, 1982

90. Goldiner PL, Carlon GC, Cvitkovic E et al: Factors influencing postoperative morbidity and mortality in patients treated with bleomycin. Br Med J 1:1664, 1978

91. Tarhan S, Lundborg RO: Effects of increased expiratory pressure on blood gas tensions and pulmonary shunting during thoracotomy with use of the Carlens catheter. Can Anaesth Soc J 17:4, 1970

92. Cohen E, Thys DM, Eisenkraft JB et al: PEEP during one lung anesthesia improves oxygenation in patients with low Pao_2. Anesth Analg 64:200, 1985

93. Alfery D, Benumof JL, Trousdale FR: Improving oxygenation during one lung ventilation: The effects of PEEP and blood flow restoration to the non-ventilated lung. Anesthesiology 55:381, 1981

94. Obara H, Tanaka O, Hoshino Y *et al:* One lung ventilation: The effect of positive end-expiratory pressure to the non-dependent and dependent lung. Anaesthesia 41:1007, 1986

95. Slinger P, Triolet W, Wilson J: Improving arterial oxygenation during one lung ventilation. Anesthesiology 68:291, 1988

96. Rees DI, Wansbrough SR: One-lung anesthesia and arterial oxygen tension during continuous insufflation of oxygen to the non-ventilated lung. Anesth Analg 61:501, 1982

97. Malmkvist G: Maintenance of oxygenation during one lung ventilation. Effect of intermittent reinflation of the collapsed lung with oxygen. Anesth Analg 68:763, 1989

98. Eisenkraft JB, Thys DM, Cohen E *et al:* CPAP and PEEP during one-lung ventilation with isoflurane. Anesthesiology 61:3A, A520, 1984

99. Hannenberg AA, Sotwicz PR, Pienes RS Jr *et al:* A device for applying CPAP to the non-ventilated upper lung during one-lung ventilation II. Anesthesiology 60:254, 1984

100. Thiagarajah S, Job C, Rao A: A device for applying CPAP to the non-ventilated upper lung during one-lung ventilation. Anesthesiology 60:253, 1984

101. Lyons TE: A simplified method of CPAP delivery to the non-ventilated lung during unilateral pulmonary ventilation. Anesthesiology 61:217, 1984

102. Arandia HY, Patel VU: PEEP and the Mapleson D Circuit. Anesthesiology 62:846, 1985

103. Brown DR, Kafer ER, Robertson VO *et al:* Improved oxygenation during thoracotomy with selective PEEP to the dependent lung. Anesth Analg 56:26, 1977

104. Nunn JF: Factors influencing the arterial oxygen tension during halothane anesthesia with spontaneous respiration. Br J Anaesth 36:327, 1964

105. Marshall BE, Cohen PJ, Klingenmaier CH *et al:* Pulmonary venous admixture before, during and after halothane: Oxygen anesthesia in man. J Appl Physiol 27:653, 1967

106. Von Euler US, Liljestrand G: Observations on the pulmonary arterial blood pressure in the cat. Acta Physiol Scand 12:301, 1946

107. Marshall BE, Marshall C, Benumof JL *et al:* Hypoxic pulmonary vasoconstriction in dogs: Effects of lung segment size and alveolar oxygen tensions. J Appl Physiol 51:1543, 1981

108. Domino KB, Wetstein L, Glasser SA *et al:* Influence of mixed venous oxygen tension (PvO$_2$) on blood flow to atelectatic lung. Anesthesiology 59:428, 1983

109. Benumof JL: One-lung ventilation and hypoxic pulmonary vasoconstriction: Implications for anesthetic management, Anesth Analg 64:821, 1985

110. Marshall C, Lindgren L, Marshall BE: Effects of halothane and isoflurane in rat lungs in vitro. Anesthesiology 60:304, 1984

111. Bjertnaes LJ: Hypoxia-induced vasoconstriction in isolated perfused lungs exposed to injectable or inhalational anaesthetics. Acta Anaesthesiol Scand 21:133, 1977

112. Mathers J, Benumof JL, Wahrenbrock EA: General anesthetics and regional HPV. Anesthesiology 46:111, 1977

113. Saidman LJ, Trousdale FR: Isoflurane does not inhibit HPV. Anesthesiology 57:A472, 1982

114. Gibbs JM, Johnson H: Lack of effect of morphine and buprenorphine on HPV in the isolated perfused cat lung and the perfused lobe of the dog lung. Br J Anaesth 50:1197, 1978

115. Domino KB, Borowec L, Alexander CM *et al:* Influence of isoflurane on HPV in dogs. Anesthesiology 64:423, 1986

116. Lumb PD, Silvay G, Weinreich AI *et al:* A comparison of the effects of continuous ketamine infusion and halothane on oxygenation during OLV in dogs. Can Anaesth Soc J 26:394, 1979

117. Bjertnaes LJ: Hypoxia-induced pulmonary vasoconstriction in man: Inhibition due to diethyl ether and halothane anaesthesia. Acta Anaesthesiol Scand 22:578, 1978

118. Jolin Carlsson A, Bindslev L, Hedenstierna G: Hypoxia-induced pulmonary vasoconstriction in the human lung. The effect of isoflurane anesthesia. Anesthesiology 66:312, 1987

119. Weinreich AI, Silvay G, Lumb PD: Continuous ketamine infusion for one-lung ventilation. Can Anaesth Soc J 27:485, 1980

120. Rees DI, Gaines GY: One-lung anesthesia—a comparison of pulmonary gas exchange during anesthesia with ketamine or enflurane. Anesth Analg 63:521, 1984

121. Rogers SM, Benumof JL: Halothane and isoflurane do not decrease Pao$_2$ during one-lung ventilation in intravenously anesthetized patients. Anesth Analg 64:946, 1985

122. Benumof JL, Augustine SD, Gibbons JA: Halothane and isoflurane only slightly impair arterial oxygenation during one-lung ventilation in patients undergoing thoracotomy. Anesthesiology 67:910, 1987

123. Marshall BE, Marshall C: Anesthesia and the pulmonary circulation. In Covino BJ, Fozzard HA, Rehder K *et al* (eds): Effects of Anesthesia, Clinical Physiology Series, p 121. Bethesda, American Physiological Society, 1985

124. Eisenkraft JB: Effects of anesthetics on the pulmonary circulation. Br J Anaesth 65:63, 1990

125. Van Keer L, Van Aken H, Vandermeersch E, Vermaut G: Propofol does not inhibit HPV in humans. J Clin Anesth 1:284, 1989

126. Chen L, Miller FL, Malmkvist G *et al:* High-dose almitrine bimesylate inhibits hypoxic pulmonary vasoconstriction in closed-chest dogs. Anesthesiology 67:534, 1987

127. Marshall C, Kim SD, Marshall BE: The actions of halothane, ibuprofen and BW 755C on hypoxic pulmonary vasoconstriction. Anesthesiology 66:537, 1987

128. Bindsley L, Cannon D, Sykes MK: Reversal of nitrous oxide-induced depression of HPV by lignocaine hydrochloride during collapse and ventilation hypoxaemia of the left lower lobe. Br J Anaesth 58:451, 1986

129. Frumin MJ, Epstein R, Cohen G: Apneic oxygenation in man. Anesthesiology 20:789, 1959

130. Fraoli RL, Sheffe LA, Steffanson JL: Pulmonary and cardiovascular effects of apneic oxygenation in man. Anesthesiology 39:588, 1973

131. Sanders RD: Two ventilating attachments for bronchoscopes. Delaware Med J 39:170, 1967

132. Giesecke AH, Gerbershagen H, Dortman C *et al:* Comparison of the ventilating and injection bronchoscopes. Anesthesiology 38:298, 1973

133. Carden E: Recent improvements in anesthetic techniques for use during bronchoscopy. Otol Rhinol Laryngol 83:777, 1974

134. Vourc'h G, Fishler M, Michon F *et al:* Manual jet ventilation vs high-frequency jet ventilation during laser resection of tracheo-bronchial stenosis. Br J Anaesth 55:973, 1983

135. Sackner MA: State of the art—bronchofiberscopy. Am Rev Respir Dis 111:62, 1975

136. Matsushima Y, Jones RL, King EG *et al:* Alterations in pulmonary mechanics and gas exchange during routine fiberoptic bronchoscopy. Chest 86:184, 1984

137. Satyanarayana T, Capan L, Ramanathan S *et al:* Bronchofiberscopic jet ventilation. Anesth Analg 59:350, 1980

138. Warner ME, Warner M, Leonard P: Anesthesia for neodymium-YAG laser resection of major airway obstructing tumors. Anesthesiology 60:230, 1984

139. Duckett JE, McDonnell TJ, Unger M *et al:* General anesthesia for Nd:YAG laser resection of obstructing endo-bronchial tumors using the rigid bronchoscope. Can Anaesth Soc J 32:67, 1985

140. Eisenkraft JB, Neustein SM: Anesthetic management of therapeutic procedures of the lungs and airway. In Kaplan JA (ed): Thoracic Anesthesia, 2nd ed, p 419. New York, Churchill-Livingstone, 1991

141. Watson CB: Fiberoptic bronchoscopy in thoracic anaesthesia. In Gotthard JW (ed): Thoracic Anaesthesia, p 33. London, Bailliere Tindall, 1987

142. Neuman G, Weingarten AE, Abramowitz RM *et al:* The anesthetic management of the patient with an anterior mediastinal mass. Anesthesiology 60:144, 1984

143. Ferrari LR, Bedford RF: General anesthesia prior to treatment of anterior mediastinal masses in pediatric cancer patients. Anesthesiology 72:991, 1990

144. Tinker TD, Crane DL: Safety of anesthesia for patients with anterior mediastinal masses: I (correspondence). Anesthesiology 73:1060, 1990

145. Zornow MH, Benumof JL: Safety of anesthesia for patients with anterior mediastinal masses: II (correspondence). Anesthesiology 73:1061, 1990

146. DeSoto H: Direct laryngoscopy as an aid to relieve airway obstruction in a patient with a mediastinal mass. Anesthesiology 67:116, 1987

147. Sibert K, Biondi JW, Hirsch NP: Spontaneous respiration during thoracotomy in a patient with a mediastinal mass. Anesth Analg 66:904, 1987

148. Carlens E: Mediastinoscopy: A method for inspection and tissue biopsy in the superior mediastinum. Dis Chest 36:343, 1959

149. Carlens E, Ericsson M, Levander-Lindgren M et al: Detector electrode introduced by mediastinoscopy for atrial triggered cardiac pacing. Br Heart J 39:1265, 1977

150. Morton JR, Guinn GA: Mediastinoscopy using local anesthesia. Am J Surg 122:696, 1971

151. Ashbaugh DG: Mediastinoscopy. Arch Surg 100:568, 1970

152. Roberts JT, Gissen AJ: Management of complications encountered during anesthesia for mediastinoscopy. Anesthesiol Rev 6:31, 1979

153. Lee J, Salvatore A: Innominate artery compression simulating cardiac arrest during mediastinoscopy. A case report. Anesth Analg 55:748, 1976

154. Barash PG, Tsai B, Kitahata LM: Acute tracheal collapse following mediastinoscopy. Anesthesiology 44:67, 1976

155. Vaughan RS: Anesthesia for mediastinoscopy. Anaesthesia 33:195, 1978

155a.Wakabayashi A: Expanded applications of diagnostic and therapeutic thoracoscopy. J Thorac Cardiovasc Surg 102:721, 1991

156. Faurschou P, Madsen G, Viskum K: Thoracoscopy: Influence of the procedure on some respiratory and cardiac values. Thorax 38:341, 1983

157. Malina JF, Nordstrom SG, Sjostrand UH et al: Clinical evaluation of high-frequency positive-pressure ventilation (HFPPV) in patients scheduled for open-chest surgery. Anesth Analg 60:324, 1981

158. Glenski JA, Crawford M, Rehder K: High-frequency small-volume ventilation during thoracic surgery. Anesthesiology 64:211, 1986

159. Wilks D, Schumann T, Riley R et al: Selective high-frequency jet ventilation of the operative lung improves oxygenation during thoracic surgery. Anesthesiology 63:A568, 1985

160. Nakatsuka M, Wetstein L, Keenan RL: Unilateral high frequency ventilation during one lung ventilation for thoracotomy. Ann Thorac Surg 46:654, 1988

161. Morgan BA, Perks D, Conacher ID et al: Combined unilateral HFJV and contralateral IPPV. Anaesthesia 42:975, 1987

162. Capan LM, Miller S, Patel KP: Pro: Application of CPAP to the non-dependent lung is preferable to HFV for optimal oxygenation during pulmonary surgery. J Cardiothorac Anesth 1:584, 1987

163. El-Baz N: Application of CPAP to the non-dependent lung is not preferable to HFV to optimize oxygenation during pulmonary surgery. J Cardiothorac Anesth 1:587, 1987

164. Rafferty TD, Palma J, Motoyama et al: Management of a bronchopleural fistula with differential lung ventilation and PEEP. Resp Care 25:654, 1980

165. Bishop MJ, Benson MS, Sato P et al: Comparison of high-frequency jet ventilation with conventional ventilation for bronchopleural fistula. Anesth Analg 66:833, 1987

166. Normandale JP: Bullous cystic lung disease. Anaesthesia 40:1182, 1985

167. McCarthy G, Coppel DL, Gibbons JR et al: High-frequency jet ventilation for bilateral bullectomy. Anaesthesia 42:411, 1987

168. Benumof JL: Sequential one-lung ventilation for bilateral bullectomy. Anesthesiology 67:268, 1987

169. Grillo HC: Carinal reconstruction. Ann Thorac Surg 34:357, 1984

170. Wilson RS: Anesthetic management of tracheal and esophageal surgery. In Kaplan JA (ed): Cardiovascular and Thoracic Anesthesia Update. Philadelphia, WB Saunders Co, 1990

171. Lippman M, Mok MS: Anesthetic management of pulmonary lavage in adults. Anesth Analg 56:661, 1977

172. Smith JC, Millen JE, Safar P et al: Intrathoracic pressure, pulmonary vascular pressures and gas exchange during pulmonary lavage. Anesthesiology 33:401, 1978

173. Cohen E, Eisenkraft JB: Bronchopulmonary lavage: Effects on oxygenation and hemodynamics. J Cardiothorac Anesth 4:119, 1990

174. Lippman M, Mok MS, Wasserman K: Anesthetic management for children with alveolar proteinosis using extracorporeal circulation. Br J Anaesth 49:173, 1977

175. Osserman KE, Genkins G: Studies in myasthenia gravis—review of a 20-year experience in over 1200 patients. Mount Sinai J Med 38:497, 1971

176. Engel AG: Myasthenia gravis and myasthenic syndromes. Ann Neurol 16:516, 1984

177. Eisenkraft JB: Myasthenia gravis and thymic surgery—anaesthetic considerations. In Gotthard JWW (ed): Thoracic Anaesthesiology, p 133. London, Bailliere Tindall, 1987

178. Buckingham JM, Howard FM, Bernatz PE: The value of thymectomy in myasthenia gravis. A computer-assisted matched study. Ann Surg 184:453, 1976

179. Papatestas AE, Genkins G, Kornfeld P et al: Effects of thymectomy in myasthenia gravis. Ann Surg 206:79, 1987

180. Eisenkraft JB, Neustein SM: Anesthesia for esophageal and mediastinal surgery. In Kaplan JA (ed): Thoracic Anesthesia, 2nd ed, p 389. New York, Churchill-Livingstone, 1991

181. Eisenkraft JB, Papatestas AE, Sivak M: Neuromuscular effects of halogenated agents in patients with myasthenia gravis. Anesthesiology 61:3A, A307, 1984

182. Nilsson E, Muller K: Neuromuscular effects of isoflurane in patients with myasthenia gravis. Acta Anaesthesiol Scand 34:126, 1990

183. Smith CE, Donati F, Bevan DR: Cumulative dose-response curves for atracurium in patients with myasthenia gravis. Can J Anaesth 36:402, 1989

184. Eisenkraft JB, Book WJ, Papatestas AE, Hubbard M: Resistance to succinylcholine in myasthenia gravis: A dose-response study. Anesthesiology 69:760, 1988

185. Baraka A, Tabboush Z: Neuromuscular response to succinylcholine-vecuronium sequence in three myasthenic patients undergoing thymectomy. Anesth Analg 72:827, 1991

186. Mora CT, Eisenkraft JB, Papatestas AE: Intravenous dantrolene in a patient with myasthenia gravis. Anesthesiology 64:371, 1986

187. Gracey DR, Divertie MB, Howard FM: Mechanical ventilation for respiratory failure in myasthenia gravis. Mayo Clin Proc 58:597, 1983

188. Eisenkraft JB, Papatestas AE, Kahn CH et al: Predicting the need for postoperative mechanical ventilation in myasthenia gravis. Anesthesiology 65:79, 1986

189. Leventhal R, Orkin FK, Hirsch RA: Prediction of the need for postoperative mechanical ventilation in myasthenia gravis. Anesthesiology 53:26, 1980

190. Younger DS, Brawn NMT, Jaretzski A: Myasthenia gravis: Determinants for independent ventilation after transsternal thymectomy. Neurology 34:336, 1984

191. Foldes FF, Nagashima H: Myasthenia gravis and anesthesia. In Oyama T (ed): Endocrinology and the Anaesthetist. Monographs in Anesthesiology, p 171. New York, Elsevier, 1983

192. Burgess FW, Wilcosky B: Thoracic epidural anesthesia for transsternal thymectomy in myasthenia gravis. Anesth Analg 69:529, 1989

193. Gorback MS: Analgesic management after thymectomy. Anesthesiol Report 2:262, 1990

194. Telford RJ, Hollway TE: The myasthenic syndrome: Anesthesia in a patient treated with 3.4 diaminopyridine. Br J Anaesth 64:363, 1990

195. Downs JB: Postoperative respiratory care. In Kaplan JA (ed): Thoracic Anesthesia, p 635. New York, Churchill-Livingstone, 1983

196. Hirschler-Schultz CJ, Hylkema BS, Beyer RW: Mechanical ventilation for acute postoperative respiratory failure after surgery for bronchial carcinoma. Thorax 40:387, 1985

197. Cane RD, Shapiro B: Mechanical ventilatory support. JAMA 254:87, 1985

198. Gallagher C, Slader RN, Lubarsky D: Thoracotomy. Postoperative complications. In Brodsky JB (ed): Thoracic Anesthesia. Probl Anesth 4:393, 1990

199. Bennett RL, Battenhorst RL, Graves D et al: Patient-controlled analgesia—a new concept of postoperative relief. Ann Surg 195:700, 1982

200. Bennett RC, Baumann TJ, Graves DA, Griffen WD Jr: Patient-controlled analgesia and analgesic outcome, nocturnal sleep, and spontaneous activity. Surg Forum 35:57, 1987

201. Lange MP, Dahn MS, Jacobs LA: Patient-controlled analgesia versus intermittent analgesia dosing. Heart Lung 17:495, 1988

202. Urquhart ML, Klapp K, White PF: Patient-controlled analgesia: A comparison of intravenous versus subcutaneous hydromorphone. Anesthesiology 69:428, 1988

203. Kaplan JA, Miller ED, Gallagher EG: Postoperative analgesia for thoracotomy patients. Anesth Analg 54:773, 1975

204. Faust RJ, Nauss LA: Postthoracotomy intercostal block: Comparison of its effects on pulmonary function with those of intramuscular meperidine. Anesth Analg 55:542, 1976

205. Fleming WH, Sarafian LB: Kindness pays dividends: The medical benefits of intercostal nerve block following thoracotomy. J Thorac Cardiovasc Surg 74:273, 1977

206. Toledo-Pereyra LH, DeMeester TR: Prospective randomized evaluation of intrathoracic intercostal nerve block with bupivacaine on postoperative ventilatory function. Ann Thorac Surg 27:203, 1979

207. Gallo JA, Lebowitz PW, Battit GE et al: Comparison of intercostal nerve blocks performed under direct vision during thoracotomy. J Thorac Cardiovasc Surg 86:628, 1983

208. Rastelli L, Movilia P, Boss L et al: Management of pain after thoracotomy: A technique of multiple intercostal nerve blocks. Anesthesiology 61:353, 1984

209. Sabanathan S, Mearns AJ, Bickford Smith PJ et al: Efficacy of continuous extrapleural intercostal nerve block on postthoracotomy pain and pulmonary mechanics. Br J Surg 77:221, 1990

210. Kolvenbach LJ, Lauven PM, Schneider B, Kunath U: Repetitive intercostal nerve block via catheter for postoperative pain relief after thoracotomy. Thorac Cardiovasc Surg 37:273, 1989

211. Safran D, Kuhlman G, Orhand EE et al: Continuous intercostal blockade with lidocaine after thoracic surgery. Clinical and pharmacokinetic study. Anesth Analg 70:345, 1990

212. Glynn CJ, Lloyd JW, Barnard JD: Cryoanalgesia in the management of pain after thoracotomy. Thorax 34:325, 1980

213. Maiwand O, Makey AR, Rees A: Cryoanalgesia after thoracotomy. Improvement of technique and review of 600 cases. J Thorac Cardiovasc Surg 92:291, 1986

214. Johannesen N, Madsen G, Ahlburg P: Neurological sequelae after cryoanalgesia for thoracotomy pain relief. Ann Chir Gynaecol 79:108, 1990

215. Shulman MS: Managing post-thoracotomy pain. In Brodsky JB (ed): Problems in Anesthesia, p 376. Vol 4, no 2, Philadelphia, JB Lippincott, 1990

216. Shafe H, Chamberlain M, Natajan KN et al: Intrapleural bupivacaine for early post-thoracotomy analgesia—comparison with bupivacaine intercostal block and cryofreezing. J Thorac Cardiovasc Surg 38:38, 1990

217. Shulman M, Sandler AN, Bradley JW et al: Post-thoracotomy pain and pulmonary function following epidural and systemic morphine. Anesthesiology 61:564, 1984

218. Whiting WG, Sandler AN, Lau LC et al: Analgesic and respiratory effects of epidural sufentanil in post-thoracotomy patients. Anesthesiology 69:36, 1988

219. Melendez J, Cirella J, Delphin E: Lumbar epidural fentanyl analgesia after thoracic surgery. J Cardiothorac Anesth 3:150, 1989

220. Whiting WG, Sandler AN, Lau LC, Choraz PM: Analgesia and respiratory effects of epidural sufentanil in post-thoracotomy patients. Anesthesiology 69:36, 1988

221. Wells DG, Davies G: Profound central nervous system depression from epidural fentanyl for extracorporeal shock wave lithotripsy. Anesthesiology 69:1017, 1988

222. Etches RC, Sandler AN, Daley MD: Respiratory depression and spinal opioids. Can J Anaesth 36:165, 1989

223. Hasenbos MA, Gielen MH, Bos J et al: High thoracic epidural sufentanil for post-thoracotomy pain: Influence of epinephrine as an adjuvant—a double blind study. Anesthesiology 69:1017, 1988

224. Shulman MS, Wakerlin G, Yamaguchi L, Brodsky JB: Experience with epidural hydromorphone for post thoracotomy pain relief. Anesth Analg 66:1331, 1987

225. Wust HS, Bromage PR: Delayed respiratory arrest after epidural hydromorphone. Anaesthesia 42:404, 1987

226. Rawal N, Schoff U, Dahlstrom B et al: Influence of naloxone infusion on analgesia and respiratory depression following epidural morphine. Anesthesiology 64:194, 1986

227. Latasch L, Probst S, Dudziak R: Reversal by nalbuphine of respiratory depression caused by fentanyl. Anesth Analg 63:814, 1984

228. Gray JR, Fromme GA, Nauss LA et al: Intrathoracic morphine for post-thoracotomy pain. Anesth Analg 65:873, 1986

229. Grant GJ, Ramanathan S, Turndorf H: Epidural fentanyl reduces isoflurane requirements during thoracotomy (Abstract). Anesthesiology 71:668, 1989

230. Cohen E, Neustein SM, Ali J, Thys DM: Intrathecal morphine reduces post thoracotomy meperidine requirements (Abstract). Anesthesiology 73:A801, 1990

231. Wynands JE, Casey WF, Ralley FE et al: The role of intrathecal morphine in the anesthetic management of patients undergoing coronary artery bypass surgery. J Cardiothorac Anesth 1:510, 1987

232. Reistad F, Stromskag KE: Interpleural catheter in the management of postoperative pain, a preliminary report. Reg Anaesth 11:89, 1986

233. Symreng T, Gomez MN, Johnson B et al: Intrapleural bupivacaine—technical considerations and intraoperative use. J Cardiothorac Anesth 3:139, 1989

234. El-Baz N, Penfield FL, Ivankovic AD et al: Intrapleural infusion of local anesthetic: A word of caution. Anesthesiology 68:809, 1988

235. Rosenberg PH, Scheinin BWA, Lepantalo MJ et al: Continuous intrapleural infusion of bupivacaine for analgesia after thoracotomy. Anesthesiology 67:811, 1987

236. Reddy Kanbam J, Hammon J, Parris WC et al: Intrapleural analgesia for post-thoracotomy pain and blood levels of bupivacaine following intrapleural injection. Can J Anaesth 36:106, 1989

237. Symreng T, Gomez MN, Rossi N: Intrapleural bupivacaine and saline after thoracotomy—effects on pain and lung function—a double blind study. J Cardiothorac Anesth 3:144, 1989

238. Bartlett RH, Gazzaniga AB, Geraghty TR: Respiratory maneuvers to prevent postoperative pulmonary complications. JAMA 224:1017, 1973

239. Iverson LI, Ecker RR, Fox HE et al: A comparison study of IPPB, the incentive spirometer and blow bottles: The prevention of atelectasis following cardiac surgery. Ann Thorac Surg 25:197, 1978

240. Andersen JB, Olesen KP, Eikard B et al: Periodic CPAP by mask in the treatment of atelectasis. Eur J Respir Dis 61:20, 1980

241. Altschule M: Reflections on Starling's laws of the heart. Chest 89:444, 1986

242. Prewitt R, Ghignone M: Treatment of right ventricular dysfunction in acute respiratory failure. Crit Care Med 5:346, 1983

243. Beck-Nielsen J, Sorenson HR, Astroup P: Atrial fibrillation following thoracotomy for noncardiac disease; in particular cancer of the lung. Acta Med Scand 193:425, 1973

244. Krowke MJ, Pairolero PC, Trustek VF et al: Cardiac dysrhythmia following pneumonectomy: Clinical correlates and prognostic significance. Chest 91:490, 1987

245. Ritchie J, Bowe P, Gibbons JRP: Prophylactic digitalization for thoracotomy: A Reassessment. Ann Thorac Surg 50:86, 1990

246. Shields TW, Uyiki GT: Digitalization for prevention of ar-

rhythmias following pulmonary surgery. Surg Gynecol Obstet 126:743, 1968

247. Burman SO: The prophylactic use of digitalis before thoracotomy. Ann Thorac Surg 14:359, 1972

248. Shields TW, Unik GT: Digitalization for prevention of arrhythmias following pulmonary surgery. Surg Gynecol Obstet 126:743, 1968

249. Morganroth J, Horowitz LN, Anderson J et al: Comparative efficacy and tolerance of esmolol to propranolol for control of supraventricular tachyarrhythmias. Am J Cardiol 56:335, 1985

250. Dyson A, Isaac PA, Pennant JH et al: Esmolol attenuates cardiovascular responses to extubation. Anesth Analg 71:675, 1990.

251. Helfman SM, Gold MI, DeLisser EA, Herrington CA: Which drug prevents tachycardia and hypertension associated with tracheal intubation: Lidocaine, fentanyl, or esmolol? Anesth Analg 72:482, 1991

252. Hankins JR, Miller JE, Atlar S et al: Bronchopleural fistula: Thirteen-year experience with 77 cases. J Thorac Cardiovasc Surg 76:755, 1978

253. Roth MD, Wright JW, Bellamy PE: Gas flow through a bronchopleural fistula: Measuring the effects of high-frequency jet ventilation and chest tube suction. Chest 93:210, 1988

254. Albeda SM, Hanssen-Flaschen JH, Taylor E et al: Evaluation of high-frequency jet ventilation in patients with bronchopleural fistulas by quantitation of the airleak. Anesthesiology 63:551, 1985

255. Feely TW, Keating D, Nishimura J: Independent lung ventilation using high-frequency ventilation in the management of bronchopleural fistula. Anesthesiology 69:420, 1988

256. Seyfer AE, Grammer NY, Bogumill GP et al: Upper extremity neuropathies after cardiac surgery. J Hand Surg 10:16, 1985

257. Khanam T, Branthwaite MA: Arterial oxygenation during one-lung anesthesia (1): A study in man. Anaesthesia 28:132, 1973

258. Aalto-Setala M, Heinonen J, Salorinne Y: Cardiorespiratory function during thoracic anesthesia: Comparison of two-lung ventilation and one-lung ventilation with and without PEEP. Acta Anesthesiol Scand 19:287, 1975

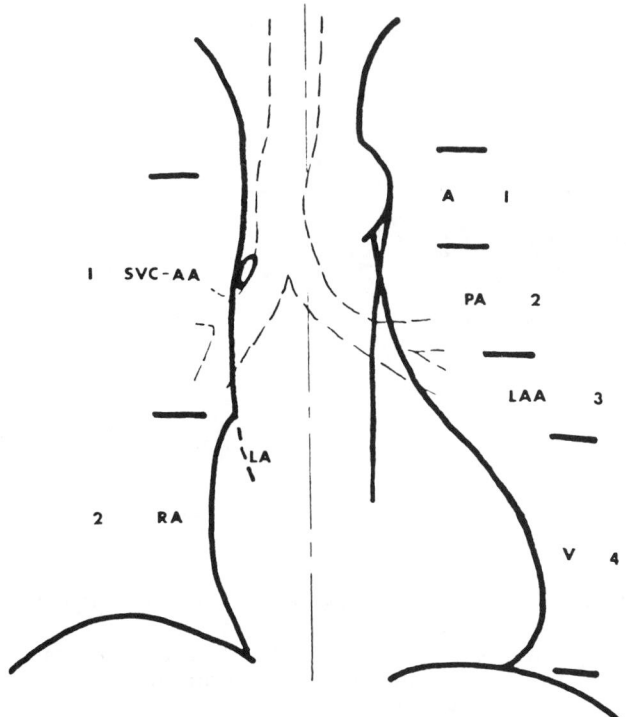

Figure 35-2. The frontal chest radiograph in a diagrammatic view. (A = the aortic arch, PA = the main pulmonary artery, V = the left ventricle, LAA = the left atrial appendage, RA = the right atrium, and SVC-AA = the superior vena cava or aortic segment.) (From New York Heart Association: Nomenclature and Criteria for Diagnosis of Disease of the Heart and Great Vessels, 8th ed. Boston, Little, Brown and Company, 1973, with permission of the New York Heart Association and the publisher. Copyright 1973.)

terior and septal papillary muscles receive chordae from the posterior and medial tricuspid valve leaflets.

Right Ventricle

The right ventricle (RV) is a pocket wrapped around one third of the left ventricle (LV). Its muscle fibers are continuous with those of the LV. Anatomically it consists of inferoposterior inflow (sinus) and anterosuperior outflow (infundibular) portions divided by the crista supraventricularis.

The inflow portion contains prominent muscle bands (moderator, septal, and parietal) and muscle bundles known as trabeculae carneae. The crista supraventricularis also joins the interventricular septum and LV to the right ventricular free wall and may be important in the integration of right and left ventricular function.[4]

Pulmonary Artery and Peripheral Pulmonary Circulation

The pulmonic valve separates the right ventricular infundibulum from the main pulmonary artery (PA). It is a trileaflet valve (right, left, and anterior cusps), normally about 4 cm^2 in area (see Fig. 35-3). As it originates from the superior portion of the RV, the PA passes backward and upward under the aorta before it bifurcates into the right and left pulmonary arteries. On the frontal chest x-ray the superior portion of the left cardiac silhouette is the aorta and just beneath is the main PA (see Fig. 35-2). The remnant of the fetal ductus arteriosus, the ligamentum arteriosum, connects the upper aspect of the bifurcation to the inferior aortic surface. The pulmonary arteries and veins of the lower lobes are normally larger and more prominent than those of the upper lobes. Pulmonary arteries branch into arterioles and thence into capillaries, which spread over the alveolar surfaces between two alveolar endothelial layers.

The size of the peripheral pulmonary vessels indicates pulmonary blood volume and flow. With left-to-right cardiac shunts, the main pulmonary artery and hilar vessels are prominent. With pulmonary hypertension, however, dilation of the main pulmonary artery and abrupt tapering of the peripheral pulmonary vessels are noted.

Left Atrium

The left atrium (LA) is slightly larger than the right and receives one or two pulmonary veins on its left and two or three on its right side. Enlargement of the LA appears on chest x-ray as a straightening of the left heart border, a double density near the right heart border, or displacement of the left mainstem bronchus (see Fig. 35-2). Normally the margins of the LA are the right main and intermediate bronchi and the left main and left lower lobe bronchi.

Leaving the LA, blood traverses the mitral valve. It consists of four cusps: (1) a large anterior (aortic) cusp; (2) a large posterior (mural) cusp; and (3) two small septal or commissural cusps. Functionally, these four cusps form two major leaflets, the anteromedial and posterolateral. The area

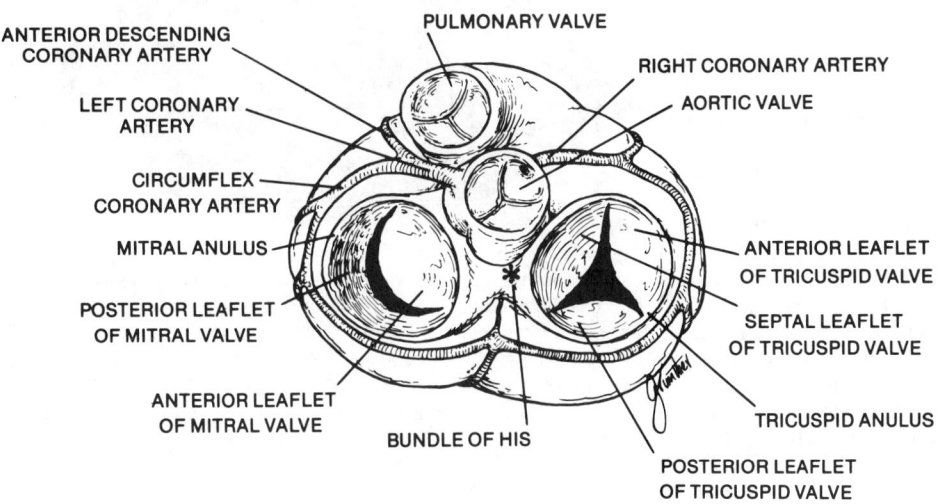

Figure 35-3. A coronal section of the heart at the level of the valves. The close association of all four cardiac valves is easily recognized. The coronary arteries, arising from the coronary cusps of the aortic valve, pass between the aorta and the pulmonic valve. The left coronary artery divides into the anterior descending and circumflex branches. (Reprinted with permission from Lowe DA: Abnormalities of the atrioventricular valves. In Lake CL (ed): Pediatric Cardiac Anesthesia, p 300. East Norwalk, Appleton and Lange, 1988.)

35

Carol L. Lake

Cardiovascular Anatomy and Physiology

A basic knowledge of cardiovascular anatomy and physiology is essential for the anesthesiologist caring for patients during either cardiac or noncardiac surgery. This chapter focuses on those aspects of cardiovascular anatomy, physiology, and pathophysiology that are important to perioperative management.

ANATOMY

Heart

The four-chambered heart is located in the middle mediastinum beneath the sternum and the 3rd through 5th ribs. It is surrounded laterally by the lungs and inferiorly by the diaphragm. Although its weight and size vary with age, gender, and other factors, the average heart weighs 275–325 g. A fibrous skeleton provides the framework for the cardiac valves and musculature. The framework includes the central fibrous body, which unites the mitral and tricuspid valves with the aortic root; the left fibrous trigone, which forms the annuli of the mitral and tricuspid valves; and the membranous portion of the interventricular septum. The functional anatomy of the heart and great vessels is easily visualized using transesophageal echocardiography[1] (Fig. 35-1).

Right Atrium

Systemic veins drain into the right atrium (RA) via the superior vena cava (SVC), inferior vena cava (IVC), and the coronary sinus. The RA consists of two parts: (1) a thin-walled trabeculated portion, the right auricle, which is separated by a ridge of muscle, the crista terminalis, from (2) the smooth-walled portion into which the SVC and IVC enter. On a frontal chest x-ray the right upper portion of the cardiac silhouette is the SVC (or ascending aorta in older patients) (Fig. 35-2). At the junction of the SVC with the RA is the sinoatrial node. The ostium of the IVC is guarded by the eustachian valve.[2] A third opening in the RA is the coronary sinus; its ostium is guarded by the thebesian valve.[3] The right and left atria are separated by the interatrial septum with its central ovoid portion, the fossa ovalis, the remnant of the fetal foramen ovale. The medial wall of

the RA is slightly indented by the torus aorticus, composed of the posterior and right coronary cusps of the aortic valve.

As blood leaves the RA, it passes through the tricuspid valve, which directs it anteriorly, inferiorly, and to the left toward the right ventricular outflow tract. As its name implies, the tricuspid valve consists of three leaflets—anterior, posterior, and medial—constituting an area of 8–11 cm^2 (Fig. 35-3). The anterior leaflet, the largest, is attached to the crista supraventricularis (described below) and controlled by the anterior papillary muscle, which originates from a prominent intraventricular muscle, the moderator band, and the anteriolateral ventricular wall. The septal leaflet attaches to the junction of the interatrial and interventricular septa.[4] The posterior leaflet originates from the diaphragmatic portion of the right ventricle. Connecting the papillary muscles to the valve leaflets are strong, fibrous structures known as the chordae tendineae. The small pos-

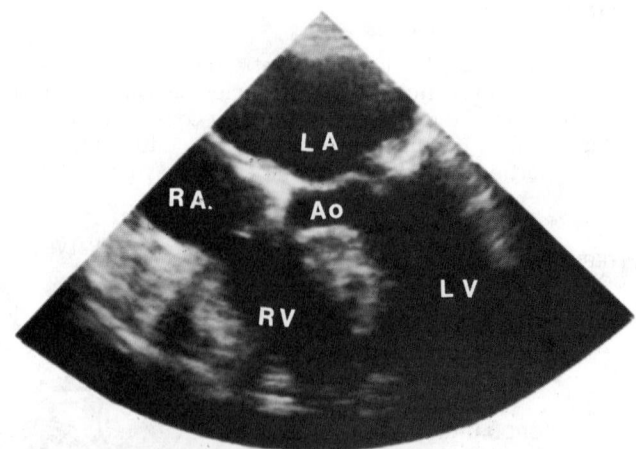

Figure 35-1. The functional anatomy of the heart is easily visualized using either transthoracic or transesophageal echocardiography. All four cardiac chambers, the atrioventricular valves, aortic outflow track, and interatrial and interventricular septa are seen in this transesophageal view. When viewed in real time, the function of both valves and ventricles can be assessed. (LA = left atrium, RA = right atrium, Ao = aorta, RV = right ventricle, and LV = left ventricle.)

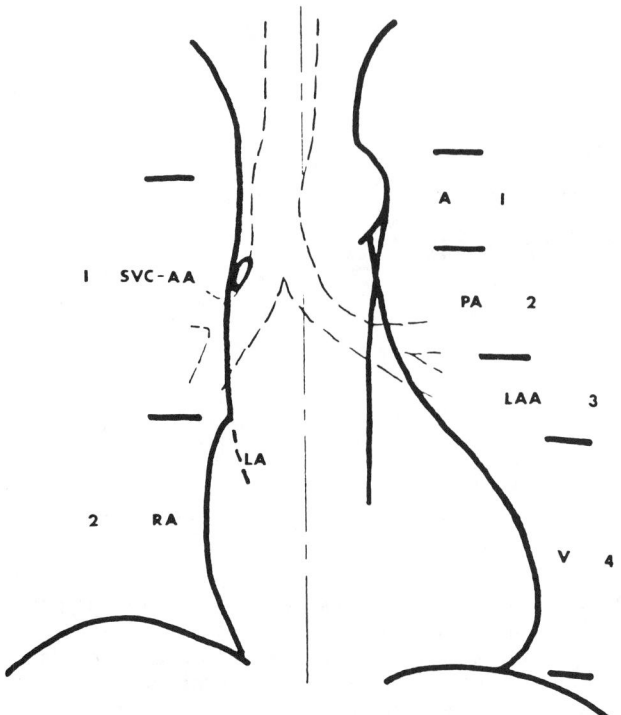

Figure 35-2. The frontal chest radiograph in a diagrammatic view. (A = the aortic arch, PA = the main pulmonary artery, V = the left ventricle, LAA = the left atrial appendage, RA = the right atrium, and SVC-AA = the superior vena cava or aortic segment.) (From New York Heart Association: Nomenclature and Criteria for Diagnosis of Disease of the Heart and Great Vessels, 8th ed. Boston, Little, Brown and Company, 1973, with permission of the New York Heart Association and the publisher. Copyright 1973.)

terior and septal papillary muscles receive chordae from the posterior and medial tricuspid valve leaflets.

Right Ventricle

The right ventricle (RV) is a pocket wrapped around one third of the left ventricle (LV). Its muscle fibers are continuous with those of the LV. Anatomically it consists of inferoposterior inflow (sinus) and anterosuperior outflow (infundibular) portions divided by the crista supraventricularis. The inflow portion contains prominent muscle bands (moderator, septal, and parietal) and muscle bundles known as trabeculae carneae. The crista supraventricularis also joins the interventricular septum and LV to the right ventricular free wall and may be important in the integration of right and left ventricular function.[4]

Pulmonary Artery and Peripheral Pulmonary Circulation

The pulmonic valve separates the right ventricular infundibulum from the main pulmonary artery (PA). It is a trileaflet valve (right, left, and anterior cusps), normally about 4 cm² in area (see Fig. 35-3). As it originates from the superior portion of the RV, the PA passes backward and upward under the aorta before it bifurcates into the right and left pulmonary arteries. On the frontal chest x-ray the superior portion of the left cardiac silhouette is the aorta and just beneath is the main PA (see Fig. 35-2). The remnant of the fetal ductus arteriosus, the ligamentum arteriosum, connects the upper aspect of the bifurcation to the inferior aortic surface. The pulmonary arteries and veins of the lower lobes are normally larger and more prominent than those of the upper lobes. Pulmonary arteries branch into arterioles and thence into capillaries, which spread over the alveolar surfaces between two alveolar endothelial layers.

The size of the peripheral pulmonary vessels indicates pulmonary blood volume and flow. With left-to-right cardiac shunts, the main pulmonary artery and hilar vessels are prominent. With pulmonary hypertension, however, dilation of the main pulmonary artery and abrupt tapering of the peripheral pulmonary vessels are noted.

Left Atrium

The left atrium (LA) is slightly larger than the right and receives one or two pulmonary veins on its left and two or three on its right side. Enlargement of the LA appears on chest x-ray as a straightening of the left heart border, a double density near the right heart border, or displacement of the left mainstem bronchus (see Fig. 35-2). Normally the margins of the LA are the right main and intermediate bronchi and the left main and left lower lobe bronchi.

Leaving the LA, blood traverses the mitral valve. It consists of four cusps: (1) a large anterior (aortic) cusp; (2) a large posterior (mural) cusp; and (3) two small septal or commissural cusps. Functionally, these four cusps form two major leaflets, the anteromedial and posterolateral. The area

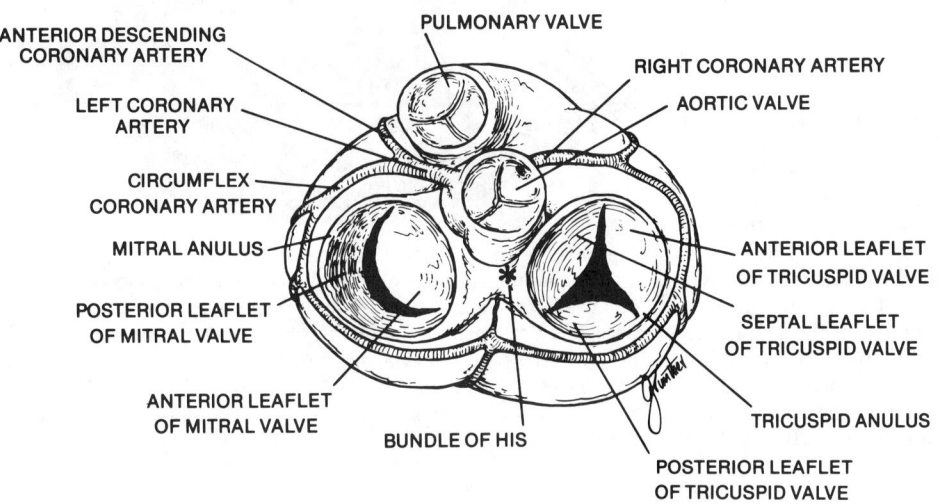

Figure 35-3. A coronal section of the heart at the level of the valves. The close association of all four cardiac valves is easily recognized. The coronary arteries, arising from the coronary cusps of the aortic valve, pass between the aorta and the pulmonic valve. The left coronary artery divides into the anterior descending and circumflex branches. (Reprinted with permission from Lowe DA: Abnormalities of the atrioventricular valves. In Lake CL (ed): Pediatric Cardiac Anesthesia, p 300. East Norwalk, Appleton and Lange, 1988.)

35

Carol L. Lake

Cardiovascular Anatomy and Physiology

A basic knowledge of cardiovascular anatomy and physiology is essential for the anesthesiologist caring for patients during either cardiac or noncardiac surgery. This chapter focuses on those aspects of cardiovascular anatomy, physiology, and pathophysiology that are important to perioperative management.

ANATOMY

Heart

The four-chambered heart is located in the middle mediastinum beneath the sternum and the 3rd through 5th ribs. It is surrounded laterally by the lungs and inferiorly by the diaphragm. Although its weight and size vary with age, gender, and other factors, the average heart weighs 275–325 g. A fibrous skeleton provides the framework for the cardiac valves and musculature. The framework includes the central fibrous body, which unites the mitral and tricuspid valves with the aortic root; the left fibrous trigone, which forms the annuli of the mitral and tricuspid valves; and the membranous portion of the interventricular septum. The functional anatomy of the heart and great vessels is easily visualized using transesophageal echocardiography[1] (Fig. 35-1).

Right Atrium

Systemic veins drain into the right atrium (RA) via the superior vena cava (SVC), inferior vena cava (IVC), and the coronary sinus. The RA consists of two parts: (1) a thin-walled trabeculated portion, the right auricle, which is separated by a ridge of muscle, the crista terminalis, from (2) the smooth-walled portion into which the SVC and IVC enter. On a frontal chest x-ray the right upper portion of the cardiac silhouette is the SVC (or ascending aorta in older patients) (Fig. 35-2). At the junction of the SVC with the RA is the sinoatrial node. The ostium of the IVC is guarded by the eustachian valve.[2] A third opening in the RA is the coronary sinus; its ostium is guarded by the thebesian valve.[3] The right and left atria are separated by the interatrial septum with its central ovoid portion, the fossa ovalis, the remnant of the fetal foramen ovale. The medial wall of

the RA is slightly indented by the torus aorticus, composed of the posterior and right coronary cusps of the aortic valve.

As blood leaves the RA, it passes through the tricuspid valve, which directs it anteriorly, inferiorly, and to the left toward the right ventricular outflow tract. As its name implies, the tricuspid valve consists of three leaflets—anterior, posterior, and medial—constituting an area of 8–11 cm^2 (Fig. 35-3). The anterior leaflet, the largest, is attached to the crista supraventricularis (described below) and controlled by the anterior papillary muscle, which originates from a prominent intraventricular muscle, the moderator band, and the anteriolateral ventricular wall. The septal leaflet attaches to the junction of the interatrial and interventricular septa.[4] The posterior leaflet originates from the diaphragmatic portion of the right ventricle. Connecting the papillary muscles to the valve leaflets are strong, fibrous structures known as the chordae tendineae. The small pos-

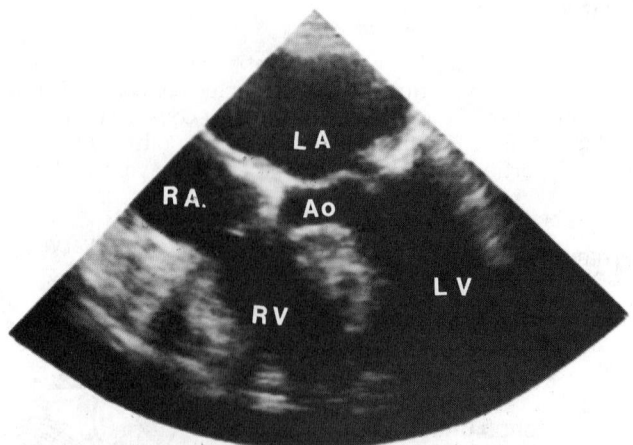

Figure 35-1. The functional anatomy of the heart is easily visualized using either transthoracic or transesophageal echocardiography. All four cardiac chambers, the atrioventricular valves, aortic outflow track, and interatrial and interventricular septa are seen in this transesophageal view. When viewed in real time, the function of both valves and ventricles can be assessed. (LA = left atrium, RA = right atrium, Ao = aorta, RV = right ventricle, and LV = left ventricle.)

of the mitral valve is about 6–8 cm² in adults. Valves of less than 1 cm² are severely stenotic. As in the tricuspid valve, two groups of papillary muscles and chordae tendineae loosely anchor the leaflets to the apical and middle left ventricular myocardium. The blood supply to the chordae and papillary muscles is often quite tenuous.[5,6]

Left Ventricle

Normally the LV is thicker (8–15 mm) and more densely trabeculated than the right. Its internal dimension is also greater, about 4.5 cm compared with 3.5 cm for the RV.[7] The interventricular septum, with its membranous superior portion near the aortic valve and muscular inferior portion, divides the RV from the LV. Separating the membranous and the muscular portions of the septum is the limbus marginalis.[8]

Aorta and Its Branches

The aortic valve is adjacent to the mitral valve within the left ventricle, separated only by the fibrous tissue framework that comprises the annuli of both valves (see Fig. 35-3). Three pocket-like structures of unequal size, the right and left (coronary) and posterior (noncoronary) cusps, form the aortic valve. A normal aortic valve is about 3–4 cm² in area, but the area, weight, and volume of the cusps increase with age and heart weight.[9] In the center of each cusp is a small nodule, the nodule of Arantius; the free edge of the cusp is termed the lunula. Coaptation of the nodules during ventricular diastole prevents regurgitation. The aorta at the level of the valve dilates to form the sinuses of Valsalva in which the coronary ostia are located.

The ascending aorta, just beyond the aortic valve, has no branches. Major branches of the aorta, the innominate, left carotid, and left subclavian arteries, arise from the aortic arch. The innominate artery subdivides into the right subclavian and right carotid arteries.

Arterial Circulation

The anatomy of many peripheral arteries is important to anesthesiologists, either for direct arterial cannulation or as a target to be avoided during venous cannulation (Fig. 35-4A). Other portions of the peripheral circulation are important to the prevention of complications arising from certain surgical procedures. Among these are the coronary, carotid, cerebral, renal, bronchial, and spinal cord circulations.

Coronary Circulation. Two coronary arteries, right and left, originating from the sinuses of Valsalva in the aortic valve, supply arterial blood to the myocardium. The left coronary artery usually has a short common or left main coronary artery before bifurcation into anterior descending and circumflex branches. The anterior descending artery courses downward over the anterior left ventricular wall and supplies the interventricular groove through its diagonal and septal perforator branches. Occlusive disease in the anterior descending distribution produces ischemic electrocardiographic changes in leads V_3 to V_5. The circumflex branch follows the atrioventricular groove, giving off the obtuse marginal branch and supplying all the posterior LV and part of the right ventricular wall.[10] Electrocardiographic changes resulting from circumflex coronary artery disease are seen in leads I and aV_L (Fig. 35-5 and Table 35-1).

From the right coronary artery the sinus node artery and atrioventricular nodal artery originate. The right atrial myocardium is also supplied by the sinus node artery. The right coronary artery terminates on the diaphragmatic surface of the heart as the posterior descending artery[11] (Fig. 35-5). The blood supply to the atrioventricular node and common bundle of His is the atrioventricular branch of the right coronary artery (in 90% of hearts) and the septal perforating branches of the left anterior descending coronary artery (in 10% of hearts).[12,13] Branches to the interatrial septum and posterior interventricular septum also arise from the atrioventricular nodal artery. The right bundle branch and the left anterior fascicle are supplied by branches of the left anterior descending artery but can be supplied by the atrioventricular nodal artery.[12,13] Both the left anterior and posterior descending coronary arteries supply the posterior fascicle.[13] Ischemic changes in electrocardiogram leads II, III, and aV_F as well as conduction abnormalities are present with significant right coronary artery occlusion. However, the amount of myocardium jeopardized by a clinically significant coronary stenosis cannot be completely determined from angiographic evaluation. Although perfusion defects usually increase with increasing stenosis, the involved myocardium is heterogeneous in different subjects.[14]

Coronary Dominance. Descriptions of the coronary circulation often refer to the dominance of one or the other coronary artery. Dominance is determined by which artery crosses the crux or junction between atria and ventricles to supply the posterior descending coronary branch. In about 50% of humans, the right coronary artery is dominant, in 20%, the left, and in 30%, a balanced pattern exists. Areas of the myocardium affected by stenosis or occlusion of individual coronary arteries are listed in Table 35-1. Collateral vessels may develop between the major coronary arteries in response to myocardial ischemia.[15]

Cerebral Circulation. The cerebral circulation consists of the anterior communicating arteries, the internal carotid arteries, the posterior communicating arteries, and the vertebral arteries. Together these vessels form the circle of Willis (Fig. 35-6). The external carotid arteries supply the face and neck but not the brain. During carotid artery surgery, a needle inserted in the internal carotid artery while the external and common carotid arteries are clamped allows measurement of the stump pressure, the arterial pressure occurring in the carotid artery as a result of blood flow through nonoccluded vessels via the circle of Willis (Fig. 35-6).

Arteries of the Upper Extremity. In the upper extremity the subclavian artery gives rise to the axillary, brachial, radial, and ulnar arteries (see Fig. 35-4). Because the brachial artery is beneath the basilic vein, it may be punctured during attempted basilic vein cannulation in the antecubital fossa. Aberrant radial arteries often traverse the radial styloid process to enter the thenar webbed space. Attempted cannulation of veins over the anatomic "snuffbox" may result in cannulation of an aberrant radial artery.

Intra-abdominal and Lower Extremity Arteries. The abdominal branches of the aorta include the superior mesenteric, inferior mesenteric, and celiac arteries, principally supplying the gastrointestinal tract (see Fig. 35-4). The kidneys receive about 20% of the cardiac output *via* a single renal artery. The aorta bifurcates into right and left iliac arteries in the lower torso. At the level of the inguinal ligament, the iliacs bifurcate into superficial and deep femoral arteries. The femoral artery can be easily cannulated just below the

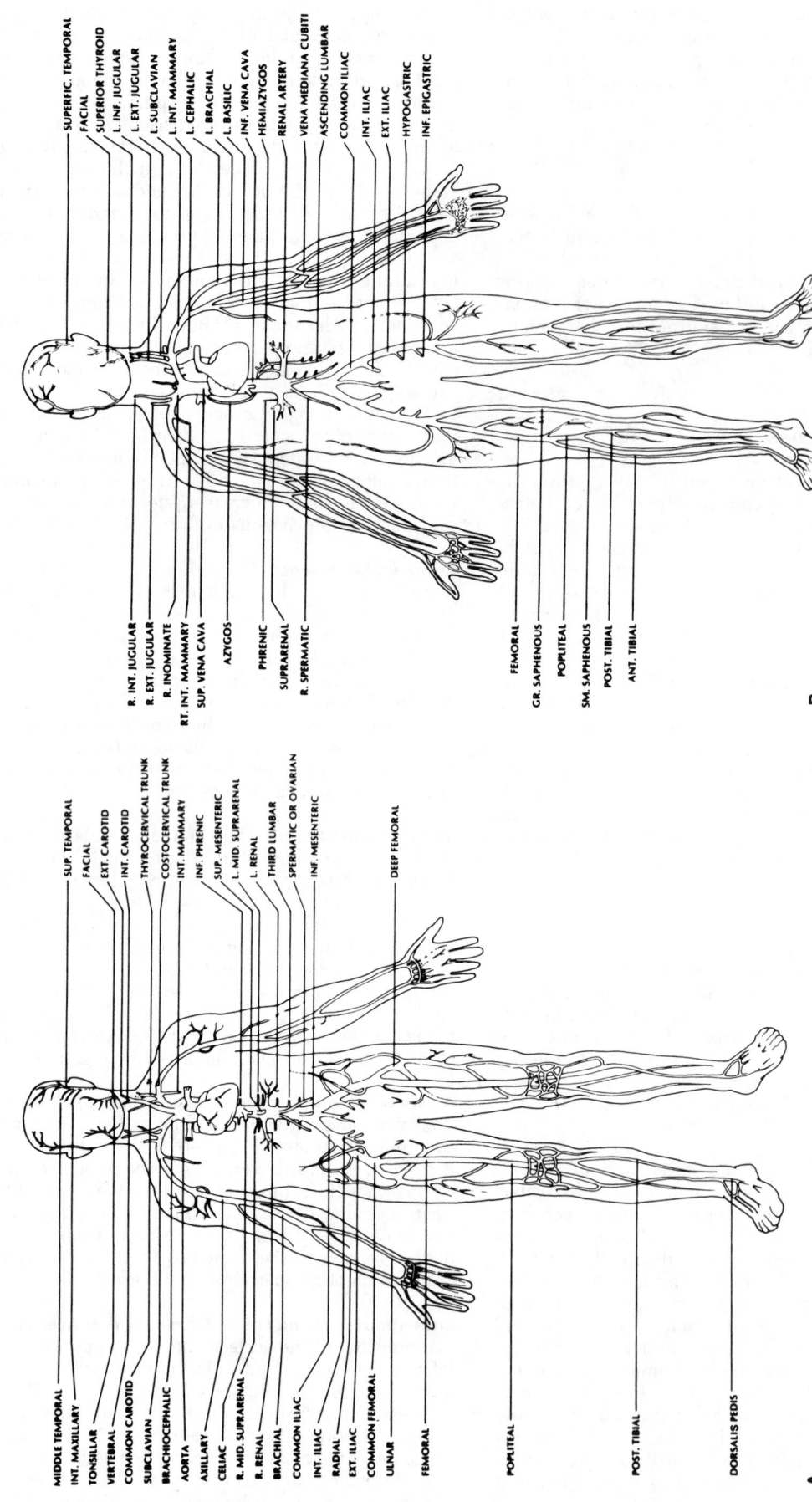

A

B

MIDDLE TEMPORAL
INT. MAXILLARY
TONSILLAR
VERTEBRAL
COMMON CAROTID
SUBCLAVIAN
BRACHIOCEPHALIC
AORTA
AXILLARY
CELIAC
R. MID. SUPRARENAL
R. RENAL
BRACHIAL
COMMON ILIAC
INT. ILIAC
RADIAL
EXT. ILIAC
COMMON FEMORAL
ULNAR
FEMORAL

POPLITEAL

POST. TIBIAL

DORSALIS PEDIS

SUP. TEMPORAL
FACIAL
EXT. CAROTID
INT. CAROTID
THYROCERVICAL TRUNK
COSTOCERVICAL TRUNK
INT. MAMMARY
INF. PHRENIC
SUP. MESENTERIC
L. MID. SUPRARENAL
L. RENAL
THIRD LUMBAR
SPERMATIC OR OVARIAN
INF. MESENTERIC

DEEP FEMORAL

SUPERFIC. TEMPORAL
FACIAL
SUPERIOR THYROID
L. INF. JUGULAR
L. EXT. JUGULAR
L. SUBCLAVIAN
L. INT. MAMMARY
L. CEPHALIC
L. BRACHIAL
L. BASILIC
INF. VENA CAVA
HEMIAZYGOS
RENAL ARTERY
VENA MEDIANA CUBITI
ASCENDING LUMBAR
COMMON ILIAC
INT. ILIAC
EXT. ILIAC
HYPOGASTRIC
INF. EPIGASTRIC

R. INT. JUGULAR
R. EXT. JUGULAR
R. INOMINATE
RT. INT. MAMMARY
SUP. VENA CAVA
AZYGOS
PHRENIC
SUPRARENAL
R. SPERMATIC

FEMORAL
GR. SAPHENOUS
POPLITEAL
SM. SAPHENOUS
POST. TIBIAL
ANT. TIBIAL

Figure 35-4. (A) The major arteries of the human body used by anesthesiologists to directly monitor arterial pressure include the radial, ulnar, femoral, brachial, axillary, dorsalis pedis, and superficial temporal. (B) The major veins of the human body accessible for cannulation include the internal and external jugular, subclavian, femoral, basilic, cephalic, median cubital, and saphenous.

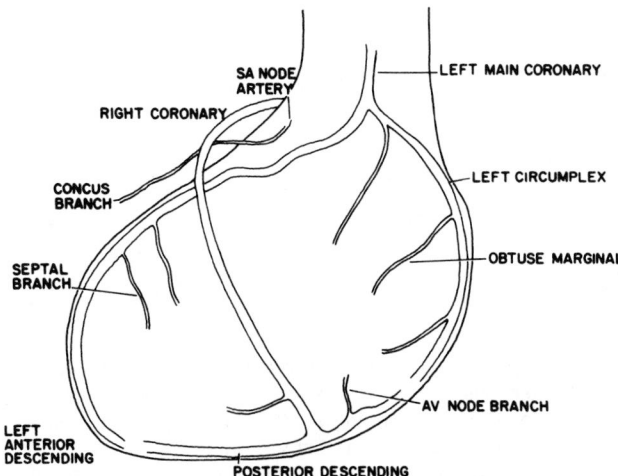

Figure 35-5. In this lateral view, the normal left coronary artery divides into the anterior descending and circumflex coronary arteries. The right coronary artery usually gives off the arteries to the sinus and atrioventricular nodes before terminating on the inferior surface of the heart as the posterior descending artery.

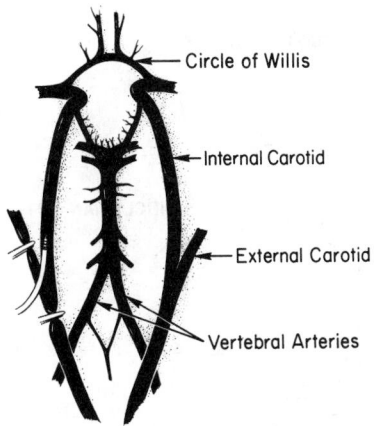

Figure 35-6. The cerebral circulation includes the internal carotid and the vertebral arteries. Together with the anterior communicating and posterior communicating arteries, the carotid arteries from both sides join to form the circle of Willis, which provides collateral circulation to the brain in the event of stenosis or occlusion of one carotid artery. The diagram also shows the position of a clamp on the carotid artery during measurement of "stump" pressure, the pressure present in the cerebral circulation during acute occlusion of the ipsilateral carotid artery. (Reprinted with permission from Lake CL: Cardiovascular Anesthesia, p 411. New York, Springer Verlag, 1985.)

inguinal ligament. Just below the knee the femoral artery bifurcates into anterior and posterior tibial arteries. In the foot, the superficial arteries are the dorsalis pedis, located just lateral to the extensor hallucis longus tendon and the posterior tibial artery behind the medial malleolus of the ankle.

Spinal Cord. The blood supply to the spinal cord consists of the anterior spinal arteries which traverse the length of the cord and arise from the vertebral arteries.[16] The anterior spinal arteries supply the majority (75%) of the cross-sectional area of the gray and white matter of the spinal cord. Only the posterior parts of the posterior columns and posterior horns are supplied by the posterior spinal artery (25%), originating from the terminal portion of the anterior spinal artery. Anastomoses between the anterior and posterior spinal arteries (circumflex arteries) are inconstant and insufficient to sustain adequate cord circulation. In addition, there are radicular arteries that are branches of the intercostal and lumbar arteries; these arteries anastomose with the anteroposterior spinal artery system (Fig. 35-7). There are usually eight (varies from four to ten) radicular

branches, at least one in the cervical, two in the thoracic, and one in the lumbar region. The largest of these is the arteria radicularis magna or artery of Adamkiewicz in the lower thoracic or upper lumbar region. When this vessel originates from the suprarenal aorta in the lower thoracic or upper lumbar region, it is generally the only significant radicular artery. However, if the origin of the arteria radicularis magna is infrarenal (lumbar segments 2 to 4), the segmental blood supply to the cord is usually good and there is another major radicular vessel in the thoracic area.

Precise radiologic verification of the spinal cord blood supply is difficult.[16] Refinement of intercostal angiography may identify the risk of spinal cord ischemia during thoracic aortic surgery.[17]

Bronchial Circulation. Three bronchial arteries (two for the left lung and one for the right lung) originate from the thoracic aorta at T5 and T6 or intercostal arteries and provide nutrients to the lung.[18] The bronchial circulation also permits heat and water exchange in the airways. Although it is normally small compared with the pulmonary circulation and receives only 1% of the cardiac output, the bronchial circulation can enlarge in response to injury, tumor growth and inadequate pulmonary blood flow (as in cyanotic congenital heart disease) and function in gas exchange.[18] Branches of the bronchial arteries accompany the bronchi down to the terminal bronchioles, where they form a plexus in the peribronchial space. They also anastomose with pulmonary alveolar microvessels and coronary, thyroid, esophageal, thymic, internal mammary, thyrocervical, vertebral, and subclavian arteries.

Hepatic and Portal Circulations. Surgery for hepatic transplantation or portal hypertension requires a knowledge of the blood supply to the liver. The liver is supplied by both the hepatic artery and the portal vein. Total hepatic blood flow is about 20% of the cardiac output and averages 100 ml·min^{-1}·100 g^{-1} of tissue. Portal venous flow supplies

---

TABLE 35-1. Coronary Artery Distribution

Left Coronary Artery

Anterior descending branch
  Right bundle branch
  Left bundle branch
  Anterior and posterior papillary muscles (mitral)
  Anterolateral left ventricle
Circumflex branch
  Lateral left ventricle

Right Coronary Artery

SA and AV nodes
Right atrium and ventricle
Posterior interventricular septum
Posterior fascicle of left bundle branch
Interatrial septum

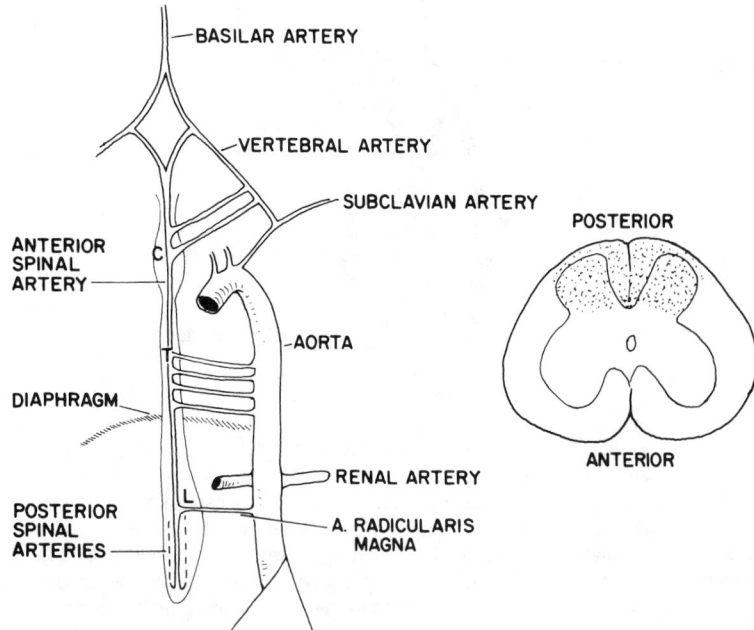

Figure 35-7. The circulation to the spinal cord is often tenuous. It consists of anterior and posterior spinal arteries arising from the vertebral arteries and radicular arteries, which originate from the intercostal and lumbar arteries. However, the radicular branches are quite variable, and ligation of a significant radicular branch causes spinal cord ischemia. In the cross-section of the spinal cord (*right*), the stippled portion indicates the posterior spinal artery distribution to the posterior columns and horns. C, T, and L are cervical, thoracic, and lumbar portions of the spinal cord.

about 65–80% of the total hepatic blood flow, with the remainder coming from the hepatic arterial system. The portal vein, which carries nutrients from the gut to the liver, arises from the superior mesenteric, splenic, and renal veins before entering the liver.

Peripheral Venous Circulation

Major veins follow a similar course to that of the arteries, and accidental arterial cannulation may occur during attempted venous cannulation. From the head, the internal and external jugular veins join the subclavian veins of either side (see Fig. 35-4). The course of the external jugular vein is often tortuous and variable, and it has two sets of valves, one at the entrance to the subclavian vein and the other about 4 cm superior to the clavicle. From the arms, the basilic (medial aspect) and cephalic veins join as the brachial vein. This vein becomes the axillary vein in the axilla and thence the subclavian. Normally, subclavian veins from both sides unite to form the SVC.

The principal cardiac veins are the great and middle cardiac veins and the posterior left ventricular vein. These veins drain into the coronary sinus. The marginal vein drains into the great cardiac vein. Near the orifice of the great cardiac vein, the oblique vein of Marshall (vein of the left atrium) enters the coronary sinus. Anterior cardiac veins and the small cardiac vein may enter the right atrium independently of the coronary sinus. Thebesian veins, which traverse the myocardium, drain into various cardiac chambers.[19] Thebesian venous flow, coupled with bronchial and pleural venous flows, contributes the normal 1–3% arteriovenous shunt.

In the legs there are both superficial and deep veins. The greater and lesser saphenous veins are the principal superficial veins. The greater saphenous vein, overlying the medial malleolus, is frequently used as a conduit during aortocoronary bypass grafting. The lesser saphenous vein is located in the posterior aspect of the calf. The saphenous vein joins the femoral vein in the thigh to enter the pelvis as the iliac vein. Right and left iliac veins unite to form the

IVC. Veins leaving the liver, the right, left and middle hepatic veins, enter the IVC.

Bronchial veins from the extrapulmonary portions of the proximal tracheobronchial tree drain into the azygos and hemiazygos veins (right side of the heart). The azygos vein also drains the perispinal areas and the esophagus. These veins assume greater importance if the IVC is occluded. Bronchial venous drainage from the intrapulmonary branches is to the pulmonary veins (left side of the heart).

Cardiac Conduction System

The system for electrical activation of the heart is termed the conduction system. It consists of the sinoatrial (SA) node, the atrioventricular (AV) node, the bundle of His, right and left bundle branches, and the Purkinje system. Pacemaker cells found in these areas include the P cells, transitional or T cells, and ameboid cells.[20] The body of the SA node lies in the right atrial wall at the junction of the RA with the SVC. Nodal cells, termed ameboid or round cells, have many mitochondria or myofibrils and little sarcoplasmic reticulum. The SA and AV nodes are connected *via* the internodal conduction system, which consists of three tracts: the anterior (Bachmann's bundle), middle, and posterior internodal systems.[21] Conduction also spreads rapidly through the atrial musculature to the left atrium *via* Bachmann's bundle. In human hearts, the AV node is located in the floor of the right atrium, near the ostium of the coronary sinus.[13] The AV node consists of three areas, the A-N zone containing cells smaller than normal atrial cells, the N region of round cells, and the N-H region, a transitional zone near the bundle of His. The fibers forming the common bundle of His pass along the superior edge of the membranous interventricular septum to the apex of the muscular portion of the septum (see Fig. 35-3). Here the bundle divides into right and left bundle branches, which extend subendocardially along the surfaces of both ventricles. The right bundle branch emerges in the right ventricular endocardium near the moderator band at the base of the anterior papillary muscle. It usually extends for some distance without dividing, but one branch passes through the moderator band and the other passes over the right ventricular endocardial surface. Subdivision of the left bundle into anterior and posterior fascicles occurs shortly after its origin. There is also a small collection of short medial fascicles that originate from the left bundle just after the anterior fascicle and activate the septal myocardium. The posterior fascicle terminates in the posterior papillary muscle.

Peripherally the fascicles of both right and left bundle branches subdivide to form the Purkinje network of large diameter fibers with few myofibrils, transverse tubules, or sarcoplasmic reticulum. The left bundle branch fascicles make their initial functional contact with the left endocardial surface of the interventricular septum below the aortic valve. Right bundle-branch fascicles contact ventricular subendocardium near the base of the anterior papillary muscle.

Cardiac and Vascular Nerves

Sympathetic System

Nerves to the heart and blood vessels originate from sympathetic neurons of the thoracolumbar region and parasympathetic nerves originate from the cervical region. Sympathetic fibers come from the stellate ganglion and the caudal halves of the cervical sympathetic trunks below the level of the cricoid cartilage. There are three major sympathetic cardiopulmonary nerves from the stellate and middle cervical ganglia bilaterally: (1) the stellate cardiopulmonary nerve; (2) the dorsal cardiopulmonary nerves (three on the left side); and (3) the right dorsal lateral and dorsal medial cardiopulmonary nerves.[22] The right dorsal medial and dorsal lateral cardiac nerves frequently unite to form one large nerve that follows the course of the left main coronary artery. It further separates into branches along the anterior descending and circumflex coronary arteries. Cholinergic fibers extend into the ventricular myocardium with considerable numbers in ventricular conducting tissue.[23] No sympathetic cardiac nerves arise from the superior cervical ganglia or the thoracic sympathetic trunks inferior to the stellate ganglia.[22] Transmission through the sympathetic ganglia occurs by release of acetylcholine, which interacts with the postsynaptic nicotinic cholinergic receptors on the postganglionic neuron. This stimulates norepinephrine release at the neuroeffector junction to activate beta$_1$-adrenergic receptors.

Parasympathetic System

Parasympathetic preganglionic neurons arise in the medulla oblongata in the dorsal vagal nucleus and the nucleus ambiguus. These fibers enter the thorax as branches from the recurrent laryngeal and thoracic vagus nerve. The dorsal and ventral cardiopulmonary plexuses between the aortic arch and the tracheal bifurcation receive both sympathetic and parasympathetic branches. From the plexuses emerge three large cardiac nerves, the right and left coronary cardiac nerves and the left lateral cardiac nerve. Smaller cardiac nerves also arise from the plexuses and the thoracic vagi.[22] Ganglia occur within the heart, usually close to the structures innervated by the short postganglionic neurons. Postganglionic transmission occurs from stimulation of nicotinic cholinergic receptors at the postganglionic junction by acetylcholine. Release of acetylcholine at the neuroeffector junction activates muscarinic receptors in the heart.

Cerebral Vasomotor Center

Afferent nerves from the heart ascend via the 10th cranial nerve (vagus) and spinal cord to the nucleus tractus solitarius and the dorsal vagal nucleus of the medullary vasomotor center. The dorsal vagal nucleus plus the nucleus ambiguus comprise the parasympathetic motor efferent system. Although the vasomotor center independently regulates arterial pressure, blood flow distribution, and cardiac contractility, influences from higher centers such as the cerebral cortex, hypothalamus, and pons are present.

Cardiac Receptors

Three types of vagal receptors located in various cardiac chambers are sensitive to changes in heart rate or chamber pressure. These include: (1) myelinated vagal afferents located at the venous-atrial junctions that indicate changes in atrial filling and heart rate; (2) unmyelinated vagal afferent nerves present in all cardiac chambers that indicate alterations of contractility, preload, and afterload; and (3) myelinated and nonmyelinated afferent nerves present in all chambers but of unknown significance.[24] These receptors may be important in coronary vasospasm, ischemia-induced dysrhythmias, maintenance of cardiac volume, perception of cardiac pain, and responses to chemical stimuli such as serotonin, bradykinin, or lactic acid.[24]

Vagal innervation affects the atrial musculature—the SA and AV nodes principally—but it also reaches the ventricular myocardium.[25] The greatest concentrations of parasympathetic nerves are in the SA node, with lesser numbers in the AV node, RA, LA, and ventricles. Parasympathetic alpha$_1$ but not alpha$_2$ receptors have been identified. Sympathetic fibers extend to all portions of the atria, ventricles, and conduction system. Both beta$_1$ and beta$_2$ subtypes of adrenergic receptors are present. Human RA contains about 74% beta$_1$ and 26% beta$_2$ receptors.[26] The proportions of beta receptors differ in the ventricle, with 86% beta$_1$ and 14% beta$_2$.

Neural Supply of the Peripheral Vasculature

Innervation of the peripheral circulation, with the exception of the cerebral and coronary vasculature, originates from the thoracolumbar sympathetic fibers. Vasodilation results from reduced sympathetic tone or activation of vasodilatory receptors. Stimulation of alpha-adrenergic fibers causes constriction in the arterial vascular beds of the skin, skeletal muscle, splanchnic organs, kidneys, and systemic veins. Stimulation of beta$_2$ receptors dilates systemic veins and arteries of the muscle, splanchnic, and renal circulations.

Pericardium

The normal pericardium consists of thick fibrous and serous visceral layers. Within the pericardial space are four areas in which pericardial fluid accumulates: transverse sinus, oblique sinus, superior sinus, and postcaval recess. Although the pericardium is nonessential, it has certain anatomic functions, among which are the isolation of the heart from other mediastinal structures, maintenance of the heart in optimal functional shape and position, minimization of cardiac dilatation, and prevention of adhesions.[27] The pericardium also contains vagal nerve branches. Finally, pericardial fluid acts as a hydrostatic system to apply a compensating hydrostatic force to the heart under conditions of acceleration and other gravitational forces.[27]

CARDIOVASCULAR CATHETERIZATION AND ANGIOGRAPHY

Abnormalities of both the anatomy and physiology of the cardiovascular system are diagnosed by invasive catheterization. However, noninvasive procedures such as echocardiography are increasingly being used to determine valvular lesions, ventricular function, and congenital defects.

Catheterization

In all age groups, cardiac catheterization is usually performed via the femoral vessels. Occasionally, the brachial vessels are used in adults if the femoral vessels cannot be entered or catheters cannot be manipulated through the abdominal aorta.[28] Direct vascular cutdowns are rarely necessary because the Seldinger technique, with various sizes of sheaths and introducers, provides adequate access in most patients.[29] The passage of catheters through either the venous or the arterial system is guided by fluoroscopy. Pressure measurements are made in each cardiac chamber or great vessel, their pressure waveforms recorded, and vascular or ventricular angiography performed. Normal pressure values and oxygen saturations are presented in Table 35-2. Oxygen saturation is greater in the IVC than in the SVC owing to the contribution of blood from the renal veins. Normal pressure waveforms are seen in Figure 35-8. Catheters can be specifically placed in virtually any major artery to demonstrate the presence of occlusion, dilation (aneurysm), or congenital abnormalities or to collect blood samples (such as renin from the renal arteries).

Angiography

Cineangiography is performed to quantitate ventricular contractility, to evaluate shunting between cardiac chambers, to demonstrate valvular regurgitation, or to delineate vascular outlines (e.g., pulmonary venous return, aortic dissection, pulmonary embolism). Iodinated dyes such as diatrizoate and ioxaglate are injected to produce contrast. The total amount of injected contrast should not exceed 5 ml·kg^{-1} body weight because contrast media are hyperosmolar sub-

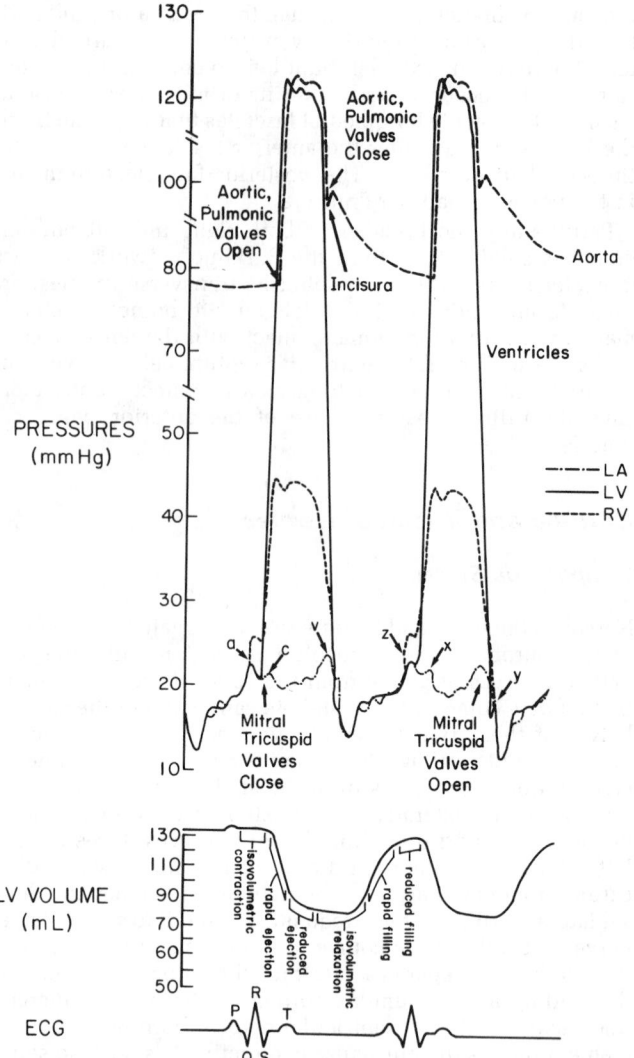

Figure 35-8. The events of the cardiac cycle from filling of the atria to ventricular emptying are demonstrated using waveforms from the aorta, pulmonary artery, right and left ventricles, and central veins. The relationship between the electrocardiogram and the phases of the cardiac cycle shows that ventricular systole occurs immediately following the QRS complex. The changes in ventricular volume coincide with ventricular ejection and filling.

stances that depress the myocardium, dilate the coronary arteries, decrease blood pH, increase serum osmolarity, and cause allergic reactions.[30] Adequate fluid replacement must be given after contrast angiography to prevent hypovolemia from the induced osmotic diuresis.

Angiography assesses the amount of valvular regurgitation by grading the amount of contrast agent re-entering the chamber preceding the valve. For instance, in the case of aortic regurgitation, 1+ regurgitation is a small amount of contrast material entering the left ventricle during diastole but clearing with each systole. The left ventricle is faintly opacified during diastole and fails to clear with systole with 2+ regurgitation. In 3+ aortic regurgitation, the left ventricle is progressively opacified during diastole and eventually completely opacified, whereas in 4+ aortic regurgitation, the left ventricle is completely opacified on the first diastole and remains opacified for several beats.

TABLE 35-2. Normal Catheterization Data

Site	Pressure (mm Hg)	Oxygen Saturation (%)
Inferior vena cava	0–8	80 ± 5
Superior vena cava	0–8	70 ± 5
Right atrium	0–8	75 ± 5
Right ventricle	15–30/0–8	75 ± 5
Pulmonary artery	15–30/4–12	75 ± 5
Pulmonary wedge	5–12 (mean)	75 ± 5
Left atrium	12 (mean)	95 ± 1
Left ventricle	100–140/4–12	95 ± 1
Aorta	100–140/60–90	95 ± 1

Coronary Arteriography

Selective coronary angiography using either the retrograde brachial technique of Sones or the percutaneous femoral approach of Amplatz or Judkins selectively evaluates each coronary artery for the presence and extent of coronary occlusive disease, aneurysm formation, or congenital anomalies (see Fig. 35-5). Coronary arteriography occasionally causes ventricular ectopy, the Bezold-Jarisch reflex, ventricular asystole, or fibrillation. More common are T-wave changes, bradycardia, and mild hypotension. Even in normal coronary arteries, injection of the right coronary artery produces T-wave inversion in lead II and injection of the left artery produces T-wave peaking in lead II.[31] These changes revert to normal when the catheter is removed from the coronary ostia or the blood pressure is increased by having the patient cough.

Determination of Cardiac Output

Cardiac output is determined by the Fick principle, dye dilution, thermodilution, or Doppler flow techniques. The Fick method requires the measurement or estimation of oxygen consumption as well as collection of arterial and venous blood.

$$\text{Cardiac output (l·min}^{-1}) = \dot{V}o_2/Cao_2 - C\bar{v}o_2 \times 100$$

where $\dot{V}o_2$ = oxygen consumption, Cao_2 = arterial oxygen content, and $C\bar{v}o_2$ = venous oxygen content. The principle of the Fick measurement is that the size of a fluid stream is calculated by the amount of substance entering or leaving the stream and the concentration difference resulting from entry or removal of the substance. Arterial and mixed venous oxygen contents are calculated using the relationship:

$$Co_2 = \text{alpha } Po_2 + 1.34 \text{ hemoglobin concentration} \\ \times \text{ \% hemoglobin saturation}$$

where alpha = the solubility of oxygen in whole blood $(0.0031 \text{ ml·100 ml}^{-1}\text{·mm Hg}^{-1})$. In the dye dilution method, the concentration of an indicator, usually indocyanine green, injected into the venous circulation, is measured by passing arterial blood through a densitometer. This method, based on the Fick principle, requires a cumbersome calculation of the area under the dye curve to measure outputs in the presence of and to detect intravascular shunts. Because recirculation of the dye occurs, some portion of the downslope of the curve must be extrapolated to near zero to eliminate redundancy.

A normal dye dilution curve has an uninterrupted build-up slope, a steep disappearance slope with a short disappearance time, and a prominent recirculation peak. In right-to-left shunts, there is a deformity on the build-up slope by the abnormal early appearance of the dye in the arterial circulation. Left-to-right shunting causes a decreased peak dye concentration, absence of the recirculation peak, and a prolongation of the disappearance time.

Doppler echocardiography permits noninvasive assessment of cardiac output by measurement of the cross-sectional area of the aorta and the velocity of blood flow from the Doppler shift of the reflected sound waves. The transesophageal ultrasound method of determining cardiac output has produced variable results when compared with thermodilution technique in experimental situations.[32,33]

Thermodilution cardiac output determinations are the most widely used in clinical situations at present. The principle for thermodilution measurements is the indicator-dilution technique. A known quantity of room temperature or cooled dextrose is injected into the central venous circulation. A thermistor in the pulmonary artery detects the bolus of injectate and records the temperature change over time only. The output of the right side of the heart is measured. Thermodilution outputs are subject to inaccuracies because of wandering baselines, improper volume or speed of injection, and pulmonary catheters placed too peripherally.

Determination of Shunts

A shunt exists when arterial and venous blood mix at some site in the circulatory system, either an intracardiac or an extracardiac location, usually as a result of a congenital cardiac malformation.

The site of a shunt can be determined by measurement of oxygen saturations in various cardiac chambers or by calculation of pulmonary and systemic flow by the Fick principle. A 10% step-up in oxygen saturation at the atrial level indicates left-to-right shunting into the right atrium. A 5% step-up at the ventricular or aorticopulmonary level indicates shunting at that site.

The measurement of pulmonary and systemic flow is performed by direct measurement or by the Fick principle using estimated oxygen consumption and measured systemic and pulmonary oxygen contents. The pulmonary (Q_p) to systemic flow (Q_s) is equal in the absence of shunting, and the flow ratio is 1. In a bidirectional shunt, the effective pulmonary flow (Q_{pe}) is $\dot{V}o_2/P\bar{v}o_2 - M\bar{v}o_2$ where $P\bar{v}o_2$ is the pulmonary venous oxygen content and $M\bar{v}o_2$ is the mixed venous oxygen content. Flow in left-to-right shunting is $Q_p - Q_{pe}$. Flow in right-to-left shunting is $Q_s - Q_{pe}$.

Calculation of Valve Areas

Valve areas and flows can be calculated from the heart rate, cardiac output, and vascular pressures.[34] The aortic valve area is calculated by determining the systolic ejection period per beat (SEP) from the pressure waveforms. The systolic ejection period per minute is calculated by multiplying the SEP per beat by the heart rate. The pressure gradient across the aortic valve is the difference between left ventricular systolic mean pressure and aortic systolic mean pressure. The aortic valve flow is cardiac output/SEP_{minute}. The aortic valve area is calculated using the following equation:

$$\text{Aortic valve area} = \frac{\text{aortic valve flow}}{1 \times 44.5 \sqrt{\text{systolic pressure gradient}}}$$

One is the empirical constant for the aortic valve, which combines the coefficient of orifice contraction (a factor to compensate for the physical reduction of the stream to an area of less than the actual orifice area), the coefficient of velocity, the conversion factor of centimeters of water to millimeters of mercury, and other factors. Recent evidence suggests that this constant varies with the transvalvular pressure gradient.[35]

A similar calculation is made for the mitral valve area, except that the diastolic filling period per beat, the diastolic gradient between left atrial and left ventricular pressures, and an empirical constant of 0.7 are used.[36] The diastolic filling period per minute is calculated by multiplying the diastolic filling period per beat by the heart rate. The mitral valve flow is cardiac output (ml·min^{-1})/diastolic filling period$_{minute}$. The mitral valve area is calculated using the following equation:

$$\text{Mitral valve area} = \frac{\text{mitral valve flow}}{0.7 \times 44.5 \sqrt{\text{diastolic pressure gradient}}}$$

PHYSIOLOGY

Cardiac Cycle

The cardiac cycle begins with the filling of the right and left atria while the tricuspid and mitral valves are closed (see Fig. 35-8). The V wave on the venous pressure waveform represents the gradual increase in atrial blood volume as blood returns from the periphery. Once the aortic valve has closed but ventricular pressure still exceeds atrial pressure, the ventricle is in the phase of isovolumetric relaxation. About 0.02–0.04 seconds after closure of the aortic valve, atrial and ventricular pressures equalize, and a small gradient develops across the AV valves as ventricular pressure decreases further. The AV valve cusps bulge into the ventricle and separate slightly. At 0.03–0.05 seconds after crossover of the atrial and ventricular pressure waves, the AV valves open completely over 0.02–0.04 seconds. The V wave of the atrial pressure waveform crests when the atria are filled, and the tricuspid and mitral valves open to initiate ventricular filling. The Y wave results from opening of the AV valves combined with ventricular relaxation. Effective atrial systole at resting heart rates contributes about 5–20% of the stroke volume. Acute atrial fibrillation increases atrial pressures, reduces atrial compliance, increases atrial oxygen consumption, and eliminates the contribution of the atria to ventricular filling.[37]

Initially there is a rapid increase in ventricular volume, the rapid filling phase of about 0.06–0.10 seconds, during which time the ventricular pressure continues to decrease because ventricular expansion exceeds filling. Peak ventricular filling in early diastole occurs at 500–700 ml·sec^{-1} as the ventricle "sucks" blood from the atria (diastolic suction). Under certain circumstances, ventricular relaxation actually produces a negative intracavitary pressure. The elastic recoil of the heart and great vessels during diastole contributes to the accelerated filling phase of the ventricle, particularly during tachycardia. The third heart sound, S$_3$, occurs at the point of transition from rapid ventricular filling to reduced filling.

The previous ventricular contraction provides much of the energy for the subsequent diastolic expansion through the energy expenditure of the gross movement and deformation of the heart during systole.[38] The nadir of the ventricular pressure curve at the end of the rapid filling phase probably marks the end of ventricular relaxation and the beginning of elastic distention of the ventricle. The third heart sound, S$_3$, occurs at the point of transition from rapid ventricular filling to reduced filling. A period of reduced ventricular filling follows the rapid filling phase. During this period, there is an upswing in the ventricular pressure that abolishes forward movement of blood and can force the AV valves into a semiclosed position unless venous return is great. Atrial systole, the A wave on the venous pressure waveform, which coincides with the P wave on the electrocardiogram, concludes ventricular filling.

Measurement of the mean right atrial pressure provides a guide to right atrial and right ventricular function. Right atrial pressure is indirectly assessed by observation of the level of jugular venous pressure, the end-expiratory peak pulsation of the internal jugular vein above the sternal angle with the subject in a 30-degree reverse Trendelenburg position. Normally, the level is <4 cm. A sustained increase in the level of more than 1 cm during abdominal compression (hepatojugular reflux) indicates abnormal right ventricular function. Only when biventricular function is normal can the central venous pressure be used as a guide of left ventricular function.

Although venous return is the most important factor contributing to ventricular filling, atrial contraction is often important to the heart with poorly functioning ventricles. In such hearts, a fourth heart sound, S$_4$, which occurs 0.04 seconds after the P wave, results from vibrations of left ventricular muscle and mitral valve. The S$_4$ is most likely to occur with vigorous atrial contraction. The adequacy of ventricular filling is determined by the distensibility (compliance) of the ventricles, the filling time, and the effective filling pressure. The effective filling pressure is the transmural ventricular pressure. Tachycardia also decreases the time available for ventricular filling, decreasing filling time from 400–500 msec at a heart rate of 60 beats per minute to 10 msec or less at 160 beats per minute. Mitral stenosis slows ventricular filling and alters the change in ventricular wall motion associated with filling. Hypertrophic cardiomyopathy slows the distention of the ventricle associated with filling. Reduced diastolic filling is also seen in patients with coronary artery disease, probably resulting from changes in compliance and regional wall motion during ischemia. The intraventricular pressure just prior to the beginning of ventricular contraction is end-diastolic pressure (see Table 35-2). However, normal end-diastolic pressures do not imply normal ventricular function. Increased end-diastolic pressures occur with hypervolemia or changes in ventricular compliance as well as decreased contractility.

The period just before the sudden increase in ventricular pressure is presystole, which includes atrial systole and the time just before isovolumetric ventricular contraction. The Z point on the venous pressure waveform is the period when atrial and ventricular pressures are essentially equal immediately preceding ventricular systole. The isovolumetric phase of ventricular contraction is marked by the C wave on the venous waveform. Isovolumetric contraction is the period between closure of the AV valves and opening of the semilunar (aortic, pulmonic) valves. Intraventricular pressure increases, but there is no change in intraventricular volume. After this point, the AV valves close, atrial diastole begins, the ventricles begin to contract, and ventricular pressure soon exceeds atrial pressure. Ventricular systole occurs immediately after the QRS complex on the electrocardiogram, about 0.12 to 0.20 seconds after atrial contraction. AV valve closure is facilitated by the increased ventricular pressure and the cessation of atrial systole. Closure of the AV valves is noted clinically by the first heart sound, S$_1$. However, some investigators suggest that S$_1$ results from reverberations of the left ventricular muscle, mitral valve, and left ventricular outflow tract in response to the acceleration and deceleration of blood during early systole.[39] Since right and left ventricular contraction are normally slightly asynchronous, S$_1$ is usually split.

The aortic and pulmonic valves open at the summit of the C wave. The atrial pressure decreases, resulting in the X descent, because blood goes into the aorta and pulmonary artery. Once the ventricular pressure exceeds the aortic pressure, the aortic and pulmonic valves open. The majority of ventricular ejection occurs during the rapid ejection phase. The pressure in the aorta is slightly lower, whereas ventricular pressure increases rapidly. Initially the output into the aorta exceeds the runoff into the peripheral circulation. Peak aortic pressure occurs slightly after peak aortic blood flow. As aortic runoff and ventricular output equilibrate, the period of reduced ventricular ejection occurs. Forward flow continues until the end of ventricular diastole—protodiastole—when a brief period of retrograde flow initiates aortic and pulmonic valve closure. On pressure waveforms, semilunar valve closure is marked by a notch or incisura. The second heart sound, S_2, which also results from rapid deceleration of blood causing vibration of the outflow tracks and great vessels and closure of the semilunar valves, is heard on auscultation.

Cardiac Electrophysiology

Cellular Electrophysiology

Cardiac pacemaker cells have an intracellular ionic composition which differs from that found in the extracellular fluid. The most important ions are calcium, sodium, and potassium. An active transport system in the cell membrane, the sodium-potassium pump, maintains normal concentration gradients for sodium and potassium by pumping three sodium ions out of the cell while pumping two potassium ions into the cell, consuming the energy released by the hydrolysis of adenosine triphosphate. Extracellular ions cross the cell membrane or sarcolemma because of special proteins or channels. Channels are characterized by their conductance, selectivity, gating, and density. Conductance is the rate (ions·msec^{-1}) at which ions pass through the channel. In a given channel, each ion has a particular conductance. Channels are named for the ion most rapidly transferred since some ions, but not others, are transported. Density is described as the number of channels per square micrometer. However, density may be variable over the cellular sarcolemma. Gating is the property of the channel that allows it to be activated or inactivated in response to voltage changes or binding of an agonist. Examples of these channels are given in Table 35-3.

Beta receptors, consisting of the receptor, the G protein (guanosine triphosphate binding protein) system,[40] and adenylate cyclase are also located in the sarcolemma. Receptors recognize and bind agonists, activating Gs (part of the G protein system), which, in turn, activates adenylate cyclase to stimulate hydrolysis of adenosine triphosphate to cyclic adenosine monophosphate. Cyclic adenosine monophosphate opens the calcium channel, permitting calcium influx. The entire complex forms a transmembrane signaling system (Fig. 35-9).

The compound action potential in cells results from local ionic transmembrane fluxes or currents through the channels (Fig. 35-10). Ionic transfer is facilitated by the energy released from the hydrolysis of adenosine triphosphate. Cardiac pacemaker cells in the unexcited state are maintained at a resting potential of -80 mV by the inward (anomalous) rectifier current I_{K1}. As the slow spontaneous depolarization of phase 4 proceeds, there is an increase in the permeability of the membrane, which permits positively charged sodium ions to move across the cell membrane into the cell, resulting in depolarization. This sodium influx (fast sodium current, I_{Na}) reverses the transmembrane potential from -80 mV to $+20-30$ mV and initiates the rapid depolariza-

TABLE 35-3. Types of Channels in Cell Membranes

Channel	Ion	Conductance (picosiemens)
Sodium	Na	13
"Slow" calcium		
L type	Ca, Ba	25
T type	Ca	8
N type	Ca	13
Potassium		
Inward rectifier (K_1)	K	5
Delayed rectifier (x_1)	K	18
Calcium activated ($K_{(Ca)}$)	K	20
Adenosine triphosphate–modulated ($K_{(ATP)}$)	K	
Muscarinic ($K_{(Ach)}$)	K	
Chloride	Cl	10
Sarcoplasmic reticulum calcium release	Ca	150

tion (phase 0) of the action potential in a cardiac pacemaker cell (Fig. 35-10). During phase 0 there is also a decrease in permeability to potassium. At about -30 mV, inward calcium transfer (I_{Ca}) begins through the L-type (long-lasting, high-threshold) channels. Although both L and T types of calcium channels actually open rapidly, the L type provides the calcium entry to sustain cellular contraction. The spread of depolarization throughout the atrial muscle results in the P wave, and the spread throughout the ventricular muscle results in the QRS complex of the electrocardiogram. After excitation, the cell membrane undergoes an initial period of rapid repolarization (phase 1), followed by a period of variable duration in which the membrane potential remains close to 0. This is termed the plateau of the action potential. The plateau is caused by decreasing sodium and calcium influx and increasing potassium efflux. The duration of the action potential is rate-dependent due to enhanced calcium entry. Phase 3, the repolarization phase that results from "delayed outward" potassium current I_{x1}, corresponds to the T wave of the electrocardiogram. During phase 4 the resting membrane potential is generated by active exchange of intracellular sodium for potassium. The resting potassium conductance that maintains the resting potential is G_{K1}, the inward (anomalous) rectifier. In the latter part of phase 4, the resting membrane potential is stable in ventricular muscle cells until the cell is excited again. In automatic cells such as the SA and AV nodes, slow, spontaneous depolarization occurs during phase 4 as a result of calcium I_f (delta I_p) and I_{K2} or pacemaker currents.

During depolarization, the cell membrane is absolutely refractory to other stimuli because almost all of the sodium channels inactivate. The end of the absolute refractory period is signaled by the earliest transient depolarization that can be elicited because sufficient numbers of activatable sodium channels are present. The absolute refractory period ends at the beginning of the T wave of the electrocardiogram. Once repolarization reaches the threshold potential, the cell is relatively refractory, since an unusually strong stimulus can produce depolarization. This period is marked by the T wave of the electrocardiogram. The earliest propagated action potential defines the end of the effective or functional refractory period.

The SA node is normally the dominant pacemaker because in it automaticity is most highly developed and im-

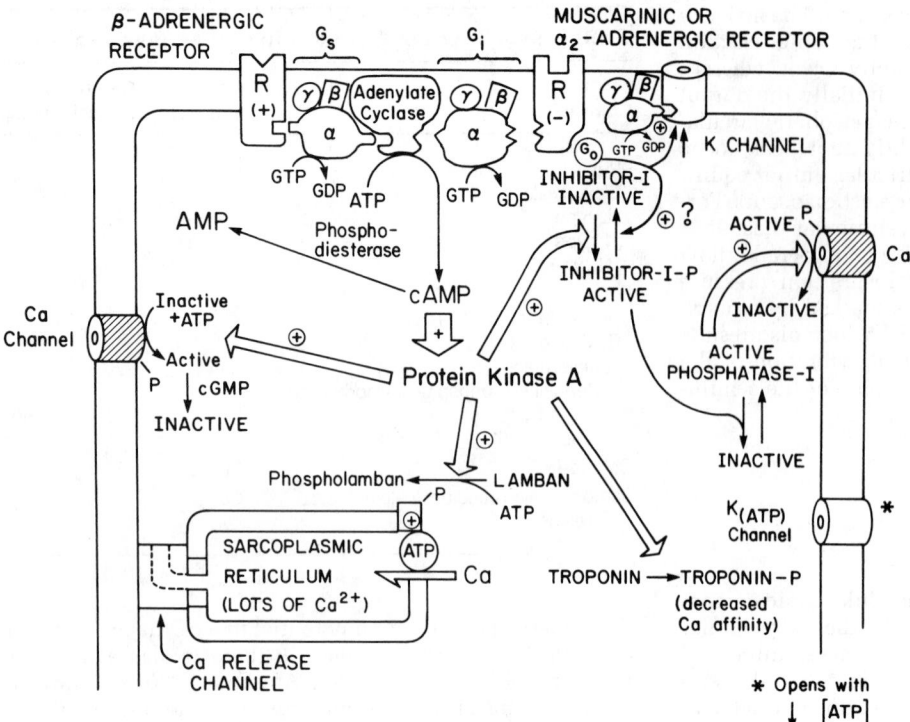

Figure 35-9. The modulation of excitation-contraction coupling requires complex interactions between the ionic channels, the G protein system, and muscarinic and beta-adrenergic receptors. Cyclic adenosine monophosphate production is controlled by adenylate cyclase activity, which can be increased by activated Gs protein or reduced by activated Gi protein. Activation of either Gs or Gi is accomplished by activation of the beta-adrenergic receptors and by the alpha₁ or muscarinic receptors, respectively. Cyclic adenosine monophosphate concentration controls the activity of the cyclic adenosine monophosphate–dependent kinase. Phosphorylation of a variety of enzymes or channels by these enzymes alters cycling of intracellular calcium. Phosphorylated calcium channels are more readily opened by depolarization and permit increased entry of calcium. Phosphorylated lamban protein enhances calcium uptake by the sarcoplasmic reticulum Ca adenosine triphosphatase (calcium pump). The net effect is a greater store of calcium in the sarcoplasmic reticulum for release. Phosphorylation of troponin results in a lower affinity for calcium, which permits faster relaxation (dissociation of calcium from troponin) but requires the increased calcium (stored in the sarcoplasmic reticulum) to activate actin-myosin; this ultimately produces development of myocardial tension. Phosphorylation of inhibitor I also decreases phosphatase I activity, so that calcium channels remain phosphorylated and active. Reduction in intracellular cyclic adenosine monophosphate results from decreased adenylate cyclase activity and breakdown of cyclic adenosine monophosphate by phosphodiesterase. Adenylate cyclase activity is reduced by activation of muscarinic or alpha-adrenergic receptors acting *via* Gi protein. Receptors may also activate other G proteins (*e.g.,* Go), which may directly enhance the activity of a K channel, responsible for repolarization. (Figure and legend by Carl Lynch III, M.D., Ph.D.)

pulses are initiated at the fastest rate. In SA nodal cells, when the internal membrane potential reaches -50 mV, the depolarization rate increases to 1–2 V·sec^{-1}, causing a slowly depolarizing action potential. The action potential of the AV node is even slower than that of the SA node. Automaticity decreases in order from SA node, AV node, His bundle, proximal Purkinje fibers, and distal Purkinje fibers. The rate of phase 4 depolarization is faster in the SA node than in the AV node and faster in the AV node than in the terminal Purkinje fibers, causing less highly developed pacemakers to be depolarized by the propagated wave from above before they spontaneously depolarize.[41] Interactions between sympathetic and parasympathetic innervations also affect the intrinsic depolarization rate.

Action Potential Alterations. Changes in the action potential itself or factors that affect the action potential alter the

rate of firing of an automatic cell. The rate of an automatic cell depends on the slope of phase 4 depolarization, the maximum diastolic potential (the maximum level of resting membrane potential achieved at the end of repolarization), and the threshold potential. If the difference between the threshold potential and the resting membrane potential is increased, a greater stimulus is needed for depolarization. A smaller stimulus is required if only a small difference exists between the resting membrane potential and the threshold potential. Other factors affecting rate include increases or decreases in the resting membrane potential, an increased or decreased rate of spontaneous phase 4 depolarization, and shifting of the threshold potential toward or away from the resting membrane potential.[42] Hypothermia decreases the slope of phase 4, whereas hyperthermia increases heart rate.[43] Hypoxia or ischemia increases the slope of phase 4 and reduces the maximum diastolic potential.[44]

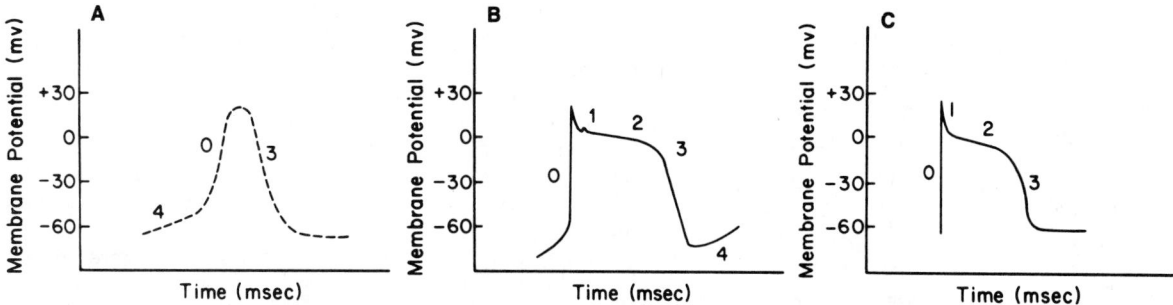

Figure 35-10. (A) The action potential of an automatic cell such as the sinoatrial node differs from that of the ventricular muscle cell in that the automatic cell slowly depolarizes spontaneously during phase 4. Phase 0 is the depolarization phase, which results from sodium ion influx through the fast channel and calcium ion influx through the slow channel. Phase 3 is the repolarization phase, which results from potassium movement through the cell membrane. (B) The action potential in a Purkinje cell has the most rapid rate of depolarization, 400–800 V·sec^{-1}. When the cell is stimulated, an action potential occurs as a result of a rapid influx of sodium ions into the cell (phase 0). Phase 1 includes a notch caused by the "early outward current" (Ieo), which is a transient K efflux, probably activated by an intracellular calcium increase. Phase 2 is the plateau of the action potential resulting principally from calcium entry through the slow channel of the cell membrane. During phase 3, repolarization of the cell occurs, whereas during phase 4, the sodium entering during phase 0 is actively pumped out of the cell. (C) The action potential in a ventricular muscle cell. Unlike what occurs in the automatic cells, there is no spontaneous phase 4 depolarization.

Acetylcholine has little effect on action potential duration in Purkinje cells but antagonizes the effect of isoproterenol and decreases action potential duration.[45] The refractory period in the Purkinje cell is prolonged by vagal and beta-adrenergic stimulation.[42]

Hypokalemia increases the rate of phase 4 depolarization in the SA node.[42] Hyperkalemia reduces the rate of phase 4 depolarization and decreases the maximum diastolic potential of Purkinje but not sinus node fibers.[46] With hyperkalemia, fewer sodium channels are available for activation, and a greater depolarization is necessary to achieve threshold.

Diastolic depolarization, conduction, and cardiac contraction are abolished at external potassium concentrations of 15–20 mM with the membrane stabilized at +20 mV, such as with cardioplegic solutions given during cardiac surgery. Decreased sodium decreases the slope of phase 4 depolarization and the height of the action potential without a change of resting membrane potential in atrial, ventricular, or Purkinje fibers.[42] Hypercalcemia decreases action potential duration, whereas hypocalcemia increases action potential duration. The changes caused by magnesium are similar to those caused by calcium.

Hypercarbia and increased pH increase the slope of phase 4 and reduce maximum diastolic potential.[42] Slow channels are selectively blocked by metabolic acidosis. Spontaneous depolarization in Purkinje fibers is enhanced by decreased bicarbonate concentrations.[47]

Clinical Electrophysiology

The first wave of the normal electrocardiogram is the P wave, which is produced by atrial depolarization resulting from an action potential in the SA node. Sinus node rate exhibits a circadian rhythm, decreasing nocturnally. Sinus node recovery time is also prolonged at night.[48] The P wave usually does not normally exceed 3 mm in height of 0.11 seconds in duration. It is usually upright, except in lead aV$_R$.

Transmission of an impulse elicited by an action potential in the SA node to the AV node takes about 0.04 seconds.

The electrical impulse travels from the SA node to the AV node via atrial tissue, specialized atrial conducting tissue, or the anterior, middle, and posterior tracts of the right atrium. Transmission is further delayed in the AV node because its conduction velocity is about 0.2 m·sec^{-1}. The effective refractory period of the AV node also demonstrates circadian rhythm and is increasingly prolonged at night.[48] The PR interval (normally 0.2 msec or less), which occupies the time between atrial and ventricular depolarization, is nearly isoelectric, because atrial repolarization is not recordable. Significant interactions between the parasympathetic and sympathetic nervous systems control the conduction through the AV node. Unlike in the SA node, sympathetic activity predominates in AV nodal conduction.[49]

Ventricular depolarization begins about 0.12–0.20 seconds in adults and 0.15–0.18 seconds in children after depolarization of the SA node.[50] Ventricular depolarization produces the QRS complex on the electrocardiogram. The first negative wave seen in the QRS complex is the Q wave, which should be 0.04 seconds or less in duration and less than one fourth of the subsequent R wave in amplitude. The first positive wave in the QRS is the R wave, and the second negative wave is the S wave. The entire QRS complex should be less than 0.10 seconds. The right and left branches of the Bundle of His connecting with the Purkinje fibers conduct the depolarizing impulse rapidly over the endocardial surface of the heart. Normally in sinus rhythm the earliest area of activation is the trabecular area on the anterior right ventricular surface about 18–25 msec after the surface QRS complex (Fig. 35-11). Activation then spreads toward the apex and base of the heart, with the latest activation at the cardiac base. Electrical activation also spreads from endocardium to epicardium.

Abnormal ventricular activation is recognized by an area exhibiting activation before the onset of the surface QRS complex. Mapping of the direct cardiac electrogram to determine such abnormal areas of activation is the basis of clinical electrophysiologic studies in patients with ventricular dysrhythmias.

On the electrocardiogram the time from the end of ven-

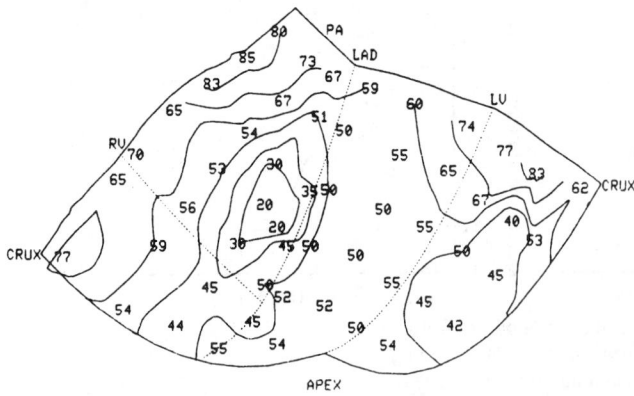

Figure 35-11. In this representation, the heart has been cut along its posterior surface from the base to the apex and laid flat. The numbers indicate the time in milliseconds after the QRS complex is seen on the electrocardiogram until electrical activity is noted. The right ventricle is activated earliest, about 19–20 msec after the QRS complex, whereas the latest activation occurs at the base of the heart at 75–80 msec. (Reprinted with permission of the author and publisher from Gallagher JJ et al: Techniques of intraoperative electrophysiologic mapping. Am J Cardiol 49:224, 1982.)

tricular depolarization to the beginning of repolarization, the ST segment, is isoelectric. More than 1 mm of elevation in the standard leads or 2 mm of elevation in the precordial leads is abnormal in this segment. No more than 0.5 mm of depression should be seen in any lead. The J point, the junction between the QRS complex and the ST segment, is depressed or elevated with the ST segment. Ventricular repolarization results in the T wave. T waves are normally upright in leads I, II, and V_3–V_6, inverted in lead aV_R, and variable in leads II, aV_L, aV_F, V_1 and V_2. The T wave should not exceed 5 mm in height in the standard leads or 10 mm in the precordial leads. The QT interval, varying inversely with heart rate, should be slightly less than one half of the RR interval.[51] The U wave, a small upright deflection after the T wave, is usually nondetectable.

Physiology of the Cardiac Nerves

Neural Regulation

Although the dominance of either the sympathetic or the parasympathetic system varies with age, situation, and physical condition, the inhibitory parasympathetic system is usually predominant.[52,53] However, neural regulation of the heart is complex. Stimulation of dorsal cardiac nerves increases or decreases heart rate and blood pressure in humans.[54] In some patients the vagal influence may be excessive, causing vagotonia.[55] Parasympathetic stimulation, particularly of the right vagus nerve, decreases heart rate by slowing the SA node. Lower pacemakers such as the AV node or His Bundle may take over, causing "nodal rhythm." Vagal stimulation tends to suppress ventricular automaticity, which may facilitate termination of ventricular dysrhythmias. Intense vagal stimulation depresses both atrial and ventricular contractility by stimulation of cardiac muscarinic receptors that alter the myocyte cyclic adenosine monophosphate level, by inhibition of norepinephrine release from nearby sympathetic nerve terminals by acetylcholine, and by inhibition of adrenergic receptor activation.[22] One of the G proteins—Gi—which inhibits

adenylcyclase, lowering the levels of cyclic adenosine monophosphate, is coupled with the muscarinic receptor to control potassium channels and decrease heart rate.

Stimulation of the stellate ganglion or other sympathetic cardiac fibers increases heart rate, contractility, and ejection fraction. The right stellate ganglion has a greater effect on heart rate, whereas the left has more effect on contractility. Abnormalities of sympathetic cardiac nerve tone occur in long QT interval syndromes.[56]

Both alpha$_1$, alpha$_2$, beta$_1$, and beta$_2$ receptors are present in the heart. The role of the cardiac alpha receptors is unclear, but their action is modulated by G protein signal transduction. Beta$_1$ receptors of the heart have positive chronotropic, inotropic, and lusitropic effects on the heart by stimulation of adenylcyclase. Action potentials may be restored by beta$_1$ stimulation owing to increased numbers of activatable calcium channels in sufficient density to permit regenerative ionic flux along a fiber. Activation of cardiac beta$_2$ receptors also increases rate and contractility, particularly in end-stage heart failure. The effects of norepinephrine on contractility are mediated by increased calcium entry through more active calcium channels and increased sarcoplasmic reticular uptake of calcium. Increased sarcoplasmic uptake of calcium has a lusitropic effect while making the increased calcium (in the sarcoplasmic reticulum) available for subsequent contractions (see Fig. 35-9).

Cardiac Receptors

There are two major types of nerve endings that interconnect in the heart: (1) the nerve net, and (2) diffuse or compact unencapsulated endings.[57]

Atrial Receptors

The atria have three types of parasympathetic receptors: Type A, Type B, and receptors innervated by Group C fibers that are less responsive than Type A or B. Atrial receptors usually reflexly alter intravascular volume or heart rate. Atrial receptor Types A and B are innervated by myelinated vagal afferent fibers. The primary location of Types A and B receptors are the cavoatrial junction, pulmonary venousatrial junction, atrial appendage, and atrial body.[57] Type A receptors discharge at the time of the A wave of the atrial pressure waveform. They may actually respond to heart rate rather than atrial pressure, since they are unaffected by the amplitude of the A wave or the rate of atrial pressure increase.[57] Type B receptors are stretch receptors that discharge during late systole, during the V wave of the atrial pressure waveform. Their discharge is closely related to atrial volume and varies with the rate of atrial pressure increase. Type B receptors are inactive during normal atrial contraction but increase their rate of discharge during tachyarrhythmias that increase atrial volume.[57]

Ventricular Receptors

Stimulation of ventricular receptors causes either cardiovascular excitation or depression. Types of ventricular receptors include the pressure-sensitive coronary baroreceptors, mechanoreceptors (innervated by nonmyelinated vagal afferent fibers), and sympathetic mechanosensitive or chemosensitive receptors.[57]

Two types of unmyelinated ventricular vagal afferent fibers are present in the heart. One type innervates chemosensitive receptors that are stimulated by capsaicin or veratridine, whereas the other type innervates mechanoreceptors that respond to aortic constriction.[57] Unmyelinated sympathetic afferent fibers with either mechanosensitive or chemosensitive receptors are present throughout the heart, great vessels, and pericardium.[57]

The Bainbridge reflex, described below, is mediated by the parasympathetic receptors. Myocardial ischemia increases discharge of both vagal and sympathetic receptors. The sympathetic afferent fibers may transmit the pain sensation associated with coronary occlusion. Postcardiotomy hypertension results from a cardiogenic reflex transmitted through the sympathetic afferent fibers of the stellate ganglion.[57] Finally, opiate receptors are found throughout the cardiovascular system (in vagus, cardiac, and sympathetic ganglia). Opiate receptors of the k type may mediate dysrhythmias, particularly during ischemia and reperfusion.[58,59]

Coronary Circulatory Physiology

About 5% of the cardiac output or 250 ml·min^{-1} perfuses the coronary arteries of a 70-kg person. Physiologically, the coronary circulation consists of large, low resistance epicardial vessels and higher resistance intramyocardial arteries and arterioles. Myocardial flow, pressure, and oxygen consumption are integrally related. Numerous methods to measure human myocardial blood flow have been described.[60] Coronary blood flow is locally regulated by metabolic, mechanical, anatomic, and possibly myogenic factors.[61] The majority of left coronary artery flow occurs in diastole because intramyocardial pressure is lowest at that time.[62] Right coronary artery flow occurs in both systole and diastole because intramyocardial pressure is lower in the thinner right ventricle. Intramyocardial pressure, although difficult to measure, affects coronary flow to a small extent because of the varying stiffness of ventricular muscle over the cardiac cycle.[62]

Coronary flow also decreases from epicardium to endocardium as a consequence of extravascular pressure. During systole about 15–25% of the coronary flow distends and is stored in the extramural coronary arteries. Only a small amount actually perfuses the myocardium. During diastole, this stored blood perfuses the myocardium[63] (Fig. 35-12).

There is a minimum coronary pressure required to initiate flow, the zero flow pressure. Normally, zero flow pressure ranges from 12–50 mm Hg. The source of this pressure includes the collapse of intramyocardial coronary microvessels at tissue pressures exceeding intraluminal pressures and the magnitude of the intracavitary back pressure. At least half of coronary vascular resistance results from vessels larger than 100 μm in diameter, whereas 10% results from coronary veins.[64] Coronary flow ceases completely at 20 mm Hg, the critical closure or critical flow pressure.[65] Coronary flow is determined by the duration of diastole and the difference between diastolic aortic pressure and left ventricular end-diastolic pressure.

Myocardial oxygen consumption is high; therefore coronary venous blood is only 30% saturated and its Po_2 of 18 or 20 mm Hg is the lowest anywhere in the body. Because oxygen extraction cannot be increased further, coronary flow must increase if the heart requires additional oxygen.

Coronary Autoregulation

Coronary perfusion is autoregulated to maintain a constant flow over a range of perfusion pressures (usually between 50 and 120 mm Hg) at any given myocardial oxygen demand.[66] Above and below these limits, coronary flow varies with perfusion pressure. The term autoregulation refers strictly to pressure-dependent changes in coronary resistance unrelated to changes in myocardial metabolism.[66] The principal site of coronary autoregulation is the coronary arteriole, a <150-μm diameter vessel, although small coronary arteries (>150 μm) can be recruited to increase flow during hypoperfusion.[67] Nevertheless, the coronary arterioles are not fully dilated even during hypoperfusion states.[67]

However, changes in myocardial oxygen demand alter autoregulation. The involved metabolite, therefore, is oxygen (specifically myocardial oxygen tension—Po_2) acting through mediators such as adenosine.[63] Adenosine-induced vasodilation is inversely related to arterial diameter, with the greatest dilation occurring in smaller vessels.[67] Hyperoxia decreases and a low Po_2 of 49 mm Hg increases coronary blood flow and myocardial oxygen consumption independently of changes in oxygen content or delivery.[68] The threshold oxygen tension for autoregulation is 32 mm Hg.[69] Coronary autoregulation is also closely coupled with coronary venous Po_2, particularly at Po_2 less than 25 mm Hg.[63,69] Decreased heart rate attenuates autoregulation, whereas pharmacologic coronary constriction augments it.[69]

The autoregulatory mechanism may even extend into different myocardial layers.[63] Autoregulation is greater in the subepicardium than in the subendocardium, possibly because of the transmural gradient to which the subendocardial vessels are exposed.[66] Autoregulation in the right coronary artery may be less than in the left coronary artery. Pressure and flow-dependent changes in myocardial oxygen consumption in the right ventricle explain these differences.[66] Reperfusion flow, immediately after occlusion of a coronary artery, increases beyond preocclusion levels. This process is termed reactive hyperemia. In a related process, reactive dilation, large coronary arteries dilate after relief of occlusion, but unlike in reactive hyperemia, the onset is delayed to 60 seconds and sustained for 150 seconds after relief of occlusion.[70]

The most important regulators of coronary vascular tone are metabolic, with adenosine being the most likely local mediator to link blood flow to oxygen consumption. Other mediators such as oxygen, potassium, pH, carbon dioxide, endothelium-derived relaxing factor, prostaglandins, prostacyclin, histamine, and adenosine triphosphate may affect coronary tone.[61] Prostaglandin E_1 dilates the coronary arteries, probably acting through adenosine as a mediator. Prostaglandin E_2, however, is a coronary vasoconstrictor.[71] Acetylcholine increases coronary flow. Acting through the H_1 receptor, histamine contracts epicardial coronary arteries, provoking spasm, but the H_2 receptor mediates vasodila-

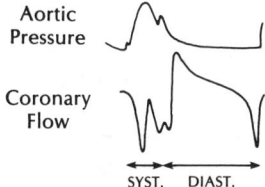

Figure 35-12. This diagrammatic relationship between aortic pressure and coronary flow demonstrates that little coronary flow occurs during systole, whereas the majority occurs during diastole. This relationship is particularly true for the left coronary artery, which supplies the left ventricle. The right ventricle, because it is thinner and develops less pressure, produces less impediment to systolic coronary flow.

tion.[72] Histamine also promotes production of prostaglandin in the heart.[72] Although norepinephrine (or sympathetic cardiac nerve stimulation) causes coronary constriction through its alpha effects, the associated increase in myocardial contractility increases coronary flow. Similarly, vagal stimulation may directly produce coronary vasodilation, but the associated decrease in heart rate and contractility causes secondary coronary vasoconstriction.

Coronary Flow Reserve

Coronary flow also increases by maximal dilation of the coronary arteries. The difference between resting and maximal coronary flow is the coronary flow reserve. Coronary flow is heterogeneous throughout the myocardium, although there is correlation between regional flow in neighboring myocardial areas.[73] Although coronary vasodilation occurs in response to ischemia or other endogenous stimuli, maximal flow, which is normally unavailable to the heart, may be achieved with pharmacologic agents. Exhaustion of autoregulatory vasodilator reserve does not necessarily mean that exhaustion of pharmacologic vasodilator reserve has occurred. Coronary flow reserve can be decreased by (1) decreased maximal flow and (2) increased regulated coronary flow.[74] Maximal coronary flow is decreased by tachycardia, increased blood viscosity, increased myocardial contractility, and myocardial hypertrophy.[63]

As epicardial coronary artery stenosis occurs, so does arteriolar vasodilation in order to maintain flow at normal levels. Once the vasodilator reserve is exhausted (usually at stenoses of greater than 90%), however, an increase in the stenosis of the coronary artery will decrease flow. Administration of a vasodilator to a vascular bed served by a normal and a stenotic coronary artery connected by collaterals will dilate the normal arterioles but produce little change in the arterioles served by the stenotic artery, since they are maximally dilated. The increased flow to the normal arterioles is termed "coronary steal."

Endocardial/Epicardial Flow Ratio

The distribution of coronary flow is as important as total flow. The ratio of flow in the endocardium to that in the epicardium, the endo/epi ratio, is used to assess flow distribution. Since subepicardial flow is usually adequate, if the endo/epi ratio remains constant, adequate subendocardial blood flow is inferred.[74] However, with maximal coronary vasodilation, the endo/epi ratio varies with the coronary perfusion pressure.[63] The ratio is minimally affected by changes in afterload but reduced by increased left ventricular preload. The latter results either from a disproportionate increase in subendocardial diastolic tissue pressure or an increase in coronary sinus pressure.[63] However, increased right ventricular preload decreases right ventricular blood flow without altering its intramyocardial distribution.[75] Transient subendocardial ischemia accompanies the onset of severe exercise. Although anemia increases coronary blood flow by autoregulation, severe anemia decreases the endo/epi ratio, indicating subendocardial ischemia.[63] Hypoxia, on the other hand, increases both coronary blood flow and the endo/epi ratio.

Neural Influences

Coronary arteries are also responsive to neural stimuli.[76] Parasympathetic and sympathetic nerves extend to the precapillary coronary vessels. Parasympathetic stimulation directly activates coronary muscarinic receptors, inducing dilation.

Sympathetic stimulation causes coronary dilatation as a result of the metabolic factors produced by increased Mvo_2 and direct beta receptor stimulation. Alpha$_2$ adrenoceptors or muscarinic receptors are present in the sympathetic nerve endings of coronary arteries. Activation of alpha$_1$ or alpha-adrenergic receptors by norepinephrine and acetylcholine (via the vagus nerve) reduces sympathetic neurotransmitter output, which would reduce the dilation of these vessels causing coronary vasoconstriction. Alpha$_2$ agonists also mediate release of endothelial-derived relaxing factor in coronary arteries. Beta$_1$-adrenergic receptors predominate over alpha$_1$ receptors in canine circumflex coronary artery.[77] Termination of the sympathetic cardiac effects results from extensive neuronal uptake of norepinephrine.[78] Only small amounts of the norepinephrine released by the heart enter the systemic circulation.[78]

Coronary artery spasm may result from unopposed alpha$_1$ adrenoceptor stimulation in the presence of beta-adrenergic blockade or when a pure alpha agonist is given. Acute coronary occlusion attenuates the baroreflex responses of heart rate and systemic vascular resistance.[79]

Cardiac Output

Cardiac output is the volume of blood pumped by the heart each minute. It is the product of the heart rate and the volume of each beat (stroke volume) but is determined by preload, afterload, heart rate, contractility, and ventricular compliance (see Table 35-4). Cardiac output measurements are usually corrected for the size of the patient by dividing the output by the body surface area to give the cardiac index. A normal cardiac index is 2.5 to 3.5 $l \cdot min^{-1} \cdot m^{-2}$ (Table 35-5). Cardiac output increases with increased heart rate, preload, or contractility and decreased afterload. Decreases in cardiac output result from decreased heart rate, contractility, or preload and increased afterload.

Determinants

Preload. Preload is defined as the end-diastolic stress on the ventricle (end-diastolic fiber length or end-diastolic volume). The determinants of preload are blood volume, venous tone, ventricular compliance, ventricular afterload, and myocardial contractility. The distribution of the blood volume between intrathoracic and extrathoracic compartments also affects preload. Extrathoracic blood volume increases with standing, whereas the negative intrathoracic pressure during inspiration increases intrathoracic blood volume.

Stroke volume is determined by the volume of blood in the heart at the beginning of systole (end-diastolic volume—EDV) and the amount of blood remaining in the ventricle at closure of the aortic valve at the end of systole

---

TABLE 35-4. Major Determinants of Cardiac Output

Preload
Afterload
Contractility
Heart rate
Compliance

TABLE 35-5. Hemodynamic Variables: Calculations and Normal Values

Variable	Calculation	Normal Values
Cardiac index (CI)	CO/BSA	$2.5-4.0$ l·min^{-1}·m^{-2}
Stroke volume (SV)	CO/HR	$60-90$ ml·beat^{-1}
Stroke index (SI)	SV/BSA	$40-60$ ml·beat^{-1}·m^{-2}
Mean arterial pressure (MAP)	Diastolic pressure + 1/3 pulse pressure	$80-120$ mm Hg
Systemic vascular resistance (SVR)	$\dfrac{\text{MAP} - \text{CVP}}{\text{CO}} \times 79.9$	$1200-1500$ dynes·cm·sec^{-5}
Pulmonary vascular resistance (PVR)	$\dfrac{\overline{\text{PAP}} - \text{PWP}}{\text{CO}} \times 79.9$	$100-300$ dynes·cm·sec^{-5}
Right ventricular stroke work index (RVSWI)	$0.0136\,(\overline{\text{PAP}} - \text{CVP}) \times \text{SI}$	$5-9$ g·m·beat^{-1}·m^{-2}
Left ventricular stroke work index (LVSWI)	$0.136\,(\text{MAP} - \overline{\text{PWP}}) \times \text{SI}$	$45-60$ g·m·beat^{-1}·m^{-2}

CVP = mean central venous pressure; BSA = body surface area; CO = cardiac output; $\overline{\text{PAP}}$ = mean pulmonary artery pressure; PWP = pulmonary wedge pressure; MAP = mean arterial blood pressure; g·m = gram meter; sec^{-5} = seconds^{-5}.

(end-systolic volume—ESV). The degree of stretch of the left ventricular fibers, determined by the amount of blood in the ventricle, determines the amount of work the ventricle can do.[80] An increase in preload increases end-diastolic volume and wall tension.

End-diastolic volume is not synonymous with end-diastolic pressure, nor are the two linearly related. The ejection fraction, normally 0.6 to 0.7, is the ratio of the stroke volume to the end-diastolic volume. Severe impairment of ventricular function is present when the ejection fraction is less than 0.4.

$$\text{Ejection fraction} = \frac{\text{EDV} - \text{ESV}}{\text{EDV}}$$

Afterload. Afterload is the wall stress or tension faced by the myocardium during ventricular ejection. It is the force opposing ventricular fiber shortening during ejection. Left ventricular afterload depends upon the shape, size, radius, and wall thickness of the ventricle, with the principal factors being the radius (related to preload and chamber volume) and aortic impedance (controlled by arterial compliance and systemic vascular resistance). Other factors involved in afterload include arterial wall stiffness (aortic), blood viscosity, and the mass of blood in the aorta. Usually the ejection phase stress is implied in discussions of afterload, although there are wall stresses during the isovolumetric contraction phase.

Clinically, systemic vascular resistance is frequently used as an estimate of afterload (see Table 35-4). However, systemic vascular resistance reflects only peripheral arteriolar tone rather than left ventricular systolic wall tension. A true measure of left ventricular afterload, such as left ventricular end-systolic wall stress, which incorporates left ventricular chamber pressure, ventricular dimensions, wall thickness, and peripheral loading conditions, should be used to accurately assess afterload.[81] However, these measurements require direct intraventricular pressure determination and echocardiographic evaluation of wall thickness and ventricular dimensions. Compared with left ventricular end-systolic wall stress, systemic vascular resistance underestimates afterload when afterload is increased or decreased or contractility is improved.[81]

When afterload is reduced, the ventricle shortens more quickly and completely.[82] An increase in afterload decreases the extent and velocity of shortening and increases active tension and the time to peak tension in cardiac muscle. Wall tension, ventricular radius, and end-diastolic volume are also increased to maintain stroke volume. In the poorly contractile heart, acute increases in afterload severely reduce stroke volume. For this reason, vasodilator therapy benefits patients with heart failure. Hearts facing chronically increased afterload adapt by hypertrophy, which returns wall stress and shortening characteristics toward normal.

Heart Rate. Heart rate is primarily determined by the automaticity of the sinus node. However, its intrinsic rate depends upon both neural and humoral influences. Neural influences are paramount, with sympathetic stimulation increasing and parasympathetic or vagal stimulation decreasing heart rate. An increase in heart rate increases cardiac output even if the stroke volume remains constant by increasing the extent and velocity of shortening and dP/dt.[83] The increase of dP/dt with heart rate is even more pronounced if end-diastolic dimensions are maintained by volume infusion.[83] This effect is often prominent during anesthesia. Between heart rates of 120 and 160 beats per minute, cardiac output increases but not as much as at more optimal heart rates (Fig. 35-13). An increase in heart rate shortens the filling time between beats, reducing end-diastolic volume. Because most cardiac filling occurs during the first half-second of the rapid filling phase, cardiac output decreases at heart rates over 160 beats per minute because of inadequate filling time.

Cardiac output is also increased during the heartbeat after a ventricular extrasystole. This extrasystolic potentiation results from increased ejection fraction, decreased left ventricular end-diastolic volume, and enhanced diastolic filling. The mechanism is probably increased availability of calcium to the contractile mechanism.[84]

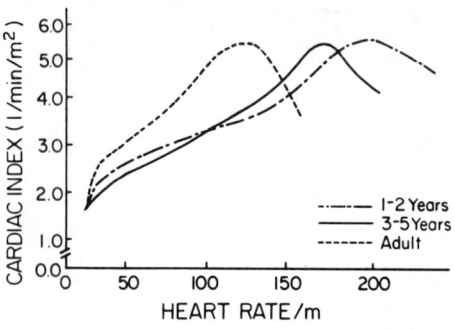

Figure 35-13. The effect of heart rate on cardiac index varies with age. In children, an increase in heart rate increases cardiac index because the immature heart is relatively noncompliant and does not increase its stroke volume in response to increased demands. In the adult, however, an increase in heart rate beyond 120 beats per minute does not increase cardiac index. (Reproduced with permission of the author and publisher from Wetsel RC: Critical Care State of the Art. Vol. 2, p 9. Fullerton, California, Society of Critical Care Medicine, 1981.)

Contractility. Contractility is the inotropic state independent of changes in preload, afterload, or heart rate.

Cardiac Systole. Myocardial contraction begins when the action potential, described previously, acting through the T-(tubule) system of the sarcoplasmic reticulum, results in calcium release into the sarcoplasm. A cyclic adenosine monophosphate–dependent protein kinase in the heart stimulates calcium transport by the vesicles of the sarcoplasmic reticulum (see Fig. 35-9). Intracellular cyclic adenosine monophosphate protein kinase is activated and transfers the terminal phosphate of adenosine triphosphate to troponin I, phospholamban, or other intracellular proteins. Troponin has three components: troponin I, the inhibitory factor inhibiting the magnesium-stimulated adenosine triphosphatase of actomyosin; troponin C, which is the calcium-sensitive factor; and troponin A, which allows attachment of the troponin complex to actin and tropomyosin. Phospholamban, a membrane-bound protein that is a calcium-stimulated magnesium adenosine triphosphatase, permits increased calcium uptake and calcium release by the sarcoplasmic reticulum.[85] Adenosine triphosphatase from the calcium pump, which couples hydrolysis of one molecule of adenosine triphosphate with the active transport of two calcium ions, is the channel through which the activator calcium is released to initiate systole. The increased free calcium is bound to troponin C, releasing the inhibition of actin-myosin interaction by the troponin-tropomyosin complex. Contraction of actin and myosin occurs. Both developed tension and relaxation depend upon the rate of calcium delivery to troponin, the quantity of available calcium, and the rate of calcium removal from troponin.[86]

Diastole. Relaxation of the heart and its return to a precontractile configuration actually begin during late systole and continue during isovolumic relaxation and rapid ventricular filling. Myocardial relaxation occurs as a result of reuptake of or binding of calcium ion by the sarcoplasmic reticulum, a lusitropic or relaxing effect of cyclic adenosine monophosphate.[87] Relaxation is a load-dependent process. In the relaxing heart, load is the premature lengthening of cardiac muscle. Myocardial relaxation depends upon internal restoring forces such as cardiac fibers, hemodynamic loading such as the impedance of the arterial system, and external restoring forces resulting from deformation of the wall of the intact heart.[88] During relaxation, load dependence indicates the dissipation of activation, and diastolic "suction" occurs as a consequence. During hypoxia, load dependence of relaxation is suppressed, probably from inhibition of the reuptake of calcium by the sarcoplasmic reticulum or impaired detachment of the force-generating site of actin and myosin.[88] These findings explain the relaxation abnormalities associated with ischemic disease.

Alterations in Contractility. Myocardial contractility is evaluated by the rate of ventricular pressure change with time (dP/dt), mean circumferential fiber shortening rate (during ejection phase), force-velocity curves, pressure-volume loops, or other derived parameters described later. The cardiac output can be increased by increasing load, either volume or pressure (heterometric autoregulation); by the Anrep effect (homeometric autoregulation), in which ventricular performance improves several beats after the initial stretching of the myocardial fibers owing to abruptly increased aortic or left ventricular pressure; by the treppe phenomenon; or by a change in the inotropic state independent of the above mechanisms. The Anrep effect occurs from increased contractility resulting from more rapid activation of the contractile process, increased developed force, and increased velocity of shortening. It is operative for only a few minutes as the initially increased ventricular end-diastolic volume and circumference decrease with recovery of stroke work.[88]

The treppe phenomenon (force-frequency relation, staircase effect, or Bowditch's phenomenon) is a progressive increase in contractile force associated with a sudden increase in heart rate. A long pause between beats also increases the force of contraction and is known as the Woodworth phenomenon or reverse (negative) staircase effect.[89] Increasing contractility increases the ejection fraction if end-systolic volume decreases while end-diastolic volume remains the same. Contractility is decreased by hypoxia, acidosis, cardiomyopathy, myocardial ischemia or infarction, and drugs such as calcium entry or beta blockers.

Compliance. Compliance is defined as the change in end-diastolic volume/change in end-diastolic pressure. The relationship between ventricular volume and diastolic pressure is nonlinear. The rapidity of diastolic filling is a major determinant of cardiac output, which is reduced by decreased compliance. Although the contractility of the ventricle may be normal, reduced relaxation from coronary artery disease, hypertrophic cardiomyopathy, cardiac tamponade, and hypertensive heart disease impairs diastolic filling which, in turn, limits cardiac output.

Myocardial Mechanics

The mechanical function of the heart is determined by evaluation of velocity of shortening, exerted force or tension, instantaneous length, and time after activation. Among the traditional indices of myocardial contractility are ventricular function (Starling) curves, ejection phase indices (force-velocity curves, ejection fraction, velocity of circumferential fiber shortening), isovolumic phase indices (rate of left ventricular pressure development [dP/dt], velocity of circumferential fiber shortening [Vcf], and maximal velocity of contractile element shortening [Vmax]), and end-systolic indices (pressure-volume or pressure-length relationship at end systole). Normal dP/dt is 800–1700 mm Hg·sec^{-1}, but measurements are affected by intrapatient variation and complicated recording equipment. Complexity of measurement is also a problem with measurement of circumferential fiber shortening, which is sensitive to acute changes in afterload. End-systolic indices are better methods of measuring contractility, less affected by either preload or afterload. End-systolic volume is independent of initial ventricular volume. However, the completeness of ventricular emptying depends on both afterload and contractility.[90] Ejection fraction is affected by changes in loading conditions independent of changes in ventricular contractility.

Starling (Ventricular Function) Curve. Myocardial contractility and function can be altered with or without changes in end-diastolic myocardial fiber length. If the cardiac muscle is stretched, it develops greater contractile tension. This observation is the basis of Starling's law, which states that "the law of the heart is therefore the same as that of skeletal muscle, namely, that the mechanical energy set free on passage from the resting to the contracted state depends . . . on the length of the muscle fibers."[91] Atrial as well as ventricular muscle obeys Starling's law. However, the Starling curve of the right ventricle is upward and to the left of the left ventricular function curve. Increased preload or initial fiber length increases resting tension, velocity of tension development, and peak tension. An increase in venous return stretches the muscle fibers to increase contractility and improve cardiac output. However, this finding appears to occur only at subnormal filling pressures. In the upright position, ventricular filling pressures decrease to about 4 mm Hg, and the normal heart operates on the ascending limb of the ventricular function curve. Peak ventricular output occurs at normal filling pressures of about 10 mm Hg in normal humans.[92] Whether the heart can fall onto a descending limb of the length-stroke volume curve like skeletal muscle is unclear.[92] On the descending limb, the heart decompensates, and further increases in end-diastolic volume decrease stroke volume, but disengagement of actin and myosin does not occur. In all probability, the heart actually moves to a different curve.

Ventricular function curves are influenced by afterload, although they incorporate the effects of preload alterations (Fig. 35-14). To ensure that a change in contractility has occurred when using Starling curves, afterload must be controlled. Starling curves are used clinically when weaning patients from cardiopulmonary bypass, to assess the effects of anesthetic agents on the heart, and to guide fluid and pharmacologic therapy in the perioperative period. The effects of both the "atrial kick" and the "idioventricular kick" on stroke volume are manifestations of Starling's law. The increased stretch and end-diastolic length produced by atrial (atrial kick) or early contracting ventricular fibers (idioventricular kick) increase ventricular stroke volume.

Pressure-Volume Loops. Another index of contractility that is less affected by preload, afterload, or other conditions is the pressure-volume loop, an end-systolic index (Fig. 35-15). At end systole, ejection ceases, and the aortic valve closes with the ventricle at minimum dimension and volume.

Although pressure-volume loops can be measured in humans using gated blood pool scintigraphy, two-dimensional echocardiography, or contrast angiocardiography and intravascular catheterization, performance is difficult and results are not immediately available for patient care.[93]

In such loops, the height and width of the loop are determined by the ventricular systolic pressure and stroke vol-

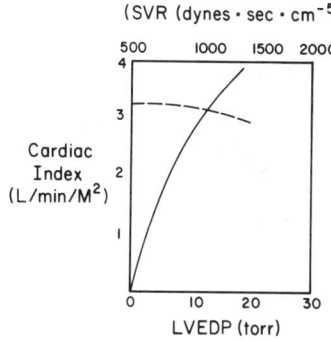

Figure 35-14. The ventricular function (Starling) curve of the normal left ventricle (solid line) is affected much more by changes in preload (left ventricular end-diastolic pressure) than by an increase in afterload (dotted line). The failing heart moves to a curve downward and to the right of the normal heart. Venodilator therapy decreases preload without increasing cardiac index (the heart moves to the left on the curve), whereas reduction of afterload increases cardiac index without a change in preload. Combined preload and afterload reduction decreases filling pressure and increases cardiac index.

ume. The area subtended by the systolic portion of the curve provides a measure of stroke work during ejection, whereas the area of the diastolic limb is a measure of diastolic work performed during ventricular filling and distention. The volume between the systolic and diastolic portions of the loop is the stroke volume. Cardiac work, the product of pressure and volume, is the area of the pressure-volume loop, which is linearly related to myocardial oxygen consumption under various hemodynamic conditions.[94] In a given ventricle, all the end systolic points are positioned on the same line, which represents the elastance of that ventricle (the change in end-systolic pressure/change in end-systolic volume). Contractility is directly proportional to elastance, with its slope becoming steeper with increased contractility and flatter with decreased contractility. The slope of the end-systolic pressure-volume relation is linear and correlates well with the ejection fraction.[95]

Pressure-volume loops also reveal information about ventricular compliance. The normal relationship between diastolic pressure and volume is curvilinear. There is a relatively gentle slope at low end-diastolic pressures (e.g., little change in pressure for large changes in volume). At end-diastolic pressures at the upper limits of normal (12 mm Hg or more), the curve becomes steeper, and pressure is almost exponentially related to end-diastolic volume. Ventricular compliance decreases under such conditions. Thus, compliance actually changes during each contraction.

The ventricular end-systolic pressure/volume relationship may be dependent on the type of loading intervention but can be used to assess left ventricular performance under various conditions[96] (Fig. 35-15). However, one limitation of pressure-volume loops is that pressure may inaccurately reflect end-systolic afterload.[90] The ratio of pressure to volume at end systole can also be used as an index of contractile function. However, this assumes that at higher pressures there are larger volumes at a given inotropic state.[90]

Pressure-Length Loops. Measurement of a pressure-length loop is a reproducible and sensitive method to evaluate total or regional systolic and diastolic myocardial function. However, it requires direct measurement of changes in myocardial length and intraventricular pressure. Ventricular segment length is plotted on the X axis and ventricular pressure

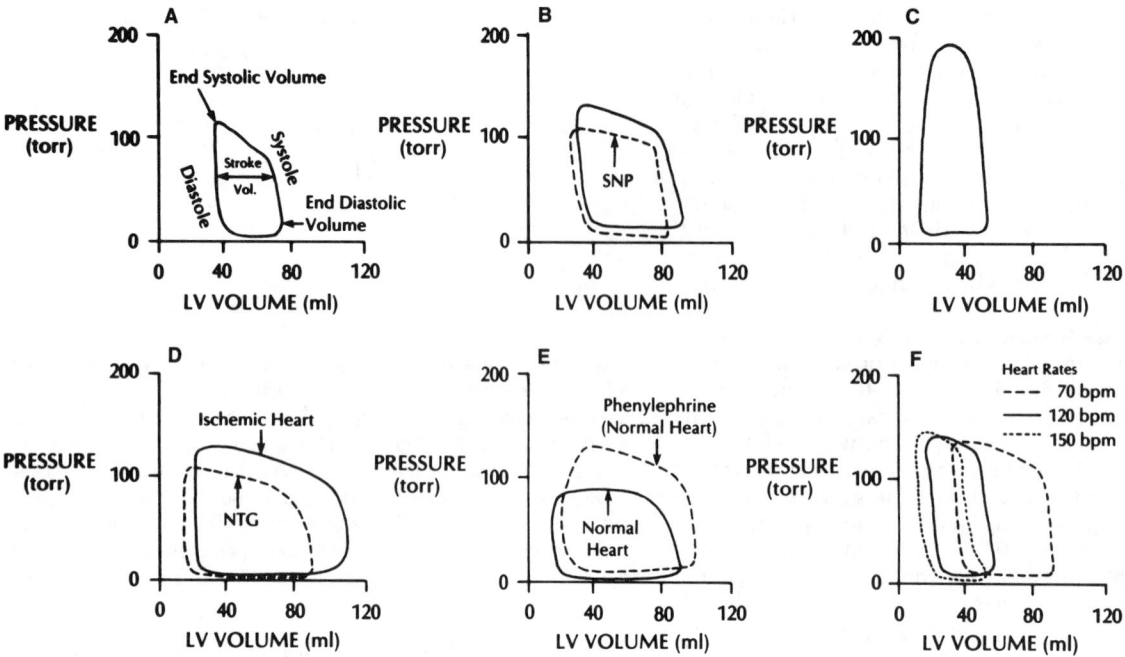

Figure 35-15. The relationship of ventricular pressure and volume over the entire cardiac cycle is the pressure-volume loop shown in (*A*). The loop begins on the bottom with opening of the mitral valve and filling of the ventricle to end-diastolic volume. An extension of the bottom portion of the loop (without ventricular systole) would give a diastolic pressure-volume curve for the ventricle. Isovolumetric contraction begins at the lower right portion of the curve with closure of the mitral valve. The aortic valve opens at the upper right portion of the loop, and ventricular ejection begins. At the upper left of the loop, the aortic valve closes (end-systolic volume), and isovolumetric relaxation returns the loop to the starting point. Stroke volume is the difference between the volume at the end of diastole and the end of systole. The effects of afterload reduction on the pressure-volume loop are shown in (*B*), whereas (*E*) shows the changes with increased afterload; (*C*) shows the changes in the pressure-volume loop in a patient with aortic stenosis, with a high peak systolic pressure and steep diastolic slope representing reduced ventricular compliance. In (*D*), an ischemic heart has its pressure/volume shifted upward and to the right. Nitroglycerin therapy moves the curve toward normal. Venodilation and coronary vasodilation improve both contractility and compliance of the ischemic heart in (*E*). In a normal heart (*F*), an increase in heart rate markedly reduces left ventricular volume.

on the Y axis. Normal loops are rectangular and include four segments: isovolumic contraction (right), ejection (top), isovolumic relaxation (left), and filling (bottom) (Fig. 35-16). The area of the loop represents ventricular stroke work.[97] Pressure-length loops are altered by changes in preload, afterload, inotropic state, and ischemia. Ischemia increases postsystolic shortening and systolic lengthening, as depicted in Figure 35-16 (inset).[98]

Force-Velocity Curve. Myocardial contractility can also increase when the myocardial fibers increase their developed force or velocity of shortening without a change in fiber length. Force-velocity curves evaluate contractility (velocity of shortening) at constant fiber length in a passively stretched muscle (preloaded), which is stimulated to contract against either no load or an afterload. Force-velocity curves are much more sensitive indicators of contractility than Starling curves and are based on the Hill model of isolated muscle.

As afterload is increased, the initial rate of shortening follows a hyperbolic relationship (Fig. 35-17). The force or tension developed during contraction is measured by dP/dt max, the maximum rate of rise of intraventricular pressure

during the isometric phase of ventricular contraction. The point of the curve where no shortening occurs, although the muscle develops maximal force, is termed Po. Extrapolation of the curve back to zero load where the maximal velocity of shortening occurs is termed Vmax. Both preload and afterload affect dP/dt max. As preload increases, the maximum isometric tension that the muscle develops increases, but the maximal velocity of shortening is unchanged. An increase in myocardial contractility increases both the developed tension and the maximum velocity of shortening, shifting the force-velocity curve upward and to the right.

Cardiac Work. Because of the difficulties in obtaining the data for pressure-volume loops or force-velocity curves under clinical conditions, cardiac work is often measured as a substitute. Cardiac work describes pump function in terms of the load carried and the distance moved. The calculation of cardiac work and its indexing to body surface area (left and right ventricular stroke work indexes) are shown in Table 35-5. The advantages of using cardiac work instead of cardiac output or stroke volume to describe pump function are (1) calculation includes heart rate, preload, and afterload, the major variables affecting cardiac function; (2)

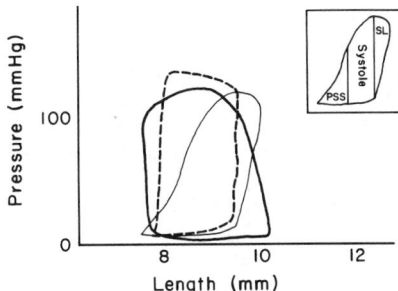

Figure 35-16. The normal pressure-length loop (*thick black line*) is a rectangle whose area indicates total ventricular work. Ischemia (*thin solid line*) causes the loop to lean toward the right because of increased systolic lengthening (SL) and postsystolic shortening (PSS) (*inset*). Increased afterload (*dashed line*) causes the loop to become taller at a similar preload. (Reprinted with permission from Lake CL: Clinical Monitoring, p 254. Philadelphia: WB Saunders, 1990.)

stroke work index defines the area of the pressure-volume loop; and (3) stroke work index measures both systolic and diastolic performance.[99]

Right Ventricular Function. The functional significance of the RV in normal circulatory homeostasis is minimal. After excitation, the wave of contraction spreads over the right ventricular free wall from the sinus to the conal (outflow) portion, with contraction of the conal portion lagging 25–50 msec behind the inflow portion.[100] Although the right ventricular spiral muscles contract during systole, direct left ventricular assistance to right ventricular contraction has been demonstrated.[101] Intraventricular pressure develops more gradually in the RV and declines more slowly during diastole. Peak ejection occurs later than in the LV. This difference in function results because the right ventricular free wall is flattened by the pull of the interventricular septum toward the LV during systole, giving a bellows-like action for expulsion of blood.[102] Because of this mechanism, right ventricular function is less likely to be impaired during right coronary arterial occlusion.[102]

During systole, right ventricular stroke volume is more sensitive to afterload than left ventricular stroke volume.

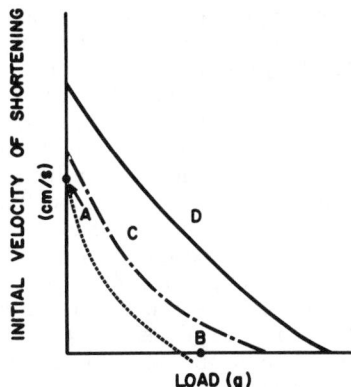

Figure 35-17. A force velocity curve of cardiac muscle shows the point of maximal shortening with no load or Vmax (point A). Point B is Po where no shortening occurs, although tension development is maximal. Curve C is a force-velocity curve with increased preload. Curve D demonstrates increased myocardial contractility. On any curve, load (afterload) increases from left to right. (Reprinted with permission from Lake CL: Cardiovascular Anesthesia, p 10. New York, Springer Verlag, 1985.)

Factors that oppose blood flow from the RV (afterload) include the resistance of the pulmonary vascular bed, pulmonary arterial impedance, the mass of the pulmonary blood, blood viscosity, and pulse wave reflection altering pulmonary artery pressure.[100]

In diastole the RV is twice as distensible (more compliant) as the LV.[103] Right ventricular pumping capability depends on (1) pressure against which it ejects, (2) filling volume, and (3) right ventricular contractility.[103] The RV obeys Starling's law except at higher end-diastolic pressures, where its response is flatter than that of the LV.[100] Increases in filling volume increase right ventricular stroke volume up to the limit imposed by the restraint of the pericardium (normally about a 20% acute increase in cardiac volume).[102] The contractility of the RV depends upon sympathetic tone, myocardial structural integrity, and the chemical content of the coronary perfusate.[103]

Normally, right ventricular systolic pressures are only 30–40 mm Hg because the recruitable vasculature of the pulmonary circulation allows between 5 and 20 l of blood to flow within it. Its ejection fraction is about 0.4. However, under conditions of pressure overload, such as increased pulmonary vascular resistance or left ventricular failure, it hypertrophies to generate systemic pressures. Although acute right ventricular failure is compatible with life, the symptoms caused by increased venous pressure suggest that right ventricular function is important for maintenance of normal venous pressures.[100,102]

Ventricular Interdependence. Because the ventricles are anatomically associated, alterations of volume and pressure in one ventricle can affect these parameters in the other.[104] During normal respiration, right ventricular end-diastolic volume increases during inspiration, left ventricular diastolic volume decreases, and left ventricular transmural pressure is unchanged. Important factors in ventricular interdependence are septal position and deformability, ventricular distensibility, and the trans-septal pressure gradient. Interdependence requires the presence of the pericardium and is enhanced during pericardial tamponade.[105]

In vitro experimental animal models confirm that when left ventricular pressure increases, both decreased diastolic compliance and depressed systolic ventricular function occur in the RV and *vice versa*. The mechanisms are (1) a Frank Starling effect caused by decreased ventricular diastolic volume, and (2) decreased systolic ventricular function.[106] The etiology of the depressed systolic function is unclear.[106]

Increased distention of either ventricle alters the compliance and geometry of the opposite ventricle. Myocardial infarction that decreases left ventricular free wall compliance causes right ventricular pressure and volume displacement to be more responsive to changes in left ventricular volume.[104] Computer models confirm that hypertrophy from right ventricular pressure overload, which increases septal thickness and decreases septal compliance, decreases transfer of pressure and volume between the ventricles, limiting ventricular interdependence.

Myocardial Metabolism

An understanding of myocardial metabolism is essential to the preservation of the heart during conditions of stress, cardiac arrest, or elective asystole during cardiac surgery. Metabolism includes both substrate utilization and oxygen consumption.

Sources of Energy. The energy supply of the heart is derived primarily from lactate and fatty acids delivered by the coronary blood. Free or nonesterified fatty acids (palmitic and oleic acids) are the preferred fuel.[107] Myocardial uptake of fatty acids is almost linear with the plasma concentration above the threshold of 345 μmol·l^{-1}.[108] Fatty acid uptake by the heart from either fatty acid–albumin complexes or lipoprotein triglyceride occurs by passive diffusion or carrier-mediated transport. During fasting, free fatty acids are always used as fuel. The heart has a limited ability to synthesize fatty acids from acetyl coenzyme A, except for the formation of structural lipids. The oxidation of fatty acids and ketone bodies inhibits uptake of glucose, pyruvate oxidation, and glycolysis while facilitating glycogen synthesis.[108] Oxidation of nonesterified fatty acids accounts for 90% of myocardial oxygen consumption.

Fuel selection by the heart probably depends on regulatory enzymes controlled by factors other than substrate availability and product removal. Myocardial lactate utilization is regulated by the arterial lactate concentrations and pyruvate oxidation in the Krebs tricarboxylic acid cycle. Glucose, pyruvate, acetate, and triglycerides can also be used by the heart as energy sources. Utilization of glucose by the myocardium depends on the arterial glucose and insulin concentrations. Glucose is normally used postprandially. However, glucose use by the myocardium as the primary energy source occurs only with high glucose levels, insulin secretion, or hypoxia. Glucose is the only substrate used by the heart anaerobically. As long as the entry of acetyl coenzyme A into the Krebs cycle is not inhibited, the heart will use as much pyruvate as it is given. Substrates such as fructose, glycogen, or proteins are used for energy only during special circumstances, such as starvation, diabetic ketoacidosis, or anoxia.[109]

Myocardial Oxygen Consumption. The heart has one of the highest metabolic rates of any organ. At rest it uses 8–10 ml of oxygen per 100 g of myocardium per minute. The subendocardium requires about 20% more oxygen than the epicardium. For this reason, the subendocardium is more vulnerable to ischemia. Myocardial oxygen consumption ($M\dot{V}O_2$) is determined by heart rate, wall tension, and myocardial contractility (Table 35-6). The relative importance of each of these factors is difficult to evaluate because they are inter-related through wall tension.[110] Less important factors include the oxygen costs of shortening of muscle fibers, electrical activation, and catecholamines as well as the basal

---

TABLE 35-6. Factors Involved in Myocardial Oxygen Supply and Demand

Myocardial Oxygen Consumption

Heart rate
Contractile state
Myocardial wall tension
Arterial oxygen content
Basal oxygen requirements
Oxygen cost of muscle fiber shortening
Oxygen cost of electrical activation

Myocardial Oxygen Supply

Aortic diastolic pressure
Left ventricular end-diastolic pressure
Coronary artery diameter
Arterial oxygen content

---

oxygen requirements and the level of arterial oxygenation. Tension development constitutes about 50% of $M\dot{V}O_2$.

Myocardial wall tension is related to the tension-time index, left ventricular end-diastolic pressure, and ventricular size. Wall tension can be divided into its components: the rate of force development, the magnitude of force development, the interval during which force is generated and maintained for each contraction, and the frequency with which force is developed per unit time.[110] Wall tension is measured according to Laplace's law:

$$T = Pr/2h$$

where radius (r) is cardiac radius, T is cardiac tension, P is interventricular pressure, and h is ventricular muscle thickness. Increases in ventricular chamber pressure or volume increase both the magnitude of force development and the force maintained during ejection.

Tachycardia is well tolerated in the normal heart, although myocardial oxygen consumption and blood flow must increase. There is little change in arteriovenous oxygen difference across the coronary bed with moderate increases in heart rate. At extremely rapid heart rates, the arteriovenous oxygen difference increases. Tachycardia shortens diastole more than systole, increases myocardial contractility, and decreases both stroke volume and ventricular volume to maintain aortic pressure.[74]

Myocardial Supply-Demand Ratio. A balance must always exist between oxygen consumption (demand) and myocardial oxygen supply if ischemia is to be avoided. Factors important to this relationship are shown in Table 35-6. Myocardial oxygen supply is dependent upon the diameter of the coronary arteries, left ventricular end-diastolic pressure, aortic diastolic pressure, and arterial oxygen content. Myocardial blood flow is determined by the blood pressure at the coronary ostia, arteriolar tone, intramyocardial pressure or extravascular resistance, coronary occlusive disease, heart rate, coronary collateral development, and blood viscosity. The epicardial coronary arteries contribute little to coronary vascular resistance, whereas the intramural coronary vessels are the principal determinants.

In the normal heart, the coronary perfusion pressure is the difference between the aortic diastolic pressure and the left ventricular end-diastolic pressure. Because in coronary occlusive disease the pressure distal to a coronary stenosis is lower than aortic diastolic pressure, this relationship is not applicable to this condition. Myocardial blood flow is also reduced by a low aortic diastolic pressure, increased pulmonary wedge pressure (both of which increase subendocardial tissue pressure), and tachycardia, which shortens diastole, reducing the duration of blood flow. Increasing preload or intracavitary pressure increases wall tension and oxygen demand while decreasing subendocardial perfusion.

Myocardial oxygen supply is also affected by the level of arterial oxygenation. Oxygen content resulting from PaO_2, hemoglobin, 2,3-diphosphoglycerate (DPG), and pH, PCO_2, or temperature effects on the oxyhemoglobin dissociation curve can be an important factor in patients with obstructive lung disease or severe anemia. Normal oxygen extraction by the heart is 60–70% and changes very little with increased cardiac work because coronary vascular resistance decreases. However, if the coronary vascular resistance response is limited, oxygen extraction can be increased to more than 90%.[110] An increase in oxygen extraction and coronary vasodilation constitutes the metabolic reserve of the heart in the case of increased demand.

Heart rate and diastolic ventricular volume are the two factors most likely to produce ischemia if either or both are increased. Increased myocardial contractility or afterload, by increasing arterial pressure and myocardial oxygen supply, offsets their tendency to increase myocardial oxygen consumption.

Distribution of Cardiac Output

The cardiac output is distributed to the organ systems as follows: brain 12%, heart 4%, liver 24%, kidneys 20%, muscle 23%, skin 6%, and intestines 8%. The total tissue blood flow in a given vascular bed is a function of the effective perfusion pressure and vascular resistance. Effective perfusion pressure is the difference between arterial and venous pressure across the vascular bed. Organ circulations that autoregulate to keep blood flow constant in the face of changes in perfusion pressure include the cerebral, renal, coronary, hepatic arterial, intestinal, and muscle circulations.

Cardiovascular Reflexes

Carotid Sinus Reflex. This reflex, also called the pressoreceptor or baroreceptor reflex, occurs when an increase in blood pressure stretches pressoreceptors in the carotid sinus or arch of the aorta to increase their frequency of discharge. The impulses are transmitted along the afferent nerve of Hering[111] to the glossopharyngeal (carotid receptors) or vagus (aortic receptors) nerve and to the cardiovascular centers in the medulla. The medullary cardiovascular center, in turn, inhibits sympathetic and increases parasympathetic activity, resulting in decreased cardiac contractility, heart rate, and vasoconstrictor tone. When the arterial pressure decreases as a result of medullary input, there are fewer afferent impulses to the cardiovascular center, sympathetic tone increases, and vagal tone decreases. The baroreceptor reflex reduces changes in arterial pressure to about one third of expected. The threshold of the reflex is about 60 mm Hg, and its limits are pressures of 175–300 mm Hg.[112] Its gain is determined by the pulse pressure.[113]

Valsalva Maneuver. The response to the Valsalva maneuver is mediated by the pressoreceptor reflex. The Valsalva maneuver is accomplished by voluntarily closing the glottis while performing a forced expiration to increase intrathoracic pressure. Venous pressure in the head and extremities increases while venous return to the right ventricle decreases. As a consequence, cardiac output and blood pressure decrease, resulting in a reflex increase in heart rate. With glottic opening, venous return to the right heart suddenly increases, causing forceful right and subsequently left ventricular contraction. The increase in blood pressure then elicits the pressoreceptor response to produce transient bradycardia.

Müller Maneuver. The Müller maneuver is an inspiratory effort against a closed airway. During this maneuver, right ventricular end-diastolic volume and left ventricular end-diastolic pressure increase, whereas left ventricular end-diastolic volume is unchanged or decreased. Ejection fraction is unchanged. Pleural pressure decreases, and the afterloading effects of decreased pleural pressure increase left ventricular volume. The net effect of these changes on left ventricular function depends on ventricular interdependence, heart rate, and contractility (position of the heart on diastolic pressure-volume curve).

In patients with coronary artery disease, ventricular akinesis may be seen during the Müller maneuver. This finding may be attributable to increased wall stress increasing myocardial oxygen demand or increased left ventricular transmural pressure decreasing motion in nonfunctional ventricular myocardium.

Bezold-Jarisch Reflex. Noxious stimuli to the ventricular wall activate left ventricular mechanoreceptors, which reflexly cause hypotension, bradycardia, and parasympathetically induced coronary vasodilation.[114-116] The afferent pathway is nonmyelinated vagal C fibers.[115] Reperfusion of previously ischemic tissue also elicits the reflex.[117]

The mirror image of the Bezold-Jarisch reflex is the cardiogenic hypertensive chemoreflex described by James.[118] The chemoreceptors are located between the aorta and pulmonary artery and supplied by the left coronary artery. The afferent reflex pathway is intrathoracic vagal branches and the efferent path is via phrenic, vagal, and sympathetic routes. In response to serotonin, arterial pressure increases markedly in 4–6 seconds owing to increased inotropy and peripheral vasoconstriction. This reflex may be responsible for hypertension during angina, myocardial infarction, and after coronary bypass grafting. It is abolished by vagotomy, atropine, local anesthesia of the intertruncal space, or cyproheptadine.[118]

Cushing's Reflex. Increased cerebrospinal fluid pressure compresses cerebral arteries, causing cerebral ischemia. The response to cerebral ischemia is an increase in arterial pressure sufficient to reperfuse the brain. Intense sympathetic activity causes severe peripheral vasoconstriction as a result of this reflex.

Atrial Reflexes. Bainbridge described a reflex increase in heart rate when vagal tone was high and the right atrium or central veins were distended. The response of the heart to atrial distention depends upon the pre-existing heart rate. There is no effect with pre-existing tachycardia, but volume loading at a slow heart rate causes progressive tachycardia.[57] Although the Bainbridge reflex is primarily mediated through vagal myelinated afferent fibers, activation of sympathetic afferent fibers may also occur.[57] Increased right atrial pressure directly stretches the SA node and enhances its automaticity, increasing the heart rate and making the existence of this reflex questionable. Experimental distention of the cavoatrial junctions or other small portions of the atria increases heart rate, but clinical conditions such as heart failure usually do not produce such locally increased atrial pressure.[119] Global atrial distention in response to high pressures causes bradycardia, hypotension, and decreased systemic vascular resistance.[120]

Chemoreceptor Reflex. Peripheral chemoreceptors sensitive to decreasing oxygen tension or increased hydrogen ion concentrations in the blood are located in the carotid and aortic bodies. Nerve fibers from the chemoreceptors pass through the nerve of Hering and the vagus nerve to the medullary vasomotor centers. Normally the peripheral chemoreceptors are minimally active. However, occlusion of the carotid artery decreases their oxygen supply and activates the reflex to increase pulmonary ventilation and blood pressure while decreasing heart rate. Stimulation of the aortic bodies causes tachycardia.

Oculocardiac Reflex. Traction on the extraocular muscles or pressure on the globe causes bradycardia and hypotension as a consequence of this reflex. Traction on the medial rectus muscle, rather than the lateral rectus muscle, is likely to elicit the reflex. Afferent fibers run with the short or long ciliary nerves to the ciliary ganglion and then with the ophthalmic division of the trigeminal nerve to the gasserian ganglion. Between 30% and 90% of patients undergoing ophthalmic surgery demonstrate the oculocardiac reflex, which can be attenuated by intravenous administration of atropine.

Celiac Reflex. Traction on the mesentery or gallbladder, stimulation of vagal nerve fibers in the respiratory tract, or rectal distention stimulates afferent vagal nerve endings to cause bradycardia, apnea, and hypotension (vagovagal reflex). Manipulation around the celiac plexus decreases systolic pressure, narrows pulse pressure, and slightly decreases heart rate.

Peripheral Circulatory Physiology

The peripheral circulation consists of resistance and capacitance vessels. The majority of the resistance is in the arterial circulation, which consists of the Windkessel vessels, the precapillary resistance vessels, and the capillary exchange vessels. The Windkessel vessels, named for the air-filled compression chamber of 18th-century fire engines, are distensible elastic arteries such as the aorta and large muscular arteries that damp the pulsatile output of the ventricle. The arterioles, the precapillary resistance vessels, are muscular vessels that provide more than 60% of the peripheral resistance. At the most distal portion of the terminal arterioles are precapillary sphincters that regulate the flow of blood into specific capillary beds. The capillary exchange vessels contribute about one fourth of the total peripheral resistance, although most capillaries consist of a single endothelial cell layer without any surrounding smooth muscle. The venous system, discussed below, is the capacitance system.

Arterial Pulses and Blood Pressure

Arterial Pulse. The arterial pulse is a wave of vascular distention resulting from the impact of the stroke volume of each beat being ejected into a closed system. The wave of distention begins at the base of the aorta and passes over the entire arterial system with each heart beat. The pulse is not caused by the passage of the blood itself. The pulse waveform is the result of the combined effects of the forward-propagating pressure wave and its reflectance back toward the heart from various parts of the vasculature. Wave reflection may occur in high resistance arterioles, branching points, or sites of changes in arterial distensibility, but the major source is the arteriole.[121] The velocity of the pulse wave depends on the elasticity of the vessel. The pulse wave velocity is most rapid in the least distensible arteries. In the aortic arch, the pulse wave travels 3–5 m·sec^{-1}, and the aortic pulse waveform precedes the brachial waveform by about 0.05 seconds. In large distensible arteries such as the subclavian, the pulse wave travels 7–10 m·sec^{-1}, whereas in the small nondistensible peripheral arteries it travels about 15–30 m·sec^{-1}. Such differences become important when timing the counterpulsation of an intra-aortic balloon.

The arterial pressure waveform changes as it moves peripherally (Fig. 35-18). In central aortic waveforms, the closure of the aortic valve is indicated by a notch or incisura

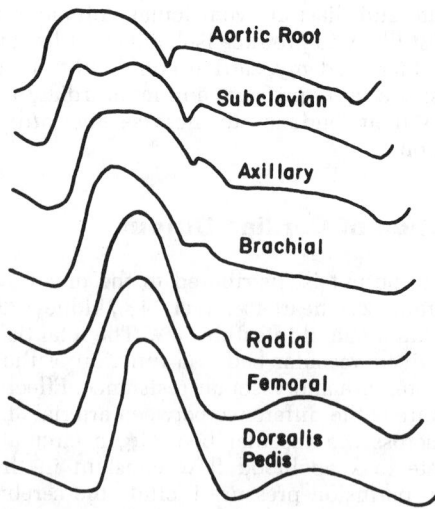

Figure 35-18. The changes in the pulse waveform as it moves from the aortic root to the dorsalis pedis artery are dramatic. These changes result from both forward wave propagation and wave reflection at branch points in the circulation. The waveform has a greater amplitude, higher systolic pressure, lower diastolic pressure, and reduced mean pressure in the peripheral circulation. (Reproduced with permission of the author and publisher from Bedford RF: Invasive blood pressure monitoring. In Blitt CD (ed): Monitoring in Anesthesia and Critical Care Medicine, p 102. New York, Churchill Livingstone, 1990.)

on the descending limb. By contrast, peripheral pulse waveforms have a greater amplitude, more pronounced diastolic wave, and lower mean pressure, and the foot of the wave is delayed.[121] The dicrotic notch, corresponding to the incisura, is more prominent. Systolic pressure is higher, whereas mean and diastolic pressures are slightly lower in the periphery. Such changes are best explained by a tubular model of the vascular system. In such a system, the contour of the pressure wave depends on the velocity of the pressure wave, the duration of the pulse, and the length of the tube.[121]

Pulse contour also changes with hemodynamic conditions. In children, wave reflection facilitates cardiac performance by a relative decrease in arterial pressure during systole and a relative increase during diastole. As aging occurs, wave reflection occurs earlier in the cardiac cycle, increasing systolic pressure and decreasing diastolic pressure. In shock, the pulse wave velocity is reduced by hypotension, increased heart rate reduces the duration of cardiac systole, and peripheral vasoconstriction increases the peripheral reflection coefficient. Pulse waveforms vary in atrial fibrillation, with beats with short systolic durations demonstrating diastolic waves and those with long durations having accentuated systolic peaks. Patients with hypertrophic cardiomyopathy have double systolic pulse waveforms because the initial systolic wave of ventricular ejection occurs during the first half of systole and the reflected wave returns during the same systole.[121]

Blood Pressure. Arterial pressure is the lateral pressure exerted by the contained blood on the walls of the vessels. Mean arterial pressure is the product of the cardiac output and the systemic vascular resistance. If a normal arterial waveform is present, mean pressure is about one third the difference between the systolic and diastolic pressures. However, mean pressure remains constant, whereas pulse pressure and systolic pressure increase as blood moves peripherally in the circulation.

Arterial pressure varies with the respiratory cycle. It normally decreases 6 mm Hg or less during inspiration because pulmonary venous capacitance increases during inspiration to a greater extent than the increase in right-sided heart venous return and output, thus causing a decrease in left ventricular stroke output and pressure. These changes are exaggerated in pericardial tamponade, causing pulsus paradoxus. Clinically, pulsus paradoxus is measured by auscultation of the blood pressure until the first heart sound is heard intermittently. Further deflation of the cuff to the pressure where all beats are heard yields the difference known as the paradoxical pulse.

Factors Controlling Peripheral Vascular Tone. Factors controlling blood pressure include central and autonomic nervous function, cardiac output, systemic vascular resistance, antidiuretic hormone, catecholamines, renin-angiotensin system, and atrial natriuretic factor. Arteriolar tone is regulated by intrinsic and extrinsic mechanisms. The intrinsic mechanism is the inherent myotonic activity of the vascular smooth muscle. Extrinsic factors include neural (sympathetic) and humoral factors. Sympathetic neural activity provides rapid alteration of tone in response to a need for greater blood flow. Humoral factors are less important in overall circulatory regulation.

ENDOTHELIUM-DERIVED RELAXING FACTOR. Endothelium-derived relaxing factor is a short-lived substance that activates soluble guanylate cyclase to increase intracellular cyclic guanosine 3',5'-monophosphate, causing relaxation of vascular smooth muscle. It appears to be nitric oxide (NO) or a similar nitrogen oxide species formed from L-arginine by a pathway requiring calcium, calmodulin, and nicotinamide adenine dinucleotide phosphate–dependent enzyme in various mammalian tissues, including vascular endothelium, macrophages, neutrophils, hepatic Kupffer cells, and cerebellum (Fig. 35-19). Numerous studies indicate that basal release of endothelium-derived relaxing factor occurs, but not in all vasculature (cerebral and coronary). Atherosclerosis impairs endothelium-dependent relaxation. Decreased production of endothelium-derived relaxing factor may also contribute to both systemic and pulmonary hypertension. Hypoxia impairs endothelium-dependent vasodilation owing to inhibition of endothelium-derived relaxing factor production and decreased half-life.[122] Endothelium-derived relaxing factor also inhibits platelet adhesion and aggregation. When internal mammary arteries are probed prior to coronary anastomosis, endothelium-derived relaxing factor is decreased, creating a potential for vasospasm, platelet aggregation, and possible graft occlusion.[122]

ATRIAL NATRIURETIC FACTOR. Atrial natriuretic factor is a peptide stored in the perinuclear granules of human atrial myocytes.[123] More storage granules are found in the right than in the left atrium.

Secretion of atrial natriuretic factor is limited to cells specialized for mechanical rather than conductive activity. Synthesis of atrial natriuretic factor begins with a 150–152 amino acid precursor, pre-proatrial natriuretic peptide, which is cleaved to a 126 amino-acid prohormone, proatrial natriuretic peptide. Proatrial natriuretic peptide is the predominant storage form and is released intact from atria.[123] After release from the granules, cleavage by a serum protease occurs to form the C-terminal hormone, atriopeptin I, circulating in the plasma.[124] Atrial natriuretic factor is released in response to increased vascular volume (atrial distention), epinephrine, vasopressin, acetylcholine (still con-

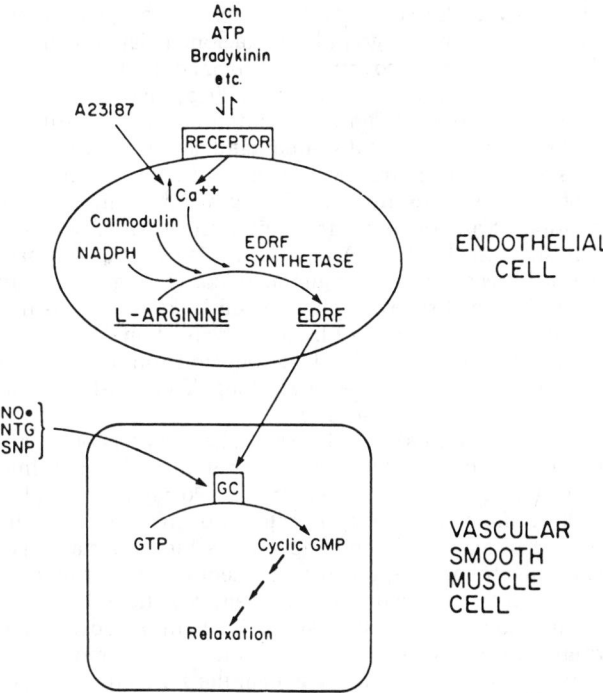

Figure 35-19. Endothelium-derived relaxing factor (EDRF) is produced from L-arginine by a process requiring calcium, calmodulin, nocotinamide adenine dinucleotide phosphate-dependent enzyme (NADPH), and EDRF synthetase. Increases in cytosolic calcium produced by agonists such as the calcium ionophore (A23187) or receptor-mediated agonists (acetylcholine, adenosine triphosphate [ATP], bradykinin) activate EDRF synthetase to produce EDRF. EDRF or other substances such as nitroprusside (SNP), nitroglycerin (NTG), or nitric oxide (NO·) produce vascular smooth muscle relaxation by activation of adenylate cyclase. (Reproduced with permission of author and publisher from Johns RA: Endothelium-derived relaxing factor: Basic review and clinical applications. J Cardiothorac Vasc Anesth 5:71, 1991.)

troversial), morphine, and increased myocardial (atrial) pressure.[123] Normal circulating plasma levels are 25–100 µg·ml⁻¹.[125]

The primary effects of atrial natriuretic factor are direct peripheral vasodilation, suppression of antidiuretic hormone release when the antidiuretic hormone is elevated by hemorrhage or dehydration, inhibition of aldosterone release, and direct renal effects such as increased glomerular filtration, natriuresis, and diuresis.[124] A renal tubular site of action mediated by guanylate cyclase appears likely.[126] Factors such as renal perfusion pressure and renal sympathetic nerve activity in conjunction with physiologic plasma concentrations of atrial natriuretic factor produce natriuresis.[126] Kaliuresis does not occur. Atrial natriuretic factor affects not only blood pressure (by decreasing cardiac output and vascular resistance) but also water and electrolyte balance and blood volume. It has no direct inotropic or chronotropic properties.

In normal volunteers, administration of atrial natriuretic factor does not cause significant changes in renin, aldosterone, cortisol, norepinephrine, or antidiuretic hormone at doses that increase urinary output, decrease blood pressure, and reduce forearm vascular resistance.[127] Disease states such as congestive heart failure and atrial tachydysrhythmias increase circulating levels of atrial natriuretic factor.[123]

RENIN-ANGIOTENSIN SYSTEM. Renin is a proteolytic enzyme produced in the granular juxtaglomerular cells of the kidney. Its release is governed by the macula densa, an intrarenal stretch-type receptor, circulating potassium, angiotensin II, epinephine, and concentrations of antidiuretic hormone, and by the renal sympathetic nerves. Renin secretion is also inversely related to renal perfusion.[128] The half-life of renin is 4–15 minutes, during which it initiates the formation of angiotensin I from angiotensinogen, which is synthesized in the liver. Angiotensin I is biologically inactive until it is cleaved by angiotensin-converting enzyme in lung and other tissues to angiotensin II.[129] Angiotensin II and angiotensin III, formed by hydrolysis of angiotensin II, stimulate the secretion of aldosterone and inhibit renin release through a negative feedback loop. The half-life of angiotensin II is about 30 seconds.

SYMPATHETIC NERVOUS SYSTEM. The receptors of the adrenergic nervous system are conveniently divided into $alpha_1$, $alpha_2$, $beta_1$, and $beta_2$ types. Postsynaptic $alpha_1$ receptors mediate smooth muscle vasoconstriction in the presence of agonist. Norepinephrine is the important agonist at the $alpha_1$ receptor. Alpha receptor stimulation constricts arteries and veins independently of neural supply. Although some investigators suggest that $alpha_1$ adrenoceptors are located preferentially on the outer media and adventitia of vascular smooth muscle, near the sympathetic nerve terminals, Tsutsui and coworkers demonstrated homogeneous distribution across aortic and vascular walls.[130] Epinephrine is more potent as a $beta_2$ receptor agonist than is norepinephrine. Beta2 receptors are located in both pre- and postsynaptic regions. Acting by stimulation of adenylcyclase, they dilate arteries.

Specific Peripheral Circulations

Pulmonary Circulation. The pulmonary circulation is a low-pressure, high-flow system that has five principal functions: (1) metabolic transport of humoral substances and drugs,[131] (2) transport of blood through the lungs, (3) reservoir for the left ventricle, (4) filtration of venous drainage, and (5) transport of gas, fluid, and solutes across the walls of exchanging vessels. Normally all circulating blood passes through the pulmonary circulation at least once each minute, but only 500 ml are present at a given time.

Metabolic Transport. The pulmonary vascular endothelium is important for removal, biosynthesis, and release of various vasoactive hormones, including biogenic amines, prostaglandins, leukotrienes, and peptides. Norepinephrine is removed by the lung by a carrier-mediated, temperature- and drug-sensitive transport process. Epinephrine, histamine, vasopressin, and dopamine, however, are unaltered by transpulmonary passage.[131] Almost complete removal of 5-hydroxytryptamine, adenosine triphosphate, and monophosphate occurs in the lungs. Acetylcholine is rapidly inactivated in the lung. Bradykinin is inactivated by the lungs, probably by an enzymatic process. Prostaglandins of the E and F series are also removed by either a carrier-mediated, energy-requiring process or by rapid degradation by 15-hydroxyprostaglandin-dehydrogenase. Prostacyclin (PGI_2) is not inactivated in the lung. Atrial natriuretic factor is rapidly removed by rabbit lung by an unknown mechanism, and the lung is ideally situated to regulate the physiologic actions of right atrial natriuretic factor.[132] Many drugs such as propranolol, lidocaine, bupivacaine, captopril, and fentanyl are removed extensively during transpulmonary passage.[132,133]

Intravascular Transport. The passage of blood and its distribution to various segments of the lung depend upon pulmonary blood flow, pulmonary vascular resistance or impedance, and left atrial pressure. They also depend on transmural distending pressure and the distensibility of the vessel walls. Blood flow to the lung apex is less than that to the base because of regional differences in pulmonary venous, alveolar, and arterial pressures. However, the pulmonary circulation accommodates a large increase in flow with little change in pressure by a substantial decrease in resistance. Pulmonary resistance is about one fifth systemic, pulmonary impedance is about one half systemic, and pulse wave reflections are stronger in the pulmonary beds owing to similar reflecting sites but the smaller size of the vascular bed.[100]

Capillary endothelium, endothelial basement membrane, interstitial space, epithelial basement membrane, and alveolar epithelium form the alveolocapillary membrane, which separates the blood and gas phases in the lung. Abundant vascular smooth muscle is present in pulmonary vessels, distributed evenly between arteries and veins. Muscular arterioles are absent in the lung. The pulmonary veins perform primarily a reservoir function, preventing pulmonary edema in the event of reduced left ventricular compliance.[134]

MEASUREMENTS OF PULMONARY TONE. Drugs and maneuvers to dilate or constrict the pulmonary vasculature have clinical applications. However, measurements of pulmonary tone are essential to therapeutic investigations. Pulmonary artery pressures are clinically measured using flow-directed catheters. Wedging of the tip of these catheters in a small branch of the pulmonary artery measures the pulmonary artery wedge pressure or occluded pressure (PAo) (see Table 35-2). As blood runs away from the tip of the catheter beyond the point of occlusion, the pressure in the pulmonary artery equilibrates with left atrial pressure. Normally left atrial pressure is similar to left ventricular end-diastolic pressure in the absence of mitral valvular stenosis. Other reasons for pulmonary artery wedge pressure that is greater than left ventricular end-diastolic pressure are increased airway pressures or the presence of an intraatrial mass. Normally, the pulmonary wedge pressure is 1–4 mm Hg lower than pulmonary end-diastolic pressure. However, with tachycardia or increased pulmonary resistance, the pulmonary wedge pressure may be the same or slightly higher than pulmonary end-diastolic pressure.

Methods for the measurement of pulmonary vascular resistance are either difficult or have limitations. Normal values for pulmonary vascular resistance are given in Table 35-5. Direct measurements of pulmonary blood flow using either isolated vessels *in vitro* or individual vessels *in situ* are affected by (1) measurements made in a single artery that may differ in size or response from those of other vessels; (2) technical factors related to vessel harvest and handling; and (3) isolated vessels unaffected by reflexes and other factors such as airway pressure and cardiac output.[135]

Indirect estimations using the classic formula in Table 35-5 have significant problems.

$$PVR = \frac{\text{mean pulmonary artery pressure} - \text{left atrial pressure}}{\text{pulmonary artery flow (cardiac output)}}$$

For example, pulmonary artery pressure is not linearly related to either flow or left atrial pressure. An increase in pulmonary flow or left atrial pressure is unaccompanied by a proportional increase in pulmonary arterial pressure. Therefore, calculated pulmonary vascular resistance decreases when either pulmonary flow or left atrial pressure increases. The nonlinearity results from distention or recruitment of vessels when flow or pressure increases. However, in Zone 3 of the lung (where left atrial pressure is greater than airway pressure), pulmonary artery pressure is the most important factor determining pulmonary blood flow.[136] Therefore, regardless of the effect on the pulmonary vascular tone, agents or manipulations that change pulmonary flow or left atrial pressure will change calculated pulmonary vascular resistance. Only if a particular intervention does not change pulmonary flow or left atrial pressure or if the changes in pulmonary resistance can be explained only by active changes in pulmonary tone (e.g., a decrease in pulmonary artery pressure accompanied by an increase in pulmonary blood flow) is pulmonary vascular resistance unchanged. However, even in these circumstances, reflex effects caused by the drug or maneuver cannot be eliminated.[137]

Another major factor affecting indirect measurements is airway pressure, since the degree of lung inflation and the ventilatory pressure directly influence pulmonary pressure-flow relationships. Either increases or decreases in lung volume beyond normal functional residual capacity increase pulmonary resistance because of compression of small intra-alveolar vessels. Baseline pulmonary tone, stimulation of pulmonary chemoreceptors, autonomic influences, and bronchospasm also directly affect the pulmonary vasculature or modify its response to drugs.

EFFECTS OF DRUGS AND MANEUVERS ON PULMONARY TONE. Various physiologic and nonphysiologic conditions alter pulmonary vascular resistance either actively or passively. These factors are summarized in Table 35-7. Alveoli in an area of lung that is poorly ventilated and contains hypoxic gas cause the precapillary arterial vessels supplying that area to constrict in order to divert blood away from the area. This process is termed *hypoxic pulmonary vasoconstriction*. Pulmonary hypertension does not occur because the hypoxia is localized. If hypoxia is generalized, pulmonary hypertension ensues.[138] Metabolic acidosis slightly enhances hypoxic pulmonary vasoconstriction, whereas respiratory acidosis has no effect.[139] Metabolic and respiratory alkalosis decreases it.[139] Drugs such as nitroprusside, nitroglycerin, and the inhalation anesthetics decrease hypoxic pulmonary vasoconstriction, resulting in worsening of venous admixture and arterial Po_2.[140] However, increased pulmonary artery pressure from whatever mechanism inhibits hypoxic pulmonary vasoconstriction.

Transvascular Transport. The filtration of fluid across the alveolocapillary membrane is described by Starling's equation:

$$\text{Fluid filtration rate} = K_f\{(\text{Pmv} - \text{Ppmv}) - \sigma(\pi\text{mv} - \pi\text{pmv})\}$$

where Pmv is the pulmonary capillary hydrostatic pressure and Ppmv is the interstitial fluid hydrostatic pressure (the hydrostatic pressures inside and outside of the pulmonary vessels); πmv is the colloid osmotic pressure inside and πpmv the interstitial colloid osmotic pressures outside the pulmonary vessels; K_f is the filtration-coefficient of the pulmonary vessel (the capillary permeability); and σ is the reflection coefficient for proteins. The reflection and filtration coefficients describe the resistance of the pulmonary vessels to passage of fluid and protein. The filtration coefficient is the product of the effective capillary surface area in a given mass of tissue and the permeability per unit surface area of the capillary wall. Normally the intravascular colloid osmotic pressure (25 mm Hg) keeps water within the capillaries, whereas the pulmonary capillary hydrostatic pressure (10 mm Hg) attempts to force water across the endothelium into the interstitial space. Fluid filtered into the interstitial compartment is removed by the lymph. Transvascular fluid movement increases if there is a decrease in resistance of the vessel wall (increased permeability) or increased filtra-

TABLE 35-7. Alterations in Pulmonary Vascular Resistance

Active Changes		Passive Changes	
Factors	*Changes*	*Factors*	*Changes*
Sympathetic stimulation	↑ or →	Pulmonary hypertension	↓
Parasympathetic stimulation	→	Left atrial hypertension	↓
Catecholamines	↑	Increased pulmonary interstitial pressure	↑
Angiotensin	↑	Increased blood viscosity	↑
Acetylcholine	↓	Increased pulmonary blood volume	↓
Histamine	↓ ↑		
Bradykinin	↓		
Serotonin	↑		
Prostaglandin E₁	↓		
Prostaglandin F	↑		
Hypoxia	↑		
Hypercarbia	↑ →		
Acidemia	↑		

Data from Murray JP: The Normal Lung, p 128. Philadelphia, WB Saunders, 1976; Perloff WH: Physiology of the heart and circulation. In Swedlow DB, Raphaely RC (eds): Cardiovascular Problems in Pediatric Critical Care, p 1. New York, Churchill Livingstone, 1986; Stalcup A et al: Inhibition of angiotensin converting enzyme activity in cultured endothelial cells by hypoxia. J Clin Invest 63:966, 1979; Hyman AL et al: Autonomic regulation of the pulmonary circulation. J Cardiovasc Pharmacol 7 (suppl 3):S80, 1985.

tion pressure (either osmotic or hydrostatic). Pulmonary edema from left-sided heart failure occurs because of an increase in Pmv, an increase in the amount of fluid filtered because of increased pulmonary venous and microvascular pressures, which overwhelms the capacity of the lymph removal system. Adult respiratory distress syndrome, on the other hand, results from increased vascular permeability rather than a change in pressure.

Bronchial Circulation. Bronchial flow depends upon the cardiac output and blood pressure and ceases at aortic pressures less than 40 mm Hg.[141] It is increased by positive airway pressure and increased by hypoxia and hypercarbia.[18] Sympathetic stimulation or epinephrine decreases bronchial flow, whereas parasympathetic or vagal stimulation increases it.[141] Bronchial veins are more responsive to autonomic influences than are bronchial arteries.[141] Histamine also increases bronchial flow, but prostaglandins decrease it.[12]

Renal Circulation. Renal blood flow is well in excess of the amount needed for renal perfusion. It is autoregulated so that glomerular filtration remains relatively constant despite changes in arterial pressure between 70 and 180 mm Hg.[142,143] Theories proposed to explain renal autoregulation include the juxtaglomerular theory (vasoactive hormonal release from the juxtaglomerular apparatus in response to the quantity or quality of filtrate reaching the macula densa) and the myogenic theory (changes in afferent arteriole tone provide the autoregulation). Of these, the myogenic theory seems most likely.[144]

The main purpose of the excessive renal flow is to provide energy for active renal tubular reabsorption of sodium. Renal oxygen consumption is high, and the arteriovenous oxygen content difference is low. Of the blood delivered to the glomeruli, about 20% is filtered to form an ultrafiltrate of plasma. The main driving force is the glomerular hydrostatic pressure, which is essentially the systemic arterial pressure modified by the renal vasculature. Glomerular capillary pressure is thus about two thirds of systemic pressure.[144] Glomerular capillary pressure is modified by afferent and efferent capillary tone. It is increased by dilation of the afferent arteriole or constriction of the efferent arteriole. Arteriolar tone is also influenced by sympathetic stimulation, catecholamines, kinins, prostaglandins, and other vasoactive substances. Other factors affecting glomerular filtration include the total surface area available for filtration and the permeability of the glomerular membrane. The ultrafiltrate collects in Bowman's space before passing into the renal tubular system.

Hepatic Circulation. Hepatic arterial flow increases in response to decreased portal venous flow. The mechanisms for this alteration (the arterial "buffer response") include myogenic, metabolic, and neural controls as well as the quantity of the portal venous blood and the washout of some endogenous substance, probably adenosine, generated by hepatic tissue.[145]

Portal flow is controlled by preportal arterioles in the splanchnic organs from which the portal vein originates. Precapillary sphincters (presinusoidal) adjust portal flow to maintain an even distribution throughout the liver. The major site of resistance to portal flow is postsinusoidal, regulated by alpha-sympathetic receptors affecting venous smooth muscle.[145] Normally the liver contains about 15% of the blood volume. Sympathetic neural activation can mobilize one half of the hepatic blood volume. Like the sys-

temic vasculature, the hepatic arteriole is the major site of resistance.

Physiology of the Venous System

Systemic veins have a conduit and a reservoir function. Since the smallest postcapillary venules lack muscular layers, and venules and small veins have only small amounts of muscle, the postcapillary resistance is usually small. However, postcapillary resistance is important because the ratio of precapillary to postcapillary resistance determines the capillary filtration pressure. The major capacitance vessels are medium and large veins as well as the venae cavae. About 60% of the systemic blood volume is in small veins and venules of 20 μm–2 mm in diameter.[146]

Venodilation to accommodate as much as 70–75% of the systemic blood volume buffers sudden increases in arterial blood pressure by allowing sequestration of blood in systemic veins. The compliance of the venous system is regulated by venomotor tone, which is controlled by cerebral autonomic impulses. Sympathetically mediated venoconstriction adds about 1 l of blood to the circulation, but passive constriction from a reduction in venous pressure contributes about two thirds of the total volume mobilized. Individual organs contribute about 30–50% of their blood volume by sympathetically mediated venoconstriction. The term vascular capacitance is used for the vascular pressure-volume relationship at a given level of venous tone. Venous tone is normally at 70% of maximum in the erect human.

Venous return, the rate of flow of blood from the periphery to the heart, is a major determinant of cardiac preload. It is determined by the pressure gradient from the peripheral vascular beds to the right side of the heart and the resistance to venous return.[146] The upstream driving pressure from the peripheral tissue to the right atrium is the mean circulatory filling pressure. The mean circulatory filling pressure is an equalization of pressures between the venous and arterial beds when flow is 0 and is usually about 10 mm Hg, similar to the mean systemic filling pressure. It is increased by catecholamines or increased sympathetic activity.[146] An increase in right atrial pressure decreases the pressure gradient and venous return. Cutaneous venous tone is determined by thermoregulatory mechanisms rather than systemic pressure regulatory mechanisms.

Loss of venous tone, as in autonomic neuropathy or during anesthesia, limits the normal compensatory increases in venous tone to changes in posture, positive airway pressure, or decreased blood volume. If these factors are excessive, ventricular preload is adversely affected. Venoconstriction induced by hypovolemia, anxiety, or exercise augments intrathoracic blood volume and preload.

Physiology of the Pericardium

The pericardium has important physiologic functions in the maintenance of normal biventricular filling.[147] Right ventricular filling and stroke volume are particularly augmented by pericardiectomy.[148] However, Mangano et al noted that neither left ventricular systolic function nor compliance is affected by the presence of the pericardium.[149] As dilatation of the left ventricle occurs, intrapericardial pressure limits right ventricular filling and reduces forward flow to the lungs, possibly preventing pulmonary edema.[105] Shifts of the left ventricular diastolic pressure-volume relationship are equal to changes in pericardial pressure and volume.[150] Thus, the role of the pericardium in the maintenance of normal ventricular systolic and diastolic functions appears to be limited.

When pathologic conditions exist, the pericardium assumes more physiologic importance. Increased intrapericardial fluid (cardiac tamponade) causes hypotension, decreased cardiac output, myocardial ischemia, and tachycardia. However, a vagally mediated depressive reflex is also operative, contributing further to the decreased cardiac output resulting from the presence of pericardial fluid.[151] Increased intrapericardial pressure results in an underfilled ventricle, which operates on the ascending limb of Starling's curve.

Lymph drainage of the myocardium occurs via the pericardium. Myocardial edema is particularly deleterious because it reduces both systolic and diastolic ventricular performance. Normally lymph flow rate adjusts rapidly to changes in myocardial interstitial fluid pressure. The relationship is defined as follows:

$$Jv = Lp \cdot A[(Pcap - Pint) - \sigma(\pi cap - \pi int)]$$

where Jv is the rate of fluid filtration, $Lp \cdot A$ is the filtration coefficient, Pcap is capillary hydrostatic pressure, Pint is interstitial hydrostatic pressure, πcap is capillary oncotic pressure, and πint is interstitial oncotic pressure.[152] Lymph, from interstitial myocardial lymphatics, collects on the epicardial surfaces and in the pericardial space before drainage into the lymphatic system *via* pericardial lymphatic vessels.[153]

REFERENCES

1. Stumper O, Fraser AG, Anderson RH et al: Transesophageal echocardiography in the longitudinal axis: Correlation between anatomy and images and its clinical implications. Br Heart J 64:282, 1990
2. Powell EDU, Mullaney JM: The Chiari network and the valve of the inferior vena cava. Br Heart J 22:579, 1960
3. Silver MA, Rowley NE: The functional anatomy of the human coronary sinus. Am Heart J 115:1080, 1988
4. James TN: Anatomy of the crista supraventricularis: Its importance for understanding right ventricular function, right ventricular infarction and related conditions. J Am Coll Cardiol 6:1083, 1985
5. Estes EH, Dalton FM, Entman ML et al: The anatomy and blood supply of the papillary muscles of the left ventricle. Am Heart J 71:356, 1966
6. Lam JHS, Ranganathan N, Wigle ED, Silver MD: Morphology of the human mitral valve. I. Chordae tendineae. Circulation 41:449, 1970
7. Byrd BF, Schiller NB, Botvinick EH, Higgins CB: Normal cardiac dimensions by magnetic resonance imaging. Am J Cardiol 55:1440, 1985
8. Rosenquist GC, Sweeney LJ: The membranous ventricular septum in the normal heart. Johns Hopkins Med J 1345:9, 1974
9. Silver MA, Roberts WC: Detailed anatomy of the normally functioning aortic valve in hearts of normal or increased weight. Am J Cardiol 55:454, 1985
10. James TN; Blood supply of the human interventricular septum. Circulation 17:391, 1958
11. Nerantzis CE, Toutouzas P, Avgoustakis D: The importance of the sinus node artery in the blood supply of the atrial myocardium. Acta Cardiol 38:35, 1983
12. Anderson KR, Murphy JG: The atrioventricular node artery in the human heart. Angiology 34:711, 1983
13. James TN: Morphology of the human atrioventricular node, with remarks pertinent to its electrophysiology. Am Heart J 62:756, 1961
14. Mahmarian JJ, Pratt CM, Boyce TM, Verani MS: The variable extent of jeopardized myocardium in patients with single vessel coronary artery disease. Quantification by thallium-201 single photon emission computed tomography. J Am Coll Cardiol 17:355, 1991
15. Fujita M, Sasayama S, Ohno A et al: Importance of myocardial ischemia for coronary collateral development in conscious dogs. Int J Cardiol 27:179, 1990
16. Adams HD, Van Geertruyden HH: Neurologic complications of aortic surgery. Ann Surg 144:574, 1956
17. Williams GM, Perler BA, Burdick JF et al: Angiographic localization of spinal cord blood supply and its relationship to postoperative paraplegia. J Vasc Surg 13:23, 1991
18. Deffebach ME, Charan NB, Lakshminarayan S, Butler J: The bronchial circulation. Am Rev Respir Dis 135:463, 1987
19. Wearn JT, Mettier SR, Klumpp TG, Zschiesche LJ: The nature of the vascular communications between the coronary arteries and the chambers of the heart. Am Heart J 9:143, 1933
20. Lowe JE, Hartwich T, Takla M, Schaper J: Ultrastructure of electrophysiologically identified human sinoatrial nodes. Basic Res Cardiol 83:401, 1988
21. Bachmann G: The inter-auricular time interval. Am J Physiol 41:309, 1916
22. Janes RD, Brandys JC, Hopkins DA et al: Anatomy of human extrinsic cardiac nerves and ganglia. Am J Cardiol 57:299, 1986
23. Rardon DP, Bailey JC: Parasympathetic effects on electrophysiologic properties of cardiac ventricular tissue. J Am Coll Cardiol 2:1200, 1983
24. Shepherd JT: The heart as a sensory organ. J Am Coll Cardiol 5:83B, 1985
25. De Geest H, Levy MN, Zieske H, Lipman RI: Depression of ventricular contractility by stimulation of the vagus nerves. Circ Res 17:222, 1965
26. Stiles GL, Taylor S, Lefkowitz RJ; Human cardiac beta adrenergic receptors: Subtype heterogeneity delineated by direct radiological binding. Life Sci 33:467, 1983
27. Spodick DH: The normal and diseased pericardium: Current concepts of pericardial physiology, diagnosis and treatment. J Am Coll Cardiol 1:240, 1983
28. Kennedy JW: Registry Committee of the Society for Cardiac Angiography: Complications associated with cardiac catheterization and angiography. Cathet Cardiovasc Diagn 8:5, 1982
29. Seldinger SI: Catheter replacement of the needle in percutaneous arteriography. Acta Radiol 39:368, 1953
30. Levin AR, Grossman H, Schubert ET et al: The effect of angiocardiography on fluid and electrolyte balance. Am J Roentgenol 105:777, 1969
31. Conti CR: Coronary arteriography. Circulation 55:227, 1977
32. Perrino AC, Fleming J, LaMantia KR: Transesophageal ultrasonography: Evidence for improved cardiac output monitoring. Anesth Analg 71:651, 1990
33. Muhuideen IA, Kuecherer HR, Lee E et al: Intraoperative estimation of cardiac output by transesophageal pulsed Doppler echocardiography. Anesthesiology 74:9, 1991
34. Gorlin R, Gorlin G: Hydraulic formula for calculation of area of stenotic mitral valve, other cardiac valves, and central circulatory shunts. Am Heart J 41:1, 1951
35. Cannon SR, Richards KL, Crawford M: Hydraulic estimation of stenotic orifice area: A correction of the Gorlin formula. Circulation 71:1170, 1985
36. Cohen MV, Gorlin R: Modified orifice equation for the calculation of mitral valve area. Am Heart J 84:839, 1972
37. White CW, Holida MD, Marcus ML: Effects of acute atrial fibrillation on the vasodilator reserve of the canine atrium. Cardiovasc Res 20:683, 1986
38. Robinson TF, Factor SM, Sonnenblick EH: The heart as a suction pump. Sci Am 254:84, 1986
39. Abrams J: Current concepts of the genesis of heart sounds. I. First and second sounds. II. Third and fourth sounds. JAMA 239:2787, 1978
40. Birnbaumer L, Brown AM: G proteins and the mechanism

of action of hormones, neurotransmitters, and autocrine and paracrine regulatory factors. Am Rev Respir Dis 141:S106, 1990

41. Durrer D, Van Dam RT, Freud GE et al: Total excitation of the isolated human heart. Circulation 41:899, 1970

42. Wendt DJ, Martin JB: Autonomic neural regulation of intact Purkinje system of dogs. Am J Physiol 258:H1420, 1990

43. Coraboeuf E, Weidman S: Temperature effects on the electrical activity of Purkinje fibers. Helv Physiol Pharmacol Acta 12:32, 1954

44. Kohlhardt M, Mnich Z, Maier G: Alteration of the excitation process of the sinoatrial pacemaker cell in the presence of anoxia and metabolic inhibitors. J Mol Cell Cardiol 9:477, 1977

45. Bailey JC, Watanabe AM, Besch HR, Lathrop DA: Acetylcholine antagonism of the electrophysiological effects of isoproterenol on canine cardiac Purkinje fibers. Circ Res 44:378, 1979

46. Fisch C, Knoebel SB, Feigenbaum H, Greenspan K: Potassium and the monophasic action potential, electrocardiogram, conduction, and arrhythmias. Prog Cardiovasc Dis 8:387, 1966

47. Von Bogaert PP, Vereecke J, Carmeliet E: Cardiac pacemaker currents and extracellular pH. Arch Intern Physiol Biochem 603, 1975

48. Cinca J, Morja A, Figueras J et al: Circadian variations in the electrical properties of the human heart assessed by sequential bedside electrophysiologic testing. Am Heart J 112:315, 1986

49. Urthaler F, Neely BH, Hageman GR, Smith LR: Differential sympathetic-parasympathetic interactions in sinus node and AV junction. Am J Physiol 250:H43, 1986

50. Hoffman BF, Moore EN, Stuckey JH et al: Functional properties of the atrioventricular conduction system. Circ Res 13:308, 1963

51. Kovacs SJ: The duration of the QT interval as a function of heart rate: A derivation based on physical principles and comparison to measured values. Am Heart J 110:876, 1985

52. de Marneffe M, Jacobs P, Haardt R, Englert M: Variations of normal sinus node function in relation to age: Role of autonomic influence. Eur Heart J 7:662, 1986

53. Evans JM, Randall DC, Funk JN, Knapp CF: Influence of cardiac innervation on intrinsic heart rate in dogs. Am J Physiol 258:H1132, 1990

54. Murphy DA, Johnstone DE, Armour JA: Preliminary observations on the effects of stimulation of cardiac nerves in man. Can J Physiol Pharmacol 63:649, 1985

55. Sapire DW, Casta A: Vagotonia in infants, children, adolescents, and young adults. Int J Cardiol 9:211, 1985

56. Medak R, Benumof JL: Perioperative management of prolonged Q-T interval syndrome. Br J Anaesth 55:361, 1983

57. Longhurst JC: Cardiac receptors: Their function in health and disease. Prog Cardiovasc Dis 27:201, 1984

58. Wong TM, Lee AY-S, Tai KK: Effects of drugs interacting with opioid receptors during normal perfusion or ischemia and reperfusion in the isolated rat heart. An attempt to identify cardiac opioid receptor subtypes involved in arrhythmogenesis. J Mol Cell Cardiol 22:1167, 1990

59. Lee AY-S: Endogenous opioid peptides and cardiac arrhythmias. Int J Cardiol 27:145, 1990

60. White CF, Wilson RF, Marcus ML: Methods of measuring myocardial blood flow in humans. Prog Cardiovasc Dis 31:79, 1988

61. Feigl EO, Neat GW, Huang AH: Interrelations between coronary artery pressure, myocardial metabolism and coronary blood flow. J Mol Cell Cardiol 22:375, 1990

62. Westerhof N: Physiological hypotheses—intramyocardial pressure. A new concept, suggestions for measurement. Basic Res Cardiol 85:105, 1990

63. Hoffman JIE: Determinants and prediction of transmural myocardial perfusion. Circulation 58:381, 1978

64. Marcus ML, Chilian WM, Kanatsuka H et al: Understanding the coronary circulation through studies at the microvascular level. Circulation 82:1, 1990

65. Rubio P, Berne RM: Regulation of coronary blood flow. Progr Cardiovasc Dis 43:105, 1975

66. Dole WP: Autoregulation of the coronary circulation. Prog Cardiovasc Dis 29:293, 1987

67. Chilian WM, Layne SM: Coronary microvascular responses to reductions in perfusion pressure. Circ Res 66:1227, 1990

68. Baron JF, Vicaut E, Hou X, Duvelleroy M: Independent role of arterial O_2 tension in local control of coronary blood flow. Am J Physiol 258:H 1388, 1990

69. Dole WP, Nuno DW: Myocardial oxygen tension determines the degree and pressure range of coronary autoregulation. Circ Res 59:202, 1986

70. Vatner SF: Regulation of coronary resistance vessels and large coronary arteries. Am J Cardiol 56:16E, 1985

71. Karmazyn M, Dhalla NS: Physiological and pathophysiological aspects of cardiac prostaglandins. Can J Physiol Pharmacol 61:1207, 1983

72. Marone G, Triggiani M, Cirillo R et al: Chemical mediators and the human heart. Prog Biochem Pharmacol 20:38, 1985

73. Austin RE, Aldea GS, Coggins DL et al: Profound spatial heterogeneity of coronary reserve. Circ Res 67:319, 1990

74. Hoffman JIE: Transmural myocardial perfusion. Progr Cardiovasc Dis 29:429, 1987

75. Dyke CM, Brunsting LA, Salter DR et al: Preload dependence of right ventricular blood flow. I. The normal right ventricle. Ann Thorac Surg 43:478, 1987

76. Vatner SF: Alpha adrenergic regulation of the coronary circulation in the conscious dog. Am J Cardiol 52:15A, 1983

77. Shepherd JT, Vanhoutte PM: Mechanisms responsible for coronary vasospasm. J Am Coll Cardiol 8:50A, 1986

78. Goldstein DS, Brush JE, Eisenhofer G et al: In vivo measurement of neuronal uptake of norepinephrine in the human heart. Circulation 78:41, 1988

79. Trimarco B, Ricciardelli B, Cuocolo A et al: Effects of coronary occlusion on arterial baroreflex control of heart rate and vascular resistance. Am J Physiol 252:H749, 1987

80. Little RC, Little WC: Cardiac preload, afterload, and heart failure. Arch Intern Med 142:819, 1982

81. Lang RM, Borow KM, Neumann A, Janzen D: Systemic vascular resistance: An unreliable index of left ventricular afterload. Circulation 74:1114, 1986

82. Prewitt RM, Wood LDH: Effect of altered resistive load on left ventricular systolic mechanics in dogs. Anesthesiology 56:195, 1982

83. Schaeffer S, Taylor AL, Lee HR et al: Effect of increasing heart rate on left ventricular performance in patients with normal cardiac function. Am J Cardiol 61:617, 1988

84. Wisenbaugh T, Nissen S, DeMaria A: Mechanics of postextrasystolic potentiation in normal subjects and patients with valvular heart disease. Circulation 74:10, 1986

85. Hathaway DR, March KL, Lash JA et al: Vascular smooth muscle. A review of the molecular basis of contractility. Circulation 83:382, 1991

86. Braunwald E, Sonnenblick EH, Ross J: Contraction of the normal heart. In Braunwald E (ed): Textbook of Cardiovascular Medicine, 2nd ed, pp 409–444. Philadelphia, WB Saunders, 1983

87. Katz AM: Cyclic adenosine monophosphate effects on the myocardium: A man who blows hot and cold with one breath. J Am Coll Cardiol 2:143, 1983

88. Brutsaert DL, Rademakers FE, Sys SU et al: Analysis of relaxation in the evaluation of ventricular function of the heart. Prog Cardiovasc Dis 28:143, 1985

89. Woodworth RS: Maximal contraction, "staircase" contraction, refractory period, and compensatory pause of the heart. Am J Physiol 8:213, 1902

90. Carabello BA, Spann JF: The uses and limitations of end-systolic indexes of left ventricular function. Circulation 69:1058, 1984

91. Starling EH: The Lineacre Lecture on the law of the heart. In Chapman CB, Mitchell JH (eds): Starling on the Heart, pp 119–147. London, Pall Mall, 1965

92. Parker JO, Case RB: Normal left ventricular function. Circulation 60:4, 1979

93. McKay RG, Aroesty JM, Heller GV et al: Left ventricular pressure-volume diagrams and end systolic pressure-volume relations in human beings. J Am Coll Cardiol 3:301, 1984

94. Chung N, Wu X, Bailey KR, Ritman EL: LV pressure-volume area and oxygen consumption. Evaluation by intact dog by fast CT. Am J Physiol 258:H1208, 1990

95. Jacob R, Kissling G: Ventricular pressure-volume relations as the primary basis for evaluation of cardiac mechanics. Return to Frank's diagram. Basic Res Cardiol 84:227, 1989

96. Van der Linden LP, Van der Wilde ET, Bruschke AVG, Baan J: Comparison between force-velocity and end-systolic pressure volume characterization of intrinsic LV function. Am J Physiol 259:H1419, 1990

97. Foex P, Francis CM, Cutfield GR, Leone B: The pressure-length loop. Br J Anaesth 60:65S, 1988

98. Safwat A, Leone BJ, Norris RM, Foex P: Pressure-length loop area: Its components analyzed during graded myocardial ischemia. J Am Coll Cardiol 17:790, 1991

99. Barash PG, Kopriva CJ: Cardiac pump function and how to monitor it. In Thomas SJ (ed): Manual of Cardiac Anesthesia, pp 1–17. New York, Churchill Livingstone, 1984

100. Piene H: Pulmonary arterial impedance and right ventricular function. Physiol Rev 66:606, 1986

101. Damino RJ, Cox JL, Lowe JE, Santamore WP: Left ventricular pressure effects on right ventricular pressure and volume outflow. Cathet Cardiovasc Diagn 19:269, 1990

102. Barnard D, Alpert JS: Right ventricular function in health and disease. Curr Probl Cardiol 12:423, 1987

103. Weber KT, Janicki JS, Shroff SG et al: The right ventricle: Physiologic and pathophysiologic considerations. Crit Care Med 11:323, 1983

104. Santamore WP, Shaffer T, Papa L: Theoretical model of ventricular interdependence: Pericardial effects. Am J Physiol 259:H181, 1990

105. Santamore WP, Li KS, Nakamoto T, Johnston WE: Effects of increased pericardial pressure on the coupling between the ventricles. Cardiovasc Res 24:768, 1990

106. Maruyama Y, Nunokawa T, Kiowa T et al: Mechanical interdependence between the ventricles. Basic Res Cardiol 78:544, 1983

107. Opie LH: Metabolism of the heart in health and disease. Am Heart J 77:100, 1969

108. Berne RM (ed): Handbook of Physiology. The Cardiovascular System, p 873. Baltimore, Williams & Wilkins, 1979

109. Merin RG: Inhalation anesthetics and myocardial metabolism. Anesthesiology 39:216, 1973

110. Weber KT, Janicki JS: The metabolic demand and oxygen supply of the heart: Physiologic and clinical considerations. Am J Cardiol 44:722, 729, 1979

111. Hering HE: Der karotisdruckversuch. Munch Med Wochenschr 70:1287, 1923

112. Aviado DM, Schmidt CF: Reflexes from stretch receptors on blood vessels, heart and lungs. Physiol Rev 35:247, 1955

113. Schmidt RM, Kumada M, Sagewa K: Cardiovascular responses to various pulsatile pressures in the carotid sinus. Am J Physiol 223:1, 1972

114. Von Bezold A, Hirt L: Uber die physiologischen wirkungen des essigsauren veratrins. Physiol Lab Wuerzburg Untersuchungen 1:75, 1867

115. Mark AL: The Bezold Jarisch reflex revisited: Clinical implications of inhibitory reflexes originating in the heart. J Am Coll Cardiol 1:90, 1983

116. Jarisch A, Richter H: Die afferenten bahnen des veratrine effektes in den herznerven. Arch Exp Pathol Pharmacol 193:355, 1939

117. Koren G, Weiss AT, Ben-David Y et al: Bradycardia and hypotension following reperfusion with streptokinase (Bezold-Jarisch reflex): A sign of coronary thrombolysis and myocardial salvage. Am Heart J 112:468, 1986

118. James TN: A cardiogenic hypertensive chemoreflex. Anesth Analg 69:633, 646, 1989

119. Ledsome JR, Linden RJ: A reflex increase in heart rate from distention of the pulmonary vein-atrial junction. J Physiol 170:456, 1964

120. Lloyd TC Jr: Control of systemic vascular resistance by pulmonary and left heart baroreflexes. Am J Physiol 225:1511, 1972

121. O'Rourke MF, Yaginuma T: Wave reflections and the arterial pulse. Arch Intern Med 144:366, 1984

122. Johns RA: Endothelium-derived relaxing factor: Basic review and clinical implications. J Cardiothorac Vasc Anesth 5:69, 1991

123. Ferrari R, Agnoletti G: Atrial natriuretic peptide: Its mechanism of release from the atrium. Int J Cardiol 25:S3, 1989

124. Needleman P, Greenwald JE: Atriopeptin: A cardiac hormone intimately involved in fluid, electrolyte, and blood-pressure homeostasis. N Engl J Med 314:828, 1986

125. de Bold AJ: Atrial natriuretic factor. A hormone produced by the heart. Science 230:767, 1985

126. Blaine EH: Atrial natriuretic factor plays a significant role in body fluid homeostasis. Hypertension 15:2, 1990

127. Richards AM, Nicholls MG, Ikram H et al: Renal, hemodynamic, and hormonal effects of human alpha atrial natriuretic peptide in healthy volunteers. Lancet 1:545, 1985

128. Reid IA: The renin-angiotensin system and body function. Arch Intern Med 145:1475, 1985

129. Ryan J, Smith U, Niemeyer R: Angiotensin I: Metabolism by plasma membrane of lung. Science 176:64, 1972

130. Tsutsui H, Tomoike H, Nakamura M: Quantitative and autoradiographic analyses of alpha-adrenergic and serotonergic receptors on aorta and coronary artery. Am J Physiol 259:H1343, 1990

131. Said SI: Metabolic functions of the pulmonary circulation. Circ Res 50:325, 1982

132. Gillis CN: Pharmacological aspects of metabolic processes in the pulmonary microcirculation. Ann Rev Pharmacol Toxicol 26:183, 1986

133. Roerig D, Bunke S, Dawson CA et al: Inhibition of fentanyl uptake in the isolated perfused rat lung by propranolol. Fed Proc 44:1758, 1985

134. Goto M, Arakawa M, Suzuki T et al: A quantitative analysis of reservoir function of the human pulmonary "venous" system for the left ventricle. Jpn Circ J 50:222, 1986

135. Kulik TJ, Lock JE: The assessment of pulmonary vascular tone: A review of experimental methodologies. Pediatr Pharmacol 4:73, 1984

136. Thorvaldson J, Ilebekk A, Loraand S, Kiil F: Determinants of pulmonary blood volume. Effects of acute changes in pulmonary vascular pressure and flow. Acta Physiol Scand 121:45, 1984

137. Rich S, Martinez J, Lam W et al: Reassessment of the effects of vasodilator drugs in primary pulmonary hypertension. Guidelines for determining a pulmonary vasodilator response. Am Heart J 105:119, 1983

138. Rudolph AM, Yuan S: Response of the pulmonary vasculature to hypoxia and H^+ ion concentration changes. J Clin Invest 45:399, 1966

139. Brimioulle S, Lejeune P, Vachiery J-L et al: Effects of acidosis and alkalosis on hypoxic pulmonary vasoconstriction in dogs. Am J Physiol 258:347, 1990

140. Marshall BE, Marshall C: Anesthesia and the pulmonary circulation. In Covino BG, Fozzard HA, Strichartz G (eds): Effects of Anesthesia, pp 121–136. Bethesda, American Physiological Society, 1985

141. Baier H: Functional adaptations of the bronchial circulation. Lung 164:247, 1986

142. Navar LG: Renal autoregulation. Perspectives from whole kidney and single nephron studies. Am J Physiol 234:F357, 1978

143. Roberts CR, Deen WM, Troy JL, Brenner BM: Dynamics of glomerular ultrafiltration in the rat. III. Hemodynamics and autoregulation. Am J Physiol 223:1191, 1972

144. Fried TA, Stein JH: Glomerular dynamics. Arch Intern Med 143:787, 1983

145. Kang YG, Gelman S: Liver transplantation. In Gelman S (ed): Organ Transplantation, pp 142–143. Philadelphia, WB Saunders, 1987

146. Rothe CF: Physiology of venous return. Arch Intern Med 146:977, 1986

147. Hoit BD, Dalton N, Bhargava V, Shabetai R: Pericardial influences on right and left ventricular filling dynamics. Circ Res 68:197, 1991

148. Reich DL, Konstadt SN, Thys DM: The pericardium exerts constraint on the right ventricle during cardiac surgery. Acta Anaesthesiol Scand 34:530, 1990

149. Mangano DT, Van Dyke DC, Hickey RF, Ellis RJ: Significance of the pericardium in human subjects: Effects on left ventricular volume, pressure, and ejection. J Am Cardiol 6:290, 1985

150. Refsum H, Junemann M, Lipton MJ et al: Ventricular diastolic pressure volume relation and the pericardium. Circulation 64:997, 1981

151. Friedman HS, Lajam F, Gomes JA et al: Demonstration of a depressor reflex in acute cardiac tamponade. J Thorac Cardiovasc Surg 73:278, 1977

152. Laine GA, Granger HJ: Microvascular, interstitial, and lymphatic interactions in normal heart. Am J Physiol 249:834, 1985

153. Miller AJ, Pick R, Johnson PJ: Lymphatic drainage of the heart. Am J Physiol 26:463, 1971

36

Doreen L. Wray   Cindy W. Hughes
Richard H. Fine   Stephen J. Thomas

Anesthesia for Cardiac Surgery

Anesthetizing patients for open heart surgery is exciting, intellectually challenging, and emotionally rewarding. Competent and skillful clinical management requires a thorough understanding of normal and altered cardiac physiology; an intimate knowledge of the pharmacology of anesthetic, vasoactive, and cardioactive drugs; and familiarity with the physiologic derangements associated with cardiopulmonary bypass and the surgical procedures themselves. This chapter presents a brief overview of the subject in order to familiarize the reader with the critical physiologic and technical considerations when caring for cardiac surgical patients. The initial discussions concerning coronary artery and valvular heart disease lay the physiologic and some of the pharmacologic groundwork upon which anesthetic planning and therapeutic decisions are based. First, we describe the balance of myocardial oxygen supply and demand, with particular reference to the patient with coronary artery disease. Next, we focus on those variables that regulate myocardial performance, specifically myocardial contractility, heart rate, and loading conditions (both preload and afterload). We then discuss the bells, whistles, and mechanics of cardiopulmonary bypass. Following this, we describe anesthetic considerations relevant to all adults undergoing open heart surgery, including preoperative evaluation, choice of monitoring techniques, selection of anesthetic drugs, and the actual conduct of the anesthetic before, during, and after bypass. The chapter concludes with some special topics as well as a brief introduction to the child with congenital heart disease. Some of the issues discussed are controversial, since the field is continuously evolving. We have tried whenever possible to suggest what is the consensus about these topics, but, inevitably, our own preferences will also be apparent.[1] For the sake of brevity, numerous tables are included in order to summarize data and to provide readily available guidelines for the various phases of the operative procedure. Many monographs are available for those who desire more detailed analysis of any aspect of cardiac anesthesia.[2-7]

CORONARY ARTERY DISEASE

The prevention or treatment of ischemia prior to cardiopulmonary bypass in patients undergoing coronary artery bypass graft surgery reduces the incidence of perioperative myocardial infarction.[8-10] The hemodynamic profile during the prebypass period, how the anesthetic is managed, and who does the managing are also important, since the avoidance or treatment of factors known to increase myocardial oxygen demand (MVo_2) reduces the frequency of pre-cardiopulmonary bypass ischemic episodes.[8,11] In addition, not only is control of MVo_2 critical, but it is now apparent that many ischemic events occur with minimal or no changes in MVo_2, suggesting that a primary reduction in oxygen supply is also a major etiologic factor for intraoperative ischemia.[8,9,11-15] Therefore, successful management of patients with coronary artery disease requires controlling the factors determining MVo_2 and, insofar as possible, optimizing oxygen delivery to the myocardium.[16] The determinants of myocardial oxygen supply and demand are listed in Table 36-1 and are also discussed in Chapter 35. A few points merit special attention.

Myocardial Oxygen Demand

Wall tension and contractility are the principal determinants of MVo_2.[17] Laplace's law states that wall tension is directly proportional to both developed intracavitary pressure and ventricular radius and inversely proportional to wall thickness. Therefore, preventing or promptly treating ventricular distention is desirable in helping to control or reduce MVo_2. Since contractility is also of major importance, myocardial depression can be very beneficial as long as such depression does not result in ischemia-producing hypotension[18] or in increases in wall tension.

Myocardial Oxygen Supply

Any increase in myocardial oxygen requirements can be met only by raising coronary blood flow. Blood oxygen content (hemoglobin concentration × O_2 saturation × 1.34) is obviously important, as is oxygen extraction by the myocardium, but these are infrequently the basis of intraoperative ischemia. Oxygenation and blood volume are usually well maintained during anesthesia. Coronary sinus Po_2 is about 27 mm Hg (50% saturation), and although extraction can be increased somewhat under conditions of stress, this is inadequate to meet the continuously changing levels of demand.[17] Therefore, the principal mechanism for matching oxygen supply to alterations in MVo_2 is exquisite regulation and control of coronary blood flow.

TABLE 36-1. Myocardial Oxygen Balance

Demand	Supply
Wall tension	Coronary blood flow
Ventricular radius	Driving pressure
Pressure generation	Diastolic time
Contractility	Arteriolar tone
Heart rate	Collaterals
	Arterial O_2 content
	Myocardial O_2 extraction

Coronary Blood Flow. The critical factors that modify coronary blood flow are diastolic time available for perfusion (namely, heart rate), perfusion pressure, coronary vascular tone, and the presence and severity of intraluminal obstructions. We are most concerned with flow to the subendocardial region of the left ventricle, since this is the area most vulnerable to ischemia. As shown in Figure 36-1 and as will become more evident in the following discussion, the subendocardium is most at risk for the development of ischemia, because metabolic requirements are greater owing to greater systolic shortening and because flow is restricted during systole.[19,20]

Perfusion of the left ventricular subendocardium takes place almost entirely during diastole; the majority of right ventricular flow occurs during systole (Fig. 36-2). This temporal disparity is explained by the differences (in the absence of pulmonary hypertension) in intracavitary pressures during systole. Since left ventricular flow is diastolic, it is evident that not only is diastolic pressure important but duration of diastole is also critical in determining the volume of left ventricular subendocardial flow. The time available for diastole decreases with increasing heart rate, with

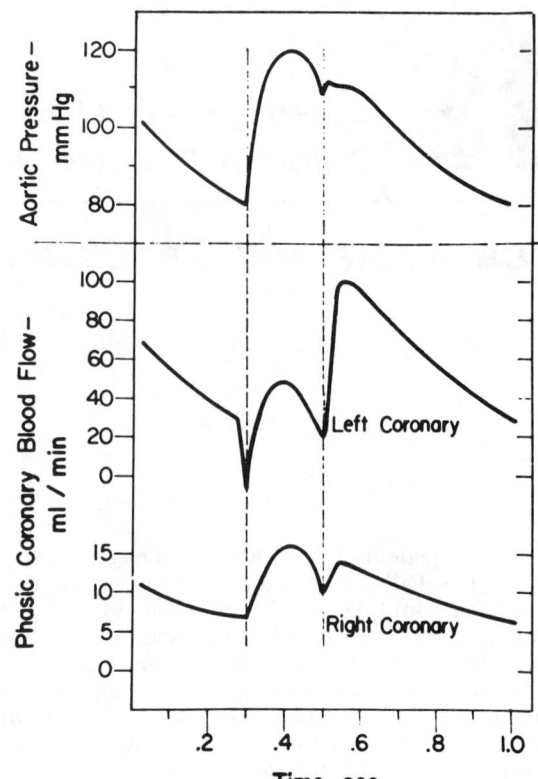

Figure 36-2. Coronary artery blood flow during a single cardiac cycle. Left ventricular flow *via* the left coronary artery occurs primarily during diastole, whereas right ventricular perfusion is predominantly systolic. (Reprinted with permission from Berne FM, Levy MN: Cardiovascular Physiology, 5th ed, p 200. St Louis, CV Mosby, 1986.)

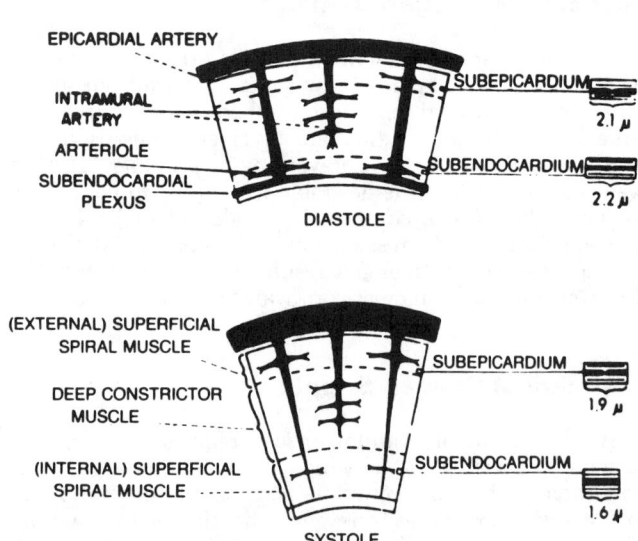

Figure 36-1. Cross-sectional views of the left ventricular wall during diastole and systole. Numbers at right represent sarcomere length. Vulnerability of the subendocardium to ischemia results from both systolic compression of blood vessels (decreased oxygen supply) and increased systolic shortening (increased oxygen demand) relative to subepicardium. (Reprinted with permission from Bell JR, Fox AC: Pathogenesis of subendocardial ischemia. Am J Med Sci 268: 2, 1974.)

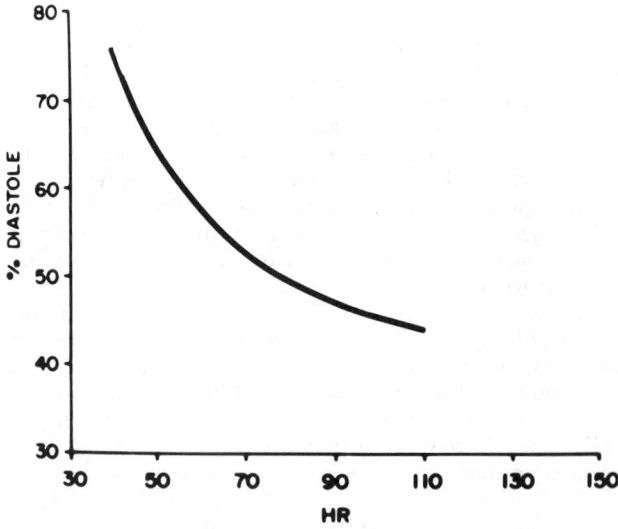

Figure 36-3. The percentage of each cardiac cycle in diastole as a function of heart rate. The time available for subendocardial perfusion decreases in nonlinear fashion as heart rate (and myocardial oxygen demand) increases. (Reprinted with permission from Boudoulas H, Rittgers SE, Lewis RP: Changes in diastolic time with various pharmacologic agents: Implication for myocardial perfusion. Circulation 60:164, 1979.)

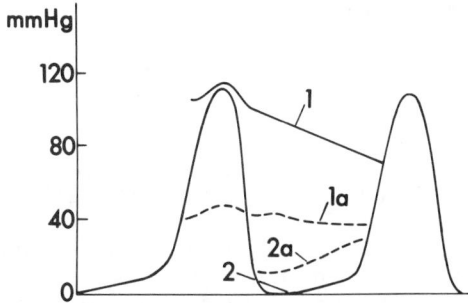

Figure 36-4. The pressure relationships between the aorta (1) and the left ventricle (2) determine coronary perfusion pressure. In coronary artery disease, myocardial perfusion may be compromised by decreased pressure distal to a significant stenosis (1a) (not quantifiable clinically) and/or by an increase in left ventricular end-diastolic pressure (2a). (Reprinted with permission from Gorlin R: Coronary Artery Disease, p 75. Philadelphia, WB Saunders, 1976.)

the greatest percentage of reductions occurring at lower heart rates[21] (Fig. 36-3).

Coronary perfusion pressure for the left ventricle is often defined as aortic diastolic pressure (AoDP) minus left ventricular end-diastolic pressure. This is an oversimplification, since there is no single AoDP. Rather, it is likely that there is a range of pressures that drive blood to the subendocardium. In the presence of intraluminal obstruction or increased vascular tone, this pressure is reduced, as depicted in Figure 36-4. The precise degree of reduction is unknown to the clinician. Although the pressure at the end of the circuit is unknown and the subject of controversy,[22,23] it is convenient and useful to consider ventricular filling pressure as this end pressure. Therefore, a low ventricular filling pressure is ideal both in terms of improving perfusion (higher pressure gradient) and of reducing MVo_2 (decreased

ventricular volume and wall tension). The consequences of altering systemic pressure are more difficult to predict, since the cost of increasing perfusion pressure is increased MVo_2. It has been shown experimentally that at any given heart rate, hypotension is more likely to induce ischemia than is hypertension.[24]

Alterations in tone of the small intramyocardial arterioles regulate diastolic vascular resistance in the absence of flow, limiting obstructions in the epicardial vessels. These adjustments, mediated primarily by adenosine, a metabolite of high-energy phosphates, allow matching of oxygen supply and metabolic demand over a wide range of perfusion pressures.[25] The difference between autoregulated supply and the amount available under conditions of maximal vasodilation is coronary vascular reserve, normally three to five times basal flow. As epicardial stenosis becomes more pronounced, progressive vasodilation of these resistance vessels allows preservation of basal flow, but at the cost of

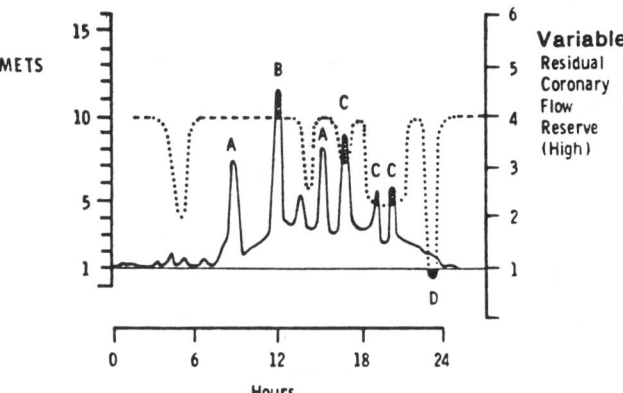

Figure 36-5. Schematic illustration of mechanisms producing myocardial ischemia. Myocardial oxygen demand is plotted on the left (as multiples of basal oxygen consumption), and oxygen supply on the right. In this example, maximal coronary flow reserve is reduced from 6 to 4 times basal levels by fixed intraluminal obstruction. As long as myocardial oxygen demand remains below this maximal limit, no ischemia occurs (A). Ischemia will develop, however, whenever oxygen demand exceeds maximal supply (B) or when supply is further compromised by coronary vasoconstriction (C). More pronounced coronary vasospasm may produce ischemia at rest (D). (Reprinted with permission from Maseri A, Chierchia S, Kaski JC: Mixed angina pectoris. Am J Cardiol 56:30E, 1985.)

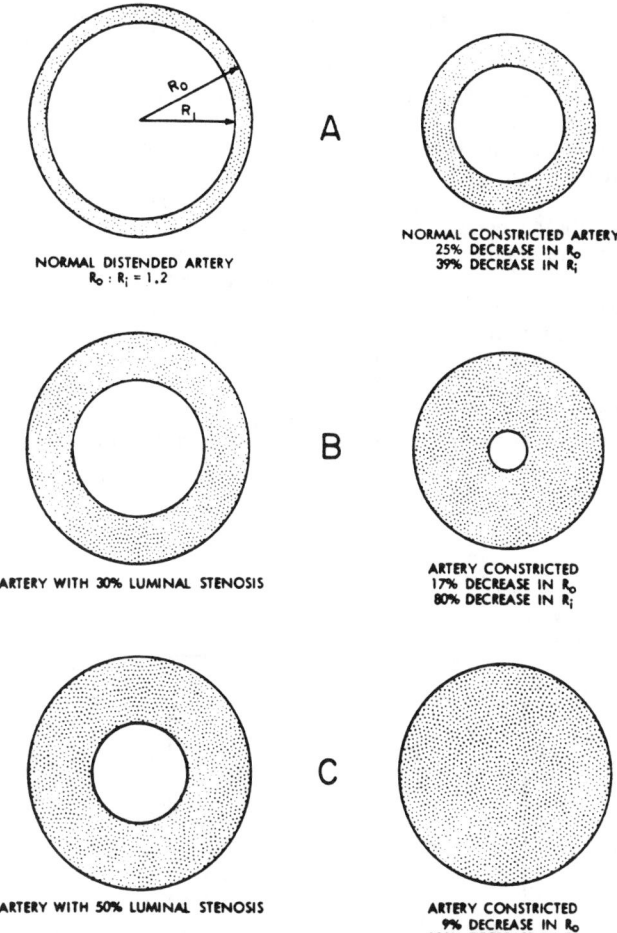

Figure 36-6. The effect of coronary vasoconstriction on luminal cross-section in normal and stenosed arteries. R_o represents the outer radius, R_i the luminal radius of the vessel. Any reduction in outer radius is associated with a substantially greater decrease in inner radius (A). This effect is magnified by pre-existing stenosis (B). A 9% decrease in R_o in a vessel with 50% stenosis completely occludes the lumen (C). (Reprinted with permission from MacAlpin R: Contribution of dynamic vascular wall thickening to luminal narrowing during coronary arterial constriction. Circulation 60:296, 1980.)

reduced reserve. Whenever demand increases above available reserve, signs, symptoms, and metabolic evidence of ischemia develop (Fig. 36-5).

Prinzmetal et al[26] first described angina and myocardial infarction in patients with angiographically normal coronary vessels. Subsequently, Maseri et al and others have emphasized repeatedly the frequency with which primary reductions in oxygen supply cause ischemia (Fig. 36-5).[26-29] Small adjustments in coronary vascular tone at the site of previous obstructions can cause substantial reductions in luminal cross-sectional area (Fig. 36-6).[30] Alterations in stenosis diameter are possible because at least two thirds of plaques or atheroma are not concentric.[31] Therefore, a certain portion of normal vessel wall, or at least reactive vessel wall, is present in the stenosis. It is now apparent that anesthesia is not protective against "supply" ischemia, which occurs frequently during surgery (Fig. 36-7).[15] The etiology of this is unclear but it may be caused by circulating catecholamines, local effects of blood components such as platelets at areas of atherosclerosis,[32] or other as yet undetermined factors. It is not uncommon during anesthesia for a patient to show signs of ischemia without any change in heart rate, blood pressure, or ventricular filling pressure. Drugs such as nitroglycerin and the calcium entry blockers may be used to prevent and/or treat such episodes of coronary spasm.[33-35]

Hypotension, vasospasm, and acute thrombosis all decrease coronary perfusion pressure, reduce coronary blood flow, and limit oxygen delivery to the myocardium. Unstable angina pectoris and/or acute coronary thrombosis is a result of plaque rupture with ensuing platelet activation and thrombus formation. The presence of potentially hyperreactive normal vessel wall adjacent to the thrombus may result in vasospasm and total occlusion of the vessel lumen in the presence of a previously nonocclusive eccentric plaque or thrombus. This type of acute thrombosis is thought to be the cause of acute myocardial infarction and sudden death (generally ischemia-induced cardiac dysrhythmias).[36]

Hemodynamic Goals

It is thus apparent that the goal of a successful anesthetic is the prevention of ischemia. Failing that, the prompt identification and treatment of new episodes are essential. As is evident from the previous discussion and from the summary in Table 36-2, anesthetic decisions are designed to reduce and control those factors that increase myocardial oxygen demand, specifically, heart rate, contractility, and wall tension. At the same time, every attempt is made to optimize coronary blood flow—notably, maintaining coronary perfusion pressure and increasing diastolic time. The buzz words for patients with coronary artery disease are "slow, small, and well perfused." Combinations of anesthetics, sedatives, muscle relaxants, and vasoactive drugs are selected to provide this hemodynamic milieu. Techniques to effectively prevent or treat alterations in coronary vascular tone are still evolving and await further clinical trial before definitive recommendations can be made.

Monitoring for Ischemia

Electrocardiogram. The ideal monitoring technique is not yet available. ST segment analysis in multiple leads (most commonly leads II and V_5) is currently the standard. In patients likely to develop right ventricular ischemia, the addition of V_{5R} might be beneficial.[37] Computerized ST segment trending and interactive monitors that alarm when the ST segment deviates from the programmed algorithm may aid in the detection of intraoperative events overlooked by even the most astute observer.[38]

Heart Rate and Blood Pressure. Multiple attempts have been made to determine ischemic thresholds using commonly measured hemodynamic variables. Among the earliest of these was the rate-pressure product,[39] obtained by multiplying heart rate by peak systolic pressure. For each patient, ischemia developed when a particular rate-pressure product was reached. The rate-pressure product was consid-

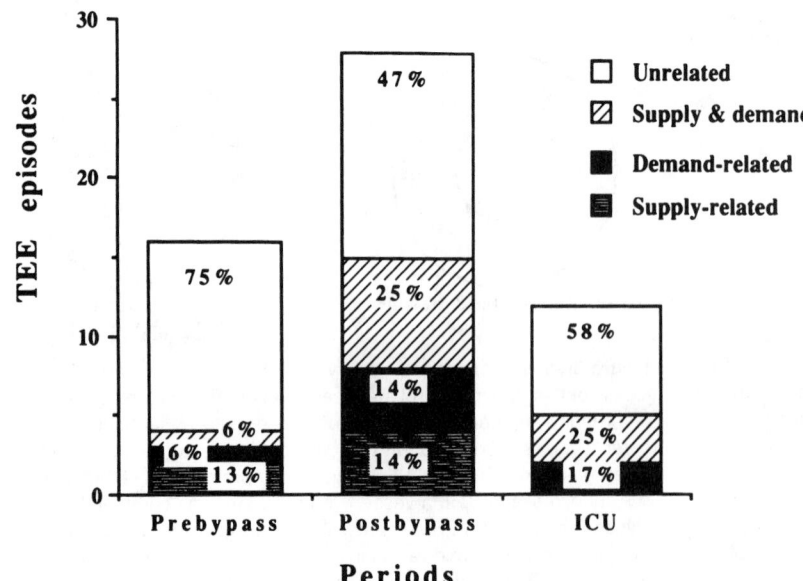

Figure 36-7. Association of transesophageal echocardiographic (TEE) wall motion changes with hemodynamic indices of supply and demand from continuous monitoring of 50 patients undergoing coronary artery bypass surgery. (Reproduced with permission from Leung JM, O'Kelly BV, Mangano DT et al: Relationship of regional wall motion abnormalities to hemodynamic indices of myocardial oxygen supply and demand in patients undergoing CABG surgery. Anesthesiology 73: 802, 1990.)

TABLE 36-2. Coronary Artery Disease—Hemodynamic Goals

P—Keep the heart small; ↓ wall tension; ↑ perfusion pressure
A—Maintain; hypertension is better than hypotension
C—Depression is beneficial when LV function is adequate
R—Slow, slow, slow
Rhy—Usually sinus
MV̇o₂—Control of oxygen demand is frequently not enough; monitor for and treat "supply" ischemia
CPB—Elevated VFP is usually not needed after CABG

P = preload; A = afterload; C = contractility; R = rate; Rhy = rhythm; MV̇o₂ = myocardial oxygen balance; CPB = pre- and post-cardiopulmonary bypass; CABG = coronary artery bypass graft; VFP = ventricular filling pressure; LV = left ventricle.

ered an easily determined index of MVo_2. Although rate-pressure product may correlate with oxygen demand, especially during exercise, it is not a sensitive or specific indicator of intraoperative ischemia. Kissin et al[40] point out that identical rate-pressure products are possible from multiple combinations of heart rate and blood pressure. Improved conditions for oxygen balance are likely with a low heart rate and high blood pressure compared with the opposite, that is, hypotension and tachycardia.[24]

In an effort to produce a more reliable predictor of ischemia, Buffington[24] devised the pressure-rate ratio. Using a canine model, he observed the effects of 20 combinations of various blood pressures and heart rates and found that no single value of either blood pressure or heart rate or the rate-pressure product was predictive of ischemia. The ischemia threshold was mutually dependent on both the heart rate and coexisting blood pressure. No ischemia occurred if mean arterial pressure (MAP) exceeded heart rate, that is, if the pressure-rate *ratio* exceeded unity (MAP/heart rate > 1). However, more recently Leung et al.,[15] using transesophageal echocardiography to detect regional wall motion abnormalities suggestive of ischemia, found that neither the rate-pressure product nor the MAP/heart rate ratio was a very sensitive predictor of ischemic changes and questioned their clinical usefulness. Furthermore, most (73%) of the ischemic episodes (detected by transesophageal echocardiography) in 50 patients undergoing coronary artery bypass graft surgery did not occur with acute changes in heart rate, blood pressure, or pulmonary arterial pressure, suggesting that most intraoperative ischemic episodes are related to decreased oxygen supply.[15] Gordon et al, using the electrocardiogram as a monitor of ischemia, also demonstrated the lack of sensitivity and specificity of the pressure-rate ratio.[42]

Pulmonary Artery Catheter. Sudden elevations in pulmonary artery or capillary wedge pressure indicating systolic and/or diastolic dysfunction, large A waves reflecting decreased ventricular compliance, and V waves signaling the development of ischemia-induced papillary muscle dysfunction and mitral regurgitation are purported signs of ischemia that may be detected with the pulmonary artery catheter.[43,44] Several recent studies contradict this long-held dogma and demonstrate that the pulmonary artery catheter is of little value as a *monitor* of myocardial ischemia. Leung et al[45] found that only 10% of all regional wall motion abnormalities were associated with an acute rise in pulmonary

capillary wedge pressure in 40 patients undergoing elective coronary artery bypass graft surgery. Haggmark et al[46] investigated 53 patients with coronary artery disease undergoing vascular surgery and compared several indicators of ischemia. They found that neither an increase in the pulmonary capillary wedge pressure nor the occurrence of an abnormal pulmonary capillary wedge pressure waveform was a sensitive indicator for myocardial ischemia. Van Daele et al[47] similarly found in 98 anesthetized patients prior to undergoing coronary artery bypass graft surgery that elevation of the pulmonary capillary wedge pressure is neither a sensitive nor a reliable indicator of ischemia. Furthermore, a large prospective study (1094 patients) by Tuman et al[48] showed that even high-risk cardiac surgical patients may be safely managed without routine use of a pulmonary artery catheter, and if a clinical need develops intraoperatively, delayed placement of a pulmonary artery catheter does not change outcome. Although pulmonary capillary wedge pressure changes are no longer considered a sensitive or reliable indicator of ischemia, the pulmonary artery catheter provides information regarding the patient's volume status and cardiac output.

Echocardiography. Transesophageal two-dimensional echocardiography permits on-line evaluation of regional wall motion and global ventricular function. Identification of new regional wall motion abnormalities may represent a very early indicator of ischemia. Recent studies using intraoperative transesophageal echocardiography to monitor left ventricular wall motion have demonstrated that it is much more sensitive than electrocardiography (and pulmonary capillary wedge pressure) in the detection of ischemia.[47,49] Furthermore, Leung et al[15] recently showed that such new regional wall motion abnormalities in the postbypass period conveyed prognostic significance in predicting adverse outcomes. Several caveats about transesophageal echocardiography must be emphasized. All regional wall motion abnormalities may not be caused by acute myocardial ischemia.[50] Other causes include "stunned" or "hibernating" myocardium, tethering, prior infarction, changes in preload/afterload, and regional temperature differences. Accurate assessment of left ventricular wall motion depends on careful attention to probe position and orientation for reproducibility and depends heavily on the skill of the operator.[51] The relationship of transesophageal echocardiography-detected regional wall motion abnormalities to ischemia is not completely validated and is based on transthoracic echocardiography data.[52] Further studies validating the transesophageal echocardiography criteria used to define ischemia and quantitative analysis of wall motion will enable transesophageal echocardiography to become more than a qualitative assessor of wall motion.

Selection of Anesthetic

Numerous reports documenting the pattern of prebypass hemodynamics and the frequency of prebypass ischemia support the conclusion that there is no "best" anesthetic for patients with coronary artery disease.[53] Two large prospective outcome studies in coronary artery bypass graft patients addressed the question of anesthetic choice. Slogoff and Keats,[54] in a prospective randomized study using various anesthetics in 1012 patients, found a perioperative incidence of myocardial infarction of 4.1% and a mortality of 1.7%. Tuman et al,[55] in a prospective nonrandomized study of five anesthetic techniques in 1094 patients, similarly found a perioperative incidence of myocardial infarction of 4.1% and a mortality of 3.1%. In neither study did anesthetic choice influence outcome. Nearly every combination of anesthetic and vasoactive drug has both favorable studies and ardent zealots promoting its use. However, the choice of anesthetic should depend primarily both upon the extent of pre-existing myocardial dysfunction and the pharmacologic properties of the drugs themselves. The fit patient who has angina only on heavy exertion and good ventricular function profits from having MVo_2 decreased with a volatile-based technique.[56,57] Conversely, the patient with severe congestive heart failure and a scarred myocardium might be better served by a less depressant technique. Clearly, there are patients who fall all along this spectrum. These examples illustrate the point that myocardial depression is only harmful in the patient whose heart cannot be further depressed without fear of precipitating overt heart failure. Most patients with mild or even moderate dysfunction may benefit from some degree of myocardial depression decreasing oxygen demand and alleviating or at least decreasing episodes of ischemia.

Opioids. The primary advantages of opioids are lack of myocardial depression, maintenance of a stable hemodynamic state, and reduction of heart rate (except for meperidine). Problems include hypertension and tachycardia during surgical stimulation[58,59] (sternotomy and aortic manipulation), especially in patients with good ventricular function, predictable hypotension when combined with benzodiazepines, lack of titratability when used in high doses, and a low incidence of intraoperative recall.[60,61] It is apparent that a primary opioid technique may be of value in the patient with severe myocardial dysfunction; in patients with normal ventricles, this may be inadequate as an anesthetic and may need to be combined with other anesthetics or vasoactive drugs.[62]

Inhalation Anesthetics. The desirable features of volatile anesthetics include dose dependence, easily reversible and titratable myocardial depression,[63,64] amnesia, and reliable suppression of sympathetic responses to surgical stress and cardiopulmonary bypass. Disadvantages include myocardial depression, systemic hypotension (whether induced by decreased contractility or vasodilation), and lack of postoperative analgesia. Combinations of narcotics and volatile anesthetics may produce the advantages of each with minimal untoward effects.

Isoflurane is a coronary vasodilator, as are the other volatile anesthetics, although to a lesser degree.[65-69] This effect is dose-related and is clinically insignificant in doses less than 1 minimum alveolar concentration. Clinical studies using isoflurane to clinical rather than pharmacologic end points do not show increased episodes of ischemia or a worsened outcome.[11]

Treatment of Ischemia

Selection of anesthetics or vasoactive drugs that will enable the heart to return to the slow, small, perfused state is frequently required during anesthesia. The principal vasoactive drugs are nitrates, beta blockers, peripheral vasoconstrictors, and calcium entry blockers. Clinical scenarios for their use are given in Table 36-3. These drugs are discussed extensively in Chapter 14 and are reviewed only briefly here. Volatile anesthetics can also be used to control blood pressure and reduce contractility.

TABLE 36-3. Treatment of Intraoperative Ischemia

Demand

↑ BP ± ↑ PCWP	TNG, ↑ anesthetic depth
↑ HR	Usual causes, then beta blocker

Supply

↓ BP	Vasoconstrictor, ↓ anesthetic depth
↓ BP and ↑ PCWP	Phenylephrine + TNG, Inotrope
NL hemodynamics	TNG, CEB

BP = blood pressure; PCWP = pulmonary capillary wedge pressure; HR = heart rate; NL = normal; TNG = nitroglycerin; CEB = calcium entry blocker.

Nitrates. Nitroglycerin is a venodilator and reduces venous return, lessening wall tension and MVo_2, and also a coronary arterial dilator, effective in coronary stenoses and in collateral beds.[71,72] Nitroglycerin is the drug of choice for the acute treatment of coronary vasospasm. The evidence for the prophylactic use of nitroglycerin for prevention of ischemic episodes is conflicting; further studies are needed to resolve this issue.[73-75] Although nitroglycerin is primarily a venodilator, at higher doses it does dilate arterial beds and may cause systemic hypotension.

Vasoconstrictors. Vasoconstrictors are useful adjuncts in the prevention and treatment of ischemia owing to their ability to increase systemic blood pressure. Administration of an alpha-adrenergic agent such as phenylephrine improves coronary perfusion pressure, although at the expense of increasing afterload and MVo_2. In addition, concomitant venoconstriction increases venous return and left ventricular preload. In most situations, the increase in coronary perfusion pressure more than offsets any increase in wall tension. Peripheral vasoconstriction is indicated during episodes of systemic hypotension, especially those caused by reduced surgical stimulation or drug-induced vasodilation. Nitroglycerin is sometimes added in order to counteract any increase in preload. Similarly, phenylephrine can be administered to patients in whom nitroglycerin results in decreased ventricular filling pressures but unacceptably low arterial pressure.

Beta Blockers. Beta-adrenergic blockade is often useful in improving myocardial oxygen balance by preventing or treating tachycardia as well as decreasing contractility. Myocardial depression can result in increased volume and wall tension, but clinically this is not a considerable problem. Indications for beta blockers include treatment of sinus tachycardia *not* resulting from the usual causes (e.g., light anesthesia, hypoxia), slowing the ventricular response to supraventricular dysrhythmias, and decreasing heart rate and contractility in hyperdynamic states. Intravenous preparations include propranolol, metoprolol, labetalol, and esmolol. Propranolol is a nonselective beta blocker with an elimination half-life from 4 to 6 hours. Metoprolol is similar to propranolol but has the advantage of beta-1 selectivity. Labetalol combines alpha-blocking properties with those of beta blockade and is useful in treating hyperdynamic situations and in controlling hypertension. Esmolol is a short-acting beta blocker that is cardioselective, with a half-life of only 9.5 minutes. It is often useful in treating momentary increases in heart rate owing to episodic sympathetic stimulation.

Calcium Channel Blockers. *In vitro,* all calcium entry blockers depress contractility, reduce coronary and systemic vascular tone, decrease sinoatrial node firing rate, and impede atrioventricular conduction. Unlike the beta blockers, which are very similar both in structure and in pharmacodynamic effect, the calcium entry blockers vary remarkably in their predominant pharmacologic action. Nifedipine is the most prominent peripheral vasodilator and, when administered sublingually, is useful intraoperatively in treating hypertension or episodes of coronary vasospasm. Verapamil's effect on coronary vascular tone is equal to that of nifedipine, but its peripheral effects are less pronounced, although still present. In addition to treating presumed coronary spasm, verapamil is very useful in the treatment of supraventricular tachycardia and in slowing the ventricular response to atrial fibrillation or flutter. Some clinicians simultaneously administer phenylephrine to counteract the peripheral vasodilation and hypotension that often accompany the use of verapamil.

VALVULAR HEART DISEASE

Alterations in loading conditions are the initial physiologic burdens imposed by valvular heart lesions, both stenotic and regurgitant. For example, the left ventricle is pressure overloaded in aortic stenosis and volume overloaded in aortic insufficiency and mitral regurgitation. However, in mitral stenosis, the left ventricle is both volume and pressure underloaded, whereas the right ventricle faces the progressively increasing left atrial and pulmonary artery pressures. The mechanisms used to compensate for these additional stresses consist of chamber enlargement, myocardial hypertrophy, and variations in vascular tone and the level of sympathetic activity.[76] These mechanisms in turn induce secondary alterations, including altered ventricular compliance, development of myocardial ischemia, chronic cardiac dysrhythmias, and progressive myocardial dysfunction. Myocardial contractility is often transiently depressed but may progress to irreversible impairment even in the absence of clinical symptoms. This is especially true in mitral regurgitation and aortic insufficiency, where markedly reduced afterload favors ejection and forward flow.[77,78] Conversely, the patient with aortic stenosis may complain of dyspnea not because of impaired systolic function but rather because of reduced ventricular compliance, increased left ventricular end-diastolic pressure, and pulmonary pressures.

When a decision for valve replacement or repair is made, we are often presented with a patient with pulmonary hypertension, severe ventricular dysfunction, and chronic rhythm disorders. Anesthetic management is predicated on understanding these altered loading conditions, preserving the compensatory mechanisms, maintaining circulatory homeostasis, and anticipating the problems that may arise during and after valve surgery. In this section, we briefly describe the pathophysiology, the desirable hemodynamic profile, and other pertinent anesthetic considerations for each valvular lesion.

Aortic Stenosis

Pathophysiology. Progressive calcification and narrowing of the aortic valve orifice are degenerative processes affecting a normal or congenitally bicuspid valve. This results in chronic obstruction to left ventricular ejection. Increased intraventricular systolic pressure with concomitant increase

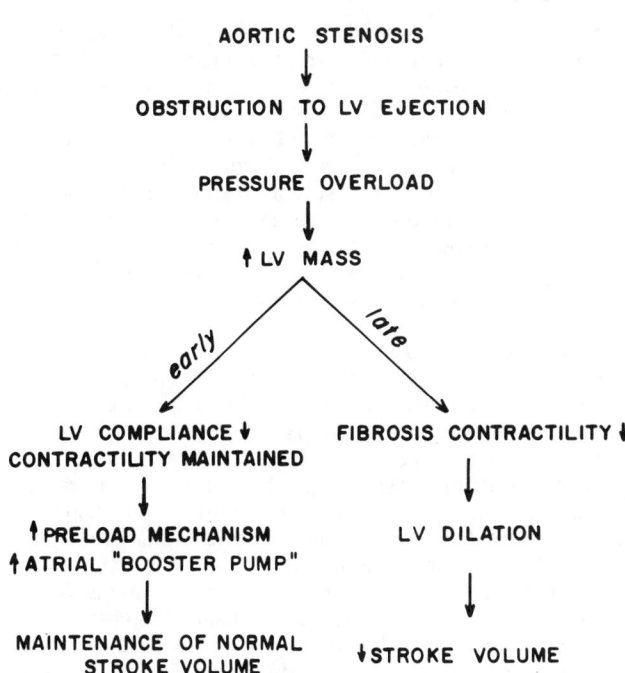

Figure 36-8. The physiologic consequences of aortic stenosis. (Reprinted with permission from Thomas SJ, Lowenstein E: Anesthetic management of the patient with valvular heart disease. Int Anesth Clin 17:67, 1979.)

in wall tension is required in order to maintain forward flow. "Concentric" ventricular hypertrophy, in which the wall gradually thickens but the chamber size remains unchanged, is the compensatory response normalizing wall tension. Contractility is preserved and ejection fraction is maintained at a normal range until late in the disease process[79] (Fig. 36-8). The normal valve area is about 3 cm²; signs and symptoms of aortic stenosis occur when this is reduced to 0.8 cm².

The cost of this concentric hypertrophy is decreased diastolic compliance and a precarious balance between myocardial oxygen supply and MVo_2. The clinical implications of the low compliance ventricle are summarized in Table 36-4. Since the ventricle is so stiff, atrial contraction is often critical for maintaining ventricular filling and stroke volume. The "atrial kick" may account for up to 40% of left ventricular end diastolic volume. Hypertrophy-induced impairment of diastolic relaxation can further impede left ventricular filling. Ventricular filling pressure is sometimes difficult to interpret, since it may vary widely yet reflect only small changes in ventricular volume.

TABLE 36-4. Clinical and Physiologic Implications of a Low Compliance Ventricle

Sensitive to volume depletion
Dependent upon atrial kick for adequate ventricular filling
Wide swings in ventricular filling pressure
PCWP underestimates LVEDP
↑ LVEDP reduces coronary perfusion pressures

PCWP = pulmonary capillary wedge pressure; LVEDP = left ventricular end-diastolic pressure.

Hypertrophied myocardium is susceptible to ischemia, even in the absence of concurrent coronary artery disease. The enlarged muscle mass increases basal myocardial oxygen requirements while demand per beat rises owing to the elevated intraventricular systolic pressure.[80] Simultaneously, supply may be impaired, perfusion pressure is reduced (aortic diastolic pressure is decreased, ventricular filling pressure is increased), capillary density is often inadequate in the hypertrophic muscle,[81] and total vasodilator reserve may be impaired.[82] This situation is compounded in the presence of coronary obstruction.

Anesthetic Considerations. The ideal hemodynamic environment for the patient with aortic stenosis is summarized in Table 36-5. Maintenance of adequate ventricular volume and sinus rhythm is crucial. Hypotension must be prevented if at all possible and treated early if it develops. Coronary perfusion pressure must be maintained to prevent the catastrophic cycle of hypotension-induced ischemia, subsequent ventricular dysfunction, and worsening hypotension. Bradycardia is a common clinical etiology for hypotension in the patient with aortic stenosis. Slowing the heart rate and increasing diastolic time will not increase stroke volume. Therefore, bradycardia will induce a fall in total cardiac output and sytemic arterial pressure. This is especially pertinent in the elderly patient, in whom sinus node disease and reduced sympathetic responses[83] may predispose to significant bradycardia.

Ischemia may be difficult to detect because the characteristic changes are often obscured by the electrocardiographic signs of left ventricular hypertrophy and strain. Unfortunately, an ideal alternative is not available. Elevated left ventricular filling pressures, although not necessarily reflecting increased volume, often require treatment in order to optimize coronary perfusion pressure. Nitroglycerin is very useful in this regard, but it must be remembered that minimal reductions in ventricular volume are required; therefore, very low doses of nitroglycerin should be used and titrated to effect.

Hypertrophic Cardiomyopathy

Hypertrophic cardiomyopathy, also known as idiopathic hypertrophic subaortic stenosis or asymmetric septal hypertrophy, is a genetically determined disease characterized by histologically abnormal myocytes and myocardial hypertro-

phy developing *a priori* and not in response to pressure or volume overload in a nondilated chamber.[84,85]

Pathophysiology. The physiologic consequences of hypertrophic cardiomyopathy are depicted in Figure 36-9. Some degree of subvalvular obstruction is present in 20–30% of patients. During systole, the left ventricular outflow tract is narrowed by apposition of the hypertrophic intraventricular septum to the anterior leaflet of the mitral valve (Fig. 36-10). Blood is ejected rapidly through this area, creating a Venturi effect, pulling the mitral valve leaflet even closer to the septum.[86] The timing and duration of septal–leaflet contact determine the severity and clinical significance of the obstruction.[87] Early prolonged contact can generate pressure gradients higher than 100 mm Hg. If the apposition occurs later, although a pressure gradient may exist, it is of little importance because most of the stroke volume has already been ejected.[88] This obstruction is dynamic and is accentuated by any intervention that reduces ventricular size, facilitating septal–leaflet contact. Therefore, increases in contractility or heart rate or decreases in either preload or afterload are detrimental in this regard. This histologically abnormal muscle demonstrates impaired diastolic relaxation and reduced ventricular compliance.[89] The clinical and hemodynamic implications are similar to those detailed for aortic stenosis.

The ventricles are hypertrophic, even in the absence of a pressure gradient. In addition, there is evidence of alterations in the small intramyocardial vessels.[90] Therefore, as expected, myocardial oxygen balance is tenuous, and the development of ischemia is an ever present possibility.

Anesthetic Considerations. Anesthetic management focuses on maintenance of ventricular filling and reduction in the factors predisposing to outflow tract obstruction or ischemia (Table 36-6). Myocardial depression is desirable,

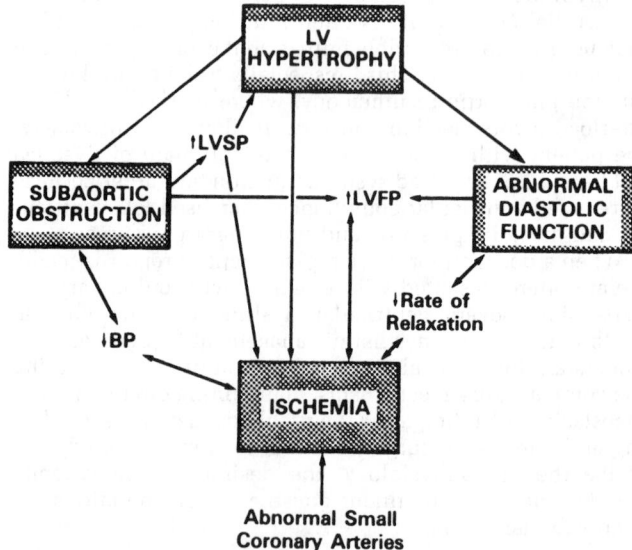

Figure 36-9. The physiologic interrelationships of primary left ventricular hypertrophy in hypertrophic cardiomyopathy. (LVSP = left ventricular systolic pressure; LVFP = left ventricular filling pressure.) (Reprinted with permission from Maron BJ, Bonow RO, Cannon RO *et al:* Hypertrophic cardiomyopathy: Interrelations of clinical manifestations, pathophysiology, and therapy. N Engl J Med 316: 344, 1987.)

TABLE 36-5. Aortic Stenosis—Hemodynamic Goals

P—Full; adequate intravascular volume to fill noncompliant ventricular chamber

A—Already elevated, but relatively fixed; coronary perfusion pressure must be maintained

C—Usually not a problem; inotropes may be helpful preinduction in end-stage aortic stenosis with hypotension

R—Not too slow (↓ CO), not too fast (ischemia)

Rhy—Sinus!! Cardioversion if hemodynamic instability from supraventricular dysrhythmia

MVo₂—Ischemia is an ever present risk; tachycardia and hypotension must be avoided

Abbreviations are defined in Table 36-2 footnote.

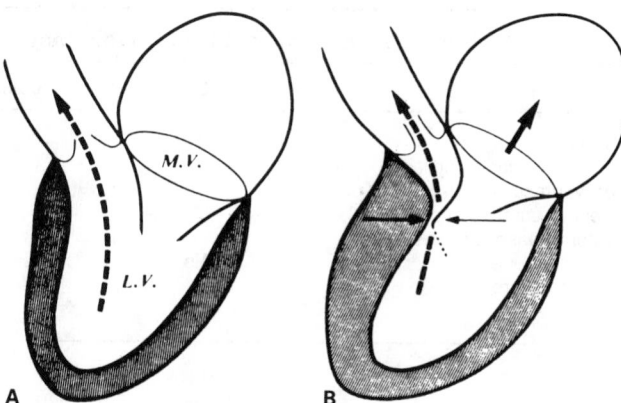

Figure 36-10. Proposed mechanism for outflow tract obstruction in hypertrophic cardiomyopathy. (*A*) The normal outflow tract is ample and offers no impedance to ejection. (*B*) The outflow tract is narrowed by the hypertrophic ventricular septum in hypertrophic cardiomyopathy. A Venturi effect is produced as blood is ejected rapidly through this area, drawing the anterior mitral leaflet toward the septum. Obstruction to forward flow (owing to mitral-septal contact) as well as mitral regurgitation can occur. (Reprinted with permission from Wigle ED, Sasson Z, Henderson MA *et al:* Hypertrophic cardiomyopathy. The importance of the site and the extent of hypertrophy. A review. Prog Cardiovasc Dis 28:1, 1985.)

and volatile anesthetics are useful, although their tendency to cause junctional rhythm is of some concern. Because of the exquisite sensitivity of preload to atrial contraction, these patients often benefit from placement of pulmonary artery catheters with atrial pacing capabilities. This permits the administration of volatile anesthetics without fear of compromising sinoatrial conduction. In addition, control of atrial rate and rhythm is very beneficial during the prebypass period.

Although infrequent, hypertrophic cardiomyopathy occasionally coexists with valvular aortic stenosis and may explain unanticipated difficulties in separating from bypass following seemingly uncomplicated aortic valve replacement. If this is suspected, measurement of the gradient between the left ventricle and the outflow tract will resolve the dilemma. In addition, dynamic left ventricular outflow obstruction is occasionally observed following mitral valve repair.[91] Anterior septal motion is observed echocardiographically. Pharmacologic management of hypotension is

---

TABLE 36-6. Hypertrophic Cardiomyopathy—Hemodynamic Goals

P—Full, full, full; volume is first prescription for hypotension
A—Up, up, up; a pure vasoconstrictor is next prescription for hypotension
C—Depression is fine
R—Not too slow, not too fast
Rhy—Sinus, sinus, sinus; consider pacing pulmonary artery catheter to better control atrial mechanism
M$\dot{V}o_2$—Usual precautions apply
CPB—Avoid inotropes post-CPB; the myocardial disease is still present; try vasoconstrictors first

Abbreviations are defined in Table 36-2 footnote.

---

with volume replacement and vasoconstrictors rather than inotropes and vasodilators.

Aortic Insufficiency

Rheumatic disease, endocarditis, or processes that dilate the aortic root such as ascending aortic aneurysms or collagen vascular diseases are the primary causes of aortic insufficiency.

Pathophysiology. The fundamental physiologic derangement is chronic volume overload (Fig. 36-11). Chamber size increases gradually, sometimes to massive proportions, increasing wall stress and inducing mural hypertrophy. This pattern of chamber enlargement and increasing ventricular wall thickness is termed *eccentric hypertrophy*. Despite these enormous increases in end-diastolic volume, end-diastolic pressures are usually within the normal range, evidence of a significant increase in chamber diastolic compliance.[89] In contrast to aortic stenosis, considerable alterations in left ventricular volume can occur with only minimal changes in left ventricular filling pressure. Although the ventricle may pump three to four times the normal cardiac output, MVo$_2$ does not increase extraordinarily, since the oxygen cost for muscle shortening is quite low. The contractile state of the myocardium is often difficult to discern from clinical signs and symptoms. Ventricular afterload is chronically reduced because of the low diastolic pressure reflecting continuing diastolic runoff as well as a moderately vasodilated state. This will allow patients to be relatively symptom-free even in the presence of reduced contractility.[92] This is important in terms of preparing the

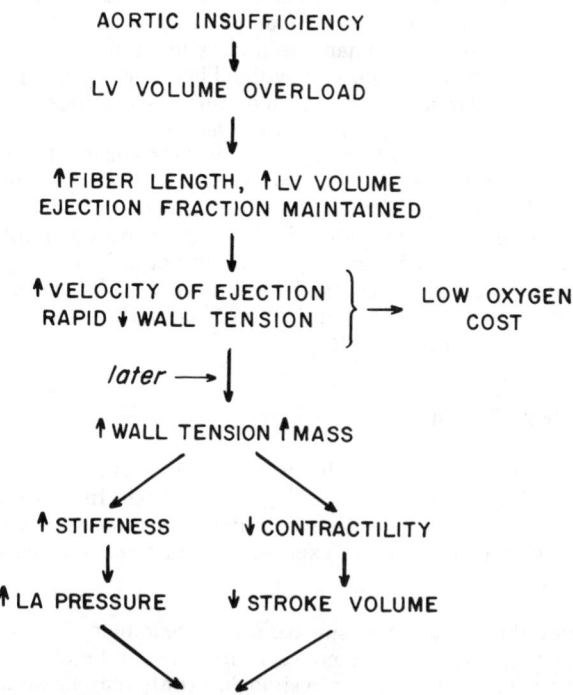

Figure 36-11. The physiologic consequences of aortic insufficiency. (Reprinted with permission from Thomas SJ, Lowenstein E: Anesthetic management of the patient with valvular heart disease. Int Anesth Clin 17:67, 1979.)

anesthetic, but perhaps even more so with respect to timing of aortic valve replacement. Ideally, the valve should be replaced just prior to the onset of irreversible myocardial damage. Therefore, continued follow-up of these patients emphasizes repeated noninvasive measurements of contractility, usually after some form of afterload stress, either pharmacologic or exercise-induced.

In contrast to chronic aortic insufficiency, acute aortic insufficiency subjects a ventricle with normal diastolic function to sudden volume overload and severe congestive heart failure dominates the clinical picture. The previously normal-sized left ventricle, with limited distensibility, is forced to handle large regurgitant volumes, rapidly elevating left ventricular end-diastolic pressure along the steep portion of the diastolic pressure-volume relation. Left ventricular end-diastolic pressure increases to alarming levels, and poor myocardial contractility becomes evident. Compensatory mechanisms include tachycardia and peripheral vasoconstriction, but occasionally hypotension and low cardiac output ensue (Table 36-7). Some patients are so acutely ill that emergency aortic valve replacement is required, whereas in less severe circumstances, mild systemic vasodilation and inotropic support can return hemodynamics toward normal.

Anesthetic Considerations. Full, mildly vasodilated, and modestly tachycardic describe the optimal cardiovascular state for patients with aortic insufficiency (Table 36-8). Vasodilation promotes forward flow, although additional intravascular volume may be necessry to maintain preload.[93] The ideal heart rate is somewhat controversial.[94,95] It is likely that changes in rate alone will not alter net forward or regurgitant flow; they will each be proportionally reduced. Tachycardia does reduce diastolic ventricular volume and wall tension and also increases diastolic blood pressure, which should improve coronary perfusion and offset the increase in oxygen demand secondary to an increased heart rate. Bradycardia should be avoided because it predisposes to ventricular distention, which causes elevations in left atrial pressure and pulmonary congestion.

Ventricular distention may occur with the onset of cardiopulmonary bypass if the heart slows or if there is unexpected ventricular fibrillation. Monitoring of the appearance of the heart, the rate and rhythm, and ventricular filling pressure if available are especially important in these patients. If distention occurs, the insertion of a left ventricular vent or the immediate application of an aortic cross-clamp should relieve the problem.

Mitral Stenosis

Stenosis of the mitral valve is usually of rheumatic origin, with clinical disease becoming manifest within 3–5 years following initial infection. Debilitating symptoms such as fatigue and dyspnea on exertion do not begin for another decade or two.

Pathophysiology. The spectrum of physiologic disruption in patients with mitral stenosis is presented in Figure 36-12. This complicated pathophysiologic profile may be simplified by grouping the changes as either proximal or distal to the obstructing mitral valve.

In mitral stenosis, unlike other valvular lesions, the left ventricle is not subject to either pressure or volume overload. In fact, it is often relatively underloaded owing to the obstruction preventing left ventricular filling. Although the

TABLE 36-7. Acute *Versus* Chronic Aortic Insufficiency

	Chronic	Acute
Left ventricular size	↑	—
Left ventricular compliance	↑	—
Left ventricular end-diastolic pressure	—	↑
Effective cardiac output	Normal	↓
Systemic vascular resistance	—	↑
Pulmonary edema	No	Yes
Pulse pressure	↑	↑/—
Heart rate	—	↑

left ventricle may be small, ventricular function is usually maintained, although one third of patients may demonstrate contractile abnormalities on angiography, presumably as a result of rheumatic carditis or involvement of the subvalvular apparatus.[96] The diminished ventricular volume precludes effective use of vasodilators to improve left ventricular flow.[97]

Increased left atrial pressure (LAP) and volume overload are inevitable consequences of the narrowed mitral orifice. The relationship between left atrial pressure and the size of the valve orifice is expressed in the formula derived by Gorlin and Gorlin:

$$\text{Valve area} = (\text{flow/K}) \times \text{pressure gradient}$$

where flow = cardiac output/diastolic filling time, pressure gradient = left atrial − left ventricular end-diastolic pressures (LVEDP), and K = hydraulic pressure constant. This calculation assumes no regurgitant flow. Assuming a constant valve area, rearranging terms and eliminating the constant provides us with a more useful expression of the clinical variables determining atrial and ventricular pressures.

$$\text{LAP} - \text{LVEDP} = (\text{cardiac output/diastolic time})^2$$

Therefore, whenever cardiac output increases or diastolic filling period decreases, the gradient across the mitral valve is altered by the square of the original changes. This explains why tachycardia or increases in forward flow, seen classically with pregnancy, thyrotoxicosis, or infection can precipitate pulmonary edema. In fact, as left atrial pressure increases, left ventricular filling pressure may actually decrease. Therefore, the development of atrial fibrillation causes hemodynamic embarrassment, not so much because of the loss of atrial kick but because of the rapid rate that

TABLE 36-8. Aortic Insufficiency—Hemodynamic Goals

P—Normal to slightly ↑
A—Reduction beneficial with anesthetics or vasodilators; increases augment regurgitant flow
C—usually adequate
R—Modest tachycardia reduces ventricular volume, raises aortic diastolic pressure
Rhy—Usually sinus; not a problem
MV̇o₂—Not usually a problem
CPB—Observe for ventricular distention (↓ HR, ↑ VFP) when going onto CPB

Abbreviations are defined in Tables 36-2 and 36-3 footnotes.

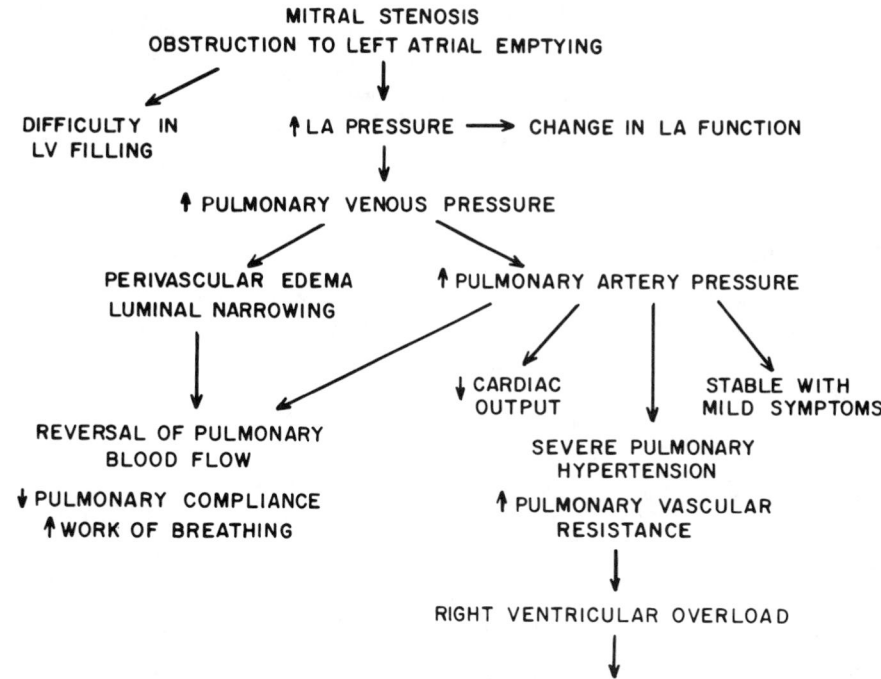

Figure 36-12. The cardiovascular and pulmonary effects of mitral stenosis. (Reprinted with permission from Thomas SJ, Lowenstein E: Anesthetic management of the patient with valvular heart disease. Int Anesth Clin 17:67, 1979.)

ensues. We are left with the paradoxical situation of a patient in pulmonary edema with a relatively empty left ventricle. The treatment in this situation is, therefore, not inotropic or vasodilator therapy but rather attempts to reduce the heart rate or diagnose and treat the cause responsible for the increased flow.

The pulmonary capillary wedge pressure can be used as an index of left ventricular filling, keeping in mind that it is higher than the true left ventricular end-diastolic pressure, at least by the amount of the pressure gradient. During episodes of tachycardia or increased flow, the wedge pressure *continues* to reflect left atrial pressure; however, this is no longer indicative of left ventricular filling pressure.

Persistent elevations in left atrial pressure are reflected back through the pulmonary circulation leading to right ventricular pressure overload with compensatory right ventricular hypertrophy and strain. The progression and severity of pulmonary hypertension are variable and reflect further narrowing of the valve orifice and irreversible reactive changes in the pulmonary vasculature. Right ventricular dysfunction may develop in response to the afterload stress. Tricuspid annular dilatation and insufficiency may climax this hemodynamic nightmare.

Chronically elevated left atrial pressure causes perivascular edema in the lung, increased vascular pressure in the dependent portions of the lung, redistribution of blood to the upper lung fields, and a somewhat increased work of breathing.

Anesthetic Considerations. Preventing trouble is the cornerstone of prebypass anesthetic management (Table 36-9), because treatment of hemodynamic derangements is sometimes difficult. Avoiding tachycardia precludes episodes of left atrial and pulmonary hypertension with potential right ventricular dysfunction as well as inadequate left ventricular filling with concomitant systemic hypotension. Preoperative maintenance of digitalis and beta blocking drugs, selection of anesthetics with no propensity to increase heart

rate, and attainment of anesthetic levels deep enough to suppress autonomic responses are methods to achieve these laudable goals. Episodes of pulmonary hypertension and potential right-sided heart failure stemming from pulmonary vasoconstriction must also be prevented. Hypoxia, hypercarbia, and acidosis are the classic offenders; follow the ancient internist's classic nostrum and avoid them.

Treatment of hypotension in patients with mitral stenosis can present a challenging dilemma. Although these patients normally take diuretics, hypovolemia is not usually the cause, and response to volume administration is often disappointing. Use of a vasoconstrictor to offset mild peripheral vasodilation is acceptable, bearing in mind the risk of pulmonary vasoconstriction and possible accentuation of right ventricular dysfunction. It is often prudent to select a drug with some inotropic effect such as ephedrine or epinephrine rather than rely on a pure vasoconstrictor.

In separating from cardiopulmonary bypass, although much is made of right ventricular failure (discussed subsequently), more commonly it is the left ventricle that is dysfunctional. This may be owing to intraoperative injury or

---

TABLE 36-9. Mitral Stenosis—Hemodynamic Goals

P—Enough to maintain flow across stenosis
A—Avoid ↑ right ventricular afterload (pulmonary vasoconstrictors) ? inotropes for systemic hypotension
C—LV usually OK until after CPB; right ventricle may be impaired if there is long-standing pulmonary hypertension
R—Slow to allow time for ventricular filling
Rhy—Often atrial fibrillation; control ventricular response
MV̇o₂—Not a problem
CPB—Vasodilators may help post-CPB right ventricular failure; control of ventricular response may be difficult

Abbreviations are defined in Table 36-2 footnote.

sudden increase in flow to and distention of the chronically underloaded left ventricle. After bypass, prominent V waves may be present in the left atrial pressure curve. This almost always reflects increased left atrial filling from the right side rather than mitral regurgitation, since cardiac output is increased after bypass when compared with preinduction values.[98]

Mitral Regurgitation

Mitral valve prolapse, chronic ischemic heart disease, rheumatic heart disease, endocarditis, and annular dilation are causes of mitral regurgitation. Acute mitral regurgitation occurs with papillary muscle dysfunction or chordal rupture following myocardial infarction and may require emergency surgical repair.

Pathophysiology. Chronic volume overload similar to that described with aortic insufficiency, is the cardinal feature of mitral regurgitation. The left atrium acts as a low pressure vent for left ventricular ejection. Total stroke volume consists of the forward flow *via* the aorta and backward flow into the left atrium. There is no period of isovolumetric contraction, since blood is immediately ejected retrograde with the onset of ventricular systole. Despite decreased contractility, patients may be minimally symptomatic despite progressive myocardial damage because of this reduced afterload. The additional oxygen lost is low, needed only for additional muscle shortening because there is little pressure development. Ventricular compliance increases, and the large end diastolic volume does not cause striking increase in left ventricular end-diastolic pressure. Atrial and ventricular chamber enlargement, ventricular wall hypertrophy, and increased blood volume are the compensatory responses. The volume of regurgitant flow is related to the size of the regurgitant orifice, the time available for retrograde flow, and the pressure gradient across the valve.[99] Regurgitant orifice size, in turn, is dependent upon ventricular size. Therefore, both increases in heart rate and preload reduction decrease the amount of regurgitant flow by diminishing ventricular volume. Arteriolar dilators, in contrast, are effective by reducing the ventriculoatrial pressure gradient.[100]

Other similarities of mitral regurgitation to aortic insufficiency include increases in ventricular chamber compliance and difficulty in evaluating left ventricular contractile function. The latter is particularly troublesome, since, in mitral regurgitation, the left ventricle is maximally unloaded. The incompetent valve acts as a low pressure vent for left ventricular ejection. There is no period of isovolumic contraction, since blood is immediately ejected retrograde with the onset of ventricular systole. This explains why many patients have minimal symptoms despite progressive myocardial damage. This reduced afterload also explains why ejection fraction, a measure heavily afterload dependent, can be misleading in patients with mitral regurgitation. Normal or minimally reduced ejection fractions can be present even with severe impairment of contractile function.[78] Repairing or replacing the valve increases afterload, and often the dysfunctional myocardium becomes apparent. Administration of inotropes and/or vasodilators may be necessary to successfully separate from bypass.

When mitral regurgitation is of acute onset, the hemodynamic picture is quite different. Volume overload of the left atrium and ventricle occurs in the absence of compensatory ventricular enlargement. Ventricular filling pressures increase dramatically, as do pulmonary pressures. Cardiac output decreases, and pulmonary edema develops. If this occurs in the setting of acute myocardial infarction, cardiac performance may be inadequate despite pharmacologic support. Intra-aortic balloon assistance as well as emergency surgery may be lifesaving.

Anesthetic Considerations. Selection of anesthetics that promote vasodilation and tachycardia are ideal in the patient with mitral regurgitation (Table 36-10). Active pharmacologic intervention is usually unnecessary, since most patients are not teetering on the brink of myocardial failure. However, in some patients, especially those with acute myocardial regurgitation, aggressive pharmacologic management may be required. In the absence of acute deterioration, difficulties in management are usually limited to the postbypass period.

The problem of unmasking depressed myocardial contractility has already been discussed. Paradoxically, after the administration of vasodilators and inotropes, a patient occasionally deteriorates even further. As mentioned earlier, in these patients, the physiologic and clinical picture is exactly that of hypertrophic cardiomyopathy. It is seen after valve repair, not replacement. Systolic anterior motion of the anterior mitral leaflet is demonstrable by echocardiography. If this scenario is suspected, a trial of volume expansion and vasoconstrictors is indicated.

CARDIOPULMONARY BYPASS

Circuits

Although there are multiple configurations used for cardiopulmonary bypass, they all incorporate essential components, including large catheters for venous drainage, an oxygenator/heat exchanger, and a pump and tubing and cannula for arterial return[101] (Fig. 36-13). In many institutions, additional components are added to this elementary circuit. These include a filter on the arterial return cannula and often on the suction catheters, alarms to detect low levels of blood in the oxygenator in order to prevent pumping of air, in-line pressure and/or blood gas monitors, and a separate circuit for infusion of crystalloid or blood cardioplegia. Vaporizers can be positioned in the gas inflow circuit so that volatile anesthetics can be administered during the bypass period.

Blood is drained into a reservoir from either a large single two-stage cannula (drains the right atrium and the inferior

---

TABLE 36-10. Mitral Regurgitation—Hemodynamic Goals

P—Usually pretty full; may need to keep that way, although preload reduction may reduce regurgitant flow
A—Decreases are beneficial; increases augment regurgitant flow
C—Unrecognized myocardial depression possible; titrate myocardial depressants carefully
R—A faster rate decreases ventricular volume
Rhy—Atrial fibrillation is occasionally a problem
MV̇o$_2$—Only if mitral regurgitation is a complication of coronary artery disease; then be careful!!
CPB—Newly competent valve post-CPB increases afterload; vasodilators may be helpful; inotropes are frequently required

Abbreviations are defined in Table 36-2 footnote.

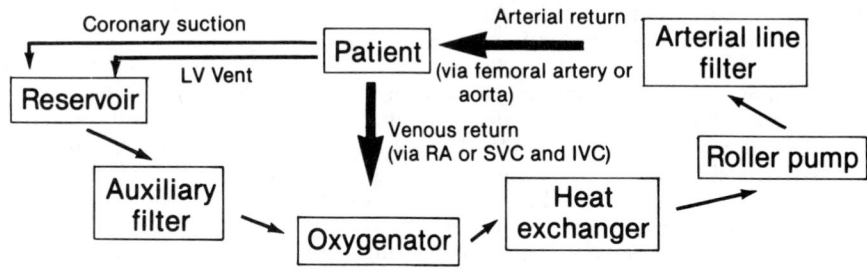

Figure 36-13. The basic circuit for cardiopulmonary bypass. See text for details. (Reprinted with permission from Tinker JH: Cardiopulmonary bypass: Technical aspects. In Thomas SJ [ed]: Manual of Cardiac Anesthesia, p 375. New York, Churchill Livingstone, 1984.)

vena cava) inserted into the right atrium or from two separate smaller cannulas placed in the superior and inferior vena cavae. The rate of venous return is dependent upon intravascular volume, the height of the patient above the reservoir, and proper placement of the cannulas. Flow can be reduced by partially or completely clamping these lines either by the surgeon or the perfusionist. Additional blood is returned from the operative field using suction generated by two small roller pumps. The first is the coronary suction that scavenges blood from the operative field, and the other is the vent suction used either to decompress the left ventricle or as an additional "coronary sucker." When used to decompress the left ventricle, this suction line is connected to either a catheter inserted across the mitral valve via the left superior pulmonary vein, to a metal or plastic tube inserted directly into the apex of the left ventricle, or to the aortic cardioplegic cannula. Many surgeons choose not to routinely vent the left ventricle during coronary artery bypass operations.

Most commonly, oxygenated blood is returned to the patient through a cannula placed in the ascending aorta. If this proves technically difficult, if emergency cannulation is necessary, or if partial bypass is used during surgery on the descending thoracic aorta, the femoral artery is usually selected.

Oxygenators

Bubble. The more commonly used and somewhat less expensive bubble oxygenators utilize direct contact between fresh gas and blood to effect transfer of oxygen (O_2) and carbon dioxide (CO_2). It is far more difficult to transfer O_2 than CO_2, since the solubility ratio is $1:25$. Foaming is an extremely efficient method of oxygenation and, in combination with high oxygen tensions, alleviates this problem. Gas is passed through a ceramic manifold to create bubbles small enough to provide sufficient total surface area for gas exchange but not so small to preclude easy removal. The smaller the bubbles, the greater the surface-to-volume ratio and the greater the oxygen transfer. In bubble oxygenators, CO_2 transfer is proportional to total gas flow, whereas oxygen transport is chiefly dependent upon bubble size. Gas flows do affect oxygen transport, and, at higher flows, CO_2 is sometimes added to the gas mixture in order to prevent unacceptable levels of hypocarbia. Critical to the function of the bubble oxygenator is the ability to reconstitute the perfusate ("defoaming") by passage through spongy polypropylene mesh impregnated with a charged silicon-containing polymer.

Bubble oxygenators are associated with time-dependent trauma to blood because of the direct blood-gas interface. Hemolysis develops with potential capillary plugging and organ damage from red blood cell debris. Platelet activity

is impaired secondary to platelet destruction, induction of aggregation, and adherence to parts of the oxygenator. Decreases in leukocyte counts have also been reported.[102,103] Additional problems associated with bubble oxygenators include activation of complement via the alternate pathway, formation of particulate and gaseous microemboli, and denaturation of blood proteins (including those of the coagulation cascade).[104-106]

Membrane. The membrane oxygenator attempts to eliminate or attenuate these problems associated with the blood-gas interface by separating the two phases by a thin silicon, Teflon, or polypropylene gas-permeable membrane. Blood flows in a thin film along the membrane, whereas gas slowly diffuses across it. The oxygen tension is controlled by the FIO_2 of the inspired gas, and CO_2 is regulated by total gas flow.

Studies comparing membrane with bubble oxygenators demonstrate less blood trauma with membranes and, in some cases, improved postoperative hemostasis.[107] However, other investigators report that these differences are clinically insignificant as long as perfusion time is less than 2 hours.[108] Differences in performance of the two types of oxygenators are also obscured by the amount of blood scavenged from the operative field, since these cells are the most severely damaged from direct mechanical trauma as well as from the turbulent blood-gas interface. Not much is known regarding the effects of the oxygenator membrane on the pharmacokinetics of inhaled anesthetics. However, it has been demonstrated in an ex vivo model of hypothermic cardiopulmonary bypass that isoflurane uptake and elimination by blood are markedly delayed by the Scimed membrane oxygenator.[109]

Pumps

Roller. Two types of pumps are used to generate the pressure required to return the perfusate to the patient (or, in the case of a membrane, to drive blood through the oxygenator and then to the patient). The first and by far the most commonly used is a roller pump. A roller pump consists of a central housing with two arms extending 180 degrees in opposite directions with smooth-faced rollers on each end. Flow is generated by compression of a heavy walled section of Silastic tubing by the rollers. Contact between one arm of the roller and the tubing begins as contact between the second roller ends, thus preventing retrograde flow. Shearing forces that would disrupt cells are minimized by ensuring that contact between the roller and tubing is nonocclusive. The roller pump head is driven by an electric motor that is designed to maintain constant speed and therefore flow despite variations in arterial inflow line resistance or power line voltage. If the motor or its power supply fails, the pump can be hand cranked in an attempt to provide adequate flow rates and systemic pressures.

Centrifugal. Centrifugal pumps are conical-shaped hardened plastic housings with rapidly rotating cones inside that impart momentum to the blood. This mechanism is pressure sensitive, and flow is determined by both inflow and outflow pressures as well as by pump head speed. An in-line electromagnetic flow meter is necessary to indicate forward flow, since, in contrast to a roller pump, direct conversion from rpms to flow rate is inaccurate. The maximal pressure generated with this pump is lower than that with a roller pump, and the likelihood of disconnects following inadvertent cannula obstruction is reduced. These are being used more frequently, especially for long-term mechanical ventricular support, because blood trauma is less than with a roller.

Pulsatile Flow. Roller pumps generate a sine wave pattern of flow, which, after dampening during transit through the inflow tubing and cannulas, results in a nonpulsatile arterial pressure wave. Selection of a different pump or insertion of additional components into a circuit allows the production of a pulsatile waveform. Theoretically, this sounds attractive and is intuitively more physiologic, but whether or not this is beneficial is controversial.[110-112] Pulsatile flow is thought to provide improved perfusion at the capillary level and is associated with lower systemic vascular resistance during bypass, improved oxygen extraction, and less production of pyruvate and lactate. Pulsatile flow has been shown to preserve pancreatic beta cell function (i.e., maintain the response of insulin secretion to hyperglycemia) during and after cardiopulmonary bypass, and thus could preserve protein anabolism in the early postoperative period.[113] A decrease in the need after bypass for pharmacologic or mechanical support as well as improved mortality has also been reported. Some investigators advocate converting to pulsatile perfusion, especially in those patients with severe preoperative impairment of ventricular function.[114] After extensive review, other investigators remain unconvinced by studies that differ significantly with regard to patient populations, the type of pumps used, and the efficiency of pulse generation.[111,115] Until noncontroversial studies demonstrate beyond doubt the superiority of pulsatile flow, the convenience and simplicity of nonpulsatility continue to make it the overwhelming choice for almost all procedures requiring cardiopulmonary bypass.

Heat Exchanger

A heat exchanger adjusts the temperature of the perfusate to provide moderate systemic hypothermia during the period of cardiac repair. Metabolic requirements are reduced approximately 8% per degree centigrade decrease in body temperature (about 50% of normal at 28°C).[116] Deliberate hypothermia provides protection during periods of hypoperfusion and potential tissue ischemia. In addition, adequate tissue oxygenation is achieved at lower flow rates, reducing trauma to the blood. Lower systemic flow also decreases flow to the heart via noncoronary collaterals (vessels arising from pericardial reflections), diminishing the rewarming and the rate of washout of cardioplegic solution. Also, by cooling the tissues surrounding the heart, reducing the rate of cardiac rewarming, hypothermia acts as an adjunct to myocardial protection.

Prime

The prime for most adult perfusions contains a balanced salt solution, since it resembles plasma in terms of osmolality and electrolyte composition. Individual recipes add albumin or hetastarch (increased oncotic pressure), mannitol (to promote diuresis), additional heparin, bicarbonate, calcium, and so on.[117] Although albumin is commonly added to prime solutions to increase oncotic pressure, it has not been shown to provide any clinical benefit in terms of outcome.[118] Blood is infrequently used except in neonates, children, and adults with significant preoperative anemia in whom profound hemodilution might decrease oxygen-carrying capacity below acceptable levels. After mixing of the patient's blood volume with the 1500–2500 ml (depending upon oxygenator and circuitry) prime, acute normovolemic hemodilution to hematocrits of 20–30 ml·dl^{-1} is normal. This offsets the increase in viscosity associated with systemic hypothermia. An asanguineous prime is not associated with metabolic acidosis and is reported to result in improved intra- and postoperative hemostasis and renal function.[119]

Anticoagulation

Prior to cannulation, systemic anticoagulation is mandatory in order to prevent catastrophic thrombus formation triggered by contact between the blood and oxygenator. Heparin, a polyanionic mucopolysaccharide extracted from bovine lung or porcine intestinal mucosa, accelerates the velocity of the reaction between antithrombin III and the activated forms of Factors II, X, XI, XII, and XIII, effectively neutralizing these factors. A tertiary complex is formed between heparin, antithrombin III, and these serine proteases. The half-life of heparin's anticoagulant effect is approximately 90 minutes in a normothermic patient, the rate of decay decreasing with hypothermia.

Anticoagulant activity varies among samples of commercially prepared heparin, as does patient response to a given dose. Patients receiving heparin in the period immediately prior to surgery and those with reduced levels of antithrombin III are notably resistant to normal precardiopulmonary bypass doses.[120] It seems prudent to assess the adequacy of heparinization prior to starting cardiopulmonary bypass because of the lack of correlation among heparin dosage, blood levels, and clinical effect as well as to ensure that heparin has in fact been given and distributed. Disagreement exists as to whether this is best done by measuring heparin levels or the effect of heparin on the coagulation process. The former utilizes a manual or automated protamine titration test or other assays for heparin level; the latter utilizes a thrombin time (not usually available) or an activated clotting time. Since heparin levels do not always correlate with effect, many centers opt for the more functional test.

The *activated clotting time*, introduced by Hattersley,[121] is the most commonly used test for the adequacy of anticoagulation. It is performed either manually or automatically and indicates the time required for thrombus formation, detected visually or magnetically, when blood is mixed with one of a variety of clotting accelerators. The exact activated clotting time value necessary before initiation of cardiopulmonary bypass to ensure absolute anticoagulation remains controversial. Many use 400 seconds, a value derived from a study in primates that found no fibrin monomer, an indicator of coagulation, as long as activated clotting time was above that level.[122] However, a recent study showed that after a single dose of 300 U·kg⁻¹ of heparin, 51 patients during cardiopulmonary bypass had an activated clotting time of less than 400 seconds (including four patients with an activated clotting time less than 300 seconds); these patients did not form clots in the oxygenator and their postoperative blood loss was not different from those patients with a higher activated clotting time.[123] This supports the belief that no minimum activated clotting time value has been determined to reflect the adequacy of heparinization during cardiopulmonary bypass.

The interpatient relationship between heparin concentration and activated clotting time is not linear nor is the sensitivity of the activated clotting time, that is, the change in activated clotting time per unit increase in heparin level.[124] However, the association between the dose of heparin administered and activated clotting time in an individual patient before cardiopulmonary bypass is somewhat linear.[125] Bull et al[125] have advocated use of such a dose-response curve to determine heparin and protamine requirements. This is often too time-consuming; it also overestimates protamine needs because hemodilution and hypothermia alter intrapatient activated clotting time sensitivity.[126] Heparin is usually given in an initial dose of 300–400 U·kg⁻¹; an activated clotting time is measured 5 minutes later, and additional heparin is given as required. The activated clotting time should be rechecked periodically, especially if the interval following initial administration is unduly protracted[127] or if the rewarming period on cardiopulmonary bypass is prolonged, since the rate of heparin decay increases.

Myocardial Protection

A wide variety of methods are used to maintain myocardial cell integrity and energy stores while the coronary circulation is interrupted. Although techniques utilizing cold cardioplegia are the most common, other techniques used include hypothermic fibrillation[128,129] and intermittent cross-clamping interspersed with periods of reperfusion.[130] The two critical elements with respect to cardioplegia are hypothermia (10–15°C) and hyperkalemia to ensure diastolic electrical arrest. Individual formulas add a variety of other ingredients, including, but not limited to, glucose as an energy substrate, buffering agents, albumin or mannitol for osmotic activity, citrate to reduce the calcium concentration, and nitroglycerin to improve distribution of the cardioplegic mixture. This solution is mixed with either crystalloid or oxygenated blood and is infused into the aortic root after the cross-clamp is applied. The cardioplegia may be injected by way of a separate cicuit on the bypass machine or manually, using a pneumatic infusion device. Direct injection into the aortic root is not feasible in patients with aortic insufficiency. The aorta must be opened and the cardioplegia injected directly into the coronary ostia with small perfusion cannulas. In patients with severe coronary ostial stenosis or multiple severe lesions preventing adequate distribution, cardioplegia may be injected retrogradely *via* the coronary sinus.[130-132] During the period of cardioplegic arrest, the anesthesiologist should monitor the electrocardiogram for return of electrical activity, the pulmonary artery pressure (if available) and/or the appearance of the heart for evidence of ventricular distention, and the operative field for return of contraction. The atria are often first to show return of contractile activity. Depending upon the duration of ischemia necessary, periodic reinjection may be necessary to maintain hypothermia and diastolic arrest and to wash out metabolic products. The variations of cardioplegic recipes and techniques are staggering. Several reviews discuss the physiologic and technologic details of cardioplegia; the interested reader is urged to consult them.[133-137]

PREOPERATIVE EVALUATION

The preoperative visit appropriately concentrates on the cardiovascular system but should also focus on the assessment of pulmonary, renal, endocrine, and hematologic functions. Equally important is a discussion with the patient of the projected events on the day of surgery, including transport to the operating room, preoperative routines (O₂ mask, vascular cannulation, anesthetic induction), and, finally, the awakening process in the recovery room or intensive care unit. The importance of communicating to the anesthesiologist any symptoms such as chest pain, shortness of breath, or the need for nitroglycerin during transport or the preinduction period should be stressed. The depth and detail of the explanation depend upon the patient's emotional state and desire to know.

Data from the history, physical examination, and laboratory investigations are used to delineate cardiovascular anatomy and functional state. Of critical importance is the assessment of severity of left or right ventricular failure. Pertinent findings suggestive of dysfunction are described in Table 36-11. Increases in the severity or frequency of anginal attacks or the presence of ischemia-induced ventricular dysfunction suggests that there are large areas of myo-

---

TABLE 36-11. Preoperative Findings Suggestive of Ventricular Dysfunction

History

History of MI, intermittent or chronic CHF
Symptoms of CHF: fatigue, DOE, orthopnea, PND, ankle swelling

Physical Examination

Hypotension/tachycardia (severe CHF).
Prominent neck veins, laterally displaced apical impulse, S₃, S₄, rales, pitting edema, pulsatile liver, ascites (tricuspid regurgitation)

Electrocardiogram

Ischemia/infarction, rhythm, or conduction abnormalities

Chest X-ray

Cardiomegaly, pulmonary vascular congestion/pulmonary edema, pleural effusion, Kerley B lines

Cardiac Testing

Cath data—LVEDP > 18, EF < 0.4, CI < 2.0 l·min⁻¹·m⁻²
Echocardiography—low EF, multiple regional wall motion abnormalities
Ventriculography—low EF, multiple areas of hypokinesis, akinesis, or dyskinesis

MI = myocardial infarction; CHF = congestive heart failure; DOE = dyspnea on exertion; PND = paroxysmal nocturnal dyspnea; LVEDP = left ventricular end-diastolic pressure; EF = ejection fraction; CI = cardiac index.

cardium at risk. A history of previous arrhythmias should be obtained, including the type, severity, associated symptoms, prior intervention, and successful treatment. Integration of this information leads to appropriate selection of monitoring devices and anesthetic techniques.

Conditions commonly associated with heart disease such as hypertension, diabetes mellitus, and cigarette smoking must also be evaluated. The last is extremely important and may be useful in differentiating whether episodes of intraoperative pulmonary hypertension are caused primarily by pulmonary or cardiac factors. Higher systemic arterial pressures may be desirable throughout surgery in patients with a history or other evidence of carotid artery disease.[138] Evidence for renal dysfunction must be sought, since the most common cause of postoperative renal failure is pre-existing renal insufficiency.[139] If renal reserve is reduced, intraoperative measures such as diuretics or the use of dopamine may be used, although data showing an improved outcome are still not available.

Current Drug Therapy

Almost without exception, cardiovascular drugs, including cardiac antidysrhythmics, beta or calcium channel blockers, and nitrates are continued until the time of surgery. Interactions between these drugs and anesthetics are rarely detrimental;[140] rather, they are more often beneficial in maintaining hemodynamic control during periods of surgical stress.

The beta blocking drugs are similar in structure and differ in degree of cardioselectivity, mode of excretion, and duration of action. Despite the known washout of these drugs during cardiopulmonary bypass, the very long-acting drugs (e.g., nadolol) may have persistent effects (either beneficial or detrimental) in the postbypass period. The calcium entry blockers have shorter elimination half-lives and somewhat different pharmacologic actions.[141] Concern about intraoperative hypotension and increased requirement for vasopressor support seems unwarranted.[142] Studies are needed to assess whether intraoperative administration might be beneficial in terms of reduction of postbypass ischemic episodes resulting from coronary vasospasm. In patients receiving calcium channel blockers without concomitant beta blockade, increases in heart rate and contractility may occur during surgical stimulation. Indeed, it has been shown that such patients have more perioperative ischemic electrocardiographic changes than patients receiving beta blocking drugs alone or in combination with calcium channel blocking drugs.[143]

Digoxin is prescribed to suppress cardiac dysrhythmias, control the ventricular response to atrial fibrillation, and improve contractility in patients with congestive heart failure. The efficacy of this last indication is sometimes difficult to discern clinically, so that discontinuation of digoxin in order to avoid digitoxic dysrhythmias seems appropriate. However, in those patients in whom it is being used for rate or rhythm control, continuation until the time of surgery seems advisable. Signs or symptoms of digoxin excess, including ventricular ectopy, atrial tachydysrhythmias, and variable degrees of atrioventricular block, should be sought. The latter is typically manifested by slowing and regularization of the ventricular response to atrial fibrillation. This represents digoxin-induced atrioventricular blockade with a regular junctional escape rhythm. Noncardiac symptoms include gastrointestinal distress or visual disturbances. Toxicity is more common in patients concomitantly receiving drugs that increase digoxin levels (e.g., nifedipine, verapamil, amiodarone) or reduce potassium levels (e.g., diuretics).

Most cardiac antidysrhythmics should also be continued to the time of surgery. Their pharmacology is well known (see Chapters 14 and 29), and they usually present little problem with anesthetic management. A newly available antidysrhythmic, amiodarone, is a notable exception.[144] This drug is a myocardial depressant with a half-life of 30 days. It can cause atropine-resistant bradycardia, severe hypotension, and atrioventricular blockade. Discontinuing it the night before surgery is obviously useless in terms of ameliorating possible side effects. Rather, suitable preparations for pacing and cardiovascular support should be readily available.

Physical Examination

As mentioned previously, the physical examination seeks to elicit signs of cardiac decompensation such as an S_3 gallop, rales, jugular venous distention, or pulsatile liver. Routes for vascular access should be assessed, and the status of peripheral arteries should be evaluated. As always, the airway should be carefully evaluated with respect to ease of mask ventilation and intubation of the trachea. Other pertinent points are described in Table 36-12.

Premedication

Even the most thorough preoperative psychological preparation is often inadequate to assuage the anxieties and apprehensions of a patient facing cardiac surgery. Premedication will assist in providing a calm, anxiety-free, but arousable and hemodynamically stable patient who is prepared, if not exactly enthusiastic, for surgery. Selection of drug and dosage is predicated on the patient's age, cardiovascular state, and level of anxiety. Heavy premedication is ideal for the fit person scheduled for coronary artery bypass grafting. Inadequate sedation may predispose to hypertension, tachycardia, or coronary vasospasm, all potential causes of myocardial ischemia. The frail, 50-kg cachectic patient with severe valvular dysfunction fares better with light premedication in order to avoid possible respiratory depression or loss of endogenous catecholamine support. Additional sedation can always be given in the operating room.

Premedication for cardiac surgery often combines the sedative and analgesic properties of an opioid (morphine, 0.1–0.2 mg·kg^{-1}) with the sedative and amnestic properties of scopolamine (0.006 mg·kg^{-1}) or a benzodiazepine (diazepam, 0.05–0.1 mg·kg^{-1}, midazolam, 0.03–0.05 mg·kg^{-1}, or lorazepam, 0.05 mg·kg^{-1}). The possibility of oversedation, hypercarbia, or hypoxia following premedication is always of concern. However, Hensley et al[145] have shown that morphine and scopolamine, when administered in standard doses, do not produce hypoxia. Rather, if hypoxia does occur after this combination, it is secondary to the additional supplementation administered in the operating room.

The choice of premedication may also affect the hemodynamic response to anesthetics. Thomson et al[146] administered a standard high-dose fentanyl anesthetic to patients premedicated with either morphine and scopolamine or lorazepam. In general, the patients receiving lorazepam were hemodynamically less responsive in that they had less hypertension, more hypotension, and a greater requirement

TABLE 36-12. Preoperative Physical Examination

Vital Signs

Current values and range while hospitalized

Height, Weight

For calculation of drug dosages and pump flows

Airway

Anatomic features that could make mask ventilation or intubation difficult

Neck

Jugular venous distention (CHF)
Carotid bruit (cerebrovascular disease)
Landmarks for jugular vein cannulation

Heart

Murmurs characteristic of valve lesions
S$_3$ (increased LVEDP)
S$_4$ (decreased compliance)
Click (MVP) or rub (pericarditis)
Lateral PMI displacement (cardiomegaly)
Precordial heave, lift (hypertrophy, wall motion abnormality)

Lungs

Rales (CHF)
Rhonchi, wheezes (COPD)

Vasculature

Sites for venous and arterial access
Peripheral pulses

Abdomen

Pulsatile liver (CHF, tricuspid regurgitation)

Extremities

Peripheral edema (CHF)

Nervous System

Motor or sensory deficits

CHF = congestive heart failure; LVEDP = left ventricular end-diastolic pressure; MVP = mitral valve prolapse; PMI = point of maximal impulse; COPD = chronic obstructive pulmonary disease.

for vasoactive drugs. This suggests that premedication may have a previously unappreciated but profound effect on intraoperative hemodynamics.

Monitoring

We will emphasize only those aspects of monitoring particularly relevant to cardiac surgery. The subject is discussed extensively in Chapter 28, and we have already reviewed techniques for identification of myocardial ischemia.

Pulse Oximeter

The need for multiple vascular cannulations and applications of numerous monitoring devices often prolongs the preinduction period. The pulse oximeter should be positioned prior to catheter insertion in order to detect clinically unsuspected episodes of hypoxemia, especially if additional intravenous sedation has been administered. Atten-

tion must be focused on the entire patient, even during the hunt for successful vascular access.

Electrocardiogram

Simultaneous observation of both a precordial lead V$_5$ and an inferior lead II for the presence of ischemia has been emphasized. If the standard leads prove inadequate for cardiac dysrhythmia detection and analysis, esophageal or epicardial leads may be used. Atrial activity can be amplified by recording bipolar atrial electrocardiograms from two atrial epicardial pacing electrodes. These may prove invaluable in diagnosing supraventricular dysrhythmias after bypass or in the postoperative period.[147] Occasionally, intraoperative myocardial injury causes substantial reductions in QRS voltage. Monitoring an electrocardiogram *via* a surgically placed ventricular pacing wire provides adequate voltage to facilitate dysrhythmia analysis or to trigger an intra-aortic balloon pump, if this is necessary. A strip-chart recorder documents and facilitates detailed analysis of both ST segment alterations and complex dysrhythmias.

Temperature

Central temperature can be measured with esophageal, tympanic, or Foley catheter probes or with a thermistor from a pulmonary artery catheter. Obviously, this last method is not reliable during the period of aortic cross-clamping when there is no flow through the heart. Rectal and toe probes record peripheral temperatures that lag behind central measurements during both cooling and rewarming.[148]

Arterial Blood Pressure

Systemic arterial pressure is always monitored invasively. The radial or femoral artery is usually cannulated, although the brachial and axillary arteries may also be used. The exact site is often the matter of personal or institutional preference. Criteria include convenience, selection of the fullest or most bounding pulse, and avoidance of the dominant hand. In addition, during dissection of the internal mammary artery, the ipsilateral pulse is often transiently occluded; therefore the radial artery opposite a planned internal mammary artery is selected.[149] Occasionally, the site of surgery dictates appropriate placement; for example, the right radial artery should be used for any procedure involving the descending thoracic aorta, since the left subclavian artery may be included in the proximal aortic clamp. Following cardiopulmonary bypass, radial artery pressure is often misleading and may be as much as 30 mm Hg lower than central aortic pressure.[150,151] The mechanism is thought to be peripheral vasodilation during rewarming.[152] Whenever such a discrepancy is suspected, aortic pressure can be estimated by palpation by the surgeon or, if direct measurement is needed, a needle may be placed directly into the aorta. The gradient between aortic and radial pressure usually disappears within 45 minutes of separation from bypass.

Central Venous Pressure/Pulmonary Artery Catheter

Access to the central circulation is mandatory for infusion of cardioactive drugs. In addition, right atrial or central venous pressure accurately reflects right ventricular filling pressure and is of critical importance whenever right ventricular dysfunction is suspected. In patients with unimpaired left ventricular function, transduced right atrial pressure is often assumed to be a reliable guide of left-sided filling.[153] This relationship is less predictable in the presence of severe left ventricular dysynergy, pulmonary hypertension, or reduced left ventricular compliance. In these instances, insertion of a pulmonary artery catheter for measurement of pulmonary capillary wedge pressure provides a more precise index of left ventricular filling. In addition, determination of cardiac output and calculation of derived hemodynamic indices offer additional information to guide hemodynamic and anesthetic management.

Indications for pulmonary artery catheterization vary greatly among institutions. In some, these catheters are used routinely, whereas in others, they are limited to patients with specific disease states such as severe left ventricular dysfunction or pronounced pulmonary hypertension. Additional indications include combined procedures (valvular plus coronary) or those that require prolonged time for dissection (cardiac reoperations or use of one or both internal mammary arteries). Insertion of a pacing pulmonary artery catheter can be very helpful whenever exact control of rate and rhythm is desirable, for example, in patients with hypertrophic cardiomyopathy or those with significant bradycardia secondary to beta blockade.[154]

When pulmonary artery catheters are used, disagreement still exists as to whether they should be placed before or after the induction of anesthesia.[155,156] In some patients, early insertion of the catheter and determination of baseline hemodynamic values can beneficially influence anesthetic selection and guide the induction sequence. However, the anxious and uncomfortable hypertensive patient is better served by a smooth induction of anesthesia followed by catheter placement. Incremental sedation followed by pre-induction placement is a suitable alternative associated with minimal, if any, hemodynamic change.[156]

It must be remembered that the catheter often migrates toward the periphery of the lung with cardiac manipulation before and during cardiopulmonary bypass.[157] Therefore, it seems wise to pull the catheter back a few centimeters prior to the initiation of bypass in order to prevent permanent wedging or possible pulmonary artery rupture.

Despite the controversy concerning the routine use of these catheters, there is no disagreement that the capability to measure both cardiac output and ventricular filling pressures must be available in any institution performing cardiac surgery. Whether this is done with a pulmonary artery catheter or with direct cannulation of the left atrium and dye dilution techniques is immaterial. The critically ill patient requires these measurements in order to determine the effectiveness of vasoactive drugs, to adjust dosage, and to evaluate the need for further pharmacologic or mechanical intervention.

Echocardiography

Two-dimensional transesophageal echocardiography is the newest, most complex, and most expensive diagnostic device. Its role in cardiac anesthesia is still evolving. Detection of ischemia by on-line evaluation of new regional wall motion abnormalities has been mentioned. Other applications specific to cardiac surgical patients may prove even more useful. It is well known that following cardiopulmonary bypass, ventricular filling pressure, irrespective of site of measurement (left ventricular end-diastolic pressure, left atrium, pulmonary capillary wedge pressure), is a poor and often misleading indicator of ventricular volume status.[158-160] Direct estimation of left ventricular volume with

two-dimensional transesophageal echocardiography may more appropriately direct fluid infusion and selection of vasoactive drugs in patients who are difficult to wean from bypass. In addition, residual valve lesions, intracardiac air, or new areas of ischemia are readily identified. Global dysfunction suggesting residual cross-clamp effect, inadequate cardioplegia, or reperfusion injury can be detected. Two-dimensional transesophageal echocardiography has already proved invaluable in detecting residual valvular insufficiency following mitral valve repair.[161]

Central Nervous System Function

Monitoring of the brain during extracorporeal bypass is still in its infancy and not yet universally used. Studies correlating postoperative neurologic or psychological outcome with changes in intraoperative "neurodynamics" have not yet been performed. In addition, definition of "normal" changes related to hemodilution or hypothermia is needed before recommendations for interventions based on central nervous system measurements can be made. The electroencephalogram has demonstrated global cerebral ischemia when perfusion pressure was reduced in order to facilitate surgical exposure.[162] A three-lead electroencephalogram was used to assess the adequacy of central nervous system depression in patients given thiopental to reduce central nervous system damage after cardiopulmonary bypass.[163] Here, the electroencephalogram was used to detect a therapeutic end point rather than for diagnosis of an intraoperative misadventure. In an attempt to prevent paraplegia, somatosensory evoked potentials have been recommended as a means of monitoring spinal cord integrity during operations on the descending thoracic aorta.[164] Once again, further studies with larger numbers of patients are required to confirm the usefulness of this technique.

Selection of Anesthetic Drugs

The task confronting the anesthesiologist is to render the patient undergoing cardiac surgery analgesic, amnesic, and unconscious while simultaneously suppressing the endocrine and autonomic responses to intraoperative stress. Equally important is preservation of compensatory cardiovascular mechanisms and prevention of perioperative episodes of myocardial ischemia. Although these goals are not unique to the cardiac surgical patient, they are sometimes a bit more difficult to accomplish because of the severity of ischemic and/or valvular disease. Although there tends to be institutional and personal bias with respect to choice of anesthetic (with preponderance favoring high-dose opioid techniques), there are no data that document superiority of any anesthetic for either coronary or valvular surgery.[165] The recent large outcome studies of Tuman et al[55] and Slogoff and Keats[54] indicate that the choice of anesthetic has no effect on outcome in coronary artery bypass graft patients. As was previously emphasized, the most critical factor governing anesthetic selection is the degree of ventricular dysfunction. Anticipated difficulties during the tracheal intubation sequence, the expected length of surgery, and the anticipated time until extubation of the trachea also influence choice of anesthetic. It is desirable to be able to alter anesthetic depth in order to accommodate the varying intensity of surgical stress. During intubation of the trachea, incision, sternotomy, pericardiotomy, and manipulation of the aorta, there is intense stimulation. The period of prepping and draping following intubation of the trachea requires minimal levels of anesthetic, as does the period of hypothermic bypass.

There is no one best technique. Familiarity with all anesthetics and their physiologic and pharmacologic effects in the patient with severe cardiac disease allows great flexibility in anesthetic selection. In addition, it provides numerous options applicable to the cardiac patient undergoing noncardiac surgery.

Potent Inhalation Anesthetics

These drugs are useful both as primary anesthetic drugs and as adjuvants to treat or prevent "breakthrough" hypertension associated with high-dose opioid techniques.[59,166-168] The balance of myocardial oxygen supply and MVo_2 is usually altered favorably by reduction in contractility and afterload. Deleterious declines in perfusion must be prevented or treated, and the possibilities of increases in wall tension must be considered. These agents have been used successfully in all types of valve surgery without untoward effects, although they are sometimes associated with more hemodynamic variability than is seen with opioids.[98,169] Use of these drugs involves no more hemodynamic intervention than upfront loading with opioids, and the ability to rapidly increase and decrease concentrations permits easy adjustment to variable levels of surgical stimulation. Volatile anesthetics can be administered during bypass through a vaporizer mounted on the pump; they are also appropriate in the postbypass period assuming that cardiac function is adequate.

Opioids

The opioids lack negative inotropic effects in the doses used clinically and have thus found widespread use as the primary agents for cardiac surgery. This era began in 1969 when high doses of morphine were used to anesthetize patients for aortic valve replacement.[170] However, hypotension, histamine release,[171] increased fluid requirements,[172] and, often, inadequate anesthesia resulted in a decline in the use of morphine in favor of the newer synthetic fentanyl derivatives. Aside from bradycardia, fentanyl and its analogues are relatively devoid of cardiovascular effects and have proved to be effective anesthetics. As a primary anesthetic agent, fentanyl (50–100 $\mu g \cdot kg^{-1}$) or sufentanil (10–20 $\mu g \cdot kg^{-1}$) and oxygen provide hemodynamic stability, although they do not consistently prevent a hypertensive response to periods of increased surgical stimulation.[59,173] In patients with good ventricular function, although high doses of opioids produce unconsciousness and characteristic electrocardiographic slowing, patient recall of intraoperative events remains a potential problem.[60,61] Adjuvant agents are frequently used to supplement the opioids—benzodiazepines to provide amnesia, and volatile anesthetics or vasodilators to control hypertension. Superiority of any one opioid has not been demonstrated for either coronary or valvular surgery.[59,174] The use of high-dose opioids prolongs the time until emergence and extubation when compared with techniques primarily based on volatile anesthetics. This is usually inconsequential for cardiac surgical patients, since mechanical ventilation of the lungs is continued for variable periods of time postoperatively. Sufentanil has been reported to result in earlier emergence and extubation of the trachea than either morphine or fentanyl.[175] Alfentanil, with an elimination half-life shorter than that of fentanyl or sufentanil, is suitable for infusion techniques and may provide optimal conditions for early extubation of the trachea.[176,177] Combinations of the fentanyl-type drugs and benzodiazepines, whether given concomitantly or as premedication, result in hypotension secondary to a fall in systemic vascular resistance.[178,179] The use of any opioid in high doses can produce excessive bradycardia. Vecuronium or atracurium may magnify this problem,[180] whereas pancuronium is often useful in preventing it. Abdominal and chest wall rigidity commonly occur with high-dose opioids and can be severe enough to render ventilation impossible. A low dose of nondepolarizing muscle relaxant should be given prior to opioid administration.[181]

Nitrous Oxide

In many centers, nitrous oxide is not used at all during cardiac surgery. In addition to the metabolic effects emphasized,[182] increases in pulmonary vascular resistance have been demonstrated, with the greatest response in patients with pre-existing pulmonary hypertension.[183,184] The drug is also a mild myocardial depressant and elicits a compensatory sympathetically mediated increase in systemic vascular resistance.[185] These minimal changes may not be well tolerated in patients with minimal cardiovascular reserve. Control of hemodynamics when nitrous oxide is added to an anesthetic prevents ischemia in dogs.[186] Using transesophageal echocardiography, Cahalan et al[187] demonstrated no ischemia when nitrous oxide was added to a fentanyl-based anesthetic.

It is well known that nitrous oxide increases the size of any air-filled cavity. The possibility of expansion of air introduced into the circulation either before or during bypass should preclude its use immediately before, during, or after bypass.

Induction Drugs

The benzodiazepines, the barbiturates, and etomidate can be used as supplements to either inhalation or opioid anesthetics and, more importantly, are excellent as sole induction drugs in patients with cardiac disease.[188,189] Obviously, dosage requirements must be altered to fit the clinical situation, but these are excellent drugs with which to begin an anesthetic.

Neuromuscular Blocking Drugs

Muscle relaxants are usually part of an anesthetic plan for cardiac surgery. Although they are not essential to surgical exposure of the heart, muscle paralysis facilitates intubation of the trachea, prevents shivering, and attenuates skeletal muscle contraction during defibrillation. In addition, muscle relaxants are necessary to prevent or treat opioid-induced truncal rigidity. The chief criteria for selection are the hemodynamic properties associated with each relaxant,[190] the patient's myocardial function, current pharmacologic regimen, and anesthetic technique. This translates into what is a desirable heart rate and blood pressure for any particular patient.[191-194] Two new, long-acting, nondepolarizing muscle relaxants, doxacurium and pipecuronium, will be particularly useful in cardiac surgical patients since they afford prolonged muscle relaxation and, unlike pancuronium, do not cause a significant increase in heart rate. Doxacurium has a superior overall hemodynamic profile in cardiac surgical patients in that it causes no significant change in systemic arterial blood pressure or cardiac output.[195] Pipecuronium has been shown to significantly decrease mean arterial pressure and cardiac output in cardiac surgical patients.[196]

Intraoperative Management

In this section, we describe the anesthetic management of a patient undergoing a cardiac surgical procedure from the time of arrival in the operating room until care is transferred to recovery room personnel. Since the physiologic and pharmacologic rationales for anesthetic selection have previously been discussed, this is rather a sequential description of what happens and what is required during surgery. Anticipation of needs specific to each stage of the procedure and ready availability of necessary equipment and drugs prevent untoward hemodynamic aberrations as well as last-minute scrambling and potentially avoidable delays.

Preparation

The operating room must be readied prior to arrival of the patient. Check the anesthesia machine, and have available all supplies necessary for management of a normal airway or any additional equipment if a difficult intubation of the trachea is anticipated. Anesthetic drugs, emergency drugs, and medicated infusions should be prepared and ready for use. Heparin must be drawn up prior to induction of anesthesia in the unlikely event of the need to "crash" onto bypass. All monitoring equipment should be switched on, working, and calibrated. Confirm that typed and cross-matched blood is available in the operating suite. Table 36-13 is a checklist to aid in proper preoperative preparation of the operating room.

Preinduction Period

A brief conversation outside the operating room serves to evaluate the patient's general status and level of anxiety and to assess the effectiveness of premedication. Remind the patient to inform you if chest pain, shortness of breath, or other symptoms occur. Angina should be promptly treated with oxygen, sublingual or iv nitroglycerin, additional sedation, or perhaps if related to anxiety-induced hypertension or tachycardia, the prompt induction of general anesthesia. Supplemental oxygen *via* nasal cannula should be given to all patients once they have been transferred to the operating table, and peripheral oxygen saturation should be monitored with a pulse oximeter during line placement. Electrocardiographic leads and blood pressure cuff are placed, and initial vital signs are recorded.

One or two large-bore iv cannulas are inserted following local anesthesia (additional routes for infusion are desirable in patients undergoing repeat cardiac surgery). In some centers, anesthesia is then induced, and following intubation of the trachea, arterial and central venous cannulas are inserted. In most institutions, however, these additional lines are inserted prior to anesthesia. Pre- or postinduction insertion of central venous or pulmonary artery catheters has been discussed previously. Once they are inserted, however, initial values for all pressures and cardiac output should be recorded, and baseline determinations of arterial blood gases, hematocrit, and activated coagulation time should be obtained.

Throughout the preinduction period, the anesthesiologist must never let preoccupation with placement of iv and pres-

---

TABLE 36-13. Anesthetic Preparation for Cardiac Surgery

Anesthesia Machine

Routine checkout

Airway Management

Nasal cannula for oxygen supplementation
Laryngoscope/blades, endotracheal tubes, airways, etc
Suction apparatus
Special equipment if difficult airway is anticipated
Inspired gas humidifier/warmer

Circulatory Access

Intravenous fluids/infusion tubing
Proper catheters for peripheral/central sites
Infusion pumps
Blood/fluid warmers

Monitoring

ECG leads, blood pressure cuff
Pulse oximeter
Esophageal stethoscope
Temperature probes (esophageal, rectal, bladder, tympanic membrane)
Central venous and/or pulmonary artery catheters
Transducers calibrated and zeroed
Strip-chart recorder
Cardiac output computer
Heparin monitoring equipment

Medications

Anesthetic and related:
  Opioids
  Barbiturates, benzodiazepines
  Neuromuscular blockers
Heparin (must be drawn up prior to starting case)
Cardioactive drugs

Syringe:	Infusion:
Atropine	Nitroglycerin/nitroprusside
Calcium chloride	Inotrope
Nitroglycerin	
Phenylephrine or	
ephedrine or ino-	
trope	

Antibiotics

Miscellaneous

Pacemaker (standard and atrioventricular sequential)
Warming blanket
Compatible blood in operating suite

---

sure monitoring catheters divert his or her attention from the patient. In addition to continuously monitoring vital signs, careful observation of the patient with periodic verbal contact facilitates detection of increased anxiety, excessive response to iv sedation, and hemodynamic or electrocardiographic abnormality.

Induction and Intubation

The exact choice and sequence of drugs are a subtle combination of art and science. The dose, speed of administration, and specific agents (e.g., sedative, opioid, volatile drug, muscle relaxant) selected depend primarily on the patient's cardiovascular reserve and desired cardiovascular profile. A smooth transition from consciousness to blissful sleep is desired without untoward airway difficulties (e.g., coughing, laryngospasm) or hemodynamic responses (either hypotension—too much drug, loss of sympathetic tone, myocardial depression; or hypertension—insertion of airway, "tugging" on the jaw). A "slow cardiac induction" sometimes creates rather than alleviates these latter problems. On the other hand, a slow, sedated, awake intubation of the trachea may be most appropriate in a bull-necked, obese patient who appears difficult to intubate and ventilate. These examples re-emphasize the necessity for an individual approach to each patient.

Deep planes of anesthesia, brief duration of laryngoscopy, and innumerable pharmacologic regimens have been proposed for eliminating the hypertension and tachycardia associated with intubation of the trachea (Chapter 26).[197] None is uniformly successful, and all drug interventions carry some degree of risk, small though they may be. In addition, in some patients, especially those with a slow heart rate prior to induction of anesthesia, the reflex response to intubation of the trachea is primarily vagal, and severe bradycardia and rarely sinus arrest can occur. Furthermore, recent evidence suggests that intubation of the trachea is a strong stimulus for coronary vasoconstriction irrespective of the anesthetic, since left ventricular blood flow is dramatically altered in the absence of hemodynamic changes.[12] Therefore, the response to tracheal intubation may be varied, although it is usually short-lived. Nevertheless, evidence for persistently abnormal hemodynamics or ischemia should be sought and treated.

After documented successful intubation of the trachea, the tube is then secured, an esophageal stethoscope is inserted, and the eyes and all pressure points are protected. The importance of frequent checks of all monitors during these busy minutes cannot be overemphasized.

Preincision Period

The period of time from intubation of the trachea until skin incision is one of minimal stimulation as the surgical team attends to insertion of a bladder catheter, temperature probe, positioning, prepping, and draping. Hypotension often occurs during this period regardless of the anesthetic technique used. It may be necessary to reduce anesthetic depth or alternatively support systemic pressure with a vasoconstrictor. The potential risks of vasoconstriction in patients with poor left or right ventricular performance must be remembered. Deeper planes of anesthesia are obviously necessary immediately prior to incision and sternotomy.

Incision to Bypass

As previously emphasized, the pre–bypass period is characterized by periods of intense surgical stimulation that may cause hypertension, tachycardia, or ischemia. Anticipating these events and deepening the anesthetic may be effective, but often a vasodilator or other adjuvant is required. This is particularly true in patients with good ventricular function when an opioid–oxygen technique is used.[70] Hypotension can occur during the less stressful moments before bypass, but it is more commonly associated with cardiac manipulation in preparation for and during atrial cannulation. This may interfere with venous return or produce episodic ectopic beats or sustained supraventricular dysrhythmias. Atrial fibrillation is not uncommon. Depending upon the blood pressure and heart rate response, appropriate treatment may range from nothing at all, to vasoconstrictors, to cardioversion, to rapid cannulation and institution of bypass. Maintenance of adequate intravascular volume may

attenuate the extent of blood pressure fall. This is a critical time; continual observation of the surgical field is essential.

During all cardiac procedures (perhaps more so than with any other type of surgery), hemodynamic change must be immediately correlated with events in the surgical field. Retracting, lifting, and in general, "mugging" the heart are sometimes necessary; the hemodynamic consequences are unpredictable. This is particularly true following cardiopulmonary bypass when grafts and suture lines are inspected and repaired if necessary. This is also true during reoperations, when dissection may be difficult, tedious, and time-consuming and when continuous retraction of the heart is often necessary. Bleeding, sometimes unexpectedly profuse, will compound the problem. In rare cases in which a cardiac chamber is entered and bleeding is uncontrollable, heparin is administered, the femoral vessels are cannulated, and cardiopulmonary bypass is begun using coronary suction from the field as a major source of venous return. Communication between the anesthesiologist and the surgeon is necessary to keep both apprised of the situation and to ensure that the heart gets a periodic "rest."

Cardiopulmonary Bypass

After heparin has been administered, the cannulas are inserted, and adequate levels of anticoagulation are checked to ensure that the patient is ready for the institution of cardiopulmonary bypass (Table 36-14). Attention is focused on adequacy of venous drainage, oxygenation, unobstructed arterial return, and provision of necessary anesthetics and

---

TABLE 36-14. Checklist Prior to Initiating Cardiopulmonary Bypass

Laboratory Values

ACT or measure of adequate heparinization
Hematocrit

Anesthesia/Machine

Adequate anesthesia and muscle relaxants given
Nitrous oxide off (if used)

Monitor

Arterial pressure—initial hypotension and then return
CVP—indication of inadequate venous drainage
PCWP—LV distention—inadequate drainage, AI
    —pull back pulmonary artery catheter 1–2 cm

Patient/Field

Cannulas in place: no air locks, clamps, or kinks; no bubbles in
    arterial cannula
Facial appearance
    Suffusion (inadequate SVC drainage)
    Unilateral blanching (innominate artery cannulation)
Heart
    Signs of distention (especially in AI, ischemia)

Support

Usually not required

The major categories for this table and Tables 36-15 and 36-16 are organized using the mnemonic LAMPS.

ACT = activated clotting time; CVP = central venous pressure; PCWP = pulmonary capillary wedge pressure; LV = left ventricle; SVC = superior vena cava; AI = aortic insufficiency.

muscle relaxants. Anesthetic requirements decrease if systemic hypothermia is used.

Once full cardiopulmonary bypass is established, it is no longer necessary to continue ventilation of the lungs. There is complete agreement on this point. However, there is no such consensus about what exactly to do with the lungs during the period of bypass. Some anesthesiologists completely disconnect the patient from the anesthesia machine; others maintain the lungs slightly inflated with low levels of positive end-expiratory pressure using 100% oxygen or various mixtures of room air. No specific method is associated with superior postoperative pulmonary function.

During the initial minutes of bypass, systemic pressure initially drops to 30–40 mm Hg as pulsatile flow ceases and the effect of the dilute prime becomes apparent. Once

TABLE 36-15. Checklist During Cardiopulmonary Bypass

Laboratory Values

ACT or measure of adequate heparinization
ABGs (uncorrected)—acidosis
Hematocrit, potassium, calcium levels

Anesthesia/Machine

Discontinue ventilation

Monitor

Arterial pressure
  Hypotension
    Venous cannula—kink, malposition, clamp, air lock
    Inadequate venous return (bleeding, hypovolemia, IVC obstruction, table too low)
    Pump—poor occlusion, low flows
    Arterial cannula—misdirected, kinked, partially clamped, dissection
    Vasodilation—anesthetics, hemodilution, idiopathic
    Transducer or monitor malfunction, stopcocks the wrong way
  Hypertension
    Pump— ↑ flow
    Arterial cannula—misdirected
    Vasoconstriction—light anesthesia, response to temperature changes
    Transducer or monitor malfunction
Venous pressure—above level of atrium—obstruction to return
  LV filling pressure—LA, PCW (if available)—any elevation?
EKG—electrical quiescence (if cardioplegia used)
EEG
Adequacy of perfusion??
  Flow and pressure??
  Acidosis
  Mixed venous oxygen saturation
Urine output
Temperature

Patient/Field

Conduct of the operation
Heart—distention, fibrillation
Cyanosis, venous engorgement, skin temperature
Movement
Breathing, diaphragmatic movement (hypercarbia, light anesthesia)

Support

Vasodilators, anesthetics, or constrictors to control blood pressure when flow is appropriate

ACT = activated clotting time; ABG = arterial blood gas; IVC = inferior vena cava; LV = left ventricle; LA = left atrium; PCW = pulmonary capillary wedge.

adequate mixing is obtained, blood pressure increases to levels primarily determined by flow rate (Table 36-15). There is no consensus as to what constitutes the ideal blood pressure or flow rate during bypass for maintenance of adequate vital organ perfusion, especially of the brain. Commonly, flow rates are maintained at approximately 50–60 ml·kg^{-1}, with systemic blood pressures in the 50–60 mm Hg range. Alternatively, some institutions believe that lower flows are beneficial (less hematologic damage, less rewarming of the heart through noncoronary collaterals) and that the need for higher flows or pressures has not been conclusively demonstrated.[198] Some surgeons believe that a higher perfusion pressure affords better myocardial protection when surgery is performed on the cold fibrillating heart rather than with cardioplegia.[128,129]

Central Nervous System Protection. Of particular concern is preservation of central nervous system function.[199] The exact etiology of postcardiopulmonary bypass neurologic and psychological injury is still unclear. Although emboli are reputed to be the leading contenders,[200] inadequate cerebral perfusion (pressure and/or flow), the duration of bypass, and age are sufficient contributing causes.

During cardiopulmonary bypass, the major factors regulating cerebral blood flow are temperature, cerebral oxygen consumption, Paco$_2$, and anesthetic depth.[201-204] Proper interpretation and management of arterial Pco$_2$ (alpha-stat versus pH-stat) remains controversial.[205] Although alpha-stat offers theoretical advantages,[206] clinical data do not yet absolutely mandate its use.[207] Cerebral blood flow appears to be autoregulated during bypass. A lower limit of 30 mm Hg has been suggested,[208] although this has not been conclusively demonstrated.[199] Data on autoregulation in patients with diabetes, untreated hypertension, and certain neurologic disorders have not been studied.

The potential for calcium or particulate emboli during cardiac surgery is enormous, especially during procedures when a chamber is opened (valve replacement, aneurysmectomy).[200] This problem persists despite the use of arterial tubing filters and meticulous maneuvers to de-air the heart. Nussmeier et al[163] reported improved neurologic outcome after administration of sufficient thiopental to completely suppress the electrocardiogram in a group of patients undergoing open ventricle procedures with normothermic bypass. The dose required averaged 40 mg·kg^{-1} and resulted in increased inotropic requirements and a prolonged time to extubation of the trachea. However, in a more recent study, Zaidan and colleagues showed no improvement with thiopental.[209] The accompanying editorial by Todd et al suggests future directions in this area.[210]

Monitoring and Management During Bypass. The common etiologies of blood pressure changes during cardiopulmonary bypass are listed in Table 36-15. Of primary importance is continuous observation of the surgical field and cannulas to ensure that nothing mechanical is awry. Attention can then be directed to other causes of hypo- or hypertension and their appropriate treatment. Other areas that require periodic monitoring and occasional intervention during bypass are also described in Table 36-15. Maintenance of adequate depths of anesthesia is obviously important during the bypass run, although clinical signs are few. Anesthetic requirements are decreased during the period of hypothermia but return toward normal when the patient is rewarmed. Continued muscle relaxation is helpful to prevent increases in oxygen consumption from shivering or massive muscle movement during defibrillation.

Arterial pH and mixed venous oxygen saturation are often used to assess the adequacy of perfusion, although changes in these values probably occur late. Urine output is also monitored, but so many variables influence this, such as arterial and venous pressure, flow rate, temperature, and diuretic history, that it is difficult to draw meaningful conclusions from this measurement. In addition, postoperative renal failure develops from either aggravation of pre-existing renal dysfunction or persistent low cardiac output following bypass. Although many institutions administer diuretics routinely, they are just as assiduously avoided elsewhere.

Rewarming. When surgical repair is nearly complete, gradual rewarming of the patient begins. A gradient of approximately 10°C is maintained between the patient and the perfusate in order to prevent formation of gas bubbles. Patient awareness becomes a possibility as the anesthetic effects of hypothermia dissipate. Volatile anesthetics are often avoided because of residual myocardial depression present at the time of separation from bypass. If adequate doses of anesthetics have not been given, administration during rewarming should be considered in order to prevent recall of intraoperative events. Upon completion of the surgical repair, a variety of maneuvers are performed to remove any residual air in the ventricles. The anesthesiologist is called upon to vigorously inflate the lungs in order to remove air from the pulmonary veins and aid in filling the cardiac chambers. The heart is defibrillated and allowed to beat and replace some of its oxygen debt. The field is tidied up, and preparations are made to separate from cardiopulmonary bypass.

Discontinuation of Cardiopulmonary Bypass

Prior to discontinuing cardiopulmonary bypass, the patient should be warmed, the surgical field dry, appropriate laboratory values checked, pulmonary compliance evaluated, and ventilation of the lungs begun (Table 36-16). Heart rate and rhythm should be regulated either pharmacologically or electrically with appropriate pacing. The venous cannulas are then incrementally occluded as bypass flow is slowly decreased and sufficient pump volume is transfused into the patient. During this time, cardiac function is continually evaluated from monitoring data and direct inspection of the heart; the need for vaso- or cardioactive drugs is assessed. The potential disparity, previously alluded to, between radial artery and aortic pressures must be kept in mind. Contractility, rhythm, and ventricular filling can all be estimated by careful observation of the beating heart. For example, the patient with a low blood pressure but a vigorously contracting, relatively empty ventricle suggests that volume and perhaps a vasoconstrictor are all that is needed to wean him or her from bypass, whereas adequate blood pressure in the presence of a sluggish and overdistended heart may be treated with a vasodilator and/or a small dose of an inotrope.

Inadequate cardiac performance must prompt a search for possible etiologies (Table 36-17); structural defects require more than mere regulation of inotropes or vasodilators. If the clinical picture is suggestive of air emboli with diffuse ST segment elevation and a hypocontractile heart, continuous support on cardiopulmonary bypass with a high perfusion pressure and an empty ventricle is indicated.

If pharmacologic support is required, an integration of cardiac physiology (Chapter 35) and pharmacology (Chapter 14) will lead to the rational selection of an appropriate drug

or drugs. Numerous algorithms are available to guide decision making; two are described in Tables 36-18 and 36-19. The first algorithm uses arterial pressure and ventricular filling pressure (central venous pressure, palpation of pulmonary artery pressure, direct left atrial measurement); the second algorithm adds cardiac output to the data base. After integrating available data, a diagnosis is made and appropriate treatment is begun. Continual reassessment of the sit-

---

TABLE 36-16. Checklist Prior to Separation from Cardiopulmonary Bypass

Laboratory Values

Hematocrit, ABGs
Potassium (? ↑ 2° cardioplegia)

Anesthesia/Machine

Lung compliance evaluated
Lungs ventilated (mechanical or manual)
Vaporizers off
Alarms on

Monitor

Temperature (37°C nasopharyngeal, esophageal; 35°C rectal)
ECG—rate, rhythm, ST segment analysis
Monitors zeroed and recalibrated
Arterial pressure, ventricular filling pressures
Strip-chart recorder on (if available)

Patient/Field

Look at the heart, look at the heart
    De-aired—aspiration, ballotment of heart
    Contractility, size, rhythm, rate
LV vent out, caval snares released
No major bleeding sites—grafts, suture lines, LV vent site

Support

As needed

ABG = arterial blood gas; LV = left ventricle.

TABLE 36-17. Etiology of Right or Left Ventricular Dysfunction After Cardiopulmonary Bypass

Ischemia

Inadequate myocardial protection
Coronary spasm
Technical difficulties
Emboli (air, thrombus, calcium)
Intraoperative infarction
Reperfusion injury

Uncorrected Structural Defects

Nongraftable vessels
Kinked or clotted grafts
Residual valve gradient
Hypertrophic cardiomyopathy
Shunts

Excess Cardioplegia

Pre-existing Dysfunction

Cardiomyopathy

TABLE 36-18. Diagnosis and Therapy of Cardiovascular Dysfunction (Arterial and Ventricular Filling Pressures)

BP	VFP	Diagnosis	Treatment
NL or ↑	↑	↑ — Too full	Take off fluid or await surgical losses
		NL — All is well	None / Wait
		↓ — ↑ SVR	Anesthesia / Vasodilate and gently add volume
↓ or ↓↓	NL	↑ — ↓↓ Contractility	CaCl₂, inotrope, vasodilator
		↓ — ↓ Contractility (? low volume)	CaCl₂, inotrope (volume challenge)
		↓ — Hypovolemia (? right heart failure)	Transfuse (Check CVP, appearance of right ventricle, inotropes, vasodilators)

BP = blood pressure; NL = normal; VFP = ventricular filling pressure; SVR = systemic vascular resistance; CVP = central venous pressure; CaCl₂ = calcium chloride.

Reprinted with permission from Thomas SJ: Manual of Cardiac Anesthesia. New York, Churchill Livingstone, 1984.

TABLE 36-19. Diagnosis and Therapy of Cardiovascular Dysfunction After Cardiopulmonary Bypass (Cardiac Output, Systemic and Ventricular Filling Pressures)

BP	VFP	CO	Diagnosis	Treatment
↑	↑	↑	Too full	Take off volume / Vasodilators
		↓	↑ SVR / ? ↓ Contractility	Slow vasodilation, then remeasure CO, inotrope if necessary
	↓	↑	Hyperdynamic	Anesthetics / ? Beta blockers
		↓	↑↑ SVR	Vasodilate, add volume
↓	↑		Vasodilated / Too full—High on Frank-Starling curve	Wait / Vasoconstrict gently
		↓	↓↓ Contractility	Inotrope / Vasodilator / IABP / LV assist
	↓	↑	↓ SVR	Vasoconstrictor
		↓	Hypovolemia / (? right heart failure)	Transfuse / (Diagnose, inotropes, vasodilators)

BP = blood pressure; VFP = ventricular filling pressure; CO = cardiac output; IABP = intra-aortic balloon pump.

Redrawn with permission from Thomas SJ: Manual of Cardiac Anesthesia. New York, Churchill Livingstone, 1984.

TABLE 36-20. Improving Systemic Flow

1. Appropriate heart rate (pacing—A, V, A/V)
2. Optimize ventricular filling
3. or 4. Reduce afterload if blood pressure is acceptable (arteriolar dilators)
4. or 3. Improve contractility (inotrope)
5. Recheck adequacy of ventricular filling
6. Combination therapy
7. IABP
8. VAD

A = atrial; V = ventricular; IABP = intra-aortic balloon pump; VAD = ventricular assist device.

uation is necessary to document the efficacy of treatment or to suggest new diagnoses and therapeutic approaches.

Our approach to patients with inadequate cardiac output is summarized in Table 36-20. Heart rate is adjusted as much as possible. Ventricular filling is then optimized by transfusing blood from the pump. It is important not to overdistend the heart by transfusing to an arbitrary level of filling pressure, since this could precipitate further myocardial dysfunction. Looking at the heart to monitor the response to small incremental volume infusions is more appropriate. If further therapy is required and systemic pressure is adequate, an arteriolar dilator may improve forward flow. If pressure is too low, precluding use of vasodilators, an inotrope should be selected. Each inotropic drug has a distinct profile with respect to its effects on rate, contractility, systemic and pulmonary vascular resistance, and cardiac dysrhythmogenic potential. By *first* defining the hemodynamic problem and *then* deciding what needs treatment and in what order, the most suitable drug for that situation may be selected rather than always selecting the standard "institutional inotrope." If these initial therapies are insufficient to promote adequate forward flow, various combinations of drugs may be tested. If systemic perfusion is still inadequate, some form of mechanical circulatory support is required.

A therapeutic approach to right ventricular failure is outlined in Table 36-21. When pulmonary arterial pressure is normal or decreased, the etiology is usually severe right ventricular ischemia owing to intraoperative damage or to air. Initially, treatment is aimed at improving perfusion on bypass and awaiting recovery and improvement in contractility. If this does not occur, inotropic and vasodilator therapy are indicated. Patients who have right ventricular fail-

TABLE 36-21. Right Ventricular Failure

PAP	Increased	Normal or Decreased
Diagnosis	? Poor right ventricular protection	Air, ischemia
Prescription	Do not ↑ preload / Inotropes / Afterload reduction (PGE₁, etc) / ? Differential infusions / RVAD	Volume / Support on CPB / High perfusion pressure / ?CABG

RVAD = right ventricular assist device; PAP = pulmonary artery pressure; CPB = cardiopulmonary bypass; CABG = coronary artery bypass graft.

ure secondary to high pulmonary vascular resistance are approached differently. Reduction of pulmonary vascular resistance with vasodilators such as prostaglandin E_1 (PGE$_1$)[211] and inotropic support is the mainstay of therapy. Overdistention of the ventricle must be assiduously avoided. Combination therapy refers to the infusion of inotropes with vasoconstrictive properties into the left side of the circulation in order to maintain systemic perfusion but avoid increasing resistance in the pulmonary circulation.[212] Persistent right ventricular failure precluding separation from cardiopulmonary bypass may require the insertion of a right ventricular assist device.

Intra-aortic Balloon Pump. The simplest and most readily available mechanical support device is the intra-aortic balloon pump. It consists of a 25-cm sausage-shaped balloon composed of nonthrombogenic polyurethane mounted on a 90-cm stiff vascular catheter. It is usually inserted into the femoral artery either percutaneously or, after surgical exposure, through a graft sutured directly to the artery and advanced so that the tip is distal to the left subclavian artery (in order to prevent emboli to the upper arterial circulation). Occasionally, peripheral vascular disease prevents passage of the balloon *via* the femoral artery and it must be placed into the ascending aorta.

The intra-aortic balloon pump does not pump blood. Rather, it utilizes the principle of synchronized counterpulsation to assist a beating, ejecting heart. Aortic blood volume is moved in a direction "counter" to normal flow. Immediately prior to systole, the intra-aortic balloon pump deflates, "removing blood," precipitously reducing blood pressure (afterload reduction), enhancing forward flow, and reducing $M\dot{V}o_2$. Proper timing of balloon deflation is necessary to reduce end-diastolic pressure as much as possible in order to maximally offload the ventricle. This blood is then "returned" during diastole as the balloon inflates, elevating aortic diastolic blood pressure (diastolic augmentation), increasing the gradient for coronary perfusion. The indications and contraindications for intra-aortic balloon pump placement are listed in Table 36-22. The primary indications for intra-aortic balloon pump in the cardiac surgical patient are inability to separate from cardiopulmonary bypass and poor hemodynamic function following cardiopulmonary bypass despite increasing drug support. Myocardial function often improves with the use of the intra-aortic balloon pump, and systemic perfusion and vital organ function are preserved.[213,214] It is crucial to control heart rate and suppress atrial and ventricular dysrhythmias in order to ensure proper balloon timing. As cardiac function returns, the assist ratio is gradually weaned from every beat to every other beat and, assuming no further cardiac deterioration, finally to 1:8, and then removed.

Complications associated with the intra-aortic balloon pump are primarily related to ischemia distal to the site of balloon insertion. Direct trauma to the vessel, arterial obstruction, and thrombosis are most common, although aortic perforation and balloon rupture occur rarely.[215,216]

Ventricular Assist Device. Infrequently (<1%), the heart is unable to meet systemic metabolic demands despite maximal pharmacologic therapy and insertion of the intra-aortic balloon pump. Under these circumstances, devices that actually pump blood and bypass either the left or right ventricle are required. These devices are effective because the injury producing myocardial dysfunction takes place intraoperatively and, more important, is often reversible. Markedly impaired cardiac function after bypass is not necessar-

---

TABLE 36-22. Intra-aortic Balloon Pump Indications and Contraindications

Indications

Complications of Myocardial Infarction

Hemodynamic—cardiogenic shock
Mechanical—mitral regurgitation, ventricular septal defect
Intractable dysrhythmias
Extension—postinfarction angina
?? Limitation of infarct size

Acute Cardiac Instability

Unstable angina—preinfarction angina
PTCA misadventure
Pretransplantation
Cardiac contusion
?? Septic shock

Open Heart Surgery

Separation from cardiopulmonary bypass
Right or left ventricular failure
Increasing inotropic requirement
Progressive hemodynamic deterioration

Contraindications

Irreversible brain damage
Severe aortic insufficiency
Inability to insert
Irreversible cardiac disease (if not a candidate for transplant)

---

ily synonymous with cell death but, rather, may represent temporary "stunning" of the myocardium.[217] Survival ranges from 20–30%, many with minimal or no decline in cardiac function.

Pierce[218] has summarized clinical guidelines when using ventricular support. He emphasizes the necessity for adequate monitoring of cardiac function, for prompt decision making and progression of therapy, and for continuously evaluating *both* ventricles. Very often, mechanical support for one ventricle unmasks previously unrecognized failure in the other ventricle, necessitating additional pharmacologic or mechanical intervention. Pennington et al[219] have emphasized the importance of diagnosing and treating right ventricular failure in patients in cardiogenic shock.

Postcardiopulmonary Bypass

The procedure is not over when the patient is safely "off pump." Continued vigilance is mandatory during decannulation, protamine administration, "drying up," and chest closure. Anesthetics are administered when clinically indicated. Although removal of the atrial cannulas may trigger cardiac dysrhythmias, they are usually transient. In fact, atrial or junctional dysrhythmias often disappear when the cannulas are out. Heparin is reversed with protamine following removal of the atrial cannulas; the arterial return remains in place for continued transfusion of pump contents. When this is completed and bleeding is controlled, the arterial cannula is removed and the chest is closed. During decannulation, the possibility exists for unexpected bleeding from the atrial or aortic suture lines, which sometimes requires rapid transfusion.

Reversal of Anticoagulation. Protamine, a polycationic protein derived from salmon sperm, is used to neutralize heparin. The initial and total dose administered vary widely. Some use a fixed ratio of protamine to heparin; others use 2–4 mg·kg^{-1}; whereas still others look to automated protamine titrations to suggest the initial dose.[220] Regardless of the method selected, further requirements are assessed by repeated measures of the activated coagulation time or other clotting assay, as well as the appearance of the surgical field.

Protamine administration is associated with a broad spectrum of hemodynamic effects.[221] Idiosyncratic responses include Type I anaphylactic reactions and both immediate and delayed anaphylactoid responses. True anaphylaxis, mercifully very rare, is characterized by increased airway pressure, decreased systemic vascular resistance with systemic hypotension, and skin flushing.[222] An increased incidence of reactions has been reported in patients sensitized to protamine from previous cadiac catheterization,[223] hemodialysis,[224] cardiac surgery,[225] or exposure to neutral protamine Hagedorn (NPH) insulin.[226] Perhaps the most devastating complication associated with protamine is sudden and profound pulmonary hypertension accompanied by an elevated central venous pressure, a flaccid distended right ventricle, and systemic hypotension.[227] This may occur in approximately 1% of patients and is mediated by release of thromboxane and C5a anaphylatoxin.[228] The reaction is extremely short-lived, and although reinstitution of bypass has been reported, it is usually not necessary. Whether protamine is administered *via* the right atrium, left atrium, or aorta or peripherally probably makes no difference.[229-231] However, slow administration into a peripheral venous site is advisable.[232]

Postbypass Bleeding. Persistent oozing following heparin reversal is not uncommon. The usual causes include inadequate surgical hemostasis and reduced platelet count or function, neither of which is identified by a prolonged activated coagulation time. Insufficient doses of protamine, dilution of coagulation factors, and, very rarely, "heparin rebound" are also in the differential diagnosis.[233-234] Definitive diagnosis is frequently difficult, since neither the activated coagulation time nor other readily available tests identify the problem.

After adequate hemostasis is obtained, the chest is closed. This is occasionally associated with transient decreases in blood pressure, which usually respond to volume infusion or "tincture of time." If hypotension persists, the chest should be reopened to rule out cardiac tamponade, a kinked graft, or other serious problems.

As the surgeon completes skin closure, the anesthesiologist prepares for an orderly, unhurried transfer of the patient from the operating room to the recovery room or intensive care unit. Medicated infusions must be regulated either manually or with portable infusion pumps. Additional syringes with emergency cardiac medications and necessary equipment for airway management should be carried. Blood pressure and electrocardiograms are monitored, and adjustments of infusions are made as clinically indicated.

Bring Backs. Postoperative re-exploration is needed in 4–10% of cases. The indications are persistent bleeding, excessive blood loss, cardiac tamponade, and, infrequently, unexplained poor cardiac performance (rule out tamponade). Surgery is usually required within the first 24 hours but may be later in cases of delayed tamponade. The possibility of cardiac tamponade must always be included in the differential diagnosis of the postoperative "dwindles," since the classic symptoms and signs (Table 36-23) are often absent.

TABLE 36-23. Cardiac Tamponade—Clinical Features

Dyspnea, orthopnea, tachycardia
Beck's triad
  Quiet heart
  ↑ Venous pressure (distended neck veins)
  ↓ Arterial pressure
Paradoxical pulse
Equalization of diastolic pressures
  RAP = RVEDP = PAEDP = LAP = LVEDP
ECG—ST segment change, electrical alternans
Chest x-ray—silhouette normal or slightly enlarged
Echocardiography—best diagnostic tool

RAP = right atrial pressure; RVEDP = right ventricular end-diastolic pressure; PAEDP = pulmonary artery end-diastolic pressure; LAP = left atrial pressure; LVEDP = left ventricular end-diastolic pressure.

Cardiac tamponade exists when intrapericardial pressure, not intravascular volume and venous pressure, determines venous return.[235] The ventricle is small and underloaded despite elevations in right and left ventricular filling pressures. These increases occur because pressures are routinely measured using atmospheric pressure as the zero reference point. Normally, this is acceptable, since the pressure surrounding the heart is within 1–3 mm Hg of atmospheric. With tamponade, this pressure is increased, transmural pressure (inside minus outside) is actually decreased, and intracardiac chamber pressures are deceptively elevated. Classically, there is equilibration of diastolic pressures across the heart. Stroke volume is limited and fixed, and cardiac output and blood pressure become dependent upon heart rate. Compensatory mechanisms include peripheral vasoconstriction to preserve venous return and systemic blood pressure and tachycardia. Also noteworthy is the potential for concurrent myocardial ischemia because of the tachycardia and reduced coronary perfusion pressure.

Clinically, patients present with dyspnea, orthopnea, tachycardia, and hypotension. The intubated, sedated, mechanically ventilated patient in the recovery room following cardiac surgery may only manifest hypotension. Ventricular filling pressures are usually elevated but not consistently so. In postoperative cardiac patients, the pericardium is no longer intact, and loculated areas of clot may compress only one chamber, causing isolated increases in filling pressure. Urine output is usually diminished. Serial chest films typically show progressive mediastinal widening.

The cure for cardiac tamponade is surgical; anesthetics can only further depress cardiac function. Therefore, drugs are selected that will preserve the compensatory mechanisms sustaining forward flow. Drugs with vasodilator (either venous or arteriolar) or myocardial depressant properties should be avoided in patients with serious hemodynamic compromise; dosages of induction agents should be appropriately reduced. Ketamine, because of its sympathomimetic effects, may be helpful in preserving heart rate and blood pressure response. It is not, however, a panacea and can induce hypotension in those patients under maximal sympathetic stress. If, upon reopening the chest, there is minimal fluid or if the patient shows little improvement, a thorough search for other causes of inadequate cardiac performance such as clotted or kinked grafts, myocardial ischemia, or valve malfunction is indicated.

CONGENITAL HEART DISEASE

In contrast to the adult with acquired cardiac disease, the anesthetic management of the child with congenital heart disease focuses on understanding those factors that determine where the blood goes, how much goes where, and why. The prevention, detection, and management of myocardial ischemia, although it does occur, are not pivotal to the care of these children. Our discussion centers on classification of these lesions, their anesthetic implications, and important clinical lessons common to any child with congenital heart disease. Other sources are available for detailed analysis of individual lesions.[236,237]

Classification

Developmental abnormalities of the heart and great vessels result in a variety of congenital anomalies—some quite complex anatomically and physiologically. The numerous anatomic combinations that occur are best understood if considered in the context of a classification system based on patterns of altered blood flow and resistances to flow (Table 36-24). Simple shunts involve shunting of blood in a left-to-right or right-to-left direction. Obstructive lesions introduce an impediment to flow through either the pulmonary or the systemic circulation. Complex shunt lesions combine an obstructive lesion with one or more shunts.

Simple Shunts. Interruptions in the normal barriers between the pulmonary and systemic circulations (atrial septal defect, ventricular septal defect, patent ductus arteriosus) result in simple shunts. Since pressure is higher on the left side of the orifice, blood is shunted from left to right. Pulmonary blood flow is increased, and the right ventricle and pulmonary vasculature become pressure and/or volume overloaded, depending on the location, size, and duration of the shunt. The ratio of pulmonary to systemic flow can be calculated using the Fick equation:

$$\dot{Q}_p = \frac{O_2 \text{ consumption}}{\text{Art } Sao_2 - \text{PA } Svo_2}$$

$$\dot{Q}_s = \frac{O_2 \text{ consumption}}{\text{Art } Sao_2 - \text{SVC } Svo_2}$$

$$\frac{\dot{Q}_p}{\dot{Q}_s} = \frac{\text{Art } Sao_2 - \text{SVC } Svo_2}{\text{Art } Sao_2 - \text{PA } Svo_2}$$

where

$\dot{Q}_p$ = pulmonary blood flow
$\dot{Q}_s$ = systemic blood flow
Sao_2 = arterial oxygen saturation
Svo_2 = venous oxygen saturation
SVC = superior vena cava
PA = pulmonary artery

Increased pulmonary blood flow may delay the normal decrease in pulmonary vascular resistance that occurs in the neonatal period and may eventually result in morphologic changes in the intimal and medial layers of the pulmonary vasculature.[238-240] The pulmonary hypertension produced is usually reversible with correction of the lesion but may persist after surgery if the increased pulmonary blood flow has

TABLE 36-24. Classification of Congenital Heart Defects

1. Increased pulmonary blood flow
   Atrial septal defect
   Ventricular septal defect
   Patent ductus arteriosus
   Endocardial cushion defect
   Aortopulmonary windows
2. Decreased pulmonary blood flow
   Tetralogy of Fallot
   Pulmonary atresia
   Tricuspid atresia
   Ebstein's anomaly
3. Complex shunts/mixing of pulmonary and systemic circulation
   Truncus arteriosus
   Transposition of the great arteries
   Total anomalous pulmonary venous drainage
   Common ventricle
4. Obstructive lesions
   Aortic stenosis
   Pulmonary stenosis
   Coarctation of the aorta
5. Airway obstruction
   Double aortic arch
   Anomalous pulmonary artery

been long-standing or very severe. Left untreated, a substantial left-to-right shunt can lead to irreversible destruction of the pulmonary vasculature, persistent pulmonary hypertension, and progressive reversal of the shunt to a right-to-left direction (Eisenmenger's complex). In these patients, the hemodynamic picture becomes one of inadequate pulmonary blood flow and systemic hypoxemia.

When the orifice of a simple shunt is small, the magnitude of flow across it is almost entirely dependent on the size of the defect and relatively independent of outflow resistance. These lesions (a small atrial or ventricular septal defect) are known as restrictive shunts (Table 36-25). The magnitude of shunt flow across a larger atrial or ventricular septal defect (a nonrestrictive shunt) is less dependent on orifice size and more dependent on the relative resistances to right and left ventricular outflow (pulmonary vascular resistance and systemic vascular resistance, respectively).[241] At the extreme of this group are lesions characterized by a common chamber (single atrium, single ventricle, truncus arteriosus) in which complete mixing of arterial and venous blood occurs. Shunting in these situations is bidirectional, with the magnitude and direction of net flow entirely dependent upon relative outflow resistances. A marked increase in pulmonary vascular resistance results in net right-to-left shunting, producing arterial oxygen desaturation and cyanosis.

Obstructive Lesions. Obstructive lesions include atrial stenosis or aortic coarctation on the left side of the circulation, pulmonic stenosis on the right. Obstruction results in pressure overloading of the corresponding ventricle. Ventricular hypertrophy is the compensating mechanism, but the immature myocardium deals poorly with pronounced afterload stress.[242] Critical atrial stenosis presents with characteristics of congestive heart failure in the newborn. These include irritability, hypotension, tachycardia, hepatic congestion, acidosis, poor peripheral perfusion, and respiratory distress. The child may appear cyanotic if the obstruction is severe and peripheral circulation is dependent upon right-

TABLE 36-25. Classifications of Shunts

	Simple Shunts			Complex Shunts	
	Restrictive (Small)	Nonrestrictive (Large)	Common Chamber (Complete Mixing)	Partial Obstruction	Total Obstruction
Pressure Gradient	Large	Small	None	Orifice size and degree of obstruction	Orifice size only
Direction	L→R*	L→R*	Bidirectional	Shunt flow dependent upon obstruction	Away from obstruction circulation
Dependence upon PVR/SVR	Independent	Dependent	Totally dependent	Minimally dependent	Independent
Examples	Small ASD, VSD Blalock	Large VSD, PDA, Waterston	Single ventricle Truncus	TOF VSD with PS	Valvular atresia

* = R→L shunt flow if severe pulmonary hypertension secondary to pulmonary vascular disease.
ASD = atrial septal defect; PDA = patent ductus arteriosus; PS = pulmonary stenosis; TOF = tetralogy of Fallot; VSD = ventricular septal defect.
Adapted with permission from Hickey PR, Wessel DL: Anesthesia for treatment of congenital heart disease. In Kaplan JA (ed): Cardiac Anesthesia, 2nd ed. Orlando, Grune & Stratton, 1987.

to-left shunting *via* the ductus arteriosus. Hypoperfusion may lead to profound acidosis and renal failure.[243] Coarctation of the aorta is the most common etiology of neonatal congestive heart failure. This usually presents as the ductus arteriosus closes. On the other hand, less severe coarctation of infancy commonly remains asymptomatic during the first two decades of life.[244] The surgical mortality of critical aortic stenosis in the neonate is greater than 50%, whereas that of a coarctation varies from 0 to 50% in neonates to 0.4% after infancy.[243]

Complex Shunts. Complex shunt lesions involve obstruction to outflow on one side of the heart with shunting to the opposite side through an associated lesion (atrial septal defect, ventricular septal defect, or patent ductus arteriosus (Table 36-25). If only partial outflow obstruction exists, the magnitude of shunt flow directed to the unobstructed circulation is somewhat dependent upon the relationship of systemic vascular resistance and pulmonary vascular resistance; the more severe the obstruction, the less the dependence on relative outflow resistance. With tetralogy of Fallot, for example, partial right outflow tract obstruction results in right-to-left shunting of blood through a ventricular septal defect. The magnitude of shunt flow increases if pulmonary vascular resistance is increased or if systemic vascular resistance is allowed to fall. As right-to-left shunting increases, so does arterial oxygen desaturation. If outflow tract obstruction is complete, all blood passes through a shunt to the opposite circulation. The magnitude and direction of shunt flow are fixed. Viability of the patient depends upon the presence of a second, more distally located shunt to return blood to the obstructed circulation. If tetralogy of Fallot is accompanied by pulmonary atresia, for example, there is shunting of all venous return across the ventricular septal defect in a right-to-left direction. Left-to-right flow through the patent ductus arteriosus then provides the entire pulmonary blood supply. In patients with mitral or aortic atresia, intracardiac left-to-right shunting occurs through an atrial septal defect or ventricular septal defect. Right-to-left shunting *via* the patent ductus provides systemic flow. Prostaglandin E_1 (PGE_1) is commonly used to maintain ductal patency in patients in whom premature closure would be life-threatening.[245]

Systemic and Pulmonary Vascular Resistance

It is essential to understand each patient's cardiac anatomy and pattern of blood flow in order to predict the effects of systemic vascular resistance and pulmonary vascular resistance on hemodynamics and arterial oxygenation. The normal circulation undergoes physiologic closure of the foramen ovale and the patent ductus arteriosus during childbirth to create "normal" blood flow. Alteration of this physiologic process by congenital heart defects may result in persistent transitional circulation with continued shunting of blood across the foramen ovale or ductus arteriosus. If especially severe, this will lead to hypoxemia, acidosis, and circulatory collapse. Conversely, in some forms of cyanotic disease ductal flow is critical and will maintain pulmonary blood flow as mentioned above.

When the direction and magnitude of shunt flow are dependent upon relative outflow resistances, hemodynamic management by the anesthesiologist affects the degree and direction of shunting. With simple left-to-right shunting, for example, further increases in pulmonary blood flow are avoided by preventing increases in systemic vascular resistance. Excessive pulmonary vasodilation can result in a marked increase in pulmonary blood flow—in extreme cases, at the expense of systemic flow.[246] This is a particular problem in the patient with a single ventricle, since shunt flow in these situations is bidirectional and entirely dependent upon systemic vascular resistance and pulmonary vascular resistance. Exacerbation of pre-existing pulmonary hypertension in patients with increased pulmonary blood flow is best prevented by avoiding maneuvers that increase pulmonary vascular resistance and utilizing for hemodynamic benefit those that decrease it (see Table 36-26). Decreasing right-to-left shunting in patients with complex shunt lesions lessens arterial oxygen desaturation. Systemic vascular resistance must be maintained in these patients because excessive hypotension will result in increased right-to-left flow. Increases in pulmonary vascular resistance promote right-to-left shunting and hypoxemia. Pulmonary vasodilation should prove beneficial. Note again that pulmonary vascular resistance/systemic vascular resistance effects are greater with a larger (nonrestrictive) shunt orifice.

TABLE 36-26. Manipulations Altering Pulmonary Vascular Resistance (PVR)

Increase PVR	Decrease PVR
Hypoxia	Oxygen
Hypercarbia	Hypocarbia
Acidosis	Alkalosis
Hyperinflation	Normal functional residual
Atelectasis	capacity
Sympathetic stimulation	Blocking sympathetic stimulation
High hematocrit	Low hematocrit
Surgical constriction	

Reprinted with permission from Hickey PR, Wessel DL: Anesthesia for treatment of congenital heart disease. In Kaplan JA (ed): Cardiac Anesthesia, 2nd ed. Orlando, Grune & Stratton, 1987.

Preoperative Evaluation

The history and physical examination should determine the presence or absence of congestive heart failure and/or cyanosis, the most significant consequences of congenital heart disease. Pump failure may result from either pressure or volume overload of a ventricle. Owing to the close association between ventricles in very young patients, univentricular failure quickly becomes biventricular.[247] The Starling curve of an infant's ventricle plateaus quickly, and heart rate becomes the primary determinant of cardiac output. Thus, tachycardia, an important compensatory mechanism, is a common finding in children with congestive heart failure. Other findings (Table 36-27) include tachypnea, dyspnea, diaphoresis, recurrent pulmonary infections, decreased exercise tolerance, and developmental delays. Cyanosis occurs with lesions resulting in right-to-left shunting and the inevitable desaturation of arterial blood. Older children with long-standing hypoxemia may develop clubbing of the fingers and toes. Polycythemia occurs in response to systemic hypoxemia as a means of increasing oxygen-carrying capacity. Hematocrits above 60 ml·dl^{-1} place the child at risk for cerebral infarction or coagulation abnormalities.[248,249]

The diagnosis of simple atrial septal defect, patent ductus arteriosus, or coarctation is often made noninvasively. When a more complicated lesion exists, the most useful data regarding the child's anatomic diagnosis are provided by echocardiography and cardiac catheterization.

With improved and more sophisticated technology, more lesions are being diagnosed solely on the basis of echocardi-ograph findings (atrial septal defect, patent ductus arteriosus, ventricular septal defect, coarctation of the aorta). Along with Doppler color flow imaging, echocardiography provides an assessment of blood flow patterns, cardiac anatomy, and shunt flow (direction and magnitude).

Cardiac catheterization remains the best available means of assessing the physiologic consequences of congenital cardiac lesions. Pressures and oxygen saturation are measured in the cardiac chambers and great vessels, and the results are used to confirm the location and direction of shunts and the presence of obstructive lesions. A step-up in oxygen saturation from the superior vena cava to the right atrium or ventricle is indicative of left-to-right shunting. Desaturation of left ventricular or aortic blood suggests right-to-left shunting of venous blood into the systemic circulation. Oxygen saturations are also used to calculate relative pulmonary and systemic resistances and flows using the Fick equation.

Premedication

Premedication is selected considering the child's age, level of activity, and the severity of the lesion. Children younger than 6 months of age and those older but critically ill usually receive no preoperative sedation. Older, active children should be sedated with intramuscular opioids and/or barbiturates prior to transport to the operating room. This is especially important with lesions resulting in right-to-left shunting. Struggling and crying increase right-to-left flow and worsen hypoxemia. The goal of premedication is a hemodynamically stable child, asleep or awake but cooperative. Table 36-28 lists appropriate doses for preoperative medications in children with congenital heart disease.

In addition, rectally administered barbiturates (methohexital 20–30 mg·kg^{-1}), iv ketamine (1–2 mg·kg^{-1}), or im ketamine (2–6 mg·kg^{-1}) have proved very effective in separating the child from the parent and are used as adjuvants to the induction. Close observation of the airway must be maintained, as apnea is poorly tolerated in the child with congestive heart disease. Rectally administered barbiturates are associated with a 1–2% risk of respiratory depression and apnea.

TABLE 36-27. Symptoms of Congenital Heart Disease

Infants	Children
Tachycardia	Tachycardia
Tachypnea	Tachypnea/dyspnea
Diaphoresis	Diaphoresis
Feeding difficulties	Poor weight gain
Failure to thrive	Repeated pulmonary infections
Pulmonary infections	Decreased exercise tolerance
Congestive heart failure	Congestive heart failure
Cyanosis	Cyanosis ± clubbing

TABLE 36-28. Premedication for Children

Anticholinergics

Scopolamine	0.01–0.02 mg·kg^{-1}	im
Atropine	0.01–0.02 mg·kg^{-1}	im

Sedatives

Diazepam	0.4 mg·kg^{-1}	im
	0.1–0.2 mg·kg^{-1}	po
Pentobarbital	2–6 mg·kg^{-1}	im/po
Diphenhydramine	0.2–0.5 mg·kg^{-1}	im/po
Hydroxyzine	0.5–1.0 mg·kg^{-1}	im/po
Midazolam	0.4 mg·kg^{-1}	im

Analgesics

Morphine	0.05–0.15 mg·kg^{-1}	im
Meperidine	1–2 mg·kg^{-1}	im

TABLE 36-29. Commonly Used Drugs for Patients With Congenital Heart Defects

Atropine	0.01–0.02 mg·kg^{-1}
Bicarbonate	1 mEq·kg^{-1}
Calcium chloride	10 mg·kg^{-1}
Calcium gluconate	30 mg·kg^{-1}
Lidocaine	1 mg·kg^{-1}
Propranolol	0.01–0.02 mg·kg^{-1}
Verapamil	0.125–0.25 mg·kg^{-1}
Digoxin	20 μg·kg^{-1} premature
	40 μg·kg^{-1} infant
	20 μg·kg^{-1} child

Common Infusions

Lidocaine	20–50 μg·kg^{-1}·min^{-1}
Sodium nitroprusside	0.5–10 μg·kg^{-1}·min^{-1}
Prostaglandin E$_1$	0.1 μg·kg^{-1}·min^{-1}
Isoproterenol	0.1–0.5 μg·kg^{-1}·min^{-1}
Epinephrine	0.1–1.0 μg·kg^{-1}·min^{-1}
Dopamine	1–20 μg·kg^{-1}·min^{-1}
Dobutamine	1–10 μg·kg^{-1}·min^{-1}
Norepinephrine	0.1–0.5 μg·kg^{-1}·min^{-1}
Phenylephrine	0.1–0.5 μg·kg^{-1}·min^{-1}

Preparation for Anesthesia

Since hypoxemia and hypotension can occur quickly, the margin for error in managing critically ill children is slim. Preparedness is essential. The anesthesiologist must have on hand all standard equipment normally used for the pediatric patient. In addition, appropriate cardioactive drugs should be available (Table 36-29). An isoproterenol infusion should be ready in case hypotension secondary to decreased heart rate occurs or if inotropy becomes a problem. It is critical that all iv catheters, injection ports, and stopcocks be meticulously cleared of bubbles to prevent systemic embolization. Aspiration should precede injection of all iv drugs. All patients are at risk regardless of the site or direction of the shunt.

Monitoring

Standard monitoring for all pediatric patients undergoing repair of congenital cardiac lesions includes an electrocardiogram, a blood pressure cuff (usually an automated device), a pulse oximeter (at a preductal site if right-to-left flow is through the patent ductus arteriosus), and appropriate temperature probes. A precordial stethoscope is essential prior to and during induction of anesthesia and intubation of the trachea. Intra-arterial blood pressure monitoring is necessary in patients requiring cardiopulmonary bypass and in those undergoing thoracotomy. A central venous catheter is necessary when the need for pharmacologic support is anticipated or monitoring of central blood volume will aid in management of the patient. A central venous pressure catheter can be inserted percutaneously after the patient is intubated or an intracardiac catheter can be placed later in the procedure. Intraoperative echocardiography has been advocated as an aid to diagnosis, assessment of repair, and pharmacologic management.[250]

Anesthetic Selection

All patients require an anesthetic regardless of age. Recent evidence documents the perception of pain in even the youngest neonate.[251,252] As with adults, anesthetic induction and maintenance must be tailored to suit the needs of each patient, with careful regard for depressant effects on the cardiovascular system and on pulmonary vascular resistance and systemic vascular resistance. Most intramuscular, iv, and inhalation drugs have been used safely in anesthetizing children with congenital heart disease.

Induction

The tracheas of neonates and premature infants are usually intubated awake after administration of atropine and following preoxygenation. Older children arriving with a functioning iv catheter can be induced with iv opioids, barbiturates, benzodiazepines, or ketamine. Atropine and a muscle relaxant can be given prior to intubation of the trachea. An inhalation induction with 1–2% halothane in nitrous oxide and oxygen is safe for patients without an intravenous access provided excessive myocardial depression is avoided. Intramuscular ketamine (5–10 mg·kg^{-1}) is useful in handling frightened or combative children. The drug has sympathetic stimulating properties and does not cause increases in pulmonary vascular resistance regardless of pre-existing pulmonary hypertension as long as airway patency and adequate oxygenation and ventilation of the lungs are ensured.[253] Theoretically, the speed of anesthetic induction can be affected by the presence of circulatory shunts.[254] The presence of a right-to-left shunt slows the equilibration between alveolar and arterial partial pressures, prolonging an inhalation induction. This effect is most evident when using less soluble gases such as nitrous oxide. The presence of concomitant left-to-right shunting attenuates this effect. In the presence of a right-to-left shunt, drugs administered intravenously reach the brain more quickly and in greater concentrations. Anesthetic effects appear rapidly. Pure left-to-right shunting has little effect on the speed of an inhalation induction provided that cardiac output is maintained. If output falls, as in any low output state, induction occurs more rapidly. The increased pulmonary blood flow associated with left-to-right shunts dilutes any iv agent. The initial peak concentration of the drug is decreased, and the effects are prolonged.

Maintenance

Drugs to be used after induction of anesthesia and airway control are chosen considering the patient's response to the induction sequence, the current hemodynamic status, the length of the procedure, and the plans for postoperative care. High-dose opioid techniques (fentanyl, 25–50 μg·kg^{-1} or sufentanil, 5–15 μg·kg^{-1}) provide cardiovascular and pulmonary vascular stability for major procedures involving cardiopulmonary bypass.[255,256] They may, however, be inappropriate for simpler repairs, after which early extubation is planned. For relatively healthy children with minimally affected cardiovascular reserve, use of an inhalation agent as the primary anesthetic with or without low-dose opioid supplementation is useful in achieving this goal. Volatile anesthetics may also be useful in sicker children receiving a high-dose opioid technique for controlling intraoperative hypertensive responses. It must be remembered that the immature myocardium and vascular system are very sensitive to the depressant effects of halothane, enflurane, and isoflurane.[257,258] Hemodynamic deterioration secondary to myocardial depression is an ongoing possibility, and the avoidance of the potent inhalation drugs in children with reduced cardiovascular reserve is warranted.

As it does in adults, nitrous oxide administered to children decreases cardiac output, heart rate, and systemic blood pressure. Contrary to findings in adults, however, its use does not increase pulmonary vascular resistance regardless of the baseline condition of the child's pulmonary vasculature.[259] Additional nitrous oxide does not result in arterial oxygen desaturation in patients with cyanotic lesions, since, with large shunts, PaO_2 becomes relatively independent of FIO_2. Concern does arise over the possibility of increasing the size of systemic air emboli. These are the primary considerations in deciding whether to use or avoid using the drug.

Cardiopulmonary Bypass

The techniques and basic circuit used for cardiopulmonary bypass in children are similar to those used for adults (components and primes are smaller). Some differences do exist. A sanguinous prime avoids excessive hemodilution in infants. Perfusion is regulated by pump flow and, in the very young, high flows (up to 150–175 ml·kg^{-1}·min^{-1}) may be required to maintain adequate perfusion. As children grow and their arterial trees mature and become less distensible, flows closer to those used for adults can be used. The presence of previous systemic-to-pulmonary shunts or significant bronchial collateral flow makes maintenance of adequate perfusion pressure more difficult, and ligation of these shunts may be necessary prior to initiation of cardiopulmonary bypass. Adequacy of perfusion is difficult to assess in children, as in adults, but can be inferred if urine output, mixed venous oxygen saturation, and pH are all normal. The temperature gradient that exists between core and peripheral sites also serves as an indicator of the adequacy of perfusion.

Deep Hypothermic Circulatory Arrest

Profound hypothermia to 10–15°C with periods of circulatory arrest is used in infants weighing less than 10 kg who are undergoing repair of complex congenital lesions. Topical cooling (ice bags, cooled room temperature) is begun immediately after induction and intubation of the trachea and supplements core cooling provided by the bypass pump and maintains deep hypothermia once the bypass pump is shut off. Deep hypothermic circulatory arrest provides a bloodless field, shortens bypass time, and aids protection of the myocardium by preventing both washout of cardioplegia solution and rewarming of the heart by contiguous organs. Circulatory arrest times are limited by the potential for central nervous system damage. Detrimental effects to other vital organs are unusual. Most centers using deep hypothermic circulatory arrest consider 60 minutes the upper limit of safe continuous arrest.[260] If more time is required for completion of the repair, a 15-minute period of reperfusion separates two 40- to 50-minute periods of arrest. Patients undergoing deep hypothermic circulatory arrest should have their temperatures monitored at multiple sites (tympanic membrane, esophagus, rectum), since significant temperature gradients between parts of the body may exist. In an attempt to prevent rewarming of the brain during the period of arrest, uniform cooling of the entire body is the goal.[261]

Separation from Bypass

Separation from the bypass pump is done using information obtained from the surgical field and, if necessary, from measurement of intracardiac pressures. Weaning is not usually a problem provided that appropriate surgical correction has occurred and that adequate ventilation and oxygenation are provided. Ischemia and residual problems with contractility are uncommon in pediatric patients, although they can occur. Low cardiac output requiring pharmacologic support after bypass is unusual but is more common when a large ventriculotomy incision has been made or if long bypass or aortic cross-clamp times have been used. Prolonged difficulty separating from bypass warrants a search for residual defects or signals a problem with the repair itself.

Timing of Extubation

Extubation of the trachea in the operative or early postoperative period is appropriate for patients undergoing repair of a simple atrial septal defect, patent ductus arteriosus, or aortic coarctation. The anesthesiologist must be certain that surgical hemostasis has been obtained, that the child is warm, that residual narcosis and paralysis are not a problem, and that spontaneous ventilation is adequate. More controversial is the timing of extubation of the trachea after correction of complex shunts. Postoperative respiratory insufficiency or failure is more likely to occur in patients in whom preoperative pulmonary blood flow was markedly increased and in those with significant pulmonary hypertension or pre-existing pulmonary infection as well as in those born prematurely, neonates, and patients younger than 6 months of age. Postoperative respiratory support is recommended in these incidences. Nasotracheal intubation, because it better maintains endotracheal tube position, is preferred when postoperative ventilation is anticipated. Extubation can be accomplished once the normal criteria have been met.

REFERENCES

1. Keats AS: The Rovenstine Lecture, 1983: Cardiovascular anesthesia: Perceptions and perspectives. Anesthesiology 60:467, 1984
2. Hensley FA Jr, Martin DE: The Practice of Cardiac Anesthesia. Boston, Little, Brown, 1990
3. Kaplan JA: Cardiac Anesthesia, 2nd ed. Orlando, Grune & Stratton, 1987
4. Lake CL: Cardiovascular Anesthesia. New York, Springer-Verlag, 1985
5. Ream AK, Fogdall RP: Acute Cardiovascular Management: Anesthesia and Intensive Care. Philadelphia, J.B. Lippincott, 1982
6. Reves JG, Hall KD: Common Problems in Cardiac Anesthesia. Chicago, Year Book Medical Publishers, Inc, 1982
7. Thomas SJ: Manual of Cardiac Anesthesia, 2nd ed, New York, Churchill Livingstone, 1992
8. Slogoff S, Keats AS: Does perioperative myocardial ischemia lead to postoperative myocardial infarction? Anesthesiology 62:107, 1985

9. Slogoff S, Keats AS: Further observations on perioperative myocardial ischemia. Anesthesiology 65:539, 1986
10. Isom OW, Spencer FC, Feigenbaum H et al: Prebypass myocardial damage in patients undergoing coronary revascularization: An unrecognized vulnerable period. Circulation 52 (suppl II):119, 1975
11. Leung JM, Goehner P, O'Kelly BF et al: Isoflurane anesthesia and myocardial ischemia: Comparative risk versus sufentanil anesthesia in patients undergoing coronary artery bypass graft surgery. Anesthesiology 74:838, 1991
12. Kleinman B, Henkin RE, Glisson SN et al: Qualitative evaluation of coronary flow during anesthetic induction using thallium-201 perfusion scans. Anesthesiology 64:157, 1986
13. Buffington CW, Ivey TD: Coronary artery spasm during general anesthesia. Anesthesiology 55:466, 1981
14. Mangano DT, Hollenberg M, Fegert G et al: Perioperative myocardial ischemia in patients undergoing noncardiac surgery—I: Incidence and severity during the 4 day perioperative period. J Am Coll Cardiol 17:843, 1991
15. Leung JM, O'Kelly BV, Mangano DT et al: Relationship of regional wall motion abnormalities to hemodynamic indices of myocardial oxygen supply and demand in patients undergoing CABG surgery. Anesthesiology 73:802, 1990
16. Merin RG, Lowenstein E, Gelman S: Is anesthesia beneficial for the ischemic heart? III. Anesthesiology 57:461, 1985
17. Weber KT, Janicki JS: The metabolic demand and oxygen supply of the heart: Physiologic and clinical considerations. Am J Cardiol 44:722, 1979
18. Buffington CW: Impaired systolic thickening associated with halothane in the presence of a coronary stenosis is mediated by changes in hemodynamics. Anesthesiology 64:632, 1986
19. Bell JR, Fox AC: Pathogenesis of subendocardial ischemia. Am J Med Sci 268:2, 1974
20. Hoffman JIE: Transmural myocardial perfusion. Prog Cardiovasc Dis 29:429, 1987
21. Boudoulas H, Rittgers SE, Lewis RP et al: Changes in diastolic time with various pharmacologic agents: Implication for myocardial perfusion. Circulation 60:164, 1979
22. Klocke FJ, Mates RE, Canty JM Jr et al: Coronary pressure–flow relationships. Controversial issues and probable implications. Circ Res 56:310, 1985
23. Hoffman JIE, Spaan JAE: Pressure-flow relations in the coronary circulation. Physiologic Rev 70:331, 1990
24. Buffington CW: Hemodynamic determinants of ischemic myocardial dysfunction in the presence of coronary stenosis in dogs. Anesthesiology 63:651, 1985
25. Feigl EO: Coronary physiology (review). Physiol Rev 63:1, 1983
26. Prinzmetal M, Kennamer R, Merliss R: Angina pectoris: A variant form of angina pectoris. Am J Med 27:375, 1959
27. Chierchia S, Brunelli C, Simonetti I et al: Sequence of events in angina at rest: Primary reduction in coronary flow. Circulation 61:759, 1980
28. Deanfield JE, Maseri A, Selwyn AP: Myocardial ischemia during daily life in patients with stable angina: Its relation to symptoms and heart rate changes. Lancet 2:753, 1983
29. Maseri A, Chierchia S: Coronary artery spasm: definition, diagnosis and consequences. Prog Cardiovasc Dis 25:169, 1982
30. McAlpin RN: Contribution of dynamic vascular wall thickening to luminal narrowing during coronary arterial constriction. Circulation 60:296, 1980
31. Freudenberg H, Lichtlen PR: The normal wall segment in coronary stenosis—a post-mortem study. Z Kardiol 70:863, 1981
32. VanHoutte PM, Houston DS: Platelets, endothelium, and vasospasm. Circulation 72:729, 1985
33. Nussmeier NA, Slogoff S: Verapamil treatment of intraoperative coronary artery spasm. Anesthesiology 62:539, 1985
34. Humphrey LS, Blanck TJJ: Intraoperative use of verapamil for nitroglycerin-refractory myocardial ischemia. Anesth Analg 64:68, 1985
35. Brown BG, Bolson EL, Dodge HJ: Dynamic mechanisms in human coronary artery stenosis. Circulation 70:917, 1984
36. Fuster V, Badimon L, Cohen M, Chesebro J: Insights into the pathogenesis of acute ischemic syndromes. Circulation 77: 1213, 1988
37. Hines RL: Monitoring for right ventricular ischemia: Is it necessary? J Cardiothorac Anesth 1:95, 1987
38. Kotrly KJ, Kotter GS, Mortara D et al: Intraoperative detection of myocardial ischemia with an ST segment trend monitoring system. Anesth Analg 63:343, 1984
39. Robinson BF: Relation of heart rate and systolic blood pressure to the onset of pain in angina pectoris. Circulation 35: 1073, 1967
40. Kissin I, Reves JG, Mardes M: Is the rate–pressure product a misleading guide? Anesthesiology 52:373, 1980
41. Buffington CW: Hemodynamic determinants of ischemic myocardial dysfunction in the presence of coronary stenosis in dogs. Anesthesiology 63:651, 1985
42. Gordon MA, Urban MK, O'Connor T, Barash PG: Is the pressure rate quotient a predictor or indicator of myocardial ischemia as measured by ST-segment changes in patients undergoing coronary artery bypass surgery? Anesthesiology 74:848, 1991
43. Kaplan JA, Wells PM: Early diagnosis of myocardial ischemia using the pulmonary artery catheter. Anesth Analg 60:789, 1981
44. Waller JL, Johnson SP, Kaplan JA: Usefulness of pulmonary artery catheters during aortocoronary bypass surgery. Anesth Analg 56:219, 1982
45. Leung JM, O'Kelly B, Browner WS et al: Prognostic importance of postbypass regional wall-motion abnormalities in patients undergoing coronary artery bypass graft surgery. Anesthesiology 71:16, 1989
46. Haggmark S, Hohner P, Ostman M et al: Comparison of hemodynamic, electrocardiographic, mechanical, and metabolic indicators of intraoperative myocardial ischemia in vascular surgical patients with coronary artery disease. Anesthesiology 70:19, 1989
47. Van Daele MERM, Sutherland GR, Mitchell MM et al: Do changes in pulmonary capillary wedge pressure adequately reflect myocardial ischemia during anesthesia? A correlative preoperative hemodynamic, electrocardiographic, and transesophageal echocardiographic study. Circulation 81:865, 1990
48. Tuman KJ, McCarthy RJ, Spiess BD et al: Effect of pulmonary artery catheterization on outcome in patients undergoing coronary artery surgery. Anesthesiology 70:199, 1989
49. Smith JS, Cahalan MK, Benefiel DJ et al: Intraoperative detection of myocardial ischemia in high-risk patients; Electrocardiography versus two-dimensional transesophageal echocardiography. Circulation 72:1015, 1985
50. Lowenstein E, Haering JM, Douglas PS: Acute ventricular wall motion heterogeneity: A valuable but imperfect index of myocardial ischemia. Anesthesiology 75:385, 1991
51. Kloner RA, Parisi AF: Acute myocardial infarction: Diagnostic and prognostic applications of two-dimensional echocardiography. Circulation 75:521, 1987
52. Vandenberg BF, Kerber RE: Transesophageal echocardiography and intraoperative monitoring of left ventricular function (editorial). Anesthesiology 73:799, 1990
53. Moffitt EA, Sethna DH: The coronary circulation and myocardial oxygenation in coronary artery disease: Effects of anesthesia (review). Anesth Analg 65:395, 1986
54. Slogoff S, Keats AS: Randomized trial of primary anesthetic agents on outcome of coronary artery bypass operations. Anesthesiology 70:179, 1989
55. Tuman KJ, McCarthy RJ, Spiess BD et al: Does choice of anesthetic agent significantly affect outcome after coronary artery surgery? Anesthesiology 70:189, 1989
56. Roizen MF, Hamilton WK, Yung JS: Treatment of stress-induced increases in pulmonary wedge pressure using volatile anesthetics. Anesthesiology 55:446, 1981
57. Tarnow J, Markschies-Hornung A, Schulte-Sasse U: Isoflurane improves the tolerance to pacing-induced myocardial ischemia. Anesthesiology 64:147, 1986
58. Bovill JG, Sebel PL, Stanley TH: Opioid analgesics in anesthesia with special reference to their use in cardiovascular anesthesia. Anesthesiology 61:731, 1984

59. Philbin DM, Rosow CE, Schneider RC et al: Fentanyl and sufentanil revisited: How much is enough? Anesthesiology 73:5, 1990

60. Hilgenberg JC: Intraoperative awareness during high-dose fentanyl oxygen anesthesia. Anesthesiology 54:341, 1981

61. Mark JB, Greenberg LM: Intraoperative awareness and hypertensive crisis during high-dose fentanyl–diazepam anesthesia. Anesth Analg 62:698, 1983

62. Hug CC Jr: Does opioid "anesthesia" exist? Anesthesiology 73:1, 1990

63. Bland JHL, Lowenstein E: Halothane-induced decrease in experimental myocardial ischemia in the nonfailing canine heart. Anesthesiology 45:287, 1976

64. Van Trigt P, Christian CC, Fagraeus L et al: Myocardial depression by anesthetic agents (halothane, enflurane and nitrous oxide): Quantitation based on end-systolic pressure-dimension relations. Am J Cardiol 53:243, 1984

65. Reiz S, Balfors E, Sorensen MB et al: Isoflurane—a powerful coronary vasodilator in patients with coronary artery disease. Anesthesiology 59:91, 1983

66. Sill JC, Bove AA, Nugent M et al: Effects of isoflurane on coronary arteries and coronary arterioles in the intact dog. Anesthesiology 66:273, 1987

67. Buffington CW, Romson JL, Levine A et al: Isoflurane induces coronary steal in a canine model of chronic coronary occlusion. Anesthesiology 66:280, 1987

68. Hickey RF, Sybert PE, Verrier ED et al: Effects of halothane, enflurane, and isoflurane on coronary blood flow regulation and coronary vascular reserve in the canine heart. Anesthesiology 68:21, 1988

69. Pagel PS, Kampine JP, Schmeling WT, Warltier DC: Comparison of the systemic and coronary hemodynamic actions of desflurane, isoflurane, halothane, and enflurane in the chronically instrumented dog. Anesthesiology 74:539, 1991

70. Leung JM, Goehner P, O'Kelly BF et al: Isoflurane anesthesia and myocardial ischemia: Comparative risk versus sufentanil anesthesia in patients undergoing coronary artery bypass graft surgery. Anesthesiology 74:838, 1991

71. Brown BG, Bolson EL, Petersen RB et al: The mechanisms of nitroglycerin action: Stenosis vasodilation as a major component of the drug response. Circulation 64:1089, 1981

72. Feldman RL, Joyal M, Conti CR et al: Effect of nitroglycerin on coronary collateral flow and pressure during acute coronary occlusion. Am J Cardiol 54:958, 1984

73. Gallagher JD, Moore RA, Jose AB et al: Prophylactic nitroglycerin infusions during coronary artery bypass surgery. Anesthesiology 64:785, 1986

74. Thomson IR, Mutch WA, Culligan JD: Failure of intravenous nitroglycerin to prevent intraoperative myocardial ischemia during fentanyl–pancuronium anesthesia. Anesthesiology 61:385, 1984

75. Coriat P, Deloz M, Bousseau D et al: Prevention of intraoperative myocardial ischemia during noncardiac surgery with intravenous nitroglycerin. Anesthesiology 61:193, 1984

76. Mason DT: Regulation of cardiac performance in clinical heart disease. Am J Cardiol 32:437, 1973

77. Ross J: Cardiac function and myocardial contractility: A perspective. J Am Coll Cardiol 1:52, 1983

78. Ross J: Afterload mismatch in aortic and mitral valve disease: Implications for surgical therapy. J Am Coll Cardiol 5:811, 1985

79. Sasayama S, Franklin D, Ross J: Hyperfunction with normal inotropic state of the hypertrophied left ventricle. Am J Physiol 232:H418, 1977

80. Marcus ML: Effects of cardiac hypertrophy on the coronary circulation. In Marcus ML (ed): The Coronary Circulation in Health and Disease. New York, McGraw-Hill, 1983

81. Rakusan K: Quantitative morphology of capillaries of the heart. Number of capillaries in animal and human hearts under normal and pathological conditions. Methods Achiev Exp Pathol 5:272, 1971

82. Marcus ML, Doty DB, Hiratzka LF et al: Decreased coronary reserve: A mechanism for angina in patients with aortic stenosis and normal coronary arteries. N Engl J Med 307:1362, 1982

83. Lakatta EG: Age-related alterations in the cardiovascular response to adrenergic mediated stress. Fed Proc 39:3173, 1980

84. Maron BJ, Bonow RO, Cannon RO 3d et al: Hypertrophic cardiomyopathy. Interrelations of clinical manifestations, pathophysiology, and therapy (2). N Engl J Med 316:844, 1987

85. Maron BJ, Bonow RO, Cannon RO 3d et al: Hypertrophic cardiomyopathy. Interrelations of clinical manifestations, pathophysiology, and therapy (1). N Engl J Med 316:780, 1987

86. Wigle ED, Sasson Z, Henderson MA et al: Hypertrophic cardiomyopathy. The importance of the site and the extent of hypertrophy. A review. Prog Cardiovasc Dis 28:1, 1985

87. Pollick C: Unlocking the mystery of systolic anterior motion: The key is timing. Can J Cardiol 1:33, 1985

88. Criley JM, Siegel RJ: Has "obstruction" hindered our understanding of hypertrophic cardiomyopathy? (review). Circulation 72:1148, 1985

89. Dodge HT, Hay RE, Sandler H: Pressure—volume characteristics of diastolic left ventricle of man with heart disease. Am Heart J 64:503, 1962

90. Maron BJ, Wolfson JK, Epstein SE et al: Intramural ("small vessel") coronary artery disease in hypertrophic cardiomyopathy. J Am Coll Cardiol 8:545, 1986

91. Galler M, Kronzon I, Slater J et al: Long-term follow-up after mitral valve reconstruction: Incidence of postoperative left ventricular outflow obstruction. Circulation 74:I99, 1986

92. Gaasch WH, Carroll JD, Levine HJ et al: Chronic aortic regurgitation: Prognostic value of left ventricular end-systolic dimension and end-diastolic radius/thickness ratio. J Am Coll Cardiol 1:775, 1983

93. Stone JG, Hoar PF, Calabro JR: Afterload reduction and preload augmentation improve the anesthetic management of patients with cardiac failure and valvular regurgitation. Anesth Analg 59:737, 1980

94. Firth BG, Dehmer GJ, Nicod P et al: Effect of increasing heart rate in patients with aortic regurgitation. Effect of incremental pacing on scintigraphic, hemodynamic, and thermodilation measurements. Am J Cardiol 49:1860, 1982

95. Judge TP, Kennedy JW, Bennet LJ et al: Quantitative hemodynamic effects of heart rate in aortic regurgitation. Circulation 44:355, 1971

96. Heller SJ, Carleton RA: Abnormal left ventricular contraction in patients with mitral stenosis. Circulation 42:1099, 1970

97. Bolen JL, Lopes MG, Harrison DC et al: Analysis of left ventricular function in response to afterload changes in patients with mitral stenosis. Circulation 52:894, 1975

98. Yared JP, Estafanous FG, Zurick AM: Anesthesia for patients with mitral valve disease secondary to rheumatic and coronary artery disease. Cleve Clin Q 51:59, 1984

99. Yoran C, Yellin EL, Becker RM et al: Dynamic aspects of acute mitral regurgitation: Effects of ventricular volume, pressure, and contractility on the effective regurgitant orifice area. Circulation 60:170, 1979

100. Chatterjee K, Parmley WW, Swan HJC et al: Beneficial effects of vasodilator agents in severe mitral regurgitation due to dysfunction of subvalvular apparatus. Circulation 48:684, 1973

101. Taylor RM: Cardiopulmonary Bypass: Principles and Management. Baltimore, Williams & Wilkins, 1986

102. Edmunds LH, Ellison N, Colman RW: Platelet function during cardiac operation—comparison of membrane and bubble oxygenators. J Thorac Cardiovasc Surg 83:805, 1982

103. Kusserow B, Larrow R, Nicholls J: Perfusion- and surface-induced injury in leukocytes. Fed Proc 30:1516, 1971

104. Cavarocchi NC, Pluth JR, Schaff HV et al: Complement activation during cardiopulmonary bypass. Comparison of bubble and membrane oxygenators. J Thorac Cardiovasc Surg 91:252, 1986

105. Chiu RC, Samson R: Complement (C3, C4) consumption in cardiopulmonary bypass, cardioplegia, and protamine administration. Ann Thorac Surg 37:229, 1984

106. vanOeveren W, Kazatchkine MD, Descamps-Latscha B et al: Deleterious effects of cardiopulmonary bypass—a prospective study of bubble vs membrane oxygenation. J Thorac Cardiovasc Surg 89:888, 1985

107. van den Dungen JJ, Karliczek GF, Brenken U et al: Clinical

study of blood trauma during perfusion with membrane and bubble oxygenators. J Thorac Cardiovasc Surg 83:108, 1982

108. Cosgrove DM, Loop FD: Clinical use of travenol TMO membrane oxygenator. In Ionescu MI (ed): Techniques in Extracorporeal Circulation, pp 85–99. London, Butterworths, 1981

109. Stern RC, Weiss CI, Steinbach JH et al: Isoflurane uptake and elimination are delayed by absorption of anesthetic by the Scimed membrane oxygenator. Anesth Analg 69:657, 1989

110. Mavroudis C: To pulse or not to pulse. Ann Thorac Surg 25:259, 1978

111. Hickey PR, Buckley MJ, Philbin DM: Pulsatile and nonpulsatile cardiopulmonary bypass: Review of a counterproductive controversy (review). Ann Thorac Surg 36:720, 1983

112. Philbin DM, Hickey PR, Buckley MJ: Should we pulse? J Thorac Cardiovasc Surg 84:805, 1982

113. Nagaoka H, Innami R, Watanabe M et al: Preservation of pancreatic beta cell function with pulsatile cardiopulmonary bypass. Ann Thorac Surg 48:798, 1989

114. Taylor KM: Pulsatile perfusion. In Taylor KM (ed): Cardiopulmonary Bypass—Principles and Management, p 184. Baltimore, Williams & Wilkins, 1986

115. Edmunds LE: Pulseless cardiopulmonary bypass. J Thorac Cardiovasc Surg 84:800, 1982

116. Blair E: Clinical Hypothermia. New York, McGraw-Hill, 1964

117. Tobias MA: Choice of priming fluids. In Taylor KM (ed): Cardiopulmonary Bypass—Principles and Management, pp 221–248. Baltimore, Williams & Wilkins, 1986

118. Marelli D, Paul A, Samson R et al: Does the addition of albumin to the prime solution in cardiopulmonary bypass affect clinical outcome? J Thorac Cardiovasc Surg 98:751, 1989

119. Verska JJ, Ludington LG, Brewer LA: A comparative study of CPB with non-blood prime. Ann Thorac Surg 18:72, 1974

120. Esposito RA, Culliford AT, Colvin SB et al: Heparin resistance during cardiopulmonary bypass. The role of heparin pretreatment. J Thorac Cardiovasc Surg 85:346, 1983

121. Hattersley PG: Activated coagulation time of whole blood. JAMA 1986:436, 1966

122. Young JA, Kisker CT, Doty DB: Adequate anticoagulation during cardiopulmonary bypass determined by activated clotting time and the appearance of fibrin monomer. Ann Thorac Surg 26:231, 1978

123. Metz S, Keats AS: Low activated coagulation time during cardiopulmonary bypass does not increase postoperative bleeding. Ann Thorac Surg 49:440, 1990

124. Esposito RA, Culliford AT, Colvin SB et al: The role of the activated clotting time in heparin administration and neutralization for cardiopulmonary bypass. J Thorac Cardiovasc Surg 85:174, 1983

125. Bull BS, Korpman RA, Huse WM: Heparin therapy during extracorporeal circulation. I. Problems inherent in existing heparin protocols. J Thorac Cardiovasc Surg 69:674, 1975

126. Culliford AT, Gitel SN, Starr N et al: Lack of correlation between activated clotting time and plasma heparin during cardiopulmonary bypass. Ann Surg 193:105, 1981

127. Gravlee GP, Angert KC, Tucker WY et al: Early anticoagulation peak and rapid distribution after intravenous heparin. Anesthesiology 68:126, 1988

128. Akins CW: Noncardioplegic myocardial preservation for coronary revascularization. J Thorac Cardiovasc Surg 88:174, 1984

129. Akins CW: Resection of left ventricular aneurysm during hypothermic fibrillatory arrest without aortic occlusion. J Thorac Cardiovasc Surg 91:610, 1986

130. Brenowitz JB, Kayser KL, Johnson WD: Results of coronary artery endarterectomy and reconstruction. J Thorac Cardiovasc Surg 95:1, 1988

131. Engleman RM: Retrograde continuous warm blood cardioplegia. Ann Thorac Surg 51:180, 1991

132. Menasche P, Kural S, Fauchot M et al: Retrograde coronary sinus perfusion: A safe alternative for ensuring cardioplegic delivery in aortic valve surgery. Ann Thorac Surg 34:647, 1982

133. Silverman NA, Levitsky S: Intraoperative myocardial protection in the context of coronary revascularization. Prog Cardiovasc Dis 29:413, 1987

134. McGoon DC: The ongoing quest for ideal myocardial protection. J Thorac Cardiovasc Surg 89:639, 1985

135. Lell WA, Huber S, Buttner EE: Myocardial protection during cardiopulmonary bypass. In Kaplan JA (ed): Cardiac Anesthesia, 2nd ed, p 927. Orlando, Grune & Stratton, 1987

136. Buckberg GD: Strategies and logic of cardioplegic delivery to prevent, avoid, and reverse ischemic and reperfusion damage. J Thorac Cardiovasc Surg 93:127, 1987

137. Buckberg GD: A proposed "solution" to the cardioplegic controversy. J Thorac Cardiovasc Surg 77:803, 1979

138. Gravlee GP, Cordell AR, Graham JE et al: Coronary revascularization in patients with bilateral internal carotid occlusions. J Thorac Cardiovasc Surg 90:921, 1985

139. Hilberman M, Myers BD, Carrie BJ et al: Acute renal failure following cardiac surgery. J Thorac Cardiovasc Surg 77:880, 1979

140. Merin RG: Calcium channel blocking drugs and anesthetics: Is the drug interaction beneficial or detrimental? Anesthesiology 66:111, 1987

141. Reves JG, Kissin I, Lell WA et al: Calcium entry blockers: Uses and implications for anesthesiologists. Anesthesiology 57:504, 1982

142. Massagee JT, McIntyre RW, Kates RA et al: Effects of preoperative calcium entry blocker therapy on alpha-adrenergic responsiveness in patients undergoing coronary revascularization. Anesthesiology 67:485, 1987

143. Chung F, Huston PL, Cheng DCH et al: Calcium channel blockade does not offer adequate protection from perioperative myocardial ischemia. Anesthesiology 69:343, 1988

144. Liberman BA, Teasdale SJ: Anaesthesia and amiodarone. Can Anaesth Soc J 32:629, 1985

145. Hensley FA, Dodson DL, Martin DE et al: Oxygen saturation during preinduction placement of monitoring catheters in the cardiac surgical patient. Anesthesiology 66:834, 1987

146. Thomson IR, Bergstrom RG, Rosenbloom M et al: Premedication and high-dose fentanyl anesthesia for myocardial revascularization: A comparison of lorazepam versus morphine–scopolamine. Anesthesiology 68:194, 1988

147. Waldo AL, MacLean WAH: Diagnosis and Treatment of Cardiac Arrhythmias Following Open Heart Surgery: Emphasis on the Use of Atrial and Ventricular Epicardial Wire Electrodes. Mount Kisco, New York, Futura Publishing Company Inc, 1980

148. Davis FM, Parimelazhagan KN, Harris EA: Thermal balance during cardiopulmonary bypass with moderate hypothermia in man. Br J Anaesth 49:1127, 1977

149. Kinzer JB, Lichtenthal PR, Wade LD: Loss of radial artery pressure trace during internal mammary artery dissection for coronary artery bypass graft surgery. Anesth Analg 64:1134, 1985

150. Mohr R, Lavee J, Goor DA: Inaccuracy of radial artery pressure measurement after cardiac operations. J Thorac Cardiovasc Surg 94:286, 1987

151. Bazaral MG, Welch M, Golding LAR et al: Comparison of brachial and radial artery pressure monitoring in patients undergoing coronary artery bypass surgery. Anesthesiology 73:38, 1990

152. Stern DH, Gerson JI, Allen FB et al: Can we trust the direct radial artery pressure immediately following cardiopulmonary bypass? Anesthesiology 62:557, 1985

153. Mangano DT: Monitoring pulmonary artery pressure in coronary artery disease. Anesthesiology 53:364, 1980

154. Latson TW, Lappas DG: Use of a pacing catheter to control heart rate in a patient with aortic insufficiency and coronary artery disease. Anesthesiology 63:712, 1985

155. Lunn JK, Stanley TH, Webster LR et al: Arterial blood pressure and pulse-rate responses to pulmonary and radial artery catheterization prior to cardiac and major vascular operations. Anesthesiology 51:265, 1979

156. Waller JL, Zaidan JR, Kaplan JA: Hemodynamic responses to preoperative vascular cannulation in patients with coronary artery disease. Anesthesiology 56:219, 1982

157. Johnston WE, Royster RL, Choplin RH et al: Pulmonary artery catheter migration during cardiac surgery. Anesthesiology 64:258, 1986

158. Douglas PS, Edmunds LH, Sutton MS et al: Unreliability of hemodynamic indexes of left ventricular size during cardiac surgery. Ann Thorac Surg 44:31, 1987

159. Hansen RM, Viquerat CE, Matthay et al: Poor correlation between pulmonary arterial wedge pressure and left ventricular end-diastolic volume after coronary artery bypass graft surgery. Anesthesiology 64:764, 1986

160. Ellis RJ, Mangano DT, Van Dyke DC: Relationship of wedge pressure to end-diastolic volume in patients undergoing myocardial revascularization. J Thorac Cardiovasc Surg 78:605, 1979

161. Cahalan MK, Litt L, Botvinick EH et al: Advances in noninvasive cardiovascular imaging: Implications for the anesthesiologist. Anesthesiology 66:356, 1987

162. Levy WJ, Parcella PA: Electroencephalographic evidence of cerebral ischemia during acute extracorporeal hypoperfusion. J Cardiothorac Anesth 1:300, 1987

163. Nussmeier NA, Arlund C, Slogoff S: Neuropsychiatric complications after cardiopulmonary bypass: Cerebral protection by a barbiturate. Anesthesiology 64:165, 1986

164. Cunningham JN, Laschinger JC, Spencer FC: Monitoring of somatosensory evoked potentials during surgical procedures on the thoracoabdominal aorta. J Thorac Cardiovasc Surg 94:275, 1987

165. Bovill JG, Warren PJ, Schuller JL et al: Comparison of fentanyl, sufentanil, and alfentanil anesthesia in patients undergoing valvular heart surgery. Anesth Analg 63:1081, 1984

166. Hess W, Arnold B, Schulte Sasse U et al: Comparison of isoflurane and halothane when used to control intraoperative hypertension in patients undergoing coronary artery bypass surgery. Anesth Analg 62:15, 1983

167. Heikkila H, Jalonen J, Arola M et al: Low-dose enflurane as adjunct to high-dose fentanyl in patients undergoing coronary artery surgery: Stable hemodynamics and maintained myocardial oxygen balance. Anesth Analg 66:111, 1987

168. Gerson JI, Hickey RF, Bainton CR: Treatment of myocardial ischemia with halothane or nitroprusside–propranolol. Anesth Analg 61:10, 1982

169. Stoelting RK, Reis RR, Longnecker DE: Hemodynamic responses to nitrous oxide—halothane in patients with valvular heart disease. Anesthesiology 37:430, 1972

170. Lowenstein E, Hallowell P, Levine FH et al: Cardiovascular response to large doses of intravenous morphine in man. N Engl J Med 281:1389, 1969

171. Rosow CE, Moss J, Philbin DM et al: Histamine release during morphine and fentanyl anesthesia. Anesthesiology 56:93, 1982

172. Stanley TH, Gray NG, Stanford W et al: The effects of high-dose morphine on fluid and blood requirements in open-heart situations. Anesthesiology 38:536, 1973

173. Sebel PS, Bovill JG, Boekhorst RAA: Cardiovascular effects of high-dose fentanyl anesthesia. Acta Anaesthesiol Scand 26:308, 1982

174. de Lange S, Boscoe MJ, Stanley TH: Comparison of sufentanil–02 and fentanyl–02 for coronary artery surgery. Anesthesiology 56:112, 1982

175. Sanford TJ, Smith NT, Dec-Silver H et al: A comparison of morphine, fentanyl, and sufentanil anesthesia for cardiac surgery: Induction, emergence, and extubation. Anesth Analg 65:259, 1986

176. de Lange S, Stanley TH, Boscoe MJ: Alfentanil–oxygen anaesthesia for coronary artery surgery. Br J Anaesth 53:1291, 1981

177. Shafer SL, Varvel JR: Pharmacokinetics, pharmacodynamics, and rational opioid selection. Anesthesiology 74:53, 1991

178. Tomicheck RC, Rosow CE, Philbin DM et al: Diazepam–fentanyl interaction—hemodynamic and hormonal effects in coronary artery surgery. Anesth Analg 62:881, 1983

179. West JM, Estrada S, Heerdt M: Sudden hypotension associated with midazolam and sufentanil. Anesth Analg 66:693, 1987

180. Starr NJ, Sethna DH, Estafanous FG: Bradycardia and asystole following the rapid administration of sufentanil with vecuronium. Anesthesiology 64:521, 1986

181. Jaffe TB, Ramsey FM: Attenuation of fentanyl-induced truncal rigidity. Anesthesiology 66:693, 1987

182. Vina JR, Davis DW, Hawkins RA: The influence of nitrous oxide on methionine, S-adenosylmethionine, and other amino acids. Anesthesiology 64:490, 1986

183. Schulte Sasse U, Hess W, Tarnow J: Pulmonary vascular responses to nitrous oxide in patients with normal and high pulmonary vascular resistance. Anesthesiology 57:9, 1982

184. Hilgenberg JC, McCammon RL, Stoelting RK: Pulmonary and systemic vascular responses to nitrous oxide in patients with mitral stenosis and pulmonary hypertension. Anesth Analg 59:323, 1980

185. Pagel PS, Kampine JP, Schmeling WT et al: Effects of nitrous oxide on myocardial contractility as evaluated by the preload recruitable stroke work relationship in chronically instrumented dogs. Anesthesiology 73:1148, 1990

186. Nathan HJ: Control of hemodynamics prevents worsening of myocardial ischemia when nitrous oxide is administered to isoflurane-anesthetized dogs. Anesthesiology 71:686, 1989

187. Cahalan MK, Prakash O, Rulf ENR et al: Addition of nitrous oxide to fentanyl anesthesia does not induce myocardial ischemia in patients with ischemic heart disease. Anesthesiology 67:925, 1987

188. Dauchot PJ, Staub F, Berzina L et al: Hemodynamic response to diazepam: Dependence on prior left ventricular end-diastolic pressure. Anesthesiology 60:499, 1984

189. Kawar P, Carson IW, Clarke RS et al: Haemodynamic changes during induction of anaesthesia with midazolam and diazepam (Valium) in patients undergoing coronary artery bypass surgery. Anaesthesia 40:767, 1985

190. Stoelting RK: Choice of muscle relaxants in patients with heart disease. Semin Anesth 4:1, 1985

191. Estafanous FG, Zurick AM: Hemodynamic effects of sufentanil/metocurine versus sufentanil/pancuronium in patients undergoing coronary artery surgery. Cleve Clin Q 52:391, 1985

192. Zaidan JR, Kaplan JA: Cardiovascular effects of metocurine in patients with aortic stenosis. Anesthesiology 56:395, 1982

193. Thomson IR, Putnins CL: Adverse effects of pancuronium during high-dose fentanyl anesthesia for coronary artery bypass grafting. Anesthesiology 62:708, 1985

194. Heinonen J, Salmenpera M, Suomivuori M: Contribution of muscle relaxant to the haemodynamic course of high-dose fentanyl anaesthesia: A comparison of pancuronium, vecuronium and atracurium. Can Anaesth Soc J 33:597, 1986

195. Stoops CM, Curtis CA, Kovach DA et al: Hemodynamic effects of doxacurium chloride in patients receiving oxygen sufentanil anesthesia for coronary artery bypass grafting or valve replacement. Anesthesiology 69:365, 1988

196. Wierda JM, Karliczek GF, Vandenbrom RHG et al: Pharmacokinetics and cardiovascular dynamics of pipecuronium bromide during coronary artery surgery. Can J Anaesth 37:183, 1990

197. Stoelting RK: Circulatory changes during direct laryngoscopy and tracheal intubation: Influence of duration of laryngoscopy with or without prior lidocaine. Anesthesiology 47:381, 1977

198. Kolkka R, Hilberman M: Neurologic dysfunction following cardiac operation with low-flow, low-pressure cardiopulmonary bypass. J Thorac Cardiovasc Surg 79:432, 1980

199. Thomson IR: Neurologic aspect of cardiopulmonary bypass. Prob Anesth 1:394, 1987

200. Slogoff S, Girgis KV, Keats AS: Etiologic factors in neuropsychiatric complications associated with cardiopulmonary bypass. Anesth Analg 61:903, 1982

201. Murkin JM, Farra JK, Tweed WA et al: Cerebral autoregulation and flow/metabolism coupling during cardiopulmonary bypass: The influence of $PaCO_2$. Anesth Analg 66:825, 1987

202. Johnsson P, Messeter K, Ryding E et al: Cerebral vasoreactivity to carbon dioxide during cardiopulmonary perfusion at normothermia and hypothermia. Ann Thorac Surg 48:769, 1989

203. Reves JG, Greeley WJ: Cerebral blood flow during cardiopulmonary bypass: Some new answers to old questions. Ann Thorac Surg 48:752, 1989

204. Govier AV, Reves JG, McKay RD et al: Factors and their influence on regional cerebral blood flow in infants and children. J Thorac Cardiovasc Surg 97:737, 1989

205. Ream AK, Reitz BA, Silverberg G: Temperature correction of

Pco$_2$ and pH in estimating acid-base status: An example of the emperor's new clothes? Anesthesiology 56:41, 1982

206. Prough DS, Stump DA, Troost BT: Paco$_2$ management during cardiopulmonary bypass: Intriguing physiologic rationale, convincing clinical data, evolving hypothesis? Anesthesiology 72:3, 1990

207. Bashein G, Townes BD, Nessly ML, et al: A randomized study of carbon dioxide management during hypothermic cardiopulmonary bypass. Anesthesiology 72:7, 1990

208. Govier AV, Reves JG, McKay RD et al: Relationship of cerebral blood flow and perfusion pressure during cardiopulmonary bypass. Anesthesiology 59:A-70, 1983

209. Zaidan JR, Klochany A, Martin WM et al: Effect of thiopental on neurologic outcome following coronary artery bypass grafting. Anesthesiology 74:406, 1991

210. Todd MM, Hindman BJ, Warner DS: Barbiturate protection and cardiac surgery: A different result. Anesthesiology 74:402, 1991

211. D'Ambra MN, Laraia PJ, Philbin DM et al: Prostaglandin E$_1$: A new therapy for refractory right heart failure and pulmonary hypertension after mitral valve replacement. J Thorac Cardiovasc Surg 89:567, 1985

212. Pearl RG, Maze M, Rosenthal MH: Pulmonary and systemic hemodynamic effects of central venous and left atrial sympathomimetic drug administration in the dog. J Cardiothorac Anesth 1:29, 1987

213. Buckley MJ, Craver JM, Gold HK et al: Intra-aortic balloon pump assist for cardiogenic shock after cardiopulmonary bypass. Circulation 48(suppl 3):90, 1973

214. Craver JM, Kaplan JA, Jones EL: What role should the intraaortic balloon have in cardiac surgery? Ann Surg 189:769, 1979

215. Rajani R, Keon WJ, Bedard P: Rupture of intraaortic balloon. J Thorac Cardiovasc Surg 79:301, 1980

216. Sanfelippo PM, Baker NH, Ewe HG et al: Experience with intraaortic balloon counterpulsation. Ann Thorac Surg 41:36, 1986

217. Braunwald E, Kloner RA: The stunned myocardium: Prolonged, postischemic ventricular dysfunction. Circulation 66:1146, 1982

218. Pierce WS: Effective clinical application of ventricular bypass. Ann Thorac Surg 39:2, 1985

219. Pennington DG, Merjavy JP, Swartz MT et al: The importance of biventricular failure in patients with postoperative cardiogenic shock. Ann Thorac Surg 39:16, 1985

220. Umlas J, Taff RH, Gauvin G et al: Anticoagulant monitoring and neutralization during open heart surgery—a rapid method for measuring heparin and calculating safe reduced protamine doses. Anesth Analg 62:1095, 1983

221. Horrow JC: Protamine: A review of its toxicity (review). Anesth Analg 64:348, 1985

222. Moorthy SS, Pond W, Rowland RG: Severe circulation shock following protamine (an anaphylactic reaction). Anesth Analg 59:77, 1980

223. Holland CL, Singh AK, McMaster PRB et al: Adverse reactions to protamine sulfate following cardiac surgery. Clin Cardiol 7:157, 1984

224. Anderson JM, Johnson TA: Hypertension associated with protamine sulfate administration. Am J Hosp Pharm 38:701, 1981

225. Doolan L, McKenzie I, Krafchek J et al: Protamine sulfate hypersensitivity. Anaesth Intensive Care 9:147, 1981

226. Stewart WJ, McSweeney SM, Kellet MA et al: Increased risk of severe protamine reactions in NPH insulin-dependent diabetics undergoing cardiac catheterization. Circulation 70:788, 1984

227. Lowenstein E, Johnston WE, Lappas DG et al: Catastrophic pulmonary vasoconstriction associated with protamine reversal of heparin. Anesthesiology 59:470, 1983

228. Morel DR, Zapol WM, Thomas SJ et al: C5a and thromboxane generation associated with pulmonary vaso- and bronchoconstriction during protamine reversal of heparin. Anesthesiology 66:597, 1987

229. Kronenfeld MA, Gaguilo R, Weinberg P et al: Left atrial injec-

tion of protamine does not reliably prevent pulmonary hypertension. Anesthesiology 67:126, 1987

230. Casthely PA, Goodman K, Fyman PN et al: Hemodynamic changes after the administration of protamine. Anesth Analg 65:78, 1985

231. Frater RWM, Oka Y, Hong Y et al: Protamine-induced circulatory changes. J Thorac Cardiovasc Surg 87:687, 1984

232. Morel DR, Costabella PMM, Pittet JF: Adverse cardiopulmonary effects and increased plasma thromboxane concentrations following the neutralization of heparin with protamine in awake sheep are infusion rate-dependent. Anesthesiology 73:415, 1990

233. Beatty N, Beatty CP, Blake DR et al: Heparin rebound studies in patients and volunteers. J Thorac Cardiovasc Surg 67:723, 1974

234. Purandare SV, Parulkar GB, Panday SR et al: Heparin rebound—a cause of bleeding following open heart surgery. J Postgrad Med 25:70, 1979

235. Reddy PS, Curtiss EL, O'Toole JD et al: Cardiac tamponade: Hemodynamic observations in man. Circulation 58:265, 1978

236. Lake CL (ed): Pediatric Cardiac Anesthesia. Norwalk, Appleton & Lange, 1988

237. Hickey PR, Wessel DL: Anesthesia for treatment of congenital heart disease. In Kaplan JA (ed): Cardiac Anesthesia, 2nd ed, p 635. Orlando, Grune & Stratton, 1987

238. Haworth SG: Normal pulmonary vascular development and its disturbance in congenital heart disease. In Godman MJ (ed): Paediatric Cardiology, pp 46–55. New York, Churchill Livingstone, 1981

239. Hoffman JIE, Rudolph AM, Heymann MA: Pulmonary vascular disease with congenital heart lesions: Pathologic features and causes. Circulation 64:873, 1981

240. Rabinovitch M, Haworth SG, Castaneda AR et al: Lung biopsy in congenital heart disease: A morphometric approach to pulmonary vascular disease. Circulation 58:1107, 1978

241. Berman W: The hemodynamics of shunts in congenital heart disease. In Johansen K, Burggran WW (eds): Cardiovascular Shunts: Phylogenic, Ontogenic, and Clinical Aspects, pp 399–410. New York, Raven Press, 1985

242. Downing SE, Talner NS, Gardner TH: Ventricular function in the newborn lamb. Am J Physiol 208:931, 1965

243. Edmunds LH, Wagner HR, Heymann MA: Aortic valvotomy in neonates. Circulation 61:421, 1980

244. Goldman S, Hernandez J, Pappas G: Results of surgical treatments of coarctation of the aorta in the critically ill neonate. J Thorac Cardiovasc Surg 91:732, 1986

245. Freed MA, Heymann MA, Lewis AB et al: Prostaglandin E$_1$ in infants with ductus arteriosus–dependent congenital heart disease. Circulation 64:899, 1981

246. Hansen DD, Hickey PR: Anesthesia for hypoplastic left heart syndrome: Use of high-dose fentanyl in 30 neonates. Anesth Analg 65:127, 1986

247. Romero T, Covell J, Friedman WF: A comparison of pressure–volume relations of the fetal, newborn, and adult. Am J Physiol 222:1285, 1972

248. Phornphutkul C, Rosenthal A, Nadas A: Cerebrovascular accidents in infants and children with cyanotic congenital heart disease. Am J Cardiol 32:329, 1973

249. Kontras S, Sirak H, Newton W: Hematologic abnormalities in children with congenital heart disease. JAMA 195:611, 1976

250. Ungerleider RM, Kisslo JA, Greeley WJ et al: Intraoperative pre and post bypass epicardial color flow in the repair of atrioventricular septal defects. J Thorac Cardiovasc Surg 98:90, 1989

251. Anand KJ, Hickey PR: Pain and its effects in the human neonate and fetus. N Engl J Med 317:1321, 1987

252. Berry FA, Gregory GA: Do premature infants require anesthesia for surgery? Anesthesiology 67:291, 1987

253. Hickey PR, Hansen DD, Cramolini GM et al: Pulmonary and systemic hemodynamic responses to ketamine in infants with normal and elevated pulmonary vascular resistance. Anesthesiology 62:287, 1985

254. Tanner GE, Angers DG, Barash PG et al: Effect of left-to-right,

mixed left-to-right, and right-to-left shunts on inhalational anesthetic induction in children. Anesth Analg 64:101, 1985

255. Hickey PR, Hansen DD, Wessel DL et al: Blunting of stress responses in the pulmonary circulation of infants by fentanyl. Anesth Analg 64:1137, 1985

256. Hickey PR, Hansen DD, Wessel DL et al: Pulmonary and systemic hemodynamic responses to fentanyl in infants. Anesth Analg 64:483, 1985

257. Friesen RH, Lichtor JL: Cardiovascular effects of inhalation induction with isoflurane in infants: A study of three induction techniques. Anesth Analg 61:42, 1982

258. Friesen RH, Lichtor JL: Cardiovascular effects of inhalation induction with isoflurane in infants. Anesth Analg 62:411, 1983

259. Hickey PR, Hansen DD, Strafford M et al: Pulmonary and systemic hemodynamic effects of nitrous oxide in infants with normal and elevated pulmonary vascular resistance. Anesthesiology 65:374, 1986

260. Tharion J, Johnson DC, Celermajer JM et al: Profound hypothermia with circulatory arrest: Nine years clinical experience. J Thorac Cardiovasc Surg 84:66, 1984

261. Hickey PR, Anderson NP: Deep hypothermic circulatory arrest: A review of pathophysiology and clinical experience as a basis for anesthetic management. J Cardiothorac Anesth 1:137, 1987

37

Michael F. Roizen
John E. Ellis

Anesthesia for Vascular Surgery

GOALS OF ANESTHESIA

The goals of anesthesia for vascular surgery are similar to those for any procedure: to minimize patient morbidity and maximize the surgical benefit. The anesthesiologist may, however, have a greater influence in reducing the morbidity from vascular surgery. The morbidity from these procedures has decreased rapidly, from a 6-day mortality of more than 25% for major aortic reconstruction in the mid-1960s to a 1–2% mortality today. This chapter discusses the major types and causes of morbidity that follow specific surgical procedures. The heart should be the major focus of the anesthesiologist's attention insofar as myocardial dysfunction is the single most important cause of morbidity following surgery for cerebrovascular, visceral, or peripheral vascular insufficiency, or following aortic reconstruction for aneurysm.

From the 1960s through the 1980s, improvements in morbidity and mortality resulted from better intraoperative care and perioperative fluid management. In the late 1980s and early 1990s the emphasis has been on patient selection and the preoperative identification of patients likely to have events related to myocardial ischemia. Although attention to the myocardial risk of the vascular surgery patient is a natural outgrowth of defining the causes of morbidity after surgery, it is not certain that such segregation benefits patients.[1] Many believe that more invasive monitoring, preoperative coronary artery bypass grafting (CABG), or percutaneous transluminal coronary angioplasty (PTCA) before vascular surgery may be survival tests that are accompanied by increased short-term morbidity; others believe that these procedures lead to a more realistic discussion of risks with the patient and to long-term survival.[2] Certainly, vascular surgery in patients who have undergone coronary revascularization is associated with a lower incidence of perioperative complications.[3] Further, because most myocardial ischemia occurs postoperatively[4-8] and because infarctions occur on postoperative days 2 and 3, the emphasis appears currently to be on more aggressive postoperative therapy.[9,10]

CAUSES OF MORBIDITY AFTER OPERATIONS FOR CEREBROVASCULAR INSUFFICIENCY

Two types of operations are used to correct cerebrovascular insufficiency: carotid endarterectomy and cerebral bypass. Extracranial to intracranial (EC-IC) bypass is performed with less than one thousandth the frequency of carotid endarterectomy (see Surgery for Cerebrovascular Insufficiency, below). The results, morbidity, and mortality following carotid endarterectomy vary directly with the preoperative neurologic and cardiac status of patients. In a large Mayo Clinic series,[11] the mortality from postoperative neurologic deficits in patients with strokes in progress or unstable neurologic status was 2.5%, and 1% died of cardiovascular complications. The mortality from myocardial ischemia in patients with a history of coronary artery disease (CAD) was 1.9%. Because more patients in this series had CAD than had unstable neurologic status, the greatest cause of morbidity and mortality following carotid endarterectomy was myocardial (Table 37-1). In four other surgical series in which routine neurologic and cardiologic examinations were performed, Hertzer and Lees[12] found that 60% of the deaths that occurred within 60 days of carotid endarterectomy were due to myocardial dysfunction, and Ennix and colleagues[13] reported an 0.8% rate of myocardial infarctions and a 1.1% rate of severe strokes in patients without symptoms of CAD, a 12.9% myocardial infarction rate and a 2.4% severe stroke rate in patients with symptomatic CAD, and a 2.6% rate of myocardial infarctions and a 1.3% rate of severe strokes in patients with a history of CAD with prior or simultaneous CABG. For asymptomatic patients (i.e., those with central nervous system [CNS] symptoms), Till and colleagues[14] discovered a 2.6% rate of myocardial infarction and a 1.2% stroke rate; for symptomatic patients, they found a 2.1% rate of myocardial infarction and a 2.6% stroke rate. Yeager and co-workers[15] found a 4% rate of myocardial infarction and a 2% stroke rate. In studies in which myocardial infarctions were not routinely sought, the stroke rate was generally greater than the myocardial infarction rate, and both were higher (6.6% and 1.7%, for example) in patients 65 years or older,[16] perhaps reflecting the quality of practices in which attention is not given to details and outcomes.

Age undoubtedly plays a role in morbidity. Glaser[17] found a strong correlation between age and both myocardial and CNS morbidity after carotid endarterectomy. The increase in morbidity may relate to an increase in co-morbidities with age.[18] Whereas Ennix et al[13] and others[2,19] have stressed the potential benefits of CABG prior to carotid endarterectomy or other surgical procedures, these studies showed no significant reduction in mortality when the mor-

TABLE 37-1. Mortality After Carotid Endarterectomy

Study, Year	No. of Patients Studied	% of Patients With Serious Morbidity or Mortality From:	
		Cardiac Causes	CNS Causes
Ennix et al,[13] 1979	1546	60	30
Sundt et al,[11] 1981	1145	50	31
Hertzer and Lees,[12] 1981	355	60	17
Burke et al,[24] 1982	1141	67	33
Graham et al,[25] 1986	105	100	0
Till et al,[14] 1987	356	67	33
Smith et al,[26] 1988	60	0	100
Yeager et al,[15] 1989	249	67	33

tality from CABG was included in the overall mortality (Fig. 37-1). Perhaps the reason for reduced morbidity and mortality after carotid endarterectomy in patients who have undergone CABG is that those patients at greatest risk experience myocardial and CNS morbidity and mortality during the first procedure (i.e., CABG). It may be that identification of high-risk patients by noninvasive tests, or better intraoperative and postoperative monitoring and management of myocardial ischemia, will alter these results.

Patients with symptomatic carotid artery disease appear to have 17 times higher risk of stroke during CABG than patients without carotid artery disease.[20,21] Such statistics have led to the simultaneous performance of carotid and coronary vascular procedures, with mortality and serious morbidity in the best series at about 9%.[21,22] In a study by Hertzer et al,[21] patients randomly assigned to receive combined procedures had a significantly lower stroke rate (2.8%) than those in whom carotid endarterectomy followed CABG (14%). No patient who had undergone prior carotid endarterectomy or who had PTCA prior to carotid endarterectomy was included in the study. However, patients with asymptomatic carotid stenosis did not have a higher stroke rate following coronary artery surgery than did those without carotid stenosis, but they did have a higher mortality

after coronary artery surgery, mostly resulting from myocardial infarction.[21]

Thus, with the exception of our series, the morbidity and mortality statistics from virtually all series documenting morbidity and mortality show that, even when a vessel to the brain is occluded, the major cause of morbidity and mortality after carotid endarterectomy is myocardial (see Table 37-1).[11-15,23-26] Even in our own series, 34% of the patients evidenced myocardial ischemia intraoperatively, but none sustained myocardial infarction or death from myocardial events during their hospital stay.[26] Perhaps the reason for the difference between our results and the outcome in other published series is that we focus on the goal of decreasing myocardial insults and on maintaining myocardial well-being perioperatively.

CAUSES OF MORBIDITY AFTER OPERATIONS FOR VISCERAL ISCHEMIA, THORACOABDOMINAL ANEURYSMS, AND AORTIC RECONSTRUCTION FOR ANEURYSM OR ATHEROSCLEROTIC DISEASE

The major cause of morbidity and mortality following these different procedures relates to the heart (Tables 37-1, 37-2).[11-15,24-36] Nevertheless, distinct pathologic and physiologic patterns exist for the different diseases.

There are three distinct patterns of occlusive peripheral vascular disease:

Type I, isolated aortoiliac disease. This pattern of atherosclerosis is characterized by disease localized to the bifurcation of the aorta and the common iliac vessels. Despite the association of this disease with smoking, the atherosclerosis tends to be absent in coronary vessels and is manifested only in symptoms of thigh and hip claudication. Type I disease is associated with a 5-year survival rate of 90% following surgery.

Type II, aortoiliac disease. This type of atherosclerotic pattern is diffuse and often involves the coronary and cerebral circulation. As in Types I and III disease, smoking is a common factor in affected patients; diabetes

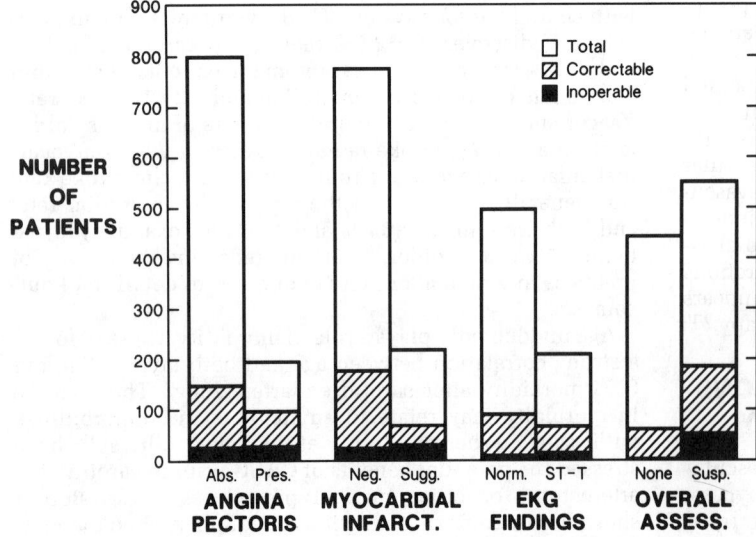

CLINICAL FEATURES (N=1000)

□ Total
▨ Correctable
■ Inoperable

NUMBER OF PATIENTS

ANGINA PECTORIS — Abs. Pres.
MYOCARDIAL INFARCT. — Neg. Sugg.
EKG FINDINGS — Norm. ST-T
OVERALL ASSESS. — None Susp.

Figure 37-1. On the basis of coronary angiograms obtained in 1000 patients prior to peripheral vascular surgical procedures, the results are stratified (correctable and inoperative) for major risk factors. For example, 19% (151 of 802) of patients in whom angina pectoris was absent had correctable coronary artery disease (CAD) and 3.5% (28 of 802) had inoperable CAD. The remaining 78% (623 of 802) patients were symptom-free. This and the other enumerated risk factors document the presence of occult CAD in this high-risk population. (Based on data from Hertzer NR, Beven EG, Young JR et al: Coronary artery disease in peripheral vascular patients: A classification of 1000 coronary angiograms and results of surgical management. Ann Surg 199:223, 1984.)

and hypertension are more common than in patients with Type I disease. The 5-year survival rate following surgery is about 80%.

Type III, atherosclerotic peripheral vascular disease. This type involves femoropopliteal and tibial atherosclerosis as well as small-vessel disease. Patients have a 60–65% 5-year survival rate following surgery.[37,38]

Although the associated conditions and prognoses for these three types of occlusive peripheral vascular diseases differ, the mortality and the factors limiting patient prognosis are the same and are related to the heart (see Table 37-2).[39-45]

Patients undergoing surgery for aneurysmal disease have higher perioperative morbidity and mortality (by a factor of 2) and a lower median survival rate (5.8 vs. 10.7 years) than do patients undergoing aortic reconstruction for occlusive disease.[46,47] Should these patients be exposed to surgery for asymptomatic aneurysms? This question was answered by Szilagyi et al[27] in 1966 when they showed that for aneurysms more than 6 cm in diameter, surgery approximately doubled a patient's life expectancy. Since then, perioperative mortality has declined from 18–25% in the mid-1960s, to 8–12% in the early 1970s, to 2–4% today. Consequently, even patients with abdominal aortic aneurysms less than 6 cm in diameter are considered candidates for aortic reconstructive surgery. This change has resulted from three factors: (1) the lower morbidity associated with elective repair today than in the 1960s; (2) the higher mortality (45–90%) associated with emergency aortic reconstruction *versus* elective reconstruction; and (3) the unpredictability of aneurysm enlargement and rupture (19% of aneurysms less than 6 cm in Szilagyi's[27] series resulted in death from rupture).[48-53]

Other causes of morbidity following vascular surgery include pulmonary infections, graft infections, renal insufficiency and failure, hepatic failure, and spinal cord ischemia resulting in paraplegia. The incidences of these other causes of morbidity have declined substantially in the past 20 years; in particular, death from renal failure has declined from 25% to less than 1% at present.[27,32,36,52-54] Much of the improvement toward elimination of renal failure has resulted from better perioperative fluid management.[55-60]

Investigators have used somatosensory-evoked potentials (SSEPs) and electroencephalograms (EEGs) to gauge spinal cord and cerebral protection, and hypothermia, magnesium, cerebrospinal fluid (CSF) drainage, papaverine, and a variety of other drugs to protect the brain and spinal cord during resection of abdominal or thoracoabdominal aneurysms or coarctation repairs.[52,53,61-65] In 1–11% of operations involving repair of the distal descending thoracic aorta, spinal cord ischemia does occur.[62-66]

Anatomy Relevant to Morbidity

The arterial blood supply to the spinal cord is generally divided into superior, midthoracic, and thoracolumbar areas (Fig. 37-2). This subdivision is better defined for the anterior spinal cord than for posterior areas, since the posterior arteries exhibit more variation in blood flow from one area to the next.[67,68] The major radiculomedullary arteries arising from the aorta terminate in three longitudinal trunks that run the length of the cord. The two posterior arteries, which together supply only 25% of the blood to the cord, are formed from the anastomoses of the posterior branch of the vertebral artery and the ascending branch of the bifurca-

TABLE 37-2. Percentages of Perioperative Mortality Related to Cardiac Events

Aortic Reconstruction Series, Year	Deaths/Total No. of Patients	% Mortality Caused by Cardiac Dysfunction
Szilagyi et al,[27] 1966	59/401	48
Young et al,[28] 1977	7/144	100
Hicks et al,[29] 1975	19/225	53
Thompson et al,[30] 1975	6/108	83
Mulcare et al,[31] 1978	14/140	79
Whittemore et al,[32] 1980	1/110	100
Crawford et al,[33] 1981	41/860	54
Hertzer,[34] 1983	22/523	64
Yeager et al,[35] 1986	4/97	100
Benefiel et al,[36] 1986	3/96	67

Adapted with permission from Roizen MF, Sohn YJ, Stoney RJ: Intraoperative management of the patient undergoing supraceliac aortic occlusion. In Wilson SE, Veith FJ, Hobson RW et al (eds): Vascular Surgery, p 312. New York, McGraw-Hill, 1986.

tion of the second posterior radicular artery. The anterior spinal artery, which supplies blood to the anterolateral 75% of the cord, is formed throughout by a series of radicular arteries. Blood does not flow from cephalad to caudad in this artery.

Each segment of the spinal cord receives its blood supply from opposing ascending and descending flows.[68] The superior area includes the cervical segment and the first two segments of the thoracic cord. The radiculomedullary arteries that supply this segment arise from the branches of the subclavian artery, but there are additional contributions of the vertebral arteries, resulting in a rich blood supply to this region. The midthoracic region, supplied by the anterior spinal artery, usually receives only one afferent vessel, which arises from a left or right intercostal vessel. The afferent arteries to the posterior spinal cord from T-2 to T-8 are also poor in collateralization. The blood supply to the thoracolumbar cord (from T-8 to the conus terminalis) is derived from the radicular artery known as the artery of Adamkiewicz. It arises from the left side in 60% of cases. In 75% of cases it joins the anterior spinal artery between T-8 and T-12, and in 10% of cases it joins between L-1 and L-2. Although other radicular arteries supply this third section, much of the blood flow in the anterior spinal artery is dependent on the artery of Adamkiewicz.

Because the flow in the spinal arteries is dependent on collateralization and is often bidirectional, the blood supply to the spinal cord can be "stolen" and "given" to the rest of the body when pressures in other areas of the body are lower. Such a situation may arise when a single high aorta-occluding clamp is applied. Thus, surgical techniques designed to minimize spinal cord ischemia include bypass shunts to supply blood to the lower extremities, femoro-femoral extracorporeal bypass techniques, double-clamping techniques, CSF drainage techniques, and preservation of the native aorta with its intercostal artery.[68,69] Only rarely will a patient develop complications from spinal cord ischemia, and this is a rare cause of morbidity and mortality in published series as well as in anecdotes. Nevertheless, the complications are so devastating that much energy is spent trying to prevent them. To date, the only definitive preventive methods are fast surgery and maintenance of normal cardiac function.[52,62-66]

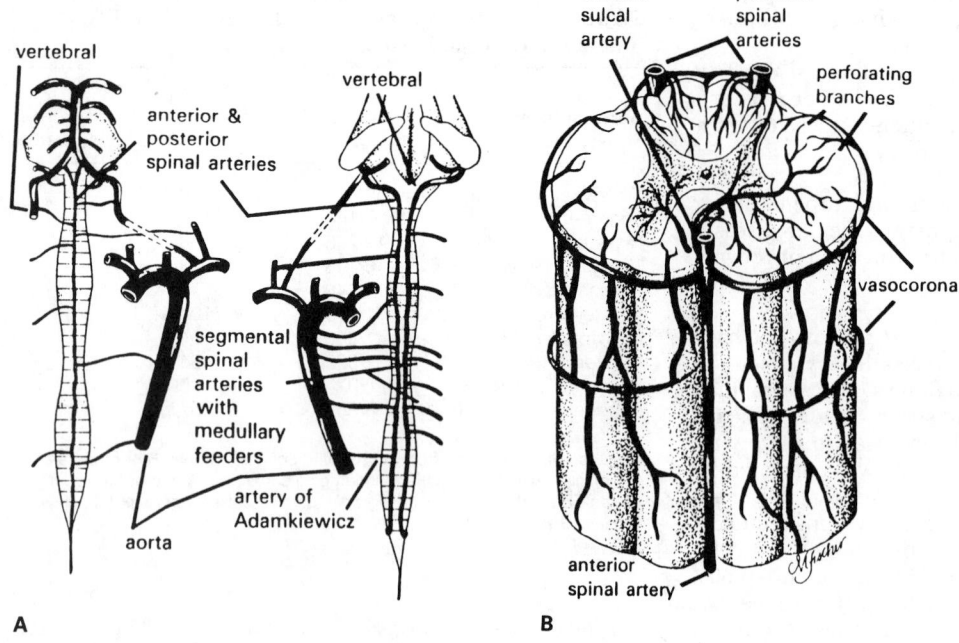

Figure 37-2. (*A*) Blood supply to spinal cord. (*B*) Segmental distribution of blood supply to spinal cord. (Reproduced with permission from Romero-Sierra C: Neuroanatomy—A Conceptual Approach. New York, Churchill Livingstone, 1986.)

Thus, in patients undergoing vascular surgery, the major cause of morbidity, and the factor limiting both perioperative and long-term survival in almost every series, relates to the heart. For this reason, the anesthetist should concentrate on preventing myocardial damage perioperatively in patients undergonig major vascular surgery. The central importance of the heart should be kept in mind when decisions are made on the management of co-morbid conditions such as hypertension, chronic obstructive lung disease, renal insufficiency, and diabetes.

THE PATIENT AND THE PATIENT'S DISORDERS

Many disorders are associated with vascular disease; however, diabetes, smoking and its sequelae, chronic pulmonary disease, hypertension and ischemic heart disease are the most common. Perhaps the most important factor in planning the perioperative management of these co-morbid conditions is understanding the end-organ effects of these diseases and understanding the appropriate drug therapy. Although it would be unusual to administer anesthesia to patients with uncontrolled hypertension, uncontrolled metabolic disease, or untreated pulmonary infections, or to patients in the first 6 months following a myocardial infarction when other portions of the myocardium are still at risk of infarction,[70-73] an expanding aneurysm, crescendo transient ischemic attacks (TIAs), or threatened limb loss can force one's hand. Attempts to control blood pressure or electrolytes rapidly may be more hazardous than leaving the condition untreated and trying to control the abnormality slowly. For example, rapid reduction of blood pressure in a patient with TIAs may precipitate cerebral ischemia and should be postponed to the postoperative period (if surgery cannot be delayed to permit gradual preoperative control of blood pressure). Similarly, stopping a drug may be more hazardous than continuing drug therapy and being cognizant of its effects.

Specific attempts have been made to identify, prior to surgical operations, patients at risk of 'myocardial insult.[1,19,70-85] An abnormal resting electrocardiograph (ECG) almost always indicates increased perioperative risk. An ECG obtained during exercise may not add substantially to the risk categorization afforded by the resting ECG.[74] Charlson et al[81] demonstrated that left ventricular hypertrophy on the ECG is associated with an increased risk of morbid cardiac events. Goldman et al[82] also reported that rhythms other than sinus rhythm indicate an increased risk.

A simple approach to preoperative evaluation is the use of Holter monitoring for detection of ischemia during daily life. Raby et al[75] found that one third of patients with preoperative ischemia had intraoperative complications, compared with only 1% of nonischemic patients. Further work may show Holter monitoring to be an inexpensive way of evaluating patients before the clinician proceeds to the tests described below.

Determination of systolic left ventricular function may provide prognostic information, because of the association of congestive heart failure with morbid postoperative events. Radionuclide angiography can define systolic and diastolic function. Most investigators attempting to predict operative risk have evaluated only systolic function; however, we are becoming increasingly aware that diastolic failure is also a problem, particularly for hypertensive patients.

Kazmers et al[76] studied 60 patients undergoing abdominal aortic aneurysm repair. Although patients with a low ejection fraction survived the operation and had no higher incidence of perioperative myocardial infarction (a tribute to modern perioperative management), their long-term survival was poor (50% vs. 86% at 20 months). When patients are selected for surgery, the relative risks of surgery, native CAD, and vascular disease are assessed, and the anesthetic risks to the patient are explained when he or she gives informed consent.

Pasternack et al[83] found that patients with an ejection fraction above 55% had no myocardial infarctions, whereas four of five patients with an ejection fraction below 35% had a myocardial infarction postoperatively within 48 hours. Their patients did not fare as well in the perioperative period as did those of Kazmers' group; still, a previous myocardial infarction predicted a 26% probability of reinfarction, and 50% of patients over 80 years of age sustained infarctions perioperatively.

Del Guercio et al[77] studied 148 elderly patients who had been cleared for major surgery by their internists. Preoperatively, patients were admitted to the intensive care unit (ICU) for insertion of a pulmonary artery (PA) catheter. Cardiac output, pulmonary capillary wedge pressure, and oxygen delivery were measured. Patients were classified into one of four stages, from normal to having severe, uncorrectable deficits. Severe hemodynamic abnormalities were detected in 34 patients, and surgery was canceled for most of these. All eight high-risk patients who underwent the planned surgical procedure died, whereas the mortality was zero for Stage 1 patients and 8.5% for Stage 2 and Stage 3 patients.

Another method advocated for preoperative risk assessment is dipyridamole-thallium scanning. Dipyridamole is a potent coronary vasodilator that produces a coronary steal by increasing blood flow to normal areas and diminishing collateral flow to poststenotic areas. Areas that are prone to ischemia are hypoperfused after dipyridamole administration; several hours later, when the steal has subsided, the areas are perfused normally. Such areas are said to have a redistribution defect. Fixed defects represent old myocardial infarctions.

The Massachusetts General Hospital's experience[78] with dipyridamole-thallium scintigraphy has yielded two important observations: an old myocardial infarction is not a risk factor in itself, and an area of redistribution (i.e., myocardium at risk) is associated with an adverse outcome. The most recent results of this group[71] suggest that dipyridamole-thallium scintigraphy is most helpful in risk stratification of patients at intermediate risk based on clinical evaluation. If a patient has a low clinical risk or a negative dipyridamole-thallium study, one might choose, given the low rate of adverse cardiac events, to forgo extensive invasive monitoring and extended ICU care, with the potential for reducing costs and iatrogenic complications.

Patients who are at high risk should probably not undergo dipyridamole-thallium scintigraphy; rather, they should undergo coronary angiography and revascularization or give informed consent that addresses the high risk of their surgery. Preoperative CABG or coronary angioplasty may be useful, although the capacity of the former to decrease perioperative mortality has been debated. Patients with uncorrected CAD, however, have greatly diminished survival after abdominal aortic aneurysm surgery (Table 37-3).

Patients with a markedly positive dipyridamole-thallium study should probably undergo myocardial revascularization. In a study of 66 patients, Lette et al[79] found that those with markedly positive scans (16 patients) were more likely to die (7 of 10 patients operated on) if surgery was not canceled. Recently, Mangano et al[84] challenged the effectiveness of dipyridamole-thallium scintigraphy for the preoperative screening of vascular surgery patients, but their view was dismissed by an accompanying editorial.[72] Further, 80% of diabetics undergoing vascular surgery have positive dipyridamole scans, and only by quantifying the degree of redistribution is it possible to stratify the risk of the diabetic patient with this scan. Lane et al[80] studied 101 diabetics and found that neither the type of anesthesia (regional vs. general), the use of PA catheters, the site of surgery (aortic vs. femoral), nor the use of nitroglycerin infusions predicted outcome. The presence of angina and a high Goldman classification did predict cardiac complications, as did the presence of more than two reversible effects, or defects in distribution in the left anterior descending artery. Thus, when patients are segregated preoperatively for either more invasive monitoring, CABG, or PTCA before vascular surgery, such procedures have been criticized as just survival tests accompanied by increased short-term morbidity. Until randomized, controlled studies are performed, we will follow the outline proposed in Figure 37-3. Until these procedures gain widespread acceptance, and until extensive trials are shown to reduce overall mortality, the goal of optimizing care and minimizing myocardial morbidity seems logical. This goal is based on both the preoperative likelihood of

TABLE 37-3. Incidence of Perioperative Myocardial Ischemia Determined with Continuous Holter Monitoring*

Study	Time Patients Were Studied/ Type of Surgery	No. of Patients	Patients with Ischemia, No. (%)	No. of Ischemic Episodes	Average Duration of Ischemia (min)
Knight et al[85]	Preoperatively/CABG	50	21 (42)	124	16
Ouyang et al[4]	Preoperatively/Vascular with CAD	24	3 (12.5)	4	20
Raby et al[75]	Preoperatively/Vascular	176	32 (18)	75	36
Ouyang et al[4]	Intraoperatively/Vascular	24	5 (21)	8	32
London et al[247]	Intraoperatively/Noncardiac Surgery with known or suspected CAD	105	25 (24)	51	10
Ouyang et al[4]	Postoperatively/Vascular	24	15 (62)	45	41

*Note that the intraoperative period does not appear more stressful than the preoperative or postoperative period.

Reproduced with permission from Ellis JE, Busse JR, Foss JF, Roizen MF: Postoperative management of myocardial ischemia. Anesthesiol Clin North Am 9(3):609, 1991.

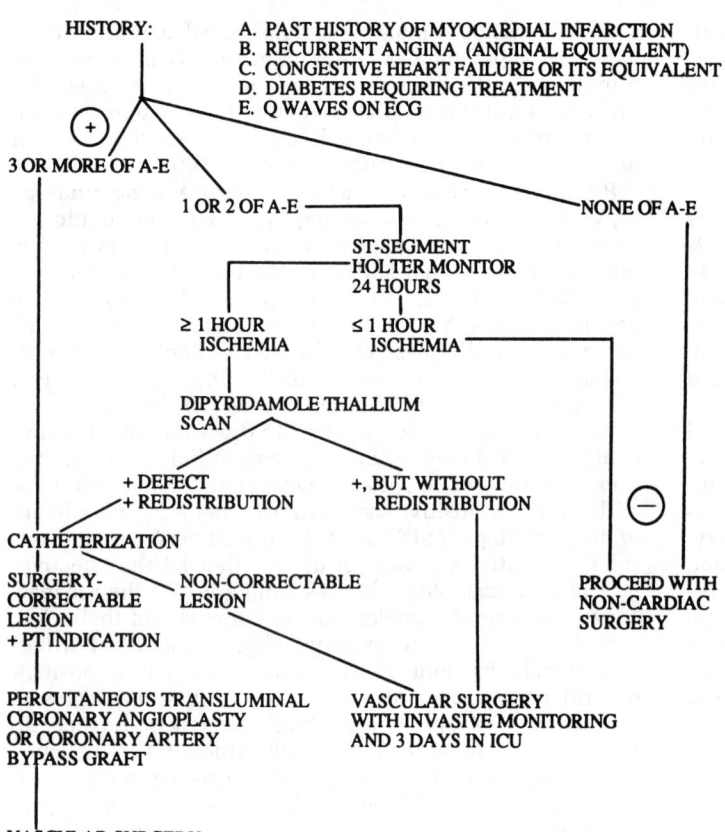

HISTORY:
A. PAST HISTORY OF MYOCARDIAL INFARCTION
B. RECURRENT ANGINA (ANGINAL EQUIVALENT)
C. CONGESTIVE HEART FAILURE OR ITS EQUIVALENT
D. DIABETES REQUIRING TREATMENT
E. Q WAVES ON ECG

3 OR MORE OF A-E

1 OR 2 OF A-E

NONE OF A-E

ST-SEGMENT
HOLTER MONITOR
24 HOURS

≥ 1 HOUR ISCHEMIA

≤ 1 HOUR ISCHEMIA

DIPYRIDAMOLE THALLIUM SCAN

+ DEFECT + REDISTRIBUTION

+, BUT WITHOUT REDISTRIBUTION

CATHETERIZATION

SURGERY- CORRECTABLE LESION + PT INDICATION

NON-CORRECTABLE LESION

PROCEED WITH NON-CARDIAC SURGERY

PERCUTANEOUS TRANSLUMINAL CORONARY ANGIOPLASTY OR CORONARY ARTERY BYPASS GRAFT

VASCULAR SURGERY WITH INVASIVE MONITORING AND 3 DAYS IN ICU

VASCULAR SURGERY

Figure 37-3. Algorithm for evaluating whether more invasive monitoring, coronary artery bypass grafting, or percutaneous transluminal coronary angioplasty should be performed before vascular surgery.

CAD in patients with vascular disorders and the fact that the major cause of morbidity and mortality following vascular surgery is related to the heart.

SURGERY FOR CEREBROVASCULAR INSUFFICIENCY

Surgical Approaches

Two groups of surgical approaches are available for the treatment and prevention of cerebrovascular insufficiency: EC-IC bypass and carotid endarterectomy. The EC-IC bypass is used to increase the collateral blood flow to a presumably focal ischemic area of the brain. In recent multicenter trials, this operation did not improve the neurologic outcome from either strokes in evolution or completed strokes.[86-88] Further, patients who underwent EC-IC bypass surgery had greater immediate disability and no better long-term prognosis than patients treated medically. Thus, it appears that the EC-IC bypass may have few indications, except possibly to prevent strokes in patients who have TIAs thought to be flow- and not embolus-related and who have bilateral occlusions or lesions located so high in the carotid artery as to preclude extracranial carotid surgery.[89] As it is therefore expected that this operation will be performed only rarely (and it has been performed with less than one-hundredth the frequency of carotid endarterectomy at our institution), we will deal with it only briefly here.

In EC-IC bypass, blood flow to the brain should be interrupted only during the short period of the EC-IC anastomosis to the recipient vessel, and shunting of the flow during such time is usually not an option. Therefore, the monitors used for making judgments about the need for shunting, the adequacy of the shunt, and the adequacy of the repair are not necessary. Otherwise, the basic goals of surgery and anesthesia, the monitoring strategies, and the anesthetic techniques are quite similar to those used in carotid endarterectomy, because the patients in both groups have similar medical and surgical problems and pose similar challenges.

In carotid endarterectomy, surgical approaches vary by surgical group, but the aim is to gain a smooth ulcer- and plaque-free vessel with smooth end points and no emboli or intraoperative neurologic ischemia.[90] To achieve these goals, most surgeons wish to have some measure of cerebral blood flow (CBF) or neurologic function, whereas others rely solely on shunting of the carotid blood flow of all patients, and still others rely on skillful general anethesia and short occlusion times. All of these techniques have been used with success by surgeons experienced in their use.[11,13,14,24-26,39,91-93]

Initially, the internal carotid artery is isolated where the plaque or ulcerative lesion has been demonstrated radiographically (usually starting near the bifurcation). Heparin is given in a dose of 2,000–20,000 units for a 70-kg person. The dose varies according to the surgical group and appears to be based on local custom, although some rationale has been sought for the dose selected.[94] The surgeon isolates the diseased carotid segment with clamps or ties placed on the proximal and distal internal carotid artery and on the external carotid artery. After a period of test occlusion during which regional cerebral blood flow (rCBF), neurologic function, EEG, processed EEG, SSEPs, stump pressure, transcranial pulsed Doppler flows, or nothing is measured, an incision is made into the artery, and a shunt is inserted (usually first in the proximal vessel and then in the distal vessel, often with clamps, sometimes with ties; often with a pressure-measuring side arm to ensure that one or more ends are not crimped or occluded). Because insertion of a shunt is associated with at least a 0.7% embolism-associated stroke rate,[95] routine shunting is not advocated by everyone.

The surgeon then endarterectomizes the ulcerated or plaque-containing area, leaving a smooth intimal surface joining the endarterectomized vessel and native vessel. Occasionally a long or tortuous region is shortened by resection and reanastomosis, or if the remaining portion of the intima is too thin, a vein (often from the leg) or a Dacron patch is used. Because suturing of the patch requires more time than suturing of the native vessel, an internal shunt is frequently used during these procedures. Time is of the essence because, at a stump pressure of 40 mm Hg, neurologic dysfunction can occur in 40 minutes, and it is common when occlusion times extend beyond 60 minutes (see Anesthetic Goals and Monitoring Techniques—Carotid Stump Pressure).[96] The future for vein patch grafts is bright with the potential for endogenous vasodilator genes vectored into the vein patch (J. Moss, pers. commun.).[97,98]

If the shunt has been used, it is then removed, and, in all cases, the arteriotomy is closed, usually with a running suture. Shunt placement and removal rarely take less than 1 minute or more than 4 minutes, and the total occlusion time rarely exceeds 40 minutes.

Most surgeons wish to have their patients awaken soon after skin closure, because a new neurologic deficit is thought by some to demand immediate re-exploration, or at least arteriography.[99] A few surgeons routinely perform arteriography after restoring blood flow, but most believe that the complications of routine arteriography (emboli, allergic reactions, vasospasm, bleeding from the puncture hole, and stroke) are greater than its benefits (the rare detection of inadequate repairs, suture lines, or flow). One approach is to use duplex ultrasonography to image the resutured vessel at the end of surgery. This approach avoids the risks of arteriography, but the benefits have not yet been established by randomized controlled trials.[100]

Anesthetic Goals and Monitoring Techniques

For minimal morbidity and mortality, the anesthetic goals are, first, to protect the heart from ischemia, and, second, to protect the brain from ischemia. Some experienced anesthesiologists believe that the order of priority of these goals should be reversed.[89,101] However, because the major cause of morbidity relates to the heart, and because anesthesiologists can have more influence over the heart than the brain, protection of the heart likely should receive a higher priority. Unfortunately, the two goals are often in conflict.

To decrease myocardial oxygen requirements, one tries to decrease the heart rate and blood pressure and the contractility of the myocardium.[102] To maintain oxygen delivery to the brain, one tries to increase the cerebral perfusion pressure and decrease the cerebral metabolic requirements. For

TABLE 37-4. Compromise Solutions That Allow Both Myocardial and Central Nervous System Protection during Carotid Endarterectomy

Hemodynamic Variable	To Protect the Heart From Ischemia	To Protect the Brain From Ischemia
Heart rate	Slow	Don't slow
Blood pressure	Decrease	Increase cerebral perfusion pressure
Contractility	Decrease	Increase

Compromise Solutions

1. Inject area of carotid bifurcation with 1% lidocaine for 10–15 min.
2. Decrease cerebral and myocardial metabolic rate and contractility.
3. Use normal findings on EEG or processed EEG to guide afterload reduction.

increased cerebral perfusion pressure, an attempt is made to increase the arterial blood pressure at least to levels above which the normal brain autoregulates.[26,96,103,104] This usually also means trying to avoid severe bradycardia or decreasing central venous pressure.

Not only blood pressure reduction and augmentation but also heart rate changes lead to conflicts in priority management of the heart versus the brain. However, certain compromise solutions allow the well-being of both heart and brain to be maintained (Table 37-4). To decrease the myocardial work, one tries to decrease the heart rate, but sudden bradycardia can occur when the surgeon stretches the baroreceptor nerve endings directly (because of atherosclerosis, these nerve endings are supersensitive, since they usually have not been stretched easily by blood pressure changes over a period of many years). Sudden bradycardia can result in substantial decreases in arterial pressure, which could compromise collateral cerebral perfusion. Injection of the area of the bifurcation with 1% lidocaine 10–15 minutes before the carotid artery is to be occluded unites the two goals by facilitating a stable heart rate of approximately 70 beats·min^{-1}. In addition, the goals of decreasing myocardial contractility and decreasing the cerebral metabolic rate are consonant, regardless of whether the major anesthetic is thiopental or isoflurane.

To maintain blood pressure, one usually uses light anesthesia (without paralysis, so that inadequate anesthesia can be detected), allowing native vasopressor substances to maintain blood pressure. This light anesthesia technique has been associated with a substantially lower incidence of myocardial ischemia than was possible with deeper anesthesia and administration of phenylephrine.[26] In fact, one of the major benefits of EEG or processed EEG monitoring is that when the EEG is normal or remains unchanged from pre- to postclamping of the carotid artery, one can decrease the blood pressure to facilitate protection of the heart.

The theoretical hemodynamic and metabolic means for facilitating the goals of protecting the heart and brain from ischemia should work in practice. It would be reassuring, however, to have monitors to ensure that these goals are actually being met. Unfortunately, the detection of both myocardial and cerebral ischemia by monitors during general or regional anesthesia is imperfect at present, with both false-negative and false-positive results confusing technicians.

Myocardial Ischemia

ST-T Segments of the ECG. Lead V_5 is usually selected as the monitor. However, in a study that we performed, ST segments of even seven leads of the ECG did not allow detection of 75% of the cases of myocardial ischemia that were detected from changes in regional wall motion and from wall-thickening defects on two-dimensional transesophageal echocardiography (2D-TEE).[105] In carotid and aortic vascular surgery, the ECG had a 40–60% sensitivity if systolic wall motion abnormalities and wall-thickening abnormalities were considered the ultimate standard.[106] In addition, lead V_5 was insensitive compared with other leads, notably II, for ischemia during carotid endarterectomy.

ECG Monitoring with ST Segment Trend Analysis (Two or Three Leads). Although these devices are purported to facilitate detection of myocardial ischemia more easily than can be obtained with simple oscilloscopic ECG traces, and although they might meet this stated goal,[106,107] one should not expect them to be as sensitive as an ECG printout or 2D-TEE. In one study, they were approximately 70–90% as sensitive as a hard-copy ECG.[106]

Changes in PCWP or Appearance of V Waves on PCWP. Although changes in pulmonary capillary wedge pressure (PCWP) in the absence of systemic pressure changes or fluid administration may be a sensitive indicator of myocardial ischemia, such changes are not specific. The appearance of v waves on the PCWP recording may be specific (indication of ischemia where it is present), but v waves are not sensitive (normal where ischemia is not present) indicators of myocardial ischemia.[108] In addition, with the 2% carotid arterial puncture rate during cannulation of the internal jugular vein that has been reported in large series, it is difficult to justify that route during this operation. Most surgeons postpone the operation to another day after disturbing the contralateral carotid. The risks of PA catheter insertion from subclavian, external jugular, arm, or femoral sites do not justify the benefit. A PA catheter is justified only in rare cases in which the patient is to undergo general anesthesia and the only evidence of myocardial ischemia is PCWP changes without ST segment changes, or in operations in which 2D-TEE is unavailable or satisfactory echograms cannot be obtained.

Angina in Patients Undergoing Regional Anesthesia. No reports on the usefulness of this symptom are available. The rates of myocardial ischemia and death from myocardial mechanisms after carotid endarterectomy performed during regional anesthesia are similar to rates following general anesthesia.[109,110]

Cerebral Ischemia

Repeated Neurologic Evaluation of the Conscious Patient. Repeated neurologic evaluation is cited as a major reason for choosing regional anesthesia. Heavily sedated patients cannot cooperate. Regional anesthesia thus requires a completely successful blockade and a surgeon who is accustomed to operating under this technique. Usually the carotid artery is occluded for a 1–4-minute trial period; if no deficit is detected on neurologic examination, the surgeon proceeds with the endarterectomy. If a new neurologic deficit occurs, the surgeon releases the clamp. After reperfusion and return of neurologic function, some surgeons immediately proceed to reocclude the vessels and try to insert a shunt and complete the surgical procedure rapidly. However, most surgeons prefer to cancel surgery at this point and return on another day to perform the procedure under general anesthesia with a shunt. Still other surgeons consider lack of tolerance for carotid occlusion to be a contraindication to any further carotid surgery on such patients.[61] The disadvantages of the technique include the need for patient cooperation; the possible loss of patient cooperation with the onset of a neurologic deficit because of confusion, panic, or seizures; the possibility that an unexpected, delayed deficit will develop at some time after the test period; the inability to administer drugs such as thiopental, which might protect the brain; and the inability to secure the airway should panic, seizure, or oversedation occur. Those surgeons who revert to general anesthesia in the event of a deficit in response to test occlusion seem to perceive general anesthesia as best for the worst cases; if this is so, as J. Michenfelder states, "It should be best for most cases."[101]

Techniques for the evaluation of neurologic function during general anesthesia are discussed next.

Electroencephalogram. The scalp-recorded EEG reflects the electrical activity of the underlying cortical tissue. Conventional recording methods provide vast amounts of information, including a voltage value at each instant in time for each pair (16 or more) of electrodes. However, interpretation of this type of information is unwieldy in the operating room (OR). Data reduction methods have been developed to describe the EEG in terms of several calculated variables, and the changes in these variables are charted over time.

Various physiologic and anesthetic manipulations have effects on the EEG. Reductions in CBF, temperature changes, hypotension, and the administration of anesthetic agents have characteristic effects on the EEG. The proper interpretation of intraoperative EEG changes requires familiarity with the effects of the commonly used anesthetic agents and of temperature on the EEG. It should be remembered, however, that the blood flow threshold for electrical failure (approximately 18 ml·100 g^{-1}·min^{-1}) is higher than the blood flow threshold for metabolic failure (approximately 10–12 ml·100 g^{-1}·min^{-1}).[111]

The EEG can be viewed in a raw form, or it can be subjected to various transformations. For example, on-line assessment of the brain's electrical activity was made simpler with the development of rapid computerized Fourier transformation of the EEG into spectral arrays of power and frequency. Generally, if focal ischemia occurs, the usual change is a localized decrease in frequency or a decrease in amplitude, or both.

How well does the EEG function as an early signal of impending ischemia? Does EEG monitoring improve outcome after carotid endarterectomy? These are quite different questions. The EEG is a sensitive early-warning device, but it is not very specific (too many false-positive results), and we have no idea whether outcome is improved by its use. However, myocardial well-being may be improved more than cerebral well-being.

In the Mayo Clinic series of 1145 patients who underwent carotid endarterectomy with monitoring by EEG and xenon blood flow measurements, no patient awoke from anesthesia with a new deficit that had not been predicted from the EEG. An analysis of the results of a series of 111 patients who underwent carotid endarterectomy monitored with a single channel of the EEG that was analyzed in real time to produce a density spectral array[112] revealed that, among patients with no preoperative neurologic deficit, new postoperative deficits appeared in only the five patients who had ischemic EEG events of 5 or more minutes' duration. However, the EEG was not as predictive of outcome in patients who had an existing preoperative neurologic deficit. One such patient without intraoperative EEG changes developed a new postoperative deficit, and one patient with EEG changes lasting 13 minutes had no demonstrable new deficit postoperatively.

The need for caution when monitoring patients with preexisting neurologic deficits was emphasized in a report of 125 patients who had had strokes or reversible ischemic neurologic deficits and who underwent carotid endarterectomy.[113] Four patients in that study awoke with new deficits, despite unchanged EEGs.

In a study of a series of 172 carotid endarterectomies,[114] EEG monitoring was undertaken in only the last 93 cases. The use of EEG monitoring was associated with a reduction in the use of indwelling shunts (from 49% to 12%) and a reduction in the combined major neurologic morbidity and mortality rates (from 2.3% to 1.1%). However, that study used historical controls and was nonrandomized. Others have cited evidence of patients without reversible ischemic neurologic deficits who awoke with abnormal neurologic status even though they had had normal EEGs.[115]

Some investigators have shown that EEG monitoring may be of limited use, because 65–95% of neurologic deficits following carotid endarterectomy are due to thromboembolic and not flow-related events. Although both can easily be detected with the EEG, no major benefit will be achieved with any therapeutic maneuver in the 65–95% of patients in whom neurologic problems are detected. In fact, if more shunts or a higher afterload result, more emboli or worsening of myocardial oxygen balance could ensue. For example, one group[116] reviewed its experience with 176 consecutive patients who underwent carotid endarterectomy without shunting but with EEG monitoring. The authors concluded that, although the majority of clamp-associated EEG changes were related to lowered rCBF, postoperative deficits were usually caused by embolism. Other studies have yielded similar results.[117]

Other issues that have been raised in the evaluation of the appropriateness of EEG monitoring for carotid endarterectomy include false-positive and false-negative results and the cost-effectiveness of EEG monitoring. Intraoperative false-positive results, that is, changes in the EEG without accompanying demonstrable deficits, may be related to several factors. First, the brain can tolerate relatively brief periods of ischemia without infarction. Thus, temporary, reversible EEG changes should not be expected in association with postoperative deficits. Second, the EEG is a sensitive but nonspecific measure of ischemia. The EEG can be affected by factors such as anesthesia or alterations in temperature and blood pressure, as well as by cerebral ischemia. Third, as stated previously, the flow threshold for electrical failure is higher than the flow threshold for metabolic failure. This means that, whereas the EEG may be viewed as an early-warning system for cerebral ischemia, not all EEG changes indicate that ischemia is taking place. Fourth, focal embolic events may not be detected by the EEG. Except as noted previously—that is, in patients with pre-existing neurologic deficits, strokes in evolution, or recent reversible ischemic neurologic deficits—there are relatively few reports of false-negative results.

In general, patients without intraoperative EEG changes do not awaken with new neurologic deficits. Because most neurologic deficits following carotid endarterectomy are not the result of flow-related ischemia, the detection of EEG changes does not guarantee reversibility upon shunt placement. In fact, shunt placement is associated with a low but definite risk of causing emboli. However, as newer agents that may be able to preserve marginal tissue surrounding an infarct become available, perhaps even some neurologic damage following an embolus can be reversed.

Evaluation of the cost-effectiveness of EEG monitoring can be thought of as a comparison of the cost of monitoring with the cost of the deficits that monitoring may prevent. Let us assume that 100,000 carotid endarterectomies are performed each year with a deficit rate of 3% (3000 new deficits each year), and that the use of monitoring devices might prevent one sixth of these deficits (500 deficits per year). One might assume that an additional 15% of patients would undergo temporary shunting of carotid flow because of EEG monitoring and that 0.7% would experience "shunt insertion–associated" neurologic deficits. This would result in an additional 106 deficits related to the monitoring, or a net 394 deficits preventable by the monitoring. If each deficit cost $100,000, on average, in medical care, loss of wages and productivity, and quality-adjusted years of life, the deficits preventable by monitoring would cost $39,400,000 per year. The break-even point for monitoring costs would be $394 per patient: at that price, the cost of monitoring would equal the cost of the deficits that monitoring would prevent. If monitoring could be provided for less than $394, it would be cost-effective.

This analysis neglects the benefit that EEG monitoring may have in preserving myocardial function. It also neglects factors to which no dollar amount can be assigned, such as human suffering. If different values are assumed for the cost per deficit, for the percentage of deficits preventable by monitoring, for the deficit rate, or for the shunt insertion–caused deficit rate, the break-even point will be higher or lower. But as long as the percentage of deficits preventable by EEG monitoring is not zero, the break-even point will also not be zero. This implies that there is some cost below which monitoring is cost-effective for large-scale application, assuming that EEG monitoring is better at prevention than other monitoring strategies, such as SSEPs or stump pressure (see the section on Carotid Stump Pressure below).

However, it is possible that EEG monitoring would allow the anesthesiologist to maintain a lower blood pressure during the period of temporary carotid occlusion than would be feasible if only stump pressure were used. Thus, EEG monitoring may provide a benefit in allowing the anesthesiologist to decrease the afterload in the patient who is at risk for myocardial ischemic events, as well as permitting an unhurried and technically superior endarterectomy, identifying delayed ischemia, and aiding in the detection of other problems such as shunt malfunction.

Unfortunately, there are no data showing that EEG demonstration of neurologic dysfunction during carotid endarterectomy results in better patient outcome than does any other method.

Somatosensory-Evoked Potential. Evoked potentials offer a method of processing the neural activity after a stimulus in which activity that is stimulus-related (signal) is separated from activity that is not stimulus-related (noise). The primary problem with evoked potentials is an unfavorable signal-to-noise ratio. The neural potentials evoked by any sensory stimulus are small compared with the spontaneous activity that is recorded at the same time. When recorded noninvasively from the scalp, evoked cerebral electrical activity (the signal) from electrical stimulation of a peripheral nerve amounts to a few microvolts in amplitude, whereas the spontaneous electrical activity (noise) of the cerebrum can be on the order of 100 μV or more. The assumption made for separating the signal from the noise is that the signal is always found after a certain latency period following the stimulation, whereas the noise bears no temporal relationship to the stimulus. By giving repeated stimuli and summing (or averaging) the resulting responses, one can average out the noise.[118]

The evoked potential used most frequently during vascular procedures is the SSEP. This evoked potential is usually elicited by electrical stimulation of a selected peripheral nerve at an intensity sufficient to cause a twitch of the muscles supplied by that nerve. The resulting afferent activity may be recorded from rostral portions of the nerve, the spinal cord and brain stem, and thalamocortical projections. The variables that describe evoked potentials are the *latency* (related to the conduction velocity characteristics of the pathway) and the *amplitude* (related to the number and synchrony of conducting fibers in the pathway) of the afferent volley recorded at successively higher levels of the nervous system. Damage to the pathways mediating these responses is manifested as alterations in these two variables.[119]

Investigators have started to examine SSEPs as a monitor of neurologic function during carotid endarterectomy. Those who have monitored SSEPs during carotid endarterectomy with both cervical plexus blockade and general anesthesia have reported that the SSEP has a sensitivity of about 60% and a specificity of 100% for cerebral ischemia and the need for a shunt.[119] The rate of shunt placement based on SSEPs was roughly the same as when selective shunting was based on the EEG—that is, about 10%. Thus, the benefit of SSEPs in monitoring of neurologic function during carotid endarterectomy is in doubt. They clearly reflect some abnormalities, and perhaps when combined with EEG have a more acceptable sensitivity and specificity.[120]

Regional Cerebral Blood Flow. Measurement of rCBF usually involves washout of a radioisotope such as ^{133}Xe after its injection into a surgically occluded carotid artery.[11] Flows above 24 ml·min^{-1}·100 g^{-1} brain are regarded as satisfactory, and those below 18 ml·min^{-1}·100 g^{-1} brain are considered to indicate the potential for cerebral ischemia. These measurements require expensive and highly technical equipment in the OR. Of the few centers that have such equipment, one has reported an excellent correlation between CBF and outcome, but flow differences representing ischemia were dependent on the anesthetic agents used.[11,121] Questions about this method of monitoring involve both its sensitivity and its specificity. As with all the other monitors of neurologic function during carotid endarterectomy, no benefit has yet been shown for it.

Middle Cerebral Artery Blood Flow. Transcutaneous pulsed Doppler has been used to monitor blood velocity in the middle cerebral artery of patients undergoing carotid endarterectomy.[122] The technique is in its infancy and requires a skilled operator's constant attention. To date, no data on its sensitivity or specificity in routine settings have been published. Because transcutaneous pulsed Doppler indicates the velocity and direction of flow, one can presume that knowledge of contralateral flow and the influence of anesthetic maneuvers on it will be forthcoming.

Carotid Stump Pressure. Stump pressure (mean blood pressure distal to the carotid clamp, sometimes termed back-pressure) is widely used for evaluation of the adequacy of cerebral perfusion during carotid surgery. Cerebral ischemia rarely occurs at stump pressures above 60 mm Hg during halothane anesthesia, presumably because of the excellent collateral circulation needed to maintain that pressure[96,123] and because of the autoregulation that is present at this level. If the stump pressure decreases below that value, the likelihood of ischemia increases. However, because pressure is not identical to flow, it is possible for stump pressures to be below 60 mm Hg and the flow to be perfectly adequate.

The major criticism of the use of stump pressure concerns the large number of false-positive results—that is, a stump pressure of less than 60 mm Hg and an rCBF of more than 24 ml·min^{-1}·100 g^{-1} brain. Such results occur in about 30% of patients.[123] Thus, a shunt may be placed when none is needed. However, the simplicity of the measurement and its validity when the pressure exceeds 60 mm Hg during anesthesia with volatile anesthetics still render it a useful clinical method for ensuring adequate perfusion during carotid endarterectomy. The stump pressure must be higher during an opioid-based anesthesia for blood flow to be adequate.[123] The technique, however, appears operator dependent.[124]

As with all other measures, no benefit has been proved for the use of stump pressure, but logic dictates that monitors that ensure adequate cerebral function at the lowest myocardial work have a role during carotid endarterectomy.

Appropriateness of Carotid Endarterectomy. A number of investigators have questioned whether carotid endarterectomy should be performed in patients with asymptomatic lesions, or for that matter in patients with symptomatic lesions. It is clear from the data available that the surgical team (including anesthesiologist and hospital setting) should know its own outcome from carotid procedures. Teams with a greater than 2% rate of stroke in asymptomatic disease or a greater than 4% rate of myocardial infarction in patients with stable angina might consider referring their patients to centers with documented lower morbidity rates.[125-127] More than 70% of patients with symptomatic disease and stenoses deserve surgical repair. Evaluation of the criteria for repair no doubt will continue during the next several years.[128,129]

Anesthesia for Surgery for Cerebrovascular Insufficiency

Many surgeons have requested general anesthesia for surgery on patients with cerebrovascular insufficiency. If the patient has no medical problem that requires optimization before surgery, the preoperative interview focuses on reducing anxiety, obtaining informed consent, and searching for the status of end-organs likely to be affected by atherosclerosis, hypertension, or other diseases. In addition, multiple blood pressure and heart rate readings are obtained while the patient is in various positions, and nurses are asked to obtain at least four additional such readings (one every 2 hours while the patient is awake and one during the night) before surgery. If multiple readings of vital signs and prehydration are not performed—for example, when carotid endarterectomy is a "come-and-stay" procedure—morbidity may increase.

Preoperative values become important in defining a range of acceptable intraoperative values. Such preoperative data are used to determine the individualized range of values considered tolerable for a particular patient during and after

surgery. For example, if the blood pressure is 180/100 mm Hg and the heart rate is 96 beats·min^{-1} on admission, with no signs or symptoms of myocardial ischemia, the patient can probably tolerate these levels during surgery. If the blood pressure decreases during the night to 80/50 mm Hg, the heart rate decreases to 48 beats·min^{-1}, and the patient does not awaken with signs of a new cerebral deficit, he or she can probably safely tolerate such levels during anesthesia. Thus, an individualized set of values is derived from preoperative data for each patient. The cardiovascular variables are kept within that range intraoperatively, and, prior to induction of anesthesia, the anesthesiologist decides which therapies to use to accomplish that goal (e.g., administration of more or less anesthesia, nitroglycerin, or nitroprusside/dopamine, dobutamine, phenylephrine, or esmolol/isoproterenol, atropine).

This type of planning is especially important for the patient with suspected cardiovascular disease, as is usual in the patient undergoing carotid endarterectomy. It is relatively unimportant for the totally healthy patient. It is unknown whether keeping cardiovascular variables within an individualized range of acceptable values improves the surgical outcome, but logic implies that using such a plan would reduce morbidity. For example, in several studies, major intraoperative deviations of the blood pressure from the preoperative level have been correlated with the occurrence of myocardial ischemia.[26,40,130]

These acceptable values are listed at the top of the anesthesia record before induction of anesthesia. Before working with surgeons who routinely used the EEG, I worked with surgeons who wanted the patient's blood pressure to be at the upper end of his ward pressure. This desire on the part of the surgeons was based on data indicating better collateral CBF distal to a carotid occlusion if the systemic blood pressure was higher.[104] On the other hand, such an increase in blood pressure increases the work that the heart has to perform and thus increases the likelihood of myocardial ischemia.[26,102] If the surgeon requires an increase in the patient's blood pressure above his or her upper limits of normal, as surgeons sometimes do for a patient whose carotid flow cannot be shunted because of the anatomy of the lesion, we do so in a test period preoperatively, asking questions about angina and examining seven ECG leads for evidence of ischemia. We rarely use a PA catheter during carotid surgery. Very few patients with myocardial ischemia have PCWP changes without ECG changes. I have tried to avoid inserting PA catheters during carotid artery surgery for two reasons: (1) there is little fluid shift during these operations, and (2) the rate of complications associated with PA catheters is reported to exceed that from carotid artery surgery at our institution.

Other data obtained during the preoperative visit and assessment are the ECG lead most likely to reveal ischemia (often found on an exercise ECG study or from evaluation of a thallium redistribution study; see above) and the patient's normal Paco$_2$. It can usually be assumed that the latter is normal if the patient's bicarbonate level on an electrolyte panel is normal or if the patient's history does not suggest chronic obstructive pulmonary disease.

Controversy exists concerning the optimal intraoperative carbon dioxide level in patients undergoing carotid endarterectomy.[104] Most practitioners now opt for slight hypocarbia or normocarbia.[89,101,104] Maintaining slight hypocarbia has the possible advantage of preferentially diverting CBF to potentially ischemic areas of the brain by constricting the nonischemic, normally reactive vessels.[89,101]

Historically, we have not given any premedication to patients about to undergo carotid artery surgery because this might delay awakening and might confuse the results of tests of mental function prior to induction of anesthesia. Although we worried about the possibility of increasing anxiety[131] and causing myocardial ischemia because of this lack of premedication, only one patient among the 1500 we "premedicated" with only an interview for this operation has arrived in the preoperative holding area or OR with angina or ECG evidence of myocardial ischemia. Either the preoperative interview is very effective[131] or there is a substantial difference between our patients and those of Slogoff and Keats.[130] Thus, local custom as well as logical considerations have led us to seek the following goals, with the techniques indicated:

1. Avoid myocardial ischemia by maintaining normal hemodynamics (especially normal heart rates). For this purpose, we usually monitor lead V$_5$ and lead II of the ECG for ST-T and heart rate changes and the transesophageal echocardiogram for wall-motion and systolic wall-thickening abnormalities.
2. Avoid cerebral ischemia by maintaining normal or high-normal blood pressure and by shunting carotid flow if an abnormal EEG develops; maintain slight hypocarbia.
3. Use general anesthesia, but have the patient awake at the end of the operation. To this end, we avoid drug premedication and "premedicate" only by interview, and we use light levels of volatile agents for general anesthesia.
4. Delay operations when there is uncontrolled hypertension, untreated pulmonary disease, myocardial infarction less than 3 months old with areas of myocardium still at risk, and uncontrolled metabolic diseases, unless crescendo TIAs are present.

Obviously, some goals are in conflict and some have been modified by study results. For example, we could provide deeper anesthesia and maintain blood pressure with an alpha$_1$-adrenergic drug such as phenylephrine. However, we found that light general anesthesia and maintenance of the same systolic pressure is associated with one-third the incidence of myocardial ischemia than that associated with deep anesthesia and the use of vasopressors to attain that blood pressure.[26] The usual procedure is described below.

After the preoperative interview, the patient is restricted from oral intake after midnight and an intravenous (iv) infusion of normal saline is begun (we now avoid dextrose; see below) through an 18-gauge plastic cannula at a maintenance rate of 100 ml·h^{-1}·70 kg^{-1}. Fluid administration is intended to ensure that the patient is not hypovolemic and thus subject to a large decrease in blood pressure during induction of anesthesia. When the patient arrives in the preoperative holding area, an 18-gauge arterial catheter is placed (after iodine preparation and lidocaine skin wheal) in the radial artery contralateral to the planned carotid surgery. This arterial catheter is 18 gauge rather than 20 gauge because no greater morbidity ensues[132] and because the 20-gauge catheter tends to have a 5–10% incidence of kinking when surgeons push on the arm with their bellies during carotid dissection. Normal saline, rather than dextrose or lactated Ringer's solution, is used because lactate is metabolized to dextrose and because animal studies indicate that increasing the blood glucose level may increase neurologic damage after global ischemia.[133] Although at least one laboratory has found different results for focal CNS ischemia,[134] and some investigators may say that survival is better with

fructose than with saline,[135] the most prudent approach at this time seems to be to maintain normoglycemia.

The patient is then brought to the OR and transferred to an operating table with an already warmed heating mattress. Here, EEG, ECG, blood pressure measurement, pulse oximetry, and other standard monitoring methods are applied, and the data are examined prior to induction of anesthesia. The heating mattress or a forced air warmer (Bair Hugger) is important for maintaining normothermia,[136] which probably helps reduce circulatory instability postoperatively.

Induction of anesthesia is then begun with a barbiturate. Some anesthesiologists titrate the dose at this time and during carotid occlusion to achieve burst suppression on the EEG.[89] This electrical suppression is associated with a reduction in cerebral metabolism to as little as 40–50% of awake levels and, at the same time, decreases the CBF and intracranial pressure. Once burst suppression occurs, barbiturates have no further cerebral metabolic effect or any effect in protecting the brain from ischemia.[137] We administer 100% oxygen, and 1–2 mg·kg^{-1} of thiopental and 3 mg of curare, followed by thiopental, 25–50 mg (for a 70-kg patient) iv, along with isoflurane at increasing concentrations in oxygen by mask. When the systolic blood pressure has been reduced by 20–30%, we administer 1.5 mg·kg^{-1} succinylcholine (assuming that the patient has no muscle or lower motor neuron dysfunction), or atracurium or vecuronium or nothing if muscle or lower motor neuron dysfunction is present (see Chapter 19), and either 100 mg of lidocaine or 100 mg of thiopental (each given iv) to blunt the cardiovascular (blood pressure and heart rate) response to laryngoscopy and tracheal intubation. After the routine checks and after verification of endotracheal intubation by end-tidal capnography, a transesophageal echocardiographic probe is inserted to obtain echocardiographic images of a cross-section of the left ventricle at the level of the papillary muscles.

Controlled ventilation of the lungs is instituted at this time, often with 50% nitrous oxide in oxygen, and at other times with oxygen alone, with the concentration of isoflurane or enflurane titrated and the table position adjusted to achieve the desired blood pressure. We avoid administering more than 10 ml·kg^{-1} of crystalloid or other fluid in this 2-hour operation, because increasing fluids may contribute to postoperative hypertension in these patients. This results from the absence of baroreceptor function, which such patients usually exhibit.[138] The lack of baroreceptor function may also account for the stability noted in these patients' heart rates intraoperatively.[26]

During the operation, light anesthesia is usually maintained, with patient movement as well as hemodynamic changes signaling that the anesthesia is inadequate. If it cannot be ensured that the patient will be anesthetized sufficiently so that he or she will not move during the period of temporary carotid occlusion, a muscle relaxant is added, the choice of which is dictated by the heart rate response one wishes to obtain (see Chapter 19).

Although the effects of anesthetics on normal CBF are known, the choice of an anesthetic for this operation appears to have no sound scientific basis. Perhaps the only information suggesting that one should choose isoflurane over other inhalational agents or opioids is that from a non-randomized study at the Mayo Clinic.[121] In this study it was evident that the CBF associated with ischemic changes in the EEG is 10 ml·min^{-1}·100 g^{-1} during isoflurane anesthesia, as opposed to about 20 ml·min^{-1}·100 g^{-1} during anesthesia with other agents, and that shunting is less frequently needed during isoflurane anesthesia than during anesthesia with other agents.

Our preference for avoiding opioids in these operations is based on a desire to have patients awaken shortly after the last stitch is placed (although this may now be possible with alfentanil) and to avoid the hemodynamic effects of naloxone and of muscle relaxant reversal, not on anecdotal reports that opioids worsen the neurologic outcome after focal or global cerebral ischemia.[139]

Before beginning carotid occlusion, the surgeon infiltrates the carotid at the bifurcation with 1% lidocaine in the hope of preventing the sudden onset of bradycardia during stretching of the baroreceptor or of the nerve from the baroreceptor. The anesthetic depth is then kept at a minimum, so that the blood pressure increases to the upper ward level. If no EEG or SSEP evidence of ischemia is found, or if the stump pressure is comfortably above 50 mm Hg, the anesthetic depth is increased somewhat and the systemic blood pressure falls slightly. If myocardial ischemia is indicated by one of the monitors, it is treated by reversing the hemodynamic cause, if any, or by administering nitroglycerin when no obvious hemodynamic cause exists. Myocardial ischemia occurred at this point in the operation in 8–35% of patients in our studies;[26] we do not know the cause at this time, because the hemodynamics did not differ substantially from those just prior to cross-clamping.

After the carotid artery repair is completed and the flow in the carotid is restored, the focus again shifts to myocardial well-being. When the muscle layer is repaired, the patient is allowed to resume spontaneous ventilation. Usually the surgeons identify the recurrent laryngeal nerve; this enables extubation of the trachea in as light a plane of anesthesia as possible, but before the gag reflex is restored. The patient usually responds to pain within 2–3 minutes after the last stitch has been placed, and before leaving the OR (usually within 4–6 minutes after the last stitch), the patient is able to follow simple commands.

The four problems feared most in the postanesthesia care unit are hemodynamic instability, respiratory insufficiency (usually as a result of vocal cord paresis), hematoma formation, and onset of new neurologic dysfunction.

Circulatory instability is usually evidenced by hypertension, but it is reported in the literature that hypotension also occurs. Since we began hydrating patients starting the night before surgery, giving antihypertensives (including diuretics) on the morning of surgery, using a heating blanket to help maintain temperature, and limiting our intraoperative administration of crystalloid to 10 ml·kg^{-1}, the incidence of postoperative hypotension has dropped to zero, and the incidence of postoperative hypertension has decreased to about 10% (from 35%). Although this change is based on historical controls and is anecdotal, any hypertension needs vigorous treatment so that the myocardial work is decreased. We often titrate combinations of nitroprusside or hydralazine and propranolol or esmolol or labetalol to achieve normotension. Such therapies have been found superior to nitroglycerin or trimethaphan in a study on post-CABG patients reported by Stinson et al.[140] Other causes of hypertension are sought (e.g., pain, a full bladder, myocardial ischemia, hypoxia, hypercarbia). However, if the patient is neurologically normal, the association of hypertension and neurologic deficit postoperatively is too strong to allow the hypertension to persist.[141]

Other authors have stated that hypotension following carotid endarterectomy is due to hypersensitivity of the carotid sinus nerve,[142] but we have found that significant hypotension (<80 mm Hg systolic) is often associated with myocardial ischemia. We routinely obtain a 12-lead ECG soon after the patient's arrival in the postanesthesia care unit, and we monitor the ECG lead(s) most likely to disclose

ischemia in these patients, which often proves to be lead II following carotid surgery (not lead V$_5$).[105,106]

Ventilatory insufficiency can appear as stridor owing to unilateral or, more often, bilateral vocal cord paresis (in the patient who has undergone bilateral carotid operations, or a thyroidectomy and a carotid operation), to hematoma, or to deficient carotid body function in patients who chronically retain carbon dioxide. In the case of stridor, the airway must be immediately secured. Hematomas can be treated by opening the suture line and applying external drainage. (This may need to be done even in the postanesthesia care unit). The chemoreceptor function of the carotid body is predictably damaged for up to 10 months following carotid endarterectomy, with complete loss of the ventilatory and circulatory response to hypoxia following bilateral endarterectomy.[138] Such loss results in an increase in the Paco$_2$ of 6 mm Hg at rest. For this reason, the routine use of supplemental oxygen is justified, at least until the patient ambulates.

Wound hematoma from venous oozing usually accumulates slowly, but both it and arterial hemorrhage can threaten the airway. This is probably the most painful part of most carotid operations. (Pain relief stronger than that provided by acetaminophen is usually not required for most patients.) Re-exploration in the OR is occasionally necessary, but rapid opening of the wound in the recovery room can be lifesaving in an emergency.

Anesthesia for Emergency Carotid Artery Revascularization

Etiology and Indications

Some recent studies indicate that reluctance to perform emergency carotid endarterectomy in patients who have fluctuating neurologic deficits may be unwarranted.[99,143] Therefore, anesthesiologists today may more frequently encounter patients with crescendo TIAs or stroke in evolution who are candidates for emergency carotid revascularization. Indications may include tight stenosis (<95%) with or without symptoms, symptomatic occlusion in the first 6–10 hours after occlusion sets in, and a recent carotid endarterectomy that either led to bleeding or has resulted in new neurologic symptoms.

Anesthetic Management

Preoperative Preparation and Induction of Anesthesia. A patient undergoing emergency carotid endarterectomy may have a full stomach and thus may require protection against aspiration of gastric contents. The main goal is to minimize the hemodynamic stress of a rapid sequence induction while maintaining adequate perfusion pressure across the stenotic lesion. The patient is allowed to breathe 100% oxygen. Venous access is secured, and peripheral arterial cannulation is performed for direct monitoring of systemic blood pressure and for obtaining blood samples for determination of gas tensions. One should then proceed with a rapid sequence iv induction with a short-acting barbiturate, a muscle relaxant, and endotracheal intubation. Before intubation of the trachea, a bolus of lidocaine (1.5 mg·kg^{-1}) or sodium nitroprusside (1–2 μg·kg^{-1}) may be administered iv for attenuation of the hypertensive response to visualization of the larynx and the intubation. Hypotension is treated by tilting the table or by iv infusion of phenylephrine or methoxamine (direct alpha$_1$-adrenergic agonists). If a PA catheter is desired (uncommonly, in the patient undergoing emer-

gency exploration of the carotid artery), a peripheral brachial or subclavian vein on the nonoperative side can be used as the site of insertion. If the patient is believed to have an empty stomach, a gentle titrated induction of anesthesia with barbiturate, followed by inhalation of increasing concentrations of a volatile anesthetic, is often used. The roles of nonparticulate antacids, histamine receptor-blocking drugs, and metoclopramide remain controversial.

General anesthesia is maintained with any of a variety of techniques aimed at attenuating hemodynamic fluctuations, achieving normocarbia (or a carbon dioxide level slightly below normal, as in elective operations), and maintaining adequate carotid artery perfusion pressure. An anesthetic technique similar to that used in elective situations is used.

If a hematoma is noted near the operative site and surgical exploration is anticipated, oxygen is given at high concentration by face mask with a reservoir bag or Ayre's T-piece. A tracheostomy or cricothyroidotomy tray should be immediately available. It may be difficult to visualize the trachea because of edema or because of deviation away from the hematoma, caused by pressure of the hematoma. In the event of acute airway obstruction, a high concentration of oxygen in the functional residual volume of the lung may provide additional protection against hypoxemia until the airway is secured by intubation or until the hematoma is evacuated surgically.

If the hematoma does not obstruct the airway and the patient is not having difficulty breathing spontaneously, induction may be accomplished as in an elective procedure. If the airway appears compromised, topical anesthesia of the lips, tongue, posterior pharynx, and epiglottis is provided. The larynx is then visualized. If no difficulty with endotracheal intubation is anticipated, induction is performed as described previously. However, if difficulty is expected, the wound is opened and drained externally, and endotracheal intubation is performed before general anesthesia is induced.

If a new neurologic deficit occurs in the postanesthesia recovery unit, most surgeons believe that immediate re-exploration is indicated, and logic would dictate utilization of pharmacologic methods of "cerebral protection," but this "logic" is controversial.

Thus, the most common causes of morbidity following carotid endarterectomy dictate the following goals:

1. To protect the heart from ischemia,
2. To protect the brain from ischemia, and
3. To enable the patient to awaken soon after the operation.

These seemingly diverse goals can result in a consonant monitoring technique (such as the EEG, which may aid both the heart and the CNS by allowing afterload reduction if normal CNS electrical activity is present) and in therapies such as injection of local anesthetic around the carotid sinus nerve to prevent increases in myocardial oxygen demand and to avoid sudden bradycardia and hypotension (see Table 37-4). As in most aspects of anesthesia, meticulous attention to details such as overnight hydration and the intraoperative use of warming mattresses or Bair Huggers in nonsurgical areas may be as important as the choice of anesthetic agents or even of monitoring techniques.

Many other techniques can be used to avoid myocardial and cerebral dysfunction postoperatively. The major postoperative complications that can lead to adverse sequelae include circulatory instability, which may be due to either myocardial or cerebral ischemia or other causes, including respiratory insufficiency resulting from edema, laryngeal nerve trauma, inadequate or too vigorous hydration, inadequate prevention of hypothermia, or deficient carotid chemoreceptor function; wound hematoma, which may compromise the airway; and a new neurologic deficit. Each of these factors may require emergency treatment.

SURGERY FOR VISCERAL ISCHEMIA AND THORACOABDOMINAL AORTIC ANEURYSMS

In vascular surgery, understanding the pathophysiology of the disease and anticipating the surgical approach and techniques allows the anesthesiologist to serve the patient most effectively. The surgical goal in these operations is to create an enduring restoration of the normal circulation to the viscera while minimizing the duration of ischemia to viscera, especially to the renal circulation. This goal is difficult to achieve: each of the possible surgical approaches compromises some aspects while optimizing others.[144] For example, the site of origin of the bypass graft to the celiac axis is an important consideration. Whereas the supraceliac aorta is usually relatively free of atheroma and a graft from this site lies anatomically so that there is antegrade flow at all times, exposure of this segment of the aorta is more difficult than exposure of the infrarenal aorta. Most surgeons have limited experience with the supraceliac region and are hesitant about working in unfamiliar areas. Probably the major concern is the need for suprarenal clamping and the subsequent risk of ischemic renal damage. This complication in an elderly patient with arterial disease may prove fatal, and it is this added potential for morbidity that prevents the routine use of supraceliac grafting. On the other hand, although the use of the infrarenal aorta as the site of origin of the bypass graft provides familiar territory for the surgeon, this infrarenal site is often diseased; also, after grafting, flow is not always antegrade, and kinking or twisting of vessels may be likely.

The pathologic conditions that give rise to chronic visceral ischemia include atherosclerotic occlusive disease, fibromuscular dysplasia, inflammatory arteriopathies, external compression, and aneurysmal atherosclerotic disease.

In most cases, symptomatic disease of the mesenteric artery is due to atherosclerotic narrowing of the origins of the three major visceral vessels: the celiac, superior mesenteric, and inferior mesenteric arteries. Disease is usually an extension of atheroma of the aorta into the origins of its branches. It rarely extends more than 1–2 cm into the visceral arteries, and it has a well-defined end point.[145] The distal thoracic aorta is often spared, but concomitant disease of the infrarenal vasculature is common. The lesion in the superior mesenteric artery may be more extensive than the celiac lesion, and propagation of thrombus to the first major collateral vessel (the inferior pancreaticoduodenal artery) often leaves a relatively long occluded segment.

A lateral aortogram is required for demonstration of the origins of the unpaired anterior aortic branches, including the celiac axis, superior mesenteric artery, and inferior mesenteric artery. The extensive collateral network of the gut is usually sufficient to maintain an adequate intestinal blood supply if one of these vessels is occluded. Morris et al[146] in 1966 were the first investigators to suggest that occlusion or major stenosis of at least two of these three arteries was necesssary for compromise of the collateral supply and production of symptoms of visceral ischemia. This concept is currently accepted, with few cases of single-vessel lesions reported as symptomatic in any series.[147,148] However,

single-vessel lesions may be important when previous intra-abdominal surgery has interrupted collateral pathways.[149,150] At one center, single-vessel lesions were present in 12% of cases.[150]

When there is occlusive disease in the celiac and superior mesenteric arteries, the major mesenteric supply often comes from the inferior mesenteric artery via the marginal artery. If the inferior mesenteric artery is not revascularized during infrarenal aortic grafting, the risk of bowel ischemia is present, with a reported incidence of colonic infarction after aortic operations of 1–2% and that of small bowel infarction of 0.15%, and with a mortality of up to 90% after the occurrence of such infarction.[149,150]

Other, less common causes of visceral ischemia include fibromuscular dysplasia in association with superior mesenteric insufficiency,[147] Takayasu's arteritis, and external compression of the celiac axis by the median arcuate ligament of the diaphragm.[145] All three of these conditions occur most commonly in women between the ages of 20 and 40 years, whereas chronic ischemia in atherosclerotic arteriopaths or in the setting of acute occlusive disease occurs more commonly in the elderly, who often are hypertensive, and in persons who have smoked cigarettes extensively. Acute mesenteric occlusion is of either embolic or thrombotic origin. If embolic, it commonly has a cardiac source and may follow a recent myocardial infarction. If thrombotic, it may occasionally be due to aortic dissection or trauma but is usually based on progressing atherosclerosis. Sudden occlusion of the superior mesenteric artery without the previous development of collateral vessels can lead to bowel infarction within a few hours. The diagnosis is often difficult to make in the early phase. The patient frequently complains of severe pain in the absence of specific signs, until peritonitis develops as a result of intestinal gangrene. The diagnosis must be strongly suspected in patients with prior cardiac disease who suddenly develop central abdominal pain, often severe, but with minimal physical signs in the first 4–6 hours.[144,150] If surgical intervention occurs before gangrene of the bowel develops, revascularization will reduce the otherwise high mortality and morbidity.

An embolus can usually be extracted by Fogarty catheter from the superior mesenteric artery by means of a direct approach to the proximal artery. Surgeons worry that fragmentation of the embolus in the attempt at catheter embolization with occlusion of the distal branches may make full revascularization impossible. However, proponents of this approach believe that clearance of major vessels will limit the extent of bowel infarction. Thrombolytic agents, angioscopy, or laser atherectomy may prove useful for removal of distal embolic fragments, but their use has not yet been established.[151]

More invasive surgery is usually attempted for both acute and chronic visceral ischemia. The long-term results of surgery for chronic visceral ischemia depend on the extent of the revascularization that is undertaken.[147] Single-vessel repair is associated with rates of recurrence of symptoms as high as 50%. In contrast, full revascularization is associated with recurrence of symptoms in only 11% of cases. These data lead to the current practice in elective procedures of performing as complete a revascularization as possible.[152,153]

Elective surgery for asymptomatic mesenteric occlusive disease is generally not justified, as the risks of surgery often outweigh the possible gains. The perioperative mortality ranges from 7.5–18%.[147,148,152] Cardiac disorders, postoperative hemorrhage, and early graft occlusion with bowel infarction are the major causes of perioperative death.

The approach to the visceral arteries is determined by the vessels involved and by the procedure contemplated for restoration of adequate blood flow. The choice may depend on the surgeon's preference for either endarterectomy or bypass or a combination of both.[144]

Generous exposure of the thoracic and abdominal aorta and its major branches is obtained with a left thoracoabdominal incision and retroperitoneal dissection. The incision is made over the eighth intercostal space and is extended obliquely across the left abdomen toward the symphysis pubis. A retroperitoneal plane of dissection anterior to the left kidney exposes the abdominal aorta and the diaphragm, which is divided circumferentially close to the rib attachments so that innervation is preserved. Good exposure of the descending aorta to the bifurcations of the iliac arteries is obtained, and all major aortic branches can be controlled with this approach. However, the dissection is more extensive than that entailed by a transabdominal approach, and the left thoracic cavity is entered, with possible added morbidity. The thoracoabdominal approach is favored for complex thoracoabdominal aortic replacement in the presence of stenotic or aneurysmal disease. In these major grafting procedures, the visceral branches are often excised from the parent aorta with a button of aortic wall. If needed, endarterectomy of these branch vessels is performed before they are attached to small openings cut in the graft at appropriate positions.[144,152] If aortic replacement is not used, endarterectomy of any or all the major branches of the aorta may be performed with this exposure.

Single-vessel endarterectomy may be carried out for either the celiac axis or the superior mesenteric artery. After exposure of these vessels, and with control of the aorta above and below, the celiac axis is opened transversely at the distal extent of the palpable atheroma. A plane of dissection is found, and a retrograde endarterectomy to the aorta is performed. The arteriotomy is then closed directly and flow is restored. It is difficult to obtain a clean end point in the distal aortic atheroma, and for this reason not many surgeons use this technique.

Two major controversies are still unresolved with respect to bypass options in the presence of mesenteric vascular disease. The first controversy concerns the choice of bypass material (autologous vs. synthetic); the second concerns the site of origin of the graft. Synthetic grafts are undesirable in cases of actual or potential bowel contamination but have long-term patency rates equal to those for autologous grafts in the conditions associated with mesenteric disease without bowel contamination.[147,152] This situation differs from that in femoropopliteal bypass, in which autologous grafts result in substantially higher patency rates.

The site of origin of the graft is usually selected on the basis of the familiarity of the surgeon; a healthy vessel is chosen, and antegrade flow is preferred. Synthetic grafts require a live tissue buffer (e.g., omentum) between them and the gut. The orientation of the graft in an anatomic position provides antegrade flow, which is considered advantageous because turbulence is minimized and development of neointima is lessened. This is best achieved with a supraceliac origin of the graft and end-to-end anastomosis of the recipient vessel(s). If the graft origin is infrarenal, a long, curved course for the graft and an end-to-end anastomosis will allow direct antegrade flow into the superior mesenteric artery.[154] A direct line to the superior mesenteric artery with end-to-side anastomosis is thought to maximize turbulence and graft kinking. An infrarenal graft origin for revascularization of the celiac axis does not allow an easy direct anastomosis to the recipient vessel. Instead, most sur-

geons choose to anastomose the graft end-to-side to the splenic or common hepatic branch of the celiac axis.[152,154]

A major problem with revascularization of the superior mesenteric artery from an infrarenal graft origin, with end-to-side anastomosis in the base of the small bowel mesentery, is the mobility of the mesentery and the tendency for such grafts to kink and thrombose. This problem does not arise with supraceliac grafts and end-to-end anastomosis. To overcome the problem of kinking from the infrarenal location, surgeons have used externally supported Gore-Tex grafts.[153] Another approach to this problem entails constructing a very short H-anastomosis from the anterior aortic wall to the proximal superior mesenteric artery in the manner of a portacaval shunt with a very short but wide (10 mm) graft.[154]

Thus, surgical problems abound in this condition. Symptomatic intestinal ischemia is uncommon because of extensive development of collaterals between the branches of the three major vessels of the mesenteric supply. At least two of these vessels are usually diseased before symptoms develop unless other surgery that interrupted the collateral network has been performed. Patients with chronic ischemia have postprandial abdominal pain, weight loss, and minimal signs apart from an epigastric bruit. Thoracoabdominal aneurysms occur in patients with hypertension or other risk factors for atherosclerotic disease. Acute mesenteric ischemia is often caused by emboli from the heart and is accompanied by acute, severe abdominal pain but minimal signs in the first 4–6 hours before bowel infarction and peritonitis develop.

Results of surgery in these conditions are improved if revascularization of all involved mesenteric vessels is performed. A transabdominal approach is satisfactory for most procedures, including supraceliac grafting. A left thoracoretroperitoneal approach is advantageous for transaortic endarterectomy of the celiac axis and superior mesenteric artery and for thoracoabdominal aneurysms. Surgery is indicated for symptomatic patients and for a small group of asymptomatic patients with proven major occlusive disease of mesenteric vessels who are to undergo a concomitant intraabdominal procedure that is likely to interrupt collateral pathways. Such procedures include aortic reconstruction for occlusive or aneurysmal disease and colonic, small bowel, or gastric resections.

Controversy exists as to the optimal surgical approach to the creation of enduring revascularizations. Both endarterectomy and grafting techniques are reported to yield satisfactory long-term results. The autogenous vein bypass does not appear to provide a clear advantage in this disease, and many surgeons prefer synthetic conduits because of their lower rate of kinking. In acute situations in which there is potential contamination of the abdominal cavity, endarterectomy or autogenous grafting are the only safe options. Transluminal balloon angioplasty for chronic situations and thrombolytic agents for acute ischemia are potentially useful new options for these patients.

SURGERY FOR INFRARENAL AORTIC RECONSTRUCTION

Reconstruction of the abdominal aorta is performed either to replace a segment in the presence of aneurysmal degenerative disease or to increase inflow to and outflow from a vessel with stenosing occlusive disease. Although the natural history of the two diseases is different, the segmental nature of the disease processes, with relatively normal vessels above and below the lesion, provides the basis for reconstruction in each.

Aneurysmal Disease

Aneurysms pose an ever-present threat to life because of their unpredictable tendency to rupture or embolize. Therefore, aggressive surgical management is warranted, even in the absence of symptoms.[155,156] Patients with aneurysms of the abdominal aorta that do not undergo operation have an 80% 5-year mortality, predominantly owing to rupture.[157-159] A larger diameter of the aneurysm is associated with a higher risk of rupture, with about a 25% 5-year incidence of rupture for lesions 4–7 cm in diameter, 45% for those 7–10 cm, and 60% for lesions larger than 10 cm.[159] The larger the aneurysm, the greater the likelihood of early rupture, with 71.8% of fatal ruptures of larger lesions occurring in the first 2 years, compared with 39.1% of fatal ruptures of smaller lesions during that time.[160]

Successful surgical repair of an abdominal aortic aneurysm is associated with prolonged life expectancy.[27,30,51,156,158] Improvements in surgical and anesthetic management have led to a steady decline in perioperative mortality, from approximately 17% before 1960 to 2–5% since 1980 in elective cases, despite broadening indications for surgery.[30,161,162] During the same period, however, mortality following surgery for ruptured aneurysms has remained high, ranging from 25% to 75%.[51,163,164]

Recommended preoperative evaluations of the patient's anatomy include palpation alone, ultrasonography, computed tomography, digital subtraction angiography, aortography, and magnetic resonance imaging. More invasive testing exposes the patient to risks and increases costs but allows determination of the presence of iliac occlusive or aneurysmal disease, juxtarenal or suprarenal extension of the aneurysm, renal artery aneurysmal or occlusive disease, and visceral artery lesions, including the presence of a "meandering mesenteric artery" (a collateral artery), horseshoe kidney, accessory renal arteries, arteriovenous fistula, and disease in other organs.

No single approach has been shown in a randomized clinical trial to yield the best results for the patient. Clinical judgment remains the basis for individualizing tests for each patient with this disease, even when it is asymptomatic.

Occlusive Disease

Occlusive disease tends to be progressive, with compromise of the distal circulation leading to disabling claudication or limb-threatening ischemia. In the case of aneurysmal disease, surgery is indicated whenever the disease is present; in the case of occlusive disease, surgical intervention is indicated only for the relief of disabling symptoms.[155]

In setting out to correct occlusive disease of the aortoiliac segment, the surgeon endeavors to return to near normal the inflow to the limbs at the groin while maintaining flow to the internal iliac and visceral branches. The mean age of patients undergoing aortoiliac reconstruction is 54 years; these patients are more than 10 years younger, on the average, than those with aneurysmal disease of the aorta.[165]

Patients who have critical limb ischemia and stenotic aortoiliac disease commonly have concomitant occlusive lesions of the femoral, popliteal, or tibial vessels. The incidence of distal femoropopliteal occlusive disease in patients undergoing repair of an abdominal aortic aneurysm is approximately 11%; for occlusive aortoiliac procedures, it is much higher (≥45%).[165-167] The patency of an aortobifemoral bypass depends on the status of distal occlusive disease in the femoral segment.[166,168] The need for subsequent femoropopliteal bypass can be reduced greatly if the profunda femoris artery is opened by profundoplasty performed concomitantly with the aortobifemoral bypass.[167,169]

Surgical Techniques

Choice of Exposure

The most popular surgical exposure for either occlusive or aortic disease is through a vertical anterior midline abdominal incision, with a transperitoneal approach to the retroperitoneal structures. This approach is versatile, providing access to all major arteries between the diaphragm and pelvis. The other major approach is a retroperitoneal one anterior to the kidney. Such an approach appears to be associated with less blood loss and lower intraoperative fluid requirements. It is gaining favor because it is also associated with less postoperative ileus, and oral intake can be resumed after a shorter period of time. Less pain is experienced, as judged by opioid requirements, and fewer pulmonary complications appear to occur with shorter hospital stays.[170] Access to renal vessels, however, may be hindered or impossible with this approach.

Graft Replacement

After the relevant portion of the aorta and the iliac arteries are exposed, the segment of the aorta involved by aneurysm is replaced by a graft. Heparin is commonly administered systemically to reduce the risk of thromboembolic complications. If the aortic graft is to be preclotted, blood for preclotting is usually harvested before the heparin is given. It is now recognized that distal ischemia complicating aortic surgery is related to dislodgment of atheroemboli from the diseased aorta. The recognition of the embolic nature of distal ischemic problems prompted Starr et al[171] to perform aneurysm resections without administration of heparin. In their series of 434 procedures, there was only one case of embolism. Thus, in the absence of major distal occlusive disease, systemic heparinization may be unnecessary in the repair of abdominal aortic aneurysms; careful technique is probably a more important factor in avoiding distal ischemia.[171,172]

A tube graft (i.e., end-to-end anastomoses on both sides) in which the graft is covered with old aorta is often used for aneurysmal resection. When the iliac vessels are not aneurysmal or stenotic, a tube graft may be used as replacement for the diseased aorta, thus making the procedure faster, with less blood loss.[172]

The standard graft material, in use since the late 1950s, has been Dacron, in either knitted or woven form.[155] More recently, polytetrafluoroethylene grafts, which are less porous, have become available. Knitted Dacron grafts are quite porous and require preclotting before implantation. These grafts develop a larger pseudointima and, as a result, may have good resistance to late infection.[173] In addition, they are relatively pliable and easy to suture, and they do not fray at the edges when cut. On the other hand, woven Dacron grafts are nonporous and do not require preclotting; this is a considerable advantage in patients with ruptured aneurysms and in those with a bleeding diathesis. A pseudointima does not form as readily, and the incidence of late infection may be greater than with knitted grafts.[173] When woven Dacron is cut by sharp instruments, its edges tend to fray, but this can be overcome by use of electrocautery for cutting the graft. Woven grafts are more rigid and not as easily manipulated as knitted grafts. Both appear to be associated with rare episodes of anaphylactic reactions, which may be related to the stabilizers used in their manufacture.[174]

Because there is no need to exclude a segment of artery from the circulation when aortoiliac occlusive disease is present, the proximal anastomosis of the graft to the aorta is often performed in an end-to-side configuration after an ellipse of anterior aortic wall has been excised. If there is any suggestion of early aneurysmal dilatation, however, this segment must be excluded. Similarly, advanced degenerative changes in the infrarenal aorta may require end-to-end placement of the graft so that subsequent embolization of atheromatous debris can be avoided. In either case, because of the expected progression of disease, the origin of any graft is usually placed as close to the renal arteries as possible.[175]

Occlusive disease may be managed by endarterectomy or angioplasty. The former procedure is now reserved for isolated lesions of iliac origin or for unusual situations in which the use of synthetic material is contraindicated, such as in sepsis. In general, bypass procedures have yielded long-lasting and very satisfactory results for treatment of occlusive disease.

In the long term, surgical resection of abdominal aortic aneurysms results in approximately double the life expectancy achieved with nonsurgical management. Bypass for occlusions in the aortoiliac region affords good long-term patency, and limb salvage rates are high. Increasing severity of distal occlusive disease is associated with poorer patency rates. Sepsis associated with groin incisions and repeat surgery remain major problems for successful treatment.

Arterial reconstructive surgery has been developed on the basis of the principle of anatomic correctness. Although this is usually the easiest and best option, situations do occur that require less advantageous revascularization procedures. Such situations include repeat surgery, surgery for graft infection, the presence of contraindications to transabdominal surgery (e.g., sepsis, adhesions, radiation therapy, malignancy), as well as less traumatic alternatives in frail, usually elderly, high-risk patients. In general, the price paid when alternative techniques are used is reduced long-term patency. Axillofemoral bypass, with the use of synthetic material in a subcutaneous tunnel, is the most popular extra-anatomic bypass for aortoiliac reconstruction.[176,177] Surgery involves exposure of relatively superficial arteries in the axilla and groin, with a long subcutaneous tract between them. The long-term patency of such grafts is significantly poorer than that for aortofemoral grafts, although surgical revision may be performed with good results.[177] The patency rate of the initial graft at 3 years is only 54% with this procedure.[176,178]

Another option for reconstruction in the presence of unilateral iliac occlusive disease is femorofemoral bypass, either alone or in combination with axillo-unifemoral or aorto-unifemoral bypass.[176] These procedures are used with the knowledge that long-term patency rates are lower. Transluminal treatments in development for occlusive disease, including the use of lasers and angioplasty, promise new horizons in this field.[179-182]

Several situations, both in patients with aneurysmal disease and in those with occlusive disease, may cause the surgeon to change from an infrarenal procedure, which is less risky to the heart and other organs, to a suprarenal procedure. (A suprarenal procedure may be precluded, hindered, or, in some hands, facilitated by the retroperitoneal approach.) Aneurysms of the abdominal aorta involve the pararenal aorta in up to 20% of cases.[183] Also, significant stenosis of the renal artery may coexist with an abdominal aortic aneurysm in an infrarenal or pararenal site, and correction of these renal artery lesions may well be contemplated in conjunction with aneurysm repair. Significant stenoses of the celiac trunk or superior mesenteric artery may similarly be addressed at the time of aortic reconstruction. Aortic surgery for a patient who has previously undergone aortic surgery will frequently necessitate revision to a higher graft origin, and problems with infection in prosthetic materials may require a clean site for a new graft origin. Ruptured aneurysms often must be controlled initially by supraceliac clamping.

In chronic aortic occlusion, even in the absence of disabling claudication, the risk of embolic disease in the kidneys is high, and surgery should be performed to re-establish distal aortic flow. During operative manipulation and clamping, great care must be taken that material is not dislodged into the renal arteries. Many surgeons first clamp the aorta above the level of the renal vessels, open the infrarenal aorta, and clear out the thrombus, then move the aortic clamp to an infrarenal position before proceeding with bypass grafting from the infrarenal aorta.[175]

Thus, many situations may arise that require aortic cross-clamping more cephalad than in the usual infrarenal position. Cardiac and renal function are most at risk in these situations, with patients known to have preoperative renal insufficiency being at greatest risk of developing postoperative renal failure. These and other concerns that the anesthesiologist can assist in managing are discussed in the following section.

ANESTHETIC GOALS IN SURGERY FOR AORTIC AND VISCERAL ARTERY RECONSTRUCTION

For minimal morbidity and mortality, the anesthetic goals are to preserve myocardial, renal, pulmonary, CNS, and visceral organ function. To meet these goals, the anesthesiologist must ensure an adequate oxygen supply to the myocardium commensurate with need, while at the same time reducing (if possible) the myocardial requirement for oxygen and maintaining adequate perfusion to all other organs. The latter objective usually requires preservation of adequate intravascular volume to maintain cardiac output.

Pathophysiologic Events

To better understand the use of specific monitors, it is helpful to be aware of the pathophysiologic events that occur on application and removal of aortic cross-clamps.

Occlusion of the aorta causes hypertension in the proximal segment and hypotension in the distal segment. During resection of a congenitally coarcted aorta, acute occlusion of the thoracic aorta has very little effect on cardiovascular variables because of the normal development, over the years, of extensive collateral vessels around the coarctation. However, in patients who have an aortic aneurysm or atherosclerosis without extensive collateral circulation, aortic occlusion increases afterload and peripheral vascular resistance in proportion to the level of the occlusion. Similarly, myocardial stress varies with the level of occlusion.[40]

Myocardial performance and circulatory variables remain within an acceptable range after the aorta is occluded at infrarenal levels.[40] This result is in agreement with many of the findings in previous work. In 1968, Perry[184] demonstrated that the increase in afterload after temporary infrarenal aortic occlusion had little effect on circulatory variables. The use of newer, more sophisticated techniques has shown that deepening anesthesia or administering vasodilating drugs at the time of infrarenal aortic occlusion maintains indices of myocardial performance within an acceptable range,[41-43,59] even in sick patients (in our series, 25% had severe left ventricular dysfunction before aortic surgery). Abnormalities of ventricular wall motion and systolic thickening, as well as changes in the ejection fraction, appear to be early signs of myocardial ischemia.[185] However, we did not detect abnormal myocardial wall motion in any patient with infrarenal occlusion.[40] Thus far, the results of only one study contradicted the view that myocardial well-being is preserved after infrarenal aortic occlusion. Attia et al[44] reported a 30% incidence (three of ten patients) of myocardial ischemia following infrarenal occlusion. Investigators from the same institution (Massachusetts General Hospital), however, later described a technique (the vasodilation already described at the time of cross-clamping) that allows infrarenal aortic occlusion without eliciting evidence of myocardial ischemia.[45] Therefore, on the basis of these data, we consider it safe to assume that aortic occlusion at the infrarenal level increases the afterload only slightly and that current techniques prevent much of the stress on the heart that is associated with such occlusion.

There are few data in published reports on myocardial and cardiovascular effects of occluding the aorta at the suprarenal-infraceliac or supraceliac level in humans. After occluding the descending thoracic aorta in eight patients, Kouchoukos et al[47] noted increases of 35%, 56%, 43%, and 90% in mean arterial, central venous, mean pulmonary arterial, and PCWPs, respectively, and a decrease of 29% in cardiac index. These hemodynamic effects are greater than those we found for supraceliac aortic occlusion and may be attributable to the more proximal level of thoracic aortic occlusion. Occlusion at the supraceliac level causes substantially more myocardial stress, as evidenced by abnormal motion of segments of the left ventricular wall, than does occlusion at the suprarenal-infraceliac or infrarenal level (Table 37-5).[40] Although systemic and PCWP pressures were kept normal at all times in 10 of 12 patients who underwent occlusion at the supraceliac level, 11 patients had abnormal motion of the left ventricular wall, suggesting ischemia. Some of the factors contributing to this increase in resistance to myocardial ejection may be the greater than 100% increase in peripheral vascular resistance, the change in aortic impedance characteristics, the release of vasoactive substances with intestinal ischemia, or the activation of hormonal systems, all of which lead to ventricular dilation. Despite low ejection fractions, these patients were able to maintain cardiac output and stroke volume *via* stretch (expansion) of the left ventricle muscle fibers. The PCWP frequently did not reflect this increased left-ventricular end-diastolic volume accurately; however, 2D-TEE allowed the identification and treatment of myocardial dysfunction that was not detected with conventional monitoring techniques.[40,105,106] The most important lesson learned from the use of two-dimensional echocardiography in patients undergoing vascular surgery is that dilating the heart by administering fluid (as is often requested by surgeons to stimulate urine output) is a likely precursor of myocardial ischemia.

These pathophysiologic changes in hemodynamic variables could result from the effect that clamping has on normal patterns of flow to the arteries. For example, 22% of the cardiac output usually goes to renal vessels and 27% to the superior mesenteric vessels and celiac trunk.[186] Thus, the expected decrease in flow and the increase in afterload and peripheral vascular resistance after supraceliac aortic occlusion could cause left ventricular dilation. Other factors that may contribute to myocardial dysfunction during operative supraceliac occlusion include release of vasoactive substances from ischemic areas and the presence of unmetabolized citrate from transfused blood.[187,188]

Results of studies on animals support the view that myocardial function is altered after occlusion of the descending thoracic aorta. Longo et al[189] studied coronary and systemic hemodynamic changes in dogs during suprarenal and infrarenal aortic clamping and unclamping. On application of the cross-clamp to the suprarenal aorta, peripheral resistance increased two- to threefold, with immediate hyperten-

TABLE 37-5. Effect of Level of Aortic Occlusion on Changes in Cardiovascular Variables

Cardiovascular Variable	% Change in Variable, by Level of Aortic Occlusion		
	Supraceliac	Suprarenal-Infraceliac	Infrarenal
Mean arterial blood pressure	54	5*	2*
Pulmonary capillary wedge pressure	38	10*	0*
End-diastolic area	28	2*	9*
End-systolic area	69	10*	11*
Ejection fraction	−38	−10*	−3*
Abnormal motion of wall, % of patients	92	33	0
New myocardial infarctions, % of patients	8	0	0

*Statistically different ($p < 0.05$) from group undergoing supraceliac aortic occlusion.

Adapted with permission from Roizen MF, Sohn YJ, Stoney RJ: Intraoperative management of the patient undergoing supraceliac aortic occlusion. In Wilson SE, Veith FJ, Hobson RW *et al* (eds): Vascular Surgery, p 312. New York, McGraw-Hill, 1986.

sion in the proximal segment, marked increases in CBF and pulse pressure, decreases in aortic blood flow and cardiac output, and little change in the pulse rate. These results were similar to ours.[40] In the study of Longo et al,[189] the canine left ventricles were dilated on application of the cross-clamp. Mandelbaum and Webb[190] showed that occluding the descending thoracic aorta in dogs decreased left ventricular function. However, occluding the infrarenal aorta was much less stressful, the cardiovascular consequences being only slight (as they are in human patients with diseased hearts).[40,190]

In normal dogs, the renal artery can be occluded for an hour before the kidneys are injured even slightly.[191] Data from a study on human subjects support this observation.[57,58] Preoperative and postoperative renal function did not differ among patients who underwent less than 40 minutes of suprarenal cross-clamping and those who underwent infrarenal aortic occlusion.[57]

Despite the negligible cardiovascular effects of temporarily applying an infrarenal aortic cross-clamp, hypotension ("declamping shock") still occurs on restoration of flow in the aorta. This hemodynamic alteration occurs even when blood flow is restored to only one leg. Although the occurrence of severe hypotension in patients is rare,[40,45,47] moderate hypotension (i.e., a decrease in systolic blood pressure of 40 mm Hg) is common.

Two hypotheses are advanced to account for this hypotension. The first suggests that myocardial depression is caused by the washout of acid, acid metabolites, and vasoactive substances from ischemic extremities when blood flow is restored. This hypothesis has not been strongly supported in recent years.[41,47,188] Our own work with 2D-TEE supports the second hypothesis, that of a relative depletion of volume. Reactive hyperemia in the freshly revascularized area decreases total vascular resistance, venous return, and blood pressure. Thus, hypotension can be ameliorated by expansion of volume without a decrease in cardiac output; in fact, the expansion may increase cardiac output. However, if hypotension persists for more than 4 minutes after removal of the clamp, and if blood deficits have been replaced, other causes should be sought. 2D-TEE of the left ventricle in these patients often reveals that venous return is still inadequate, sometimes as a result of hidden persistent bleeding or misjudged replacement of blood deficits, or that a rare allergic reaction to graft material has occurred.[174]

Because of these complications, we stress, in our monitoring practices, preservation of myocardial, pulmonary, and renal function as well as intravascular volume. We almost always insert a catheter in the radial artery of the nondominant hand. We also monitor urinary output and some form of ventricular filling pressure, the latter usually via a PA catheter. This catheter allows monitoring of systemic vascular resistance, cardiac output, and PCWP. For its insertion, we prefer the external jugular route, although many anesthesiologists use the internal jugular or subclavian route. We use a modified chest lead to monitor the ECG during the operation, except in patients who have demonstrated myocardial ischemia in areas other than the anterior myocardial wall. In addition, body temperature is monitored and maintained by warming all fluids (starting preoperatively), and by the use of heating mattresses on the OR table. If necessary, we humidify the anesthetic gases. We have found 2D-TEE an invaluable tool for monitoring the myocardial consequences of cross-clamping and unclamping of the aorta, and we now use it routinely for such procedures as temporary aortic occlusion at the supraceliac level. A short-axis cross-sectional view of the left ventricle provides an

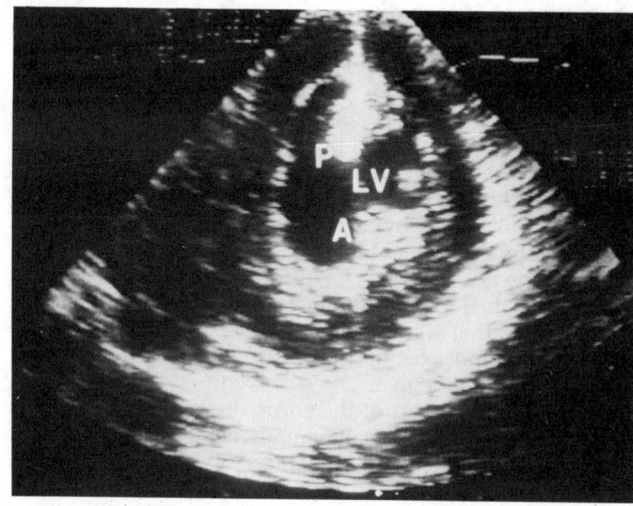

Figure 37-4. Left ventricular echocardiograph obtained from a transesophageal echocardiogram. The transesophageal echocardiogram originates in the esophagus, the small piece of the pie-shaped wedge shown at the top of the picture. The area marked "LV" is the inside of the heart, where blood is normally shown. The whiteness surrounding the LV cavity that is not marked "A" or "P" is the endocardium. The "A" and "P" represent the anterior and posterior papillary muscles, respectively. At the bottom of the image is the anterior wall of the myocardium. To the right is the left ventricular free wall; to the left is the septum; and to the top is the posteroinferior portion wall of the myocardium.

excellent qualitative assessment of left ventricular filling volumes, global ventricular contractility, and regional ventricular function (Fig. 37-4).[191] When a discrepancy exists between pulmonary capillary filling pressures and end-diastolic dimension (volume) as determined from 2D-TEE, we have found the latter to be more reliable and useful.[40,192]

To reduce the incidence of organ ischemia and pulmonary dysfunction, fluid administration is managed with the aim of preventing intraoperative hypotension and minimizing cardiac dilation. Although there are no supporting data at present, it is strongly believed that prehydration of patients undergoing vascular reconstructive surgery minimizes the hemodynamic fluctuations that occur with induction of anesthesia, by ensuring that perfusion of vital organs is adequate. During the early period of dissection, intravascular volume is maintained at normal levels by noting ventricular filling on 2D-TEE or by sustaining a normal PCWP. To accomplish this, blood losses of less than 10 ml·kg^{-1} and insensible losses (assumed to be 5–7 ml·kg^{-1} during this dissection phase) are replaced with Ringer's lactate or saline solution.

The following indicators are used for assessing perfusion of the organs before cross-clamping: (1) for the heart, *myocardial contractility*, as judged by global and regional motion of the wall on 2D-TEE,[40,105,185] by ST segments on modified chest lead V of the ECG, and by cardiac output; (2) for the kidney, *urinary output* (2 ml per half hour per 70 kg is adequate, although with 20–30 ml per half hour per 70 kg, it may be easier to convince surgeons of adequacy); urinary flow almost always decreases during dissection around the renal vessels; (3) for the central nervous system, *eye signs* (although the EEG or sensory-evoked potentials or both[61] can be used, we have had little experience with these monitors); and (4) for the lung, *gas exchange*.

Protection of Myocardium

In the half hour immediately preceding cross-clamping and aortic occlusion, we keep the patient slightly hypovolemic by examining the ventricular volume with 2D-TEE, or by keeping pulmonary arterial pressure at 5–12 mm Hg. At the time of occlusion, we are prepared to give a vasodilating drug through an iv catheter available specifically for that purpose. This avoids hypotension secondary to an accidental bolus of vasodilator. This infusion site is often the third lumen of the PA catheter. The difference in our management of aortic occlusion at different levels (e.g., supraceliac vs. infrarenal) is that we rigorously and meticulously plan the management and execute that procedure in all occlusions at renal vessels or above.

During the early part of the aortic dissection, the heart is protected by maintenance of hemodynamic variables within the range of the preoperative values.[70] Without evidence to the contrary, it is assumed that a little hypertension is just as harmful as a little hypotension. For example, in extreme cases, we might permit the systolic blood pressure of a patient whose preoperative range was 110–170 mm Hg to fall as low as 90 mm Hg, or to rise as high as 190 mm Hg. If values approach or exceed these limits, we have a contingency treatment plan. If the blood pressure reaches 150 mm Hg, the amount of anesthetic is increased; at approximately 160 mm Hg, nitroprusside is infused; at 165 or 175 mm Hg, the table is tilted. If the systolic blood pressure drops to 110 mm Hg, the anesthetic is decreased and the possible causes of hypotension are reviewed. At 105 mm Hg, the amount of anesthetic is decreased even more, and the patient is placed in a head-down position. At 100 mm Hg, more fluid is infused, the patient is tilted to a more steeply head-down position, the possible causes of hypotension are reviewed again, and, if possible, the cause is corrected. At 90 mm Hg, a dilute infusion of phenylephrine (10 mg in 500 ml, infused at a rate that restores systolic blood pressure to approximately 100 mm Hg) is added.

The range of acceptable values in heart rate is similarly based on preoperative determinations. If a preoperative range of 60–90 beats·min^{-1} is established, treatment would be initiated once these limits were exceeded intraoperatively. It is assumed that tachycardia is of greater concern than bradycardia and must be avoided more aggressively. At 95 beats·min^{-1}, the level of anesthesia might be increased, more opioid given, or an iv infusion of a beta-adrenergic receptor blocking drug added. At 100 beats·min^{-1}, a bolus is given or an iv infusion of a beta-adrenergic receptor blocker is begun, if the intravascular fluid volume is acceptable. At 45 beats·min^{-1}, the anesthetic might be decreased or a dilute solution of dopamine (200 mg in 500 ml) administered to keep the heart rate within the acceptable range. Bradycardia is better tolerated than tachycardia during these operations, because minimizing the myocardial oxygen demand should be of primary importance. Imaging with 2D-TEE allows some latitude in the range of acceptable values before intervention must be undertaken. However, PA pressures are not allowed to remain abnormal, that is, below 5 mm Hg or above 15 mm Hg, during this procedure, assuming that these values correlate with the echocardiographic values. Increases in PA pressure are treated aggressively by administering nitroglycerin or nitroprusside, depending on whether the suspected cause is an increase in preload or an increase in afterload.[193] For low pressures, more fluid is infused except in the 1- or 2-minute interval immediately before application of the aortic cross-clamp.

The application of a cross-clamp to the supraceliac aorta probably produces the greatest hemodynamic stress ever experienced by a patient. In fact, 92% of the patients whom we studied had ischemia, as evidenced by abnormal motion and thickening of the wall (Fig. 37-5; see Table 37-5).[40] More distal levels of temporary occlusion are less stressful hemodynamically. Stabilizing PA pressure and systemic blood pressure by administering vasodilating drugs before and during suprarenal cross-clamping may not be sufficient. When myocardial ischemia was indicated by abnormal global or regional motion of the wall in patients in our study, we gave more vasodilating drugs, to the point of bringing the systolic blood pressure toward the low end of the normal preoperative range. Once the blood pressure is as low as possible (achieved by reducing afterload with the administration of nitroprusside), we often attempt to decrease the preload with nitroglycerin and, if necessary, to decrease the heart rate with iv esmolol. If, despite these maneuvers, myocardial dysfunction is evident on placement of the cross-clamp, the surgeon is asked (before he has actually incised the aorta or its branches) to unclamp the aorta partially until myocardial function is more stable. In our study, despite myocardial dysfunction in 11 of the 12 patients who underwent supraceliac cross-clamping, only one of the 11 had perioperative myocardial infarction.[40] Therefore, myocardial contractile function seems to be affected most by ventricular size and by maintenance of vital signs within the normal preoperative range.

Administration of exogenous vasoconstrictors is avoided if possible. Although coronary and cerebral vessels are not prominently innervated, alpha$_1$- and alpha$_2$-adrenergic agents can induce cerebral vasoconstriction. In addition, alpha-adrenergic vasoconstriction appears to be important in maintaining an appropriate distribution of flow between the outer and inner myocardium.[194] Perhaps because of this, or perhaps for other reasons, patients who are deeply anesthetized and whose systemic pressure is maintained with an infusion of phenylephrine have more than twice the incidence of myocardial ischemia than patients whose blood pressure is maintained simply by light anesthesia and endogenous vasoconstrictors.[26] The ischemia appears to be related to the myocardial dilation induced by these agents (the problem of a stretched, dilated myocardium).[26]

During unclamping of the aorta, a different set of maneuvers is performed to achieve the same goals. To ensure adequate volume when the cross-clamp is removed, blood losses are replaced during occlusion by administering warmed blood, milliliter for milliliter. We normally have only 4 units of packed cells available during this procedure. (We are progressively using autologous predeposit, with or without erythropoietin treatment.) The packed cells are diluted with normal saline or lactated Ringer's solution. Although we would prefer to administer whole blood, as that is what is lost, we are unable to obtain it routinely at our institution.

When greater blood loss is anticipated (e.g., in patients previously operated on for the same condition), autotransfusion is often available and a second person (usually a technician) to operate it. After the 6th unit of blood has been given and if more blood loss is anticipated, or after 8 units of blood have been administered, 10 units of platelets are requested for the patient (and occasionally 2 units of fresh frozen plasma). After giving 8 to 10 units of packed cells, we routinely administer a unit of fresh frozen plasma for each unit of packed cells. When no more blood is at hand, and if it is absolutely necessary (i.e., when colloid or crystalloid cannot be used), the best available type-specific, washed packed cells are administered. For example, if B-negative blood is needed but not available, we give B-posi-

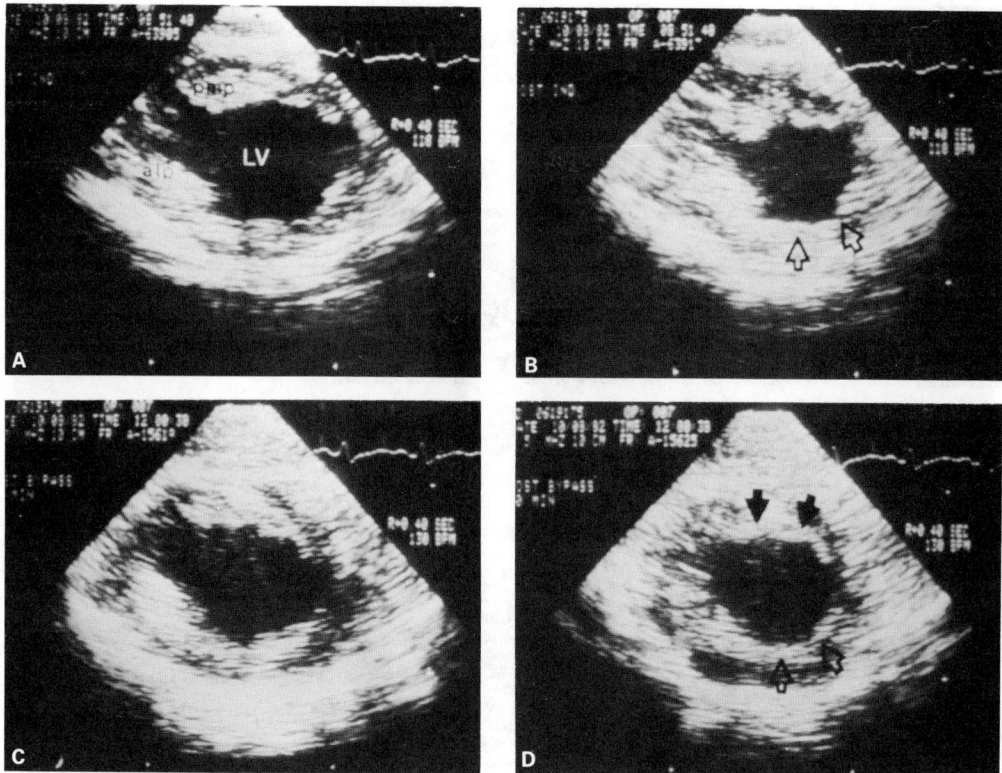

Figure 37-5. Echocardiographic view of the left ventricle with the papillary muscles on the left side of the figure. A and C are end-diastolic views; the end-systolic views are shown in B and D. The *arrows* in B indicate an area of permanent myocardial infarction with no contraction occurring. Note that the placement of the anterior wall or the wall in the bottom part of the image where the arrows are is no different from where it was end-diastole. In D, one sees that the posterior part or the part toward the uppermost part of that figure is also not moving. That is different from B and indicates a new area of ischemia. This wall motion abnormality, coupled with the absence of thickening of the wall in this area, is a sign of myocardial ischemia and illustrates a way that the echocardiogram can aid in the diagnosis of myocardial ischemia.

tive blood. Blood filters are changed after every 2 units when the blood for transfusion is more than 10 days old, and after every 4 units when it is less than 10 days old.

Because a large part of the vascular tree is excluded from circulation during temporary aortic occlusion, blood loss can be considerable during supraceliac cross-clamping without onset of hypotension or tachycardia.

Because maintenance of volume status is so important, more than just PA pressures or PCWP is monitored. Observation of the surgical field is of key importance. When any blood vessel is dissected, the anesthesiologist and surgeon must communicate closely; blood loss can occur with astonishing rapidity, and the attention of the anesthesiologist may not be directed at the operative field. Watching the volumes in the suction bottles supplements the data, as does observation of left ventricular cavity size on 2D-TEE.

Blood loss into the pleural or retroperitoneal cavity may not be detected in the amounts that are measured every 5–10 minutes. In addition, evisceration of bowel, often necessary for optimal exposure of the thoracoabdominal aorta, further depletes the intravascular volume. Thus, one must be guided closely by PA pressures or echocardiographic estimates of left ventricular filling volumes, or both. Just before opening of the aorta, we allow blood pressure, PCWP, and filling volumes to go as high as possible without the occurrence of myocardial ischemia (Fig. 37-6). The surgeon then opens the aorta gradually to ensure that overly severe

hypotension does not develop and that there is not too much bleeding from the suture line.

Pathophysiologic events on removal of the aortic cross-clamp (see previous discussion) are associated with inadequate return of volume to the heart (i.e., inadequate preload). Thus, immediately before and during removal of the cross-clamp, we stop infusing nitroprusside and start infusing crystalloid or blood; usually, 2 units of whole blood are pressured into venous access sites. Guided by filling pressures or echocardiographic estimates of volume, or both, we are careful not to dilate the left ventricle to an abnormal size. Another technique for maintaining normal volumes during cross-clamping is controlled volume depletion, that is, the removal of a specific amount of blood from the patient just before or during application of the cross-clamp for a short period of time. During the minutes remaining just before the cross-clamp is removed, this amount is replaced. Although we have used this technique, we do not advocate its routine use.

A third technique for maintaining normal hemodynamic values involves the use of halothane, enflurane, or isoflurane, rather than nitroglycerin or nitroprusside, as the vasodilating agent. This is an interesting technique that is usually effective,[195] but it requires very close observation of PA pressures, the echocardiogram, or both, to ensure that myocardial dilation and dysfunction do not occur. This technique is not recommended for routine use.

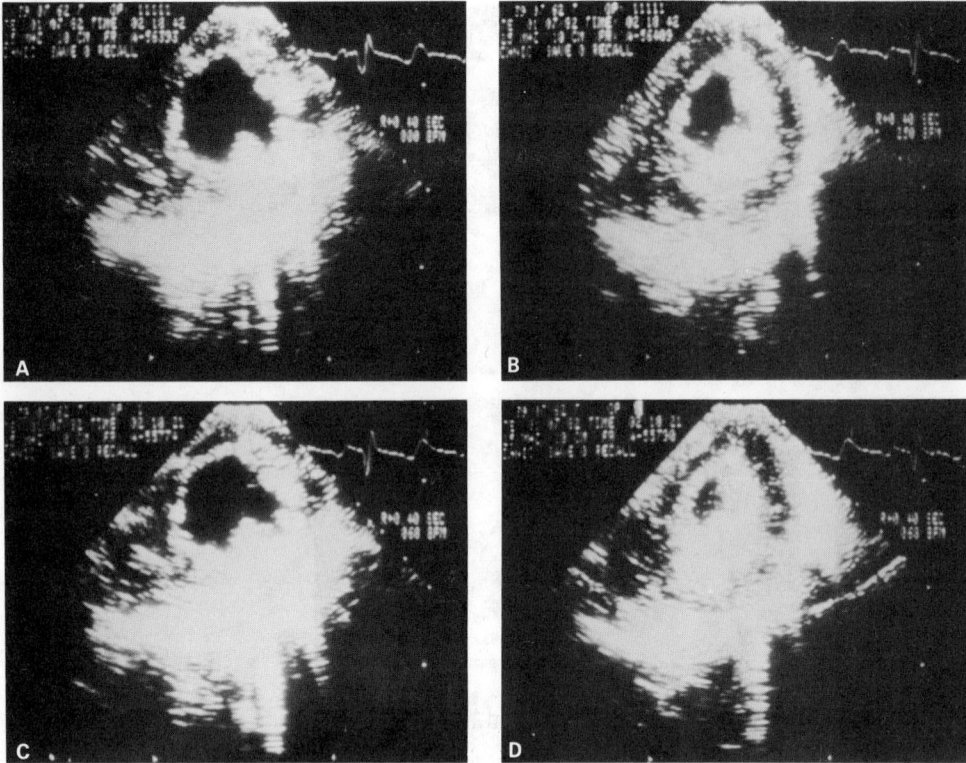

Figure 37-6. Set of echocardiograms with the papillary muscles shown on the right. *A* and *C* are end-diastolic images; *B* and *D* are end-systolic. All the walls of the heart are contracting symmetrically and come in so that there is almost no volume at end-systole in the left ventricular cross-section at the area of the papillary muscles. This picture of hypovolemia can be seen often when one releases the cross-clamp, as occurred between *A* and *B* and *C* and *D*.

It is common for moderate hypotension (*i.e.*, decreases in systolic pressure of 40–60 mm Hg) to occur on removal of the aortic cross-clamp, regardless of whether the clamp is replaced infrarenally or in such a way that blood flow to only one leg is obstructed. Our anecdotal impressions, gained in work with 2D-TEE, support the view that such hypotension is caused mainly by relative depletion of volume. Reactive hyperemia in the freshly revascularized area decreases vascular resistance, venous return, and systemic blood pressure. If hypotension persists for more than 4 minutes following removal of the clamp and the pressure does not return toward normal levels after blood deficits have been replaced, other causes should be sought. These include myocardial dysfunction caused by inadequate metabolism of the citrate present in replacement blood; such blood has not yet gone to the liver, where citrate is metabolized. This problem can be treated by administration of calcium, which antagonizes the effect of citrate.[187] Other causes include hidden, persistent bleeding or misjudged replacement of blood deficits; on the echocardiogram, the ventricular cavity is devoid of volume, and on the oscilloscope, filling pressures reflecting PA pressures are low. If necessary, the surgeon can reclamp or occlude the aorta, preferably below the renal arteries. Thus, replacement and maintenance of volume are mainstays of therapy before, during, and immediately after removal of the supraceliac cross-clamp. When blood flow is restored to the first extremity, replacement of volume should also be considered. Removal of the clamp from the second leg usually causes few hemodynamic effects, presumably because of collateral blood vessels across the pelvis.

Central Nervous System Protection

Other investigators have used sensory-evoked potentials and the EEG to gauge protection of the spinal cord and cerebrum.[61] We have found no benefit in examining the EEG and no evidence that stroke is a predictable consequence of aortic reconstruction, even of supraceliac aortic reconstruction. However, in rare instances, spinal cord ischemia is a predictable consequence of this procedure. Spinal cord sensory-evoked potentials may prove useful, but there has not been much experience in the use of this technique.[62-65,119] Experiments on animals indicate that isoflurane may allow longer periods of temporary occlusion of the blood supply to the spinal cord before development of permanent neurologic injury than are possible with other anesthetic agents. Other halogenated anesthetics and iv anesthetics decrease the interval during which the spinal cord can be ischemic before permanent neurologic damage sets in in this animal model.[196] CSF drainage and hypothermia also may prove useful and are used commonly, but fast surgery remains a mainstay of therapy.[62-65]

Renal Protection

Intraoperative urinary output is not predictive of postoperative renal function.[57,58] In 137 patients undergoing aortic reconstruction (38 at the supraceliac level), we measured the urine output hourly and calculated each patient's lowest and mean urinary outputs. The PCWP was kept within normal limits in each patient. If urinary output was less than $0.125 \ ml \cdot kg^{-1} \cdot h^{-1}$, patients were given either crystalloid (to

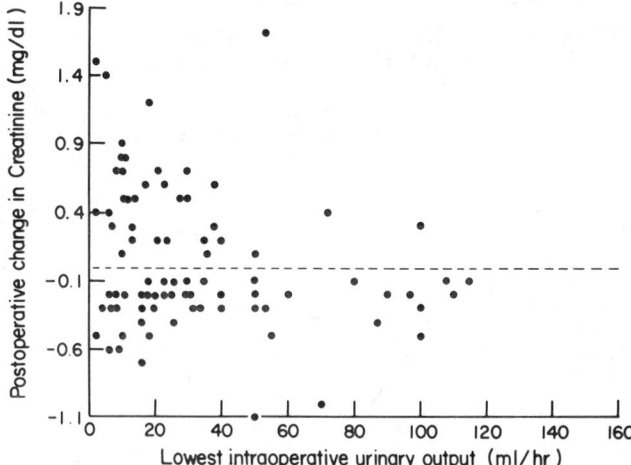

Figure 37-7. Lowest hourly intraoperative urinary output and maximal adverse change in renal function as assayed by change in creatinine from preoperatively to 7 days postoperatively; there was no correlation between lowest intraoperative urinary output and change in renal function postoperatively. (Modified with permission from Alpert RA, Roizen MF, Hamilton WK et al: Intraoperative urinary output does not predict postoperative renal function in patients undergoing abdominal aortic revascularization. Surgery 95:707, 1984.)

increase PCWP to a high-normal level) or furosemide, mannitol, or nothing. For each patient, serum creatinine and blood urea nitrogen (BUN) levels were assayed on the first, third, and seventh postoperative days. There was no significant correlation between intraoperative mean urinary output, or lowest hourly urinary output, and changes from preoperative to postoperative levels of creatinine or BUN (Fig. 37-7). Thus, urinary output, which is believed to be an index of perfusion and therefore is monitored routinely during surgery, was not predictive of postoperative renal function in normovolemic patients.

When patients who underwent aortic occlusion at the suprarenal level were compared with those who underwent occlusion at the infrarenal level, there was no difference in postoperative renal function.[57]

Our results in patients who underwent aortic reconstruction conflict with those reported in older studies but have been confirmed.[58] In investigations in which a period of renal ischemia was imposed on patients and animal models, pretreatment with mannitol lessened postischemic increases in creatinine.[197-200] Direct infusion of mannitol into the renal artery sustained renal cortical perfusion (as assayed by the xenon washout technique) in mongrel dogs after infrarenal aortic occlusion.[197] In rabbits, pretreatment with mannitol prevented an increase in serum creatinine levels after 60 minutes of renal artery occlusion.[200] In dogs subjected to aortic clamping and unclamping, adequate replacement of blood with saline prevented a decrease in renal blood flow, consistent with the findings of Alpert et al.[57] In addition, furosemide and ethacrynic acid significantly increase both the total and the cortical components of renal blood flow, as demonstrated by studies of ^{133}Xe washout.[197] The use of mannitol, furosemide, or ethacrynic acid, however, has not been clearly shown to prevent renal failure. The difference between the results of Alpert et al[57] and those of others[197-200] may be due to variations among species, the maintenance of normal intravascular volume by Alpert et al, the insensitivity of urinary output as a measure of the adequacy of renal perfusion, or a combination of these

factors. We believe that preoperative renal function and the maintenance of an appropriate intravascular volume and normal myocardial function are the most important determinants of postoperative renal function.

It is important to monitor renal function, because the development of acute renal failure after aortic reconstruction is associated with a high morbidity and a mortality of more than 30%.[54] This complication is most frequent in patients with ruptured aneurysms who have significant hypotensive episodes, and in those for whom suprarenal aortic clamping is required. Despite our aforementioned data, infusion of mannitol prior to clamping of the renal arteries is believed by some to be beneficial and is commonly used.[144,201] Furosemide, vasodilators, and angiotensin-converting enzyme inhibitors may also have a place before renal artery clamping. If prolonged renal ischemia is anticipated, selective profound hypothermia of the kidneys may decrease the incidence of postoperative renal impairment. Recently, it was suggested that infusion of verapamil into the renal arteries just before reperfusion may also be beneficial,[201] although the question has been raised as to whether anything better than good surgical technique exists.[57,58] Our management, however, is biased by the results of our own studies. Thus, when intraoperative urinary output is less than 0.125 $ml \cdot kg^{-1} \cdot h^{-1}$, we ensure that no mechanical problems in urine collection are present and that left-sided cardiac filling volumes or pressures are adequate. We then continue to monitor but do not treat. Urinary output usually returns to acceptable levels within 2 hours. If it does not, or if we are uneasy about low urinary output, 2–5 mg of furosemide is administered iv to stimulate urine production.[57]

Thus, virtually all investigators have concluded that maintenance of adequate intravascular volume and myocardial function largely prevents renal insufficiency and insufficiency of other organs from being major clinical problems and that it is the key to intraoperative perfusion of critical organs.

ANESTHETIC AGENTS AND TECHNIQUES FOR AORTIC RECONSTRUCTION

Virtually all anesthetic techniques and drugs have been used for aortic reconstructive surgery. For this operative procedure, as for other types of vascular surgery, maintaining hemodynamic equilibrium and attending to detail appear to be more crucial to outcome than is the choice of drugs.[202] Although it is now believed that the choice of the agent or technique is important to the outcome,[36,202-204] the quality and attentiveness of the anesthesiologist are much more important than the choice of agent.

Inhalational Anesthetics

Halothane, enflurane, and isoflurane are halogenated hydrocarbons that exhibit negative inotropic properties when administered to volunteers not undergoing surgery. However, during surgery these agents act as vasodilators,[195] isoflurane being the most potent. Vasodilation is both advantageous and disadvantageous. It provides an additional means (besides administration of nitroglycerin or nitroprusside) of controlling afterload and preload but can lead to an increased need for intravascular volume. The resultant increase in intravascular volume can be detrimental at the end of the procedure. As the amount of the anesthetic is decreased, intravascular volume could return to the central compartment and cause relative hypervolemia and even pulmonary edema. To prevent this problem in patients who are still receiving a volatile anesthetic or an epidural anesthetic, increase in central blood volume that occurs with awakening is simulated for the 30–45 minutes of closure by tilting the patient (head lower than feet), and the patient is then slowly returned to the level position while the concentration of the anesthetic agent is gradually reduced, if it is a volatile agent, or the effects of the epidural anesthetic are dissipating. The tilting allows one to predict the patient's postanesthetic volume status and make appropriate adjustments.

Volatile drugs have several other advantages. They permit careful, deliberate induction, manipulation and monitoring of hemodynamic variables, and adjustment of dose. In addition, by providing a moderate degree of muscle relaxation, they decrease the need for muscle relaxants and increase the ease of reversing paralysis.

With the use of volatile hydrogen anesthetics, extubation of the trachea is usually accomplished by the end of surgery, and the patient is allowed to breathe spontaneously. Thus, the stressful stimuli and hypertension associated with continued intubation of the trachea are avoided, and early assessment of neurologic function is facilitated, allowing evaluation of motor function and limb sensation before placement of an epidural catheter to facilitate postoperative analgesia. Also, because tracheal extubation occurs at the end of surgery, the patient is able to complain of angina (if it is present), for which nitroglycerin can be administered.

Since isoflurane was introduced, we have tried to avoid using halothane; occlusion of the aorta at the supraceliac level tends to make the liver hypoxic for a time, and in this situation, halothane can in theory create a hepatitis-like condition.[205] However, 20 of the first 40 patients whom we anesthetized for supraceliac aortic revascularization received halothane without any adverse effect attributable to the drug.

Opioids

All commonly used opioids produce similar cardiovascular effects unless they are administered rapidly in large doses.[202] Induction of anesthesia with opioids can be accomplished quickly and decreases the cardiac index by a small but statistically significant amount. In sufficient doses, opioids produce analgesia and hypnosis, with only slight decreases in cardiac contractility and blood pressure.[202] Higher doses predictably decrease peripheral vascular resistance[206] especially when administered after benzodiazepines. With continual infusion of opioids or other drugs, anesthesia can be maintained throughout the surgical procedure. Surgical stimulation after such induction significantly increases the heart rate, arterial blood pressure, and systemic vascular resistance. Nitroglycerin, nitroprusside, or a volatile anesthetic can be added to the opioid for manipulation of the circulation during cross-clamping and unclamping.

Nitrous oxide can be used with opioids, as with the inhalational drugs. It increases afterload and myocardial work while depressing myocardial inotropic performance and output, and it decreases renal and splanchnic blood flows.[207,208] In addition, nitrous oxide may have a long-lasting toxic effect by causing nutritional, neurologic, and immunologic deficits.[209] It can also contribute to bowel distention.

A disadvantage to the opioids is that they linger into the postoperative period. Until opioids that provide pain relief

TABLE 37-6. Morbidity After Aortic Reconstruction With Either of Two Different Anesthetic Agents

Morbidity	Isoflurane-Based Anesthetic ($n = 50$)	Sufentanil-Based Anesthetic ($n = 46$)
Renal insufficiency	16	4*
Congestive heart failure	13	4*
Ventilation > 24 hr	9	4
Pneumonia	2	1
Renal failure	3	1
Stroke	2	0
Myocardial ischemia	0	1
Death	2	1
Important or severe complications	20	9*
Important or severe complications and failure	17	7*

*$p < 0.05$ by Fisher's exact test.

Modified with permission from Benefiel DJ, Roizen MF, Lampe GH et al: Morbidity after aortic surgery with sufentanil versus isoflurane anesthesia. Anesthesiology 65:A516, 1986.

without affecting the respiratory drive are produced, the likelihood increases that controlled ventilation of the lungs will be required in the postoperative period. However, in more than 50% of the opioid–nitrous oxide anesthetic techniques used for suprarenal aortic reconstruction, Benefiel et al[36] were able to extubate the trachea in the OR. An advantage to high-dose opioids as the anesthetic is the continued, excellent postoperative analgesia.

In a prospective controlled study, patients who consented and were about to undergo aortic reconstruction were randomly assigned to receive either a volatile anesthetic (isoflurane) or an opioid (sufentanil)-based anesthetic.[36] Intraoperatively and postoperatively, systemic and pulmonary capillary blood pressures and heart rates were kept within 20% of mean preoperative (baseline) values. Sufentanil anesthesia alone was associated with less major morbidity than isoflurane anesthesia in patients undergoing aortic reconstruction (Table 37-6). Because published data[27-37] indicate that the complication rates in patients who undergo aortic reconstruction are as high as or higher than those for the isoflurane group of Benefiel et al,[36] we postulate that sufentanil has a protective effect. Further study is needed to determine whether all opioids are protective, or whether the combination of sufentanil and isoflurane can produce an outcome equivalent to or better than that achieved with sufentanil alone.

Epidural Anesthetics

Epidural anesthesia has been used successfully for resection of infrarenal aortic aneurysms and aortic reconstruction,[210] and it can be combined with general anesthesia for supraceliac aortic reconstruction. A significant risk with epidural anesthetics is that administration of heparin might create an epidural hematoma and subsequent neurologic deficit.[211-213] Such a deficit could be confused with that caused by spinal cord ischemia, thereby delaying the correct diagnosis, evacuation of the hematoma, and return of neurologic function. Thus, we are reluctant to use epidural anesthesia for supraceliac aortic reconstruction. In addition, the absence of sensation and leg movement postoperatively might create undue worry for the patient. This disadvantage can be ameliorated by the use of concentrations of epidural anesthetic agents at the end of the operation that affect sensory but not motor fibers. Another disadvantage of epidural anesthesia is the possibility of a relative overload of fluid toward the end of the procedure. As with inhalational agents, we tilt the patient (head lower than feet) near the end of the procedure so that the fluid status is normal as the anesthetic wears off. A number of studies, including a large series reported by Rao and El-Etr[211] and a study on use of epidural anesthesia even after full heparinization in cardiac surgery,[214] indicate that this potential problem is of more theoretical than actual concern. Thus, use of heparin does not appear to contraindicate the use of epidural anesthesia, or even continuous epidural anesthesia.

Rao and El-Etr[211] stated that proper patient selection and atraumatic technique for regional anesthesia were important for a low complication rate. Their protocol included postponement of the planned elective vascular surgery procedure for 24 hours if blood returned from the epidural needle. This protocol was intended to allow clot formation in the epidural space before intraoperative anticoagulation. Other groups use a "single-shot" epidural or intrathecal technique with a 25- or 26-gauge needle to reduce the risk of postponement of surgery and to provide for postoperative pain relief by addition of an opioid.[215] To reduce the incidence of pruritus and respiratory depression from such epidural or intrathoracic analgesia, some anesthesiologists routinely infuse naloxone (2 mg in 250 ml saline, which equals $8 \mu g \cdot ml^{-1}$, given at a rate of $0.5-1.5 \mu g \cdot kg^{-1} \cdot h^{-1}$, or about $7 ml \cdot h^{-1}$).[215,216] Since urinary catheters are typically left in place for at least 36 hours following aortic reconstruction surgery, retention of urine, another side-effect of spinal or epidural opioids, is not a major issue.

The advantages of epidural anesthesia include a potential decrease in myocardial ischemia,[214] although it may also make myocardial ischemia worse;[195] excellent muscle relaxation; a smaller bowel (because of sympathectomy) that tends not to obstruct the operative field; and hemodynamic stability once the blockade is fully achieved. However, most studies suggesting a potential decrease in myocardial ischemia with epidural anesthesia included a comparison group that received a fixed dose of isoflurane, rather than an individualized dose based on the patient's hemodynamic variables.[214] The initiation of epidural anesthesia often causes a decrease in blood pressure, cardiac output, and possibly perfusion to the gut and kidney, which, in the stenotic state, may be pressure dependent. During crossclamping and unclamping in a patient under epidural anesthesia, the circulation can be controlled by administration of volatile anesthetics or iv drugs that reduce the afterload.

In addition, Yeager et al[204] compared outcomes after epidural anesthesia with outcomes after general anesthesia in 48 surgical patients, some of whom underwent vascular operations. The patients who received epidural anesthesia and analgesia postoperatively had fewer cardiovascular and infectious disease complications and lower medical care costs than those receiving general anesthesia. Similar results were obtained for those receiving epidural analgesia postoperatively.[217] Thus, the data may imply that epidural anesthesia is not only *not* a risky technique, but that it may even be an advantageous one for providing anesthesia for aortic reconstruction. Further, prophylaxis of stress and pain by any mechanism—epidural anesthetics, opiate infusion, or alpha$_2$ agonists—may result in lower morbidity in those

least able to tolerate the myocardial and cardiovascular demands of stress.[218-222]

Muscle Relaxants

The choices of muscle relaxants for use during aortic reconstruction are succinylcholine as a continuous infusion or, in bolus injections, d-tubocurarine, metocurine, pancuronium, vecuronium, or atracurium. Vecuronium and atracurium have shorter half-lives and provide more hemodynamic stability than do the other agents. d-Tubocurarine is preferable to metocurine or pancuronium when the degree of hypertension is significant, the vagolytic effect of pancuronium is not desired, or renal insufficiency is great enough to prolong the excretion of metocurine or pancuronium. We do not yet have enough experience with doxacurium or pipecuronium to recommend their use. We routinely titrate the muscle relaxant to the chronotropic cardiovascular effect that we want to achieve.

In view of the small number of patients in general and of vascular patients in particular, and the detail provided about the general anesthesia technique in the study of Yeager et al,[204] another study verifying these findings similar to our study, which showed a benefit for sufentanil compared with inhalational anesthetics, would be helpful.[36]

Anesthesia for Aortic Reconstruction

As soon as all oral intake is stopped, prehydration is begun at maintenance rates. Although we are unable to prove this with specific data, we believe that maintenance of a normal hydration status reduces variations in blood pressure on induction of anesthesia.

After the patient's preoperative condition has been optimized, the range of hemodynamic variables for that patient is determined. The anesthetic management is then planned to keep the patient within 20% of this range, as long as the PCWP does not exceed 15 mm Hg, the heart rate does not exceed 100 beats·min^{-1}, and signs of organ ischemia are absent. Premedication consisting of a benzodiazepine and an opioid is requested (usually 0.015 mg·kg^{-1} of diazepam 1.5–2 hours before the planned incision and 0.01 mg·kg^{-1} of morphine sulfate im 1 hour before the planned incision; these dosages are reduced for old age, debility, pulmonary disease, and so on) in addition to all the patient's usual medications. Any drug therapy needed before major vascular surgery most probably will also be needed during the operative period. Omitting chronic drug therapy can result in a worsened disease condition in the postoperative period. For example, tachycardia, angina, or both may occur if propranolol, atenolol, or other beta-adrenergic receptor blocking drugs are omitted; aspiration may occur if L-dopa is omitted; and accelerated hypertension may result if clonidine is omitted. The patient should be given antihypertensive medication, including diuretics, before being brought to the OR.[70] Many diabetic patients who require insulin are given an insulin infusion throughout surgery. Preoperative considerations and drug therapy for diabetic patients are described in Chapters 21 and 45.[70] However, because no particular premedication seems indicated or contraindicated for most patients, the patient's anesthesiologist should determine what is appropriate. Anticholinergic drugs might be avoided because they produce a dry mouth and tachycardia, which increases myocardial oxygen consumption.

In the preoperative holding area or in the OR, those monitors and catheters that are needed for induction of anesthesia are placed—usually an 18-gauge radial artery catheter in the nondominant hand, a manual blood pressure cuff, pulse oximeter, ECG (leads II and MCL 5), ST segment trend monitor, precordial stethoscope, 16-gauge iv line, and, occasionally, a PA catheter (or central venous catheter if the patient shows no evidence of myocardial, pulmonary, or renal disease), although placement of the PA catheter can usually wait until induction of anesthesia is completed. Then, after 3 mg of d-tubocurarine is given, an infusion of 750 μg of sufentanil in 100 ml of saline is begun at a rate of about 15 to 50 $\mu g \cdot min^{-1} \cdot 70 \ kg^{-1}$, and the patient is coached to breathe 100% oxygen from a face mask. After about 3 minutes, 75 mg of thiopental iv is administered, and 0.1 $mg \cdot kg^{-1}$ pancuronium or vecuronium is given over 3–5 minutes, depending on whether one wishes the heart rate to increase or stay the same. Other drugs are chosen if the patient has renal insufficiency with a creatinine level above 2 $mg \cdot dl^{-1}$.

When the depth of anesthesia is judged adequate by the lack of response to Foley catheter insertion or placement of another iv line or by pinpoint pupils, and when muscle relaxation is adequate, the trachea is intubated and mechanical ventilation with 0–60% nitrous oxide in oxygen is begun. The remainder of the pre-cross-clamping phase is devoted to meticulous attention to details of maintaining temperature homeostasis (by a heating mattress and heating of all fluids and, if necessary, heating of ventilatory gases); maintaining volume homeostasis as judged by heart rate, blood pressure, pulmonary capillary or central venous pressure; maintaining left ventricular end-diastolic volume as assessed by 2D-TEE; ensuring absence of organ ischemia; monitoring (but usually not treating) urine output; and keeping systemic and pulmonary blood pressures and heart rate in the patient's usual range. Every increase in blood pressure or heart rate is either anticipated or treated as soon as it occurs with 25–50 μg of sufentanil. Further increases are treated with repeated doses, or with the addition of nitroglycerin or nitroprusside, enflurane, isoflurane, esmolol, or propranolol, depending on the event and the suspected cause. The remainder of the patient's course is managed according to the physiologic principles described earlier in this chapter.

For the half hour immediately before cross-clamping and aortic occlusion, the patient is kept slightly hypovolemic by examining the ventricular volume (end-diastolic dimension) by means of 2D-TEE or by keeping PCWP at 5–12 mm Hg. At the time of occlusion one should be prepared to give a vasodilating drug through an iv line placed specifically for that purpose in order to avoid hypotension secondary to an accidental bolus of vasodilator. This catheter site is often the third lumen of the PA catheter.

Stabilizing the PA pressure and systemic blood pressure with more sufentanil (25–50 μg) and vasodilating drugs before and during cross-clamping may not be enough. When myocardial ischemia is evidenced by regional wall motion abnormalities or ST segment changes, or by new v waves on PCWP transduction, more vasodilating drugs are given, to the point of bringing the systolic blood pressure toward the low end of the normal preoperative range. Once the blood pressure is made as low as possible (by reducing afterload with nitroprusside), we often attempt to decrease the preload with nitroglycerin and, if necessary, to decrease the heart rate with propranolol or esmolol given iv. If, despite these maneuvers, myocardial dysfunction is evident on placement of the cross-clamp, the surgeon can be asked

to unclamp the aorta partially until myocardial function is more stable before he has incised the aorta or its branches. Close communication with the surgeon and a mutual appreciation of what the other physician is doing are key factors in facilitating the patient's course. We try to avoid the use of exogenous vasoconstrictors at this time.

To ensure adequate volume at the time of cross-clamp removal, blood lost during occlusion is replaced with warmed blood, milliliter for milliliter, to keep the hematocrit slightly above 30%. (It will fall to 30% in the postocclusion period.) It is my personal belief, substantiated by some data, that this is the minimal acceptable value for patients in this risk group.[223-225] Although most patients can tolerate hematocrits in the 20–25% range intraoperatively, it has been my experience that vascular patients have a worse postoperative course and a longer convalescence with a hematocrit of 20% than with one of 30%. No randomized, controlled study has been done, however, to substantiate that impression. Much of the transfused blood administered is from either predeposited blood or autotransfusion of blood salvaged from the operative field. Immediately before and during removal of the cross-clamp, we stop infusing the vasodilator and start infusing crystalloid or blood; usually, 2 units of whole blood are pressured into venous access sites. Guided by filling pressures or echocardiographic estimates of volume, we are careful not to dilate the left ventricle to an abnormal size.

It is not uncommon for moderate hypotension (i.e., a decrease in systolic pressure of 40–60 mm Hg) to occur on removal of the aortic cross-clamp, regardless of whether the clamp is replaced infrarenally or such that blood flow to only one leg is obstructed. On observations with 2D-TEE, we believe that such hypotension is caused mainly by relative volume depletion. If hypotension persists for more than 4 minutes after removal of the clamp and does not return toward normal after blood deficits have been replaced, we search for other causes, including myocardial dysfunction, hidden blood loss, and so on. If necessary, the surgeon can reclamp or occlude the aorta, preferably below the renal arteries. Thus, volume replacement and maintenance are mainstays of therapy before, during, and immediately after removal of the aortic cross-clamp. When blood flow to the first extremity is opened up, volume replacement should also be considered.

During closure, we again ensure adequate organ perfusion as well as hemodynamic and temperature homeostasis, and we reverse the effects of muscle relaxants. Nitroglycerin and esmolol infusions should be available at this time, and hemodynamic variations outside the patient's normal range are not allowed. If the patient demonstrates adequate ventilation (as is common 6 hours after our initial dose of sufentanil), the trachea is extubated; otherwise, controlled ventilation is maintained until spontaneous ventilation is judged adequate. If an inhalational anesthetic technique is used, I often place an epidural catheter in the OR at the end of the operation, after the patient has demonstrated bilateral foot movement (with light anesthesia during closure). Epidural opioids are administered to this group of patients, but rarely is other pain therapy needed for 24 hours when the sufentanil-based technique described here is used. Continuing care into the postoperative period is very important for patient outcome.

The outcome after infrarenal aortic reconstructive surgery has improved. Hicks et al[29] reported a decrease in mortality from 22% during 1955–1960 (for 41 patients) to 12.5% during 1966–1970, and to 4.2% during 1970–1973. In the series of Scobie and Masters,[226] the perioperative mortality for elective repair of an abdominal aneurysm decreased from 12% during 1961–1969 to 4.1% during 1971–1975, and to 1.8% during 1976–1980. Accompanying this decrease in mortality was an increase in the use of venous pressure (fluid) monitoring devices: from 13% for the period 1961–1969 to 100% after 1971. After 1975, the use of PA thermodilution catheters also increased.[226] Thus, overall, the mortality and morbidity from aortic reconstructive surgery have decreased greatly in the past three decades. Crawford et al[33] attributed most of the reduction in morbidity in patients who had infrarenal resections before 1971 to improvement in operative techniques and, after 1981, to improvements in anesthesia, monitoring, and supportive care. However, the perioperative mortality from supraceliac aneurysms still exceeds 4%.

An 8% incidence rate of myocardial infarction with no mortality, which occurred in 12 patients who were studied with 2D-TEE, is possible in patients who have severe myocardial dysfunction.[40] However, we believe that aiming for the 4% mortality reported by Crawford et al[33] and the even lower rate reported by Benefiel et al[36] is the best one can do with current techniques. In patients who have isolated celiac artery disease and little dysfunction in other organs, mortality and morbidity should be negligible.

On the other hand, most morbidity is myocardial, and most myocardial morbidity occurs postoperatively (see Table 37-3).[1-10] Rao et al[7] indicated that intensive normalization of hemodynamics postoperatively might result in better outcome. A number of other studies have implied that preventing postoperative pain and stress may decrease adverse events.[36,204,215,218-222] Improved outcomes in the next decade may result not only from better patient segregation for prophylactic and therapeutic procedures (see Fig. 37-4), but also from better postoperative care.

ANESTHESIA FOR EMERGENCY AORTIC RECONSTRUCTION

Causes and Indications

The most common cause of emergency aortic reconstruction is a leaking or ruptured aortic aneurysm. Patients with symptoms of acute ischemia are discussed in the following section. Ruptured aneurysms can be atherosclerotic, mycotic, syphilitic, or inflammatory, or may occur in patients with the marfanoid syndrome.[159] These ruptures are 10 times more common in male than in female patients, whereas aortic aneurysms in general have a 4:1 male-female preponderance.

Ruptures most commonly occur into the retroperitoneum.[227-231] This site permits tamponade of the hemorrhage; however, retroperitoneal hemorrhage and subsequent hematoma can displace the left renal vein, inferior vena cava, and intestine, possibly leading to damage to these structures during the surgical approach. Venous hemorrhage is often much more difficult to control than arterial hemorrhage.

Approximately 25% of aneurysms rupture into the peritoneal cavity, a site associated with a great degree of exsanguination. Other sites of rupture include adjacent structures after formation of fistulae with the inferior vena cava, iliac veins, or renal veins.[232-235]

Aortoenteric fistulae most commonly rupture into the fixed third portion of the duodenum.[236] These fistulae usually occur between the overlying bowel and a portion of the aorta that has previously undergone resection and grafting for an existing aneurysm. The mortality from these fistulae is high, often exceeding 50%. An abdominal aortic aneurysm may dissect proximally, resulting in hemopericardium.[237] The overall mortality rates vary in published series from 15% to 90%, and the time from the onset of symptoms to control of bleeding appears to be the key to determining outcome. This gives credence to the inescapable sense of urgency that accompanies such events. Other factors that adversely affect outcome[228,231] are a history of chronic hypertension, heart disease, or renal insufficiency, a hematocrit below 32.5% at diagnosis, hypotension at diagnosis, surgery lasting more than 400 minutes, and blood loss greater than 11,000 ml. Factors associated with a poor outcome that may be influenced by anesthetic management are hypotension lasting longer than 110 minutes and a systolic blood pressure below 100 mm Hg at the end of the operation.

The interval from the onset of symptoms to arrival at the hospital ranges from 0.3 to 22.5 hours, the mean interval being approximately 7 hours.[231] Among 100 patients with ruptured abdominal aortic aneurysms, Ottinger[229] found the following distribution of symptoms: pain, 92 patients; collapse, 17 patients; faintness, 13; vomiting, 13; numbness in leg, 3; inability to void, 2; and weakness in leg, 1. In 8 patients an adequate history could not be obtained. Pain in the back, abdomen, or both was almost always present. This pain resulted from "dissection of the aortic wall and retroperitoneal spaces by blood." Therefore, many surgeons believe that pain in combination with a known abdominal aortic aneurysm or pulsatile abdominal mass indicates dissection or rupture and the immediate need for surgical exploration until proved otherwise.

Shock also frequently accompanies rupture. May et al[163] reported that 56% of patients with ruptured abdominal aortic aneurysms were in shock at the time of admission, with cold and clammy extremities or blood pressures of 100/60 mm Hg or less. However, the absence of hypotension does not rule out the possibility of rupture, and shock may occur suddenly. Patients with dissection may have severe hypertension, which must be controlled immediately if rupture is to be prevented.

Rapid diagnosis with immediate laparotomy and control of the proximal aorta are of the highest priority. If systolic blood pressure is less than 90 mm Hg, some clinicians advocate the administration of oxygen by face mask, with endotracheal intubation performed only after proximal control of the aorta has been achieved.[228] Because experienced anesthesia personnel can usually intubate the trachea rapidly, and because of the substantial threat of aspiration pneumonitis, we usually do not follow the procedure of Lawrie et al.[228] Initially, a rapid sequence endotracheal intubation is performed. We believe that this causes little morbidity, creates only a slight delay, and prevents a potentially serious complication. The probability of rupture into the free peritoneal cavity is high if loss of consciousness or mental aberration occurs along with marked hypotension that is unresponsive to rapid volume infusion. In this case, the trachea is immediately intubated in a rapid sequence fashion, usually with the aid of muscle relaxants and with only small doses of barbiturates, opioids, or etomidate (and a steroid); ventilation with 100% oxygen is also started. Almost simultaneously, laparotomy is begun so that the surgeon can clamp the aorta.

I attempt to replace volume to the point of normalizing the systemic blood pressure (at this time, often the only guide to volume replacement in the patient with an uncontained rupture). A difference from elective surgery is that heparin is not administered before aortic cross-clamping.

The patient is resuscitated quickly (before induction of anesthesia, if possible) with type-specific non-cross-matched blood and crystalloid administered via large-bore venous catheters by roller pumps or pressured bags. If type-specific blood is not available, O-negative washed red blood cells may be given.

Once the aorta is controlled with a cross-clamp and blood pressure and perfusion are restored, additional venous access is obtained if necessary. It is often helpful, indeed necessary, to have a second anesthesiologist secure vascular access while the first is securing the airway, monitoring blood pressure, and administering volume into the iv sites that have been established. Peripheral arterial and PA catheters are then inserted. Even more quickly, a 2D-TEE probe can be inserted, and left ventricular volume assayed by left ventricular area (see Fig. 37-6). At this point, volume administration is guided by means of filling pressures obtained from PA catheter readings or by the area on the echocardiographic representation of the left ventricle.

We do not administer diuretics routinely, although many clinicians do. If intraoperative oliguria (urinary output of $0.125 \, ml \cdot kg^{-1} \cdot h^{-1}$ or less) is noted, patency of the urinary catheter and collection system and adequate left-sided cardiac filling pressures are first ensured. If hypotension has occurred secondary to rupture, and perhaps low-output acute tubular necrosis is present, 12.5–25 g of mannitol or 40–120 mg of furosemide is administered in an attempt to increase the urinary output.

We do not hesitate to paralyze and administer large doses of opioids to these patients if they are hemodynamically stable, because these patients usually need postoperative mechanical ventilation of the lungs and sedation to minimize cardiovascular stress.

In a second group are patients with pain and shock reversible with volume administration. In such patients, it may be assumed that hemorrhage has been at least partially contained. However, because rapid exsanguination can occur at any time, patients are transported immediately to the OR for emergency laparotomy, and the same urgency is maintained.

If the blood pressure and heart rate are stable when the patient arrives, sterile preparation of the abdomen is begun. The intravascular volume status may be assessed by observation of the patient for a decrease in systemic blood pressure or an increase in the heart rate when the head is raised 10–15 degrees. Administration of a 50-mg bolus of thiopental iv may also aid in the assessment of volume. Induction of anesthesia is delayed until the patient's abdomen is prepared and draped and the surgeon is ready. Venous access is ensured, and positive indications of acceptable volume loading are demonstrated by the tilt test or administration of small doses of thiopental, or measurements from a PA catheter (rapidly placed) are sought. Thus, in this situation, minimal extra time is spent on inserting and attaching monitors.

Preoxygenation is followed by rapid sequence induction of anesthesia with small doses of fentanyl or sufentanil, small to moderate doses of thiopental ($0.5–5 \, mg \cdot kg^{-1}$, depending on the response to the test dose of thiopental), a rapidly acting muscle relaxant, application of cricoid pressure, and endotracheal intubation. To blunt the hemodynamic effects of laryngeal visualization and endotracheal intubation, one may administer an iv bolus of lidocaine,

sodium nitroprusside, nitroglycerin, esmolol, or additional fentanyl, sufentanil, or thiopental.

If hypotension occurs following induction, administer 100% oxygen, elevate the patient's legs, and rapidly administer blood and fluids. If these measures fail to produce adequate blood pressure and perfusion, we infuse phenylephrine or dopamine until the aorta can be occluded.

During temporary aortic occlusion we insert a PA catheter (if it is not already in place) to guide volume administration. High-normal filling pressures are desirable for attenuation of hypotension following removal of the aortic clamp.

Because of the site of aortic occlusion, replacement blood may not pass through the liver in amounts adequate to allow for metabolism of citrate.[187] Therefore, if hypotension due to poor myocardial contractility or to coagulopathy develops, administration of calcium may be therapeutic.

A third possibility is the patient who was initially treated with a military antishock trouser (MAST) suit. This temporizing measure allows transport of the patient to the OR with less hemorrhage and, some believe, with clot formation and temporary sealing of the aortic rent. If possible, pressure should be removed in stages (e.g., from the epigastrium, then one leg, then the other leg) rather than all at once, and only after the surgeons are scrubbed and ready to begin immediately if necessary. Reducing all pressure at once increases blood flow (reactive hyperemia) in all areas simultaneously, thereby causing a large and precipitous decrease in blood pressure and filling volumes of the heart.

We routinely use autotransfusion in patients with actual or suspected rupture of an aortic aneurysm. However, a separate team is available to set up and operate autotransfusion devices, as the primary anesthesiologist should direct all of his or her attention to the patient's volume status, gas exchange, and depth of anesthesia. Our mnemonic for treatment of such patients is "wovcath," for *w*onder what anesthetic to give, or *w*onder whether the patient can tolerate an anesthetic, *o*xygen, *v*ecuronium, *c*oagulation, *a*cid-base change, *t*emperature change, and *h*emodynamic change. This mnemonic lists, in reverse order, the important aspects of patient care that we try to remember when everything about these patients invites disorganization.

Because cardiovascular complications account for more than 50% of all deaths associated with elective aortic reconstruction,[27-36] the most important determinant of outcome is the maintenance of cardiac well-being, but hypotension because of exsanguination is the primary cause of death if rupture occurs.[226-231] Therefore, when rupture is suspected, rapid control of the proximal portion of the aorta is probably more important than is optimizing the patient's preoperative condition.

The primary goal of aortic reconstruction is an enduring restoration of normal visceral and limb perfusion. The complications that occur during aortic occlusion can usually be linked to the heart, CNS, or kidneys. I believe that organ dysfunction, which involves the heart, can be minimized by maintenance of intraoperative values for hemodynamic variables within the normal preoperative range, ensuring that cardiac dilation does not occur at any point, and minimizing episodes of tachycardia. Attention to details of preoperative drug therapy, preoperative hydration, and temperature homeostasis may also promote an improved outcome. Further, vigilance must continue into the postoperative period if morbidity and mortality are to be minimized. As opposed to elective aortic reconstruction, in which preserving myocardial function is the primary goal, in emergency resection the crucial factor for patient survival is initial rapid control of blood loss and reversal of hypotension, and then preservation of myocardial function.

SURGERY FOR PERIPHERAL VASCULAR INSUFFICIENCY

There are three clinical indications for elective surgery for chronic peripheral occlusive disease: (1) claudication, (2) ischemic rest pain or ulceration, and (3) gangrene.[238] Patients with claudication have symptoms on walking that are relieved by rest. Such patients are not at significant risk for imminent limb loss. Patients with rest pain, ulceration, or gangrene are at variable risk for imminent limb loss and may have severe progressive ischemia. Thus, reconstruction is semiurgent or urgent. Vascular reconstruction procedures are generally categorized as either inflow or outflow procedures. Inflow reconstruction involves bypass of the obstruction in the aortoiliac segment, whereas outflow procedures are those performed distal to the inguinal ligament for bypass of femoropopliteal or distal obstructions.

The most common inflow reconstruction procedure for obstructions in the aortoiliac segment is aortofemoral bypass. This method was discussed in the previous section. The usual vascular reconstruction below the inguinal ligament is a bypass graft that originates in the common femoral artery and extends to the popliteal or tibial artery. Such a bypass may be performed with a reversed saphenous vein, the saphenous vein *in situ*, or a prosthetic graft.[239] For the vascular surgeon, the differences among these procedures involve different technical aspects of vessel dissection and exposure, of anastomosis, and of tunneling.

The complexity of femoropopliteal and femorotibial bypass varies widely. The site for distal anastomosis and the quality of the outflow vessels are assessed by preoperative angiography. The best short- and long-term results are achieved when the saphenous vein is used;[240,241] however, this requires longer operative time and greater technical expertise than are needed for prosthetic grafts. The duration and complexity of the operation are usually determined by the quality of the saphenous vein and the quality and size of the distal outflow vessels. Operative arteriography is commonly used for evaluation of the adequacy of the surgical repair. Major blood loss or hemodynamic changes are not usually encountered with distal reconstruction, but the procedure tends to be lengthy, making intraoperative urinary drainage advisable. Because the major morbidity and mortality with this procedure are related to the cardiovascular system, with rates above 8% and 2%, respectively, the noninvasive nature and the absence of hemodynamic alterations should not lull the anesthesiologist into taking a casual attitude.[239-241]

In a reversed saphenous vein bypass, the vein is dissected from its entrance into the common femoral vein to the level of the distal anastomosis. All branches of the saphenous vein are ligated and divided, and the vein is excised and inspected. After exposure of the proximal and distal vessels, the direction of the saphenous vein is reversed to permit blood flow in the direction of the valves, and the vein is tunneled from the femoral artery to the distal vessel. In this process, the surgeon tries to avoid damaging, injuring, or twisting the vein. After the proximal and distal anastomoses are completed, the adequacy of flow is determined from the quality of pulse and ultrasound signals, and from angiographic images obtained upon completion.

The use of the vein *in situ* offers significant advantages over the reversed-vein bypass. The large proximal saphenous vein is sutured to the large common femoral vein, and the small distal vein is sutured to the small distal artery. The size match is particularly important for tibial artery bypass, which permits the use of small saphenous veins that were previously judged unsuitable. In addition, because the vein is not removed from its bed, it is subjected to little trauma; twisting or kinking is unlikely. These advantages have resulted in improved patency rates.[242,243]

For bypass procedures in which the saphenous vein *in situ* is used, the vein in its bed is dissected, and side branches are ligated. The proximal saphenous vein is then sutured end-to-side to the common femoral artery, and arterial flow is introduced into the vein. The valves that obstruct retrograde flow in the saphenous vein are lysed with a valvulotome or valve cutter introduced through side branches. When all valves have been rendered incompetent, blood is seen flowing from the distal end of the vein. This distal end is then anastomosed to the appropriate arterial site. The quality of the repair is determined from the pulse quality, Doppler ultrasound studies, and completion angiography.

Prosthetic bypasses can be performed more quickly and require less dissection than the saphenous vein bypass, because it is not necessary to make multiple incisions for vein harvest. Prosthetic bypasses, however, have significantly lower patency rates than saphenous vein bypasses, particularly when they extend below the knee.[242] Incisions are made for exposure of the proximal and distal arteries, and a tunneling instrument is used for tunneling of the graft between the incisions. After completion of the proximal and distal anastomoses, the quality of the anastomoses and the blood runoff to the foot are judged by intraoperative angiography or Doppler ultrasound. (The latter technique is not yet accepted at all institutions, because of the importance of smooth intimal junctions.) The patient is usually given heparin during the procedure. In most cases the heparin effect is not antagonized, since bleeding problems are rare.

Emergency surgery for peripheral vascular insufficiency is required when acute arterial occlusion results in severe ischemia and threatens the viability of a limb. Immediate operation and restoration of blood flow are needed if limb loss is to be avoided. Depending on the etiology of the occlusion, the patient may or may not be at very high risk.

With acute arterial occlusion, the involved extremity suddenly becomes cold and pulseless. Patients usually complain of coldness, pain, numbness, and paresthesias, and they may lose motion and sensation. The severity of ischemia and the urgency of immediate operation can be assessed by examination of leg motion and sensation. Abnormal sensation in the toes, feet, and legs in response to light touch and pinprick, as well as abnormal proprioception and loss of motor function in the feet and toes, are hallmarks of acute ischemia and nonviability. If the ischemia is not reversed in a matter of hours, irreversible loss of viability is likely to result.

Acute arterial occlusion may develop in patients with pre-existing peripheral occlusive or aneurysmal disease caused by thrombosis of a stenotic or ulcerated atherosclerotic artery. Acute arterial occlusion can also occur in patients with normal peripheral arteries that contain emboli. Such embolism is usually of cardiac origin in patients with cardiac dysrhythmias, recent myocardial infarctions, or ventricular aneurysms.[244,245]

The cause is important in planning operative treatment. If the cause is an arterial embolus, Fogarty embolectomy through a groin incision, angioscopy, or laser atherectomy under local anesthesia may suffice.[179-182] However, if the cause is thrombosis of severely diseased atherosclerotic arteries, bypass reconstruction will be required. Preoperative angiography may be of help in the differential diagnosis; often the cause is not uncovered until the vessel is opened. Thus, the anesthesiologist must be prepared for either a simple procedure or a complex, extended procedure.

Patients with acute ischemia (arterial insufficiency) may be very ill. Significant fluid losses can be anticipated when the artery is flushed during thrombectomy and fluid is sequestered in edematous revascularized tissue. Serum potassium levels can change quickly, since cell death and release of intracellular potassium into the circulation can be anticipated. Myoglobin may also be released into the circulation, and the development of a compartment syndrome is a possibility.

An incision in the groin is usually made for exposure of the femoral artery. Attempts to pass Fogarty catheters proximally and distally are made in the effort to establish flow and extract the thrombus. If flow is not restored in this manner, more complex reconstructive procedures such as aortofemoral, axillofemoral, or femoropopliteal bypass may be required. Femoral venous drainage on restoration of flow to the femoral artery can aid in management by wasting the initial venous effluent from an acutely ischemic extremity. This may entail significant blood loss.

Anesthetic Goals and Management

There is perhaps no other disease entity in which the anesthesiologist can be misled so easily. One is apt to hear, "Oh, it's just a local procedure," or, "Just put a spinal in and let's get on with it; you don't have to read the chart." However, the morbidity and mortality following distal operations approach those following infra-aortic reconstruction and are mainly of cardiac origin. Thus, although I tend to use epidural anesthesia and epidural opioids for pain relief, attention to body temperature, oxygen delivery, and hemodynamic homeostasis should be just as intense during peripheral vascular procedures as during aortic procedures that involve much greater hemodynamic fluctuations. The devices and the concerns previously described apply, with special attention to the postoperative period. It is during the postoperative period that most cardiac problems arise and pain relief and correction of hemodynamic and fluid dysequilibria are most likely to be needed. Care must be taken not to allow overhydration to occur intraoperatively in support of blood pressure, and then to cause congestive heart failure as the epidural sympathectomy wears off. As is done for patients with aortic disease, I routinely tilt the patient's head down (while monitoring gas exchange closely) for the last hour of the planned surgery. Dye loads given for completion angiography also contribute to fluid shifts; thus, monitoring of left ventricular filling volumes is important for a successful outcome.

The surgeons' concerns for patients with peripheral vascular insufficiency include not only those involving the cardiovascular system, but also specific problems related to the operative repair. Graft patency is evaluated carefully in the recovery room. Most surgeons believe that the patient's feet should be kept warm and that the patient should be well hydrated so that peripheral vasoconstriction, which may limit outflow from the new graft, is prevented. If graft thrombosis develops early in the postoperative period, the patient is promptly returned to the OR for graft thrombectomy and

for evaluation and correction of the cause of the thrombosis. It can be anticipated that, during graft thrombectomy, significant blood loss will occur with flushing of the graft.

Anesthesia for Emergency Surgery for Peripheral Vascular Insufficiency

Acute peripheral vascular occlusion must be attended to quickly. Although this problem may appear to be localized to an extremity, the occluding material may originate in the heart or in major arteries. Therefore, peripheral vascular occlusion may be the result of a more serious cardiovascular problem. In fact, some patients with peripheral vascular occlusion are the sickest patients I have ever anesthetized.

Anticoagulants are commonly administered to patients suspected of having peripheral vascular occlusion. If a patient has received anticoagulants, the appropriateness of using a major conduction block (subarachnoid or epidural block with or without catheter placement) is controversial. Cunningham et al[210] described the effect of continuous epidural anesthesia in 100 patients who underwent resection of abdominal aortic aneurysms and operations for aortoiliac occlusion. No epidural hematoma was encountered. Another group reported on the results of continuous epidural anesthesia in 3168 patients and continuous subarachnoid anesthesia in 841 patients undergoing peripheral vascular surgery of the lower extremities.[211] Patients who received anticoagulants or who had leukemia, thrombocytopenia, hemophilia, or traumatic insertion of the catheter were given a general anesthetic. In this series also no hematomas or neurologic sequelae were reported. Similar results have been reported in other large series.[213,221] If patients with acute peripheral occlusion who are to undergo emergency surgery have received anticoagulants before arriving in the OR, we avoid giving major conduction blockade anesthesia. This rule is based on anecdotal case reports of epidural hematomas that caused paraplegia in similar situations.[213-215,246]

In addition, these patients often have hyperkalemia and acidosis as a result of ischemic extremities, and myoglobin may be released into the circulation. Although the surgical procedure may be only a peripheral one, cardiac causes, generalized atherosclerosis, electrolyte and acid-base balance disturbances, and fluid shifts, as well as the high morbidity and mortality associated with these procedures, will bring the cavalier anesthesiologist to his knees. Getting away with no care or little care for such patients is just a matter of luck. Skill and intensive care as meticulous as that given patients with visceral ischemia may also benefit patients with peripheral vascular insufficiency.

CONCLUSION

The skills of the anesthesiologist can greatly influence outcome in vascular surgery. The considerations for preoperative patient evaluation are the same as for patients with cardiac disease undergoing other noncardiac procedures. Patients undergoing vascular reconstruction are generally elderly. Vascular disease is a generalized process; thus, patients having surgery for a specific vascular disorder are likely to have atherosclerotic disease elsewhere in the vascular system. Most of the patients have CAD. Many have a history of smoking, and chronic obstructive pulmonary disease, renal insufficiency, and lipid abnormalities are frequently present. Although blood flow to many different organs may be interrupted, the stress of clamping and unclamping of vessels differs in different operations, and the co-morbid conditions, typically encountered are not similar in different operations. The major morbidity in each of the operations relates to myocardial well-being; therefore, the heart should be the major focus of the anesthesiologist's attention.

Attempts have been made to segregate patients who have significant CAD by use of Holter monitoring, hand exercises, dipyridamole-thallium scanning, coronary angiography, or other means, and then to have patients at high risk for myocardial events undergo coronary artery bypass surgery before vascular surgery. However, it has not been proved that such approaches reduce morbidity. Critics claim that such segregation is useful for identification of high-risk patients but that coronary angiography and surgery are simply "survival tests" preparatory to vascular surgery.[247]

In cerebrovascular surgery, the goals in anesthesia management—i.e., ensuring adequate myocardial and brain perfusion and a rapidly arousable patient—may be facilitated with the use of EEG as a guide to afterload reduction. In aortic reconstruction, ensuring intact myocardial function is probably the best way of making certain that spinal cord, visceral, and renal perfusion will be adequate.

In the case of peripheral occlusive disease, the absence of hemodynamic changes should not lull the anesthesiologist into loss of vigilance with regard to myocardial well-being. In addition, vigilance in ensuring routine prehydration and use of a warming mattress is probably more important to outcome than is occasional brilliance. If I needed vascular surgery, I would prefer the diligent, compulsive practitioner to the occasionally brilliant one. Nowhere is such diligence needed more than in the postoperative period, when most morbidity related to the heart occurs. Perhaps it is most important to remember that the best patient results are achieved when intraoperative vigilance is extended to the preoperative and postoperative periods as well.

REFERENCES

1. Hertzer NR, Young JR, Beven EG et al: Late results of coronary bypass in patients with infrarenal aortic aneurysms: The Cleveland Clinic Study. Ann Surg 205:360, 1987
2. Reul GJ Jr, Cooley DA, Duncan JM et al: The effect of coronary bypass on the outcome of peripheral vascular operations in 1093 patients. J Vasc Surg 3:788, 1986
3. Roger VL, Ballard DJ, Hallett JW et al: Influence of coronary artery disease on morbidity and mortality after abdominal aortic aneurysmectomy: A population-based study, 1971–1987. J Am Coll Cardiol 14:1245, 1989
4. Ouyang P, Gerstenblith G, Furman WR et al: Frequency and significance of early postoperative silent myocardial ischemia in patients having peripheral vascular surgery. Am J Cardiol 64:1113, 1989
5. Plumlee JE, Boettner RB: Myocardial infarction during and following anesthesia and operation. South Med J 65:886, 1972
6. Tarhan S, Moffitt EA, Taylor WF, Giuliani ER: Myocardial infarction after general anesthesia. JAMA 220:1451, 1972
7. Rao TLK, Jacobs KH, El-Etr AA: Reinfarction following anesthesia in patients with myocardial infarction. Anesthesiology 59:499, 1983
8. Becker RC, Underwood DA: Myocardial infarction in patients undergoing noncardiac surgery. Cleve Clin J Med 54:25, 1987
9. Mangano DT, Browner WS, Hollenberg M et al: Association of perioperative myocardial ischemia with cardiac morbidity and mortality in men undergoing noncardiac surgery. N Engl J Med 323:1781, 1990
10. Ellis JE, Busse JR, Foss JF, Roizen MF: Postoperative management of myocardial ischemia. Anesthesiol Clin North Am 9(3):609, 1991
11. Sundt TM, Sharbrough FW, Piepgras DG et al: Correlation of cerebral blood flow and electroencephalographic changes during carotid endarterectomy with results of surgery and hemodynamics of cerebral ischemia. Mayo Clin Proc 56:533, 1981
12. Hertzer NR, Lees CD: Fatal myocardial infarction following carotid endarterectomy: Three hundred thirty-five patients followed 6-11 years after operation. Ann Surg 194:212, 1981
13. Ennix CL, Lawrie GM, Morris GC: Improved results of carotid endarterectomy in patients with symptomatic coronary artery disease: An analysis of 1,546 consecutive carotid operations. Stroke 10:122, 1979
14. Till JS, Toole JF, Howard VJ et al: Declining morbidity and mortality of carotid endarterectomy. The Wake Forest Center experience. Stroke 18:823, 1987
15. Yeager RA, Moneta GL, McConnell DB et al: Analysis of risk factors for myocardial infarction following carotid endarterectomy. Arch Surg 124:1142, 1989
16. Brook RH, Park RE, Chassin MR et al: Carotid endarterectomy for elderly patients: Predicting complications. Ann Intern Med 113:747, 1990
17. Glaser RB: Morbidity and mortality resulting from major vascular surgery. In Roizen MF (ed): Anesthesia for Vascular Surgery, p 1. New York, Churchill Livingstone, 1990
18. Maxwell JG, Rutherford EJ, Covington DL et al: Community hospital carotid endarterectomy in patients over age 75. Am J Surg 160:598, 1990
19. Hertzer NR, Beven EG, Young JR et al: Coronary artery disease in peripheral vascular patients: A classification of 1000 coronary angiograms and results of surgical management. Ann Surg 199:223, 1984
20. Kartchner MM, McRae LP: Carotid occlusive disease as a risk factor in major cardiovascular surgery. Arch Surg 117:1086, 1982
21. Hertzer NR, Loop FD, Beven EG et al: Surgical staging for simultaneous coronary and carotid disease: A study including prospective randomization. J Vasc Surg 9:455, 1989
22. Maki HS, Kuehner ME, Ray JF III: Combined carotid endarterectomy and myocardial revascularization. Am J Surg 158:443, 1989
23. Barnes RW, Marsalek PG: Asymptomatic carotid disease in the cardiovascular surgical patient: Is prophylactic endarterectomy necessary? Stroke 12:497, 1981
24. Burke PA, Callow AD, O'Donnell TF et al: Prophylactic carotid endarterectomy for asymptomatic bruit. Arch Surg 117:1222, 1982
25. Graham AM, Gewertz BL, Zarins CK: Predicting cerebral ischemia during carotid endarterectomy. Arch Surg 121:595, 1986
26. Smith JS, Roizen MF, Cahalan MK et al: Does anesthetic technique make a difference? Augmentation of systolic blood pressure during carotid endarterectomy: Effects of phenylephrine versus light anesthesia and of isoflurane versus halothane on the incidence of myocardial ischemia. Anesthesiology 69:846, 1988
27. Szilagyi DE, Smith RF, Derusso FJ et al: Contribution of abdominal aortic aneurysmectomy to prolongation of life. Ann Surg 164:678, 1966
28. Young AE, Sandberg GW, Couch NP: The reduction of mortality of abdominal aortic aneurysm resection. Am J Surg 134:585, 1977
29. Hicks GL, Eastland MW, Deweese JA et al: Survival improvement following aortic aneurysm resection. Ann Surg 181:863, 1975
30. Thompson JE, Hollier LH, Patman RD et al: Surgical management of abdominal aortic aneurysms: Factors influencing mortality and morbidity—a 20-year experience. Ann Surg 181:654, 1975

31. Mulcare RJ, Royster TS, Lynn RA et al: Long-term results of operative therapy for aortoiliac disease. Arch Surg 113:601, 1978

32. Whittemore AD, Clowes AW, Hechtman HB et al: Aortic aneurysm repair. Reduced operative mortality associated with maintenance of optimal cardiac performance. Ann Surg 192:414, 1980

33. Crawford ES, Saleh SA, Babb JW III et al: Infrarenal abdominal aortic aneurysm. Factors influencing survival after operation performed over a 25-year period. Ann Surg 193:699, 1981

34. Hertzer NR: Myocardial ischemia. Surgery 93:97, 1983

35. Yeager RA, Weigel RM, Murphy SS et al: Application of clinically valid cardiac risk factors to aortic aneurysm surgery. Arch Surg 121:278, 1986

36. Benefiel DJ, Roizen MF, Lampe GH et al: Morbidity after aortic surgery with sufentanil versus isoflurane anesthesia. Anesthesiology 65:A516, 1986

37. Nevelsteen A, Suy R, Daenen MD et al: Aortofemoral grafting: Factors influencing late results. Surgery 88:642, 1980

38. Martinez BD, Hertzer NR, Beven EG: Influence of distal arterial occlusive disease on prognosis following aortobifemoral bypass. Surgery 88:795, 1980

39. Roizen MF, Ellis JE, Smith JS et al: Anesthesia for major vascular surgery. In Estafanous FG (ed): Anesthesia and the Heart Patient, p 183. Stoneham, Massachusetts, Butterworth Publishers, 1989

40. Roizen MG, Beaupre PN, Alpert RA et al: Monitoring with two-dimensional transesophageal echocardiography: Comparison of myocardial function in patients undergoing supraceliac, suprarenal-infraceliac, or infrarenal aortic occlusion. J Vasc Surg 1:300, 1984

41. Carroll RM, Laravuso RB, Schauble JF: Left ventricular function during aortic surgery. Arch Surg 111:740, 1976

42. Lunn JK, Dannemiller FJ, Stanley TH: Cardiovascular responses to clamping of the aorta during epidural and general anesthesia. Anesth Analg 58:372, 1979

43. Meloche R, Pottecher T, Audet J et al: Haemodynamic changes due to clamping of the abdominal aorta. Can Anaesth Soc J 24:20, 1977

44. Attia RR, Murphy JD, Snider M et al: Myocardial ischemia due to infrarenal aortic cross-clamping during aortic surgery in patients with severe coronary artery disease. Circulation 53:961, 1976

45. Silverstein PR, Caldera DL, Cullen DJ et al: Avoiding the hemodynamic consequences of aortic cross-clamping and unclamping. Anesthesiology 50:462, 1979

46. Plecha FR, Avellone JC, Beven EG et al: A computerized vascular registry: Experience of the Cleveland Vascular Society. Surgery 86:826, 1979

47. Kouchoukos NT, Lell WA, Karp RB et al: Hemodynamic effects of aortic clamping and decompression with a temporary shunt for resection of the descending thoracic aorta. Surgery 85:25, 1979

48. DeBakey ME, Creech O Jr, Morris GC Jr: Aneurysm of thoracoabdominal aorta involving the celiac, superior mesenteric, and renal arteries. Report of four cases treated by resection and homograft replacement. Ann Surg 144:549, 1956

49. Denlin A, Ohlsen H, Swedenborg J: Growth rate of abdominal aortic aneurysms as measured by computed tomography. Br J Surg 72:530, 1985

50. Darling RC: Ruptured arteriosclerotic abdominal aortic aneurysms: A pathologic and clinical study. Am J Surg 119:397, 1970

51. Collin J, Murie J, Morris PJ: Two year prospective analysis of the Oxford experience with surgical treatment of abdominal aortic aneurysm. Surg Gynecol Obstet 169:527, 1989

52. Svensson LG, Crawford ES, Hess KR et al: Dissection of the aorta and dissecting aortic aneurysms: Improving early and long-term surgical results. Circulation 82:IV-24, 1990

53. Schmidt CA, Wood MN, Gan KA, Razzouk AJ: Surgery for thoracoabdominal aortic aneurysms. Am Surg 56:745, 1990

54. Berisa F, Beaman M, Adu D et al: Prognostic factors in acute renal failure following aortic aneurysm surgery. Q J Med 76:689, 1990

55. Barry KG, Mazze RI, Schwartz FD: Prevention of surgical oliguria and renal-hemodynamic suppression by sustained hydration. N Engl J Med 270:1371, 1964

56. Wheeler CG, Thompson JE, Kartchner MM et al: Massive fluid requirement in surgery of the abdominal aorta. N Engl J Med 275:320, 1968

57. Alpert RA, Roizen MF, Hamilton WK et al: Intraoperative urinary output does not predict postoperative renal function in patients undergoing abdominal aortic revascularization. Surgery 95:707, 1984

58. Knos GB, Berry AJ, Isaacson IJ, Weitz FI: Intraoperative urinary output and postoperative blood urea nitrogen and creatinine levels in patients undergoing aortic reconstructive surgery. J Clin Anesth 1:181, 1989

59. Bush HL Jr, LoGerfo FW, Weisel RD et al: Assessment of myocardial performance and optimal volume loading during elective abdominal aortic aneurysm resection. Arch Surg 112:1301, 1977

60. Moyer JH, Heider C, Morris GC Jr et al: Renal failure: I. The effect of complete renal artery occlusion for variable periods of time as compared to exposure to subfiltration arterial pressures below 30 mm Hg for similar periods. Ann Surg 145:41, 1957

61. Laschinger JC, Cunningham JN Jr, Catinella FP et al: Detection and prevention of intraoperative spinal cord ischemia after cross-clamping of the thoracic aorta: Use of somatosensory evoked potentials. Surgery 92:1109, 1982

62. Svensson LG, Grum DF, Bednarski M et al: Appraisal of cerebrospinal fluid alterations during aortic surgery with intrathecal papaverine administration and cerebrospinal fluid drainage. J Vasc Surg 11:423, 1990

63. McCullough JL, Hollier LH, Nugent M: Paraplegia after thoracic aortic occlusion: Influence of cerebrospinal fluid drainage. Experimental and early clinical results. J Vasc Surg 7:153, 1988

64. Coles JG, Wilson GJ, Sima AF et al: Intraoperative management of thoracic aortic aneurysm: Experimental evaluation of perfusion cooling of the spinal cord. J Thorac Cardiovasc Surg 85:292, 1983

65. Svensson LG, Rickards E, Coull A et al: Relationship of spinal cord blood flow to vascular anatomy during thoracic aortic cross-clamping and shunting. J Thorac Cardiovasc Surg 91:71, 1986

66. Crawford ES, Walker HSJ, Saleh SA et al: Graft replacement of aneurysm in descending thoracic aorta: Results without bypass or shunting. Surgery 89:73, 1981

67. Djindjian R, Hurth RM, Houdart M et al: Arterial supply of the spinal cord. In: Angiography of the Spinal Cord, p 3. Baltimore, University Park Press, 1970

68. Connolly JE: Prevention of paraplegia secondary to operations on the aorta. J Cardiovasc Surg 27:410, 1986

69. Wadouh F, Arndt C-F, Oppermann E et al: The mechanism of spinal cord injury after simple and double aortic cross-clamping. J Thorac Cardiovasc Surg 92:121, 1986

70. Roizen MF: Anesthetic implications of concurrent diseases. In Miller RD (ed): Anesthesia, 3rd ed, vol 1, p 793. New York, Churchill Livingstone, 1990

71. Eagle KA, Coley CM, Newell JB et al: Combining clinical and thallium data optimizes preoperative assessment of cardiac risk before major vascular surgery. Ann Intern Med 110:859, 1989

72. Pohost GM: Dipyridamole thallium test: Is it useful for predicting coronary events after vascular surgery? Circulation 84:931, 1991

73. Shah KB, Kleinman BS, Sami H et al: Reevaluation of perioperative myocardial infarction in patients with prior myocardial infarction undergoing noncardiac operations. Anesth Analg 71:231, 1990

74. Carliner NH, Fisher ML, Plotnick GD et al: Routine preoperative exercise testing in patients undergoing major noncardiac surgery. Am J Cardiol 56:51, 1985

75. Raby KE, Goldman L, Creager MA et al: Correlation between preoperative ischemia and major cardiac events after peripheral vascular surgery. N Engl J Med 321:1296, 1989

76. Kazmers A, Cerqueira MD, Zierler RE: The role of preoperative radionuclide ejection fraction in direct abdominal aortic aneurysm repair. J Vasc Surg 8:128, 1988

77. Del Guercio LRM, Cohn JD: Monitoring operative risk in the elderly. JAMA 243:1350, 1980

78. Eagle KA, Singer DE, Brewster DC et al: Dipyridamole-thallium scanning in patients undergoing vascular surgery: Optimizing preoperative evaluation of cardiac risk. JAMA 257:2185, 1987

79. Lette J, Waters D, Lassonde J et al: Postoperative myocardial infarction and cardiac death: Predictive value of dipyridamole-thallium imaging and five clinical scoring systems based on multifactorial analysis. Ann Surg 211:84, 1990

80. Lane SE, Lewis SM, Pippin JJ et al: Predictive value of quantitative dipyridamole-thallium scintigraphy in assessing cardiovascular risk after vascular surgery in diabetes mellitus. Am J Cardiol 64:1275, 1989

81. Charlson ME, MacKenzie CR, Gold JP et al: The preoperative and intraoperative hemodynamic predictors of postoperative myocardial infarction or ischemia in patients undergoing non-cardiac surgery. Ann Surg 210:637, 1989

82. Goldman L, Caldera DL, Southwick FS et al: Cardiac risk factors and complications in non-cardiac surgery. Medicine 57:357, 1978

83. Pasternack PF, Imparato AM, Bear G et al: The value of radionuclide angiography as a predictor of perioperative myocardial infarction in patients undergoing abdominal aortic resection. J Vasc Surg 1:320, 1984

84. Mangano DT, London MJ, Tubau JF et al: Dipyridamole thallium-201 scintigraphy as a preoperative screening test. A reexamination of its predictive potential. Circulation 84:493, 1991

85. Knight AA, Hollenberg M, London MJ et al: Myocardial ischemia in patients awaiting coronary artery bypass grafting. Am Heart J 117:1189, 1989

86. Samson D, Boone S: Extracranial-intracranial (ED-IC) arterial bypass. Past performance and current concepts. Neurosurgery 3:79, 1978

87. EC/IC Bypass Study Group: Failure of extracranial-intracranial arterial bypass to reduce the risk of ischemic stroke: Results of an international randomized trial. N Engl J Med 313:1191, 1985

88. Haynes RB, Mukherjee J, Sackett DL et al: Functional status changes following medical or surgical treatment for cerebral ischemia: Result of the Extracranial-Intracranial Bypass Study. JAMA 257:2043, 1987

89. Larson CP Jr: Anesthesia for emergency surgery for cerebrovascular insufficiency: One approach at Stanford. In Roizen MF (ed): Anesthesia for Vascular Surgery, p 135. New York, Churchill Livingstone, 1990

90. Lusby RJ: Surgery for cerebrovascular disease. Surgical goals and methods. In Roizen MF (ed): Anesthesia for Vascular Surgery, p 85. New York, Churchill Livingstone, 1990

91. Baker WH, Dorner DB, Barnes RW: Carotid endarterectomy: Is an indwelling shunt necessary? Surgery 82:321, 1977

92. Ferguson GG: Intra-operative monitoring and internal shunts: Are they necessary in carotid endarterectomy? Stroke 13:287, 1982

93. West H, Burton R, Roon AJ et al: Comparative risk of operation and expectant management for carotid artery disease. Stroke 10:117, 1979

94. Donaldson MC, Weinberg DS, Belkin M et al: Screening for hypercoagulable states in vascular surgical practice: A preliminary study. J Vasc Surg 11:825, 1990

95. Stundt TM, Houser OW, Sharbrough FW et al: Carotid endarterectomy: Results, complications, and monitoring techniques. Adv Neurol 16:97, 1977

96. Wylie EJ: Is an asymptomatic carotid stenosis a surgical lesion? Presidential Address, Society of Cardiovascular Surgeons, 1982

97. Husain M, Moss J: Endothelium-dependent vascular smooth muscle control. J Clin Anesth 1:135, 1988

98. Vane JR, Änggard EE, Botting RM: Regulatory functions of the vascular endothelium. N Engl J Med 323:27, 1990

99. Koslow AR, Ricotta JJ, Ouriel K et al: Reexploration for thrombosis in carotid endarterectomy. Circulation 80:III-78, 1989

100. Bandyk DF, Hermann HW, Adams MB, Towne JB: Turbulence occurring after carotid bifurcation endarterectomy: A harbinger of residual and recurrent carotid stenosis. J Vasc Surg 7:261, 1988

101. Michenfelder JD: Anesthesia and surgery for cerebrovascular insufficiency: One approach at the Mayo Clinic. In Roizen MF (ed): Anesthesia for Vascular Surgery, p 123. New York, Churchill Livingstone, 1990

102. Hamilton WK: Do let the blood pressure drop and do use myocardial depressants! Anesthesiology 45:273, 1976

103. Boysen G, Engell HC, Henriksen H: The effect of induced hypertension on internal carotid artery pressure and regional cerebral blood flow during temporary carotid clamping for endarterectomy. Neurology 22:1133, 1972

104. Ehrenfeld WK, Hamilton WK, Larson CP et al: Effect of CO_2 and systemic hypertension on downstream cerebral arterial pressure during carotid endarterectomy. Surgery 67:87, 1970

105. Smith JS, Cahalan MK, Benefiel DJ et al: Intraoperative detection of myocardial ischemia in high-risk patients: Electrocardiography versus two-dimensional transesophageal echocardiography. Circulation 872:1015, 1985

106. Ellis JE, Roizen MF, Aronson S et al: Comparison of two automated ST-segment analysis systems, EKG (including T wave analysis), and transesophageal echocardiography for the diagnosis of intraoperative myocardial ischemia. Anesth Analg, in press

107. Kotrly KJ, Kotter GS, Mortara D et al: Intraoperative detection of myocardial ischemia with an ST segment trend monitoring system. Anesth Analg 63:343, 1984

108. Pichard AD, Diaz R, Marchant E et al: Large V waves in the pulmonary capillary wedge pressure tracing without mitral regurgitation: Influence of pressure/volume relationship on the V wave size. Clin Cardiol 6:534, 1983

109. Riles TS, Kopelman I, Imparato AM: Myocardial infarction following carotid endarterectomy: A review of 683 operations. Surgery 85:249, 1979

110. Palmer MA: Comparison of regional and general anesthesia for carotid endarterectomy. Am J Surg 157:329, 1989

111. McCaffrey MT: Monitoring of the electroencephalogram during carotid endarterectomy. In Roizen MF (ed): Anesthesia for Vascular Surgery, p 373. New York, Churchill Livingstone, 1990

112. Rampil IJ, Holzer JA, Quest DO et al: Prognostic value of computerized EEG analysis during carotid endarterectomy. Anesth Analg 62:186, 1983

113. Rosenthal D, Stanton PE, Lamis PA: Carotid endarterectomy: The unreliability of intraoperative monitoring in patients having had stroke or reversible ischemic neurological deficit. Arch Surg 116:1569, 1981

114. Cho I, Smullens SN, Streletz LJ et al: The value of intraoperative EEG monitoring during carotid endarterectomy. Ann Neurol 20:508, 1986

115. Kresowik TF, Worsey MJ, Khoury MD et al: Limitations of electroencephalographic monitoring in the detection of cerebral ischemia accompanying carotid endarterectomy. J Vasc Surg 13:439, 1991

116. Blume WT, Ferguson GG, McNeil DK: Significance of EEG changes at carotid endarterectomy. Stroke 17:891, 1986

117. Morawetz RB, Zeiger HE, McDowell HA et al: Correlation of cerebral blood flow and EEG during carotid occlusion for endarterectomy (without shunting) and neurologic outcome. Surgery 96:184, 1984

118. McCaffrey MT: Monitoring and predictive value of somatosensory and motor evoked potentials for peripheral vascular surgery. In Roizen MF (ed): Anesthesia for Vascular Surgery, p 383. New York, Churchill Livingstone, 1990

119. Horsch S, De Vleeschauwer P, Ktenidis K: Intraoperative assessment of cerebral ischemia during carotid surgery. J Cardiovasc Surg 31:599, 1990

120. Lam AM, Manninen PH, Ferguson GG, Nantau W: Monitoring electrophysiologic function during carotid endarterectomy: A

comparison of somatosensory evoked potentials and conventional electroencephalogram. Anesthesiology 75:15, 1991

121. Messick JM Jr, Casement B, Sharbrough FW et al: Correlation of regional cerebral blood flow (rCBF) with EEG changes during isoflurane anesthesia for carotid endarterectomy: Critical rCBF. Anesthesiology 66:344, 1987

122. Padayachee TS, Bishop CCR, Gosling RG, Browse NL: Monitoring cerebral perfusion during carotid endarterectomy. J Cardiovasc Surg 31:112, 1990

123. McKay RD, Sundt TM, Michenfelder JD et al: Internal carotid artery stump pressure and cerebral blood flow during carotid endarterectomy: Modification by halothane, enflurane and innovar. Anesthesiology 45:390, 1976

124. Beebe HG, Starr C, Slack D: Carotid artery stump pressure: Its variability when measured serially. J Cardiovasc Surg 30:419, 1989

125. Winslow CM, Solomon DH, Chassin MR et al: The appropriateness of carotid endarterectomy. N Engl J Med 318:721, 1988

126. Leape LL, Park RE, Solomon DH et al: Relation between surgeons' practice volumes and geographic variation in the rate of carotid endarterectomy. N Engl J Med 321:653, 1989

127. AbuRahma AF, Boland J, Robinson P: Complications of carotid endarterectomy: The influence of case load. South Med J 81:711, 1988

128. Mayo Asymptomatic Carotid Endarterectomy Study Group: Effectiveness of carotid endarterectomy for asymptomatic carotid stenosis: Design of a clinical trial. Mayo Clin Proc 64:897, 1989

129. Asymptomatic Carotid Atherosclerosis Study Group: Study design for randomized prospective trial of carotid endarterectomy for asymptomatic atherosclerosis. Stroke 20:844, 1989

130. Slogoff S, Keats AS: Further observations on perioperative myocardial ischemia. Anesthesiology 65:539, 1986

131. Egbert LD, Battit GE, Turndorf H et al: The value of the preoperative visit by an anesthetist. JAMA 185:553, 1963

132. Bedford RF: Radial arterial function following percutaneous cannulation with 18- and 20-gauge catheters. Anesthesiology 47:37, 1977

133. Lanier WL, Stangland KJ, Scheithauer BW et al: The effects of dextrose infusion and head position on neurologic outcome after complete cerebral ischemia in primates: Examination of a model. Anesthesiology 66:39, 1987

134. Zasslow MA, Pearl RG, Shuer LM et al: Hyperglycemia decreases acute neuronal ischemic changes after middle cerebral artery occlusion in cats. Stroke 20:519, 1989

135. Farias LA, Willis M, Gregory GA: Effects of fructose-1,6-diphosphate, glucose, and saline on cardiac resuscitation. Anesthesiology 65:595, 1986

136. Roizen MF, Sohn YJ, L'Hommedieu CS et al: Operating room temperature prior to surgical draping: Effect on patient temperature in recovery room. Anesth Analg 59:852, 1980

137. Nehls DG, Todd MM, Spetzler RF et al: A comparison of the cerebral protective effects of isoflurane and barbiturates during temporary focal ischemia in primates. Anesthesiology 66:453, 1987

138. Wade JG, Larson CP, Hickey RF et al: Effect of carotid endarterectomy on carotid chemoreceptor and baroreceptor function in man. N Engl J Med 282:823, 1970

139. Hosobuchi Y, Baskin DS, Woo SK: Reversal of induced ischemic neurologic deficit in gerbils by the opiate antagonist naloxone. Science 215:69, 1982

140. Stinson EB, Holloway EL, Derby G et al: Comparative hemodynamic responses to chlorpromazine, nitroprusside, nitroglycerin, and trimethaphan immediately after open-heart operations. Circulation 53:I-26, 1974

141. Assiddao CB, Donegan JH, Whitesell RC et al: Factors associated with perioperative complications during carotid endarterectomy. Anesth Analg 61:631, 1982

142. Tarlov E, Schmidek H, Scott RM et al: Reflex hypotension following carotid endarterectomy: Mechanism and management. J Neurosurg 39:323, 1973

143. Mentzer RM Jr, Finkelmeier BA, Crosby IK et al: Emergency carotid endarterectomy for fluctuating neurologic deficits. Surgery 89:60, 1981

144. Lusby RJ: Visceral ischemia: Surgical goals and methods. In Roizen MF (ed): Anesthesia for Vascular Surgery, p 155. New York, Churchill Livingstone, 1990

145. Stoney RJ, Lusby RJ: Surgery of celiac and mesenteric arteries. In Haimovici H (ed): Vascular Surgery—Principles and Techniques. Norwalk, Connecticut, Appleton-Century-Crofts, 1984

146. Morris GC, DeBakey ME, Bernhard V: Abdominal angina. Surg Clin North Am 46:919, 1966

147. Hollier LH, Bernatz PE, Pairolero PC et al: Surgical management of chronic intestinal ischaemia: A reappraisal. Surgery 90:940, 1981

148. Baur GM, Millay DJ, Taylor LM Jr et al: Treatment of chronic visceral ischemia. Am J Surg 148:138, 1984

149. Bergqvist D, Bowald S, Eriksson I et al: Small bowel necrosis after aorto-iliac reconstruction. Br J Surg 73:28, 1986

150. Zelenock GB, Strodel WE, Knol JA et al: A prospective study of clinically and endoscopically documented colonic ischemia in 100 patients undergoing aortic reconstructive surgery with aggressive colonic and direct pelvic revascularization, compared with historic controls. Surgery 106:771, 1989

151. Boley SJ, Borden EB: Acute mesenteric vascular disease. In Wilson SE, Veith FJ, Hobson RW et al (eds): Vascular Surgery—Principles and Practice, p 659. New York, McGraw-Hill, 1987

152. Crawford ES, Morris GC Jr, Myhre HO et al: Celiac axis, superior mesenteric artery, and inferior mesenteric artery occlusion: Surgical considerations. Surgery 82:856, 1977

153. Jaxheimer EC, Jewell ER, Persson AV: Chronic intestinal ischemia. The Lahey Clinic approach to management. Surg Clin North Am 64:123, 1985

154. Eidemiller LR, Nelson JC, Porter JM: Surgical treatment of chronic visceral ischemia. Am J Surg 138:264, 1979

155. DeBakey ME: Changing concepts in vascular surgery. J Cardiovasc Surg 27:367, 1986

156. Hollier LH, Reigel MM, Kazmier FJ et al: Conventional repair of abdominal aortic aneurysm in the high-risk patient: A plea for abandonment of non-resective treatment. J Vasc Surg 3:712, 1986

157. Estes E: Abdominal aortic aneurysm: A study of one hundred and two cases. Circulation 2:258, 1950

158. Foster JH, Bolashy BL, Gobbel WG Jr: Comparative study of elective resection and expectant treatment of abdominal aortic aneurysm. Surg Gynecol Obstet 129:1, 1969

159. Darling RC, Messina CR, Brewster DC et al: Autopsy study of unoperated abdominal aortic aneurysms. The case for early resection. Circulation 56:II-161, 1977

160. Szilagyi DE, Elliott JP: Clinical fate of the patient with asymptomatic abdominal aortic aneurysm and unfit for surgical treatment. Arch Surg 104:600, 1972

161. Thurmond AS, Semler HJ: Abdominal aortic aneurysm: Incidence in a population at risk. J Cardiovasc Surg 27:457, 1986

162. Reigel MM, Hollier LH, Kazmier EJ et al: Late survival in abdominal aortic aneurysm patients: The role of selective myocardial revascularization on the basis of clinical symptoms. J Vasc Surg 5:222, 1987

163. May AG, DeWeese JA, Frank I et al: Surgical treatment of abdominal aortic aneurysms. Surgery 63:711, 1968

164. Lambert ME, Baguley P, Charlesworth D: Ruptured abdominal aortic aneurysms. J Cardiovasc Surg 27:256, 1986

165. Brewster DC, Darling RC: Optimal methods of aortoiliac reconstruction surgery. Surgery 84:739, 1978

166. Szilagyi DE, Elliott JP Jr, Smith RF et al: A thirty-year survey of the reconstructive surgical treatment of aorto-iliac occlusive disease. J Vasc Surg 3:421, 1986

167. Simma W, Bassiouny H, Haril P et al: Evaluation of profundoplasty in reconstructions of combined aorto-iliac and femoro-popliteal occlusive disease. J Cardiovasc Surg 27:141, 1986

168. Sladen JG, Gilmour JL, Wong RW: Cumulative patency and actual palliation in patients with claudication after aorto-femoral bypass. Prospective long-term follow-up of 100 patients. Am J Surg 152:190, 1986

169. Poulias GE, Polemis L, Skoutas B et al: Bilateral aorto-femoral bypass in the presence of aorto-iliac occlusive disease and

factors determining results. Experience and long-term follow-up with 500 consecutive cases. J Cardiovasc Surg 26:527, 1985

170. Gregory RT, Wheeler JR, Snyder SO et al: Retroperitoneal approach to aortic surgery. J Cardiovasc Surg 30:185, 1989

171. Starr DS, Lawrie GM, Morris GC Jr: Prevention of distal embolism during arterial reconstruction. Am J Surg 138:764, 1979

172. Burnett JR, Gray-Weale AC, Byrne K et al: The place of systemic heparin in elective aortic aneurysm repair. J Cardiovasc Surg 28:7, 1987

173. Williams GM, Ricotta J, Zinner M et al: The extended retroperitoneal approach for treatment of extensive atherosclerosis of the aorta and renal vessels. Surgery 88:846, 1980

174. Roizen MF, Rodgers GM, Valone FH et al: Anaphylactoid reactions to vascular graft material presenting with vasodilation and subsequent disseminated intravascular coagulation. Anesthesiology 71:331, 1989

175. Wylie EJ, Stoney RJ, Ehrenfeld WK: Aorto-iliac atherosclerosis. In: Manual of Vascular Surgery, vol 1, p 107. New York, Springer-Verlag, 1980

176. Donaldson MC, Louras JC, Bucknam CA: Axillofemoral bypass: A tool with a limited role. J Vasc Surg 3:757, 1986

177. Moore WS: Thrombosis of aortofemoral, axillofemoral, or femorofemoral grafts. In Veith FJ (ed): Critical Problems in Vascular Surgery, p 445. Norwalk, Connecticut, Appleton-Century-Crofts, 1982

178. Kazman PG, Hosang M, Cina C et al: Current indications for axillounifemoral and axillobifemoral bypass grafts. J Vasc Surg 5:828, 1987

179. Grundfest WS, Litvack F, Glick D et al: Intraoperative decisions based on angioscopy in peripheral vascular surgery. Circulation 78:I-13, 1988

180. Wilson SE, Wolf GL, Cross AP: Percutaneous transluminal angioplasty versus operation for peripheral arteriosclerosis: Report of a prospective randomized trial in a selected group of patients. J Vasc Surg 9:1, 1989

181. Eugene J, Ott RA, Baribeau Y et al: Initial trial of argon ion laser endarterectomy for peripheral vascular disease. Arch Surg 125:1007, 1990

182. Hinohara T, Selmon MR, Robertson GC et al: Directional atherectomy: New approaches for treatment of obstructive coronary and peripheral vascular disease. Circulation 81:IV-79, 1990

183. Qvarfordt PG, Stoney RJ, Reilly LM et al: Management of pararenal aneurysms of the abdominal aorta. J Vasc Surg 3:84, 1986

184. Perry MO: The hemodynamics of temporary abdominal aortic occlusion. Ann Surg 168:193, 1968

185. Pandian NG, Kerber RE: Two-dimensional echocardiography in experimental coronary stenosis. I. Sensitivity and specificity in detecting transient myocardial dyskinesis: Comparison with sonomicrometers. Circulation 66:597, 1982

186. Guyton AC: Textbook of Medical Physiology, 8th ed. Philadelphia, WB Saunders, 1991

187. Olinger GN, Hottenrott C, Mulder DG et al: Acute clinical hypocalcemic myocardial depression during rapid blood transfusion and postoperative hemodialysis. A preventable complication. J Thorac Cardiovasc Surg 72:503, 1976

188. Bengtson A, Lannsjö W, Heideman M: Complement and anaphylatoxin responses to cross-clamping of the aorta: Studies during general anesthesia with and without extradural blockade. Br J Anaesth 59:1093, 1987

189. Longo T, Marchetti G, Vercellio G: Coronary hemodynamic changes induced by aortic cross-clamping. J Cardiovasc Surg 10:36, 1969

190. Mandelbaum I, Webb MK: Left ventricular function during cross-clamping of the descending thoracic aorta. JAMA 186:229, 1963

191. Schlüter M, Langenstein BA, Polster J et al: Transesophageal cross-sectional echocardiography with a phased array transduced system. Technique and initial clinical results. Br Heart J 48:67, 1982

192. Beaupre PN, Cahalan MK, Kremer PF et al: Does pulmonary artery occlusion pressure adequately reflect left ventricular filling during anesthesia and surgery? Anesthesiology 59:A3, 1983

193. Gerson JI, Allen FB, Seltzer JL et al: Arterial and venous dilation by nitroprusside and nitroglycerin: Is there a difference? Anesth Analg 61:256, 1982

194. Feigl EO: The paradox of adrenergic coronary vasoconstriction. Circulation 76:737, 1987

195. Roizen MF, Hamilton WK, Sohn YJ: Treatment of stress-induced increases in pulmonary capillary wedge pressure using volatile anesthetics. Anesthesiology 55:446, 1981

196. Koike M, Roizen MF, Zivin J et al: Naloxone ameliorates adverse effects of some anesthetics on CNS injury. Anesthesiology 59:A333, 1983

197. Abbott WM, Austen WG: The reversal of renal cortical ischemia during aortic occlusion by mannitol. J Surg Res 16:482, 1974

198. Barry KG, Cohen A, Knochel JP et al: Mannitol infusion. II. The prevention of acute functional renal failure during resection of an aneurysm of the abdominal aorta. N Engl J Med 264:967, 1961

199. Flores J, DiBona DR, Beck CH et al: The role of cell swelling in ischemic renal damage and the protective effect of hypertonic solute. J Clin Invest 51:118, 1972

200. Hanley MJ, Davidson K: Prior mannitol and furosemide infusion in a model of ischemic acute renal failure. Am J Physiol 241:F556, 1981

201. Miller DC, Myers BD: Pathophysiology and prevention of acute renal failure associated with thoraco-abdominal or abdominal-aortic surgery. J Vasc Surg 5:518, 1987

202. Roizen MF: Does choice of anesthetic (narcotic vs inhalational) significantly affect cardiovascular surgery? In Estafanous FG (ed): Opioids in Anesthesia, p 180. Boston, Butterworths, 1984

203. Reiz S, Bålfors E, Sørensen MB et al: Isoflurane: A powerful coronary vasodilator in patients with coronary artery disease. Anesthesiology 59:91, 1983

204. Yeager MP, Glass DD, Neff RK et al: Epidural anesthesia and analgesia in high-risk surgical patients. Anesthesiology 66:729, 1987

205. Shingu K, Eger El II, Johnson BH et al: Effect of oxygen concentration, hypothermia, and choice of vendor on anesthetic-induced hepatic injury to rats. Anesth Analg 62:146, 1983

206. White DA, Reitan JA, Kien ND, Thorup SJ: Decrease in vascular resistance in the isolated canine hindlimb after graded doses of alfentanil, fentanyl, and sufentanil. Anesth Analg 71:29, 1990

207. Smith NT, Eger EL II, Stoelting RK et al: The cardiovascular and sympathomimetic responses to the addition of nitrous oxide to halothane in man. Anesthesiology 32:410, 1970

208. Eisele JH, Smith NT: Cardiovascular effects of 40 percent nitrous oxide in man. Anesth Analg 51:956, 1972

209. Koblin DD, Watson JE, Deady JE et al: Inactivation of methionine synthetase by nitrous oxide in mice. Anesthesiology 54:318, 1981

210. Cunningham FO, Egan JM, Inahara T: Continuous epidural anesthesia in abdominal vascular surgery. A review of 100 consecutive cases. Am J Surg 139:624, 1980

211. Rao TLK, El-Etr AA: Anticoagulation following placement of epidural and subarachnoid catheters: An evaluation of neurologic sequelae. Anesthesiology 55:618, 1981

212. Dickman CA, Shedd SA, Spetzler RF et al: Spinal epidural hematoma associated with epidural anesthesia: Complications of systemic heparinization in patients receiving peripheral vascular thrombolytic therapy. Anesthesiology 72:947, 1990

213. Horlocker TT, Wedel DJ, Offord KP: Does preoperative antiplatelet therapy increase the risk of hemorrhagic complications associated with regional anesthesia? Anesth Analg 70:631, 1990

214. Reiz S, Bålfors E, Sørensen MB et al: Coronary hemodynamic effects of general anesthesia and surgery: Modification by epidural analgesia in patients with ischemic heart disease. Reg Anesth 7:S8, 1982

215. Isaacson IJ, Weitz FI, Berry AJ et al: Intrathecal morphine's

effect on the postoperative course of patients undergoing abdominal aortic surgery. Anesth Analg 66:S86, 1987

216. Jones ROM, Jones JG: Intrathecal morphine: Naloxone reverses respiratory depression but not analgesia. Br Med J 281:645, 1980

217. Smith JS, Cahalan MK, Benefiel DJ et al: Fentanyl versus fentanyl and isoflurane in patients with impaired left ventricular function. Anesthesiology 63:A18, 1985

218. Tuman KJ, McCarthy RJ, Spiess BD et al: Does choice of anesthetic agent significantly affect outcome after coronary artery surgery? Anesthesiology 70:189, 1989

219. Slogoff S, Keats AS: Randomized trial of primary anesthetic agents on outcome of coronary artery bypass operations. Anesthesiology 70:179, 1989

220. Siliciano D, Hollenberg M, Goehner P, Mangano D: Use of continuous vs intermittent narcotic after CABG surgery: Effects on myocardial ischemia. Anesth Analg 70:S371, 1990

221. Tuman KJ, McCarthy RJ, Spiess BD, Ivankovich AD: Epidural anesthesia and analgesia decreases postoperative hypercoagulability in high-risk vascular patients. Anesth Analg 70:S414, 1990

222. Quintin L, Roux C, Macquin I et al: Clonidine blunts the endocrine and circulatory surge during recovery of aortic surgery. Anesthesiology 71:A155, 1989

223. Lundsgaard-Hansen P: Hemodilution: New clothes for an anemic emperor. Vox Sang 36:321, 1979

224. Most AS, Ruocco NA, Gerwirtz H: Effect of a reduction in blood viscosity on maximal myocardial oxygen delivery distal to a moderate coronary stenosis. Circulation 74:1085, 1986

225. Weisel RD, Charlesworth DC, Mickleborough LL et al: Limitations of blood conservation. J Thorac Cardiovasc Surg 88:26, 1984

226. Scobie TK, Masters RG: Changing factors influencing abdominal aortic aneurysm repair. J Cardiovasc Surg 23:309, 1982

227. Friedman SA: The evaluation and treatment of patients with arterial aneurysms. Med Clin North Am 65:83, 1981

228. Lawrie GM, Morris GC Jr, Crawford ES et al: Improved results of operation for ruptured abdominal aortic aneurysm. Surgery 85:483, 1979

229. Ottinger LW: Ruptured arteriosclerotic aneurysms of the abdominal aorta: Reducing mortality. JAMA 233:147, 1975

230. Thompson JE, Garrett WV: Peripheral-arterial surgery. N Engl J Med 302:491, 1980

231. Wakefield TW, Whitehouse WM Jr, Shu-Chen W et al: Abdominal aortic aneurysm rupture: Statistical analysis of factors affecting outcome of surgical treatment. Surgery 91:586, 1982

232. Merrill WH, Ernst CB: Aorta-left renal vein fistula: Hemodynamic monitoring and timing of operation. Surgery 89:678, 1981

233. Savrin RA, Gustafson R: Spontaneous aorto-vena caval fistula: Hemodynamic monitoring. J Cardiovasc Surg 22:88, 1981

234. Schramek A, Hashmonai M, Better OS et al: Aortocaval fistula due to rupture of abdominal aortic aneurysm. Isr J Med Sci 16:733, 1980

235. Cohen LJ, Sukov RJ, Boswell W et al: Spontaneous aortocaval fistula. Radiology 138:357, 1981

236. Connolly JE, Kwaan JHM, McCart PM et al: Aortoenteric fistula. Ann Surg 194:402, 1981

237. Snow N: Hemopericardium from retrograde dissection of an abdominal aortic aneurysm. Am Surg 46:589, 1980

238. Zarins CZ: Surgery for peripheral vascular insufficiency: surgical goals and methods. In Roizen MF (ed): Anesthesia for Vascular Surgery, p 317. New York, Churchill Livingstone, 1990

239. Veith FJ, Gupta SK, Ascer E: Femoral, popliteal, and tibial occlusive disease. In Wilson SE, Veith FJ, Hobson RW et al (eds): Vascular Surgery—Principles and Practice, p 353. New York, McGraw-Hill, 1987

240. Mannick JA, Jackson BT, Coffman JD: Success of bypass vein grafts in patients with isolated popliteal artery segments. Surgery 61:17, 1967

241. Reichle FA, Tyson R: Comparison of long-term results of 364 femoropopliteal or femorotibial bypasses for revascularization of severely ischemic lower extremities. Ann Surg 182:449, 1975

242. Leather RP, Shah DM, Karmody AM: Infrapopliteal arterial bypass for limb salvage: Increased patency and utilization of the saphenous vein used in-situ. Surgery 90:1000, 1981

243. Buchbinder D, Singh JK, Karmody AM et al: Comparison of patency rate and structural change of in-situ and reversed vein arterial bypass. J Surg Res 30:213, 1981

244. Abbott WM, Maloney RD, McCabe RD et al: Arterial embolism: A 44-year perspective. Am J Surg 143:460, 1982

245. Connett MC, Murray DH Jr, Denneker WW: Peripheral arterial emboli. Am J Surg 148:14, 1984

246. Brem SS, Hafler DA, Van Uitert RL et al: Spinal subarachnoid hematoma: A hazard of lumbar puncture resulting in reversible paraplegia. N Engl J Med 304:1020, 1981

247. London MJ, Hollenberg M, Wong MG et al: Intraoperative myocardial ischemia: Localization by continuous 12-lead electrocardiography. Anesthesiology 69:232, 1988

38
Kathryn E. McGoldrick

Anesthesia and the Eye

Anesthesia for ophthalmic surgery presents many unique challenges (Table 38-1). In addition to possessing technical expertise, the anesthesiologist must have detailed knowledge of ocular anatomy, physiology, and pharmacology. It is essential to appreciate that ophthalmic drugs may significantly alter the reaction to anesthesia and that, concomitantly, anesthetic drugs and maneuvers may dramatically influence intraocular dynamics. Patients undergoing ophthalmic surgery may represent extremes of age and coexisting medical diseases (e.g., diabetes mellitus, coronary artery disease, essential hypertension, chronic lung disease), but they are likely to be in the elderly age group. Apprehension is predictable in blind or potentially blind patients awaiting surgery.

It is mandatory to be knowledgeable about the numerous surgical procedures unique to the specialty of ophthalmology. Whereas the list of ocular surgical interventions is lengthy, these procedures may, in general, be classified as extraocular or intraocular. This distinction is critical since anesthetic considerations are different for these two major surgical categories. For example, with intraocular procedures, profound akinesia (relaxation of recti muscles) and meticulous control of intraocular pressure (IOP) are requisite. However, with extraocular surgery, the significance of IOP fades, whereas concern about elicitation of the oculocardiac reflex assumes prominence.

OCULAR ANATOMY

The anesthesiologist should be knowledgeable about ocular anatomy in order to enhance his or her understanding of surgical procedures and to aid the surgeon in the performance of regional blocks when needed (Fig. 38-1).[1,2] Salient subdivisions of ocular anatomy include the orbit, the eye itself, the extraocular muscles, the eyelids, and the lacrimal system.

The orbit is a bony box, or pyramidal cavity, housing the eyeball and its associated structures in the skull. The walls of the orbit are composed of the following bones: frontal, zygomatic, greater wing of the sphenoid, maxilla, palatine, lacrimal, and ethmoid. A familiarity with the surface relationships of the orbital rim is mandatory to the skilled performance of regional blocks.

The optic foramen, located at the orbital apex, transmits the optic nerve, artery, and vein as well as sympathetic nerves from the carotid plexus. The superior orbital fissure transmits the superior and inferior branches of the oculomotor nerve, the lacrimal, frontal, and nasociliary branches of the trigeminal nerve, as well as the trochlear and abducens nerves and the superior and inferior ophthalmic veins. The inferior orbital or sphenomaxillary fissure contains the infraorbital and zygomatic nerves and a communication between the inferior ophthalmic vein and the pterygoid plexus. The infraorbital foramen, located about 4 mm below the orbital rim in the maxilla, transmits the infraorbital nerve, artery, and vein. In the superior temporal orbit, one finds the lacrimal fossa, which contains the lacrimal gland. The supraorbital notch, located at the junction of the medial one third and temporal two thirds of the superior orbital rim, transmits the supraorbital nerve, artery, and vein. The supraorbital notch, the infraorbital foramen, and the lacrimal fossa are clinically palpable and function as major landmarks for administration of regional anesthesia.

The eye itself is actually one large sphere with part of a smaller sphere incorporated in the anterior surface, constituting a structure with two different radii of curvature. The coat of the eye is composed of three layers: sclera, uveal tract, and retina. The fibrous outer layer, or sclera, is protective, providing sufficient rigidity to maintain the shape of the eye. The anterior portion of the sclera, the cornea, is transparent, permitting light to pass into the internal ocular structures. The double spherical shape of the eye exists because the corneal arc of curvature is steeper than the scleral arc of curvature. The focusing of rays of light to form a retinal image commences at the cornea.

The uveal tract, or middle layer of the globe, is vascular and in direct apposition to the sclera. A potential space, known as the suprachoroidal space, separates the sclera from the uveal tract. This potential space, however, may become filled with blood during an expulsive or suprachoroidal hemorrhage, often associated with surgical disaster. The iris, ciliary body, and choroid compose the uveal tract. The iris includes the pupil, which, by contractions of three sets of muscles, controls the amount of light entering the eye. The iris dilator is sympathetically innervated; the iris sphincter and the ciliary muscle have parasympathetic innervation. Posterior to the iris lies the ciliary body, which produces aqueous humor (see the section on Formation and Drainage of Aqueous Humor). The ciliary muscles, situated in the ciliary body, adjust the shape of the lens to accommodate focusing at various distances. Large vessels and a network of small vessels and capillaries known as the choriocapillaris constitute the choroid, which supplies nutrition to the outer part of the retina.

The retina is a neurosensory membrane composed of ten layers that convert light impulses into neural impulses. These neural impulses are then carried through the optic nerve to the brain. Located in the center of the globe is the vitreous cavity, filled with a gelatinous substance known as vitreous humor. This material is adherent to the most anterior 3 mm of the retina as well as to large blood vessels and the optic nerve. The vitreous humor may pull on the retina, thus causing retinal tears and retinal detachment.

The crystalline lens, located posterior to the pupil, refracts rays of light passing through the cornea and pupil to focus images on the retina. The ciliary muscle, whose contractile state causes tautness or relaxation of the lens zonules, regulates the thickness of the lens.

In addition, six extraocular muscles move the eye within the orbit to various positions. The bilobed lacrimal gland provides the majority of the tear film, which serves to maintain a moist anterior surface on the globe. The lacrimal drainage system, composed of the puncta, canaliculi, lacrimal sac, and lacrimal duct, drains into the nose below the inferior turbinate. Blockage of this system occurs not infrequently, necessitating procedures ranging from lacrimal duct probing to dacryocystorhinostomy, which involves anastomosis of the lacrimal sac to the nasal mucosa.

Covering the surface of the globe and lining the eyelids is a mucous membrane called the conjunctiva. Since drugs are absorbed across the membrane, it is a popular site for administration of ophthalmic drugs.

The eyelids consist of four layers: (1) the conjunctiva, (2) the cartilaginous tarsal plate, (3) a muscle layer composed mainly of the orbicularis and the levator palpebrae, and (4) the skin. The eyelids protect the eye from foreign objects; through blinking, the tear film produced by the lacrimal gland is spread across the surface of the eye, keeping the cornea moist.

Blood supply to the eye and orbit is by means of branches of both the internal and external carotid arteries. Venous drainage of the orbit is accomplished through the multiple anastomoses of the superior and inferior ophthalmic veins. Venous drainage of the eye is achieved mainly through the central retinal vein. All these veins empty directly into the cavernous sinus.

The sensory and motor innervations of the eye and its adnexa are very complex, with multiple cranial nerves supplying branches to various ocular structures. A branch of the oculomotor nerve supplies a motor root to the ciliary ganglion, which in turn supplies the sphincter of the pupil and the ciliary muscle. The trochlear nerve supplies the

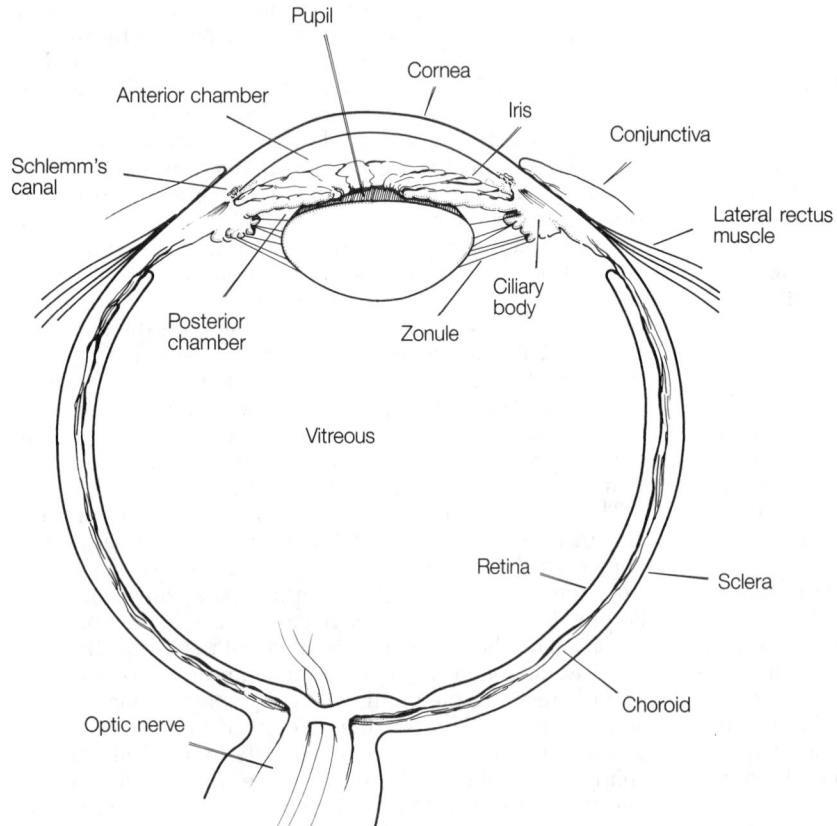

Figure 38-1. Diagram of ocular anatomy.

superior oblique muscle. The abducens nerve supplies the lateral rectus muscle. The trigeminal nerve constitutes the most complex ocular and adnexal innervation. In addition, the zygomatic branch of the facial nerve eventually divides into an upper branch, supplying the frontalis and the upper lid orbicularis, whereas the lower branch supplies the orbicularis of the lower lid.

OCULAR PHYSIOLOGY

Despite its relatively diminutive size, the eye is a complex organ, concerned with many intricate physiologic processes. The formation and drainage of aqueous humor and their influence on IOP in both normal and glaucomatous eyes are among the most important functions, especially from the anesthesiologist's perspective. An appreciation of the effects of various anesthetic manipulations on IOP requires an understanding of the fundamental principles of ocular physiology.

Formation and Drainage of Aqueous Humor

Two thirds of the aqueous humor is formed in the posterior chamber by the ciliary body in an active secretory process involving both the carbonic anhydrase and the cytochrome oxidase systems (Fig. 38-2). The remaining third is formed by passive filtration of aqueous humor from the vessels on the anterior surface of the iris.

At the ciliary epithelium, sodium is actively transported into the aqueous humor in the posterior chamber. Bicarbonate and chloride ions passively follow the sodium ions. This active mechanism results in the osmotic pressure of the aqueous being many times greater than that of plasma. It is this disparity in osmotic pressure that leads to an average rate of aqueous humor production of 2 μl·min^{-1}.

Aqueous humor flows from the posterior chamber through the pupillary aperture into the anterior chamber, where it mixes with the aqueous formed by the iris. During its journey into the anterior chamber, the aqueous humor bathes the avascular lens, providing essential metabolic materials and removing metabolic wastes. Once in the anterior chamber, the aqueous also bathes the corneal endothelium, maintaining healthy corneal metabolism. Then the aqueous

flows into the peripheral segment of the anterior chamber and exits the eye via the trabecular network, Schlemm's canal, and the episcleral venous system. A network of connecting venous channels eventually leads to the superior vena cava and the right atrium. Thus, obstruction of venous return at any point from the eye to the right side of the heart impedes aqueous drainage, elevating IOP accordingly.

Maintenance of Intraocular Pressure

IOP normally varies between 10 and 22 mm Hg and is considered abnormal above 25 mm Hg. This level varies 1–2 mm Hg with each cardiac contraction. Also, a diurnal variation of 2–5 mm Hg is observed, with a higher value noted on awakening. This higher awakening pressure has been ascribed to vascular congestion, pressure on the globe from closed lids, and mydriasis—all of which occur during sleep.

IOP far exceeds not only tissue pressure (2–3 mm Hg) but also intracranial pressure (7–8 mm Hg). Apparently the maintenance of such a relatively high pressure in the eye is demanded by the optical properties of refracting surfaces; the corneal surface should be kept at a constant curvature, and the stroma must be under constant high pressure to maintain a uniform refractive index.[3] However, an abnormally high pressure may result in opacities by interfering with normal corneal metabolism.

During anesthesia, a rise in IOP can produce permanent visual loss. If the IOP is already elevated, a further increase can trigger acute glaucoma. If penetration of the globe occurs when the IOP is excessively high, rupture of a blood vessel with subsequent hemorrhage may transpire. Intraocular pressure becomes atmospheric once the eye cavity has been entered, and any sudden rise in pressure may lead to prolapse of the iris and lens, and loss of vitreous. Thus, proper control of IOP is critical.

Three main factors influence IOP: (1) external pressure on the eye by the contraction of the orbicularis oculi muscle and the tone of the extraocular muscles, venous congestion of orbital veins (as may occur with vomiting and coughing), and conditions such as orbital tumor; (2) scleral rigidity; and (3) changes in intraocular contents that are semisolid (lens, vitreous, or intraocular tumor) or fluid (blood and aqueous humor). Although these factors are significant in affecting IOP, the major control of intraocular tension is exerted by the fluid content, especially the aqueous humor.

Sclerosis of the sclera, not uncommonly seen in the aged, may be associated with decreased scleral compliance and increased IOP. Other degenerative changes of the eye linked with aging can also influence IOP, the most significant being a hardening and enlargement of the crystalline lens. When these degenerative changes occur, they may lead to anterior displacement of the lens–iris diaphragm. A resultant shallowness of the anterior chamber angle may then occur, reducing access of the trabecular meshwork to aqueous. This process is usually gradual, but, if rapid lens engorgement occurs, angle closure glaucoma may transpire.

Changes in the nature of the vitreous that affect the amount of unbound water also influence IOP. Myopia, trauma, and aging produce liquefaction of vitreous gel and a subsequent increase in unbound water, which may lower IOP by facilitating fluid removal. However, under different circumstances, the opposite may occur, that is, the hydration of more normal vitreous may be associated with elevation of IOP. Hence, it is often prudent to produce a slightly dehydrated state in the surgical glaucoma patient.

Intraocular blood volume, determined primarily by vessel

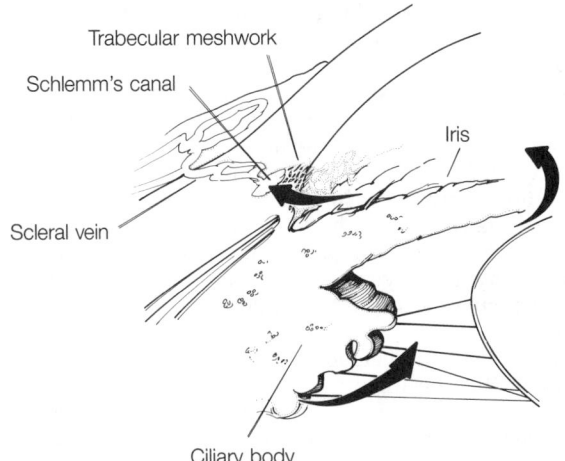

Figure 38-2. Ocular anatomy concerned with control of intraocular pressure.

Trabecular meshwork

Schlemm's canal

Iris

Scleral vein

Ciliary body

dilation or contraction in the spongy layers of the choroid, contributes significantly to IOP. Although changes in both arterial or venous pressure may secondarily affect IOP, excursions in arterial pressure have much less importance than do venous fluctuations. In chronic arterial hypertension, ocular pressure returns to normal levels after a period of adaptation brought about by compression of vessels in the choroid as a result of increased IOP. Thus, a feedback mechanism reduces the total volume of blood, keeping IOP relatively constant in patients with systemic hypertension.[4]

However, if venous return from the eye is disturbed at any point from Schlemm's canal to the right atrium, IOP increases substantially. This is due to both increased intraocular blood volume and distention of orbital vessels, as well as to interference with aqueous drainage. Straining, vomiting, or coughing greatly increase venous pressure and will raise IOP as much as 40 mm Hg or greater. The deleterious implications of these activities cannot be overemphasized. Laryngoscopy and tracheal intubation may also elevate IOP, even without any visible reaction to intubation, but especially when the patient coughs. Topical anesthetization of the larynx may attenuate the hypertensive response to laryngoscopy but does not reliably prevent associated increases in IOP.[5] Ordinarily, the pressure elevation from such increases in blood volume or venous pressure dissipates rapidly. However, if the coughing or straining occurs during ocular surgery when the eye is open, as in cataract extraction or in penetrating keratoplasty, the result may be a disastrous expulsive hemorrhage, at worst, or a disconcerting loss of vitreous, at best.

Despite the significant role of venous pressure, scleral rigidity, and vitreous composition, maintenance of IOP is determined *primarily* by the rate of aqueous formation and the rate of aqueous outflow. The most important influence on formation of aqueous humor is the difference in osmotic pressure between aqueous and plasma.[3] This fact is illustrated by the equation

$$IOP = K \left[(OPaq - OPpl) + CP \right] \qquad (38\text{-}1)$$

where

$$K = \text{coefficient of outflow}$$
$$OPaq = \text{osmotic pressure of aqueous humor}$$
$$OPpl = \text{osmotic pressure of plasma}$$
$$CP = \text{capillary pressure}$$

The fact that a small change in solute concentration of plasma can markedly influence the formation of aqueous humor and hence IOP is the rationale for using hypertonic solutions, such as mannitol, to lower IOP.

Fluctuations in aqueous outflow may also produce a dramatic alteration in IOP. The most significant factor controlling aqueous humor outflow is the diameter of Fontana's spaces[6] as illustrated by the equation:

$$A = \frac{r^4 \times (Piop - Pv)}{8 \eta L} \qquad (38\text{-}2)$$

where

$$A = \text{volume of aqueous outflow per unit of time}$$
$$r = \text{radius of Fontana's spaces}$$
$$Piop = \text{intraocular pressure}$$
$$Pv = \text{venous pressure}$$
$$\eta = \text{viscosity}$$
$$L = \text{length of Fontana's spaces}$$

When the pupil dilates, Fontana's spaces narrow, resistance to outflow is increased, and IOP rises. Because mydriasis is undesirable in both narrow- and wide-angle glaucoma, miotics such as pilocarpine are applied conjunctivally in patients with glaucoma.

Glaucoma

Glaucoma is a condition characterized by elevated IOP, resulting in impairment of capillary blood flow to the optic nerve with eventual loss of optic nerve tissue and function. Two different anatomic types of glaucoma exist: open-angle or chronic simple glaucoma, and closed-angle or acute glaucoma. (Other variations of these processes occur but are not especially germane to anesthetic management.)

With open-angle glaucoma, the elevated IOP exists with an anatomically open anterior chamber angle. It is thought that sclerosis of trabecular tissue results in impaired aqueous filtration and drainage. Treatment consists of medication to produce miosis and trabecular stretching. Commonly used eyedrops are epinephrine, timolol, dipivefrin, and betaxolol.

Closed-angle glaucoma is characterized by the peripheral iris moving into direct contact with the posterior corneal surface, mechanically obstructing aqueous outflow. People who have a narrow angle between the iris and posterior cornea are predisposed to this condition. In these patients, mydriasis can produce such increased thickening of the peripheral iris that corneal touch occurs and the angle is closed. Another mechanism producing acute, closed-angle glaucoma is swelling of the crystalline lens. In this case, pupillary block occurs, with the edematous lens blocking the flow of aqueous from the posterior to the anterior chamber. This situation can also develop if the lens is traumatically dislocated anteriorly, thus physically blocking the anterior chamber.

It was previously thought by some clinicians that patients with glaucoma should not be given atropine premedication. However, this claim is untenable. Atropine premedication in the dose range used clinically has no effect on IOP in either open- or closed-angle glaucoma. When 0.4 mg of atropine is given to a 70-kg person, approximately 0.0001 mg is absorbed by the eye.[7] Garde et al[8] reported, however, that scopolamine has a greater mydriatic effect than atropine and recommended not using scopolamine in patients with known or suspected *narrow*-angle glaucoma.

Equation 38-2, describing the volume of aqueous outflow per unit of time, clearly demonstrates that outflow is exquisitely sensitive to fluctuations in venous pressure. Because a rise in venous pressure produces an increased volume of ocular blood as well as decreased aqueous outflow, it is obvious that considerable elevation of IOP occurs with any maneuver that increases venous pressure. Hence, in addition to preoperative instillation of miotics, other anesthetic goals for the patient with glaucoma include perioperative avoidance of venous congestion and of overhydration. Furthermore, hypotensive episodes are to be avoided, because these patients are allegedly vulnerable to retinal vascular thrombosis.

Primary congenital glaucoma is classified according to age of onset, with the infantile type presenting any time after birth until 5 years of age. The juvenile type presents between the ages of 6 and 30 years. Moreover, childhood glaucoma may also occur in conjunction with various eye diseases or developmental anomalies such as aniridia, mesodermal dysgenesis syndrome, and retinopathy of prematurity.[9]

Successful management of infantile glaucoma is crucially dependent on early diagnosis. Presenting symptoms include epiphora, photophobia, blepharospasm, and irritability. Ocular enlargement, termed *buphthalmos*, or "ox eye," and corneal haziness secondary to edema are common. Buphthalmos is rare, however, if glaucoma develops after 3 years of age because by then the eye is much less elastic.

Because infantile glaucoma is frequently associated with obstructed aqueous outflow, management of it often requires surgical creation, via goniotomy or trabeculotomy, of a route for aqueous humor to flow into Schlemm's canal. However, advanced disease may be unresponsive to even multiple goniotomies, and the more radical trabeculectomy or some other variety of filtering procedure may be necessary.

The juvenile form of glaucoma, in which the cornea and eye size are normal, is commonly associated with a family history of open-angle glaucoma and is treated similarly to primary open-angle glaucoma.

In cases of pediatric secondary glaucoma, goniotomy and filtering may be unsuccessful, whereas cyclocryotherapy may effect a reduction in IOP, pain, and corneal edema. The ciliary body is destroyed with a cryoprobe, cooled to $-70°C$, thus dramatically decreasing aqueous formation.

It is essential to appreciate that the high IOP frequently encountered in infantile glaucoma can be reduced by more than 15 mm Hg when surgical anesthesia is achieved. (Some clinicians maintain that ketamine is a useful drug to use for examination under anesthesia when infantile glaucoma is part of the differential diagnosis, because ketamine does not appear to reduce IOP, giving a spuriously low reading.) Moreover, even normal infants will sporadically have pressures in the mid-20s. Hence, diagnosis is not based exclusively on the numerical pressure recorded under anesthesia. Other factors such as corneal edema and increased corneal diameter, tears in Descemet's membrane, and cupping of the optic nerve are considered in making the diagnosis. If these aberrations are noted, surgical intervention may be mandatory, even in the setting of a reputedly normal IOP.

EFFECTS OF ANESTHESIA AND ADJUVANT DRUGS ON INTRAOCULAR PRESSURE

Central Nervous System Depressants

Inhalation anesthetics purportedly cause dose-related decreases in IOP.[10] The exact mechanisms are unknown, but postulated etiologies include depression of a central nervous system (CNS) control center in the diencephalon,[4] reduction of aqueous humor production, enhancement of aqueous outflow, or relaxation of the extraocular muscles.[7] Moreover, virtually all CNS depressants, including barbiturates,[11,12] neuroleptics,[13] opioids,[14] tranquilizers,[7] and hypnotics,[15] lower IOP in both normal and glaucomatous eyes. It is interesting that etomidate, despite its proclivity to produce pain on intravenous (iv) injection and skeletal muscle movement, is associated with a significant reduction in IOP.[16] However, etomidate-induced myoclonus may be hazardous in the setting of a ruptured globe.

Controversy, however, surrounds the issue of ketamine's effect on IOP. Administered iv or intramuscularly (im), ketamine initially was thought to increase IOP significantly, as measured by indentation tonometry.[17] Corssen and Hoy[18] had also reported a slight but statistically significant increase in IOP that appeared unrelated to changes in blood pressure or depth of anesthesia. However, nystagmus made proper positioning of the tonometer difficult and may have resulted in less than accurate measurements.

Conflicting results arose from a study in which 2 mg·kg^{-1} of ketamine given iv to adults failed to reflect a significant effect on IOP.[19] Furthermore, a pediatric study reported no increase in IOP following an im ketamine dose of 8 mg·kg^{-1}. Indeed, values obtained were similar to those reported with halothane and isoflurane.[20,21]

Some of the confusion may arise from differences in premedication practices and from the use of different instruments to measure IOP. (More recent studies have used applanation tonometry rather than indentation tonometry.) However, even if future studies should confirm that ketamine has minimal or no effect on IOP, it is important to appreciate that ketamine's proclivity to cause nystagmus and blepharospasm makes it a less than optimal agent for many types of ophthalmic surgery.

Ventilation and Temperature

Hyperventilation decreases IOP, whereas asphyxia, administration of carbon dioxide, and hypoventilation have been shown to elevate IOP.[3,22]

Hypothermia lowers IOP. On superficial musing, one might expect a rise in IOP with hypothermia because of the associated increase in viscosity of aqueous humor. However, hypothermia is linked with decreased formation of aqueous humor and with vasoconstriction; hence, the net result is a reduction in IOP.

Adjuvant Drugs: Ganglionic Blockers; Hypertonic Solutions; Acetazolamide

Ganglionic blockers such as tetraethylammonium[23] and pentamethonium both effect a dramatic decrease in IOP. Trimethaphan also significantly lowers IOP in normal subjects, despite mydriasis.

Intravenous administration of hypertonic solutions such as dextran, urea, mannitol, and sorbitol elevate plasma osmotic pressure, thereby decreasing aqueous humor formation and reducing IOP.[24] As effective as urea is in reducing IOP, iv mannitol has the advantage of fewer side-effects. Mannitol's onset, peak (30–45 minutes), and duration of action (5–6 hours) are similar to those of urea. Moreover, both drugs may produce acute intravascular volume overload. Sudden expansion of plasma volume secondary to efflux of intracellular water into the vascular compartment places a heavy workload on the kidneys and heart, often resulting in hypertension and dilution of plasma sodium. Furthermore mannitol-associated diuresis, if protracted, may trigger hypotension in volume-depleted persons.

Glycerin has the advantage of being effective orally. However, the ocular hypotensive effect is said to be less predictable than that of mannitol. Onset usually occurs within 10 minutes of ingestion, and peak action is noted at 30 minutes. The duration of action is 5 to 6 hours. Unfortunately, glycerin may trigger nausea or vomiting, and gastric fluid trapping increases the risk of aspiration.

Intravenous administration of acetazolamide inactivates carbonic anhydrase and interferes with the sodium pump. The resultant decrease in aqueous humor formation lowers IOP. However, the action of acetazolamide is not limited to the eye, and systemic effects include loss of sodium, potassium, and water secondary to the drug's renal tubular effects. Such electrolyte imbalances may then be linked to cardiac dysrhythmias during general anesthesia.

An advantage of acetazolamide is its relative ease of administration. Whereas large volumes of hypertonic solutions must be infused to reduce IOP, acetazolamide is easily given as a typical adult dose of 500 mg dissolved in 10 ml of sterile water. Acetazolamide may also be given orally, and topical carbonic anhydrase inhibitors may soon be commercially available.

Neuromuscular Blocking Drugs

Neuromuscular blocking drugs have both direct and indirect actions on IOP. Hence, a paralyzing dose of *d*-tubocurarine directly lowers IOP by relaxing the extraocular muscles.[25] The same is true of equipotent doses of the other nondepolarizing drugs, including pancuronium[26] (Fig. 38-3). However, if paralysis of the respiratory muscles is accompanied by alveolar hypoventilation, the latter secondary effect may supervene to increase IOP.

In contrast to nondepolarizing drugs, the depolarizing drug succinylcholine elevates IOP. Lincoff *et al*[27] reported extrusion of vitreous following succinylcholine administration to a patient with an open eye injury. An average peak IOP increase of about 8 mm Hg is produced within 1–4 minutes of an iv dose. Within 7 minutes, return to baseline usually transpires.[28] The ocular hypertensive effect of succinylcholine has been attributed to several mechanisms, including tonic contraction of extraocular muscles,[7] choroidal vascular dilation, and relaxation of orbital smooth muscle.[29] Of note, ocular muscles differ anatomically from skeletal muscles in having a population of muscle fibers with multiple motor nerve endings. Whereas skeletal muscle responds to depolarizing drugs with flaccid paralysis, the ocular response to succinylcholine is one of sustained tonic contracture. It has been postulated that this action results from a summation of the local depolarizing effects of succinylcholine on the numerous postjunctional membrane areas of these fibers.[30]

A variety of methods have been advocated to prevent succinylcholine-induced elevations in IOP. In truth, although some attenuation of the increase results, none of these techniques consistently and completely blocks the ocular hypertensive response. Prior administration of such drugs as acetazolamide,[31] propranolol, and nondepolarizing neuromuscular blocking drugs has been suggested. The efficacy of pretreatment with nondepolarizing drugs is controversial.

In 1968 Miller *et al*,[32] using indentation tonometry, reported that pretreatment with small amounts of gallamine or *d*-tubocurarine prevented succinylcholine-associated increases in IOP. However, in 1978 Meyers and colleagues,[33] using the more sensitive applanation tonometer, were unable to consistently circumvent the ocular hypertensive response following similar pretreatment therapy (Table 38-2). Additionally, Verma[34] in 1979 had claimed that a "self-taming" dose of succinylcholine was protective, but Meyers *et al*[35] in 1980, in a controlled study using applanation tonometry, challenged this claim. Although iv pretreatment with lidocaine, 1–2 mg·kg^{-1}, may blunt the hemodynamic response to laryngoscopy,[5,36] such therapy does not reliably prevent the ocular hypertensive response associated with succinylcholine and/or intubation.[37] However, Grover and associates[38] recently claimed that pretreatment with lidocaine, 1.5 mg·kg^{-1} iv, 1 minute prior to induction with thiopental and succinylcholine offered protection from IOP increases due to succinylcholine and may therefore be of value in rapid sequence induction for open eye injuries.

Certainly, no one would disagree that succinylcholine—if unaccompanied by pretreatment with a nondepolarizing neuromuscular blocking drug—is contraindicated in patients with penetrating ocular wounds and should not be given for the first time after the eye has been opened. Nonetheless, it no longer is valid to recommend that succinylcholine be used only with extreme reluctance in ocular surgery. Clearly, any succinylcholine-induced increment in IOP is usually dissipated before surgery is started. Of concern, however, is Jampolsky's warning that succinylcholine be avoided in patients undergoing repeat strabismus surgery, because the forced duction test does not return to baseline for approximately 30 minutes after administration of the drug.[39] More recent and quantitatively sophisticated studies by France *et al*[40] have supported this caveat, although the latter investigators suggest waiting only 20 minutes after administration of succinylcholine before performing forced duction testing.

OCULOCARDIAC REFLEX

Bernard Aschner and Guiseppe Dagnini first described the oculocardiac reflex in 1908. This reflex is triggered by pressure on the globe and by traction on the extraocular muscles as well as on the conjunctiva or on the orbital structures. Moreover, the reflex may also be elicited by performance of a retrobulbar block,[41] by ocular trauma, and by direct pressure on tissue remaining in the orbital apex after enucleation.[42] The afferent limb is trigeminal and the efferent limb is vagal. Although the most common manifestation of the oculocardiac reflex is sinus bradycardia, a wide spectrum of cardiac dysrhythmias may occur, including junctional rhythm, ectopic atrial rhythm, atrioventricular blockade, ventricular bigeminy, multifocal premature ventricular contractions, wandering pacemaker, idioventricular rhythm, asystole, and ventricular tachycardia.[43-45] This reflex may appear during either local or general anesthesia; however, hypercarbia and hypoxemia are thought to augment the in-

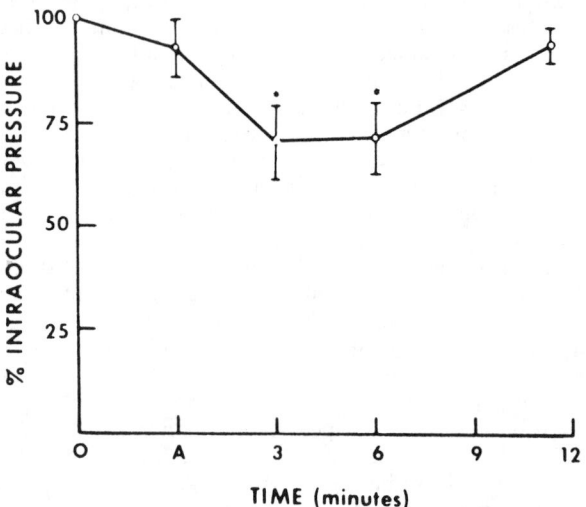

Figure 38-3. Mean intraocular pressure following administration of thiopental, 3–4 mg·kg^{-1}, and pancuronium, 0.08 mg·kg^{-1} at 0. A = loss of lid reflex. *$p < 0.05$. (Reprinted with permission from Litwiller RW, DeFazio CA, Rushia EF: Pancuronium and intraocular pressure. Anesthesiology 42:750, 1975.)

TABLE 38-2. Effects of Succinylcholine (SCh) on Intraocular Pressure: Double-Blind *d*-Tubocurarine or Gallamine Pretreatment

Pretreatment*	Mean Age (yr)	Intraocular Pressure (mm Hg, mean ± SE)		
		Baseline	*3 Minutes After Pretreatment*	*1 Minute After SCh†*
d-Tubocurarine	13.4	13.0 ± 1.0	12.3 ± 1.2	24.0 ± 1.3
Gallamine	8.7	10.9 ± 1.1	10.6 ± 1.0	23.4 ± 2.3

* *d*-Tubocurarine, 0.09 mg·kg⁻¹, or gallamine, 0.3 mg·kg⁻¹.

† 1 to 1.5 mg·kg⁻¹ iv.

Reprinted with permission from Meyers EF, Krupin T, Johnson M et al: Failure of nondepolarizing neuromuscular blockers to inhibit succinylcholine-induced increased intraocular pressure: A controlled study. Anesthesiology 48:149, 1978.

cidence and severity of the problem, as may inappropriate anesthetic depth.

Reports on the alleged incidence of the oculocardiac reflex are remarkable in their striking variability. Berler's study[41] reported an incidence of 50%, but other sources quote rates ranging from 16% to 82%.[43,46] Commonly, those articles disclosing a higher incidence included children in the study population, and children tend to have more vagal tone.

A variety of maneuvers to abolish or obtund the oculocardiac reflex have been promulgated. None of these methods has been consistently effective, safe, and reliable. Inclusion of im anticholinergic drugs such as atropine or glycopyrrolate in the usual premedication regimen for oculocardiac reflex prophylaxis is ineffective.[47] Nearly complete vagolytic blockade in the adult mandates 2–3 mg of atropine or 0.03–0.05 mg·kg⁻¹.[48] Insofar as the peak action of im atropine occurs approximately 30 minutes after administration, it is not surprising that studies of the usual, routine, much smaller doses of atropine administered more than 1 hour prior to surgery have shown inconsistent protection against the oculocardiac reflex.

For the young child who is extremely apprehensive about "shots," giving oral atropine, 0.04 mg·kg⁻¹, with a small amount of water 60–90 minutes preoperatively is an alternative.[49] However, the oral route has not enjoyed tremendous popularity with anesthesiologists because of its slower absorption and more erratic efficacy.

Atropine given iv within 30 minutes of surgery[46] is thought to effect a reduced incidence of the reflex. However, reports differ concerning dosage and timing. Moreover, it must be pointed out that some anesthesiologists claim that prior iv administration of atropine may yield more serious and refractory cardiac dysrhythmias[50] than the reflex itself. Clearly, atropine may be considered a potential myocardial irritant. A variety of cardiac dysrhythmias[51,52] and several conduction abnormalities,[53] including ventricular fibrillation, ventricular tachycardia, and left bundle-branch block, have been attributed to iv atropine.

Although administration of retrobulbar anesthesia may provide some cardiac antidysrhythmic value by blocking the afferent limb of the reflex arc, such a regional technique is not devoid of potential complications, which include, but are not limited to, optic nerve damage, retrobulbar hemorrhage, and stimulation of the oculocardiac reflex arc by the retrobulbar block itself.

It is generally believed that, in adults, the aforementioned prophylactic measures, laced with inherent hazards, are usually not indicated. If a cardiac dysrhythmia appears, initially the surgeon should be asked to cease operative manipulation. Next, the patient's anesthetic depth and ventilatory status are evaluated. Commonly, heart rate and rhythm will return to baseline within 20 seconds following institution of these measures. Moreover, Moonie et al[54] noted that, with repeated manipulation, bradycardia is less likely to recur, probably secondary to fatigue of the reflex arc at the level of the cardioinhibitory center. However, if the initial cardiac dysrhythmia is especially serious or if the reflex tenaciously recurs, atropine should be administered iv, but only after the surgeon stops ocular manipulation.

During pediatric strabismus surgery, however, current popular practice favors administration of iv atropine, 0.02 mg·kg⁻¹, prior to commencing surgery.[55] Alternatively, glycopyrrolate, 0.01 mg·kg⁻¹ administered iv, may be associated with less tachycardia than atropine in this setting.

Clearly, considerable controversy surrounds the issues of incidence and prophylaxis of the oculocardiac reflex. Nonetheless, there is consensus that continuous monitoring of the electrocardiogram (ECG) is important during all types of eye surgery in order to detect potentially dangerous cardiac rhythm disturbances.

ANESTHETIC RAMIFICATIONS OF OPHTHALMIC DRUGS

There is considerable potential for drug interactions during administration of anesthesia for ocular surgery. Topical ophthalmic drugs may produce undesirable systemic effects or may have deleterious anesthetic implications. Systemic absorption of topical ophthalmic drugs may occur from either the conjunctiva or the nasal mucosa following drainage through the nasolacrimal duct. Additionally, some percutaneous absorption, from spillover, through the immature epidermis of the premature infant may transpire.[56] Occluding the nasolacrimal duct by pressing on the inner canthus of the eye for a few minutes after each instillation greatly decreases systemic absorption.

Some of the potentially worrisome topical ocular drugs include acetylcholine, anticholinesterases, cocaine, cyclopentolate, epinephrine, phenylephrine, and timolol. In addition, intraocular sulfur hexafluoride and other intraocular gases have important anesthetic ramifications. Furthermore, certain ophthalmic drugs given systemically may produce untoward sequelae germane to anesthetic management. Drugs in this category include glycerol, mannitol, and acetazolamide.

Acetylcholine

Acetylcholine is commonly used intraocularly following lens extraction to produce miosis. The local use of this drug may occasionally result in such systemic effects as bradycardia, increased salivation, and bronchial secretions, as well as bronchospasm. The side-effects, including hypotension and bradycardia,[57] that may develop in patients given acetylcholine after cataract extraction may be rapidly reversed with iv atropine. Furthermore, one might anticipate that vagotonic anesthetic agents such as halothane could accentuate the effects of acetylcholine.

Anticholinesterase Agents

Echothiophate is a long-acting anticholinesterase miotic that lowers IOP by decreasing resistance to the outflow of aqueous humor. Useful in the treatment of glaucoma, echothiophate is absorbed into the systemic circulation after instillation in the conjunctival sac. Any of the long-acting anticholinesterases may prolong the action of succinylcholine,[58] because, after a month or more of therapy, plasma pseudocholinesterase activity may be less than 5% of normal.[59] It is said, moreover, that normal enzyme activity does not return until 4–6 weeks after discontinuance of the drug.[60] Hence, the anesthesiologist should anticipate prolonged apnea if these patients are given a usual dose of succinylcholine. In addition, a delay in metabolism of ester local anesthetics should be expected.

Cocaine

Cocaine, introduced to ophthalmology in 1884 by Koller, has limited topical ocular use, because it can cause corneal pits and erosion. However, as the only local anesthetic that inherently produces vasoconstriction and shrinkage of mucous membranes, cocaine is commonly used in a nasal pack during dacryocystorhinostomy. The drug is so well absorbed from mucosal surfaces that plasma concentrations comparable to those following direct iv injection are achieved.[61] Because cocaine interferes with catecholamine uptake, it has a sympathetic nervous system potentiating effect.[61]

Historically, epinephrine had often been mixed with cocaine in hopes of augmenting the degree of vasoconstriction produced. This practice is both superfluous and deleterious, as cocaine is a potent vasoconstrictor in its own right, and the combination of epinephrine with cocaine may trigger dangerous cardiac dysrhythmias. It has been shown that cocaine used alone, without topical epinephrine, to shrink the nasal mucosa in conjunction with halothane or enflurane does not sensitize the heart to *endogenous* epinephrine during halothane or enflurane anesthesia.[62] However, animal studies have shown that following pretreatment with *exogenous* epinephrine, cocaine facilitates the development of epinephrine-induced cardiac dysrhythmias during halothane anesthesia.[63]

The usual maximal dose of cocaine used in clinical prac-

tice is 200 mg for a 70-kg adult, or 3 mg·kg^{-1}. However, 1.5 mg·kg^{-1} is preferable, because this lower dose has been shown not to exert any clinically significant sympathomimetic effect in combination with halothane.[64] Although 1 g is considered to be the usual lethal dose for an adult, considerable variation occurs. Furthermore, systemic reactions may appear with as little as 20 mg.

Meyers[65] described two cases of cocaine toxicity during dacryocystorhinostomy, underscoring that cocaine is contraindicated in hypertensive patients or in patients receiving drugs such as guanethidine, reserpine, tricyclic antidepressants, or monoamine oxidase inhibitors. Additionally, sympathomimetics such as epinephrine or phenylephrine should not be given with cocaine.

Obviously, before administering cocaine or another potent vasoconstrictor for dacryocystorhinostomy, the physician should carefully search out possible contraindications. In order to avoid toxic levels, doses of dilute solutions should be meticulously calculated and carefully administered. If serious cardiovascular effects occur, labetalol should be used to counteract them.[66] In the past, propranolol was widely used to control cocaine-induced hypertension,[67] but a lethal hypertensive exacerbation has been ascribed to unopposed alpha stimulation.[68] Labetalol offers the advantage of combined alpha and beta blockade.

Cyclopentolate

Despite the popularity of cyclopentolate as a mydriatic, it is not without side-effects, which include CNS toxicity. Manifestations include dysarthria, disorientation, and frank psychotic reactions. Purportedly, CNS dysfunction is more likely to follow use of the 2% solution, as opposed to the 1% solution.[69] Furthermore, cases of convulsions in children following ocular instillation of cyclopentolate have been reported.[70] Hence, for pediatric usage, 0.5–1.0% solutions are recommended. Cyclopentolate, at higher concentrations, also causes cycloplegia.

Epinephrine

Although topical epinephrine has proved useful in some patients with open-angle glaucoma, the 2% solution has been associated with such systemic effects as nervousness, hypertension, angina pectoris, and tachycardia and with cardiac dysrhythmias.[71]

Some anesthesiologists have maintained that it is unwise to use epinephrine in patients being anesthetized with a halogenated hydrocarbon. However, Smith and colleagues[72] reported on the administration of epinephrine into the anterior chamber of patients undergoing cataract surgery by phacoemulsification and aspiration. They concluded it is safe to administer epinephrine into the anterior chamber in doses up to 68 μg·kg^{-1} under these circumstances. It was postulated that the iris, with its rich supply of adrenergic receptors, may be able to capture with extreme rapidity the epinephrine given into the eye. Apparently, there is not much systemic absorption from the globe.

Phenylephrine

Pupillary dilation and capillary decongestion are reliably produced by topical phenylephrine. Although systemic effects secondary to topical application of prudent doses are rare,[73] severe hypertension, headache, tachycardia, and tremulousness have been reported.[71]

Persons with coronary artery disease may develop severe myocardial ischemia, cardiac dysrhythmias, and even myocardial infarction following topical 10% eyedrops. Those with cerebral aneurysms may be susceptible to cerebral hemorrhage following phenylephrine in this concentration. In general, a safe systemic level follows absorption from either the conjunctiva or the nasal mucosa after drainage by the tear ducts. However, phenylephrine should not be given in the eye after surgery has begun and venous channels are patent.

Children are especially vulnerable to overdose and may respond in a dramatic and adverse fashion to phenylephrine drops. Hence, the use of only 2.5%, rather than 10%, phenylephrine is recommended in infants and the elderly, and the frequency of application should be strictly limited in these patient populations.

Timolol

Timolol, a nonselective beta-adrenergic blocking drug, is a popular antiglaucoma drug. Because significant conjunctival absorption may occur, timolol should be administered with caution to patients with known obstructive airways disease, congestive heart failure, or greater than first-degree heart block. Life-threatening asthmatic crises have been reported following the administration of timolol drops to some patients with chronic, stable asthma.[74] Not unexpectedly, the development of severe sinus bradycardia in a patient with cardiac conduction defects (left anterior hemiblock, first degree atrioventricular block, and incomplete right bundle-branch block) has been reported following timolol.[75] Moreover, timolol has been implicated in the exacerbation of myasthenia gravis[76] and in the production of postoperative apnea in neonates and young infants.[77,78]

In contrast to timolol, an even newer antiglaucoma drug, betaxolol, a beta$_1$-blocker, is said to be more oculospecific and have minimal systemic effects. However, patients receiving an oral beta blocker and betaxolol should be observed for potential additive effect on known systemic effects of beta blockade. Caution should be exercised in patients receiving catecholamine-depleting drugs. Although betaxolol has produced only minimal effects in patients with obstructive airways disease, caution should be exercised in the treatment of patients with excessive restriction of pulmonary function. Moreover, betaxolol is contraindicated in patients with sinus bradycardia, congestive heart failure, greater than first-degree heart block, cardiogenic shock, and overt myocardial failure.

Intraocular Sulfur Hexafluoride

For a patient with a retinal detachment, intraocular sulfur hexafluoride[79] or other gases such as certain perfluorocarbons may be injected into the vitreous in order to mechanically facilitate reattachment. These recommendations do not apply to open eye procedures during which volume and pressure changes are readily compensated for by fluid and gas leak.

Stinson and Donlon[80] suggest terminating nitrous oxide 15 minutes before gas injection in order to prevent significant changes in the size of the intravitreous gas bubble. The patient is then given virtually 100% oxygen (admixed with a small percentage of volatile agent) for the balance of the

TABLE 38-3. Differential Solubilities of Gases

	Blood Gas Partition Coefficients
Sulfur hexafluoride	0.004
Nitrogen	0.015
Nitrous oxide	0.468

operation without adversely affecting intravitreous gas dynamics. Furthermore, if a patient requires reoperation and general anesthesia after intravitreous gas injection, nitrous oxide should be avoided for 5 days subsequent to air injection and for 10 days following sulfur hexafluoride injection (Table 38-3).[81]

Perfluoropropane and octafluorocyclobutane may also be employed in vitreoretinal surgery to support the retina. Like sulfur hexafluoride, these gases are relatively insoluble and require discontinuance of nitrous oxide at least 15 minutes prior to injection. Should the patient require reoperation, it must be remembered that perfluoropropane lingers in the eye for longer than 30 days.[82]

Systemic Ophthalmic Drugs

In addition to topical therapies, various ophthalmic drugs given systemically may result in complications of concern to the anesthesiologist. These systemic drugs include glycerol, mannitol, and acetazolamide. For example, oral glycerol may be associated with nausea, vomiting, and risk of aspiration. Hyperglycemia or glycosuria, disorientation, and seizure activity may occur following oral glycerol.

The recommended iv dose of mannitol is 1.5–2 g·kg^{-1} given over a 30- to 60-minute interval. However, serious systemic problems may result from rapid infusion of large doses of mannitol. These complications include renal failure, congestive heart failure, pulmonary congestion, electrolyte imbalance, hypotension or hypertension, myocardial ischemia, and, rarely, allergic reactions. Clearly, the patient's renal and cardiovascular status must be thoroughly evaluated prior to mannitol therapy.

Acetazolamide, a carbonic anhydrase inhibitor with renal tubular effects, should be considered contraindicated in patients with marked hepatic or renal dysfunction or in those with low sodium levels or abnormal potassium values. As is well known, severe electrolyte imbalances can trigger serious cardiac dysrhythmias during general anesthesia. Furthermore, persons with chronic lung disease may be vulnerable to the development of severe acidosis with long-term acetazolamide therapy. Topically active carbonic anhydrase inhibitors have recently been developed[83] and may be commercially available soon. Such topical agents might well be expected to be relatively free of clinically significant systemic effects.

PREOPERATIVE EVALUATION

Establishing Rapport and Assessing Medical Condition

Preoperative preparation and evaluation of the patient begins with the establishment of rapport and communication among the anesthesiologist, the surgeon, and the patient.

Most patients realize that surgery and anesthesia entail inherent risks, and they appreciate a candid explanation of potential complications, balanced with information concerning probability, or frequency, of permanent adverse sequelae. Such an approach, furthermore, fulfills the medicolegal responsibilities of the physician to obtain informed consent.

A thorough history of the patient and physical examination are the *sine qua non* of safe patient care. A complete list of medications that the patient is currently taking, both systemic and topical, must be obtained so that potential drug interactions can be anticipated and, additionally, so that essential medication will be administered during the hospital stay. Naturally, a history of any allergies to medicines, foods, or tape should be documented. Clearly, knowledge of any personal or family history of adverse reactions to anesthesia is mandatory. The requisite laboratory data will vary, depending on the age and physical status of the patient. An ECG is often obtained in patients older than 40 years of age and on younger patients if their medical history suggests the possibility of cardiovascular disease.

The anesthesiologist must be aware of the anesthetic implications of congenital and metabolic diseases with ocular manifestations. Diabetics often present with ocular complications, and the anesthesiologist must be knowledgeable about the systemic disturbances of physiology that affect these patients. Indeed, the list of congenital and metabolic diseases with ocular pathology that have significant anesthetic implications is lengthy. A partial summary includes such syndromes as Crouzon's, Apert's, Goldenhar's (oculoauriculovertebral dysplasia), Sturge-Weber, Marfan's, Lowe's (oculocerebrorenal syndrome), Down's (trisomy 21), Wagner-Stickler, and Riley-Day (familial dysautonomia). Other diseases in this category are homocystinuria, malignant hyperthermia, myotonia dystrophica, and sickle cell disease.[84]

Furthermore, eye patients are often at the extremes of age—ranging from premature babies to nonagenarians. Hence, special age-related considerations, such as altered pharmacokinetics and pharmacodynamics, apply. In addition, elderly patients not infrequently suffer from thyroid dysfunction and cardiopulmonary and renal diseases.

Selection of Anesthesia

The requirements of ophthalmic surgery include safety, akinesia, profound analgesia, minimal bleeding, avoidance or obtundation of the oculocardiac reflex, prevention of intraocular hypertension, awareness of drug interactions, and a smooth emergence devoid of vomiting, coughing, or retching (see Table 38-1). Moreover, the exigencies of ophthalmic anesthesia mandate that the anesthesiologist be positioned remote from the patient's airway, and this necessity sometimes creates certain logistic problems.

Most ophthalmic procedures may be performed in adults under either local or general anesthesia. (In children, general anesthesia is almost always selected.) When local anesthesia is elected, the ophthalmologist usually administers the local or regional blockade, and the anesthesiologist is present to continually monitor the patient's ECG, routinely check vital signs, and administer sedation appropriately. If a mature, cooperative patient and a gentle, communicative surgeon are involved, local anesthesia should provide satisfactory conditions for almost any ophthalmic operation of reasonable length. Local anesthesia is especially popular for anterior segment surgery of 2 hours' duration or less. Many

TABLE 38-4. Factors Influencing Choice of Anesthesia

Nature and duration of procedure
Coagulation status
Patient's ability to communicate and cooperate
Personal preference

retina operations of similar length, however, may also be done under local anesthesia.

The choice of anesthesia should be individualized according to the nature and duration of the procedure, the coagulation status of the patient, the ability of the patient to communicate and cooperate, and the personal preference of the surgeon (Table 38-4). Patients who are deaf or who speak a foreign language and those with claustrophobia or excessive anxiety are poor candidates for local anesthesia. Other relative contraindications include tremors, chronic coughing, and inability to lie flat.

Retrobulbar block is a practical means to achieve akinesis of the globe. Deep general anesthesia or nondepolarizing muscle relaxants also produce a motionless eye. Retrobulbar block entails injection of local anesthesia behind the eye into the muscle cone. In the past, patients were typically asked to gaze superonasally while the block was being performed. This maneuver theoretically freed the inferior oblique muscle from the course of the needle. More recently, however, Unsold and colleagues[85] found that the eye was more vulnerable to optic nerve or ophthalmic artery injury in this position. Hence, they suggest performing the injection with the eye in neutral position or looking slightly downward and outward, as these positions move the optic nerve sheath farther away from the path of the needle. A 25-gauge needle is then introduced through the lower lid in the inferotemporal quadrant, just nasal to the junction of the lateral and inferior rim of the orbit. The needle is advanced approximately 1.5 cm along the inferotemporal wall of the orbit and is then directed upward and nasally toward the orbital apex. The plunger of the syringe is withdrawn to reveal an unwanted intravascular location, and 4 ml of local anesthetic is then injected. The retrobulbar injection should be followed by gentle massage of the globe to enhance dispersion of the local anesthetic.

Akinesia of the eyelids is then obtained by blocking the branches of the facial nerve supplying the orbicularis muscle. Since first used for ophthalmic surgery by Van Lint in 1914,[86] numerous methods of facial nerve blockade have been described. All these techniques block the facial nerve either proximally or distally to its exit point from the skull by the stylomastoid foramen.

Available data have failed to demonstrate a significant difference in complications such as iris prolapse or vitreous loss between local and general anesthesia for cataract surgery,[87] and local anesthesia has proved safe for patients with certain types of cardiovascular disease such as a relatively recent myocardial infarction.[88] Nonetheless, the use of general anesthesia for intraocular surgery has increased significantly in the past two decades.

One must not be lulled into a false sense of security with local anesthesia, because this technique does not necessarily involve less physiologic trespass than does general anesthesia. Complications associated with retrobulbar block may be local or systemic and may result in blindness and even death (Table 38-5). The most common complication is retrobulbar hemorrhage secondary to puncture of vessels within the retrobulbar space. This misadventure is characterized by the simultaneous appearance of an excellent mo-

TABLE 38–5. Complications of Retrobulbar Blockade

Stimulation of oculocardiac reflex arc
Retrobulbar hemorrhage
Puncture of posterior globe, resulting in retinal detachment
  and vitreous hemorrhage
Central retinal artery occlusion
Penetration of optic nerve
Inadvertent brain stem anesthesia
Inadvertent intraocular injection

tor block of the globe, closing of the upper lid, proptosis, and a palpable increase in IOP. If this develops, it is prudent to defer the proposed intraocular procedure and monitor the patient for several hours after the hemorrhage to follow central retinal artery pulsations to rule out retinal artery occlusion and to watch for the possible appearance of the oculocardiac reflex as blood extravasates from the muscle cone.

Other complications of retrobulbar block include direct intravascular injection, with all the attendant CNS and cardiovascular effects of excessive drug levels; stimulation of the oculocardiac reflex; inadvertent intraocular injection; inadequate blockade of extraocular muscles with compression of the globe and extrusion of intraocular contents; puncture of the posterior segment of the globe, producing a posterior retinal tear resulting in retinal detachment and vitreous hemorrhage; and penetration of the optic nerve. Furthermore, central retinal artery occlusion, a potentially blinding situation, may result either after a retrobulbar hemorrhage or if the dura around the optic nerve has been penetrated and local anesthetic solution is accidently injected into the subarachnoid space. An initially insidious but potentially lethal complication may also develop when accidental access to cerebrospinal fluid during performance of a retrobulbar nerve block occurs secondary to perforation of the meningeal sheaths that surround the optic nerve. One case report[89] described the gradual onset of unconsciousness and apnea over 7 minutes without any accompanying seizures or cardiovascular collapse. Hence, anesthesiologists and ophthalmologists should be exquisitely aware of the possibility of accidental brain stem anesthesia following retrobulbar block. In a series of 6000 retrobulbar blocks, Nicoll[90] reported 16 cases of apparent brain stem anesthesia; 8 of the 16 patients developed respiratory arrest. Other symptoms included agitation, contralateral ophthalmoplegia and amaurosis, ptosis, mydriasis, dysphagia, and cardiac arrest. It is axiomatic that persons skilled in airway maintenance and in ventilatory and circulatory support should be immediately available whenever retrobulbar block is administered.

Because the complications of retrobulbar block can be both vision-threatening and life-threatening, alternative approaches have been developed. Since the late 1980s, peribulbar block has become popular. The advantages of this technique include its safety and the fact that a lid block is generally superfluous, as the relatively large volume of injected local anesthetic usually diffuses into the eyelids. Two injections are required; these are placed inferotemporally and then superonasally, just below and medial to the supraorbital notch. For both injections, the needle is held in a plane parallel to the orbit, careful aspiration is performed, and 4–5 ml of anesthetic solution is injected in each site. Onset is generally slower than with retrobulbar blockade and may be delayed for as long as 15–20 minutes. However, pH adjustment of a lidocaine-bupivacaine mix-

ture or of plain bupivacaine with bicarbonate will accelerate the onset.[91] Another disadvantage includes increased forward pressure on the eyeball consequent to the larger volume of local anesthetic deposited in the orbit compared to retrobulbar block. However, no cases of either retrobulbar hemorrhage or of brain stem anesthesia associated with peribulbar block have been documented to date. Indeed, Hamilton et al[92] recently reported 5714 peribulbar blocks without a single case of brainstem anesthesia or respiratory arrest.

Many advocate the administration of approximately 10–30 mg of methohexital iv immediately prior to performance of ocular regional anesthesia, provided that no contraindications to the use of this drug exist. Such a practice is usually quite satisfactory, affording considerable comfort and amnesia. What should be avoided at all costs, however, is the combination of local anesthesia with heavy sedation in the form of high doses of opioids, benzodiazepines, and hypnotics. This polypharmacology is highly unsatisfactory because of the pharmacologic vagaries in the geriatric population and the attendant risks of respiratory depression, airway obstruction, hypotension, CNS aberrations, and prolonged recovery time. This undesirable technique has all the disadvantages of a general anesthetic in the absence of a tracheal tube without the advantage of controllability that general anesthesia offers. The patient should be relaxed but awake, to avoid head movement associated with snoring or sudden abrupt movement upon awakening. Clearly, patients under conscious sedation must be capable of responding rationally to commands and must be able to maintain airway patency. Undersedation should likewise be avoided, because tachycardia and hypertension may have deleterious effects, especially in patients with coronary artery disease. Moreover, patients with orthopedic deformities or arthritis must be meticulously positioned and given comfortable padding on the operating table. Adequate ventilation about the face is essential for all patients to avoid carbon dioxide accumulation, and each must be comfortably warm. (The hazards of shivering in patients with cardiac disease and, for that matter, in any patient having delicate eye surgery are well known.) Continuous ECG monitoring is vital, lest performance of the retrobulbar block, pressure on the orbit, or tugging on the extraocular muscles stimulate the oculocardiac reflex arc and produce dangerous cardiac dysrhythmias. Likewise, pulse oximetry is essential.

A question that is frequently asked is whether, for cardiac patients, epinephrine may be safely combined with local anesthetics in order to achieve vasoconstriction and increased anesthetic duration. Donlon and Moss[93] emphasize that release of endogenous catecholamines secondary to suboptimal analgesia may greatly exceed the relatively minute amount of injected exogenous catecholamine. Specifically, they mention that 0.06 mg epinephrine (12 ml of 1:200,000) produces some systemic uptake but no untoward clinical effects.[93]

ANESTHETIC MANAGEMENT IN SPECIFIC SITUATIONS

General Concepts and Objectives

The majority of patients undergoing eye surgery are either younger than 10 years of age or older than 55 years of age. In children, operations on the ocular adnexa, including lid surgery, repair of lacrimal apparatus, and adjustment of extraocular muscles, are common. However, surgery on the anterior segment, such as cataract removal, glaucoma procedures, and trauma repair, is definitely not limited to the adult population. Nor are posterior segment operations such as scleral buckling and vitrectomy the exclusive domain of geriatrics.

Most ocular procedures demand profound analgesia but minimal skeletal muscle relaxation. The airway must be protected from obstruction, and the anesthesiologist must distance himself or herself—along with anesthetic apparatus—from the surgical field. Depending on whether the patient is a child or an adult and various other factors previously discussed, a decision is reached regarding whether to select local or general anesthesia. Additional preparation must include, of course, identification of underlying diseases, such as asthma, diabetes mellitus, or nephropathy. The patient should also be prepared emotionally for the recovery period, when he or she will awaken with one or both eyes closed by bandages. This is important not only to spare him or her fear and anxiety but also to prevent much of the thrashing about that fright might produce, to the detriment of the eye.

Preoperative sedation is chosen carefully. Except for strabismus correction, retinal detachment surgery, and cryosurgery, ophthalmic procedures are generally associated with little pain. Thus, the routine use of opioid premedication, replete with emetic potential, is ill-advised. Rather, premedication should be prescribed with a view toward amnesia, sedation, and antiemesis. Reasonable selections would include a benzodiazepine, for sedative-hypnotic effect, or the phenothiazine promethazine or the antihistaminic hydroxyzine for their sedative and antiemetic properties.

Analgesia and akinesis are then secured through either local or general anesthesia, with careful attention paid to proper control of IOP and to the possible appearance of the oculocardiac reflex. The anesthesiologist strives to provide a smooth intraoperative course and to prevent coughing, retching, and vomiting, lest harmful increases in IOP transpire that could hinder successful surgery. If general anesthesia is elected, extubation of the trachea should be accomplished before there is a tendency to cough. The administration of iv lidocaine, $1.5-2$ mg·kg^{-1}, prior to extubation of the trachea is helpful in attentuating coughing. Likewise, prophylactic iv droperidol is valuable in reducing the incidence and severity of nausea and vomiting.[94,95]

"Open Eye, Full Stomach" Encounters

The anesthesiologist involved in caring for a patient with a penetrating eye injury and a full stomach confronts special challenges. He or she must weigh the risk of aspiration against the risk of blindness in the injured eye that could result from elevated IOP and extrusion of ocular contents.

As in all cases of trauma, attention should be given to the exclusion of other injuries, such as skull and orbital fractures, intracranial trauma associated with subdural hematoma formation, and the possibility of thoracic or abdominal bleeding.

Although regional anesthesia or an awake intubation are often valuable alternatives for the management of trauma patients who have recently eaten, such options are not available for patients with penetrating eye injuries. Retrobulbar blockade is ill-advised in this setting, because extrusion of intraocular contents may ensue. Moreover, although it is conceivable that a well-conducted, extremely smooth awake intubation following topical anesthesia might not increase

IOP, it seems much more probable that coughing or straining will occur in this setting, resulting in an increased IOP.

Preoperative prophylaxis against aspiration may involve administering H$_2$ receptor antagonists to elevate gastric fluid pH and to reduce gastric acid production.[96,97] Metoclopramide may be given to induce peristalsis and enhance gastric emptying.

Not infrequently, a barbiturate, nondepolarizing neuromuscular blocking drug technique is described as the method of choice for the emergency repair of an open eye injury; the nondepolarizing drug pancuronium in a dose of 0.15 mg·kg^{-1} has been shown to lower IOP. However, this method has its disadvantages, including risk of aspiration and death during the relatively lengthy period—ranging from 75 seconds[98] to 150 seconds[99]—that the airway is unprotected. (Performance of the Sellick maneuver during this interval affords some protection.) Furthermore, a premature attempt at intubation of the trachea will produce coughing, straining, and a dramatic rise in IOP, emphasizing the need to confirm the onset of drug effect with a peripheral nerve stimulator while appreciating, nonetheless, that muscle groups vary in their response to muscle relaxants. Moreover, the cardiovascular side-effects of tachycardia and hypertension may prove worrisome in patients with coronary artery disease. Also, the long duration of action of intubating doses of pancuronium may mandate postoperative mechanical ventilation of the lungs. Intermediate-acting nondepolarizing drugs such as vecuronium and atracurium have briefer durations of action, less dramatic, if any, circulatory effects, and lack cumulative tendency but nevertheless have an onset of action similar to that of pancuronium.[100,101]

Several studies have explored the use of extremely large doses of nondepolarizing muscle relaxants to accelerate the onset of adequate relaxation for endotracheal intubation. Using vecuronium doses of 0.2 and 0.4 mg·kg^{-1}, Casson and Jones[102] found mean onset times of 95 and 87 seconds, respectively. Recently Ginsberg et al[103] found comparable albeit slightly longer onset times. Ginsberg's group reported that the administration of high dose (0.4 mg·kg^{-1}) vecuronium reduced the onset from 208 ± 41 seconds, as seen with the usual intubating dose of 0.1 mg·kg^{-1}, to 106 ± 35 seconds. However, the design of this study did not eliminate the possibility of bias being introduced by factors that could influence the quality of intubating conditions. For example, the doses of diazepam, fentanyl, and thiopental given prior to intubation of the trachea varied greatly among patients.

Succinylcholine offers the distinct advantages of swift onset, superb intubating conditions, and brief duration of action. If administered after careful pretreatment with a nondepolarizing drug and an induction dose of thiopental (4 mg·kg^{-1}), succinylcholine produces only small increases in IOP.[104,105] Although the advisability of this technique has been debated vociferously, there are no published reports of loss of intraocular contents from a pretreatment–barbiturate–succinylcholine sequence when used in this setting.[106] Upon completion of surgery and return of spontaneous ventilation, an awake extubation of the trachea may be performed with the patient in a lateral, head-down position.

In managing certain pediatric patients in this situation, a reasonable approach might be to perform an inhalation induction with cricoid pressure and intubation of the trachea under deep halothane anesthesia.[107] In these cases, attempting to start an iv infusion prior to induction of anesthesia can trigger struggling, sobbing, and screaming, and optimal visual outcome may be compromised. Moreover, it is important to keep in mind that much damage to the eye may already have occurred as a result of vomiting owing to pain or as a result of eye-rubbing and eye-squeezing by the child. The anesthesiologist cannot be held accountable for every insult to the eye.

What about the so-called priming principle?[108,109] This concept involves using approximately one tenth of an intubating dose of nondepolarizing drug, followed 4 minutes later by an intubating dose. Then, after waiting an additional 90 seconds, intubation of the trachea may be performed. However, studies in this area demonstrate wide variability and disconcerting scatter of data. Future investigations should use a randomized, double-blind design, because studies of intubating conditions are notoriously difficult to interpret. Moreover, priming is not devoid of risk; a case of pulmonary aspiration after a priming dose of vecuronium has been reported.[110]

Perhaps the wisest approach to the management of open eye–full stomach situations is summarized by Baumgarten and Reynolds,[111] who wrote in 1985:

It may be possible to devise a combination of intravenous anesthetics and nondepolarizing relaxants that totally prevents coughing after rapid intubation. Until this combination is devised and confirmed in a large, controlled double-blind series, clinicians should not apply the priming principle to the open eye–full stomach patient. Use of a blockade monitor to predict intubating conditions may be unreliable, since muscle groups vary in their response to nondepolarizing relaxants. At this time, succinylcholine with precurarization probably remains the most tenable compromise in the open eye–full stomach challenge.

Strabismus Surgery

Approximately 5% of the population have malalignment of the visual axes, which may be accompanied by diplopia, amblyopia, and loss of stereopsis (Table 38-6).[112] Indeed, strabismus surgery is the most common pediatric ocular operation performed in the United States, and it entails a variety of techniques to weaken an extraocular muscle by moving its insertion on the globe (recession) or to strengthen an extraocular muscle by eliminating a short strip of the tendon or muscle (resection).[113]

Infantile strabismus occurs within the first 6 months of life and is often observed in the early neonatal period. Although the majority of patients with strabismus are healthy, normal children, the incidence of strabismus is increased in those with CNS dysfunctions such as cerebral palsy and meningomyelocele with hydrocephalus. Moreover, strabismus may be acquired secondary to oculomotor nerve trauma or to sensory abnormalities such as cataracts or refractive aberrations.

In addition to the well-known propensity of strabismus surgery to trigger the oculocardiac reflex (previously discussed), there is also an increased incidence of malignant hyperthermia in patients with conditions such as strabismus or ptosis. This observation is consistent with the impression that persons susceptible to malignant hyperthermia often have localized areas of skeletal muscle weakness or other musculoskeletal abnormalities.[114-116] Other aspects of strabismus surgery of interest to anesthesiologists include succinylcholine-induced tonic contracture of the extraocular muscles and an increased incidence of post-operative nausea and vomiting.

In formulating a surgical treatment plan for incomitant strabismus, ophthalmologists often find the forced duction test (FDT) to be exquisitely helpful in differentiating between a paretic muscle and a restrictive force preventing ocular motion. To perform the FDT, the surgeon grasps the sclera of the anesthetized eye with a forceps near the corneal limbus and moves the eye into each field of gaze, concomitantly assessing tissue and elastic properties. This simple test provides valuable clues to the presence and site of mechanical restrictions of the extraocular muscles.

France et al[40] quantitated the magnitude and duration of change of the FDT following succinylcholine administration. They demonstrated that quantitation of the force necessary to rotate the globe remained significantly elevated over control for 15 minutes, even though the rise in IOP and the skeletal muscle paralysis lasted less than 5 minutes. Because succinylcholine interferes with FDT, its use is contraindicated less than 20 minutes prior to testing. Hence, France suggests performing the FDT on the anesthetized patient either while mask inhalation anesthesia is being administered, prior to intubation of the trachea, and then using succinylcholine to expedite intubation; or, after intubation, facilitated by nondepolarizing neuromuscular blocking drugs; or after intubation under moderately deep inhalation anesthesia, unaided by succinylcholine. However, when deep inhalational anesthesia is elected, atropine (0.02 mg · kg^{-1}, administered iv) should be given before or in the early stage of induction of anesthesia to prevent the fall in cardiac output that may accompany the significant dose-dependent depression of left ventricular function in children.[117,118] Additionally, the use of iv atropine at this time affords some protection against elicitation of the oculocardiac reflex. For these reasons, many anesthesiologists administer iv atropine routinely to children scheduled for strabismus surgery.

Once intubation of the trachea has been accomplished, anesthesia is commonly maintained with halothane or isoflurane, nitrous oxide, and oxygen. The patient is carefully monitored with a precordial stethoscope, ECG, blood pressure device, pulse oximeter, and temperature probe. If bradycardia occurs, the surgeon is asked to discontinue ocular manipulation, and the patient's ventilatory status and anesthetic depth are quickly assessed. If additional iv atropine is deemed indicated, it is not given while the oculocardiac reflex is active, lest even more dangerous cardiac dysrhythmias be triggered.

Vomiting after eye muscle surgery is common, giving credibility to the existence of the oculogastric reflex. Abramowitz et al[94,95] reported that prophylactic iv adminis-

TABLE 38-6. Concerns With Various Ocular Procedures

Procedure	Concerns
Strabismus repair	Forced duction testing Oculocardiac reflex Oculogastric reflex Malignant hyperthermia
Intraocular surgery	Proper control of IOP Akinesia Drug interactions Associated systemic disease
Retinal detachment surgery	Oculocardiac reflex Proper control of IOP Nitrous oxide interaction with air or sulfur hexafluoride

tration of 0.075 mg·kg^{-1} of droperidol 30 minutes prior to termination of surgery was "highly effective" in reducing the frequency and severity of vomiting in pediatric patients undergoing repair of strabismus. (The incidence was decreased from 85% to 43%.) Fortunately, since strabismus surgery is commonly performed on an ambulatory basis, no significant prolongation of recovery time was observed with this protocol. More recently, the administration of droperidol, 0.075 mg·kg^{-1} at induction of anesthesia before manipulation of the eye, has been claimed to reduce the incidence of vomiting after strabismus surgery to a more clinically acceptable level of approximately 10%.[119] Moreover, a low dose of droperidol, 0.01–0.02 mg·kg^{-1} iv, administered immediately after anesthetic induction in strabismus patients may decrease both the incidence and severity of nausea and vomiting (Wetchler, personal communication).

Although Warner and associates[120] reported an incidence of vomiting of approximately 16% when lidocaine, 2 mg·kg^{-1}, was given iv prior to tracheal intubation, others have not been able to document such favorable results following lidocaine prophylaxis.[121,122]

Perhaps ondansetron, a selective serotonin Type 3 antagonist, will prove useful in reducing nausea and vomiting following pediatric strabismus surgery.

Intraocular Surgery

Advances in both anesthesia and in technology now permit a level of controlled intraocular manipulation not possible a quarter of a century ago (see Table 38-6).

Proper control of IOP is crucial for such intraocular procedures as glaucoma drainage surgery, open eye vitrectomy, penetrating keratoplasty (corneal transplantation), and traditional intracapsular cataract extraction. Prior to scleral incision (when IOP then becomes equal to atmospheric pressure), a low-normal IOP is essential, as abrupt decompression of a hypertensive eye could result in iris or lens prolapse, vitreous loss, or expulsive choroidal hemorrhage. Although available data[87] have not demonstrated a major difference in the rate of complications such as vitreous loss and iris prolapse between local anesthesia and general anesthesia, and although local anesthesia has proved to be a safe technique for eye patients with a recent myocardial infarction,[88] utilization of general anesthesia for intraocular surgery has increased impressively in the past 20 years.

Premedication is selected with a view toward antiemesis. Furthermore, atropine may be given safely, if desired, for antisialagogue properties. In the usual systemic premedicating dose, atropine is not harmful to glaucoma patients.[123]

Many anesthetic techniques may be safely used for elective intraocular surgery. If general anesthesia is selected, virtually any of the inhalation drugs may be given following iv induction of anesthesia with a barbiturate and neuromuscular blocking drug and topical laryngeal lidocaine. Because complete akinesia is essential for delicate intraocular surgery, nondepolarizing drugs are administered, followed by neuromuscular function monitoring to ensure a 90–95% twitch suppression level during surgery. Because proper control of IOP is critical, controlled ventilation of the lungs is used, along with end-tidal carbon dioxide monitoring to ensure avoidance of hypercarbia.

Maximal pupillary dilation is important for many types of intraocular surgery and can be induced by continuous infusion of epinephrine 1:200,000 in a balanced salt solution, delivered through a small-gauge needle placed in the anterior chamber. Almost simultaneous with its administration, the drug is removed by aspirating it from the anterior chamber. The iris usually dilates immediately on contact with the epinephrine infusion, and drug uptake is presumably limited by the associated intense vasoconstriction of the iris and ciliary body. However, epinephrine may also be potentially absorbed by drainage through Schlemm's canal into the venous system or by spillover of the infusion into the conjunctival vessels or drainage to the nasal mucosa.

Clearly, the extent of systemic absorption of epinephrine is of concern to the anesthesiologist, especially in view of the drug's cardiac dysrhythmogenic potential when given concomitantly with potent inhalation drugs. However, plasma catecholamine levels during epinephrine infusion into the anterior chamber have not been investigated extensively. Nonetheless, under halothane anesthesia, in both children and adults, Smith et al[72] were unable to show any increased incidence of cardiac dysrhythmias or signs of systemic effects following instillation of 1:1000 epinephrine (0.4–68 µg·kg^{-1}) directly into the anterior chamber during cataract surgery. (However, all patients were given lidocaine, 2 mg·kg^{-1}, as topical laryngeal anesthesia.) The authors postulated that the globe is not a fertile site for systemic absorption. Hence, general guidelines for subcutaneous injection may not be germane for intraocular injection.[72]

At the completion of surgery, any residual neuromuscular blockade is reversed. Upon resumption of spontaneous ventilation, the patient's trachea is extubated (often in the lateral position) still deeply anesthetized and following iv administration of lidocaine to prevent coughing. Of note, atropine and neostigmine may be safely used to reverse neuromuscular blockade even in patients with glaucoma, because this combination of drugs, in conventional doses, will have minimal effects on pupil size and IOP.[124]

Retinal Detachment Surgery

Surgery to repair retinal detachments involves procedures affecting intraocular volume, frequently using a synthetic silicone band or sponge to produce a localized or encircling scleral indentation (see Table 38-6). Furthermore, internal tamponade of the retinal break may be accomplished by injecting an expandable gas such as sulfur hexafluoride into the vitreous. Owing to blood gas partition coefficient differences, the administration of nitrous oxide may enhance the internal tamponade effect of sulfur hexafluoride intraoperatively, only to be followed by a dramatic drop in IOP and volume upon discontinuance of nitrous oxide. The injected sulfur hexafluoride bubble, in the presence of concomitant administration of nitrous oxide, can cause a rapid and dramatic rise in IOP, reaching a peak within 20 minutes[79-81] (see the section on Intraocular Sulfur Hexafluoride). Because the resultant rise in IOP may compromise retinal circulation, Stinson and Donlon[80] recommend cessation of nitrous oxide administration 15 minutes before gas injection in order to prevent significant changes in the volume of the intravitreous gas bubble. Furthermore, Wolf et al[81] state that if a patient requires anesthesia after intravitreous gas injection, nitrous oxide should be omitted for 5 days following an air injection, and for 10 days following sulfur hexafluoride injection. Perfluoropropane, moreover, remains in the eye longer than 30 days.

Alternatively, silicone oil, a vitreous substitute, may be injected to achieve internal tamponade of a retinal break.

Retinal detachment operations are basically extraocular but may briefly become intraocular if the surgeon elects to perforate and drain subretinal fluid. Furthermore, rotation of the globe with traction on the extraocular muscles may elicit the oculocardiac reflex, so the anesthesiologist must be vigilant about potential cardiac dysrhythmias. Additionally, because it is desirable to have a soft eye while the sclera is being buckled, iv administration of acetazolamide or mannitol is common during retinal surgery to lower IOP.

These patients are generally managed in the same manner as those having intraocular surgery except that maintenance of intraoperative skeletal muscle paralysis is not as critical as during intraocular surgery. Hence, inhalational anesthetics need not be accompanied intraoperatively by nondepolarizing neuromuscular blocking drugs.

POSTOPERATIVE OCULAR COMPLICATIONS

Postoperative complications include corneal abrasion, chemical injuries, thermal injury, minor visual disturbances, and serious visual disturbances, including visual loss. The latter, serious misadventures may be due to such diverse conditions as acute corneal epithelial edema,[125] central retinal artery occlusion,[126] ketamine,[127] Valsalva hemorrhagic retinopathy,[128] glycine toxicity, retinal ischemia, and acute glaucoma.

Corneal Abrasion

Although the most common ocular complication of general anesthesia is corneal abrasion,[129] the incidence varies widely, depending on the perioperative circumstances. Cucchiara et al[130] found a 0.17% incidence of corneal abrasion in 4652 neurosurgical patients whose eyes were protected, while Batra and Bali[129] one decade earlier reported a 44% incidence of corneal abrasion when eyes were left unprotected and partly open. A variety of mechanisms can result in corneal abrasion, including damage caused by the anesthetic mask, surgical drapes, and spillage of solutions. During intubation of the trachea, moreover, the end of plastic watch bands or hospital ID cards clipped to the laryngoscopist's vest pocket can injure the cornea.[131] Ocular injury may also occur owing to loss of pain sensation, obtundation of protective corneal reflexes, and decreased tear production during anesthesia.

Taping the eyelids closed,[132] applying protective goggles, and instilling petroleum-based ointments (artificial tears) into the conjunctival sac may provide protection. Disadvantages of ointments include occasional allergic reactions; flammability, which may make their use undesirable during surgery around the face and contraindicated during laser surgery; and blurred vision in the early postoperative period.[132] Interestingly, the blurring and foreign body sensation associated with ointments may actually increase the incidence of postoperative corneal abrasions if they trigger excessive rubbing of the eyes while the patient is still emerging from anesthesia. Moreover, halothane absorption into paraffin-based ointments can damage the cornea,[133] and even water-based (methylcellulose) ointments may be irritating and cause scleral erythema. It would seem prudent, therefore, during general anesthesia for procedures away from the head and neck to close the eyelids with tape. For certain procedures on the face, ocular occluders or tarsorrhaphy may be indicated. Special attention should also be devoted to frequent checking of the eyes during procedures on a prone patient.

Patients with corneal abrasion usually complain of a foreign body sensation, pain, tearing, and photophobia. The pain is typically exacerbated by blinking and ocular movement. It is wise to have an ophthalmologic consultation immediately. Treatment consists of the prophylactic application of antibiotic ointment and patching the injured eye. Although permanent sequelae are possible, healing usually occurs within 24 hours.

Chemical Injury

Spillage of solutions during skin preparation may result in chemical damage to the eye. Recently, the Food and Drug Administration reported serious corneal damage due to eye contact with Hibiclens, a 4% chlorhexidine gluconate solution formulated with a detergent.[134] Again, with meticulous attention to detail, this misadventure is preventable. Treatment consists of liberal bathing of the eye with water to remove the offending agent. Postoperatively, it may be desirable to have an ophthalmologist examine the eye to document any residual injury or lack thereof.

Thermal Injury

The potential for thermal injury to the cornea or retina from certain laser beams requires that the patient's eyes be protected with moist gauze pads and metal shields and that operating room personnel wear protective glasses.[135] These goggles must be appropriately tinted for the specific wavelength they are intended to block. One may wear clear goggles when working with the carbon dioxide laser, whereas for work with the argon, Nd-YAG, or Nd-YAG-KTP laser the goggles must be tinted orange, green, and orange-red, respectively.

Mild Visual Symptoms

After anesthesia, mild visual disturbances such as photophobia or diplopia are not uncommon.[136] Blurred vision in the early postoperative period may reflect residual effects of petroleum-based ophthalmic ointments or ocular effects of anticholinergic drugs administered in the perioperative period (see Corneal Abrasion, above). Dhamee et al[137] reported an incidence (7–14%) of benign, transient visual disturbances after gynecologic procedures.

By contrast, the complaint of visual loss postoperatively is rare and is cause for alarm. Several of the following conditions may be associated with visual loss after anesthesia and surgery and should be included in the differential diagnosis: hemorrhagic retinopathy, retinal ischemia, and acute glaucoma.

Hemorrhagic Retinopathy

Retinal hemorrhages that occur in otherwise healthy persons secondary to hemodynamic changes associated with turbulent emergence from anesthesia or protracted vomiting are termed *Valsalva retinopathy*.[138] Fortunately, these venous hemorrhages are usually self-limiting and resolve completely in a few days to a few months.

Because no visual changes occur unless the macula is involved, the vast majority of cases are asymptomatic. However, if bleeding into the optic nerve occurs, resulting in optic atrophy, or if the hemorrhage is massive, permanent visual impairment may ensue.[139] In some instances of massive hemorrhage, vitrectomy may offer some improvement.

Retinal Ischemia

Retinal bleeding may also originate from the arterial circulation. This bleeding may be associated with extraocular trauma. Fundoscopic examination shows cotton-wool exudates,[140] and this condition is known as Purtscher's retinopathy. Purtscher's retinopathy should be ruled out when a trauma patient complains of postanesthetic visual loss. This condition is associated with a poor prognosis, and the majority of patients afflicted sustain permanent visual impairment.

Retinal ischemia or infarction may also result from direct ocular trauma secondary to pressure exerted by an ill-fitting anesthetic mask, especially in a hypotensive setting, as well as from embolism during cardiac surgery[141] or from the intraocular injection of a large volume of sulfur hexafluoride in the presence of high concentrations of nitrous oxide.

The importance of carefully positioning patients and scrupulously monitoring external pressure on the eye cannot be overemphasized, especially when the patient is in the prone or jack-knife positions. When the head is dependently positioned, venous pressure may be elevated. If external pressure is applied to the globe from improper head support, perfusion pressure to the eye is likely to be reduced. An episode of systemic hypotension in this setting could further decrease perfusion pressure and thereby decrease intraocular blood flow, resulting in possible retinal ischemia.

Acute Glaucoma

Although *topical* application of such mydriatic-inducing drugs as atropine and scopolamine is contraindicated in patients with glaucoma, the systemic use of anticholinergics in usual premedicating doses is safe for glaucomatous eyes.[123] The use of atropine-neostigmine combination for reversal of neuromuscular blockade is also safe in patients with glaucoma.[124] Topical ophthalmic medications that are being administered to control glaucoma should be continued through the perioperative period.

Acute angle-closure glaucoma, caused by pupillary block, is a serious, multifactorial disease. Risk factors include genetic predispostion,[142] shallow anterior chamber depth,[143] increased lens thickness,[143] small corneal diameter,[143] female sex,[143] and advanced age.[142] A recent study[144] explored possible precipitating events in at-risk persons and found no evidence that the type of anesthetic agent, the duration of surgery, the volume of parenteral fluids, or the intraoperative blood pressure were related to the development of acute angle-closure glaucoma.

Despite its seriousness, acute angle-closure glaucoma may be difficult to recognize. However, physicians should be knowledgeable about this potential complication, as diagnostic delay may detrimentally affect visual outcome. Fazio et al[144] recommend that the preoperative evaluation include a thorough ocular history as well as a penlight examination to detect a shallow anterior chamber. Those patients considered at risk should then undergo a preoperative ophthalmic evaluation as well as perioperative miotic therapy. Postoperatively, these patients should be scrupulously watched for red eye or for complaints of pain and blurred vision.

REFERENCES

1. Bruce RA: Ocular anatomy. In Bruce RA, McGoldrick KE, Oppenheimer P: Anesthesia for Ophthalmology, p 3. Birmingham, Alabama, Aesculapius, 1982
2. Wolff E: Anatomy of the Eye and Orbit, 7th ed, p 1. Philadelphia, WB Saunders, 1976
3. Aboul-Eish E: Physiology of the eye pertinent to anesthesia. In Smith RB (ed): Anesthesia in Ophthalmoloy, p 1. Boston, Little, Brown & Co, 1973
4. Adler FH: Physiology of the Eye: Clinical Application, 5th ed, p 249. St. Louis, CV Mosby, 1970
5. Stoelting RK: Circulatory changes during direct laryngoscopy and tracheal intubation: Influence of duration of laryngoscopy with or without prior lidocaine. Anesthesiology 47:381, 1977
6. Hill DW: Physics Applied to Anaesthesia. Norwalk, Connecticut, Appleton-Century-Crofts, 1968
7. Duncalf D, Foldes FF: Effect of anesthetic drugs and muscle relaxants on intraocular pressure. In Smith RB (ed): Anesthesia in Ophthalmology, p 21. Boston, Little, Brown & Co, 1973
8. Garde JF, Aston R, Endler GC et al: Racial mydriatic response to belladonna preparations. Anesth Analg 57:572, 1978
9. Lee P: Congenital glaucoma. In Femann SS, Reinecke RD (eds): Handbook of Pediatric Ophthalmology. New York, Grune & Stratton, 1978
10. Al-Abrak MH, Samuel JR: Effects of general anesthesia on intraocular pressure in man: Comparison of tubocurarine and pancuronium in nitrous oxide and oxygen. Br J Ophthalmol 58:806, 1974
11. Joshi C, Bruce DL: Thiopental and succinylcholine: Action on intraocular pressure. Anesth Analg 54:471, 1975
12. Everett WG, Vey EK, Veenis CY: Factors in reducing ocular tension prior to intraocular surgery. Trans Am Acad Ophthalmol 64:286, 1959
13. Presbitero JV, Ruiz RS, Rigor BM et al: Intraocular pressure during enflurane and neuroleptic anesthesia in adult patients undergoing ophthalmic surgery. Anesth Analg 59:50, 1980
14. Leopold IH, Comroe JH: Effect of intramuscular administration of morphine, atropine, scopolamine, and neostigmine on the human eye. Arch Ophthalmol 40:285, 1948
15. Famewo CE, Odugbesan CO, Osuntokun OO: Effect of etomidate on intraocular pressure. Can Anaesth Soc J 24:712, 1977
16. Thompson MF, Brock-Utne JG, Bean P et al: Anaesthesia and intraocular pressure: A comparison of total intravenous anaesthesia using etomidate with conventional inhalational anaesthesia. Anaesthesia 37:758, 1982
17. Yoshikawa K, Murai Y: Effect of ketamine on intraocular pressure in children. Anesth Analg 50:199, 1971
18. Corssen G, Hoy JE: A new parenteral anesthetic—CI581: Its effect on intraocular pressure. J Pediatr Ophthalmol 4:20, 1967
19. Peuler M, Glass DD, Arens JF: Ketamine and intraocular pressure. Anesthesiology 43:575, 1975
20. Ausinsch B, Rayburn RL, Munson ES et al: Ketamine and intraocular pressure in children. Anesth Analg 55:773, 1976
21. Ausinsch B, Graves SA, Munson ES et al: Intraocular pressure in children during isoflurane and halothane anesthesia. Anesthesiology 42:167, 1975
22. Duncalf D, Weitzner SW: Ventilation and hypercapnia on intraocular pressure in children. Anesth Analg 43:232, 1963
23. Drucker AP, Sadove MS, Unna KR: Ocular manifestations of intravenous tetraethylammonium chloride in man. Am J Ophthalmol 33:1564, 1950
24. Galin MA, Aizawa F, McLean JM: Intravenous urea in the treatment of acute angle glaucoma. Am J Ophthalmol 50:379, 1960
25. Agarwal LP, Mathur SP: Curare in ocular surgery. Br J Ophthalmol 36:603, 1952
26. Litwiller RW, Difazio CA, Rushia EL: Pancuronium and intraocular pressure. Anesthesiology 42:750, 1975
27. Lincoff HA, Ellis CH, DeVoe AG et al: Effect of succinylcholine on intraocular pressure. Am J Ophthalmol 40:501, 1955
28. Pandey K, Badolas RP, Kumar S: Time course of intraocular hypertension produced by suxamethonium. Br J Anaesth 44:191, 1972
29. Bjork A, Hallidin M, Wahlin A: Enophthalmus elicited by succinylcholine. Acta Anaesthesiol Scand 1:41, 1957
30. Bach-y-rita P, Lennerstrand G, Alvarado J et al: Extraocular muscle fibers: Ultrastructural identification of iontophoretically labeled fibers contracting in response to succinylcholine. Invest Ophthalmol Vis Sci 16:561, 1977

31. Carballo AS: Succinylcholine and acetazolamide in anesthesia for ocular surgery. Can Anaesth Soc J 12:486, 1965
32. Miller RD, Way WL, Hickey RF: Inhibition of succinylcholine-induced increased intraocular pressure by nondepolarizing muscle relaxants. Anesthesiology 29:123, 1968
33. Meyers EF, Krupin T, Johnson M et al: Failure of nondepolarizing neuromuscular blockers to inhibit succinylcholine-induced increased intraocular pressure: A controlled study. Anesthesiology 48:149, 1978
34. Verma RS: "Self-taming" of succinylcholine-induced fasciculations and intraocular pressure. Anesthesiology 50:245, 1979
35. Meyers EF, Singer P, Otto A: A controlled study of the effect of succinylcholine self-taming on IOP. Anesthesiology 53:72, 1980
36. Stoelting RK: Blood pressure and heart rate changes during short duration laryngoscopy for tracheal intubation: Influences of viscous or intravenous lidocaine. Anesth Analg 57:197, 1978
37. Smith RB, Babinski M, Leano N: Effect of lidocaine on succinylcholine-induced rise in IOP. Can Anaesth Soc J 26:482, 1979
38. Grover, VK, Lata K, Sharma S et al: Efficacy of lignocaine in the suppression of the intraocular pressure response to suxamethonium and tracheal intubation. Anaesthesia 44:22, 1989
39. Jampolsky A: Strabismus: Surgical overcorrections. Highlights Ophthalmol 8:78, 1965
40. France NK, France TD, Woodburn JD et al: Succinylcholine alteration of the forced duction test. Ophthalmoloy 87:1282, 1980
41. Berler DK: Oculocardiac reflex. Am J Ophthalmol 12:56, 954, 1963
42. Kirsch RE, Samet P, Kugel V et al: Electrocardiographic changes during ocular surgery and their prevention by retrobulbar injection. Arch Ophthalmol 58:348, 1957
43. Bosomworth PP, Ziegler CH: The oculocardiac reflex in eye muscle surgery. Anesthesiology 19:7, 1958
44. Alexander JP: Reflex disturbances of cardiac rhythm during ophthalmic surgery. Br J Ophthalmol 59:518, 1975
45. Smith RB, Douglas H, Petruscak J: The oculocardiac reflex and sino-atrial arrest. Can Anaesth Soc J 19:138, 1972
46. Taylor C, Wilson FM, Roesch R et al: Prevention of the oculocardiac reflex in children: Comparison of retrobulbar block and intravenous atropine. Anesthesiology 24:646, 1963
47. Mirakur RK, Clarke RSJ, Dundee JW et al: Anticholinergic drugs in anaesthesia—a survey of their present position. Anaesthesia 33:133, 1978
48. Gaviotaki A, Smith RM: Use of atropine in pediatric anesthesia. Int Anesthesiol Clin 1:97, 1962
49. Joseph MC, Vale RJ: Premedication with atropine by mouth. Lancet 2:1060, 1960
50. Katz RL, Bigger JT: Cardiac arrhythmias during anesthesia and operation. Anesthesiology 33:193, 1970
51. Massumi RA, Mason DT, Amsterdam EA et al: Ventricular fibrillation and tachycardia after intravenous atropine for treatment of bradycardias. N Engl J Med 287:336, 1972
52. Horgan J: Atropine and ventricular tachyarrhythmias. JAMA 223:693, 1973
53. McGoldrick KE: Transient left bundle branch block during local anesthesia. Anesthesiol Rev 8(6):36, 1981
54. Moonie GT, Rees DI, Elton D: Oculocardiac reflex during strabismus surgery. Can Anaesth Soc J 11:621, 1964
55. Steward DJ: Anticholinergic premedication for infants and children. Can Anaesth Soc J 30:325, 1983
56. Nachman RL, Esterly NB: Increased skin permeability in preterm infants. J Pediatr 79:628, 1971
57. Rongey KA, Weisman H: Hypotension following acetylcholine. Anesthesiology 36:412, 1972
58. Humphreys JA, Holmes JH: Systemic effects produced by echothiophate iodide in treatment of glaucoma. Arch Ophthalmol 69:737, 1963
59. DeRoeth A, Detbarn W, Rosenberg P et al: Effect of phospholine iodide on blood cholinesterase levels of normal and glaucoma subjects. Am J Ophthalmol 59:586, 1965
60. Ellis EP, Esterdahl M: Echothiophate iodide therapy in children; effect upon blood cholinesterase levels. Arch Ophthalmol 77:598, 1967
61. Ritchie JM, Greene NM: Local anesthetics. In Gilman AG, Goodman LS, Rall TW et al (eds): The Pharmacological Basis of Therapeutics, 7th ed, p 302. New York, Macmillan, 1985
62. Chung B, Naraghi M, Adriani J: Sympathetic effects of cocaine and their influence on halothane and enflurane anesthesia. Anesthesiol Rev 5:16, 1978
63. Koehntop DE, Liao J, Van Bergen FH: Effects of pharmacologic alterations of adrenergic mechanisms by cocaine, tropolone, aminophylline, and ketamine on epinephrine-induced arrhythmias during halothane-N_2O anesthesia. Anesthesiology 46:83, 1977
64. Barash PG, Kopriva CJ, Langou R et al: Is cocaine a sympathetic stimulant during general anesthesia? JAMA 243:1437, 1980
65. Meyers EF: Cocaine toxicity during dacryocystorhinostomy. Arch Ophthalmol 98:842, 1980
66. Gay GR, Loper KA: Control of cocaine-induced hypertension with labetalol (letter). Anesth Analg 67:92, 1988
67. Rappolt RT, Gay GR, Inaba DS: Propranolol: A specific antagonist to cocaine. Clin Toxicol 10:265, 1977
68. Ramoska E, Sacchetti AD: Propranolol-induced hypertension in treatment of cocaine intoxication. Ann Emerg Med 14:1112, 1985
69. Binkhorst RD, Weinstein GW, Baretz RM et al: Psychotic reaction induced by cyclopentolate: Results of pilot study and a double-blind study. Am J Ophthalmol 55:1243, 1963
70. Kennerdell JS, Wucher FP: Cyclopentolate associated with two cases of grand mal seizure. Arch Ophthalmol 87:634, 1972
71. Lansche RK: Systemic effects of topical epinephrine and phenylephrine. Am J Ophthalmol 49:95, 1966
72. Smith RB, Douglas H, Petruscak J et al: Safety of intraocular adrenaline with halothane anaesthesia. Br J Anaesth 44:1314, 1972
73. Brown MM, Brown GC, Spaeth GL: Lack of side effects from topically administered 10% phenylephrine eye drops: A controlled study. Arch Ophthalmol 98:487, 1980
74. Jones FL, Eckberg NL: Exacerbation of asthma by timolol. N Engl J Med 301:170, 1979
75. Kim JW, Smith PH: Timolol-induced bradycardia. Anesth Analg 59:301, 1980
76. Shavitz SA: Timolol and myasthenia gravis. JAMA 242:1612, 1979
77. Olson RJ, Bromberg BB, Zimmerman TJ: Apneic spells associated with timolol therapy in a neonate. Am J Ophthalmol 88:120, 1979
78. Bailey PL: Timolol and postoperative apnea in neonates and young infants. Anesthesiology 61:622, 1984
79. Fineberg E, Machemer R, Sullivan P et al: Sulfur hexafluoride in owl monkey vitreous cavity. Am J Ophthalmol 79:67, 1975
80. Stinson TW, Donlon JV: Interaction of SF6 and air with nitrous oxide. Anesthesiology 51:S16, 1979
81. Wolf GL, Capriano C, Hartung J: Effects of nitrous oxide on gas bubble volume in the anterior chamber. Arch Ophthalmol 103:418, 1985
82. Chang S, Lincoff HA, Coleman DJ et al: Perfluorocarbon gases in vitreous surgery. Ophthalmology 92:651, 1985
83. Lippa EA, Aasved H, Airaksinen PJ et al: Multiple-dose, dose-response relationship for the topical carbonic anhydrase inhibitor MK-927. Arch Ophthalmol 109:46, 1991
84. McGoldrick KE: Anesthetic implications of congenital and metabolic diseases. In Bruce RA, McGoldrick KE, Oppenheimer P (eds): Anesthesia for Ophthalmology, p 139. Birmingham, Alabama, Aesculapius, 1982
85. Unsold R, Stanley JA, DeGroot J: The CT-topography of retrobulbar anesthesia. Graefes Arch Clin Exp Ophthalmol 217:125, 1981
86. Van Lint: Paralysis palperbrale temporaire provoquee dans l'operation de la cataracte. Ann Occul 151:420, 1914
87. Lynch S, Wolf GL, Berlin I: General anesthesia for cataract surgery: A comparative review of 2217 consecutive cases. Anesth Analg 53:909, 1974
88. Backer CL, Tinker JH, Robertson DM: Myocardial reinfarction following local anesthesia. Anesthesiology 51:S61, 1979

89. Chang J-L, Gonzalez-Abola E, Larson CE: Brain stem anesthesia following retrobulbar block. Anesthesiology 61:789, 1984

90. Nicoll JMV, Acharya PA, Ahlen K et al: Central nervous system complications after 6000 retrobulbar blocks. Anesth Analg 66:1298, 1987

91. Zahl K, Jordan A, McGroarty J et al: The use of pH-adjusted bupivacaine/hyaluronidase for peribulbar anesthesia. Anesthesiology 72:230, 1990

92. Hamilton RC, Gimbel HV, Strunin L: Regional anesthesia for 12,000 cataract extractions and intraocular lens implantation procedures. Can J Anaesth 35:615, 1988

93. Donlon JV, Moss J: Plasma catecholamine levels during local anesthesia for cataract operations. Anesthesiology 51:471, 1979

94. Abramowitz MD, Epstein BS, Friendly DS et al: Effect of droperidol in reducing vomiting in pediatric strabismic outpatient surgery. Anesthesiology 55:A329, 1981

95. Abramowitz MD, Oh TH, Epstein BS: Antiemetic effect of droperidol following outpatient strabismus surgery in children. Anesthesiology 59:579, 1983

96. Dobb G, Jordan MJ, Williams JG: Cimetidine in prevention of pulmonary acid aspiration syndrome. Br J Anaesth 51:967, 1979

97. Williams JG: H$_2$ receptor antagonists and anaesthesia. Can Anaesth Soc J 30:264, 1983

98. Brown EM, Krishnaprasad D, Smiler BG: Pancuronium for rapid induction technique for tracheal intubation. Can Anaesth Soc J 26:489, 1979

99. Goudsouzian NG, Liu LMP, Coté CJ: Comparison of equipotent doses of nondepolarizing muscle relaxants in children. Anesth Analg 60:862, 1981

100. Savarese JJ: New neuromuscular blocking drugs are here. Anesthesiology 55:1, 1981

101. Basta SJ, Ali HH, Savarese JJ et al: Clinical pharmacology of atracurium besylate (BW33A): A new nondepolarizing muscle relaxant. Anesth Analg 61:723, 1982

102. Casson WR, Jones RM: Vecuronium induced neuromuscular blockade. Anaesthesia 41:354, 1986

103. Ginsberg B, Glass PS, Quill T et al: Onset and duration of neuromuscular blockade following high-dose vecuronium administration. Anesthesiology 71:201, 1989

104. Konchiergeri HN, Lee YE, Venugopal K: Effect of pancuronium on intraocular pressure changes induced by succinylcholine. Can Anaesth Soc J 26:479, 1979

105. Smith RB, Leano N: Intraocular pressure following pancuronium. Can Anaesth Soc J 20:742, 1973

106. Libonati MM, Leahy JJ, Ellison N: The use of succinylcholine in open eye surgery. Anesthesiology 62:637, 1985

107. McGoldrick KE: Pediatric anesthesia for ophthalmic surgery. In Bruce RA, McGoldrick KE, Oppenheimer P (eds): Anesthesia for Ophthalmology, p 75. Birmingham, Alabama, Aesculapius, 1982

108. Foldes FF: Rapid tracheal intubation with nondepolarizing neuromuscular blocking drugs: The priming principle. Br J Anaesth 56:663, 1984

109. Schwarz S, Ilias W, Lackner F et al: Rapid tracheal intubation with vecuronium: The priming principle. Anesthesiology 62:388, 1985

110. Musich J, Walts LF: Pulmonary aspiration after a priming dose of vecuronium. Anesthesiology 64:517, 1986

111. Baumgarten RK, Reynolds WJ: Priming principle and the open eye–full stomach. Anesthesiology 63:561, 1985

112. Reinecke RD: Current concepts in ophthalmology: Strabismus. N Engl J Med 300:1139, 1979

113. Isenberg SJ: New techniques in the treatment of strabismus. Surg Rounds 12, 1980

114. Beasley H: Hyperthermia associated with ophthalmic surgery. Am J Ophthalmol 77:76, 1974

115. Dodd MJ, Phattiyakul P, Silpasuvan S: Suspected malignant hyperthermia in a strabismus patient. Arch Ophthalmol 99:1247, 1981

116. Sessler DI; Malignant hyperthermia. J Pediatr 109:9, 1986

117. Barash PG, Katz JD, Firestone S et al: Cardiovascular performance in children during induction: An echocardiographic comparison of enflurane and halothane. Anesthesiology 51 (3S):315, 1979

118. Barash PG, Glanz S, Katz D et al: Ventricular function in children during halothane anesthesia: An echocardiographic evaluation. Anesthesiology 49:79, 1978

119. Lerman MD, Eustis S, Smith DR: Effect of droperidol pretreatment on postanesthetic vomiting in children undergoing strabismus surgery. Anesthesiology 65:322, 1986

120. Warner LO, Rogers GL, Marino JD et al: Intravenous lidocaine reduces the incidence of post-strabismus vomiting in children. Anesthesiology 68:618, 1988

121. Christensen S, Farrow-Gillespie A, Lerman J: Incidence of emesis and postanesthetic recovery after strabismus surgery in children: A comparison of droperidol and lidocaine. Anesthesiology 70:251, 1989

122. Woelfel SK: Intravenous lidocaine does not prevent postoperative vomiting in pediatric strabismus patients. Anesthesiology 73(3A): A7, 1990

123. Schwartz H, de Roeth A, Papper EM: Pre-anesthetic use of atropine in patients with glaucoma. JAMA 165:144, 1957

124. Rawstron RE, Hutchinson BR: Pupillary and circulatory changes at the termination of relaxant anesthesia. Br J Anaesth 35:795, 1963

125. Richardson RB, McBride CM, Berkely RG et al: An unusual ocular complication after anesthesia. Anesthesiology 43:357, 1975

126. Givner I, Jaffe N: Occlusion of the central retinal artery following anesthesia. Arch Ophthalmol 43:197, 1950

127. Fine J, Weissman J, Finestone SC: Side effects after ketamine anesthesia: Transient blindness. Anesth Analg 53:72, 1974

128. Boldner PM, Norton MI: Retinal hemorrhage following anesthesia. Anesthesiology 61:595, 1984

129. Batra YK, Bali M: Corneal abrasions during general anesthesia. Anesth Analg 56:363, 1977

130. Cucchiara R, Black S: Corneal abrasion during anesthesia and surgery. Anesthesiology 69:978, 1988

131. Watson W, Moran R: Corneal abrasion during induction. Anesthesiology 66:440, 1987

132. Siffring PA, Poulton TJ: Prevention of ophthalmic complications during general anesthesia. Anesthesiology 66:569, 1987

133. Boggild-Madsen N, Bundgard-Nielson P, Hammer U, Jakobsen B: Comparison of eye protection with methylcellulose and paraffin ointments during general anesthesia. Can Anaesth Soc J 28:575, 1981

134. Tabor E, Bostwick DC, Evans CC: Corneal damage due to eye contact with chlorhexidine gluconate (letter). JAMA 261:557, 1989

135. Kalhan SB, Cascorbi HF: Anesthetic management of laser microlaryngeal surgery. Anesth Rev 8:23, 1981

136. Conway C: Neurological and ophthalmic complications of anaesthesia. In Churchill-Davidson HC (ed): A Practice of Anaesthesia, 4th ed, p 1021. Philadelphia, WB Saunders, 1978

137. Dhamee MS, Ghandi SK, Callen KM et al: Morbidity after outpatient anesthesia: A comparison of different endotracheal anesthetic techniques for laparoscopy. Anesthesiology 57:A375, 1982

138. DeVoe AG, Norton EWD, Kearns TP et al: Valsalva hemorrhagic retinopathy: Discussion. Trans Am Ophthalmol Soc 70:307, 1972

139. Madsen PH: Traumatic retinal angiopathy. Ophthalmologica 165:453, 1972

140. McLeod D: Reappraisal of the retinal cotton-wool spot. J R Soc Med 74:682, 1981

141. Gutman FA, Zegarra H: Ocular complications in cardiac surgery. Surg Clin North Am 51:1095, 1971

142. Drance SM: Angle-closure glaucoma among Canadian Eskimos. Can J Ophthalmol 8:252, 1973

143. Alsbirk PH: Angle-closure glaucoma surveys in Greenland Eskimos. Can J Ophthalmol 8:260, 1973

144. Fazio DT, Bateman JB, Christensen RE: Acute angle-closure glaucoma associated with surgical anesthesia. Arch Ophthalmol 103:360, 1985

39

Robert Feinstein
William D. Owens

Anesthesia for Ear, Nose, and Throat Surgery

Like many other areas of medicine, anesthesia has evolved into subspecialties. Otorhinolaryngology (ENT) anesthesia might be regarded as the parent of all anesthesia, because it was for an ENT procedure that the first public demonstration of anesthesia took place in the ether dome in 1846. Thus, while anesthesia has adapted to the changing needs of surgery and the surgical subspecialties, many of the surgical advances we take for granted today were made possible by comparable adaptations in anesthetic techniques.

Anesthesia for ENT surgery poses many unique problems for the anesthesiologist, some of which are examined in this chapter. The functional anatomy of the head and neck is reviewed in relation to anesthesia for ENT procedures. The discussion considers the implications of a shared airway by the anesthesia and surgical teams. As in other areas of surgery, laser technology is being applied at an ever increasing rate to various ENT problems. This chapter also examines the special problems created for the anesthesiologist by this technology. Finally, mastery of some of the techniques routinely used in anesthesia for ENT surgery carries over to other areas of anesthetic practice, and this interrelationship is highlighted at various points in the discussion.

ANATOMY OF THE HEAD AND NECK

A discussion of the salient features of head and neck anatomy will be presented to better enable us to conceptually deal with the procedures and problems presented to us by patients' pathology and surgical approaches.[1-4]

The visceral tube consists of the pharynx and larynx. These structures are continuous with the trachea and esophagus. The pharynx is a muscular tube that extends from the base of the skull to the esophagus. It serves as a passageway for both air and food. The pharynx is always open for passage of air except during swallowing. Because this passageway serves the transport of both air and liquids and solids, a complex control system enables the pharynx to serve as a conduit for the intake of food at one time and for air at another. The pharynx also serves as a modulating chamber for vocalization generated by the larynx. Figure 39-1 shows the anatomic relationships of many of the structures of the pharynx and larynx.

The pharynx is a midline structure. Just lateral to the pharynx, on both sides of the neck, lie the carotid sheath and its contents (internal jugular vein, common carotid artery, vagus nerve, and internal carotid artery). The nasopharynx communicates with the pharynx by the choanae, which are approximately 2.5 cm by 1.25 cm oblong openings.[1] The accessory sinuses all drain into the nasopharynx, as does the eustachian tube. Because of this anatomy, patients whose trachea is nasally intubated are prone to sinus infections, especially of the maxillary sinuses, and middle ear infections.

The oropharynx lies posterior to the mouth. The most prominent structure is the base of the tongue, which lies in the posterior part of the mouth. At the same level as the base of the tongue and forming an arch at this level are the palatine tonsils and other lymphoid structures, which form Waldeyer's ring. The palatine tonsils project into the pharynx for a variable distance, depending on their size. This tonsilar bed lies in close relation to the facial artery and the internal carotid artery. The tonsils are richly supplied with blood by branches of the external carotid artery, the maxillary artery, and the facial artery, as well as others. Posterior and caudad to this lymphoid ring lies the larynx.

The larynx is a hollow organ that provides a direct connection between the pharynx and the trachea. The larynx is made up of three larger unpaired cartilages, the thyroid, cricoid, and epiglottic cartilages, and three paired cartilages, the arytenoid, corniculate, and cuneiform cartilages. The thyroid cartilage forms an open shield, with the shield facing anteriorly. The epiglottic cartilage is a leaf-shaped structure that extends superiorly and posteriorly from the thyroid cartilage. Beneath the thyroid cartilage lies the cricoid cartilage, which is broader posteriorly than anteriorly. The cricoid is the only complete cartilaginous ring found in the respiratory system. Because of this property the cricoid cartilage can be used to compress the esophagus, which lies posterior to it, when there is an increased risk of aspiration of oral or gastric contents during the induction and intubation phase of anesthesia. This is known as Sellick's maneuver.[5]

The arytenoid cartilages attach at the posterior portion of the cricoid cartilage. A membrane connects the arytenoids with the epiglottic cartilage, forming the beginning of the tube that becomes the trachea. The true vocal cords are found at this level in the larynx. The membrane that joins

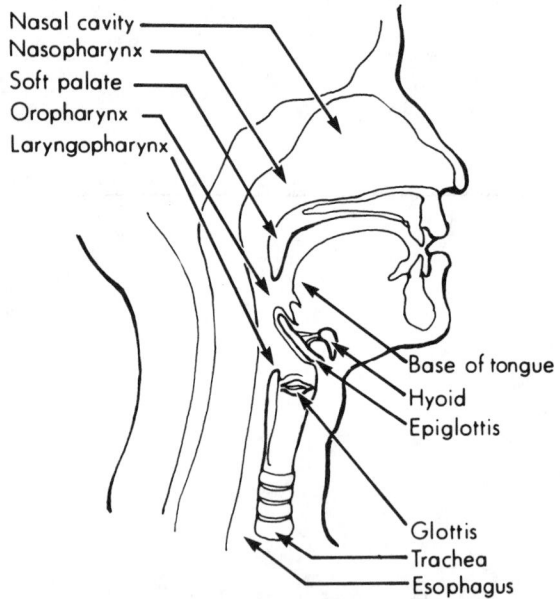

- Nasal cavity
- Nasopharynx
- Soft palate
- Oropharynx
- Laryngopharynx
- Base of tongue
- Hyoid
- Epiglottis
- Glottis
- Trachea
- Esophagus

Figure 39-1. Schematic representation of significant anatomic features of human head and neck anatomy. Note especially the space between the hyoid bone and the mandible.

the thyroid and cricoid cartilages anteriorly is a common site for the anesthesiologist to obtain emergency access to the airway. The trachea is located inferior to the true vocal cords. Superior to the thyroid cartilage is the hyoid bone, which, like the thyroid cartilage, is wishbone-shaped, with the open portion facing posteriorly. The membrane connecting the thyroid cartilage and the hyoid bone is the thyrohyoid membrane; it is pierced by the superior laryngeal nerve. The junction of the thyroid cartilage and the posterior portion of the hyoid bone serves as a landmark for a superior laryngeal nerve blockade.

The nerve supply to the larynx can be divided into sensory innervation to the mucous membrane, which is responsible for inducing the cough reflex when something other than air enters the larynx, and the motor nerve supply to the intrinsic muscles. The sensory nerve supply to the mucous membrane from the epiglottis to and including the vocal cords is from the superior laryngeal branch of the vagus nerve. The external branch of the superior laryngeal nerve, which comes off just before the point at which the nerve pierces the thyrohyoid membrane, provides motor innervation to the cricothyroid muscle and to a portion of the transverse arytenoid muscle. The mucous membrane beneath the vocal cords to the trachea is innervated by the recurrent laryngeal nerve, which also provides motor innervation to all the intrinsic muscles of the larynx except the cricothyroid muscle. The cricothyroid muscle is the only tensor of the vocal cords, and it is also the only intrinsic muscle to lie outside the cartilaginous framework of the larynx. This pattern of innervation explains why the vocal cords in humans tend to close if both recurrent laryngeal nerves are accidentally cut during surgery. Because the only remaining muscles are the cricothyroid muscles, whose action is to tense the vocal cords, and the transverse arytenoid muscle, which will bring the vocal cords closer together, severing both recurrent laryngeal nerves would be expected to result in tensing and approximation of the vocal cords. In actuality, however, the vocal cords are flaccid and approximated, likely because the cricothyroid muscles cannot tense the

cords without eliciting resistance from other intrinsic muscles. This can result in a closed glottis and inability of the patient to breathe; a tracheostomy should be done immediately. However, if only one of the recurrent laryngeal nerves is cut, the corresponding cord is flaccid and midline but the other cord functions normally. The patient is usually hoarse, and aspiration can be a significant problem, because the nonfunctional flaccid cord sags below the level of the innervated cord, resulting in an incompetent glottis.

In the adult, the vocal cords constitute the narrowest portion of the larynx, whereas in children less than 5 years old, the cricoid cartilage is the narrowest portion of the larynx. Because of this anatomy, uncuffed tubes may be preferentially used in children, because the cuff is more likely to cause subglottic edema and damage than in older patients.[6]

Control of the structures of the pharynx and larynx requires a complex control system to sort out the appropriate contents for the esophagus and trachea. For food to pass into the esophagus, three openings must be closed: the opening to the nasal pharynx, the opening to the mouth, and the opening to the larynx. The opening to the nose is closed by elevating the soft palate and approximating the walls of the pharynx to meet the raised soft palate. The oral cavity is closed by elevating the tongue against the hard palate. The larynx is closed during swallowing by raising the larynx so that it meets the epiglottis. The larynx actually forces the epiglottis into the base of the tongue. In addition, breath-holding occurs, which results in closing of the vocal cords.[1] Thus, the epiglottis does not serve as a leaflet valve that falls over the laryngeal opening; rather, the larynx is elevated onto it. Recall that this passageway, pharynx–larynx, is open except during swallowing.

Other salient anatomic features that anesthesiologists make use of in everyday practice should be noted. As shown in Figure 39-1, the tongue lies superior to the hyoid bone. The space between the hyoid and the mandible is commonly used to evaluate the adequacy of a patient's airway.[7-11] It is into this space that the tongue is displaced during laryngoscopy. Thus, tracheal intubation of patients with a short mandible or large tongue, for example those with Pierre Robin syndrome or acromegaly, will be difficult because there is inadequate room to displace the tongue during laryngoscopy.

Notice from Figure 39-1 that if a tube is inserted through the nasopharynx into the oropharynx, it will lie directly above the pharynx and the larynx. If the tube is an endotracheal tube, it will be in an excellent position for a blind nasotracheal intubation; or, if it is a fiberoptic laryngoscope, it will provide a view of the supraglottic structures—the epiglottis, vocal cords, and the esophagus.

The external anatomy of the head and neck also is relevant to the practice of ENT anesthesia. The facial nerve runs in a groove that is in close proximity to the middle ear; it then exits the skull through the stylomastoid foramen. Just before leaving the skull, it sends forth the chorda tympani, which conveys taste from the anterior two thirds of the tongue. After giving off the posterior auricular nerve, the facial nerve passes over the external carotid artery; it then enters the posterior median portion of the parotid gland. The nerve then quickly divides into branches that supply the muscles of facial expression. The trigeminal nerve conveys sensory information from the face and also provides motor innervation to the muscles of mastication. The glossopharyngeal nerve carries somatic sensory information from the base of the tongue and the pharynx. The recurrent laryngeal branches of the vagus nerve run along the posterolateral portion of the thyroid gland and are intimately associated with the gland and its blood supply. Because many of these nerves are intimately involved with the structures of the head and neck, the ENT surgeon is always concerned with their identification and preservation. For this reason the use of muscle relaxants, other than transiently, is usually restricted in ENT anesthesia.

ANESTHETIC CONSIDERATIONS IN COMMON OTORHINOLARYNGOLOGIC PROCEDURES

The following discussion highlights the unique features of anesthesia with regard to ENT procedures. Emphasis is placed on the concept of the shared airway and on the rapidly changing field of laser laryngoscopy.

Laryngoscopy and Microlaryngoscopy

As in other areas of medicine, endoscopy is used as a diagnostic tool for direct visualization of internal structures under consideration and as a means of obtaining biopsy specimens for diagnosis or for performing excisional biopsies for therapy. Many patients who present for endoscopic procedures are hoarse or stridorous or have pharyngeal or laryngeal pathology that is already compromising their airway. Adequate lung ventilation, vital in any patient, is especially critical in these patients. Pulse oximetry assesses oxygenation, but oxygenation can take place in the absence of ventilation, and adequate oxygenation does not equate with adequate ventilation.[12-14] For these reasons, it would be prudent to avoid sedation from preoperative medication in such patients with existing pathology or obstruction.

A dry immobile field with minimal intrusion by implements will facilitate the surgeon's task. Oral secretions can be effectively minimized with the use of an antisialagogue as a premedicant. There are many ways to immobilize the surgical site. The mouth, pharynx, larynx, and trachea can be anesthetized with a local anesthetic technique so that any of the endoscopic procedures can be carried out on a cooperative, awake patient. The local anesthesia is usually supplemented with some sedation. With proper patient selection and surgical skill, many of the minor airway procedures, for example vocal cord stripping, excision of vocal cord nodules, biopsies of the vocal cords and of other pharyngeal and laryngeal structures, and Teflon injections, can be safely performed under local anesthesia.[15] Local anesthesia can be effected by superior laryngeal nerve blockade, glossopharyngeal nerve blockade, or transtracheal injection.[16-18] The gag reflex can be obliterated and sufficient local anesthesia achieved by spraying the appropriate structures with a local anesthetic solution. Lidocaine is the most frequently used anesthetic. The toxic dose is approximately $5 \text{ mg} \cdot \text{kg}^{-1}$, and absorption from mucosal surfaces is almost as rapid after administration by this route as after intravenous (iv) administration.[19] Any contraindication to obliteration of the pharyngeal reflexes would most likely preclude the use of a purely local technique, and patients who have had their airways locally anesthetized should be fasted for at least 2 hours afterward or until their reflexes have returned. Often, because of the patient's preference, the surgeon's preference, or the chance of bleeding or gastric reflux (with resultant aspiration), a general anesthetic technique with a relatively protected and controlled airway is preferred.

Once a general anesthetic technique is elected, there are several methods available for providing adequate surgical exposure and ventilation of the patient's lungs.[20-24] The necessary immobilization of the patient may be achieved with or without the use of muscle relaxants. Immobility is important not only for the surgeon's benefit: coughing can result in a positive feedback condition, invoking both airway and cardiovascular reflexes, that can be life-threatening.[25-28] For laryngoscopy, esophagoscopy, and rigid bronchoscopy, muscle relaxation provides good operating conditions for the surgeon. Induction of anesthesia can be done in any acceptable, safe manner; iv or inhalation techniques are common. Muscle relaxation can be achieved with intermittent doses or continuous infusions of succinylcholine or the intermediate-acting muscle relaxants atracurium or vecuronium.[29] Neuromuscular blockade must be monitored, and the patient's airway reflexes must be intact before the patient leaves the operating room. Maintenance of anesthesia can be accomplished by any acceptable method, with the anesthesiologist keeping in mind that endoscopic procedures are usually of short duration—5 to 60 minutes—and that the patient's airway reflexes must be intact at the end of the procedure.

Tracheal intubation with a small-diameter endotracheal tube will permit ventilation of the patient's lungs and still afford the surgeon adequate visualization. A 5- or 6-mm internal diameter cuffed endotracheal tube will provide an adequate airway; however, higher than normal pressures will be needed to ventilate the lungs, owing to the increased resistance associated with the small-bore endotracheal tube.[30] Most surgeons prefer to have the endotracheal tube taped to the left side of the patient's mouth because the surgeon's laryngoscope will be inserted on the right side of the mouth. Because both anesthesiologist and surgeon will be working in the patient's airway, it is vital that they communicate with each other. The surgeon's and anesthesiologist's objectives and concerns are different, and it is only through adequate communication that both can arrive at a safe means of achieving both sets of objectives. The use of an endotracheal tube will provide adequate ventilation of the lungs and good direct visualization of the glottis in most cases. However, for posterior commissure laryngeal lesions, the endotracheal tube will obstruct the surgeon's field of view, and something other than the standard endotracheal tube must be used. A special endotracheal tube, developed by Coplans,[31] has an asymmetric cuff that allows the tube to clear the posterior commissure.

If the endotracheal tube interferes with the surgeon's field of view, an alternative method of ventilating the lungs must be used. Alternative techniques may leave an unprotected airway and do not always ensure adequate ventilation. The Carden tube is a short flexible cuffed tube that is inserted in its entirety below the level of the vocal cords.[32-34] Gas mixtures can be instilled into the tube through a small-diameter tube comparable in size to the tubing used for the endotracheal tube cuff. Because the vocal cords are above the tube, it is possible to ventilate the patient's lungs through such a device using jet ventilation. Others have used a catheter and tube, with the catheter connected to a gas supply either to ventilate the patient's lungs with both an inspiratory and expiratory phase or just to insufflate gas mixtures through the catheter. Adequacy of ventilation is assessed by observing the rise and fall of the chest, and adequacy of oxygenation is assessed by pulse oximetry or an equivalent. Both jet ventilation and constant gas insufflation use the Venturi effect to entrain room air, thereby diluting the delivered gas mixture. For that reason, most investigators use 100% oxygen or at most a 50:50 mixture of nitrous oxide and oxygen. Many of the operating laryngoscopes used by ENT surgeons have side arms that can be used to provide jet ventilation to the patient. By using high-pressure gas jets, as high as 60 psi, it is possible to adequately ventilate the lungs.[35-38] Inspiration is achieved through the instillation of a jet of gas, whereas exhalation is accomplished by passive relaxation of the chest wall and lungs. Studies have also examined the use of high-frequency jet ventilation for laryngoscopy (Fig. 39-2).[39-42] At present, it is not clear whether high-frequency ventilation techniques have any advantage over traditional ventilation techniques. The aforementioned techniques are contraindicated in patients in whom an unprotected airway would be contraindicated. All of the jet ventilation techniques carry some significant risks. The jets must be directed at or through the glottic opening or the patient will not receive the desired gas, and the gas jets will go into structures other than the trachea. Cases of pneumothorax, subcutaneous air, mediastinal air, gastric distention, and respiratory acidosis (hypoventilation) have been reported.[43]

The only significant difference between laryngoscopy and microlaryngoscopy is the use of a microscope in microlaryngoscopy. Often the laryngoscope is suspended from a Mayo stand or a specially designed bracket attached to the operating room table. This frees both of the surgeon's hands. Whenever the patient's head is flexed or extended, the rela-

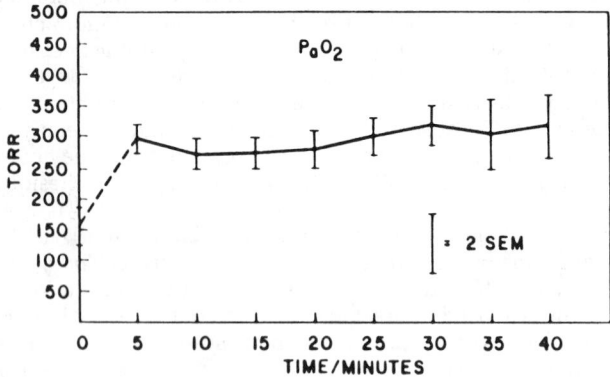

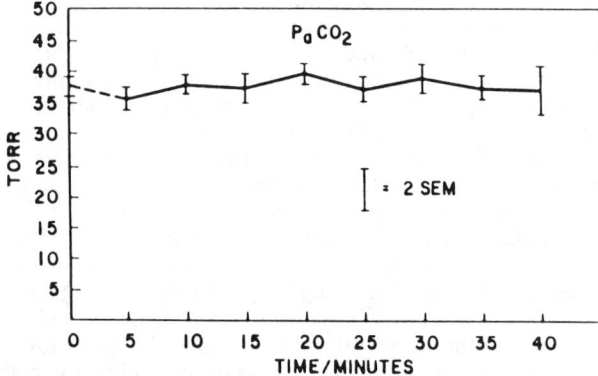

Figure 39-2. Mean Pao$_2$ and Paco$_2$ values in 18 adult patients whose lungs were ventilated at a rate of 100 breaths·min^{-1} by a 3.5-mm internal diameter tube placed in the trachea. Because of air entrainment, the inspired concentration of oxygen was less than 100%. Exhalation occurred around the tracheal tube. (Reprinted with permission from Babinski M, Smith RB, Klain M: High-frequency jet ventilation for laryngoscopy. Anesthesiology 52:178, 1980.)

tive position of the endotracheal tube with respect to the carina changes. Therefore, after each manipulation of the patient's head and airway by the surgeon, the location of the endotracheal tube should be verified.

Laser Laryngoscopy

The laser (light amplification by stimulated emission of radiation) is now more than 25 years old. The first demonstration of this phenomenon was by T. H. Maiman in 1960, with a ruby laser. Since that time lasers have been developed that span the electromagnetic spectrum from the infrared to the threshold of the x-ray region.

Lasers have been used in medicine almost since their inception.[44] They provide the surgeon with several advantages and are capable of providing very high-intensity outputs that can be collimated, resulting in spot sizes on the order of the wavelength of light, having extremely high-energy densities. Laser output is monochromatic; thus, substances that absorb at specific wavelengths can be selectively targeted while others are spared. Absorption of the laser's energy is essential; it is the key to all laser tissue interactions. It is possible to precisely control the duration of the laser pulses, and this is critical for the spatial confinement of the heat produced in tissue by the laser, thus sparing surrounding healthy tissue while destroying target tissue.

Laser output is either continuous wave or pulsed. The mode used is a function of energy output and the desired result. Most lasers used in ENT surgery are carbon dioxide (CO$_2$) lasers, which are operated in the continuous wave mode with intermittent bursts delivered to the tissues. Lasers have the advantages of extreme precision, almost no blood loss (the heat generated produces immediate coagulation), and minimal edema.

CO$_2$ lasers emit energy with a wavelength of 10.6 μm, which lies in the infrared portion of the electromagnetic spectrum and is invisible to the unaided eye. Most medical CO$_2$ lasers have a helium-neon (He-Ne) laser built into them. The radiation of the He-Ne laser is visible, is poorly absorbed by tissues, is of low energy, and serves as a means of directing the CO$_2$ laser beam, which is invisible. The wavelength of energy at which CO$_2$ emits energy is strongly absorbed by water. Because tissue is approximately 80% water, the tissue is rapidly heated, boiled, and finally vaporized, resulting in a clean cut through the tissue with little tissue penetration. Argon lasers, on the other hand, emit radiation at approximately 500 nm, which is in the visible portion of the spectrum and is highly absorbed by hemoglobin and poorly absorbed by water. Thus, the argon laser can be used to coagulate blood vessels in the back of the eye and passes harmlessly and without attenuation through the humors of the eye.

Recent years have seen a greatly expanded application of lasers in surgery, including ENT surgery. With the advent of new lasers the versatility of their use in surgery has increased. Neodymium-doped yttrium-aluminum-garnet (Nd:YAG) lasers produce energy at 1.06 μm, which has a greater ability to penetrate tissue than does the CO$_2$ laser. Nd:YAG lasers produce a rim of denatured tissue 1–2 mm thick. These lasers have been used in the treatment of intraluminal bronchial tumors, bladder tumors, and gastric lesions. Another laser that has come into recent use in ENT surgery is the potassium-titanyl-phosphate(KTP) laser. It emits energy at 532 nm and has little tissue penetration, but is highly absorbed by hemoglobin. Surgeons are now using the KTP laser to perform tonsillectomies, claiming a reduction in blood loss and postoperative pain. There are no studies to substantiate these claims to date. As technology produces new modalities of laser energy, they will find their way into the operating room environment.

The primary anesthetic consideration in laser surgery is the safety of the patient and the operating room personnel. The energy of the laser must be absorbed with sufficient energy density over a long enough period of time to cause tissue damage. If the energy is dispersed before it encounters viable tissue, or if the dispersed energy is delivered in short bursts, the chance of unintentional injury can be greatly reduced. The operating room should have a sign posted cautioning all who enter that a laser is in use and that protective eyewear should be worn. All operating room personnel should wear goggles that absorb the radiation frequency of the laser being used, because the eye is the organ most susceptible to damage. The goggles should wrap around the face to protect the eyes from the side as well as from the front. The patient's eyes should be closed and protected with moistened eye pads. If possible, viable tissue within the surgical field should be protected with moistened sponges, so that if the laser beam is inadvertently diverted, it will be absorbed harmlessly. Another means of protecting adjacent tissues and operating room personnel is to dissipate and disperse the laser's energy in case it inadvertently strays from the desired target and strikes a reflective surface (e.g., the laryngoscope or suction device). Thus, instruments used for laser surgery should be nonreflective, should have rough surfaces that will not act as a mirror for the laser beam, and should be nonflammable. These features will help disperse the beam and hence reduce the energy density.

The most serious danger during any laser surgery is fire; this is especially true in laser surgery in the airway.[45] There are numerous case reports of endotracheal tube fires in laser surgery in the airway, and there is a report of an endotracheal tube fire ignited by electrocautery.[46,47] When a fire is started in an endotracheal tube, the tube becomes a blowtorch because of the high oxygen content and the high gas flows that occur during ventilation of the lungs. Such a fire can cause great devastation to the tracheobronchial tree. The prevalence of endotracheal tube fire has been reported to be as high as 1.5% in patients undergoing laryngeal surgery with the CO_2 laser.[48] Endotracheal tube fires can be avoided by using other means to ventilate the patient's lungs. Jet and Venturi ventilation have been successfully used for such procedures[49,50]; however, in addition to all the limitations previously described for these techniques, in laser laryngoscopy procedures these techniques can result in instillation of debris, tumor, genetic material, and smoke inhalation. In an attempt to provide some degree of protection, several special-purpose endotracheal tubes have been designed, all with a similar objective: to provide a nonflammable airway capable of either harmlessly absorbing the laser's energy or reflecting and dispersing the energy. Polyvinylchloride (PVC) is the compound most frequently used to make endotracheal tubes. It is highly flammable, and PVC endotracheal tubes ideally should not be used during laser airway surgery.[51,52] Tubes used especially for laser airway surgery are made of other compounds, ranging from rubber and silicone to metal. All endotracheal tubes not made from metal will ignite in an enriched oxygen atmosphere.[53-55] Nitrous oxide will also support combustion and thus does not provide any protection.[54] Studies suggest that the substitution of helium, an inert gas, for nitrous oxide will significantly increase the amount of energy required to produce combustion in PVC endotracheal tubes.[56,57] Thus, many anesthesiologists substitute helium for nitrous oxide during laser laryngoscopy. Helium, however, interferes with the proper operation of anesthetic mass spectrometers and produces false readings.[58]

A popular method of producing a "laser-proof" tube is to wrap a red rubber tube with a foil tape. Selection of the correct tape is critical, because some tapes have the aluminized surface on the back, so that the laser beam must pass through a clear layer of plastic compound before encountering the reflective surface.[59,60] The plastic compound is likely to be flammable. The correct metal tape is a metal ribbon with no surface coating but with an adhesive coating on the back. Proper wrapping technique is essential or gaps will exist, exposing the underlying endotracheal tube to the laser; in addition, rough edges can damage laryngeal structures.

A tube manufactured by Xomed and made from silicone and metallic particles provides some advantages over the red rubber tube, especially for its cuff. Silicone tube fires have occurred,[61-63] even though the silicone tube requires substantially more energy for ignition than either PVC or rubber tubes. Xomed has now discontinued manufacture of this silicone tube and has introduced a new tube that appears to be a foil tape–wrapped tube covered with Teflon tape. Preliminary testing by this author indicates that it is suitable for use with the CO_2 laser. A Japanese firm is importing a modified silicone tube, the Fuji tube, which from preliminary tests appears to have no advantage over the older Xomed tube. An all-metal endotracheal tube, the Norton tube, is available but has no cuff. A sponge-coated, silver foil adhesive sheet, Laser Guard, is available to wrap tubes and provides excellent protection for most laser modalities. However, the sponge coating must be kept moist or it may ignite when exposed to laser energy.

The weak link in all cuffed tubes is the vulnerability of the cuff itself to puncture by the laser beam.[55] Some tubes are provided with two cuffs, each with a separate pilot, so that if one cuff is made incompetent by laser penetration, the back-up cuff beneath it can maintain a sealed airway. Figure 39-3 shows a wrapped red rubber tube and the Mallinckrodt Laser Flex tube with the redundant cuffs. This tube has been shown to be superior for use with CO_2 and KTP lasers. Other special-purpose tubes have been developed for laser laryngoscopy, but no study has shown any clear advantage to any one of them.[48,64]

The cuffs of all tubes should be filled with either saline or water.[52] The liquid allows the cuff to absorb more energy before becoming hot or disrupted, and, if the cuff should be penetrated by the laser beam, the escaping liquid will help extinguish any fire. Some anesthesiologists have suggested adding methylene blue to the solution used to inflate the endotracheal tube cuff. Thus, if the cuff were pierced by the laser beam, a visible stream of liquid would be seen by the surgeon. Observing these precautions will greatly reduce the risk of endotracheal tube fires. These precautions should also be observed in patients who have tracheostomies. The trachea should be fitted with a protected tube before the laser procedure is begun. If the cuff of any of the single-cuffed endotracheal tubes is penetrated, the endotracheal tube should be changed.

No one type of endotracheal tube protection is suitable for all forms of laser energy. For example, Nd:YAG lasers will easily cut through metal tubes. Thus, if a new laser modality is to be used, the vulnerability of the endotracheal tube must be determined beforehand.

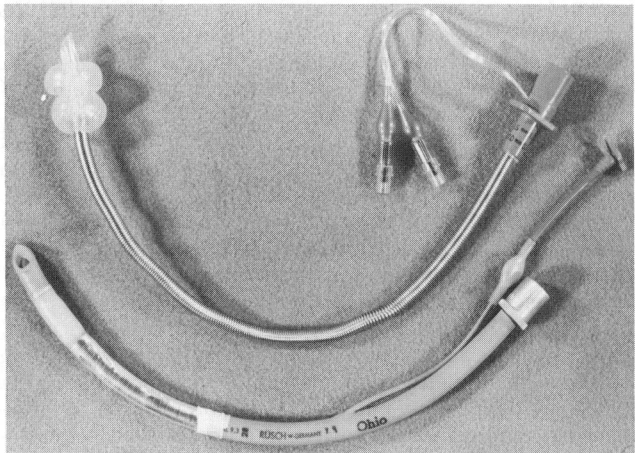

Figure 39-3. Two types of endotracheal tubes used for laser laryngoscopy. The lowermost endotracheal tube is the familiar red rubber tube, which has been wrapped with aluminum foil tape. The end of the aluminum tape is wrapped with a small piece of silk tape to prevent unraveling. The uppermost endotracheal tube is the Laser Flex, manufactured by Mallinckrodt. It is made of flexible stainless steel spiral tubing with a soft silicone tip. Note that this endotracheal tube has two independent cuffs. If the upper cuff is punctured by the laser beam, the lower cuff will still protect the airway.

If an endotracheal tube fire does occur, it is vital that a well-thought-out plan be followed. The most important steps to take are: to stop ventilation, turn off the oxygen, remove the flaming endotracheal tube from the airway, and extinguish the fire with sterile water or saline. The water is for the endotracheal tube, not the patient, unless flaming remnants of the tube remain in the patient's airway, in which case some of the liquid should be used to extinguish these fragments before they are removed. Thus, an ample quantity of sterile water or saline must be kept in the sterile field at all times during laser laryngoscopy. Bronchoscopy with both rigid and flexible scopes should then be performed to determine the extent of the damage and to remove any debris from the airway. Ventilation of the lungs should be performed during these maneuvers, either with jet ventilation through a ventilating bronchoscope or through an endotracheal tube of as small a diameter as possible to minimize further airway trauma. Depending on the extent of damage, tracheostomy and assisted ventilation of the lungs may be required. The administration of steroids[64] and humidification of inhaled gases should be accomplished. A chest radiograph should be taken and the patient admitted to an intensive care unit for observation, even if no significant damage is suspected.

The anesthetic considerations for laser laryngoscopy are the same as those for other forms of laryngoscopy.[65-67] The only possible exception is that immobility is mandatory to prevent inadvertent laser damage to healthy tissue if the patient moves. This can be accomplished with the use of muscle relaxants or deep anesthesia. At the end of the procedure, after the trachea has been extubated, the endotracheal tube should be inspected to ensure that no piece of foil tape or other protective covering is missing and presumed left in the airway. If something is missing, laryngoscopy and bronchoscopy are mandatory to retrieve it. Recently, some surgeons have started to resect tracheal and bronchial lesions with a laser, using either a rigid scope or a fiberoptic scope. The considerations for the anesthesiologist are the same as those for any other bronchoscopy. If a fiberoptic bronchoscope is used, a PVC endotracheal tube may be used, because the laser will be active at a point below the end of the endotracheal tube.

Adenotonsillectomy

Many consider adenotonsillectomy to be an innocuous procedure. The patients, for the most part, are children and young adults who are usually classified as American Society of Anesthesiologists physical status I or II. Many institutions are now performing this procedure on an outpatient basis. Indications for the surgical procedure are varied and controversial.[68] In the mid-1970s, it was estimated that approximately 750,000 young Americans underwent this surgical procedure or a variant thereof. Estimates of mortality associated with various forms of tonsillectomies are difficult to determine, but, in 1963, it was reported as being one in 10,000 patients in England.[69,70] Most of the deaths were associated with hypovolemia or a compromised airway and occurred as a result of postoperative bleeding. The reported mortality in patients requiring reoperation for postoperative bleeding was approximately one in 500 patients.[71,72] In another study, there were no deaths in 9409 children undergoing adenoidectomy, tonsillectomy, or adenotonsillectomy over a 4-year period.[73]

The population undergoing tonsillectomies is also changing. The operation is now part of a surgical procedure used to alleviate *obstructive sleep apnea*, of which patients with Pickwickian syndrome are a subset. During rapid eye movement sleep, the pharyngeal muscles relax, along with the other muscles of the body. In patients with obstructive sleep apnea, this relaxation produces airway obstruction, which can lead to episodes of hypoxia, eventually resulting in pulmonary hypertension, cor pulmonale, and congestive heart failure, if left untreated.[74] Adults with this syndrome are usually obese and have short, thick necks, relatively large tongues, and redundant soft tissue in the oropharynx. Children with obstructive sleep apnea usually have obstruction secondary to a congenital anomaly such as Pierre-Robin or Treacher Collins syndromes. It is also possible to produce obstructive sleep apnea in children with cleft palates who have undergone pharyngeal flap corrections, which have a tendency to decrease the anteroposterior oropharyngeal distance and can result in airway obstruction when the pharyngeal muscles relax during sleep. Sudden death during sleep in patients with sleep apnea is probably caused by fatal arrhythmias that occur secondary to asphyxia.[74] In adults, this condition can be surgically remedied by performing a uvulopharyngopalatoplasty, which consists of a tonsillectomy, uvulectomy, and limited pharyngectomy with resection of the redundant soft tissue of the soft palate and oropharynx.[75,76] In children in whom the obstruction is secondary to one of the previously mentioned syndromes, correction of the skeletal abnormality will usually correct the obstruction. The tonsils and adenoids sometimes become so hypertrophic in children that they can significantly encroach on the airway, and removal may be indicated to alleviate the obstruction.[77] In extreme cases, or if the patient's medical condition warrants, a tracheostomy may be performed to relieve the obstruction. The tracheostomy can be plugged during the day for normal laryngeal function while the patient is awake.

In all patients being considered for adenotonsillectomy, the clinician must consider whether or not airway obstruction is a significant factor. If it is a factor, sedative-hypnotics should be avoided as preoperative medications. Because it is an intraoral procedure, an antisialagogue would be a good choice for premedication. In children, recurrent tonsillitis is an indication for tonsillectomy; however, the procedure should not be performed on an elective basis if signs and symptoms of upper respiratory infection or tonsillitis are present. This admonition is also true for adults. Adults with obstructive sleep apnea should be in stable cardiovascular condition before the operation. As with any other anesthetic procedure, the anesthesiologist should look for signs and symptoms of cor pulmonale and congestive heart failure preoperatively. These conditions should be optimally managed medically before surgery is initiated.

Induction of anesthesia in patients without a history of airway obstruction and in whom airway assessment indicates normal airway anatomy can take place either by iv or inhalation routes, as appropriate, depending on the age of the patient. In patients with a history of obstruction during sleep and in whom airway assessment indicates that oral intubation of the trachea should present no significant problem, preoxygenation and an iv induction of anesthesia with an ultra-short-acting barbiturate is appropriate. These patients are usually more sensitive to hypnotics, analgesics, and anesthetics, and these drugs should be titrated for effect in each patient. Often, insertion of an oral or nasal airway is all that is required to be able to ventilate the lungs. By providing topical anesthesia of the mouth and nasal passages, it is possible to insert an airway and use a reduced dose of barbiturate, thereby reducing the time needed for spontaneous breathing to return in case it is not possible to adequately ventilate the lungs. A lighter plane of anesthesia, however, will increase the likelihood of positive pressure–induced laryngospasm. The anesthesiologist should have instruments at hand for difficult tracheal intubations; these instruments include a stylet, an assortment of laryngoscope blades, and a fiberoptic laryngoscope. Equipment should also be available for performing a cricothyrotomy and ventilating through it if necessary. If the assessment of the patient's airway indicates that tracheal intubation will be difficult, an awake intubation should be performed in adults and a spontaneously breathing inhalation induction should be done in children. In all cases, blood oxygen saturation should be measured with a pulse oximeter during the entire procedure.

Once the airway has been secured, the surgeon inserts a mouth gag into the patient's mouth. A variety of mouth gags are available; all require that the endotracheal tube be located in the midline. The endotracheal tube is usually held in place by being pressed between the tongue blade of the mouth gag and the tongue. The most popular gag is a modification of the Crowe-Davis mouth gag. The tongue blade of this gag has a groove so that it will accept an endotracheal tube. The endotracheal tube can be moved while the surgeon is placing the mouth gag; however, it can also be compressed between the tongue blade and the tongue to the point of kinking, especially if the endotracheal tube is not entirely within the groove. Thus, it is essential to check breath sounds after gag placement, and to check the pressure needed to ventilate the patient. The tube can be taped in place, or a piece of tape can be placed on the tube to serve as a visual marker indicating whether or not the surgeon has inserted or withdrawn the tube during placement of the mouth gag. Maintenance of anesthesia can be accomplished with either additional drugs or solely with the use of inhalation drugs. The use of muscle relaxants is acceptable if indicated. All muscle relaxation should be completely reversed prior to extubation of the trachea. As in laryngoscopy and bronchoscopy, the goal is to have an awake patient at the end of the procedure whose protective airway reflexes are intact. Thus, the use of long-acting iv drugs is probably unwise in these patients. At the end of the surgical procedure, many surgeons will relax the tension on the mouth gag to determine whether or not the gag itself has been compressing vessels, which will bleed when the tension on the tissues is released. When this is done, be aware that if the endotracheal tube has not been taped in place, it is only loosely held in place by the mouth gag and can easily become dislodged.

It is difficult to determine exact blood loss during these procedures, because a significant amount of blood can enter the gastrointestinal tract and be undetected. A graduated suction should be used by the surgical team, and blood loss should be adequately replaced with crystalloid or, if sufficient volume is lost, by blood transfusion. The anesthesiologist should make a habit of requesting that the surgeon insert an orogastric tube at the end of the procedure and empty the stomach with suction. This will reduce the likelihood of nausea and emesis, because blood in the stomach is a potent stimulus for nausea. Before awakening the patient, the anesthesiologist should inspect the mouth for the presence of blood, blood clots, debris, and active bleeding and should take proper action. Carefully suction the nasopharynx through the nares, as a significant amount of blood can be lodged there and can slowly ooze into the oropharynx, resulting in laryngospasm[78-80] after extubation of the trachea.

When the patient is awake and breathing adequately with intact airway reflexes, the trachea may be extubated. Patients are often transported to the recovery room in the lateral head-down position, the "tonsil position," and kept in this position until they are fully awake. This will help to prevent aspiration of blood from either the nasopharynx or the tonsillar bed, and also prevents blood and secretions from dripping onto the vocal cords, resulting in laryngospasm. In patients with sleep apnea, the use of steroids to help reduce tissue edema is worth considering. Patients with obstructive sleep apnea should be admitted to the intensive care unit overnight, where their breathing, oxygen saturation, and electrocardiogram can be monitored, since relief of the obstruction does not always immediately relieve apnea but may unmask an underlying central apneic component. It may also take several weeks before central mechanisms have readjusted.

The most frequent complication associated with adenotonsillectomy is postoperative bleeding, with resultant hypovolemia and airway obstruction. There are two likely periods for postoperative bleeding. The first period is in the immediate 4–6 hours postoperatively. A study by Crysdale indicated that 76% of postoperative bleeding episodes occurred within the first 6 hours, and 87% occurred within 9 hours.[73] Only 0.06% of the patients bled postoperatively, and of these, only 3% required reoperation. Other studies have reported reoperation rates as high as 0.9% of all patients undergoing one of the variants of adenotonsillectomy. Most of the postoperative bleeding that occurs is of a slow oozing nature, and it is not until the patient vomits a large amount of blood, which he has been swallowing, that anyone realizes the problem. At this point the patient may be hypovolemic and should be adequately rehydrated so that at least no orthostatic blood pressure changes are present. Airway obstruction may be present, and the stomach should be presumed full of blood. If the surgeon believes that the bleeding cannot be controlled through application of electrocautery, silver nitrate, or topical vasoconstrictors, preparations should be made to return the patient to the operating room. The patient should have an adequate iv line in place, and preferably two lines. An awake intubation of the trachea is often preferable if at all possible. If not, a rapid sequence induction of anesthesia with adequate preoxygenation and use of the Sellick maneuver is indicated. In children, an inhalation induction can be accomplished by administering halothane in oxygen and adding cricoid pressure as soon as consciousness is lost. With the patient breathing spontaneously, a gentle laryngoscopy can be performed, and only when the glottis is visualized can succinylcholine be administered. If bleeding is active, the patient's head can be held in the lateral position during induction of anesthesia. Laryngoscopy and endotracheal intubation are surprisingly easy in this position but should be practiced in patients when they are not necessary so that the clinician can acquire some skill. It is probably wise to avoid thiopental as the induction drug since the patient's intravascular status may be tenuous at best. Ketamine, 1 to 2 mg·kg^{-1}, or etomidate, 0.2 to 0.4 mg·kg^{-1}, may be a better choice for an induction drug. The important point is to maintain intravascular volume status. Most patients undergoing tonsillectomy will tolerate transient anemia. The hematocrit will help determine whether or not a blood transfusion is advisable.

After the bleeding has been stopped, the stomach should be emptied with suction through an orogastric tube. The criteria for extubation of the trachea are the same as for the first extubation. Through this conservative approach, it is possible to greatly reduce the mortality associated with adenotonsillectomy.

The second common period for postoperative tonsillar bleeding is approximately 5–10 days postoperatively. Bleeding at this time is usually attributable to infection with the persistence of fever and sore throat in the postoperative period.

Cancer of the Head and Neck

Most cancers of the head and neck structures are associated with a history of chronic cigarette smoking and alcohol use. As a result, most patients presenting with tumors of the head and neck are in their fifth or sixth decade of life. In addition to having cancer, they also have acquired other sequelae of heavy smoking and drinking, such as some degree of chronic obstructive pulmonary disease (COPD) and coronary artery disease (CAD). Many of these patients are hypertensive. There should be high suspicion of alcohol withdrawal, and treatment with a long-acting hypnotic such as diazepam should be initiated if a history of heavy drinking is elicited. Obviously, this does not apply if any degree of sedation would be contraindicated owing to a compromised airway. If airway compromise prevents preoperative use of delirium tremens precautions, a long-acting hypnotic should be administered once the airway has been secured. Often, the patient's nutritional status will be poor secondary to dysphagia. If the tumor involves the vocal cords, either directly or indirectly, there may be evidence of aspiration pneumonia.

A thorough history and physical examination should be performed with special emphasis on the respiratory and cardiac systems. Neoplasms often cause inflammation and resultant edema. Thus, a careful search for signs and symptoms of airway compromise should be performed. Many patients with head and neck cancer who present for ENT surgery will already have undergone radiation therapy,

which produces fibrosis. A thin patient with normal-appearing external airway anatomy may be difficult to intubate, because the fibrosed tissue is unyielding. In most cases the surgeon has performed an indirect laryngoscopy and has formed an opinion of the likelihood of successful tracheal intubation. If the surgical procedure will require a tracheostomy, an awake tracheostomy under local anesthesia should be discussed with the surgeon. An awake tracheostomy should be done if the lesion is considered extremely friable or exophytic, thereby avoiding the dislodgement of cancerous tissue into the tracheobronchial tree and the possibility of starting significant bleeding in the airway. If the patient's trachea can be intubated, even though there is airway compromise or distortion, an awake intubation, either by direct laryngoscopy or by fiberoptic laryngoscopy, should be seriously considered. If there is any reservation about the ability to intubate the patient's trachea by direct oral laryngoscopy after induction of anesthesia, it is advisable to be aggressive about awake intubations. Once the airway has been traumatized after several unsuccessful attempts at intubation of the trachea in an anesthetized patient, it is much more difficult to then perform a fiberoptic laryngoscopy, with a bloody field added to the already distorted anatomy.

Pulmonary function tests, baseline arterial blood gases, chest radiographs, and computed tomographs of the neck should be obtained. In addition to a routine 12-lead electrocardiograph, other studies may be indicated to evaluate the cardiovascular status of these patients, because it is often difficult to differentiate between pulmonary and cardiac causes of symptoms in patients with head and neck cancer. If consultations are indicated, the anesthesiologist should discuss any concerns with the surgeon and the consultant prior to the consult, so that the consultant's response will directly address the anesthesiologist's concerns. The patient should be in optimal medical condition before surgery. Unless airway obstruction is imminent, none of the oncology procedures are emergencies.

Whether the procedure is a glossectomy, pharyngectomy, or laryngectomy, with or without an accompanying neck dissection, it will take anywhere from 3 to 8 hours to complete, and significant blood loss of 1000 ml or more is not uncommon. Blood loss during these procedures is difficult to estimate because much of it is hidden from view, pooling under the patient's head, saturating the surgical sheets, and eventually dripping onto the floor.

The choice of an induction drug should be based on the patient's medical condition; for example, a patient with severe coronary artery disease is not likely to benefit from an induction with ketamine. Monitoring during ENT procedures in patients with head and neck cancers entails the use of routine monitors as well as a Foley catheter to monitor urine output. Depending on the patient's pulmonary and cardiac status, and on whether or not a neck dissection will be part of the procedure, monitoring of blood pressure by an arterial catheter may be indicated. If for no other reason than the need for repeated arterial blood gas determinations in patients with significant COPD, an arterial line is appropriate. Also, depending on cardiac function, expected blood loss, and length of procedure, a central venous line or pulmonary artery catheter may be indicated.[6] If central venous access is required, preoperative placement is indicated. Internal jugular vein access is denied by most of the head and neck procedures because the access line would be in the operative field. Antecubital access can be achieved at the time of the procedure; however, it is frequently difficult to pass the line around the shoulder and into the central circulation. Subclavian access can be achieved at the time of the surgical procedure; however, after line placement, a chest radiograph may be useful to ensure that no pneumothorax exists prior to induction of anesthesia, positive pressure ventilation of the lungs, and the use of nitrous oxide. Subclavian access can be obtained the night before surgery, and a radiograph can be taken and read by a radiologist before the patient arrives in the operating room the next morning, thus avoiding unnecessary delay in the operating room.

Intraoperative management requires consideration of the patient's pre-existing medical problems. Several authors have discussed the anesthetic management of specific procedures[81-85]; however, there is no one anesthetic technique that has been shown to be superior to others for any of these procedures. Use of muscle relaxants may be limited by the need to evaluate the intactness of nerves during neck dissection or parotid surgery. If the procedure will involve a tracheostomy, it may be useful to avoid muscle relaxants for this portion of the procedure and try to maintain spontaneous respiration. Administration of 100% oxygen prior to the actual tracheotomy is advised, so that if the airway is lost, there will be some oxygen reserve before hypoxia results. During tracheostomy, it is possible to produce a tracheoesophageal fistula, a false passage, damage to the recurrent laryngeal nerve, subcutaneous emphysema, pneumothorax, bleeding, and blood aspiration.[86,87] If the procedure involves a neck dissection, manipulation of the carotid sinus can result in cardiac dysrhythmias and wide fluctuations in blood pressure. If this occurs, the anesthesiologist should request that the surgeon stop his manipulation and infiltrate the tissues surrounding the carotid sinus with a local anesthetic. Cardiac dysrhythmias associated with a prolonged QT interval and cardiac arrest have been described in patients undergoing radical neck dissection (Fig. 39-4).[88] Open neck veins can serve to entrain air into the venous system and result in significant venous air embolism. Venous air embolism can be reduced, if not eliminated, by keeping the patient in a slight head-down position. Tumor can involve the major vessels of the neck and may require sacrifice of one or both internal jugular veins. If this occurs, cerebral perfusion pressure may be decreased, and the increased intracerebral venous pressure can result in cerebral edema. Some authors have advocated induced hypotension for these procedures to help reduce the blood loss and provide a drier surgical field. The use of induced hypotension in these patients is controversial. Because most of these patients will have, at best, silent CAD, and because the chance of compromising cerebral blood flow is present, it is difficult to predict a priori what degree of hypotension would be tolerated.[89,90]

Occasionally, a tumor may involve the carotid artery, requiring sacrifice of the carotid artery on the side of the lesion. The radiologist can temporarily occlude the involved vessel with a balloon during angiography in an awake patient to determine whether or not the patient will tolerate loss of blood flow from the involved vessel. Regardless of the outcome of the temporary occlusion, the electroencephalogram should be monitored intraoperatively if there is any chance that the surgeon will sacrifice the carotid artery. It would also be prudent to maintain normal systemic blood pressure and normocarbia to preserve cerebral blood flow in these patients. These functions can be facilitated by the use of an arterial pressure monitor, arterial blood gases, and an end-tidal carbon dioxide monitor.

If a tracheostomy is part of the procedure, the cuffed tracheostomy tube will help protect the airway. The portion of trachea lying superior to the tracheostomy site should be

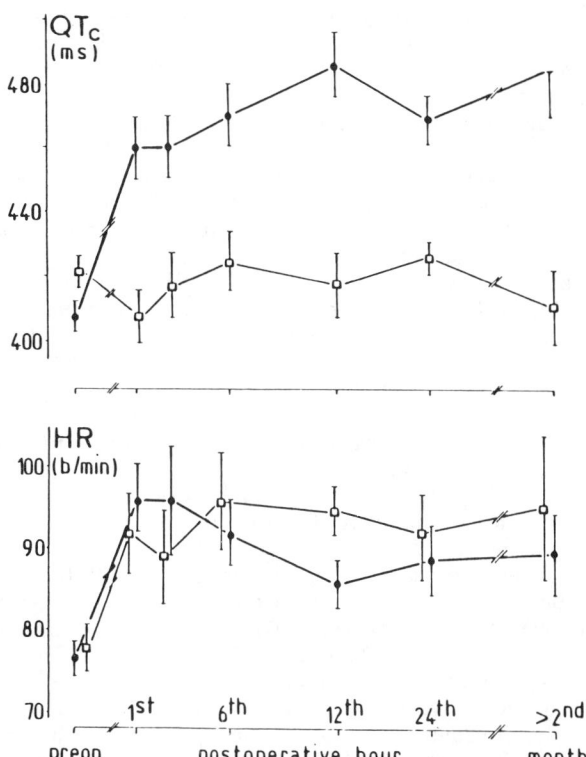

Figure 39-4. Corrected QT interval (QT$_c$) and heart rate (HR) as measured before and after right (*solid symbols*) or left (*clear symbols*) radical neck dissection. Right radical neck dissection increased QT$_c$ when compared with left radical neck dissection ($p < 0.001$). Mean ± SE. (Reprinted with permission from Otteni JC, Pottecher T, Bronner G *et al:* Prolongation of the Q-T interval and sudden cardiac arrest following right radical neck dissection. Anesthesiology 59:358, 1983.)

suctioned before the temporary tracheostomy tube is exchanged for a permanent tube, because a significant amount of blood can be sequestered there. If it is necessary to ventilate the patient's lungs in the postoperative period, a cuffed tracheal tube can be used. If no tracheostomy was done, the anesthesiologist and surgeon must decide whether or not the surgical procedure produced sufficient edema and distortion to compromise the patient's airway in the immediate postoperative period. If there is any doubt, the patient's trachea should remain intubated in the immediate postoperative period, and one should continue to evaluate the airway postoperatively. Administration of steroids early on may help to minimize tissue edema.

Surgical Procedures Involving the Ear

The majority of procedures done on the ear involve the middle ear, its contents, and the mastoid air cells. Usually these procedures are performed to correct hearing loss in patients who are young and otherwise healthy. Chronic infection can cause scarring of the tympanic membrane, fibrosis, and cholesteatoma involving the ossicular chain, all resulting in hearing loss. Involvement of the labyrinth will result in vertigo, nystagmus, nausea, and vomiting. The facial nerve is intimately associated with the structures of the ear, and its preservation is always a consideration. Disease processes in the middle ear often involve the facial nerve, and surgical procedures expressly for facial nerve decompression are done. There are three aspects of surgery of the ear that are controversial: (1) the use of nitrous oxide, (2) induced hypotension, and (3) the use of muscle relaxants.

The fact that nitrous oxide is approximately 34 times more soluble in blood than nitrogen can present a problem in closed spaces in the body. Because nitrous oxide will enter the closed space at a faster rate than nitrogen can be removed, the volume of any gas contained within a closed space can significantly expand.[91] The middle ear represents an air-filled noncompliant space within the body. Numerous studies have documented the increase in middle ear pressure that occurs during the use of nitrous oxide and the harmful effects associated with its use (Fig. 39-5).[92-99] Cases of actual rupture of the tympanic membrane have been reported and attributed to the use of nitrous oxide.[100] Tympanic membrane grafts have been dislodged through the use of nitrous oxide. The other consideration is that when the nitrous oxide is discontinued and a previously open space is closed, the withdrawal of nitrous oxide will produce a negative pressure.

In operative procedures on the middle ear, until the surgeon begins to close the middle ear, there is no closed space. It has been proposed that the use of nitrous oxide be discontinued approximately 30 minutes before the tympanic membrane graft is placed.[101] In practice, if the nitrous oxide is discontinued for approximately 15 minutes before the graft is placed, it usually does not present a problem for the surgeon. If the surgeon packs the middle ear with Gelfoam, this will usually prevent significant retraction of the graft postoperatively. Surgeons have their own individual biases with respect to the use of nitrous oxide during middle ear surgery. At the start of the case, the anesthesiologist should ask whether or not the surgeon is concerned about the use of nitrous oxide. If he or she is concerned, the nitrous oxide can be discontinued several minutes before placement of the graft. If for any reason the surgeon appears to be having difficulty with the graft, discontinue the nitrous oxide.

Many surgeons believe that a bloodless operative field is a requirement for the successful performance of microsurgical procedures on the ear. Much of the anesthesia literature supports this position.[6,89] Profound hypotension has been advocated, with systolic blood pressure reduced to 50 mm Hg for significant periods of time with spontaneous breathing and with no means of monitoring the adequacy of cerebral perfusion other than the regularity of the respiratory pattern.[102,103] Interestingly, Eltringham and colleagues[103] found no correlation between the degree of hypotension and the surgeon's assessment of the adequacy of the surgical conditions. Many surgeons infiltrate the tissues of the ear with epinephrine-containing solutions to help achieve hemostasis. Most patients needing these procedures are young and healthy, with no history or evidence of pulmonary or cardiovascular disease, and will tolerate hypotension well. Adequate measures must be taken to ensure the adequacy of vital organ perfusion during hypotension. An arterial catheter to measure blood pressure and obtain samples for arterial blood gas analysis, end-tidal carbon dioxide measurement, an electroencephalogram, and other monitors have been proposed as standards of care during induced hypotension.[79] Spontaneous ventilation has been advocated during the hypotensive anesthetic so as to reduce cerebral venous pressure.[77] It has also been suggested that the operating table be positioned so that the head is elevated 15 to 30 degrees in order to aid in venous drainage and reduce cerebral venous pressure.[79] Elevating the operative field above the level of the heart increases the risk of venous air embolism. Is profound hypotension in addition to the use of potent vasoconstrictors necessary or greatly beneficial in microsurgical procedures of the ear? There is no definitive answer at this time.

Identification and preservation of the facial nerve is always a consideration in surgical procedures on the ear. It is known that different muscle groups possess different sensitivities to muscle relaxants[104] and that it is possible to provide skeletal muscle relaxation without complete paralysis, thus enabling the surgeon to elicit a response from direct nerve stimulation, even though the patient has only a small percentage of neuromuscular function intact. Theoretically, there is no logical reason why neuromuscular blocking drugs cannot be used, even when nerve preservation is a significant consideration. Practically speaking, if for any reason there is facial nerve dysfunction postoperatively and if muscle relaxants were used other than as an aid to intubation of the trachea, it could create an awkward situation for the anesthesiologist and the surgeon.

As in all surgical procedures, patient safety is the anesthesiologist's prime concern. For microsurgery on the ear, the patient must be immobile. This can be accomplished by producing an adequate level of anesthesia without the use of muscle relaxants. Volatile inhalation anesthestics provide some degree of muscle relaxation, can easily produce an adequate level of anesthesia, do not require nitrous oxide for their effective use, and can be used to induce hypotension. Thus, volatile inhalation anesthesia is a logical choice as a primary anesthetic technique for microsurgery of the ear. In addition, the incidence of nausea is less with a pure inhalation technique than when opioids are used.[105] Nausea and dizziness are always postoperative problems in patients undergoing ear surgery. Avoidance of opioids as well as prophylactic administration of antiemetics such as droperidol or promethazine are useful in these patients.[106,107]

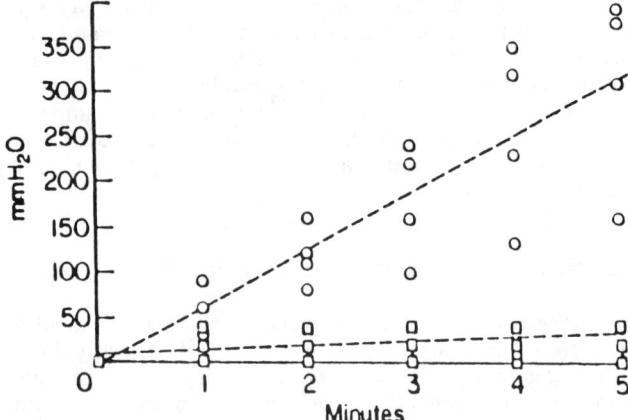

Figure 39-5. Rate of increase of middle ear pressure in children (5 to 12 years of age) during assisted ventilation of the lungs with halothane and nitrous oxide in oxygen (*circles*) compared with children breathing halothane in oxygen (*squares*). (Reprinted with permission from Casey WF, Drake-Lee AB: Nitrous oxide and middle ear pressure. Anaesthesia 37:896, 1982.)

CONCLUSIONS

For most anesthetic procedures the anesthesiologist is at the patient's head and is in control of the airway. This can produce a false sense of security. In anesthesia for ENT procedures, the anesthesiologist is almost never at the head and normally does not have easy access to the airway. Patients undergoing ENT surgery frequently have intraoral lesions that will make direct oral laryngoscopy and intubation of the trachea difficult if not impossible. The ENT anesthesiologist must learn to accurately assess the patient's airway and, as part of that assessment, to communicate with the surgeon, who has knowledge of the patient's pathology. Communication is the key to safe anesthesia in ENT surgery. It is vital for good patient care that the anesthesiologist know what the surgeon is doing at all times, and it is vital for the surgeon to know what technique the anesthesiologist is using.

REFERENCES

1. Crafts RC: A Textbook of Human Anatomy. New York, Ronald Press, 1966
2. Goss CM: Gray's Anatomy of the Human Body, 28th ed. Philadelphia, Lea & Febiger, 1966
3. Anderson JE: Grant's Atlas of Anatomy, 7th ed. Baltimore, Williams & Wilkins, 1978
4. Clemente CD: Anatomy. A Regional Atlas of the Human Body. Philadelphia, Lea & Febiger, 1978
5. Sellick BA: Cricoid pressure to control regurgitation of stomach contents during induction of anaesthesia. Lancet 2:404, 1961
6. Miller RD: Anesthesia, 2nd ed. New York, Churchill Livingstone, 1986
7. Bhagwandas G, McDonald JS: The difficult airway. Hosp Physician 22:65, 1986
8. Spoerel WE: Problems of the upper airway. Int Anesthesiol Clin 10:1, 1972
9. Salem MR, Mathrubhutham M, Bennett EJ: Difficult intubation. N Engl J Med 295:879, 1976
10. Ament R: A systematic approach to the difficult intubation. Anesthesiol Rev 5:12, 1978
11. White A, Kander PL: Anatomical factors in difficult laryngoscopy. Br J Anaesth 47:468, 1975
12. Rah KH, Salzberg AM, Boyan CP et al: Respiratory acidosis with small Storz-Hopkins bronchoscopes: Occurrence and management. Ann Thorac Surg 27:197, 1979
13. Eger EI, Severinghaus JW: The rate of rise of Pa_{CO_2} in the apneic anesthetized patient. Anesthesiology 22:419, 1968
14. Neil SG, Lam AM, Turnbull KW et al: Monitoring of oxygen. Can J Anaesth 34:56, 1987
15. Calcaterra TC, House J: Local anesthesia for suspension microlaryngoscopy. Ann Otol 85:71, 1976
16. Moore DC: Regional Block. A Handbook for Use in the Clinical Practice of Medicine and Surgery, 4th ed. Springfield, Illinois, Charles C Thomas, 1965
17. Eriksson E: Illustrated Handbook in Local Anesthesia, 2nd ed. Philadelphia, WB Saunders, 1980
18. Barton S, Williams JD: Glossopharyngeal nerve block. Arch Otolaryngol 93:186, 1971
19. Covino BG, Vassello HG: Local Anesthetics. Mechanisms of Action and Clinical Use. New York, Grune & Stratton, 1976
20. Rajagopalan R, Smith F, Ramachandran PR: Anaesthesia for microlaryngoscopy and definitive surgery. Can Anaesth Soc J 19:83, 1972
21. Raj PP, Forestner J, Watson TD et al: Technics for fiberoptic laryngoscopy in anesthesia. Anesth Analg 53:708, 1974
22. Glenski JA, MacKenzie RA, Maragos NE et al: Assessing tidal volume and detecting hyperinflation during Venturi jet ventilation for microlaryngeal surgery. Anesthesiology 63:554, 1985
23. Webster AC: Anesthesia for operations on the upper airway. Int Anesthesiol Clin 10:61, 1972
24. Spoerel WE, Narayanan PS, Singh NP: Transtracheal ventilation. Br J Anaesth 43:932, 1971
25. Strong MS, Vaughan CW, Mahler DL et al: Cardiac complications of microsurgery of the larynx: Etiology, incidence and prevention. Laryngoscope 84:908, 1974
26. Elguindi AS, Harrison GN, Abdulla AM et al: Cardiac rhythm disturbances during fiberoptic bronchoscopy: A prospective study. J Thorac Cardiovasc Surg 77:557, 1979
27. Katz AS, Michelson EL, Stawicki J et al: Cardiac arrhythmias: Frequency during fiberoptic bronchoscopy and correlation with hypoxemia. Arch Intern Med 141:603, 1981
28. Pereira W, Kovnat DM, Snider GL: A prospective cooperative study of complications following flexible fiberoptic bronchoscopy. Chest 73:813, 1978
29. Carnie J: Continuous suxamethonium infusion for microlaryngeal surgery. Br J Anaesth 54:11, 1982
30. Bolder PM, Healy TEJ, Bolder AR et al: The extra work of breathing through adult endotracheal tubes. Anesth Analg 65:853, 1986
31. Coplans MP: A cuffed nasotracheal tube for microlaryngeal surgery. Anaesthesia 31:430, 1976
32. Carden E, Schwesinger WB: The use of nitrous oxide during ventilation with the open bronchoscope. Anesthesiology 39:551, 1973
33. Carden E, Vest HR: Further advances in anesthetic techniques for microlaryngeal surgery. Anesth Analg 53:584, 1974
34. Carden E, Ferguson GB, Crutchfield WM: A new silicone elastomer tube for use during microsurgery on the larynx. Ann Otol Rhinol Laryngol 83:360, 1974
35. Pybus DA, O'Connor AF, Henville JD: Anaesthesia for laryngoscopy: A technique using the Nuffield anaesthetic ventilator. Br J Anaesth 50:501, 1978
36. Keen RI, Kotak PK, Ramsden RT: Anaesthesia for microsurgery of the larynx. Ann R Coll Surg Engl 64:111, 1982
37. Carden E, Galido J: Foot-pedal control of jet ventilation during bronchoscopy and microlaryngeal surgery. Anesth Analg 54:405, 1975
38. Frederickson JM, Haight JS, Soder CM: Ventilation during laryngoscopy in chronic obstructive lung disease. Laryngoscope 94:1606, 1984
39. Eng UB, Eriksson I, Sjostrand U: High-frequency positive-pressure ventilation (HFPPV): A review based upon its use during bronchoscopy and for laryngoscopy and microlaryngeal surgery under general anesthesia. Anesth Analg 59:594, 1980
40. Eriksson I, Sjostrand U: A clinical evaluation of high-frequency positive-pressure ventilation (HFPPV) in laryngoscopy under general anesthesia. Acta Anaesthesiol Scand 64:101, 1977
41. Rogers RC, Gibbons J, Cosgrave J et al: High-frequency jet ventilation for tracheal surgery. Anaesthesia 40:32, 1985
42. Babinski M, Smith RB, Klain M: High-frequency jet ventilation for laryngoscopy. Anesthesiology 52:178, 1980
43. Chang JL, Meeuwis H, Bleyaert A et al: Severe abdominal distention following jet ventilation during general anesthesia. Anesthesiology 49:216, 1978
44. Walsh JT, Parrish JA: Lasers: The healing tool of the future. IEEE Potentials 4:36, 1985
45. Sosis MB: Hazards of laser surgery. Semin Anesth 9:90, 1990
46. Simpson JI, Wolf GL: Endotracheal tube fire ignited by pharyngeal electrocautery. Anesthesiology 65:76, 1986
47. Sommer RM: Preventing endotracheal tube fire during pharyngeal surgery. Anesthesiology 66:439, 1987
48. Hermens JM, Bennett MJ, Hirshman CA: Anesthesia for laser surgery. Anesth Analg 62:218, 1983
49. Ruder CB, Rapheal NL, Abramson AL et al: Anesthesia for carbon dioxide laser microsurgery of the larynx. Otolaryngology 89:732, 1981
50. Gussack GS, Evans RF, Tacchi EJ: Intravenous anesthesia and jet ventilation for laser microlaryngeal surgery. Ann Otol Rhinol Laryngol 96:29, 1987
51. Sosis MB, Dillon FX: Saline-filled cuffs help prevent laser-induced polyvinylchloride endotracheal tube fires. Anesth Analg 72:187, 1991
52. Simpson JI, Wolf GL: Flammability of esophageal stethoscopes, nasogastric tubes, feeding tubes, and nasopharyngeal

airways in oxygen- and nitrous oxide-enriched atmospheres. Anesth Analg 67:1093, 1988

53. Hayes DM, Gaba DM, Goode RL: Incendiary characteristics of a new laser-resistant endotracheal tube. Otolaryngology 95:37, 1986

54. Wolf GL, Simpson JI: Flammability of endotracheal tubes in oxygen and nitrous oxide enriched atmosphere. Anesthesiology 67:236, 1987

55. LeJeune FE, Guice C, LeTard F et al: Heat sink protection against lasering endotracheal cuffs. Ann Otol Rhinol Laryngol 91:606, 1982

56. Pashayan AG, Gravenstein JS: Helium retards endotracheal tube fires from carbon dioxide lasers. Anesthesiology 62:274, 1985

57. Pashayan AG, Gravenstein JS, Cassisi NJ et al: The helium protocol for laryngotracheal operations with CO_2 laser: A retrospective review of 523 cases. Anesthesiology 68:801, 1988

58. Siegel M, Gravenstein N: Evaluation of helium interference with mass spectrometry. Anesth Analg 67:887, 1988

59. Sosis M, Heller S: An evaluation of five metallic tapes for protection of endotracheal tubes during CO_2 laser surgery. Anesthesiology 69:A252, 1988

60. Sosis M, Dillon F: What is the safest foil tape for endotracheal tube protection during Nd-YAG laser surgery? A comparative study. Anesthesiology 72:553, 1990

61. Sosis M: Airway fire during CO_2 laser surgery using a Xomed laser endotracheal tube. Anesthesiology 72:747, 1990

62. Brown B: Anesthesia and ENT Surgery. Philadelphia, FA Davis, 1987

63. Giffin B, Shapshay SM, Bellack GS et al: Flammability of endotracheal tubes during Nd-YAG laser application in the airway. Anesthesiology 65:54, 1986

64. Patil V, Stehling LC, Zauder HI: A modified endotracheal tube for laser microsurgery. Anesthesiology 51:571, 1979

65. Paes ML: General anaesthesia for carbon dioxide laser surgery within the airway. Br J Anaesth 59:1610, 1987

66. Perera ER, Mallon JS: General anaesthetic management for laser resection of central airway lesions in 85 procedures. Can J Anaesth 34:383, 1987

67. North C, Marsh B, Hirshman CA: Anesthetic management of a patient with reactive airway disease for carbon dioxide laser debulking of a laryngeal tumor. Anesth Analg 65:1225, 1986

68. Orkin FK, Cooperman LH: Complications in Anesthesiology. Philadelphia, JB Lippincott, 1983

69. Carden TS: Tonsillectomy: Trials and tribulations. JAMA 240:1961, 1978

70. Tate N: Deaths from tonsillectomy. Lancet 2:1090, 1963

71. Keenan RL, Boyan CP: Cardiac arrest due to anesthesia. JAMA 253:2373, 1985

72. Davies DD: Re-anaesthetizing cases of tonsillectomy and adenoidectomy because of persistent postoperative haemorrhage. Br J Anaesth 36:244, 1964

73. Crysdale WS: Complications of tonsillectomy and adenoidectomy in 9409 children observed overnight. Can Med Assoc J 135:1139, 1986

74. Hall JB: The cardiopulmonary failure of sleep-disordered breathing. JAMA 255:930, 1986

75. Bradley TD, Phillipson EA: Pathogenesis and pathophysiology of the obstructive sleep apnea syndrome. Med Clin North Am 69:1169, 1985

76. Chung F, Crago RR: Sleep apnea syndrome and anaesthesia. Can Anaesth Soc J 29:439, 1982

77. Tobin MJ, Cohn MA, Sackner MA: Breathing abnormalities during sleep. Arch Intern Med 143:1221, 1983

78. Weinberg S, Kravath R, Phillips L et al: Episodic complete airway obstruction in children with undiagnosed obstructive sleep apnea. Anesthesiology 60:356, 1984

79. Rex MAE: A review of the structural and functional basis of laryngospasm and a discussion of the nerve pathways involved in the reflex and its clinical significance in man and animals. Br J Anaesth 42:891, 1970

80. Suzuki M, Saski CT: Laryngeal spasm: A neurophysiologic redefinition. Ann Otol 86:150, 1977

81. Donlon JV: Anesthetic management of patients with compromised airways. Anesthesiol Rev 7:22, 1980

82. Davies RM, Scott JG: Anaesthesia for major oral and maxillofacial surgery. Br J Anaesth 40:202, 1968

83. Geffin B, Bland J, Grillo HC: Anesthetic management of tracheal resection and reconstruction. Anesth Analg 48:884, 1969

84. Ellis RH, Hinds CJ, Gadd LT: Management of anaesthesia during tracheal resection. Anaesthesia 31:1076, 1976

85. Kamvyssi-dea S, Kritikou P, Exharhos N et al: Anaesthetic management of reconstruction of the lower portion of the trachea. Br J Anaesth 47:82, 1975

86. Kirchner JA: Tracheotomy and its problems. Surg Clin North Am 60:1093, 1980

87. Greenway RE: Tracheostomy: Surgical problems and complications. Int Anesthesiol Clin 10:151, 1972

88. Otteni JC, Pottecher T, Bronner G et al: Prolongation of the Q-T interval and sudden cardiac arrest following right radical neck dissection. Anesthesiology 59:358, 1983

89. Morrison JD, Mirakur RK, Craig HJL: Anaesthesia for Eye, Ear, Nose and Throat Surgery, 2nd ed. Edinburgh, Churchill Livingstone, 1985

90. Enderby GEH: Hypotensive Anaesthesia. Edinburgh, Churchill Livingstone, 1985

91. Eger EI: Anesthetic Uptake and Action. Baltimore, Williams & Wilkins, 1974

92. Shaw JO, Stark EW, Gannaway SD: The influence of nitrous oxide anaesthetic on middle-ear fluid. J Laryngol Otol 92:131, 1978

93. Marshall FPF, Cable HR: The effect of nitrous oxide on middle-ear effusions. J Laryngol Otol 96:893,1982

94. Patterson ME, Bartlett PC: Hearing impairment caused by intratympanic pressure changes during general anesthesia. Laryngoscope 86:399, 1976

95. Davis I, Moore JRM, Lahiri SK: Nitrous oxide and the middle ear. Anaesthesia 34:147, 1979

96. Matz GJ, Rattenborg CG, Holaday DA: Effects of nitrous oxide on middle ear pressure. Anesthesiology 28:948, 1967

97. Thomsen KA, Terkildsen K, Arnfred I: Middle ear pressure variations during anesthesia. Arch Otolaryngol 82:609, 1965

98. Casey WF, Drake-Lee AB: Nitrous oxide and middle ear pressure. Anaesthesia 37:896, 1982

99. Waun JE, Sweitzer RS, Hamilton WK: Effect of nitrous oxide on middle ear mechanics and hearing acuity. Anesthesiology 28:846, 1967

100. Owens QD, Gustave F, Sclaroff A: Tympanic membrane rupture with nitrous oxide anesthesia. Anesth Analg 57:283, 1978

101. Jahrsdoerfer RA: Anesthesia in otologic surgery. Otolaryngol Clin North Am 14:699, 1981

102. Kerr AR: Anaesthesia with profound hypotension for middle ear surgery. Br J Anaesth 49:447, 1977

103. Eltringham RJ, Young PN, Fairbairn MD et al: Hypotensive anaesthesia for microsurgery of the middle ear: A comparison between enflurane and halothane. Anaesthesia 37:1028, 1982

104. Caffrey RR, Warren ML, Becker KE: Neuromuscular blockade monitoring comparing the orbicularis oculi and adductor pollicis muscles. Anesthesiology 65:95, 1986

105. Clarke RSJ: Nausea and vomiting. Br J Anaesth 56:19, 1984

106. Palazzo MGA, Strunin L: Anaesthesia and emesis: I. Etiology. Can Anaesth Soc J 31:178, 1984

107. Palazzo MGA, Strunin L: Anaesthesia and emesis: II. Prevention and management. Can Anaesth Soc J 31:407, 1984

40

Donald S. Prough
Arthur S. Foreman

Anesthesia and the Renal System

Prevention of perioperative morbidity and mortality depends in part upon an understanding of renal physiology and pharmacology and the effects of alterations in renal function on the excretion of drugs administered during and after surgery. Many patients, particularly those who are elderly, present for surgery with substantial alterations in renal function. Such patients are not only subject to prolonged duration of renally excreted drugs but also are at risk for further deterioration of renal function, especially in procedures in which renal perfusion is threatened, such as vascular and cardiac operations. Therefore, this chapter provides a physiologic and pharmacologic basis for management of patients with chronic or acute renal disease.

ANATOMY AND PHYSIOLOGY OF THE RENAL EXCRETORY SYSTEM

Anatomy of the Kidneys, Ureters, and Bladder

The kidneys are bilateral, paired organs weighing 115–160 g each and are located retroperitoneally just beneath the diaphragm. Medially, the kidneys are bounded by the psoas muscles; superiorly, they lie adjacent to the adrenal glands and the diaphragm; and anterolaterally, the right kidney borders the liver, colon, and ileum, whereas the left kidney borders the stomach, pancreas, and ileum. The center of each kidney approaches the level of the second lumbar vertebra. Vasomotor and pain fibers innervating the kidney originate in the 4th through 12th thoracic segments, the vagus nerves (through the celiac axis), and the splanchnic nerves.

The kidneys' blood supply originates from the aorta via the renal arteries. A single renal artery supplies two out of three kidneys; one third have multiple renal arteries. Each renal artery divides into five interlobar arteries, each an end artery. At the junction of the renal medulla and cortex the interlobar branches divide into arcuate arteries, which course at right angles to the interlobar arteries. The interlobular arteries arise at right angles to the arcuate arteries and penetrate through the renal cortex (Fig. 40-1). The afferent arterioles, which arise from the interlobular arteries, divide within the cortical tissue to form the glomerular capillary

network (Fig. 40-2). The capillaries then reunite to form the efferent arterioles. The subsequent course of the efferent arterioles varies, depending upon whether they are located superficially in the cortex or are situated in the juxtamedullary cortex. Superficial efferent arterioles feed a plexus of peritubular venous capillary vessels, which supply the proximal and distal tubules and portions of the loops of Henle and the collecting ducts before joining the interlobular veins and returning to the inferior vena cava through the arcuate, interlobar, and renal veins. Juxtamedullary efferent arterioles also supply the venous capillary network and give rise to the vasa recta, small-diameter vessels that penetrate deeply into the medulla and that provide most of the oxygen supply to the loop of Henle and then return to the arcuate veins. The juxtaglomerular apparatus is formed by the angle between the afferent and efferent arterioles and the macula densa, a specialized group of cells in the distal convoluted tubule.

The glomerular capillaries course within Bowman's capsule, the beginning of the tubular system. Bowman's capsule empties into the proximal convoluted tubule, which, in turn, joins the loop of Henle. The loop of Henle feeds the distal convoluted tubule, which empties into the collecting duct. The collecting ducts from many glomeruli join within the medulla to form the minor and major calyces before emptying into the renal pelvis. Each renal pelvis empties into a ureter, which courses retroperitoneally to join the urinary bladder. The ureters, each about 28–30 cm long and 5 mm in diameter, develop cyclic peristaltic waves, which raise intraluminal pressure as high as 30 mm Hg. Because of the highly anastomotic blood supply from multiple sources, the ureters may be extensively mobilized during surgery with minimal risk of ischemic injury.

Physiology of Urine Formation

The kidneys perform three major functions: filtration, reabsorption, and secretion. Trauma, surgical stress, and anesthesia alter renal function primarily by altering filtration and reabsorption.[1] The kidneys receive 20–25% of the total cardiac output—1000 ml·min^{-1} to 1250 ml·min^{-1} in the average adult. Ten percent of renal blood flow (or about 20%

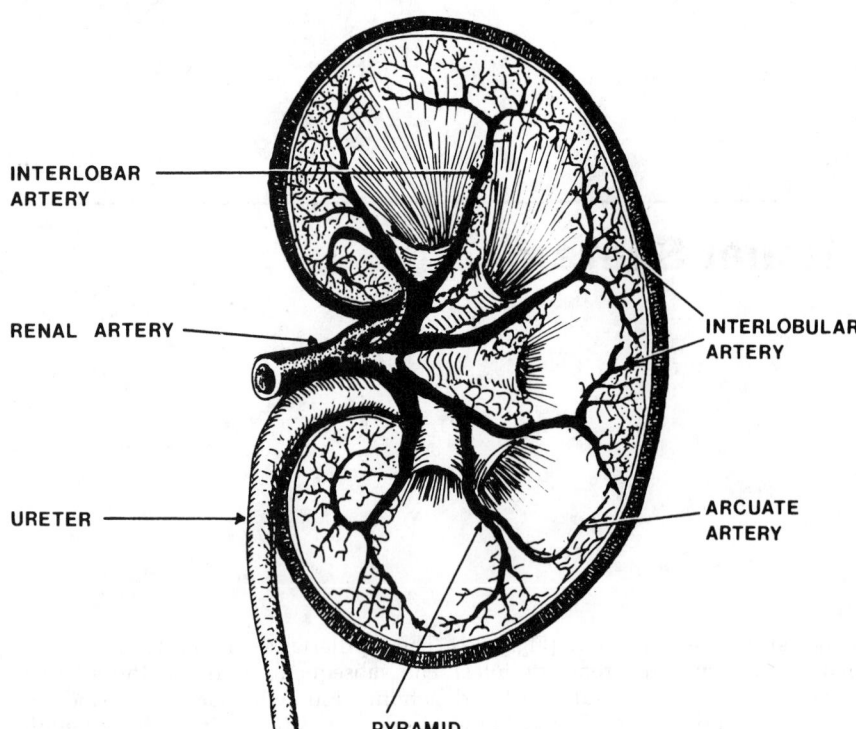

INTERLOBAR ARTERY

RENAL ARTERY

URETER

INTERLOBULAR ARTERY

ARCUATE ARTERY

PYRAMID

Figure 40-1. The distribution of the arteries in the kidney. (Reproduced with permission from Goudsouzian N, Karamanian A: The kidneys. In Goudsouzian N, Karamanian A [eds]: Physiology for the Anesthesiologist, 2nd edition, p 434. Norwalk, Connecticut: Appleton-Century-Crofts, 1984.)

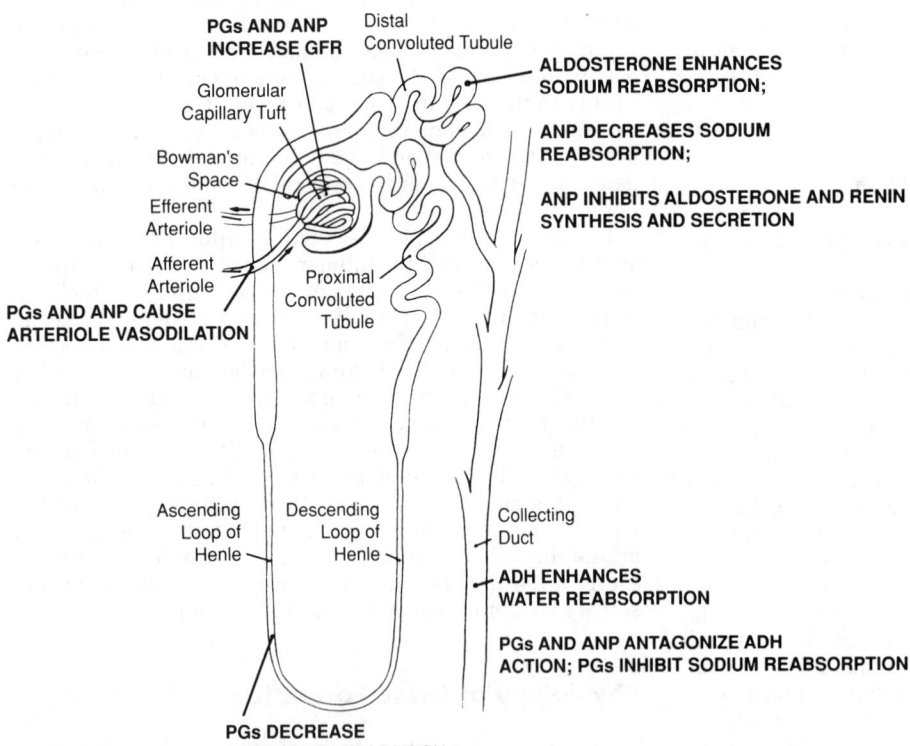

PGs AND ANP INCREASE GFR

Distal Convoluted Tubule

Glomerular Capillary Tuft

Bowman's Space

Efferent Arteriole

Afferent Arteriole

PGs AND ANP CAUSE ARTERIOLE VASODILATION

Proximal Convoluted Tubule

ALDOSTERONE ENHANCES SODIUM REABSORPTION;

ANP DECREASES SODIUM REABSORPTION;

ANP INHIBITS ALDOSTERONE AND RENIN SYNTHESIS AND SECRETION

Ascending Loop of Henle

Descending Loop of Henle

Collecting Duct

ADH ENHANCES WATER REABSORPTION

PGs AND ANP ANTAGONIZE ADH ACTION; PGs INHIBIT SODIUM REABSORPTION

PGs DECREASE SODIUM REABSORPTION

Figure 40-2. Schematic diagram of renal glomerulus and tubule. Constriction of the afferent arteriole decreases pressure within the glomerular capillary bed, thereby decreasing the GFR. In contrast, an increase in the efferent arteriolar resistance increases pressure within the glomerular capillary bed, thereby increasing GFR. (PGs = prostaglandins; ANP = atrial natriuretic peptide; ADH = antidiuretic hormone.)

of renal plasma flow) is filtered, producing a glomerular filtration rate (GFR) of 125 ml·min^{-1} in healthy young adults. The total filtration volume of approximately 180 l·day^{-1} contrasts strikingly with the renal volume of urine excreted, which averages only 1–2 l·day^{-1} (Table 40-1). The tubules and collecting ducts of the kidney reabsorb approximately 99% of the filtered solute.

Sodium Filtration and Reabsorption

Urinary sodium excretion decreases if the GFR decreases or if sodium reabsorption increases. The concentration of sodium in the glomerular filtrate approximates that in plasma. Thus, normal adult kidneys filter more than 25,000 mEq of sodium per day, of which roughly 65% is reabsorbed by the proximal renal tubule. Because water reabsorption occurs at nearly the same rate, the concentration of sodium remains similar throughout the proximal tubule.

An additional 25% of filtered sodium is actively reabsorbed as the filtrate passes through the ascending loop of Henle. Thus, only 10% of the originally filtered sodium enters the distal tubule, within which aldosterone regulates sodium reabsorption. Usually, the distal tubules and collecting ducts reabsorb most of the remaining sodium; only 1% of filtered sodium is ultimately excreted in the urine.

Water Filtration and Reabsorption

As noted previously, the proximal tubular epithelium reabsorbs 65% of filtered water in conjunction with sodium reabsorption. In the loop of Henle, water is reabsorbed to a lesser extent than is sodium. Nonetheless, the fluid leaving the loop remains isosmotic because urea has replaced about half of the total osmolar load originally contributed by sodium and chloride. Subsequently, water is reabsorbed to a variable extent in the distal tubules, the cortical collecting tubules, and the medullary collecting ducts. Antidiuretic hormone (ADH) regulates the amount of water reabsorbed in the collecting ducts.

The countercurrent multiplier system in the loop of Henle is a vital component of the kidney's ability to conserve salt and water. Reabsorption of sodium and water critically depends upon the presence of a hypertonic medullary interstitium. Increasing or decreasing blood flow within the vasa recta diminishes the interstitial gradient. The rate of filtrate flow through the loop of Henle also influences the ability of the kidney to produce a concentrated urine, since a high filtrate flow rate (such as is produced by the administration of mannitol) may "wash out" the concentrating gradient. Table 40-2 summarizes urine flow and sodium and osmolar excretion.

Physiologic Control of Glomerular Filtration and Solute Reabsorption

GFR (the rate at which fluid is filtered through the glomerular capillaries into Bowman's space) is described by the equation

$$GFR = K_f \times (P_{GC} - P_{BC} - \pi_{GC})$$

The permeability of the glomerular membrane and the surface area of that membrane together constitute the glomerular filtration coefficient (K_f). The hydraulic gradient across the endothelium is determined by the pressure within the glomerular capillary bed (P_{GC}) and by the pressure outside the capillary bed in Bowman's capsule (P_{BC}). The hydraulic

TABLE 40-1. Overview of Renal Function (Euvolemic, Young Adult)

Cardiac output	$\approx$5000 ml·min^{-1}
Renal blood flow	$\approx$1250 ml·min^{-1}
Renal plasma flow	$\approx$750 ml·min^{-1}
Glomerular filtration rate	$\approx$125 ml·min^{-1}
Urinary flow	$\approx$2 ml·min^{-1}

gradient works in opposition to the plasma oncotic pressure (π_{GC}).

Acute changes in the GFR most commonly result from changes in P_{GC}, although K_f may be reduced by active contraction of glomerular mesangial cells, a physiologic response that decreases glomerular surface area. The P_{GC} declines if the resistance increases in the afferent arterioles (the input vessels for the glomerulus) and increases if the resistance in efferent arterioles rises (see Fig. 40-2).

Neurohumoral Regulation of Renal Function

The major physiologic influences determining the reabsorption of filtered sodium and water are the hormonal factors aldosterone, ADH, atrial natriuretic factor, and the renal prostaglandins.

Aldosterone. This important hormonal regulator of sodium-potassium homeostasis and blood pressure is produced by the adrenal cortex as a result of a chain of endocrine events: (1) Renin is released from the granular cells of the juxtaglomerular apparatus in response to activation of the sympathetic nervous system, stimulation of intrarenal baroreceptors, or reduced delivery of sodium chloride to the macula densa. (2) After entering the systemic circulation, renin catalyzes the release of angiotensin I from angiotensinogen. (3) Angiotensin I transformation to angiotensin II then follows, catalyzed by angiotensin-converting enzyme in the lungs. (4) Angiotensin II stimulates the cells of the adrenal cortex to produce aldosterone. Acting primarily in the distal tubules and collecting ducts, aldosterone regulates the excretion of about 2% of filtered sodium. Through the renin-angiotensin-aldosterone system, the kidney can maintain sodium balance despite variations in daily sodium intake from 10–250 mmol.[2] Table 40-2 illustrates the effects of maximal aldosterone stimulation.

Antidiuretic Hormone. Release of ADH from the posterior pituitary gland occurs in response to stimulation of the osmoreceptors (located primarily in the hypothalamus) by increased blood osmolarity. ADH release is inhibited by increased stretch of atrial baroreceptors when atrial volume is increased. Thus, the secretion of ADH responds both to changes in osmolarity and to changes in intravascular volume. ADH acts primarily on the cortical collecting tubules and medullary collecting ducts to increase water permeability. Hence, high circulating levels of ADH produce rapid reabsorption of water as the urine flows through the collecting ducts, resulting in the excretion of small volumes of highly concentrated urine. Urinary volume may vary 100-fold, depending upon ADH concentration. Table 40-2 summarizes the range of urine flow rates and osmolarities produced by minimal and maximal ADH secretion.

Atrial Natriuretic Peptide. Atrial natriuretic peptide, a hormone secreted by the cardiac atria (although it has been

TABLE 40-2. Sodium, Water, and Osmolar Excretion

	Flow Rate (ml·min^{-1})	[Na+] (mEq·l^{-1})	Osmolality (mOsm·kg^{-1})
Plasma	750	140	290
Filtrate	125	140	290
Final urine			
Euvolemic, young adult	2	100	300
Maximal aldosterone secretion	2	1.0	100
Minimal ADH secretion	20	10	50
Maximal ADH secretion	0.2	300	1400
"Average" perioperative patient	0.5	20	800

identified in a variety of other organ systems, including the brain) in response to intravascular volume expansion, acts on the arterial and venous systems, adrenals, and kidneys to reduce intravascular volume and decrease blood pressure.[3-6] Atrial natriuretic peptide reduces blood pressure by relaxing vascular smooth muscle and reducing sympathetic vascular stimulation and by extravasation of intravascular fluid into the interstitial space.[3] Atrial natriuretic peptide also inhibits renin and aldosterone secretion, thereby antagonizing sodium retention.[3,4] Within the kidney, atrial natriuretic peptide increases hydraulic pressure in the glomerular capillaries by dilating the afferent arterioles and, to a certain extent, by constricting efferent arterioles.[5] Atrial natriuretic peptide also inhibits sodium uptake in the inner medullary collecting ducts, although controversy regarding the relative importance of its glomerular and tubular effects continues.[5]

Prostaglandins. The kidneys synthesize large quantities of prostaglandin (PG) metabolites, including PGE_2 and thromboxane A_2, which appear to modulate the renal effects of other hormones.[7-10] For instance, the vasodilator PGE_2 decreases the contraction of glomerular mesangial cells produced by angiotensin II.[7] Thromboxane A_2, in contrast, produces mesangial contraction.[7] Renal prostaglandins appear to influence renal water excretion and sodium excretion, particularly in sodium-depleted states.[8] In patients with congestive heart failure, cirrhosis, nephrotic syndrome, and mild chronic renal failure, PGE_2 and prostacyclin (PGI_2) are produced endogenously to maintain renal perfusion and GFR.[9,10]

Neuroendocrine Response to Trauma. The physiologic stress of trauma and surgery is associated with reduced urinary excretion of sodium and water, which occurs in response to changes in intravascular and extracellular volume and to secondary neuroendocrine effects, especially the release of ADH, catecholamines, and aldosterone. The kidneys and the neuroendocrine factors that influence renal function represent a tightly integrated system that acts to preserve intravascular volume and maintain GFR. In response to a decrease in effective arterial blood volume, whether secondary to decreased cardiac output or peripheral arterial vasodilation, ADH secretion increases renal water retention, activation of the renin-angiotensin-aldosterone system stimulates renal sodium retention, and sympathetic activation increases peripheral and renal arterial vascular resistance (Fig. 40-3).[11]

In response to renal hypoperfusion, three major regulatory mechanisms support renal function. These include afferent arteriolar dilation (increasing the proportion of cardiac output that perfuses the kidney), increased resistance in the efferent arterioles (which increases the filtration fraction), and activation of the renin-angiotensin-aldosterone system (which improves renal perfusion by increasing intravascular volume, thereby indirectly increasing cardiac output) (Fig. 40-4).[12] Vasodilator prostaglandins appear to function primarily by reducing resistance in the afferent arterioles, whereas angiotensin II appears to be particularly important in increasing efferent arteriolar resistance. However, despite the wealth of information available regarding renal neuroendocrine responses to hypotension and renal hypoperfusion, remarkably few data describe the integrity of these responses in animals or patients during anesthesia. Limited data suggest that renal vasodilation in response to hemorrhage is impaired in anesthetized as opposed to conscious animals subjected to similar amounts of hemorrhage,[13,14] a difference that is attributable, at least in part, to more profound hypotension associated with hemorrhage in anesthetized animals.[14]

RENAL PHARMACOLOGY

Comparative Renal Pharmacology of Inhaled and Injected Anesthetics

Anesthetic drugs may alter renal function directly by changing renal vascular resistance and renal blood flow, GFR, or renal tubular function. Anesthetics also indirectly influence renal function by producing changes in cardiovascular function and/or neuroendocrine activity. For example, an anesthetic could alter renal blood flow indirectly by reducing cardiac output, by activating the sympathetic nervous system to increase renal vascular resistance, or by increasing endogenous secretion of ADH to produce renal vasoconstriction.

Anesthetic drugs exert diverse cardiovascular effects, many of which could adversely affect renal function. These include myocardial depression, decreases in effective arterial blood volume, and changes in peripheral vascular resistance. Commonly used potent inhalation agents decrease

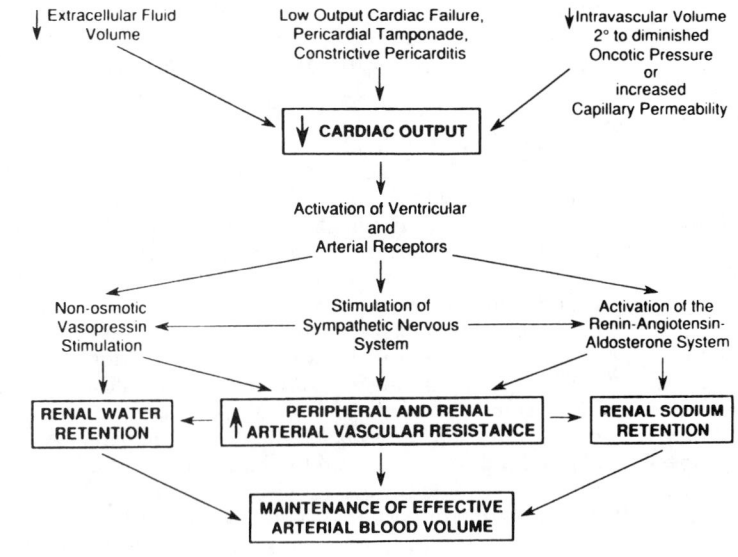

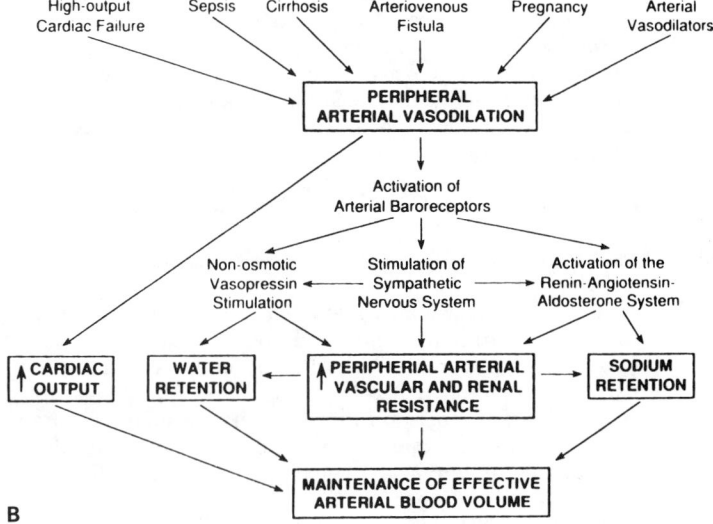

Figure 40-3. (A) Schematic diagram of the changes in water and sodium retention produced by reduction in cardiac output. (B) Changes in total body water and sodium produced by peripheral arterial vasodilation. (Reproduced with permission from Schrier RW: Body fluid volume regulation in health and disease: A unifying hypothesis. Ann Intern Med, 113:156, 1990.)

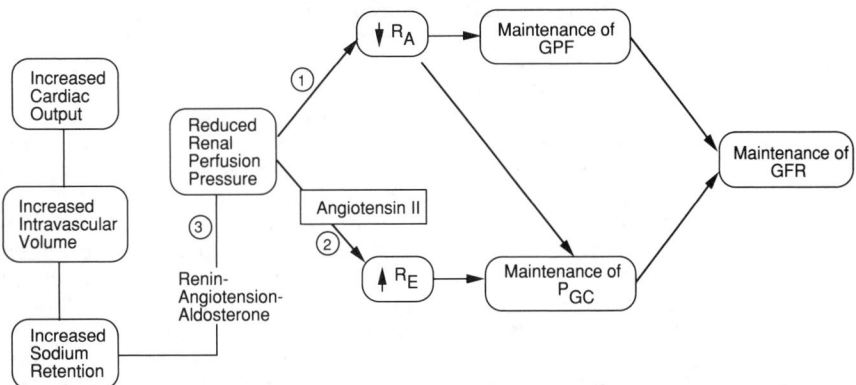

Figure 40-4. In response to hypotension, highly efficient homeostatic mechanisms come into play to maintain the GFR. This is accomplished (1) by a marked reduction in afferent arteriolar resistance (R_A), and (2) by an increase in efferent arteriolar resistance (R_E) in response to locally released angiotensin II. By maintaining the glomerular plasma flow rate (GPF) and glomerular capillary hydraulic pressure (P_{GC}), these arteriolar adjustments preserve GFR. Concomitantly, increased release of renin (3) initiates the renin-angiotensin-aldosterone sequence, resulting in sodium retention and increased intravascular volume. (Modified with permission from Badr KF, Ichikawa I: Prerenal failure: A deleterious shift from renal compensation to decompensation. N Engl J Med 319:625, 1988.)

stroke volume in a dose-dependent fashion. At higher concentrations, these drugs reduce cardiac output sufficiently to decrease renal blood flow. High levels of spinal or epidural anesthesia can impair venous return, thereby diminishing cardiac output to levels that compromise renal perfusion. Either an increase or a decrease in peripheral vascular resistance may indirectly reduce renal blood flow. Anesthetics such as diethyl ether and cyclopropane stimulate catecholamine secretion, increase total peripheral resistance, and decrease renal blood flow.[15]

Surgical stress and anesthesia alter autonomic and neuroendocrine function. Norepinephrine and epinephrine, released by sympathetic postganglionic fibers and by the adrenal medulla in response to noxious stimulation or hypovolemia, cause both renal vasoconstriction and renin release from the juxtamedullary apparatus. Renin release is also stimulated by atrial baroreceptors and, in the kidney, by a low ratio of serum sodium to serum potassium. Anesthetics are associated with numerous changes in endocrine function, including increased secretion of ADH and aldosterone. It is unclear whether anesthetics directly cause ADH and aldosterone release or whether the release is the result of changes in blood pressure or cardiac output. However, stress, whether preoperative, intraoperative, or postoperative, triggers ADH and aldosterone secretion.

In addition to the direct and indirect effects of the anesthetic agents themselves, other intraoperative interventions may also directly and indirectly modify renal function. The initiation of mechanical ventilation of the lungs and positive end-expiratory pressure are associated with reduced urinary output. This form of renal dysfunction accompanies decreased cardiac output, increased sympathetic outflow, and the release of renin. ADH apparently is not responsible for reduced renal function during ventilation with positive end-expiratory pressure;[16] both animal and human data suggest that the reduced urinary volume and sodium excretion may be secondary to decreased release of atrial natriuretic peptide.[17,18]

The technical difficulties involved in determining renal blood flow certainly contribute to the conflicting reports of anesthetic effects on renal function. In experimental animals, direct measurement techniques, including cannulation of venous vessels and placement of circumferential arterial probes, permit repeated analyses. Potential errors introduced by direct measurement techniques include changes in flow caused by the probes as well as the possible effects of inadvertent surgical renal denervation.

Several techniques measure renal blood flow indirectly by clearance of inert filtered substances, washout of inert gases, and distribution of radioactive microspheres. Para-amino hippurate is filtered by the glomeruli and secreted to a limited extent by the tubules. Clearance of para-amino hippurate is proportional to renal plasma flow and renal blood flow. Inert gas washout permits inferences regarding the intrarenal distribution of flow, whereas radioactive microsphere techniques allow more precise quantification of variations in intraorgan blood flow. These methods, however, also have several limitations. The clinical pharmacology of anesthetic drugs would be markedly advanced by a minimally invasive measurement of renal blood flow that permitted repeated assessment of renal perfusion in humans.

Effects of Inhaled Anesthetics on Renal Function

Methoxyflurane nephrotoxicity offers a classic example of an alteration in renal function produced by an anesthetic drug. The clinical manifestations of methoxyflurane nephrotoxicity include hyposmotic diuresis, azotemia, hypernatremia, and hyperosmolality.[19] Although the impairment usually resolves in 10–20 days, some deficits persist for a year or longer. Inorganic fluoride ion, the methoxyflurane metabolite responsible for renal dysfunction,[20] produces dose-related toxicity. Greater exposure to methoxyflurane is associated with higher fluoride levels; clinical toxicity occurs consistently at serum inorganic fluoride levels exceeding 50 $\mu M \cdot l^{-1}$.[21] Likely mechanisms for fluoride ion toxicity include impaired ultratransport in the ascending loop of Henle, increased solute washout by enhanced medullary blood flow, and swelling and destruction of the proximal convoluted tubule mitochondria.[22,23]

Significant amounts of fluoride ion are also released from enflurane but not from halothane or isoflurane (Fig. 40-5).[23] Some volunteers receiving enflurane for more than 9.5 hours have peak serum inorganic fluoride levels in the 30–40 $\mu M \cdot l^{-1}$ range.[24] Clinically, this correlates with decreased urinary concentrating ability and with decreased responsiveness to vasopressin (Fig. 40-6).[24] Although this is probably not important in healthy patients, it is not known what effects such levels of inorganic fluoride have on renal function in patients with minimal reserve. Concentrations of fluoride ion in excess of 50 $\mu M \cdot l^{-1}$ have been observed in some patients treated with isoniazid after enflurane anesthesia[25] and in obese patients after prolonged exposure to enflurane. Experimental administration of enflurane to obese rats also results in higher levels of inorganic fluoride than in nonobese animals.[26] Enflurane appears to enhance the nephrotoxic potential of aminoglycosides in humans, as evidenced by greater urinary excretion of alanine aminopeptidase.[27]

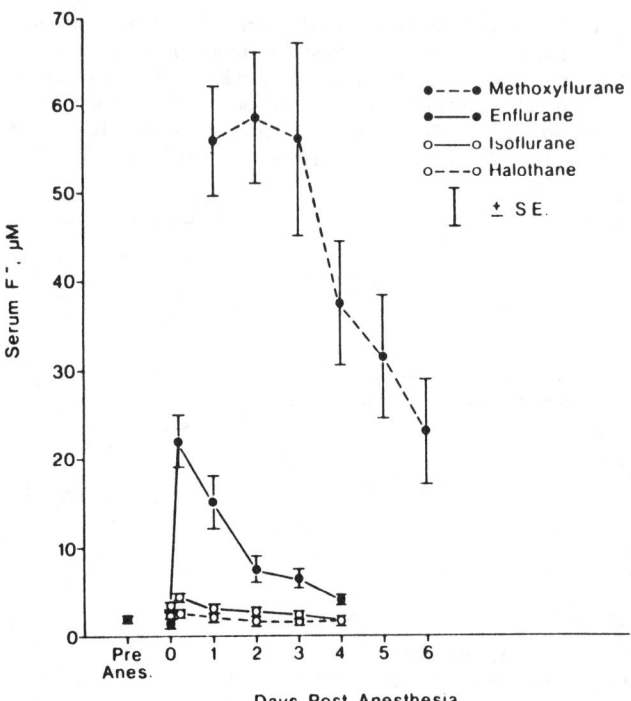

Figure 40-5. Serum inorganic fluoride (F$^-$) concentrations prior to and following administration of methoxyflurane, enflurane, isoflurane, or halothane to adult patients. (Reproduced with permission from Cousins MJ, Greenstein LR, Hitt BA, Mazze RI: Metabolism and renal effects of enflurane in man. Anesthesiology 44:48, 1976.)

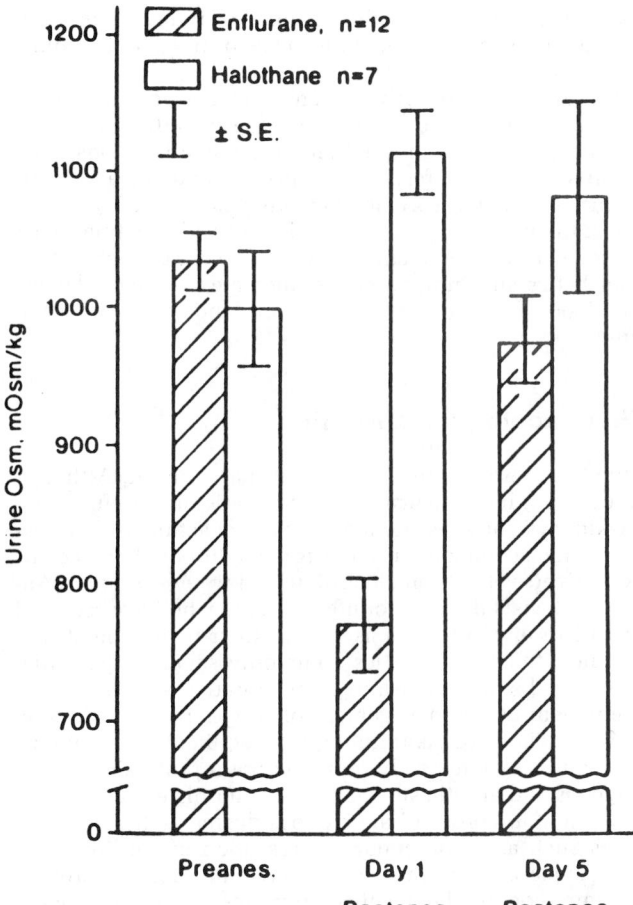

Figure 40-6. Histogram showing maximum urinary osmolarities before and after administration of vasopressin to volunteers. One group had received enflurane for an average of 9.6 minimum alveolar concentration hours, and the second group had received halothane for 13.7 minimum alveolar concentration hours. The ability to concentrate urine was decreased on day 1 following administration of enflurane. (Reproduced with permission from Mazze RI, Calverley RK, Smith NT: Inorganic fluoride nephrotoxicity: Prolonged enflurane and halothane anesthesia in volunteers. Anesthesiology 46:267, 1977.)

With the possible exception of methoxyflurane, halothane remains the best studied anesthetic agent with regard to effects on renal function. Although most investigators agree that halothane decreases GFR and urinary output,[28] studies of the responses of renal blood flow to halothane anesthesia have yielded conflicting results. Reasons for this include difficulty in controlling other factors influencing renal blood flow, such as circulating catecholamine levels, as well as methodologic problems with the measurement of renal blood flow. Initial studies, using techniques based on the clearance of inert filtered substances, concluded that halothane reduces renal blood flow.[29] Later, direct measurement techniques indicated that clinical doses of halothane decrease renal vascular resistance but have little effect on renal blood flow.[30] In isolated, perfused canine kidneys, halothane markedly increases renal blood flow.[31] Renal autoregulatory responses to hypotension are not impaired by low to moderate doses of halothane (Fig. 40-7).[32] Even when administering halothane under conditions of acute hemorrhagic hypovolemia, autoregulation remains intact

and decreased renal vascular resistance maintains renal blood flow at normal levels.[33]

Only fragmentary data characterize changes in tubular function associated with halothane anesthesia. In the toad urinary bladder, which shares many physiologic characteristics of mammalian cortical collecting tubules, halothane does not change basal levels of water transport but decreases the response to ADH.[34] Like most other inhalation and intravenous anesthetics tested, halothane stimulates sodium transport in low doses and inhibits sodium transport in higher doses.[34] Halothane also produces a dose-dependent, reversible inhibition of organic acid transport, as do other anesthetics.[34] However, the in vivo effects of halothane and other anesthetics on renal blood flow, sodium excretion, osmolal clearance, and urinary volume are complex, influenced not only by the direct effects of the anesthetics but by sympathetic innervation, the renin-angiotensin system, release of ADH, and release of catecholamines.[34]

Data describing the renal effects of other inhaled anesthetics remain scarce. Enflurane decreases GFR, renal blood flow, and urinary output.[23,34] Isoflurane produces little change in renal blood flow but decreases GFR and urinary output.[35,36] Even prolonged isoflurane-induced hypotension is associated with preservation of GFR and renal blood flow and prompt postoperative return of renal function.[37] When added to halothane, nitrous oxide potentiates the reduction in urine flow.[38] Nitrous oxide and halothane in combination, however, do not appear to adversely affect the autoregulation of renal blood flow.[39] The new anesthetic desflurane appears to produce no evidence of renal toxicity;[40] in fact, renal blood flow is well maintained even during administration of high concentrations of desflurane.[41]

Effects of Intravenous Induction Agents on Renal Function

Thiopental, delivered in either high- or low-dose regimens, does not alter renal blood flow. Following low doses, systemic blood pressure, renal resistance, and renal blood flow change little from baseline.[42] Initially, thiopental administration can even produce a transient elevation of systemic blood pressure and a rise in renal blood flow. This may be caused by sympathetic nervous system activation as the subject senses the onset of anesthesia. At high doses, thiopental's cardiovascular depressant properties, which in-

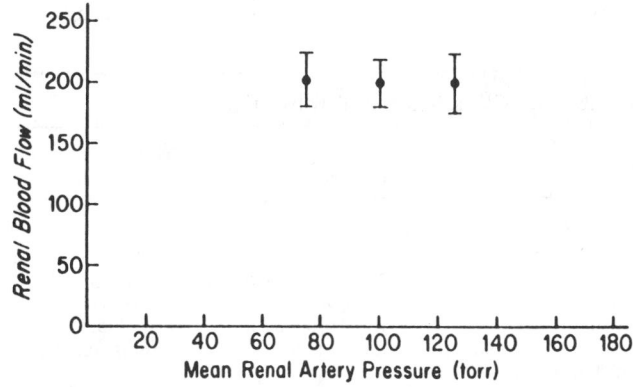

Figure 40-7. Renal blood flow in dogs remained unchanged in the presence of 0.9% end-expired halothane. (Reproduced with permission from Bastron RD, Perkins FM, Pyne JL: Autoregulation of renal blood flow during halothane anesthesia. Anesthesiology 46:143, 1977.)

clude venodilation, decreased myocardial contractility, and decreased cardiac preload, reduce blood pressure and induce a reflex increase in peripheral vascular resistance.[43] Despite increased systemic vascular resistance and decreased cardiac output, renal blood flow remains unchanged because of reduced renal vascular resistance.[43]

When administered directly into a renal artery in unanesthetized rabbits, sodium thiopental produces a dose-dependent increase in urinary volume and urinary sodium, although renal blood flow is unaffected. Renal vein concentrations of renin and norepinephrine are decreased, suggesting inhibition of renal sympathetic activity or direct tubular effects.[44] In contrast, an intravenously administered anesthetic dose of sodium thiopental decreases blood pressure, renal blood flow, GFR, and urinary volume.[44] In rats, the impairment of renal hemodynamics during pentobarbital anesthesia appears to be mediated by the renin-angiotensin system.[45] In pentobarbital-anesthetized dogs, infusion of human atrial natriuretic peptide produces greater natriuresis than in awake animals, a response that is attenuated by renal denervation.[46]

Most of the data regarding the effects of other intravenous drugs on renal blood flow and renal function also derive from animal models. In dogs, systemic blood pressure, renal blood flow, and renal vascular resistance increase after ketamine administration.[43] Other animal studies of the effects of ketamine and diazepam on renal blood flow have yielded conflicting results.[47,48] Variations in measurement techniques and in experimental preparation probably explain the differences. Morphine, even when given in doses that lower blood pressure, does not reduce renal blood flow.[49] Fentanyl decreases urinary flow and GFR while renal blood flow appears to increase or decrease, depending upon whether direct or indirect measurement techniques are used.[50,51] Although propofol reduces systemic clearance of both meperidine[52] and organic anions such as cefoxitin,[53] renal blood flow appears to be minimally affected.[54]

The effects of regional anesthesia on renal physiology have been evaluated in moderate detail. In humans, spinal anesthesia only slightly decreases GFR and renal blood flow, despite levels of spinal blockage to the first thoracic dermatome.[55] Thoracic levels of epidural block using epinephrine-containing local anesthetics cause moderate reductions in GFR and renal blood flow that parallel decreases in mean arterial pressure.[56] Epidural block performed with epinephrine-free solutions generates little change in systemic hemodynamics and only a small decrease in GFR and renal blood flow.[57] In clinical practice, the pre-existing in-

travascular volume and the quantity of intravenous fluids strongly influence the renal response to spinal and epidural anesthesia.

In summary, virtually all anesthetic agents and techniques are associated with a decrease in GFR and urinary output. The effects on renal blood flow are less consistent. Results vary with respect to species studied, anesthetic methods, and measurement techniques. In clinical situations, the net effect on renal perfusion and function represents a complex interaction between the direct effects of the anesthetics and indirect effects mediated through changes in blood pressure, cardiac output, and neuroendocrine function.

Pharmacology of Diuretics

Diuretics are drugs that increase urinary output. Although all diuretics increase urinary flow in patients with functioning kidneys, the sites and mechanisms of action differ markedly among commonly used drugs. In addition, these agents exert diverse effects on electrolyte and water excretion. Anesthesiologists daily encounter patients who have received or will receive diuretics as part of their management. For instance, thiazide diuretics commonly serve as the initial treatment for hypertension, loop diuretics are an integral component of the management of congestive heart failure, and furosemide or mannitol or both facilitate neurosurgical procedures by effectively reducing brain protrusion. Many surgeons and anesthesiologists also administer mannitol in an attempt to "protect" the kidneys during high-risk procedures such as aortic aneurysm resection or cardiopulmonary bypass. Both intraoperatively and postoperatively, patients commonly receive diuretics to relieve acute intravascular overload and, based on simplistic physiologic reasoning, to increase urinary output. Because these drugs are a ubiquitous part of perioperative management, anesthesiologists must possess an understanding of their use and potential for misuse.

Classification of Diuretics

The pharmacologic classification of diuretics (Table 40-3) includes the following: osmotic diuretics, loop or "high-ceiling" diuretics, benzothiadiazides and related agents, carbonic anhydrase inhibitors, aldosterone antagonists, xanthines, other potassium-sparing diuretics, and uricosuric diuretics.[58,59]

TABLE 40-3. Classification of Diuretic Drugs

Class	Examples	Principal Site of Action	Mechanism of Action
Osmotic	Mannitol, glycerol	Loop of Henle, distal nephron	Limit water reabsorption
Loop	Furosemide, ethacrynic acid, bumetanide	Ascending limb of loop of Henle	Inhibit NaCl reabsorption
Thiazide	Hydrochlorothiazide	Distal tubule	Inhibit Na reabsorption
Carbonic anhydrase inhibitors	Acetazolamide	Proximal tubular lumen	Inhibit hydrogen ion secretion into the lumen
Aldosterone antagonists	Spironolactone	Collecting duct, distal tubule	Oppose aldosterone
Xanthines	Theophylline	Renal blood flow	Increase cardiac output (some tubular effects)

Osmotic diuretics, agents that are filtered at the glomerulus but not reabsorbed in the tubules, hold water within the tubular lumen, thereby limiting water reabsorption in the loop of Henle and in the distal nephron. *"High-ceiling"* or *loop diuretics* inhibit sodium chloride reabsorption in the thick ascending limb of the loop of Henle.[58-60] *Benzothiadiazides* act at the distal convoluted tubule to inhibit the reabsorption of sodium.[58,59] In some patients who become resistant to loop diuretics or benzothiadiazides because of contraction of extracellular fluid and intrarenal compensatory processes, a combination of a benzothiadiazide and a loop diuretic appears to exert synergistic effects.[60] The *carbonic anhydrase inhibitors* are weak diuretics that act by limiting the secretion of hydrogen ions into the proximal tubular lumen, thereby promoting the loss of bicarbonate in the urine.[58,59] Clinicians rarely use carbonic anhydrase inhibitors as diuretics but rather use them for their inhibitory effect on cerebrospinal fluid production and aqueous humor secretion and their ability to reduce serum bicarbonate concentration. *Aldosterone antagonists,* as the name implies, exert potassium-sparing effects by opposing the action of aldosterone on the late distal tubule and collecting system.[61] *Xanthines,* such as aminophylline, induce diuresis partly by increasing cardiac output and partly by direct effects on the renal tubules. Other potassium-sparing diuretics include triamterine and amiloride, agents that interfere with ion transport in the principal cells of the collecting duct to reduce the excretion of potassium.[60] *Uricosuric diuretics,* none of which are currently available, increase the urinary excretion of urate.

Osmotic diuretics are employed during neurosurgical procedures to reduce brain bulk,[62] and in surgical procedures that threaten renal function they are often used prophylactically or therapeutically, with the hope of attenuating renal ischemic injury. During osmotic diuresis, sodium is lost to a lesser extent than water. Available in the form of 50-ml ampules containing 12.5 g (25% solution) and in 500-ml bottles containing 100 g (20% solution), mannitol is usually given in doses of $0.25-1.5$ g·kg^{-1} intravenously. The lower dose is appropriate for use in patients with acute oliguria that is unresponsive to volume expansion and other hemodynamic support. Higher doses are given acutely to produce brain dehydration in patients with intracranial hypertension. Administration of an osmotic load has the immediate hemodynamic effect of increasing intravascular volume and cardiac output.[63] Consequently, mannitol should not be administered to patients with congestive heart failure or established oliguric renal failure because of the risk of precipitating acute pulmonary edema.

The loop diuretics, such as furosemide, ethacrynic acid, and bumetanide, limit the reabsorption of sodium chloride in the ascending loop of Henle.[58,59] Renal vasodilation is produced to some extent by the acute administration of loop diuretics; however, rapid depletion resulting from excessive diuresis of intravascular volume may lead to a secondary reduction in GFR.

Benzothiadiazides, which are rarely used during anesthesia, are commonly used for the management of chronic hypertension. During preoperative evaluation, anesthesia personnel should recall the tendency of benzothiadiazides to produce hypokalemia and metabolic alkalosis. In addition, the thiazides slightly increase or decrease GFR, especially when given intravenously, and decrease the excretion of calcium.[58] Hyperuricemia and hyperglycemia are other occasional complications.

The carbonic anhydrase inhibitors decrease bicarbonate reabsorption and reduce the secretion of aqueous humor in the eye and cerebrospinal fluid. However, the utility of the carbonic anhydrase inhibitor acetazolamide for the reduction of intracranial pressure is diminished by the transient increase in cerebral blood flow.[64] From a clinical standpoint, anesthesiologists should be aware of the potential for potassium loss and hyperchloremic metabolic acidosis if patients have received carbonic anhydrase inhibitors for more than a few days.

Aldosterone antagonists and other potassium-sparing agents are rarely used acutely in the perioperative period. These agents reduce the hypokalemia that otherwise occurs with the chronic use of potassium-wasting diuretics such as the loop diuretics and the benzothiadiazides. Controversy continues regarding whether potassium-sparing diuretics reduce morbidity when used in this fashion.[65] Spironolactone is also used to counteract the intense hyperaldosteronism that accompanies cirrhosis. Because of the potential for producing hyperkalemia, the anesthesiologist should be wary of rapid administration of potassium to patients who have recently received potassium-sparing diuretics.

CHRONIC RENAL FAILURE

Clinical Characteristics

Chronic renal failure produces a wide variety of pathophysiologic conditions.[66,67] In the past few decades, a progressively better understanding of these abnormalities has led to more successful management of patients with renal disease. Improved dialysis techniques have extended life expectancy for those with chronic renal failure. Concomitantly, the number of surgical procedures required in dialysis-dependent patients has increased.[67] Although renal failure results from a variety of specific disease processes, the common denominator is the progressive loss of nephron function.

Chronic renal failure is not an "all or nothing" phenomenon. As the number of functioning nephrons declines, the signs, symptoms, and biochemical abnormalities pass through several stages (Table 40-4). Until fewer than 40% of normal functioning nephrons remain, there are no signs, symptoms, or laboratory abnormalities. This stage is described as decreased renal reserve. Function of as few as 10–40% of nephrons is associated with only mild signs of renal failure, such as nocturia, which occurs secondary to a decrease in concentrating capability. In this stage of renal insufficiency, patients seem well compensated when excretory capacity is unstressed but they possess little or no renal reserve. The metabolism and excretion of certain drugs are impaired,[68] as is the ability to eliminate an unusually large quantity of protein catabolic products. In this stage, the preservation of remaining functional nephrons is at a premium, since toxic substances (e.g., aminoglycosides) can worsen renal insufficiency.

The loss of approximately 95% of functioning nephrons culminates in the uremic syndrome, which includes all of the problems of overt renal failure, including fluid overload and congestive heart failure. The concentrating and diluting properties of the kidney are severely compromised. Electrolyte, hematologic, and acid-base disturbances are common. The uremic syndrome usually requires dialysis.

The Uremic Syndrome

Patients with dialysis-dependent renal failure have several disease manifestations, including metabolic acidosis, platelet dysfunction, fluid overload, electrolyte disorders, central nervous system abnormalities, and gastrointestinal disor-

TABLE 40-4. Stages of Chronic Renal Failure

	GFR (ml·min^{-1})	Signs/Symptoms	Laboratory Abnormalities
Normal	125	None	None
Decreased renal reserve	50–80	None	None
Renal insufficiency	12–50	Nocturia	Increased BUN, serum creatinine levels, especially when stressed
Uremia	<12	Uremic syndrome	Multiple

ders. These components of the uremic syndrome are controlled to a variable extent by dialysis. The accumulation each day of about 50 mEq of hydrogen ion, normally excreted by the kidneys, produces metabolic acidosis. Dialysis returns pH to normal or near-normal values. Renal failure results in the accumulation of waste products that inhibit platelet function by interfering with the process by which platelets release and respond to adenosine diphosphate.[69] A further qualitative defect in platelet function results from a decline in platelet Factor III activity. Although there are other defects in the coagulation cascade, the prothrombin time and the partial thromboplastin time usually remain normal.

Excretory failure results in a wide variety of other complications. Fluid overload occurs, since free water and sodium are not excreted. Resulting signs and symptoms include congestive heart failure, hypertension, and, if hypertension is severe and chronic, left ventricular hypertrophy. Several common electrolyte disturbances that accompany renal failure are listed in Table 40-5. Hyperkalemia is one abnormality of paramount anesthetic importance because of its potential to precipitate fatal cardiac dysrhythmias. Neurologic complications include central, peripheral, and autonomic dysfunction. Fatigue, malaise, and intellectual impairment are common. If left untreated, uremic encephalopathy progresses to coma. Paresthesias, burning, and itching of the lower extremities are the most frequent peripheral neuropathic symptoms. Autonomic dysfunction, including postural hypotension, may be present. Orthostasis may be aggravated by the wide swings in intravascular volume that accompany renal failure and dialysis. Common gastrointestinal disorders associated with uremia include nausea and vomiting, gastrointestinal bleeding, anorexia, and hiccups. Most of the platelet, fluid and electrolyte, nervous system, and gastrointestinal system manifestations of uremia improve with dialysis. However, dialytic treatment does not adequately resolve some uremic complications. Chronic anemia, with hemoglobin levels of 5–7 g·dl^{-1}, results from decreased production of erythropoietin and diminished red blood cell survival time. Recently, human recombinant

TABLE 40-5. Common Electrolyte Disturbances in Chronic Renal Failure

Hyperkalemia
Hyponatremia
Hypercalcemia
Hypocalcemia
Hypermagnesemia
Hyperphosphatemia

erythropoietin has been used to manage anemia.[70,71] Despite the threat of tissue hypoxia from decreased oxygen-carrying capacity of red blood cells, patients usually tolerate such anemia relatively well because the onset is slow and because tissue blood flow increases secondary to decreased blood viscosity and increased stroke volume. Heart rate usually remains in the normal range. Tissue oxygenation is aided somewhat by a rightward shift of the oxyhemoglobin dissociation curve owing to metabolic acidosis and an increased concentration of 2,3 diphosphoglycerate.[72] Nevertheless, if anemia is corrected using erythropoietin, patients with chronic renal failure show a striking improvement in cognitive function and quality of life.[71]

In the chronic renal failure patient, an altered immune system confers greater susceptibility to infection. Sepsis, the leading cause of death in uremic patients, is even more likely to occur in the post-transplant period owing to the use of immunosuppressive therapy. Additionally, there is a greater incidence of hepatitis B in patients with renal failure.

Dialytic Treatment

Seventy-two thousand patients in the United States undergo chronic dialytic therapy. Of these, a substantial percentage require hospitalization each year; many require surgery, if only for maintenance of dialytic access.

The replacement of renal excretory and homeostatic functions poses a complex technical challenge. The normal kidneys eliminate waste products, especially the waste products of protein catabolism, and they also regulate total body water, total body sodium, and the serum concentrations of sodium, potassium, phosphate, magnesium, and calcium. Although even a small percentage of residual renal function is superior to any form of dialytic therapy, much of the function of the normal kidney can be replaced by artificial means. Hemodialysis, peritoneal dialysis, continuous arteriovenous hemofiltration, and continuous arteriovenous hemodialysis are techniques that can process large quantities of water and solutes and eliminate waste products.[73-79]

Hemodialysis

Dialysis refers to diffuse transport of solute down an osmotic gradient across a semipermeable membrane. Accumulated waste solutes such as urea and potassium move across the membrane into a chemically prescribed dialysate. Substances such as the bicarbonate substrate, acetate, move from higher concentrations in the dialysate into blood. Specific solutes are added to or removed from blood based on the relative concentrations in blood and dialysate. Blood and dialysate flow rapidly in opposite directions through the dialyzer (blood inside and dialysate outside the hollow fibers) to achieve maximal effective solute exchange. Both diffusive and convective (i.e., hydrostatic pressure-driven) transport occur during this countercurrent flow.

The semipermeable membrane that separates blood from the dialysate during hemodialysis must have a large surface area to be efficient. Solute is transported in direct relationship to the surface area and permeability of the membrane and to the difference in molecular concentrations on either side of the membrane, as expressed by the equation:

$$J_S = DA(C_B - C_D)$$

where J_S = solute flux, D = diffusion coefficient of the membrane for the solute, which varies, depending on size and charge, A = area of membrane, C_B = concentration of the solute in blood, and C_D = concentration of the solute in the dialysate.

Substances move across the dialyzer membrane in a manner quite different from the transport of substances across the renal glomerular membrane. The glomerulus quantitatively filters substances up to a molecular weight of 7000–10,000 daltons. As molecular weight increases further, glomerular filtration progressively falls, until the upper limit of filtration size (approximately 100,000 daltons) is attained. In contrast, dialytic clearance relates inversely to molecular weight across the entire range of 0–100,000 daltons. Small molecules, such as urea, are cleared readily by dialysis. In comparison to glomerular filtration, dialytic clearance is least efficient for molecules with molecular weights of 300–5000 daltons, the so-called middle molecules.[79]

Systemic or regional heparinization during hemodialysis counteracts the activation of the coagulation cascade brought on by contact between blood and the surface of the dialyzer. In regional heparinization, heparin is added to the blood in the arterial line and is neutralized with protamine in the venous line before being returned to the patient, thereby limiting the consequences of systemic heparinization. With either systemic or regional heparinization, careful monitoring of anticoagulation is required.

Hemodialysis requires vascular access sufficient to provide adequate blood flow. Emergency hemodialysis, now performed rarely through arteriovenous shunts, frequently proceeds through a Shaldon catheter inserted percutaneously in a femoral vein. Blood is returned through a peripheral vein or, when necessary, through a second Shaldon catheter inserted in the same or the contralateral femoral vein. Similar catheters, inserted in the subclavian vein, may be superior to femoral catheterization for temporary access for hemodialysis.[80] Chronic hemodialysis, in contrast, is usually performed through an arteriovenous fistula. Patients requiring chronic hemodialysis often undergo numerous surgical procedures to revise or replace failed fistulae, particularly in the first month after the shunt is placed.[81] The necessity for maintaining vascular access represents a major cause of morbidity in patients with chronic renal failure.

Peritoneal Dialysis

This intracorporeal diffusive method uses the natural semipermeable membrane consisting of the tissue layers that separate peritoneal capillary blood from the dialysate. Peritoneal dialysis begins with the surgical placement of an indwelling peritoneal catheter.[82] Percutaneous insertion, an alternative, introduces the risk of bowel perforation or catheter loss. Dialysate is infused into and drained from the peritoneal cavity in a tidal fashion. The large capillary network in the peritoneal cavity provides contact between blood and dialysate.[83]

Peritoneal dialysis clears small molecules such as urea more slowly than hemodialysis and clears larger molecules such as insulin more rapidly. Clearance of solutes depends upon the volume and composition of the dialysate, the rate of blood flow in the peritoneal capillaries, the permeability of the peritoneal tissue layers, the area of the peritoneal membrane, and the circulation of the fluid film in the peritoneal cavity.[83] The volume of dialysate infused per exchange in adults is usually 2 l. Higher volumes increase the efficiency of dialysis but may restrict diaphragmatic motion. The composition of the dialysate may be modified to increase or decrease blood concentrations of solute. The tonicity of the dialysate may be increased by increasing the concentration of dextrose, which will then increase the rate of ultrafiltration of water and solute out of the capillary bed.

Acute peritoneal dialysis is used for correction of severe accumulation of water or solutes. Intermittent peritoneal dialysis, used to maintain chronic renal failure patients, consists of three to seven treatments per week, each requiring 8 to 12 hours of cyclic infusion and removal of dialysate. Continuous ambulatory peritoneal dialysis (CAPD), a strategy developed to facilitate the activities of daily living for patients on chronic peritoneal dialysis,[84] is performed throughout each day. Compared with intermittent peritoneal dialysis, dwell time (the duration of time during which the dialysate is permitted to remain in the peritoneal cavity) is much longer. Three to five exchanges are performed daily, generally allowing an uninterrupted night of sleep. Peritonitis remains the major complication of long-term peritoneal access.[85]

Continuous Arteriovenous Hemofiltration

Ultrafiltration is a process whereby water and solutes are transported convectively from blood through a semipermeable membrane by hydrostatic pressure or by the osmotic force exerted by a hypertonic solution on the side of the membrane opposite the blood compartment.

Continuous arteriovenous hemofiltration (CAVH), an innovative technique for the purely convective removal of fluid and solute, uses the hydraulic driving pressure generated by systemic arterial pressure or a blood pump.[86-89] The apparatus consists of an arterial cannula connected to a high solvent flux filter, which empties into a venous return cannula (Fig. 40-8). The rate of ultrafiltration is described by the following equation:

$$QF = KA(P_{tm} - P_{onc})$$

where QF = flow of filtrate, K = filtration characteristics of the membrane, A = membrane area, P_{tm} = transmembrane hydrostatic pressure gradient, and P_{onc} = serum oncotic pressure.

The addition of a blood pump to raise P_{tm} may increase formation of ultrafiltrate from 300–1000 ml·h^{-1} (the range achievable using arterial hydraulic pressure) to as much as 2400 ml·h^{-1}.[85] The application of negative pressure to the ultrafiltrate line also increases P_{tm}. CAVH removes fluid containing the same concentrations of solutes present in serum; solute concentrations are not changed by the filtration process but rather by the infusion of replacement fluid (see Fig. 40-8) that dilutes waste solutes or increases the concentration of desired solutes. Because of its considerable

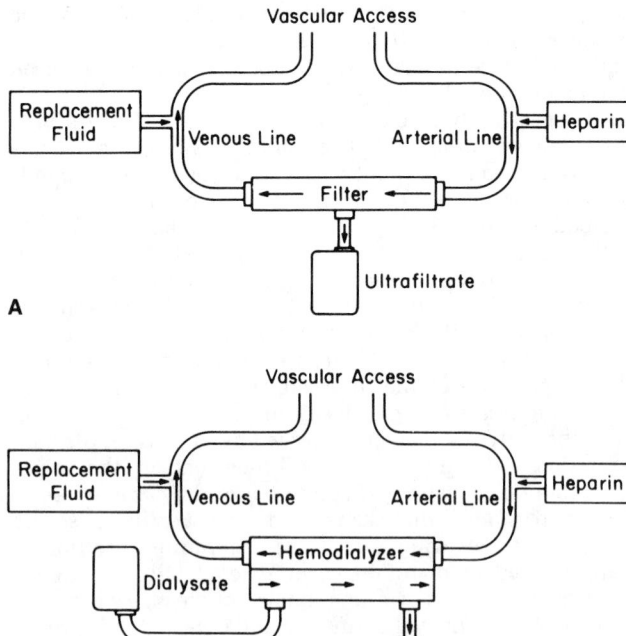

Vascular Access

A

Vascular Access

B

Figure 40-8. Schematic representation of (*A*) continuous arteriovenous hemofiltration (CAVH) and (*B*) continuous arteriovenous hemodialysis (CAVHD). (Reproduced with permission from Nahman NS, Middendorf DF: Continuous arteriovenous hemofiltration. Med Clin North Am 74:977, 1990.)

capacity for removing salt and water, CAVH has been used to permit full-calorie, high-protein nutritional support of critically ill patients.[89] Critically ill patients have also undergone CAVH as part of the treatment for acute renal failure associated with sepsis[90] and to speed removal of fluid in noncardiac pulmonary edema.[91] Continuous arteriovenous hemodialysis (CAVHD), a modification of CAVH, adds the capacity for diffusive transport to the convective transport achieved by CAVH (see Fig. 40-8).[89,92-94]

Table 40-6 lists the relative indications for and limitations of hemodialysis, peritoneal dialysis, CAVH, and CAVHD.

TABLE 40-7. Complications of Dialysis and Ultrafiltration

Central nervous system
  Disequilibrium syndrome
  Dialysis dementia
  Progressive intellectual dysfunction
Cardiovascular system
  Hypotension
Respiratory system
  Hypoxemia
Neuromuscular
  Cramping
Nutritional
  Protein depletion
  Hyperglycemia
  Peritonitis

Physiologic Effects and Complications of Dialysis and Ultrafiltration

In most instances, renal replacement therapy improves the profound physiologic abnormalities induced by renal failure, *i.e.*, fluid overload, pericarditis, electrolyte abnormalities, coagulopathy, and uremic encephalopathy. However, despite major advances over the past 25 years, the complications of hemodialysis, peritoneal dialysis, CAVH, and CAVHD still represent problems in the management of patients with acute or chronic renal failure.[95,96] The most important physiologic effects and complications of renal replacement therapy involve the central nervous system, the cardiovascular system, the respiratory system, the striated musculature, and nutritional status (Table 40-7).

Central Nervous System Effects

The disequilibrium syndrome is an uncommon but potentially severe complication of acute hemodialysis.[97] Predisposing factors include severe azotemia (blood urea nitrogen concentration greater than 150 mg·dl^{-1}), hypernatremia, profound acidemia, and pre-existing brain disease. The syndrome may be mild or may progress to stupor, coma, and seizures. Proposed mechanisms for the syndrome include transient cerebral intracellular hypertonicity and cerebral

TABLE 40-6. Selection of Renal Replacement Therapy

	Indications	Limitations
Hemodialysis	Rapid catabolism Severe volume, electrolyte, or acid-base disorders	Hypotension Anticoagulation risk Need for vascular access
Peritoneal dialysis	Lower cost Anticoagulation risk Difficult vascular access Hypotension Infants and small children	Rapid catabolism Diaphragmatic defects Severe volume, electrolyte, or acid-base disorders
CAVH	Hemodynamic instability Inexpensive equipment	Rapid catabolism Severe volume, electrolyte, or acid-base disorders Constant supervision
CAVHD	Hemodynamic instability Inexpensive equipment	Constant supervision

intracellular acidosis.[97] Management is primarily preventive, that is, the avoidance of rapid simultaneous reduction of urea and sodium concentrations in high-risk patients.

Dialysis dementia, another central nervous system complication of hemodialysis, occurs in a small number of patients. Fraser and Arieff[97] list three forms of dialysis dementia: sporadic, epidemic, and the type associated with pediatric renal disease. Elimination of aluminum from the dialysate has been associated with a gradual clearance of symptoms in some but not in all patients.[97] Dialysis dementia does not appear to be due to abnormalities of cerebral perfusion.[98]

Cardiovascular Effects

Symptomatic hypotension complicates 25% of individual hemodialysis treatments.[99] Critically ill septic patients are particularly prone to develop hypotension during dialysis.[100] Hypotension appears to result from a combination of decreased intravascular volume and impaired compensatory responses to hypovolemia. Intravascular volume is certainly reduced by dialysis, although mobilization of interstitial fluid into plasma volume can help to offset dialytic losses. Hemofiltration alone (performed using a conventional dialysis machine) produces a similar reduction in volume but less hypotension than hemodialysis.[101] During hemodialysis, the vasoconstrictor response often cannot adequately compensate for reductions in plasma volume and cardiac output. In healthy persons, mild plasma volume reduction results in venoconstriction; if hypovolemia is more severe, the venoconstriction is followed by the catecholamine-induced effects of arterial constriction and increased myocardial contractility. In contrast, uremic patients appear to have defective carotid and aortic body reflex arcs.[102] Peripheral resistance declines during hemodialysis despite a decreased pulmonary capillary wedge pressure and hypotension.[103] The impairment of compensatory vasoconstriction may be owing to the presence of acetate in the dialysate, which is hepatically metabolized to bicarbonate and is added to dialysate to replace bicarbonate consumed by buffering unexcreted hydrogen ions. As a vasodilator, acetate interferes with reflex vasoconstriction.[104] Replacement of acetate with bicarbonate in the dialysate reduces hemodynamic instability, especially in critically ill septic patients.[104,105]

Dialysis with either acetate or bicarbonate modestly improves left ventricular function,[106,107] most markedly in those patients in whom predialysis ventricular function is impaired.[108] Increasing the calcium concentration of dialysate from 5.5 to 7.5 $mg \cdot dl^{-1}$ improves left ventricular function and produces substantially higher intradialytic blood pressure.[109]

The management of hemodialysis-induced hypotension is based on maneuvers designed to decrease the rapidity and magnitude of plasma volume reduction. Transfusion sufficient to maintain a hematocrit higher than 20 $ml \cdot dl^{-1}$ may decrease the incidence of hypotension.[77] Leg elevation, intravenous fluid administration, and, occasionally, vasoconstrictors can be used for the short-term management of hypotension. When hypotension remains a persistent problem despite these maneuvers, substitution of bicarbonate for acetate in the dialysate often permits adequate dialytic therapy, even in patients with underlying hemodynamic instability.[100] In general, hypotension occurs less commonly during peritoneal dialysis and CAVH than during hemodialysis.

Respiratory System Effects

Dialytic therapy produces a complex, incompletely understood series of changes in Pa_{O_2}, Pa_{CO_2}, pH, and $[HCO_3^-]$. Although oxygenation may improve as hypervolemia is resolved,[110,111] hemodialysis more commonly results in hypoxemia. Two general mechanisms may contribute to hypoxemia during hemodialysis: ventilation-perfusion mismatch and hypoventilation.

Because neutropenia consistently occurs shortly after the initiation of hemodialysis,[112] some investigators have attempted to explain hypoxemia on the basis of ventilation-perfusion mismatch secondary to leukocyte-mediated pulmonary dysfunction.[113] However, more precise measurements suggest that during dialysis, the alveolar-arterial oxygen gradient remains unchanged.[112,114,115] These data support the hypothesis, first proposed by Aurigemma and colleagues,[116] that patients may hypoventilate during hemodialysis without becoming hypercarbic because CO_2 is lost across the dialyzer membrane.[115] The attendant decrease in Pa_{O_2} can be explained in terms of the alveolar gas equation:

$$PA_{O_2} = PI_{O_2} - \frac{Pa_{CO_2}}{RE}$$

where PA_{O_2} = alveolar oxygen tension, PI_{O_2} = $FI_{O_2} \times$ (barometric pressure − 47), Pa_{CO_2} = arterial carbon dioxide tension, and RE = CO_2 excretion by the lung divided by oxygen consumption.

Under circumstances other than hemodialysis, RE equals the respiratory quotient (RQ), which is CO_2 production divided by oxygen consumption. However, when dialysis proceeds against a bath containing acetate, CO_2 is both excreted by the lung and transported through the dialyzer membrane into the dialysate. Therefore, CO_2 excretion by the lung becomes less than CO_2 production, thereby decreasing RE and necessarily decreasing Pa_{O_2} if the $P(A-a)_{O_2}$ remains the same. The decrement in Pa_{O_2} is similar in patients with and without chronic obstructive pulmonary disease.[117]

Hypoxemia during hemodialysis is easily treated by increasing the inspired oxygen concentration. In reference to the alveolar gas equation, as FI_{O_2} increases, the term by which Pa_{CO_2} is multiplied progressively decreases toward one, regardless of the value of the RQ (or RE). In rare cases, bicarbonate rather than acetate dialysis may be necessary. Occasionally, a less rapid rate of plasma volume reduction may be used if a decrease in cardiac output is contributing to hypoxemia through the production of a lower mixed venous oxygen content.

During peritoneal dialysis, hypoxemia occurs if upward displacement of the diaphragm is poorly tolerated or if fluid traverses the diaphragm. Hypoxemia seldom occurs during CAVH or CAVHD.

Muscular Complications

Skeletal muscle cramping occasionally complicates hemodialysis but rarely occurs during other forms of renal replacement therapy. Because approximately 30% of dialysis procedures are associated with skeletal muscle cramping if the dialysate contains only 130 $mEq \cdot l^{-1}$ of sodium,[77] clinicians often prefer to dialyze against a bath containing a higher sodium concentration (132–140 $mEq \cdot l^{-1}$). When skeletal muscle cramping does occur, treatment consists of slowing the rate of reduction of serum sodium concentration and intravascular volume.

Nutritional Complications

Disease processes that produce chronic or acute renal failure are associated with nutritional depletion. Dietary restriction may produce a tasteless diet, leading to a decrease in nutritional intake. Patients with acute renal failure frequently have severe catabolic illnesses. Hemodialysis, CAVH, and CAVHD produce few additional nutritional complications. To a limited extent, amino acids are lost into the dialysate during hemodialysis, and some filtration of amino acids presumably occurs during CAVH and CAVHD. Usually, however, nutritional status improves during dialysis, because removal of excess fluid permits more aggressive nutritional support.

In contrast, peritoneal dialysis may actually result in an increase in caloric intake because of absorption of dextrose from the dialysate.[118] However, peritoneal dialysis induces marked protein losses into the dialysate.[81] Peritonitis, a frequent complication of peritoneal dialysis, further increases protein wasting.[85] Although the losses do not preclude effective peritoneal dialytic therapy, they do produce hypoalbuminemia and have been implicated in immunocompromise. In order to prevent progressive protein loss, patients undergoing peritoneal dialysis should consume 1.5 g·kg^{-1}·day^{-1} of protein.

ANESTHETIC MANAGEMENT OF THE PATIENT WITH CHRONIC RENAL FAILURE

Preoperative Evaluation

A comprehensive preoperative evaluation of overall physiologic reserve should include an assessment of renal function.[67,119] Renal function tests are influenced not only by intrinsic renal disease but also by intravascular and extracellular volume, by cardiovascular function, and by neuroendocrine factors. The greater the magnitude and duration of the expected surgical insult, the greater the likelihood of perioperative renal compromise and the greater the urgency of adequate preoperative identification of risk. The choice of monitoring devices and of anesthetic techniques depends upon these factors.

Unfortunately, there is no simple, inexpensive test that adequately quantifies renal function. The readily available tests fail to accurately reflect the status of the kidneys in a large percentage of patients, especially the elderly, the malnourished, and the dehydrated (Table 40-8). The commonly obtained tests of renal function include urinalysis and determination of blood urea nitrogen (BUN), serum creatinine, and creatinine clearance. The urinalysis provides qualitative information that must be cautiously interpreted. Hematuria (more than one to two red blood cells per high-power field in a concentrated sediment) suggests glomerular disease or, in a trauma patient, injury to the kidneys or the lower urinary tract. Pyuria (more than four white blood cells per high-power field) suggests urinary tract infection. Although urine may normally contain hyaline and granular casts, cellular casts represent a pathologic finding. Red blood cell casts indicate active glomerulonephritis, whereas white blood cell casts suggest interstitial nephritis, including pyelonephritis. Urinary pH, although difficult to interpret on a spot urine sample, may assist in the diagnosis of some acid-base disturbances. The presence of proteinuria on a routine dipstick examination may be "normal" or it may suggest severe renal disease. In a concentrated urine

sample, trace or 1+ proteinuria is a nonspecific finding, whereas 3+ or 4+ proteinuria suggests glomerular disease.

Both BUN and serum creatinine levels offer rapid but inexact estimates of creatinine clearance. The actual measurement of creatinine clearance constitutes the best overall indicator of GFR. However, all three measurements require careful interpretation. A product of protein metabolism, BUN is increased by high-protein intake, blood in the gastrointestinal tract, and accelerated catabolism (e.g., as occurs in traumatized or septic patients). The normal range is between 8.0–20 mg·dl^{-1}. Because urea is synthesized in the liver, hepatic dysfunction decreases urea production and, therefore, BUN concentration. Most important, BUN fails a key criterion as a reliable estimate of GFR. Although urea is freely filtered at the glomerulus, it is reabsorbed to a large and variable extent. The reabsorption of urea is greater (approximately 60% of the filtered load) when urinary flow is low; in comparison, only about 40% is reabsorbed when flow is high.

Creatinine, a product of skeletal muscle protein catabolism, is produced at a lower rate in elderly than in young adults and in females than in males. Consequently, serum creatinine levels may fail to accurately reflect the magnitude of nephron loss. Similarly, patients with muscle wasting from chronic disease may manifest misleadingly low serum creatinine measurements. In contrast, heavily muscled or acutely catabolic patients may have serum creatinine values greater than the normal range (0.5–1.5 mg·dl^{-1}) because of more rapid muscle breakdown.

Combining the evaluation of BUN and serum creatinine may provide more information than either alone. If the BUN:serum creatinine ratio exceeds the normal upper limit of 20:1, dehydration or one of the individual factors that alters the serum concentration of the two metabolites should be suspected.

Measurements of creatinine clearance are superior to BUN or serum creatinine alone or to the combination for the quantification of renal reserve. Creatinine clearance often is estimated using the equation:

$$GFR = \frac{(140 - age)wt^*}{72 \times serum\ creatinine}$$

where wt = weight in kilograms. However, that estimate is subject to the same limitations as the measurement of serum creatinine. Precise measurements of creatinine clearance require collection of timed urine samples, using the following formula:

$$GFR = \frac{UV}{P}$$

where U = urinary concentration of creatinine (mg·dl^{-1}), V = volume of urine (ml·min^{-1}), and P = plasma concentration (mg·dl^{-1}).

Although 24-hour specimens are usually used, a 2-hour sample, collected through a urinary catheter, provides acceptable accuracy (Fig. 40-9).[120] Varying hydration of the patient invalidates short-term determinations of GFR,[121,122] as does failure to accurately record urinary volume.[123]

The preoperative evaluation of patients with chronic renal failure should include consideration of the physiologic problems associated with loss of renal function and the adequacy of recent dialytic therapy in addition to the usual

---

*Multiplied by 0.8 for women.

TABLE 40-8. Preoperative Assessment, Renal Function

Test	Normal Range	Limitations
BUN	8–20 mg·dl^{-1}	Dehydration Variable protein intake Gastrointestinal bleeding Catabolic state
SCr	0.5–1.2 mg·dl^{-1}	Advanced age Muscle mass Catabolic state
CCr (estimated)*	120 ml·min^{-1}	Advanced age Muscle mass Catabolic state
CCr (measured)†	120 ml·min^{-1}	Weight-dependency Inaccurate urine volume measurement

SCr = serum creatinine; CCr = creatinine clearance.

* Using the formula:

$$CCr = \frac{(140 - age)wt}{72 \times SCr}$$

where weight is given in kilograms; multiplied by 0.8 for women.

† Using the formula:

$$CCr = \frac{UV}{P}$$

where U = urinary creatinine concentration, V = urinary volume, and P = plasma creatinine concentration.

history, physical examination, and laboratory evaluation. Questioning a patient about exercise tolerance can be as important as knowing the absolute hemoglobin concentration in determining whether to transfuse red blood cells preoperatively. Information regarding a patient's usual and recent weight may provide insights into nutritional status or recent fluid gain. Dialysis is usually advisable shortly before anesthesia and surgery. Blood transfusion, if necessary, can proceed during dialysis without adding to the patient's intravascular volume. Because renal failure produces neuropathy and decreases gastric emptying, a premedicant that decreases gastric pH and volume may prove beneficial. Usually, premedication with sedatives or opioids should be given in a reduced dose because of the possibility of exaggerated effects.

Intraoperative Management

Monitoring

The selection of monitoring techniques for patients with diminished or absent renal function should be based on the same physiologic considerations as would be appropriate if the same patient were to undergo nonrenal surgery (Table 40-9). Frequent recording of the blood pressure and continuous recording of the body temperature, heart rate, and electrocardiogram are essential. Electrocardiography allows early detection of hyperkalemia. Since in the presence of chronic anemia a further reduction in oxygen delivery ow-

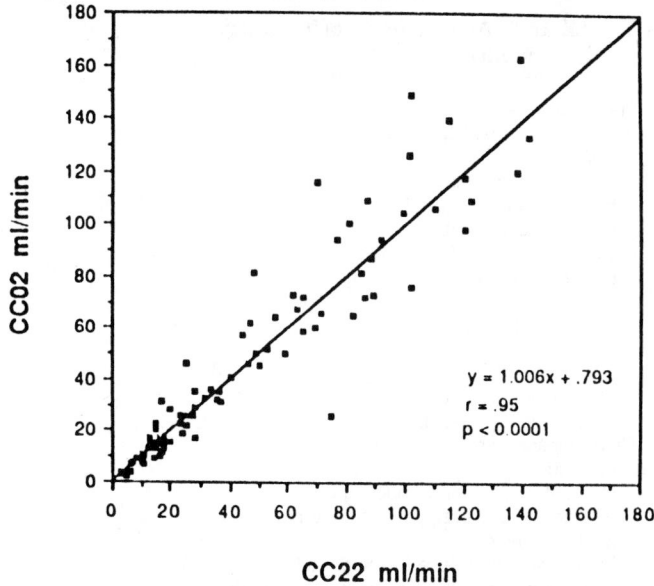

2 vs. 22 hr Creatinine Clearance

$y = 1.006x + .793$
$r = .95$
$p < 0.0001$

CC02 ml/min

CC22 ml/min

Figure 40-9. Correlation between the 2-hour creatinine clearance (CC02) and 22-hour creatinine clearance (CC22). (Reproduced with permission from Sladen RN, Endo E, Harrison T: Two-hour versus 22-hour creatinine clearance in critically ill patients. Anesthesiology 67:1015, 1987.)

ing to hypoxemia could be extremely hazardous, pulse oximetry is especially desirable. Capnometry may also be valuable. Because of the chronic metabolic acidosis present in many patients with chronic renal failure, hypercarbia will reduce pH to a greater extent than in a patient with normal bicarbonate levels. Acid-base assessment provides sensitive information regarding superimposition of additional disturbances in these fragile patients. The decision to use an arterial or a pulmonary artery catheter depends on the patient's functional cardiac reserve and the severity of hypertension. These devices may facilitate evaluation of the status of cardiac performance, intravascular volume, and venous capacitance. In the future, the further development of continuous monitors of blood pressure and cardiac output may simplify monitoring decisions. Additionally, vascular access ports such as shunts and fistulas must be identified and protected, because malfunction may occur as a consequence of diminished flow in the perioperative period. The patient's extremities should be well padded.

Perioperative fluid management must take into account the inability of the kidney to excrete excess sodium and water, including water produced by catabolic body processes. Nevertheless, relative hypovolemia, combined with intraoperative vasodilation and cardiac depressants, results in organ hypoperfusion and frank hypotension. If necessary intraoperative fluid administration increases intravascular volume to a level that is unsatisfactory in the postoperative period, or if acid-base or electrolyte problems develop intraoperatively, dialysis can be repeated in the immediate postoperative period.

Selection of Anesthetic Agents

Formulation of a satisfactory intraoperative anesthetic plan for a renal failure patient requires an understanding of pharmacology and the judicious use of anesthetic drugs. The action and elimination of several anesthetic and nonanesthetic drugs can affect a patient's perioperative course.

TABLE 40-9. Anesthetic Considerations for the Anephric Patient

Preoperative evaluation
  Adequacy of dialytic therapy
    Volume status
    Acid-base status
  Hemoglobin concentration
  Cardiovascular status
Monitoring
  Blood pressure
  Heart rate
  Electrocardiogram
  Pulse oximeter
  Capnometer
  Peripheral nerve stimulator
  Invasive cardiovascular monitoring as needed
Fluid management
  Cautious
  No contraindication to packed red blood cells
  If necessary, dialyze patient postoperatively
Anesthetic choice
  Lower induction dose of thiopental
  Exaggerated response to benzodiazepines
  Prolonged morphine effect
  Avoid succinylcholine if serum K^+ exceeds 6.0 mEq·l^{-1}
  Delayed excretion of pancuronium, d-tubocurarine
  Prolonged effect of anticholinesterase agents

Intravenous Agents. Because renal failure reduces protein binding, highly protein-bound drugs may cause exaggerated and prolonged effects. For example, intravenous administration of short-acting barbiturates (with a high affinity for protein) to renal failure patients leads to a larger fraction of unbound, bioavailable drug.[124] In addition, the acidemic pH of renal failure increases the proportion of thiopental circulating in the non-ionized, unbound form, the state in which tissue availability, particularly to the brain, is greatest. Further, uremia alters the blood-brain barrier, which increases the sensitivity to intravenous induction agents such as thiopental. Hence, uremic patients require a lower dose of thiopental for the induction of anesthesia.[125] However, thiopental clearance, after adjusting for the altered protein binding, volume of distribution, and tissue binding, is similar in patients with and without renal failure. Although the initial dose should be lower and given more cautiously than in patients with normal renal function, the same total dose of short-acting barbiturate induction agents may be necessary.[126]

Because ketamine and the benzodiazepines are less heavily protein-bound than the barbiturates, induction doses require less alteration. Ketamine frequently increases blood pressure and cardiac output, effects that may aggravate pre-existing hypertension. Benzodiazepines, given in doses that usually exert minimal respiratory or cardiovascular effects, may profoundly affect a generally debilitated renal failure patient.

Morphine-induced respiratory depression is prolonged in some renal failure patients.[127] However, careful pharmacokinetic studies demonstrate that the elimination half-life and clearance of morphine are no different in patients with and without renal failure.[128,129] Hepatic glucuronidation by glucuronyl transferase represents the major route of morphine biotransformation. Very little unchanged morphine undergoes urinary excretion, and patients with and without renal disease have similar morphine plasma concentrations.[130] Morphine glucuronides alone can cause analgesia and respiratory depression.[128,129] Therefore, the increased accumulation of morphine glucuronides accounts for the prolonged respiratory depression observed in patients with renal failure.

The elimination of fentanyl is also largely accomplished through hepatic metabolism, with subsequent renal excretion of metabolites. Whether renal failure can cause prolonged narcosis as a result of metabolite activity remains unclear. In theory, low doses of fentanyl should represent a good analgesic choice because rapid tissue redistribution should preserve the short duration of action observed in normal persons. Despite an individual case report of prolonged respiratory depression after administration of sufentanil to a patient with chronic renal failure,[131] the clearance of sufentanil appears to be similar in patients with normal renal function and those with chronic renal failure.[132,133] However, clearance may be more variable among patients with chronic renal failure.[134] Alfentanil appears to be pharmacokinetically and pharmacodynamically similar in patients with renal insufficiency and normal individuals.[135,136]

Inhalational Anesthetics. Unlike the intravenous drugs, elimination of inhalation anesthetics does not rely on adequate renal function, although to varying degrees biotransformation may produce renally excreted metabolites. Inhalation agents with low blood gas solubility coefficients, such as desflurane and nitrous oxide, may permit quicker recovery and return of ventilatory and cognitive functions. In addition, inhalation agents can be administered without nitrous oxide, permitting high inspired oxygen concentrations. To a limited extent, this may offset the decrease in arterial oxygen content resulting from anemia. Although the direct nephrotoxicity of some of the inhalation agents restricts their selection for patients with remaining renal function, avoidance of nephrotoxic agents is not a major consideration in dialysis-dependent renal failure. Potent inhalation agents may also facilitate neuromuscular blockade, thereby allowing lower doses of neuromuscular blockers.

Neuromuscular Blocking Agents. Succinylcholine, administered to normal patients, transiently increases serum potassium by approximately 0.5 mEq·l^{-1}. Serum potassium levels increase similarly in response to succinylcholine in patients who have renal failure.[137] Renal failure is not associated with the dramatic increases in serum potassium values that lead to serious cardiac dysrhythmias in patients with burns, trauma, and neuromuscular disease. Uremic patients with normal serum potassium levels can receive succinylcholine; however, if the potassium concentration is already elevated, an additional increase of 0.5–0.7 mEq·l^{-1} may be sufficient to induce cardiac dysrhythmias. If life-threatening cardiac dysrhythmias occur, the general debility of chronic renal failure patients may then render resuscitation more difficult. Serum cholinesterase levels appear adequate in renal failure patients, whether or not they are undergoing dialysis.[138] Repeated doses of succinylcholine in these patients do not incrementally elevate serum potassium levels or prolong muscle relaxation.

Historically, most nondepolarizing muscle relaxants have had a prolonged elimination half-life in patients with chronic renal failure because they have been primarily excreted through the kidneys. Some clinicians have preferred d-tubocurarine to pancuronium, metocurine, and gallamine in uremic patients, since d-tubocurarine's elimination half-life is less prolonged. Chronic renal failure increases the duration of action of d-tubocurarine slightly in the low-dose range and considerably at higher doses.[139] Although evidence suggests that renal failure accelerates the onset of neuromuscular blockade with d-tubocurarine, this effect is probably not secondary to changes in plasma protein binding because binding is approximately 40% in both normal and renal failure patients.[140]

The intermediate-duration nondepolarizing muscle relaxants qualify as suitable adjunctive agents in patients with chronic renal failure. Atracurium has an elimination half-life of less than 30 minutes in patients with and without renal failure.[141] There is little, if any, difference between patients with normal renal function and those with renal impairment with respect to pharmacokinetics and pharmacodynamics of atracurium. Ester hydrolysis and Hoffmann elimination, neither of which depend upon renal function, clear atracurium from the blood. Similarly, renal disease causes little alteration of the duration of action of single doses of vecuronium.[142-145] However, lower doses of vecuronium are required for maintenance in patients with end-stage renal disease than in normal individuals.[146] The tendency toward accumulation of vecuronium in patients with renal failure suggests that caution should be employed when the drug is used in such patients.[147] Because they have a shorter duration of action than d-tubocurarine, atracurium and vecuronium are more easily titrated in fragile patients.

The two new long-acting muscle relaxants, doxacurium and pipecuronium, have been studied in patients with normal and absent renal function. Doxacurium has a signifi-

cantly prolonged duration of action in patients with renal failure.[148] In contrast, the average duration of action of pipecuronium is not prolonged; however, the more variable duration of action suggests that pipecuronium may be less appropriate for use in such patients than the intermediate-acting muscle relaxants.[149]

Neostigmine, pyridostigmine, and edrophonium, three anticholinesterase agents commonly used to reverse nondepolarizing muscle relaxants, undergo elimination primarily through the kidney; therefore renal failure prolongs their duration of action at least 100%.[150-152] Thus, these agents effectively counteract the lingering nondepolarizing effects of d-tubocurarine in renal failure patients, making recurarization theoretically unlikely. Anticholinesterase reversal of atracurium or vecuronium seems especially safe because the duration of action of these neuromuscular blockers is not prolonged.

Despite the longer half-lives of the anticholinesterases, the clinician must consider several other factors that contribute to the ease of reversal of neuromuscular blockade, such as temperature, the depth of the blockade, the acid-base status, and the concomitant use of potentiating drugs such as diuretics or antibiotics. Because of the marked variability among patients, clinical assessment of depth of neuromuscular blockade should be supplemented by the use of a peripheral nerve stimulator to quantitate the response to train-of-four and tetanic stimulation.

ACUTE RENAL FAILURE

Incidence

Acute renal failure (ARF) is a frequently lethal, distressingly common complication of critical surgical illness. Perioperative ARF accounts for one half of all patients requiring acute dialysis.[153] Despite the rapid development of sophisticated techniques to replace renal function over the past 25 years, ARF is still associated with a mortality in excess of 50%.[154-156] Even intensive dialytic therapy, once thought to improve outcome in comparison with less aggressive dialysis,[157] appears to produce no significant benefit in patients with ARF.[158]

Mild to moderate renal dysfunction is surprisingly common after surgery. Charlson et al studied renal function after nonemergency general, vascular, or gynecologic surgery in 278 patients, 76% of whom had hypertension and 38% of whom had diabetes.[159] Within the first 6 postoperative days, 65 of 278 patients demonstrated an increase of serum creatinine level ≥20%. Thirty-two of seventy-eight patients had increases that were sustained for ≥48 hours; in half of those patients, creatinine clearance had not returned to baseline levels by the time of discharge. In 9 of 32 patients, renal function continued to deteriorate, although only 2 developed frank ARF. The risk of suffering a 20% increase in serum creatinine level was greatest on the first postoperative day, after which it rapidly declined (Fig. 40-10).[159]

Acute elevations of BUN and serum creatinine occur in approximately 5% of all general hospital admissions and in up to 20% of intensive care unit patients. In traumatized patients, the risk of ARF increases as the severity and number of injuries increase. Cardiovascular surgery (e.g., valvular heart surgery, coronary artery bypass grafting, and aortic aneurysm repair) is now the most common etiology of postoperative ARF.[160] Vascular surgical procedures threaten renal perfusion because of extensive tissue manipulation, loss of plasma volume into the interstitium, and variable and

A

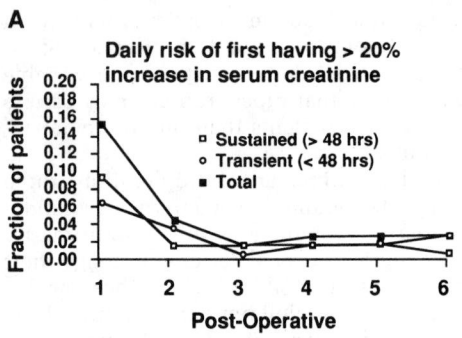

Daily risk of first having > 20% increase in serum creatinine

□ Sustained (> 48 hrs)
○ Transient (< 48 hrs)
■ Total

Post-Operative

B

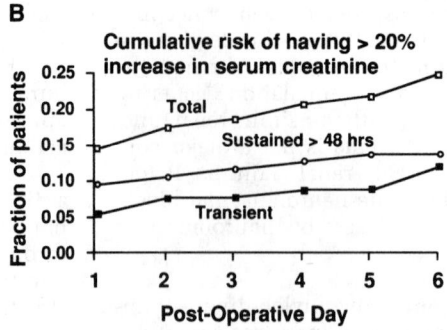

Cumulative risk of having > 20% increase in serum creatinine

Total
Sustained > 48 hrs
Transient

Post-Operative Day

Figure 40-10. Postoperative risk of developing an increase in serum creatinine > 20%; daily risk (*A*) and cumulative risk (*B*). Overall, 65 of 278 patients developed such an increase. (Reproduced with permission from Charlson ME, MacKenzie CR, Gold JP: Postoperative changes in serum creatinine. When do they occur and how much is important. Ann Surg 209:330, 1989.)

sometimes massive hemorrhage. Aortic and renal vascular procedures also reduce renal perfusion[161,162] as a result of suprarenal or infrarenal aortic cross-clamping or temporary renal artery occlusion.

In patients who undergo thoracic aortic cross-clamping, the incidence of ARF is 2.7–13.8%,[163-165] whereas less severe renal dysfunction occurs in 50% of patients.[164] After infrarenal aortic cross-clamping, 15% of patients develop an increase ≥ 0.5 mg·dl^{-1} in serum creatinine level.[166] Of 47 patients who developed ARF after aortic aneurysm surgery, 79% died, 15% regained renal function, and the remainder required chronic hemodialysis.[160] Although aggressive medical management of patients with ARF after repair of ruptured abdominal aortic aneurysms has been associated with improved survival in some small series,[167] larger series report poor survival,[168] most commonly as a consequence of infection related to the necessity for prolonged intensive physiologic and nutritional support.

ARF also occurs frequently in patients undergoing extensive nonvascular abdominal procedures,[169] in patients with hepatic insufficiency, and in patients with sepsis or volume depletion. McMurray et al[168] reported that gastrointestinal surgery was responsible for 32% of postoperative ARF. Ten to fifty percent of intensive care unit patients suffering from respiratory failure, sepsis, or hepatic failure develop ARF; the majority of those affected succumb.

Pathophysiology

Oliguria

Although ARF commonly develops without antecedent oliguria, the occurrence of intraoperative oliguria continues to represent an ominous sign in patients at risk for ARF. Oliguric states are conventionally defined as prerenal, renal, and postrenal. Prerenal refers to oliguria produced by hemodynamic or endocrine factors; renal refers to parenchymal disease; postrenal denotes obstructive oliguria. For reference purposes, oliguria usually is defined in acutely stressed patients as a urinary output of less than 0.5 ml·kg^{-1}·h^{-1}. This urinary volume (30 ml·h^{-1} on the average) exceeds that which defines oliguria in unstressed patients, i.e., 17 ml·kg^{-1}·h^{-1}. The higher limit is necessary in acutely stressed patients because many such patients are unable to maximally concentrate urine.

Prerenal Oliguria. The conditions producing prerenal oliguria include an acute reduction in GFR, an acute increase in

the reabsorption of salt and water, and both mechanisms acting in concert. Increased circulating levels of exogenous or endogenous alpha-adrenergic agonists, increased concentrations of ADH, and increased concentrations of aldosterone represent major systemic physiologic factors that can decrease urinary output. Frank hypotension need not occur for the production of severe prerenal oliguria. If not treated promptly, prerenal oliguria may progress to parenchymal renal failure.

Experience with military trauma convincingly demonstrates the crucial link between the severity (i.e., magnitude and duration) of prerenal insults and the subsequent development of parenchymal renal failure. In World War II, the overall incidence of ARF was 5% in all wounded combatants and 42% in those with severe wounds. During the Korean conflict, the overall incidence of ARF declined to 35% of severely wounded soldiers. The incidence further declined in the Vietnam War to 0.17% of those severely wounded.[169,170] Rapid, effective resuscitation and transport produced the improvement. For those wounded combatants who did develop ARF, the mortality decreased from 90% (World War II) to 53% (Korea) and 77% (Vietnam).[170] The introduction of dialytic therapy accounted for this decrease in mortality, an improvement of far less clinical importance than the dramatic reduction in incidence of ARF.

Renal Oliguria. ARF, frequently termed acute tubular necrosis, may be produced by a variety of factors that interfere with glomerular filtration and tubular reabsorption. The pathogenesis of ARF conventionally is divided into an initiation period, a maintenance period (Table 40-10), and a recovery period.[171]

Renal hypoperfusion, nephrotoxic insults, or both may initiate ARF. In surgical patients, hypoperfusion, produced by external or internal fluid loss or sepsis, constitutes a frequent cause. Experimental renal hypoperfusion, whether induced by intrarenal norepinephrine infusion or hemor-

TABLE 40-10. Pathogenesis of Acute Renal Failure

Initiation	Maintenance
Renal hypoperfusion	Tubular dysfunction
Hemodynamic factors	Tubular obstruction
Nephrotoxins	Decreased glomerular filtration
	Decreased renal blood flow

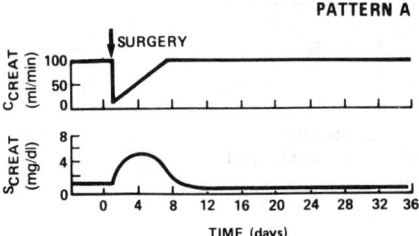

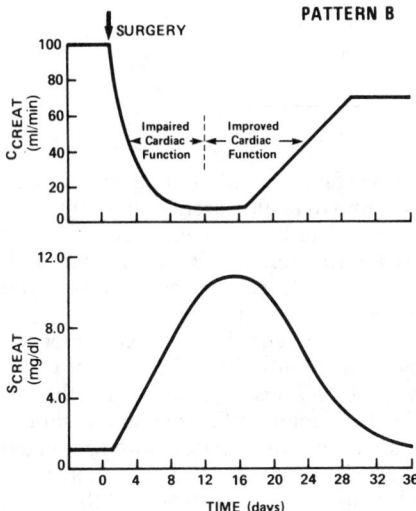

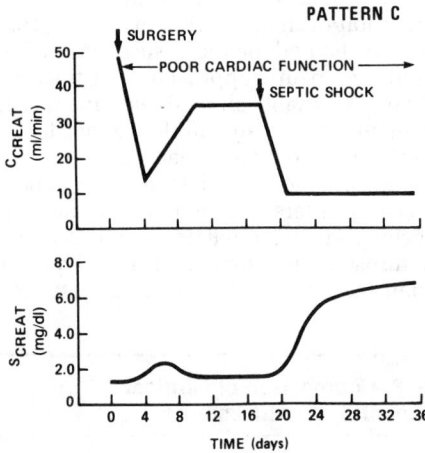

Figure 40-11. Three patterns of hemodynamically mediated ARF occur after major trauma or surgery. Pattern A (ARF) consists of acute reduction in creatinine clearance (C_{Creat}) with prompt recovery. Serum creatinine (s_{Creat}) may be increasing even as C_{Creat} recovers. Pattern B (overt ARF) consists of concurrent, mirror-image decreases in C_{Creat} and increases in S_{Creat}, usually in association with compromised cardiac function followed by recovery. Pattern C (protracted ARF) develops as a consequence of prolonged hemodynamic compromise, often complicated by systemic sepsis. (Reproduced with permission from Myers BD, Moran SM: Hemodynamically mediated acute renal failure. N Engl J Med 314:100, 1986.)

rhagic shock, impairs renal function in proportion to the depletion of high-energy phosphates.[172,173] One promising hypothesis states that the renal medulla, because of its low baseline flow, is particularly at risk for damage if total renal blood flow is reduced.[174]

The initiating insult ultimately culminates in the development of one or more of the maintenance factors (e.g., decreased tubular function, tubular obstruction, decreased glomerular filtration, and decreased renal blood flow) that reduce urine flow and osmolar excretion. Although decreased renal blood flow characterizes both the initiation and the maintenance phases of ARF, once the maintenance phase begins, pharmacologic improvement in renal blood flow will not reverse ARF. In contrast, the hemodynamic factors that initiate perioperative ARF often prove amenable to acute therapeutic intervention during the period when the anesthesiologist is directly responsible for the patient's welfare.

In general, improved management of acute prerenal oliguria has resulted in both a decreasing incidence of ARF and an increase in the proportion of patients with ARF who remain nonoliguric.[175] Myers and Moran[175] proposed a practical, clinical classification of hemodynamically mediated ARF, dividing it into abbreviated, overt, and protracted ARF on the basis of (1) the pattern of reduction in creatinine clearance and (2) the increase in serum creatinine level (Fig. 40-11). This classification is clinically pertinent because it emphasizes the role of secondary insults, such as sepsis, in protracted ARF. Sepsis often complicates the course of patients with protracted critical illness.[175,176] Myers and Moran's[175] classification emphasizes the frequency of nonoliguric ARF and provides a useful framework for grouping patients with similar prognoses.

Diagnostic Tests

Clinical investigators have expended considerable effort to develop tools to evaluate laboratory tests that could clearly differentiate prerenal from renal oliguria, predict the outcome of acute oliguric states, and direct therapy intended to prevent ARF. Unfortunately, none of the tools is sufficiently sensitive or specific to predict which patients will or will not respond to therapy. Consequently, the physician usually must treat the acutely oliguric patient without information that could accurately determine whether a patient has already developed or will develop ARF.

Table 40-11 summarizes typical laboratory findings in patients with prerenal and renal oliguria. Prerenal oliguria is

TABLE 40-11. Diagnostic Tests in Acute Oliguria

Test	Prerenal	Renal
Urine osmolality (mOsm·kg⁻¹)	>500	<350
Urine/plasma osmolality	>1.3	<1.1
Urine sodium (mEq·l⁻¹)	<20	>40
Urine/plasma urea	>8	<3
Urine/plasma creatinine	>40	<20
FENa (%)*	<1	>2

* FENa = fractional excretion of sodium, calculated as

$$\frac{U/P_{Na}}{U/P_{Cr}} \times 100$$

where U = urinary concentration, P = plasma concentration, Na = sodium, and Cr = creatinine.

TABLE 40-12. Characteristics of Urinary Diagnostic Tests in Oliguric Postoperative Patients

	Avid Water Conservation; Without Sodium Conservation (Normovolemic)	Avid Water and Sodium Conservation (Hypovolemic)
n	11	7
Urinary output (ml·h^{-1})	13 ± 2	17 ± 2
Urinary osmolality (mOsm·kg^{-1} H$_2$O)	522 ± 36	525 ± 34
Urinary Na$^+$ (mEq·l^{-1})	83 ± 12*	11 ± 2
FENa	1.15 ± 0.2*	0.15 ± 0.3

FENa = fractional excretion of sodium.

* $p < 0.05$ compared with hypovolemic group.

Reprinted with permission from Zaloga GP, Hughes SS: Oliguria in patients with normal renal function. Anesthesiology 72:598–602, 1990.

associated with physiologic mechanisms that conserve salt and water, resulting in excretion of waste products in a minimal volume of urine; therefore, patients with prerenal oliguria classically produce urine with high osmolality and low sodium. However, in patients with a chronic reduction in concentrating ability owing to pre-existing renal disease, urinary sodium and osmolality may not achieve "prerenal" values during acute prerenal insults. In addition, diuretics increase urinary sodium and decrease urinary osmolality.

In an effort to clarify ambiguous laboratory findings, several investigators have proposed the fractional excretion of sodium as a laboratory guide that can more accurately differentiate patients according to those with prerenal oliguria and those with renal oliguria. The fractional excretion of sodium is calculated by dividing the urine-to-plasma sodium ratio by the urine-to-plasma creatinine ratio, and then multiplying by 100.[177] Values less than 1% suggest prerenal azotemia. Despite early enthusiasm for this derived index, it is now apparent that it has limited diagnostic and prognostic use in the acute situation.[178,179] The most critical limitation of these derived indices is that they may suggest established parenchymal ARF at a time when hemodynamically mediated prerenal factors are still reversible. Moreover, these tests are unreliable in sodium-avid patients (those with liver failure, nephrotic syndrome, and cirrhosis) in whom urinary sodium levels may be low despite inexorably progressive renal failure.[180]

Recently, Zaloga and Hughes reported data suggesting that postoperative oliguria could result from avid water conservation in the absence of sodium conservation.[181] Of 100 prospectively studied patients admitted to a surgical intensive care unit, seven developed oliguria associated with increased urinary osmolality, low urinary sodium, and a fractional excretion of sodium well below 1.0%. Eleven patients, in contrast, developed a similar picture of oliguria and high urinary concentration but without evidence of sodium conservation and with calculated fractional excretion of sodium averaging 1.15 ± 0.2 (Table 40-12).[181]

Experimental *versus* Clinical Acute Renal Failure: Therapeutic Implications

Many therapeutic approaches to ARF have their origins in animal models that differ substantially from clinical ARF. The development of clinical ARF involves moderate-to-severe prerenal hemodynamic insults, often in combination with nephrotoxic factors, which progress over a highly variable period of time to acute parenchymal injury. In contrast, experimental renal failure is generated by very severe insults, usually administered over a short period of time. The differences between typical clinical and experimental ARF are summarized in Table 40-13.

At present, the most widely used experimental models of ARF employ a 40- to 60-minute interval of complete renal ischemia to produce a lesion physiologically and prognostically similar to human ARF. Ischemia of shorter duration does not cause reproducible ARF; more prolonged ischemia produces irreversible injury.[182] The majority of interventions proved to alleviate experimental ARF must be administered before or immediately after an ischemic insult, and their magnitude and duration must be precisely defined. Clinicians, in interpreting the results of such studies, must bear in mind that the clinical setting, in contrast to the animal laboratory, provides the opportunity to limit the magnitude and duration of the initiating insult by promptly providing adequate hemodynamic resuscitation. Table 40-14 lists potential therapeutic approaches for treating fixed experimental versus variable clinical renal insults. The potential management options are similar except for the critical role of effective hemodynamic management.

Most clinical approaches to the reduction of perioperative ARF are based on inferences from animal models of acute, norepinephrine-induced renal ischemia. Mannitol, dopamine, and furosemide promote urinary flow and reduce the renal damage produced by experimental renal ische-

TABLE 40-13. Comparison of Clinical and Experimental Renal Ischemia

Fixed Insult	Variable Insult
Animal Models	***Animal Models***
Complete renal ischemia	Profound hemorrhagic shock
Intrarenal norepinephrine	
Renal artery occlusion	***Clinical Models***
Nephrotoxin	Shock
Uranyl nitrate	Sepsis
	Multifactorial (often including
Clinical Insult	nephrotoxic antibiotics)
Complete surgical ischemia	
Suprarenal aortic cross-clamp	

TABLE 40-14. Treatment Strategies for Acute Renal Insults

Fixed Experimental Insult	Variable Clinical Insult

Increase solute excretion
  Mannitol[184-186]
  Furosemide[185,186]
  Dopamine[188,189]
Increase renal blood flow
  Mannitol[184-186]
  Furosemide[185,186]
  Dopamine[188,189]
Decrease substrate consumption
  Hypothermia[211]
Antagonize calcium entry
  Calcium entry blockers[212-214]
Antagonize free radicals[219,220]
Vasodilatory prostaglandins
  PGI_2[225]
  PGE_1[223,224]
  PGE_2[221,222]
Antagonize vasoconstrictor
  prostaglandins[227,228]
Enhance cellular metabolism
  Adenosine triphosphate-magnesium
    chloride[207,208]
  5' Nucleotidase[209]
  Fructose-1,6-diphosphate[210]
  Thyroxine[232]
	Limit magnitude and duration
	  Hemodynamic support
	Increase renal blood flow
	  Dopamine
	  Mannitol
	  Furosemide
	Increase solute excretion
	  Dopamine
	  Mannitol
	  Furosemide
	Decrease substrate consumption
	  Hypothermia
	Enhance cellular metabolism
	  Adenosine triphosphate-magnesium chloride

mia.[183-193] Mannitol improves renal cortical blood flow and may exert a renal cellular protective effect.[183-186] By maintaining high tubular flow, it may decrease the incidence and severity of ARF secondary to contrast media or pigmenturia. However, mannitol is ineffective in reversing profound reductions in GFR and renal blood flow induced by suprarenal aortic cross-clamping for 60 minutes in dogs.[187] Dopamine, used in doses of 1–3 $\mu g \cdot kg^{-1} \cdot min^{-1}$ to achieve selective renal vasodilation, increases renal cortical blood flow with minimal systemic effects.[188] Dopamine induces natriuresis, increases GFR, improves urinary flow,[188,189] and is a useful adjunct to the treatment of oliguria. Dopamine, like mannitol, is ineffective in reversing the renal injury produced by thoracic aortic cross-clamping.[187] Fenoldopam, a novel dopamine$_1$ receptor agonist, substantially enhances urinary flow, sodium excretion, and creatinine clearance while reducing systemic vascular resistance.[194-197] Although fenoldopam will likely become a valuable perioperative adjunct in the treatment of ARF, its precise role remains to be demonstrated.

Furosemide is effective in experimental models of complete renal ischemia,[185,186] although generally less effective than mannitol. Used by some clinicians in an attempt to convert established oliguric ARF to nonoliguric ARF, furosemide does not improve outcome or reduce the frequency of dialysis requirement.[190,193] In an effort to combine the potentially beneficial effects of both dopamine and furosemide, Lindner and colleagues infused both dopamine and furosemide in a canine model of nephrotoxic ARF and demonstrated a synergistic renal protective effect.[191] Subsequently, in an uncontrolled trial in a small group of patients who had oliguric ARF, the combination of furosemide and low-dose dopamine (1–3 $\mu g \cdot kg^{-1} \cdot min^{-1}$) resulted in production of a brisk diuresis and stabilization of renal function.[192] However, this has not been duplicated in a controlled, randomized trial.

In addition to the commonly discussed renal protective

effects of volume expansion and of mannitol, dopamine, and furosemide, a variety of agents demonstrate efficacy in experimental models of ARF. Perhaps effective pharmacologic therapy will be available within the decade. Numerous recent reviews address potential mechanisms that may lead to therapeutic progress.[198-203]

Because renal hypoperfusion reduces renal concentrations of high-energy phosphate,[173] one of the consequences of renal ischemia to which the thick ascending limb of Henle's loop may be most vulnerable,[174,204-206] infusion of adenine nucleotides in combination with magnesium chloride preserves experimental postischemic renal function.[207,208] Inhibition of 5'-nucleotidase similarly enhances metabolic and functional recovery following renal ischemia.[209] Infusion of fructose-1,6-diphosphate, a high-energy metabolite, also enhances the ability of the kidney to withstand ischemic injury.[210] Presumably, the renal protective effects of hypothermia are also dependent upon preservation of high-energy phosphate.[211]

Depletion of high-energy phosphates initiates a pathophysiologic sequence involving a variety of potentially toxic biochemical intermediates. In the kidneys, as in other organs, ischemia causes an increase in intracellular calcium ion. Pretreatment with calcium entry blockers limits renal injury produced by experimental complete renal ischemia,[212-214] although additional clinical evidence is necessary before calcium entry blockers can be added to management of patients who must undergo complete renal ischemia.[215] In partial renal ischemia, calcium entry blockers may produce salutary or deleterious effects, depending upon the magnitude of drug-induced blood pressure decline and the etiology of the renal hypoperfusion.[216-218]

Oxygen free radicals, arachidonate, leukotrienes, and neutrophils have also been implicated in ischemic renal damage. Oxygen free radicals appear to be produced in large quantities following renal ischemia,[219] an observation that may explain why superoxide dismutase or allopurinol reduces renal experimental ischemic injury when administered prophylactically.[220] Evidence suggests that renal vascular tone depends in part on the balance between the vasodilator prostaglandin (PG)I_2 and the vasoconstrictor thromboxane A_2. That balance may be disrupted by ischemic renal injury. The administration of exogenous vasodilator prostaglandins such as PGE_2,[221,222] PGE_1,[223,224] and PGI_2[225] reduces experimental injury. Leukotrienes, presumably derived from neutrophils, appear to partially mediate ischemic renal injury; neutrophil depletion improves postischemic renal function.[226] Inhibition of thromboxane A_2 synthesis protects against tubular necrosis following experimental ischemia in the rat.[227] Surprisingly, scavengers of oxygen free radicals also inhibit synthesis of thromboxane A_2 and improve renal outcome.[228] Clinically, selective antagonism of thromboxane A_2 synthesis improves renal function in patients with nephritis secondary to lupus erythematosus.[229]

A variety of other interventions, only a few of which are mentioned here, have also been used in experimental attempts to attenuate ARF. On the assumption that tubuloglomerular feedback is involved in the pathogenesis of renal ischemic injury, Koelz and colleagues administered enalapril, an angiotensin-converting enzyme inhibitor, to rats with renal ischemia and found no evidence of protection.[230] Sodium bicarbonate, administered before renal ischemia, partially attenuates the subsequent rise in serum creatinine levels in rats.[231] Pretreatment with thyroxine partially protects against experimental nephrotoxic ARF, possibly because of effects mediated at the level of the plasma membrane.[232] The phosphodiesterase inhibitor theophylline improves inulin clearance after renal ischemia or nephrotoxic myoglobinuric injury in rats.[233,234] The mechanism may be antagonism of the renal vasoconstrictor effects of endogenous adenosine. Pentoxifylline, both a phosphodiesterase inhibitor and a hemorrheologically active agent, also attenuates nephrotoxic ARF, although the mechanism is not known.[235] Finally, epidermal growth factor, an agent that accelerates replication of DNA, appears to accelerate recovery when administered following renal ischemia.[236]

Although a variety of agents appear to offer promise for amelioration of ARF, application in the clinical arena requires cumbersome clinical testing. Clinical ARF is more heterogeneous than experimental ARF, frequently involving elderly patients with reduced renal reserve and highly variable degrees of renal ischemia. Two experimental studies particularly emphasize the extent to which small differences in preischemic status could affect the subsequent course of ARF. Andrews and Bates demonstrated that protein intake in the weeks prior to renal ischemia profoundly affected renal function and survival in rats.[237] Rats maintained on no or low-protein diets survived, whereas those maintained on normal or high-protein diets before ischemia had a much higher mortality.[237] Postischemic protein ingestion did not affect recovery. Seguro and colleagues demonstrated that preischemic potassium depletion markedly accentuated renal injury secondary to ischemia.[238]

The clinician should avoid the uncritical application of results from animal studies of ARF to the clinical setting. Experimental data demonstrating the protective effects of dopamine, mannitol, and furosemide may not apply to clinical acute oliguria in which hypovolemia typically is an etiologic factor. The diuresis produced by any of these agents, singly or in combination, may further complicate hemodynamic management, thereby increasing the magnitude and the duration of the prerenal insult.[239] However, it can reasonably be concluded from experimental and clinical data that the addition of dopamine, mannitol, or furosemide to appropriate hemodynamic support and monitoring may improve the results beyond what could be obtained with hemodynamic management alone. The experimental demonstration of the renal protective effects of various pharmacologic intervention holds promise. However, the reduction in blood pressure associated with many potential interventions, such as calcium entry blockers, suggests that their clinical application may be limited to patients with ensured hemodynamic stability.

Comparison of Oliguric and Nonoliguric Acute Renal Failure

Nonoliguric ARF, once uncommon, now appears frequently. In contrast to oliguric ARF, nonoliguric ARF is somewhat easier to manage clinically, since it requires less scrupulous control of fluid and electrolyte intake. The first extensive clinical description of nonoliguric ARF stressed its lower mortality rate.[240] In that study, a larger percentage of patients with nonoliguric ARF had a nephrotoxic injury, whereas a larger group of oliguric patients had ARF in association with surgery, with prolonged volume depletion, or with impaired cardiac output. Therefore, it appears that nonoliguric ARF, occurring spontaneously in a hospitalized population, is associated with a lower mortality rate. Nonoliguric ARF occurring as a complication of trauma may also carry a better prognosis. Shin et al[241] reported on two consecutive groups (Groups 1 and 2) of trauma patients. In Group 2, more liberal fluid administration and less frequent diuretic administration increased the incidence of nonoliguric ARF and decreased the incidence of oliguric ARF in comparison with Group 1, which received fluid in lower volumes and underwent chemical diuresis more frequently. The mortality and morbidity in Group 2 were substantially less than in Group 1.[241]

Because ARF represents a syndrome that includes both oliguric patients and a heterogeneous group of nonoliguric patients, the accurate characterization and classification of clinical ARF should improve prognosis and treatment. Myers et al extensively studied hemodynamically mediated ARF in surgical patients, using a combination of clinical variables and creatinine kinetic modeling to describe the key pathogenetic features.[175,242-246] They defined three patterns (see Fig. 40-11). The first type, abbreviated ARF, is characterized by an abrupt decrement in creatinine clearance, followed by a steady improvement in renal function. The second type, overt ARF, represents a sustained prerenal insult, recovery from which is contingent upon hemodynamic improvement. Protracted ARF, the third type, represents the net effects of multiple episodes of renal injury. Prognostically, low mortality in abbreviated ARF and high mortality in protracted ARF can be anticipated.[175]

Because of the reported improved mortality and morbidity in patients with nonoliguric ARF, several investigators have attempted to convert established oliguric ARF to nonoliguric ARF using diuretic drugs with or without dopamine. Uncontrolled series emphasize the efficacy of induced diuresis.[192,247] However, controlled randomized trials have failed to demonstrate that conversion of oliguric ARF to nonoliguric ARF improves mortality, morbidity, the duration of renal failure, or the number of necessary dialyses.[190,193] In addition, direct intrarenal administration of furosemide (275 mg over 30 minutes) failed to improve renal function or renal blood flow in patients with ARF.[248] The aforementioned data support the conclusion that early, aggressive hemodynamic support of the patient with prerenal oliguria may produce a better outcome, even if nonoliguric ARF develops. Conversely, the chemical conversion of oliguric to nonoliguric ARF does not improve outcome.

Therapeutic Conflicts in the Management of Acute Oliguria

Effective treatment of oliguria requires not only an understanding of the effects of various therapeutic interventions on the kidney but also an assessment of the effects of those interventions on the lungs and the heart.

Kidney-Lung Therapeutic Conflicts

Aggressive expansion of intravascular volume, a common strategy in the hemodynamic management of prerenal oliguria, increases pulmonary microvascular pressure, thereby potentially increasing pulmonary edema. In a healthy person, clinical pulmonary edema occurs at a pulmonary microvascular pressure exceeding 25 mm Hg. However, in patients with decreased serum oncotic pressure or increased pulmonary capillary permeability, pulmonary edema may occur at lower pulmonary microvascular pressures.[249] Consequently, the clinician treating a patient with prerenal oliguria frequently confronts the question of whether to risk ARF or acute respiratory failure.[250] Approximately 40% of patients with ARF develop pulmonary complications.[251-253] Conversely, more than 50% of patients with the adult respiratory distress syndrome develop ARF.[254] In a broader cross-section of patients with respiratory failure resulting from a variety of medical and surgical illnesses, 11–33% develop ARF.[255,256]

In general, the argument in favor of sacrificing pulmonary function to save renal function rests on the ease with which mechanical ventilation can support the patient with deteriorating pulmonary function. One can defend this position by noting that the mortality from ARF ranges from 50–70%.[154,250] The counterargument, less often heard, states that it is better to sacrifice renal function, since dialysis can effectively support patients with acute ARF. One can defend this approach by noting that the mortality from adult respiratory distress syndrome also ranges from 50–70%.[257]

Certainly, in the course of providing hemodynamic support for the oliguric patient, the two extremes of frank hypovolemia and inappropriate overhydration should be avoided. However, the practical definition of these two terms presents a problem. In everyday terms, the pulmonary artery occlusion pressure, although imperfect, may be the best single estimate. In choosing an upper limit for the pulmonary artery occlusion pressure, the clinician decides which extreme to risk. The lower the limit, the greater the chance of inadequate resuscitation and the more frequent the need for inotropic support; the higher the pulmonary artery occlusion pressure limit, the greater the risk of pulmonary edema. Nevertheless, pulmonary edema does not occur simply because of fluid administration. For example, Shin et al[241] reported that post-traumatic respiratory failure occurred less often in patients receiving a greater amount of fluid and less frequent diuretics. More thorough resuscitation from shock may limit the pathophysiologic responses that produce adult respiratory distress syndrome.

Kidney-Heart Therapeutic Conflicts

Just as aggressive volume expansion may worsen pulmonary edema, so may it lead to increased left ventricular end-diastolic pressure and wall tension, thereby increasing myocardial oxygen consumption. Because left ventricular end-diastolic pressure limits left ventricular subendocardial perfusion, increases in filling pressure may also limit myocardial oxygen availability. The production of myocardial ischemia by aggressive volume loading represents a more subtle, less easily appreciated complication of volume resuscitation than does the production of pulmonary edema. Unfortunately, limiting volume expansion to a lower pulmonary artery occlusion pressure limit and using positive inotropic agents or vasodilators earlier in the course of hemodynamic resuscitation do not necessarily reduce the cardiac risk. Rather, positive inotropic agents, by increasing heart rate and myocardial contractility, may increase myocardial oxygen consumption. Vasodilators may precipitate sudden hypotension and myocardial ischemia, particularly if used in the setting of inadequate intravascular volume. However, when used with careful augmentation of intravascular volume, vasodilators such as nitroprusside may substantially improve both hemodynamic and renal function.[258]

Suggested Management

No specific guidelines exist that routinely and simultaneously produce the least compromise to the kidneys, lungs, and heart. Instead, therapy needs to be individualized, based on the apparent risk to each of the systems. Although we lack an easy "cookbook" approach to preventing the progression from acute prerenal oliguria to ARF, the following generalizations form the basis of a logical approach.

1. The most common cause of ARF is prolonged renal hypoperfusion.
2. The prevention of ARF reduces mortality more effectively than does dialytic therapy.
3. The duration and magnitude of the initiating renal insult are critical in determining the severity of ARF.

Based on those generalizations, the following strategies can be applied:

1. *Limit the magnitude and duration of renal ischemic insults that might initiate ARF.* This constitutes the key strategy in limiting the incidence of renal failure. In the majority of patients, oliguria signals inadequate systemic perfusion, and carefully monitored efforts to improve perfusion, including volume expansion, pulmonary artery catheterization, inotropic support (ideally with dopamine), and vasodilation, should be used.

However, oliguria and other monitors of intraoperative renal function are insufficiently sensitive and specific to detect hypoperfusion in all patients.[259] Moreover, several important studies of high-risk surgical patients[260-262] suggest that certain postoperative surgical complications, such as renal failure, hepatic failure, and sepsis, may result from unrecognized, subclinical tissue hypoperfusion during the immediate perioperative period. Average cardiac output (CO) and systemic oxygen transport ($CO \times CaO_2$) are greater in high-risk surgical patients who survive than in those who succumb to critical illness.[260,261] Therefore, Shoemaker et al adjusted hemodynamic therapy to achieve the higher values for CO and systemic oxygen delivery previously associated with improved survival.[262] In the first of two studies they compared conventional management of a control surgical group to a protocol that utilized hemodynamic values of previous survivors as goals for therapy. In the protocol group, in which cardiac output and oxygen delivery were elevated above control values as guided by pulmonary artery catheterization, survival was improved and complications were reduced.[262] The control group received conventional monitors, including a central venous pressure catheter. In a second study, combined with the first study for publication, an additional control group received conventional monitoring, supplemented by pulmonary artery catheterization without specific management guidelines. As in the first series, the protocol group demonstrated improved mortality and reduced complications. The control group that underwent pulmonary artery catheterization and treatment without specific hemodynamic goals had mortality and complication rates equal to those of the group managed without a pulmonary artery catheter.[262] These data suggest that aggressive, goal-directed hemodynamic support avoids clinically inapparent hypoperfusion and as a consequence limits the incidence of mortality and morbidity secondary to that process. Confirmation, however, is essential before this concept can be applied routinely. Figure 40-12 summarizes three possible approaches to prevention of ARF.

2. *Promote solute excretion.* When aggressive attempts to restore perfusion have failed to establish adequate urinary output, dopamine, mannitol, and/or furosemide should be added. Earlier use, although theoretically attractive, further compromises the value of urinary output as a monitor of the adequacy of resuscitation. No evidence exists that small "test" doses of diuretics decrease either morbidity or mortality in patients with uncertain volume status. At best, there is no effect; at worst, production of short-term increases in urine output delays effective therapy and potentiates the development of volume deficits.[239] However, in the special circumstance of rhabdomyolysis-induced pigmenturia, early diuresis may limit the incidence of ARF.[263] The use of diuretics earlier in the course of prerenal oliguria would be easier to defend if an appropriate monitor of renal function were available to permit ongoing assessment of changes in renal function.

3. *Consider diagnostic data with caution.* Urinary output, although an extremely crude estimate of renal function, offers the most consistently useful diagnostic information in the acute intraoperative management of potential renal failure. Hemodynamic data prove useful in situations in which empirical volume expansion does not restore urine flow or may be used to prevent clinically inapparent tissue hypoperfusion.[262] In the acute situation, most therapeutic decisions should not rely on urinary sediment, electrolytes, osmolality, or complex formulas derived from urinary and plasma sodium and creatinine measurements. The discriminatory value of those measurements is too limited for application in the perioperative setting. Unfortunately, the readily available tests are insufficiently sensitive and specific, require excessive time for completion, and provide little information that can guide therapy. All acutely oliguric patients at risk for ARF should receive fluids and should undergo monitoring and hemodynamic support in the same fashion, using the same end points, regardless of the results of those tests. The resuscitation of patients with perioperative oliguria should be sufficiently aggressive to restore urinary flow and systemic perfusion or should be continued until oliguria persists despite a pulmonary artery

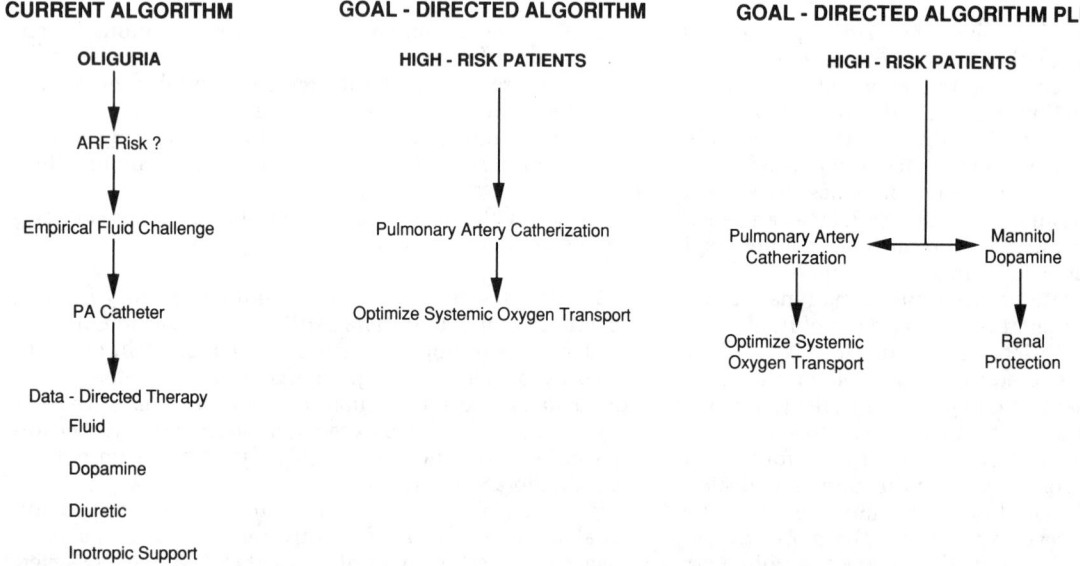

Figure 40-12. Three possible approaches to prevention of ARF. The left-hand algorithm is derived from the approach used by many clinicians. Once oliguria is recognized, the diagnostic and therapeutic approach consists of empirical volume expansion, supplemented if necessary by pulmonary artery catheterization with subsequent data-directed therapy consisting of fluid, dopamine, inotropic support, mannitol, or furosemide. In contrast, the goal-directed algorithm is based upon identification of high-risk patients. Such patients would undergo pulmonary artery catheterization with subsequent support of systemic oxygen transport (cardiac output × arterial oxygen content) at levels associated with improved survival in high-risk surgical patients.[254] The right-hand figure combines goal-oriented therapy with early pharmacologic support.

occlusion pressure of 18 mm Hg or greater following the administration of dopamine and diuretics.

Excessive reliance on the determination of urinary electrolytes, osmolality, or specialized indices may lead to the delay, interruption, or premature termination of appropriate, timely therapy, thereby increasing the chance that a patient will suffer the high morbidity and mortality of ARF.

MANAGEMENT OF ACUTE RENAL FAILURE

When renal replacement therapy proves necessary despite intensive efforts to prevent ARF, several aspects of care deserve special consideration. Occasionally, controversy exists regarding optimal therapy. The physicians caring for the patient must consider the timing and selection of renal replacement techniques, review the patient's pharmacologic management, make careful plans regarding fluid and electrolyte therapy and nutritional support, intensify surveillance for infection, and maintain an appropriate level of monitoring.

Timing and Technique of Renal Replacement Therapy

After establishing the diagnosis of ARF, the clinician must decide how soon to begin renal replacement therapy and must choose from among the various available modalities the most suitable technique for the individual patient. At this point in the patient's care, conflicts are likely. Because many of these patients have undergone extensive fluid resuscitation for the management of traumatic, surgical, or septic sequestration of sodium and water, the health care team often attempts to aggressively remove fluid. Unfortunately, the processes resulting in fluid sequestration frequently persist at the time when renal failure becomes manifest. Aggressive attempts to remove sodium and water with hemodialysis, peritoneal dialysis, or CAVH frequently result in intravascular volume depletion. At such times, the indications for acute dialytic therapy should be kept in mind: intravascular volume overload, azotemia, hyperkalemia, and severe acid-base disturbances. In addition, dialysis may facilitate the improvement of white blood cell function and permit more aggressive nutritional support.[73,91]

Review Pharmacologic Therapy

A large number of drugs are excreted by the kidney. Other drugs are removed by dialytic therapy or by CAVH. At the time of initiation of renal replacement therapy, the clinician should review all pharmacologic therapy and should adjust that therapy appropriately for the patient's acute change in renal status. Bennett et al have comprehensively described drug dosages for adults with renal failure.[264]

Because of the high incidence of stress gastritis in critically ill patients, particularly in those with ARF, some form of stress ulcer prophylaxis should be considered. The three approaches to the prophylaxis of stress ulceration include aggressive antacid titration,[265] the administration of an H$_2$ receptor antagonist, and the administration of sucralfate.[266,267] Although aggressive titration of antacids represents the gold standard for prophylaxis,[265] the frequent requirement for large quantities of antacids has prompted a search for a more convenient form of treatment. H$_2$ receptor antagonists appear to be most effective in patients with few risk factors for stress gastritis, but they are less effective in patients with renal failure.[267-269] Sucralfate, originally introduced for the management of duodenal ulceration, seems to compare favorably with either antacids or cimetidine for the prevention of gastrointestinal bleeding in critically ill patients.[266,267]

Carefully Monitor Fluid and Electrolyte Therapy

Patients with ARF do not easily tolerate excessive intravascular volume expansion. In those who are hemodynamically stable, fluid administration can be restricted to that necessary to provide adequate nutritional intake. Patients with sepsis or multiple system failure, however, often require continued sodium and water administration despite the cessation of renal function. Serum potassium, calcium, magnesium, and phosphate levels should be monitored carefully. In general, potassium excretion is a function of urinary flow rate rather than of GFR. Magnesium may accumulate in patients receiving magnesium-containing antacids. Hyperphosphatemia may occur as a consequence of excretory failure; conversely, hypophosphatemia may become a problem in patients receiving aggressive nutritional support and phosphate-binding antacids. Dialysis best manages metabolic acidosis. Some patients with nonoliguric renal failure develop a hyperchloremic acidosis, which responds to the administration of sodium bicarbonate.

Nutritional Support

The recovery of patients with ARF may depend, in part, upon the adequacy of their nutritional support. Inadequate nutrition will result in muscle wasting and immune compromise. One of the goals of renal replacement therapy should be to remove sufficient excess fluid to permit the provision of an adequate number of calories and an adequate amount of protein.

Surveillance of Infection

Infection remains the most common cause of death in patients with ARF. In addition, ARF constitutes one of the earliest manifestations of multiple system organ failure, the cause of which is usually sepsis and the mortality of which is prohibitively high.[270-272] The control of apparent infection, the search for occult sepsis, and vigilance regarding the development of new infectious complications must be intensive and persistent. The clinician must realize that ARF may be followed by failure of other organ systems, which in patients with severe infections may in turn require aggressive support.

Monitoring

The indications for pulmonary artery catheterization in patients with ARF are similar to those indications in other critically ill patients. Hemodynamic monitoring proves especially useful for those patients in whom a conflict exists regarding the need for aggressive dialytic removal of sodium and water. The estimation of pulmonary artery occlusion pressure before and during dialysis may assist the dialysis personnel in managing fluid removal during dialysis and in determining appropriate therapy if hypotension develops.

One of the greatest limitations of current monitoring techniques is the lack of an effective means for determining the rate of recovery of renal function in patients with ARF. The inability to accurately estimate renal blood flow and GFR means that dialysis frequently continues for an unnecessarily long period of time. Myers and Moran[175] suggest that limiting the number of dialysis sessions, and their attendant risk of hypotension would hasten recovery from renal failure in some patients.

REFERENCES

1. Sladen RN: Effect of anesthesia and surgery on renal function. Crit Care Clin 3:373, 1987
2. Laragh JH: Atrial natriuretic hormone, the renin-aldosterone axis, and blood pressure-electrolyte homeostasis. N Engl J Med 313:1330, 1985
3. Zeidel ML: Renal actions of atrial natriuretic peptide: Regulation of collecting duct sodium and water transport. Annu Rev Physiol 52:747, 1990
4. Shenker Y: Atrial natriuretic hormone and aldosterone regulation in salt-depleted state. Am J Physiol 257:E583, 1989
5. Cogan MG: Renal effects of atrial natriuretic factor. Annu Rev Physiol 52:699, 1990
6. Goetz KL: Physiology and pathophysiology of atrial peptides. Am J Physiol 254:E1, 1988
7. Scharschmidt LA, Lianos E, Dunn MJ: Arachidonate metabolites and the control of glomerular function. Fed Proc 42:3058, 1983
8. Raymond KH, Lifschitz MD: Effect of prostaglandins on renal salt and water excretion. Am J Med 80(1A):22, 1986
9. Whelton A, Stout RL, Spilman PS, Klassen DK: Renal effects of ibuprofen, piroxicam, and sulindac in patients with asymptomatic renal failure. A prospective, randomized, crossover comparison. Ann Intern Med 112:568, 1990
10. Makhoul RG, Gewertz BL: Renal prostaglandins. J Surg Res 40:181, 1986
11. Schrier RW: Body fluid volume regulation in health and disease: A unifying hypothesis. Ann Intern Med 113:155, 1990
12. Badr KF, Ichikawa I: Prerenal failure: A deleterious shift from renal compensation to decompensation. N Engl J Med 319:623, 1988
13. Vatner SF, Braunwald E: Cardiovascular control mechanisms in the conscious state. N Engl J Med 293:970, 1975
14. Vatner SF: Effects of hemorrhage on regional blood flow distribution in dogs and primates. J Clin Invest 54:225, 1974
15. Price HL, Linde HW, Jones RE et al: Sympathoadrenal responses to general anesthesia in man and their relation to hemodynamics. Anesthesiology 20:563, 1959
16. Payen DM, Farge D, Beloucif S, De La Coussaye JE: No involvement of antidiuretic hormone in acute antidiuresis during PEEP ventilation in humans. Anesthesiology 66:17, 1987
17. Kharasch ED, Yeo KT, Kenny MA, Buffington CW: Atrial natriuretic factor may mediate the renal effects of PEEP ventilation. Anesthesiology 69:862, 1988
18. Andrivet P, Adnot S, Brun-Buisson C et al: Involvement of ANF in the acute antidiuresis during PEEP ventilation. J Appl Physiol 65:1967, 1988
19. Crandell WB, Pappas SG, Macdonald A: Nephrotoxicity associated with methoxyflurane anesthesia. Anesthesiology 27:591, 1966
20. Mazze RI, Trudell JR, Cousins MJ: Methoxyflurane metabolism and renal dysfunction: Clinical correlation in man. Anesthesiology 35:247, 1971
21. Cousins MJ, Mazze RI: Methoxyflurane nephrotoxicity. A study of dose response in man. JAMA 225:1611, 1973
22. Whitford GM, Taves DR: Fluoride-induced diuresis: Renal-tissue solute concentrations, functional, hemodynamic, and histologic correlates in the rat. Anesthesiology 39:416, 1973
23. Cousins MJ, Greenstein LR, Hitt BA, Mazze RI: Metabolism and renal effects of enflurane in man. Anesthesiology 44:44, 1976
24. Mazze RI, Calverley RK, Smith NT: Inorganic fluoride nephrotoxicity: Prolonged enflurane and halothane anesthesia in volunteers. Anesthesiology 46:265, 1977
25. Mazze RI, Woodruff RE, Heerdt ME: Isoniazid-induced enflurane defluorination in humans. Anesthesiology 57:5, 1982
26. Rice SA, Fish KJ: Anesthetic metabolism and renal function in obese and nonobese Fischer 344 rats following enflurane or isoflurane anesthesia. Anesthesiology 65:28, 1986
27. Motuz DJ, Watson WA, Barlow JC et al: The increase in urinary alanine aminopeptidase excretion associated with enflurane anesthesia is increased further by aminoglycosides. Anesth Analg 67:770, 1988
28. Mazze RI, Schwartz FD, Slocum HC, Barry KG: Renal function during anesthesia and surgery. I. The effects of halothane anesthesia. Anesthesiology 24:279, 1963
29. Blackmore WP, Erwin KW, Wiegand OF, Lipsey R: Renal and cardiovascular effects of halothane. Anesthesiology 21:489, 1960
30. Theye RA, Maher FT: The effects of halothane on canine renal function and oxygen consumption. Anesthesiology 35:54, 1971
31. Bastron RD, Pyne JL, Inagaki M: Halothane-induced renal vasodilation. Anesthesiology 50:126, 1979
32. Bastron RD, Perkins FM, Pyne JL: Autoregulation of renal blood flow during halothane anesthesia. Anesthesiology 46:142, 1977
33. Priano LL: Effect of halothane on renal hemodynamics during normovolemia and acute hemorrhagic hypovolemia. Anesthesiology 63:357, 1985
34. Mujais SK: Transport and renal effects of general anesthetics. Semin Nephrol 6:251, 1986
35. Lundeen G, Manohar M, Parks C: Systemic distribution of blood flow in swine while awake and during 1.0 and 1.5 MAC isoflurane anesthesia with or without 50% nitrous oxide. Anesth Analg 62:499, 1983
36. Gelman S, Fowler KC, Smith LR: Regional blood flow during isoflurane and halothane anesthesia. Anesth Analg 63:557, 1984
37. Lessard MR, Trépanier CA: Renal function and hemodynamics during prolonged isoflurane-induced hypotension in humans. Anesthesiology 74:860, 1991
38. Hill GE, Lunn JK, Hodges MR et al: N_2O modification of halothane-altered renal function in the dog. Anesth Analg 56:690, 1977
39. Leighton KM, Macleod BA, Bruce C: Renal blood flow: Differences in autoregulation during anesthesia with halothane, methoxyflurane, or alphaprodine in the dog. Anesth Analg 57:389, 1978
40. Jones RM, Koblin DD, Cashman JN et al: Biotransformation and hepato-renal function in volunteers after exposure to desflurane (I-653). Br J Anaesth 64:482, 1990
41. Merin RG, Bernard J-M, Doursout M-F et al: Comparison of the effects of isoflurane and desflurane on cardiovascular dynamics and regional blood flow in the chronically instrumented dog. Anesthesiology 74:568, 1991
42. Lebowitz PW, Cote ME, Daniels AL, Bonventre JV: Comparative renal effects of midazolam and thiopental in humans. Anesthesiology 59:381, 1983
43. Priano LL: Alteration of renal hemodynamics by thiopental, diazepam, and ketamine in conscious dogs. Anesth Analg 61:853, 1982
44. Kyung WC, Suhn HK, Gou YK et al: Renal and renin effects of sodium thiopental in rabbits. Renal Physiol 10:261, 1987
45. Walker LA, Gellai M, Valtin H: Renal response to pentobarbital anesthesia in rats: Effect of interrupting the renin-angiotensin system. J Pharmacol Exp Ther 236:721, 1986
46. Madwed JB, Wang BC: Pentobarbital anesthesia alters renal action of α-hANP in dogs. Am J Physiol 258:R616, 1990
47. Hirasawa H, Yonezawa T: The effects of ketamine and Innovar on the renal cortical and medullary blood flow of the dog. Anaesthesist 8:349, 1975
48. Idvall J, Aronsen KF, Stenberg P: Tissue perfusion and distri-

bution of cardiac output during ketamine anesthesia in nor-movolemic rats. Acta Anaesthesiol Scand 24:257, 1980

49. Bidwai AV, Stanley TH, Bloomer HA, Blatnick RA: Effects of anesthetic doses of morphine on renal function in the dog. Anesth Analg 54:357, 1975

50. Hunter JM, Jones RS, Utting JE: Effect of anaesthesia with nitrous oxide in oxygen and fentanyl on renal function in the artificially ventilated dog. Br J Anaesth 52:343, 1980

51. Priano LL: Effects of high-dose fentanyl on renal haemody-namics in conscious dogs. Can Anaesth Soc J 30:10, 1983

52. Mather LE, Selby DG, Runciman WB: Effects of propofol and of thiopentone anaesthesia on the regional kinetics of pethi-dine in the sheep. Br J Anaesth 65:365, 1990

53. Selby DG, Mather LE, Runciman WB: Effects of propofol and of thiopentone anaesthesia on the renal clearance of cefoxitin in the sheep. Br J Anaesth 65:360, 1990

54. Runciman WB, Mather LE, Selby DG: Cardiovascular effects of propofol and of thiopentone anaesthesia in the sheep. Br J Anaesth 65:353, 1990

55. Kennedy WF Jr, Sawyer TK, Gerbershagen HU et al: Simulta-neous systemic cardiovascular and renal hemodynamic mea-surements during high spinal anaesthesia in normal man. Acta Anaesthesiol Scand 37(suppl):163+, 1969

56. Kennedy WF Jr, Sawyer TK, Gerbershagen HY et al: Systemic cardiovascular and renal hemodynamic alterations during peridural anesthesia in normal man. Anesthesiology 31:414, 1969

57. Sivarajan M, Amory DW, Lindbloom LE: Systemic and re-gional blood flow during epidural anesthesia without epi-nephrine in the rhesus monkey. Anesthesiology 45:300, 1976

58. Weiner IM, Mudge GH: Diuretics and other agents employed in the mobilization of edema fluid. In Gilman AG, Goodman LS, Rall TW, Murad F (eds): Goodman and Gilman's The Phar-macologic Basis of Therapeutics, 7th ed, p 887. New York, Macmillan, 1985

59. Stoelting RK: Diuretics. In Stoelting RK (ed): Pharmacology and Physiology in Anesthetic Practice, p 423. Philadelphia, JB Lippincott, 1987

60. Ellison DH: The physiologic basis of diuretic synergism: Its role in treating diuretic resistance. Ann Intern Med 114:886, 1991

61. Corvol P, Claire M, Oblin ME et al: Mechanism of the antimin-eralocorticoid effects of spirolactones. Kidney Int 20:1, 1981

62. Schettini A, Stahurski B, Young HF: Osmotic and osmotic-loop diuresis in brain surgery: Effects on plasma and CSF electrolytes and ion excretion. J Neurosurg 56:679, 1982

63. Warren SE, Blantz RC: Mannitol. Arch Intern Med 141:493, 1981

64. Hjer-Pedersen E: Effect of acetazolamide on cerebral blood flow in subacute and chronic cerebrovascular disease. Stroke 18:887, 1987

65. Moser M: Diuretics in the management of hypertension. Med Clin North Am 71:935, 1987

66. Bastron RD: Anesthetic considerations for patients with end-stage renal disease. In Barash PG (ed): Refresher Course in Anesthesiology, p 13. Philadelphia, JB Lippincott, 1985

67. Kaufman BS, Contreras J: Preanesthetic assessment of the pa-tient with renal disease. Anesthesiol Clin North Am 8:677, 1990

68. Gibson TP: Renal disease and drug metabolism: An overview. Am J Kidney Dis 8:7, 1986

69. Dodds A, Nicholls M: Haematological aspects of renal disease. Anaesth Intensive Care 11:361, 1983

70. Erslev AJ: Erythropoietin. N Engl J Med 324:1339, 1991

71. Nissenson AR, moderator. Recombinant human erythropoie-tin and renal anemia: Molecular biology, clinical efficacy, and nervous system effects. Ann Intern Med 114:402, 1991

72. Lichtman MA, Murphy MS, Byer BJ, Freeman RB: Hemoglo-bin affinity for oxygen in chronic renal disease: The effect of hemodialysis. Blood 43:417, 1974

73. Prough DS, Adams PL, Hamilton RW: Complications of renal replacement therapy. In Lumb PD, Bryan-Brown CW (eds): Complications in Critical Care Medicine, p 145. Chicago, Year Book Medical Publishers, 1988

74. Levey AS, Harrington JT: Continuous peritoneal dialysis for chronic renal failure. Medicine 61:330, 1982

75. Nolph KD: Continuous ambulatory peritoneal dialysis. Am J Nephrol 1:1, 1981

76. Kliger AS: Complications of dialysis: Hemodialysis, perito-neal dialysis, CAPD. In Arieff AI, DeFronzo RA (eds): Fluid, Electrolyte, and Acid-Base Disorders, vol II, p 777. New York, Churchill Livingstone, 1985

77. Cogan MG, Garovoy MR: Introduction to Dialysis. New York, Churchill Livingstone, 1985

78. Jameson MD, Wiegmann TB: Principles, uses, and complica-tions of hemodialysis. Med Clin North Am 74:945, 1990

79. Alfred HJ, Cohen AJ: Use of dialytic procedures in the inten-sive care unit. In Rippe JM, Irwin RS, Alpert JS et al (eds): Intensive Care Medicine, p 562. Boston, Little, Brown & Co, 1985

80. Dorner DB, Stubbs DH, Shadur CA, Flynn CT: Percutaneous subclavian vein catheter hemodialysis—impact on vascular access surgery. Surgery 91:712, 1982

81. Palder SB, Kirkman RL, Whittemore AD et al: Vascular access for hemodialysis. Patency rates and results of revision. Ann Surg 202:235, 1985

82. Tenckhoff H, Schechter H: A bacteriologically safe peritoneal access device. Trans Am Soc Artif Intern Organs 14:181, 1968

83. Maher JF: Physiology of the peritoneum. Implications for peri-toneal dialysis. Med Clin North Am 74:985, 1990

84. Kurtz SB, Wong VH, Anderson CF et al: Continuous ambula-tory peritoneal dialysis. Three years' experience at the Mayo Clinic. Mayo Clin Proc 58:633, 1983

85. Saklayen MG: CAPD peritonitis. Incidence, pathogens, diag-nosis, and management. Med Clin North Am 74:997, 1990

86. Kaplan AA, Longnecker RE, Folkert VW: Continuous arterio-venous hemofiltration. A report of six months' experience. Ann Intern Med 100:358, 1984

87. Lauer A, Saccaggi A, Ronco C et al: Continuous arteriovenous hemofiltration in the critically ill patient. Clinical use and operational characteristics. Ann Intern Med 99:455, 1983

88. Nahman NS Jr, Middendorf DF: Continuous arteriovenous he-mofiltration. Med Clin North Am 74:975, 1990

89. Bartlett RH, Mault JR, Dechert RE et al: Continuous arteriove-nous hemofiltration: Improved survival in surgical acute renal failure? Surgery 100:400, 1986

90. Ossenkoppele GJ, van der Meulen J, Bronsveld W, Thijs LG: Continuous arteriovenous hemofiltration as an adjunctive therapy for septic shock. Crit Care Med 13:102, 1985

91. Gotlieb L, Barzilay E, Shustak A, Lev A: Sequential hemofil-tration in nonoliguric high capillary permeability pulmonary edema of severe sepsis: Preliminary report. Crit Care Med 12:997, 1984

92. Gibney RT, Stollery DE, Lefebvre RE et al: Continuous arterio-venous hemodialysis: An alternative therapy for acute renal failure associated with critical illness. Can Med Assoc J 139:861, 1988

93. DiCarlo JV, Dudley TE, Sherbotie JR et al: Continuous arterio-venous hemofiltration/dialysis improves pulmonary gas ex-change in children with multiple organ system failure. Crit Care Med 18:822, 1990

94. Voerman HJ, Strack van Schijndel RJ, Thijs LG: Continuous arterial-venous hemodiafiltration in critically ill patients. Crit Care Med 18:911, 1990

95. Twardowski ZJ, Nolph KD: Blood purification in acute renal failure. Ann Intern Med 100:447, 1984

96. Freeman RB: Treatment of chronic renal failure: An update (editorial). N Engl J Med 312:577, 1985

97. Fraser CL, Arieff AI: Nervous system complications in uremia. Ann Intern Med 109:143, 1988

98. Mathew RJ, Rabin P, Stone WJ, Wilson WH: Regional cerebral blood flow in dialysis encephalopathy and primary degenera-tive dementia. Kidney Int 28:64, 1985

99. Henderson LW: Symptomatic hypotension during hemodialy-sis. Kidney Int 17:571, 1980

100. Huyghebaert MF, Dhainaut JF, Monsallier JF, Schlemmer B: Bicarbonate hemodialysis of patients with acute renal failure and severe sepsis. Crit Care Med 13:840, 1985

101. Wehle B, Asaba H, Castenfors J et al: Hemodynamic changes

during sequential ultrafiltration and dialysis. Kidney Int 15:411, 1979

102. Lazarus JM, Hampers CL, Lowrie EG, Merrill JP: Baroreceptor activity in normotensive and hypertensive uremic patients. Circulation 47:1015, 1973

103. Endou K, Kamijima J, Kakubari Y, Kikawada R: Hemodynamic changes during hemodialysis. Cardiology 63:175, 1978

104. Graefe U, Milutinovich J, Follette WC et al: Less dialysis-induced morbidity and vascular instability with bicarbonate in dialysate. Ann Intern Med 88:332, 1978

105. Leunissen KM, Hoorntje SJ, Fiers HA et al: Acetate versus bicarbonate hemodialysis in critically ill patients. Nephron 42:146, 1986

106. Hung J, Harris PJ, Uren RF et al: Uremic cardiomyopathy—effect of hemodialysis on left ventricular function in end-stage renal failure. N Engl J Med 302:547, 1980

107. Nixon JV, Mitchell JH, McPhaul JJ Jr, Henrich WL: Effect of hemodialysis on left ventricular function. Dissociation of changes in filling volume and in contractile state. J Clin Invest 71:377, 1983

108. Ruder MA, Alpert MA, Van Stone J et al: Comparative effects of acetate and bicarbonate hemodialysis on left ventricular function. Kidney Int 27:768, 1985

109. Maynard JC, Cruz C, Kleerekoper M, Levin NW: Blood pressure response to changes in serum ionized calcium during hemodialysis. Ann Intern Med 104:358, 1986

110. Susini G, Zucchetti M, Bortone F et al: Isolated ultrafiltration in cardiogenic pulmonary edema. Crit Care Med 18:14, 1990

111. Lamer C, Valleaux T, Plaisance P et al: Continuous arteriovenous hemodialysis for acute renal failure after cardiac operations (letter). J Thorac Cardiovasc Surg 99:175, 1990

112. Francos GC, Besarab A, Burke JF Jr et al: Dialysis-induced hypoxemia: Membrane dependent and membrane independent causes. Am J Kidney Dis 5:191, 1985

113. Craddock PR, Fehr J, Brigham KL et al: Complement and leukocyte-mediated pulmonary dysfunction in hemodialysis. N Engl J Med 296:769, 1977

114. De Backer WA, Verpooten GA, Borgonjon DJ et al: Hypoxemia during hemodialysis: Effects of different membranes and dialysate compositions. Kidney Int 23:738, 1983

115. Sherlock J, Ledwith J, Letteri J: Determinants of oxygenation during hemodialysis and related procedures. A report of data acquired under varying conditions and a review of the literature. Am J Nephrol 4:158, 1984

116. Aurigemma NM, Feldman NT, Gottlieb M et al: Arterial oxygenation during hemodialysis. N Engl J Med 297:871, 1977

117. Pitcher WD, Diamond SM, Henrich WL: Pulmonary gas exchange during dialysis in patients with obstructive lung disease. Chest 96:1136, 1989

118. Manji S, Shikora S, McMahon M et al: Peritoneal dialysis for acute renal failure: Overfeeding resulting from dextrose absorbed during dialysis. Crit Care Med 18:29, 1990

119. Burke JF Jr, Francos GC: Surgery in the patient with acute or chronic renal failure. Med Clin North Am 71:489, 1987

120. Sladen RN, Endo E, Harrison T: Two-hour versus 22-hour creatinine clearance in critically ill patients. Anesthesiology 67:1013, 1987

121. Wilson RF, Soullier G: The validity of two-hour creatinine clearance studies in critically ill patients. Crit Care Med 8:281, 1980

122. Preece MJ, Richardson JA: The effect of mild dehydration on one-hour creatinine clearance rates. Nephron 9:106, 1972

123. Wheeler LA, Sheiner LB: Critical estimation of creatinine clearance. Am J Clin Pathol 72:27, 1979

124. Ghoneim MM, Pandya H: Plasma protein binding of thiopental in patients with impaired renal or hepatic function. Anesthesiology 42:545, 1975

125. Dundee JW, Richards RK: Effect of azotemia upon the action of intravenous barbiturate anesthesia. Anesthesiology 15:333, 1954

126. Burch PG, Stanski DR: Decreased protein binding and thiopental kinetics. Clin Pharmacol Ther 32:212, 1982

127. Don HF, Dieppa RA, Taylor P: Narcotic analgesics in anuric patients. Anesthesiology 42:745, 1975

128. Sear JW, Hand CW, Moore RA, McQuay HJ: Studies on mor-

phine disposition: Influence of renal failure on the kinetics of morphine and its metabolites. Br J Anaesth 62:28, 1989

129. Woolner DF, Winter D, Frendin TJ et al: Renal failure does not impair the metabolism of morphine. Br J Clin Pharmacol 22:55, 1986

130. Chauvin M, Sandouk P, Scherrmann JM et al: Morphine pharmacokinetics in renal failure. Anesthesiology 66:327, 1987

131. Wiggum DC, Cork RC, Weldon ST et al: Postoperative respiratory depression and elevated sufentanil levels in a patient with chronic renal failure. Anesthesiology 63:708, 1985

132. Fyman PN, Reynolds JR, Moser F et al: Pharmacokinetics of sufentanil in patients undergoing renal transplantation. Can J Anaesth 35:312, 1988

133. Sear JW: Sufentanil disposition in patients undergoing renal transplantation: Influence of choice of kinetic model. Br J Anaesth 63:60, 1989

134. Davis PJ, Stiller RL, Cook DR et al: Pharmacokinetics of sufentanil in adolescent patients with chronic renal failure. Anesth Analg 67:268, 1988

135. Van Peer A, Vercauteren M, Noorduin H et al: Alfentanil kinetics in renal insufficiency. Eur J Clin Pharmacol 30:245, 1986

136. Davis PJ, Stiller RL, Cook DR et al: Effects of cholestatic hepatic disease and chronic renal failure on alfentanil pharmacokinetics in children. Anesth Analg 68:579, 1989

137. Miller RD, Way WL, Hamilton WK, Layzer RB: Succinylcholine-induced hyperkalemia in patients with renal failure? Anesthesiology 36:138, 1972

138. Ryan DW: Preoperative serum cholinesterase concentration in chronic renal failure. Clinical experience of suxamethonium in 81 patients undergoing renal transplant. Br J Anaesth 49:945, 1977

139. Gibaldi M, Levy G, Hayton WL: Tubocurarine and renal failure. Br J Anaesth 44:163, 1972

140. Orko R, Heino A, Rosenberg PH, Alanen T: Dose-response of tubocurarine in patients with and without renal failure. Acta Anesthesiol Scand 28:452, 1984

141. Fahey MR, Rupp SM, Fisher DM et al: The pharmacokinetics and pharmacodynamics of atracurium in patients with and without renal failure. Anesthesiology 61:699, 1984

142. Fahey MR, Morris RB, Miller RD et al: Pharmacokinetics of Org NC45 (norcuron) in patients with and without renal failure. Br J Anaesth 53:1049, 1981

143. Bencini AF, Scaf AH, Sohn YJ et al: Disposition and urinary excretion of vecuronium bromide in anesthetized patients with normal renal function or renal failure. Anesth Analg 65:245, 1986

144. Orko R, Heino A, Björkstén F et al: Comparison of atracurium and vecuronium in anaesthesia for renal transplantation. Acta Anaesthesiol Scand 31:450, 1987

145. Lynam DP, Cronnelly R, Castagnoli KP et al: The pharmacodynamics and pharmacokinetics of vecuronium in patients anesthetized with isoflurane with normal renal function or with renal failure. Anesthesiology 69:227, 1988

146. Lepage JY, Malinge M, Cozian A et al: Vecuronium and atracurium in patients with end-stage renal failure. A comparative study. Br J Anaesth 59:1004, 1987

147. Pollard BJ, Doran BR: Should vecuronium be used in renal failure? (letter). Can J Anaesth 36:602, 1989

148. Cashman JN, Luke JJ, Jones RM: Neuromuscular block with doxacurium (BW A938U) in patients with normal or absent renal function. Br J Anaesth 64:186, 1990

149. Caldwell JE, Canfell PC, Castagnoli KP et al: The influence of renal failure on the pharmacokinetics and duration of action of pipecuronium bromide in patients anesthetized with halothane and nitrous oxide. Anesthesiology 70:7, 1989

150. Cronnelly R, Stanski DR, Miller RD et al: Renal function and the pharmacokinetics of neostigmine in anesthetized man. Anesthesiology 51:222, 1979

151. Cronnelly R, Stanski DR, Miller RD, Sheiner LB: Pyridostigmine kinetics with and without renal function. Clin Pharmacol Ther 28:78, 1980

152. Morris RB, Cronnelly R, Miller RD et al: Pharmacokinetics of edrophonium in anephric and renal transplant patients. Br J Anaesth 53:1311, 1981

153. Kasiske BL, Kjellstrand CM: Perioperative management of patients with chronic renal failure and postoperative acute renal failure. Urol Clin North Am 10:35, 1983

154. Abreo K, Moorthy AV, Osborne M: Changing patterns and outcome of acute renal failure requiring hemodialysis. Arch Intern Med 146:1338, 1986

155. Lordon RE, Burton JR: Post-traumatic renal failure in military personnel in Southeast Asia. Experience at Clark USAF Hospital, Republic of the Philippines. Am J Med 53:137, 1972

156. Hou SH, Bushinsky DA, Wish JB et al: Hospital-acquired renal insufficiency: A prospective study. Am J Med 74:243, 1983

157. Conger JD: A controlled evaluation of prophylactic dialysis in post-traumatic acute renal failure. J Trauma 15:1056, 1975

158. Gillum DM, Dixon BS, Yanover MJ et al: The role of intensive dialysis in acute renal failure. Clin Nephrol 25:249, 1986

159. Charlson ME, MacKenzie CR, Gold JP, Shires GT: Postoperative changes in serum creatinine. When do they occur and how much is important? Ann Surg 209:328, 1989

160. Gornick CC Jr, Kjellstrand CM: Acute renal failure complicating aortic aneurysm surgery. Nephron 35:145, 1983

161. Gamulin Z, Forster A, Morel D et al: Effects of infrarenal aortic cross-clamping on renal hemodynamics in humans. Anesthesiology 61:394, 1984

162. Gamulin Z, Forster A, Simonet F et al: Effects of renal sympathetic blockade on renal hemodynamics in patients undergoing major aortic abdominal surgery. Anesthesiology 65:688, 1986

163. Crawford ES, Walker HS III, Salch SA, Normann NA: Graft replacement of aneurysm in descending thoracic aorta: Results without bypass or shunting. Surgery 89:73, 1981

164. Carlson DE, Karp RB, Kouchoukos NT: Surgical treatment of aneurysms of the descending thoracic aorta: An analysis of 85 patients. Ann Thorac Surg 35:58, 1983

165. Najafi H, Javid H, Hunter J et al: Descending aortic aneurysmectomy without adjuncts to avoid ischemia. Ann Thorac Surg 30:326, 1980

166. Alpert RA, Roizen MF, Hamilton WK et al: Intraoperative urinary output does not predict postoperative renal function in patients undergoing abdominal aortic revascularization. Surgery 95:707, 1984

167. Sinicrope RA, Serra RM, Engle JE et al: Mortality of acute renal failure after rupture of abdominal aortic aneurysms. Am J Surg 141:240, 1981

168. McMurray SD, Luft FC, Maxwell DR et al: Prevailing patterns and predictor variables in patients with acute tubular necrosis. Arch Intern Med 138:950, 1978

169. Schrier RW: Acute renal failure. JAMA 247:2518, 1982

170. Tilney NL, Lazarus JM: Acute renal failure in surgical patients. Causes, clinical patterns, and care. Surg Clin North Am 63:357, 1983

171. Wilkes BM, Mailloux LU: Acute renal failure. Pathogenesis and prevention. Am J Med 80:1129, 1986

172. Sinsteden TD, O'Neil TJ, Hill S et al: The role of high-energy phosphate in norepinephrine-induced acute renal failure in the dog. Circ Res 49:93, 1986

173. Ratcliffe PJ, Moonen CT, Holloway PA et al: Acute renal failure in hemorrhagic hypotension: Cellular energetics and renal function. Kidney Int 30:355, 1986

174. Brezis M, Rosen S, Silva P, Epstein FH: Renal ischemia: A new perspective. Kidney Int 26:375, 1984

175. Myers BD, Moran SM: Hemodynamically mediated acute renal failure. N Engl J Med 314:97, 1986

176. Wardle N: Acute renal failure in the 1980s: The importance of septic shock and of endotoxaemia. Nephron 30:193, 1982

177. Espinel CH, Gregory AW: Differential diagnosis of acute renal failure. Clin Nephrol 13:73, 1980

178. Oken DE: On the differential diagnosis of acute renal failure. Am J Med 71:916, 1981

179. Pru C, Kjellstrand CM: The FE^{Na} test is of no prognostic value in acute renal failure. Nephron 36:20, 1984

180. Diamond JR, Yoburn DC: Nonoliguric acute renal failure associated with a low fractional excretion of sodium. Ann Intern Med 96:597, 1982

181. Zaloga GP, Hughes SS: Oliguria in patients with normal renal function. Anesthesiology 72:598, 1990

182. Cronin RE, Erickson AM, de Torrente A, Schrier RW: Norepinephrine-induced acute renal failure: A reversible ischemic model of acute renal failure. Kidney Int 14:187, 1978

183. Cronin RE, de Torrente A, Miller PD et al: Pathogenic mechanisms in early norepinephrine-induced acute renal failure: Functional and histological correlates of protection. Kidney Int 14:115, 1978

184. Burke TJ, Cronin RE, Duchin KL et al: Ischemia and tubule obstruction during acute renal failure in dogs: Mannitol in protection. Am J Physiol 238:F305, 1980

185. Patak RV, Fadem SZ, Lifschitz MD, Stein JH: Study of factors which modify the development of norepinephrine-induced acute renal failure in the dog. Kidney Int 15:227, 1979

186. Hanley MJ, Davidson K: Prior mannitol and furosemide infusion in a model of ischemic acute renal failure. Am J Physiol 241:F556, 1981

187. Pass LJ, Eberhart RC, Brown JC et al: The effect of mannitol and dopamine on the renal response to thoracic aortic cross-clamping. J Thorac Cardiovasc Surg 95:608, 1988

188. Henderson IS, Beattie TJ, Kennedy AC: Dopamine hydrochloride in oliguric states. Lancet 2:827, 1980

189. Schwartz LB, Gewertz BL: The renal response to low dose dopamine. J Surg Res 45:574, 1988

190. Kleinknecht D, Ganeval D, Gonzales-Duque LA, Fermanian J: Furosemide in acute oliguric renal failure. A controlled trial. Nephron 17:51, 1976

191. Lindner A, Cutler RE, Goodman G: Synergism of dopamine plus furosemide in preventing acute renal failure in the dog. Kidney Int 16:158, 1979

192. Lindner A: Synergism of dopamine and furosemide in diuretic-resistant, oliguric acute renal failure. Nephron 33:121, 1983

193. Brown CB, Ogg CS, Cameron JS: High dose frusemide in acute renal failure: A controlled trial. Clin Nephrol 15:90, 1981

194. Elliott WJ, Weber RR, Nelson KS et al: Renal and hemodynamic effects of intravenous fenoldopam versus nitroprusside in severe hypertension. Circulation 81:970, 1990

195. Allison NL, Dubbs JW, Ziemniak JA et al: The effect of fenoldopam, a dopaminergic agonist, on renal hemodynamics. Clin Pharmacol Ther 41:282, 1987

196. Murphy MB, McCoy CE, Weber RR et al: Augmentation of renal blood flow and sodium excretion in hypertensive patients during blood pressure reduction by intravenous administration of the dopamine-1 agonist, fenoldopam. Circulation 76:1312, 1987

197. Hughes JM, Ragsdale NV, Felder RA et al: Diuresis and natriuresis during continuous dopamine-1 receptor stimulation. Hypertension 11:I–69, 1988

198. Bonventre JV: Mediators of ischemic renal injury. Annu Rev Med 39:531, 1988

199. Corwin HL, Bonventre JV: Acute renal failure. Med Clin North Am 70:1037, 1986

200. Cronin RE: Drug therapy in the management of acute renal failure. Am J Med Sci 292:112, 1986

201. Corwin HL, Bonventre JV: Acute renal failure in the intensive care unit. Part 2. Intensive Care Med 14:86, 1988

202. Epstein FH, Brown RS: Acute renal failure: A collection of paradoxes. Hosp Pract 23:171, 1988

203. Mandal AK, Lightfoot BO, Treat RC: Mechanisms of protection in acute renal failure. Circ Shock 11:245, 1983

204. Vetterlein F, Petho A, Schmidt G: Distribution of capillary blood flow in rat kidney during postischemic renal failure. Am J Physiol 251:H510, 1986

205. Ratcliffe PJ, Endre ZH, Tange JD, Ledingham JG: Ischaemic acute renal failure: Why does it occur? Nephron 52:1, 1989

206. Mason J, Torhorst J, Welsch J: Role of the medullary perfusion defect in the pathogenesis of ischemic renal failure. Kidney Int 26:283, 1984

207. Hirasawa H, Odaka M, Soeda K et al: Experimental and clinical study on ATP-MgCl$_2$ administration for postischemic acute renal failure. Clin Exp Dial Apheresis 7:37, 1983

208. Siegel NJ, Glazier WB, Chaudrey IH et al: Enhanced recovery from acute renal failure by the postischemic infusion of adenine nucleotides and magnesium chloride in rats. Kidney Int 17:338, 1980

209. van Waarde A, Stromski ME, Thulin G et al: Protection of the kidney against ischemic injury by inhibition of 5′-nucleotidase. Am J Physiol 256:F298, 1989

210. Didlake R, Kirchner KA, Lewin J et al: Protection from ischemic renal injury by fructose-1,6-diphosphate infusion in the rat. Circ Shock 16:205, 1985

211. Zager RA, Gmur DJ, Bredl CR, Eng MJ: Degree and time sequence of hypothermic protection against experimental ischemic acute renal failure. Circ Res 65:1263, 1989

212. Wait RB, White G, Davis JH: Beneficial effects of verapamil on postischemic renal failure. Surgery 94:276, 1983

213. Goldfarb D, Iaina A, Serban I et al: Beneficial effect of verapamil in ischemic acute renal failure in the rat. Proc Soc Exp Biol Med 172:389, 1983

214. Silverman M, Rose H, Puschett JB: Modifications in proximal tubular function induced by nitrendipine in a rat model of acute ischemic renal failure. J Cardiovasc Pharmacol 14:799, 1989

215. Russell JD, Churchill DN: Calcium antagonists and acute renal failure. Am J Med 87:306, 1989

216. Leahy AL, Galla J, Fitzpatrick JM, Wait RB: The canine kidney in haemorrhagic shock: Effect of verapamil. Eur Urol 13:401, 1987

217. Loutzenhiser RD, Epstein M: Renal hemodynamic effects of calcium antagonists. Am J Med 82:23, 1987

218. Diamond JR, Cheung JY, Fang LS: Nifedipine-induced renal dysfunction. Alterations in renal hemodynamics. Am J Med 77:905, 1984

219. Canavese C, Stratta P, Vercellone A: The case for oxygen free radicals in the pathogenesis of ischemic acute renal failure. Nephron 49:9, 1988

220. Ratych RE, Bulkley GB: Free-radical-mediated postischemic reperfusion injury in the kidney. J Free Radic Biol Med 2:311, 1986

221. Mauk RH, Patak RV, Fadem SZ et al: Effect of prostaglandin E administration in a nephrotoxic and a vasoconstrictor model of acute renal failure. Kidney Int 12:122, 1977

222. Mandal AK, Miller J: Protection against ischemic acute renal failure by prostaglandin infusion. Prostaglandins Leukotrienes Med 8:361, 1982

223. Tobimatsu M, Konomi K, Saito S, Tsumagari T: Protective effect of prostaglandin E$_1$ on ischemia-induced acute renal failure in dogs. Surgery 98:45, 1985

224. Torsello G, Schror K, Szabo Z et al: Effects of prostaglandin E$_1$ (PGE$_1$) on experimental renal ischaemia. Eur J Vasc Surg 3:5, 1989

225. Lifschitz MD, Barnes JL: Prostaglandin I$_2$ attenuates ischemic acute renal failure in the rat. Am J Physiol 247:F714, 1984

226. Klausner JM, Paterson IS, Goldman G et al: Postischemic renal injury is mediated by neutrophils and leukotrienes. Am J Physiol 256:F794, 1989

227. Lelcuk S, Alexander F, Kobzik L et al: Prostacyclin and thromboxane A$_2$ moderate postischemic renal failure. Surgery 98:207, 1985

228. Kaufman RP Jr, Klausner JM, Anner H et al: Inhibition of thromboxane (Tx) synthesis by free radical scavengers. J Trauma 28:458, 1988

229. Pierucci A, Simonetti BM, Pecci G et al: Improvement of renal function with selective thromboxane antagonism in lupus nephritis. N Engl J Med 320:421, 1989

230. Koelz AM, Bertschin S, Hermle M et al: The angiotensin converting enzyme inhibitor enalapril in acute ischemic renal failure in rats. Experientia 44:172, 1988

231. Atkins JL: Effect of sodium bicarbonate preloading on ischemic renal failure. Nephron 44:70, 1986

232. Cronin RE, Brown DM, Simonsen R: Protection by thyroxine in nephrotoxic acute renal failure. Am J Physiol 251:F408, 1986

233. Lin JJ, Churchill PC, Bidani AK: Effect of theophylline on the initiation phase of postischemic acute renal failure in rats. J Lab Clin Med 108:150, 1986

234. Bidani AK, Churchill PC, Packer W: Theophylline-induced protection in myoglobinuric acute renal failure: Further characterization. Can J Physiol Pharmacol 65:42, 1986

235. Vadiei K, Brunner LJ, Luke DR: Effects of pentoxifylline in experimental acute renal failure. Kidney Int 36:466, 1989

236. Humes HD, Cieslinski DA, Coimbra TM et al: Epidermal growth factor enhances renal tubule cell regeneration and repair and accelerates the recovery of renal function in postischemic acute renal failure. J Clin Invest 84:1757, 1989

237. Andrews PM, Bates SB: Dietary protein prior to renal ischemia dramatically affects postischemic kidney function. Kidney Int 30:299, 1986

238. Seguro AC, Shimizu MH, Monteiro JL, Rocha AS: Effect of potassium depletion on ischemic renal failure. Nephron 51:350, 1989

239. Lucas CE, Zito JG, Carter KM et al: Questionable value of furosemide in preventing renal failure. Surgery 82:314, 1977

240. Anderson RJ, Linas SL, Berns AS et al: Nonoliguric acute renal failure. N Engl J Med 296:1134, 1977

241. Shin B, Mackenzie CF, McAslan TC et al: Postoperative renal failure in trauma patients. Anesthesiology 51:218, 1979

242. Moran SM, Myers BD: Pathophysiology of protracted acute renal failure in man. J Clin Invest 76:1440, 1985

243. Hilberman M, Derby GC, Spencer RJ, Stinson EB: Sequential pathophysiological changes characterizing the progression from renal dysfunction to acute renal failure following cardiac operation. J Thorac Cardiovasc Surg 79:838, 1980

244. Hilberman M, Myers BD, Carrie BJ et al: Acute renal failure following cardiac surgery. J Thorac Cardiovasc Surg 77:880, 1979

245. Moran SM, Myers BD: Course of acute renal failure studies by a model of creatinine kinetics. Kidney Int 27:928, 1985

246. Myers BD, Miller DC, Mehigan JT et al: Nature of the renal injury following total renal ischemia in man. J Clin Invest 73:329, 1984

247. Krasna MJ, Scott GE, Scholz PM et al: Postoperative enhancement of urinary output in patients with acute renal failure using continuous furosemide therapy. Chest 89:294, 1986

248. Epstein M, Schneider NS, Befeler B: Effect of intrarenal furosemide on renal function and intrarenal hemodynamics in acute renal failure. Am J Med 58:510, 1975

249. Prewitt RM, Matthay MA, Ghignone M: Hemodynamic management in the adult respiratory distress syndrome. Clin Chest Med 4:251, 1983

250. Miller SB, Anderson RJ: The kidney in acute respiratory failure. J Crit Care 2:45, 1987

251. McMurray SD, Luft FC, Maxwell DR et al: Prevailing patterns and predictor variables in patients with acute tubular necrosis. Arch Intern Med 138:950, 1978

252. Frankel MC, Weinstein AM, Stenzel KH: Prognostic patterns in acute renal failure: The New York Hospital, 1981–1982. Clin Exp Dial Apheresis 7:145, 1983

253. Bullock ML, Umen AJ, Finkelstein M, Keane WF: The assessment of risk factors in 462 patients with acute renal failure. Am J Kidney Dis 5:97, 1985

254. Bell RC, Coalson JJ, Smith JD, Johanson WG Jr: Multiple organ system failure and infection in adult respiratory distress syndrome. Ann Intern Med 99:293, 1983

255. Bartlett RH, Morris AH, Fairley HB et al: A prospective study of acute hypoxic respiratory failure. Chest 89:684, 1986

256. Kraman S, Khan F, Patel S, Seriff N: Renal failure in the respiratory intensive care unit. Crit Care Med 7:263, 1979

257. Montgomery AB, Stager MA, Carrico CJ, Hudson LD: Causes of mortality in patients with the adult respiratory distress syndrome. Am Rev Respir Dis 132:485, 1985

258. Maseda J, Hilberman M, Derby GC et al: The renal effects of sodium nitroprusside in postoperative cardiac surgical patients. Anesthesiology 54:284, 1981

259. Prough DS, Zaloga GP: Monitoring renal function. Crit Care Clin 4:573, 1988

260. Bland RD, Shoemaker WC, Abraham E, Cobo JC: Hemodynamic and oxygen transport patterns in surviving and nonsurviving postoperative patients. Crit Care Med 13:85, 1985

261. Bland RD, Shoemaker WC: Probability of survival as a prognostic and severity of illness score in critically ill surgical patients. Crit Care Med 13:91, 1985

262. Shoemaker WC, Appel PL, Kram HB et al: Prospective trial

of supranormal values of survivors as therapeutic goals in high-risk surgical patients. Chest 94:1176, 1988

263. Honda N: Acute renal failure and rhabdomyolysis. Kidney Int 23:888, 1983

264. Bennett WM, Aronoff GR, Morrison G et al: Drug prescribing in renal failure: Dosing guidelines for adults. Am J Kidney Dis 3:155, 1983

265. Hastings PR, Skillman JJ, Bushnell LS, Silen W: Antacid titration in the prevention of acute gastrointestinal bleeding. A controlled, randomized trial in 100 critically ill patients. N Engl J Med 298:1041, 1978

266. Borrero E, Bank S, Margolis I et al: Comparison of antacid and sucralfate in the prevention of gastrointestinal bleeding in patients who are critically ill. Am J Med 79(2C):62, 1985

267. Tryba M, Zevounou F, Torok M, Zenz M: Prevention of acute stress bleeding with sucralfate, antacids, or cimetidine. A controlled study with pirenzepine as a basic medication. Am J Med 79(2C):55, 1985

268. Priebe HJ, Skillman JJ, Bushnell LS et al: Antacid versus cimetidine in preventing acute gastrointestinal bleeding. A randomized trial in 75 critically ill patients. N Engl J Med 302:426, 1980

269. Zinner MJ, Zuidema GD, Smith PL, Mignosa M: The prevention of upper gastrointestinal tract bleeding in patients in an intensive care unit. Surg Gynecol Obstet 153:214, 1981

270. Tilney NL, Bailey GL, Morgan AP: Sequential system failure after rupture of abdominal aortic aneurysms: An unsolved problem in postoperative care. Ann Surg 178:117, 1973

271. Fry DE, Pearlstein L, Fulton RL, Polk HC Jr: Multiple system organ failure. The role of uncontrolled infection. Arch Surg 115:136, 1980

272. Knaus WA, Draper EA, Wagner DP, Zimmerman JE: Prognosis in acute organ-system failure. Ann Surg 202:685, 1985

41

Wen-Shin Liu
K. C. Wong

Anesthesia for Genitourinary Surgery

Important advances in surgery of the genitourinary system have occurred in recent years. Especially notable are the use of shock wave lithotripsy for the nonsurgical removal of urinary calculi and the availability of high-quality flexible ureteroscopes that complement their rigid counterparts and extend indications for upper urinary tract endoscopy. With improved health care and diet, the elderly population is increasing and now constitutes more than a quarter of the surgical patients. Prostatectomy, a surgical intervention in the middle-aged to elderly man, is being performed with increasing frequency. To meet these challenges, sophisticated and invasive monitors have also become more common in the operating room.

An appreciation of the pathology that can alter normal genitourinary physiologic functions and the nonphysiologic insults (such as unusual positions, and absorption of irrigating fluid in open transurethral resective procedures) to which the patient might be subjected in the surgical procedure will help the anesthesiologist optimize preoperative preparation and intraoperative anesthetic management of these patients.

REGIONAL ANESTHESIA IN GENITOURINARY PROCEDURES

Regional anesthesia has a particular place in urologic surgery because the majority of procedures are in the lower abdomen and the perineum and thus are easily performed under regional anesthesia. However, some patients who receive regional anesthesia still need supplemental sedation or light general anesthesia because of either exaggerated position or prolonged surgery.

Surgical procedures on the kidney with the patient placed in the lateral position and the kidney elevator beneath the 12th rib can be performed under epidural blockade in selected patients. But the kidney position may not only be uncomfortable for a conscious patient but may also cause serious cardiovascular and respiratory embarrassment. The anesthesiologist also must be wary of the potential problems of accidental opening of the pleura and lung with a subcostal incision in a spontaneously breathing patient.

Deep vein thrombosis of the legs occurs more often in patients undergoing genitourinary surgery. Lumbar epidural blockade was significantly better than general anesthesia in reducing the incidence of deep vein thrombosis.[1] It is probable that both the increased circulation produced by epidural blockade and the reduced blood loss with a decreased need for blood transfusion in the patients receiving epidural anesthesia may have contributed to the reduced occurrence of deep vein thrombosis.

Regional anesthesia may cause a higher incidence of postoperative urinary retention and the need for catheterization than does general anesthesia. The mechanism is presumed to be delayed recovery of autonomic and somatic nerve functions, eventually leading to overdistention and atony of the bladder under regional anesthesia. The inability to empty the bladder is also exaggerated by overdistention if intravenous (iv) fluid therapy is overzealous. The site of operation, however, may be more important than the type of anesthesia in determining whether urinary retention would occur. Operative trauma to the detrusor muscle of the bladder or pelvic nerves, edema around the bladder neck, and pain-induced reflex spasm of the urethral sphincters may contribute to postoperative urinary retention. An indwelling catheter should be inserted prophylactically to minimize urinary retention from bladder dysfunction or vesical neck obstruction following surgery.

POSITIONS IN GENITOURINARY PROCEDURES

The positions required for surgery on the genitourinary system are anatomically unusual. They include the Trendelenburg position for intrapelvic surgeries, the lithotomy position for cystoscopic and transurethral procedures, the exaggerated lithotomy position for perineal prostatectomy, the flank or lateral decubitus position with the kidney rest elevated for renal and upper ureteric surgical procedures, and sometimes a semisitting position in a water bath for extracorporeal shock wave lithotripsy. These positions have adverse physiologic effects on patients (see Chapter 27).

ANESTHESIA FOR URETHRAL, BLADDER, AND URETERAL PROCEDURES

Endourologic Procedures

Since the late 1970s, endourologic procedures have been performed with increasing frequency and have comprised a significant part of urologic procedures. Many patients undergoing cystoscopy and related procedures performed with rigid instrumentation and accessories generally need general or regional anesthesia. In the past decade a new generation of endoscopes designed specifically for use in the lower urinary tract have gained widespread use. Flexible cystoscopy has many applications and can be used for procedures previously performed with rigid cystoscopes. Flexible endoscopy of the lower urinary tract has become the preferred method of cystoscopy for many urologists. The ability to navigate the flexible cystoscope more gently around anatomic angles increases patient acceptance of the examination and allows cystoscopy to be performed in some patients with local anesthesia or sedation only.

More recently, rigid and flexible ureteroendoscopes have afforded endoscopic access to the upper urinary tract for retrieval or manipulation of calculi, removal of foreign bodies and migrated stents, diagnostic endoscopy and biopsy, fulguration of tumors or suspicious lesions, and laser treatment. In order to pass the instrument, the ureteral orifice must be dilated, which requires general or regional anesthesia.

Urethral Procedures

Simple procedures such as external urethrostomy or dilation of the urethra can sometimes be performed with topical anesthesia using 2% lidocaine jelly in addition to premedication or iv sedation, especially in older patients with poor risk status and in patients with neurogenic bladder dysfunction from spinal injury. Penile block also offers good analgesia for procedures on the distal urethra.

Internal urethrotomies are usually performed with the patient in the lithotomy position, and a good sacral block with some lumbar analgesia for muscle relaxation of the legs is needed to keep the legs in the stirrups. A caudal or spinal block is suitable for these procedures and, with supplemental iv sedation, patients can be kept comfortable. Because urethroplasties are generally done with the patient in the exaggerated lithotomy position and usually are long procedures, general anesthesia is preferable. However, in selected patients spinal block with hyperbaric tetracaine with epinephrine or continuous lumbar epidural block with 0.5% bupivacaine has been used with success. Supplemental sedation is usually necessary.

Bladder and Ureteral Procedures

Diagnostic or therapeutic cystoscopic procedures are relatively minor and are generally performed on an outpatient basis. There is a wide variation in anesthetic techniques for cystoscopy, including intramuscular opioid premedication, topical anesthetic jelly, iv sedation (diazepam or midazolam), regional blockade, and general anesthesia. Most surgeons still prefer routine general anesthesia or regional anesthesia to ensure analgesia and relaxation of the surgical field. Sensations aroused by bladder distention are mediated by sensory fibers accompanying the sympathetic and parasympathetic nerves that arise from the T9 to L2 segments of the spinal cord. Therefore, a level of blockade to T9 is usually required. Spinal, lumbar epidural, or caudal blockade with the common local anesthetics have all proved satisfactory.

Quadriplegics or paraplegics are a special group of patients who may undergo repeated cystoscopies and stone manipulations. Care must be taken to avoid autonomic hyperreflexia if the injured cord level is above T5.[2] Autonomic hyperreflexia is a disorder limited primarily to spinal cord–injured patients, occurring in 66–85% of quadriplegics and high paraplegics.[3] It is manifested by acute generalized sympathetic hyperactivity (e.g., paroxysmal hypertension, bradycardia, cardiac dysrhythmias) in response to stimuli below the level of transection, such as catheterization or irrigation of the bladder. For full-blown paroxysmal hypertension to develop, the lesion of the spinal cord injury must be above the splanchnic outflow (from T4 or T6). Lesions between T5 and T10 result in mild elevations of blood pressure.[2] General anesthesia, epidural blockade, or spinal blockade all are effective in preventing this phenomenon, although regional anesthesia may be technically difficult to perform in spinal cord–injured patients.[4]

Endoscopic Treatment of Bladder Tumors

Bladder tumors are generally resected by endoscopic transurethral resection. Bladder perforation has been reported from jerking of the patient's legs during surgery. In addition to inadequate anesthesia, electrical stimulation of the obturator nerve by the resectoscope can also cause leg movements, which can be abolished by muscle relaxants under general anesthesia or by regional block (spinal, caudal, or epidural).

Vesicoureteral Reflux

Vesicoureteral reflux (VUR) denotes reflux of urine into the ureter secondary to an incompetent valve mechanism at the ureterovesicular junction. VUR is the most frequent urinary tract problem other than urinary tract infection and is usually a congenital anomaly, frequently manifested in children. Anesthesia is needed for the diagnostic evaluation or the surgical treatment of these children.

The usual diagnostic studies include cystoscopy, retrograde or iv pyelography, and various urodynamic studies, including urethral pressure profiles and voiding cystourethrography. It has been found that sedative and all inhalation anesthetics except nitrous oxide decrease sphincter pressure to such a degree as to invalidate the results.[5] Urodynamic studies are difficult to perform in awake children; therefore, some anesthesia is needed to facilitate the study. Light general anesthesia, however, may lead to laryngospasm associated with instrumentation of the urethra; therefore, the anesthesiologist should be prepared to provide deeper anesthesia to carry out urethral instrumentation and later lighten the anesthesia so that the voiding studies can be performed. If urodynamic studies are delayed for an appropriate period of time following induction of anesthesia and if instrumentation is performed under deeper anesthesia, reliable results can be obtained by lightening anesthesia, using nitrous oxide and oxygen only in children.[6] Although atropine may be a desirable antisialagogue drug and is effective in preventing bradycardia during induction of anesthesia in children, it relaxes the smooth muscle of the bladder and invalidates urodynamic studies. Therefore, premedication with atropine should be avoided.

The major medical problems associated with VUR are renal damage and hypertension. These problems have been documented in 10–20% of children with VUR and renal scarring. Hypertension resulting from VUR may occur in the absence of altered renal function because it is associated more with vascular damage than with any particular amount of parenchymal damage. Also, the frequency of urinary tract infection and the need for antibiotics may result in the administration of certain antibiotics that could induce renal toxicity and enhance, or by themselves may cause, neuromuscular blockade.

Suprapubic Cystostomy

Regional anesthesia in the form of spinal, epidural, caudal, or field block can be used for suprapubic cystostomy. Field block or local infiltration, which are used by some surgeons, may be inadequate because of the limited muscular relaxation and analgesia achieved.

Radical Cystectomy with Ileal Conduit Formation

The removal of the bladder and its replacement by an ileal conduit for bladder cancer is a major operation that carries a high morbidity and mortality. Preoperatively, patients are frequently undernourished and often have undergone radiation therapy, making surgical dissection more difficult. Preoperative nutritional supplementation with iv hyperalimentation has been advocated. Patients may be dehydrated from extensive bowel preparation and enemas preoperatively; thus, particular care should be taken to hydrate these patients before instituting anesthesia, especially if spinal or epidural block is used. Notable intraoperative problems including bleeding, prolonged operative time, intravascular fluid loss to third space compartments, and the heat loss that is frequently associated with bowel surgery. Manipulation of the bowel during surgery can cause significant fluid loss to third space compartments, and this, combined with the inability to measure urine output, makes the use of a central venous pressure catheter important in monitoring changes in intravascular volume.

Regional anesthesia alone is unsuitable for most patients undergoing this surgery because of the long duration and extent of surgery. Continuous epidural blockade combined with light general endotracheal anesthesia has been shown to reduce intraoperative blood loss.[7] Other advantages to the use of this technique are early extubation and continued postoperative analgesia, which can be achieved with epidural opioids or local anesthetics. Because blood loss may be considerable, hypotensive anesthesia has been advocated to minimize blood loss.

ANESTHESIA FOR OPERATIONS ON THE EXTERNAL GENITALIA

These procedures are done in patients of various age groups. High reflexogenic sensitivity is present in the genital and perineal areas; therefore, when general anesthesia is used, deep planes of anesthesia are generally necessary to prevent undesirable autonomic reflexes such as laryngospasm and hypertension. Laryngospasm is a common occurrence secondary to urethral instrumentation or dilation of the rectum in a lightly anesthetized patient.[8] Regional anesthesia in the form of penile, caudal, saddle, or epidural blockade suppresses these responses completely. Another major reason for consideration of regional techniques is to provide postoperative pain relief and obviate the need for analgesics during the immediate postoperative period.

Surgical procedures on the scrotum, testicles, and epididymis and reconstructive operations on the vas deferens can be done under spinal or epidural blockade, depending on the duration and extent of surgery. Testicular innervation can be traced up to the T10 segment; thus, a T10 level blockade may be required to prevent pain from testicular traction or manipulation. Vasectomies performed in clinics are usually done under local infiltration anesthesia with 1% lidocaine or mepivacaine. Reconstructive surgery on the vas deferens, however, requires longer surgical time, and regional anesthesia is required. Penile prosthetic surgery requires several hours of analgesia and can be done under spinal, continuous lumbar epidural, or caudal blockade.

Hypospadias is one of the most frequent genitourinary anomalies. It is associated with hernias and hydroceles but does not appear to carry an increased risk of upper urinary tract anomalies. The potential psychological difficulty and concerns about toilet training usually favor surgical repair at the age of 1 year under general anesthesia.

Orchiopexy is increasingly being performed on an outpatient basis.[9,10] General anesthesia should be used in children because the procedure may be lengthy and abdominal musculature relaxation is often helpful. The operation is associated with considerable postoperative pain and a high incidence of nausea and vomiting. Caudal blockade (0.25% bupivacaine, 0.5 ml·kg^{-1}) or ilioinguinal/iliohypogastric nerve blockade (0.25% bupivacaine in dosages up to 2 mg·kg^{-1}) have been shown to provide highly effective postoperative analgesia following orchiopexy in children under general anesthesia.[10]

Surgical procedures on the penis, such as circumcision and hypospadias correction, are most commonly performed in children. Postoperative analgesia may be especially important in children because agitation and restlessness with pain may cause unwanted manipulation of the operative site by the patient, resulting in postoperative hemorrhage. Caudal or penile blockade has been applied immediately after children are induced with iv drugs or light general anesthesia by mask, or at the completion of the surgical procedure. These techniques of combining general anesthesia and regional anesthesia have proved valuable in decreasing the amount of general anesthetic needed intraoperatively and providing postoperative analgesia.

Caudal blockade provides excellent postoperative analgesia following a wide variety of surgical procedures such as hypospadias repair, orchiopexy, and circumcision. The blockade is performed with the child in a lateral or semiprone position after induction with general inhalational technique or with ketamine or a barbiturate. Bupivacaine 0.25% (1.25–1.5 mg·kg^{-1}) is injected through the sacrococcygeal membrane with a 20-gauge needle. Caudal blockade (1.25–1.5 mg·kg^{-1}, 0.25% bupivacaine) appears significantly better than intramuscular morphine (0.15 mg·kg^{-1}) or buprenorphine for immediate postoperative analgesia and is associated with a lower frequency of postoperative vomiting after circumcision in boys.[11,12]

Penile blockade may be used for most surgical procedures performed on the penis, such as circumcision, and for insertion of a penile prosthesis. It is a simple and safe procedure to perform in adults and children, with fewer associated complications than caudal blockade. To perform this block-ade for penile surgery in adults, a 25- or 27-gauge needle is inserted through the skin at the 2:00 o'clock and 10:00 o'clock positions at the base of the penis until the lower border of the symphysis pubis is contacted. The needle is withdrawn slightly and moved progressively in a caudal direction until bone is no longer contacted. A "pop" may be felt as the deep (Buck's) fascia of the penis is pierced. Local anesthetics are injected, typically 1 ml of 1% lido-caine at each side. A triangular ring of local anesthetic (about 10–15 ml of 1% lidocaine) is also formed subcutane-ously at the base of the penis, with the pubic tubercles and the median raphe of the scrotum at the base of the penis as the corners of the triangle.[13] A blockade of the dorsal nerves of the penis only (1–4 ml of 0.25% bupivacaine) has also been found to provide good postoperative analgesia (lasting more than 6 hours) in 96% of children after circumcision or correction of hypospadias and has proved to be a good alternative to opioid analgesics.[14] For postoperative analge-sia, the local anesthetic used most often is 0.25% bupiva-caine without epinephrine; volumes range from 0.8 ml in the neonate to 10 ml in the adult. Epinephrine-containing solutions should not be used because of the risk of penile ischemia.

Topical analgesia has also been used successfully for pain relief after circumcision in children. A thin film of lidocaine spray, 10–20 mg of 10% solution, lidocaine ointment (0.5–1 ml of a 5% preparation), or lidocaine jelly (0.5–1 ml of a 2% preparation) can be applied to the surgical wound post-operatively but before the child is awake. Topical lidocaine has the advantage of being noninvasive and simple to apply and provides an extended period of analgesia.[15]

ANESTHESIA FOR PROSTATIC SURGERY

Benign prostatic hypertrophy is a common disease of middle-aged and elderly men that necessitates surgical re-section of the prostatic gland when obstruction of urinary outflow through the prostatic urethra becomes symptom-atic. It has been estimated recently that a 50-year-old man has a 20–25% chance of having a prostatectomy during his lifetime.[16] It is the second most common surgical procedure (after cataract extraction) in men over age 65.[17,18] This pa-tient population generally carries greater anesthetic risk be-cause of the greater prevalence of coexisting cardiovascular or pulmonary problems.

In addition to the increased prevalence of cardiopulmo-nary disease in elderly men, the physiologic changes of aging will reduce the anesthetic or drug requirement and contribute to intraoperative and postoperative morbidity and mortality (see Chapter 49).

Transurethral Resection of the Prostate (TURP)

TURP currently is the most commonly performed procedure in men with symptomatic bladder outlet obstruction sec-ondary to benign prostatic hyperplasia, cancer, or bladder neck contracture. In the United States, more than 90% of patients with bladder outlet obstruction from benign pros-tatic hyperplasia undergo transurethral correction.[19] It has been the predominant major surgical procedure performed by American urologists for at least three decades. More than 350,000 of these procedures are now performed annually in the United States.[18]

TURP generally is a safe procedure. There has been a gradual reduction in the mortality associated with TURP, from 1.3% in 1974[20] to 0.2% in 1989.[21] It is preferred over suprapubic, retropubic, and perineal approaches, which af-ford better surgical access to large prostate glands but carry a higher morbidity and mortality. TURP carries unique com-plications because of the need to use large volumes of irri-gating fluid for the endoscopic resection. The anatomy of the pathologic hypertrophic gland, the size of the gland, and the skill of the resectionist all contribute to the morbidity associated with this surgical procedure. Therefore, it is ger-mane to describe the pathologic changes of benign prostatic hypertrophy to better understand the pathophysiology asso-ciated with TURP and anesthetic management.

The prostate is a pear-shaped gland surrounding the pros-tatic urethra at the base of the bladder. Although anatomi-cally the prostate has five lobes (one anterior, two lateral, one median, and one posterior), only the median and lateral lobes are enlarged and surgically excised in primary idio-pathic prostatic hypertrophy (Fig. 41-1). In the majority of men over 50 years of age, the submucosal glands and the smooth muscle of the prostatic urethra undergo glandular and leiomyomatous hyperplasia. This growth is stimulated by testicular hormones and presses the normal prostatic tis-sue against the fibrous capsule, forming a "surgical capsule" consisting of compressed normal prostatic tissue and veins, infiltrated by nodular new growth. It is sometimes unavoid-able that these compressed prostatic veins (sinuses) are en-tered during TURP and that irrigating fluid is absorbed into the intravascular compartment. However, fibrosis can some-times occur in the hypertrophic prostatic gland and reduce the vascularity of the gland. Resection of a fibrotic gland is associated with less bleeding and less fluid access into the circulation.

TURP is performed through a resectoscope. The hypertro-phied lateral and median lobes of the prostate gland are

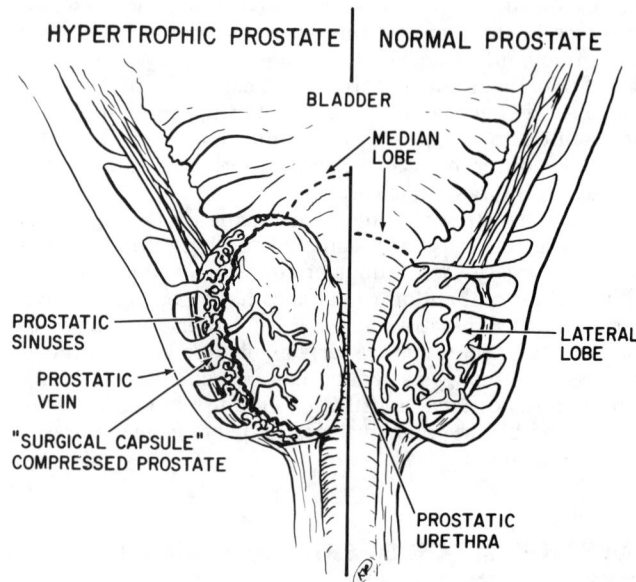

Figure 41-1. Anatomy of hypertrophic prostate. The hypertrophic gland represents glandular and leiomyomatous hyperplasia of the submucosal glands and the smooth muscle of the prostatic urethra, thus pushing the normal prostatic tissue to create a "surgical cap-sule." (Reprinted with permission from Stoelting RK, Barash PG, Gallagher TJ: Advances in Anesthesia, vol III, p 379. Chicago, Year Book Medical Publishers, 1986.)

excised with an electrically energized wire loop; bleeding is controlled with a coagulating current. The procedure usually brings about complete excision of the prostatic adenoma, exposing the fibers of surgical capsule throughout the entirety of the prostatic fossa. Continuous irrigation is used to distend the bladder and to wash away blood and dissected prostatic tissue. Distilled water interferes least with visibility; however, absorption of large quantities of water can lead to water intoxication with hypo-osmolality, excessive dilutional hyponatremia, which results in intravascular hemolysis, acute renal failure, and central nervous system (CNS) symptoms ranging from confusion to convulsions and coma. Because of this, today probably 80% of surgeons use a nonelectrolyte iso-osmotic or near iso-osmotic solution for TURP.[19] Although electrolytic solutions such as normal saline or Ringer's lactate do least harm when absorbed into the circulation, they are highly ionized and promote dispersion of high current from the resectoscope, thereby inhibiting its cutting properties. Therefore, nonelectrolytic solutions consisting of sorbitol and mannitol (Cytal), or of glycine 1.5%, which are slightly hypo-osmolar to the blood, have been used most often.[22,23]

Because the prostate gland contains large venous sinuses, it is inevitable that irrigating solution will be absorbed. The amount of absorption is governed mainly by the hydrostatic pressure driving fluid into prostatic veins and sinuses, which is determined by the height of the container of irrigating fluid above the patient. The amount of irrigating fluid absorbed during TURP is proportional to the duration of resection. On average, 10 to 30 ml of fluid is absorbed per minute of resection time, with as much as 6 to 8 l absorbed in some cases when resection lasted up to 2 hours.[24,25] In addition, the number and sizes of the venous sinuses opened during resection influence vascular absorption.[25] Although water intoxication is not totally preventable, limiting the resecting time to less than 1 hour is desirable.[26,27]

Optimizing the patient's preoperative condition is essential to the anesthetic management. Men over 60 years of age generally are at greater risk for anesthesia-related problems because they are more likely to be debilitated from multisystem disease. In the American Urological Association cooperative study of almost 4000 patients, only 23% of the patients who underwent TURP did not have significant prior medical problems. The most common problems were pulmonary (14.5%), gastrointestinal (13.2%), myocardial infarction (12.5%), cardiac arrhythmias (12.4%), and renal insufficiency (9.8%).[21] In the past the most common cause of death after TURP was cardiovascular complications.[20] However, in recent years the most common cause of death has been sepsis occurring in patients who were debilitated and had other systemic disease processes.[21] Today, many patients are admitted on the day of surgery, and therefore their preoperative evaluation must be completed on an outpatient basis. Common findings in these elderly patients are chronic obstructive pulmonary disease, hypertension, angina, congestive heart failure, presence of a cardiac pacemaker, diabetes mellitus, infection, stroke, and renal insufficiency. Because TURP is generally an elective procedure, these patients should be in the best condition possible before surgery.

Complications of TURP

A summary of intraoperative and immediate postoperative complications of TURP which are of concern to anesthesiologists is listed in Table 41-1. In the 1989 American Urological Association cooperative study,[21] the incidence of com-

---

TABLE 41-1. Complications of TURP of Particular Interest to Anesthesiologists

Intravascular absorption of irrigating fluid
  Fluid overload
  Serum hypo-osmolality
  Hyponatremia
  Hyperglycinemia and hyperammonemia
  Hemolysis
  Hypothermia
  Bacteremia
Excessive bleeding and coagulopathy
Perforation of bladder or urethra with extravasation
  Extraperitoneal
  Intraperitoneal

---

plications occurring intraoperatively was 6.9%. The most common intraoperative complications were bleeding requiring transfusion (2.5%), TURP syndrome (2%), myocardial arrhythmia (1.1%), and extravasation (0.9%). In the immediate postoperative period, the complication rate was 18%. The most common complications were failure to void (6.5%), bleeding requiring transfusions (3.9%), clot retention (3.3%), and genitourinary infections documented by culture (2.3%).

TURP Syndrome. During or immediately following TURP, a few patients may exhibit overt signs (including bradycardia) of increasing circulating blood volume and dilution of serum electrolytes, and increases in systolic, diastolic, and pulse pressure. If the patient is awake he may show symptoms of restlessness, nausea and vomiting, mental confusion, skeletal muscle twitching, and visual disturbance. These signs and symptoms may progress to hypotension, with cyanosis, dyspnea, cardiac dysrhythmias, lethargy, seizures, and occasionally death.[19,24,26,28] This clinical syndrome has been termed the "TURP syndrome" or "TURP reaction."

A major component of the TURP syndrome is severe hyponatremia. Intravascular absorption of irrigating fluid can lead to a significant increase in the blood volume (hypervolemia), dilutional hyponatremia, and decreased serum osmolality (hypo-osmolality) and adverse hemodynamic and CNS changes.[26,29,30]

As previously noted, the ideal irrigating fluid for TURP should be optically satisfactory, iso-osmolar, nonhemolytic, nonelectrolytic or very weakly ionized, nontoxic when administered iv, and inexpensive. Today, glycine and Cytal are the two most commonly used irrigating fluids for TURP. Cytal is a mixture of 2.7% sorbitol and 0.54% mannitol. It is nonelectrolytic, iso-osmolar, and cleared from the plasma rapidly, but it is more expensive than glycine. Currently glycine 1.5% in water is most commonly used because of its low cost. It is a slightly hypo-osmolar solution (230 mOsm/l). Nevertheless, using it as irrigating fluid has eliminated hemolysis and reduced renal failure associated with TURP, compared with the use of distilled water as the irrigating fluid. However, the other major problem associated with absorption of large volumes of irrigating fluid— overhydration—still remains even when a nonhemolytic fluid is used as the irrigating fluid. Moreover, recent data suggest there are potential chemical toxicities associated with the absorption of glycine and its metabolic product, ammonia.[31-33]

The irrigating fluid used during TURP is absorbed through open venous sinuses of the gland; the amount absorbed varies considerably, depending on the area of raw surface exposed by the surgeon, the hydrostatic pressure exerted by the irrigating fluid, and the duration of the procedure.[24] When irrigating fluid rapidly enters the vascular compartment, the load on the circulation as well as myocardial work are increased. The nonelectrolytic solution (glycine 1.5%) dilutes blood proteins as well as electrolytes. The additive effects of increased intravascular pressure and decreased protein oncotic pressure favor the movement of fluid from the vascular compartment to the interstitial compartment.[34] Under usual conditions, only 20–30% of a load of crystalloid solution remains in the intravascular space; the remainder enters the interstitial space. For every 100 ml of fluid entering the interstitial compartment, 10 to 15 mEq of sodium also moves with it.[22] Desmond described a patient who gained 2.2 kg by the end of the operation but whose blood volume had increased only 500 ml. The other 1500 ml of fluid presumably moved into the interstitial compartment and carried with it 100 to 150 mEq of sodium.[22] Whether patients will develop symptoms of circulatory overload depends on their cardiovascular status, the amount and rapidity of absorption of the irrigating fluid, and the extent of surgical blood loss. Therefore, it is imperative to monitor patients carefully. In this regard, spinal or epidural blockade, supplemented with only light iv sedation, has the advantage of allowing the patient to verbalize potential cardiopulmonary and CNS problems during surgery. In addition, the cardiovascular depression associated with the administration of potent volatile anesthetics is avoided. Regional anesthesia also produces sympathetic blockade and increases venous capacitance, which tends to reduce the likelihood of intraoperative fluid overload during TURP. However, when the blockade dissipates, venous capacity acutely decreases, and circulatory overload could occur during the postoperative period.

If dilutional hyponatremia develops rapidly, serum osmolality also falls, promoting efflux of intravascular fluid into other compartments. Signs of cerebral and pulmonary edema may appear. All patients who undergo TURP will have some degree of dilutional hyponatremia, but only those in whom the heart is incapable of handling the fluid overload will manifest cerebral edema, increased intracranial pressure, and pulmonary edema. CNS symptoms, including apprehension, irritability, confusion, headache, seizures, visual disturbance, and coma, have usually been attributed to dilutional hyponatremia and water intoxication with hypo-osmolality. Hyponatremia can disturb electrophysiology. The concentration of extracellular sodium must be in a physiologic range for effective depolarization of excitable cells and for production of action potentials. When brain cells are incapable of producing effective impulses, CNS symptoms ensue. When myocardial cells are incapable of producing effective impulses, cardiac dysrhythmias may develop. Hyponatremia also contributes to negative inotropic effects and hypotension. A serum sodium level of 120 mEq·l^{-1} appears to be borderline for the development of severe TURP syndrome. When extracellular sodium levels drop below 120 mEq·l^{-1}, CNS symptoms, usually restlessness and confusion, may occur. Electrocardiographic (ECG) changes are seen when the serum sodium falls below 115 mEq·l^{-1} and are characterized by widening of the QRS complex and ST segment elevation. Seizures occur at serum sodium levels of 102 mEq·l^{-1}. Cardiac dysrhythmias, hypotension, and pulmonary edema may also occur.[35] At levels below 100 mEq·l^{-1}, consciousness is often lost.[36] However, it is impossible to separate the latter events from those resulting from fluid overload alone.

The degree of irrigating fluid absorption is usually assessed from the serum sodium concentration measured at the end of the resection or from the volumetric irrigating fluid balance and blood loss.[37,38] A fall in the plasma sodium concentration indicates fluid absorption but does not necessarily correlate well with the volume absorbed.[24,25,39] Fluid may enter the intracellular space rapidly, and serum sodium may not accurately reflect the true dilution that has occurred. None of the available methods of measuring volumetric balance and blood loss has proved of great practical value to be widely adopted for use during surgery.[37] Recently a simple, noninvasive method that relies on ethanol marking of the irrigating fluid (1.5% glycine + 1% ethanol) has been introduced to detect irrigating fluid absorption.[40] The presence and volume of irrigating fluid absorbed can be determined immediately from measurement of the ethanol content of the expired breath so that treatment and steps to prevent further absorption can be instituted immediately.

There have been some case reports of temporary visual disturbance following TURP, and attention has turned to the absorption of glycine, a nonessential amino acid, and its metabolic by-product, ammonia, as possible causes of visual impairment and other CNS symptoms associated with TURP.[31,41] Glycine is known to be an inhibitory neurotransmitter in the mammalian CNS, where it acts in the same manner as γ-aminobutyric acid on chloride ion channels.[42] Ovassapian and colleagues[31] suggested glycine as the possible cause of visual impairment due to interruption of retinal synapses by high glycine concentrations. Others[32,43] have identified ammonia as a toxic metabolite of glycine metabolism and have implicated other possible harmful breakdown products. It is possible that both glycine and ammonia[32] can produce CNS symptoms, which vary from mild depression, confusion, and transient blindness to coma. Wang et al have demonstrated in laboratory animals[33] and in patients undergoing TURP[44] the association between increased glycine levels and inhibition of the visual evoked potentials. Normal plasma glycine levels are 13 to 17 mg·l^{-1}, whereas levels as high as 1029 mg·l^{-1} were measured during one episode of blindness in one patient.[31] Twelve hours later the glycine level in this patient had fallen to 143 mg·l^{-1} and vision had returned. In one report, encephalopathy after TURP was noted in three patients in association with elevated blood ammonia concentrations.[41] Each patient had blood ammonia levels more than 10 times the upper limit of normal. A high ammonia concentration in the CNS after neutral amino acid metabolism can result in the production of false neurotransmitters and the suppression of norepinephrine and dopamine release. This has been the proposed pathologic etiology of encephalopathy in a subset of patients who developed TURP syndrome.[41] Marked elevation in blood ammonia from metabolism of absorbed glycine solution may enhance or act independently of dilutional hyponatremia to produce encephalopathy common to TURP syndrome.[41] The data are far from conclusive, but hyperglycinemia and hyperammonemia could be the potential causes of problems during TURP.

In summary, fluid overload, hypo-osmolarity, and hyponatremia are the recognized factors contributing to the TURP syndrome; however, glycine and ammonia may also contribute to this complex clinical problem.

If the early signs of TURP syndrome appear, immediate treatment is essential. The operation should be terminated as soon as possible. Oxygenation should be optimized. Serum sodium and arterial blood gas values should be determined. Circulatory collapse should be carefully evaluated, as hypotension is often a result of circulatory overloading rather than hypovolemia. Invasive monitoring of arterial blood pressure, central venous pressure, and pulmonary pressure is very helpful in patients with cardiovascular instability or with pulmonary edema. Diuretics and hypertonic saline (3–5%), infused at a rate not to exceed 100 ml/hour, may be required if serum sodium is low.[36] Serum sodium and osmolality should be carefully monitored. The use of hypertonic saline still seems to be controversial.[45] Some feel that hyponatremia in TURP syndrome is not a true sodium deficit, as if the patient is merely overloaded with water, no hypertonic saline is needed. If significant blood loss is evident, red blood cells should be administered. In the American Urological Association cooperative study,[21] the incidence of the intraoperative TURP syndrome was 2%, and in 66% of cases it was corrected simply with diuretics and observation. Maintaining accurate fluid balance intraoperatively is difficult in these patients but should be achieved postoperatively.

Postoperatively these patients need a good diuresis to prevent clot formation as well as to remove excessive water and glycine from the body.

Excessive Bleeding in TURP. Blood loss during TURP has been correlated with the vascularity of the prostate gland, the weight of the prostate resected, the length of resection time, and the surgeon's experience and technique.[46-51] In a recent nationwide study, the incidence of bleeding, defined as the percentage of patients needing a blood transfusion, was 2.5% intraoperatively and 3.7% immediately postoperatively.[21] The same study found that the probability of bleeding was increased in patients with larger prostates (greater than 45 g) or who underwent procedures lasting 90 minutes or more. There is disagreement concerning the relation between the technique of anesthesia and the blood loss, and also the relation between intraoperative hypotension and the blood loss in TURP. Some authors have reported a significant reduction in blood loss when epidural blockade was compared with general anesthesia.[46,50] However, others noted no difference in blood loss between epidural blockade versus general anesthesia[51] or spinal blockade versus general anesthesia.[48] Some studies showed no correlation between blood pressure and blood loss either in the epidural group or in the general anesthesia group[46,51] while others showed less bleeding coincident with a significantly lower blood pressure under epidural blockade.[50]

Assessment of blood loss is difficult during TURP because the irrigating fluid dilutes the blood. Visual estimations of blood loss are often grossly inaccurate,[52,53] and the usual hemodynamic responses indicative of blood loss (e.g., tachycardia, hypotension) are unreliable owing to the increased circulating volume accompanying absorption of irrigating fluid. The hematocrit may appear to be decreased or unchanged intraoperatively, depending on the amount of fluid that is absorbed in the intravascular space at the time of measurement. Generally, intraoperative blood transfusion has not been necessary until more reliable indices of blood loss are ascertained in the postoperative period. In the study by Mebust et al,[21] patients with glands larger than 45 g had a significantly higher incidence of intraoperative transfusions (10%) than patients with glands weighing less than 45 g (0.9%). If the surgeon is experienced and the estimated prostatic weight is less than 30 g, preoperative cross-matching should not be necessary. Blood transfusion intraoperatively should be based on the preoperative hematocrit, the duration and difficulty of the resection, and the clinical assessment of the patient's condition. Continuous excessive bleeding postoperatively may indicate a coagulation prob-

lem. Excessive bleeding after TURP has never been directly correlated with the degree of activation of the fibrinolytic mechanism in the general circulation.[54] ε-Amino caproic acid, an inhibitor of plasminogen activation, has been demonstrated to produce a statistically significant but minimal reduction in hematuria in TURP patients as well as in those undergoing perineal and suprapubic prostatectomy.[55] Disseminated intravascular coagulation appeared to be responsible for many of the instances of severe postoperative hematuria in TURP patients.[56] The coagulation profiles that supported this diagnosis were thrombocytopenia, marked shedding of red blood cells from the blood clot, decreased concentration of fibrinogen, high titer of fibrin degradation products in the serum, decreased one-stage prothrombin activity, and decreased concentrations of multiple clotting factors, particularly factors V and VIII.[56] Successful treatment of postprostatectomy bleeding depends on rapid assessment of the degree and nature of the coagulation disorder.

Hypothermia During TURP. Elderly patients have an age-related decline in the function of the autonomic nervous system that leads to progressive thermoregulatory impairment.[57] The ability to increase mean body temperature by increasing heat production decreases with age.[58] These patients tolerate hypothermia poorly. Hypothermia could be another intraoperative cause of mental confusion in patients who have undergone TURP. Hypothermia can cause shivering with increased oxygen consumption and cardiac irritability. Administration of iv fluid at ambient temperature and the constant irrigation of cold fluid through the bladder together with its intravascular absorption will rapidly lower the core body temperature of patients undergoing TURP, especially in cold operating rooms. It has been shown that intraoperative hypothermia is not influenced by the anesthetic technique used.[58,59] General anesthesia reduces heat production, whereas heat production is uninfluenced by lumbar epidural blockade.[58] But after termination of general anesthesia, oxygen uptake and plasma catecholamines increased; no such changes could be detected when epidural blockade was used. Increasing the operating room temperature and the use of warming mattresses, a reflective blanket, warming of both iv fluid and irrigating fluids, and heating of humidified respiratory gases can minimize this problem.[60-62] Nasal administration of oxygen or mask oxygen supplementation should be provided along with regional anesthesia to these elderly patients. Shivering is also a common postoperative sequela that in turn increases venous pressure and promotes hemorrhage. Hypothermia and pain are common causes of postoperative increases in body metabolism; maintaining body temperature and ensuring postoperative analgesia are important measures for providing optimal care of these patients.

Bacteremia. Bacteremia is a common occurrence following TURP. Infection of the prostate should be controlled prior to surgery. Sudden cardiovascular collapse after TURP is most commonly a manifestation of bacteremia, and no time should be lost in obtaining blood cultures. Broad-spectrum antibiotic therapy is usually given preoperatively and postoperatively on the basis of the preoperative urine culture results. In addition, antibiotics are usually used prophylactically in the majority of patients postoperatively.[21]

Bladder Perforation. Another complication of TURP is bladder perforation.[63] Perforations usually occur during difficult resections and are most often made by the cutting loop or knife electrode. Some, however, are made by the tip of the resectoscope or result from overdistention of the bladder with irrigating fluid. Most perforations are extraperitoneal and, in the conscious patient, result in pain in the periumbilical, inguinal, or suprapubic regions. Perforation of the prostatic capsule should be suspected if the irrigation fluid fails to return as it should. Less often the perforation is through the wall of the bladder and is intraperitoneal, or a large extraperitoneal perforation may extend into the peritoneum. In such cases, pain may be generalized in the upper abdomen or referred from the diaphragm to the precordial region or the shoulder. Subdiaphragmatic irritation from intraperitoneal irrigating fluid may induce hiccupping and shortness of breath. Other signs and symptoms such as pallor, diaphoresis, abdominal rigidity, nausea, vomiting, hypotension, and hypertension have been reported. These symptoms and their severity depend on the location and size of the perforation and the type of irrigating fluid. Generally, intraperitoneal fluid will eventually be excreted by the kidneys without the need for operative intervention. A small perforation can be managed conservatively with catheter drainage, but if significant extravasation has occurred, it should be drained suprapubically.[64] When hemodynamic embarrassment occurs, suprapubic drainage is the most efficient manner of eliminating the excess intraperitoneal fluid. The incidence of perforation is estimated at 0.9–1.1%.[21,65]

Choice of Anesthetic Techniques

The choice of anesthetic technique for TURP is a matter for individual assessment and is tailored to the specific needs of the patient. Regional anesthesia has the advantages of early warning of fluid overload and possibly decreased blood loss, but occasional difficulties in placement of the local anesthetics because of vertebral disease, and the desire of many patients to be asleep, make general anesthesia just as acceptable.

General anesthesia may mask the early signs and symptoms of TURP syndrome but may be more desirable than regional anesthesia in patients who need pulmonary support, who cannot tolerate iv infusion of fluids to compensate for the rapid loss of sympathetic tone from regional anesthesia, or who need invasive monitoring. Provided that 1.5% glycine solution is used, hemolysis is generally avoided, but fluid overload can still occur with hyponatremia. Central venous pressure monitoring is helpful under such situations. Although increases in systolic and diastolic blood pressures are considered to be the classic signs of hypervolemia, abrupt falls in blood pressure can occur in response to dilutional hyponatremia and hypervolemia.

Spinal anesthesia has been advocated as the anesthetic technique of choice for TURP, and in a recent nationwide study, the majority of TURP procedures were done under spinal anesthesia.[21] With spinal blockade, the patient is awake and capable of aiding the anesthesiologist in the early recognition of intravascular absorption of irrigating fluid and can describe early signs of fluid overload and water intoxication. Also, the early diagnosis and treatment of inadvertent urinary bladder perforation with extravasation of irrigating fluid can be recognized promptly. But if the blockade level is higher than T10, the capsular sign (pain on perforation of the capsule of the prostate) may not be preserved. The amount of local anesthetic agent used for spinal anesthesia is small, and a solid blockade is generally predictable. Epidural or caudal anesthetic techniques do not offer much advantage over spinal anesthesia because of a generally lower success rate with the extradural approaches.

Furthermore, the controllability of continuous epidural anesthesia for the level and duration of anesthesia is usually not necessary for TURP. Sacral segments may be missed with lumbar epidural blockade, and caudal blockade may be more suitable if the patient has previously undergone spinal surgery or has an osteoarthritic spine. The use of regional techniques for TURP is believed by some to reduce blood loss, compared with general anesthetic techniques.[18] Others, however, have found no difference in blood loss between spinal or epidural blockade and general anesthesia. The mode of breathing (spontaneous or mechanical ventilation) in the latter did not affect the overall results.[48,51] Postoperatively a significant cause of blood loss may be a rise in venous pressure brought about by straining or coughing as a result of a partially obstructed upper airway or from painful stimuli. The abolition of both these factors by regional anesthesia or maintenance of a patent upper airway could decrease bleeding. There is no place for controlled hypotension as a technique to limit blood loss in these patients. Regardless of whether general or regional anesthesia is selected, careful monitoring of cardiopulmonary parameters is vital. Anesthesia and surgery for patients undergoing TURP require a high degree of expertise and vigilance.

In 1986 it was reported that TURP could be performed successfully under local anesthesia with iv supplementation with sedatives in the majority of patients with small to moderate-sized prostate glands.[66] Local anesthetics (0.25% bupivacaine, 1% lidocaine, or both) were injected into the prostate transurethrally, and a lidocaine-bupivacaine mixture was infiltrated transperineally into the gland.

With improved fiberoptics, perioperative management, and anesthesia, TURP can be performed in selected patients in an outpatient setting.[66-68]

Open Prostatectomy

Open prostatectomy can be performed through a suprapubic (transvesical) approach, a retropubic approach, or a perineal approach. Open prostatectomy is usually preferable to TURP if the prostate gland is excessively enlarged, if other intravesical pathologic conditions are present that warrant open exploration, or if previous hip fixation prevents placement of the patient in the lithotomy position. Prostates greater than 100 g are more conveniently removed by open prostatectomy and with less morbidity than that associated with the transurethral approach.

Open prostatectomy can be performed under either general or regional anesthesia. Considerations that influence the choice of regional or general anesthesia are (1) the status of the patient's cardiopulmonary system, (2) the position of the patient during surgery, and (3) the patient's mental status. The patient with significant cardiopulmonary problems often cannot tolerate fluid overload and electrolyte imbalance. Having control of ventilation of the lungs and ensuring adequate oxygenation will favor general anesthesia for such patients. Uncooperative patients, especially elderly persons who are mentally confused or disoriented, are also more easily managed by general anesthesia. On the other hand, regional anesthesia, especially spinal blockade, has the advantage of being simple to administer and allows the patient to be relatively pain free during the recovery period. Furthermore, this approach lessens the postoperative agitation and restlessness that frequently follow general anesthesia in elderly patients. In addition, the use of epidural or spinal blockade has been shown to reduce operative blood loss during lower abdominal or TURP procedures.[46,69,70] Because the patient is supine during suprapubic retropubic prostatectomy, spinal or epidural blockade with light sedation is well accepted by patients and provides adequate anesthesia.

For perineal prostatectomy the patient is placed in an exaggerated lithotomy position with some flexion of the trunk and a moderate head-down tilt. This position can cause marked impairment of the cardiovascular and respiratory systems. Although a continuous epidural blockade combined with a light general anesthesia with endotracheal intubation and controlled ventilation of the lungs using nitrous oxide–oxygen has been successfully used, most anesthesiologists prefer general anesthesia in such patients so that they may better control the cardiopulmonary system and intravascular fluid volume.

Balloon Dilation of the Prostate

Some of the alternatives to prostatectomy, such as transurethral incision, urethral stents, and balloon dilation, usually can be done under iv sedation, perineal injection of local anesthetics, or intraurethral viscous 2% lidocaine jelly anesthesia on an outpatient basis. But many patients still need short-acting spinal or light general anesthesia for balloon dilation.[71]

ANESTHESIA FOR OTHER UROLOGIC PROCEDURES

Lithotripsy

Percutaneous ultrasonic lithotripsy and extracorporeal shock wave lithotripsy (ESWL) represent new techniques in urologic surgery. The anesthetic management for these procedures may be different from routine general and regional anesthesia.

Percutaneous Ultrasonic Lithotripsy

In percutaneous ultrasonic lithotripsy a nephroscope is introduced through a small flank incision, and a hollow metal probe is inserted through the nephroscope to contact the calculus. Ultrasonic energy is delivered by this metal probe through the percutaneous nephrostomy track and into the renal pelvis to fracture renal or upper ureteral stones. The stone fragments are flushed out with large quantities of irrigating fluids such as normal saline. This technique has been widely adopted by urologists, and, with the advent of ESWL, it is predicted that open renal surgery for stones will become an uncommon event.[64] Acute hyponatremia, acute hemolysis with hyperkalemia owing to sudden absorption of a bolus of water, and air embolism are possible complications in percutaneous ultrasonic lithotripsy. Because the irrigating fluid is likely to be absorbed, the use of normal saline for irrigation is recommended.[72] In contrast to electroresection of the prostate, electrolytic irrigating solution does not interfere with percutaneous ultrasonic lithotripsy.

General, regional, and local anesthesia techniques have been successfully used for this procedure.

Extracorporeal Shock Wave Lithotripsy (ESWL)

ESWL has revolutionized the treatment of urinary calculi. The method has been considered the procedure of choice for small renal calculi and for the majority of ureteral calculi. Larger renal calculi or impacted ureteral calculi may be managed by endoscopic techniques with or without adjunctive (ultrasonic or electrohydraulic) lithotripsy or laser fragmentation. ESWL is a technique for pulverizing urinary stones, without surgical intervention, by means of shock waves so that the disintegrated pieces of stones can be passed in the urine. Shock waves impose mechanical stresses that exceed the strength of brittle material such as kidney stones, and shock waves can be transmitted through water and propagated through the body without energy loss. In conjunction with suitable reflectors, shock waves can be focused and reproduced reliably.

Anesthesia is required for ESWL performed with earlier models of lithotriptors, because the shock wave causes pain. Although local infiltration of the entry site with high doses of local anesthetic and iv sedatives has been effective in selected patients,[73] in the majority of patients some form of regional (spinal, epidural) or general anesthesia is required. With earlier models of lithotriptors, anesthesiologists are confronted with the problem of anesthetizing a patient who is partly submerged in a stainless steel tank of warm water with only the head and arms out of the bath, and with the relative inaccessibility of the patient's airway (Fig. 41-2). The patient must be positioned properly so that the shock waves will travel harmlessly through the water until they hit the kidneys and disintegrate the stones, but not reach the lungs. Immersion has been shown to augment cardiac preload as a result of compression of peripheral vessels by hydrostatic pressure and a shift of blood volume into the central vascular compartment. Administration of anesthesia, immersion in water, or ESWL may all cause hemodynamic changes.[74-76] All these hemodynamic changes can be detrimental to patients with cardiac insufficiency and valvular heart diseases. Patients with dilated hearts, a dilated left atrium, paroxysmal tachycardia, frequent extrasystoles, or syncope should be properly evaluated and treated preoperatively before subjected to anesthesia and ESWL with an immersion tub system.

Epidural blockade has been used in many centers for ESWL. Continuous epidural blockade has the following advantages: (1) Many patients undergoing ESWL require cystoscopy with stone manipulation just prior to ESWL, and the same epidural catheter can be used for both procedures. (2) An awake patient can cooperate to a certain extent and facilitate positioning onto the frame; thus, brachial plexus injury due to positioning can be avoided. Compared with general anesthesia, epidural blockade also requires less an-

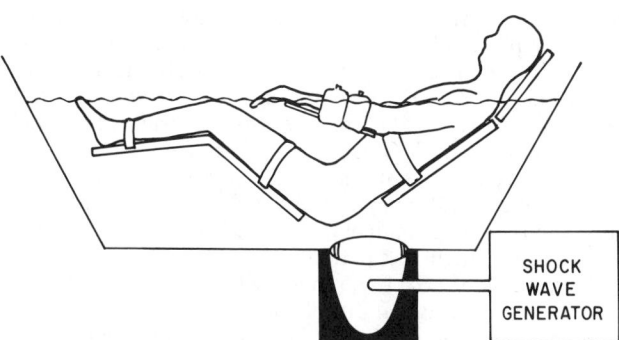

Figure 41-2. Patient position for ESWL. The patient is positioned in the frame and is partially immersed in or emersed out of the water bath by moving the frame in and out of the bath. Arm floats are used for arm support.

esthetic equipment attached to the patient in the bath. (3) The length of the ESWL treatment is often quite variable. Under continuous epidural blockade, analgesia can be extended as long as desired. If a regional technique is contraindicated for medical or psychological reasons, general endotracheal anesthesia can be performed. The latter is also preferred for high-risk patients because it enables closer cardiopulmonary control of patients. Regional anesthesia is not recommended for apprehensive patients who need high doses of sedative drugs. Analgesia to T6 is usually required for ESWL, and epidural anesthesia is preferable to spinal anesthesia because it is more easily controlled. Spinal blockade produces more profound sympathetic blockade than epidural blockade and can produce more pronounced circulatory changes during positioning.

Fluid regimens during ESWL are aimed at adequate urine formation to ensure passage of disintegrated stones and to maintain acceptable hemodynamics during anesthesia. This goal is complicated in the setting of significant cardiac problems (e.g., coronary artery disease, pump failure, and valvular insufficiency). Continuous arterial and central venous pressure monitoring is needed in critically ill patients in order to carefully monitor changes and to titrate vasopressors for circulatory support.

A problem unique to ESWL is the sudden exaggerated peripheral vasodilation and hypotension after sympathetic blockade under regional or general anesthesia as the patient is emerging from the bath. Caution should be exercised at the time of transferring the patient out of the bath. During immersion or emerging, cardiac dysrhythmias occasionally occur, even in healthy patients. The cause is an acute change in the right atrial and right ventricular wall tensions as a result of the rapid increase and decrease in preload.

At present, the following conditions are contraindications to ESWL with immersion in the tub: aortic aneurysm, hemangioma in the vertebral canal (intra- and extradural), orthopedic implants in the lumbar region, pregnancy, morbid obesity, and the presence of an artificial cardiac pacemaker. Coagulation disturbances may also contraindicate the use of ESWL.[77]

Intraoperative complications of ESWL include (1) a high incidence of cardiac dysrhythmias from the discharge of shock waves independent of the cardiac cycle (cardiac dysrhythmias have been minimized by coupling the lithotriptor to the patient's continuously monitored ECG so that shock waves are triggered by the R waves); (2) renal subcapsular hematoma; (3) myocardial ischemia and infarction; and (4) cerebrovascular accident.

The optimal anesthetic management of patients undergoing ESWL should include the following: (1) If regional anesthesia is administered, all equipment for airway control should be present in the ESWL room. (2) A cardiac defibrillator and a well-stocked emergency cart should be easily accessible. (3) The ECG tracing must be of good quality, because the R wave of the tracing is used to trigger the shock waves. Waterproof ECG pads and properly positioned leads are necessary to prevent burns. (4) The use of a pulse oximeter is essential. (5) Invasive lines such as radial artery, central venous, and pulmonary artery catheters may be indicated in some high-risk patients.

The success of ESWL, coupled with the complexity and expense of the original lithotriptor, stimulated intensive technical development in the field. In recent years several new machines have become available, such as the Dornier modifications and the piezoelectric lithotriptor, which is painless and can be combined with real-time sonography for stone localization; the tubless lithotriptor; and several other devices that are in various stages of development.[78] These second-generation lithotriptors incorporate several modifications that result in a reduction of pressure, a broader wave front where the shock wave enters the skin, and a reduction in the dimensions of the focal spot. Most patients regard treatment with these new machines as pain free or easily tolerated with oral premedication. Particular to these new machines are lack of radiation exposure, no need for anesthesia, applicability in an outpatient setting, no ECG problems, and a high degree of safety. Some machines are designed as a universal urologic table with fluoroscopy and radiographic capability that allows a full array of diagnostic and therapeutic endourologic procedures to be performed. However, young children or patients undergoing preoperative stone manipulations before ESWL may still need general anesthesia.

Laser Procedures

Lasers, especially the neodymium-doped yttrium-aluminum-garnet laser, have been increasingly used to treat tumors of the bladder and external genitalia.[79] For endoscopic procedures, if extensive or numerous tumors are present, the operation is generally performed under spinal or general anesthesia. For treatment of benign and malignant lesions of the external genitalia, lasers may prove to have a significant advantage over existing methods of treatment. Local infiltration of local anesthetic agents provides sufficient analgesia for the treatment of small penile or vulvar lesions, but extensive lesions or perianal lesions require regional (spinal or epidural) or general anesthesia.

REFERENCES

1. Hendolin H, Mattila MAK, Poikolainen E: The effect of lumbar epidural analgesia on the development of deep vein thrombosis of the legs after open prostatectomy. Acta Chir Scand 147:425, 1981
2. Guttmann L, Whitteridge D: Effects of bladder distention on autonomic mechanisms after spinal cord injuries. Brain 70:361, 1947
3. Bors E: The challenge of quadriplegia. Bull LA Neurol Soc 21:105, 1956
4. Lambert DH, Deane RS, Mazuzan JE: Anesthesia and the control of blood pressure in patients with spinal cord injury. Anesth Analg 61:344, 1982
5. Doyl PT, Briscoe CE: The effects of drugs and anaesthetic agents on the urinary bladder and sphincters. Br J Urol 48:329, 1976
6. Stehling LC, Patil U, Patil V: Anesthesia for urodynamic studies in children. Anesthesiol Rev 6:13, 1969
7. Ryan DW: Anaesthesia for cystectomy. Anaesthesia 37:554, 1982
8. Stephen CR, Ahlgren EW, Bennett EJ: Elements of Pediatric Anesthesia, p 8. Springfield, Illinois, Charles C Thomas, 1970
9. Cloud DT: Outpatient pediatric surgery. Int Anesthesiol Clin 20:99, 1982
10. Hannallah RS, Broadman LM, Belman AB et al: Comparison of caudal and ilioinguinal/iliohypogastric nerve blocks for control of post-orchiopexy pain in pediatric ambulatory surgery. Anesthesiology 66:832, 1987
11. Lunn JN: Postoperative analgesia after circumcision. Anaesthesia 34:552, 1979
12. May AE, Wandless J, James RD: Analgesia for circumcision in children. Acta Anaesthesiol Scand 26:331, 1982
13. Katz J: Atlas of Regional Anesthesia, p 138. Norwalk, Connecticut, Appleton-Century-Crofts, 1985
14. Soliman MG, Tramblay NA: Nerve block of the penis for postoperative pain relief in children. Anesth Analg 57:495, 1978

15. Tree-Trakarn T, Pirayavaraporn S: Postoperative pain relief for circumcision in children: Comparison among morphine, nerve block and topical analgesia. Anesthesiology 62:519, 1985

16. Birkhoff JD: Natural history of benign prostatic hypertrophy. In Hinman F Jr, Boyarsky S (eds): Benign Prostatic Hypertrophy, p 5. New York, Springer-Verlag, 1983

17. Graves EJ: Detailed diagnoses and procedures. National Hospital Discharge Survey: 1987. Vital and Health Statistics, Series 13, No. 100, p 295. Washington, DC, US Government Printing Office, 1989

18. Health—United States, 1989. US Department of Health and Human Services, PHS-90-1232. Washington, DC, US Government Printing Office, 1983

19. Mebust WK: Transurethral prostatectomy. Urol Clin North Am 17:575, 1990

20. Melchior J, Valk WL, Foret JD et al: Transurethral prostatectomy: Computerized analysis of 2,223 consecutive cases. J Urol 112:634, 1974

21. Mebust WK, Holtgrewe HL, Cockett ATK et al: Transurethral prostatectomy—immediate and postoperative complications: A cooperative study of 13 participating institutions evaluating 3,885 patients. J Urol 141:243, 1989

22. Desmond J: Serum osmolality and plasma electrolytes in patients who develop dilutional hyponatremia during transurethral resection. Can J Surg 13:116, 1970

23. Nesbitt TE, Carter OW, Tudor JM et al: Complications of transurethral prostatectomy and their management. South Med J 59:361, 1966

24. Marx GF, Orkin LR: Complications associated with transurethral surgery. Anesthesiology 23:802, 1962

25. Hagstrom RS: Studies on fluid absorption during transurethral prostatic resection. J Urol 73:852, 1955

26. Harrison RH, Boren JS, Robinson JR: Dilutional hyponatremia shock: Another concept of the transurethral prostatic resection reaction. J Urol 75:95, 1956

27. Fillman EM, Hanson OL, Gilbert LO: Radioisotopic study of effects of irrigation fluid in transurethral prostatectomy. JAMA 171:1488, 1959

28. Norris HT, Aasheim GM, Sherrard DJ et al: Symptomatology, pathophysiology, and treatment of the transurethral resection of the prostate syndrome. Br J Urol 45:420, 1973

29. Wakim KG: The pathophysiologic basis for the clinical manifestations and complications of transurethral prostatic resection. J Urol 106:719, 1961

30. Hurlbert BJ, Wingard DW: Water intoxication after fifteen minutes of transurethral resection of the prostate. Anesthesiology 50:355, 1979

31. Ovassapian A, Joshi CW, Brunner EA: Visual disturbance: An unusual symptom of transurethral prostatic resection reaction. Anesthesiology 57:332, 1982

32. Roesch RP, Stoelting RK, Lingeman JE et al: Ammonia toxicity resulting from glycine absorption during a transurethral resection of the prostate. Anesthesiology 58:577, 1983

33. Wang JM, Wong KC, Creel DJ et al: Effects of glycine on hemodynamic responses and visual evoked potentials in the dog. Anesth Analg 64:1071, 1985

34. Mani M, Keh E, Kartha RK et al: Transurethral prostatic surgery revisited. Anesthesiol Rev 3(11):15, 1976

35. Aasheim GM: Hyponatremia during transurethral surgery. Can Anaesth Soc J 20:247, 1973

36. Henderson DJ, Middleton RG: Coma from hyponatremia following transurethral resection of prostate. Urology 15:267, 1980

37. Madsen P, Kuni H, Naber K: Various methods of determining irrigating fluid absorption during transurethral resection of the prostate. Urol Res 1:70, 1973

38. Hahn RG: Influence of variations in blood haemoglobin concentration on the calculation of blood loss and volumetric irrigating fluid balance during transurethral resection of the prostate. Br J Anaesth 59:1223, 1987

39. Taylor RO, Maxson ES, Carter FH et al: Volumetric gravimetric and radio-isotopic determination of fluid transfer in transurethral prostatectomy. J Urol 79:490, 1958

40. Hahn RG: Early detection of the TURP syndrome by marking the irrigating fluid with 1% ethanol. Acta Anaesthesiol Scand 33:146, 1989

41. Hoekstra PT, Kahnoski R, McCamish MA et al: Transurethral prostatic resection syndrome—a new perspective: Encephalopathy with associated hyperammonemia. J Urol 130:704, 1983

42. Snyder SH: The glycine synaptic receptor in the mammalian central nervous system. Br J Pharmacol 53:473, 1975

43. Ryder KW, Olson JF, Kahnoski RJ et al: Hyperammonemia after transurethral resection of the prostate: A report of 2 cases. J Urol 132:995, 1984

44. Creel DJ, Wang JML, Wong KC: Transient blindness associated with transurethral resection of the prostate. Arch Ophthalmol 105:1537, 1987

45. Goble NM, Hammonds JC: Water intoxication. Br Med J 292:59, 1986

46. Abrams PH, Shah PJR, Bryning K et al: Blood loss during transurethral resection of the prostate. Anaesthesia 37:71, 1982

47. Levin K, Nyren O, Pompeius R: Blood loss, tissue weight and operating time in transurethral prostatectomy. Scand J Urol Nephrol 15:197, 1981

48. McGowan SW, Smith GFN: Anaesthesia for transurethral prostatectomy. Anaesthesia 35:847, 1980

49. Perkins JB, Miller HC: Blood loss during transurethral prostatectomy. J Urol 101:93, 1969

50. Madsen RE, Madsen PO: Influence of anaesthesia form on blood loss in transurethral prostatectomy. Anesth Analg 46:330, 1967

51. Nielsen KK, Andersen K, Asbjorn J et al: Blood loss in transurethral prostatectomy: Epidural versus general anesthesia. Int Urol Nephrol 19:287, 1987

52. Desmond J: A method of measuring blood loss during transurethral prostatic surgery. J Urol 109:453, 1973

53. Jansen H, Berseus O, Johansson JE: A simple photometric method for determination of blood loss during transurethral surgery. Scand J Urol Nephrol 12:1, 1978

54. Elliot JS, MacDonald JK, Fowell AH: Blood loss and fibrinolysin levels during transurethral prostatic resection. J Urol 89:462, 1963

55. McNicol GP, Fletcher AP, Alkjaersig N et al: Impairment of hemostasis in the urinary tract: The role of urokinase. J Lab Clin Med 58:34, 1961

56. Friedman NJ, Silvija Hoag M, Robinson AJ et al: Hemorrhagic syndrome following transurethral prostatic resection for benign adenoma. Arch Intern Med 124:341, 1969

57. Collins KJ, Dore C, Exoton-Smith AN et al: Accidental hypothermia and impaired temperature homeostasis in the elderly. Br Med J 1:353, 1977

58. Stjerstrom H, Henneberg S, Eklund A et al: Thermal balance during transurethral resection of the prostate: A comparison of general anesthesia and epidural analgesia. Acta Anaesthesiol Scand 29:743, 1985

59. Jenkins J, Fox J, Sharwood-Smith G: Changes in body heat during transvesical prostatectomy. Anaesthesia 38:748, 1983

60. Dyer PM, Heathcote PS: Reduction of heat loss during transurethral resection of the prostate. Anaesth Intensive Care 14:12, 1986

61. Morrison RC: Hypothermia in the elderly. Int Anesthesiol Clin 26:124, 1988

62. Harioka T, Murakawa M, Dona J et al: Effect of continuously warmed irrigating solution during transurethral resection. Anaesth Intensive Care 16:324, 1988

63. Kenyon HR: Perforation in transurethral operations: Technique for immediate diagnosis and management of extravasations. JAMA 142:798, 1950

64. Whitfield HN, Hendry WF: Endoscopic surgery. In Whitfield HN, Hendry WF (eds): Textbook of Genito-Urinary Surgery, vol 2, p 1373. New York, Churchill Livingstone, 1985

65. Holtgrewe HL, Valk WL: Factors influencing the mortality and morbidity of transurethral prostatectomy: A study of 2015 cases. J Urol 87:450, 1962

66. Sinha B, Haikel G, Lange PH et al: Transurethral resection of the prostate with local anesthesia in 100 patients. J Urol 135:719, 1986

67. Moffat NA: Transurethral resection of prostate and bladder tumors. Urol Clin North Am 14:115, 1987

68. McLoughlin MG, Kinahan TJ: Transurethral resection of the prostate in the outpatient setting. J Urol 143:951, 1990

69. Moir DD: Blood loss during major vaginal surgery: A statistical study of the influence of general anaesthesia and epidural analgesia. Br J Anaesth 40:233, 1968

70. Donald JR: The effect of anaesthesia, hypotension, and epidural analgesia on blood loss in surgery for pelvic floor repair. Br J Anaesth 41:155, 1969

71. Dawd JB, Smith JJ III: Balloon dilatation of the prostate. Urol Clin North Am 17:671, 1990

72. Bennett MJ, Smith RW, Fuchs E: Sudden cardiac arrest during percutaneous ultrasonic nephrostolithotomy. Anesthesiology 60:245, 1984

73. Loening S, Karamolowsky EV, Willoughby B: Use of local anesthesia for extracorporeal shock wave lithotripsy. J Urol 137:626, 1987

74. Arborelius M, Balldin UL, Lilja B et al: Hemodynamic changes in man during immersion with the head above water. Aviat Space Environ Med 43:592, 1972

75. Begin R, Epstein M, Sackner MA et al: Effects of water immersion to the neck on pulmonary circulation and tissue volume in man. J Appl Physiol 40:293, 1976

76. Loellgen H, Von Nieding G, Horres R: Respiratory and hemodynamic adjustment during head out water immersion. Int J Sports Med 1:25, 1980

77. Drach GW, Dretler S, Fair W et al: Report of the United States cooperative study of extracorporeal shock wave lithotripsy. J Urol 135:1127, 1986

78. Wilson WT, Preminger GM: Extracorporeal shock wave lithotripsy: An update. Urol Clin North Am 17:231, 1990

79. Staehler G, Chaussey C, Jocham D et al: The use of neodymium-YAG lasers in urology: Indications, technique and critical assessment. J Urol 134:1155, 1985

42

F. Peter Buckley

Anesthesia and Obesity and Gastrointestinal Disorders

OBESITY

Obesity is usually defined in relation to ideal body weight (IBW) derived from actuarial tables, or in relation to height using indices such as the body mass index (BMI). The BMI is defined as weight (kg) divided by height (m) squared (wt/ht^2). For example, a 70-kg, 1.7-m patient has a BMI of 24. Patients who weigh 20% above IBW or have a BMI of greater than 28 are regarded as obese. Some 10–15% of the general population meet one of these definitions of obesity.[1,2] The very obese, usually termed the morbidly obese, weigh more than 45 kg above IBW or have a BMI of greater than 35.

Obesity is associated with a number of anatomic, physiologic, and biochemical deviations from normality. These abnormalities can affect all body systems and have implications for the health of individuals and for their anesthetic management.[3] Much of the information about obese patients and their anesthetic management has come from studies of morbidly obese patients with no systemic clinical disease. Caution should therefore be used when applying such information to the less heroically obese or to the morbidly obese population as a whole, which has a high prevalence of systemic clinical disease.

Not all body fat is the same. Fat in different anatomic distributions appears to be associated with different physiologic and pathophysiologic consequences. Android obesity, or obesity that is primarily of truncal distribution (with a waist-hip circumference ratio of 0.9 in men and 0.8 in women), is associated with increased oxygen consumption ($\dot{V}o_2$) and an increased incidence of cardiovascular disease. In gynecoid obesity, in which fat is distributed primarily on the buttocks and thighs, the fat is metabolically less active and less closely associated with cardiovascular disease.[4] Fat distributed intra-abdominally appears to be particularly associated with cardiovascular risk[5] and left ventricular (LV) dysfunction.[6]

Pathophysiology of Obesity

Respiratory System

Obese persons have increased $\dot{V}o_2$ and carbon dioxide production ($\dot{V}co_2$), but the basal metabolic rate, because it is related to body surface area (BSA), is usually normal.[7-9]

Contributing to the increased $\dot{V}o_2$ are the metabolic activity of fat, an increase in energy expenditure for locomotion and breathing (to move the mass-loaded chest and abdomen, and to maintain a high minute volume to remain normocarbic in the setting of an increased $\dot{V}co_2$). With exercise, $\dot{V}o_2$ and $\dot{V}co_2$ rise more sharply than in persons of normal body weight, as does the oxygen cost of respiration, implying respiratory muscle inefficiency.

As a consequence of fat producing mass loading, chest wall compliance is reduced, but lung compliance remains relatively normal. Mass loading also results in a fall in static lung volumes. In the upright position, residual volume remains normal, but expiratory reserve volume and functional residual capacity (FRC) are often reduced so that tidal ventilation may fall within the range of closing capacity, with ensuing ventilation-perfusion (V/Q) abnormalities, or frank right-to-left shunt, with ensuing hypoxemia (Fig. 42-1). As mass loading is increased by adopting the supine position, FRC often falls further within the range of closing capacity, with worsening hypoxemia (see Fig. 42-1). The usual clinical tests of respiratory function (e.g., forced vital capacity [FVC], forced expiratory volume in 1 sec [FEV$_1$], and peak expiratory flow rate [PEFR]) are usually normal in the healthy obese patient.

The majority of obese patients maintain a sufficient minute volume of ventilation ($\dot{V}E$) to remain normocarbic and preserve a normal response to carbon dioxide challenge. However, with increasing obesity, intercurrent lung disease, and the changes wrought by pulmonary hypertension, their condition may deteriorate to the obesity hypoventilation syndrome (loss of hypercarbic drive, sleep apnea, hypersomnolence, and potential or overt airway difficulties) or to the worst end of the spectrum, the Pickwickian syndrome (hypercarbia, hypoxemia, polycythemia, hypersomnolence, pulmonary hypertension, and biventricular failure).[10] The interactions of the respiratory and cardiovascular effects of obesity that lead to these conditions are shown schematically in Figure 42-2.

Cardiovascular System

In obese persons, circulating blood volume, plasma volume, and cardiac output increase proportionately with rising weight and $\dot{V}o_2$. Cerebral and renal blood flows are similar to those in normal persons, but splanchnic blood flow is

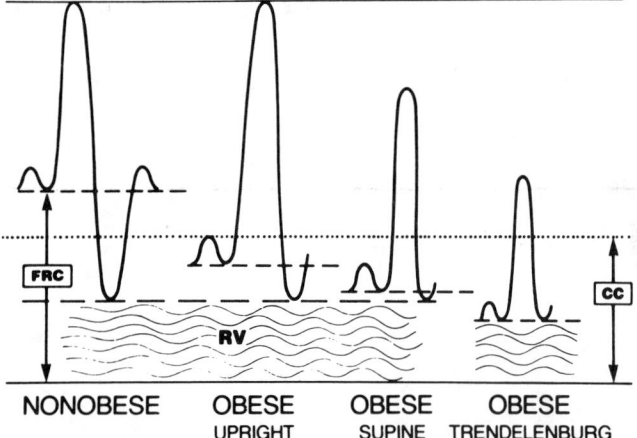

Figure 42-1. The effect of change in position on various lung volumes in nonobese and morbidly obese patients (FRC = functional residual capacity; RV = residual volume; CC = closing capacity). (Reprinted with permission from Vaughan RW: Pulmonary and cardiovascular derangements. In Brown BR [ed]: Anesthesia and the Obese Patient. Contemporary Anesthesia Practice Series, p 19. Philadelphia, FA Davis, 1982.)

20% higher than in normal-weight persons.[9,11,12] At rest, blood flow to fat is 2–3 ml per 100 g tissue; thus, for a patient with a fat mass of 50 kg, blood flow to this fat mass will account for an extra cardiac output of $1.5–2.0 \, l \cdot min^{-1}$. The increase in cardiac output parallels the rise in $\dot{V}O_2$; thus, systemic arteriovenous oxygen difference remains normal or slightly above normal. The pulse rate in the obese person is usually within normal limits; thus, with an increased cardiac output, stroke volume is increased.

Arterial hypertension occurs frequently in the morbidly obese. It is severe in 5–10% of the obese population and moderate in 50%. The increase in cardiac output in response to exercise is more abrupt than in normal-weight persons and may be accompanied by increases in LV end-diastolic pressure and pulmonary capillary wedge pressure.[12] Changes similar to those seen during exercise have been observed in the perioperative period.[13] Thus, patients with any degree of cardiovascular compromise are particularly at risk in the perioperative period.

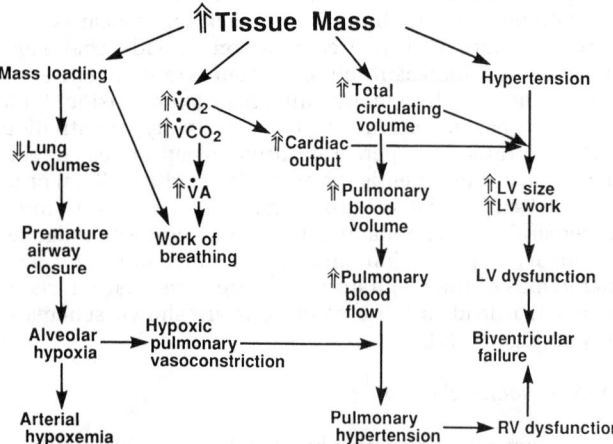

Figure 42-2. A schema interrelating the cardiovascular and respiratory abnormalities in morbidly obese patients to the pathophysiologic changes found in such patients.

The pathophysiologic effects of obesity on cardiac function are complex. Normotensive morbidly obese patients without evidence of coronary artery disease show normal myocardial performance, but raised preloads and afterloads.[14] In 20–50% of the morbidly obese population, cardiac diameter is increased on a chest radiograph, but a substantial proportion of patients maintain normal LV function in the setting of elevated circulating blood volume, plasma volume, cardiac output, and systemic blood pressure. Hypertension is associated with an increased LV mass. The quality of LV function in morbidly obese people is somewhat uncertain. Early studies reported that patients with both an increased LV wall thickness and an increased LV chamber size maintained normal LV systolic function in response to chronic circulatory overload. Those patients without an increased LV wall thickness had impaired LV systolic function.[12] More recent studies of the morbidly obese (mean weight, 170% of IBW) with increased LV wall thickness but without other demonstrable cardiac disease found that such subjects have normal ejection fractions at rest but cannot mount an increase in ejection fraction in response to exercise.[15] Thus in the old, morbidly obese patients and in those with demonstrable cardiac disease, a low threshold for performing detailed cardiac investigations is appropriate.

The pulmonary circulation is also vulnerable to the pathophysiologic changes produced by obesity. An increase in pulmonary blood volumes and flows predisposes obese patients to pulmonary hypertension, which may be accentuated or precipitated by hypoxic pulmonary vasoconstriction, which in turn occurs secondary to the static lung volume changes found in the morbidly obese (see Fig. 42-2).

Endocrine and Metabolic Systems

To maintain a stable weight, morbidly obese patients have to maintain a greater than normal caloric intake.[16] But, as with $\dot{V}O_2$, when this intake is related to BSA, the values are similar to those of normal-weight persons. Glucose tolerance is frequently impaired, with pancreatic islet cell hypertrophy and hyperinsulinemia, irrespective of the state of carbohydrate tolerance, and is reflected in a high prevalence of diabetes mellitus in the morbidly obese. Abnormal serum lipid profiles are often found and may be associated with an increased prevalence of ischemic heart disease.

Gastrointestinal System

Morbidly obese patients have an increased prevalence of hiatal hernia and a linear increase in intra-abdominal pressure with increasing weight. At the time of induction of anesthesia, 90% of fasted morbidly obese patients presenting for elective surgery have a gastric fluid volume in excess of 25 ml and a gastric fluid pH of less than 2.5.[17] Such volume and pH figures are generally accepted as being indicative of a high risk of acid aspiration pneumonitis if the gastric fluid reaches the airway. Because both intra-abdominal pressure and the volume of gastric content increase during pregnancy, the pregnant morbidly obese woman is at particular risk for aspiration pneumonitis.

There is an increase in liver fat content in 90% of morbidly obese patients[16,18] that may not show up on the usual clinical tests of hepatic function.[18] The increase appears to reflect the duration rather than the degree of obesity. The prevalence of hepatic dysfunction is particularly high in patients who have undergone intestinal bypass operations.

The effect of gastric partitioning operations on hepatic function is uncertain.

Airway

Obesity produces a number of anatomic changes that can affect the airway. Flexion of the cervical spine and the atlantoaxial joint may be limited by numerous "chins" and by thoracic wall or breast fat, and extension of these joints may be limited by low cervical or upper thoracic fat pads. Mouth opening may be restricted by submental fat. Fleshy cheeks, a large tongue, and copious flaps of palatal, pharyngeal, and supralaryngeal soft tissue may narrow the airway. Moreover, the laryngeal aperture may occupy a "high and anterior" infantile position. The morbidly obese have a high prevalence of obstructive apnea syndrome.[19] Such patients often present particular airway difficulties when anesthetized.

Psychology of the Obese

Although the prevalence of psychopathology in the obese population as a whole is similar to that in the normal-weight population, it may be somewhat higher in the morbidly obese.[20] Obese patients have a reputation among medical professionals for being difficult to manage, intolerant of discomfort, noncompliant with therapies, and prone to outbursts of anger or hysteria. Whether these characteristics are inherent to the obese state or result from individuals' interactions with their environment and its "thin-thinking" inhabitants is uncertain. There is evidence that obese people are the victims of prejudice and discrimination from an early age and are characterized by others as ugly, slothful, lacking in self-control, and prone to depression and self-consciousness. Physicians are not exempt from such prejudices. However, the alleged behavior may be largely a consequence of obese subjects' interactions with those around them, not exempting physicians. In my experience with a number of morbidly obese patients about to undergo gastric stapling operations, the patients were compliant with management regimens and conducted themselves normally throughout the perioperative period.[21] However, much time and effort were expended with this group, and the patients were obviously highly selected and motivated, having decided on a very dramatic course of action in an attempt to reduce their obesity.

Pharmacokinetics in the Obese

While there are few direct data on drug kinetics in the obese, certain inferences may be drawn from the known pathophysiologic changes in obesity.[22] Because obese persons have a larger than normal fat compartment, the proportion of body water and muscle mass in relation to total body weight will be less than normal. Drug biotransformation may be altered by hepatic disease, diabetes, or changes in splanchnic blood flow. Renal drug excretion may be changed as a result of alterations in glomerular filtration, and biliary excretion may be changed by the presence of gallstones or pancreatitis. Finally, the high incidence of hyperlipoproteinemia may affect drug binding.

Lipophilic drugs such as benzodiazepines[23] and thiopental[24] have an increased volume of distribution, more selective distribution to fat stores, and a longer elimination half-life in obese subjects than in normal-weight persons, but clearance values are similar in both groups. The implication of these findings is that fat-soluble volatile anesthetic agents may have a prolonged elimination time, with a consequent slow recovery. However, theoretical studies have shown that for prolonged recovery to occur, such agents would have to be administered for periods in excess of 24 hours.[25] Clinical studies of volatile agents administered to morbidly obese patients for commonly encountered operative times (2–4 hours) have shown normal recovery times.[26]

When administered to the obese patient on a mg·kg^{-1} body weight basis, fentanyl has similar pharmacokinetic parameters as in normal-weight subjects.[27] When administered on a mg·kg^{-1} body weight basis, sufentanil shows a large volume of distribution and a similar mean elimination half-life that is very variable.[28] When administered on a mg·kg^{-1} lean body weight basis, alfentanil has a similar volume of distribution in obese patients as in normal-weight patients but a longer elimination half-life secondary to reduced clearance.[29]

Hydrophilic drugs have similar volumes of distribution, elimination half-life, and clearance times in obese and nonobese patients. Morbidly obese patients have a higher pseudocholinesterase activity than nonobese subjects,[30] and dosages of 1.2–1.5 mg·kg^{-1} of succinylcholine are advised. To produce a given degree of neuromuscular blockade, a larger dose of pancuronium must be given to morbidly obese patients than to normal-weight patients. However, when this dose is related to BSA, it is similar to the dose in normal-weight patients.[31] When vecuronium[32] and metocurine[33] are administered on a mg·kg^{-1} body weight basis, recovery in the morbidly obese is slower than in normal-weight subjects. In contrast, when atracurium is administered on a mg·kg^{-1} body weight basis, the speed of recovery is similar in both populations,[32,36] even though blood levels of atracurium at the time of recovery are higher in the morbidly obese patients.[34]

Preoperative Evaluation

Although obese persons have a reputation for being difficult to handle, this difficulty can be minimized by a suitable preoperative evaluation and visit. The anesthesiologist should be aware of his or her own feelings, attitudes, and prejudices toward obesity and avoid condescension. Obese patients should be evaluated in a thorough, nonjudgmental fashion, with particular emphasis on the difficulties that obesity presents to the anesthesiologist. As for any patient, time should be allowed for the patient to detail previous adverse experiences with anesthetics and operations, as well as any fears and anxieties about the upcoming experience. The various potential difficulties that the patient presents should be enumerated, and the specific anesthesia plan that is to be used to minimize or avoid such difficulties should be discussed with the patient. The likely postoperative course should be discussed, and the patient should be allowed some degree of input and choice in the management plan.

Cardiovascular System

The evaluation should be directed toward the abnormalities detailed in the pathophysiology section. Hypertension, signs of LV or right ventricular (RV) failure, and signs of pulmonary hypertension should be sought. Sites for venous access and, if needed, sites for arterial cannulation should be identified. The electrocardiogram (ECG) and chest radiograph should be scrutinized for evidence of ischemic heart disease, LV or RV hypertrophy, an increase in cardiac size, and pulmonary congestion. The finding of any of these abnormalities should lead to appropriate detailed investigations such as exercise ECGs, echocardiography, LV ejection fraction, or pulmonary artery catheterization.[15] For patients with evidence of the obesity hypoventilation syndrome or the Pickwickian syndrome, a cardiologist's opinion should be sought, both to define the magnitude of the problem and for advice on how best to optimize the patient's condition prior to operation.

Respiratory System

The clinical history should seek to identify symptoms indicative of severe degrees of respiratory disease (e.g., orthopnea), obesity hypoventilation syndrome, or sleep apnea syndrome and should elicit any history of upper airway obstruction, especially if associated with previous anesthesia and surgery. In young, morbidly obese patients, the results of routine pulmonary function tests such as FVC, FEV_1, and PEFR are usually normal, but, in older patients and those who smoke, the results may uncover unsuspected bronchospastic disease. Chest radiographs should be obtained and blood gases should be measured with the patient seated and supine to rule out carbon dioxide retention and to provide guidelines for preoperative and postoperative oxygen administration. More detailed pulmonary investigations should be reserved for those with severe disease. Because the degree of respiratory compromise in the postoperative period is often pronounced, it is imperative to optimize the patient's pulmonary status prior to embarking on anesthesia or surgery.

Endocrine, Metabolic, and Gastrointestinal Systems

Fasting blood glucose levels should be determined and the urine should be tested for ketones. If gross carbohydrate intolerance, diabetes, or ketosis is found, it should be corrected before either elective or emergency operations are begun. The patient should be closely questioned for symptoms of esophageal reflux and for a previous history of investigations or therapies that might be aimed at such a problem. Routine liver function tests should be performed.

Airway

A history of airway difficulties during previous anesthetics and operations should be obtained from the patient or previous anesthetic records. The patient should be questioned about symptoms suggestive of obstructive sleep apnea (excessive nocturnal snoring, with or without apneic episodes), which may suggest a potential for mechanical airway obstruction when the level of consciousness is decreased. Patients with such histories, and those presenting for operations (tracheostomy, palatoplasty) designed to alleviate such conditions, should be scrutinized especially closely, as they may present formidable airway difficulties. Physical examination of the patient should include range of motion testing of the atlantoaxial joint and cervical spine, the degree to which the mouth can open, and the distance between the tip of the chin and the hyoid cartilage. The interior of the mouth and pharynx should be scrutinized for excessive folds of tissue. The Mallampati classification, based on an ability to visualize the uvula, may help identify those with potentially difficult laryngeal visualization.[35] Lateral soft-tissue radiographs of the neck in neutral and extended positions, computed tomographs of the pharynx, hypopharynx, and the larynx, or consultation with an otolaryngologist for a specialized workup[36] may help delineate airway difficulties preoperatively.

Perioperative Management

Premedication

Premedication, if any, should be given intravenously (iv) or orally. Attempts to give an intramuscular (im) injection will usually result in an intra-fat injection, which leads to unpredictable absorption. Because the effects of central nervous system (CNS) active drugs on the morbidly obese are not predictable and because of the high prevalence of respiratory disease in the morbidly obese, premedication should not be administered until the patient is in a safely monitored environment (e.g., the holding area or the operating room). This is particularly true for any patient with a history of airway obstruction or cardiovascular or respiratory disease. Even when such drugs are administered in the operating room, the patient should be monitored diligently. If an awake or a fiberoptic intubation of the trachea is anticipated, anticholinergic drugs should be given in an attempt to reduce secretions.

Because the risk of gastric regurgitation is high in obese patients, specific measures should be taken to guard against it. If a large volume of gastric contents is suspected (e.g., in an emergency situation), an attempt should be made to empty the stomach with a nasogastric tube. The tube should be removed prior to induction of anesthesia for fear of making a likely difficult tracheal intubation even more difficult. For elective cases, the preoperative administration of a clear antacid, metoclopramide, and H_2 (histamine) blockers is advisable both to lower the volume and to increase the pH of gastric contents.[37-40] Suggested doses would be metoclopramide, 10 mg iv; cimetidine, 300 mg; or ranitidine, 50 mg iv, given 1 hour before operation.

Operating Room Preparation

It is important to ensure that equipment such as gurneys, operating tables, and lithotomy stirrups are capable of bearing the weight of the obese patient. The heels, buttocks, and shoulders of obese persons are at risk of developing decubitus ulcers. All vulnerable areas should be padded. The distribution of body fat may make the usual operating table positions hazardous to the obese. For example, excessive posterior extension of the shoulder with the potential for brachial plexus injury may occur when a patient with a large posterior thoracic fat pad is placed supine with arms abducted at 90 degrees to the body.

Monitoring

If cuff blood pressure monitoring is to be used, the cuff should be of an appropriate size (the bladder should enclose 70% of the arm). Cuff blood pressure monitoring may be both difficult and inaccurate in obese patients, and intra-arterial monitoring is advised for all but the shortest and simplest cases. Paradoxically, although it is often difficult to secure venous access in the obese, intra-arterial cannulation is usually no more difficult than in nonobese persons. A V_5 or equivalent ECG lead should be used on all patients. Monitoring of patients with cardiovascular disease will be dictated by their specific problem. Pulmonary artery catheterization may be indicated in patients with LV compromise or pulmonary hypertension.[15]

Perioperative hypoxia is a constant threat in obese patients; therefore, oxygenation should be monitored by pulse oximetry and by frequent arterial blood gas measurements. End-tidal carbon dioxide monitoring should be used to ensure adequacy of mechanical ventilation and to confirm correct endotracheal tube placement.

To ensure that any nondepolarizing neuromuscular blockade is adequate intraoperatively and fully reversed at the conclusion of the operation, such blockade must be monitored with a peripheral nerve stimulator. It may be difficult to achieve adequate peripheral nerve stimulation with skin electrodes, as considerable amounts of tissue may separate skin electrodes from the relevant nerve. This problem may be circumvented by the use of percutaneous needle electrodes.

Because obese patients are no less likely than normal-weight patients to lose heat intraoperatively, body temperature should be monitored and maintained. It is particularly important to avoid postoperative shivering in obese patients, because this may produce further mixed venous hypoxia and subsequently arterial hypoxia in patients who may be borderline normal in this regard.

Intraoperative Management

Airway Maintenance

Other than for the shortest general anesthetics in highly selected patients, general anesthesia should be delivered by an endotracheal tube. This is advocated because

1. It may be difficult or impossible to maintain a gastight fit with a mask while maintaining an adequate airway and attending to the manual tasks necessary during anesthesia,
2. Obese patients are at high risk for aspiration of gastric contents, and
3. Obese patients, if allowed to breathe spontaneously under general anesthesia, will hypoventilate and become undesirably hypoxic or hypercarbic. Mechanical ventilation via an endotracheal tube is almost mandatory.

Difficulties with endotracheal intubation should be anticipated in all obese patients, and *the person doing the intubation* should thoroughly evaluate the patient and define all risks at the preoperative visit. All appropriate airway management equipment should be available, including a selection of oropharyngeal and nasopharyngeal airways, endotracheal tubes with introducers, intubation stylets, and laryngoscope blades of different patterns and sizes. If chest wall or breast fat is likely to obstruct the usual laryngoscope handles, a "polio blade" laryngoscope, which has a handle in the reverse of the usual direction, may be helpful. Fiberoptic intubation devices or bronchoscopes should also be available (see also Chapter 26).

A carefully considered choice as to whether the patient's trachea should be intubated awake or asleep should be made in each case, bearing in mind the anticipated difficulties and the expertise of the anesthesiologist. An estimated 13% of morbidly obese patients pose difficulties for tracheal intubation.[21] Awake tracheal intubation has been recommended for all patients more than 75% above IBW,[41] but difficulties may also be encountered at weights below that cutoff point. Inability to visualize the patient's uvula with the mouth open may be helpful in identifying those patients in whom intubation is likely to be difficult.[35,42]

A useful practice is to topically anesthetize the mouth, pharynx, and supralaryngeal area with a local anesthetic and then gently introduce a standard laryngoscope and attempt to visualize the epiglottis and the larynx. If it is possible to see these structures, it is likely that intubation of the trachea after induction of anesthesia can be performed; if not, an awake intubation should be performed. If in doubt, the anesthesiologist should err on the side of caution and perform an awake intubation. Awake intubations should be accomplished with a fiberoptic laryngoscope or bronchoscope after suitable topical anesthesia. Any CNS depressant drug used to provide patient comfort should be kept to a minimum and its effects monitored closely. Supplemental oxygen should be given for awake intubations.

Patients with a history suggestive of obstructive sleep apnea and those who are to undergo operations designed to alleviate such conditions almost invariably pose formidable endotracheal intubation difficulties. Endotracheal intubation attempted under general anesthesia in such patients frequently fails. The difficulty with bag and mask ventilation subsequent to a failed tracheal intubation, and the ensuing hypoxia, dictate that many of these patients should be intubated while awake.

If tracheal intubation under general anesthesia is to be performed, it is a useful policy to have two pairs of experienced hands available. If the initial attempt at intubation is not successful and it is necessary to resort to bag and mask ventilation, one person may have to maintain a gastight fit with the mask and an airway while the second person squeezes the bag. A second pair of educated hands is also useful to cope with other difficulties.

Intubation under general anesthesia should be performed in a manner designed to avoid hypoxia and the aspiration of vomited or regurgitated gastric contents. Cricothyroid pressure (Sellick maneuver) should be applied in all cases. Thorough preoxygenation/denitrogenation by a conventional 3-minute period or a four-breath technique[43] is essential, because intubation may take longer than usual, and obese patients have smaller than normal oxygen stores in their lungs (low FRC) and a high $\dot{V}o_2$ and therefore become hypoxic much faster than normal-weight patients.[35,44] As with all tracheal intubations, the routine use of a pulse oximeter will provide early warning of hypoxia.

Irrespective of the method used to place the endotracheal tube, special care should be taken to ensure its correct placement, as chest wall fat may render unfeasible the usual auscultatory methods of confirming placement. Correct endotracheal placement should be confirmed by capnometry, and fiberoptic bronchoscopy should be considered to rule out a bronchial intubation.

Choice of Anesthetic Technique

General Anesthesia

The doses of induction drugs used for the obese patient should be larger than for normal-weight patients (e.g., thiopental, 7.5 mg·kg^{-1} IBW), but allowance should be made for any cardiovascular dysfunction. Nitrous oxide is a logical choice for maintenance anesthesia—it is fat insoluble, has a rapid onset and decrement of action, and is subject to little metabolism. However, even in fit morbidly obese patients, it may be necessary to use an FIo_2 in excess of 0.5 to maintain an adequate Pao_2;[45] thus, the usefulness of nitrous oxide is limited.

Obese patients metabolize volatile anesthetics to a greater extent than do normal patients. The blood levels of fluoride after methoxyflurane, halothane, and enflurane and the blood levels of bromide after halothane are higher in the morbidly obese than in normal-weight patients.[16] Moreover, as the incidence of "halothane hepatitis" is allegedly higher in the obese, and because obese subjects metabolize some halothane by a potentially hepatotoxic reductive pathway,[46] this drug should be used with caution. However, simple tests of hepatic function are similarly marginally impaired after either halothane or enflurane anesthesia. Morbidly obese patients metabolize isoflurane to a minimal extent, and therefore isoflurane is the agent of choice.[47]

The supposition that recovery from fat-soluble volatile anesthetics may be prolonged in the obese, as such drugs may take a long time to leach out of fat stores, has been elegantly disproved in theory[25] and in clinical studies of speed of awakening[26] (see section on Pharmacokinetics in the Obese).

Great care should be exercised when giving opioids to obese patients. Unless the patient's trachea is to be left intubated and the patient provided with ventilator support in the immediate postoperative period, it is wise to keep the dose of opioid to a minimum. Maintenance of normal ventilation is already difficult for obese patients, and further respiratory depression with opioids could predispose to hypoxia or hypercarbia in the recovery room.

For neuromuscular blockade, atracurium appears to be the logical choice of drug. When administered on a $mg \cdot kg^{-1}$ basis, its duration of action is similar in morbidly obese and normal-weight subjects.[34]

Paramount among the changes in the physiology of obese patients produced by general anesthesia are respiratory abnormalities. With the induction of anesthesia, there is further disruption of the already altered FRC-closing capacity relationship, with a further deterioration in V/Q relations or the development of a frank right-to-left shunt. The impairment of pulmonary hypoxic vasoconstriction by volatile agents will contribute further to such changes. All obese patients should be considered at risk of hypoxia under general anesthesia. Obese patients should initially receive an F_{IO_2} of 1.0. Then, based on Sa_{O_2} or Pa_{O_2}, the F_{IO_2} may be titrated downward, slowly. The application of positive end-expiratory pressure (PEEP) may improve Pa_{O_2}.[48]

Even in fit obese patients, intraoperative events that influence lung volumes may produce changes in oxygenation. The Trendelenburg or lithotomy position and the placement of subdiaphragmatic packs or retractors may lead to further decreases in Sa_{O_2} and Pa_{O_2}.[9] Given these findings, it is important that particular attention be paid to oxygenation at the time of positional changes and various surgical maneuvers. Morbidly obese patients may, however, be safely maintained by one-lung anesthesia performed via a double-lumen endobronchial tube during transthoracic operations.[49]

Because of the hypoventilation produced by general anesthesia, spontaneous respiration during general anesthesia is relatively contraindicated. Intermittent positive pressure ventilation (IPPV) is best accomplished with large tidal volumes* at a rate of 8–10 breaths·min^{-1}. Hypocarbia with a

Pa_{CO_2} of less than 30 mm Hg is best avoided, as this may result in a rise in shunt fraction.[50] Ventilation may also be judged by end-tidal capnography or sampling of arterial blood gases.

At the conclusion of the operation any neuromuscular blockade must be totally reversed, as judged by the response to peripheral nerve stimulation, and the parameters for extubation must be fulfilled. The trachea should not be extubated until the patient is fully awake and in control of the airway, in order to avoid hazards of pulmonary aspiration or airway obstruction. Before extubating the patient the anesthesiologist should ensure, either by pulse oximetry or by arterial blood gas measurements, that hypoxia is not present.

Regional Anesthesia

Regional anesthesia would appear to be a useful alternative to general anesthesia but is accompanied by its own constellation of difficulties. The considerable body fat and the indistinct nature of bony landmarks make regional anesthesia techniques difficult. For peripheral nerve blocks, these difficulties may be circumvented by the use of insulated needles and a peripheral nerve stimulator to ensure correct needle and drug placement.

Subarachnoid blockade may be more difficult to perform in obese patients than in normal-weight patients, but the difficulties are not insurmountable. The midline of the back in the lumbar region generally does not have as thick a layer of fat as does the more lateral portions, and subarachnoid puncture may be made easier by having the patient sit up. Often needles longer than usual may be needed. For a given age and height of a patient, the dose requirement for subarachnoid anesthesia is approximately 75–80% of that of normal,[52-54] and with more variability than in normals.[54] Evidence from case reports implies that the level of blockade produced by subarachnoid local anesthetics is not predictable and that the blockade is of slow onset and creeps insidiously higher over the first 30 minutes.[55] Anecdotal reports have implied that a high subarachnoid blockade tends to produce respiratory compromise, especially if patients are sedated.[55] However, in obese patients with a blockade at T5, both respiratory volume[56] and blood gases[57] show minimal change from baseline. If the blockade does extend higher in the thoracic area than T5 there is a distinct possibility of respiratory compromise, particularly in obese patients with respiratory disease. Moreover, the high extension of the blockade, with the variable extent of the autonomic blockade above the somatic blockade,[58] may lead to cardiovascular compromise, which can also be precipitated by panniculus retraction.[59] A strong case can be made for the use of a continuous subarachnoid block. This could provide all the benefits of regional anesthesia, and yet allow careful titration of the drug to the desired effect, thus circumventing the potential unpredictability of "single-shot" subarachnoid blocks.

Although technically more exacting than subarachnoid anesthesia, epidural anesthesia has been widely used and described in obese patients,[21,60,61] particularly for abdominal operations. The technique usually consists of a high lumbar or thoracic puncture, followed by the introduction of a catheter and the induction of a segmental block. Catheter placement may be easier with fluoroscopic guidance.[61] The technique is usually used in combination with a light general anesthetic delivered by an endotracheal tube, and IPPV. Such a technique bypasses many of the problems of general anesthesia, reduces the volatile drug requirement,

---

*By rearranging the BMI equation (BMI = wt [kg]/ht^2 [m]) to BMI × ht^2 (m) = wt (kg), one may calculate various body weights for the individual. Thus, a patient with a true body weight of 139 kg and a height of 1.77 m has a BMI of $139/1.77^2 = 44.4$. At IBW, BMI = 25, and at low body weight (LBW), BMI = 30. Thus, for this patient, IBW = $25 \times 1.77^2 = 78$ kg. LBW = $30 \times 1.77^2 = 94$ kg. IPPV at a rate of 12 ml·kg^{-1} at the LBW at a rate of 8–10 breaths·min^{-1} achieves a Pa_{CO_2} of approximately 30 mm Hg.[51]

eliminates the need for neuromuscular blocking drugs, and permits rapid postoperative mobilization. As is true for subarachnoid anesthesia, the dose requirement for epidural anesthesia for operative procedures is approximately 75–80% of that for normal-weight patients.[21,62] The use of epidural analgesia may confer some benefits on morbidly obese patients intraoperatively and postoperatively (decreased shunt fraction, LV work, A-Vdo$_2$, and $\dot{V}o_2$).[63,64] The catheter used to provide epidural anesthesia may be used again to provide postoperative analgesia either with local anesthesia[21,42] or with opioids,[64] which may be particularly beneficial in morbidly obese patients.[21,64] The epidural dose requirement for analgesia in obese patients appears to be similar to that in normal-weight patients, for both local anesthetics[21,65] and opioids.[64]

Because it may be difficult to deal with respiratory or cardiovascular emergencies in the obese, any such potential hazards must be detected as early as possible and dealt with vigorously. The obese patient receiving a regional anesthetic should receive supplemental oxygen, minimal sedation or analgesia, and must be monitored in the same fashion as if the patient were receiving a general anesthetic. The anesthesiologist should not choose regional anesthesia for a patient unless prepared to convert to general anesthesia, if the regional anesthesia is unsatisfactory for the surgical procedure or if the patient develops respiratory difficulties.

Postoperative Care

Obese patients with a previous history of respiratory disease, those with obesity hypoventilation syndrome or Pickwickian syndrome, and those who have undergone major abdominal and thoracic operations are likely to have a high incidence of respiratory complications. Thus, it may be wise to admit these patients electively to an intensive care unit (ICU). Their management in the ICU will depend on the individual patient but should include IPPV if necessary and aggressive prophylaxis against the development of respiratory complications. Obese patients are highly immobile postoperatively; measures should be taken to assist them in moving by the provision of an adjustable bed, overhead trapeze, and sufficient nursing staff.

Respiratory Function

Even in healthy obese patients, postoperative hypoxemia is a universal hazard. Supplemental oxygen should be given during transport from the operating room to the recovery room. Respiratory monitoring should be particularly aggressive in the recovery room and should include pulse oximetry and/or arterial blood gas monitoring. Patients should not be discharged to the ward until they have been shown not to be hypoxemic, and it may be appropriate to use long-term oxygen therapy on the ward. Following intra-abdominal operations, arterial hypoxemia may last 4–6 days[66] and is of greater magnitude with vertical than with horizontal incisions. Postoperative hypoxemia can be minimized by having patients sit in bed. There is some evidence that the use of regional anesthesia techniques intraoperatively and postoperatively will reduce the incidence of postoperative respiratory complications.[21,66]

Immobilization

Obese patients have a high incidence of postoperative deep vein thrombosis and pulmonary emboli. The use of mini-heparin or intermittent leg compression prophylaxis may be appropriate. The use of regional anesthesia techniques may decrease the incidence of deep vein thrombosis and pulmonary emboli.[21,66]

Analgesia

Obese patients may have lesser need for postoperative analgesics than normal-weight patients.[67] For previously stated reasons, the use of opioid analgesics can be hazardous in obese patients. Moreover, the routine use of im injections may not result in predictable blood levels of the opioid. If opioids are to be used, they should probably be delivered directly into the intravascular compartment using devices such as patient-controlled analgesia machines. An anecdotal report implies that patient-controlled anesthesia may be hazardous in patients with obstructive sleep apnea.[68]

If an epidural catheter was placed for operative anesthesia, it may be used as the route for injecting either local anesthetic or opioid to provide analgesia postoperatively. The use of local anesthesia[21] or opioids[64] is associated with faster postoperative recovery and a lesser incidence of respiratory complications than is the use of conventional opioid techniques. The doses of either local anesthetic[21,65] or opioid[64] necessary to provide postoperative epidural analgesia are similar to those in normal-weight patients. Epidural opioid analgesia may result in delayed respiratory depression, and, because of the difficulty of maintaining or securing the airway in obese patients, those receiving epidural opioids should probably be nursed in a closely monitored environment (e.g., an ICU) until the potential for such a complication has passed.

GASTROINTESTINAL DISORDERS

Functional Anatomy and Physiology

The mouth and pharyngeal musculature are under voluntary control as boluses of food and fluid are swallowed and delivered to the esophagus. Such boluses are lubricated by saliva, which amounts to approximately 1200 ml·day^{-1}.[69]

Esophagus

The esophageal musculature is under involuntary control[70] and is innervated by the vagus nerve and a sympathetic component derived from segments T6–T10. Waves of esophageal contraction pass boluses of food down to the gastroesophageal junction, which relaxes to allow them to enter the stomach.

At the gastroesophageal junction, reflux is prevented by a number of means, including the esophagus acting as a flap valve and the diaphragmatic crura pinching off the esophagus. The major barrier to gastroesophageal reflux is now believed to be the lower esophageal sphincter (LES).[71] The LES is histologically similar to the rest of the esophagus but is functionally quite different. It may be identified by gastroesophageal manometry, in which a series of transducers is drawn from the stomach back through the gastroesophageal junction into the esophagus. The LES appears as an area of increased pressure (Fig. 42-3). It is usually 2–3 cm long and extends above and below the diaphragm. Peak pressure occurs just above the diaphragm and varies with respiration. The LES relaxes on swallowing, in contrast to the rest of the esophagus, which exhibits peristalsis.

The tendency for esophageal reflux is related to some de-

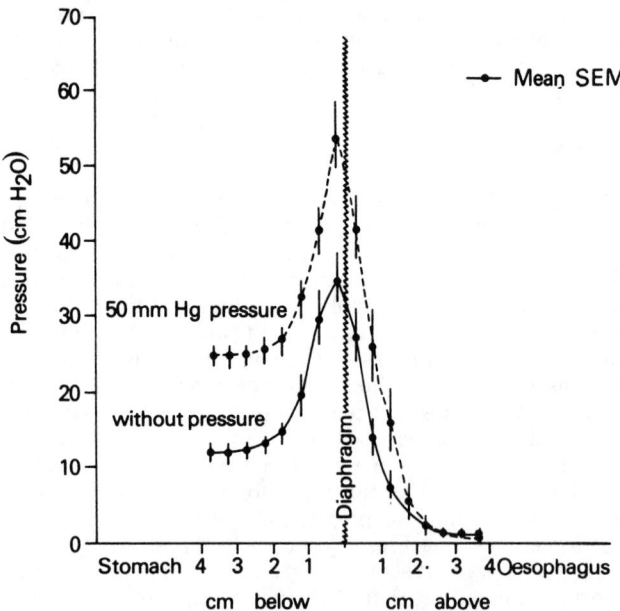

Figure 42-3. The pressures found by lower esophageal manometry, illustrating the relationship of the lower esophageal sphincter to the diaphragm. Note also the effect of increasing intraabdominal pressure causing a concurrent rise in lower esophageal sphincter pressure. (Reprinted with permission from Colton BR, Smith G: The lower esophageal sphincter and anaesthesia. Br J Anaesth 56:37, 1984.)

TABLE 42-1. Lower Esophageal Sphincter Effect of Drugs Used in Anesthesia

Increase	Decrease	No Change
Metoclopramide	Atropine	Propranolol
Domperidone	Glycopyrrolate	Oxprenolol
Prochlorperazine	Dopamine	Cimetidine
Cyclizine	Sodium nitroprusside	Ranitidine
Edrophonium	Ganglion blockers	Atracurium
Neostigmine	Thiopental	?Nitrous oxide
Histamine	Tricyclic antidepressants	
Suxamethonium	Halothane	
Pancuronium	Enflurane	
Metoprolol	Opioids	
Antacids	?Nitrous oxide	

gree to LES tone but more to the barrier pressure, that is, the difference between the LES pressure and the gastric pressure.[71] Thus, if intragastric pressure is sufficiently high, it may surmount the LES to produce reflux. However, in health, the LES pressure usually rises in response to a rise in intragastric pressure. The LES tends to relax during pregnancy; thus, the tendency for reflux to occur is greater at that time. Patients with hiatal hernia may have a normal LES pressure, although in such patients the LES is nearly always above the diaphragm. Patients with gastroesophageal reflux tend to have lower barrier pressures, ranging from low to near normal rather than exhibiting a distinct cutoff point. The LES is innervated by both vagal and sympathetic nerves, but the role of the innervation is uncertain; vagal denervation does not affect resting tone or active function. Clinical circumstances associated with reduced LES tone include pregnancy, obesity, and hiatal hernia. Patients with gastroesophageal reflux may also have reduced LES tone. A number of drugs may increase or decrease LES tone (Table 42-1).

The Stomach

The stomach has various functions. As a distensible receptacle, it allows the storage of large amounts of food and fluids (it may accept 1–1.5 l of fluid with minimal rises in intragastric pressure). As a chamber, it is the site for mixing of ingested food and gastric secretions, and where digestion begins; and as a system, it expels small and manageable amounts of gastric contents into the duodenum.[72,73]

The proximal part of the stomach is functionally a receptacle, exhibiting little mobility and in which little mixing occurs. Mixing occurs primarily in the distal stomach, with

electrical activity originating from a "pacemaker," usually located near the midpoint of the greater curvature. The electrical activity and resulting mechanical activity spread circumferentially and longitudinally toward the pylorus. Pyloric relaxation occurs in response to the waves of gastric activity, permitting expulsion of small amounts of gastric contents into the duodenum. In health, gastric emptying occurs at a rate that closely approximates an exponential curve, although varying from this curve when the stomach is full or nearly empty.

The rate of gastric emptying can be influenced by physiologic factors such as the type of intake—liquids leave the stomach more quickly than solids—and by the volume, pH, and osmotic qualities of the gastric contents.[73] The customary 4-hour preoperative fast does not guarantee that the stomach is empty, and evidence is accumulating that modest feeding or intake of small amounts of fluid during the preoperative period may be associated with lower volumes of gastric contents and may shorten the usual NPO waiting period prior to elective surgery.[74,75] Certain groups of patients tend to have a high resting gastric content volume, including pregnant persons, the obese, and the bedridden (Table 42-2). Pathologic states associated with high resting gastric content volume include pain, shock, and trauma. Laparotomy will slow the rate of gastric emptying for approximately 24 hours, although this is probably the result of a combination of the mechanical effects of bowel handling and the postoperative use of opioids. A number of drugs may influence the rate of gastric emptying (see Table 42-2).

Gastric secretions are produced at a rate of nearly 2000 ml·day^{-1}. They have a pH of 1.0–3.5, are isotonic with extracellular fluid, and consist predominantly of hydrochloric acid, with a higher potassium content than extracellular fluid. The pH of gastric contents may be raised by the administration of antacids or H_2-blocking drugs.

The Duodenum

In the duodenum, secretions of the pancreas and the biliary tract are mixed with the gastric contents. Secretions of the pancreas and biliary tract are predominantly alkaline, with pH values in the region of 7.8–8.3 and daily volumes of 1200 and 700 ml, respectively. The pH of the resultant mix of gastric contents and duodenal secretions will be a function of the respective volumes and pH of the gastric contents and the pancreatic and biliary tract secretions.

TABLE 42-2. Some Factors Influencing Gastric Emptying Rate

	Accelerate	Delay
Physiologic	Gastric distention Neuroticism	Food Acid High osmotic pressure Posture Pregnancy
Pathologic	Thyrotoxicosis	Shock Trauma and pain Myocardial infarction Pyloric stenosis Crohn's disease Celiac disease Diabetic autonomic neuropathy
Pharmacologic	Metoclopramide Neostigmine Propranolol Sodium bicarbonate Cigarette smoking	Anticholinergics Tricyclic antidepressants Aluminum hydroxide Alcohol Isoprenaline Opioid analgesics

Small Intestine

At rest, the activity of the small intestine is governed by the migrating myoelectric complex (MMC). This complex has two components, electromyographic and manometric. Four phases may be seen: phase I, with slow-wave electrical activity with quiescent intestine; phase II, characterized by slow-wave activity with some spikes, accompanied by periodic intestinal contractions; phase III, characterized by intense spiking accompanied by slow waves electrically with vigorous mechanical contractions; and phase IV, which reverts from phase III to phase I and is associated with rapid subsidence of contractions.

When food is taken the MMC is disrupted and there is contractile activity throughout the whole intestine. Postprandial intestinal activity can be divided into a cephalic phase, which may be abolished by vagotomy, a gastric phase, which is promoted by gastric distention, and an intestinal phase, which is provoked by perfusion of the intestine with nutrients.

The mode of control of small intestinal activity is not known with certainty. The parasympathetic system plays a role, because parasympathetic stimulation results in increased activity and suppression of the parasympathetic system results in decreased activity. The sympathetic nervous system also plays a role, as sympathetic suppression causes an increase in activity and stimulation causes a decrease in activity, with the changes mediated by both catecholamines and dopaminergic receptors. However, with bowel denervation, there appears to be little change in activity, and it is likely that humoral secretions, especially pancreatic polypeptides and somatostatin, play a major role in mediating activity. Small intestinal activity is suppressed for 24–48 hours following laparotomy and may also be decreased by peritonitis and a reduction in serum potassium levels.

The small intestine secretes 2000 ml of fluid a day with a pH of 7.0–8.0.[76] The small intestine is the site of the majority of the absorption of fluid and nutrients in the gastrointestinal (GI) tract. It is presented with 5500 ml of fluid a day (2000 ml from the stomach, 1500 ml from the pancreas and biliary tract, and 2000 ml from the small intestine) but passes on only 500 ml to the colon. Thus, the net turnover of fluid in the small intestine is of the order of about 5000 ml·day^{-1}. The absorptive abilities of the small intestine are impaired for approximately 36 hours following laparotomy.

The Colon

Approximately 500–700 ml of bowel content is presented to the colon each day.[77] The colon expels only 100–200 ml·day^{-1}; therefore, its function is predominantly absorptive. Colonic motility is controlled by a pacemaker located in the transverse colon. Three types of activity can be observed: (1) antiperistalsis from the transverse colon to the cecum, which permits maximal exposure of the feces for absorption of fluid; (2) peristalsis, which pushes feces forward to the distal parts of the colon; and (3) a powerful peristaltic movement that is responsible for the evacuation of fecal content; this movement proceeds anally in a series of large mass movements.

Parasympathetic neural control of the colon as far as the splenic flexure is furnished by the vagus nerve; beyond that point, it is furnished by the sacral parasympathetic outflow.[77] The sympathetic supply is from segments T6–T10. Parasympathetic stimulation increases motility, whereas sympathetic stimulation decreases activity. Administration of neostigmine increases activity in terms of both activity and tone, whereas morphine decreases activity.[78]

Splanchnic Blood Flow

Splanchnic oxygenation can be influenced by changes in the blood oxygen-carrying capacity (such as anemia) and by changes in blood flow to the bowel. There is anecdotal evidence that anemia may lead to poor rates of wound healing in areas of relatively compromised blood flow such as the colon.[79] The optimal hematocrit is thought to be in the mid-30s.

In normal circumstances of a normal cardiac output, splanchnic blood flow remains relatively stable, being regulated by the splanchnic vascular resistance through mechanisms similar to those regulating hepatic blood flow. Splanchnic vascular resistance is largely regulated by the sympathetic nervous system, with sympathectomy decreasing splanchnic vascular resistance, alpha-adrenergic stimulation promoting vasoconstriction, and beta-adrenergic stimulation promoting vasodilation. Dopamine may act in the splanchnic vascular bed through two receptors, with alpha-adrenergic vasoconstriction predominating over the mild vasodilation produced by beta-adrenergic stimulation. Parasympathetic stimulation results in an increase in blood flow and an increase in motor activity.

In stress states, a number of humoral agents may influence splanchnic blood flow, including catecholamines, vasopressin, and angiotensin II. With hemorrhage, splanchnic vascular resistance rises, presumably as a teleologic mechanism to permit the diversion of cardiac output to organs more vital to survival. A modest hemorrhage of 10–15% of circulating blood volume, which does not affect systemic arterial pressure, may markedly impair splanchnic blood flow. The restoration of circulating volume does not result in a rapid restortion of splanchnic blood flow, which may remain decreased for several hours. Although blood loss and hypotension are not particularly critical for the blood supply to the stomach and small bowel, which have a liberal vascular supply, such circumstances may be associated with an increased rate of colonic anastomotic dehiscence.[79,80]

A number of perioperative factors may alter splanchnic blood flow. Following trauma, there may be an increase in splanchnic blood flow, but laparotomy alone produces little change. Morphine decreases splanchnic vascular resistance and therefore increases splanchnic blood flow. There is almost a linear relationship between splanchnic blood flow and $Paco_2$, with hypocapnia decreasing flow and hypercapnia increasing flow. Halothane and isoflurane decrease splanchnic blood flow.[81] Regional anesthesia with high levels of sympathetic blockade results in an increase in splanchnic blood flow owing to a decrease in splanchnic vascular resistance, both as a consequence of the sympathectomy itself and of the fall in catecholamine levels associated with sympathetic blockade. However, if such a sympathectomy results in a fall in cardiac output, splanchnic blood flow may fall. Sympathectomy does not influence the changes in splanchnic blood flow produced by changes in $Paco_2$.[82] Neostigmine will reduce mesenteric blood flow by 30–50% in association with the exaggerated motor activity of the intestine. Such decreases in blood flow may be somewhat ameliorated by the prior administration of atropine.[80]

General Considerations for Anesthesia and the GI Tract

Irrespective of the target of the surgery in the GI tract, a number of factors bearing on patient evaluation and management must be taken into consideration.

Airway Management and Protection

The oral, pharyngeal, and hypopharyngeal areas may be distorted by a number of pathologic processes, including tumor, infection, obstruction by an ingested foreign body, thermal or chemical damage, and nonmalignant variations on normal anatomy such as pharyngeal pouches. Thus, it is necessary to carefully evaluate the patient with respect to the site, type, and magnitude of the distortion and the pathologic process producing the airway abnormality. The choice of airway management and method of securing the airway should be based on clinical findings, supplemented as necessary by investigations such as direct or indirect laryngoscopy, soft-tissue radiography, and computed tomography or magnetic resonance imaging of the abnormal area (see Chapter 26).

A major consideration in anesthesia for surgery on the GI tract is the prevention of inadvertent airway soiling by aspiration of GI contents during induction and maintenance of anesthesia. During the maintenance of routine anesthesia, in the absence of risk factors, the incidence of regurgitation of gastric contents into the perilaryngeal area is approximately 8%. In approximately 1% of the total operative population, gastric contents can be shown to reach the airway.[83] Aspiration is most likely to occur during the induction of anesthesia, when the airway is not securely protected by an endotracheal tube and when active vomiting is most likely. The consequences of regurgitation and subsequent aspiration of gastric contents into the airway will depend on the character and volume of the aspirate. Solid matter will produce an anatomic obstruction of the airway, and fluid of neutral pH will produce the clinical picture of near drowning, whereas the aspiration of even small amounts of acidic fluid may be associated with the aspiration syndrome (Mendelson syndrome). The incidence of the latter is estimated at 0.05%.[84] It is generally accepted that a gastric content in excess of 25 ml with a pH of less than 2.5 implies a special risk of producing an aspiration syndrome if such fluid is aspirated.[85] However, there is also opinion that acid aspiration syndromes can be produced by aspirates with a higher pH. Therefore, it is incumbent upon anesthesiologists to attempt to reduce the volume and increase the pH of any gastric contents.

If the volume of gastric contents is suspected to be high, this volume may be reduced by emptying the stomach with a nasogastric tube or by inducing vomiting with apomorphine.[86] Gastric emptying can also be facilitated by using drugs to increase gastric motility. Several pharmacologic agents that hasten gastric emptying are listed in Table 42-2. However, the use of such maneuvers does not guarantee an empty stomach and should not lull the anesthesiologist into a false sense of security. Application of these techniques does not absolve the anesthesiologist of the responsibility of taking other precautions to prevent regurgitation and possibly aspiration of GI tract contents.

A major thrust in reducing the potential for acid aspiration syndrome has been to raise the pH of gastric contents. This may be done effectively with particulate antacids such as aluminum hydroxide or magnesium trisilicate. However, such drugs may cause lung damage if they are aspirated;[87] thus, it is preferable to use nonparticulate antacids such as sodium citrate (0.3 mM).[88] Drugs that reduce acid secretion, such as the H_2 blockers cimetidine and ranitidine, in iv doses of 300 and 50 mg, respectively, will effectively raise the pH.[39,40,89] Ranitidine and famotidine are probably the drugs of choice, as they are associated with fewer side-effects and have a longer duration of action than cimetidine.[90] Some anticholinergics, particularly glycopyrrolate, will also reduce gastric acidity. The volume of the gastric content can be reduced by use of motility-stimulating drugs such as metoclopramide.[89]

Studies of the acid aspiration syndrome have shown that a high proportion of patients who suffer from this problem have an LES dysfunction.[84] Thus, it is important to maintain LES function. Circumstances associated with a lowered LES tone were discussed in an earlier section. Drugs that raise LES tone are listed in Table 42-1.

Prior to induction of anesthesia, the risk of regurgitation and pulmonary aspiration may be reduced by the following measures:

Reducing the volume of the stomach content:
  By using nasogastric tubes
  By inducing vomiting
  By accelerating gastric emptying with drugs such as metoclopramide
Raising the gastric content pH with clear antacids and H_2 blockers
Increasing LES tone with metoclopramide

Once the anesthesiologist has attempted to reduce the likelihood of regurgitation and aspiration, the airway should be secured coincident with the induction of anesthesia by the expeditious passage of an endotracheal tube and with the use of maneuvers designed to prevent gastric contents from reaching the airway, such as application of cricoid pressure (Sellick maneuver).

Fluid and Electrolyte Balance

Patients with GI disease may be in fluid or electrolyte imbalance for a number of reasons, some of which are listed below.

1. *Inadequate intake.* Patients awaiting surgery are often kept from oral intake (NPO) for varying periods of time preoperatively. This is especially likely to be a problematic factor in children, small adults, and patients in a hot environment or with pyrexia, in whom insensible fluid losses may be high. In the chronically ill patient there may be a long period of inadequate intake, or oral intake may be prevented by anorexia or GI tract obstruction.

2. *Sequestration of water and electrolytes into abdominal structures,* for example, the bowel lumen, bowel wall, and peritoneum, in patients with inflammatory bowel disease or intestinal obstruction.

3. *Extracorporeal loss of fluid* such as from vomiting, diarrhea, or loss through fistulae.

Frequently the etiology of the fluid deficit will be an amalgam of these three causes. The magnitude of the fluid and electrolyte deficit reflects the duration of the problem and the site of the fluid loss. Deficient intake and salivary loss, for example, in a patient with a pharyngeal tumor, is primarily water loss with minimal electrolyte loss.

Loss of fluid that is primarily gastric contents (which, in a patient with pyloric stenosis, may reach 2000 ml·day^{-1}) will result in a hypochloremic alkalosis and hypokalemia. Not only is potassium lost in the gastric fluid, it will also be excreted by the kidney in response to the alkalosis.

If fluid is lost externally from the lower GI tract, the resulting deficit will be predominantly a metabolic acidosis and hypochloremia. The loss may be up to 3000 ml·day^{-1}.

When small bowel obstruction occurs, a complex series of events takes place. The segment of bowel proximal to the obstruction dilates and will contain gas (primarily swallowed gas) and fluids. The fluids result from bowel contents upstream and an increase in small bowel secretion with a decrease in fluid absorption. As bowel dilation increases, fluid is lost into the bowel wall and peritoneal cavity. Progressive dilation and edema of the bowel or of a volvulus may lead to impaired bowel blood supply, with potential bowel necrosis and perforation. In these circumstances, further rapid fluid loss will occur and the patient may develop bacterial toxemia or septicemia. The usually encountered abnormalities include hemoconcentration, a fall in circulating blood volume, and a fall in total body potassium.

Large bowel obstruction tends to occur more slowly and manifests less dramatically than does small bowel obstruction. The effects of the obstruction depend on the competence of the ileocecal valve. If the valve is competent, the closed obstruction will result in large bowel dilation, particularly of the right colon and cecum, with the potential for progression to impairment of colonic blood supply and necrosis and perforation. However, if the ileocecal valve is not competent, the bowel contents will reflux into the small bowel and will ultimately result in feculent vomiting. The speed of progression of symptoms in large bowel obstruction tends to be slower than in small bowel obstruction, but the fluid and electrolyte disturbances may be just as severe, with similar intravascular and extracellular fluid consequences.

Diarrhea may result from impaired intestinal absorption of water and electrolytes, from abnormal bowel motility, or from an increase in the osmotically active substances in the bowel lumen. The fluid and volume deficit reflects the hypotonic, potassium-containing nature of the stools and tends to produce a hypokalemic metabolic acidosis.

Preoperative evaluation of the patient's fluid and electrolyte deficit includes assessment of clinical parameters such as skin turgor, peripheral circulation, heart rate, blood pressure, and urine output. Useful laboratory studies include hematocrit, serum electrolytes, and blood urea nitrogen. If necessary, invasive monitoring such as central venous pressure and pulmonary artery pressure measurements should be used to further assess the patient's vascular volume. The speed with which resuscitation and rehydration should be accomplished will depend on the urgency of the surgical procedure. Small bowel obstruction, which may rapidly progress to bowel ischemia and perforation, necessitates urgent operation. Therefore, resuscitation should be swift and aggressive and aimed at rendering the patient fit for operation in a brief period of time. Resuscitation for large bowel obstruction or for a more chronic fluid loss, from whatever source, may be accomplished in a somewhat more leisurely fashion. The type of fluid resuscitation will depend on the volume of loss and the clinical and laboratory findings. This subject is also discussed in Chapter 9.

Malabsorption and Malnutrition

The GI tract is responsible for absorbing all nutrients; therefore, bowel abnormalities may be associated with malabsorption of nutrients and consequent malnutrition. The malabsorption may be of one element only, but more commonly it is of multiple elements and is usually associated with chronic rather than acute disease.

Gastric lesions and gastric resections are commonly associated with a poorly understood iron deficiency anemia and with megaloblastic vitamin B_{12} deficiency anemia owing to either lack of intrinsic factor or overgrowth of vitamin B_{12}-consuming bacteria in a blind loop. A deficiency of bile salt secretion impairs fat absorption, leading to steatorrhea and deficiencies of the fat-soluble vitamins A, D, and K, and of calcium. Pancreatic insufficiency may lead to protein and fat malabsorption with steatorrhea and fat-soluble vitamin deficiency. Intestinal malabsorption may occur owing to motility disorders, a reduction in absorptive area, mucosal abnormalities, or bacterial overgrowth. The severity of the malabsorption and malnutrition will be related to the magnitude, site, and duration of the disease and the magnitude of the decrease in absorptive surface. Malabsorption is generally of protein, fats, and vitamins; carbohydrate absorption is relatively well preserved.

Malnutrition may also result from loss of bowel contents through fistulae or from intestinal loss of protein into the bowel lumen in diseases such as regional enteritis, ulcerative colitis, and allergic enteropathies.

Although the correction of malnutrition in the preoperative period is relatively unimportant for acute diseases, it may be extremely important in chronic disease states. Experience with preoperative elemental diets or hyperalimentation has shown that correction of malnutrition improves both wound healing and the overall outcome of surgical procedures for chronic bowel diseases. Postoperatively, adequate nutrition is also important to improve healing and to reduce the incidence of complications. After abdominal operations, most patients have increased needs for calories and protein, particularly patients with major abdominal infections (see Chapter 12).

Special Anesthesia Considerations for Bowel Surgery

Use of Nitrous Oxide

The solubility of nitrous oxide in blood is much greater than that of nitrogen. The blood-gas partition coefficient of nitrous oxide is 34 times that of nitrogen. In consequence, nitrous oxide in the bloodstream will enter gas-containing body cavities much faster than the nitrogen in those cavities can be removed by the circulation. If this occurs in the bowel, the gas-containing bowel will distend.[91] The amount of distention depends on the following factors:

1. *The amount of gas within the bowel.* In health, the bowel contains about 100 ml of gas, the majority of which is swallowed; therefore, distention is relatively unimportant. However, with obstruction or aerophagy, the bowel may contain much larger amounts of gas, and the potential for expansion is much greater.

2. *The duration of administration.* During the initial administration of nitrous oxide, there will be a linear increase in bowel gas cavity size. By about 100 minutes after the commencement of administration of nitrous oxide, bowel gas cavity size will have increased by 75–100%, and, at that time, the ratio of bowel nitrous oxide to end-tidal nitrous oxide will be about 0.5.

3. *The concentration of nitrous oxide.* If the alveolar concentration is only 50%, the maximum possible increase in bowel gas would be twofold. At 80%, the increase could potentially be fivefold.[91]

The distention of bowel by nitrous oxide may produce a number of problems. In a critical situation with an already distended bowel, for example, in bowel obstruction, the increases in size and intraluminal pressure may tip the balance toward bowel ischemia and necrosis. More commonly, the increase in size will cause difficulties for the surgeon intraoperatively, especially during abdominal closure. One study also suggests that nitrous oxide will prolong hospitalization.[92] Therefore, it is best to avoid nitrous oxide when the bowel contains much gas. It is probably safe to use nitrous oxide, limiting its concentration to 50% for a brief period of time (e.g., 10–15 minutes), at the start of an operation in order to facilitate induction of anesthesia with a volatile drug. The nitrous oxide should be withdrawn thereafter and anesthesia should be maintained with oxygen and a volatile drug—a technique that leads to little or no increase in the size of gas-containing cavities.

Neostigmine

Parasympathetic activity results in increased bowel peristalsis. Thus, drugs that increase parasympathetic effects, for example, cholinesterase inhibitors such as neostigmine, will also increase bowel activity.[78] In normal bowel, neostigmine increases the frequency and magnitude of the pressure waves, particularly in the colon, and this effect is magnified in diseased bowel. Such effects may be reduced by the presence of anesthetic drugs or the previous administration of atropine or glycopyrrolate.[93] There is anecdotal evidence that the administration of neostigmine to patients with a large bowel anastomosis may lead to an increased incidence of anastomotic disruption.[78] Thus, if neostigmine is to be used in these circumstances, it should be used with caution.

Specific Disease States

Esophageal Perforation. Patients with this anomaly may be extremely ill, fluid depleted, and septic. They may have pneumomediastinum, pneumothorax, and pleural effusions. The patient's inability to swallow may complicate airway management.

Acute Pancreatitis. This entity is commonly associated with chronic alcohol ingestion; thus, the patient is usually suffering from the effects of alcoholism. The patient may be malnourished with impaired liver function and possibly an alcohol withdrawal syndrome. More acute problems include a fluid deficit, hypocalcemia, hyperglycemia, pleural effusions, and the adult respiratory distress syndrome.

Pancreatic Cysts and Pseudocysts. These cysts are usually a consequence of acute or chronic pancreatitis. Patients are usually malnourished and often septic.

Crohn's Disease. Patients with Crohn's disease are chronically ill, malnourished, and dehydrated owing to bowel obstruction, malabsorption, or loss of fluids and nutrients via fistulae. They are often very ill, taking large doses of steroids or immunosuppressive therapy.

Ulcerative Colitis. This chronic disease often results in electrolyte and fluid imbalance, vitamin B_{12} and folate deficiency, and extracolonic manifestations such as arthritis, iritis, and hepatitis. Operations in the quiescent phases are often undertaken for precancerous lesions. Acute problems that may necessitate urgent operation include hemorrhage, bowel perforation, bowel obstruction, and toxic megacolon. Patients undergoing operations in the acute phase are often very ill, taking large doses of steroids, and undergoing extensive operations, for example, total colectomy or total proctocolectomy. Careful resuscitation and intensive monitoring may be required.

Carcinoid Tumors. Although carcinoid tumors may occur at other anatomic sites, the GI tract is the source of most of them.[94] The tumors are usually small and frequently multiple. Fifty percent occur in the appendix, 25% in the ileum (these are usually the source of metastatic tumors), and 20% in the rectum. The hormones secreted by nonmetastatic carcinoid tumors reach the liver by way of the portal vein and are usually inactivated there. However, once metastases to the liver have occurred, the hormones secreted by the hepatic metastases may have direct access to the systemic circulation, to produce the symptoms and signs of the carcinoid syndrome. Approximately 35% of patients with carcinoid tumors and metastases have symptoms of the carcinoid syndrome. The classic presentation of the carcinoid syndrome is not evident in all patients: 75% have cutaneous flushing, 70% exhibit an increase in GI motility, 40% have cardiovascular symptoms, and 20% experience bronchospasm.

Carcinoid tumors produce a variety of hormones, and the symptoms produced in each case will probably depend on the hormone(s) secreted. A summary of the hormones secreted, their physiologic effects, and suggested treatments is given in Table 42-3.

TABLE 42-3. Hormones Released by Carcinoid Tumors and Their Management

	Physiologic Effects	Treatment		
		Inhibiting Synthesis	Hormone Depletion	Receptor Blockers
Serotonin	Vasoconstriction Vasodilation Increased motility Tryptophan depletion	Parachlorophylalamine	Fenluranine	Methysergide Cyproheptadine Ketanserin
Kinins	Vasodilation Histamine release Bronchoconstriction	Steroids Aprotinin		
Histamine	Vasodilation H_1 = extravascular smooth muscle contraction H_2 = extravascular smooth muscle relaxation			H_2 antagonists Phenothiazines

Although carcinoid tumors are relatively rare, patients with carcinoid tumors who present for surgery are usually the worst affected and pose a number of problems. Carcinoid heart disease occurs in about one third of the patients, but its etiology is somewhat uncertain. The pathologic findings are predominantly right-sided fibrinous plaques deposited on the RV wall and on the tricuspid valve, producing incompetence or, less frequently, stenosis or deposition on the pulmonary valve. Such plaques are rarely found on the left side of the heart. Invasive or noninvasive cardiologic evaluation is necessary to determine the magnitude and the effects of heart disease.

It is difficult to give blanket recommendations for the management of all patients with carcinoid syndrome, as it is likely that the extent and proportion of hormonal secretion and the hormones' effects will vary from person to person. The majority of information on the carcinoid syndrome comes from anecdotal reports; there are no good published series of large numbers of patients dealing with overall management. When anesthetizing a patient with a carcinoid syndrome, it may be possible to get clues to likely intraoperative events from the previous history, although this is not necessarily so (e.g., 50% of the patients with intraoperative bronchospasm may have no previous history). Likely problems that one may encounter include the following:

1. *Bronchospasm.* This may be quite severe. It can be provoked by the use of histamine-releasing drugs such as morphine and d-tubocurarine. Because adrenergic drugs are likely to cause release of histamine, these should also be avoided. The prophylactic use of H_1 and H_2 blockers and steroids is advised. If the bronchospasm occurs intraoperatively, the use of steroids, diphenhydramine, halothane, ketanserin, or somatostatin has been recommended.

2. *Hypotension.* Hypotension may be a consequence of the disease causing a generated fluid deficit, but hypotension that occurs acutely may be secondary to hormone release. It is important to have the patient adequately volume resuscitated preoperatively. The measurement of central venous pressure or pulmonary artery pressure to assess cardiovascular status may be helpful. Prophylactic measures to minimize hypotension include administration of steroids, administration of H_1 and H_2 blockers, cautious titration of volatile anesthetics, avoiding histamine-releasing drugs such as morphine and d-tubocurarine, and avoiding succi-

nylcholine, which can cause abdominal wall fasciculations, pressure on the tumor, and hormone release. If hypotension occurs intraoperatively, it is important to give volume and avoid the use of catecholamines. The use of angiotensin in a dose of 1.5 mg·kg^{-1} may improve the hypotension.

3. *Hypertension.* Hypertension is usually an acute intraoperative phenomenon, often associated with bronchospasm, and is probably due to tumor release of serotonin. Prophylactic treatment with ketanserin has been described.[95] If hypertension occurs acutely, the use of methotrimeprazine, conventional vasodilating agents such as sodium nitroprusside and nitroglycerin, or ketanserin has been described.

REFERENCES

1. Rosenbaum S, Skinner RF, Knight AB et al: A survey of height and weight in Great Britain 1980. Ann Hum Biol 12:115, 1985
2. Van Itallie TB: Health implications of overweight and obesity in the United States. Ann Intern Med 103:983, 1985
3. Fisher A, Waterhouse TD, Adams AP: Obesity: Its relation to anaesthesia. Anaesthesia 30:633, 1975
4. Bray GA, Gray DS: Obesity: Part 1. Pathogenesis. West J Med 149:429, 1988
5. Peiris AN, Sothmann MS, Hoffman RG et al: Adiposity, fat distribution and cardiovascular risk. Ann Intern Med 110:867, 1989
6. Nakajima T, Fujioka S, Tokunaga K et al: Correlation of intraabdominal fat accumulation and left ventricular function in obesity. Am J Cardiol 64:369, 1989
7. Farebrother MJB: Respiratory function and cardiorespiratory response to exercise in obesity. Br J Dis Chest 73:211, 1979
8. Luce JM: Respiratory complications of obesity. Chest 78:626, 1980
9. Vaughan RW: Pulmonary and cardiovascular derangements in the obese patient. In Brown BR (ed): Anesthetics and the Obese Patient, p 19. Contemporary Anesthesia Practice Series. Philadelphia, FA Davis, 1982
10. Burwell CS, Robin ED, Whaley RD et al: External obesity associated with alveolar hypoventilation: A Pickwickian syndrome. Am Med 21:811, 1956
11. Reisin E, Frolich ED: Obesity: Cardiovascular and respiratory pathophysiological alterations. Arch Intern Med 141:431, 1981
12. Alexander JK: The cardiomyopathy of obesity. Prog Cardiovasc Dis 28:325, 1985
13. Paul DR, Hoyt IL, Boutros AR: Cardiovascular and respiratory

changes in response to change of posture in the obese. Anesthesiology 45:73, 1976

14. Corrello BA, Gittens L: The cardiac mechanisms and function in obese normotensive persons with normal coronary arteries. Am J Cardiol 59:469, 1987

15. Alper MA, Singh A, Terry BE et al: Effect of exercise on left ventricular systolic function and reserve in morbid obesity. Am J Cardiol 63:1478, 1989

16. Vaughan RW: Biochemical and biotransformation alterations in obesity. In Brown BR (ed): Anesthesia and the Obese Patient, p 55. Contemporary Anesthesia Practice Series. Philadelphia, FA Davis, 1982

17. Vaughan RW, Bauer S, Wise L: Volume and pH of gastric juice in obese patients. Anesthesiology 43:686, 1975

18. Nomura F, Ohnishi K, Satomura Y et al: Liver function in moderate obesity: Study in 536 moderately obese subjects among 4613 male company employees. Int J Obes 10:349, 1986

19. Wittels EH, Thompson S: Obstructive sleep apnea and obesity. Otolaryngol Clin North Am 23:751, 1990

20. Wadden TA, Stunkard AJ: Social and psychological consequences of obesity. Ann Intern Med 103:1062, 1985

21. Buckley FP, Robinson NB, Simonowitz DA et al: Anesthesia in the morbidly obese: A comparison of anesthetic and analgesic regimens for upper abdominal surgery. Anaesthesia 38:840, 1983

22. Abernathy DR, Greenblatt DS: Pharmacokinetics of drugs in obesity. Clin Pharmacokinet 7:108, 1981

23. Abernathy DR, Greenblatt DS, Divoll M et al: The influence of obesity on the pharmacokinetics of oral alprazolam and triazolam. Clin Pharmacokinet 9:177, 1984

24. Mayersohn M, Calkins JM, Perrier DG et al: Thiopental kinetics in obese patients. Anesthesiology 55:A178, 1981

25. Ladergaard-Pederson MJ: Recovery from general anesthesia in obese patients. Anesthesiology 55:720, 1981

26. Cork RC, Vaughan RW, Bentley JB: General anesthesia for morbidly obese patients: An examination of postoperative outcomes. Anesthesiology 54:310, 1981

27. Bentley JB, Borel JD, Gillespie TS et al: Fentanyl pharmacokinetics in obese and nonobese patients. Anesthesiology 55:A177, 1981

28. Schwartz AE, Matteo RS, Ornstein E et al: Pharmacokinetics of sufentanil in the obese. Anesthesiology 65:A652, 1986

29. Bentley JB, Finley JM, Humphrey LR et al: Obesity and alfentanil pharmacokinetics. Anesth Analg 62:251, 1983

30. Bentley JB, Bond JB, Vaughan RW et al: Weight, pseudocholinesterase activity and succinylcholine requirements. Anesthesiology 57:48, 1982

31. Tseueda K, Warren JE, McCafferty LA: Pancuronium bromide requirement during anesthesia for the morbidly obese. Anesthesiology 48:483, 1978

32. Weinstein JE, Matteo RS, Ornstein E et al: Pharmacodynamics of vecuronium and atracurium in the obese surgical patient. Anesth Analg 65:684, 1986

33. Schwartz AE, Matteo RS, Ornstein E et al: Pharmacokinetics and dynamics of metocurine in the obese. Anesthesiology 65:A295, 1986

34. Varin F, Ducharme J, Thoret Y et al: The influence of extreme obesity on body disposition and neuromuscular blocking effect of atracurium. Clin Pharmacol Ther 48:18, 1990

35. McCarroll SM, Bras P, Edmiston LK et al: A prospective study to identify features associated with difficulty in laryngoscopy and intubation in the obese patient. Anesth Analg 70:S261, 1990

36. Norton ML, Brown ACD: Evaluating the patient with a difficult airway for anesthesia. Otolaryngol Clin North Am 23:771, 1990

37. Wilson SL, Manaltea NR, Malvesa JD: Effects of atropine, glycopyrrolate and cimetidine on gastric secretions in markedly obese patients. Anesth Analg 60:37, 1981

38. Goldberg ME, Rosenberg FL, Everts EA Jr et al: Metoclopramide and cimetidine pretreatment does not reduce the risk of acid aspiration in the morbidly obese patient. Anesthesiology 63:A279, 1985

39. Lam AM, Grace DM, Penny FJ et al: Prophylactic IV cimetidine reduces the risk of acid aspiration in morbidly obese patients. Anesthesiology 65:684, 1986

40. Manchikanti L, Roush JR, Colliver JR: Effect of preanesthetic ranitidine and metoclopramide on gastric contents of morbidly obese patients. Anesth Analg 65:195, 1986

41. Lee JJ, Larson RM, Buckley JJ et al: Airway maintenance in the morbidly obese. Anesthesiol Rev 7:33, 1980

42. Mallampati SR, Gatt SP et al: A clinical sign to predict difficult tracheal intubation: A prospective study. Can Anaesth Soc J 32:429, 1985

43. Moyer GA, Rein P: Preoxygenation in the morbidly obese patient. Anesth Analg 65:S106, 1986

44. Jense HG, Dubin SA, Silverstein PI et al: Effect of obesity on safe duration of apnoea in anesthetised humans. Anesth Analg 72:89, 1991

45. Vaughan RW, Wise L: Intraoperative hypoxemia in obese patients. Ann Surg 184:35, 1976

46. Bentley JB, Vaughan RW, Gandolfi J et al: Halothane biotransformation in obese and nonobese patients. Anesthesiology 57:94, 1982

47. Strube PJ, Hulands GM, Halsey MJ: Serum fluoride levels in morbidly obese patients: Enflurane compared with isoflurane. Anaesthesia 42:685, 1987

48. Salem MR, Joseph N, Lim R et al: Respiratory and hemodynamic response to PEEP in grossly obese patients. Anesthesiology 61:A511, 1984

49. Brodsky JB, Wyner J, Ehrenwerth S et al: One lung ventilation anesthesia in morbidly obese patients. Anesthesiology 57:32, 1982

50. In-amani M, Kikuta Y, Nagai H et al: The increase in pulmonary venous admixture by hypocapnia is enhanced in obese patients. Anesthesiology 63:A520, 1985

51. Ferguson CL, Sivashankaran S, Dauchot PJ: Ventilator settings to mitigate hypocarbia in the obese patient. Anesth Analg 65:53, 1986

52. McCullough WJD, Littlewood DG: Influence of obesity on spinal analgesia with bupivacaine. Br J Anaesth 58:610, 1984

53. Pitkanen MJ: Body mass and the spread of spinal analgesia with bupivacaine. Anesth Analg 66:127, 1987

54. Taivainen T, Tuominen M, Rosenberg PM: Influence of obesity on the spread of spinal analgesia after injection of plain 0.5% bupivacaine at the L3–4 or L4–5 interspace. Br J Anaesth 64:542, 1990

55. Catennacci AJ, Anderson JD, Boersma D: Anesthetic hazards of obesity. JAMA 175:657, 1961

56. Catennacci AJ, Sampathakar DR: Ventilation studies in the obese patient during spinal anesthesia. Anesth Analg 48:48, 1969

57. Blass NM: Regional anesthesia in the morbidly obese. Reg Anaesth 5(3):20, 1979

58. Chamberlain DD, Chamberlain BDL: Changes in skin temperature and their relationship to sympathetic blockade during spinal anesthesia. Anesthesiology 65:139, 1986

59. Hodgkinson R, Hussein FJ: Caesarian section associated with gross obesity. Br J Anaesth 52:919, 1980

60. Fox GS, Whalley DG, Bevan DR: Anaesthesia for the morbidly obese: Experience with 110 patients. Br J Anaesth 53:811, 1981

61. Gelman S, Vitek JJ: Thoracic epidural catheter placement under fluoroscopic control in morbidly obese patients. Reg Anaesth 4(4):19, 1980

62. Hodgkinson R, Hussein FJ: Obesity and the spread of analgesia following epidural administration of bupivacaine for caesarian section. Anesth Analg 59:89, 1980

63. Gelman S, Laws ML, Potzick J et al: Thoracic epidural vs. balanced anaesthesia in morbid obesity: An intraoperative and postoperative hemodynamic study. Anesth Analg 59:902, 1980

64. Rawal N, Sjostrand V, Christofferson E et al: Comparison of intramuscular and epidural morphine for postoperative analgesia in the grossly obese: Influence on postoperative ambulation and pulmonary function. Anesth Analg 63:583, 1986

65. Milligan KR, Cramp P, Schatz L et al: The effect of positioning and obesity on epidural analgesic spread. Anesth Analg 72:S185, 1991

66. Vaughan RW, Wise L: Intraoperative hypoxemia in obese patients. Ann Surg 180:872, 1974

67. Rand CSW, Kuldau JM, Yost RL: Obesity and postoperative pain. J Psychosom Res 29:43, 1985

68. Vandercar DH, Martinez AP, De Lisser EA: Sleep apnea syndromes: A potential contraindication for patient controlled analgesia. Anesthesiology 74:623, 1991
69. Scratcherd T, Grundy O: The physiology of intestinal motility and secretion. Br J Anaesth 56:3, 1984
70. Diamant NE: Physiology of esophageal motor function. Gastroenterol Clin North Am 18:179, 1989
71. Colton BR, Smith G: The lower oesophageal sphincter and anaesthesia. Br J Anaesth 56:37, 1984
72. Read NW, Houghton LA: Physiology of gastric emptying and pathophysiology of gastroparesis. Gastroenterol Clin North Am 18:359, 1989
73. Nimmo WS: Effect of anaesthesia on gastric motility and emptying. Br J Anaesth 56:29, 1984
74. Maltby JR, Sutherland AP, Sace JP et al: Preoperative oral fluids: Is a five-hour fast justified prior to elective surgery? Anesth Analg 65:1112, 1986
75. Shevde K, Trivedi N: Effects of clear liquids on gastric volume and pH in healthy volunteers. Anesth Analg 72:528, 1991
76. Sharna SK, Otterson MF: Small intestine physiology and pathophysiology. Gastroenterol Clin North Am 18:375, 1989
77. Gonella J, Bouvier M, Balnquet F: Extrinsic control of small and large intestines and related sphincters. Physiol Rev 67:902, 1990
78. Aitkenhead AR: Anaesthesia and bowel surgery. Br J Anaesth 56:95, 1984
79. Schrock TR, Deveney CW, Dunphy JE: Factors contributing to leakage of colonic anastomosis. Ann Surg 173:515, 1973
80. Whittaker BL: Observations on the blood flow in the inferior mesenteric artery and the healing of colonic anastomosis. Ann Surg 43:89, 1968
81. Gelman S, Fowler KC, Smith LR: Regional blood flow during isoflurane and halothane anesthesia. Anesth Analg 63:557, 1986
82. Aitkenhead AR, Gilmour PS, Hothersall AP et al: Effects of subarachnoid nerve block and arterial Pco2 on colon blood flow. Br J Anaesth 52:1071, 1980
83. Blitt CD, Gutman ML, Cohen DD et al: Silent regurgitation and aspiration during general anesthesia. Anesth Analg 49:707, 1970
84. Olsson GL, Hallen B, Hambraeus-Jonzn K: Aspiration during anesthesia: A computer-aided study. Acta Anaesthesiol Scand 30:844, 1970
85. Roberts RB, Shirley MA: Reducing the risk of acid aspiration during caesarian section. Anesth Analg 53:859, 1976
86. Holdsworth JS, Furness RMB, Ralston RG: A comparison of apomorphine and stomach tubes for emptying the stomach before general anesthesia in obstetrics. Br J Anaesth 46:526, 1974
87. Eyler SW, Cullen BF, Murphy ME et al: Antacid aspiration in rabbits: A comparison of Mylanta and Bicitra. Anesth Analg 61:288, 1982
88. Gibbs CP, Banner TC: Effectiveness of Bicitra as a preoperative antacid. Anesthesiology 61:97, 1984
89. Manchikanti L, Colliver JA, Marrero T et al: Ranitidine and metoclopramide for prophylaxis of aspiration pneumonitis in elective surgery. Anesth Analg 63:903, 1984
90. Kazuo A, Masahiko S, Demizu A et al: Effect of oral and intramuscular famotidine on pH and volume of gastric contents. Anesth Analg 68:541, 1989
91. Eger EL III, Saidman LJ: Hazards of nitrous oxide in bowel obstruction and pneumothorax. Anesthesiology 26:61, 1965
92. Scheinin B, Lindgren L, Scheinin TM: Perioperative nitrous oxide delays bowel function after colonic surgery. Br J Anaesth 64:154, 1990
93. Childes CS: Prevention of neostigmine induced colonic activity. Anaesthesia 39:1083, 1984
94. Longnecker M, Roizen MF: Patients with carcinoid syndrome. Anesthesiol Clin North Am 51:313, 1987
95. Castholy PA, Jablons M, Griepp RB et al: Ketanserin in the preoperative and intraoperative management of a patient with carcinoid tumor undergoing tricuspid valve replacement. Anesth Analg 65:809, 1986

43 Simon Gelman

Anesthesia and the Liver

INCIDENCE OF POSTOPERATIVE HEPATIC COMPLICATIONS

The incidence of postanesthesia and surgery complications related to hepatic dysfunction varies greatly.[1-9] These differences result, not only from the different populations of patients, but also from the different criteria authors use to define postoperative hepatic dysfunction. Most patients having hepatic dysfunction demonstrate only a transient increase in the serum concentration of liver enzymes or bilirubin. The latter change may be related to an excessive load of bilirubin resulting from blood transfusions rather than to hepatic dysfunction. Some studies have demonstrated relatively high incidences (as high as 20%) of temporary jaundice without any signs of preoperative liver disease.[7-9] For example, Evans et al[7] analyzed the results of 218 major surgical procedures in a prospective study and found an incidence of 3.7% for severe jaundice and 16.5% for mild jaundice. The causes were varied, but it seems that the primary one was a bilirubin overload, which resulted mainly from blood transfusions, apparently combined with disturbances in hepatic cellular metabolism that compromised the ability of the liver cells to excrete bilirubin. Those authors did not find any correlation between the incidence and severity of jaundice on the one hand and the incidence and severity of arterial hypotension on the other. It is noteworthy that the majority of their patients did not have any preoperative liver disease, neither could the authors demonstrate a statistically significant association between jaundice and halothane anesthesia. However, it is also interesting that the few cases of severe postoperative jaundice and of jaundice accompanied by abnormal liver function tests were observed only in patients who received halothane anesthesia. In addition to hyperbilirubinemia, approximately one third of these patients demonstrated a temporary increase in the plasma concentrations of hepatic enzymes. Thus, it appears that in a rather large part of the surgical population, hyperbilirubinemia is secondary to blood transfusion, resorption of hematomas from the operating field, or both.

Dykes and Walzer[4] concluded in 1967 that the incidence of postoperative hepatic dysfunction ranges from 1:239 to 1:1091 administrations of a general anesthetic. Later analysis revealed that approximately 0.15% of completely asymptomatic patients actually have significant liver disease before anesthesia and surgery,[10,11] and such patients who are scheduled for elective surgical procedures may be at risk of manifesting hepatic disease, including acute viral hepatitis, perioperatively. Schemel[10] reported that 1 of 700 patients admitted for elective surgery without any notable symptomatic disease showed unexpected and unexplained abnormalities in liver blood tests during routine preoperative evaluations and that one third of these patients had jaundice a short time after cancellation of the scheduled operation. If these patients had undergone the elective surgical procedures as planned, the anesthetic administered in these cases—halothane, isoflurane, or anything else—would surely have been deemed guilty of induction of the jaundice.

The issue of severe hepatic necrosis after a halothane anesthetic is intriguing. The National Halothane Study reviewed more than 850,000 surgical cases from 1959 to 1962. Extensive hepatic necrosis occurred in 0.01%, but the majority of these complications could be attributed to shock, prolonged use of vasopressors, infection, congestive heart failure, or existing hepatic disease. Only nine cases were of unknown origin.[12]

It is important to realize that a laparotomy with liver biopsy (without major abdominal surgery) in patients with liver disease carries an extremely high mortality rate. The immediate postoperative mortality rate was rather high two decades ago,[13,14] and despite the rather impressive developments in anesthesia care since then, the mortality rate has not decreased substantially. A 1982 report from Britain documents a 31% and 61% 30-day mortality and morbidity rate, respectively, after laparotomy and liver biopsy.[15] In that study, all the patients with viral or alcoholic hepatitis died, as did the majority of the patients with ascites (13 of 15).[15] The results in the United States in 1986 were not very different: the 30-day mortality rate in patients with severe hepatic disease and ascites approached 83%, and prolongation in prothrombin time by more than 2.5 seconds was associated with a 30-day mortality rate as high as 91%.[16]

ANATOMY AND PHYSIOLOGY OF THE LIVER AND BILIARY TRACT

The liver lies in the right upper quadrant of the abdominal cavity and is attached to the diaphragm. It is the largest gland in the human body, weighing approximately 1.5 kg and representing 2% of body weight in the adult. In the neonate, the liver accounts for approximately 5% of body weight. The liver is divided into four lobes, which are supplied by right and left branches of the portal vein and hepatic artery; bile drains into the right and left hepatic ducts. The liver is covered by a thin connective tissue layer called Glisson's capsule. Under normal conditions, the liver contains relatively little connective tissue; however, such tissue provides an internal supporting framework for the hepatic parenchyma and intrahepatic vessels and nerves.

The hepatic blood flow equals approximately 100 ml·min^{-1}·100 g^{-1}, which represents about 25% of the cardiac output. The liver is supplied by two large vessels. The hepatic artery brings blood to the liver and accounts for approximately 25% of the total hepatic blood flow but 45 to 50% of the oxygen supply, whereas the portal vein provides 75% of the total hepatic blood supply and only 50 to 55% of the oxygen supply because this blood is partially deoxygenated in the preportal organs and tissues (stomach, intestines, spleen, and pancreas) (Fig. 43-1). In contrast, portal venous blood is rich in nutrients and other substances absorbed in the gastrointestinal tract. Its flow is controlled primarily by the arterioles in the preportal splanchnic organs. This flow, combined with the resistance to portal flow within the liver, determines the portal pressure (7–10 mm Hg). Presinusoidal (precapillary) sphincters determine the relatively uniform distribution of flow through the liver and play a certain, although rather limited, role in the regulation of portal blood flow. There are data, however, suggesting that the principal site of venous resistance within the liver is postsinusoidal. The sinusoidal pressure is determined by the tone of presinusoidal and postsinusoidal sphincters and by blood flow. Smooth muscles in the wall of the venules

regulate venous compliance and blood volume. Both resistance and compliance are controlled predominately by the sympathetic innervation mediated through alpha-adrenoceptors. Changes in hepatic venous compliance play an essential part in the overall regulation of cardiac output, whereas the myogenic and metabolic intrinsic regulation of hepatic venous compliance plays a very small role, if any, in controlling the hepatic venous resistance. The main controlling mechanism seems to be sympathetic innervation mediated through alpha-adrenoceptors.

The liver vasculature has a vital role as a blood reservoir. An increase or a decrease in the resistance in the hepatic veins is accompanied by rather dramatic changes in the blood volume within the liver. This reservoir function is mediated mainly through the sympathetic nervous system. For example, during hemorrhage, the liver may "squeeze" an additional 500 ml of blood into the systemic circulation. Anesthetics that suppress sympathetic nervous system function may interfere with such compensatory responses and lead to decompensation if lost blood is not replaced immediately. Patients with liver disease have a decreased sensitivity to catecholamines, probably as a result of an increase in glucagon concentration. Therefore, these patients may have an impaired ability to compensate for hemorrhage and hypovolemia by sympathetic mechanisms: (1) to develop vasoconstriction to divert blood to the heart and brain from the muscles and splanchnic circulation; (2) to expel blood from the splanchnic reservoir into the systemic circulation; and (3) to constrict the capacitance vasculature.

The principal site of resistance in the hepatic arterial vasculature is the arterioles. Regulation of the tone in these vessels is achieved mainly by local and intrinsic mechanisms that adjust hepatic arterial flow to compensate for

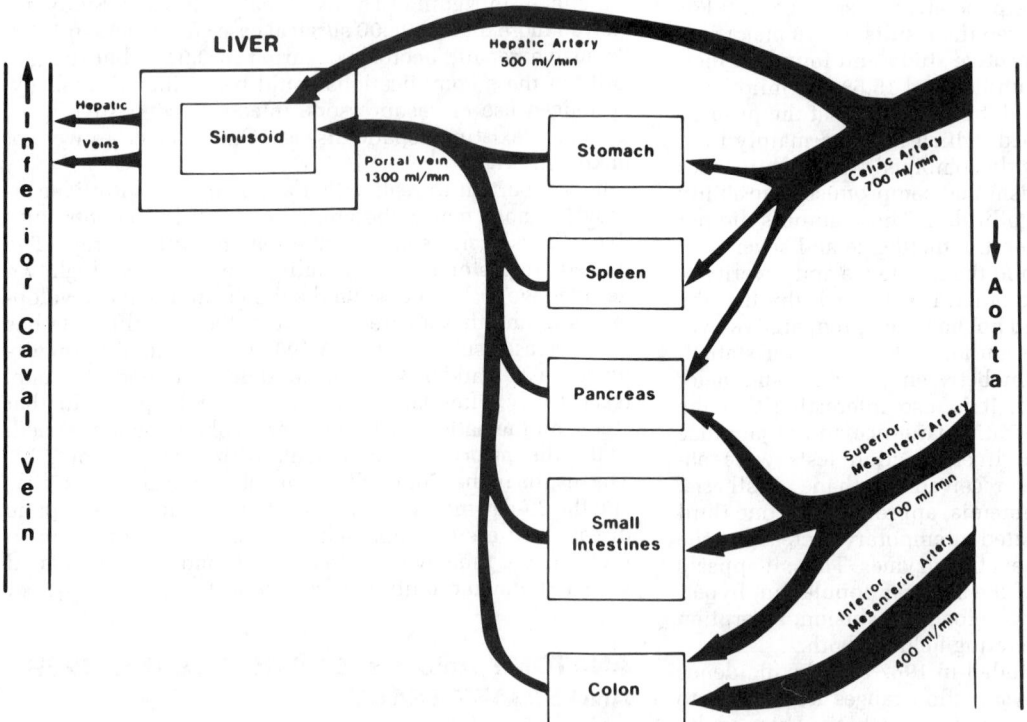

Figure 43-1. Schematic representation of splanchnic circulation. (Reprinted with permission from Gelman S: Effects of anesthetics on splanchnic circulation. In Altura BM, Halevy S [eds]: Cardiovascular Action of Anesthetics and Drugs Used in Anesthesia, p 127. Basel, Karger Publishing, 1986.)

changes in portal blood flow, a phenomenon referred to as the "arterial buffer response." Decreases in portal blood flow usually are associated with an increase in hepatic arterial blood flow,[17,18] which may be considered an attempt to maintain the hepatic oxygen supply (which is essential for hepatocyte function) and the total hepatic blood flow (which, in turn, is essential for clearance of exogenous and endogenous compounds with a high hepatic extraction). The mechanisms of hepatic arterial flow autoregulation involve neural, myogenic, and metabolic controls, as well as the content of portal blood and the washout effect.[17,18] A decrease in portal blood pH or oxygen content is accompanied by an increase in hepatic arterial blood flow, even when portal blood flow is intentionally maintained unaltered.[17] The washout theory suggests that a substance, apparently adenosine, is generated within the liver tissue; when portal blood flow decreases, this vasodilator accumulates and subsequently leads to hepatic arterial dilation. Increased portal blood flow causes an effective washout of this substance and a reduction in the vasodilating effect on the hepatic arterial vasculature.

The liver and hepatic vasculature also play an extremely important role in fluid homeostasis. With even small increases in hepatic venous pressure, excessive amounts of fluid transude into the lymph and leak through the outer surface of the liver capsule into the peritoneal cavity. This fluid contains 80–90% of the normal plasma protein.

Bile ducts accompany the hepatic arteries and the portal veins. Bile flows from the bile canaliculi of the liver to enter ductules, the larger interhepatic bile ducts, and, finally, the right and left hepatic bile ducts, which form the hepatic duct proper (Fig. 43-2). The common hepatic duct is formed at the porta hepatis from the right and left hepatic lobular ducts. It is approximately 3 cm long and is joined by the cystic duct from the gallbladder to create the common bile duct, ductus choledochus, which is approximately 7 cm long and empties into the duodenum.

The gallbladder is located under the surface of the right lobe of the liver. It is very distensible and may contain 30–50 ml of bile. The cystic artery, which usually arises from the right hepatic artery, provides the arterial supply to the gallbladder.

Structural Concepts of Liver Lobulation

Small histologic units, or lobules, of the liver have been recognized since the 17th century. Two primary models have been developed to describe these histologic and functional units.

The classic lobule is a polyhedral prism of liver tissue about 1–2 mm in diameter. The lobule is roughly hexagonal, and at the angles of the hexagon, there are interlobular portal canals containing some connective tissue and a portal triad. The central vein, which is actually the terminal hepatic venule, lies in the center of this lobule. The parenchyma lies between blood-carrying vascular channels of the sinusoids. The parenchymal cells form plates that radiate from the central vein to the portal canals at the periphery of the lobule (Fig. 43-3).

Approximately 30 years ago, Rappaport and colleagues[19] defined the liver lobule as an acinus. According to this concept, parenchymal cells are grouped into zones surrounding the terminal afferent vessels (Fig. 43-4). Zone 1 cells receive blood and oxygen first, are usually the last to undergo necrosis, and regenerate first. Cells in Zones 2 and 3, particularly the latter, are located more distal to the afferent vessels and

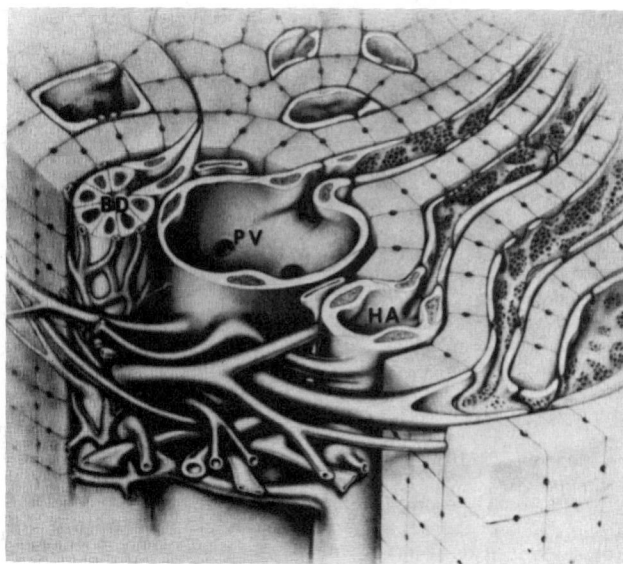

Figure 43-2. Relations of branches of the portal vein (PV), hepatic artery (HA), and bile duct (BD). Notice the peribiliary capillary plexus associated with the bile duct. (Reprinted with permission from Jones AL: Anatomy of the normal liver. In Zakim D, Boyer TD [eds]: Hepatology: A Textbook of Liver Disease. Philadelphia, WB Saunders, 1982.)

so receive blood with a lesser amount of oxygen and nutrients. They therefore are probably less resistant to hepatotoxins and oxygen deprivation.

The smallest branches of the biliary tree are the canaliculi, which are located between a few hepatocytes. Bile proceeds down the canaliculi, moving from the centrilobular cells toward the perilobular and interlobular portal triads (from Zone 3 to Zone 1). The bile then enters the small terminal ductules or canals of Hering. From the terminal ductules, bile passes to the interlobular bile ducts, which form a continuous passageway with increasing size and wall complexity.

Ultrastructure of Hepatocytes

Hepatocytes, or hepatic parenchymal cells, represent approximately 80% of the cytoplasmic mass within the liver. These cells are relatively large, approximately 20–30 μm, and their function is extremely diverse and complex. They absorb digestive material from the portal venous blood, and they store proteins, vitamins, carbohydrates, and lipids, which they release into the blood in bound or unbound forms. They excrete bile salts, which facilitate the absorption of fat from the intestines, and synthesize plasma proteins, glucose, cholesterol, fatty acids, and phospholipids. They also metabolize, detoxify, and inactivate exogenous and endogenous compounds, including drugs, some poisons, steroids, and the majority of other hormones. Hepatocytes may also play an important role in the immune system.

A system of intracellular organelles is needed to perform these multiple and complex functions. Approximately 800 mitochondria can be found in every liver cell, occupying about 18% of the hepatocyte volume and playing a crucial role in oxidative phosphorylation and the oxidation of fatty acids. Lysosomes are usually located in the pericanalicular

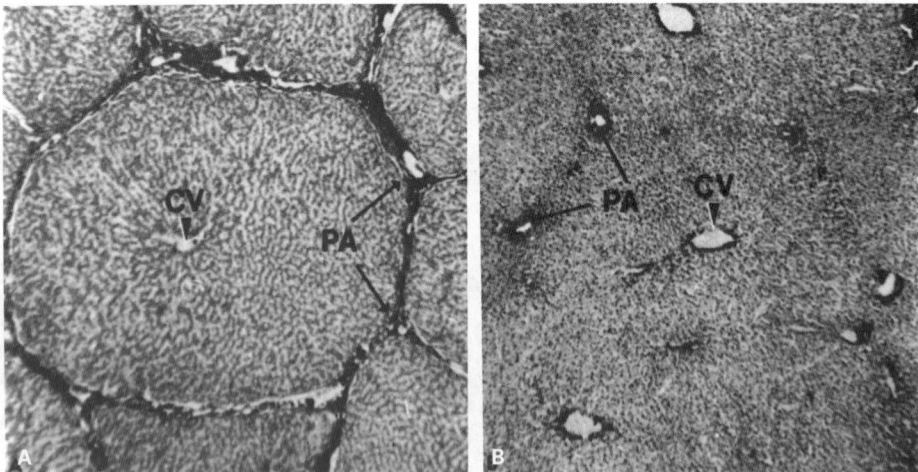

Figure 43-3. Structure of the hepatic lobule. (*A*) Cross-section of a pig lobule, illustrating the boundaries of the classic lobule. (*B*) A classic lobule of normal human liver. The boundaries are poorly seen because of the absence of connective tissue septa. (PA = portal area; CV = central vein; ≃ × 100.) (Reprinted with permission from Jones AL, Schmucker DL: Current concepts of liver structure as related to function. Gastroenterology 73:833, 1977. Copyright 1977 by The American Gastroenterological Association.)

region and interact in the digestion and catabolism of many exogenous substances. Both rough and smooth endoplasmic reticulum probably is involved in essentially every function of the liver cells. For example, hepatic drug-metabolizing activities, as well as the conversion of cholesterol to bile acids and certain steps in cholesterol biosynthesis, appear

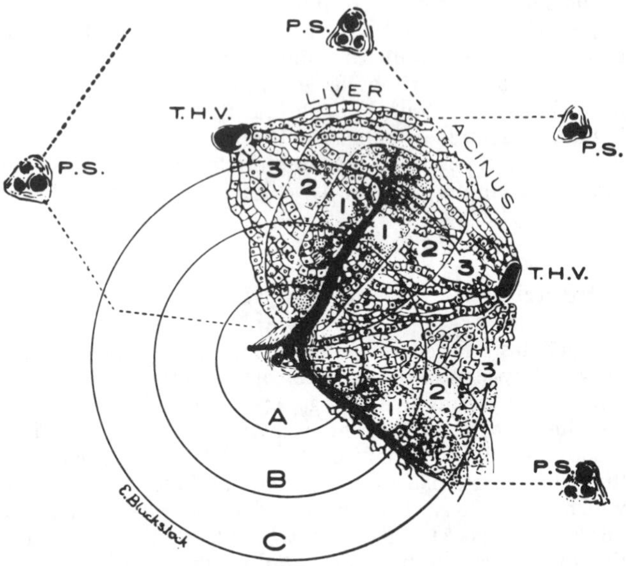

Figure 43-4. The blood supply of the hepatic structural unit, which occupies adjacent sectors of neighboring hexagonal fields. Zones 1, 2, and 3 represent areas supplied with blood of first, second, and third quality, respectively, with regard to oxygen and nutrients. These zones cluster about the terminal afferent vascular twigs and extend into the periportal field from which these twigs originate. Zones 1', 2', and 3' designate corresponding areas in a portion of an adjacent structural unit. In Zones 1 and 1', the afferent vascular twigs empty into the sinusoids. The circles A, B, and C delimit concentric bands of the hepatic parenchyma arranged around a small portal field. (Reprinted with permission from Rappaport AM, Borowy ZJ, Lougheed WM *et al:* Subdivision of hexagonal liver lobules into a structural and functional unit. Anat Rec 119:16, 1954.)

to occur within the endoplasmic reticulum. The Golgi complex is involved in the production of very low-density lipoproteins, in glycoprotein synthesis, and in albumin secretion. The Golgi complex may also play a role in bile secretion. Other cellular inclusions store fat droplets and other compounds, including the stores of glycogen that first appear in Zone 1 and disappear from Zone 3 (centrilobular areas) of the acinus.

The liver contains large reticuloendothelial Kupffer's cells, which primarily phagocytize bacteria and other foreign matter in the blood. In addition to hepatocytes and Kupffer's cells, the liver contains endothelial cells, sinusoidal lining cells, and lipocytes.

Metabolic Functions of the Liver

The liver synthesizes and excretes many different substances. Among the most important is bilirubin. When the cell membranes of erythrocytes rupture, the released hemoglobin is phagocytized by the reticuloendothelial cells, which split the hemoglobin into globin and heme. The latter provides a substrate from which the bile pigments are formed. The first pigment is biliverdin, which is reduced to free bilirubin and released into the plasma. Free bilirubin combines strongly with the plasma albumin and is transported throughout the blood and intestinal fluids. Bilirubin is then released from the plasma albumin and subsequently absorbed by hepatocytes. Within the liver cells, bilirubin is conjugated with different substances, primarily glucuronic acid. In conjugated forms, bilirubin is excreted by active transport into the bile. A small portion of the conjugated bilirubin returns to the plasma directly into the sinusoids and indirectly by absorption from the bile ducts and lymphatics. Bilirubin is converted into urobilinogen in the intestine by bacteria. Some of the urobilinogen, being very soluble, is reabsorbed through the intestinal mucosa into the blood and is then re-excreted by the liver into the intestine. About 5% of the urobilinogen is excreted by the kidneys. When exposed to air, urobilinogen is oxidized to urobilin in the urine or to stercobilin in the feces.

Hyperbilirubinemia can be the result of an overproduction of bilirubin (unconjugated hyperbilirubinemia) as a consequence of hemolysis, large hematomas, or ineffective erythropoiesis or of defective elimination of bilirubin. The latter can result from inadequate hepatobiliary elimination of conjugated bilirubin (conjugated hyperbilirubinemia), which primarily reflects cholestatic diseases of the liver and biliary obstruction. Also, defective hepatic removal of bilirubin can result in unconjugated hyperbilirubinemia. These disorders include all diseases interfering with hepatic bilirubin uptake or conjugation, such as neonatal hyperbilirubinemia, breast milk jaundice of the newborn, and conditions such as the hereditary Gilbert's disease (cholemia) and Crigler-Najjar syndrome (congenital nonhemolytic jaundice). Unconjugated hyperbilirubinemia may cause severe neurologic dysfunction, including a rapidly fatal encephalopathy,[20-22] whereas conjugated hyperbilirubinemia is not accompanied by apparent neurotoxicity.

Bilirubin is toxic for many enzymes.[23] This effect usually occurs with very high concentrations of bilirubin and can be modified by the addition of albumin.[24] Bilirubin may play a role in uncoupling oxidative phosphorylation in mitochondria, but it seems that such metabolic disturbances occur only with very high concentrations. Alternative mechanisms proposed to explain the neurotoxicity of hyperbilirubinemia include bilirubin-mediated changes in ATPase and inhibition of protein synthesis and cellular growth. Bilirubin may also interfere with membrane function.[25]

The main function of the liver in carbohydrate metabolism consists of storing glycogen, converting galactose to glucose, gluconeogenesis, and forming many of the intermediate compounds of carbohydrate biotransformation. The liver plays a critical role in maintaining normal blood glucose levels, which is termed the "glucose buffer function." Specific functions of the liver in fat metabolism consist of beta-oxidation of fatty acids; formation of acetoacetic acid, lipoproteins, cholesterol, and phospholipids; and conversion of carbohydrates and proteins into fat. Its most important functions in protein metabolism consist of deamination of amino acids, formation of urea for removal of ammonia, synthesis of plasma proteins, and interconversions among the different amino acids and other compounds.

Other metabolic functions of the liver include production of blood coagulation factors and storage of iron, vitamins, and some other compounds.

Pharmacokinetics and Pharmacodynamics

The involvement of the liver in pharmacokinetics is reflected in the elimination of exogenous, as well as endogenous, compounds by biotransformation or excretion of unchanged compounds into the bile.[26,27] The hepatic elimination of a drug can be affected by different mechanisms. The main ones are changes in hepatic blood flow and in the ability of the liver cells to biotransform or excrete a given compound. The latter process is called intrinsic clearance. These two mechanisms, hepatocyte function and hepatic blood flow, are important considerations in patients with liver disease, as well as in patients with relatively normal liver function that may deteriorate temporarily during anesthesia and surgery. Other mechanisms of altered pharmacokinetics include changes in the binding of drugs—in other words, changes in the ratio of bound to (free) unbound drugs, and changes in the volume of distribution. These mechanisms often play an extremely important role in patients with advanced liver disease. Some specific information regarding the pharmacokinetics of certain drugs relative to anesthesia practice is presented later in a discussion of the comparative pharmacology of anesthetics and of anesthetic management for patients with liver disease.

Pharmacodynamic observations in patients with hepatic disease are limited, as, unfortunately, the pharmacologic effects of drugs in these patients have attracted relatively little attention from researchers. The reasons for this neglect are multifactorial; however, some of them are relatively clear. A study of this type would necessitate concurrent pharmacokinetic studies; otherwise, interpretation of the pharmacologic effects would become impossible, because it would never be clear which effects were related to altered pharmacodynamics and which were the result of changed pharmacokinetics. In other words, a changed response that resulted from an altered interaction between the drug and its receptors (pharmacodynamics) would not be distinguished from one that resulted from a change in the concentration of drug available to the receptors (pharmacokinetics).

Despite certain methodologic limitations, some studies suggest that patients with liver cirrhosis, particularly those with histories of hepatic coma, are much more sensitive to morphine[28] and chlorpromazine[29,30] than are normal persons. It also has been demonstrated that equal plasma concentrations of diazepam result in much more pronounced encephalographic alterations in patients with severe hepatic disease than in normal persons.[31] However, there are reasons to believe that the response to catecholamines in patients who have hepatic cirrhosis and portal hypertension is substantially decreased. Patients, as well as animals, with portal hypertension have an increased plasma glucagon concentration,[32] and glucagon substantially reduces the response of the different vessels to catecholamines.[33] Thus, it is not surprising that cirrhotic patients do not respond to catecholamines as do normal persons. It seems, therefore, that the dose of drugs such as morphine and chlorpromazine should be decreased, whereas either the dose of any needed catecholamines should be increased or a different vasopressive drug, such as vasopressin, should be used.

The pharmacokinetic and pharmacodynamic interactions can be complex, and an ideal choice of one or another drug may not be possible. As an illustration, it was observed more than 20 years ago that patients with hepatic cirrhosis require higher doses of d-tubocurarine to achieve a similar degree of muscle relaxation than do normal persons.[34] This effect seems to be related purely to pharmacokinetic deviations: patients with hepatic cirrhosis have a larger volume of distribution for d-tubocurarine, primarily related to an increased gamma-globulin fraction with a subsequent greater binding of d-tubocurarine and a smaller free fraction. On the other hand, all drugs, including muscle relaxants, that are excreted with the bile are excreted much more slowly in patients with hepatic cirrhosis or obstructive jaundice–cholestasis. These observations suggest the advisability of the use of gallamine or, particularly, atracurium, because these relaxants are not excreted with the bile.[35] However, the overall judgment should consider not only the pharmacokinetics but also the pharmacodynamics of a drug or, in this case, the side effects of muscle relaxants. For example, the clearance and half-life of vecuronium is prolonged in patients with severe liver disease compared with normal persons, whereas the clearance of gallamine is not significantly altered. This does not mean that one should not use vecuronium in patients with hepatic cirrhosis: if a drug is cautiously titrated against effect, it can be used safely; however, gallamine, which induces tachycardia, may not be a drug of choice.

The lesson is clear. Owing to pharmacodynamic and

pharmacokinetic alterations, the response of any patient to a drug is virtually unpredictable. Therefore, each drug must be carefully selected and, probably more importantly, carefully titrated to the desirable effect.

PATHOPHYSIOLOGY OF LIVER DISEASE

For practical clinical purposes, anesthesiologists may divide patients with liver disease into two large heterogeneous groups: those with parenchymal disease, including acute and chronic viral hepatitis, hepatic cirrhosis with or without portal hypertension, and some other disorders; and those with cholestasis, including obstruction of the extrahepatic biliary pathway.

Parenchymal Disease (Viral Hepatitis, Cirrhosis)

For simplicity, we will discuss the pathophysiology of parenchymal liver disease with an example of hepatic cirrhosis as it relates to the practice of anesthesia. The most common clinical features of cirrhosis are an enlarged spleen and liver, often ascites, mild to moderate jaundice, weakness, large esophageal varices, spider nevi, anorexia, nausea, vomiting, encephalopathy, and, sometimes, abdominal pain. Practically, the function of every organ and body system is altered in a patient with advanced parenchymal hepatic disease.

Cardiovascular Function in Cirrhosis

Systemic Circulation. Systemic cardiovascular function in patients with liver cirrhosis and portal hypertension is characterized by a hyperdynamic state, including high cardiac output, low peripheral vascular resistance, and normal filling pressure, heart rate, and arterial pressure (Table 43-1). The circulating blood volume is usually increased, and peripheral blood flow is substantially increased above the metabolic oxygen requirements. Therefore, oxygen tension and saturation in the peripheral and mixed venous blood are usually increased, whereas the arteriovenous difference in oxygen content is narrowed. This clinical and pathophysiologic syndrome mimics the usual picture of a peripheral arteriovenous fistula. Patients with liver cirrhosis and portal

---

TABLE 43-1. Cardiovascular Function in Hepatic Cirrhosis

Decreased vascular resistance (peripheral vasodilation, increased arteriovenous shunting)
Increased circulating blood volume
Increased cardiac output
Maintained arterial blood pressure, filling pressures, and heart rate (deterioration is late)
Possible cardiomyopathy
Decreased arteriovenous oxygen content difference and increased venous oxygen content
Decreased responsiveness to catecholamines
Increased splanchnic (except the liver), pulmonary, muscle, and skin blood flow
Decreased portal blood flow to the liver
Maintained or decreased hepatic arterial blood flow
Maintained or decreased renal blood flow

---

hypertension have developed arteriovenous collaterals in many organs and tissues, including the splanchnic organs, lungs, skin, muscles, and probably others. The reasons for such development are multifactorial and not completely understood. In rats with experimentally induced portal stenosis, an increase in arteriovenous shunting and blood flow in preportal tissues, at least by 40%, is secondary to an increase in the glucagon concentration of the blood.[32] It has yet to be established which factors are responsible for the remaining 60% increase. Other substances such as ferritin and vasoactive intestinal polypeptide may also be responsible for peripheral vasodilation, decreased vascular resistance, and increased arteriovenous shunting.

Arterial vasodilation decreases the vascular resistance and aortic pressure, which may increase stroke volume and cardiac output even with certain degrees of cardiomyopathy. Thus, the majority of patients with hepatic cirrhosis have high cardiac output despite some degree of cardiomyopathy. Patients with hepatic cirrhosis have a reduced ability to develop vasoconstriction, as well as tachycardia, in response to appropriate stimuli. This distorted response is probably related to circulating vasodilating factors but may also be attributable to an impairment in baroreceptor-mediated responses.

The responsiveness of the cardiovascular system to sympathetic discharge or catecholamines is reduced.[28] The mechanism of this change is not completely clear; however, it seems that the increased glucagon concentration in blood plays an important role. Experimentally, glucagon (the concentration of which is always increased in patients with liver cirrhosis and portal hypertension) decreases the vasculature responsiveness to infused catecholamines and other vasopressors.[36,37] Clinically, however, patients with liver cirrhosis and portal hypertension who are already decompensated and would not respond well to an infused α-adrenoceptor agonist may still respond better to vasopressin.

The decompensation of cardiovascular function in patients with liver cirrhosis often starts with an increase in ventricular filling pressures or a decrease in stroke volume, with a subsequent increase in heart rate. This change is often associated with a further increase in mixed venous oxygen tension and saturation and a decrease in oxygen consumption. The state of decompensation becomes similar to that observed in septic shock.

Ascites can be one of the important complications aggravating cardiovascular function abnormalities in patients with liver cirrhosis. With an increase in intra-abdominal pressure and a shift of the diaphragm upward, the intrathoracic pressure increases, with a subsequent reduction in the transmural pressure gradient across the heart. As fluid accumulates, venous return and cardiac output decrease. Removal of the intra-abdominal fluid decreases the intra-abdominal pressure, often with a subsequent improvement in overall cardiovascular function. Obviously, if paracentesis is performed, the ascitic fluid should be removed slowly while carefully observing cardiovascular function.

Alcohol decreases myocardial contractile force *in vitro* and myocardial contractility *in vivo*. Alcohol ingestion is usually accompanied by an increase in the concentration of catecholamines. Therefore, the direct depressive effect of alcohol on contractile force often is masked by a catecholamine-mediated stimulation of myocardial contractility. Chronic alcoholism is often accompanied by cardiomyopathy, which may eventually develop into low-output congestive heart failure. Often, alcoholics develop either cardiomyopathy or cirrhosis, but these two conditions usually do not coexist. Episodes of disorders in cardiac rhythm are sometimes observed after heavy weekend or holiday drinking and are even called "holiday heart syndrome."[38]

Renal Circulation. Renal blood flow is normal in patients with portal hypertension, and there is no obvious renal dysfunction. A decrease in renal cortical blood flow is probably one of the first signs of impairment of renal function. Renal circulatory disturbances play an important role in the pathogenesis of the hepatorenal syndrome, which sometimes complicates liver cirrhosis. Renal blood flow, especially in the cortex, can be decreased as a result of an increase in renal vascular resistance despite a relatively high cardiac output and low total peripheral vascular resistance. Other organs and tissues are hyperperfused, whereas the kidneys suffer from hypoperfusion. In fact, blood flow through preportal organs and tissues, as well as through the skin, lungs, and muscles (although to a lesser extent) is often increased. An increase in renal vascular resistance is secondary to an increase in resistance in the afferent, more than the efferent, arterioles. There are different humoral substances involved in the pathogenesis of renal circulatory disorders in patients with liver cirrhosis and portal hypertension.

Hepatic Circulation. Portal hypertension is the main feature of the splanchnic circulatory disorders in hepatic cirrhosis. Theoretically, portal pressure is determined by one or any combination of three factors: blood flow into the portal system, resistance to portal flow, and resistance in the portacaval collaterals. The classic "backward theory" proposes that fibrotic tissue within the liver, formed during cirrhosis, increases the resistance to portal flow, with subsequent development of portal hypertension. However, many clinical and experimental observations do not fit the backward theory. For example, in experimental animals, restriction of transhepatic portal flow does not always produce portal hypertension comparable to that encountered clinically, nor does it produce bleeding from esophageal varices. In addition, acute portal hypertension induced by specific narrowing of the portal vein is accompanied by a substantial decrease in splanchnic venous oxygen saturation, an increase in the arteriomesenteric venous oxygen content difference, an increase in mesenteric vascular resistance, and a decrease in mesenteric arterial flow. Completely opposite changes are observed in patients with hepatic cirrhosis and portal hypertension.

To explain the clinical and physiologic features of patients with hepatic cirrhosis that do not fit the backward theory, a "forward theory" has been introduced.[39] This theory suggests that certain factors (glucagon and some other vasodilating compounds) lead to vasodilation and formation of arteriovenous fistulae in the intestine and the spleen, which produce a hyperdynamic state with increased splanchnic blood flow and cardiac output. Concerning the hepatic circulation itself, portal blood flow to the liver is substantially decreased, whereas hepatic arterial blood flow is maintained or even increased. Therefore, in the majority of situations, the hepatic oxygen supply is maintained, while the total hepatic blood flow is decreased. A decrease in total hepatic blood flow has certain pharmacokinetic implications: compounds, exogenous as well as endogenous, with high hepatic clearance are eliminated more slowly than in normal persons.

Circulatory Effects of Some Modalities of Treatment for Portal Hypertension. In an attempt to stop acute bleeding from esophageal varices in patients with hepatic cirrho-

sis and portal hypertension, a triple-lumen Sengstaken–Blakemore tube, which has a gastric and an esophageal balloon, can be inflated to compress the varices. One lumen of this tube provides the opportunity to remove gastric contents. Many different surgical procedures still are used to stop or prevent variceal bleeding. Some procedures, such as ligation of the varices, portal vein–azygos vein disconnection, or transposition of the spleen, are rarely performed, whereas other procedures, such as sclerosing the varices or the creation of portasystemic shunts (including portacaval shunt, end-to-end or end-to-side), as well as mesocaval, mesorenal, or splenorenal peripheral shunts, are used more often.

Surgical and pharmacologic treatment of portal hypertension produces important alterations in systemic and regional hemodynamics, and it is important that the anesthesiologist be cognizant of these pathophysiologic changes. Surgical formation of a portacaval shunt immediately redistributes the blood flow from the portal vein through the surgical shunt to the inferior vena cava, with an apparent increase in the flow in the inferior vena cava and venous return. Surgical portacaval shunts also lead to an immediate decrease in the resistance to portal flow, which, in turn, leads to a decrease in arterial resistance in the intestine and spleen with a subsequent increase in the flow through these organs. However, this increase in the preportal blood flow is associated with both increased flow through the surgical shunt and decreased portal blood flow to the liver. In the majority of patients, this decrease is associated with some increase in hepatic arterial blood flow, which maintains the hepatic oxygen supply. Total hepatic blood flow is apparently decreased, which is probably responsible, at least partially, for the increase in the concentrations of circulating glucagon and other vasodilating substances. Total peripheral vascular resistance is decreased, and the ejection fraction may subsequently be increased, which, in combination with an increase in venous return, causes a further increase in cardiac output (Fig. 43-5).

Many patients with portal hypertension undergoing portacaval shunt surgery are given specific medications to stop or prevent bleeding from esophageal varices. Vasopressin is commonly used in this situation. The beneficial effect of vasopressin is related to vasoconstriction in the preportal area, with a subsequent decline in portal blood flow and portal pressure. Hepatic arterial blood flow is often slightly increased. However, vasopressin has certain adverse effects related mainly to systemic vasoconstriction, including coronary vasoconstriction, with subsequent arterial hypertension. The combination of vasopressin with a vasodilating drug such as sodium nitroprusside or nitroglycerin is beneficial, as it produces a further reduction in portal pressure, an increase in hepatic arterial blood flow, and possibly an improvement in coronary circulation.[40-42] Somatostatin can also be successful in controlling bleeding from esophageal varices. Somatostatin decreases portal blood flow and portal pressure by a considerable reduction in glucagon activity and intestinal motility, resulting in a substantial decrease in mesenteric blood flow.[43]

Propranolol has gained popularity recently in preventing gastrointestinal bleeding in patients with portal hypertension. Experimentally, propranolol decreases portal hypertension by both beta$_1$- and beta$_2$-adrenergic blockade. Beta$_1$-adrenergic blockade is associated with a reduction in cardiac output and a subsequent decrease in portal blood flow. Beta$_2$-adrenergic blockade results in splanchnic vasoconstriction and a decrease in blood flow through portacaval collaterals.[44] The antirenin activity of propranolol prob-

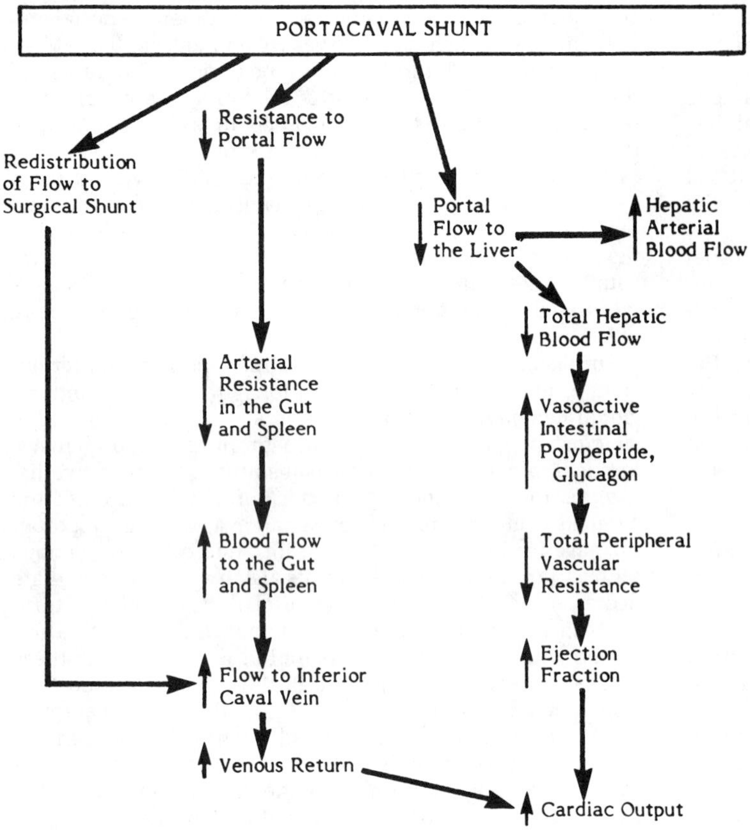

Figure 43-5. Schematic representation of the cardiovascular consequences of a portacaval shunt. (Reprinted with permission from Kang YG, Gelman S: Liver transplantation. In Gelman S [ed]: Anesthesia and Organ Transplantation, p 150. Philadelphia, WB Saunders, 1987.)

ably also plays a role in the effectiveness of this drug. The beneficial effect of propranolol is partially attributed also to a decrease in anxiety and the degree of alcohol abuse. The adverse effects of propranolol include a decrease in the efficacy of diuretic therapy, an increase in the ammonia concentration in blood with signs of encephalopathy, sometimes hypoglycemia, and decreased clearance of other drugs. Severe withdrawal syndrome and gastrointestinal bleeding may result from termination of propranolol treatment. Conn has stated, "Once treatment with propranolol is begun, it is a lifetime sentence."[45] Some controlled trials were unable to demonstrate that propranolol is effective in the prevention of variceal rebleeding in patients with liver cirrhosis.[46]

Respiratory Function and Pulmonary Circulation in Cirrhosis

Patients with liver cirrhosis and portal hypertension usually have an increased red blood cell content of 2,3-diphosphoglycerate (2,3DPG), which is accompanied by reduced affinity of hemoglobin for oxygen and a shift of the oxyhemoglobin dissociation curve to the right.

Patients with liver cirrhosis commonly demonstrate different degrees of arterial oxygen desaturation. There are many reasons for these observations (Table 43-2). Collaterals between the portal venous and pulmonary vasculature systems have been well documented, but they probably do not play a clinically significant role. Intrapulmonary shunting is most likely a result of an increase in the concentration of vasodilating substances (glucagon, vasoactive intestinal polypeptide, ferritin), which apparently play a substantial role in the development of hypoxemia. These and

some other vasodilating substances are probably responsible for impaired hypoxic pulmonary vasoconstriction. A decrease in the inspired fraction of oxygen is usually accompanied by an increase in pulmonary vascular resistance in healthy volunteers but not in patients with liver cirrhosis.[47]

In patients with cirrhosis complicated by ascites, an increase in closing volume, which may exceed the functional residual capacity, is often observed.[48] This change leads to gas trapping in the lower lung zones and a decrease in the ventilation/perfusion ratio, with subsequent hypoxemia.

Patients with hepatic cirrhosis sometimes develop pulmonary hypertension, the pathogenesis of which is not clear. The mechanisms probably involve increased cardiac output and circulating blood volume, which may secondarily involve the pulmonary vasculature leading to pulmonary hypertension. An increase in the activity of some circulating vasoconstricting substances may also be involved.

TABLE 43-2. Hypoxemia in Hepatic Cirrhosis

Rightward shift of the oxyhemoglobin dissociation curve
Ventilation/perfusion abnormalities (impaired hypoxic pulmonary vasoconstriction)
Hypoventilation owing to ascites
Decrease in pulmonary diffusing capacity owing to an increase in extracellular fluid
Right-to-left shunt across the lungs owing to:
  Spider angiomas in the lungs
  Portapulmonary venous communications
  Humoral factors (e.g., vasodilation—glucagon, ferritin, vasointestinal polypeptide)

Blood and Coagulation in Cirrhosis

Hematocrit values in patients with liver cirrhosis are usually decreased owing to an increased plasma volume and, obviously, to blood loss when gastrointestinal bleeding occurs. Megaloblastic anemia resulting from vitamin B_{12} and other vitamin deficiencies is not uncommon, especially in alcoholics, because of malnutrition. An increased rate of hemolysis contributes to the anemia. The hemolytic activity is proportional to the size of the spleen but not to the degree of portal hypertension[49,50] and is related to reticulocytosis and splenomegaly. Leukopenia and thrombocytopenia, usually related to hypersplenism and ethanol-induced depression of the marrow, are not uncommon in patients.

The majority of patients with liver cirrhosis have some mild abnormalities in coagulation processes. The most common is a reduction in the concentration of Factor VII, and then of Factors V, X, and II (prothrombin); the concentration of Factor I (fibrinogen) is also often decreased. Usually, the concentration of fibrin degradation products is not increased; however, increased fibrinogen consumption may be observed. Occasionally, severe disseminated intravascular coagulation (DIC) develops after LeVeen shunt surgery. Hepatic failure is associated with a substantial decrease in the synthesis of clotting factors, resulting in prolongation of the prothrombin and partial thromboplastin times. Factors II, VII, IX, and X are vitamin K–dependent, whereas Factors I and V are not. Factor VIII, which is not synthesized in the liver, can even be increased in patients with hepatic cirrhosis. Owing to the relatively short half-life of Factor VII, it decreases earlier and to a greater extent than the other liver-produced clotting factors.[51] Factor I (fibrinogen) synthesis deteriorates last. Changes in the prothrombin time usually reflect well the extent of liver dysfunction.

The plasma concentration of albumin in patients with liver cirrhosis is usually decreased. The reasons are relatively complex but are related to a decrease in the rate of albumin synthesis, as well as to an increase in total body water and other factors.

Endocrine Disorders

The growth hormone concentration usually increases in patients with liver cirrhosis, which may be partially responsible for their intolerance of carbohydrates. Many patients have abnormal glucose utilization; the mechanism of this phenomenon is rather complex and includes an increased plasma concentration of fatty acids, which interfere with the insulin effect on glucose uptake by skeletal muscles. An increased plasma glucagon concentration also plays a role in the disorders of carbohydrate metabolism observed.

Abnormal sex hormone metabolism may cause gonadal function disorders in both sexes and feminization in men, as evidenced by microscopic pictures of testicular dystrophy, a decrease in testicular size, a higher frequency of impotence, and hypospermia in those who can still produce and ejaculate semen. Gynecomastia is not uncommon, and the prostate gland is small. Oligomenorrhea or amenorrhea is common among women.

Encephalopathy

Patients with hepatic encephalopathy usually appear obtunded and confused. An increase in the blood concentration of nitrogenous compounds resulting from gastrointestinal bleeding or an overdose of diuretics can be found in such patients. It is believed that the increased blood ammonia concentration is responsible for the severity of hepatic encephalopathy. However, the severity of encephalopathy does not seem to be directly related to the blood ammonia concentration. That is, some patients with hepatic encephalopathy do not have an increased blood ammonia concentration, whereas others with an increased blood ammonia concentration do not have detectable encephalopathy.

The pathogenesis of hepatic encephalopathy involves insufficient hepatic elimination of nitrogenous compounds (ammonia is one of them) ingested (e.g., meat) or formed (from the blood during bleeding) in the gastrointestinal tract. Hepatic encephalopathy may result from inadequate hepatocyte function, as well as from reduced blood flow and increased collaterals; that is, portacaval blood flow. The portacaval collaterals include those of the esophageal, rectal, and other areas that usually develop in patients with hepatic cirrhosis, as well as surgically created portacaval shunts. There are some data suggesting that the central nervous system (CNS) of patients with advanced hepatic disease is more sensitive to functional interference by nitrogenous compounds than is the neural tissue of normal subjects. Many recent studies have been devoted to elucidating the precise role of different substances, including ammonia, in the pathogenesis of hepatic encephalopathy.

It has been suggested that certain mercaptans, short-chain fatty acids, play a significant role in the pathogenesis of hepatic encephalopathy. Further, it has been theorized that in patients with encephalopathy, biogenic amines are formed within the CNS and then released along with normal neurotransmitters or instead of them in response to neural stimulation. Structurally, these amines are similar to norepinephrine or dopamine, but they are much less active in eliciting a response from the effector. Thus, the false neurotransmitter displaces the normal one from the nerve endings, which results in nervous system dysfunction manifested as hepatic encephalopathy. At present, the false-neurotransmitter hypothesis, even though it looks very attractive, requires more evidence to be accepted. In certain experimental models, hepatic encephalopathy may be accompanied by an increased gamma-aminobutyric acid (GABA) concentration. However, the significance of these findings to clinical hepatic encephalopathy requires further studies.

The treatment of hepatic encephalopathy mainly involves minimization of factors that lead to its worsening. For example, all attempts should be made to stop gastrointestinal bleeding, to control infection (neomycin is usually the drug of choice), and to titrate diuretic drugs and the fluid load. Acid–base and electrolyte balance should be normalized. A specific diet is used to reduce the intake of food containing nitrogen (protein). Lactulose has been successful in the treatment of hepatic encephalopathy: this product traps ammonia in the acidified fecal stream and makes it unavailable for absorption. Thus, lactulose would promote ammonia excretion from the body. Dopamine agonists and L-dopa also have been used successfully. The hypothetical mechanism of action is a displacement of false neurotransmitters in the CNS. It has been suggested that L-dopa also facilitates renal excretion of ammonia.

The effects of anesthesia on patients with hepatic encephalopathy have not been thoroughly studied. However, some data suggest clinically significant alterations in this regard. Cerebral uptake of benzodiazepines is substantially increased, which may indicate an increase in the density or affinity of benzodiazepine receptors. Alternatively, the observed increase in cerebral uptake may result from enhanced permeability of the blood–brain barrier.[52] The lesson from this observation is clear: any drug administered to a patient with advanced hepatic disease must be carefully titrated against effect.

The pathogenesis and management of hepatic encephalopathy is described in detail elsewhere.[53]

Renal Function in Patients with Liver Disease

Renal dysfunction and electrolyte imbalance often accompany advanced liver disease. Disorders of sodium, potassium, and water metabolism and excretion are often observed. Certain forms of glomerulopathy and disorders of renal acidification, as well as acute renal failure and hepatorenal syndrome, are observed in patients with cirrhosis and other forms of severe liver disease.

Ascites and Edema. Patients with liver disease frequently excrete urine that is virtually free of sodium. It is not surprising that this failure to excrete sodium sufficiently leads to extracellular fluid accumulation, with subsequent ascites and edema. It is important to realize that ascites and edema in patients with liver cirrhosis are related mainly to disturbances in sodium rather than in water excretion. Such patients can excrete very large volumes of dilute urine when a large amount of water without sodium is administered.

The pathogenesis of sodium retention in these patients is rather complex and currently is explained by a decrease in "effective" blood volume or by the so-called overflow hypothesis,[54] as represented schematically in Figure 43-6. The theory of reduced effective blood volume involves an imbalance of Starling forces in the hepatic sinusoids and splanchnic capillaries, resulting in excessive lymph formation. Subsequently, lymph accumulates in the peritoneal cavity as ascites. This, in turn, leads to a reduction in circulating plasma volume. The total plasma volume may be normal or even increased at that time, and the reduction in the

effective plasma volume is attributable mainly to a redistribution of fluid. The reduced effective (circulating) plasma volume is sensed by the renal tubule, resulting in increased sodium and water resorption. Thus, this hypothesis explains renal sodium retention as a secondary rather than a primary phenomenon.

In contrast, the overflow hypothesis assumes that the primary factor in the pathogenesis of sodium retention in patients with liver cirrhosis is inappropriate retention of excessive sodium *per se*, resulting in increased plasma volume. Conditions of high hydrostatic pressure (portal hypertension), in conjunction with a reduced plasma colloid osmotic pressure and an expanded plasma volume (supposedly owing to sodium retention), lead to the formation of ascites. Thus, according to the overflow hypothesis, renal sodium retention and plasma volume expansion, rather than a reduction in plasma volume, are responsible for ascites formation.

These two hypotheses are not necessarily exclusive. It is conceivable that the primary defect in sodium excretion plays a more important role in the early stages of cirrhosis, whereas a reduced circulating plasma volume may be more important in patients with advanced liver cirrhosis.[54]

Several neural, hemodynamic, and hormonal factors are important in the pathogenesis of sodium retention in patients with hepatic cirrhosis. When the effective plasma volume is decreased, the sympathetic nervous discharge is increased, probably through stimulation of volume receptors. This is accompanied by a rise in renin activity, which, through the angiotensin system, stimulates aldosterone secretion. An increase in both sympathetic nervous tone and aldosterone activity leads to enhanced tubular resorption of sodium. This effect is aggravated by a redistribution of intrarenal blood flow, a result of increased vasoconstricting influences such as sympathetic nervous tone and activity of the renin–angiotensin system. Prostaglandins and the

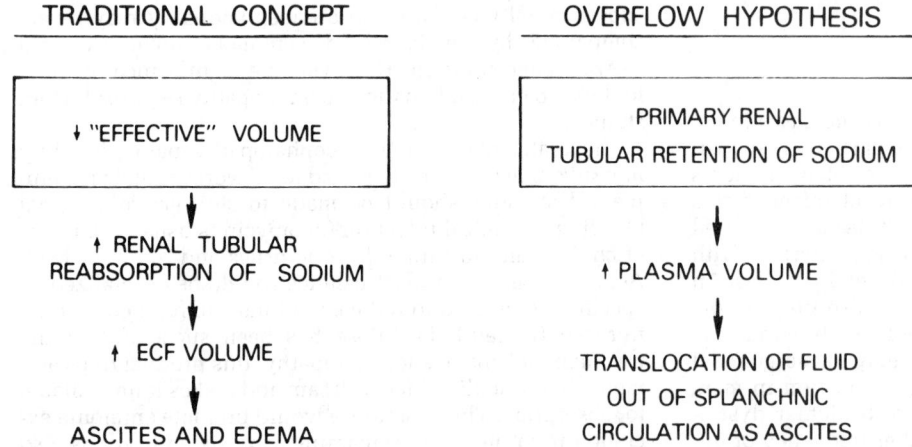

Figure 43-6. The presumed sequences of events resulting in ascites formation according to two theories: the traditional and the overflow. The primary events are shown within the boxes. According to the traditional concept, the primary event is a diminution in effective volume attributable to the development of abnormal Starling forces in the portal venous circulation with a maldistribution of circulating volume. The diminished "effective" volume is thought to constitute an afferent signal to the renal tubule to augment salt and water reabsorption. The attempt to replenish the diminished effective volume results in an expansion of the total blood volume to values far in excess of normal, with resultant ascites and edema formation. The overflow hypothesis holds that retention of excessive sodium by the kidneys is the primary event. In the setting of abnormal Starling forces in the portal venous bed, the expanded plasma volume is sequestered preferentially in the peritoneal sac. (Reprinted with permission from Epstein M: Renal functional abnormalities in cirrhosis: Pathophysiology and management. In Zakim D, Boyer TD [eds]: Hepatology: A Textbook of Liver Disease, p 448. Philadelphia, WB Saunders, 1982.)

kallikrein–kinin system also participate in modulating sodium retention. An interesting study by Perez–Ayuso et al[55] suggested that prostaglandins and the kallikrein–kinin system probably play a compensatory, counteracting role in renal circulation and function. As the concentration of these vasodilating substances ceases to rise, decompensation occurs, and different degrees of renal insufficiency develop.

Diuretics are often given to patients with hepatic cirrhosis and ascites to increase urine output and decrease ascites. However, diuretic therapy is often accompanied by complications, such as hypovolemia, azotemia, sometimes hyponatremia, and encephalopathy. It is conceivable that diuretic therapy without proper fluid volume management decreases the effective plasma volume, with a subsequent deterioration of renal function and development of the hepatorenal syndrome.

A peritoneovenous LeVeen shunt is another modality for treating severe ascites in patients with hepatic cirrhosis. The idea behind this treatment is rather simple and logical: if the abnormality in ascites is a maldistribution of extracellular fluid, an attempt to reverse such a maldistribution of body fluids between compartments seems to be justified. The shunt between the peritoneal cavity and the central venous system has a one-way valve activated by a pressure gradient that allows the ascites fluid to move into the venous system. Treatment with a LeVeen shunt is used mainly in patients with ascites refractory to dietary and diuretic measures.

The pathogenesis of water retention in patients with hepatic cirrhosis is complex. The mechanisms include increased secretion of antidiuretic hormone, as well as a reduced delivery of filtrate to the diluting segments of the nephron.[52] The causes of the observed hypokalemia include inadequate diet, vomiting, diarrhea, hyperaldosteronemia, and diuretic therapy.

Hepatorenal Syndrome. The hepatorenal syndrome usually develops in patients with classic symptoms of hepatic cirrhosis, portal hypertension, and, particularly, ascites. These patients usually maintain urine output, although it is somewhat decreased; however, the urine, even if concentrated, contains almost no sodium. The blood creatinine and BUN concentrations progressively increase. Actually, the characteristics of urine from patients with hepatorenal syndrome are similar to those of urine from patients with hypovolemia. Apparently, the renal damage in hepatorenal syndrome is reversible: kidneys transplanted from patients with the syndrome can resume normal function in recipients.[56]

The pathogenesis of hepatorenal syndrome has not been clearly established, but it is believed that renal vasoconstriction, with a subsequent decrease in renal blood flow, is primarily responsible. The renin–angiotensin system, the sympathetic nervous system, alterations in prostaglandins and the kallikrein–kinin system, as well as endotoxemia, all play a certain role. The crucial role of prostaglandins in maintaining renal function in patients with advanced liver disease is well illustrated by the observation that drugs impairing renal prostaglandin synthesis; e.g., nonsteroidal anti-inflammatory agents, reduce the glomerular filtration rate and renal plasma flow and can precipitate acute renal insufficiency. Cirrhotic patients without ascites do not seem to be susceptible to this side effect; however, cirrhotic patients with ascites might experience a sharp 50% decrease in creatinine clearance, indicating a substantial decrease in glomerular filtration rate. These observations strongly suggest that renal blood flow in the patient with ascites is vitally dependent on the vasodilatory actions of prostaglandins synthesized in the kidney.[57]

Because hepatorenal syndrome seems to develop in the hospital rather than before the patient is admitted, one must wonder what events in the hospital affect its development. This coincides with the impression from some studies that hepatorenal syndrome follows a reduction in plasma volume, as in vigorous diuretic therapy, gastrointestinal bleeding, and paracentesis. The majority of patients with hepatorenal syndrome die; therefore, the prevention of this syndrome with very carefully managed diuretic therapy and volume status is mandatory.

Acute renal failure, acute tubular necrosis, or both may also develop in patients with hepatic cirrhosis and often complicates arterial hypotension and infection. Acute tubular necrosis appears more often during or after the release of obstructive jaundice compared with similar operations performed on nonjaundiced patients.[58] It is conceivable that patients with hepatic disease or obstructive jaundice have a very limited ability to mobilize blood from the splanchnic (including hepatic) vasculature to increase the central blood volume.[59] Thus, in response to even moderate hemorrhage, such patients may develop severe hypotension with subsequent acute tubular necrosis. Some studies also demonstrated that circulating conjugated bilirubin exercises a toxic effect on the renal tubule and may be responsible for the development of acute tubular necrosis in jaundiced patients.[60]

The differential diagnosis between hepatorenal syndrome and acute tubular necrosis is usually relatively simple (Table 43-3). The treatment of hepatorenal syndrome, as well as that of acute tubular necrosis, is complex and includes identification of the underlying causes of renal insufficiency, supportive therapy, and careful maintenance of the necessary circulating blood volume, particularly when bleeding occurs or when diuretics are used.

It is clear that the pathogenesis of hepatic cirrhosis and

TABLE 43-3. Differential Diagnosis of Acute Azotemia in the Patient With Liver Disease—Important Differential Urinary Findings

	Prerenal Azotemia	Hepatorenal Syndrome	Acute Renal Failure (ATN)
Urinary sodium concentration	<10 mEq·l^{-1}	<10 mEq·l^{-1}	>30 mEq·l^{-1}
Urine-to-plasma creatinine ratio	>30:1	>30:1	<20:1
Urinary osmolality	At least 100 mOsm > plasma osmolality	At least 100 mOsm > plasma osmolality	Equal to plasma osmolality
Urinary sediment	Normal	Unremarkable	Casts, cellular debris

Reproduced with permission from Epstein M: Renal functional abnormalities in cirrhosis: Pathophysiology and management. In Zakim D, Boyer TD (eds): Hepatology: A Textbook of Liver Disease, p 460. Philadelphia, WB Saunders, 1982.

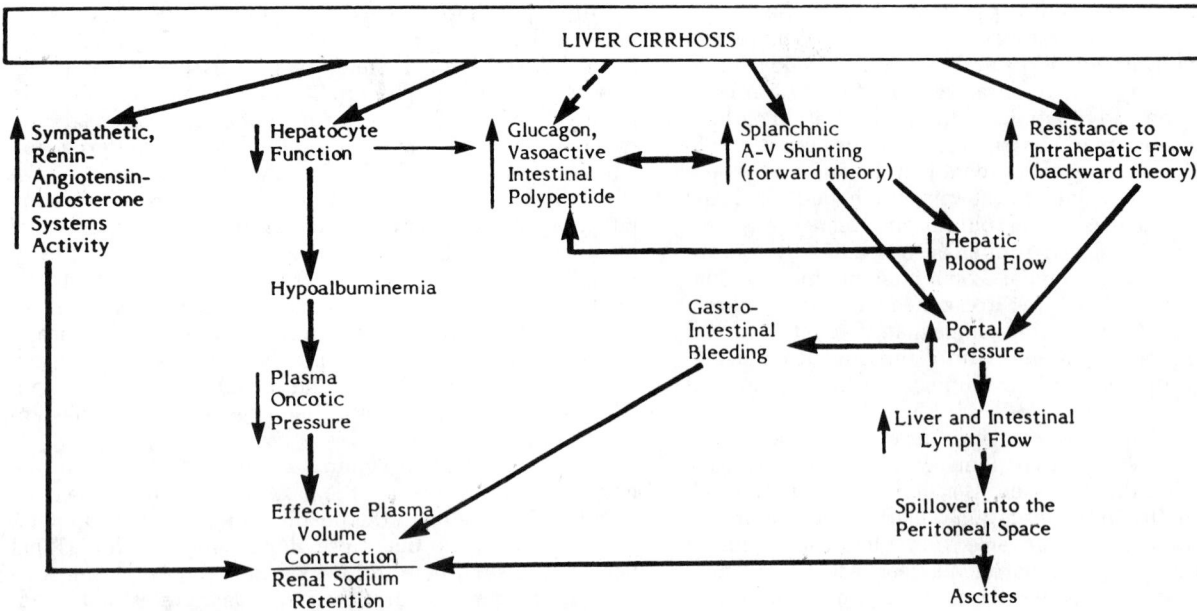

Figure 43-7. Pathogenesis of liver cirrhosis—schematic representation. (Reprinted with permission from Kang YG, Gelman S: Liver transplantation. In Gelman S [ed]: Anesthesia and Organ Transplantation, p 145. Philadelphia, WB Saunders, 1987.)

portal hypertension is extremely complex and is still not clearly understood. A schematic representation is provided in Figure 43-7.

Ischemic Hepatitis

Respiratory or cardiovascular dysfunction may result in a condition termed "ischemic hepatitis,"[61] a relatively rare form of hepatic disease that may be particularly interesting to anesthesiologists. Typically, ischemic hepatitis is diagnosed when a patient with cardiac disease develops acute changes in liver function tests mimicking acute hepatitis. Usually, there is a moderate increase in the bilirubin and alkaline phosphatase concentrations in the blood, moderate jaundice, and a dramatic increase in both aspartate and alanine aminotransferases. Histologically, centrilobular hepatic necrosis may be seen. An interesting feature of ischemic hepatitis is that despite a rather extreme increase in hepatic enzymes, severe hepatic dysfunction does not develop. If cardiovascular function is normalized, ischemic hepatitis resolves by itself without serious sequelae. It seems that ischemic hepatitis is associated more with a decrease in hepatic blood and oxygen supply than with hepatic congestion.[62,63] The concentration of aminotransferases usually returns to relatively normal values within 5–10 days, much faster than in patients with viral hepatitis. Also, patients with ischemic hepatitis usually develop an increase in lactic dehydrogenase, whereas this enzyme changes little in the majority of patients with viral hepatitis.

Cholestasis (Obstructive Jaundice)

In most patients with cholestasis, the presence of bile in liver tissue is identifiable histologically, most often in the canaliculi in Zone 3 of the liver acinus, the tissue surrounding the terminal hepatic venules or central vein. Phys-

iologically, cholestasis means a reduction in the hepatic secretion of bile. It is always accompanied by an accumulation in the blood of substances such as bilirubin, cholesterol, and bile acids that normally are excreted with the bile.

Most cases of cholestasis that require surgical intervention are caused by extrahepatic biliary obstruction. On the other hand, there are many forms of cholestasis that result from hepatocyte dysfunction deriving from certain alterations in the structure and enzymatic activity of cell membranes, dysfunction of microfilaments and microtubules, alterations in canalicular permeability, and abnormal interactions between chemical substances (including bile acids) and biliary solutes.

Bilirubin is toxic for many enzyme systems, including those of respiration and oxidative phosphorylation, glycolysis, glycogenesis, and the tricarboxylic acid cycle, as well as those involved in heme biosynthesis and lipid, amino acid, and protein metabolism.[23] This effect occurs at high concentrations of bilirubin and can be modified by additional albumin.[24] Bilirubin may also interfere with membrane function.[25]

Cardiovascular Function

There are data strongly suggesting that cholemia per se impairs myocardial contractility.[64-66] Cholemia also blunts the response to norepinephrine, angiotensin II, and isoproterenol,[67] probably by interfering with the binding of these agents to membrane receptors. It has been suggested that bile acids interfere either with the entry of calcium into or the exit of potassium from the myocardial cells.[66]

Cardiovascular dysfunction in patients with biliary obstruction mimics to a lesser degree the pattern observed in patients with hepatic cirrhosis, namely, peripheral vascular resistance decreases while cardiac output increases; portal venous blood flow decreases while portal venous pressure increases; and hepatic arterial blood flow does not change significantly while portacaval shunting increases substantially.[68]

Patients with liver disease, both parenchymal and cholestatic, have a reduced sensitivity to vasopressor drugs. The reasons for this resistance have not been clarified. However, experiments in vitro and in vivo strongly suggest that bile acids contribute to the vasodilation and hypotension often observed in patients with biliary obstruction.[66] An increase in the blood concentrations of vasoactive substances such as ferritin, vasoactive intestinal polypeptide, and glucagon contributes to the vasodilating and hyperdynamic state.

It is conceivable that the decreased sensitivity of patients with biliary obstruction to vasoactive substances, including catecholamines, is responsible for the rather interesting and clinically important observation that these patients do not seem to tolerate even small blood losses as well as do normal persons. In normal animals, moderate loss, that is, 10% of the estimated blood volume, does not substantially decrease the mean arterial pressure, whereas in animals with experimentally induced biliary obstruction, such a blood loss leads to severe (approximately 50%) arterial hypotension (Fig. 43-8). Moreover, this study demonstrated that in intact animals, the pulmonary and splanchnic blood volumes decrease by approximately 15% in response to blood loss, but in animals with biliary obstruction, the pulmonary blood volume decreases by only 7%, whereas the splanchnic blood volume does not change (Fig. 43-9). If we can extrapolate these results to humans, these observations imply that patients with biliary obstruction would not respond sufficiently to blood loss by expelling blood into the systemic circulation to compensate for bleeding as would normal persons. Further, the results imply that it is necessary to replace volume losses in these patients immediately during the perioperative period. The anesthesiologist should be aware that biliary decompression may be accompanied by severe cardiovascular collapse.[69]

Blood Coagulation

Patients with biliary obstruction develop certain coagulation disorders. Usually, at least during short-lasting biliary obstruction, coagulopathy is secondary to a deficiency of vitamin K–dependent coagulation factors, because absorption of vitamin K depends on the absorption of fat and therefore on the excretion of bile into the gastrointestinal tract. Later, with long-lasting biliary obstruction, a parenchymal component develops, with a subsequent deterioration in the hepatic synthesis of protein, including coagulation factors. Usually, the coagulation disorders are moderate and can be restored relatively easily by parenteral vitamin K. However, if this treatment is not effective, which probably would mean that the patient has parenchymal liver disease or a parenchymal component in his or her cholestasis, or if surgery is urgent and coagulopathy should be treated immediately, fresh frozen plasma is indicated. If the prolonged prothrombin time does not respond to vitamin K therapy, significant depression of hepatic parenchymal function is present, which coincides with a poor prognosis.

Renal Function

It has been suggested that bilirubin or bile salts sensitize the kidneys to hypoxic–ischemic damage.[60,70] Bile duct ligation actually increases the glomerular filtration rate and renal blood flow in the dog.[71] Some recent studies suggest that in the dog, intrarenal infusion of dilute bile increases the renal

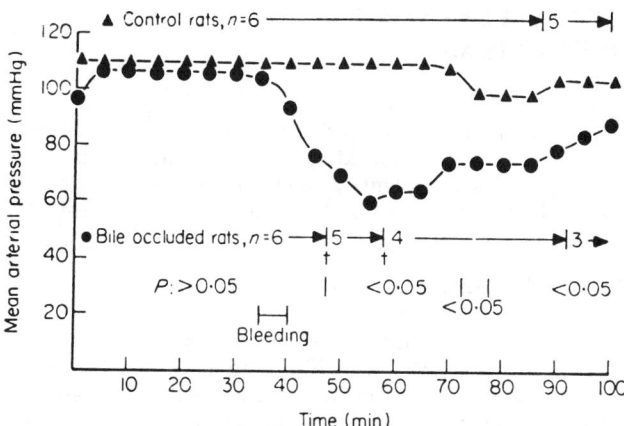

Figure 43-8. Effect of a 10% blood loss on mean arterial pressure in anesthetized rats. ●, bile duct occluded 7 days previously. ▲, sham operated. Two of the bile-occluded animals died immediately after the blood loss. The level of significance between the groups is given. In response to similar blood loss, animals with an occluded bile duct developed more severe arterial hypotension than did control rats. (Reprinted with permission from Aarseth S, Bergan A, Aarseth P: Circulatory homeostasis in rats after bile duct ligation. Scand J Clin Lab Invest 39:93, 1979.)

production of prostaglandin E_2 (PGE_2). Moreover, indomethacin abolishes both the natriuresis and the increase in renal PGE_2 synthesis associated with intrarenal infusion of bile.[66] It is currently believed that moderate cholemia is not nephrotoxic, nor are even high bilirubin concentrations. However, the increase in jaundice can be considered a prelude to the hepatorenal syndrome.[66] Deterioration of renal function in patients with biliary obstruction may result from endotoxin produced in the intestines. Some toxemia is related to a reduction in bile salts, with a subsequent change in the intestinal flora in patients with biliary obstruction, as well as to a reduction in the reticuloendothelial function of the liver.

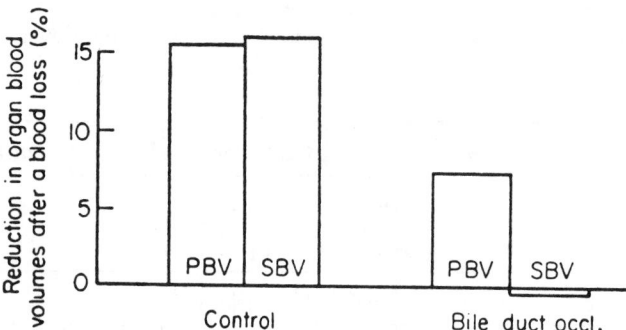

Figure 43-9. Effect of a 10% blood loss on pulmonary (PBV) and splanchnic (SBV) blood volume in anesthetized rats. The blood loss resulted in a 15% decrease in both PBV and SBV in control animals, whereas PBV decreased only 7% and SBV did not change in animals with an occluded bile duct. The observation suggests a decrease in reservoir function (response to hypovolemia) of the pulmonary and, particularly, the splanchnic vasculature. (Reprinted with permission from Aarseth S, Bergan A, Aarseth P: Circulatory homeostasis in rats after bile duct ligation. Scand J Clin Lab Invest 39:93, 1979.)

BLOOD TESTS FOR PATIENTS WITH LIVER DISEASE

Hepatic function is extremely complex; therefore, it is not surprising that many different biochemical tests are used to evaluate it. Generally speaking, some tests characterize liver function and some identify liver damage, whereas others deal with specific markers of hepatic disease (Table 43-4).

Serum Enzymes

High serum concentrations of enzymes such as aspartate aminotransferase (AST or SGOT) and alanine aminotransferase (ALT or SGPT) may be, and usually are, indicative of hepatocellular injury. However, both of these enzymes are present in tissues other than the liver, for example, in skeletal muscles, kidneys, and the heart. Therefore, an increase in their concentrations in the blood may reflect damage to these other tissues, not necessarily the liver. These enzymes are simply released when a liver cell is damaged or dies. Alanine aminotransferase is considered to be more specific for the liver than is AST. The degree of increase in the concentrations of these enzymes in the blood reflects the acuteness and extent of injury but by no means characterizes liver function or the prognosis. Moreover, a decrease in the high plasma concentration of the enzymes may not reflect recovery, but, to the contrary, a decreased ability of hepatocytes to synthesize enzymes and, therefore, possibly implies a poor prognosis. The concentrations of serum aminotransferases in chronic liver disease often are considerably less than those seen in acute liver disease, and it is not uncommon to observe a perfectly normal or low concentration of these enzymes in patients with severe hepatic parenchymal disease or even liver failure.

Alkaline phosphatase is another serum enzyme frequently measured when hepatic disease is suspected. This enzyme may be released, not only from the hepatobiliary system, but also from the intestinal tract, bones, and placenta. Therefore, the concentration may be increased during normal pregnancy, growth (in teenagers), and, in the case of bone metastasis, certain forms of hepatobiliary disease, mainly extrahepatic biliary obstruction. Elevation of this enzyme in the blood is not considered a reflection of deterioration in liver function or liver damage. Some other enzymes such as 5'-nucleotidase, leucine aminopeptidase,

and gamma-glutamyl transpeptidase are considered to be more specific and better reflections of cholestasis and biliary obstruction.

Serum Bilirubin and Bile Acids

Serum bilirubin concentrations reflect the efficacy of hepatic uptake and excretion relative to the production rate (i.e., hemolysis) of bilirubin. An increase in conjugated versus unconjugated bilirubin in the plasma (see discussion of the metabolism of bilirubin) often helps to differentiate jaundice related to parenchymal disease from jaundice resulting from biliary obstruction. The measurement of serum bile acids seems to be a more accurate and useful way of characterizing this hepatic function and is more sensitive than the dynamics of the bilirubin concentration in the blood. Determination of bile acids is especially useful in the diagnosis of the different forms of cholestasis and biliary obstruction. After all, the definition of cholestasis is impaired bile excretion with subsequently increased plasma bile acid concentrations.

Prothrombin Time and Serum Proteins

The serum concentration of proteins synthesized in the liver reflects its protein-synthesizing ability and therefore this particular hepatic function. One such protein is prothrombin. Prolongation of prothrombin time is not highly specific for hepatic disease. One of the most common other reasons for this abnormality is vitamin K deficiency, which may result from a specific medication for antagonizing the prothrombin complex (bishydroxycoumarin). Other reasons for prolongation of prothrombin time include incomplete clearing of activated clotting factors and coagulation inhibitors from the plasma by the liver, impaired plasminogen synthesis by the liver, primary fibrinolysis, and DIC. However, if all these reasons are ruled out (the differential diagnosis is seldom difficult and is based on other clinical and laboratory data), prolongation of the prothrombin time is considered a relatively sensitive test characterizing liver function. Prothrombin time is probably one of the most accurate qualitative, rather than quantitative, estimates of hepatic function in patients with hepatic disease. However, "it gives the liver more of a pass or fail than a numerical grade on its

TABLE 43-4. Blood Tests and the Differential Diagnosis of Hepatic Dysfunction

	Bilirubin Overload (Hemolysis)	Parenchymal Dysfunction	Cholestasis
Bilirubin	Unconjugated	Conjugated	Conjugated
Aminotransferases	Normal	Increased (may be normal or decreased in advanced stages)	Normal (may be increased in advanced stages)
Alkaline phosphatase	Normal	Normal	Increased
Prothrombin time	Normal	Prolonged	Normal (may be prolonged in advanced stages)
Serum proteins	Normal	Decreased	Normal (may be decreased in advanced stages)
BUN	Normal	Normal (may be decreased in advanced stages)	Normal
BSP/ICG (dye)	Normal	Retention	Normal or retention

performance."[72] Prolongation of the prothrombin time confirms a rather significant depression of hepatic parenchymal function.

Albumin is synthesized by the liver; thus, a low plasma albumin concentration may, but not necessarily does, reflect depressed hepatic function. Despite certain deficiencies, the determination of albumin concentration in the plasma may have a predictive value for survival in patients with advanced hepatic disease, basically cirrhosis, after major surgery. Many hepatic diseases are accompanied by a decrease in albumin and an increase in different fractions of globulin in the blood. Hyperglobulinemia usually indicates a chronic hepatic disease but says very little about hepatic reserves or the degree of hepatic dysfunction.

Metabolizing Function of the Liver

The BUN is not considered a blood test characterizing liver function; however, low BUN concentrations in the plasma, for example, below 5 mg·dl^{-1}, may indicate a severely depressed hepatic ability to synthesize urea. This test seems to be especially valid in patients with alcoholic cirrhosis. The metabolizing function of the liver also can be evaluated by galactose elimination and metabolism and by the excretion of different drugs.

The liver removes many lipophilic substances from the plasma and excretes them into bile. Some of these substances are excreted unchanged, whereas others are excreted after conversion to more polar forms. These forms include mainly organic anions and, to a lesser extent, organic cations and neutral organic compounds. Dyes such as sulfobromophthalein (BSP) and indocyanine green (ICG) are organic anions that characterize the metabolic and excretory function of the liver. The BSP and ICG tests require the injection of dye into the bloodstream with subsequent evaluation of the rate of disappearance from or the degree of retention of the dye in the blood. There are many different approaches to using these tests. At present, their clinical application is somewhat limited, because interpretation of the results is difficult and often questionable.

The metabolism of some drugs can be used as an indicator of the metabolizing function of the liver. The most common tests at present are antipyrine clearance and the aminopyrine breath test. However, these tests cannot be considered very sensitive, as they become abnormal only with relatively advanced liver disease. Thus, a substantial reduction in the metabolism of these substances would indicate an already severe hepatic dysfunction, whereas relatively normal results may be found in patients with limited hepatic reserves.

The galactose elimination test is even less sensitive than the BSP and ICG tests, probably because BSP and ICG are distributed mainly in plasma volume, whereas galactose is distributed in the extracellular space. Extracellular volume can vary rather substantially from patient to patient, and this would be reflected in the test results.

Specific Tests

Certain immunologic and serologic tests can be of some value in patients with parenchymal hepatic disease. Antigens and antibodies may help identify viral hepatitis. The diagnosis of halothane hepatitis is sometimes suggested by specific serologic tests.[73] There are many other tests that may verify certain common and uncommon hepatic diseases.[74]

In summary, the determination of aminotransferases and alkaline phosphatase is extremely useful in differentiating cholestasis from acute parenchymal disease. Aminotransferases are substantially increased in acute parenchymal hepatic disease, whereas alkaline phosphatase is increased in cholestatic disease. The severity and prognosis of hepatic disease are best evaluated by determinations of serum albumin and the prothrombin time. The diagnosis of hepatobiliary disease, as well as assessment of the degree of hepatic dysfunction, are extremely difficult and should be made by an experienced and knowledgeable hepatologist. Detailed information regarding the tests characterizing different hepatic functions as well as various hepatic diseases is available in the literature.[74]

ANESTHESIA, SURGERY, AND LIVER FUNCTION

Comparative Pharmacology and Hepatotoxicity of Anesthetics

Different anesthetics affect hepatic function in various directions and to different degrees. Perioperative hepatic dysfunction may result from the direct effect of an anesthetic on hepatocyte function or from the indirect effect of decreased oxygen and blood supply to the liver, accumulation of certain hormones and other substances that affect liver function, and the initiation of more complex mechanisms such as the formation of antibodies and the involvement of immunologic mechanisms.

Halothane

Halothane is probably the anesthetic best studied for hepatotoxicity. The National Halothane Study analyzed approximately 850,000 anesthesia cases, with halothane administered to only 250,000 of these patients.[12] Eighty-two patients had fatal hepatic necrosis. Only nine cases were unexplainable on grounds other than anesthesia; seven of these nine patients received halothane; therefore, the true incidence of unexplained fatal hepatic necrosis after halothane anesthesia is 7 of 250,000, or 1 per 35,000 anesthetics. This number is often misquoted and misinterpreted: the number 1 per 10,000 persons is frequently, unjustifiably quoted.[75,76] Later studies have shown that severe hepatic dysfunction follows halothane anesthesia in approximately 1 of 6000 to 1 of 20,000 administrations.[77,78] Schemel[10] found that 11 of 7620 patients of ASA I status scheduled for elective surgery had elevated plasma concentrations of hepatic enzymes preoperatively. The surgery was postponed in these cases, yet three patients developed jaundice. If these patients had undergone surgery, their jaundice would have been attributed to the anesthesia. Moreover, surgery and anesthesia could have aggravated the condition, and these three patients might have suffered from more severe hepatic dysfunction than they developed without surgery.

It is extremely difficult to differentiate halothane hepatitis from viral hepatitis that develops in the postoperative period.[15] Simple calculations show that approximately 100 of the 1 million anesthetized patients may have unrecognized viral A hepatitis prior to anesthesia and surgery and may develop signs of this hepatitis postoperatively.[79]

There is relatively strong evidence in the literature that

certain factors substantially enhance the risks of halothane-induced hepatotoxicity. These factors include multiple exposure to halothane, obesity, gender (females are more susceptible than are males), middle age, and certain ethnic origins (Mexican-Americans seem to be more susceptible than others).[73] There are data that strongly suggest a familial constitutional susceptibility factor.[80] A recent article by Japanese investigators posited that genetic susceptibility to halothane hepatitis may be associated with certain alterations in a region of chromosome 6.[81]

There are three proposed mechanisms for halothane-induced hepatotoxicity: (1) a direct effect of the intermediates of halothane metabolism, a view that assumes that halothane undergoes reductive metabolism in conditions of oxygen deprivation and that the products of this biotransformation are toxic for the liver cells; (2) hepatic oxygen deprivation resulting from respiratory, systemic circulatory, or regional circulatory disturbances induced by halothane; and (3) immunologically mediated necrosis. This last mechanism assumes that the oxidative metabolism of halothane, without hepatic oxygen deprivation, results in the formation of a haptene, which then reacts with protein and lipoprotein of hepatocyte membranes, with subsequent autoimmune-mediated injury to liver cells.

Metabolic Theory. The metabolic theory of halothane-induced hepatotoxicity assumes that particular animals (rats) and some patients developing halothane-induced liver damage possess an enhanced ability to biotransform the anesthetic by the reductive pathway, thereby producing toxic reactive intermediates.[82] The primary function of the cytochrome P450 oxygenase system is to transfer electrons from nicotinamide adenine dinucleotide phosphate hydrogenase (NADPH) to oxygen, activating oxygen, which then oxidizes a drug. During hepatic oxygen deprivation, the cytochrome P450 system transfers an electron directly to certain substrates, thereby reducing them. All volatile anesthetics undergo some degree of metabolism, and the cytochrome P450 system plays the main role in this biotransformation. Exposure to many drugs and chemicals induces the cytochrome P450 system, increasing the amount of enzymes with a subsequent increase in the turnover rate of substrate into product.

Enflurane and, particularly, isoflurane undergo very limited metabolism in the liver compared with halothane.[83] The latter can undergo oxidative metabolism when the oxygen supply is adequate and reductive metabolism when hepatic oxygen deprivation develops. The reductive metabolism of halothane results in the release of inorganic fluoride and some other intermediates. Free radicals have been proposed as potentially harmful intermediates in the reductive metabolism of halothane.

It is interesting that patients with cyanotic congenital heart disease have a greater reductive metabolism of halothane than do acyanotic patients, yet the two groups demonstrate similar rates of postoperative hepatic and renal dysfunction.[84] This observation does not fit the contention that the reductive metabolism of halothane is particularly important in the development of halothane-induced hepatic injury. The supporters of the metabolic theory collected some valuable data that probably better fit this theory than prove it, and many observations are still difficult to explain. For example, similar degrees of reductive metabolism of halothane may be accompanied by different degrees of hepatic injury.[85] Also, the end-products of the reductive metabolism of halothane have never been found to be hepatotoxic: liver damage could not be reproduced by exposure to these products, namely, fluoride; 2-chloro-1,1,1-trifluoroethane (CTF); and 2-chloro-1,1-difluorethylene (CDF).[76] Free radical intermediates have also been blamed for halothane-induced hepatic damage; however, the extent of free radical formation is not reflected in the degree of hepatotoxicity.[76] Moreover, the evidence suggests that hepatic injury occurs during exposure, before metabolism takes place and before the binding of reactive metabolites, either to lipids or proteins, is at its peak.[83] It seems that hepatotoxicity is initiated without the full impact of metabolism, suggesting that reductive metabolism plays only a limited role, if any, in the mechanism of hepatotoxicity. Detailed critical analyses of the results of experimental studies in this area are provided elsewhere.[76,83,86]

Some data suggest that even in the model of phenobarbital-pretreated rats exposed to hypoxia and halothane, which was used primarily to collect the data supporting the metabolic theory of halothane-induced hepatotoxicity, injury is related not so much to the reductive metabolism of halothane as to hepatic oxygen deprivation.[87,88] An interesting model for studying anesthesia-induced hepatotoxicity was introduced in Australia.[89] The authors of that article demonstrated that guinea pigs not pretreated with phenobarbital and exposure to hypoxia developed hepatic necrosis after exposure to halothane but not to isoflurane when similar degrees of arterial hypotension (50%) were achieved.[89] Those authors assumed that equal degrees of arterial hypotension are accompanied by equal degrees of hepatic oxygen deprivation and that the hepatic injury observed after halothane anesthesia was attributed to the reductive metabolism of halothane. However, a subsequent study in our laboratory demonstrated that equal degrees of arterial hypotension (50%, exactly as in the Australian study[89]), were accompanied by very different degrees of hepatic oxygen deprivation: a 50% decrease in arterial blood pressure achieved by halothane was associated with a 65% decrease in the hepatic oxygen supply, whereas the same degree of arterial hypotension achieved with isoflurane led to a 35% decrease in the hepatic oxygen supply.[90] Thus, the role of reductive metabolism of halothane in hepatotoxicity is still questionable.

Hepatic Oxygen Deprivation. Hypoxia might play an important, if not leading, role in some forms of halothane-induced hepatic injury.[87] Many experimental observations on halothane-induced hepatotoxicity in animals that have been explained by the metabolic theory can be attributed to hepatic oxygen deprivation alone without direct involvement of reductive biotransformation of halothane. This issue has been thoroughly reviewed.[83,91] It is interesting that halothane apparently decreases hepatic oxygen demand,[92,93] which suggests some protective mechanisms possessed by halothane that might decrease the damage induced by oxygen deprivation. However, the available evidence suggests that halothane decreases the hepatic oxygen supply to a greater extent than the oxygen demand and therefore does not offer any noticeable protection for the liver against oxygen deprivation.[92,94] It is important to realize, though, that hepatic oxygen deprivation might be responsible for certain forms of anesthesia-associated hepatic damage. However, it appears highly unlikely that hepatic oxygen deprivation can be responsible for fulminant halothane hepatitis.

Immunologic Theory. The involvement of hypersensitivity and idiosyncrasy in halothane hepatitis has been postulated on the basis of several important observations.[73,95] These observations include the frequent association of halothane hepatitis with multiple exposures to halothane, mild fever after the first exposure followed by severe jaundice on re-exposure, an association with fever and eosinophilia, a frequent history of other drug allergy, positive challenge tests, and demonstration of circulating antibodies to liver microsomes. It was believed that halothane hepatitis does not develop in children; however, recently, five cases were reported among children, one of whom died.[96]

The immunologic theory of halothane hepatitis assumes that one of the possible mechanisms of injury involves intermediates produced in the oxidative pathway of halothane metabolism[97,98] that can bind covalently to liver tissue (proteins or lipoproteins) as haptens, forming complexes that can induce an immunologic response in susceptible persons. Thus, it seems that, in part, halothane hepatitis is secondary to specific cellular susceptibility. Another part of the response appears to be multifactorial. A suggested sequence of events is as follows. Trifluoroacetyl chloride, which is produced by the oxidative biotransformation of halothane, covalently binds to the lysine residues of proteins. This distorted protein may then act as an antigen, with subsequent production of antibodies.[99-101]

Circulating antibodies that would bind to the membrane surface of halothane-altered rabbit hepatocytes were detected in 9 of 14 samples from 11 patients with halothane hepatitis.[101] Halothane-related antibodies have been detected in other patients with hepatitis after halothane administration.[102,103] There has been clear success in the development of assays for specific antibodies in patients sensitized to halothane.[104]

Contrary to the metabolic theory, which implies the involvement of the reductive pathway of halothane metabolism, the halothane-altered membrane antigen is produced by the oxidative pathway of metabolism.[97] Thus, according to the immunologic theory, the role of the reductive metabolism of halothane or hepatic oxygen deprivation in the development of halothane hepatitis is probably negligible or nonexistent.

Regarding inhalational anesthetic toxicity, an interesting hypothetical mechanism was proposed by Van Dyke and associates from the Mayo Clinic.[105-107] They demonstrated that halothane, enflurane, and isoflurane affect phosphorylase activity in isolated rat hepatocytes. Their observations suggest that all three of these anesthetics, even at low concentrations, raise intracellular calcium concentrations, which may result in hepatocellular injury.

In their recent review, Stock and Strunin[76] came to the following conclusions. First, halothane has a very low risk potential for liver damage in children, even when used repeatedly. Second, there is no contraindication to the use of halothane in the presence of compensated liver disease provided this disease does not relate to a previous anesthetic. The outcome here will be determined by the degree of preoperative liver dysfunction and the extent of the surgical procedure. Third, severe liver damage is unlikely to follow a single exposure to halothane. Fourth, repeated exposure to halothane in adult humans, particularly obese, middle-aged women, and over a short period of time (probably 4–8 weeks), may result in severe liver damage in only a few persons. Fifth, if repeated halothane anesthesia is contemplated, the anesthesiologist should document the reason for using halothane on the second occasion. Sixth, the mechanism of hepatitis associated with halothane is unclear but probably involves an immunologic response. Finally, at present, there is no reliable specific test for halothane-induced liver damage.

It is important to focus on the effects of halothane on liver function even when hepatitis does not develop, because the drug does affect hepatic function. As an example, halothane suppresses the synthesizing ability of the liver: in isolated perfused liver, halothane decreases protein synthesis in a dose-related fashion.[108] Experimental data on the effects of halothane on hepatic function are not very elaborate; however, most of the available data suggest that halothane, compared with other widely used inhalational anesthetics (enflurane and isoflurane), is probably the worst in its influence on liver function. For example, prolonged enflurane or isoflurane anesthesia in volunteers did not affect BSP elimination, whereas halothane significantly increased BSP retention.[109,110]

Drug biotransformation is one of the most important and sensitive functions of the liver. Aminopyrine half-life is prolonged and for a longer time postanesthetically with halothane administration than with enflurane or isoflurane. With the latter two agents, the prolongation of aminopyrine half-life was observed for a short period of time or not at all.[111] Clinical observations are in agreement with the aforementioned experimental data: halothane anesthesia is accompanied by a substantial release of hepatic glutathione S-transferase (GST), whereas patients anesthetized with isoflurane do not demonstrate any increase in the blood concentration of this hepatic enzyme.[112] The excretory function of the liver is impaired during halothane, whereas it is well maintained during isoflurane anesthesia, even when the anesthetics are used in equipotent doses according to MAC values, as well as according to the degree of arterial hypotension.[88] The reasons for these differences in the extent of impairment of hepatic function are not clear but may be related to the direct effect of halothane but not the other two agents on hepatic function. However, other mechanisms may be involved: halothane decreases the hepatic oxygen supply to a much greater extent than does isoflurane or enflurane when used in equipotent doses.[91,113,114] Portal blood flow usually decreases in parallel with the reduction in cardiac output, while hepatic arterial blood flow compensates for this decrease in an attempt to meet the oxygen requirement or to maintain total blood flow. Enflurane and, particularly isoflurane, preserve the ability of the hepatic arterial blood flow to increase when portal blood flow is decreased; halothane preserves this autoregulation ability to a very limited extent and only when it is used in relatively small doses. This ability is completely abolished when halothane is used in doses that decrease arterial blood pressure by approximately 20–25%.[91,113]

An appropriate comment on this subject appeared in a recent editorial in the *British Medical Journal*: "the revolution that resulted from the introduction of halothane is likely to be replaced by another—the use of the more expensive but less hazardous enflurane and isoflurane."[96]

Enflurane

The incidence of hepatitis after enflurane anesthesia is much lower than with halothane. Lewis et al[115] reviewed the observations on hepatic damage associated with enflurane anesthesia and concluded that the anesthetic caused the injury in 24 patients. The authors based their conclusions on the following speculations. Enflurane is a halogenated organic compound similar to halothane; therefore, enflurane may, and even should, cause liver injury similar to that observed with halothane. The authors could not find any other obvious explanation for the liver injury. They also believed that the clinical and histologic pictures in these patients were similar to those seen with halothane hepatitis.

TABLE 43-5. Differences Between Inhalational Anesthetics Relevant to Hepatotoxicity

	Halothane	Enflurane	Isoflurane
Stable in sunlight	No	Yes	Yes
Stable in soda lime	No	Yes	Yes
Toxic breakdown products?	Yes	—	—
Metabolism	15–20%	2.4%	0.2%
Reductive metabolism	Yes	No	No
Metabolism to free radicals	Yes	No	No
Tissue binding of metabolites?	Yes	No	—
Hepatic oxygen delivery	Decreased	Slightly decreased	Unchanged

Modified with permission from Eger EI II: IARS Review Course Lectures 116, 1986.

These arguments appear to be weak, as enflurane does not undergo biotransformation as does halothane and because the physical and biological properties of these two anesthetics are very different (Table 43-5). In 9 of these 24 cases, rational explanations other than enflurane were suggested.[110,116] It seems at present that the known incidence of hepatic injury with enflurane anesthesia is too small to suggest any association. Even if enflurane may be hepatotoxic on rare occasions, its toxicity is much less than that attributed to halothane.

There is no specific histologic picture in patients who develop hepatic injury after enflurane anesthesia.[110] Eger et al,[110] who examined 88 cases of postoperative liver dysfunction attributed to enflurane, could say that only 15 cases were possibly related to the drug and that this group did not present any consistent pathology or clinical picture.

In contrast to halothane administration, repeated administrations of enflurane do not increase the incidence of liver blood test abnormalities.[117] The incidence of hepatic damage after halothane anesthesia, as defined by the authors of published case reports, increased dramatically approximately 5 years after halothane was introduced into clinical practice,[110] whereas such an increase has not occurred with enflurane anesthesia (Fig. 43-10).[118] This difference in patterns of hepatic injury can be explained by the need to develop a pool of previously exposed patients; that is, patients sensitized to an anesthetic. It happened with halothane but has not happened with enflurane. Within the first 4 years after the introduction of halothane, more than 350 cases of unexplained postoperative jaundice were reported and attributed to the anesthetic. Eight years after the introduction of enflurane, Lewis et al[115] described 24 patients with postoperative liver disorders that were possibly attributable to the anesthetic. More than 20 million enflurane anesthetics had been administered by that time. If the rate of "enflurane hepatitis" were 1 per 800,000 administrations, this would still be remarkably low, much lower even than the rate of viral hepatitis. Antibodies generated by one of these anesthetics may cross-react with antigens generated by another one. Therefore, although administering enflurane after exposure to halothane probably will reduce the incidence of hepatic damage, it will not necessarily prevent an occurrence.[119,120] Thus, one cannot completely rule out the possibility that enflurane can cause hepatic injury. However, the incidence of such injury, if it occurs at all, is so small that an accurate estimation seems to be impossible. There is no evidence of crossover sensitivity between halothane- and enflurane-induced hepatic injury.

Isoflurane

As of 1987 there were 45 reports of hepatic injury associated with isoflurane anesthesia.[121] The estimated incidence of such injury therefore is 0.00032%—45 cases from 14 million anesthetics administered, with an approximate 25% mortality rate. The incidence of viral hepatitis in apparently healthy patients having anesthesia and surgery may be as great as 1 per 1000,[10,11] which is much higher than the incidence of unexplained hepatic injury after anesthesia. A subcommittee of the Anesthetic and Life Support Advisory Committee of the U.S. Food and Drug Administration evaluated all available reports to determine whether an association exists between administration of isoflurane and subsequent hepatic dysfunction. The committee concluded that "current evidence does not indicate a reasonable likelihood of an association between the use of isoflurane and the occurrence of postoperative hepatic dysfunction."[121]

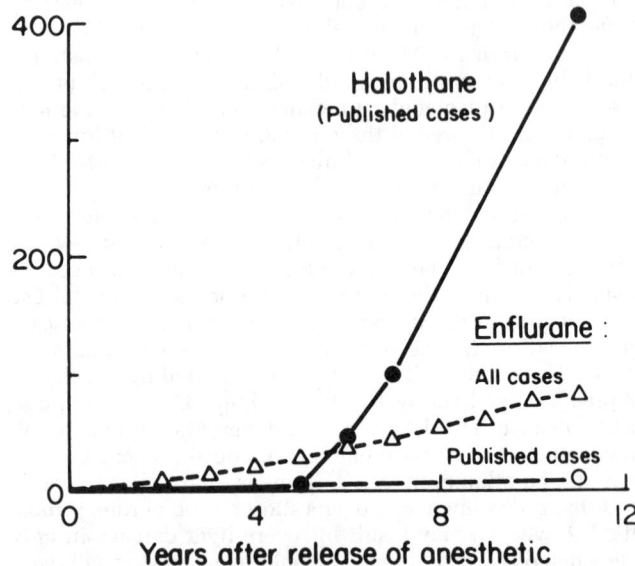

Figure 43-10. Total reported cases of hepatic injury since commercial release of halothane and enflurane. The number of published reports of injury after halothane anesthesia increased dramatically about 5 years after its introduction (●). No such upturn has appeared in the 11-year period since the release of enflurane (▲ and ○). (Reprinted with permission from Eger EI II, Smuckler EA, Ferrell LD et al: Is enflurane hepatotoxic? Anesth Analg 65:21, 1986.)

Enflurane and isoflurane undergo little or no biotransformation, whereas substantial amounts of halothane are metabolized.[122-124] Halothane undergoes reductive metabolism, whereas enflurane and isoflurane do not. As discussed earlier, the metabolism of halothane may be accompanied by the formation of free radicals and also of some metabolites that bind to lipids or proteins within the tissue. This is not the case with enflurane or isoflurane. Finally, halothane decreases the hepatic blood and oxygen supply to a much greater extent than does either enflurane[114] or isoflurane[88,90,113] when used in equipotent doses, titrated by MAC values or similar decreases in blood pressure or cardiac output. Other hepatic functions seem to be affected by halothane to a greater extent than by enflurane or isoflurane, as mentioned earlier. The effects of newer volatile anesthetics, such as desflurane and sevoflurane, await thorough evaluation, but some preliminary data suggest that desflurane probably does not seriously affect hepatic function.[125]

Nitrous Oxide

Nitrous oxide by itself usually is not associated with significant changes in blood pressure and cardiac output. Hepatic circulation is not disturbed when nitrous oxide is used in trained animals without any baseline anesthesia or surgical preparation.[126] However, a significant decrease in both portal and hepatic arterial blood flows, 15% and 24%, respectively, is observed when nitrous oxide is used in conditions of barbiturate anesthesia and laparotomy.[127] In the rat, nitrous oxide decreases cardiac output and intestinal, splenic, and total hepatic blood flow.[128] It has not been proved whether this decrease subjects the liver to ischemic injury.

Nitrous oxide in clinically used concentrations decreases methionine synthetase activity in the livers of animals and humans.[129] This decrease becomes greater with longer exposure. It is not clear whether this decrease in enzyme activity is detrimental to liver function. One study clearly demonstrated that persons anesthetized with halothane and nitrous oxide had a significant increase in serum liver enzymes compared with patients anesthetized with halothane in oxygen.[130] The difference can be attributed to a somewhat better hepatic oxygenation in the group of patients who did not receive nitrous oxide, but also by the absence or presence of nitrous oxide per se. Other studies could not demonstrate significant liver dysfunction during nitrous oxide anesthesia supplemented with methohexital.[131] Currently, there is no convincing evidence that nitrous oxide causes hepatotoxicity.[132]

Intravenous Anesthetics

Pharmacodynamics. The effect of intravenous anesthetics and opioids on the liver has not been thoroughly studied. A time-related reduction in hepatic arterial blood flow during a constant infusion of etomidate is observed in dogs.[133] These changes, however, probably result from systemic hemodynamic disturbances, mainly a decrease in cardiac output, as etomidate and althesin produce dose-dependent reductions in cardiac output and mean arterial pressure.[134] Doses of etomidate and althesin that are not sufficient to induce significant changes in cardiac output or mean arterial pressure still lead to a significant decrease in hepatic arterial blood flow. These data are partially in agreement with the results observed in isolated perfused rat livers.[135] In those experiments, althesin and ketamine added to the perfusate caused constriction of the hepatic arterial vasculature. All three drugs studied by Thomson and associates increased the resistance in the hepatic arterial and mesenteric vasculatures when infused at low rates. Higher infusion rates were accompanied by systemic hemodynamic disturbances, with a subsequent decrease in hepatic blood flow.[134]

Liver blood tests were found to be unchanged in patients after minor surgery with etomidate, propofol, thiopental, midazolam, and althesin, whereas similar surgery under ketamine anesthesia was associated with a moderate increase in the serum concentration of some liver enzymes.[136-139] Major surgical procedures under similar kinds of intravenous anesthetics supplemented with nitrous oxide were accompanied by a significant increase in the plasma concentrations of liver enzymes.[131,140] Sear,[141] in his review of the toxicity of intravenous anesthetics, concluded that, "it appears that single infusions of all the iv hypnotic agents (with the possible exceptions of thiopentone and ketamine) cause only minimal alterations in plasma concentrations of the routinely measured liver function tests."

Opioids can induce spasm of the sphincter of Oddi, with a subsequent increase in intrabiliary pressure, as well as severe abdominal pain. Such spasms may be responsible for false results on intraoperative cholangiography. It is important to realize that such spasm is observed in approximately 3% of patients receiving opioids.[142] It seems that with equipotent doses, the largest increase in intrabiliary pressure is associated with fentanyl and morphine; meperidine (pethidine) and pentazocine are associated with smaller increases (Fig. 43-11).[143-145] However, nalbuphine probably does not cause spasm of the sphincter of Oddi.[146]

Pharmacokinetics. Data concerning the pharmacokinetics of midazolam in patients with advanced liver disease are conflicting. One study[147] demonstrated a significant decrease in clearance and elimination half-life, whereas another study[148] demonstrated only slightly impaired disposition in cirrhotic patients. Pharmacokinetics of single doses of sufentanil,[149] and propofol[150] were found to be similar in patients with hepatic cirrhosis and patients with normal hepatic function, but some differences in elimination time were observed. These findings imply that during use of multiple doses of intravenous infusion of the drugs, delayed elimination, and therefore increased pharmacologic effect, should be expected in patients with advanced hepatic disease. The differences in the results of these studies are probably a consequence of certain differences in the binding proteins, as well as accumulation of endogenous binding inhibitors such as bilirubin. This might explain a smaller degree of midazolam protein binding in cirrhotic individuals, with a subsequent increase in the free fraction of the drug and enhancement of the pharmacologic effect in patients with advanced hepatic disease.

For thiopental, total plasma clearance and total apparent volume of distribution at the steady state are unchanged in patients with hepatic cirrhosis. Therefore, the elimination half-life is not prolonged.[151] Thiopental has a low extraction ratio; therefore, its clearance is independent of hepatic blood flow. However, an increase in the unbound fraction of the drug may enhance the activity of a single dose and therefore may increase the incidence of an acute harmful effect during anesthesia induction.

The plasma clearance of fentanyl is significantly lower in patients with hepatic cirrhosis than in controls. The total apparent volume of distribution is not changed, whereas the elimination half-life is prolonged owing to the decreased plasma clearance. The plasma free fraction of alfentanil is

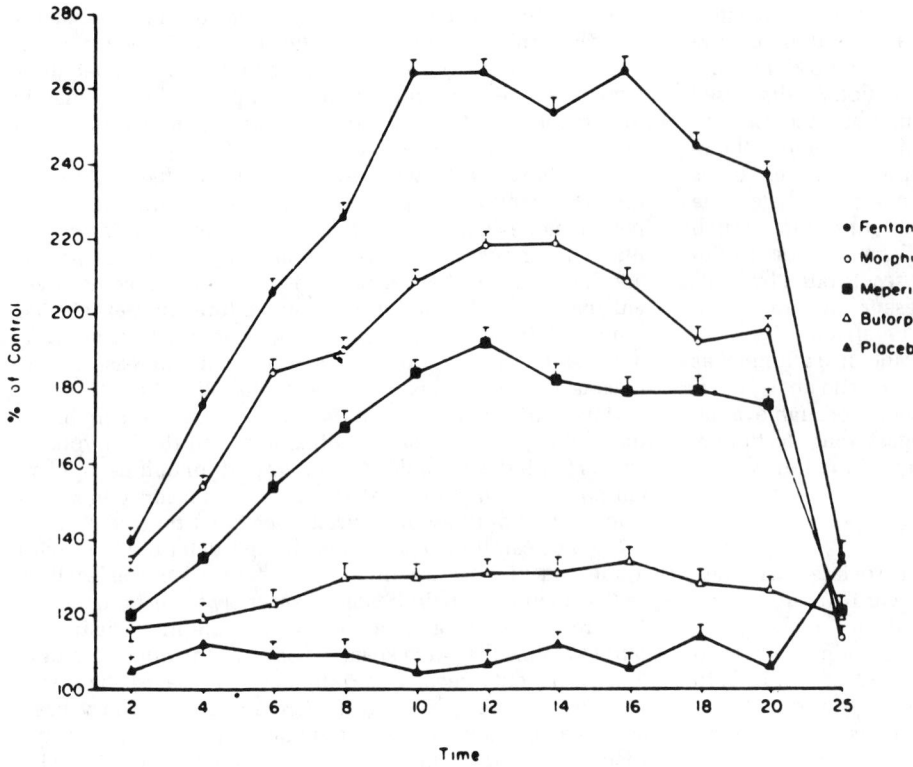

Figure 43-11. The effect of opioids and placebo on common bile duct pressure and the response to naloxone administered at 20 minutes. (Reprinted with permission from Radnay PA, Duncalf D, Novakovic M *et al:* Common bile duct pressure changes after fentanyl, morphine, meperidine, butorphanol, and naloxone. Anesth Analg 63:441, 1984.)

likewise increased in patients with hepatic cirrhosis.[152] It is clear that alfentanil exerts a prolonged and pronounced effect in patients with advanced liver disease.

The data regarding morphine pharmacokinetics in patients with hepatic cirrhosis are contradictory. For example, Patwardhan *et al*[153] did not find a significant difference in morphine pharmacokinetics in patients with hepatic cirrhosis compared with healthy persons and suggested that "reported intolerance to the central effects of morphine cannot be explained by impaired drug elimination and increased availability of morphine to cerebral receptors."[153] However, a more recent French study found a somewhat decreased clearance and a prolonged half-life of free morphine, as well as of morphine metabolites, in patients with liver cirrhosis compared with healthy controls.[154]

It seems that opioids and intravenous anesthetics *per se* do not affect hepatic function to any extent provided they do not jeopardize the hepatic blood and oxygen supply. Hepatic function, as evaluated by the serum concentrations of intracellular enzymes, depends much more on the severity of surgical stress than on the specific anesthetic chosen.[6,155] The hepatic oxygen supply–demand relation can be different during different anesthetics when anesthesia is superimposed on surgery. The pertinent question that may be raised is to what extent one or another anesthetic protects the liver from surgical stress. In other words, it is important to know whether the combination of one or another anesthetic with surgical intervention results in different degrees of hepatic dysfunction.

Effects of Anesthetics on Drug Pharmacokinetics

Anesthetics can decrease the elimination of many other drugs, mainly by a decrease in intrinsic clearance (i.e., a decrease in the ability of the liver cells to metabolize or excrete the drug) or by a decrease in hepatic blood flow (for drugs with a high hepatic extraction ratio). For example, halothane substantially decreases the intrinsic clearance of diazepam,[156] as well as of propranolol.[157] Clearance of lidocaine is also substantially decreased during halothane anesthesia.[158] On the other hand, elimination of aminophylline is not significantly altered by enflurane or halothane.[159] There are approximately three dozen reports demonstrating a reduction of drug clearance by halothane.

Enflurane has no significant effect on the pharmacokinetics of thiopental.[160-162] Isoflurane has not been extensively studied in this regard; however, it has been reported that this anesthetic inhibits the oxidative metabolism of halothane.[163] Nitrous oxide prolongs the half-life of etomidate,[164] whereas diazepam prolongs the half-life of ketamine.[165]

Effects of Surgical Stress on Liver Function

Surgical intervention induces certain, sometimes rather severe, disorders in homeostasis, including alterations in hepatic circulation and function. The general response to stress has been well studied, and certain responses to surgical stress, such as an increase in circulating catecholamines, cortisol, growth hormone, antidiuretic hormone, and aldosterone and activation of the renin–angiotensin system, are well known. However, the specific effects of stress on hepatic function have been studied to a lesser degree. Available data strongly suggest that laparotomy by itself reduces blood flow through the intestine and the liver.[166,167] The mechanisms responsible for such disorders have not been directly studied. Traction and manipulation of the viscera probably play a significant role; however, a general biologic response to stress is also important. For example, laparotomy is associated with marked mesenteric vasoconstriction and a decrease in gastrointestinal blood flow, which can be abolished by hypophysectomy.[168] Surgical stress is usually accompanied by the release of several hormones and other substances, including catecholamines, renin–angiotensin, and vasopressin, that can and do disturb the splanchnic circulation. The concentration of these circulating compounds may be increased for many hours or even days after surgery.[169,170]

One study demonstrated that phenobarbital-pretreated (liver enzyme-induced) rats anesthetized with halothane developed liver necrosis after laparotomy alone or after laparotomy with ligation of the hepatic artery.[171] Under similar conditions, halothane anesthesia without laparotomy was not associated with hepatic necrosis. This finding suggests that laparotomy may be accompanied by a reduction in the liver oxygen supply severe enough to cause hepatic necrosis under these particular experimental conditions. Actually, this is not surprising considering the sensitivity of the liver to oxygen deprivation.

In patients with chronic lung disease, when blood oxygen content is decreased below 9 ml·dl^{-1}, liver injury develops in all patients, without obvious myocardial or cerebral damage.[172] There are experimental and even clinical data substantiating the detrimental effect of oxygen deprivation on the perioperative hepatic function when otherwise similar anesthetic management is provided.[173] There is a specific term, "ischemic hepatitis," for relatively moderate injury that results from mild hepatic oxygen deprivation.

Hepatic function may be compromised when hepatic blood flow is reduced; major surgery is associated with a substantial increase in the concentration of enzymes supposedly released from the liver. The degree of such an increase depends on the type of surgery rather than the anesthesia provided; such an increase is rarely observed during minor surgery, even under the same type of anesthesia.[6,174] Other studies have likewise demonstrated that postoperative liver dysfunction results mainly from the operation itself rather than from the selected anesthetic technique.[175-177] Thus, surgery, particularly laparotomy, does affect liver function but usually without detrimental consequences. However, in patients with advanced hepatic disease, laparotomy carries extremely high postoperative morbidity and mortality rates. In the 1960s, the immediate mortality rate from laparotomy alone in patients with acute hepatitis approached 10–11% in certain groups.[13,14] During the last 20 years, the situation has not significantly improved: as was mentioned at the beginning of this chapter, the British and American literature both report extremely high 30-day postoperative morbidity and mortality rates after laparotomy and liver biopsy in patients with advanced hepatic disease.[15,16]

As mentioned previously, all anesthetics, particularly inhalational ones, decrease total hepatic blood flow to a variable degree in a dose-related fashion. When surgical intervention is superimposed, hepatic blood flow is further decreased[167] to a degree that depends on the specific type of intervention. That is, minor peripheral procedures are accompanied by a relatively small reduction in hepatic blood flow, whereas major procedures, especially upper abdominal laparotomy, are associated with a much larger decrease.[167] These data demonstrate that anesthesia may play a modifying role in the complex of surgery and anesthesia: similar surgical interventions are associated with different degrees of hepatic circulatory disturbances when different types of anesthesia are administered.[167] Therefore, the modifying role of anesthesia in the development of hepatic cir-

culatory disorders, as well as of hepatic dysfunction during surgery, can be more important clinically than the effect of one or another anesthetic *per se*. A question that is probably of paramount importance in this regard is which kind of anesthesia administered for similar surgical procedures would be accompanied by minimal hepatic circulatory disturbances and hepatic dysfunction.

During surgical stress, even a 30% reduction in the mean arterial pressure induced by isoflurane is not associated with a deterioration in hepatic oxygen supply, whereas in pigs, a similar degree of arterial hypotension achieved by halothane reduces the hepatic oxygen supply and supply-uptake ratio during severe surgical stress (thoracotomy, laparotomy, and extensive surgical preparation).[178] Fentanyl anesthesia in a porcine model maintains the hepatic oxygen supply at least at baseline levels but is accompanied by hepatic oxygen requirements somewhat higher than those observed during isoflurane or halothane anesthesia. Therefore, the hepatic oxygen supply-uptake relation during anesthesia with fentanyl is maintained rather than increased, and halothane is less desirable than isoflurane or fentanyl anesthesia.[178] The reasons for the fentanyl-associated increase in hepatic oxygen uptake are not clear. It seems conceivable that the stress response to surgical intervention is accompanied by increased metabolism within the liver, yielding a subsequent increase in oxygen demand. This increase in demand (followed by an increase in supply) is not blocked by fentanyl but was substantially modified by isoflurane as well as by halothane.

ANESTHESIA FOR PATIENTS WITH LIVER DISEASE

Preoperative Evaluation

During the preoperative visit, the anesthesiologist should determine the current drug therapy, previous and present jaundice, history of blood transfusions and gastrointestinal bleeding, previous operations, and anesthetic managements. The physical examination should include, in addition to the routine examination of organs and systems, a careful review of the patient's appearance, as well as of the degree of ascites and encephalopathy. The physical evaluation of a patient with chronic liver disease is particularly valuable: the patient may feel and look unwell a long time before hepatic dysfunction can be revealed by certain changes in blood tests. Abnormal values of blood tests may have somewhat limited importance if the patient feels well, because the tests are relatively nonspecific.[179]

Blood tests should include determinations of hemoglobin and hematocrit; platelet count; serum bilirubin; serum electrolytes, particularly sodium and potassium; creatinine and BUN; arterial blood gases; serum proteins; prothrombin time; and several enzymes, including aminotransferases, alkaline phosphatase, lactate dehydrogenase, and hydroxybutyrate dehydrogenase (lactate dehydrogenase isoenzyme being more specific for liver function).

The function of the coagulation system should be evaluated and properly treated before surgery. In patients with obstructive jaundice, demonstrating abnormal prothrombin and partial thromboplastin times, a trial of vitamin K (10 mg intramuscularly three times a day for a few days) may prove to be beneficial. If a trial of vitamin K is not successful or if there is no time for correction of hypocoagulation with vitamin K, treatment with fresh frozen plasma should be considered. Thrombocytopenia, which often accompanies advanced liver disease, must be corrected if possible prior to surgery by an appropriate transfusion of platelet concentrates. The platelet count should be 100,000 per mm³; each unit of platelets increases the count approximately 10,000 per mm³ in an average adult. The diagnosed coagulopathy must be corrected before spinal or epidural anesthesia.

The blood glucose concentration should be checked. If there is hypoglycemia, which sometimes develops in patients with advanced liver disease, glucose solution should be infused with periodic monitoring of the blood concentration.

The surgical procedure that the patient is undergoing is important in planning the anesthetic management. Even procedures that are relatively short and considered to be "safe" for average patients can be extremely dangerous for the patient with advanced liver disease. It has been stated earlier in this chapter that even simple laparotomy without other major interventions is accompanied by extremely high perioperative morbidity and mortality rates in this population.

If there are no clotting abnormalities and the patient is scheduled for peripheral surgery, a regional blockade can be the anesthetic management of choice. However, for surgical procedures involving the abdomen and in patients with obvious coagulopathy, regional anesthesia is usually contraindicated. For some relatively minor procedures, such as sclerotherapy, local anesthesia with sedation can be used successfully. Benzodiazepines, for example, midazolam, can be a drug of choice for sedation and may be combined with small doses of fentanyl. It is noteworthy that midazolam is a highly protein-bound compound; therefore, if the patient has a decreased protein concentration in blood, a relative overdose can occur. Also, a relative overdose of benzodiazepines may result from a greater affinity of the CNS, possibly owing to an increased population of specific receptors to benzodiazepines in patients with advanced hepatic disease compared with normal persons.[52] Therefore, all drugs, including sedatives, should be carefully titrated against their effect.

Preoperative treatment for patients with severe liver disease should be devoted to normalization of coagulopathy; the treatment may be based on changes in prothrombin time. Assurance of adequate hydration and adequate diuresis (approximately 1 ml·kg⁻¹·h⁻¹) is also of paramount importance. Inadequate diuresis should be treated by appropriate fluid load—volume and content are equally important. The volume load should be titrated against ventricular filling pressures, central venous pressure if myocardial and pulmonary function is adequate, or pulmonary capillary wedge pressure, if needed. Proper fluid content should be ensured by analysis of blood electrolytes (mainly sodium and potassium, as well as ionized calcium), hematocrit, and glucose. Patients with liver disease require infusion of albumin more often than do other patients. Diuretic therapy should include furosemide, mannitol, or both and a low dose of dopamine (2–4 μg·kg⁻¹·min⁻¹) owing to its renal vasodilation and antialdosterone effect. In chronic situations, spironolactone may be a diuretic of choice because of its strong antialdosterone activity.

Premedication

All medications needed to control the diseased state should be administered. Considering the reduced ability of the liver to metabolize drugs, sedatives should be omitted or the dose decreased.

Patients with advanced liver disease may have a full stomach, even if they have not taken food or fluid for several hours, because of hiatal hernia, massive ascites, and decreased gastric and intestinal motility. Therefore, premedication may include an H2 histamine-receptor blocker (e.g., ranitidine), metoclopramide, as well as sodium citrate.

Monitoring

Routine monitoring, including electrocardiogram, blood pressure, precordial or esophageal stethoscope, temperature, F_{IO_2}, end-expired carbon dioxide, and pulse oximeter, should be used. Cannulation of an artery is important for direct blood pressure monitoring, as well as for periodic sampling for determinations of blood gases, electrolytes, hematocrit, and other tests as needed during surgery. Fluid load should be carefully titrated in patients with advanced liver disease. Therefore, insertion of a pulmonary artery catheter, or at least a central venous catheter, is often necessary. Monitoring with a pulmonary artery catheter may be important if, in addition to advanced hepatic disease, the patient has compromised left ventricular function, pulmonary disease, or severe renal dysfunction. Urine output should always be monitored in patients with advanced liver disease who are undergoing surgery longer than 1 or 2 hours. Surgical procedures associated with extensive blood loss (e.g., liver transplantation) require monitoring of the blood coagulation status, which should include periodic determinations of prothrombin time, partial thromboplastin time, and platelet count. Thromboelastography seems to be helpful.[180] A transcutaneous nerve stimulator is helpful in titrating muscle relaxants in every patient, but particularly in patients with advanced liver disease, in whom the effects of muscle relaxants are unpredictable.

Anesthesia Induction

Rapid-sequence induction (or awake intubation of the trachea) should be provided if a full stomach is suspected. All widely used intravenous anesthetics for induction have been administered in patients with advanced hepatic disease. The chosen drug has to be carefully titrated until the desired effect is achieved. Depolarizing muscle relaxants may be used to facilitate endotracheal intubation. Succinylcholine activity is usually relatively normal, despite some decrease in plasma cholinesterase. In patients with severely decreased cholinesterase activity, the effect of succinylcholine can last longer than it does in normal persons. Nondepolarizing muscle relaxants chosen to facilitate endotracheal intubation (e.g., d-tubocurarine) have a high affinity with gamma-globulin, and the volume of distribution for such a drug can be increased; therefore, the dose required to achieve total relaxation can be higher than in normal persons. The volume of distribution of pancuronium also is increased in patients with advanced liver disease, although the reasons are not clear and probably differ from those for d-tubocurarine. Pancuronium is poorly bound to plasma protein, and there is no correlation between the volume of distribution and the plasma gamma-globulin concentration.[181] The volume of distribution of atracurium also is increased,[182] possibly owing to a substantial increase in extracellular fluid. However, the volume of distribution of vecuronium is not significantly altered;[183] therefore, a substantial change in the requirement for the effective dose of this muscle relaxant should not be expected. However, the titration of the muscle relaxant using a transcutaneous nerve stimulator is still desirable.

Maintenance of Anesthesia

Intraoperative liver injury can develop from oxygen deprivation, the stress response, drug toxicity, blood transfusion, and infection. It is important to realize that the hepatic oxygen supply can be jeopardized at any step of oxygen transport to the liver: (1) hypoxic hypoxia may result from inadequate FIO_2 or hypoventilation; (2) anemic hypoxia may develop if the oxygen-carrying capacity of the blood (adequate hematocrit) is not ensured; (3) circulatory hypoxia may result from systemic (hypovolemia, arterial hypotension, reduction in cardiac output) or regional (decrease in hepatic blood and oxygen supply) hemodynamic disorders. The decrease in hepatic blood and oxygen delivery may follow systemic circulatory disturbances or may result from manipulations around the liver as well as from the effects of many endogenous vasoconstrictive substances (e.g., renin–angiotensin, catecholamines, antidiuretic hormone; and (4) interference of anesthetics with electron transport at the cellular level may lead to a histotoxic hypoxia; however, the clinical relevance of this mechanism has not been demonstrated.

The concept of the oxygen supply–demand relations in the liver should be kept in mind. For example, in a 1987 study in pigs, severe surgical stress under anesthesia with moderate doses of fentanyl was accompanied by a somewhat higher hepatic oxygen supply and uptake than identical stress under isoflurane anesthesia, which resulted in similar values of hepatic oxygen supply–uptake ratio.[178] Taking this into consideration, the main rule is to maintain adequate pulmonary ventilation and cardiovascular function, including cardiac output, blood volume, and perfusion pressures. Arterial hypotension, owing to inadequate blood and volume replacement, a relative overdose of inhalational anesthetics, or controlled drug-induced hypotension, should be avoided, because vasodilation and a decrease in perfusion pressure accompanied by a decrease in blood velocity would unavoidably cause an increase in oxygen extraction in all tissues, including the preportal area. Decreased blood velocity and increased oxygen extraction result in a decrease in venous oxygen content—in this case, decreased oxygen content in the portal venous blood. A reduction in portal blood oxygen content or flow is usually accompanied by a compensatory increase in hepatic arterial blood flow. Thus, hepatic injury after moderate arterial hypotension is a relatively rare event. However, in animals with severe liver dysfunction, the autoregulatory ability of hepatic arterial blood flow to increase is diminished or abolished.[184] Therefore, in such animals, and probably in patients with severe hepatic disease, the hepatic arterial blood flow would not increase when the portal blood flow or the oxygen content of the portal venous blood decreased. This might lead to a decrease in hepatic blood and oxygen supply, with subsequent hepatic oxygen deprivation. Thus, the lesson is clear: arterial hypotension, as well as states with reduced cardiac output, should be avoided.

Regional anesthesia should be used whenever possible in patients with advanced liver disease. Keeping in mind the comparative pharmacology of inhalational anesthetics, it seems that halothane should be avoided, because this anesthetic is accompanied by the most prominent decrease in hepatic blood and oxygen supply and postoperative hepatic dysfunction; rarely will severe postoperative hepatitis fol-

low halothane anesthesia, however. Enflurane, particularly isoflurane, seems to be the anesthetic of choice if an inhalational technique is selected. Nitrous oxide has been used for many years in patients with advanced hepatic disease and thus far has not been incriminated in an increased incidence of anesthesia-related postoperative hepatic complications. However, the well-known sympathomimetic effect of nitrous oxide and some possibility of jeopardized oxygenation render the routine use of nitrous oxide undesirable in patients with advanced liver disease according to some experts. It is important to remember that long operations under anesthesia with nitrous oxide may result in the accumulation of the gas in the intestinal lumen, with subsequent intestinal distention.

Opioids can also be successful in patients with hepatic disease. Despite certain pharmacokinetic consequences (decreased clearance and prolonged half-life), fentanyl probably should be considered the opioid of choice. Interestingly, fentanyl does not decrease the hepatic oxygen and blood supply; however, neither does it prevent an increase in hepatic oxygen requirements when used in moderate doses. Therefore, the hepatic oxygen supply–demand relation during anesthesia with fentanyl is not much better than that during anesthesia with isoflurane.[178] It seems at present that anesthetic management using inhalational agents (isoflurane would probably be the drug of choice) alone or in combination with small doses of fentanyl can be considered as the method of choice provided adequate pulmonary ventilation, cardiac output, and arterial pressures are maintained. Other drugs also can be used successfully in patients with advanced hepatic disease.

When administering drugs to patients with hepatic disease, one must appreciate the substantially changed pharmacokinetics. For example, the half-life of lidocaine may be increased by more than 300%, that for benzodiazepines by more than 100%, and so on. For drugs binding to albumin (e.g., sodium pentothal), the volume of distribution can be decreased, and, therefore, the dose should be decreased. On the other hand, the volume of distribution of many drugs can be substantially increased for different reasons, including an increase in gamma-globulin or edema, dictating an increase in the first effective dose of the drug; however, owing to a decrease in hepatic blood flow and metabolic and excretory functions, as well as impairment of renal function, the clearance of such drugs can be decreased, and therefore the effect can be prolonged (e.g., d-tubocurarine, pancuronium). It seems that advanced hepatic disease does not significantly affect the pharmacokinetics of vecuronium, although some dose-dependent pharmacokinetic alterations have been observed.[183] This is possibly the result of a limited hepatic uptake capacity, which is usually exceeded after doses of vecuronium greater than $0.15 \ mg \cdot kg^{-1}$. With a smaller dose, hepatic dysfunction does not affect the pharmacokinetics or duration of action of vecuronium.[183]

Actually, any muscle relaxant can be used in patients with advanced liver disease. Atracurium has a theoretical advantage, because its elimination is determined mainly by Hofmann decomposition and therefore is relatively independent of renal or hepatic function. Thus, it is not surprising that the clearance and elimination half-life of atracurium in patients with liver cirrhosis and impaired renal function is not particularly different from that of persons who have normal hepatorenal function. However, volumes of distribution are larger, and accordingly, the distribution half-life is shorter in patients with severe hepatorenal dysfunction compared with normal persons.[182] This study also demonstrated that the only situation that prolongs the elimination half-life of atracurium is marked metabolic acidosis, which may decrease the rate of Hofmann decomposition.[182] The pharmacokinetics of many muscle relaxants in conditions of cholestasis and obstructive jaundice may also be altered: prolonged duration of action has been demonstrated.[185] However, if it is planned to continue controlled ventilation of the lungs postoperatively, vecuronium, atracurium, and pancuronium can be used successfully. Titration of any relaxant according to transcutaneous nerve stimulation monitoring is beneficial.

It is noteworthy that although pharmacokinetic studies in patients with hepatic cirrhosis provide interesting results that are helpful in understanding the pathogenetic aspects of chronic liver disease, the results do not have significant value for predicting the safety of a drug. The degree of hepatic dysfunction affects the degree of pharmacokinetic disorder; therefore, again, the best way to avoid complications is to titrate drugs against effect.

Renal function must be maintained by administering proper fluid load (volume and content) and diuretics, if needed. It is extremely difficult, if not impossible, to maintain the proper fluid load without monitoring filling pressures. Therefore, insertion of a pulmonary artery catheter, or at least a central venous catheter, is often mandatory. The content of infused solutions should be chosen and, often, adjusted according to periodic analysis of the blood for electrolytes. For example, normal or, especially, high serum concentrations of sodium require an infusion of a solution such as 5% glucose in water, whereas a decrease in sodium concentration below 130–135 mEq·l^{-1} allows an infusion of a solution such as Normosol. Furosemide or mannitol should be considered effective diuretics in these patients. A small dose of dopamine (2–4 μg·kg^{-1}·min^{-1}) can be beneficial owing to many different effects, including improvement in renal perfusion and the antialdosterone effect.

The parameters of controlled ventilation should be carefully selected in order to avoid an unnecessary increase in intrathoracic pressure, which may impede venous return, thereby decreasing cardiac output. Hypocarbia should probably be avoided, because it can aggravate hepatic encephalopathy. It has been mentioned previously that opioids can induce spasm of the sphincter of Oddi (see Fig. 43-11). The incidence of such spasm does not exceed 3%.[142] Spasm induced by opioids can be relieved with many different drugs, one of which is atropine.[145] The clinical disadvantage of this treatment is the accompanying tachycardia. Another drug that relaxes the sphincter of Oddi is naloxone;[186,187] a potential problem with this drug is that the analgesic effect of the opioid is reversed (together with relaxation of the sphincter); some other means of anesthesia–analgesia should be provided. The possible cardiovascular complications of naloxone treatment should also be kept in mind. Glucagon is effective in producing relaxation of the sphincter;[188,189] however, this might not be the drug of choice, as it has many different side effects, including hyperglycemia and a hyperdynamic cardiovascular state. Finally, nitroglycerin is effective in relieving opioid-induced spasm of the sphincter of Oddi. Volatile anesthetics attenuate the response of the sphincter to opioids.[190]

Coagulopathy can develop during surgery, and monitoring of the coagulation state can be important, particularly during liver transplantation. Treatment may include administration of platelets, fresh frozen plasma, cryoprecipitate, and sometimes epsilon-aminocaproic acid and protamine sulfate. Interestingly, some coagulopathies that develop during liver transplantation may be related to heparin sequestered in and then washed out from the graft when circu-lation is re-established to include the graft in the systemic circulation. Protamine sulfate effectively reverses this effect of heparin.[191] Some authors observed DIC.[192] Sometimes, fibrinolysis can also be identified.[191] A detailed description of the monitoring and treatment of hepatic coagulopathy during liver transplantation is available elsewhere.[180]

POSTOPERATIVE HEPATIC DYSFUNCTION

Many different forms of hepatic disorder may develop during the postoperative period (Table 43-6). Fortunately, most clearly identified postoperative hepatic dysfunctions will resolve without treatment. However, certain precautions should be taken in the event that liver function deteriorates. Gas exchange and cardiovascular function should be optimized and appropriate viral studies initiated. All medications should be examined, and their potential harm to the liver should be weighed against potential benefits. Infection should be treated vigorously. A diagnosis of cholestatic jaundice versus parenchymal jaundice should be established. A hepatic biopsy does not always provide answers to questions in such situations. However, to determine whether the patient has developed hepatic injury during the perioperative period, this observer agrees with the statement that "most importantly, the patient feels and looks unwell."[179] When a patient develops severe hepatic injury, the symptoms are striking enough to make the diagnosis simple; however, diagnosing the exact cause of injury is difficult. It may be compared to a house that is in flames: it is easy to see that the house is burning but impossible to determine the cause and origin of the fire.

Postoperative jaundice, as any other jaundice, can be the result of one or any combination of three causes: (1) overproduction–overload of bilirubin; (2) impaired excretion of bilirubin resulting from hepatocellular injury; and (3) biliary obstruction (Fig. 43-12). An increased load of bilirubin can be secondary to blood transfusion, resorption of extravasated blood accumulations (e.g., hematomas, hemothorax), hemolytic anemia, and a prosthetic heart valve.[1] Excessive blood transfusions, as well as resorption of hemoglobin from hematomas, represent a classic and probably the most common cause of postoperative jaundice related to overproduction–overload of bilirubin. Approximately

---

TABLE 43-6. Etiology of Postoperative Liver Dysfunction

Hepatic O$_2$ deprivation
  Hypoxia
  Decreased arterial pressure or cardiac output
  Decreased hepatic blood flow
Viral hepatitis, acute
Aggravated chronic hepatitis
  Immunity depression by anesthesia and/or surgery
  Respiratory/circulatory depression resulting in liver hypoxia
  Deteriorated hepatic artery blood flow autoregulation
  Relative overdose (altered pharmacokinetics)
Fulminant hepatitis with specific halothane-related antibodies
Free radicals produced by reductive metabolism of halothane
Specific drug therapy
Blood transfusion
Infection

Modified with permission from Kang YG, Gelman S: Liver transplantation. In Gelman S (ed): Anesthesia and Organ Transplantation, p 152. Philadelphia, WB Saunders, 1987.

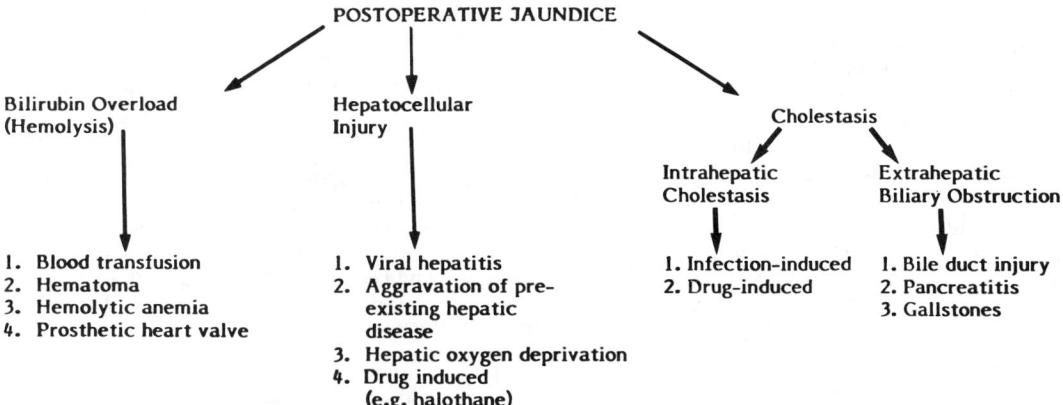

Figure 43-12. Etiology of postoperative jaundice.

10% of stored blood undergoes hemolysis within 24 hours after transfusion, and a transfusion of 500 ml results in the production of approximately 250 mg of bilirubin. The normal liver excretes this load easily, without any increase in the plasma bilirubin concentration. However, if a seriously ill patient undergoing a major surgical procedure receives a transfusion load much greater than 500 ml of blood, the hemolysis that follows is reflected in an increase, mainly in indirect or unconjugated bilirubin. If the extrabilirubin pigment is conjugated but not excreted enough, an increase also is observed in the direct or conjugated fraction of bilirubin. Unconjugated hyperbilirubinemia may result in severe neurologic dysfunction, including rapidly developing fatal encephalopathy.[20-22] On the other hand, conjugated hyperbilirubinemia is not accompanied by apparent neurotoxicity. This subject is discussed in more detail earlier in this chapter.

Hemolytic anemia as a cause of postoperative jaundice is relatively rare but should be considered, especially if the indirect/unconjugated bilirubin represents 90% or more of the total. Sickle cell anemia (and maybe some forms of autoimmune hemolytic anemia) is probably the most common cause of hemolytic anemia observed postoperatively. Some patients with congenital deficiencies of glucose-6-phosphate dehydrogenase develop hemolysis after surgical stress and also after administration of certain drugs such as sulfonamides, chloramphenicol, nitrofurantoin, and aspirin. Patients with prosthetic heart valves, particularly aortic valves, develop hemolytic jaundice, apparently as a result of the damage of the erythrocytes resulting from contact with the prosthesis. Some patients demonstrate a positive Coombs' test, which suggests an autoimmune component in the hemolytic process.

Hepatocellular injury is characterized primarily by an increased concentration of liver enzymes, as well as prolonged prothrombin time, decreased albumin concentrations, increased ammonia concentration, and different degrees of hepatic encephalopathy. Alkaline phosphatase can also be elevated, even though this is usually a sign of a cholestatic disorder; however, in the case of hepatocellular injury, the primary abnormalities are observed in the synthesizing functions of the liver.

Postoperative viral hepatitis can be the result of an infection the patient had before surgery—unknown chronic hepatitis or incubating acute hepatitis. Postoperative viral hepatitis can also be a complication of blood transfusion; this type usually develops somewhere between 30 and 70 days after transfusion.

Pre-existing hepatic disease, known or unknown, probably plays a substantial role in postoperative hepatic dysfunction, including jaundice. Deterioration in existing hepatic disease can result from a stress response to surgery, with an increase in the concentration of hormones and substances affecting hepatic blood and oxygen supply, as well as cellular function. Hepatic oxygen deprivation may develop in these patients, because they may not be able to increase hepatic arterial blood flow in response to a decrease in the portal blood flow or oxygen content that usually accompanies severe stress.[167,193] The inability of hepatic arterial blood flow to increase may jeopardize oxygen supply to the liver.

The most common cause (fortunately usually without clinically detrimental consequences) of postoperative hepatic dysfunction probably is hepatic oxygen deprivation, which can be induced by all anesthetics at any step of oxygen transport to the liver tissue. Any kind of hypoxic hypoxia (decrease in F_{IO_2}, hypoventilation, including inadvertent disconnection between the endotracheal tube and the respirator) may lead to hypoxic ischemic damage to any organ, including the liver. Most commonly, however, hepatic oxygen deprivation develops as a result of a decreased cardiac output or systemic arterial pressure, as well as regional disturbances in the hepatic blood supply, even when blood pressure is maintained at acceptable levels. Regional (splanchnic and hepatic) circulatory disturbances may result from a decrease in cardiac output, as well as from manipulations in the surgical field near the liver. Circulating vasoconstricting substances such as antidiuretic hormone, renin–angiotensin, and catecholamines apparently play a significant role in hepatic circulatory disturbances during surgery. Hepatic oxygen deprivation resulting from hypoxia and hypovolemia is usually associated with a relatively modest increase in bilirubin concentrations, up to 20 $mg \cdot dl^{-1}$ within 2–12 days after surgery. A moderate increase in the concentration of liver enzymes is often observed. The most common histologic finding in such situations is centrilobular congestion, sometimes with necrosis. Often, this type of hepatic dysfunction heals by itself without apparent sequelae.

Severe hepatocellular injury may be induced by different drugs used during anesthesia. Halothane is one of them. Halothane hepatitis is rare but is associated with an extremely high mortality rate. It appears that the severity of halothane hepatotoxicity is increased with repeated exposure to the drug within relatively short periods of time. Clinically, halothane hepatitis can be manifested by fever, jaundice, an increase in the serum concentration of liver enzymes, and eosinophilia. It seems that female, as well as obese, patients are more susceptible than are other groups of persons. Children are much less susceptible than are adults. Typically, halothane hepatitis develops after minor surgery without any episodes of hypoxia. The clinical picture appears a few days after the anesthetic administration. At the beginning, the increases in hepatic enzymes and bilirubin concentrations are relatively minor. However, if extensive hepatic necrosis follows, it is accompanied by a very dramatic increase in the plasma concentration of hepatic enzymes and bilirubin. Associated coagulation abnormalities and hepatic encephalopathy may follow. Liver biopsy or autopsy often reveals acute yellow atrophy and widespread hepatocellular necrosis, practically indistinguishable from the picture of fulminant viral hepatitis. Specific serologic tests may help confirm the diagnosis of halothane hepatitis.[73] The mortality rate fluctuates between 20% and 50%. The mechanism of halothane hepatitis has not been clarified. The issue is addressed in a previous section of this chapter.

Cholestasis is another possible cause of postoperative jaundice. Extrahepatic biliary obstruction can be caused by stones in the common duct, postoperative bile duct stricture, or pancreatitis. Postoperative cholestasis can also be intrahepatic in origin and can be induced by drugs or infection. This type of liver dysfunction is characterized primarily by deterioration of excretory function of the liver and is accompanied clinically by a dramatic increase in bilirubin and alkaline phosphatase concentrations in blood, whereas other hepatic enzymes, prothrombin time, and albumin concentrations are relatively normal or just slightly decreased.

Some patients with arterial hypotension and hypoxemia develop postoperative jaundice that clinically mimics that of biliary obstruction. This condition usually occurs in patients who underwent major surgical procedures, often complicated by episodes of severe hypotension or hypoxemia, extensive blood transfusion, and sometimes cardiac failure, renal failure, or sepsis. Despite the seeming severity of the disorder, it heals by itself without apparent sequelae. It has therefore been named "benign postoperative intrahepatic cholestasis."[89,194] The nature of this type of cholestasis has not been clarified.

Different kinds of infection can and do lead to postoperative hepatic dysfunction with jaundice of cholestatic origin. Many drugs such as erythromycin, tetracycline, chloramphenicol, and sulfonamides can induce cholestasis. Some other relatively rare disorders such as Gilbert's syndrome and Dubin–Johnson syndrome should also be kept in mind.

The differential diagnosis of postoperative hepatic injury may be extremely difficult. It usually is necessary to go through a rather elaborate evaluation, with the final conclusion being based on meticulous attention to small, sometimes seemingly unimportant, details related to the medical history, physical examination, laboratory tests, and perioperative course of each patient.

REFERENCES

1. LaMont JT: Postoperative jaundice. Surg Clin North Am 54:637, 1974
2. Craver WL, Johnson G Jr, Beal JM: Alterations in serum glutamic–oxalacetic transaminase activity following operations. Surg Forum 8:77, 1957
3. Dunlap RW, Dockerty MB, Waugh JM: Hepatic changes occurring during upper abdominal operations: Biopsy studies. Surg Gynecol Obstet 99:220, 1954
4. Dykes MHM, Walzer SG: Preoperative and postoperative hepatic dysfunction. Surg Gynecol Obstet 124:747, 1967
5. Morgenstein L: Postoperative jaundice, miscellaneous disorders, part 2. In Schiff L (ed): Diseases of the Liver, 4th ed, p 1353. Philadelphia, JB Lippincott, 1975
6. Clarke RSJ, Doggart JR, Lavery T: Changes in liver function after different types of surgery. Br J Anaesth 48:119, 1976
7. Evans C, Evans M, Pollock AV: The incidence and causes of postoperative jaundice. Br J Anaesth 46:520, 1974
8. Koff RS, Gardner RC, Harinasuta U et al: Profile of hyperbilirubinemia in three hospital populations. Clin Res 18:680, 1970
9. Cahalan MK, Mangano DT: Liver function and dysfunction with anesthesia and surgery. In Zakim D, Boyer TD (eds): Hepatology: A Textbook of Liver Disease, p 1250. Philadelphia, WB Saunders, 1982
10. Schemel WH: Unexpected hepatic dysfunction found by multiple laboratory screening. Anesth Analg 55:810, 1976
11. Wataneeywech M, Kelly KA Jr: Hepatic diseases unsuspected before surgery. NY State J Med 75:1278, 1975
12. National Research Council: In Bunker JP, Forrest WH Jr, Mosteller F et al: National Halothane Study: A Study of the Possible Association Between Halothane Anesthesia and Postoperative Hepatic Necrosis. Washington, DC, National Institute of General Medical Sciences, US Government Printing Office, 1969
13. Harville DD, Summerskill WHJ: Surgery in acute hepatitis: Causes and effects. JAMA 184:257, 1963
14. Keeri–Szanto M, Lafleur F: Postanaesthetic liver complications in a general hospital: A statistical study. Can Anaesth Soc J 10:531, 1963
15. Powell–Jackson P, Greenway B, Williams R: Adverse effects of exploratory laparotomy in patients with suspected liver disease. Br J Surg 69:449, 1982
16. Aranha GV, Greenlee HB: Intraabdominal surgery in patients with advanced cirrhosis. Arch Surg 121:275, 1986
17. Gelman S, Ernst E: Role of pH, PCO_2 and O_2 content of portal blood in hepatic circulatory autoregulation. Am J Physiol 233:E255, 1977
18. Lautt WW: Mechanism and role of intrinsic regulation of hepatic arterial blood flow: Hepatic arterial buffer response. Am J Physiol 249:G549, 1985
19. Rappaport AM, Borowy ZJ, Lougheed WM et al: Subdivision of hexagonal liver lobules into a structural and functional unit. Anat Rec 119:16, 1954
20. Scheidt PC, Mellits ED, Hardy JB et al: Toxicity of bilirubin in neonates: Infant development during first year in relation to maximum neonatal serum bilirubin concentration. J Pediatr 1:292, 1977
21. Naeye RL: Amniotic fluid infections, neonatal hyperbilirubinemia, and psychomotor impairment. Pediatrics 62:497, 1978
22. Haymaker W, Margoles C, Pentschew A et al: Pathology of kernicterus and posticteric encephalopathy: Presentation of 87 cases, with a consideration of pathogenesis and etiology. In Cerebral Palsy, p 221. Springfield, Illinois, Charles C Thomas, 1961
23. Karp WB: Biochemical alterations in neonatal hyperbilirubinemia and bilirubin encephalopathy: A review. Pediatrics 64:361, 1979
24. Odell GB: The distribution of bilirubin between albumin and mitochondria. J Pediatr 68:164, 1966
25. Sanchez E, Tephly TR: Activation of hepatic microsomal glucuronyl transferase by bilirubin. Life Sci 13:1483, 1973
26. Wilkinson GR, Schenker S: Drug disposition and liver disease. Drug Metab Rev 4:139, 1975
27. Williams RL, Benet LZ: Hepatic function and pharmacokinetics. In Zakim D, Boyer TD (eds): Hepatology: A Textbook of Liver Disease, p 230. Philadelphia, WB Saunders, 1982
28. Laidlaw J, Read AE, Sherlock S: Morphine tolerance in hepatic cirrhosis. Gastroenterology 40:389, 1961

29. Read AE, Laidlaw J, McCarthy CF: Effects of chlorpromazine in patients with hepatic disease. Br Med J 3:497, 1969
30. Maxwell JD, Carrella M, Parkes JD et al: Plasma disappearance and cerebral effects of chlorpromazine in cirrhosis. Clin Sci 43:143, 1972
31. Branch RA, Morgan MH, James J et al: Intravenous administration of diazepam in patients with chronic liver disease. Gut 17:975, 1976
32. Benoit JN, Granger DN: Splanchnic hemodynamics in chronic portal hypertension. Semin Liver Dis 6:287, 1986
33. Bomzon A, Blendis LM: Vascular reactivity in experimental portal hypertension. Am J Physiol 252:G158, 1987
34. Baraka A, Gabali F: Correlation between tubocurarine requirements and plasma protein pattern. Br J Anaesth 40:89, 1968
35. Parker CJR, Hunter JM: Pharmacokinetics of atracurium and laudanosine in patients with hepatic cirrhosis. Br J Anaesth 62:177, 1989
36. Bomzon A, Blendis LM: Vascular reactivity in experimental portal hypertension. Am J Physiol 252:G158, 1987
37. Richardson PDI, Withrington PG: The inhibition by glucagon of the vasoconstrictor actions of noradrenaline, angiotensin and vasopressin on the hepatic arterial vascular bed of the dog. Br J Pharmacol 57:93, 1976
38. Ettinger PO, Wu CF, DeLaCruz C Jr et al: Arrhythmias and the "holiday heart": Alcohol-associated cardiac rhythm disorders. Am Heart J 95:555, 1978
39. Witte CL, Witte MH: Splanchnic circulatory and tissue fluid dynamics in portal hypertension. Fed Proc 42:1685, 1983
40. Gelman S, Ernst E: Nitroprusside prevents adverse hemodynamic effects of vasopressin. Arch Surg 113:1465, 1978
41. Groszmann RJ, Kravetz D, Bosch J et al: Nitroglycerin improves the hemodynamic response to vasopressin in portal hypertension. Hepatology 2:757, 1982
42. Changler JG: Vasopressin and splanchnic shunting. Ann Surg 195:543, 1982
43. Price BA, Jaffe BM, Zinner MJ: Effect of exogenous somostatin infusion on gastrointestinal blood flow and hormones in the conscious dog. Gastroenterology 88:80, 1985
44. Bosch J, Mastai R, Kravetz D et al: Measurement of azygos venous blood flow in the evaluation of portal hypertension in patients with cirrhosis. J Hepatol 1:125, 1985
45. Conn HO: Propranolol in portal hypertension: Problems in paradise? Hepatology 4:560, 1984
46. Villeneuve JP, Pomier–Layragues G, Infante–Rivard C et al: Propranolol for the prevention of recurrent variceal hemorrhage: A controlled trial. Hepatology 6:1239, 1986
47. Daoud FS, Reeves JT, Schaefer JW: Failure of hypoxic pulmonary vasoconstriction in patients with liver cirrhosis. J Clin Invest 51:1076, 1972
48. Ruff F, Hughes JMB, Stanley N et al: Regional lung function in patients with hepatic cirrhosis. J Clin Invest 50:2403, 1971
49. Maennl HFK, Matzander U, Tkocz HJ et al: Surgery of portal hypertension in cirrhotics. J Abdominal Surg 18:17, 1976
50. Paumgartner G, Richter H, Brunner H et al: Enterohepatic vascular dimensions and the erythrocyte survival time in patients with cirrhosis of the liver. Wein Z Inn Med 51:278, 1970
51. Dymock IW, Tucker JS, Woolf IL et al: Coagulation studies as a prognostic index in acute liver failure. Br J Haematol 29:385, 1975
52. Samson Y, Bernuau J: Cerebral uptake of benzodiazepine measured by positron emission tomography in hepatic encephalopathy. N Engl J Med 316:414, 1987
53. Black M: Hepatic detoxification of endogenously produced toxins and their importance for the pathogenesis of hepatic encephalopathy. In Zakim D, Boyer TD (eds): Hepatology: A Textbook of Liver Disease, p 397. Philadelphia, WB Saunders, 1982
54. Epstein M: Renal functional abnormalities in cirrhosis: Pathophysiology and management. In Zakim D, Boyer TD (eds): Hepatology: A Textbook of Liver Disease, p 446. Philadelphia, WB Saunders, 1982
55. Perez–Ayuso RM, Arroyo V, Camps J et al: Renal kallikrein excretion in cirrhotics with ascites: Relationship to renal hemodynamics. Hepatology 4:247, 1984
56. Koppel MH, Coburn JW, Mims MM et al: Transplantation of cadaveric kidneys from patients with hepatorenal syndrome: Evidence for the functional nature of renal failure in advanced liver disease. N Engl J Med 280:1367, 1969
57. Epstein M: The hepatorenal syndrome. Hosp Practice, April 15, 1989, p 65
58. Dawson JL: The incidence of postoperative renal failure in obstructive jaundice. Br J Surg 52:663, 1965
59. Aarseth S, Bergan A, Aarseth P: Circulatory homeostasis in rats after bile duct ligation. Scand J Clin Lab Invest 39:93, 1979
60. Baum M, Stirling GA, Dawson JL: Further study into obstructive jaundice and ischaemic renal damage. Br Med J 2:229, 1969
61. Gibson PR, Dudley FJ: Ischaemic hepatitis: Clinical features, diagnosis and prognosis. Aust NZ J Med 14:822, 1984
62. Cohen JA, Kaplan MM: Left-sided heart failure presenting as hepatitis. Gastroenterology 74:583, 1978
63. Bynum TE, Boitnott JK, Maddrey WC: Ischemic hepatitis. Dig Dis Sci 24:129, 1979
64. Garrard CL Jr, Weissler AM, Dodge HT: The relationship of alterations in systolic time intervals to ejection fraction in patients with cardiac disease. Circulation 42:455, 1970
65. Weissler AM, Harris WS, Schoenfeld CD: Systolic time intervals in heart failure in man. Circulation 37:149, 1968
66. Better OS: Renal and cardiovascular dysfunction in liver disease. Kidney Int 29:598, 1986
67. Bomzon A, Monies–Chass I, Kamenetz L, Blendis L: Anesthesia and pressor responsiveness in chronic bile–duct–ligated dogs. Hepatology 11:551, 1990
68. Bosch J, Enriquez R, Groszmann RJ et al: Chronic bile duct ligation in the dog: Hemodynamic characterization of a portal hypertensive model. Hepatology 3:1002, 1983
69. Tamakuma S, Wada N, Ishiyama M et al: Relationship between hepatic hemodynamics and biliary pressure in dogs: Its significance in clinical shock following biliary decompression. Jpn J Surg 5:255, 1975
70. Aoyagi T, Lowenstein L: The effect of bile acid and renal ischemia on renal function. J Lab Clin Med 71:686, 1968
71. Levy M, Finestone H: Renal response to four hours of biliary obstruction in the dog. Am J Physiol 244:F516, 1983
72. Galambos JT: Cirrhosis, vol 17, p 191. Philadelphia, WB Saunders, 1979
73. Brown BR Jr, Gandolfi AJ: Adverse effects of volatile anaesthetics. Br J Anaesth 59:14, 1987
74. Kaplowitz N, Eberle D, Yamada T: Biochemical tests for liver disease. In Zakim D, Boyer TD (eds): Hepatology: A Textbook of Liver Disease, p 583. Philadelphia, WB Saunders, 1982
75. Strunin L: The Liver and Anaesthesia. Philadelphia, WB Saunders, 1977
76. Stock JGL, Strunin L: Unexplained hepatitis following halothane. Anesthesiology 63:424, 1985
77. Inman WHW, Mushin WW: Jaundice after repeated exposure to halothane: An analysis of reports to the Committee on Safety of Medicines. Br Med J 1:5, 1974
78. Bottinger LE, Dalen E, Hallen B: Halothane-induced liver damage: An analysis of the material reported to the Swedish Adverse Drug Reaction Committee 1966–1973. Acta Anaesthesiol Scand 20:40, 1976
79. Johnstone M: Letter: Halothane hepatitis. Lancet 2:526, 1978
80. Farrell G, Prendergast D, Murray M: Halothane hepatitis: Detection of a constitutional susceptibility factor. N Engl J Med 313:1310, 1985
81. Otsuka S, Yamamoto M, Kasuya S et al: HLA antigens in patients with unexplained hepatitis following halothane anesthesia. Acta Anaesthesiol Scand 29:497, 1985
82. McLain GE, Sipes IG, Brown BR: An animal model of halothane hepatotoxicity: Roles of enzyme induction and hypoxia. Anesthesiology 51:321, 1979
83. Van Dyke RA: Halogenated anaesthetic hepatotoxicity—Is the answer close at hand? Clin Anaesthesiol 1:485, 1983

84. Moore RA, McNicholas KW, Gallagher JD et al: Halothane metabolism in acyanotic and cyanotic patients undergoing open heart surgery. Anesth Analg 65:1257, 1986

85. Plummer J, Hall P de la M, Jenner MA et al: Sex differences in halothane metabolism and hepatotoxicity in a rat model. Anesth Analg 64:563, 1985

86. Gelman S: Halothane hepatotoxicity—Again? Anesth Analg 65:831, 1986

87. Shingu KI, Eger EI II, Johnson BH: Hypoxia per se can produce hepatic damage without death in rats. Anesth Analg 61:820, 1982

88. Gelman S, Rimerman V, Fowler KC et al: The effect of halothane, isoflurane, and blood loss on hepatotoxicity and hepatic oxygen availability in phenobarbital-pretreated hypoxic rats. Anesth Analg 63:965, 1984

89. Lunam CA, Cousins MJ, Hall P: Guinea pig model of halothane-associated hepatotoxicity in the absence of enzyme induction and hypoxia. J Pharmacol Exp Ther 232:802, 1985

90. Hursh D, Gelman, Bradley EL Jr: Hepatic oxygen supply during halothane and isoflurane anesthesia in guinea pigs. Anesthesiology 67:701, 1987

91. Gelman S: General anesthesia and hepatic circulation. Can J Physiol Pharmacol 252:G648, 1987

92. Nagano K, Gelman S, Parks D, Bradley E: Hepatic oxygen supply—uptake relationship and metabolism during anesthesia in miniature pigs. Anesthesiology 72:902, 1990

93. Rock P, Beattie C, Kimball AW, et al: Halothane alters the oxygen consumption—oxygen delivery relationship compared with conscious state. Anesthesiology 73:1186, 1990

94. Nagano K, Gelman S, Parks D, Bradley EL Jr: Hepatic circulation and oxygen supply—uptake relationships after hepatic ischemic insult during anesthesia with volatile anesthetics and fentanyl in miniature pigs. Anesth Analg 70:53, 1990

95. Klatskin G, Kimberg DV: Recurrent hepatitis attributable to halothane sensitization in an anesthetist. N Engl J Med 280:515, 1969

96. Blogg CE: Halothane and the liver: The problem revisited and made obsolete. Br Med J 292:1691, 1986

97. Neuberger N, Mieli–Vergani G, Tredger JM et al: Oxidative metabolism of halothane in the production of altered hepatocyte membrane antigens in acute halothane-induced necrosis. Gut 22:669, 1981

98. Rice SA, Maze M, Smith CM et al: Halothane hepatotoxicity in Fischer 344 rats pretreated with isoniazid. Toxicol Appl Pharmacol 87:411, 1987

99. Callis AH, Brooks SD, Waters SJ et al: Evidence for a role of the immune system in the pathogenesis of halothane hepatitis. In Roth SH, Miller KW (eds): Molecular and Cellular Mechanisms of Anesthetics. New York, Plenum, 1986

100. Satoh H, Fukada Y, Anderson DK et al: Immunological studies on the mechanisms of halothane-induced hepatotoxicity: Immunohistochemical evidence of trifluoroacetylated hepatocytes. J Pharmacol Exp Ther 233:857, 1985

101. Vergani D, Mieli–Vergani G, Alberti A et al: Antibodies to the surface of halothane-altered rabbit hepatocytes in patients with severe halothane-associated hepatitis. N Engl J Med 303:66, 1980

102. Neuberger J, Vergani D, Mieli–Vergani G et al: Hepatic damage after exposure to halothane in medical personnel. Br J Anaesth 53:1173, 1981

103. Lewis RB, Blair M: Halothane hepatitis in a young child. Br J Anaesth 54:349, 1982

104. Martin J, Kenna JG, Pohl LR: Antibody assays for the detection of patients sensitized to halothane. Anesth Analg 70:154, 1990

105. Van Dyke RA, Madson TH: Stimulation of phosphorylase activity by volatile anesthetics in isolated rat hepatocytes. Fed Proc 45:699, 1986

106. Gelman S, Van Dyke R: Mechanisms of halothane-induced hepatotoxicity: Another step on a long path. Anesthesiology 68:479, 1988

107. Iaizzo PA, Seewald MJ, Powis G, Van Dyke RA: The effects of volatile anesthetics on Ca^{++} mobilization in rat hepatocytes. Anesthesiology 72:504, 1990

108. Flaim KE, Jefferson LS, McGwire JB et al: Effect of halothane on synthesis and secretion of liver proteins. Mol Pharmacol 24:277, 1983

109. Eger EI II, Calverley RK, Smith NT: Changes in blood chemistries following prolonged enflurane anesthesia. Anesth Analg 55:547, 1976

110. Eger EI II, Smuckler EA, Ferrell LD et al: Is enflurane hepatotoxic? Anesth Analg 65:21, 1986

111. Wood M, Wood AJJ: Contrasting effects of halothane, isoflurane, and enflurane on in vivo drug metabolism in the rat. Anesth Analg 63:709, 1984

112. Allan LG, Howie J, Smith AF et al: Hepatic glutathione S-transferase release after halothane anaesthesia: Open randomized comparison with isoflurane. Lancet 1:771, 1987

113. Gelman S, Fowler KC, Smith LR: Liver circulation and function during isoflurane and halothane anesthesia. Anesthesiology 61:726, 1984

114. Hughes RL, Campbell D, Fitch W: Effects of enflurane and halothane on liver blood flow and oxygen consumption in the greyhound. Br J Anaesth 52:1079, 1980

115. Lewis JH, Zimmerman HJ, Ishak KG et al: Enflurane hepatotoxicity. A clinico-pathologic study of 24 cases. Ann Intern Med 98:984, 1983

116. Eger EI II: Anesthetic-induced hepatitis. IARS Review Course Lectures 116, 1986

117. Fee JPH, Black GW, Dundee JW et al: A prospective study of liver enzyme and other changes following repeat administration of halothane and enflurane. Br J Anaesth 51:1133, 1979

118. Zimmerman HJ: Hepatotoxicity: The Adverse Effects of Drugs and Other Chemicals on the Liver, p 370. Norwalk, Connecticut, Appleton-Century-Crofts, 1978

119. Hubbard AK, Gandolfi AJ, Brown BR, Jr: Immunological basis of anesthetic-induced hepatotoxicity. Anesthesiology 69:814, 1988

120. Christ DD, Kenna JG, Kammerer W et al: Enflurane metabolism produces covalently bound liver adducts recognized by antibodies from patients with halothane hepatitis. Anesthesiology 69:833, 1988

121. Stoelting RK, Blitt CD, Cohen PJ et al: Hepatic dysfunction after isoflurane anesthesia. Anesth Analg 66:147, 1987

122. Rehder K, Forbes J, Alter H et al: Halothane biotransformation in man: A quantitative study. Anesthesiology 28:711, 1967

123. Chase RE, Holaday DA, Fiserova–Bergerova V et al: The biotransformation of Ethrane in man. Anesthesiology 35:262, 1972

124. Holaday DA, Fiserova–Bergerova V, Latto IP et al: Resistance of isoflurane to biotransformation in man. Anesthesiology 43:325, 1975

125. Holmes MA, Weiskopf RB, Eger EI et al: Hepatocellular integrity in swine after prolonged desflurane (IG53) and isoflurane anesthesia: evaluation of plasma alanine aminotransferase activity. Anesth Analg 71:249, 1990

126. Lundeen G, Manohar M, Parks C: Systemic distribution of blood flow in swine while awake and during 1.0 and 1.5 MAC isoflurane anesthesia with and without 50% nitrous oxide. Anesth Analg 62:499, 1983

127. Thomson IA, Fitch HW, Campbell D: Effects of nitrous oxide on liver haemodynamics and oxygen consumption in the greyhound. Anaesthesia 37:548, 1982

128. Ellis JE, Longnecker DE: Nitrous oxide decreases renal and splanchnic blood flow in rats. Anesthesiology 61:A26, 1984

129. Koblin DD, Waskell L, Watson JE et al: Nitrous oxide inactivates methionine synthetase in human liver. Anesth Analg 61:75, 1982

130. Pratilas V, Pratila MG, Bramis J et al: The hepatoprotective effect of oxygen during halothane anesthesia. Anesth Analg 57:481, 1978

131. Prys–Roberts C, Sear JW, Low JM et al: Hemodynamic and hepatic effects of methohexital infusion during nitrous oxide anesthesia in humans. Anesth Analg 62:317, 1983

132. Brodsky JB: Toxicity of nitrous oxide. In Eger EI II (ed): Nitrous Oxide/N_2O, p 265. New York, Elsevier, 1985

133. Van Lambalgan AA, Bronsveld W, van den Bos GC et al:

Cardiovascular and biochemical changes in dogs during etomidate–nitrous oxide anaesthesia. Cardiovasc Res 16:599, 1982

134. Thomson IA, Fitch W, Hughes RL et al: Effects of certain i.v. anaesthetics on liver blood flow and hepatic oxygen consumption in the greyhound. Br J Anaesth 58:69, 1986

135. Sear JW: Ph.D. thesis: The metabolism of steroid intravenous anaesthetic agents, and their modification by liver disease. University of Bristol, 1981

136. Blunnie WP, Zacharias M, Dundee JW et al: Liver enzyme studies with continuous infusion anaesthesia. Anaesthesia 36:152, 1981

137. Kawar PK, Briggs LP, Bahar M et al: Liver enzyme studies with disoprofol (ICI 35868) and midazolam. Anaesthesia 37:305, 1982

138. Robinson FP, Patterson CC: Changes in liver function tests after propofol (Diprivan). Postgrad Med J 61(suppl 3):160, 1985

139. Dundee JW, Fee JPH, Moore J et al: Changes in serum enzyme levels following ketamine infusions. Anaesthesia 35:12, 1980

140. Sear JW, Prys–Roberts C, Dye A: Hepatic function after anaesthesia for major vascular reconstructive surgery: A comparison of four anaesthetic techniques. Br J Anaesth 55:560, 1983

141. Sear JW: Toxicity of i.v. anaesthetics. Br J Anaesth 59:24, 1987

142. Jones RM, Detmer M, Hill AB et al: Incidence of choledocho-duodenal sphincter spasm during fentanyl-supplemented anesthesia. Anesth Analg 60:638, 1981

143. Economou G, Ward–McQuaid JN: A crossover comparison of the effect of morphine, pethidine, and pentazocine on biliary pressure. Gut 12:218, 1971

144. Tremblay PR, Poncelet P, Dinh DK: Le fentanyl et la pression dans les voies biliaires. Can Anaesth Soc J 20:747, 1973

145. Arguelles JE, Franatovic Y, Romo–Salas F et al: Interbiliary pressure changes produced by narcotic drugs and inhalation anesthetics in guinea pigs. Anesth Analg 58:120, 1979

146. Vatashsky E, Haskel Y: Effect of nalbuphine on intrabiliary pressure in the early postoperative period. Can Anaesth Soc J 33:433, 1986

147. MacGilchrist AJ, Birnie GG, Cook A et al: Pharmacokinetics and pharmacodynamics of intravenous midazolam in patients with severe alcoholic cirrhosis. Gut 27:190, 1986

148. Trouvin JH, Farinotti R, Haberer JP et al: Pharmacokinetics of midazolam in anaesthetized cirrhotic patients. Br J Anaesth 60:762, 1988

149. Chauvin M, Ferrier C, Haberer JP et al: Sufentanil pharmacokinetics in patients with cirrhosis. Anesth Analg 68:1, 1989

150. Servin F, Desmonts JM, Haberer JP et al: Pharmacokinetics and protein binding of propofol in patients with cirrhosis. Anesthesiology 69:887, 1988

151. Pandele G, Chaux F, Salvadori C et al: Thiopental pharmacokinetics in patients with cirrhosis. Anesthesiology 59:123, 1983

152. Ferrier C, Marty J, Bouffard Y et al: Alfentanil pharmacokinetics in patients with cirrhosis. Anesthesiology 62:480, 1985

153. Patwardhan RV, Johnson RF, Hoyumpa A Jr et al: Normal metabolism of morphine in cirrhosis. Gastroenterology 81:1006, 1981

154. Maziot JX, Sandouk P, Zerlaoui P et al: Pharmacokinetics of morphine in normal and cirrhotic patients. Anesthesiology 61:A244, 1984

155. Ghoneim MM, Pandya H: Plasma protein binding of thiopental in patients with impaired renal or hepatic function. Anesthesiology 42:545, 1975

156. Bell LE, Slattery JT, Calkins DF: Effect of halothane–oxygen anesthesia on the pharmacokinetics of diazepam and its metabolites in rats. J Pharmacol Exp Ther 233:94, 1985

157. Reilly CS, Wood AJJ, Koshakji RP et al: The effect of halothane on drug disposition: Contribution of changes in intrinsic drug metabolizing capacity and hepatic blood flow. Anesthesiology 63:70, 1985

158. Burney RG, DiFazio CA: Hepatic clearance of lidocaine during N_2O anesthesia in dogs. Anesth Analg 55:322, 1976

159. Berger JM, Stirt JA, Sullivan SF: Enflurane, halothane, and aminophylline—Uptake and pharmacokinetics. Anesth Analg 62:733, 1983

160. Duthie DJR, Nimmo WS: The pharmacokinetics of fentanyl by constant rate IV infusion for pain relief after surgery. Anesthesiology 63:A282, 1985

161. Ghoneim MM, van Hamme MJ: Pharmacokinetics of thiopentone: Effects of enflurane and nitrous oxide anaesthesia and surgery. Br J Anaesth 50:1237, 1978

162. Runciman WB, Mather LE: Effects of anaesthesia on drug disposition. In Feldman SA, Scurr CF, Paton SW (eds): Drugs in Anaesthesia: Mechanisms of Action, p 87. London, Edward Arnold, 1987

163. Fiserova–Bergerova V: Inhibitory effect of isoflurane upon oxidative metabolism of halothane. Anesth Analg 63:399, 1984

164. Sear JW, Walters FJM, Wilkins DG et al: Etomidate by infusion for neuroanaesthesia. Anaesthesia 39:12, 1984

165. Idvall J, Aronsen KF, Stenberg P et al: Pharmacodynamic and pharmacokinetic interactions between ketamine and diazepam. Eur J Clin Pharmacol 24:337, 1983

166. Gelman S: Effects of anesthetics on splanchnic circulation. In Altura BM, Halevy S (eds): Cardiovascular Action of Anesthetics and Drugs used in Anesthesia, p. 126. Basel, Karger Publishing, 1986

167. Gelman S: Disturbances in hepatic blood flow during anesthesia and surgery. Arch Surg 111:881, 1976

168. McNeill JR, Pang CC: Effect of pentobarbital anesthesia and surgery on the control of arterial pressure and mesenteric resistance in cats: Role of vasopressin and angiotensin. Can J Physiol Pharmacol 60:363, 1982

169. Johnston IDA: Endocrine aspects of the metabolic response to surgical operation. Ann R Coll Surg Engl 35:270, 1964

170. Oyama T: Endocrine response to general anesthesia and surgery. Monogr Anaesthesiol 11:1, 1983

171. Harper MH, Collins P, Johnson BH et al: Postanesthetic hepatic injury in rats: Influence of alterations in hepatic blood flow, surgery, and anesthesia time. Anesth Analg 61:79, 1982

172. Refsum HE: Arterial hypoxaemia, serum activity of GO-T, GP-T and LDH, and central lobular liver cell necrosis in pulmonary insufficiency. Clin Sci 25:369, 1963

173. Sims JL, Morris LE, Orth OS et al: The influence of oxygen and carbon dioxide levels during anesthesia upon postsurgical hepatic damage. J Lab Clin Med 38:388, 1951

174. Viegas O, Stoelting RK: LDH5 changes after cholecystectomy or hysterectomy in patients receiving halothane, enflurane, or fentanyl. Anesthesiology 51:556, 1979

175. Zinn SE, Fairley HB, Glenn JD: Liver function in patients with mild alcoholic hepatitis, after enflurane, nitrous oxide–narcotic, and spinal anesthesia. Anesth Analg 64:487, 1985

176. Loft S, Boel J, Kyst A et al: Increased hepatic microsomal enzyme activity after surgery under halothane or spinal anesthesia. Anesthesiology 62:11, 1985

177. Oikkonen M, Rosenberg PH, Neuvonen PJ: Hepatic metabolic ability during anaesthesia. Anaesthesia 39:660, 1984

178. Gelman S, Dillard E, Bradley EL Jr: Hepatic circulation during surgical stress and anesthesia with halothane, isoflurane, or fentanyl. Anesth Analg 66:936, 1987

179. Strunin L, Davies JM: The liver and anaesthesia. Can Anaesth Soc J 30:208, 1983

180. Kang YG, Gelman S: Liver transplantation. In Gelman S (ed): Anesthesia and Organ Transplantation, p 139. Philadelphia, WB Saunders, 1987

181. Duvaldestin P, Agoston S, Henzel D et al: Pancuronium pharmacokinetics in patients with liver cirrhosis. Br J Anaesth 50:1131, 1978

182. Ward S, Neill EAM: Pharmacokinetics of atracurium in acute hepatic failure (with acute renal failure). Surv Anesth 28:364, 1984

183. Arden JR, Cannon JC, Lynam DP et al: Vecuronium pharmacokinetics and pharmacodynamics in hepatocellular disease. Anesth Analg 66:S3, 1987

184. Gelman S, Ernst EA: Hepatic circulation during sodium nitroprusside infusion in the carbon tetrachloride–treated dog. Ala J Med Sci 19:371, 1982

185. Westra P, Houwertjes C, DeLange AR et al: Effect of experimental cholestasis on neuromuscular blocking drugs in cats. Br J Anaesth 52:747, 1980

186. McCammon RL, Viegas OJ, Stoelting RK et al: Naloxone reversal of choledochoduodenal sphincter spasm associated with narcotic administration. Anesthesiology 48:437, 1978

187. Lang DW, Pilon RN: Naloxone reversal of morphine-induced biliary colic. Anesth Analg 59:619, 1980

188. Bordley J, Alson JE: The use of glucagon in operative cholangiography. Surg Gynecol Obstet 149:583, 1979

189. Jones RM, Fiddian–Green R, Knight PR: Narcotic-induced choledochoduodenal sphincter spasm reversed by glucagon. Anesth Analg 59:946, 1980

190. Tigerstedt I, Turunen MT, Hastbacka J: Effect of anaesthesia on fentanyl-induced changes in human intracholedochal pressure. Ann Clin Res 16:204, 1984

191. Belani KG, Estrin JA, Ascher NL et al: Reperfusion coagulopathy during human liver transplantation. Anesth Analg 66:S10, 1987

192. Groth CG: Changes in coagulation. In Starzl TE (ed): Experience in Hepatic Transplantation, p 54. Philadelphia, WB Saunders, 1969

193. Boher SL, Rogers EL, Koehler RC et al: Effect of hypovolemic hypotension and laparotomy on splanchnic and hepatic arterial blood flow in dogs. Curr Surg Sept–Oct 1981, p 325

194. Schmid M, Hefti ML, Gattiker R et al: A benign postoperative intrahepatic cholestasis. N Engl J Med 272:545, 1965

Theodore C. Smith

Anesthesia and Orthopaedic Surgery

Orthopaedic surgery has undergone a quiet revolution as advances in medicine have changed the orthopaedist's focus. Diseases previously responsible for large numbers of orthopaedic operations have become uncommon. Rickets and scurvy are usually detected and cured before they reach a stage that requires surgery. Poliomyelitis is nearly eradicated, and tuberculosis can be detected early and treated effectively with drugs. Antibiotics and prompt care have radically changed the character of operations for chronic osteomyelitis and septic arthritis. Early detection often results in effective nonoperative treatment for congenital hip dysplasia, clubfoot, idiopathic scoliosis, and Legg-Calvé-Perthes disease, or permits simpler surgery, as in the case of slipped femoral capital epiphysis.

Concomitantly, demographic changes and changes in health care delivery have broadened the scope of orthopaedic interests. Automobile and industrial accidents have resulted in an increase in trauma surgery. As the population ages, there are more age-related orthopaedic problems. Oncology and pain clinics are generating increasing demands for orthopaedic consultations and collaboration. Rehabilitation after stroke, spinal cord injury, and some muscular and neuromuscular disorders[1] demands new and more inventive procedures. The increasing practice of joint replacements for fingers, knees, shoulders, and especially hips has contributed to improved function and the relief of pain and suffering.[2] Sports medicine has grown from an occasional interest to a subspecialty in its own right.[3] New materials from space age technology such as carbon ribbons and carbon-reinforced plastics have invited new applications.[4,5] New sensors and controls from computer technology provide electronic assistance to paralyzed or prosthetic limbs,[6,7] which, although not yet the equivalent of television's "bionic" Six Million Dollar Man, have certainly progressed beyond Captain Hook's wildest dream. Magnetic and electromagnetic field studies have opened new investigations and new therapies in the field of bone growth and healing.[8] Piezoelectric effects and bone chemistry are adding to detailed knowledge of bone repair and remodeling under strain.

The new orthopaedics has increased the anesthesiologist's need to understand the patient, the wide variety of problems, and the complicated apparatus and procedures that appear in the modern operating room.

PREOPERATIVE CONSIDERATIONS

As in other areas of anesthesia, the preoperative period should be used for discovery and planning of orthopaedic procedures, with the anesthesiologist learning as much as possible about the patient and the procedure within the time available. In the acutely traumatized patient who needs emergency surgery, only a survey of the three most important systems—central nervous, circulatory, and respiratory—is possible. True emergencies include dislocated hip,[9] digital replantation, and the compartment syndrome. For elective procedures such as implantation or removal of prostheses, the anesthesiologist spends as long as necessary in preoperative preparation. Even in an urgent situation—for example, an elderly patient with an acute fractured hip—it may be judicious to spend 12–48 hours properly preparing the patient for surgery. Careful preoperative evaluation facilitates a rational and safe choice of anesthetic technique. It may also uncover serious systemic disease requiring further diagnostic and therapeutic measures prior to operation.[10]

Some orthopaedic patients present special considerations. The pediatric patient, the acutely traumatized patient, the arthritic patient, and the elderly patient are examples of patients in whom frequently recurring problems are met by common solutions (Table 44-1).

Pediatric Patients

Special problems in pediatric anesthesiology include the small airway diameter, high cardiac index, and small blood volume of young children, a sensitivity to certain drugs and resistance to others, and lack of cooperation, especially when pain is present (see Chapter 48). Children may be distressed from acute injury or from recollection of prior hospitalizations and anesthetic episodes. The patient's history is commonly taken from a parent or guardian. The physical examination and various laboratory tests are easier if rapport can be established with the child and cooperation achieved. Good rapport improves the likelihood that subsequent inductions of anesthesia will be pleasant in children with cerebral palsy, muscular dystrophy, and other diseases that may necessitate multiple procedures.[11] The mentally

TABLE 44-1. Common Patients and Problems in Orthopaedics

Patient	Airway	Circulation	Pain	Medication	Allied
Pediatric	Narrow diameter	Small blood volume	Uncooperative	Varied tolerance	Congenital anomalies
Traumatized	Facial injury	Blood loss	Severe pain	Prior opioids	Hidden injuries
Arthritic	Difficult intubation	Cardiac dysrhythmia	Chronic pain	Aspirin steroids	Limits to positioning
Elderly	Edentulous, sleep apnea	Ischemic diseases	Disorientation	Multiple interactions	Multisystem afflictions

Certain problems such as noted here occur so frequently that experienced anesthesiologists develop a well-thought-out approach to their management. Although it is economical timewise to have such routines, the measures should not be applied unless they are appropriate and consistent with the management of other concurrent problems. Common practice may be routine, but routine is never mandatory.

retarded child may pose particular problems in gaining rapport and cooperation, but no unusual problems exist in sensitivity to anesthetic drugs.[12] Regional anesthesia is increasingly used in children.[13,14]

Traumatized Patients

Patients who have sustained acute trauma must undergo a careful evaluation of all systems by a multidisciplinary team. Modern trauma care requires the institution of emergency treatment for potentially lethal events before the initial evaluation is complete (see Chapter 51). Diagnostic steps are initiated in an order that will detect life-threatening injuries first. Entities that require immediate attention, such as hypotension, respiratory obstruction or depression, facial and neck lesions that affect airway patency, severed blood vessels, pneumothorax, hemothorax, hemopericardium, ruptured viscus, nervous system injury, and peridural hematoma, should be detected and treated immediately.[15] In the absence of life-threatening problems, relief of severe pain can be addressed. The possibility of prior administration of opioids should be considered, and the dosage should be adjusted if necessary. On resuscitation, a previously ineffective intramuscular dose may unexpectedly exert its several effects.

After important occult injuries have been ruled out, relatively urgent intervention may be needed for some fractures. Immobilization will help prevent secondary injury to other organs, minimize pain, and decrease the incidence of fat embolism. Rapid treatment of femoral, pelvic, and some open fractures can help limit the amount of bleeding. If a period of more than 6 hours separates the traumatic incident and surgery, the risk of infection may mandate that an open wound not be closed primarily. Delaying an orthopaedic procedure may result in excessive soft-tissue swelling, which can make closed reduction of a fracture more difficult or the compartment syndrome more likely.

Under stress, in the presence of severe pain, or after opioid administration, gastric emptying time may be prolonged severalfold. Early treatment with cimetidine (doses of 300 mg given 6 hours apart) helps to decrease hydrogen ion secretion. Antacids neutralize existing acid. Soluble salts such as sodium citrate are less damaging than particulate suspensions if aspirated. Metoclopramide (10 mg given over 1 hour prior to induction, or given intravenously [iv] over 1–2 minutes) can decrease gastric emptying time. However, even waiting 6–8 hours for gastric emptying to occur will not ensure an empty stomach, and precautions against regurgitation and aspiration must be taken.

In patients with cervical vertebral fracture, dislocation, or subluxation, the possibility of spinal cord damage with neck motion must be considered. When the nature of the procedure and the patient's desires permit, regional anesthesia is preferable. When general anesthesia is elected, a clear airway must be ensured prior to induction of anesthesia.

Arthritic Patients

Arthritic patients often present with chronic pain and fixation of the joints, making positioning difficult. Because tracheal intubation is often difficult, physical examination should include evaluation of the patient's airway, focusing on the range of motion of the neck, temporomandibular joint function, and jaw motion.[16,17] A hoarse, thin voice may be a clue to cricoarytenoid dysfunction. Instability at the first or second cervical vertebra may prove problematic during positioning and tracheal intubation and may warrant lateral spine radiography or computed tomography (CT). Cervical myelopathy may exist even if plain radiographs of the axis and atlas appear normal.[18] Tracheal intubation may be difficult in patients with ankylosing spondylitis (Marie-Strümpell disease) because of cervical fixation in flexion, unsuspected fracture, or cord compression.[19,20] When tracheal intubation is necessary, special aids (e.g., modified laryngoscopes, lighted stylets, and flexible fiberoptic laryngoscopes) can be helpful (see Chapter 26). In rare cases, tracheostomy under local anesthesia must be performed before anesthesia can be safely induced. If tracheal intubation is not necessary, oral or nasal airways may aid in maintaining unobstructed breathing. Topical anesthesia produced before induction facilitates the introduction of an airway under light anesthesia, with decreased respiratory and circulatory consequences.

The specific arthritic condition frequently suggests associated problems that may be of importance to the anesthesiologist. Osteoarthritis may relate to obesity or to repetitive occupational stress. The gouty arthritic patient may have renal disease. The traumatic arthritic patient may have other sequelae of the accident. The patient with infectious arthritis may have bacteremia or metastatic infections. The patient with rheumatoid arthritis usually has multiple manifestations that may include airway limitation, pleural effusion, pulmonary fibrosis with alveolar capillary block syndrome, cardiac dysrhythmias and conduction defects, valvular involvement, coronary insufficiency, renal amyloid disease, and anemia.[21]

The arthritic patient is likely to be taking a variety of medications of significance to the anesthesiologist. Aspirin depresses platelet function, with the attendant risk of increased bleeding. Steroid therapy is frequent and carries the risk of adrenal cortical insufficiency in the setting of surgical and anesthetic stress. The characteristic thin skin and decreased subcutaneous fat may make venipuncture difficult, and infiltration around even a soft venous catheter is a frequent problem. Steroids prescribed for arthritis are selected for their anti-inflammatory efficacy and relative lack of mineralocorticoid effect. Steroid replacement intraoperatively and postoperatively should be chosen to ensure both glucocorticoid and mineralocorticoid effects. A common regimen for a patient undergoing an extensive surgical procedure includes a preoperative dose of hydrocortisone, 100 mg, followed by a 100-mg dose every 6 hours for the first postoperative day, with tapering of the daily dose by 100 mg each day thereafter.

Elderly Patients

Elderly patients have decreased reserve in every body system (see Chapter 49). Even in the absence of disease there is progressive loss of brain cells, nephrons, alveoli, muscle fibers, and even subcellular organelles, as well as stiffening of heart and skeletal muscles, lung tissue, ligaments, and tendons.[22] Not only is there a general decrease in the number of functioning cells, but the capabilities of the remaining cells and systems also slowly decrease (Fig. 44-1). Mental quickness and acuity, arterial oxygen tension, cardiac index, and gastrointestinal motility diminish. Special senses are obtunded, with presbyopia, presbyacusia, hyposmia, and failing taste commonplace. Lack of dentition makes airway maintenance more difficult.

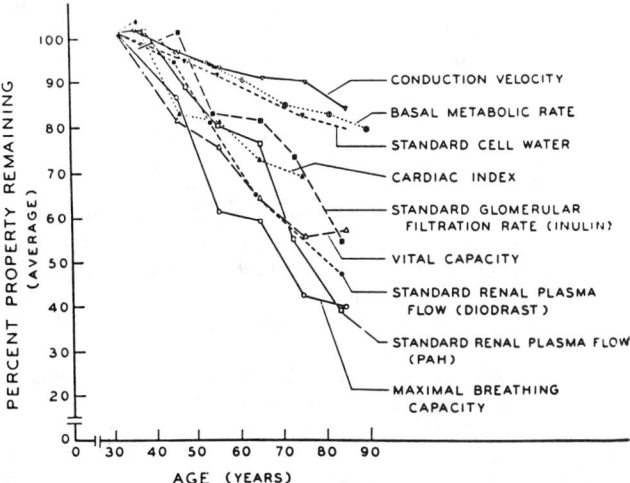

Figure 44-1. Changes in physiologic functions with aging. For each function, values are expressed as the percentage of the mean value for subjects aged 25–35 years. All subjects were men. Whereas deterioration occurs at different rates for different functions, measures of reserve such as maximum breathing capacity (now called maximum voluntary ventilation) fall faster than resting values such as basal metabolic rate. (Reproduced by permission from Jeffers FC [ed]: The science of gerontology. In Proceedings of Seminars 1959–61, p 123. Durham, Duke University Press, 1962.)

Mental status is an important factor in the evaluation of elderly patients. There is a great difference between a septuagenarian who fractures a hip canvassing door to door during a political campaign and another who fractures a hip while stumbling to an adjacent bathroom in a nursing home. Disorientation in the elderly can result from the absence of familiar people and surroundings, from pain, or from multiple medications. The potential interactions of these medications with anesthetic drugs must be kept in mind.

The elderly also have a high prevalence of degenerative diseases, including Alzheimer's disease, ischemic cerebral and cardiovascular problems, and emphysema. Thus, hypoxia is more likely and more dangerous in these patients.[23] The elderly are also prone to become confused in the postoperative period. Although the incidence does not appear to be related to the choice of anesthetic, preoperative depression and premedication with anticholinergic drugs can be contributory factors.[24] Nonetheless, with care, even nonagenarians may undergo anesthesia and surgery with a mortality approaching that of age- and sex-matched nonoperate cohorts.[25]

INTRAOPERATIVE MANAGEMENT

Choice of Anesthetic Technique

Although the final choice of anesthesia depends on the usual interplay of patient and surgical factors, one can build a strong argument for consideration of specific nerve blockades, iv regional anesthesia, plexus anesthesia, and spinal or epidural blockade in orthopaedic anesthesia. Even though there are potential complications of spinal and epidural anesthesia, several studies provide data favoring these methods over general anesthesia for high-risk patients[26] and those having hip procedures.[27-32] Larger studies show that the 6% mortality 1 month after a regional block can be equaled with general anesthesia.[33-35] Newer agents continue to appear, offering broader and potentially better choices.[36] In operations in which low regional blockade can be used, abdominal motor power and hence cough are preserved, and a number of potential advantages may be realized, including profound skeletal muscle relaxation,[29] normal respiratory mechanics,[37] no maldistribution of ventilation-perfusion matching,[38] blockade of the stress response,[39] decreased blood loss,[27,40] decreased venous thromboembolism without additional anticoagulants,[41-49] decreased serum enzymes,[50] preservation of monocyte function,[51] postoperative analgesia,[52] and lower immediate mortality,[47] although studies differ on the possible benefit in terms of long-term mortality.[25,32] An extensive review by Scott and Kehlet of 86 reports in the literature favored regional anesthesia on balance for infraumbilical procedures, although a formal meta-analysis was not attempted.[53] The active beneficial effects of spinal or epidural anesthesia may even accrue in patients with cardiac problems.[54] Upper abdominal procedures are associated with about the same incidence of pulmonary complications after regional anesthesia as after general anesthesia,[55] probably because of equivalent diaphragmatic dysfunction in either case.

Use of regional anesthesia is sometimes limited because of lack of patient acceptance. Some anesthesiologists feel repugnance about "selling" patients on spinal, epidural, or peripheral nerve blockade anesthesia. It takes time and tact to explain that general anesthesia is not equivalent to sleep, and that spinal anesthesia does not require that the patient remain wide awake with full perception. It may be instructive to recall that John Lundy, in 1926, coined the term "balanced anesthesia" to describe major nerve blockade or spinal anesthesia combined with light general obtundation.[56]

A patient's desires and expectations may be satisfactorily met only if time and effort are expended to understand them. Inaz et al,[57] in a study of European practice, found that patients brought an "out-dated and distorted attitude toward anesthesia, but that overall they [were] comparably satisfied with regional and general anesthesia." Specific suggestions for specific procedures are given below.

Positioning

No other surgical specialty uses such varied positions as orthopaedics. The positions, chosen primarily to facilitate operative exposure of bones and joints, are secondarily modified for physiologic considerations. Increasingly complex "fracture tables" with special attachments often replace the typical operating room table (Fig. 44-2). Because the patient may be in pain preoperatively or may suffer pain during positioning on the fracture table, anesthetization before final positioning may be necessary. This places an additional burden on the surgeon and anesthesiologist—that of ensuring safety for the unconscious or paralyzed patient during positioning. Surgeons, operating room staff, and anesthesiologists should discuss and agree on the positioning procedure. A compromise between optimal exposure, optimal circulation, and ventilation may be needed, but the anesthesiologist must be able to protect the airway and monitor ventilation and circulation at all times.

The supine position is usually safe and simple. For some arthroscopies, a leg-holder may support the thigh.[58] This should be placed so as not to injure muscle, nerve, or vessels or to place unusual strain on joints that will be unsupported when anesthesia or paralysis decreases skeletal muscle tone. The leg-holder may be tried just before induction of anesthesia to be sure that it is reasonably comfortable. When a fracture table is used, the supine position offers more of a challenge. The trunk is usually supported by a sacral plate and post, which must be properly padded, and a biscapular shelf. Arm supports must protect against brachial plexus stretch. On many tables the Trendelenburg position is neither quickly nor easily achieved, making treatment of vomiting or hypotension more difficult. Two people may be needed to support and elevate the patient's legs when the lock is released to provide head-down tilt. A special key or wrench may be needed to operate the lock. The vagaries and mechanisms of specific tables must be familiar to the operating room team preoperatively.

The prone position is used primarily for spinal operations, with the goal of preserving thoracic kyphosis and reversing lumbar lordosis without increasing abdominal pressure. Pressure not only compromises ventilation but decreases venous return, contributing to hypotension and increased venous bleeding in the wound. Various mattresses, frames, and supports have been devised for these purposes. Ventilation is usually adequate if the chest and abdomen are free to move laterally or anteriorly. Frames that support the trunk by the sides and that can be arched after the patient is placed on them are useful, simple, and stable.[59] Supporting the patient with upper thoracic rolls or supports placed under the acromioclavicular joint and with iliac supports is better, in theory, for abdominal pressure and excursion, but in practice may be less stable.

Flexing the supine patient's thighs past a 90-degree angle

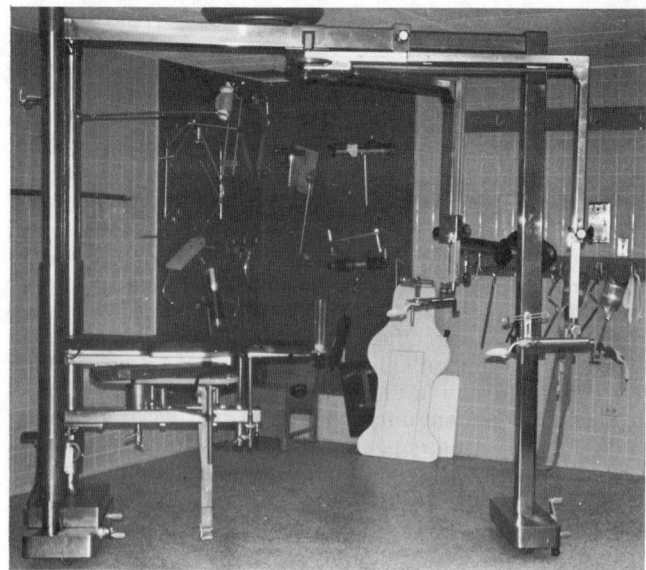

Figure 44-2. This orthopaedic fracture table is one of many available for complex operative approaches to pelvic, hip, and leg fractures. In this model, a single-foot–operated hydraulic pump raises the two posts at the head and the single post at the foot simultaneously with the back plate and arm board supports. Two buttons release the head and foot pillars separately to allow either tilting or lowering. Two separate foot supports provide adjustable distraction. A hand crank at the head end provides side tilt, while a foot treadle at the other end locks the wheels. In the background are other typical appliances such as a hand table, thigh and knee supports, and weights tourniquets.

puts sufficient tension on the relaxed gluteal muscles to reverse the lordosis optimally. This may be overdone in the "Mohammedan praying position"; Dinmore describes one of several buttock supports that are safe, comfortable, and effective.[60] Failure to flex the thighs more than 90 degrees leads to instability, allowing for shifts during operation. If a body cast has been applied preoperatively, the anesthesiologist should be certain he or she can remove part or all of it if resuscitation is necessary.

The sitting position is occasionally used for operations on the shoulder and neck. The anesthesiologist should be wary of orthostatic hypotension after induction of anesthesia and should elevate the patient's back slowly, with frequent checking of blood pressure. Elastic bandaging of the lower limbs before moving the patient to the sitting position helps to avoid hypotension. The hips may be flexed 20–45 degrees and the knees 15–20 degrees to achieve a *chaise lounge* effect for stability and to decrease venous pooling. Care should be taken to keep the head supported, which will avoid neck injuries and airway obstruction.

Spontaneous ventilation is more effective if the patient is sitting than if the patient is supine. The incidence of air embolism and pneumothorax is small for operations on the shoulder performed with the patient sitting. Air embolism may occur during cervical laminectomy in the sitting position. An esophageal stethoscope, transthoracic Doppler device, and end-tidal carbon dioxide monitor are helpful in diagnosis. In high-risk patients, a right atrial catheter permits removal of air.

The lateral position is commonly used for prosthetic hip replacement and occasionally for laminectomy. The problems associated with this position are primarily comfort for the awake patient and stability for the unconscious patient. Extra mattresses or a layer of "egg crate" foam over the usual mattress are appreciated by the awake patient. Pillows rather than folded sheets or blankets are always more comfortable when the patient must lie on his ear and not move for hours. The extremities should be moderately flexed for comfort. When hypobaric spinal anesthesia is used, a small additional injection of hyperbaric drug will often promote comfort in the dependent parts. The use of ribbed hypo-hyperthermia blankets under the patient is rarely effective in this position because of the decreased area of contact. If body temperature decreases, a smaller water blanket draped over the thorax is additionally effective in rewarming.

Stability may be promoted with side-to-side 7.5-cm adhesive straps, but these must be applied carefully. The upper arm and elbow may be included in the strapping of the shoulder girdle. Better and safer support is achieved with appliances, attached to the table, that cradle the pelvis and shoulder girdle, or with individually moldable bean bags, which are set by vacuum. An axillary roll is often routinely placed, presumably to prevent nerve and vascular compression in this position. However, neurovascular compression is a problem in the lateral position only when obesity causes a roll of fat to compress axillary structures. A palpable pulse, visual inspection, and a free-flowing iv infusion in the dependent arm are sufficient evidence of adequate circulation. The other arm is reserved for blood pressure measurement and the starting of a second iv infusion if necessary. Paresthesia, edema, myonecrosis, and vascular accident may also follow groin compression. Arterial disease and obesity are risk factors.[61] Dependent limbs may be monitored with a pulse oximeter.

Occasionally, tracheal intubation is necessary while the patient is in the lateral position. Tracheal intubation is made easier with the following technique. An assistant pulls the upper shoulder back and down, so that the shoulder girdle rotates around the spinal axis about 45 degrees. The laryngoscope is initially inserted in the superior side of the mouth (the left side in patients in the right lateral decubitus position), so that the tongue falls away from the path of visualization. This may be easier than elevating the tongue. If the anesthesiologist then bends laterally at the waist, the usual view of the larynx is obtained.

Prevention of Blood Loss

Tourniquets

Orthopaedic procedures on limbs with tumors or major skeletal muscle and bone dissections may be quite bloody. In these cases, tourniquets can be useful in minimizing blood loss. The width of the inflated cuff should be more than half the limb diameter, and the cuff should be applied over limited smooth padding or none at all. Padding can promote irritation because of its wrinkles and folds, or by absorbing soap or iodophor. During skin preparation, the cuff and padding may be protected with temporary absorbent padding or with an impermeable plastic drape placed just distal to the cuff. The cuff should more than encircle the limb to ensure circumferentially uniform pressure, and the point of overlap should be placed 180 degrees from the neurovascular bundle, because there is some area of decreased compression at the overlap point (Fig. 44-3). Pressure is maintained by compressed gas (air or oxygen), a volatile refrigerant (Freon), or a dedicated pump and must be monitored continually while the tourniquet is in use.

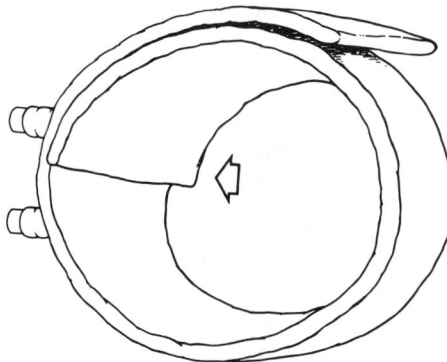

Figure 44-3. Typical modern pneumatic tourniquet. Note the point of overlap (*arrow*) where the pressure exerted by the cuff on the underlying tissue is uncertain but lower than that opposite it. This area of overlap should be opposite the neurovascular bundle of a limb rather than over it.

Deliberately squeezing the inflated cuff should produce visible oscillations on the cuff pressure monitor, which itself should be regularly checked for accuracy, linearity, hysteresis,[62] and pressure creep from faulty regulators.[63] The limb should be elevated for about 1 minute and tightly wrapped with an Esmarch bandage distally to proximally immediately before the cuff is inflated. Since compressive exsanguination may be unwise when there is infection or tumor, limb tourniquets are relatively contraindicated in these situations.

Opinions differ as to the pressure required in tourniquets to prevent bleeding. Some gauges are marked with average arm and leg pressures, but it is irrational to expect that all patients will be average. Leg tourniquets are often pressurized more than arm tourniquets, on the theory that larger limbs require more pressure than smaller limbs. Shaw and Murray[64] have shown that deep tissue pressure is 70–95% of intracuff pressure, depending mainly on the diameter of the limb. Femoral systolic pressure is slightly higher than brachial pressure, owing to complex hemodynamic factors. If the cuff is applied loosely, there may be a big pressure drop across the noncompliant cuff wall itself. A cuff pressure 100 mm Hg above a patient's measured systolic pressure is adequate for the thigh, and 50 mm Hg above systolic pressure is adequate for the arm, with the understanding that if hypertensive episodes occur, the cuff pressure should be increased. Various techniques to determine the optimal cuff pressure from the concurrent blood pressure give widely varying results.[65] Continued oozing after cuff inflation may rarely be due to inadequate occlusion of the major arterial inflow, which is corrected by cuff reapplication and use of the proper degree of inflation. Oozing is more commonly due to intramedullary blood flow in the long bones, particularly in the skeletally immature, and to small arterial vessels between the two bones of distal extremities. In neither of these cases will overinflation stop the oozing.

A properly maintained, properly applied, and properly monitored pneumatic tourniquet is reasonably safe. There are reports of fatal pulmonary embolus, apparently caused solely by inflation of a tourniquet on a traumatized limb, and there are several reports of emboli following Esmarch bandaging.[66-68] The duration of safe tourniquet inflation is unknown.[69] Recommendations range from 30 minutes to 4 hours. Five minutes of intermittent perfusion between 1- and 2-hour inflations, followed by repeated exsanguination through elevation and compression, may allow more extended use by resupplying intracellular high-energy me-tabolites.[70] But reperfusion may also supply more substrate for free radical production. Local hypothermia protects muscle from ischemia,[71,72] and lack of tonic muscle activity after motor block is also likely protective. When tourniquets are used at multiple sites, it is wise to loosen or remove underlying padding at one site before starting at the next site.

There are a few reports of damage to underlying vessels, nerves, and skeletal muscles.[73] The injury is a function of both inflation pressure and duration of inflation.[63,74] The pressure under the cuff is more damaging than the distal ischemia.[74,75] Arterial spasm, venous thrombosis, and nerve injury are all demonstrable after many hours, depending on the technique used to search for injury. Electron microscopy performed after 1 hour of ischemia shows only depletion of glycogen granules in sarcoplasm, with some extracellular edema.[76] After 2 hours there are lesions of acidosis: mito-chondrial swelling, myelin degeneration, and Z-line lysis (Fig. 44-4).[74] Clinical examination, electromyography, and effluent blood analysis all show completely reversible changes for inflations of 1 to 2 hours.[77,78] Heppenstall and co-workers showed that for similar periods of compression, tourniquet ischemia is more easily reversible than high tis-sue pressure ischemia (compartment syndrome).[79]

Transient systemic metabolic acidosis and increased arte-rial carbon dioxide levels after tourniquet deflation do not cause deleterious effects in healthy patients.[80-82] Measurable changes include a 10–15% increase in heart rate, a 5–10% increase in serum potassium, and a rise of 1–8 mm Hg in carbon dioxide tension in blood, depending on whether or not the patient is mechanically ventilated. There is also the expected acidosis, generally representing a fall of 0.1 pH unit or less. Prolonged inflation or the simultaneous release of two tourniquets may produce clinically significant acido-sis, particularly in previously acidotic patients.[80] There is one report of a severe increase in intracranial pressure after release.[83] An increase of 20–50% in controlled minute vol-ume will avoid the acidosis and the arousal seen in general anesthesia.[81]

Rarely, neuralgia paresthetica has been reported, which reverses within weeks to months. Sickling of red cells in properly exsanguinated limbs is not a problem.[84] Alteration in clotting factors does not occur. Reactive hyperemia in the limb lasts no more than 30–45 minutes after tourniquet deflation. When the tourniquet is released, potassium and acid metabolites, which are washed out, become diluted with the rest of the cardiac output and usually cause no serious systemic changes.[80,85] However, foreign material ad-ministered iv in a Bier block has caused loss of a forearm.[86] Washout of local anesthetic drug may produce rapid return of sensation after lidocaine anesthesia, or toxic blood levels after bupivacaine anesthesia. Studies have *not* established a protocol for intermittent cuff release that yields lower sys-temic drug concentrations.[87] Prilocaine is reportedly a suit-able compromise, giving long enough analgesia following tourniquet release to permit surgical hemostasis and closure without toxicity.[88,89] An alternative approach that avoids prilocaine and its risk of methemoglobinemia is the use of low-dose iv regional blockade, with the blockade repeated by infusion through an indwelling catheter.[90]

When a pneumatic tourniquet is used with regional anes-thetic techniques, a number of patients complain of dull aching pain or become restless, even though seemingly ade-quate analgesia exists for the operation itself. Patient dis-comfort appears about 45 minutes after the tourniquet is inflated and becomes more intense with time. No satisfac-tory explanation for its genesis has been found. Two early

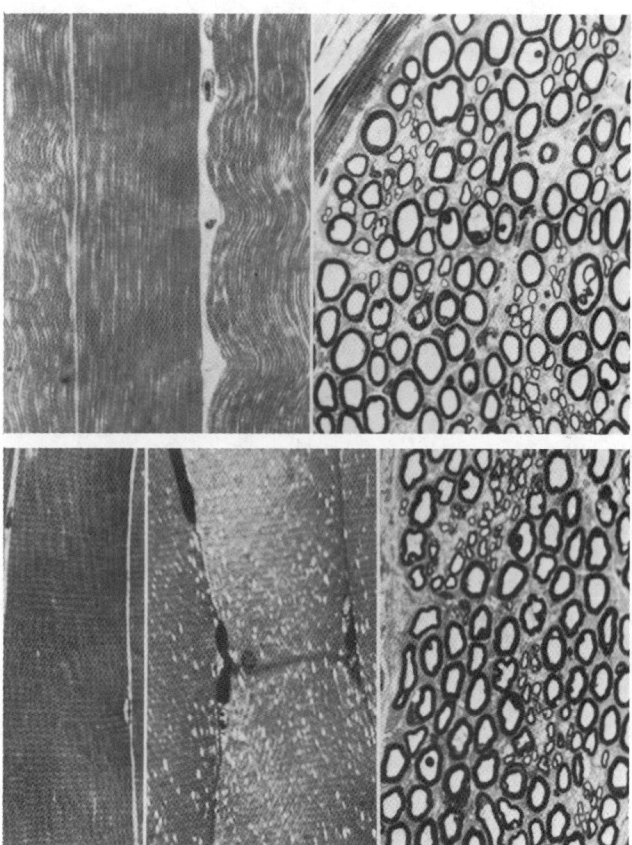

Figure 44-4. Electron micrographs of nerve (*top*) and muscle (*bottom*). After 3 hours of ischemia, the muscle was normal in appear-ance (*left panel*). After 4 hours, small vacuoles began to appear. Also noted in other sections were swelling of mitochondria and di-lation of sarcoplasmic reticulum, but the nerve was normal. (Re-printed with permission from Tountas CP, Bergman RA: Tourniquet ischemia: Ultrastructural and histochemical observations of is-chemic human muscle and of monkey muscle and nerve. J Hand Surg 2:31, 1977.)

hypotheses were suggested: (1) the pain is transmitted by large fibers that can be completely blocked only by greater concentrations of local anesthetic than are generally used[91,92]—a theory for which no anatomic evidence has been presented, and (2) the pain is transmitted by small unmyelinated fibers that travel with the sympathetic nerves and enter the spinal cord at a higher segment than that of cutaneous analgesia.[93,94] But Farah and Thomas gave stellate ganglion blocks in upper limb surgery and were unable to prevent tourniquet pain during Bier blockade.[95]

Current explanations involve pain transmission through both A delta and C fibers, and its modulation in the dorsal horn synapses. The C (slow pain) fibers recover faster as the block wanes. Supporting observations include the follow-ing: (1) bupivacaine produces less tourniquet pain than tet-racaine,[96] (2) glucose increases the incidence of pain,[97] (3) increasing the dose of local anesthetic decreases or delays the onset of pain,[94] (4) agents promoting frequency-dependent C fiber block reduce pain,[98] and (5) intrathecal morphine decreases the incidence but not the severity of tourniquet pain.[99]

Analogous phenomena may be observed under general anesthesia: 45–50 minutes after tourniquet inflation signs of light anesthesia (increase in blood pressure and pulse rate) often appear, even though the same concentrations of anesthetic are being delivered.[100,101] Hypotension may ensue when the tourniquet is subsequently deflated.[102]

The definitive treatment for tourniquet pain is release of the tourniquet. Relief of pain is prompt and complete, too rapid to be explained by anaerobic metabolite washed out by restored perfusion,[101] since increased blood lactate levels and ischemia both blunt somatosensory-evoked potentials.[103] During surgery, however, analgesics and hypnotics are usually administered. Sometimes only a general anesthetic will relieve the patient's discomfort and circulatory effects will persist. If excessive iv medications have been given, with or without general anesthesia, the anesthesiologist must be prepared for sudden central depression when the tourniquet is deflated and the afferent arousal ceases.

Deliberate Hypotension

Hypotension as a means of reducing surgical blood loss has been recommended when the benefits can be expected to outweigh the risks. In hip and scoliosis surgery, deliberate hypotension has proved to be beneficial.[104] In Jehovah's Witnesses, it may be the only option available.[105] In a comparative study, average blood loss during induced nitroprusside hypotension with nitrous oxide–halothane anesthesia for hip arthroplasty was 1.3 liters, whereas neuroleptanalgesia or nitrous oxide–halothane without hypotension yielded blood losses of 2.6 and 2 liters, respectively.[30] Epidural anesthesia with no attempt to alter blood pressure was associated with an intermediate blood loss, 1.6 liters. Preliminary reports suggest that low-dose epinephrine can be used to support cardiac output without hypertension or increased bleeding.[106,107] In adolescents undergoing scoliosis correction, Knight and colleagues,[108] using ganglionic blockade and propranolol during nitrous oxide–morphine anesthesia, achieved a dry field with a mean blood pressure of 40–55 mm Hg. There was no tachycardia, the cardiac index was near normal, and no increases in plasma renin, angiotensin II, norepinephrine, or dopamine levels were seen. McNeil and colleagues,[109] in another study of scoliosis surgery, found that deliberate hypotension achieved with pentolinium, trimethaphan, or deep halothane anesthesia was associated with a blood loss that was 900 ml less than that during normotension. Hypotension also shortened the operative time by 33 minutes. Diltiazem, nitroprusside with and without captopril, and nitroglycerin have also been used to induce hypotension.[110]

Replacement of Blood Loss

Despite efforts to reduce bleeding, some orthopaedic procedures can be associated with major blood loss, sometimes approximating the patient's blood volume.[111] This is especially true for patients with rheumatoid arthritis, Paget's disease, tumor metastases to bone, and those undergoing operations at the site of previous surgery. In such cases, blood loss should be continually calculated by weighing sponges, measuring the suction bottle contents, estimating the amount of blood on the drapes, and subtracting the amount of irrigating fluid.

The aim of intraoperative fluid therapy is to maintain normal circulating blood volume with adequate amounts of hemoglobin. The complications of homologous blood transfusion may be avoided by use of autologous blood or hemodilution. Several methods of autologous transfusion have been used: (1) storing the patient's blood removed 1–2 weeks preoperatively (earlier if the blood is frozen);[112-114] (2) removing blood from the patient before the procedure, replacing it with crystalline or albumin solutions, and reinfusing the blood at the end of the operation;[115] and (3) reinfusing blood removed from the operative field, especially in major trauma surgery.[116] In orthopaedic procedures, the presence of marrow fat and bone chips in the lost blood has limited the use of reinfusion techniques, but orthopaedic surgeons are increasing their use of these "cell-saving" techniques.[117-119] A theoretically attractive but complicated method for autotransfusion involves removing 1 unit of blood at the beginning of week 1, removing 2 units of blood at the beginning of week 2 and reinfusing the single unit removed the previous week, removing 3 units of blood at the beginning of week 3 and reinfusing the 2 units removed the previous week, and so on. At N + 1 weeks, N units of patient blood are available for transfusion during surgery—all 1 week old!

Moderate hemodilution is emerging as beneficial rather than tolerable. Oxygen transport has been shown to be maximal at hematocrits around 30%. Except in patients with fixed arterial resistance (e.g., severe coronary artery disease), peripheral tissue oxygenation is not compromised at even lower hematocrits.[120,121] Albumin, plasma protein fraction, cellulose, and starch solutions have been found useful in decreasing blood transfusions. Emulsions of fluorocarbons and stroma-free hemoglobin solutions offer the hope for simultaneous maintenance of vascular volume and oxygen-carrying capacity. However, the fluorocarbons have a straight-line hemoglobin dissociation curve, requiring very high oxygen tension, and dilute stroma-free hemoglobins have a markedly left-shifted dissociation curve, interfering with tissue unloading of their oxygen content. Dextran solutions find little favor today because of the possibility of bleeding and anaphylaxis,[122] although the use of haptens has reduced the incidence of the latter markedly.[41]

In choosing among the available fluids, cost, convenience, availability, and personal preference are all factors to be considered. Since full intravascular replacement of 1 ml of shed blood requires 5–7 ml of crystalloid solution or 1 ml of colloid, there is little difference in net cost between balanced salt solutions and hetastarch. However, an increased incidence of pulmonary edema may be seen after excessive infusion of electrolyte solutions unless the more conservative 3 ml for 1 ml replacement formula is used. Such a 3:1 ratio has been rationalized on the basis of the extracellular fluid to blood volume ratio, which is about 3:1, but it neglects the facts that red cell volume is a part of the intracellular space, and that the extracellular to plasma volume ratio is between 5:1 and 7:1.

Deliberate isovolemic hemodilution requires careful estimation of continuing loss, volume replacement, and maintenance of an adequate hematocrit. Since intra-anesthetic oxygen demand is lower than oxygen demand in the awake convalescing patient, many anesthesiologists believe that it is safe and in fact preferable to delay transfusion with red cell concentrates to the postoperative period if at all possible. Intraoperative hemoglobin concentrations of 8 g·dl^{-1} are probably adequate in most patients. Postoperative hemoglobin concentrations of 9–10 g·dl^{-1} can be achieved by red cell replacement in the recovery room and convalescent ward. It is safer to transfuse an awake patient, in whom signs of a transfusion reaction are more easily identifiable, and it is reasonable to allow loss of relatively low hematocrit blood intraoperatively in preference to losing recently transfused red blood cells.

With continued blood loss, replacement of red blood cells eventually becomes necessary. As with cold fluids, transfusions should be warmed before infusion, and the use of microfilters for multiple transfusions of blood should be considered (see Chapter 11).

Intraoperative Radiography

Protection from radiation should be available to the anesthesiologist. The internal shields of the x-ray generator are used to cone down the primary beam as much as possible. The secondary (scattered) radiation is inherently softer (longer wave length, less penetrating, and therefore absorbed in tissues to a greater extent). A number of practices serve to protect against this exposure. The anesthesiologist should wear the standard lead apron, be positioned as far from the axial beam of the x-ray tube as possible, and turn away at the moment of exposure to minimize thyroid and lens dosage.[123] Leaded eyeglasses and thyroid shields are available for those who are frequently exposed.[124] The greatest protection lies in the inverse square law: doubling the distance from the ionizing radiation source reduces the dose fourfold. The doors and walls of most operating suites provide little additional attenuation.

Intraoperative fluoroscopy and arthroscopy require darkened rooms. The anesthesiologist can use a flashlight to check machine settings and to observe the patient. Often a surgical light can be directed at the anesthesia machine and floor beyond the patient's head, so that the illuminated area is shielded from the surgeon's dark-adapted peripheral vision by the drapes. Even in the dark, heart tones, oxygen saturation, and electrocardiogram (ECG) may be continuously monitored. The use of anesthesia machines with a lighted display and use of videofluoroscopic equipment materially reduces the problems of radiation and patient care in the dark.

Control of Infection

Postoperative infections can be disastrous in orthopaedic surgery patients, for several reasons. They delay healing and destroy the operative repair, resulting in potentially worse function than before the corrective procedure was performed. Implanted devices or prostheses may have to be removed. Eradication of an osteomyelitis is extremely difficult, time-consuming, and expensive. Finally, subsequent surgery, even after cure of a deep infection, is more likely to become complicated by infections.[125]

Prevention of infection must be constantly kept in mind. The most common sources of wound infection are the patient's skin and oropharyngeal bacteria, airborne bacteria originating from the head and neck of operating room personnel, cross-infection from other patients, and bacteria harbored on dust and lint particles. Crow and Greene[126] showed that anesthesiologists commit aseptic transgressions at a rate twice that of surgeons. The measures available to reduce infection rates include preoperative baths and showers, meticulous skin preparation,[127] multilayered draping with impervious sterile materials,[128] use of double gloves,[129] meticulous attention to covering of the head and neck of personnel, and limiting conversation and traffic in the operating room.[130,131]

There is general acceptance that operating room attire (cap, mask, suit, and shoe covers) should be of nonlinting materials that are effective bacterial barriers, provide maxi-

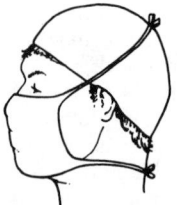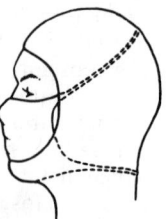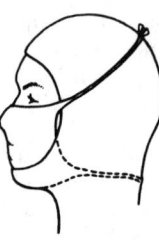

Figure 44-5. Complete coverage of facial hair is best achieved with a full hood. Although mask-inside-hood (*center*) is recommended rather than mask-over-cap (*left*), it is difficult to tie the mask directly over hair. An alternate method (*right*) involves tying the top ends over the hood and the bottom ones around the neck under the hood before tying the hood neck bands.

mal skin coverage, are comfortable, provide freedom of movement, transmit heat and water vapor, are nonflammable or flame retardant, and, although not necessarily conductive, do not accumulate static electric charge. Shirt and drawstrings should be tucked into the waistband of the trousers. Shoe covers are preferable to operating room—dedicated shoes, because the latter need but usually do not receive frequent cleaning. Face masks worn inside head hoods reduce the number of bacterial colony-forming units per cubic foot of air (Fig. 44-5).[132] The prophylactic use of antibiotics when prostheses are implanted lowers infection rates; overuse, however, leads to the development of antibiotic-resistant bacteria.

More extreme measures have been studied and recommended but have not achieved uniform acceptance. These include continuous ultraviolet radiation, high-efficiency particulate air (HEPA) filtration combined with laminar flow ventilation, and complete enclosure of the head or entire body of operating room personnel in a "space" suit supplied with an air filter system that protects not only the patient from the personnel, but the personnel from the patient. With each of these measures, more inconvenience is introduced. For example, ultraviolet light at an intensity of 25 watt·cm^{-2} at the wound reduces the infection rate[133,134] but requires that personnel wear head gear, goggles, and protective cream to protect against eye and skin damage. Lowell et al[135] suggest that it is vital to germicidal effect to control operating room humidity closely—a detail neglected in previous studies of germicidal lamps.

Application of laminar flow ventilation to operating rooms is notable because of its vast literature and remarkable cost.[136-140] HEPA filters produce a 1000-fold reduction of airborne particles larger than one-half micron in the air supply. By virtue of a great increase in ventilation at the operative site (up to 500 air exchanges per hour, as opposed to the 12–15 exchanges in ordinary operating rooms) with HEPA filters, particles shed by the operating team are excluded from the wound. Although this procedure can reduce bacterial counts, it is estimated that more than 5000 matched cases would be required in a clinical study to show a real reduction in the incidence of surgical infection caused by a single intervention such as laminar air flow. It is clear that the cost-benefit ratio would be most favorable in patients with prosthetic implants or reduced resistance to infection owing to age, disease, or therapy.

The flow of air in laminar air flow rooms may be horizontal or vertical from a plenum (a chamber in which the air is under slight pressure and emitted to the operating room through multiple adjacent orifices). In the horizontal design, the plenum is mounted on one wall and the gas flow sweeps across the operative site horizontally. This design is generally cheaper and easier to install in existing operating rooms than the vertical type, but in practice it is less easy to ensure laminar flow at the operative site. The more effective design involves a ceiling plenum that provides a high rate of laminar flow over the entire operative field. Large quantities of air must be blown through large surfaces of the HEPA filters and swept through the room in a single pass. Thus, one might expect noise and drafts. The drafts are not serious, as a linear air velocity of approximately 33 m·min^{-1} is perceived as only a gentle zephyr. As an additional feature, the Allander air curtain provides a peripheral frame of still higher flow of filtered air, which tends to entrain bacterial particles from the center of the field and prevents particles in the rest of the room from entering the operative field when they are stirred up by personnel walking about.[136]

Thoughtlessly entering a room without a cap and mask is not a serious break in technique in a laminar air flow room, but turbulence can be generated by picking up objects from the floor and depositing them within the laminar air flow area, transiently defeating the laminar flow design. In general, these rooms reinforce good sterile technique rather than compensate for carelessness.

Since most rooms recirculate air through the HEPA filters, the overflow scavengers of anesthesia machines should exhaust by a separate route. The increased air flow at the operative site promotes drying of the operative field and increases patient cooling. Noise may obscure some of the auditory clues that the anesthesiologist relies on subliminally. The overhead surgical light may materially interfere with the designed laminar flow, as may operating room microscopes, radiograph machines, and other equipment. There should be regular checks of pressure, temperature, and humidity in laminar air flow rooms.

There have been many previous studies of infection rates in operating rooms that are obsolete by present standards. Multi-institutional surveys usually disclose a wound infection rate of about 5% in all patients.[141] However, numerous studies of infection rates in rooms equipped with special devices report rates lower than 1%. This may be due to the device or to the increased consciousness of sterile technique associated with the study, or both.

Autonomic Hyperreflexia

Patients with spinal cord injuries often require orthopaedic intervention for debridement of pressure sores, ischiotomies, osteotomies, or spinal fusions.[142] Depending on the level and completeness of the cord transection, the patient may need no anesthesia. When completeness of the lesion is not certain or autonomic hyperreflexia is possible, anesthesia is necessary. Autonomic hyperreflexia, a sudden massive sympathetic discharge with severe hypertension, results from reflex stimulation of the sympathetic neurons in the anterolateral column of the cord below the lesion which are not under higher control of the central nervous system.[143] Hypotension and marked heart rate changes in either direction may also be encountered. A lesion at or above the midthoracic segments may be associated with this condition. Autonomic hyperreflexia may be treated with drugs that block the sympathetic system at the central, ganglionic, or peripheral levels.

Adequate spinal or general anesthesia usually prevents occurrence of the syndrome. Some might think that the obvious central nervous system disease would serve as a con-

traindication to spinal anesthesia, but most anesthesiologists believe that if the lesion has not been progressing or improving, no harm will result from spinal anesthesia. Gentle handling of the spinal cord–injured patient is necessary to prevent hypotension resulting from a lack of vasomotor control. Massive potassium release may follow the use of succinylcholine; this drug is usually avoided.

POSTOPERATIVE CONSIDERATIONS

Positioning and Immobilization

Immobilization is an important part of orthopaedic treatment during the weeks necessary for bone and ligament healing. General anesthesia should be maintained until the desired postoperative immobilization is ensured by cast, splint, sling, or bulky dressing. Smooth emergence is important, with avoidance of coughing and bucking during extubation of the trachea. Early use of postoperative analgesics is often of value. Emergence delirium should be detected and treated early. After a patient has received regional anesthesia, the recovery room staff should be made aware of the patient's motor status and the importance of protecting a paralyzed limb from injury. To minimize postoperative edema and circulatory embarrassment, it is often desirable to keep the operate part of the body elevated. Careful padding and positioning of an extremity may be necessary to avoid nerve damage. The ulnar nerve may be predisposed to injury, augmented by pressure resulting from the Gardner elevator (Fig. 44-6).[144] The recovery room and nursing staff must be apprised of the proper postoperative positioning for each patient.

Relief of Pain

Postoperative pain is frequent in patients who have undergone orthopaedic surgery. The basic armamentarium for the treatment of pain consists of immobilization, systemic and spinal analgesics, and local anesthetics. Immobilization and rest of the affected part is more practical for extremities than

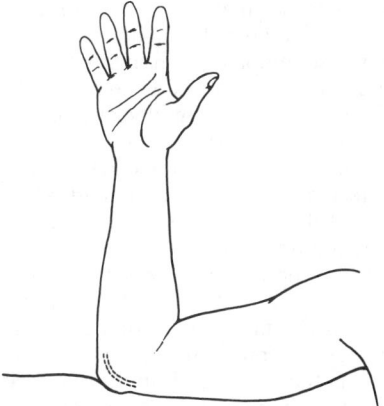

Figure 44-6. After hand surgery, the forearm is often kept elevated to decrease swelling and pain by suspending it from an iv pole or other device. Care must be taken to either pad the ulnar nerve in the olecranon groove or elevate the hand enough to keep pressure off the nerve. The abducted humerus should be allowed to rotate caudad rather than let the hand go cephalad, to protect the ulnar nerve and the brachial plexus.

for the trunk, because of the respiratory movements of the trunk. Systemic opioids in adequate doses are still the mainstay of postoperative pain relief.[145] In patients of advanced age and infirmity, prudence and caution in dosage are necessary, but it is important to ensure that sufficient drug is given to achieve the desired effect.[146] Initial routine orders must be tempered by observation of the patient's response, and the dose should be adjusted accordingly. One major concern in the use of opioid drugs is depression of ventilation. Opioids of the agonist-antagonist type may minimize the risk of severe ventilatory depression, but these drugs (e.g., buprenorphine, butorphanol, nalbuphine) do not always provide total relief for severe pain (see Chapter 16).

Both pharmacokinetic principles and experience suggest that initial loading and frequent multiple small doses given iv are more likely to achieve smooth and safe analgesia than 6-hourly intramuscular or oral administrations. Parenteral administration by continuous infusion and on-demand injection into a continuous infusion have produced good results.[147-149] Patient-controlled analgesia has proved highly effective and been given a firm pharmacokinetic basis by Tamsen et al[150,151] (see Chapter 57).

Nerve blockade with opioids or local anesthetics, as an alternate to systemic analgesics, may be particularly useful after extremity surgery.[152,153] The lipid-soluble drugs such as fentanyl and meperidine act more quickly than morphine, but their duration of action is shorter. Doses from 2 to 10 mg of morphine have been recommended, but good pain relief usually necessitates doses in the upper half of that range.[154] Despite considerable enthusiasm, not all patients gain adequate relief. In addition to occasional severe respiratory depression, there may be annoying pruritis, distressing nausea and vomiting, and acute urinary retention.[149,154-157] Epidural anesthesia, by removing the important symptom of pain, can mask postoperative compartment syndrome.[158]

Embolic Phenomena

Fat Embolism

Fat embolism is a threat in patients with pelvic or long bone fractures[159-161] or intramedullary instrumentation.[162] The etiology seems to be related to mobilization of marrow fat from the cavity of fractured long bones. An important result of pulmonary fat embolism is hypoxia,[163-165] often signaled by tachypnea and tachycardia. The affected lungs suffer a number of changes, including blockage of small pulmonary arterioles, interstitial pulmonary edema, epithelial damage, leakage of proteins into the interstitial and then the alveolar spaces, a decrease in surfactant, and alveolar collapse. There is frequently a diphasic clinical course, with initial disability attributed to mechanical effects of the blockade in the lesser circulation. Subsequent effects are caused by hydrolysis of the neutral fat to irritating free fatty acids and by migration of the fat to systemic circulatory beds. Signs include change in consciousness, petechial hemorrhages, fat globules in the urine and sputum, elevation of serum triglyceride and lipase levels, progressive anemia, and thrombocytopenia. In the late stages, the diseased lung becomes stiff (decreased compliance) and the vital capacity decreases.[160]

Blood gas analysis is a useful diagnostic measure. A PaO_2 below 60 mm Hg, a pH below 7.3 units, or a respiratory rate above 35 breaths per minute or evident dyspnea with the use of accessory muscles of breathing should alert the observer.[165] Early correction of hypoxia with increased inspired oxygen to produce a PaO_2 in the range of 70–100 mm Hg, intubation of the trachea, and ventilation of the lungs with positive end-expiratory pressure are routine in the respiratory care of this syndrome. Other treatment measures that have been suggested include high doses of corticosteroids and the use of heparin, low molecular weight dextran, and iv alcohol.[159,166]

Thromboembolism

Venous thrombosis and pulmonary embolism are common complications in the postoperative period. The mechanism of development of venous thrombosis is not totally clear, but contributing factors include increased platelet adhesiveness, hypercoagulability of blood owing to activation of clotting factors, vessel wall lesions, and stagnation of blood in the venous system. The source of pulmonary emboli is usually the iliofemoral segment or the deep veins of the calf, where thrombosis may develop without obvious signs.

The risk of postoperative thromboembolism is increased with advanced age, immobilization, lack of muscle contraction in the lower extremities, a history of previous thromboembolism, congestive heart failure, decreased arterial flow to the extremities, estrogen therapy, gram-negative sepsis, carcinoma of the lung or pancreas, blood groups other than O, and trauma. It is clear that orthopaedic patients share many of these risk factors. Conventional prophylactic measures include the use of pneumatic devices and administration of heparin, coumadin, dextran, and aspirin.[167] Only recently has the surgical community paid heed to reports of regional anesthesia as thrombotic prophylaxis.[168]

In patients with pre-existing venous thrombosis, the anesthesiologist should avoid succinylcholine fasciculation to prevent mobilization of a thrombus. In the recovery room and throughout the postoperative period, the operate part should be examined to ensure that an immobilizing cast or dressing does not produce pressure and ischemia or cause undue obstruction to venous return.

The treatment of established venous thrombosis entails elevation, rest, and administration of analgesics, anticoagulants, and antiplatelet agents to prevent extension. Administration of thrombolytic substances such as streptokinase or urokinase, or surgical removal is sometimes considered. Attempts to reduce the incidence of thrombosis by early ambulation, limb elevation, bed exercise, and support garments have had incomplete success. Surprisingly, prolonged or continuous regional anesthesia may be desirable in preventing thromboembolism.[169] The increased blood flow secondary to sympathetic block is usually credited with the observed decrease,[170] especially as it persists postoperatively, in contrast to any flow increase during general anesthesia.[171,172]

Other preventive methods include the use of high molecular weight dextran and aspirin, with varying degrees of success. A reduction in the prevalence of anaphylactic reactions with hapten dextran of 1000 daltons molecular weight has spurred a resurgence of interest in dextran prophylaxis.[41,173] Coumadin and heparin in low doses have produced good results in general surgical patients but may not be similarly effective in orthopaedic patients. Anticoagulant treatment is probably more effective if initiated before surgery. Some surgeons, however, hesitate to operate on patients who are anticoagulated because of the increased incidence of bleeding and wound hematoma. The anesthesiologist may similarly be loath to administer an otherwise indicated regional anesthetic. Thus, initiation of anticoagulant therapy is often delayed until the postoperative period.

Xenobiotic Gas

Air embolism is rare during orthopaedic procedures, as most incisions are below the hydrostatic pressure level of the right atrium. Postoperatively, however, gas from several interesting sources has been found in tissues. Gas may be forced into tissues during long bone reaming and rodding; during hip arthroplasty, from malfunction of nitrogen-powered tools; and even from the extensive use of hydrogen peroxide.[174-176] Carbon dioxide used to distend the knee joint can dissect to the abdomen and even to the pericardium.[177] Cryogenic use of liquid nitrogen[178] and air injection during aspiration of a bone cyst[179] have produced unexpected gas emboli.

SPECIAL CONSIDERATIONS FOR SPECIFIC PROCEDURES

Hip Fractures

Hip fractures occur most often in elderly persons and may result from an apparently minor fall. When hip fractures occur in younger persons, they are usually due to motorcycle, automobile, and other high-impact accidents. Haljamae et al[180] found important nonorthopaedic findings in 92% of elderly patients, the majority of which required treatment or correction preoperatively. The average patient had correctable abnormalities in two major organ systems, which underscores the importance of careful preoperative evaluation. Whereas adequate preparation of the elderly or the traumatized patient is essential,[181] protracted delay without active therapy is associated with a greater incidence of aseptic necrosis of the head of the femur and a significant increase in mortality, largely due to respiratory causes.

Preoperative evaluation and preparation of the patient for hip surgery should include careful assessment of blood volume. An apparently normal hemoglobin concentration may be a sign of dehydration, since many elderly patients exhibit low normal values. Hematomas containing more than a liter of blood may be unrecognized after fracture of the hip. In the absence of adequate fluid replacement, such a hematoma may not result in a decreased hemoglobin or hematocrit. Evaluation and monitoring of fluid status may be facilitated by central venous pressure measurement, tilt table testing, evaluation of urine output, and determination of urine sodium and osmolarity. The frequency of intraoperative hypothermia in these procedures makes temperature monitoring advisable.

The choice of anesthetic technique for urgent hip fractures remains controversial,[33,182] but increasingly studies recommend spinal or epidural anesthesia,[183] and even femoral nerve blockade is espoused.[184] Wickstrom et al[185] found a lower immediate mortality after regional anesthesia than after dissociative or inhalational anesthesia, but after 1 month there was no difference. The mortality was similar to that reported by others—about 7%.[33] Although the patient's age, physical status, and the type of fracture seem to be the most important determinants for survival, careful attention to details intraoperatively and postoperatively (including thrombosis prophylaxis, oxygen therapy, continued hemodilution, and pain relief with nerve blockade) are also

important factors.[186] The combination of trauma and age may produce extraordinarily long gastric emptying times and the possibility of a full stomach. Continuous spinal anesthesia is often useful in such patients.[29,187] The technical problems of lumbar puncture and insertion of a subarachnoid catheter in the elderly are compounded by the patient's pain, but this can be minimized with traction on the limb. After the first few milliliters of spinal solution (hypobaric if the fractured hip is up, hyperbaric if it is down) are injected, the pain is sufficiently relieved that the patient can be moved to the fracture table, with traction maintained on the fractured limb. Once the patient is supine, a hypobaric solution best maintains or augments the blockade.[188] In a supine patient, the lumbar nerve roots are highest in the spinal canal. Isobaric solutions are also useful, as are rapid injections of heavy solutions through a catheter; turbulence minimizes spread "down" the canal to higher spinal levels.

If the lateral decubitus position is desired, hypobaric spinal anesthesia may be induced with the patient in the operative position, eliminating the need for further movement. Gentle traction on the injured limb and a pillow between the legs will decrease discomfort. The incidence of post-lumbar puncture headache is low in elderly people, as these individuals are rarely nursed in an upright position immediately postoperatively.

Gentle handling is a must, since hypotension may occur with either regional or general anesthesia, especially in debilitated and elderly patients. To lie awake, immobile, for several hours of operation is difficult. Light planes of general anesthesia may be maintained during positioning. Small iv doses of ketamine (25-mg increments until the sensorium is depressed) usually permit safe and easy positioning without hypotension or airway obstruction. Benzodiazepines are widely used for both sedation and amnesia.

Hip Joint Replacement

Disabling pain and limitation of motion are produced by a variety of diseases such as osteoarthritis, traumatic arthritis, rheumatoid arthritis, aseptic necrosis of the femoral head, and congenital hip disease. Smith-Peterson's concept of a mold arthroplasty brought remarkable relief to some patients (Fig. 44-7).[189] The cup, which was originally of glass and later of vitallium, induced the formation of fibrous cartilage, and even a synovium-like lining of a joint space in some patients, after which it was removed. However, unsatisfactory results in some patients included continued pain despite good motion, aseptic necrosis with bone collapse, cup migration, and infection. Moore and Thompson introduced prostheses that were essentially balls on stalks. These implants, however, could result in pain and acetabular erosion.

A number of biomechanical principles were appreciated and applied by Charnley in the 1960s.[190] He pioneered total replacement of the hip joint with a low-friction bearing, a small ball so that more material could be placed in the acetabular component to provide for wear, a small neck diameter relative to the ball to improve mobility, a flexible shaft to simulate the flexibility of bone, and, in particular, the use of acrylic bone cement to transmit forces from the prosthesis to a broad surface of the femoral cortex, thus minimizing loosening and postoperative failure.[191] It is now recognized that the ultimate success or failure of any surgical implant depends on many elements, including the phys-

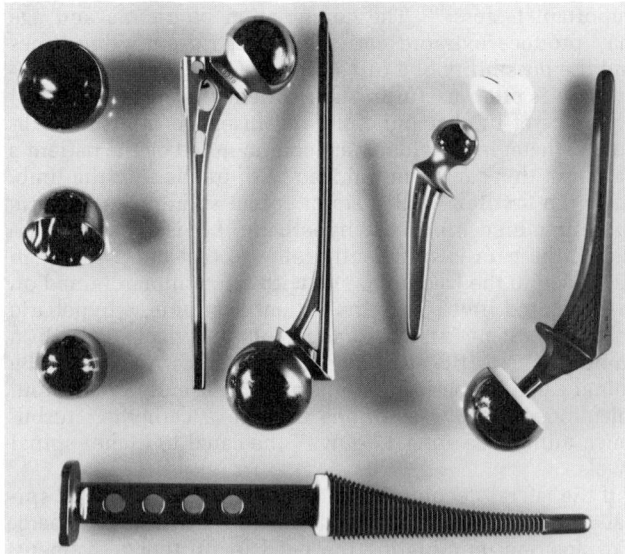

Figure 44-7. Three generations of hip prostheses. *Left,* three Smith-Peterson arthroplasty cups; *center,* two sizes of Austin-Moore nails; *right,* two modern bipolar prostheses, a Charnley with a small ball and plastic acetabular component, and a modification showing the figuring on the humeral stem to aid fixation with cement. *Below,* a precision reamer.

ical, mechanical, and biochemical properties of the implant material; the design, construction, and surface finish of the implant; operative technique; and postoperative management of the patient. Charnley further highlighted the importance of measures to prevent infection. His published series show a decrease in the infection rate from 5% to well below 1%.

Attempts to improve on his results with other bearing materials (such as Teflon and nylon, which unfortunately abraded to produce increased tissue reaction) or with different bearing surfaces such as trunnion joints (which wore out-of-round irregularly) have not added substantially to progress in hip prostheses. They have, however, stimulated the development of artificial joints for knees and shoulders and other joint improvements. Currently, materials for implants are chosen with a view to the yield strength, tensile strength, ductility, and resistance to fatigue. The bulk of metal prostheses are cobalt chromium alloys or stainless steel, but titanium, tantalum, and an occasional exotic alloy have been used. The materials and methods of manufacture have been chosen to produce high corrosion resistance, low crevice formation, and little or no local irritation. High-density polyethylene, chosen for low friction, and silicone elastomers, chosen for high flexibility, are examples of materials chosen for special properties.

Surgery is generally performed with the patient in the lateral decubitus position. As is the case with hip fracture, there is no general agreement as to the preferred method of anesthesia.[182] In more than 200 operations, Sculco and Ranawat[32] found that complications were less frequent with spinal anesthesia. In a prospective study of 157 consecutive patients, Rosenberg et al[31] found that surgical blood loss could be related directly to blood pressure, with the least loss following general anesthesia with deliberate hypotension, using nitroprusside. Somewhat more blood loss occurred with epidural anesthesia, and the most blood was lost during normotensive general anesthesia.[30] The reduc-

tion in the frequency of thrombotic and embolic events after epidural block was matched with the use of high molecular weight dextran and neurolept anesthesia.[192] Hole *et al*[28,51,193,194] report clear-cut advantages for epidural versus general anesthesia in the postoperative course. In regard to postoperative ventilatory function and mental recovery, studies have not been able to show that either general or regional anesthesia is preferable.[24,195,196] Similarly, urine retention may occur after either anesthetic regimen, probably more related to preoperative obstruction than to anesthesia.[136] As in the patient with hip fracture, good management includes slow, accurate induction of the anesthetic level, gentle handling of the patient, attention to comfort of the shoulder and upper limbs, and the judicious use of iv drugs from the sedative and dissociative classes.

Methyl Methacrylate Cement

Acrylic bone cement is commonly used in hip replacement operations. The anesthesiologist must understand its function, its complications, and their treatment. Acrylic bone cement is a self-polymerizing methyl methacrylate used as a space-filling mortar to transmit compressive loads from bone to prosthesis to bone.[190] It is not a glue. It helps to achieve fixation of the prosthesis by entering osseous interstices and engulfing small trabeculae of the bone surface and deliberate irregularities in the prosthesis, producing a tight fit. Available preparations consist of two parts: (1) granular polymerized methyl methacrylate with an activator and anti-inhibitor to initiate polymerization, and sometimes other additives such as carbon fibers for strength or barium sulfate for radiopacity;[197] and (2) liquid methyl methacrylate monomer with a polymerization inhibitor such as hydroquinone. The exothermic polymerization process is begun by mixing as little liquid as possible with the powder to achieve a semisolid that can be squeezed or injected into desired cavities. Within minutes after mixing (the time may vary slightly with ambient temperature and humidity), the cement loses its tacky surface and is ready to be implanted. Hardening occurs in the next few minutes and is accompanied by the release of heat, the extent of which depends on the amount of liquid used. The temperature of a ball of cement with a radius of 1 cm may reach over 100°C in the interior. Thus, there is a potential for tissue necrosis in the vicinity of large globs.

During mixing, the odor of the monomer permeates the entire room. It is not known to be a biologic hazard, but it is objectionable to some. Shrouded mixing bowls attached to suction or the scavenging system in the operating room can minimize this problem.

Insertion of the cement has been associated with sudden episodes of hypotension. During nitrous oxide–opioid–muscle relaxant anesthesia, mean rises in pressure were reported, although one fourth of the patients had an initial fall in blood pressure.[198] The hypotension is attributed to the vasodilating effects of the absorbed volatile monomer,[199-202] to emboli forced into the circulation as the prosthesis is inserted into a reamed and curetted medullary bone,[174,203] to effects of heating of bone marrow and blood cells, with release of thrombotic and vasoactive substances,[204] and to hydrolysis of the methyl methacrylate to methacrylate acid.[205]

All of the postulated mechanisms probably play a role in one patient or another, judging from the variability in time and extent of hypotension.[206] The degree of hypotension probably depends on the condition of capacitance vessels in a particular patient. If these vessels are constricted, as is the case in hypovolemic patients, sudden vasodilation results in a significant decrease in arterial blood pressure. If the patient is normovolemic and the vasculature is well filled, or if the vessels are dilated through the use of deliberate hypotension, the decrease in blood pressure may be minimal. The hypotensive effect may appear within 30–60 seconds after insertion of the cement, or up to 10 minutes after the prosthesis is inserted. It usually terminates spontaneously in less than 5 minutes. The hypotension may be prevented or treated with vasopressor drugs such as ephedrine. Cardiac arrest with less than a 50% recovery rate was reported following application of bone cement in the femoral shaft, but this is a grossly higher mortality than is currently experienced. Autopsy reports have revealed severe degrees of pulmonary fat and bone marrow emboli.[166,207] Such pulmonary embolism results from the high femoral medullary pressure generated during cement insertion and may be prevented by venting the femoral shaft during insertion of the cement and prosthesis.[208]

In addition to hypotension, hypoxemia, presumably resulting from fat and marrow emboli, occurs in some patients.[206,209] This can be prevented by maximizing alveolar oxygen tension before femoral cement insertion. Pulmonary artery hypertension has been seen after the use of femoral shaft cement.[210] This was a more sensitive indicator than capnography in detecting emboli in dogs.[211] In one patient, cement intended to stabilize cervical spine surgery extruded anteriorly, obstructing the airway.[212]

The cement may be subjected to centrifugation, which eliminates air bubbles and improves the mechanical strength of the prosthetic-bone interface,[213] but the process is controversial.[214] Cement with antibiotic added may be useful in infected operative sites.[215] In the future, the cement may be replaced with prostheses that allow bony growth into the appliance, as with sintered metal coatings, but such coated prostheses are accompanied by their own problems, which usually manifest late after implantation.[216,217]

Procedures on the Extremities

Operations on the Upper Limb

In orthopaedics, regional anesthesia is most frequently used for surgery on the hand, forearm, elbow, or arm. A variety of techniques are described in detail in Chapter 31, including iv (Bier) blockade, specific nerve blockades of the digital, ulnar, median, radial, musculocutaneous, or intercostobrachialis nerves, and brachial plexus nerve block. There is no substitute for thorough anatomic grounding in performing these procedures. Each limb should be individually examined before the final approach is selected. The descriptions of axillary blockade by Thompson in Seattle, Winnie in Chicago, and Murphy in Philadelphia are nearly as different as the home cities. All can produce satisfactory working conditions. The aim is to reduce failure to a low level.

The anesthesiologist should be prepared to "rescue" a blockade by supplementation with another, usually more distal blockade. Early detection of partial failure by sensory and motor observation will permit rescue by a specific blockade of the missed nerve (Fig. 44-8). In fact, combined plexus and peripheral nerve blockade is recommended by

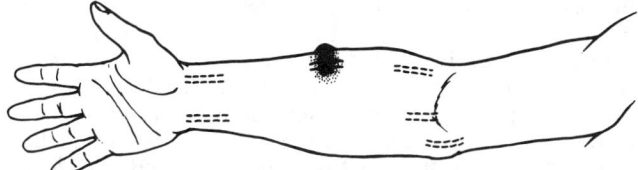

Figure 44-8. Diagram of arm with suggestions for blockade of radial (at elbow and forearm), ulnar (at elbow and forearm), and median nerve (at elbow and forearm). Either the anesthesiologist or surgeon may be able to forestall a general anesthetic by supplemental blockade of a distal nerve.

some.[218] To perform a serial blockade accurately, the anesthesiologist must have sufficient experience and insistence to be able to differentiate a slow onset of blockade from a missed nerve before the orthopaedic prepping and draping is complete. Sensory testing with a sterile needle can continue through the scrub without violating aseptic principles. Motor function may be tested during the prep as well. The anesthesiologist can also perform the blockade early to permit 30 minutes or more of "soak" time, reducing the number of failed blockades. Lidocaine diffuses better through tissue than does mepivacaine or bupivacaine.

Appreciating three facts about axillary approaches to the nerves of the brachial plexus reduces failures. First, palpating excessively high in the axilla is ill-advised. It is harder to feel the axillary artery, and the pressure of the probing finger distorts the anatomy. When the finger is withdrawn, the sheath moves back to the normal position, so that the needle is effectively placed too deep. Second, the nerves as well as vessels can often be felt distal to the crossing of the coracobrachialis by the pectoralis major. The patient's arm should be abducted 70–80 degrees flat on a table or armboard, with the forearm flexed 90 degrees and pointing upward (ventrad, not cephalad). The anesthesiologist can then pluck the structures in the sheath much as a guitarist plucks the instrument's strings. Even a 90-degree abduction of the arm may distort the distribution of injected local anesthetic, with an incomplete block as a consequence. Third, the sheath is relatively superficial just dorsal (below in this position) to the coracobrachialis. If the tip of the needle is placed subcutaneously and the skin is moved slightly back and forth as the needle is advanced, one can often appreciate a scratching sensation and the fixation of the point of the needle in the investing fascia at a depth about equal to a skin fold pinched at the site—1.5–2.25 cm is the range in the majority. Any insertion much deeper has probably passed through the sheath to provide a solid blockade of the muscle fibers of the triceps.

An added benefit of brachial plexus blockade is the ability to extend the anesthetic into the postoperative period. Use of a catheter and repeated instillation of local anesthetic can provide pain relief and increased blood flow to replanted digits on the hand.[219]

Closed Reduction of Fractures or Dislocations

These procedures present a special set of considerations. They are usually of short duration, especially reductions of dislocated joints, and usually require analgesia and nearly complete skeletal muscle paralysis. Most closed reductions are performed as emergency procedures to avoid loss of blood supply and aseptic necrosis. Previous attempts to reduce a dislocation with the muscle-relaxing effects of diazepam or morphine, if unsuccessful, bring a depressed patient to the anesthesiologist. Patients may have recently had a full meal. Thus, Bier blockades are useful for distal dislocations;[220] or plexus anesthesia may be used when it is not contraindicated by vascular or nerve damage. Traditionally, Colles fractures of the wrist have been reduced after local anesthetic infiltration of the hematoma. But Kongsholm and Olerud found an increased incidence of neurologic sequelae.[221] When closed reduction is performed as an elective procedure, a brief general anesthetic technique with succinylcholine for skeletal muscle relaxation is efficient. Fasciculation may further dislocate or fracture long bone segments or result in vascular or nerve damage. Although a slow iv drip of succinylcholine or "self-taming" may be used instead of bolus injections to avoid violent muscular movements, more commonly pretreatment with a nondepolarizing neuromuscular paralysant in a small dose blocks fasciculation.

Operations on the Shoulder

Perhaps the most frequent use of general anesthesia in orthopaedic surgery is for shoulder operations. The proximity of the awake patient's head to the operative site suggests that unpleasant sensory inputs will be more annoying than those from more distant operative sites. For brief procedures such as examination and manipulation, a general anesthetic is often used because of the brevity of the procedure.[222] Furthermore, an adequate regional procedure requires either a supraclavicular blockade, such as Winnie's subclavian perivascular approach, or a paravertebral plus other blockades, which are relatively unfamiliar to many anesthesiologists.[223] Nonetheless, we may confidently recommend a blockade, secure in the knowledge that any procedure in the orthopaedic repertoire for the shoulder can be done painlessly with a regional technique.[224] Some recommend either deep cervical plexus block[225] or thoracic paravertebral blocks[223] in addition to a supraclavicular approach, but I have not found either helpful or necessary. Preoperative informative interviews, analgesic and sedative adjuvants, and intraoperative support are solutions to the largely perceptual problems. Patient satisfaction can be high.[225]

Operations on the Knee

A variety of anesthetic techniques are available for procedures on the knee. Arthroscopy may be done with field blockade and intra-articular local anesthetic,[226-228] with the "three-in-one block" plus lateral femoral cutaneous nerve blockade,[229] with a limited epidural, and with hypobaric spinal tetracaine. Tetracaine is relatively easy to confine to low thoracic levels (T10) by very slowly (>60 seconds) injecting 10–12 mg in 5–6 ml of sterile water, with the patient in a 2–4 degrees head-down position. This technique provides 3–4 hours of analgesia. Intraoperative tourniquet pain, described in an earlier section, may be encountered and is treated with opioid analgesics. Instrumentation of the femoral marrow cavity during knee arthroplasty, as with hip arthroplasty, can produce marrow cell, bone, fat, and cement emboli.[230,231]

Amputations

Amputation is required after traumatic injury or when insufficient blood supply results in gangrene. The patient undergoing amputation may have important systemic diseases (diabetes, cardiovascular disease, sepsis) that necessitate careful preoperative evaluation and consultation to ensure optimal preparation. Analgesic drugs are often administered for pain control and should be continued until anesthesia is induced. Cryoanesthesia, achieved by packing the limb in ice for 12–24 hours, is an old but still occasionally useful method, conferring pain control, surgical anesthesia, and remission of toxemia as absorption from the gangrenous limb is decreased.

Spinal anesthesia is often preferred for lower extremity amputations if there are no contraindications, although the advantages are demonstrable only in the first 24 hours.[232] A hypnotic dose of a short-acting barbiturate may be given just before the bone is sawed, to spare the patient psychological trauma. An amnestic state from diazepam, lorazepam, or midazolam injection is not entirely reliable in this regard, resulting in an incidence of true amnesia of 50–80%. Tourniquets may be used in younger patients for post-traumatic amputation, but they are generally omitted when the surgeon wishes to identify viable tissue or fears damage to sclerotic vessels in elderly patients.

Regional anesthesia produces in some patients a subjective sensation that the blocked extremity occupies a position different from the actual one. This phantom limb syndrome[233] is named after the phantom limb pain that some amputees experience long after the amputation. The patient has the impression that the extremity is floating up, slightly flexed, often in the same position as it was when afferent conduction was interrupted. The phantom sensation disappears after nerve conduction is restored. There is no established explanation for the phantom sensation.

Phantom limb sensations occur in almost all amputees but dissipate with time. Severe postoperative phantom limb pain is rare and of unknown etiology, but the incidence may be reduced through the use of perioperative regional anesthetic techniques.[234,235]

Joint Manipulation and Examination

Joints with limited range of motion are sometimes manipulated to break up adhesions. The procedure is short and almost always elective and may be performed under thiopental–nitrous oxide anesthesia. Succinylcholine, 0.5 mg·kg^{-1}, suffices, and tracheal intubation is not necessary. Opioid premedication together with a reduction in the iv barbiturate dosage is helpful in relieving postmanipulation pain without significantly prolonging emergence.

Operations on the Lower Limb

There are many anesthetic approaches to the lower extremity, but common to almost all is the pneumatic tourniquet on the thigh. Low spinal or epidural anesthesia is the most common anesthetic technique. There are several approaches to the sciatic, femoral, and obturator nerves, but they are used infrequently. Intravenous regional anesthesia is frequently discouraged, for several reasons: the veins are few, a large dose of drug is needed, there is oozing through inter- and intraosseous vessels, and tourniquet pain is very common and severe. However, a standard pneumatic tourniquet can be successfully applied just above the ankle, and block of the five distal nerves to the foot is simple, safe, and eminently satisfactory for most invasive podiatric procedures, with the added benefit of prolonged postoperative analgesia. Even successful iv regional block is possible with care.[236,237]

Replantation of Limbs and Grafts

Microsurgical anastomosis of vessels and nerves permits remarkable salvage of traumatic amputations. The anesthetic problems are largely related to the extraordinary duration of some of these operations.[238,239] Sympathetic denervation is thought to be important, giving rise to the use of catheter techniques for continuous blockade.[219] Adequate sedation and analgesia are challenges often best met by light continuous general anesthesia. More than usual attention must be given to positioning in order to avoid necrosis at pressure points, to the humidification of inspired gas, and to fluid intake and output, all because of the prolonged procedures. A team of anesthesiologists may be needed to provide maintained vigilance.[238] Hypothermia should be avoided, since vasoconstriction and shivering postoperatively may jeopardize the reimplanted tissue.

Major homologous bone grafts or autologous grafts of bone, muscle, subcutaneous tissue, skin, and their nutrient vessels involve similar meticulous surgery.[240,241] They may be used after major extirpation of cancer (to fill defects), after long bone excision (to provide support), or after control of indolent ulcer (to cover the wound). To the considerations cited above are added those of large blood loss and replacement, cardiovascular support, and the consequences of inanition and malnutrition.

Operations on the Spine

The most common procedures on the spine include spinal fusion (for scoliosis, vertebral fracture, or spine instability) and operations for herniated intervertebral disk, including laminectomy, microdiskectomy, and chemonucleolysis. Common to the majority of these procedures is the necessity for the prone position,[242] although, rarely, surgeons may use the lateral position (see Chapter 27). The sitting position is used for some posterior cervical laminectomies, and the supine position is used for anterior cervical fusion.[243] Fiberoptic-assisted intubation of the trachea is advantageous in patients with severe or unstable spines.[244] In positioning the patient, one weighs the conflicting needs for surgical exposure, freedom of ventilation and venous return, and patient comfort and safety.

Several methods have been developed for prone positioning. Older methods include use of the Wilson and Relton frames[59] and the Georgia prone position.[245] Other devices place the weight of the buttocks on a seat or support with the thighs flexed ("Mohammedan praying position"),[60] or on a pelvic frame.[246] In most instances the surgeon's aim is to flatten or reverse the lumbar lordosis and the anesthesiologist's aim is to provide free excursion, either laterally or ventrally, for the abdomen. Both specialists are interested in preventing engorgement of the epidural venous system, which results in increased venous oozing. These aims can be met if the iliac crest can be held securely and if the pelvis is allowed to tilt, or the thighs flexed more than 90 degrees, creating tension in the gluteal muscles, which achieves the same end result.

The neck should be kept in the same plane as the back and slightly flexed to avoid strain and postanesthetic discomfort. The arms should be well padded and pointing cephalad, with the elbows at the level of the head and rotated anteriorly. The head must be supported, with attention paid to avoid injuring the eyes or kinking the airway. Sufficient help must be available during positioning to avoid exceeding a patient's normal range of motion of the spine

and extremities. A useful technique is neuroleptanalgesia plus topical anesthesia for awake intubation, so that the patient may pronate comfortably and safely before losing consciousness.[247]

Spinal Fusion

Scoliosis is a deformity of the thoracolumbar spine and rib cage caused by lateral deviation and rotation of the vertebral bodies. One hemithorax is compressed toward residual volume, and the other is expanded toward total lung capacity. When the angle of the deformity exceeds 65 degrees, there is severe functional change in the respiratory system as both hemithoraces are on flattened (e.g., stiff) portions of their pressure-volume curves.[248] Decreasing lung volumes and mechanical impairments lead to an increase in the work of breathing and alveolar hypoventilation.[249] Ventilation-perfusion mismatch with increased physiologic shunting and dead space increases the functional severity of the deformity. A decrease in Pao_2, an increase in the alveolar-arterial oxygen difference, and an increase in $Paco_2$ result (Fig. 44-9).

The kyphoscoliotic patient with chronic hypercapnia responds subnormally to further elevations in $Paco_2$, hypoventilates when inhaling a high inspired oxygen concentration, and may be unusually sensitive to depressant drugs (e.g., opioids and barbiturates). Pulmonary vascular resistance is elevated, leading to right ventricular hypertrophy and cor pulmonale. In such a patient with significant curvature, preoperative pulmonary function testing and arterial blood gas analysis should determine the severity of the impairment. The ECG is helpful in detecting cor pulmonale. When nonoperative treatment is unsuccessful in arresting the progression of deformity, and when the deformity has progressed to a degree that will predictably cause severe

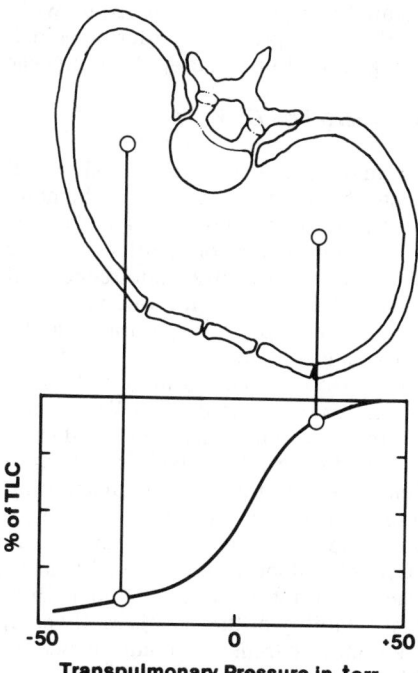

Figure 44-9. Pressure-volume diagram of chest wall and lung (*top*) and approximate position at end-expiratory lung volume of the hyperinflated (convex) and hypoinflated (concave) hemithorax. Note that both are on flattened (less compliant) portions of the pressure-volume curve.

respiratory or cardiovascular embarrassment, surgery becomes mandatory.[250] Postoperative ventilatory support in an intensive care unit may be necessary, since respiratory deterioration in the immediate postoperative period is common. Risk factors include mental retardation, anterior approaches, age over 20 years, preoperative hemoglobin desaturation, and obstructive or restrictive lung disease.[251]

Regional and general anesthesia techniques may be used separately or combined for scoliosis surgery.[252] It is more important to attend to ventilatory and cardiovascular function than to search for a single best anesthetic. The anesthesiologist must closely follow estimates of blood loss, fluid requirements, and the changing effects of mechanical ventilation of the lungs.

In patients who are undergoing spinal fusion for scoliosis, the anesthesiologist faces problems of blood loss and spinal cord function. Deliberate hypotension is widely accepted for minimizing blood loss. A variety of hypotensive techniques have been used.[108,109,253,254] Hemodynamic and hormonal analysis suggests that sodium nitroprusside produces safe hypotension with preservation of central nervous system blood flow and oxygen consumption, and maintenance of some degree of autoregulation of spinal cord blood flow.[255] Assurance that cord function has not been impaired can be provided by two different techniques. Waldman et al[256] have described a wake-up technique before closure to ensure that voluntary motion of the lower extremity remains. Grundy et al[257] have shown that the somatosensory-evoked response can be used in a nearly continuous fashion for the same purpose. Neither technique is foolproof.[258] A continuous opioid infusion technique has been adapted to either method.[259]

Patients with kyphoscoliosis who are to undergo anesthesia for other surgical procedures (e.g., labor and delivery, abdominal surgery) are prepared for surgery and managed in a similar way.[260] Scoliosis may be associated with a high risk of malignant hyperpyrexia in the patient with myotonia dystrophica. However, previous posterior spinal fusion is not a contraindication to lumbar epidural blockade.[261]

Herniated Intervertebral Disk

This problem may be treated with extensive laminectomy, microlaminectomy and diskectomy, or chemonucleolysis. In the first two procedures, positioning for optimal surgical exposure without circulatory or ventilatory embarrassment is the major problem. Generally, endotracheal inhalational anesthesia is supplemented with a variety of muscle relaxants and adjuvants, but spinal,[31] epidural,[262] and local anesthesia have been successfully used. Muscle relaxants facilitate surgical exposure in laminectomy but abolish muscle movement on nerve root stimulation. When this type of response is desired, relaxants must be avoided or their effects allowed to dissipate. Partial paralysis facilitates surgical exposure without deep anesthesia, but total abolition of neuromuscular transmission is not essential.

Blood loss is rarely sufficient to necessitate deliberate hypotension. Cyanotic blood in the surgical field may be due to venous stasis and not to hypoxia.[263] Especially after microdiskectomy, stability of the back is rarely compromised, and the patient may be transported and nursed in any position thought desirable.

Smith began testing chemonucleolysis in 1963,[264] but a variety of events slowed approval of chymopapain[265] in the United States. Following use in Canada and England it was approved by the Food and Drug Administration in 1982.[266] The drug lyses mucopolysaccharides, but not the annular ring of the ruptured disk. A rapid decrease in size of the herniated mass is attributed to loss of the mucopolysaccharide's ability to bind water. Local capillary dissolution leads to the possibility of hematoma formation in muscle, intrathecally, or in the disk itself. Alpha$_2$-macroglobulins in the plasma inactivate the drug if it is given systemically.

With the patient in the lateral decubitus position, a needle is introduced into the disk under fluoroscopic guidance, and a diskogram is obtained to demonstrate pathology. It is desirable to avoid cerebrospinal fluid puncture and injection of the dye or drug into the epidural space. General anesthesia is most frequently used, despite some advantages claimed for local anesthesia.[267] The anesthetic management is uneventful except for the occurrence of uncommon but severe allergic reactions,[268] signs of which include flushing, tachycardia, hypotension, wheezing, and edema of the skin, larynx, and lung. The treatment is administration of epinephrine, which aborts degranulation of mast cells and histamine release. Anticipating this treatment, most anesthesiologists avoid the use of halothane and choose enflurane, isoflurane, or a balanced anesthetic with nitrous oxide. Steroids and aminophylline should be available for immediate parenteral use, but their prophylactic use has not been validated. A rational but also unvalidated treatment would be the use of both histamine-1, and histamine-2 blockers in premedication (e.g., diphenhydramine, cimetidine).

The final New Drug Application reported 909 patients treated with chymopapain, with nine cases of anaphylaxis, the majority in women with erythrocyte sedimentation rates greater than 20 mm·h^{-1}. A multicenter double-blind study demonstrated clinical efficacy of chymopapain, with 90% successful outcomes and no anaphylaxis.[269] The surgical procedure was taught in a training course sponsored jointly by the American Academy of Orthopaedic Surgeons and the American Association of Neurological Surgeons. A Diagnostic and Therapeutic Technology Assessment—1988 probably sounded the death-knell for chymopapain,[270] although proponents continue their support.[271] The enthusiasm for chemonucleolysis evident in the early 1980s is clearly waning, as evidenced by the paucity of published papers since the 1980–1983 period.

REFERENCES

1. Dresner DL, Ali HH: Anaesthetic management of a patient with facioscapulohumeral muscular dystrophy. Br J Anaesth 62:331, 1989
2. Office for Medical Applications of Research, National Institutes of Health: Consensus Conferences. Total Hip-Joint Replacement. JAMA 243:1817, 1982
3. Farfan HF: Major sports injury. Clin Orthop 164:2, 1982
4. Merz B: Try a carbon ribbon 'round the old hurt knee (and shoulder). JAMA 248:1681, 1982
5. Freedman LS, Jenkins AIR, Jenkins DHR: Carbon fibre reinforcement for chronic lateral ankle instability. Injury 19:25, 1988
6. Law HT: Engineering of upper limb prostheses. Orthop Clin North Am 12:929, 1981
7. Solomonow M: Restoration of movement by electrical stimulation. Orthopedics 7:245, 1984
8. Connelly JF (ed): Clinical application of bioelectrical effects. Clin Orthop 161:2, 1981
9. Pietrafesa CA, Hoffman JR: Traumatic dislocation of the hip. JAMA 249:3342, 1983
10. Banks HH: Symposium on Care of the Critically Ill Orthopedic Patient. Orthop Clin North Am 9:3, 1978
11. Scott DB: Regional anesthesia for pediatric surgery. Anesth Analg 69:697, 1989

12. Stehling L: Anesthesia for children requiring orthopedic surgery. Anesthesiol Rev 5:19, 1978

13. Olney BW, Lugg PC, Turner PL et al: Outpatient treatment of upper extremity injuries in childhood using intravenous regional anesthesia. J Pediatr Orthop 8:576, 1988

14. Audenaert SM, Vickers H, Burgess R: Axillary block for vascular insufficiency after repair of radial club hands in an infant. Anesthesiology 74:368, 1991

15. Pavlin EG: Anaesthesia for the traumatized patient. Can Anaesth Soc J 30(3):S27, 1983

16. Marbach JJ, Spiera H: Rheumatoid spondylitis and systemic lupus erythematosus with temporomandibular joint changes. NY State Med J 69:2908, 1969

17. Phelps JA: Laryngeal obstruction due to cricoarytenoid arthritis. Anesthesiology 27:518, 1966

18. Calabro JJ, Maltz BA: Ankylosing spondylitis. N Engl J Med 282:606, 1970

19. Salthe M, Johr M: Unsuspected cervical fractures: A common problem in ankylosing spondylitis. Anesthesiology 70:869, 1989

20. Stevens JM, Kendall BE, Crockard HA: The spinal cord in rheumatoid arthritis with clinical myelopathy: A computed myelographic study. J Neurol Neurosurg Psychiatry 49:140, 1986

21. Edelist G: Principles of anesthetic management in rheumatoid arthritic patients. Anesth Analg 43:227, 1964

22. Ellison N, Mull TD: Unique anesthetic problems in the elderly patient coming to surgery for fracture of the hip. Orthop Clin North Am 5:493, 1974

23. Sari A, Miyauchi Y, Yamashita S et al: The magnitude of hypoxemia in elderly patients with fractures of the femoral neck. Anesth Analg 65:892, 1986

24. Berggren D, Gustafson Y, Eriksson B et al: Confusion after anesthesia in elderly patients with femoral neck fractures. Anesth Analg 66:497, 1987

25. Hosking MP, Lobdell CM, Warner MA et al: Anaesthesia for patients over 90 years of age: Outcomes after regional and general anaesthetic techniques for two common surgical procedures. Anaesthesia 44:142, 1989

26. Yaeger MP, Glass DD, Neff RK et al: Epidural anesthesia and analgesic in high-risk surgical patients. Anesthesiology 66:729, 1987

27. Davis FM, Laurenson VG: Spinal anaesthesia or general anaesthesia for emergency hip surgery in elderly patients. Anaesth Intensive Care 9:352, 1981

28. Hole A, Terjesen T, Breivik H: Epidural versus general anaesthesia for total hip arthroplasty in elderly patients. Acta Anaesthesiol Scand 24:279, 1980

29. Kallos T, Smith TC: Continuous spinal anesthesia with hypobaric tetracaine for hip surgery in lateral decubitus. Anesth Analg 51:766, 1972

30. Rosberg B, Fredin H, Gustafson C: Anesthetic techniques and surgical blood loss in total hip arthroplasty. Acta Anaesthesiol Scand 26:189, 1982

31. Rosenberg MK, Berner G: Spinal anesthesia in lumbar disc surgery: Review of 200 cases, with a case history. Anesth Analg 44:419, 1965

32. Sculco TP, Ranawat C: The use of spinal anesthesia for total hip-replacement arthroplasty. J Bone Joint Surg 57A:173, 1975

33. Valentin N, Lomholt B, Jensen JS et al: Spinal or general anaesthesia for surgery of the fractured hip? Br J Anaesth 58:284, 1986

34. Davis FM, Woolner DF, Frampton C et al: Prospective multicentre trial of mortality following general or spinal anaesthesia for hip fracture surgery in the elderly. Br J Anaesth 59:1080, 1987

35. McKenzie PJ, Wishart HY, Smith G: Long-term outcome after repair of fractured neck of femur: Comparison of subarachnoid and general anaesthesia. Br J Anaesth 56:581, 1984

36. Brown DL, Carpenter RL, Thompson GE: Comparison of 0.5% ropivacaine and 0.5% bupivacaine for epidural anesthesia in patients undergoing lower-extremity surgery. Anesthesiology 72:633, 1990

37. Mebius C, Hedenstierna G: Airway closure and gas distribution during hip arthroplasty. Acta Anaesthesiol Scand 26:72, 1982

38. Hedenstierna G, Mebius C, Bygdeman S: Ventilation-perfusion relationship during hip arthroplasty. Acta Anaesthesiol Scand 27:56, 1983

39. Engquist A, Brandt MR, Fernandes A et al: The blocking effect of epidural analgesia on the adrenocortical and hyperglycemic responses to surgery. Acta Anaesthesiol Scand 21:330, 1977

40. Modig J: Beneficial effects on intraoperative and postoperative blood loss in total hip replacement when performed under lumbar epidural anesthesia. Acta Chir Scand [Suppl] 550:95, 1988

41. Fredin H, Gustafson C, Rosberg B: Hypotensive anesthesia, thromboprophylaxis and postoperative thromboembolism in total hip arthroplasty. Acta Anaesthesiol Scand 28:503, 1984

42. Modig J, Borg T, Bagge L et al: Role of extradural and of general anesthesia in fibrinolysis and coagulation after total hip replacement. Br J Anaesth 55:625, 1983

43. Modig J, Malberg P, Karlstrom G: Effect of epidural versus general anaesthesia on calf blood flow. Acta Anaesthesiol Scand 24:305, 1980

44. Coon WW: Thrombosis prophylaxis following total hip replacement. JAMA 260:3508, 1988

45. Modig J, Borg T, Karlstrom G et al: Thromboembolism after total hip replacement: Role of epidural and general anesthesia. Anesth Analg 62:174, 1983

46. Thornburn R, Louden JR, Vallance R: Spinal and general anesthesia in total hip replacement: Frequency of deep vein thrombosis. Br J Anaesth 52:1117, 1980

47. Davis FM, Laurenson VG, Gillespie WJ et al: Deep vein thrombosis after total hip replacement. J Bone Joint Surg 71B:181, 1989

48. Modig J: The role of lumbar epidural anaesthesia as antithrombotic prophylaxis in total hip replacement. Acta Chir Scand 151:589, 1985

49. McKenzie PJ, Wishart HY, Gray I et al: Effects of Anaesthetic technique on deep vein thrombosis: A comparison of subarachnoid and general anesthesia. Br J Anaesth 57:853, 1985

50. Benoni G, Johnell O, Rosberg B: Postoperative course of serum aminotransferases after total hip arthroplasty. J Bone Joint Surg 69A:255, 1987

51. Hole A, Unsgaard G, Breivik H: Monocyte functions are depressed during and after surgery under general anaesthesia but not under epidural anaesthesia. Acta Anaesthesiol Scand 26:301, 1983

52. Scott DB, Schweitzer S, Thron J: Epidural block in postoperative pain relief. Reg Anaesth 7:135, 1982

53. Scott NB, Kehlet H: Regional anaesthesia and surgical morbidity. Br J Surg 75:299, 1988

54. Amaranath L, Esfandiari S, Lockrem J et al: Epidural analgesia for total hip arthroplasty in a patient with dilated cardiomyopathy. Can Anaesth Soc J 33:84, 1986

55. Jayr C, Mollie A, Bourgain JL et al: Postoperative pulmonary complications: General anesthesia with postoperative parenteral morphine compared with epidural analgesia. Surgery 104:58, 1987

56. Lundy JS: Balanced anesthesia. Minn Med 9:399, 1926

57. Inaz E, Theiss D, Emmerich EA et al: Regional versus general anesthesia: Attitudes and experiences of patients. Reg Anaesth 7:S163, 1982

58. Rosenberg TD, Wong HC: Arthroscope knee surgery in a freestanding outpatient center. Orthop Clin North Am 13:277, 1982

59. Relton JES, Hall JE: An operation frame for spinal fusion: A new apparatus designed to reduce hemorrhage during operation. J Bone Joint Surg 49B:327, 1967

60. Dinmore P: A new operating position for posterior spinal surgery. Anaesthesia 32:377, 1977

61. Smith JW, Pellicci PM, Sharrock N et al: Complications after total hip replacement. J Bone Joint Surg 71A:528, 1989

62. McEwen JA, Auchinleck GF: Advances in surgical tourniquets. AORN J 36:889, 1982

63. Hurst LN, Weinglein O, Brown WF et al: The pneumatic tour-

niquet: A biomechanical and electrophysiologic study. Plast Reconstr Surg 67:648, 1981

64. Shaw JA, Murray DG: The relationship between tourniquet pressure and underlying soft-tissue pressure in the thigh. J Bone Joint Surg 64A:1148, 1982

65. Wilson JK, Lyon GD: Bier block tourniquet pressure. Anesth Analg 68:823, 1989

66. Hofman AA, Wyatt RWB: Fatal pulmonary embolism following tourniquet inflation. J Bone Joint Surg 67A:633, 1985

67. Pollard BJ, Lovelock HA, Jones RM: Fatal pulmonary embolism secondary to limb exsanguination. Anesthesiology 58:373, 1983

68. San Juan AC, Stanley TH: Pulmonary embolism after tourniquet inflation. Anesth Analg 63:371, 1982

69. Klenerman L: Tourniquet time: How long? Hand 12:231, 1980

70. Sapega A, Heppenstall RB, Chance B et al: Optimizing tourniquet application and release times in extremity surgery. J Bone Joint Surg 67A:303, 1985

71. Irving GA, Noakes TD: The protective role of local hypothermia in tourniquet-induced ischaemia of muscle. J Bone Joint Surg 67B:297, 1985

72. Ikemoto Y, Kobayashi H, Usui M et al: Changes in serum myoglobin levels caused by tourniquet ischemia under normothermic and hypothermic conditions. Clin Orthop Relat Res 234:296, 1987

73. Hamilton WK, Sokoll MD: Tourniquet paralysis. JAMA 199:37, 1967

74. Patterson S, Klenerman L: The effect of pneumatic tourniquets on ultrastructure of skeletal muscle. J Bone Joint Surg 61B:178, 1979

75. Miller SH, Price G, Buch D et al: Effects of tourniquet ischemia and postischemic edema on muscle metabolism. J Hand Surg 4:547, 1979

76. Jozsa L, Renner A, Santha E: The effect of tourniquet ischaemia on intact, tenotomized and motor nerve–injured human hand muscles. Hand 12:235, 1980

77. Heppenstall RB, Balderston R, Goodwin C: Pathophysiologic effects distal to a tourniquet in the dog. J Trauma 19:234, 1979

78. Tountas CP, Bergman RA: Tourniquet ischemia: Ultrastructural and histochemical observations of ischemic human muscle and of monkey muscle and nerve. J Hand Surg 2:31, 1977

79. Heppenstall B, Scott R, Sapega A: A comparative study of the tolerance of skeletal muscle to ischemia. J Bone Joint Surg 68A:820, 1986

80. Lynn AM, Fischer T, Brandford HG et al: Systemic responses to tourniquet release in children. Anesth Analg 65:865, 1986

81. Bourke DL, Silberberg MS, Ortega R et al: Respiratory responses associated with release of intraoperative tourniquets. Anesth Analg 69:541, 1989

82. Brustowicz RM, Moncorge C, Koka BV: Metabolic responses to tourniquet release in children. Anesthesiology 67:792, 1987

83. Conaty KR, Klemm MS: Severe increases of intracranial pressure after deflation of a pneumatic tourniquet. Anesthesiology 71:294, 1989

84. Stein RE, Urbaniak J: Use of tourniquet during surgery in patients with sickle cell hemoglobinopathy. Clin Orthop 151:231, 1980

85. Klenerman L, Biswas M, Hulands GH et al: Systemic and local effects of the application of a tourniquet. J Bone Joint Surg 62A:385, 1980

86. Luce EA, Mangubat E: Loss of hand and forearm following Bier block: A case report. J Hand Surg 8:280, 1983

87. Sukhani R, Garcia CJ, Munhall RJ et al: Lidocaine disposition following intravenous regional anesthesia with different tourniquet deflation technics. Anesth Analg 68:633, 1989

88. Tryba M, Zenz M, Hausmann E: Prolonged analgesia after cuff release following IV regional analgesia with prilocaine. Br J Anaesth 55:631, 1983

89. Robinson DA, Shimmings KI: Uncomplicated accidental early tourniquet deflation during intravenous regional anaesthesia with prilocaine. Anaesthesia 44:83, 1984

90. Drexler H, Felman B, Finsterbusch A et al: Low-dose intravenous regional anesthesia in a case of multistaged, bilateral hand surgery. Anesth Analg 65:812, 1986

91. Egbert LD, Deas TC: Cause of pain from a pneumatic tourniquet during spinal anesthesia. Anesthesiology 23:287, 1962

92. Egbert LD: Tourniquet pain. Anesthesiology 25:247, 1964

93. DeJong RH: Tourniquet pain during spinal anesthesia: Anesthesiology 23:881, 1962

94. DeJong RH: Letter to the editor. Anesthesiology 25:248, 1964

95. Farah RS, Thomas PS: Sympathetic blockade and tourniquet pain in surgery of the upper extremity. Anesth Analg 66:1033, 1987

96. Concepcion MA, Lambert DH, Welch KA et al: Tourniquet pain during spinal anesthesia: A comparison of plain solutions of tetracaine and bupivacaine. Anesth Analg 67:828, 1988

97. Bridenbaugh PO, Hagenouw RR, Gielen MJM et al: Addition of glucose to bupivacaine in spinal anesthesia increases incidence of tourniquet pain. Anesth Analg 65:1181, 1986

98. Stewart A, Lambert DH, Concepcion MA et al: Decreased incidence of tourniquet pain during spinal anesthesia with bupivacaine. Anesth Analg 67:833, 1988

99. Valli TH, Kalso E, Rosenberg PH: Efficacy of 0.3 mg morphine intrathecally in preventing tourniquet pain during spinal anesthesia with hyperbaric bupivacaine. Acta Anaesthesiol Scand 32:113, 1988

100. Valli H, Rosenberg PH: Effects of three anaesthetic methods on haemodynamic responses connected with the use of thigh tourniquets in orthopaedic patients. Acta Anaesthesiol Scand 29:142, 1985

101. Hagenouw RPM, Bridenbaugh PO, van Egmond J et al: Tourniquet pain: A volunteer study. Anesth Analg 65:1175, 1986

102. Kahn RL, Marino VG, Urquhart B et al: Hemodynamic changes associated with tourniquet use under epidural anesthesia for total knee arthroplasty. Anesthesiology 71:A77, 1989

103. Benzon HT, Tolelkis JR, Meagher LL et al: Changes in venous blood lactate, venous blood gases and somatosensory evoked potentials after tourniquet application. Anesthesiology 69:677, 1988

104. Lambert DH, Deane RS, Mazuzan JE: Anesthesia and the control of blood pressure in patients with spinal cord injury. Anesth Analg 61:344, 1982

105. Nelson CL, Bowen WS: Total hip arthroplasty in Jehovah's Witnesses without blood transfusion. J Bone Joint Surg 68A:350, 1986

106. Sharrock NE, Mineo R: Hemodynamic response to low dose epinephrine infusions under hypotensive epidural anesthesia for total hip replacement. Anesth Analg 68:S255, 1989

107. Sharrock NE, Mineo R: The effects of low dose epinephrine and phenylephrine infusions on the hemodynamic response to epidural anesthesia. Anesth Analg 70:S366, 1990

108. Knight PR, Lane GA, Nichols MG et al: Hormonal and hemodynamic changes induced by pentolinium and propranolol during surgical correction of scoliosis. Anesthesiology 53:127, 1980

109. McNeil TW, DeWald RL, Kuo KN et al: Controlled hypotensive anesthesia in scoliosis surgery. J Bone Joint Surg 56A:1167, 1974

110. Bernard JM, Pinaud M, Carteau S et al: Hypotensive actions of diltiazem and nitroprusside compared during fentanyl anaesthesia for total hip arthroplasty. Can Anaesth Soc J 33:308, 1986

111. Gardner RC: Blood loss in orthopedic operations: Comparative studies in 19 major orthopedic procedures utilizing radioisotope labeling and an automatic blood volume computer. Surgery 68:489, 1970

112. Cowell HR, Swickard JW: Autotransfusion in children's orthopaedics. J Bone Joint Surg 56A:908, 1974

113. Thompson JD, Callaghan JJ, Savory CG et al: Prior deposition of autologous blood in elective orthopaedic surgery. J Bone Joint Surg 69A:320, 1987

114. Woolson ST, Marsh JS, Tanner JB: Transfusion of previously deposited autologous blood for patients undergoing hip replacement surgery. J Bone Joint Surg 69A:325, 1987

115. Ochsner JL, Mills NL, Leonard GL et al: Fresh autologous blood transfusions with extracorporeal circulation. Ann Surg 177:811, 1973

116. Rakower SR, Worth MH, Lackner H: Massive intraoperative autotransfusion of blood. Surg Gynecol Obstet 137:633, 1973

117. Bailey TE, Mahoney OM: The use of autologous blood in patients undergoing surgery for spinal deformity. J Bone Joint Surg 69A:329, 1987

118. Goulet JA, Bray TJ, Timmerman LA et al: Intraoperative autologous transfusion in orthopaedic patients. J Bone Joint Surg 71A:3, 1989

119. Wilson WJ: Intraoperative autologous transfusion in revision total hip arthroplasty. J Bone Joint Surg 71A:8, 1989

120. Messmer K, Lewis DH, Sunder-Plassman L et al: Acute normovolemic hemodilution: Changes of central hemodynamics and microcirculatory flow in skeletal muscle. Eur Surg Res 4:55, 1972

121. Messmer K, Sunder-Plassman L, Jesch F et al: Oxygen supply to the tissues during limited normovolemic hemodilution. Res Exp Med 159:152, 1973

122. Kallos T, Smith TC: Replacement for intraoperative blood loss. Anesthesiology 41:293, 1974

123. Cullings HM, Hendee WR: Radiation risks in the orthopaedic operating room. Contemp Orthop 8:48, 1984

124. Miller ME, Davis ML, MacClean CR et al: Radiation exposure and associated risks to operating room personnel during use of fluoroscopic guidance for selected orthopaedic surgical procedures. J Bone Joint Surg 65A:1, 1983

125. Nelson JP, Glassburn AR, Talbott RD et al: The effect of previous surgery, operating room environment, and preventive antibiotics on postoperative infection following total hip arthroplasty. Clin Orthop 147:167, 1980

126. Crow S, Greene VW: Aseptic transgressions among surgeons and anesthesiologists: A quantitative study. Arch Surg 117:1012, 1982

127. Alexander JW, Fisher JE, Boyojian M et al: The influence of hair removal methods on wound infections. Arch Surg 118:347, 1983

128. Ha'eri GB, Wiley AM: Wound contamination through drapes and gowns: A study using "tracer particles." Orthopedics 154:181, 1981

129. McCue SF, Berg EW, Saunders EA: Efficacy of double-gloving as a barrier to microbial contamination during total joint arthroplasty. J Bone Joint Surg 63A:811, 1981

130. Fitzgerald RH, Washington JA: Contamination of the operative wound. Orthop Clin North Am 6:1105, 1975

131. Letts RM, Doemer E: Conversation in the operation theater as a cause of airborne bacterial contamination. J Bone Joint Surg 65A:357, 1983

132. Ha'eri GB, Wiley AM: The efficacy of standard surgical face masks: An investigation using "tracer particles." Clin Orthop 148:160, 1980

133. Hart D: Bacterial ultraviolet radiation in the operating room: Twenty-nine-year studies for control of infections. JAMA 172:1019, 1960

134. Howard JM, Barker WF, Culbertson MR et al: Postoperative wound infections: The influence of ultraviolet irradiation on the operating room and various other factors. Ann Surg 160S:1, 1964

135. Lowell JD, Kundsin RB, Schwartz CM et al: Ultraviolet radiation and reduction of deep wound infection following hip and knee arthroplasty. Ann NY Acad Sci 353:285, 1980

136. Allander C, Abel E: Investigation of a new ventilating system for clean rooms. Med Res Engl 7:28, 1980

137. Charnley J, Eftekhar N: Postoperative infection in total prosthetic replacement arthroplasty of the hip joint, with special reference to the bacterial content of the air. Br J Surg 56:641, 1969

138. Coriell LL, Blackmore WS, McGarrity GJ: Medical applications of dust-free rooms: II. Elimination of airborne bacteria from an operating theater. JAMA 203:1038, 1968

139. Ha'eri GB, Wiley AM: Total hip replacement in a laminar flow environment, with special reference to deep infections. Clin Orthop 148:163, 1980

140. Haslam KR: Laminar air-flow air conditioning in the operating room: A review. Anesth Analg 53:194, 1974

141. Cruse RJ, Ford R: A five-year prospective study of 23,649 surgical wounds. Arch Surg 107:206, 1973

142. Fraser A, Edmonds-Seal J: Spinal cord injuries: A review of the problems facing the anaesthetist. Anaesthesia 37:1084, 1982

143. Caron CF, Bors E: A study of vascular changes during surgery of paraplegic patients. Paraplegia 7:292, 1970

144. Alvine FG, Schurrer ME: Postoperative ulnar nerve palsy. J Bone Joint Surg 69A:255, 1987

145. Mather LE: Parenteral opiates for postoperative analgesia. Reg Anesth 7:144, 1982

146. Griffen WO, Bennett RL: Inadequate treatment of pain in hospitalized patients (letter). N Engl J Med 307:56, 1982

147. Bennett RL, Batenhorst RL, Bivins B et al: Patient-controlled analgesia: A new concept of postoperative pain relief. Ann Surg 195:700, 1982

148. Check WA: Results are better when patients control their own analgesia. JAMA 247:945, 1982

149. Scott DB: Postoperative pain relief. Reg Anesth 7:S110, 1982

150. Tamsen A, Hartvig P, Fagerlund C et al: Patient-controlled analgesic therapy. Part I. Pharmacokinetics of pethedine in the pre- and postoperative periods. Clin Pharmacokinet 7:149, 1982

151. Dahlstrom B, Tamsen A, Pallzow L: Patient-controlled analgesic therapy. Part IV. Pharmacokinetics and analgesic plasma concentrations of morphine. Clin Pharmacokinet. 7:266, 1982

152. Ready LB, Oden R, Chadwick HS et al: Development of an anesthesiology-based postoperative pain management service. Anesthesiology 68:100, 1988

153. McQuay HJ, Carol D, Moore RA: Postoperative orthopaedic pain: The effects of opiate medication on local anesthetic blocks. Pain 33:291, 1988

154. Martin R, Salbaing J, Bloise G et al: Epidural morphine for postoperative pain relief: A dose-response curve. Anesthesiology 56:423, 1982

155. Barron DW, Strong JE, Postoperative analgesia in major orthopaedic surgery: Epidural and intrathecal opiates. Anaesthesia 36:937, 1981

156. Bromage PR, Camporesi EM, Durant PAC et al: Rostral spread of epidural morphine. Anesthesiology 56:431, 1982

157. Busch EK, Stedman PM: Epidural morphine for postoperative pain on medical-surgical wards: A clinical review. Anesthesiology 67:101, 1987

158. Strecker WB, Wood MB, Bieber EJ: Compartment syndrome masked by epidural anesthesia for postoperative pain. J Bone Joint Surg 68A:1447, 1986

159. Gossling HR, Ellison LH, Degraff AC: Fat embolism: The role of respiratory failure and its treatment. J Bone Joint Surg 56A:1327, 1974

160. Gossling HR, Pellegrini VD: Fat embolism syndrome: A review of the pathophysiology and physiological basis of treatment. Clin Orthop 165:68, 1982

161. Levy D: The fat embolism syndrome: A review. Clin Orthop 261:281, 1990

162. Hagley SR, Lee FC, Blumbergs PC: Fat embolism syndrome with total hip replacement. Med J Aust 145:541, 1986

163. Weisz GM, Steiner E: The cause of death in fat embolism. Chest 59:511, 1971

164. Wilson RF, McCarthy B, LeBlanc LP et al: Respiratory and coagulation changes after uncomplicated fractures. Arch Surg 106:395, 1973

165. Lindeque BGP, Shoeman HS, Dommisse GF et al: Fat embolism and the fat embolism syndrome. J Bone Joint Surg 69B:128, 1987

166. Gresham GA, Kuczynski A, Rosborough D: Fatal fat embolism following replacement arthroplasty for transcervical fractures of femur. Br Med J 2:617, 1971

167. Reilly DT: Prophylactic methods against thromboembolism. Acta Chir Scand [Suppl] 550:115, 1988

168. Hull RD, Raskob GE: Hip surgery and venous thrombosis: Effect of anesthesia. JAMA 264:2072, 1990

169. Saltzman EW, Harris WM: Prevention of venous thromboembolism in orthopaedic patients. J Bone Joint Surg 58A:903, 1976

170. Modig J: Influence of regional anesthesia, local anesthetics, and sympathicomimetics on the pathophysiology of deep vein thrombosis. Acta Chir Scand [Suppl] 550:119, 1988

171. Davis FM, Laurenson VG, Gillespie WJ et al: Leg blood flow during total hip replacement under spinal or general anaesthesia. Anaesth Intensive Care 17:136, 1989

172. Wille-Jorgensen P, Christensen W, Bjerg-Nielsen A et al: Prevention of thromboembolism following elective hip surgery. Clin Orthop Relat Res 247:163, 1989

173. Consensus Conference: Prevention of Venous Thrombosis and Pulmonary Embolism. JAMA 256:744, 1986

174. Anderson KH: Air aspirated from the venous system during total hip replacement. Anaesthesia 38:1175, 1983

175. Friedman RJ, Gumley GJ: Crepitation simulating gas gangrene. J Bone Joint Surg 67A:646, 1985

176. Whitehall R, Moskal JT, Scully KS et al: Nitrogen-gas injection from a power reamer: A complication of closed intramedullary nailing of the femur. J Bone Joint Surg 65A:860, 1983

177. Shupak RC, Shuster H, Funch RS: Airway emergency in a patient during CO_2 arthroscopy. Anesthesiology 60:171, 1984

178. Dwyer DM, Thorne AC, Healey JH et al: Liquid nitrogen installation can cause venous gas embolism. Anesthesiology 73:179, 1990

179. Rusheen JM, Hsu D, Lee C et al: Venous air embolism during surgical manipulation of femoral bone cyst. Anesthesiology 72:200, 1990

180. Haljamae H, Stefansson T, Wickstrom I: Preanesthetic evaluation of the female geriatric patient with hip fracture. Acta Anaesthesiol Scand 26:393, 1982

181. Davie IT, MacRae WR, Malcom-Smidi NA: Anesthesia for the fractured hip: A survey of 200 cases. Anesth Analg 49:165, 1970

182. Covert CR, Fox GS: Anaesthesia for hip surgery in the elderly. Can J Anaesth 36:311, 1989

183. Nightingale PJ, Marstrand T: Subarachnoid anaesthesia with bupivacaine for orthopaedic procedures in the elderly. Br J Anaesth 53:369, 1981

184. Howard CB, Mackie IG, Fairclough J et al: Femoral neck surgery using a local anaesthetic technique. Anaesthesia 38:993, 1983

185. Wickstrom I, Holmberg I, Stefansson T: Survival of female geriatric patients after hip fracture surgery: A comparison of five anaesthetic methods. Acta Anaesthesiol Scand 26:607, 1982

186. Groucke CR: Mortality following surgery for fracture of the neck of the femur. Anaesthesia 40:578, 1985

187. Hurley RJ: Continuous spinal anesthesia. Int Anesthesiol Clin 27:46, 1989

188. Van Gessel EF, Forster A, Gamulin Z: Surgical repair of hip fracture using continuous spinal anesthesia: A comparison of hypobaric solutions of tetracaine and bupivacaine. Anesth Analg 68:276, 1989

189. Smith-Peterson MN: Evolution of mould arthroplasty of the hip joint. J Bone Joint Surg 30B:59, 1948

190. Charnley J: Acrylic Cement in Orthopaedic Surgery. Baltimore, Williams & Wilkins, 1970

191. Eftekhar N: Low-friction arthroplasty: Indications, contraindications and complications. JAMA 218:705, 1971

192. Fredin H, Gustafson C, Rosberg B: Anaesthetic techniques and thromboembolism in total hip arthroplasty. Acta Anaesthesiol Scand 28:503, 1984

193. Hole A: Pre- and postoperative monocyte and lymphocyte function: Effects of combined epidural and general anaesthesia. Acta Anaesthesiol Scand 28:367, 1984

194. Hole A, Unsgaard G: The effect of epidural anaesthesia on lymphocyte functions during and after major orthopaedic surgery. Acta Anaesthesiol Scand 27:135, 1983

195. Hedenstierna G, Lofstrom J: Effect of anaesthesia on respiratory function after major lower extremity surgery. Acta Anaesthesiol Scand 29:55, 1985

196. Riis J, Lomholt B, Haxholdt O et al: Immediate and long-term mental recovery from general versus epidural anesthesia in elderly patients. Acta Anaesthesiol Scand 27:44, 1983

197. Combs SP, Greenwald AS: The effects of barium sulfate on the polymerization temperature and sheer strength of surgical simplex P. Clin Orthop 145:287, 1979

198. Svartling N, Lehtinen AM, Tarkkanen L: The effect of anaesthesia on changes in blood pressure and plasma cortisol levels induced by cementation with methylmethacrylate. Acta Anaesthesiol Scand 30:247, 1986

199. Ellis RH, Mulvein J: The cardiovascular effects of methylmethacrylate. J Bone Joint Surg 56B:59, 1974

200. Peebles DJ, Ellis RH, Stide SDK et al: Cardiovascular effects of methylmethacrylate cement. Br Med J 1:349, 1972

201. Samii K, Elmehk E, Goutaher D et al: Hemodynamic effects of prosthesis insertion during knee replacement without tourniquet. Anesthesiology 52:271, 1980

202. Samii K, Elmelik E, Mourtada MB et al: Intraoperative hemodynamic changes during total knee replacement. Anesthesiology 50:239, 1979

203. Weissman BN, Sosman JL, Braunstein EM et al: Intravenous methylmethacrylate after total hip replacement. J Bone Joint Surg 66A:44, 1984

204. Bengtson A, Larsson M, Gammer W et al: Anaphylatoxin release in association with methylmethacrylate fixation of hip prostheses. J Bone Joint Surg 69A:46, 1987

205. Crout DHG, Corkill JA, James ML et al: Methylmethacrylate metabolism in man: The hydrolysis of methylmethacrylate to methacrylate acid during total hip replacement. Clin Orthop 141:90, 1979

206. Modig J, Busch C, Olerud S et al: Arterial hypotension and hypoxemia during total hip replacement: The importance of thromboplastic procedures, fat embolism and acrylic monomers. Acta Anaesthesiol Scand 19:28, 1975

207. Sevitt S: Fat embolism in patients with fractured hips. Br Med J 2:257, 1972

208. Kallos T, Enis JE, Gollan F et al: Intramedullary pressure and pulmonary embolism of femoral medullary contents in dogs during insertion of bone cement and a prosthesis. J Bone Joint Surg 56A:1363, 1974

209. Kallos T: Impaired oxygenation associated with use of bone cement in the femoral shaft. Anesthesiology 42:210, 1975

210. Sharrock NE, Sanborn KV, Castellano P et al: Pulmonary hypertension following insertion of femoral prosthesis during total hip replacement. Anesth Analg 70:S367, 1990

211. Byrick J, Kay JC, Mullen JB: Capnography is not as sensitive as pulmonary artery pressure monitoring in detecting marrow microembolism. Anesth Analg 68:98, 1989

212. Cromwell TH: Methylmethacrylate airway obstruction. Anesthesiology 52:89, 1980

213. Burke DW, Gates ET, Harris WH: Centrifugation as a method of improving tensile and fatigue properties of acrylic bone cement. J Bone Joint Surg 66A:1265, 1984

214. Rimnac CM, Wright TM, McGill DL: The effect of centrifugation on the fracture properties of acrylic bone cements. J Bone Joint Surg 68A:281, 1986

215. Trippel SB: Current concept review: Antibiotic-impregnated cement in total joint arthroplasty. J Bone Joint Surg 68A:1297, 1986

216. Buchert PK, Vaughn BK, Mallory TH et al: Excessive metal release due to loosening and fretting of sintered particles on porous-coated hip prostheses. J Bone Joint Surg 68A:606, 1986

217. Turner TM, Sumner DR, Urban RM et al: A comparative study of porous coatings in a weight-bearing total hip arthroplasty model. J Bone Joint Surg 68A:1396, 1986

218. Smith BE, Challands JF, Suchak M et al: Regional anaesthesia for surgery of the forearm and hand. Anaesthesia 44:747, 1989

219. Rosenblatt R, Pepitone-Rockwell F, McKillop MJ: Continuous axillary analgesia for traumatic hand injury. Anesthesiology 51:565, 1979

220. Schiller MG: Intravenous regional anesthesia for closed treatment of fractures and dislocations of upper extremities. Clin Orthop 118:25, 1976

221. Kongsholm J, Olerud C: Neurologic complications of dynamic reduction of Colles' fractures without anesthesia compared with traditional manipulation after local infiltration anesthesia. J Orthrop Trauma 1:43, 1987

222. Cofield RH, Irving JF: Evaluation and classification of shoulder instability. Clin Orthop Relat Res 223:32, 1987

223. Peterson DO: Shoulder block anesthesia for shoulder reconstruction surgery. Anesth Analg 64:373, 1985

224. Roch J, Sharrock NE, Neudachin L: Interscalene brachial plexus block for shoulder surgery: Significance of paresthesia site. Anesthesiology 73:A849, 1990

225. Conn RA, Cofield RH, Byer DE et al: Interscalene block anesthesia for shoulder surgery. Clin Orthop Relat Res 216:94, 1987

226. Ericksson E, Haggmark T, Saartok T et al: Knee arthroscopy with local anesthesia in ambulatory patients. Orthopaedics 9:186, 1986

227. Kirkeby OJ, Aase S: Knee arthroscopy and arthrotomy under local anesthesia. Acta Orthop Scand 58:133, 1987

228. Carnes RS III, Butterworth JF IV, Poehling GS et al: Safety and efficacy of intra-articular bupivacaine and epinephrine anesthesia for knee arthroscopy. Anesthesiology 71:A729, 1989

229. Patel NJ, Flashburg MH, Paskin S et al: A regional anesthetic technique compared to general anesthesia for outpatient knee arthroscopy. Anesth Analg 65:185, 1986

230. Tartiere J, Berthelin C, Jehan C et al: Hemodynamic changes during total knee replacement surgery with total condylar prosthesis. Anesthesiology 67:838, 1987

231. Fahmy W, Danylchuk K, Chandler HP et al: Changes in the circulation and gas exchange during total knee replacement: A detailed study of intramedullary rodding of the femur. Anesthesiology 69:A823, 1988

232. Mann RAM, Bisset WLK: Anaesthesia for lower limb amputation. Anaesthesia 38:1185, 1983

233. Bromage PR, Melzack R: Phantom limbs and the body schema. Can Anaesth Soc J 21:267, 1974

234. Bach S, Noreng M, Tjellden NU: Phantom limb pain in amputees during the first 12 months following limb amputation, after preoperative lumbar epidural blockade. Pain 33:297, 1988

235. Jacobsen L, Chabal C: Prolonged relief of acute postamputation phantom limb pain with intrathecal fentanyl and epidural morphine. Anesthesiology 71:984, 1989

236. Akturk G, Baki C, Ozen I et al: Intravenous prilocaine (Citanest) for anesthesia in the lower extremity. Isr J Med Sci 24:716, 1988

237. Cox P: Intravenous regional analgesia: A new modification. Acta Anaesthesiol Scand 33:336, 1989

238. Bird TM, Strunin L: Anaesthetic considerations for microsurgical repair of limbs. Can Anaesth Soc J 31:51, 1984

239. Caplan RA, Long MC: Prolonged anesthesia-management and sequelae of a two-day general anesthetic. Anesth Analg 63:353, 1984

240. Friedlander GE: Bone grafting. Orthop Clin North Am 18:179, 1987

241. MacDonald DJF: Anaesthesia for microvascular procedures. Br J Anaesth 57:904, 1985

242. Taylor AR, Gleadhill CA, Bilsland WL et al: Posture and anaesthesia for spinal operations with special reference to intervertebral disc surgery. Br J Anaesth 28:213, 1956

243. Santavirta S, Slatis P, Kankaanpaa U et al: Treatment of the cervical spine in rheumatoid arthritis. J Bone Joint Surg 70A:65, 1988

244. Ovassapian A, Land P, Schafer NF et al: Anesthetic management for surgical correction of severe flexion deformity of the cervical spine. Anesthesiology 58:370, 1983

245. Smith RH, Gramling ZW, Volpitto PP: Problems related to the prone position for surgical operations. Anesthesiology 22:189, 1961

246. Smith RH: One solution to the problem of the prone position for surgical procedures. Anesth Analg 53:221, 1974

247. Lee C, Barnes A, Nagel EL: Neuroleptanalgesia for awake pronation of surgical patients. Anesth Analg 56:276, 1977

248. Bergofsky EH, Turino GM, Fishman AP: Cardiorespiratory failure in kyphoscoliosis. Medicine 38:263, 1959

249. Baydur A, Swank SM, Stiles CM et al: Respiratory elastic load compensation in anesthetized patients with kyphoscoliosis. J Appl Physiol 67:1024, 1989

250. Harrington PR: Treatment of scoliosis. J Bone Joint Surg 44A:591, 1962

251. Anderson PR, Puno MR, Lovell SL et al: Postoperative respiratory complications in non-idiopathic scoliosis. Acta Anaesthesiol Scand 29:186, 1985

252. Wills DG: Anaesthetic management of posterior lumbar osteotomy. Can Anaesth Soc J 32:248, 1985

253. Mandel RJ, Brown MD, McCollough NC et al: Hypotensive anesthesia and autotransfusion in spinal surgery. Clin Orthop 154:27, 1981

254. Marshall WK, Bedford RF, Arnold WP et al: Effects of propranolol on the cardiovascular and renin-angiotensin systems during hypotension produced by sodium nitroprusside in humans. Anesthesiology 55:277, 1981

255. Hoffman WE, Albrecht RT, Miletich DJ: Cardiovascular and metabolic effects of SNP-induced hypotension in young and aged hypertensive rats. Anesthesiology 56:427, 1982

256. Waldman J, Kaufer H, Hensinger RN et al: Wake-up technique to avoid neurologic sequelae during Harrington rod procedure: A case report. Anesth Analg 56:733, 1977

257. Grundy BL, Nash CL, Brown RH: Deliberate hypotension for spinal fusion: Prospective randomized study with evoked potential monitoring. Can Anaesth Soc J 29:452, 1982

258. Pathak KS, Brown RH, Nash CL Jr et al: Continuous opioid infusion for scoliosis fusion surgery. Anesth Analg 62:841, 1983

259. Diaz JH, Lockhart CH: Postoperative quadriplegia after spinal fusion for scoliosis with intraoperative awakening. Anesth Analg 66:1039, 1987

260. Kafer ER: Respiratory and cardiovascular functions in scoliosis and the principles of anesthetic management. Anesthesiology 52:339, 1980

261. Feldstein G, Ramanathan S: Obstetrical lumbar epidural anesthesia in patients with previous posterior spinal fusion for kyphoscoliosis. Anesth Analg 64:83, 1985

262. Matheson D: Epidural anaesthesia for lumbar laminectomy and spinal fusion. Can Anaesth Soc J 7:149, 1960

263. Brown EM, Gass H, Noe FD et al: Oxygen tension during laminectomy. JAMA 205:882, 1968

264. Smith L, Brown JE: Treatment of lumbar intervertebral disc lesions by direct injection of chymopapain. J Bone Joint Surg 49B:502, 1967

265. Nordby EJ, Brown MD: Present status of chymopapain and chemonucleolysis. Clin Orthop 129:79, 1977

266. Department of Health and Human Services: Chymopapain approved. FDA Drug Bull 12:17, 1982

267. Spencer CW: Chemonucleolysis under local anesthesia. Orthopedics 6:1617, 1983

268. Hall BB, McCulloch JA: Anaphylactic reaction following the intradiscal injection of chymopapain under local anesthesia. J Bone Joint Surg 65A:1215, 1983

269. Javid MJ, Nordby EJ, Ford LT et al: Safety and efficacy of chymopapain (Chymodiactin) in herniated nucleus pulposus with sciatica: Results of a randomized, double-blind study. JAMA 249:2489, 1983

270. Allison CW, Wardlaw D: Anaphylaxis and chymopapain. Anaesthesia 45:164, 1990

271. Smith L: Chymopapain. JAMA 265:215, 1991

45

George Graf
Stanley Rosenbaum

Anesthesia and the Endocrine System

THYROID GLAND

The thyroid hormones, thyroxine (T_4) and 3,5,3'-1-triiodothyronine (T_3), are the major regulators of cellular metabolic activity. Thyroid hormones influence a variety of proteolytic reactions by regulating the synthesis and activity of various proteins. They are necessary for proper cardiac, pulmonary, and neurologic function during both health and illness.

Thyroid Metabolism and Function

The production of thyroid hormone is initiated by the active uptake and concentration of iodide within the thyroid gland (Fig. 45-1). Iodine is absorbed and reduced to iodide in the gastrointestinal (GI) tract. Circulating iodide is taken up and concentrated in the thyroid gland, where the iodide is oxidized by a peroxidase reaction to form iodine. It is then bound to tyrosine residues to form various iodotyrosines. After organification, mono- or diiodotyrosine are coupled enzymatically (thyroid peroxidase) to form either T_3 or T_4. These hormones are attached to the thyroglobulin protein and stored as colloid within the gland. The release of T_3 and T_4 from the gland is accomplished through proteolysis from the thyroglobulin and diffusion into the circulation. Thyrotropin (TSH) is produced in the anterior pituitary gland, and its secretion is regulated by thyrotropin-releasing hormone (TRH), produced in the hypothalamus. Thyrotropin is responsible for maintaining the uptake of iodide and proteolytic release of thyroid hormone.[1] Excess iodine inhibits the synthesis and secretion of thyroid hormone.[2] The thyroid gland is solely responsible for the daily secretion of T_4 (80–100 $\mu g \cdot day^{-1}$).[3] The half-life of T_4 in the circulation is 6–7 days.

Approximately 80% of T_3 is produced by the extrathyroidal deiodination of T_4 and 20% by direct thyroid secretion. The half-life of T_3 is 24–30 hours. Most of the effects of thyroid hormones are mediated by the more potent and less protein bound T_3. The degree to which these hormones are protein bound in the circulation is the major factor influencing their activity and degradation. T_4 is metabolized by monodeiodination to either T_3 or reverse T_3 (rT_3). T_3 is biologically active, whereas rT_3 is inactive. The major fraction of circulating hormone is bound to thyroid-binding globulin (TBG), with a smaller fraction bound to thyroid-binding prealbumin. Changes in serum binding protein concentrations have a major effect on total T_3 and T_4 serum concentrations. The plasma normally contains 5–12 $\mu g \cdot dl^{-1}$ of T_4 and 80–220 $ng \cdot dl^{-1}$ of T_3. The secretion of TRH and TSH appears to be regulated by a negative feedback loop, which is dependent on circulating levels of T_4 and T_3. T_3 probably exerts its numerous effects through interaction with nuclear receptors. This nuclear binding stimulates messenger RNA synthesis, which in turn controls protein synthesis.

Although the thyroid hormone is important to many aspects of growth and function, the anesthesiologist is most often concerned with the cardiovascular manifestations of thyroid disease. Thyroid hormones affect tissue responses to sympathetic stimuli and increase the intrinsic contractile state of cardiac muscle.[4] Beta-adrenergic receptors are increased in number and cardiac alpha-adrenergic receptors are decreased by thyroid hormone.[5] It has been proposed that thyroid hormone may modulate the conversion of alpha to beta receptors without affecting the overall affinity of these receptors. Two possible explanations for the "hyperadrenergic" state of thyrotoxicosis or the decreased tone of hypothyroidism are an increased or decreased number of sympathetic receptors, or possibly an alteration in the beta-adrenergic signal between hormone and receptor.[6]

Tests of Thyroid Function

Total Serum Thyroxine

The serum T_4 assay is the standard screening test for evaluation of thyroid gland function (Table 45-1). The total T_4 will be elevated in about 90% of patients with hyperthyroidism, and it will be low in 85% of those who are hypothyroid. The concentration of T_4 is measured by radioimmunoassay (RIA). The serum T_4 concentration is influenced by thyroid hormone protein-binding capacity. An increase or decrease in TBG levels or in protein binding may therefore alter the total T_4. Elevations in the TBG concentration are the most common cause of hyperthyroxinemia in euthyroid patients. Increases in TBG due to acute liver disease, pregnancy, or drugs (oral contraceptives, exogenous estrogens, clofibrate, opioids) may be responsible. Because a total T_4 can be mis-

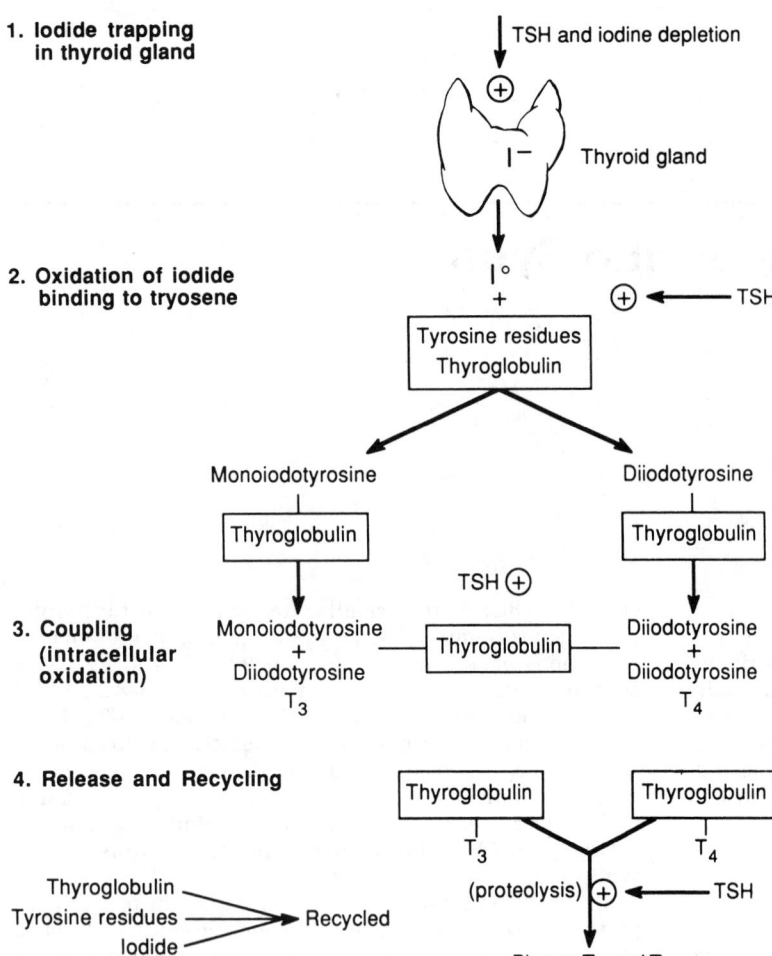

1. **Iodide trapping in thyroid gland**

2. **Oxidation of iodide binding to tryosene**

3. **Coupling (intracellular oxidation)**

4. **Release and Recycling**

Figure 45-1. Thyroid hormone biosynthesis consists of four stages: (1) organification, (2) binding, (3) coupling, and (4) release.

leadingly high in euthyroidism or normal in hypothyroidism, some measure of free thyroid hormone activity (free T_4) must also be used.

Free T_4 (FT$_4$) and Free T_3 (FT$_3$)

The percentage of FT_4 (normal, 1.5–5.0 ng·dl^{-1}) or FT_3 is currently measured by equilibrium dialysis. A small quantity of radiolabeled T_4 or T_3 is added to the patient's serum. The percentage of the labeled hormone that crosses a dialysis membrane represents the percentage of free hormone in the serum. This volume is multiplied by the total serum T_4 or T_3 to give the amount of free hormone in the plasma. An RIA for FT_4 has recently become available and may soon replace the older method of analysis.[1] This test is independent of the plasma concentration of TBG.

Serum Triiodothyronine

The serum T_3 is also measured by RIA. The normal range is 80–200 ng·dl^{-1}. Serum T_3 levels are often determined to detect disease in patients with clinical evidence of hyperthyroidism in the absence of elevations of T_4. T_3 may be the only thyroid hormone produced in excess. T_3 concentrations may be depressed by factors that impair the peripheral conversion of T_4 to T_3 (sick euthyroid syndrome). In 50% of hypothyroid patients, the serum T_3 concentration is low; in the remaining 50% it is normal.[7]

T_3 Resin Uptake (RT$_3$U)

RT_3U is an indirect measure of the unbound plasma concentration of thyroxine. Radiolabeled T_3 is added to the patient's serum. Some of this T_3 binds to available protein-binding sites. A resin is then added that binds to the remaining unbound T_3. Resin uptake of radiolabeled T_3 varies indirectly with the number of free binding sites. In normal patients, RT_3U is 25–35%. RT_3U is not related to serum T_3 levels since the affinity of TBG for T_3 is low compared with that of T_4. RT_3U is high in hyperthyroidism, when protein binding sites are occupied by other substances (salicylates) or when TBG is decreased (nephrotic syndrome, chronic liver disease). RT_3U is decreased when fewer binding sites are occupied by T_4 (hypothyroidism) or when TBG is increased.

In general, if both the total T_4 and T_3 resin uptake are high or if both are low, the patient probably has hyperthyroidism or hypothyroidism, respectively. When the T_4 and T_3 resin uptake are in opposite directions, a binding abnormality is probable.

Free Thyroxine Index

The free thyroxine index (FTI) is calculated by multiplying the total FT_4U and FT_3U. Normal values range from 1.6 to 5.7 µg·dl^{-1}. The free T_4 index is frequently used to distinguish alterations in binding from true metabolic abnormalities.

TABLE 45-1. Tests of Thyroid Gland Function

	T_4	RT_3U	T_3	TSH
Hyperthyroidism	Elevated	Elevated	Elevated	Normal or low
Primary hypothyroidism	Low	Low	Low or normal	Elevated
Secondary hypothyroidism	Low	Low	Low	Low
Sick euthyroidism (decreased peripheral conversion of T_4 to T_3)	Normal	Normal	Low	Normal
Pregnancy	Elevated	Low	Normal	Normal

T_4 = total serum thyroxine, RT_3U = T_3 resin uptake, T_3 = serum triiodothyronine, TSH = thyroid-stimulating hormone.

Thyroid-Stimulating Hormone

The RIA for this hormone has proved most useful in detecting patients who are hypothyroid. It is often higher than 20 $\mu IU \cdot ml^{-1}$ in primary hypothyroidism (normal, <8 $\mu IU \cdot ml^{-1}$). TSH assays are not sensitive enough to discriminate between hyperthyroid and euthyroid states. A low TSH level in the hypothyroid patient indicates disease at the pituitary or hypothalamic level. Starvation, fever, stress, corticosteroids, and T_3 or T_4 can all depress TSH levels.

Thyroid-Releasing Hormone Testing

The administration of TRH (400 μg) increases the serum TSH level within 30 minutes in normal subjects. Hypothyroid patients have an exaggerated response, whereas hyperthyroid patients have a subnormal response or no response. This illustrates the exquisitely sensitive response of the hypothalamic-pituitary axis to T_3 or T_4. Other conditions that may blunt the response to TRH include fasting glucocorticoid administration, dopamine, some psychiatric disorders, and advanced age.

Radioactive Iodine Uptake

The thyroid gland has the ability to concentrate large amounts of inorganic iodide. The oral administration of radioactive iodine (^{131}I) can be used to indicate thyroid gland activity. Thyroid uptake is elevated in hyperthyroidism unless the hyperthyroidism is caused by thyroiditis, in which case the uptake is low or absent. Because of overlap in values, it is difficult to distinguish euthyroid from hypothyroid persons. Radioactive iodide uptake (RAIU) may be increased by a variety of factors, including dietary iodine deficiency, renal failure, and congestive heart failure. Because uptake is under TSH control, elevated FT_4 levels, corticosteroids, and dopamine will all decrease RAIU. Functioning thyroid tissue ("hot") is rarely malignant. Nonfunctioning ("cold") tissue may be malignant or benign.

Hyperthyroidism

Hyperthyroidism results from the exposure of tissues to excessive amounts of thyroid hormone. The most common etiology is the multinodular diffuse goiter of Graves' disease (Table 45-2). This typically occurs between the ages of 20 and 40 years and is predominant in females. The majority of these patients demonstrate a syndrome characterized by diffuse glandular enlargement, ophthalmopathy, dermopathy, and clubbing of the fingers. A thyroid-stimulating autoantibody (LATS) may be present.[8] Thyroiditis is another cause of increased thyroid hormone synthesis.[9] Subacute thyroiditis frequently follows a respiratory illness[10] and is characterized by a viral-like illness with a firm painful gland. This type of thyroiditis is frequently treated with anti-inflammatory agents alone. Rarely, subacute thyroiditis may occur in a patient with a normal-sized painless gland.[11] Hashimoto's thyroiditis is a chronic autoimmune disease that usually produces hypothyroidism but may occasionally produce hyperthyroidism. Hyperthyroidism may also be associated with pregnancy,[12] thyroid adenoma, ^{131}I therapy, thyroid carcinoma, trophoblastic tumors, or solely from a TSH-secreting pituitary adenomas. Iatrogenic hyperthyroidism may follow thyroid hormone replacement or may occur following iodide exposure[13] (angiography dye) in patients with chronically low iodide intake (Jod-Basedow's phenomenon). The antiarrhythmic agent amiodarone is iodine rich and is another cause of iodine-induced thyrotoxicosis.[14]

TABLE 45-2. Causes of Hyperthyroidism

Intrinsic Thyroid Disease

Hyperfunctioning thyroid adenoma
Toxic multinodular goiter

Abnormal TSH Stimulator

Graves' disease
Trophoblastic tumor

Disorders of Hormone Storage or Release

Thyroiditis

Excess Production of TSH

Pituitary thyrotropin (rare)

Extrathyroidal Source of Hormone

Struma ovarii
Functioning follicular carcinoma

Exogenous Thyroid

Iatrogenic
Iodine-induced

The major manifestations of hyperthyroidism are weight loss, diarrhea, skeletal muscle weakness, warm moist skin, heat intolerance, and nervousness. Hypercalcemia, thrombocytopenia, and a mild anemia may be present. Elderly patients may present with heart failure owing to papillary muscle dysfunction, atrial fibrillation, or other cardiac dysrhythmias without other systemic signs or symptoms of hyperthyroidism (apathetic hyperthyroidism).[15,16] Patients with Graves' disease may have a number of extrathyroidal manifestations, including ophthalmopathy and clubbing of the fingers.

"Thyroid storm" is a life-threatening exacerbation of hyperthyroidism seen during periods of stress (e.g., infection, injury, surgery).[17-19] Its manifestations include hyperpyrexia, tachycardia, anorexia, extreme anxiety, altered consciousness, and cardiovascular instability.[20] Although FT_4 levels are often markedly elevated, no laboratory test is diagnostic.[21] The potential for significant perioperative morbidity with uncontrolled hyperthyroidism necessitates postponing elective surgery until the patient has been made clinically euthyroid. Therapy takes several directions: suppression of thyroid hormone synthesis through the use of antithyroid drugs; blocking the release of preformed hormone; inhibition of the peripheral conversion of T_4 to T_3; and supportive therapy, including correction of fluid and electrolyte imbalances and, most importantly, when thyroid storm is a consideration in the treatment of the precipitating (nonthyroidal) cause.

Treatment and Anesthetic Considerations

The drugs propylthiouracil and methimazole are thiourea derivatives that inhibit the synthesis of thyroid hormone. Propylthiouracil also decreases the peripheral conversion of T_4 to T_3. Both drugs are well absorbed from the GI tract. Normal thyroid glands usually contain a store of hormone that is large enough to maintain a euthyroid state for several months, even if all synthesis is abolished.[22] Therefore, hyperthyroid patients are unlikely to be regulated to a euthyroid state with antithyroid drugs alone in less than 6–8 weeks. Once a euthyroid state is achieved, the dosage of these drugs should be reduced in order to avoid hypothyroidism. Toxic reactions from these drugs are uncommon but include skin rash, nausea, fever, agranulocytosis, hepatitis, and a lupus-like syndrome.

Inorganic iodide inhibits iodide organification and thyroid hormone release. Oral iodide is supplied as a potassium iodide solution (Lugol's solution), which is usually given about an hour after the administration of antithyroid drugs so that thyroidal accumulation of iodide may be avoided. Iodide is also effective in reducing the size of the hyperplastic gland.

Beta-adrenergic antagonists are effective in attenuating the manifestations of excessive sympathetic activity. For example, propranolol given over 12–24 hours improves tachycardia, heat intolerance, anxiety, and tremor. Beta-adrenergic blockade alone does not inhibit hormone synthesis, but it does impair the peripheral conversion of T_4 to T_3 over a period of 1–2 weeks. The combination of propranolol (in doses titrated to effect) plus potassium iodide (2–5 drops every 8 hours) is frequently used preoperatively to ameliorate cardiovascular symptoms and reduce circulating concentrations of T_4 and T_3.[23] Preoperative preparation usually requires 7–14 days. Beta-adrenergic antagonists should not be used routinely in patients with symptoms of congestive heart failure or bronchospasm. Heart failure secondary to poorly controlled paroxysmal atrial fibrillation may improve with slowing of the ventricular rate, but abnormalities of left ventricular function secondary to hyperthyroidism may not be corrected with the use of beta antagonists.[24] If a hyperthyroid patient with clinically apparent disease requires emergency surgery, propranolol is administered in 0.5 mg intravenous (iv) boluses. As an alternative, the ultra-short-acting beta antagonist esmolol may be delivered as a continuous infusion, which is adjusted to maintain a heart rate less than 90 beats·min^{-1}. T_4 can also be removed from the circulation by means of blood exchanges, plasmapheresis, or peritoneal dialysis. These methods should be considered if conventional pharmacologic methods fail to improve the patient's condition and emergency surgery is necessary.

Other drugs infrequently used to combat the symptoms of hyperthyroidism are the catecholamine-depleting drugs reserpine and guanethidine. Glucocorticoids such as dexamethasone (8–12 mg·day^{-1}) reduce thyroid hormone secretion in Graves' disease and reduce the peripheral conversion of T_4 to T_3. The mild hypercalcemia often seen in hyperthyroid patients is also reduced by glucocorticoids through an inhibition of bone resorption.

Radioactive iodine therapy is an effective treatment for some patients with thyrotoxicosis. It should not, however, be administered to pregnant patients, because it crosses the placenta and may destroy the fetal thyroid. A side-effect of RAI therapy includes hypothyroidism; 10–60% of cases occur in the first year of therapy, and an additional 2% occur per year thereafter.[25]

Surgery

Subtotal thyroidectomy as an alternative to prolonged medical therapy is used less frequently today than in the past. Patients are rendered euthyroid prior to thyroid surgery through the use of a combination of beta blockers plus potassium iodide for 7–14 days or antithyroid medication for 6–8 weeks. Potassium iodide may be added to the antithyroid medication for the 7–10 days prior to surgery to facilitate shrinking of the gland. All antithyroid medications are continued through the morning of surgery.

A variety of anesthetic techniques and drugs have been used for hyperthyroid patients undergoing surgery.[26] The key to the management of these patients is delaying the stress of surgery until the patient has been brought to a euthyroid state. The goal of intraoperative management in the hyperthyroid patient is achieving a depth of anesthesia that prevents an exaggerated sympathetic response to surgical stimulation while avoiding the administration of medication that stimulates the sympathetic nervous system. It is best to avoid using ketamine even when a patient is clinically euthyroid.[27] Hypotension that occurs during surgery is best treated with direct-acting vasopressors rather than a medication that provokes the release of catecholamines. The appropriate selection of neuromuscular blocking drug deserves mention. Pancuronium has the ability to increase the heart rate and should probably be avoided; drugs that provide greater cardiovascular stability (vecuronium, atracurium) should be used. The incidence of myasthenia gravis is increased in hyperthyroid patients; thus, the initial dose of muscle relaxant should be reduced and a twitch monitor should be used to guide all subsequent administration of neuromuscular blocking agents. Regional anesthesia is an excellent alternative when appropriate; however, epinephrine-containing solutions are avoided.

Complications of surgery in hyperthyroid patients occur more frequently when preoperative preparation has been inadequate. Airway obstruction is a potential problem in the patient with a large goiter. Computed tomography (CT) of the neck preoperatively provides valuable information about airway anatomy.[28] Thyroid storm, "thyrotoxicosis," may occur intraoperatively or in the immediate postoperative period. Hyperthermia, tachycardia, and dysrhythmias may mimic the onset of malignant hyperthermia.[29] In addition to the various antithyroid medications mentioned previously, supportive measures to control fever and restore intravascular volume should be used. Hemodynamic monitoring (pulmonary artery catheter, arterial catheter) is especially useful in guiding the treatment of patients with significant left ventricular dysfunction. Again, it is essential to remove or treat the precipitating event.

The complications following subtotal thyroidectomy include recurrent laryngeal nerve damage, tracheal compression secondary to hematoma or tracheomalacia, and hypoparathyroidism.[30] Hypoparathyroidism secondary to the inadvertent surgical removal of parathyroid glands is most frequently seen after total thyroidectomy. The symptoms of hypocalcemia develop within the first 24–48 hours following surgery. Laryngeal stridor progressing to laryngospasm may be one of the first indications of hypocalcemic tetany. The iv administration of calcium chloride or calcium gluconate is warranted in this situation. Bilateral recurrent laryngeal nerve injury is an extremely rare injury and necessitates reintubation. Unilateral nerve injury is more common and often goes unnoticed. Unilateral damage to the recurrent laryngeal nerve is characterized by hoarseness and a paralyzed vocal cord, while bilateral injury causes aphonia. It is wise to evaluate vocal cord function preoperatively and postoperatively by laryngoscopy or by asking the patient to phonate by saying the letter "e." Postoperative extubation of the trachea should be performed under optimal conditions. Intraoperative laryngeal nerve injury or collapse of the tracheal rings from previous weakening may mandate emergency reintubation.[31]

Hypothyroidism

Hypothyroidism is a relatively common disease (0.5–0.8% of the adult population) that results from inadequate circulating levels of T_4 or T_3, or both. The development of hypothyroidism is often slow and progressive, making the clinical diagnosis difficult, especially in the more subtle cases. Hypofunctioning of the thyroid gland has many causes (Table 45-3).[32] Primary failure of the thyroid gland refers to decreased production of thyroid hormone despite adequate TSH production and accounts for 95% of all cases of thyroid dysfunction. The remainder are caused by either hypothalamic or pituitary disease (secondary hypothyroidism).

Clinical Manifestations

A lack of thyroid hormone produces a variety of signs and symptoms. These early findings are often nonspecific and difficult to recognize. A history of RAI therapy, external neck irradiation, or the presence of a goiter are all helpful in making a diagnosis. There is a generalized reduction in metabolic activity, resulting in lethargy, slow mental functioning, cold intolerance, and slow movements. The cardiovascular manifestations of hypothyroidism reflect the importance of the thyroid hormone on myocardial contractility and catecholamine function. These patients exhibit bradycardia and depressed myocardial contractility.[33] The accumulation of a cholesterol-rich pericardial fluid produces

---

TABLE 45-3. Causes of Hypothyroidism

Primary Hypothyroidism

Autoimmune
Irradiation to the neck
Previous ^{131}I therapy
Surgical removal
Thyroiditis (Hashimoto's)
Severe iodine depletion
Medications (iodines, propylthiouracil, methimazole)
Hereditary defects in biosynthesis
Congenital defects in gland development

Secondary or Tertiary Hypothyroidism

Pituitary
Hypothalamic

Reproduced with permission from Petersdorf RG (ed): Harrison's Principles of Internal Medicine, 10th ed. New York, McGraw-Hill, 1983.

---

low voltage on the electrocardiogram (ECG).[34] Impaired myocardial contractility generally correlates with the severity of hypothyroidism, but, interestingly, myxedema rarely produces congestive heart failure in the absence of coexisting heart disease.[35] Autopsy findings of more advanced coronary artery disease in myxedematous hypertensive patients compared with euthyroid hypertensive controls may reflect the abnormal lipid profile of hypothyroidism.[36] Angina pectoris itself is unusual in hypothyroidism and usually appears when thyroid hormone treatment is initiated (catecholamine hypersensitivity). Peripheral vasoconstriction may lead to hypertension and a cool dry skin. Hypothyroidism with amyloidosis is associated with cardiac conduction abnormalities, renal dysfunction, and enlargement of the tongue. Zwilich and colleagues[37] have reported that the ventilatory responsiveness to hypoxia and hypercapnia is depressed in hypothyroid patients. This depression is potentiated by sedatives, opioids, and general anesthesia. It should be noted that postoperative ventilatory failure requiring prolonged ventilation is rarely seen in hypothyroid patients in the absence of coexisting lung disease, obesity, or myxedema coma.[37] Other abnormalities found in hypothyroidism include various coagulation abnormalities, reduced platelet adhesiveness, GI bleeding, anemia, hypothermia, and impaired renal concentrating ability.[38,39] Basal plasma levels of cortisol are usually normal in hypothyroidism; however, in long-standing or severe disease, the stress response may be blunted and adrenal depression may occur.

In addition to these clinical findings, laboratory analysis is used to confirm the diagnosis of hypothyroidism and to aid the clinician in determining the severity of the disease. "Severe" hypothyroidism denotes cases of extreme clinical abnormalities, including "myxedema coma" and T_4 levels as low as 1 μg·dl^{-1} or less and TSH levels in the range of 50–100 μIU·ml^{-1}. When the diagnosis of hypothyroidism is suspected, a blood sample is obtained for T_4, TSH, RT$_3$U, and cortisol determination. Thyroid replacement may be started while the clinician is awaiting results. Primary hypothyroidism is characterized by low T_4 and RT$_3$U levels and an elevated TSH. Secondary hypothyroidism is evidenced by low T_4, RT$_3$U, and TSH levels. A thorough evaluation of other pituitary function should be undertaken when this condition exists; entities to be identified or excluded include pituitary tumor and postpartum pituitary necrosis.

Treatment and Anesthetic Considerations

Controversy remains regarding the preoperative anesthetic management of the hypothyroid patient. Although it seems logical to recommend that all surgical candidates who are hypothyroid be restored to a euthyroid state prior to surgery, such a recommendation is in general based on individual case reports. There have been few controlled studies to support the position that most hypothyroid patients are unusually sensitive to anesthetic drugs, have prolonged recovery times, or suffer from a higher incidence of cardiovascular instability or collapse.

Two controlled studies investigated the subject of surgery in the hypothyroid patient. Weinberg et al[40] conducted a retrospective analysis of 59 hypothyroid patients who were matched with 59 euthyroid controls. All patients underwent surgery with general anesthesia and endotracheal intubation. The hypothyroid patients were divided into three subsets ($T_4 < 1$ $\mu g \cdot dl^{-1}$, $T_4 < 3$ $\mu g \cdot dl^{-1}$, $T_4 \geq 3$ $\mu g \cdot dl^{-1}$). Of the 59 study patients, 52 were classified as mildly or moderately hypothyroid ($T_4 > 1$ $\mu g \cdot dl^{-1}$). Analysis of the three subsets of hypothyroid patients and their matched controls disclosed no significant differences with regard to fluid and electrolyte imbalances, hemodynamic stability, time to extubation of the trachea, or length of postoperative hospitalization. There were no significant differences in the incidence of complications between the groups. Because the number of patients with severe hypothyroidism was small (seven patients), no conclusions can be drawn with regard to the proper management of this group. The authors did recommend that it was safe to proceed with anesthesia and surgery before thyroid hormone replacement in those patients with mild or moderate hypothyroidism. Ladenson et al[41] retrospectively reviewed 40 hypothyroid patients undergoing surgery and compared them with 80 euthyroid controls. Although 33 of the hypothyroid patients received thyroid hormone replacement therapy preoperatively, all of the test patients had persistent chemical hypothyroidism at the time of surgery. A comparison of partially treated patients with untreated hypothyroid patients showed no significant differences in the frequency of complications. Despite a higher incidence of intraoperative hypotension and postoperative GI and neuropsychiatric complications among hypothyroid patients undergoing noncardiac surgery, the authors did not believe there were compelling clinical reasons to postpone surgery in mildly or moderately hypothyroid patients. They further concluded that conventional clinical or biochemical criteria may not accurately define a subgroup of hypothyroid patients with increased operative risk. They recommended that surgery be postponed when possible in severely hypothyroid patients until these patients are at least partially treated.

The management of hypothyroid patients with symptomatic coronary artery disease has been a subject of controversy. The need for thyroid hormone replacement therapy must be weighed against the risk of precipitating myocardial ischemia. Drucker and Burrow[42] prospectively studied ten patients with mild to moderate hypothyroidism who underwent cardiac surgery requiring cardiopulmonary bypass. No patient received thyroid replacement therapy preoperatively. There were no significant differences in the frequency of intraoperative or postoperative complications when the study patients were compared with a large control group. Drucker and Burrow concluded that there was no justification for postponing coronary artery bypass surgery in the ischemic patient with mild or moderate hypothyroidism. Hay and associates[43] retrospectively reviewed 18 hypo-

thyroid patients with coronary artery disease who underwent coronary artery bypass graft surgery. Nine patients were rendered euthyroid preoperatively and nine received no preoperative treatment. The authors noted no significant differences between the groups with regard to complications or outcome. An extensive literature review by Becker[44] supports the position that cardiac catheterization or coronary artery bypass surgery can be safely performed without preoperative thyroid hormone replacement therapy. In symptomatic patients or unstable patients with cardiac ischemia who are surgical candidates, thyroid replacement should probably be delayed until the postoperative period in order to avoid the risk of precipitating acute myocardial ischemia or infarction.

On the basis of recent investigations, there appears to be little reason to postpone elective surgery in patients who have mild or moderate hypothyroidism. Thyroid replacement therapy is, however, indicated for patients with severe hypothyroidism or myxedema coma and for pregnant patients who are hypothyroid. Untreated hypothyroidism in pregnant patients is associated with an increased incidence of spontaneous abortion and mental and physical abnormalities in the offspring.[45]

Myxedema coma represents a severe form of hypothyroidism characterized by stupor or coma, hypoventilation, hypothermia, hypotension, and hyponatremia. This is a medical emergency with a high mortality ($>50\%$) and as such requires aggressive therapy. Intravenous thyroid replacement is initiated as soon as the clinical diagnosis is made. An iv loading dose of T_4 (sodium levothyroxine, 400–500 μg) is given initially and followed by a maintenance dose of T_4, 50–200 $\mu g \cdot day^{-1}$ iv.[46,47] Alternatively, an iv loading dose of T_3 (50–200 μg bolus) is given, followed by a maintenance dose.[48] Initial treatment with T_3 is preferred because it has a more rapid onset of activity. Improvements in heart rate, blood pressure, and body temperature may occur within 24 hours. Because parenteral T_3 is not available commercially in the United States, the oral or nasogastric route is the only option available.[49] This route may be suboptimal because of ileus or unpredictable GI absorption accompanying myxedema coma. Although the use of T_3 remains controversial, it should be noted that replacement therapy with either form of thyroid hormone may precipitate myocardial ischemia. There is also an increased likelihood of acute primary adrenal insufficiency in these patients, and they should receive 100–300 $mg \cdot day^{-1}$ of hydrocortisone by infusion. Steroid replacement continues until normal adrenal function can be confirmed.

A number of anesthetic medications have been used without difficulty in hypothyroid patients. More than two thirds of the patients in the study of Weinberg et al[40] received an opioid premedication without problems. Although ketamine has been proposed as the ideal induction agent, thiopental has also been used in the hypothyroid patient. The suggestion that thiopental may decrease the peripheral conversion of T_4 to T_3 does not appear to be clinically relevant.[50] The maintenance of anesthesia may be safely achieved with either iv or inhaled anesthetics. To date, there are no controlled studies addressing the specific questions of increased opioid potency and prolonged depression of ventilation in hypothyroid patients. Inhaled volatile anesthetics have also been used in hypothyroid patients without difficulty. There appears to be little if any decrease in the minimum alveolar concentration (MAC) for volatile agents (Fig. 45-2).[51]

Regional anesthesia is a good choice in the hypothyroid patient provided that the intravascular volume is well main-

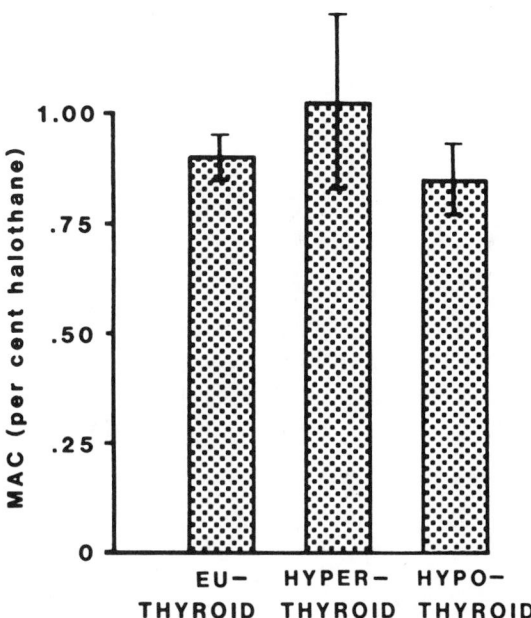

Figure 45-2. The minimum alveolar concentration of halothane (MAC, mean ± SD) was determined in euthyroid, hyperthyroid, and hypothyroid dogs. There was no significant difference in MAC between euthyroid and either hyperthyroid or hypothyroid animals. MAC in hyperthyroid dogs was greater than MAC in hypothyroid dogs (p < 0.05). (Data adapted from Babad AA, Eger EI: The effects of hyperthyroidism and hypothyroidism on halothane and oxygen requirements in dogs. Anesthesiology 29:1087, 1968.)

tained. Monitoring is directed toward the early recognition of hypotension, congestive heart failure, and hypothermia. Scrupulous attention should be paid to maintaining normal body temperature.

PARATHYROID GLANDS

Calcium Physiology

The normal adult body contains approximately 1000 g of calcium (Ca^{2+}), of which 99% is in the skeleton and 1% is elsewhere. Plasma calcium is present in three forms: (1) a protein-bound fraction (40%), (2) an ionized fraction (50%), and (3) a diffusible but nonionized fraction (10%) that is complexed with phosphate, bicarbonate, and citrate. This division is of interest, because it is the ionized fraction that is physiologically active and homeostatically regulated. The normal total serum calcium concentration is 8.8–10.4 $mg \cdot dl^{-1}$. Albumin binds about 90% of the protein-bound fraction of calcium, and total serum Ca^{2+} is consequently dependent on albumin levels.[52] In general, an increase or decrease in albumin of 1 $g \cdot dl^{-1}$ is associated with a parallel change in total serum Ca^{2+} of 0.8 $mg \cdot dl^{-1}$. The serum ionized Ca^{2+} concentration is affected by temperature and blood pH through alterations in Ca^{2+} protein binding to albumin. Acidosis decreases protein binding (increases ionized Ca^{2+}), and alkalosis increases protein binding (decreases ionized Ca^{2+}). The concentration of free Ca^{2+} ion is of critical importance in regulating skeletal muscle contraction, coagulation, neurotransmitter release, endocrine secretion, and a variety of other cellular functions. As a conse-

quence, the maintenance of serum Ca^{2+} concentration is subject to exquisite hormonal control by parathyroid hormone (PTH) and vitamin D (Fig. 45-3).

PTH acts to maintain the extracellular fluid Ca^{2+} concentration through direct effects on bone resorption and renal Ca^{2+} resorption (distal tubule) and indirectly through its effects on the synthesis of 1,25-dihydroxyvitamin D.[53] The renal effects of PTH include phosphaturia and bicarbonaturia, in addition to enhanced Ca^{2+} and magnesium resorption.[54] Most evidence suggests that rapid changes in blood Ca^{2+} levels are primarily due to hormonal effects on bone and to a lesser extent are due to renal Ca^{2+} clearance, whereas maintenance of Ca^{2+} balance is more dependent on the indirect effects of the hormone on intestinal calcium absorption. The effects of PTH are mediated by specific hormone–target cell membrane interaction. Hormone-receptor activation of adenylate cyclase leads to increased intracellular cyclic adenosine monophosphate (cAMP). Presumably, the rapid rise in cAMP promotes an increase in protein kinase, leading to a phosphorylation of key effector proteins that initiate the hormonal effect. Following the administration of PTH, there is a rise in urinary cAMP. This "nephrogenous-cAMP" leaks from renal tubular cells and provides an index of the biologic activity of PTH.[55]

PTH secretion is primarily regulated by the serum ionized Ca^{2+} concentration.[56] This negative feedback mechanism is exquisitely sensitive in maintaining calcium levels in a normal range. Release of PTH is also influenced by phosphate, magnesium, and catecholamine levels. Acute hypomagnesemia directly stimulates PTH release, whereas chronic magnesium depletion appears to inhibit proper functioning of the parathyroid gland.[57] The plasma phosphate concentration has an indirect influence on PTH secretion by causing reciprocal changes in the serum ionized Ca^{2+} concentration.

Vitamin D Metabolism

Vitamin D is absorbed from the GI tract and can be produced enzymatically by ultraviolet irradiation of the skin.[56] Vitamin D (cholecalciferol) is made from cholesterol metabolites and is inactive. Calciferol is hydroxylated in the liver to 25-hydroxycholecalciferol (25-OHD) and in the kidney is further hydroxylated to 1,25-dihydroxycholecalciferol (1,25(OH)$_2$D) or 24,25-dihydroxycholecalciferol (24,25(OH)$_2$D). 25-OHD is the major circulating form of vitamin D. The synthesis of this hormone is not regulated by a hormone or by Ca^{2+} or phosphate levels. 1,25(OH)$_2$D and 24,25(OH)$_2$D are the major active metabolites of vitamin D, and their production is reciprocally regulated at the kidney. Hypocalcemia and hypophosphatemia cause an increased production of 1,25(OH)$_2$D and a decreased production of 24,25(OH)$_2$D. 1,25(OH)$_2$D stimulates bone, kidney, and intestinal absorption of calcium and phosphate.[56] Vitamin D deficiency can lead to decreased intestinal absorption of Ca^{2+} and secondary hyperparathyroidism.

Hyperparathyroidism

Primary hyperparathyroidism increases with age and female sex, reaching its highest incidence in women older than 60 years of age. Primary hyperparathyroidism is most commonly due to a benign parathyroid adenoma (90% of cases) or hyperplasia (9%) and very rarely to a parathyroid carcinoma. Primary hyperparathyroidism may also exist as part of a multiple endocrine neoplastic (MEN) syndrome. Hyper-

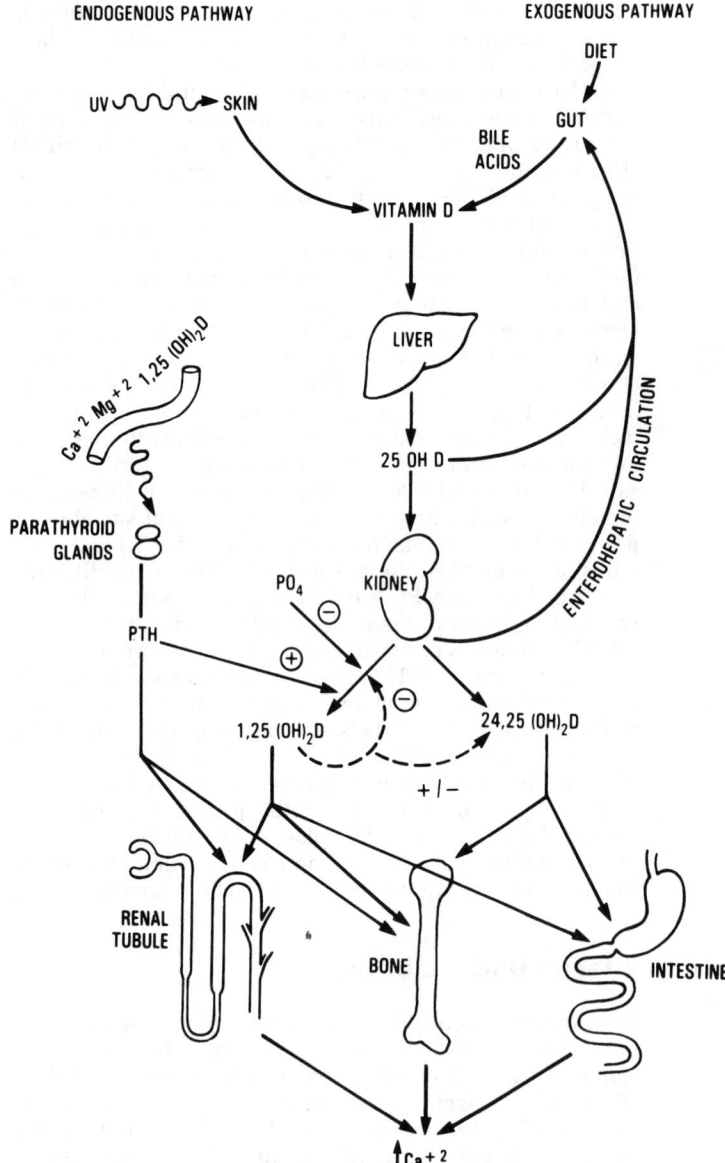

ENDOGENOUS PATHWAY   EXOGENOUS PATHWAY

Figure 45-3. Parathyroid hormone and vitamin D metabolism and action. (Reproduced with permission from Geelhoed GW, Chernow B [eds]: Endocrine Aspects of Acute Illness. New York, Churchill Livingstone, 1985.)

plasia usually involves all four glands. Although the majority of patients with primary hyperparathyroidism are hypercalcemic, most are asymptomatic at the time of diagnosis. When symptoms occur, they usually result from the hypercalcemia that accompanies the disease. Primary hyperparathyroidism occurring during pregnancy is associated with a high maternal and fetal morbidity (50%). The placenta allows the fetus to concentrate calcium, promoting hypercalcemia in the fetus and leading to hypoparathyroidism in the newborn. Pregnant women with primary hyperparathyroidism should be treated with surgery.

Hypercalcemia is responsible for a broad spectrum of signs and symptoms. Nephrolithiasis is the most common manifestation, occurring in 60–70% of patients.[58] Polyuria and polydipsia are also common complaints. An increase in bone turnover may lead to generalized demineralization and subperiosteal bone resorption; however, only a small group of patients (10–15%) develop clinically significant bone disease. Patients may experience generalized skeletal muscle weakness and fatigability, epigastric discomfort, peptic ulceration, and constipation. Psychiatric manifesta-

tions include depression, memory loss, confusion, or psychosis. Between 20% and 50% of patients are hypertensive, but this usually resolves with successful treatment of the disease. Consequently, the ECG may reveal a shortened QT interval. Cardiac function is enhanced in the early stages of hypercalcemia. Calcium flux into the cells is reflected in the plateau phase of the action potential (phase 2). As extracellular calcium increases, the inward flux is more rapid, and phase 2 is shortened. The corresponding ECG change is a shorter QT interval. Cardiac contractility may increase until a level between 15 and 20 mg·dl^{-1} is reached. At this point, there is a prolongation of the PR segment and QRS complex that can result in heart block or bundle-branch block. Bradycardia also occurs.[59,60]

An elevated serum Ca^{2+} concentration is a valuable diagnostic indicator of primary hyperparathyroidism. The serum phosphate concentration is nonspecific, with many patients having normal or near-normal levels. The reported incidence of hyperchloremic acidosis varies widely in primary hyperparathyroidism, but most patients usually have a serum chloride concentration in excess of 102 mEq·l^{-1}.[61]

Rarely does a patient with hypercalcemia secondary to ectopic PTH production (malignancy) present with hyperchloremic acidosis. The definitive diagnosis of primary hyperparathyroidism is made by RIA demonstration of an elevation in PTH levels in the presence of hypercalcemia. An elevated nephrogenous cAMP is noted in more than 90% of patients with primary hyperparathyroidism.

Hypercalcemia may also result from the ectopic production of PTH or PTH-like substances from lung, genitourinary, breast, GI, and lymphoproliferative malignancies.[62,63] Tumors may also produce hypercalcemia through direct bone resorption or the production of osteoclast-activating factor.[64] In the absence of a clinically obvious neoplasm, there may be difficulty in differentiating between PTH-producing malignancies and primary hyperparathyroidism. PTH fragments from malignant tissue differ from native PTH and aid in distinguishing between ectopic PTH production and primary hyperparathyroidism.

Secondary hyperparathyroidism represents an increase in parathyroid function as a result of conditions that produce hypocalcemia or hyperphosphatemia. Chronic renal disease is a common cause of hyperphosphatemia (due to decreased phosphate excretion) and decreased vitamin D metabolism. The hypocalcemia that results leads to an increased production of PTH. GI disorders accompanied by malabsorption may also lead to a secondary increase in parathyroid activity.

Tertiary hyperparathyroidism refers to the development of hypercalcemia in a patient who has had prolonged secondary hyperparathyroidism that is suddenly corrected (renal transplantation). The usually mild and transient hypercalcemia reflects an inability of the hyperactive parathyroid glands to adapt to the normal handling of renal calcium phosphorylate and vitamin D.

Treatment and Anesthetic Considerations

Surgery is the treatment of choice for the patient with symptomatic disease. Considerable controversy, however, surrounds the choice of treatment in the asymptomatic patient.[65] It is not clear that mild primary hyperparathyroidism decreases longevity. Surgery is often chosen over medical therapy because it offers definitive treatment and is generally safe.

Preoperative preparation focuses on the correction of intravascular volume and electrolyte irregularities. It is particularly important to evaluate the patient with chronic hypercalcemia for abnormalities of the renal, cardiac, or central nervous systems. Emergency treatment of hypercalcemia is undertaken preoperatively when the serum Ca^{2+} concentration exceeds 15 mg·dl^{-1} (7.5 mEq·l^{-1}). Lowering of the serum Ca^{2+} concentration is initially accomplished by expanding the intravascular volume and establishing a sodium diuresis. This is achieved with the iv administration of normal saline and furosemide. Rehydration alone is capable of lowering the serum Ca^{2+} level by 2 mg · dl^{-1} or more. Hydration dilutes the serum Ca^{2+}, and a sodium diuresis promotes Ca^{2+} excretion through an inhibition of sodium and Ca^{2+} resorption in the proximal tubule. Another element in the treatment of hypercalcemia is the correction of hypophosphatemia. Hypophosphatemia increases GI absorption of Ca^{2+}, stimulates the breakdown of bone, and impairs the uptake of Ca^{2+} by bone. Low serum phosphate levels impair cardiac contractility and may contribute to congestive heart failure.[66] Hypophosphatemia also causes skeletal muscle weakness, hemolysis, and platelet dysfunction.

Other medications that have a role in lowering the serum Ca^{2+} include mithramycin, calcitonin, and glucocorticoids. Mithramycin, a cytotoxic agent administered in a dose of 25 μg·kg^{-1}, inhibits PTH-induced osteoclast activity and can lower the serum Ca^{2+} levels by 2 mg·dl^{-1} or more in 24–48 hours.[67] Toxic effects include azotemia, hepatotoxicity, and thrombocytopenia. Calcitonin is useful in transiently lowering the serum Ca^{2+} level 2–4 mg·dl^{-1} through direct inhibition of osteoclastic bone resorption. The advantages of calcitonin are that side-effects are mild (urticaria, nausea) and the onset of activity is rapid. Calcitonin resistance usually develops within 24–48 hours.[68] Glucocorticoids are effective in lowering the serum Ca^{2+} concentration in several conditions (sarcoidosis, some malignancies, hyperthyroidism, vitamin D intoxication) through its actions on osteoclast bone resorption, GI absorption of calcium, and the urinary excretion of calcium. Glucocorticoids are usually of no benefit in the treatment of primary hypercalcemia. Finally, hemodialysis or peritoneal dialysis can be used to lower the serum Ca^{2+} level when alternative regimens are ineffective or contraindicated.

There is no evidence that a specific anesthetic drug or technique has advantages over another. A thorough knowledge of the clinical manifestations attributable to hypercalcemia is of the greatest value in choosing an anesthetic technique. Special monitoring is usually not required. Because of the unpredictable response to neuromuscular blocking drugs in the hypercalcemic patient, a conservative approach to muscle paralysis makes sense. Careful positioning of the osteopenic patient is necessary to avoid pathologic bone fractures.

Postoperative complications include recurrent laryngeal nerve injury, bleeding, and transient or complete hypoparathyroidism. Unilateral recurrent laryngeal nerve injury is characterized by hoarseness and usually requires no intervention. Bilateral recurrent laryngeal nerve injury is a rare complication, producing aphonia and requiring immediate endotracheal intubation. Following successful parathyroidectomy, one should observe a decrease in the serum Ca^{2+} level within 24 hours. Patients with significant preoperative bone disease may develop hypocalcemia following removal of the PTH-secreting glands. This "hungry bone" syndrome comes as a result of the rapid remineralization of bone. Thus, serum Ca^{2+}, magnesium, and phosphorus levels should be closely monitored until stable. The serum Ca^{2+} nadir usually occurs within 3–7 days.

Hypoparathyroidism

An underproduction of PTH or resistance of the end-organ tissues to PTH results in hypocalcemia (<8 mg·dl^{-1}). The normal physiologic response to hypocalcemia is an increase in PTH secretion and 1,25(OH)$_2$D synthesis with an increase in Ca^{2+} mobilization from bone, GI absorption, and renal tubule reclamation. The most common cause of acquired PTH deficiency is inadvertent removal of the parathyroid glands during thyroid or parathyroid surgery. Other causes of acquired hypoparathyroidism include ^{131}I therapy for thyroid disease, neck trauma, granulomatous disease, or an infiltrating process (malignancy or amyloidosis). Idiopathic hypoparathyroidism is rare and may occur as an isolated disease or as part of an autoimmune polyglandular process (hypothyroidism, adrenal insufficiency). Pseudohypoparathyroidism is an inherited disorder in which parathyroid gland function is normal but the end-organ response to the PTH is deficient.[56] Affected patients have hypocalcemia and hyperphosphatemia. They are characterized by mental retardation, a short stature, obesity, and shortened metacarpals. Pseudopseudohypoparathyroid patients are characterized by the same physical findings but have normal serum calcium and phosphate levels. Severe hypomagnesemia (<0.8 mEq·l^{-1}) from any cause can produce hypocalcemia by suppressing PTH secretion. Renal insufficiency leads to phosphorus retention and impaired 1,25(OH)$_2$D synthesis, and this results in hypocalcemia. These patients are commonly treated with vitamin D, which increases intestinal calcium absorption and suppresses secondary increases in PTH secretion. Hypocalcemia resulting from pancreatitis and burns results from the suppression of PTH and from the sequestration of calcium.[69]

Clinical Features and Treatment

The clinical features of hypoparathyroidism are a manifestation of hypocalcemia. Neuronal irritability and skeletal muscle spasms, tetany, or seizures reflect a reduced threshold of excitation. Latent tetany may be demonstrated by eliciting Chvostek's or Trousseau's signs. Chvostek's sign is a contracture of the facial muscle produced by tapping the facial nerve as it passes through the parotid gland. Trousseau's sign is contraction of the fingers and wrist following application of a blood pressure cuff inflated above the systolic blood pressure for approximately 3 minutes. Other common complaints of hypocalcemia include fatigue, depression, paresthesias, and skeletal muscle cramps. The acute onset of hypocalcemia following thyroid or parathyroid surgery may manifest as stridor and apnea. Cardiovascular manifestations of hypocalcemia include congestive heart failure, hypotension, and a relative insensitivity to the effects of beta-adrenergic agonists.[70,71] Delayed ventricular repolarization results in a prolonged QT interval on the ECG. Although prolongation of the QT interval may be a reliable sign of hypocalcemia in an individual patient, the ECG is relatively insensitive for the detection of hypocalcemia.[72]

The treatment of hypoparathyroidism consists of electrolyte replacement. The objective is to have the patient's clinical symptoms under control prior to anesthesia and surgery. Hypocalcemia caused by magnesium depletion is treated by correcting the magnesium deficit. Serum phosphate excess is corrected by the removal of phosphate from the diet and the oral administration of phosphate-binding resins (aluminum hydroxide). The urinary excretion of phosphate can be increased with a saline volume infusion.[73] Ca^{2+} deficiencies are corrected with Ca^{2+} supplements and/or vitamin D analogues. Patients with severe symptomatic hypocalcemia are treated with iv calcium gluconate (10–20 ml of 10% solution) given over several minutes and followed by a continuous infusion (1–2 mg·kg^{-1}·h^{-1}) of elemental Ca^{2+}. The correction of serum Ca^{2+} levels should be monitored by measuring serum Ca^{2+} concentrations and following clinical symptoms. When oral or iv calcium is inadequate to maintain a normal serum ionized calcium level, vitamin D is added to the regimen.

ADRENAL CORTEX

The adrenal cortex functions to synthesize and secrete three types of hormones. Endogenous and dietary cholesterol is utilized in the adrenal biosynthesis of glucocorticoids (cortisol), mineralocorticoids (aldosterone and 11-deoxycorticosterone), and androgens (dehydroepiandrosterone) (Fig. 45-4). Cortisol and aldosterone are the two essential hormones, whereas adrenal androgens are of relatively minor physiologic significance in adults. The major biologic effects of adrenal cortical hyperfunction or hypofunction occur as a result of cortisol or aldosterone excess or deficiency. Abnormal function of the adrenal cortex may render a patient unable to respond appropriately during a period of surgical stress or critical illness.

Glucocorticoid Physiology

Cortisol (hydrocortisone) is the most potent glucocorticoid produced by the inner portions of the adrenal cortex (zona fasciculata, zona reticularis). Cortisone is a glucocorticoid produced in small amounts. Cortisol is produced under the control of adrenocorticotropic hormone (ACTH), a polypeptide synthesized and released by the anterior pituitary gland. Glucocorticoids exert their biologic effects by diffusing into the cytoplasm of target cells and combining with specific high-affinity receptor proteins. The steroid receptor protein complex influences the transcription of new RNA by attaching to the nuclear chromatin. The synthesis of new proteins ultimately mediates the expression of the hormone.[74]

The daily production of endogenous cortisol is about 20 mg. Most of the circulating hormone is bound to the alpha-globulin transcortin (cortisol-binding globulin). It is the relatively small amount of free hormone that exerts the biologic effects. Glucocorticoids such as cortisol are inactivated primarily by the liver and are excreted in the urine as 17-hydroxycorticosteroids. Cortisol is also filtered at the glomerulus and may be excreted unchanged in the urine. Although the rate of cortisol secretion is decreased by about 30% in the elderly patient, plasma cortisol levels remain in a normal range because of a corresponding decrease in hepatic and renal clearance.

Cortisol has multiple effects on intermediate carbohydrate, protein, and fatty acid metabolism. Glucocorticoids enhance gluconeogenesis, elevate blood glucose, and promote hepatic glycogen synthesis.[75,76] The catabolic effect of glucocorticoids is partially blocked by insulin. The net effect on protein metabolism is enhanced degradation of muscle tissue and negative nitrogen balance. In supraphysiologic amounts, glucocorticoids suppress growth hormone secretion and impair somatic growth. The anti-inflammatory actions of cortisol relate to its effect in stabilizing lysosomes and promoting capillary integrity. Cortisol also antagonizes leukocyte migration inhibition factor (MIF), thus reducing white cell adherence to vascular endothelium and diminishing leukocyte response to local inflammation.[77] Phagocytic activity does not decrease, although the killing potential of macrophages and monocytes is diminished.[78] Other diverse actions include the facilitation of free water clearance, maintenance of blood pressure, a weak mineralocorticoid effect, promotion of appetite, stimulation of hematopoiesis, and induction of liver enzymes.

Control of Glucocorticoid Secretion

Cortisol secretion is directly controlled by ACTH, which in turn is regulated by the corticotropin-releasing factor (CRF). ACTH is synthesized in the pituitary gland from a precursor molecule that also produces beta-lipotropin and beta-endorphin. The secretion of ACTH and CRF is governed chiefly by cortisol-like steroids, the sleep-wake cycle, and stress. Cortisol is the most potent regulator of ACTH secre-

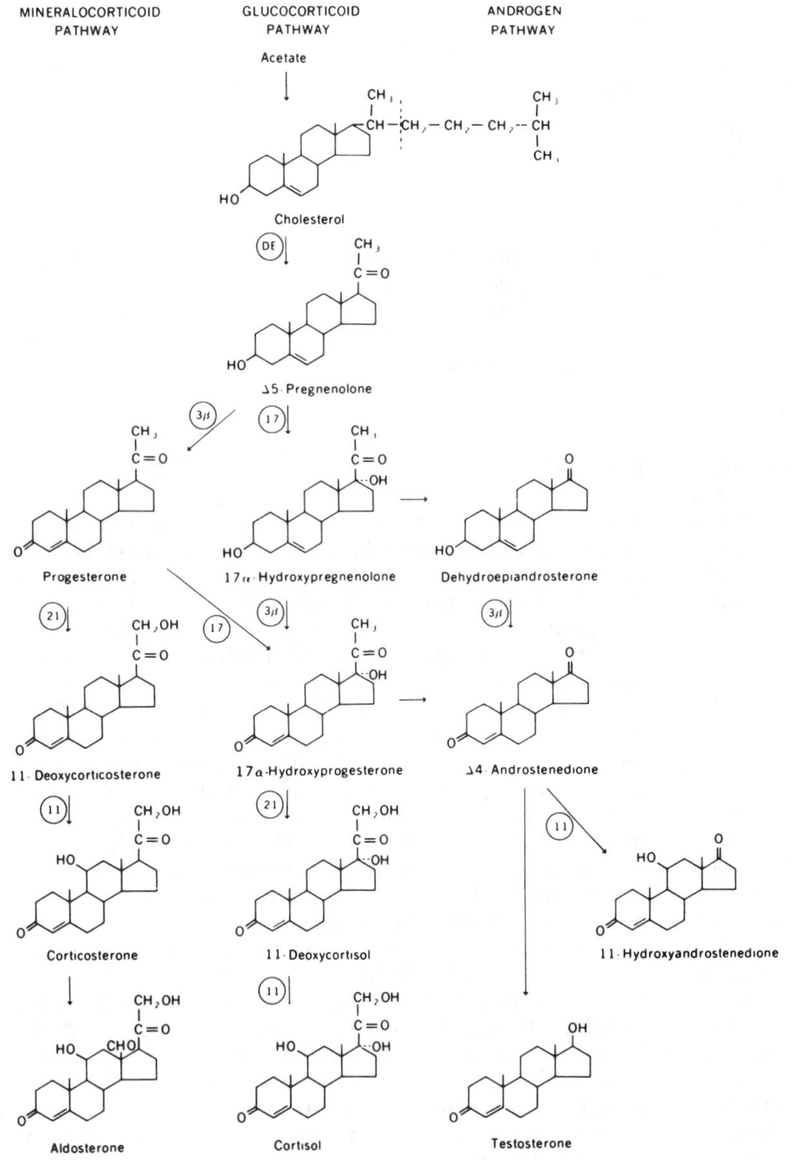

Figure 45-4. Biosynthetic pathways for adrenal steroid production: major pathways for mineralocorticoids, glucocorticoids, and androgens. Circled letters and numbers denote specific enzymes: DE = debranching enzyme; 3β = 3β-ol-dehydrogenase with 4,5 isomerase; 11 = C-11 hydroxylase; 17 = C-17 hydroxylase; 21 = C-21 hydroxylase. (Reproduced with permission from Petersdorf RG [ed]: Harrison's Principles of Internal Medicine, 10th ed. New York, McGraw-Hill, 1983.)

tion, acting by a negative feedback mechanism to maintain cortisol levels in a physiologic range. There is some evidence that cortisol may also feed back on higher neuronal centers. ACTH acts within minutes to elicit adrenal secretion by activating adenylate cyclase and the production of cAMP. ACTH release follows a diurnal pattern, with maximal activity occurring soon after awakening. This diurnal pattern of activity occurs in normal subjects as well as in those with adrenal insufficiency. Psychological or physical stress (trauma, surgery, intense exercise) also promotes ACTH release regardless of the level of circulating cortisol or the time of day.[79]

Mineralocorticoid Physiology

Aldosterone is the most potent mineralocorticoid produced by the zona glomerulosa of the adrenal gland. This hormone binds to receptors in sweat glands, the alimentary tract, and the distal convoluted tubule of the kidney. Aldosterone is a major regulator of extracellular volume and potassium homeostasis through the resorption of sodium and the secretion of potassium by these tissues.[76,80] The major regulators

of aldosterone release are the renin-angiotensin system, serum potassium, and ACTH (Fig. 45-5). The juxtaglomerular apparatus that surrounds the renal afferent arterioles produces renin in response to decreased perfusion pressures (hypovolemia), sympathetic stimulation, and hypokalemia. Renin splits the hepatic precursor angiotensinogen to form the decapeptide, angiotensin I, which is then altered enzymatically by converting enzyme (primarily in the lung) to form the octapeptide angiotensin II. Angiotensin II is the most potent vasopressor produced in the body. It directly stimulates the adrenal cortex to produce aldosterone. The renin-angiotensin system is the body's most important protector of volume status. Other stimuli that increase the production of aldosterone include hyperkalemia and, to a limited degree, ACTH.

Androgen Physiology

Dehydroepiandrosterone and androstenedione are weak androgens produced in the adrenal cortex. These adrenal androgens are converted outside of the adrenal gland to testosterone, which is inactivated in the liver to form 17-

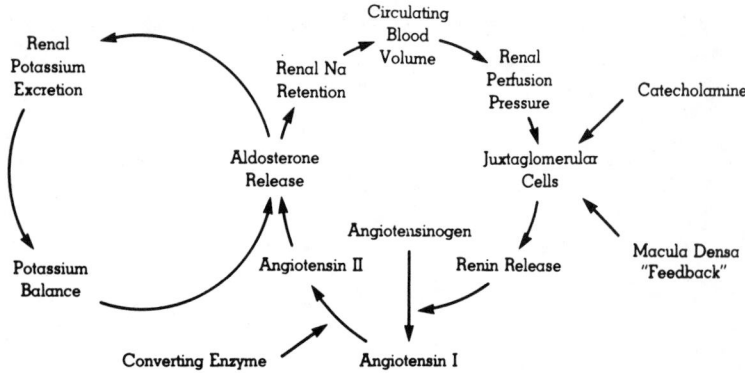

Figure 45-5. The interrelationship of the volume and potassium feedback loops on aldosterone secretion. (Reproduced with permission from Petersdorf RG [ed]: Harrison's Principles of Internal Medicine, 10th ed. New York, McGraw-Hill, 1983.)

ketosteroids. Dehydroepiandrosterone serves as the major precursor of urinary 17-ketosteroids. There is a progressive decline in adrenal androgen production with age. Some congenital defects in adrenal enzyme activity are associated with alterations in adrenal androgen production and cortisol deficiency. The release of adrenal androgens is stimulated by ACTH, not by gonadotropins.

Glucocorticoid Excess (Cushing's Syndrome)

The overproduction of cortisol by the adrenal cortex results in a syndrome characterized by truncal obesity, hypertension, hyperglycemia, increased intravascular fluid volume, hypokalemia, fatigability, abdominal striae, osteoporosis, and muscle weakness.[81] The majority of cases of Cushing's syndrome that occur spontaneously are due to bilateral adrenal hyperplasia secondary to ACTH produced by an anterior pituitary microadenoma or nonendocrine tumor (e.g., of the lung, kidney, or pancreas). The incidence of adrenal hyperplasia secondary to pituitary overproduction of ACTH is three times higher in women than in men. The primary overproduction of cortisol and other adrenal steroids is caused by an adrenal neoplasm in approximately 20–25% of patients with Cushing's syndrome. These tumors are usually unilateral, and about half are malignant. Spontaneously occurring Cushing's disease is more common in younger patients, with a peak incidence in the 3rd decade of life. When Cushing's syndrome occurs in patients older than 60 years of age, the most likely cause is an adrenal carcinoma or ectopic ACTH produced from a nonendocrine tumor. Finally, an increasingly common cause of Cushing's syndrome is the prolonged administration of exogenous glucocorticoids to treat a variety of illnesses.

The signs and symptoms of Cushing's syndrome follow from the known actions of glucocorticoids. Truncal obesity and thin extremities reflect increased muscle wasting and a redistribution of fat in facial, cervical, and truncal areas. Impaired calcium absorption and a decrease in bone formation may result in osteopenia.[82] Sixty percent of patients have hyperglycemia, but overt diabetes mellitus occurs in less than 20%. Hypertension and fluid retention are seen in a majority of patients. Profound emotional changes ranging from emotional lability to frank psychosis may be present. An increased susceptibility to infection reflects the immunosuppressive effects of corticosteroids. If adrenal androgen secretion is increased, acne and hirsutism are frequent in women. Hypokalemic alkalosis without distinctive physical findings is common when adrenal hyperplasia is caused by ectopic ACTH production from a nonendocrine tumor.[83]

Diagnosis

The biochemical diagnosis of hyperadrenocorticism is based on a variable elevation in plasma and urinary cortisol levels, urinary 17-hydroxycorticosteroids, and plasma ACTH. The diagnosis can be established by failure to normally suppress endogenous cortisol secretion following the exogenous administration of dexamethasone. The initial screening test for hyperadrenocorticism is a low-dose dexamethasone suppression test (0.5 mg every 6 hours for 48 hours). As an aid to diagnosing the specific type of Cushing's disease, a high-dose dexamethasone suppression test (2 mg every 6 hours for 48 hours) may follow. Patients with pituitary adenomas frequently show a marked depression in cortisol and 17-hydroxycorticosteroid levels when a high dose of dexamethasone is administered. The ectopic production of ACTH by a nonendocrine tumor usually shows no suppression with low- or high-dose dexamethasone. The administration of metyrapone, a drug that suppresses cortisol production by inhibiting the conversion of 11-deoxycortisol to cortisol (11-beta-hydroxylase inhibition), is useful in differentiating adrenal tumors from adrenal hyperplasia. When metyrapone is given to the patient with an adrenal tumor, the suppressed pituitary fails to release ACTH in an appropriate manner. In contrast, patients with adrenal hyperplasia display a normal or hyperactive response. At the current time, CT is the radiologic technique most commonly used to identify abnormalities of the adrenal glands. Magnetic resonance imaging (MRI) is becoming popular as a method to study the pituitary.

Treatment and Anesthetic Management

Adrenalectomy is the traditional treatment for hyperadrenocorticism. General considerations for the preoperative preparation of the patient include regulating hypertension and diabetes and normalizing intravascular fluid volume and electrolyte concentrations. Diuresis with the aldosterone antagonist spironolactone helps to mobilize fluid and normalize the potassium concentration. Careful positioning of the osteopenic patient is very important. Intraoperative monitoring is planned after evaluation of the patient's cardiac reserve and consideration of the site and extent of the proposed surgery. In general, excision of a pituitary tumor carries less morbidity than either unilateral or bilateral adrenalectomy. The incidence of postoperative complications and perioperative mortality is highest in the patient undergoing bilateral adrenalectomy. When unilateral or bilateral adrenalectomy is planned, glucocorticoid replacement therapy is initiated at a dose equal to full replacement of adrenal output during periods of extreme stress (see the section on Steroid Replacement During the Perioperative Period). The total dosage is reduced by about 50% per day until a daily maintenance dose of steroids is achieved (20–30 mg·day^{-1}). Hydrocortisone given in doses of this magnitude exerts significant mineralocorticoid activity, and additional exogenous mineralocorticoid is generally not necessary during the perioperative period. The oral administration of mineralocorticoid is usually started on day 5. Following bilateral adrenalectomy, most patients need 0.05–0.1 mg·day^{-1} of fludrocortisone (9-alpha-fluorohydrocortisone). Slightly higher doses may be needed if prednisone is used for glucocorticoid maintenance (little intrinsic mineralocorticoid activity). The fludrocortisone dose is reduced if congestive heart failure, hypokalemia, or hypertension develops. For the patient with a solitary adrenal adenoma, unilateral adrenalectomy may be followed by normalization of function in the contralateral gland over time. Treatment plans should therefore be individualized, and adjustments in dosage may be necessary. The production of glucocorticoids or ACTH by a neoplasm may not be eliminated if the tumor is unresectable. These patients often need continuous medical therapy with steroid inhibitors such as metyrapone to control their symptoms.

There are no recommendations regarding the use of a particular anesthetic technique or medication in patients with hyperadrenocorticism. When significant skeletal muscle weakness is present, a conservative approach to the use of muscle relaxants is warranted.

Mineralocorticoid Excess

Hypersecretion of the major adrenal mineralocorticoid aldosterone increases the renal tubular exchange of sodium for potassium and hydrogen ions. This leads to potassium depletion, skeletal muscle weakness, fatigue, and hypokalemic alkalosis.[84,85] Approximately 1% of unselected hypertensive patients have primary hyperaldosteronism. The increase in renal sodium reabsorption and extracellular volume expansion is in part responsible for the high incidence of diastolic hypertension in these patients.[86] Patients with primary hyperaldosteronism (Conn's syndrome) characteristically do not have edema; however, in long-standing cases, a nephropathy may occur, and, in rare instances, it is associated with congestive heart failure and pretibial edema. The majority of cases are caused by a unilateral adenoma; however, bilateral adrenal hyperplasia is another possible etiology. The diagnosis of primary or secondary hyperaldosteronism should be entertained in the nonedematous hypertensive patient with persistent hypokalemia who is not receiving potassium-wasting diuretics. Hyposecretion of renin that fails to increase appropriately during volume depletion is an important finding in primary aldosteronism. Secondary aldosteronism results from an elevation in renin production. The measurement of plasma renin levels is useful in distinguishing these two from one another; however, it is of limited value in differentiating patients with primary aldosteronism from those with other causes of hypertension, because renin activity is also suppressed in about 25% of patients with essential hypertension. The hypersecretion of aldosterone that is not suppressed during volume expansion (salt loading) is the final diagnostic criterion.[87] The most common diagnostic problem is distinguishing between an adenoma and bilateral adrenal hyperplasia as the cause of hypersecretion. Although patients with bilateral adrenal hyperplasia tend to have

lower aldosterone levels and less severe hypokalemia, differentiation is impossible on clinical or biochemical grounds. CT is useful in this situation.[88] This distinction is particularly important because the hypertension associated with an adenoma is usually markedly improved or cured following surgical excision of the tumor. In contrast, hypertension associated with bilateral hyperplasia usually does not benefit from bilateral adrenalectomy. Surgery is indicated only when symptomatic hypokalemia cannot be controlled with medical therapy.

Anesthetic Considerations

Preoperative preparation for the patient with primary aldosteronism is directed toward restoring the intravascular volume and the electrolyte concentrations to normal. Hypertension and hypokalemia may be controlled by restricting sodium intake and administration of the aldosterone antagonist spironolactone. This diuretic works slowly to produce an increase in potassium levels, with dosages in the range of 25–100 mg every 8 hours. Total body potassium deficits are difficult to estimate and may be in excess of 300 mEq. Whenever possible, potassium is replaced over a 24- to 48-hour period in order to allow equilibration between intracellular and extracellular potassium stores. Extended medical management is possible, but chronic therapy with spironolactone is limited by the occurrence of gynecomastia and impotence.

Adrenal Insufficiency

The undersecretion of adrenal steroid hormones may develop as the result of a primary inability of the adrenal gland to elaborate sufficient quantities of hormone or as the result of a secondary deficiency in the production of ACTH.

Clinically, primary adrenal insufficiency is usually not apparent until at least 90% of the adrenal cortex has been destroyed. The predominant cause of primary adrenal insufficiency during the early part of the century was tuberculosis; however, at the present time, the most frequent cause of Addison's disease is idiopathic adrenal insufficiency secondary to an autoimmune destruction of the gland (Table 45-4).[89] The autoimmune destruction of the adrenal cortex causes both a glucocorticoid and a mineralocorticoid deficiency. A variety of other conditions presumed to have an autoimmune pathogenesis may also occur concomitantly with idiopathic Addison's disease. Hashimoto's thyroiditis in association with autoimmune adrenal insufficiency is termed Schmidt's syndrome.[90] Other possible causes of adrenal gland destruction include certain bacterial or fungal infections, cancer, and hemorrhage.

Secondary adrenal insufficiency occurs when the anterior pituitary fails to secrete sufficient quantities of ACTH. The most important cause of hypothalamic-pituitary-adrenal axis suppression confronting the anesthesiologist is the exogenous administration of glucocorticoids. Pituitary failure may also result from tumor, infection, surgical ablation, or radiation therapy.[91]

Clinical Presentation

Several important differences exist between primary adrenal insufficiency and hypopituitarism. The cardinal symptoms of idiopathic Addison's disease include asthenia,

TABLE 45-4. Classification of Adrenal Insufficiency

Primary Adrenal Insufficiency

Anatomic destruction of gland (chronic and acute)
"Idiopathic" atrophy (autoimmune)
Surgical removal (metastatic breast cancer)
Infection (tuberculosis, fungus)
Hemorrhage
Invasion: metastatic

Metabolic Failure in Hormone Production

Congenital adrenal hyperplasia
Enzyme inhibitors (metyrapone)
Cytotoxic agents (OP1–DDD)

Secondary Adrenal Insufficiency

Hypopituitarism due to pituitary disease
Suppression of hypothalamic-pituitary axis
  Exogenous steroid
  Endogenous steroid from tumor

weight loss, anorexia, abdominal pain, nausea, vomiting, diarrhea, and constipation. Hypotension is almost always encountered in the disease process. Diffuse hyperpigmentation occurs in most patients with primary adrenal insufficiency and is secondary to the compensatory increase in ACTH and beta-lipotropin. These hormones stimulate an increase in melanocyte production. Mineralocorticoid deficiency is characteristically present in primary adrenal disease, and, as a result, there is a reduction in urine sodium conservation and a decreased pressure response to circulating catecholamines. Hyperkalemia may be a cause of life-threatening cardiac dysrhythmias. Female patients may exhibit decreased axillary and pubic hair growth owing to the loss of adrenal androgen secretion. Adrenal insufficiency secondary to pituitary suppression is not associated with cutaneous hyperpigmentation or mineralocorticoid deficiency. Salt and water balance are usually maintained unless severe fluid and electrolyte losses overwhelm the subnormal aldosterone secretory capacity. Organic lesions of pituitary origin require a diligent search for coexisting hormone deficiencies.

It is important to recognize the patient with adrenal insufficiency secondary to exogenous steroid therapy, because it is possible for acute adrenal crisis to occur if high-dose glucocorticoids are abruptly withdrawn or if deficient patients are subjected to even minor stress.[92-94] Because patients who have received exogenous glucocorticoids may exhibit pituitary-adrenal suppression for up to 12 months following cessation of therapy, these patients receive supplemental glucocorticoid coverage during periods of increased stress (e.g., trauma, surgery, infection).[95] Patients receiving inhaled or topical steroids may also exhibit pituitary-adrenal suppression for up to 9 months following the cessation of therapy.

Diagnosis

The patient's pituitary adrenal responsiveness should be determined when the diagnosis of primary or secondary adrenal insufficiency is first suspected. Biochemical evidence of impaired adrenal or pituitary secretory reserve will unequivocally confirm the diagnosis. Patients who are clinically stable may undergo testing before treatment is initi-

ated. Those thought to have acute adrenal insufficiency should receive immediate therapy.

Plasma cortisol levels are measured before and 30 and 60 minutes after the iv administration of 250 μg of synthetic ACTH. In patients with adequate adrenal reserve, plasma cortisol will rise at least 7 $\mu g \cdot dl^{-1}$ (or to a total greater than 18 $\mu g \cdot dl^{-1}$) 60 minutes following the injection of the synthetic ACTH. Patients with adrenal insufficiency usually demonstrate little or no adrenal response. When extended ACTH testing is used, both plasma ACTH (measured by RIA) and urinary metabolites (17-hydroxycorticosteroids) are measured to avoid diagnostic errors. Endogenous pituitary ACTH reserve may be further tested through the administration of metyrapone. Patients with primary adrenal insufficiency exhibit elevated ACTH levels, whereas those with secondary adrenal insufficiency have either a subnormal or absent ACTH response to the administration of metyrapone. The value of metyrapone testing is limited in many clinical settings (e.g., exogenous steroid administration, hypothyroidism, pregnancy) and has largely been replaced by ACTH stimulation tests. In addition, the metyrapone test may precipitate adrenal crisis in a patient with primary adrenal insufficiency.

Treatment

Normal adults secrete 20 mg of cortisol (hydrocortisone) and 0.1 mg of aldosterone per day. Glucocorticoid therapy is usually given twice daily in sufficient dosage to meet physiologic requirements. A typical regimen may consist of prednisone, 5 mg in the morning and 2.5 mg in the evening, or hydrocortisone, 20 mg in the morning and 10 mg in the evening. The daily glucocorticoid dosage is typically 50% higher than basal adrenal output in order to cover the patient for mild stress. Replacement dosages are adjusted in response to the patient's clinical symptoms or the occurrence of intercurrent illnesses. Addisonian patients should be instructed to increase glucocorticoid medication to three or four times their usual daily dosage during periods of increased stress. Mineralocorticoid replacement is also administered on a daily basis; most patients require 0.05–0.1 $mg \cdot day^{-1}$ of fludrocortisone. The mineralocorticoid dose may be reduced if severe hypokalemia, hypertension, or congestive heart failure develops, or it may be increased if postural hypotension is demonstrated. Children with Addison's disease receive lesser daily amounts of steroids. Twelve milligrams of cortisol per square meter of body surface area is usually sufficient.

Secondary adrenal insufficiency often occurs in the presence of multiple hormone deficiencies. A decrease in ACTH production results in the decreased secretion of cortisol and adrenal androgens, but aldosterone control by more dominant mechanisms remains intact. A liberal salt diet is encouraged. Glucocorticoid substitution follows the same guidelines previously outlined for primary adrenal insufficiency.

Acute Adrenal Insufficiency

Acute adrenal insufficiency is usually precipitated by sepsis, trauma, or surgical stress in the setting of hypovolemic shock and severe electrolyte imbalance. Immediate therapy is mandatory regardless of the etiology. Minimal therapy consists of fluid and electrolyte resuscitation and steroid replacement.

Initial therapy begins with the rapid iv administration of an isotonic crystalloid solution (D5NS). When emergency ACTH testing is being carried out, methylprednisolone (20 mg) is initially given. (Methylprednisolone is not detected by either RIA or protein displacement methods for steroid measurements.) If ACTH testing is not being performed, 200–300 mg of hydrocortisone is administered as an iv bolus over several minutes. Steroid replacement is continued during the first 24 hours with 100 mg iv hydrocortisone given every 6 hours. If the patient is stable, the steroid dose is reduced starting on the second day. Following adequate fluid resuscitation, if the patient continues to be hemodynamically unstable, inotropic support may be necessary. Invasive monitoring is extremely valuable as a guide to both diagnosis and therapy. When primary adrenal insufficiency is diagnosed, mineralocorticoid replacement is also initiated. Once again, it is important to individualize therapy.

Mineralocorticoid Insufficiency

Isolated mineralocorticoid insufficiency has been reported as a congenital biosynthetic defect following unilateral adrenalectomy for removal of an aldosterone-secreting adenoma, during protracted heparin therapy, and in patients with a deficiency in renin production.[96] This syndrome is commonly seen in patients with mild renal failure and long-standing diabetes mellitus. A feature common to all patients with hypoaldosteronism is a failure to increase aldosterone production in response to salt restriction or volume contraction.

Most patients present with hyperkalemia and a metabolic acidosis that is out of proportion to the degree of coexisting renal impairment. Most patients are hypotensive, and the hyperkalemia may be life-threatening. Patients with low renin secretion, hypoaldosteronism, and renal dysfunction will respond to ACTH stimulation. Nonsteroidal anti-inflammatory drugs, which inhibit prostaglandin synthesis, may further inhibit renin release and exacerbate the condition.[97] Patients with isolated hypoaldosteronism are given fludrocortisone orally in a dose of 0.05–0.1 mg·day^{-1}. Patients with low renin secretion usually require higher doses to correct the electrolyte abnormalities. Caution should be

observed in patients with hypertension or congestive heart failure. An alternative approach in these patients is the administration of furosemide alone or in combination with mineralocorticoid.

Exogenous Glucocorticoid Therapy

The therapeutic utilization of supraphysiologic doses of glucocorticoids has expanded, and, as a consequence, the clinical implications of such therapy are important. The relative glucocorticoid and mineralocorticoid properties of the various preparations are listed in Table 45-5. Dexamethasone, methylprednisolone, and prednisone have less mineralocorticoid effect than do cortisone and hydrocortisone. The anti-inflammatory activity of a glucocorticoid depends on the hydroxyl group at the carbon 11 position. Therefore, glucocorticoids such as cortisone and prednisone must undergo hepatic conversion from 11-keto compounds to 11-beta-hydroxyl compounds before anti-inflammatory activity can occur. Consequently, prednisone and cortisone should probably be avoided in the presence of severe liver disease. Since most side-effects from steroids are related to the dose and duration of administration, the smallest effective dose is used for the shortest period of time.

Patients at particular risk for developing complications related to steroid therapy include those with diabetes mellitus, pre-existing infection, hypertension, or congestive heart failure. Aseptic necrosis of the bones, subcapsular cataracts, pancreatitis, benign intracranial hypertension, and glaucoma are complications associated with exogenous steroid administration. Although the overall prevalence of steroid-associated peptic ulceration is small (2%), patients receiving exogenous steroids have approximately twice the risk of developing peptic ulceration or GI hemorrhage as do controls.[98]

Steroid Replacement During the Perioperative Period

The normal adrenal gland secretes somewhat less than 200 mg of cortisol per day during the perioperative period. During periods of extreme stress, the adrenal gland may be ex-

TABLE 45-5. Glucocorticoid Preparations

Generic Name	Trade Name	Relative Potency* Anti-inflammatory	Relative Potency* Mineralocorticoid	Approximate Equivalent Dose (mg)
Short-Acting				
Hydrocortisone (cortisol)	Cortef	1.0	1.0	20.0
Cortisone	Cortigen	0.8	0.8	25.0
Prednisone	Deltasone	4.0	0.25	5.0
Prednisolone	Hydeltrasol	4.0	0.25	5.0
Methylprednisolone	Medrol	5.0	±	4.0
Intermediate-Acting				
Triamcinolone	Aristocort	5.0	±	4.0
Long-Acting				
Dexamethasone	Decadron	30.0	±	0.75

*Relative milligram comparisons with cortisol. The glucocorticoid and mineralocorticoid properties of cortisol are set as 1.

ogenously stimulated to secrete between 200 and 500 mg·day^{-1} of cortisol.[99] The pituitary-adrenal axis is generally considered to be intact if plasma cortisol greater than 22 µg·dl^{-1} is measured during acute stress.[100] Plumpton et al[101] correlated the degree of adrenal responsiveness with the duration of surgery and the extent of surgical trauma. The mean maximal plasma cortisol level measured during major surgery (colectomy, hip osteotomy) was 47 µg·dl^{-1}. Minor surgical procedures (herniorrhaphy) resulted in mean maximal plasma cortisol levels of 28 µg·dl^{-1}. Adrenal activity may also be affected by the anesthetic technique used. Engquist et al[102] demonstrated the effectiveness of regional anesthesia in postponing the elevation in cortisol levels during surgery of the lower abdomen and extremities. Deep general anesthesia may also suppress the elevation of stress hormones such as ACTH and cortisol during the surgical procedure.[103-106]

Although symptoms indicative of clinically significant adrenal insufficiency have been reported during the perioperative period, these clinical findings have rarely been documented in direct association with glucocorticoid deficiency.[92,94,107] Because acute adrenal crisis is life-threatening, and because there is relatively little risk in providing steroid coverage for isolated periods of stress, supplemental steroids are empirically administered to all patients who have received daily steroid replacement for at least 1 week in the year prior to surgery.[95]

A controlled study by Udelsman et al[108] demonstrated the life-threatening consequences of inadequate glucocorticoid replacement during a period of surgical stress. Nonhuman primates were maintained on physiologic doses of glucocorticoids for 4 months following bilateral adrenalectomy. The adrenalectomized animals were then separated into three groups receiving, respectively, subphysiologic, physiologic, and supraphysiologic doses of steroid replacement. After 4 days the animals underwent cholecystectomy. Those primates that received subphysiologic doses of steroid perioperatively were hemodynamically unstable and had a significantly higher mortality than did sham-operated controls. Monkeys that received physiologic or supraphysiologic replacement doses of steroids had similar hemodynamic profiles and mortality rates as the sham-adrenalectomized controls. Wound healing and metabolic profiles were no different for animals receiving physiologic or supraphysiologic doses of steroids. Although there was no apparent advantage in providing supraphysiologic coverage, it was clear from the results that subphysiologic corticosteroid replacement was associated with an increase in cardiovascular instability and a higher mortality.

Symreng et al[109] advocate the iv infusion of 25 mg of cortisol before the induction of anesthesia, followed by a continuous infusion of cortisol (100 mg) in the next 24 hours. This "low-dose" cortisol replacement program was used in patients with proven adrenal insufficiency and resulted in plasma cortisol levels as high as those seen in healthy control subjects subjected to a similar operative stress (Fig. 45-6). Although the "low-dose" approach appears logical, many clinicians are unwilling to adopt this regimen until further trials have been undertaken in patients receiving physiologic steroid replacement. A popular regimen calls for the administration of 200–300 mg per 70 kg body weight of hydrocortisone in divided doses on the day of surgery. The lower dose is adjusted upward for longer and more extensive surgical procedures. Patients who are using steroids at the time of surgery receive their usual dose on the morning of surgery and are supplemented at a level

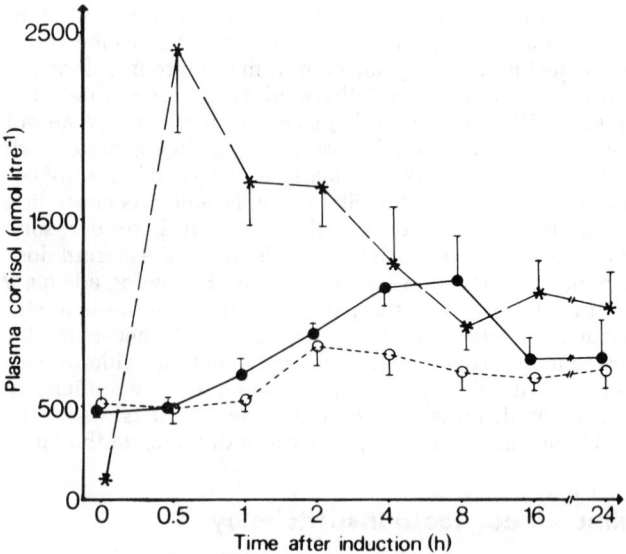

Figure 45-6. Plasma cortisol concentrations (mean ± SEM) were measured in three groups of patients undergoing elective surgery. Group I, control patients, $n = 8$ (●—●), had never received corticosteroids. Group II, $n = 8$ (○—○), patients received corticosteroids preoperatively with a normal response to ACTH (corticotropin) stimulation testing preoperatively. These patients and controls received no corticosteroid substitution during the perioperative period. Group III, $n = 6$ (*—*), consisted of patients receiving long-term corticosteroid therapy with an abnormal response to ACTH stimulation testing during the perioperative period. These patients (Group III) received intravenous cortisol, 25 mg, following the induction of anesthesia plus a continuous intravenous infusion of cortisol, 100 mg, during the next 24 hours. Plasma cortisol levels in Group III were significantly lower than in the other two groups before the induction of anesthesia. Following intravenous administration of cortisol to Group III patients, plasma concentrations were significantly higher than in Groups I and II for the next 2 hours (p < 0.01). Thereafter, the mean plasma concentrations were similar for all groups. There were no clinical signs of circulatory insufficiency in any group. (Reproduced with permission from Symreng T, Karlberg BE, Kagedol B, Schildt B: Physiological cortisol substitution of long-term steroid-treated patients undergoing major surgery. Br J Anaesth 53:949, 1981.)

that is at least equivalent to the usual daily replacement.[110] Glucocorticoid coverage is reduced to the patient's normal maintenance dosage during the postoperative period. Although there is no conclusive evidence supporting an increased incidence of infection or abnormal wound healing when supraphysiologic doses of supplemental steroids are used acutely, the goal of therapy is to use the minimal drug dosage necessary to adequately protect the patient.

ADRENAL MEDULLA

The adrenal medulla is derived embryologically from neuroectodermal cells. As a specialized part of the sympathetic nervous system, the adrenal medulla synthesizes and secretes the catecholamines epinephrine (80%) and norepinephrine (20%). Preganglionic fibers of the sympathetic nervous system bypass the paravertebral ganglia and pass directly from the spinal cord to the adrenal medulla. The adrenal medulla is analogous to a postganglionic neuron,

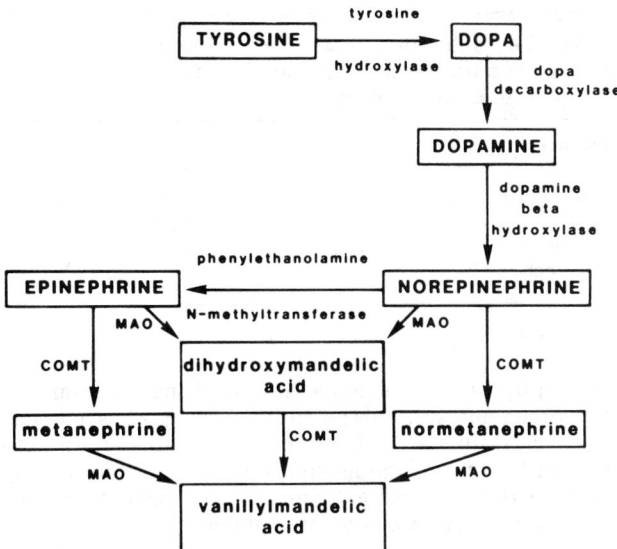

Figure 45-7. The synthesis and metabolism of endogenous cate-cholamines. (Reproduced with permission from Stoelting RK, Dierdorf SF [eds]: Anesthesia and Co-Existing Disease. New York, Churchill-Livingstone, 1983.)

although the catecholamines secreted by the medulla function as hormones, not as neurotransmitters.

The biosynthetic pathway for catecholamines produced in the adrenal medulla is outlined in Figure 45-7. The synthesis of norepinephrine begins with hydroxylation of tyrosine to DOPA. This rate-limiting step in catecholamine biosynthesis is regulated so that synthesis is coupled to release. In the adrenal medulla and in those rare central neurons utilizing epinephrine as a neurotransmitter, the majority of norepinephrine is converted to epinephrine by the enzyme phenylethanolamine-N-methyltransferase. It is likely that the capacity of the adrenal medulla to synthesize epinephrine is influenced by the flow of glucocorticoid-rich blood from the adrenal cortex through the intra-adrenal portal system, since it is known that high concentrations of glucocorticoid are able to induce the enzyme phenylethanolamine-N-methyltransferase.

In the adrenal medulla, catecholamines are stored in chromaffin granules complexed with adenosine triphosphate (ATP) and Ca^{2+}. The normal adrenal releases epinephrine and norepinephrine by exocytosis in response to stimulation by preganglionic sympathetic neurons. The circulatory half-life (10–30 seconds) of these catechols is considerably longer than the brief receptor activity of norepinephrine released as a neurotransmitter from postganglionic sympathetic nerve endings. Biotransformation of circulating norepinephrine and epinephrine is accomplished chiefly by the enzyme catechol-O-methyltransferase, located in the liver and kidney. Monoamine oxidase is of less importance in the metabolism of circulating catechols. Metanephrines and vanillylmandelic acid (VMA) are the major end products of catecholamine metabolism. These metabolites and a small amount of unchanged catecholamine (less than 1%) appear in the urine.

The outflow of postganglionic sympathetic neurotransmitters and circulating catecholamine from the adrenal medulla is coordinated by higher cortical centers connected to the brain stem. The intrinsic activity of the brain stem sympathetic areas is modulated by higher cortical functions,

emotional reactions (anger, fear), and various physiologic stimuli, including changes in the physical and chemical properties of the extracellular fluid (hypoglycemia, hypotension). The adrenal medulla and sympathetic nervous system are often stimulated together in a generalized fashion, although many physiologic conditions exist in which they act independently.

Pheochromocytoma

The only important disease process associated with the adrenal medulla is pheochromocytoma. These tumors produce, store, and secrete catecholamines. Most pheochromocytomas secrete both epinephrine and norepinephrine, with the percentage of secreted norepinephrine being greater than that secreted by the normal gland. Although pheochromocytomas occur in fewer than 0.1% of hypertensive patients, it is important to aggressively evaluate the patient with clinically suspect symptoms, because surgical extirpation is curative in more than 90% of patients[111,112] and because complications are often lethal in undiagnosed cases. Postmortem series have reported high perioperative mortality rates in undiagnosed patients undergoing relatively minor surgical procedures.[113,114] The majority of deaths are from cardiovascular causes.[115] Of particular importance to the anesthesiologist is that anesthetic drugs can exacerbate the life-threatening cardiovascular effects of the catecholamines secreted by these tumors.

The majority (85–90%) of pheochromocytomas are solitary tumors localized to a single adrenal gland, usually the right. Approximately 10% of adults and 25% of children have bilateral tumors. The tumor may originate in extra-adrenal sites (10%) anywhere along the paravertebral sympathetic chain; however, 95% are located within the abdomen, and a small percentage are located in the thorax, urinary bladder, or neck. Malignant spread of these highly vascular tumors occurs in about 10% of cases.[116]

In about 5% of cases, this tumor is inherited as a familial autosomal dominant trait. It may be part of the polyglandular syndrome referred to as multiple endocrine neoplasia (MEN) Type IIA or IIB. Type IIA includes medullary carcinoma of the thyroid, parathyroid hyperplasia, and pheochromocytoma; Type IIB consists of medullary carcinoma of the thyroid, pheochromocytoma, and neuromas of the oral mucosa. Pheochromocytomas may also arise in association with von Recklinghausen's neurofibromatosis or von Hippel–Lindau disease (retinal and cerebellar angiomatosis). The pheochromocytoma of the familial syndromes is rarely extra-adrenal or malignant. Bilateral tumors occur in approximately 75% of cases. When these patients present with a single adrenal pheochromocytoma, the chances of subsequent development of a second adrenal pheochromocytoma are sufficiently high that bilateral adrenalectomy should be considered. Every member of a MEN family should be screened periodically for pheochromocytoma.

Clinical Presentation

Pheochromocytoma may occur at any age, but it is most common in young to mid-adult life. The clinical manifestations are mainly due to the pharmacologic effects of the catecholamines released from the tumor. These tumors are not innervated, and catecholamine release is independent of neurogenic control. Although most patients (90%) are hypertensive, the blood pressure profile is labile in half of these cases. Forty percent have paroxysmal hypertension that occurs only during an attack. When true paroxysms occur, the blood pressure may rise to alarmingly high levels, placing the patient at risk for cerebrovascular hemorrhage, heart failure, dysrhythmias, or myocardial infarction. Headache, palpitations, tremor, profuse sweating, and either pallor or flushing may accompany an attack. There are reports of pheochromocytoma manifesting as malignant hyperthermia.[117] Orthostatic hypotension, probably resulting from a reduction in plasma volume, is a frequent finding. Physical examination of the patient with pheochromocytoma may be unrevealing during the period between attacks unless the patient presents with symptoms and signs of sequelae related to long-standing hypertension. A well-described catecholamine-induced cardiomyopathy may manifest as myocarditis accompanied by heart failure and cardiac dysrhythmias.[118,119] Paroxysms are commonly not associated with clearly defined events but may be precipitated by displacement of the abdominal contents or, in the case of a bladder tumor, by micturition.

Diagnosis

Biochemical determination of free catecholamine concentration and catecholamine metabolites in the urine is the most common screening test used to establish the diagnosis of pheochromocytoma. Urinary VMA and unconjugated norepinephrine and epinephrine levels are measured in a 24-hour urine collection and are expressed as a function of the creatine clearance (Table 45-6). The VMA level is elevated in most cases.[120] Urinary metanephrine is not quantified because it is not predictably elevated in pheochromocytoma. Free catecholamines represent less than 1% of the originally released hormone, and urinary levels are not always elevated to a significant degree. Hence, differentiation from normals may be difficult. A change in the ratio of unconjugated epinephrine to norepinephrine may be the only biochemical finding. In addition, certain drugs interfere with urinary assays,[121] and some patients with paroxysmal hypertension have normal values between attacks. The sensitivity of the urine assay has been greatly increased through the use of high-pressure liquid chromatography. The yield is further improved when multiple 24-hour urine specimens are collected. Although the distinction between "normal" and pheochromocytoma levels of urinary catecholamines may be difficult, provocative testing (with glucagon or histamine) or suppression testing (with clonidine) is seldom utilized. The RIA determination of plasma catecholamine levels has been advocated by some investigators as a more reliable diagnostic tool than urine assays; however, plasma catecholamine determinations have not gained widespread acceptance because of problems with the interpretation of results.[122,123]

Although routine laboratory data are unlikely to provide specific diagnostic insight, the ECG, chest radiograph, and complete blood cell count can provide valuable information to the clinician who entertains the diagnosis. Left ventricular hypertrophy and nonspecific T-wave changes are two of the more common ECG findings.[124,125] Evidence of acute myocardial infarction or tachyarrhythmia has also been reported.[115] The chest radiograph may reveal cardiomegaly, and the blood count often shows an elevated hematocrit consistent with a reduced intravascular volume and hemoconcentration. Standardized imaging methods such as CT and MRI are used in the noninvasive localization of these tumors.[126] Ultrasound and MRI are especially useful in pregnant patients. ^{131}I-metaiodobenzylguanidine ([131]IMIBG)

TABLE 45-6. Reference Values for Normal Daily Urinary Excretion of Catecholamines and Catecholamine Metabolites

Substance	Value
Vanillylmandelic acid	$<5.0-6.0$ mg·24 h^{-1}
Norepinephrine	<80 mg·24 h^{-1}
Epinephrine	<20 mg·24 h^{-1}
Total catecholamines	<100 mg·24 h^{-1}

scintigraphy is also effective in localizing recurrent or extra-adrenal masses. This guanidine analogue has a molecular structure similar to that of norepinephrine and is concentrated in catecholamine storage vesicles. Arteriography must be performed with extreme care in these patients, because a pressor crisis can be precipitated.

Anesthetic Considerations

Preoperative Preparation. The reduction in perioperative mortality from a high of 45% to between zero and 3% with the excision of pheochromocytoma followed the introduction of alpha-antagonists for preoperative therapy. Perioperative blood pressure fluctuations, myocardial infarction, congestive heart failure, cardiac dysrhythmias, and cerebral hemorrhage all appear to be reduced in frequency when the patient has been treated preoperatively with alpha blockers and the intravascular fluid compartment has been re-expanded.[127,128] Extended treatment with alpha antagonists is also effective in treating the clinical manifestations of catecholamine myocarditis.[118,129] A list of drugs frequently used in the management of pheochromocytoma is given in Table 45-7.

Alpha-adrenergic blockade is initiated once the diagnosis of pheochromocytoma is established. The patient receives phenoxybenzamine, a long-acting (24–48 hours) noncompetitive presynaptic (alpha$_2$) and postsynaptic (alpha$_1$) blocker, at doses of 10 mg every 8 hours. Increments are added until the blood pressure is controlled and paroxysms disappear. Most patients need between 80 and 200 mg·day^{-1}. The absorption following oral administration is variable, and side-effects are common. Certain cardiovascular reflexes, such as the baroreceptor reflex, are blunted, and postural hypotension is common. Alpha-adrenergic blockade also causes nasal stuffiness and impairs ejaculation. Prazosin, a postsynaptic (alpha$_1$) blocking agent with a shorter half-life than phenoxybenzamine, has also been used effectively. Because postural hypotension can be pronounced with the commencement of therapy, the initial 1-mg dose is given at bedtime. Postural changes are also seen with maintenance therapy (6–10 mg·day^{-1}). A comparison of patients receiving phenoxybenzamine and prazosin has shown both drugs to be equally effective in controlling the blood pressure in patients with pheochromocytoma. A case report of severe hypertension in a prazosin-treated patient following the initiation of beta blocker therapy suggested that a less selective blockade of both alpha$_1$ and alpha$_2$ receptors (phenoxybenzamine) might be preferable in patients with severe hypertension.[130] Although the optimal period of preoperative treatment has not been established, most clinicians recommend beginning alpha blockade therapy at least 10–14 days before the proposed surgery. During this time, the contracted intravascular volume returns toward

TABLE 45-7. Drugs Used in the Management of Pheochromocytoma

Drug	Action	Pressor Crisis		Preoperative Blood Pressure Control		Comment
		Route	Dose	Route	Dose	
Phentolamine	Alpha blocker	IV	2–5 mg	—	—	Rapid onset, short-acting; give bolus every 5 min or infuse initially 1 mg·min^{-1}
Phenoxybenzamine	Alpha blocker	—	—	Oral	30 mg·day^{-1}, increasing daily dosage by 30 mg	Long half-life; may accumulate; give twice or three times daily
Prazosin	Alpha blocker	—	—	Oral	1.0 mg single dose, increasing to t.i.d. regimen	First dose phenomenon; may cause syncope, so start with low dose before bedtime
Propranolol	Beta blocker	IV	1.0 mg bolus to total of 10 mg	Oral	40 mg b.i.d.; increase to 480 mg·day^{-1}	When used alone may cause syncope, so start with low dose
Atenolol	Beta blocker	—	—	Oral	50 mg·day^{-1} initially; may increase to 100 mg·day^{-1}	Long-acting selective beta$_1$ antagonist eliminated unchanged by kidney
Esmolol	Beta blocker	IV	500 μg·kg^{-1}·min^{-1} loading followed by maintenance infusion		—	Ultra-short-acting selective beta$_1$ antagonist, may be used during anesthesia
Labetalol	Alpha and beta blocker	IV	10 mg bolus to 150 mg	Oral	200 mg t.i.d.	A much weaker alpha blocker than beta blocker; may cause pressor response in pheochromocytoma
Nitroprusside	Vasodilator	IV	Infusion initially 0.5–1.5 μg·kg^{-1}·min^{-1}	—	—	Powerful vasodilator; short-acting; may be used during anesthesia
Alpha-methyl-tyrosine	Inhibitor of biosynthesis of catecholamines	—	—	Oral	1–4 g·day^{-1}	Suitable for patients not amenable to surgery; may be nephrotoxic

normal and the blood pressure is stabilized. Despite the real possibility of hypotension following vascular isolation of the tumor, we continue alpha blockers up until the morning of surgery.

Beta-adrenergic blockade is often added after alpha blockade has been established. This addition is considered in patients with persistent tachycardia or cardiac dysrhythmias that may be exacerbated by alpha blockade. Beta blockers should not be given until adequate alpha blockade is ensured in order to avoid the possibility of unopposed alpha-mediated vasoconstriction. There is no clear advantage of one beta antagonist over another. We have effectively used both propranolol and atenolol. Labetalol, a beta antagonist with alpha-blocking activity, is effective as a second-line medication, but there are reports of increases in blood pressure when this drug is used alone.[131] In our opinion, inadequate postsynaptic alpha-blocking properties disqualify this medication as a first choice in the preoperative preparation of the patient.

Acute hypertensive crises are treated with iv infusions of nitroprusside or phentolamine. Phentolamine is a short-acting alpha-adrenergic antagonist that may be given as an iv bolus (2–5 mg) or by continuous infusion. Tachydysrhythmias are controlled with iv boluses of propranolol (1-mg increments) or by a continuous infusion of the ultrashort-acting selective beta$_1$-adrenergic antagonist esmolol.

Alpha-methyl tyrosine is an agent that inhibits the enzyme tyrosine hydroxylase, the rate-limiting step in cate-

cholamine biosynthesis. This medication is currently reserved for patients with metastatic disease or for situations in which surgery is contraindicated and long-term medical therapy is required. When alpha-methyl tyrosine is used in combination with alpha-adrenergic-blocking agents, there is a significant reduction in catecholamine biosynthesis.[121]

Unrecognized pheochromocytoma during pregnancy may be life-threatening to the mother and fetus. Although the safety of adrenergic-blocking agents during pregnancy has not been established, these agents probably improve fetal survival in pregnant patients with pheochromocytoma. There is no reason to terminate an early pregnancy, but the patient should be aware of the risk of spontaneous abortion resulting from abdominal surgery to remove the tumor. When pheochromocytoma is diagnosed during the third trimester, the mother is treated in the usual manner, and, when the fetus is sufficiently mature, the child is electively delivered by cesarean section, and the tumor is excised.[132]

Perioperative Anesthetic Management. Symptomatic patients continue to receive medical therapy until tachycardia, cardiac dysrhythmias, and paroxysmal elevations in blood pressure are well controlled. Occasionally, a patient with pheochromocytoma unaccompanied by hypertension is referred for consultation prior to surgery. These patients are difficult to manage with alpha blockade therapy on an outpatient basis because of the fear of clinically significant orthostatic hypotension. These patients are admitted to the hospital at least 24 hours before surgery in order to institute bed rest, "prophylactic" alpha-adrenergic blockade (prazosin), and fluid therapy. Central venous and peripheral artery pressure monitoring is routinely used to guide preoperative intervention. Because of the unpredictable and potentially lethal nature of the patient response to the stress of anesthesia and surgery, all patients presenting for pheochromocytoma surgery should receive a preoperative anesthesiology consultation and alpha blocker therapy. Experience suggests that pretreated patients have fewer cardiac dysrhythmias and less fluctuation in blood pressure and heart rate during the induction of anesthesia than other, "normotensive" patients who do not receive preoperative alpha blockade therapy. If it is not possible to initiate alpha-blocking therapy prior to surgery, or if the patient has received less than 48 hours of intensive treatment, it is frequently necessary to infuse phentolamine or nitroprusside during the induction of anesthesia. A low-dose infusion is often initiated in anticipation of the marked blood pressure elevations that can occur with laryngoscopy and surgical stimulation.

Although there is no clear advantage to one anesthetic technique over another, drugs that are known to liberate histamine are avoided.[128] Because of the potential for ventricular irritability, halothane is not administered. Pulmonary artery and peripheral artery pressure monitoring are used in all adult patients. Good patient sedation facilitates the placement of these monitoring devices before the induction of anesthesia. A potent sedative-hypnotic in combination with an opioid analgesic is used for induction. It is extremely important to achieve an adequate depth of anesthesia before proceeding with laryngoscopy in order to minimize the sympathetic nervous system response to this maneuver. Maintenance is provided with an opioid analgesic and either isoflurane or enflurane. A recent report of pheochromocytoma surgery with sevoflurane is noted.[133] Manipulation of the tumor may produce marked elevations in blood pressure, which are controlled with nitroprusside and, if necessary, phentolamine. Tachydysrhythmias are treated with iv beta blockers (e.g., propranolol, labetalol, esmolol). The reduction in blood pressure that may occur following ligation of the tumor's venous supply should be anticipated through close communication with the surgical team. Restitution of any intravascular fluid deficit is the initial therapy in this situation. Following replenishment of the intravascular volume, if the patient remains hypotensive, phenylephrine is administered. Postoperatively, catecholamine levels return to normal over several days. Approximately 75% of patients become normotensive within 10 days.[134]

DIABETES MELLITUS

Diabetes mellitus is the most commonly occurring endocrine disease found in surgical patients.[135,136] It has a broad spectrum of severity, and its manifestations can be altered in reaction to the patient's metabolic stress. Although the most serious complications of diabetes mellitus are related to its character as a chronic disease, it can cause difficulties in the short-term management of acute illness. Occasionally, diabetes remains clinically inapparent until exacerbated by the stress of trauma or surgery.

The principles of the treatment of diabetes will be easier to understand if we review the physiology of glucose metabolism and the stress response and then consider some of the specific pathologic entities that make up the clinical picture of diabetes mellitus. The reader is also referred to Chapter 15.

Classification

Diabetes mellitus is primarily a disease of carbohydrate metabolism; however, it has numerous manifestations and interactions with a large range of hormonal and endocrinologic functions. Despite a variety of etiologic factors, its hallmark is a deficiency, either absolute or relative, in the amount of insulin available to the tissues.

Diabetes is often divided into two broad types.[137] Type I, or insulin-dependent diabetes mellitus (IDDM), is distinguished from Type II, or non-insulin-dependent diabetes mellitus (NIDDM). The patient with IDDM typically experienced the onset of disease early in life. Consequently, this form is also referred to as juvenile-onset diabetes. Generally, the patient with IDDM is not obese, had an abrupt onset of the disease, and has very low levels of circulating insulin. Disease in these patients cannot be controlled with diet or oral hypoglycemic agents and mandates treatment with insulin. Patients in this group are often difficult to maintain in good glucose balance, are more likely to become ketotic, and are likely to develop the end-organ complications of diabetes if they live long enough.

Patients with NIDDM, also called maturity-onset diabetes, typically experience a gradual onset of the disease later in life. They are often obese and have some degree of resistance to the effects of insulin. They may have normal or even elevated levels of insulin. In milder forms, this version of diabetes can often be treated with diet or oral hypoglycemic agents. Because these patients are relatively resistant to ketosis, their disease may be clinically inapparent until exacerbated by the stress of surgery or intercurrent illness.

This classification of diabetes mellitus is only a generalization. The milder NIDDM form occasionally occurs in young people, and many older adults develop a severe and brittle form of IDDM. Diabetes can also be a secondary result of a disease that damages the pancreas and thus impairs insulin secretion. Pancreatic surgery, chronic pancreatitis, cystic fibrosis, and hemochromatosis can damage the pancreas and thus impair insulin secretion to produce clinical diabetes. Diabetes can result from one of the endocrine diseases that produces a hormone that opposes the action of insulin. Hence, a patient with a glucagonoma, pheochromocytoma, or acromegaly may be diabetic. An increased effect of glucocorticoids, either from Cushing's disease or steroid therapy, may also oppose the effect of insulin enough to elicit clinical diabetes and would certainly complicate the management of pre-existing diabetes. Patients with circulating anti-insulin receptor antibodies in association with other autoimmune processes are also diabetics. Finally, there is a clinical triad of severe insulin resistance in young hirsute women with polycystic ovaries who have decreased insulin receptors.

Physiology

Insulin has multiple and complex interactions with lipid, protein, and glucose metabolism.[138-140] For present purposes, it is easiest to regard the effects of insulin on glucose metabolism as primary and to view its effects on other metabolic functions only as they relate to glucose.

Insulin is a small protein produced by the beta cells of the islets of Langerhans in the pancreas. Normal production in the adult human is about 40–50 units·day^{-1}. Insulin acts through receptor sites on cells. The half-life of insulin in the circulation is only a few minutes. However, it may clinically appear to have a longer duration of action, owing to delays in binding and release from the cellular receptors. These facts lead us to the important principle that once a high level of insulin saturates all the binding sites, insulin will not have a more potent effect, just a more long-lasting effect. This is key to understanding insulin therapy, which is discussed in the following paragraphs.

Insulin is metabolized in the liver and kidney. In patients with hepatic dysfunction, the loss of gluconeogenesis as well as a prolongation of insulin effect increases the risk of hypoglycemia. Renal disease is another risk factor for hypoglycemia and is an important consideration in managing the use of exogenous insulin in diabetic patients.

Insulin release is related to a number of events. First is the direct effect of glucose (and amino acids) to stimulate insulin release. The mechanism involves interaction with hormones from the GI tract released during enteral feeding. The autonomic nervous system, also *via* vagal stimulation, will increase insulin release, as will beta-adrenergic stimulation and alpha-adrenergic blockade.

The most fundamental action of insulin is to cause increased uptake of glucose into the cells. This is particularly important in skeletal muscle cells, where muscle activity will also increase glucose uptake and is an important variable in the management of the physically active diabetic. (The brain and liver are exceptional areas where insulin does not affect glucose transport). Hence, the diabetic patient has hyperglycemia because of inadequate cellular uptake of glucose. Along with glucose, potassium enters the cells under the influence of insulin, so the diabetic patient is also likely to have an imbalance of potassium concentrations across the cell membranes.

Other important metabolic functions of insulin include the stimulation of glycogen formation and the depression of gluconeogenesis and lipolysis. The patient with insulin deficiency will have low glycogen stores and active gluconeogenesis. This implies that in the diabetic, owing to an absence of glycogen, protein will have to be broken down to make glucose. Insulin also increases the uptake of amino acids into muscle cells. Hence, an insulin deficiency will lead to catabolism and negative nitrogen balance.

Fat metabolism is also abnormal in the diabetic state, with acceleration of lipid catabolism and increased formation of ketone bodies.[141] A deficiency of insulin leads to increased fatty acid liberation from adipose tissue. These fatty acids have multiple metabolic effects, including interference with carbohydrate phosphorylation in muscle, which leads to further hyperglycemia. Low concentrations of insulin, which may be inadequate to prevent hyperglycemia, are often sufficient to block lipolysis. This effect explains the common clinical situation in which a patient is hyperglycemic without being ketotic.

Glucagon is a polypeptide released from the alpha cells of the pancreas and acts both to stimulate the release of insulin and to oppose some of the effects of insulin. Hence, it has both a direct and an indirect ability to increase circulating glucose levels. In some patients, after total pancreatic resection, glucose balance is not as poor as might be expected because of the concomitant absence of glucagon. Glucagon release is stimulated by hypoglycemia as well as by epinephrine and cortisol, and is suppressed by glucose ingestion.[142]

Diabetes and Stress

The metabolic effects of stress are intricately involved with the same pathways as those involved in diabetes mellitus (Fig. 45-8).[143] During stress, elevations in the circulating levels of cortisol, glucagon, catecholamines, and growth hormones all act to cause hyperglycemia at the tissue level. In addition, glucagon and epinephrine exert a suppressive effect on insulin release. Hyperglycemia is common in the stressed patient who does not have diabetes mellitus. In the diabetic patient, stress will make the diabetes more difficult to control. In a patient with minimal or subclinical diabetes prior to the stressful episode, the glucose balance may become quite difficult to manage during the stress-related event. Thus, in the stressed diabetic patient, the catabolic effects of the stress may not be adequately countered by the anabolic effects of an inadequate insulin response.

The induction of anesthesia will increase the levels of circulating catecholamines and is a form of metabolic stress. Regional anesthesia may block part of the metabolic stress response during surgery, probably by blockade of the neural communications from the surgical area. It is theorized that the persistently high levels of circulating catecholamines in trauma and critical illness lead to stress hyperglycemia through a direct inhibition of insulin release. The bypass of the gut hormonal actions in patients receiving iv glucose feedings, especially if given in large amounts, contributes to the impairment of insulin release during illness and can create a particularly difficult management problem for diabetics.

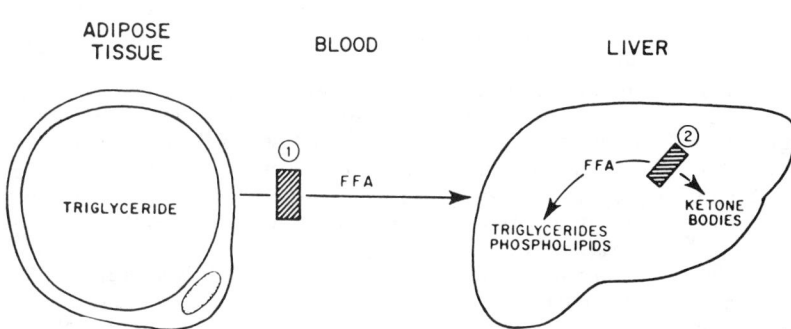

Figure 45-8. Ketone production is increased in diabetes by augmented release (1) of free fatty acids (FFA) from adipose tissue, and (2) beta oxidation of these FFA into ketones in the liver. (Illustration from McGarry JD, Foster DW: Arch Intern Med 137:496, 1977, with permission. Copyright 1977, American Medical Association.)

Hyperglycemia

Many diabetic patients, especially those with NIDDM, have circulating levels of insulin that in normal patients would be considered adequate or even excessive. Because insulin resistance at the cellular level is typical of diabetics, such patients have difficulty with glucose homeostasis and have elevated blood sugar concentrations. Nevertheless, they often have enough insulin effect present to prevent ketosis. Such patients, especially with a therapeutic boost from sulfonylureas, diet, or exercise, are often able to control their metabolism enough to avoid severe swings in blood glucose concentrations and to avoid ketoacidosis. With more severe disease or with added stress, their metabolism may become quite disarrayed; insulin plus aggressive therapy of the concomitant disease may be required.

The insulin-dependent diabetic may have enough endogenous insulin present after the initial boost provided by a therapeutic dose of exogenous insulin. In such circumstances, the patient is likely to remain in good diabetic control, avoiding large swings in blood sugar and ketosis. However, when the amount of endogenous insulin available continues to be much less than what is metabolically required, additional therapeutic dosing is required to match the body's varying needs. The use of computerized insulin pumps with continuously reading glucose meters is more precise than other approaches to insulin therapy.

Hypoglycemia

Hypoglycemia is the clinical occurrence most feared when dealing with diabetic patients.[144] The precise level at which symptomatic hypoglycemia occurs is variable. The normal, fasted patient may have blood sugar levels lower than 50 mg·dl^{-1} without symptoms. However, the diabetic patient who has a chronically elevated blood sugar level may be symptomatic at levels quite above this glucose concentration. Hypoglycemia is almost impossible to diagnose clinically in the unconscious patient.

In the awake patient, hypoglycemia will often produce central nervous system (CNS) changes ranging from lightheadedness to coma with seizures. Often the patient recognizes the symptoms and can tell that the blood sugar is low before any overt clinical signs develop. With hypoglycemia, there is a reflex catecholamine release that produces overt sympathetic hyperactivity causing tachycardia, lacrimation, diaphoresis, and hypertension. In the anesthetized patient, these signs of sympathetic hyperactivity can easily be misinterpreted as inadequate or "light" anesthesia. In the anesthetized, sedated, or seriously ill patient, the mental changes of hypoglycemia will also be unrecognizable. Furthermore, in patients being treated with beta-adrenergic blocking agents or in patients with advanced diabetic autonomic neuropathy, the sympathetic hyperactivity of hypoglycemia may be obscured. Thus, the clinical diagnosis of hypoglycemia in the surgical patient may be quite difficult to make.

Hypoglycemia is more likely to occur in the diabetic surgical patient under certain circumstances. With renal insufficiency, the action of insulin and oral hypoglycemic agents is prolonged. This is a common problem, due to the prevalence of renal disease in the diabetic. Because the effect of some of the oral agents, especially chlorpropamide, can be long-lasting, an accurate medical history with attention to medications taken in the past day or two is essential. A frequent and totally avoidable cause of inadvertent hypoglycemia is the administration of insulin to a patient who is not receiving sufficient oral or iv caloric input. For the purpose of preventing hypoglycemia, transfused blood has a low glucose concentration (even with citrate-phosphate-dextrose added, it contains only about 2 g of glucose per unit); lactated Ringer's solution is also inadequate (the lactate is metabolized to produce about 9 kcal·l^{-1}).

The anesthesiologist must recognize that hypoglycemia in the critically ill or anesthetized patient is a serious hazard that may be difficult to diagnose. It is therefore quite reasonable to aim for mild hyperglycemia as the goal in diabetes management in these patients. There is considerable discussion by endocrinologists as to how close to normal the blood sugar level should be maintained (chronic management) in long-standing diabetes in order to avoid the end-organ damage that diabetes can produce in the eyes, kidneys, nerves, and blood vessels.[145] In the perioperative period it is unlikely that such chronic damage is exacerbated by mild hyperglycemia.

Patients with chronic diabetes will often develop autonomic neuropathies that can cause bladder atony, postural hypotension, impotence, and delayed gastric emptying. There have also been rare reports of sudden death under anesthesia that are associated with autonomic cardiac dysfunction.[146,147] Although all of these phenomena are of concern, there is no reason to believe that they are effected by short-term glucose fluctuations.

Even if mild hyperglycemia is the "ideal" for the perioperative patient, the clinician should be alert to problems associated with hyperglycemia. There is the potential for an increased risk of infection. The alert patient may complain of some changes in vision consequent to osmotic changes in the lens. The likely result is an osmotic diuresis that leads to hypovolemia and washout of potassium. If the hyperglycemia is severe, the plasma will be hyperosmolar, and stupor or even coma could occur. Therefore, even if hyperglycemia is the intended goal, blood sugar levels above 500–600 mg·dl^{-1} are to be avoided. Hyperglycemia is likely if, in an overly eager attempt to avoid hypoglycemia, all the replacement fluids given to a perioperative patient contain dextrose. Such therapy will result in a large dextrose load that will cause significant hyperglycemia.

There is good evidence that hyperglycemia augments the damage caused by cerebral ischemia. The mechanism may be increased tissue acidosis due to anaerobic glucose metabolism during ischemia. Hence, it seems wise to recommend that hyperglycemia be especially avoided whenever there is a significant risk of cerebral ischemia, such as during neurosurgical procedures or cardiopulmonary bypass.[148,149]

Hyperosmolar Nonketotic Coma

An occasional elderly patient with minimal or mild diabetes may present with remarkably high blood glucose levels and profound dehydration.[150] Such patients usually have enough endogenous insulin activity to prevent ketosis; even with blood sugar concentrations above 1000 mg · dl^{-1}, they are not in ketoacidosis. Presumably it is the combination of an impaired thirst response and mild renal insufficiency that allows the hyperglycemia to develop. The marked hyperosmolarity may lead to coma and seizures, with the increased plasma viscosity producing a tendency to intravascular thrombosis. It is characteristic of this syndrome that the metabolic disturbance responds quickly to rehydration and small doses of insulin. With rapid correction of the hyperosmolarity, cerebral edema is a risk, and recovery of

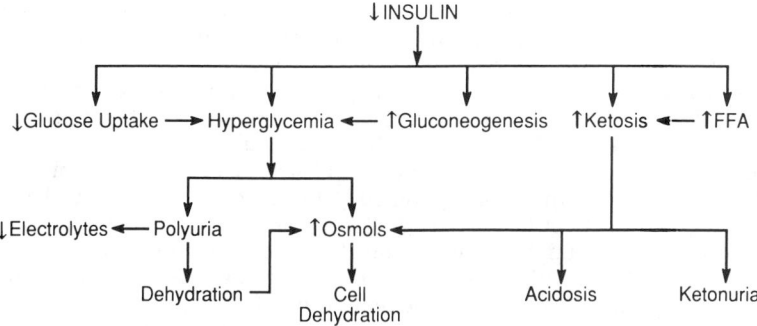

Figure 45-9. Pathophysiology of diabetic ketoacidosis starting from relative insulin deficiency. (Adapted with permission from Olefsky JM: In Wyngaarden JB, Smith LH [eds]: Cecil Textbook of Medicine, p. 1375. Philadelphia, WB Saunders, 1988.)

mental acuity may be delayed after the blood glucose level and circulating volume have been normalized.

Diabetic Ketoacidosis

If the diabetic patient has insufficient insulin effect to block the mobilization and metabolism of free fatty acids, the metabolic byproducts acetoacetate and beta-hydroxybutyrate will accumulate (Fig. 45-9).[151] These ketone bodies are organic acids and will cause a metabolic acidosis with an increased unmeasured anion gap. Clinically, the patient often presents because of intercurrent illness, trauma, or the untoward cessation of insulin therapy. Although hyperglycemia is almost always present, the degree of hyperglycemia does not correlate with the severity of the acidosis. Blood sugar levels are often in the 300–500 mg·dl^{-1} range. The patient is always dehydrated because of the combination of the hyperglycemia-induced osmotic diuresis and the nausea and vomiting typical of this syndrome. Because leukocytosis, abdominal pain, GI ileus, and mildly elevated amylase levels are all common in ketoacidosis, an occasional patient is misdiagnosed as having an intra-abdominal surgical problem.

Potassium replacement is a key concern in patients with diabetic ketoacidosis. Because of the diuresis, the total body potassium stores are reduced. However, acidosis by itself causes a shift of potassium ions out of the cell. Thus, the serum potassium concentration may be normal or even slightly elevated while the patient is acidotic. As soon as the metabolic acidosis is corrected, the potassium ions shift back into the cells. Consequently, the serum potassium concentration can decline acutely. Therefore, early and vigorous potassium replacement is required in these patients, the exception being those patients with renal failure. Hypophosphatemia also occurs with the correction of the acidosis and, if severe, may cause impairment of ventilation resulting from skeletal muscle weakness in the vulnerable patient. Instead of diabetic ketoacidosis, the diabetic patient with a metabolic acidosis may have lactic acidosis, which results from poor tissue perfusion or sepsis. It is diagnosed by the presence of an increased serum lactate concentration without an elevated ketone concentration.

Diabetic ketoacidosis must also be distinguished from the syndrome of alcoholic ketoacidosis.[152] This typically occurs in the poorly nourished alcoholic patient following acute intoxication. Except for the presence of chemical ketoacidosis, alcoholic ketoacidosis is not clinically related in any way to diabetes mellitus. The alcoholic patient may be hypoglycemic or mildly hyperglycemic. The predominant ketone in this syndrome is beta-hydroxybutyrate, which tends to react less sensitively in the standard laboratory nitroprus-

side reaction measurement of ketones. Hence, the diagnosis may be obscured. Administration of dextrose and parenteral fluids is the specific treatment for alcoholic ketoacidosis; insulin is not indicated (except in the rare circumstance in which the patient also has clear-cut diabetes mellitus). Although unrelated to the ketoacidosis, early thiamine supplementation to prevent the development of Wernicke-Korsakoff syndrome may be the most important part of the treatment of any poorly nourished alcoholic.

Perioperative Monitoring

The anesthesiologist must usually determine in advance the types of physiologic monitoring that will be used during surgery. For the diabetic patient, fluid output and metabolic measurements are likely to be particularly important. It is reasonable to request that all diabetic surgical patients undergo preoperative determination of blood glucose and potassium levels and urine glucose and ketone levels, and that these tests be repeated immediately after surgery. For operations of short duration in patients without brittle diabetes, it is unlikely that much metabolic dysfunction can occur. However, for longer surgical procedures, changes may be very significant, and blood glucose measurements should be obtained every 2–4 hours. A urinary catheter allows frequent re-evaluation of glucose and ketone levels. Another argument for the use of a urinary catheter is to prevent bladder distention, which can cause serious bladder dysfunction in the diabetic, who may already have a neurogenic bladder. This is further potentiated by the presence of a large urine output caused by a hyperglycemic osmotic diuresis. The urinary catheter may, however, cause a bladder infection in the susceptible diabetic.

On the basis of a preoperative osmotic diuresis, the diabetic patient may reach the operating room with clinically significant dehydration. In addition to the usual principles of perioperative fluid management, it is important to note the amount of glucose administered iv to avoid a massive overdose of glucose. The standard glucose dosage for an adult patient is 5–10 g·h^{-1} (100–200 ml of 5% dextrose solution hourly). It is best to monitor and record the dextrose administered separately from the fluids given. It would be wrong to give large amounts of dextrose (contained in the iv solutions) just because that patient needed vigorous fluid replacement. If this happens, the patient is likely to be very hyperglycemic in the postanesthesia care unit. It is difficult to determine the proper dose of insulin to correct this iatrogenic hyperglycemia, and prolonged observation and therapy may be required.

Management of the patient who arrives in the operating room with significant metabolic impairment, such as diabetic ketoacidosis, is very similar to management in the medical intensive care unit, including hourly determinations of blood glucose, arterial pH, electrolytes, and fluid balance. Frequent reassessments with medical consultation as necessary guide the use of fluids, electrolytes (especially potassium), insulin, phosphate, and glucose.[153,154]

Another area of patient monitoring that is extremely important in the diabetic patient is positioning on the operating table. Injuries to the limbs or nerves are more likely in the patient who arrives in the operating room already suffering from diabetic peripheral vascular disease or neuropathy. The peripheral nerves may already be partly ischemic and therefore particularly vulnerable to pressure or stretch injuries.[155]

Management Regimens

Several different regimens can be used to provide an appropriate balance of insulin and glucose in the diabetic patient undergoing anesthesia and surgery.[156-159] These approaches use different combinations of iv and subcutaneous insulin and seem, in general, to be equally satisfactory in the hands of experienced clinicians. However, regardless of the approach used, the basic principles of diabetic management must be recognized. First, and most obvious, it is important to avoid hypoglycemia. Second, since hypoglycemia may develop insidiously and be difficult to detect quickly, insulin and glucose therapy is administered to bring about a mild, transient hyperglycemia that can be gradually corrected in the postoperative period. Mild hyperglycemia is not an acute problem, and there is no need for it to be corrected rapidly. It is never simple to determine the precise dose of insulin needed to correct hyperglycemia. Excessively rapid correction may lead to glucose instability and fluctuations that can persist for hours to days.

For some diabetic patients, the best method of diabetic management is to give no insulin. For short procedures in unstressed patients, especially if they are not chronically receiving insulin, there may be enough endogenous production of insulin to maintain reasonable glucose balance in the unfed state. Glucose should still be given during surgery as protection against the delayed effects of prior oral hypoglycemic agents or long-acting insulin and to prevent the occurrence of mild ketosis.

Another common method of management is to administer a fraction of the patient's usual morning NPH insulin dose the morning of the day of surgery. Often, half the usual NPH dose will suffice to maintain the patient through the day. It is critical for the patient who is NPO and receiving insulin to also receive an iv infusion of a dextrose solution. If 5–10 $g \cdot h^{-1}$ of dextrose (100–200 $ml \cdot h^{-1}$) of 5% dextrose solution) is administered to the adult, the risk of hypoglycemia is small. Nevertheless, the patient's usual dosage depends on caloric intake and physical activity, which are very different in the hospital setting.

The "sliding scale" regimen for insulin administration is one that is very popular and easy to use. Varying doses of regular insulin are administered on a 4- to 6-hour schedule, depending on the blood or urine glucose levels and the patient's prior responses to insulin. This method of management guarantees that the glucose levels are checked frequently. Large fluctuations in blood glucose can occur if insulin is administered in the presence of high glucose levels and no insulin is given for normal or intermediate levels. This can be avoided if some insulin is always present. Small doses of insulin can be prescribed for all but the lowest levels of blood glucose, or the sliding scale can be combined with a small morning dose of long-acting NPH insulin.

Although regular insulin may also be given intramuscularly, a continuous infusion of insulin may be the only method that is effective in the hypotensive or hypothermic patient. Intravenous boluses of insulin have a rapid onset of action but a short duration because of the rapid clearance of insulin from the blood (10 units of iv insulin will have an effect lasting about an hour). Except in the patient with renal failure, in whom insulin effects are difficult to predict, the continuous infusion method has the advantage of allowing rapid adjustment of the insulin effect by changing the rate of infusion. If the insulin is mixed with a 5% dextrose solution, the balance of insulin and dextrose can be maintained. In the adult with normal renal function, 7–10 units of regular insulin in 1 liter of 5% dextrose, infused at a rate of 75–100 $ml \cdot h^{-1}$, provides 0.5–1 $unit \cdot h^{-1}$ of insulin. This tends to be a low dose, and many patients will need more insulin, which can be given either as an increased insulin concentration in the infusion or as a sliding scale subcutaneous regimen. To this regimen must be added the standard amount of water and electrolytes needed for maintenance and replacement. A small amount of iv insulin will be lost by adherence to the wall of the tubing and containers, but this loss is not clinically significant and should not be a deterrent to this route of administration.[160]

PITUITARY GLAND

The pituitary gland is located below the base of the brain in a bony structure, the sella turcica. The pituitary gland and the hypothalamus together form a central unit that regulates the release of various hormones. The pituitary gland is divided into two components. The anterior pituitary (adenohypophysis) secretes prolactin, growth hormone, gonadotropins (luteinizing hormone and follicle-stimulating hormone), TSH, and ACTH. The posterior pituitary (neurohypophysis) secretes the hormones vasopressin and oxytocin. Hormone release from the anterior and posterior pituitary is regulated by the hypothalamus. Regulatory peptides or preformed hormones from the hypothalamus are transported to the pituitary gland through vascular or tissue connections.

Hyposecretion of anterior pituitary hormones is usually due to compression of the gland by tumor. This may begin as an isolated deficiency, but it usually develops into multiglandular dysfunction. Male impotence or secondary amenorrhea in the female is an early manifestation of panhypopituitarism. Panhypopituitarism following postpartum hemorrhagic shock (Sheehan's syndrome) is due to necrosis of the anterior pituitary gland.[161] Radiation therapy delivered to the sella turcica or nearby structures and surgical hypophysectomy are other causes of panhypopituitarism. Panhypopituitarism is treated with specific hormone replacement therapy.

The hypersecretion of various anterior pituitary hormones is usually caused by an adenoma. Excess prolactin secretion with galactorrhea is a common hormonal abnormality associated with pituitary adenoma.[162] Cushing's disease may occur secondary to excess ACTH production, and giantism or acromegaly may occur as a consequence of excess growth hormone production in the child or adult, respectively. Excessive secretion of TSH is rare.

Acromegaly in the adult patient may pose several problems for the anesthesiologist. Excess hypertrophy occurs in skeletal, connective, and soft tissues.[163] The tongue and epiglottis are enlarged, making the patient susceptible to upper airway obstruction. Hoarseness may reflect thickening of the vocal cords or paralysis of a recurrent laryngeal nerve due to stretching. Dyspnea or stridor is associated with subglottic narrowing. Peripheral nerve and/or artery entrapment, hypertension, and diabetes mellitus are other common findings. The anesthetic management of these patients is complicated by distortion of the facial anatomy and upper airway. Induction of general anesthesia may put the patient at increased risk if mask placement or vocal cord visualization is impaired. When the preoperative history suggests upper airway or vocal cord involvement, it is prudent to consider intubation of the trachea while the patient is awake.

Posterior Pituitary

The posterior pituitary, or neurohypophysis, is composed of terminal nerve endings that extend from the ventral hypothalamus. Vasopressin (antidiuretic hormone, ADH) and oxytocin are the two principal hormones secreted by the posterior pituitary. Both hormones are synthesized in the supraoptic and paraventricular nuclei of the hypothalamus. They are bound to inactive carrier proteins, neurophysins, and transported by axons to membrane-bound storage vesicles located in the posterior pituitary. ADH is a nonapeptide that circulates as a free peptide after its release. The primary functions of ADH are the maintenance of extracellular fluid volume and regulation of plasma osmolality. Oxytocin elicits contraction of the uterus and promotes milk secretion and ejection by the mammary glands.

Vasopressin

ADH promotes resorption of solute-free water by increasing cell membrane permeability to water alone. Target sites for ADH are the collecting tubules of the kidneys. A decrease in free water clearance causes a fall in serum osmolality and a corresponding increase in circulating blood volume. Under normal conditions, the primary stimulus for the release of ADH is an increase in serum osmolality.[164] Osmoreceptors located in the hypothalamus are sensitive to changes in the normal serum osmolality of as little as 1% (normal osmolality is about 285 mOsm·l^{-1}). Stretch receptors in the left atrium and perhaps pulmonary veins, which are sensitive to moderate reductions in the blood volume, are also capable of stimulating ADH secretion. The need to restore plasma volume may at times override osmotic inhibition of ADH release. Various physiologic and pharmacologic stimuli also influence the secretion of ADH. Positive pressure ventilation of the lungs, stress, anxiety, hyperthermia, beta-adrenergic stimulation, and any histamine-releasing stimulus can promote the release of ADH.

ADH also has other actions. ADH can increase blood pressure by constricting vascular smooth muscle.[165] This activity is most significant in the splanchnic, renal, and coronary vascular beds and provides the rationale for administering exogenous vasopressin in the management of hemorrhage due to esophageal varices (decreased portal venous pressure).[166] Caution must be observed when this drug is used in patients with coronary artery disease. ADH (even in small doses) can precipitate myocardial ischemia through vasoconstriction of the coronary arteries. It is unclear whether selective arterial infusion is safer than systemic administration with regard to cardiac and vascular side-effects.[167]

ADH also promotes hemostasis through an increase in the level of circulating von Willebrand factor and factor VIII. Desmopressin (DDAVP), an analogue of ADH, administered to patients following cardiopulmonary bypass in a dose of 0.3 µg·kg^{-1} significantly decreased blood loss and reduced transfusion requirements in comparison to a group of patients who did not receive the drug.[168] ADH may also have a place in the management of bleeding during major vascular surgery.[169]

Diabetes Insipidus

This disorder results from inadequate secretion of ADH or resistance on the part of the renal tubules to the ADH hormone (nephrogenic diabetes insipidus).[170] Failure to secrete adequate amounts of ADH results in polydipsia, hypernatremia, and a high output of poorly concentrated urine. Hypovolemia and hypernatremia may become so severe as to be life-threatening. This disorder usually occurs following destruction of the pituitary gland by intracranial trauma, infiltrating lesions, or surgery. Patients who develop diabetes insipidus secondary to head trauma usually recover after a short period of time. The treatment of diabetes insipidus depends on the extent of the hormonal deficiency. Intraoperatively, the patient with complete diabetes insipidus receives an iv infusion of aqueous ADH (100–200 milliunits·h^{-1}) combined with the administration of an isotonic crystalloid solution. The serum sodium and plasma osmolality are measured on a regular basis, and therapeutic changes are made accordingly. ADH may also be given intramuscularly (as vasopressin tannate in oil). DDAVP administered intranasally has prolonged antidiuretic activity (12–24 hours) and is associated with a low incidence of pressor effects. As a consequence of the large outpouring of ADH in response to surgical stress, patients with residual functioning gland usually do not need parenteral ADH during the perioperative period unless the plasma osmolality rises above 290 mOsm·l^{-1}. Nonhormonal agents that have efficacy in the treatment of incomplete diabetes insipidus include the oral hypoglycemic chlorpropamide (200–500 mg·day^{-1}). This drug stimulates the release of ADH and sensitizes the renal tubules to the hormone. Hypoglycemia is a serious side-effect that limits the usefulness of the drug. Clofibrate, a hypolipidemic agent, is also capable of stimulating ADH release and has been used in the outpatient setting. None of these medications is effective in the patient with nephrogenic diabetes insipidus. Paradoxically, the thiazide diuretics exert an antidiuretic action in patients with this disorder.

Inappropriate Secretion of ADH

The inappropriate and excessive secretion of ADH may occur in association with a number of diverse pathologic processes, including head injuries, intracranial tumors, pulmonary infections, small cell carcinoma of the lung, and hypothyroidism. The clinical manifestations occur as a result of a dilutional hyponatremia, decreased serum osmolality, and a reduced urine output with a high osmolality.[171] Weight gain, skeletal muscle weakness, and mental confusion or convulsions are presenting symptoms. Peripheral edema and hypertension are rare. The diagnosis of the syndrome of inappropriate antidiuretic hormone (SIADH) secretion is one of exclusion, and other causes of hyponatremia must first be ruled out. The prognosis is related to the underlying cause of the syndrome.

The treatment of patients with mild or moderate water intoxication is restriction of fluid intake to 800 ml·day^{-1}. Patients with severe water intoxication associated with hyponatremia and mental confusion may require more aggressive therapy, with the iv administration of a hypertonic saline solution. This may be administered in conjunction with furosemide. Isotonic saline is substituted for hypertonic solutions once the serum sodium is brought into a safe range. Caution must be observed in patients with poor left ventricular function. Other drugs that may be used in the patient with SIADH are demeclocycline and lithium. Demeclocycline interferes with the ability of the renal tubules to concentrate urine and is frequently used in outpatients. Lithium is generally not used because of the high incidence of toxicity.

THE ENDOCRINE RESPONSE TO SURGICAL STRESS

Anesthesia and surgery elicit a generalized endocrine metabolic response characterized by an increase in the plasma levels of cortisol, ADH, renin, catecholamines, and endorphins and by metabolic changes such as hyperglycemia and a negative nitrogen balance. Various neural and humoral factors (e.g., pain, anxiety, acidosis, local tissue factors, hypoxia) play a role in activating this stress response.

Endorphins are a group of endogenous peptides with opioid activity that have been isolated from the CNS. It is well documented that beta-endorphin is released from the anterior pituitary, where it is contained as part of beta-lipoprotein, a 91-chain amino acid, which is a cleavage product of the precursor peptide for ACTH. Large increases in the CNS and plasma concentrations of endorphins in response to emotional or surgical stimuli suggest that these substances play a role in the body's response to stress. These substances modulate painful stimuli by binding to opiate receptors located throughout the brain and spinal cord.[172]

Numerous experiments have focused on the stress response and its relationship to the depth of anesthesia. Regional and general anesthesia appear to blunt the release of various stress hormones during the period of surgical stimulation in a dose-dependent fashion. Historically, anesthesiologists have relied on the indirect measurement of hemodynamic variables such as blood pressure and heart rate to evaluate the level of autonomic activity in response to anesthesia and surgery. It is assumed that the physiologic manifestations of stress are potentially harmful, especially in patients with limited functional reserve. As such, our anesthetic techniques and pain management strategies are designed to limit this neurohormonal response, in the hope of providing the patient with some benefit. Further investigations are needed to assess the impact of these efforts on perioperative morbidity and mortality.

REFERENCES

1. Larsen PR: Thyroid-pituitary interaction. N Engl J Med 306:23, 1982
2. Sherwin JR, Tong W: The actions of iodide and TSH on thyroid cells showing a dual control system for the iodide pump. Endocrinology 94:1465, 1974
3. Brennan MD: Thyroid hormones. Mayo Clin Proc 55:33, 1980
4. Chernow B, O'Brien JT: Overview of catecholamines in selected endocrine disorders. In Lake CR, Ziegler M (eds): Norepinephrine, vol 2. Baltimore, Williams & Wilkins, 1984
5. Bilezikian J, Loeb JN. The influence of hyperthyroidism and hypothyroidism on alpha and beta adrenergic receptor systems and adrenergic responsiveness. Endocr Rev 4:378, 1983
6. Sterling K: Thyroid hormone action at the cell level. N Engl J Med 300:173, 1979
7. Melmed S, Geola FL, Reed AW et al: A comparison of methods for assessing thyroid function in non-thyroidal illness. J Clin Endocrinol Metab 54:300, 1982
8. McKenzie JM, Zakarija M, Soto A: Humoral immunity in Graves' disease. Clin Endocrinol Metab 7:31, 1978
9. Volpe R: Thyroiditis: Current views of pathogenesis. Med Clin North Am 59:1163, 1975
10. Greene JW: Subacute thyroiditis. Am J Med 51:97, 1971
11. Woolf PD, Daly R: Thyrotoxicosis with painless thyroiditis. Am J Med 60:73, 1976
12. Amino N, Morik H, Iwantani Y et al: High prevalence of transient post partum thyrotoxicosis and hypothyroidism. N Engl J Med 306:849, 1982
13. Fradkin JE, Wolff J: Iodide induced thyrotoxicosis. Medicine 62:1, 1983
14. Brennan MD, van Heeden JA, Carney JA: Amiodarone associated thyrotoxicosis: Expertise with surgical management. Surgery 102:1062, 1987
15. Channick BJ, Aldin EV, Marks AD et al: Hyperthyroidism and mitral valve prolapse. N Engl J Med 305:497, 1981
16. Davis PJ, Davis FB: Hyperthyroidism in patients over the age of 60 years: Clinical features in 85 patients. Medicine 53:161, 1974
17. Carter JN, Eastman CJ, Kilham HA et al: Rational therapy for thyroid storm. Aust NZ J Med 5:458, 1975
18. Mackin JE, Canary JJ, Pittman CS: Thyroid storm and its management. N Engl J Med 291:1396, 1974
19. Mazzaferri EL, Skillman TG: Thyroid storm. Arch Intern Med 124:684, 1969
20. Howton JC: Thyroid storm presenting as coma. Ann Emerg Med 17:343, 1988
21. Brooks MH, Waldstein SS: Free thyroxine concentration in thyroid storm. Ann Intern Med 93:694, 1980
22. Greer MA: Antithyroid drugs in the treatment of thyrotoxicosis. Thyroid Today 3:1, 1980
23. Feek CM, Sawers JS, Irvine WJ et al: Combination of potassium iodide and propranolol in preparation of patients with Graves' disease for thyroid surgery. N Engl J Med 302:883, 1980
24. Eriksson M, Rubenfeld S, Garber AJ et al: Propranolol does not prevent thyroid storm. N Engl J Med 296:263, 1977
25. Dunn JT, Chapman EM: Rising incidence of hypothyroidism after radioactive iodine therapy in thyrotoxicosis. N Engl J Med 271:1037, 1964
26. Stehling LC: Anesthetic management of the patient with hyperthyroidism. Anesthesiology 41:585, 1974
27. Kaplan JA, Cooperman LH: Alarming reactions to ketamine in patients taking thyroid medication treatment with propranolol. Anesthesiology 35:229, 1971
28. Wade JSH: Respiratory obstruction in thyroid surgery. Ann Coll Surg Engl 62:15, 1980
29. Peters KR, Nance P, Wingard DW: Malignant hyperthyroidism or malignant hyperthermia? Anesth Analg 60:613, 1981
30. Waldstein SS: Medical complications of thyroid surgery. Otolaryngol Clin North Am 13:99, 1981
31. Green WER, Sheppard HWH: Tracheal collapse after thyroidectomy. Br J Surg 66:544, 1979
32. Hall R, Scanlon MF: Hypothyroidism: Clinical features and complications. Clin Endocrinol Metab 8:29, 1979
33. Amidi M, Leon DF, de Groot WJ et al: Effect of the thyroid state on myocardial contractility and ventricular ejection rate in man. Circulation 38:229, 1968
34. Zondek H: The electrocardiogram in myxedema. Br Heart J 26:227, 1964
35. Aber CP, Thompson GS: Factors associated with cardiac enlargement in myxedema. Br Heart J 25:421, 1963
36. Kannel WB, Dowler TR: Factors of risk in the development of coronary heart disease. Ann Intern Med 55:33, 1961
37. Zwilich CW, Pierson DJ, Hofeldt FD et al: Ventilatory control

in myxedema and hypothyroidism. N Engl J Med 292:662, 1975

38. Edson JR, Feeber DR, Doc RP: Low platelet adhesiveness and other hemostatic abnormalities in hypothyroidism. Ann Intern Med 82:342, 1975

39. Tudhope GR, Wilson GM: Anemia in hypothyroidism: Incidence, pathogenesis, and response to treatment. Q J Med 29:513, 1960

40. Weinberg AD, Brennan MD, Gorman CA et al: Outcome of anesthesia and surgery in hypothyroid patients. Arch Intern Med 143:893, 1983

41. Ladenson PW, Levin AA, Ridgway EC et al: Complications of surgery in hypothyroid patients. Am J Med 77:261, 1984

42. Drucker DJ, Burrow GN: Cardiovascular surgery in the hypothyroid patient. Arch Intern Med 145:1585, 1985

43. Hay ID, Duick DS, Vlietstra RE et al: Thyroxine therapy in hypothyroid patients undergoing coronary revascularization: A retrospective analysis. Ann Intern Med 95:456, 1981

44. Becker C: Hypothyroidism and atherosclerotic heart disease: Pathogenesis, medical management, and the role of coronary artery bypass surgery. Endocr Rev 6:432, 1985

45. Cohen SE, Wyner J: Endocrine disease. In James F III, Wheeler AS (eds): Obstetric Anesthesia: The Complicated Patient, p 160. Philadelphia, FA Davis, 1982

46. Braverman LB: Treatment of hypothyroidism: A practical guide. Thyroid Today 2:1, 1979

47. Weinberg AD, Ehrenwerth J: Anesthestic considerations and perioperative management of patients with hypothyroidism. Adv Anesth 4:185, 1987

48. Chernow B, Burman KD, Johnson DL et al: T3 may be a better agent than T4 in the critically ill hypothyroid patient. Crit Care Med 11:99, 1983

49. McCudlock W, Price P, Hinds CJ et al: Effects of low dose oral triiodothyronine in myxedema coma. Intensive Care Med 11:259, 1985

50. Murkin JM: Anesthesia and hypothyroidism: A review of thyroxine physiology, pharmacology and anesthetic implications. Anesth Analg 61:371, 1982

51. Babad AA, Eger EI: The effects of hyperthyroidism and hypothyroidism on halothane and oxygen requirements in dogs. Anesthesiology 29:1087, 1968

52. Robertson WG: Measurement of ionized calcium in body fluids: A review. Ann Clin Biochem 13:540, 1976

53. Habener JF, Potts JT: Biosynthesis of parathyroid hormone: Parts I and II. N Engl J Med 299:580, 635, 1978

54. Nordin BEC, Peacock M: Role of kidney in regulation of plasma calcium. Lancet 2:1280, 1969

55. Broadus AE, Mahaffey JE, Bartter FC et al: Nephrogenous cyclic adenosine monophosphate as a parathyroid function test. J Clin Invest 60:771, 1977

56. Broadus AE: Mineral metabolism. In Felig P, Baxter JD, Broadus AE, Frohman LA (eds): Endocrinology and Metabolism, p 953. New York, McGraw-Hill, 1981

57. Buckle RH, Care AD, Cooper CW et al: The influence of plasma magnesium concentration on parathyroid hormone secretion. J Endocrinol 42:529, 1968

58. Mazzaferri EL: The parathyroid glands, calcium metabolism, and disorders of calcium homeostasis. In Mazzaferri EL (ed): Endocrinology. New York, Medical Examination Publishing Company, 1974

59. Ellman H, Dembin H, Seriff N: The rarity of the QT interval in patients with hypercalcemia. Crit Care Med 10:320, 1982

60. Weidmann P, Massry SG, Coburn WJ et al: Blood pressure effects of acute hypercalcemia. Ann Intern Med 76:741, 1972

61. Wills MR: Value of plasma chloride concentration and acid base status in the differential diagnosis of hyperparathyroidism from other causes of hypercalcemia. J Clin Pathol 24:219, 1971

62. Buckle R: Ectopic PTH syndrome, pseudohyperparathyroidism, hypercalcemia of malignancy. J Endocrinol Metab 3:237, 1974

63. Stewart AF, Horst R, Deftos LJ et al: Biochemical evaluation of patients with cancer associated hypercalcemia. N Engl J Med 303:1377, 1980

64. Mundy GR, Raisz LG, Cooper RA et al: Evidence for the secretion of an osteoclast stimulating factor in myeloma. N Engl J Med 291:1041, 1974

65. Purnell DC, Scholz DA, Smith LH et al: Treatment of primary hyperparathyroidism. Am J Med 56:800, 1974

66. Chopra RA, Janson P, Sawin CT: Insensitivity to digoxin associated with hypocalcemia. N Engl J Med 296:917, 1977

67. Perlia CP, Gubisch NJ, Wolter J et al: Mithramycin treatment of hypercalcemia. Cancer 25:389, 1970

68. Deftos LJ, First BP: Calcitonin as a drug. Ann Intern Med 95:192, 1981

69. Condon JR, Ives D, Knight MJ et al: The etiology of hypocalcemia in acute pancreatitis. Br J Surg 62:115, 1975

70. Brenton DP, Pollard AB, Gonzales J: Hypocalcemic cardiac failure. Postgrad Med 54:633, 1978

71. Chaimowitz C, Abinader E, Benderly A et al: Hypocalcemia hypotension. JAMA 22:86, 1972

72. Rumancik WM, Denlinger JK, Nahrwold ML et al: The QT interval and serum ionized calcium. JAMA 240:366, 1978

73. Zaloga GP, Chernow B: Divalent ions: Calcium, magnesium and phosphorus. In Chernow B (ed): The Pharmacologic Approach to the Critically Ill Patient, 2nd ed, p 603. Baltimore, Williams & Wilkins, 1988

74. McPartland RP: Metabolic and pharmacologic actions of glucocorticoids. In Mulrow PJ (ed): The Adrenal Gland, p 85. New York, Elsevier, 1986

75. Munck A, Guyre PM: Glucocorticoid physiology, pharmacology and stress. Adv Exp Med Biol 196:81, 1986

76. Fischer JE, Hasselgren PO: Cytokines and glucocorticoids in the regulation of the "hepato-skeletal muscle axis" in sepsis. Am J Surg 161:266, 1991

77. Fauci AS, Dale DC, Balow JE: Glucocorticosteroid therapy: Mechanisms of action and clinical consideration. Ann Intern Med 84:304, 1976

78. Hirsch JG, Church AB: Adrenal steroids and infection: The effect of cortisone administration on polymorphonuclear leukocyte functions and on serum opsonins and bacteriocidins. J Clin Invest 40:794, 1961

79. Sainsberg JRC, Stoddard JC, Watson MJ: Plasma cortisol levels: A comparison between sick patients and volunteers given intravenous cortisol. Anaesthesia 36:16, 1981

80. Hollenberg NK, Williams GH: Hypertension, the adrenal and the kidney: lessons from pharmacologic interruption of the renin-angiotensin system. Adv Intern Med 25:327, 1980

81. Gold EM: The Cushing syndromes: Changing views of diagnosis and treatment. Ann Intern Med 90:829, 1979

82. Avioli LV: Effects of chronic corticosteroid therapy on mineral metabolism and calcium absorption. Adv Exp Biol Med 171:80, 1984

83. Narins RG, Jones ER, Stom MC et al: Diagnostic strategies in disorders of fluid, electrolyte and acid-base homeostasis. Am J Med 72:496, 1982

84. Herf SM, Teates DC, Tegtmeyer CJ et al: Identification and differentiation of surgically correctable hypertension due to primary aldosteronism. Am J Med 67:397, 1979

85. Weinberger MH, Grim CE, Hollifield JW et al: Primary aldosteronism: Diagnosis, localization, and treatment. Ann Intern Med 90:386, 1979

86. Izenstein BZ, Dluhy RG, Williams GH: Endocrinology. In Vandam LD (ed): To Make the Patient Ready for Anesthesia: Medical Care of the Surgical Patient, p 112. Menlo Park, California, Addison-Wesley, 1980

87. Holland OB, Brown H et al: Further evaluation of saline infusion for the diagnosis of primary aldosteronism. Hypertension 6:717, 1984

88. White EA, Schambelan M et al: The use of computed tomography in diagnosing the cause of primary aldosteronism. N Engl J Med 303:1503, 1980

89. Nerup J: Addison's disease—clinical studies. A report of 108 cases. Acta Endocrinol 76:127, 1974

90. Anderson P: Familial Schmidt's syndrome. JAMA 244:2068, 1980

91. Moore T: Adrenal insufficiency. In Hare JW (ed): Signs and

Symptoms in Endocrine and Metabolic Disorders, p 121. Philadelphia, JB Lippincott, 1986

92. Sampson PA, Brooke BN, Winstone NE: Biochemical confirmation of collapse due to adrenal failure. Lancet 1:1377, 1961

93. Sampson PA, Winstone NE, Brooke BN: Adrenal function of surgical patients after steroid therapy. Lancet 2:322, 1962

94. Knudsen L, Christiansen LA, Lorentzen JE: Hypotension during and after operation in glucocorticoid-treated patients. Br J Anaesth 53:295, 1981

95. Meakin J: Pituitary-adrenal function following long-term steroid therapy. Am J Med 29:459, 1960

96. Schambelan M, Sebastian A: Hyporeninemic hypoaldosteronism. Adv Intern Med 24:385, 1979

97. Zusman RM: Prostaglandins and water excretion. Annu Rev Med 32:359, 1981

98. Spiro HM: Is the steroid ulcer a myth? N Engl J Med 309:45, 1983

99. Chin R: Adrenal crisis. Crit Care Clin 7:23, 1991

100. Byyny RL: Preventing adrenal insufficiency during surgery. Postgrad Med 67:219, 1980

101. Plumpton FS, Besser GM, Cole PV: Corticosteroid treatment and surgery: I. An investigation of the indications for steroid cover. Anesthesia 24:3, 1969

102. Engquist A, Brandt MR, Fernandes A et al: The blocking effect of epidural analgesia on the adrenocortical and hyperglycemic responses to surgery. Acta Anaesthesiol Scand 21:330, 1977

103. Cooper GM, Paterson JL, Ward ID et al: Fentanyl and the metabolic response to gastric surgery. Anesthesiology 36:667, 1981

104. Lehtinen AM, Fyhrquist F, Kivalo I: The effect of fentanyl on arginine, vasopressin and cortisol secretion during anesthesia. Anesth Analg 63:25, 1984

105. Namba Y, Smith JB, Fox GS et al: Plasma cortisol concentrations during cesarean section. Br J Anaesth 52:1027, 1980

106. Oyama T, Taniguchi K, Jin T et al: Effects of anesthesia and surgery on plasma aldosterone concentration and renin activity in man. Br J Anaesth 51:747, 1979

107. Oyama T: Hazards of steroids in association with anaesthesia. Can Anaesth Soc J 16:361, 1969

108. Udelsman R, Ramp J, Gallucci WT et al: Adaptation during surgical stress: A reevaluation of the role of glucocorticoids. J Clin Invest 77:1377, 1986

109. Symreng T, Karlberg BE, Kagedal B et al: Physiological cortisol substitution of long-term steroid-treated patients undergoing major surgery. Br J Anaesth 53:949, 1981

110. Axelrod L: Glucocorticoid therapy. Medicine 55:39, 1976

111. Scott HW Jr, Oates JA, Nies AS et al: Pheochromocytoma: Present diagnosis and management. Ann Surg 183:587, 1976

112. Manger WN, Gifford RW: Current concepts of pheochromocytoma. Cardiovasc Med 3:289, 1978

113. St. John Sutton N, Sheps SG, Lie JT: Prevalence of clinically unsuspected pheochromocytoma: Review of a 50-year autopsy series. Mayo Clin Proc 56:354, 1981

114. Cross DA, Meyer JS: Postoperative deaths due to unsuspected pheochromocytoma. South Med J 70:1320, 1977

115. Kaul U, Mohan J, Rao P et al: Pheochromocytoma presenting as recurrent syncope resulting from ventricular tachycardia: An annual presentation. Indian Heart J 36:118, 1984

116. ReMine WH, Chong GC, vanHeerden JA et al: Current management of pheochromocytoma. Ann Surg 179:740, 1974

117. Allen GC, Rosenberg H: Pheochromocytoma presenting as acute malignant hyperthermia, a diagnostic challenge. Can J Anaesth 37(5):593, 1990

118. Ram CVS: Pheochromocytoma. Cardiol Clin 6(4):517, 1988

119. Schaffer MS, Zuberbuhler P, Urlson G et al: Catecholamine cardiomyopathy: An unusual presentation of pheochromocytoma in children. J Pediatr 99:276, 1981

120. Engelman K: Pheochromocytoma. Clin Endocrinol Metab 6(3):769, 1977

121. Ram CVS, Engelman K: Pheochromocytoma—recognition and management. Curr Probl Cardiol 4(1), 1979

122. Henry DT, Starman BJ, Johnson DG et al: A sensitive radioenzymatic assay for norepinephrine in tissues and plasma. Life Sci 16:375, 1975

123. Bravo EL, Tarazi RC, Gifford RW et al: Circulating and urinary catecholamines in pheochromocytomas. N Engl J Med 301:682, 1979

124. Shub C, Cueto-Garcia L, Sheps SG et al: Echocardiographic findings in pheochromocytoma. Am J Cardiol 57:971, 1986

125. Dunn EJ, Wolff RK, Wright CB et al: Presentation of undiagnosed pheochromocytoma during coronary artery bypass surgery. J Cardiovasc Surg 30:284, 1989

126. Samaan NA, Hickey RC, Shutts PE: Diagnosis, localization and management of pheochromocytoma. Cancer 62:2451, 1988

127. Desmonts JM, LeHouelleur J, Remond P et al: Anaesthetic management of patients with pheochromocytoma: A review of 102 cases. Br J Anaesth 49:991, 1977

128. Roizen MF, Horrigan RW, Koike M et al: A perspective randomized trial of four anesthetic techniques for resection of pheochromocytoma. Anesthesiology 57:A43, 1982

129. Roizen MF, Hunt TK, Beaupre PN et al: The effect of alpha adrenergic blockade on cardiac performance and tissue oxygen delivery during excision of pheochromocytoma. Surgery 94:941, 1983

130. Knapp HR, Fitzgerald GA: Hypertensive crisis in prazosin-treated pheochromocytoma. South Med J 77:535, 1984

131. Briggs RSJ, Birtwell AJ, Pohl JEF: Hypertensive response to labetalol in pheochromocytoma. Lancet 1:1045, 1978

132. Hopkins PM, MacDonald R, Lyons G: Cesarean section at 27 weeks gestation with removal of pheochromocytoma. Br J Anaesth 63:121, 1989

133. Doi M, Ikeda K: Sevoflurane anesthesia with adenosine triphosphate for resection of pheochromocytoma. Anesthesiology 70:360, 1989

134. Jovenich JJ: Anesthesia in adrenal surgery. Urol Clin North Am 16:583, 1989

135. Gusberg RJ, Moley J: Diabetes and abdominal surgery. Yale J Biol Med 56:285, 1983

136. Alberti KGMM, Thomas DJB: The management of diabetes during surgery. Br J Anaesth 51:693, 1979

137. National Diabetes Group: Classification and diagnosis of diabetes mellitus and other categories of glucose intolerance. Diabetes 28:1039, 1979

138. Allison SP, Tomlin PJ, Chamberlain MJ: Some effects of anaesthesia and surgery on carbohydrate and fat metabolism. Br J Anaesth 41:588, 1969

139. Clarke RSJ, Johnston H, Sheridan B: The influence of anaesthesia and surgery on plasma cortisol, insulin and free fatty acids. Br J Anaesth 42:295, 1970

140. Stevens A, Roizen MF: Patients with diabetes mellitus and disorders of glucose metabolism. Anesthesiol Clin North Am 5:339, 1987

141. McGarry JD, Foster DW: Ketogenesis and its regulation. Am J Med 61:9, 1976

142. Unger RH, Orci L: Glucagon and the A cell (two parts). N Engl J Med 304:1518, 1575, 1981

143. Cryer PE, Gerich JE: Glucose counter-regulation, hypoglycemia, and intensive insulin therapy in diabetes mellitus. N Engl J Med 313:232, 1985

144. Fischer KF, Lees JA, Newman JM: Hypoglycemia in hospitalized patients. N Engl J Med 315:1245, 1986

145. Raskin P, Rosenstack J: Blood glucose control and diabetic complications. Ann Intern Med 105:254, 1986

146. Page MM, Watkins PJ: Cardiorespiratory arrest and diabetic autonomic neuropathy. Lancet 1:14, 1978

147. Bhatnagar SK, Al-Yusuf AR, Al-Asfoor AR: Abnormal autonomic function in diabetic and non-diabetic patients after first acute myocardial infarction. Chest 92:5, 1987

148. Sieber FE, Smith DS, Traystman RH, Wollman H: Glucose: A reevaluation of its intraoperative use. Anesthesiology 67:72, 1987

149. Lanier WL: Glucose management during cardiopulmonary bypass: Cardiovascular and neurologic implications. Anesth Analg 72:423, 1991

150. Foster DW: Insulin deficiency and hyperosmolar coma. Adv Intern Med 19:159, 1974

151. Foster DW, McGarry JD: The metabolic derangements and treatment of diabetic ketoacidosis. N Engl J Med 309:159, 1983

152. Fulop M, Hoberman HD: Alcoholic ketosis. Diabetes 24:785, 1975
153. Cefalu WT: Diabetic ketoacidosis. Crit Care Clin 7:89, 1991
154. Morris LR, Murphy MB, Kitabchi AE: Bicarbonate therapy in severe diabetic ketoacidosis. Ann Intern Med 105:836, 1986
155. Harati Y: Diabetic peripheral neuropathies. Ann Intern Med 107:546, 1987
156. Hirsch IB, McGill JB, Cryer PE, White PF. Perioperative management of surgical patients with diabetes mellitus. Anesthesiology 74:346, 1991
157. Woodruff RE, Lewis SB, McLeskey CH et al: Avoidance of surgical hyperglycemia in diabetic patients. JAMA 244:166, 1980
158. Podolsky S: Management of diabetes in the surgical patient. Med Clin North Am 66:1361, 1982
159. Meyers EF, Alberts D, Gordon MD: Perioperative control of blood glucose in diabetic patients—A two-step protocol. Diabetes Care 9:40, 1986
160. Weisenfeld S, Podolsky S, Goldsmith L et al: Adsorption of insulin to infusion bottles and tubing. Diabetes 17:766, 1968
161. Sheehan HL, Stanfield JP: A pathogenesis of post-partum necrosis of the anterior lobe of the pituitary gland. Acta Endocrinol Scand 37:479, 1961
162. Kleinberg DL, Noel GL, Frantz AG: Galactorrhea: A study of 235 cases including 48 with pituitary tumors. N Engl J Med 296:589, 1977
163. Kitahata LM: Airway difficulties associated with anaesthesia in acromegaly. Br J Anaesth 43:1187, 1971
164. Dunn FL, Brennan TJ, Nelson AE et al: The role of blood osmolality and volume in regulating vasopressin secretion in the rat. J Clin Invest 52:3212, 1973
165. Corliss RJ, McKenna DH, Sialer S et al: Systemic and coronary hemodynamic effects of vasopressin. Am J Med 256:293, 1968
166. Edmunds R, West JB: A study on the effect of vasopressin on portal and systemic blood pressure. Surg Gynecol Obstet 114:458, 1962
167. Getzen LC, Brink RR, Wolfman EF: Survival following infusion of pitressin into the superior mesenteric artery to control bleeding esophageal varices in cirrhotic patients. Ann Surg 187:337, 1978
168. Salzman EW, Weinstein MJ, Weintraub RM et al: Treatment with desmopressin acetate to reduce blood loss after cardiac surgery: A double-blind randomized trial. N Engl J Med 314:1402, 1986
169. Lethagen S, Rugarn P, Bergqvist D: Blood loss and safety with desmopressin or placebo during aorto-iliac graft surgery. Eur J Vascular Surg 5:173, 1991
170. Ober KP: Diabetes insipidus. Crit Care Clin 7:109, 1991
171. Robinson AG: Disorders of the posterior pituitary. In Kelley WN (ed): Textbook of Internal Medicine, p 2176. Philadelphia, JB Lippincott, 1989
172. Pleuvry BJ: Opioid receptors and their ligands: Natural and unnatural. Br J Anaesth 66:370, 1991

46

Alan C. Santos   Mieczyslaw Finster
Hilda Pedersen

Obstetric Anesthesia

THE PHYSIOLOGIC CHANGES OF PREGNANCY

During pregnancy, with the increasing metabolic and nutritional demands of the growing fetus, there are major alterations in nearly every maternal organ system. These changes are initiated by hormonal secretions from the corpus luteum and placenta. The mechanical effects of uterine size and compression of surrounding structures play an increasing role in the second and third trimesters. This "altered physiologic state" has important implications for the anesthesiologist in treatment of the pregnant patient. The most pertinent changes, involving hematologic, cardiovascular, ventilatory, metabolic, and gastrointestinal functions, will be considered here (Table 46-1).

Hematologic Alterations

Increased mineralocorticoid activity during pregnancy produces sodium retention and increased body water content and plasma volume.[1] Thus, under hormonal influence, plasma volume begins to increase between the 6th and 12th gestational weeks, resulting in a total increase of 40–50% and a 25–40% increase in total blood volume at term. The relatively lesser increase in red blood cell volume (20%) accounts for a reduction in hemoglobin (to 11–12 g·dl^{-1}) and hematocrit (to 35%).[2] The leukocyte count remains 8,000–10,000 per mm^3 throughout pregnancy, whereas the platelet count shows no remarkable change. Plasma fibrinogen concentrations increase during normal pregnancy by about 50%, whereas some clotting factor activities increase and others decrease.[3]

Serum cholinesterase activity declines to a level of 20% below normal at term and into the puerperium.[4] However, there is no structural malformation of the enzyme molecule, and it is doubtful that moderate succinylcholine doses can lead to prolonged apnea in otherwise normal circumstances.[5]

Plasma proteins show changes similar to those seen in erythrocytes, namely, their total concentration declines (to less than 6 g·dl^{-1} at term), whereas the total amount in the circulation increases.[6] The albumin-globulin ratio declines because of the relatively greater reduction in albumin concentration. Fibrinogen increases in both absolute and relative concentrations. During gestation, alterations in protein content, especially albumin, may be clinically significant, in that the free fractions of protein-bound drugs can be expected to increase.[7]

In the first 2–3 weeks after delivery, the blood volume slowly decreases, whereas the hematocrit increases to nonpregnant levels.[1]

Cardiovascular Changes

As oxygen consumption increases during pregnancy, the maternal cardiovascular system adapts to meet the metabolic demands of the growing fetus.[8] Decreased vascular resistance may be the initiating factor. For example, the administration of various estrogens to nonpregnant ewes leads to increased cardiac output and reduced vascular resistance, whereas the decrease in vascular resistance and vasodilation in normal human pregnancy may also be related, in part, to the increased production of prostacyclin.[9,10]

Lowered resistance is found in the uterine, renal, and other vascular beds; at term the heart rate (92–95 beats·min^{-1}), cardiac output, and blood volume are increased. Arterial blood pressure decreases slightly because the decrease in peripheral resistance exceeds the increase in cardiac output. Cardiac output, increasing from the 8th week, reaches its plateau of 30–50% above the normal nonpregnant state at approximately the 30th to 34th weeks. Additional increases occur during labor (when cardiac output may reach 12–14 l·min^{-1}) and in the immediate postpartum period.

From the second trimester, aortocaval compression by the enlarged uterus becomes progressively more important. Studies of cardiac output, measured with the patient in the supine position during the last weeks of pregnancy, have indicated a decrease to nonpregnant levels; the decrease was not seen when patients were in the lateral decubitus position.[11,12] In another group of patients reductions were seen while they were in the supine, sitting, or lateral decubitus positions, with the greatest reduction occurring when they were supine.[13] Vena caval compression can develop from the second trimester and becomes maximal at 36–38 weeks, after which it may decrease as the fetal head de-

TABLE 46-1. Summary of Physiologic Changes of Pregnancy at Term

Variable	Change	Amount
Total blood volume	Increase	25–40%
Plasma volume	Increase	40–50%
Fibrinogen	Increase	50%
Serum cholinesterase activity	Decrease	20–30%
Cardiac output	Increase	30–50%
Minute ventilation	Increase	50%
Alveolar ventilation	Increase	70%
Functional residual capacity	Decrease	20%
Oxygen consumption	Increase	20%
Arterial carbon dioxide tension	Decrease	10 mm Hg
Arterial oxygen tension	Increase	10 mm Hg
Minimum alveolar concentration	Decrease	32–40%

scends into the pelvis. Radiographs have shown complete vena caval obstruction in as many as 90% of supine pregnant women at term, venous blood being shunted to the superior vena cava by the intervertebral plexus and the azygos vein.[12] Nevertheless, most women maintain a normal or near-normal brachial artery pressure by increasing peripheral resistance, although this may indirectly be harmful to the fetus through a reduction in uteroplacental blood flow.[14] As has been known for a long time, obstructed venous return can lead to maternal tachycardia, arterial hypotension, faintness, and pallor, the so-called supine hypotensive syndrome, which occurs in approximately 10% of pregnant patients near term when placed supine.[15] Compression of the lower aorta in this position, as demonstrated by aortography, may also lead to decreased uteroplacental perfusion and fetal distress.[16] Therefore, left uterine displacement or lateral pelvic tilting should be used during the second and third trimesters of pregnancy, regardless of the lack of maternal arterial hypotension. Shortly after delivery, the increased cardiac output probably results from the addition of 500–600 ml of blood to the central circulation by contraction of the evacuated uterus; cardiac output gradually decreases over the next 24–72 hours.

Changes in the electrocardiogram (ECG) result from the shift in the position of the heart (left axis deviation), resulting from the upward displacement of the diaphragm by the gravid uterus. There is also a tendency toward premature contractions, sinus tachycardia, and paroxysmal supraventricular tachycardia, the cause of which is unknown. In the absence of organic heart disease, these cardiac dysrhythmias do not alter the normal course of pregnancy, and there is no significant hazard to the mother.

Ventilatory Changes

The increased extracellular fluid and vascular engorgement typical of gestation may not only lead to edema of the extremities but may also compromise the upper airway. Many pregnant women complain of difficulty in nasal breathing, and the friable nature of the mucous membranes can cause severe bleeding, especially on insertion of nasopharyngeal airways or nasogastric and endotracheal tubes.[17] Airway edema may be particularly severe in patients with pre-eclampsia, in patients placed in the Trendelenburg position for prolonged periods, or with the use of tocolytic agents. It is also difficult to perform laryngoscopic examination in

obese, short-necked parturients with enlarged breasts. Use of a short-handled laryngoscope has proved helpful.[18]

The level of the diaphragm rises as the uterus increases in size, but diaphragmatic breathing remains unimpeded.[19] The upward shift is compensated for by an increase in the anteroposterior and transverse diameters of the thoracic cage, through flaring of the ribs.

Progesterone-induced relaxation of bronchiolar smooth muscle decreases airway resistance, whereas lung compliance remains unchanged.[20] This in turn paves the way for the increase in minute ventilation ($\dot{V}E$) necessary to meet the increasing metabolic demand for oxygen. $\dot{V}E$ increases from the beginning of pregnancy to a maximum of 50% above normal at term.[21] This is accomplished by an approximately 40% increase in tidal volume and an approximately 15% increase in respiratory rate. Because dead space does not change significantly, alveolar ventilation is increased by 70% at term.

With enlarging uterine size, lung volumes change. From the 5th month, the expiratory reserve volume (ERV), residual volume (RV), and functional residual capacity (FRC) decrease, the latter to 20% less than in the nonpregnant state.[22] However, there is a concomitant increase in inspiratory reserve volume (IRV), so that total lung capacity (TLC) remains unchanged. In most parturients decreased FRC does not cause problems, but those with pre-existing alterations in closing volume as a result of smoking, obesity, or scoliosis may experience early airway closure leading to hypoxemia as pregnancy advances. The Trendelenburg and supine positions also exacerbate the abnormal relationship between closing volume and FRC.[23] RV and FRC quickly return to normal after delivery. As blood progesterone levels decline, ventilation returns to normal within 1–3 weeks.[22]

Metabolism

The fetus depends on the mother for nutritional substances such as amino acids, glucose, and iron. Basal oxygen consumption increases during early pregnancy, with an overall increase of 20% at term.[8] However, increased alveolar ventilation—probably resulting from the effects of progesterone—leads to a reduction in the partial pressure of carbon dioxide in arterial blood ($Paco_2$) to 32 mm Hg and an increase in the partial pressure of oxygen in arterial blood (Pao_2) to 106 mm Hg.[21] The plasma buffer base decreases from 47 to 42 mEq$\cdot$l^{-1} so that the pH remains practically unchanged.[24]

Increased alveolar ventilation, along with the decreased FRC, enhances maternal uptake and elimination of inhalational anesthetics.[25] On the other hand, the decreased FRC and increased metabolic rate predispose the mother to hypoxemia during endotracheal intubation or airway obstruction.[26]

Human placental lactogen (hPL) and cortisol increase the tendency to hyperglycemia and ketosis, which may unmask or exacerbate pre-existing diabetes mellitus. The patient's ability to handle a glucose load is decreased, and the transplacental passage of glucose may stimulate fetal secretion of insulin, leading in turn to neonatal hypoglycemia in the immediate postpartum period.[27]

Gastrointestinal Changes

Enhanced progesterone production causes decreased gastrointestinal motility, slower absorption of food, and a lower volume of intestinal secretions.[28,29] The gastric juice is more acidic, and lower esophageal sphincter (LES) tone is decreased.[30] A delay in gastric emptying can already be demonstrated by the end of the first trimester.[31] Uterine growth leads to upward displacement and rotation of the stomach, with increased pressure and a further delay in gastric emptying. By the 34th week, evacuation of a watery meal may be prolonged by 60%.[32] Pain, anxiety, and administration of opioids and belladonna alkaloids may further exacerbate this delay.

In patients near term, the lithotomy and Trendelenburg positions will increase intragastric pressure. The risk of regurgitation, leading to aspiration pneumonitis on induction of general anesthesia, depends on the gradient between the intragastric and LES pressures. In most patients the gradient increases after succinylcholine administration, because the increase in LES pressure exceeds the increase in intragastric pressure.[33] However, in parturients with "heartburn," the LES tone is greatly reduced.[34] The current requirement for consideration as being "at risk" for aspiration is gastric juice with a pH less than 2.5 and volume greater than 25 ml. The efficacy of prophylactic nonparticulate antacids is reduced by inadequate mixing with gastric contents, improper timing of administration, and the tendency for antacids to increase gastric volume. Administration of H_2 receptor antagonists, such as cimetidine and ranitidine, requires careful timing and dose schedules. There are many drug interactions and side-effects, including aplastic anemia, anaphylaxis, bradycardia, hypotension, cardiac dysrhythmias, cardiac arrest, and inhibition of cytochrome P-450, with impaired elimination of many drugs currently used in anesthesia, e.g., diazepam, theophylline, and amide local anesthetics.[35] A good case can be made for the administration of intravenous (iv) metoclopramide before elective cesarean section. This dopamine antagonist hastens gastric emptying and increases resting LES tone in both nonpregnant and pregnant women.[36] However, conflicting reports have appeared on its efficacy and on the frequency of side-effects such as extrapyramidal reactions and postoperative neurologic dysfunction.[37-39] It seems that no routine prophylactic regimen can be recommended, although the available agents may all be useful. A rapid sequence induction of anesthesia with cricoid pressure, and intubation of the trachea with a cuffed tube are necessary for all pregnant patients receiving general anesthesia from the 12th week of gestation.[31]

There is some doubt as to when the gastric volume of the postpartum patient has returned to normal; a nonparticulate antacid and a rapid sequence induction of anesthesia should be used in women undergoing general anesthesia within 48 hours after delivery.

Altered Drug Responses

In pregnancy many anesthetic drugs have a reduced dose requirement. The minimum alveolar concentration (MAC) for halothane, isoflurane, and methoxyflurane is decreased by 32–40% in pregnant ewes, which may be related to the gestational increase in progesterone levels.[40,41] It has also been noted that lower doses of local anesthetics were needed per segment of epidural or spinal block. This was originally attributed to venous engorgement reducing the volume of the epidural and subarachnoid spaces. However, more recent investigations of conduction blockade induced in the vagus nerve excised from pregnant and nonpregnant rabbits indicate that in pregnancy there is a greater sensitivity to local anesthetics.[42] This explains the reduced local anesthetic requirement found as early as the first trimester.[43]

FETAL EXPOSURE TO DRUGS USED IN OBSTETRIC ANESTHESIA

It is generally accepted that most drugs, including anesthetic agents, readily cross the placenta. We have learned more about this area from the development of highly sensitive and specific techniques for drug analysis in biologic fluids and tissues, as well as from a better understanding of the fetal circulation.

Placental Transfer

Several factors influence the placental transfer of drugs, including the physicochemical characteristics of the drug itself, maternal drug concentrations in the plasma, properties of the placenta, and hemodynamic events within the feto-maternal unit.

Drugs cross biologic membranes by simple diffusion, the rate of which is determined by the Fick principle, which states that

$$Q/t = \frac{KA\,(C_m - C_f)}{D}$$

where

Q/t = rate of diffusion
K = diffusion constant
A = surface area available for exchange
C_m = concentration of free drug in maternal blood
C_f = concentration of free drug in fetal blood
D = thickness of diffusion barrier

The diffusion constant (K) of the drug depends on physicochemical characteristics such as molecular size, lipid solubility, and degree of ionization.

Compounds with a molecular weight less than 500 daltons are unimpeded in crossing the placenta, whereas those with molecular weights of 500–1000 daltons are more restricted. Most drugs commonly used by the anesthesiologist have molecular weights that permit easy transfer.

Drugs that are highly lipid soluble cross biologic membranes more readily, and the degree of ionization is important because the un-ionized moiety of a drug is more lipophilic than the ionized one. Local anesthetics and opioids are weak bases, with a relatively low degree of ionization and considerable lipid solubility. In contrast, muscle relaxants are less lipophilic and more ionized. Their placental transfer is more limited.[44,45]

The relative concentrations of drug existing in the un-ionized and ionized forms can be predicted from the Henderson-Hasselbalch equation:

$$pH = pK_a + \log\frac{(base)}{(cation)}$$

The ratio of base to cation becomes particularly important with local anesthetics because the un-ionized form penetrates tissue barriers, whereas the ionized form is pharmacologically active in blocking nerve conduction.

The pK_a is the pH at which the concentrations of free base

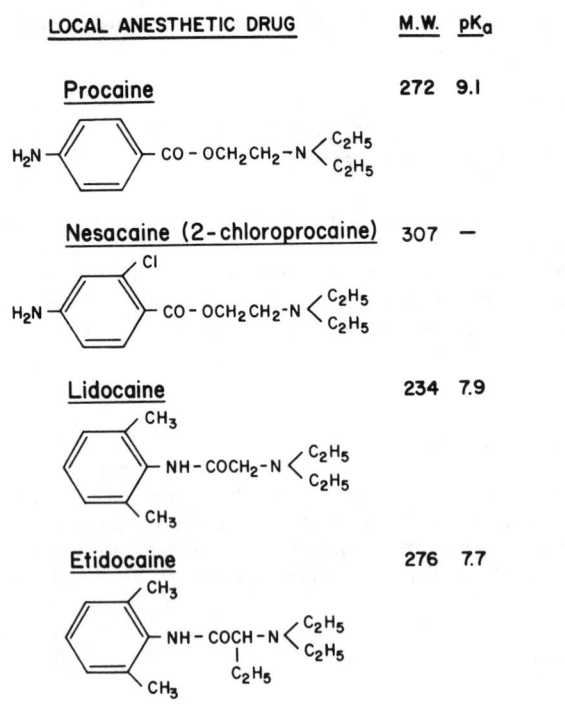

Figure 46-1. Chemical structures, pK_a, and molecular weights of commonly used local anesthetics. (Reprinted with permission from Finster M, Pedersen H: Placental transfer and fetal uptake of local anesthetics. Clin Obstet Gynecol 556, 1975.)

and cation are equal. For the amide local anesthetics, the pK$_a$ values (7.7–8.1) are sufficiently close to physiologic pH that changes in maternal or fetal biochemical status may significantly alter the proportion of ionized and un-ionized drug present (Fig. 46-1). At equilibrium, the concentrations of un-ionized drug in the fetal and maternal plasma are equal. In the case of the acidotic fetus, a greater tendency for drug to exist in the ionized form, which cannot diffuse back across the placenta into the maternal plasma, causes a larger total amount of drug to accumulate in the fetal plasma. This is the mechanism for the phenomenon described as "ion trapping."[46] It also causes enhanced accumulation of local anesthetic in the tissues of acidotic fetuses (Fig. 46-2).[47] Fetal acidosis should also increase the uptake of other basic drugs such as opioids.

The effects of maternal plasma protein binding on the rate and amount of drug transferred to the fetus are not so well understood. One would assume that highly bound drugs, having a lesser fraction in the unbound form, would be more restricted in crossing the placenta. Animal studies have shown that the transfer rate is slower for drugs that are extensively bound to maternal plasma proteins, such as bupivacaine.[48,49] In sheep, the low fetomaternal ratio of bupivacaine plasma concentrations has been attributed to the difference between the fetal and maternal plasma protein binding rather than to extensive fetal tissue uptake.[50] However, if enough time is allowed for fetomaternal equilibrium to be approached, substantial accumulation can occur in the fetus. Indirect evidence in humans was provided by the observation that neonates exposed *in utero* to the drug administered for epidural anesthesia had measurable plasma concentrations and urinary excretion of bupivacaine for at least 3 days after delivery.[51]

As already stated, the driving force for placental drug transfer is the concentration gradient of free drug between the maternal and fetal blood. On the maternal side the following factors interact: the dose administered, the mode and site of administration, and, in the case of local anesthet-

ics, the use of vasoconstrictors. The rate of distribution, metabolism, and excretion of the drug, which may vary at different stages of pregnancy, as well as interactions with other drugs, such as cimetidine, are equally important.

Generally speaking, higher doses result in higher maternal blood concentrations. This effect is illustrated by a study in which thiamylal was administered by iv injection to mothers undergoing elective cesarean section while under general anesthesia.[52] In the group of patients receiving thiamylal, 4 mg·kg^{-1}, the peak maternal arterial and umbilical vein barbiturate concentrations at the time of birth were approximately 50 mg·l^{-1} and 14 mg·l^{-1} respectively. Dou-

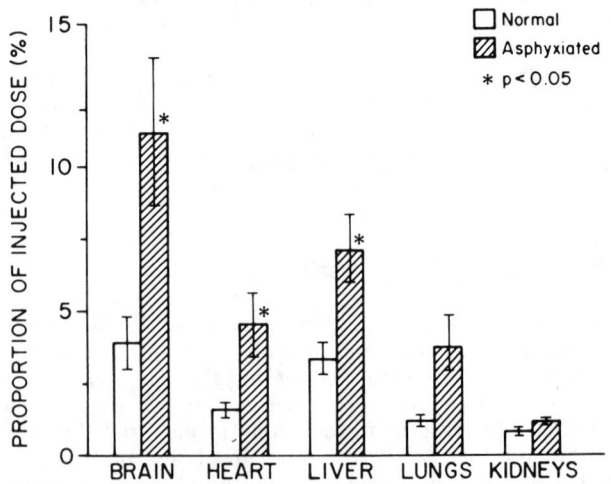

Figure 46-2. Mean (±SE) values for the proportions of injected lidocaine dose found in the brain, heart, liver, lungs, and kidneys in nonasphyxiated and asphyxiated fetuses. (Reprinted with permission from Morishima HO, Covino BG: Toxicity and distribution of lidocaine in nonasphyxiated and asphyxiated baboon fetuses. Anesthesiology 54:182, 1981.)

bling the dose resulted in an almost double maternal drug concentration (84 mg·l^{-1}) and an increase in the umbilical vein concentration of thiamylal (18 mg·l^{-1}).

The absorption rate varies with the site of drug injection. Compared with other forms of administration, an iv bolus results in the highest blood concentrations. This was documented in a study comparing maternal and fetal plasma levels of meperidine after iv, intramuscular (im), or epidural injection (2 mg·kg^{-1} over 60 seconds) to pregnant ewes.[53] A mean peak concentration of 1623 ng·ml^{-1} was measured in the maternal plasma 2 minutes after iv injection, whereas a mean peak concentration of 500 ng·ml^{-1} occurred at 15 minutes after im or epidural administration. Fetuses whose mothers had received the drug iv had significantly higher plasma concentrations of meperidine for at least 30 minutes, compared with those whose mothers had received the drug by the other two routes. It has also been shown that, after an iv injection of meperidine during labor, a greater proportion of the dose administered is transferred to the fetus than after an im injection.[54]

It was believed that intrathecal administration of local anesthetics resulted in negligible plasma concentrations because of the small doses used and the relatively poor vascularity of this area. However, in a study of pregnant patients undergoing cesarean section with spinal anesthesia (induced with lidocaine, 75 mg), maternal plasma concentrations of the drug were similar to those reported by others after epidural anesthesia.[55] Furthermore, significant levels of the drug were found in the umbilical vein at birth.

Increased maternal blood concentrations after repeated administration of a drug greatly depend on the dose and frequency of reinjection as well as on the kinetic character-

istics of the drug. The elimination half-life of amide local anesthetic agents is relatively long, so that repeated injection may lead to accumulation in the maternal plasma[56] (Fig. 46-3). On the other hand, 2-chloroprocaine, an ester local anesthetic, undergoes rapid enzymatic hydrolysis in the presence of pseudocholinesterase. *In vitro* studies have shown the half-life of this drug to be 21 seconds in the maternal serum.[57] After epidural injection, the mean half-life in the mother was 3.1 minutes.[58] After reinjection, 2-chloroprocaine could be detected in the maternal plasma for only 5–10 minutes, and no accumulation of this drug was evident (Fig. 46-4).[59] The discrepancy in the half-life between *in vivo* and *in vitro* studies can be ascribed to continued absorption of 2-chloroprocaine from the epidural space.

Pregnancy is associated with physiologic changes that may influence maternal pharmacokinetics and the action of anesthetic drugs. These changes may be progressive during the course of gestation and are often difficult to predict. Kinetic studies after thiopental injection for induction of anesthesia at cesarean section showed a longer elimination half-life and a larger volume of distribution than were noted by the same authors in a group of nonpregnant women.[60] In contrast, the elimination half-life of bupivacaine after epidural injection was similar in pregnant and nonpregnant women.[61]

Alterations in ventilation and lung volumes have a significant effect on the rate of uptake and excretion of inhalation agents. Of most concern to the anesthesiologist is a 20% reduction in FRC. As a result, the equilibration time between the alveolar and inspired concentrations of inhalation agents is shortened.

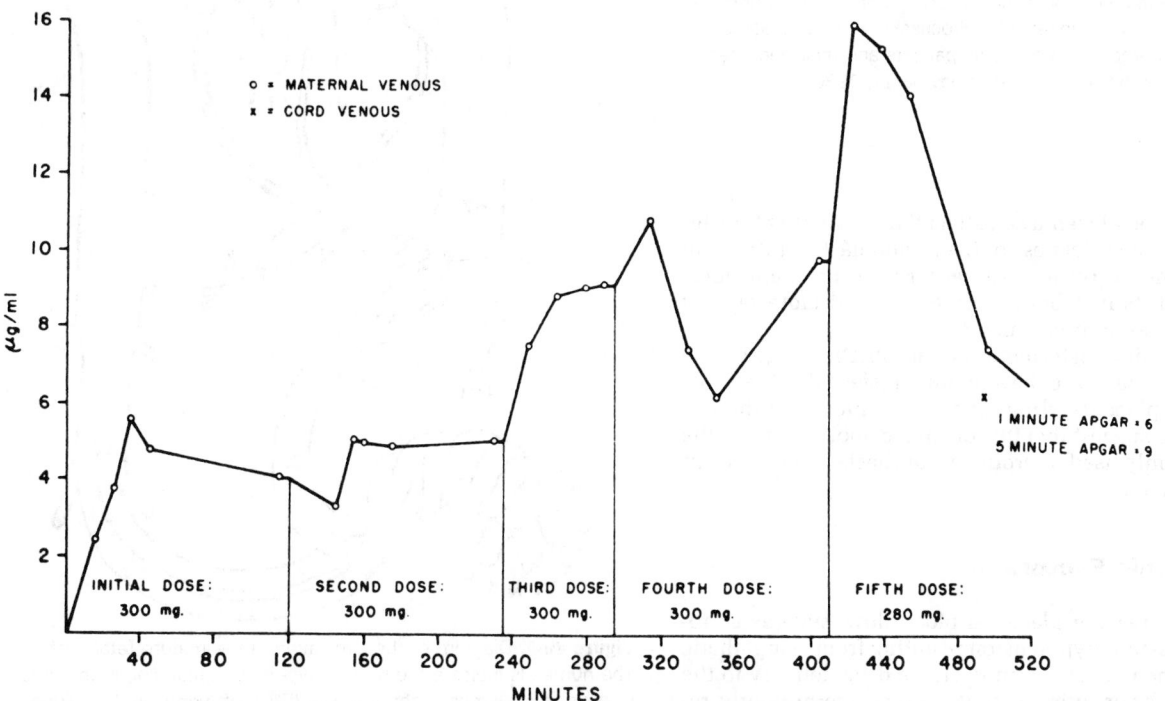

Figure 46-3. Increased levels of mepivacaine with each reinforcing dose in a patient receiving continuous caudal anesthesia during parturition. (Reprinted with permission from Moore DC, Bridenbaugh LD, Bagdi PA *et al:* Accumulation of mepivacaine hydrochloride during caudal block. Anesthesiology 29:585, 1968.)

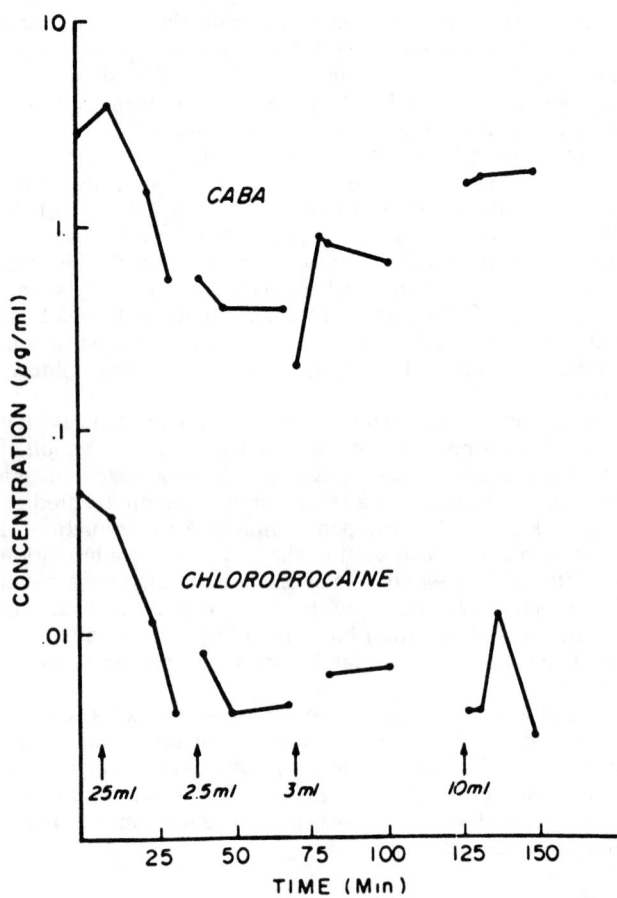

Figure 46-4. Plasma concentrations of chloroprocaine and chloro-aminobenzoic acid (CABA) in a typical patient after epidural anesthesia (multiple injections) for vaginal delivery. (Reprinted with permission from Kuhnert BR, Kuhnert PM, Prochaska AL *et al:* Plasma levels of 2-chloroprocaine in obstetric patients and their neonates after epidural anesthesia. Anesthesiology 53:21, 1980.)

Placenta

Maturation of the placenta can affect the rate of drug transfer to the fetus, as the thickness of the trophoblastic epithelium decreases from 25 μm to 2 μm at term. In pregnant mice, diazepam and its metabolites are transferred more rapidly in late than in early pregnancy.[62]

Uptake and biotransformation of anesthetic drugs by the placenta would decrease the amount transferred to the fetus. However, the placental drug uptake is limited, and there is no evidence to suggest that this organ metabolizes any of the agents commonly used to produce anesthesia or analgesia in pregnant women.

Hemodynamic Factors

Any factor decreasing placental blood flow, such as aorto-caval compression, hypotension resulting from sympathetic blockade, or hemorrhage, can decrease drug delivery to the fetus. During labor, uterine contractions intermittently reduce perfusion of the placenta. If a uterine contraction coincides with a rapid decline in plasma drug concentration after an iv bolus injection, by the time perfusion has returned to normal, the concentration gradient across the placenta will have been greatly reduced. When women were

given an iv injection of diazepam—administered at the onset of contraction in one group and during uterine diastole in the other—less drug was found in infants born to mothers in the former group.[63]

Several characteristics of the fetal circulation delay the equilibration between the fetal arterial and venous blood and thus delay the depressant effects of anesthetic drugs (Fig. 46-5). The liver is the first fetal organ perfused by umbilical vein blood, which carries drug to the fetus. Substantial uptake by this organ has been demonstrated for a variety of drugs, including thiopental, lidocaine, and halothane. During its transit to the arterial side of the fetal circulation, the drug is progressively diluted as blood in the umbilical vein becomes admixed with fetal venous blood from the gastrointestinal tract, the lower extremities, the head and upper extremities, and, finally, the lungs. Because of this unique pattern of fetal circulation, administration of anesthetic concentrations of nitrous oxide or cyclopropane during elective cesarean sections caused newborn depression only if the induction-to-delivery interval exceeded 5–10 minutes. On the other hand, because of the rapid decline in maternal plasma drug concentrations, administration of

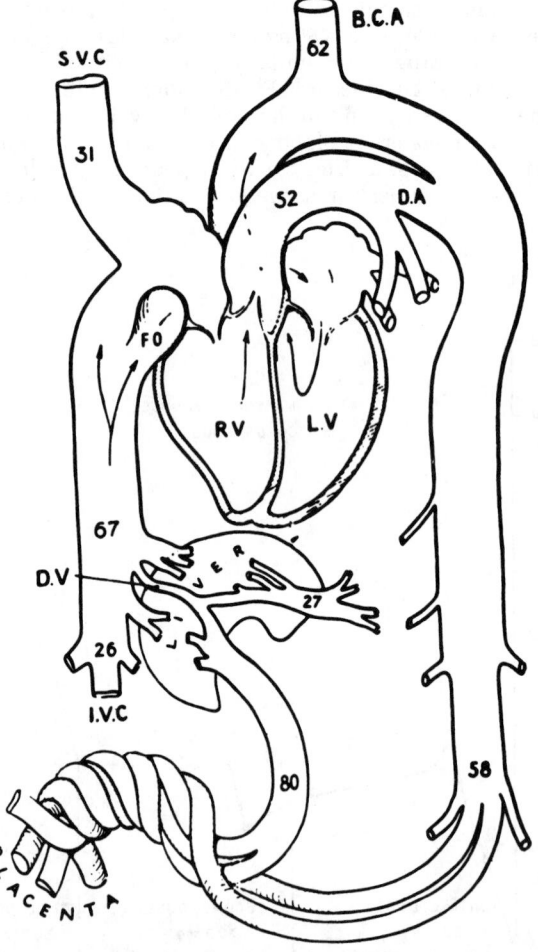

Figure 46-5. Diagram of the circulation in the mature fetal lamb. The numerals indicate the mean oxygen saturation (%) in the great vessels of six lambs: right ventricle (RV); left ventricle (LV); superior vena cava (SVC); brachiocephalic artery (BCA); foramen ovale (FO); ductus arteriosus (DA); ductus venosus (DV). (Reprinted with permission from Born GVR, Dawes GS, Mott JC *et al:* Changes in the heart and lungs at birth. Cold Spring Harbor Symp Quant Biol 19:103, 1954.)

thiopental or thiamylal, not in excess of 4 mg·kg^{-1}, resulted in fetal arterial concentrations of barbiturate below a level that would result in neonatal depression (Fig. 46-6).[52]

Fetal regional blood flow changes can also affect the amount of drug taken up by individual organs. For example, during asphyxia and acidosis, a greater proportion of the fetal cardiac output perfuses the fetal brain, heart, and placenta. Infusion of lidocaine to asphyxiated baboon fetuses resulted in increased drug uptake in the heart, brain, and liver, compared with uptake in nonasphyxiated controls.[47]

Fetus and Newborn

Any drug that reaches the fetus will be subjected to metabolism and excretion. In this respect the fetus has an advantage over the newborn in that it can excrete the drug back to the mother once the concentration gradient of the free drug across the placenta has been reversed. With the use of local anesthetics, this may occur even though the total plasma drug concentration in the mother may exceed that in the fetus, because there is lower protein binding in fetal plasma.[49] One drug, 2-chloroprocaine, is metabolized in the fetal blood so rapidly ($T_{1/2} = 43$ seconds) that substantial accumulation in the fetus is avoided even in acidosis.[57,59]

In the term as well as preterm newborn, the liver contains enzymes essential for the biotransformation of amide local anesthetics.[64] A study comparing the pharmacokinetics of lidocaine among adult ewes and fetal and neonatal lambs showed that the metabolic clearance in the newborn was similar to, and renal clearance greater than, that in the adult.[65] Nonetheless, the elimination half-life was more prolonged in the newborn. This was attributed to a greater volume of distribution and tissue uptake of the drug, so that at any given time the neonate's liver and kidneys were exposed to a smaller fraction of lidocaine accumulated in the body. Similar results were reported in another study involving lidocaine administration to human infants in a neonatal intensive care unit.[64] Prolonged elimination half-lives in the newborn compared with the adult have been noted for other amide local anesthetics.

The question remains whether the fetus and newborn are more sensitive to the depressant and toxic effects of drugs than is the adult. Laboratory investigations have shown that the newborn is, in fact, more sensitive to the depressant effects of opioids. With local anesthetics, neonatal depression occurred at blood concentrations of mepivacaine or lidocaine that were approximately 50% less than those producing toxic manifestations in the adult. However, infants accidentally injected with mepivacaine in utero (intended for maternal caudal anesthesia) stopped convulsing when the drug concentration decreased below the threshold level for convulsions in the adult.[66] The relative central nervous and cardiorespiratory toxicity of several local anesthetics has been studied in adult ewes and fetal and newborn lambs.[67,68] The sequence of toxic manifestations was similar in the three groups: convulsions, followed by hypotension, apnea, and circulatory collapse. The doses required to produce toxicity in the fetus and newborn were significantly higher than those required in the adult. In the fetus this difference was attributed to placental clearance of drug into the mother and better maintenance of blood gas tensions during convulsions. In the newborn, the larger volume of distribution is probably responsible for the higher doses needed to induce toxic effects.

Bupivacaine has been implicated as a possible cause of neonatal jaundice.[69] It was postulated that high affinity of the drug for fetal erythrocyte membranes led to a decrease in filterability and deformability, rendering red blood cells more prone to hemolysis.[70] However, a recent study failed to show increased bilirubin production in newborns whose mothers received bupivacaine for epidural anesthesia during labor and delivery.[71]

Lastly, neurobehavioral studies revealed subtle changes in newborn neurologic and adaptive function. In the case of most anesthetic agents, these changes are minor and transient, lasting for only 24–48 hours.[72,73]

ANESTHESIA FOR LABOR AND VAGINAL DELIVERY

Most women experience moderate to severe pain during parturition. In the first stage of labor it is caused by uterine contractions, associated with dilation of the cervix and stretching of the lower uterine segment. Impulses generated in this process are carried in visceral afferent Type C fibers

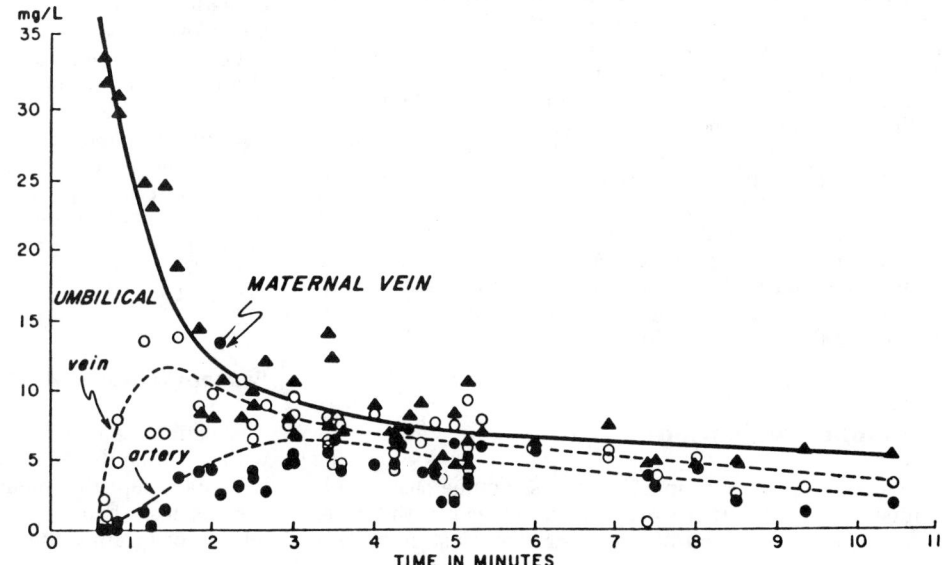

Figure 46-6. Cesarean section. Thiamylal concentrations in maternal vein (▲—▲), umbilical vein (○—○), umbilical artery (●—●). Curves drawn by inspection. (Reprinted with permission from Kosaka Y, Takahashi T, Mark LS: Intravenous thiobarbiturate anesthesia for cesarean section. Anesthesiology 31:489, 1969.)

accompanying the sympathetic nerves. Pain is referred to the corresponding dermatomal segments where these fibers enter the spinal cord. In early labor, only the lower thoracic dermatomes (T11–12) are affected, but with progressing cervical dilation in the transition phase, adjacent dermatomes may be involved and pain referred from T10 to L1. In the second stage, because of the descent of the fetal presenting part, additional impulses arise from distention of the vaginal vault and perineum. These impulses are carried by the pudendal nerves, composed of lower sacral fibers (S2–4).

Well-conducted obstetric analgesia, in addition to relieving pain and anxiety, may benefit the mother. For instance, in animal models pain has been shown to result in maternal hypertension and reduced uterine blood flow.[74,75] During the first and second phases of labor, epidural analgesia blunts the increases in maternal cardiac output, heart rate, and blood pressure that occur with painful uterine contractions and "bearing-down" efforts.[76] In reducing maternal secretion of catecholamines, epidural analgesia may convert a previously dysfunctional labor pattern to normal.[77] Maternal analgesia may also benefit the fetus. It may eliminate maternal hyperventilation, which often leads to a reduced fetal arterial oxygen tension consequent on the leftward shift of the maternal oxygen-hemoglobin dissociation curve.[78]

The most frequently chosen methods for relieving the pain of parturition are psychoprophylaxis, systemic medication, and epidural or spinal analgesia. Inhalational analgesia, intrathecal opioids, or paracervical blockade are less commonly used. General anesthesia is rarely necessary but may be indicated for uterine relaxation in some deliveries.

Psychoprophylaxis

The philosophy of prepared childbirth maintains that lack of knowledge, misinformation, fear, and anxiety can heighten a patient's response to pain and consequently increase the need for analgesics. Although there is no question that an informed patient is better equipped for the stresses of parturition, few women are able to withstand labor without some pharmacologic analgesia.[79] The most popular method of prepared childbirth is that introduced by Lamaze. It provides an educational program on the physiology of parturition and attempts to diminish cortical pain perception by encouraging responses such as specific patterns of breathing and focused attention on a fixed object. This approach is usually successful through the latent and early active phase, but not if labor is prolonged or augmented with the use of oxytocin. The advantage of the method is that well-prepared patients generally need less medication.[80] Neonatal outcome appears to be similar for women who deliver babies solely with the Lamaze technique and for women who receive appropriate supplementary analgesia. A realistic attitude is to encourage the mother in the Lamaze method while recognizing individual variations in pain tolerance and need for medication. Of course, medication should not be withheld if required.

Systemic Medication

The advantages of systemic analgesics include ease of administration and patient acceptability. However, the drug, dose, time, and method of administration must be chosen carefully so as to avoid maternal or neonatal depression. Drugs used for systemic analgesia are opioids, tranquilizers, and occasionally ketamine.

Opioids

Meperidine is the most commonly used systemic analgesic and is reasonably effective in ameliorating pain during the first stage of labor. It has virtually replaced morphine, because in equianalgesic doses morphine appears to cause greater neonatal ventilatory depression.[81] Meperidine can be administered by iv injection (effective analgesia in 5–10 minutes) or im (peak effect in 40–50 minutes). The major side-effects of this drug are a high incidence of nausea and vomiting, dose-related depression of ventilation, and orthostatic hypotension. Placental transmission is rapid, and fetal blood and tissue levels depend on the dose, mode, and frequency of administration.[54] Meperidine may cause transient alterations of the fetal heart rate, such as decreased beat-to-beat variability and tachycardia. Among other factors, the risk of neonatal depression is related to the interval from the last drug injection to delivery.[82] The placental transfer of the active metabolite, normeperidine, has also been implicated in contributing to neonatal depression.[83] Subtle neonatal neurobehavioral dysfunction may be related to the long elimination half-life of normeperidine in the neonate (62 hours).[84]

Experience with the newer synthetic opioids, such as fentanyl and alfentanil, has been limited. Although they are potent, their use during labor is restricted by the short duration of analgesia consequent on a very brief distribution phase. An iv injection of fentanyl, up to 1 $\mu g \cdot kg^{-1}$, results in prompt pain relief without severe neonatal depression.[85] These drugs offer an advantage in situations in which analgesia of rapid onset but short duration is necessary (such as with forceps application).

Opioid agonists-antagonists such as butorphanol and nalbuphine have also been used for obstetric analgesia. Those drugs have the proposed benefits of a lower incidence of nausea, vomiting, and dysphoria, as well as a "ceiling effect" on depression of ventilation. However, studies for the most part have not demonstrated a clear advantage in parturition.[86] Butorphanol is probably most popular; unlike meperidine, it is biotransformed into inactive metabolites and has a ceiling effect on depression of ventilation in doses exceeding 2 mg. A potential disadvantage is the high incidence of maternal sedation. The recommended dose is 1–2 mg by iv or im injection. Nalbuphine, 10 mg iv or im, is an alternative to butorphanol.

To prevent neonatal ventilatory depression, naloxone, a pure opioid antagonist, should not be administered to the mother shortly before delivery. Although the technique is effective in this regard, it reverses analgesia at a time when it is most needed and in some instances has caused maternal pulmonary edema and cardiac arrest.[87] If necessary, the drug should be given directly to the newborn (0.1 $mg \cdot kg^{-1}$).

Patient-Controlled Analgesia

The patient can regulate the iv administration of opioids with a device that she can trigger to release a preset dose. Patients accept this method, and the total amount of drug used is less than that needed for conventional analgesia with iv or im injections.[88]

Tranquilizers

Tranquilizers are principally used during labor to control maternal anxiety and as adjuvants to opioids. Promethazine is most commonly used to provide sedation and diminish nausea and vomiting. Its addition to meperidine resulted in no greater neonatal depression than when meperidine was given alone.[89] Barbiturates are no longer popular because of their antianalgesic effects and neonatal depression. Diazepam should not be used routinely because it results in transient hypotonia and impaired thermoregulation in the newborn.[90]

Ketamine

Ketamine is a potent analgesic capable of producing profound amnesia. The latter is a disadvantage in routine obstetrics, because most mothers want to remember the birthing process. However, ketamine is a useful adjuvant to incomplete regional analgesia during vaginal delivery or obstetric manipulations. In low doses ($0.2–0.4$ mg·kg^{-1}), ketamine provides adequate analgesia without causing neonatal depression.[91]

Regional Anesthesia

The following techniques of regional anesthesia are used in obstetrics: continuous lumbar or sacral (caudal) epidural block, paracervical and pudendal block, and spinal anesthesia. Regional blocks have several advantages that make them preferable to other modalities of analgesia during labor and delivery. They can provide excellent pain relief without obtunding the mother or fetus and, if properly applied, should not affect the progress of labor or the mother's ability to bear down during the second stage.

Spinal and Epidural Anesthesia

Because of the profound motor paralysis it produces, the use of spinal anesthesia is limited to delivery itself. It is particularly useful to provide rapid, reliable anesthesia for operative delivery, such as midforceps or vacuum extraction, and for perineal repair. To reduce the incidence of post-dural puncture headache, 25- or 26-gauge spinal needles, preferably with a pencil point, should be used routinely.[92] Local anesthetics, prepared as hyperbaric solution, are lidocaine 5% (30–50 mg), tetracaine 0.5% (4–5 mg), and bupivacaine 0.75% (5–6 mg). Lidocaine is the drug of choice because of its shorter duration of action.

In contrast to spinal anesthesia, segmental epidural analgesia can be provided for labor as well as delivery. For adequate pain relief with the smallest amount of drug, only T10–L1 segments need to be blocked during the first stage of labor. For the second stage, the block should be extended to the S2–4 segments. Unless the patient receives oxytocin stimulation, epidural block is usually induced when labor has been well established and the cervix is dilated to 5–6 cm in the primipara and 3–4 cm in a multipara. The first stage of labor is usually not prolonged by administration of epidural anesthesia, as long as aortocaval compression is avoided.[93,94] In contrast, the second stage is often lengthened when adequate blockade is maintained.[95] This led the American College of Obstetricians and Gynecologists to define an abnormally prolonged second stage as greater than 3 hours in nulliparous and greater than 2 hours in multiparous parturients receiving epidural analgesia.[96]

The most frequent complication of spinal and epidural anesthesia is maternal hypotension (systolic blood pressure less than 100 mm Hg, or a 20% decrease in systolic pressure). Therefore, maternal blood pressure and heart rate must be checked frequently, typically every 2–5 minutes for 15–20 minutes immediately after induction of the block and every 5–10 minutes thereafter. In most instances, hypotension can be prevented by acute plasma volume expansion (prehydration) and proper positioning of the parturient to avoid aortocaval compression. Prehydration should be accomplished by rapid iv infusion of a balanced salt solution, 500–1000 ml. Unless the mother is hypoglycemic, use of glucose-containing solutions is better avoided to prevent neonatal hypoglycemia.[27] If hypotension occurs, the iv infusion rate should be increased. If the blood pressure is not restored within 1–2 minutes, ephedrine should be administered iv in 5–10 mg increments.

Spinal or epidural anesthesia can be induced with the patient in the lateral decubitus or sitting position. We prefer to use the sitting position because the midline of the back is easier to identify in pregnant women, who frequently have sacral edema, and because, with the common use of narrow-gauge spinal needles, cerebrospinal fluid (CSF) flows more readily in this position. For epidural anesthesia, the loss of resistance technique is more reliable than the hanging drop technique, because epidural pressures tend to be positive during parturition. Once the catheter has been threaded, its placement should be carefully determined to rule out intrathecal or iv penetration. Aspiration of the catheter may not be diagnostic because the thin-walled epidural veins collapse easily. A more reliable method is to inject 0.5–1.0 ml of saline through the catheter to distend the vessel if the placement was indeed iv, hold the catheter in the dependent position, and observe for back flow of blood. Thereafter, a test dose must be administered. Bupivacaine, 7.5 mg, lidocaine, 45 mg, or 2-chloroprocaine, 60 mg, are effective in the detection of intrathecal injection. The inclusion of 15 μg of epinephrine, with careful blood pressure and heart rate monitoring (by ECG), may help indicate intravascular injection because it causes a transient increase in both parameters within 30–90 seconds.[97] However, the use of epinephrine is controversial in obstetrics because false-positive results do occur with uterine contractions, and the drug may reduce uteroplacental perfusion.[98,99] Isoproterenol (5 μg) may be a useful alternative to epinephrine since it induces maternal tachycardia after iv injection but is devoid of alpha-adrenergic effects.[100] Safety and efficacy studies should precede its clinical application. Injection of air (1 cc) in conjunction with the use of precordial Doppler appears to be a reliable indicator of iv placement of an epidural catheter.[101] Lastly, the addition of fentanyl to local anesthetic solution may result in altered sensorium after unintended intravascular injection of a test dose.[102] After a test dose with negative results, adequate first-stage analgesia is usually achieved with an additional injection of 5 ml of lidocaine 1.0%, bupivacaine 0.25%, or 2-chloroprocaine 2%. The dose may be repeated as necessary or may be followed immediately by a continuous epidural infusion of a more dilute solution: 0.33% lidocaine, 10–15 ml·h^{-1}; 0.125% bupivacaine, 8–12 ml·h^{-1}; or 1.0% 2-chloroprocaine, 20–25 ml·h^{-1}. For the second stage of labor, analgesia can be extended to include the sacral segments by administration of an additional 5–10 ml of the originally used local anesthetic solution with the patient in a semirecumbent position. Significant motor blockade should be avoided.

Patient-controlled epidural analgesia is a safe and effective alternative to conventional "top-up" or continuous infusion techniques.[103-105] Patient acceptance is excellent and anesthesia manpower demands are reduced. Effective analgesia is usually established using boluses of 0.25% bupivacaine. A maintenance infusion of bupivacaine 0.125% is then set at 6 ml·h⁻¹. As required, patient-triggered boluses of 4 ml may be obtained, separated by a 10-minute lockout period.[105] The addition of fentanyl (1 μg·ml⁻¹) to bupivacaine may reduce local anesthetic requirement.

Mepivacaine and etidocaine are other local anesthetics currently available for epidural anesthesia. Neither has been popular in obstetrics because of the untoward effects of mepivacaine on neonatal neurobehavioral adaptation and because of the profound motor blockade caused by etidocaine in the mother.[106,107] However, a recent study refutes the untoward effects of mepivacaine on the neonate.[108]

Caudal anesthesia is used infrequently. It does not allow for a selective blockade of lower thoracic segments in the first stage of labor. Consequently, larger doses of local anesthetics are necessary from the outset. However, caudal anesthesia may be preferable to epidural block when rapid onset of perineal anesthesia is desired, as with midforceps delivery. To avoid accidentally injecting the fetus, the mother's rectum must be examined when the needle is still in place and before administration of the test dose.[66]

Spinal and epidural (lumbar or sacral) blocks are generally contraindicated in the presence of coagulopathy, acute hypovolemia, or infection at the site of needle puncture.

Paracervical Block

Although paracervical block effectively relieves pain during the first stage of labor, the technique has fallen out of favor because it is associated with a high incidence of fetal distress and poor neonatal outcome, particularly with the use of bupivacaine. This may be related to uterine artery constriction or increased uterine tone.[109,110] The technique is basically simple and involves a submucosal injection of local anesthetic at the vaginal fornix, in the proximity of those fibers innervating the uterus. All local anesthetics except bupivacaine may be used for that purpose.

Pudendal Nerve Block

The pudendal nerves, derived from the lower sacral nerve roots (S2–4), supply the vaginal vault, perineum, and rectum and parts of the bladder. The nerves are easily anesthetized transvaginally because they loop around the ischial spines. Ten milliliters of local anesthetic deposited behind each sacrospinous ligament provides adequate anesthesia for outlet forceps delivery and episiotomy repair.

Epidural and Intrathecal Opioids

The use of epidural opioids to relieve labor pain has been disappointing. Although morphine, 4–5 mg, provides prolonged and intense analgesia after cesarean section, it is not as consistently beneficial during labor.[111,112] Better pain relief may be obtained with higher drug doses (7.5 mg), but the risk of delayed depression of ventilation and the fetal effects after placental transfer preclude its routine use.[113] However, the addition of fentanyl, 2–5 μg·ml⁻¹, sufentanil, 1 μg·ml⁻¹, or butorphanol, 0.2 mg·ml⁻¹, to dilute solutions of bupivacaine (0.0625–0.125%) has proved quite valuable.[114-117] This combination achieves a solid block with a greatly reduced dose of local anesthetic. In contrast, opioids very effectively relieve the pain of uterine contractions when injected intrathecally: morphine, 0.5–1.5 mg, fen-

tanyl, 37.5–50 μg, or a combination of fentanyl, 25 μg, and morphine, 0.25 mg, provides profound analgesia of rapid onset and long duration.[118-120] A pudendal block or local infiltration of the perineum may be required at delivery. Intrathecal opioids are particularly useful in parturients with severe heart disease in whom sympathetic blockade should be strongly avoided. Complications of epidural and intrathecal opioids in obstetric patients are the same as in the general surgical population, viz., pruritus, urinary retention, and delayed ventilatory depression. Prophylactic oral naltrexone (6 mg) may diminish the incidence of side-effects observed with intrathecal morphine but may also shorten the duration of analgesia.[121]

Inhalation Analgesia

Inhalation analgesia is easy to administer and, although it does not relieve pain completely, it makes uterine contractions more tolerable. During delivery, a combination of inhalation analgesia with a pudendal block or infiltration of the perineum with a local anesthetic can be very satisfactory. A particular advantage of inhalation analgesia pertains to the uptake and excretion of the drugs. The desired level of analgesia can be easily and rapidly achieved or terminated. The neonate can also excrete inhalation agents through the lungs. A serious disadvantage is the need for a scavenging system. The potential for fluoride nephrotoxicity is greatest with methoxyflurane and much less so with enflurane. However, nephrotoxicity with methoxyflurane has not been a problem in laboring patients so long as the total dose does not exceed 15 ml of the agent.[122] Use of either drug should probably be avoided in the setting of compromised renal function.

Inhalation drugs can be administered by trained personnel or by the patient herself, with adequate supervision. A conventional anesthesia circuit can be used, and a methoxyflurane inhaler is commercially available for self-administration. The system must be able to deliver a precise concentration of the agent over a wide range of inspiratory flow rates. The parturient is instructed to breathe deeply from the inhaler when she detects the onset of uterine contraction, so that analgesia will be established at its peak. Commonly used inhalation drugs for analgesia during labor are nitrous oxide, up to 50 vol%, methoxyflurane, 0.25–0.4 vol%, or enflurane, 0.5–1.0 vol%. A mixture of either potent drug in nitrous oxide and oxygen has also been used. The inspired concentration of oxygen in nitrous oxide–containing mixtures should be monitored. Halothane is a poor analgesic.[123]

General Anesthesia

General anesthesia is rarely used for vaginal delivery and always with precautions against aspiration. It may be required when time constraints prevent induction of regional anesthesia, as in acute fetal distress. If uterine relaxation is necessary for obstetric maneuvers, potent inhalation drugs can provide a dose-related response.[124] This may be at delivery of the second twin or breech or after delivery, for manual removal of a retained placenta. Nitroglycerin (50–500 μg) has been successfully used as an alternative to general anesthesia during manual extraction of a retained placenta.[125,126] If general anesthesia is used, an inhaled concentration of 2 MAC is usually adequate. In all cases, preoxygenation and rapid iv induction of anesthesia with the use of cricoid pressure and placement of a cuffed tube in the trachea are mandatory. High inspiratory flows ensure quick delivery of the drug. The mother must not be overdosed during controlled ventilation of the lungs. Immediately after the obstetric procedure is completed, the potent drug should be discontinued or its concentration reduced, to minimize the risk of hemorrhage resulting from continued uterine relaxation. Oxytocin, 20–30 units, should be added to the iv infusion. The patient's trachea should not be extubated until she is awake and airway reflexes have returned.

ANESTHESIA FOR CESAREAN SECTION

The frequency of cesarean section has steadily increased in recent decades, reaching the high incidence of 20–25% of all deliveries. The most frequent indications include failure to progress, fetal distress, cephalopelvic disproportion, malpresentation, prematurity, and prior uterine surgery. The choice of anesthesia should depend on the urgency of the procedure, as well as on the condition of the mother and fetus. In the absence of specific indications, the mother's wishes should be seriously considered.

Regional Anesthesia

A 1986 survey of obstetric anesthesia practices in the United States revealed that most patients undergoing cesarean section do so under spinal or epidural anesthesia.[127] Regional techniques have several advantages: a lessened risk of gastric aspiration, fulfillment of the mother's wish to remain awake, and avoidance of depressant anesthetic drugs. It has also been suggested that operative blood loss is less with regional than general anesthesia.[128] The time required for induction of regional anesthesia makes the technique less suitable for urgent cesarean section. The induction-to-delivery interval averages 15–20 minutes with spinal anesthesia and 30–40 minutes with epidural anesthesia. In elective cesarean sections, the duration of antepartum anesthesia does not affect the neonatal outcome as long as there is no protracted aortocaval compression or hypotension.[129] The risk of hypotension is greater than during vaginal delivery because the block must extend to the T4 segment. Therefore, proper positioning and prehydration are critical. At least 1500–2000 ml of a crystalloid solution is required. In this regard, epidural anesthesia is advantageous, because of its slower onset and progression. If hypotension occurs despite these measures, left uterine displacement should be increased, the rate of iv infusion augmented,

and ephedrine, in 10–15 mg increments, administered by iv injection.

Spinal Anesthesia

Subarachnoid block is the more commonly administered regional anesthetic for cesarean delivery.[127] It is popular partially because of the simplicity and reliability of the technique, as well as the relative rapidity with which adequate anesthesia can be established. In fact, it has been suggested as a reasonable alternative to general anesthesia for emergency cesarean section.[130]

Solutions of lidocaine 5%, tetracaine 1.0%, or bupivacaine 0.75% are available. The doses and duration of action of these local anesthetics are listed in Table 46-2. Using 0.75% hyperbaric bupivacaine, Norris et al have shown that it is not necessary to adjust the dose of drug based on patient's height.[131]

Blood pressure, ventilation, and ECG should be monitored throughout, and hemoglobin oxygen saturation (pulse oximeter) should be monitored when possible. Before delivery, oxygen should be routinely administered by face mask to improve fetal oxygenation.[132]

Despite a block extending to the T4 segment, patients experience varying degrees of visceral discomfort, particularly with exteriorization of the uterus, and traction on abdominal viscera. Improved perioperative analgesia can be provided by the addition of fentanyl, 6.25 μg, or 0.1 mg of preservative-free morphine to the local anesthetic solution.[133-135] Supplementary analgesia may be provided by the incremental iv injection of 2–3 mg of morphine, 20–30 mg of meperidine, or 25 μg of fentanyl. The patient can be sedated by the addition of 2.5–5 mg of diazepam. Midazolam is a less desirable sedative in the obstetric setting because of its strong amnestic properties. Nausea and vomiting may be alleviated by the administration of a small dose of droperidol or metoclopramide.[136,137] One should take care not to oversedate the mother and blunt her airway reflexes.

Lumbar Epidural Anesthesia

Lumbar epidural anesthesia is also popular for use with cesarean sections. In contrast to spinal anesthesia, more time and drug are required to establish an adequate sensory block. The advantages are the lessened risk of post-dural puncture headache and the ability to titrate the dose of local anesthetic through an indwelling epidural catheter. The usual precautions must be taken to ensure proper placement

TABLE 46-2. Local Anesthetics Commonly Used for Cesarean Section with Subarachnoid Block

	Lidocaine 5% in 7.5% Dextrose	Tetracaine 1% in Equal Volume of 10% Dextrose	Bupivacaine 0.75% in 8.25% Dextrose
Dosage (mg) according to height (cm):			
150–160	65	8	8
160–182	70	9	10
182 and taller	75	10	12
Onset of action (min)	1–3	3–5	2–4
Duration of action (min)	45–75	120–180	120–180

of the needle and catheter to prevent inadvertent intrathecal or intravascular injection. This is especially important because the drug requirements for cesarean section are greater than for labor and vaginal delivery.

The most commonly used agents are 2-chloroprocaine 3%, bupivacaine 0.5%, and lidocaine 2% with epinephrine 1:200,000. Adequate anesthesia is usually achieved with 15–25 ml of the solution, given in divided doses. The patient should be monitored as with spinal anesthesia.

Because of its extremely high rate of metabolism in the maternal and fetal plasma, 2-chloroprocaine provides a rapid-onset, reliable block with minimal risk of systemic toxicity.[57] It is the local anesthetic of choice in the presence of fetal acidosis and when a pre-existing block is to be rapidly extended for an urgent cesarean section.[138] Reports of transient neurologic deficits after massive inadvertent intrathecal administration of the drug have somewhat diminished enthusiasm for its use.[139,140] The formulation containing a relatively high concentration of sodium bisulfite, at a low pH, has been implicated as neurotoxic.[141] In the current formula of 2-chloroprocaine, ethylene diaminotetraacetate (EDTA) has been substituted for sodium bisulfite. Severe spasmodic back pain may occur after epidural injection.[142] This complication has been attributed to EDTA-induced leaching of calcium from paravertebral muscles. In one reported case, iv infusion of calcium chloride ameliorated the symptoms.[143]

Bupivacaine 0.5% provides profound anesthesia for cesarean section, of slower onset but longer duration than the other two drugs. Considerable attention has focused on the drug since it was reported that unintentional intravascular injection could result not only in convulsions, but also in an almost simultaneous cardiac arrest, often refractory to resuscitation.[144] The greater cardiotoxicity of bupivacaine (and etidocaine) in comparison with other amide local anesthetics has been well demonstrated in various animal models.[69,145] Pregnancy itself appears to enhance the cardiotoxic effects of the drug.[146] This may be related to a reduction in plasma protein binding and to the enhanced myocardial depressant effects of bupivacaine during pregnancy.[147,148]

Lidocaine has an onset and duration intermediate between those of 2-chloroprocaine and bupivacaine. The need to include epinephrine (1:200,000) in the local anesthetic solution to ensure adequate lumbosacral anesthesia limits its use in the setting of maternal hypertension and reduced uteroplacental perfusion.

With epidural anesthesia, prolonged pain relief also can be provided in the postoperative period by intraspinal administration of an opioid. The following opioids have been used successfully: 5 mg morphine, 2 mg butorphanol, 1 mg hydromorphone, 50 μg fentanyl, and 20–30 μg sufentanil.[111,149-153] All were diluted to a volume of 10 ml with normal saline. Because delayed depression of ventilation may occur, particularly with the use of morphine, the patient must be monitored carefully in the postoperative period.[154]

General Anesthesia

The advantages of general anesthesia are the rapidity and reliability with which the patient can be prepared for surgery. It is the technique of choice for emergency cesarean section and when substantial hemorrhage is anticipated (placenta previa, fibromyomas). We also prefer to use general anesthesia in situations in which uterine relaxation will facilitate delivery, as in prematurity, breech presentation, and transverse lie, and in patients with multiple gestation or polyhydramnios, who frequently have dyspnea and supine hypotension syndrome. General anesthesia should be used cautiously in patients with asthma, upper respiratory infection, or a history of difficult tracheal intubation. The airway should be evaluated carefully during the preoperative visit, because inability to intubate the trachea is one of the leading causes of maternal death.[155] If difficulties are anticipated, one should consider using a regional technique, an awake tracheal intubation, or a fiberoptic bronchoscope. Preoperative medication is usually not necessary, except for oral administration of 15–30 ml of a nonparticulate antacid within 30 minutes of induction of anesthesia. On the operating table, the patient's pelvis should be tilted to prevent aortocaval compression. Routine monitoring is the same as with regional anesthetic techniques, with the addition of a capnometer, pulse oximeter, nerve stimulator, inspired oxygen concentration monitor, and temperature probe.

Preoxygenation is an important step that should be carried out for 3–5 minutes with the use of a tight-fitting mask. In an emergency situation, four deep breaths with 100% oxygen will suffice.[156] A "defasciculating" dose of a nondepolarizing muscle relaxant is not necessary. Rapid induction of anesthesia is achieved with an iv injection of thiopental (4 mg·kg^{-1}), ketamine (up to 1 mg·kg^{-1}), or a combination of thiopental (2–3 mg·kg^{-1}) and ketamine (0.5 mg·kg^{-1}). If the patient is in labor, and time constraints permit, induction drugs should be administered at the onset of uterine contraction to decrease fetal drug exposure.[63] Succinylcholine (1–1.5 mg·kg^{-1}) is then injected while cricoid pressure is applied by a trained assistant until the airway is properly secured with a cuffed endotracheal tube. If there is difficulty in securing the airway, cricoid pressure should be maintained throughout and the mother ventilated with 100% oxygen before a subsequent attempt at tracheal intubation is made. It is safer to permit the mother to awaken and to reassess the method of induction than to persist with traumatic efforts at tracheal intubation, which may result in loss of the airway because of edema and bleeding. Once the endotracheal tube placement is confirmed, preferably with a capnometer, the obstetrician may proceed with skin incision. In the predelivery interval, anesthesia is maintained with a 50:50 mixture of nitrous oxide in oxygen and 0.5 MAC of a potent agent. An infusion of succinylcholine may only be added when there is evidence that neuromuscular function has returned. Severe maternal hyperventilation should be avoided, because it may reduce uterine blood flow. A study performed in pregnant sheep established that placental hypoperfusion results from the mechanical effect of hyperventilation, because it could not be corrected by restoring Paco$_2$ to normal or above-normal levels.[157] A few minutes before delivery is anticipated, the concentration of the potent agent may be increased temporarily to 2 MAC, when uterine relaxation is desired.

The newborn's condition after cesarean section with general anesthesia is comparable to that with regional techniques.[158] The uterine incision-to-delivery interval seems to be more important to neonatal outcome than induction of anesthesia-to-delivery interval. Lower Apgar scores at 1 minute and acidosis were reported in cases in which the uterine incision-to-delivery time interval exceeded 180 seconds, whereas anesthesia for up to 30 minutes before delivery appears to have no adverse effects on the infant.[159,160] This is in contrast to the earlier practice of using 70–75% nitrous oxide in oxygen, which resulted in neonatal depression within approximately 10 minutes of anesthesia.[161] The increase to 50% in the oxygen concentration inhaled by the mother also benefits the fetus by increasing its PaO$_2$.[162]

After delivery of the infant, 20 units of oxytocin is added to the infusion, and anesthesia is deepened with adjuvants such as an opioid. At the end of the procedure, the mother's trachea is extubated once she is awake. The usual blood loss at a cesarean section is 750–1000 ml, and transfusion is rarely necessary.

MANAGEMENT OF HIGH-RISK PARTURIENTS

Pregnancy or parturition are considered "high risk" when accompanied by conditions unfavorable to the well-being of the mother or fetus, or both. Maternal problems may be related to pregnancy, such as pre-eclampsia–eclampsia and other hypertensive disorders of pregnancy, or antepartum hemorrhage resulting from placenta previa (literally, "the placenta going ahead") or abruptio placentae ("breaking away of the placenta"). Diabetes mellitus; cardiac, chronic renal, neurologic, or sickle cell disease; and asthma, obesity, and drug abuse are not related to pregnancy but often are affected by it. Prematurity (gestation of less than 37 weeks), postmaturity (42 weeks or longer), intrauterine growth retardation, and multiple gestation are fetal conditions associated with high risk. During labor and delivery, fetal malpresentation (breech, transverse lie), placental abruption, compression of the umbilical cord (prolapse, nuchal cord), precipitous labor, or intrauterine infection (prolonged rupture of membranes) may enhance the risk to the mother or the fetus.

In general, the anesthetic management of the high-risk parturient is based on the same maternal and fetal considerations as the management of healthy mothers and fetuses. These include maintenance of maternal cardiovascular function and oxygenation, maintenance and possibly improvement of the uteroplacental blood flow, and creation of optimal conditions for a painless, atraumatic delivery of an infant without significant drug effects. However, there is less room for error, because many of the above functions may be compromised before the induction of anesthesia. For example, significant acidosis is prone to develop in fetuses of diabetic mothers when delivered by cesarean section with spinal or epidural anesthesia complicated by even brief maternal hypotension.[163] Because the high-risk parturient may have received a variety of drugs, anesthesiologists must be familiar with potential interactions between these drugs and the anesthetic drugs they plan to administer.

Pre-eclampsia–Eclampsia

Hypertensive disorders, which occur in approximately 7% of all late pregnancies, are among the major causes of maternal mortality, accounting for approximately one fifth of maternal deaths, and have been estimated to result in 30,000 neonatal deaths and stillbirths per year in the United States alone. Pre-eclampsia is diagnosed on the basis of development of hypertension with proteinuria or edema, or both. The added appearance of convulsions and coma makes for the diagnosis of eclampsia.

Pre-eclampsia–eclampsia is a disease unique to human pregnancy, occurring predominantly in young nulliparas. Symptoms usually appear after the 20th week of gestation, occasionally earlier than that if in association with a hydatidiform mole. Thus, the condition requires the presence of a trophoblast but not a fetus.

The origin of pre-eclampsia–eclampsia is unknown. One proposed theory invokes immunologic rejection of fetal tissues by the mother, which causes a placental vasculitis and ischemia.[164] This theory explains why the disease is more common among nulliparas (no previous exposure to a trophoblast) and in conditions associated with an abnormally large mass of trophoblastic tissues, as in hydatidiform mole, multiple pregnancy, diabetes, and Rh incompatibility. Various studies have demonstrated an abnormal maternal immune responsiveness in pre-eclampsia. Placental ischemia would result in a release of uterine renin and an increase in angiotensin activity (Fig. 46-7).[165] This would lead to a widespread arteriolar vasoconstriction, causing hypertension, tissue hypoxia, and endothelial damage. Adherence of platelets at sites of endothelial damage would result in coagulopathies, occasionally in disseminated intravascular coagulation (DIC). Enhanced angiotensin-mediated aldosterone secretion would lead to an increased sodium reabsorption and edema. Proteinuria, another symptom of pre-eclampsia, may also be attributed to placental ischemia, which would lead to local tissue degeneration and a release of thromboplastin with subsequent deposition of fibrin in constricted glomerular vessels and increased permeability to albumin and other plasma proteins. Furthermore, there is thought to be a decreased production of prostaglandins E, potent vasodilators secreted in the trophoblast, which normally would balance the hypertensive effects of the renin-angiotensin system.

A 1985 study suggested that many of the symptoms associated with pre-eclampsia, including placental ischemia, systemic vasoconstriction, and increased platelet aggregation, may result from an imbalance between the placental production of prostacyclin and thromboxane (Fig. 46-8).[166] During normal pregnancy the placenta produces equivalent

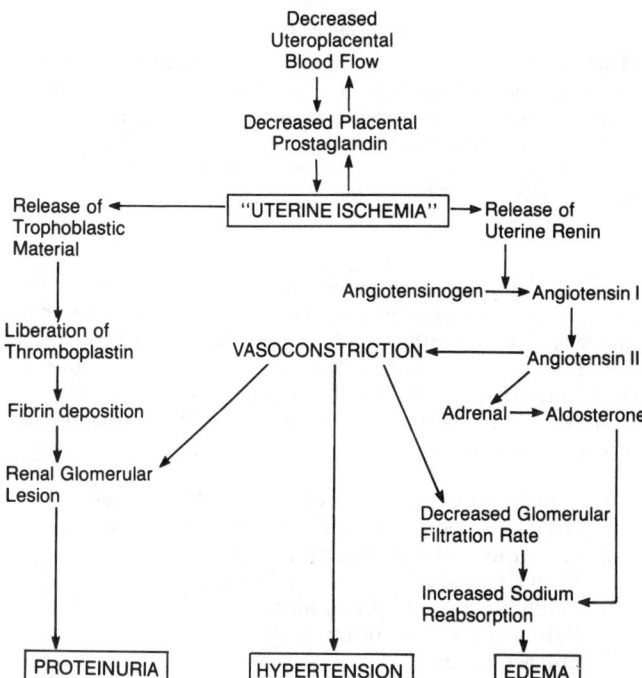

Figure 46-7. Proposed scheme of pathophysiologic changes in toxemia of pregnancy. (Reprinted with permission from Speroff L: Toxemia of pregnancy: Mechanism and therapeutic management. Am J Cardiol 32:582, 1973.)

NORMAL PREGNANCY

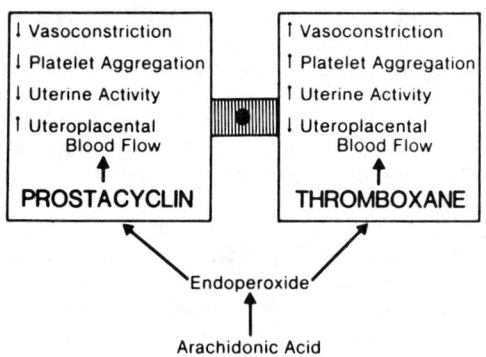

PREECLAMPSIA

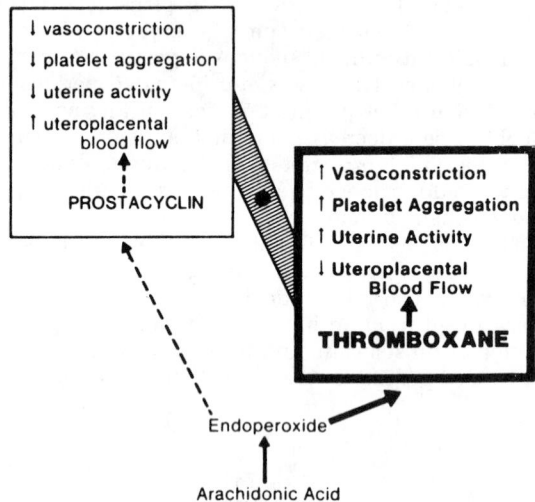

Figure 46-8. Comparison of the balance in the biologic actions of prostacyclin and thromboxane in normal pregnancy with the imbalance of increased thromboxane and decreased prostacyclin in preeclamptic pregnancy. (Reprinted with permission from Walsh SW: Preeclampsia: An imbalance in placental prostacyclin and thromboxane production. Am J Obstet Gynecol 152:335, 1985.)

quantities of these prostaglandins, whereas in pre-eclamptic pregnancy there is seven times more thromboxane than prostacyclin. In another study, a significant correlation was found between intervillous blood flow and the ratio of placental productions of thromboxane and prostacyclin.[167]

Pre-eclampsia is classified as severe if it is associated with any of the following:

1. Systolic blood pressure of 160 mm Hg or greater
2. Diastolic blood pressure of 110 mm Hg or greater
3. Proteinuria of 5 g or more per 24 hours
4. Oliguria (400 ml or less per 24 hours)
5. Cerebral or visual disturbances
6. Pulmonary edema or cyanosis
7. Epigastric pain
8. Intrauterine growth retardation

In severe pre-eclampsia–eclampsia, all major organ systems are affected because of widespread vasospasm. Overall cerebral blood flow is not diminished, but focal hypoperfu-

sion cannot be ruled out. Indeed, postmortem examination has revealed hemorrhagic necrosis in the proximity of thrombosed precapillaries, suggesting intense vasoconstriction. Edema and small foci of degeneration have been attributed to hypoxia. Petechial hemorrhages are common after the onset of convulsions. Symptoms related to the above changes include headache, vertigo, cortical blindness, hyperreflexia, and convulsions. The extent of blood pressure elevation correlates poorly with the incidence of seizures, which are commonly generalized. In a 1984 study, 50% of pre-eclamptic and 75% of eclamptic women were found to have abnormal electroencephalograms (EEGs) consisting of diffuse slowing in the form of theta and delta waves.[168] Cerebral hemorrhage and edema are the leading causes of death in pre-eclampsia–eclampsia, together accounting for approximately 50% of deaths.[169]

In the eyes, intense arteriolar constriction may result in blurred vision, even temporary blindness.

Heart failure may occur in severe cases as a result of peripheral vasoconstriction and increased blood viscosity secondary to hemoconcentration. Changes described in autopsy specimens include left ventricular hypertrophy, subendocardial hemorrhages, cloudy swelling, and fatty and hyaline degeneration.

Decreased blood supply to the liver may result in periportal necrosis of variable extent and severity. Subcapsular hemorrhages account for the epigastric pain encountered in severe cases. Rarely, there is a rupture of the overstretched liver capsule and massive hemorrhage into the abdominal cavity. Hepatic function tests have shown elevated plasma levels of serum glutamic-oxaloacetic transaminase (SGOT), lactic dehydrogenase (LDH), and alkaline phosphatase, whereas bilirubin levels were unaltered.[170]

In the kidneys, swelling of glomerular endothelial cells and deposition of fibrin leading to a constriction of the capillary lumina have been described. Renal blood flow and glomerular filtration rate decrease, resulting in reduced uric acid clearance and, in severe cases, reduced clearance of urea and creatinine.[170] As already stated, oliguria and proteinuria are among the characteristic symptoms of severe pre-eclampsia. The severity of renal involvement is reflected in the degree of proteinuria, which may reach nephrotic levels of 10–15 g·24 h^{-1}.

A mild degree of pulmonary ventilation-perfusion imbalance has been reported in severe cases. It is not believed to be clinically important because the arterial oxygen tension was within normal limits.[171] In contrast, airway edema, which may also occur in severe pre-eclampsia, is of great concern because it may lead to respiratory embarrassment and difficulty in endotracheal intubation. Pulmonary edema is commonly found at autopsy in fatal cases. It may result from heart failure, circulatory overload, or aspiration of gastric contents during convulsions.

In the placenta, a reduction in the intervillous blood flow may result from vasoconstriction or the development of occlusive lesions in decidual arteries, despite the elevated maternal blood pressure. Histologic examination of the placenta often reveals nodular ischemia and varying stages of infarction. Necrosis of the supporting tissues may lead to a rupture of fetal cotyledonary vessels and hemorrhage. If the hemorrhage is extensive, it may extend retroplacentally, initiating the process of abruption. Reduced placental blood flow leads to chronic fetal hypoxia and malnutrition. The risks of intrauterine growth retardation, premature birth, and perinatal death are substantially higher than in normal pregnancies and correlate with the severity of pre-eclampsia.[172]

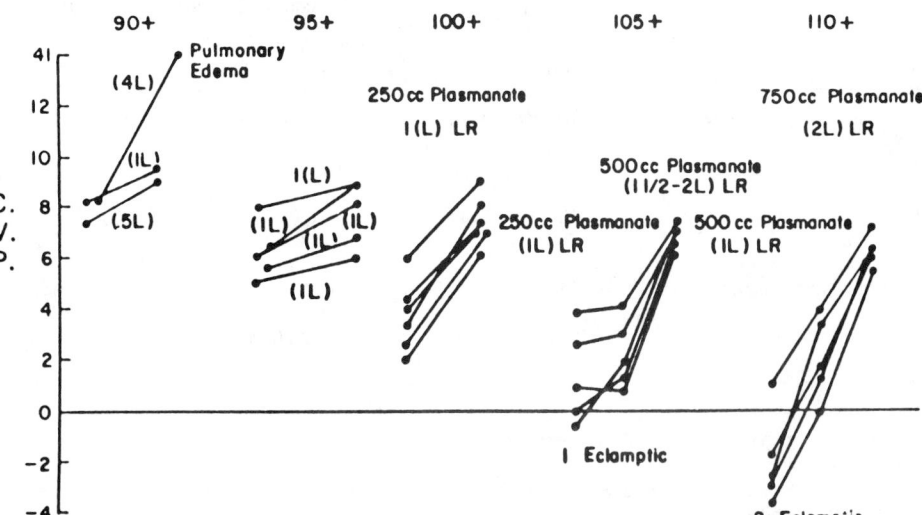

Figure 46-9. Initial central venous pressure measurements (three or more recordings of maternal diastolic pressure) and intravenous volume replacement required to attain the range of 6–8 cm H₂O in five groups of women with pre-eclampsia classified according to the severity of the disease. (Reprinted with permission from Joyce TH III, Debnath KS, Baker, EA: Pre-eclampsia—Relationship of CVP and epidural analgesia. Anesthesiology 51:S297, 1979.)

Although pre-eclampsia is accompanied by exaggerated retention of water and sodium, the shift of fluid and proteins from the intravascular into the extravascular compartment may result in hypovolemia, hypoproteinemia, and hemoconcentration. This phenomenon may be further aggravated by proteinuria. The risk of uteroplacental hypoperfusion and poor fetal outcome has been shown to correlate with the degree of maternal plasma and protein depletion.[173] The mean plasma volume in women with pre-eclampsia was found to be 9% less than normal, and in those with severe disease it was as much as 30–40% below normal.[174] The inverse relationship between the intravascular volume and the severity of hypertension was confirmed with measurements of central venous pressure (CVP) (Fig. 46-9).[175] Patients with a diastolic pressure of 110 mm Hg or greater may have a CVP as low as −4 cm H₂O and may require an infusion of approximately 3 liters volume to increase the CVP to the normal range. It has also been shown that a significant reduction in the maternal plasma volume may precede the clinical appearance of pre-eclampsia in previously normotensive patients.[176]

Earlier studies involving the use of a pulmonary artery flow-directed catheter suggested that patients with severe pre-eclampsia were in a hyperdynamic state.[177] However, these investigations were performed when patients were in labor or in the postpartum period, after treatment had been instituted. More recently, hemodynamic data were obtained in 10 pre-eclamptic and four healthy pregnant women near term.[178] None were in labor. In the pre-eclamptic women, measurements were made before treatment, after volume expansion, and, finally, after vasodilation was achieved with a continuous iv infusion of dihydralazine (Table 46-3). The initial measurements revealed a low pulmonary capillary wedge pressure, a low cardiac index, a high systemic vascular resistance, and an increased heart rate, indicating the existence of a low output state in untreated pre-eclamptic women. Volume expansion resulted in a significant increase in pulmonary capillary wedge pressure and cardiac index, whereas the systemic vascular resistance and maternal heart rate decreased. The mean arterial pressure was significantly reduced, mainly because of a decrease in systolic pressure. Others have also documented this benefi-

cial effect of volume expansion on systemic blood pressure.[175] Subsequent infusion of dihydralazine did not alter the capillary wedge pressure but led to an additional increase in cardiac index and a decrease in systemic vascular resistance. These data indicate that volume expansion may improve maternal tissue perfusion in severe pre-eclampsia.

Simultaneous determinations of CVP and pulmonary capillary wedge pressure were obtained in another group of 18 patients with severe pre-eclampsia.[179] In approximately half of cases, there was a linear relation between the two modalities, but even in these women it was impossible to predict the pulmonary capillary wedge pressure from the CVP because of wide interindividual variations.

Adherence of platelets at sites of endothelial damage may result in consumption coagulopathy, which develops in approximately 20% of patients with pre-eclampsia. Thrombocytopenia is the most frequent finding. It is usually mild, with the platelet count in the range of 100,000–150,000 per mm³. Elevated levels of fibrin degradation products are found less frequently, and plasma fibrinogen concentrations remain normal unless there is a placental abruption. Prolongation of prothrombin and partial thromboplastin times indicates consumption of procoagulants. Bleeding time, which was found to be prolonged in approximately 25% of patients with normal platelet counts,[180] is no longer considered a reliable test of clotting.[181]

General Management

Because the origin of pre-eclampsia–eclampsia is not known, management is symptomatic. Its goals are to prevent or control convulsions, improve organ perfusion, normalize blood pressure, and correct clotting abnormalities. Delivery is indicated in refractory cases or if the pregnancy is close to term. In severe cases, aggressive management should continue for at least 24–48 hours after delivery.

The mainstay of anticonvulsant therapy in the United States is magnesium sulfate. Although its efficacy in preventing seizures has been well substantiated, its mechanism of action remains controversial. In pre-eclamptic–eclamptic patients who had serial EEG recordings, the EEG abnormalities noted during an iv infusion of magnesium sulfate were

TABLE 46-3. Hemodynamic Variables (Mean and Range) in Pre-eclamptic Patients and Control Subjects

| Variable | Pre-eclamptic Patients (n = 10) | | | | | | Control Subjects (n = 4) |
	Initial	After Volume Expansion	p*	After Vasodilation	p†	
Diastolic blood pressure (mm Hg)	106 (100–120)	102 (90–120)	NS‡	85 (75–100)	<0.01	77 (70–90)
Mean arterial pressure (mm Hg)	121 (113–136)	116 (103–136)	<0.02	102 (97–116)	<0.01	95 (93–106)
Heart rate (beats·min^{-1})	100 (90–130)	81 (60–110)	<0.01	82 (70–100)	NS	84 (70–90)
Pulmonary capillary wedge pressure (mm Hg)	3.3 (1–5)	8 (7–10)	<0.01	8 (7–9)	NS	9 (6–12)
Systemic vascular resistance (dynes·s^{-1}·cm^{-5})	1,943 (1,480–2,580)	1,284 (1,073–1,600)	<0.01	947 (782–1,028)	<0.01	886 (805–1,021)
Cardiac index (l·min^{-1}·m^{-2})	2.75 (1.97–3.33)	3.77 (3.26–4.05)	<0.01	4.40 (3.94–5.00)	<0.01	4.53 (3.96–4.97)

Wilcoxon signed-rank test (two-tailed).

*As compared with initial values.

†As compared with values after volume expansion.

‡NS = not significant.

Reproduced with permission from Groenendijk R, Trimbos MJ, Wallenberg HCS: Hemodynamic measurements in preeclampsia: Preliminary observations. Am J Obstet Gynecol 150:232, 1984.

similar to those occurring in the absence of magnesium sulfate therapy.[168] The patient usually receives an iv loading dose of 4 g in a 20% solution, administered over 5 minutes. Therapeutic blood levels are maintained by continuous infusion of 1–2 g·h^{-1}. In addition to its anticonvulsant properties, by causing peripheral arterial vasodilation, magnesium sulfate may affect the maternal hemodynamic state.[182] Magnesium ions cross the placenta readily and may lead to fetal and neonatal hypermagnesemia. There is a poor correlation between magnesium concentrations in the umbilical cord blood and the incidence of low Apgar scores and depression of ventilation at birth. It appears that the depression attributed to magnesium in earlier studies resulted from asphyxia or prematurity.[183]

Magnesium potentiates the duration and intensity of action of depolarizing and nondepolarizing muscle relaxants by decreasing the amount of acetylcholine liberated from the motor nerve terminals, diminishing the sensitivity of the end-plate to acetylcholine, and depressing the excitability of the skeletal muscle membrane.

The aim of fluid therapy is to increase the CVP and pulmonary capillary wedge pressure to the normal range (4–6 cm H_2O and 5–10 mm Hg, respectively) and to increase the urine output to 1 ml·kg^{-1}·h^{-1}. As already mentioned, this has been shown to improve the cardiac index and, interestingly, to decrease the mean systemic arterial pressure as well as systemic vascular resistance.[178] Approximately one third of the fluid infused may consist of 5% albumin solution to correct the decreased colloid osmotic pressure. The infusion should be administered slowly, over a period of several hours, to avoid fluid overload. In severe cases, careful monitoring of arterial pressure, central venous pressure, pulmonary artery and pulmonary capillary wedge pressure, urine output, and specific gravity should be started as soon as possible. Monitoring should be carried out in the postpartum period as well, preferably in the recovery room or intensive care setting. In patients with blood clotting abnormalities, the risk of inadvertent puncture of the carotid artery associated with internal jugular cannulation may be averted by inserting the line in the basilic or external jugular vein.

The antihypertensive therapy in pre-eclampsia is used to lessen the risk of cerebral hemorrhage in the mother while maintaining, even improving, tissue perfusion. Plasma volume expansion combined with vasodilation will fulfill these goals.[178] Hydralazine is the most commonly used vasodilator in pre-eclampsia because it increases uteroplacental and renal blood flows. It can be given orally, im, or iv. Nitroprusside, a potent vasodilator of resistance and capacitance vessels, having an immediate but evanescent action, is useful in preventing dangerous elevations in systemic and pulmonary blood pressure during laryngoscopy and intubation and is ideal for treatment of hypertensive emergencies. Its infusion can be decreased gradually in the interim when a longer-acting agent, such as hydralazine, is beginning to take effect. Infusion rates of nitroprusside less than 5–10 μg·kg^{-1}·min^{-1}, depending on the length of administration, can be maintained without undue risk of cyanide toxicity in the mother and fetus.[184] Trimethaphan, a ganglionic blocking agent, is particularly useful in hypertensive emergencies when cerebral edema and increased intracranial pressure are of particular concern, because it will not cause vasodilation in the brain. Other agents used less frequently to control maternal blood pressure in pre-eclampsia include alpha-methyldopa and clonidine (acting in the central nervous system), as well as nitroglycerin, ketanserin (a serotonin receptor antagonist), atenolol (a beta-adrenoreceptor antagonist), and labetalol (a nonselective beta blocker with some alpha$_1$-blocking effects).

Consumption coagulopathy may require corrective measures involving infusion of fresh whole blood, platelet concentrates, fresh frozen plasma, and cryoprecipitate. The administration of conduction anesthesia is contraindicated in patients with coagulation failure because of the increased risk of formation of an epidural hematoma, leading to permanent neurologic damage.

Anesthetic Management

Epidural anesthesia for labor and delivery should no longer be considered contraindicated, providing there is no clotting abnormality or plasma volume deficit. In volume-repleted patients positioned with left uterine displacement, epidural anesthesia does not cause unacceptable reduction in blood pressure and leads to a significant improvement in placental perfusion.[175,185] With the use of radioactive xenon, it was shown that the intervillous blood flow increased by approximately 75% after the induction of epidural analgesia (10 ml of bupivacaine 0.25%).[186] However, the total maternal body clearance of amide local anesthetics is prolonged in pre-eclampsia, and repeated administration of these drugs can lead to higher blood concentrations than in normotensive patients.[187] Spinal anesthesia should be used with great caution, if at all, because it produces severe alterations in cardiovascular dynamics resulting from sudden sympathetic blockade.

For cesarean section, the sensory level of regional anesthesia must extend to T3–4, making adequate fluid therapy and left uterine displacement even more vital. If hypotension occurs, its correction will require a reduced dose of ephedrine in view of the increased sensitivity to vasopressors.

General anesthesia in pre-eclamptic patients has its particular hazards. The rapid sequence induction of anesthesia and intubation of the trachea necessary to avoid aspiration are occasionally difficult because a swollen tongue, epiglottis, or pharynx distort the anatomy. In patients with impaired coagulation, laryngoscopy and intubation of the trachea may provoke profuse bleeding. Marked systemic and pulmonary hypertension occurring at intubation and extubation enhance the risk of cerebral hemorrhage and pulmonary edema (Fig. 46-10).[188,189] However, these hemodynamic changes can be minimized with appropriate antihypertensive therapy, such as administration of a trimethaphan or nitroprusside infusion. The use of ketamine and ergot alkaloids should be avoided. As already mentioned, magnesium sulfate may prolong the effects of all muscle relaxants through its actions on the myoneural junction. Therefore, relaxants should be administered with caution (using a nerve stimulator) to avoid overdosage. General anesthesia is indicated in acute emergencies, such as abruptio placentae, and in patients who do not meet the criteria for epidural anesthesia.

Antepartum Hemorrhage

Antepartum hemorrhage occurs most commonly in association with placenta previa (abnormal implantation on the lower uterine segment, and partial to total occlusion of the internal cervical os) and abruptio placentae.

Placenta previa occurs in 0.1–1.0% of all pregnancies, resulting in up to a 0.9% incidence of maternal and a 17–26% incidence of perinatal mortality.[190] Its presence occasionally leads to an abnormality in fetal presentation, such as transverse lie or breech. Placenta previa should be suspected in a patient presenting with painless bright red bleeding, usually after the 7th month of pregnancy. The diagnosis is confirmed by ultrasonography. Obstetric management is conservative if the bleeding is not profuse and the fetus is immature, in order to prolong pregnancy. In severe cases, or if the fetus is mature at the onset of symptoms, prompt delivery is indicated, usually by cesarean section. Hemorrhage may be severe even after delivery of the placenta because of poor contractility of the lower uterine segment, occasionally necessitating an emergency hysterectomy. The risk of severe hemorrhage following an attempted removal of a placenta previa is greatly increased in patients who have undergone prior uterine surgery, including cesarean section.[191,192] This is due to a higher incidence of placenta accreta, which results from the penetration of myometrium by placental villi. Following four or more previous cesarean deliveries, placenta accreta was reported to occur in 67% of patients with placenta previa.[191]

Abruptio placentae occurs in 0.2–2.4% of pregnant women, usually in the final 10 weeks of gestation. Approximately 50% of affected women are hypertensive.[193] Compli-

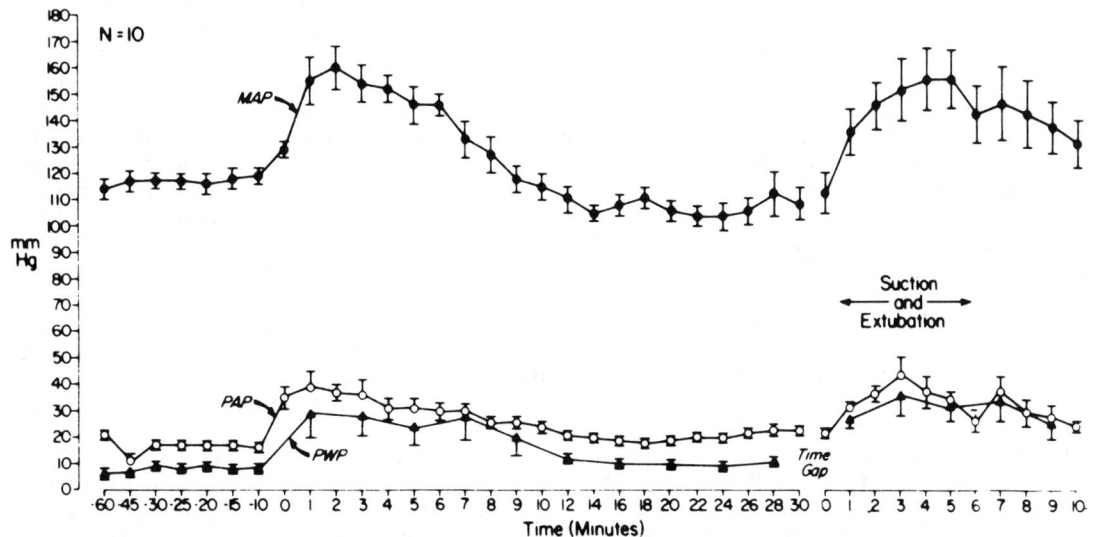

Figure 46-10. Mean and SE of mean arterial pressure (MAP), mean pulmonary artery pressure (PAP), and pulmonary wedge pressure (PWP) in patients with severe pre-eclampsia receiving thiopental and nitrous oxide (40%) with 0.5% halothane anesthesia for cesarean section. (Reprinted with permission from Hodgkinson R, Husain FJ, Hayashi RH: Systemic and pulmonary blood pressure during cesarean section in parturients with gestational hypertension. Can Anaesth Soc J 27:389, 1980.)

cations include Couvelaire uterus (*i.e.*, when extravasated blood dissects between the myometrial fibers), renal failure, DIC, and anterior pituitary necrosis (Sheehan syndrome). The maternal mortality is high, 1.8–11.0%, and the perinatal mortality is even higher, in excess of 50%.[190] The diagnosis of abruptio placentae is based on the presence of uterine tenderness and hypertonus and vaginal bleeding of dark, clotted blood. Bleeding may be concealed if the placental margins have remained attached to the uterine wall. If the blood loss is severe (2 liters or more), there may be changes in the maternal blood pressure and pulse rate indicative of hypovolemia. Fetal movements may increase in acute hypoxia or decrease if hypoxia is gradual. Fetal bradycardia and death may ensue, usually if maternal blood loss exceeds 2.5 liters.[194] Management of milder cases of abruption includes artificial rupture of amniotic membranes and oxytocin augmentation of labor, if required. In the presence of fetal distress, an emergency cesarean section should be performed.

The anesthesiologist plays a dual role in acute hemorrhage. He or she acts as a resuscitator of the mother. This may include the establishment of invasive monitoring (an arterial and central venous catheter are usually adequate) and blood volume replacement, preferably through 14- or 16-gauge cannulae. To correct clotting abnormalities, blood components such as fresh-frozen plasma, cryoprecipitate, and platelet concentrates may be required. The anesthesiologist also performs the traditional role of providing appropriate anesthesia for a cesarean section or, occasionally, a hysterectomy. General anesthesia is indicated in most cases because of the high risk of postpartum hemorrhage and clotting disorders. As usual, it should be preceded by adequate denitrogenation. In hypovolemic patients, induction should be accomplished with ketamine, 0.75–1.0 mg·kg^{-1}. As in all obstetric patients, proper precautions should be taken to prevent aspiration of gastric contents. These include the administration of a clear antacid, rapid sequence induction of anesthesia, and tracheal intubation with the application of cricoid pressure.

Heart Disease

Heart disease during pregnancy occurs in 0.4–4.1% of patients and is the leading nonobstetric cause of maternal mortality, ranging from 0.4% among patients in Class I or II of the New York Heart Association's functional classification to 6.8% among those in Classes III and IV.[195-197] The following lesions pose the greatest risk for the mother: pulmonary hypertension, particularly in Eisenmenger's syndrome; mitral stenosis with atrial fibrillation; tetralogy of Fallot; Marfan's syndrome; and coarctation of the aorta. Cardiac decompensation and death occur most commonly at the time of maximum hemodynamic stress, *i.e.*, in the third trimester of pregnancy, during labor and delivery, and during the immediate postpartum period. During labor, cardiac output increases above antepartum levels. Between contractions this increase is approximately 15% in the early first stage, about 30% during the late first stage, about 45% during the second stage, and, after delivery, 30–50%.[76] With each uterine contraction about 200 ml of blood is squeezed out of the uterus into the central circulation. Consequently, stroke volume, cardiac output, and left ventricular work increase, and each contraction consistently increases cardiac output by 10–25% above that between contractions.[198] The greatest increase occurs immediately after delivery of the placenta, when cardiac output increases to an average of 80% above

prepartum values, and in some patients it may increase by as much as 150%. These changes in cardiac output can be reduced by administration of regional anesthesia. In patients managed with continuous caudal anesthesia, cardiac output increased only 24% above prepartum control values during the second stage and 59% immediately post partum.[76]

Until 1960, rheumatic fever was responsible for almost 90% of the heart disease encountered in pregnant women.[199] Since that time, with improved medical care and surgical techniques, more patients with congenital disease survive to reach child-bearing age. Simultaneously, better living conditions and antibiotic treatment have reduced the incidence of rheumatic heart disease, and the ratio of rheumatic to congenital heart disease among the parturients has declined to 3 : 1.[199]

Rheumatic Heart Disease

Mitral stenosis is the sole or predominant valvular lesion in most parturients with rheumatic heart disease. The primary defect is obstruction to the diastolic blood flow from the left atrium to the left ventricle. This becomes hemodynamically significant when the valve orifice is diminished or the rate of blood flow through the constricted orifice is increased sufficiently to raise left atrial pressure and, consequently, pressure in the pulmonary veins and capillaries.

The physiologic changes of pregnancy usually aggravate the problems of mitral stenosis. The increased pulse rate necessitates a higher diastolic flow rate across the mitral orifice to maintain cardiac output. The flow rate is also augmented by the increased cardiac output that pregnancy demands. In the presence of significant mitral stenosis, these increases in flow rate can only be accomplished by an increase in left atrial and pulmonary venous pressure. The increased blood volume within the lungs that occurs in pregnancy may also add to the distention of pulmonary capillaries. Atrial fibrillation may occur in the presence of an enlarged left atrium, leading to pulmonary edema with an associated maternal mortality as high as 17%.[200] Cardioversion should be undertaken if drug therapy does not decrease the ventricular rate.[201] Mitral commissurotomy may be necessary because of symptoms of congestive heart failure or, less frequently, because of hemoptysis or emboli. When performed in the second or early third trimester, closed as well as open commissurotomies have been reported to be well tolerated by the mother and were accompanied by fetal survival in excess of 80%.[202] Fortunately, 90% of pregnant women with mitral stenosis are in functional Classes I and II. These patients generally tolerate child-bearing well. The relatively small number in functional Classes III and IV account for most maternal cardiac deaths.

Other valvular diseases, namely mitral regurgitation, aortic stenosis, or regurgitation, are much less frequent in pregnant cardiac patients. Together they account for 10–35% of all cases. Pure mitral regurgitation is rarely a problem. Properly managed patients can have repeated pregnancies without serious complications.[199] Similarly, pure aortic insufficiency rarely causes disability in the absence of bacterial endocarditis. Aortic stenosis is frequently associated with aortic insufficiency and mitral stenosis. Myocardial failure secondary to pure aortic stenosis is rare in patients of childbearing age because symptoms develop in most patients when they are in their 5th or 6th decades. Left ventricular hypertrophy and a relatively fixed stroke volume develop in those with significant aortic stenosis. These changes reduce their tolerance to decreases in systemic vascular resistance, bradycardia, and decreased venous return (and left ventricular filling).[203]

Continuous epidural block offers particular advantages to the pregnant cardiac patient. It not only eliminates pain and tachycardia throughout labor and delivery, but it also prevents the progressive increase in cardiac output and stroke volume that normally occurs in parturition.[76] It also abolishes the bearing-down reflex. In view of these advantages, continuous lumbar epidural analgesia is recommended for most pregnant women with rheumatic valvular diseases, whether they are to have vaginal or cesarean section deliveries, except for those with severe, symptomatic aortic stenosis. In patients with this condition, even transient episodes of hypotension may cause serious coronary hypoperfusion, arrhythmias, and even cardiac arrest. Intrathecal opioids have been used in an attempt to provide adequate obstetric analgesia without the risk of hypotension.[118,204] Morphine, 0.5–1.5 mg, or fentanyl, 37.5–50 μg, alone or in combination relieve the pain of uterine contractions. Pudendal block will be needed for delivery. Should general anesthesia be deemed necessary for cesarean section, the standard thiopental–nitrous oxide–halogenated anesthetic–muscle relaxant technique is recommended. In cases of severe mitral stenosis, etomidate, 0.2–0.3 mg·kg^{-1}, or a slow induction with halothane or iv fentanyl is preferred. In patients with severe aortic stenosis and evidence of left ventricular compromise, halogenated agents should be avoided.[203]

Congenital Heart Diseases

Patent ductus arteriosus, atrial septal defect, and ventricular septal defect are the more common congenital cardiovascular abnormalities. In all these conditions, anomalous communicating channels exist between the cardiac chambers or the great vessels. Normally, pressures on the left side of the circulation are higher than those on the right and there is a left-to-right shunt. Late in the natural history of these diseases, pulmonary hypertension may develop, causing a reversal of the shunt (Eisenmenger's syndrome).[205] Patients with Eisenmenger's syndrome rarely live beyond the age of 40. Pregnancy is poorly tolerated, because the gestational decrease in systemic vascular resistance in the presence of fixed pulmonary vascular resistance results in a significant increase in the right-to-left shunt.[206] Changes in systemic and pulmonary pressures are also likely to occur with the aortocaval compression near the end of pregnancy, hypotension caused by epidural or spinal anesthesia, and bearing-down efforts of parturition. Severe shunt disturbances induced by these changes may lead to further cyanosis, even death.

Tetralogy of Fallot is the most common cyanotic congenital heart defect.[205] It consists of an interventricular septal defect, pulmonary stenosis, displacement of the aortic orifice so that it overlies the ventricular septal defect, and right ventricular hypertrophy. The pulmonary stenosis leads to increases in right ventricular systolic pressure with dilation and hypertrophy of that chamber. Blood from the right ventricle is shunted through the septal defect, and the overriding aorta receives venous blood from this source and oxygenated blood from the left ventricle. Reduced arterial oxygenation leads to cyanosis, polycythemia, and clubbing. Symptoms develop in patients during the first few months of life, their severity being related to the degree of the pulmonic stenosis. However, the introduction of cardiac surgery has increased the number of patients surviving to child-bearing age.

Anesthesia for parturients with cyanotic heart disease should provide effective pain relief while avoiding hypotension, struggling, or coughing and eliminating bearing-down efforts, all of which could increase the right-to-left shunt. For labor, intrathecal opioids rather than epidural anesthesia should be administered. Light planes of general anesthesia are usually well tolerated for cesarean section.[203]

Preterm Delivery

Preterm labor and delivery present a significant challenge to the anesthesiologist, because the mother and the infant may be at risk.

The definition of prematurity was altered recently to distinguish between the preterm infant, born before the 37th week of gestation is completed, and the "small for gestational age" infant, who may be born at term but whose weight is more than 2 SD below the mean. Although preterm deliveries occur in 8–10% of all births, they account for approximately 80% of early neonatal deaths.[207] In general, the mortality and morbidity are higher among preterm infants than among small for gestational age babies of comparable weight.

Severe problems, including the respiratory distress syndrome, intracranial hemorrhage, hypoglycemia, hypocalcemia, and hyperbilirubinemia, are prone to develop in preterm infants. Fortunately, with improved neonatal intensive care, severe lasting impairment, such as cerebral palsy, mental retardation, or chronic lung disease, has become infrequent among the survivors.[208]

Obstetricians frequently try to inhibit preterm labor to enhance fetal lung maturity. Delaying delivery by even 24–48 hours may be beneficial if glucocorticoids are administered to the mother. Various agents have been used to suppress uterine activity (tocolysis), including ethanol, magnesium sulfate, prostaglandin inhibitors, beta-sympathomimetics, and calcium channel blockers. Beta-adrenergic drugs, such as ritodrine and terbutaline, are the most commonly used tocolytics. These agents are initially administered by an iv infusion at the rate of 0.05–0.1 mg·min^{-1} for ritodrine and 0.01 mg·min^{-1} for terbutaline.[209] Their predominant effect is beta$_2$-receptor stimulation, resulting in myometrial inhibition, vasodilation, and bronchodilation. Numerous maternal complications have been reported: hypotension, hypokalemia, hyperglycemia, myocardial ischemia, pulmonary edema, and death.[210] Complications also may occur because of interactions with anesthetic drugs and techniques. With the use of regional anesthesia, peripheral vasodilation caused by beta-adrenergic stimulation enhances the risk of hypotension. Acute prehydration must be managed carefully to avoid pulmonary edema. General anesthesia may be risky in the presence of pre-existing tachycardia, hypotension, and hypokalemia. It is better to avoid using halothane (cardiac dysrhythmias) as well as atropine and pancuronium (tachycardia). In nonemergency situations, delay of anesthesia by at least 3 hours from the cessation of tocolysis will allow beta-mimetic effects to dissipate. Potassium supplementation is not necessary.[211]

It has become axiomatic that the premature infant is more vulnerable than the term newborn to the effects of drugs used in obstetric analgesia and anesthesia. However, there have been few systematic studies to determine the maternal and fetal pharmacokinetics and dynamics of drugs throughout gestation. There are several postulated causes of enhanced drug sensitivity in the preterm newborn: less protein available for drug binding; higher levels of bilirubin, which may compete with the drug for protein binding; greater drug access to the central nervous system because of a poorly developed blood-brain barrier; greater total body water and lower fat content; and a decreased ability to metabolize and excrete drugs. However, these deficiencies of the preterm infant should not be as serious as we have been led to believe. Although the serum albumin and alpha$_1$-acid glycoprotein concentrations are lower in the preterm fetus, this would primarily affect drugs that are highly bound to these proteins. However, most drugs used in anesthesia exhibit only low to moderate degrees of binding in the fetal serum: approximately 50% for etidocaine and bupivacaine, 25% for lidocaine, 52% for meperidine, and 75% for thiopental.

The placenta efficiently eliminates fetal bilirubin. Thus, the hyperbilirubinemia of prematurity normally occurs in the postpartum period. With the exception of diazepam, bilirubin will not compete with anesthetic drugs because most are bound to other serum proteins, e.g., meperidine and local anesthetics to alpha$_1$-glycoproteins, d-tubocurarine to gamma-globulin.

It seems likely that the human blood-brain barrier develops substantially in early gestation.[212] Thus, factors such as tissue affinity changes may account for differences between immature and mature animals in brain uptake of highly lipid-soluble drugs.

Greater total body water in the preterm fetus results in a greater volume of distribution for drugs. Thus, to achieve equal blood concentrations, the immature fetus will have to receive a greater amount of drug transplacentally than will the mature fetus. A study of age-related toxicity of lidocaine in sheep showed that the greater the volume of distribution, the greater the dose required to achieve toxic blood concentrations of the drug.[67]

Decreased ability to metabolize or excrete drugs, associated with prematurity, is certainly not a universal phenomenon. In a study comparing the pharmacokinetics of lidocaine in preterm newborns and adults, plasma clearance was similar in both groups.[64] Neonates excreted much more unchanged lidocaine than did adults. Similarly, although meperidine metabolism is more limited in the neonate than in the adult, urinary excretion of the unchanged drug is greater in the neonate.

Another factor is gestational changes in maternal serum albumin and alpha$_1$-acid glycoprotein concentrations, which tend to decrease. Serial determinations of protein binding of diazepam, phenytoin, and valproic acid in the maternal serum, performed in early (8–16 weeks), mid- (17–32 weeks), and late pregnancy, showed a progressive increase in the unbound fraction of these drugs.[213] That would increase drug availability for placental transfer. Placental permeability itself increases as pregnancy progresses because of the increased area and decreased thickness of tissue barriers.[62]

In a largely ignored, prospective study of more than 1000 premature labors, during which mothers received meperidine alone or with scopolamine, medication had no effect on the perinatal death rate, the incidence of respiratory distress syndrome, Apgar scores, the need for resuscitation, and the incidence of severe neurologic defects within 1 year.[214]

Therefore, it appears that in selection of the anesthetic drugs and techniques for delivery of a preterm infant, concerns regarding drug effects on the newborn are far less important than prevention of asphyxia and trauma to the fetus. For labor and vaginal delivery, well-conducted epidural anesthesia is advantageous in providing good perineal relaxation. One should ascertain that the fetus is neither hypoxic nor acidotic prior to induction of epidural blockade. Asphyxia results in a redistribution of fetal cardiac output, which increases oxygen delivery to vital organs such as the brain, heart, and adrenals. The preterm fetus exposed to local anesthetics, particularly lidocaine, may lose its cardiovascular adaptation to asphyxia and its condition may deteriorate further.[215] Preterm infants with breech presentation are usually delivered by cesarean section. General anesthesia with uterine relaxation, provided by a halogenated drug, will facilitate delivery of the aftercoming head.

FETAL AND MATERNAL MONITORING

The development of biophysical and biochemical monitoring of the fetus during labor and delivery has had a tremendous impact on obstetric practice over the last 20 years. Monitoring procedures are now performed routinely, and it is important that the anesthesiologist understand the basic principles of the technology, as well as the interpretation of results, because they relate to both mother and fetus.

During the same period there has been an explosion in monitoring technology in the fields of anesthesiology and intensive care. The mother with serious medical problems requiring intensive care or the one whose baby is delivered in an operating room under an anesthesiologist's care is subject to the same standards of monitoring as any other surgical patient. It is generally agreed that the use of intensive peripartum monitoring is appropriate in a "high-risk" pregnancy. In contrast, patients with routine labor are frequently observed in the same way that patients were many generations ago, i.e., with intermittent blood pressure readings. With the growing sophistication of electronic devices, and specifically the science of telemetry, we can look forward to better surveillance of both mother and fetus without the loss of maternal freedom and activity that monitoring currently entails.

The importance of maternal ECG and blood pressure recording during induction and maintenance of epidural anesthesia has already been discussed. Noninvasive maternal oxygen saturation monitoring (by pulse oximetry) during labor and delivery is easily performed and should provide useful information about the degree of pain and adequacy of analgesia.[216]

The early reports of continuous fetal heart rate monitoring came from Hon in 1958, who also recognized variable decelerations associated with umbilical cord compression. In 1971 and 1972, those working in this field met at two international conferences and agreed on nomenclature and standards that are still in use today.[217]

Biophysical Monitoring

A fetal monitor is a two-channel recorder of fetal heart rate and uterine activity. In the direct system, the fetal ECG is obtained from an electrode attached to the presenting part. Intrauterine pressure is measured continuously with a transducer connected to a saline-filled catheter that is inserted transcervically. Direct monitoring is quantitative but requires rupture of the membranes and a cervical dilation of at least 1.5 cm. In addition, the presenting part must dip into the true pelvis. Indirect fetal monitoring uses data obtained from transducers secured to the mother's abdomen with adjustable straps. The following three systems can be used to obtain fetal heart signals: ECG, phonocardiography, and ultrasound cardiography. The first two approaches are impractical. Fetal QRS complexes obtained with abdominal electrodes are too small to distinguish from the maternal tracing, whereas phonocardiography provides a poor signal-to noise ratio. Thus, ultrasound cardiography is the most commonly used indirect method today. Uterine activity is monitored with a tocodynamometer triggered by the changing shape of the uterus during the contraction. Indirect monitoring is mostly quantitative. Its advantage is that it can be applied without rupture of membranes, even before the onset of labor.

The following variables are taken into account when fetal well-being is determined: baseline heart rate, beat-to-beat variability, periodic patterns, and uterine activity.

The baseline fetal heart rate is measured between contractions. It is 120–160 beats·min^{-1} in the normal fetus. An acceleration of fetal heart rate in response to fetal stimulation, such as during vaginal examination or fetal capillary blood sampling, is a reassuring sign that the fetus is not acidotic. Persistently elevated rates may be associated with chronic fetal distress, maternal fever, or administration of drugs such as ephedrine and atropine. Abnormally low rates may be encountered in fetuses with congenital heart block or as a late occurrence during the course of fetal hypoxia and acidosis.

The baseline fetal heart rate tracing normally is not flat. The variability reflects the beat-to-beat adjustments of the parasympathetic and sympathetic nervous systems to a variety of internal and external stimuli. When these divisions of the nervous system are functioning normally, variability is also normal, with the fetus being in good condition. Fetal central nervous system depression by asphyxia may decrease baseline variability. Therefore, a smooth fetal heart rate tracing may be an ominous finding. Studies comparing beat-to-beat variability with fetal acid-base analysis indicate a good correlation between the two parameters.[218] However, drugs can also decrease fetal heart rate variability by depressing mechanisms in the central nervous system that integrate cardiac control (tranquilizers, opioids, barbiturates, anesthetics) or by blocking the transmission of control impulses to the cardiac pacemaker (atropine). In contrast, ephedrine administration increases beat-to-beat variability.[219]

Periodic fetal heart rate patterns consist of decelerations or accelerations, of relatively brief duration, in association with uterine contractions (Fig. 46-11). There are three major forms of fetal heart rate deceleration: early, late, and variable. Early decelerations are U-shaped, with the heart rate usually not decreasing to less than 100 beats·min^{-1}. The fetal heart begins to slow with the onset of the contraction, the low point coincides with the peak of the contraction, and the rate generally returns to the baseline as the uterus relaxes. This type of deceleration has been attributed to fetal head compression, leading to increased vagal tone. It is not ameliorated by increasing fetal oxygenation but is blocked

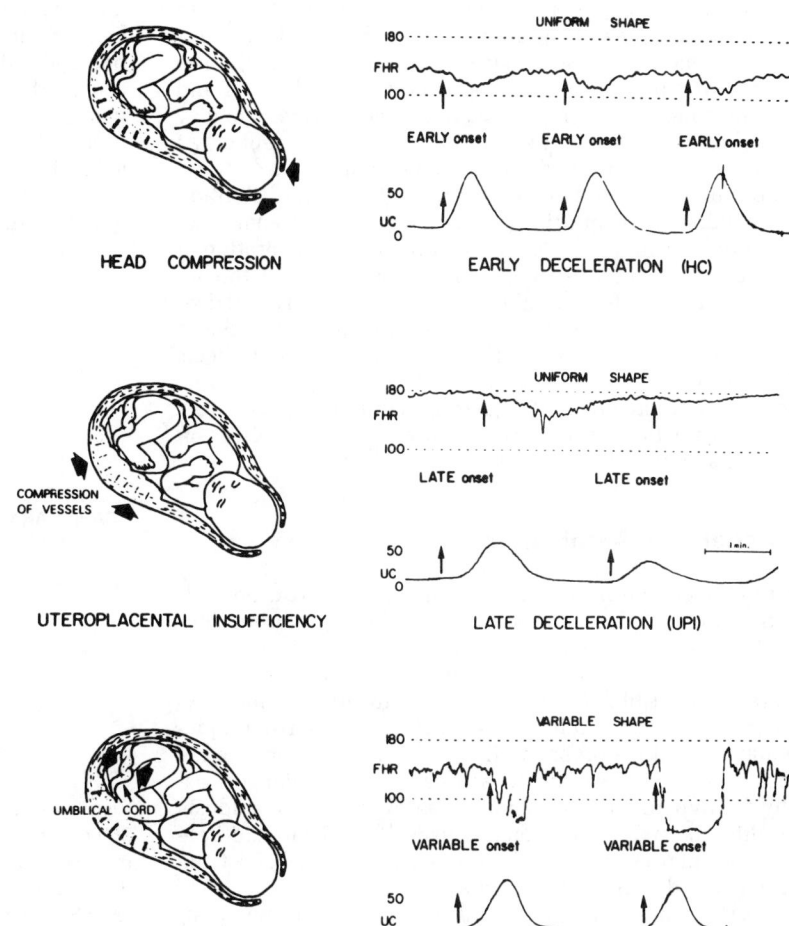

Figure 46-11. Classification and mechanism of fetal heart rate patterns. (Reprinted with permission from Hon EH: An Introduction to Fetal Heart Rate Monitoring, p 29. New Haven, Harty Press, 1969.)

by atropine administration. Early decelerations are transitory and well tolerated by the fetus because there is no systemic hypoxemia or acidosis.[220]

Late decelerations are also U-shaped. They begin 20–30 seconds or more after the onset of uterine contraction, and the low point of the deceleration occurs well after the peak of the contraction. Myocardial ischemia resulting from uteroplacental insufficiency is believed to cause this pattern. The pattern of late deceleration can be corrected by improving fetal oxygenation, which may be accomplished with oxygen administration to the mother, correction of maternal hypotension, or aortocaval compression, or by taking measures that decrease uterine activity. If this pattern is repetitive, continuous, and progressive in severity, there is a significant correlation with fetal acidosis. Uncorrectable late decelerations, or late decelerations that worsen despite corrective measures, are an indication for prompt delivery.[217]

Variable decelerations, which result from umbilical cord compression, are the most common periodic patterns observed in the intrapartum period. They are variable in shape and onset, the rate usually decreasing to less than 100 beats·min^{-1}. Although the initial fetal heart rate changes are of reflex origin, if the cord compressions are frequent or prolonged, fetal asphyxia may result in direct myocardial depression.

Cervical dilation and descent of the presenting part during the first stage of labor result primarily from uterine contractions. During the active phase, contractions should occur every 2–3 minutes, with peak intrauterine pressures of 50–80 mm Hg and resting pressures of 5–20 mm Hg. Uterine activity may be abnormally elevated in association with abruptio placentae or the injudicious use of oxytocics. Tetanic uterine contractions have been reported after the use of methoxamine, a pure alpha agonist.[221] In the first and second trimesters of pregnancy, increased uterine tone may be induced with ketamine in a dose-dependent manner. At term, ketamine does not appear to have this effect.[222]

Poor uterine contractility may result from overdistention (polyhydramnios, multiple pregnancy) or maintenance of the supine position.[223] During early labor, administration of opioids, sedatives, or regional anesthesia may delay the onset of the active phase by diminishing uterine activity. However, in large, well-controlled studies, regional anesthesia instituted during the active phase had no untoward effects on uterine activity as long as hypotension and the supine position were avoided.[224] The addition of epinephrine to a local anesthetic solution may have an inhibitory effect on uterine activity.[225]

Biochemical Monitoring

Before labor, the normal fetus is neither hypoxic nor acidotic. During labor many events, including uterine contractions, cord compression, aortocaval compression, and maternal hypotension from any cause, may decrease uteroplacental blood flow sufficiently to produce fetal hypoxia and acidosis. Acidosis associated with short-term placental hypoperfusion primarily results from carbon dioxide accumulation ("respiratory acidosis"). In prolonged asphyxia, hypercarbia is accompanied by metabolic acidosis resulting from anaerobic metabolism. Thus, fetal acid-base indices, such as Pco_2 and base deficit, usually reflect the degree and duration of asphyxia.

Assessment of acid-base status of the fetus became possible in the early 1960s, when Saling developed a fetal capillary blood-sampling technique.[226] Blood is usually obtained

from the scalp but may also be sampled from the breech. It is collected into a heparinized glass capillary tube, and pH, Pco_2, Po_2, and base deficit are determined immediately with an appropriate electrode system adapted to small sample size.

This technique has been validated in animal and clinical studies. It has been shown in fetal monkeys that the blood values obtained from the scalp are closely correlated with those in simultaneously obtained samples from the carotid artery and jugular vein.[227] A fetal capillary blood pH of 7.25 is the lowest limit of normal. Values between 7.24 and 7.20 are considered "preacidotic," whereas a pH below 7.20 indicates fetal acidosis. Several studies correlated the last predelivery fetal pH with the Apgar score at 1 or 2 minutes after birth.[228,229] Ninety-two per cent of infants scored 7 or better when the pH was above 7.25. With the pH below 7.16, 80% of babies scored 6 or less.[228] In general, when the pH is normal immediately before delivery, one can assume that the baby will be in good condition. However, there is a small incidence of false-positive and false-negative results. In one study, normal pH was associated with low Apgar scores (false-positive results) in approximately 10% of cases (Fig. 46-12).[229] In approximately 8% of cases (false-negative results), a vigorous infant was born despite a low capillary scalp pH. The major factors contributing to false-positive outcomes are administration of sedative drugs or anesthetics, infection, airway obstruction, and congenital anomalies. False-negative outcomes are usually associated with maternal acidosis, which may occur after prolonged labor, excessive muscular activity, or inadequate fluid and caloric intakes. Obtaining a maternal sample (arterial or free-flowing venous blood) for the evaluation of the acid-base status helps identify this group. If the fetal acidosis is of maternal origin, the mother's blood will show a large base deficit value, and the difference between the fetal and maternal base deficit values (ΔBD) will be small. In contrast, fetal acidosis resulting from prolonged asphyxia is reflected in a large fetal but a normal maternal base deficit value; consequently, ΔBD will be large. Fetal acidosis of maternal origin

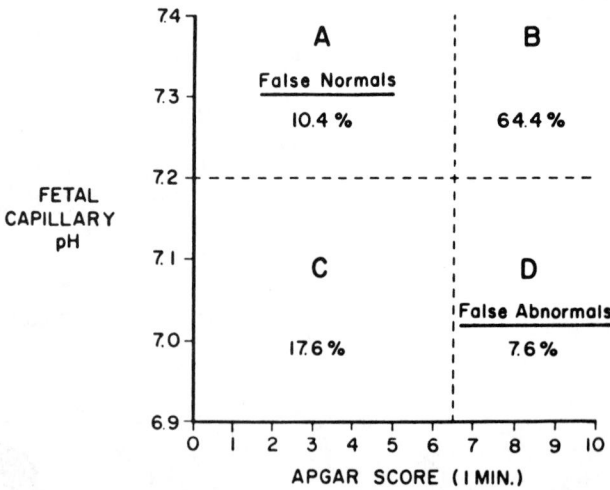

Figure 46-12. Fetal pH as an index of infant's condition at birth in 355 patients during labor. Segment *A*: depressed infants with normal pH; segment *B*: vigorous infants with normal pH; segment *C*: depressed infants with low pH; segment *D*: vigorous infants with low pH. (Reprinted with permission from Bowe ET, Beard RW, Finster M et al: Reliability of fetal blood sampling. Am J Obstet Gynecol 107:279, 1970.)

can be treated by correcting the maternal acid-base imbalance.

Complications

There are data correlating direct fetal monitoring with maternal infection.[230,231] However, conclusions from these reports are tenuous because most of the affected patients had prolonged rupture of membranes. A less frequent complication of internal monitoring is uterine perforation. The firm plastic cannula used to introduce the intra-amniotic pressure catheter has been implicated.

Fetal complications related to scalp electrodes are ecchymoses, lacerations, leakage of CSF, osteomyelitis of the skull, sepsis, scalp abscesses, and a case of meningitis with ventriculitis and hydrocephalus. The overall incidence of these complications is unknown. Scalp abscess is the most commonly reported. One publication indicates that with the use of a coil electrode, it occurs in 5.4% of cases.[232] In most reviews the incidence is less than 1%.[233]

Scalp capillary blood sampling can also lead to fetal complications. The two major ones are hemorrhage and abscess formation. Bleeding from the sampling site is usually self-limited, but massive hemorrhage resulting in severe anemia and, rarely, neonatal death has been reported. After a sample has been obtained, pressure should be applied to the scalp with a sponge through at least two contractions. Occasionally, prolonged pressure or a skin clip may be necessary to achieve hemostasis. Prenatal and postnatal bleeding from a sampling incision may be the first manifestation of a severe coagulation disorder.[234] Excessive bleeding from the vagina after scalp capillary blood sampling may be of fetal origin. Thus, testing for fetal hemoglobin is advised in these circumstances.

The costs and benefits of fetal monitoring are still being questioned. There is a conflict between the desire for a "natural" childbirth experience and the physician's concern for maternal and fetal safety. It is generally agreed that the use of intensive intrapartum monitoring is appropriate in high-risk pregnancies. Debate continues concerning the benefits of these methods to low-risk fetuses. A recent large randomized controlled trial comparing continuous electronic fetal monitoring with traditional intermittent auscultation of the fetal heart (with an option to measure fetal scalp capillary blood pH) showed that neonatal seizures and abnormal neurologic signs occurred twice as frequently in the group with intermittent auscultation. In addition, the study showed no difference in the cesarean section rate between the two groups.[235]

ANESTHETIC COMPLICATIONS

General Anesthesia

The changes in the respiratory tract associated with pregnancy, such as lowered FRC and mucosal congestion, may enhance problems in the patient awakening from anesthesia. These may include laryngeal spasm or edema after extubation, rapid desaturation secondary to soft-tissue airway obstruction or opioid depression of respiration, and the ever-present chance of vomiting or regurgitation, with aspiration of gastric contents. The anesthesiologist may be deceived by the patient's restlessness and agitation on emergence from anesthesia when she is frequently anxious, in

pain, and relatively unsedated. Before extubation of the trachea she should be observed carefully until she is conscious and pharyngeal and laryngeal reflexes have fully returned.

Pulmonary Aspiration

As already described, aspiration of gastric contents contributes seriously to maternal complications and deaths. To decrease the incidence of this complication, efforts should be directed toward careful preoperative assessment of obstetric patients, the training of obstetric anesthesia personnel, and the use of regional anesthesia where appropriate, as well as the measures already outlined in the section on the physiologic changes of pregnancy.[236]

Regional Anesthesia

Complications of regional anesthesia can be separated into those that occur concurrently with the block, such as hypotension, total spinal anesthesia, convulsions induced by local anesthetics, nausea, vomiting, and breathing difficulties, and those arising later, such as headache or effects of nerve injury.

Hypotension

Hypotension is the most likely side-effect to occur on induction of either spinal or epidural anesthesia, although the rapidity of onset and severity are more controllable in the case of epidural block, with which a test dose and subsequent slow incremental injections of drug are usually used. The best method of decreasing the incidence and morbidity of this complication is to institute preventive measures before induction, such as prehydration, left uterine displacement, and administration of ephedrine. Treatment includes increased displacement of the uterus, rapid iv infusion of fluids, small iv doses of ephedrine (5–10 mg), oxygen given by face mask, and placement of the patient in the Trendelenburg position. Rapid reversal of hypotension usually prevents serious sequelae in either mother or neonate.[237]

Total Spinal Anesthesia

High or total spinal anesthesia is relatively rare, occurring after excessive spread of local anesthetic in the subarachnoid or epidural space. Accidental puncture of the dura during attempted or continuous epidural block (catheter migration) may also lead to this complication, especially when the aberrant catheter position is not recognized. Most important is prompt diagnosis and treatment, which mandates the presence of trained personnel in the labor suite. The airway should be quickly established and protected by means of an endotracheal tube while ventilation with oxygen is applied. Left uterine displacement and the Trendelenburg position should be used and fluids and ephedrine given to maintain normal blood pressure. With proper management, the outcome for mother and baby should be good.

Convulsions

High blood levels of local anesthetics may result from accidental intravascular injection (through a needle or catheter), accumulation of drugs after repeated epidural or caudal injection, or rapid absorption of local anesthetic from a highly vascular site of injection. Thus, paracervical and pudendal blocks can be implicated, as well as epidural techniques.

When any major nerve block is undertaken, the equipment and drugs needed for resuscitation (including means for establishing the airway and administering positive pressure ventilation with 100% oxygen, a laryngoscope, endotracheal tubes, oral airways, an oxygen source, and an ambu bag with mask) should always be available. In addition, a suction device should be on hand, as well as the following drugs: thiopental or diazepam, atropine, and succinylcholine. It is necessary to establish a venous access for these drugs before the local anesthetic is injected. The best way of preventing systemic toxic reactions is to adhere strictly to recommended dosages and avoid intravascular injection, as outlined previously. Despite precautions, a few patients may have life-threatening convulsions and, more rarely, cardiovascular collapse. Convulsions should be treated by protecting the airway and establishing effective ventilation of the lungs, because hypoxia and acidosis develop very rapidly. If thiopental or diazepam is administered iv to stop convulsions, very small doses (50–100 mg and 5–10 mg, respectively) are adequate and will help avoid cardiorespiratory depression. If cardiovascular collapse occurs, cardiopulmonary resuscitation and cesarean delivery should be started immediately, the latter to relieve aortocaval compression and ensure the effectiveness of cardiac massage.[238]

Headache

Unfortunately, later development of headache, resulting from puncture of the dura mater and subsequent leakage of CSF from the subarachnoid space, is quite common in parturients. The incidence is related to the diameter of the puncture hole, being very high after use of a 16-gauge needle (more than 70%) and as little as 1% with a small spinal needle (25 or 26 gauge). The shape of the needle tip is also of importance. As already stated, the incidence of cephalalgia is reduced with the use of a pencil-point (Whitacre) needle as compared with the diamond-shaped (Quincke) tip.[92] Bed rest, hydration, and analgesics are beneficial when the discomfort is mild to moderate, but severe headaches that do not respond to conservative measures are best treated by an autologous blood patch in the epidural space. With an aseptic technique, 10–15 ml of the patient's blood is injected epidurally near the site of the dural tear. This procedure has a success rate of more than 90%.[239] The iv injection of caffeine sodium benzoate in doses of 500 mg has been shown to alleviate headache in 70% of cases.[240] When an epidural catheter is in place after delivery, 40–60 ml of preservative-free saline or 10–15 ml of autologous blood may be injected through it, before its removal. This effectively lowers the incidence of severe headache.[241]

Nerve Injury

Although rare, neurologic sequelae have been reported after administration of major regional blocks with all the known local anesthetics. Pressure exerted by a needle or catheter on spinal roots produces immediate pain, and the irritant should be withdrawn quickly. Infections such as epidural or caudal abscess or meningitis are very rare and may be secondary to infection at another site. Epidural hematoma can occur as a result of coagulation defects. Unfortunately, recovery from trauma to the nerve roots may be prolonged for weeks or months. Other causes of nerve injury, such as

fetal compression of the lumbosacral trunk or prolonged use of the lithotomy position for bearing down in the second stage of labor, should be kept in mind.

NEWBORN RESUSCITATION IN THE DELIVERY ROOM

Of the approximately 3.5 million babies born in the United States each year, 6% require resuscitation in the delivery room. Among those weighing 1500 g or less, the incidence is approximately 80%.[242]

The following factors may contribute to depression of the newborn: drugs used in labor or during delivery, including anesthetic agents; trauma of precipitate labor and operative obstetrics; and birth asphyxia, meaning hypoxia and hypercapnea with acidosis.

Fetal Asphyxia

Fetal asphyxia, the best-studied cause of neonatal depression, generally develops as a result of interference with maternal or fetal perfusion of the placenta. As stated previously, the normal fetus is neither hypoxic nor acidotic before labor. Experimental data have revealed that transplacental gradients for pH and P_{CO_2} are approximately 0.05 pH units and 5 mm Hg, respectively.[243] Although oxygen tension is low, oxygen saturation is relatively high (80–85%) by virtue of the shift to the left of the fetal dissociation curve for hemoglobin.

During labor, uterine contractions decrease the blood flow through the intervillous space of the placenta or may stop it completely. On the fetal side, cord compression occurs during the final stages of approximately one third of vaginal deliveries. Thus, mild degrees of hypoxia and acidosis occur even during normal labor and delivery and play an important role in initiation of ventilation.[244] On average, healthy vigorous infants (at birth) have an oxygen saturation of 21%, a pH of 7.24, and a $Paco_2$ of 56 mm Hg.

Severe fetal asphyxia occasionally develops as a result of fetal and maternal complications such as a tight nuchal cord, prolapsed cord, premature separation of the placenta, uterine hyperactivity, or maternal hypotension.

During asphyxia, changes in blood gases and hydrogen ion concentration are rapid. Investigations performed on newborn animals have shown that the oxygen content of arterial blood decreases to near zero in 2.5 minutes, whereas pH declines by nearly 0.1 pH unit·min^{-1}.[245] The decrease in pH results from accumulation of carbon dioxide as well as of end products of anaerobic glycolysis. After oxygen stores are exhausted, the documented ability of fetal brain and myocardium to derive energy from anaerobic metabolism is essential for survival. However, anaerobic glycolysis is pH dependent, and its rate is greatly diminished when the pH decreases below 7.0.[246] Other untoward effects of severe hypoxia and acidosis include depression of the myocardium resulting from a decrease in its responsiveness to catecholamines; a shift to the right of the fetal dissociation curve for hemoglobin, resulting in reduced oxygen-carrying capacity; and an increase in pulmonary vascular resistance, which plays an important role during circulatory readjustment after birth.

Ventilatory and cardiovascular responses to controlled experimental asphyxia have been investigated extensively in newborn monkeys (Fig. 46-13).[247] During the initial phase of asphyxia, the unanesthetized animal exhibits respiratory

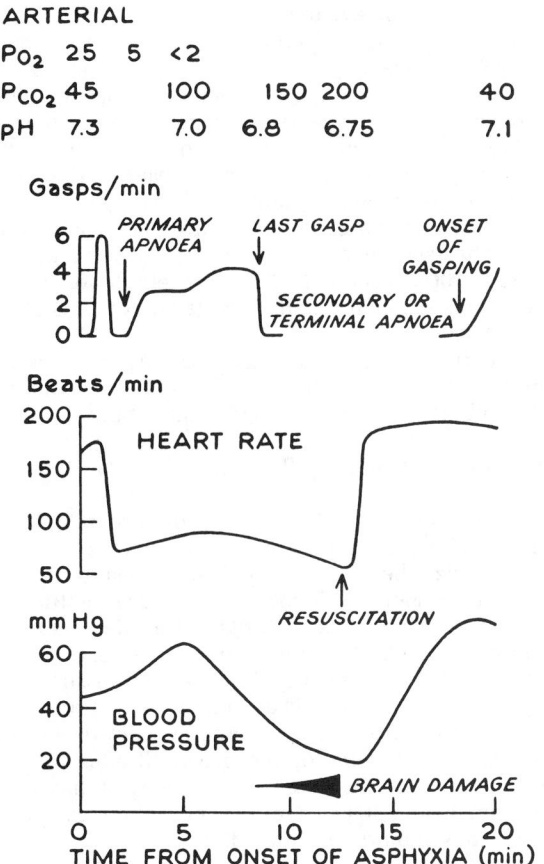

Figure 46-13. Schematic diagram of changes in rhesus monkeys during asphyxia and with resuscitation by positive pressure ventilation. Brain damage was assessed by histologic examination some weeks or months later. (Reprinted with permission from Dawes GS: Foetal and Neonatal Physiology: A Comparative Study of the Changes at Birth, p. 149. Chicago, Year Book Medical Publishers, 1968.)

efforts that increase in depth and frequency for up to 3 minutes. This period, called primary hyperpnea, is followed by primary apnea, which lasts for approximately 1 minute. Rhythmic gasping then begins and is maintained at a fairly constant rate of about 6 gasps·min⁻¹ for 4–5 minutes. Thereafter, the gasps become weaker and slower. Their cessation at approximately 8.5 minutes after the onset of asphyxia marks the beginning of secondary apnea. Administration of opioids and systemic anesthetic agents to the mother can abolish the period of primary hyperpnea and prolong primary apnea.

There is a linear relationship between the duration of asphyxia and the onset of gasping and rhythmic spontaneous breathing. In the newborn monkey, for each minute of asphyxia beyond the last gasp, 2 additional minutes of artificial ventilation are required before gasping begins again and 4 minutes before rhythmic breathing is established.[248] This indicates that the longer artificial ventilation of the lungs is delayed during secondary apnea, the longer it will take to resuscitate the infant. Furthermore, in the newborn monkey, prolongation of asphyxia for 4 minutes beyond the last gasp is accompanied by extensive damage to brain stem nuclei, whereas animals resuscitated before the last gasp show little or no brain damage. Thus, a relatively short delay in resuscitation can have serious sequelae.

Neonatal Adaptations at Birth

During this period, and through the early hours and days of life, many morphologic and functional changes take place, with the cardiovascular and ventilatory systems undergoing the most dramatic alterations. In the normal newborn, two events occur almost simultaneously, and within seconds of delivery: the arrest of umbilical circulation through the placenta and expansion of the lungs. These events change the fetal circulation toward the adult type. Survival of the neonate depends primarily on prompt expansion of the lungs and establishment of effective ventilation.

The onset of ventilation and expansion of the lungs opens up the pulmonary vascular bed, resulting in decreased resistance and a significant increase in pulmonary blood flow. A fetal pulmonary blood flow of 30–40 ml·kg⁻¹·min⁻¹ increases to approximately 300 ml·kg⁻¹·min⁻¹ shortly after birth, not only because of the mechanical effects of lung expansion, but also because of the direct effects of oxygen and carbon dioxide on the blood vessels. Pulmonary vascular resistance decreases as oxygen tension increases and carbon dioxide levels decrease. As soon as pulmonary perfusion increases, the foramen ovale, which constitutes a communication between the inferior vena cava and the left atrium, undergoes functional closure because of pressure changes across the valve of the foramen (see Fig. 46-5). Cessation of the umbilical circulation reduces pressure in the inferior vena cava and right atrium, whereas the increase in pulmonary blood flow increases venous return and pressure in the left atrium. The ductus arteriosus does not constrict completely or abruptly after birth; functional closure may take hours, even days. Thus, shunting still occurs in the neonatal period, its direction depending on relative resistances in the pulmonary and systemic vascular beds. The smooth muscle of the ductus arteriosus constricts in response to increased oxygen tension in the newborn's blood. Catecholamines, which exist in increased concentrations in the newborn, particularly during the first 3 hours of life, also constrict the ductus arteriosus. In contrast, prostaglandins PGI_2 and PGE_2, produced by the wall of the ductus arteriosus, relax the ductal smooth muscle. Administration of prostaglandin synthesis inhibitors to fetal animals promotes constriction of the ductus arteriosus. Thus, control of the ductus arteriosus involves a balance between constricting and relaxing substances.[249]

Cardiac output and its distribution also increase; left ventricular output increases from approximately 150 to 400 ml·kg⁻¹·min⁻¹, whereas right ventricular output increases less significantly. Cardiac output changes closely parallel the increase in oxygen consumption.[250] The redistribution of cardiac output also leads to increases in myocardial, renal, and gastrointestinal blood flow and decreases in cerebral, adrenal, and carotid flows.

During fetal life, respiratory gas exchange takes place through the placenta. Delivery of the infant's trunk relieves the thoracic compression that occurs as the infant passes through the birth canal, and the thorax and the lungs expand. Most infants initiate respiratory efforts a few seconds after birth. After the first inspiration, a cry usually results, as the infant exhales against a partially closed glottis, thus increasing intrathoracic pressure significantly. Negative pressures in excess of 40 cm H_2O bring about the initial entry of air into fluid-filled alveoli. In the mature, normal neonate, the lungs expand almost completely after the first few breaths, and the pressure-volume changes achieved with each respiration resemble those of the adult. After lung expansion, the FRC approximates 70 ml in the term newborn and changes little over the first 6 days of life. The tidal volume varies between 10 and 30 ml, the breathing frequency ranges from 30 to 60 breaths·min^{-1}, and minute ventilation exceeds 500 ml.

It has been difficult to evaluate the factors responsible for the initial respiratory efforts to achieve expansion of the lungs and for the subsequent maintenance of rhythmic respiration because many stimuli contribute simultaneously. Asphyxia is considered the principal driving force.

After delivery and prompt lung expansion, reoxygenation is rapid, but it takes 2 or 3 hours to achieve a relatively normal acid-base balance, primarily by pulmonary excretion of carbon dioxide. By 24 hours the healthy newborn infant has reached the same acid-base state as that of the mother before labor.

Resuscitation

The delivery room must be prepared for adequate and prompt treatment of severe depression at birth. All members of the delivery room team should be trained in resuscitation methods because both mother and baby may have difficulty at the same time.[251] Every piece of apparatus necessary for emergency resuscitation should be checked carefully before delivery (Table 46-4). An overview of resuscitation in the delivery room is depicted in Figure 46-14.[251]

Initial Treatment and Evaluation of All Infants

Immediately after delivery, the baby should be held head down while the cord is clamped and cut. The infant should then be placed supine under a radiant heat source, the head kept low with a slight lateral tilt, and its skin should be dried promptly. A nurse or assistant should listen to the heart beat immediately, indicating the rate by finger movement. If help is not available, the rate can be detected from pulsation of the umbilical cord. At the same time, the resuscitator should aspirate the mouth, pharynx, and nose with a catheter. This suction should be brief, not exceeding 30 seconds. Slapping the infant's soles lightly or rubbing its back frequently aids in initiating a deep breath or cry.

The initial appraisal of the newborn should start from the moment of birth, with particular attention paid to the first

---

TABLE 46-4. Resuscitation Equipment in the Delivery Room

Radiant warmer
Suction with manometer and suction trap
Suction catheters
Wall oxygen with flow meter
Resuscitation bag (≤750 ml)
Infant face masks
Infant oropharygeal airways
Endotracheal tubes, 2.5, 3.0, 3.5, and 4.0 mm
Endotracheal tube stylets
Laryngoscope(s) and blade(s)
Sterile umbilical artery catheterization tray
Needles, syringes, three-way stopcocks
Medications and solutions:
    1:10,000 epinephrine
    Naloxone hydrochloride
    Sodium bicarbonate
    Volume expanders

---

few breaths and the evenness and ease of respiration. Most infants are vigorous and cough or cry within seconds of delivery. Their heart rate is above 100 beats·min^{-1}. The administration of free-flowing oxygen will rapidly improve their oxygenation and decrease pulmonary vascular resistance. Mildly to moderately depressed infants constitute the largest group requiring some form of resuscitation at birth. These infants are pale or cyanotic, they have not established sustained respiration even at 1 minute after delivery, and they may be nearly flaccid. However, their heart rate is usually above 100 beats·min^{-1}. The severely depressed infant is flaccid, unresponsive, and pale; its heart rate is often below 100 beats·min^{-1}.

The scoring system introduced by Apgar is a useful method of clinically evaluating the baby, particularly at 1 and 5 minutes after delivery (see Table 46-5).[252]

Treatment of Moderately Depressed Infants

If initial resuscitative methods, including rubbing the back or slapping the feet once or twice, have produced no response—viz., the infant is apneic or its heart rate remains below 100 beats·min^{-1}—positive pressure ventilation by bag and mask should be instituted at a rate of 40 breaths per minute. The initial breath may require pressures of 30–40 cm H_2O. Subsequently the inflation pressures should be reduced to 15–20 cm H_2O in an infant with normal lungs. A small plastic oropharyngeal airway may be needed to maintain patency of the upper airway. If after 15–30 seconds of ventilation the heart rate is below 60 beats·min^{-1}, or between 60 and 80 beats·min^{-1} and not increasing, chest compressions should be initiated.

Treatment of Severely Depressed Infants

Ventilation should be established without delay. The glottis should be inspected immediately with the laryngoscope. If meconium or thick meconium-stained mucus has been aspirated into the trachea, it must be suctioned out at once via an endotracheal tube before the lungs are inflated. It is usually possible to accomplish this within 1–2 minutes of delivery. Severely depressed infants may require 3–8 minutes of artificial ventilation before a spontaneous gasp is taken. The endotracheal tube can be removed as soon as quiet and sustained respiration is established.

Use of Cardiac Massage

If the blood pressure is unduly low at the beginning of resuscitation, positive pressure ventilation is unlikely to be successful unless cardiac massage is employed. The technique preferred by the authors consists of intermittent compression of the lower third of the sternum 120 times per minute with the index and middle fingers. During chest compressions, positive pressure ventilation with 100% oxygen should be performed at a rate of 40–60 per min^{-1}. Cardiac massage and ventilation should be maintained until the heart rate exceeds 100 beats·min^{-1}.

Rapid Correction of Acidosis

Experiments on newborn monkeys have shown that maintenance of a normal pH during asphyxia by rapid infusion of base together with glucose prolongs gasping and delays cardiovascular collapse.[245] Furthermore, the rapid correction or maintenance of pH during asphyxia can reduce or prevent morphologically detectable brain damage. Resusci-

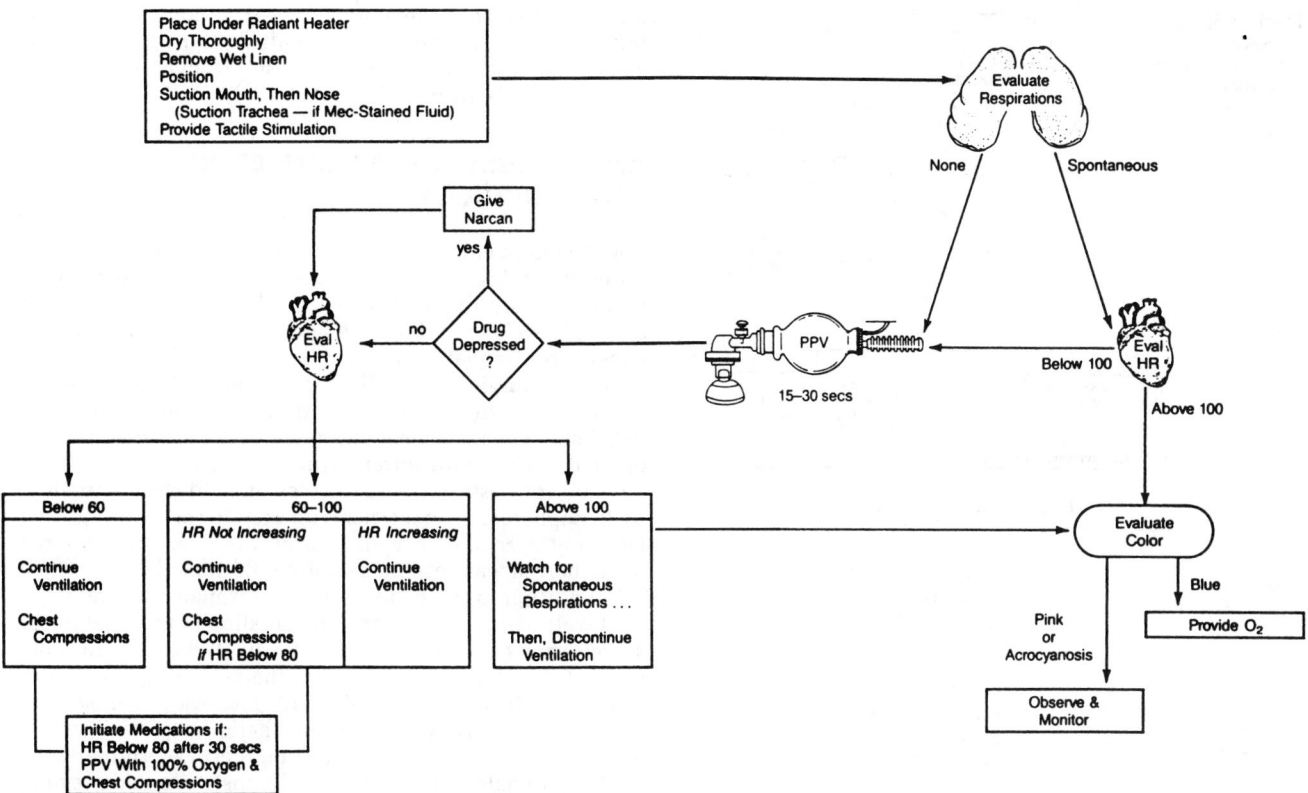

Figure 46-14. Overview of resuscitation in the delivery room. (Reprinted with permission from Bloom RS, Cropley C: Textbook on Neonatal Resuscitation. American Heart Association/American Academy of Pediatrics, Elk Grove Village, Illinois, 1990.)

tation is also facilitated if alkali and glucose are infused when artificial ventilation is started; oxygen consumption is greater and the time needed to establish spontaneous breathing is shorter.[248] In clinical practice, severe acidosis (pH less than 7.0 or a base deficit in excess of 15 mEq·l^{-1}) should be corrected promptly to improve pulmonary perfusion and oxygenation.[253] For that purpose, a 3.5 or 5.0 French catheter should be inserted, under sterile conditions, into the umbilical vein and advanced until the tip of the catheter is just below the skin level. A solution of sodium bicarbonate, 0.5 mEq·ml^{-1} (4.2%), is then infused over at least 2 minutes, up to a total dose of 2 mEq·kg^{-1} (Fig. 46-15). Adequate pulmonary ventilation should be assured during the infusion.

Other Drugs and Fluids

If it is believed that persistent depression has resulted from maternal opioid medication, naloxone should be given after adequate ventilation has been established (Table 46-6). The recommended dose of 0.1 mg·kg^{-1} may be injected iv, im, subcutaneously or *via* an endotracheal tube. The initial dose may be repeated as needed. Naloxone should be avoided in infants born to opioid-addicted mothers in order not to precipitate acute withdrawal. A severely asphyxiated newborn might require cardiotonic drugs during early resuscitation. Epinephrine should be used to treat asystole or persistent bradycardia despite adequate ventilation and external cardiac massage. A dose of 0.1–0.3 ml·kg^{-1} of 1:10,000 so-

TABLE 46-5. Apgar Scores

Sign	0	1	2
Heart rate	Absent	Less than 100 beats·min^{-1}	More than 100 beats·min^{-1}
Respiratory effort	Absent	Slow, irregular	Good, crying
Muscle tone	Limp	Some flexion of extremities	Active motion
Reflex irritability	No response	Grimace	Cough, sneeze, or cry
Color	Pale, blue	Body pink, extremities blue	Completely pink

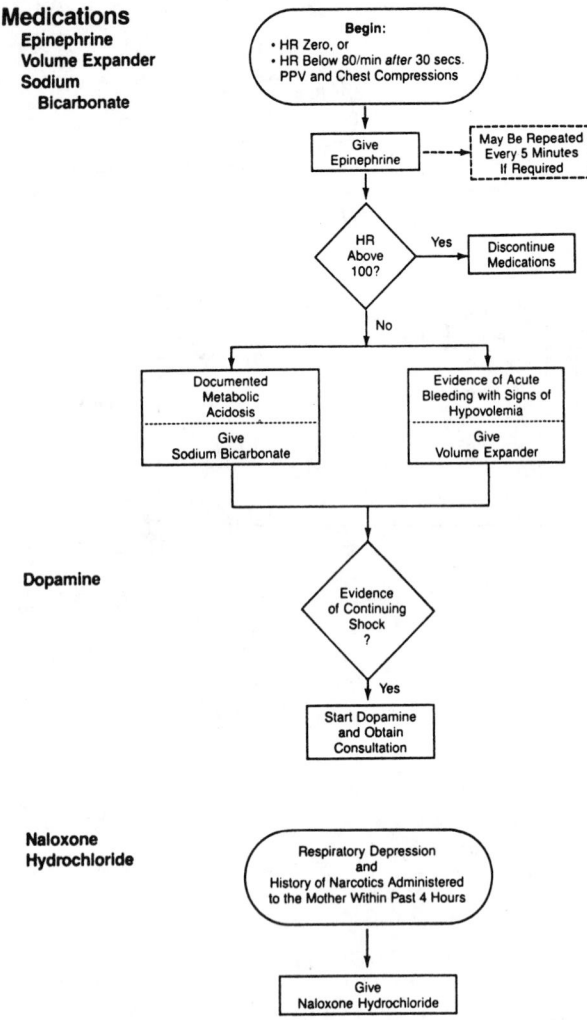

Medications

Epinephrine
Volume Expander
Sodium
   Bicarbonate

Begin:
• HR Zero, or
• HR Below 80/min *after* 30 secs.
  PPV and Chest Compressions

Give
Epinephrine

May Be Repeated
Every 5 Minutes
If Required

HR
Above
100?

Yes → Discontinue
Medications

No

Documented
Metabolic
Acidosis

Give
Sodium Bicarbonate

Evidence of Acute
Bleeding with Signs of
Hypovolemia

Give
Volume Expander

Dopamine

Evidence
of Continuing
Shock
?

Yes

Start Dopamine
and Obtain
Consultation

Naloxone
Hydrochloride

Respiratory Depression
and
History of Narcotics Administered
to the Mother Within Past 4 Hours

Give
Naloxone Hydrochloride

Figure 46-15. Drug sequence for neonatal resuscitation. (From Bloom RS, Copley C, Drew CR: Textbook of Neonatal Resuscitation. Reproduced with permission of the American Heart Association, Academy of Pediatrics, Dallas, 1987.)

lution should be injected iv or by endotracheal tube, and repeated every 5 minutes if necessary.

Hypovolemia frequently follows severe birth asphyxia, because a greater than normal portion of fetal blood remains in the placenta. The infant appears pale and has low arterial pressure, tachycardia, and tachypnea. Acute blood volume expansion may be accomplished with the iv administration of the following solutions over 5–10 minutes: O-negative blood, cross-matched with the mother's blood, 10 ml·kg^{-1}; 5% albumin, 10 ml·kg^{-1}; and normal saline or Ringer's lactate, 10 ml·kg^{-1}.

Diagnostic Procedures

After the neonate is successfully resuscitated and stabilized, several diagnostic procedures are indicated. To rule out choanal atresia, each nostril should be obstructed. Because newborn babies must breathe through their noses, occlusion of the nostril on the patent side would cause respiratory obstruction. To rule out esophageal atresia, a suction cathe-

ter is inserted into the stomach. Gastric contents are aspirated: volume in excess of 12 ml after vaginal delivery and 20 ml after cesarean section may result from an abnormality of the upper gastrointestinal tract.

ANESTHESIA FOR INTRAUTERINE FETAL SURGERY

The development of invasive as well as noninvasive procedures, involving amniocentesis, amniography, fetoscopy, fetal blood sampling, and real-time ultrasonography, has enabled physicians to diagnose and, in some cases, treat fetal anomalies. Neonatal morbidity and mortality may be improved by surgical procedures performed while the fetus is still *in utero* when there is a correctable anatomic lesion or deficiency state impairing normal organ growth and development. At present, intrauterine surgery on a fetus can be justified for obstructive lesions, such as hydronephrosis or hydrocephalus, or in a fetus with conditions resulting from failure of normal embryonic tissues to close, e.g., diaphragmatic hernia, gastroschisis, and neural tube defects.[254-257]

In addition to the usual concerns for maternal safety and fetal well-being, anesthetic considerations for prenatal fetal surgery must include fetal anesthesia and adequate relaxation of the uterus. The fetus has the sensitivity and ability to respond to varying stimuli with increases in motor and sympathetic activity.[258] The anesthetic drug effect in the fetus is greater than that in the mother. Determination of the MAC of halothane in chronically instrumented pregnant ewes and their fetuses has shown that it is lower in the fetus—0.33%, compared with 0.69% in the mother.[259] Because of the unique pattern of the fetal circulation, accumulation of effective anesthetic concentrations is delayed in the fetal brain. Neonatal depression was seen after cesarean sections with general anesthesia only when anesthetic concentrations of nitrous oxide were used for approximately 10 minutes.[161] An anesthetic agent with a higher lipid solubility than nitrous oxide may take longer to anesthetize the fetus.[260,261]

The use of nondepolarizing neuromuscular blocking agents as adjuvants to fetal anesthesia has recently been investigated. Because these drugs do not cross the placenta readily, *d*-tubocurarine, 1.5 mg·kg^{-1} of estimated fetal weight, or pancuronium, 0.3 mg·kg^{-1}, was injected into the fetal buttocks under ultrasonic guidance.[262] Paralysis was achieved approximately 5 minutes after *d*-tubocurarine and 4 minutes after pancuronium administration. The mean duration of neuromuscular blockade, estimated from maternal perception of the return of fetal movements, was 3.8 and 6.8 hours in the *d*-tubocurarine and pancuronium-treated groups, respectively. For minor surgical procedures on the fetus that involve minimal pain but require fetal immobilization (e.g., fetal transfusion), maternal sedation combined with fetal paralysis may be adequate.

Fetal surveillance during intrauterine surgical procedures has been difficult because invasive monitoring techniques often are not feasible. At present, continuous fetal heart rate monitoring in conjunction with determination of blood pH and gas tensions appear to be good indicators of fetal well-being. A continuous oxygen saturation monitor (pulse oximeter) may also be applied to an accessible fetal extremity.[263]

Intraoperative management should include techniques that induce uterine relaxation. In this respect, the use of potent halogenated agents is advantageous, not only in inducing and maintaining fetal anesthesia, but also in providing dose-related inhibition of uterine tone and contractions.

TABLE 46-6. Therapeutic Guidelines for Neonatal Resuscitation

Drug or Volume Expander	Concentration to Administer	Preparation (Based on Recommended Concentration)	Dosage	Route/Rate
Epinephrine	1:10,000	1 ml in a syringe Can dilute 1:1 with normal saline if giving IT	0.1–0.3 ml·kg⁻¹	iv or IT Give rapidly
Volume expanders	Whole blood 5% albumin/ saline solution Normal saline Ringer's lactate	40 ml to be given by syringe or iv drip	10 ml·kg⁻¹	Give over 5–10 minutes
Sodium bicarbonate	0.5 mEq·ml⁻¹ (4.2% solution)	20 ml in a syringe or two 10-ml prefilled syringes	2 mEq·kg⁻¹	iv Give slowly over at least 2 minutes (1 mEq·kg⁻¹·min⁻¹)
Naloxone hydrochloride	NARCAN Neonatal 0.02 mg·ml⁻¹	2 ml in a syringe	0.5 ml·kg⁻¹	iv, im, sc, or IT Give rapidly

im = intramuscular; iv = intravenous; IT = intratracheal; sc = subcutaneous.

Adapted from Bloom RS, Cropley C, Drew CR: Textbook of Neonatal Resuscitation. Reproduced with permission of the American Heart Association, American Academy of Pediatrics, Dallas, 1987.

Because the onset of preterm labor is a major complication of intrauterine procedures, postoperative administration of tocolytic agents, such as ritodrine, terbutaline, or magnesium sulfate, is recommended. In some reported cases, indomethacin, a prostaglandin synthetase inhibitor, was given with preoperative medication to prevent early labor.[255,264]

NONOBSTETRIC SURGERY IN THE PREGNANT WOMAN

Some 1.6% to 2.2% of pregnant women undergo surgery for reasons unrelated to parturition.[265,266] Apart from trauma, the most common emergencies are abdominal, involving torsion or rupture of an ovarian cyst and acute appendicitis, but breast tumors are not uncommon, and serious conditions such as intracranial aneurysms, cardiac valvular disease, and pheochromocytoma have been described.[267,268] Surgery to correct an incompetent cervix with Shirodkar or McDonald sutures is more related to the pregnancy itself.

When the necessity for surgery arises, anesthetic considerations are related to the alterations in maternal physiologic condition with advancing pregnancy, the teratogenicity of anesthetic drugs, the indirect effects of anesthesia on uteroplacental blood flow, and the potential for abortion or premature delivery. The risks must be balanced to provide the most favorable outcome for mother and child.

Four major studies have attempted to relate surgery and anesthesia during human pregnancy to fetal outcome as determined by anomalies, premature labor, or intrauterine death.[265,266,269,270] Although they failed to correlate surgery and anesthetic exposure with congenital anomalies, all of them demonstrated an increased incidence of fetal deaths, particularly after operations during the first trimester. No particular anesthetic agent or technique was implicated, and it seemed that the condition that necessitated surgery was the most relevant factor, with fetal mortality highest after pelvic surgery.

A 1963 report on a large population of pregnant women, of whom 67 had operations during pregnancy, showed a fetal mortality of 11.2%. Survival was poorest when the procedure was performed for cervical incompetence.[269] In 1965, a study of approximately 9000 parturients, of whom 1.6% had undergone surgery, found an 8.8% incidence of premature labor (and a perinatal mortality of 7.5%) in the surgical group, compared with only 2% in the control group.[265] More recently, pregnancy outcome after surgery in 287 women of a population of approximately 13,000 dental assistants or dentists' wives, showed that surgery during pregnancy was associated with a significant increase in spontaneous abortion rates compared with those not having surgery (8% vs. 5.1%).[266] In an attempt to answer the questions raised by these findings, a review was taken of the entire population of the province of Manitoba between the years 1971–1978.[270] State health insurance records were used to identify approximately 2500 pregnant women who had undergone surgery during this period. Each patient was matched with a woman of similar age, living in the same area, with a pregnancy-related condition but no surgical intervention. As in earlier studies, there was no increase in the incidence of congenital anomalies in the offspring of mothers who had had surgery. However, there was an increased risk of spontaneous abortion in women who had received general anesthesia during the first or second trimesters. This was most evident after gynecologic operations. Few of the surgical group had had procedures to treat cervical incompetence, suggesting that factors other than the obstetric condition itself might be important. The results also might have been influenced by the fact that a small number of gynecologic procedures were performed with anesthesia other than general, so that the effect of the surgical site alone could not be evaluated. The authors emphasized the multiplicity of factors other than choice of anesthetic agent (e.g., diagnostic radiologic procedures, antibiotics, analgesics, infection, decreased uterine perfusion, and stress) that might have been responsible for the increased risk of abortion.

The largest study to date regarding reproductive outcome after surgery during pregnancy is a Swedish registry review covering the years 1973–1981.[271] During this period there was a total of 720,000 births, 5405 of them after anesthesia and surgery during pregnancy. The results of this study are reassuring in that there was no increased incidence of congenital anomalies or stillbirths among infants exposed *in utero* to maternal surgery and anesthesia. However, in this group there was an increased frequency of very low and low birth weights, and of deaths within 168 hours after delivery. The reasons for this are unclear and are not related to any specific type of operation. The authors postulated that the maternal illness itself may have been a major contributor to adverse neonatal outcome.

The study of the effects of chronic exposure to subanesthetic concentrations of inhalation agents on pregnancy offers a different approach to the question of outcome. Evidence originates from animal studies and from epidemiologic surveys performed on operating room personnel and their children. A nationwide survey conducted by the American Society of Anesthesiologists found a higher incidence of cancer among female anesthesia personnel as well as increased rates of abortion and congenital abnormalities in their infants.[272] Furthermore, the last of these misfortunes also applied, although to a lesser degree, to unexposed wives of male operating room personnel. Another study, involving nurse anesthetists, suggested a higher than expected incidence of cancer.[273] These studies have been disputed because of possible statistical inaccuracies and inappropriate choices of control groups.[274,275] Another survey conducted among dentists and their female assistants compared the incidence of spontaneous abortions and congenital abnormalities among those exposed to inhalation anesthetics and those using only local anesthetics in their daily practices.[276] A significant increase in these complications occurred among assistants and wives of dentists exposed to inhalation drugs. Because of the controversy surrounding this issue, the American Society of Anesthesiologists commissioned an independent review by a team of epidemiologists.[277] This group found the data from most of the surveys to be flawed for a variety of reasons. These included responder bias, inappropriate control groups, failure to document exposure levels or verify medical data, and inability to ascertain which of the many environmental factors present in operating rooms might be blamed. The group concluded that, although exposed women appeared to have an increased risk of abortion (and to a much lesser extent, congenital anomalies), the increase was small enough to be accounted for by bias and uncontrolled variables. Some of these problems are absent in two subsequent studies in which questionnaire information was matched with information obtained from medical records or registries of abortions, births, and congenital malformations.[278,279] Neither of these studies found significant deviations from expected rates of threatened abortion in exposed women. In addition, no differences in birth weight distribution, perinatal mortality, or congenital malformations in the infants of exposed and nonexposed women were detected.[279] The authors point out that their results do not indicate that there is no reproductive hazard relating to working in operating rooms; effects that might have been missed include very early abortions not requiring hospitalization, congenital abnormalities not apparent at birth, and infertility.

Physiologic Changes in Pregnancy

Because these changes have been described earlier in the chapter, only a few points will be emphasized. The lesser increase in red blood cell volume relative to total blood volume leads to a decline in red blood cell count, hemoglobin, and hematocrit.[2] Serum cholinesterase activity declines moderately.[4] Cardiac output and heart rate gradually increase to a peak of 30–50% above normal at 30–34 weeks. From this time on, inferior vena caval compression becomes increasingly important.[15] Drug requirement for regional anesthesia may be reduced by 25–30%. Capillary engorgement throughout the respiratory tract makes nasal breathing more difficult and intubation of the trachea more hazardous.[17] From the 5th month, FRC decreases, and, at term, alveolar ventilation exceeds that of the nonpregnant state by about 70%.[21,22] These two factors enhance maternal uptake and elimination of inhalation anesthetics.[25] The low FRC and increased metabolic rate predispose the mother to hypoxemia, especially during airway obstruction or endotracheal intubation.[26] The stomach and intestines are gradually pushed upward by the enlarging uterus. Evacuation of a watery meal may be delayed by as much as 60% from the 34th week onward.[32] Pain and opioids will potentiate this delay. The administration of general anesthesia enhances the risk of regurgitation and aspiration during pregnancy, making rapid induction with cricoid pressure and endotracheal intubation mandatory in all patients having general anesthesia from the 12th week of gestation onward.

Direct Effects of Anesthetic Agents on Embryo and Fetus

The idea that surgical anesthesia, although deemed necessary for the patient, might have detrimental effects on the growth and development of the human fetus has led to a great deal of investigation, both *in vitro* and in experimental animals. These studies present difficulties in interpretation because the concentrations of anesthetic and the duration of exposure are frequently far in excess of what is clinically used and because most of the studies were performed in lower animals. The first test of embryotoxicity of an anesthetic agent (nitrous oxide) was made in the chick embryo.[280] Subsequent studies mostly have been on mammalian models, such as the rat, in which pregnancy lasts for a few weeks and organogenesis lasts for only a few days.

Animals exposed to toxic substances and anesthetics show a dose-related response, the first change being decreased fertility and increased fetal death. With increasing dose, the number of surviving fetuses with anomalies begins to increase, the peak incidence occurring at a dose that causes a 50% incidence of fetal death.[281] The teratogenic effects between species and also within the same species vary significantly. The developmental stage is crucial, with dramatic sensitivity to exposure at certain times and little or no effect at a later time.[281,282] The period of organogenesis is most critical. In humans it corresponds to the 15th–56th days of gestation.

Several experiments have demonstrated that brief intrauterine exposure of rats to halothane adversely affects postnatal learning behavior and causes central nervous system cellular degeneration and decreased brain weight; the findings with enflurane have been inconsistent.[283-285]

Many congenital malfunctions show a pattern of multifactorial inheritance. In this mode, maldevelopment may result from a combination of factors within one person, such as hereditary predisposition, sensitivity to a given drug, and exposure at a vulnerable time in development. There are numerous other factors contributing to the potential teratogenicity of anesthesia. The cytotoxicity of anesthetic agents is closely associated with biodegradation, which, in turn, is influenced by oxygenation and hepatic blood flow. Thus, the complications associated with anesthesia, such as maternal hypoxia, hypotension, administration of vasopressors, hypercarbia, hypocarbia, electrolyte disturbances, etc., may possibly be a greater cause for concern as regards teratogenesis than the use of the agents themselves.[286-288] Hypoxia is certainly a well-documented teratogen in the incubating chick embryo.[289] The role of maternal carbohydrate metabolism on embryonic development is also very important. For example, the effects of 48 hours of fasting and administration of insulin to pregnant rats have included a large number of skeletal deformities.[290]

Experimental evidence on exposure to specific drugs and agents will be highlighted very briefly, with the consideration that it is difficult to extrapolate laboratory data to the clinical situation as seen in humans. Very large numbers of patients must be exposed to a suspected teratogen before its safety can be ascertained. Complicating factors include the frequency of maternal exposure to a multiplicity of drugs; the difficulty in separating the effects of the underlying disease process and surgical treatment from those of the drug administered; differing degrees of risk with stage of gestation; and the variety, rather than the consistency, of anomalies that appear in association with one agent. Of the premedicants, anticholinergics have not been found to be teratogenic, whereas tranquilizers and sedatives such as phenothiazines and barbiturates produce anomalies in some species.[282,291-293] Several reports have described a specific relationship between diazepam and oral clefts, but another study has not confirmed this.[294-296] Intravenous agents such as thiopental, methohexital, and ketamine, in doses normally used in the operating room, have not been associated with birth defects. Only one study has shown musculoskeletal deformities involving the joints after infusion of a muscle relaxant (d-tubocurarine) in the chick embryo between the 7th and 15th day of incubation.[297] Although local anesthetics have not been shown to be teratogenic in animals or humans, procaine, lidocaine, and bupivacaine affected cultures of hamster lung fibroblasts by decreasing cell survival with ED_{50} values at concentrations as low as one-tenth of those used clinically.[298] Halogenated inhalation drugs have produced conflicting results. Pregnant rats exposed to halothane 0.8% for 12 hours at various times during gestation have increased incidences of anomalous skeletal development and fetal death.[299] Other investigations have failed to show teratologic effects of halothane in rats, rabbits, and mice exposed to subanesthetic concentrations for brief periods. Subanesthetic concentrations of enflurane do not appear to be teratogenic. However, mice exposed to 1% enflurane for 4 hours·day^{-1} on days 6–15 of gestation showed an increased incidence of cleft palates and minor skeletal and visceral abnormalities.[300] In a subsequent study by the same authors, teratogenic changes after exposure to 0.6% isoflurane in mice were similar to those found with enflurane, but the incidence of cleft palate was six times more frequent (12% vs. 1.9%).[301] Because cleft palate readily develops in mice, its occurrence as an isolated finding suggests that this might be a species-specific response. So that the results from earlier studies could be clarified, rats were exposed to 0.75 MAC halothane, isoflurane, or enflurane; 0.55 MAC nitrous oxide; or a known teratogen, retinoic acid, for two 6-hour periods at three different stages of pregnancy.[302] No major morphologic abnormalities occurred in any of the anesthetic-exposed groups.

Nitrous oxide has been the most extensively investigated agent since the 1955 observation that patients with tetanus developed leukopenia after inhaling nitrous oxide for several days. Numerous studies have demonstrated significant effects on fetal growth, skeletal development, and death rate in both pregnant rats and incubating chicks exposed to concentrations of from 50% to 80% for periods ranging from hours to days.[303,304] The question arises whether adverse effects at such high doses resulted from the anesthetic itself or from the accompanying physiologic derangements. After prolonged exposure of rats to subanesthetic concentrations of nitrous oxide or room air, 1000 ppm of nitrous oxide resulted in a higher incidence of fetal resorptions, skeletal malformations, and smaller fetuses than did air.[305] Because these concentrations do not produce anesthesia, this study supports the conclusion that nitrous oxide itself may be teratogenic. In contrast to the above findings with high dosage or prolonged exposure, concentrations of 50% or less for periods of less than 24 hours resulted in no adverse fetal effects.[306,307]

Although the mechanism of the teratogenic effect of nitrous oxide has not been determined, it may be related to the inhibitory effect of the agent on methionine synthetase activity.[308] Vitamin B_{12}, a cofactor of this enzyme, is irreversibly oxidized to an inactive form. Inhibition of methionine synthetase has been detected in liver biopsy specimens obtained from surgical patients after exposure to 50–70% nitrous oxide for 1.25–2.75 hours.[309] A dose-dependent decrease in both maternal and fetal methionine synthetase activity occurred in pregnant rats receiving 10% or 50% nitrous oxide for periods ranging from 60 to 240 minutes.[310] It is possible that failure of this enzyme to convert homocysteine to the essential amino acid methionine may lead to abnormalities of myelination of nerve fibers (Fig. 46-16). Furthermore, inhibition of methionine synthesis results in decreased thymidine production, which in turn can lead to decreased DNA synthesis and inhibition of cell division. Because there is evidence that nitrous oxide adversely affects methionine synthetase activity, it has been recommended that it not be administered to pregnant women in the first two trimesters.[311,312] However, a recent human study demonstrated no significant changes in plasma methionine concentrations after anesthesia with 60–70% nitrous oxide for up to 4 hours.[313] Two other reviews of exposure to this agent, this time for cervical cerclage procedures, showed no effects on fetal outcome.[314-315] Further, in the already mentioned Swedish birth registry study, nitrous oxide was administered to almost all of 2929 patients receiving general anesthesia, without adverse fetal consequences.[271] In rats, the teratogenic effects of nitrous oxide could be prevented by the concomitant administration of isoflurane or halothane.[316] It is controversial whether pretreatment with folinic acid, the concentration of which is reduced when methionine synthetase is inhibited, affords protection against the effects of nitrous oxide.[316,317] Because a single exposure to anesthetic agents seems unlikely to result in fetal abnormality, the selection of agent should be based on specific surgical requirements.

Indirect Effects of Agents and Techniques

The adequacy of the uteroplacental circulation, so vital to the well-being of the fetus, is easily affected by drugs and anesthetic procedures. As discussed previously, perfusion of the intervillous space of the placenta may be diminished consequent on maternal systemic hypotension, which in turn may result from the use of epidural or spinal anesthesia, from aortocaval compression with the patient in the

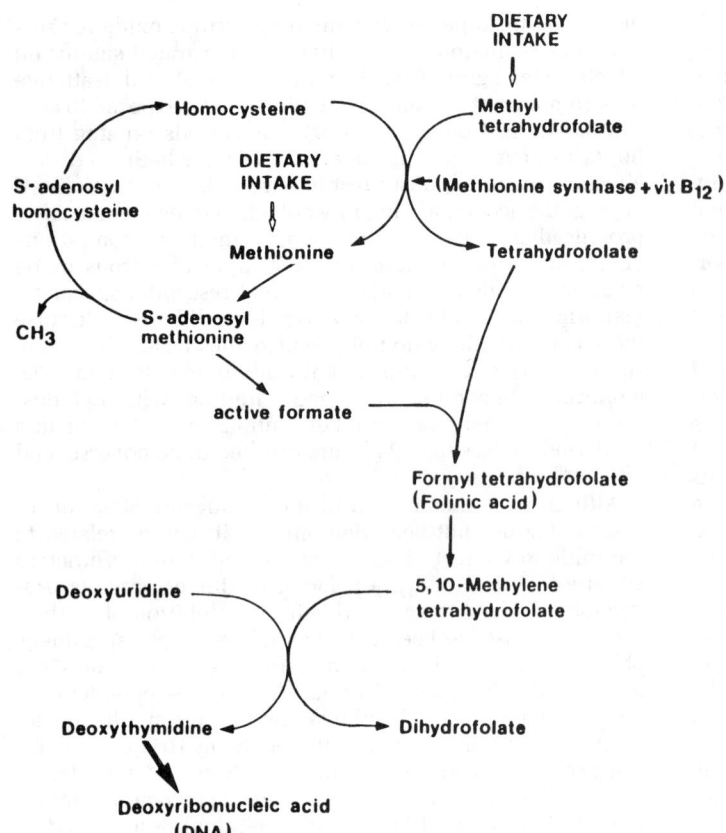

Figure 46-16. Abridged metabolic map showing the relationship between methionine and deoxythymidine syntheses. (Reprinted with permission from Nunn JF: Interaction of nitrous oxide and vitamin B_{12}. Trends Pharmacol Sci 5:225, 1984.)

supine position, or from hemorrhage. Similarly, increased uterine activity may result in reduced placental perfusion. Thus, the use of alpha-adrenergic drugs to correct maternal hypotension and anesthetics such as ketamine (in doses above 1 mg·kg^{-1}) may produce increased uterine tone sufficient to endanger the fetus.[221,318] Severe hyperventilation of the mother may also reduce uterine blood flow.[157] Finally, it has been shown in experimental animals that epinephrine or norepinephrine infusion results in decreased uterine blood flow and deterioration of fetal condition. Maternal pain and apprehension may similarly affect the fetus.[319,320]

Practical Suggestions

It is generally agreed that only emergency surgery should be performed during pregnancy, particularly in the first trimester. The possibility of pregnancy should be considered in all female surgical patients of reproductive age. Based on the maternal and fetal hazards already described, the following approach to anesthesia seems indicated:

1. The patient's apprehension should be allayed as much as possible by personal reassurance during the preanesthetic visit and by adequate sedation and premedication. It is important to discuss the hazards of anesthesia with the patient and her family, because they are likely to have many fears for the unborn baby.
2. Pain should be relieved whenever present.
3. Administration of an antacid, 15–30 ml, within half an hour before induction of anesthesia will usually increase the pH of the gastric fluid above the critical level. Ranitidine and metoclopramide may be useful.
4. Beginning in the second trimester, mothers should not be transported or placed in the supine position on the operating table. The lateral decubitus position or left uterine displacement will minimize the risk of aortocaval compression.
5. Hypotension related to spinal or epidural anesthesia should be prevented as much as possible by rapid iv infusion of crystalloid solution before induction. If the mother becomes hypotensive despite this pretreatment, a predominantly beta-adrenergic vasopressor, such as ephedrine, should be promptly administered iv.
6. General anesthesia should be preceded by careful denitrogenation.
7. The risk of aspiration should be minimized by application of cricoid pressure and rapid tracheal intubation with a cuffed tube.
8. To reduce fetal hazard, particularly during the first trimester, it appears preferable to choose drugs with a long history of safety; these drugs include thiopental, morphine, meperidine, muscle relaxants, and low concentrations of nitrous oxide. However, ketamine, 0.5–0.75 mg·kg^{-1}, might be preferable to thiopental as an induction agent in the face of severe hypovolemia. Halothane or other volatile drugs may offer the specific advantage of relaxing the uterus during procedures involving the pelvic organs, particularly the uterus itself, e.g., cervical cerclage (Shirodkar or McDonald procedure).
9. To avoid maternal hyperventilation, one should monitor end-expiratory P_{CO_2} or arterial blood gases.

10. Fetal heart rate should be monitored continuously throughout surgery and anesthesia, providing that the placement of the transducer does not encroach on the surgical field.[321,322] Using the directional Doppler apparatus, this monitoring becomes technically feasible from the 16th week of pregnancy. Uterine tone may also be monitored with an external tocodynamometer if the uterus has grown enough to reach the umbilicus or above.

11. Monitoring of uterine activity should be continued after operation, and tocolytic agents should be administered, if necessary, to inhibit uterine contractions.

12. Special procedures such as hypothermia and induced hypotension might be necessary to facilitate surgery, despite the potential fetal hazard. It is reassuring to know that there was successful fetal outcome after both procedures for intracranial operations.[323,324] There are numerous reports of cardiopulmonary bypass being performed during pregnancy, with generally good maternal and fetal results.[202,325-327] A frequent finding was a persistent fetal bradycardia and loss of beat-to-beat variability throughout the period of bypass, despite acceptable maternal oxygenation and acid-base balance. One survey reported only one maternal death in 86 procedures in which extracorporeal circulation was used, and a more than 80% survival rate of fetuses.[202] It was suggested that the procedures might be safer when fetal heart and uterine monitoring was used and perfusion hypothermia avoided. At this time, little work has been done to determine the fetal effects of cardiopulmonary bypass.

REFERENCES

1. Ueland K: Maternal cardiovascular dynamics. VII. Intrapartum blood volume changes. Am J Obstet Gynecol 126:671, 1976

2. Lund CJ, Donovan JC: Blood volume during pregnancy. Am J Obstet Gynecol 98:393, 1967

3. Maternal adaptation to pregnancy. In Pritchard JA, Macdonald PC (eds): Williams Obstetrics, p 236. New York, Appleton-Century-Crofts, 1980

4. Hazel B, Monier D: Human serum cholinesterase: Variations during pregnancy and post-partum. Can Anaesth Soc J 18:272, 1971

5. Wildsmith JAW: Serum pseudocholinesterase, pregnancy and suxamethonium. Anaesthesia 27:90, 1972

6. De Alvarez RR, Afonso JF, Sherrard DJ: Serum protein fractionation in normal pregnancy. Am J Obstet Gynecol 82:1096, 1961

7. Levy G: Protein binding of drugs in the maternal-fetal unit and its potential clinical significance. In Krauer B, Krauer F, Hytten FE et al (eds): Drugs and Pregnancy, p 29. London, Academic Press, 1984

8. Pernoll ML, Metcalf J, Schlenker TL et al: Oxygen consumption at rest and during exercise in pregnancy. Respir Physiol 25:285, 1975

9. Ueland K, Parer JT: Effects of estrogens on the cardiovascular system of the ewe. Am J Obstet Gynecol 96:400, 1966

10. Goodman RP, Killom AP, Brash AR et al: Prostacyclin production during pregnancy—Comparison of production during normal pregnancy and pregnancy complicated by hypertension. Am J Obstet Gynecol 142:817, 1982

11. Hamilton HFH: Cardiac output in normal pregnancy. J Obstet Gynaecol Br Commonw 56:548, 1949

12. Kerr MG, Scott DB, Samuel E: Studies of the inferior vena cava in late pregnancy. Br Med J 1:532, 1964

13. Ueland K, Novy MJ, Peterson EN: Maternal cardiovascular dynamics. IV. The influence of gestational age on the maternal cardiovascular response to posture and exercise. Am J Obstet Gynecol 104:856, 1969

14. Humphrey MD, Chang A, Wood EC et al: A decrease in fetal pH during the second stage of labour when conducted in the dorsal position. J Obst Gynaecol Br Commonw 81:600, 1974

15. Howard BK, Goodson JH, Mengert WF: Supine hypotensive syndrome in late pregnancy. Obstet Gynecol 1:371, 1953

16. Bieniarz J, Crottogini JJ, Curuchet E et al: Aortocaval compression by the uterus in late human pregnancy. II. An angiographic study. Am J Obstet Gynecol 100:203, 1968

17. Bonica JJ: Principles and Practice of Obstetric Analgesia and Anesthesia, p 21. Philadelphia, FA Davis, 1967

18. Datta S, Briwa J: Modified laryngoscope for endotracheal intubation of obese patients. Anesth Analg 60:120, 1981

19. Kruttgen HG, Emerson K Jr: Physiological response to pregnancy at rest and during exercise. J Appl Physiol 36:549, 1974

20. Gee JBL, Packer BS, Miller JE et al: Pulmonary mechanics during pregnancy. J Clin Invest 46:945, 1967

21. Andersen GJ, James GB, Mathers NP et al: The maternal oxygen tension and acid-base status during pregnancy. J Obstet Gynaecol Br Commonw 76:16, 1969

22. Cugell DW, Frank NR, Gaensler EA et al: Pulmonary function in pregnancy. I. Serial observations in normal women. Ann Rev Tuberc 67:568, 1953

23. Bevan DR, Holdcroft A, Loh L et al: Closing volume and pregnancy. Br Med J 1:13, 1974

24. Prowse CM, Gaensler EA: Respiratory and acid-base changes during pregnancy. Anesthesiology 26:381, 1965

25. Moya F, Smith BE: Uptake, distribution and placental transport of drugs and anesthetics. Anesthesiology 26:465, 1965

26. Archer GW, Marx GF: Arterial oxygenation during apnaea in parturient women. Br J Anaesth 46:358, 1974

27. Datta S, Kitzmiller JL, Naulty JS et al: Acid-base status of diabetic mothers and their infants following spinal anesthesia for cesarean section. Anesth Analg 61:662, 1982

28. Murray FA, Eskine JP, Fielding J: Gastric secretions in pregnancy. J Obstet Gynaecol Br Commonw 64:313, 1957

29. Taylor G, Pryse-Davies J: The prophylactic use of antacids in the prevention of the acid-pulmonary aspiration syndrome (Mendelson's syndrome). Lancet 1:288, 1966

30. Lind JF, Smith AM, McIver DR et al: Heartburn in pregnancy—A manometric study. Can Med Assoc J 98:571, 1968

31. Simpson KH, Stakes AF, Miller M: Pregnancy delays paracetamol absorption and gastric emptying in patients undergoing surgery. Br J Anaesth 60:24, 1988

32. Davison JS, Davison MC, Hay DM: Gastric emptying time in late pregnancy and labour. J Obstet Gynaecol Br Commonw 77:37, 1970

33. Smith G, Dalling R, Williams TIR: Gastro-oesophageal pressure gradient changes produced by induction of anaesthesia and suxamethonium. Br J Anaesth 50:1137, 1979

34. Brock-Utne JG, Dow TGB, Dimopoulos GE et al: Gastric and lower oesophageal sphincter (LOS) pressures in early pregnancy. Br J Anaesth 53:381, 1981

35. Coombs DW: Aspiration pneumonia prophylaxis (editorial). Anesth Analg 62:1055, 1983

36. Wyner J, Cohen SE: Gastric volume in early pregnancy: Effect of metoclopramide. Anesthesiology 57:209, 1982

37. Cohen SE, Woods WA, Wyner J: Antiemetic efficacy of droperidol and metoclopramide. Anesthesiology 60:67, 1984

38. Murphy DF, Nally B, Gardiner J et al: Effect of metoclopramide on gastric emptying before elective and emergency cesarean section. Br J Anaesth 56:1113, 1984

39. Scheller MS, Sears KL: Post-operative neurologic dysfunction associated with preoperative administration of metoclopramide. Anesth Analg 66:274, 1987

40. Palahniuk RJ, Shnider SM, Eger EI: Pregnancy decreases the requirements for inhaled anesthetic agents. Anesthesiology 41:82, 1974

41. Datta S, Migliozzi RP, Flanagan HL et al: Chronically administered progesterone decreases halothane requirements in rabbits. Anesth Analg 68:46, 1989

42. Datta S, Lambert DH, Gregus et al: Differential sensitivities of mammalian nerve fibers during pregnancy. Anesth Analg 62:1070, 1983

43. Fagraeus L, Urban BJ, Bromage PR: Spread of epidural analgesia in early pregnancy. Anesthesiology 58:184, 1983

44. Drabkova J, Crul JF, Van Der Kleijn E: Placental transfer of ^{14}C labelled succinylcholine in near-term Macaca mulatta monkeys. Br J Anaesth 46:1087, 1973

45. Duvaldestin P, Demetriou M, Henzel D et al: The placental transfer of pancuronium and its pharmacokinetics during caesarean section. Acta Anaesthesiol Scand 22:327, 1978

46. Brown WU, Bell GC, Alper MH: Acidosis, local anesthetics and the newborn. Obstet Gynecol 48:27, 1976

47. Morishima HO, Covino BG: Toxicity and distribution of lidocaine in nonasphyxiated and asphyxiated baboon fetuses. Anesthesiology 54:182, 1981

48. Hamshaw-Thomas A, Rogerson N, Reynolds F: Transfer of bupivacaine, lignocaine and pethidine across the rabbit placenta: Influence of maternal protein binding and fetal flow. Placenta 5:61, 1984

49. Morishima HO, Pedersen H, Santos A et al: Maternal and fetal uptake of bupivacaine vs. lidocaine at steady state plasma drug concentrations. Anesthesiology 67:A437, 1987

50. Kennedy RL, Miller RP, Bell JU et al: Uptake and distribution of bupivacaine in fetal lambs. Anesthesiology 65:247, 1986

51. Kuhnert PM, Kuhnert BR, Stitts BS et al: The use of a selected ion monitoring technique to study the disposition of bupivacaine in mother, fetus and neonate following epidural anesthesia for cesarean section. Anesthesiology 55:611, 1981

52. Kosaka Y, Takahashi T, Mark LC: Intravenous thiobarbiturate anesthesia for cesarean section. Anesthesiology 31:489, 1969

53. Finster M, Morishima HO, Pedersen H et al: Meperidine: Placental transfer after epidural, intramuscular, and intravenous injection. Anesthesiology 55:A321, 1981

54. Crawford JS, Rudofsky S: The placental transmission of pethidine. Br J Anaesth 37:929, 1965

55. Kuhnert BR, Philipson EH, Pimental R et al: Lidocaine disposition in mother, fetus, and neonate after spinal anesthesia. Anesth Analg 65:139, 1986

56. Morishima HO, Daniel SS, Finster M et al: Transmission of mepivacaine hydrochloride (Carbocaine) across the human placenta. Anesthesiology 27:147, 1966

57. O'Brien JE, Abbey V, Hinsvark O et al: Metabolism and measurement of 2-chloroprocaine, an ester type local anesthetic. J Pharm Sci 68:75, 1979

58. Kuhnert BR, Kuhnert PM, Philipson EH et al: The half-life of 2-chloroprocaine. Anesth Analg 65:273, 1986

59. Kuhnert BR, Kuhnert PM, Prochaska AL et al: Plasma levels of 2-chloroprocaine in obstetric patients and their neonates after epidural anesthesia. Anesthesiology 53:21, 1980

60. Morgan DJ, Blackman GL, Paul JD et al: Pharmacokinetics and plasma binding of thiopental. II. Studies at cesarean section. Anesthesiology 54:474, 1981

61. Pihlajamäki K, Kanto J, Lindberg R et al: Extradural administration of bupivacaine: Pharmacokinetics and metabolism in pregnant and non-pregnant women. Br J Anaesth 64:556, 1990

62. Idanpaan-Heikkila JE, Taska RJ, Allen HA et al: Placental transfer of diazepam—^{14}C in mice, hamsters and monkeys. J Pharmacol Exp Ther 176:752, 1971

63. Haram K, Bakke OM, Johannessen KH et al: Transplacental passage of diazepam during labor: Influence of uterine contractions. Clin Pharmacol Ther 24:590, 1978

64. Mihaly GW, Moore RG, Thomas J et al: The pharmacokinetics and metabolism of the anilide local anaesthetics in neonates. Eur J Clin Pharmacol 13:143, 1978

65. Morishima HO, Finster M, Pedersen H et al: Pharmacokinetics of lidocaine in fetal and neonatal lambs and adult sheep. Anesthesiology 50:431, 1979

66. Finster M, Poppers PJ, Sinclair JC et al: Accidental intoxication of the fetus with local anesthetic drug during caudal anesthesia. Am J Obstet Gynecol 92:922, 1965

67. Morishima HO, Pedersen H, Finster M et al: Toxicity of lidocaine in adult, newborn and fetal sheep. Anesthesiology 55:57, 1981

68. Morishima HO, Pedersen H, Finster M et al: Etidocaine toxicity in the adult, newborn and fetal sheep. Anesthesiology 58:342, 1983

69. Campbell N, Harvey D, Norman AP: Increased frequency of neonatal jaundice in a maternity hospital. Br Med J 2:548, 1975

70. Clark DA, Landaw SA: Bupivacaine alters red blood cells properties: A possible explanation for neonatal jaundice associated with maternal anesthesia. Pediatr Res 19:341, 1985

71. Gale R, Ferguson JE II, Stevenson D: Effect of epidural analgesia with bupivacaine hydrochloride on neonatal bilirubin production. Obstet Gynecol 70:692, 1987

72. Hodgkinson R, Marx GF, Kim SS et al: Neonatal neurobehavioral tests following vaginal delivery under ketamine, thiopental and extradural anesthesia. Anesth Analg 56:548, 1977

73. Amiel-Tison C, Barrier G, Shnider SM et al: A new neurologic and adaptive capacity scoring system for evaluating obstetric medications in full term newborns. Anesthesiology 56:340, 1982

74. Morishima HO, Yeh M-N, James LS: Reduced uterine blood flow and fetal hypoxemia with acute maternal stress: Experimental observation in the pregnant baboon. Am J Obstet Gynecol 134:270, 1979

75. Shnider SM, Wright RG, Levinson G et al: Uterine blood flow and plasma norepinephrine changes during maternal stress in the pregnant ewe. Anesthesiology 50:524, 1979

76. Ueland K, Hansen JM: Maternal cardiovascular dynamics. III. Labor and delivery under local and caudal analgesia. Am J Obstet Gynecol 103:8, 1969

77. Moir DD, Willocks J: Management of incoordinate uterine action under continuous epidural analgesia. Br Med J 2:396, 1967

78. Miller FC, Petrie RH, Arce JJ et al: Hyperventilation during labor. Am J Obstet Gynecol 120:489, 1974

79. Melzack R, Taenzer P, Feldman P et al: Labour is still painful after prepared childbirth training. Can Med Assoc J 125:357, 1981

80. Scott JR, Rose NB: Effect of psychoprophylaxis (Lamaze preparation) on labor and delivery in primiparas. N Engl J Med 294:1205, 1976

81. Way WL, Cortley EC, Way EL: Respiratory sensitivity of the newborn infant to meperidine and morphine. Clin Pharmacol Ther 6:454, 1965

82. Shnider SM, Moya F: Effects of meperidine on the newborn infant. Am J Obstet Gynecol 89:1009, 1964

83. Kuhnert BR, Kuhnert PM, Philipson EH et al: Disposition of meperidine and normeperidine following multiple doses during labor. II. Fetus and neonate. Am J Obstet Gynecol 151:410, 1985

84. Kuhnert BR, Linn PL, Kennard MJ et al: Effect of low doses of meperidine on neonatal behavior. Anesth Analg 64:335, 1985

85. Eisele JH, Wright R, Rogge P: Newborn and maternal fentanyl levels at cesarean section. Anesth Analg 61:179, 1982

86. Maduska AL, Hajghassemali M: A double blind comparison of butorphanol and meperidine in labor: Maternal pain relief and effect on newborn. Can Anaesth Soc J 25:398, 1978

87. Clark RB: Transplacental reversal of meperidine depression in the fetus by naloxone. J Arkansas Med Soc 68:128, 1971

88. Evans JM, Rosen M, MacCarthy J et al: Patient-controlled intravenous narcotic administration during labor. Lancet 1:906, 1976

89. Powe CE, Kiem IM, Fromhagen C et al: Propiomazine hydrochloride in obstetrical analgesia. JAMA 181:280, 1962

90. Cree IE, Meyer J, Hailey DM: Diazepam in labour: Its metabolism and effect on the clinical condition and thermogenesis of the newborn. Br Med J 4:251, 1973

91. Akamatsu TJ, Bonica JJ, Rehmet R et al: Experiences with the use of ketamine for parturition. I. Primary anesthetic for vaginal delivery. Anesth Analg 53:284, 1974

92. Snyder GE, Person DL, Flor CE et al: Headache in obstetrical patients: Comparison of Whitacre needle versus Quincke needle. Anesthesiology 71:A860, 1989

93. Read MD, Hunt LP, Anderson JM et al: Epidural block and

the progress and outcome of labour. J Obstet Gynaecol 4:35, 1983

94. Schellenberg JC: Uterine activity during lumbar epidural analgesia with bupivacaine. Am J Obstet Gynecol 127:26, 1977

95. Chestnut DH, Bates JN, Choi WW: Continuous infusion epidural analgesia with lidocaine: Efficacy and influence during the second stage of labor. Obstet Gynecol 69:323, 1987

96. American College of Obstetrics and Gynecology: Obstetric Forceps. ACOG Committee on Obstetrics, Maternal and Fetal Medicine, Committee Opinion No. 71, 1989

97. Moore DC, Batra MS: The components of an effective test dose prior to epidural block. Anesthesiology 55:694, 1984

98. Cartwright PD, McCarroll SM, Antzaka C: Maternal heart rate changes with plain epidural test dose. Anesthesiology 65:226, 1986

99. Hood DD, Dewan DM, James FM III: Maternal and fetal effects of epinephrine in gravid ewes. Anesthesiology 64:610, 1986

100. Leighton BL, DeSimone CA, Norris MC et al: Isoproterenol is an effective marker for intravenous injection in laboring women. Anesthesiology 71:206, 1989

101. Leighton BL, Norris MC, Desimone CA et al: The air test as a clinically useful indicator of intravenously placed epidural catheters. Anesthesiology 73:610, 1990

102. Freeman AB, Hicks L: Epidural fentanyl as a test dose. Anesthesiology 68:187, 1989

103. Lysak SZ, Eisenach JC, Dobson CE: Patient-controlled epidural analgesia during labor: A comparison of three solutions with a continuous infusion control. Anesthesiology 72:44, 1990

104. Gambling DR, McMorland GH, Yu P et al: Comparison of patient-controlled epidural analgesia and conventional intermittent "top-up" injections during labor. Anesth Analg 70:256, 1990

105. Viscomi C, Eisenach JC: Patient-controlled epidural analgesia during labor. Obstet Gynecol 77:348, 1991

106. Scanlon JW, Brown WV Jr, Weiss JB et al: Neurobehavioral responses of newborn infants after maternal epidural anesthesia. Anesthesiology 40:121, 1974

107. Bromage PR, Datta S, Dunford LA: Etidocaine: An evaluation in epidural analgesia for obstetrics. Can Anaesth Soc J 21:535, 1974

108. Abboud TK, Kern S, Jacobs J et al: The neonatal neurobehavioral effects of mepivacaine for epidural anesthesia during labor. Reg Anesth 11:143, 1986

109. Baxi LV, Petrie RH, James LS: Human fetal oxygenation following paracervical block. Am J Obstet Gynecol 135:1109, 1979

110. Thiery M, Vroman S: Paracervical block analgesia during labor. Am J Obstet Gynecol 113:988, 1972

111. Kotelko DM, Dailey PA, Shnider SM et al: Epidural morphine analgesia after cesarean delivery. Obstet Gynecol 63:409, 1984

112. Husemeyer RP, O'Connor ML, Davenport HT: Failure of epidural morphine to relieve pain in labour. Anaesthesia 35:161, 1980

113. Hughes SC, Rosen MA, Shnider SM et al: Maternal and neonatal effects of epidural morphine for labor and delivery. Anesth Analg 63:319, 1984

114. Cohen SE, Tan S, Albright GA et al: Epidural fentanyl/bupivacaine mixtures for obstetric analgesia. Anesthesiology 67:403, 1987

115. Chestnut DH, Laszewski LJ, Pollack KL et al: Continuous epidural infusion of 0.0625% bupivacaine–0.0002% fentanyl during the second stage of labor. Anesthesiology 72:613, 1990

116. Vertommen JD, Vandermeulen E, Van Aken H et al: The effects of the addition of sufentanil to 0.125% bupivacaine on the quality of analgesia during labor and on the incidence of instrumental deliveries. Anesthesiology 74:809, 1991

117. Hunt CO, Naulty JS, Malinow AM et al: Epidural butorphanol–bupivacaine for analgesia during labor and delivery. Anesth Analg 68:323, 1989

118. Baraka A, Noueihid R, Hajj S: Intrathecal injection of morphine for obstetric analgesia. Anesthesiology 54:136, 1981

119. Abboud TK, Shnider SM, Dailey PA et al: Intrathecal administration of hyperbaric morphine for the relief of pain in labour. Br J Anaesth 56:1351, 1984

120. Leighton BL, DeSimone CA, Norris MC et al: Intrathecal narcotics for labor revisited: The combination of fentanyl and morphine intrathecally provides rapid onset of profound, prolonged analgesia. Anesth Analg 69:122, 1989

121. Abboud TK, Lee K, Zhu J et al: Prophylactic oral naltrexone with intrathecal morphine for cesarean section: Effects on adverse reactions and analgesia. Anesth Analg 71:367, 1990

122. Creasser CW, Stoelting RK, Krishna G et al: Methoxyflurane metabolism and renal function after methoxyflurane analgesia during labor and delivery. Anesthesiology 41:62, 1974

123. Dundee JW, Moore J: Alterations in response to somatic pain associated with anaesthesia. IV. The effects of sub-anaesthetic concentrations of inhalation agents. Br J Anaesth 32:453, 1960

124. Munson ES, Embro WJ: Enflurane, isoflurane and halothane and isolated human uterine muscle. Anesthesiology 46:11, 1977

125. Peng ATC, Gorman RS, Shulman SM et al: Intravenous nitroglycerin for uterine relaxation in the postpartum patient with retained placenta. Anesthesiology 71:172, 1989

126. DeSimone CA, Norris MC, Leighton BL: Intravenous nitroglycerin aids manual extraction of a retained placenta. Anesthesiology 73:787, 1990

127. Gibbs CP, Krischer J, Peckam BM et al: Obstetric anesthesia: A national survey. Anesthesiology 65:298, 1986

128. Gilstrap LC III, Hauth JC, Hankins GDV et al: Effect of type of anesthesia on blood loss at cesarean section. Obstet Gynecol 69:328, 1987

129. Shnider SM, Levinson G: Anesthesia for cesarean section. In Shnider SM, Levinson G (eds): Anesthesia for Obstetrics, 2nd ed, p 159. Baltimore, Williams & Wilkins, 1987

130. Marx GF, Luykx WM, Cohen S: Fetal-neonatal status following cesarean section for fetal distress. Br J Anaesth 56:1009, 1984

131. Norris MC: Height, weight and the spread of subarachnoid hyperbaric bupivacaine in the term parturient. Anesth Analg 67:555, 1988

132. Ramanathan S, Gandhi S, Arismendy J et al: Oxygen transfer from mother to fetus during cesarean section under epidural anesthesia. Anesth Analg 61:576, 1982

133. Hunt CO, Naulty S, Bader AM et al: Perioperative analgesia with subarachnoid fentanyl-bupivacaine for cesarean delivery. Anesthesiology 71:535, 1989

134. Abboud TK, Dror A, Mosaad P et al: Mini-dose intrathecal morphine for the relief of post-cesarean section pain: Safety, efficacy and ventilatory responses to CO_2. Anesthesiology 67:A464, 1987

135. Abouleish E, Rawal N, Fallon K et al: Combined intrathecal morphine and bupivacaine for cesarean section. Anesthesiology 67:A619, 1987

136. Santos A, Datta S: Prophylactic use of droperidol for control of nausea and vomiting during spinal anesthesia for elective cesarean section. Anesth Analg 63:85, 1984

137. Chestnut DH, Vandewalker GE, Owen CL et al: Administration of metoclopramide for prevention of nausea and vomiting during epidural anesthesia for elective cesarean section. Anesthesiology 66:563, 1987

138. Philipson EH, Kuhnert BR, Syracuse CD: Fetal acidosis, 2-chloroprocaine, and epidural anesthesia for cesarean section. Am J Obstet Gynecol 151:322, 1985

139. Ravindran RS, Bond VK, Fasch MD et al: Prolonged neural blockade following regional analgesia with 2-chloroprocaine. Anesth Analg 59:447, 1980

140. Reisner LS, Hochman BN, Plumer MH: Persistent neurologic deficit and adhesive arachnoiditis following intrathecal 2-chloroprocaine injection. Anesth Analg 59:452, 1980

141. Gissen AJ, Datta S, Lambert D: The chloroprocaine controversy: Is chloroprocaine neurotoxic? Reg Anaesth 9:135, 1984

142. Hynson JM, Sessler DI, Glosten B: Back pain in volunteers after epidural anesthesia with chloroprocaine. Anesth Analg 72:253, 1991

143. Dirkes J: Treatment of Nesacaine-MPF-induced back pain with calcium chloride (letter). Anesth Analg 70:461, 1990

144. Albright GA: Cardiac arrest following regional anesthesia with etidocaine or bupivacaine. Anesthesiology 51:285, 1979

145. Tanz RD, Heskett T, Loehning RW et al: Comparative cardiotoxicity of bupivacaine and lidocaine in the isolated perfused mammalian heart. Anesth Analg 63:549, 1984

146. Morishima HO, Pedersen H, Finster M et al: Bupivacaine toxicity in pregnant and nonpregnant ewes. Anesthesiology 63:134, 1985

147. Santos AC, Pedersen H, Harmon TW, et al: Does pregnancy alter the systemic toxicity of local anesthetics? Anesthesiology 70:991, 1989

148. Moller RA, Datta S, Fox J et al: Progesterone-induced increase in cardiac sensitivity to bupivacaine. Anesthesiology 69:A675, 1988

149. Chambers WA, Mowbray A, Wilson J: Extradural morphine for the relief of pain following caesarean section. Br J Anaesth 55:1201, 1983

150. Abboud TK, Moore M, Zhu J et al: Epidural butorphanol or morphine for the relief of post-cesarean section pain: Ventilatory responses to carbon dioxide. Anesth Analg 66:887, 1987

151. Chestnut DH, Choi WW, Isbell TJ: Epidural hydromorphone for post-cesarean analgesia. Obstet Gynecol 68:65, 1986

152. Naulty JS, Datta S, Ostheimer GW et al: Epidural fentanyl for post-cesarean delivery pain management. Anesthesiology 63:694, 1985

153. Madej TH, Strunin L: Comparison of epidural fentanyl with sufentanil. Analgesia and side effects after a single bolus dose during elective caesarean section. Anaesthesia 42:1156, 1987

154. Leicht CH, Hughes SC, Dailey PA et al: Epidural morphine sulphate for analgesia after cesarean section: A prospective report of 1000 patients. Anesthesiology 65:A366, 1986

155. Morgan M: Anaesthetic contribution to maternal mortality. Br J Anaesth 59:842, 1987

156. Norris MC, Dewan DM: Preoxygenation for cesarean section: A comparison of two techniques. Anesthesiology 81:A400, 1984

157. Levinson G, Shnider SM, deLorimier AA et al: Effects of maternal hyperventilation on uterine blood flow and fetal oxygenation and acid-base status. Anesthesiology 40:340, 1974

158. James FM III, Crawford JS, Hopkinson R et al: A comparison of general anesthesia and lumbar epidural analgesia for elective cesarean section. Anesth Analg 56:228, 1977

159. Datta S, Ostheimer GW, Weiss JB et al: Neonatal effect of prolonged anesthetic induction for cesarean section. Obstet Gynecol 58:331, 1981

160. Crawford JS, James FM, Crawley M: A further study of general anaesthesia for caesarean section. Br J Anaesth 48:661, 1976

161. Finster M, Poppers PJ: Safety of thiopental used for induction of general anesthesia in elective cesarean section. Anesthesiology 29:190, 1968

162. Marx GF, Mateo CV: Effects of different oxygen concentrations during general anaesthesia for elective caesarean section. Can Anaesth Soc J 18:587, 1971

163. Datta S, Brown WU: Acid-base status in diabetic mothers and their infants following general or spinal anesthesia for cesarean section. Anesthesiology 47:272, 1977

164. Willems J: The etiology of preeclampsia: A hypothesis. Obstet Gynecol 50:495, 1977

165. Speroff L: Toxemia of pregnancy: Mechanism and therapeutic management. Am J Cardiol 32:582, 1973

166. Walsh SW: Preeclampsia: An imbalance in placental prostacyclin and thromboxane production. Am J Obstet Gynecol 152:335, 1985

167. Makila U-M, Jouppila P, Kirkinen P et al: Placental thromboxane and prostacyclin in the regulation of placental blood flow. Obstet Gynecol 68:537, 1986

168. Sibai BM, Spinnato JA, Watson DL et al: Effect of magnesium sulfate on electroencephalographic findings in preeclampsia-eclampsia. Obstet Gynecol 64:261, 1984

169. Hibbard LT: Maternal mortality due to acute toxemia. Obstet Gynecol 42:263, 1973

170. Sibai BM, Anderson GD, McCubbin JH: Eclampsia II. Clinical significance of laboratory findings. Obstet Gynecol 59:153, 1982

171. Wright JP: Anesthetic considerations in preeclampsia-eclampsia. Anesth Analg 63:590, 1983

172. Lin CC, Lindheimer MD, River P et al: Fetal outcome in hypertensive disorders of pregnancy. Am J Obstet Gynecol 142:255, 1982

173. Soffronoff EC, Kaufmann BM, Connaughton JF: Intravascular volume determinations and fetal outcome in hypertensive diseases of pregnancy. Am J Obstet Gynecol 127:4, 1977

174. Chesley LC: Plasma and red cell volumes during pregnancy. Am J Obstet Gynecol 112:440, 1972

175. Joyce TH III, Debnath KS, Baker EA: Preeclampsia—relationship of CVP and epidural analgesia. Anesthesiology 51:S297, 1979

176. Hays PM, Cruickshank DP, Dunn LJ: Plasma volume determination in normal and preeclamptic pregnancies. Am J Obstet Gynecol 151:958, 1985

177. Rafferty TD, Berkowitz RL: Hemodynamics in patients with severe toxemia during labor and delivery. Am J Obstet Gynecol 138:263, 1980

178. Groenendijk R, Trimbos MJ, Wallenburg HCS: Hemodynamic measurements in preeclampsia: Preliminary observations. Am J Obstet Gynecol 150:232, 1984

179. Cotton DB, Gonik B, Dorman K et al: Cardiovascular alterations in severe pregnancy-induced hypertension. Relationship of central venous pressure to pulmonary capillary wedge pressure. Am J Obstet Gynecol 151:762, 1985

180. Kelton JG, Hunter DJS, Neame PB: A platelet function defect in preeclampsia. Obstet Gynecol 65:107, 1985

181. Rodgers RPC, Levin J: A critical reappraisal of the bleeding time. Semin Thromb Hemost 161:1, 1990

182. Cotton DB, Gonik B, Dorman KF: Cardiovascular alterations in severe pregnancy-induced hypertension: Acute effects of intravenous magnesium sulfate. Am J Obstet Gynecol 148:162, 1984

183. Green KW, Key TC, Coen R et al: The effects of maternally administered magnesium sulfate on the neonate. Am J Obstet Gynecol 146:29, 1983

184. Shoemaker CT, Meyers M: Sodium nitroprusside for control of severe hypertensive disease of pregnancy: A case report and discussion of potential toxicity. Am J Obstet Gynecol 149:171, 1984

185. Newsome LR, Bramwell RS, Curling PE: Severe preeclampsia: Hemodynamic effects of lumbar epidural anesthesia. Anesth Analg 65:31, 1986

186. Jouppila P, Jouppila R, Hollmen A et al: Lumbar epidural analgesia to improve intervillous blood flow during labor in severe preeclampsia. Obstet Gynecol 59:158, 1982

187. Ramanathan J, Botorff M, Jeter JN et al: The pharmacokinetics and maternal and neonatal effects of epidural lidocaine in preeclampsia. Anesth Analg 65:120, 1986

188. Hodgkinson R, Husain FJ, Hayashi RH: Systemic and pulmonary blood pressure during cesarean section in parturients with gestational hypertension. Can Anaesth Soc J 27:389, 1980

189. Connell H, Dalgleish JG, Downing JW: General anaesthesia in mothers with severe pre-eclampsia/eclampsia. Br J Anaesth 59:1375, 1987

190. Abdul-Karim RW, Chevli RN: Antepartum hemorrhage and shock. Clin Obstet Gynecol 19:533, 1976

191. Clark SL, Koonings PP, Phelan JP: Placenta previa/accreta and prior cesarean section. Obstet Gynecol 66:89, 1985

192. Greene AT, Ostheimer GW, Datta S et al: Risks of placenta previa/accreta in patients with previous cesarean deliveries. Anesthesiology 69:A659, 1989

193. Pritchard JA, Mason R, Corley M et al: Genesis of severe placental abruption. Am J Obstet Gynecol 108:22, 1970

194. Pritchard JA: Haematological problems associated with delivery, placental abruption, retained dead fetus and amniotic fluid embolism. Clin Haematol 2:562, 1973

195. Perloff JK: Pregnancy and cardiovascular disease. In Braunwald E (ed): Heart Disease: Textbook of Cardiovascular Medicine, 2nd ed, p 1763. Philadelphia, WB Saunders, 1984

196. Hibbard LT: Maternal mortality due to cardiac disease. Clin Obstet Gynecol 18:27, 1975

197. Sugrue D, Blake S, MacDonald D: Pregnancy complicated by maternal heart disease at the National Maternity Hospital, Dublin, Ireland, 1969–1978. Am J Obstet Gynecol 139:1, 1981

198. Ueland K, Hansen JM: Maternal cardiovascular dynamics. II. Posture and uterine contractions. Am J Obstet Gynecol 103:1, 1969

199. Szekely P, Snaith L: Heart Disease and Pregnancy, p 29. London, Churchill Livingstone, 1974

200. Sullivan JM, Ramanathan KB: Management of medical problems in pregnancy—Severe cardiac disease. N Engl J Med 313:304, 1985

201. Schroeder JS, Harrison DC: Repeated cardioversion during pregnancy: Treatment of refractory paroxysmal atrial tachycardia during 3 successive pregnancies. Am J Cardiol 27:445, 1971

202. Becker RM; Intracardiac surgery in pregnant women. Ann Thorac Surg 36:453, 1983

203. Mangano DT: Anesthesia for the pregnant cardiac patient. In Shnider SM, Levinson G (eds): Anesthesia for Obstetrics, 2nd ed, p 345. Baltimore, Williams & Wilkins, 1987

204. Abboud TK, Raya J, Noueihid R et al: Intrathecal morphine for relief of labor pain in patients with severe pulmonary hypertension. Anesthesiology 59:477, 1983

205. Campbell M: The incidence and later distribution of malformations of the heart. In Watson H (ed): Paediatric Cardiology, p 71. London, Lloyd-Luke, 1968

206. Jones AM, Howitt G: Eisenmenger's syndrome in pregnancy. Br Med J 1:1627, 1965

207. Rush RW, Davey DA, Segall ML: The effect of pre-term delivery on perinatal mortality. Br J Obstet Gynaecol 85:806, 1978

208. Allen MC, Jones MD: Medical complications of prematurity. Obstet Gynecol 67:427, 1986

209. Dailey PA: Anesthesia for preterm labor. In Shnider SM, Levinson G (eds): Anesthesia for Obstetrics, 2nd ed, p 243. Baltimore, Williams & Wilkins, 1987

210. Benedetti TJ: Maternal complications of parenteral beta-sympathomimetic therapy for premature labor. Am J Obstet Gynecol 145:1, 1983

211. Young DC, Toofanian A, Leveno KJ: Potassium and glucose concentration without treatment during ritodrine tocolysis. Am J Obstet Gynecol 145:105, 1983

212. Saunders NR: Development of blood-brain barrier in the fetus. In Bossart H (ed): Perinatal Medicine, p 54. Bern, Hans Huber, 1973

213. Krauer B, Krauer F, Hytten F: Drug Prescribing in Pregnancy, Vol 7, Current Reviews in Obstetrics and Gynaecology, p 44. Edinburgh, Churchill Livingstone, 1984

214. Kaltreider DF: Premature labor and meperidine analgesia. Am J Obstet Gynecol 99:989, 1967

215. Morishima HO, Pedersen H, Santos AC et al: Adverse effects of maternally administered lidocaine on the asphyxiated preterm fetal lamb. Anesthesiology 71:110, 1989

216. Deckardt R, Fembacher PM, Schneider KTM et al: Maternal arterial oxygen saturation during labor and delivery: Pain-dependent alterations and effects on the newborn. Obstet Gynecol 70:21, 1987

217. Freeman RK, Garite TJ: Fetal Heart Rate Monitoring, p 1. Baltimore, Williams & Wilkins, 1981

218. Martin CB, Gingerich B: Factors affecting the fetal heart rate: Genesis of FHR patterns. JOGN (Nurs) 5(suppl):30S, 1976

219. Wright RG, Shnider SM, Levinson G et al: The effect of maternal administration of ephedrine on fetal heart rate and variability. Obstet Gynecol 57:734, 1981

220. Finster M, Petrie RH: Monitoring of the fetus. Anesthesiology 45:198, 1976

221. Vasicka A, Hutchinson HT, Eng M et al: Spinal and epidural anesthesia, fetal and uterine response to acute hypo- and hypertension. Am J Obstet Gynecol 90:800, 1964

222. Oats JN, Vasey DP, Waldron BA: Effects of ketamine on the pregnant uterus. Br J Anaesth 51:1163, 1979

223. Caldeyro-Barcia R, Noriega-Guerra L, Cibils LA et al: Effect of position changes on the intensity and frequency of uterine contractions during labor. Am J Obstet Gynecol 80:284, 1960

224. Ralston DH, Shnider SM: The fetal and neonatal effects of regional anesthesia in obstetrics. Anesthesiology 48:34, 1978

225. Matadial L, Cibils LA: The effect of epidural anesthesia on uterine activity and blood pressure. Am J Obstet Gynecol 125:846, 1976

226. Goodlin RC: History of fetal monitoring. Am J Obstet Gynecol 133:323, 1979

227. Adamsons K, Beard RW, Cosmi EV et al: The validity of capillary blood in the assessment of the acid-base state of the fetus. In Adamsons K (ed): Diagnosis and Treatment of Fetal Disorders, p 175. New York, Springer-Verlag, 1968

228. Beard RW. Fetal blood sampling. Br J Hosp Med 3:523, 1970

229. Bowe ET, Beard RW, Finster M et al: Reliability of fetal blood sampling. Am J Obstet Gynecol 107:279, 1970

230. Gibbs RS, Listwa HM, Read JA: The effect of internal monitoring on maternal infection following cesarean section. Obstet Gynecol 48:653, 1976

231. Gassner CB, Ledger WJ: The relationship of hospital-acquired maternal infection to invasive intrapartum monitoring techniques. Am J Obstet Gynecol 126:33, 1976

232. Sola A, Bednarek FJ, Davidson R et al: Meningitis, ventriculitis, and hydrocephalus: A complication of fetal monitoring. Obstet Gynecol 56:663, 1980

233. Lang-Gee C, Ledger WJ: Maternal and fetal morbidity associated with intrapartum monitoring. JOGN (Nurs) 5:(suppl)65S, 1976

234. Modanlou HD, Linzey M: An unusual complication of fetal blood sampling during labor. Obstet Gynecol 51(suppl):7S, 1978

235 MacDonald D, Grant A, Sheridan-Pereira M et al: The Dublin randomized controlled trial of intrapartum fetal heart rate monitoring. Am J Obstet Gynecol 152:524, 1985

236. Cohen SE: The aspiration syndrome. Clin Obstet Gynaecol 9:235, 1982

237. Brizgys RV, Dailey PA, Shnider SM et al: The incidence and neonatal effects of maternal hypotension during epidural anesthesia for cesarean section. Anesthesiology 67:782, 1987

238. Kasten GW, Martin ST: Resuscitation from bupivacaine-induced cardiovascular toxicity during partial inferior vena cava occlusion. Anesth Analg 65:341, 1986

239. DiGiovanni AJ, Galbert MW, Wahle WM: Epidural injection of autologous blood for postlumbar puncture headache. II. Additional clinical experiences and laboratory investigation. Anesth Analg 51:226, 1972

240. Jarvis AP, Greenwalt JW, Fagraeus L: Intravenous caffeine for postdural puncture headache. Anesth Analg 65:313, 1986

241. Brownridge P: The management of headache following accidental dural puncture in obstetric patients. Anaesth Intensive Care 11:4, 1983

242. Standards and guidelines for cardiopulmonary resuscitation (CPR) and emergency cardiac care (ECC). Part VI: Neonatal advanced life support. JAMA 255:2969, 1986

243. Adamsons K, James LS, Towell ME et al: Physiologic observations during induced anemia in utero in the rhesus monkey. J Pediatr 67:1042, 1965

244. James LS, Weisbrot IM, Prince CE et al: The acid-base status of human infants in relation to birth asphyxia and the onset of respiration. J Pediatr 52:379, 1958

245. Adamsons K, Behrman R, Dawes GS et al: The treatment of acidosis with alkali and glucose during asphyxia in foetal rhesus monkey. J Physiol 169:679, 1963

246. Birmingham MK, Elliot KAC: Effects of pH, bicarbonate and cofactors on the metabolism of brain suspensions. J Biol Chem 189:73, 1951

247. James LS, Adamsons K: Respiratory physiology of the fetus and newborn. N Engl J Med 271:1352, 1964

248. Adamsons K, Behrman R, Dawes GS et al: Resuscitation by positive pressure ventilation and Tris-hydroxymethylaminomethane of rhesus monkeys asphyxiated at birth. J Pediatr 65:807, 1964

249. Heymann MA, Iwamoto HS, Rudolph AM: Factors affecting changes in the neonatal systemic circulation. Annu Rev Physiol 43:371, 1981

250. Klopfenstein HS, Rudolph AM: Postnatal changes in the cir-

culation and responses to volume loading in sheep. Circ Res 42:839, 1978

251. Bloom RS, Cropley C: Textbook of Neonatal Resuscitation. Elk Grove Village, Illinois, American Heart Association/American Academy of Pediatrics, 1990

252. Apgar V: A proposal for a new method of evaluation of the newborn infant. Anesth Analg 32:260, 1953

253. Rudolph AM, Yuen S: Response of the pulmonary vasculature to hypoxia and H⁺ ion concentration changes. J Clin Invest 45:399, 1966

254. Harrison MR, Golbus MS, Filly RA et al: Fetal surgical treatment. Pediatr Ann 11:896, 1982

255. Harrison MR, Golbus MS, Filly RA et al: Fetal surgery for congenital hydronephrosis. N Engl J Med 306:591, 1982

256. Clewell WH, Johnson ML, Meier RR et al: A surgical approach to the treatment of fetal hydrocephalus. N Engl J Med 306:1320, 1982

257. Harrison MR, Golbus MS, Filly RA; Management of the fetus with a correctable congenital defect. JAMA 246:774, 1981

258. Anand KJS, Hickey PR: Pain and its effects in the human neonate and fetus. N Engl J Med 317:1321, 1987

259. Gregory GA, Wade JG, Biehl DR et al: Fetal anesthetic requirement (MAC) for halothane. Anesth Analg 62:9, 1983

260. Marx GF, Joshi CW, Orkin LR: Placental transmission of nitrous oxide. Anesthesiology 32:429, 1970

261. Siker ES, Wolfson B, Dubnonsky J et al: Placental transfer of methoxyflurane. Br J Anaesth 40:588, 1968

262. Moise KJ, Carpenter RJ, Deter RL et al: The use of fetal neuromuscular blockade during intrauterine procedures. Am J Obstet Gynecol 157:874, 1987

263. Rosen MA: Anesthesia for fetal surgery. In Shnider SM, Levinson G (eds): Anesthesia for Obstetrics, 2nd ed, p 206. Baltimore, Williams & Wilkins, 1987

264. Harrison MR, Anderson J, Rosen MA et al: Fetal surgery in the primate. I. Anesthetic, surgical and tocolytic management to maximize fetal-neonatal survival. J Pediatr Surg 17:115, 1982

265. Shnider SM, Webster GM: Maternal and fetal hazards of surgery during pregnancy. Am J Obstet Gynecol 92:891, 1965

266. Brodsky JB, Cohen EN, Brown BW Jr et al: Surgery during pregnancy and fetal outcome. Am J Obstet Gynecol 138:1165, 1980

267. Levine W, Diamond B: Surgical procedures during pregnancy. Am J Obstet Gynecol 81:1046, 1962

268. Babaknia A, Parsa H, Woodruff JD: Appendicitis during pregnancy. Obstet Gynecol 50:40, 1977

269. Smith BE: Fetal prognosis after anesthesia during gestation. Anesth Analg 42:521, 1963

270. Duncan PG, Pope WDB, Cohen MM et al: Fetal risk of anesthesia and surgery during pregnancy. Anesthesiology 64:790, 1986

271. Mazze RI, Köllén B: Reproductive outcome after anesthesia and operation during pregnancy: A registry study of 5405 cases. Am J Obstet Gynecol 161:1178, 1989

272. Ad Hoc Committee on the Effect of Trace Anesthetics on the Health of Operating Room Personnel, American Society of Anesthesiologists: Occupational disease among operating room personnel: A national study. Anesthesiology 41:321, 1974

273. Corbett TH, Cornell RG, Lieding K et al: Incidence of cancer among Michigan nurse-anesthetists. Anesthesiology 38:260, 1973

274. Walts LF, Forsythe AB, Moore JG: Critique: Occupational disease among operating room personnel. Anesthesiology 42:608, 1975

275. Fink BR, Cullen BF: Anesthetic pollution: What is happening to us? Anesthesiology 45:79, 1976

276. Cohen EN, Brown BW, Wu M: Anesthetic health hazards in the dental operatory. Anesthesiology 51:S256, 1976

277. Buring JE, Hennekens CH, Mayrent SL: Health experiences of operating room personnel. Anesthesiology 62:325, 1985

278. Axelsson G, Rylander R: Exposure to anesthetic gases and spontaneous abortion: Response bias in postal questionnaire study. Int J Epidemiol 11:250, 1982

279. Ericson HA, Källén AJB: Hospitalization for miscarriage and delivery outcome among Swedish nurses working in operating rooms, 1973–1978. Anesth Analg 64:981, 1985

280. Rector GHN, Eastwood DW: The effects of nitrous oxide and oxygen on the incubating chick. Anesthesiology 25:109, 1964

281. Smith BE: Teratogenicity of inhalation anesthetics. In: Progress in Anesthesiology, p 589. London, Excerpta Medica, 1970

282. Smith BE: Teratogenic capabilities of surgical anesthesia. Adv Teratol 3:127, 1968

283. Chalon J, Hillman D, Gross S et al: Intrauterine exposure to halothane increases murine postnatal autotolerance to halothane and reduced brain weight. Anesth Analg 62:565, 1983

284. Chalon J, Tang C-K, Ramanathan S et al: Exposure to halothane and enflurane affects learning function of murine progeny. Anesth Analg 60:794, 1981

285. Peters MA, Hudson PM: Postnatal development and behavior in offspring of enflurane exposed pregnant rats. Arch Int Pharmacodyn Ther 256:134, 1982

286. Heinonen OP, Slone O, Shapiro S: Birth Defects and Drugs in Pregnancy, p 516. Littleton, Massachusetts, Publishing Sciences Group, 1977

287. Hodach RJ, Gilbert EF, Fallon JF: Aortic arch anomalies associated with administration of epinephrine in chick embryos. Teratology 9:203, 1974

288. Haring OM: Cardiac malformations in rats induced by exposure of the mother to carbon dioxide during pregnancy. Circ Res 8:1218, 1960

289. Grabowski CT, Paar JA: The teratogenic effects of graded doses of hypoxia on the chick embryo. Am J Anat 103:313, 1958

290. Hannah RS, Moore KL: Effects of fasting and insulin on skeletal development in rats. Teratology 4:135, 1971

291. Shepard TH: Catalog of Teratogenic Agents, 3rd ed. Baltimore, Johns Hopkins University Press, 1980

292. Roux C: Action tératogène de la prochlorpérazine. Arch Fr Pediatr 16:968, 1959

293. Hartz SC, Heinonen OP, Shapiro S et al: Antenatal exposure to meprobamate and chlordiazepoxide in relation to malformations, mental development and childhood mortality. N Engl J Med 292:726, 1975

294. Sáxen I, Sáxen L: Association between maternal intake of diazepam and oral clefts. Lancet 2:498, 1975

295. Safra MJ, Oakley GP: Association between cleft lip with or without cleft palate and prenatal exposure to diazepam. Lancet 2:478, 1975

296. Rice SA, Pellegrini M: Teratology of fixed agents. In Baden JM, Brodsky JB (eds): The Pregnant Surgical Patient, p 53. Mt Kisco, New York, Futura, 1985

297. Drachman DB, Coulombre AJ: Experimental clubfoot and arthrogryposis multiplex congenita. Lancet 2:523, 1962

298. Sturrock JE, Nunn JF: Cytotoxic effects of procaine, lignocaine and bupivacaine. Br J Anaesth 51:273, 1979

299. Basford AB, Fink BR; The teratogenicity of halothane in the rat. Anesthesiology 29:1167, 1968

300. Wharton RS, Mazze RI, Wilson AI: Reproduction and fetal development in mice chronically exposed to enflurane. Anesthesiology 54:505, 1981

301. Mazze RI, Wilson AI, Rice SA et al: Effects of isoflurane on reproduction and fetal development in mice. Anesth Analg 63:249, 1984

302. Mazze RI, Fujinaga M, Rice SA et al: Reproductive and teratogenic effects of nitrous oxide, halothane, isoflurane and enflurane in Sprague-Dawley rats. Anesthesiology 64:339, 1986

303. Fink BR, Shepard TH, Blandau RJ: Teratogenic activity of nitrous oxide. Nature 214:146, 1967

304. Smith BE, Gaub MI, Moya F: Teratogenic effects of anesthetic agents: Nitrous oxide. Anesth Analg 44:726, 1965

305. Vieira E, Cleaton-Jones P, Austin JC et al: Effects of low concentrations of nitrous oxide on rat fetuses. Anesth Analg 59:175, 1980

306. Pope WDB, Halsey MJ, Lansdown ABG et al: Fetotoxicity in rats following chronic exposure to halothane, nitrous oxide or methoxyflurane. Anesthesiology 48:11, 1978

307. Mazze RI, Wilson AI, Rice SA et al: Reproduction and fetal

development in mice chronically exposed to nitrous oxide. Teratology 26:11, 1982

308. Chanarin I: Cobalamins and nitrous oxide: A review. J Clin Pathol 33:909, 1980

309. Koblin DD, Waskell L, Watson JE et al: Nitrous oxide inactivates methionine synthetase in human liver. Anesth Analg 61:75, 1982

310. Baden JM, Serra M, Mazze RI: Inhibition of fetal methionine synthase by nitrous oxide. Br J Anaesth 56:523, 1984

311. Nunn JF, Chanarin I: Nitrous oxide inactivates methionine synthetase. In Eger EI II (ed): Nitrous Oxide/N_2O, p 221. New York, Elsevier-Dutton, 1985

312. Eger EL II: Should we not use nitrous oxide? In Eger EI II (ed): Nitrous Oxide/N_2O, p 339. New York, Elsevier-Dutton, 1985

313. Nunn JF, Sharer NM, Battiglieri T et al: Effect of short-term administration of nitrous oxide on plasma concentration of methionine, tryptophan, phenylalanine, and S-adenosyl methionine in man. Br J Anaesth 58:1, 1986

314. Crawford JS, Lewis M: Nitrous oxide in early human pregnancy. Anaesthesia 41:900, 1986

315. Aldridge LM, Tunstall ME: Nitrous oxide and the fetus: A review and the results of a retrospective study of 175 cases of anaesthesia for insertion of Shirodkar suture. Br J Anaesth 58:1348, 1986

316. Fujinaga M, Baden JM, Yhap EO et al: Halothane and isoflurane prevent the teratogenic effects of nitrous oxide in rats, folinic acid does not. Anesthesiology 67:A456, 1987

317. Nunn JF, Chanarin I, Tanner AG et al: Megaloblastic bone marrow changes after repeated nitrous oxide anaesthesia. Reversal with folinic acid. Br J Anaesth 58:1469, 1986

318. Galloon S: Ketamine for obstetric delivery. Anesthesiology 44:522, 1976

319. Adamsons K, Mueller-Heubach E, Myers RE: Production of fetal asphyxia in the rhesus monkey by administration of catecholamines to the mother. Am J Obstet Gynecol 109:148, 1971

320. Rosenfeld CR, Barton MD, Meschia G: Effects of epinephrine on distribution of blood flow in the pregnant ewe. Am J Obstet Gynecol 124:156, 1976

321. Katz JD, Hook R, Barash PG: Fetal heart rate monitoring in the pregnant patients under surgery. Am J Obstet Gynecol 125:267, 1976

322. Liu PL, Warren TM, Ostheimer GW et al: Foetal monitoring in parturients undergoing surgery unrelated to pregnancy. Can Anaesth Soc J 32:525, 1985

323. Hehre RW: Hypothermia for operations during pregnancy. Anesth Analg 44:424, 1965

324. Kofke WA, Wuest HP, McGinnis LA: Cesarean section following ruptured cerebral aneurysm and neuroresuscitation. Anesthesiology 60:242, 1984

325. Estafanous FG, Buckley S: Management of anesthesia for open heart surgery during pregnancy. Cleve Clin Q 43:121, 1976

326. Trimakas AP, Maxwell KD, Berkay S et al: Fetal monitoring during cardiac pulmonary bypass for removal of a left atrial myxoma during pregnancy. Johns Hopkins Med J 144:156, 1979

327. Bahary CM, Ninio A, Gorokesky IG et al: Tococardiography in pregnancy during extracorporeal bypass for mitral valve replacement. Isr J Med Sci 16:395, 1980

47

Frederic A. Berry

Neonatal Anesthesia

PHYSIOLOGY OF THE INFANT AND THE TRANSITION PERIOD

The first year of life is characterized by an almost miraculous growth in size and maturity. The body weight alone changes by a factor of 3, and there is no other period in extrauterine life when changes occur so rapidly. Before birth, fetal growth and development depend on the genetic composition of the fetus, the mother's placental function, and potential exposure to chemicals or infectious agents that can affect mother, fetus, or both. The journey down the birth canal (or through the abdominal wall)—called the most dangerous trip in a person's life—ends the fetal period, and the newborn must adapt to extrauterine life. This change from fetal to extrauterine life is called the period of transition or adaptation.

The newborn infant is an infant in the first 24 hours of life. This chapter focuses on the neonatal period, which is defined as the first 30 days of extrauterine life and includes the newborn period. The most significant part of transition occurs in the first 24 to 72 hours after birth. All systems of the body change during transition, but the most important to the anesthesiologist are the circulatory, pulmonary, and renal systems. The circulatory and pulmonary systems are so interdependent that they will be discussed together.

Transition of the Cardiopulmonary System

Fetal Circulation

Fetal circulation is characterized by the presence of three main shunts (Fig. 47-1A). These shunts are the placenta, foramen ovale, and ductus arteriosus. The relatively low pressure in the left atrium and the high pressure in the right atrium result in the foramen ovale being open. The pulmonary vascular bed has a high vascular resistance because the alveoli are relatively closed and filled with fluid and the blood vessels are compressed. In addition, the low partial pressure of oxygen in arterial blood (Pao_2) and pH increase pulmonary vascular resistance. On the other hand, the ductus arteriosus represents a low-resistance system because it is dilated secondary to a low Pao_2. Therefore, the blood that leaves the right ventricle by the pulmonary artery is shunted preferentially (90%) through the ductus arteriosus and down the descending aorta, whereas only 10% of the output of the right ventricle flows through the pulmonary artery into the pulmonary vascular bed. The pulmonary vascular bed requires only enough blood flow to assure growth and development of the pulmonary tissue, including surfactant production.

The placenta oxygenates the blood, which then courses up the inferior vena cava into the right atrium. The right atrium is divided by a structure called the crista dividends, so that this relatively well-oxygenated blood is shunted from the right atrium through the foramen ovale into the left atrium, thereby bypassing the right ventricle and the pulmonary vascular bed. This blood, the best oxygenated in the fetus, progresses from the left atrium to the left ventricle and out the ascending aorta to provide oxygenation for the brain and upper extremities. Blood returns from the upper body to the right heart by the superior vena cava, where it is directed by the crista dividends into the right ventricle, where it is then pumped out the pulmonary artery.

Clamping of the umbilical cord and initiation of ventilation produce enormous circulatory changes in the newborn (Fig. 47-1B). The transition of the alveoli from a fluid-filled to an air-filled state has a mechanical effect on the pulmonary circulation, resulting in a reduced compression of the pulmonary alveolar capillaries with a reduction in pulmonary vascular resistance; however, the decrease in pulmonary vascular resistance is relatively slow. It takes 3 to 4 days for the pulmonary vascular resistance to decrease to the eventual level that it will achieve during the neonatal period. The initial moderate decrease in pulmonary vascular resistance is accompanied by constriction of the ductus arteriosus secondary to oxygenation. This results in an increase in pulmonary blood flow and an increase in left atrial pressure, so that the foramen ovale functionally closes. Closure of these two neonatal shunts (i.e., the ductus arteriosus and the foramen ovale) is initially only a functional closure. Both shunts usually close permanently in the first several months of life. However, an autopsy study of normal hearts has demonstrated an approximately 30% incidence of patent foramen ovale during the first 30 years of life and an approximately 20% incidence for persons aged 30 years and older. The size of the patent foramen ovale was found to increase with age.[1]

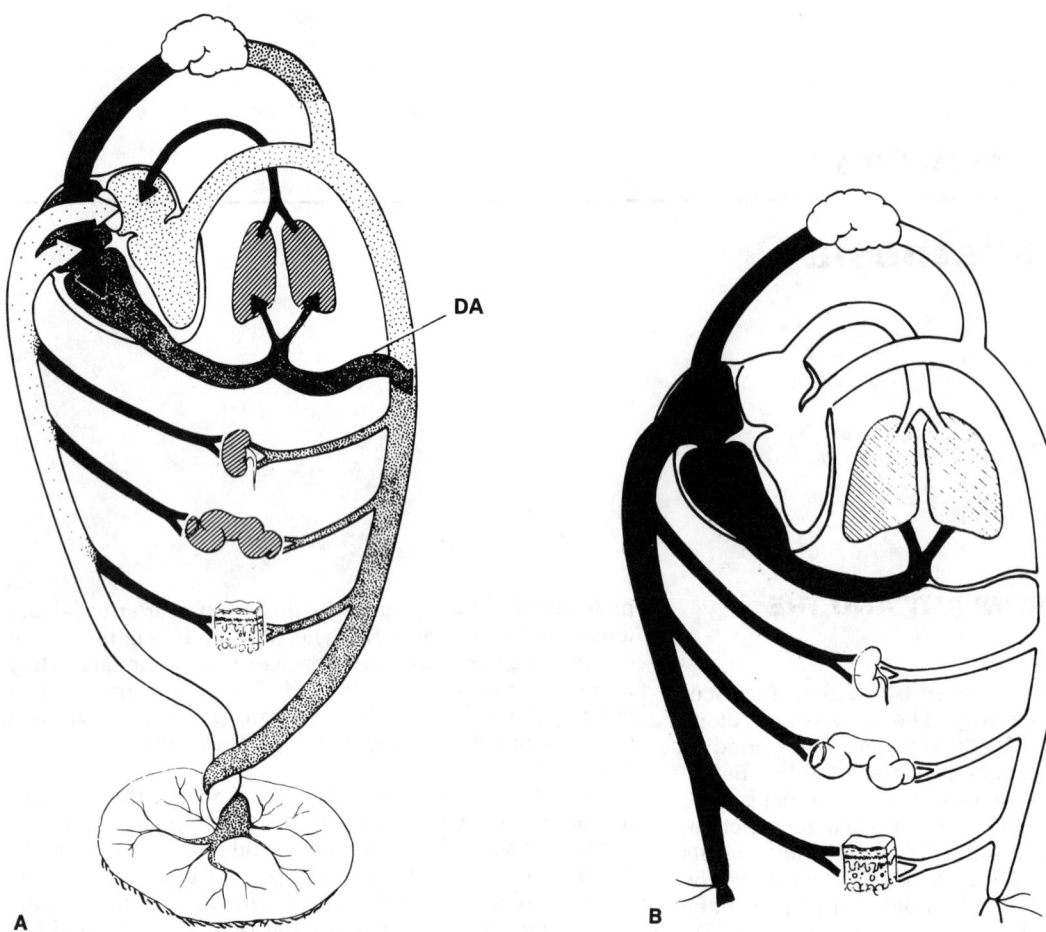

Figure 47-1. (*A*) Schematic representation of the fetal circulation. Oxygenated blood leaves the placenta in the umbilical vein (*vessel without stippling*). Umbilical vein blood joins blood from the viscera (*represented here by the kidney, gut, and skin*) in the inferior vena cava. Approximately half of the inferior vena cava flow passes through the foramen ovale to the left atrium, where it mixes with a small amount of pulmonary venous blood, and this relatively well oxygenated blood (*light stippling*) supplies the heart and brain by way of the ascending aorta. The other half of the inferior vena cava stream mixes with superior vena cava blood and enters the right ventricle (blood in the right atrium and ventricle has little oxygen, which is denoted by *heavy stippling*). Because the pulmonary aterioles are constricted, most of the blood in the main pulmonary artery flows through the ductus arteriosus (DA), so that the descending aorta's blood has less oxygen (*heavy stippling*) than does blood in the ascending aorta (*light stippling*). (*B*) Schematic representation of the circulation in the normal newborn. After expansion of the lungs and ligation of the umbilical cord, pulmonary blood flow and left atrial and systemic arterial pressures increase. When left atrial pressure exceeds right atrial pressure, the foramen ovale closes so that all the inferior and superior vena cava blood leaves the right atrium, enters the right ventricle, and is pumped through the pulmonary artery toward the lung. With the increase in systemic arterial pressure and decrease in pulmonary artery pressure, flow through the ductus arteriosus becomes left-to-right and the ductus constricts and closes. The course of circulation is the same as in the adult. (Reprinted with permission from Phibbs R: Delivery room management of the newborn. In Avery GB [ed]: Neonatology, Pathophysiology and Management of the Newborn, p 184. Philadelphia, JB Lippincott, 1981.)

Transition of the Pulmonary System

The pulmonary system transition occurs more quickly than the circulatory system transition. The primary event of the pulmonary system transition is the initiation of ventilation, which changes the alveoli from a fluid-filled to an air-filled state. During the first 5 to 10 minutes of extrauterine life, normal ventilatory volumes develop and a normal tidal ventilation is established. The initial negative intrathoracic pressures that the newborn generates are often in the range of 40 to 60 cm H_2O. By 10 to 20 minutes of life, the newborn has achieved its near normal functional residual capacity and the blood gases are well stabilized. Table 47-1 lists the normal blood gases for the various periods of life.

Persistent Pulmonary Hypertension (Persistent Fetal Circulation)

The major pulmonary system transition occurs over the first hour of life, whereas the major transition of the circulatory system occurs over the first 2 or 3 days of life. Figure 47-2 illustrates the correlation of the mean pulmonary artery pressure with age during the first 3 days of life. The pulmonary circulation is extremely sensitive to oxygenation and pH. Hypoxia and acidosis, along with unknown factors, may cause pulmonary artery pressure either to persist at a high level, or, after having been at a low level, to increase. The result is termed "persistent pulmonary hypertension." It

TABLE 47-1. Normal Blood Gas Values in the Newborn

Subject	Age	Po₂ (mm Hg)	Pco₂ (mm Hg)	pH
Fetus (term)	Before labor	25	40	7.37
Fetus (term)	End of labor	10–20	55	7.25
Newborn (term)	10 min	50	48	7.20
Newborn (term)	1 h	70	35	7.35
Newborn (term)	1 week	75	35	7.40
Newborn (preterm, 1,500 g)	1 week	60	38	7.37

was previously called persistent fetal circulation, but this is a misnomer, because the fetal circulation is characterized by the presence of a placental shunt that is no longer present. The pathophysiologic characteristics of persistent pulmonary hypertension comprise a spectrum, ranging from normal pulmonary vasculature to completely abnormal pulmonary vasculature that is characterized by extension of smooth muscle into the distal respiratory units (Fig. 47-3). There are all degrees in between. In some situations, the pulmonary vessels initially appear to vasodilate normally and later vasoconstrict. This situation is seen in some infants after repair of a congenital diaphragmatic hernia: the "honeymoon period" during and immediately after operation is followed by episodes of vasoconstriction that may or may not be amenable to therapy. This results in pulmonary hypertension with a right-to-left shunt through the foramen ovale and the ductus arteriosus (Fig. 47-4). The persistence of pulmonary hypertension occurs in three main situations in which the anesthesiologist may become involved: meconium aspiration, respiratory failure of the neonate, and congenital diaphragmatic hernia.

Meconium Aspiration

Interference with the normal maternal placental circulation in the third trimester may cause chronic fetal hypoxia. Fetal hypoxia can result in an increase in the amount of muscle in the blood vessels of the distal respiratory units.[2] Figure

47-3 illustrates the muscle increase found in blood vessels of a series of 11 infants who died of persistent pulmonary hypertension. Chronic fetal hypoxia leads to the passage of meconium *in utero*. The fetus swallows the meconium, which ends up in the pulmonary system. It is thought that the meconium *per se* does not cause the extension of the muscle of the pulmonary vascular system but that such muscle extension along pulmonary arterial branches is due to fetal hypoxia. Meconium aspiration can be a marker of chronic fetal hypoxia in the third trimester. This condition is quite different from the meconium aspiration that occurs during delivery, when again fetal hypoxia leads to the pas-

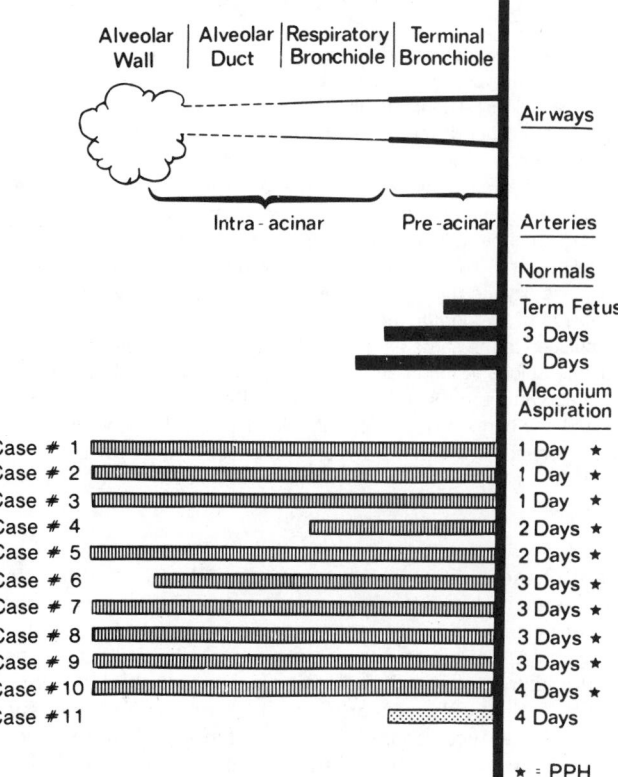

Figure 47-3. Diagram of muscle extension along pulmonary arterial branches (*shaded bars*). In the normal newborn infant, virtually no intraacinar artery is muscular. In 9 of 10 infants with meconium aspiration and persistent pulmonary hypertension (PPH), muscle extended into the most peripheral arteries; the infant with meconium aspiration without PPH (case #11) had normal intraacinar arteries. (Reprinted with permission from Murphy JD *et al*: Pulmonary vascular disease in fetal meconium aspiration. J Pediatr 104:758, 1984.)

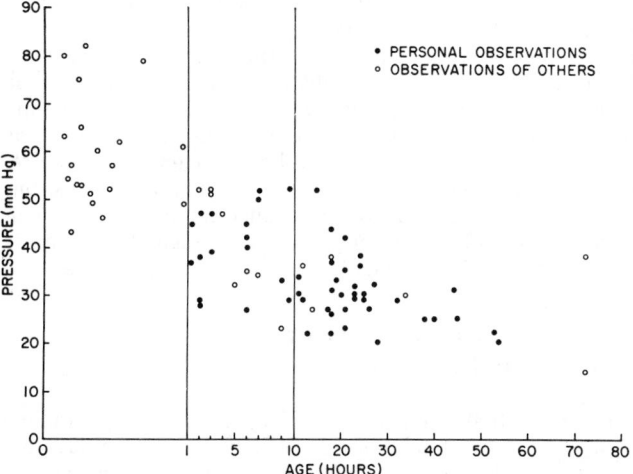

Figure 47-2. Correlation of mean pulmonary arterial pressure with age in 85 normal term infants studied during the first 3 days of life. (Reprinted with permission from Emmanouilides GC *et al*: Pulmonary arterial pressure changes in human newborn infants from birth to 3 days of age. J Pediatr 65:327, 1964.)

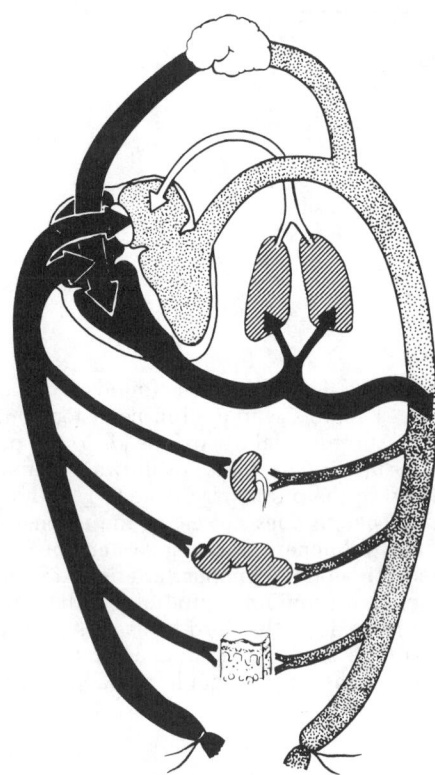

Figure 47-4. Schematic representation of the circulation in an asphyxiated newborn with incomplete expansion of the lungs. Pulmonary vascular resistance is high, pulmonary blood flow is low (note the small caliber of the pulmonary vein), and flow through the ductus arteriosus is high. With little pulmonary venous flow, left atrial pressure decreases below right atrial pressure, the foramen ovale opens, and vena cava blood flows through the foramen into the left atrium. This partially venous blood flows to the brain by the ascending aorta. The descending aorta blood that flows to the viscera has less oxygen than that of the ascending aorta (*heavy stippling*) because of the right-to-left flow through the ductus arteriosus. The circulation is the same as in the fetus except that there is no oxygenated blood in the inferior vena cava from the umbilical vein. (Reprinted with permission from Phibbs R: Delivery room management of the newborn. In Avery GB [ed]: Neonatology, Pathophysiology and Management of the Newborn. Philadelphia, JB Lippincott, 1981.)

sage of meconium. This meconium at birth is quite thick and tenacious and mechanically obstructs the tracheobronchial system. It is evident that the presence of meconium may be a marker of chronic fetal hypoxia and may cause acute airway obstruction of the tracheobronchial system.

Until relatively recently tracheal intubation and suctioning was recommended for all infants with frank meconium aspiration or meconium staining (approximately 10% of newborns). Now a more conservative approach should be used because routine intubation may cause unnecessary respiratory complications. Routine oral oropharyngeal suctioning is recommended immediately at the time of delivery, but tracheal intubation and suctioning should be performed selectively, depending on the condition of the infant. Infants with a high Apgar score (*i.e.*, 8 or 9) need no further airway management. Infants with a low Apgar score or who are clinically obstructed with meconium should have the appropriate resuscitative measures taken.

In summary, there are two potential clinical problems associated with meconium. The first is that of thick meconium which at birth obstructs the airway and causes mechanical obstruction. The second, termed the meconium aspiration syndrome, is a condition in which the infant has some degree of respiratory failure with persistent pulmonary hypertension secondary to chronic intrauterine hypoxia.

Persistent Pulmonary Hypertension and Respiratory Failure

Any infant with respiratory failure of any cause and in whom hypoxia, carbon dioxide retention, and acidosis develop may have persistent pulmonary hypertension. Persistent pulmonary hypertension and respiratory failure have been treated in several ways.[3] There was initial enthusiasm for the use of hyperventilation to reduce the partial pressure of carbon dioxide (Pco_2) to between 20 and 30 mm Hg. These infants often require inflating pressures of 40 to 50 cm H_2O, with rates of 100 to 150 breaths·min^{-1}. However, there is controversy over this therapeutic technique, the concern being that it will cause barotrauma and increase the incidence of residual lung disease. Alternative treatments have been used. One of these is based on the belief that oxygenation of the infant is the major concern and carbon dioxide control is secondary.[4] Therefore, if the infant can maintain a Pao_2 between 50 to 70 mm Hg with 5 to 8 cm H_2O positive end-expiratory pressure (PEEP), then $Paco_2$ levels of up to 60 to 70 mm Hg are accepted. This therapeutic approach has apparently increased the number of survivors and decreased the incidence of residual lung disease, but the issue has yet to be settled.

A number of reports have discussed the use of extracorporeal membrane oxygenation (ECMO).[5,6] The therapy is aimed at resting the infant's lungs while providing adequate oxygenation for survival and lung repair. It is hoped that the rested lung will be able to recover its function by repairing the pulmonary parenchyma and restructuring the pulmonary vascular bed. The lung is ventilated with low pressures, *i.e.*, 20 cm H_2O pressure with 5 cm H_2O of PEEP and an FIO_2 of 0.21 to 0.3. As the infant's pulmonary function improves, evidenced by increasing Pao_2 levels, the ECMO is reduced accordingly. This is an extremely expensive and high-risk technique that requires an experienced and talented team. The vascular shunt is performed through either a venovenous or a venoarterial circuit. Heparin must be administered to the infants, and this may increase the chance of intracranial bleeding.[7] The use of ECMO therapy has increased tremendously in the past several years. It has proved to be quite successful in the management of respiratory failure. There are no long-term outcome studies, but the short-term results are quite encouraging. The use of ECMO in infants with congenital diaphragmatic hernia is discussed later in the chapter.

Transition and Maturation of the Renal System

The fetal kidneys and the fetal lungs have certain similarities. During the fetal period, both have a relatively low blood flow compared with that during the newborn and neonatal periods because both organs need only enough blood flow for growth and development. The maternal placenta removes fetal waste material. The major function of the fetal kidneys is the passive production of urine, which contributes to the formation of amniotic fluid, which is important for the normal development of the fetal lung and acts as a shock absorber for the fetus. The fetal kidney is characterized by a low renal blood flow (RBF) and glomerular filtration rate (GFR).[8] There are four major reasons for the low RBF and GFR: low systemic arterial pressure, high renal vascular resistance, low permeability of the glomerular capillaries, and the small size and number of glomeruli. The low systemic arterial pressure and high vascular resistance are the two characteristics that are similar to those found in the fetal lung. This results in a low RBF, which in turn results in a low GFR. Transition changes the first two factors: the systemic arterial pressure increases and the renal vascular resistance decreases. Again, this is similar to what occurs in the lung. The other two factors are changed through maturation. The limited ability of the newborn's kidney to concentrate or dilute urine results from the low GFR at birth. However, during the first 3 to 4 days, the circulatory changes increase RBF and GFR and improve the neonate's renal function. By 3 to 4 days, there is a significant improvement in the ability to concentrate and dilute the urine. The maturation continues, and by the time the normal full-term infant is 1 month of age, the kidneys are approximately 70% mature. This is sufficient renal function to handle almost any contingency.

The neonatal kidney does have certain limitations. The renin-angiotensin-aldosterone system is the primary compensatory system for the reabsorption of sodium and water to compensate for the loss of plasma, blood, gastrointestinal tract fluid, and third-space fluid (Fig. 47-5). Although the neonate has a normal renin-angiotensin-aldosterone system, the neonatal kidney cannot completely conserve sodium, even with a severe sodium deficit. Aldosterone facilitates the reabsorption of sodium in the distal tubule. The immature tubular cells cannot completely reabsorb sodium under the stimulus of aldosterone, so that the neonate will continue to excrete sodium in the urine even in the presence of a severe sodium defect. For this reason, the neonate is considered an "obligate sodium loser." In the mature state, the distal tubule can reabsorb essentially all of the sodium, so that the urine will have less than 5 to 10 mEq of sodium per liter of urine. In the neonate, this figure may be as high as 20–25 mEq·l^{-1} of urine.

Fluid and Electrolyte Therapy in the Neonate

The neonatal kidney matures rapidly. In the mature state, the kidney's ability to fully conserve sodium and water compensates for fluid and electrolyte deficits. The inability of the neonatal distal tubule to fully respond to aldosterone results in the obligatory sodium loss in the urine. Therefore, fluids given intravenously (iv) to the neonate must contain sodium. Most operations on neonates involve loss of blood and extracellular fluid, which must be replaced with a fluid of similar electrolyte content, such as lactated Ringer's solution. When considering blood transfusion it is important to consider that the neonate needs a higher hematocrit (approximately 35%) because of a high oxygen demand and relatively limited ability to increase cardiac output, whereas the 3-month-old infant can easily tolerate a hematocrit of 25%.

The other problems of the neonate are those of appropriate glucose administration. Infants of diabetic mothers and those small for gestational age have particular problems with hypoglycemia. These infants need to have their blood glucose values monitored until stable. Neonates scheduled for surgery who have been receiving hyperalimentation flu-

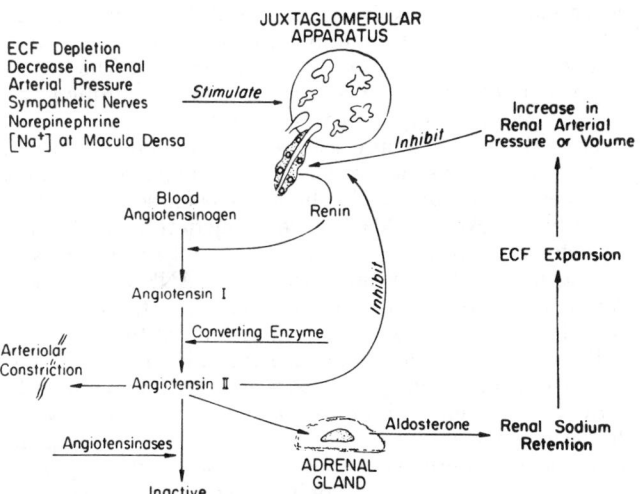

Figure 47-5. The juxtaglomerular apparatus and control of renin secretion. (Reprinted with permission from Mulrow PJ, Siegel NJ: Mechanisms in hypertension. In Edelmann CM Jr [ed]: Pediatric Kidney Disease. Boston, Little, Brown & Co, 1978.)

ids or supplementary glucose must continue to receive that fluid intraoperatively or must have their glucose levels monitored because of concern over hypoglycemia. This concern must be balanced against the potential augmentation of ischemic injury by the administration of glucose. The issue of glucose metabolism has not been well studied.[9] A recent symposium that addressed the issue of hypoglycemia in infants suggested that a blood glucose level of less than 20 mg·dl^{-1} represented hypoglycemia in premature and small for gestational age babies, whereas a blood glucose level above 36 mg·dl^{-1} represented hypoglycemia in the full-term infant.[10]

Premature infants and neonates must receive full-strength, balanced salt solution for the replacement of third-space and blood losses during the perioperative period. There is a misconception that these infants cannot tolerate the salt load, and therefore they are often given hypotonic fluids. It is not unusual to see premature infants with postoperative sodium values of 125–130 mEq·l^{-1}. Alone, these levels may not be a major problem, but when added to the residual effects of muscle relaxants and antibiotics in a sick infant, they may result in depression of neuromuscular function.

Premature infants and those with bronchopulmonary dysplasia have problems with increased pulmonary lung water, and furosemide has been shown to acutely decrease airway resistance in chronic bronchopulmonary dysplasia.[11] Fluid therapy should be administered conservatively, i.e., 2–3 ml·kg^{-1}·h^{-1} of maintenance requirement plus the replacement fluid for trauma and blood loss.[12] These infants need balanced salt solution for replacement fluid and more than the usual dose if they are being treated with a diuretic. Lung function will improve as these infants age and mature.[13]

Atrial Natriuretic Factor

There has been recent interest in the role of atrial natriuretic factor (ANF, a peptide) in sodium homeostasis of the infant.[14] ANF is released from the atria and reduces sodium overload in the body. ANF affects renal function by altering renal hemodynamics and increasing urinary sodium and water excretion; it also increases the GFR, which results in a significant natriuresis without an alteration in total RBF. In addition, ANF opposes the renin system. The renin-angiotensin-aldosterone system is a tightly controlled system that immediately activates when there is a challenge to arterial blood pressure as well as a deficit of sodium. Sometimes this system overshoots and the patient acquires an excessive sodium load. There has been some question about blood levels of ANF and the function of ANF in the neonate. It has been found that in the first several days of life, the neonate has elevated ANF levels. ANF has also been found to be present in the premature infant, and it may provide a sensitive and important system for the control of sodium balance in the premature and full-term infant and play a role in reducing the extracellular fluid volume to normal. Water and sodium balance are usually negative in the early neonatal period. The role of ANF in this fluid shift is unknown. The newborn infant, particularly the premature infant, has a relatively high extracellular fluid volume. This volume is reduced from 50% of body weight in the premature infant and 40% of body weight in the newborn to approximately 20% of body weight in the 18-month-old infant.

ANATOMIC AND MATURATIONAL FACTORS OF NEONATES AND THEIR CLINICAL SIGNIFICANCE

The anatomic and maturational factors unique to the neonate have far-reaching clinical implications (Fig. 47-6). The anatomic differences of the neonatal head and airway are as follows: narrow nares, a large tongue, a high glottis, slanting vocal cords, a narrow cricoid ring, and a large occiput. Neonates must breathe through the nose because they cannot coordinate the usual swallowing and breathing mechanics. Therefore, anything that obstructs the nares will compromise the neonate's ability to breathe. For this reason, choanal atresia is a life-threatening surgical problem for the infant. The large tongue occupies space in the infant's airway and makes it difficult to use the laryngoscope and intubate the infant's trachea. In the normal adult, the glottis is at the level of C5. In the full-term infant, the glottis is at the

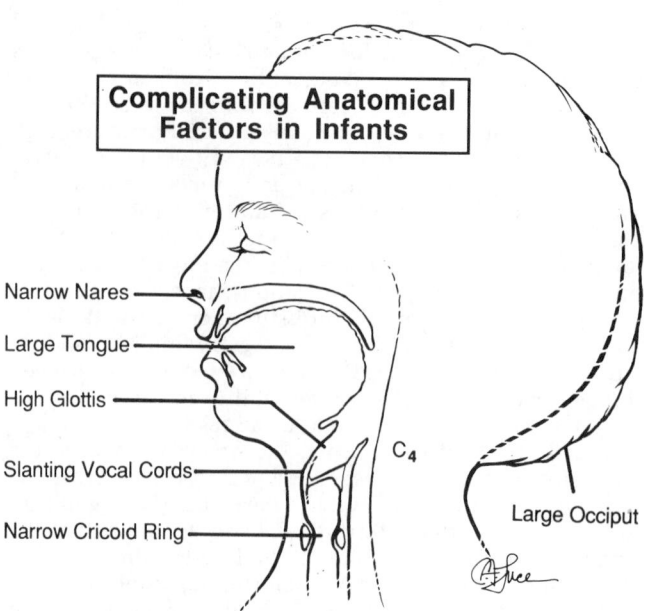

Figure 47-6. Complicating anatomic factors in infants. (Modified with permission from Smith RM: Anesthesia for Infants and Children, 4th ed. St Louis, CV Mosby, 1980.)

level of C4, and in the premature infant it is at the level of C3. The combination of a large tongue and a relatively high glottis means that on laryngoscopic examination it is more difficult to establish a line of vision between the mouth and larynx: there is relatively more tissue in less distance. Therefore, the infant's larynx appears to be anterior. When combined with the anterior slanting vocal cords, the result is a more difficult laryngoscopic examination and intubation. Application of cricoid pressure by the anesthesiologist or an assistant will help visualization of the neonate's larynx. If the anesthesiologist's hand is large enough, cricoid pressure can be applied with the little finger (Fig. 47-7). This is more effective than having an assistant apply pressure because the anesthesiologist can determine the best position for intubation.

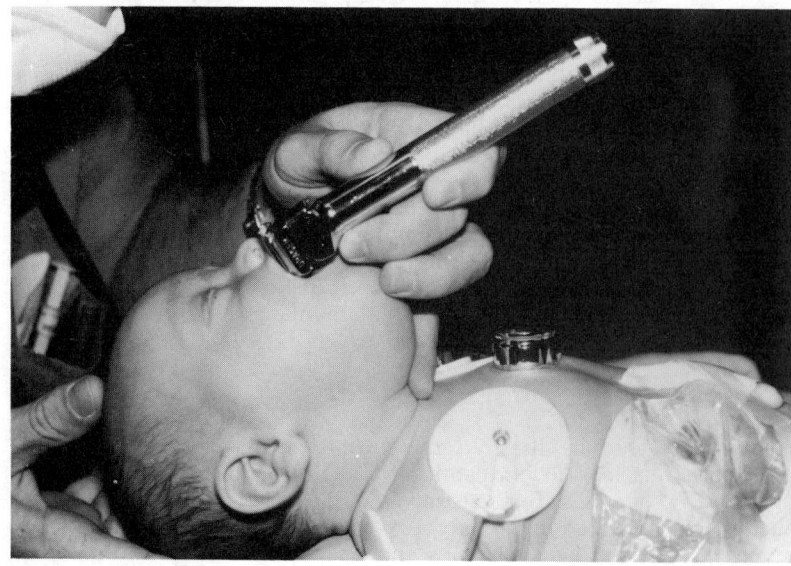

Figure 47-7. Cricoid pressure applied with little finger. (Reprinted with permission from Berry FA [ed]: Anesthetic Management of Difficult and Routine Pediatric Patients. New York, Churchill Livingstone, 1990.)

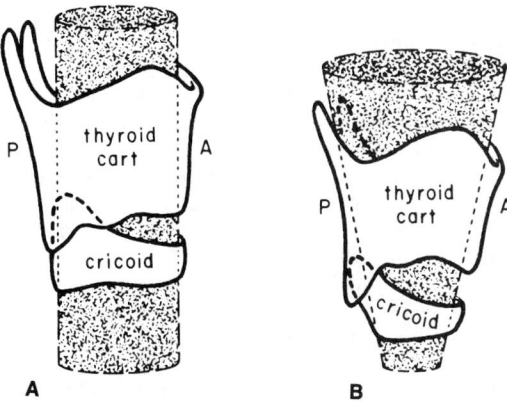

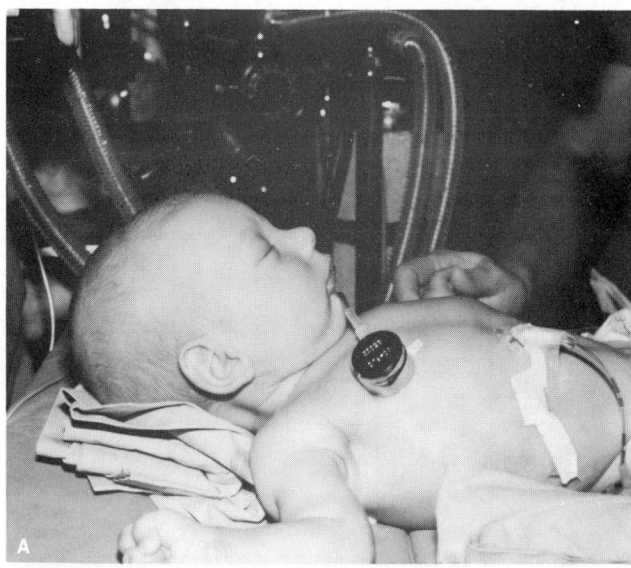

Figure 47-8. Configuration of the adult (*A*) *versus* the infant larynx (*B*). The adult larynx has a cylindric shape. The infant larynx is funnel shaped because of the narrow, undeveloped cricoid cartilage. (Reprinted with permission from Ryan JF, Todres ID, Cote CJ et al [eds]: A Practice of Anesthesia for Infants and Children. Orlando, Grune & Stratton, 1986.)

A narrow cricoid ring is significant because it means that the narrowest portion of the neonate's airway is not the vocal cords but the cricoid ring. In the mature state, the airway from the vocal cords down the trachea is of equal dimensions (Fig. 47-8). If the endotracheal tube passes comfortably through the vocal cords, it will not be tight within the cricoid cartilage. However, the neonate's laryngeal structures resemble a funnel; even though the endotracheal tube may pass through the vocal cords, which are at the midpoint of the funnel, the endotracheal tube may be tight within the cricoid ring.[15] This tight fit may cause temporary or permanent damage to the cricoid cartilage, resulting in short- or long-term airway difficulties. When the infant has a large occiput, the head will flex forward onto the chest when the infant is lying supine with its head in the midline (Fig. 47-9A). Extreme extension can also obstruct the airway, so that a midposition of the head with slight extension is preferred for airway maintenance. This is accomplished by placing a small roll at the base of the neck and shoulders (Fig. 47-9B).

Anatomic and Physiologic Factors of the Pulmonary System

Anatomically and physiologically, the neonate's pulmonary system differs in at least four respects from that of the mature infant: a high oxygen consumption, high closing volumes, a high minute ventilation to functional residual capacity (FRC) ratio, and pliable ribs. The oxygen consumption of the infant is 7–9 ml·kg^{-1}·min^{-1}, whereas in the mature state it is 3 ml·kg^{-1}·min^{-1}. Therefore, varying degrees of airway obstruction have more impact on oxygen delivery and reserve in the neonate. The neonate, infant, and child require high oxygen consumption for growth and development, but in terms of supplying oxygen during periods of airway compromise, it is a distinct disadvantage. Because of the high oxygen consumption, apnea in an infant uses up the residual oxygen in the lungs much more quickly than in the older child and adult.

The high closing volumes of the neonate's lungs are within the lower range of the normal tidal volume (Fig.

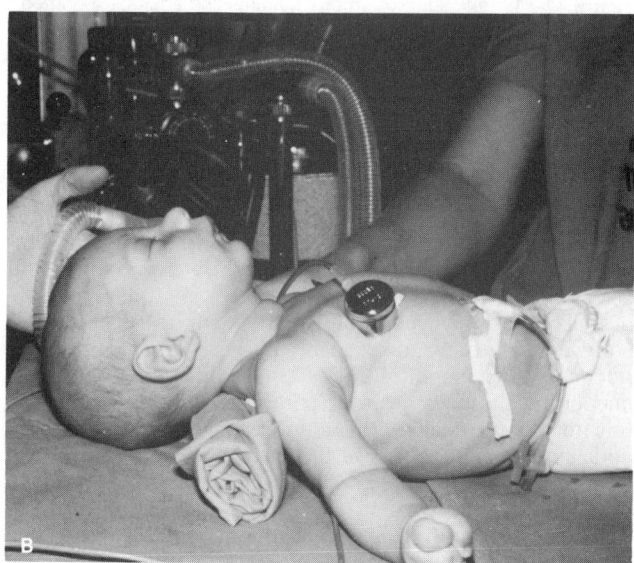

Figure 47-9. (*A*) Pad under occiput in an attempt to achieve the "sniffing" position obstructs the infant's airway. (Reprinted with permission from Berry FA [ed]: Anesthetic Management of Difficult and Routine Pediatric Patients. New York, Churchill Livingstone, 1990.) (*B*) Pad is placed under infant's neck to improve the airway patency and for laryngoscopic examination. (Reprinted with permission from Berry FA [ed]: Anesthetic Management of Difficult and Routine Pediatric Patients. New York, Churchill Livingstone, 1990.)

47-10). This is also true of the elderly patient. Closing volumes are the lung volumes at which alveoli close, resulting in the shunting of blood by a closed alveolus. If an infant experiences mild laryngospasm and a reduction in lung volume, the high closing volume will contribute to shunting of blood and rapid desaturation. When a high oxygen consumption is combined with a high closing volume in the presence of laryngospasm, the rapidity with which desaturation occurs is breathtaking not only for the infant but also for the anesthesiologist. When coughing, breath-holding, and so on occur when an endotracheal tube is in place, the situation is not much different, because there is an inability

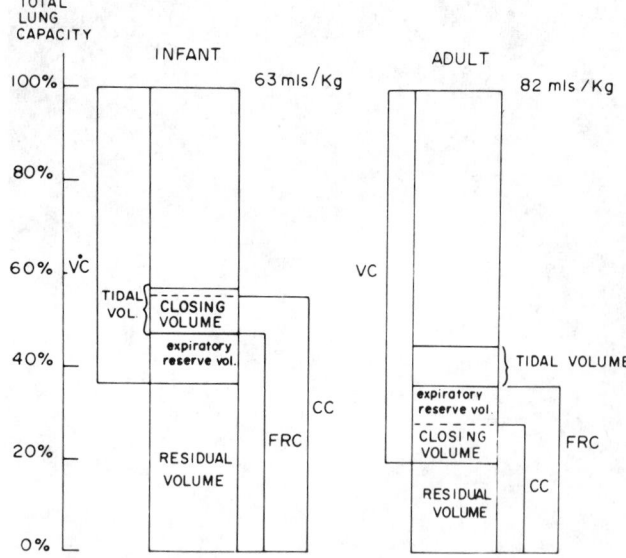

Figure 47-10. Static lung volumes of infants and adults. (Reprinted with permission from Smith CA, Nelson NM: Physiology of the Newborn Infant, 4th ed. Springfield, Illinois, Charles C Thomas, 1976.)

to ventilate the alveoli. Positive pressure will ventilate the large airways, but there will be no oxygen delivery to the closed alveoli. Therefore, even though an endotracheal tube may be in the appropriate anatomic location, severe desaturation can occur in infants who are lightly anesthetized and are coughing on the endotracheal tube. At times, because of inability to oxygenate the infant, it might be incorrectly believed that the endotracheal tube has come out of the trachea. Management of the patient in this situation entails deepening the anesthesia or paralysis. The bottom line is that the infant needs either depression of the central nervous system or paralysis of the muscles. This can be done with either small iv doses of succinylcholine, 0.5 mg·kg^{-1}, or iv lidocaine, 1.5 mg·kg^{-1}. Caution must be taken not to exceed this dose of lidocaine in the neonate. One neonate who received 2 mg·kg^{-1} of lidocaine in a similar situation developed a high-grade atrioventricular heart block and a ventricular rate of 40.[16]

The third unique pulmonary feature of the neonate is the high minute ventilation to FRC ratio, which is similar to that of the term pregnant woman but occurs for different reasons. The pregnant woman has a reduction in FRC because of elevation of the diaphragm by the uterus. The neonate has an increased alveolar ventilation because of the need to increase oxygen delivery secondary to the high oxygen consumption. Table 47-2 compares the normal respiratory values for newborns and adults.

It is important to remember that the tidal ventilation for an infant is the same, in ml·kg^{-1}, as for the adult; therefore, with an oxygen consumption that is three times greater, the respiratory rate must be three times greater, which results in an alveolar ventilation that is three times greater. Consequently, the ratio of minute ventilation to FRC is 5:1 in the neonate, whereas in adults it is 1.5:1. The clinical implication of the high minute ventilation to FRC ratio is that there is a much more rapid induction of inhalational anesthesia, as well as more rapid awakening from inhalational anesthesia. The more rapid induction of anesthesia also results from a higher percentage of the neonate's body weight consisting of vessel-rich tissues.[17] Figure 47-11 compares the predicted *vs.* observed ratio of end-tidal to inspired halothane in infants and adults. The practical implication of the data is that clinicians who use the adult curve and the usual overpressure of halothane (approximately 3% inspired) for induction will find the neonate more rapidly induced and perhaps at risk for an overdose of anesthetic. This subject is discussed later in the chapter, under Uptake and Distribution of Anesthetic Agents.

The fourth anatomic difference of the neonate is a pliable rib cage. Normal, quiet ventilation in the neonate physically resembles that in the older child. However, if there is a need for increased minute ventilation, requiring an increase in respiratory frequency or tidal volume, the pliable ribs of the neonate will be a disadvantage. The neonate's diaphragm is the major ventilatory muscle. In order to increase oxygen delivery by either an increase in frequency or excursion, the contraction of the diaphragm results in greater negative intrathoracic pressures. In mature individuals with a fixed rib cage, this results in an increase in air movement. However, with a pliable rib cage, the resulting increase in negative intrathoracic pressure results in retractions of ribs as well as retraction in the subcostal and supraclavicular area. This results in less efficient ventilation and a high energy price for the effort involved. This is one of the reasons why neonates are susceptible to fatigue with airway obstruction,

TABLE 47-2. Comparison of Normal Respiratory Values in Infants and Adults

Parameter	Infant	Adult
Respiratory frequency	30–50	12–16
Tidal volume (ml·kg^{-1})	7	7
Dead space (ml·kg^{-1})	2–2.5	2.2
Alveolar ventilation (ml·kg^{-1}·min^{-1})	100–150	60
Functional residual capacity (ml·kg^{-1})	27–30	30
Oxygen consumption (ml·kg^{-1}·min^{-1})	7–9	3

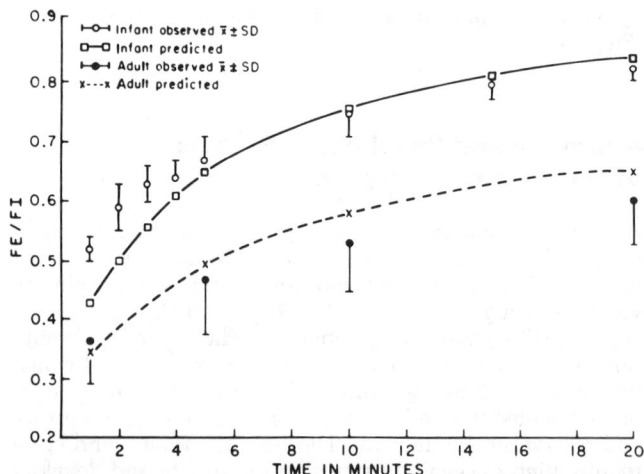

Figure 47-11. Predicted *vs.* observed FE/FI for halothane in infants and adults. Predicted FE/FI values are those generated by a computed program of anesthetic uptake and distribution. In infants, the minute ventilation averaged 1.9 l; in adults, 6.9 l. The inspired fraction of halothane was 0.5% in both cases. (Reprinted with permission from Brandom BW, Brandom RB, Cook DR: Uptake of halothane in infants. Anesth Analg 62:404, 1983.)

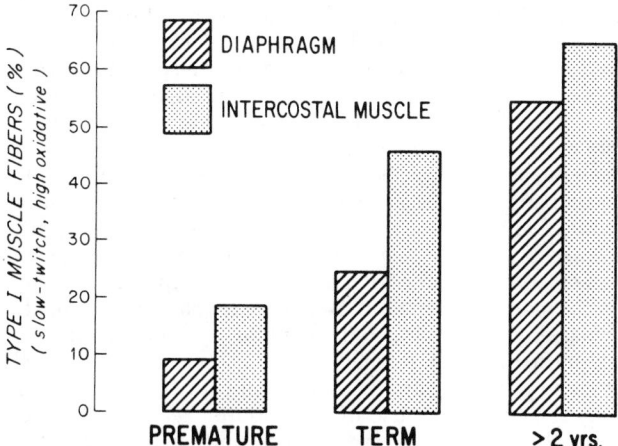

Figure 47-12. Muscle fiber composition of diaphragm and intercostal muscles related to age. The premature infant's diaphragm and intercostal muscles have fewer Type I fibers compared with those of newborns and older children. The data suggest a possible mechanism for early fatigue in premature and term infants when the effort of breathing is increased. (Reprinted with permission from Ryan JF, Todres ID, Coté CJ et al [eds]: A Practice of Anesthesia for Infants and Children. Orlando, Grune & Stratton, 1986.)

pneumonia, and any other condition that results in interference with pulmonary function; another reason is the immaturity of the muscles.

Maturation of Respiratory Muscles

There are two types of muscles: Type 1, slow-twitch, high oxidative muscles, which are necessary for sustained muscle activity; and Type 2, fast-twitch, low oxidative muscles, which have an immediate but short activity.[18] The development of Type 1 muscles is necessary for sustained ventilatory activity. The premature infant has 10% Type 1 and the newborn 25% Type 1 muscles in the diaphragm, which is the primary muscle for ventilation (Fig. 47-12). The infant achieves maturity of Type 1 muscles at approximately 8 months of age. At that point, he or she will have approximately 55% Type 1 muscles. The intercostal muscles are the other ventilatory muscles. The premature infant has 20% Type 1 intercostal muscles and the newborn, 46%. The age of maturity for these muscles is 2 months, when there will be 65% Type 1 muscles.

Maturation of the Cardiovascular System

The Heart and Sympathetic Nervous System

The ability of the neonate's immature cardiovascular system to respond to stress is limited by the relatively low contractile mass per gram of cardiac tissue, which results in a limited ability to increase myocardial contractility, as well as a reduction in the compliance of the ventricle.[19] The clinical implication of this limited stretchability or compliance of the ventricle means that, although there may be some ability to increase stroke volume, it is extremely limited. Therefore, any increase in cardiac output must be accomplished by an increase in heart rate. For this reason, the infant is said to be rate dependent for its cardiac output. Thus, any slowing of the heart rate is reflected in a reduction in cardiac output. This is why bradycardia has such serious consequences for

the infant. The major cause of bradycardia in an infant is hypoxia. The second major cause is vagal stimulation. Even in the absence of stress, the neonatal heart has limited ability to increase cardiac output as compared with the mature heart (Fig. 47-13). The resting cardiac output of the immature heart is very close to the maximal cardiac output, so there is a very limited reserve. The mature heart can increase cardiac output by 300%, whereas the immature heart can only increase cardiac output by 30–40%.

In summary, the neonatal heart has some significant limitations. The resting cardiac output is much higher relative to body weight than in the adult. The neonatal heart is less able to handle a volume or pressure change. Stimulation of the myocardium produces a limited increase in contractility and cardiac output. The sympathetic nervous system, which usually provides the important chronotropic and inotropic

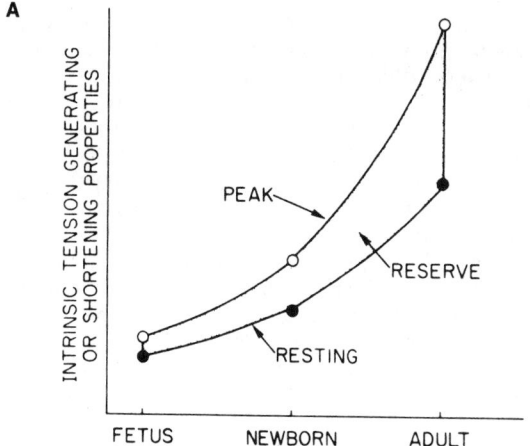

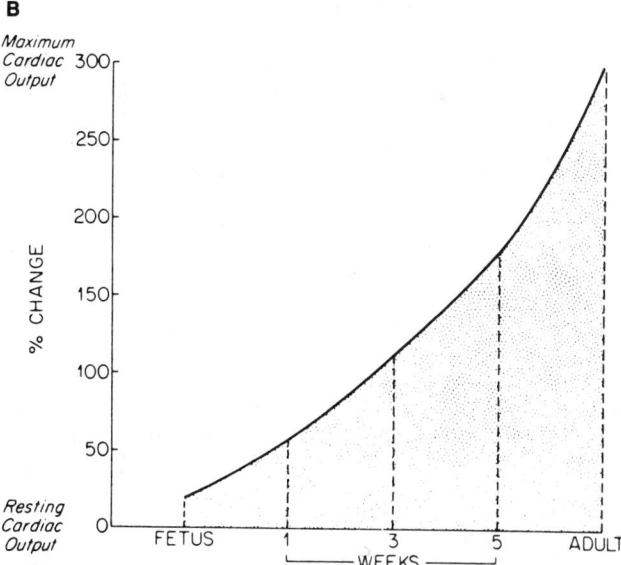

Figure 47-13. Schema of reduced cardiac reserve in fetal and newborn animal hearts compared with adult hearts. (*A*) In the newborn infant, resting cardiac muscle performance is close to a peak of ventricular function because of limitations in diastolic, systolic, and heart rate reserve. (*B*) Similarly, pump reserve early in life is limited by these factors as well as by much higher resting cardiac output relative to body weight, compared with that in adults. (Reprinted with permission from Friedman WF, George BL: Treatment of congestive heart failure by altering loading conditions of the heart. J Pediatr 106:700, 1985.)

support to the mature circulation during stress, owing to its immaturity, is severely limited in the neonate.

The Baroresponse

Immaturity of the baroresponse, which results in a reflex tachycardia in response to hypotension, has been demonstrated in baby rabbits.[20] Therefore, the immaturity of this reflex would limit the neonate's ability to compensate for hypotension. In addition, the baroresponse of the neonate is more depressed than that of the adult at the same level of anesthesia.

ANESTHESIA FOR THE NEONATE

Premedication

There is controversy about the need for premedication with anticholinergics. Many clinicians only administer anticholinergics to patients older than 6 months and for a specific indication, such as a sensitive airway, asthma, or a reactive airway. However, two special concerns in the neonate distinguish it from the more mature child: an active vagal reflex and secretions. Because of these concerns, most anesthesiologists routinely administer anticholinergics either preoperatively or intraoperatively to infants less than 6 months old.

Certainly one of the major indications for anticholinergics is to reduce secretions. The management of the combination of a difficult infant airway and excessive secretions can be simplified by reducing secretions. The dose of atropine in the neonate is 0.02 mg·kg^{-1}; for glycopyrrolate it is 0.01 mg·kg^{-1} given intramuscularly (im).

Endotracheal Intubation

One of the frequently asked questions about the anesthetic management of neonates is whether or not endotracheal intubation is routinely needed. The answer to this question depends on the skill of the anesthesiologist and the surgical procedure, but in most clinical situations, the neonate should be intubated because of various anatomic and physiologic considerations. If the anesthesiologist is skilled and the surgery is short, intubation may not be necessary. This is a clinical judgment that must be determined individually by each anesthesiologist and in each situation. Another question is whether or not to control the ventilation of all neonates. If the overall condition of the neonate is healthy and the procedure is short, then spontaneous ventilation is certainly acceptable. However, if the neonate is debilitated, has had a relatively long-standing illness, has circulatory instability, and requires muscle relaxation for the surgery, then intraoperative controlled ventilation of the lungs is certainly indicated.

Opinion on whether or not to perform awake tracheal intubation in the neonate has changed in the last several years. There is concern that awake tracheal intubation causes hypertension and that the hypertension can rupture the fragile intracerebral vessels, particularly in premature infants. There are times when awake tracheal intubation would seem to be the technique of choice, such as in neonates who are critically ill and need resuscitation. Neonates who are persistently vomiting and in whom the stomach cannot be emptied should have an awake tracheal intubation if at all possible. An awake tracheal intubation can be accomplished with topical anesthesia of the oropharynx

and lidocaine, 1.5 mg·kg^{-1} iv, in order to blunt the response to the intubation. If problems of a full stomach and the resulting concern for aspiration are not present, the current trend is to perform endotracheal intubation after the induction of anesthesia. This topic is discussed more fully in the section on anesthetic techniques.

The question of extubation of the trachea is considerably easier to answer. The awake state is associated with control of the airway reflexes. Partially anesthetized infants are susceptible to laryngospasm and its associated apnea. Laryngospasm, apnea, and a high oxygen consumption are a devastating combination that is best avoided. Therefore, the trachea should be extubated when the neonate is awake and reacting to the endotracheal tube. An awake neonate will open its eyes, grasp the endotracheal tube, and cry. Crying cannot be heard because of the endotracheal tube but can be readily visualized. Any of these findings indicates that the infant is ready for extubation. If there is any doubt, however, the neonate should remain intubated until the clinician feels comfortable that the neonate can be extubated.

Does the Neonate Need Anesthesia?

There was some question in past years about whether the premature infant needed anesthesia for surgery. However, today the neonate and premature infant should be considered as any other patient who needs anesthesia.[21] Infants perceive pain and react to pain.[22] There is a concern that the hypertensive response to pain may cause intracranial bleeding in susceptible infants. The selection of anesthetic techniques for the neonate is based on the same criteria as for any patient, while at the same time recognizing the pharmacokinetic and pharmacodynamic differences.

Which Anesthetic Technique Is Best?

Which anesthetic agent or anesthetic technique is best: regional, general, or a combination? The answer depends on the knowledge, skills, and experience of the anesthesiologist and the surgeon, and the surgical needs of the patient. Rarely is a situation encountered in which one anesthetic agent or technique is indicated to the exclusion of all others. On the other hand, anesthetic agents and techniques do not have identical effects, and careful thought should be given to the selection of the best anesthetic for each patient and operation.

Impact of Surgical Requirements on Anesthetic Technique

Blood loss and muscle relaxation are two areas of concern for the surgeon and anesthesiologist. Parents and health care workers also are concerned about the transmission of acquired immunodeficiency syndrome (AIDS) and hepatitis through transfusion of blood and blood products. The use of blood and blood products should be minimized whenever possible. One way to minimize blood replacement is to minimize blood loss. This can be achieved through the control of blood pressure by the various anesthetics and muscle relaxants. The anesthetic techniques used can be directed toward preventing hypertension, which often occurs with the use of nitrous oxide or a low-dose opioid plus muscle relaxant, or toward inducing controlled normovolemic hypotension. Therefore, it is extremely important for the anesthesiologist and surgeon to discuss the impact of blood pressure on the surgical procedure, as well as the potential for loss of blood. Blood replacement is indicated if the neonate has demonstrated circulatory instability and considerable blood loss is anticipated. However, if the neonate is basically healthy and the anticipated blood loss is less than 25–30% of the blood volume, then blood transfusion probably can be avoided. This topic is discussed more fully in the section on fluid and blood therapy. The anesthesiologist can tailor the anesthetic to control the blood pressure and thereby reduce blood loss. This requires an appreciation of the cardiovascular effects of anesthetics and muscle relaxants.

Cardiovascular Effects of Muscle Relaxants

Although d-tubocurarine does have a dose-related histamine release that causes peripheral vasodilation, the incremental administration of d-tubocurarine will minimize, if not eliminate, any effect on the blood pressure. The same is true for atracurium. Pancuronium has vagolytic and sympathomimetic actions that will cause tachycardia and an increase in blood pressure (Table 47-3).[23] If a neonate is moribund or in shock, or there is concern about the volume status, then pancuronium may well be the muscle relaxant of choice. However, in a relatively normal neonate with a normal blood pressure and normal blood volume, the use of pancuronium may result in hypertension, which has the potential to increase blood loss. In such an infant atracurium would be a more logical choice of muscle relaxant for short surgical cases, or perhaps d-tubocurarine for longer cases. Atracurium has certain advantages over vecuronium in the infant younger than 1 year of age. The duration of action of vecuronium is approximately twice that observed in older children, either because of liver immaturity or because of an increased volume of distribution.[24,25] The length of action of atracurium in the neonate is similar to that in the older infant or child. The infant's neuromuscular junction is more sensitive to muscle relaxants, and the infant has a larger volume of distribution because of a large extracellular fluid volume. These two effects tend to balance each other, so that, roughly speaking, the dose of a nondepolarizing muscle relaxant for an infant is quite similar to that for a child on a mg·kg^{-1} basis. The major difference in neonates is the great variability in response to the nondepolarizing muscle relaxants, so that dose-response effects must be carefully observed to avoid either overdose or underdose.

However, there is some increase in succinylcholine requirement in the infant compared with the older child.[26] The im dose of succinylcholine is 5 mg·kg^{-1} in the infant, whereas the dose for children is 4 mg·kg^{-1}. The iv dose of succinylcholine in the infant and child is 2 mg·kg^{-1}.

A concern about the administration of succinylcholine in the neonate is the development of bradycardia. Succinylcholine (two molecules of acetylcholine) results in stimulation of the acetylcholine receptors; if the muscarinic receptor predominates, cardiac slowing occurs; if the nicotinic receptor predominates, tachycardia occurs. More often than not, the cause of the bradycardia is either laryngoscopy or hypoxia. The use of a pulse oximeter will clarify the issue. Bradycardia will develop in a small number of infants and children with the first iv dose of succinylcholine. Intramuscular succinylcholine is not associated with muscle fasciculation or cardiovascular effects. The bradycardia is self-limited and of no consequence unless the patient is hypoxic at the time. However, some believe that atropine should be administered before iv succinylcholine.

Atracurium appears to be the drug of choice among the intermediate-acting, nondepolarizing muscle relaxants. As already mentioned, it does not have a prolonged effect in the neonate. Its metabolism is by Hofmann elimination, ester hydrolysis, and the liver and kidney.[27] There is some controversy over the dose of atracurium needed for tracheal intubation. The recommended doses have varied from 0.6 to 0.9 mg·kg^{-1}. The recovery time from the action of atracurium depends on whether or not a volatile drug is used along with the atracurium, because volatile drugs will increase the neuromuscular blocking effects of atracurium. The use of nondepolarizing muscle relaxants should be guided by monitoring of neuromuscular function with a nerve stimulator. There is some controversy about the routine reversal of nondepolarizing muscle relaxants, because a nerve stimulator indicates only 75–80% return of function.[28] One opinion is that if the usual time period for the spontaneous reversal of neuromuscular function has been exceeded by a factor of 2, and if neuromuscular function is determined to be normal, there is no need for reversal. The other opinion is that, regardless of time, there is relatively little risk in administering neuromuscular reversal drugs.

Reversal of Nondepolarizing Neuromuscular Blocking Agents

Edrophonium in a dose of 1 mg·kg^{-1} will achieve a 90% reversal of a neuromuscular block in 2 minutes, whereas neostigmine in a dose of 0.06 mg·kg^{-1} will require 10 minutes for a 90% reversal of neuromuscular block.[29] This difference in time to peak effect allows the anesthesiologist to decide which agent is needed. A word of caution: when

---

TABLE 47-3. Cardiovascular Effects of Muscle Relaxants

Drug	Mechanism of Action on Circulation	Circulatory Changes
Curare	Histamine release	Slow administration—minimal Rapid administration—20–30% decrease in blood pressure
Atracurium	Histamine release	Rapid administration, high dose—20% decrease in blood pressure
Metocurine	None	Minimal change
Vecuronium	None	No change
Pancuronium	Vagal blockade, indirect adrenergic stimulation	Increased pulse and blood pressure

edrophonium is used to reverse neuromuscular blockade, the effect is so rapid that atropine should be administered before the edrophonium; and there is some opinion that atropine is superior to glycopyrrolate for this reversal. The dose of atropine is 0.01–0.02 mg·kg^{-1}. Neostigmine is a suitable alternative for reversal of nondepolarizing muscle relaxants in neonates. The muscarinic effects of neostigmine can be blocked with glycopyrrolate (0.01 mg·kg^{-1}), and the two can be given concurrently. The two advantages of edrophonium over neostigmine are a more rapid reversal and fewer muscarinic side-effects.

Cardiovascular Effects of the Anesthetic Drugs

Opioids are vasodilators but have little effect on cardiac function. If the neonate is hypovolemic, the administration of opioids may well decrease blood pressure. On the other hand, if the infant is adequately volume resuscitated, then the administration of opioids should have little if any effect on the blood pressure.[30-32] Ketamine has mild α-adrenergic agonist activity and may cause tachycardia and a mild degree of vasoconstriction. Ketamine is a useful agent for the infant who has an unstable cardiovascular system or in whom there is some question about volume repletion.[33-35] The iv induction dose of ketamine is 1–2 mg·kg^{-1} in titrated doses, followed by 0.5–1 mg·kg^{-1} every 15 to 30 minutes.

Nitrous oxide usually is considered a reasonably benign anesthetic drug from the standpoint of the cardiovascular system. However, in adult patients, when nitrous oxide is combined with opioids, the cardiac index and arterial pressure decrease because of myocardial depression.[36,37] Nitrous oxide has mild depressant effects on systemic hemodynamics in sedated infants, similar to those reported in adults, but does not produce the elevations in pulmonary artery pressure and pulmonary vascular resistance that are seen in adults.[38] Therefore, it would appear that nitrous oxide is a reasonable drug in neonates if there is no concern for expanding gas pockets within the body (i.e., pneumoencephalograms, intestinal obstruction, pneumothorax) and no need for a high F$_{IO_2}$ to maintain saturation.

All of the volatile anesthetics are myocardial depressants. Halothane has little effect on peripheral vascular resistance; therefore, the decrease in blood pressure that accompanies the administration of halothane results from myocardial depression. On the other hand, isoflurane decreases systemic vascular resistance so that the major effect on blood pressure is a decrease in peripheral vascular resistance. Desflurane has cardiovascular and metabolic effects similar to those of halothane but tends to cause coughing and laryngospasm when inhaled.[39] In the presence of heart disease or a compromised circulation, all of the volatile drugs may have a profound effect on myocardial contractility, and their administration should be monitored carefully.

Anesthetic Dose Requirements of Neonates

Neonates and premature infants have lower anesthetic requirements than older children.[40] The minimum alveolar concentration (MAC) of halothane for the premature infant is 0.6%; it is 0.89% for full-term neonates and 1.12% for 2- to 4-month-old infants.[40,41] The reasons for the lower MAC requirements are thought to be an immature nervous system, progesterone, and elevated blood levels of endorphins, coupled with an immature blood-brain barrier. The neonate

has an immature central nervous system with attenuated responses to nociceptive cutaneous stimuli. These responses rapidly mature in the first several months of an infant's life, along with an increase in the MAC. Progesterone has been shown to reduce the MAC of the pregnant mother. The newborn infant has elevated progesterone levels similar to those of the mother. In a study in lambs, Gregory et al showed that the MAC increased progressively over the first 12 hours of life, with a concomitant decrease in progesterone levels.[42] Elevated levels of β-endorphin and β-lipotropin have been demonstrated in newborns and in the first few days of postnatal life. The levels returned to adult concentrations by the time the infants were 24 days old. Endorphins do not cross the blood-brain barrier in adults; however, it is thought that the neonate's blood-brain barrier is more permeable and that the endorphins might well pass into the central nervous system, thus elevating the pain threshold and reducing the MAC requirement.

ANESTHETIC MANAGEMENT OF THE NEONATE

The anesthesiologist has a host of anesthetic techniques from which to choose and can tailor the anesthetic to the requirements of the surgery and the condition of the neonate. The neonate who is moribund or who has a severely compromised cardiovascular status needs resuscitation. If muscle relaxants are needed, pancuronium is the relaxant of choice. As the neonate's status improves, anesthetic drugs may be titrated in. The neonate with a questionable cardiovascular and volume status needs anesthetic drugs such as ketamine or an opioid. On the other hand, in neonates who have a stable cardiovascular state, the choice of drugs depends on the type of surgery and on whether or not the neonate will be extubated at the end of surgery.

The three major factors to consider in selecting an anesthetic technique are (1) whether or not it is anticipated that the neonate will be extubated at the end of surgery or shortly thereafter, (2) the need to control blood pressure, and (3) the need for postoperative pain relief. The drugs and techniques available to achieve these goals are many and include inhalational anesthetics, regional techniques, muscle relaxants, opioids, and ketamine. If extubation is anticipated at the end of surgery or shortly thereafter, the anesthetic must be tailored so that there will be minimal residual effects from inhalational agents and muscle relaxants, thereby allowing the infant to be awake and in control of its airway reflexes, which promotes early extubation. The muscle relaxant of choice in this situation is atracurium because of its moderate duration of action (30 to 45 minutes), which is the same in the neonate as it is in the older child and adult. Vecuronium, by contrast, is metabolized by the liver and in the neonate is a long-acting muscle relaxant. The use of a regional anesthesia technique, such as a caudal technique, will reduce the need for inhalational agents, opioids, and muscle relaxants. There are great advantages to using a combined general and regional technique when early extubation is anticipated. On the other hand, if the management plan is to leave the infant intubated and ventilated for a period of time, then the choice of anesthetic technique and muscle relaxant will depend on other factors, such as the need to control blood pressure to reduce bleeding and the need for postoperative pain management.

Nitrous oxide can be added so long as oxygenation is closely monitored and expansion of any gas pockets within the body is considered. In the case of intestinal obstruction, the use of air along with appropriate concentrations of oxygen and a volatile drug is indicated. The normal full-term neonate has a systolic blood pressure between 60 and 70 mm Hg. For purposes of controlled hypotension, a blood pressure of 40–50 mm Hg is desired. If there is any problem with oxygen saturation or the development of metabolic acidosis, blood pressure should be increased and a fluid bolus of 10 ml·kg^{-1} of lactated Ringer's solution should be given. All neonates with an arterial pressure below 40 mm Hg should be vigorously resuscitated (with fluids, controlled ventilation, oxygenation, or relaxation with pancuronium), and when the patient responds to the resuscitation with an increase in blood pressure, ketamine should be administered in titrated doses of 0.5 mg·kg^{-1}. As the blood pressure increases further, opioids can be administered incrementally. The use of opioids and a muscle relaxant can be advantageous when caring for the hemodynamically unstable infant. A study on the dose response of fentanyl in neonates having surgery demonstrated that, in doses of 10–12.5 μg·kg^{-1}, fentanyl produced a stable hemodynamic state and reliable anesthesia as determined by the heart rate and blood pressure.[32] The muscle relaxant used was metocurine, because it was believed that pancuronium with its tachycardia would mask the autonomic response to pain. The doses were given in increments of 2.5 μg·kg^{-1}. In all infants in the study, heart rate and systolic blood pressure decreased with the administration of fentanyl. One of the concerns with the administration of opioids in neonates is the altered pharmacokinetics and pharmacodynamics.[43-45] In one study, 25–50 μg·kg^{-1} of fentanyl was given to infants, which resulted in an unpredictable effect and postoperative respiratory depression.[43] Four of 14 neonates studied, none of whom had any respiratory impairment secondary to surgery or disease, needed ventilatory support for 11 to 40 hours after operation. All infants had a rebound of fentanyl blood levels. There was a prolonged metabolism of the fentanyl, particularly in those with an increase in intra-abdominal pressure. It was believed that there might be a reduction in liver blood flow and hence metabolism of fentanyl. This is evidence of altered pharmacokinetics. In addition, it also appeared that newborns were more sensitive at the same plasma level to the respiratory depressant effects of fentanyl. This is evidence of altered pharmacodynamics.

Regional Anesthesia

There has been a tremendous increase in the use of regional anesthesia in children.[46-48] In general, the regional techniques are combined with general anesthesia to permit early extubation and for postoperative pain relief. Spinal anesthesia has been reported to be effective when used as the sole anesthetic technique in premature and high-risk infants, but this technique requires excellent cooperation between anesthesiologist and surgeon, an experienced surgeon, and relative speed. Even at a dose of 0.5 mg·kg^{-1}, tetracaine lasts for only approximately 90 minutes in the neonate. Total spinal anesthesia, produced either with a primary spinal technique or secondary to an attempted epidural, presents as respiratory insufficiency rather than as hypotension.[49,50] The reason for this is the lack of sympathetic tone in infants.[51] The first indication of trouble is a falling oxygen saturation rather than a falling blood pressure. Sedation can be added to regional anesthesia but may cause problems of apnea in ex-premature infants.[52]

The techniques of caudal, spinal, brachial plexus, and other blocks should be considered in all neonates. Another block that has become popular is a simple ring block of the penis for circumcision.[53] Bupivacaine, 0.5% or 0.25%, is injected subcutaneously in a ring about the base of the penis. This way there is no danger of causing a hematoma occasionally found with a penile block.

Postoperative Ventilation

The choice of an anesthetic drug should also be determined by the need for postoperative management of ventilation and by the drug's effects on the circulation. If the surgical procedure or the neonate's condition is such that postoperative ventilation of the lungs is indicated, the prolonged respiratory effects of opioids or any other drug are of little concern. However, if the surgical procedure is relatively short and by itself would not require postoperative ventilation, the clinician should carefully select drugs and doses of anesthetic drugs and relaxants that will not necessitate prolonged postoperative ventilation of the lungs or intubation of the trachea. Postoperative ventilation places the neonate at added risk because of the problems associated with mechanical ventilation, the trauma to the subglottic area, and the potential development of postoperative subglottic stenosis or edema.[54] On the other hand, if there is any question about the neonate's ability to maintain protective airway reflexes or normal ventilation after anesthesia, the neonate should be returned to the recovery room or newborn intensive care unit with the trachea intubated, and either ventilated or treated with a small amount of PEEP (2–4 cm H_2O).

Postoperative Pain Management

The concepts of postoperative pain management are well known to most anesthesiologists. The use of epidural anesthesia intraoperatively followed by postoperative epidural opioids has been very popular in older children and adults, and these techniques are being applied to neonates.[48] In addition, most neonatologists are quite experienced with the iv administration of opioids for patient comfort. Every technique has its risks, and these risks will be better defined in the next several years.

Uptake and Distribution of Anesthetics in Neonates

Rapid induction of anesthesia with volatile drugs can cause a greater degree of hypotension in young infants than in older infants and children.[55-57] However, no adverse effects from this blood pressure were reported. There are several possible reasons for this observation. One reason for the hypotension may be that younger infants have a higher end-tidal halothane or isoflurane concentration than may be appreciated, because the uptake of anesthetic drugs is more rapid in infants than in adults.[58,59] Brandom et al reported a study of both computer-simulated and measured halothane concentrations in infants (see Fig. 47-11).[60] Whereas in the adult it takes 15 to 20 minutes to arrive at approximately a 50–60% equilibration of the end-tidal to the inspired halothane concentration, the infant will be 70–80% equilibrated in the same period. The computer simulation similarly showed a higher concentration of halothane in the heart

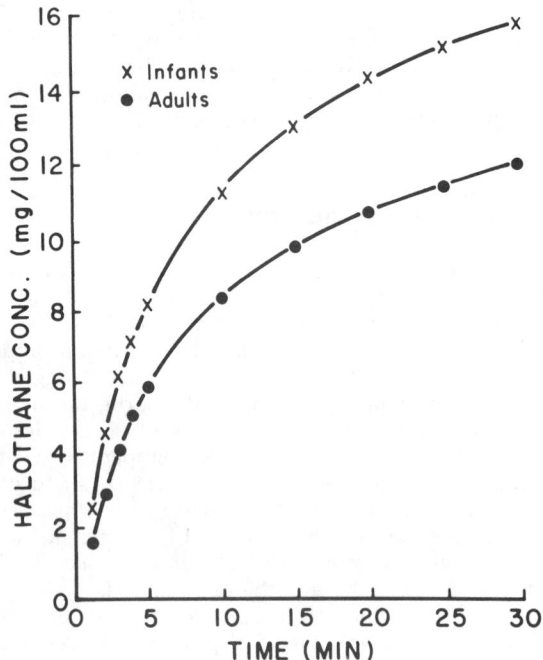

Figure 47-14. Predicted concentration of halothane in the heart. The values were derived from a computerized model of anesthetic uptake and distribution. The model infant weighed 4 kg; the model adult weighed 70 kg. In both cases normal ventilation and a constant inspired fraction of 0.5% halothane were used. Tissue levels are given in milligrams per 100 ml of tissue. (Reprinted with permission from Brandom BW, Brandom RB, Cook DR: Uptake of halothane in infants. Anesth Analg 62:404, 1983.)

of infants (Fig. 47-14). The same anesthetic concentration would also be present in the brain.

Various reasons for the faster uptake of anesthetics in infants have been proposed: (1) The ratio of alveolar ventilation to FRC is 5:1 in the infant and 1.5:1 in the adult. (2) In the neonate, more of the cardiac output goes to the vessel-rich group of organs, which includes the heart and brain. (3) The neonate has a greater cardiac output per kilogram of body mass. (4) The infant has a lower blood gas partition coefficient for volatile anesthetics. In addition, neonates have lower anesthetic requirements than older infants.[41] An appreciation of the lower MAC in neonates, along with recognition of the more rapid uptake, suggests that care must be taken not to "overpressure" the concentration of the volatile drugs to as great a degree or for as long before intubation as would be done with an older infant or adult. The use of end-tidal gas measurements to determine both inspired and end-tidal anesthetic concentrations of the various volatile drugs can be helpful.

SURGICAL PROCEDURES IN NEONATES

For the purposes of discussion, surgical procedures in neonates will be divided into two time periods: those performed in the first week and those performed in the first month. This time difference is somewhat arbitrary because most of the procedures done during the first week are performed in the first 24 to 48 hours, but postoperative care, when the anesthesiologist is often still involved, may extend for several days.

Surgical Procedures in the First Week of Life

The five most frequent major surgical procedures performed in the first week of life are for congenital diaphragmatic hernia (CDH), omphalocele and gastroschisis, tracheoesophageal fistula (TEF), intestinal obstruction, and meningomyelocele. Some of these conditions, such as CDH, omphalocele and gastroschisis, and meningomyelocele, are obvious at birth. It may take hours or days for a TEF or intestinal obstruction to become manifest.

Two confounding factors in neonatal surgery are prematurity and associated congenital anomalies. The presence of one congenital anomaly increases the likelihood that another congenital anomaly will be present. In conditions such as TEF, the mortality from the associated congenital anomaly may be far higher than the mortality from the surgical correction of the TEF.[61,62] Prematurity, particularly when associated with the respiratory distress syndrome, may adversely affect surgical outcome.[63] A neonatologist should be consulted in the case of any neonate with a congenital defect who is considered for surgery. All of these neonates need a chest radiograph and an echocardiogram. The most serious associated congenital lesion is that of the cardiovascular system. About 25–30% of infants with CDH have a cardiac anomaly.[64] Some 15–25% of infants with TEF have an associated congenital cardiac anomaly, and the congenital heart defect is the major cause of death in neonates with a TEF.[65]

Maternal Cocaine Use During Pregnancy

Maternal cocaine use during pregnancy leads to a host of problems for the neonate. Cocaine results in a reduced catecholamine reuptake, which may result in the accumulation of catecholamines and activation of the sympathetic nervous system. This has circulatory effects on the uterus, the umbilical blood vessels, and the fetal cardiovascular system. The three major problems affecting the infant are premature birth, intrauterine growth retardation, and cardiovascular abnormalities.[66] A recent report documented a decrease in cardiac output in infants of mothers who abused cocaine.[67] The cardiac output and stroke volume were reduced on the first day of life but had returned to normal by the second day of life. The clinical implication of this finding is that in infants of mothers who have abused cocaine, it may be advantageous to postpone any surgery until the second or third day of life. A recent study on cardiovascular abnormalities in infants who were prenatally exposed to cocaine revealed an increase in structural cardiovascular malformations and electrocardiographic abnormalities.[67] The most frequent lesions were peripheral pulmonic stenosis, right ventricular conduction delay, right ventricular hypertrophy, and ST and T wave changes.

Congenital Diaphragmatic Hernia

CDH occurs in an incidence of approximately 1 in 4000 live births. Despite intensive, often heroic postoperative measures, the mortality from CDH remains in the range of 40–50% because of severe underdevelopment of the lung. A brief discussion of the embryologic characteristics of CDH will help the clinician understand the potentially enormous postoperative problems that may be encountered. It will become evident that the defect is more than a hernia of the diaphragm.

Early in fetal development, the pleuroperitoneal cavity is a single compartment. The gut is herniated or extruded to

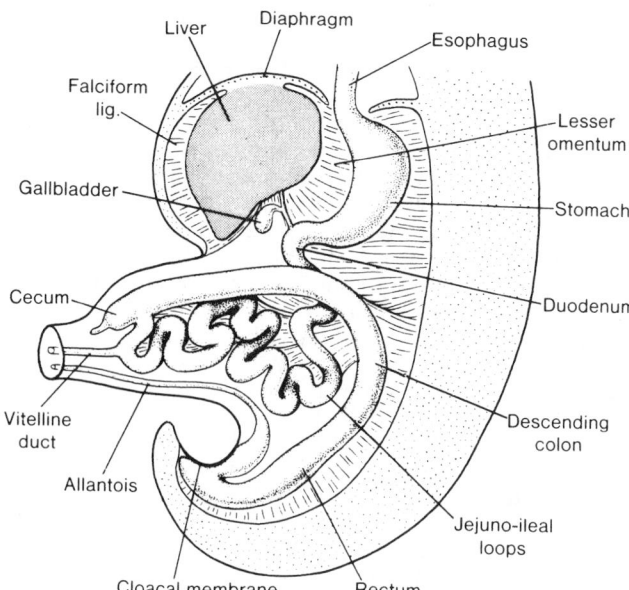

Figure 47-15. Umbilical herniation of the intestinal loops in an embryo of approximately 8 weeks' gestation (crown–rump length, 35 mm). Coiling of the small intestinal loops and formation of the cecum occur during the herniation. (Reprinted with permission from Sadler TW: Langman's Medical Embryology, 5th ed. Baltimore, Williams & Wilkins, 1985.)

the extraembryonic coelom during the fifth to tenth weeks of fetal life (Fig. 47-15). During this period the diaphragm develops to separate the thoracic and abdominal cavities (Fig. 47-16). The development of the diaphragm is usually completed by the seventh fetal week. In the ninth to tenth weeks, the developing gut returns to the peritoneal cavity. If there is delay or incomplete closure of the diaphragm, or if the gut returns early and prevents normal closure of the diaphragm, a diaphragmatic hernia will develop, producing varying degrees of herniation of the intestinal contents into the chest. The left side of the diaphragm closes later than the right side, which results in the higher incidence of left-sided diaphragmatic hernias (foramen of Bochdalek). Approximately 90% of hernias detected in the first week of life are on the left side.

The clinical presentation and the outcome from a diaphragmatic hernia are quite varied. At one end of the spectrum, the diaphragmatic hernia may develop early in fetal life so that the abdominal contents compress the developing lung bud, resulting in an extremely small, hypoplastic lung with no chance for survival. At the other end of the spectrum, a moderately small diaphragmatic hernia may develop late in fetal life, so that the lung is normal but compressed by the abdominal viscera. In between is a large range of possibilities. At the mild end of the scale the infant might have a relatively normal pulmonary vascular bed that develops varying degrees of persistent pulmonary hypertension that may revert to normal. At the more serious end of the spectrum are severe pulmonary hypoplasia and abnormal pulmonary vasculature with a very low chance for survival.

After closure of the pleuroperitoneal membrane, muscular development of the diaphragm occurs. Incomplete muscularization of the diaphragm results in the development of a hernia sac because of intra-abdominal pressure. The condition is known as eventration of the diaphragm, and the diaphragm may extend well up into the thoracic cavity. The other possibility is that the innervation of the diaphragm is incomplete and the muscle atonic. Eventration of the diaphragm usually is not observed in the first week of life.

Antenatal Diagnosis. An increased awareness of the potential of congenital defects has resulted in intrauterine diagnosis of many congenital defects. Because 30% of cases of diaphragmatic hernia are associated with polyhydramnios, one can suspect it while the fetus is *in utero*. Also, with the increasingly sophisticated diagnostic capabilities of ultrasound, some diaphragmatic hernias are being diagnosed in this manner as well. This has led to explorations in fetal surgery. Fetal surgery is a young discipline, and the results and risk-benefit ratio still need to be defined. Theoretically, however, early repair of CDH with decompression of the lung bud should allow the lung to partially repair itself during the remainder of fetal life.

The other advantage of antenatal diagnosis is that if a CDH is suspected *in utero*, the mother can be transferred to a center where extracorporeal membrane oxygenation (ECMO) is available. Some infants with severe CDH and bilateral pulmonary hypoplasia die immediately after delivery, so that there is an irreducible mortality in this condition.

Clinical Presentation. Because the infant's status immediately at birth is determined primarily by the oxygenation of the placenta, the 1-minute Apgar score may well be normal. The occurrence of symptoms depends on the degree of her-

Figure 47-16. Schematic drawings illustrating the development of the diaphragm. (*A*) The pleuroperitoneal folds appear at the beginning of the sixth week. (*B*) The pleuroperitoneal folds have fused with the septum transversum and the mesentery of the esophagus in the seventh week, thus separating the thoracic cavity from the abdominal cavity. (*C*) In a transverse section at the fourth month of development, an additional rim derived from the body wall forms the most peripheral part of the diaphragm. (Reprinted with permission from Sadler TW: Langman's Medical Embryology, 5th ed. Baltimore, Williams & Wilkins, 1985.)

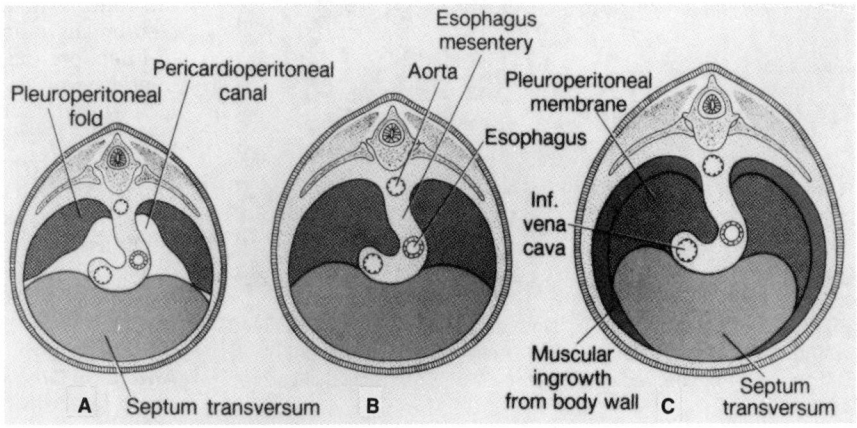

niation and interference with pulmonary function. At times the degree of interference is so great that the neonate's clinical condition begins to deteriorate immediately, whereas in other situations it may be several hours before the infant's condition is fully appreciated. In the severely involved newborn, the initial clinical findings are usually classic and readily discerned. The infant has a scaphoid abdomen secondary to the absence of intra-abdominal contents, which have herniated into the chest (Fig. 47-17). Breath sounds on the affected side are reduced or absent. The diagnosis can be confirmed with an immediate radiograph. Immediate supportive care entails endotracheal intubation and control of the airway, along with decompression of the stomach. Excessive airway pressure carries a high risk for pneumothorax and worsening of a bad situation.

Anesthetic Considerations for CDH. Considerable progress has been made in the preoperative and postoperative management of neonates with CDH. Several studies have shown the value of delaying surgery for 24 to 48 hours while the infant's condition is being stabilized.[68,69] In one study, surgery resulted in a decrease in compliance of the lungs, which may further complicate surgery.[69] In several centers the newborn infant with severe pulmonary dysfunction is being treated with ECMO preoperatively, then weaned from ECMO and scheduled for surgery.[70-72] In some institutions, infants with severe CDH are being operated on while on ECMO and are maintained on ECMO for periods of up to 25 to 30 days.[73] This technique has produced discouraging results.

The anesthetic considerations for the infant with CDH depend on pulmonary function and the ability to close the abdominal incision. The anesthetic techniques are chosen according to the criteria listed previously.

After repair of the diaphragmatic hernia, it may be difficult to return all of the abdominal contents to the abdominal cavity. For that reason, use of nitrous oxide should be avoided. After the intestinal contents have been removed from the chest, the lung should be gently re-expanded under direct vision using pressures no greater than 30 cm H_2O. The involved lung may not re-expand because it is so hypoplastic that it cannot expand. High-pressure attempts to expand the lung may cause a contralateral pneumothorax.

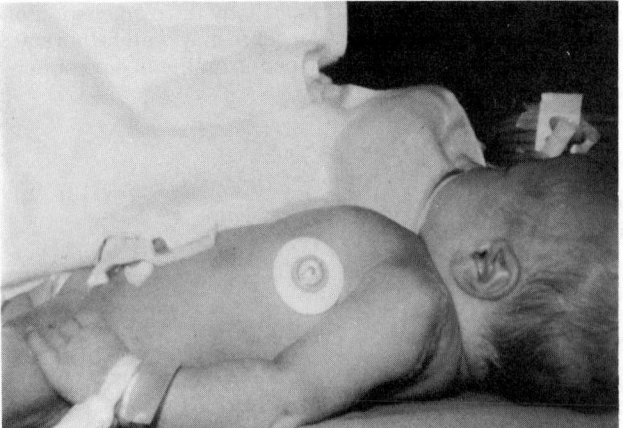

Figure 47-17. Infant with CDH. Note scaphoid abdomen. (Reprinted with permission from Berry FA [ed]: Anesthetic Management of Difficult and Routine Pediatric Patients. New York, Churchill Livingstone, 1990.)

This condition should be suspected in any infant in whom a sudden decrease in oxygen saturation or vital signs develops after the application of positive pressure ventilation.

Postoperative Care. Intensive postoperative care is critical. After surgical repair of a CDH, infants will have various types of recovery, depending on the condition of the lung and the pulmonary vasculature. In addition, the infant may be premature or may have an associated cardiac anomaly. For purposes of discussion, these infants will be placed into three groups: infants in Group 1 have normal lungs and pulmonary vasculature and will do quite well; those in Group 2 have mildly hypoplastic lungs and reactive pulmonary vasculature and may experience episodes of decreased oxygenation; those in Group 3 have severely hypoplastic lungs and abnormal vasculature. The latter have severe problems with oxygenation and hypercarbia from the outset.

Group 2 infants may enjoy a "honeymoon period" of improved oxygenation during surgery and in the immediate postoperative period. However, for unknown reasons, these infants may have episodes of pulmonary vascular constriction leading to a decrease in oxygen saturation.

All of these infants remain intubated and sedated with ventilatory support. Infants in Group 2 who have deteriorating pulmonary function and infants in Group 3 currently are being treated with ECMO in many medical centers.

Omphalocele–Gastroschisis

Although omphalocele and gastroschisis sometimes appear similar and may be confused, they have entirely different origins and associated congenital anomalies.[74] During the fifth to tenth weeks of fetal life, the abdominal contents are extruded into the extraembryonic coelom, and the gut returns to the abdominal cavity at approximately the tenth week (see Fig. 47-15). Failure of part or all of the intestinal contents to return to the abdominal cavity results in an omphalocele that is covered with a membrane called the amnion. The amnion protects the abdominal contents from infection and the loss of extracellular fluid. The umbilical cord is found at approximately the apex of the sac (Fig. 47-18). Gastroschisis, by contrast, develops later in fetal life, after the intestinal contents have returned to the abdominal cavity. It results from interruption of the omphalomesenteric artery, which results in dissolution of the various layers of the abdominal wall at the base of the umbilical cord.[75] The gut then herniates through this tissue defect (Fig. 47-19). The degree of herniation may be slight, or almost all of the abdominal viscera may be found outside the peritoneal cavity. The umbilical cord is found to one side of the intestinal contents. The intestines and viscera are not covered by any membrane and therefore are highly susceptible to infection and loss of extracellular fluid. There is a high incidence of associated congenital anomalies with omphalocele but not with gastroschisis. The Beckwith-Wiedemann syndrome is a collection of problems consisting of mental retardation, hypoglycemia, congenital heart disease, a large tongue, and an omphalocele. Congenital heart lesions are found in approximately 20% of infants with omphalocele. Other associated congenital defects are found with gastroschisis and omphalocele; most involve the gastrointestinal tract and consist primarily of intestinal atresia or stenosis and malrotation.

Antenatal Diagnosis. α-Fetoprotein (AFP) is a protein present in fetal tissues during fetal development. Closure of the

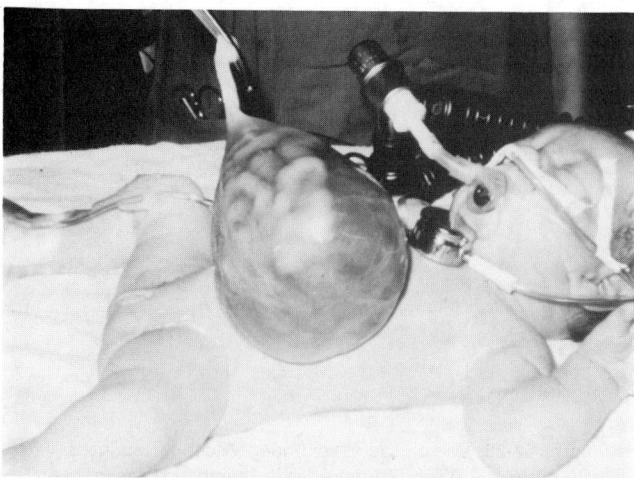

Figure 47-18. Omphalocele. (Reprinted with permission from Berry FA [ed]: Anesthetic Management of Difficult and Routine Pediatric Patients. New York, Churchill Livingstone, 1990.)

abdominal wall and the neural tube (see section on Meningomyelocele) prevents release of large quantities of this protein into the amniotic fluid. High levels of AFP in the amniotic fluid can cross the placenta and be detected in maternal blood. Thus, abnormal levels of AFP in the mother raise concerns over the possibility of either an abdominal wall defect or a neural tube defect in the fetus, as do high levels of AFP in fluid obtained during amniocentesis. Ultrasonography is reliable in helping to diagnose either condition.

Delivery Room Management. There is controversy over the appropriate mode of delivery, vaginal or cesarean section, in parturients in whom the antenatal diagnosis has been

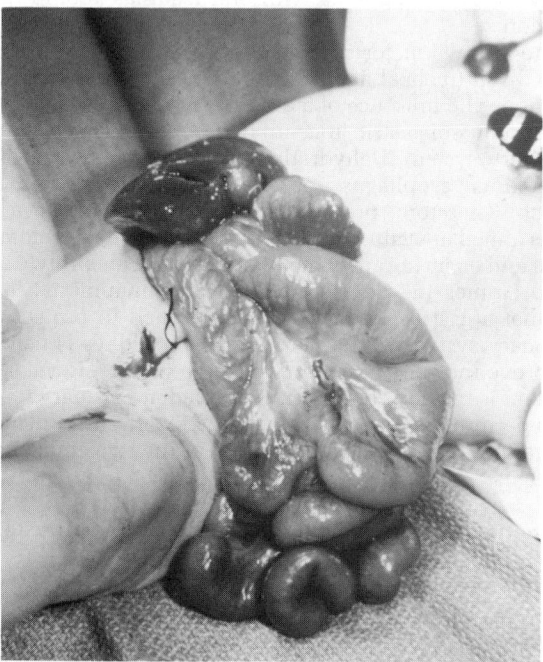

Figure 47-19. Gastroschisis. (Reprinted with permission from Berry FA [ed]: Anesthetic Management of Difficult and Routine Pediatric Patients. New York, Churchill Livingstone, 1990.)

made. Advocates of operative delivery maintain that it is necessary to prevent trauma to the exposed bowel and that it allows better coordination of the various medical specialities needed for immediate surgical management of the defect. Advocates of vaginal delivery point out that most infants with abdominal wall defects are born without the obstetrician's prior knowledge of the defect, that injury to the bowel has not been shown to be a problem, and that the convenience of surgeons and anesthesiologists should not be a factor in decisions regarding mode of delivery.

The aspect of delivery room care unique to an infant with gastroschisis is the need to protect the exposed bowel and minimize fluid and temperature loss. This is best achieved by "bagging" the neonate—that is, by placing its lower body in a sterile, clear plastic bag. The bag is then filled with warm saline, and a drawstring is used to tighten the bag against the infant's body. This fluid must be maintained at body temperature to prevent hypothermia. Use of a fluid-filled bag helps protect against infection and the massive fluid loss that can occur with exposed bowel. This procedure is not necessary with omphalocele because the bowel is still enclosed by amnion.

Perioperative Concerns. The perioperative concerns are fluid loss, infection, associated congenital anomalies, and postoperative hypertension and ventilation. The preoperative preparation of the infant with gastroschisis primarily focuses on controlling infection and ensuring that the infant has a normal extracellular fluid volume. The fluid volume management of the infant often entails provision of enormous amounts of full-strength balanced salt solution. The adequacy of the peripheral circulation and urine output is an indicator of the adequacy of the volume resuscitation. Both conditions may present an intraoperative challenge to the anesthesiologist, because with an omphalocele, after the amniotic membrane is removed, large volumes of fluid may transudate or exudate from the exposed abdominal viscera. The fluid that is lost is extracellular fluid, which should be replaced with full-strength balanced salt solution.

If the defect in the abdominal wall is small, a primary repair of the deficit can be accomplished. However, it may be difficult to return the abdominal viscera to the peritoneal cavity. Because of concern for the increase in the volume of gas in the intestine, nitrous oxide should not be used. Excellent skeletal muscle relaxation is necessary to allow closure of the abdomen. With moderate-sized abdominal wall defects, it may not be possible to close the peritoneum, but there may be sufficient skin to close the defect. With large defects the peritoneal cavity may be too small to contain the viscera, and attempted closure can impair circulation to the bowel and lower extremities as well as compromise respiration.[76,77]

Attempts have been made to find objective criteria by which to determine whether the infant will tolerate the primary closure of the defect and to avoid or minimize the circulatory and ventilatory problems. One study that measured intragastric pressure in infants who underwent primary closure found that if the intragastric pressure was 20 mm Hg or more, the infant needed reoperation and placement of a Dacron silo (Fig. 47-20) within 24 hours of the primary closure.[78] If the intragastric pressure was less than 20 mm Hg, the defect was successfully closed primarily. Intragastric pressure is measured by placing a nasogastric tube in the stomach and using a column of saline to measure the pressure. A value of 20 mm Hg is approximately 27 cm H_2O. Studies in dogs revealed a close correlation between bladder pressure and intra-abdominal pressure; thus, blad-

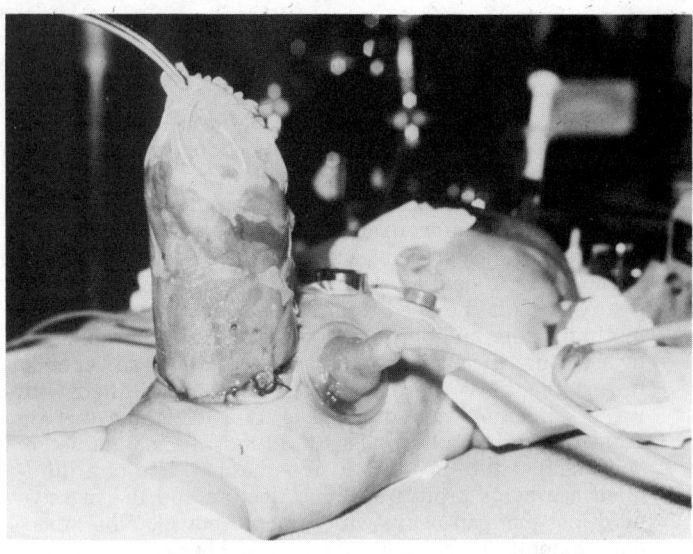

Figure 47-20. Dacron silo for extruded viscera. (Reprinted with permission from Berry FA [ed]: Anesthetic Management of Difficult and Routine Pediatric Patients. New York, Churchill Livingstone, 1990.)

der pressure can be used as an alternative measurement of intra-abdominal pressure.[79]

If primary closure is impossible, a silo is incorporated into the abdominal wall to contain and cover the abdominal viscera. The repair is then staged from this point onward. Every 2 or 3 days the size of the silo is reduced, in much the same fashion that a tube of toothpaste is squeezed. The infant may feel some degree of discomfort as the peritoneum and skin are stretched. Small doses of ketamine, 0.5–1.0 mg·kg^{-1}, are titrated as the silo is reduced in size. The infant is allowed to breathe spontaneously and without intubation. Oxygen saturation should be monitored with a pulse oximeter, and the infant's pulse and blood pressure are also monitored. These measurements help the surgeon and anesthesiologist determine the appropriate silo reduction that allows adequate ventilation and circulation. This is a situation that requires clinical judgment. After several stages of silo reduction, the final operation is complete closure of the abdominal wall defect under full anesthesia with complete muscle relaxation.

Postoperative Care. The postoperative care of infants with omphalocele or gastroschisis is critical. Some need tracheal intubation and assisted ventilation of the lungs for as long as 3 to 7 days. Additional complications include postoperative hypertension and edema of the extremities.[80] The increased abdominal pressure can reduce the circulation to the kidneys, which results in a release of renin. Renin activates the renin-angiotensin-aldosterone system, which is thought to cause the hypertension. Obstruction of the venous circulation of the lower body may cause a large amount of edema of the legs. These infants need large amounts of extracellular fluid resuscitation.

Tracheoesophageal Fistula (TEF)

The treatment of esophageal atresia and TEF can be both challenging and satisfying for the anesthesiologist. Death in the perioperative period typically results from prematurity or from an associated congenital heart defect. TEF occurs in approximately 1 in 3000 live births. Approximately 85% consist of a fistula from the distal trachea to the esophagus and a blind proximal esophageal pouch. In 10% of cases there is a blind proximal esophageal pouch with no TEF.

The embryologic defect results from imperfect division of the foregut into the anteriorly positioned larynx and trachea and the posteriorly positioned esophagus; the division should occur between the fourth and fifth weeks of intrauterine life. Fifty percent of affected infants have associated congenital anomalies, of which approximately 15–25% involve the cardiovascular system.

Clinical Presentation. Atresia of the esophagus leads to inability of the fetus to swallow amniotic fluid and the subsequent development of polyhydramnios. For that reason, if polyhydramnios is present, attempts should be made to pass a nasogastric tube shortly after delivery. Passing a nasogastric tube is not routine in the delivery room, and therefore the diagnosis may not become apparent until the infant is fed. Cyanosis and choking with oral feedings should raise suspicion.

There are two major complications of esophageal atresia with a distal tracheal fistula: aspiration pneumonia and dehydration. The presence of a distal TEF increases the likelihood of reflux of gastric juice up the esophagus and into the pulmonary system. Dehydration results from the fact that the proximal esophagus does not communicate with the stomach. Therefore, preoperative preparation of these infants is aimed at evaluation and treatment of the pulmonary system and ensuring adequate hydration and electrolyte balance. At times the degree of reflux and pneumonia is so great that a gastrostomy must be performed to protect the pulmonary system, and a period of several days is needed to improve the general condition of the infant. However, if the infant is in good condition, an immediate primary repair can be performed. This consists of ligation of the fistula and a primary repair with approximation of the two ends of the esophagus.

Anesthetic Considerations. The presence of a gastrostomy reduces the potential for reflux of gastric juice during the surgical procedure. If a gastrostomy is present, the gastrostomy tube should be open to air and left at the head of the table under the anesthesiologist's observation to avoid kinking and obstruction. Not all patients need a gastrostomy, however.[83] There is some difference of opinion concerning the technique for intubation of the trachea. Some prefer to intubate the trachea with the patient awake, others prefer intubation after induction of anesthesia. The important issue is to avoid positive pressure ventilation, which will distend the stomach, thereby increasing the risk for reflux and ventilatory compromise. If an awake tracheal intubation is done, it can be facilitated by the topical administration of lidocaine and with the use of 1 mg·kg^{-1} of lidocaine iv 1 to 2 minutes before laryngoscopic examination.

There are two approaches to tracheal intubation after induction of anesthesia. One is to use an inhalation induction, followed by topical application of lidocaine and intubation while the infant is breathing spontaneously. The other technique is to use an iv or inhalation induction and intubate the trachea after muscle paralysis. This technique may lead to distention of the fistula and stomach with positive pressure ventilation. With either technique, topical anesthesia of the larynx may be achieved with 3–4 mg·kg^{-1} of 2% lidocaine sprayed on the larynx and vocal cords. Lidocaine 2% is preferred to higher concentrations in these small infants because it is easier to control the dose. When controlled ventilation of the lungs is used, attempts must be made to minimize the distention of the stomach and the potential for reflux. If a gastrostomy tube is in place, the point is moot. Alternatively, because the fistula is usually located just above the carina on the posterior wall of the trachea, the endotracheal tube can be placed just distal to the TEF.[81] To do this, the endotracheal tube is inserted until it enters one or the other main-stem bronchus. This is judged by unilateral expansion of the chest and unilateral breath sounds. The endotracheal tube is then slowly withdrawn until bilateral chest movement and breath sounds are present. Or, if there is a gastrostomy tube in place, constant pressure can be placed on the rebreathing bag while it is attached to the endotracheal tube. The gastrostomy tube is placed under water seal so that the gas bubbles can be seen easily. While the endotracheal tube is above the fistula, the excess gas will course through the fistula into the gastrostomy and out the gastrostomy tube. The endotracheal tube is advanced and, as it passes the fistula, there will be a reduction or stoppage in the gas bubbles (Fig. 47-21).

The endotracheal tube might inadvertently enter the fistula either during the initial tracheal intubation of the infant, when the infant is turned, or during surgical manipulation. The clinical indications that this may have happened are increased difficulty in ventilation of the lungs and decreased oxygen saturation. Because these findings are also present when the lung is packed away to perform the surgery, and because there are other explanations for these findings, intubation of the fistula should always be included in the differential diagnosis. Any time ventilation is difficult and desaturation is occurring, the surgeon must stop the procedure and the lungs should be ventilated. The surgeon will be able to palpate the tip of the tube in the fistula if this is the problem.

TEF may occur in a premature infant with respiratory distress syndrome for whom tracheal intubation and ventilation of the lungs may be necessary. Treatment of the pulmonary condition can be greatly complicated by the presence of TEF. The relatively low compliance of the pulmonary system, coupled with the high compliance of the fistula and the stomach, may result in the anesthetic gas preferentially traversing the fistula into the stomach and upper gastrointestinal system. The result is a decrease in ventilation, the possibility of regurgitation and aspiration, and the potential for gastric and intestinal distention and perforation. A gastrostomy will reduce the chances of the latter problem occurring. At times, however, these infants may require ligation of the fistula in order to improve ventilation for respiratory distress syndrome. A technique has been described for placement of a Fogarty catheter in the fistula until ligation can be accomplished.[82]

Postoperative Care. Although there have been great advances in the treatment of TEF and esophageal atresia, postoperative care can be complicated by associated congenital heart disease, respiratory distress syndrome, and a need for continued postoperative ventilation. The compression of the lung for several hours, along with the pre-existing aspiration pneumonia that many of these infants have, suggests the need in the more difficult cases for a short period of postoperative ventilation, or at least intubation with PEEP, as the most conservative technique for postoperative airway management. Some infants are in excellent condition at the time of surgery and have no complicating factors, and therefore should be considered for extubation immediately at the end of surgery or shortly thereafter. If extubation of the trachea is planned for the end of surgery, the anesthetic technique must be tailored accordingly. Caudal anesthesia as part of the technique is quite useful in these situations.

A very high percentage of infants with esophageal atresia have residual difficulties of the tracheobronchial tree and

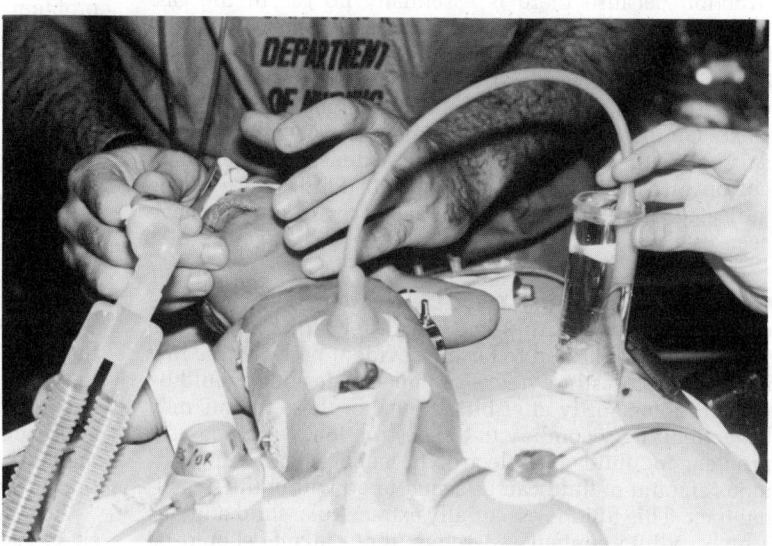

Figure 47-21. Gastrostomy tube under water seal. (Reprinted with permission from Berry FA [ed]: Anesthetic Management of Difficult and Routine Pediatric Patients. New York, Churchill Livingstone, 1990.)

esophagus for many years.[83] These include tracheomalacia, gastroesophageal reflux, and esophageal stricture.[84]

Intestinal Obstruction

For purposes of discussion, obstruction of the gastrointestinal system can be arbitrarily divided into obstruction of the upper gastrointestinal tract (*i.e.*, duodenum) and obstruction of the lower gastrointestinal tract (*i.e.*, terminal ileum, colon, imperforate anus). Obstruction of the upper gastrointestinal tract usually is evident within the first 24 hours of life, with the institution of feedings, whereas obstruction of the lower gastrointestinal tract manifests somewhere between 2 and 7 days of age, as the infant becomes progressively distended, little or no stool is passed, and there is vomiting.

Upper Gastrointestinal Tract Obstruction. If there has been persistent vomiting, upper intestinal obstruction usually means that a major deficit of fluids or electrolytes will develop in the infant. The stomach contains approximately 100–130 mEq·l^{-1} of sodium and 5–10 mEq·l^{-1} of potassium. The greatest deficit will be for sodium. The major concern in the infant with upper gastrointestinal tract obstruction is aspiration of gastric contents. Therefore, awake tracheal intubation is often preferred. Because of concern that awake tracheal intubation will cause hypertension, and intracranial hemorrhage in premature infants with immature cerebral blood vessels, several techniques have been described for modifying the discomfort and ensuing hypertension of awake intubation. These techniques include topical anesthesia and iv lidocaine. Topical anesthesia of the tongue and hypopharynx with lidocaine will reduce but not eliminate the discomfort of awake intubation. Intravenous administration of lidocaine in a dose of 1 mg·kg^{-1} also acts to depress the central nervous system and reduces the stimulation associated with awake tracheal intubation. There is the theoretical concern that any amount of sedation or topical anesthesia will increase the risk of aspiration of gastric contents. This appears to be more of a theoretical than a practical concern.

The anesthetic management of these patients is directed toward ensuring adequate relaxation for abdominal exploration, repair of the congenital defect, and closure of the abdomen. Nitrous oxide can be used in high intestinal obstruction because there is essentially no gas in the gastrointestinal tract. The next concern is whether or not the infant's trachea should be extubated at the end of surgery. If the infant is robust and the incision is relatively small, extubation of the trachea at the end of surgery can be anticipated. On the other hand, if the infant is moderately debilitated or if the surgical incision is extensive, a period of postoperative tracheal intubation with PEEP may well be indicated, particularly if moderate doses of opioids have been used.

Lower Gastrointestinal Tract Obstruction. The problems usually develop within 2 to 7 days after birth. It may take this long for the lesion to become evident because it is low in the gastrointestinal tract. An imperforate anus should be recognizable shortly after birth. Some of these infants may have vomiting secondary to the obstruction, which poses a problem for fluid and electrolyte management. An enormous amount of fluid can be sequestered within the intestinal tract. This fluid is essentially extracellular fluid and has a high sodium content. Therefore, these infants should be prepared carefully for surgery and have a serum sodium

level greater than 130 mEq·l^{-1} and a urine volume of 1–2 ml·kg^{-1}·h^{-1}.

The trachea of these infants may need to be intubated while awake. If the infant has had minimal or no vomiting, rapid-sequence induction of anesthesia and tracheal intubation can be done. Rapid-sequence induction in an infant is the same as in an adult, with iv barbiturate, muscle relaxant, cricoid pressure, and oxygenation. If the infant has had vomiting, the most conservative approach would be an awake tracheal intubation after gastric decompression. Although a nasogastric tube is in place, there is no guarantee that the stomach is empty. Therefore, in the face of vomiting, an awake tracheal intubation is the usual technique of choice, which is performed as described above. Although there is little difference in choice between anesthetic drugs for upper and lower gastrointestinal tract obstruction, nitrous oxide should not be used in any infant who has a gaseous distention of the intestine. This is easily determined from the preoperative radiograph. Providing adequate muscle relaxation for surgery is also a consideration. This can be done with various anesthetic techniques.

The criteria for tracheal extubation at the end of surgery are the same as those described for upper gastrointestinal tract obstruction. In general, however, these infants may have a greater degree of debilitation because they have had intestinal obstruction for a longer period of time. The caveat about timing of tracheal extubation is, "When in doubt, leave the endotracheal tube in place with PEEP." This is not to suggest that prolonged endotracheal intubation is benign. It is not. There is a small but significant risk for the development of subglottic stenosis; but this is a situation in which the risk of subglottic stenosis and other airway trauma must be weighed against the risk of too early tracheal extubation with vomiting and aspiration, airway obstruction, fatigue, and so on.

Meningomyelocele

Although the incidence of meningomyelocele has decreased in the past 20 years, it still occurs in a significant number of infants. There are five major concerns with a meningomyelocele: infection, fluids, positioning for tracheal intubation, the presence of the Arnold-Chiari malformation, and hydrocephalus. The meningomyelocele is very susceptible to trauma, leakage, and hence infection. Positioning alone can cause enough trauma to the meningomyelocele to cause this problem. The delivery process may also cause rupture and leakage of fluid. Spinal fluid is extracellular fluid with serum levels of sodium and potassium. Leakage of this fluid can create a preoperative and intraoperative volume and electrolyte problem. Replacement of spinal fluid with full-strength, balanced salt solution is indicated. If the surgical procedure is extensive because of a large meningomyelocele, there may be additional intraoperative third-space and blood loss.

A second concern is appropriate positioning for tracheal intubation. Endotracheal intubation in the supine infant with meningomyelocele necessitates the use of padding, which will prevent contact of the meningomyelocele with the operating table. The trachea can be intubated when the infant is in the lateral position with the left side down, but it is more difficult than a supine intubation. If a lateral approach to intubation is attempted, provision must be made to immediately turn the infant into the supine position if the intubation is unsuccessful.

Virtually all infants with a meningomyelocele also have an associated anomaly of the brain stem known as the Arnold-Chiari malformation. The Arnold-Chiari malformation is characterized by a caudal displacement of the brain stem and the cerebellar tonsils into the cervical spinal canal. This is associated with an obliteration of the normal exit foramina of the fourth ventricle and in more than 90% of cases will result in progressive hydrocephalus necessitating a shunting procedure. This is usually not a problem at the time the meningomyelocele is repaired but may occur in the postoperative period. Any unusual breathing or blood pressure patterns should immediately raise the suspicion of increased intracranial pressure.

Hydrocephalus

Hydrocephalus may occur after closure of a meningomyelocele because of the Arnold-Chiari malformation. The cranial sutures in the neonate are open, so that intracranial pressure increases are blunted or minimized. However, infants with hydrocephalus eventually have an increase in head size and sometimes in intracranial pressure, resulting in lethargy, vomiting, and cardiorespiratory problems. The anesthetic approach and the technique for tracheal intubation depend on the infant's condition. The major concern is protection of the airway and control of intracranial pressure. Awake tracheal intubation, crying, struggling, and straining can increase intracranial pressure, but this increase will be blunted by the open sutures. I prefer to perform a rapid sequence induction of anesthesia in order to control the airway and intracranial pressure. A rapid sequence induction with 4–5 mg·kg^{-1} of thiopental, 2 mg·kg^{-1} of succinylcholine, and cricoid pressure can lead to rapid control of the airway. Hyperventilation, along with the barbiturate, will rapidly control intracranial pressure. Volatile drugs, nitrous oxide, and opioids are all reasonable choices for maintenance of anesthesia. Noninvasive intracranial pressure measurements in neurologically normal preterm neonates have shown a decrease in intracranial pressure with all drugs, including ketamine, fentanyl, isoflurane, and halothane. The blood pressure decreased with the volatile drugs but not with ketamine or fentanyl. The failure of volatile anesthetics and ketamine to increase intracranial pressure as in adults is attributed to the compliance of the neonate's open-sutured cranium.

After operation, the trachea of these infants should remain intubated and they should receive PEEP for a period of time if they were experiencing periods of apnea or bradycardia before operation because of the intracranial abnormalities. If not, the trachea can be extubated as soon as the protective reflexes have recovered.

Surgical Procedures in the First Month of Life

Surgical procedures in the first month also are considered emergent, or at least urgent, surgery. The six most frequent surgical procedures in the first month are exploratory laparotomy for necrotizing enterocolitis (NEC), inguinal hernia repair, correction of pyloric stenosis, patent ductus arteriosus ligation, a shunt procedure for hydrocephalus, and placement of a central venous catheter.

Necrotizing Enterocolitis

NEC is a disease that affects premature infants who have survived the first days of life. It often occurs at the time when feedings are introduced. It primarily affects the very low birth weight infant, but it may also affect the larger premature and occasionally full-term neonates. The incidence of NEC among very low birth weight infants varies

between 5% and 15%.[85] It has been postulated that because the use of surfactant increases the survival of very small premature infants with respiratory distress syndrome, it may also increase the incidence of NEC.[85-87]

The exact origin of NEC has yet to be determined.[88-90] Kosloske proposed the hypothesis that NEC occurs by the coincidence of two of three pathologic events: intestinal ischemia, colonization by pathogenic bacteria, and excess protein substrate in the intestinal lumen.[90] NEC is more likely to appear after quantitative extremes (i.e., severe ischemia, highly pathogenic flora, or significant excess of substrate). NEC develops only if a threshold of injury sufficient to initiate intestinal necrosis is exceeded. The condition is characterized by a cascade of pathologic events, beginning with an immature intestine that has a decreased ability to absorb substrate, leading to stasis. Stasis encourages bacterial proliferation, which leads to local infection. The picture is complicated by further pooling of fluid. The ischemia and infection may lead to necrosis of the intestinal mucosa, followed by perforation. The perforation leads to gangrene, fluid loss, peritonitis, septicemia, and disseminated intravascular coagulation. The first signs that NEC may be developing are abdominal distention, irritability, and the development of metabolic acidosis. NEC is primarily a medical disease and is treated by cessation of oral intake and administration of antibiotics and supportive care, particularly fluid and electrolyte therapy. In nonresponsive cases, the infant becomes more septic with severe peritonitis, and the only solution is to perform an exploratory laparotomy to remove the gangrenous bowel and perform an ileostomy.[91]

The preoperative problems are an acute abdomen with severe peritonitis, necrosis and gangrene of the intestine, septicemia, metabolic acidosis, and hypovolemia. Preparation of the patient must include stabilization of the circulation. Often the septicemia, coupled with the distended abdomen and the overall clinical deterioration of the infant, also necessitates the use of intubation and ventilation in the nursery. The anesthetic requirements are continuation of resuscitation, provision of excellent abdominal relaxation for the surgery, and careful titration of anesthetic drugs. These infants are often so critically ill that they tolerate minimal anesthesia. One choice is to start with small doses of ketamine, 0.5–1 mg·kg^{-1}. This can be administered every 20 to 30 minutes. If the condition improves, fentanyl, 2–3 μg·kg^{-1}, can be administered, up to a total dose of 10–12 μg·kg^{-1}. If the infant's condition improves dramatically, small doses of volatile drug can be added as well. The use of nitrous oxide should be avoided because of the gas pockets within the abdomen.

These infants represent one of the most challenging cases in all of pediatric anesthesia. Monitoring of intra-arterial pressure, central venous pressure, and arterial blood gases is usually indicated. The fluid loss can be enormous.[92] They need full-strength, balanced salt solution for maintenance of blood pressure and urine output. If the hematocrit is below 30–35%, whole blood should be administered. These infants must be returned to the intensive care unit with their tracheas intubated and lungs ventilated, and their postoperative care must be coordinated carefully with the surgeon, neonatologist, or pediatrician.

Inguinal Hernia Repair in the Neonate

The development of a hernia in the premature infant or neonate is a different clinical problem from the development of a hernia in an infant older than 1 year of age.[93-95] Of 100 infants less than 2 months old who needed inguinal hernia repair,[94] 30% were premature, 42% had a history of respiratory distress syndrome, 16% had been ventilated, and 19% had congenital heart disease. Furthermore, 31% of the infants had incarcerated hernias, 9% had an intestinal obstruction, and 2% had gonadal infarction. These data preclude waiting until a premature infant or neonate is 6 months or 1 year old before performing "elective" surgery. The potential for emergent or urgent intervention is so great that surgical repair should be accomplished within a reasonable amount of time after an inguinal hernia is discovered. The "reasonable" time depends on the infant's condition. If the infant is normal and has no other life-threatening medical problems, repair can be done within several days or weeks. If the infant has another problem such as respiratory distress syndrome, the waiting period should be longer, in order to maximally improve the infant's status.

Perioperative complications are frequent in these infants.[96-98] In the 100 patients reported by Rescorla and Grosfeld, two had apnea and bradycardia, four needed postoperative ventilatory support, one had a cardiac arrest resulting from digoxin toxicity, and one developed *Klebsiella* sepsis.[94] It has long been recognized that premature infants undergoing elective surgery have a higher rate of complications than full-term infants undergoing the same type of surgery. Steward reported that complications developed in 13 of 33 premature infants who underwent elective inguinal hernia repair, whereas only 1 of 38 full-term infants having the same type of surgery had complications.[96] Five of the complications occurred intraoperatively and eight occurred postoperatively.

Postoperative Apnea. A major concern in the premature infant is the development of apnea in the postoperative period. The presence of an endotracheal tube in any infant leads to the development of short periods of apnea; however, the apnea that develops in premature infants can be quite prolonged and associated with bradycardia. Most of the time this apnea and bradycardia can be treated by conservative methods, such as the administration of oxygen and stimulation. Rarely, the condition may alarm the clinician to the point where the infant's trachea is reintubated or remains intubated after operation. There are individual case reports of apnea developing as long as 12 hours after operation.[98] Therefore, questions arise as to whether or not these infants are candidates for same-day surgery, what type of monitoring they need, and how long they need to be monitored. The consensus today is that infants who were born prematurely and who are younger than 50 weeks postconceptual age should not be operated on as ambulatory surgical patients. They should be admitted to the hospital and monitored with an apnea monitor and a cardiac monitor until the morning after surgery.[97,98]

Premature infants at particular risk are those with a history of apnea, although premature infants without a history of apnea may have apneic episodes after anesthesia. The exact origin of postoperative apnea is not known, although it may involve lingering effects of anesthetics. A study in adult volunteers showed that subanesthetic concentrations of halothane (0.15% inspired) profoundly depressed the peripheral chemoreflex pathway.[99] There is no reason to think that the premature infant and the neonate might not respond in the same way. Subjects were somewhat drowsy, but they remembered everything and were coherent and talked to the investigators. The peripheral chemoreflex pathway protects the body from hypoxia through the carotid bodies, which, when stimulated, initiate a cascade of protective physiologic defense mechanisms. These mechanisms include an increase in minute ventilation, hypertension, a favorable redistribution of cardiac output, and an arousal of the patient. The anesthetic implications of this study, combined with the anatomic and physiologic handicaps of the infants, suggest that infants should remain intubated until completely awake and active at the end of surgery and that they should be monitored very carefully. In addition, because the premature infant and neonate are particularly susceptible to laryngospasm, oral feedings should be delayed for at least 2–3 hours after tracheal extubation. Laryngospasm is a protective reflex of the airway. The closure of the glottic opening is accompanied by apnea.

Anesthetic Techniques for Hernia Repair. Surgical procedures below the umbilicus can be performed with either general or regional anesthesia. There is no consensus about which is preferred. Local or regional anesthesia can be used entirely for the surgery or as an adjunct to reduce general anesthetic requirements and produce postoperative analgesia.[100] Ilioinguinal-iliohypogastric nerve block with 0.5% bupivacaine, 3 mg·kg^{-1}, with epinephrine, can be administered either shortly after the induction of anesthesia or at the end of surgery; it affords excellent postoperative analgesia without the need for opioids.

Caudal anesthesia is also very effective when combined with general anesthesia. It will increase muscle relaxation and decrease the concentration of inhalation anesthetic needed so that the infant more rapidly regains control of its airway reflexes at the end of surgery. Spinal anesthesia has been used as the sole anesthetic in these patients. Infants less than 50 weeks' postconceptual age are still susceptible to apnea. If spinal anesthesia is used in this high-risk group of infants, it should not be combined with a sedative, because this combination greatly increases the incidence of postoperative apnea, to the same level as is found with general anesthesia.[52]

There remains considerable debate regarding when to operate on graduates of the premature nursery as ambulatory patients, what types of postoperative monitors to use, the length of time they should be monitored, the anesthetic techniques, and whether or not surgery should be delayed for some length of time. The current consensus is that ambulatory surgery is appropriate for infants who are at least 50 conceptual weeks of age (gestational age + postnatal age). The infant less than 50 weeks' postconceptual age should be hospitalized and postoperative apnea monitoring should be used for approximately 18 hours.

Pyloric Stenosis

Pyloric stenosis is a relatively frequent surgical disease of the neonate and infant. It can appear as early as the second week of life. The pathologic characteristics include hypertrophy of the pyloric smooth muscle with edema of the pyloric mucosa and submucosa. This process, which develops over a period of days to weeks, leads to progressive obstruction of the pyloric valve, causing persistent vomiting. The vomiting leads to varying losses of fluids and electrolytes. Pediatricians are now adept at diagnosing pyloric stenosis, so it is rare to find an infant with severe fluid and electrolyte derangements. However, an infant is occasionally seen whose problem has developed slowly over a period of weeks, resulting in severe fluid and electrolyte derangements. The stomach contents contain sodium, potassium, chloride, hydrogen ions, and water. The infant may have a hyponatremic, hypokalemic, hypochloremic metabolic alkalosis with a compensatory respiratory acidosis. The anesthesiologist, pediatrician, and surgeon are all responsible for preparing these infants before operation. Pyloric stenosis is a medical emergency and should not be converted into an anesthetic nightmare by premature surgical repair before adequate fluid and electrolyte homeostasis has been achieved. The infant should have normal skin turgor, and the correction of the electrolyte imbalance should produce a sodium level that is greater than 130 mEq·l^{-1}, a potassium level that is at least 3 mEq·l^{-1}, a chloride level that is greater than 85 mEq·l^{-1} and increasing, and a urine output of at least 1–2 ml·kg^{-1}·hr^{-1}. These patients need a resuscitation fluid of full-strength, balanced salt solution and, after the infant begins to urinate, the addition of potassium chloride.

Anesthestic Management. The major concern in the anesthetic management of patients with pyloric stenosis is the aspiration of gastric contents. Affected infants are usually older and stronger than those in whom an intestinal obstruction appears in the first day or so of life. For this reason, a slightly different approach is used. A large orogastric tube is passed and the stomach contents aspirated. Then, 5 to 7 ml of sodium bicarbonate (the iv solution will suffice) is administered down the orogastric tube. The infant is gently agitated to distribute the fluid. The tube is suctioned and removed. This procedure greatly reduces the quantity of gastric fluid and increases the pH to 6 or 7. Intubation of the trachea can be done while the patient is awake or after induction of anesthesia. I prefer to first anesthetize these infants. If an iv line is not in place and cannot be placed with reasonable ease, then, after the above regimen is followed to adequately prepare the stomach, an inhalation induction of anesthesia is done with nitrous oxide and halothane. Use of nitrous oxide should be discontinued as soon as the infant loses the lid reflex. If a vein becomes evident, an iv line is placed and rapid intubation of the trachea accomplished with the use of succinylcholine or atracurium and cricoid pressure. If an iv line still cannot be placed easily, two options exist: one should either deepen inhalation anesthesia with 3–4% halothane, perform laryngoscopic examination, topically anesthetize the vocal cords with 2–3 mg·kg^{-1} of lidocaine, and intubate the trachea; or administer 5 mg·kg^{-1} of succinylcholine im before intubation. If iv access has already been obtained, a rapid sequence tracheal intubation technique is preferred. The infant is preoxygenated with high-flow oxygen; atropine, 0.01 mg·kg^{-1}, is given, followed by thiopental, 3–4 mg·kg^{-1}, and succinylcholine, 2 mg·kg^{-1}, or atracurium, 0.8 mg·kg^{-1}. Cricoid pressure is applied as soon as tolerated and the infant's trachea is intubated. Anesthesia can be maintained by almost any technique that the clinician prefers. The point to remember is that surgeons will need skeletal muscle relaxation at two times: when they deliver the pylorus at the beginning of surgery and when they replace the pylorus into the abdomen at the end of surgery, shortly before closing the peritoneum. Atracurium, as both an intubating relaxant and a maintenance relaxant, seems to be a useful drug. I also prefer to use a volatile drug plus 70% nitrous oxide, along with controlled ventilation of the lungs. The halothane or isoflurane is discontinued as soon as the peritoneum is closed. The atracurium is reversed and the nitrous oxide discontinued as the last two or three skin sutures are placed. Another technique is to administer a caudal (1.25 ml·kg^{-1} of 0.25% bupivacaine) after the induction of general anesthesia with tracheal intubation. Caudal anesthesia will provide intraoperative relaxation, reduce the anesthetic requirement, and provide postoperative analgesia. The infant's trachea should remain intubated until he or she is awake with eyes opened and is reaching for the endotracheal tube, or is crying.

Ligation of a Patent Ductus Arteriosus (PDA)

As the number of small premature infants that are surviving has increased, so also has the number of infants who have PDA with heart failure and respiratory failure. Prostaglandins (PGE$_2$ and PGI$_2$) relax the smooth muscle of the ductus so that it cannot constrict. Indomethacin, a prostaglandin synthetase inhibitor, is administered to encourage closure of the ductus. However, indomethacin is often unsuccessful in the small premature infant because of the lack of muscle within the ductus. Infants with a PDA and heart failure need maximal medical management with fluid restriction and diuretics. These infants are at special risk because of the reduced blood volume and precarious cardiopulmonary system. Fentanyl with pancuronium is a frequent choice for anesthesia. The clinician must be prepared to augment volume rapidly with 10–15 ml·kg^{-1} of lactated Ringer's solution. If the lactated Ringer's solution accompanies the administration of 20–25 μg·kg^{-1} of fentanyl and pancuronium, the pressure changes will be minimal and the infant will be appropriately anesthetized.[101] The tracheas of these infants usually remain intubated and the lungs ventilated in the postoperative period, so concern about the length of action of muscle relaxants and opioids is minimized.

Placement of a Central Venous Catheter

The use of a central venous catheter for monitoring central venous pressure, serum electrolytes, and blood gases. For hyperalimentation, and for administering medications is increasing. It can be done either as part of the surgical procedure or at some other time as a separate procedure. The three major concerns in central venous line placement are airway management, pneumothorax, and bleeding. The airway must be secured by an endotracheal tube in small infants because of the difficulty in sharing the head, neck, and upper chest with the surgeon and as an adjunct for treating complications such as pneumothorax and bleeding. The anesthetic technique depends upon the infant's condition, but the neonate must be motionless for the procedure. A pneumothorax may occur with attempts at subclavian vein puncture. The first signs of trouble may be a decreasing oxygen saturation or difficulty with ventilation of the lungs. Because a fluoroscope is often used for central venous line placement, it can be used to rapidly diagnose a pneumothorax. If not, the chest must be rapidly aspirated for both diagnostic and therapeutic reasons. Bleeding is an unusual but serious complication of central venous line placement. It usually becomes manifest in the postoperative period as a hemothorax or as hypovolemia with a decreasing hematocrit.

Respiratory Distress Syndrome

Because of the enormous technical ability of the neonatologist and the resources of newborn intensive care units, many very small infants will survive who need surgery. One of the frequent problems of these infants is the occurrence of the respiratory distress syndrome secondary to a deficiency of surfactant. Respiratory distress syndrome is not an all-or-none disease. There are varying degrees of the disease, and various treatments for it. Exogenous surfactant has been widely used in premature infants of low birth weight either to prevent or to treat respiratory distress syndrome.[86,87] As a result, fewer infants now die of this entity, and the incidence of bronchopulmonary dysplasia in survivors has fallen. However, the use of exogenous surfactant appears to have had little impact on other complications of prematurity such as patent ductus arteriosus, necrotizing enterocolitis, or intraventricular hemorrhage. In fact, with the increase in survivors of respiratory distress syndrome, there may be an increase in the number of babies with necrotizing enterocolitis. The use of surfactant might also greatly assist in the perioperative management of infants with respiratory distress syndrome who are in need of urgent or emergency surgery. This area remains to be investigated.

The Retinopathy of Prematurity

With the increasing ability to support the life of an extremely premature infant (*i.e.*, infants weighing less than 1000 g) has come an increase in the number of infants with residual unpreventable central nervous system and visual deficits. The apparent "epidemic" of retinopathy of prematurity is likely due to the better survival of infants weighing less than 1000 g.[102] The anesthesiologist may be faced with the issues of oxygenation for surgery on premature infants. Infants weighing more than 1500 g and without other complicating medical conditions have a very low incidence of retinopathy of prematurity. However, in today's legal climate, caution is always warranted. The technological advancements of the past 5 years allow the contemporary anesthesiologist to monitor oxygen saturation and inspired and expired concentrations of gases. It has been suggested that the incidence of the retinopathy of prematurity can be decreased if the Pao_2 is maintained below 90 mm Hg. This is an arbitrary figure, and there is little scientific support for this type of suggestion. Even lacking solid data, however, the clinician must still do something about the inspired oxygen concentration in an infant at risk for retinopathy of prematurity. It would appear that it would be appropriate to maintain the oxygen saturation of infants below 40 weeks of conceptual age in the neighborhood of 95%. However, if the infant is experiencing episodes of hypotension and problems with ventilation, fluid resuscitation, or any other ventilatory or circulatory problem, maximum saturation values are indicated until the clinical situation stabilizes.

Sudden Infant Death Syndrome

Prematurity and congenital defects cause most infant deaths in the first month of life. Sudden infant death syndrome (SIDS) is the most frequent cause of death in infants between the ages of 1 month and 1 year.[103] Death from SIDS is relatively rare in the first month of life, with the peak occurring at the third to fourth months of life. SIDS remains a mystery in many ways; its exact causes are unknown. It appears, however, that certain groups of infants may be more at risk for SIDS; these groups include premature infants, infants who have had bronchopulmonary dysplasia, and infants with the "infant apnea syndrome."[104] The infant apnea syndrome is the new designation for what was previously termed the "near-miss sudden infant death syndrome."[105] It was previously believed that SIDS might be more frequent among siblings of SIDS victims, but a report by Peterson *et al* suggests that the risk of SIDS in siblings of SIDS victims is inflated.[106] There are reports that infants who have had episodes of infant apnea syndrome have a defect in the regulation of alveolar ventilation.[107] They have

slightly increased levels of carbon dioxide and an impaired response to carbon dioxide breathing. Elevated levels of β-endorphin have also been detected in the cerebrospinal fluid of infants with the infant apnea syndrome.[105] This syndrome should not be confused with apnea resulting from prematurity, which disappears as the infant matures. There is currently no evidence that general anesthesia might trigger SIDS or the infant apnea syndrome.[103] Premature infants with or without a history of apnea are at increased risk for apnea in the postoperative period, and this risk may persist until the infant is 50 weeks' postconceptual age (gestational age plus postnatal age). For this reason, ex-premature infants who need surgery should be admitted to the hospital after surgery and monitored with an apnea and cardiac monitor for approximately 18 hours. Families of SIDS victims also are reported to have a higher incidence of malignant hyperthermia and other serious reactions to anesthetics.[108,109]

POSTOPERATIVE MANAGEMENT OF THE NEONATE

Neonates undergoing surgery still have the handicaps of immature skeletal muscles, an immature nervous system, and an immature cardiovascular system. In addition, they may have severe physiologic derangements secondary to congenital defects. The postoperative care of these infants requires considerable teamwork among surgeon, anesthesiologist, pediatrician, or neonatologist. The anesthetics should be tailored for one of two situations: immediate tracheal extubation in the perioperative period or postoperative intubation of the trachea with a need for ventilation. If the infant has a surgical problem that does not impair ventilation to any great extent and the infant is in good condition, attempts should be made to extubate the trachea, either at the end of surgery or in the immediate postoperative period. In this situation, the anesthetics should be tailored so that the infant recovers its protective reflexes, has full neuromuscular function, and is awake. The endotracheal tube should be left in place until the infant makes purposeful attempts to remove it. When older infants and children move their extremities, it is usually a sign that the trachea can be extubated. This may not be true for the neonate. A purposeful move toward the endotracheal tube and opening of the eyes or crying usually signifies that the infant will be able to maintain spontaneous ventilation without laryngospasm.

REFERENCES

1. Hagen PT, Scholz DG, Edwards WD: Incidence and size of patent foramen ovale during the first 10 decades of life: An autopsy study of 965 normal hearts. Mayo Clin Proc 59:17, 1984
2. Murphy JD, Vawter GF, Reid LM: Pulmonary vascular disease in fetal meconium aspiration. J Pediatr 104:758, 1984
3. Avery ME, Tooley WH, Keller JB et al: Is chronic lung disease in low birth weight infants preventable? A survey of eight centers. Pediatrics 79:26, 1987
4. Wung J-T, James LS, Kilchevsky E et al: Management of infants with severe respiratory failure and persistence of the fetal circulation, without hyperventilation. Pediatrics 76:488, 1985
5. O'Rourke PP, Crone RK, Vacanti JP et al: Extracorporeal membrane oxygenation and conventional medical therapy in neo-

nates with persistent pulmonary hypertension of the newborn: A prospective randomized study. Pediatrics 84:957, 1989

6. Boedy RF, Howell CG, Kanto WP: Hidden mortality rate associated with extracorporeal membrane oxygenation. J Pediatr 117:462, 1990

7. Cilley RE, Zwischenberger JB, Andrews AF et al: Intracranial hemorrhage during extracorporeal membrane oxygenation in neonates. Pediatrics 78:699, 1986

8. Berry FA: The renal system. In Gregory GA (ed): Pediatric Anesthesia, vol 1, p 93. New York, Churchill Livingstone, 1989

9. Larsson LE, Nilsson K, Niklasson A et al: Influence of fluid regimens on perioperative blood-glucose concentrations in neonates. Br J Anaesth 64:419, 1990

10. Cornblath M, Schwartz R, Aynsley-Green A et al: Hypoglycemia in infancy: The need for a rational definition. Pediatrics 85:834, 1990

11. Kao LC, Warburton D, Sargent CW et al: Furosemide acutely decreases airway resistance in chronic bronchopulmonary dysplasia. J Pediatr 103:624, 1983

12. Berry FA: Practical aspects of fluid and electrolyte therapy. In Berry FA (ed): Anesthetic Management of Difficult and Routine Pediatric Patients, p 89. New York, Churchill Livingstone, 1990

13. Blayney M, Kerem E, Whyte H, O'Brodovich H: Bronchopulmonary dysplasia: Improvement in lung function between 7 and 10 years of age. J Pediatr 118:201, 1991

14. Tulassay T, Rascher W, Seyberth HW et al: Role of atrial natriuretic peptide in sodium homeostasis in premature infants. J Pediatr 109:1023, 1986

15. Cote CJ, Todres ID: The pediatric airway. In Ryan JF, Todres ID, Cote CJ et al (eds): A Practice of Anesthesia for Infants and Children, p 35. New York, Grune & Stratton, 1985

16. Garner L, Stirt JA, Finholt DA: Heart block after intravenous lidocaine in an infant. Can Anaesth Soc 32:425, 1985

17. Cook DR: Pharmacology of pediatric anesthesia. In Katz J, Steward DJ (eds): Anesthesia and Uncommon Pediatric Diseases, p 12. Philadelphia, WB Saunders, 1987

18. Keens TG, Bryan AC, Levison H et al: Developmental pattern of muscle fiber types in human ventilatory muscles. J Appl Physiol 44:909, 1978

19. Friedman WF, George BL: Treatment of congestive heart failure by altering loading conditions of the heart. J Pediatr 106:697, 1985

20. Wear R, Robinson S, Gregory GA: The effect of halothane on the baroresponse of adult and baby rabbits. Anesthesiology 56:188, 1982

21. Berry FA, Gregory GA: Do premature infants require anesthesia for surgery? Anesthesiology 67:3, 1987

22. Anand KJS, Brown MJ, Causon RC et al: Can the human neonate mount an endocrine and metabolic response to surgery? J Pediatr Surg 20:41, 1985

23. Cabal LA, Siassi B, Artal R et al: Cardiovascular and catecholamine changes after administration of pancuronium in distressed neonates. Pediatrics 75:284, 1985

24. Miller RD, Rupp SM, Fisher DM et al: Clinical pharmacology of vecuronium and atracurium. Anesthesiology 61:444, 1984

25. Fisher DM, Miller RD: Neuromuscular effects of vecuronium (ORG NC45) in infants and children during N$_2$O, halothane anesthesia. Anesthesiology 58:519, 1983

26. Meakin G, McKiernan EP, Morris P, Baker RD: Dose-response curves for suxamethonium in neonates, infants and children. Br J Anaesth 62:655–658, 1989

27. Fisher DM, Canfell PC, Fahey MR et al: Elimination of atracurium in humans: Contribution of Hofmann elimination and ester hydrolysis versus organ-based elimination. Anesthesiology 65:6, 1986

28. Goudsouzian NG: Relaxants in paediatric anaesthesia. Clin Anaesthesiol 3:539, 1985

29. Meakin G, Sweet PT, Bevan JC et al: Neostigmine and edrophonium as antagonists of pancuronium in infants and children. Anesthesiology 59:316, 1983

30. Hickey PR, Hansen DD, Wessel DL et al: Pulmonary and sys-

31. Hickey PR, Hansen DD, Wessel DL et al: Blunting of stress responses in the pulmonary circulation of infants by fentanyl. Anesth Analg 64:1132, 1985

32. Yaster M: The dose response of fentanyl in neonatal anesthesia. Anesthesiology 66:433, 1987

33. Morray JP, Lynn AM, Stamm SJ et al: Hemodynamic effects of ketamine in children with congenital heart disease. Anesth Analg 63:895, 1984

34. Hickey PR, Hansen DD, Gramolini GM et al: Pulmonary and systemic hemodynamic responses to ketamine in infants with normal and elevated pulmonary vascular resistance. Anesthesiology 62:287, 1985

35. Greeley WJ, Bushman GA, Davis DP et al: Comparative effects of halothane and ketamine on systemic arterial oxygen saturation in children with cyanotic heart disease. Anesthesiology 65:666, 1986

36. Lappas GD, Buckley MJ, Daggett WM et al: Left ventricular performance and pulmonary circulation following addition of nitrous oxide during coronary artery surgery. Anesthesiology 43:61, 1975

37. Maretoja OA, Tukkunen OK, Heikkila H et al: Haemodynamic response to nitrous oxide during high-dose fentanyl pancuronium anaesthesia. Acta Anaesthesiol Scand 29:137, 1985

38. Hickey PR, Hansen DD, Strafford M et al: Pulmonary and systemic hemodynamic effects of nitrous oxide in infants with normal and elevated pulmonary vascular resistance. Anesthesiology 65:374, 1986

39. Welborn L, Zwass M, Coté C et al: Comparison of desflurane and halothane anesthesia in pediatric ambulatory patients. Anesth Analg 72:S320, 1991

40. LeDez KM, Lerman J: The minimum alveolar concentration (MAC) of isoflurane in preterm neonates. Anesthesiology 67:301, 1987

41. Lerman J, Robinson S, Willis MM et al: Anesthetic requirements for halothane in young children 0–1 month and 1–6 months of age. Anesthesiology 59:421, 1983

42. Gregory GA, Wade JG, Beihl DR et al: Fetal anesthetic requirement (MAC) for halothane. Anesth Analg 62:9, 1983

43. Koehntop DE, Rodman JH, Brundage DM et al: Pharmacokinetics of fentanyl in neonates. Anesth Analg 65:227, 1986

44. Davis PJ, Cook R, Stiller RL et al: Pharmacodynamics and pharmacokinetics of high-dose sufentanil in infants and children undergoing cardiac surgery. Anesth Analg 66:203, 1987

45. Gauntlett IS, Fisher DM, Hertzka RE et al: Pharmacokinetics of fentanyl in neonatal humans and lambs: Effects of age. Anesthesiology 69:683, 1988

46. Mazoit JX, Denson DD, Samii K: Pharmacokinetics of bupivacaine following caudal anesthesia in infants. Anesthesiology 68:387, 1988

47. Yaster M, Maxwell LG: Pediatric regional anesthesia. Anesthesiology 70:324, 1989

48. Valley RD, Bailey AG: Caudal morphine for postoperative analgesia in infants and children: A report of 138 cases. Anesth Analg 72:120, 1991

49. Baily A, Valley R, Bigler R: High spinal anesthesia in an infant. Anesthesiology 70:560, 1989

50. Wright TE, Orr RJ, Haberkern CM, Walbergh EJ: Complications during spinal anesthesia in infants: High spinal blockade. Anesthesiology 73:1290, 1990

51. Dohi S, Naito H, Takahasi T: Age-related changes in blood pressure and duration of motor block in spinal anesthesia. Anesthesiology 50:319, 1979

52. Welborn LG, Rice LJ, Hannallah RS et al: Postoperative apnea in former preterm infants: Prospective comparison of spinal and general anesthesia. Anesthesiology 72:838, 1990

53. Broadman LM, Hannallah RS, Belman AB et al: Postcircumcision analgesia: A prospective evaluation of subcutaneous ring block of the penis. Anesthesiology 67:399, 1987

54. Jones R, Bodnar A, Roan Y et al: Subglottic stenosis in newborn intensive care unit graduates. Am J Dis Child 135:367, 1981

55. Friesen RH, Lichtor JL: Cardiovascular depression during hal-

othane anesthesia in infants: A study of three induction techniques. Anesth Analg 61:42, 1982

56. Diaz JH, Lockhart CH: Is halothane really safe in infancy? Anesthesiology 51:S313, 1979

57. Friesen RH, Lichtor JL: Cardiovascular effects of inhalation induction with isoflurane in infants. Anesth Analg 62:411, 1983

58. Salanitre E, Rackow M: The pulmonary exchange of nitrous oxide and halothane in infants and children. Anesthesiology 30:388, 1969

59. Steward DJ, Creighton RE: The uptake and excretion of nitrous oxide in the newborn. Can Anaesth Soc J 25:215, 1978

60. Brandom BW, Brandom RB, Cook DR: Uptake and distribution of halothane in infants: In vivo measurements and computer simulations. Anesth Analg 62:404, 1983

61. Koop CE, Schnaufer L, Broeule AM: Esophageal atresia and tracheoesophageal fistula: Supportive measures that affect survival. Pediatrics 54:558, 1974

62. Louhimo I, Lindahl H: Esophageal atresia: Primary results of 500 consecutively treated patients. J Pediatr Surg 18:217, 1983

63. Holmes SJK, Kiely EM, Spitz L: Tracheoesophageal fistula and respiratory distress syndrome. Pediatr Surg Int 2:16, 1987

64. Greenwood RD, Rosenthal A, Nadas AS: Cardiac anomalies associated with congenital diaphragmatic hernia. Pediatrics 57:92, 1976

65. Greenwood RD, Rosenthal A: Cardiovascular malformations associated with tracheoesophageal fistula and esophageal atresia. Pediatrics 57:87, 1976

66. Lipshultz SE, Frassica JJ, Orav EJ: Cardiovascular abnormalities in infants prenatally exposed to cocaine. J Pediatr 118:44, 1991

67. van de Bor M, Walther FJ, Ebrahimi M: Decreased cardiac output in infants of mothers who abused cocaine. Pediatrics 85:30, 1990

68. Bohn D, Tamura M, Perrin D et al: Ventilatory predictors of pulmonary hypoplasia in congenital diaphragmatic hernia, confirmed by morphologic assessment. J Pediatr 111:423, 1987

69. Sakai H, Tamura M, Hosokawa Y et al: Effect of surgical repair on respiratory mechanics in congenital diaphragmatic hernia. J Pediatr 111:432, 1987

70. Newman KD, Anderson KD, Van Meurs K et al: Extracorporeal membrane oxygenation and congenital diaphragmatic hernia: Should any infant be excluded? J Pediatr Surg 25:1048, 1990

71. Connors RH, Tracy T, Bailey PV et al: Congenital diaphragmatic hernia repair on ECMO. J Pediatr Surg 25:1043, 1990

72. Van Meurs KP, Newman KD, Anderson KD et al: Effect of extracorporeal membrane oxygenation on survival of infants with congenital diaphragmatic hernia. J Pediatr 117:954, 1990

73. Truog RD, Schena JA, Hershenson MB: Repair of congenital diaphragmatic hernia during extracorporeal membrane oxygenation. Anesthesiology 72:750, 1990

74. Grosfeld JL, Weber TR: Congenital abdominal wall defects: Gastroschisis and omphalocele. Curr Probl Surg 19:158, 1982

75. Hoyme HE, Higginbottom MC, Jones JL: The vascular pathogenesis of gastroschisis: Intrauterine interruption of the omphalomesenteric artery. Pediatrics 98:228, 1981

76. Masey SA, Buck JR, Koehler RC et al: Effects of increased intra-abdominal pressure of regional blood flow in newborn lambs. Anesthesiology 59:A425, 1983

77. Masey SA, Buck JR, Koehler RC: Cardiovascular and metabolic effects of increased intra-abdominal pressure in newborn lambs. Anesthesiology 59:A426, 1983

78. Yaster, Buck JR, Dudgeon DL et al: Hemodynamic effects of primary closure of omphalocele/gastroschisis in human newborns. Anesthesiology 69:84, 1988

79. Iberti TJ, Lieber CE, Benjamin E: Determination of intra-abdominal pressure using a transurethral bladder catheter: Clinical validation of the technique. Anesthesiology 70:47, 1989

80. Harman PK, Kron IL, McLachlan HD et al: Elevated intra-abdominal pressure and renal function. Ann Surg 196:90, 1982

81. Salem MR, Wong AY, Lin YH et al: Prevention of gastric distention during anesthesia for newborns with tracheoesophageal fistulas. Anesthesiology 38:82, 1973

82. Filston HC, Chitwood WR, Schkolne B et al: The Fogarty balloon catheter as an aid to management of the infant with esophageal atresia and tracheoesophageal fistula complicated by severe RDS or pneumonia. J Pediatr Surg 17:149, 1982

83. Leendertse-Verloop K, Tibboel D, Hazebroek FWJ et al: Postoperative morbidity in patients with esophageal atresia. Pediatr Surg Int 2:2, 1987

84. Jolley SG, Johnson DG, Roberts CC et al: Patterns of gastroesophageal reflux in children following repair of esophageal atresia and distal tracheoesophageal fistula. J Pediatr Surg 15:857, 1980

85. Kliegman RM: Neonatal necrotizing enterocolitis: Bridging the basic science with the clinical disease. J Pediatr 117:833, 1990

86. Bose C, Corbet A, Bose G et al: Improved outcome at 28 days of age for very low birth weight infants treated with a single dose of a synthetic surfactant. J Pediatr 117:947, 1990

87. Fujiwara T, Konishi M, Chida S: Surfactant replacement therapy with a single postventilatory dose of a reconstituted bovine surfactant in preterm neonates with respiratory distress syndrome. Final analysis of a multicenter, double-blind, randomized trial and comparison with similar trials. Pediatrics 86:753, 1990

88. Ostertag SG, LaGamma EF, Reisen CE et al: Early enteral feeding does not affect the incidence of necrotizing enterocolitis. Pediatrics 77:275, 1986

89. Milner ME, de la Monte SM, Moore GW et al: Risk factors for developing and dying from necrotizing enterocolitis. J Pediatr Gastroenterol Nutr 5:359, 1986

90. Kosloske AM: Pathogenesis and prevention of necrotizing enterocolitis: A hypothesis based on personal observation and a review of the literature. Pediatrics 74:1086, 1984

91. Buras R, Guzzetta P, Avery G et al: Acidosis and hepatic portal venous gas: Indications for surgery in necrotizing enterocolitis. Pediatrics 78:273, 1986

92. Buntain WL, Conner E, Emrico J et al: Transcutaneous oxygen (tcPO$_2$) measurements as an aid to fluid therapy in necrotizing enterocolitis. J Pediatr Surg 14:728, 1979

93. Puri P, Guiney EJ, O'Donnell B: Inguinal hernia in infants: The fate of the testis following incarceration. J Pediatr Surg 19:44, 1984

94. Rescorla FJ, Grosfeld JL: Inguinal hernia repair in the perinatal period and early infancy: Clinical considerations. J Pediatr Surg 19:832, 1984

95. Peevy KJ, Speed FA, Hoff CJ: Epidemiology of inguinal hernia in preterm neonates. Pediatrics 77:246, 1986

96. Steward DJ: Preterm infants are more prone to complications following minor surgery than are term infants. Anesthesiology 56:304, 1982

97. Liu LMP, Coté CJ, Coudsouzian NG et al: Life-threatening apnea in infants recovering from anesthesia. Anesthesiology 59:506, 1983

98. Kurth CD, Spitzer AR, Broennle AM et al: Postoperative apnea in former premature infants. Anesthesiology 66:483, 1987

99. Knill RL, Clement JL: Site of selective action of halothane on the peripheral chemoreflex pathways in humans. Anesthesiology 61:121, 1984

100. Melman E, Pennelas J, Maruffo J: Regional anesthesia in children. Anesth Analg 54:387, 1975

101. Robinson SR, Gregory GA: Fentanyl-air-oxygen anesthesia for ligation of patent ductus arteriosus in preterm infants. Anesth Analg 60:331, 1981

102. Gibson DL, Sheps SB, Hong S et al: Retinopathy of prematurity-induced blindness: Birth weight-specific survival and the new epidemic. Pediatrics 86:405, 1990

103. Steward DJ: Is there a risk of general anesthesia triggering SIDS? Possibly not! Anesthesiology 63:326, 1985

104. Werthhammer J, Brown ER, Neff RK et al: Sudden infant death syndrome in infants with bronchopulmonary dysplasia. Pediatrics 69:301, 1982

105. Orlowski JP: Cerebrospinal fluid endorphins and the infant apnea syndrome. Pediatrics 78:233, 1986

106. Peterson DR, Sabotta EE, Daling JR: Infant mortality among subsequent siblings of infants who died of sudden infant death syndrome. Pediatrics 108:911, 1986

107. Shannon DC, Kelly DH, O'Connell K: Abnormal regulation of ventilation in infants at risk of sudden-infant-death syndrome. N Engl J Med 297:747, 1977

108. Denborough MA, Galloway GJ, Hopkinson KC: Malignant hyperpyrexia and sudden infant death. Lancet 2:1068, 1982

109. Peterson DR, Davis N: Malignant hyperthermia diathesis and sudden infant death syndrome. Anesth Analg 65:209, 1986

48

D. Ryan Cook

Pediatric Anesthesia

Pediatric anesthesia involves the anesthetic management of patients in the process of rapid growth and development. The anatomic, physiologic, pharmacologic, and psychological characteristics of the infant or child influence anesthetic care. Thus, appropriate anesthetic management of the pediatric surgical patient must be considered within the context of the patient's maturity and the severity of the surgical problem. The purpose of this chapter is to provide an overview of the important issues in pediatric anesthesia. Several pediatric anesthesia and specialized texts are available to fill the gaps.[1-8]

Rapid growth, development, and maturation of organ function occur during the first several months of life. Circulatory and ventilatory adaptation are completed, thermoregulation processes change, the sizes of body fluid compartments are shifting to adult values, skeletal muscle mass is developing, hepatic enzyme systems responsible for the metabolism of drugs are developing, and renal function is maturing (Table 48-1). By the time an infant is 3 months of age, the major tasks of maturation have been accomplished. Over the next 1–1.5 years the infant gradually is physically transformed into a miniature adult; psychological maturation may take years. Between 6 months and 1 year of age, the infant begins to show sufficient awareness of his or her surroundings so that the psychological aspects of hospitalization and surgery must be considered. At this age, therefore, sedative drugs may be used in preoperative preparation. The preschool aged child (2–6 years old) presents relatively few technical problems to the anesthesiologist. However, the child's fear, apprehension, and lack of cooperation are of particular concern to the anesthesiologist. For good anesthetic management, children at this age need to be prepared psychologically by both parent and anesthesiologist and may need preoperative medication. Children of school age (6–18 years old) may be considered to be small adults from a physiologic and, to a lesser extent, a psychological point of view. Fear and apprehension are still problems, but it becomes more likely that the child of this age will be cooperative.

PREANESTHETIC EVALUATION AND PREPARATION

Before surgery, the anesthesiologist should visit the patient and, when possible, the patient's parents. The primary purpose of the visit should be to obtain information about the surgical problem and medical history and to make an estimate of the patient's personality and response to hospitalization. Parental anxieties concerning the surgical procedure may be profound and may be transmitted to the child. These fears and anxieties, whether rational (realistic) or irrational (unrealistic), may stress the family unit. In addition, children may have age-related fears of their own.[9-13] To prepare the child psychologically for elective surgery, educational booklets, movies, slide shows, puppet shows, and preoperative hospital tours may be useful. The anesthesiologist and other health care workers should also reinforce the information. Unified, coherent, noncontradictory teaching materials and information should be developed. The goal is to have calm parents and calm children. Outpatient surgery or same-day surgery programs, in addition, minimize separation anxieties of the younger child. Such programs provide support to the parents and child. Ordinarily, it is best to give a simple explanation of what the patient can expect before induction of anesthesia. This reduces the element of surprise and can be used to reinforce preoperative teaching materials. In the older child, the preoperative visit allows the anesthesiologist to establish a personal rapport, which aids in a smoother anesthetic induction. Some children who have had previous hospitalizations or whose parents or friends have told them about operations may show interest in or anxiety about the anesthesia. These children deserve a frank explanation without too many details and forthright

TABLE 48-1. Body Composition During Growth

Body Compartment	Percentage of Body Weight	
	Infant	Adult
Total body water	73	60
Extracellular fluid	44	15–20
Blood volume	8–10	7
Intracellular water	33	40
Muscle mass	20	50
Fat	12	18

answers to their questions. In some clinics it is common to have parents actively participate in the anesthetic induction process.[12-13] For some parents and preschool children, this joint experience attenuates a multitude of fears and anxieties and is, thus, a positive experience. However, for other parents, participation is emotionally traumatic. The psychodynamics of these experiences are poorly understood. Anesthesiologists are constantly amazed at how well many preschool children adapt to stressful situations if provided with information in advance. This adaptation does not necessarily require active parental participation but most likely is a complex reflection of general parenting. For example, pediatric dentists commonly perform routine dental care with limited or no fuss in preschool children without the parents present; for many children, this is an immense source of pride.

Minimum Hemoglobin Values

There is controversy as to what constitutes the minimum acceptable hemoglobin value for elective pediatric surgery and if, indeed, such a minimum should be considered at all.[11,14-15] The arbitrary figure of 10 g·dl^{-1} has been used extensively for patients older than 3 months, with appropriately higher values for the younger infant. The use of an arbitrary value as a minimum requirement for elective surgery is useful as a simple screening procedure, but it should not be used as the final criterion for deciding if a patient may be anesthetized for elective surgery. Anemia is defined dynamically in infants and children because a normal "physiologic" anemia occurs within the first several months. Cardiac output, oxygen-carrying capacity, type of anesthesia, and type of surgery are factors other than hematocrit that help define allowable blood loss. Neonates have 60–90% hemoglobin F, and it is not until they are 6 months of age that the adult hemoglobin A–hemoglobin F ratio is achieved. Hemoglobin F has a high affinity for oxygen, and the oxygen dissociation curve is shifted to the left. Thus, oxygen delivery to the tissues at a given oxygen tension is decreased. As the infant matures from 1 to 6 months, the arterial to venous difference in oxygen content and tissue oxygen delivery progressively increases. A full-term infant's hematocrit rarely decreases below 50% during the first several weeks of life. It takes about 3 months for the hematocrit to reach its nadir at 30%. This decrease in hematocrit results from decreased erythropoietin production, a shorter red blood cell survival time, and increased plasma volume.

Patients whose hemoglobin values are found to be below the arbitrary standard should be investigated and the cause of the anemia determined. The decision to proceed with surgery and anesthesia should then be based on the findings and not merely on a numeric value. Patients with low hemoglobin values that result from chronic dietary iron deficiency present less anesthetic risk than do those whose anemia results from blood loss or hemoglobinopathies. There seems little reason not to proceed with elective surgery in patients with iron-deficiency anemia if the anticipated surgical procedure is to be short and no significant blood loss is anticipated. Major surgical procedures in which transfusion is planned also may be started in this type of patient. Elective major surgery in which transfusion is not anticipated is better postponed until the anemia has been corrected. In elective procedures, preoperative blood transfusion is never justified simply to treat uncomplicated iron-deficiency anemia or to increase a hemoglobin value to some arbitrary standard. Patients with sickle cell anemia require special preoperative preparation. These patients run the risk of intravascular sickling and thrombosis if subjected to hypoxia, hypothermia, or acidosis.[15]

Hydration and Restriction of Fluids

The safety of an anesthetic depends to a large extent on the patient's stomach being empty. On the other hand, it is desirable that the patient have anesthesia and surgery under conditions of optimal hydration. These two goals are not incompatible or difficult to achieve. The patient who is fed at the usual meal times and sleeps through the night presents no particular problems. The preoperative orders should include the scheduled time of operation, the instruction that food or fluids be offered or encouraged until a specific time 8 hours before the scheduled surgery, and the instruction that the patient have "nothing by mouth" after that hour. The traditional "nothing by mouth after midnight" then applies only to early morning cases. Infants and younger children scheduled for later surgery may have clear liquids 3–4 hours before their operation.[16-25] In the case of the infant who is fed more frequently or still has fourth-hour feedings, the preoperative orders should distinguish between solid food and clear liquids. (The term solid food includes not only the usual foods but also milk and pulp-containing fruit juices—in short, anything other than clear liquids.) The preoperative orders should include the time of the scheduled surgery, the instruction that no solid food or milk be allowed after a specific time 4 hours before the scheduled surgery, the instruction that clear liquids be offered until a specific time 2 hours before surgery, and the instruction that the patient have nothing by mouth after that hour.

If these details are not clearly stated in a positive, itemized fashion with stated hours, the child, particularly the infant, inadvertently may not be given fluids for excessively long periods. Although these facts are well known to surgeons and anesthesiologists, pediatric patients nevertheless are occasionally subjected to unnecessarily long periods without fluid intake. This sometimes arises from improper case scheduling and delays in the surgical schedule, but it results most often from carelessly written preoperative orders. In general, the youngest infant should be first on the operating schedule or at least should be scheduled and operated on at a specific time. Both the surgeon and the anesthesiologist must be alert to delays and make sure that the infant's fluid restriction is revised accordingly.

Preanesthetic Medication

Preanesthetic medication can play an important part in the anesthetic care of infants and children. It is unclear whether sedation is a substitute for or a supplement to rapport. Key reasons for the use of preanesthetic medications are to help decrease apprehensiveness; to induce quiescence; to control secretions in the airway; to prevent vagal reflexes, which may be stimulated by the anesthetic agent or by anesthetic or surgical maneuvers; to reduce gastric volume and increase gastric pH. Sedative-hypnotics, opioids, or ataractic drugs, either alone or in combination, are generally used for the first two objectives; anticholinergic drugs for the next two; and antacids, H_2 receptor blockers, and metoclopramide for the last. It is not necessary, and sometimes not desirable, to achieve all these goals. The relative importance of

TABLE 48-2. Preoperative Medication

Age	Weight		Morphine (mg)	Atropine or Scopolamine (mg)	Seco-barbital (mg)
	Kilograms	*Pounds*			
Premature	Less than 2.5	Less than 5½		Atropine 0.075	
0–1 mo	2.5–3.0	5½–7		Atropine 0.1	
1–3 mo	3.0–5.5	7–12		Atropine 0.15	
3–6 mo	5.5–7	12–15		Atropine 0.2	
6–12 mo	7–9	15–20	0.6	Scopolamine 0.1	20
12–18 mo	9–11	20–25	0.8	Scopolamine 0.15	25
18–24 mo	11–14	25–30	1.0	Scopolamine 0.15	30
2–3 yr	14–16	30–35	1.5	Scopolamine 0.15	40
3–5 yr	16–20	35–45	2.0	Scopolamine 0.15	50
5–8 yr	20–30	45–65	3.0	Scopolamine 0.2	75
8–10 yr	30–40	65–80	4.0	Scopolamine 0.2	75
10–12 yr	40–45	80–100	5.0	Scopolamine 0.3	100
12–14 yr	45–60	100–130	8.0	Scopolamine 0.3	100
Older than 14 yr	More than 60	More than 130	10.0	Scopolamine 0.3	100

each one varies with the age and condition of the patient and with the type of anesthesia to be used.

It is desirable to induce sleep (or quiescence) and freedom from apprehension for the child who is to have anesthesia and surgery. However, such states may sometimes be achieved at the price of some degree of respiratory depression or hypoxemia. Anesthesiologists must decide not only the degree of sedation they desire for their patients but also how much sedation patients can "afford." The type of anesthesia to be used, the duration of the procedure, and the quality of the postanesthetic care must be considered. The heavily sedated patient will have no memory of the surgical experience and is likely to have a smooth induction. However, this type of premedication may produce prolonged emergence and residual central nervous system depression, especially after relatively short procedures. Return of protective airway reflexes may also be delayed.

Atropine and Scopolamine

Certain drugs (e.g., halothane, succinylcholine, fentanyl) have a cholinergic effect and may cause vagally induced bradycardia. This effect is most prominent in infants, especially those younger than 3 months. Atropine is superior to scopolamine in controlling bradycardia and other dysrhythmias in infants younger than 6 months of age. A vagolytic dose of atropine ($0.02~mg \cdot kg^{-1}$) provides complete protection against a cholinergic challenge in infants; relatively lower doses of atropine provide adequate protection in older infants and children. These seemingly high doses are well tolerated by the infant and may be used safely. In general, we prefer to administer atropine intravenously in the operating room rather than as an intramuscular or oral preanesthetic medication. The effect by the oral route is generally less certain, and much higher doses must be used. At the age when sedative drugs are added to the preanesthetic medication, many prefer scopolamine to atropine because it contributes additional sedation, amnesia, and effective suppression of secretions in the airway. When scopolamine is combined with narcotic, delirium is seldom seen.

Sedatives and Opioids

Many drugs and combinations of drugs have been tried, but in our view none is much better than the combination of opioid, barbiturate, and scopolamine. Table 48-2 shows a

dosage schedule for preoperative medication that may be used as a guide. The doses of barbiturate and opioid given in this table are quite conservative. With scopolamine, they provide adequate sedation in most situations. However, either the opioid or the barbiturate dose may safely be increased for the particularly apprehensive child if heavier sedation is needed.

Although the intramuscular route does not appear to be unduly traumatic and is by far the most reliable, many children have an innate, profound fear of needles. For this reason many offer preanesthetic medication orally, nasally, transorally, or by rectum.[26-32] A number of commonly used barbiturates and sedatives are available as suppositories or flavored syrups. Absorption from the rectum is uneven and unpredictable, and oral preparations may be refused or vomited.

Sedative drugs can be effective only if sufficient time is allowed for the full effect to be achieved. The various drugs reach their maximum effect at different times and therefore theoretically should be given separately. However, in most cases this is impractical, and usually all drugs are administered at the same time. They should be given at least 45 minutes to 1 hour before anesthesia. It is our practice to call on each patient twice: 1 hour before surgery, for medication, and a second time just before anesthesia is begun. This requires planning and the cooperation of the surgical, nursing, and anesthesia staffs, but it is well worth the effort because the sedation is more effective and anesthetic inductions are made easier for both patient and anesthesiologist.

Antacids, H₂ Blockers, and Metoclopramide

Children may be at slightly greater risk than adults for acid aspiration syndrome because they have a greater gastric residual volume and nearly all have a gastric pH of less than 2.5.[33] Specific H_2 receptor antagonists such as cimetidine or ranitidine, clear antacids, or metoclopramide may play an important role in reducing the likelihood of gastric aspiration in patients having elective or emergency surgery.[34-36]

ANESTHETIC DRUGS AND RELATED DRUGS

The choice of anesthetic drugs for infants and children is not strikingly different from that for adults. There appears to be no specific contraindication to any of the commonly used anesthetic drugs on the basis of age alone. Likewise, no contraindications on the basis of age alone have been demonstrated for any of the commonly used anesthetic induction techniques—inhalation, intravenous, or rectal. Selection of drugs and techniques is based on the individual anesthesiologist's experience, preference, and skill. Nevertheless, the anesthesiologist should use special care in choosing the optimal method for each patient. Nitrous oxide reinforced by potent inhalation drugs or intravenous drugs is frequently used to maintain anesthesia in pediatric patients; muscle relaxants are common adjuncts.

Inhalation Agents

Induction of general anesthesia in the infant may be difficult no matter what technique is selected. Inhalation inductions are frequently complicated by breath-holding, laryngospasm, and distention of the stomach with anesthetic gases. Difficulty in maintaining a good mask fit is common. The procedure must be performed gently, cautiously, and with close attention to vital signs and indications of deepening anesthesia.

Young infants usually are not upset at induction of anesthesia with a loosely applied face mask. With increasing age, the induction process becomes progressively easier. Older children may prefer to hold the mask for themselves if they have chosen an inhalation method over a "shot." In general, halothane allows the most rapid and smooth induction compared with enflurane and isoflurane. The ether anesthetics are pungent and produce airway irritation. Flavored lip gloss or scented oils applied to the inside of the mask can be used to hide the pungency of these agents.[37-38] A single-breath method for induction of anesthesia with halothane has been described; the patient exhales to residual volume and then takes a full inspiration from a reservoir bag containing 5% halothane in 70% nitrous oxide with oxygen. The halothane concentration is then reduced to continue the induction process.

The incidence of bradycardia, hypotension, and cardiac arrest during induction of inhalation anesthesia is higher in infants and small children than in adults.[39] This greater incidence of untoward effects from potent drugs can be attributed to age-related differences in uptake, anesthetic requirements, and sensitivity of the cardiovascular system. The uptake of inhalation anesthetics is more rapid in infants and small children than in adults because of major differences in blood-gas solubility coefficients, blood-tissue solubility coefficients, body composition, the ratio of alveolar ventilation to functional residual capacity, and the distribution of cardiac output.[40-42] Thus, early in anesthetic induction the infant has higher tissue concentrations of anesthetic than the adult (e.g., in brain, heart, muscle).[43]

Intracardiac shunts, common in infants and children, can also alter the uptake of inhalation anesthetics.[44] A right-to-left shunt slows the uptake of anesthetic because its tension or concentration in the arterial blood increases more slowly; induction of anesthesia is prolonged. The influence of a left-to-right shunt on anesthetic uptake depends on the size of the shunt and on whether a right-to-left shunt exists. A large (greater than 80%) left-to-right shunt increases the rate of anesthetic transfer from the lungs to the arterial blood; smaller shunts (less than 50%) have a negligible effect on uptake. A left-to-right shunt may speed induction when it coexists with a large right-to-left shunt. Increases in pulmonary vascular resistance or decreases in systemic vascular resistance occasionally can reverse left-to-right shunts.

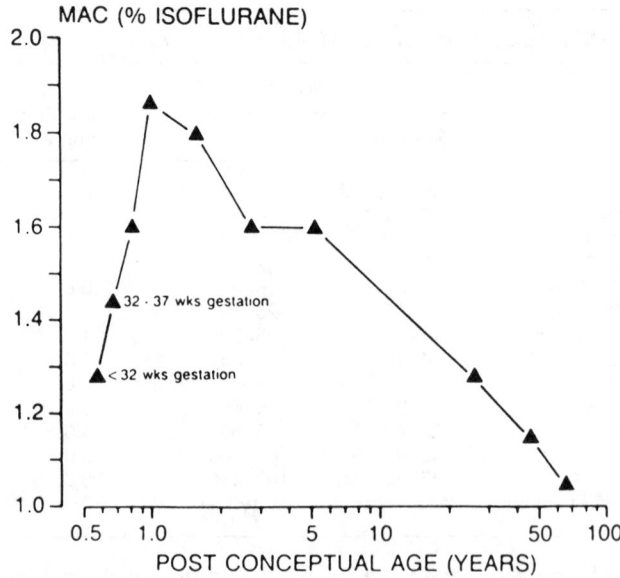

Figure 48-1. The MAC of isoflurane and postconceptual age. (Data from LeDez KM, Lerman J: The minimum alveolar concentration [MAC] of isoflurane in preterm neonates. Anesthesiology 67:301, 1987.)

The anesthetic requirements for various inhalation anesthetics (e.g., halothane, isoflurane, and enflurane) are generally inversely related to age (Fig. 48-1).[45-47] Thus, higher inspired concentrations (overpressure) are often used early in an anesthetic induction to compensate for the age-related differences in anesthetic requirements.

Isoflurane has fewer adverse cardiovascular effects than equipotent halothane concentrations.[48-55] Although the drugs similarly reduce contractility and heart rate in vitro, isoflurane reduces peripheral resistance several fold but halothane does not. The resulting reduction in cardiac index with isoflurane is only half that with halothane. Isoflurane may, thus, permit greater hemodynamic stability than halothane. The alarming reduction in blood pressure caused by isoflurane may reflect only a decrease in peripheral resistance with near-normal cardiac output. Anesthetic drugs blunt baroreceptor reflexes in a concentration-dependent manner to a greater degree in infants than in older patients.[56-59] The reasons why anesthetics depress the baroreceptor reflexes more in infants are unknown. Most likely they are related to developmental differences in the autonomic nervous system. The separation between minimum alveolar concentration and the lethal concentration of a potent inhalation anesthetic defines the safety margin or therapeutic ratio. Isoflurane has a higher therapeutic ratio than does halothane in older animals but not in young animals.[51-54]

Intravenous Drugs

In older children, intravenous infusions are more readily started, and induction with an intravenous anesthetic is frequently used. Intravenous drugs can be administered to small infants with very little discomfort if a skilled, "concealed" technique using a fine (27-gauge) needle is used. Dermal lidocaine patches (EMLA) may facilitate intravenous catheter insertion.[60-61] Thiopental, methohexital, propofol, and ketamine may be used for induction of an-

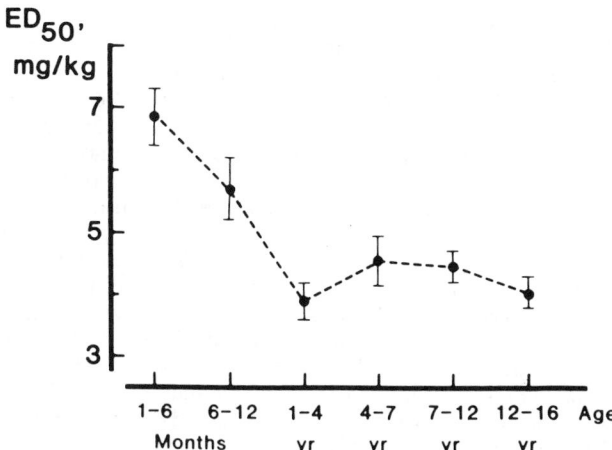

Figure 48-2. Estimated ED_{50} of thiopental in various age groups of children. (Data from Jonmarker C, Westrin P, Larsson S *et al:* Thiopental requirements for induction of anesthesia in children. Anesthesiology 67:104, 1987.)

esthesia.[62-73] Rarely, each may be given intramuscularly.[64] Infants generally need more thiopental than older children or adults to minimize the reaction to application of a face mask or intubation of the trachea; however, "sleep" doses may be little different (Fig. 48-2).[65-69] Midazolam may be unreliable as an intravenous induction drug.[70]

Thiopental, methohexital, and ketamine have been used by the rectal route to induce anesthesia in pediatric patients. Methohexital (15–25 mg·kg^{-1}) is now more commonly used and is probably the drug of choice in view of its more rapid metabolism.[71] Hiccough is a common side effect. Clinical recovery from rectal methohexital occurs in 30–40 minutes and shows some correlation with plasma concentrations of the drug.

A variety of sedative-hypnotic drugs appear to have increased duration of effects in the infant; in older children higher doses may be needed. The mechanism of this change in sensitivity has been elucidated for some of the barbiturates and benzodiazepines.[72] The dose of ketamine required to prevent gross movements is four times greater in infants younger than 6 months than in 6-year-old children.[73] Acute studies show little metabolism of ketamine by the newborn. In the "anesthetic" state associated with ketamine, respiration and blood pressure are usually well maintained. However, use of ketamine in infants, particularly at the high doses required for lack of movement, has been associated with depression of ventilation and apnea, generalized extensor spasm with opisthotonus, an increase in intracranial pressure in infants with hydrocephalus, and acute increases in pulmonary artery pressure in infants with congenital heart disease.[74-77] Recent studies suggest that pulmonary vascular resistance is not changed by ketamine in infants with either normal or elevated pulmonary vascular resistance as long as the airway and ventilation are maintained.[78-79]

Opioids

Meperidine (0.5–1 mg·kg^{-1}), morphine (0.05–0.1 mg·kg^{-1}), or fentanyl (3–5 µg·kg^{-1}), sufentanil (1–2 µg·kg^{-1}), or alfentanil (100 µg·kg^{-1}) is used to reinforce nitrous oxide–oxygen anesthesia in the infant or small child. Such doses attenuate the cardiovascular responses to surgical stress.

High-dose morphine (1.0 mg·kg^{-1}), fentanyl (25–50 µg·kg^{-1}), or sufentanil (10–15 µg·kg^{-1}) anesthesia is given with oxygen-air to critically ill infants or children, particularly those requiring palliative heart surgery. The cardiovascular effects of those opioids seem minimal.

Bradycardia and chest wall rigidity are potential features of opioid anesthesia. To ameliorate these side effects, it is common to administer a muscle relaxant with desired cardiovascular countereffects (*e.g.*, pancuronium). The cardiovascular effects of high-dose fentanyl or sufentanil (with pancuronium) are minimal.[80-82] The cardiovascular and ventilatory effects of fentanyl (without relaxant) depend on concentration. The dose of fentanyl needed to guarantee satisfactory anesthesia for infants is unknown. Age-related differences in the kinetics and sensitivity to fentanyl and changes in kinetics associated with profound pathophysiologic conditions make generalizations difficult.[83-84] However, fentanyl clearance in the infant seems comparable to that in the older child or adult; it is significantly reduced in the premature infant. Sufentanil is approximately seven times more potent than fentanyl and has minimal cardiovascular effects. Bradycardia is an uncommon feature.[85-86] Alfentanil is one third as potent as fentanyl and has a shorter duration of action. Because of its relatively short duration of action, alfentanil may be particularly useful in anesthesia for infants and children, particularly for short surgical procedures.[87-92]

Muscle Relaxants

Muscle relaxants are common adjuncts to nitrous oxide–opioid anesthesia. Throughout infancy and early childhood, the neuromuscular junction matures physically and biochemically, the contractile properties of skeletal muscle change, the amount of muscle in proportion to body weight increases, and the neuromuscular junction is variably sensitive to relaxants.[93-94] In addition, the apparent volume of distribution of relaxants, their redistribution and excretion (clearance), and possibly their rate of metabolism change throughout life. These factors influence the dose-response relationship of relaxants and the duration of neuromuscular blockade. When allowances are made for differences in the volume of distribution and for the type and concentration of anesthetic, infants appear relatively resistant to succinylcholine and relatively sensitive to nondepolarizing relaxants. However, the response of children to relaxants differs little from that of adults.[95-114]

ENDOTRACHEAL INTUBATION

The advantages of endotracheal intubation for any patient having anesthesia are beyond question. The endotracheal tube has become an indispensable part of all intrathoracic, neurosurgical, and other surgical procedures involving unusual positions or distortion of the airway or in which the anesthesiologist does not command access to the airway. In a number of other situations, endotracheal intubation is not absolutely necessary but facilitates airway maintenance and ventilation of the lungs. In such cases tracheal intubation is elective and may be considered as an aid to both the anesthesiologist and the surgeon. In patients presenting little or no difficulty with the airway, endotracheal intubation is probably unjustified or at least unnecessary.

Indications

The indications for tracheal intubation are the same for patients of any age, but the young infants' anatomic and physiologic problems raise the question of whether infancy itself may not be an indication for endotracheal intubation. At this age the airway is difficult to maintain, mask fit is difficult, and assisted or controlled ventilation of the lungs is essential in view of the poor respiratory reserve of the infant. These problems are all greatly simplified by endotracheal anesthesia.

The suggestion that all infants should have endotracheal anesthesia has led to controversy among anesthesiologists. All agree that a finite morbidity accompanies endotracheal intubation and that this morbidity and its potential consequences are greater in the infant. There is also agreement that endotracheal intubation in the infant requires knowledge and skills that the average anesthesiologist may not have. The debate therefore centers around the relative advantages *versus* the risks of tracheal intubation. Nevertheless, routine intubation of the trachea of infants and children can be achieved with an exceedingly low morbidity.

Over a number of years we have used endotracheal anesthesia virtually routinely in all patients younger than 6 months of age, except in very short procedures. There are many advantages in standardizing not so much the technique but the philosophy of good anesthetic care of small infants. When endotracheal intubation becomes a part of standard care, the skill with which the technique is performed by the various members of the department is increased, and there is no need for debate in borderline situations about whether the technique should be used.

Intubation of the infant's trachea is not more difficult than that of the adult, but the anesthesiologist must be familiar not only with the anatomic differences of the infant larynx but also with the specialized equipment required. Trauma can be minimized in tracheal intubation by working gently and by ensuring adequate relaxation either with a sufficiently deep plane of anesthesia or with muscle relaxants. At least three tube sizes should be available for each patient. The tube should pass the glottis and cricoid without resistance, and gas should leak around the tube when positive pressure of approximately 20 cm H_2O is applied to the airway (Table 48-3).

TABLE 48-3. Approximate Sizes of Endotracheal Tubes for Infants and Children*

Age	Weight (kg)	Internal Diameter (mm)†	French†
6 mo	6	4.0	16
9 mo	9	4.5	18
1 yr	12	5.0	20
2 yr	14	5.5	22
4 yr	16	6.0	24
6 yr	20	6.5	26
8 yr	28	7.0	28
10 yr	30	7.5	30

*These suggested endotracheal tube sizes produce a snug fit with a minimal leak during positive pressure ventilation. Smaller sizes may be used if a moderate leak is desired.

†French size is the outside circumference of the endotracheal tube; Fr = $\pi \times$ outside diameter.

Use of cuffed endotracheal tubes in children younger than 10 years is neither necessary nor good practice; a suitably large tube in patients younger than this age will make sufficiently good contact at the level of the cricoid to prevent significant air leak. If a cuffed tube is used, a smaller size with correspondingly higher air flow resistance may be necessary. Finally, there is an increased likelihood of trauma to the tracheal mucosa from the pressure of the inflated cuff.

Tube selection also is important in controlling the complications of endotracheal intubation. Tubes should be sterile and free of any material that might be irritating or toxic to the mucosa. Sterile, prepackaged, disposable vinyl plastic tubes are recommended. Lubricants must be used carefully. Tubes of ointment or jelly may become contaminated, and lubricants containing local anesthetics may be irritating or allergenic. Sterile water is usually an adequate lubricant except for nasal or cuffed tubes.

PEDIATRIC BREATHING CIRCUITS

An optimal breathing circuit system for the pediatric patient provides minimal dead space and minimal resistance to breathing and permits accurate, rapid control of anesthetic depth, inspired oxygen concentration, and inspired carbon dioxide concentration. Such systems should be small, light, and as free as possible from malfunction. Although many types of pediatric devices have been developed, modifications of the simple T-piece are the most popular for infants. For older children (*i.e.*, 6–8 years of age), modified or traditional circle systems with a carbon dioxide absorber are more reasonable.

A number of combinations of T-piece tubing, breathing bag, and sites of fresh gas entry and overflow are possible. Mapleson classified the various combinations into five types (Fig. 48-3). The Jackson Rees modification is functionally identical to the Mapleson Type D. Types B and C are not used clinically. Carbon dioxide is removed more effectively in the D configuration when controlled ventilation is used. In recent years the Mapleson D device has emerged in a new guise, the coaxial circuit. It is virtually identical in principle but much different in design. The lightweight disposable inspired and expired gas conduits are usually arranged coaxially with the inspiratory tubing running within the expiratory tubing. The rebreathing bag and expiratory pop-off valve are permanently mounted on a bracket clamped to the gas machine. Scavenging of expired and excess gases is thus easily accomplished. The unit can be used for patients of any size and age provided that suitable volumes of fresh gases are chosen. The coaxial arrangement permits some heat exchange between the warm expired and unwarmed inspired gases, thus preventing some degree of heat loss from the airway.

The T-piece systems, although they incorporate neither directional valves nor soda lime, were originally conceived of as non–rebreathing systems. Thus, early attention was directed toward removal of expired carbon dioxide from the system rather than from the patient. In the spontaneously breathing patient, a fresh gas flow of three times the minute volume is necessary to flush the expiratory limb completely (regardless of its volume) and thus prevent rebreathing. With controlled ventilation of the lungs, it is not necessary to completely eliminate expired carbon dioxide from the expiratory limb to maintain eucapnia. Arterial carbon dioxide tension ($Paco_2$) is determined by fresh gas flow and minute ventilation (see Chapter 25). The introduction of the coaxial circuit has rekindled interest in establishing suitable

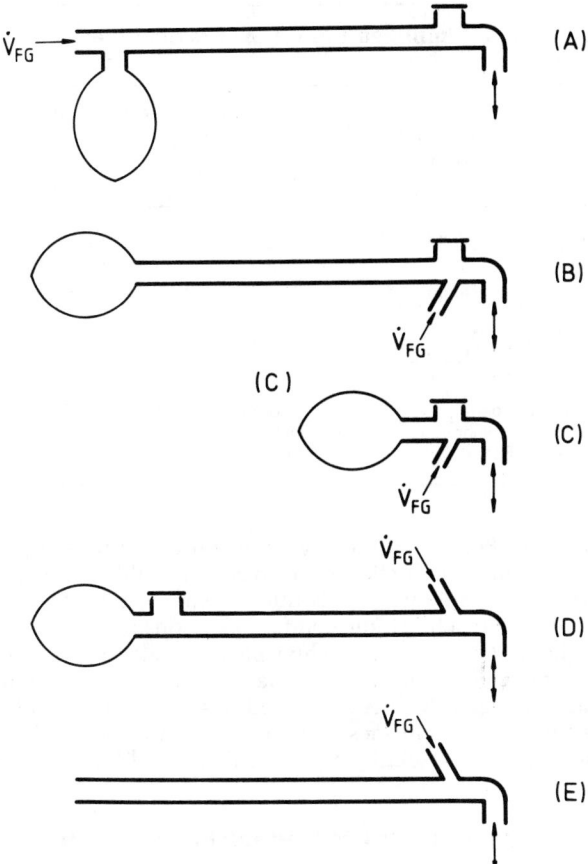

Figure 48-3. Mapleson classification (A–E) of some rebreathing systems. $\dot{V}_{FG}$ is the fresh gas flow. (Reprinted by permission of the publisher from Mushin WW, Jones PL: Physics for the Anaesthetist, 4th ed, p 375. Boston, Blackwell Scientific, 1987.)

values for minute ventilation and fresh gas flow in semi-closed systems, particularly for infants and children. Complete non–rebreathing occurs with fresh gas flows two to three times the minute volume. Maximum permissible rebreathing occurs with fresh gas flows in the range of 0.6–1.0 times the minute volume. With increasing rebreathing, maintenance of sufficient minute volume ventilation becomes increasingly critical. In large children, an obvious advantage of the partial rebreathing approach is the economy of fresh gas flow. Another advantage for patients of all ages is the ability to set fixed ventilatory volumes (on a mechanical ventilator, for instance) and to control $Paco_2$ simply by adjustment of fresh gas flow. Dangers of the rebreathing approach for infants are implicit in the "safe" minimum fresh gas flow settings recommended by several authors. In the smallest patients the accuracy of flow meters is critical and the risk of hypercarbia is acute unless there is scrupulous $Paco_2$ monitoring.

Circle Absorption

The circle absorption system potentially eliminates the problems of carbon dioxide control, humidification, and scavenging of waste gases seen with Mapleson D systems. High-resistance valves, the large dead space of the Y-pieces, and the large, heavy tubing make the standard adult circle system unsuitable for infants and small children. With im-

proved low-resistance valves, infants can maintain normal blood gas values even with spontaneous ventilation. With controlled ventilation of the lungs, resistance across valves is moot.

The Foregger-Bloomquist and Ohio infant absorbers, Columbia circle absorber, and Revell Cirqulator were developed in an attempt to tailor a circle absorption system to the needs of the very small patient. The canisters and tubing are reduced in size. Better-designed directional valves and chimney Y-pieces with minimal dead space are substituted. The Ohio and the Foregger-Bloomquist absorbers became quite popular, especially among anesthesiologists who wanted to use closed or semiclosed techniques. The presence of directional valves, however, always raised the specter of possible incompetence or increased airway resistance. The Columbia circle absorber is an adult absorber modifiable for pediatric use by interchangeable smaller canister tubing and fittings and, most important, it has an especially designed low-resistance and low dead space (concentric) valve mount (Fig. 48-4). Smaller tubing and fittings are most important. The Revell Cirqulator reduced dead space and valve resistance of the standard absorber (Fig. 48-5) by constant circulation and mixing of gases within the circuit, independent of ventilatory flow. A septate Y piece used in conjunction with the circulator directed the moving gases into the mask to provide better mixing and thus reduce dead space. The constant flow of gases within the circuit tended to keep the directional valves unseated and thus reduce air flow resistance by reducing or eliminating opening pressures. More practically, the nuisance of setting up a separate absorber and finding a suitable location for these extra pieces of equipment on or around the anesthesia machine discouraged many anesthesiologists from using these systems. Thus, most such systems are of historical interest only.

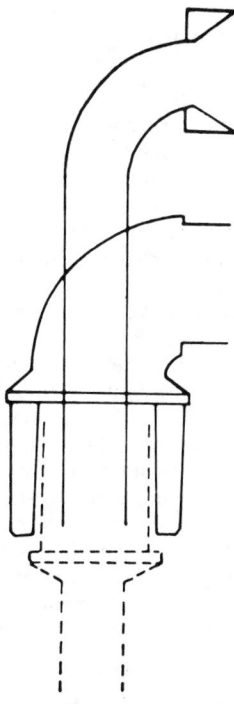

Figure 48-4. Divided airway adapter. The Columbia Pediatric Circle Valve is shown. Dead space is 0.5 ml, significantly less than the 40-ml dead space of a conventional airway adapter. (Reprinted with permission from Rackow H, Salanitre E: A new pediatric circle valve. Anesthesiology 29:833, 1968.)

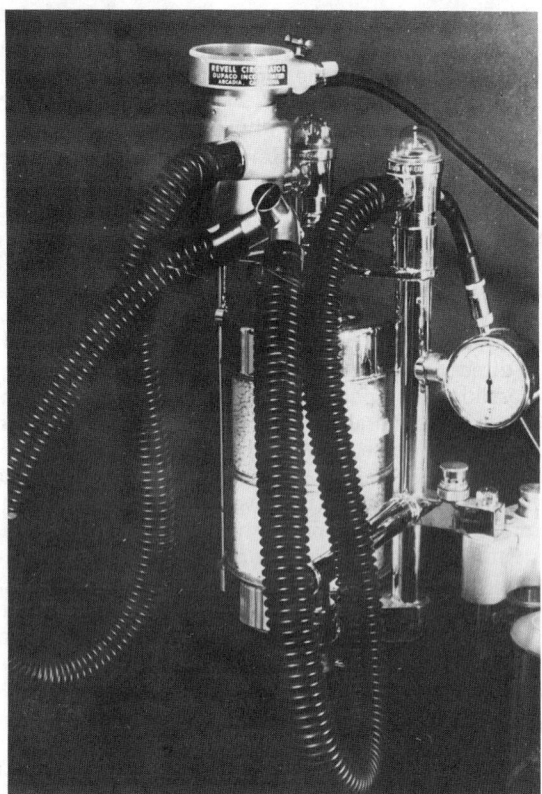

Figure 48-5. The Revell Cirqulator and septate Y piece are used in conjunction to reduce dead space of the face mask. Circuit diagram: The patient and the rebreathing bag are not included in the circulation. The bag moves normally, reflecting the tidal exchange between the patient and the bag.

REGIONAL ANESTHESIA

Regional anesthetic techniques (e.g., axillary block, combined ilioinguinal and iliohypogastric block, penile block, epidural block, and subarachnoid block) are becoming more popular for infants and children to supplement general anesthesia, as the sole anesthetic, or for postoperative analgesia.[115-131] In general, the anatomy and principles of regional anesthesia are the same in infants and children as in adults. Regional anesthesia can provide good relaxation, a reduction in the amount of potent anesthetic needed, safe, rapid recovery, early pain relief, and minimal complications. The use of regional anesthesia is limited, however, because of the lack of cooperation, the child's fear of needles, and the conscious child's apprehension in the atmosphere of the operating room. Heavy sedation or even light general anesthesia may be needed prior to adolescence to maintain the necessary quiescence while the block is being performed. In young infants, little or no sedation may be needed; in school-aged children, light sedation is required. Despite the potential problems, the anesthesiologist who is skilled in nerve blocks will find many occasions in which this type of anesthesia is useful.

Brachial Plexus Block and Intravenous Regional Block

The axillary approach to the brachial plexus block is the most popular one in children. However, the selection of the site of the block should depend on the location of the

TABLE 48-4. Simplified Dosage for Brachial Plexus Blocks

Age (yr)	Formula for Determining Volume (ml)	Concentration (%)	
		Lidocaine Mepivacaine	Bupivacaine
0–4	$\dfrac{\text{Height (cm)}}{12}$	1	0.25
5–8	$\dfrac{\text{Height (cm)}}{10}$	1	0.25
9–16	$\dfrac{\text{Height (cm)}}{7}$	1	0.25

Adapted with permission from Lanz E: Blockaden des Plexus brachialis im Kindesalter. In Kuhn K, Hausdorfer J (eds): Regional Anaesthesie im Kindesalter, p 24. Berlin, Springer Verlag, 1984.

operation. For operations on the forearm and outer upper arm, including reduction of dislocated shoulders, a supraclavicular technique, usually interscalene, is indicated. The axillary approach is indicated for operations on the forearm and hand. Continuous brachial plexus analgesia has been recommended to follow revascularization procedures of the hands or digits.[132-133] A simplified dose schedule to calculate the dose of local anesthetics is useful (Table 48-4). Intravenous regional techniques also may be used.[134-135]

Ilioinguinal and Iliohypogastric Nerve Block

The ilioinguinal and iliohypogastric nerves eventually pierce the internal oblique muscle just below and 1–2 cm medial to the anterior superior spine and come to lie between the internal oblique and the aponeurosis of the external oblique muscle. They supply the skin of the lower abdomen and the inguinal region. Thus, the combined block is useful to provide intraoperative or postoperative analgesia for inguinal surgery. If the block is to be used for surgery as well as postoperative analgesia, it is also necessary to infiltrate the hernial sac. Bupivacaine (0.5%) is used for this purpose at a dose of 0.5 ml per year of age.

Penile Block

The penile block is a useful alternative to caudal anesthesia for providing intraoperative and postoperative analgesia for circumcision.[136] This block can be applied with the patient lying in the supine position. The dorsal nerves of the penis enter from under the symphysis pubis and run below the deep (Buck's) fascia and superficial to the corpora cavernosa. The nerves are blocked just at their point of entry before they divide to also supply the anterior parts. Bupivacaine (0.5%) is used at a maximum dose of 1.0 ml·kg^{-1}. Epinephrine-containing solutions must never be used because of the risk of ischemia of the penis. The only complications of penile block are intravascular injection or extensive hematoma.

Spinal Anesthesia

The patient's size and age do not contraindicate the use of spinal anesthesia. In older, cooperative children and adolescents, the indications for its use are identical to those of adults. Its use for infants and young children was initially limited to those who had liver, kidney, or pulmonary disease and were having surgical procedures below the diaphragm; its use is now advocated for healthy infants.[137-141] The spinal cord may end as low as L3 in the infant. Thus, spinal punctures should be performed at the L4–5 or L5–S1 level. With spinal anesthesia the circulation of infants or children tends to be more stable than that of adults. Therefore, use of vasopressor drugs is seldom necessary to maintain the blood pressure.

Although any of the accepted spinal anesthetic drugs may be used, tetracaine has been the most popular. The duration of action of any given spinal anesthetic agent is somewhat less in the infant than in the adult, and for this reason epinephrine is nearly always added to the injected mixture of drugs. The dose of tetracaine may be estimated at roughly 0.4 mg·kg^{-1} or at 1 mg per year of age. A minimum dose of 1.5 mg to 2.0 mg is usually required for even the smallest infant.

Caudal-Epidural Anesthesia

Caudal anesthesia for perineal or lower abdominal procedures has been effective and relatively easy to administer in infants and small children.[141-158] Caudal blocks placed after the induction of general anesthesia reduce the amount of potent anesthetic agent required and, more important, reduce postoperative agitation and opioid requirements. Administration of 1.0 ml·kg^{-1} of bupivacaine (0.25%) with epinephrine (1:200,000) provides adequate postoperative analgesia; a maximum dose of 3.0 mg·kg^{-1} is used. Takasaki et al have described formulas for calculating the dose of lidocaine and other local anesthetics for caudal analgesia in infants and children.[147] Because infants and children have limited epidural fat, caudal catheters may be positioned easily at the lumbar or thoracic level. Alternatively, lumbar or thoracic epidural catheters can be inserted for intraoperative and postoperative pain control.

MONITORING

Although most pediatric surgical patients can be monitored adequately by the intelligent use of a few simple devices, the advent of more sophisticated equipment allows moment-to-moment monitoring of oxygenation, blood pressure, electrocardiogram, central venous pressure, intracranial pressure, and end-tidal gases.[159]

The infant or child should be monitored continuously with a precordial or esophageal stethoscope. The anesthesiologist can thus detect changes in the rate, quality, and intensity of the heart sounds, which may be helpful in evaluating blood loss, depth of anesthesia, or failing circulation or in diagnosing air emboli. Continuous noninvasive monitoring of arterial oxygen saturation can be accomplished by pulse oximetry.[160-161] The amplitude of the constantly varying detected signal depends on the magnitude of the pulse, wavelength, and oxygen saturation of the arterial hemoglobin. Artifact from blood, skin, connective tissue, or bone is completely eliminated. The technique has been shown to be accurate with oxygen saturations from 70 to 100%. Reduction in vascular pulsation diminishes the instrument's ability to calculate saturations in such conditions as hypothermia or hypotension or with use of vasoconstrictive drugs. In addition to continuous indication of arterial oxygen saturation, the pulse oximeter provides a continuous readout of pulse rate and amplitude. There are several obvious advantages of pulse oximetry over transcutaneous oxygen measurement in the patient having anesthesia: no special site preparation is necessary and application is extremely simple. The risk of burns is eliminated because it is not necessary to heat the sensor. Plethysmographic monitors attached to the finger or toe are helpful but are subject to artifacts and are frequently unreliable in the very young. Doppler monitors are also reliable audible pulse indicators. Electrocardiographic monitoring is useful in determining pulse rate and the presence of cardiac arrhythmias. The value of the electrocardiographic tracing in evaluating cardiac function is limited, however, because it indicates only electrical activity and gives no indication of cardiac output.

Blood Pressure

Systolic blood pressure may be determined in virtually all patients by the oscillometric method with use of a suitable cuff and an aneroid manometer. However, several relatively simple electronic devices have greatly facilitated the indirect determination of blood pressure in small patients. The first of these entails the use of Doppler ultrasonography to detect the equivalent arterial wall motion or red blood cell movement of the Korotkoff sounds. Electronic oscillometers (e.g., Dinamap) detect transmitted pulsatile oscillation of the pressure cuff itself.[162-163] Because oscillations of the cuff itself are being detected, careful positioning of the cuff is not necessary, but a loose fit or residual air severely attenuates the signal. Motion, dysrhythmias, and heart rates greater than 200 beats per minute also render the device useless. Long deflation and cycle times are necessary with this technique, and because inflation occurs automatically by means of an electric pump, unrecognized runaway or prolonged inflation may cause ischemic nerve damage.[164-165]

Cannulation of the radial artery or dorsalis pedis artery allows continuous measurement of blood pressure and permits frequent serial determinations of blood gases and pH, hematocrit, electrolytes, and osmolality. With a translumination technique, either 22- or 24-gauge plastic cannulas can be placed percutaneously in infants; rarely, a cutdown may be necessary.

Central Venous Pressure

Central venous pressure catheters can be used to estimate mean intrathoracic pressure during mechanical ventilation, estimate adequacy of blood replacement or venous return, and extract air embolism from the right side of the heart. Catheters can be inserted from the antecubital fossa or external or internal jugular vein. Because the position of the catheter is critical if it is to be used to extract air (venous air embolus), a chest roentgenogram must be taken to confirm its position. Monitoring changes in the P waves of the electrocardiogram can assist in correct placement of a right atrial catheter.

Ventilation

The anesthesiologist has few direct aids to measure tidal volume in infants and must depend to a large extent on clinical observation. Standard ventilation meters such as the Wright respirometer are useful for older children, but they either do not respond or are grossly inaccurate in the ranges required for infants. When available, arterial pH,

Pa_{CO_2}, and Pa_{O_2} determinations are the most reliable indices of adequate ventilation.

Capnography and Mass Spectrometry

End-tidal carbon dioxide monitors (capnographs) or mass spectrometers can be used to assess the adequacy of ventilation.[166] Most modern capnographs display the carbon dioxide waveform as well as the numeric readings. The adaptation of the mass spectrometer as a clinical respiratory monitor can now provide continuous on-line analysis of oxygen, carbon dioxide, nitrogen, nitrous oxide, and the major volatile anesthetic drugs in the anesthetized patient. The mass spectrometer can be used as a sensitive detector of air emboli.

A capnographic tracing is usually displayed as well as an alpha-numeric reading of inspired and end-tidal values of each gas expressed in volumes percent or torr, the respiratory rate, and I:E ratio. Trending can be displayed as well. A computer interprets as inspired and end-tidal values those occurring at the instants of minimal and maximal carbon dioxide concentrations, respectively. Thus, the accuracy of the displayed inspired and end-tidal values depends crucially upon the faithfulness of the capnographic tracing. Mapleson D circuits, particularly coaxial circuits, provide continuous fresh gas flow near the airway. Mixing of this fresh gas with expired gases may dilute the end-tidal concentrations, degrade the capnograph tracing, and yield inaccurately low results.[167-169] These problems can be minimized by using an elbow connector and sampling near the endotracheal tube. In essence, the elbow connector separates the jet stream of the breathing circuit from the expired gases.

Temperature

Because of their high surface area to body mass ratio, small children are particularly susceptible to rapid heat loss. The thermistor thermometer and heat-sensitive strips have greatly facilitated continuous temperature determination during anesthesia. Temperature monitoring should be routine in virtually all surgical patients. Its importance is unquestioned in the management of all infants and in major cases with patients of any age.

PEDIATRIC FLUID THERAPY

Maintenance Fluids

Various calculations involving body weight, surface area, or caloric expenditure have been used to determine fluid therapy for infants and children.[170-172] Body weight, caloric expenditure, and estimates of insensible water loss, renal water requirements, stool water loss, and water needed for growth determine the volume of fluid needed for maintenance. Caloric expenditure is size-related: infants 1–10 kg require 100 calories·kg^{-1}; small children (10–20 kg) require 1000 calories·day^{-1} plus 50 calories·kg^{-1}·day^{-1} over 10 kg; older children (weighing more than 20 kg) require 1500 calories·day^{-1} plus 25 calories for each kg·day^{-1} over 20 kg. For every 100 calories consumed, 67 ml of water are needed for solute excretion; an additional 50 ml·100 $calories^{-1}$ are associated with insensible loss but 17 ml·100 $calories^{-1}$ are produced by oxidation. Thus, the infant needs 100 ml of water for 100 calories. This simple relationship can be used to calculate the maintenance fluid needed by healthy full-term infants and children; its simplicity may explain the popularity of the method.

If it is assumed that each day is 25 hours, the hourly fluid needs of the infant can be estimated at 4 ml·kg^{-1}·h^{-1}. For every 100 ml of water, the infant needs 3 mEq Na^+, 2 mEq K^+, 2 mEq Cl^-, and 5 g glucose. It is more convenient to equalize the sodium and chloride requirements at 3 mEq. For routine use, 5% dextrose in 0.25 normal saline adequately provides this.

Intraoperative Fluids and Blood Loss Replacement

Intraoperative fluid therapy may involve the initiation of fluid management or alternatively may be a continuation of ongoing fluid therapy. It can be as simple as replacing the deficits from the preoperative fast and providing maintenance fluids or as complex as correcting preoperative abnormal deficits, intraoperative translocated fluids, and variable blood loss in addition to providing maintenance fluids. It is best to consider each of these factors separately before discussing general guidelines.

Fasting Deficit

Because infants have a high metabolic rate and water turnover, significant hypoglycemia and dehydration may occur in those who are allowed to fast for prolonged periods of time. The fasting period before induction of anesthesia should be adjusted by timing feeding and surgery to minimize both the risk of dehydration and the risk of aspiration. However, delays in the surgical schedule may place the infant at risk for hypoglycemia and dehydration. In these instances, intravenous administration of fluids is prudent. The fluid deficit incurred during fasting should be replaced during anesthesia. Assuming that a healthy infant is in water and electrolyte balance at the time oral feedings stop, the fluid deficit at the start of anesthesia can be estimated by multiplying the infant's hourly maintenance fluid requirement (MFR) by the number of hours since the last feeding. This deficit may be replaced by giving half of the calculated volume during the first hour of anesthesia and the other half over the next 2 hours, in addition to intraoperative maintenance fluids.[173]

Thus, in the first 3 hours, in an infant having a superficial surgical procedure with minimal or no third-space losses, fluid would be given as follows:

Estimated fluid deficit (EFD)	= hours NPO × MFR (ml·kg^{-1}·h^{-1})
First hour fluids	= MFR + ½ EFD
Second hour fluids	= MFR + ¼ EFD
Third hour fluids	= MFR + ¼ EFD

Five percent dextrose in quarter-normal saline (5% dextrose/0.25 normal saline or 2.5% glucose/0.5 normal saline) is frequently used for maintenance fluid. Currently, there is a trend to using 2.5% glucose in 0.5 normal saline or lactated Ringer's solution as the maintenance fluid.[174-178] Minimal deficits can be replaced more rapidly during short surgical procedures. These approaches minimize the hazards of hyperglycemia and maintain the blood glucose level between 100 and 150 mg·dl^{-1}. The stress of surgery and anesthesia usually increases the blood glucose.

Third-Space Intraoperative Losses

Surgical trauma, blunt trauma, burns, infections, and a host of surgical conditions are associated with isotonic transfer of fluids from the extracellular fluid compartment and to a lesser extent from the intracellular compartment to a nonfunctional interstitial compartment.[179] This acute sequestration of edema fluid to a nonfunctional compartment has been called third-space loss. Plasma volume may be decreased. The magnitude of third-space loss varies with the surgical procedure and is usually highest in infants having intra-abdominal, intestinal surgery. In addition, failure to cover the exposed intestine and the use of heat lamps may increase evaporative loss. In infants, estimated third-space loss during intra-abdominal surgery varies from 6 to 10 $ml \cdot kg^{-1} \cdot h^{-1}$; in intrathoracic surgery it is less (4–7 $ml \cdot kg^{-1} \cdot h^{-1}$); in superficial surgery or neurosurgery it is trivial (1–2 $ml \cdot kg^{-1} \cdot h^{-1}$). Translocated fluids are a finite functional loss and contribute to the magnitude of dehydration. Thus, clinical signs of the extent of dehydration may be used to estimate needed fluid replacement. Generally, lactated Ringer's solution is used to restore third-space losses. In cases of massive volume replacement, some advocate using 5% albumin to restore one third to one fourth of the loss. The end point of third space replacement therapy is sustained adequate blood pressure (appropriate for the patient's age and weight), tissue perfusion, and urine volume.

Isotonic fluid also may be translocated in hypovolemic shock. When blood is lost, some interstitial fluid moves into the central circulation to restore plasma volume, but some moves intracellularly, perhaps because of altered membrane permeability. In severe shock, intracellular fluid volume expands to as much as 6% of body weight. Maintenance of adequate circulating volume and avoidance of hypoperfusion during periods of massive volume replacement may prevent these intracellular shifts.

Conceptually, two types of fluids may be indicated for long procedures with moderate to extensive third-space loss: 2.5% dextrose/0.5 normal saline, or 5% dextrose/0.25 normal saline, should be used for normal maintenance, and balanced salt solution should be used to compensate for third-space losses. For short surgical procedures with minimal to moderate third-space losses, one type of fluid usually suffices (e.g., 5% dextrose/lactated Ringer's solution or 5% dextrose/0.9 normal saline). These relatively hypertonic fluids are used for a dual purpose, but large volumes can lead to profound hyperglycemia and hyperosmolality; an osmotic diuretic effect is common. This diuresis may cause cellular dehydration in the brain. Balanced salt solution used as a substitute for blood or packed red blood cells should not contain glucose.

Blood Replacement

All blood loss in infants and children should be replaced in some way. Accurately measuring blood loss and assessing the acceptable blood loss in the infant are vital to any replacement regimen. Weighing sponges, using calibrated miniaturized suction bottles, and visually estimating (combined with a guess factor) will define the magnitude of the blood loss. The concept of allowable blood loss that considers the starting blood volume and hemoglobin or hematocrit of the patient is a good guide to blood replacement.[173,180] Normovolemic hemodilution to a predetermined hematocrit can be achieved with crystalloid or, more rarely, with colloid solutions.

Estimating Allowable Blood Loss

Several methods have been proposed for estimating allowable blood loss (ABL) from the blood volume, weight, and hematocrit. The formulas range from the simple to the complex, but all involve an estimate of blood volume. Allowable blood loss (ABL) equation calculated from the following can be:

$$ABL = Wt \times EBV \times \frac{[HO\text{-}HL]}{\overline{H}}$$

where Wt is weight (kg), EBV is the estimated blood volume, HO is the original hematocrit, HL is the lowest acceptable hematocrit, and $\overline{H}$ is the average hematocrit (HO + HL)/2; all hematocrits are decimal values (i.e., 0.6, 0.5). This equation assumes that blood loss and replacement were gradual and exponential. This equation has general applicability for all age groups, but the lowest acceptable hematocrit should be age-adjusted.

This method can be illustrated by estimating the ABL for a 6-kg infant with a 100 $ml \cdot kg^{-1}$ blood volume and an original hematocrit of 50%; HL was 40%.

$$ABL = 6 \text{ kg} \times \frac{100 \text{ ml}}{\text{kg}} \times \frac{(0.5 - 0.4)}{(0.5 + 0.4)/2} = 133 \text{ ml}$$

There is controversy over how the blood volume should be supported while the hematocrit is being allowed to decrease. Data are nonexistent, and several approaches are possible. If ongoing blood loss is replaced milliliter for milliliter with 5% colloid (i.e., albumin, fresh frozen plasma), with the use of the equation given above the hematocrit will be within 1–3 volume $\% \cdot dl^{-1}$ of the desired level; others replace blood loss with three to four times the volume of lactated Ringer's solution. Although this volume of clear crystalloid fluid may be needed in patients in shock, it seems excessive in patients with well-perfused tissues. Hypoproteinemia may result. We replace gradual blood loss with volumes of crystalloid 1.5 times the measured or calculated loss.

In major surgery involving one to two body cavities, intravascular albumin may be transiently depleted or translocated. If 25% salt-poor albumin is used to replace these losses, its hypertonicity will mobilize fluids from the extracellular compartment; if the patient's third space is depleted, fluid will be mobilized from the intracellular compartment, leading to intracellular dehydration. Therefore, serum albumin should be replaced with 5% albumin.

Blood component therapy depends on the clinical setting and the availability of various blood products. Fresh whole blood (less than 4 hours old) has a limited availability. The septic infant benefits from its clotting factors, platelets, and white blood cells. If predicted blood loss is greater than or equal to 40% of blood volume, fresh whole blood is helpful in supplying platelets and clotting factors. However, component therapy is usually the rule.[181] Packed red blood cells have a hematocrit between 55% and 65%. On the average, 1 $ml \cdot kg^{-1}$ of packed cells will increase the hematocrit by 1.5%. Units of packed cells can be subdivided into pediatric packs of 80–100 ml. The fluid of these cells is relatively hyperkalemic (K = 15–20 $mEq \cdot l^{-1}$), acidotic (pH < 7.0), and low in ionized calcium. With rapid administration of packed red blood cells, each of these factors is significant.

When blood loss approaches one blood volume, labile clotting factors are greatly reduced; normal clotting requires 5–20% of Factor V and 30% of Factor VIII. All the coagulation factors except platelets are present in normal quantities in fresh frozen plasma. We prefer to provide near equal volumes of fresh frozen plasma and packed cells to patients (hematocrit = 35–40%) with massive blood loss (i.e., greater than or equal to one blood volume). The ratio of cells and plasma can be varied to produce any desired hematocrit. The intraoperative need for platelets may be predicted from the preoperative platelet count. Platelets can be mobilized from the spleen and bone marrow as bleeding occurs. An infant with a high preoperative count (greater than 250,000 per mm³) may not need a platelet transfusion until two to three blood volumes are lost, whereas an infant who has a low count (less than 150,000 per mm³) may need platelets after only one blood volume is lost. One platelet pack per 10 kg is usually adequate. Rapid administration of cold, citrated blood products can be hazardous; obviously, all such products should be warmed before infusion. Fresh frozen plasma contains the greatest amount of citrate per unit volume of any blood product; rapid infusion of fresh frozen plasma should cause the greatest change in ionized calcium. Under most circumstances, the mobilization of calcium and hepatic metabolism of citrate are sufficiently rapid to prevent precipitous decreases in ionized calcium. However, because infants' stores of calcium are small and a larger fraction of their blood volume can be replaced more rapidly, they are at special risk for hypocalcemia. For example, transient decreases in ionized calcium are seen in infants with jaundice during exchange transfusion. Coté et al demonstrated that fresh frozen plasma infusion at rates of 1–2.5 $ml \cdot kg^{-1} \cdot min^{-1}$ was associated with transient decreases in ionized calcium and occasional significant decreases in arterial blood pressure.[182] Equipotent doses of calcium chloride (2.5 $mg \cdot kg^{-1}$) or calcium gluconate (7.5 $mg \cdot kg^{-1}$) effectively increased calcium and ameliorated the hemodynamic changes. Empirical buffering of blood may lead to profound metabolic alkalosis as citrate loads are metabolized.

OUTPATIENT AND SAME-DAY SURGERY

Many pediatric surgical procedures are brief, and the patients require little preoperative preparation. The rapidity with which healthy young patients recover from the effects of anesthesia and surgery has been mentioned already. For these reasons, many procedures are handled easily and safely on an outpatient basis. There are many advantages to this approach. Children need not spend one or more nights away from their homes and families, and their exposure to hospital nosocomial-acquired infections is reduced. The convenience to parents of small children is considerable and much appreciated, especially if there are other children in the family. In many cases, the hospital costs for outpatient surgery are less than for inpatients. The surgeon and the patient benefit from quicker and easier scheduling. Finally, outpatient surgery keeps hospital beds available for more seriously ill patients.

Selection of Patients

The types of operation to be managed on an outpatient basis must be chosen and agreed upon by the surgeon, anesthesiologist, and hospital administration. There are no universal criteria, although in general only procedures that can reasonably be completed within an hour are permitted. Patients with major medical problems such as juvenile diabetes or cystic fibrosis are best excluded, as are those who

will require blood transfusion or other special preoperative preparation. Limitations of health insurance are another possible inducement to outpatient status.

Preoperative Preparation

The preoperative history, physical examination, and laboratory work should be completed before the day of surgery. Special forms may be developed to facilitate this aspect of preparation. A hematocrit or hemoglobin determination is the only routine laboratory study required, and depending on the type of surgery, this may not be necessary.[183] At the last clinic or office visit, the parents should be given information (preferably printed) on time, place, and administrative details, and, most important, instructions for withholding food and fluids.

On the patient's admission to the outpatient unit, a nurse or clerk determines that all necessary paperwork is completed, including the history, physical examination, laboratory work, and operative permit. Parents are questioned about the possibility of fever or upper respiratory infection within the past few days and about when the patient last ingested food or drink.

Of course, preoperative psychological preparation is just as desirable for outpatients as for inpatients, but sedatives and opioids should be used with caution. Their effect continues long after completion of the surgery, thus prolonging recovery time and delaying discharge. Allowing parents to remain with children until they go to the operating room allays the children's apprehension to some extent, especially because they know they may return immediately to their parents after operation and will not have to remain in the hospital.

Anesthesia

The type of anesthesia used for outpatients does not differ significantly from that already described for inpatients. Nitrous oxide–halothane is most common, and ketamine may be used if repeated doses are not required. We use endotracheal intubation if it is indicated. In the event that tracheal intubation is required, discharge is delayed for 4 hours to ensure that there are no complications. If there is any question about the airway, the patient is admitted overnight.

Recovery and Discharge

Outpatients receive the same immediate postoperative care as do other patients in the postanesthesia care unit. After recovery from anesthesia, they are returned to the outpatient unit, where they rejoin their parents. They are discharged when they are fully awake, have retained fluids, have no respiratory problems, and can walk.[184-185]

To be successful, an outpatient surgery program must be primarily designed to ensure patient safety. The quality of medical care must not be sacrificed for expediency. Preoperative preparation, anesthesia, the surgical procedure, and postoperative care must meet the same standards as for hospitalized patients. Time is the only factor that is altered. The other requirements are good organization and communication between all concerned parties—the parents, surgeon, surgeon's office, hospital business office, outpatient unit, operating room, and, of course, the anesthesiologist.

POSTANESTHETIC CARE

Infants and children generally recover more quickly from the stress of anesthesia and surgery, have less postoperative pain, and are less disturbed by minor complications than adults. Nevertheless, the immediate postoperative period may be as hazardous as the operation and anesthetic. The end of the operation should not signal the end of the intensive minute-to-minute observation and care that the patient received while under anesthesia. More and more attention is being directed to continuing intensive care in the postoperative period and to a large extent, such care is the anesthesiologist's responsibility.

Conclusion of Surgery

In addition to regaining of consciousness recovery from anesthesia involves many factors, including the restoration of normal body temperature, return of protective reflexes and neuromuscular function if muscle relaxants have been used, ability to maintain a patent airway without dependence on a mechanical device, and re-establishment of adequate spontaneous ventilation. Stringent criteria should be used in evaluating infants' recovery. The incompletely reacted infant may appear to breathe adequately when stimulated but may fall asleep again and have very shallow respirations or apnea. Infants should be kept in the operating room until they are fully conscious and active, as indicated by a lusty cry.

Immediate Postanesthetic Care

The airway should be maintained and the anesthesiologist should monitor pulse oxygenation and respiration during transportation from the operating room and provide supplemental oxygen as needed.[186] In some patients this may entail the continued use of a precordial or esophageal stethoscope and positive-pressure ventilation with oxygen and self-inflating bag.

On the patient's arrival in the postanesthesia care unit or intensive care unit, attention should first be directed to the assurance of adequate ventilation, either spontaneous or by artificial means if necessary. The vital signs should be ascertained by recovery room personnel and reported to the anesthesiologist as soon as possible. The anesthesiologist, in turn, should report any special problems. Only after these precautions are observed should attention be directed to other aspects of the patient's care.

It appears that in most instances pain can simply be controlled with nonopioid analgesics. However, if they are necessary, judicious use of more potent opioid analgesics should not be withheld.

Emergence delirium is occasionally seen in children, particularly in those in whom scopolamine has been used for premedication. A dose of 0.01–0.02 mg·kg^{-1} of physostigmine salicylate (Antilirium) has been dramatically effective in treating this condition.[187]

Management of Subglottic Edema

Croup or subglottic edema after extubation of the trachea usually is manifested within 2–4 hours; in severe cases, the signs occur earlier. In most cases only a brassy cough and stertorous respirations are observed. With more severe edema there may be labored respirations, suprasternal retractions, tachypnea, restlessness, and sweating.

Mild cases require little or no therapy other than high concentrations of humidified oxygen. The most effective treatment of subglottic edema is that described by Jordan et al.[188] Racemic epinephrine (0.5 ml of a 2% solution diluted to a volume of 3.5 ml) is usually administered by a nebulizer rather than with an intermittent positive-pressure breathing apparatus. As yet, there is no clear-cut evidence that steroids are effective in the management of postintubation croup, but they seem to be so in some cases. There appears to be no harm in a single high dose; therefore we have not hesitated to use dexamethasone intravenously in single doses of 4 mg for infants younger than 1 year of age and 8 mg for older children.

When it results from trauma, untreated subglottic edema reaches its peak in 6–8 hours. If the process does not respond to treatment, the patient must be watched very closely. Preparations necessary for tracheostomy should be made, and tracheostomy should not be delayed if airway obstruction is severe or progressing rapidly. If the edema is infectious in origin, the recovery process is much slower and respiratory difficulty may continue for 48 hours or more.

REFERENCES

1. Cook DR, Marcy JH (eds): Neonatal Anesthesia. Pasadena, California, Appleton Davies Inc, 1988
2. Motoyama EK, Davis PJ (eds): Smith's Anesthesia for Infants and Children. St Louis, CV Mosby, 1990
3. Gregory GA: Pediatric Anesthesia, 2nd ed. New York, Churchill Livingstone, 1989
4. Katz J, Steward D: Anesthesia and Uncommon Pediatric Diseases. Philadelphia, WB Saunders Co, 1987
5. Ryan JF, Coté CJ, Todres ID, Goudsouzian N: A Practice of Anesthesia for Infants and Children. Orlando, Grune & Stratton, 1986
6. Lake CL: Pediatric Cardiac Anesthesia. San Mateo, California, Appleton and Lange, 1988
7. Berry FA: Anesthetic Management of Difficult and Routine Pediatric Patients. New York, Churchill Livingstone, 1986
8. McLaurin RL, Schut L, Venes JL, Epstein F: Pediatric Neurosurgery, 2nd ed. Philadelphia, WB Saunders Co, 1989
9. Visintainer MA, Wolfer JA: Psychological preparation for surgical pediatric patients: The effect on children's and parents' stress responses and adjustment. Pediatrics 56:187, 1975
10. Wolfer JA, Visintainer MA: Prehospital psychological preparation for tonsillectomy patients: Effects on children's and parents' adjustment. Pediatrics 64:646, 1979
11. Berry FA: Preoperative assessment and general management of outpatients. Int Anesthesiol Clin 20:3, 1982
12. Hannallah RS, Rosales JK: Experience with parents' presence during anesthesia induction in children. Can Anaesth Soc J 30:286, 1983
13. Bevan JC, Johnston C, Haig MJ, Tausignant G et al: Preoperative parental anxiety predicts behavioral and emotional responses to induction of anaesthesia in children. Can J Anaesth 37:177, 1990
14. Herbert W, Hammond D: Preoperative evaluation of the anemic child. Am Surg 29:660, 1963
15. Janik AR, Seeler RA: Perioperative management of children with hemoglobinopathy. J Pediatr Surg 15:117, 1980
16. Sandhar BK, Goresky GV, Maltby JR, Shaffer EA: Effect of oral liquids and ranitidine on gastric fluid volume and pH in children undergoing outpatient surgery. Anesthesiology 71:327, 1989
17. Coté CJ, Goudsouzian NG, Liu LMP, et al: Assessment of risk

factors related to the acid aspiration syndrome of pediatric patients—gastric pH and residual volume. Anesthesiology 56:70, 72, 1982

18. Sutherland AD, Maltby JR, Sale JP, et al: The effect of preoperative oral fluid and ranitidine on gastric fluid volume and pH. Can J Anaesth 34:117, 1987

19. McGrady EM, MacDonald AG: Effect of the preoperative administration of water on gastric volume and pH. Can J Anaesth 34:117, 1987

20. Splinter WM, Stewart JA, Muir JG: Large volumes of apple juice preoperatively do not affect gastric pH and volume in children. Can J Anaesth 37:36, 1990

21. Schreiner MS, Triebwasser A, Keon TP: Ingestion of liquids compared with preoperative fasting in pediatric outpatients. Anesthesiology 72:593, 1990

22. Splinter WM, Schaefer JD: Clear fluids three hours before surgery do not affect the gastric fluid contents of children. Can J Anaesth 37:498, 1990

23. Coté CJ: NPO after midnight—a reappraisal (Editorial). Anesthesiology 72:589, 1990

24. Miller BR et al: Gastric residual volume in infants and children following a 3-hour fast. J Clin Anesth 2:301, 1990

25. Splinter WM, Schaefer JD: Ingestion of clear fluids is safe for adolescents up to 3 h before anesthesia. Br J Anaesth 66:48, 1991

26. Henderson JM, Brodsky DA, Fisher DM et al: Pre-induction of anesthesia in pediatric patients with nasally administered sufentanil. Anesthesiology 68:671, 1988

27. Nicolson SC, Betts EK, Jobes DR et al: Comparison of oral and intramuscular preanesthetic medication for pediatric inpatient surgery. Anesthesiology 71:8, 1989

28. Rita L, Seleny FL, Mazurek A et al: Intramuscular midazolam for pediatric preanesthetic sedation: A double-blind controlled study with morphine. Anesthesiology 63:528, 1985

29. Saint-Maurice C, Meistelman C, Rey E et al: The pharmacokinetics of rectal midazolam for premedication in children. Anesthesiology 65:536, 1986

30. Shafer A, White P, Urquhart ML et al: Outpatient premedication: Use of midazolam and opioid analgesics. Anesthesiology 71:495, 1989

31. Wilton NCT, Leigh J, Rosen DR et al: Preanesthetic sedation of preschool children using intranasal midazolam. Anesthesiology 69:972, 1988

32. Goldstein-Dresner MC, Davis PJ, Kretchman E et al: Double-blind comparison of oral transmucosal fentanyl citrate with oral meperidine, diazepam, and atropine as preanesthetic medication in children with congenital heart disease. Anesthesiology 74:28, 1991

33. Coté CJ, Goudsouzian NG, Liu LMP et al: Assessment of risk factors related to the acid aspiration syndrome in pediatric patients—gastric pH and residual volume. Anesthesiology 56:70, 1982

34. Goudsouzian N, Coté CJ, Liu LMP et al: The dose-response effects of oral cimetidine on gastric pH and volume in children. Anesthesiology 55:533, 1981

35. Manchikanti L, Marrero TC, Roush JR: Preanesthetic cimetidine and metoclopramide for acid aspiration prophylaxis in elective surgery. Anesthesiology 61:48, 1984

36. Henderson JM, Spence DG, Clarke WN et al: Sodium citrate in paediatric outpatients. Can Anaesth Soc J 34:560, 1987

37. Hinkle AJ: Scented masks in pediatric anesthesia. Anesthesiology 66:104, 1987

38. Yamashita M, Motokawa K: "Fruit-flavored" mask induction for children. Anesthesiology 64:837, 1986

39. Friesen RH, Lichtor JL: Cardiovascular depression during halothane anesthesia in infants: A study of three induction techniques. Anesth Analg 61:42, 1982

40. Steward DJ, Creighton RE: The uptake and excretion of nitrous oxide in the newborn. Can Anaesth Soc J 25:215, 1978

41. Brandom BW, Brandom RB, Cook DR: Uptake and distribution of halothane in infants: In vivo measurements and computer simulations. Anesth Analg 62:404, 1983

42. Lerman J, Gregory GA, Willis MM et al: Age and solubility of volatile anesthetics in blood. Anesthesiology 61:139, 1984

43. Cook DR, Brandom BW, Shiu G et al: The inspired median effective dose, brain concentration at anesthesia, and cardiovascular index for halothane in young rats. Anesth Analg 60:182, 1981

44. Tanner G, Angers D, Barash PG et al: Does a left-to-right shunt speed the induction of inhalational anesthesia in congenital heart disease? Anesth Analg 64:101, 1985

45. Lerman J, Robinson S, Willis MM et al: Anesthetic requirements for halothane in young children 0–1 month and 1–6 months of age. Anesthesiology 59:421, 1983

46. Gregory GA, Wade JG, Beihl DR et al: Fetal anesthetic requirement (MAC) for halothane. Anesth Analg 62:9, 1983

47. LeDez KM, Lerman J: The minimum alveolar concentration (MAC) of isoflurane in preterm neonates. Anesthesiology 67:301, 1987

48. Rao CC, Bayer M, Krishna G et al: Effects of halothane, isoflurane and enflurane on the isometric concentration of the neonatal isolated rat atria. Anesthesiology 61:A424, 1984

49. Boudreaux JP, Schieber RA, Cook DR: Hemodynamic effects of halothane in the newborn piglet. Anesth Analg 63:731, 1984

50. Bailie MD, Alward CT, Sawyer DC et al: Effect of anesthesia on cardiovascular and renal function in the newborn piglet. J Pharmacol Exp Ther 208:298, 1979

51. Wolfson B, Kielar CM, Lake C et al: Anesthetic index—a new approach. Anesthesiology 38:583, 1973

52. Wolfson B, Hetrick WD, Lake C et al: Anesthetic indices—further data. Anesthesiology 48:187, 1978

53. Kissen I, Morgan PL, Smith LR: Comparison of isoflurane and halothane safety margins in rats. Anesthesiology 58:556, 1983

54. Schieber RA, Namnoum A, Sugden A et al: Hemodynamic effects of isoflurane in the newborn piglet. Comparison with halothane. Anesth Analg 65:633, 1986

55. Murray D, Vandewalker G, Matherne GP et al: Pulsed doppler and two-dimensional echocardiography: Comparison of halothane and isoflurane on cardiac function in infants and small children. Anesthesiology 67:211, 1987

56. Gootman PM, Gootman N, Buckley BJ: Maturation of central autonomic control of the circulation. Fed Proc 42:1648, 1983

57. Gregory GA: The baroresponses of preterm infants during halothane anesthesia. Can Anaesth Soc J 29:105, 1982

58. Duncan P, Gregory GA, Wade JA: The effects of nitrous oxide on the baroreceptor response of newborn and adult rabbits. Can Anaesth Soc J 18:339, 1981

59. Wear R, Robinson S, Gregory GA: The effect of halothane on the baroresponse of adult and baby rabbits. Anesthesiology 56:188, 1982

60. Maunuksela EL, Korpela R: Double-blind evaluation of a lignocaine-prilocaine cream (EMLA) in children. Br J Anaesth 58:1242, 1986

61. Soliman IE, Broadman LM, Hannallah RS et al: Comparison of the analgesic effects of EMLA (eutectic mixture of local anesthetics) to intradermal lidocaine infiltration prior to venous cannulation in unpremedicated children. Anesthesiology 68:804, 1988

62. Hamza J, Ecoffey C, Gross JB: Ventilatory response to CO_2 following intravenous ketamine in children. Anesthesiology 70:422, 1989

63. Johnston R, Noseworthy T, Anderson B et al: Propofol versus thiopental for outpatient anesthesia. Anesthesiology 67:431, 1987

64. Hannallah RS, Patel RI: Low-dose intramuscular ketamine for anesthesia pre-induction in young children undergoing brief outpatient procedures. Anesthesiology 70:598, 1989

65. Coté CJ, Goudsouzian NG, Liu LMP et al: The dose response of intravenous thiopental for the induction of general anesthesia in unpremedicated children. Anesthesiology 55:703, 1981

66. Jonmarker C, Westrin P, Larsson S et al: Thiopental requirements for induction of anesthesia in children. Anesthesiology 67:104, 1987

67. Brett CM, Fisher DM: Thiopental dose-response relations in unpremedicated infants, children, and adults. Anesth Analg 66:1024, 1987

68. Purcell-Jones G, Yates A, Baker JR et al: Comparison of the

induction characteristics of thiopentone and propofol in children. Br J Anaesth 59:1431, 1987

69. Westrin P, Jonmarker C, Werner O: Thiopental requirements for induction of anesthesia in neonates and in infants one to six months of age. Anesthesiology 71:344, 1989

70. Salonen M, Kanto J, Lisalo E et al: Midazolam as an induction agent in children: A pharmacokinetic and clinical study. Anesth Analg 66:625, 1987

71. Liu LMP, Goudsouzian NG, Liu PL: Rectal methohexital premedication in children, a dose-comparison study. Anesthesiology 53:343, 1980

72. Sorbo S, Hudson RJ, Loomis JC: The pharmacokinetics of thiopental in pediatric surgical patients. Anesthesiology 61:666, 1984

73. Lockhart CH, Nelson WL: The relationship of ketamine requirements to age in pediatric patients. Anesthesiology 40:507, 1974

74. Eng M, Bonica JJ, Akamatsu TJ et al: Respiratory depression in newborn monkeys at cesarean section following ketamine administration. Br J Anaesth 47:917, 1975

75. Radney PA, Badola RP: Generalized extensor spasm in infants following ketamine anesthesia. Anesthesiology 39:459, 1973

76. Lockhart CH, Jenkins JJ: Ketamine-induced apnea in patients with increased intracranial pressure. Anesthesiology 37:92, 1972

77. Gasser S, Cohen M, Aygen M: The effect of ketamine on pulmonary artery pressure. Anaesthesia 29:141, 1974

78. Morray JP, Lynn AM, Stamm SJ et al: Hemodynamic effects of ketamine in children with congenital heart disease. Anesth Analg 63:895, 1984

79. Hickey PR, Hansen DD, Cranolini GM: Pulmonary and systemic hemodynamic responses to ketamine in infants with normal and elevated pulmonary vascular resistance. Anesthesiology 61:A438, 1984

80. Hickey PR, Hansen DD: Fentanyl- and sufentanil-oxygen-pancuronium anesthesia for cardiac surgery in infants. Anesth Col 63:117, 1984

81. Hickey PR, Hansen DD, Wessell D: Responses to high dose fentanyl in infants: Pulmonary and systemic hemodynamics. Anesthesiology 61:445, 1984

82. Koren G, Goresky G, Crean P et al: Pediatric fentanyl dosing based on pharmacokinetics during cardiac surgery. Anesth Analg 65:577, 1984

83. Koehntop D, Rodman J, Brundage D et al: Pharmacokinetics of fentanyl in neonates. Anesth Analg 65:227, 1986

84. Singleton MA, Rosen JI, Fisher DM: Pharmacokinetics of fentanyl for infants and adults. Anesthesiology 61:A440, 1984

85. Davis PJ, Cook DR, Stiller RL et al: Pharmacodynamics and pharmacokinetics of high-dose sufentanil in infants and children undergoing cardiac surgery. Anesth Analg 66:203, 1987

86. Greeley WJ, de Bruijn NP, Davis DP: Sufentanil pharmacokinetics in pediatric cardiovascular patients. Anesth Analg 66:1067, 1987

87. Roure P, Jean N, Leclerc AC et al: Pharmacokinetics of alfentanil in children undergoing surgery. Br J Anaesth 59:1437, 1987

88. Goresky GV, Koren G, Sabourin MA et al: The pharmacokinetics of alfentanil in children. Anesthesiology 67:654, 1987

89. Meistelman C, Saint-Maurice C, Lepaul M et al: A comparison of alfentanil pharmacokinetics in children and adults. Anesthesiology 66:13, 1987

90. Davis PJ, Chopyk JB, Kretchman E et al: Continuous alfentanil infusions in children undergoing general anesthesia for complete oral rehabilitation. J Clin Anesth 3:125, 1991

91. Mulroy JJ Jr, Davis PJ, Rymer DB et al: Safety and efficacy of alfentanil and halothane in pediatric surgical patients. Can J Anaesth 38:4:445, 1991

92. Davis PJ, Stiller RL, Cook DR et al: Effects of cholestatic hepatic disease and chronic renal failure on alfentanil pharmacokinetics in children. Anesth Analg 68:568, 1989

93. Goudsouzian NG: Maturation of neuromuscular transmission in the infant. Br J Anaesth 52:205, 1980

94. Crumrine RS, Yodlowski EH: Assessment of neuromuscular function in infants. Anesthesiology 54:29, 1981

95. Goudsouzian NG, Liu LMP, Coté CJ: Comparison of equipotent doses of nondepolarizing muscle relaxants in children. Anesth Analg 60:862, 1981

96. Goudsouzian NG, Martyn JJA, Liu LMP: The dose response effect of long-acting non-depolarizing neuromuscular blocking agents in children. Can Anaesth Soc J 3:246, 1984

97. Cook DR: Clinical use of muscle relaxants in infants and children. Anesth Analg 60:335, 1981

98. Fisher DM, O'Keefe C, Stanski DR et al: Pharmacokinetics and pharmacodynamics of d-tubocurarine in infants, children, and adults. Anesthesiology 57:2030, 1982

99. Brandom BW, Rudd GD, Cook DR: Clinical pharmacology of atracurium in pediatric patients. Br J Anaesth 55:117S, 1983

100. Brandom BW, Woelfel SK, Cook DR et al: Clinical pharmacology of atracurium in infants. Anesth Analg 63:309, 1984

101. Brandom BW, Cook DR, Stiller RL et al: Pharmacokinetics of atracurium in infants and children. Clin Pharmacol Ther 62:404, 1983

102. Goudsouzian NG, Liu L, Coté CJ et al: Safety and efficacy of atracurium in adolescents and children anesthetized with halothane. Anesthesiology 60:97, 1984

103. Goudsouzian NG, Liu LMP, Gionfriddo M et al: Neuromuscular effects of atracurium in infants and children. Anesthesiology 62:75, 1985

104. D'Hollander AA, Luyckx C, Barvais L et al: Clinical evaluation of atracurium besylate requirement for a stable muscle relaxation during surgery: Lack of age-related effects. Anesthesiology 59:2327, 1983

105. Fisher DM, Miller RD: Neuromuscular effects of vecuronium (ORG NC45) in infants and children during N₂O, halothane anesthesia. Anesthesiology 58:519, 1983

106. Rupp SM, Miller RD, Gencarelli PJ: Vecuronium-induced neuromuscular blockade during enflurane, halothane, and isoflurane in humans. Anesthesiology 60:102, 1984

107. Fisher DM, Castagnoli K, Miller RD: Vecuronium kinetics and dynamics in anesthetized infants and children. Clin Pharmacol Ther 37:402, 1985

108. Goudsouzian NG, Alifimoff JK, Eberly C et al: Neuromuscular and cardiovascular effects of mivacurium in children. Anesthesiology 70:237, 1989

109. Goudsouzian NG: Atracurium infusion in infants. Anesthesiology 68:267, 1988

110. Laycock JRD, Baster MK, Bevan JC et al: The potency of pancuronium at the adductor pollicis and diaphragm in infants and children. Anesthesiology 68:908, 1988

111. Pittet JF, Tassonyi E, Morel DR et al: Pipecuronium-induced neuromuscular blockade during nitrous oxide-fentanyl, isoflurane, and halothane anesthesia in adults and children. Anesthesiology 71:210, 1989

112. Brandom BW, Sarner JB, Woelfel SK et al: Mivacurium chloride (BW B1090U) infusion requirements in pediatric surgical patients during nitrous oxide-halothane and nitrous oxide-narcotic anesthesia. Anesth Analg 71:16, 1990

113. Sarner JB, Brandom BW, Dong ML et al: Clinical pharmacology of pipecuronium in infants and children during halothane anesthesia. Anesth Analg 71:362, 1990

114. Woelfel SK, Dong ML, Brandom BW et al: Vecuronium infusion requirements in children during nitrous oxide-halothane, nitrous oxide-isoflurane, and nitrous oxide-narcotic anesthesia. Anesth Analg 73:33, 1991

115. Shandling B, Steward DJ: Regional analgesia for postoperative pain in pediatric outpatient surgery. J Pediatr Surg 15:447, 1980

116. Shapiro LA, Jedeikin RJ, Shaley D et al: Epidural morphine and analgesia in children. Anesthesiology 61:210, 1984

117. Jones SEF, Beasley JM, MacFarlane DWR et al: Intrathecal morphine in postoperative pain relief in children. Br J Anaesth 56:137, 1984

118. Tree-Trakarn T, Pirayavaraporn S: Postoperative pain relief for circumcision in children: Comparison among morphine, nerve block, and topical analgesia. Anesthesiology 62:519, 1985

119. Broadman LM, Hannallah R: Regional anesthesia in children. Reg Anesth 10:33, 1985

120. Blaise G, Roy WL: Postoperative pain relief after hypospadias repair in pediatric patients: Regional analgesia versus systemic analgesics. Anesthesiology 65:84, 1986

121. Dalens B, Tanguy A, Haberer JP: Lumbar epidural anesthesia for operative and postoperative pain relief in infants and young children. Anesth Analg 65:1069, 1986

122. Hannallah RS, Broadman LM, Belman AB et al: Comparison of caudal and ilioinguinal/iliohypogastric nerve blocks for control of post-orchiopexy pain in pediatric ambulatory surgery. Anesthesiology 66:832, 1987

123. Hinkle AJ: Percutaneous inguinal block for the outpatient management of post-herniorrhaphy pain in children. Anesthesiology 67:411, 1987

124. Tree-Trakarn T, Pirayavaraporn S, Lertakyamanee J: Topical analgesia for relief of post-circumcision pain. Anesthesiology 67:395, 1987

125. Broadman LM, Hannallah RS, Belman AB et al: Post-circumcision analgesia—a prospective evaluation of subcutaneous ring block of the penis. Anesthesiology 67:399, 1987

126. Warner MA, Kunkel SE, Offord KO et al: The effects of age, epinephrine, and operative site on duration of caudal analgesia in pediatric patients. Anesth Analg 66:995, 1987

127. Desparmet J, Meistelman C, Barre J et al: Continuous epidural infusion of bupivacaine for postoperative pain relief in children. Anesthesiology 67:108, 1987

128. Murat I, Delleur MM, Esteve C et al: Continuous extradural anaesthesia in children. Br J Anaesth 69:1441, 1987

129. Krane EJ, Jacobson LE, Lynn AM et al: Caudal morphine for postoperative analgesia in children: A comparison with caudal bupivacaine and intravenous morphine. Anesth Analg 66:647, 1987

130. Tyler DC: Respiratory effects of pain in a child after thoracotomy. Anesthesiology 70:873, 1989

131. Yaster M, Maxwell LG: Pediatric regional anesthesia. Anesthesiology 70:324, 1989

132. Miranda DR: Continuous brachial plexus block. Acta Anaesthesiol Belg 4:323, 1977

133. Selander D: Catheter technique in axillary block. Acta Anesthesiol Scand 21:316, 1977

134. Carell ED, Eyring EJ: Intravenous regional anesthesia for childhood fractures. Trauma 11:301, 1971

135. Fitzgerald B: Intravenous regional anesthesia in children. Br J Anaesth 48:485, 1976

136. Yeoman PM, Cooke R, Hain WR: Penile block for circumcision? Anaesthesia 38:862, 1983

137. Dohi S, Seino H: Spinal anesthesia in premature infants: Dosage and effects of sympathectomy (correspondence). Anesthesiology 65:559, 1986

138. Harnik EV, Hoy GR, Potolicchio S et al: Spinal anesthesia in premature infants recovering from respiratory distress syndrome. Anesthesiology 64:95, 1986

139. Blaise GA, Roy WL: Spinal anesthesia for minor paediatric surgery. Can Anaesth Soc J 33:227, 1986

140. Abajian JC, Melish RWP, Browne AF et al: Spinal anesthesia for surgery in the high risk infant. Anesth Analg 63:359, 1984

141. Schulte-Steinberg O, Rahlfs WR: Caudal anaesthesia in children and spread of 1 percent lignocaine. Br J Anaesth 42:1093, 1970

142. Lourey CJ, McDonald IH: Caudal anesthesia in infants and children. Anaesth Intensive Care 1:547, 1973

143. Kay B: Caudal blockade for postoperative pain relief in children. Anaesthesia 29:610, 1974

144. Melman E, Peneulas J, Marrufo J: Regional anesthesia in children. Anesth Analg 54:387, 1975

145. Hassan SZ: Caudal anesthesia in infants. Anesth Analg 56:686, 1977

146. Schulte-Steinberg O, Rahlfs WR: Spread of extradural analgesia following caudal injection in children. Br J Anaesth 49:1027, 1977

147. Takasaki M, Dohi S, Kawabata Y et al: Dosage of lidocaine for caudal anesthesia in infants and children. Anesthesiology 47:527, 1977

148. Soliman MG, Ansara S, Laberge R: Caudal anaesthesia in paediatric patients. Can Anaesth Soc J 25:226, 1978

149. McGown RG: Caudal analgesia in children. Anaesthesia 37:806, 1982

150. Bramwell RGB, Bullen C, Radford P: Caudal block for postoperative analgesia in children. Anaesthesia 37:1024, 1982

151. Eyres RL, Bishop W, Oppenheim RC et al: Plasma bupivacaine concentrations in children during caudal epidural analgesia. Anaesth Intensive Care 11:20, 1983

152. Satoyoski M, Kamiyama Y: Caudal anesthesia for upper abdominal surgery in infants and children: A simple calculation of the volume of local anaesthetic. Acta Anaesth Scand 28:57, 1984

153. Ecoffey C, Desparmet J, Maury M et al: Bupivacaine in children: Pharmacokinetics following caudal analgesia. Anesthesiology 63:447, 1985

154. Matsumiya N, Dohi S, Takahashi H et al: Cardiovascular collapse in an infant after caudal anesthesia with lidocaine-epinephrine solution. Anesth Analg 65:1074, 1986

155. Bosenberg AT, Bland BAR, Schulte-Steinberg O et al: Thoracic epidural anesthesia via caudal route in infants. Anesthesiology 69:265, 1988

156. Krane EJ, Tyler DC, Jacobson LE: The dose response of caudal morphine in children. Anesthesiology 71:48–52, 1989

157. Rosen KR, Rosen DA: Caudal epidural morphine for control of pain following open heart surgery in children. Anesthesiology 70:418, 1989

158. Wolf AR, Valley RD, Fear DW et al: Bupivacaine for caudal analgesia in infants and children: The optimal effective concentration. Anesthesiology 69:102, 1988

159. Ward CF: An update on pediatric monitoring. J Clin Monit 1:172, 1985

160. Yelderman M: Evaluation of pulse oximetry. Anesthesiology 59:349, 1983

161. Coté CJ, Goldstein EA, Cote MA et al: A single-blind study of pulse oximetry in children. Anesthesiology 68:184, 1988

162. Zmyslowski WP, Lena DM: Dinamap adaptation for neonatal blood pressure determination. Anesthesiology 58:583, 1983

163. Kochansky SW: Potential deficiencies in modifying the Dinamap for use in the neonate. Anesthesiology 60:171, 1984

164. Sy WP: Ulnar nerve palsy possibly related to use of automatically cycled blood pressure cuff. Anesth Analg 60:687, 1981

165. Showman A, Betts EK: Hazard of automatic non-invasive blood pressure monitoring. Anesthesiology 55:717, 1981

166. Coté CJ, Liu LMP, Szytelbein SK et al: Intraoperative events diagnosed by expired carbon dioxide monitoring in children. Can Anaesth Soc J 33:315, 1986

167. Gravenstein N, Lampotang S, Beneken JEW: Factors influencing capnography in the Bain Circuit. J Clin Monit 1:6, 1985

168. Beneken JEW, Gravenstein N, Gravenstein JS et al: Capnography and the Bain Circuit I: A computer model. J Clin Monit 1:103, 1985

169. Schieber RA, Namnoum A, Sugden A et al: Accuracy of expiratory carbon dioxide measurements using the coaxial and circle breathing circuits in small subjects. J Clin Monit 1:149, 1985

170. Roy RN, Sinclair JC: Hydration of the low-birth-weight infant. Clin Perinatol 2:393, 1975

171. Bell EF, Oh W: Fluid and electrolyte balance in very low birth weight infants. Clin Perinatol 6:139, 1979

172. Holliday MA, Segar WE: The maintenance need for water in parenteral fluid therapy. Pediatrics 19:823, 1957

173. Furman EB, Roman DG, Lemmer LAS et al: Specific therapy in water, electrolyte and blood-volume replacement during pediatric surgery. Anesthesiology 42:187, 1975

174. Sieber FE, Smith DS, Traysman RJ et al: Glucose: A re-evaluation of its intraoperative use. Anesthesiology 67:72, 1987

175. Welborn LG, Hannallah RS, McGill WA et al: Glucose concentrations for routine intravenous infusion in pediatric outpatient surgery. Anesthesiology 67:427, 1987

176. Doze VA, White PF: Effects of fluid therapy on serum glucose levels in fasted outpatients. Anesthesiology 66:223, 1987

177. Lindahl SGE: Energy expenditure and fluid and electrolyte requirements in anesthetized infants and children. Anesthesiology 69:377, 1988

178. Welborn LG, McGill WA, Hannallah RS et al: Perioperative

blood glucose concentrations in pediatric outpatients. Anesthesiology 65:543, 1986

179. Rowe MI, Arango A: Colloid versus crystalloid resuscitation in experimental bowel obstruction. J Pediatr Surg 11:635, 1976
180. Bourke DL, Smith TC: Estimating allowable hemodilution. Anesthesiology 41:609, 1974
181. Buchholz DH: Blood transfusion: Merits of component therapy. J Pediatr 84:1, 1974
182. Coté CJ, Drop LJ, Daniels AL et al: Calcium chloride versus calcium gluconate: Comparison of ionization and cardiovascular effects in children and dogs. Anesthesiology 66:465, 1987
183. Mayhew JF, Kaplan RM: Should hemoglobin-hematocrit be routinely measured in children undergoing minor surgery? Anesthesiology 72:1100, 1990

184. Christensen S, Farrow-Gillespie A, Lerman J: Incidence of emesis and postanesthetic recovery after strabismus surgery in children: A comparison of droperidol and lidocaine. Anesthesiology 70:251, 1989
185. Patel RI, Hannallah RS: Anesthetic complications following pediatric ambulatory surgery: A 3-yr study. Anesthesiology 69:1009, 1988
186. Motoyama EK, Glazener CH: Hypoxemia after general anesthesia in children. Anesth Analg 65:267, 1986
187. Greene LT: Physostigmine treatment of anticholinergic drug depression in postoperative patients. Anesth Analg 50:222, 1971
188. Jordan WS, Graves CL, Elwyn RA: A new therapy for postintubation laryngeal edema and tracheitis (croup) in children. JAMA 212:585, 1970

49

Charles H. McLeskey

Anesthesia for the Geriatric Patient

What is a geriatric patient? An absolute definition is not possible because arbitrary limits constantly change. For example, many studies of surgery in the elderly have been published since the early 1900s, but the definition of "elderly" has changed continually. An early report in 1907 described 167 operations performed on patients older than age 50 and described this advanced age as a contraindication to surgery.[1] Twenty years later, Ochsner suggested that "an elective operation for inguinal hernia in a patient older than 50 years was not justified."[2] In 1937, Brooks reported a series of 293 operations in patients older than age 70, and subsequently most authors have considered patients older than the ages of 65–70 years as elderly.[3] For convenience in this chapter, geriatric patients are considered those 65 years of age or older. However, with the not infrequent recent reports of anesthesia and surgery performed on patients older than age 80, there is no consensus today as to the definition of "geriatric" in medical practice, and very likely the arbitrary age defining a geriatric patient will increase in the near future.[4,5] Catlic reported on six patients older than the age of 100 who had anesthesia and surgery, and he reflected on the changed mood of medicine today when he stated that "elective surgery should not be deferred nor emergency surgery denied [even for] centenarians on the basis of chronologic age."[6]

Nevertheless, far more important than chronologic age is the patient's physiologic age. Because the aging process varies from person to person and from one organ system to another within a given person, elderly patients are not a homogeneous entity. There is little correlation between chronologic age and biologic age. People appear to reach their peak physiologic function in their late 20s or early 30s and from then on it is, in general, a "downhill course" (Fig. 49-1).[7] The amount of physiologic function that remains varies among people with advancing age. Physiologically, some patients may appear as relatively young octogenarians compared with others who appear physiologically as relatively old septuagenarians. Rowe and Kahn have defined this concept more elegantly.[8] They suggest that persons who age with minimal impairment of physiologic function undergo what is known as "successful aging," whereas other persons, who have a deterioration of physiologic function (what we have grown to associate with the aging process in many persons), are labeled as having undergone "usual aging." Again, those elderly persons who have aged while retaining most physiologic functions associated with youth are regarded as having aged successfully.

From an anesthetic perspective, the most important concept to gain from Figure 49-1 is that younger patients tend to be more similar and older patients tend to be more dissimilar, making individualization of the anesthetic technique mandatory.

Figure 49-2 illustrates that in 1900 only 4% of Americans were 65 years of age or older. Today, people older than 65 constitute approximately 11% of the United States population, which is the fastest growing segment of our society. Interestingly, from Figure 49-3 we can see that a subset of the population older than 65, those persons older than age 75 (sometimes referred to as the "old old"), is growing at an even faster rate than the geriatric group as a whole. If life spans continue to lengthen in our society at the current rate, it is projected that the elderly segment will increase to 13% of the population by the year 2000 and that, by the year 2030, fully 52,000,000 Americans, or 17% of the population, will be older than age 65 (Fig. 49-2).[9,10]

This dramatic increase in the number of geriatric Americans has not occurred without social consequence. For example, an article in the November 1985 issue of *Money Magazine* stated that in 1945 there were 50 times as many

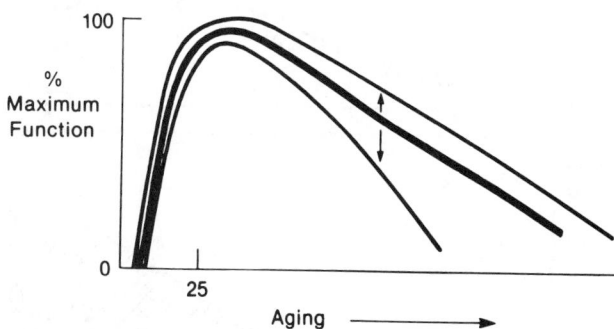

Figure 49-1. The age-related change in physiologic function. Maximum physiologic capacity is usually achieved in the late 20s or early 30s. The physiologic function that remains becomes increasingly variable as people advance in age. (Reprinted with permission from McLeskey CH: Anesthesia for the geriatric patient. In Stoelting RK, Barash PG, Gallagher TJ [eds]: Advances in Anesthesia, p 31. Chicago, Year Book Medical Publishers, 1985.)

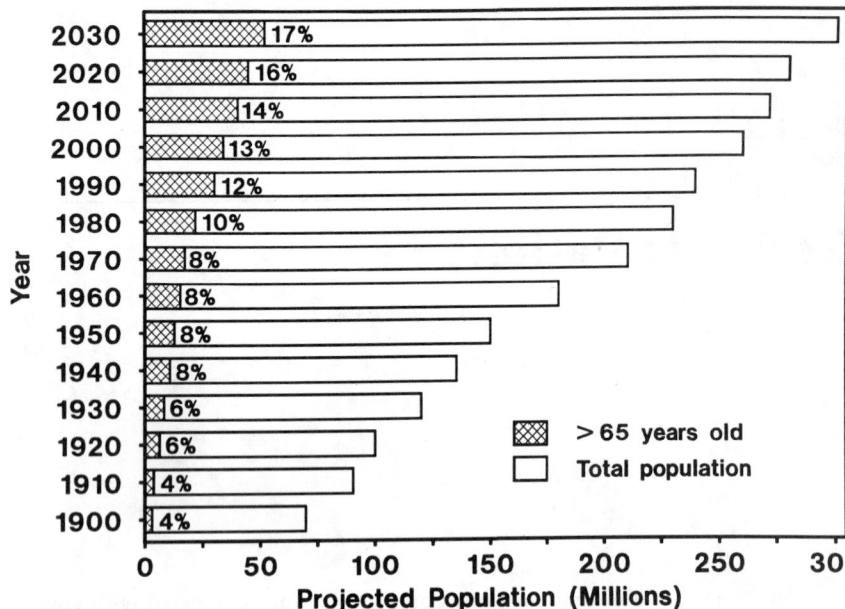

Figure 49-2. The increasing population in the United States from the year 1900 to 1990, with projections to the year 2030. People who are now older than 65 (*left portion of bars*) represent approximately 11–12% of the overall population. This portion is expected to increase to 17–18% by the year 2030. (Reprinted with permission from the U.S. Census Bureau.)

working Americans contributing to the Social Security system as there were elderly persons deriving pension benefits from it. In 1985 the ratio decreased to only 3.3 working Americans contributing for each person receiving pension benefits, and it was projected that by the year 2030 each beneficiary would be receiving benefits from a system in which contributions will be made by only two working Americans per beneficiary. Legislative changes regarding the Social Security system must be made if the system is to survive.

Why has the average American's life expectancy increased so dramatically? In Figure 49-4, Fries and Crapo have illustrated the gains in life expectancy that have been made from 1900 to 1980 in United States citizens and how the life span of the average American has advanced toward the proposed "ideal."[11] In the described ideal curve of survival for a society, the death rate is low and life is extended until approximately age 85, when death is preceded by a very short period of illness. The progress that has been made in the United States in extending the average life expectancy of our citizens probably results from a combination of improved medical care and improved nutrition of our society as a whole. However, it can be seen in Figure 49-4 that most improvement in life expectancy has resulted from a dramatic improvement in reducing the effects of childhood diseases. Perhaps this improvement can be attributed to advances such as the development of antibiotics and childhood immunizations. Significantly fewer gains have been made in curing the diseases of old age, such as heart disease and cancer. Although it appears that the average life expec-

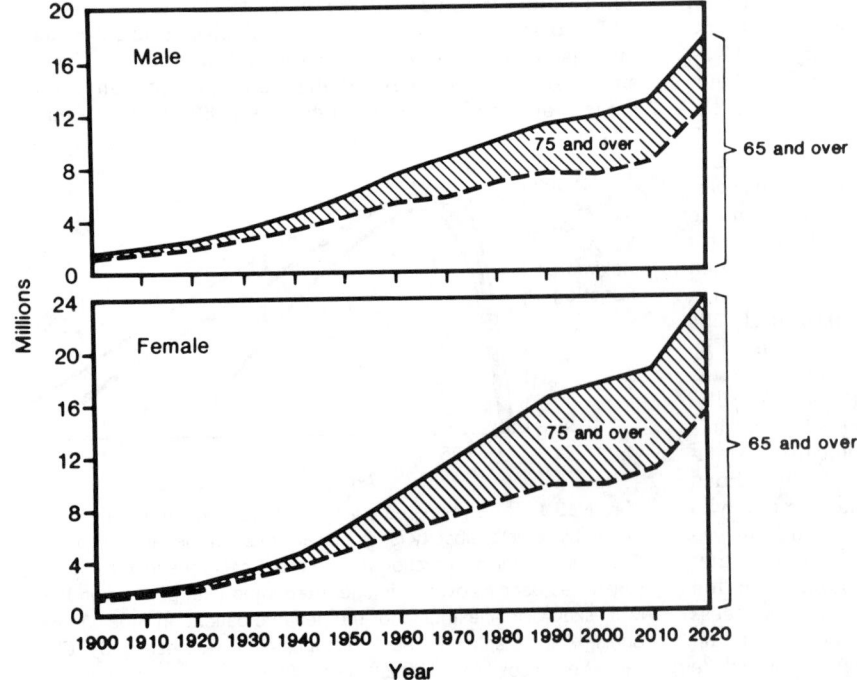

Figure 49-3. Growth from 1900 to 2020 of the population age 65 years and older. (Reprinted with permission from the Bureau of the Census: Current Population Reports, series P-23, no. 43.)

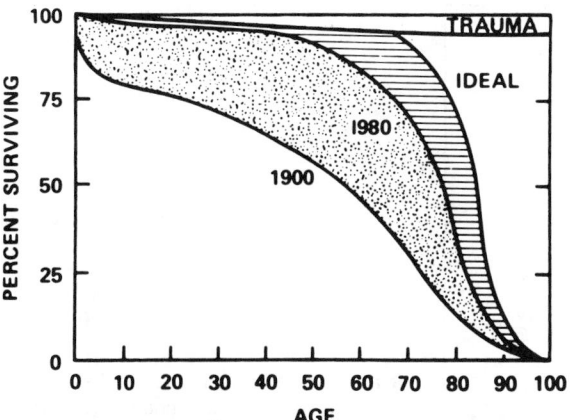

Figure 49-4. A comparison of the survival curve of Americans observed in the years 1900 and 1980 *versus* the "ideal" survival curve. By the year 1980, more than 80% improvement toward the "ideal" had occurred. (Reprinted with permission from Fries JF, Crapo LM: The sharp downslope of natural death. In Fries JF, Crapo LM [eds]: Vitality and Aging, p 73. San Francisco, WH Freeman and Company, 1981.)

tancy of an American from 1900 to 1980 has increased, the maximum length of life has not been prolonged nearly as dramatically. It has been suggested, however, that modest improvement has also been made in this area. For example, in 1980 the United States Census Bureau reported that 32,194 people were at least 100 years of age or older.[12] Rowe and Kahn now encourage health care practitioners to attempt to match the past gains in life span by improving health span, defined as the allowance for maintenance of unchanged physiologic function as near as possible to the end of life.[8]

Because the average life expectancy has been extended, increasing numbers of elderly patients are having surgery. It is estimated that at least 50% of Americans older than the age of 65 will have at least one operative procedure before death. This chapter summarizes the risks of anesthesia and surgery in the elderly patient, identifies the physiologic changes that occur during the aging process, and suggests how these changes affect anesthetic management of these

patients. It is hoped that the risk of age, *per se*, in increasing the hazards of anesthesia and surgery, may be minimized by a better understanding of the physiologic changes occurring during the aging process.

ANESTHESIA RISKS

It is widely believed that, compared with younger patients, elderly patients (even those free of concomitant disease) having major surgery have a significantly higher incidence of complications or death.[13] In an English survey, approximately 50% of intraoperative deaths occurred in geriatric patients, although this group of patients represented only 5% of the overall surgical population.[14] As shown in Table 49-1, age, *per se*, appears to predict increased perioperative morbidity and mortality.[15] Similarly, in a large clinical series of patients, Mircea *et al* found that the three most important factors leading to pulmonary complications after operation were duration of surgery, obesity, and a patient age older than 70 years.[16] A large study from Cardiff of 108,878 administered anesthetics also supported the concept of a higher mortality for both men and women of older age groups (Table 49-2).[17]

However, not all studies agree with the notion that patients who are older necessarily have a higher complication rate during the perioperative period. For instance, in a series of 500 patients having anesthesia and surgery, Djokovic and Hedley-Whyte found no consistent increase in the incidence of death as patients' ages increased from 80 to 95 years (Fig. 49-5).[4] In 1983, Filzweiser and List reported a prospective study of 500 consecutive patients older than 70 and did not find a single intraoperative death.[18] In view of this controversy, is there possibly a factor other than age that better predicts potential complications and deaths in geriatric patients undergoing the stress of anesthesia and surgery?

When the role that age plays as a risk factor for geriatric patients having anesthesia and surgery is examined, the distinction between physiologic age and chronologic age becomes important. Compared with younger patients, elderly patients may be at greater risk for perioperative complications and deaths because of two factors: first, an increased prevalence of age-related, concomitant disease, and second, a decline in basic organ function (independent of disease) resulting from aging *per se*. Let us examine each of these factors.

TABLE 49-1. Mortality Within Seven Days of Anesthesia in Consecutive Surgical Patients

Age (yr)	Patients	Deaths No.(%)
<1	3,396	56 (1.6)
1–10	3,650	30 (0.8)
11–20	5,608	25 (0.45)
21–30	5,192	41 (0.8)
31–40	3,962	55 (1.4)
41–50	4,129	97 (2.3)
51–60	4,063	126 (3.1)
61–70	2,941	130 (4.4)
71–80	1,162	79 (6.8)
>81	73	6 (8.2)
Total	34,140	645 (1.9)

Reprinted with permission from Marx GF, Mateo CV, Orkin LR: Computer analysis of postanesthetic deaths. Anesthesiology 39:54, 1973.

TABLE 49-2. Mortality by Age and Sex

	Males			Females		
Age (yr)	Deaths	Total	Mortality (%)	Deaths	Total	Mortality (%)
0–14	105	8,041	1.3	59	4,601	1.3
15–24	46	5,695	0.8	27	9,683	0.3
25–44	121	9,488	1.3	94	22,411	0.4
45–64	428	14,174	3.0	331	15,925	2.1
>65	578	9,749	5.9	612	9,111	6.7

Reprinted with permission from Farrow SC, Fowkes FGR, Lunn JN *et al*: Epidemiology in anaesthesia. II: Factors affecting mortality in hospital. Br J Anaesth 54:811, 1982.

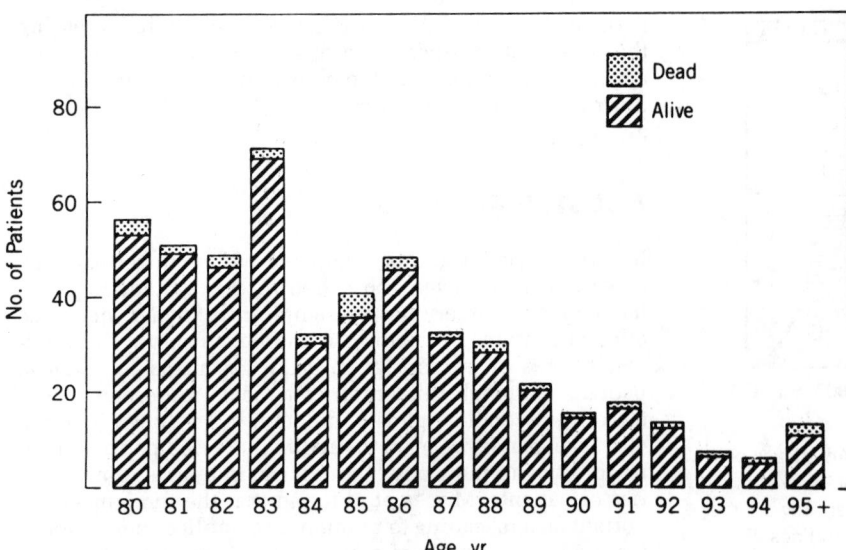

Figure 49-5. Mortality in patients having anesthesia and surgery who range in age from 80 to older than 95 years. (Reprinted with permission from Djokovic JL, Hedley-Whyte J: Prediction of outcome of surgery and anesthesia in patients over 80. JAMA 242:2301, 1979. Copyright 1979, American Medical Association.)

Effects of Concomitant Disease

Multiple concomitant diseases are the rule rather than the exception in elderly patients. A current surgical illness is likely to be present in patients in whom old injuries, prior illnesses, past operations, and a variety of chronic disorders, including cataracts, osteoarthritis, anemia, osteoporosis, and diabetes mellitus, may be observed. Malignancy, cerebral vascular accidents, parkinsonism, dementia, and fractures of the femur are observed with increased frequency in this patient group. Figure 49-6 illustrates the incidence of four common disease states by patient age and shows how much more commonly these disease processes occur as people become age 65 or older.[19] In another study, pathologic findings were observed on medical examination in 92% of patients 81 years of age or older.[20] Of these, cardiovascular abnormalities, including arteriosclerosis and hypertension, were seen in 78% of patients, whereas mental dysfunction occurred in 30% and pulmonary, endocrine, and neurologic abnormalities were observed in 14%, 12%, and 10% of patients, respectively. Stephen has reported on the frequency of abnormalities encountered in 1000 patients older than age 70 (Table 49-3).[21] Once again, hypertension, atherosclerosis, and renal disease led the list of concomitant disease states in patients interviewed before operation.

Which of the common pre-existing conditions correlates most closely with an increased risk of perioperative complications and death in elderly patients? Rowe et al found that ischemic heart disease, dementia, and diabetes mellitus seem to correlate most closely with an increased risk.[22] On the other hand, Farrow et al found that cardiac failure, impaired renal function, and angina were the preoperative conditions most indicative of a high risk of perioperative death.[17] These conditions were associated with mortality 10–30 times greater than the overall 0.5% mortality observed in patients without preoperative medical conditions (Table 49-4).

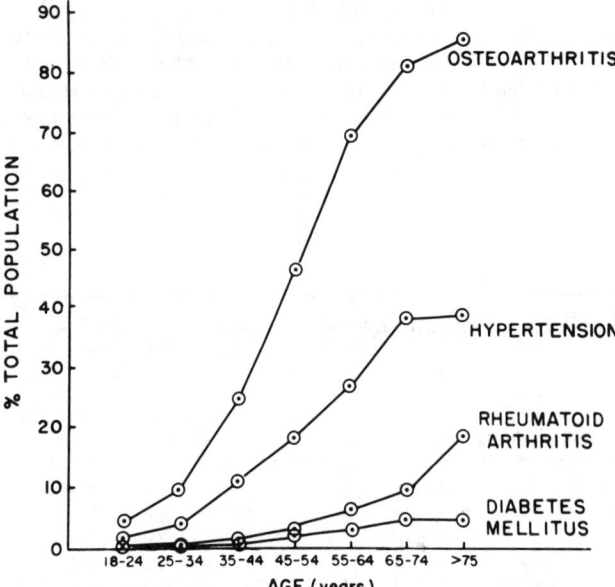

Figure 49-6. Comparison of the prevalence of four common diseases by age of United States citizens. (Reprinted with permission from Ellison N: Problems in geriatric anesthesia. Surg Clin North Am 55:929, 1975.)

TABLE 49-3. Preanesthetic Complications Encountered in 1000 Elderly Patients

Complications	Incidence (%)
Hypertension	46.6
Renal disease	31.4
Atherosclerosis	26.9
Myocardial infarction	18.5
Chronic obstructive pulmonary disease	14.0
Cardiomegaly	13.6
Diabetes	9.2
Liver disease	8.5
Congestive heart failure	7.5
Angina	6.4
Cerebrovascular accident	5.8

Reprinted with permission from Stephen CR: The risk of anesthesia and surgery in the geriatric patient. In Krechel SE (ed): Anesthesia and the Geriatric Patient, p 231. New York: Grune & Stratton, 1984.

TABLE 49-4. Mortality by Selected Preoperative Condition

Condition	Deaths	Operations	Mortality (%)
Cardiac failure	186	1175	15.8
Impaired renal function	84	779	10.8
Angina, arteriosclerosis, or ischemic heart disease	544	7776	7.0
Diabetes	82	1452	5.7
Chronic lower respiratory tract infection	408	8060	5.1
No preoperative condition	206	43483	0.5

Reprinted with permission from Farrow SC, Fowkes FGR, Lunn JN *et al:* Epidemiology in anaesthesia. II: Factors affecting mortality in hospital. Br J Anaesth 54:811, 1982.

The number of associated diseases also may be important in determining the rate of perioperative complications. A prospective French survey of 198,103 anesthetics appeared to demonstrate once again that the rate of anesthesia-related complications correlates directly with patients' ages (Fig. 49-7).[23] However, on closer examination (Fig. 49-8), it is clear that the complication rate relates far more closely to the patient's number of associated diseases than to the patient's age. Stephen observed the same phenomenon.[22] Although he reported an overall mortality of 5.8% in elderly patients, of those who died, 84% had more than three preexisting medical conditions. Likewise, Denney and Denson reported a mortality of 29% among patients older than age 90 who had disease in multiple organ systems, compared with a mortality of 4.9% in a group of healthy persons of similar age.[24] The Goldman study of cardiac risk factors also suggests that the pre-existing medical condition is more important than a patient's age when attempting to predict the risks associated with anesthesia and surgery.[25] "Points" in the Goldman risk index are assigned to patients before operation, with greater point values given to those criteria more likely to result in perioperative complications and death. Age older than 70 years is assigned a point value, indicating that age, *per se*, may be a risk. However, it is a lesser value than that assigned to certain preoperative medical conditions, such as a recent myocardial infarction or signs of congestive heart failure.

The American Society of Anesthesiologists (ASA) physical status classification is not affected by patients' ages but rather by the number and severity of pre-existing medical conditions. The ASA classification system predicts with reasonable accuracy the risks of elderly patients having anesthesia and surgery. For instance, in a study of 500 patients older than 80 years, only one of 187 ASA Class II patients died in the perioperative period, whereas 14 of 56 (25%) ASA Class IV patients died (Fig. 49-9).[4] Similarly, a prospective French study of almost 200,000 anesthetics demonstrated an incidence of complications that related very closely to the patient's ASA physical status (Fig. 49-10).[23] Del Guercio and Cohn have also shown in patients older than age 65 that ASA physical status relates directly to perioperative mortality.[26] In their patients, preoperative assignment of a patient to ASA Class II resulted in a mortality of less than 10%. However, ASA Class III patients had an increased mortality between 10 and 15% and ASA Class IV patients had a mortality greater than 20%. More recently, Hosking and colleagues have shown in 795 patients over age 90 that a close correlation exists between short- and

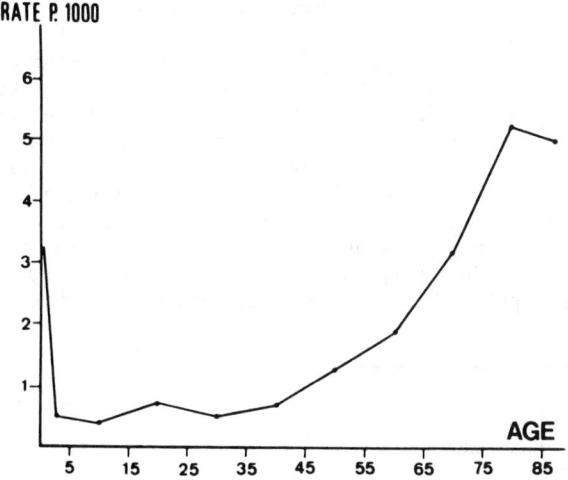

Figure 49-7. Complication rate per 1000 anesthetics, related to patient age from ages 5 to 85. (Reprinted with permission from Tiret L, Desmonts JM, Hatton F *et al:* Complications associated with anaesthesia—A prospective study in France. Can Anaesth Soc J 33:336, 1986.)

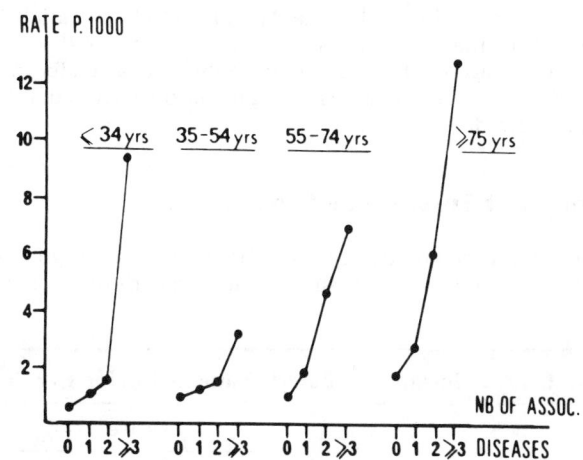

Figure 49-8. Complications rate per 1000 anesthetics, related to number of associated diseases in patients of four different age groups. (Reprinted with permission from Tiret L, Desmonts JM, Hatton F *et al:* Complications associated with anaesthesia—A prospective study in France. Can Anaesth Soc J 33:336, 1986.)

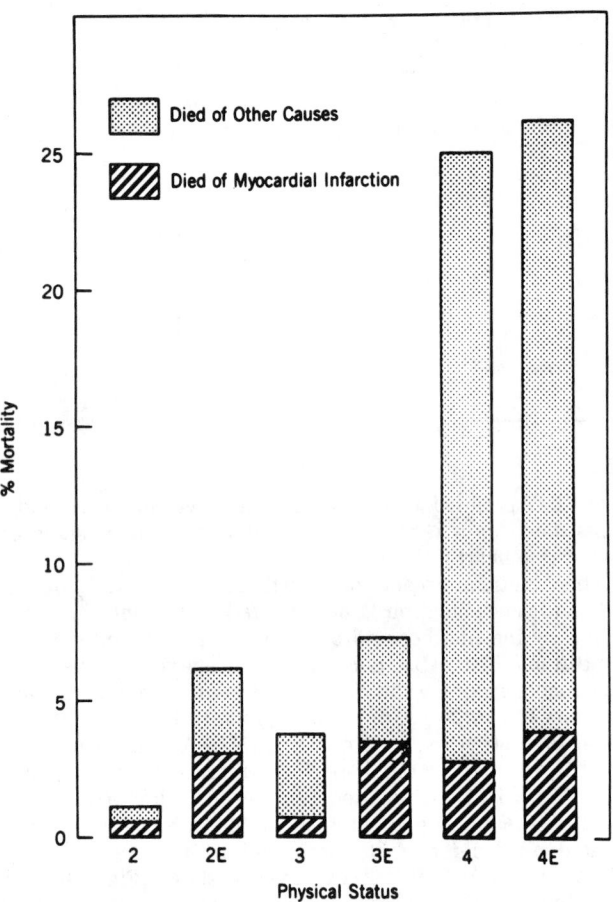

Figure 49-9. The relationship of ASA physical status to percentage of deaths after anesthesia and surgery in patients older than age 80. Perioperative mortality increases significantly as physical status increases. In patients of the same physical status, emergency procedures are generally associated with a higher incidence of death. (Reprinted with permission from Djokovic JL, Hedley-Whyte J: Prediction of outcome of surgery and anesthesia in patients over 80. JAMA 242:2301, 1979. Copyright 1979, American Medical Association.)

long-term morbidity and mortality and ASA classification.[27] From all of the information presented, it appears that the presence of age-related disease probably plays a greater role than does age itself in contributing to perioperative complications and death.

Effects of Emergency Procedures

The risk of perioperative complications and death is greatly increased in the elderly if surgery must be performed on an

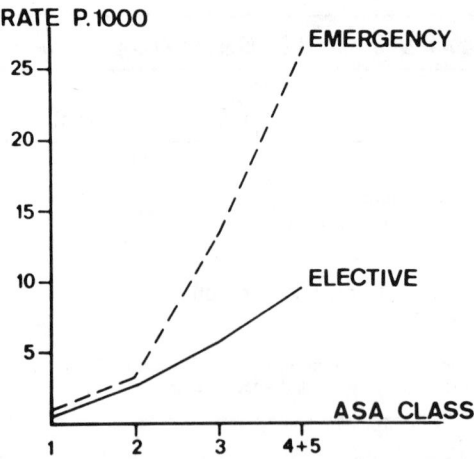

Figure 49-10. Complications rate per 1000 anesthetics related to ASA physical status (class) for elective and emergency surgical procedures. Higher ASA classes of surgical patients and surgical procedures performed on an emergency basis exaggerate the risks of perioperative complications and death. (Reprinted with permission from Tiret L, Desmonts JM, Hatton F *et al:* Complications associated with anaesthesia—A prospective survey in France. Can Anaesth Soc J 33:336, 1986.)

emergency basis.[26-30] Gibson *et al* suggested that death is four times more frequent in the elderly patient with coexistent disease compared with the healthy elderly patient and 20 times more frequent in those requiring emergency surgery.[30] Farrow *et al* also showed that the crude mortality increased 3.5-fold if procedures were performed on an emergency rather than an elective basis.[17] Table 49-5 lists findings in three separate studies in elderly patients that illustrate the dramatic increase in mortality associated with emergency herniorrhaphy compared with the mortality when the same procedures were performed electively.[31-33] Tiret's French study has also demonstrated that performing surgical procedures in elderly patients on an emergency basis significantly increases the risks of perioperative complications and death (Fig. 49-10).[23]

Perhaps the best explanations for why elderly patients requiring emergency surgery have a higher incidence of perioperative complications and death are that they may have delayed seeking health care and may have more advanced pathologic conditions. Also, presentation for emergency surgery allows little time for control of pre-existing disease. Although apparently healthy elderly patients may tolerate an elective operation, the additional stress of an emergency procedure, because of an acute exacerbation of pre-existent disease or an unexpected complication, can tax their limited physiologic reserve and lead to disastrous consequences. In general, it is wise to adequately prepare an elderly patient for elective surgery but unwise to defer sur-

TABLE 49-5. Mortality in Elderly Patients Having Herniorrhaphy

Study	Elective		Emergency	
	Percentage	*Total No.*	*Percentage*	*Total No.*
Nehme[31]	1.3	1044	7.5	235
Williams and Hale[32]	2		16	
Tingwald and Cooperman[33]	0	44	22	18

gery simply because of age. An unnecessary delay may result in complications that necessitate surgery under even more adverse emergency conditions, with a significantly increased risk of associated perioperative complications and death.

PATHOPHYSIOLOGY OF AGING

We have previously discussed the increased risks that age-related diseases produce. In this section we discuss the pathophysiologic changes of aging that affect major organ systems and that subsequently influence our anesthetic techniques.

Cardiovascular System

Perhaps the most important age-related physiologic changes that affect the anesthetic management of the elderly patient are those that occur in the cardiovascular system. Many of these physiologic changes that were once thought to reflect the aging process itself now appear to be manifestations of age-related disease or a lifestyle resulting in prolonged deconditioning. Because major lifestyle changes occur and the prevalence of disease increases sharply with advancing age, it is difficult to determine the effects of the aging process alone on the cardiovascular system. All three processes are closely interrelated.[34]

Cardiovascular changes associated with aging are summarized in Table 49-6. These changes include the concept that with aging there may be impaired myocardial pump function and reduced cardiac output. For example, variable degrees of myocardial fiber atrophy occur during aging with replacement by connective tissue. However, heart wall thickness may increase modestly with age because of an increase in myocyte size.[35] When this process develops in an area of the myocardium adjacent to the sinoatrial pacemaker, the heart rate may be affected in elderly patients. Increasing fibrosis of the endocardial lining of the cardiac chambers and valves leads to progressive endocardial thickening and rigidity. Calcification of valves, especially in the region of the annulus, may produce distortion of valvular leaflets, resulting in progressive valvular incompetence. In addition, loss of elasticity throughout the vascular tree with age produces a progressive loss of arterial distensibility and increased impedance to left ventricular output, resulting in a progressive compensatory hypertrophy of the left ventricle. With age-induced diminished caliber and elasticity of

TABLE 49-6. Cardiovascular Changes Associated With Aging

Sign	Change
Maximum coronary blood flow	Decrease
Cardiac index	No change or a decrease
Resting heart rate	No change
Maximum heart rate	Decrease
Arterial distensibility	Decrease
Peripheral vascular resistance	Increase
Impedance to left ventricular output	Increase
Systolic blood pressure	Increase
Stroke volume	No change or an increase
Ejection fraction	No change or a decrease

coronary arteries as well, maximum coronary perfusion decreases. Not surprisingly, many of these factors combine to contribute to an increased incidence of hypertension and ischemic heart disease in elderly patients.

Vascular Elasticity and Blood Pressure Changes During Aging

In general, large artery elasticity is reduced during the aging process, resulting in stiffening of the arterial vasculature. The histologic and morphologic changes seen in the aging aorta and arterial tree resemble those in younger patients who have essential hypertension.[34] Consequently, there is an age-related increased impedance to ejection of blood with each contraction of the heart, resulting in increased systolic blood pressure. Probably as an adaptive mechanism to maintain normal wall stress, an approximately 30% concentric hypertrophy of the left ventricular wall develops in people between 30 and 80 years of age. Further, the decrease in early diastolic filling rate and the increase in left atrial dimension observed with advanced age may be consequences of a thicker walled, less compliant left ventricle. The thoracic aorta is thought to contribute approximately half of the total capability of the arterial tree to buffer the energy released with each ejection of the heart. Partial compensation for the age-related arterial stiffening is provided by an approximate 6% aortic dilatation that develops between the 4th and 8th decades of life.[36] Despite this partial compensation by the elderly, long-term longitudinal studies of patients, such as that reported in the Framingham study, demonstrated an increased systolic blood pressure of 25–35 mm Hg (Fig. 49-11).[37] Hypertension in the elderly is frequently inadequately treated, and if diastolic blood pressure is chronically greater than 100–110 mm Hg, plasma volume depletion is likely.[38] Pre-existent hypovolemia in poorly treated elderly hypertensive patients makes intraoperative blood pressure lability likely and also renders the patient less tolerant of sudden changes in posture, intrathoracic pressure, or blood loss.

Pulmonary artery pressures and vascular resistance also increase with age. Although multiple explanations, including coronary artery disease, have been advanced, Davidson and Fee have demonstrated in patients without coronary artery disease or ventricular dysfunction an age-induced increase in pulmonary systolic pressure from 20 mm Hg in young patients to 26 mm Hg in older patients, an increase in pulmonary artery diastolic pressure from 9 mm Hg to 11 mm Hg, and an increase in pulmonary vascular resistance from 70 to 124 dynes·sec·cm^{-5}.[39] Thus, if age-related changes in pulmonary hemodynamics are not taken into account, the clinical severity of an elevation in measured pulmonary artery pressure in an elderly patient might be overestimated.

Coronary Artery Disease

The age-associated replacement of elastic tissue by less resilient fibrous connective tissue occurs not only in the peripheral vascular system but also in the coronary arteries, reducing maximum available coronary flow. Coronary artery disease progressively increases in severity over the entire adult age span, but clinical symptoms may not be seen until a critical threshold is reached. Although a high percentage of elderly persons have coronary stenosis at autopsy, a much lower percentage demonstrate clinical manifestations such as angina pectoris or myocardial infarction. Thus, coronary artery disease may be occult in many elderly persons. As illustrated in Figure 49-12, an estimate of the

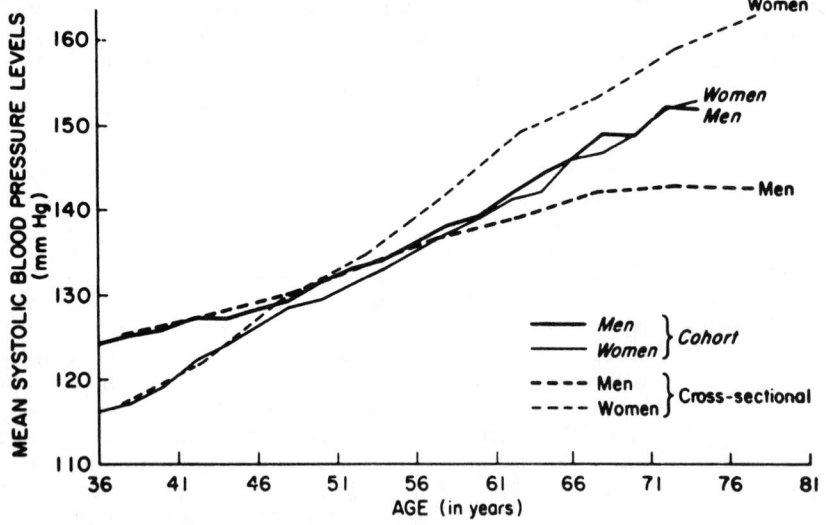

Figure 49-11. Increases in systolic blood pressure of 25–35 mm Hg occur in both men and women during the aging process. (Reprinted with permission from Kannel WB, Gordon T: Evaluation of cardiovascular risk in the elderly: The Framingham study. Bull NY Acad Med 54:573, 1978.)

prevalence of coronary artery disease in men ages 51–90 will be significantly low and inaccurate if only resting criteria are relied upon, such as a history of angina pectoris or previous myocardial infarction or an abnormal electrocardiogram.[34] On the other hand, with more intensive evaluation of coronary perfusion, such as with the use of radionuclide imaging of the myocardium, coupled with electrocardiographic monitoring during a treadmill stress test, many more cases of significant coronary artery disease may be identified. In fact, it appears that people who are 70 years of age or older have at least a 50% chance of developing significant coronary artery disease, whether or not they have symptoms.

Cardiac Output

Cardiac output is thought to decrease by approximately 1% per year beyond age 30 (Fig. 49-13).[40] As a consequence, in elderly patients it should take longer for intravenously administered drugs to reach receptor sites, thus delaying the onset of pharmacologic action. An example of this might be the patient's response to the administration of a test dose of thiopental (approximately 50 mg) before a complete induction dose is administered. Some believe that administration of a test dose of thiopental is a useful technique in elderly patients because it allows an assessment of the patient's sensitivity to the drug and enables an estimation of the eventual proper dose required to complete the induction of anesthesia. However, allowing 30–45 seconds for observation of a response to this test dose (which may be an adequate time in a younger patient) may not be an adequate

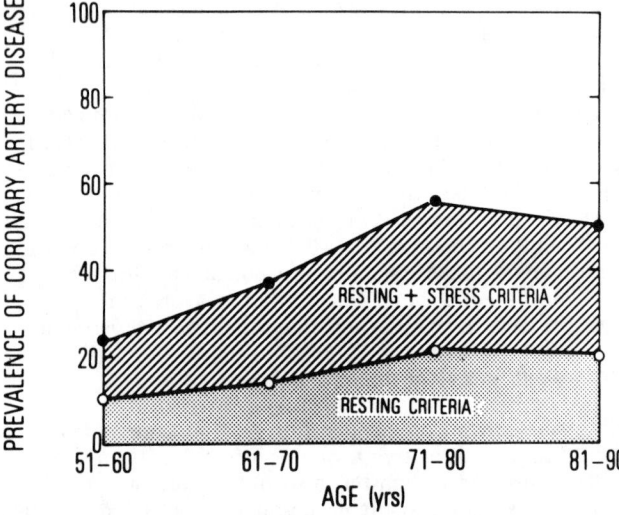

Figure 49-12. Estimate of the prevalence of coronary artery disease in men ages 51–90. Resting criteria represent a history of angina pectoris or myocardial infarction or an abnormal ECG. Stress criteria represent an abnormal exercise ECG or a thallium scan perfusion defect during exercise. (Reprinted with permission from Lakatta EG: Health, disease, and cardiovascular aging. In The Aging Society: The Burden of Long-term Illness and Disability. Washington DC, National Academy Press, 1986.)

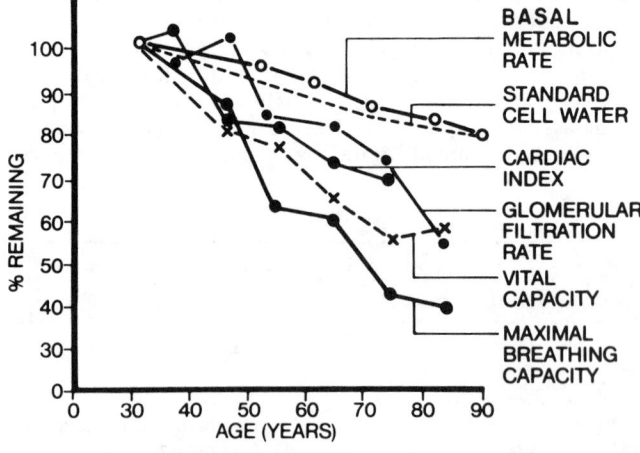

DECLINE IN PHYSIOLOGICAL MEASUREMENTS WITH AGE

Figure 49-13. The classically held concept is that various physiologic functions decline as a person ages. Most functions decrease by approximately 1–1.5% per year after age 30. (Reprinted with permission from Evans TI: The physiological basis of geriatric general anaesthesia. Anaesth Intensive Care 1:319, 1973.)

time in an elderly patient with a reduced cardiac output and a prolonged circulation time. Reduced cardiac output and a slower circulation time in the elderly also affect induction of inhalation anesthesia. A faster induction of anesthesia with inhalation drugs would be expected. If cardiac output is slow, uptake of inhalation drugs from the alveoli is reduced and results in a higher partial pressure of anesthetic in the alveoli. This higher partial pressure is, in turn, reflected as a higher partial pressure of the agent in the blood, the heart, and, in turn, the brain. Profound hypotension may result.

Succinylcholine may theoretically be less effective in the elderly in the presence of a reduced cardiac output. A slower circulation time would permit a longer exposure of the injected drug to plasma pseudocholinesterase, allowing greater metabolism and reduced effectiveness of the drug before its eventual delivery to the effector sites at the neuromuscular junction.

Many studies support the belief that cardiac output gradually declines with advancing age. A typical example is a study by Brandfonbrener et al, in which a 50% decline in cardiac index from ages 20–80 was observed.[41] Unfortunately, the population tested in many of these classic studies was composed of patients who were housed in hospital wards and were being treated for acute or chronic disease. A large percentage of these patients may have been sedentary and may have been convalescing from a variety of illnesses. Thus, it may have been lifestyle or age-associated disease that produced the observed decrease in cardiac output, and it may be incorrect to conclude that aging itself produces a predetermined obligatory decline in cardiac output.

The Baltimore Longitudinal Study on Aging is a program that, on a longitudinal basis, follows volunteer subjects who are carefully screened and are viewed as healthy and not affected by disease or deconditioning. These subjects return to Baltimore every other year for a complete physical evaluation. Recently, data from this study have yielded a divergent view of the change that has classically been thought to occur in resting cardiac output as a result of age. Rodeheffer et al demonstrated that there is no significant age-associated decline in cardiac output at rest or during exercise in healthy adults between the ages of 25 and 79 (Fig. 49-14).[42] Therefore, it appears that elderly people may have a decline in cardiac output with age if they have maintained a sedentary lifestyle or if they are affected by age-related disease. On the other hand, healthy elderly people who have maintained an active lifestyle do not necessarily have a predetermined obligatory decline in cardiac output with age.

Cardiac Reserve

It has been believed for a long time that elderly patients have a reduced myocardial reserve, making them less capable of responding to stress. Traditional studies in exercise physiology have shown that maximum exercise performance is reduced with age. Specifically, declines have been identified in maximum aerobic capacity, heart rate, stroke volume, and cardiac output. For example, when tested with the stress of exercise, healthy young subjects increased their ejection fraction and stroke volume 10–24% compared with resting values.[43] However, elderly people did not respond with an increase in ejection fraction, and many actually had a reduced ejection fraction in response to this stress. Another study suggesting reduced cardiovascular reserve in elderly people demonstrated a diminished cardiovascular

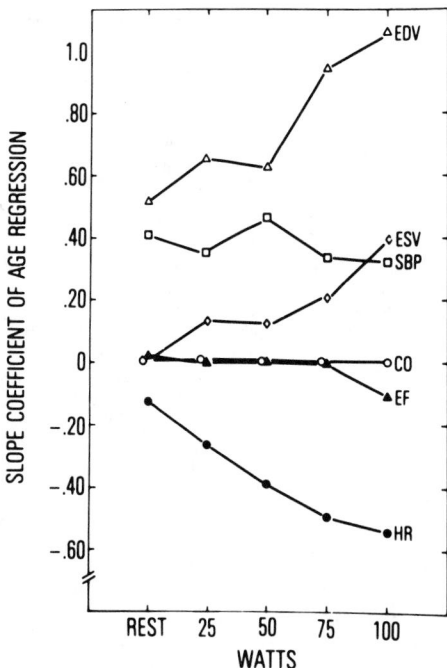

Figure 49-14. The slope coefficients of the regression functions of age for cardiac parameters in persons tested at rest and at four different exercise workloads. An increase or decrease in the slope coefficient with increasing workloads indicates a respective increasing or decreasing age effect. During exercise, older persons demonstrate a reduced heart rate (HR) and ejection fraction (EF) compared with younger subjects. Despite this, when older persons exercise, they generate a cardiac output (CO) similar to that of youth. This is accomplished by increasing end-diastolic volume (EDV) to a greater extent than the increase in end-systolic volume (ESV), resulting in an age-related increase in stroke volume during increased workloads. (Reprinted with permission of the American Heart Association, Inc. Rodeheffer RJ, Gerstenblith G, Becker LC et al: Exercise cardiac output is maintained with advancing age in healthy human subjects: Cardiac dilatation and increased stroke volume compensate for a diminished heart rate. Circulation 69:203, 1984.)

response to the stress of acute hemodilution.[44] More specifically, during neurolept anesthesia, acute normovolemic hemodilution from a hematocrit of 38 to 28 resulted in a significant increase in cardiac output in young patients. However, no such increase was observed in elderly patients; rather, oxygen extraction from hemoglobin increased, resulting in a diminished central venous oxygen tension. This study suggests that acute hemodilution does not seem to trigger appropriate reflex mechanisms in the elderly but instead results in a reduced oxygen transport capacity. Caution should be used when this technique is used to reduce surgical blood loss during surgical procedures in geriatric patients.

Data from the Baltimore Longitudinal Study on Aging have suggested that the older notion that the elderly have a reduced myocardial reserve in response to stress may be incorrect. When carefully screened in order to exclude coronary disease and other age-associated cardiac diseases, elderly subjects demonstrated no decrease in cardiac output in response to the stress of exercise when compared with younger subjects (Fig. 49-14).[42]

However, physiologic differences in elderly patients allow an increase in cardiac output in response to exercise

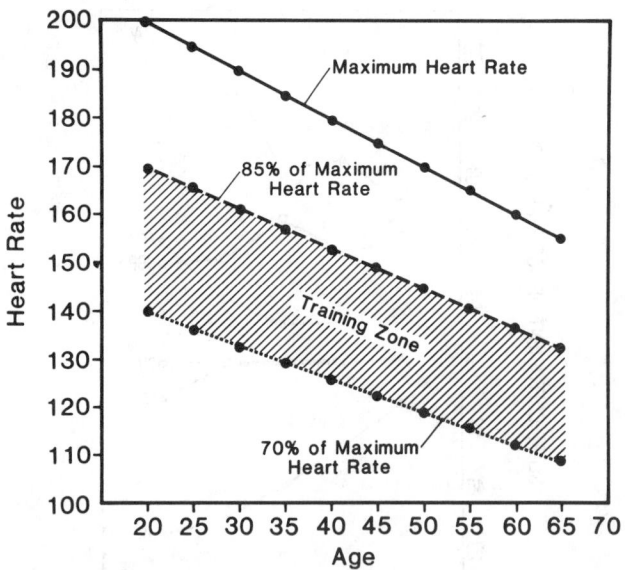

Figure 49-15. An exercise chart typical of that posted in many exercise facilities demonstrates the decrease in maximum heart rate observed at an increased age. The maximum heart rate may be determined by this formula: maximum heart rate = 220 − age.

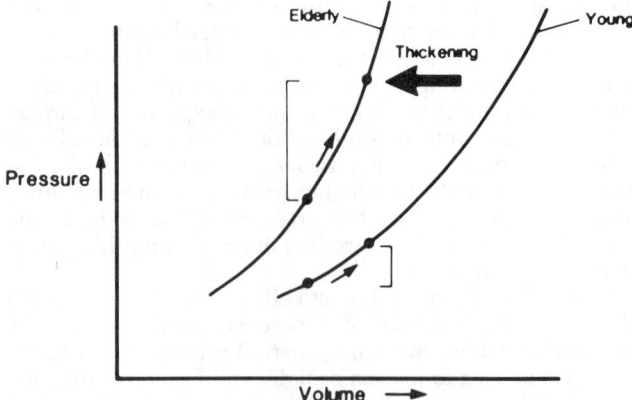

Figure 49-16. The aged myocardium, after years of pumping against an increased afterload, hypertrophies, resulting in a steeper pressure/volume slope. As a result, when elderly persons increase cardiac output during exercise (primarily by increasing filling volumes of the left ventricle), a much greater filling pressure is required than that for younger persons. Therefore, this compensatory mechanism is more limited in elderly persons and predisposes them to congestive heart failure if large filling volumes are required.

(and presumably to other stresses as well) by a mechanism different from that observed in younger subjects. For example, the maximum heart rate generated by an elderly person is less than that of younger subjects.[42,45] Maximum attainable heart rate in persons of different ages is predicted by the following equation:

$$\text{Maximum heart rate} = 220 - \text{age} \qquad (49\text{-}1)$$

Thus, 20-year-old people have an approximate maximal heart rate of 200 beats·min⁻¹, whereas those who are 60 have an approximate maximal heart rate of 160 beats·min⁻¹.

The principle of reduced maximum attainable heart rate with age is well known and used in exercise facilities. A typical example of an exercise chart posted in many exercise facilities is shown in Figure 49-15. Many exercise instructors promote the concept that an aerobic benefit is achieved only if heart rate is increased by exercise to the "target zone" that lies somewhere between 70 and 85% of maximal attainable heart rate.

If exercise increases cardiac output in healthy elderly people as much as in young people, yet maximal attainable heart rate and enhancement of ejection fraction are reduced, how do healthy elderly patients increase cardiac output in response to exercise or other challenges? As shown in Figure 49-14, the major mechanism by which older people enhance cardiac output is by an increased reliance on the Frank-Starling mechanism. An increase in end-diastolic volume, which becomes more pronounced as exercise levels increase, results in a larger stroke volume.[44] Although end-systolic volume also increases to some extent, the increase in end-diastolic volume is significantly greater, resulting in an augmentation of stroke volume. Thus, despite the age-associated attenuation in maximal heart rate and a sluggish enhancement of ejection fraction in response to stress, healthy, nonsedentary elderly patients are able to enhance cardiac output when demands are placed upon them primarily by an enhancement of stroke volume resulting from an increase in end-diastolic volume.

This compensatory increase in end-diastolic volume necessarily requires an increase in filling pressure. As shown in Figure 49-16, the elevation in left ventricular filling pressure necessary to produce an increase in end-diastolic volume in elderly people may be even more dramatic than in young people because older people have a steeper pressure/volume curve as a result of the progressive myocardial hypertrophy that accompanies age. Thus, the primary compensatory mechanisms that healthy elderly people use to improve cardiac output in response to stress may make them less able to tolerate fluid loads and predispose them to congestive heart failure.

Heart Rate and Adrenoreceptor Responsiveness of the Elderly Cardiovascular System

Although the resting heart rate and heart rate response to submaximal exercise loads in the elderly are similar to those of younger patients, the maximum heart rate that can be generated by an elderly patient is considerably less (see Equation 49-1).[45] Regulation of chronotropic and inotropic cardiac function depends partly on a catecholamine effect. During exercise, serum catecholamine levels in elderly subjects exceed those seen in younger subjects.[46] Thus, failure to elaborate and release catecholamines during stress cannot explain the elderly patient's apparent diminution in adrenergic response, manifested by a reduced maximal heart rate and ejection fraction. Instead, an age-related decrease in target organ responsiveness, whether resulting from a reduced number of receptors or a reduced receptor sensitivity, has been suggested.[47,48] Thus, catecholamine effects that enhance calcium ion transport in the myocardium and improve calcium ion availability are less pronounced in elderly patients, partly explaining the reduced myocardial contractility and the reduced maximum heart rate in elderly subjects.

Many studies in the elderly have also demonstrated a reduced chronotropic response to a variety of exogenously administered drugs. For example, older patients have a reduced tachycardic response to atropine in comparison with younger patients.[49] When a person is age 50 or older, the heart rate is increased by only 4–5 beats·min^{-1} after atropine administration, whereas the same dose produces a far more dramatic response in younger subjects. Similarly, a multicenter clinical study demonstrated a greater increase in the heart rates of younger patients compared to the elderly in response to the administration of isoflurane.[50]

Chronotropic and inotropic effects of beta-agonist drugs are also significantly reduced in elderly patients. The decrease in beta receptor–mediated responsiveness suggests an alteration in beta receptor numbers or affinity or an alteration in the dose–response curve of the beta receptor adenylate cyclase system, resulting in the generation of less cyclic adenosine monophosphate after beta receptor stimulation.[47,48,51] Isoproterenol produces a far greater increase in heart rate in young subjects compared with older subjects.[52] Terbutaline, another beta adrenoreceptor agonist with relative beta$_2$ selectivity, also produces less tachycardia in elderly patients compared with younger patients.[53] Interestingly, the sensitivity of elderly patients to the beta blocker propranolol is also reduced, as shown by a greater reduction in heart rate in patients younger than age 35 as compared with those older than age 50.[54]

The response of the autonomic nervous system to stress is less effective in the elderly, making stress-related cardiac decompensation more likely in this patient population.[55,56] For example, healthy elderly subjects in whom blood pressure was reduced by the administration of the alpha$_1$ antagonist, prazosin, demonstrated significantly less tachycardia in response to the associated hypotension.[57] Younger subjects responded with a heart rate increase to 103 beats·min^{-1}, whereas there was no change observed in the heart rate in elderly patients from the resting rate of 80 beats·min^{-1}. We have also previously seen that elderly patients respond to the stress of acute hemodilution with far less of a compensatory increase in heart rate and cardiac output than that observed in young patients.[44] This reduced compensatory cardiac response to hypotension or hemodilution is compatible with the phenomenon of reduced responsiveness of cardiac beta receptors and reduced baroreflex mechanisms in elderly patients.

Responsiveness of the vascular adrenoreceptors also seems to be reduced in the elderly. For example, the dose of the alpha$_1$ agonist phenylephrine required to increase mean arterial pressure by 20 mm Hg is almost twice as great in the elderly as that required in younger patients.[57] When injected intra-arterially, isoproterenol produces a lesser increase in forearm blood flow in older subjects compared with that seen in young subjects.[52] Younger patients also demonstrate a greater plasma renin response to the administration of beta agonists.[52] Thus, there appears to be an age-related parallel reduction in cardiac, peripheral vascular, and renal beta adrenoreceptor–mediated responses. All of these studies indicate a generalized diminution of adrenoreceptor sensitivity in elderly patients. An attractive hypothesis to explain the hemodynamic profiles of a decreased maximum heart rate, increased preload, and reduced ejection fraction at maximum effort, despite elevated levels of circulating catecholamines, is an age-associated decrease in end-organ response, similar to progressive, nonpharmacologically induced beta-adrenergic blockade.

Dysrhythmias

The prevalence of cardiac dysrhythmias at rest, during normal routine activity, and during vigorous exercise has been shown to increase with age. With continuous electrocardiographic monitoring, isolated supraventricular and ventricu-

lar ectopic beats, usually less than 1 every hour, were found in 88 and 78% of elderly men and women, respectively.[58] Seventeen percent of the subjects demonstrated more than 100 ventricular ectopic beats over a 24-hour period, and supraventricular tachydysrhythmias were observed in 33% of subjects. The incidence of ventricular dysrhythmias in elderly patients is also greater than that observed in the young.[59] Other common electrocardiographic abnormalities in elderly patients include decreased T wave amplitude and T wave inversions, especially in leads I, aV$_L$, V$_5$, and V$_6$. First-degree heart block, left anterior hemiblock, and right bundle-branch block are also commonly seen.

In summary, it may be difficult to determine on an initial examination if an elderly patient has maintained his or her cardiac function during the aging process. To make this decision, a skilled anesthesiologist should try to determine if an elderly patient has age-related cardiac disease or has allowed a sedentary lifestyle to interfere with the maintenance of long-term cardiovascular fitness. It is reassuring to know that a significant percentage of elderly patients may have surprisingly well maintained cardiac function and an ability to compensate to meet demands of stressful situations, primarily by increasing end-diastolic volume. However, it is unnerving to realize that it is difficult to determine on superficial evaluation what sort of cardiac reserve the average elderly patient may have. More than half of elderly people have significant coronary artery disease, regardless of whether they have symptoms.

Ventilatory System

In general, aging is associated with reduced ventilatory volumes and decreased efficiency of gas exchange. From age 20 to age 70, total lung capacity is reduced by approximately 10%, in part as a consequence of narrowing of the intervertebral disk spaces with shortening of overall body height. Stiffening of cartilage and replacement of elastic tissue in the costal, intercostal, and intervertebral areas produce rigidity of the thoracic cage, which impairs the bellows function of the lung. Progressive kyphosis or scoliosis produces upward and anterior rotation of the ribs and sternum, which leads to increased anterior-posterior chest diameter, further restricting chest expansion. The gradual loss of skeletal muscle mass with aging results in diaphragm and intercostal muscle wastage, further reducing an elderly person's ability to ventilate. All these changes contribute to an age-related reduction in vital capacity, total lung capacity, and maximum breathing capacity (Figs. 49-13, 49-17, and 49-18).[60-62]

As seen in Figure 49-17, at age 20 maximum voluntary ventilation is approximately 100 l·min^{-1} or 12–15 times that needed to meet basal metabolic needs. However, at age 80 maximum voluntary ventilation decreases to approximately 30–40 l·min^{-1}, representing a ventilatory reserve of approximately sevenfold. This is more than adequate to meet ventilatory needs for the average nonstressed healthy elderly person. However, if other age-related diseases or the effects on ventilation of anesthesia and surgery are superimposed on this pattern, ventilatory reserve may, in fact, be quite limited. For instance, following an emergency abdominal operation, a patient with pre-existent pulmonary infection and postoperative pain is predisposed to respiratory failure. Residual effects of anesthetic drugs and muscle relaxants may further reduce the patient's ventilatory capability. Similarly, a patient who is septic, with increased ventilatory requirements to meet the needs of an increased basal

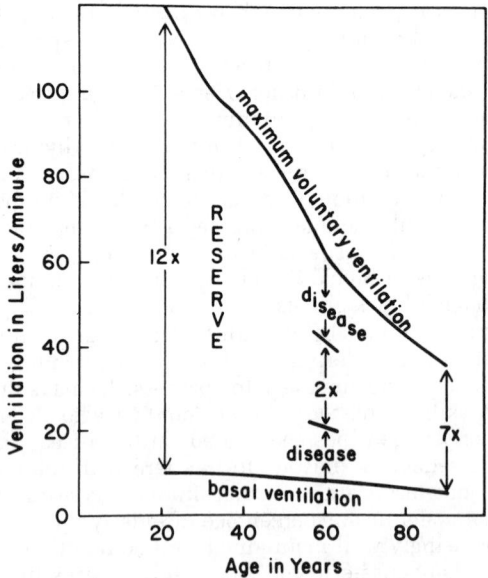

Figure 49-17. Basal ventilation needs decrease with age primarily because of a reduction in basal metabolic rate. Maximum voluntary ventilation at age 20 is 12–15 times that needed to meet basal metabolic needs. During aging, with loss of elasticity of the chest cage and lung parenchyma, maximum voluntary ventilation declines steeply. Although a healthy elderly person has a ventilatory reserve of approximately sevenfold, this reserve is quickly eroded if disease processes reduce a person's ability to ventilate or increase ventilatory requirements to meet increased metabolic needs. As a result, elderly persons more likely will require postoperative ventilatory support compared with their younger counterparts. (Reprinted with permission from Smith TC: Respiratory effects of aging. Semin Anesth 5:14, 1986.)

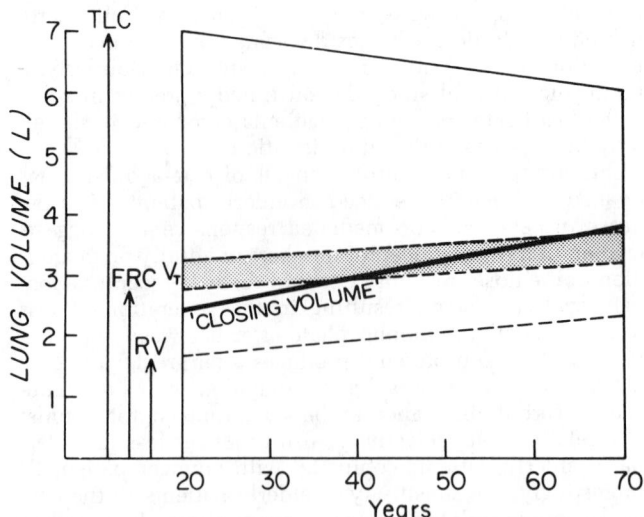

Figure 49-18. A comparison of pulmonary capacities and volumes at different ages. Total lung capacity (TLC) decreases with age. The reduction in alveoli and alveolar septa reduces tethering of terminal bronchioles and results in an increase in closing volume with advancing age. As closing volume increases with age, greater portions of tidal ventilation occur at lung volumes below closing volume, resulting in air trapping, V/Q mismatch, and an associated decrease in resting Pao2. (Reprinted with permission from Pontoppidan H, Geffins B, Lowenstein A: Acute respiratory failure in the adult. N Engl J Med 287:690, 1972.)

metabolic rate, who arrives in the recovery room hypothermic and shivering is also at risk for ventilatory failure. Therefore, it is easy to understand why elderly patients with reasonably adequate ventilatory reserve under normal preoperative conditions may have inadequate pulmonary reserves after operation. Not surprisingly, therefore, elderly patients more commonly require ventilatory support after operation until their metabolic needs are reduced and their ability to ventilate returns to preoperative levels.

Age-induced parenchymal changes of the lung mimic those of emphysema.[63] With aging, the pores of Kohn enlarge and coalesce into fenestrae, alveolar septa are lost, and alveolar spaces expand, producing decreased alveolar surface area and diminished pulmonary capillary bed density.[62] The progressive diminution in functional alveoli with age reduces elastic recoil of the lung, resulting in an increase in the ratio of residual volume to total lung capacity and the ratio of functional residual capacity to total lung capacity. In addition, because alveolar septa produce radial traction or tethering of the terminal bronchioles, a reduction in their quantity during aging makes the support framework for the terminal bronchioles less stable in geriatric patients. Thus, small airways will collapse at greater and greater lung volumes, producing an age-related increase in the "closing volume" of the lung (Fig. 49-18).[62] As closing volume increases with age, greater portions of tidal ventilation occur at lung volumes below closing volume, thus producing air trapping and ventilation-perfusion ratio (V/Q) mismatch. Other major contributors to the decline in gas exchange efficiency during aging include the reduced surface area of alveoli, increased alveolocapillary membrane thickness, re-

duced membrane permeability, and reduced pulmonary capillary blood volume. As a result, resting Pao2 normally declines with age at a rate described by the following equation:[64-66]

$$Pao_2 = 100 - (0.4 \times age\ [yr])\ mm\ Hg \qquad (49-2)$$

The normal decline in Pao2 with age is described by the "pre-op" line in Figure 49-19.[65] For the reasons described above, patients of all ages demonstrate a lower Pao2 value after operation compared with preoperative levels. As shown in Figure 49-19, this difference becomes more exaggerated as people age. The problem is particularly evident

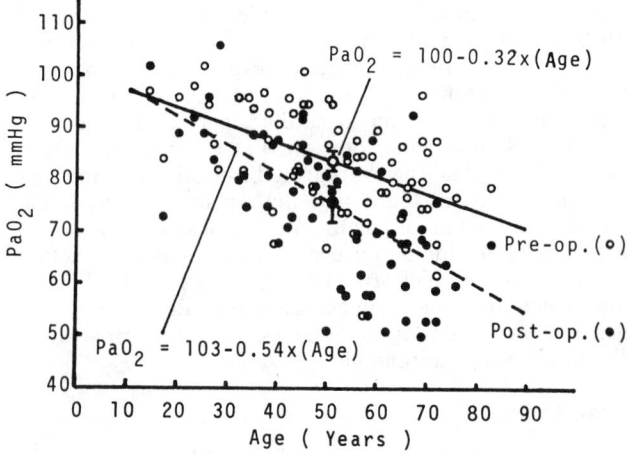

Figure 49-19. Relationship between Pao2 and age during room air breathing. (Reprinted with permission from Kitamura H, Sawa T, Ikezono E: Postoperative hypoxemia: The contribution of age to the maldistribution of ventilation. Anesthesiology 36:244, 1972.)

after upper abdominal and thoracic operations, in which there is significant postoperative splinting, causing an exaggeration in V/Q mismatch and dramatic decreases in PaO_2 after operation.[65] A change in position from sitting to supine will cause a 10 mm Hg decline in PaO_2 because of a reduced functional residual capacity and increased V/Q mismatch. The assumption of a supine posture after operation may partially explain the reduced Po_2 values observed in elderly patients after surgery.[67] In addition, the response to hypoxia or hypercapnia in healthy geriatric patients is approximately half that seen in younger persons.[69] This is further impaired by opioid premedication and by anesthetic drugs in a dose-related fashion.

For all of these reasons, elderly patients must be observed more closely after operation because their protective mechanisms against hypoxia and hypercapnia are less effective than those of younger patients. Elderly patients may require higher inspired intraoperative concentrations of oxygen because of their lower resting PaO_2 values and reduced efficiency of ventilatory exchange. Supplemental inspired oxygen should be considered for as long as 24 hours after operation or until adequate oxygenation is assured while the patient is breathing room air.

Central Nervous System

Classically, it has been thought that the physiologic function of most organs, including the central nervous system (CNS) undergoes a gradual decline during the aging process. Cross-sectional comparisons between age groups have shown significantly lower scores in many cognitive capacities for older age groups, commonly interpreted as reflecting a decline in CNS performance with advancing age. However, it now appears likely that a decline in mental function with age, should it occur, may be related more to nutritional or educational differences that occur as people age rather than to the aging process itself. Much of the loss of cognitive function in later life that has been considered intrinsic to aging may, in fact, be caused by extrinsic factors and therefore may be preventable with better nutrition and stimulation of mental function in the elderly population.[68]

On the other hand, age-related CNS disease is not uncommon in elderly patients. Dementia may result from localized areas of microemboli or from organic brain syndrome (a neuropsychiatric disorder associated with impaired brain tissue function). A common variety of this, Alzheimer's disease, is associated with cerebral atherosclerosis, which results in a gradual reduction of cerebral blood flow and CNS activity.

Although the presence of an obligatory age-induced decline in cerebral cognitive function remains controversial, it is generally agreed that geriatric patients have a reduced requirement for anesthetic agents. This may not be distinguishable in any given patient, but it is observed in cross-sectional studies comparing elderly patients with younger people and is believed to result, at least in part, from a reduction in pre-existent CNS activity. Muravchick suggests that we think of anesthetic requirement as resistance to loss of consciousness and that elderly people may have a reduced anesthetic requirement because of a decrement in this resistance.[70] An example of reduced CNS activity in the elderly is the age-dependent reduced sensitivity to painful stimuli (e.g., electrical stimulation).[71] A corollary to this is reported in a double-blind study of 712 patients in which the magnitude of pain relief after administration of either 10 mg morphine or 20 mg pentazocine correlated with age.[72]

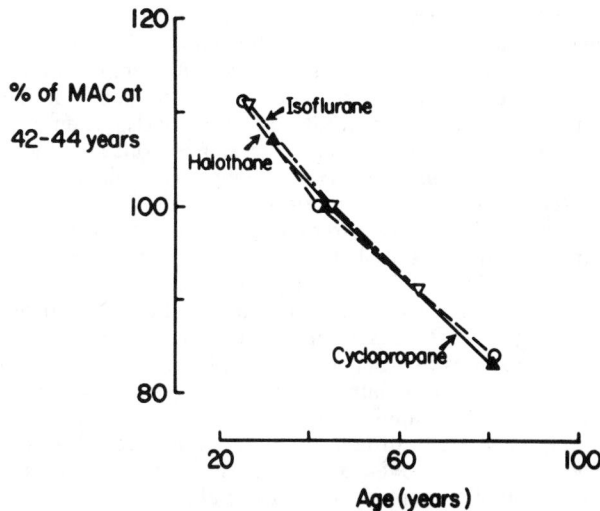

Figure 49-20. The relationship between anesthetic requirement (MAC) and age. MAC values are noted for persons of different ages receiving isoflurane, halothane, or cyclopropane. The parallelism of the three slopes indicates similar age-related effects on anesthetic requirements for all three inhalation agents. (Reprinted with permission of the International Anesthesia Research Society. From Munson ES, Hoffman JC, Eger EI: Use of cyclopropane to test generality of anesthetic requirement in the elderly. Anesth Analg 63:998, 1984.)

Evidence of an age-related reduced anesthetic requirement is the reduced minimum alveolar concentration (MAC) necessary to produce anesthesia in elderly patients with cyclopropane, halothane, or isoflurane.[73-75] The requirement for these inhalation agents decreases linearly with patient age (Fig. 49-20).

The reduced anesthetic requirement for geriatric patients applies not only to inhalation anesthetics but also to local anesthetics, opioids, barbiturates, benzodiazepines, and other intravenous anesthetic agents. Elderly patients achieve a comparable level of sedation at diazepam plasma concentrations significantly lower than those required in young adults. Equivalent electroencephalogram suppression occurs at lower plasma concentrations of both fentanyl and alfentanil in elderly patients.[76] As with opioids, the induction dose of barbiturates required in 70-year-old adults is approximately 30% less than that required for patients 4–5 decades younger. Arden et al found that the dose of etomidate required to reach a uniform electroencephalogram end point, indicative of anesthesia, decreased significantly with patients of increased age.[77] However, for the barbiturates and etomidate, it has been suggested that elderly patients' increased sensitivity to the drugs may relate more to differences in pharmacokinetics than to pharmacodynamics. For example, Christensen et al found that, in elderly patients, thiopental left the central compartment and entered the peripheral compartment at a slower rate.[78] This might allow the blood-brain barrier to be exposed to a greater concentration of drug for a longer period of time, thus permitting greater drug availability at receptor sites in the brain, producing enhanced pharmacologic action. Homer and Stanski, using the "spectral edge" determination of EEG frequencies as a measure of anesthetic depth, found that the serum concentration of thiopental required to induce anesthesia in elderly patients was no different from that of younger patients.[79] They explained elderly patients' greater sensitivity to a given dose of thiopental on the basis of a reduced volume of distribution, resulting in a higher plasma concentration. Similarly, for etomidate, a comparison of plasma concentrations of the drug to depth of anesthesia, as measured by electroencephalogram, demonstrated no increased brain sensitivity in the elderly when contrasted with the young. Rather, a greater response in elderly patients to a given dose of etomidate was explained by a decreased volume of distribution for this drug.[77]

Elderly patients may also demonstrate greater sensitivity to drugs on the basis of pharmacodynamic factors associated with aging. The CNS and peripheral nervous system undergo progressive anatomic and functional changes during the aging process that may influence the dose-response relationship to anesthetic agents. Multiple observations have been proposed to explain the enhanced responsiveness of elderly patients to anesthetic drugs.

First, there is a continual loss of neuronal substance with advancing age. On average, a daily attrition of perhaps as many as 50,000 neurons from an initial neuron pool of approximately 10,000,000,000 occurs during a person's life span. Cortical regions of the brain representing the peak of evolutionary development and those subcortical regions responsible for synthesis of neurotransmitters appear to have the most severe degree of age-related loss.[69,80] The gray matter fraction of human brain decreases from 45 to 35% of total brain weight during the time span between the ages of 20 and 80 years, and neuronal density of the occipital cortex decreases 48% during this time period.[81,82] By the time people reach age 80, brain weight has declined at least 15% from its maximal value of approximately 1400 g achieved at age 30 to a weight of between 1100 and 1200 g. Sapolsky et al reported a similar loss of neurons in the hippocampus of rats, a loss they believe eventually results in functional impairments typical of senescence.[83] Interestingly, their study revealed that exposure to corticosteroids accelerated the process of neuronal loss. They therefore concluded that age-related loss of neurons, resulting in an acceleration of the process of senescence, is exaggerated by stress or exposure to chronically elevated levels of corticosteroids. The reduction in neuronal density that occurs with age is accompanied by a parallel reduction in cerebral blood flow and cerebral oxygen consumption ($CMRO_2$) (Fig. 49-21).[84-86] Regional cerebral blood flow remains as tightly coupled to cerebral metabolic activity in the healthy elderly person as it does in young adults. Interestingly, Baughman et al, utilizing a unilateral cerebral ischemia model in rats, failed to demonstrate age-related differences in neurologic outcome following carotid artery ligation.[87] They concluded that cerebrovascular reactivity and neuronal viability may not be reduced by aging. The absence of a quantitative relationship between age-related brain atrophy (accompanied by reduced cerebral blood flow) and general level of mental function, however, suggests that at the time of maximum brain weight, there is considerable redundancy of neuronal function within each cortical, subcortical, and spinal region.

Peripherally, in nerve axons there is a loss of myelin, a reduction in the number of axons and synapses, and a diminished number of fibers in each tract. The reduction in axonal population may explain the decrease in nerve conduction velocity reported with increased age.[88] This, in turn, may be partially responsible for decreased function of feedback mechanisms that control hormone and enzyme release in response to various stimuli and also reduced baroreflex capability in elderly patients.

A second and closely related explanation for the greater sensitivity of elderly patients to anesthetics is a reduced number of receptor sites or a decrease in receptor affinity

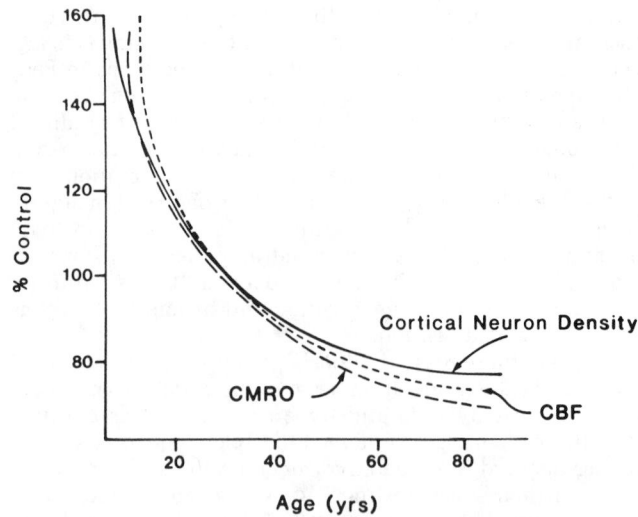

Figure 49-21. Cerebral blood flow (CBF), cerebral metabolic rate of oxygen consumption ($CMRO_2$), and cortical neuron density expressed as a percentage of control values at age 25 years. (Reprinted with permission from Hilgenberg JC: Inhalation and intravenous drugs in the elderly patient. Semin Anesth 5:44, 1986.)

for hormones and drugs in the brain. For example, the pharmacologic characteristics of the autonomic nervous system are altered, necessitating increased plasma norepinephrine levels in elderly patients to produce the same effects as lower levels in younger patients.[89] Beta-receptor density has also been observed to decrease in the cerebrum and cerebellum of rats and humans. The reduced sensitivity of the elderly to beta-adrenergic agents has been suggested to result from a functional alteration in beta receptor affinity or uncoupling of the beta receptor–adenylate cyclase system.[51] These age-related observations in the CNS parallel the changes in the cardiovascular system of the elderly that have been mentioned previously (see the section on Cardiovascular System).

A third theory proposed for the reduced anesthetic requirements of the elderly involves the rate of synthesis of neurotransmitters. A progressive and significant decrease in the concentration of enzymes that synthesize neurotransmitters is consistently seen in aging neural tissues.[90] Corresponding reductions in brain levels of neurotransmitters have been observed.[91] Reduced brain levels of dopamine, norepinephrine, tyrosine, and serotonin have also been observed.[92]

Although the exact explanation for why elderly people may be more sensitive to anesthetics remains unclear, the observation of their greater sensitivity to most agents is not in doubt. The anatomic and functional changes occurring in the CNS with aging that result in a reduced anesthetic requirement may also increase patients' risk for postoperative deterioration of mental function. This may be an issue of equal or even greater importance affecting the quality of an elderly patient's perioperative experience and is discussed more fully in the section on Regional Anesthesia Versus General Anesthesia.

Change in Body Compartments

Important age-related changes in body composition include a loss of skeletal muscle (lean body mass), an increase in percentage of body fat, and intracellular dehydration (Fig.

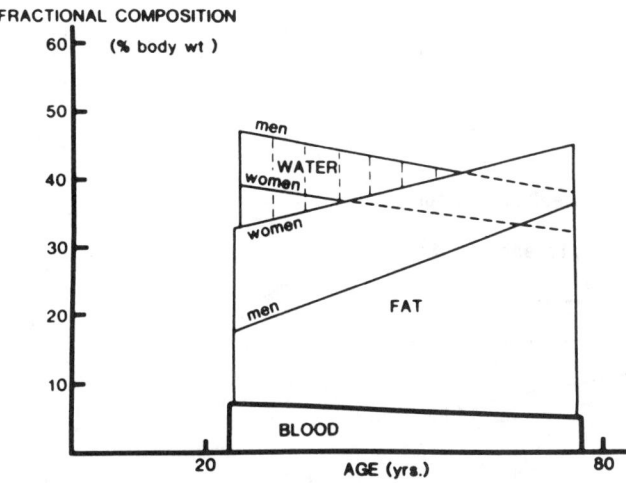

Figure 49-22. Change in fractional body composition with age. (Reprinted with permission from Muravchick S: Current concepts: Anesthetic pharmacology in geriatric patients. Prog Anesthesiol I:2, 1987.)

49-22).[70] The gradual decline in intracellular water content with aging simultaneously occurs with a comparable and slightly greater increase in percentage of body fat (Fig. 49-23).[7] These changes are more exaggerated in women. The reduction in total body water primarily represents intracellular dehydration and a reduction of blood volume. It has been suggested that a 20–30% reduction in blood volume occurs by age 75 (see Standard Cell Water, Fig. 49-13). Therefore, injection of anesthetic drugs is initially dispersed in a contracted blood volume in the elderly patient, producing a higher than expected initial plasma drug concentration (Fig. 49-24).

There is an approximate 10% decline in skeletal muscle mass (lean body mass) with aging. The average loss of muscle mass with age is estimated to be 6 kg at age 80, with more dramatic changes observed in women. Therefore, one might predict that the requirement for muscle relaxants

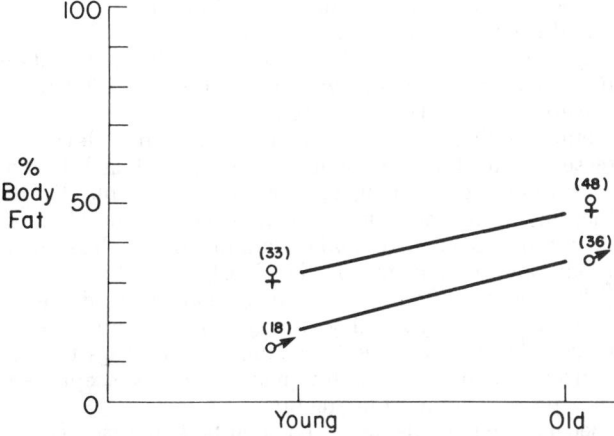

Figure 49-23. Age-related changes in percentage of body fat in nonobese subjects. At all ages, women tend to have a higher percentage of body fat than do men. The percentage of body weight that is fat increases with age. (Modified with permission from McLeskey CH: Anesthesia for the geriatric patient. In Stoelting RK, Barash PG, Gallagher TJ [eds]: Advances in Anesthesia, p 31. Chicago, Year Book Medical Publishers, 1985.)

would also be reduced and a lower initial dose might be required. However, in a variety of experimental studies, this has not been found to be the case. It has been proposed that, although there are reduced numbers of skeletal muscles available, there is similarly a reduced number of muscle receptors present to bind with exogenous muscle relaxants; on the whole, this makes elderly patients' sensitivity to muscle relaxants no different from that of younger patients. There are pharmacokinetic changes that affect the elimination of muscle relaxants, suggesting that the total dose of muscle relaxants should be reduced, but the initial sensitivity of elderly patients to muscle relaxants seems to be no different from that of a younger patient population.

The increase in percentage of body fat that occurs with age results in an increased availability of lipid-storage sites and a greater reservoir for deposition of lipid-soluble anesthetic drugs (see Fig. 49-23). The sequestration of anesthetics in lipid tissues of the elderly slows the elimination of drugs, results in greater residual plasma concentrations of drug, and prolongs anesthetic effects.

Protein Binding

All anesthetic agents are bound to plasma proteins to some extent. The portion of the drug that is bound to protein is unable to cross membranes, including the blood-brain barrier, and to produce an effect. Protein binding of anesthetic drugs is reduced in the elderly. As illustrated in Figure 49-24, a theoretical, highly lipid-soluble drug (that can cross the blood-brain barrier readily and be measured in cerebrospinal fluid) has been administered in the same intravenous bolus dose to a typical elderly person and a typical young adult. As discussed in the section on Change in Body Compartments, the smaller initial volume of distribution of elderly patients results in a higher initial plasma concentration. Also, because protein binding of anesthetic drugs is decreased in elderly patients, the cerebrospinal fluid or brain concentration more closely approaches the plasma concentration. Thus, for a given plasma concentration, one would predict a higher cerebrospinal fluid or brain level of anesthetic in elderly patients and a more profound anesthetic effect. The reduced protein binding of anesthetic drugs by elderly patients affects not only the distribution of those drugs but also their elimination. For the period of time a drug is bound to plasma protein, it is not available for metabolism or excretion. Thus, a decrease in binding of anesthetics to plasma proteins with aging should make more drug available for elimination and would have a minor effect in enhancing drug clearance.

Four factors may explain the reduced drug binding to serum protein in elderly patients. First, with aging, the circulating level of serum protein, especially albumin, decreases in quantity, reducing available protein binding sites. Second, qualitative changes may occur in circulating protein, which reduce the binding effectiveness of the available protein. Third, coadministered drugs may interfere with the ability of anesthetic drugs to bind to available serum protein-binding sites. Fourth, certain disease states may inhibit plasma protein binding of anesthetic drugs.

As mentioned above, during the aging process the circulating level of serum protein, especially albumin, and the binding effectiveness of those proteins are gradually reduced. Most drugs are bound to serum albumin, although other plasma proteins and erythrocytes contribute protein binding sites to a lesser degree. Although at one time controversial, it is now well documented that the concentration

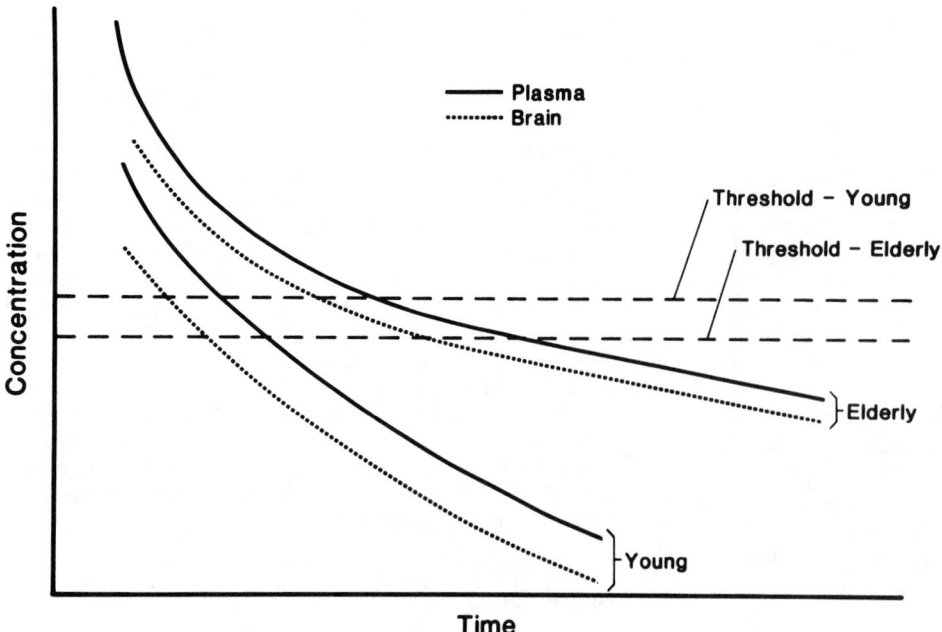

Figure 49-24. Pharmacokinetic and pharmacodynamic differences resulting from age-related physiologic changes. The curves represent the theoretical processes occurring in a typical young *versus* an elderly patient after receiving an identical intravenous bolus dose of an anesthetic. Elderly persons in general have a higher initial plasma drug concentration because of a contracted intravascular volume decreasing the initial volume of distribution of injected drugs. Elderly persons also in general have brain concentrations more closely approaching plasma concentrations because of less effective protein binding. The enhanced protein binding of anesthetic drugs in younger persons keeps more of the drug in the plasma, making it unavailable for transfer across the blood–brain barrier, and results in a lower brain concentration for a given plasma concentration. It is believed that for many drugs, such as opioids, a reduced plasma concentration and in turn a reduced brain concentration produce the same CNS effect in the elderly patient as that resulting from higher plasma and brain concentrations in the young. This is represented as a reduced "threshold" concentration in elderly persons. The end result of all these changes is that, for the same dose of a drug administered to an elderly person, a more profound and more prolonged drug effect may be expected compared with the effect on young patients.

of plasma albumin gradually declines during the aging process. For instance, in subjects younger than 50 years of age, the average plasma albumin concentration is 4.0 g·dl⁻¹, whereas in subjects older than 50 years of age, the albumin concentration is reduced to only 3.4 g·dl⁻¹.[93] In a study by Wallace et al,[94] young patients had an albumin concentration of 4.2 g·dl⁻¹, which reduced to 3.6 g·dl⁻¹ in healthy older patients. In a large, tightly controlled study, Greenblatt demonstrated a gradual decrease in plasma albumin concentration from approximately 4.0 g·dl⁻¹ in patients younger than 40 years of age to approximately 3.6 g·dl⁻¹ in patients 80 years of age or older.[95]

With the age-related quantitative decline in serum protein concentration, is there a simultaneous decrement in qualitative binding characteristics? Many authors believe that age is not associated with a major qualitative defect in the binding capacity of serum proteins.[93] In most studies in which there has been a reduced qualitative binding of drugs observed during aging, there has also been a simultaneous, parallel decrease in plasma albumin concentration, which explains the bulk of the observed decrement in protein binding.[96] A notable exception to this was observed for etomidate, where a qualitative difference in its binding by serum albumin exists between young adults and elderly patients. Old patients were observed to bind 4.1 mol of etomi-

date/mmol of albumin, whereas young patients bound almost 4.5 mol of etomidate/mmol of albumin.[97]

Acid drugs are bound primarily to albumin, while basic drugs may be preferentially bound to a different protein, alpha₁ acid glycoprotein, which was once thought to increase with age.[98] However, new data suggest that age has no effect on this protein although serum albumin levels decrease.[99] Thus, the binding of basic drugs such as lidocaine and propranolol is unchanged in elderly patients. On the other hand, most acid drugs, such as meperidine, thiopental, and diazepam, are bound to albumin and are less highly protein-bound on average in the elderly patient.[100]

The presence of one or more exogenous drugs decreases the protein binding of salicylates, sulfadiazine, and phenylbutazone.[94] Elderly patients consume more drugs than do younger patients and therefore may be more susceptible to this type of drug–drug interaction.

Because the incidence of concomitant diseases significantly increases in the elderly patient population (see the section on Effects of Concomitant Disease), the effect of these diseases on plasma protein binding should be considered. For example, Andreason demonstrated that the reduced protein binding of many drugs to the plasma proteins of patients with acute renal failure was explained only partially by the reduced albumin concentration present.[101] He

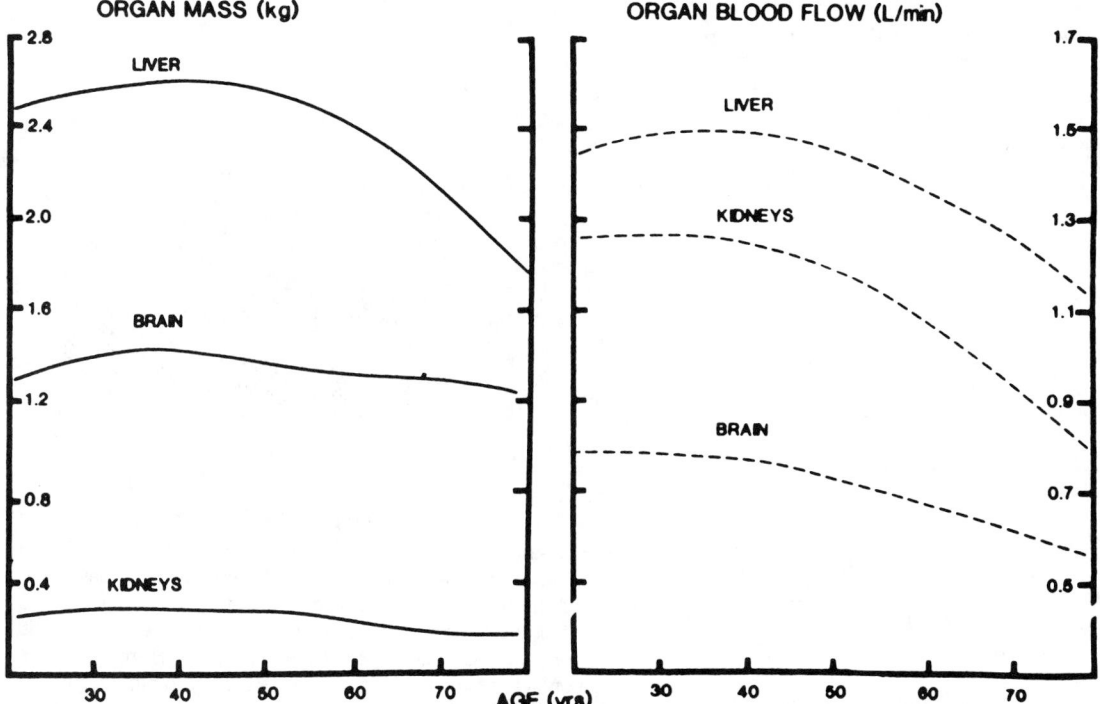

Figure 49-25. Age-related loss of organ mass and organ blood flow for the liver, kidneys, and brain. Reduction in hepatic metabolism with age results from loss of hepatic tissue and from reduced hepatic blood flow. (Reprinted with permission from Muravchick S: The aging patient and age related disease. ASA Annual Refresher Course Lecture 151, 1987.)

suggested that renal failure caused a structural change in plasma protein or resulted in an accumulation of bound substances to the protein, either of which would interfere with the qualitative effectiveness of albumin for drug binding.[102] Uremic patients generally have less effective binding of acidic drugs, whereas patients with hypoproteinemia resulting from any cause demonstrate reduced binding of both acidic and basic drugs.[103,104]

To summarize, because elderly patients have reduced quantities of circulating protein, may have qualitative defects in the binding capacity of their circulating proteins, are susceptible to drug interactions because of increased drug consumption, and may have an increased incidence of age-related pathologic conditions, an exaggerated clinical effect may be expected when drugs are administered that are highly protein-bound. As an example, consider a theoretical drug that is 98% protein-bound in a young healthy patient. Let us assume, because of the effects of aging on serum albumin, that protein binding decreases to 90% in an elderly patient. This seemingly minor 8% reduction in the amount of drug bound actually results in an increase in free drug availability from 2 to 10%, or a fivefold increased availability.

Renal Function

As other organ functions deteriorate, the number of effective renal glomeruli decreases with age. The glomerular filtration rate is reduced about 1 ml·min^{-1}·yr^{-1}, or about 1–1.5% per year (see Fig. 49-13).[105] In addition to reductions in glomerular function (filtration), tubular function (excretion) shows a parallel decline during aging. As a result, renal clearance of drugs and their metabolites is adversely affected.

The decrease in glomerular filtration rate is far more dramatic than the modest age-associated loss of renal tissue mass (Fig. 49-25), suggesting that reduced renal plasma flow may be the primary explanation for loss of renal function with age.[106] The reduced renal plasma flow associated with increased age may result from an overall age-associated decrease in cardiac output or, more important, from a reduction in the magnitude of the renal vascular bed. There is a disproportionately large loss of cortical renal tissue mass (glomeruli) with aging.

Creatinine, a normal metabolic by-product of muscle creatine, is excreted less efficiently in elderly patients, measured as a decrease in creatinine clearance rate (Table 49-7).[107] However, healthy geriatric patients have approximately the same circulating level of serum creatinine as do younger patients because there is less skeletal muscle and less creatinine production.[22] Measurement of serum creatinine levels in an attempt to determine renal function is therefore inaccurate; clearance of creatinine or another substance is a more appropriate test for accurately assessing renal function. Elevated serum creatinine levels in an elderly patient imply a decrement in renal function even greater than that normally observed with aging. The reduced capacity for renal clearance in elderly people also affects their ability to clear some anesthetic drugs and may contribute to a longer duration of action of these drugs.

There is sufficient residual renal function to prevent gross uremia, but renal functional reserve needed to withstand gross water or electrolyte imbalance is minimal in elderly patients. In addition, alterations in renal blood flow produced by dehydration, congestive heart failure, or excess

Age (yr)	Creatinine Clearance (ml·min^{-1}·1.73 m^{-2})	
	Men	Women
20	120	110
30	113	104
40	107	98
50	193	93
60	87	87
70	80	81
80		76

Reprinted with permission from Hicks R, Dysken MW, Davis JM et al: The pharmacokinetics of psychotropic medication in the elderly: A review. J Clin Psychiatry 42:374, 1981.

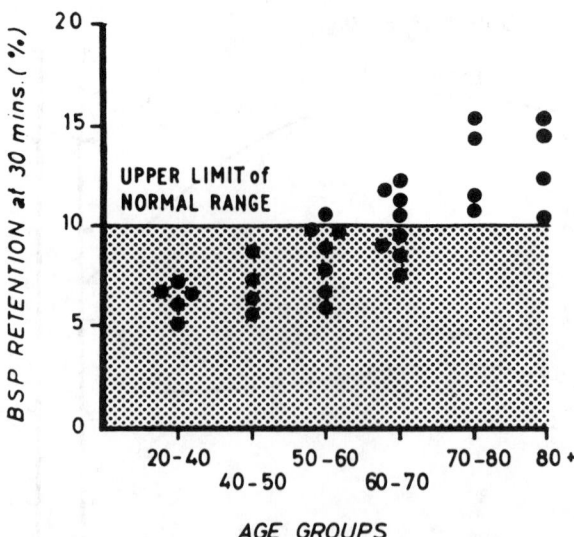

Figure 49-26. Percentage of administered bromsulphalein (BSP) retained after 30 minutes in patients of different ages. Increased BSP retention indicates reduced hepatic ability to clear this material and indicates a decline in hepatic function in patients older than age 50. (Reprinted with permission from Thompson EN, Williams R: Effect of age on liver function with particular reference to bromsulphalein excretion. Gut 6:266, 1965.)

sodium or water loads can easily lead to renal failure. Acute renal failure is responsible for a very high percentage of perioperative mortality seen in elderly surgical patients. The best way to protect the kidney during operation is to monitor and maintain urine output at a level of at least 0.5 ml·kg^{-1}·h^{-1}. It is interesting that, because of the reduced renal blood flow of aging, the renal threshold for serum glucose that results in glycosuria is also elevated in elderly patients. Two factors determine if glucose will spill from plasma to urine: the plasma glucose concentration and the amount of renal blood flow. In situations in which there is a reduced renal blood flow (such as that which occurs with aging), a higher plasma glucose concentration is required to reach the renal threshold, which will result in glycosuria. As a result, glycosuria, when present in an elderly patient, implies a far higher blood glucose concentration than that of younger glycosuric patients.

Hepatic Function

Lipid-soluble anesthetics filtered by the glomerulus are readily reabsorbed by the renal tubules and not excreted. The liver converts lipid-soluble drugs into water-soluble metabolites by many processes, including conjugation and oxidation. A water-soluble metabolite that is filtered by the glomerulus will be minimally reabsorbed through the tubules and, as a result, will be significantly excreted. Although results of standard liver function tests, notably serum bilirubin, albumin, and alkaline phosphatase levels, may be normal in geriatric patients, other tests reveal the decrement in hepatic function that parallels age. For example, impaired bromsulphalein (BSP) excretion may first be observed in patients older than 50 years of age and become progressively worse with increasing age (Fig. 49-26).[108]

The most likely explanation for reduced hepatic clearance of a variety of substances in elderly patients is the significant reduction in hepatic size that occurs with the aging process.[10,106] As shown in Figure 49-25, 40–50% of hepatic tissue may be lost by the age of 80, with a proportional reduction in hepatic blood flow. Hepatic blood flow is particularly important when considering drugs with extensive first-pass metabolism, such as propranolol. Compared with young patients, the elderly have been observed to have five-fold greater plasma levels of propranolol despite a lack of clinical evidence of hepatic, renal, or cardiac disease.[109]

Microsomal and nonmicrosomal hepatic enzyme concen-

tration or function appears to be maintained with aging. However, there are isolated reports that microsomal enzyme activity is reduced.[110] Age-related decreases in hepatic microsomal mixed function oxidase enzymes, especially cytochrome P-450, have been observed in aging rats.[111] These enzymes stimulate metabolism of toxic or potentially toxic substances to which all of us are exposed. The age-associated changes in this enzyme system may be partially responsible for the age-related increase in the incidence of tumors and deaths from cancer in our society.[112]

The effect of an age-associated reduction of hepatic blood flow and a potential reduction in microsomal enzyme function impair the liver's ability to metabolize anesthetics and nondepolarizing muscle relaxants. This, combined with the reduced filtration and excretory capability of the aging kidney, results in a more gradual decline in plasma concentration of drugs used in anesthesia in elderly patients (a prolonged beta elimination half-life) and contributes to a longer duration of effect (Fig. 49-24).

Basal Metabolic Rate and Thermoregulation

As seen in Figure 49-13, basal metabolic rate declines approximately 1% per year beyond age 30. Thus, drugs may be expected to be metabolized and excreted more slowly in elderly patients. In addition, the incidence of intraoperative hypothermia is explained at least in part by the decrease in metabolic rate with aging. Goldberg and Roe, in a study of 101 adult surgical patients, have shown that the difficulty in maintaining normothermia during general anesthesia is age-related.[113] Elderly patients had a greater decrease in rectal temperature than did young patients, even during short and relatively minor surgical procedures (Fig. 49-27). Not surprisingly, the development of intraoperative hypothermia also correlated with the length of operation. The ability of young patients to maintain intraoperative body tempera-

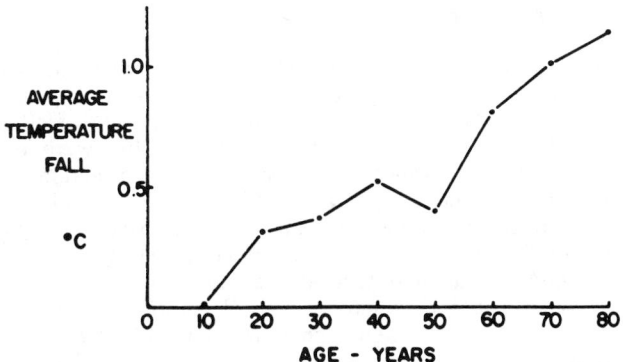

Figure 49-27. The relationship between patient age and intraoperative decline in rectal temperature. (Reprinted with permission from Goldberg MJ, Roe F: Temperature changes during anesthesia and operations. Arch Surg 93:365, 1966. Copyright 1966, American Medical Association.)

ture has been attributed, in part, to their higher basal metabolic rate and greater endogenous heat production (Fig. 49-28).

Elderly patients also experience more intraoperative hypothermia because of an impaired thermoregulatory system, which includes decreased heat production (as discussed above), increased heat loss, and deficient thermostat control.[114] Heat loss is common in all patients during general anesthesia because anesthetics alter thermoregulation, prevent shivering, and produce peripheral vasodilation. Healthy younger persons, exposed to a cold environment, reduce their heat loss to the environment by intense cutaneous vasoconstriction. The reduced autonomic peripheral vascular control of the elderly may lessen the effectiveness of this protective ability during anesthesia.

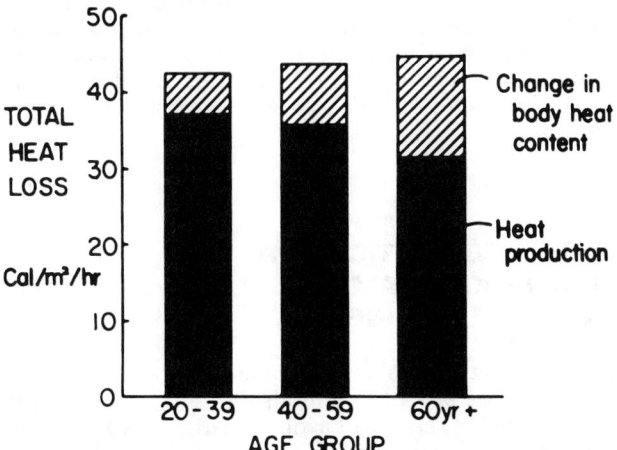

Figure 49-28. Intraoperative heat loss per unit time is slightly greater in older subjects. This is explained by a reduced basal heat production (*solid bars*), primarily resulting from a reduced basal metabolic rate in the elderly and a greater change in body heat content (*hatched bars*) as a result of lesser ability to vasoconstrict when placed in a cool environment (reduced autonomic neuronal function). When combined, these changes lead to a greater total intraoperative heat loss in elderly patients. (Reprinted with permission from Goldberg MJ, Roe F: Temperature changes during anesthesia and operations. Arch Surg 93:365, 1966. Copyright 1966, American Medical Association.)

Thus, because of elderly patients' impaired heat production and reduced ability to thermoregulate, it is not surprising that Vaughn *et al* have shown that patients older than 60 years of age are admitted to and discharged from the postanesthesia care unit with a lower measured body temperature than that of younger patients (Fig. 49-29).[115] The lower temperatures in elderly patients on discharge from the postanesthesia care unit relate to the fact that there is no difference in the rate of temperature rise in older compared with younger patients. Older subjects thus demonstrated a longer duration of hypothermia in the postanesthesia care unit than that seen in young patients.

Several adverse effects can result from hypothermia. The first problem is shivering. Postoperative shivering may represent a particular risk to the elderly patient because it significantly increases basal metabolic rate. Oxygen consumption must increase, perhaps as much as 400–500%, which increases demands on the cardiac and pulmonary systems.[116,117] In the elderly patient, if either system cannot adequately compensate for the increased demand produced by shivering, arterial hypoxemia may result. In addition, shivering may cause myocardial ischemia in geriatric patients (who frequently have occult coronary artery disease) because of the requirement for an increased cardiac output in the presence of peripheral vasoconstriction. It is fortunate to some extent that hypothermic patients between the ages of 60 and 80 years cannot increase their oxygen demands to the same degree by shivering as do younger patients.[121] However, this increases the time period required for elderly patients to return to normothermia. Protracted postoperative hypothermia also reduces elimination of anesthetics and prolongs awakening.

Another and longer lasting adverse effect of intraoperative hypothermia has been demonstrated by Carli et al.[118] In this study, urinary protein loss during the first 48 hours after operation was determined to quantitate postoperative catabolism. Elderly patients in whom normothermia was maintained during the intraoperative period had only minimal protein catabolism after operation. However, a similar group of elderly patients having a similar anesthetic, but who were

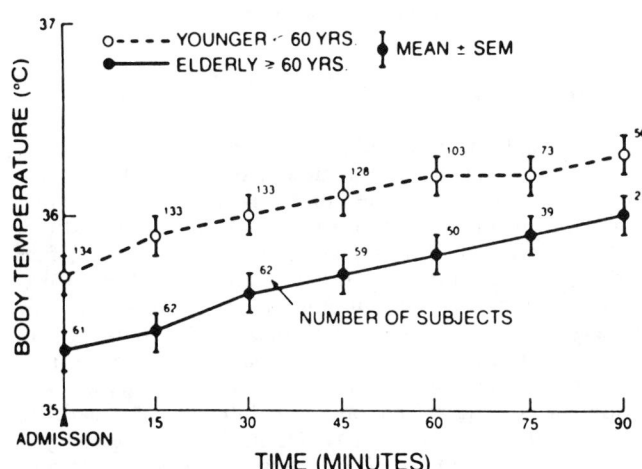

Figure 49-29. Tympanic membrane temperature in 198 patients measured at time of admission fo the postanesthesia care unit and at 15-minute intervals thereafter. (Reprinted with permission of the International Anesthesia Research Society. From Vaughn MS, Vaughn RW, Cork RC: Postoperative hypothermia in adults: Relationship of age, anesthesia and shivering to rewarming. Anesth Analg 60:746, 1981.)

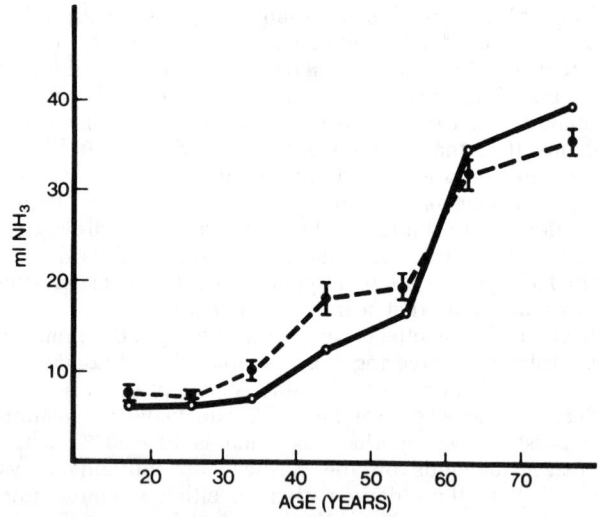

Figure 49-30. The volume of inhaled ammonia vapor required to cause volunteers of varying ages to hold their breath. Required volumes increase after age 30, indicating an age-related gradual decline in protective airway reflexes. (Reprinted with permission from Pontoppidan H, Beecher HK: Progressive loss of protective reflexes in the airway with the advance of age. JAMA 174:2209, 1960. Copyright 1960, American Medical Association.)

allowed to become hypothermic during operation, spilled significantly greater amounts of urinary nitrogen after surgery, indicating dramatically larger degrees of postoperative catabolism.

It is important to concentrate on maintaining intraoperative body temperature in all patients, but it is especially crucial in geriatric patients. Methods to reduce temperature loss include administering humidified and warmed inspired gases. In elderly patients undergoing joint replacement surgery, use of a heated humidifier has been shown to be superior to a heat and moisture exchanger (artificial nose) in maintaining core temperature intraoperatively and reducing shivering postoperatively.[119] Other methods such as reducing radiation losses by providing adequate blankets and maintaining a warm room are also beneficial.

Airway Reflexes

Laryngeal, pharyngeal, and airway reflexes are less effective in older patients. Pontoppidan and Beecher[120] have illustrated the gradual decline in protective airway reflexes that accompanies the aging process (Fig. 49-30). In their study, elderly patients had to inhale a much larger volume of an irritant gas, ammonia vapor, before airway protection was demonstrated. Thus, the blunting of laryngeal and airway reflexes in older patients makes these patients less able to protect their airways from foreign material and makes pulmonary aspiration more likely. A clinical corollary is that a patient who requires endotracheal intubation to facilitate surgical anesthesia should have tracheal extubation delayed during emergence until airway reflexes are as close to normal as possible. Older patients also have fewer cilia in their tracheobronchial tree and are less able to mobilize secretions. Coughing is less efficient in terms of volume, force, and flow rate compared with that of younger patients. For all these reasons, anesthesia and recovery room personnel must be very attentive to the state of an elderly person's airway to reduce the likelihood of pulmonary aspiration.

Endocrine System

It has been known for more than 60 years that advancing age is associated with progressive impairment in the capacity to metabolize a glucose load.[121] After patients with fasting hyperglycemia indicative of diabetes mellitus were excluded, elderly patients demonstrated an age-related increase in the 2-hour postprandial blood glucose level after oral or intravenous glucose administration. The same glucose intolerance has been demonstrated in a study in which intravenous infusion of glucose at a rate of 4 mg·kg^{-1}·min^{-1} produced a blood glucose level of approximately 200 mg·dl^{-1} in elderly patients, compared with 150 mg·dl^{-1} in young patients.[122]

It has been thought that pancreatic function declines during aging, explaining the increased incidence of glucose intolerance and diabetes mellitus that is observed in patients 60–70 years of age. The variability of insulin responsiveness and glucose tolerance increases substantially in people in successive age groups. In elderly patients, insulin liberation is sluggish in response to hyperglycemia. However, resistance to the effect of insulin at peripheral sites appears to play the major role in the genesis of glucose intolerance among older people without diabetes.[123] As with other insulin-resistant states, aging is associated with progressive increases in postprandial insulin levels.[124] As observed in other organ systems, much of the carbohydrate intolerance of older people may be caused by factors other than biologic aging. It has therefore been suggested that dietary or exercise modifications may substantially blunt the emergence with age of carbohydrate intolerance and insulin resistance.[125]

A variety of other endocrine changes occur during aging. For example, plasma renin concentration or activity is diminished 30–50% in elderly patients, which, in turn, results in a reduction in the plasma concentration of aldosterone. Alterations in the renin–aldosterone system contribute to an elderly person's increased risk of development of hyperkalemia in a variety of clinical settings, especially when potassium salts are administered intravenously. Van Brummelen *et al* have provided evidence of an age-related reduction in renin response to beta-adrenergic agents.[52] It is suggested that a less responsive beta adrenoreceptor contributes to the decrease in plasma renin activity with age.

PHARMACOKINETICS AND PHARMACODYNAMICS RELATIVE TO AGING

Pharmacokinetic variables determine the relationship between the dose of a drug administered and the concentration delivered at the site of action. Pharmacodynamic variables determine the relationship between the concentration of drug at the site of action and the intensity and duration of effect produced. Pharmacokinetics has been described as what the body does to the drug, whereas pharmacodynamics has been described as what the drug does to the body (see Chapter 13).

Aging significantly changes anesthetic drug distribution and elimination such that the elimination half-life ($T_{1/2\beta}$) for a drug may be significantly increased in an elderly patient.[126] The primary factors affecting $T_{1/2\beta}$ are the volume of distribution (VD) and clearance (Cl), as described by the equation that follows:

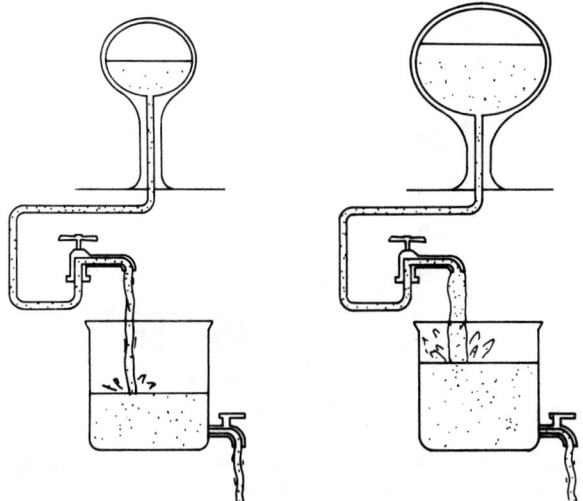

Figure 49-31. Relationship of volume of distribution of lipid-soluble drugs to emergence from anesthesia. The volume of distribution of these drugs can be viewed as a reservoir that is in equilibrium with the plasma. In the figure, the level of fluid in the beaker represents the plasma concentration of a given lipid-soluble drug. The *left panel* represents the clinical situation of young patients, whereas the *right panel* represents that of older patients. Elderly persons, with a greater percentage of body weight that is fat, may be thought of as having a larger reservoir for lipid-soluble drugs. These drugs administered to elderly persons are sequestered to a greater extent than in younger patients by filling to a greater capacity a larger reservoir. At the completion of an anesthetic, greater elution of drugs from larger lipid-storage sites in elderly patients tends to result in higher plasma concentrations for longer periods of time, producing delayed emergence from anesthesia.

$$T_{1/2\beta} = \frac{0.693 \times VD}{Cl} \qquad (49\text{-}3)$$

Volume of distribution relates to protein binding and, for a lipid-soluble drug, to the percentage of body weight that is lipid. Because elderly patients have increased body fat, as shown in Figure 49-23, they have a larger volume of distribution for lipid-soluble anesthetics. This can delay emergence from anesthesia. As illustrated in Figure 49-31, volume of distribution can be viewed as a reservoir of drugs that is in equilibrium with the plasma. With a larger volume of distribution and a greater drug sequestration, the plasma concentration of a lipid-soluble anesthetic decreases more slowly at the end of a surgical procedure because of constant movement of drug from the storage site into the bloodstream, even if clearance is rapid. Thus, according to Equation 49-3, the increased volume of distribution of anesthetic drugs in elderly patients will significantly prolong the beta elimination half-life, assuming no change in clearance occurs, and the prolonged beta elimination half-life will contribute to an overall extended duration of action of anesthetics. Once the storage sites for a lipid-soluble anesthetic are saturated, elution of drugs from this storage site will be relatively constant. In this situation, if a fixed plasma concentration of a drug is desired, it can be given by incremental administrations at greater intervals or by a continuous infusion at a slower rate. Thus, any of the highly lipid-soluble anesthetic drugs, e.g., barbiturates, benzodiazepines, and opioids, have an increased steady-state plasma

concentration in elderly patients, resulting from a prolonged beta elimination half-life.

On the other hand, clearance of a drug, expressed in units of volume per unit time, represents the hypothetical volume of blood from which a drug would be completely cleared in a given period of time. Clearance is inversely related to the beta elimination half-life of drugs (Equation 49-3). Clearance thus indicates a person's ability to remove or eliminate a drug and usually relates to the efficiency of hepatic metabolism and renal elimination. For the inhalation anesthetics, clearance relates primarily to the efficiency of the cardiovascular system in delivering stored anesthetics to the lung and, in turn, to the efficiency of the pulmonary system in their removal to the atmosphere.

As illustrated in Figure 49-13, hepatic and renal functions are reduced about 1% per year beyond age 30. The effect of these age-related changes on hepatic clearance of drugs is complex. A useful scheme categorizing the biotransformation reactions in the liver characterizes reactions as either Phase I (preparative) or Phase II (synthetic). Phase I activity includes reactions such as oxidation, reduction, and hydrolysis. These preparative reactions generally constitute minor molecular modifications, yielding products that may be slightly more water-soluble than the parent compound but that may retain part of its pharmacologic activity. Phase II reactions involve conjugation or attachment of a drug molecule to a larger component, such as glucuronide, making the compound more polar and more available for renal excretion. Aging appears to have little effect on Phase II reactions but impairs Phase I reactions, leading to a reduced total drug clearance and higher steady-state plasma concentration of drugs. As discussed above, hepatic function is impaired because of loss of cellular function and reduced hepatic blood flow (see Figure 49-25). Hepatic blood flow declines with age partly because of reduced cardiac output but primarily because of a reduced mass of hepatocytes, with an overall 40–50% reduction in hepatic mass and hepatic perfusion in the elderly. For drugs that are metabolized readily by the liver, hepatic blood flow is the major factor determining clearance rate.

Renal blood flow similarly decreases by about 1% per year beyond age 30 and is accompanied by a gradual loss of functioning glomeruli. The combination of these changes produces a predictable decline in glomerular filtration rate in older people that is only 60% of that found in younger people. Because of these renal changes elderly patients have a reduced ability to excrete drugs and their metabolites.

Pharmacodynamics describes the responsiveness of receptors at the effector site. It is quantitated by determining the plasma concentration–drug response relationship when equilibrium has been achieved between the drug and the receptor. The pharmacodynamics of anesthetic drugs in elderly patients is difficult to determine and has not been extensively studied. The age-associated decline in CNS function, accompanied by a decrease in neuronal and synaptic density, would probably cause elderly patients to be more sensitive to anesthetics and, in turn, to have reduced anesthetic requirements (see the section on Central Nervous System).

Although it is generally agreed that geriatric patients require reduced quantities of anesthetics compared with younger patients, the overlap between pharmacokinetics and pharmacodynamics makes it difficult to substantiate a primary pharmacodynamic explanation for this difference. The next section addresses the pharmacokinetic and pharmacodynamic differences of the elderly patient regarding specific anesthetic drugs.

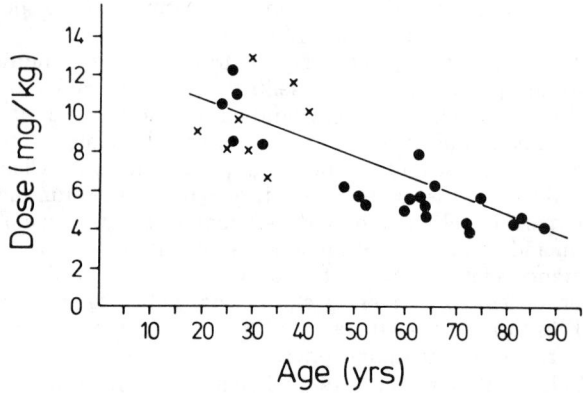

Figure 49-32. The dose of thiopental required to induce anesthesia (quantitated by burst suppression on EEG) decreases with age. Because the arterial plasma concentration of thiopental required to produce this effect is not different in elderly patients from that in younger patients, the reduced dose requirement for thiopental in elderly patients must reflect a pharmacokinetic difference. Elderly patients have a reduced initial volume of distribution, which results in a higher plasma concentration after any given administered thiopental dose. Thus, a lower dose is required in these patients to achieve the same anesthetic effect. (Reprinted with permission from Homer, TD, Stanski DR: The effect of increasing age on thiopental disposition and anesthetic requirement. Anesthesiology 62:714, 1985.)

Intravenous Agents

Barbiturates

Numerous studies have shown that the dose of thiopental required to induce anesthesia in elderly patients is less than that for younger patients.[77-79] The lowest dose of thiopental necessary to produce loss of consciousness (failure to "open eyes" on command) in geriatric patients is only 1.26 mg·kg^{-1} compared with 2.24 mg·kg^{-1} in young adult patients.[77] The dose required to abolish the ciliary reflex in elderly patients (3.9 mg·kg^{-1}) is significantly less than that for younger patients (5.3 mg·kg^{-1}).[78] Similarly, as shown in Figure 49-32, the dose of thiopental required to produce early burst suppression on the EEG (Stage III) decreases with advancing age.[79] Instead of the age-related decrease in thiopental dose requirements shown by others, Christensen and Andreason found that most adult patients premedicated with diazepam, meperidine, and atropine required about the same dose of thiopental for induction of anesthesia until age 60. At that age, a permanent step change occurred whereby the dose requirement for anesthesia was significantly less.[127]

Several authors have determined that the arterial plasma concentration of thiopental required to induce anesthesia is not different in elderly patients *versus* younger patients.[79,128] Using a 50% decrease in "spectral edge" EEG frequency as a measure of anesthetic depth, Homer and Stanski found that despite a reduced dose of thiopental required to produce this response in elderly patients, the serum concentration of thiopental was no different in the two groups.[79] Thus, it appears that the lower dose of thiopental required in elderly patients has a pharmacokinetic rather than a pharmacodynamic explanation. Elderly people have a reduced initial volume of distribution, a larger volume of distribution at steady state, and reduced clearance. Very likely, the smaller initial volume of distribution results in

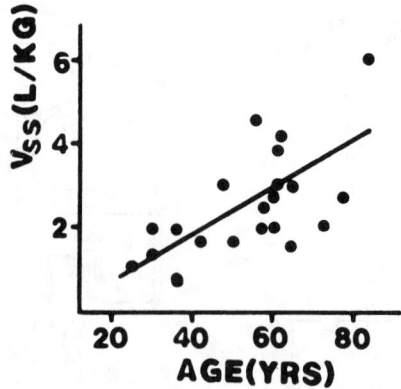

Figure 49-33. Relationship between the volume of distribution at steady state (Vss) for thiopental *versus* patient age. The greater percentage of body weight that is fat in elderly patients explains the greater volume of distribution of the lipid-soluble drug thiopental in this age group. (Reprinted with permission from Jung D, Mayersohn M, Perrier D *et al*: Thiopental disposition as a function of age in female patients undergoing surgery. Anesthesiology 56:263, 1982.)

a higher plasma concentration in the elderly after any given thiopental dose.

In addition, barbiturates have a longer duration of effect in elderly patients. For example, rats receiving hexobarbital at 3-month intervals have a duration of hypnosis that increases linearly with age.[129] In humans, recovery from thiopental anesthesia requires 28.5 minutes in young patients compared with more than 45 minutes in elderly patients.[130] The age-related increased duration of hypnosis with barbiturates may result from a decline in hepatic enzyme function but more likely results from age-related changes in volume of distribution.[129] The steady-state volume of distribution of the lipid-soluble drug thiopental increases 35% in geriatric patients (Fig. 49-33), largely explaining the 20% increase in beta elimination half-life (see Equation 49-3).[131]

The onset of action of barbiturates is also delayed in the elderly. Muravchick demonstrated that loss of eyelash reflex after thiopental administration to geriatric patients required 48 seconds compared with 39 seconds in younger patients.[132] This may be a consequence of a decreased cardiac index and prolonged circulation time seen with advancing age. Also, it may result from the fact that the cardiovascular system of elderly patients is more sensitive to thiopental.[128] After an intravenous barbiturate induction technique, cardiac output, determined by impedance cardiography, was reduced 6% in young patients and 13% in elderly patients. This effect of barbiturates on cardiac output can contribute both to a delay in onset of action and a prolonged clinical effect because of reduced clearance.

Benzodiazepines

The elderly patient is pharmacodynamically more sensitive to benzodiazepines.[133,134] The initial dose and resultant plasma concentration of diazepam preventing response to verbal stimulation, before cardioversion, is significantly lower in elderly patients. In addition, the dose of diazepam producing sedation (grip relaxation) for endoscopic and dental procedures averages 10 mg in 80-year-old patients and 30 mg in 20-year-old patients. A similar observation has been made by Bell *et al* in that the dose of midazolam

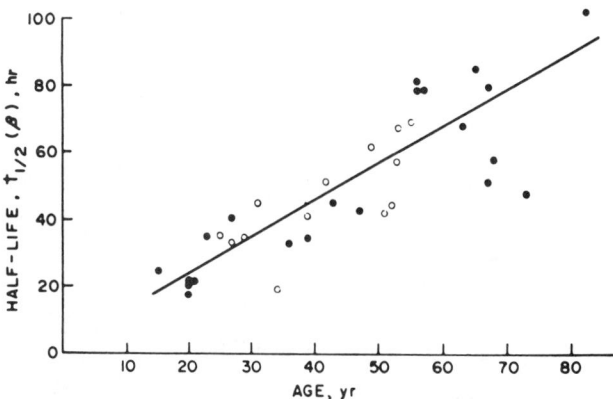

Figure 49-34. The relationship of the beta elimination half-life for diazepam with age. The deterioration with age in metabolism of diazepam results in an age-dependent prolongation of diazepam's effect. (Reprinted with permission of the American Society for Clinical Investigation. From Klotz U, Avant GR, Hoyumpa A et al: The effects of age and liver disease on the disposition and elimination of diazepam in adult man. J Clin Invest 55:347, 1975.)

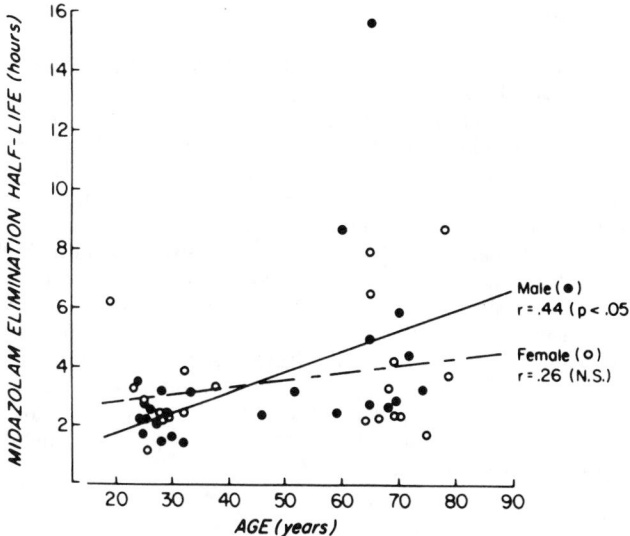

Figure 49-35. The relationship of age to midazolam's elimination half-life in men and women. Because midazolam is metabolized by hepatic microsomal oxidation, its clearance rate is reduced with age. As a result, the elimination half-life of this drug is more than twice as long in elderly men as it is in younger volunteers. The age-related prolongation of midazolam's elimination half-life is less dramatic, although quite variable, in women. (Reprinted with permission from Reves JG, Fragen RJ, Vinik HR et al: Midazolam: Pharmacology and uses. Anesthesiology 62:310, 1985.)

required to induce ptosis in upper gastrointestinal endoscopy patients averages 10 mg in patients age 20 vs. only 2 mg in patients age 85.[135]

Age also affects the pharmacokinetics of benzodiazepines. An age-related impairment of hepatic microsomal oxidation of benzodiazepines results in a prolonged beta elimination half-life for these drugs in elderly patients. As shown in Figure 49-34, a rule of thumb for diazepam is that the beta elimination half-life in hours is approximately the same as the patient's age in years.[136] This is borne out by clinical observations of prolonged sedative effects after relatively low doses of diazepam in the elderly. Because diazepam impairs performance for almost 24 hours in healthy young patients, its prolonged beta elimination half-life in elderly patients emphasizes the need to administer this drug very carefully to older patients.[86]

Newer benzodiazepines have the advantage of a more rapid metabolism to inactive metabolites, resulting in a shorter beta elimination half-life and a shorter duration of pharmacologic action. For this reason, midazolam may have a potential advantage in elderly patients, but, as with other benzodiazepines, it also has greater pharmacodynamic activity in this group. In a dose of 0.3 mg·kg^{-1}, midazolam induces sleep in 100% of unpremedicated elderly patients (62–76 years), whereas a higher dose of 0.5 mg·kg^{-1} successfully induces anesthesia in only 60% of younger adults (29–40 years).[137] Reports of adverse reactions to midazolam in elderly patients (as a result of an enhanced sensitivity to this drug) have prompted a change in its product labeling, with more conservative dosage recommendations for elderly patients. Because midazolam is also metabolized by hepatic microsomal oxidation, its clearance rate is reduced with age. As a result, the elimination half-life for this drug is more than twice as long in elderly patients compared with that for young, male volunteers.[138] In women, the age-related prolongation of the beta elimination half-life of midazolam is less evident (Fig. 49-35).

Opioids

Age-related pharmacokinetic and pharmacodynamic differences exist for opioids as well. The beta elimination half-life

of morphine is 4.5 hours in older patients, significantly longer than the 2.9 hours observed in younger adults.[139] This primarily results from an increased volume of distribution and only secondarily from decreased clearance. Reduced protein binding with age also has importance for the opioids, especially meperidine. For example, the unbound fraction of meperidine increases from 30% at age 30 to approximately 70% at age 70. This may result in an exaggerated drug effect in elderly patients.[72,140]

Of all the currently available opioids, fentanyl and its analogues may be best suited for geriatric patients. These drugs have a shorter beta elimination half-life compared with their predecessors, and they appear to be better able to blunt the cardiovascular and hormonal responses to intraoperative noxious stimuli. In addition, they are less depressant to myocardial function and cardiac output. However, as with most other drugs, the beta elimination half-life for fentanyl, alfentanil, and other newer opioids is also prolonged in elderly patients. For example, fentanyl has a beta elimination half-life of 265 minutes in young patients compared with 945 minutes in elderly patients, whereas alfentanil has an extension of its 83-minute beta elimination half-life in young patients to 137 minutes in the elderly.[141,142]

As with the barbiturates and benzodiazepines, elderly patients also demonstrate a greater sensitivity to opioids. Scott and Stanski have shown that the dose requirement for fentanyl or alfentanil is decreased approximately 50% in elderly patients.[143] They observed only minor pharmacokinetic differences in this age group and concluded that brain sensitivity (as determined by the "spectral edge" on an EEG) was significantly enhanced in the elderly because of pharmacodynamic factors. Thus, unlike with barbiturates, pharmacodynamic factors appear to explain why fentanyl and its analogues may have a greater effect in elderly patients.

Etomidate

Etomidate, an imidazole intravenous hynotic drug, is associated with hemodynamic stability, which may offer an advantage for induction of anesthesia in elderly patients, especially those with limited cardiovascular reserve. However, pharmacokinetic differences also exist for this drug in elderly patients. Plasma clearance is reduced 37% and beta elimination half-life is increased 61% in elderly patients.[77] Reduced hepatic blood flow and metabolism explain this alteration. The dose of etomidate required to reach uniform EEG depression, an end point of anesthesia, significantly decreases with age.[77] Thus, etomidate is similar to thiopental. There is no change in the drug's pharmacodynamics in elderly people, but a smaller initial volume of distribution results in the development of a higher initial plasma concentration and the need for a reduced dosage requirement in elderly patients.

Propofol

Propofol, a diisopropylphenol, is touted as providing a more rapid and lucid emergence from anesthesia when compared with other intravenous anesthetics. It is a reasonable agent for consideration in the geriatric patient. However, because of the pharmacokinetic changes accompanying the aging process, dosing of this drug in the elderly needs to be altered from the technique utilized in a younger patient population. Kirkpatrick et al have demonstrated a central compartment for propofol that is significantly smaller in patients 65–80 years old compared with those 18–35 years of age.[144] As a result, in spite of reducing the intravenous induction dose from 2.5 mg·kg^{-1} in younger patients to 2.0 mg·kg^{-1} in older patients, a higher average plasma propofol concentration developed in the older patients. Very likely as a result, Dundee et al have shown clinically that the induction dose of propofol in patients under age 60 is 2.25–2.50 mg·kg^{-1}, compared with an average induction dose of 1.5–1.75 mg·kg^{-1} in patients over age 60.[145] They emphasized that side-effects, especially hypotension, were more marked in the elderly if propofol was injected rapidly and in a dose exceeding 1.75 mg·kg^{-1}. Clearance rates of propofol have also been shown to be reduced in the elderly[146] and this probably explains why clinically lower maintenance infusion rates are recommended in the elderly.[147]

Inhalation Drugs

The MAC of potent inhalation drugs decreases with advancing age (see Fig. 49-20).[75] A rough estimate for the true MAC value in elderly patients may be obtained by decreasing the published MAC values approximately 4% for each decade of life over age 40. Age-related changes in cerebral metabolism correspond to changes in MAC requirements, emphasizing the pharmacodynamic correlation between cerebral metabolic function and anesthetic requirements for inhalation drugs (Fig. 49-36).[86]

Many of the physiologic changes of aging discussed earlier suggest that desflurane and isoflurane have a number of advantages for geriatric patients compared with other inhalation drugs. Because geriatric patients metabolize drugs less readily, any anesthetic that requires metabolism to terminate its activity would be expected to have a more prolonged effect in the elderly. Desflurane and isoflurane are less metabolized than other potent inhalation anesthetics. Similarly, potentially toxic metabolites, such as fluoride,

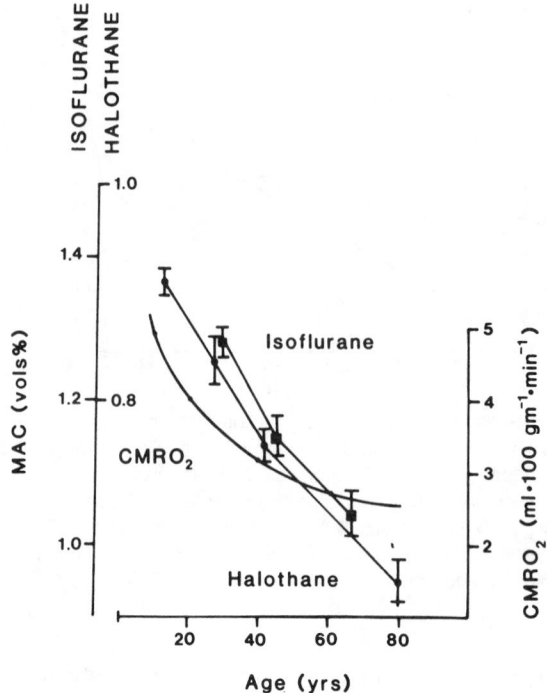

Figure 49-36. Alveolar concentrations of inhalation anesthetics required to produce anesthesia (minimum alveolar concentration) decrease with age. Age-related changes in cerebral metabolism reflected as changes in cerebral metabolic requirements for oxygen (CMRo$_2$) are similar to changes in minimum alveolar concentration requirements, emphasizing the pharmacodynamic correlation of cerebral metabolic function to anesthetic requirement. (Reprinted with permission of Grune & Stratton, Orlando. From Hilgenberg JC: Inhalation and intravenous drugs in the elderly patient. Semin Anesth 5:44, 1986.)

exist in lower concentrations after desflurane and isoflurane anesthesia than after enflurane or methoxyflurane anesthesia. This may be even more important in obese elderly patients, in whom (like the younger obese patient) the percentage of body fat is increased. Desflurane and isoflurane's low solubility in blood, relative to other potent inhaled anesthetics, not only increases the speed of recovery from anesthesia but also permits somewhat easier control of depth of anesthesia. Because geriatric patients tend to have greater intraoperative blood pressure lability compared with younger normotensive patients, a drug that can be added and removed rapidly is advantageous. All inhalation anesthetics reduce myocardial contractility and produce peripheral vasodilation. However, studies in human volunteers suggest that desflurane and isoflurane produce substantially less depression of myocardial contractility and left ventricular ejection fraction than either halothane or enflurane.[148] Preexisting congestive heart failure exaggerates the myocardial depression produced by inhalation anesthetics.[149] In young adults, the decreased stroke volume produced by isoflurane is offset by a compensatory increase in heart rate such that cardiac output is not significantly altered. In contrast, isoflurane reduces cardiac output in elderly patients because there is a smaller compensatory increase in heart rate.

A decreased cardiac output in elderly patients would be expected to produce a more rapid increase in the alveolar, arterial, and tissue concentrations of inhalation anesthetics during induction of anesthesia. The increased V/Q mismatch that occurs with aging should accelerate the rate of

TABLE 49-8. Pharmacokinetics of Nondepolarizing Relaxants in Elderly Patients

	Volume of Distribution ($l \cdot kg^{-1}$)	Plasma Clearance ($ml \cdot kg^{-1} \cdot min^{-1}$)	Elimination Half-Life (min)	Reference
Alcuronium	0.29	1.2	182	151
Metocurine	0.26	0.4	530	152
Pancuronium	0.26	1.28	204	154
d-Tubocurarine	0.22	0.8	268	152
Vecuronium	0.18	3.7	58	155
Atracurium	0.16	5.5	20	158

rise of end-tidal partial pressures of inhalation anesthetics, whereas the rate of increase of arterial partial pressures should be retarded. However, very little pharmacokinetic investigation of inhalation anesthetics in elderly patients has been performed. Lerman et al have shown that, with aging, volatile anesthetic drugs are more soluble in blood and body tissues, which tends to delay induction of anesthesia with inhalation agents.[150] Overall, however, there appear to be no obvious clinically significant differences in the pharmacokinetics of inhalation drugs resulting from age-related changes.

Muscle Relaxants

Skeletal muscles, the neuromuscular junction, and nerves deteriorate with age. As a result, the volumes of distribution for metocurine, d-tubocurarine, and vecuronium are all decreased in elderly patients (Table 49-8). Because elderly patients have a reduced skeletal muscle mass compared with younger patients, one might expect that the initial requirements for neuromuscular blocking agents would be reduced. However, these results have not been obtained in clinical studies. For example, the potency of d-tubocurarine was no different in patients older than 66 years of age than in younger patients.[152,153] The response of elderly patients (older than 75 years of age) to a given pancuronium dose was comparable to that of patients younger than 60 years of age.[154] Similarly, no correlation has been observed between age and maximum effect from a given dose of vecuronium[155-157] or atracurium.[158] Thus, in general, there is no difference in original dosing requirements for nondepolarizing muscle relaxants in elderly patients compared with younger patients.

Nondepolarizing muscle relaxants (with the exception of atracurium) are usually highly polarized, relatively fat-insoluble, and dependent on urinary excretion for elimination from the body. Metabolism and direct biliary excretion, although important, play lesser roles. Because elderly patients metabolize and eliminate most drugs more slowly, a longer duration of action of nondepolarizing relaxants may be expected. With the exception of atracurium, there is a reduction in clearance and an increase in elimination half-life for most nondepolarizing relaxants.

Pancuronium clearance has been shown to be significantly reduced in a geriatric group, necessitating its administration at less frequent intervals than with younger patients. When administered by continuous infusion, pancuronium is effective at lower infusion rates in elderly patients. The time for recovery of twitch tension to 25% of control after pancuronium administration was prolonged from 44 to 73 minutes in elderly patients. This is principally due to a 35% decrease in plasma clearance, resulting in an elimination half-life of 204 minutes compared with 107 minutes in younger adult patients.[154] It is therefore perhaps fortunate that the reversal agents neostigmine and pydostigmine appear to have a prolonged duration of effect in the elderly compared with younger patients.[159]

Vecuronium clearance is also decreased in elderly patients. Lien et al have demonstrated a vecuronium clearance of 5.6 $ml \cdot kg^{-1} \cdot min^{-1}$ in patients with an average age of 41 years compared with a clearance rate less than 50% as rapid in patients with an average age of 77 years.[160] As might be expected, recovery time after vecuronium administration correlates directly with age.[156] After steady-state infusion, elderly patients require 45 minutes for recovery as compared with 17 minutes in young adults.[155] In general, in the elderly, the reduction in requirements for nondepolarizing relaxants administered by infusion is explained on a pharmacokinetic basis (reduced clearance) rather than on a pharmacodynamic basis.

The time to onset of action with nondepolarizing muscle relaxants is also age-related, as is the time for maximal effect. This implies that there is a slower circulation time in elderly people or that receptor site sensitivity is reduced.[156]

Atracurium is different from other nondepolarizing relaxants in that its action and elimination in elderly patients are very similar to that in younger patients.[161,162] Although atracurium is eliminated by both organ-dependent and nonorgan-dependent mechanisms, the total clearance rate of atracurium in older adults (average age 75) does not appear to be statistically different from that in younger adults (average age 33).[158] Other authors have also not shown significant age-related changes in steady-state dose requirements for atracurium, indicating that inactivation of the drug by Hofmann elimination or plasma ester hydrolysis is independent of age.[163]

Two long-acting nondepolarizing neuromuscular blocking drugs, doxacurium and pipecuronium, require hepatic and renal function for elimination. One would expect less effective clearance and longer duration of effect of both of these agents in the elderly patient. However, surprisingly, these differences are relatively small. For example, the $T_{1/2\beta}$ of doxacurium in older subjects is 96 minutes compared with 86 minutes in younger subjects.[164] Similar observations have been made for pipecuronium with a $T_{1/2\beta}$ of 122 minutes in older subjects, compared with 113 minutes in younger subjects.[165]

With aging there is the suggestion that trophic support for the neuromuscular junction decreases. There is a loss of peripheral nerve axons, resulting in a net proliferation of muscle end plates and an increase in the number of acetylcholine receptors. This fact, along with the observation of a reduced level of plasma cholinesterase in elderly patients, may explain why the same degree of muscle blockade can be produced in the elderly from a lower dose of succinylcholine.[166,167]

Mivacurium, a short-acting, nondepolarizing neuromuscular blocking drug, also requires plasma cholinesterase for elimination and may have a slightly longer duration of effect in the elderly. On the other hand, if cardiac output is reduced significantly in elderly patients, succinylcholine may be less effective because a slower circulation time would permit a longer exposure of succinylcholine to plasma cholinesterase and allow greater metabolism and inactivation of the drug before its delivery to the neuromuscular junction. Overall, the pharmacokinetic and pharmacodynamic differences observed in elderly people produce minimal clinical differences in succinylcholine dose requirements.

Local/Regional Anesthesia Techniques

Controversy surrounds the question of reduced local anesthetic requirements for epidural, spinal, and regional anesthesia in elderly patients compared with younger patients. There are anatomic changes that occur with aging that suggest a generalized reduction in the requirement for local anesthetic drugs. For example, there is a decrease in the quantity and a change in the configuration of myelinated fibers in the dorsal and ventral roots of the spinal cord. By age 90, only approximately one third of the original neuronal population remains.[167] In general, the number of axons in peripheral nerves decreases, similar to the decline in CNS neuronal concentration.[168] Functional changes also occur that result in increased permeability of extraneural tissues with advanced age.[169] As myelin sheaths deteriorate and nerve fibers decrease in number, it is reasonable to postulate a reduced requirement for local anesthetics.

Because there is a narrowing of intervertebral spaces and osteophytic growth in elderly patients, Bromage suggested that local anesthetics injected during epidural anesthesia would be less likely to spread outward (transforaminal escape) and would be more likely to spread upward in the spinal canal, producing an increased level of block.[170] Park et al confirmed this concept when they found that local anesthetic requirements declined from 0.69 ml·segment^{-1}·m^{-1} of patient height to a dose of 0.62 ml·segment^{-1}·m^{-1} in patients older than age 40.[171] Although not all authors agree, studies also suggest greater segmental spread of analgesia in elderly patients with epidural anesthesia produced either by bupivacaine or lidocaine (Fig. 49-37).[172,173] Similar to epidural anesthesia, the correlation between age and dose requirements for subarachnoid anesthesia may be more closely related to change in vertebral column height with age rather than to age itself. Racle et al have demonstrated that subarachnoid injection of hyperbaric bupivacaine, 15 mg, resulted in a shorter time to onset and slightly greater spread of block in older patients.[174] However, because of great individual variation, the clinical significance of these differences may be unimportant. Of more concern is the fact that older patients demonstrate a greater decrease in arterial blood pressure from resting value, despite customary prehydration.

Although they do not achieve statistical significance, higher plasma concentrations of local anesthetics after epidural anesthesia have been observed in elderly people.[172,173] This may reflect reduced plasma clearance with age and a prolonged elimination half-life. Although CNS toxicity in a rhesus monkey model occurs at the same threshold serum bupivacaine concentration in both old and young ani-

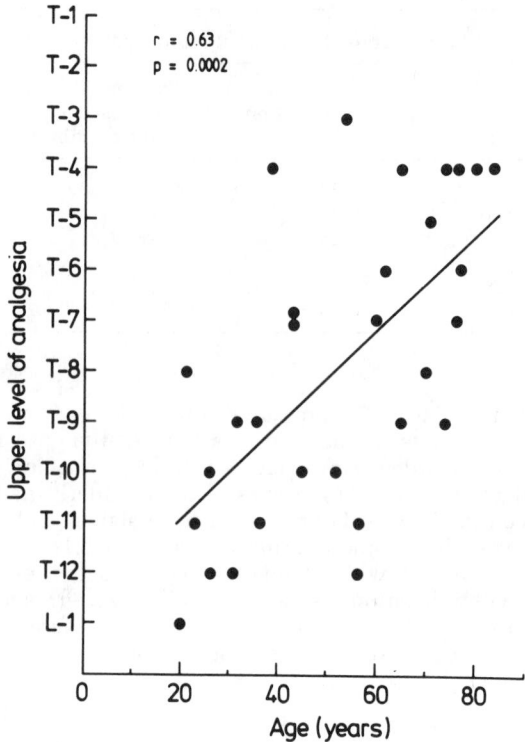

Figure 49-37. The relationship between age and the upper level of analgesia achieved after epidural administration of 0.5% bupivacaine. Greater segmental spread of analgesia appears to occur in elderly patients after epidural administration of local anesthetic drugs. (Reprinted with permission of the International Anesthesia Research Society. From Veering BT, Burm AGL, van Kleef JW et al: Epidural anesthesia with bupivacaine: Effects of age on neural blockade and pharmacokinetics. Anesth Analg 66:589, 1987.)

mals,[175] because of reduced clearance, toxic plasma concentrations may result from lower doses of local anesthetic drugs in elderly patients.

UNIQUE ANESTHETIC CONSIDERATIONS

Premedication

When visiting elderly patients before operation, the anesthesiologist need not alter his or her normal practice. Elderly people generally have their emotions under good control and are frequently placid. Having seen many of life's problems over a long life span, these patients generally are less intimidated by the threat of upcoming surgery than younger patients. Nevertheless, verbal reassurance is still important for allaying anxiety.

In general, premedicant drugs must be administered with caution to elderly patients, who will manifest a greater sensitivity and a longer duration of drug effect compared with their younger counterparts. Normal adult premedication doses may produce an exaggerated effect in elderly patients and can create unwanted confusion and agitation. For example, midazolam given as in im premedicant is recommended in a dose of approximately 5 mg for an average 70-kg adult. However, this dose will produce excessive sedation in the elderly. Wong et al found that giving midazolam in doses of 1, 2, or 3 mg resulted in adequate sedation and amnesia in patients from 60 to 69 years old.[176] In fact, at these doses, 3% of patients became unresponsive. If there is doubt, premedication should be light or omitted.

No single premedication regimen is ideal for all elderly patients. Temazepam, triazolam, and diphenhydramine have been suggested as effective premedicant agents for elderly patients.[177] Compared with diazepam, triazolam's far shorter beta elimination half-life of 1.5–5 hours has a theoretical advantage in elderly people. Also, in contrast to diazepam, temazepam has been shown to not delay postoperative recovery and not produce excessive sedation 2 hours after operation in elderly patients.[177] Diphenhydramine, an antihistamine, exerts sedative and hypnotic effects but minimal psychomotor effects in adults. Kinetic analysis in elderly people has demonstrated a volume of distribution, clearance, and plasma elimination half-life similar to that of younger patients.[178] Ghignone and colleagues suggest that clonidine ought to be considered as an effective premedicant for elderly patients, especially those undergoing eye surgery.[179] When compared with elderly patients receiving po diazepam, 0.1 mg·kg^{-1}, 90–120 minutes prior to arrival in the operating room, patients receiving clonidine, po, 5 mg·kg^{-1}, demonstrated attenuated cardiovascular responses to the stresses of laryngoscopy and endotracheal intubation and significantly reduced intraoperative lability and anesthetic requirements. In addition, clonidine produced satisfactory intraoperative sedation in 85% of patients compared with a similar response in only 50% of diazepam-treated patients.

Monitoring

Because of limited physiologic reserves and a reduced margin for error in elderly patients, monitoring generally should be more intense for this patient group than for younger patients. Del Guercio et al have shown that preoperative invasive monitoring helped predict the elderly patients' tolerance to major operations.[26] Frequently, intensive preoperative monitoring revealed a much worse physical status than suspected on the basis of standard clinical observations. Djokovic et al concluded that invasive monitoring allowed earlier recognition and treatment of intraoperative problems in elderly patients, which resulted, in turn, in a lower mortality rate than previously reported.[4] Although these studies demonstrate positive results with enhanced invasive monitoring, it is not mandatory to monitor every geriatric patient invasively; each patient must be evaluated individually.

In deciding on the intensity of monitoring for any given elderly patient, it is important to weigh the fact that complications from invasive monitoring are also more likely to be observed in elderly people. For instance, ischemic complications from invasive arterial monitoring are more likely to occur in an elderly person when atherosclerosis reduces the luminal diameter of the artery. Similarly, cardiac dysrhythmias associated with flow-directed pulmonary artery catheters are observed more frequently in elderly patients who more likely have myocardial ischemia and irritability. Thus, every monitoring technique has a cost-benefit relationship that must be assessed individually in view of the patient's age, physical status, and proposed surgical procedure. Inserting invasive monitoring devices before induction of anesthesia allows the establishment of baseline values before induction and surgical stimulation and enhances proper intraoperative interpretation of monitored values. If patients are adequately informed and sedated, invasive devices can be inserted before induction of anesthesia without untoward hemodynamic alterations.[180]

Endotracheal Intubation

Airway management is frequently difficult in elderly patients. If they are not edentulous, remaining teeth may be loose with poor supportive structure because of resorption of the alveolar ridges of the jaws. Facial shape is also altered by alveolar bone resorption and loss of dentition, leading to concave cheeks. Because of these changes, it may be difficult to adequately ventilate the lungs of an elderly patient by mask. The use of an oropharyngeal airway may partially restore the shape of the face and alleviate this problem. Markedly loose teeth should be removed before laryngoscopic examination is attempted. Temporomandibular joint dysfunction, which reduces anterior advancement of the mandible and mouth opening, combined with cervical arthritis, makes exposure of the larynx more difficult in the elderly patient. Care should be taken during laryngoscopic examination to avoid overextension of the neck because of the increased likelihood of vertebrobasilar arterial insufficiency. In addition, when rapid-sequence endotracheal intubation is performed, cricoid pressure should be applied directly over the cricoid cartilage and not lateral to it, where contact with the carotid artery can loosen an atherosclerotic plaque and possibly result in a cerebrovascular accident.

It is well known that laryngoscopic examination and tracheal intubation are accompanied by tachycardia and hypertension if performed in a lightly anesthetized patient. These changes are normally of short duration and are usually well tolerated by patients who do not have cardiovascular disease. However, myocardial ischemia, ventricular ectopy, left ventricular failure, and cerebral hemorrhage have been reported in response to the stresses of laryngoscopic examination and tracheal intubation. Administration of opioids, local anesthetics, or short-acting vasodilators and antihypertensive agents immediately before induction of anesthesia lessens the severity of cardiovascular responses to placement of an endotracheal tube.

Regional Anesthesia *Versus* General Anesthesia

No single anesthetic technique has been shown to be superior for elderly patients. In addition to the significant cardiopulmonary complications associated with anesthesia and surgery, the risk of postoperative mental deterioration in this patient group may be of equal or even greater importance in affecting their quality of life after operation.

Selection of the anesthetic technique should be influenced not only by the patient's clinical condition and surgical requirements but also by the anesthesiologist's skill and experience. In general, a fragile geriatric patient should be handled gently and the anesthetic achieved in as simple a fashion as possible. Evidence suggests that geriatric patients have an improved prognosis if minor surgical procedures are performed with local anesthesia rather than general anesthesia or major regional anesthesia.[31,181] During certain surgical procedures, regional anesthesia in elderly patients may have the advantages of reduced postoperative negative nitrogen balance, amelioration of endocrine stress responses to surgery, reduction in blood loss, and a reduced incidence of postoperative thromboembolic complications.[182-185]

During hip surgery, regional anesthesia is associated with

TABLE 49-9. Complications of Emergency Hip Surgery

Parameter	Subarachnoid Block (n = 37)	General Anesthesia (n = 39)
Incidence deep vein thrombosis (%)	46	77
Intraoperative blood loss (ml)	304	468
Total blood loss (ml)	513	714
Postoperative decrease in Pao$_2$ (mm Hg)	1.2	6.5
Deaths within 4 weeks of surgery (no.)	3	9

Reprinted with permission from Davis FM, Laurenson VG: Spinal anaesthesia or general anaesthesia for emergency hip surgery in elderly patients. Anaesth Intensive Care 9:352, 1981.

TABLE 49-10. Complications of Total Hip Arthroplasty

Parameter	Epidural (0.75% Bupivacaine) (n = 29)	General Anesthesia (n = 31)
Pao$_2$ first postoperative day (mm Hg)	75	68
Patients describing persistent mental changes 3 months after operation	0	7
Patients describing change in quality of life 3 months after operation	0	5

Reprinted with permission from Hole A, Terjesen T, Breivik H: Epidural versus general anaesthesia for total hip arthroplasty in elderly patients. Acta Anaesthesiol Scand 24:279, 1980.

a reduced incidence of deep vein thrombosis (Table 49-9).[186] A potential explanation for this phenomenon is that sympathectomy produced by spinal anesthesia produces vasodilation and increases lower limb blood flow, whereas general anesthesia reduces cardiac output and peripheral blood flow. Further, stress hormones released during general anesthesia may enhance the coagulation process. As observed in Table 49-9, use of regional anesthesia also resulted in reduced intraoperative blood loss and less postoperative hypoxemia. Deaths occurring within 4 weeks of surgery happened less often in patients receiving regional anesthesia. In a similar study comparing mortality in patients over age 50 undergoing correction of upper femoral fractures, Valentin et al noted reduced mortality following regional anesthesia (spinal anesthesia) versus general anesthesia 30 days after surgery.[187] However, 6 months to 2 years after surgery the mortality rate was identical in patients receiving either regional or general anesthesia. High long-term mortality was more closely related to ASA physical status than to selection of anesthetic technique. In a similar study, greater hypoxemia was observed after operation in patients receiving general anesthesia compared with epidural anesthesia for total hip arthroplasty.[188] The development of V/Q mismatch and pulmonary shunt appeared to be greater in patients who required general anesthesia with controlled ventilation versus those who maintained spontaneous ventilation with epidural anesthesia. Intraoperative pulmonary changes may have been exaggerated after operation by splinting and reduced coughing in patients receiving general anesthesia.

Mental changes lasting months or years after administration of general anesthesia to elderly patients having major surgery have been reported.[189] Possible explanations for this deterioration in mental function include the stress of the operation, intraoperative or perioperative episodes of hypoxemia, perioperative episodes of hypotension, and prolonged action of administered drugs. As shown in Table 49-10, Hole et al have observed persistent postoperative mental changes in more than 20% of patients receiving general anesthesia, whereas no patients receiving epidural anesthesia demonstrated this problem. Five of 31 patients receiving general anesthesia observed a change in quality of life for as long as 3 months after the date of surgery.[188] If it could be reproducibly shown that mental dysfunction occurred in elderly patients to a greater extent after general anesthesia, regional anesthetic techniques would be of obvious benefit. However, comparisons of groups of elderly patients who have had the same surgical procedure with general anesthesia compared with regional or local anesthesia are not universal in this conclusion. For example, Riis et al found identical patterns of altered mental function in elderly patients, regardless of type of anesthesia for hip arthroplasty, and concluded that the transient mental impairment that occurred during the first postoperative week was caused by factors other than the selection of anesthesia.[189] Similarly, Karhunen and Jonn found a comparable incidence of postoperative memory loss after cataract extraction whether general or local anesthesia was used.[190] Mann and Bisset have shown no difference in postoperative mental dysfunction whether general or spinal anesthesia was used for surgery of the lower limbs.[191] Berggren et al demonstrated no difference in the incidence of postoperative confusion in patients receiving general or epidural anesthesia for repair of femoral neck fractures.[192] Instead, they correlated postoperative confusion with the patient's history of mental depression and use of anticholinergic medication.

Perhaps part of the confusion regarding postoperative mental dysfunction has been resolved by Chung et al. In a study comparing spinal anesthesia versus general anesthesia in elderly patients undergoing transurethral resection of the prostate, patients managed with a spinal anesthetic had demonstrably less mental dysfunction postoperatively than those receiving a general anesthetic.[193] In addition, in a separate study of older patients undergoing cataract surgery via local anesthesia with sedation, patients found to have impaired cognitive function preoperatively were more likely to develop exaggerated postoperative mental dysfunction.[194] However, in a separate study in which patients managed with spinal anesthesia also received relatively low doses of adjuvant parenteral sedative/analgesic drugs, there was absolutely no difference in mental dysfunction compared with patients managed with general anesthesia.[195] Regional anesthesia may result in somewhat less mental impairment postoperatively, but only if very low doses of supplemental sedative/analgesic agents are employed.

In summary, it is difficult to recommend regional anesthesia over general anesthesia for all kinds of surgical procedures in the geriatric patient group. The selection of anesthesia must be based on the patient's individual circumstances. Spinal anesthesia has particular advantages for certain types of surgery, including transurethral resection of the prostate, during which the patient remains awake and can give early warning of surgical complications. Similarly, allowing a patient to remain conscious during regional

TABLE 49-11. Incidence of Spinal Headache in Relation to Age

Age (yr)	Patients (no.)	Incidence of Headaches (%)
20–29	23	17
30–39	36	11
40–49	32	9
50–59	29	7
60–69	14	0
70–79	8	0

Reprinted with permission from Benzon HT, Linde HW, Molloy RE *et al:* Post-dural puncture headache in patients with chronic pain. Anesth Analg 59:772, 1980. Reprinted with permission of the International Anesthesia Research Society.

anesthesia permits patient recognition of an anginal attack or acute cerebral changes resulting from a variety of causes. Spinal anesthesia also has a lower incidence of postpuncture headaches in older patients (Table 49-11).[196] This is thought to result from age-related anatomic changes in the intervertebral foramina, which inhibits leakage of cerebrospinal fluid from the dural rent produced by the spinal needle. Fink has suggested that this may also be a result of a generalized loss of elasticity in the elderly.[197] Less elasticity in the dura may result in reduced puncture hole size in the dura following needle placement.

For older patients who are cooperative, regional techniques, especially subarachnoid and epidural blockade, can be used effectively and safely for procedures requiring anesthesia below the T8 determatome. Regional blockade also may be used effectively for various procedures on the extremities. However, use of a regional anesthetic in an elderly patient who becomes agitated, excited, or uncomfortable because of awkward positioning tempts the anesthesiologist to provide supplemental sedation. Injudicious use of supplemental drugs may actually result in a pseudo-general anesthetic for a patient that obviates some of the advantages of a regional anesthetic technique. Oversedation of a patient may lead to hypoventilation, an unprotected airway, and the possibility of mental changes after operation resembling those with general anesthesia.[189]

Positioning

Aging is associated with a progressive decrease in bone density in both men and women after maturity. Losses in bone density so severe as to result in fractures after minimal trauma define the disease of osteoporosis, which accounts for more than one million fractures in the United States each year.[8] Osteoporosis is of staggering importance in the elderly and contributes to the observation that, by age 65, one third of women will have had vertebral fractures and, by age 81, one third of women and one sixth of men will have had a hip fracture. This loss of bony matrix not only explains many of the orthopedic injuries for which elderly patients are seen for surgery but also emphasizes the fragility of elderly patients and indicates the importance of positioning patients gently for surgical procedures (see Chapter 27). After receiving either regional or general anesthesia, elderly patients must be placed in a neutral position, with

consideration of their decreased range of motion. If possible, the patient's neck should be kept in a position that was comfortable when he or she was awake in order to avoid compromising cerebral blood flow. Great care must be used when turning elderly patients in order to prevent pathologic fractures. Placing elderly patients in the lithotomy position is known to produce postoperative back pain. For example, after a spinal anesthetic is administered to an elderly man for transurethral surgery, it is very easy to place his legs in a position very much more exaggerated than he would have permitted had analgesia and relaxation not been produced as a result of the spinal anesthetic. A postoperative backache incorrectly attributed to the spinal technique more likely results from inadequate attention to positioning.

Senile atrophy, with loss of subcutaneous elastic tissue, makes the skin of elderly patients sensitive to injury from adhesive tape or application of monitoring electrodes. Because elderly patients have fragile skin and decreased subcutaneous elastic tissue, careful padding is essential. Bony prominences such as elbows, ankles, and trochanters must be padded with sheepskin, foam, or other suitable padding, and tape should be removed very carefully.

Drug Interactions

Geriatric patients have more illnesses and invariably take more medications than do younger patients, thus exposing them to an increased risk of adverse drug reactions. Although patients 65 years of age and older make up only 12% of the United States population, 30% of all prescriptions are written for people of this age group.[9] Almost 70% of elderly patients regularly use over-the-counter drugs, compared with approximately 10% of the general adult population.[198] Over-the-counter drugs account for approximately 40% of all drugs taken by elderly patients.[199]

Because of the larger number and variety of drugs prescribed for and consumed by elderly patients, these patients have an approximate threefold increased potential for adverse drug reactions. For example, in a study of 714 hospitalized patients at Johns Hopkins University, patients aged 41–50 had an 11.8% incidence of adverse drug reactions, whereas patients aged 80 or greater had a 24.9% incidence.[200] Similarly, in a study by Hurwitz, patients aged 40–49 years had a 7% incidence of adverse drug effects, whereas patients aged 70–79 years had an incidence three times as great.[201]

Delirium following general surgery may occur in 10–15% of older patients or in up to 50% of older patients undergoing repair of femoral neck fracture.[202] However, the most common single cause of delirium in later life may be adverse effects from medications, especially the anticholinergic drugs.[203] Theoretically, arousal time after general anesthesia with neuromuscular block reversal might be affected by the anticholinergic agent selected. Glycopyrrolate, a quarternary ammonium compound that does not cross the blood-brain barrier, may have theoretical advantages over atropine when administered for this purpose. However, Malling and colleagues were unable to demonstrate a difference in emergence from anesthesia as a result of anticholinergic drug selection.[204]

Many of these problems with drug interaction in the elderly population simply reflect polypharmacy, resulting from the additive or synergistic action of multiple drugs. However, they also may reflect discrepancies in duration of drug action or may represent the decreased clearance of one drug because of the hepatic effects of another. This last situation has been described for the interaction of cimetidine with beta blocking drugs, and benzodiazepines.[205]

Before operation, one must inquire into the patient's corticosteroid, antihypertensive, anticoagulant, beta blocker, monoamine oxidase inhibitor, tricyclic antidepressant, and antidiabetic drug use. In general, patients should continue to take all cardiovascular medications up until the time of surgery. Also, elderly patients use alcohol in greater quantities than do young patients, with a significant percentage of elderly patients reported as alcoholics. To minimize the risks of hazardous drug interactions, the anesthetic should be kept simple in elderly patients.

Outpatient Anesthesia for Elderly Patients

In our current system of health care, cost containment has been greatly emphasized. This has brought the geriatric patient into the outpatient setting. As discussed in the section on Regional Anesthesia Versus General Anesthesia, postoperative confusion and mental dysfunction are of great concern in the elderly patient. These side-effects may be reduced by allowing elderly patients to have surgery in an ambulatory setting, where they are given fewer medications and they can return more quickly to normal surroundings with their relatives and friends nearby. As Rowe and Kahn have suggested, the maintenance of control or autonomy for elderly patients (where they make decisions regarding choice of activity, timing, pace, and so on) is very important.[8] Lack of control has adverse effects on their emotional state, performance, subjective well-being, and physiologic function. As a result, it may be beneficial for elderly patients to have surgery in an outpatient setting, where there is a smaller loss of autonomy and control.

Obviously, not all geriatric patients should have surgery in an ambulatory setting. Many of these patients have more than one disease or a significant physiologic decrement in function that prevents them from being candidates for ambulatory surgery. However, if elderly patients pass routine preoperative screening visits, there is no reason why age alone should prevent them from being considered candidates for outpatient procedures. Meridy found that age does not affect the duration of recovery from anesthesia or the rate of complications after outpatient surgery.[206] However, others have observed that more time was required for older patients to successfully complete a manipulative skill test when they were emerging from thiopental, halothane, and nitrous oxide anesthesia for cervical dilation and curettage.[130] Also, Gold et al reported that as the patient age increased 30 years the likelihood for unscheduled admission of outpatients increased 2.6 fold.[207]

The anesthesiologist's preoperative screening visit before surgery is of prime importance and should take place before the day of surgery. This enables anesthesia personnel to make rational judgments as to the patient's acceptability for surgery as an outpatient, permits treatment of pre-existent diseases, contributes to more efficient scheduling, allows appropriate laboratory testing to be performed, enhances the visibility of the anesthesiologist in the overall medical practice scheme, and enables an interview with the "responsible adult" who will not only ensure the patient's delivery from the hospital back home but will also stay with the patient and assist with recovery in the home setting. In a special study sponsored by the Federated Ambulatory Surgery Association, Natof reviewed 87,492 patients having outpatient procedures and found a relationship between the

TABLE 49-12. Complications Related to Operating Room Time

Operating Room Time	Patients	Complications	Incidence
1 hour or less	69,461	449	1/155 patients
1–2 hours	11,971	142	1/84 patients
2–3 hours	2481	46	1/54 patients
More than 3 hours	729	21	1/35 patients

Reprinted with permission from Natof HE: FASA Special Study I. Alexandria, VA: Federated Ambulatory Surgery Association, 1985.

incidence of complications and the length of the surgical procedure (Table 49-12).[208] As a result, the type and difficulty of the surgical procedure should be taken into consideration before a complex and protracted surgical procedure is allowed to be performed on an elderly patient on an outpatient basis. Similarly, the relationship of complication rate to pre-existent disease demonstrates again the importance of preanesthesia screening in determining whether elderly patients with one or more pre-existent medical conditions should be allowed to have their surgical procedures on an outpatient basis (Table 49-13). Finally, the selection of anesthesia for the geriatric patient depends on the anticipated surgical procedure, the patient's state of health, and the anesthesiologist's skill and experience. Many elderly patients fear general anesthesia more than regional or local anesthesia and believe that they have a greater sense of control if they do not receive a general anesthetic. Again, in the large study of the Federated Ambulatory Surgery Association, a much lower incidence of complications was observed in patients who received local anesthesia or regional techniques. A higher incidence of complications was observed in those who received local anesthesia with sedation or general anesthesia (Table 49-14).[208]

Not all elderly patients have multiple medical problems. Physiologic age is obviously more important than chronologic age, and a profile of the patient's medical history and current level of physical activity far better indicates his or her ability to tolerate a surgical procedure as an outpatient than does age alone. A patient should not be denied ambulatory surgery solely on the basis of age.

TABLE 49-13. Complications Related to Pre-existing Disease

Pre-existing Disease	Incidence
Cardiac disease	1/74 patients
Hypertension	1/87 patients
Chronic lung disease	1/112 patients
Asthma	1/139 patients
None	1/156 patients

Reprinted with permission from Natof HE: FASA Special Study I. Alexandria, VA: Federated Ambulatory Surgery Association, 1985.

TABLE 49-14. Complications Related to Anesthetic Technique

Technique	Incidence
Local and sedation	1/106 patients
General	1/120 patients
Local only	1/268 patients
Regional blockade	1/277 patients

Reprinted with permission from Natof HE: FASA Special Study I. Alexandria, VA: Federated Ambulatory Surgery Association, 1985.

POSTOPERATIVE MANAGEMENT

The elderly patient needs special attention immediately after operation. Elderly patients have increased V/Q mismatch after operation, which contributes to a greater degree of postoperative hypoxemia compared with that in young patients.[66] Because even young patients are known to experience reduced oxygenation during transfer from the operating room to the postanesthesia care unit, elderly patients are at greater risk for hypoxia both during transfer to the postanesthesia care unit and during the recovery room stay. For this reason, supplemental oxygen is useful during transport to the postanesthesia care unit and while the patient is in the postanesthesia care unit.[209] Monitoring oxygen saturation with a pulse oximeter enables a rational decision to be made as to the need for supplemental oxygen. Frequently, ventilatory depression from residual anesthetic, ventilatory compromise (from splinting), or pre-existent pulmonary disease necessitates the administration of supplemental oxygen for the first 24 hours. Like other patients, elderly patients need to be encouraged to breathe deeply and cough and may benefit from elevation of the head of the bed. As discussed in the section on Airway Reflexes, because of a reduction in airway protective reflexes, elderly patients require increased observation to protect them from passive aspiration.

Because elderly patients lose more body heat during operation and arrive in the postanesthesia care unit cooler than their younger counterparts (see Fig. 49-29), it may be necessary to apply exogenous heat to speed rewarming.[116] Placing them in a warm environment during their recovery room stay reduces the likelihood of shivering with its associated problems. Some of what may be interpreted as slow emergence or delayed return of orientation may be pharmacologically induced. For example, elderly patients are at risk for confusion, memory loss, and an impaired ability to concentrate as a side-effect of antimuscarinic drugs administered. Elderly patients are probably at greater risk for such side-effects than younger patients because of decreased cholinergic activity in the brain.[210] Elderly patients also benefit from reassurance and additional measures to assist them with orientation to reality. They may need to be reminded at frequent intervals with statements such as "your operation is over and you are doing fine" or "you are not at home; you are in the hospital." These comments help them to regain their sense of awareness and of their surroundings. In addition, when they are provided with their dentures, glasses, hearing aids, and other personal items, they gain additional psychological security while remaining in the postanesthesia care unit.

Postoperative pain management in the elderly needs to be judiciously managed as a result of the pharmacokinetic and pharmacodynamic changes associated with aging. The same factors that affect intraoperative dosing of opioids (see the section on Opioids) also affect their postoperative dosing. In addition to demonstrating greater sensitivity to postoperatively administered opioids,[211] elderly patients also require repeat dosing at less frequent intervals. For example, older patients managed with epidural morphine administered in a dose of 0.07 mg·kg^{-1} required redosing toward the end of their first postoperative day (13–24 hours following initial injection), whereas most younger patients required redosing less than 12 hours after initial injection.[212]

REFERENCES

1. Smith OC: Advanced age as a contraindication to operation. Med Rec (NY) 72:642, 1907
2. Ochsner A: Is risk of operation too great in the elderly? Geriatrics 22:121, 1927
3. Brooks B: Surgery in patients of advanced age. Ann Surg 105:481, 1937
4. Djokovic JL, Hedley-Whyte J: Prediction of outcome of surgery and anesthesia in patients over 80. JAMA 242:2301, 1979
5. Miller R, Marlar K, Silvay G: Anesthesia for patients aged over 90 years. NY State J Med 77:1421, 1977
6. Catlic MR: Surgery in centenarians. JAMA 253:3139, 1985
7. McLeskey CH: Anesthesia for the geriatric patient. In Stoelting RK, Barash PG, Gallagher TJ (eds): Advances in Anesthesia, p 31. Chicago, Year Book Medical Publishers, 1985
8. Rowe JW, Kahn RL: Human aging: Usual and successful. Science 237:143, 1987
9. Thompson TL, Moran MG, Nies AS: Psychotropic drug use in the elderly. N Engl J Med 308:134, 1983
10. Vestal RE: Drug use in the elderly: A review of problems and special consideration. Drugs 16:382, 1978
11. Fries JF, Crapo LM: The sharp downslope of natural death. In Fries JF, Crapo LM (eds): Vitality and Aging, p 73. San Francisco, WH Freeman and Company, 1981
12. 1980 Census of Population: General population characteristics, p 26. Washington, DC, United States Census Bureau, 1983
13. Renck H: The elderly patient after anaesthesia and surgery. Acta Anaesthesiol Scand [Suppl] 13:9, 1969
14. Davenport HT: Anesthesia for the geriatric patient. Can Anaesth Soc J 30:S51, 1983
15. Marx GF, Mateo CV, Orkin LR: Computer analysis of postanesthetic deaths. Anesthesiology 39:54, 1973
16. Mircea N, Constantinescu C, Jianu E et al: Risk of pulmonary complications in surgical patients. Resuscitation 10:33, 1982
17. Farrow SC, Fowkes FGR, Lunn JN et al: Epidemiology in anaesthesia. II: Factors affecting mortality in hospital. Br J Anaesth 54:811, 1982
18. Filzweiser G, List WF: Morbidity and mortality in elective geriatric surgery. In Vickers MD, Lunn JN (eds): Mortality and Anesthesia, p 75. Berlin, Springer-Verlag, 1983
19. Ellison N: Problems in geriatric anesthesia. Surg Clin North Am 55:929, 1975
20. Haljamae T, Stefannsson T, Wickstrom I: Preanesthetic evaluation of the female geriatric patient with hip fracture. Acta Anaesthesiol Scand 26:393, 1982
21. Stephen CR: The risk of anesthesia and surgery in the geriatric patient. In Krechel SE (ed): Anesthesia and the Geriatric Patient, p 231. New York, Grune & Stratton, 1984
22. Rowe JW, Adres R, Tobin JD et al: The effect of age on creatinine clearance in man: A cross-sectional and longitudinal study. J Gerontol 31:155, 1976
23. Tiret L, Desmonts JM, Hatton F et al: Complications associated with anaesthesia—a prospective survey in France. Can Anaesth Soc J 33:336, 1986
24. Denney JH, Denson JS: Risk of surgery in patients over 90. Geriatrics 27:115, 1972

25. Goldman L, Caldera DL, Nussbaum SR et al: Multifactorial index of cardiac risks in non-cardiac surgical procedures. N Engl J Med 297:845, 1977

26. Del Guercio LRN, Cohn JD: Monitoring operative risk in the elderly. JAMA 243:1350, 1980

27. Hosking MP, Warner MA, Lobdell CM et al: Outcomes of surgery in patients 90 years of age and older. JAMA 261:1909, 1989

28. Johnson JC: The medical evaluation and management of the elderly surgical patient. J Am Geriatr Soc 31:621, 1983

29. Goldman L, Caldera DL, Southwick FS et al: Cardiac risk factors and complications in non-cardiac surgery. Medicine 57:357, 1978

30. Gibson JR, Mendelhall MK, Axel NJ: Geriatric anesthesia: Minimizing the risk. In Brindly GU (eds): Clinics in Geriatric Medicine, p 313. Philadelphia, WB Saunders, 1985

31. Nehme AE: Groin hernias in elderly patients. Am J Surg 146:257, 1983

32. Williams JS, Hale HW: The advisability of inguinal herniorrhaphy in the elderly. Surg Gynecol Obstet 122:100, 1966

33. Tingwald GR, Cooperman M: Inguinal and femoral hernia repair in geriatric patients. Surg Gynecol Obstet 154:704, 1982

34. Lakatta EG, Fleg JL: Aging of the adult cardiovascular system. In Stephen CR, Assaf RAE (eds): Geriatric anesthesia: Principles and Practices, p 1. Boston, Butterworths, 1986

35. Lakatta EF: Changes in cardiovascular function with aging. Eur Heart J 11 (suppl C):22, 1990

36. Ensor RE, Fleg JL, Kim YC et al: Longitudinal chest x-ray changes in normal men. J Gerontol 38:307, 1983

37. Kannel WB, Gordon T: Evaluation of cardiovascular risk in the elderly: The Framingham study. Bull NY Acad Med 54:573, 1978

38. Tarazi RC, Frohlich ED, Dustan HP: Plasma volume in men with essential hypertension. N Engl J Med 278:762, 1968

39. Davidson WR, Fee EC: Influence of aging on pulmonary hemodynamics in a population free of coronary artery disease. Am J Cardiol 65:1454, 1990

40. Evans TI: The physiological basis of geriatric general anesthesia. Anaesth Intensive Care 1:319, 1973

41. Brandfonbrener M, Landowne M, Shock NW: Changes in cardiac output with age. Circulation 69:557, 1955

42. Rodeheffer RJ, Gerstenblith G, Becker LC et al: Exercise cardiac output is maintained with advancing age in healthy human subjects: Cardiac dilatation and increased stroke volume compensate for a diminished heart rate. Circulation 69:203, 1984

43. Port S, Cobb FR, Coleman RE et al: Effect of age on the responses of the left ventricular ejection fraction to exercise. N Engl J Med 303:1133, 1980

44. Rosberg B, Wulff K: Hemodynamics following normovolemic hemodilution in elderly patients. Acta Anaesthesiol Scand 25:402, 1981

45. Skinner JS: The cardiovascular system with aging and exercise. In Brunner D, Jake E (eds): Medicine and Science in Sport, vol 4, p 100. Baltimore, University Park Press, 1970

46. Tuzankoff ST, Fleg JL, Norris AH et al: Age-related increase in serum catecholamine levels during exercise and healthy adult men. Physiologist 23:50, 1980

47. Shocken DD, Roth GS: Reduced beta-adrenergic receptor concentrations in aging man. Nature 267:856, 1977

48. Dillon N, Chung S, Kelly J et al: Age and beta adrenoreceptor mediated function. Clin Pharmacol Ther 27:769, 1980

49. Grollman A, Grollman EF: Pharmacology and therapeutics, 7th ed, p 269. Philadelphia, Lea & Febiger, 1970

50. Forrest JB: Clinical evaluation of isoflurane: Pulse and blood pressure. Can Anaesth Soc J 29:S15, 1982

51. Feldman RD, Limbird LE, Nadeau J et al: Alterations in leukocyte-receptor affinity with aging: A potential explanation for altered-adrenergic sensitivity in the elderly. N Engl J Med 310:815, 1984

52. Van Brummelen P, Buhler FR, Kiowski W et al: Age-related decrease in cardiac and peripheral vascular responsiveness to isoprenaline: Studies in normal subjects. Clin Sci 60:571, 1980

53. Kendall MJ, Woods KL: Responsiveness to alpha-adrenergic receptor stimulation: The effects of age are cardioselective. Br J Clin Pharmacol 14:821, 1982

54. Conway J, Wheeler R, Sannerstedt R: Sympathetic nervous activity during exercise in relation to age. Cardiovasc Res 5:577, 1971

55. Lakatta EG: Age-related alterations in the cardiovascular response to adrenergic mediated stress. Fed Proc 39:3171, 1980

56. Kennedy RD, Claird FI: Physiology of aging of the heart. Cardiovasc Clin 12:1, 1981

57. Elliott HL, Sumner DJ, McLean K et al: Effect of age on the responsiveness of vascular alpha-adrenoreceptors in man. J Cardiovasc Pharmacol 4:388, 1982

58. Fleg JL, Kennedy HL: Cardiac arrhythmias in a healthy elderly population: Detection by 24-hour ambulatory monitoring. Chest 81:302, 1982

59. Levy W: Clinical evaluation of isoflurane: Cardiac arrhythmias. Can Anaesth Soc J 29:S28, 1982

60. Goldman HL, Becklake MR: Respiratory function tests: Normal values at median altitudes and the prediction of normal results. Am Rev Tuberculosis 79:457, 1959

61. Smith TC: Respiratory effects of aging. Semin Anesth 5:14, 1986

62. Pontoppidan H, Geffins B, Lowenstein A: Acute respiratory failure in the adult. N Engl J Med 287:690, 1972

63. Pump KK: Emphysema and its relation to age. Am Rev Respir Dis 114:5, 1976

64. Raine JM, Bishop MJ: A-a difference in O_2 tension and physiological dead space in normal man. J Appl Physiol 18:284, 1963

65. Kitamura H, Sawa T, Ikezono E: Postoperative hypoxemia: The contribution of age to the maldistribution of ventilation. Anesthesiology 36:244, 1972

66. Wahba W: Body build and preoperative arterial oxygen tension. Can Anaesth Soc J 22:653, 1972

67. Ward RJ, Tolas AG, Benveniste RJ et al: Effect of posture on normal arterial blood gas tensions in the aged. Geriatrics 21:139, 1966

68. Labouvie-Vief G: Intelligence and cognition. In Birren JE, Schaie KW (eds): Handbook of the Psychology of Aging, p 500. New York, Van Nostrand Reinhold, 1985

69. Kronenberg RS, Drage GW: Attenuation of the ventilatory and heart rate responses to hypoxia and hypercapnia with aging in normal man. J Clin Invest 52:1812, 1973

70. Muravchick S: Current concepts: Anesthetic pharmacology in geriatric patients. Prog Anesthesiol 1:2, 1987

71. Hess GD, Joseph JA, Roth GS: Effect of age on sensitivity to pain and brain opiate receptors. Neurobiol Aging 2:49, 1981

72. Bellville JW, Forrest WH, Miller E: Influence of age on pain relief from analgesics: A study of postoperative patients. JAMA 217:1835, 1971

73. Gregory GA, Eger El II, Munson ES: The relationship between age and halothane requirement in man. Anesthesiology 30:488, 1969

74. Stevens WC, Dolan WM, Gibbons RT et al: Minimum alveolar concentrations (MAC) of isoflurane with and without nitrous oxide in patients of various ages. Anesthesiology 42:197, 1975

75. Munson ES, Hoffman JC, Eger EI: Use of cyclopropane to test generality of anesthetic requirement in the elderly. Anesth Analg 63:998, 1984

76. Kaiko RF, Wallenstein SL, Rogers AG et al: Narcotics in the elderly. Med Clin North Am 66:1079, 1982

77. Arden JR, Holley FO, Stanski DR: Increased sensitivity to etomidate in the elderly: Initial distribution versus altered brain response. Anesthesiology 65:19, 1986

78. Christensen F, Andreasen F, Jansen JA: Influence of age and sex on the pharmacokinetics of thiopentone. Br J Anaesth 53:1189, 1981

79. Homer TD, Stanski DR: The effect of increasing age on thiopental disposition and anesthetic requirement. Anesthesiology 62:714, 1985

80. Lytle LD, Altar A: Diet, central nervous system, and aging. Fed Proc 38:2017, 1979

81. Naritomi H, Meyer JS, Sakai F et al: Effect of advancing age on regional cerebral blood flow. Arch Neurol 36:410, 1979

82. Devaney KO, Johnson HA: Neuron loss in the aging visual cortex of man. J Gerontol 35:836, 1980

83. Sapolsky RM, Krey LC, McEwen BS: Prolonged glucocorticoid exposure reduces hippocampal neuron number: Implications for aging. J Neurosci 5:1222, 1985

84. Melamed E, Lavy S, Bentin S et al: Reduction in regional cerebral blood flow during normal aging in men. Stroke 11:31, 1980

85. Kety SS: Human cerebral blood flow and oxygen consumption as related to aging. J Chronic Dis 3:478, 1956

86. Hilgenberg JC: Inhalation and intravenous drugs in the elderly patient. Semin Anesthesia 5:44, 1986

87. Baughman UL, Hoffman WE, Thomas C et al: Neurologic outcome in aged rats after incomplete cerebral ischemia. Anesth Analg 67:677, 1988

88. Dorfman LJ, Bosley TM: Age-related changes in peripheral and central nerve conduction in men. Neurology 29:38, 1979

89. Lake CR, Ziegler MG, Coleman MD et al: Age-adjusted plasma norepinephrine levels are similar in normotensive and hypertensive subjects. N Engl J Med 296:208, 1977

90. McGeer EG, McGeer PL: Age changes in the human for enzymes associated with metabolism of catecholamine, GABA, and acetylcholine. Adv Behav Biol 16:287, 1975

91. Gibson GE, Peterson C: Aging decreases oxidative metabolism and the release and synthesis of acetylcholine. J Neurochem 37:978, 1981

92. McGeer EG, McGeer PL: Neurotransmitter metabolism in the aging brain. In Terry RD, Gershon S (eds): Neurobiology of Aging, p 389. New York, Raven Press, 1976

93. Bender AD, Post A, Meier JP et al: Plasma protein binding of drugs as a function of age in adult human subjects. J Pharm Sci 64:1711, 1975

94. Wallace S, Whiting B, Runcie J: Factors affecting drug binding in plasma of elderly patients. Br J Clin Pharmacol 3:3270, 1976

95. Greenblatt DJ: Reduced serum albumin concentration in the elderly: A report from the Boston collaborative drug surveillance program. J Am Geriatr Soc 27:20, 1979

96. Hayes MJ, Langman MJS, Short AH: Changes in drug metabolism with increasing age. 1. Warfarin binding and plasma proteins. Br J Clin Pharmacol 2:69, 1975

97. Carlos R, Calvo R, Erill S: Plasma protein binding of etomidate in different age groups and in patients with chronic respiratory insufficiency. Int J Clin Pharmacol Ther Toxicol 19:1714, 1981

98. Taxton JW, Briant RH: Alpha-1 acid glycoprotein concentration and propranolol binding in elderly patients with acute illness. Br J Clin Pharmacol 18:806, 1984

99. Veering BR, Burm AG, Souverish JH et al: The effect of age on serum concentration of albumin and alpha 1-acid glycoprotein. Br J Clin Pharmacol 29:201, 1990

100. Chan K, Kendall MJ, Wells WD et al: Factors influencing the excretion and relative physiological availability of pethidine in man. J Pharm Pharmacol 27:235, 1975

101. Andreasen F: Protein binding of drugs in plasma from patients with acute renal failure. Acta Pharmacol Toxicol 32:417, 1973

102. Andreasen F: The effect of dialysis on the protein binding of drugs in the plasma of patients with acute renal failure. Acta Pharmacol Toxicol 34:284, 1974

103. Reidenberg MM: The binding of drugs to plasma proteins from patients with poor renal function. Clin Pharmacokinet 1:121, 1976

104. O'Malley K, Velasco M, Pruitt A et al: Decreased plasma protein binding of diazoxide in uremia. Clin Pharmacol Ther 18:53, 1975

105. Hollenberg NK, Adams DF, Solomon HS et al: Senescence and the renal vasculature in normal man. Circ Res 34:309, 1974

106. Muravchick S: The aging patient and age related disease. ASA Annual Refresher Course Lecture #151. Park Ridge, Illinois, American Society of Anesthesiologists, 1987

107. Hicks R, Dysken MW, Davis JM et al: The pharmacokinetics of psychotropic medication in the elderly: A review. J Clin Psychiatry 42:374, 1981

108. Thompson EN, Williams R: Effect of age on liver function with particular reference to bromosulphalein excretion. Gut 6:266, 1965

109. Castleden CM, Kaye CM, Parsons RL: The effect of age on plasma levels of propranolol and practolol in man. Br J Clin Pharmacol 2:303, 1975

110. Greenblatt DJ, Sellers EM, Shader RI: Drug disposition in old age. N Engl J Med 306:1081, 1982

111. McMartin DN, O'Connor JA, Fasco MJ et al: Influence of aging and induction on rat liver and kidney microsomal mixed function oxidase systems. Toxicol Appl Pharmacol 54:411, 1980

112. Baird MB, Birnbaum LS: Increased production of mutagenic metabolites of carcinogens by tissues from senescent rodents. Cancer Res 39:4752, 1979

113. Goldberg MJ, Roe F: Temperature changes during anesthesia and operations. Arch Surg 93:365, 1966

114. Collins KJ, Exton-Smith AN: Thermal homeostasis in old age. American Geriatric Society J 31:519, 1983

115. Vaughn MS, Vaughn RW, Cork RC: Postoperative hypothermia in adults: Relationship of age, anesthesia and shivering to rewarming. Anesth Analg 60:746, 1981

116. Roe CG, Goldberg MJ, Blair CS et al: Influence of shivering on early post-operative oxygen consumption. Surgery 60:85, 1966

117. Bay J, Nunn JF, Prys-Roberts C: Factors influencing arterial PO_2 during recovery from anaesthesia. Br J Anaesth 40:398, 1968

118. Carli F, Clark MM, Woollen JW: Investigation of the relationship between heat loss and the nitrogen excretion in elderly patients undergoing major abdominal surgery under general anaesthesia. Br J Anaesth 54:1023, 1982

119. Yam PC, Carli F: Maintenance of body temperature in elderly patients who have joint replacement surgery. Anaesthesia 45:563, 1990

120. Pontoppidan H, Beecher HK: Progressive loss of protective reflexes in the airway with the advance of age. JAMA 174: 2209, 1960

121. Minaker KL, Meneilly GS, Rowe JW: Endocrine systems. In Finch CE, Schneider EL (eds): Handbook of the Biology of Aging, p 433. New York, Van Nostrand Reinhold, 1985

122. Robert JJ, Cummins JC, Wolfe RR et al: Quantitative aspects of glucose production and metabolism in healthy elderly subjects. Diabetes 31:203, 1982

123. Defronzo RA: Glucose intolerance and aging: Evidence for tissue insensitivity to insulin. Diabetes 28:1095, 1979

124. Davidson MB: The effects of aging on carbohydrate metabolism: A review of the English literature and a practical approach to the diagnosis of diabetes mellitus in the elderly. Metabolism 28:688, 1979

125. Tonino RP, Nedde WH, Robbins DC et al: Effect of physical training on the insulin resistance of aging. Clin Res 34:557, 1986

126. Mitenko PA: Geriatric anesthesia: Changes in drug disposition. Can J Anaesth 34:159, 1987

127. Christensen JH, Andreason F: Individual variation in response to thiopental. Acta Anaesthesiol Scand 22:303, 1978

128. Christensen JH, Andreason F, Jansen JA: Pharmacokinetics and pharmacodynamics of thiopentone: A comparison between young and elderly patients. Anaesthesia 37:398, 1982

129. Baird MB: A longitudinal study of the relationship between aging and the duration of hexobarbital hypnosis in male CFN rats. Exp Gerontol 18:47, 1983

130. Sear JW, Cooper GM, Kumar V: The effect of age on recovery. Anaesthesia 38:1158, 1983

131. Jung D, Mayersohn M, Perrier D et al: Thiopental dispostion as a function of age in female patients undergoing surgery. Anesthesiology 56:263, 1982

132. Muravchick S: Effect of age and premedication on thiopental sleep dose. Anesthesiology 61:333, 1984

133. Reidenberg MM, Levy M, Warner H et al: Relationship between diazepam dose, plasma level, age, and central nervous system depression. Clin Pharmacol Ther 23:371, 1978

134. Kanto J, Aaltone L, Himberg JJ et al: Midazolam as an intravenous induction agent in the elderly. A clinical and pharmacokinetic study. Anesth Analg 65:15, 1986

135. Bell GD, Spichett GP, Reeve PA et al: Intravenous midazolam for upper gastrointestinal endoscopy: A study of 800 consecutive cases relating dose to age and sex of patient. Br J Clin Pharmacol 23:241, 1987

136. Klotz U, Avant GR, Hoyumpa A et al: The effects of age and liver disease on the disposition and elimination of diazepam in adult man. J Clin Invest 55:347, 1975

137. Reves JG, Fragen RJ, Vinik HR et al: Midazolam: Pharmacology and uses. Anesthesiology 62:310, 1985

138. Greenblatt DJ, Abernathy DR, Locniskar A et al: Effect of age, gender, and obesity on midazolam kinetics. Anesthesiology 61:27, 1984

139. Stanski DR, Greenblatt DJ, Lowenstein E: Kinetics of intravenous and intramuscular morphine. Clin Pharmacol Ther 24:52, 1978

140. Mather LE, Tucker GT, Pflug AE et al: Meperidine kinetics in man: Intravenous injection in surgical patients and volunteers. Clin Pharmacol Ther 17:21, 1975

141. Bentley JB, Borel JE, Nenad RE: Influence of age on the pharmacokinetics of fentanyl. Anesth Analg 61:171, 1982

142. Helmers H, Van Peer A, Woestenborghs R et al: Alfentanil kinetics in the elderly. Clin Pharmacol Ther 36:239, 1984

143. Scott JC, Stanski DR: Decreased fentanyl and alfentanil dose requirements with age. A simultaneous pharmacokinetic and pharmacodynamic evaluation. J Pharmacol Exp Ther 240:159, 1987

144. Kirkpatrick T, Cockshott ID, Douglas EJ et al: Pharmacokinetics of propofol ("Diprivan") in elderly patients. Br J Anaesth 60:146, 1988

145. Dundee JW, Robinson FP, McCollum JSC et al: Sensitivity to propofol in the elderly. Anaesthesia 41:482, 1986

146. Shafer A, Doze VA, Shafer SL et al: Pharmacokinetics and pharmacodynamics of propofol infusions during general anesthesia. Anesthesiology 69:348, 1988

147. Scheepstra GL, Boois LHDJ, Rutter CLG et al: Propofol for induction and maintenance of anaesthesia: Comparison between younger and older patients. Br J Anaesth 62:54, 1989

148. Merin IG, Basch S: Are the myocardial functional and metabolic effects of isoflurane really different from those of halothane and enflurane? Anesthesiology 55:398, 1981

149. Kemmosetsu O, Hasimoto Y, Shimosata S: Inotropic effects of isoflurane on mechanics of contraction in isolated cat papillary muscles from normal and failing hearts. Anesthesiology 39:470, 1973

150. Lerman J, Schmitt-Bantel BI, Gregory GA et al: Effect of age on the solubility of volatile anesthetics in human tissues. Anesthesiology 65:307, 1986

151. Stephens ID, Po PC, Holloway AM et al: Pharmacokinetics of alcuronium in elderly patients undergoing total hip replacement of aortic reconstructive surgery. Br J Anaesth 56:45, 1984

152. Matteo RS, Backus WW, McDaniel ZD et al: Pharmacokinetics and pharmacodynamics of d-tubocurarine and metocurarine in the elderly. Anesth Analg 64:23, 1985

153. Dundee JW: Relationship of dosage of d-tubocurarine chloride and laudolissin to body weight, sex and age. Br J Anaesth 26:174, 1954

154. Duvaldestin P, Saada J, Berger JL et al: Pharmacokinetics, pharmacodynamics, and dose-response relationships of pancuronium in control and elderly subjects. Anesthesiology 56:36, 1982

155. Rupp SM, Fisher DM, Millers RD et al: Pharmacokinetics and pharmacodynamics of vecuronium in the elderly. Anesthesiology 59:A270, 1983

156. d'Hollander AA, Nevelsteen M, Barvais L et al: Effect of age on the establishment of muscle paralysis induced in anaesthetized adult subjects by ORG NC 45. Acta Anaesthesiol Scand 27:108, 1983

157. O'Hara DA, Fragen RJ, Shanks CA: The effects of age on the dose-response curves for vecuronium in adults. Anesthesiology 63:542, 1985

158. Kitts JB, Fisher DM, Canfell PC et al: Pharmacokinetics and pharmacodynamics of atracurium in the elderly. Anesthesiology 72:272, 1990

159. Young WL, Matteo RS, Ornstein E et al: Duration of action of neostigmine and pyridostigmine in the elderly. Anesth Analg 67:775, 1988

160. Lien CA, Matteo RS, Ornstein E et al: Distribution, elimination and action of vecuronium in the elderly. Anesth Analg 73:33, 1989

161. deBros FM, Lai A, Scott R et al: Pharmacokinetics and pharmacodynamics of atracurium under isoflurane anesthesia in normal and anephric patients. Anesth Analg 64:207, 1985

162. Fahey MR, Rupp SM, Fisher DM et al: Pharmacokinetics and pharmacodynamics of atracurium in patients with and without renal failure. Anesthesiology 61:699, 1984

163. d'Hollander AA, Luyckx C, Barvais L et al: Clinical evaluation of atracurium besylate requirement for a stable muscle relaxation during surgery: Lack of age-related effects. Anesthesiology 59:237, 1983

164. Dresner DL, Basta SS, Ali H et al: Pharmacokinetics and pharmacodynamics of doxacurium for young and elderly subjects during isoflurane anesthesia. Anesth Analg 71:498, 1990

165. Matteo S: Pharmacokinetics and pharmacodynamics of pipecuronium in elderly surgical patients. Anesth Analg 72:S172, 1991

166. Shanor SP, Van Hees GR, Baart N et al: The influence of age and sex on human plasma and red cell cholinesterase. Am J Med Sci 242:357, 1961

167. Rexed B: Contributions to the knowledge of the postnatal development of the peripheral nervous system in man. Acta Psychiatr Scand 31(suppl):33, 1944

168. LaFratta CW, Canestrani RE: A comparison of sensory and motor nerve conduction velocities as related to age. Arch Phys Med Rehabil 47:286, 1966

169. Kirk JR, Laursen TJS: Diffusion coefficients of various solutes for human aortic tissue with special reference to variation to tissue permeability with age. J Gerontol 10:288, 1955

170. Bromage PR: Aging and epidural dose requirements. Br J Anaesth 41:1016, 1969

171. Park WY, Massengale M, Kim S et al: Age and the spread of local anesthetic solutions in the epidural space. Anesth Analg 59:768, 1980

172. Veering BT, Burm AGL, van Kleef JW et al: Epidural anesthesia with bupivacaine: Effects of age on neural blockade and pharmacokinetics. Anesth Analg 66:589, 1987

173. Finucane BT, Hammonds WD, Welch MB: Influence of age on vascular absorption of lidocaine from the epidural space. Anesth Analg 66:843, 1987

174. Racle JP, Benkhadra A, Poy JY et al: Spinal analgesia with hyperbaric bupivacaine: Influence of age. Br J Anaesth 60:508, 1988

175. Veering BT, Denson DD, Burm AG et al: Threshold serum concentrations of bupivacaine associated with early CNS toxicity and pharmacokinetics of bupivacaine in young versus old rhesus monkeys. Reg Anaesth 14:288, 1989

176. Wong HY, Fragen RJ, Dunn K: Dose-finding study of intramuscular midazolam anesthetic medication in the elderly. Anesthesiology 74:675, 1991

177. Clark G, Erwin D, Yate P et al: Temazepam as premedication in elderly patients. Anaesthesia 37:421, 1982

178. Berlinger WG, Goldberg MJ, Spector R et al: Diphenhydramine: Kinetics and psychomotor effects in elderly women. Clin Pharmacol Ther 32:387, 1982

179. Ghignone M, Noe C, Calvillo O et al: Anesthesia for ophthalmic surgery in the elderly: The effects of clonidine on intraocular pressure, perioperative hemodynamics, and anesthetic requirement. Anesthesiology 68:707, 1988

180. Waller JL, Zaidan SR, Kaplan JA et al: Hemodynamic responses to preoperative vascular cannulation in patients with coronary artery disease. Anesthesiology 56:219, 1982

181. Backer CL, Tinker JH, Robertson DM et al: Myocardial reinfarction following local anesthesia for ophthalmic surgery. Anesth Analg 59:257, 1980

182. Brandt MR, Fernandes A, Mordhorst R et al: Epidural analgesia improves postoperative negative nitrogen balance. Br Med J 1:1106, 1978

183. Kehlet H: Influence of epidural analgesia on endocrine metabolic response to surgery. Acta Anaesthesiol Scand [Suppl] 70:39, 1978

184. Keith I: Anaesthesia and blood loss in total hip replacement. Anaesthesia 32:444, 1977

185. Modig J, Malmberg P: Pulmonary and circulatory reactions during total hip replacement surgery. Acta Anaesthesiol Scand 19:219, 1975

186. Davis FM, Laurenson VG: Spinal anaesthesia or general anaesthesia for emergency hip surgery in elderly patients. Anaesth Intensive Care 9:352, 1981

187. Valentin N, Lomholt B, Jensen JS et al: Spinal or general anaesthesia for surgery of the fractured hip? Br J Anaesth 58:284, 1986

188. Hole A, Terjesen T, Breivik H: Epidural versus general anaesthesia for total hip arthroplasty in elderly patients. Acta Anaesthesiol Scand 24:279, 1980

189. Riis J, Lomholt B, Haxholdt O et al: Immediate and long-term mental recovery from general versus epidural anesthesia in elderly patients. Acta Anaesthesiol Scand 23:44, 1983

190. Karhunen U, Jonn G: A comparison of memory function following local and general anaesthesia for extraction of senile cataracts. Acta Anaesthesiol Scand 26:291, 1982

191. Mann RAM, Bisset WIK: Anaesthesia for lower limb amputation. Anaesthesia 38:1185, 1983

192. Berggren D, Gustafson Y, Eriksson B et al: Postoperative confusion after anesthesia in elderly patients with femoral neck fractures. Anesth Analg 66:497, 1987

193. Chung FF, Meier R, Lautenschlager E et al: General or spinal anesthesia: Which is better in the elderly? Anesthesiology 67:422, 1987

194. Chung F, Lavelle PA, McDonald S et al: Cognitive impairment after neuroleptanalgesia in cataract surgery. Anesth Analg 68:614, 1989

195. Chung FF, Chung A, Meier RH et al: Comparison of perioperative mental function after general anaesthesia and spinal anaesthesia with intravenous sedation. Can J Anaesth 36:382, 1989

196. Benzon HT, Linde HW, Molloy RE et al: Postdural puncture headache in patients with chronic pain. Anesth Analg 59:772, 1980

197. Fink BR: Postspinal headache. Anesth Analg 71:208, 1990

198. Guttman D: Patterns of legal drug use by older Americans. Addict Behav 3:337, 1977

199. Chien CT, Townsend EJ, Ross-Townsend A: Substance use and abuse among the community elderly: The medical aspect. Addict Behav 3:357, 1978

200. Seidl LG, Thornton GF, Smith JW et al: Studies on the epidemiology of adverse drug reactions: III. Reactions in patients on a general medical service. Bull Johns Hopkins Hosp 119:299, 1966

201. Hurwitz N: Predisposing factors in adverse reactions to drugs. Br Med J 1:536, 1969

202. Berggren D, Gustafson Y, Eriksson B et al: Postoperative confusion after anesthesia in elderly patients with femoral neck fractures. Anesth Analg 66:497, 1987

203. Lipowski ZJ: Delirium in the elderly patient. N Engl J Med 320:578, 1989

204. Malling BVG, Nissen LR, Larsen KB et al: Postanesthetic arousal time in elderly patients: A double-blind study of glycopyrrolate and atropine. Br J Anaesth 60:426, 1988

205. Seymour G: Medical assessment of the elderly surgical patient. Rockville, MD: Aspen Systems, 1986

206. Meridy HW: Criteria for selection of ambulatory surgical patients and guidelines for anesthesia management. A retrospective study of 1553 cases. Anesth Analg 61:921, 1982

207. Gold BS, Kitz DS, Lecky JH et al: Unanticipated admission to the hospital following ambulatory surgery. JAMA 262:3008, 1989

208. Natof HE: FASA Special Study I. Alexandria, VA: Federated Ambulatory Surgery Association, 1985

209. Tyler IL, Tantisira B, Winter PM et al: Continuous monitoring of arterial oxygen saturation with pulse oximetry during transfer to the recovery room. Anesth Analg 64:1108, 1985

210. Peters NL: Snipping the thread of life—antimuscarinic side effects of medications in the elderly. Arch Intern Med 149:2414, 1989

211. Ready LB, Chadwick HS, Ross B: Age predicts effective epidural morphine dose after abdominal hysterectomy. Anesth Analg 66:1215, 1987

212. Moore AK, Vilderman S, Lubensky W et al: Differences in epidural morphine requirements between elderly and young patients after abdominal surgery. Anesth Analg 70:316, 1990

50

Bernard V. Wetchler

Outpatient Anesthesia

Outpatient surgery came into existence in the 20th century and has slowly proved itself a reasonable alternative to hospitalization for quality care. The American Hospital Association predicts that by 1995, 60% of all operations will be performed on an outpatient basis. Physicians and patients now accept outpatient surgery readily. Anesthesiologists entering practice today can anticipate that a substantial proportion of their practice may be devoted to outpatient cases.

Outpatient surgery has a longer history than is generally realized. In 1909 James H. Nicoll described the practice of outpatient surgery when he presented to the British Medical Association the results of 8988 operations on outpatients performed at the Glasgow Royal Hospital for Sick Children between the years 1899 and 1909.[1] In the same era, in 1916, Ralph M. Waters opened the Down-Town Anesthesia Clinic in Sioux City, Iowa, for minor surgery and dental cases. His was the prototype of the modern freestanding center. In an article in the Anesthesia Supplement of the *American Journal of Surgery* he wrote, "When the war is over, I trust many of you may develop down-town minor surgery and dental clinics of much larger scope."[2]

These early reports failed to spur an upsurge of national interest in outpatient surgery, however. There was a hiatus in the reporting of large series until 1937, when G. Hertzfeld reported on more than 1000 outpatient pediatric hernia repairs performed with the use of general anesthesia.[3] In 1959 Webb and Graves reported their experiences with outpatient surgery.[4] Finally, in 1962, an outpatient surgical program was initiated at the University of California at Los Angeles (J. B. Dillon, pers. commun., 1987), followed shortly by the opening of a formal outpatient surgical facility at George Washington University in 1966 (M.-L. Levy, pers. commun., 1987).

In 1968 the Dudley Street Ambulatory Surgical Center opened in Providence, Rhode Island. Lacking support from the state health department, which considered it to be no more than a physician's office, and finding no support from third-party insurance carriers, the Dudley Street facility could not maintain itself financially.

In 1970 the Phoenix Surgicenter, a freestanding facility, opened in Phoenix, Arizona. Ralph Waters's message had finally been heard. A plaque in its lobby proclaims, "Dedicated to the principle that high quality outpatient surgical care can be provided in a caring, personal environment, in a free-standing ambulatory facility at a lower cost than other alternatives."

In 1974 the Society for the Advancement of Freestanding Ambulatory Surgical Centers was established. It is now known as the Federated Ambulatory Surgery Association. In 1983 Porterfield and Franklin advocated office outpatient surgery. Of 18,000 procedures, 5038 were performed with the use of general anesthesia.[5]

In 1984 the Society for Ambulatory Anesthesia was organized. Outpatient anesthesia was becoming recognized as a subspecialty. In 1988, hospital-affiliated ambulatory surgery accounted for more than 10 million operations performed in a hospital setting. By 1989 there were 984 Medicare-participating, freestanding outpatient surgery centers in the United States performing almost 2 million procedures annually.

SELECTION CRITERIA FOR OUTPATIENT ANESTHESIA

Are the lists of "appropriate outpatient procedures" being generated by governmental bodies, corporations, and third-party payers designed only to inform the medical community that reimbursement may be limited or nonexistent unless the stipulated procedure is performed on an outpatient basis? Are physicians being deprived of the right to exercise medical judgment in determining the appropriateness of patients for outpatient surgery? Are selection criteria for outpatient surgery becoming too liberal? All three questions can be answered with a qualified no.

Determining which patient and which procedure is suitable for outpatient surgery generates considerable discussion. The selection of appropriate patients and procedures will limit the number of unanticipated hospitalizations after outpatient procedures.

Patient Factors

The surgeon should provide the patient with information about the outpatient procedure, the type of facility in which the procedure will be performed (hospital or freestanding center), laboratory studies that will be ordered, and dietary restrictions. The patient must understand that he or she will be going home the day of surgery, must want to have surgery on an outpatient basis, and must be willing to follow instructions.[6] Patients who are unable to follow instructions may be appropriate candidates for outpatient surgery as long as a responsible person who understands and can follow instructions is available to provide care.

Dietary Restrictions

If conventional guidelines are followed (Table 50-1), preoperative fasting, even for periods of 13–15 hours, does not result in hypoglycemia in healthy outpatients up to 5 years old.[7] Studies in patients aged 6 months to 9 years have confirmed this finding, although asymptomatic hypoglycemia has been reported[8-12] following prolonged fasting (i.e., fasting overnight for surgery on the following afternoon). Meakin et al determined the effects of decreasing the traditional period of fasting and of giving oral premedicants before anesthesia to 224 healthy children.[13] Fasting for less than 4 hours increased the volume of gastric aspirate. Oral premedicants and their vehicles (capsule vs. elixir) significantly affected the increase in gastric volume. A positive correlation was noted between the duration of fasting and gastric pH (the longer the fast, the more alkaline the contents) when the volume of gastric contents was measured after anesthesia induction in patients scheduled for either morning or afternoon surgery.[14] Crawford et al have shown that healthy children may receive 2 ml·kg^{-1} of water up to 2 hours before elective surgery without a decrease in gastric fluid pH or an increase in gastric fluid volume beyond values obtained after fasting for 6 hours.[15]

In adult patients, Maltby et al examined the effect on residual gastric fluid volume and pH of 150 ml of water taken orally, with or without ranitidine, between 2 and 3 hours before operation.[16] Prolonged fasting did not provide a safe gastric environment, and the ingestion of 150 ml of water actually reduced residual gastric volume, probably by reflex contraction of the stomach when it was stimulated by a bolus of liquid. The addition of oral ranitidine, 150 mg, further reduced residual gastric volume and acidity. In a follow-up study, patients were given various fluids or premedicants 2–3 hours before the scheduled time of surgery: 150 ml of coffee or orange juice with 150 mg ranitidine orally, 150 ml of coffee or orange juice with placebo, 150 mg ranitidine, or placebo only. The effect of ranitidine on gastric volume and pH appeared to override all other variables investigated.[17] A routine "NPO after midnight" order ignores both differences in the rates of gastric emptying of solid foods and clear liquids and differences in scheduled times for surgery.[18] When more than 2 hours have elapsed following ingestion of clear fluids, endogenous gastric secretion is the principal determinant of the pH and volume of gastric contents. A longer fluid fast does not improve the gastric environment.

The Canadian Anaesthetists' Society, which previously recommended a 5-hour fast for patients undergoing elective surgery, now recommends that each department of anesthesia formulate its own policies regarding preoperative fasting.[19] Goresky and Maltby suggest that the following regimen be followed in healthy patients scheduled for elective surgery:[18]

1. No solid food should be ingested on the day of surgery.
2. Unrestricted intake of clear liquids should be permitted until 3 hours before the scheduled time of surgery, and oral medication should be taken with 30 ml of water up to 1 hour before surgery.
3. The preoperative administration of an H$_2$ receptor blocker should be considered for patients at increased risk of regurgitation and aspiration of gastric contents.

Preoperative Screening

Each outpatient facility should develop its own method of preoperative screening, to be conducted before the day of surgery. The patient may visit the facility, or staff members of the facility may call the patient by telephone. Screening allows facility staff to obtain necessary information about the patient, including a complete medical and family history, information about medications the patient is taking, and problems the patient or patient's family may have had with anesthesia. The process also provides the staff with an opportunity to remind patients of their arrival time, clothes to wear, and restrictions (i.e., nothing to eat or drink after midnight, no jewelry or makeup). Staff members can determine if there is a problem with transportation and if a responsible person is available to escort the patient to and from the facility and care for the patient at home after surgery. The anesthesiologist should review the screening record and determine whether additional laboratory studies must be completed, whether the patient is medically stable, what precautions must be taken, and whether the patient's medical or family history (problems with anesthesia) warrants an anesthesiologist's evaluation several days before surgery, or if the evaluation can be done on the day of surgery. Preoperative screening provides staff members with the opportunity to reassure the patient, answer questions, and determine whether any support services are needed (e.g., transportation, visiting nurse).[20]

The following are simple questions whose answers correlated with a consensus of fitness for anesthesia:[21]

1. Do you feel sick?
2. Have you had any serious illnesses?
3. Do you get more short of breath on exertion than others of your age?
4. Do you have a cough?
5. Do you have a wheeze?
6. Do you have chest pain on exertion?
7. Do you have ankle swelling?
8. Have you taken any medications in the last 3 months?
9. Do you have any allergies?
10. Have you had an anesthetic in the past 2 months?

TABLE 50-1. NPO Orders at Children's National Medical Center (Washington, D.C.)

Age	Interval Between Solid Food*	Interval Between Clear Liquids†
<1 yr	6 h	4 h
1–6 yr	Midnight	6 h
>6 yr	Midnight	8 h

* Includes milk or milk products.

† Includes breast milk.

Reproduced with permission from Hannallah RS, Epstein BS: The pediatric patient. In Wetchler BV (ed): Anesthesia for Ambulatory Surgery, 2nd ed, p 144. Philadelphia, JB Lippincott, 1991.

11. Have you or your relatives had problems with anesthesia?

Wilson *et al* concluded, "Patients who are thought to be perfectly fit on the basis of simple questions, usually prove to be so after the traditional preoperative history and investigations," and they suggested that a questionnaire could be developed to aid in selecting appropriate patients for ambulatory surgery.[21] Sample telephone screening questionnaires for children and adults are given in Tables 50-2 and 50-3.

Automated history taking may prove beneficial. Health Quiz, a computer software program that automates the taking of patient histories, also flags problem areas and suggests laboratory tests to be ordered.[22] When used in an initial multicenter evaluation, this lap-top computer program, invented by Michael F. Roizen, averaged savings of $68.70 by more efficient use of laboratory testing (M. F. Roizen, pers. commun., 1990).

Additional factors to be considered in determining whether a patient is a suitable candidate for outpatient surgery include the distance the patient lives from the hospital and the length of time it will take the patient to get care if problems arise. "Reasonable" distance and time are not easily defined. These areas must be addressed by each facility on an individual patient basis.

Physical Status

Outpatient surgery is no longer restricted to patients of the American Society of Anesthesiologists (ASA) Physical Status 1 and 2. Patients of ASA Physical Status 3 (or 4) are appropriate candidates if their systemic diseases are medically stable. Anesthesiologists want to know from the patient's primary physician if the patient's medical problem is in optimal control. We don't want to hear "maintain blood pressure, monitor ECG, give plenty of oxygen."

Does physical status classification predict complications after an outpatient procedure? Is there a relationship between physical status and unanticipated hospitalization? In 1980 the Phoenix Surgicenter reported that their overall hospital transfer rate of 0.2% increased to 0.59% for patients older than age 64 and increased to 1.41% for patients of ASA Physical Status 3.[23] Natof monitored the correlation of

complications with pre-existing medical problems.[24,25] The incidence of major complications (1.12%) in patients with no pre-existing disease was comparable to the incidence of major complications (1.16%) in patients with pre-existing disease.

In a study encompassing 87,492 patients, the Federated Ambulatory Surgery Association concluded the following: (1) certain surgical procedures are associated with a higher established incidence of complications, (2) there appears to be little or no cause-and-effect relationship between pre-existing disease and the incidence of complications, and (3) the incidence of complications increases with increasing length of operation.[26] Gold and co-workers examined the rate of unanticipated hospital admissions following ambulatory surgery among 9616 patients at a university hospital and identified several factors that were associated with unanticipated admission.[27] The admission rate was 1%, and factors independently associated with an increased likelihood of admission were general anesthesia, type of procedure (specifically, lower abdominal procedures), lengthy procedures (i.e., lasting more than 1 hour), postoperative vomiting, and age (Table 50-4). In an 8-year period (1981–1988), the Methodist Ambulatory SurgiCare recorded an unanticipated admission rate of 1.2% for patients older than

---

TABLE 50-3. Adult Preanesthesia Telephone Interview

The following items are discussed in a telephone interview with an adult scheduled for ambulatory surgery:

1. Serious past illness
2. Heart problems
3. High blood pressure
4. Chest pain
5. Asthma/emphysema
6. Allergies
7. Diabetes
8. Medications
9. Problems with anesthesia in the past
10. Possibility of pregnancy (where applicable)

Source: Methodist Medical Center of Illinois Ambulatory SurgiCare, Peoria. Reproduced with permission from Wetchler BV: Patient selection criteria 1987. AORN J 45:30, 1987.

TABLE 50-2. Pediatric Preanesthesia Telephone Interview

The following items are discussed in a telephone interview with the parent of a child scheduled for ambulatory surgery:

1. Breath-holding spells
2. Cardiac, respiratory, or other problems
3. History of prematurity:
   If yes:
   Was oxygen used?
   Was the child's trachea intubated?
   Any lasting effects?
4. Muscular problems
5. Developmental delays
6. Asthma or frequent colds
7. Sickle cell disease or trait
8. Medications
9. Recent exposure to contagious disease

Source: Children's National Medical Center, Washington, DC. Reproduced with permission from Wetchler BV: Patient selection criteria 1987. AORN J 45:30, 1987.

TABLE 50-4. Multivariate Logistic Regression Analysis of Factors Associated with Hospital Admission Following Same-Day Surgery

Factor	Odds Ratio	95% Confidence Interval
General anesthesia	5.18*	2.60–10.30
Emesis	3.03*	1.35– 6.81
Abdominal surgery	2.89*	1.07– 7.79
Operating room time >1 hour	2.72*	1.46– 5.08
Age (30-yr intervals)	2.56*	1.32– 4.94
Laparoscopy	1.71	0.69– 4.22
Patient lives >1 hour from hospital	1.49	0.79– 2.80

*$p < 0.05$.

Reproduced with permission from Gold B, Kitz D, Lecky J *et al*: JAMA 262:3008, 1989.

60, compared with an overall unanticipated admission rate of 0.8%. For patients older than age 60 receiving inhalational anesthesia, the admission rate was 4.6%, compared with a 1.4% admission rate for all patients receiving inhalational anesthesia.[28]

Age

The Very Old. The acceptability of very old and very young patients for outpatient surgical procedures is well documented. For geriatric patients, chronological age is not a deterrent. The factors that determine the acceptability of a geriatric patient for outpatient surgery are physiologic age, physical status, surgical procedure, anesthetic technique, and quality of care available at home.[28]

Two factors must be considered in providing anesthesia for the elderly patient—the patient's pre-existing diseases and the physiologic changes associated with aging. A primary concern for elderly patients is to keep hospitalization as brief as possible. More than half of hospitalized geriatric patients experience transient confusion after operation.[29] Because of a quicker return to normal surroundings following outpatient surgery, the elderly patient is exposed to fewer hypnotic, narcotic, and tranquilizing medications, with a resultant decrease in the incidence of postoperative confusion. The older patient is less able to cope with a new environment and frequently has fewer psychological and physiologic defenses than younger patients for coping with stress. It is important that staff members actively engage and relate to the geriatric patient.

The superiority of a specific anesthetic technique in the elderly has not been demonstrated. Opinions are frequently based on impressions and tradition, not on prospective studies. The consequences of different types of anesthesia are difficult to assess. Chung and co-workers found that mental function in the elderly population was better maintained after spinal anesthesia than after general anesthesia.[30] For certain procedures, regional anesthesia may be a better choice in the elderly ambulatory surgery patient, providing less deterioration of mental function, a lower incidence of postoperative confusion, and a reduced risk of drug interactions.

Geriatric patients have more problems than younger patients, and the problems are of a wholly different nature. Elderly patients show significantly poorer comprehension of information relevant to informed consent. They must be treated with gentle patience; they should not be rushed or made to feel as though they are keeping everyone waiting.

The Very Young. Infants considered at risk are best handled as inpatients. An infant with a hemoglobin or hematocrit level below the lower limits of normal for its age group is at risk and needs further medical workup before anesthesia for an elective procedure. If an infant with a history of respiratory distress syndrome is intubated and needs ventilatory support, it may take up to a year to outgrow symptoms and have normal blood gas values. If bronchopulmonary dysplasia develops, the at-risk period extends until the infant has no symptoms. The patient with bronchopulmonary dysplasia is more likely to die of sudden infant death syndrome (SIDS). A history of prematurity, apnea, or aspiration with feeding places the infant at risk. Is an infant at risk if a sibling has died of SIDS? In this situation, a prudent decision would be to monitor the infant for apnea on an inpatient basis for 24 hours after surgery.[20]

When is the infant who was born prematurely considered acceptable for outpatient surgery? Several studies have doc-umented an increased incidence of apnea for 12 hours after anesthesia in ex-premature infants. Steward found that preterm infants of less than 10 weeks' postnatal age developed apnea during anesthesia and up to 12 hours after operation, compared with no incidence of apnea in full-term infants.[31] Liu et al reported an increased incidence of apneic episodes after anesthesia in preterm infants younger than 41–46 weeks' postconceptual age.[32] Kurth et al suggested monitoring for postoperative apnea for 12–24 hours in patients younger than 60 weeks' postconceptual age.[33] Welborn et al studied infants younger than 12 months' postnatal age who had general anesthesia for herniorrhaphy.[34] Premature infants younger than 44 weeks' postconceptual age were found to be at high risk for the development of postoperative ventilatory dysfunction. Mestad et al noted that patients older than 40 weeks' postconceptual age and who did not have a prior history of apnea or lung disease did not develop apnea postoperatively.[35]

There is no universal agreement as to the acceptable postconceptual age (gestation plus postnatal age) at which an ex-premature infant may undergo outpatient surgery. As the infant matures, the tendency to apnea greatly diminishes, but no one knows the age at which all babies may be safely anesthetized. The age at which the ex-premature infant attains physiologic maturity and no longer is at increased risk must be considered individually, with attention given to growth and development, persistent problems during feeding, time to recover from upper respiratory infections, apneic history, and the presence of metabolic, endocrine, neurologic, or cardiac disorders.

Infants at greatest risk appear to be those younger than 46 weeks' postconceptual age and who have a preoperative history of apnea. Obviously, there must be a middle ground between the conservative 60 weeks recommended by Kurth and co-workers and the recommendations by Liu et al and Welborn et al of 44–46 weeks.[32-34]

Inappropriate Candidates for Ambulatory Surgery

There are no published guidelines and few data with which to identify patients who are inappropriate candidates for ambulatory surgery. In almost every instance we must individualize; with few exceptions, we must address a combination of the following factors: the patient, surgical procedure, anesthetic technique, and the anesthesiologist's comfort level. The following list, provided by the Methodist Ambulatory SurgiCare facility, divides inappropriateness into medical and social reasons. Abnormal laboratory values that may cause postponement of the procedure are a separate consideration.

I. Medical contraindications to ambulatory surgery
   A. The infant at risk
      1. A healthy infant who was born prematurely and is younger than 50 weeks' postconceptual age.
      2. An infant still experiencing apneic episodes, difficulty with feeding, and delayed growth and development (failure to thrive).
      3. An infant who had respiratory distress syndrome and was intubated and on ventilatory support. The infant should have no wheezing or bronchospasm at the time of surgery. It may take 6 months or more before the infant has no symptoms and may undergo surgery. Using blood gas values as an indication that the infant is asymptomatic is a matter of individual preference (the Children's

National Medical Center in Washington, DC, does not routinely check blood gases). There should have been no recent or recurrent episodes (in the previous 2–3 months) of wheezing, bronchospasm, or apnea, and the infant should not have a history of wheezing or bronchospasm that was not precipitated by an upper respiratory infection. The infant's ability to handle an upper respiratory tract infection should be considered. The patient should be symptom free at the time of surgery and when discharged from the facility (no wheezing) (R. S. Hannallah, pers. commun., 1987). Pulse oximetry may be a useful indicator of the patient's status in the postanesthesia care unit (PACU).

   4. If an infant has had bronchopulmonary dysplasia, it must be free of symptoms before surgery and when discharged from the facility. Again, the use of blood gas values is an individual decision. The infant who has had bronchopulmonary dysplasia is at increased risk of SIDS.

   5. An infant whose sibling has died of SIDS is not an acceptable candidate when younger than 6 months (with a more conservative approach, possibly up to 1 year of age).

B. Patients with malignant hyperthermia or who are susceptible to malignant hyperthermia. Most facilities take the position that a patient with malignant hyperthermia requires overnight observation, but this period has not been substantiated by specific data. When a patient has only a history (masseter spasm or an episode of malignant hyperthermia in the family), some facilities administer a trigger-free anesthetic, watch the patient for 6–8 hours, and consider discharge that evening. Gronert believes that malignant hyperthermia is not a contraindication to outpatient surgery but advises that "all centers must have dantrolene for immediate use" (G. Gronert, pers. commun., 1991).

C. Patients with uncontrolled seizure activity are considered inappropriate by some; however, other facilities do not consider this an absolute contraindication (the patient is observed for 4–8 hours and may be sent home if seizure free). If the patient with uncontrolled seizure activities is sent home, two responsible individuals must be in attendance, one to drive the car and the other to sit next to the patient and provide care should a seizure occur.

D. Medically unstable ASA Physical Status 3 (or 4) patient.

E. Morbidly obese patient with other systemic diseases. The obese patient is acceptable if there is no other systemic disease that would cause any patient to be classified as ASA Physical Status 3.[36]

F. Patient being treated with monoamine oxidase inhibitors. The patient must have stopped taking medication for 10 days. The need for this has been questioned.[37,38]

G. Acute substance abuser.

II. Social contraindications to ambulatory surgery

A. Uncooperative patient

   1. Patient refuses to have ambulatory procedure.

   2. Patient is unwilling to follow instructions. Patients who are unable to follow instructions (handicapped) are acceptable if they have a responsible person to monitor their care following discharge.

B. No responsible person at home. A responsible person

is defined as someone who is physically and intellectually capable of taking care of the patient.

Procedure Related Factors

Parameters established in the early 1970s for procedure selection included the following: the procedure should take less than 90 minutes, the risk of postoperative complications should be reliably low, transfusion should not be anticipated, and the surgeon should be skillful and speedy because outpatient procedures do not lend themselves to resident teaching or performance by a trainee.[39] Are these parameters still appropriate today? The limits on the duration of surgery no longer appear warranted, particularly because the relationship between anesthesia time and recovery time is weak. The length of time for a procedure is a consideration, but one must also look at many other variables, including the patient's physical status, the surgeon's ability, whether the procedure is superficial or deep, the type of anesthesia, and whether local anesthesia will be used to supplement inhalational technique.

We should still be interested in performing procedures with a reliably low rate of postoperative complications. However, the definition of a reliably low rate appears to depend on the relative aggressiveness of the facility, surgeon, patient, and payer. For example, cholecystectomy, vaginal hysterectomy, reduction mammaplasty, open arthrotomy with ligament repair, and thyroidectomy are all being performed on an outpatient basis.

The potential need for a transfusion is no longer an absolute contraindication to performance of a procedure on an outpatient basis. Autologous blood transfusion is being used in a small percentage of patients undergoing extensive liposuction procedures (W. A. Reed, pers. commun., 1987).

The stipulation that the procedures should take less than 90 minutes was made in the belief that skillful and speedy surgeons were essential to the success of ambulatory surgery and that the time factor precluded resident training. Today, more than 10 million outpatient surgical procedures are performed each year by qualified surgeons and residents in training.

Three statements can serve as the basis of procedure acceptability as we approach the 21st century:

1. Procedures are not "acceptable" in and of themselves. The procedure cannot be separated from the patient having the procedure. Pediatric inguinal hernia surgery is a good example; it is an acceptable procedure for outpatient surgery, but one must be aware of the high-risk patient. This is a good reason why lists of procedures cannot be allowed to undermine medical judgment.[40]

2. Dawson and Reed stated, "Any procedure which does not require a major intervention in the cranial vault, abdomen or thorax can be considered acceptable."[23]

3. Orkin wrote, "The actual list of acceptable procedures in a given ambulatory unit is established in an evolutionary process. . . . On a periodic basis, the medical director of the unit must decide which procedures (and which patients) are appropriate for the unit, given its equipment, staff and their capabilities, ability and reliability of the given surgeon and medical condition of the particular patient."[41]

Facility

Outpatient surgery occurs in a variety of settings, both within a hospital and in freestanding facilities. In the hospital setting, ambulatory surgery is categorized as integrated (performed in the hospital operating suite), separated (away from the hospital operating suite), or freestanding (a satellite facility located away from the hospital campus).[42] The freestanding label is also given to a surgery center when it is distinct and independent from the hospital campus. This facility can maintain its autonomy but be affiliated with the hospital. These facilities are usually owned and managed by physicians, by a for-profit subsidiary of a hospital, or by a multifacility health care corporation.

Physicians office-based surgery is performed in a physician's office where there is an established surgical suite.

Hospital
  Integrated
  Separated
Freestanding
  Hospital affiliated
  Independent
  Hospital corporate chain
Physicians office-based surgery

Some believe that hospital facilities can be more liberal in their selection process than can freestanding facilities because of the ease of consultation as well as of obtaining inpatient services should the need arise.

OUTPATIENT ANESTHESIA MANAGEMENT

Standaert has stated that "everyone involved with therapeutic agents, patient, physician, medicinal chemist, wants a magic bullet, a drug that does exactly what is expected of it and does nothing else."[43] As we continue our search for the magic bullet, we should keep the useful drugs and discard those with adverse effects. The same applies to the drugs used in outpatient anesthesia.

Premedication

There are special premedication considerations that anesthesiologists should be aware of when managing the outpatient. Like outpatient surgery and outpatient anesthesia, outpatient premedication represents a break from tradition. We must tailor both our psychological and pharmacologic preparation to be a part of the compacted perioperative care the outpatient receives. The medications, dosages, and routes of administration chosen should be practical and should not prolong the patient's stay in the PACU.

Meridy found that the use of premedicants other than opioids did not prolong recovery.[44] Premedication had a marginal effect on recovery time, although patients given opioids (morphine, meperidine) had a significantly longer recovery time than nonmedicated patients. Preanesthesia medication is based on tradition and is influenced by the anesthesiologist's training, clinical experience, and inpatient medication routine. Past practice dictates the use of no or limited premedication for outpatient surgery. Is this practice appropriate today? Can we modify our choice of drugs, doses, and routes of administration to limit the outpatient's apprehension without significantly increasing length of stay? Can new drugs supplant old favorites?

In 1967 Dillon wrote, "We find that a great deal of premedication is unnecessary. We frequently give our premedication intravenously, which assures its prompt action in a predictable time and in a predictable manner."[45]

In 1974 Epstein stated, "Minimal or no premedication is advisable. All physicians recognize that the greater the dose and the more long-acting the depressant medication, the greater the chance of prolongation of recovery and coincident drowsiness, dizziness, hypotension, or vomiting. At George Washington University Hospital no premedication is used. In some centers only belladonna drugs are administered."[39]

According to Reed, "Heavy, long-lasting premedication, an additional 100 mg to 200 mg of barbiturate, or extra depth with an inhalation drug may cause no deleterious effect in the healthy patient. The resulting increase in recovery time, however, will have an unfavorable impact on the surgical outpatient who would otherwise safely ambulate; it could even create an anesthetic inpatient out of what was meant to be an outpatient surgical procedure."[46]

Levy and Weintraub believe the outpatient is frequently more apprehensive about the anesthetic, which is perceived as major, compared with "minor surgery," which is thought to be non-life-threatening.[47] They recommend that the anesthesiologist have a frank discussion with the patient and explain the anesthetic, monitoring, and after-effects of anesthesia and surgery to help relieve patient apprehension. Twersky and colleagues compared the effect of early (1–7 days prior to surgery) and day-of-surgery preanesthetic assessment and noted no advantage to early presurgical evaluation in reducing anxiety levels or perioperative anesthetic and analgesic requirements.[48] Contrary to conventional teaching, a preanesthesia interview may not lower preoperative anxiety in outpatients.[49]

During the preanesthesia interview, the intelligent, well-informed patient will understand and accept the rationale of forgoing traditional methods of providing premedication.

Patient apprehension can be minimized by the following measures:

Keeping the waiting time before surgery short.
Providing an attractive waiting room with reading materials and television.
Providing games for children.
Reducing the time the patient must be separated from family or friends.
Having the patient change to a hospital gown just before surgery.

Although a preanesthesia evaluation may have limited benefits in diminishing patient anxiety, there is a distinct advantage to every facility having its own screening mechanism. Effective prescreening of patients will help limit last-minute postponements and cancellations.

The routine of using little or no premedication is advisable.[23,39] Others, however, believe the patients' time in the holding unit can be made more pleasant with the use of premedicant drugs.[50,51] Premedicant drugs may be used if needed by the patient and if the drug and dosage are chosen carefully. Drugs used as premedicants for outpatients include anticholinergics, H_2 receptor antagonists and antacids, opioids, sedative-hypnotics, and gastrokinetics.

The use of preinduction agents is becoming increasingly popular in pediatric anesthesia.[52,53] Preinduction anesthesia refers to the use of rapidly acting medications as a last-minute premedication. The drug and dose selected should ensure a rapid onset of sedation (3–10 minutes) with minimal or no prolongation of recovery time.[54] Several preinduction techniques are claimed to achieve cooperation in children during induction with inhalational agents. Low-dose intramuscular (im) ketamine (2 mg·kg^{-1})[53] or oral midazolam (0.5–0.75 mg·kg^{-1})[55] are frequently chosen. Rectal methohexital (25 mg·kg^{-1} of the 2% solution, 25 mg·kg^{-1} of the 1% solution) is also an effective preinduction medication.[56,57]

Anticholinergics

Tradition dictates the use of anticholinergic drugs as part of preanesthetic medication for their antisialagogic and vagolytic actions. More satisfactory conditions as a result of decreased secretions are likely to be achieved during inhalational anesthesia when an anticholinergic is administered as a premedicant, particularly when an endotracheal tube is in place.[58]

Currently used inhalational drugs are considerably less irritating than the anesthetics used earlier (diethyl ether), and routine anticholinergic premedication is not needed for the outpatient. Furthermore, drying of mucous membranes by anticholinergics can contribute to a sore throat and complaints of a dry mouth postoperatively.[50] Elderly patients have decreased salivary gland production and do not need antisialagogues. The blocking of vagal reflexes requires larger doses than those given as premedication. Vagal reflexes are best treated by intravenous (iv) administration of an appropriate anticholinergic if and when they occur. Glycopyrrolate may be of limited use for short outpatient procedures because of its more prolonged and intense drying effect compared with that of atropine.[59]

Clarke and Hurtig found that a combination of meperidine (1 mg·kg^{-1}) and atropine (0.01 mg·kg^{-1}), given im as a premedicant, did not prolong recovery in an outpatient population.[50]

In pediatric outpatients, oral diazepam (0.1 mg·kg^{-1}), hydroxyzine (0.5 mg·kg^{-1}), or a combination of diazepam (0.2 mg·kg^{-1}), meperidine (1.5 mg·kg^{-1}), and atropine (0.02 mg·kg^{-1}) did not prolong recovery time.[60,61]

H$_2$ Receptor Antagonists and Antacids

Outpatients and inpatients have the potential for aspiration pneumonitis. This potential is increased in patients who are obese or pregnant (second and third trimesters), have peptic ulceration, hiatal hernia, or diabetes mellitus, or have undergone upper abdominal procedures. The Trendelenburg and prone positions and fasciculation after the use of succinylcholine may increase regurgitation.[62]

Is the outpatient at greater risk for acid aspiration than the inpatient? With risk potential considered as a pH less than 2.5 and a gastric volume greater than 25 ml, Ong et al found pH values to be similar in both groups, but 86% of outpatients had volumes greater than 0.4 ml·kg^{-1}, compared with only 57% of inpatients.[63] Although an initial study did not find an increased potential for aspiration in outpatients, a more recent study by Manchikanti and colleagues reported a significant number of outpatients to have a decreased pH and an increased gastric volume.[64,65] Wyner and Cohen found no significant difference in residual gastric volume between pregnant (mean gestational age, 15 ± 3 weeks) and nonpregnant outpatients at induction of anesthesia.[66]

Patients undergoing emergency surgery are at increased risk for aspiration. In a computer-assisted study of 185,358 anesthetics, 87 cases of aspiration were identified, and aspiration was six times more common during the night than during the day.[67]

In a multicenter study (181 outpatient facilities), there were 90 documented cases of aspiration (1.7 per 10,000).[68] Of 266 suspected cases during the past decade reported by the survey respondents, 54.1% required hospital admission and 27.4% of patients were hospitalized more than 1 day; there were no reported deaths. Natof et al prospectively reviewed the cases of 32,001 outpatients and found only one case of suspected aspiration and no deaths.[69]

Of the various drug therapies suggested, suspension antacids are no longer recommended because they may cause significant pulmonary damage if aspirated. Antacids reduce gastric acidity but increase gastric fluid volume. Martin et al studied the effects of oral Bicitra and im cimetidine in patients undergoing outpatient breast biopsy.[70] The potential for aspiration pneumonitis in the various treatment groups was as follows: in the control group, 80% (pH 1.68 ± 0.30, volume 44.67 ± 14.1 ml); in the group given Bicitra, 26% (pH 3.20 ± 1.00, volume 61.80 ± 25.4 ml); and in the group given cimetidine, 0% (pH 6.3 ± 1.06, volume 12.33 ± 8.5 ml). In this study, Bicitra (15 ml) was administered orally 15 minutes before induction and cimetidine (300 mg) was administered im 30 minutes before induction of anesthesia.

Oral administration of cimetidine (300 mg) 1–4 hours before anesthesia induction resulted in a pH above 2.5 in 84% of patients and a gastric volume less than 20 ml in 88% of patients.[64] Glycopyrrolate alone had no effect on volume or acidity, and the addition of glycopyrrolate to cimetidine added no protective effect. Despite convincing evidence that cimetidine increases gastric fluid pH, there are no data to demonstrate that there will be no pulmonary damage if gastric contents are inhaled by patients pretreated with cimetidine or that the use of cimetidine reduces anesthetic mortality from aspiration.[71,72] Oral administration of ranitidine (150 mg) the evening before and the morning of surgery decreased the incidence of risk from 47% to zero for outpatients.[73] An oral regimen of either ranitidine (150 mg), cimetidine (400 mg), or placebo given approximately 5 hours before induction of anesthesia showed both H$_2$ receptor blockers to be significantly better than placebo at reducing gastric acidity and volume. The potential for acid aspiration in the group treated with placebo was 100%, in the group given cimetidine it was 46%, and in the group given ranitidine it was 15%.[74] Oral ranitidine appears to be as effective as oral cimetidine in reducing the potential for aspiration pneumonitis without the side-effects and adverse drug interactions associated with cimetidine.[75,76]

Somori and Kallar administered cimetidine syrup orally (7.5 mg·kg^{-1}) to pediatric outpatients 1 hour before surgery.[77] Cimetidine-treated patients had a pH of 5.06 ± 0.35 and a volume of 4.5 ml ± 0.35; the control group had a pH of 1.55 ± 0.09 and volume of 9.5 ml ± 2.00. When ranitidine (2.0 mg·kg^{-1}) was administered orally 1 hour before surgery, patients had a pH of 5.1 ± 0.5 and a volume of 0.10 ml·kg^{-1} ± 0.05. A control group had a pH of 2.0 ± 0.3 and a volume of 0.31 ml·kg^{-1} ± 0.07.[78] Oral administration of sodium citrate, 0.4 ml·kg^{-1}, to children 30 minutes before induction of anesthesia was equally as effective in increasing gastric pH as oral administration of cimetidine (10 mg·kg^{-1}) 60 minutes before induction of anesthesia.[79]

Both ranitidine and cimetidine appear to be effective agents for reducing the potential for aspiration pneumonitis. Ranitidine can be considered slightly superior to cimetidine because of its longer duration of action.

Cohen et al did not find any significant antiemetic effect when metoclopramide was administered to outpatients.[80] Rao et al found that outpatients who received the combination of a 300-mg cimetidine tablet and a 10-mg metoclopramide tablet with 20 ml of water 2 hours before induction had both a significantly lower gastric volume and a significantly higher pH than those who received cimetidine alone or metoclopramide alone, or patients in a control group.[81]

Alka Seltzer Effervescent (two tablets dissolved in 20 ml of water), a non-aspirin-containing preparation, will increase gastric pH as well as if not better than magnesium trisilicate or sodium citrate. The solution should not be administered until all effervescence has ceased.[82]

Antacids, anticholinergics, gastrokinetics, and H_2 receptor blocking drugs have been used to limit the potential for aspiration pneumonitis in outpatients. The use of any of these drugs individually or in combination does not eliminate the need for careful anesthetic technique to protect the airway during induction, maintenance, and emergence from anesthesia.

Opioids

Long-acting opioids such as meperidine and morphine are not recommended for premedication in outpatients.[44] In comparing the use of fentanyl, 1.5 μg·kg^{-1} iv, and meperidine, 1 mg·kg^{-1} iv, 2–5 minutes before induction for outpatient dilation and extraction, White and Chang found recovery times decreased by opioid premedication because of the decreased requirement for an iv induction agent.[83] Neither drug significantly increased the incidence of postanesthetic side-effects. Although the use of opioid premedication in its traditional form has been questioned, opioid premedication given iv just before anesthesia induction can be advantageous in the outpatient setting.

Epstein et al evaluated a group of patients undergoing voluntary interruption of pregnancy or dilation and curettage (D&C).[84] Patients were given thiopental plus nitrous oxide and oxygen or thiopental plus nitrous oxide and oxygen with supplemental fentanyl. Fentanyl-treated patients recovered statistically earlier than those who did not receive opioid premedication. Hunt et al added a single dose of fentanyl (75–125 μg) iv immediately before induction of anesthesia in a group of outpatients.[85] The addition of fentanyl significantly reduced the frequency of pain in the PACU and during the first evening at home. In outpatients undergoing suction termination of pregnancy, Sanders et al found that patients receiving alfentanil as a supplement to iv inhalational anesthesia recovered statistically earlier than those anesthetized with iv inhalational drugs alone.[86]

Pandit and Kothary compared the use of equianalgesic iv premedicant doses of morphine, meperidine, fentanyl, and sufentanil with normal saline, administered 15–30 minutes before induction, for their effects on anxiety, sedation, ease of anesthetic induction and maintenance, requirement for postoperative analgesic, recovery time, and frequency of side-effects.[87] Opioid premedication generally afforded more satisfactory induction and maintenance than did placebo premedication. Opioid premedication did not prolong recovery time significantly (mean discharge time for all groups was greater than 3 hours). The prevalence of side-effects in the PACU was comparable in all treatment groups (Table 50-5).

Sedative-Hypnotics

Diazepam, lorazepam, and midazolam are the currently available benzodiazepines; lorazepam and diazepam are available in oral preparation. The duration of action of lorazepam is too long for it to be useful for the ambulatory surgical patient, and when it is given parenterally it can produce prolonged amnesia for 6 to 8 hours. Because of its prolonged sedative and amnesic effect, lorazepam should not be used by any route to premedicate the outpatient.

In nonpremedicated outpatients, the frequency of awareness after general anesthesia has been reported to be as high as 9%.[51] Epstein found that diazepam, 0.15 mg·kg^{-1} (up to a total dose of 5 mg), given iv 2–3 minutes before induction of anesthesia, significantly reduced the rate of awareness experienced with a balanced anesthetic technique for laparoscopy (B. S. Epstein, pers. commun., 1982). Without diazepam, 4.9% of patients could recall conversation, 2.1% extubation of the trachea, and 0.7% pain. Oral administration of diazepam (0.25 mg·kg^{-1}) significantly decreased preoperative discomfort and apprehension without extending the length of stay for outpatients undergoing a variety of surgical procedures.[88] Jansen et al objectively measured postural stability after oral diazepam premedication (0.2 mg·kg^{-1}). Because patients exhibited decreased stability with a tendency to fall, the authors believed patients should not be allowed to walk after administration of this premedication dose.[89]

Other benzodiazepines were tried as oral premedicants for outpatients. Temazepam, 20 mg given 1 hour before surgery, resulted in satisfactory sedation and anxiolysis in outpatients.[90] Recovery was faster than after premedication with diazepam, 10 mg.[91]

Intramuscular midazolam is a satisfactory premedicant in both adult and pediatric outpatients. Fragen et al compared the effects of midazolam (0.08 mg·kg^{-1}) and hydroxyzine (1.5 mg·kg^{-1}) as im premedicants.[92] Midazolam resulted in a quicker onset of action, greater anxiolysis for the first hour, greater amnesia, less local irritation, and a higher overall rating by the patients. Drowsiness, while greater with midazolam than with hydroxyzine, was neither significant nor prolonged. When midazolam was given im, sedative effects occurred within 15 minutes but started to wear off between 60 to 90 minutes after injection. In comparing midazolam (0.07 mg·kg^{-1}) or hydroxyzine (1.0 mg·kg^{-1}) with a placebo, Vinik et al found that midazolam and hydroxyzine reduced anxiety more significantly than did placebo, with the peak effect appearing 30 to 60 minutes after drug administration in both treatment groups.[93] There was significantly less evidence of tissue irritation at the injection site in the midazolam-treated patients than in the hydroxyzine-treated patients. Rita et al compared im midazolam premedication (starting with 0.04 mg·kg^{-1} and increased in 0.01 mg·kg^{-1} increments until a dose of 0.1 mg·kg^{-1} was reached) in a wide dosage range for pediatric patients.[94] The 0.08 mg·kg^{-1} dose produced the highest percentage of drowsy or sleeping patients in the holding area, smooth induction of anesthesia, calm awakening in the PACU, and overall satisfactory ratings from anesthesia staff. All children appeared drowsy within 15 minutes of receiving the im injection, and the

TABLE 50-5. Recovery Time (min) Following Premedication with Various Opioids

Premedicant	Orientation	Ambulation	Discharge
Morphine	21.4 ± 6.63	148.4 ± 49.33	210.3 ± 65.84
Meperidine	19.2 ± 6.54	135.2 ± 30.02	187.0 ± 50.87
Fentanyl	19.9 ± 7.41	145.8 ± 51.73	187.9 ± 67.73
Sufentanil	19.7 ± 8.19	134.2 ± 44.05	181.5 ± 62.01
Placebo	20.2 ± 7.69	156.0 ± 54.04	200.0 ± 69.12

Statistical method: ANOVA; no significant differences among groups.

Reproduced with permission from Pandit SK, Kothary SP: Intravenous narcotics for premedication in outpatient anaesthesia. Acta Anaesthesiol Scand 33:353, 1989.

degree and duration of drowsiness were dose dependent. Midazolam as an oral premedicant (unlabeled use—an approved drug for a nonapproved indication) is gaining acceptance in the United States. To allay anxiety and facilitate separation of children from their parents, Feld and colleagues recommend 0.5–0.75 mg·kg^{-1} 30 minutes prior to induction of anesthesia.[55]

Hydroxyzine, a nonphenothiazine (antihistamine) tranquilizer, does not prolong recovery from anesthesia. In addition to its sedative effects, it has antihistaminic, antiemetic, and antisialagogic effects.

The careful use and appropriate timing of administration of sedative hypnotics and analgesic premedications in outpatients can relieve anxiety without prolonging a patient's stay in the PACU.

Techniques and Drugs

Anesthetic techniques and drugs are discussed fully in other chapters in this book. The sections that follow—on regional, conscious sedation, injectable, and inhalational anesthesia—discuss anesthetic techniques only with regard to their use in the outpatient population.

Regional Techniques

Local and regional anesthesia have long been used for ambulatory surgery. At the University of California, Los Angeles, during 1963 and 1964, 56% of ambulatory procedures were performed with the use of these techniques.[95] Mulroy believes that successful outpatient anesthesia depends on four postanesthesia and postsurgical requirements: alertness, ambulation, analgesia, and alimentation.[96] Although regional anesthetic techniques have a reputation for prolonged induction time and delay in recovery, these techniques can offer significant advantages for outpatients. The additional time needed to perform many regional blocks, as well as time to allow the anesthetic to take effect, is a potential drawback when procedures are short and turnover time between cases is rapid. Use of a regional technique that requires more time than the procedure itself (i.e., an epidural for D&C) should be limited to situations in which it is the indicated technique for the patient. Meridy[44] and Bridenbaugh and Soderstrom[97] found significantly shorter recovery times after local and regional anesthesia than after general anesthesia.

If regional anesthesia is contemplated, the surgeon must be aware of it because he or she must encourage the patient to accept a regional technique. Of 116 appropriately chosen patients who received good preoperative instructions, 98% could complete a laparoscopic procedure while under local anesthesia.[98] When preanesthesia education and premedication are limited, anxiety may be a major drawback to performing a regional anesthetic technique. Small doses of short-acting sedative drugs can be used to overcome simple anxieties without prolonging PACU stay after the procedure. A satisfactory outpatient regional anesthesia experience depends on appropriate selection of the patient, appropriate use of sedatives, local anesthetics, and a specific regional technique, and the anesthesiologist's skill.

Sedatives must be selected carefully, whether they are used for premedication or intra-anesthetic sedation. Small doses of short-acting drugs should be used.[99] Midazolam is an excellent sedative for the moderately anxious patient; it is better than diazepam because of its shorter duration of action and lack of venous irritation.[100,101] The amnesia it produces does not correlate with the apparent level of sedation; fully conscious patients may have no awareness of perianesthetic events. "Awake" patients have completely failed to recall talking to the surgeon or anesthesiologist during the operation.[102] Propofol infusion appears to be an excellent alternative to midazolam for sedation.[103] Where intraoperative amnesia is desired in addition to a rapid recovery, administration of a small dose of midazolam (1–3 mg iv) prior to a propofol infusion may offer advantages over either drug alone.

The analgesic properties of a short-acting opioid (e.g., fentanyl, alfentanil) are especially useful if paresthesia is sought during a regional technique and obtundation is undesirable. Either of these opioid analgesics can be combined with midazolam (adding the potential for amnesia) and allow excellent cooperation with blocks.[96] The combination must be used carefully to avoid oversedation, which blunts or delays the response to paresthesia.

Verbal reassurance and explanation should continue throughout the operation, thereby decreasing the need for supplemental medication. Philip and Covino reported using music through headphones to supplement regional anesthesia, asking the patient to bring in tapes of preferred music.[104]

Although inpatient regional anesthesia may require the longest possible local anesthetic block to provide postoperative analgesia, outpatient surgery necessitates careful selection of shorter-acting agents (typically chloroprocaine or lidocaine) for most blocks, particularly for procedures begun late in the day.[96] Reliance on local wound infiltration with long-acting local anesthetic will provide prolonged postoperative analgesia.

Certain block techniques in themselves may be inappropriate in an outpatient setting. A sciatic–femoral nerve block may delay discharge because of prolonged loss of motor strength and coordination in the affected lower extremity. A supraclavicular or intrascalene brachial plexus block may be contraindicated because of a potential for pneumothorax, and spinal anesthesia may be relatively contraindicated because of the potential for post-dural puncture headache after discharge. For example, this would pose a disadvantage for patients living a great distance from the hospital or contemplating air travel shortly after surgery.[105]

When a hand or foot is still numb after a peripheral nerve block and the patient is ready for discharge, the patient must be carefully instructed in the care of the extremity and warned that the normal sensation that protects against injury is still lacking. The patient should be reassured that sensation will return after discharge and that it is not a problem to be concerned about.

Lumbar epidural anesthesia is suitable for pelvic, lower abdominal, and lower extremity surgery. Epidural anesthesia may delay a patient's ability to walk because of motor block of the legs; however, the use of a short-acting local anesthetic in a continuous catheter technique will reduce this problem to a minimum while allowing the duration of anesthesia to match the sometimes unpredictable duration of surgery. At the Mason Clinic, epidural anesthesia is administered to 50% of patients undergoing a laparoscopic procedure.[96] In a series of patients receiving lumbar epidural compared with general anesthesia for laparoscopy, the incidence of nausea and vomiting was reduced from 38% (general) to 4% (epidural).[97] Mulroy states that not all patients having laparoscopic procedures are suitable candidates for an epidural block.[96] Some are too anxious about the procedure, whereas others cannot tolerate the respiratory compromise of abdominal distention in the head-down position. When epidural anesthesia is used for laparoscopic examination, the patient should be forewarned that she may experience shoulder pain. This referred diaphragmatic irritation can be minimized with appropriate explanation and sedation.

For the outpatient, spinal anesthesia is superior to an epidural technique for lower extremity and perianal surgery because of the absence of sacral nerve root sparing. Long-acting local anesthetics that may be acceptable for spinal anesthesia in inpatients may be problematic in outpatients. Drugs such as bupivacaine and tetracaine, whose length of action may preclude the patient from ambulating and being transferred from the PACU to home care in less than 6–8 hours, are not acceptable. This is too long a time and is frequently followed by a variety of problems such as orthostatic hypotension and urinary retention.

Harris believes that spinal anesthesia has a distinct advantage over epidural anesthesia because of the long induction time for epidural anesthesia; he therefore considers spinal anesthesia the only practical major regional anesthetic technique for ambulatory patients.[106] Spinal anesthesia does not impair operating room efficiency and, because of a lesser incidence of nausea and vomiting, can result in higher rates of discharge home on the day of surgery relative to general anesthesia. Although there may be some intraoperative and PACU advantages to the use of spinal anesthesia, the increased incidence of post-dural puncture headache in outpatients must be taken into consideration. Neal and co-workers evaluated 366 patients undergoing spinal anesthesia for a variety of surgical procedures, both as inpatients and as outpatients.[107] The incidence of post-dural puncture headache was higher in outpatients (6.6%) than in inpatients (1.4%). Half the patients sustaining a post-dural puncture headache required epidural blood patch therapy.

Bed rest does not reduce the frequency of headache.[108-110] The seemingly increased incidence of post-dural puncture headache in outpatients as compared with inpatients has yet to be explained. Whereas post-dural puncture headache might be an acceptable complication in an inpatient who anticipates 3–4 days of hospitalization, it is a serious setback for a young, healthy, active outpatient anticipating a rapid return to work or resumption of other daily activities. For younger patients (less than age 50) who have a higher incidence of headache (slightly greater in females) and who have an urgent need to return to full ambulatory function within 24 hours after the surgical procedure, spinal anesthesia for an ambulatory surgical procedure is far from ideal.

In 160 outpatients who received spinal anesthesia, the incidence of post-dural puncture headache after puncture with a 25-gauge needle was nearly four times greater than when a 26-gauge needle was used.[111] The occurrence of post-spinal puncture headache in patients over the age of 45 years was significantly lower than in younger patients.

With good technique, an appropriate choice of needle (25 or 26 gauge), and an appropriate direction of bevel, the incidence of post-dural puncture headache should be less than 2% in most outpatient facilities.[112] The patient should be advised to avoid straining at home and to maintain good oral fluid intake. If a headache occurs, it can be treated on an outpatient basis with an epidural blood patch. Cohen instructs the patient to rest quietly for 1 hour after injection of 10 ml of blood before being discharged.[113] Electrolyte infusion is not started before the procedure, and the patient is not encouraged to drink large quantities of fluid afterward; this does little to increase cerebrospinal fluid production "while necessitating multiple, uncomfortable expeditions to urinate."[113]

For those patients who do receive a spinal anesthesia, it

is incumbent upon the anesthesiologist and the facility to have follow-up contact (telephone calls) to make certain that no disabling symptoms of headache have developed.[114] If the headache does not respond to bed rest, analgesics, and oral hydration, the patient must return to the hospital for a course of caffeine iv therapy or an immediate epidural blood patch. Further study is needed to assess the relative risk-benefit ratio of spinal anesthesia as a technique for the ambulatory surgery patient. Currently it should be reserved for older patients, patients in whom follow-up can be maintained for at least 72 hours, and patients who live close enough to the facility that they can easily return for an epidural blood patch.

Randel and co-workers consider epidural anesthesia superior to spinal or general anesthesia for outpatient knee arthroscopy.[115] Patients given epidural anesthesia had significantly faster recovery times than those given spinal or general anesthesia, and there were significantly more severe headaches in the spinal group (5.2%) versus the epidural (0.0%) or general group (0.0%). There was no significant difference in the incidence of moderate to severe backaches between the spinal and epidural groups, but in both groups the incidence was significantly higher than in the general anesthesia group.

Mulroy thinks spinal anesthesia is one of the most useful techniques in outpatient regional anesthesia. The advantages are ease of administration, rapid onset of action, and high reliability and predictability.[116] These advantages must be weighed against the possible disadvantages, which range from urine retention to postspinal headache. If the incidence of these side-effects in a specific clinical setting does not differ widely from the 2% probability of unplanned overnight hospital admission following outpatient general anesthesia, Mulroy believes the choice of technique becomes a matter of preference.

Conscious Sedation

Because many patients undergoing surgery with local or regional anesthesia prefer to be sedated and to have no recollection of the procedure, a variety of adjuncts to these techniques have been recommended. Supplemental agents commonly used for sedation include sedative-hypnotics, opioids, and inhalational agents (Table 50-6).

Outpatient anesthesia is not limited to ASA Physical Status 1 or 2 patients; an increasing number of Physical Status 3 and elderly patients are presenting for surgery. Some of these patients are unsuitable for outpatient general anesthesia, but surgery can often be performed if local or regional anesthesia is supplemented with a combination of hypnotics and analgesics in subanesthetic doses, a technique known as *conscious sedation*.

TABLE 50-6. Supplemental Agents for Regional or Local Anesthesia

Sedative-hypnotics	Opioids
Diazepam	Fentanyl
Midazolam	Alfentanil
Thiopental	Sufentanil
Methohexital	
Ketamine	*Inhalational Agents*
Propofol	Nitrous oxide
	Enflurane
	Isoflurane

Conscious sedation is an art not easily learned.[117] Originally developed by dentists and oral surgeons for office use, conscious sedation is quickly becoming an important technique in the outpatient surgical anesthesia armamentarium. As defined by the American Dental Association Council on Dental Education, conscious sedation emphasizes that the patient must be able to respond rationally to commands and to maintain his or her own airway patency.[118] Shane has described an "intravenous amnesia" technique entailing a combination of opioid, anticholinergic, ataractic, and barbiturate medications given in small incremental doses.[117,119] The term "conscious sedation," first used by Bennett, referred to the administration of iv agents as supplements to regional and local anesthetics that minimally depressed consciousness while maintaining protective reflexes intact.[120] The challenge lies in selecting appropriate drugs and titrating their doses.

The definitions of conscious sedation and related terms proposed by the American Dental Association Council on Dental Education[121] are listed in Table 50-7. The objectives of conscious sedation have been outlined by Scamman and co-workers as follows:[122]

1. Maintain adequate sedation with minimal risk. The patient's ability to communicate verbally is preserved. Usual monitoring is employed and emergency resuscitation equipment is on hand.
2. Relieve anxiety and produce amnesia. These objectives are accomplished by means of good preoperative communication and instruction and low levels of visual and auditory stimuli (including concealed instruments and minimal conversation) in the operating room and by keeping the patient warm and covered (preserving the patient's modesty).
3. Provide relief from pain and other noxious stimuli. Opioids are given to supplement local or topical anesthetics and to block pain sensations remote from the operative site.

The technique must be suited to the individual patient and to the individual surgeon as well as to the specific surgical procedure. While experienced surgeons readily perform

---

TABLE 50-7. Definitions of Conscious Sedation (and Related Terms) Proposed by the American Dental Association Council on Dental Education

Analgesia Diminution or elimination of pain in the conscious patient

Local anesthesia Elimination of sensations, especially pain, in one part of the body by the topical application or regional injection of a drug

Conscious sedation Minimally depressed level of consciousness that retains the patient's ability to independently and continuously maintain an airway and respond appropriately to physical stimulation and verbal command, produced by a pharmacologic or non-pharmacologic method, or a combination

General anesthesia (includes deep sedation) Controlled state of depressed consciousness or unconsciousness, accompanied by partial or complete loss of protective reflexes, including the ability to independently maintain an airway and respond purposefully to physical stimulation or verbal command, produced by a pharmacologic or nonpharmacologic method, or a combination

Reproduced with permission from McCarthy FM, Solomon AL, Jastak J et al: Conscious sedation: Benefits and risks. J Am Dental Assoc 109:46, 1984.

---

laparoscopic tubal sterilizations or breast biopsies using local infiltration anesthesia with sedation, surgical residents are rarely able to perform similar procedures without a general anesthetic. Similarly, an intelligent, mature adult who has been given a thorough explanation of the planned anesthetic, the rationale behind it, and the advantages of it will often readily accept sedation. An uninformed, anxious patient who is facing the stress of surgery and is filled with the fear of pain and complications will more frequently choose to be "all the way out."[123]

The numbers and types of outpatient procedures that are being managed with varying drug and dosage modifications of conscious sedation are increasing rapidly. At the Medical College of Virginia Ambulatory Surgery Center, conscious sedation was used in more than 7000 outpatient procedures from 1981 to 1988 to supplement local or regional anesthesia for removal of external skeletal fixation, removal of percutaneous Kirschner wires, excision of Morton's neuroma, laser conization of the cervix, cervical dilation and evacuation of the uterus, diagnostic D&C, myringotomy with tube insertion in adults, laparoscopic tubal sterilization, knee arthroscopic examination (in selected patients), breast biopsy, and a variety of plastic surgical procedures.[124]

During conscious sedation, the anesthesiologist primarily concentrates on monitoring patient awareness or level of consciousness by speaking to the patient frequently, being reassuring, responding to any evidence of distress or discomfort, and warning of stimulating events about to take place (i.e., injection of local anesthetic, laparoscope insertion, tourniquet inflation). The expected event is less stimulating than the same event that is not anticipated. Patient responsiveness can best be evaluated from the patient's ability to obey frequent simple commands that do not require verbal response (i.e., "take a deep breath"). Verbal responses by the patient require a higher level of arousal than a mere nod or finger movement or the passive obeying of a command.[120]

Important pharmacokinetic properties of drugs used for conscious sedation include a high clearance rate and a short elimination half-life. This allows blood concentration and therefore clinical responses to be altered quickly and minimizes the problem of drug accumulation during surgery and prolonged postoperative recovery. The newer sedative-hypnotics and analgesics with these properties are midazolam, propofol, and alfentanil.

Because of the ever-present risk of synergistic interactions between sedative and analgesic drugs with respect to respiratory and cardiovascular depression, there is need for specific and diligent monitoring to minimize potentially serious side-effects. Pulse oximetry is an easy-to-use noninvasive method of assessing oxygen saturation that provides an early indication of impending desaturation prior to the development of clinical signs of hypoxemia.[125] The ASA Standards for Basic Intraoperative Monitoring apply to sedation techniques that are a part of monitored anesthesia care.[126]

Epstein raises the issue, "When does conscious sedation become general anesthesia?"[127] From the definitions provided by the American Dental Association, conscious sedation clearly lies on a dose-dependent continuum leading from minimal sedation to general anesthesia. Moving from a conscious sedated state to an unconscious state can be a dramatic and life-threatening experience. Epstein believes this is often a difficult concept to understand for those who administer sedation/analgesia in more than a calming dose. The ASA, unlike the American Dental Association, has not attempted to define the state of CNS depression produced by adjunctive drugs. The potential for organ depression is what is important. Cohen *et al* reviewed approximately 100,000 anesthetics and reported that monitored anesthesia care was associated with the highest rate of mortality (209 deaths per 10,000 anesthetic episodes).[128]

In the 7000 procedures performed under conscious sedation at the Medical College of Virginia Ambulatory Surgery Center, there were no deaths or serious complications.[124] Transient but significant hypoxemia (digital pulse oximetry < 90%) was noted in 28% of patients undergoing elective termination of pregnancy, but no significant clinical sequelae were observed. Supplemental nasal oxygen is provided to all patients receiving conscious sedation at the Medical College of Virginia Ambulatory Surgery Center. Forty reports of apnea and respiratory or cardiac arrest in patients receiving midazolam for sedation for endoscopy and other procedures have been received by the US Food and Drug Administration.[129] Most occurred in older patients who were receiving other drugs and had concomitant diseases.

Injectable Drugs

Selection of injectable drugs plays a greater role in determining whether adult patients can go home on the same day as surgery than does the choice of inhalational agents. The properties of an ideal injectable agent are listed in Table 50-8.

Thiopental/Methohexital. Despite a long elimination half-life (10–12 hours) that can contribute to a prolonged recovery time, thiopental is the standard against which other iv induction drugs are measured. In studying the pharmacokinetics of thiopental and methohexital in patients undergoing short surgical procedures, Hudson *et al* evaluated the following: disposition of a single iv bolus of methohexital followed by other agents for maintenance of anesthesia, the pharmacokinetics of thiopental and methohexital in surgical patients, and the relative importance of metabolism compared to redistribution in the recovery process after use of both iv induction agents.[130]

Although the distribution phase kinetics of thiopental and methohexital appear similar, redistribution is a major factor determining the duration of sedation after a single bolus dose of either drug. The more rapid recovery of complete psychomotor function seen after methohexital administration probably results from its more rapid metabolism.

TABLE 50-8. Physical and Pharmacologic Properties of an Ideal Intravenous Agent

1. High therapeutic (safety) index
2. Water-soluble, stable in solution, and long shelf-life
3. Nonirritating after intramuscular or intravenous administration
4. No hypersensitivity (or anaphylactoid) reactions
5. Rapid, smooth onset of action after intramuscular or intravenous administration
6. No depression of cardiovascular and respiratory systems
7. Rapid degradation to inactive, nontoxic metabolites
8. Short elimination half-life ($T_{1/2\beta}$) value
9. Analgesia at subanesthetic levels
10. Rapid, smooth emergence without side-effects

Reproduced with permission from White PF, Shafer AS: Clinical pharmacology and uses of injectable anesthetic and analgesic drugs. In Wetchler BV (ed): Outpatient Anesthesia, vol 2, p 38. Philadelphia, JB Lippincott, 1988.

The authors concluded that methohexital would be preferable to thiopental whenever more rapid recovery from anesthesia is desired, particularly if large or repeated doses are necessary. Others have found methohexital to be associated with a shorter awakening and recovery time than thiopental.[131,132]

Elliott *et al* assessed coordination in methohexital-treated and thiopental-treated patients. Not only did coordination return more quickly in the methohexital-treated patients, but the subjects themselves reported being less sedated and clearer mentally than thiopental-treated patients.[133]

After patients were given a single iv bolus dose of thiopental, electroencephalography (EEG) showed a rapid return to consciousness; however, at 2.5 hours and 3.5 hours after induction, drowsiness appeared, and at 4.5 hours a sleep tracing appeared on the EEG that lasted up to 12 hours.[134] Although initial recovery after thiopental is fairly fast, patients experience a hangover for several hours, even after induction for short anesthetics. The outpatient should be made aware of this probable return of drowsiness before he or she is discharged.

Although methohexital is associated with a faster return to consciousness, greater stability in solution, less tissue irritation, and shorter periods of hypotension than is thiopental, Dundee found that methohexital produced a higher incidence of excitatory phenomena, cough, and hiccoughing when used as an induction agent.[135]

Etomidate. A short-acting iv hypnotic drug without any analgesic action, etomidate is associated with remarkable cardiovascular stability and lacks histamine release.[136-138] Pain on injection (occurring in up to 50% of patients) and involuntary myoclonic movements (to 70% of patients) are two of the major side-effects of this drug.[137] Pain can be severe enough that patients refuse a second etomidate induction.[136] Involuntary movements are minimized by the iv administration of midazolam, 0.07 mg·kg^{-1}, or diazepam, 0.15 mg·kg^{-1}, and fentanyl, 1.5 µg·kg^{-1} or by a preinduction dose of alfentanil (7 µg·kg^{-1}).[139-141] Melnick *et al* completely abolished pain on injection related to etomidate.[142] Just before induction, 25–100 mg of lidocaine is administered through an injection port attached directly to the iv catheter. The iv drip is turned off for 30 seconds, and etomidate is then injected.

Fragen and Caldwell found no difference in quality of patient recovery following induction with etomidate or thiopental; however, etomidate-treated patients had a threefold increase in nausea and vomiting.[137] White compared PACU time and side-effects in outpatients receiving thiopental, methohexital, or etomidate continuous infusions as adjuvants to nitrous oxide for outpatient anesthesia (Table 50-9).[143] The methohexital-treated patients were awake, oriented, and discharged significantly faster than those in the other two groups. The incidence of nausea was significantly higher in the etomidate-treated patients.

A single induction dose of methohexital can produce transient postoperative suppression (approximately 8 hours in duration) of adrenocortical function; however, this does not necessitate steroid supplementation.[144] Etomidate does not appear to offer any advantage over barbiturates for outpatient anesthesia.

Ketamine. The role of ketamine in adult outpatient anesthesia is questionable. In comparing ketamine with thiopental as induction agents for outpatient anesthesia, Thompson *et al* found that ketamine-treated patients were less alert, had more headaches and dizziness, and complained of

TABLE 50-9. Recovery Times and Side-Effects After Continuous Infusions of Thiopental, Methohexital, or Etomidate

Agent	Recovery Times (min), Mean ± SD			Postoperative Side-Effects (%)			
	Awake	Oriented	Ambulatory	Nausea	Dizziness	Drowsiness	Pain
Thiopental	8 ± 7	12 ± 9	84 ± 9	15	10	50	25
Methohexital	2 ± 2*	3 ± 2*	45 ± 4*	10	10	5*	20
Etomidate	5 ± 3	6 ± 4	67 ± 8	45*	5	20	15

*Significantly different from thiopental-treated group ($p < 0.05$).

Reproduced with permission from White PF: Continuous infusions of thiopental, methohexital or etomidate as adjuvants to nitrous oxide for outpatient anesthesia. Anesth Analg 63:282, 1984.

"weird dreams" when discharged.[51] Two thirds of the ketamine-treated patients reported that their unpleasant dreams were frightening; none of the thiopental-treated patients had strange dreams. Although the administration of diazepam or droperidol can decrease the incidence of unpleasant dreams, the addition of these drugs may further delay the patient's recovery. In the PACU, ketamine-treated patients had a significant increase in nausea and vomiting. Ketamine-treated patients also reported an increased awareness of perianesthetic events (9%) compared with thiopental-treated patients (4%). As with other rapid and short-acting iv drugs, the continuous infusion of ketamine may offer considerable advantages over the traditional intermittent bolus technique in the outpatient setting.[145] Ketamine appears to fall short of the requirements for an ideal outpatient anesthetic drug and has not found wide acceptance in the management of adult patients in an ambulatory setting. Its main role may be as a pediatric induction agent in doses of $2-3$ mg·kg^{-1} im.[146] In a recent study comparing recovery and discharge time following ketamine preinduction or pure inhaled anesthesia in young children undergoing brief surgical procedures, recovery time was not prolonged by ketamine. Even though the total discharge time was statistically longer when ketamine was used, the actual delay was less than 15 minutes.[147] This technique is useful for children aged 1–5 years and will provide satisfactory conditions for a mask induction within 3–7 minutes. When children receive low-dose im ketamine as an induction drug, hallucinations and nightmares do not appear to be a problem.[148] Koka compared four induction techniques in nonpremedicated pediatric outpatients: ketamine im (2 mg·kg^{-1} in the deltoid area), halothane by mask, methohexital rectally (25 mg·kg^{-1}), and thiopental iv (4–5 mg·kg^{-1}).[152] Early recovery was faster with halothane; at 1 hour in the PACU recovery was comparable, regardless of the induction technique used (B. V. Koka, pers. commun., 1988).

Propofol. A member of the sedative-hypnotic group, propofol produces dose-dependent CNS, cardiovascular, and ventilatory depression very similar to that produced by the barbiturate induction drugs. Onset of action is almost identical to that of thiopental or methohexital; in the PACU, recovery from propofol is much faster and is associated with few postanesthetic side-effects.[149-151] Pain on injection depends on the site of administration (dorsal hand veins) and is minimized if forearm or larger antecubital veins are used.[149,152] Thrombophlebitis does not appear to be a problem after iv administration of this agent. The addition of 1 ml lidocaine (10 mg) to 19 ml propofol significantly reduces the incidence and severity of pain on injection.[153] The use of iv lidocaine immediately before propofol injection only partially reduced the incidence of pain when dorsal hand veins were used.[150] The elimination half-life of propofol (1–3 hours) is shorter than that of methohexital (6–8 hours) or thiopental (10–12 hours). Although Youngberg et al, Doze and White, and Johnston et al concluded that the cardiovascular depressant activities of propofol were similar to those of thiopental, others have found it to produce greater cardiovascular depression, typically manifested by decreases in arterial pressure and cardiac index without a significant change in heart rate.[154-159]

When equivalent doses of propofol (2.5 mg·kg^{-1}), methohexital (1.5 mg·kg^{-1}), and thiopental (5 mg·kg^{-1}) were compared as induction agents, propofol induction was smoother but was associated with greater cardiorespiratory depression; the speed and quality of recovery were superior with propofol.[149,160] The propofol induction dose should be decreased in patients aged 60 years or older. Korttila et al compared recovery following propofol induction and maintenance with thiopental-isoflurane.[161] Propofol-treated patients tolerated oral fluid intake significantly earlier, experienced fewer emetic symptoms (none of the propofol patients vomited in the PACU), and were ready for discharge significantly sooner (Table 50-10). Emetic symptoms were significantly less severe with propofol than with thiopental-isoflurane anesthesia.

TABLE 50-10. Recovery Times After Propofol or Thiopental-Isoflurane Anesthesia

N$_2$O off to:	Propofol (min), Mean ± SD	Thiopental-Isoflurane (min), Mean ± SD
Response to commands	3.7 ± 3.0*	6.2 ± 2.9
Spontaneous eye opening	4.2 ± 3.2*	6.7 ± 2.8
Orientation	5.7 ± 3.3*	10.0 ± 5.6
Able to stand	66 ± 24*	92 ± 38
Tolerates fluids orally	61 ± 20*	129 ± 101
Able to void	103 ± 67*	184 ± 95
"Home-ready"	136 ± 77*	204 ± 101

*$p < 0.05$, propofol vs. thiopental-isoflurane.

Reproduced with permission from Korttila K, Ostman P, Faure E et al: Randomized comparison of recovery after propofol–nitrous oxide versus thiopentone–isoflurane–nitrous oxide anaesthesia in patients undergoing ambulatory surgery. Acta Anaesthesiol Scand 34:400, 1990.

Propofol may also be used for sedation during local or regional anesthesia.[103,162,163] After an initial dose of 1–2 mg·kg^{-1}, patients can be kept lightly asleep but easily arousable by a continuous infusion of 3–4 mg·kg^{-1}·h^{-1}. Propofol may have an advantage over other sedation techniques because of the ease with which the infusion can be increased and the anesthetic management converted to a general anesthetic from which awakening will be rapid.[162]

Because of the rapid awakening times, minimal side-effects, and no return of sedation, propofol appears to be an ideal iv agent for the ambulatory surgery patient. An economic model comparing propofol with thiopental-isoflurane for all cases in a given surgical day noted that 18.8 minutes less of intense nursing care would be needed for the propofol patients, there would be less waiting time to get into the PACU, and utilization of PACU nurses could be reduced by 25%.[164] This type of cost savings could more than offset the higher price of propofol compared with thiopental.

Succinylcholine. Many short outpatient procedures require no neuromuscular blocking drug, whereas some require an ultra-short-acting agent to facilitate tracheal intubation, and other procedures require muscle relaxation during the procedure. Succinylcholine, a depolarizing relaxant, is the relaxant used most widely in outpatient anesthesia to facilitate tracheal intubation and provide a short period of profound relaxation. A significant drawback to using succinylcholine for outpatient procedures is the occurrence of postanesthesia skeletal muscle aches and pains. Myalgia may occur up to the fourth postoperative day and may be more painful than the surgery itself. The incidence of myalgia is significantly higher in patients who walk shortly after surgery (66%) than in inpatients who remain resting in bed (13.9%).[165] Pretreatment with a variety of drugs (d-tubocurarine, 0.05 mg·kg^{-1}; diazepam, 0.05 mg·kg^{-1}; calcium gluconate, 1000 mg; succinylcholine, 10 mg) has been reported to lessen and even eliminate the myalgia that occurs after administration of succinylcholine. In an outpatient study comparing the varying pretreatment regimens, the incidence of moderate to severe complaints of postanesthesia myalgia was never less than 8% in any group (d-tubocurarine, 0.05 mg·kg^{-1}).[166] Although d-tubocurarine has been shown to be a better defasciculant than atracurium, postanesthesia myalgia was significantly less in patients pretreated with atracurium (0.025 mg·kg^{-1}).[167] In the healthy outpatient undergoing an elective procedure, the onset time of skeletal muscle relaxation to facilitate intubation of the trachea or surgery is less important than eliminating postanesthesia myalgia and the potential problem of prolonged apnea after succinylcholine administration. Short duration of effect after intubation of the trachea is more important. Succinylcholine is far from being an ideal muscle relaxant for the outpatient.

Atracurium/Vecuronium. These intermediate-acting drugs are valuable new clinical options, affording greater flexibility and safety than were available before. They have an important place in outpatient anesthesia for procedures lasting longer than 20 minutes. Atracurium has the shortest elimination half-life of all clinically available nondepolarizing relaxants, but the duration of effect after an initial dose is similar to that of vecuronium. Although the recommended intubating dose of 0.4–0.5 mg·kg^{-1} produces good intubating conditions (2.5–3 minutes), its duration of action (50–70 minutes to 95% recovery) may be too long for some shorter outpatient procedures. Sokoll et al found that 0.3 mg·kg^{-1} of atracurium produced a block lasting 44 minutes with an opioid anesthetic, compared with 67 minutes with isoflurane.[168] Stirt et al consider atracurium an acceptable alternative to succinylcholine when speed of tracheal intubation is not critical.[169] The volatile anesthetics potentiate atracurium (20%) and vecuronium (20–40%). Enflurane (minimum alveolar concentration [MAC] = 1.25) potentiates both muscle relaxants more than either isoflurane or halothane does.[170,171]

The duration of effect of these intermediate-acting drugs is dose dependent and can be lengthened or shortened, depending on the dose chosen. The lowest dose of atracurium compatible with adequate intubating conditions is 0.25 mg·kg^{-1}.[172] In 18 patients undergoing oral surgery, intubating conditions were excellent in ten, good in seven, and inadequate in one. Fragen and Shanks administered vecuronium (0.045 mg·kg^{-1}) for outpatient gynecologic laparoscopic procedures.[173] Time to maximum blockade (condition suitable for intubation of the trachea) was approximately 5 minutes. The duration of action was longer when vecuronium was used with inhalational agents than when it was used with opioids. With opioid anesthesia, recovery to 50% depression of twitch height was seen at 15 minutes, and with isoflurane anesthesia, at 20 minutes.

When desirable, the time to intubation of the trachea after administration of vecuronium or atracurium can be shortened by use of the priming principle (Francis Foldes is associated with its development).[174] The technique entails administration of a subclinical priming dose of a relaxant (for atracurium, 0.05–0.075 mg·kg^{-1}; for vecuronium, 0.01–0.015 mg·kg^{-1}), followed in approximately 2–2.5 minutes by an induction dose of anesthetic, and immediately thereafter by a slightly smaller than usual intubating dose of a relaxant (for atracurium, 0.25–0.3 mg·kg^{-1}; for vecuronium, 0.04–0.05 mg·kg^{-1}). Induction of anesthesia should continue (i.e., with nitrous oxide and oxygen plus a major inhalational drug). Satisfactory intubation of the trachea can be performed 2–2.5 minutes after administration of the intubating dose.

Patient variability and sensitivity (skeletal muscle weakness evidenced by diplopia, difficulty in swallowing, and difficulty in breathing) can occur with the priming dose.[175] The longer one waits after the priming dose, the more likely it is that symptoms will occur. By applying the priming principle to the outpatient, time to intubation of the trachea, as well as length of action, can be shortened (i.e., vecuronium, 0.05 mg·kg^{-1}, provides 15–25 minutes of surgical muscle relaxation, whereas 0.1 mg·kg^{-1} provides 30–45 minutes). The effects of these nondepolarizing relaxants must be completely reversed at the conclusion of the procedure.

Mivacurium. This nondepolarizing relaxant has been under clinical investigation since 1985. The ED$_{95}$ dose of 0.1 mg·kg^{-1} produces maximum blockade in approximately 4 minutes; recovery to 95% depression of twitch height requires about 25 minutes. The recommended intubating dose of 0.2–0.25 mg·kg^{-1} shortens the time to maximum blockade to approximately 2.5 minutes; recovery to 95% twitch height takes only 30 minutes.[176] Intubating doses of mivacurium are about twice as long-acting as those of succinylcholine and half as long-acting as those of atracurium or vecuronium.[177] If a priming dose of 0.03 mg·kg^{-1} is followed by an intubating dose of 0.2 mg·kg^{-1} in a well-anesthetized patient, the intubation time can be shortened to 90 seconds.[178] At the completion of surgery, residual blockade, if present, is easily antagonized.

Org 9426. Under clinical investigation since 1989, Org 9426 is an intermediate-acting (similar to vecuronium in length of action), nondepolarizing, monoquaternary compound (David Savage Memorial Interface Symposium, London, 1990). The ED_{95} dose (0.3 mg·kg^{-1}) produces maximum blockade more rapidly than vecuronium. There is a virtual absence of autonomic side-effects and no release of histamine. Org 9426 is stable in solution and is supplied in liquid form.

Fentanyl. A preinduction iv dose of an opioid analgesic immediately before induction of anesthesia can reduce sedative-hynotic and inhalational anesthesia requirements and lessen the postsurgical analgesia requirement with a resultant decrease in PACU stay. However, small preduction doses of opioid analgesic drugs can increase the incidence of PACU emesis.[83,138] Although longer acting opioid analgesics (i.e., morphine and meperidine) have been used for outpatient anesthesia, neither is as acceptable as the more potent and shorter-acting opioid analgesics fentanyl, sufentanil, and alfentanil. As a supplement to thiopental plus nitrous oxide and oxygen anesthesia, fentanyl not only provided a smoother intra-anesthetic course, it also decreased postoperative pain and length of PACU stay.[84] Fentanyl, 1–3 μg·kg^{-1}, is highly effective when included as part of the anesthetic regimen. It decreased the incidence of involuntary movement and hiccoughing when added to a methohexital plus nitrous oxide and oxygen anesthetic.[179]

Pollard compared the clinical differences between an iv technique using fentanyl-droperidol and an inhalational technique using isoflurane in procedures lasting 30 minutes or less.[180] The fentanyl-droperidol-treated group had a more rapid recovery to consciousness and orientation and less need for postoperative analgesics. The clinician should be aware that somnolence, respiratory depression requiring ventilatory support, and respiratory arrest have occurred up to 4 hours after apparent recovery from fentanyl.[181] However, these respiratory depressant effects are unlikely to occur with the smaller doses (1–2 μg·kg^{-1}) commonly used in ambulatory surgery.

Sufentanil. The optimal preinduction dose of sufentanil for short outpatient procedures is 10–15 μg iv.[182] At doses equipotent with fentanyl (sufentanil is 10 times more potent), it produces shorter depression of ventilation and longer analgesia.[183] When compared with isoflurane-treated patients, sufentanil-treated patients were significantly more awake on arrival in the PACU and had less need for postoperative pain medication; after 90 minutes the level of recovery was the same in both groups.[184] The incidence of nausea was approximately the same for both groups. After outpatient arthroscopic surgery, awakening was more rapid after sufentanil preinduction than after isoflurane preinduction, although after 2 hours there was no difference between the groups.[185] Both anesthetic techniques provided satisfactory operating conditions, but the sufentanil-treated group had a higher incidence of nausea and vomiting (45%) than the isoflurane-treated group (15%). In outpatients who underwent laparoscopic examination (sufentanil versus isoflurane), the opioid compound significantly decreased PACU analgesia requirements and length of stay.[184] In 50 outpatients undergoing D&C who received either fentanyl or sufentanil infusion as an adjunct to thiopental plus nitrous oxide and oxygen anesthesia, the incidence of nausea and pain requiring analgesics was significantly less in the sufentanil-treated group.[186]

Alfentanil. White and others believe the potency ratio of fentanyl to alfentanil, based on administered dose, is 8:1.[187,188] Alfentanil may have advantages over fentanyl in the outpatient surgery setting; an equianalgesic dose of alfentanil may be associated with less depression of ventilation.[189] Awakening from anesthesia was more rapid with alfentanil than with isoflurane after outpatient arthroscopic procedures and short urologic and gynecologic procedures.[190,191] When compared with halothane- or enflurane-treated patients, alfentanil-treated patients recovered more rapidly; postanesthesia side-effects (nausea, vomiting, drowsiness) were the same for each group.[192] DeChene found alfentanil to be well suited as an adjunct to nitrous oxide and thiopental in short surgical procedures.[193] Minor chest wall rigidity was a consistent side-effect that was eliminated by pretreatment with d-tubocurarine. Coe et al see alfentanil as a clinically superior iv adjuvant for ambulatory anesthesia.[194] In a study comparing fentanyl and alfentanil in patients who underwent termination of pregnancy, they found a higher incidence of chest wall rigidity and ventilatory depression in the fentanyl-treated group, a higher incidence of mild bradycardia and moderate hypotension in the alfentanil-treated group, and no significant between-group differences in the incidence of nausea, vomiting, dizziness, or excessive drowsiness. The fentanyl-alfentanil potency ratio was 6:1, based on total dose administered. Kallar and Keenan compared recovery times after use of alfentanil and fentanyl in 43 patients in whom pregnancies were terminated.[195] The median time to establish alertness was significantly shorter for the alfentanil-treated group (16 minutes) than for the fentanyl-treated group (25 minutes). Although the percentage of completely recovered alfentanil-treated patients was significantly greater than the percentage of completely recovered fentanyl-treated patients at 20 and 30 minutes after operation, at 60 minutes after anesthesia recovery room scores indicating alertness were the same in both groups. White compared recovery times in outpatients who received fentanyl as a bolus, fentanyl by infusion, alfentanil as a bolus, and alfentanil by infusion.[188] The patients who received alfentanil by either method were awake, oriented, and able to walk significantly sooner than the fentanyl-treated patients (Table 50-11). There appears to be no return of depressant effects (4–6 hours after iv administration) when alfentanil is used.

Zelcer and co-workers compared alfentanil with fentanyl to determine which agent best blunted the hemodynamic response to laryngoscopy.[196] They concluded that alfentanil and propofol anesthesia more effectively attenuated the cardiovascular response to laryngoscopy and intubation than fentanyl and propofol, and that the combination was associated with a rapid recovery without adverse side-effects. Erythromycin apparently interferes with the metabolism of alfentanil, resulting in prolonged effects.[197] No other important drug interactions have been reported.

Butorphanol. Discharge time from the PACU and the most common side-effects after anesthesia were compared in a series of outpatients who received fentanyl (3 μg·kg^{-1}), butorphanol (60 μg·kg^{-1}), or nalbuphine (300 μg·kg^{-1}) as part of a balanced anesthesia technique.[198] Fentanyl-treated patients had the shortest awakening time and needed no hospital admission, whereas there was one hospital admission in the nalbuphine-treated group and three in the butorphanol-treated group because of excessive drowsiness. In a study comparing butorphanol (40 μg·kg^{-1}) and fentanyl (2 μg·kg^{-1}), the butorphanol-treated patients were more drowsy but also had less pain in the PACU.[199] The incidence

TABLE 50-11. Postoperative Recovery Times and Side-Effects After Use of Either Fentanyl or Alfentanil an Adjuvant to Nitrous Oxide Anesthesia

Agent, Method	Recovery Times (min), Mean ± SEM			Side-Effects (%)			
	Awake	Oriented	Ambulatory	Nausea	Vomiting	Dizziness	Drowsiness
Fentanyl bolus (FB)	5.2 ± 0.9	7.7 ± 1.1	67 ± 5	60	48	52	36
Fentanyl infusion (FI)	3.7 ± 0.8*	6.1 ± 1.2	55 ± 5	68	60	24	28
Alfentanil bolus (AB)	2.5 ± 0.3†	3.5 ± 0.4†	48 ± 4†	52	36	24	16
Alfentanil infusion (AI)	1.2 ± 0.1*†	2.6 ± 0.3*†	41 ± 3†	68	60	28	8†

*AI or FI group significantly different from AB or FB group ($p < 0.05$), respectively.

†AB or AI group significantly different from FB or FI group ($p < 0.05$), respectively.

Reproduced with permission from White PF, Coe V, Shafer A et al: Comparison of alfentanil with fentanyl for outpatient anesthesia. Anesthesiology 64:99, 1986.

of nausea and vomiting was comparable in both groups. When used as preinduction iv drugs (butorphanol, 20 $\mu g \cdot kg^{-1}$ and 40 $\mu g \cdot kg^{-1}$, vs. fentanyl, 2 $\mu g \cdot kg^{-1}$), no significant differences were found between butorphanol, 20 $\mu g \cdot kg^{-1}$, and fentanyl, 2 $\mu g \cdot kg^{-1}$.[200] Statistically significant variation ($p < 0.05$) was found in both length of recovery time and in the symptoms of nausea and dizziness when butorphanol, 40 $\mu g \cdot kg^{-1}$, was compared with fentanyl. Butorphanol administered by transnasal spray resulted in satisfactory postoperative pain relief.[201]

Nalbuphine. Garfield et al compared nalbuphine, 300 $\mu g \cdot kg^{-1}$ or 500 $\mu g \cdot kg^{-1}$, with fentanyl, 1.5 $\mu g \cdot kg^{-1}$ and found a significantly longer recovery phase for both nalbuphine-treated groups (three patients who received nalbuphine were admitted because of excessive disorientation and sedation), a higher degree of anxiety in the 500 $\mu g \cdot kg^{-1}$ group at the time of discharge, and a significantly higher incidence of unpleasant dreams in the nalbuphine-treated groups.[202] For day surgery patients, there were no significant differences in recovery times, levels of nausea and vomiting, or patient acceptance when either nalbuphine (150 $\mu g \cdot kg^{-1}$ or 300 $\mu g \cdot kg^{-1}$) or fentanyl (1.5 $\mu g \cdot kg^{-1}$ or 3 $\mu g \cdot kg^{-1}$) were given (D. M. Robinson et al, pers. commun., 1987). In response to specific directed questioning, the nalbuphine-treated patients reported having bad dreams. In both studies, those having unpleasant dreams ranged from 20% to 38% of nalbuphine-treated patients, compared with 0–6% of fentanyl-treated patients.

Benzodiazepines. Diazepam, lorazepam, and midazolam were discussed in the sections on premedication, regional anesthesia, and conscious sedation. Lorazepam is not acceptable for the outpatient, and the use of injectable diazepam may now be limited because of the availability of injectable midazolam.

Does midazolam have a role as an induction drug for outpatient anesthesia? Concerns have been raised regarding delayed recovery times and residual amnesia.[203,204] Midazolam, 0.15 $mg \cdot kg^{-1}$, was not sufficient to induce anesthesia reliably in healthy unpremedicated volunteers.[205] Anterograde amnesia (40 ± 3 minutes' duration) and drowsiness (lasting 128 ± 23 minutes) were observed in all subjects. In a randomized study of 100 women undergoing pregnancy termination as an outpatient procedure, the combination of midazolam–fentanyl–nitrous oxide was compared with

thiopental–fentanyl–nitrous oxide.[206] Midazolam (0.2–0.3 $mg \cdot kg^{-1}$) iv induction of anesthesia resulted in a lesser degree of awareness 30 minutes after the termination of anesthesia; at 60 and 180 minutes the scores were equal. Fragen and Caldwell, when comparing midazolam (0.2 $mg \cdot kg^{-1}$) with thiopental (4 $mg \cdot kg^{-1}$) for induction and maintenance of anesthesia along with 67% nitrous oxide for short gynecologic procedures, found prolongation to orientation and cognition in the midazolam-induced group.[207] Midazolam produced a profound period of amnesia for 1–2 hours; important instructions could not be given to patients during that time. Vomiting was less frequent after midazolam. All patients were awake enough to be discharged from the hospital 200 minutes after the last dose of hypnotic was given.

The use of midazolam for the induction of anesthesia for outpatient surgery may depend entirely on how long the outpatient surgical procedure lasts and the dose of the drug to be given.[208] For very short outpatient procedures it may be best not to use midazolam: not only will patients be drowsy in the postoperative period, they will also be very amnesic and not likely to remember any instructions given them during that period.

Flumazenil, a specific benzodiazepine antagonist, can reverse benzodiazepine-induced sedation without producing toxic side-effects. Sixty women who underwent laparoscopic surgery were treated with flumazenil or placebo after the surgical procedure. Flumazenil reversed the hypnotic effect of midazolam within a few minutes.[209] The patients were alert, cooperative, and oriented and had good recall of events after awakening; effects were statistically better than with placebo for up to 30 minutes after administration. Of those outpatients undergoing upper gastrointestinal endoscopy who received flumazenil 0.5 mg iv 30 minutes after administration of midazolam iv, the flumazenil group had a significant improvement in assessments of memory function, psychomotor performance, and coordination.[210] At 3½ hours following administration of flumazenil or placebo, no difference could be detected between groups. The flumazenil-treated group, however, reported a subjective feeling of alertness at the time of discharge which was greater than that reported by the patients given placebo. The duration of action of flumazenil is shorter than that of most benzodiazepines, and in the outpatient setting patient observation must be of sufficient length to preclude the recurrence of significant sedation in a noncontrolled setting (i.e., during transport home or at home).

Inhalational Techniques

As Apfelbaum has written, "In theory, therefore, if all other factors are held constant (inspired partial pressure, ventilation, blood flow, cardiac output, etc.), inhalation agents with low blood/gas partition coefficients (i.e., low solubility) would be preferable for outpatient anesthesia because these agents achieve equilibrium with the brain most rapidly, allowing for fast induction and emergence."[211]

Nitrous Oxide. Lacking pungency, and having a pleasant odor, nitrous oxide is used as an adjunct for beginning the induction of inhalational anesthesia in both pediatric and adult outpatients who dislike needles. The use of nitrous oxide as a maintenance adjunct can significantly decrease the MAC, substantially reducing requirements for other anesthetic drugs and thereby resulting in more rapid emergence from anesthesia.[212] The combination of nitrous oxide plus halothane, enflurane, or isoflurane appears to produce less depression at a given MAC than either of the potent drugs alone.[213-215] This can be of particular importance in the anesthetic management of an outpatient of ASA Physical Status 3.

A major drawback to the use of nitrous oxide in outpatients is the unresolved question of its possible contribution to postoperative nausea and vomiting. Nitrous oxide may be associated with a higher incidence of postoperative nausea and vomiting following laparoscopic surgery.[216,217] Other investigators do not consider nitrous oxide to be a prime causative factor in the occurrence of postoperative nausea and vomiting.[218,219] Despite any potential drawback, nitrous oxide continues to be the mainstay of inhalational anesthesia in the ambulatory setting.

Halothane. Halothane is the most commonly used potent inhalational drug in pediatric outpatient anesthesia; it allows a smooth mask induction with the lowest incidence of excitement.[220,221] Halothane or isoflurane was used to induce anesthesia in children scheduled for outpatient surgical procedures.[222] Anesthesia induction and time to intubation of the trachea were protracted in patients who received isoflurane. Recovery times were similar in patients who received either anesthetic drug. Induction and maintenance of anesthesia were satisfactory when isoflurane was compared with halothane for outpatient dental extractions in 80 children, although there was a higher incidence of coughing, salivation, and laryngospasm in the group receiving isoflurane.[223] Immediate recovery was slower in patients who received isoflurane. Recovery from halothane anesthesia is usually rapid and uneventful, although postoperative shivering, headache, and nausea and vomiting have been reported and may affect time to discharge in outpatients.[224,225] Compared with the use of enflurane or isoflurane, during halothane anesthesia ventricular cardiac dysrhythmias are far more likely to occur, especially in female and younger outpatients.[226-229]

Enflurane. Unlike halothane, enflurane can provide skeletal muscle relaxation sufficient for most outpatient surgical procedures. Additionally, enflurane enhances the effect of many nondepolarizing neuromuscular blocking agents. Theoretically, the use of less muscle relaxant should provide additional safety after operation and allow the surgical outpatient to return more rapidly to street fitness.[211]

After 7 minutes of 2 MAC enflurane or halothane for D&C,

patients who received enflurane could respond after 5.7 minutes when their names were spoken, compared with 7.6 minutes for those who received halothane.[230] Postoperative physical complaints and intellectual or perceptual-motor function appear comparable between groups treated with the two anesthetic agents.[231-233] Jellicoe evaluated recovery time in 60 outpatients given either alfentanil, halothane, or enflurane.[192] The alfentanil-treated group recovered more rapidly, but there was no difference between halothane and enflurane in terms of recovery time. In a study comparing enflurane, isoflurane, and continuous fentanyl infusion for outpatient anesthesia, all three agents provided satisfactory intraoperative conditions.[234] There was no between-group difference in PACU time. The isoflurane and enflurane techniques were equal and were superior to the fentanyl infusion technique in regard to the incidence of postoperative nausea and vomiting.

In patients undergoing outpatient procedures, recovery appears to be quicker after use of enflurane versus halothane.[230,235] Azar et al found that awakening times were not significantly different in patients who underwent short outpatient procedures with either isoflurane or enflurane.[236]

Isoflurane. In high enough concentrations, isoflurane, like enflurane, can produce profound skeletal muscle relaxation and can substantially potentiate the effects of many nondepolarizing muscle relaxants.[237-239] This effect is reversible when isoflurane is withdrawn and allows the anesthesiologist to use lower intraoperative doses of relaxant.

Because of its pungent smell and irritating effects on the airway, isoflurane is associated with a higher incidence of excitement, breath holding, coughing, and laryngospasm than either enflurane or halothane.[221,240,241]

Short et al evaluated indices of recovery in unpremedicated patients who underwent brief urologic and gynecologic procedures.[191] Although patients in the alfentanil-treated group opened their eyes and gave their names and dates of birth significantly faster after operation than those in the isoflurane-treated group, there were no significant differences between the groups on later tests of recovery. Zuurmond and van Leeuwen compared alfentanil given by continuous iv infusion with isoflurane as anesthetic drugs for outpatient arthroscopic procedures.[185] Although awakening from anesthesia was more rapid in the alfentanil-treated patients, both anesthetic techniques provided satisfactory anesthesia and rapid recovery. The patients who received isoflurane scored better on all early recovery tests, but after 3 hours there was no difference between the groups. The alfentanil-treated group had a higher incidence of nausea and vomiting (45%) than the isoflurane-treated group (14%). Rising et al compared isoflurane versus fentanyl for outpatient laparoscopic procedures and found that immediate recovery was more rapid in the fentanyl-treated group, although reaction times in the isoflurane-treated patients returned to levels seen in control patients by 3 hours, whereas fentanyl-treated patients were still 10% slower than control patients at 4 hours after anesthesia.[242] Nausea and vomiting were more frequent in the fentanyl-treated group. Both anesthetic techniques afforded satisfactory operating conditions, but isoflurane appeared to provide a better recovery with fewer side-effects than fentanyl.

Korttila and Valanne found that lengthy enflurane anesthesia (longer than 90 minutes) was associated with significantly slower recovery than shorter enflurane anesthesia (less than 40 minutes).[243] The rapidity of recovery did not depend on the duration of anesthesia when isoflurane was used, which suggests that isoflurane may have significant advantages in regard to rapidity of recovery in patients undergoing ambulatory surgical procedures lasting longer than 90 minutes.

Sixty unpremedicated outpatients undergoing D&C were randomly allocated to receive one of three inhalational agents (halothane, enflurane, or isoflurane) to supplement 67% nitrous oxide–oxygen after induction of anesthesia with methohexital.[244] After anesthesia there was no difference between the groups in time to eye opening or return of preoperative level of manipulative skill. The p-deletion test, which indicates the subject's ability to concentrate, was completed more quickly by patients in the isoflurane-treated group. The differences among the three inhalational drugs (after iv induction) when used for short procedures are insufficient to allow recommendation of any one over the other two.

Desflurane. Desflurane's physicochemical properties suggest that it may become the inhalational anesthetic of choice for the outpatient. Hemodynamics, emergence, and recovery from desflurane vs. alfentanil anesthesia were not significantly different in a small group of outpatients.[245] Fletcher and colleagues compared psychomotor recovery in the postoperative period in desflurane- and isoflurane-treated patients.[246] Recovery of choice reaction time performance was faster following desflurane anesthesia than following isoflurane anesthesia. Paradoxically, patients who received nitrous oxide with desflurane performed better than those who received a desflurane plus oxygen anesthetic. Psychomotor performance at 1 hour following desflurane was significantly better in volunteers than in a propofol infusion group.[247]

No single agent or technique affords ideal anesthetic conditions for outpatient surgery. Apfelbaum believes that "unless specific circumstances require or exclude a specific technique, most anesthesiologists combine the advantages of several types of drugs (intravenous induction agents, opioids, potent inhaled agents, nitrous oxide); this approach typically requires smaller amounts of each agent."[211]

POSTANESTHESIA CARE UNIT MANAGEMENT

Managing common PACU problems quickly and effectively is equally as important as appropriate patient selection and choice of anesthetic technique if the patient is to return home on the same day that surgery is performed. Unanticipated admission rates after an outpatient procedure vary from 0.1% to 5%.[23,44,248,249] Depending on the type of surgery, pain (i.e., after orchiopexy) or nausea and vomiting (i.e., after strabismus correction) can be a significant reason for hospital admission.

Pain

Postsurgical pain must be treated quickly and effectively. Medications given in the PACU should be monitored closely and given in small, immediately effective doses. Intramuscular opioid analgesic injection for pain control in the PACU is probably more a custom than a thoroughly considered process.[250] Appropriate control of postoperative pain includes the following:

1. Supplementation of inhalational anesthesia with opioid analgesics or a nonsteroidal anti-inflammatory drug
2. Supplementation of inhalational anesthesia with local or regional block
3. Administration of opioid analgesics in the PACU

Epstein et al found a significantly higher incidence of pain and a slightly higher incidence of excitement during recovery in outpatients who did not receive an opioid analgesic intra-anesthetically than in those who did.[84] Although there was a higher incidence of nausea in the fentanyl-treated group, patients recovered statistically sooner than those who did not receive opioid supplementation during anesthesia. The opioid-supplemented patients had a shorter time to walk without support and stand, with a negative Romberg test, and they spent less time in the PACU. The use of a longer-acting opioid, meperidine (1–1.5 mg·kg^{-1}), compared with fentanyl (2 µg·kg^{-1}), administered intraoperatively did not delay recovery from anesthesia or patient discharge.[251] Anesthesia techniques that provided the best pain relief in the first 2 hours after surgery were associated with a lower incidence of overall complications and more rapid recovery. Sanders et al administered alfentanil or halothane to patients who had received either etomidate or methohexital plus nitrous oxide and oxygen anesthesia for termination of pregnancy. Patients who received alfentanil recovered faster.[86] In short urologic and gynecologic procedures, alfentanil-treated patients recovered more rapidly than halothane-, enflurane-, or isoflurane-treated patients.[191,192] Late recovery scores as well as subjective feelings of drowsiness and unsteadiness were the same in all four groups.

Nonsteroidal anti-inflammatory drugs have been shown to reduce postoperative pain following laparoscopic tubal ligation.[252] Ketorolac (30–60 mg im) provides analgesia comparable to that seen with morphine (6–12 mg) and meperidine (50–100 mg).[253-255] Ketorolac is peripherally acting, associated with few CNS side-effects (drowsiness was comparable for groups receiving Ketorolac or placebo), and has no potential to cause physical addiction. For ambulatory surgery patients weighing over 50 kg and less than 65 years of age, 60 mg given by im injection in the deltoid muscle following induction of anesthesia will provide satisfactory pain relief in the immediate postsurgical period.

A decrease in pain, analgesic requirements, and minor complications in the PACU; earlier home readiness; and more rapid return to normal activity can be achieved by combining many simple (sensory) nerve blocks with inhalational anesthesia.[256]

Shandling and Steward believe that children older than 6 months of age almost invariably need postoperative analgesics after inguinal hernia repair.[257] When ilioinguinal and iliohypogastric nerves were infiltrated with bupivacaine during surgery, pain and vomiting decreased during the recovery period. The extended duration of action of bupivacaine can produce postoperative analgesia for 8–12 hours.

The incidence of postoperative complications after laparoscopic tubal sterilization is low and is primarily related to pain. There is minimal incisional pain, but abdominal discomfort, shoulder pain, and nausea and vomiting frequently delay discharge. The level of discomfort will vary, depending on the type of sterilization performed; there is less pain and cramping after cautery than after sterilization with the Yoon fallopian ring.[258,259] Infiltration of the mesosalpinx with 0.5% bupivacaine in the area of placement of the Yoon ring at the conclusion of surgical sterilization significantly decreased patients' pain subsequently in the PACU.[260,261]

McGlinchy et al supplemented general anesthesia with regional block of the dorsal nerve of the penis (0.5% bupivacaine) in a group of adult outpatients undergoing circumcision.[262] None of the patients needed analgesia in the 6 hours after surgery, whereas in a control group all patients needed strong opioid analgesic supplementation during the recovery stage. Topical anesthesia (lidocaine spray 10%, 10–20 mg; lidocaine jelly 2%, 0.5–1 ml; lidocaine ointment 5%, 0.5–1 ml) has provided postoperative pain relief after pediatric circumcision.[263] The duration of analgesia (4–5 hours) approximated that produced by supplemental dorsal nerve block or im morphine. Pain relief was comparable with all topical techniques; however, children preferred lidocaine spray if repeated application was necessary. Subcutaneous ring block of the penis with 0.25% bupivacaine is another simple and effective method of providing postcircumcision analgesia without delaying discharge from the hospital.[264]

Caudal block supplementation has been used to limit postsurgical pain not only after pediatric circumcision but also after correction of hypospadias and orchiopexy.[265,266] Caudal block performed with 0.25% bupivacaine containing epinephrine 1:200,000 produces effective postoperative analgesia. There does not appear to be any advantage to using more concentrated solutions.[267] The optimum concentration of local anesthetic should provide effective analgesia, minimal motor blockade, and few side-effects. Wolf and co-workers noted that 0.0625% bupivacaine was ineffective for caudal analgesia.[268] However, 0.125% bupivacaine (with epinephrine 1:200,000) in a volume of 0.75 ml·kg^{-1} provided equipotent analgesia and significantly less motor blockade than 0.25% bupivacaine (with epinephrine 1:200,000). The key to the safety of caudal analgesia is knowledge of children's anatomy and how it differs from that of adults (the dural sac extends more caudad in children), meticulous attention to detail in site selection and preparation, and careful aspiration to be certain that neither a vessel nor a subarachnoid space has been entered.[269]

Caudal analgesia has consistently been shown to be superior to systemic opioid analgesics administered at the time of surgery in respect to a more tranquil early recovery period, superior analgesia during the early postoperative period, a significantly lower incidence of vomiting, and a swifter resumption of normal activities.[270-273] Dorsal nerve block, when compared with caudal analgesia, provided good pain relief after circumcision; micturition occurred earlier, patients stood unaided sooner, and patients had a lower incidence of vomiting.[274] Ilioinguinal nerve block is a satisfactory alternative to caudal block for patients undergoing herniorrhaphy or orchiopexy.[275]

When the anesthesiologist and postanesthesia care nurse communicate problem-solving techniques to the surgeon, patients can be provided with a smoother course in the PACU and the immediate postoperative period at home.

Although the choice of opioid analgesic is usually a matter of individual judgment, drugs such as morphine and meperidine are generally believed to be too long acting for outpatient use. Potent opioid analgesics given in the PACU may contribute significantly to postoperative drowsiness, nausea and vomiting, and delay in discharge home. A delicate balance must be struck in order to provide a postoperative period as free of pain as possible.

At the Methodist Ambulatory SurgiCare facility, pain in both adults and children is managed with a short-acting opioid analgesic. Intravenous fentanyl (0.35 μg·kg^{-1}) is given at the first sign of discomfort and administration is repeated at 5-minute intervals until pain is controlled. For children, we also use an elixir of acetaminophen containing codeine (120 mg acetaminophen, 12 mg codeine, in each 5 ml of solution). Five milliliters is administered to children between the ages of 3 and 6, and 10 ml to children between the ages of 7 and 12. Children are returned to parental care as soon as they are awake.

At the Children's National Medical Center (Washington, DC), infants younger than 6 months of age usually only need to be reunited with their parents and be nursed (or fed from a bottle) after a procedure not associated with severe pain. For older infants and young children, acetaminophen, 60 mg per year of age (given orally or rectally), is one of the drugs most commonly given to relieve mild pain while they are in the PACU. Intravenous fentanyl (up to a dose of 2 μg·kg^{-1}) is the drug of choice for more severe pain. Meperidine (0.5 mg·kg^{-1}) and codeine (1–1.5 mg·kg^{-1}) can be given im if an iv route has not been established.[276]

Outpatient facilities should establish a minimum length of time that patients must be observed in the PACU before discharge after administration of any depressant medication.

Nausea and Vomiting

Protracted vomiting (occurring in 36% of patients) is the leading reason for patient admission to the hospital from the short-stay recovery unit at the Children's National Medical Center (Table 50-12).[277] Nausea (30%) and vomiting (20%) are the most common complications occurring in the PACU at the Phoenix Surgicenter.[43] Contributing factors are a history of motion sickness, sudden movement or position changes, pain, administration of opioid analgesic drugs, choice of anesthetic agent, obesity, and site of surgical procedure. Laparoscopic surgery performed around the time of menses resulted in a fourfold increase in the incidence of nausea and vomiting.[278] Pataky and co-workers evaluated the incidence of postoperative nausea and vomiting (general anesthesia) for the five most common procedures in the day-surgery unit at the University of Pennsylvania.[279] Depending on the procedure, 12–54% of patients experienced emetic symptoms (D&C, 12%; dental, 16%; arthroscopy, 22%; laparoscopy, 35%; ovum retrieval, 54%). Nausea and

TABLE 50-12. Reasons for Hospital Admission Following Same-Day Surgery

| Reason | Cases | |
	Number	Percent
Protracted vomiting	26	36
Croup	8	11
Family request	6	8
Fever	6	8
Bleeding	3	4
Complicated surgery	3	4
Sleepiness	2	2
Other reasons	18	25
Total	72	

Reproduced with permission from Patel RI, Hannallah RS, Murphy LS et al: Pediatric outpatient anesthesia—A review of postanesthetic complications in 8995 cases. Anesthesiology 65:A435, 1986.

vomiting prolonged PACU stay and increased per-patient labor costs.[280] Korttila and co-workers noted a decrease in the occurrence and severity of emetic symptoms when propofol for induction and maintenance was compared with thiopental isoflurane for outpatient anesthesia.[161]

A relationship between postoperative pain and the frequency of nausea in the early postsurgical period has been established.[281] Relief of pain without relief of nausea was unusual, regardless of the analgesic used for pain control. Nausea often accompanies pain in the postoperative period and can be relieved in many patients when pain relief is achieved by the iv use of opiates. Using traditional Chinese acupuncture, Dundee et al significantly reduced postoperative nausea and vomiting.[282]

An important part of the preanesthesia interview is identification of the nausea-susceptible patient and awareness on the part of the anesthesiologist of those procedures that are associated with an increased frequency of emetic symptoms following surgery. During the preanesthesia interview, eliciting a history of motion sickness or emesis after a prior anesthetic episode should alert the anesthesiologist to establish an "anesthesia game plan." When faced with this type of patient, the anesthesiologist must carefully prioritize use of the following: antiemetics, gastrokinetics, nitrous oxide, opioid analgesics, regional block supplementation, or regional anesthesia.

Nausea-susceptible patients should:

Receive positive reassurance by all members of the staff to alleviate anxiety.

Be moved slowly at all times to avoid motion sickness.

Have a warm blanket placed over them to add to their sense of security.

Have limited suction at the conclusion of the procedure (to avoid stimulation of the gag reflex).

Be allowed to wake up slowly in the PACU.

Antiemetics

Benzquinamide, trimethobenzamide, prochlorperazine, and hydroxyzine have all been used with limited success in efforts to control postanesthetic nausea and vomiting.[283,284] Droperidol has been found to be an effective antiemetic in iv doses as low as 0.25 mg in a group of ambulatory surgery patients undergoing D&C (E. S. Shelley, H. A. Brown, pers. commun., 1978). When droperidol (0.625–1.25 mg) was administered iv immediately after intubation of the trachea, it proved to be an effective antiemetic in outpatients undergoing laparoscopic tubal surgery.[285] Patients who received droperidol during anesthesia had a lower prevalence of nausea and vomiting in the PACU and consequently a shorter stay than patients in the control group.

Valanne and Korttila administered droperidol, 0.014 mg·kg^{-1}, 5 minutes after induction of anesthesia. The frequency of nausea (18%) or vomiting (7%) was lower in droperidol-treated patients than in patients given saline (27% and 11%), respectively.[286]

Droperidol can potentiate drowsiness and, if administered during the final phases of recovery care, may extend the patient's stay. In an outpatient setting, as the dose is increased above 1.25 mg, drowsiness becomes more noticeable.

Pandit and co-workers evaluated droperidol (5, 10, and 20 μg·kg^{-1}) iv, metoclopramide (5 and 10 mg) orally, and a combination of the two drugs in adult women undergoing outpatient laparoscopy under general anesthesia.[287] Oral metoclopramide alone did not reduce the frequency of nau-

sea and vomiting. Droperidol (10 and 20 μg·kg^{-1}) and a combination of metoclopramide (10 mg) and droperidol (10 μg·kg^{-1}) significantly decreased the frequency of nausea and vomiting in the PACU; however, only droperidol-treated (20 μg·kg^{-1}) patients required no additional antiemetic therapy in the PACU. Rao et al found that outpatients who underwent laparoscopic procedures and received metoclopramide (10 mg alone or in combination with cimetidine, 300 mg) had a significant decrease in nausea and vomiting compared with a control group or a group treated with cimetidine alone.[288] Patients were instructed to fast from midnight and to take their tablets with a sip of water on the day of surgery just before leaving home to the outpatient facility. Rao et al believe that metoclopramide, 10 mg iv, relieves postoperative nausea and vomiting within 5–10 minutes and does not prolong the PACU stay. In the PACU, we administer droperidol iv (10–20 μg·kg^{-1}) to patients who have persistent nausea or after a second emesis.

The prevalence of postoperative nausea and vomiting is significantly higher (up to 85%) in children who undergo strabismus surgery.[289-292] When droperidol was given iv 30 minutes before termination of surgery, 75 μg·kg^{-1} reduced vomiting to 43%, compared with 85% in the control group. When droperidol (75 μg·kg^{-1}) was administered during induction of anesthesia and before manipulation of the extraocular muscles, the prevalence of vomiting was reduced from 75% in the control group to 10% in the droperidol-treated group.[291] Brown and colleagues recommend conservative management of children during and after strabismus surgery, involving gastric suctioning prior to extubation, complete replacement of preoperative fluid deficits, avoidance of narcotics, and a small dose of droperidol (20 μg·kg^{-1}) given iv during induction of anesthesia.[293]

When using doses of 75 μg·kg^{-1}, the anesthesiologist should be prepared for a PACU stay of several hours. A recovery time of 4–6 hours after surgery would be considered prolonged in children after myringotomy or herniotomy, but, because of nausea and vomiting, it is not an unusual length of stay after strabismus or orchiopexy surgery. Intraoperative use of droperidol is recommended for these patients. After orchiopexy, up to 5% of patients may have to be admitted because of drowsiness or nausea and vomiting, or because surgery was more extensive than planned.[249]

Nitrous Oxide

The possible contribution of nitrous oxide to postoperative nausea and vomiting has not been fully established. Studies implicating nitrous oxide as a causative factor in postoperative nausea and vomiting are matched by those refuting it as a potential cause.[216-219]

Transdermal Scopolamine

When evaluating this method of preventing or treating nausea and vomiting, we are faced with many anecdotal comments but lack significant outpatient studies. In a non-outpatient study, a 72-hour application of transdermal scopolamine effectively limited postoperative nausea and emesis.[294] The scopolamine dot was applied to the posterior auricular skin 12 hours before surgery and removed 48 hours after surgery. Insignificant benefits were seen in reducing postoperative emesis after pediatric eye surgery.[295] An unacceptable incidence of behavioral side-effects (hallucination, extreme agitation) was reported. The routine use of scopolamine as a transdermal preparation for the prophylaxis of vomiting in the child undergoing eye surgery is not recommended.

DISCHARGE CRITERIA

When can the patient safely leave the outpatient facility? Outpatient surgical facilities must develop practical criteria for patient discharge that in no way compromise patient safety. Although various psychomotor tests yield some information that can be used in developing practical criteria, most tests are too complex, time-consuming, and cumbersome to be used in a busy clinical setting.

To be ready for the ride home, Phoenix Surgicenter patients must be accompanied by a responsible person and must meet the following:

1. Stable vital signs for at least 30 minutes.
2. No new signs or symptoms after operation that may threaten a safe recovery (e.g., the patient with mild shoulder pain after a laparoscopic procedure will be released home, but a patient with more than mild abdominal pain after a diagnostic D&C will be detained for further observation).
3. Cessation of oozing or bleeding when bleeding was a feature of the operation.
4. No nausea or emesis for 30 minutes, or evidence that it is waning.
5. Good circulation in and return of sensation to the operate extremity when a tourniquet has been used.
6. No evidence of swelling or impaired circulation in an extremity when a cast has been applied.
7. Clear urine voided after a cystoscopic examination.
8. Ability to recognize time and place.
9. Little or no dizziness after changing clothes and sitting for 10 minutes.
10. No pain not controllable by oral analgesics.

After a state of home readiness has been established, the responsible nurse notifies the anesthesiologist and together they make sure that the applicable requirements of the Surgicenter's postoperative checklist and satisfied. This is known as informed discharge.[296]

1. Dietary instructions are given. Clear liquids are allowed until the patient's stomach is settled; then he or she can progress to regular feedings. The patient should not have alcohol (unless by physician's order) for at least 12 hours.
2. Pain medication appropriate to need is provided.
3. Prescriptions are checked. The patient or responsible person has prescriptions for all medications ordered by the surgeon.
4. The surgeon's instructions are reviewed, including limitations on activity, elevation of an operate extremity, when to return to the office, anticipated complications, and whom to call in the event of unanticipated complications.
5. The anesthesiologist's instructions are given:
   a. "You may feel sleepy and somewhat sluggish for several hours." "Don't drive until tomorrow." "Postpone important decisions until tomorrow."
   b. "You may have a sore throat for a few hours" (if patient's trachea was intubated). The patient should be instructed in the use of salt-water gargles, humidifying devices, aspirin, or acetaminophen and advised to call if soreness persists more than a day.
   c. "You may have some muscular soreness for a day or two" (soreness, which follows the use of succinylcholine, may be more pronounced than any other discomfort). It is often, but not always, relieved by the medication prescribed to relieve pain at the operative site. Aspirin is recommended to relieve this soreness, and a warm bath is suggested if not contraindicated by the surgical procedure.
6. Dentures, valuables, and clothes are returned.
7. The patient is reassured that he or she has behaved properly. The patient should be informed that dreaming often occurs, and an opportunity should be afforded for the patient to discuss any dream that may be remembered.
8. The patient is informed that a follow-up call is routine and is to be expected.

Methodist Ambulatory SurgiCare patients must meet predetermined discharge criteria:[297]

1. Stable vital signs: Temperature, pulse, respiration, and blood pressure must be stable when appropriate. Vital signs should remain stable (i.e., blood pressure ±20 mm Hg) for a period of at least 30 minutes and should be consistent with the patient's age and preanesthesia levels.
2. Ability to swallow and cough: The patient must demonstrate ability to swallow fluids and be able to cough.
3. Ability to walk: The patient must demonstrate ability to move consistent with age and development level (sit, stand, and walk).
4. Minimal nausea, vomiting, and dizziness
   a. Minimal nausea: No nausea, or, if nausea is present, the patient can still swallow and retain some fluids.
   b. Minimal vomiting: No vomiting, or, if vomiting is present, it does not require treatment. After vomiting that requires treatment, the patient should be able to swallow and retain fluids.
   c. Minimal dizziness: Dizziness is either absent or present only on sitting, and the patient can still move consistent with his or her age.
5. Absence of respiratory distress: The patient exhibits no signs of snoring, obstructed respiration, stridor, retractions, or croupy cough.
6. Alertness and orientation: The patient is aware of surroundings and what has taken place and is interested in returning home.

Scoring systems used in the PACU immediately after anesthesia determine the patient's recovery progression but do not evaluate home readiness for ambulatory surgery patients. Chung and colleagues have developed a postanesthetic discharge score that uses numerical values to assess patient recovery and discharge readiness.[298]

When is it safe to permit patients to walk after spinal or epidural anesthesia? The generally accepted sequence of return of function is motor, sensory, and finally sympathetic. Several studies examining the sequence of return of function have found recovery of sympathetic activity to occur before complete regression of the subarachnoid block.[299-301] Pflug et al considered the ability to urinate a final indication of reversal of sympathetic paralysis because an intact, functioning sympathetic nerve supply to the bladder and urethra is necessary for this function.[300]

Suitable criteria for walking after spinal anesthesia include normal perianal (S_{4-5}) pinprick sensation, plantar flexion of the foot, and proprioception of the big toe. Discharge criteria after spinal anesthesia include normal sensation, ability to walk (return of strength and proprioception), and ability to urinate (return of sympathetic nervous function).

Patients who have had spinal anesthesia do not need to remain flat in bed for 24 hours after returning home as a means of preventing post-dural puncture headache. After discharge, our patients who have had spinal anesthesia are instructed to rest in bed for 24 hours; they may be propped up on pillows, sit up to eat, and have bathroom privileges, but they must wait until the next day before resuming appropriate normal activities. They are instructed to call the facility if they have a headache not relieved by acetaminophen, a stiff neck, or an elevated temperature. Similar instructions are given to patients who have epidural anesthesia, but we are more liberal in allowing them to be up and out of bed.[297] At the outpatient facilities of both the Brigham and Women's Hospital and the Virginia Mason Hospital, patients are instructed not to lift heavy objects or strain, but walking, activity, and position are not otherwise limited.

Before a patient is discharged, dressings should be checked and the patient should attempt to urinate. Urination as a criterion for discharge is usually mandated for patients who have had spinal or epidural anesthesia, but it may also be applicable to patients who have undergone urologic intervention. It is wise to include the responsible person in all discharge instructions, and these instructions are best made available on printed forms. Patients and responsible parties should be reminded that the patient should not drive a car, operate power tools, or be involved in major business decisions for up to 24 hours after sedation, iv or inhalational anesthesia.

Before being discharged home, patients should be informed that they may experience pain, headache, nausea, vomiting, dizziness, and muscle aches and pains not related to the incision (if succinylcholine was used) for at least 24 hours after surgery and anesthesia. The well-informed patient will be less stressed if any of the above symptoms occur after return to home.

In 100 consecutive outpatients who were given no written instructions at discharge, Ogg found that 31% of patients went home unaccompanied by a responsible adult; 73% of car owners drove within 24 hours of surgery, and 30% drove within 12 hours; 9% of patients drove themselves home; and a bus driver returned to work on the same day, driving a busload of passengers a distance of 95 miles.[302] Patients in this study reported postoperative symptoms of headache (27%), drowsiness (26%), nausea (22%), and dizziness (11%). Fifty percent of medical outpatients do not follow physicians' instructions, but the addition of written and verbal education techniques at discharge has a significant impact on improving compliance.[303]

For patients with whom there is a language barrier (i.e., in a population with a high percentage of immigrants), consent forms, procedural explanation, and discharge information may have to be written in appropriate languages and the services of an interpreter may be necessary.

Nursing staff should assess the adult who will take the patient home to determine whether he or she is in fact a responsible person. A responsible person is someone who is physically and intellectually capable of taking care of the patient at home.

The Joint Commission on the Accreditation of Healthcare Organizations (JCAHO) 1991 edition of the *Accreditation Manual for Hospitals* (AMH) standards states the following: "A licensed independent practitioner who has appropriate clinical privileges and who is familiar with the patient is responsible for the decision to discharge a patient from a postanesthesia recovery area or, when the surgical or anesthesia services are provided on an ambulatory basis, from the hospital. When the responsible licensed independent practitioner is not personally present to make the decision to discharge or does not sign the discharge order, the name of the licensed independent practitioner responsible for the discharge is recorded in the patient's medical record; and relevant discharge criteria are rigorously applied to determine the readiness of the patient for discharge. The discharge criteria are approved by the medical staff."

Facilities should develop a method of follow-up after the patient has been discharged. Staff members at some facilities telephone the patient the next day to determine how they are recovering from surgery and anesthesia; others use follow-up postcards.

INNOVATIVE APPROACHES TO POSTOPERATIVE CARE

Whenever we become innovative in the management of our outpatients, we must carefully assess how different and more compacted care affects patient safety. We must determine what we can do for the patient who lives alone, the patient whose responsible person is unable to manage his or her needs, the patient without any means of transportation, and the patient with limited insurance coverage. Some innovative approaches to postoperative care are described below.

Observation beds in hospital: Patients going into an observation bed after an ambulatory surgical procedure are still considered outpatients. There is an hourly charge for time spent in the observation area.

Hospital hotel/medical motel services: Hospitals are establishing in-hospital hotel guest services or are joining with management firms to have a hospital hotel or medical motel built and managed close to the hospital itself. The ambulatory hotel, usually a nonmedical facility, offers the outpatient a comfortable, inexpensive, and convenient place to recuperate while they are cared for by family or health care nurses.

Home health care nursing: After surgical procedures such as reduction mammaplasty, abdominoplasty, vaginal hysterectomy, and major open ligament repairs of the knee, Texas Outpatient Surgicare (Houston) uses home health care nursing services. Patients are transported home in an ambulance with a registered nurse who stays with the patient (administering iv fluids, antibiotics, opioid analgesics) for periods of 12–48 hours.

Surgical recovery facility: In Phoenix, Arizona, the freestanding Surgical Recovery Center accepts patients transferred directly from hospital PACUs, freestanding outpatient centers, and physicians' offices and patients from hospitals on the first or second postoperative day for additional nursing care. The California legislature approved a demonstration project that allows freestanding, hospital, and skilled nursing facilities to add or utilize up to 20 beds for recovery of surgical patients. Patients may occupy these beds for up to 3 days following their surgical procedure. If it is demonstrated that freestanding surgery centers can perform inpatient-type surgical procedures and provide postoperative care more economically than hospitals, without compromising care or safety, it is estimated that 30% of all surgeries currently performed in California on an inpatient basis could be transferred to ambulatory surgery care utilizing this innovative recovery concept.

The varying outpatient observation and home health care services stand today where outpatient surgery stood in the health care delivery system 20 years ago. Prospective studies must be done to assess the quality of care and the effect these innovative approaches have on patient safety.

Patient, procedure, availability (including quality) of aftercare, and anesthetic technique must be individually and collectively assessed in determining acceptability for ambulatory surgery. A definite balance exists between physical status of patient, proposed surgical procedure, and appropriate anesthetic technique, to which must be added the comfort level of the anesthesiologist caring for that patient.

REFERENCES

1. Nicoll JH: The surgery of infancy. Br Med J 2:753, 1909
2. Waters RM: The down-town anesthesia clinic. Am J Surg (Anesth Suppl) 33:71, 1919
3. Herzfeld G: Hernia in infancy. Am J Surg 39:422, 1938
4. Webb E, Graves H: Anesthesia for the Ambulant Patient. Philadelphia, JB Lippincott, 1966
5. Porterfield HW, Franklin LT: The use of general anesthesia in the office surgery facility. Clin Plast Surg 10:292, 1983
6. Wetchler BV: Outpatient general and spinal anesthesia. Urol Clin North Am 14:31, 1987
7. Stafford M, Jeon A, Pascucci R: Pre- and post-induction blood glucose concentrations in healthy fasting children. Anesthesiology 63:A350, 1985
8. Jensen BH, Wernberg M, Adersen M: Preoperative starvation and blood glucose concentrations in children undergoing inpatient and outpatient anesthesia. Br J Anaesth 54:1071, 1982
9. Welborn LG, McGill WA, Hannallah RS et al: Perioperative blood glucose concentrations in pediatric outpatients. Anesthesiology 65:543, 1986
10. Redfern N, Addison GM, Meakin G: Blood glucose in anaesthetised children. Anaesthesia 41:272, 1986
11. Thomas DKM: Hypoglycaemia in children before operation: Its incidence and prevention. Br J Anaesth 46:66, 1974
12. Graham IFM: Preoperative starvation and plasma glucose concentrations in children undergoing outpatient anaesthesia. Br J Anaesth 51:161, 1979
13. Meakin G, Dingwall AE, Addison GM: Effect of fasting and oral premedication on the pH and volume of gastric aspirate in children. Br J Anaesth 59:678, 1987
14. Hutchinson BR, Merry AF, Wild CJ: The relationship of duration of fast to the volume and pH of gastric contents. Anaesth Intensive Care 14:128, 1986
15. Crawford M, Lerman J, Christensen S et al: Effects of duration of fasting on gastric fluid pH and volume in healthy children. Anesth Analg 71:400, 1990
16. Maltby JR, Sutherland AD, Sale JP et al: Preoperative oral fluids: Is a five-hour fast justified prior to elective surgery? Anesth Analg 65:1112, 1986
17. Maltby JR, Sutherland AD, Sale JP et al: Preoperative oral fluids: Is "NPO after midnight" justified? Anesthesiology 65:A244, 1986
18. Goresky GV, Maltby JR: Fasting guidelines for elective surgical patients. Can J Anaesth 37:493, 1990
19. Guidelines to the Practice of Anaesthesia as Recommended by the Canadian Anaesthetists' Society. Toronto, Canadian Anaesthetists' Society, 1987
20. Wetchler BV: Patient and procedure selection. In Wetchler BV (ed): Outpatient Anesthesia. Probl Anesth 2:9, 1988
21. Wilson ME, Williams NB, Baskett PJF et al: Assessment of fitness for surgical procedures and the variability of anaesthetists' judgments. Br Med J 1:509, 1980
22. Wetchler BV: Forms and policies. In Wetchler BV (ed): Anesthesia for Ambulatory Surgery, 2nd ed, p 662. Philadelphia, JB Lippincott, 1991
23. Dawson B, Reed WA: Anaesthesia for adult surgical outpatients. Can Anaesth Soc J 27:409, 1980
24. Natof HE: Complications associated with ambulatory surgery. JAMA 244:1116, 1980
25. Natof HE: Ambulatory surgery: Patients with pre-existing medical problems. Ill Med J 166:101, 1984
26. FASA Special Study 1. Alexandria, Virginia, Federated Ambulatory Surgery Association, 1987
27. Gold B, Kitz DS, Lecky JH et al: Unanticipated admission to the hospital following ambulatory surgery. JAMA 262:3008, 1989
28. Wetchler BV: The geriatric outpatient. In Wetchler BV (ed): Outpatient Anesthesia. Probl Anesth 2:128, 1988
29. Vandam LD: To make the patient ready for anesthesia. In: Medical Care of the Surgical Patient, 2nd ed. Reading, Massachusetts, Addison-Wesley, 1983
30. Chung F, Meier R, Lautenschlager E et al: General or spinal anesthesia: Which is better in the elderly? Anesthesiology 67:422, 1987
31. Steward DJ: Preterm infants are more prone to complications following minor surgery than are term infants. Anesthesiology 56:304, 1982
32. Liu LMP, Cote CJ, Goudsouzian NG et al: Life-threatening apnea in infants recovering from anesthesia. Anesthesiology 59:506, 1983
33. Kurth CD, Spitzer AR, Broennle MD et al: Postoperative apnea in former premature infants. Anesthesiology 63:A475, 1985
34. Welborn LG, Ramirez N, Oh TH et al: Postanesthetic apnea and periodic breathing in infants. Anesthesiology 65:658, 1986
35. Mestad PH, Glenski JA, Binda RE: When is outpatient surgery safe in preterm infants? Anesthesiology 69:744, 1988
36. Jensen S, Wetchler BV: The obese patient: An acceptable candidate for outpatient anesthesia. AANA J 50:369, 1982
37. El-Ganzouri AR, Ivankovich AD, Braverman B et al: Monoamine oxidase inhibitors: Should they be discontinued preoperatively? Anesth Analg 64:592, 1985
38. Ebrahim Z, O'Hara J, Tetzlaff J: Should monoamine oxidase inhibitors be discontinued preoperatively? Anesth Analg 72:S62, 1991
39. Epstein BS: Outpatient anesthesia. American Society of Anesthesiologists Refresher Courses in Anesthesiology, vol 2, p 81. Philadelphia, JB Lippincott, 1974
40. Wetchler BV: Patient and procedure selection. In Wetchler BV (ed): Outpatient Anesthesia. Probl Anesth 2:13, 1988
41. Orkin FK: Selection. In Wetchler BV (ed): Anesthesia for Ambulatory Surgery, 2nd ed, p 81. Philadelphia, JB Lippincott, 1991
42. Henderson JA: Ambulatory surgery: Past, present, and future. In Wetchler BV (ed): Anesthesia for Ambulatory Surgery, 2nd ed, p 6. Philadelphia, JB Lippincott, 1991
43. Standaert FG: Magic bullet, science and medicine. Anesthesiology 63:577, 1985
44. Meridy HW: Criteria for selection of ambulatory surgical patients and guidelines for anesthetic management: A retrospective study of 1,553 cases. Anesth Analg 61:921, 1982
45. Dillon JB: Anesthetic management of the outpatient. Ayrest Anesth Rounds 2:3, 1967
46. Reed WA: Recovery from anesthesia and discharge. In Shultz R (ed): Outpatient Surgery, p 45. Philadelphia, Lea & Febiger, 1979
47. Levy ML, Weintraub HD: Premedication: Yes or no? In Wetchler BV (ed): Outpatient Anesthesia. Probl Anesth 2:23, 1988
48. Twersky RS, Lewis M, Lebovits AH: Early ambulation of patients in an ambulatory surgical setting: Does it really help? Anesthesiology 71:A1186, 1989
49. Rosenblatt MA, Bradford C, Miller R et al: A preoperative interview by an anesthesiologist does not lower preoperative anxiety in outpatients. Anesthesiology 71:A926, 1989
50. Clark AJM, Hurtig JB: Premedication with meperidine and atropine does not prolong recovery to street fitness after outpatient surgery. Can Anaesth Soc J 28:390, 1981
51. Thompson GE, Remington JM, Millman BS et al: Experiences with outpatient anesthesia. Anesth Analg 52:881, 1973
52. Henderson JM, Brodsky DA, Fisher DM et al: Pre-induction

of anesthesia in pediatric patients with nasally administered sufentanil. Anesthesiology 68:671, 1988

53. Hannallah RS, Patel RI: Low-dose intramuscular ketamine for anesthesia pre-induction in young children undergoing brief outpatient procedure. Anesthesiology 70:598, 1989

54. Hannallah RS, Epstein BS: The pediatric patient. In Wetchler BV (ed): Anesthesia for Ambulatory Surgery, 2nd ed, p 131. Philadelphia, JB Lippincott, 1991

55. Feld LH, Negus JB, White PF: Oral midazolam preanesthetic medication in pediatric outpatients. Anesthesiology 73:831, 1990

56. Forbes RB, Vandewalker GE: Two percent rectal methohexital for induction of anesthesia in children. Anesthesiology 65:A420, 1986

57. Khalil SN, Nuutinen LS, Rawal N: Sigmodorectal methohexital as an inducing agent for general anesthesia in children. Anesth Analg 67:S113, 1988

58. Falick YS, Smiler BG: Is anticholinergic premedication necessary? Anesthesiology 43:472, 1975

59. Wyant GM, Kao E: Glycopyrrolate methobromide: Effect on salivary secretion. Can Anaesth Soc J 21:230, 1974

60. Desjardins R, Ansara S, Charest J: Preanesthetic medication in paediatric day-care surgery. Can Anaesth Soc J 28:141, 1981

61. Brzustowicz RM, Nelson DA, Betts EK et al: Efficacy of oral premedication for pediatric outpatient surgery. Anesthesiology 60:475, 1984

62. Miller RD, Way WL: Inhibition of succinylcholine-induced increased intragastric pressure by non-depolarizing muscle relaxants and lidocaine. Anesthesiology 34:185, 1971

63. Ong BY, Palahniuk RJ, Cumming M: Gastric volume and pH in outpatients. Can Anaesth Soc J 25:36, 1978

64. Manchikanti L, Roush JR: Effect of pre-anesthetic glycopyrrolate and cimetidine on gastric fluid pH and volume in outpatients. Anesth Analg 63:40, 1984

65. Manchikanti L, Canella MG, Hohlbein LJ et al: Assessment of effect of various modes of premedication on acid aspiration risk factors in outpatient surgery. Anesth Analg 66:81, 1987

66. Wyner J, Cohen SE: Gastric volume in early pregnancy—Effect of metoclopramide. Anesthesiology 57:209, 1983

67. Olsson GL, Hallen B, Hambraeus Jonzon K: Aspiration during anaesthesia: A computer aided study of 185,358 anaesthetics. Acta Anaesthesiol Scand 30:84, 1986

68. Kallar SK: Aspiration pneumonitis: Fact or fiction? In Wetchler BV (ed): Outpatient Anesthesia. Probl Anesth 2:29, 1988

69. Natof HE, Gold B, Kitz DS: Complications. In Wetchler BV (ed): Anesthesia for Ambulatory Surgery, 2nd ed, p 437. Philadelphia, JB Lippincott, 1991

70. Martin CC, Kallar SK, Ciresi SA: The effect of oral Bicitra compared with intramuscular cimetidine on gastric volume and pH in outpatient surgery. Am Assoc Nurse Anesth J 56(6):515, 1988

71. Stoelting RK: Gastric fluid pH in patients receiving cimetidine. Anesth Analg 57:675, 1978

72. Manchikanti L, Marrero TC: Effect of cimetidine and metoclopramide on gastric contents in outpatients. Anesthesiol Rev 10:9, 1983

73. Manchikanti L, Colliver JA, Marrero TC et al: Ranitidine and metoclopramide for prophylaxis of aspiration pneumonitis in elective surgery. Anesth Analg 63:903, 1984

74. Gonzalez ER, Butler SA, Jones MK et al: Cimetidine versus ranitidine: Single-dose, oral regimen for reducing gastric acidity and volume in ambulatory surgery patients. Drug Intell Clin Pharm 21:192, 1987

75. Gillett GB, Watson JD, Langford RML: Ranitidine and single-dose antacid therapy as prophylaxis against acid aspiration syndrome in obstetric practice. Anaesthesia 39:638, 1984

76. Zeldis JE, Friedman LS, Isselbacher KJ: Ranitidine: A new H$_2$ receptor antagonist. N Engl J Med 309:1368, 1983

77. Somori GJ, Kallar SK: The effects of cimetidine on gastric pH and volume in pediatric patients in an ambulatory surgical center. Anesthesiology 61:3A, 1984

78. Young ET, Goudsouzian NG, Shah A: Effect of ranitidine on intragastric pH in children. Anesth Analg 65:S170, 1986

79. Solamki DR, Nicholas DA, Williams KR: Comparative effects of oral sodium citrate and oral cimetidine on gastric pH in pediatric patients. Anesth Analg 65:S147, 1986

80. Cohen SE, Woods WA, Wyner J: Antiemetic efficacy of droperidol and metoclopramide. Anesthesiology 60:67, 1984

81. Rao TLK, Madhavareddy S, Chinthagada M et al: Metoclopramide and cimetidine to reduce gastric fluid pH and volume. Anesth Analg 63:1014, 1984

82. Murrell GC, Rosen M: In vitro buffering capacity of Alka Seltzer Effervescent. Anesthesiology 41:138, 1986

83. White PF, Chang T: Effect of narcotic premedication on the intravenous anesthetic requirement. Anesthesiology 61:A389, 1984

84. Epstein BS, Levy ML, Thein MH et al: Evaluation of fentanyl as an adjunct to thiopental–nitrous oxide–oxygen anesthesia for short surgical procedures. Anesthesiol Rev 2(3):24, 1975

85. Hunt TM, Plantevin OM, Gilbert JR: Morbidity in gynaecological day-case surgery: A comparison of two anaesthetic techniques. Br J Anaesth 51:785, 1979

86. Sanders RS, Sinclair ME, Sear JW: Alfentanil in short procedures. Anaesthesia 39:1202, 1984

87. Pandit SK, Kothary SP: Should we premedicate ambulatory surgical patients? Anesthesiology 65:A352, 1986

88. Jakobsen H, Hertz JB, Johansen JR et al: Premedication before day surgery: A double-blind comparison of diazepam and placebo. Br J Anaesth 57:300, 1985

89. Jansen EC, Wachowiak-Andersen G, Munster-Swendsen J et al: Postural stability after oral premedication with diazepam. Anesthesiology 63:557, 1985

90. Greenwood BK, Bradshaw EG: Preoperative medication for day-case surgery. Br J Anaesth 55:933, 1983

91. Clark G, Erwin D, Yate P et al: Temazepam as premedication in elderly patients. Anaesthesia 37:421, 1982

92. Fragen RJ, Funk DI, Avram MJ et al: Midazolam versus hydroxyzine as intramuscular premedicant. Can Anaesth Soc J 30:136, 1983

93. Vinik HR, Reves JG, Wright D: Premedication with intramuscular midazolam: A prospective randomized double-blind controlled study. Anesth Analg 61:933, 1982

94. Rita L, Seleny FL, Goodarzi M et al: Dose-finding study of intramuscular midazolam in children. Anesthesiol Rev 12:40, 1985

95. Cohen DD, Dillon JB: Anesthesia for outpatient surgery. JAMA 196:98, 1966

96. Mulroy MF: Regional anesthesia: When, why, why not? In Wetchler BV (ed): Outpatient Anesthesia. Probl Anesth 2:82, 1988

97. Bridenbaugh LD, Soderstrom RM: Lumbar epidural block anesthesia for outpatient laparoscopy. J Reprod Med 23:85, 1979

98. Coupland GAE, Townsend DM, Martin CJ: Peritoneoscopy—Use in assessment of intraabdominal malignancy. Surgery 89:645, 1981

99. Philip BK: Supplemental medication for ambulatory procedures under regional anesthesia. Anesth Analg 64:1117, 1985

100. Reeves JG, Fragen RJ, Vinik HR et al: Midazolam: Pharmacology and uses. Anesthesiology 62:310, 1985

101. White PF: The role of midazolam in outpatient anesthesia. Anesthesiol Rev 12:55, 1985

102. Philip BK: Hazards of amnesia after midazolam in ambulatory surgical patients. Anesth Analg 66:97, 1987

103. White PF, Negus JB: Sedative infusions during local and regional anesthesia: A comparison of midazolam and propofol. J Clin Anesth 3:32, 1991

104. Philip BK, Covino BG: Local and regional anesthesia. In Wetchler BV (ed): Anesthesia for Ambulatory Surgery, 2nd ed, p 309. Philadelphia, JB Lippincott, 1991

105. Mulroy MF: Spinal headache and air travel. Anesthesiology 51:479, 1979

106. Harris AP: Spinal anesthesia: It works. Anesthesiol Rep 3:56, 1990

107. Neal JM, Bridenbaugh LD, Mulroy MF: Incidence of post dural puncture headache is similar between 22g Greene and 26g Quincke spinal needles. Anesthesiology 71:A678, 1989

108. Carbaat P, van Crevel H: Lumbar puncture headache: Con-

trolled study on the preventive effect of 24 hours' bed rest. Lancet 2:1131, 1981

109. Jones RJ: The role of recumbency in the prevention and treatment of postspinal headache. Anesth Analg 53:788, 1974

110. Vandam LD, Dripps RD: Long-term follow-up of patients who received 10,098 spinal anesthetics: Syndrome of decreased intracranial pressure. JAMA 161:586, 1956

111. Sarma VJ, Bostrom U: Intrathecal anesthesia for day-care surgery. Anaesthesia 45:769, 1990

112. Burke RK: Spinal anesthesia for laparoscopy: A review of 1,063 cases. J Reprod Med 21:59, 1978

113. Cohen SE: Epidural blood patch in outpatients: A simpler approach. Anesth Analg 64:458, 1985

114. Wetchler BV: Spinal anesthesia: Handle with care. Anesthesiol Rep 3:57, 1990

115. Randel GI, Levy L, Kothary SP et al: Epidural anesthesia is superior to spinal or general for outpatient knee arthroscopy. Anesthesiology 71:A769, 1987

116. Mulroy MF: Regional anesthesia for adult outpatients. In White PF (ed): Outpatient Anesthesia. New York, Churchill Livingstone, 1990

117. Shane SM: Conscious-Sedation for Ambulatory Surgery, p 1. Baltimore, University Park Press, 1983

118. McCarthy FM, Solomon AL, Jastak JT et al: Conscious sedation: Benefits and risk. J Am Dent Assoc 109:546, 1984

119. Shane SM: Intravenous amnesia for total dentistry in one sitting. J Oral Surg 24:27, 1966

120. Bennett CR: Conscious-Sedation in Dental Practice, 2nd ed, p 12. St Louis, CV Mosby, 1978

121. McCarthy FM, Solomon AL, Jastak J et al: Conscious sedation: Benefits and risks. J Am Dental Assoc 109:46, 1984

122. Scamman FL, Klein SL, Choi WW: Conscious sedation for procedures under local or topical anesthesia. Ann Otol Rhinol Laryngol 94:21, 1985

123. Apfelbaum JL, Kallar SK, Wetchler BV: Adult and geriatric patients. In Wetchler BV (ed): Anesthesia for Ambulatory Surgery, 2nd ed, p 197. Philadelphia, JB Lippincott, 1991

124. Kallar SK, Dunwiddie WC: Conscious sedation. In Wetchler BV (ed): Outpatient Anesthesia. Probl Anesth 2:93, 1988

125. Cohen DE, Downes JJ, Raphaely RC: What difference does pulse oximetry make? Anesthesiology 68:181, 1988

126. Standards for Basic Intraoperative Monitoring. Approved by the House of Delegates, American Society of Anesthesiologists, Oct 21, 1989

127. Epstein BS: Controversies in outpatient anesthesia. In White PF (ed): Outpatient Anesthesia, p 486. New York, Churchill Livingstone, 1990

128. Cohen MM, Duncan PG, Tate RB: Does anesthesia contribute to operative mortality? JAMA 260:2859, 1988

129. Food and Drug Administration: Warning re-emphasized in midazolam labeling. FDA Drug Bull 27:5, 1986

130. Hudson RJ, Stanski DR, Burch PG: Pharmacokinetics of methohexital and thiopental in surgical patients. Anesthesiology 59:215, 1983

131. Carson IW: Recovery from anaesthesia—A review of methods for evaluation of recovery from anaesthesia. Proc R Soc Med 68:108, 1975

132. Hannington-Kiff JG: Measurement of recovery from outpatient general anaesthesia with a simple ocular test. Br Med J 3:132, 1970

133. Elliott CJR, Green R, Howells TH et al: Recovery after intravenous barbiturate anaesthesia. Lancet 1:68, 1962

134. Doneicke A, Kugler J, Laub M: Evaluation of recovery and "street-fitness" by EEG and psychodiagnostic tests after anaesthesia. Can Anaesth Soc J 14:567, 1967

135. Dundee JW: Clinical studies of induction agents. VII. A comparison of eight intravenous anaesthetics as main agents for a standard operation. Br J Anaesth 35:784, 1963

136. Lees NW, Hendry JGB: Etomidate in urological outpatient anaesthesia. Anaesthesia 32:592, 1977

137. Fragen RJ, Caldwell N: Comparison of a new formulation of etomidate with thiopental—Side effects and awakening times. Anesthesiology 50:242, 1979

138. Horrigan RW, Moyers JR, Johnson BH et al: Etomidate vs. thiopental with and without fentanyl—A comparative study of awakening in man. Anesthesiology 52:362, 1980

139. White PF, Shafer A: Clinical pharmacology and uses of injectable anesthetic and analgesic drugs. In Wetchler BV (ed): Outpatient Anesthesia. Probl Anesth 2:37, 1988

140. Giese JL, Stanley TH, Pace NL: Fentanyl pretreatment reduces side effects associated with etomidate anesthesia induction. Anesthesiology 59:A320, 1983

141. Collin RIW, Drummond GB, Spence AA: Alfentanil supplemented anaesthesia for short procedures: A double-blind study of alfentanil used with etomidate and enflurane for day cases. Anaesthesia 41:477, 1986

142. Melnick BM, Phitayakorn P, McKenzie R: Abolishing pain on injection of etomidate. Anesthesiology 66:444, 1987

143. White PF: Continuous infusions of thiopental, methohexital, or etomidate as adjuvants to nitrous oxide for outpatient anesthesia. Anesth Analg 63:282, 1984

144. Wagner RL, White PF: Etomidate inhibits adrenocortical function in surgical patients. Anesthesiology 61:647, 1984

145. White PF: Use of continuous infusion versus intermittent bolus administration of fentanyl or ketamine during outpatient anesthesia. Anesthesiology 59:294, 1983

146. Wetchler BV: For ambulatory surgery patients, use ketamine with caution. Same-Day Surg 8(1):11, 1984

147. Hannallah RS, Patel RI: Low-dose intramuscular ketamine for anesthesia pre-induction in young children undergoing brief outpatient procedure. Anesthesiology 70:598, 1989

148. Krantz EM: Low-dose intramuscular ketamine and hyaluronidase for induction of anesthesia in nonpremedicated children. S Afr Med J 58:506, 1983

149. Mackenzie N, Grant IS: Comparison of the new emulsion formulation of propofol with methohexitone and thiopentone for induction of anaesthesia in day cases. Br J Anaesth 57:725, 1985

150. Jones DF: Recovery from day-care anaesthesia—Comparison of a further four techniques including the use of the new induction agent Diprivan. Br J Anaesth 54:629, 1982

151. Doze VA, Westphal LM, White PF: Comparison of propofol with methohexital for outpatient anesthesia. Anesth Analg 65: 189, 1986

152. McCulloch MJ, Lees NW: Assessment and modification of pain on induction with propofol (Diprivan). Anaesthesia 40: 1117, 1985

153. Helbo-Hansen S, Westergaard V, Krogh BL et al: The reduction of pain on injection of propofol: The effect of addition of lignocaine. Acta Anaesthesiol Scand 32:592, 1988

154. Youngberg JA, Texitor MS, Smith DE: A comparison of induction and maintenance of anesthesia with propofol to induction with thiopental and maintenance with isoflurane. Anesth Analg 66:S191, 1987

155. Doze VA, White PF: Comparison of propofol with thiopental-isoflurane for induction and maintenance of outpatient anesthesia. Anesthesiology 65:A544, 1986

156. Johnston RG, Anderson BJ, Noseworthy TW: Diprivan versus thiopentone for outpatient surgery. Can Anaesth Soc J 33: S106, 1986

157. Henricksson BA, Carlsson P, Hallen B et al: Propofol versus thiopenton as anaesthetic agents for short operative procedures. Acta Anaesthesiol Scand 31:63, 1987

158. Dundee JW, McCollum JSC, Milligan KR et al: Thiopental and propofol as induction agents. Anesthesiology 65:A545, 1986

159. Fahy LT, van Mourik GA, Utting JE: A comparison of the induction characteristics of thiopentone and propofol. Anaesthesia 40:939, 1985

160. O'Toole DP, Milligan KR, Howe JP et al: A comparison of propofol and methohexitone as induction agents for day case isoflurane anaesthesia. Anaesthesia 42:373, 1987

161. Korttila K, Ostma P, Faure E et al: Randomized comparison of recovery after propofol—nitrous oxide versus thiopentone—isoflurane—nitrous oxide anaesthesia in patients undergoing ambulatory surgery. Acta Anaesthesiol Scand 34:400, 1990

162. Mackenzie N, Grant IS: Propofol for intravenous sedation. Anaesthesia 42:3, 1987

163. Jessop E, Grands RM, Morgan M et al: Comparison of infu-

sions of propofol and methohexitone to provide light general anesthesia during surgery with regional blockade. Br J Anaesth 57:1173, 1985

164. Marais ML, Maher MW, Wetchler BV et al: Reduced demands on recovery room resources with propofol (Diprivan) compared to thiopental–isoflurane. Anesthesiol Rev 16:29, 1989

165. Churchill-Davidson HC: Suxamenthonium chloride and muscle pains. Br Med J 1:74, 1954

166. Perry J, Wetchler BV: Outpatient anesthesia: The effects of diazepam pretreatment of succinylcholine on fasciculation and postoperative myalgia. AANA J 52:48, 1984

167. Sosis M, Broad T, Larijani GE et al: Comparison of atracurium and d-tubocurarine for prevention of succinylcholine myalgia. Anesth Analg 66:657, 1987

168. Sokoll MD, Gergis SD, Mehta M et al: Safety and efficacy of atracurium (BW33A) in surgical patients receiving balanced or isoflurane anesthesia. Anesthesiology 58:450, 1983

169. Stirt JA, Katz RL, Murray AL et al: Intubation with atracurium in man. Anesthesiology 59:A266, 1983

170. Rupp SM, McChristian JW, Miller RD: Neuromuscular effects of atracurium during halothane–nitrous oxide and enflurane–nitrous oxide anesthesia in humans. Anesthesiology 63:16, 1985

171. Rupp SM, Miller RD, Gencarelli PJ: Vecuronium-induced neuromuscular blockade during enflurane, isoflurane and halothane anesthesia in humans. Anesthesiology 60:102, 1984

172. Pearce AC, Williams JP, Jones RM: The use of atracurium for short surgical procedures in day-case patients. Anesthesiology 59:A265, 1983

173. Fragen RJ, Shanks CA: Neuromuscular recovery after laparoscopy. Anesth Analg 63:51, 1984

174. Gergis SD, Sokoll M, Mehta O et al: Intubation conditions after atracurium and suxamethonium. Br J Anaesth 55:835, 1983

175. Glass P, Wilson W, Mace J et al: Assessment of the optimal priming dose for atracurium, pancuronium and vecuronium to obtain rapid onset muscle relaxation. Anesth Analg 66:S69, 1987

176. Basta SJ, Savarese JJ, Ali HH et al: The neuromuscular pharmacology of BW B1090U in anesthetized patients. Anesthesiology 63:A318, 1985

177. Ali HH, Savarese JJ, Embree PB et al: Clinical pharmacology of BW B1090U continuous infusion. Anesthesiology 65:A282, 1986

178. Savarese JJ, Ali HH, Basta SJ et al: Clinical conditions with and without priming after fentanyl-thiopental induction. Anesthesiology 65:A283, 1986

179. Goroszeniuk T, Whitwam JG, Morgan M: Use of methohexitone, fentanyl and nitrous oxide for short surgical procedures. Anesthesiology 32:209, 1977

180. Pollard J: Clinical evaluation of intravenous vs inhalational anesthesia in the ambulatory surgical unit: A multicenter study. Curr Ther Res 36:617, 1984

181. Adams AP, Peybus DA: Delayed respiratory depression after use of fentanyl during anaesthesia. Br Med J 1:278, 1978

182. White PF, Sung ML, Doze VA: Use of sufentanil in outpatient anesthesia—Determining an optimal preinduction dose. Anesthesiology 63:A202, 1985

183. Bailey PL, Streisand JB, Pace NL et al: Sufentanil produces shorter lasting respiratory depression and longer lasting analgesia than equipotent doses of fentanyl in human volunteers. Anesthesiology 65:A493, 1986

184. Wasudev G, Kambam JR, Hazlehurst WM et al: Comparative study of sufentanil and isoflurane in outpatient surgery. Anesth Analg 66:S186, 1987

185. Zuurmond WWA, van Leeuwen L: Recovery from sufentanil anaesthesia for outpatient arthroscopy: A comparison with isoflurane. Acta Anaesthesiol Scand 31:154, 1987

186. Phitayakoran P, Melnick BM, Vicinie AF: Comparison of continuous sufentanil and fentanyl infusions for outpatient anesthesia. Can J Anaesth 34:242, 1987

187. Andrews CJH, Sinclair M, Prys-Roberts C et al: Ventilatory effects during and after continuous infusion of fentanyl or alfentanil. Br J Anaesth 55:S211, 1983

188. White PF, Coe V, Shafer A et al: Comparison of alfentanil with fentanyl for outpatient anesthesia. Anesthesiology 64:99, 1986

189. Scamman FL, Ghoneim MM, Korttila K: Ventilatory and mental effects of alfentanil and fentanyl. Acta Anaesthesiol Scand 28:63, 1984

190. Zuurmond WWA, van Leeuwen L: Alfentanil v. isoflurane for outpatient arthroscopy. Acta Anaesthesiol Scand 30:329, 1986

191. Short SM, Rutherfoord CF, Sebel PS: A comparison between isoflurane and alfentanil supplemented anaesthesia for short procedures. Anaesthesia 40:1160, 1985

192. Jellicoe JA: A comparison of alfentanil, halothane and enflurane for day-case gynaecological surgery. Anaesthesia 40:810, 1985

193. Dechene JP: Alfentanil as an adjunct to thiopentone and nitrous oxide in short surgical procedures. Can Anaesth Soc J 32:346, 1985

194. Coe V, Shafer A, White PF: Techniques for administering alfentanil during outpatient anesthesia—A comparison with fentanyl. Anesthesiology 59:A347, 1983

195. Kallar SK, Keenan RL: Evaluation and comparison of recovery time from alfentanil and fentanyl for short surgical procedures. Anesthesiology 61:A379, 1984

196. Zelcer J, Tyres M, White PF et al: Comparison of alfentanil and fentanyl as adjuvants to propofol and nitrous oxide anesthesia. Anesthesiology 71:A28, 1989

197. Bartkowski RR, Larijani GE, Goldberg ME et al: Erythromycin treatment inhibits alfentanil metabolism. Anesthesiology 69:A590, 1988

198. Fine J, Finestone SC: A comparative study of the side-effects of butorphanol, nalbuphine and fentanyl. Anesthesiol Rev 8:13, 1981

199. Pandit SK, Kothary SP, Pandit UA et al: Comparison of fentanyl and butorphanol for outpatient anaesthesia. Can J Anaesth 34:130, 1987

200. Wetchler BV, Alexander CD, Shariff MS et al: A comparison of recovery in patients receiving fentanyl vs those receiving butorphanol. J Clin Anesth 1:339, 1989

201. Chu G, Cool M, Wetchler BV: Transnasal butorphanol following ambulatory surgical procedures: A pilot study (abstr). Presented at a meeting of the Joint American and Canadian Pain Society, Toronto, 1988

202. Garfield JM, Garfield FB, Philip B et al: A comparison of clinical and psychologic effects of fentanyl and nalbuphine in ambulatory surgical patients. Anesth Analg 66:1303, 1987

203. Berggren L, Eriksson I: Midazolam for induction of anaesthesia in outpatients—A comparison with thiopentone. Acta Anaesthesiol Scand 25:492, 1981

204. Verma R, Ramasubramanian R, Sachar RM: Anesthesia for termination of pregnancy: Midazolam compared with methohexital. Anesth Analg 64:792, 1985

205. Forster A, Gardaz JP, Suter PM et al: I.V. midazolam as an induction agent for anaesthesia: A study in volunteers. Br J Anaesth 52:907, 1980

206. Crawford ME, Andersen CP, Mikkelson BO: Comparison between midazolam and thiopentone-based balanced anaesthesia for day-case surgery. Br J Anaesth 56:165, 1984

207. Fragen RJ, Caldwell NJ: Awakening characteristics following anesthesia induction with midazolam for short surgical procedures. Arzneim Forsch 31:2261, 1981

208. Fragen RJ: The uses of midazolam. Anesthesiol Rev 12:29, 1986

209. Alon E, Baitella L, Hossli G: Double-blind study of the reversal of midazolam-supplemented general anaesthesia with Ro15-1788. Br J Anaesth 59:455, 1987

210. Andrews PJD, Wright DJ, Lamont MC: Flumazenil in the outpatient. Anaesthesia 45:458, 1990

211. Apfelbaum JL: Inhalational agents in anesthesia for ambulatory surgery. In Wetchler BV (ed): Outpatient Anesthesia. Probl Anesth 2:55, 1988

212. Saidman LJ, Eger EI II: Effect of nitrous oxide and of narcotic premedication on the alveolar concentration of halothane required for anesthesia. Anesthesiology 25:302, 1964

213. Bahlman SH, Eger EI II, Smith NT et al: The cardiovascular

effects of nitrous oxide-halothane anesthesia in man. Anesthesiology 35:274, 1971

214. Smith NT, Calverley RK, Prys-Roberts C et al: Impact of nitrous oxide on the circulation during enflurane anesthesia in man. Anesthesiology 48:345, 1978

215. Dolan WM, Stevens WC, Eger EI II et al: The cardiovascular and respiratory effects of isoflurane-nitrous oxide anesthesia. Can Anaesth Soc J 21:557, 1974

216. Alexander GD, Skupski JN, Brown EM: The role of nitrous oxide in postoperative nausea and vomiting. Anesth Analg 63:175, 1984

217. Lonie DS, Harper NJN: Nitrous oxide anaesthesia and vomiting. Anaesthesia 41:703, 1986

218. Sengupta P, Plantevin OM: Nitrous oxide and day-case laparoscopy: Effects on nausea, vomiting and return to normal activity. Br J Anaesth 60:570, 1988

219. Hovorka J, Korttila K, Erkola O: Nitrous oxide does not increase nausea and vomiting following gynaecological laparoscopy. Can J Anaesth 36:145, 1989

220. Hannallah RS: Pediatric outpatient anesthesia. Urol Clin North Am 14:51, 1987

221. Fisher DM, Robinson S, Brett CM et al: Comparison of enflurane, halothane and isoflurane for diagnostic and therapeutic procedures in children with malignancies. Anesthesiology 63:647, 1985

222. Kingston HGG: Halothane and isoflurane anesthesia in pediatric outpatients. Anesth Analg 65:181, 1986

223. McAteer PM, Carter JA, Cooper GM et al: Comparison of isoflurane and halothane in outpatient paediatric dental anaesthesia. Br J Anaesth 58:390, 1986

224. Jones HD, McLaren AB: Postoperative shivering and hypoxaemia after halothane, nitrous oxide, oxygen anaesthesia. Br J Anaesth 37:35, 1965

225. Tyrell MF, Feldman S: Headache following halothane anaesthesia. Br J Anaesth 40:99, 1968

226. Miller JR, Redish CH, Fisch C et al: Factors in arrhythmia during dental outpatient general anesthesia. Anesth Analg 49:701, 1970

227. Ryder W, Wright PA: Halothane and enflurane in dental anaesthesia. Anaesthesia 36:492, 1981

228. Johnston RR, Eger EI II, Wilson C: A comparative interaction of epinephrine with enflurane, isoflurane, and halothane in man. Anesth Analg 55:709, 1976

229. Sigurdsson GH, Lindahl S: Cardiac arrhythmias in intubated children during adenoidectomy. A comparison between enflurane and halothane anesthesia. Acta Anaesthesiol Scand 27:484, 1983

230. Stanford BJ, Plantevin OM, Gilbert JR: Morbidity after day-case gynaecological surgery—Comparison of enflurane with halothane. Br J Anaesth 51:1143, 1979

231. Kreienbuhl G: Subjektive Beschwerden nach Halothan- und nach Enfluraneanaesthesie bei ambulanten (tagesklinik-) Patienten. Anaesthetist 27:533, 1978

232. Tracey JA, Holland AJC, Unger L: Morbidity in minor gynaecological surgery: A comparison of halothane, enflurane and isoflurane. Br J Anaesth 54:1213, 1982

233. Storms LH, Stark AH, Calverley RK et al: Psychological functioning after halothane or enflurane anesthesia. Anesth Analg 59:245, 1980

234. Melnick BM, Chalasani J, Hy NTL: Comparison of enflurane, isoflurane and continuous fentanyl infusion for outpatient anesthesia. Anesthesiol Rev 11:36, 1984

235. Padfield A: Recovery comparison between enflurane and halothane technique. A study of outpatients undergoing cystoscopy. Anaesthesia 35:508, 1980

236. Azar I, Karambelkar DJ, Lear E: Neurologic state and psychomotor function following anesthesia for ambulatory surgery. Anesthesiology 60:347, 1984

237. Miller RD, Eger EI II, Way WL et al: Comparative neuromuscular effects of forane and halothane alone and in combination with d-tubocurarine in man. Anesthesiology 35:38, 1971

238. Rupp SM, Fahey MR, Miller RD: Neuromuscular and cardiovascular effects of atracurium during nitrous oxide–fentanyl and nitrous oxide–isoflurane anaesthesia. Br J Anaesth 55:67S, 1983

239. Rupp SM, Miller RD, Gencarelli PJ: Vecuronium-induced neuromuscular blockade during enflurane, isoflurane, and halothane anesthesia in humans. Anesthesiology 60:102, 1984

240. Homi J, Konchigeri HN, Eckenhoff JE: A new anesthetic agent—Forane: Preliminary observation in man. Anesth Analg 41:439, 1972

241. Buffington CW: Clinical evaluation of isoflurane. Reflex actions during isoflurane anesthesia. Can Anaesth Soc J 29:S35, 1982

242. Rising S, Dodgson MS, Steen PA: Isoflurane v fentanyl for out-patient laparoscopy. Acta Anaesthesiol Scand 29:251, 1985

243. Korttila K, Valanne J: Recovery after outpatient isoflurane and enflurane anesthesia. Anesth Analg 64:239, 1985

244. Carter JA, Dye AM, Cooper GM: Recovery from day-case anaesthesia. The effect of different inhalational agents. Anaesthesia 40:545, 1985

245. Battito MF, Langner R, Bradley EL: Desflurane and alfentanil in surgical outpatients: Comparative hemodynamics, emergence and recovery. Anesth Analg 72:S14, 1991

246. Fletcher JE, Sebel PS, Murphy MR et al: Psychomotor recovery after desflurane in outpatients. Anesth Analg 72:S78, 1991

247. Lichtor JL, Apfelbaum JL, Lane B et al: Long-term recovery: Desflurane vs propofol. Anesth Analg 72:S163, 1991

248. Faculty expert explains steps to low hospital admission rates. Same-Day Surg 6:136, 1982

249. Caldamone AA, Rabinowitz R: Outpatient orchiopexy. J Urol 127:286, 1982

250. Aldrete JA: Are intramuscular injections obsolete in the recovery room? Curr Rev Recovery Room Nurses 5:147, 1983

251. Soni V, Burney R: Anesthetic techniques for laparoscopic tubal ligation. Anesthesia 55:A145, 1981

252. Rooney ME, Code WE: Can the NSAID naproxen reduce postoperative pain in laparoscopic tubal ligation? Anesth Analg 72:S227, 1991

253. O'Hara DA, Fragen RJ, Kinzer M et al: Ketorolac tromethamine as compared with morphine sulphate for treatment of postoperative pain. Clin Pharmacol Ther 41:556, 1987

254. Yee JP, Koshiver JE, Allbon C et al: Comparison of intramuscular ketorolac tromethamine and morphine sulphate for analgesia of pain after major surgery. Pharmacotherapy 6:253, 1986

255. Brown CR, Moodie JE, Dickie G et al: Analgesic efficacy and safety of single-dose oral and intramuscular ketorolac tromethamine for postoperative pain. Pharmacotherapy 10:59, 1990

256. Wetchler BV: Managing pain in the postanesthesia care unit. J Postanesth Nurs 1:52, 1986

257. Shandling B, Steward D: Regional analgesia for post-operative pain in pediatric outpatient surgery. J Pediatr Surg 15:477, 1980

258. Yoon F: Fallope ring offers safety, limited tubal damage. Same-Day Surg 4:85, 1980

259. Burnhill MS: Pitfalls of the fallope ring. Same-Day Surg 4:86, 1980

260. Thompson RE, Wetchler BV, Alexander CD: Infiltration of the mesosalpinx for pain relief after laparoscopic tubal sterilization with Yoon rings. J Reprod Med 32:537, 1987

261. Alexander CD, Wetchler BV, Thompson RE: Bupivacaine infiltration of the mesosalpinx in ambulatory surgical laparoscopic tubal sterilization. Can J Anaesth 34:362, 1987

262. McGlinchey J, McLean P, Walsh A: Day case penile surgery with penile block for postoperative pain relief. Ir Med J 76:319, 1983

263. Tree-trakarn T, Pirayavaraporn S: Postoperative pain relief for circumcision in children: Comparison among morphine, nerve block, and topical analgesia. Anesthesiology 62:519, 1985

264. Elder PT, Belman AB, Hannallah RS et al: Postcircumcision pain—A prospective evaluation of subcutaneous ring block of the penis. Reg Anaesth 9:48, 1984

265. Hannallah RS, Broadman LM, Belman AB et al: Control of post-orchidopexy pain in pediatric outpatients: Comparison of two regional techniques. Anesthesiology 61:A429, 1984

266. Takasaki M, Dohi S, Kawahata Y et al: Dosage of lidocaine for caudal anesthesia in infants and children. Anesthesiology 47:527, 1977

267. Broadman LM, Hannallah RS, Norrie WC et al: Caudal analgesia in pediatric outpatient surgery: A comparison of three different bupivacaine concentrations. Anesth Analg 66:S19, 1987

268. Wolf AR, Valley RD, Fear DW et al: Bupivacaine for caudal analgesia in infants and children: The optimum concentration. Anesthesiology 69:102, 1988

269. Broadman LM, Hannallah RS, Norden JM et al: Kiddie caudals: Experience with 1,154 consecutive cases without complications. Anesth Analg 66:S18, 1987

270. Lunn JW: Post-operative analgesia after circumcision. Anaesthesia 34:552, 1979

271. Bramwell RGB, Bullen C, Radford P: Caudal block for postoperative analgesia in children. Anaesthesia 37:1024, 1982

272. May AE, Wandless J, James RH: Analgesia for circumcision in children. Acta Anaesthesiol Scand 26:331, 1982

273. Yeoman PM, Cooke R, Hain WR: Penile block for circumcision. Anaesthesia 38:862, 1983

274. Vater M, Wandless J: Caudal or dorsal nerve block? A comparison of two local anaesthetics for postoperative analgesia following day case circumcision. Acta Anaesthesiol Scand 29:175, 1985

275. Markham SJ, Tomlinson J, Hain WR: Ilioinguinal nerve block in children: A comparison with caudal block for intra- and postoperative analgesia. Anaesthesia 41:1098, 1986

276. Hannallah RS, Epstein BS: The pediatric patient. In Wetchler BV (ed): Anesthesia for Ambulatory Surgery, 2nd ed, p 131. Philadelphia, JB Lippincott, 1991

277. Patel RI, Hannallah RS, Murphy LS et al: Pediatric outpatient anesthesia—A review of post-anesthetic complications in 8,995 cases. Anesthesiology 65:A435, 1986

278. Lindblad T, Beattie WS, Buckley DN et al: Increased incidence of postoperative nausea and vomiting in menstruating women. Can J Anaesth 36:S78, 1989

279. Pataky AO, Kitz DS, Andrews RS et al: Nausea and vomiting following ambulatory surgery: Are all procedures created equal? Anesth Analg 67:S163, 1988

280. Metter SE, Kitz DS, Young ML et al: Nausea and vomiting after outpatient laparoscopy: Incidence impact on recovery room stay and cost. Anesth Analg 66:S116, 1987

281. Anderson R, Crohg K: Pain as a major cause of postoperative nausea. Can Anaesth Soc J 23:366, 1976

282. Dundee JW, Chestnutt WN, Ghaly RG et al: Traditional Chinese acupuncture: A potentially useful antiemetic. Br Med J 293:583, 1986

283. Wheaton NE: Comparison of benzquinamide hydrochloride and droperidol in preventing postoperative nausea and vomiting following general outpatient anesthesia. AANA J 53:322, 1985

284. McKenzie R, Wadhwa RK, Uy NTL et al: Antiemetic effectiveness of intramuscular hydroxyzine compared with intramuscular droperidol. Anesth Analg 60:783, 1981

285. Wetchler BV, Collins IS, Jacob L: Antiemetic effects of droperidol on the ambulatory surgery patient. Anesth Rev 9:23, 1982

286. Valanne J, Korttila K: Effect of a small dose of droperidol on nausea, vomiting and recovery after outpatient enflurane anaesthesia. Acta Anaesthesiol Scand 29:359, 1985

287. Pandit SK, Kothary SP, Pandit UA et al: Dose-response study of droperidol and metoclopramide as antiemetics for outpatient anesthesia. Anesth Analg 68:798, 1989

288. Rao TLK, Madhavareddy S, Chinthagada M et al: Metoclopramide and cimetidine to reduce gastric fluid pH and volume. Anesth Analg 63:1014, 1984

289. Abramowitz MD, Oh TH, Epstein BS et al: The antiemetic effect of droperidol following outpatient strabismus surgery in children. Anesthesiology 59:579, 1983

290. Abramowitz MD, Epstein BS, Friendly DS et al: The effect of droperidol in reducing vomiting in pediatric strabismic outpatient surgery. Anesthesiology 55:A329, 1981

291. Lerman J, Eustis S, Smith DR: Effect of droperidol pretreatment on postanesthetic vomiting in children undergoing strabismus surgery. Anesthesiology 65:322, 1986

292. Hardy JF, Charest J, Girouard G et al: Nausea and vomiting after strabismus surgery in preschool children. Can Anaesth Soc J 33:57, 1986

293. Brown RE, James DJ, Weaver RG et al: Low-dose droperidol vs. standard-dose droperidol for prevention of vomiting after pediatric strabismus surgery. Anesth Analg 70:S37, 1990

294. Jackson SH, Schmidt MN, McGuire J et al: Transdermal scopolamine as a preanesthetic drug and postoperative antinauseant and antiemetic. Anesthesiology 57:A330, 1982

295. Gibbons PA, Nicolson SC, Betts EK et al: Scopolamine does not prevent post-operative emesis after pediatric eye surgery. Anesthesiology 61:A435, 1984

296. Reed WA: Recovery from anesthesia and discharge. In Shultz R (ed): Outpatient Surgery, p 45. Philadelphia, Lea & Febiger, 1979

297. Wetchler BV: Problem solving in the postanesthesia care unit. In Wetchler BV (ed): Anesthesia for Ambulatory Surgery, 2nd ed, p 375. Philadelphia, JB Lippincott, 1991

298. Chung F, Ong D, Seyone C et al: A new postanesthetic discharge scoring system for ambulatory surgery. Anesth Analg 72:S42, 1991

299. Daos FG, Virtue RW: Sympathetic block persistence after spinal or epidural analgesia. JAMA 183:285, 1963

300. Pflug AE, Aasheim GM, Foster C: Sequence of return of neurological function and criteria for safe ambulation following subarachnoid block (spinal anaesthetic). Can Anaesth Soc J 25:133, 1978

301. Roe CF, Cohn FL: Sympathetic blockade during spinal anesthesia. Surg Gynecol Obstet 136:265, 1973

302. Ogg TW: An assessment of post-operative outpatient cases. Br Med J 4:573, 1972

303. Blackwell B: Treatment adherence. Br J Psychiatry 129:510, 1976

51

Lawrence L. Priano

Trauma and Burns

The prominence of trauma as a major health hazard cannot be argued. Trauma is the leading cause of death in the United States in people 38 years of age and younger.[1,2] Because most trauma occurs during the victims' peak productivity years, it is the leading cause of lost years of life and lost income to families.[1,2] Approximately 175,000 people die from trauma annually in the United States, and for every death there are two permanent disabilities.[1,2] Since 1960, while deaths from cancer, heart disease, and stroke have decreased, deaths from trauma have increased.[2,3]

Death following an accident usually occurs during one of three periods. Fifty percent of deaths from trauma are classified as "immediate"; they occur at the scene and generally are not preventable. Causes of immediate death include lacerations of the brain, brain stem, spinal cord, heart, and great vessels. Thirty percent of trauma deaths are classified as "early" and occur within 3 hours of the accident. Causes of death in this period include expanding intracranial masses, exsanguination, and hypoxia secondary to airway obstruction, tension pneumothorax, and the like. The 20% of trauma deaths classified as "late" occur days to weeks after injury and result primarily from sepsis and multiple organ failure. The organ systems most commonly involved are the renal, pulmonary, and coagulation systems.[3]

Improved prehospital care of the trauma victim has contributed to a reduction in mortality.[4] Paramedical personnel are trained to establish an airway, ventilate the patient's lungs, and perform a number of other life-saving measures at the scene of an accident.[5,6] The efficacy of such intervention has been debated, with some people advocating a "scoop and run" approach and others advocating a delay in transport until the patient has been stabilized in the field. For critically ill trauma victims, endotracheal intubation, vigorous fluid resuscitation, immobilization of the spine, and rapid transport by paramedics have proved effective.[7] The military antishock trousers, favored by some emergency personnel, probably are helpful only in tamponading wounds, stabilizing long bone or pelvic fractures, and preventing hypotension secondary to vasodilation with spinal cord injury.[3,8]

Expedient transport of a trauma victim directly to a regional trauma center rather than to the nearest hospital results in improved outcome for the victim.[9] A trauma center is most simply defined as an institution that has made a commitment of personnel and facilities to the care of trauma victims. Functionally, this involves the in-house, immediate availability of trauma surgeons, anesthesiologists, emergency room (ER), operating room (OR), and critical care (ICU) nurses, as well as the availability of ER, OR, and ICU beds, diagnostic x-ray facilities, and blood bank support at all times. The specifics of acceptable variations in the availability of such personnel and facilities have been spelled out by the American College of Surgeons Committee on Trauma.[10]

Proper care of the trauma victim at the hospital requires detailed, advanced planning, an orderly protocol, and efficiency. A team of physicians, nurses, and support personnel must be capable of rapid mobilization, and each member of the team should have preassigned duties that are performed under the direction of a team leader. In addition, the radiology department must have portable equipment and personnel who are immediately available for the ER, and a computed tomography (CT) scanner available. A stat laboratory must be ready for determination of a complete blood count, coagulation screen, blood gas analysis, serum electrolytes and toxicologies. The blood bank must be well supplied and capable of supplying large quantities of blood products quickly. Finally, the anesthesiologist must have available, prepared, and checked-out an assortment of supplies and equipment for the ER and OR (Tables 51-1 and 51-2).

INITIAL ASSESSMENT AND MANAGEMENT OF THE TRAUMA PATIENT

The anesthesiologist can play a major role in assessing the trauma victim and therefore should be knowledgeable about acute trauma and how it may affect perioperative management. Many anesthesiologists have become certified in Advanced Trauma Life Support (ATLS), a course developed by the Committee on Trauma of the American College of Surgeons.[11] Although some of the principles taught may be controversial, the course presents a highly organized and practical approach to the diagnosis and management of trauma.

Ideally, the first notification of the impending arrival of a trauma victim should include information on the patient's circulatory, ventilatory, and neurologic function. Some centers use a trauma score to periodically quantify the patient's

TABLE 51-1. Suggested Anesthesia Supplies for the Trauma Emergency Room

1. Laryngoscopes with assorted adult and pediatric size blades
2. Assorted face masks
3. Assorted endotracheal tubes and stylets
4. Oral and nasal airways
5. Suction, with a rigid, large-orifice tip
6. A source of 100% oxygen
7. A means of providing positive pressure ventilation with 100% oxygen, such as with a self-inflating resuscitation bag with a tail or an Ayre's T-piece circuit with a Jackson-Rees modification
8. A large needle, catheter, and knife for emergency cricothyrotomy
9. Succinylcholine, vecuronium, pancuronium, thiopental, etomidate
10. Assorted catheters and cutdown equipment for establishment of large-bore intravenous access
11. Prewarmed bags of crystalloid solutions
12. Pressurized intravenous infusion devices
13. Monitor and transducer for arterial pressure measurements
14. Electrocardiographic capability

status.[12] The neurologic portion of this score is based on the Glasgow Coma Scale, which examines eye opening and verbal and motor functions (see Table 32-14). A high score indicates a good condition, whereas a low score signals a poor condition and possible poor outcome.

Upon the patient's arrival, the airway, breathing, circulation, and neurologic status must be quickly assessed. This initial assessment can be done in less than a minute. A first step is to ask the patient to take a deep breath. If no breath is taken, ventilate the patient's lungs and prepare to secure the airway with an endotracheal tube. Simultaneously, palpate a radial pulse for fullness and rate, and determine the blood pressure as soon as possible. A conscious, normotensive, moving patient without stridor, tachypnea, tachycardia, or neck pain is temporarily stable, and a slower, more thorough diagnostic approach may be undertaken.

TABLE 51-2. Suggested Anesthesia Supplies and Equipment for the Trauma Operating Room

1. Airway equipment as detailed in items 1 through 7 in Table 51-1
2. Properly checked out anesthesia machine with tubing and rebreathing bag attached
3. A mechanical ventilator, capable of delivering PEEP and tidal volume at high inspiratory pressures, preset to normal adult values (e.g., $V_T = 800$ ml, F = 10 breaths·min^{-1})
4. Heated humidifier
5. Warming blanket
6. Primed blood infusion sets routed through fluid warmers
7. Pressurized fluid and blood infusion devices
8. Physiologic monitor with transducers attached, filled, and calibrated (infection potential is small[107])
9. Prefilled and labeled syringes of drugs for induction and intubation
10. Defibrillator and resuscitation drugs in the room
11. Extra supplies (catheters, tubing, etc.)
12. Supplies for placement of arterial, central venous, and pulmonary artery catheters
13. Capability of increasing the OR temperature

Airway Injuries

All trauma victims must be considered to have a full stomach and to be at high risk for vomiting and aspiration. In an unconscious but spontaneously breathing patient with a patent airway, it is probably wise to take time to obtain a radiograph of the cervical spine to rule out a fracture before proceeding with tracheal intubation. If the patient is not ventilating adequately, the clinician must establish an airway and ventilate the lungs prior to obtaining a radiograph of the neck.

Early endotracheal intubation has been a major factor in reducing mortality from trauma. Indications for intubation of the trachea include protection of the airway, airway obstruction, positive pressure ventilation, tracheal toilet, coma, and shock. If a patient is semiconscious, combative, or uncontrollable, skeletal muscle paralysis and tracheal intubation may be necessary to facilitate diagnosis and/or treatment (i.e., to obtain a head CT scan to assess CNS injury).

When performing oral tracheal intubation, an assistant should apply axial head and neck traction, being careful to leave the neck in a neutral position. The intubation should be done in rapid sequence fashion. That is, after preoxygenation, muscle paralysis, and application of cricoid pressure, an endotracheal tube (with a stylet inserted) should be placed under direct vision. Nasotracheal intubation is rarely indicated in the acute management of an unconscious trauma patient. Blind attempts are particularly dangerous in an unconscious patient because of the risk of vomiting from stimulation of the gag reflex. Tubes placed through the nose may also penetrate the brain in patients with certain skull or facial fractures.[13-15] Administration of muscle relaxants for tracheal intubation should only be done by those skilled in bag and mask ventilation of the lungs, in the unusual event that intubation of the trachea cannot be accomplished. Rarely, needle or surgical cricothyroidotomy may be necessary. The administration of sedative-hypnotic drugs prior to tracheal intubation should be reserved for patients who are awake and hemodynamically stable, or for some patients with elevated intracranial pressure (ICP).

Initial management of the airway depends on the clinical situation at hand. In some situations endotracheal intubation is contraindicated or not possible—for example, in patients with massive facial trauma and laryngeal or tracheal trauma. If external tracheal or laryngeal damage is not obvious, it should be suspected if hoarseness, stridor, dysphagia, subcutaneous emphysema, or dyspnea in the recumbent position are present.[16,17] Alternative methods for airway management, other than direct oral tracheal intubation, include blind oral intubation, use of a flexible fiberoptic bronchoscope, use of a catheter guide placed retrograde through the larynx, jet ventilation by way of a cricothyroid catheter, and tracheostomy.[18] The use of an esophageal obturator airway should be discouraged. Complications of the device include accidental tracheal intubation, esophageal perforation, an inability to provide adequate ventilation, difficulty in performing tracheal intubation around the esophageal tube, and a nearly 100% prevalence of emesis on removal of the tube.

Cervical Spine and Neck Injuries

Injury to the cervical spinal cord should be suspected when one observes flaccidity (especially of the rectal sphincter), diaphragmatic breathing, priapism, or hypotension with a

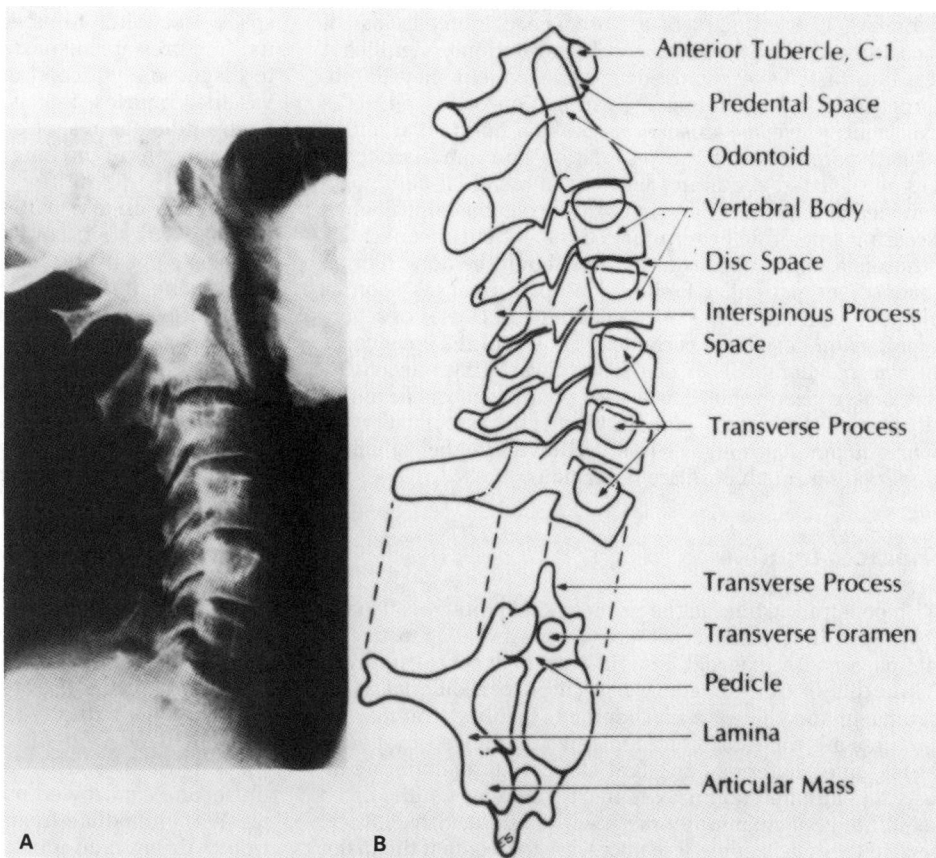

Figure 51-1. (*A*) Lateral radiograph of the cervical spine. (*B*) Diagram: anatomy of the spine, lateral and superior view. (Reprinted with permission from Blaisdell FW, Trunkey DD: Cervicothoracic Trauma. Trauma Management Series, Vol III. New York, Thieme Medical Publishers, 1985.)

A   B

Labels on diagram:
- Anterior Tubercle, C-1
- Predental Space
- Odontoid
- Vertebral Body
- Disc Space
- Interspinous Process Space
- Transverse Process
- Transverse Process
- Transverse Foramen
- Pedicle
- Lamina
- Articular Mass

slow pulse and warm extremities. Complete evaluation of the cervical spine may require CT and/or multiple radiographs, including flexion-extension films. However, a lateral view of the cervical spine is quick and reveals most unstable fractures (Fig. 51-1). All seven cervical vertebrae must be seen, as C-7 is the most common site of injury.[19] An excellent review of cervical anatomy and its impact on airway management in health and disease is definitely suggested reading.[20] The cervical spine should be lordotic in attitude. Kyphosis is indicative of spasm and should raise suspicion of injury. Prevertebral soft tissues should be less than 7 mm at C3 and less than 20 mm at C5. These tissue thicknesses cannot be evaluated with nasogastric or nasotracheal tubes in place. The disk interspaces should be similar at all levels, and narrowing should raise suspicion of an injury. The clinician should check for vertical alignment along the pre- and postvertebral and spinolaminar lines. Although a single normal lateral radiograph does not "clear" the neck, given a careful approach it makes neck injury from tracheal intubation very unlikely. Lack of neck pain and an ability to move all extremities also make a cervical spine injury unlikely, although not ruled out. Evaluation for a cervical spine injury is more complicated in patients with altered levels of consciousness who cannot be easily assessed, such as those with head injury or acute intoxication. Adequate neck evaluation must be delayed until the patient is alert or additional radiologic studies have been performed. In the continuing care of a trauma patient, it is often necessary to perform semielective operative procedures within several days of the original accident. By that time the status of the cervical spine should be known and recorded in the chart unless there is good medical reason

for not completing the evaluation (e.g., continued critical status and altered levels of consciousness). Until complete "clearance" is obtained, a rigid collar should be left in place.

The patient should also be evaluated for trauma to the anterior neck, because a number of structures can be damaged.[21] Blunt or penetrating trauma to the anterior neck can lead to a high likelihood for damage. In order of decreasing frequency, the structures most often injured are the veins, arteries, larynx and trachea, pharynx and esophagus, brachial plexus, cranial nerves, and the spinal cord.[22] Arterial hemorrhage in the neck can produce rapid and severe airway obstruction necessitating immediate tracheal intubation and/or decompression of the hematoma. Cervical subcutaneous air, pneumothorax, and pneumomediastinum can result from tracheal or laryngeal injury, whereas dysphagia is more common with pharyngeal and esophageal trauma. If airway damage or a hematoma is compromising the airway, it may be advisable not to paralyze the patient with muscle relaxants prior to securing the airway. Neither tracheal intubation nor mask ventilation may be possible under such circumstances. It is safer to leave the patient with the muscle power to breathe until the airway is secured.

Head Injuries

Brain damage resulting from a head injury is a common cause of mortality and morbidity. With early institution of ventilation, restoration of cerebral perfusion, and reduction of an elevated ICP, the outcome is much more favorable. The hallmark of a closed head injury is loss of consciousness. With severe scalp lacerations, significant bleeding may have occurred and the patient may be obtunded due to hypovolemia. Examination of the pupils is important; however, anisocoria can be a normal variant in a small percentage of the population and can also occur with an isolated eye injury without intracranial pathology. Knowledge of the mechanism of injury can be helpful when assessing a possible head injury. If the patient is conscious, a thorough neurologic examination should be done. For an unconscious patient, CT should be performed as soon as adequate ventilation has been ensured and causes of severe hypotension have been corrected. Time is of the essence, as intracranial hemorrhage can have devastating effects. Severe closed head injury has a very poor prognosis in multiple trauma patients.[23] Hyperglycemia is associated with poor outcome, although it is not known whether attempts to reduce serum glucose are efficacious.[24]

Thoracic Injuries

With penetrating trauma the primary site of injury is usually obvious. Blunt trauma presents a greater diagnostic dilemma because external examination may reveal nothing. While this is true for all injuries, it is particularly so for trauma to the thorax and abdomen. In blunt trauma, rib fractures are the most common injury, followed by hemothorax, pneumothorax, and flail chest. With penetrating injury, a hemopneumothorax is most common, with isolated hemothorax or pneumothorax seen less frequently.[25]

With thoracic trauma it is necessary to decide if the major injury involves the lungs, the cardiovascular system, or both. Because the majority of intrathoracic volume is air, it is not surprising that a high percentage of chest injuries can be treated conservatively with a tube thoracostomy and observation. If treating only a pneumothorax, a 26–32 French tube is adequate. For a hemothorax or hemopneumothorax, a larger (30–40 French) tube should be placed. In either case, the tube should be placed in the fourth or fifth interspace in the midaxillary line and directed posteriorly. The tubes should be placed to -15 to -20 cm H_2O suction until there has been no leak and/or less than 100 ml blood evacuated for 24 hours. If 1000 ml of blood is obtained after initial chest tube placement, or if bleeding exceeds 1500 ml in 24 hours, surgical exploration is indicated.

A severe chest injury, penetrating or blunt, is the primary cause of death in approximately 50% of trauma victims who die. In those patients who die, the most common findings are rib fractures, hemothorax, lung lacerations, and great vessel rupture. There is a lower incidence of lung contusion, lacerated diaphragm, or tracheal and myocardial injury. Signs that frequently correlate with severe pulmonary or vascular injuries include fracture of the first or second ribs (15–20% incidence of vascular injury), a widened mediastinum (33% incidence of vascular injury), flail chest (almost 100% incidence of lung contusion), and massive hemothorax (surgical bleeding requiring immediate thoracotomy). Although the injury may appear to be limited to the thorax, if it is below the sixth rib the major pathology is most likely intra-abdominal.[26]

Chest radiography is an essential diagnostic tool for thoracic trauma. An upright inspiratory film is preferred (although expiratory films also show pneumothorax) because there is better overall contrast between structures. More common is an anteroposterior supine film, but significant pneumothoraces can be missed. Cross-table lateral radiographs may be used to help find free fluid in the pleural space. Decubitus films are contraindicated if pelvic or spinal fractures are suspected. Angiography may be necessary to diagnose a widened mediastinum or clinically apparent vascular injuries, that is, a pulseless arm. Angiography is contraindicated if shock or expanding head injuries coexist.

Contusions of the lung are not uncommon and are usually associated with multiple rib fractures, with or without flail chest. The injury pattern results from high-force blunt trauma with subsequent hemorrhage into lung tissue. Changes appear on radiographs within the first few hours. Thus, if the initial chest radiograph is clear and a new radiopacity appears late, it is most likely aspiration pneumonitis, atelectasis, or pneumonia. The most life-threatening aspect of a lung contusion is severe hypoxia. Ventilation and oxygenation need to be supported mechanically with high FIO_2 and PEEP, if necessary. A pulmonary artery catheter may be needed to assist the caregivers in optimizing tissue oxygenation and oxygen transport. Chest tubes are also often necessary either therapeutically or prophylactically. Contusions usually begin to resolve in 2–5 days if other pulmonary complications are not superimposed.[27]

Direct cardiac trauma can be either blunt or penetrating. With the exception of high-force missiles, penetrating trauma to the heart usually has a better prognosis than blunt trauma, as there is less tissue damage. The three most common cardiac injuries are tamponade, contusion, and rupture. Patients with myocardial tamponade may have hypotension, neck vein distention, and muffled heart sounds (Beck's triad), and, in addition, tachycardia, paradoxical pulse, and a narrowed pulse pressure. If the patient is hypotensive, immediate treatment should consist of fluids, inotropic drugs, and open surgical drainage. Patients with myocardial contusions can develop cardiac dysrhythmias and angina pectoris that do not respond to nitrates. The diagnosis may be difficult to establish. Any patient with a suspected myocardial contusion and abnormal ventricular function and who is unstable should probably be managed with a pulmonary artery catheter. Myocardial ruptures usually result in death at the scene, although isolated knife injuries have a better prognosis.

Aortic injuries are rare, yet it is important to have a high index of suspicion for this injury when other associated conditions exist, that is, sternal, clavicular, and upper rib fractures; a rightward-shifted trachea or blunting of the aortic knob; or head, cervical, or thoracic spine trauma. The ultimate diagnostic tool is arch aortography, although a high percentage of studies for widened mediastinum will not show arterial injury. In the monitoring of patients with suspected aortic injuries, radial artery cannulation should be performed on the right side, as the survivable injuries are usually distal to the left subclavian artery.

Abdominal Injuries

Injury to organs in the peritoneal cavity can be difficult to diagnose when the patient has sustained blunt trauma. The most common injuries are splenic rupture or laceration of the liver, resulting in significant hemorrhage. Bowel perforation can occur with blunt or penetrating injuries. Because radiographs of the abdomen are unreliable, the diagnosis of intra-abdominal hemorrhage is done with peritoneal lavage or CT.[28,29]

Urinary and pelvic injuries can be difficult to evaluate. If there is bleeding from the urethra, a retrograde urethrogram is indicated before a bladder catheter is inserted. Continued hematuria after the catheter has been inserted indicates a possible bladder injury and the need for a cystogram or intravenous pyelogram. Pelvic fractures are present in 10–12% of patients who have sustained blunt torso injury. The mortality rate in this set of circumstances is 20–30%, owing to hemorrhage.[30]

Traumatic injuries to abdominal vessels (aorta, vena cava, portal vein) are unusual. However, abdominal aortic injuries carry a 50% mortality. Abdominal vascular injuries result primarily from gunshot and stab wounds and less often follow blunt trauma.[27] They are detected by deterioration of vital signs, by positive peritoneal lavage, or at laparotomy. Peritoneal lavage is considered by some to be too sensitive, giving false positive results. In addition, it is not organ specific, does not evaluate the retroperitoneum, and is probably contraindicated in patients who have undergone prior abdominal surgery.[29] However, it does have a place in unstable patients, in whom rapid diagnosis of a hemorrhagic abdominal injury may be preferred.[31]

Extremity Injuries

Perhaps the most important aspect of evaluation of the injured extremity is to realize that significant hemorrhage (1000–1500 ml of blood) can occur and not be obvious. This is particularly true with proximal leg injuries. The clinician should pay attention to distal pulses, visual symmetry of two extremities, and distention or tightness of the skin, especially in the thigh areas after femur fractures. Early immobilization of obvious fractures is indicated.

The urgency with which long bone fractures devoid of neurovascular compromise need to be surgically addressed is not clear. Urgency usually relates to open fractures. The severity of an open fracture is classified by the size of the wound, the degree of contamination, and the amount of soft tissue and bone injured.[32,33] With grade III-C injuries, which involve vascular compromise and are the most severe, the incidence of limb loss greatly increases if vascularity is not re-established within 6 hours of injury.[34] The incidence of wound infection correlates with the extent of soft-tissue damage, the extremity injured (lower extremity wounds become infected more frequently than upper extremity wounds), the type of fixation used, the amount of blood transfused, the mechanism of injury, and the use of prophylactic antibiotics.[33] Although it seems intuitively true that expedient wound cleansing should lower the infection rate, existing data do not validate this belief for open fractures up to 6 hours.[33,35] Data are not available on the infection outcome of fractures left open more than 6 hours before treatment is instituted. For the anesthesiologist, perhaps the greatest risk attendant on proceeding hastily is the possibility of vomiting and aspiration. The key question is, "Could this risk be lessened by allowing more time for gastric emptying?" Normal adult gastric emptying time is 4–6 hours and varies with the nature of gastric contents, patient emotional status, and other factors.[36] Injuries prolong this time, as do medications such as opioids given for pain. How much these influences delay emptying of the stomach is not known for sure. Surgeons and anesthesiologists must exercise judgment when deciding on the best time for operative intervention.

Burns

Care of the burn patient places tremendous demands on the medical team, and is costly. Each year about 100,000 patients are hospitalized for a total of 2 million days.[37] The severity of a burn depends on the body surface area (BSA)

involved and the thickness of the burn. Partial-thickness burns may only involve the superficial dermis, are exquisitely painful, and usually heal in 2–3 weeks without skin grafting. Full-thickness burns involve destruction of all dermal appendages and do not heal properly unless the destroyed skin is excised and replaced with grafts. The mortality from burns increases with the severity of the burn and with advancing age. The prognosis for patients with a greater than 50% BSA full-thickness burn is poor, but patients have survived a 90% BSA burn.

As is true for any patient who sustains trauma, initial treatment of the burned patient should involve attention to the airway, breathing, and circulation. If the patient is apneic, the face is burned, the patient has stridor or is hoarse, or the patient inhaled steam, smoke, or toxic fumes, the trachea should be intubated immediately. Intubation of the trachea is much easier if done earlier rather than later, when there is glottic and/or facial edema. Oral or nasotracheal intubation is preferable to tracheostomy in the burned patient, as the latter is associated with a high mortality rate.[38]

Inhalation of carbon monoxide is a frequent cause of hypoxia in burned patients. Carbon monoxide has 200 times more affinity for hemoglobin than oxygen, and although the patient's arterial oxygen pressure (Pa_{O_2}) may be normal, the oxygen content of the blood may be quite low. Measurement of oxygen content or carboxyhemoglobin levels (or both) is indicated. Carbon monoxide inhalation should be treated with inhalation of 100% oxygen by mask or an endotracheal tube. Hyperbaric oxygen is generally not indicated because transport of a severely burned patient to a chamber is hazardous. Damage to the subglottic airway is rare, unless the patient has inhaled live steam. If sloughing of the tracheal epithelium occurs, bronchoscopy may be necessary.[39]

After the airway has been secured and other life-threatening injuries have been treated, the burn patient must be resuscitated with large volumes of fluid. A burn causes a generalized increase in capillary permeability, with a considerable loss of fluid and protein into the interstitial tissue, plus an increase in evaporative losses. Fluid loss is greatest in the first 12 hours and subsides after about 24 hours.[40] One of several formulae to determine replacement needs was developed for adults at Parkland Hospital and calls for administration of 4 $ml \cdot kg^{-1}$ of balanced salt solution for every 1% BSA burned in the first 24 hours[40] (considerations for burned children differ[41]). However, volume replacement should be determined more by urine output and hemodynamic variables than by a fixed formula.

Within hours after a burn and until it has nearly healed, the patient is hypermetabolic. This is manifested in hyperthermia, increased catabolism, increased oxygen consumption, tachypnea, tachycardia, and increased serum catecholamine levels. As a result, the patient should be given oxygen, ventilation proportionate to the increase in carbon dioxide production, and parenteral nutrition.

The mortality, morbidity, and cosmetic outcome following thermal injury have improved considerably with the introduction of early excision of burned tissue and skin grafting.[42] Providing anesthesia for this operation is challenging and involves the following considerations:[42-44]

Access for monitoring can be difficult. Needle electrodes may be required for the ECG and nerve stimulator. A blood pressure cuff can be applied over burned tissue, but an arterial catheter is probably preferable in patients with large burns.

Accurate measurement and maintenance of body temperature is essential. Because of hypermetabolism, evaporative fluid loss, and exposure, the burned patient is particularly susceptible to hypothermia. As a consequence, the OR should be warmed to 28–30°C, intravenous (iv) solutions should be warmed, and a heated humidifier should be placed in the anesthetic circuit.

Blood loss can be prodigious. This loss should be anticipated, pressurized infusion devices should be available, and the anesthesiologist should be prepared to encounter all the complications associated with massive transfusion (such as a loss of clotting factors).

The selection of anesthetic drugs is not critical as long as they are used rationally. Opioids should usually be a part of any technique, as excruciating pain can be expected in the postoperative period. Halothane may not be a good choice because epinephrine-soaked pads are applied after excision of the burn and cardiac dysrhythmias may result. Ventilation of the lungs should usually be controlled, as increased carbon dioxide production or respiratory failure may exist. Common anesthesia ventilators may not deliver a sufficient minute volume to maintain normocarbia.

Burned patients do not respond normally to muscle relaxants.[45] After about 24 hours following the burn and until the wound has healed, succinylcholine administration can result in a rapid rise in the serum potassium level and cardiac arrest. On the other hand, burned patients are resistant to nondepolarizing muscle relaxants, and doses must be adjusted upward and administered more frequently. The mechanism for this altered response to muscle relaxants is not known, although it is likely to involve a change in receptors rather than a pharmacokinetic factor.[45,46]

The principles for the care of a patient with an electrical burn are similar to those for patients with a thermal burn, with two exceptions. First, the extent of burn can be misleading. Small cutaneous lesions may overlie extensive areas of devitalized skeletal muscle and other deep tissues. Consequently, the patient should be watched for myoglobinuria and renal failure. Second, patients may suffer spinal cord injury with an electrical burn.

Shock

Shock may be defined as a state of generalized inadequate tissue perfusion.[47] Although hypotension usually accompanies shock, shock can be present with a normal blood pressure, and hypotension can exist without shock. Shock can result from hypovolemia, poor cardiac function, sepsis, and blood flow obstruction (e.g., pulmonary embolism). Anaphylactic and neurogenic (spinal) shock are variants of hypovolemic shock. Hypovolemic shock is characteristic of the trauma patient immediately after injury, whereas septic shock, if it occurs, usually develops after several days of hospitalization.

The clinical manifestations of shock include pallor, cyanosis, sweating, disorientation, tachycardia, cardiac dysrhythmias, pump failure, tachypnea, increased wasted ventilation, venous admixture, low cardiac output, hypotension, oliguria, sludging of blood, disseminated intravascular coagulation (DIC), and acidosis.[47,48]

Hypovolemic shock is usually the result of hemorrhage. The body's normal homeostatic reflexes are geared to vigorously defend blood pressure and vital organ perfusion. As hemorrhage ensues, there is an elevation of plasma renin levels, antidiuretic hormone secretion, and sympathetic nervous system activity to produce tachycardia and arterio-

lar vasoconstriction. These mechanisms maintain blood pressure until about 30–40% of the blood volume has been lost. Thus, a patient may be severely hypovolemic yet have reasonably normal blood pressure. Significant hypovolemia should be suspected if tachycardia, diaphoresis, pallor, and other signs of shock are present, or if there is evidence of orthostatic hypotension. Testing for orthostatic changes is best accomplished with a tilt test on the OR table.[49] With the patient supine, baseline blood pressures and heart rate are recorded. With a safety belt firmly secured across the pelvis, the table and patient are then turned to a 45- to 60-degree head-up position. After 60 seconds these variables are again measured. Normovolemic patients will show no change or a slight increase (5 mm Hg) in diastolic pressure, no change or a slight decrease (10 mm Hg) in systolic pressure, and a 10–15 beat·min^{-1} increase in heart rate.[50] The tilt test only shows significant changes if blood loss of greater than 1000 ml has occurred.[49] Central venous pressure is more sensitive to hypovolemia, with a decline of more than 5 mm Hg (7 cm H_2O), or to values below zero, indicative of substantial hypovolemia. Once blood loss exceeds 40% of the blood volume, compensatory mechanisms fail and shock may become irreversible. Prolonged inadequate tissue perfusion results in vital organ ischemia, loss of membrane integrity, and progressive cellular death.

The key to treatment of hypovolemic shock is aggressive iv fluid therapy.[51] Large-bore iv catheters should be placed and warm crystalloid solutions or blood infused. Although the issue remains controversial, colloid solutions are probably of little advantage in the resuscitation of hypovolemic patients.[52] If type-specific blood is not available, type O, Rh negative blood can be given on a temporary basis.

Spinal shock is seen with high spinal cord injuries (i.e., C6–7) and results from mechanical disruption of sympathetic nervous system outflow as sympathetic preganglionic fibers emanate from T1–L2. These patients feel warm and dry to the touch and have a slow pulse despite being relatively hypotensive. They are functionally hypovolemic; that is, intravascular capacity is greater than intravascular volume, because of an inability to venoconstrict. The pulse is slow because sympathetic supply to the heart is also interrupted. Organ perfusion may or may not be normal in this state. Systemic vascular resistance is low, offering little impedance to flow; however, if venous return is inadequate, cardiac output and organ perfusion may be inadequate. The patient should be left flat with slight leg elevation. Fluids should be given iv to restore adequate intravascular volume, venous return, and cardiac output. If arterial pressure is so low that vital organ perfusion is threatened, mixed inotropic-vasoconstrictor type drugs can be used, that is, ephedrine, epinephrine, or metaraminol. Because these patients cannot vasoconstrict to conserve body heat, they are very susceptible to hypothermia. Spinal injuries can also affect breathing. Patients with very high lesions (C3–C4 and above) usually die of asphyxia at the accident scene. With lower and more common cord injuries (C6–C7), diaphragmatic action is spared and normal tidal volumes are possible despite loss of intercostal muscle activity. Ventilation may become compromised, however, if injury-related edema of the spinal cord spreads to higher levels or if diaphragmatic breathing efficiency wanes due to abdominal injury, distention of abdominal contents, and loss of lung volumes. Eventually tracheal intubation, and positive pressure ventilation of the lungs, may be needed.[53]

Septic shock is a late complication of trauma. The presence of microorganisms or their products in blood produces circulatory insufficiency and defects in oxygen exchange.

There is a reduction in peripheral resistance to flow and a maldistribution of blood flow to tissues.[54] Myocardial depression may also exist. Patients with septic shock have enormous fluid requirements caused by vasodilation and capillary leak. Patients may respond early to fluids and vasopressors, but if progress of the disease is not halted, renal, hepatic, and cerebral failure may ensue. A normal cardiac output predicts reversal of septic shock and a favorable outcome.[47]

Monitoring and Fluid Resuscitation

Patients who have sustained a major injury and who are about to undergo an emergency surgical procedure should have at least two large-bore iv catheters and a urinary catheter in place. If time permits, an arterial and central venous catheter are also indicated. When the patient is unstable, the anesthesiologist needs to prioritize regarding the necessity for these additional monitors. It may be preferable to call for additional help so that the anesthesiologist's attention can be directed to assuring the adequacy of ventilation, sorting out lines, giving drugs, monitoring the patient, and infusing fluids. A pulmonary artery catheter is rarely indicated in the acute management of trauma, although it may be placed at the end of surgery to facilitate postoperative care. The preferred site for monitoring central venous pressure is the internal jugular vein, as there is a lower incidence of pneumothorax with this approach than with the subclavian approach. However, this may vary with individual skills. The antecubital or femoral veins are alternative sites. An arterial catheter not only facilitates continuous and instantaneous assessment of blood pressure, but it is invaluable for frequent blood sampling (such as for serial hematocrits, blood gases, electrolytes, and coagulation studies). It can also provide valuable information regarding intravascular volume status if there has been insufficient time to place a central line.[55]

Providing adequate access for rapid infusion of fluids is crucial. Poisseuille's law states that the flow of fluid is proportional to the 4th power of the radius of the vein and, more important, the iv catheter. Venous catheters should be at least 16 gauge or larger. Introducers for pulmonary artery catheters, particularly if in a central vein,[56] or placement of iv tubing in an antecubital or saphenous vein by surgical cutdown are also effective. The infusion of large volumes of fluid and blood can be facilitated by pressurizing the container. In addition to the traditional hand-inflated blood transfusion pumps, there are now several automated devices available that can infuse up to 1000 ml of fluid or blood per minute. However, damage to blood cells can result if infused at high pressure through too small a catheter and rapid infusion of banked blood can cause a serious elevation in serum potassium.[57]

ADMINISTERING THE ANESTHETIC

Aspiration of Gastric Contents

If the trachea has not been intubated prior to the patient's arrival in the ER or OR, it is necessary to protect the patient from pulmonary aspiration of gastric contents while inducing anesthesia. Several measures can be taken to achieve this goal. One is to attempt to empty the stomach by inserting a nasogastric tube. However, the stomach cannot be completely emptied in this way. Passing a nasogastric tube can decompress the stomach by drainage of fluid and gas but is ineffective for chunks of solid material. Induced vomiting can be more effective at emptying the stomach and is achieved by the simultaneous iv administration of 0.1 mg·kg^{-1} apomorphine and 0.01 mg·kg^{-1} atropine. This should not be done in the presence of eye, head and neck, thoracic, or abdominal injuries because of the increased pressures or motions in those areas associated with retching.

To prevent pulmonary damage should the patient aspirate, the clinician can attempt to neutralize gastric contents with 30–45 ml of a nonparticulate antacid, such as a 0.3 molar solution of sodium citrate given orally 15–20 minutes prior to induction of anesthesia. Alternatively, gastric contents can be neutralized and the volume reduced with H_2 histamine blockers[58] and/or gastric motility-stimulating drugs.[59] The use of gastric motility-stimulating drugs is contraindicated in a patient with an acute abdomen. Recommended doses of H_2 blockers are 300 mg of cimetidine or 50 mg of ranitidine given iv 30–60 minutes prior to induction. A gastric motility-stimulating agent, such as 10 mg iv metoclopramide, can be given 30–60 minutes prior to induction of anesthesia. Even if there is not enough time for these drugs to have an effect prior to induction of anesthesia, they probably should be given if extubation of the trachea is anticipated immediately postoperatively, as they may have a beneficial effect by that time. Antimuscarinic drugs such as atropine and glycopyrrolate should not be used as they decrease gastroesophageal sphincter tone and thereby facilitate gastric reflux and silent regurgitation.[60] If a nasogastric tube is in place it is best to remove it prior to induction of anesthesia as it serves as a wick to allow passive reflux of gastric contents and is a mechanical hindrance during tracheal intubation.

Endotracheal intubation in the presence of a full stomach can be done awake or with a rapid sequence technique using induction agents and muscle paralysis. Awake tracheal intubation can be done either orally or nasally. For the oral approach the base of the tongue should be topically anesthetized with a local anesthetic. Benzocaine or 10% lidocaine are good choices because of their rapid onset of action. The patient is coached to breathe rapidly and to continue to do so during laryngoscopy. Breathing and gagging are mutually exclusive and if the patient focuses on breathing rapidly he or she will not gag. If the vocal cords can be exposed, an endotracheal tube is placed between them and an induction drug given rapidly after inflation of the cuff. For the nasal approach, the nasal passage should be topically anesthetized and a small, warmed, lubricated tube passed into the pharynx and then positioned either blindly or under direct vision with a laryngoscope (after topicalization of the base of the tongue) into the trachea. Passage of tubes through the nose is not safe if there are facial fractures or a basilar skull fracture. Oral or nasal awake tracheal intubation can be attempted with a fiberoptic bronchoscope; however, this is frequently ungratifying under emergency conditions. Success is limited because of the lack of proper patient preparation and the presence of secretions that blur the field. Adequate topical anesthesia of the lower airway (i.e., superior laryngeal nerve blocks or transtracheal blocks), which greatly facilitate successful fiberoptic bronchoscopy, is contraindicated in patients with full stomachs, as is heavy sedation as both potentially create conditions that could result in aspiration from either active vomiting or reflux. As a final comment, awake tracheal intubation should be attempted with caution if there is evidence of a brain injury or penetrating eye or neck injuries.

The rapid sequence induction technique with muscle paralysis and oral tracheal intubation is preferred in most acute trauma situations. The patient may breathe 100% oxygen for 3–5 minutes, at normal tidal volumes, to denitrogenate the functional residual capacity of the lungs. If time is limited, almost the same degree of preoxygenation can be accomplished with three to five vital capacity breaths of 100% oxygen. However, preoxygenation by the "quick method" does not sustain arterial oxygen saturation as long, once apnea ensues—at least in the elderly.[61] An induction dose of one of several iv anesthetic drugs is then given rapidly, followed immediately by an appropriate dose of a rapid-acting muscle relaxant. After the patient loses consciousness, cricoid pressure (the Sellick maneuver)[62] is applied and maintained until the trachea is intubated and the cuff inflated. It is important not to apply cricoid pressure too early as it may stimulate a gag reflex and result in vomiting at a most inopportune time. If extubation is planned at the end of the case, it should not occur until the patient is fully awake and able to protect his or her airway. How awake is safely awake is difficult to assess. Experience has shown that it is probably safe to extubate when the patient responds with a "yes" motion when asked "do you want the tube removed," and then will volitionally reach for the tube and extubate himself or herself when instructed to do so.

Induction

Induction of anesthesia is one of the more critical aspects of management of the trauma patient. A short-acting iv induction agent is normally used; it can be selected from one of several pharmacologic categories. Most common is thiopental, in a usual dose of 3–4 mg·kg^{-1}. It can cause venodilation with a subsequent decrease in venous return, cardiac output, and blood pressure. In the presence of moderate hypovolemia, thiopental has been shown to increase renal blood flow.[63] Thiopental can also be a cardiac depressant when the myocardium is compromised, and can depress baroreceptor function.[64] Therefore, in hypovolemic patients one may want to decrease the dose or use a different drug. Ketamine is one of the few drugs in the anesthesiologist's armamentarium that is a cardiovascular stimulant. It normally raises blood pressure secondary to a rise in heart rate and cardiac output, mediated by a central anticholinergic mechanism.[65] When this drug is used to induce anesthesia in severely hypovolemic patients, the normal iv dose of 1–2 mg·kg^{-1} should be reduced to 0.25–0.5 mg·kg^{-1}. The drug can be a myocardial depressant in patients whose sympathetic nervous system is already maximally stressed. Ketamine also has excellent amnestic properties. It should be avoided, however, in patients with elevated ICP or open eye injury. Benzodiazepines have been used for induction of anesthesia after trauma; however, diazepam can cause hypotension if hypovolemia exists. Midazolam may have less effect on the cardiovascular system[66] but it has not been adequately tested in severe hypovolemic states.

Perhaps the safest drug from a hemodynamic standpoint is etomidate. This drug, in iv doses of 0.1–0.3 mg·kg^{-1}, produces minimal change in cardiovascular variables.[67,68] It has three drawbacks, none of which should contraindicate its use as a single bolus in a hemodynamically unstable patient. It can produce a transient burning on iv administration, it can produce myoclonus, and it can, after a single bolus, produce up to 4 hours of adrenal cortical suppression.[69] Though noteworthy, this latter effect has not been demonstrated to be detrimental to patient outcome. Supplemental cortisol can be used if necessary. A newer induction agent, propofol, has become available.[70] Propofol causes a 20–30% decrease in systemic vascular resistance in normal subjects with a subsequent decrease in blood pressure. Data on propofol's action in hypovolemic subjects are not available, but in injured patients surviving on maximum sympathetic drive, the use of this agent would be unwise, owing to the potential for severe decreases in blood pressure. It might have application if given by iv drip in conjunction with muscle relaxants for maintenance of unconsciousness and amnesia in injured patients who cannot tolerate deep anesthesia.

A major decision in performing a rapid sequence induction of anesthesia is the selection of a muscle relaxant. The drug of choice is succinylcholine, 1–1.5 mg·kg^{-1}, unless otherwise contraindicated. Succinylcholine is not recommended if there is a risk of massive potassium release, if there is a history of malignant hyperthermia, or in certain neuromuscular disorders. Its use in patients with a lacerated cornea is controversial. Pretreatment with a nondepolarizing relaxant may reduce the likelihood of vitreous extrusion.[70a] Vecuronium is the preferred alternative to succinylcholine because it is relatively devoid of hemodynamic effects.[71] However, it is not as rapid in onset as succinylcholine unless large doses are used (0.15–0.2 mg·kg^{-1}) or a priming principle is followed. Both approaches make vecuronium almost as fast in onset as succinylcholine. If one desires to increase the heart rate with the muscle relaxant, pancuronium, 0.12–0.15 mg·kg^{-1} iv, can be employed with an onset time almost as fast as succinylcholine. An important principle of a rapid sequence induction is "never paralyze someone you do not know you can ventilate." If endotracheal intubation does not appear to be easy, an awake intubation of the trachea or tracheostomy under local anesthesia should be entertained. Despite our best efforts to assess the airway, the law of averages means that tracheal intubation occasionally cannot be accomplished after induction. If this occurs, and if succinylcholine has been used, gentle mask ventilation of the lungs, with maintenance of cricoid pressure, should be instituted. At that point, repeat attempts at tracheal intubation can be undertaken, or the patient can be allowed to awaken. If the endotracheal tube has inadvertently been placed into the esophagus, it can be left in place with the cuff inflated and the patient's lungs ventilated with a mask around the esophageal tube. The patient can then be allowed to awaken or repeated attempts at tracheal intubation can be performed with another endotracheal tube. If repeat tracheal intubation is attempted, flaccid skeletal muscle paralysis and cricoid pressure should be maintained. As a last measure, if the patient is hypoxic due to an inability to intubate the trachea or ventilate the lungs, an emergency cricothyroidotomy or tracheostomy should be performed.

Maintenance

Once the patient's airway has been secured, the essential monitors placed, and induction of anesthesia accomplished, the anesthesiologist must remember several issues of importance during the maintenance phase of anesthesia. The mnemonic CATHUR may be helpful in that process (Table 51-3).

The first priority in anesthetizing the trauma patient continues to be respiration (R). With a few exceptions, such as with tracheal injuries, it is best to mechanically control ventilation of the lungs. This permits the anesthesiologist

TABLE 51-3. Analysis of CATHUR Mnemonic for Prioritization of Care in Trauma Patients

Order of Importance

R—Respiration (airway, ventilation, oxygenation)
H—Hemodynamics
A—Acid-base balance
U—Urine output
T—Temperature
C—Coagulation

to have an extra hand for infusing blood and drugs. It is also advisable to have a ventilator available that is capable of generating high inspiratory pressure (e.g., >60 cm H_2O) and PEEP. An ordinary anesthesia ventilator may not be effective if there has been pulmonary aspiration or a severe lung contusion. For many patients, insertion of an arterial catheter and frequent monitoring of arterial blood gases is advisable.

The next important priority is preservation of hemodynamic (H) stability. This can be influenced by a number of factors, but two main ones are the anesthetic drug and the patient's intravascular volume.

There is no perfect anesthetic drug or technique for trauma. Regional anesthesia may be useful for some isolated limb injuries, but techniques associated with major sympathetic nervous system blockade are relatively contraindicated in the face of hypovolemia.[72] Studies in dogs suggest that epidural anesthesia may have a beneficial effect and reduce the mortality from hypovolemic shock, but this has not yet been demonstrated in humans.[73] Use of regional anesthesia does not obviate the need for concern about aspiration and the full stomach.

In most instances, general anesthesia is preferred. When severe hypovolemic shock or a reduced level of consciousness exists, there may be no need for administration of an anesthetic drug. Skeletal muscle paralysis and ventilation of the lungs will suffice. However, when the patient is awake and an anesthetic is necessary, the choice of drugs is less important than titrating their administration carefully. There is a natural tendency to choose an anesthetic for patients in shock that is an adrenergic agonist and associated with the least hypotension when administered to healthy people. Thus, the sympathetic nervous system stimulation associated with cyclopropane made it a popular choice several years ago, and ketamine is popular now. However, there are limited data to support the efficacy of these drugs in hypovolemic shock. Studies have shown that cyclopropane, in comparison with halothane or isoflurane, shortens the survival time and causes excess lactate production when given to hemorrhaged dogs.[74] Ketamine is a potent analgetic and amnestic agent, but when given to hypovolemic pigs, its cardiovascular effects are not different from those of thiopental, and it causes a metabolic acidosis.[75] Similarly, nitrous oxide offered no hemodynamic advantage over halothane in hypovolemic pigs.[76] Because trauma patients frequently have pulmonary contusions, increased venous admixture, and other causes for a large alveolar-arterial oxygen gradient, nitrous oxide probably should not be used unless the adequacy of oxygenation is confirmed, preferably by blood gas analysis or at the least pulse oximetry. It should also be used with caution whenever there may be a pneumothorax.[77]

To minimize the hypotension produced by anesthetics in the presence of hypovolemia, it is common practice to administer only small quantities and to prevent patient movement by administration of a muscle relaxant. Unfortunately, patients may not be completely anesthetized and may have recall of events during surgery. In a series of 14 severely injured patients who were given no anesthetic for endotracheal intubation and for at least 20 minutes during a subsequent operation, 6 (43%) had recall of intraoperative events. Conditions that might normally be expected to reduce anesthetic requirements, such as alcohol in the blood, acidosis, hypothermia, and hypotension, did not reliably prevent recall.[78] To establish amnesia in the setting of shock, one might consider administration of small iv doses of scopolamine (0.1–0.2 mg), midazolam (1 mg), or ketamine (0.25 mg·kg^{-1}).

Some general guidelines for the administration of anesthetics to severely injured patients include the following:

1. For conscious, hypovolemic patients, induce anesthesia with small doses of ketamine, etomidate, a benzodiazepine, or thiopental.
2. Avoid prolonged use of drugs that stimulate the sympathetic nervous system. A need for continued use of vasopressors should be interpreted as hypovolemia or cardiac tamponade until proven otherwise.
3. Avoid nitrous oxide until the adequacy of oxygenation is assured.
4. Use opioids if necessary for analgesia.
5. Titrate volatile anesthetics as soon as feasible.
6. Recognize that blood pressure alone is an unreliable index of blood volume, tissue perfusion, or the level of consciousness.
7. Resort to oxygen and skeletal muscle paralysis, alone, only if the patient will not tolerate any anesthetic drugs.

Hemodynamic stability also results from control of surgical bleeding by the surgeon and restoration of blood volume by the anesthesiologist. Several choices of fluids are available for use by the anesthesiologist. With hemorrhage there is a contraction of extracellular volume as the patient attempts to autotransfuse the intravascular compartment with his or her own interstitial fluid.[79,80] Initially, administration of a physiologic salt solution such as lactated Ringer's solution restores this depletion and also expands intravascular volume to help maintain venous return and cardiac output. Physiologic salt solutions remain intravascular for only 30–60 minutes before redistributing throughout the entire extracellular fluid volume.[81] Other plasma expanders, such as colloid solutions, maintain intravascular volume for 2–5 hours but are fraught with certain hazards. Protein solutions can impair pulmonary function if they extravasate into a damaged lung,[82] and they can cause vasodilation.[83] Dextran solutions can cause bleeding disorders and severe allergic reactions.[84] Fresh frozen plasma should be reserved for treatment of specific, documented coagulation disorders.[85] Hydroxyethyl starch, a glucose polymer in a 6% solution, has proved useful as a volume expander. It has a long plasma half-life (1.5 days) and does not affect coagulation when given in recommended doses. The dose should be limited to no more than 20 ml·kg^{-1}.[86-88] Finally, hypertonic saline has been effective as a volume expander in preliminary studies in animals[89] and humans[90] but there are data to question its use on a routine basis.[91] Despite the availability of all of these forms of intravascular volume expansion, and the continuation of a "colloid *vs.* crystalloid" controversy,[92,93] the mainstay of therapy should be lactated Ringer's solution.

Most trauma victims are young, with good cardiac and renal function, so that severe degrees of anemia can be well tolerated if intravascular volume is supported. Nevertheless, with extreme blood loss, red cells eventually must be given. Fresh whole blood (less than 6 hours old) is preferable, if available. After 1 day of storage, only 12% of the original platelets remain in whole blood. Regardless of its age, whole blood is preferable to packed red blood cells. Trauma patients need cells and volume. If there is no time for a crossmatch, type-specific whole blood, type-specific red cells, or, as a last resort, type O negative red cells will suffice. Red cells today are stored and suspended in a solution of citrate, adenine, saline, and mannitol. This formulation, unlike the older "packed cells," has an average hematocrit of 40–45, vs. 75–80 for packed cells. It has a viscosity resembling that of whole blood, and the need for reconstitution with normal saline is obviated.

The C of the CATHUR mnemonic refers to coagulation. When whole blood or red cells are given as a massive transfusion (defined as replacement of one or more patient blood volumes), platelets may be necessary to correct a dilutional thrombocytopenia.[95] It is best to perform coagulation studies at regular intervals, but as a general rule, one should administer 10–20 units of platelets per 10 units of replaced blood. Stored whole blood is deficient in factors V and VIII, but whole blood usually contains adequate levels of these clotting factors for the coagulation process to occur. This may not be the case if most of the replaced blood consisted of packed red blood cells with the plasma components removed. In that case, fresh frozen plasma (2–3 units) in addition to platelets may be needed for each 10 units of transfused red cells.

Two other coagulation disorders can be seen in shock— DIC, a consumption coagulopathy with secondary fibrinolysis, and primary fibrinolysis. In both conditions, serum fibrinogen is decreased and fibrin split products, prothrombin time, and partial thromboplastin time are increased. Thrombocytopenia, relative or absolute, usually exists with DIC, but not primary fibrinolysis. Fibrin degradation products can result from lysis of either fibrinogen or fibrin and thus do not discriminate between DIC and primary fibrinolysis. A new coagulation study, D-dimers, is now available. D-dimers can only be elevated when fibrin is lysed, and thus this test is now more specific for the presence of DIC than thrombocytopenia.[94] If DIC is diagnosed, small doses of heparin can be tried (50 units·kg^{-1}) while also replacing clotting factors and platelets. If the diagnosis of primary fibrinolysis is secure, epsilon-aminocaproic acid can be given to inhibit fibrinolysis. However, this will aggravate DIC, and if doubt exists as to which pathology exists, it should not be used.[95] In acute trauma the large majority of clotting disorders are secondary to dilutional thrombocytopenia. If a more complicated picture is encountered, testing the patient's coagulation profile is indicated and consultation with a hematologist should be considered.

Although citrate is the anticoagulant in most stored blood, clinically significant citrate intoxication and hypocalcemia are not seen unless blood is infused exceedingly fast and in vast quantities. Serum ionized calcium can decrease during massive transfusion[96] but should not be clinically significant unless the volume of infused blood exceeds 100 ml·min^{-1} in the adult patient.[97,98] The clinical signs of hypocalcemia are those of poor myocardial function.

Assessment of blood loss and the adequacy of replacement can be very difficult in the trauma patient. Lost blood can be on the floor, under drapes, on sponges and gowns, and in the suction canisters. In such a situation, the physician must rely on the patient's vital signs, urine output, acid-base balance, and serial hematocrits as an indication that satisfactory replacement has been achieved. Signs of success will be a reasonable heart rate (less than 100 beats· min^{-1}), a reasonable pulse pressure (greater than 30 mm Hg), urine output greater than 0.5–1 ml·kg^{-1}·hr^{-1}, no metabolic acidosis, and a lack of large swings in heart rate and blood pressure with positive pressure ventilation of the lungs.

The standard pore size of filters on blood administration sets is 170 microns. These filters catch a significant portion of the cellular debris from blood products, but some of this material does bypass the filter, enter the patient, and lodge in the lung. It has been suggested that this may be one of the contributing factors to "shock lung" or adult respiratory distress syndrome (ARDS).[99] Micropore filters, with 20–40 micron pore size, can be placed in line and filter out a significantly greater percentage of cellular debris. Some data indicate a pulmonary benefit from the use of micropore filters[99] while others do not.[100] If transfusions are massive, some benefit probably results. The trade-off is that the finer filters offer a great deal of in-line resistance to flow and can make it difficult to keep up with intravascular volume if blood loss is swift. Platelets should not be infused through a micropore filter.

The A of CATHUR refers to acid-base and electrolyte balance. Not uncommonly, trauma victims have a metabolic acidosis due to shock, hypothermia, hypoxia, and generalized stress. Mechanical ventilation of the lungs can be used to normalize blood pH over the short term by manipulation of Paco$_2$. With time, restoration of tissue perfusion and renal and hepatic function should resolve the problem. However, if the metabolic acidosis does not resolve, or if it is so severe that ventilatory mechanisms are inadequate, it can be treated with sodium bicarbonate as a temporizing measure. Treatment with bicarbonate should be reserved for instances in which the acidosis is severe. Studies suggest that bicarbonate may be detrimental in the treatment of lactic acidosis, as it leads to a deterioration of blood pressure and cardiac output.[101,102] The most important treatment for metabolic acidosis is fluid/blood resuscitation, ventilation, and rewarming. It is not necessary to administer sodium bicarbonate prophylactically in these situations. Patients with normal liver function who have received a large volume of lactated Ringer's solution or blood products containing citrate often develop a metabolic alkalosis 6–24 hours later.[103]

The T of CATHUR is for temperature. A maximum effort must be made to maintain patient body temperature at normal values. Hypothermia is associated with a number of undesirable effects such as reduced glomerular filtration, poor platelet function, lowered glucose utilization, postoperative shivering with increased oxygen demand, postoperative vasoconstriction with increased peripheral and pulmonary vascular resistance, metabolic acidosis, and decreased metabolism of drugs. Because of exposure and shock, trauma victims are usually hypothermic. This can be compounded if cool resuscitation fluids are also administered. All fluids must be warm, by using prewarmed, non-glucose-containing crystalloid solutions or blood warmers. Not only does warming help maintain patient temperature, but it reduces blood viscosity and improves tissue blood flow. When selecting blood warming devices be sure they are capable of efficient warming at high rates of infusion.[104] Of perhaps equal benefit in maintaining body temperature is a warm OR, particularly at the outset until the patient is draped.[105] A warming blanket under the patient is not beneficial, especially if the patient is already hypothermic, because an inadequate area of well-perfused body surface is in contact with it. Because the body loses heat in the course of warming and humidifying inspired gases, the use of a humidifier in the anesthetic circuit helps to maintain normothermia and in fact can actively warm a patient, given enough time.

The final letter to recall from the mnemonic CATHUR is U, for urine. Maintenance of good urine output after trauma is important for several reasons. The greatest concern is the prevention of acute oliguric renal failure which can result from hypoperfusion and hypotension. Unfortunately, there is no formula to predict how much hypoperfusion or hypotension, for how long, will result in renal failure. Certainly acute renal failure can occur without apparent hypotension and sometimes does not occur despite the presence of hypotension. If a closed head injury has occurred, maintenance of urine output is important for control of ICP. If skeletal muscle crush injuries or electrocution have occurred, myoglobinuria must be treated with a vigorous diuresis. Mannitol is the diuretic of choice in all of the above cases. The same concerns apply to the hemoglobinuria that occurs after a hemolytic transfusion reaction. The initial dose should be $0.25 \mathrm{~g \cdot kg^{-1}}$ given as a drip or as a bolus, and the total dose should be limited to $1-1.5 \mathrm{~g \cdot kg^{-1}}$. If the patient has undergone angiography, renal function must be preserved to avert the toxic effects of contrast media on the kidney. Mannitol or fluids also work well for this. A healthy renal system contributes significantly to the favorable outcome of patients who survive severe trauma. This concern becomes greater in the postoperative period, when primary parenchymal renal failure can occur from toxins (antibiotics) or sepsis.[106] It is helpful if a prior prerenal insult has been avoided.

REFERENCES

1. Trunkey DD: The nature of things that go bang in the night. Surgery 92:123, 1982
2. Trunkey DD: Trauma. Sci Am 249:28, 1983
3. Trunkey DD: Shock trauma. Can J Surg 27:479, 1984
4. Klauber MR, Marshall LF: Cause of decline in head-injury mortality rate in San Diego County, California. J Neurosurg 62:528, 1985
5. Jacobs LM, Berrizbeitia LD, Bennett B et al: Endotracheal intubations in the prehospital phase of emergency medical care. JAMA 250:2175, 1983
6. Smith JP, Bodai BI: The urban paramedic's scope of practice. JAMA 253:544, 1985
7. Copass MK, Oreskovich MR, Bladengroen MR et al: Prehospital cardiopulmonary resuscitation of the critically injured patient. Am J Surg 148:20, 1984
8. Mattox KL, Bickell WH, Pepe PE et al: Prospective randomized evaluation of antishock MAST in post-traumatic hypotension. J Trauma 26:779, 1986
9. West JG, Cales RH, Gazzaniga AB: Impact of trauma regionalization: The Orange County experience. Arch Surg 118:740, 1983
10. American College of Surgeons Committee on Trauma: Hospital resources for optimal care of the trauma patient. Bull Am Coll Surg 64(8):43, 1979
11. American College of Surgeons Committee on Trauma: Advanced Trauma Life Support Course for Physicians, Student Manual. Chicago, American College of Surgeons, 1984
12. Champion HR, Sacco WJ, Carnazzo AJ et al: Trauma score. Crit Care Med 9:672, 1981
13. Muzzi DA, Losasso TJ, Cucchiara RF: Complications from a nasopharyngeal airway in a patient with a basilar skull fracture. Anesthesiology 74:366, 1991
14. Fremstad JD, Martin SH: Lethal complication for insertion of a nasogastric tube after severe basilar skull fracture. J Trauma 18:820, 1978
15. Gregory JA, Tarter PT, Reynolds AF: A complication of nasogastric intubation: Intracranial penetration. J Trauma 18:822, 1978
16. Butler RM, Moser FH: The padded dash syndrome: Blunt trauma to the larynx and trachea. Laryngoscope 78:1172, 1968
17. Green R, Stark P: Trauma of the larynx and trachea. Radiol Clin North Am 16:309, 1978
18. Benumof JL: Management of the difficult adult airway. Anesthesiology 75:1087, 1991
19. Parks RE, Livoni JP: Detection of cervical spine injury in the multi-trauma patient. In Blaisdell FW, Trunkey DD (eds): Trauma Management III: Cervical Thoracic Trauma, p 56. New York, Thieme, 1986
20. Crosby ET: The adult cervical spine: Implications for airway management. Can J Anaesth 37:77, 1990
21. Campbell FC, Robbs JV: Penetrating injuries of the neck: A prospective study of 108 patients. Br J Surg 67:582, 1980
22. Goodnight JE Jr: Cervical injury. In Blaisdell FW, Trunkey DD (eds): Trauma Management III: Cervical Thoracic Trauma, p 94. New York, Thieme, Inc, 1986
23. Baker CC, Coronna JJ, Trunkey DD: Neurologic outcome after emergency room thoracotomy for trauma. Am J Surg 139:677, 1980
24. Lam AM, Winn HR, Cullen BF, Sundling N: Hyperglycemia and neurological outcome in patients with head injury. J Neurosurg 75:545, 1991
25. Blaisdell FW: Initial assessment of thoracic injuries. In Blaisdell FW, Trunkey DD (eds): Trauma Management III: Cervical Thoracic Trauma, p 1. New York, Thieme, 1986
26. Blaisdell FW: Pneumothorax and hemothorax. In Blaisdell FW, Trunkey DD (eds): Trauma Management III: Cervical Thoracic Trauma, p 150. New York, Thieme, 1986
27. Wiot JF: The radiologic manifestations of blunt chest trauma. JAMA 231:500, 1975
28. Brinton M, Miller SE, Lim RC et al: Acute abdominal aortic injuries. J Trauma 22:481, 1982
29. Trunkey DD, Federle MP: Computed tomography in perspective. J Trauma 26:660, 1986
30. Trunkey DD: Torso trauma. Curr Probl Surg 24:211, 1987
31. Federle MP, Crass RA, Jeffrey RB et al: Computed tomography in blunt abdominal trauma. Arch Surg 117:645, 1982
32. Chapman NW: The role of intramedullary fixation in open fractures. Clin Orthop 212:26, 1986
33. Dellinger EP, Miller SD, Wertz MJ et al: Risk of infection after open fracture of the arm or leg. Arch Surg 123:1320, 1988
34. Gustillo RB, Markow RL, Templeman D: The management of open fractures. J Bone Joint Surg 72A:299, 1990
35. Roth AI, Fry DE, Polk HC: Infectious morbidity in extremity fractures. J Trauma 26:757, 1986
36. Hunt JN: Gastric emptying and secretion in man. Physiol Rev 39:491, 1959
37. Lamb JD: Anaesthetic considerations for major thermal injury. Can Anaesth Soc J 32:84, 1985
38. Eckhauser FE, Billote J, Burke JF: Tracheostomy complicating massive burn injury: A plea for conservation. Am J Surg 127:418, 1974
39. Trunkey DD: Inhalation injury. Surg Clin North Am 58:1133, 1978
40. Baxter CR, Shires T: Physiological responses to crystalloid resuscitation of severe burns. Ann NY Acad Sci 150:874, 1968
41. Caravajal HF: A physiologic approach to fluid therapy in severely burned children. Surg Gynecol Obstet 150:379, 1980

42. Heimbach D, Engrav L: Surgical Management of the Burn Wound. New York, Raven Press, 1984

43. Szyfelbein SK: Anesthetic considerations for major burn surgery. ASA Refresher Courses in Anesthesiology 8:201, 1980

44. De Campo T, Aldrete JA: Anesthetic management of the severely burned patient. Intens Care Med 7:55, 1981

45. Martyn J: Clinical pharmacology and drug therapy in the burned patient. Anesthesiology 65:67, 1986

46. Marathe PH, Pavlin EG: Effect of thermal injury on the pharmacokinetics and pharmacodynamics of atracurium in humans. Anesthesiology 70:752, 1989

47. Houston MC, Thompson WL, Robertson D: Shock. Diagnosis and management. Arch Intern Med 144:1433, 1984

48. Moss GS, Saletta JD: Traumatic shock in man. N Engl J Med 290:724, 1974

49. Knopp R, Claypool R, Leonardi D: Use of the tilt test in measuring acute blood loss. Ann Emerg Med 9:72, 1980

50. Currens JH: A comparison of blood pressure in lying and standing positions: A study in 500 men and women. Am Heart J 35:646, 1948

51. Shires GT: Management of hypovolemic shock. Bull NY Acad Sci 55:139, 1979

52. Gallagher TJ, Banner MJ, Barnes PA: Large volume crystalloid resuscitation does not increase extravascular lung water. Anesth Analg 64:323, 1985

53. Fraser A, Edmonds-Seal J: Spinal cord injuries. A review of problems facing the anaesthetist. Anaesthesia 37:1084, 1982

54. Parrillo JE: Septic shock in humans: Advances in the understanding of pathogenesis, cardiovascular dysfunction and therapy. Ann Intern Med 113:227, 1990

55. Perel A, Pizov R, Cotev S: Systolic blood pressure variation is a sensitive indicator of hypovolemia in ventilated dogs subjected to graded hemorrhage. Anesthesiology 67:498, 1987

56. Richey JV, Wilson RD: IV equipment for massive transfusions. Anesthesiol Rev 7:36, 1980

57. Jameson LC, Popic PM, Harms BA: Hyperkalemic death during use of a high-capacity fluid warmer for massive transfusion. Anesthesiology 73:1050, 1990

58. Stoelting RK: Gastric fluid pH in patients receiving cimetidine. Anesth Analg 57:675, 1978

59. Solanki DR, Suresh M, Ethridge HC: The effects of intravenous cimetidine and metoclopramide on gastric volume of pH. Anesth Analg 63:599, 1984

60. Brock-Utne JG, Rubin J, Welman S: The effect of glycopyrrolate on lower esophageal sphincter. Canad Anaesth Soc J 25:144, 1978

61. Valentine SJ, Marjot R, Monk R: Preoxygenation in the elderly: A comparison of the four maximal breath and three minute techniques. Anesth Analg 71:516, 1990

62. Sellick BA: Cricoid pressure to control the regurgitation of stomach contents during induction of anesthesia. Lancet 2:404, 1961

63. Priano LL: Renal hemodynamic alterations following administration of thiopental, diazepam or ketamine in conscious hypovolemic dogs. Adv Shock Res 9:173, 1983

64. Priano LL, Bernards C, Marrone B: Effect of anesthetic induction agents on cardiovascular neuroregulation in dogs. Anesth Analg 68:344, 1989

65. Traber DL, Wilson RD, Priano LL: A detailed study of the cardiopulmonary response to ketamine and its blockade by atropine. South Med J 63:1077, 1970

66. Reves JG, Fragen RJ, Vinik HR et al: Midazolam: Pharmacology and uses. Anesthesiology 62:310, 1985

67. Gooding JM, Corssen G: Effect of etomidate on the cardiovascular system. Anesth Analg 56:717, 1977

68. Kettler D, Sonntag H, Donath U: Hemodynamic myocardmechanic Sowrstuff bedard und Sowrstuff Versorgum des menschen Herzens unter Narcosienlitung mit Etomidate. Der Anaesthetist 23:116, 1974

69. Fragen RJ, Shanks CA, Molteni A et al: Effects of etomidate on hormonal responses to surgical stress. Anesthesiology 61:652, 1984

70. Sebel PS, Lowdon JD: Propofol, a new intravenous anesthetic. Anesthesiology 71:260, 1989

70a. Miller RD, Way WL, Hickey RF: Inhibition of succinylcholine-induced increased intraocular pressure by non-depolarizing muscle relaxants. Anesthesiology 29:123, 1968

71. Lennon RL, Olson RA, Gronert GA: Atracurium or vecuronium for rapid sequence endotracheal intubation. Anesthesiology 64:510, 1986

72. Kennedy WF, Bonica JJ, Akamatsu TJ et al: Cardiovascular and respiratory effects of subarachnoid block in the presence of acute blood loss. Anesthesiology 29:29, 1968

73. Shibata K, Yamamoto Y, Kobayashi T et al: Beneficial effect of upper thoracic epidural anesthesia in experimental hemorrhagic shock in dogs: Influence of circulating catecholamines. Anesthesiology 74:303, 1991

74. Theye RA, Perry LB, Brzica SM: Influence of anesthetic agent on response to hemorrhagic hypotension. Anesthesiology 40:32, 1974

75. Weiskopf RB, Bogetz MS, Roizen MF et al: Cardiovascular and metabolic sequelae of inducing anesthesia with ketamine or thiopental in hypovolemic swine. Anesthesiology 60:214, 1984

76. Weiskopf RB, Bogetz MS: Cardiovascular action of nitrous oxide on halothane in hypovolemic swine. Anesthesiology 63:509, 1985

77. Eger EI, Saidman LJ: Hazards of nitrous oxide anesthesia in bowel obstruction and pneumothorax. Anesthesiology 26:61, 1965

78. Bogetz MS, Katz JA: Recall of surgery for major trauma. Anesthesiology 61:6, 1984

79. Shires T: The role of sodium containing solutions in the treatment of oligemic shock. Surg Clin North Am 45:365, 1965

80. Shires T, Coln D, Carrico J et al: Fluid therapy and hemorrhagic shock. Arch Surg 88:688, 1964

81. Cervera LA, Moss G: Crystalloid distribution following hemorrhage and hemodilution. J Trauma 14:506, 1974

82. Holcroft JW, Trunkey DD, Carpenter MA: Sepsis in the baboon: Factors affecting resuscitation and pulmonary edema in animals resuscitated with Ringer's lactate versus plasmanate. J Trauma 17:600, 1977

83. Bland JHL, Laver MB, Lowenstein E: Vasodilator effect of commercial 5% plasma protein fraction solutions. JAMA 224:1721, 1973

84. Giesecke AH, Jenkins MT: Fluid therapy. Clin Anesth 11:57, 1976

85. Bove JR: Fresh-frozen plasma: Too few indications, too much use. Anesth Analg 64:849, 1985

86. Lee WH, Cooper N, Weidner MG et al: Clinical evaluation of a new plasma expander, hydroxyethyl starch. J Trauma 8:381, 1968

87. Solanke TF, Khwaja MS, Madojemu EI: Plasma volume studies with four different plasma volume expanders. J Surg Res 11:140, 1971

88. Munoz E, Raciti A, Dove DB et al: Effect of hydroxyethyl starch versus albumin on hemodynamic and respiratory function in patients in shock. Crit Care Med 8:255, 1980

89. Layon J, Duncan D, Gallager TJ et al: Hypertonic saline as a resuscitation solution in hemorrhagic shock. Anesth Analg 66:154, 1987

90. De Felippe J, Timenor J, Velasco IT et al: Treatment of refractory hypovolemic shock by 7½% sodium chloride injections. Lancet 2:1002, 1980

91. Gross D, Landau EH, Klin B, Krausz MM: Treatment of uncontrolled hemorrhagic shock with hypertonic saline solution. Surg Gynecol Obstet 170:106, 1990

92. Twigley AJ, Hillman KM: The end of the crystalloid era? Anaesthesia 40:860, 1985

93. Virgilio RW, Rice CL: Crystalloid vs colloid resuscitation: Is one better? A randomized clinical study. Surgery 85:129, 1979

94. Gaffney PJ, Perry MJ: Unreliability of current serum fibrin degradation products (FDP) assays. Thromb Haemost 53:301, 1985

95. Miller RD: Complications of massive blood transfusions. Anesthesiology 39:82, 1973

96. Carpenter MA, Trunkey DD, Holcroft J: Ionized calcium and

magnesium in the baboon: Hemorrhagic shock and resuscitation. Circ Shock 5:163, 1978

97. Denlinger JK, Nahrwold ML, Gibbs PS *et al:* Hypocalcemia during rapid blood transfusion in anaesthetized man. Br J Anaesth 48:995, 1976

98. Kahn RC, Jascott D, Carlon GC *et al:* Massive blood replacement: correlation of ionized calcium, citrate and hydrogen ion concentration. Anesth & Analg 58:274, 1979

99. Reul GJ, Greenberg SD, Lefrak EA *et al:* Prevention of post-traumatic pulmonary insufficiency with fine screen filtration of blood. Arch Surg 106:386, 1973

100. Grindlinger GA, Vegas AM, Churchill WH *et al:* Is respiratory failure a consequence of blood transfusion? J Trauma 20:627, 1980

101. Graf H, Leach W, Arieff AI: Evidence for a detrimental effect of bicarbonate therapy in hypoxic lactic acidosis. Science 227:754, 1985

102. Cooper D, Walley K: Bicarbonate doesn't improve hemodynamics of critically ill patients who have lactic acidosis. Ann Intern Med 112:492, 1990

103. Wilson RF, Gibson D, Percinel AK *et al:* Severe alkalosis in critically ill surgical patients. Arch Surg 105:197, 1972

104. Russell WJ: A review of blood warmers for massive transfusion. Anaesth Intens Care 2:109, 1974

105. Priano LL, Solanki D: Operating room temperature. Anesth Analg 60:226, 1981

106. Mazze RI: Critical care of the patient with renal failure. Anesthesiology 47:138, 1977

107. Tenold R, Priano L, Kim K *et al:* Infection potential of nondisposable pressure transducers prepared prior to use. Crit Care Med 15:582, 1987

52

Jerrold H. Levy

The Allergic Response

The immune system represents a series of complex cellular and humoral elements that can interact with many different types of foreign molecular structures called antigens to provide host defense against foreign substances. These foreign substances (antigens) represent molecular configurations located on cells, bacteria, viruses, circulating proteins, or complex macromolecules. Immunologic mechanisms have two major characteristics: (1) they involve interaction of both antigens with antibodies and/or specific effector cells, and (2) they are reproducible when the subject is rechallenged with specific antigens. In addition, they are specific and adaptive, capable of distinguishing among a host of foreign substances and amplifying reactivity to produce a specific immunologic memory.

The immune system protects the body against external microorganisms and toxins and internal threats from neoplastic cells. The immune system can also respond inappropriately and cause *hypersensitive (allergic) reactions*. Life-threatening allergic reactions to drugs and other foreign substances observed perioperatively may represent different aspects of the immune response.[1,2] Therefore, basic immunologic principles are reviewed here to elucidate the complex interplay of cells and molecules.

BASIC IMMUNOLOGIC PRINCIPLES

Host defense systems of the immune organs are usually divided into cellular and humoral elements.[3] The humoral system includes the circulating protein antibodies, complement, and other serum proteins that provide host defense against most bacteria. Cellular immunity, on the other hand, is mediated by specific lymphocytes of the T-cell series and provides a host defense against intracellular organisms, viruses, fungi, and tumor cells. Lymphocytes are components of the cellular immune system. They have highly specific receptors that distinguish between antigens of normal host origin and those that are foreign. When lymphocytes react with foreign antigens, they respond to orchestrate immunosurveillance, regulate immunospecific antibody synthesis, and destroy foreign invaders. Individual aspects of the immune response and their importance are considered separately.

Antigens

Molecules capable of stimulating an immune response when injected (immunospecific antibody production or lymphocyte stimulation) are called *antigens*. The specificity of the immunologic response in producing antibodies directed against the chemical structure is an important characteristic.[4] A molecule's ability to act as an antigen to stimulate an immune response is called its immunogenicity, and antigens are often referred to as immunogens. Only a few drugs used by anesthesiologists, such as large polypeptides (chymopapain) and other large macromolecules (dextrans), are complete antigens (Table 52-1). Most commonly used drugs are simple organic compounds of low molecular weight, usually less than 1000 daltons. For such a small molecule to become immunogenic, it must form a stable bond with circulating albumin or tissue micromolecules to result in a complete antigen (hapten-macromolecular complex). Small molecular weight substances such as drugs or drug metabolites that bind to host proteins or cell membranes to sensitize patients are called *haptens*. Haptens are not antigenic by themselves. Often, a reactive drug metabolite (e.g., penicilloyl derivative of penicillin) is thought to bind with macromolecules to become antigens, but for most drugs this has not been proved.

Thymus-Derived Lymphocytes (T-Cell Lymphocytes)

The thymus of the fetus influences the differentiation of immature lymphocytes into thymus-derived cells (T cells). T cells are the most abundant type of circulating lymphocytes in the adult. On the surface of T cells are specific receptors that are activated by binding with foreign antigens. Once activated, these cells secrete specific mediators that regulate the immune response. The subpopulations of T cells that exist in man include helper, suppressor, cytotoxic, and killer cells.[5] The two types of regulatory T cells are helper cells (OKT4) and suppressor cells (OKT8). Helper cells are important for normal antibody production and for key effector cell response. Suppressor cells, on the other hand, retard both of these functions. For instance, the ac-

TABLE 52-1. Agents Administered During Anesthesia That Act as Antigens

Haptens	Macromolecules
Penicillin and its derivatives	Blood products
Anesthetic drugs(?)	Chymopapain
	Colloid volume expanders
—Protamine(?)—	

quired immunodeficiency syndrome (AIDS) that is produced by infection of helper T cells with a retrovirus known as the human immunodeficiency virus (HIV) (also known as human T-cell lymphotrophic virus Type III and the lymphadenopathy virus) produces a specific increase in the number of suppressor cells. Another important function of T cells is their destruction of foreign cells, including mycobacteria, fungi, and viruses, by cytotoxic T cells activated by antigen from these pathogens. Other lymphocytes, called natural killer cells, do not require specific antigen stimulation to initiate their function. Both the cytotoxic T cells and natural killer cells participate in defense against tumor cells as well as in the rejection of transplanted tissues. T cells produce a spectrum of mediators that influence the response of other cell types involved in the recognition and destruction of foreign substances. T cells activated by antigenic exposure synthesize molecules called lymphokines that regulate the immune response by (1) communicating with other lymphocytes (both T and B cells), (2) inducing inflammation and mononuclear cell infiltration, and (3) modulating phagocytic function.

Bursa-Derived Lymphocytes (B-Cell Lymphocytes)

B cells represent a specific lymphocyte cell line that, when activated, can differentiate into specific plasma cells that synthesize antibodies. The differentiation of B cells into plasma cells is controlled by both helper and suppressor T-cell lymphocytes.[5] B cells are also called bursa-derived cells because in birds the bursa of Fabricius is important in producing cells responsible for antibody synthesis.

Antibodies

Antibodies are specific proteins called immunoglobulins that can recognize and bind to a specific antigen.[6] The basic structure of the antibody molecule is illustrated in Figure 52-1. Each antibody has at least two heavy chains and two light chains that are bound together by disulfide bonds. The Fab fragment has the ability to bind antigen while the Fc or crystalizable fragment is responsible for the unique biologic properties of the different classes of immunoglobulins (cell binding and complement activation).

Antibodies function as specific receptor molecules located on different immune cell surfaces. When antigen binds covalently to the Fab fragment on the cell, the antibody undergoes conformational changes to activate the Fc receptor. The results of antigen-antibody binding depend on the cell type, which causes a specific type of activation (e.g., lymphocyte proliferation and differentiation into antibody-secreting cells, mast cell degranulation, and complement activation).

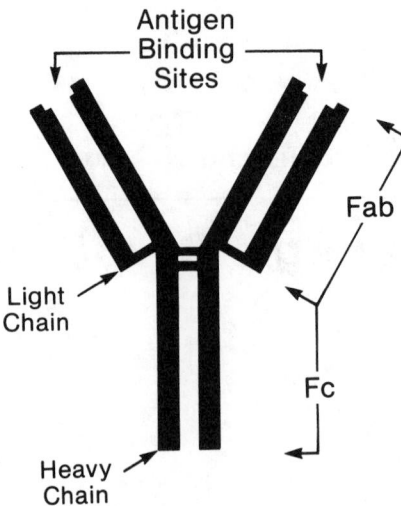

Figure 52-1. Basic structural configuration of the antibody molecule representing human immunoglobulin G (IgG). Immunoglobulins are composed of two heavy chains and two light chains bound by disulfide linkages (represented by *crossbars*). Papain cleaves the molecule into two Fab fragments and one Fc fragment. Antigen binding occurs on the Fab fragments, whereas the Fc segment is responsible for membrane binding or complement activation. (Reproduced with permission from Levy JH: Anaphylactic Reactions in Anesthesia and Intensive Care. Boston, Butterworths, 1986.)

Five major classes of antibodies occur in man: IgG, IgA, IgM, IgD, and IgE. The heavy chain determines the structure and the function of each molecule. The basic properties of each antibody are listed in Table 52-2.

Effector Cells and Proteins of the Immune Response

Monocytes, neutrophils (polymorphonuclear leukocytes, or PMNs), and eosinophils represent important effector cells that migrate into areas of inflammation in response to specific chemotactic factors, including lymphokines, bacterial products, and complement-derived mediators. Foreign organisms or cells are recognized specifically by circulating antibody to their component protein system. The deposition of antibody or complement fragments on the surface of foreign cells is called *opsonization*, a process that facilitates phagocytic ingestion. Subsequently, a series of metabolic processes is activated that enable the phagocytes to kill the foreign cell. In addition, lymphokines and other mediators released from lymphocytes produce chemotaxis of other inflammatory cells in a manner described in the following paragraphs. The role of each cell type in effecting the immune response is considered separately.

Monocytes and Macrophages

Macrophages play a central role not only in regulating immune responses by processing and presenting antigens to T-cell lymphocytes, but also in effecting inflammatory, tumoricidal, and microbicidal functions. Macrophages arise from circulating monocytes or may be confined to specific organs such as the lung. They are recruited and activated by lymphokines produced in response to microorganisms or other causes of tissue injury. Macrophages ingest antigens before they interact with receptors on the lymphocyte sur-

TABLE 52-2. Biologic Characteristics of Immunoglobulins

	IgG	IgM	IgA	IgE	IgD
Heavy chain	γ	μ	α	ε	δ
Molecular weight	160,000	900,000	170,000	188,000	184,000
Subclasses	1,2,3,4	1,2	1,2		
Serum concentration, mg·dl⁻¹	6–14	0.5–1.5	1–3	$< -.5 \times 10^3$	<0.1
Complement activation	All but IgG$_4$	+	–	–	–
Placental transfer	+	–	–	–	–
Serum half-life (days)	23	5	6	1–5	2–8
Cell binding	Mast cells (IgG$_4$) Neutrophils Lymphocytes Mononuclear cells Platelets	Lymphocytes		Mast cells Basophils Lymphocytes	Neutrophils Lymphocytes

Modified with permission from Levy J: Anaphylactic Reactions in Anesthesia and Intensive Care. Boston, Butterworths, 1986.

face to regulate their action. In addition, macrophages synthesize mediators to facilitate both B-cell and T-cell lymphocyte response. Macrophages and lymphocytes are the predominant cells at sites of chronic inflammation, and their interaction seems important for defense mechanisms.

Neutrophils

The first cells to appear in an acute inflammatory reaction are probably neutrophils (PMNs). These cells contain specific lysosomal granules that fuse with ingested material or are extruded into the extracellular environment. The granules contain a variety of enzymes, including acid hydrolases, neutral proteases, and lysosomes. In addition, activated neutrophils produce hydroxyl radicals, superoxide, and hydrogen peroxide that aid in microbial killing.

Eosinophils

The exact function of the eosinophil in host defense is unclear; however, these cells are associated with parasitic infections. Mast cells, basophils, and lymphocytes synthesize eosinophilic chemotactic factors to recruit eosinophils to accumulate at sites of parasitic infections, tumors, and allergic reactions. Eosinophils secrete enzymes such as arylsulfatase and histaminase that may limit the response of other inflammatory cells, including basophils and mast cells.[7]

Basophils

Basophils constitute less than 0.5–1% of circulating granulocytes in the blood.[7] On the surface of basophils are IgE receptors that release a spectrum of physiologically active mediators following activation. Basophils function similarly to mast cells but have the capacity for chemotactic migration in response to other stimuli.

Mast Cells

Mast cells are important mediators of immediate hypersensitivity responses. They are tissue fixed, located in the perivascular spaces of the skin, lung, and intestine.[7] Also on the surface of mast cells are IgE receptors that bind to specific antigens. Once activated, these cells release a spectrum of physiologically active mediators important to immediate hypersensitivity responses (see below, Anaphylactic Reactions: IgE Mediated).

Complement

The primary humoral response to antigen and antibody binding is activation of the complement system.[8] Analogous to the clotting cascade, the complement system consists of approximately 20 different proteins that bind to activated antibodies, other complement proteins, and cell membranes. The complement system is an important effector system of inflammation.

Two pathways activate the complement system, either with or without the aid of antibodies. Activation can be initiated by IgG or IgM binding to antigen, by plasmin through the classical pathway, by endotoxin, or by drugs through the alternate (properdin) pathway (Fig. 52-2).[8] Spe-

COMPLEMENT CASCADE

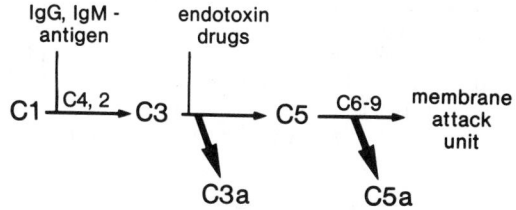

Figure 52-2. Diagram of complement activation. Complement system can be activated by either the classical pathway (IgG, IgM-antigen interaction) or the alternate pathway (endotoxin, drug interaction). Small peptide fragments of C3 and C5 called anaphylatoxins (C3a, C5a) released during activation are potent vasoactive mediators. Formation of the complete complement cascade produces a membrane attack unit that lyses cell walls and membranes. An inhibitor of the complement cascade, the C1 esterase inhibitor (C1 INH), ensures that the complement system is turned off most of the time.

cific fragments released during complement activation of the native complement proteins are important in host defense and hypersensitivity reactions. Breakdown products include C3a, C4a, C5a, which have important humoral and chemotactic properties (see below, Non-IgE-Mediated Reactions). The major function of the complement system is to recognize bacteria both directly and indirectly by the attraction of phagocytes (chemotaxis), as well as the increased adherence of phagocytes to antigens (opsonization), and cell lysis by activation of the complete cascade.

As with most biologic systems, a series of inhibitors regulate activation to ensure that the complement system is turned off most of the time. Hereditary (autosomal dominant) or acquired (associated with lymphoma, lymphosarcoma, chronic lymphatic leukemia, macroglobulinemia) angioneurotic edema is an example of a deficiency in an inhibitor of the C_1 complement system (C_1 esterase deficiency). This syndrome is characterized by recurrent increased vascular permeability of specific subcutaneous and serosal tissues (angioedema) producing laryngeal obstruction and respiratory and cardiovascular abnormalities following tissue trauma and surgery, or even without any obvious precipitating factor.[9]

Effects of Anesthesia on Immune Function

Exposure to both anesthesia and surgery depresses both T-cell and B-cell responsiveness as well as nonspecific host resistance mechanisms, including phagocytosis.[6] Various anesthetic drugs depress immune responses; however, the effects are short-lived and may be modified by multiple other factors occurring perioperatively. Immune competence during surgery can be affected by direct and hormonal effects of anesthetic drugs, by immunologic consequences of other drugs used, by the type of surgery, and by coincident infections. Although multiple studies demonstrate *in vitro* alterations of immune function, no studies have ever demonstrated the actual importance.[6] Furthermore, such alterations are likely of minor importance when compared with the hormonal aspects of stress responses.

HYPERSENSITIVITY RESPONSES (ALLERGY)

The scheme proposed in 1963 by Gell and Coombs for classifying immune responses still provides a useful basis for understanding specific diseases mediated by immunologic processes. The immune pathway functions as a protective mechanism but can also react inappropriately to produce a hypersensitivity or allergic response. The Gell and Coombs scheme defines four basic types of hypersensitivity, Types I through IV. It is useful first to review all four mechanisms to understand the different immune reactions that occur in man.

Type I Reactions

Type I reactions are also known as anaphylactic or immediate-type hypersensitivity reactions and are discussed in more detail in the following section (Fig. 52-3). They are produced by the release of physiologically active mediators released primarily from mast cells and basophils following specific antigen binding with IgE antibodies bound to the membranes of these cells. Clinically recognized Type I hy-

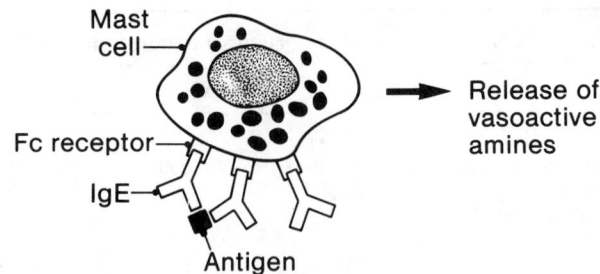

Figure 52-3. Type I immediate hypersensitivity reactions (anaphylaxis) involve IgE antibodies binding to mast cells or basophils by way of their Fc receptors. On encountering immunospecific antigens, the IgE becomes cross-linked, inducing degranulation, intracellular activation, and release of mediators. This reaction is independent of complement.

persensitivity reactions include anaphylaxis, extrinsic asthma, and allergic rhinitis.

Type II Reactions

Type II reactions are also known as antibody-dependent cytotoxic hypersensitivity or cytotoxic reactions (ADCC) (Fig. 52-4). These reactions are mediated by either IgG or IgM antibodies directed against antigens on the surface of foreign cells. These antigens may be either integral cell membrane components (A or B blood group antigens in ABO incompatibility reactions) or haptens that absorb to the surface of a cell, stimulating the production of antihapten antibodies (autoimmune hemolytic anemia). The actual damage in Type II reactions can be produced by different mechanisms, including (1) direct cell lysis following complete complement cascade activation, (2) increased phagocytosis by macrophages, or (3) killer T-cell lymphocytes producing ADCC effects. Systemic effects associated with Type II reactions are produced by release of complement anaphylatoxins. Common examples of Type II reactions in man are ABO-incompatible transfusion reactions, drug-induced im-

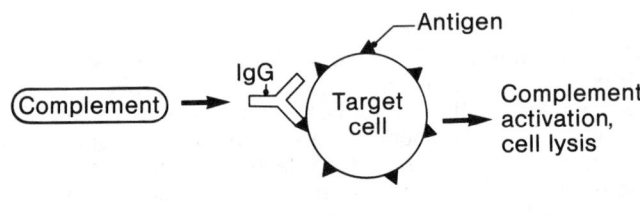

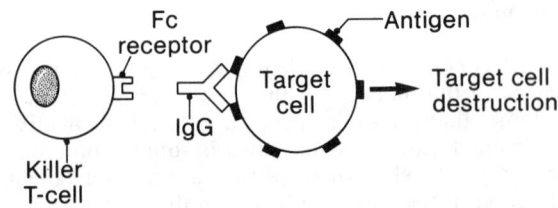

Figure 52-4. Type II or cytotoxic reactions. Antibody of an IgG or IgM class is directed against antigens on an individual's own cells (target cell). The antigens may be integral membrane components or foreign molecules that have been absorbed. This may lead to complement activation, including cell lysis (*upper figure*), or to cytotoxic action by killer T-cell lymphocytes (*lower figure*).

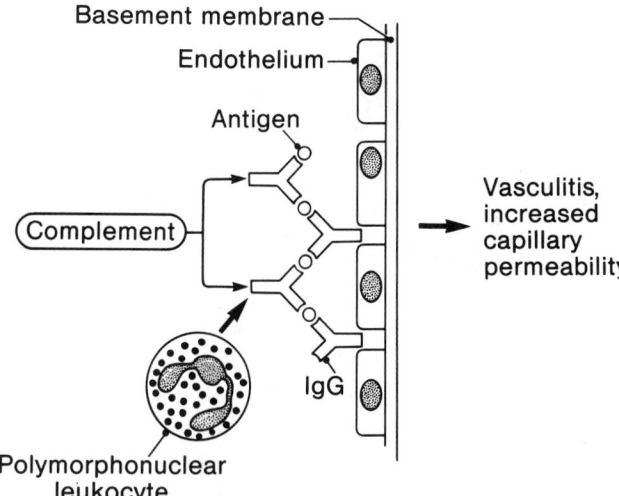

Figure 52-5. Type III immune complex reactions. Antibodies of an IgG or IgM type bind to the antigen in the soluble base and subsequently are deposited in the microvasculature. Complement is activated, resulting in chemotaxis and activation of polymorphonuclear leukocytes at the site of antigen-antibody complexes and subsequent tissue injury.

mune hemolytic anemia, and heparin-induced thrombocytopenia.

Type III Reactions (Immune Complex Reactions)

Type III reactions result from circulating soluble antigens and antibodies that bind to form insoluble complexes, which subsequently lodge in the microvasculature of different organ systems (Fig. 52-5). Complement is subsequently activated, producing leukocyte chemotaxis at the site of the inflammatory stimulus. The PMNs localized to the site of complement deposition release potent inflammatory mediators producing tissue damage. Examples of Type III reactions include classic serum sickness observed following snake antisera or antithymocyte globulin, and immune complex nephritis (post-streptococcal infections).

Type IV Reactions (Delayed Hypersensitivity Reaction, or Cell-Mediated Immunity)

Type IV reactions result following the interactions of sensitized lymphocytes to specific antigens (Fig. 52-6). The reactions result without complement or antibody involvement. Delayed hypersensitivity reactions are predominantly mononuclear in character and are slow to develop, first appearing in 18–24 hours, reaching a maximum in approximately 40–80 hours, and disappearing in 72–96 hours. The antigen binding to specific key lymphocytes produces lymphokine synthesis, lymphocyte proliferation, and generation of cytotoxic T cells. These activated lymphocytes stimulate the migration of macrophages and other mononuclear and polymorphonuclear leukocytes to the site of inflammatory stimulus. In addition, cytotoxic T cells are generated to specifically kill target cells that bear antigens identical to those that triggered the reaction. This form of immunity is important in tissue rejection, graft-vs.-host reactions, contact dermatitis (e.g., poison ivy), and tuberculin immunity.

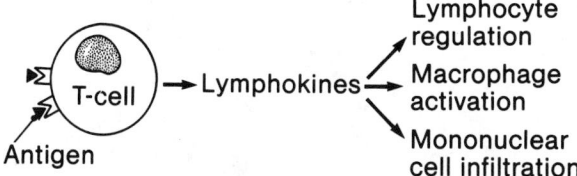

Figure 52-6. Type IV immune complex reactions (delayed hypersensitivity or cell-mediated immunity). Antigen binds to sensitized T-cell lymphocytes to release lymphokines following a second contact with the same antigen. This reaction is independent of circulating antibody or complement activation. Lymphokines induce inflammatory reactions and activate as well as attract macrophages and other mononuclear cells to produce delayed tissue injury.

INTRAOPERATIVE ALLERGIC REACTIONS

It is estimated that intraoperative allergic reactions occur once in every 5000–25000 anesthetics with a 3.4% mortality.[10,11] More than 90% of the allergic reactions evoked by drugs administered intravenously (iv) occur within 3 minutes of administration. In the anesthetized patient, the most common life-threatening manifestation of an allergic reaction is circulatory collapse, reflecting peripheral vasodilation with resulting decreased venous return (Table 52-3). In some anesthetized patients the only manifestation of an allergic reaction may be refractory hypotension.[12]

Portier and Richet first used the word anaphylaxis (ana—against, prophylaxis—protection) to describe the profound shock and subsequent death that sometimes occurred in dogs immediately following a second challenge

TABLE 52-3. Recognition of Anaphylaxis During Regional and General Anesthesia

Systems	Symptoms	Signs
Respiratory	Dyspnea Chest discomfort	Coughing Wheezing Sneezing Laryngeal edema Decreased pulmonary compliance Fulminant pulmonary edema Acute respiratory distress
Cardiovascular	Dizziness Malaise Retrosternal oppression	Disorientation Diaphoresis Loss of consciousness Hypotension Tachycardia Dysrhythmias Decreased systemic vascular resistance Cardiac arrest Pulmonary hypertension
Cutaneous	Itching Burning Tingling	Urticaria (hives) Flushing Periorbital edema Perioral edema

Reproduced with permission from Levy JH: Anaphylactic Reactions in Anesthesia and Intensive Care. Boston, Butterworths, 1986.

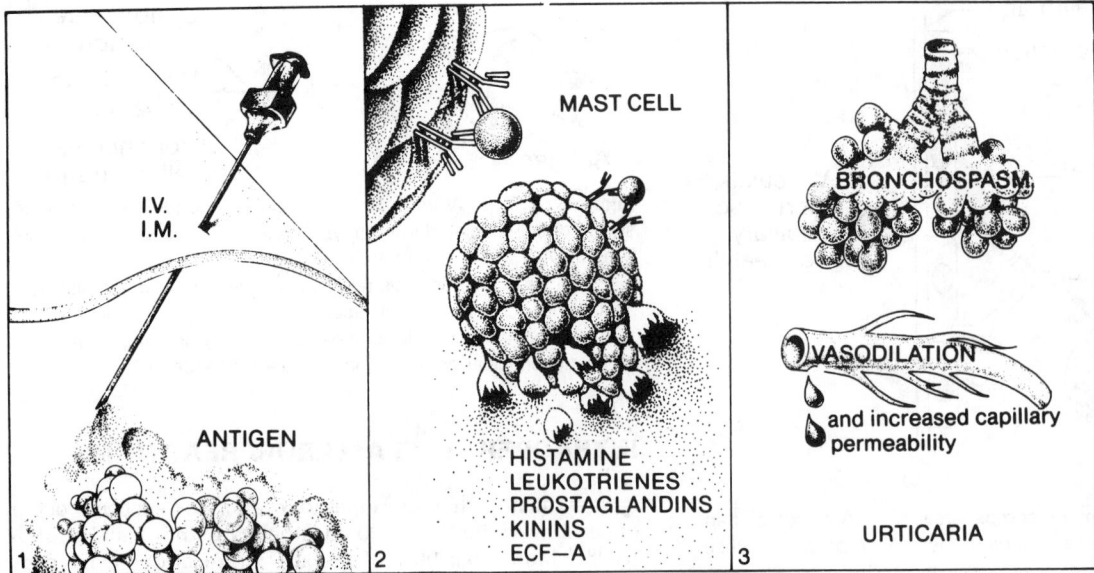

Figure 52-7. During anaphylaxis (Type I immediate hypersensitivity reaction), (*1*) antigen enters a patient during anesthesia through a parenteral route. (*2*) It bridges two IgE antibodies on the surface of mast cells or basophils. In a calcium- and energy-dependent process, cells release various substances—histamine, eosinophilic chemotactic factor of anaphylaxis, leukotrienes, prostaglandins, and kinins. (*3*) These released mediators produce the characteristic effects in the pulmonary, cardiovascular, and cutaneous systems. The most severe and life-threatening effects of the vasoactive mediators occur in the respiratory and cardiovascular systems. (Reproduced with permission from Levy JH: Identification and Treatment of Anaphylaxis: Mechanisms of Action and Strategies for Treatment Under General Anesthesia. Chicago, Smith Laboratories.)

with a foreign antigen.[13] When life-threatening allergic reactions mediated by antibodies occur, they are defined as "anaphylactic." When antibodies are not responsible for the reaction or when we are unable to prove antibody involvement in the reaction, the reaction is called *anaphylactoid*.[14] Anaphylactic or anaphylactoid reactions cannot be distinguished from one another on the basis of clinical observation.

Anaphylactic Reactions: IgE Mediated

Pathophysiology

Antigen binding to IgE antibodies initiates anaphylaxis (Fig. 52-7). Prior exposure to the antigen or to a substance of similar structure is required to produce sensitization, although an allergic history may be unknown to the patient. On re-exposure, binding of the antigen to bridge two immunospecific IgE antibodies located on the surfaces of mast cells and basophils liberates histamine and chemotactic factors of anaphylaxis.[15,16] These preformed mediators are released by a calcium- and energy-dependent process.[17] Other chemical mediators, including arachidonic acid metabolites (leukotrienes and prostaglandins) and kinins, subsequently are synthesized and released in response to cellular activation.[18] The liberated mediators produce a symptom complex of bronchospasm and upper airway edema in the respiratory system, vasodilation and increased capillary permeability in the cardiovascular system, and urticaria in the cutaneous system. Different mediators are released from mast cells and basophils following activation.

Chemical Mediators of Anaphylaxis

Histamine. Histamine, a beta-imidazolethylamine, stimulates H_1 and H_2 receptors. H_1 receptor activation causes increased capillary permeability, bronchoconstriction, and smooth muscle contraction.[19,20] H_2 receptor activation causes gastric secretion and inhibits mast cell activation.[19] Vasodilation results from stimulation of both H_1 and H_2 receptors. When injected into skin, histamine produces the classic wheal (increased capillary permeability producing tissue edema) and flare (cutaneous vasodilation) response in man (Fig. 52-8).[21] Histamine undergoes rapid metabolism in humans by the enzymes histamine N-methyltransferase and diamine oxidase located in endothelial cells.[1]

Chemotactic Factors of Anaphylaxis. Factors are released from mast cells and basophils that cause granulocyte migration (chemotaxis) and collection at the site of the inflammatory stimulus.[18] Eosinophilic chemotactic factor of anaphylaxis (ECF-A) is a small molecular weight peptide chemotactic for eosinophils.[22] Although the exact role of ECF-A or the eosinophil in the acute allergic response is unclear, eosinophils release enzymes that can inactivate histamine and leukotrienes.[18] In addition, a neutrophilic chemotactic factor is released that causes chemotaxis and activation.[18,23] Granulocyte activation may be responsible for recurrent manifestations of anaphylaxis.

Leukotrienes (Slow-Reacting Substance of Anaphylaxis). Various leukotrienes are synthesized following mast cell activation from arachidonic acid metabolism of phospholipid cell membranes via the lipoxygenase pathway.[24] The slow-reacting substance of anaphylaxis is a combination of leukotrienes C4, D4, and E4.[25] Leukotrienes produce bronchoconstriction, increased capillary permeability, vasodilation, coronary vasoconstriction, and myocardial depression.[25]

Prostaglandins. Prostaglandins are the products of arachidonic acid metabolism by way of the cyclo-oxygenase pathway.[25] Prostaglandins are potent mast cell mediators that produce vasodilation, bronchospasm, pulmonary hypertension, and increased capillary permeability.[18,25] Prostaglan-

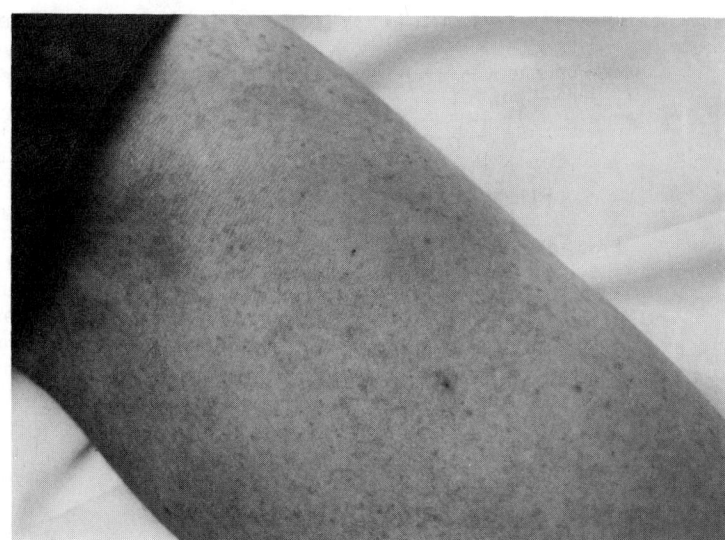

Figure 52-8. Histamine-induced wheal-and-flare response in man. The injection of a small dose of histamine, 10 μg, produces a profound wheal or localized tissue edema, caused by an increased capillary permeability, and a flare response, characterized by erythema due to cutaneous vasodilation. This patient demonstrated a profound wheal of 14 mm and a larger flare of 28 mm following the injection of 10 μg of histamine intradermally.

din D_2, the major metabolite of mast cells, produces bronchospasm and vasodilation.[25] Elevated plasma levels of thromboxane B_2 (the metabolite of thromboxane A_2), also a prostaglandin synthesized by mast cells as well as by PMNs, have been demonstrated following protamine reactions associated with pulmonary hypertension.[26,27]

Kinins. Small peptides called kinins are synthesized in mast cells and basophils to produce vasodilation, increased capillary permeability, and bronchoconstriction.[18,28]

Platelet-Activating Factor. Platelet-activating factor (PAF), an unstored lipid synthesized in activated human mast cells, is an extremely potent biologic material, producing physiologic effects at concentrations as low as 10^{-10} molar.[18] PAF aggregates and activates human platelets, and perhaps leukocytes, to release inflammatory products. PAF causes a profound wheal-and-flare response, smooth muscle contraction, and increased capillary permeability.[18]

Recognition of Anaphylaxis

The onset and severity of the reaction relate to the mediator's specific end-organ effects. Antigenic challenge in a sensitized individual usually produces immediate clinical manifestations of anaphylaxis, but the onset may be delayed 2–20 minutes.[29,30] The reaction may include some or all of the symptoms and signs listed in Table 52-3. Individuals vary greatly in their manifestations and course of anaphylaxis.[31,32] A spectrum of reactions exists, ranging from minor clinical changes to the full-blown syndrome leading to death.[31,33] The enigma of anaphylaxis lies in the unpredictability of occurrence, the severity of the attack, and the lack of a prior allergic history.

Non-IgE-Mediated Reactions

Other immunologic and nonimmunologic mechanisms liberate many of the mediators previously discussed independent of IgE, creating a clinical syndrome identical to anaphylaxis. Specific pathways important in producing the same spectrum of clinical manifestations are considered later.

Complement Activation

Complement activation follows both immunologic (antibody-mediated, *i.e.*, classic pathway) or nonimmunologic (alternative) pathways to include a series of multimolecular, self-assembling proteins that liberate biologically active complement fragments of C3 and C5.[10,34] C3a and C5a are called anaphylatoxins because they release histamine from mast cells and basophils, contract smooth muscle, and increase capillary permeability (Table 52-4). In addition, C5a interacts with specific high-affinity receptors on white blood cells and platelets, initiating leukocyte chemotaxis, aggregation, and activation.[35] Aggregated leukocytes embolize to various organs, producing microvascular occlusion and liberation of inflammatory products such as arachidonic acid metabolites, oxygen free radicals, and lysosomal enzymes (Fig. 52-9). Antibodies of the IgG class directed against antigenic determinants or granulocyte surfaces can also produce leukocyte aggregation.[36] These antibodies are called leukoagglutinins. Investigators have implicated complement activation and PMN aggregation in producing the clinical manifestations of transfusion reactions,[36,37] pulmonary vasoconstriction following protamine reactions,[27] adult respiratory distress syndrome,[36] and septic shock.[38]

Nonimmunologic Release of Histamine

Many diverse molecules administered during the perioperative period release histamine in a dose-dependent, nonimmunologic fashion (Table 52-5; Fig. 52-10).[39-43] The mechanisms involved in nonimmunologic histamine release

TABLE 52-4. Biologic Effects of Anaphylatoxins

Biologic Effects	C3a	C5a
Histamine release	+	+
Smooth muscle contraction	+	+
Increased vascular permeability	+	+
Chemotaxis		+
Leukocyte and platelet aggregation		+

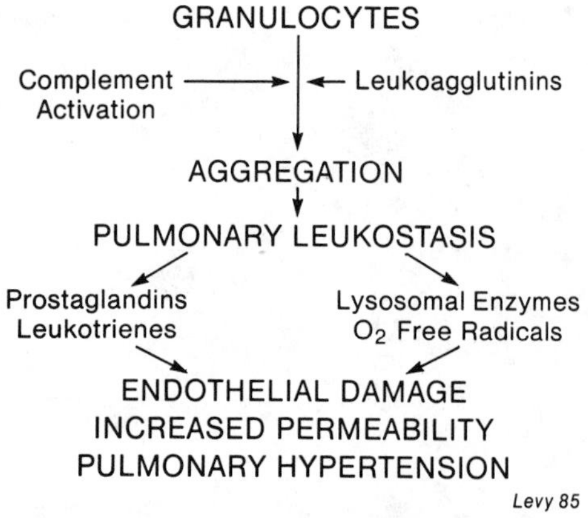

GRANULOCYTES

Complement ⟶ | ← Leukoagglutinins
Activation

AGGREGATION

PULMONARY LEUKOSTASIS

Prostaglandins   Lysosomal Enzymes
Leukotrienes   O₂ Free Radicals

ENDOTHELIAL DAMAGE
INCREASED PERMEABILITY
PULMONARY HYPERTENSION

Levy 85

Figure 52-9. Sequence of events producing granulocyte aggregation, pulmonary leukostasis, and cardiopulmonary dysfunction. (Reproduced with permission from Levy JH: Anaphylactic Reactions in Anesthesia and Intensive Care. Boston, Butterworths, 1986.

are not well understood but appear to represent noncytotoxic degranulation of mast cells but not basophils (Fig. 52-11).[43,44] A variety of endogenous neuropeptides can also release histamine from cutaneous mast cells. Human cutaneous mast cells are the only cell population that releases histamine in response to both exogenous and endogenous stimuli. Nonimmunologic histamine release is different from antigen- or anti-IgE-mediated histamine release because histamine alone, and not the other arachidonic acid and lipid mediators, is released (Fig. 52-12).[43,44] A number of different molecular structures release histamine in man, which suggests that different mechanisms are involved. Histamine release is not dependent on the mu receptor, as previously suggested, because fentanyl and sufentanil, the most potent mu receptor agonists clinically available, do not release histamine in human skin.[39] Although the newer muscle relaxants may be more potent at the neuromuscular junction, it appears that all drugs that are mast cell degranulators are equally capable of releasing histamine.[39,40] We have shown that on equimolar basis, atracurium is as potent as *d*-tubocurarine or metocurine in its ability to release histamine from human skin.[40]

Antihistamine pretreatment (*e.g.*, with H_1 blockers such as diphenhydramine or H_2 blockers such as cimetidine) prior to administration of drugs that are known to release histamine in man does not inhibit histamine release; rather, the antihistamine competes with histamine at the receptor and may attenuate decreases in systemic vascular resistance.[45] However, the effect of any drug on systemic vascular resistance may be dependent on other factors in addition to histamine release.[46,47]

TABLE 52-5. Drugs Capable of Nonimmunologic Histamine Release

---

Antibiotics (vancomycin, pentamidine)
Basic compounds
Hyperosmotic agents
Muscle relaxants (*d*-tubocurarine, metocurine, atracurium, miracurium, doxacurium)
Opioids (morphine, meperidine, codeine)
Thiobarbiturates

Treatment Plan

A plan for the treatment of anaphylactic or anaphylactoid reactions must be established before the event. Airway maintenance, 100% oxygen administration, intravascular volume expansion, and epinephrine are essential to treat the hypotension and hypoxia that result from vasodilation, increased capillary permeability, and bronchospasm.[1] Table 52-6 lists a protocol for the management of anaphylaxis during general anesthesia, with representative doses for a 70-kg adult. The treatment plan is the same for life-threatening anaphylactic or anaphylactoid reactions. Therapy must be titrated to desired effects with careful monitoring. Severe reactions require aggressive therapy and may be protracted, with persistent hypotension, pulmonary hypertension, lower respiratory obstruction, or laryngeal obstruction that may persist 5–32 hours despite vigorous therapy.[48] All patients who have experienced an anaphylactic reaction should be admitted to an intensive care unit for 24 hours of monitoring, as manifestations may recur following successful treatment.

Initial Therapy

Stop Administration of Antigen. In practice, this may not always be possible. Limiting antigen administration may prevent further recruitment of activated mast cells and basophils.

Maintain Airway and Administer 100% Oxygen. Profound ventilation-perfusion abnormalities producing hypoxemia can occur with anaphylactic reactions.[49] Always administer 100% oxygen along with ventilatory support as needed. Arterial blood gas values should be followed during resuscitation.

Discontinue All Anesthetic Drugs. Inhalational anesthetic drugs are not the bronchodilators of choice in treating bronchospasm following anaphylaxis, especially during hypotension. These drugs interfere with the body's compensatory response to cardiovascular collapse. Furthermore, halothane sensitizes the myocardium to catecholamines, which must be administered in severe reactions.

Provide Volume Expansion. Hypovolemia rapidly ensues during anaphylactic shock.[50] Fisher has reported an up to 40% loss of intravascular fluid into the interstitial space during reactions, as demonstrated by hemoconcentration.[50] Therefore, volume expansion is extremely important in conjunction with epinephrine in correcting the acute hypotension. Initially, 2–4 l of lactated Ringer's solution and/or colloid or normal saline should be administered, with the clinician keeping in mind that an additional 25–50 ml·kg⁻¹ may be necessary if hypotension persists. Refractory hypotension following volume and epinephrine administration requires additional hemodynamic monitoring, including pulmonary and radial arterial catheterization for accurate assessment of intravascular volume and to guide rational therapeutic interventions. Fulminant noncardiogenic pulmonary edema with loss of intravascular volume can occur following anaphylaxis. This condition requires intravascular volume repletion with careful hemodynamic monitoring until the capillary defect improves. Colloid volume expansion has not proved to be more effective than crystalloid volume expansion for treating anaphylactic shock.

Give Epinephrine. Epinephrine is the drug of choice when resuscitating patients during anaphylactic shock. Alpha-

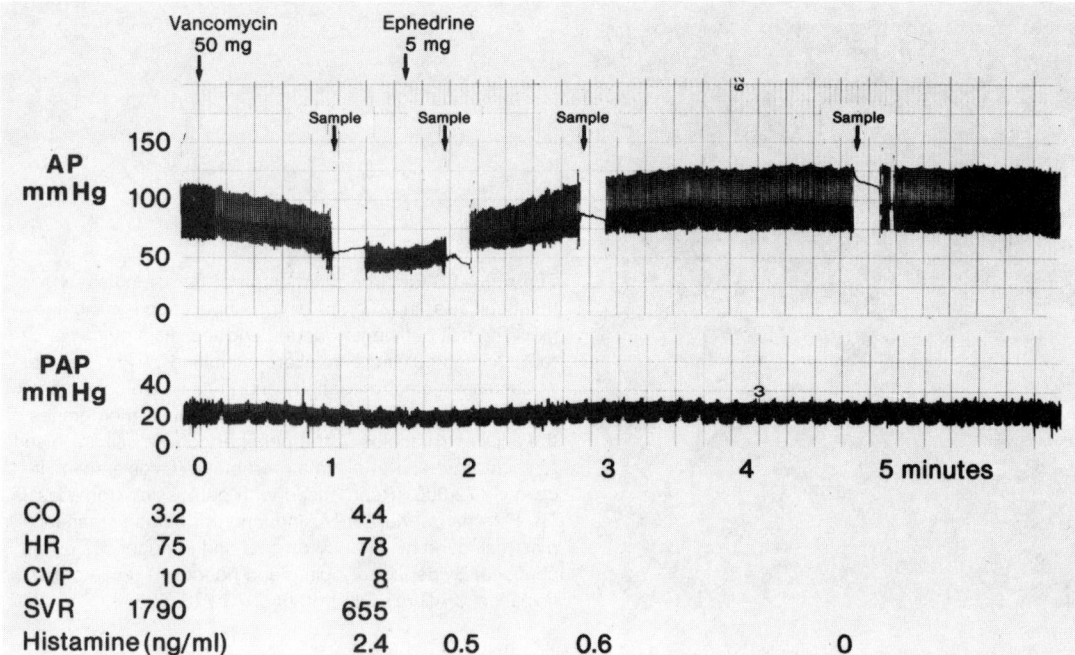

Figure 52-10. Example of an anaphylactoid reaction following rapid vancomycin administration in a patient. Hypotension is associated with an increased cardiac output and decreased calculated systemic vascular resistance. Plasma histamine levels 1 minute after the vancomycin administration were 2.4 ng·ml^{-1} and subsequently decreased to zero. The patient was given ephedrine, 5 mg, and blood pressure returned to baseline values. (Reproduced with permission from Levy JH, Kettlekamp N, Goertz P *et al:* Histamine release by vancomycin: A mechanism for hypotension in men. Anesthesiology 67:122, 1987.)

adrenergic effects vasoconstrict to reverse hypotension; beta$_2$ receptor stimulation bronchodilates and inhibits mediator release by increasing cyclic adenosine monophosphate (cAMP) in mast cells and basophils.[32] *The route of epinephrine administration and the dose depend on the patient's condition. Rapid and timely intervention is important when treating anaphylaxis.* Furthermore, patients under general anesthesia may have altered sympathoadrenergic responses to acute anaphylactic shock, whereas the patient under spinal or epidural anesthesia may be partially sympathectomized and may need even larger doses of catecholamines.[51]

In hypotensive patients, 5–10 μg boluses of epinephrine should be administered and incrementally titrated to restore blood pressure.* Additional volume and incrementally increased doses of epinephrine should be administered until hypotension is corrected. Although epinephrine infusion is an ideal method of administering epinephrine, it is usually impossible to infuse the drug through peripheral iv access lines during acute volume resuscitation. With cardiovascular collapse, full iv cardiopulmonary resuscitative doses of epinephrine, 0.1–1.0 mg, should be administered and repeated until hemodynamic stability resumes. Patients with laryngeal edema without hypotension should receive subcutaneous epinephrine. Epinephrine should not be administered iv to patients with normal blood pressures.[52]

Secondary Treatment

Antihistamines. Because H$_1$ receptors mediate many of the adverse effects of histamine, the iv administration of 0.5–1 mg·kg^{-1} of an H$_1$ antagonist such as diphendydramine may

*This dose of epinephrine can be obtained with 0.05–0.1 ml of a 1:10,000 dilution (100 μg·ml^{-1}) or by mixing 2 mg epinephrine with 250 ml of fluid to yield an 8 μg·ml^{-1} solution.

be useful in treating acute anaphylaxis. Antihistamines do not inhibit anaphylactic reactions or inhibit histamine release but compete with histamine at receptor sites. H$_1$ antagonists are indicated in all forms of anaphylaxis. The H$_1$ antagonists presently available for parenteral administration may have antidopaminergic effects and should be given slowly to prevent precipitous hypotension in potentially hypovolemic patients.[1] The indication for administering an H$_2$ antagonist once anaphylaxis has occurred remains unclear.

Catecholamines. Epinephrine infusions may be useful in patients with persistent hypotension or bronchospasm after initial resuscitation.[1] Epinephrine infusions should be started at 0.05–0.1 μg·kg^{-1}·min^{-1} (4–8 μg·min^{-1}) and titrated to correct hypotension.

Norepinephrine infusions may be needed in patients with refractory hypotension due to decreased systemic vascular resistance. It may be started at 0.05–0.1 μg·kg^{-1}·min^{-1} (4–8 μg·min^{-1}) and adjusted to correct hypotension.

Isoproterenol infusions can be used in patients with refractory bronchospasm, pulmonary hypertension, or right ventricular dysfunction. The usual starting dose is 0.01 to 0.02 μg·kg^{-1}·min^{-1} (0.5–1 μg·min^{-1}). Isoproterenol has profound beta$_2$-adrenergic effects that can produce systemic vasodilation; therefore, it must be used cautiously in hypotensive or hypovolemic patients.

Aminophylline. Aminophylline, a nonspecific phosphodiesterase inhibitor, bronchodilates and decreases histamine release from mast cells or basophils in part by increasing intracellular cAMP. In addition, it increases right and left ventricular contractility and decreases pulmonary vascular resistance. Aminophylline should be considered in patients with persistent bronchospasm and hemodynamic stability, although beta$_2$-specific adrenergic drugs are the first-line

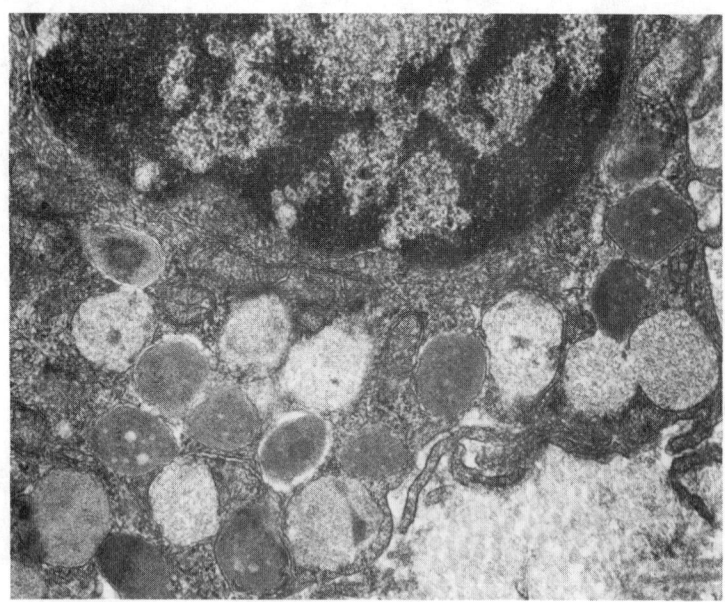

Figure 52-11. Electron micrograph of human cutaneous mast cell after injection of dynorphin, a kappa opioid agonist. The cell outline is rounded and the majority of the cytoplasmic granules are swollen, exhibiting varying degrees of decreased electron density and flocculence consistent with ongoing degranulation. The perigranular membranes of the adjacent granules at the periphery of the cell are fused to each other and to plasma membrane. Original magnification ×72,000. (Reproduced with permission from Casale TB, Bowman S, Kaliner M: Induction of human cutaneous mast cell degranulation by opiates and endogenous opioid peptides: Evidence for opiate and nonopiate receptor participation. J Allergy Clin Immunol 73:778, 1984.)

drugs of choice. An iv loading dose of 5–6 mg·kg^{-1} of aminophylline given over 20 minutes should be followed by an infusion of 0.5–0.9 mg·kg^{-1}·h^{-1}.

Corticosteroids. Indications for corticosteroid administration during anaphylaxis are not well defined. Experimental evidence suggests that they will decrease arachidonic acid metabolites by inducing synthesis of nuclear regulatory proteins to inhibit phospholipid membrane breakdown.[53] In addition, they may alter the activation and migration of other inflammatory cells (*i.e.*, PMNs) following an acute re-

action.[54] Corticosteroids may require 12–24 hours to work and, despite their unproven usefulness in treating acute reactions, they are often administered as adjuncts to therapy when refractory bronchospasm or refractory shock occurs following resuscitative therapy.[55] Although the exact corticosteroid dose and preparation are unclear, investigators have recommended 0.25–1 g of hydrocortisone in IgE-mediated reactions. Alternately, 1–2 g of methylprednisolone (30–35 mg·kg^{-1}) may be useful in reactions thought to be complement mediated, such as catastrophic pulmonary vasoconstriction following protamine transfusion reac-

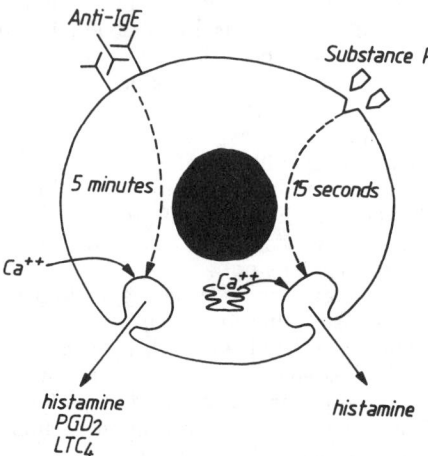

Figure 52-12. Different mechanisms of mediator release from human cutaneous mast cells stimulated immunologically by anti-IgE and by nonimmunologic stimuli with substance P. Anti-IgE stimulation, like antigen stimulation, initiates the release of histamine, PGD$_2$, and LTC$_4$ by a mechanism that takes 5 minutes to reach completion and requires the influx of extracellular calcium. Nonimmunologic activation with drugs or substance P releases histamine but not PGD$_2$ or LTC$_4$ by a mechanism that is complete within 15 seconds and uses calcium mobilized from intracellular sources. (Reproduced with permission from Caulfield JP *et al:* Dissociated human foreskin mast cells degranulate in response to anti-IgE and substance P. Lab Invest 63:502, 1990.)

TABLE 52-6. Management of Anaphylaxis During General Anesthesia

Initial Therapy

1. Stop administration of antigen
2. Maintain airway and administer 100% O$_2$
3. Discontinue all anesthetic agents
4. Start intravascular volume expansion (2–4 l of crystalloid/colloid with hypotension)
5. Give epinephrine (5–10 µg iv bolus with hypotension, titrate as needed; 0.1–1.0 mg iv with cardiovascular collapse)

Secondary Treatment

1. Antihistamines (0.5–1 mg·kg^{-1} diphenhydramine)
2. Catecholamine infusions (starting doses: epinephrine, 4–8 µg· min^{-1}; norepinephrine, 4–8 µg·min^{-1}; or isoproterenol, 0.5–1 µg·min^{-1} as a drip; titrated to desired effects)
3. Aminophylline (5–6 mg·kg^{-1} over 20 minutes with persistent bronchospasm)
4. Corticosteroids (0.25–1 g hydrocortisone; alternatively, 1–2 g methylprednisolone)*
5. Sodium bicarbonate (0.5–1 mEq·kg^{-1} with persistent hypotension or acidosis)
6. Airway evaluation (prior to extubation)

*Methylprednisolone may be the drug of choice if the reaction is suspected to be mediated by complement.

Reproduced with permission from Levy JH: Anaphylactic Reactions in Anesthesia and Intensive Care, p 104. Boston, Butterworths, 1986.

tions.[56] Administering corticosteroids after an anaphylactic reaction may also be important in attenuating the late-phase reactions reported to occur 12–24 hours after anaphylaxis.[48]

Bicarbonate. Acidosis develops rapidly in patients with persistent hypotension. This diminishes the effect of epinephrine on the heart and systemic vasculature. Therefore, with refractory hypotension or acidemia, sodium bicarbonate, 0.5–1 mEq·kg^{-1}, should be given and repeated every 5 minutes or as dictated by arterial blood gas valves.

Airway Evaluation. Because profound laryngeal edema may be the sequela of anaphylactic reactions, the airway should be evaluated before extubation of the trachea.[29] Persistent facial edema suggests airway edema. The trachea of these patients should remain intubated until the edema subsides. The development of a significant air leak after endotracheal tube cuff deflation and before extubation of the trachea is useful in assessing airway patency. If there is any question of airway edema, direct laryngoscopy should be performed before the trachea is extubated.

PERIOPERATIVE MANAGEMENT OF THE PATIENT WITH ALLERGIES

Allergic Drug Reactions

Allergic drug reactions account for 6–10% of all adverse reactions.[57] DeSwarte suggests that the risk of an allergic drug reaction occurring is approximately 1–3% for most drugs, and that approximately 5% of adults in the United States may be allergic to one or more drugs.[58] Unfortunately, patients often refer to adverse drug effects as being allergic in nature. For example, opioid administration can produce nausea, vomiting, or even local release of histamine along the vein of administration. Patients will say they are allergic to a specific drug when in fact their adverse reaction is independent of allergy. Approximately 15% of adults in the United States believe they are allergic to specific medication(s), and therefore may be denied treatment with an indicated drug. To understand allergic reactions, the spectrum of adverse reactions to drugs needs to be considered.

Predictable adverse drug reactions account for approximately 80% of adverse drug effects. They are often dose dependent and related to the known pharmacologic actions of the drug, and typically occur in otherwise normal patients. Most serious predictable adverse drug reactions are toxic and are directly related to the amount of drug in the body (overdosage) or to an inadvertent route of administration (e.g., lidocaine-induced seizures). Side-effects are the most common adverse drug reactions and are undesirable but often unavoidable pharmacologic actions of the drugs occurring at usual prescribed dosages. Most anesthetic drugs exhibit multiple side-effects that can produce precipitous hypotension. For example, morphine dilates the venous capacitance bed, thereby decreasing preload; releases histamine from cutaneous mast cells, thereby producing arterial and venodilation; slows the heart rate; and decreases sympathetic tone. However, the net effects of morphine on blood pressure and myocardial function depend on the patient's blood volume, sympathetic tone, and ventricular function. A volume-depleted trauma patient in pain who is given morphine rapidly develops hypotension. In addition, drug interactions represent important predictable adverse drug reactions. Intravenous fentanyl or sufentanil adminis-

tration to a patient who has just received iv benzodiazepines or other sedative-hypnotic drugs may produce precipitous hypotension that results from decreased sympathetic tone.[59] This represents a dose-dependent, predictable adverse drug reaction that is independent of allergy.

Unpredictable adverse drug reactions are usually dose-independent and usually not related to the drugs' pharmacologic actions, but are often related to the immunologic response (allergy) of the individual. On occasion, adverse reactions can be related to genetic differences (i.e., idiosyncratic) occurring in susceptible individuals who have an isolated genetic enzyme deficiency. The most common example of an idiosyncratic reaction is the hemolytic anemia that occurs in patients whose erythrocytes lack the enzyme glucose-6-phosphate dehydrogenase, when such patients are exposed to chloramphenicol, sulfonamides, or other oxidant drugs. Allergic reactions are also quantitatively aberrant and cannot be explained in terms of the normal pharmacology of the drug given in the usual therapeutic doses but are related to the individual's immune response.

In most allergic drug reactions an immunologic mechanism is present or, more often, presumed. Such a mechanism may be impossible to establish with most anesthetic drugs. Proving that the initiating event involves a reaction between the drug or drug metabolites with drug-specific antibodies or sensitized T lymphocytes is often costly and time-consuming, and may be inaccurate. Even in the absence of direct immunologic evidence, however, criteria are available that may be helpful in distinguishing an allergic reaction from other adverse reactions; these criteria are detailed below.

Allergic reactions occur in only a small percentage of patients receiving the drug. In addition, the observed clinical manifestations do not resemble known pharmacologic actions of the drug. In the absence of prior drug exposure, allergic symptoms rarely appear after less than 1 week of continuous treatment. Following sensitization, even years previously, the reaction will develop rapidly on re-exposure to the drug. In general, drugs that have been administered without complications for several months or longer are rarely responsible for producing drug allergy. The time span between exposure to the drug and noticed manifestations is often the most vital information in determining which drugs administered were the cause of a suspected allergic reaction.

Although the reaction may produce a life-threatening response in the cardiopulmonary system (anaphylaxis), a variety of cutaneous manifestations, fever, and pulmonary reactions have been attributed to drug hypersensitivity. Usually the reaction may be reproduced by very small doses of the suspected drug or other agents possessing similar or cross-reacting chemical structures. On occasion, drug-specific antibodies or lymphocytes have been identified that react with the suspected drug, although the relationship is seldom diagnostically useful in practice. Even when an immune response to a drug is demonstrated, it may not be associated with a clinical allergic reaction. As with adverse drug reactions in general, the reaction usually subsides within several days following discontinuation of the drug.

Immunologic Mechanisms of Drug Allergy

Different immunologic responses to any antigen can occur. Drugs have been associated with all of the immunologic mechanisms proposed by Gell and Coombs. Although more than one mechanism may contribute to a particular reaction,

Anesthetic Agents Implicated in Allergic Reactions

Induction agents (cremophor solubilized drugs, barbiturates, etomidate, propofol)
Local anesthetics (para-aminobenzoic ester agents)
Muscle relaxants (succinylcholine, gallamine, pancuronium, d-tubocurarine, metocurine, atracurium, vecuronium, mivacurium, doxacurium)
Opioids (meperidine, morphine, fentanyl)

Other Agents Implicated in Allergic Reactions

Antibiotics (cephalosporins, penicillin, vancomycin)
Blood products (whole blood, packed cells, fresh frozen plasma, platelets, cryoprecipitate)
Bone cement
Chymopapain
Cyclosporin
Drug additives
Mannitol
Methylmethacrylate
Protamine
Radiocontrast dye
Latex (natural rubber)
Vascular graft material
Colloid volume expanders (dextrans, protein fractions, albumin, hydroxyethyl starch)

Reproduced with permission from Levy JH: Anaphylactic Reactions in Anesthesia and Intensive Care. Boston, Butterworths, 1986.

any one can in fact occur. Penicillin may produce different reactions in different patients or a spectrum of reactions in the same patient. In one patient penicillin can produce anaphylaxis (Type I reaction), hemolytic anemia (Type II reaction), serum sickness (Type III reaction), and contact dermatitis (Type IV reaction).[58] Therefore, any one antigen has the ability to produce a diffuse spectrum of allergic responses in man. Why some patients develop localized rashes or angioneurotic edema in response to penicillin while others develop complete cardiopulmonary collapse is unknown.

Most anesthetic drugs and agents administered perioperatively have been reported to produce anaphylactic/anaphylactoid reactions (Table 52-7).[31,39-45,60-81] Muscle relaxants are the most common drugs responsible for evoking intraoperative allergic reactions.[67] In this regard, there is crosssensitivity between succinylcholine and the nondepolarizing muscle relaxants. Unexplained intraoperative cardiovascular collapse has been attributed to anaphylaxis triggered by latex (natural rubber).[68] Even vascular graft material has been reported as a cause of intraoperative allergic reactions.[69]

Life-threatening allergic reactions are more likely to occur in patients with a history of allergy, atopy, or asthma. Nevertheless, because the incidence is low, the history is not a reliable predictor that an allergic reaction will occur and does not mandate that such patients should be investigated or pretreated, or that specific drugs be selected or avoided.[60] Although different mechanisms have been proposed, no one hypothesis has been proved.[1] The drugs and foreign substances listed in Table 52-7 may have both immunologic and nonimmunologic mechanisms for adverse drug reactions in man.

EVALUATION OF PATIENTS WITH ALLERGIC REACTIONS

Identifying the drug responsible for a suspected allergic reaction still depends on circumstantial evidence indicating the temporal sequence of drug administration. Conventional *in vivo* and *in vitro* methods of diagnosing allergic reactions to most anesthetic drugs are unavailable or not applicable for supporting an allergic reaction. The most important factor in diagnosis is the awareness of the physician that an untoward event may be related to a drug that the patient received. The physician must always be aware of the ability of any drug to produce an allergic reaction. The history is extremely important when evaluating whether an adverse drug reaction is allergic and whether the drug can be readministered. Although a prior allergic reaction to the drug in question is important, this is rarely the case. Direct challenge of a patient with a test dose of drug is the only way to establish reaction, but this is potentially hazardous and not recommended. Although the anesthesiologist commonly administers small test doses of anesthetic drugs, these are pharmacologic test doses and have nothing to do with immunologic dosages.

The demonstration of drug-specific IgE antibodies is generally accepted as evidence that the patient may be at risk for anaphylaxis if the drug is administered.[58] Different clinical tests are available to confirm or diagnose drug allergy; several are considered below.

Testing for Allergy

Following an anaphylactoid reaction, it is important to identify the causative agent to prevent readministration. When one particular drug has been administered and there is a clear correlation between the time of administration and the occurrence of a reaction, testing may be unnecessary and general avoidance of the drug should occur. However, when patients have simultaneously received multiple drugs (e.g., an opioid, muscle relaxant, hypnotic, and antibiotic), it is often difficult to establish which particular drug caused the reaction. Furthermore, the reaction might have been caused by the vehicle or by one of the preservatives. For patients who desire to know which drug was responsible and for patients scheduled for subsequent procedures, some degree of allergy evaluation should be undertaken to evaluate the drug at risk. Unfortunately, very few *in vitro* tests exist for anesthetic drugs; therefore, the presently available allergy tests are discussed.

Leukocyte Histamine Release

Leukocyte histamine release simulates an *in vivo* anaphylactoid reaction by incubating the patient's own leukocytes with different concentrations of the offending drug and measuring histamine release as a marker for basophil activation. Similar to intradermal testing, a positive test identifies the causative agent, suggesting a potential IgE mechanism, but false positive results can occur.[31] However, in some instances it is possible to sensitize leukocytes from a nonallergic patient, then challenge them *in vitro* to determine whether the reaction is IgE-mediated. This test is not easy to perform and requires large quantities of fresh leukocytes and tedious isolation techniques. Modifications of this test allow the use of whole blood instead of isolated PMNs.[76,82]

Radioallergosorbent Test (RAST)

The RAST allows *in vitro* detection of specific IgE directed toward particular antigens.[83] In this test, antigens are linked to insoluble material such as cellulose or paper to make an immunoabsorbent.[83,84] When incubated with the serum in question, antibodies of different classes directed toward the antigen bind to it. After washing, the antigen-antibody complex on the immunoabsorbent is incubated with radiolabeled antibodies directed against human IgE. With the anti-IgE-bound human complex, the complex may be easily counted in a scintillation counter. A numerical value reflects the concentration of specific IgE in the patient's serum that is directed toward the allergen. The RAST uses a blood sample to give similar information as the skin test. The RAST is more quantitative than skin tests and avoids the potential of re-exposure to an antigen in a patient who previously had a life-threatening anaphylactic reaction.[84] Furthermore, it avoids the discomfort of skin testing. However, it is more expensive, and the antigens available for RASTs to anesthetic drugs are limited. RAST testing has been used to detect the presence of antibodies to meperidine,[49] succinylcholine,[85] and thiopental.[86] Two major limitations to this test include the commercial availability of the drug prepared as an antigen, and false positive test results in patients with elevated IgE levels.[87]

Enzyme-Linked Immunosorbent Assay (ELISA)

The ELISA measures antigen-specific antibodies. The basis of the ELISA is similar to the RAST; however, immunospecific IgE directed against the antigen in question is determined by the addition of an anti-IgE coupled to an enzyme such as peroxidase that acts as a chromogen.[5] A colorless substrate is acted on by peroxidase to produce a colored byproduct. The ELISA has been used to demonstrate IgE antibodies to chymopapain and protamine and has been developed to screen for other antibodies to diverse agents such as the human T-cell lymphotrophic virus Type III (the AIDS virus). At present, there are no clinically available ELISA tests for anesthetic drugs.

Intradermal Testing (Skin Testing)

Skin testing is the method generally used to confirm specific sensitivity in patients following anaphylactic reaction to anesthetic drugs after the history has suggested the relevant antigens for testing.[88,89] Within minutes after antigen introduction, histamine released from cutaneous mast cells causes vasodilation (flare) and localized edema from increased vascular permeability (wheal). Fisher suggests that this is a simple, safe, and useful method in establishing a diagnosis in most cases of anaphylactoid reactions occurring in the perioperative period.[67,88] If strict protocols established by Fisher are used, intradermal reactions can be very helpful.[88] Intradermal testing is of no value in reactions to contrast media or colloid volume expanders. Furthermore, cross-sensitivity between drugs of similar structures can often be evaluated on the basis of skin testing. Skin testing to local anesthetics is considered a direct challenge or provocative dose testing.[90] Local anesthetic drugs are injected in increasing quantities under controlled circumstances. This testing determines if the individual can safely receive amide derivatives (e.g., lidocaine) and can also be used to determine if the individual is sensitive to the paraaminobenzoic ester agents (e.g., procaine; Fig. 52-13).

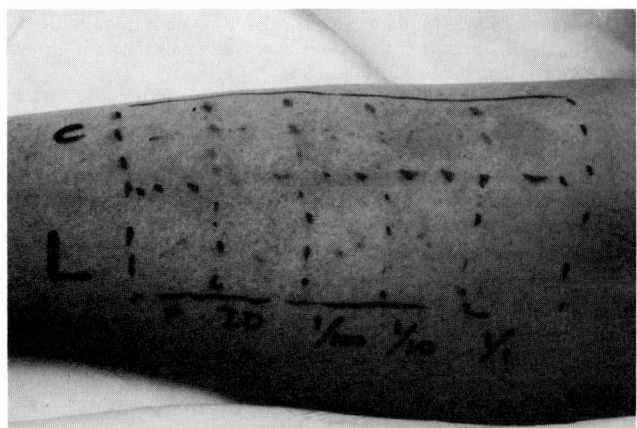

Figure 52-13. Skin testing in a man with a suspected history of a local anesthetic reaction. Skin testing is used to identify what agents a patient may be allergic to as well as what agents he may safely receive. C represents procaine and L lidocaine, tested without preservatives. The patient exhibited a positive wheal-and-flare response to procaine at a 1:10 dilution, but no response to lidocaine. (P = prick test, ID = intradermal; 1:100, 1:10, 1:1 = local anesthetic drug dilutions.)

SUMMARY

Although the immune system functions to provide host defense, it can respond inappropriately to produce hypersensitivity or allergic reactions. A spectrum of life-threatening allergic reactions to any drug or agent can occur in the perioperative period. The enigma of these reactions lies in their unpredictable nature. However, a high index of suspicion, prompt recognition, and appropriate and aggressive therapy can help to avoid a disastrous outcome.

REFERENCES

1. Levy J: Anaphylactic Reactions in Anesthesia and Intensive Care. Boston, Butterworths, 1986
2. Watkins J: Hypersensitivity response to drugs and plasma substitutes used in anesthesia and surgery. In Watkins J, Salo M (eds): Trauma, Stress and Immunity in Anaesthesia and Surgery, p 254. London, Butterworth & Co, 1982
3. Gell PGH, Coombs RRA, Lachmann PJ (eds): Clinical aspects of Immunology, 3rd ed. Oxford, Blackwell Scientific Publications, 1975
4. Butler VP Jr, Beiser SM: Antibodies to small molecules: Biologic and clinical applications. Adv Immunol 17:255, 1973
5. Roitt I, Brostoff J, Male D (eds): Immunology. St. Louis, CV Mosby, 1985
6. Stevenson GW, Hall SC, Rudnick S et al: The effects of anesthetic agents on the human immune response. Anesthesiology 72:144, 1990
7. Metcalf DD: Effector cell heterogeneity in immediate hypersensitivity reactions. Clin Rev Allergy 1:311, 1982
8. Frank MM: Complement: A brief review. J Allergy Clin Immunol 84:411, 1988
9. Wall RT, Frank M, Hahn M: A review of 25 patients with hereditary angioedema requiring surgery. Anesthesiology 71:309, 1989
10. Fisher MMcD, More DG: The epidemiology and clinical features of anaphylactic reactions in anaesthesia. Anaesth Intensive Care 9:226, 1981
11. Weiss ME, Adkinson NF, Hirshman CA: Evaluation of allergic reactions in the perioperative period. Anesthesiology 71:438, 1989

12. Laxenaire MC, Moneret-Vautrin DA, Boileau S, Moeller R: Adverse reactions to intravenous agents in anaesthesia in France. Klin Wochenschr 60:1006, 1982
13. Portier MM, Richet C: De l'action anaphylactique de certains venins. C R Soc Biol 54:170, 1902
14. Watkins J: Anaphylactoid reactions to I.V. substances. Br J Anaesth 51:51, 1979
15. Ishizaka T: Analysis of triggering events in mast cells for immunoglobulin E-mediated histamine release. J Allergy Clin Immunol 67:90, 1981
16. Kazimierczak W, Diamant B: Mechanisms of histamine release in anaphylactic and anaphylactoid reactions. Prog Allergy 4:295, 1978
17. Winslow CM, Austen KF: Enzymatic regulation of mast cell activation and secretion by adenylate cyclase and cyclic AMP-dependent protein kinases. Fed Proc 41:22, 1982
18. Wasserman SI: Mediators of immediate hypersensitivity. J Allergy Clin Immunol 72:101, 1983
19. Reinhardt D, Borchard V: H_1 receptor antagonists: Comparative pharmacology and clinical use. Klin Wochenschr 60:983, 1982
20. Ginsburg R, Bristow MR, Stinson EB et al: Histamine receptors in the human heart. Life Sci 26:2245, 1980
21. Majno G, Palade GE: Studies on inflammation: I. The effect of histamine and serotonin on vascular permeability. An electron microscopic study. J Biophys Biochem Cytol 11:571, 1961
22. Wasserman SI, Goetzl EJ, Austen KF: Preformed eosinophil chemotactic factor of anaphylaxis (ECF-A). J Immunol 112:351, 1974
23. Mathe AA, Hedqvist P, Strandberg K et al: Aspects of prostaglandin function in the lung. N Engl J Med 296:850, 910, 1977
24. Parker CW: Leukotrienes: Their metabolism, structure, and role in allergic responses. In Samuelsson B, Paoletti R (eds): Leukotrienes and Other Lipoxygenase Products, pp 115–126. New York, Raven Press, 1982
25. Stenson WF, Parker CW: Metabolites of arachidonic acid. Clin Rev Allergy 1:369, 1983
26. Schulman ES, Newball HH, Demers LM et al: Anaphylactic release of thromboxane A_2, prostaglandin D_2, and prostacyclin from human lung parenchyma. Am Rev Respir Dis 124:402, 1981
27. Morel DR, Zapol WM, Thomas SJ et al: C5a and thromboxane generation associated with pulmonary vaso- and bronchoconstriction during protamine reversal of heparin. Anesthesiology 66:597, 1987
28. Meier HL, Kaplan AP, Lichtenstein LM et al: Anaphylactic release of a prekallikrein activator from human lung in vitro. J Clin Invest 72:574, 1983
29. Delage C, Irey NS: Anaphylactic deaths: A clinicopathologic study of 43 cases. J Forensic Sci 17:525, 1972
30. Smith Laboratories: Chymodiactin post marketing surveillance report, 1984
31. Laxenaire MC, Moneret-Vautrin DA, Vervloet D et al: Accidents anaphylactoides graves peranesthesiques. Ann Fr Anesth Reanim 4:30, 1985
32. Kelly JF, Patterson R: Anaphylaxis: Course, mechanisms and treatment. JAMA 227:1431, 1974
33. Pavek K, Wegmann A, Nordström L et al: Cardiovascular and respiratory mechanisms in anaphylactic and anaphylactoid shock reactions. Klin Wochenschr 60:941, 1982
34. Atkinson JP, Frank MM: Role of complement in the pathophysiology of hematologic disease. Prog Hematol 10:211, 1977
35. Jacob HS, Craddock PR, Hammerschmidt DE et al: Complement-induced granulocyte aggregation: An unsuspected mechanism of disease. N Engl J Med 302:789, 1980
36. Dubois M, Lotze MT, Diamond WI et al: Pulmonary shunting during leukoagglutinin-induced noncardiogenic pulmonary edema. JAMA 244:2186, 1980
37. Teissner B, Brandslund I, Grunnet N et al: Acute complement activation during an anaphylactoid reaction to blood transfusion and the disappearance rate of C3c and C3d from the circulation. J Clin Lab Immunol 12:63, 1983
38. Hammerschmidt DE, Weaver LJ, Hudson LD et al: Association of complement activation and elevated plasma-C5a with adult respiratory distress syndrome. Lancet 1:947, 1980
39. Levy JH, Brister NW, Shearin A et al: Wheal and flare responses to opioids in humans. Anesthesiology 70:756, 1989
40. Levy JH, Adelson DM, Walker BF: Wheal and flare responses to muscle relaxants in humans. Agents Actions, in press
41. Hirshman CA, Edelstein RA, Eastman CL: Histamine release by barbiturates in human mast cells. Anesthesiology 63:353, 1985
42. Levy JH, Kettlekamp N, Goertz P et al: Histamine release by vancomycin: A mechanism for hypotension in man. Anesthesiology 67:122, 1987
43. Caulfield JP, El-Lati S, Thomas G, Church MK: Dissociated human foreskin mast cells degranulate in response to anti-IgE and substance P. Lab Invest 63:502, 1990
44. Casale TB, Bowman S, Kaliner M: Induction of human cutaneous mast cell degranulation by opiates and endogenous opioid peptides: Evidence for opiate and nonopiate receptor participation. J Allergy Clin Immunol 73:775, 1984
45. Philbin DM, Moss J, Akins CW et al: The use of H_1 and H_2 histamine antagonists with morphine anesthesia: A double-blind study. Anesthesiology 55:292, 1981
46. Levy JH, Hug CC: Cardiopulmonary bypass as a model to study the effects of drugs on myocardial function. Br J Anaesth 60:35S, 1988
47. Hirshman CA, Downes H, Butler J: Relevance of plasma histamine levels to hypotension. Anesthesiology 57:424, 425, 1982
48. Stark BJ, Sullivan TJ: Biphasic and protracted anaphylaxis. J Allergy Clin Immunol 78:76, 1986
49. Levy JH, Rockoff MR: Anaphylaxis to meperidine. Anesth Analg 61:301, 1982
50. Fisher MM: Blood volume replacement in acute anaphylactic cardiovascular collapse related to anaesthesia. Br J Anaesth 49:1023, 1977
51. Barnett A, Hirshman CA: Anaphylactic reaction to cephapirin during spinal anesthesia. Anesth Analg 58:337,1979
52. Levy JH: Anaphylactic/anaphylactoid reactions during cardiac surgery. J Clin Anesthesiol 1:426, 1989
53. Austen KF: Tissue mast cells in immediate hypersensitivity. Hosp Pract 17:98, 1981
54. Hammerschmidt DE, White JG, Craddock PR et al: Corticosteroids inhibit complement-induced granulocyte aggregation: A possible mechanism for their efficacy in shock states. J Clin Invest 63:798, 1979
55. Halevy S, Altura BM: Pathophysiological basis for the use of steroids in the treatment of shock and trauma. Klin Wochenschr 60:1021, 1982
56. Sheagren JN: Septic shock and corticosteroids. (editorial). N Engl J Med 305:456, 1981
57. Borda IT, Slone D, Jick H: Assessment of adverse reactions within a drug surveillance program. JAMA 205:645, 1968
58. DeSwarte RD: Drug allergy: Problems and strategies. J Allergy Clin Immunol 74:209, 1984
59. Tomicheck RC, Rosow CG, Philbin DM et al: Diazepam-fentanyl interaction: Hemodynamic and hormonal effect in coronary artery surgery. Anesth Analg 62:881, 1983
60. Fisher M McD, Outhred A, Bowey CJ: Can clinical anaphylaxis to anaesthetic drugs be predicted from allergic history? Br J Anaesth 59:690, 1987
61. Christman D: Immune reaction to propanidid. Anaesthesia 39:470, 1984
62. Watkins J, Clarke SJ: Report of a symposium: Adverse responses to intravenous agents. Br J Anaesth 50:1159, 1978
63. Driggs RL, O'Day RA: Acute allergic reaction associated with methohexital anaesthesia: Report of six cases. J Oral Surg 30:906, 1972
64. Watkins J, Salo M: Incidence of immediate adverse response to intravenous anaesthetic drugs. In Trauma, Stress and Immunity in Anaesthesia and Surgery, p 272. London, Butterworth & Co, 1982
65. Schwartz HJ, Sher TH: Bisulfite sensitivity manifesting as allergy to local dental anaesthesia. J Allergy Clin Immunol 75:525, 1985
66. Brown DT, Beamins D, Wildsmith JAW: Allergic reaction to an amide local anesthetic. Br J Anaesth 53:435, 1981
67. Fisher M McD, Munro I: Life-threatening anaphylactoid reactions to muscle relaxants. Anesth Analg 62:559, 1983

68. Swartz J, Braude BM, Gilmour RF et al: Intraoperative anaphylaxis to latex. Can J Anaesth 37:589, 1990

69. Roizen MF, Rodgers GM, Valone FH et al: Anaphylactoid reactions to vascular graft material presenting with vasodilation and subsequent disseminated intravascular coagulation. Anesthesiology 71:331, 1989

70. Laxenaire MC, Moneret-Vautrin DA, Watkins J: Diagnosis of the causes of anaphylactoid anaesthetic reactions. Anaesthesia 38:147, 1983

71. Vervloet D, Nizankowska E, Arnaud A et al: Adverse reactions to suxamethonium and other muscle relaxants under general anesthesia. J Allergy Clin Immunol 71:552, 1983

72. Harle DG, Baldo BA, Fisher MM: Detection of IgE antibodies to suxamethonium after anaphylactoid reactions during anaesthesia. Lancet 1:930, 1984

73. Zucker-Pinchoff B, Ramanathan S: Anaphylactic reaction to epidural fentanyl. Anesthesiology 71:599, 1989

74. Hilgard P: Immunological reactions to blood and blood products. Br J Anesth 51:45, 1979

75. Sheffer AL, Pennoyer DS: Management of adverse drug reactions. J Allergy Clin Immunol 74:580, 1984

76. Levy JH, Zaidan JR, Faraj B: Prospective evaluation of risk of protamine reactions in NPH insulin-dependent diabetics. Anesth Analg 65:739, 1986

77. Levy JH, Schwieger IM, Zaidan JR et al: Evaluation of patients at risk for protamine reactions. J Thorac Cardiovasc Surg 98:200, 1989

78. Goldberg M: Systemic reactions to intravascular contrast media: A guide for the anesthesiologist. Anesthesiology 60:46, 1984

79. Isbister JP, Fisher M McD: Adverse effects of plasma volume expanders. Anaesth Intensive Care 8:145, 1980

80. Colman WR: Paradoxical hypotension after volume expansion with plasma protein fraction. N Engl J Med 299:97, 1978

81. Ring K, Messmer K: Incidence and severity of anaphylactoid reactions to colloid volume substitutes. Lancet 1:466, 1977

82. Grant JA, Cooper JR, Arens JF et al: Anaphylactic reactions to protamine in insulin-dependent diabetics during cardiovascular surgery. Anesthesiology 59:A74, 1983

83. Berg TLO, Johansson SGO: Allergy diagnosis with the radioallergosorbent test: A comparison with the results of skin and provocation tests in an unselected group of children with asthma and hay fever. J Allergy Clin Immunol 54:209, 1974

84. Johansson SGO: In vitro diagnosis of reagin-mediated allergic diseases. Allergy 33:292, 1978

85. Baldo BA, Fisher MM: Detection of serum IgE antibodies that react with alcuronium and tubocurarine after life-threatening reactions to muscle relaxants. Anaesth Intensive Care 11:194, 1983

86. Harle DG, Baldo BA, Smal MA et al: Detection of thiopentone-reactive IgE antibodies following anaphylactoid reactions during anesthesia. Clin Allergy 16:493, 1986

87. Dueck R, O'Connor RD: Thiopental: False positive RAST in patient with elevated serum IgE. Anesthesiology 61:337, 1984

88. Fisher MM: Intradermal testing after anaphylactoid reaction to anaesthetic drugs: Practical aspects of performance and interpretation. Anaesth Intensive Care 12:115, 1984

89. Sage D: Intradermal drug testing following anaphylactoid reactions during anesthesia. Anaesth Intensive Care 9:381, 1981

90. Shatz M: Skin testing and incremental challenge in the evaluation of adverse reactions to local anesthetics. J Allergy Clin Immunol 74:606, 1984

53

Christine S. Rinder

Cancer Therapy and Its Anesthetic Implications

Cancer therapy has evolved dramatically over the last four decades. Combination chemotherapy, surgery, and radiotherapy are now coordinated in complex treatments for malignancy, with increasing success. Newer modalities such as biologic therapy hold promise for the future, and therapies such as bone marrow transplantation are now becoming widely instituted. These advances, coupled with the increasing number of patients who survive longer or are cured of their disease, ensure that cancer patients will present for surgery with increasing frequency. Anesthesiologists will not only be asked to manage patients currently undergoing therapy for cancer but also to manage those manifesting early or late toxicities associated with their treatment. This chapter offers a review of the major complications of chemotherapy, radiation therapy, and cancer issues of special concern to the anesthesiologist. Some of the newer treatment modalities whose toxicities are still evolving are also introduced. The major classes of chemotherapeutic agents are shown in Table 53-1, along with some of the more widely used drugs.

PULMONARY COMPLICATIONS

Overview

The relationship between chemotherapeutic agents and pulmonary damage is often difficult to conclusively demonstrate. Frequently, patients receive a regimen of several antineoplastic agents with potential for lung toxicity, as well as radiation therapy. In addition, they may have lung infiltrates that may be infectious or neoplastic. The evaluation of these patients as possible surgical candidates requires knowledge of the specific chemotherapeutic agents and the effects of their cumulative doses.

Currently, 19 different chemotherapeutic agents in routine use have been linked to pulmonary syndromes.[1] Proposed cytotoxic mechanisms common to many of these agents are summarized here, and more specific toxicities are reviewed as the different agents are discussed below (Table 53-2).

Some cytotoxic agents may produce pulmonary injury by altering the balance between the formation of reactive oxygen metabolites such as the superoxide anion (O_2^-), hydro-

gen peroxide (H_2O_2), the hydroxyl radical (OH·) and their antioxidant systems.[2] High concentrations of these oxidant species may induce pulmonary damage by participating in redox reactions and fatty acid oxidation, ultimately producing membrane disruption. Agents such as carmustine and cyclophosphamide reduce glutathione stores, thereby limiting the body's antioxidant defenses.[3] Other agents, such as bleomycin,[4] have been demonstrated to produce chemotactic substances, promoting polymorphonuclear leukocyte and monocyte infiltration of lung parenchyma. These cells have the potential to amplify pulmonary injury by release of their oxidant species and their proteolytic enzymes such as elastase.

Risk factors predisposing to the development of pulmonary toxicity vary for the different agents but include total dose, patient age, prior or concomitant radiation therapy, oxygen exposure, other cytotoxic medications, and prior pulmonary disease. Table 53-3 shows these risk factors and the drugs with which they have been implicated. For many of these agents, however, the incidence of toxicity is such that large studies would be necessary to reliably identify their risk factors.

Clinical Syndromes

In general, the pulmonary syndromes developing after exposure to these drugs fall into three major categories. The clinical syndrome most frequently associated with chemotherapeutic agents is a chronic pneumonitis and progressive pulmonary fibrosis. This picture has been seen with virtually all classes of agents listed in Table 53-1, although it is atypical for some groups such as the antimetabolites. Symptoms include progressive dyspnea on exertion, a nonproductive cough, and fatigue developing over weeks to months. The radiographic picture is nonspecific and may primarily reflect either the underlying neoplastic process or infection. Although no test is 100% predictive, pulmonary function tests may be useful. The single breath carbon monoxide diffusion capacity (DL_{CO}) is considered to be the most sensitive indicator of early pulmonary fibrosis induced by a variety of antineoplastic agents such as bleomycin.[5] A progressive fall in DL_{CO} during therapy with bleomycin may antedate the development of arterial hypoxemia and symp-

TABLE 53-1. Classes of Chemotherapeutic Agents and Immunotherapeutic Agents

Class of Compound	Type of Agent	Nonproprietary Names
Alkylating agents	Nitrogen mustards	Mechlorethamine
		Cyclophosphamide
		Melphalan
		Uracil mustard
		Chlorambucil
	Ethylenimine derivatives	Thiotepa
	Alkyl sulfonates	Busulfan
	Nitrosoureas	Carmustine (BCNU)
		Lomustine (CCNU)
		Semustine (Methyl CCNU)
		Streptozocin
	Triazenes	Dacarbazine
Antimetabolites	Folic acid analogues	Methotrexate
	Pyrimidine analogues	Fluorouracil
		Cytarabine (cytosine arabinoside)
	Purine analogues	Mercaptopurine
		Thioguanine
Natural products	Vinca alkaloids	Vinblastine
		Vincristine
	Antibiotics	Dactinomycin
		Daunorubicin
		Doxorubicin (Adriamycin)
		Bleomycin
		Mithramycin
		Mitomycin C
	Enzymes	L-Asparaginase
Miscellaneous agents	Substituted urea	Hydroxyurea
	Methyl hydrazine derivative	Procarbazine
	Adrenocortical suppressant	Mitotane
	Cisplatinum	Cisplatinum
Hormones	Adrenocorticosteroids	Prednisone
	Progestins	Hydroxyprogesterone caproate (Dalalutin)
		Medroprogesterone acetate
		Megestrol acetate (Provera)
	Estrogens	Diethylstilbestrol
		Ethinyl estradiol (Estinyl)
	Androgens	Testosterone propionate
		Fluoxymesterone (Halotestin)
Immunotherapy		Vaccines from BCG (bacille Calmette-Guérin)
		Vaccines from *Corynebacterium parvum*

Reprinted with permission from Chung F: Cancer, chemotherapy, and anaesthesia. Can Anaesth Soc J 29:365, 1982.

toms of dyspnea. Spirometry may show a pattern typical for restrictive lung disease, including decreases in forced vital capacity.

A second syndrome often associated with antineoplastic agents is an acute hypersensitivity reaction.[6] In most cases, this is an IgE-mediated reaction in which the drug appears to directly degranulate mast cells. Some agents may stimulate the alternative complement activation pathway, resulting in release of vasoactive substances. Symptoms include dyspnea, a nonproductive cough, and a peripheral eosinophilia. More severe reactions typically are manifested by wheezing, fevers, and possibly hypotension. Treatment includes corticosteroid treatment and discontinuation of the offending agent.

A third entity, noncardiogenic pulmonary edema, is a relatively rare occurrence after administration of methotrexate, cyclophosphamide, cytosine arabinoside, and teniposide (VM-26).[1] Its clinical symptoms and treatment are identical to those of adult respiratory distress syndrome, and the clinical course is unpredictable.

Toxicities of Specific Agents

Bleomycin

Bleomycin belongs to the antibiotic class of antineoplastic agents and is used primarily for treatment of lymphomas, testicular tumors, and squamous cell carcinomas.[7] It may produce all three syndromes of pulmonary toxicity, particularly pulmonary fibrosis, and lung toxicity is the dose-limiting side-effect. The incidence of pulmonary fibrosis varies between 2 and 40%, although some form of pulmonary disease develops in approximately 4% of all patients.[8,9] The pulmonary fibrosis syndrome carries a mortality rate estimated at 10%.

The risk of pulmonary toxicity is dose-related, and above a cumulative dose of 450–500 mg, the incidence increases exponentially (Fig. 53-1). Fatal pulmonary toxicity has been seen with doses as low as 100 mg,[10] however, particularly in the presence of other risk factors. Age appears to predispose to toxicity, as does combined use of bleomycin with other potential pulmonary toxins, especially cyclophosphamide.[1] Chest irradiation during bleomycin administration may sensitize the patient to the toxic effects of bleomycin, particularly at radiation doses above 3300 rads; this may affect the contralateral lung as well as the lung within the radiation port. Prior thoracic irradiation may also increase the risk of bleomycin toxicity in a "radiorecall" fashion. One review found that 10% of patients who received both irradiation and bleomycin therapy died from pulmonary complications.[11] Smoking may also potentiate bleomycin-induced pulmonary damage *via* enhanced release of hydrogen peroxide from alveolar macrophages.[12]

Early reports of postoperative complications in bleomycin-treated patients suggested that either hyperoxia or excessive crystalloid administration played a role in the exacerbation of pulmonary fibrosis.[13-16] Subsequent case reports also implicated high inspired oxygen concentrations in the pathophysiology of postoperative respiratory failure. The role of excessive crystalloid administration has not received as careful scrutiny. Several retrospective studies have challenged the need to limit oxygen administration to bleomycin-treated patients.[17,18] These studies, however, involved relatively small numbers of younger patients with testicular tumors having short operations after a wide range of bleomycin dosages. These findings cannot necessarily be extended to all patients who have been exposed to bleomycin. Clearly, with the availability of pulse oximetry to monitor tissue oxygenation, it is prudent to maintain low inspired oxygen concentrations whenever possible in a patient with any prior history of bleomycin therapy, since pulmonary fibrosis has been reported to manifest over 1 year after the last bleomycin dose.

Studies using pulmonary function tests for early detection of pulmonary fibrosis after bleomycin have met with variable success. A decrease in the forced vital capacity may herald the onset of pulmonary fibrosis,[19] but this is not a universal finding. The $D_{L_{CO}}$ has been proposed as a more sensitive test for pulmonary damage before the onset of clinical symptoms,[1] although this finding has been disputed.[20] A careful history and examination are probably the most reliable indicators of pulmonary disease. A low $D_{L_{CO}}$ aids in the diagnosis except in the setting of anemia, where results may be artificially low and a normal test does not exclude occult fibrosis. Sequential studies of the $D_{L_{CO}}$ may also be of use in following patients being treated with bleomycin.

The mechanism of lung injury with bleomycin has been the most widely studied among all chemotherapeutic agents. Bleomycin is concentrated preferentially in the lung[21] and is inactivated by a hydrolase enzyme, which is relatively deficient in lung tissue.[22] Initially, it produces pulmonary capillary endothelial damage, progressing to alveolar epithelial injury with necrosis of Type I and proliferation of Type II alveolar cells (Fig. 53-2). Interstitial fibrosis develops and may progress to involve the entire lung.[1] Bleomycin may cause pulmonary injury *via* production of reactive oxygen metabolites. When incubated *in vitro* with iron in the presence of oxygen, bleomycin generates superoxide anions (O_2^-),[23] which hypoxia protects against the effects of bleomycin in animals.[24] This may explain the reported potentiation of bleomycin toxicity associated with high concentrations of oxygen. A similar mechanism of free radical injury has been proposed for radiation therapy, possibly explaining its apparent synergistic toxicity.[25] Bleomycin may also stimulate chemotaxis of neutrophils and lymphocytes to the lung, where they may act to aggravate the direct bleomycin insult by release of additional oxygen radicals and lymphokines.[4,26]

Nitrosoureas

As a class, these agents are used largely in the treatment of intracranial tumors, melanomas, and gastrointestinal and hematologic malignancies. Carmustine (BCNU) is the agent in greatest clinical use and has been associated with interstitial pneumonitis and fibrosis much like that produced by bleomycin.[27] The incidence of toxicity is in the range of 20–30%, with a mortality in those affected of between 24 and 90%. The major risk factor is the cumulative dose, with between 1200–1500 $mg \cdot m^{-2}$ associated with a significantly high incidence and 50% of patients exhibiting toxicity at doses above that range.[28] Associated risk factors are not as well delineated as for bleomycin. Concurrent use of other agents exhibiting pulmonary toxicity, particularly cyclophosphamide,[29] and pre-existing lung disease[28] appears to increase the potential for toxicity. The histologic similarity between the lesions produced by BCNU and those found with bleomycin and mitomycin toxicity raise the possibility that thoracic irradiation and oxygen therapy might have synergistic toxicity with the nitrosoureas, much as they do with bleomycin.[29] Case reports have linked other nitrosoureas with lung toxicity, but the incidence appears to be low, particularly in the dose ranges used for these agents.

Mitomycin

Mitomycin is another agent of the antibiotic class capable of inducing pulmonary fibrosis.[30] Its incidence ranges between 3 and 12%,[31] and like bleomycin, it appears to act synergistically with thoracic radiation and oxygen therapy. Therefore, inspired oxygen concentrations in patients undergoing mitomycin treatment should be kept to a minimum, as for bleomycin.

Alkylating Agents

Busulfan, cyclophosphamide, chlorambucil, and melphalan have the potential for pulmonary toxicity. *Busulfan* is used in the treatment of myeloproliferative disorders, particularly chronic myelogenous leukemia. Busulfan produces progressive pulmonary fibrosis similar to that seen with bleomycin.[5] The $D_{L_{CO}}$ is decreased, and patients may exhibit a restrictive deficit with hypoxemia. The incidence of busulfan-induced fibrosis is 4%, but subclinical fibrosis was reported at autopsy in 46% of patients treated with the drug.[32] The risk factors predisposing to development of lung disease are less clear than for bleomycin. Although no clear relationship between incidence and total dose exists, toxicity has not been reported at doses less than 500 mg unless other potentially toxic treatments (such as radiation therapy) or other chemotherapeutic agents have been used in combination with busulfan. The duration of treatment also appears to be a risk factor, with a mean treatment time of

(*Text continues on page 1452*)

TABLE 53-2. Clinical and Pathologic Features of Chemotherapy-Induced Toxicity

Drug	Mechanism of Injury	Histopathology	Clinical Features	Chest Roentgenogram	Diagnosis	Treatment
Alkylating Agents						
Busulfan	No studies, but direct toxicity to epithelial lining cells is suggested.	Pneumocyte dysplasia (degeneration of Type I cells; atypical hyperplastic Type II cells), atypical bronchial lining cells, mononuclear cell infiltration, fibrosis.	4% incidence; no direct dose-dependent toxicity; may be threshold dose (>500 mg); radiation and alkylating agents may enhance toxicity. Insidious onset after 4 years (8 months–10 years). Dyspnea, cough, weight loss, weakness, fever; crepitant basilar rales, pigmentation. Prognosis: poor.	Most common bibasilar reticular pattern; rarely pleural effusion, pulmonary ossification, normal chest radiograph.	Suggested by history and bizarre pneumocytes in sputum or lavage fluid. Definitive diagnosis by open lung biopsy.	Withdrawal of the drug; anecdotal reports of improvement with high-dose steroids. Mean survival after diagnosis is 5 months.
Cyclophosphamide	May be toxic through production of reactive oxygen species.	Endothelial swelling, pneumocyte dysplasia, lymphocytic and histiocytic infiltration, fibrosis.	Less than 1% incidence; does not appear to be dose-dependent, but synergy with oxygen and other agents possible. Subacute onset 3 weeks–8 years after initiation of therapy, up to 8 years after stopping therapy. Cough, dyspnea, fever; basilar rales.	Commonly, bibasilar reticular pattern; diffuse pulmonary edema pattern also reported.	As above.	Drug withdrawal; corticosteroids may hasten improvement, but no documented effect on mortality. Overall recovery about 65%.
Antibiotics						
Bleomycin	Several possible mechanisms: (a) direct toxicity through generation of reactive oxygen metabolites; (b) leukocyte influx and lung injury from release of proteases; (c) increased collagen synthesis and subsequent pulmonary fibrosis.	Endothelial blebbing; interstitial edema, necrosis of Type I cells and metaplastic Type II cells; inflammation with polymorphonuclear cells; fibroblast proliferation and fibrosis; occasionally eosinophilic infiltration.	Incidence 2–40%; age- and dose-related (>500 mg); synergy seen with oxygen therapy, radiation, and other agents. Occurs during and after stopping therapy. Cough, dyspnea, fever; tachypnea, rales. Hypersensitivity pneumonitis variant.	Bibasilar reticular pattern; multiple nodules similar to metastatic disease; acinar pattern, especially with hypersensitivity reaction; rarely, localized infiltrate.	Bronchoalveolar lavage might suggest diagnosis (polymorphonuclear alveolitis). Transbronchial or open lung biopsy required for diagnosis, especially to rule out other causes.	Drug withdrawal. In bleomycin hypersensitivity reactions, definite role for steroids; in other forms of bleomycin toxicity, efficacy less clear. Mortality estimated at 50%.
Mitomycin	No studies, but probably similar to the alkylating agents.	Similar to bleomycin; in patients with microangiopathic anemia, prominent vascular changes are present.	3–12% incidence; does not appear to be dose-related but possible synergy with oxygen, radiotherapy, and other agents. Dry cough and dyspnea; fever not seen; bibasilar rales.	Diffuse reticular pattern; pleural effusions seen.	Lung biopsy for definitive diagnosis; no bronchoalveolar lavage studies reported.	Drug withdrawal; steroids may alter outcome. Mortality approaches 50%.

Nitrosoureas*

Drug	Mechanism	Pathology	Clinical Features	Radiograph	Diagnosis	Treatment
BCNU (carmustine)	Few studies; direct injury through generation of toxic oxidant molecules possible.	Similar to bleomycin; fibrosis predominates.	20–30% incidence; dose-related; increased risk with pre-existing lung disease and tobacco use; possible synergism with other agents; can be seen after drug stopped. Dry cough, dyspnea, bibasilar rales.	Bibasilar reticular pattern; may be normal.	As above.	Early recognition and withdrawal of the drug; steroids not beneficial since most patients are on the drug for intracranial processes when toxicity develops. Mortality reported between 24 and 90%.

Antimetabolites

Drug	Mechanism	Pathology	Clinical Features	Radiograph	Diagnosis	Treatment
Methotrexate	Direct toxic effect may play a role but mechanism not known; hypersensitivity suggested by occurrence of eosinophils and presence of increased helper T lymphocytes in lavage fluid.	Interstitial and alveolar infiltrate of lymphocytes, eosinophils, and plasma cells; occasional poorly formed noncaseating granuloma; fibrosis unusual.	8% incidence; synergism with other agents possible; occurs 12 days to 18 years after beginning therapy. Fever, chills, malaise, headache—a prodrome for days and weeks; cough, dyspnea, rales common. Skin rash in 17% and blood eosinophilia in 40%.	Early interstitial infiltrates; later, alveolar infiltrates; hilar and mediastinal adenopathy, pleural effusions described; chest radiography can be normal.	Clinical history suggestive; bronchoalveolar lavage might suggest diagnosis (helper T cells in fluid), but lung biopsy required for diagnosis.	Discontinue drug, but reports of reinstitution without recurrence of the abnormality. Dramatic responses to steroids reported. Mortality 1%; outlook favorable.
Cytosine arabinoside	Unknown.	Pulmonary edema; proteinaceous exudate with extravasation of red blood cells, no inflammatory cells.	If given within 30 days of death, high incidence of pulmonary edema. Abrupt onset of dyspnea; GI toxicity coexists.	Diffuse interstitial and alveolar pattern.	Clinical picture suggests diagnosis.	Supportive; no studies.

Miscellaneous

Drug	Mechanism	Pathology	Clinical Features	Radiograph	Diagnosis	Treatment
Procarbazine	Hypersensitivity.	Mononuclear cell infiltration and scattered foci of eosinophils; fibrosis in one case.	Acute onset within hours to days of first dose. Nausea, fevers, chills, arthralgias, urticaria, dry cough, and dyspnea. Blood eosinophilia common.	Interstitial infiltrates; pleural effusion.	Clinical picture highly suggestive of diagnosis.	Rapid recovery following discontinuation of drug. Role of steroids not known.
Vinca alkaloids—vinblastine and vindesine	Unknown.	Dysplasia of alveolar lining cells; interstitial and alveolar influx of inflammatory cells; fibrosis.	Most common reports in association with mitomycin. Dyspnea and wheezing seen with vindesine. Obstructive pattern on pulmonary function testing in one patient.	Diffuse interstitial and alveolar infiltrates with combination drugs; normal chest radiograph with vinca alkaloid alone.	Clinical history suggests diagnosis.	Drug withdrawal; steroids probably beneficial. Prognosis poor if pulmonary infiltrates develop.

* Pulmonary toxicity has been reported with all other nitrosoureas, including CCNU (lomustine), methyl-CCNU (semustine), and DCNU (chlorozotocin).
Reprinted with permission from Stover DE: Adverse effects of treatment. In DeVita VT, Hellman S, Rosenberg SA (eds): Cancer: Principles and Practice of Oncology, 3rd ed, pp 2166–2168. Philadelphia: JB Lippincott, 1989.

TABLE 53-3. Risk Factors Predisposing to Development of Cytotoxic Drug-Induced Pulmonary Disease

Risk Factor	Drug(s) Implicated
Cumulative dose	Bleomycin, busulfan, carmustine
Age	Bleomycin
Concurrent or previous radio-therapy	Bleomycin, busulfan, mitomycin
Oxygen therapy	Bleomycin, cyclophosphamide, mitomycin
Other cytotoxic drug therapy	Carmustine, mitomycin, cyclo-phosphamide, bleomycin, methotrexate
Pre-existing pulmonary disease	Carmustine

Reprinted with permission from Cooper JA, White DA, Matthay RA: Drug-induced pulmonary disease. Am Rev Respir Dis 133:324, 1986.

3.5 years in patients reported to exhibit toxicity.[5] Enhanced toxicity with oxygen therapy has not been noted. The onset of symptoms is insidious, beginning with dyspnea, cough, and fever, but the prognosis after the appearance of clinical symptoms is poor, with a median survival after diagnosis of 5 months.

Cyclophosphamide

Cyclophosphamide is an alkylating agent used in treatment of a wide range of cancers and inflammatory diseases. Both hypersensitivity reactions[5] and fibrosing pneumonitis[33] have been noted with this drug, although the incidence is less than 1%. Age, underlying disease, radiation therapy, and drug dosage have not been clearly associated with enhanced toxicity, and synergistic effects with other agents are anecdotal. Animal studies have shown that high inspired oxygen concentrations increase the risk of pulmonary toxicity,[34] but no comparable relationship has been found in humans. Symptoms of dyspnea and cough may develop months to years after initiation of the drug. Symptomatic patients demonstrate a reduced $D_{L_{CO}}$ similar to that seen with bleomycin. Chlorambucil and melphalan have also been associated with pulmonary fibrosis in isolated cases,[5] but no clear incidence or risk factors have been noted.

Methotrexate

Methotrexate belongs to the antimetabolite category of chemotherapeutic agents. It is widely used in the treatment of malignant and some nonmalignant disorders. Pulmonary toxicity may take the form of fulminant noncardiogenic edema[35] or a more progressive inflammation, with interstitial infiltrates and pleural effusions.[36] The incidence of pulmonary toxicity attributed to methotrexate is in the range of 8%, but its frequent use in combination with other chemotherapeutic agents with potential lung toxicity makes this number uncertain.[1] There are no known risk factors, and although toxicity does not appear to be related to total dose, there may be a threshold because toxicity is rare at weekly doses of less than 20 mg. Leucovorin rescue does not protect against the development of this toxicity. Mortality owing to lung toxicity is low (approximately 1%), and

symptoms generally respond to corticosteroid administration.[37]

Radiation

Thoracic radiation may induce a syndrome of radiation pneumonitis independent of concurrent chemotherapy. The incidence of radiation pneumonitis occurs in as many as 5–15% of patients receiving thoracic irradiation.[38] Risk factors for the development of clinically significant injury include the size of the radiation field, the total dose, and the doses used in individual fractions. The same total radiation dose applied over a larger number of fractions appears to cause a lesser degree of damage with each exposure and a greater potential for lung repair.

The pathogenesis of radiation damage may relate to production of OH^-, H_2O_2, and other free radicals, which produce DNA damage such as single-strand breaks and cross-links.[25] Capillary endothelial cells and Type I epithelial cells appear particularly susceptible to this type of damage, but the basis for the delay often seen between irradiation and the onset of symptoms is unclear.

Clinical features of radiation pneumonitis include dyspnea and arterial hypoxemia.[38] Restrictive changes occur in the irradiated lung segments, and these are matched by a fall in $D_{L_{CO}}$ and a reduction in blood flow to the affected area. These changes typically occur 6–12 weeks after radiation treatment and in most cases resolve spontaneously over a few months. In a small percentage of patients, symptoms progress and death is usually caused by respiratory failure and cor pulmonale. Radiation fibrosis of the irradiated field typically develops progressively, beginning 6–12 months after radiation exposure and becoming stable 1–2 years later. Fibrosis may be associated with an additional decrease in pulmonary compliance.

Head and neck irradiation can produce airway edema with the potential for severe laryngeal fibrosis and airway obstruction, particularly after combined radical neck dissection and radiation therapy.[39,40] These complications may be stable and may first be evidenced as difficulty with airway management after induction of anesthesia. The total dose of radiation appears to be the best predictor of these complications.

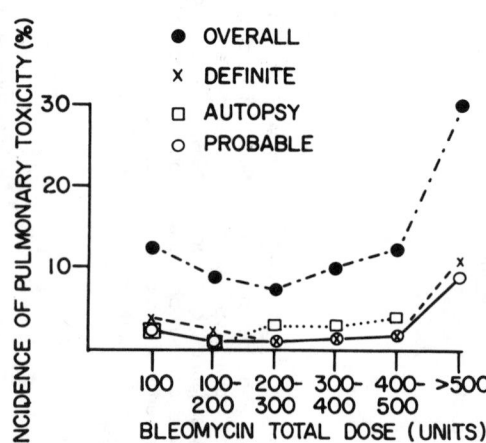

Figure 53-1. The relationship between the total cumulative bleomycin dose and pulmonary toxicity. (Reprinted with permission from Ginsberg SJ, Comis RL: The pulmonary toxicity of antineoplastic agents. Semin Oncol 9:35, 1982.)

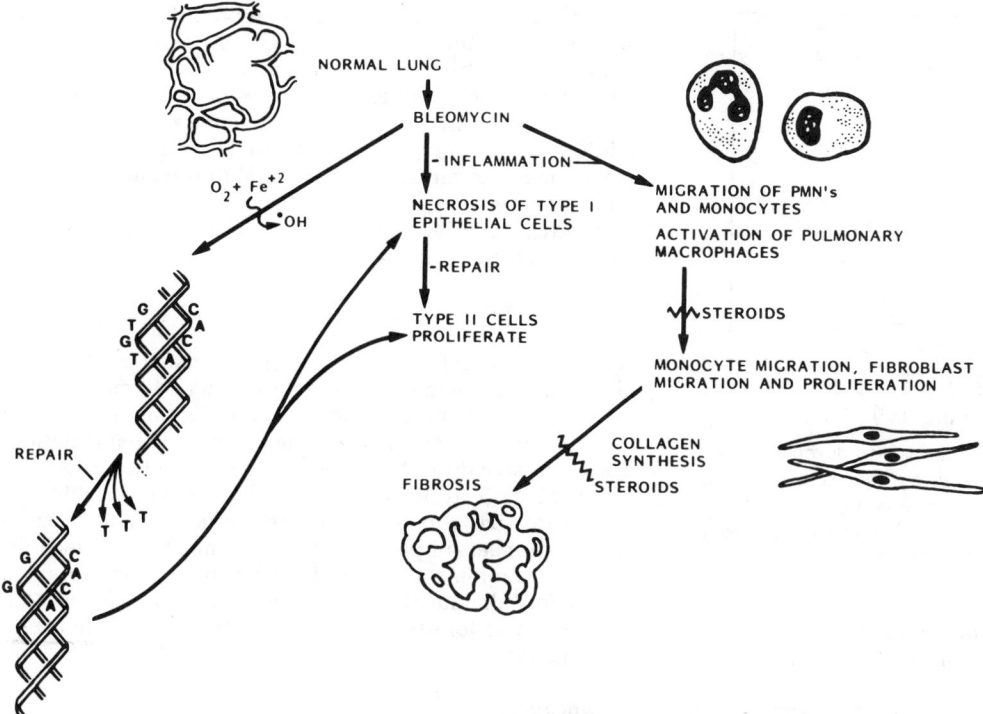

Figure 53-2. Schematic representation of the steps in the pathogenesis of bleomycin-induced lung injury and fibrosis. (Reprinted with permission from Eigen H, Wyszomierski D: Bleomycin lung injury in children: Pathophysiology and guidelines for management. Am J Pediatr Hematol Oncol 7:73, 1985.)

CARDIAC COMPLICATIONS

Overview

Antineoplastic agents have the potential to produce a wide spectrum of cardiac toxicity, which may include electrocardiographic changes and life-threatening arrhythmias, pericarditis, myocardial ischemia, cardiomyopathies, and congestive heart failure. The interaction of these toxicities with volatile anesthetics and other agents in common use in the operative setting has not been well studied. The anesthesiologist must therefore be well acquainted with the nature of the cardiac toxicity associated with certain chemotherapeutic agents, the risk factors that increase the likelihood of toxicity, and the most sensitive tests for functional impairment.

Toxicities of Specific Agents

Doxorubicin (Adriamycin)

This anthracycline has significant antitumor effects against leukemias, lymphomas, and solid tumors such as breast cancer and soft-tissue sarcomas. The cardiac toxicity of doxorubicin is typically its dose-limiting side-effect, even in patients whose malignancy responds well to the drug.

Acutely, up to 33% of patients develop some electrocardiographic changes, most commonly nonspecific ST-T wave changes and premature ventricular and atrial contractions.[41] These changes do not appear to be dose-related and are generally transient and benign. The one possible exception is a depressed QRS voltage, which does appear to be both dose-related and irreversible. QRS voltage decreases of greater than 30% have been associated with an increased risk of subsequent cardiomyopathy.[42]

The most serious toxicity associated with doxorubicin is cardiomyopathy, which is clinically indistinguishable from cardiomyopathy due to other causes. Symptoms develop anywhere from days to years after cessation of treatment but typically within the first 3–4 months.[43] The incidence of cardiomyopathy associated with doxorubicin varies widely among studies, ranging from 2–32%, with an associated mortality as high as 61%.[44]

A number of risk factors have been identified that may increase the potential for development of doxorubicin cardiomyopathy. The most important predictor is the cumulative dose. Patients receiving total doses less than 550 $mg \cdot m^{-2}$ have an incidence of drug-induced congestive heart failure of less than 1%,[45] whereas at doses above 550 $mg \cdot m^{-2}$ the incidence rises to between 15 and 30%.[44] Some oncologists advocate empirically stopping the drug at 550 $mg \cdot m^{-2}$, although the relationship between drug dose and risk of cardiomyopathy (Fig. 53-3) does not demonstrate a sharp rise in incidence at this point but rather more of a continuum of dose-response.

Prior or concurrent mediastinal irradiation is another risk factor for the development of cardiomyopathy.[42,46] This risk is particularly prominent at radiation doses greater than 2000 rads. The age-related risk appears to be bimodal. The very young and the elderly appear to be at increased risk for the development of cardiomyopathy.[44] Patients over the age of 40 may also be more likely to have a rapid, progressive deterioration of cardiac function, whereas patients under 40 stabilize or even improve with time after cessation of the drug. Although case reports of synergistic toxicity

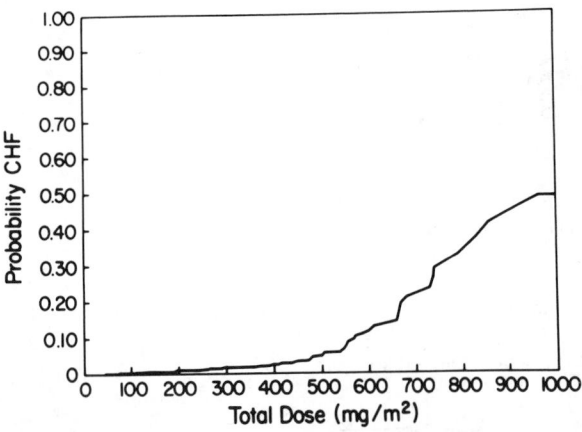

Figure 53-3. Cumulative probability of developing doxorubicin-induced congestive heart failure (CHF) versus total cumulative dose of doxorubicin. (Reprinted with permission from Von Hoff DD, Layard MW, Basa P et al: Risk factors for doxorubin-induced congestive heart failure. Ann Intern Med 91:712, 1979.)

with other antineoplastic agents have been published,[47] none of these agents have reliably been demonstrated to augment doxorubicin toxicity.

The pathophysiologic basis for this cardiotoxicity is uncertain. The anthraquinone nucleus of doxorubicin has been shown to reversibly convert to a free radical semiquinone, capable of donating an electron to molecular oxygen, thereby forming superoxide.[48] The heart may be particularly susceptible to such free radical injury because of its low levels of superoxide dismutase.

Monitoring for the development of doxorubicin-induced cardiomyopathy has been directed at identifying patients who can tolerate higher doses of the drug and at detecting toxicity before it becomes clinically evident. Endomyocardial biopsy is the most accurate method for determining subclinical cardiomyopathy.[49] Less invasive techniques have included systolic time intervals and serial echocardiography, but these methods have not been shown capable of detecting disease before the onset of clinical symptoms. Radionuclide angiography has proved to be the best noninvasive procedure for identifying early cardiomyopathy before the development of overt congestive heart failure. In 32 asymptomatic patients receiving a cumulative doxorubicin dose between 480 and 550 mg·m^{-2}, 25% had an abnormal resting ejection fraction and an additional 38% had an abnormal left ventricular response to exercise[50] (Fig. 53-4). In patients being evaluated preoperatively for surgery, exercise radionuclide angiography appears to be the most sensitive test for the detection of impaired cardiac reserve.

Daunorubicin (Cerubidine)

This anthracycline is also used in antileukemia regimens. Like doxorubicin, its dose-limiting toxicity is its cardiotoxic effect. Acutely, daunorubicin has been associated with electrocardiographic changes ranging from tachycardia to nonspecific ST-T wave changes. These electrocardiographic changes are typically benign and resolve spontaneously after the drug is discontinued.[51]

Daunorubicin cardiomyopathy, like doxorubicin, shows a dose-related incidence. One large retrospective study (5613 patients) found an incidence of congestive heart failure of 1.5% at doses <600 mg·m^{-2}, a 12% incidence at 1000 mg·m^{-2}, and a mortality of 79% after development of symp-

toms.[52] The influence of age on daunorubicin-induced congestive heart failure is less clear. Other risk factors such as thoracic irradiation and concurrent chemotherapy have not been as thoroughly investigated as with doxorubicin.

At present other investigational anthracyclines are in clinical trials, aiming for decreased cardiotoxicity with maintenance of antitumor effects. Unfortunately, no drug has yet proved entirely free of cardiac toxicity, and patients presenting for surgery must therefore be evaluated for any signs of cardiomyopathy.

Cyclophosphamide

Cyclophosphamide is in common use in many combination chemotherapy regimens. High doses (120–240 mg·kg^1) may be used in the therapy of some solid tumors and for marrow ablation in preparation for bone marrow transplantation. These massive doses have been associated with a 33% incidence of pericarditis and pericardial effusion, which in some cases has progressed to cardiac tamponade.[53] Much smaller numbers of patients show a hemorrhagic myocarditis with symptoms of congestive heart failure, and rarely, a fatal myocardial necrosis may occur.[54] This latter syndrome may not occur for up to 2 weeks after the last dose of cyclophosphamide.

5-Fluorouracil

5-Fluorouracil-induced myocardial ischemia is a rare cardiac toxicity that may lead to myocardial infarction anywhere from 3 hours–1 week after treatment. The incidence is low (1.1%) in patients without underlying heart disease but may rise to 4.5% in patients with pre-existing coronary artery disease.[55] The etiology of this ischemia is unclear. Approximately one half of patients with angina have no evidence of coronary artery disease at cardiac catheterization, suggesting coronary artery spasm as a mechanism, but response to calcium channel blockers has been variable. As many as 17% of patients reported have suffered a myocardial infarction.[56] The vinca alkaloids, vincristine and vinblastine, have similarly been associated with coronary artery disease, including vasospasm, angina, and myocardial infarction,[57-59] but the connection is less clear and the incidence even rarer as compared to 5-FU.

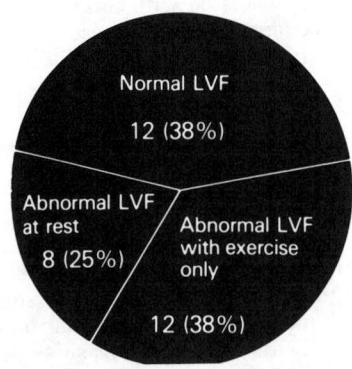

Figure 53-4. Distribution of rest and exercise left ventricular functional (LVF) abnormalities in 32 patients after doxorubicin. Exercise enhances detection of abnormal LVF in these patients. (Reprinted with permission from Gottdiener JS, Mathiesen DJ, Borer JS et al: Doxorubicin cardiotoxicity: Assessment of late left ventricular dysfunction by radionuclide cineangiography. Ann Intern Med 94:433, 1981.)

Reprinted with permission from Lancaster LD, Ewy GA: Cardiac consequences of malignancy and their treatment. Adv Intern Med 30:288, 1984.

TABLE 53-4. Forms of Radiation-Induced Heart Disease

Acute pericarditis
  Effusion, tamponade
Chronic pericarditis
  Effusion, constriction
Myocardial fibrosis
Valvular dysfunction
Conduction disturbances
Accelerated coronary arteriosclerosis
  Myocardial infarction

Radiation

Exposure of the heart to radiation in high doses may result in a number of clinically important forms of heart disease (Table 53-4). Accelerated atherosclerotic coronary artery disease has been of particular concern, occurring in up to 53% of patients who received radiation doses higher than 3500 rads.[60] This number has decreased significantly in the past 10–15 years with the use of subcarinal blockers and equally weighted anterior and posterior radiation fields. One study of 377 patients with Hodgkin's disease revealed only a single myocardial infarction in a 2-year follow-up study of patients receiving 4400 rads using these techniques.[61] Patients who received their radiation therapy before the advent of these protective techniques continue to demonstrate decreased functional cardiac reserve.[62] These patients may warrant further evaluation of their left ventricular function preoperatively.

Cardiac toxicity reported with other antineoplastic agents is sufficiently rare that a clear association cannot be made in most cases. Nonetheless, the possibility of a chemotherapy-induced cardiac dysfunction must always be considered in the cancer patient presenting for surgery.

CENTRAL NERVOUS SYSTEM COMPLICATIONS

Overview

Neurologic toxicities arising from chemotherapy, radiotherapy, or the malignancy itself often occur in cancer patients. Because of the potential for neurotoxicity with many chemotherapies, this section is limited to agents in common use with a relatively high incidence of neurologic complications. Assessment of neurologic status remains an important part of the preoperative assessment of all cancer patients on any therapeutic regimen to guide both intraoperative management and postoperative evaluation.

Specific Agents

Methotrexate

Neurologic toxicity of methotrexate (MTX) varies considerably with the route of administration. Intrathecal MTX provokes symptoms of meningeal irritation within hours of administration in up to 61% of patients.[63] Headache, stiff neck, nausea, and lethargy may persist for 12–72 hours after injection. Far more rare is a transient or permanent paraplegia beginning soon after intrathecal administration and resolving as late as 2–5 months afterward.[64] A similar paraplegia has been reported with intrathecal administration of cytosine arabinoside (ara-C).[65]

More chronic toxicities of MTX include encephalopathic syndromes. These syndromes can occur after intrathecal or iv administration[66] and may be transient or permanent. As noted in Figure 53-5, the frequency of encephalopathy increases exponentially when intrathecal or iv administration of MTX and cranial irradiation are combined.[67] Ara-C may similarly potentiate the toxicity of MTX, given either intravenously or intrathecally. The clinical picture typically develops insidiously as early as a few weeks or as late as 2 years after cranial irradiation. Prominent among symptoms are confusion, somnolence, ataxia, and tremors. Symptoms may also be focal, including quadriparesis, slurred speech, and seizure activity. Methotrexate leukoencephalopathy is often fatal, but most patients survive for months and even years with chronic neurologic deficits. The mechanism of MTX toxicity is unclear, but the finding of higher cerebrospinal fluid MTX concentrations in patients with signs of neurotoxicity[68] suggests a direct toxicity caused by prolonged exposure of nerve tissue to the drug. Histopathologically, demyelinization is often found in affected nerves[69] and is independent of the diluent or the preservative. Whether the presence of MTX neurotoxicity lowers the threshold for toxicity from other potential neurotoxins is unclear but justifies some concern over subarachnoid administration of any drug in these patients.

Vinca Alkaloids

Neurotoxicity from vincristine and its relatives, vinblastine and vindesine, is often the dose-limiting symptom.[70,71] The earliest clinical finding, occurring before any overt symptoms, is loss of the Achilles tendon reflex. Paresthesias are generally the first symptoms to appear, typically in the feet or hands, and are found in approximately 57% of patients. Continued drug administration often results in progression of this toxicity to muscle pain, weakness, and sensory impairment. Weakness has been reported to progress to quadriparesis. Findings are largely symmetric and dose-related. Paresthesias typically disappear gradually after the drug is discontinued; however, the more severe symptoms may persist for months, and resolution may be incomplete.

Cranial nerves may also be affected by the vinca alkaloids, and recurrent laryngeal nerve palsy is prominent among these.[72] Bilateral facial nerve and oculomotor nerve palsies have also been described.[73] Cranial nerve toxicity is found in up to 10% of patients and occasionally is the first sign of vinca toxicity. Fortunately, this toxicity is usually reversible with discontinuation of therapy.

Autonomic neuropathy is another manifestation of vinca neurotoxicity, occurring in 46% of patients in one large series.[74] Symptoms are largely those of paralytic ileus, or bladder atony, but orthostatic hypotension has also been reported by a number of authors.[74,75]

Symptoms of encephalopathy accompanied in some cases by seizures have been reported in children after treatment with vincristine. Many of these were probably a result of hyponatremia stemming from the syndrome of inappropriate secretion of antidiuretic hormone.[76,77] This syndrome may be a result of a direct effect of the vinca alkaloids on the posterior pituitary gland. Symptoms generally develop

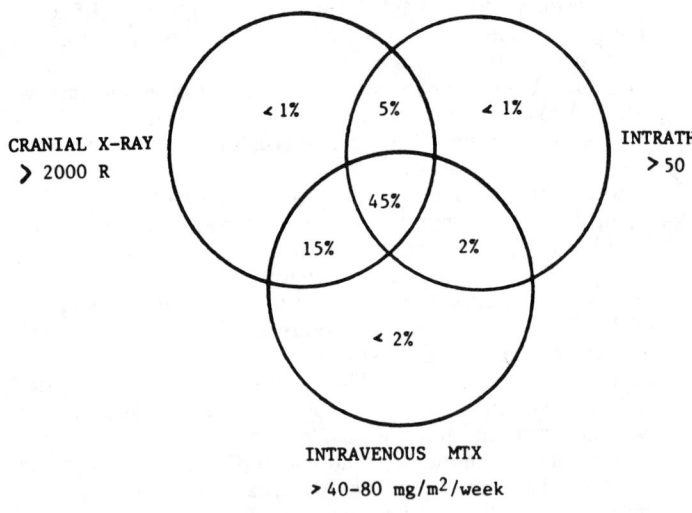

Figure 53-5. Approximate risk of methotrexate (MTX)-induced leukoencephalopathy as a function of three treatment modalities. (Reprinted with permission from Bleyer WA, Griffin TW: White matter necrosis, mineralizing microangiopathy, and intellectual abilities in survivors of childhood leukemia: Associations with central nervous system irradiation and methotrexate therapy. In Gilber HA, Kagan AT [eds]: Radiation Damage to the Nervous System. New York, Raven Press, 1980.)

within the first 10 days of treatment and resolve 1–2 weeks after discontinuation of therapy.

All of the vinca alkaloids have the potential to produce neurotoxicity, differing only slightly in their frequency of such effects, with vincristine having the highest frequency, followed by vindesine and then vinblastine. Histologic examination shows primary axonal degeneration as the principal finding associated with toxicity.[78] The vinca alkaloids inhibit microtubule formation in the mitotic spindle, thus arresting cell division in metaphase. Microtubules also function in axoplasmic transport, and the observed axonal degeneration may stem from disruption of this process.

L-Asparaginase

L-Asparaginase is an enzyme that hydrolyzes the amino acid L-asparagine to aspartic acid and ammonia. Most of the asparaginases have some activity against L-glutamine as well. Selected tumors such as acute lymphoblastic leukemia have no asparagine synthetase activity and require exogenous asparagine to proliferate.

Encephalopathy is the major manifestation of neurotoxicity produced by L-asparaginase, occurring in 33–60% of patients in larger series.[70] Symptoms appear to be dose-related, and adults are more susceptible than children. Mild symptoms of confusion or drowsiness are common and well tolerated and do not require halting therapy. Even the more severe syndrome of stupor and coma generally clears within a few days of drug discontinuation. A less common neurotoxicity (≈10%) is a delayed encephalopathy that begins about 1 week following L-asparaginase treatment and persists for several weeks.[79] The acute syndrome is most likely a result of the accumulation of the products of amino acid metabolism, such as L-glutamate and ammonia. The delayed form may be a result of L-asparagine depletion, and "rescue" infusions of L-asparagine have shown some promise.[79,80]

Procarbazine

Procarbazine was originally synthesized as a monoamine oxidase inhibitor but was found to have antineoplastic effects against Hodgkin's lymphoma and certain brain tumors. The mechanism for its anticancer effect is uncertain but may involve blocking DNA synthesis.

The most common neurotoxicity attributable to procarbazine is central nervous system depression, occurring in as many as 31% of patients,[70] with symptoms ranging from mild drowsiness to confusion, agitation, and profound stupor. Procarbazine potentiates the sedative effects of other drugs, such as the phenothiazines, which are often administered to control the nausea and vomiting frequently associated with procarbazine. Some of the reported toxicity may be a result of this synergistic central nervous system depression between procarbazine and other sedative medications.[81]

Procarbazine may cause a peripheral neuropathy in 10–20% of patients, largely manifested by paresthesias in the extremities and proximal muscle myalgias.[66] These symptoms are completely reversible, and the myalgias may resolve despite continuation of treatment.

Other toxicities such as orthostatic hypotension can be attributed to the monoamine oxidase inhibition. Procarbazine shows the same potential for profound hypertension with administration of indirect sympathomimetic agents as is found with other monoamine oxidase inhibitors.

Platinum

The most common neurotoxicity attributable to platinum is its ototoxicity. Tinnitus occurs in about 9% of patients and is usually reversible.[82] Symptomatic hearing loss is slightly less frequent, occurring in about 6% of patients, although 24–50% of all patients demonstrate some abnormalities on audiographic examination.[83]

Peripheral neuropathies have also been associated with platinum administration, taking the form of sensory neuropathies primarily of a "stocking and glove" distribution.[84] Paresthesias and loss of vibratory and position sense are common findings. Motor neuropathy is not typical, although some ataxia has been reported.[85] Symptoms occur in approximately 4% of patients tested[86] and appear to be dose-related. In most cases symptoms are reversible, although they may persist for months.

Many other chemotherapeutic agents have been associated with neurotoxicity in an idiosyncratic fashion. Some may be the result of a direct neurotoxicity, whereas others have complications secondary to the agent's antitumor action. Studies assessing the safety of different anesthetic techniques and specific anesthetic agents in the presence of such neurotoxicities are lacking. The anesthesiologist is faced with the task of carefully assessing the neurologic status of the patient presenting for surgery, tailoring the technique to the specific needs of the patient, and avoiding agents with any known neurotoxic potential.

HEMATOLOGIC COMPLICATIONS

Malignancy and chemotherapy are capable of bringing about diverse and often complex hematologic changes. Anemia may result from blood loss or hemolysis, and myelosuppression may ensue from bone marrow invasion or chemotherapy. Anemia in a cancer patient being readied for surgery cannot be assumed to be the result of chemotherapy or the underlying malignancy. Diagnostic studies should be initiated preoperatively where possible, as surgery may considerably confound and even exacerbate the anemia.

The myelosuppressive effects of chemotherapy are well known and largely dose- and time-related. Likewise, malnutrition, malabsorption, and direct effects of tumors themselves may contribute to the marrow suppression in these patients. The need for vigilance with respect to infection prophylaxis is self-evident. The topic of the immunosuppressed patient is too broad for discussion here, but several principles are relevant to the anesthesiologist, particularly in the critical care setting. Fever should never be assumed to be secondary to malignancy until all reasonable causes are ruled out. In addition, fever should be treated aggressively as if it were due to infection, since these patients are susceptible to fatal, overwhelming gram-negative sepsis. Because of neutropenia, localizing signs such as pain, erythema, or swelling may be absent.

Of immediate concern to the anesthesiologist are problems with hemostasis in cancer patients presenting for surgery. These patients should have preoperative evaluation of their platelet count and routine coagulation assays such as prothrombin time and partial thromboplastin time. More specialized studies, e.g., fibrinogen levels, may be warranted when abnormalities are noted. Some specific coagulopathies associated with certain cancers and their treatment are discussed.

Fibrinolysis

Operative bleeding after prostatectomy is a classic example of a fibrinolytic state. Surgery of the prostate gland for cancer or other pathology may result in release of urokinase, which infiltrates the operative field and dissolves clots. This generally causes only local fibrinolysis, and several studies indicate that therapy with epsilon-aminocaproic acid, which prevents plasmin from binding to fibrin, may arrest the fibrinolysis.[87] Epsilon-aminocaproic acid should be used only when there is excessive operative bleeding, since its administration can cause thromboembolic complications. The priming dose of epsilon-aminocaproic acid is 0.1 $g \cdot kg^{-1}$ given intravenously over 30 minutes, followed by an infusion of 0.5–1.0 $g \cdot h^{-1}$.

Platelet Dysfunction

Qualitative platelet defects that occur in the myeloproliferative syndromes may complicate the intra- and postoperative management of these patients. This dysfunction may take the form of either a hypercoagulable state or a bleeding diathesis, neither of which can reliably be predicted by *in vitro* platelet function tests.[88] Bleeding complications are most common with two particular types of myeloproliferative syndromes: essential thrombocythemia and myeloid metaplasia. The hemorrhagic problems may resolve after lowering the platelet count with chemotherapy. In contrast, polycythemia vera is often associated with thromboembolic manifestations. Chemotherapy or phlebotomy is the treatment of choice but is not uniformly successful. Patients with polycythemia vera also have a high risk of thrombotic complications associated with major surgery; reduction of the preoperative hematocrit to 40–50 $ml \cdot dl^{-1}$ is desirable, and minidose heparin has also been shown to further decrease the risk of thrombosis.[88]

Disseminated Intravascular Coagulation

Acute promyelocytic leukemia may exhibit a baseline coagulopathy that is exacerbated by chemotherapy. The primary granules of the leukemic cells have thromboplastic activity that causes a consumptive coagulopathy. Patients may present with disseminated intravascular coagulation at the time of diagnosis, and placement of indwelling catheters for chemotherapy may be complicated by severely compromised hemostasis.

With induction chemotherapy for promyelocytic leukemia, cell destruction and release of additional granule contents may worsen the disseminated intravascular coagulation. The intravascular coagulation usually subsides within 1 week after successful induction chemotherapy. Bleeding, especially intracranial hemorrhage, is the major complication. The use of heparin in this situation is a matter of controversy,[89] but if the patient is not bleeding and has established disseminated intravascular coagulation, low-dose heparin may be a useful adjunct to replacement of fibrinogen and platelets.[90] Heparin at an infusion rate of 7.5 $U \cdot kg^{-1} \cdot h^{-1}$, accompanied by aggressive transfusions of platelets and cryoprecipitate, may serve as baseline therapy and can be adjusted as needed. Frequent monitoring of the platelet count, reptilase time, and fibrinogen level is critical. Fresh frozen plasma can be used to replace low levels of antithrombin III; epsilon-aminocaproic acid can counter the unbalanced fibrinolysis when alpha$_2$-antiplasmin levels are low.

METABOLIC COMPLICATIONS

Tumor Lysis Syndrome

In patients with tumors that have a high growth fraction or a rapid rate of growth, such as Burkitt's lymphoma, acute lymphocytic leukemia, or non-Hodgkin's lymphoma, chemotherapy may cause significant cell death, resulting in the release of intracellular contents into the extracellular fluid, analogous to the granule release seen with promyelocytic leukemia.[91] This complication is rarely seen in solid tumors. Tumor lysis may cause hyperuricemia, hyperkalemia, and hyperphosphatemia and may precipitate acute renal failure. Hyperphosphatemia may result in a secondary decrease in serum calcium.[92] These electrolyte abnormalities should be corrected preoperatively when possible, and may be ongoing, necessitating intraoperative testing and appropriate adjustments in electrolyte replacement.

Hypercalcemia

Multiple myeloma and solid tumors with skeletal metastases, particularly cancers of the breast, kidney, and small cell of the lung, are often complicated by hypercalcemia. As many as 40–50% of breast cancer patients may have hypercalcemia. This may be the result of direct bone resorption, or indirectly through mediators such as interleukin-1 or tumor necrosis factor, which are produced by tumor cells in bone.[93]

Large-cell lung cancer and renal carcinoma are the most common solid tumors in which hypercalcemia develops in the absence of skeletal spread. This humoral hypercalcemia may be secondary to the production of osteoclast-activating factor,[94] either by the tumor itself or by tumor-stimulated normal osteocytes. In addition, there is evidence that growth factors derived from tumors may directly resorb bone.[95] Osteoclast-activating factor is also found with the severe bone destruction seen in multiple myeloma.

Serum calcium levels should be routinely checked in patients with malignancy. Patients with moderate hypercalcemia have no special perioperative difficulties; hypovolemia is common with severe hypercalcemia and requires preoperative hydration. Diuretics may be used in conjunction with hydration to help lower serum calcium levels. If hypercalcemia is chronic, there is a significant incidence of renal calculi and loss of urinary concentrating ability as well as the potential for cardiac arrhythmias. Besides adequate hydration, preoperative therapy of hypercalcemia may include steroids, phosphates, mithramycin, or calcitonin. The diphosphonates also appear to effectively lower the serum calcium level in association with malignancy.[96,97]

Paraneoplastic Syndromes

The term paraneoplastic syndrome refers to manifestations of cancer at sites not directly affected by malignant disease. Humoral hypercalcemia, as described above, is one of the most common of these syndromes. Ectopic Cushing's syndrome[94] is another in which adrenocorticotropic hormone is synthesized by tumor cells. Clinical signs and symptoms include hypokalemia, hyperglycemia, hypertension, edema, and muscle weakness. Small-cell lung cancer is the malignancy most commonly associated with ectopic Cushing's syndrome, followed by other neuroendocrine tumors. Therapy is directed against the underlying tumor, but inhibition of adrenal steroid synthesis is also important. Aminoglutethimide and metyrapone are used to stop all steroid synthesis, and maintenance corticosteroids then are added to avoid hypoadrenalism. Stress doses are required with surgical procedures.

Another syndrome typically found with small-cell lung cancer is that of secretion of inappropriate antidiuretic hormone, either at baseline or as a side-effect of chemotherapy with vincristine or cyclophosphamide.[94] Secretion of inappropriate antidiuretic hormone results in hyponatremia and hypo-osmolality, with the associated (often life-threatening) neurologic sequelae. Fluid restriction alone may be successful in mild cases. Severe, acute secretion of inappropriate antidiuretic hormone is treated with iv furosemide or demeclocycline.[98,99]

A variety of tumors are associated with paraneoplastic syndromes that impair neurologic function. The central nervous system may be principally affected, as in the case of lung cancer, which can cause dementia and cerebellar degeneration. Alternatively, lung and renal cancers may produce a myelopathy of the spinal cord characterized by ascending sensory and motor paralysis. Non-Hodgkin's lymphoma can result in a lower motor neuron degeneration with a highly variable course. Both pure and mixed sensory and motor neuropathies may be present with malignancies, occasionally as the presenting complaint. Autonomic dysfunction with orthostatic hypotension, impaired gastrointestinal motility, and neurogenic bladder also may be encountered.[100] Lung cancer, especially small cell, has many neurologic manifestations, and a thorough neurologic evaluation is critical in these patients, as these disorders may profoundly complicate their intraoperative management.

Small-cell lung cancer and occasionally stomach and ovarian cancer are also linked to Eaton-Lambert syndrome, a myasthenic variant that differs from true myasthenia gravis in that it predominantly involves peripheral weakness rather than facial or bulbar muscles. Paresthesias, dysarthria, and dysphagia may be seen, but respiratory muscle weakness is rare.[91] There is less fatigability than with myasthenia gravis as well as a poorer response to anticholinesterases. Successful chemotherapy of the underlying malignancy usually relieves the neurologic symptoms. Potentiation of neuromuscular blockade occurs in Eaton-Lambert syndrome with nondepolarizing muscle relaxants, and the doses of these agents must be reduced accordingly.[101]

Profoundly debilitated cancer patients may have prolonged muscular relaxation with succinylcholine owing to decreased synthesis of pseudocholinesterase. Another cause of increased duration of neuromuscular blockade after succinylcholine is the depression of pseudocholinesterase activity associated with cyclophosphamide.[102-104] Cases of prolonged apnea following succinylcholine have been reported in patients receiving cyclophosphamide. Both in vitro and in vivo studies of cyclophosphamide have demonstrated significant inhibition of pseudocholinesterase, occurring up to several weeks after its discontinuation. It is prudent in patients recently treated with cyclophosphamide either to decrease the dose of succinylcholine or to choose a nondepolarizing agent in its place. In either case, awareness of the potential for prolonged muscular paralysis with succinylcholine is critical.

RENAL COMPLICATIONS

Overview

Renal toxicity is a major side-effect of several chemotherapeutic agents. The most prominent among these is cisplatin, for which renal toxicity is the dose-limiting complication.

Cis-(II) Platinum Diamminedichloride (Cisplatin)

Cisplatin is a common component of combination chemotherapy of ovarian, testicular, bladder, and head and neck cancer. Beginning as early as 3 to 5 days after administration, there may be a progressive fall in glomerular filtration rate and development of acute tubular necrosis.[105] Along with rising blood urea nitrogen and creatinine levels, proteinuria, and hyperuricemia, there is a magnesium-wasting defect in up to 50% of patients manifesting some degree of renal impairment.[106] The acute tubular necrosis may progress to acute renal failure requiring hemodialysis.

The mechanism for the renal toxicity is not entirely understood but is possibly related to prolonged retention of platinum.[107] Other experimental platinum-containing agents have shown variable degrees of renal injury in animal models, and the toxicity seen in animals and humans resembles the renal injury produced by mercury. However, metal chelators do not reduce the toxicity of cisplatin,[108] and the *trans* form of the compound does not produce renal tubular damage,[109] suggesting that a metabolite specific to the cisplatin stereoisomer may be responsible.

The implications of recent cisplatin administration for anesthesiologists include attention to hydration and possible electrolyte abnormalities. Hydration and diuresis with mannitol and furosemide may protect against the development of renal toxicity by dilution of the tubular urinary concentration. The hypomagnesemia that is associated with cisplatin's tubular injury may predispose to cardiac arrhythmias and decrease the response to neuromuscular blockers, and it should be corrected prior to elective operations.

Methotrexate is also associated with renal toxicity, with an incidence approaching 10% in higher doses.[110] Renal insufficiency may be prevented by hydration and urinary alkalinization. Mithramycin also causes a hemorrhagic diathesis in as many as 60% of patients.[111] This complication is associated with renal and hepatic dysfunction, probably related to volume depletion from hemorrhage. Mithramycin is currently used principally for testicular cancer. Mitomycin C and streptozocin are other agents for which renal toxicity has been infrequently described.

LIVER COMPLICATIONS

Overview

Many antineoplastic agents have the potential for hepatic toxicity. These are often related to nonspecific hepatitis and may be difficult to distinguish from metastatic disease and infectious complications of the cancer. Some agents have been directly implicated in different forms of liver toxicity (Table 53-5).

Methotrexate

Methotrexate is one chemotherapeutic agent that is clearly implicated in hepatic complications. Methotrexate binds to dihydrofolate reductase and prevents the conversion of folic acid to its active form, folinic acid, thereby blocking the synthesis of nucleic acids. Although it is widely used in the treatment of hematologic malignancies, methotrexate has also been included in the treatment of psoriasis and other rheumatologic disorders. From this experience, the relationship between methotrexate therapy and chemically and histologically defined liver damage has emerged. Short-term or intermittent therapy with methotrexate results in elevations of liver function test results, particularly serum glutamic-pyruvic transaminase, which generally returns to normal by 1 to 2 weeks after cessation of therapy.[112] More intensive therapy, typical in the treatment of malignancies, is associated with hepatic fibrosis in up to 30% of patients, and a small number of these go on to develop cirrhosis.[110] Preexisting liver disease may predispose to more severe enzyme derangements and a slower recovery of hepatic function. The etiology of methotrexate's toxicity may involve inhibition of lipid metabolism by impaired choline synthesis, resulting in fatty liver and portal inflammatory reactions.

With regard to hepatotoxicity, the experience with anesthesia in patients receiving methotrexate is limited. However, preoperative attention to liver function tests is advisable. Use of drugs requiring hepatic metabolism should be modified by the results of these tests.

TABLE 53-5. Chemotherapeutic Agents Producing Hepatic Toxicity

Drug	Effect
Nitrosoureas	
BCNU (carmustine)	Elevated liver enzymes
CCNU (lomustine)	Elevated liver enzymes
Streptozocin	Elevated liver enzymes
Antimetabolites	
Methotrexate	Fibrosis, cirrhosis
6-Mercaptopurine	Cholestasis, necrosis
Azathioprine	Cholestasis, necrosis
Cytosine arabinoside	Elevated liver enzymes
Antibiotics	
Mithramycin	Acute necrosis
Enzymes	
L-Asparaginase	Fatty metamorphosis

Reprinted with permission from Perry MC: Hepatotoxicity of chemotherapeutic agents. Semin Oncol 9:66, 1982.

VASCULAR COMPLICATIONS

Overview

In recent years, the vascular toxicity of antineoplastic agents (Table 53-6) has become manifested by a heterogeneous group of syndromes whose etiology is unclear. These toxicities may result from drug-induced endovascular damage, platelet and hemostatic abnormalities, or even autonomic dysfunction. All of these mechanisms may have an impact on the intraoperative management of affected patients and may account for some postoperative complications.

Pulmonary

Pulmonary vascular occlusive disease is a relatively rare cause of pulmonary hypertension characterized by fibrotic narrowing of pulmonary veins and venules. The lack of associated coagulation defects in these patients suggests a drug-induced endothelial injury. Bleomycin and mitomycin C are the agents most associated with development of this syndrome;[113] pulmonary vascular endothelial damage may be one manifestation of the spectrum of pulmonary toxicities associated with bleomycin and mitomycin C noted earlier. Treatment of pulmonary vascular occlusive disease with vasoactive agents has not been very successful, and the diagnosis is often made post mortem. However, high pulmonary artery pressures in one patient were reported to respond to hydralazine.[113]

Hepatic

Hepatic veno-occlusive disease (HVOD), like its pulmonary counterpart, shows progressive, nonthrombotic occlusion of small veins by loose connective tissue. Necrosis in hepatocytes occurs in centrilobular areas. The diagnosis is made

TABLE 53-6. Vascular Complications Associated With Antineoplastic Agents

Complications	Drug
Pulmonary veno-occlusive disease	Bleomycin
	Mitomycin
Hepatic veno-occlusive disease	Cyclophosphamide, carmustine, cisplatin
	Cyclophosphamide, busulfan
	Cyclophosphamide, total body irradiation
	Cyclophosphamide, high-dose cytosine arabinoside
	Dacarbazine
	Carmustine, etoposide (VP-16-213)
	Urethane
	Mitomycin
	Azathioprine
	6-Thioguanine
Budd-Chiari syndrome	Dacarbazine
	6-Thioguanine
	Cytosine arabinoside
	Methotrexate
Cerebrovascular accidents	Cisplatin-based chemotherapy
Raynaud's phenomenon	Bleomycin
	Bleomycin and vinca alkaloid
	Bleomycin, cisplatin, vinca alkaloid
Myocardial infarction	Vinca alkaloids
	Etoposide (VP-16-213)
	Vinblastine, bleomycin
	Cisplatin, bleomycin, vinca alkaloid
	5-Fluorouracil
Thrombotic microangiopathy	Mitomycin
	Cisplatin-based chemotherapy
Venous thrombosis	Cytoxan, methotrexate, vincristine, 5-fluorouracil, prednisone
Hypotension	Etoposide (VP-16-213)
	Teniposide (VM-26)
	Dacarbazine
	Homoharringtonine
	Vincristine
	Carmustine
Hypertension	Cisplatin
	Procarbazine
Acral erythema	Cytosine arabinoside
	Hydroxyurea
	Protracted infusion of 5-fluorouracil or doxorubicin
Retinal toxicity	Carmustine (carotid infusion)
	Cisplatin (carotid infusion and intravenous high dose)

Reprinted with permission from Doll DC, Ringenberg QS, Yarbro JW: Vascular toxicity associated with antineoplastic agents. J Clin Oncol 4:1406, 1986.

on clinical grounds, since liver biopsy has a high rate of false-negative results.[114]

Until recently, HVOD was a rare diagnosis made in association with conventional doses of cytotoxic drugs. With the larger numbers of bone marrow transplantations being performed and the high doses of chemotherapy required for bone marrow ablation, HVOD is being recognized with increasing frequency. The incidence of HVOD following either autologous or allogeneic transplant in most centers is about 20%.[115] The mortality from the disease ranges from 7–50% and was thought to be a contributing factor in another 30% of deaths following transplant in one series.[116]

The classic picture of HVOD includes jaundice, hepatomegaly or right upper quadrant pain, and ascites or unexplained weight gain; two of these symptoms are considered sufficient to make the diagnosis.[114] As mentioned earlier, liver biopsies are insensitive. Other causes of liver disease must be excluded, particularly viral, bacterial, and fungal infections. Alkylating agents, such as cyclophosphamide, carmustine (BCNU), lomustine, busulfan, and mitomycin C, have been associated with HVOD, principally at the elevated doses used in bone marrow transplantation.[113] A small number of antimetabolites at conventional doses have also been linked to HVOD, including 6-mercaptopurine, cytosine arabinoside, azathioprine, and 6-thioguanine.

Therapy for HVOD parallels therapy used for ascites, including sodium restriction, use of spironolactone rather than furosemide for diuresis, and attempts to maintain plasma oncotic pressure with plasma expanders when possible. These patients have a decreased effective blood volume, and invasive monitoring with a central venous or pulmonary artery catheter may be necessary to ensure adequate filling volumes during surgery. Drugs requiring hepatic metabolism or elimination should be given cautiously or avoided.

BIOLOGIC THERAPY OF CANCER

With the advent of recombinant DNA technology, therapy for malignancy using pharmacologic doses of human lymphokines and growth factors is rapidly progressing. Recombinant interleukin-2 has been given with some success to patients with refractory metastatic cancer and melanoma.[117] In these studies, infusion of interleukin-2 induced a vascular leak with hypotension and cardiac indices typical for septic shock in 65% of patients.[118] Decreases in left ventricular ejection fraction, oliguria, and noncardiogenic pulmonary edema requiring intubation were also seen. Other complications, including bronchospasm, coma, angina, and arrhythmias, may occur as well. These patients often require pressor support[119] (usually dopamine, phenylephrine, or norepinephrine) for as long as the interleukin-2 infusion continues. Fluid boluses may be ineffective and may aggravate the vascular leak. Monitoring with a flow-directed pulmonary catheter is often necessary. The etiology of the vascular leak and decrease in systemic vascular resistance may be a direct effect of the interleukin-2 or a result of further release of cytokines, such as tumor necrosis factor.[120,121] There is no current therapy available to prevent these side-effects of interleukin-2.

Other forms of biologic therapy include the hematopoietic growth factors, which are used to stimulate the bone marrow of patients undergoing chemotherapy. Granulocyte-macrophage colony-stimulating factor (GM-CSF) has been shown to increase the rate at which the leukocyte count rises after chemotherapy,[122] thus decreasing the number of days that the patient has fever and the need for antibiotics. GM-CSF itself rarely produces major limiting side-effects at the doses employed. The most severe complications are bone pain and pleuropericarditis, with occasional effusions.[123,124] The vascular leak and hypotension seen with interleukin-2 do not appear to occur with the colony-stimulating factors. With amelioration of the myelosuppressive effects of chemotherapy, GM-CSF may allow the use of more intensive chemotherapy regimens to attempt a cure. At these higher doses, solid organ toxicities as described above are likely to become more prominent, and currently occult toxicities may emerge.

BONE MARROW TRANSPLANTATION

Allogeneic bone marrow transplantation is now well established as a therapy for malignancy or genetic disease. It is indicated when total ablation of the diseased marrow is necessary for cure of the recipient's disease. Reconstitution of the hematopoietic and immune systems is accomplished with an HLA-identical donor marrow. Autologous bone marrow transplant is performed in patients with solid tumors and certain hematologic malignancies. These patients often require very high doses of chemotherapy, with resultant severe and prolonged myelosuppression; prior harvesting and infusion of their bone marrow permits autologous rescue and more rapid hematopoietic recovery. The harvested marrow may also be subjected to in vitro antineoplastic treatment in cases in which the cancer involves the marrow. Anesthetic management of these patients falls into two categories: (1) anesthesia for bone marrow harvesting, and (2) anesthetic care of the patient who has already received an allogeneic or autologous transplant.

Marrow Harvest

When allogeneic harvesting is done, the donor is usually healthy and often young. As older patients become eligible for allogeneic transplant, the average age of marrow donors will probably increase, with a concomitant increase in the incidence of hypertension, heart disease, and other unrelated illnesses. Volume management is critical in marrow donors, especially children, in whom the marrow harvest may equal up to one third of their blood volume.[125] The volume of marrow removed should be carefully monitored and replaced with crystalloid (and transfusion where appropriate) as though it were hemorrhagic blood loss. The volume of marrow required is dictated by the size of the recipient and usually amounts to 10 ml·kg^{-1} of the recipient's ideal body weight.

Similar volume considerations apply in autologous marrow harvesting. In addition, these patients may be older and chronically or acutely ill from their malignancy, metastatic disease, radiation, or chemotherapy. Anesthetic management must be carefully tailored to each patient in autologous harvesting.

Specific anesthetic plans for harvesting should be formulated in conjunction with the transplant team. Typically, the harvesting begins with the patient in the supine position, and repeated bone marrow aspirations are performed bilaterally on the anterior iliac crests. When marrow yields at this site decrease, the patient is turned to the prone position and the procedure is repeated on the posterior iliac spine. On average three hundred bone marrow aspirations through less than a dozen incisions are necessary. Either general anesthesia or regional techniques may be employed. The duration of harvesting depends on the volume of marrow to be aspirated and the difficulty in obtaining marrow; the latter may be important in autologous transplant patients who have received previous radiation or chemotherapy or have very dense bone. In most adults, about 2 hours are required for the procedure.

The only anesthetic that may be considered controversial in bone marrow harvesting is nitrous oxide. Nitrous oxide inhibits methionine synthetase and may result in megaloblastic hematopoiesis, depending on the duration and dose of the agent. Currently, there is no evidence that use of nitrous oxide during harvesting adversely affects marrow engraftment, subsequent hematopoiesis, or survival of the patient. However, it may be prudent to avoid nitrous oxide in harvests lasting longer than 2 hours, in patients currently receiving methotrexate, and in those who, because of chronic illness, may be folate- or vitamin B$_{12}$-deficient.

Postharvesting management is usually uncomplicated. In allogeneic cases, the principal difficulties are nausea, emesis, and hypotension caused by volume depletion, occurring in less than 10% of cases.[125] Pain management can be accomplished with routine use of narcotics, patient-controlled analgesia, or epidural narcotics. When large hematomas are avoided during harvesting, allogeneic donors are usually ready for discharge 1 or 2 days after the procedure; autologous donors may be more chronically ill and can require a longer hospitalization.

Anesthetic Care of the Marrow Transplant Recipient

The complications following bone marrow transplantation may have significant bearing on the anesthetic management of recipients presenting for subsequent surgery, both in the acute and in the long-term setting. These sequelae depend on the conditioning regimen used for bone marrow ablation (total body irradiation and/or high-dose chemotherapy), the severity of subsequent graft-versus-host disease, and the time interval since the transplantation. Depending on the disease and the age of the recipient, mortality in the first 100 days following bone marrow transplant may reach 30%.

The toxicities of chemotherapies used in bone marrow transplantation have been described earlier in this section. Cyclophosphamide is the most common agent employed and is associated with pulmonary, gastrointestinal, hepatic, and renal toxicity. Total body irradiation may result in hypothyroidism,[126] which was found in approximately 50% of patients at 13 months after transplant in one study.

Graft-versus-host disease represents one of the major complications in the area of transplant-related illness. The sequelae of acute graft-versus-host disease are related to organ dysfunction, especially the lungs, liver, and gastrointestinal system, and to infections and other complications of the immunosuppressive therapy to treat graft-versus-host disease[127] (Fig. 53-6).

Acute pulmonary complications usually occur within 3 months after marrow transplantation but may appear 1–2 years after transplant. Interstitial pneumonitis, characterized by hypoxemia and infiltrates on chest roentgenogram, may be the result of acute graft-versus-host disease, total body irradiation, or viral infection, often cytomegalovirus.[128] In two thirds of patients with interstitial pneumonitis, no specific etiologic agent can be found. The diagnosis is usually made by exclusion of other infections, hemorrhage, or fluid overload. In one series,[128] the incidence of interstitial pneumonitis after transplant was as high as 50%, and the mortality may reach 50–75% in affected patients. These patients often require intubation for ventilatory failure and may undergo bronchoscopy or open lung biopsy for diagnosis. Treatment is primarily supportive, with careful fluid management and treatment of graft-versus-host disease with steroids and immunosuppressive agents, such as methotrexate and cyclosporine. Stress doses of steroids may be needed for surgery.

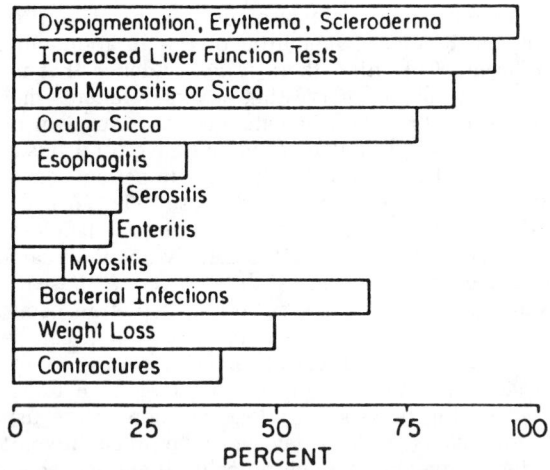

Figure 53-6. Incidence of clinical manifestations of extensive chronic graft-versus-host disease. (Reprinted with permission from Deeg HJ, Storb R, Thomas ED: Bone marrow transplantation: A review of delayed complications. Br J Haematol 57:188, 1984.)

Investigators have also noted more insidious pulmonary changes after marrow transplant. Pulmonary function tests show a decrease in vital capacity, total lung volume, and DL_{CO} in survivors of transplantation at 1 year;[129,130] this is more likely to occur in patients who had early interstitial pneumonitis. By 3–4 years after transplant, these restrictive changes were largely resolved. By contrast, there is an increasing number of survivors with obstructive pulmonary indices at 3 years after transplant. By that time, 8% of survivors have been reported to have a reduction in the ratio of forced expiratory volume in 1 second to vital capacity (FEV_1/FVC) to less than 50%. Unlike the earlier restrictive changes, late obstructive pulmonary disease is not associated with previous interstitial pneumonitis; the etiology of these late obstructive changes is not known.

Cancer and its therapies present unique challenges for the anesthesiologist. In addition to knowledge of the particular neoplasm and its spread, the anesthesiologist needs an understanding of the treatment modalities used, their cumulative doses, and duration of therapy. Specific studies investigating the interaction between anesthetics and different forms of chemotherapy are lacking, but knowledge of the complications of cancer therapy may aid in the anesthetic management of these complex patients.

REFERENCES

1. Cooper JA Jr, White DA, Matthay RA: Drug-induced pulmonary disease. Am Rev Respir Dis 133:321, 1986
2. Freeman BA, Crapo JD: Biology of disease: Free radical and tissue injury. Lab Invest 47:412, 1982
3. Smith AC, Boyd MR: Preferential effects of 1,3-bis(2-chloroethyl)-1-nitrosoureas (BCNU) on pulmonary glutathione/glutathione disulfide ratios: Possible implications for lung toxicity. J Pharmacol Exp Ther 76:128, 1984
4. Wesswlius LJ, Catanzaro A, Wasserman SI: Neutrophil chemotactic activity macrophages after bleomycin injury. Am Rev Respir Dis 129:485, 1984
5. Ginsberg SJ, Comis RL: The pulmonary toxicity of antineoplastic agents. Semin Oncol 9:34, 1982
6. Weiss RB: Hypersensitivity reactions to cancer chemotherapy. Semin Oncol 9:5, 1982
7. Yagoda A, Mukherji B, Young C et al: Bleomycin, an antitumor antibiotic. Clinical experience in 274 patients. Ann Intern Med 77:861, 1972
8. De Lena M, Guzzon A, Monfardini L, Bonodonna G: Clinical, radiologic, and histopathologic studies on pulmonary toxicity induced by treatment with bleomycin. Cancer Chemother Rep 56:343, 1972
9. Luce JK, Freireich EJ, Luna MA et al: Clinical trials with daily IV bleomycin (abstract). Proc Am Assoc Cancer Res 12:83, 1971
10. Iacovino JR, Leitner J, Abbas AK et al: Fatal pulmonary reaction from low doses of bleomycin. An idiosyncratic tissue response. JAMA 235:1253, 1976
11. Catane R, Schwade JG, Turrist AT et al: Pulmonary toxicity after radiation and bleomycin: A review. Int J Radiat Oncol Biol Phys 5:1513, 1979
12. Waid-Jones MI, Coursin DB: Perioperative considerations for patients treated with bleomycin. Chest 99:993, 1991
13. Goldiner PL, Carlon GD, Cvitkovic E et al: Factors influencing postoperative morbidity and mortality in patients treated with bleomycin. Br Med J 1:1664, 1978
14. Allen SC, Riddell GS, Butchart EG: Bleomycin therapy and anesthesia. The possible hazards of oxygen administration to patients after treatment with bleomycin. Anesthesia 60;121, 1981
15. Hulbert JC, Grossman JE, Cummings KB: Risk factors of anesthesia and surgery in bleomycin-treated patients. J Urol 130:163, 1983
16. Eigen H, Wyszomierski D: Bleomycin lung injury in children: Pathophysiology and guidelines for management. Am J Pediatr Hematol Oncol 7:71, 1985
17. Douglas JF, Coppin CML: Bleomycin and subsequent anaesthesia: A retrospective study at Vancouver General Hospital. Can Anaesth Soc J 27:449, 1980
18. LaMantia KR, Glick JH, Marshall BE: Supplemental oxygen does not cause respiratory failure in bleomycin-treated surgical patients. Anesthesiology 60:65, 1984
19. Blum RH, Carter SK, Agre KA: A clinical review of bleomycin: A new antineoplastic agent. Cancer 31:903, 1973
20. Piotti P, Genitoni V, Comazzi R et al: Relationship between pulmonary function tests and morphologic changes in the lung in bleomycin-treated patients. Tumori 70:439, 1984
21. Ishizuka M, Takayama H, Takeuchi T, Umezawa J: Activity and toxicity of bleomycin. J Antibiot (Tokyo) 20:15, 1967
22. Ohnuma T, Holland JF, Masuda J et al: Microbiological assay of bleomycin: Inactivation, tissue distribution, and clearance. J Cancer 33:1230, 1974
23. Oberley LW, Buettner GR: The production of hydroxyl radical by bleomycin and iron (II) (letter). Fed Exp Biol Soc 97:47, 1979
24. Berend N: Protective effect of hypoxia on bleomycin lung toxicity in the rat. Am Rev Respir Dis 130:307, 1984
25. Gross NJ: The pathogenesis of radiation-induced lung damage. Lung 159:115, 1981
26. Mosely PL, Shasby DM, Brady M, Hunninghake GW: Lung parenchymal injury induced by bleomycin. Am Rev Respir Dis 130:1082, 1984
27. Weiss RB, Poster DS, Penta JS: The nitrosoureas and pulmonary toxicity. Cancer Treat Rev 8:111, 1991
28. Aronin PA, Mahaleu MS, Rudnick SA et al: Prediction of BCNU pulmonary toxicity in patients with malignant gliomas. An assessment of risk factors. N Engl J Med 303:183, 1980
29. Weiss RB, Muggia FM: Pulmonary effects of carmustine (BCNU). Ann Intern Med 91:131, 1979
30. Gunstream SR, Seidenfeld JJ, Sobonya RE, McMahon LJ: Mitomycin-associated lung disease. Cancer Treat Rev 67:301, 1983
31. Orwoll ES, Kiessling P, Patterson R: Interstitial pneumonia from mitomycin. Ann Intern Med 89:352, 1978
32. Heard BE, Cooke RA: Busulphan lung. Thorax 23:187, 1968
33. Patel AR, Shah PC, Rhee HL et al: Cyclophosphamide therapy and interstitial pulmonary fibrosis. Cancer 38:1542, 1979
34. Hakkinen PJ, Whitely JW, Witschi HR: Hyperoxia, but not thorac x-irradiation, potentiates bleomycin and cyclophosphamide-induced lung damage in mice. Am Rev Respir Dis 126:281, 1982
35. Lascari AD, Strano AJ, Johnson WW et al: Methotrexate induced sudden fatal pulmonary reaction. Cancer 40:1393, 1977

36. White DA, Orenstein M, Godwin TA, Stover DE: Chemotherapy-associated pulmonary toxic reactions during treatment for breast cancer. Arch Intern Med 144:953, 1984

37. Zusman J, Frentz J, Waring W: Rapid resolution of "methotrexate lung" with preoperative steroids. Proc Am Assoc Cancer Res Am Soc Clin Oncol 20:412, 1979

38. Gross NJ: Pulmonary effects of radiation therapy. Ann Intern Med 86:81, 1977

39. Wang CC: Dental care of patients with head and neck cancer receiving radiation therapy. In Wang CC (ed): Radiation Therapy for Head and Neck Neoplasms: Indications, Techniques and Results, p 19. Littleton, Mass, John Wright PSG Inc, 1983

40. Parsons JT: The effect of radiation on normal tissues of the head and neck. In Million RR, Cassisi NJ (eds): Management of Head and Neck Cancer. A Multidisciplinary Approach, p 173. Philadelphia, JB Lippincott, 1984

41. Dindogru A, Barcos M, Henderson ES, Wallace HJ Jr: Electrocardiographic changes following Adriamycin treatment. Med Pediatr Oncol 5:65, 1978

42. Minow RA, Benjamin RS, Lee ET, Gottlier JA: Adriamycin cardiomyopathy—risk factors. Cancer 39:1397, 1977

43. Dresdale A, Bonow RO, Wesley R et al: Prospective evaluation of doxorubicin-induced cardiomyopathy resulting from postsurgical adjuvant treatment of patients with soft tissue sarcomas. Cancer 52:51, 1983

44. Von Hoff DD, Layard MW, Basa P et al: Risk factors for doxorubicin-induced congestive heart failure. Ann Intern Med 91:710, 1979

45. Praga C, Beretta G, Vigo PL et al: Adriamycin cardiotoxicity: A survey of 1273 patients. Cancer Treat Rep 63:827, 1979

46. Bristow MR, Billingham ME, Mason JW, Daniels JR: Clinical spectrum of anthracycline antibiotic cardiotoxicity. Cancer Treat Rep 62:873, 1978

47. Appelbaum F, Strauchen JA, Graw RG et al: Acute lethal carditis caused by high-dose combination chemotherapy: A unique clinical and pathological entity. Lancet 1:58, 1976

48. Unverferth DV, Magorien RD, Leier CV, Balcerzak SP: Doxorubicin cardiotoxicity. Cancer Treat Rev 9:149, 1982

49. Bristow MR, Lopez MB, Mason JW et al: Efficacy and cost of cardiac monitoring in patients receiving doxorubicin. Cancer 50:32, 1982

50. Gottdiener JS, Mathiesen DJ, Borer JS et al: Doxorubicin cardiotoxicity: Assessment of late left ventricular dysfunction by radionuclide cineangiography. Ann Intern Med 94:430, 1981

51. Von Hoff DD, Rozenweig M, Piccart M: The cardiotoxicity of anticancer agents. Semin Oncol 9:23, 1982

52. Von Hoff DD, Rozenweig M, Layard M et al: Daunomycin-induced cardiotoxicity in children and adults: A review of 110 cases. Am J Med 16:226, 1977

53. Gottdiener JS, Appelbaum FR, Ferrans VJ et al: Cardiotoxicity associated with high-dose cyclophosphamide therapy. Arch Intern Med 141:758, 1981

54. Cazin B, Gorin NC, Laporte JP et al: Cardiac complications after bone marrow transplantation. Cancer 57:2061, 1986

55. Labianca R, Beretta G, Clerici M et al: Cardiac toxicity of 5-fluorouracil: A study on 10083 patients. Tumori 68:505, 1982

56. Torti FM, Lum BL: Cardiac toxicity. In DeVita VT, Hellman S, Rosenberg SA (eds): Cancer, Principles and Practice of Oncology, p 2155. Philadelphia, JB Lippincott Co, 1990

57. Harris AL, Wong C: Myocardial ischemia, radiotherapy, and vinblastine. Lancet 1:787, 1981

58. Lejonc JL, Vernant JP, Macquin I et al: Myocardial infarction following vinblastine treatment. Lancet 2:692, 1980

59. Mandel EM, Lewinski U, Djaldetti M: Vincristine-induced myocardial infarction. Cancer 36:1979, 1975

60. Slanina J, Mussoff K, Rahner I, Stiasny R: Long-term side effects in irradiated patients with Hodgkin's disease. Int J Radiat Oncol Biol Phys 2:1, 1977

61. Carmel RJ, Kaplan HS: Mantle irradiation in Hodgkin's disease. Cancer 37:2813, 1976

62. Gottdiener JS, Katin MJ, Borer JS et al: Late cardiac effects of therapeutic mediastinal irradiation. N Engl J Med 308:569, 1983

63. Duettera MJ, Bleyer WA, Pomeroy TC et al: Irradiation, methotrexate toxicity, and the treatment of meningeal leukemia. Lancet 2:703, 1973

64. Babliano RG, Costanzi JJ: Paraplegia following intrathecal methotrexate. Cancer 37:1663, 1976

65. Breuer AC, Pitman SW, Dawson DM, Schoene WC: Paraparesis following intrathecal cytosine arabinoside. Cancer 40:2817, 1977

66. Kaplan RS, Wienik PH: Neurotoxicity of antineoplastic drugs. Semin Oncol 9:103, 1982

67. Bleyer WA, Griffin TW: White matter necrosis, mineralizing microangiopathy, and intellectual abilities in survivors of childhood leukemia: Associations with central nervous system irradiation and methotrexate therapy. In Gilber HA, Kagan AT (eds): Radiation Damage to the Nervous System, p 155. New York, Raven Press, 1980

68. Bleyer WA, Drake JC, Chabner BA: Neurotoxicity and elevated cerebrospinal-fluid methotrexate concentrations in meningeal leukemia. N Engl J Med 289:770, 1973

69. Saiki JH, Thompson S, Smith F, Atkinson R: Paraplegia following intrathecal chemotherapy. Cancer 29:370, 1972

70. Weiss HD, Walker MD, Wiernic PH: Neurotoxicity of commonly used antineoplastic agents. N Engl J Med 291:75, 1974

71. Hildebrand J: Lesions of the Nervous System in Cancer Patients, p 49. New York, Raven Press, 1978

72. Whittaker JA, Griffith IP: Recurrent laryngeal nerve paralysis in patients receiving vincristine and vinblastine. Br Med J 1:1251, 1977

73. Holland JF, Scharlab C, Gailani S et al: Vincristine treatment of advanced cancer: A cooperative study of 392 cases. Cancer Res 33:1258, 1973

74. Sandler SG, Tobin W, Henderson ES: Vincristine-induced neuropathy: A clinical study of fifty leukemic patients. Neurology 19:610, 1969

75. Carmichael SM, Eagleton L, Ayers CR et al: Orthostatic hypotension during vincristine therapy. Arch Intern Med 126:290, 1970

76. Slater DM, Weiner RA, Serpick AA: Vincristine neurotoxicity with hyponatremia. Cancer 23:122, 1969

77. Suskind RM, Brusilow SW, Zehr J: Syndrome of inappropriate secretion of antidiuretic hormone produced by vincristine toxicity (with bioassay of ADH level). J Pediatr 81:699, 1972

78. Moress GR, D'Agostino AN, Jarcho LW: Neuropathy in lymphoblastic leukemia treated with vincristine. Arch Neurol 16:377, 1967

79. Ohnuma T, Holland JF, Freeman A, Sinks LF: Biochemical and pharmacological studies with asparaginase in man. Cancer Res 30:2297, 1970

80. Riccardi R, Holcenberg J, Glaubiger D, Poplack D: L-asparaginase pharmacokinetics and L-asparaginase in the cerebrospinal fluid. Proc Am Assoc Cancer Res 21:336, 1980

81. Lee IP, Lucier GW: The potentiation of barbiturate-induced narcosis by procarbazine. J Pharmacol Exp Ther 196:586, 1976

82. Von Hoff DD, Schilsky R, Reichert CM et al: Toxic effects of Cis-dichlorodiammineplatinum (II) in man. Cancer Treat Rep 63:1527, 1979

83. Piel IJ, Meyer D, Perlia CP, Wolfe VI: Effects of cis-diamminedichloroplatinum on hearing function in man. Cancer Chemother Rep 58:871, 1974

84. Hadley D, Herr HW: Peripheral neuropathy associated with cis-dichlorodiamine platinum (II) treatment. Cancer 44:2026, 1979

85. Kedar A, Cohen ME, Freeman AI: Peripheral neuropathy as a complication of cis-dichlorodiaminoplatinum (II) treatment: A case report. Cancer Treat Rep 62:819, 1978

86. Panettieire FJ: Cis-platinum toxicity. An analysis based on 3 SWOG studies. Proc Am Assoc Cancer Res 22:157, 1981

87. Marder VJ, Butler FO, Barlow GH: Anti-fibrinolytic therapy. In Colman RW, Hirsh J, Marder VJ et al (eds): Hemostasis and Thrombosis, p 380. Philadelphia, JB Lippincott, 1987

88. Carvalho ACA, Rao AK: Acquired qualitative platelet defects. In Colman RW, Hirsh J. Marder VJ, et al (eds): Hemostasis and Thrombosis, p 750. Philadelphia, JB Lippincott, 1987

89. Goldberg MA, Ginsberg D, Mayer RJ et al: Is heparin administration necessary during induction chemotherapy for patients with acute promyelocytic leukemia? Blood 69:187, 1987

90. Feinstein DI: Disseminated intravascular coagulation: How to intervene in a complex process. J Crit Illness 4:21, 1989

91. Chung F: Cancer, chemotherapy and anaesthesia. Can Anaesth Soc J 29:364, 1982

92. Fields ALA, Josse RG, Bergsagel DE: Metabolic emergencies. *In* DeVita VT Jr, Hellman S, Rogenberg SA (eds): Cancer: Principles and Practice of Oncology, 2nd ed, p 1866. Philadelphia, JB Lippincott, 1985

93. Broadus AE, Mangin M, Ikeda K *et al*: Humoral hypercalcemia of cancer. N Engl J Med 319:556, 1988

94. Ihde DC: Paraneoplastic syndromes. Hosp Pract Aug 15:79, 1987

95. Mundy GR: Hypercalcemia of malignancy revisited. J Clin Invest 82:1, 1988

96. Hasling C, Charles P, Mosekilde L: Etidronate disodium in the management of malignancy-related hypercalcemia. Am J Med 82(suppl 2A):51, 1987

97. Ryzen E, Martodam RR, Troxell M *et al*: Intravenous etidronate in the management of malignant hypercalcemia. Arch Intern Med 145:449, 1985

98. Decaux G, Waterlot Y, Genette F *et al*: Treatment of the syndrome of inappropriate secretion of antidiuretic hormone with furosemide. N Engl J Med 304:329, 1981

99. Forrest JN Jr, Cox M, Hong C *et al*: Superiority of demeclocycline over lithium in the treatment of chronic syndrome of inappropriate secretion of antidiuretic hormone. N Engl J Med 298:173, 1978

100. Bunn PA Jr, Minna JD: Paraneoplastic syndromes. *In* DeVita VT Jr, Hellman S, Rosenberg SA (eds): Cancer, Principles and Practice of Oncology, pp 1797–1842. Philadelphia, JB Lippincott, 1985

101. Dierdorf SF: Rare and co-existing diseases. *In* Barash PG, Cullen BF, Stoelting RK (eds): Clinical Anesthesia, 2nd ed, p 563. Philadelphia, JB Lippincott, 1992

102. Colhoun EH, Rylett BJ: Further facts about neuromuscular blockades by nitrogen mustard and by thio-tepa. Anesthesiology 48:381, 1978

103. Zsigmond EK, Robins F: The effect of a series of anti-cancer drugs on plasma cholinesterase activity. Can Anaesth Soc J 19:75, 1972

104. Walker IR, Zapf PW, Mackay IR: Cyclophosphamide, cholinesterase and anaesthesia. Aust NZ J Med 3:247, 1972

105. Goldstein RS, Mayor GH: The nephrotoxicity of cisplatinum. Life Sci 32:685, 1983

106. Schilsky RL, Anderson T: Hypomagnesemia and renal magnesium wasting in patients receiving cis-platinum. Ann Intern Med 90:929, 1979

107. Choie DD, Delcampo AA, Guarino AM: Subcellular localizations of cis-dichlorodiammineplatinum(II) in rat kidney and liver. Toxicol Appl Pharmacol 55:245, 1980

108. Grazanio J, Jones B, Piscotto P: The effect of heavy metal chelators on the renal accumulation of platinum after cis-dichlorodiammineplatinum II administration to the rat. Br J Pharmacol 73:649, 1981

109. Hoeschele JD, Van Camp L: Whole body counting and the distribution of cis-platinum-195M diammine dichloride in the major organs of Swiss white mice. Adv Antimicrob Antineopl Chemother 2:241, 1972

110. Chabner BA, Donehower RC, Schilsky J: Clinical pharmacology of methotrexate. Cancer Treat Rep 65:51, 1981

111. Kennedy BJ: Metabolic and toxic effects of mithramycin during tumor therapy. Am J Med 49:494, 1970

112. Hersh EM, Wong VG, Henderson ES *et al*: Hepatotoxic effects of methotrexate. Cancer 4:600, 1966

113. Doll DC, Ringengerg QS, Yarbro JW: Vascular toxicity associated with antineoplastic agents. J Clin Oncol 4:1405, 1986

114. Schulman HM, McDonald GB, Matthews D *et al*: An analysis of hepatic veno-occlusive disease and centrilobular hepatic degeneration following bone marrow transplantation. Gastroenterology 79:1178, 1980

115. McDonald GB, Sharma P, Matthews D *et al*: Veno-occlusive disease of the liver after bone marrow transplantation: Diagnosis, incidence, and predisposing factors. Hepatology 4:123, 1984

116. D'Cruz CA, Wimmer RS, Harcke HT *et al*: Veno-occlusive disease of the liver in children following chemotherapy for acute myelocytic leukemia. Cancer 52:1803, 1983

117. Rosenberg SA, Lotze MT, Mule JJ: New approaches to the immunotherapy of cancer using interleukin-2. Ann Intern Med 108:853, 1988

118. Gaynor ER, Vitek L, Stickin L *et al*: The hemodynamic effects of treatment with interleukin-2 and lymphokine-activated killer cells. Ann Intern Med 109:953, 1988

119. Lee RE, Lotze MT, Skibber JM *et al*: Cardiorespiratory effects of immunotherapy with interleukin-2. J Clin Oncol 7:7, 1989

120. Isner JM, Dietz WA: Cardiovascular consequences of recombinant DNA technology: Interleukin-2. Ann Intern Med 109:933, 1988

121. Herberman RB: Interleukin-2 therapy of human cancer. Potential benefits versus toxicity. J Clin Oncol 7:1, 1989

122. Brandt SJ, Peters WP, Atwater SK *et al*: Effect of recombinant human granulocyte-macrophage colony-stimulating factor on hematopoietic reconstitution after high-dose chemotherapy and autologous bone marrow transplantation. N Engl J Med 318:869, 1988

123. Gabrilove JL, Jakubowski A, Scher H *et al*: Effect of granulocyte colony-stimulating factor on neutropenia and associated morbidity due to chemotherapy for transitional-cell carcinoma of the urothelium. N Engl J Med 318:1414, 1988

124. Vadhan-Raj S, Keating M, LeMaistre A *et al*: Effects of recombinant human granulocyte-macrophage colony-stimulating factor in patients with myelodysplastic syndromes. N Engl J Med 317:1545, 1987

125. Filshie J, Pollock AN, Hughes RG *et al*: The anaesthetic management of bone marrow harvest for transplantation. Anaesthesia 39:480, 1984

126. Sklar CM, Kim TH, Ramsay NKC *et al*: Thyroid dysfunction among long-term survivors of bone marrow transplant. Am J Med 73:688, 1982

127. Vogelsang GB, Hess AD, Santos GW: Acute graft-versus-host disease: Clinical characteristics in the cyclosporine era. Medicine 67:163, 1988

128. Wingard JR, Mellits ED, Sostrin MB *et al*: Interstitial pneumonitis after allogeneic bone marrow transplantation. Medicine 67:175, 1988

129. Deeg HJ, Storb R, Thomas ED: Bone marrow transplantation: A review of delayed complications. Br J Haematol 57:185, 1984

130. Springmeyer SC, Flournoy N, Sullivan KM *et al*: Pulmonary function changes in long-term survivors of allogeneic marrow transplantation. *In* Gale RP (ed): Recent Advances in Bone Marrow Transplantation, p 343. New York, Alan R Liss, 1983

54

Bruce S. Gillies

Anesthesia Outside the Operating Room

The environment outside the operating room offers a unique challenge to the anesthesiologist. With the increasing number of diagnostic and therapeutic procedures performed every year, there is a greater need for patient monitoring and assurance of quality care. Technologic advancements as well as new equipment requiring specialized environments have provided an expansion of anesthetic care to the nonoperative location. The role of the anesthesiologist in this setting is to ensure the safety and comfort of the patient and to facilitate the performance of the procedure. Fundamental anesthetic principles apply to all patient care whether the procedures are within or outside of the operating room.

GENERAL PRINCIPLES

Monitoring capabilities and anesthesia equipment may not be as sophisticated outside the operating room as in the operating room. Although uniformity of anesthesia equipment would enhance safety, many anesthesia machines in locations outside the operating room may be outdated and not adapted to meet the needs of the frequently restricted environments in which they are used. Constant maintenance of this equipment is essential because the remote location of the procedure often makes immediate help from operating room personnel unavailable. Thorough preoperative or preprocedural preparation is a must. The anesthesiologist unfamiliar with the anesthesia machines and layout in the nonoperating room location should spend additional time ensuring proper function of this equipment.

Several problems may be encountered in the nonoperative location. Most facilities for nonsurgical procedures were not designed to meet the needs of anesthetic care for the patient. There is often limited space. In addition, access to the patient may be limited, which may pose a significant safety risk. In certain procedures, e.g., radiation therapy, the anesthesiologist may not even be present in the same room as the patient. Room lighting may not be optimal. Darkness may be required for radiologic procedures; this increases the likelihood of unrecognized airway obstruction, circuit disconnections, and possible exhaustion of gas cylinders. In addition to routine anesthesia equipment, self-inflating bags, extra oxygen cylinders, a defibrillator, and emergency drugs must be readily accessible. If suction is not available, portable vacuum devices will be necessary.

Usual standards for monitoring should be followed just as in the operating room, including determination of blood pressure and heart rate every 5 minutes. An electrocardiogram should be continuously displayed. Continuous monitoring of ventilation and circulation during general anesthesia with qualitative end-tidal carbon dioxide measurement and pulse oximetry should be performed. Ventilation controlled mechanically mandates continuous use of a breathing system disconnection device. In addition, oxygen concentration should be monitored by an oxygen analyzer equipped with a low-concentration alarm.

The nonoperative environment may be hazardous to both the anesthesiologist and the patient. Increased exposure to radiation during radiologic procedures can occur. Anesthesia personnel who are involved in these procedures, even on an infrequent basis, should consider wearing badges to measure cumulative exposure.

Electrical equipment used for monitoring should be evaluated for electrical safety and line isolation. Electrical outlets should be identified and checked for adequate grounding. Proper equipment for scavenging of anesthetic gases should be available. Lack of scavenging capability has led to the exclusion of volatile anesthetic gases for certain procedures at some centers.[1]

Reliance on sophisticated monitors has become a necessary part of anesthetic management. In the nonoperative location, monitoring must play an even greater role because of the frequent need for separation of patient from anesthesiologist. When restrictions on space limit monitoring capabilities, reliance on tactile and auditory signs during anesthesia assume increased importance.

ANESTHESIA FOR EXTRACORPOREAL SHOCK WAVE LITHOTRIPSY

Extracorporeal shock wave lithotripsy (ESWL) was developed over the latter part of the 1970s as an outgrowth of research on shock waves. ESWL provides a truly noninvasive method for the treatment of nephrolithiasis.[2-4] The first clinical use of ESWL was in 1980 with an electrohydraulic lithotriptor described by Chaussy.[5] Today ESWL is the most common form of treatment for urinary calculi.

The first-generation lithotriptors used patient submersion in water, which was used as a cushion and a medium for generating and propagating a focused shock wave. This method is commonplace today. A number of second-generation lithotriptors are also in use.[3,6-9] They have the advantage of not requiring patient submersion in water and a decreased level of anesthesia or analgesia is required.[9-11] This is because a lower energy density shock wave is felt at the skin surface. Experience shows that this newer therapy results in an increased need for repeated treatments.[3] ESWL has expanded to the treatment of cholelithiasis. Both immersion and nonimmersion techniques have been used with success.[10-13]

The commonly used first-generation lithotriptor requires patient immersion in water, as noted previously. After radiographic or fluoroscopic localization of the renal calculus, high-voltage energy is released across a spark gap, causing the evaporation of water between the electrodes. This results in a powerful high-pressure shock wave focused on the stone by an ellipsoidal reflector (Fig. 54-1). Five hundred to 2,500 shocks are delivered at each session. The energy lost as the focused shock waves cross from the surrounding tissue to the stone results in the eventual fragmentation of the stone. The patient can easily pass the stone once it has been pulverized into small fragments. The second-generation lithotriptors differ with respect to generation of the shock waves. Electromagnetic, piezoelectric, and microexplosive are several of the newer energy sources used.[3,6-8,11] The newer lithotriptors also differ in the methodology for stone localization. While fluoroscopic techniques are still common, ultrasound localization is being used with many of the newer instruments, and stone identification may actually be enhanced and exposure to radiation reduced.[6]

Several important features are unique to immersion ESWL. The immersion of the body in the head-out position results in physiologic changes that can be considerable.[14-16] Hemodynamic changes include an increase in central circulatory volume by as much as 500–700 ml.[14] Stroke volume and cardiac output are enhanced. Systemic vascular resistance is decreased by one-third. Pulmonary changes include a decrease in functional residual capacity and an increase in diffusing capacity.[15-17] Diffusion improves owing to favorable changes in pulmonary blood flow. Airway resistance increases because of external pressure on extrathoracic airways. The work of breathing is markedly increased.[18] Hormonal changes with prolonged immersion include decreased renin, aldosterone, and antidiuretic hormones. The role of atrial natriuretic factor with respect to these changes is unknown.

Immersion of patients may lead to undesirable shivering caused by hypothermia, unless the water bath temperature is maintained at body temperature. Shivering may interfere with the localization of the renal calculus or may cause an artifact on the ECG. This is important because the shock wave must be triggered from the ECG signal. Various disturbances of cardiac conduction and rhythm can be seen when the shock wave is initiated during the RT interval. These include premature ventricular and atrial contractions as well as supraventricular tachycardia. This problem is resolved by initiating the shock wave 0.20–0.22 msec after the R wave during the absolute refractory period.

Indications for lithotripsy depend on the size, number, and composition of the stones. Approximately 70% of all patients with urinary tract stones can be treated with ESWL. Contraindications for ESWL are outlined in Table 54-1. ESWL for gallstones can be undertaken with either immersion or nonimmersion techniques. A recent addition is a multipurpose device for the treatment of both urinary and biliary stones. Shock waves from the lithotriptor are usually

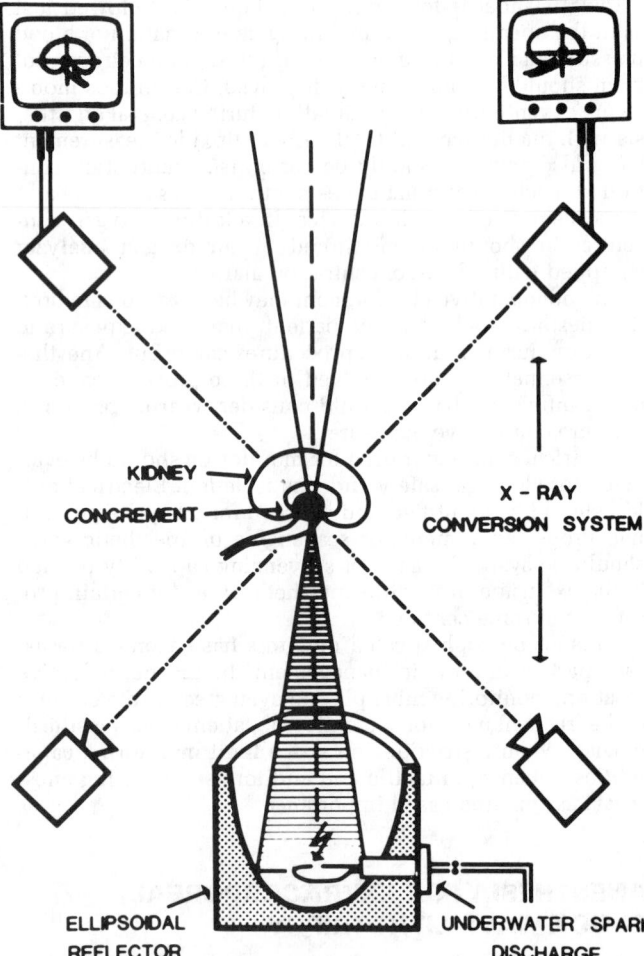

Figure 54-1. Schematic drawing of extracorporeally induced destruction of kidney stone with two integrated x-ray conversion systems. (Reproduced with permission from Chaussey C, Schmiedt E, Jocham D *et al:* First clinical experience with extracorporeally induced destruction of kidney stones by shock waves. J Urol 127:417, 1982.)

KIDNEY
CONCREMENT
X – RAY CONVERSION SYSTEM
ELLIPSOIDAL REFLECTOR
UNDERWATER SPARK DISCHARGE

TABLE 54-1. ESWL

Contraindications

Bleeding disorders
Pregnancy
Aortic or renal artery calcifications
Aortic or renal artery aneurysms
Unstable medical status

Relative Contraindications

Pacemakers
Obesity
Abnormalities of body habitus
Ectopic kidney or other anatomic anomaly

focused on the stone with the patient prone. The pathway for the shock wave must avoid bone and the lungs. Contraindications to biliary lithotripsy in addition to those in Table 54-1 are acute cholecystitis, cholangitis, biliary obstruction, gastric or duodenal ulcers, and pancreatitis.[12]

Anesthetic Considerations

The preoperative assessment is similar to that for any patient scheduled to receive anesthesia. Routine history, physical exam, and laboratory results should be obtained. Patients for ESWL should be stable medically, as lithotripsy is usually elective. Patients with preexisting disease or considerable variance in body habitus may present an even greater challenge to the anesthesiologist. Patients should be well hydrated and fluids continued throughout the case. Radiographs of the abdomen are usually obtained prior to the procedure to assess stone position.

Adequate monitoring during ESWL is essential. Once the patient has been lowered into the water bath, access to the patient may be difficult. Blood pressure cuff, ECG, and pulse oximetry are essential. All leads of the ECG should be checked to provide a good quality signal. The shock wave is triggered from the R wave and artifact or poor signal may predispose the patient to dysrhythmias. Waterproof ECG pads or occlusive dressings are recommended. Supplemental oxygen may be necessary due to the changes in ventilation and work of breathing. A method of detecting end-tidal carbon dioxide is necessary if general anesthesia is used. Temperature monitoring is useful to help prevent hypothermia and shivering. Intravenous hydration that results in a modest diuresis throughout the procedure is helpful for passage of stone fragments.

Electrohydraulic lithotripsy (water bath) is painful. The arrival of the focused shock wave at the skin–water interface is associated with a release of energy dissipated at the skin. Patients who undergo ESWL often have significant ecchymosis at the entry site. A single session may use as many as 2,500 shocks to disrupt the calculus. A major claim of the newer energy source lithotriptors is that they may be used without anesthesia.[9-11] In fact, considerable intravenous analgesia is required, and often these newer methods are associated with significant pain.[13] The benefits of lower anesthetic requirements are usually obtained at the expense of an increased number of shocks per session and repeat treatment.

Lithotriptors have been characterized as sound hazards.[19] The noise emitted from a lithotriptor during shock wave generation is in the range of 90–110 dB. A patient that is anxious or nervous may feel even more uncomfortable with this sound level. Patient preparation will improve the tolerance of the procedure. Some method of attenuating the noise for the patient as well as the anesthesiologist is recommended.

Patient positioning for submersion lithotripsy is crucial. In order to obtain adequate imaging and focusing of the shock wave, the patient must remain motionless. With the awake patient, comfort must be assured prior to lowering the patient into the water bath.

Several different methods of anesthesia have been used to facilitate performance of ESWL. The most commonly used method is continuous epidural anesthesia, which has been shown to provide adequate pain relief.[20-22] The patient is positioned with his arms raised above his head and strapped in place (Fig. 54-2). The awake patient can aid in determining a comfortable position. Numerous studies have

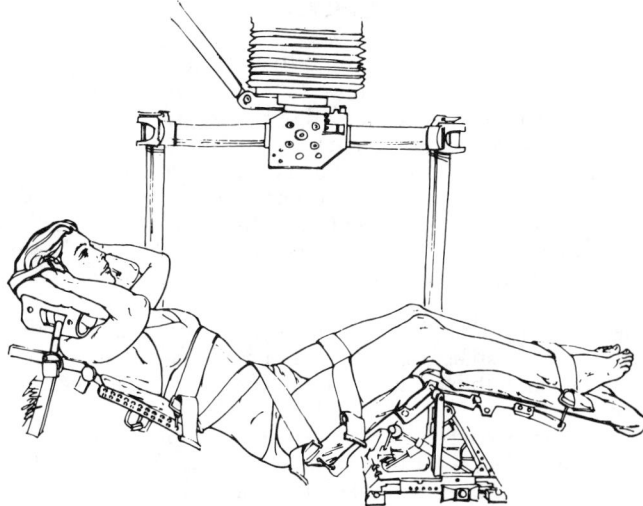

Figure 54-2. Patient positioning for immersion extracorporeal shock wave lithotripsy. Note that brachial plexus injury can occur with arms extended in this fashion. (Reproduced with permission from Duvall JO, Griffith DP: Epidural anesthesia for extracorporeal shock wave lithotripsy. Anesth Analg 64:544, 1985.)

examined the choice of local anesthetic for regional anesthesia.[20-23] Because many ESWL procedures are performed on an outpatient basis, the choice of local anesthetic may influence recovery time. A recent study has shown that 2-chloroprocaine and lidocaine decrease the admission rate and length of stay in this setting.[21]

Care must be taken with placement and securing of the epidural catheter. Foam tape, which is often used for securing the epidural catheter to the back, may trap gas between the patient and the tape, possibly decreasing the effectiveness of the shock waves.[24] Waterproof, occlusive dressings are recommended to avoid contamination of the epidural catheter in the water bath. Loss of resistance techniques for localizing the epidural space without air are recommended. Possible complications of epidural anesthesia include dural punctures and moderate to severe hypotension. Adequate hydration prior to the procedure can attenuate this.

General anesthesia has the advantage of providing rapid induction of anesthesia and may allow for a shorter turnover time. Patients may prefer general anesthesia because of the discomfort of submersion and the exposure to loud noise associated with the procedure. The method of ventilation has been the subject of controversy. Many centers advocate the use of high-frequency jet ventilation to minimize movement of the stone, which allows for rapid localization and more precise focusing of the shock wave.[25-28] However, when compared with conventional ventilation or epidural anesthesia, stone movement has not been shown to be a problem influencing successful fragmentation of the calculus.[29] A novel method for ECG-controlled ventilation has been described, allowing for shock wave initiation during exhalation without respiratory movement, which can cause stone excursion.[30] A number of intravenous sedation and analgesia regimens have been used with both first- and second-generation ESWL.[31-36] Adequate sedation and analgesia must be carefully titrated to provide analgesia adequate for pain control yet without causing respiratory depression. Combinations of midazolam with alfentanil or ketamine and propofol infusions have also been used with success.[31-33,36]

Complications of ESWL

Most patients who undergo ESWL will have some degree of hematuria after the procedure.[3,4,37] Long-term complications of perirenal hematomas include fibrosis and possible compression of renal parenchyma, causing hypertension.[3,37,38] Dysrhythmias can occur during ESWL due to incorrect timing of the shock wave and its occurrence during the RT interval on the ECG. Correct timing and an enhanced quality ECG trace will alleviate this problem.

Sepsis following ESWL may lead to septic shock.[25,39] This unusual event may occur in patients having preexisting urosepsis or pyelonephritis.[39] Positive urine cultures should alert the anesthesiologist to this possibility. ESWL is not associated with bacteremia in the absence of positive urine cultures.[40]

Only recently has ESWL been adapted for the treatment of biliary stones. Further studies are needed to assess the incidence of side effects associated with this procedure.

RADIOLOGY AND RADIATION THERAPY

Diagnostic and therapeutic radiology constitute the major requirement for anesthesia outside the operating room. Diagnostic procedures can be both invasive and noninvasive, including angiography, magnetic resonance imaging (MRI), and computed tomography (CT). Therapeutic radiology includes embolization during angiography, external beam radiation, and intraoperative radiation therapy. Cardiac catheterization and angioplasty are other invasive procedures commonly performed.

Most adult patients with adequate instruction and preparatory guidance are able to tolerate noninvasive procedures even without sedation. Imaging will be satisfactory in most cases; however, some patients may require an increased level of care. Monitoring of the patient with trauma, intracranial hypertension, or a compromised airway may be necessary. Anesthesiology consultation may be needed for confused or combative patients and for patients who are unwilling or unable to remain still because of neuromuscular movement disorders. Pediatric patients have special needs. Fear, anxiety, and separation from parents make it difficult to perform radiologic procedures without anesthesia.

Contrast agents are used routinely during angiographic and other radiologic procedures. Frequently, anesthesiologists are asked to monitor or care for patients at risk for adverse reactions to contrast media. The incidence of adverse reactions to intravascular injection of contrast dye is approximately 5–8%.[41-43] Many factors contribute to development of such adverse reactions. The method of injection (either slow infusion or bolus), the type of dye used, and dose may influence the risk of systemic reactions.[41] Type of technique or site to be studied also have a significant influence on the incidence of adverse reactions. For example, both coronary artery and cerebral angiography are associated with a high risk of reactions.[41] Patients with a prior history of atopy or known allergy to shell fish or seafood are more prone to contrast-related adverse reactions.[41,43] Obviously, patients with prior reactions to contrast media should be treated very cautiously.[44] Adverse reactions can be mild, moderate, or severe (Table 54-2).

Although nausea and vomiting are classified as mild reactions to contrast dye injection, they occur as prodromal symptoms in as many as 20% of all anaphylactoid and fatal

TABLE 54-2. Manifestations of Adverse Reactions to Radiologic Contrast Media

Mild	Moderate	Severe
Urticaria	Tissue edema	Prolonged hypotension
Chills	Bronchospasm	Cyanosis
Fever	Hypotension	Anoxia
Facial flushing	Seizures	Pulmonary edema
Nausea		Angina
Vomiting		Dysrhythmias

Adapted from Goldberg M: Systemic reactions to intravascular contrast media. Anesthesiology 60:45, 1984.

reactions.[41] Direct vasoactive substance release and complement activation stimulated by contrast media have been proposed as mechanisms for many adverse reactions including hypotension, urticaria, flushing, and bronchospasm.[41,45,46] Hypotension frequently occurs and, although mild, is often preceded by a transient period of systemic hypertension. In addition to systemic hypertension, increases in central venous, pulmonary artery, and left atrial pressure may occur. In patients with compromised cardiac function, this may precipitate pulmonary edema.[41,47] The hypertension is thought to be related to the hyperosmolarity of contrast media.[41] Contrast dyes are made of iodine-containing anions linked ionically to various cations including magnesium, calcium, and methylglucamine. The dyes are hyperosmolar with respect to blood plasma with osmolarities ranging from 600–2100 $mOsm·l^{-1}$. Patients undergoing contrast procedures usually have an induced diuresis from the osmotic load. Adequate hydration of these patients should be assured to prevent aggravation of preexisting azotemia. Patients with renal dysfunction should be approached with particular caution.[48]

Treatment of adverse reactions often depends on the severity of the reaction. Often supportive care is all that is necessary. Fluids, intravenous access, and careful monitoring of the patient are essential. Access to oxygen and drugs, including epinephrine, atropine, diphenhydramine, steroids, benzodiazepines, and methylxanthines (such as aminophylline), is recommended. Prophylaxis with diphenhydramine 25–50 mg iv and/or steroids (methylprednisolone 100–1000 mg iv) has been shown to be of benefit.[41,44,49-51]

Most radiologic procedures entail exposure of the physician, other health care workers, and patient to ionizing radiation, usually in the form of x-rays. Infrequent exposure to gamma radiation, or rarely alpha or beta radiation, from radioactive isotopes may also occur during radiation implantation or removal procedures. Radiation dosage and terminology are shown in Table 54-3.

The greatest source of radiation exposure is usually fluoroscopy. The dose delivered to the patient's skin during a routine procedure may be greater than 8000 mrem.[52,53] During fluoroscopy for cardiac angiography, the delivered dose may be greater than 75,000 mrem.[52] A single CT scan exposes the patient to approximately 1–3 rad.[52] The exposure of health care workers to the ionizing radiation emitted from CT scanners is relatively low because the radiation is highly focused. Radiation exposure during fluoroscopy is most often from scatter. X-rays will pass through most materials; however, as with all other sources of radiation, some

TABLE 54-3. Radiation Terminology and Dosage

Term	Definition
Radiation absorbed dose (rad)	A measure of an absorbed dose equal to 100 ergs·g^{-1} of any absorber (SI units Gray (GY): 1 GY = 100 rad)
Roentgen (R)	Total dosage absorbed of either x-rays or gamma rays. One roentgen is equal to 86.9 ergs·g^{-1} of dry air
Roentgen-equivalent-man (rem)	The dose of ionizing radiation with the same biologic tissue effect as 1 rad of x-rays

Maximum Dose Recommended by the National Council of Radiation Protection

Exposure	<100 mrem·wk^{-1} <5000 mrem·yr^{-1}

Adapted from Davies D: Subspecialty monitoring techniques—miscellaneous. In Gravenstein N (ed): Problems in Anesthesia Monitoring, pp 138–156. Philadelphia, JB Lippincott, 1987.

scatter occurs. Radiation intensity decreases with the inverse square of the distance from the emitting source.[54] A minimum of 1–2 meters is recommended. With this precaution and the use of a lead apron and thyroid shield, exposure to ionizing radiation can be kept at a safe level.

Anesthetic care is required in radiology suites for a number of different procedures. Pediatric patients most commonly require anesthesia. In addition, patients who cannot remain still during imaging for cardiac catheterization, angioplasty, valvuloplasty, or who require an increased level of care due to severity of disease may need anesthesia care. Monitored anesthesia care ("stand by") for angioplasty or valvuloplasty is also common.

Several important considerations for management of children during cardiac catheterization should be noted.[55] Catheterization is usually performed for congenital heart disease (CHD). Cyanosis, dyspnea, failure to thrive, and congestive heart failure are common presenting signs and symptoms. In addition, anxiety and increased activity may exacerbate preexisting cardiopulmonary problems. Premedication and sedation play an important role in alleviating anxiety and fear. The level of analgesia and sedation or general anesthesia must be adequate to prevent tachycardia, hypertension, and changes in cardiac function. Large changes in existing shunts should be avoided. These may occur due to excess myocardial depression or alterations in preload and afterload, due to fluid balance or excessive stimulation. Both hypercarbia and hypocarbia should be avoided with ventilation. In patients dependent on a patent ductus arteriosis (e.g., coarctation of the aorta), caution must be exercised to avoid high oxygen tension, which may lead to ductal closure. Prostaglandin E$_1$ infusions are often used to prevent this. Polycythemia is common in pediatric patients with cyanotic CHD. While a high hematocrit causes problems with viscosity, coagulopathy, and an increased risk of thrombosis, lowering the hematocrit can be detrimental to oxygen delivery in these patients.

The onset of action of many anesthetic drugs is influenced by the presence of left to right or right to left shunts as well as preexisting congestive failure. Dysrhythmias can frequently occur and are an important cause of morbidity in the pediatric and adult patient. Atropine premedication for children, especially those with cyanotic disease, is important.

During cardiac catheterization monitoring of the pediatric patient is usually adequately performed using an ECG, pulse oximeter, blood pressure cuff, and actual catheterization data. Blood gases may be obtained as necessary.

Adult patients rarely require anything more than sedation for catheter insertion and performance of the procedure. Some recent studies have shown benefit from general anesthesia during angioplasty procedures for acute myocardial infarction, but the main benefit was improved patient satisfaction.[56]

Monitoring and management of ischemic episodes and dysrhythmias are important problems that require the attention of the anesthesiologist in the catheterization laboratory. Dysrhythmias occur in almost 4% of patients. Conduction block can occur during catheter insertion but is rarely permanent or of hemodynamic significance. Ventricular tachycardia or fibrillation may worsen ischemia and complicate administration of contrast media. Prompt access to a defibrillator and resuscitative drugs is required. Oxygen therapy and availability of nitroglycerin, vasopressors, and inotropes for all patients is recommended. If acute cardiorespiratory decompensation occurs and CPR is necessary, access to patients during catheterization procedures may be difficult because of the presence of fluoroscopic equipment. Protective clothing must be worn during the procedure, as even scatter from the ionizing radiation may result in a significant exposure.

Angiography

Most contrast angiography studies do not require anesthetic care. Adept use of local anesthesia, with or without light sedation, is all that is usually required. Anesthesiology services may be requested to facilitate procedures involving pediatric patients. Most children will not be able to tolerate the large catheters required for angiography, even under local anesthesia. General anesthesia is usually required. Careful attention to standard monitoring, including ECG, blood pressure, and pulse oximetry, is required. Anesthesia care for adults may include monitored anesthesia care or general anesthesia. Choice of technique is dictated by the needs and medical condition of the patient. Provision of adequate hydration is essential. The osmotic load from contrast dyes can create a significant diuresis.[41] In addition, patients will have been fasted, usually from midnight the previous day.

Cerebral angiography deserves special attention. Indications for cerebral angiography include cerebrovascular disease, tumors, arteriovenous malformations, and aneurysms with or without subarachnoid hemorrhage. Patients may also present with a history of seizures. Monitoring for these patients should be standard. Although sedation may be required to facilitate catheter placement, it is advantageous to keep the patient as awake as possible so as to facilitate neurologic assessment during the procedure. General anesthesia may be required in patients who are unable to cooperate or who require airway protection. Many patients presenting for cerebral angiography are at risk for intracranial hypertension. Control of arterial blood pressure, carbon dioxide tension, and prudent use of anesthetic agents and vasodilators is recommended.[57,58] Intubation without adequate depth of anesthesia or improper positioning leading to increased CVP can elevate ICP and should thus be avoided. Once the patient is intubated, hyperventilation may improve study quality by causing cerebral vasoconstriction, which slows cerebral circulation, reducing dye washout and increasing dye concentration.

Hypotension and bradycardia can occur during cerebral angiography with contrast dye injection and will usually respond to volume and atropine, respectively.[58] Because contrast material can cross the blood–brain barrier, a higher concentration of dye in the brain may result, causing seizures. Whether this is a result of direct toxicity or chemoreceptor trigger-zone stimulation is unclear.[41,57,58] Other complications including embolization of plaques, bleeding, thrombosis, or puncture site hematomas have been reported.[57,59] The overall incidence of complications from cerebral angiography has been reported to be 8–12%.[57,60,61]

Several preexisting conditions increase the risk of complications associated with angiography. These include a history of cerebrovascular disease, stroke, diabetes, and transient ischemic attacks. Obtaining a good patient history is important.

Embolization Procedures

Angiographic embolization is usually undertaken for vascular malformations, aneurysms, cavernous sinus fistulas, or tumors. A successfully staged artery embolization may offer a safe, nonsurgical cure. Patients requiring an embolization are managed in a manner similar to those needing angiographic procedures. Choice of sedation and use of either regional or general anesthesia depends on the clinical indication. Analgesia or anesthesia is often required since embolization can be quite painful. Closely monitored awake but sedated patients may help with detection and avoidance of neurologic complications during intracranial embolization. Regional anesthesia may be useful for procedures in the lower body and extremities, as well as in the upper extremities.

Embolizations are carried out by stimulatory intravascular thrombosis with introduction of a foreign body. Small pieces of polymeric plastics, small detachable balloons or threads are commonly used. Sclerosing agents, such as bucrylate or alcohol, are often used. Patients must be watched carefully for disruption of vessel integrity and flow in other vascular beds. Again, routine basic monitoring standards should be followed.

Because the dose of contrast dye used during these procedures is high, with a resultant diuresis, adequate hydration is necessary. Nausea and vomiting are common. Metoclopramide, ranitidine, droperidol, or, more recently, ondansetron may be useful.

Computed Tomography

CT scanning is essentially noninvasive and painless. The most frequent use of CT scanning today is for imaging of the head[62] to diagnose intracranial bleeding, neoplasms, or hydrocephalus.[60] Thoracic and abdominal scanning is also becoming more common. Interventional CT-scanning, including biopsy and needle aspiration, can be performed as well.[62] Early CT scanners generated a cross-sectional image of the patient over several minutes.[58] A motionless patient was essential. More recently cross-sectional images can be obtained in a few seconds, although motion artifact can still be a problem. The majority of adult patients will tolerate CT scanning without anesthesia. If the patient is anxious, sedation and emotional support are usually all that is necessary. Sedation or general anesthesia is usually required only for procedures with children, for long and uncomfortable procedures, and for patients who have difficulty remaining motionless. Patients requiring a more intensive level of care, e.g., trauma patients, may also require an anesthesiologist.

Modern CT-scanning facilities are equipped with hospital-piped oxygen, nitrous oxide, air, vacuum, and suction. Additional oxygen tanks should still be available. Often the anesthesia machines in radiology suites are older models. The anesthesiologist must be familiar with the operation of all anesthesia equipment. Routine monitoring equipment may be used with CT scanning. Older imaging suites may lack space and compromise access to the patient during the scan.

Pediatric patients may experience fear and separation when inside the scanning room. Induce these patients away from the scanner and position them once they are anesthetized. Temperature monitoring in pediatric patients is mandatory. CT suites are often colder than 25°C to allow for optimal function of the equipment.[58]

During CT scanning of adult patients requiring general anesthesia or sedation, the primary concerns of the anesthesiologist are airway management and oxygenation. Positioning and movement of the gantry during the procedure may result in kinking or disconnection of the anesthesia circuit. Patients for emergency procedures, as well as patients who receive contrast agents orally or through a nasogastric tube, should be considered to have a full stomach.[63]

Stereotactic-guided surgery is possible using CT scanning. Most stereotactic procedures involve biopsies or aspirations, usually of intracranial masses. The stereotactic procedure is used to minimize injury to adjacent structures. The procedure involves placement of a radiolucent frame around the head. Since drilling for the pins of the frame can be painful, deep sedation or general anesthesia is often used in combination with local anesthetic. Heavy sedation must be used with caution in patients with suspected intracranial hypertension because of possible elevation of CO_2, which can further increase ICP. Once the frame has been attached to the skull, the patient may be positioned on the gantry to ensure a motionless field for precise localization. Well-informed, cooperative patients will often tolerate this procedure with minimal sedation and good local anesthesia.

Magnetic Resonance Imaging

Magnetic resonance imaging (MRI) entails placing the patient in a magnetic field oriented in the longitudinal axis.[25,64] Once established, magnetic pulses are applied in a transverse plane. The magnetic pulses are discontinued with relaxation of magnetism in the transverse plane to zero. Relaxation back to the initial magnetic field in the longitudinal plane also occurs.

During this time, radiofrequency pulses are emitted and used to generate the image. The relaxation times obtained from the change in magnetic fields are specific for a given tissue and, in theory, may even be discriminating at the cellular level.[64] The magnetic field is of such high energy that use of ferromagnetic equipment near the scanner is not allowed.[65-67] Standard monitoring equipment must be modified to prevent distortion of the imaging study. Of note, bank cards, credit cards, and other belongings containing electromagnetic strips should not come near the scanner, as they can become demagnetized. Several authors have described ventilators, equipment, and anesthesia machines that are compatible to use within the MRI suite.[68-70] This equipment is made of aluminum or nonmagnetic steel. Current contraindications for MRI scanning include patients with a pacemaker, aneurysm clips, or intravascular wires.[67,71-73]

The imaging capabilities of MRI are similar to CT scanning. MRI is also noninvasive and has the advantage of producing no ionizing radiation. Most magnetic imaging uses magnetic properties of proton environments. More sophisticated MRI scanning using ^{13}C, ^{19}F, ^{23}Na, and ^{31}P may be possible.[62] Women in the first trimester of pregnancy have been shown to have an increased probability of developmental problems in the child. Patients with large metal implants should be monitored for implant heating.[65]

Anesthesiology involvement with MRI scanning is similar to CT scanning. Most adult patients will tolerate MRI scanning with little or no sedation. Anesthesia will be primarily used for improved patient immobility and for children. The patient environment is significantly different from the CT scanner. With MRI, the patient is positioned on a long, thin table. Once the patient has been placed in the scanner, access to the patient is difficult (Fig. 54-3). Careful attention to position and anesthesia circuitry is required. As the magnetic field is not dangerous, the anesthesiologist can stay close to the patient. Procedures of long duration may be very uncomfortable for the patient in the scanner.

Constant reassurance of the awake patient is helpful. ECG, oscillometric blood-pressure monitoring, pulse oximetry, and esophageal or precordial stethoscopes may be used. Be careful when using pulse oximetry, as burns from heating of the probe in the MRI have occurred. ECG telemetry and capnography systems have been used to minimize distortion of the signal.[74] With awake, alert patients monitoring is usually performed outside the room to minimize the possibility of distortion of the signal. Laryngoscopy may be difficult in the MRI suite because of the magnetic properties of batteries.

Radiation Therapy

The two major types of radiation therapy requiring anesthesia care are external beam radiation, usually in children, and intraoperative radiation therapy. Anesthetic management of the child for radiation therapy is a challenge. External beam radiation is useful for a number of radiosensitive tumors as shown in Table 54-4.

These patients are usually scheduled for a series of treatments extended over several weeks. Radiation doses are in the range of 180–250 rad per treatment. For this reason, all personnel must leave the room during the treatment period. Special capabilities are necessary to provide safe and ade-

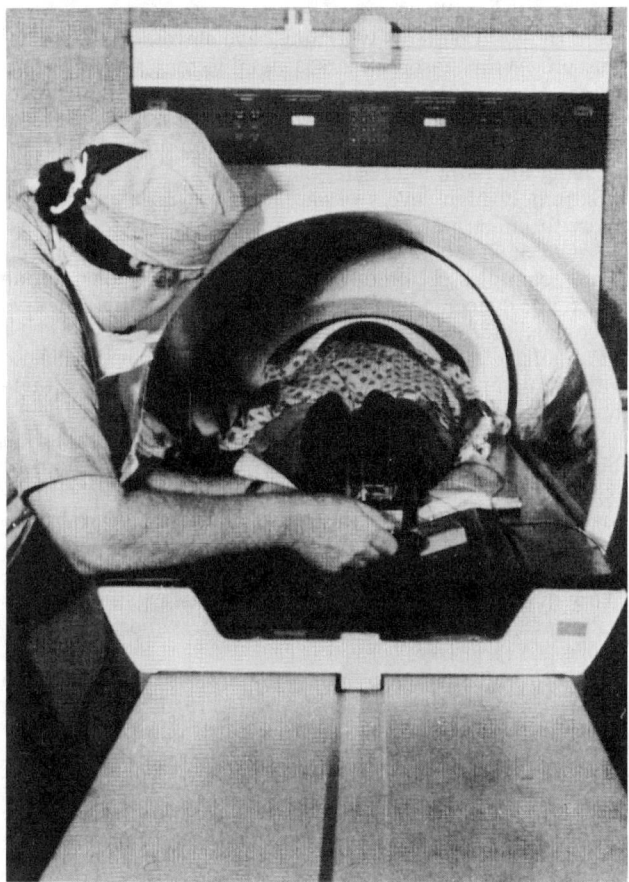

Figure 54-3. Illustration of difficult patient accessibility during magnetic resonance imaging. (Reproduced with permission from Roth J, Nugent M, Gray J *et al:* Patient monitoring during magnetic resonance imaging. Anesthesiology 62:80, 1985.)

quate monitoring.[52,75,76] Although the anesthesiologist is some distance from the patient, with closed-circuit television and equipment capable of even intensive-care application, the quality of care can approach that of the standard operating room.[38] Standard monitoring is interfaced with the remote location. Television cameras may be mounted so that observation of equipment and the patient are possible. In the event of patient problems or circuit disconnections, access to the patient should be rapid (20–30 sec).[77]

Patient immobility is the primary reason anesthesia is required. Fairly large doses of radiation are used, and this must be precisely focused to minimize surrounding tissue damage. General anesthesia may be facilitated with a number of techniques that must be appropriate for the short duration of the procedure. Many patients have indwelling

---

TABLE 54-4. Radiation-Sensitive Tumors

Neuroblastoma
Wilms Tumor
Medulloblastoma
Rhabdomyosarcoma
Retinoblastoma

catheters that will facilitate induction. Caution should be exercised with patients who may have elevated intracranial pressure. With these patients, ketamine may not be appropriate. After induction, the airway may be secured by placement of an aquaplast immobilization mask. This serves two purposes: improvement of immobilization and marking for focusing the radiation beam.

Extremely high levels of radiation are used intraoperatively to effect palliative treatment of a variety of tumors. Doses of 5000–6000 rad may be used during a single treatment. Examples of tumors treated by this method include pancreatic cancer, colon or rectal cancer, radiation-sensitive sarcomas, and many gynecologic cancers.

Patients with advanced cancer will often be cachectic with many nutritional deficiencies: dehydration, electrolyte imbalances, and coagulation problems.

Hospitals may be equipped with combination radiation therapy–operating room suites. In other centers, surgical exploration must be done in the operating room with subsequent transfer of the patient to the radiation therapy room. This may require transporting the patient considerable distances. Portable monitoring equipment and methods for delivery of oxygen and anesthetics are necessary. Intravenous techniques may avoid the difficulties of transporting inhalation agent vaporizers.[77]

Monitoring for intraoperative radiation is much the same as described for external beam radiation. Personnel must leave the room during the radiation treatment. Equipment interfaced to an external control desk allows adequate monitoring. Observation of the patient is by closed-circuit television. After treatment, patients are transported back to the operating room or to the postanesthesia care unit, if combination suites are used.

CARDIOVERSION

Anesthesiologists are often needed to manage the airway and to provide adequate sedation for patients undergoing elective cardioversion. Most cardioversions are scheduled in advance, which allows for adequate preparation. Occasionally, sedation for cardioversion is required emergently, owing to hemodynamic instability. In this situation, adherence to basic ACLS protocols is satisfactory. This discussion will focus on elective cardioversion.

A number of disturbances of cardiac rhythm are commonly treated with elective cardioversion. Uncomplicated atrial fibrillation and atrial flutter, often subsequent to prior coronary artery bypass, are probably the most common dysrhythmias treated by elective cardioversion. Supraventricular tachycardias refractory to medical management can also be treated in this way.

Elective cardioversion is best performed near the operating room for a number of reasons. Often these are additions to a busy operating schedule. Because of the short duration of the procedure, they can easily be facilitated if the anesthesiologist is nearby. Proximity to additional airway management equipment and anesthetic medications is also helpful. Cardioversion can be easily performed in holding areas or in the postanesthesia care unit (PACU).

A patient history and physical examination should be performed with all patients receiving anesthesia. Current health status and concurrent medications, including heparin, history of reflux, and npo status are important considerations. Many patients may have coexisting cardiovascular disease. Sedation for cardioversion is recommended as a way to attenuate anxiety and pain associated with an elec-

tric shock. Success with a number of intravenous sedation techniques has been reported using benzodiazepines, thiopental, methohexital, and etomidate.[78-82] Thiopental and methohexital are thought to be superior to benzodiazepine.[79,82] Etomidate myoclonus may preclude its use with cardioversion.[79,80] Methods of assessing amnesia for the determination of countershock timing have been described.[78,81,82]

ECG, blood pressure, and pulse oximetry should be used routinely. Invasive monitoring is usually not required for cardioversion, however, physical status and condition should dictate monitoring needs. Intubating equipment, drugs, supplemental oxygen, methods for ventilation, suction, and resuscitation equipment must be readily available. Induction of anesthesia or amnesia should follow adequate preoxygenation. Onset of amnesia is often delayed due to an increased circulation time. This may occur because of the low cardiac output associated with the dysrhythmia. The appropriate synchronized charge is delivered once adequate sedation has occurred. The airway is maintained and ventilation supported until the patient regains consciousness. The patient should be closely monitored after cardioversion for recurrence of the dysrhythmia or other rhythm disturbance, and until awake and alert. Discharge to a monitored bed is usually at the discretion of the referring service.[78]

ELECTROCONVULSIVE THERAPY

Electroconvulsive therapy (ECT) was introduced in 1937 as an alternative to pharmacologically induced seizures for the treatment of a number of major affective disorders, including severe depression.[83,84] The most common use of ECT is for the treatment of major depressive illness in patients who have failed a trial of antidepressant medications. ECT may be used as initial treatment in patients with recurrent depression, associated schizophrenic disorders, or for the acutely suicidal patient.

Depression is both a psychologic and biologic disorder.[85-87] Associated symptoms include feelings of worthlessness, anorexia or hyperphagia, depressed mood, and insomnia or hypersomnia.[86,87] Depression may occur as the primary illness or as a secondary manifestation of another disease, e.g., Parkinson's disease, Cushing's disease, or intracranial tumors.[88] Depression is often associated with terminal illness. In addition to these symptoms, signs of poor nutritional status and dehydration may be present. Noncompliance with medications is common.[86,87]

Patients presenting for ECT may be taking a variety of antidepressants and also drugs for concurrent medical problems. The mainstays of psychopharmacotherapy for depression are the monoamine oxidase (MAO) inhibitors and the tricyclic antidepressants. Examples of the commonly used drugs are in Table 54-5.[89] MAO inhibitors block the action of monoamine oxidase, which selectively deaminates amine neurotransmitters by oxidation. These include epinephrine, norepinephrine, dopamine, and serotonin. As a result of deamination by MAO inhibitors, these neurotransmitters accumulate in nerve terminals. Indirectly acting sympathomimetics can precipitate hypertensive crises through the release of accumulated neurotransmitters.[90] To a lesser extent MAO inhibitors exaggerate the effects of direct acting sympathomimetics.[90] As an example, reduced doses of phenylephrine would be recommended if used to treat hypotension.[89]

Tricyclic antidepressants block the re-uptake of catechol-

TABLE 54-5. Commonly Used Antidepressants

Monoamine Oxidase Inhibitors	Tricyclic Antidepressants
Deprenyl	Amitryptyline
Isocarboxazid	Desipramine
Phenelzine	Doxepin
Tranylcypromine	Imipramine
	Nortriptyline
	Protriptyline

Adapted from Stoelting RK: Drugs used in the treatment of psychiatric disease. In Stoelting RK (ed): Pharmacology and Physiology in Anesthetic Practice. Philadelphia, JB Lippincott, 1991.

amines at the presynaptic-nerve terminal and as a result increase circulatory catecholamines. This results in an increase in adrenergic tone.[84,89] Administration of sympathomimetic drugs such as ephedrine will result in an exaggerated pressor response in patients taking these antidepressants.[84,89]

The exaggerated pressor responses to MAO inhibitors or tricyclic antidepressants may lead to hypertensive crises. Because of this risk, several authors have recommended that they be discontinued up to two weeks prior to ECT or surgery.[84,91] Other authors have suggested that this may not be necessary.[92]

Lithium is used to treat manic depressive illness as well as recurrent depression. Lithium acts by interrupting the cell membrane sodium–potassium pump, disrupting the transmembrane potential, and by interfering with production of cAMP.[89] ECG changes may occur as a result of lithium therapy.[83] It has been suggested that ECT and concurrent lithium therapy may have a negative interaction and patients should be lithium-free prior to treatment.[83]

The electrically induced grand mal seizure produced by ECT is responsible for the therapeutic effect rather than the electrical stimulus.[83,93] Bilateral grand mal seizures are more effective than unilateral seizures.[93] The actual cellular mechanism for the therapeutic effect is unknown, but many theories have been suggested.[83] Duration of seizure is important. Seizures lasting less than 30 seconds are usually not therapeutic. The therapeutic window for duration is thought to be 210–1000 seconds.[94] Electrical stimulation results in production of a grand mal seizure lasting up to several minutes and consisting of a short 10–15 second tonic phase followed by a more prolonged clonic phase. The

TABLE 54-6. Physiologic Effects of ECT Seizure

Cardiovascular Effects	Cerebral Effects
Initial Phase	Increased cerebral blood flow
Bradycardia	Elevated ICP
Hypotension	Increased oxygen consumption
Later Phase	*Other Effects*
Tachycardia	Elevated intraocular pressure
Dysrhythmia	Increased intragastric pressure
Hypertension	
Increased systemic and myocardial oxygen consumption	

Adapted from Gaines GY, Rees DI: Electroconvulsive therapy and anesthetic considerations. Anesth Analg 65:1345, 1986.

seizure causes a wide range of physiologic effects outlined in Table 54-6.

The initial phase results in a transient vagal predominance with bradycardia and often some degree of hypotension. Rarely does this need to be treated. A secondary phase, one of sympathetic dominance, follows and lasts up to 1 minute and corresponds to the onset of the clonic phase of the seizure. Tachycardia and elevations in blood pressure are seen. ECG changes resembling that of acute myocardial infarction can also be observed. The hypertension after ECT is common and may be treated with a beta-blocker or short-acting vasodilator.[83,88,95] Other physiologic changes are shown in Figure 54-4.

Anesthetic Considerations

Several medical conditions relative to ECT deserve special consideration. Patients with preexisting cardiac or cardiovascular disease may require consultation prior to ECT. The benefits of successful treatment often outway the risk of exacerbating preexisting disease owing to the physiologic effects of ECT. Invasive monitoring may be necessary to assess myocardial function and allow for more sensitive blood-pressure control. Close monitoring throughout an extended post-ECT treatment period is recommended.[83,88] Patients with a recent myocardial infarction, history of congestive heart failure, valvular heart disease, or thoracic aneurysm should have prior medical or cardiology consultation. Patients with pheochromocytoma should not undergo ECT because of the increased risk for hypertensive crises.[83] Pacemaker function has not been shown to be affected.[88]

ECT should not be performed on patients with intracranial mass lesions due to the risk of elevated intracranial pressure and possible herniation. ECT should await surgical therapy if possible.[83] Patients with recent cerebrovascular accidents should await resolution of the acute insult. A period of 3 months has been recommended prior to undergoing ECT.[83,84] Other relative contraindications to ECT include pregnancy, presence of long bone fractures, thrombophlebitis, and acute or severe pulmonary disease.[83,84,88] If a pregnant patient is treated, close monitoring of the fetus should be performed with an obstetrician present.[83] Esophageal reflux and hiatal hernia are common findings in patients receiving ECT.[84,88] Pretreatment with H_2 antagonists or metoclopramide may be helpful.

The anesthetic requirements for ECT include amnesia, airway management, prevention of bodily injury due to the seizure, control of hemodynamic changes, and smooth, rapid emergence.[83,84,88,95] As the therapeutic effects of ECT are affected by multiple treatments, accurate records documenting therapy and effect are necessary. Complete records will allow different anesthesiologists to deliver appropriate care and minimize undue risk from changing an effective regimen.

Oxygen should be administered before, during, and after ECT.[96-98] Barbiturates are most often employed (methohexital 0.5–1 mg·kg^{-1} or thiopental 1.5–3 mg·kg^{-1}). Methohexital is reported to have a decreased incidence of dysrhythmias compared with other induction agents. Etomidate may be associated with longer duration seizures. The use of muscle relaxants has been advocated to prevent injury to the patient during onset of the grand mal seizure.[83,84,98] Succinylcholine is most widely used. Even though a number of patients may be susceptible to the malignant neuroleptic syndrome, succinylcholine is probably still safe to use. Atracurium may also be used as an alternative.[83,84,99] Doses

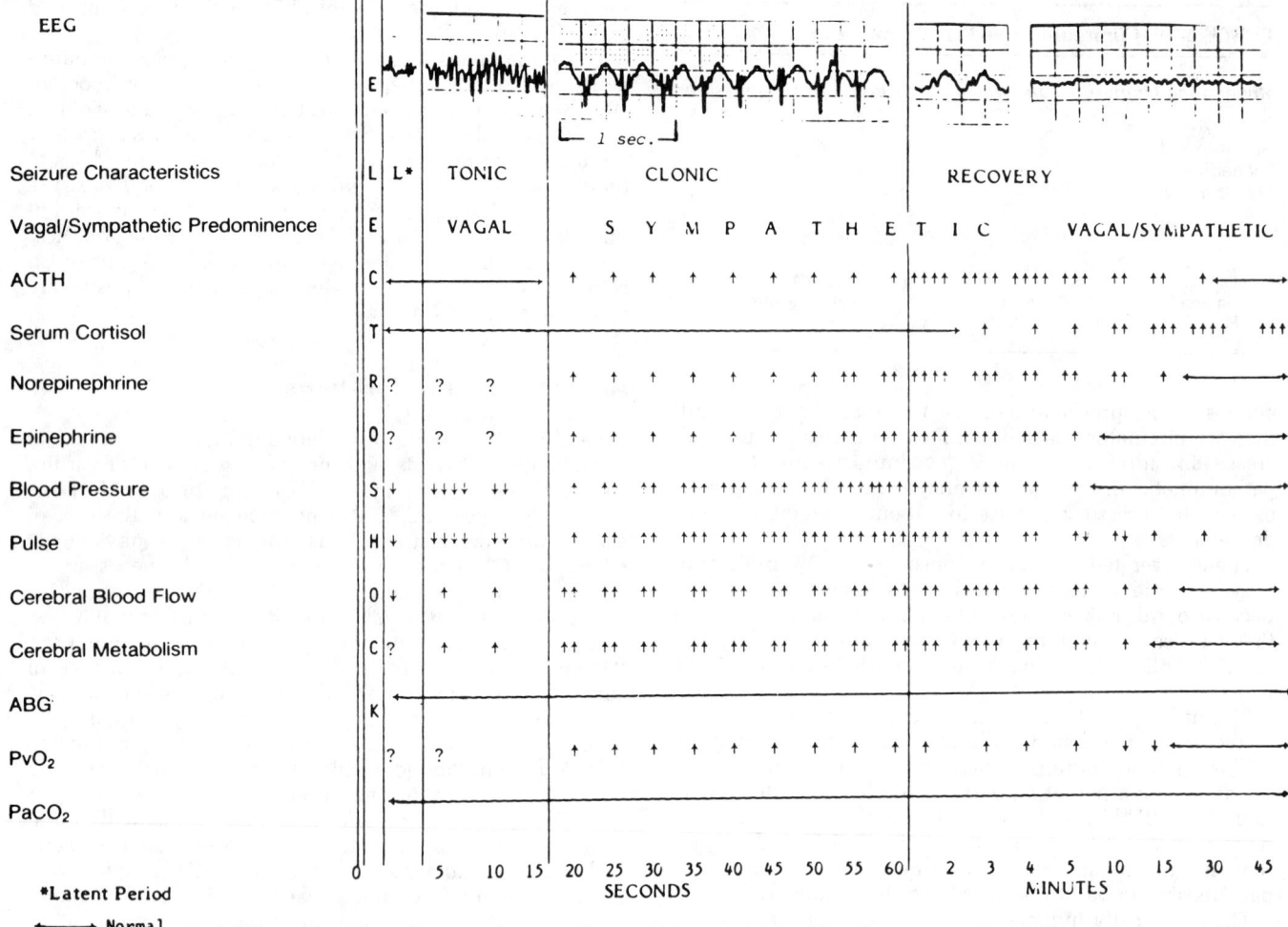

Figure 54-4. Overview of physiologic events related to ECT (modified). (Reproduced with permission from Selvin BL: Electroconvulsive therapy. Anesthesiology 67:367, 1987.)

of succinylcholine range from 0.5 to 1.0 mg·kg^{-1} but should be titrated to minimize injury from the seizure. Monitoring should include blood pressure cuff, ECG, and pulse oximetry, at a minimum. More invasive monitoring may be required if indicated from the patient's clinical condition. A blood pressure cuff is often used to occlude the circulation to one arm or lower leg to accurately assess the duration of the seizure. Obviously this is used to occlude blood flow prior to administration of muscle relaxants. ECT should be carried out in quiet, somewhat isolated areas, away from distraction to prevent undue anxiety in the depressed patient. The postanesthesia care unit is ideal for the initial treatment and recovery phases of the procedure. Adequate monitoring, oxygen supply, airway equipment, and suction should be present.

ANESTHESIA FOR DENTAL SURGERY

The majority of dental procedures may be done in the office, usually without supplemental sedation or anesthesia. More complicated procedures and patients who are uncooperative or phobic may require anesthetic care in the operating room. Procedures for healthy adult patients can usually be facilitated with routine anesthetic care. Anesthesia for the mentally retarded, combative, or pediatric patient presents a unique challenge.

For children or the mentally retarded patient, the increased fear and anxiety produced by separation from familiar surroundings and parents or guardians often leads to aggressive, noncompliant, or combative behavior. The association of previous visits to health care facilities with pain, needles, or unpleasant odors contributes to this anxiety. Apprehension in the guardian or parent significantly affects patient behavior.[100] In all cases, communication, preoperative education, and desensitization of the patient and parent or guardian have proven helpful.[100,101]

Mentally retarded patients frequently have a number of associated medical problems of importance to the anesthesiologist. Cardiac disease, including conduction abnormalities or structural defects, are associated with trisomy 21. Patients with neuromuscular diseases may have a history of aspiration and chronic pneumonitis. Macroglossia, hypoplastic maxilla, palatal abnormalities, or mandibular protrusion are airway anomalies often seen in trisomy-21 patients.[102] If the sitting position in the dental chair is used, the vasodilatory and depressive effects of anesthetic agents may be more pronounced in patients with preexisting cardiovascular disease.

The ideal technique for anesthesia should allow for a

smooth, rapid induction, easy airway management, stable procedural course, and prompt uncomplicated emergence. Standard monitoring should be employed including ECG, BP monitoring, pulse oximetry and capnography. Temperature monitoring is particularly important in children because of the risk of malignant hyperthermia. Both the anesthesiologist and the dentist should assure that the airway is protected from aspiration of blood, saliva, and other fluid or debris. Obstruction can also occur, particularly from throat packs, which are used to prevent the swallowing of blood. The importance of using a properly functioning suction apparatus cannot be overemphasized.

A number of anesthetic strategies have been suggested to facilitate induction and maintenance of anesthesia.[103-106] Ketamine has been recommended for use as a primary anesthetic agent or to facilitate induction.[103-106] It has the advantage of administration through oral (po), intramuscular (im), or intravenous (iv) routes. In addition, preservation of some laryngeal and oropharyngeal reflexes make it ideally suited for dental surgery procedures. Intravenous access for all procedures is ideal; however, it may be difficult to achieve prior to induction in anxious or hostile patients. In such cases, small im doses of ketamine, 2 mg·kg^{-1}, provide sufficient anesthesia for iv access to be achieved.[104] Oral premedication has also been used. Oral ketamine in doses of 0.5–8 mg·kg^{-1} has been used successfully in uncooperative or mentally retarded patients. Oral midazolam is also becoming popular.[103-107] While midazolam has a bitter taste, 0.5 mg·kg^{-1} dissolved in a small amount of a sugar-based drink mix (e.g., Kool-Aid), provides sufficient amnesia and sedation.[108] Administration in this manner avoids needle sticks or masks, which normally cause anxiety or pain.

A number of intravenous techniques have been described using ketamine, barbiturates, and alfentanil.[104-106] A disadvantage of using ketamine is the overstimulation of the sympathetic nervous system and possible adverse cardiovascular stimulation, particularly if atropine is used to control excessive salivary secretions. Alternative antisialagogues, including glycopyrrolate or scopolamine, may be used. Dissociative emergence can also be a problem with the use of ketamine. This may be difficult to assess in the confused or mentally retarded patient. Barbiturates, including methohexital, thiopental, and thiamylal, are ideally suited for induction of anesthesia rather than maintenance. Methohexital has the advantage of being approximately two times more potent than thiopental and it has rapid onset and recovery times. Propofol is also ideal for short outpatient procedures. Anesthesia can be supplemented with a number of drugs including inhalation agents. Alfentanil infusion has been described as a successful iv technique for oral restorations in children, providing smooth induction, maintenance, and rapid emergence. However, iv access was required and a significant amount of postoperative nausea and vomiting was noted.[106] Inhalation techniques can also be useful in patients without iv access; however, excitement during induction can be a problem, particularly in the larger combative patient.[109] Combinations of iv techniques with inhalational techniques, particularly with barbiturate or ketamine supplementation, may significantly prolong awakening and recovery.[109] Obviously the technique that provides the safest, smoothest induction and emergence should be used. Tracheal intubation, usually through the nose, is recommended in lengthy or unusually bloody procedures.

Because of bleeding and the routine use of oropharyngeal packing during dental procedures, close observation of these patients during emergence and recovery is essential. Emergence excitation, shivering, and residual sedation may compound any respiratory obstruction. Additional personnel and equipment, including suction and airway devices, should be readily available during recovery.

TRANSPORT OF PATIENTS

Patients who receive anesthesia or sedation for procedures outside the operating room should be monitored during transfer to the PACU since this often means traveling significant distances and through crowded hallways. The ASA standards for postoperative care require that the patient be accompanied by a member of the anesthesia team and that evaluation, monitoring, treatment, and support appropriate to the patient's medical condition be maintained.[110] Constant vigilance is necessary as hypoxemia after anesthesia or even with sedation is relatively frequent.[111-113] In addition, recognition of hypoxemic episodes may be difficult. This is especially important, as some attention must be diverted to directing the bed or gurney. Supplemental oxygen has been shown to be helpful for both children and adults during transport and the immediate postoperative period.[114-115] Monitoring of the relatively healthy patient, in addition to auditory and tactile awareness, may include noninvasive BP monitoring, ECG, and pulse oximetry. For critically ill patients more sophisticated methods of monitoring may be necessary, including continuous arterial pressure monitoring with transducers. Although central venous pressure monitoring may be useful in critically ill patients, continuous monitoring during transfer is rarely necessary. The ECG will allow detection of serious rhythm changes or dysrhythmias but, because of motion artifact or poor monitor resolution, ischemia or ST-T wave changes may be difficult to detect.[25]

Emergency drugs including vasopressor agents, drugs for resuscitation, and a portable defibrillator should accompany any severely injured or critically ill patient. Battery power and access to wall power should be assessed prior to transportation.

The transport stretcher should be equipped with an iv pole and have access for iv pumps, transducers, and oxygen tanks. Oxygen tanks must be checked for adequate supply and functioning regulators. A self-inflating breathing bag should be available with several mask sizes, if necessary, as well as equipment needed to maintain an airway. Most critically ill patients requiring ventilatory support can be transported with a self-inflating bag or Mapleson-type circuit, but several types of portable ventilators are available if manual ventilation is not adequate.

REFERENCES

1. Henneberg S, Nilsson A, Hok B et al: Anesthesia and monitoring during whole body radiation in children. J Clin Anes 2:76, 1990
2. Chaussy C, Brendel W, Schmiedt E: Extracorporeally induced destruction of kidney stones by shock waves (abstract). Lancet 2:1265, 1980
3. Chaussy CG, Fuch GJ: Current state and future developments of noninvasive treatment of human urinary stones with extracorporeal shock wave lithotripsy. J Urol Part 2. 141:782, 1989
4. Gissen, D: Anesthesia for extracorporeal shock wave lithotripsy. Semin Anesth VI:57, 1987
5. Chaussy C, Schmiedt E, Jocham D et al: First clinical experience with extracorporeally induced destruction of kidney stones by shock waves. J Urol 127:417, 1982

6. Tailly GG: Experience with the Dornier HM4 and MPL 9000 lithotriptors in urinary stone treatment. J Urol 144:622, 1990
7. Ryan PC, Jones BJ, Kay EW et al: Acute and chronic bioeffects of single and multiple doses of piezoelectric shock waves (EDAP LT.01). J Urol 145:399, 1991
8. El-Damanhoury H, Scharfe T, Ruth J et al: Extracorporeal shock wave lithotripsy or urinary calculi: Experience in treatment of 3,278 patients using the Siemens Lithostar and Lithostar Plus. J Urol 145:484, 1991
9. Pettersson B, Tiselius HG, Andersson A et al: Evaluation of extracorporeal shock wave lithotripsy without anesthesia using a Dornier HM3 lithotriptor without technical modifications. J Urol 142:1189, 1989
10. Sackmann M, Weber W, Delius M et al: Extracorporeal shockwave lithotripsy of gallstones without general anesthesia: First clinical experience. Ann Intern Med 107:347, 1987
11. Ell C, Kerzel W, Heyder N et al: Shock wave lithotripsy of gallbladder stones (letter to the editor). N Engl J Med 319:371, 1988
12. Sackmann M, Delius M, Sauerbruch T et al: Shock wave lithotripsy of gallbladder stones: the first 175 patients. N Engl J Med 318:393, 1988
13. Staritz M: Is extracorporeal biliary lithotripsy painless? My experience with three shock-wave sources (abstract). N Engl J Med 320:811, 1989
14. Epstein M: Cardiovascular and renal effects of head-out water immersion in man. Circ Res 39:619, 1976
15. Craig AB, Ware DE: Effect of immersion in water on vital capacity and residual volume of the lungs. J Appl Physiol 23:423, 1967
16. Agostoni E, Gurtner G, Torri G et al: Respiratory mechanics during submersion and negative-pressure breathing. J Appl Physiol 21:251, 1966
17. Begin R, Epstein M, Sackner MA et al: Effects of water immersion to the neck on pulmonary circulation and tissue volume in man. J Appl Physiol 40:293, 1976
18. Hong S, Cerretelli P et al: Mechanics of respiration during submersion in water. J Appl Physiol 27:535, 1969
19. Arnold WP, Ruth RA, Ross WT et al: The lithotriptor as a sound hazard (abstract). Anesthesiology 63:A179, 1985
20. Duvall JO, Griffith DP: Epidural anesthesia for extracorporeal shock wave lithotripsy. Anesth Analg 64:544, 1985
21. Kopacz DJ, Mulroy MF: Chloroprocaine and lidocaine decrease hospital stay and admission rate after outpatient epidural anesthesia. Reg Anesth 15:19, 1990
22. Stromskag KE, Steen PA: Comparison of interpleural and epidural anesthesia for extracorporeal shock wave lithotripsy. Anesth Analg 67:1181, 1988
23. London R, Kudlak T, Riehle R: Immersion anesthesia for extracorporeal shock wave lithotripsy. Review of two hundred twenty treatments. Urology 28:86, 1986
24. Pandit SK, Powell RB, Crider B et al: Epidural fentanyl is not effective for analgesia for ESWL. Anesthesiology 68:176, 1988
25. Gallagher TJ: Anesthesia outside the operating room. In Stoelting RK, Barash PG, Gallagher TJ. Advances in Anesthesia, pp 25–46. Chicago, Yearbook Medical Publisher, 1987
26. Perel A, Hoffman B, Podeh D et al: High frequency positive pressure ventilation during general anesthesia for extracorporeal shock wave lithotripsy. Anesth Analg 65:1231, 1986
27. Carlson CA, Gravenstein JS, Banner MJ et al: Monitoring techniques during anesthesia and HFJV for extracorporeal shock wave lithotripsy (abstract). Anesthesiology 63:A178, 1985
28. Carlson CA, Boyston PG, Banner MJ et al: Conventional versus high frequency jet ventilation for extracorporeal shock wave lithotripsy (abstract). Anesthesiology 63:A530, 1985
29. Zeitlin GL, Roth RA: Effect of three anesthetic techniques on the success of extracorporeal shock wave lithotripsy. Anesthesiology 68:272, 1988
30. Perel A, Segal E, Pizov R et al: QRS-Activated ventilation during general anesthesia for extracorporeal shock wave lithotripsy. J Clin Anesth 4:268, 1988
31. Monk TG, Rater JM, White PF: Comparison of alfentanil and ketamine infusions in combination with midazolam for outpatient lithotripsy. Anesthesiology 74:1023, 1991
32. Connelly NR, Weinstock AD: Continuous alfentanil infusion for extracorporeal shock wave lithotripsy of gallbladder stones. Anesth Analg 70:299, 1990
33. Monk TG, Boure B, White PF et al: Comparison of intravenous sedative–analgesic techniques for outpatient immersion lithotripsy. Anesth Analg 72:616, 1991
34. Schelling G, Weber W, Sackmann M et al: Pain control during extracorporeal shock wave lithotripsy of gallstones by titrated alfentanil infusion (letter to the editor). Anesthesiology 70:1022, 1989
35. Freilich JD, Brull SJ, Schiff S et al: Anesthesia for lithotripsy: Efficacy of monitored anesthesia care with alfentanil (abstract). Anesth Analg 70:S115, 1990
36. Harries A, Bagley G, Lim M: Anaesthesia for extracorporeal shock-wave lithotripsy. A comparison of propofol and methohexitone infusions during high frequency jet ventilation. Anaesthesia 43:100, 1988
37. Lingeman JE, Woods J, Toth PD et al: The role of lithotripsy and its side effects. J Urol, Part 2 141:793, 1989
38. Finlayson B, Ackermann D: Overview of surgical treatment of urolithiasis with special reference to lithotripsy. J Urol, Part 2 141:778, 1989
39. Silber N, Kremer I, Gaton DD et al: Severe sepsis following extracorporeal shock wave lithotripsy. J Urol 45:1045, 1991
40. Westh H, Knudsen F, Hedengran AM et al: Extracorporeal shock wave lithotripsy of kidney stones does not induce transient bacteremia. A prospective study. J Urol 144:15, 1990
41. Goldberg M: Systemic reactions to intravascular contrast media. Anesthesiology 60:45, 1984
42. Shehadi W, Toniolo G: Adverse reactions to contrast media. Radiology 136:299, 1980
43. Shehadi W: Adverse reactions to intravascularly administered contrast media. Am J Roentgenol 124:145, 1975
44. Greenberger P, Patterson R, Kelly J et al: Administration of radiographic contrast media in high risk patients. Invest Radiol 15:540, 1980
45. Rockoff S, Brasch R, Kuhn C et al: Contrast media as histamine liberators. Invest Radiol 5:503, 1970
46. Simon R, Schatz M, Stevenson D et al: Radiographic contrast media infusions. J Allergy Clin Immunol 63:281, 1973
47. Morisette M, Gagnon R, Lamourent J et al: Effects of angiographic contrast media on oncotic pressure. Am J Hematol 100:319, 1980
48. Anto H, Chon S, Porush J et al: Infusion intravenous pyelography and renal function: Effects of hypertonic mannitol in patients with chronic renal insufficiency. Arch Intern Med 141:1652, 1981
49. Kalmer M, Orange R, Ansten K: Immunological release of histamine and slow reacting substance of an aphylaxis from the human lung. J Exp Med 136:556, 1972
50. Zweiman B, Mishkin M, Mildreth E: An approach to the performance of contrast studies in contrast sensitive persons. Ann Intern Med 83:159, 1975
51. Lasser E, Lang J, Sovak M et al: Steroids: Theoretical and experimental basis for utilization in prevention of contrast media reactions. Radiology 125:1, 1977
52. Davies D: Subspecialty monitoring techniques—miscellaneous. In Gravenstein N (ed): Problems in Anesthesia Monitoring, pp 138–156. Philadelphia, JB Lippincott, 1987
53. Carmichael J, Henshaw E: Radiation hazards of diagnostic radiology. In Ansell GE, Wilkins RA (eds): Complications in Diagnostic Imaging, p 457. Oxford, Blackwell Scientific Publications, 1987
54. Barkar D: Protection and safety in the x-ray department. Radiography 44:45, 1978
55. Steward D: Cardiac surgery and cardiologic procedures. In Steward D (ed): Manual of Pediatric Anesthesia, 2nd ed, pp 213–247. New York, Churchill Livingstone, 1985
56. DeBruijn N, Hlatky M et al: General anesthesia during percutaneous transluminary coronary angioplasty for acute myocardial infarction. Anesth Analg 68:201, 1989
57. Earnest F, Forbes G, Samdok D et al: Complications of cerebral angiography. AJR 142:247, 1984
58. Wolfson B, Hetrick W: Anesthesia for neuroradiologic proce-

dures. In Cottrell JE, Turndorf H, (eds). Anesthesia and Neurosurgery, pp. 104–113. St Louis, CV Mosby, 1986

59. Feild J, Robertson J, DeSaussure R: Complications of cerebral angiography in 2000 consecutive cases. J Neurosurg 19:775, 1962

60. Fanjht E, Trader S, Hanna G: Cerebral complications of angiography for transient ischemia and stroke. Neurology 29:4, 1979

61. Dion J, Gates P, Fox A et al: Clinical events following neuroangiography. Stroke 18:997, 1987

62. Weston G, Strunin L, Amundson G: Imagery for anesthetists: A review of the methods and anaesthetic implications of diagnostic imagery techniques. Can Anaesth Soc J 32:552, 1985

63. Forestner J: Anesthesia for radiologic procedures. In Murphy C, Murphy M (eds): Radiology for Anesthesia and Critical Care, p 239. New York, Churchill Livingstone, 1987

64. Bydder GM: Magnetic resonance imagery of the brain. Radiol Clin North Am 22:779, 1984

65. New P, Rosen B et al: Potential hazards and artifacts of ferromagnetic and nonferromagnetic surgical and dental materials and devices in NMR imaging. Radiology 147:139, 1983

66. Shellock F: Monitoring during MRI evaluation of the effect of high field MRI on various patient monitors. Medical Electronics 17:93, 1986

67. Davis P, Crooks L, Arakawa M et al: Potential hazard in NMR. AJR 137:857, 1981

68. Rao C, Krishna G, Emhardt J: Anesthesia machine for use during magnetic resonance imagery. Anesthesiology 73:1054, 1990

69. Rao C, McNiece W, Emhardt J: Modification of an anesthesia machine for use during magnetic resonance imagery. Anesthesiology 68:640, 1988

70. Ramsay J, Gale L, Sykes M: A ventilator for use in nuclear magnetic resonance studies. Br J Anaesth 58:1181, 1986

71. Roth J, Nugent M, Gray J et al: Patient monitoring during magnetic resonance imaging. Anesthesiology 62:80, 1985

72. Pavlicek W, Geisiuiger M, Castle L et al: The effects of nuclear magnetic resonance on patients with cardiac pacemakers. Radiology 147:149, 1983

73. Fetter J, Aram G, Holmes D et al: Nuclear magnetic resonance imagery of external and implantable cardiac pacemakers. Chest 84:345, 1983

74. Nixon C, Hirsch N, Ormerod I et al: Nuclear magnetic resonance: Its implications for the anesthetist. Anesthesia 41:131, 1986

75. Glanber D, Audenaert S: Anesthesia for children undergoing craniospinal radiotherapy. Anesthesiology 56:801, 1987

76. Pandya J, Martin J: Improved remote cardiorespiratory monitoring during radiation therapy. Anesth Analg 65:529, 1986

77. Bashein G, Russell A, Momil S: Anesthesia and remote monitoring for intraoperative radiation therapy. Anesthesiology 64:805, 1986

78. Orko R: Anaesthesia for cardioversion: A comparison of diazepam, thiopentone, and propranidid. Br J Anaesth 48:257, 1976

79. Shulman MS, Edelmann R: Use of etomidate for elective cardioversion (letter to the editor). Anesthesiology 68:656, 1988

80. Lind GH, Kamaya H: Minimum drug dose to obtain adequate amnesia for cardioversion (letter to the editor). Anesthesiology 68:475, 1988

81. White PF: Use of a thiopental-lidocaine combination for elective cardioversion (letter to the editor). Anesthesiology 60:511, 1984

82. Ford SR, Maze M, Gaba DM: Etomidate vs. thiopental anesthesia for elective cardioversion. Anesthesiology 67:A143, 1987

83. Selvin BL: Electroconvulsive therapy. Anesthesiology 67:367, 1987

84. Gaines GY, Rees DI: Electroconvulsive therapy and anesthetic considerations. Anesth Analg 65:1345, 1986

85. American Psychiatric Association: Diagnostic and Statistical Manual of Mental Disorders: DSMIII-R, 3rd ed. Washington, DC, 1987

86. Gold P, Goodwin F, Chronsos G: Clinical and biochemical

manifestations of depression. Part 1. Relation to the neurobiology of stress. N Engl J Med 319:348, 1988

87. Gold P, Goodwin F, Chronsos G: Clinical and biochemical manifestations of depression. Part 2. Relation to the neurobiology of stress. N Engl J Med 319:413, 1988

88. McPherson R, Lipsey J: Electroconvulsive therapy. In Rodgers M (ed): Current Practice in Anesthesiology, pp 212–217. Philadelphia, BC Decker, 1988

89. Stoelting RK: Drugs used in treatment of psychiatric disease. In Stoelting RK (ed): Pharmacology and Physiology in Anesthetic Practice, pp 347–364. Philadelphia: JB Lippincott, 1987

90. Stack C, Rogers P, Linter S: Monoamine oxidase inhibitors and anaesthesia. Br J Anaesth 60:222, 1988

91. Consensus Conference: Electroconvulsive therapy. JAMA 254:2103, 1985

92. El-Ganzouri A, Ivankovich A, Braverman B, McCarthy R: Monoamine oxidase inhibitors: Should they be discontinued preoperatively? Anesth Analg 64:592, 1985

93. Fink M, Johnson L: Monitoring the duration of electroconvulsive therapy seizures: Cuff and EEG methods compared. Arch Gen Psychiatry 39:1189, 1982

94. Maletzky B: Seizure duration and clinical effect in electroconvulsive therapy. Compr Psychiatry 19:541, 1978

95. Jones R, Knight P: Cardiovascular and hormonal responses to electroconvulsive therapy. Anaesthesia 36:795, 1981

96. Lew J, Eastley R, Hanning C: Oxygenation during electroconvulsive therapy: A comparison of two anesthetic techniques. Anaesthesia 41:1092, 1986

97. Swindells S, Simpson K: Oxygen saturation during electroconvulsive therapy. Br J Psychol 150:695, 1987

98. Riley R: Preoxygenation and electroconvulsive therapy. Anesth Analg 66:1049, 1987

99. Guiduschek J, Cohen SA, Khan A et al: Repeated anesthesia for a patient with neuroleptic malignant syndrome. Anesthesiology 68:134, 1988

100. Wright G, Alpern G, Leake J: The modifiability of maternal anxiety as it relates to children's cooperative dental behavior. J Dent Child 40:265, 1973

101. Johnson R, Machen JB: Behavior modification techniques and maternal anxiety. J Dent Child 40:272, 1973

102. Gullikson J: Oral findings in children with Down's syndrome. J Dent Child 40:293, 1973

103. Bragg C, Miller B: Oral ketamine facilitates induction in a combative mentally retarded patient. J Clin Anesth 3:121, 1990

104. Carrel R: Ketamine: A general anesthetic for manageable ambulatory patients. J Dent Child 40:288, 1973

105. Bamber D, Ratcliffe R, McEwan T: Ketamine for out patient dental conservation in children. Anaesthesia 28:446, 1973

106. Davis P, Chopyk JB, Mazif M: Continuous alfentanil infusion in pediatric patients undergoing general anesthesia for complete oral restoration. J Clin Anesth 3:125, 1991

107. Rosen D, Rosen K, Elkins T et al: Outpatient sedation: an essential addition to gynecologic care for persons with mental retardation. Am J Obstet Gynecol 164:825, 1991

108. Clarke WR: Personal communication

109. White P: Anesthesia for ambulatory surgery. In Stoelting RK (ed): Advances in Anesthesia, vol 2, pp 1–29. Chicago, Yearbook Medical Publishers, 1985

110. ASA Newsletter: American Society of Anesthesiologists. December:7, 1988

111. Motoyama E, Glazener C: Hypoxemia after general anesthesia in children. Anesth Analg 65:267, 1986

112. Bailey P, Pace N, Ashbury M et al: Frequent hypoxemia and apnea after sedation with midazolam and fentanyl. Anesthesiology 73:826, 1990

113. Moller J, Wittrap M, Johansen S: Hypoxia in the postanesthesia care unit: An observer study. Anesthesiology 73:890, 1990

114. Murray R, Raemer D, Morris R: Supplemental oxygen after ambulatory surgical procedures. Anesth Analg 67:967, 1988

115. Chripko D, Bevan J, Archer D et al: Decreases in arterial oxygen saturation in pediatric outpatients during transfer to the postanesthesia recovery room. Anesthesiology 65:180, 1986

55

Leonard Firestone
Susan Firestone

Anesthesia for Organ Transplantation

Transplantation of a variety of tissues is now routine in clinical practice. Bone, tendon, cartilage, and fascia readily provide a partially inert framework for the ingrowth of healthy native cells. Cornea, blood vessels, heart valves, and certain endocrine tissues such as parathyroid are also, to some extent, immunologically privileged and have been successfully transplanted. Bone marrow can be used to replace the entire hematopoietic and lymphopoietic systems. More recently, transplantation of vital organs with distinct vasculature, including the kidneys, liver and heart, has achieved the status of preferred therapeutic option for end-stage visceral disease. Technical and biological factors have thus far prevented widespread introduction of lung, pancreas, and small bowel transplantation, but the intensity of current research suggests that important advances will be forthcoming.

Anesthesiologists' role in transplantation may involve caring for organ donors, prospective recipients, or patients who have already received transplants but require further surgery. To do so, specialized knowledge is required in a multitude of disciplines as diverse as organ preservation, biomedical ethics, transplantation immunology, and the physiology of brain death.

ANESTHESIA CARE OF ORGAN DONORS

In the United States, the majority of viscera for transplantation are derived from brain-dead organ donors through voluntary programs established by state and federal law. To supplement these programs, many states have also enacted "required request" legislation, obliging hospital personnel to ask the family of a brain-dead patient to grant permission for organ donation. Organs are distributed through a nation-wide organ and transplantation network developed, under federal contract, by the United Network for Organ Sharing (UNOS). UNOS is also responsible for collecting data, reporting statistics, and educating the public about organ donation and transplantation.[1]

Brain death is usually a consequence of catastrophic neurologic injury following blunt head trauma (most often from motor vehicle accidents); penetrating head injury (from gunshot wounds); or, intracranial hemorrhage (cerebrovascular accidents). In general, suitable donors will not have suffered prolonged periods of circulatory compromise or septicemia.

Donors are screened for serologic evidence of hepatitis-B or the human immunodeficiency virus (HIV) infection, as well as active toxoplasmosis, herpes, or tuberculosis. All of these infectious processes would disqualify organ donation. In contrast, most transplant centers will use organs obtained from donors with prior cytomegalovirus (CMV) infection when recipients have previously had CMV exposure. At present, autoimmune disease has not been a criterion for disqualification of donors, but the report that idiopathic thrombocytopenic purpura can be transmitted by liver transplantation has renewed debate.[2] Cardiac donors are usually under age 50 years and without pre-existing myocardial or coronary artery disease. Myocardial contractility must be adequate as judged by echocardiography, and there should be no history of use of intracardiac injections or high doses of inotropes. Hepatic function tests are useful to screen potential liver donors who may have abused drugs or alcohol. Urinalysis and cultures, and blood urea nitrogen and creatinine levels are standard tests for potential kidney donors.

Viscera for transplantation are also obtained from living donors. Almost all viscera derived from living donors are kidneys, although recently, partial liver and lung resections have been performed to create reduced-size allografts for relatively few recipients. Living donors must be closely related to recipients if there is to be any benefit. The strategy underlying living-related kidney transplantation is that HLA identity between donor and recipient results in significantly greater graft survival than even a partially matched organ.[3] Because all individuals possess two sets of genes coding for HLA antigens, and one is inherited from each parent, there is a finite probability of HLA identity among close family members. For example, parents share one haplotype with their child, and siblings have a 50% chance of sharing one haplotype and 25% chance of sharing both haplotypes. Discussion of the perioperative care of living donors is continued in the kidney transplantation section.

Diagnosis of Brain Death

The need for a uniform definition of brain death arose with the advent of heart transplantation in the late 1960s. Prior to this time, retrieval of kidneys, which are tolerant of a

TABLE 55-1. Criteria for the Diagnosis of Brain Death

Loss of Cerebral Cortical Function

No spontaneous movement
Unresponsive to external stimuli

Loss of Brain-stem Function

Absent respiratory reflex (apnea test)
Absent cranial nerve reflexes
    Pupillary light reflex
    Corneal reflex
    Oculocephalic reflex
    Oculovestibular reflex
    Atropine resistance

Supporting Studies

EEG
Cerebral flow studies
    Angiography
    Transcranial Doppler exam
    Xenon CT scan

---

short period of warm ischemia, was performed following cessation of the donor's heartbeat. Following several legislative efforts to address the issue, a special panel of medical consultants to the President's Commission for the Study of Ethical Problems in Medicine and Biomedical and Behavior Research issued a report that defined brain death as "irreversible cessation of all function of the entire brain, including the cortex and brain stem, determined in accordance with accepted medical standards."[4] The concept of brain death is now widely recognized in society, although the medical standards of its determination have been the subject of much debate.[5]

Cerebral cortical function is deemed absent when no spontaneous movement or response to noxious external stimuli can be elicited by an experienced physician (Table 55-1). However, studies supporting these physical findings are often obtained in accordance with local "medical standards," which may include electroencephalography (EEG) and/or cortical blood-flow determinations. An electrically silent (flat) EEG is consistent with the diagnosis of brain death, although residual activity may still be found after cessation of cerebral blood-flow.[6] Four-vessel cerebral angiography has been used to establish brain death,[7] but less invasive methods, e.g., transcranial Doppler[8] and xenon-enhanced computerized tomography,[9] are gaining popularity.

Brain-stem infarction is indicated by loss of reflexes mediated by bulbar cranial nerve and respiratory nuclei. These include the direct pupillary light reflex (absent when bright light fails to constrict the homolateral pupil); the oculocephalic reflex (absent when ocular position is fixed during rotation of the head ("doll's eyes")); the corneal reflex (absent when lightly touching the cornea fails to elicit a blink); and, the oculovestibular reflex (absent when irrigation of the external auditory canal with ice water fails to produce nystagmus ("cold caloric test")). Respiratory reflexes are assessed by the apnea test.[10] In most protocols, following a period of mechanical ventilation on 100% oxygen, the ventilator is disconnected (although oxygen is still supplied) and respiratory effort is judged by serial determinations of $Paco_2$. By this means, an accurate assessment of respiratory brain-stem function can be obtained in 10 minutes of obser-

vation, if the patient remains otherwise physiologically stable.[11]

Irreversibility is implicit in the diagnosis of brain death and is established by the lack of improvement in the neurologic examination for 12–24 hours. Factors that may confound this diagnosis include generalized seizures, centrally active drug effects, hypothermia, and cardiovascular or metabolic instability, since all may reversibly depress brain function. Therefore it is also important that the cause of brain death is known and sufficient to account for this diagnosis. In children, the potential for recovery from neurologic insults may be less predictable than in adults, so it has been recommended that an experienced pediatrician be consulted when evaluating young brain-injured patients.[12]

Physiologic Derangements with Brain Death

Brain death is frequently accompanied by marked physiologic instability, and treatment is often necessary to maintain the viability of donor organs (Table 55-2). Hypotension, hypoxemia, or arrhythmias may be part of the pathogenesis of brain death or else a consequence of brain-stem infarction. Hypotension results from the loss of descending vasomotor control and is exacerbated by hemorrhage, massive diuresis from diabetes insipidus or radiographic dyes, or dehydration therapy for cerebral edema. Treatment consists of restoration of intravascular volume with colloid and crystalloid solutions, and if necessary, vasopressin administration ($0.5–15$ $U \cdot h^{-1}$) or vasoactive drug infusion. Since phenylephrine may diminish splanchnic perfusion and thereby jeopardize abdominal donor organs, dopamine ($2–5$ $\mu g \cdot kg^{-1} \cdot min^{-1}$) is recommended for blood pressure support in this setting. Hypoxemia may follow from overzealous fluid administration during resuscitation attempts, atelectasis, aspiration, pneumothorax, pulmonary contusion, or pneumonia. The Fio_2, minute volume of ventilation, and positive end-expiratory pressure (PEEP) are usually adjusted to maintain systemic arterial saturation in excess of 95%. Atrial and ventricular arrhythmias, as well as varying degrees of conduction blockade have been noted after brain death.[13] Etiologies include intracranial hypertension, vagal nucleus infarction, myocardial ischemia or contusion, hy-

TABLE 55-2. Common Physiologic Derangements After Brain Death

Condition	Cause
Hypotension	Hypovolemia (diabetes insipidus; hemorrhage) Neurogenic shock
Hypoxemia	Neurogenic pulmonary edema Pulmonary contusion Pneumonia Gastric aspiration Fluid overload
Hypothermia	Hypothalamic infarction Exposure
Dysrhythmia (especially bradycardia)	Intracranial injury or herniation Hypothermia Hypoxia Electrolyte abnormality Myocardial contusion, ischemia

pothermia, and abnormal pH or serum electrolytes. Bradycardia is resistant to atropine[14] but responds to direct-acting chronotropic agents (e.g., dopamine, isoproterenol).

Numerous endocrine responses have been associated with brain death, including diabetes insipidus. This diagnosis is confirmed when polyuria is accompanied by relative hypoosmolarity of the urine (<300 mOsm·l^{-1}) despite serum hyperosmolarity (>310 mOsm·l^{-1}) and hypernatremia (serum sodium > 150 mEq·l^{-1}). Treatment consists of replacement of free water losses while restoring normal serum electrolyte and osmolarity values, and infusion of aqueous vasopressin (Pitressin, 0.5–15 U·h^{-1} iv). Infrequently, catecholamine and cortisol levels are markedly elevated, and thyroid hormone (T3) or insulin activity reduced following brain death. However, there is no consistent pattern and therefore replacement therapies are not routinely used.

Donor Operation

Anesthesia care for multiple organ retrieval should continue the focus on maintenance of donor organ perfusion and oxygenation begun in the ICU. Although cortical and brain-stem function are absent, both visceral and somatic reflexes that can lead to physiologic responses during the procedure may be present.[14a] For example, reflex pressor responses may accompany surgical stimuli and can jeopardize the renal microvasculature. Vasodilator infusion is sufficient treatment, because general anesthetics are unnecessary under these circumstances. Reflex neuromuscular activity mediated by spinal somatic reflexes is suppressed with relaxants.

After surgical preparation in the supine position, a midline incision is made from the suprasternal notch to the pubic symphysis, followed by sternotomy. Once exposed, the liver is freed of its ligamentous attachments to the diaphragm. In order to minimize warm ischemic time and surgical trauma to the harvested viscera, most recent approaches to the donor operation involve regional cooling and preservation of organs *in situ*, followed by en bloc removal (Fig. 55-1).[15] Thus, after the abdominal aorta is encircled with a ligature above the celiac artery, either the splenic or inferior mesenteric vein is cannulated and the liver is flushed through the portal system with cold preservative solution. The donor is then systemically heparinized and the abdominal aorta is cannulated, cross clamped, and perfused with cold preservative. This cools the donor's kidneys and liver, and once the ureters are dissected and divided, en bloc graft nephrectomy can be accomplished by transecting the aorta and inferior vena cava above and below the renal pedicles. The hepatic artery and common bile duct are then divided and the donor liver can now be removed. Donor cardiectomy begins once *in situ* preservation of the abdominal viscera is begun; further details about the cardiac donor procedure are found in the section on Heart Transplantation below. After all donor organs are removed, ventilatory and circulatory support is discontinued and the anesthesiologist's involvement ends. Death is always certified prior to the donor procedure and is not considered to have occurred in the operating room.

ORGAN PRESERVATION

Organ transplantation depends on the temporary separation of a donor organ from blood supply and protection from ischemia while *ex vivo*. Organ sharing networks are based on distant procurement, which may extend the period of

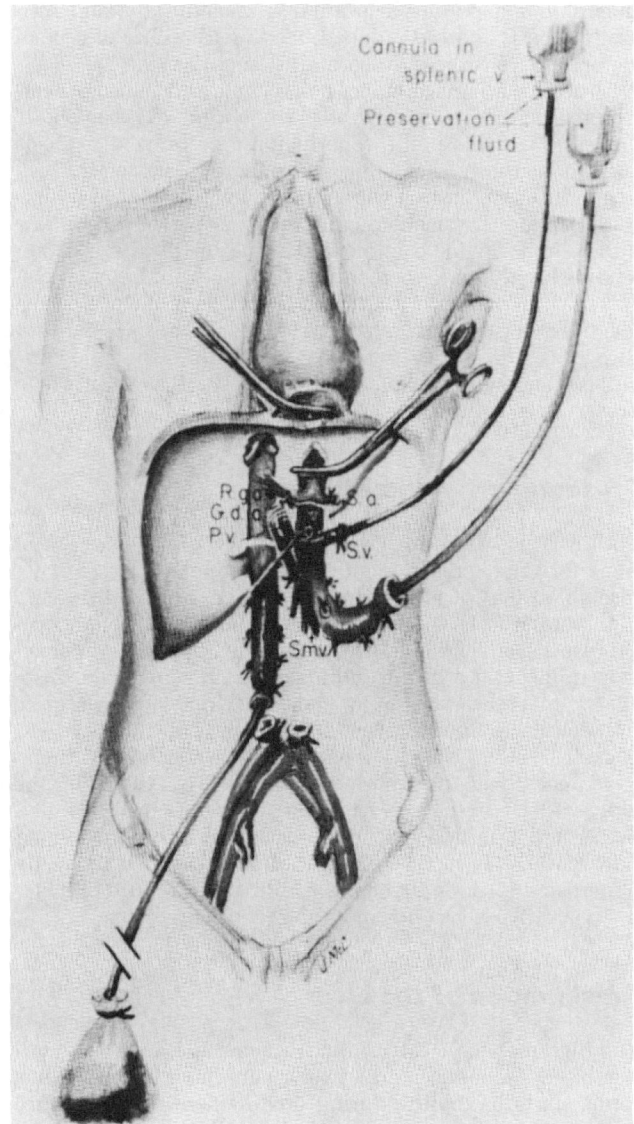

Figure 55-1. *In situ* infusion technique for preservation of both the liver and kidneys. Preservative fluid is infused by gravity into both the portal and systemic circulations, and drained via the inferior vena cava to prevent venous congestion of the organs. (R.g.a. = right gastric artery; G.d.a. = gastroduodenal artery; S.a. = splenic artery; S.v. = splenic vein; P.v. = portal vein; S.m.v. = superior mesenteric vein.) (Reprinted with permission from Starzl TE, Hakala TR, Shaw BW *et al:* A flexible procedure for multiple cadaveric organ procurement. Surg Gyn Obstet 158:223, 1984.)

ischemia to the biologically tolerable limit. Currently, the strategy to provide protection combines hypothermia to decrease metabolism with preservative solutions of specific electrolyte composition to maintain cellular integrity. These solutions may also contain chemical additives that are cryoprotective and prevent cellular swelling, vasospasm, buildup of toxic metabolites, and provide a source of energy.

Preservation strategies are based on the control of the adverse cellular events that follow ischemia and reperfusion. Shortly after disruption of the blood supply, the intracellular oxygen tension precipitously falls. Since metabolism can only proceed by anaerobic glycolysis, lactic acid and other anaerobic metabolites accumulate intracellularly, and ATP production is sharply reduced, leading to failure of crucial membrane ion-transport proteins such as the N^+-K^+-ATPase. As a consequence, cells swell and become overwhelmed with Ca^{2+}, which is toxic to numerous metabolic processes. At this point, reperfusion may prevent necrosis but can lead to further injury by generating oxygen-derived free radicals, including superoxides, hydroxyls, and hydrogen peroxide. These chemically reactive species can initiate intracellular chain reactions, resulting in liberation of numerous highly toxic metabolites derived from native cellular constituents, including free fatty acids and lipid peroxides. Preventing these chain reactions is the rationale for using free radical scavengers (e.g., mannitol, superoxide dismutase) and synthesis blockers (allopurinol) as additives to preservative solutions.

Preservation of the Kidney

Collins[16] first developed a series of isotonic flushing solutions for renal preservation. Their compositions generally resembled that of intracellular fluid (i.e., low sodium and high potassium), which was shown to diminish renal cortical respiration. Other additives included heparin, phenoxybenzamine, and procaine, all meant to prevent agonal vasospasm and thrombosis in cadaver kidneys. Hypertonic intracellular solutions were subsequently developed (e.g., Sacks', >400 mOsm)[17] but seemed to confer no additional advantages over the isotonic regimens. Today, among the most widely used kidney flushing solutions in the United States and Europe is a modified Collins solution, termed Euro-Collins (Table 55-3). Euro-Collins solution is modestly hyperosmotic, does not contain additives, and supports kidney viability ex vivo for more than 48 hours.[55]

Preservation of the Liver

The high metabolic rate of the liver makes it relatively vulnerable to ischemia, and its relatively large bulk prevents rapid, uniform cooling during procurement. Probably as a consequence of these two factors, the most common cause of postoperative hepatic graft dysfunction is ischemic injury. Recently, UW (University of Wisconsin) solution[18] was shown to extend hypothermic preservation of donor livers for at least 24 hours ex vivo, and possibly longer.[18,19] The key additives in UW solution (Table 55-3) include lactobionate and raffinose, which are used as impermeants to suppress hypothermia-induced cellular swelling.

Preservation of the Heart

Myocardial protection is based on cellular metabolic arrest and uniform cooling, both of which prevent the generation of cytotoxic free radicals.[20] Techniques that provide myocardial protection, particularly cardioplegia, developed in parallel with heart transplantation and greatly facilitated distal procurement.[21] Compared with other preservative regimens, cardioplegia solutions (Table 55-3) were shown to reduce the need for inotropic support following implantation[21] and are now generally used for ex vivo myocardial preservation. Under laboratory conditions, cardioplegia is able to preserve cardiac function for up to 24 hours.[22] However, in humans, the practical limit of ischemic time is 4–6 hours.[21,23]

TABLE 55-3. Common Organ Preservation Solutions

Solution	Amount per Liter
Euro-Collins Solution*	
Potassium	115 mEq
Sodium	10 mEq
Chloride	15 mEq
Bicarbonate	10 mEq
Dihydrogen phosphate	15 mEq
Monohydrogen phosphate	85 mEq
Measured osmolality	375 mOsm
pH (4°C)	7.25
University of Wisconsin (UW) or Belzer's Solution†	
K^+ Lactobionate	100 mmol
KH_2PO_4	25 mmol
Adenosine	5 mmol
$MgSO_4$	5 mmol
Glutathione	3 mmol
Raffinose	30 mmol
Allopurinol	1 mmol
Insulin	100 Units
Penicillin	40 Units
Dexamethasone	8 mg
Hydroxyethyl starch	50 g
Osmolality	320–330 mOsm
pH (4°C)	7.4
Crystalloid Cardioplegia‡	
Potassium	30 mEq
Sodium	25 mEq
Chloride	30 mEq
Bicarbonate	25 mEq
Dextrose	50 g
Mannitol	12.5 g
Osmolality	440 mOsm
pH (4°C)	8.1–8.4

* "Modified" Euro-Collins contains 5 cc·l^{-1} of 50% glucose and 1 g·l^{-1} of magnesium sulfate. Adapted with permission from Collins GM, Bravo-Schuarman M, Teraskai PI: Kidney preservation for transplantation. Initial perfusion and 30 hours ice storage. Lancet 2:1219, 1969.

† Adapted with permission from Belzer FO, Southard JH: Principles of solid organ preservation by cold storage. Transplant 45:673, 1988.

‡ Adapted with permission from Hardesty RL, Griffith BP, Deep GM et al: Improved cardiac function using cardioplegia during procurement and transplantation. Transplant Proc 15:1253, 1983.

TRANSPLANTATION IMMUNOLOGY

Tissue derived from a (nontwin) donor of the same species for transplantation is termed an *allograft*. When an immunocompetent recipient is confronted with foreign antigens present on the cell surfaces of an allograft, an immune response occurs. All elements of a recipient's immune system contribute to the response provoked by transplanted tissue; these include humoral factors (immunoglobulins secreted by B-lymphocytes as well as complement proteins) and cellular elements (T cells, other leukocytes, and macrophages). T-lymphocytes play a primary role in the immune response by initial antigen recognition and ultimate allograft destruction. On the basis of their specific reactivity to certain monoclonal antibodies or their cell-surface antigens, T-lymphocytes can be subdivided into at least four subpopulations:[24] cytotoxic T-cells, helper T-cells, delayed hypersensitivity

T-cells, and suppressor T-cells. All are important participants in the reaction to foreign tissue.

The cell surface glycoproteins that establish the immunologic identity of donor tissues are termed the major histocompatibility complex (MHC) antigens. Class I MHC antigens, also called *human leucocyte antigens* or HLA-A, -B and -C, are found on all nucleated cells. These are the classic transplantation antigens as well as the primary targets for cytotoxic cells.[25] Class II MHC antigens, also termed HLA-DR, -DQ, and -DP, are located on activated T cells, B cells, and macrophages, and are the primary targets for helper T-cells.[26] There is an enormous diversity of alleles at the chromosomal loci encoding for the HLA antigens, and this accounts for the varying degrees of HLA matching observed. Finally, the major blood group antigens (ABO) are particularly potent transplantation antigens, such that organs transplanted into patients with known preformed

isohemagglutinins against the donor blood type can be expected to provoke the most violent of immune responses.

Mechanisms of Allograft Rejection

Unless suppressed, the immune response to transplanted tissue begins with the recognition of the donor antigens as foreign or "nonself," proceeds with proliferation of immunocompetent cells, and culminates in an effector phase. Briefly, recognition involves a binding reaction between an immunogenic histocompatibility antigen present on the surface of the allogeneic (donor) cell and a receptor on the surface of a helper or cytotoxic T cell (Fig. 55-2, *top*). After T cells are bound, accessory macrophages secrete "monokines," notably interleukin-1 (IL-1), to further enhance T-cell activation. Interleukin-2 (IL-2) and other lymphokines

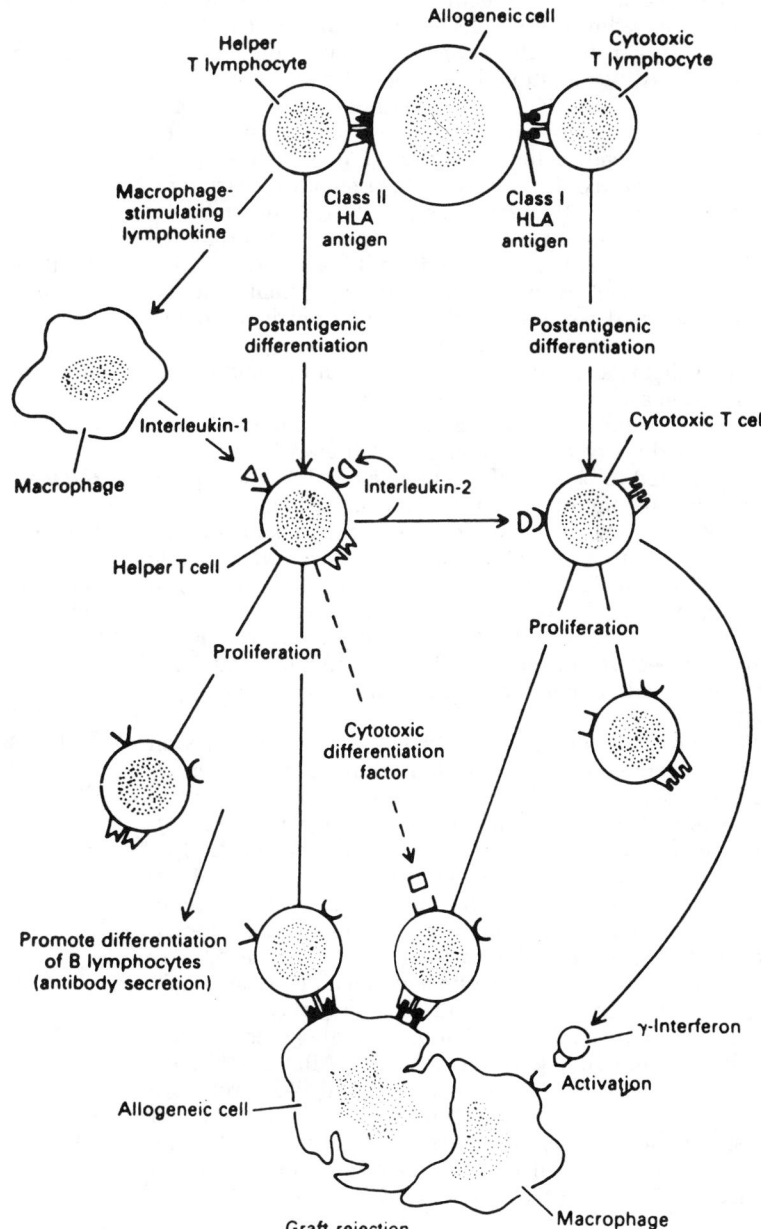

Figure 55-2. Immune response to allogeneic tissue. The cellular and humoral events that comprise the immune cascade are illustrated, starting with recognition of an allogenic (foreign) cell by T-lymphocytes at the top of the figure. See text for details. (Reprinted with permission from Strom TB: Immunosuppressive agents in renal transplantation. Kidney Int 26:353, 1984.)

are secreted by helper T cells, promoting lymphocyte proliferation and differentiation. Differentiated lymphocytes, in turn, secrete effector molecules including γ-interferon, which activate and enlist macrophages and leukocytes to cooperate in the process of graft rejection.

Clinical Immunology of Visceral Transplantation

Hyperacute rejection of renal allografts, characterized by microvascular thrombosis rapidly followed by graft necrosis, occurs in the presence of major blood-group (ABO) incompatibilities.[27] However, like blood transfusion, kidneys from type O donors can be transplanted into compatible, nonidentical (A, B, or AB) recipients. In some centers, ABO-incompatible living-related donor kidney transplants are performed with good results, but only under special immunosuppression protocols that include splenectomy, plasmapheresis, donor-specific platelet transfusion and cyclosporine administration. The importance of HLA histocompatibility matching in kidney transplantation is controversial; HLA-incompatible living-related donor transplants yield excellent results, but survival rates of HLA-matched cadaver allografts are superior. The presence of preformed cytotoxic antibodies to the donor's T-lymphocytes (antilymphocyte antibodies) increases the risk of hyperacute rejection and generally precludes kidney transplantation.[28] One other immunologic parameter that may affect renal allograft survival is the panel reactive antibody (PRA). In this test, cross-match testing is done between patient sera and donor cells to detect the presence of preformed antibodies. It has been reported that patients with lymphocytotoxic antibodies that react against more than 50% of the random test panel have a greater rate of rejection.[29]

Donor-specific ABO isoagglutinins may induce hyperacute reactions of cardiac allografts,[30] thus ABO matching is considered to be essential. The role of HLA matching in heart transplantation is more controversial. Some studies indicate that HLA mismatching does not correlate with the number of cardiac rejection episodes or survival,[31] while others find that HLA mismatching has clinically important consequences.[32] However, until the tolerable donor-heart ischemic time is extended beyond the present 4–6 hours, full prospective histocompatibility matching and PRA screening will remain impractical and limit their application.

In contrast to the heart and kidneys, hyperacute rejection has not been reported to occur in liver allografts,[33] supporting the assertion that the liver is resistant to such antibody-mediated injury.[34] Consequently, liver transplantation is often performed in spite of major ABO incompatibility, although the risk of subsequent rejection is elevated.[27,35] When ABO matching is done, short-term survival is better with ABO-identical than with ABO-compatible, nonidentical allografts,[27] and the longer-term trend is similar.[36] There does not seem to be any relation between either HLA matching[37] or T-cell crossmatch[38] and allograft survival.

In summary, the distribution of renal allografts depends mostly on immunologic factors such as ABO match, HLA histocompatibility, T-cell crossmatch, and PRA profile. In contrast, except for ABO matching, the distribution of donor livers and hearts depends more on factors such as size compatibility and medical urgency than on immunologic criteria.

Mechanisms of Immunosuppression

In clinical practice, the immune response must be controlled to avoid allograft rejection. Immunosuppressant drugs have been developed for this purpose but their use is accompanied by significant morbidity. Because of side effects and toxicities (as discussed below in Evaluation of Patients with Prior Organ Transplant), immunosuppression is warranted only for grafts essential for life. For example, a thyroid allograft would be inappropriate because it is easily substituted by a medication.

Ideally, immunosuppressants should inhibit only that lymphocyte subset directed against donor-specific alloantigens, but in fact, the drugs in current use are immunologically nonspecific. Antirejection regimens usually combine low doses of several agents to provide superior immunosuppression and to minimize side effects.

Glucocorticoids

Glucocorticoids (Table 55-4) are potent anti-inflammatory agents and have been a mainstay in almost all immunosuppressive regimens. These agents decrease macrophage production of IL-1, a critical factor in helper T-cell development.[39] In addition, T-cell secretion of IL-2 is also diminished, preventing clonal expansion of helper and cytotoxic T-cells.[40]

Azathioprine

Azathioprine is an imidazole derivative of 6-mercaptopurine (6-MP), an analog of the purine, hypoxanthine. Thioinosinic acid, a metabolite of azathioprine, competes with inosinic acid for conversion to xanthylic acid, an essential substrate for de novo purine synthesis required for production of both DNA and RNA. As a result, protein synthesis and both T- and B-lymphocyte proliferation is inhibited.[41]

Cyclosporine, FK506, and Rapamycin

Cyclosporine is a lipophilic undecapeptide antibiotic isolated from a soil fungus, that virtually revolutionized viscera transplantation by making it feasible to routinely achieve results comparable to those obtained in transplants

TABLE 55-4. Mechanisms of Immunosuppressants Action

Agent	Main Effect(s)
Glucocorticoids	Decrease IL-1 production from macrophages (reducing effectiveness of T helper cells) Decrease IL-2 production from T cells (reducing clonal expansion of T helper and cytotoxic cells)
Azathioprine	Inhibits DNA and RNA synthesis (reducing lymphocyte proliferation)
Cyclosporine	Prevents T helper cell activation by antigen Inhibits elaboration of T cell derived factors, particularly IL-2
Antilymphocyte globulin	Diminishes populations of both T and B lymphocytes
OKT3	Inactivates T cells and prevents reactivation

between identical twins. Its major target is the T cell, which is inhibited from elaborating key lymphokines such as IL-2.[42] Cyclosporine also prevents activation of helper T-cells by foreign antigens and inhibits the production of IL-1 by macrophages.

FK506 and rapamycin are newer macrolide antibiotic immunosuppressants currently undergoing clinical trials. Both are highly potent and may have somewhat more immunospecificity and less toxicity than cyclosporine. These agents diminish activation and proliferation of T cells as well as lymphokine production, but do so through distinct intracellular signaling pathways.

Antilymphocyte Globulin and OKT3

Antilymphocyte globulin (ALG) is a polyclonal antibody produced by immunizing animals with human lymphoid cells and isolating the IgG fraction from resulting antisera. ALG seems to rapidly diminish the availability of activated T-lymphocytes, interrupting the chain of events leading to rejection. ALG may also have a sustained effect on T-cell proliferation, perhaps by promoting formation of nonspecific suppressor T-cells.[43] Similarly, the OKT series of murine monoclonal antibodies directed against T-cell surface antigens are added to some immunosuppression regimens to treat rejection. OKT3 is specifically directed against the T3 (CD3) complex on the surface of mature T-lymphocytes. The T3 complex is located adjacent to the T-cell receptor involved in recognition of foreign antigens; binding of OKT3 blocks the recognition of MHC antigens and, consequently, the immune response cascade.[44] Administration of OKT3 also results in removal of opsonized T-cells by the reticuloendothelial system.

Transfusion and Immunosuppression

Multiple blood transfusions prior to renal transplantation have been shown to have a significant beneficial effect on graft survival,[45,46] perhaps by inducing some degree of specific immunologic nonreactivity to the transfused histocompatibility antigens. The combination of azathioprine–prednisone with deliberate transfusion markedly improves cadaveric renal allograft survival, but the beneficial effects are not as apparent since the introduction of cyclosporine. In any case, many centers encourage transfusion of uremic patients awaiting transplantation, and a few perform deliberate transfusions from either the prospective living-related donor or from random donors. Cyclosporine may be administered during pretransplant transfusions to promote the development of tolerance.

GENERAL PREANESTHETIC EVALUATION OF TRANSPLANT CANDIDATES

The general indication for organ transplantation is failure of medical or other surgical management to enhance the quality of life for patients with end-stage organ disease or to significantly improve their chances for long-term survival. Since major organ transplantation procedures are now associated with reasonably low perioperative mortalities, this option is currently considered in virtually all such cases.

The major contraindications to organ transplantation are incurable malignancy; the presence of another systemic dis-

TABLE 55-5. General Contraindications to Viscera Transplantation

1. Incurable malignancy
2. Other major systemic illness
3. Old ("physiologic") age
4. Active systemic or incurable infection
5. Significant obesity
6. Current alcohol, drug, or tobacco abuse
7. Evidence of emotional instability or lack of supportive social milieu

ease; active, poorly controlled infection; and physical or social factors that would either impede recovery or lead to recurrent disease (Table 55–5). Rather than being considered absolute, these criteria are under continuous evolution in light of new information. For example, diabetes mellitus was formerly felt to contraindicate organ transplantation, but many diabetics have now undergone renal transplantation and 1-year allograft survival is the same as for nondiabetics. In fact, patients with diabetic nephropathy now comprise the largest segment of adults who undergo renal transplantation. Similarly, many elderly patients have undergone heart transplantation with results that are comparable to those for younger subpopulations.

Candidates for organ transplantation often manifest physical findings or laboratory abnormalities indicative of secondary organ involvement (e.g., hepatomegaly consequent to right ventricular failure). It is important to verify that such findings do not represent a coexistent primary disease process (which might disqualify potential recipients) and to bear in mind that compromised organs may be especially vulnerable to acute insults. Because recipients will be immunosuppressed, occult infection (e.g., tuberculosis) should assiduously be ruled out. For the same reason, it is standard to order CMV negative blood for transfusion unless recipients are seropositive. On occasion, technical feasibility may become the overwhelming source of concern (e.g., with atypical vascular anatomy or body habitus, or multiple previous surgeries).

Because of the shortage of suitable donor organs, patients may remain on a waiting list for many months while their conditions continue to deteriorate. Interval changes, as well as corresponding alterations in their medical regimens, should be ascertained. The urgency of surgery may, by necessity, influence the acceptability of an available donor organ.

With organs for which the safe ischemic time is less than 24 hours, transplant procedures are usually performed under emergency circumstances. The patient to receive the organ may have eaten recently and will arrive in the operating room without the benefit of premedication. The remaining management considerations are specific to the particular type of transplant procedure, as discussed in the following sections.

KIDNEY TRANSPLANTATION

Presently nearly 9,000 renal transplants are performed each year in the United States. This comprises about 10% of patients with end-stage renal disease who are otherwise dependent on dialysis. Dialysis is clearly effective in prolonging life, but considerable morbidity and mortality is

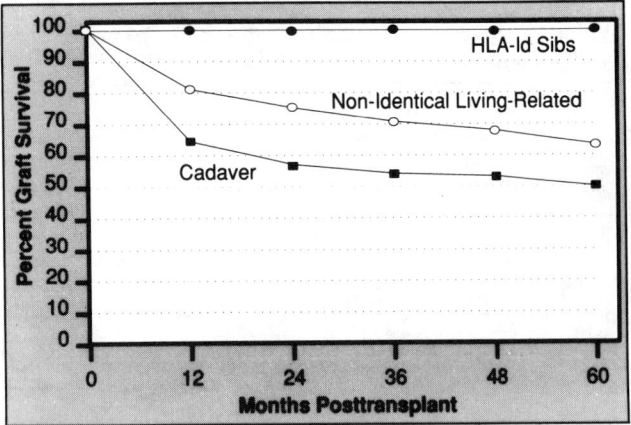

Figure 55-3. Actuarial survival of renal allografts obtained from cadaver, nonidentical living-related, and HLA-identical sibling donors. (Reprinted with permission from Chavers BM, Matas AJ, Nevins TE *et al:* Results of pediatric kidney transplantation at the University of Minnesota. In Terasaki P (ed): Clinical Transplants, pp 253–266. Los Angeles, UCLA Tissue Typing Laboratory, 1989.)

TABLE 55-6. Etiologies of End-Stage Renal Disease in Renal Transplant Recipients*

Etiology	Total Cases (%)
Diabetic glomerulonephropathy	43.6
Other glomerulonephritides	23.2
Polycystic kidney disease	5.8
Chronic pyelonephritis	5.4
Obstructive uropathy	3.4
Alport's syndrome	2.1
Lupus nephritis	1.6
Miscellaneous, including unknown	14.9

*Data derived from 2,591 cases at the University of Minnesota performed between 1963 and 1990.

Adapted with permission from Belani KG, Palahniuk RJ: Kidney transplantation. In Firestone LL (ed): Anesthesia and Organ Transplantation, pp 17–39. Boston, Little, Brown and Co, 1991.

associated with its use. For example, in 1988 the 1-year mortality after renal transplantation was 5%; in some studies the yearly mortality of patients on chronic dialysis is at least twice as high.[47,48]

Renal transplantation is a highly successful procedure. According to recent data from the national organ procurement and transplantation network, UNOS (United Network for Organ Sharing), cadaveric renal allografts have a 1-year survival rate of 81%, while the same statistic for living-related donor organs is 91%.[49] Studies from large centers indicate that longer-term graft survival is also comparably favorable (Fig. 55-3), as are other measures of outcome. In adults with end-stage renal disease, kidney transplantation improves the quality of life[50] while remaining cost-effective,[51] and for children, transplantation provides superior growth and development.[52,53] For these reasons, renal transplantation has become the treatment of choice for end-stage renal disease, with its growth limited only by the supply of available donor organs.[54]

Pathophysiology of End-Stage Renal Disease

End-stage renal disease can result from numerous causes (Table 55-6), all of which ultimately lead to the uremic syndrome. In uremia, patients are unable to regulate the volume and composition of their body fluids, resulting in fluid overload, acidemia, and imbalance of electrolytes such as potassium, phosphorous, magnesium, and calcium. In addition, there is usually evidence of secondary dysfunction in other organ systems (Table 55-7). Even patients maintained by dialysis may have peripheral neuropathy, pericardial or pleural effusions, renal osteodystrophy, and gastrointestinal as well as immunologic dysfunction.

Specific Indications and Contraindications

A large proportion of adults with end-stage renal disease are candidates for kidney transplantation. Aside from the general contraindications to viscera transplantation

(see Table 55-5), relative contraindications specific to renal transplantation are disease processes likely to recur in the transplanted kidney. Hemolytic uremic syndrome, membranoproliferative glomerulonephritis, and metabolic derangements that produce toxic deposits in the kidney (e.g., gout, oxalosis, cytinosis) fall into this group. In practice, however, patients with such disorders may derive years of benefit from transplantation, and thus at many centers are still considered eligible. Similarly, diabetic nephropathy can also recur in allografts, but diabetes mellitus is no longer considered a contraindication to venal transplantation.

Preanesthetic Considerations

Since the tolerable ischemic time for kidneys is at least 48 hours,[55] cadaver allografts may be transplanted semielectively. With living-related donation, renal transplantation is an elective procedure. In either case, sufficient time is available for ABO matching, crossmatching of the recipient's serum with donor lymphocytes, and at some institutions, HLA-tissue typing. Likewise, dialysis may precede transplantation to correct serious electrolyte and volume derangements. Following dialysis, it is important to ascertain the net volume status of patients; the final hematocrit, electrolyte, and bicarbonate levels; and whether there is any residual heparin effect. The serum potassium should be normal, and the serum calcium supplemented if less than 7 mg% to prevent tetanus. Most uremic patients, even those on dialysis, will have hemoglobin levels in the 6–8 g·dl^{-1} range. However, in chronically anemic patients, compensatory changes promote tissue oxygen unloading, and, on this basis alone, preoperative transfusion is not mandatory. But transfusion may enhance allograft survival (see the Transplantation Immunology section). Thus it has become a standard part of the preoperative regimen at some centers. On occasion, pleural or pericardial effusions may require treatment if there is functional impairment; in patients on chronic steroids, preoperative administration of full replacement doses of glucocorticoids should be considered.

Since many adult recipients are diabetics, the possibility of coexistent ischemic heart disease is usually evaluated by exercise stress testing and, if indicated, coronary angiography.[56] Diffuse, inoperable coronary disease has not been

TABLE 55-7. Common Pathophysiologic Consequences of End-Stage Renal Disease

Organ System	Consequence
Nervous system	Peripheral neuropathy Lethargy → coma
Hematologic	Anemia Diminished erythrocyte survival Platelet dysfunction Shift in P_{50} of oxyhemoglobin dissociation curve
Cardiovascular	Congestive heart failure Pericarditis Hypertension Dysrhythmias (abnormal electrolytes) Capillary fragility
Pulmonary	Pleural effusions Pulmonary edema
Musculoskeletal	Generalized muscle weakness Renal osteodystrophy Metastatic calcification Gout, pseudogout
Gastrointestinal	Nausea, vomiting Ileus Peptic and colonic ulceration
Endocrine	Pancreatitis Glucose intolerance
Integument	Pruritus Hyperpigmentation
Immunologic	Impaired cellular immunity

Adapted with permission from Belani KG, Palahniuk RJ: Kidney transplantation. In Firestone LL (ed): Anesthesia and Organ Transplantation, pp 17–39. Boston, Little, Brown and Co, 1991.

considered a contraindication to renal transplantation, providing ventricular function is not seriously diminished and the patient is willing to assume the added risk. In such patients, appropriate invasive monitoring (arterial and pulmonary artery catheters) is warranted; in all others, a central venous pressure catheter is sufficient to monitor intravascular volume for optimal renal perfusion. Finally, transplanted kidneys, particularly those derived from cadaver donors, may not be functional immediately, so it is vital to protect existing arteriovenous fistulas or other routes for postoperative hemo- or peritoneal dialysis.

Donor Procedure and Related Considerations

The procedure employed for harvesting abdominal viscera from cadaver donors is reviewed in the section Anesthesia Care of Organ Donors. If the cadaver is brain dead but the circulation is intact, harvesting may procede at leisure through the transperitoneal route. If the circulation fails, however, the kidneys must be rapidly removed and flushed with preservative solution to minimize warm ischemic time.

Living donors are the source of one-fifth of the kidneys transplanted in the United States and 60% of those in Europe. Because results with unrelated donors are no better than those achieved with cadaver donors, living donors are virtually always close relatives. Most are healthy adults,

since any significant systemic disease would increase the risk of general anesthesia and surgery, giving rise to ethical conflicts. For similar reasons, donors who are age 45 years (male) or 50 years (female) usually undergo noninvasive studies to detect occult coronary ischemia. The use of living-related donors has gained widespread acceptance because the overall incidence of serious perioperative morbidity in this population is small (2% or less), and mortalities are extremely rare.[57,58] Furthermore, long-term follow-up studies indicate that donors have no greater risk of renal failure or hypertension.[59]

Preoperatively, donors undergo renal arteriography, intravenous pyelography and are screened for ABO blood-group compatibility and CMV titer. Then, 2–4 weeks before the procedure, several units of blood are donated for autologous transfusion. During the night preceding harvesting, donors are hydrated with crystalloid solutions to promote an active diuresis, and at the time of nephrectomy, a minimum urine output of 1 ml·min^{-1} is achieved by means of mannitol and furosemide. The timing of the donor and recipient procedures is coordinated so that the kidney's ischemic interval is minimized. Heparin is administered systemically before removal of the organ from the donor, which is then flushed free of blood with a cold crystalloid solution and transplanted immediately.

Anesthesia Induction for Recipients

Diabetic patients can have delayed gastric emptying,[60] and therefore rapid induction may be warranted. Provided the serum potassium is normal after recent dialysis, there is no contraindication to the use of succinylcholine. Drugs that are highly protein bound (e.g., Thiopental) should be administered in reduced dosages. Further discussion of the kinetics and dynamics of drugs in renal failure patients is found in Chapter 40.

Central venous catheters are useful for the reasons discussed earlier but are usually inserted after induction. Many renal transplant recipients are moderately hypertensive and maintained on combinations of appropriate medications. Most have recently been dialyzed and are volume depleted. Thus the possibility of synergistic interactions between strongly vasodilating anesthetics (e.g., isoflurane, fentanyl), antihypertensives (e.g., hydralazine, diltiazem, captopril), and hypovolemia should be considered.

Anesthesia and Surgical Procedures

Although regional anesthetic techniques have been advocated by some,[61,62] the use of general anesthesia is more common.[63,64] With general anesthesia, there is superior control of ventilation, which becomes particularly important when surgical retraction is close to the diaphragm. In addition, the duration of renal transplant procedures in most centers makes regional techniques impractical. Enflurane is seldom chosen since its biotransformation results in inorganic fluoride that is nephrotoxic. Nitrous oxide is often omitted to avoid distension of the bowel, particularly in children, so either opioids and benzodiazepines are used in combination, or a potent inhaled agent is used alone. Atracurium and vecuronium are the preferred muscle relaxants because they are least dependent upon renal metabolism, although laudanosine, a metabolite of atracurium, may accumulate in patients with end-stage renal disease.[65] Laudanosine increases the MAC of halothane in laboratory ani-

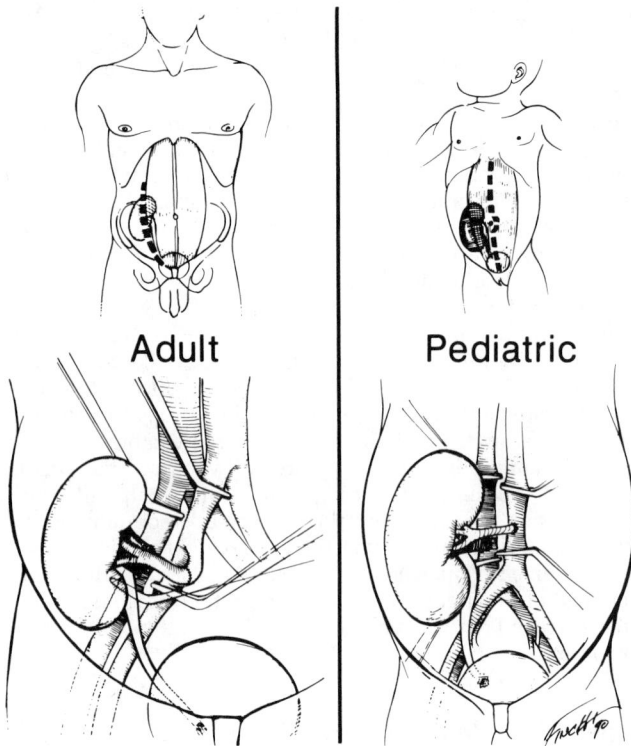

Figure 55-4. Surgical approach and vascular anastomoses for adult and pediatric renal transplantation. (Reprinted with permission from Belani KG, Palahniuk RJ: kidney transplantation. In Firestone LL (ed): Anesthesia and Organ Transplantation, pp 17–39. Boston, Little, Brown and Co, 1991.)

mals[66] but does not seem to cause an analogous clinical effect in humans.[67] The response to vecuronium may be quite variable in renal failure,[68] and since it is not clear precisely when renal metabolic function is restored following transplantation, neuromuscular monitoring is highly recommended.

In adults, the kidney is implanted retroperitoneally in the upper pelvis using a paramedian lower-abdominal approach; in children weighing less than 20 kg, abdominal implantation is the rule. Revascularization of the allograft in adults involves anastomoses of the renal vessels to an iliac vein and artery (Fig. 55-4). This necessitates clamping the common iliac vessels, resulting in lower extremity ischemia for usually less than 60 minutes. After the anastomoses are complete, the circulation is restored to the allograft and lower extremities. To promote renal perfusion, a high-normal blood pressure is achieved by reducing the depth of anesthesia, bolus administration of crystalloid, and/or temporary dopamine infusions. When the vascular clamps are released, renal preservative solution and the venous drainage from the legs are also released into the circulation. These effluents are relatively rich in potassium and acid metabolites, but in adults, have little systemic effect. The final stage of the procedure involves ureteral implantation for urinary drainage.

Postoperative Management

Varying periods of oliguria or anuria due to acute tubular necrosis are associated with cadaveric renal transplantation in about one-third of cases,[69] thus fluids must be adminis-

tered judiciously to reduce the risk of postoperative pulmonary edema. In contrast, the ischemic time for organs derived from living-related donors is minimal and urine flow is usually immediate. Emergence is often accompanied by both pain and hypertension, which are particularly hazardous in diabetic patients with coexistent ischemic heart disease. In such cases, preparations should be made to administer potent analgesics (e.g., via epidural catheter) and antihypertensives in the recovery room, if myocardial ischemia is to be avoided. Other early postoperative complications include atelectasis, bleeding and thrombosis of vascular anastomoses, urinary obstruction or leak, and rarely, gastric aspiration. Hyperacute rejection may also occur and lead to anuria; definitive diagnosis requires a renal biopsy. This complication has become rare since both ABO matching and crossmatching of the recipient's serum to donor lymphocytes are routinely performed.

Immunosuppression with "triple therapy" (cyclosporine, azathioprine, prednisone) is usually begun prior to transplantation of living-related donor organs or following transplantation of cadaveric kidneys. Long-term complications of renal transplantation related to immunosuppression are discussed in the section on Evaluation of Patients With Prior Organ Transplant, below.

LIVER TRANSPLANTATION

Medical treatment for chronic end-stage liver disease is generally supportive, but does little to prolong or improve the quality of life, particularly after serious complications (e.g., GI bleeding, coma, uremia) develop. In acute hepatic failure, the salvage rate with medical treatment is between 5% and 20%.[70] In contrast, in the cyclosporine era, the overall 1-year survival of orthotopic liver recipients is 76% with an allograft survival rate of 69%.[49] Longer-term survival is also comparatively high (Fig. 55-5). Moreover, the quality of life for a high proportion of transplant survivors is markedly improved.[71,72]

The yearly rate of liver transplantations in the United States has reached approximately 2,500, although it has

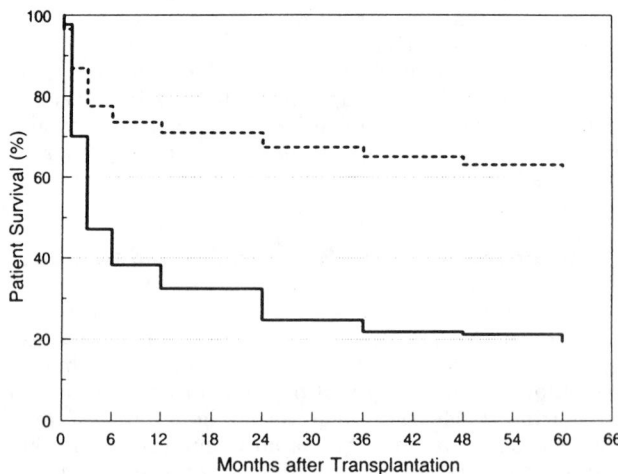

Figure 55-5. Survival of liver transplant recipients treated before and after the availability of cyclosporine. Data are derived from 170 "before" (*solid line*) and 1258 "after" (*dashed line*) recipients. Survival is calculated using the life-table method. (Reprinted with permission from Starzl TE, Demetris AJ, van Thiel DH: Liver transplantation. N Engl J Med 321:1014, 1092, 1989.)

been argued that more than twice that number are needed.[72] The overwhelming majority of these procedures are orthotopic, involving native hepatectomy and implantation of the donor organ in anatomic position in the right upper quadrant. Heterotopic (also called auxiliary) transplantation, where the donor liver is implanted adjacent to the native liver, which is left *in situ,* has been used on rare occasion for reversible hepatic failure and in patients too frail for the orthotopic procedure.[73]

Pathophysiology of End-Stage Liver Disease

The liver has numerous synthetic and metabolic functions (see Chapter 43), thus end-stage liver disease has ramifications that extend to virtually every other organ system (Table 55-8). In disease processes that destroy the normal hepatic architecture, portal hypertension results and extensive venous collaterals develop in the abdominal wall, mesentery, retroperitoneum, and GI tract. Aside from the significant morbidity associated with hemorrhage from esophageal varices, the extensive network of arteriovenous communications results in low systemic vascular resistance and high cardiac output. Intrapulmonary shunting is also seen frequently in patients with end-stage liver disease,[74] leading to hypoxemia that is exacerbated by pleural effusions and bibasilar atelectasis from abdominal distension. Renal function may be impaired from hepatorenal syndrome or prerenal azotemia. Ascites develops as a result of venous hypertension, decreased albumin synthesis, and sodium and water retention from a relative excess of aldosterone and antidiuretic hormone. Treatment often consists of diuretics,

TABLE 55-8. Common Pathophysiologic Consequences of End-Stage Liver Disease

Organ System	Consequence
Central nervous system	Encephalopathy (mild confusion → coma)
	Brain edema (fulminant hepatitis)
Cardiovascular	Hyperdynamic circulation
	Reduced systemic resistance
	Increased plasma volume
	Pericardial effusion
Pulmonary	Pleural effusion
	Interstitial edema (hypoalbuminemia)
	Atelectasis
	Ventilation–perfusion mismatch and shunting
Gastrointestinal	Esophageal varices
	Ascites
	Portal hypertension
	Delayed gastric emptying
Hematologic	Reduced clotting factor levels
	Anemia
	Thrombocytopenia (hypersplenism)
	Reduced clearance of fibrinolytic substances and tissue plasminogen activators
Endocrine	Glucose intolerance
	Diminished glycogen stores
Renal	Oliguria (hepatorenal syndrome, prerenal azotemia)
	Hyponatremia (diuretics, increased antidiuretic hormone activity)
	Hypokalemia (poor nutrition, diuretics, GI losses)

which in turn may cause electrolyte and acid-base derangements and intravascular volume depletion. Blood coagulation is abnormal, since synthesis of the hepatically derived clotting factors (I [fibrinogen], II [prothrombin], V, VII, IX, X) and clearance of fibrinolytic factors is compromised. Hypersplenism may markedly diminish the platelet count. Eventually, even the central nervous system is affected, resulting in a progressive toxic encephalopathy and cerebral edema, which presages death.

Specific Indications and Contraindications

The decision to transplant is difficult to base on objective liver function tests, since these values will vary considerably according to the specific pathologic process. Instead, the degree of medical, social, and psychological impairment are considered in combination, then balanced against the mortality associated with conservative management.[72] Ideally, liver transplantation is undertaken before the degree of organ failure becomes severe, to reduce perioperative morbidity.

There is little debate that liver transplantation is indicated for nonmalignant end-stage liver disease that will not recur in the hepatic graft. Most often, this procedure is used to treat benign parenchymal diseases including postnecrotic cirrhosis and any of the causes of acute liver failure, or cholestatic processes, e.g., primary biliary cirrhosis or biliary atresia in children (Table 55-9). In all, more than 60 disease entities have now been successfully treated by liver transplantation.[72] Transplanting in the presence of a disease when recurrence is a possibility is somewhat more controversial, considering the limited supply of donor organs. Alcoholic cirrhosis was once considered an absolute contraindication to transplantation, but multidisciplinary care and careful selection has led to results with Laennec's cirrhosis that are comparable to those with other liver diseases.[75] Similarly, transplantation for cirrhosis from hepatitis B virus has proven to be beneficial for many patients[72] despite the inability to prevent infection in the donor liver. Advanced age was also once a contradiction, but recipients over age 50 years have been shown to have a 5-year survival after transplantation, comparable to that of younger adults.[76]

Treatment of hepatic cancers by transplantation is being studied at several centers, and is the subject of considerable debate. Patients with primary liver and bile duct cancers, as well as hepatic metastases from GI and endocrine tumors, have undergone liver transplantation with varying duration of remission.[77-79] But recurrence of tumor is the rule, so transplantation is generally reserved for selected cases with isolated tumors and deteriorating liver function. If hepatic function remains preserved in the presence of a liver tumor, major hepatic resection is the recommended alternative.

Other possible contraindications relate to specific surgical obstacles, including thromboses of major abdominal veins and scarring from multiple abdominal procedures. However, the successful use of vein grafts and accumulation of practical experience with the transplantation procedure have rendered even these contraindications obsolete.

Preanesthetic Considerations

Candidates for liver transplantation present a broad clinical spectrum, ranging from chronic fatigue with mild jaundice, to coma with multiorgan failure. Hepatic encephalopathy

TABLE 55-9. Preoperative Pathologic Diagnoses in Liver Transplant Recipients*

Disease	No. of Cases
Parenchymal	
Postnecrotic cirrhosis	348
Alcoholic cirrhosis	76
Acute liver failure	54
Budd–Chiari syndrome	18
Congenital hepatic fibrosis	9
Cystic fibrosis	6
Neonatal hepatitis	8
Hepatic trauma	3
Cholestatic	
Biliary atresia	217
Primary biliary cirrhosis	186
Sclerosing cholangitis	100
Secondary biliary cirrhosis	25
Familial cholestasis	16
Inborn errors of metabolism	114
Tumors	
Benign	10
Primary malignant	60
Metastatic	8
Total	1,258

* Data are derived from 400 pediatric and 858 adult recipients of liver transplants at the University of Pittsburgh, 1981–1988.
Adapted with permission from Starzl TE, Demetris AJ, van Thiel DH: Liver transplantation. N Engl J Med 321:1014, 1092, 1989.

may be reversible, thus the timing of liver transplantation can be critical to outcome. Emergency transplantation for fulminant hepatic failure can have a salvage rate of 55–75%[80,81] provided symptoms have not progressed to Grade 4 encephalopathy.[72] Without transplantation, most causes of fulminant hepatic failure are associated with much poorer prognoses.[82,83]

Certain uncommon diseases treated by liver transplantation have additional implications for anesthesiologists. For example, following transplantation for Budd–Chiari syndrome, which typically is associated with extensive hepatic venous thrombosis, patients may require anticoagulation.[84] In children with an even rarer disorder, Crigler–Najjar syndrome (bilirubin UDP-glucuronyl transferase deficiency), drugs that interfere with bilirubin binding to albumin (e.g., barbiturates) should be avoided.[85]

Many of the physiologic derangements associated with end-stage liver disease are not correctable until after transplantation. Therefore the major emphasis in the preanesthetic evaluation should be on identifying the most important areas of physiologic compromise and treating only those that threaten the safe induction of anesthesia. For example, pleural effusions may be responsible for profound hypoxemia, and despite clotting abnormalities, preoperative thoracentesis may be a necessity. However, defects in coagulation are usually not corrected at this point unless there is active hemorrhage.

Preparation of fluid warming units, gas circuit humidifiers, warming blankets, and nonconductive wraps for the head and extremities is essential prior to induction, otherwise hypothermia will rapidly result from transfusion, convective and evaporative losses from exposure of abdominal organs, diminished hepatic energy production, and implantation of a cold donor-organ of large thermal mass. A thrombelastograph instrument is also prepared at many centers, as a relatively rapid means to elucidate a need for specific blood product replacement under conditions of massive transfusion.[86]

Finally, as a result of the primary disease process or subsequent multiple transfusions, recipient serologies may be positive for hepatitis A, B, or C. The health care team should be aware of the potential for infectious contamination and take appropriate precautions.

Anesthesia Induction

Liver transplantation involves transection and reanastomosis of several major venous structures (portal vein and inferior vena cava (IVC)), and the ability to rapidly transfuse is vital to successful outcome.[87] At the University of Pittsburgh, at least two large-bore peripheral venous cannulae are inserted, one of which is 8.5 Fr to facilitate the use of a rapid transfusion device (discussed below). Because major shifts in intravascular volume are common and reperfusion of the donor liver has been associated with hypotension,[88] invasive monitoring with arterial and pulmonary artery catheters is standard. Both radial and femoral artery catheters are often placed, since distal arterial flow may be compromised by aortic clamps during hepatic artery anastomoses. The balance of the monitoring array is similar to that used for any critically ill patient undergoing a major general surgical procedure.

Patients with end-stage liver disease have numerous reasons for delayed gastric emptying, such as ascites or active upper GI bleeding. Therefore, aspiration precautions are mandatory and induction of general anesthesia should proceed by either a rapid sequence technique or, in patients with hemodynamic instability or significant hypovolemia, awake intubation.

Anesthesia and Surgical Procedures

Anesthesia is maintained by agents that preserve splanchnic flow (e.g., opioids or isoflurane) combined with muscle relaxants, except in cases of fulminant hepatic failure where the possibility of intracranial hypertension contraindicates potent inhaled agents. Nitrous oxide is not contraindicated but is usually avoided because of its ability to distend the bowel and increase the size of gas bubbles entrained in the circulation. Pharmacokinetic alterations associated with end-stage liver disease are complex, and are described in Chapter 43. The net effect of these factors for nondepolarizing muscle relaxants is to increase the loading dose requirements and prolong the durations of action. In contrast, fentanyl kinetics are not markedly changed.[89] Although well-preserved liver allografts can rapidly begin to metabolize drugs,[90] many of the pharmacokinetic changes (e.g., diminished serum albumin, enlarged volumes of distribution) persist beyond the transplant procedure.

The orthotopic procedure involves replacing the diseased native liver with a cadaveric organ in the most anatomic position possible. It consists of three stages: the preanhepatic, anhepatic, and neohepatic stages (Table 55-10).

The *preanhepatic* stage involves dissection of the structures of the porta hepatis and mobilization of the native liver. Cardiovascular instability is common during this phase, due to hypovolemia from acute third-space losses (ascites) and hemorrhage from venous collaterals in the body wall and mesentery. Citrate-induced hypocalcemia,[91] hyperkalemia from rapid transfusion and hemolysis, embarrassment of venous return from retraction, or precipitous drops in intra-abdominal pressure and consequent venous pooling also contribute to hemodynamic instability. During sudden volume shifts, previously asymptomatic pericardial effusions may reduce cardiac output, so they are often drained under direct vision. Hemorrhage may be exacerbated by clotting factor deficiencies or hemodilution, and fibrinolysis.[92] These defects should be treated as specifically as is feasible using either conventional studies (prothrombin time, partial thromboplastin time, bleeding time, fibrinogen, fibrin split product levels, and platelet count), or thromboelastography. At the University of Pittsburgh, a rapid infusion system designed to deliver prewarmed fluids or blood products at a rate of up to 1.5 l·min^{-1} is routinely employed (Fig. 55-6). Line pressure monitors, filters, air detectors and fluid-level sensors are built into the device to minimize trauma to the blood and to prevent transfusion of air. Blood salvaging ("autotransfusion") systems, which collect and wash extravasated blood are also used, provided that there is no active infection or malignancy.[93]

Metabolic acidosis may accompany hypotension and persist in the absence of hepatic metabolic function. Sodium bicarbonate is used for treatment, although if acidosis is severe, THAM (tromethamine (tris[hydroxymethyl]aminomethane)) is an alternative that avoids hyperosmolar hypernatremia.[87] Oliguria is also common in this phase, and once prerenal causes are ruled out, aggressive treatment with os-

TABLE 55-10. Overview of the Orthotopic Liver Transplantation Procedure

Phase	Surgical Procedures	Physiologic Changes
Preanhepatic	Dissection of porta hepatis Release of hepatic attachments	Third space losses (ascites) Hemorrhage (venous collaterals)
Anhepatic	Clamp hepatic a, portal v Venovenous bypass (adults) Clamp IVC Retraction on diaphragm	Obstruction of venous return Oliguria (venous congestion) Atelectasis, decreased compliance
Neohepatic	Anastomosis of IVC Flush hepatic allograft Anastomosis of portal v, hepatic a Biliary drainage procedure	Hemorrhage (coagulopathy) Citrate intoxication Hyperkalemia Hypothermia Metabolic acidosis

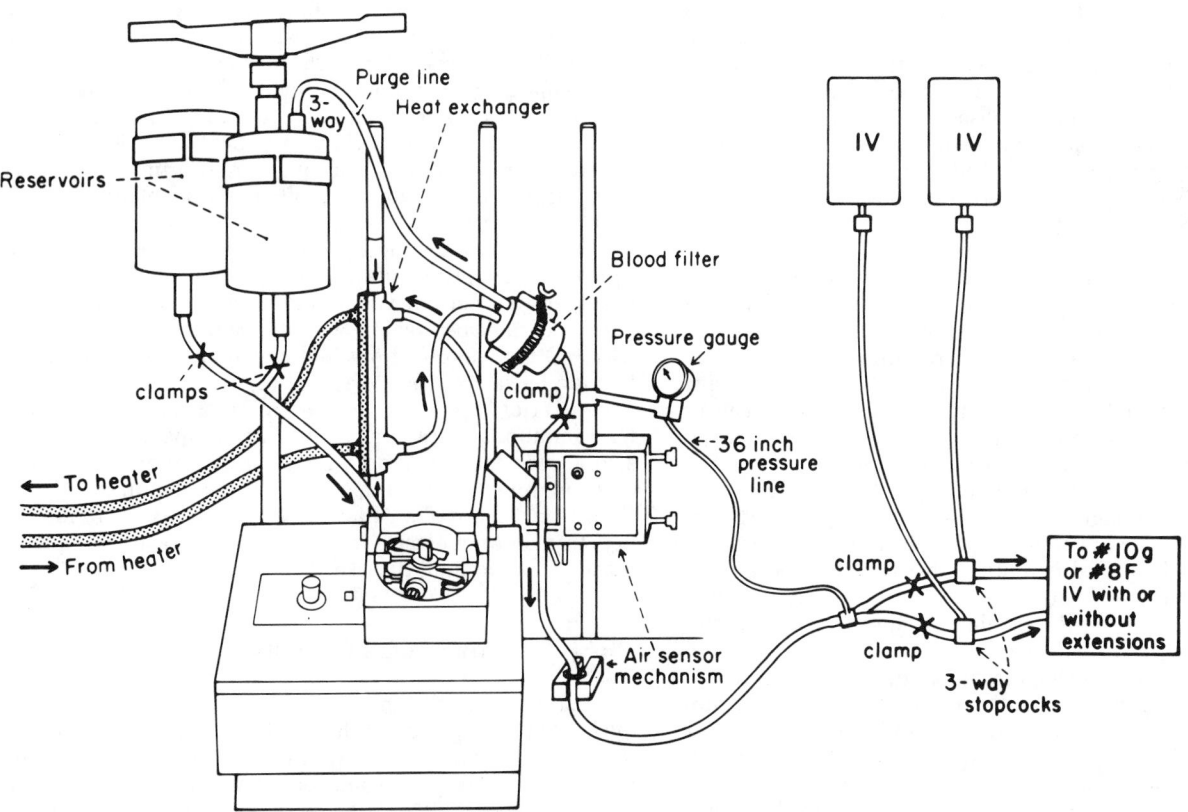

Figure 55-6. Rapid infusion system used during liver transplantation at the University of Pittsburgh. See text for explanation. (Reprinted with permission from Kang YG, Martin DJ, Marquez J *et al:* Intraoperative changes in blood coagulation and thomboelastogastric monitoring in liver transplantation. Anesth Analg 64:888, 1985.)

motic or potent loop diuretics, as well as "renal-dose" dopamine (2.5 $\mu g \cdot kg^{-1} \cdot min^{-1}$), is begun.

The *anhepatic stage* begins when the native diseased liver is removed after transection of its blood supply (hepatic artery and portal vein) as well as occlusion of the supra- and infrahepatic portions of the IVC. If large esophageal varices seem at high risk for rupturing during IVC clamping, a Sengstaken–Blakemore tube may be temporarily placed. To avoid drastic falls in venous return and cardiac output, as well as venous congestion in the lower body, bowel, and kidneys,[94] many centers employ a venovenous bypass system. The venovenous circuit drains blood from the portal and femoral veins and routes it extracorporeally to the axillary vein. A centrifugal pump propels blood through the circuit at a flow rate 20%–50% of usual total systemic flow. The circuit makes use of heparin-bonded tubing, which at the flow rates typically used, obviates the need for systemic heparinization.[95] Although venous bypass may help to preserve renal function,[94] it may not improve overall morbidity and mortality[96] and can lead to venous air embolism[97] and thrombosis. In addition, the use of venous bypass can prolong the procedure and contribute to heat loss.[98] Moreover, support of cardiac output with positive inotropes may still be required.

Removal of the native liver and implantation of the allograft usually require vigorous retraction near the diaphragm, decreasing respiratory compliance and causing atelectasis and hypoventilation. Adding PEEP and raising inspiratory pressures may help minimize these effects. Due to the lack of liver metabolic function during the anhepatic phase, citrate intoxication from rapid transfusion is a more likely possibility, and calcium must be infused to maintain the ionized calcium level above 1.0 mM. Calcium chloride is often chosen, but even in the absence of hepatic function, calcium gluconate has effectively treated ionized hypocalcemia.[99] Progressive hyperkalemia may be treated with an insulin infusion, despite the absence of liver, but metabolic acids, including lactate, remain largely uncleared during the anhepatic period.

The *neohepatic* or postreperfusion stage begins with reanastomoses of the major vascular structures. Prior to removal of all clamps, the allograft is flushed of air, debris, and preservative solution with blood released from the portal vein. Despite this, subsequent final unclamping can cause release of a large load of potassium and metabolic acids into the circulation.[100] Dysrhythmias, hypotension, and cardiac arrest may ensue, and the anesthesiologist should be prepared to treat the underlying metabolic causes specifically. Inotropic support may be needed to treat hypotension stemming from myocardial depression by putative vasoactive mediators,[88] or right heart failure from venous air embolism.[101,102] Appearance of significant end-tidal nitrogen from venous air embolism by mass spectroscopy is useful to differentiate between these alternatives. Pulmonary thromboembolism has also been reported to be a cause of cardiovascular collapse during reperfusion.[102,103]

Once the allograft begins to function, hemodynamic and metabolic stability is gradually restored. The need for inotropic support usually diminishes, and urine output improves even in patients with prior hepatorenal syndrome.[104] Clotting parameters can usually be normalized with specific replacement therapy, and fibrinolysis controlled with epsilon-amino-caproate (Amicar). The procedure ends with some form of biliary reconstruction, either direct bile duct anastomosis, or a Roux-en-Y choledochojejunostomy (Fig. 55-7).

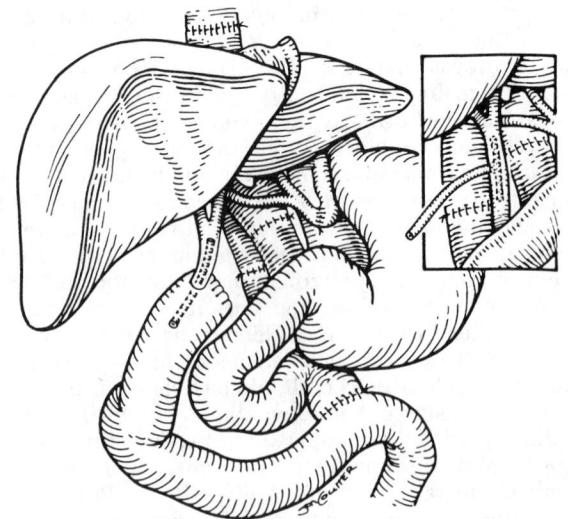

Figure 55-7. Biliary reconstruction following orthotopic liver transplantation. Biliary drainage can be accomplished *via* a Roux-en-Y (choledochojejunostomy) or "duct-to-duct" anastomosis (*insert*). (Reprinted with permission from Starzl TE, Demetris AJ, van Thiel DH: Liver transplantation. N Engl J Med 321:1014, 1092, 1989.)

Postoperative Management

In a well-functioning allograft, metabolic acids including lactate will continue to be metabolized and systemic alkalosis may result. Meticulous postoperative pulmonary toilet is vital and may be complicated by injury to the diaphragm, nosocomial pneumonia, adult respiratory distress syndrome from massive transfusion, and weakness from nutritional deficiencies. Primary nonfunction of the allograft is now a rare complication of liver transplantation, perhaps because of the widespread use of University of Wisconsin (UW) solution for preservation.[105] Recovery from primary nonfunction has occurred, but most often, retransplantation has been necessary.[106]

The full immunosuppression regimen of cyclosporine or FK506, azathioprine, and prednisone is begun in the early postoperative period, yet rejection episodes are still common and may be treated with the monoclonal antibody, OKT3. Other complications include biliary or vascular anastomotic leaks, abdominal abscesses, and thrombosis of the hepatic artery or portal vein. As in other patients on long-term immunosuppression with cyclosporine, recipients are also at risk for developing lymphoproliferative malignancies and opportunistic infections (see Evaluation of Patients With Prior Organ Transplant). Cases of transplantation for hepatitis B or neoplasms may also be complicated by recurrence of the original disease.[107]

HEART TRANSPLANTATION

It is estimated that as many as 14,000 patients per year in the United States alone could benefit from heart transplantation.[108] However, after rapid growth in the mid-1980s, the number of heart transplants per year has now reached a plateau of about 3,000 cases worldwide, due to the limited availability of donor organs. The orthotopic procedure has accounted for the overwhelming majority of cases.[109]

Growth in heart transplantation has been encouraged by dramatic increases in survival. Prior to the introduction of

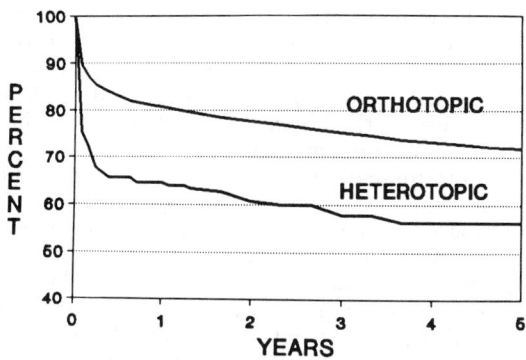

Figure 55-8. Actuarial survival for cardiac recipients according to the International Society for Heart Transplantation Registry. (Reprinted with permission from Kriett JM, Kaye MP: The Registry of the International Society for Heart Transplantation. Seventh Official Report—1990. J Heart Transplant 9:323, 1990.)

cyclosporine, 1-year survival was about 40%.[110] In the past decade, cyclosporine, coupled with intensive immunologic surveillance by endomyocardial biopsy and aggressive anti-rejection treatment with lymphocyte-specific monoclonal antibodies, has boosted overall survival of orthotopic recipients worldwide to more than 80% at 1 year, and more than 70% at 5 years (Fig. 55-8).[109] Individual centers have reported survival to be as high as 90% at 4 years.[111] Other outcome variables, such as patients' quality of life,[112] are quite favorable as well.

Pathophysiology of End-Stage Heart Disease

End-stage heart disease may result from either congenital or acquired diseases of the heart or vascular system. The leading causes include ischemic and valvular disease and primary cardiomyopathy. Depending on the cause, a varying period of physiologic adaptation precedes the onset of decompensation, which is usually manifested by congestive heart failure. Once this symptom is present, overall 5-year survival is less than 50%, although patients with rapidly progressive symptoms seem even less likely to survive.[113] Dysrhythmias and laboratory evidence of pump failure (e.g., low ejection fraction) are also associated with a relatively poorer prognosis.

As the left ventricle fails, the main compensatory mechanism is an increase in left ventricular end diastolic volume,[114] which enhances resting myocardial fiber length and promotes more effective fiber shortening. Such changes restore stroke volume, at the cost of increasing left atrial pressure and producing pulmonary venous congestion. Other compensations include elevation in catecholamine levels[115] and increased renin production resulting in salt and water retention.

Progression of the underlying pathophysiology eventually reduces ejection fraction, and results in severe congestive heart failure refractory to conventional drug therapy. At this point, some patients may still be ambulatory but have little functional reserve; others are not ambulatory due to dyspnea or dependence on intravenous inotropes, mechanical circulatory support, and/or mechanical ventilation. Protracted periods of low cardiac output compromise other vital organ functions (e.g., passive congestion of the liver and prerenal azotemia) and may culminate in inadequate perfusion to the heart itself, initiating a final, irreversible downward spiral. Patients may enter a transplant program during

any of these stages, or even after mechanical circulatory support with an intra-aortic balloon or ventricular assist device becomes necessary. Interestingly, survival rates remain relatively high in patients requiring mechanical circulatory support as a bridge to transplantation,[116] even those receiving a temporary artificial heart.[117]

Specific Indications and Contraindications

The indication for heart transplantation is fulfilled when New York Heart Association Class IV status (severely compromised) and prognosis (guarded despite therapy) persist despite maximal medical therapy. The typical candidate is a 40–60-year-old male with a pretransplant diagnosis of ischemic cardiomyopathy and left ventricular ejection fraction of less than 20%. The other common diagnoses are idiopathic cardiomyopathy and viral cardiomyopathy, while end-stage congenital heart disease accounts for the remainder. In the latter group, the congenital defect is often associated with a cardiomyopathy secondary to longstanding cyanosis and/or myocardial hypertrophy, making further palliation impossible.[118]

The list of contraindications has undergone considerable evolution in the last decade and will probably continue to do so. For example, the upper age limit was formerly 50 years. However, substantial numbers of older patients have now undergone this procedure without disproportionate morbidity and as a consequence, "physiologic" rather than chronologic age is now emphasized when deciding upon candidacy. Diabetes mellitus had also been an absolute contraindication; however, it now seems that even insulin-dependent diabetics can be successfully immunosuppressed without the aid of steroids, and short-term results are favorable.[119] A history of cancer was once an absolute contraindication as well, but strict exclusion on this basis became obsolete as true long-term cures for certain malignancies (e.g., Hodgkin's lymphoma) were demonstrated. The presence of certain systemic diseases may also contraindicate heart transplantation; for example, the cardiomyopathy accompanying sarcoidosis could respond to medical therapy, and amyloidosis might recur in the donor organ.

Severe, irreversible pulmonary hypertension remains one of the few absolute contraindications to orthotopic heart transplantation, since the right ventricle of a normal donor heart is unable to acutely cope with a markedly elevated, fixed pulmonary vascular resistance and rapidly decompensates.[120] The precise level of pulmonary hypertension deemed unacceptable is still a matter of debate: the traditional values are greater than 6–8 Wood units (6–8 mm Hg·[l·min]$^{-1}$, or in metric resistance units, 480–640 dynes·sec·cm^{-5}), or a transpulmonary gradient (mean pulmonary artery pressure − mean pulmonary capillary wedge pressure) of 10–15 mm Hg. If irreversible pulmonary hypertension is present, heterotopic heart transplantation is one option, although more recently, provided suitable organs are available, heart–lung transplantation would be preferred.

Preanesthetic Considerations

Given the candidacy criteria, the recipient's other vital organs are usually not seriously impaired. However, low cardiac output may lead to chronic passive liver congestion and oliguria, and there may be corresponding physical signs and abnormal laboratory values (Table 55-11).

TABLE 55-11. Pathophysiologic Consequences of Dilated Cardiomyopathy

Organ System	Consequence
Pulmonary	Pulmonary venous congestion Interstitial edema
Renal	Prerenal azotemia Oliguria
Hepatic	Chronic passive congestion Hepatomegaly Ascites
Central nervous	Confusion (low cardiac output)
Endocrine	Elevated serum catecholamines Elevated renin levels

Candidates for heart transplantation are usually maintained on oral or intravenous inotropes (e.g., digoxin, amrinone), vasodilators (captopril, amrinone), and diuretics, and when appropriate, antidysrhythmics. Patients with large, dilated hearts and low cardiac output are prone to form intracardiac thrombi and thus are anticoagulated with warfarin. In such cases, fresh frozen plasma is required following cardiopulmonary bypass, and appropriate arrangements should be made prior to induction. Blood products should be CMV-free for patients without antibody evidence of prior exposure, considering the likelihood and morbidity of CMV sepsis in immunosuppressed recipients.[121] Bacterial pneumonia is relatively common early after heart transplantation,[122] so preparation of the anesthesia machine with a fresh, sterile breathing circuit and bacterial filter seems prudent. It has not been found necessary to sterilize tracheal intubation equipment, although at most institutions, factory-sterilized disposable endotracheal tubes are standard.

Some transplant candidates have previously undergone coronary bypass or other thoracic or mediastinal procedures. If so, they are likely to require more than the usual time for insertion of vascular catheters and cannulation for cardiopulmonary bypass. To avoid unnecessary prolongation of donor organ ischemic times, the surgical and anesthesia teams must factor in these potential sources of delay.

Donor Procedure and Related Considerations

General principles of the donor operation were outlined earlier. It is worth emphasizing that cardiac harvesting is best done simultaneously with the harvesting of abdominal viscera. This approach, which involves local perfusion with preservative solutions after cross-clamping the abdominal and thoracic aortae, avoids inadvertent cardiac arrest before cardiectomy and damage to the allograft.

Donor cardiectomy begins with pericardiotomy; then the epicardial coronary arteries are grossly palpated for plaques. The aorta and both cavae are dissected, and after systemic heparinization, the superior vena cava is ligated and the inferior vena cava and a pulmonary vein is transected. The heart is then exsanguinated, and cardioplegia is administered via the aortic root. After cardiac arrest, the aorta is cross-clamped, the heart is topically cooled, and the remaining pulmonary veins are individually transected. Finally, the great arteries are divided, the heart is rinsed and examined for a patent foramen ovale or valvular lesions,

and then placed in a sterile plastic bag containing cold saline which, in turn, is placed inside an insulated cooler.[123] In laboratory studies, hearts have been preserved for as long as 24 hours with excellent subsequent graft function.[124] Presently, however, the generally accepted limit on human donor heart ischemic time (measured from the time the cross-clamp is applied, to the time of cross-clamp removal after implantation) is 4–6 hours.[125,126] In view of this limited duration, the only immunologic matching performed prospectively is ABO compatibility.

Cardiac trauma, cardiac arrest, hypoxemia, and excessive requirement for exogenous catecholamines may render a potential donor's heart unacceptable for transplantation. However, as long as there is echocardiographic evidence of good contractility, such criteria do not necessarily mandate exclusion.[127] In most transplant centers, there is no absolute age limit for eligibility as a heart donor, but in donors older than 40 years, careful physical examination at the time of harvest is essential to avoid transplanting organs with significant coronary lesions.

Anesthesia Induction

Candidates are often on the transplant list for extended periods and build up considerable apprehension. Despite this, preoperative sedation must be used judiciously, since residual cardiac performance depends on elevated endogenous catecholamines. The monitoring regimen employed by most heart transplant centers includes intra-arterial and pulmonary artery pressure monitoring. While avoidance of sepsis is important, conventional aseptic techniques have proven to be sufficient.[128] At the University of Pittsburgh, pulmonary artery catheterization is routinely performed via the right internal jugular vein, and does not seem to jeopardize access for future endomyocardial biopsies. Correct catheter positioning is often more difficult in this population, owing to severe orthopnea (necessitating a semi-sitting position), cardiac dilatation (promoting intraventricular coiling), tricuspid regurgitation, atrial fibrillation or other arrhythmias, or vascular congenital anomaly. Once placed, a long, sterile sheath is always used, since the pulmonary artery catheter is pulled back to "CVP position" prior to caval cannulation.

Whether hospital inpatients or newly admitted through the emergency room, most of these patients have recently eaten and thus require rapid inductions. There have been numerous descriptions of anesthetic techniques under these circumstances,[129-134] all based on agents compatible with the pathophysiology of end-stage heart disease. In one study of induction regimens, a combination of etomidate 0.3 mg·kg^{-1}, fentanyl 10 μg·kg^{-1}, and succinylcholine 1.5 mg·kg^{-1} iv was shown to rapidly produce adequate intubating conditions without significant cardiovascular depression.[135] Anesthesia can then be maintained using a regimen compatible with extremely poor ventricular function (e.g., O_2 – fentanyl 35–75 μg·kg^{-1} iv (total) + scopolamine 0.3 mg iv).

Following induction, tracheal intubation is accomplished without specially sterilized laryngoscopy equipment, and broad-spectrum prophylactic antibiotics and the immunosuppressant azathioprine are infused. Patients with end-stage heart disease are often exquisitely sensitive to changes in preload or afterload, thus hypotension may stem from relatively small degrees of hypovolemia or alterations in systemic vascular resistance. Since one or both ventricles are usually extremely noncompliant, filling pressures may not accurately reflect intracavitary volumes, so transesophageal echocardiography can be especially helpful in maintaining cardiovascular stability.

Surgery and Cardiopulmonary Bypass

In the prepump phase of the orthotopic procedure, manipulation of the heart is minimized to avoid dislodging any intracardiac thrombi. After individual cannulation of the cavae as well as the aorta, cardiopulmonary bypass is initiated and patients are cooled as for conventional cardiac procedures (26–28°C). During cooling, the diseased heart is excised, leaving an atrial cuff containing the caval and pulmonary venous orifices and long remnants of the aorta and pulmonary artery. The donor heart's back wall (atria) is trimmed appropriately and anastomosed with the recipient's atrial remnant. Special care must be taken to keep the anterior wall of the donor heart cold, even during posterior wall anastomoses, since warming may contribute to poor right ventricular function later. The heart is then filled with cold saline to displace most of the air, the aorta is anastomosed, and after de-airing once again, the crossclamp is removed (ending the ischemic time). Often, electromechanical activity resumes spontaneously, and finally, the pulmonary artery anastomosis is completed (Fig. 55-9).

For the heterotopic procedure (Fig. 55-10), after sternotomy, a right pleuropericardial flap is created. When cardiopulmonary bypass is initiated, the native heart undergoes cardioplegic arrest for myocardial protection, and the donor heart is placed in the right thorax anterior to the collapsed lung. The donor and recipient superior vena cavae and right atriae are incised and sutured together, and the donor's aorta is sutured end-to-side to the recipient's ascending aorta. The donor's pulmonary artery is then connected to the recipient's main pulmonary artery by means of a Dacron graft.

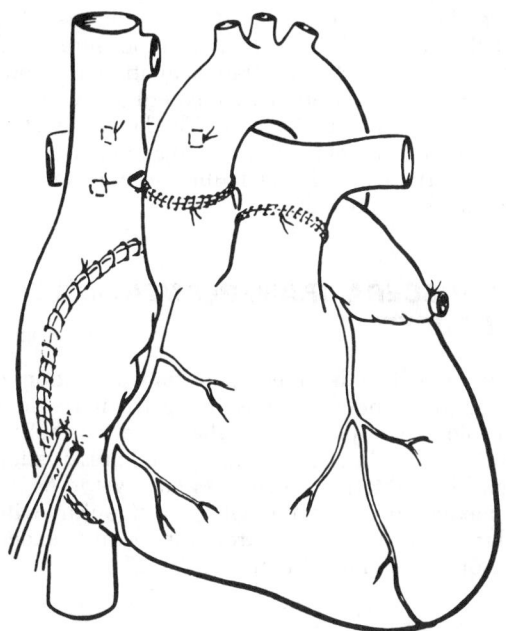

Figure 55-9. Sites of anastomoses following the midatrial excision orthotopic cardiac transplantation procedure. (Reprinted with permission from Reitz BA, Fowles RE, Ream AK: Cardiac transplantation. In Ream AK, Fogdall RP (eds): Acute Cardiovascular Management, pp 549–567. Philadelphia, JB Lippincott, 1982.)

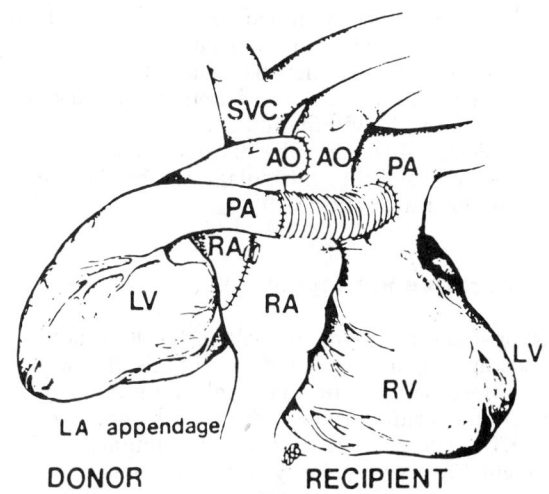

Figure 55-10. Heterotopic transplantation of a donor heart. Abbreviations are standard. (Reprinted with permission from Cooper DKC, Lanza LP: Heart Transplantation: The Present Status of Orthotopic and Heterotopic Heart Transplantation. MTP Press, Lancaster, England, 1984.)

Since many patients with end-stage heart disease are maintained on diuretics, mannitol or furosemide may be necessary to maintain a urine flow. In some cases, these patients may have markedly expanded blood volumes and benefit from hemoconcentration on bypass. At many centers, just prior to release of the aortic crossclamp, to modulate the possibility of "hyperacute" immune response, methylprednisolone 500 mg iv is administered. Immediately after release of the aortic crossclamp, slow junctional rhythms or AV nodal dysfunction are relatively common. An infusion of either isoproterenol or another catecholamine with positive chronotropic effects is often begun to temporarily support heart rate. Most of these dysrhythmias resolve, but a small percentage do persist postoperatively, even in the absence of rejection. Ultimately, some 5% of recipients require implantation of a permanent pacemaker, although the balance of survivors do not seem particularly prone to other serious dysrhythmias.

Immediately prior to weaning from cardiopulmonary bypass, the posterior anastomosis is rechecked because leaks in this area are difficult to repair later on. After final de-airing, the superior vena caval cannula is removed, the pulmonary artery catheter advanced and repositioned, and the serum ionized calcium restored to normal. If heart rate is less than 60–70 beats per minute (bpm), epicardial electrodes are placed and pacing is begun.

Cardiac performance is often mildly compromised immediately following heart transplantation, and many transplant centers routinely use inotropic infusions to wean from cardiopulmonary bypass. Although there have been reports of exaggerated effects,[136] in practice, responses to catecholamine infusions seem qualitatively similar to those in other cardiac surgical patients. Further discussion of the physiology and pharmacology of cardiac denervation is found in the section on Evaluation of the Patient With Prior Organ Transplant.

Markedly elevated pulmonary vascular resistance is a contraindication to orthotopic transplantation. But transient pulmonary vasospasm can occur during weaning, even in patients with previously normal pulmonary artery pressures, producing life-threatening right heart failure. Prostaglandin E_1 (PGE_1), at infusion rates of between 0.025–0.2

$\mu g \cdot kg^{-1} \cdot min^{-1}$, has been shown to effectively unload the right heart[137] although simultaneous norepinephrine or phenylephrine infusion may be required to support systemic vascular resistance. Elevated pulmonary vascular resistances often fall within hours of the procedure,[138,139] allowing PGE_1 infusions to be discontinued, but as a last resort, mechanical right ventricular assist has been used for varying periods with success.[140]

Postoperative Management

The short-term management goals in the ICU include cardiovascular support and prevention of rejection and infection.[122] Most patients receive triple immunosuppression (cyclosporine-azathioprine-prednisone)[109] and, at some centers, OKT3. The sources of fever or pulmonary infiltrates are sought aggressively. Early in the postoperative period, bacterial pneumonias with typical nosocomial organisms are encountered. Later, opportunistic infection with CMV, Pneumocystis, or Legionella[141] may occur, and transbronchoscopic brushing may be necessary to establish the etiology. There may be bradydysrhythmias and/or AV block in this period, and temporary pacing may be required. Persistently low cardiac output may result from rejection or from reperfusion injury, and endomyocardial biopsy may be the only means to establish the diagnosis.

Excessive mediastinal bleeding and coagulopathy may be encountered in patients who had previously undergone a cardiac surgical procedure(s), and are treated in the conventional fashion. If hemodynamic stability is maintained, evidence of mild organ compromise present before transplantation, will gradually disappear. If, however, the transplanted heart functions poorly, organs with preoperative impairment may rapidly decompensate.

Heart–Lung Transplantation

Heart–lung transplantation is the procedure of choice for patients with end-stage lung disease complicated by right ventricular failure, or end-stage congenital heart disease with secondary pulmonary vascular involvement (Eisenmenger's syndrome). Specific pathologic diagnoses in recipients have included primary pulmonary hypertension, emphysema, multiple pulmonary emboli, cystic fibrosis, and granulomatous and fibrotic diseases of the lung. Suitable donor blocs are in extremely short supply, since both the lungs and heart must fulfill the criteria for acceptability (see the section on Other Viscera Transplantation Procedures, below). Such blocs consist of the entire heart and lungs, including a tracheal segment long enough to facilitate anastomosis. Distal procurement is made feasible by flushing the harvested bloc with modified Euro-Collins or UW solution, to which PGE_1 or other pulmonary vasodilators may be added.

Considerations for monitoring and induction of anesthesia are generally similar to those for heart transplantation, but air trapping and pulmonary hypertension are additional factors that may lead to hemodynamic instability. Difficulty with the airway during induction can result in hypercarbia or hypoxia and elevate pulmonary vascular resistance. Patients with congenital heart disease may have bidirectional intracardiac shunts, which can become predominantly right-to-left and lead to profound hypoxemia. Such shunts may also lead to paradoxical air emboli, so bubbles in intravenous tubing should be scrupulously avoided. Chronically cyanotic patients are frequently severely polycythemic (hematocrit >60%) and manifest clotting derangements. Under these circumstances, phlebotomy and hemodilution are beneficial. In all recipients, large-sized endotracheal tubes are preferred to facilitate therapeutic bronchoscopies.

In the prebypass phase, surgical dissections may be complicated by extensive pleural adhesions: however, once on bypass, en bloc implantation is relatively straightforward and accomplished by sequential tracheal, right atrial, and aortic anastomoses. Note that the phrenic, vagus, and recurrent laryngeal nerves may be damaged by both dissection and topical cooling, and that the tracheal anastomosis generally involves some technique to prevent dehiscence, for example, wrapping the suture line with vascularized omentum. Re-expansion of transplanted lungs may require bronchoscopy to relieve mechanical obstruction by secretions, and occasionally, bronchodilators will be useful to treat bronchospasm.[142] Due to the extensive mediastinal and pleural dissection, the early postbypass period may be complicated by hemorrhage leading to coagulopathy. Pulmonary compliance and gas exchange may deteriorate during this same period, due to pulmonary hemorrhage or to inadequate preservation, and the use of PEEP is often required.

Postoperatively, rejection episodes are relatively common and are characterized by infiltrates, fever, and deteriorating gas exchange. Pulmonary allografts may be rejected without significant abnormalities in endomyocardial specimens,[143] so low cardiac output is not necessarily a symptom of rejection. Recipients are also highly susceptible to bacterial pneumonia, which presents with the same clinical picture as rejection, bronchoalveolar lavage or transbronchial biopsy may be necessary for definitive diagnosis. A dreaded problem soon after heart–lung transplantation is dehiscence of the tracheal suture line, which can lead to fatal mediastinitis. Later on, a significant proportion of survivors develop bronchiolitis obliterans. The etiology is as yet unknown, but this condition is associated with a progressive decline in exercise tolerance. Bronchiolitis obliterans and the physiology of transplanted lungs are discussed further in the Other Viscera Transplantation Procedures section.

In the future, heart–lung transplantation will probably have even fewer indications, as experience with isolated lung transplantation accumulates. The latter operation will then be used in patients with end-stage lung disease, *before* the onset of right ventricular failure necessitates the combined heart–lung procedure.

OTHER VISCERA TRANSPLANTATION PROCEDURES

There is considerable interest in transplantation of the lungs, pancreas, and small intestine, particularly in view of the sizeable patient populations that stand to benefit. These are relatively fragile viscera, and optimal preservation regimens and implantation procedures have yet to be defined. Clinical experience is accumulating most rapidly with lung transplantation, as it evolves from the realm of experiment to a reasonable therapeutic option.[144]

Lung Transplantation

End-stage lung disease from destruction of the pulmonary parenchyma or vasculature is a leading cause of disablement and death among adults. Several lung transplanta-

TABLE 55-12. Pathologic Diagnoses in Lung Transplant Recipients*

Diagnosis	Number
Chronic obstructive pulmonary disease	20
Alpha$_1$ antitrypsin deficiency	19
Cystic fibrosis	8
Pulmonary hypertension	8
Pulmonary fibrosis	7
Bronchiectasis	2
Eosinophilic granuloma	1
Lymphangiomyomatosis	1

*Data derived from 66 consecutive patients who underwent lung transplantation at Barnes Hospital, St Louis, between July 1988 and January 1991.

Adapted with permission from Trulock EP, Cooper JD, Kaiser LR et al: The Washington University–Barnes Hospital experience with lung transplantation. JAMA 266:1943, 1991.

tion operations have been developed to treat end-stage lung disease, each having certain conceptual and practical advantages. These include the heart–lung, en bloc double-lung, single-lung, and bilateral sequential single-lung procedures. In the setting of chronically elevated pulmonary vascular resistance with right ventricular failure, heart–lung transplantation is generally chosen. However, when cardiac performance is preserved, isolated lung transplantation has been shown to be of benefit to carefully selected patients with end-stage lung disease (Table 55-12).[145]

End-stage pulmonary parenchymal diseases are either restrictive, obstructive, or infectious in nature. Briefly, *restrictive* lung *diseases* are characterized by interstitial fibrosis with a loss of lung elasticity and compliance. Most fibrotic diseases are idiopathic in nature, but they may also be caused by an inhalation injury or immune process. Interstitial lung disease may affect the blood vessels as well, so pulmonary hypertension is often found. Functionally, diseases in this category are associated with diminished lung volumes and diffusion capacity, but preserved air-flow rates. Respiratory muscle strength is usually excellent because the work of breathing is chronically elevated. The most common cause of end-stage *obstructive lung disease* is smoking-induced emphysema, but other causes include asthma and several comparatively rare congenital disorders. Among these, alpha$_1$ antitrypsin deficiency is associated with severe bullous emphysema in the fourth or fifth decade of life. With obstructive diseases, airway resistance is elevated, expiratory flow rates are diminished, air trapping may be prominent, and ventilation–perfusion mismatching severe. The common *infectious* etiologies of end-stage lung disease include cystic fibrosis and bronchiectasis. Cystic fibrosis, which occurs in 1 of every 2,000 live births in the United States, produces mucous plugging of peripheral airways, chronic bronchitis, and bronchiectasis. Smoking and environmental exposures may also lead to bronchiectasis. End-stage *pulmonary vascular disease* may be a consequence of primary pulmonary hypertension, which is a relatively rare disease of unknown etiology characterized by marked elevation of pulmonary vascular resistance from hyperplasia of the muscular pulmonary arteries and fibrosis of smaller arterioles. Congenital heart disease with Eisenmenger's syndrome, and diffuse arteriovenous malformations, are other causes of destruction of the pulmonary arterial bed.

The general indications for transplantation with any of the end-stage lung diseases are progressive exercise intolerance, increasing oxygen requirements, and carbon dioxide retention. Other factors favoring the transplantation option are recurrent need for phlebotomy and increasing physical and social debilitation. The timing of surgery depends on the rate of functional deterioration and ability of the right ventricle to tolerate the progression of pulmonary hypertension. Considering the limited supply of donor organs, specific contraindications to lung transplantation include severe debilitation, neuromuscular disease or mechanical ventilator-dependence (since respiratory muscle strength is crucial to recovery); severe chest deformity or pleural disease (complicating surgical procedures and postoperative ventilation); advanced right ventricular failure; or, glucocorticoid dependence (because healing of airway anastomoses is impeded by steroids).

The choice of lung transplantation procedure is based largely on the consequences of leaving the native lung *in situ*. For example, single-lung transplantation is not an option if infection or severe bullous emphysema are present in the contralateral lung. Infection would cross-contaminate the healthy transplanted lung, and severe bullous disease in the native lung could lead to gross ventilation–perfusion mismatching and shifting of the mediastinum. Instead, double-lung transplantation would be chosen for such cases. Similarly, double-lung transplantation may also lead to better functional outcomes in the treatment of end-stage pulmonary hypertension.[145,146] The other major factor influencing the choice of procedure is the relative rate of perioperative complications. For example, single-lung transplantation is feasible without cardiopulmonary bypass and is seldom complicated by bleeding diatheses. In contrast, en bloc double-lung transplantation mandates cardiopulmonary bypass with full systemic heparinization and extensive mediastinal dissection—both risk factors for developing coagulation defects postoperatively. Another advantage of single-lung transplantation is that it makes use of bronchial anastomoses, which heal with significantly fewer complications than the tracheal repairs integral to the en bloc double-lung procedure. Bilateral sequential lung transplantation, a recently introduced alternative to en bloc double-lung transplantation, combines advantages by employing bibronchial anastomoses and avoiding cardiopulmonary bypass.

Donor Lungs

Donor lungs may be jeopardized by massive fluid resuscitation, aspiration, contusion, and exposure to nonphysiologic oxygen tensions, because most organ donors are trauma victims. Ideally, the donor's history should indicate early endotracheal intubation with no evidence of aspiration, minimal fluid administration in the course of resuscitation, and absence of chest tubes, pleural diseases, or tracheostomy at any time. Suitable donors should have a minimal alveolar–arterial O_2 gradient (i.e., a Pao$_2$ of >400 mm Hg while breathing 100% O_2, or 100 mm Hg on 40% O_2/5 cm H_2O PEEP), as well as a clear chest x-ray and sputum examination within 2 hours of harvesting.[147] If bronchoscopy fails to elucidate any pathology, iv glucocorticoids and antibiotics are administered and the lungs harvested. Because both the heart and lungs may be harvested from the same donor, a method has been developed for cardiectomy without jeopardizing the use of the lungs.[148] First, the heart is removed but a cuff of left atrium is left attached to the donor lungs. The trachea is then stapled and divided at its midpoint, and the lungs removed en bloc and immersed in cold preservation solution. In some centers, prior to removal, the donor is treated with a pulmonary vasodilator (e.g., PGE₁) to improve the distribution of a large volume of either a blood-based or intracellular-type cold-crystalloid preservative solution, infused *via* the pulmonary artery. Finally, the lungs may be inflated before immersion in preservation solution and stored for transportation.

Preanesthetic Considerations

Preanesthetic considerations for lung recipients have been described.[149-152] Briefly, size matching is achieved by comparing the vertical and transverse radiologic chest dimensions of the donor and recipient. Organs are also matched on the basis of ABO compatibility, but because the need for histocompatibility is still unknown and the tolerable ischemic time for the lung is relatively short (approximately 4 hours), HLA matching is only done in retrospect. Preoperative pulmonary function and right heart catheterization studies, ventilation–perfusion scans, and arterial blood gas values are helpful to predict the difficulties likely to be encountered during and after induction. For example, diminished expiratory flow rates and air trapping may exacerbate hypoxemia and hypercapnia and lead to hemodynamic instability during mask ventilation and after tracheal intubation. Elevated pulmonary artery pressures may indicate a likelihood that cardiopulmonary bypass will be necessary, because right ventricular failure can suddenly result when one-lung ventilation or ligation of a pulmonary artery is begun. Even in the absence of pulmonary hypertension, many centers recommend "pump standby" for these cases, because gas exchange is so precarious. Clearly, both systemic and pulmonary arterial pressure monitoring are vital during lung transplantation procedures, although profound dyspnea may make internal jugular cannulation difficult prior to induction. Pulmonary artery catheters should be inserted through a sterile sleeve to allow withdrawal during the anastomosis and subsequent repositioning. Finally, candidates may have recently undergone weaning from glucocorticoids, but "stress doses" are avoided in the perioperative period to protect from systemic sepsis or suture line dehiscence.

Single-Lung Transplantation

The single-lung transplantation procedure involves pneumonectomy and implantation of a new lung, frequently preceded by mobilization of omentum with its vascular pedicle for bronchial wrapping. If the native lungs are equally impaired and no pleural scarring is present, the left lung is often chosen for transplantation for technical reasons; the native right pulmonary veins are less accessible than those on the left, the recipient's left bronchus is longer, and the left hemithorax can more easily accommodate a somewhat oversized donor lung. Most surgeons prefer that the lung to be removed is collapsed during dissection; both bronchial blockers and double-lumen endobronchial tubes have been used for this purpose. Because the right upper lobe bronchial orifice is relatively close to the origin of the mainstem bronchus, left-sided endobronchial double-lumen tubes have been recommended for both right and left single-lung transplants as well as for the bilateral sequential operation.

For the induction of anesthesia by the rapid sequence technique, drugs that do not release histamine or depress the myocardium are generally preferred (e.g., etomidate, vecuronium). Nitrous oxide is avoided in patients with bullae or elevated pulmonary vascular resistance and when 100% oxygen is needed to maintain acceptable arterial satu-

ration. Both high-dose opioids and potent inhaled agents, supplemented with long-acting relaxants, have been used successfully for the maintenance of anesthesia. With the onset of one-lung ventilation, acute deterioration in gas exchange and/or hemodynamics is the rule. Strategies for improving oxygenation under these circumstances are discussed in detail in Chapter 34, but briefly, include the use of PEEP in the dependent lung, CPAP or high-frequency ventilation in the nondependent lung, or ligation of the (nondependent) pulmonary artery. If pulmonary artery pressures rise sharply at this point, right ventricular failure may ensue. Vasodilators and/or inotropes may diminish right heart strain; if not, one-lung ventilation should be abandoned. Similarly, if hemodynamics or systemic arterial saturations deteriorate when the pulmonary artery is clamped in anticipation of pneumonectomy, cardiopulmonary bypass may be necessary.

Immediately before implantation, the donor lung is trimmed to match the size of the recipient bronchus, branch pulmonary artery, and atrial cuff containing the orifices of the pulmonary veins. While attempting to keep the allograft cold, the atrial, pulmonary artery, and bronchial anastomoses are completed in sequence. The circulation is then restored to the donor lung, ending the ischemic interval, but until ventilation to the allograft is restarted, systemic arterial saturation will suffer. Flexible bronchoscopy may be required at this stage to reinflate the allograft by removing secretions or blood from the airway. Once the anastomosis is secure, a pedicle of omentum with its blood supply intact may be brought into the chest and wrapped around the bronchial anastomosis. This practice is based on work in experimental animals, where omental collaterals can improve anastomotic healing after transplantation.[153,154] Finally, after the chest is closed, the supine position can be restored and the endobronchial tube exchanged for a standard endotracheal type (except if "split" ventilation is planned, as discussed below).

Double-Lung Transplantation

Double-lung transplantation is most often used in patients with primary pulmonary hypertension or cystic fibrosis. The en bloc operation is performed in the supine position, and because both lungs are replaced at once, cardiopulmonary bypass is mandatory. Cardioplegic arrest is used to accomplish anastomosis of the left atrial cuff containing all four pulmonary venous orifices. The airway is interrupted at the level of the trachea, so a standard endotracheal tube is suitable. Since systemic arterial supply to the trachea is permanently interrupted, an omental wrap is added. The extensive retrocardiac dissection required often leads to cardiac denervation, and postoperative bleeding that is difficult to control.[155]

Bilateral sequential single-lung transplantation was introduced to treat the same spectrum of patients as the en bloc procedure, but obviates the need for cardiopulmonary bypass and tracheal anastomosis. Access to the hilar structures is gained in the supine position *via* a rather extensive incision that includes a transverse sternotomy ("clamshell" incision, Fig. 55-11). Another relative disadvantage is that serial implantation results in a longer ischemic time for the second allograft.

Postoperative Management

Postoperative management of patients after isolated lung transplant involves intensive respiratory support and differentiating between lung infection and rejection using trans-

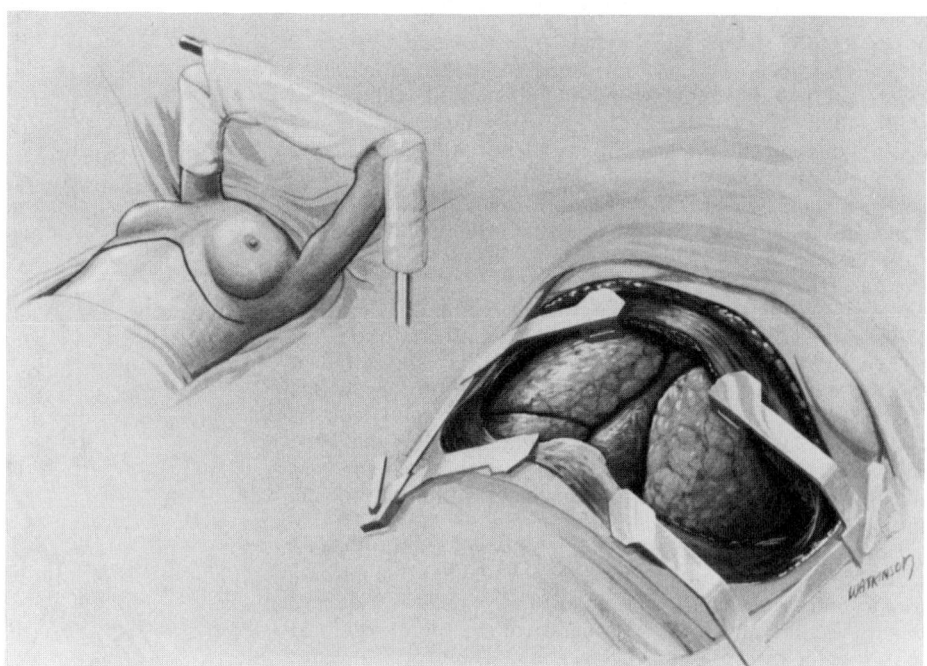

Figure 55-11. Positioning and surgical approach for bilateral sequential lung transplantation. The incision consists of bilateral anterior thoracotomies with a transverse sternotomy. Following insertion of vascular catheters, the patient's arms are wrapped and suspended from the ether screen. (Reprinted with permission from Cooper JD, Patterson GA: Isolated lung transplantation. In Kapoor AS, Laks H, Schroeder JS *et al* (eds): Cardiomyopathies and Heart–Lung Transplantation, pp 429–440. New York, McGraw-Hill, 1991.)

bronchial biopsies obtained by flexible bronchoscopy.[156] Early respiratory insufficiency may be due to preservation or reperfusion injury, and characterized by large alveolar–arterial oxygen gradients, poor pulmonary compliance, and parenchymal infiltrates in spite of low cardiac filling pressures. Mechanical ventilation with PEEP is essential, but in consideration of new airway anastomoses, inflation pressures are kept to a minimum. FiO$_2$s are also maintained at the lowest levels compatible with acceptable oxygen saturation. After single-lung transplantation for an obstructive disease, the endobronchial tube may be left in place for several days, and special respiratory support in the form of "split" (individual lung) ventilation used to avoid overinflation of the native lung, gross ventilation–perfusion mismatching, and shifting of the mediastinum.[157]

The lung is unique among transplanted viscera because it is exposed to the external environment. Lymphatic disruption, poor mucociliary function, and the presence of suture lines across the airway are other factors increasing the susceptibility of transplanted lungs to infection. In the first postoperative month, bacteria are the most frequent cause of pneumonia; nosocomial gram-negative organisms comprise the bulk of isolates.[158] After this period, CMV pneumonitis becomes more common, particularly if lungs from a CMV seropositive donor are used in a seronegative recipient.[147] There is a high rate of acute rejection episodes after lung transplantation, which on clinical grounds alone are often difficult to distinguish from infection. This distinction is vital, however, since steroid boluses used to treat rejection may worsen pneumonia or promote systemic sepsis. Bronchoalveolar lavage fluid or sputum specimens obtained by fiberoptic bronchoscopy may be helpful in diagnosing an infectious etiology; transbronchial or, occasionally, open-lung biopsy is needed to establish the diagnosis of rejection.[156]

Hemorrhage is a complication that most frequently occurs after en bloc double-lung transplantation, particularly in patients with pleural disease or Eisenmenger's syndrome with extensive mediastinal vascular collaterals. The recurrent laryngeal, phrenic, and vagal nerves are jeopardized during

lung transplantation, and injury will complicate the process of weaning from mechanical ventilation. Primary healing occurs with most bronchial anastomoses; rarely, bronchial fistulae lead to stenoses that can be successfully treated by silicone stents and dilatation. In contrast, tracheal anastomotic leaks often lead to fatal mediastinitis. Long-term complications include lung infections with opportunistic organisms such as *Pneumocystis* carinii and *Candida* albicans. Bronchiolitis obliterans, a pathologic condition characterized by lumenal destruction of small respiratory bronchioles, has been noted after heart–lung transplantation,[159] but so far seems less common after single-lung transplantation.

Outcome studies of lung transplantation series are beginning to reach publication, and results from specialized centers are promising. The Washington University Lung Transplantation Group has reported[145] on a series of 69 procedures and found the actuarial survival after single-lung transplantation to be 90% at 1 year, and 82% after the bilateral sequential operation. Pulmonary function tests, pulmonary arterial pressure and resistance, arterial blood gases, and exercise capacities all improved significantly following operation. In an earlier analogous series from Toronto, there were no ventilatory limitations noted in lung transplant survivors nor significant desaturation during exercise testing.[146]

Pancreas Transplantation

There are as many as 20,000 new cases of Type I (juvenile onset, insulin-dependent) diabetes mellitus in the United States each year.[160] This disease destroys the insulin-producing pancreatic beta cells by an inflammatory process. The microangiopathy that results from diabetes is among the leading causes of blindness and renal failure.

Pancreatic transplantation by surgical means was first attempted in the mid-1960s, and by 1989 the annual rate of such cases reported to the International Pancreas Transplantation Registry was 554.[161] At specialized centers, the operative mortality was low (1% or less), 1-year survival was at least 90%, and normoglycemia and insulin-independence was achieved in 50–70% of cases at 1 year.[162] In many of these cases, patients received both kidney and pancreas allografts, which seemed to prevent the recurrence of diabetic nephropathy in the transplanted kidney[163] as well as some of the other microvascular complications.

Pancreatic transplantation is usually reserved for diabetics with the severest, most rapidly progressive complications, in view of the considerable side effects of immunosuppression. Preoperative screening consists of thorough evaluation of the organ systems most affected by diabetes; metabolic studies, including a glucose tolerance test; and urine and serum C-peptide levels ("connecting peptide" is cleaved from pro-insulin before secretion into the circulation); glycosylated hemoglobin levels (an index of glycemic control during preceding months); and insulin and islet cell antibodies. Ultrasound of the gallbladder is conducted to rule out cholelithiasis. In addition to tight preoperative plasma glucose control, mechanical and antibiotic bowel preparation is usually undertaken.

Currently, most pancreatic transplants are accomplished using the bladder drainage technique.[164] This involves extraperitoneal pancreatic placement and exocrine drainage *via* duodenocystostomy. Postoperatively, patients seldom require intensive care, although assiduous control of plasma glucose using an insulin infusion is recommended. Once oral feeding is resumed, insulin is unnecessary unless allograft function is lost. A major advantage of the bladder drainage technique is the ability to monitor allograft exocrine function, which deteriorates during episodes of rejection. Urinary pH may fall, reflecting a decrease in pancreatic bicarbonate secretion, and urinary amylase may diminish. Other postoperative complications include graft thrombosis and intra-abdominal infection.

Pancreatic islet transplantation, in which only the required cell type is introduced, has recently undergone clinical trials.[165] In this procedure, which does not require surgical intervention, just the islets are isolated by cell-separation techniques then infused into the portal vein. In some cases, islet cells may become fully functional over several weeks and restore insulin-independence;[165] in others, insulin requirement has been reduced but not eliminated.

Multiviscera Transplantation

Simultaneous replacement of multiple digestive organs, known as the "cluster operation," has been introduced to treat two diseases: short-gut syndrome and locally confined GI tumors.[166] With short-gut syndrome from any cause, parenteral feeding may lead to liver failure, and en bloc transplantation of the liver combined with the pancreas, stomach, duodenum and jejunum (Fig. 55-12) has met with some success.[167] In children, multiviscera transplantation is performed primarily for short-gut syndrome resulting from necrotizing enterocolitis or midgut volvulus.

Tumors such as hepatomas and cholangiocarcinomas, as well as carcinomas of the proximal GI tract or pancreas, have also been treated by cluster operation after upper abdominal exenteration. Without surgery, the prognosis for these cancers is uniformly dismal, and even partial resections combined with chemotherapy or radiation offers little improvement in overall survival. In contrast, although experience is still limited, multiviscera transplantation is associated with 1-year survivals of 70% (with sarcomas or GI-derived neuroendocrine tumors) or 44% (primary liver cancers).[168]

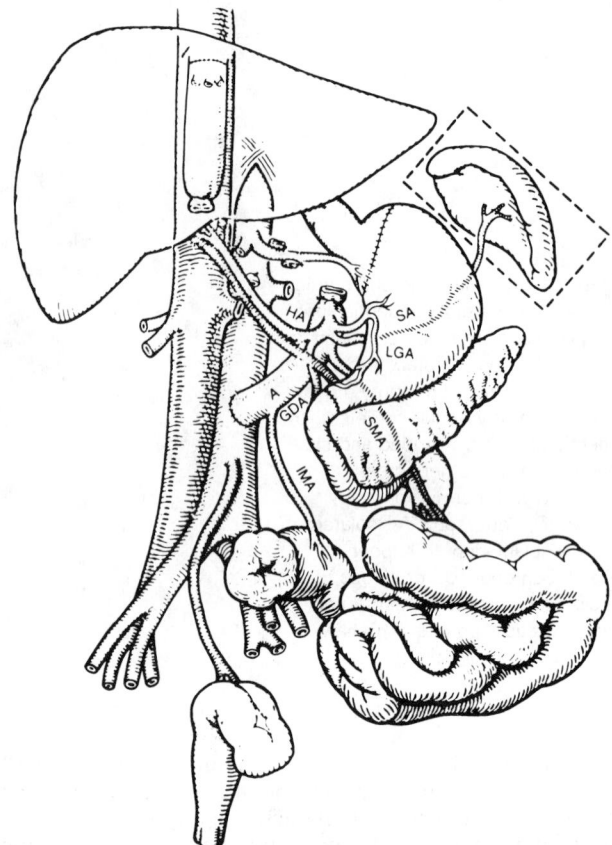

Figure 55-12. Schematic representation of the recipient procedure for multiviscera transplantation. (A = donor aorta, HA = hepatic artery, SA = splenic artery, LGA = left gastric artery, SMA = superior mesenteric artery, IMA = inferior mesenteric artery, GDA = gastroduodenal artery.) (Reprinted with permission from Starzl TE, Rowe MI, Todo S *et al:* Transplantation of multiple abdominal viscera. JAMA 261:1449, 1989.)

Anesthetic management of cluster surgery has recently been reviewed in detail.[169] Briefly, the types and doses of previous chemotherapy should be ascertained during the preoperative visit, since some agents have long-lasting toxic effects on the heart or kidneys. Hormone-secreting tumors, producing "carcinoid crisis," can be suppressed with octreotide acetate, a somatostatin analogue; ketanserin, a serotonin antagonist; or by arterial embolization. During surgery, the management issues are similar to those for liver transplantation alone, namely massive transfusion, coagulopathies, hypothermia, electrolyte abnormalities, and the use of venovenous bypass for systemic venous return. Postoperative complications include a high incidence of rejection, particularly of the small bowel, sepsis from loss of the intestinal barrier, and graft-versus-host disease (GVHD). The likelihood of GVHD is proportional to the length of intestine transplanted, presumably reflecting the quantity of lymphoid tissue contained in the wall of this organ.[170]

VISCERA TRANSPLANTATION IN CHILDREN

The clinical manifestations of end-stage organ disease in children are generally similar to those found in adults; however, the pathologic processes leading to organ failure often differ. For example, the etiologies of end-stage renal disease noted in the pediatric population (Table 55-13) differ mark-

TABLE 55-13. Etiology of End-Stage Renal Disease in Children

	Total Cases (%)
Urinary tract malformations	29
Chronic glomerulonephritis	24
Renal dysplasia/hypoplasia	23
Hereditary nephropathies	14
Miscellaneous	10

Adapted with permission from Turcotte JG, Campbell DA, Dafoe DC et al: Pediatric renal transplantation, pp 349–360. In Cerilli GJ (ed): Organ Transplantation and Replacement. Philadelphia, JB Lippincott, 1988.

edly from those for the general population (Table 55-6). During childhood, developmental anomalies and genetic defects, both anatomic or functional (*i.e.*, inborn errors of metabolism), may lead to end-stage organ disease. Congenital anomalies may be confined to a single organ system (e.g., reflux nephropathy) or be part of a constellation of abnormalities. For example, in Alagille's syndrome, end-stage liver disease is accompanied by congenital heart disease, hypercholesterolemia, and renal dysfunction. Clearly, awareness of such syndromes is necessary to anticipate coexistent pathology in other organ systems.

Ethical Considerations

The ethics of transplantation are also somewhat different in the pediatric age group. For example, the legally adopted criteria for brain death are not deemed applicable in the immediate neonatal period,[171,172] so organ donation from this population is controversial. Size considerations place additional constraints on the organ-matching process in children, exacerbating the shortages. To remedy this, living-related donor operations have been developed and applied to kidney transplantation, and more recently, liver[173,174] and lung[175] transplantation. Although living-related renal transplantation has gained acceptance because of its particular benefits for children (*vide supra*), the liver and lung procedures are more controversial owing to higher morbidity and mortality in the donors. Other ethical dilemmas, such as whether transplanted organs grow and develop normally in children, remain unresolved. In addition, long-term immunosuppression with cyclosporine increases the risk of developing a lymphoproliferative malignancy, perhaps related to Epstein-Barr virus infection or reactivation.[176] While the overall incidence is reasonably low, the shift to earlier presentation of aggressive malignancies raises new concerns.[177]

Renal Transplantation

Although pharmacologic agents combined with dialysis can be used to treat end-stage renal disease in children, medical management has an overall high morbidity and adversely affects growth and development.[178,179] Children treated medically during their maximum growth years show a marked decrease in eventual height and weight,[180] as well as retarded cognitive development,[181] when compared with controls. Early transplantation seems to prevent these problems,[182,183] justifying the current recommendation to "ex-

pectantly" transplant children with progressive renal insufficiency, sometimes even before dialysis is required.[184]

The most common diseases leading to renal transplantation in children are related to congenital anomalies; acquired nephropathies and a group of miscellaneous diseases account for the remainder (Table 55-14). Living-related renal transplantation is most often done in children and confers significant advantages: both short- and long-term mortality is improved, and graft survival is superior[184,185] perhaps because the risk of minor antigenic mismatch is reduced. Organ survival in children receiving a living-related kidney approaches 100% at 1 year and 70% at 10 years.[184,185] Because perioperative mortality and renal rejection is greater in infants,[186] current practice is to avoid transplantation until early childhood.

In contrast to adults, pediatric renal transplantation relies on intra-abdominal placement of the organ (Fig. 55-4). This allows adult-sized kidneys to be transplanted into very small children and increases the size of the donor pool. But intraoperatively, placement of the allograft can acutely cause hypothermia and sequester relatively large proportions of the child's blood volume. As a consequence, hypotension can occur at the very time when adequate perfusion is critical. To prevent this, fluid boluses and vasoactive infusions are used to maintain systemic blood pressure in the high-normal range. As in adults, living-related donor kidneys usually function at once, while cadaver kidneys may take hours to resume urine production. Fluid management must take this into account. In either case, adult kidneys will initially produce adult-sized volumes of urine, so maintenance fluids must be adjusted accordingly.

Liver Transplantation

Some 20% of the orthotopic liver transplants performed worldwide are in children and the majority of recipients are under 5 years of age.[187] Biliary atresia is by far the most common cause of liver failure in this population (Table 55-15), followed by inborn errors of metabolism, which include disorders such as alpha$_1$ antitrypsin deficiency, glycogen storage diseases, Wilson's disease, and tyrosinemia. The latter three conditions primarily involve biochemical de-

TABLE 55-14. Pathologic Diagnoses in Pediatric Renal Transplant Recipients at the University of Minnesota*

	Total Cases (%)
Obstructive uropathy	16.8
Renal hypoplasia	15.3
Glomerulonephritis	15.3
Congenital nephrotic syndrome	8.5
Steroid-resistant nephrotic syndrome	7.2
Medullary cystic disease	4.5
Pyelonephritis	4.1
Hemolytic uremic syndrome	4.0
Alport's syndrome	2.6
Oxalosis	2.3
Miscellaneous, including unknown	19.4

*Data are derived from a total of 531 cases performed between 1963 and 1990.

Adapted with permission from Belani K, Palahniuk R: Kidney transplantation. In Firestone L (ed): Anesthesia and Organ Transplantation, pp 17–39. Boston, Little, Brown and Co, 1991.

TABLE 55-15. Pathologic Diagnoses in Pediatric Orthotopic Liver Transplant Recipients*

	Total Cases (%)
Biliary atresia	44
Alpha$_1$ antitrypsin deficiency	20
Other inborn errors of metabolism	10
Other obstructive diseases (e.g., Allagille's and Byler's syndromes)	12
Miscellaneous	14

*Data derived from 50 pediatric orthotopic liver transplant patients at Children's Hospital of Pittsburgh between 1981 and 1983.

Adapted with permission from Borland LM, Roule M, Cook DR: Anesthesia for pediatric orthotopic liver transplantation. Anesth Analg 64:117, 1985.

fects in hepatocytes and are therefore considered cured by liver transplantation.

Several aspects of the orthotopic liver transplant procedure are unique to children. For example, patients with biliary atresia have usually undergone prior decompression with a Kasai (choledochojejunostomy) procedure, and this may complicate abdominal dissection during the preanhepatic phase of liver transplantation, as well as later biliary reconstruction. Venovenous bypass is not feasible in patients under 20 kg, so the lower body venous congestion that accompanies portal and IVC occlusion often leads to oliguria and intestinal complications in this group. An oversized allograft may sequester a substantial proportion of the blood volume, increase the risk of excessive potassium release after reperfusion, and lead to severe hypothermia. In children whose temperature falls below 34°C, lavage of the peritoneal cavity with warm saline is effective in raising core temperature.

The limited availability of suitably sized organs for small patients has prompted the development of techniques for transplanting part of a liver. Figure 55-13 illustrates the technique that is used to create a reduced-size ("split") liver and enable one donor liver to be used for multiple patients. There is a significantly higher complication rate with this method, including greater blood loss,[188] risk of organ necrosis, and diminished patient survival,[188,189] so it is usually reserved for patients who are rapidly deteriorating. Living-related (partial) liver donation has also been promoted by the contention that up to one-half of pediatric liver transplant candidates die while awaiting a suitable organ. However, other studies have suggested that more effective allocation of available organs would solve this problem.[174] In view of the potential for donor morbidity and the relatively reduced survival of recipients of reduced-size livers, very few centers offer this option.

The overall 1-year survival in children after orthotopic liver transplantation is 70–75%, but results for younger (less than 3 yr) and smaller (less than 12 kg) patients are not as good (45–50% 1-year survival).[187,189] This discrepancy probably stems from the two factors: the greater incidence of hepatic artery thrombosis in small children, which in turn is related to arterial size, and the use of reduced-size livers.[173,190]

Heart Transplantation

Recently, cardiac transplantation for congenital heart disease overtook dilated cardiomyopathy as the major indication for this procedure in children, so that the majority of recipients are under 5 years of age.[191] However, overall mortality for these young children is higher than in older children and adults (76% vs 81% 1-year survival, respectively).[191] Cardiac-related complications are responsible for the majority of early deaths, stemming from the presence of complex vascular anatomy, previous cardiac surgery, and elevation of pulmonary vascular resistance (PVR). The latter factor is a well-recognized contraindication to heart transplantation in adults, but it is often difficult to accurately quantify the "fixed" component of PVR in infants. If PVR is fixed at a high level, the normal allograft's right ventricle will not be able to acutely adjust to the afterload, and refractory right-heart failure ensues. Long-term survival may be limited by an accelerated form of coronary atherosclerosis,[192] as is seen in adults.

In contrast to the case for the other commonly transplanted viscera, there are generally accepted indications for

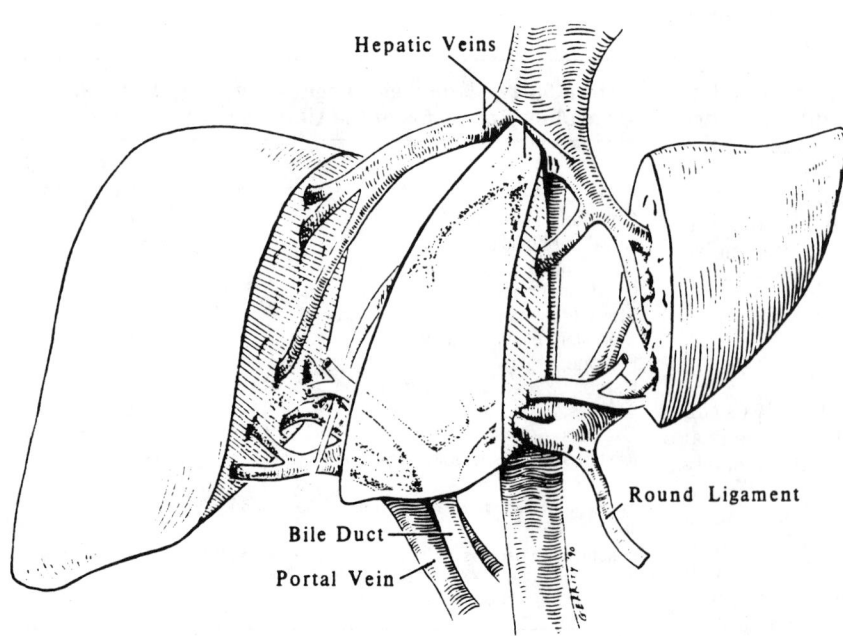

Hepatic Veins

Bile Duct

Portal Vein

Round Ligament

Figure 55-13. A schematic for *ex vivo* dissection of an adult liver to create reduced-size liver allografts with vascular supplies and biliary orifices. Donor iliac arteries or veins are used as needed to extend the vessels. (Adapted and reprinted with permission from Broelsch CE, Emond JC, Whitington PF *et al:* Application of reduced-size liver transplants as split grafts, auxiliary orthotopic grafts, and living related segmental transplants. Ann Surg 212:368, 1990.)

heart transplantation in newborns, specifically, aortic atresia and hypoplastic left-heart syndrome. If reconstruction of the aortic arch is required, profound hypothermia and circulatory arrest is usually necessary. Positional or size discrepancies of the great vessels and abnormal arrangements of systemic and/or pulmonary venous return can complicate these procedures, and have so far limited overall survival for neonates to 66% at 1 year.

A scientifically provocative aspect of transplantation unique to neonates is that the immature immune system seems relatively tolerant of foreign antigens.[193,194] By several criteria, the neonatal immune response to allograft tissue is attenuated, although the response to infective organisms and active immunization is comparatively intact. The mechanisms responsible are currently unclear, but may involve neonatal suppressor cells or maternal cells that enter the circulation during gestation.

Other Viscera Transplantation Procedures

Rarely, heart–lung transplantation is indicated prior to early adulthood for cystic fibrosis, Eisenmenger's syndrome, or primary pulmonary hypertension.[195,196] Isolated lung transplantation may offer the only chance of survival to children with severe developmental anomalies of the lung, including cystadenomatous malformations and congenital diaphragmatic hernia with pulmonary hypoplasia. The scarcity of suitable donor organs has led to instances of living-related lung donation,[175] but the merits of this approach have yet to be fully evaluated. Multiviscera transplantation, which combines liver and small bowel transplantation, has been tried in children with short-gut syndrome (as a result of necrotizing enterocolitis or midgut volvulus) further complicated by hepatic failure after long-term hyperalimentation. So far, intra-abdominal infection and repeated episodes of bowel rejection have limited survival, and thus the approach is still considered experimental.

EVALUATION OF PATIENTS WITH PRIOR ORGAN TRANSPLANT

Transplant recipients may return for a staged repair (e.g., bile duct reconstruction after liver transplantation) or for entirely unrelated surgery. They may also present with a surgical illness superimposed on organ rejection, where the usual signs and symptoms are masked.

Immunosuppression increases the risk of opportunistic infection, so many recipients are maintained on a fixed-dose combination of trimethoprim/sulfamethoxazole, which is effective in preventing such illnesses.[197] Postoperative bacterial infections are also more common in this group, so an attempt should be made to minimize exposure to nosocomial sources, such as urinary bladder and intravascular catheters, and mechanical ventilators. Immunosuppressants also have numerous other adverse effects that can influence perioperative management.

Immunosuppressant Side Effects and Toxicities

Although immunosuppressants are usually administered in combination to diminish the risk of dose-related toxicity from any single agent, significant morbidity is still associated with their use (Table 55-16).

TABLE 55-16. Immunosuppressant Side-Effects and Toxicities

Agent	Side-Effect/Toxicity
Glucocorticoids	Adrenal suppression
	Glucose intolerance
	Cushingoid appearance
	Integument fragility
	Aseptic necrosis
	Peptic ulceration
Azathioprine	Anemia
	Thrombocytopenia
	Leukopenia
	Pancreatitis
	Hepatitis
	Decrease nondepolarizing relaxant requirement
Cyclosporine	Glomerulosclerosis (elevation of BUN, creatinine)
	Hypertension
	Hepatotoxicity
	Neurotoxicity
	Enhanced renal "sensitivity" to insults
Antilymphocyte globulin	Leukopenia
	Thrombocytopenia
	Systemic symptoms
OKT3	Systemic symptoms
	Increased susceptibility to CMV infections

Glucocorticoids

Glucocorticoids produce glucose intolerance, cushingoid habitus, fragility of the integument, aseptic necrosis, and exacerbation of peptic ulcer disease. Yet attempts to eliminate them from immunosuppression regimens have generally not met with success,[198] with the possible exception of neonatal heart-transplant recipients. Chronic glucocorticoid use is also associated with adrenal suppression. Although some authors advocate administration of "stress doses" of glucocorticoids preoperatively, this was shown to be unnecessary in at least one large series of patients who underwent a surgical procedure following renal transplantation.[199]

Azathioprine

Azathioprine is a myelosuppressant, producing anemia, thrombocytopenia and occasionally marrow aplasia. It has also been associated with hepatitis, alopecia, and gastrointestinal upset, and through an allergic mechanism, pancreatitis. Azathioprine has been reported to increase the requirement for nondepolarizing relaxants to a modest degree, probably by presynaptic inhibition of phosphodiesterase in the motor nerve terminal.[200]

Cyclosporine

Cyclosporine is both acutely and chronically nephrotoxic, producing interstitial renal fibrosis and tubular atrophy. Chronic toxicity is common, leading to mild elevations in blood urea nitrogen and creatinine levels, as well as systolic and diastolic hypertension.[201] Management with conventional antihypertensives is usually successful, but the kidneys of such patients may be more vulnerable to acute insults, such as radiographic dye- or hypotension-induced nephropathy. Cyclosporine may be hepatotoxic, producing hyperuricemia, gingival hypertrophy, or seizures and neurotoxicity at high serum levels.

Antilymphocyte Globulin and OKT3

Antilymphocyte globulin is a polyclonal antibody, and as such is "contaminated" with antibodies other than those directed against lymphocytes. These may give rise to marked leukopenia and thrombocytopenia, and systemic symptoms such as fever, chills, pruritis, GI upset, and even frank serum sickness. The first dose of OKT3 is frequently followed by systemic symptoms such as fever, dyspnea, and nausea, unless patients are pretreated with hydrocortisone, acetaminophen, and diphenhydramine. Subsequent reactions are less pronounced. OKT3 has also been associated with episodes of pulmonary edema, aseptic meningitis, and an unusually high incidence of CMV infection.

Early after transplantation, bacterial infections related to wound infection, urinary catheters, and pneumonia are most common (e.g., with S. aureus, E. coli, and S. pneumoniae, respectively). After 1 month, immunosuppressed patients become vulnerable to opportunistic infections (Pneumocystis carinii pneumonia, Herpes zoster infections, and CMV sepsis).[121] These episodes need not be fatal and can be overcome if diagnosis is rapid and treatment specific.[202] The most common viral infection is CMV,[203] which can occur as a primary infection from contaminated blood or allograft tissue in seronegative recipients, or as a reactivated infection in seropositive patients.[204]

Immunosuppressed patients are also more likely to develop one of several histologically distinct types of lymphoproliferative malignancy. For example, the incidence of B-cell lymphoma in patients with renal allografts is some 350-fold higher than that seen in the normal age-matched population, and the same will probably be true for cardiac recipients. Some studies have documented a causal role for Epstein–Barr virus,[205] and it is speculated that cyclosporine may diminish the cytotoxic response of suppressor T-cells to autologous Epstein–Barr virus-infected B cells. Unfortunately, mortality associated with these malignancies is relatively high; in one series, the 5-year mortality rate was 37%.[206]

Other Preanesthetic Considerations

Transplant recipients depend on immunosuppressants to avoid rejection, and these regimens must be restarted soon after surgery. If oral intake is expected to be delayed, a transplant consultant should be asked to recommend appropriate parenteral formulations. Certain drugs used in the perioperative period may inhibit the cytochrome P-450 system and interfere with metabolism of cyclosporine (e.g., cimetidine), while others may induce the P-450 enzymes and decrease cyclosporine levels (e.g., phenobarbital and phenytoin). Cyclosporine increases the hypnotic duration of pentobarbital in laboratory animals,[207] but because it does not increase the requirement for inhaled agents,[208] such an effect may be pharmacokinetic in origin. Cyclosporine has also been reported to prolong the action of pancuronium,[209] but controlled data are lacking.

The transplant population is also particularly prone to bacterial pneumonia and CMV sepsis,[121] so early extubation of the trachea is an important goal following any surgical procedure, and the use of CMV-negative blood is mandatory. In addition, intravascular catheterization is used only when specifically indicated, although standard aseptic cannulation techniques seem sufficient.

Anesthesia After Kidney Transplantation

Although renal transplantation is usually highly successful, some recipients still require dialysis. Thus it is important to ascertain the degree of residual renal impairment and treat such patients accordingly. If the allograft is functional, renal excretion of drugs may be expected to be comparable to that through native kidneys.

Many of these patients are diabetics who return to the operating room for ophthalmologic or peripheral vascular procedures. Perioperative complications leading to loss of the renal allograft are uncommon,[199,210] but sepsis is a major cause of morbidity. Management of blood sugars may be complicated by steroid immunosuppressants and fever; in such cases, insulin infusions are often necessary.

Since kidney recipients are maintained on cyclosporine, other agents with nephrotoxic potential (e.g., enflurane) are usually avoided. Cyclosporine may render allografts particularly sensitive to insults, so maintaining a brisk urine flow during anesthesia is recommended. During long procedures, this may justify the use of central venous pressure and urinary catheters.

Anesthesia After Liver Transplantation

In a well-functioning liver allograft, common biochemical pathways for drug metabolism are unimpaired.[211] Provided that the metabolic and synthetic functions of the transplanted liver are also intact, the anesthetic care of these patients differs little from that of any other visceral transplant patient. Within the first 2 months following liver transplantation, the most common surgical procedures are exploratory laparotomy for biliary leak or abscess drainage, or open liver biopsy. Regional anesthesia is avoided unless the coagulation profile has returned to normal, and the likelihood of ileus or elevated intra-abdominal pressure indicates the use of rapid-sequence inductions. Later on, patients may require biliary reconstruction procedure.

Anesthesia After Heart Transplantation

Heart-transplant recipients return to the operating room for noncardiac surgery with some regularity. Such procedures do not always follow the transplant immediately, but instead, may occur months or even years later. Overall, 25–30% of these patients will require a general surgical procedure (Table 55-17) within 2 years of transplantation.[212-215] Infectious causes for surgery (e.g., drainage of abscesses) can clearly be attributed to immunocompromise, but a relatively high incidence of cholecystitis is unexplained. In addition to these common general surgical problems, orthopedic procedures are frequently required secondary to joint complications arising from chronic steroid use.[216] Despite numerous case reports of cardiac recipients undergoing noncardiac surgery,[217-224] there are no prospective data addressing the risks of anesthesia in this physiologically unique population.

During orthotopic heart transplantation, the aorta and the main pulmonary artery are transected (Fig. 55-9). As a result, the cardiac plexus is divided, resulting in autonomic afferent and efferent denervation. Myocardial tissue ob-

TABLE 55-17. General Surgical Diagnoses in Patients After Heart Transplantation

Diagnosis	Time After Transplantation
Perforated sigmoid diverticulum	8 mo; 29 mo; 39 mo
Small bowel perforation	4 mo; 5 mo
Free intraperitoneal air	3 days; 5 wks
Cholecystitis	2 wk; 21 mo
Vagus nerve injury	3 mo
Ventral hernia	26 mo
Inguinal hernia	7 mo
Perirectal abscess	20 mo
Pancreatitis	18 mo; 1 mo; 2 mo
Diverticulitis	18 mo

Adapted with permission from Steed DL, Brown B, Reilly JJ et al: General surgical complications in heart and heart–lung transplantation. Surgery 98:739, 1985.

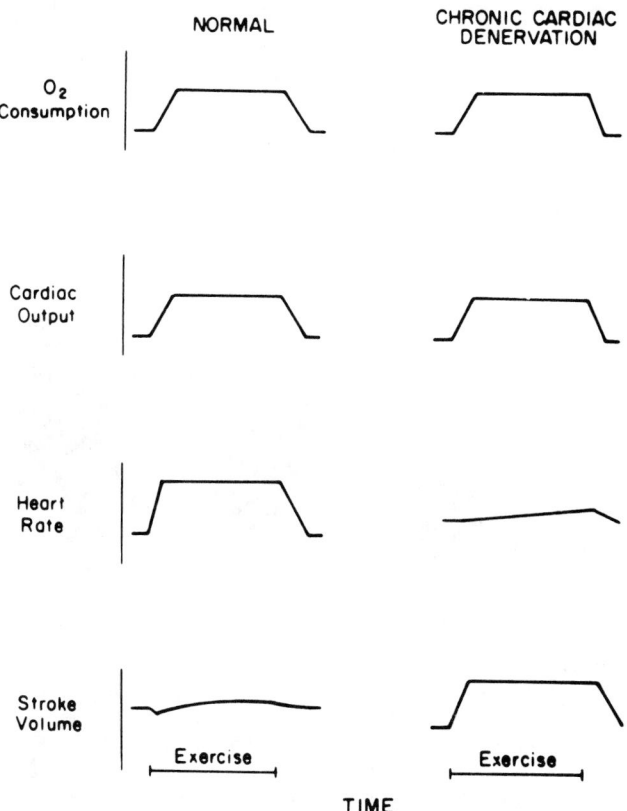

Figure 55-14. Schematic representation of the cardiac physiologic responses to moderate supine exercise in humans. Responses of normal subjects are represented on the left; those following cardiac denervation are on the right. (Reprinted with permission from Kent KM, Cooper T: The denervated heart: A model for studying autonomic control of the heart. N Engl J Med 291:1017, 1974.)

tained from hearts transplanted for as long as 12 years fails to reveal evidence of reinnervation.[225] Although some nerve cells may be present in the ultrastructure of transplanted specimens, they probably represent postganglionic parasympathetics because significant amounts of acetylcholine do remain.[226] While early canine studies indicated that implanted hearts underwent efferent reinnervation and thus regained autonomic control,[227] in humans, with rare exception,[228,228a] studies of transplanted heart-rate responses to exercise and respiratory stimuli[226,229-231] indicate that autonomic efferent denervation is permanent.

In the absence of rejection or significant pulmonary hypertension, long-term follow-up studies after heart transplantation have demonstrated that despite denervation, the resting stroke volume and indices of myocardial contractility are often normal[232] or only subtly reduced.[233] However, with demands for increased cardiac output (e.g., during exercise), the response of the denervated heart is demonstrably different (Fig. 55-14). In the normally innervated heart, immediate increases in cardiac output are mediated by elevation in heart rate with little change in stroke volume. In contrast, the denervated heart responds to such demands by increases in stroke volume rather than in heart rate. Cardiac recipients are thus preload-dependent, and must have adequate central volume to meet the demands of stress or anesthetic techniques that redistribute vascular volume to the periphery.

The denervated heart eventually can manifest increases in heart rate, albeit with some delay (Fig. 55-15). In cardiac-transplant recipients, the maximal achievable pulse rate during exercise develops more slowly than in controls, and the return of heart rate to baseline is slower. The delay in achieving a maximal heart rate seems to correspond to the time required for secretion and circulation of adrenal catecholamines, and the slow return is probably related to the absence of vagal input.

As a consequence of the midatrial orthotopic surgical technique, the transplant recipient retains remnants of the native atria, and the electrocardiogram (ECG) may contain both donor and native P waves. Because the sinus node is normally under the continual influence of autonomic (vagal) nerves,[234] the rate of the transplanted atria generally exceeds that of the native atria.[235] With parasympathetic activation (e.g., via visceral traction including laryngoscopy or drug effects), the native atrial rate may diminish but the

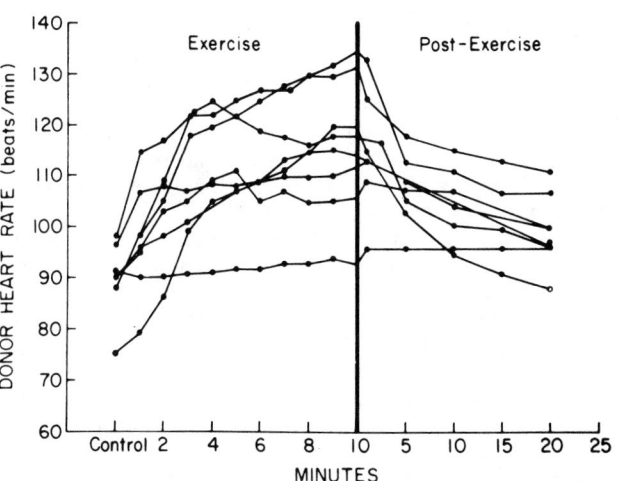

Figure 55-15. Donor heart rates during supine bicycle exercise by eight patients 1 year following heart transplantation. The rates of achieving a maximal pulse are slower than in patients with innervated hearts. "Control" refers to measurements made at the start of exercise. The postexercise scale is compressed. (Reprinted with permission from Stinson EB, Griepp RB, Schroeder JS et al: Hemodynamic observations one and two years after cardiac transplantation in man. Circulation 45:1183, 1972.)

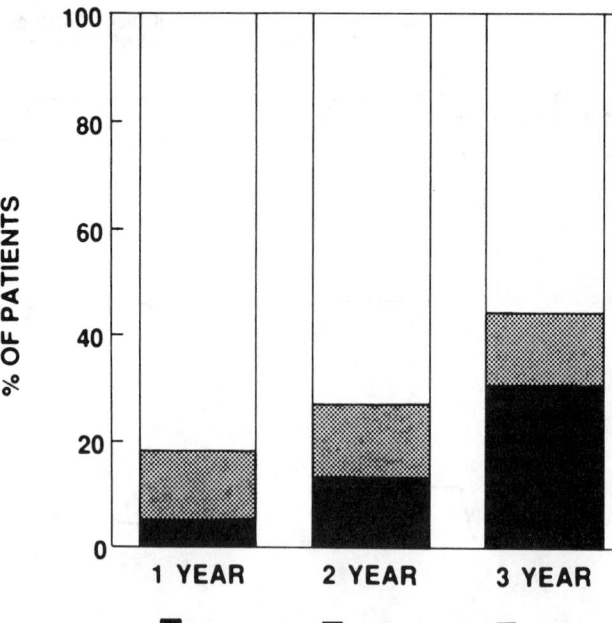

Figure 55-16. Life table analysis showing the risk, in humans, of developing coronary artery disease over the first 3 years after cardiac transplantation. (Reprinted with permission of the authors and the American Heart Association. From Uretsky BF, Murali S, Reddy PS et al: Development of coronary artery disease in cardiac transplant patients receiving immunosuppressive therapy with cyclosporine and prednisone. Circulation 76:827 1987.)

transplanted heart rate remains unchanged, because vagal input is absent. In contrast, sympathetic stimulation (whether from hypoxemia, hypercapnia, hypotension, or pain) can still increase the transplant's sinus rate, although importantly, such responses are delayed. In contrast to effects on the SA node, denervation generally does not alter the AV conduction time[235,236] or affect ventricular conduction.

By 3 years, some 30% of survivors have multivessel coronary stenoses (Fig. 55-16).[237] These lesions are diffuse, concentric narrowings of the coronary lumen,[238] and are thought to arise from areas of immune-mediated endothelial damage. In some cases, lesions are amenable to angioplasty or surgical bypass, but often, myocardial ischemia and infarction limit the useful life of the allograft. Although a recent report has documented the ability to perceive angina pectoris in a small group of these patients,[239] afferent innervation seems to be lacking in most, rendering episodes of myocardial ischemia silent. Thus, diagnostic ECG monitoring is essential throughout the perioperative period, and paroxysmal dyspnea, which may be the only indication of ischemia, should be regarded as an ominous symptom.

Clearly, drugs that act indirectly on the heart will fail to produce their typical effects after denervation, so that administration of atropine, pancuronium, and neostigmine will not affect heart rate (Table 55-18). In contrast, agents that act directly on myocardium or cardiac conduction tissues will manifest their usual effects; for example, isoproterenol will increase contractility and heart rate, while propranolol will have the opposite effects. Digoxin, which has mixed direct–indirect actions,[240] will only act directly after transplantation. An IV bolus of digoxin fails to alter either the functional or effective refractory periods of the AV node,[241] whereas it significantly increases the refractory pe-

TABLE 55-18. Altered Responses to Common Cardioactive Drugs After Cardiac Denervation

Drug	Response
Atropine	No vagolytic effect
Pancuronium	No vagolytic effect
Edrophonium	No vagotonic effect
Ephedrine	Less cardiostimulatory effect
Nifedipine	No depression of nodal conduction
Digoxin	No acute vagotonic effect
Norepinephrine	Enhanced beta-stimulatory effect
Phenylephrine	Diminished vasoconstrictive effects with long-standing heart failure

riod in normal patients. This suggests that digoxin's *acute*, chronotropic effects are vagotonic, dependent on intact autonomic innervation. When treated *chronically* with digoxin, cardiac transplant patients will demonstrate an inotropic response from a direct effect independent of autonomic innervation. Norepinephrine is another cardioactive drug with somewhat atypical effects in this population. Infusions at conventional doses may be accompanied by more pronounced chronotropic effects than usual, through a direct beta-adrenergic receptor-mediated effect on the sinus node that is normally masked by vagal reflexes. Cardiac transplant recipients with previous longstanding heart failure may also have a persistently blunted response to alpha$_1$-adrenergic agonists.[242] This probably results from adjustment of the peripheral vasculature or the baroreceptors to chronically elevated catecholamine levels.

Finally, it is worth remembering that cardiac rejection may be superimposed on the surgical illness and may be the cause of low cardiac output and arrythmias. Rejection can thus impair responses to the stress of surgery and anesthesia. Endomyocardial biopsy may be necessary for definitive diagnosis of rejection, and aggressive immunotherapy with high-dose steroids and/or antilymphocyte globulin may be started in the perioperative period.

FUTURE TRENDS

Since its inception, viscera transplantation has been limited by a shortage of suitable donor organs. For patients with end-stage renal disease, this has meant longer periods on dialysis with greater costs and morbidity. But for cardiac and liver patients, there is a 10–40% mortality while awaiting transplantation.[243] One remedy lies in further improvements in organ preservation, because prolonging tolerable organ ischemic time increases the potential donor pool.[244] The size of this pool will also increase as the criteria for donor acceptability expand (e.g., to include older donors, donors with certain systemic diseases, and terminally ill and fetal donors). Other approaches to deal with the limited supply of organs include cellular transplantation, where healthy allograft cells derived from one organ may be infused into multiple recipients, and xenotransplantation from genetically "humanized" animals.[245]

Optimizing use of the available donor organs will also be important. For example, early application of isolated lung transplantation could make the heart–lung procedure obsolete and allow each heart–lung bloc to serve several patients. Accelerated atherosclerosis is a major factor limiting the useful lifespan of donor hearts; development of an effective therapy would represent a major breakthrough.

For the forseeable future, immunosuppressant drugs will continue to be necessary to prevent the response to foreign tissue antigens. Development of agents with greater immunoselectivity and reduced toxicity is of the highest priority. Noninvasive methods to diagnose organ rejection would also substantially improve the quality of life for transplant survivors. Longer-term approaches to the problem of rejection currently under investigation include induction of tolerance to foreign antigens, definition of the most critical elements for histocompatibility, and development of better "rescue" drugs once rejection has begun.

REFERENCES

1. UNOS receives federal contract to develop OPTN. UNOS Update 2:1(Oct), 1986
2. Friend PJ, McCarthy LJ, Filo RS et al: Transmission of idiopathic (autoimmune) thrombocytopenic purpura by liver. Ann Thorac Surg 41:520, 1986
3. Simmons RL, Canafax DM, Fryd DS et al: New immunosuppressive drug combinations for mismatched and cadaveric renal transplantation. Trans Proc 18(Suppl 1):76, 1986
4. Guidelines for the determination of death: Report of the medical consultants on the diagnosis of death to the President's Commission for the Study of Ethical Problems in Medicine and Biomedical and Behavioral Research. JAMA 246:2184, 1981
5. Black PM: Brain death. New Engl J Med 299:338, 1978
6. Grigg MM, Kelly MA, Celesia GG et al: Electroencephalographic activity after brain death. Arch Neurol 44:948, 1987
7. Lynn J: Diagnosis of brain death. JAMA 250:612, 1983
8. Ropper AH, Kehne SM, Wechsler L: Transcranial Doppler in brain death. Neurology 37:1733, 1987
9. Ashwal S, Schneider S, Thompson J: Xenon computed tomography measuring cerebral blood flow in the determination of brain death in children. Ann Neurol 25:539, 1989
10. Earnest MP, Beresford HR, McIntyre HB: Testing for apnea in suspected brain death: Methods used by 129 clinicians. Neurology 36:542, 1986
11. Belsh JM, Blatt R, Schiffman PL: Apnea testing in brain death. Arch Intern Med 146:2385, 1986
12. Report of special task force. Guidelines for determination of brain death in children. Pediatrics 80:298, 1988
13. Logigian EL, Ropper AH: Terminal electrocardiographic changes in brain-dead patients. Neurology 35:915, 1985
14. Vaghadia H. Atropine resistance in brain dead organ donors. Anesthesiology 65:711, 1986.
14a. Conci F, Procaccio F, Arosio M et al: Viscero-somatic and viscero-visceral reflexes in brain death. J Neurol Neurosurg Psychiatry 9:695, 1986
15. Starzl TE, Miller C, Broznick B et al: An improved technique for multiple organ harvesting. Surg Gynecol Obstet 165:343, 1987
16. Collins GM, Bravo-Shuarman M, Teraskai PI: Kidney preservation for transplantation. Initial perfusion and 30 hours ice storage. Lancet 2:1219, 1969
17. Sacks SA, Petritsch PH, Kaufman JJ: Canine kidney preservation using a new perfusate. Lancet 1:1024, 1973
18. Belzer FO, Southard JH: Principles of solid organ preservation by cold storage. Transplant 45:673, 1988
19. Todo S, Nery J, Yanaga K et al: Extended preservation of human liver grafts with UW solution. JAMA 261:711, 1989
20. Downey JM: Free radicals and their involvement during long-term myocardial ischemia and reperfusion. Ann Rev Physiol 52:487, 1990
21. Hardesty RL, Griffith BP, Deep GM et al: Improved cardiac function using cardioplegia during procurement and transplantation. Transplant Proc 15:1253, 1983
22. Guerraty A, Alivizatos P, Warner M et al: Successful orthotopic canine heart transplantation after 24 hours in vitro preservation. J Thorac Cardiovasc Surg 82:531, 1981
23. Watson DC, Reitz BA, Baumgartner WA et al: Distant heart procurement for transplantation. Surgery 86:56, 1979
24. Reinherz EL, Sclossman SF: The differentiation and function of human T-lymphocytes. Cell 19:821, 1980
25. Harris HW, Gill TJ III: Expression of class I transplantation antigens. Transplantation 42:109, 1986
26. Bach FH, Sach DH: Current concepts: Transplantation immunology. N Engl J Med 317:489, 1987
27. Iwaki Y, Ashizaqa T, Cook D et al: ABO matching in liver transplantation. Transplant Proc 20(Suppl 1):564, 1988
28. Patel R, Terasaki PI: Significance of the positive cross-match test in kidney transplantation. N Engl J Med 14:735, 1969
29. Opelz G: Effect of HLA matching, blood transfusions, and presensitization in cyclosporine-treated kidney transplant recipients. Transplant Proc 17:2179, 1985
30. Weil R, Clarke DR, Iwaki Y et al: Hyperacute rejection of a transplanted human heart. Transplantation 32:71, 1981
31. Stinson EB, Payne R, Griepp RB et al: Correlation of histocompatibility matching with graft rejection and survival after cardiac transplantation in man. Lancet 2:459, 1971
32. Zerbe T, Arena V, Kormos R et al: Role of major histocompatibility complex (HLA) matching in cardiac allograft rejection. Transplant Proc 20(Suppl 1):74, 1988
33. Starzl TE, Tzakis A, Makowka L et al: The definition of ABO factors in transplantation: Relation to other hymoral antibody states. Transplant Proc 19:4492, 1987
34. Gordon RD, Iwatsuki S, Esquivel CO et al: Liver transplantation across ABO blood groups. Surgery 100:342, 1986b
35. Demetris AJ, Jaffe R, Tzakis A et al: Antibody-mediated rejection of human orthotopic liver allografts: a study of liver transplantation across ABO blood group barriers. Am J Pathol 132:489, 1988
36. Gordon RD, Fung JJ, Markus B et al: The antibody crossmatch in liver transplantation. Surgery 100:705, 1986a
37. Markus BH, Duquesnoy RJ, Gordon RD et al: Association of HLA compatibility and decreased liver transplant survival. Transplant Proc 20(Suppl 1):43, 1988
38. Iwatsuki S, Rabin BS, Shaw BW Jr et al: Liver transplantation against T cell-positive warm crossmatches. Transplant Proc 16:1427, 1984
39. Snyder DS, Unanue ER: Corticosteroids inhibit immune macrophage's Ia expression and interleukin-1 production. J Immunol 129:1803, 1982
40. Dupont E, Wybran J, Toussant C: Glucocorticosteroids and organ transplantation. Transplantation 37:331, 1984
41. Keown PA, Stiller CR: Kidney transplantation. Surg Clin North Am 66:517, 1986
42. Kahane BD: Cyclosporine. N Engl J Med 321:1725, 1989
43. Maki T, Simpson M, Monaco MP: Development of suppressor T cells by antilymphocyte serum treatment in mice. Transplantation 34:376, 1982
44. Acuto O, Reinherz EL: The human T cell receptor: Structure and function. N Engl J Med 312:1100, 1985
45. Opelz G, Gengar DPS, Mickey MR et al: The effect of blood transfusions on subsequent kidney transplants. Transplant Proc 5:253, 1973
46. de Waal LP, van Truyver E: Blood transfusion and allograft survival. Crit Rev Immunol 10:417, 1991
47. Hull AR, Parker TF: Proceedings from the Morbidity, Mortality and Prescription of Dialysis Symposium, Dallas, TX, Sept 15–17, 1989. Am J Kidney Dis 15:375, 1990
48. Hellerstedt WL, Johnson WJ, Axher NL et al: Survival rates of 2728 patients with end-stage renal disease. Mayo Clin Proc 59:776, 1984
49. United Network for Organ Sharing Newsletter, Richmond, VA, January 21, 1991
50. Evans RW, Manninen DL, Garrison LP et al: The quality of life of patients with end-stage renal disease. N Engl J Med 312:553, 1985
51. Eggers PW: Effect of transplantation on the Medicare end-stage renal disease program. N Engl J Med 318:223, 1988
52. Inglefinger J, Grupe W, Harmon W et al: Growth acceleration

following renal transplantation in children less than 7 years of age. Pediatrics 68:255, 1981

53. Miller LC, Bock GH, Lum CT et al: Transplantation of the adult kidney into the very small child: Long-term outcome. J Pediatr 100:675, 1982

54. Elick BA, Sutherland DER, Gillingham K et al: Use of distant relatives and living unrelated donors: A strategy to increase the application of kidney transplantation to treat chronic renal failure. Transplant Proc 22:343, 1990

55. Baron P, Heil J, Condie R et al: 96-Hour renal preservation with silica gel precipitated plasma cold storage versus pulsatile perfusion. Transplant Proc 22:464, 1990

56. Velez RL, Vergne-Marini P: Pretransplantation evaluation. In Toledo-Pereyra LH (ed): Kidney Transplantation, pp 50–60. Philadelphia, FA Davis, 1988

57. Najarian JS, Weiland D, Chavers B et al: Studies on living related kidney donors at a single institution. Proc Eur Dial Transplant Assoc Eur Ren Assoc 21:911, 1985

58. Bay WH, Herbert LA: The living donor in kidney transplantation. Ann Intern Med 106:719, 1987

59. Spital A, Spital M, Spital R: The living kidney donor: Alive and well. Arch Intern Med 146:1993, 1986

60. Minami H, McCallum RW: The physiology and pathophysiology of gastric emptying in humans. Gastroenterology 86:1592, 1984

61. Vandam LD, Harison JH, Murray JE et al: Anesthetic aspects for renal transplantation in man. Anesthesiology 23:783, 1962

62. Lincke CL, Merin RG: A regional anesthetic approach for renal transplantation. Anesth Analg 55:69, 1976

63. Heino A, Orko R, Rosenberg PH: Anaesthesiological complications in renal transplantation: A retrospective study of 500 transplantations. Acta Anaesthesiol Scand 30:574, 1986

64. Graybar GB: Choice of anesthesia. In Graybar GB, Bready LL (eds): Anesthesia for renal transplantation, pp 139–155. Boston, Martinus Nijhoff, 1987

65. Fahey MR, Rupp SM, Canfell C et al: Effect of renal failure on laudanosine excretion in man. Br J Anaesth 57:1049, 1985

66. Shi WZ, Fahey MR, Fisher DM et al: Laudanosine (a metabolite of atracurium) increases the minimum alveolar concentration of halothane in rabbits. Anesthesiology 63:584, 1985

67. Belani KG, Palahniuk RJ: Kidney transplantation. In Firestone LL (ed): Anesthesia and Organ Transplantation, pp 17–39. Boston, Little, Brown and Co, 1991

68. Fahey MR, Morris RB, Miller RD et al: Pharmacokinetics of ORG NC45 (Norcuron) in patients with and without renal failure. Br J Anaesth 53:1049, 1981

69. Chapman JR, Allen RD: Dialysis and transplantation. In Morris PJ (ed): Kidney Transplantation: Principles and Practice, pp 37–69. Philadelphia, WB Saunders, 1988

70. Bernuau J, Rueff B, Benhamou JP: Fulminant and subfulminant liver failure: Definition and causes. Semin Liver Dis 6:97, 1986

71. Tarter RE, Erb S, Biller PA et al: The quality of life after liver transplantation: A preliminary report. Gastroenterol Clin North Am 17:207, 1988

72. Starzl TE, Demetris AJ, van Thiel DH: Liver transplantation. N Engl J Med 321:1014, 1092, 1989

73. Terpstra OT, Schalm SW, Weimar W et al: Auxiliary partial liver transplantation for end-stage chronic liver disease. N Engl J Med 319:1507, 1988

74. Krowka MJ, Cortese DA: Pulmonary aspects of chronic liver disease and liver transplantation. Mayo Clin Proc 60:407, 1985

75. Starzl TE, van Thiel DH, Tzakis AG et al: Orthotopic liver transplantation for alcoholic cirrhosis. JAMA 260:2542, 1988

76. Starzl TE, Todo S, Gordon R et al: Liver transplantation in older patients. N Engl J Med 316:484, 1987

77. Starzl TE, Todo S, Tzakis A et al: Abdominal organ cluster transplantation for the treatment of upper abdominal malignancies. Ann Surg 210:374, 1989b

78. Iwatsuki S, Gordon RD, Shaw BW Jr et al: Role of liver transplantation in cancer therapy. Ann Surg 202:401, 1985

79. Makowka L, Tzakis AG, Massaferro V et al: Transplantation of the liver for metastatic endocrine tumors of the intestine and pancreas. Surg Gynecol Obstet 168:107, 1989

80. Iwatsuki S, Esquivel CO, Gordon RD et al: Liver transplantation for fluminant hepatic failure. Semin Liver Dis 5:325, 1985

81. Bismuth H, Samuel D, Gugenheim J et al: Emergency liver transplantation for fulminant hepatitis. Ann Intern Med 107:337, 1987

82. Gimson AE, White YS, Eddleston AL et al: Clinical and prognostic differences in fulminant hepatitis type A, B, and non-A non-B. Gut 24:1194, 1983

83. Rakela J, Kurtz SB, McCarthy JT et al: Fulminant Wilson's disease treated with postdilution hemofiltration and orthotopic liver transplantation. Gastroenterology 90:2004, 1986

84. Campbell DA, Rolles K, Jamieson N et al: Hepatic transplantation and long-term anticoagulation as treatment for Budd-Chiari syndrome. Surg Gynecol Obstet 166:511, 1988

85. Pett S, Mowat AP: Crigler-Najjer syndrome types I and II: Clinical experience—King's College Hospital 1972–1978. Phenobarbitone, phototherapy, and liver transplantation. Mol Aspects Med 9:473, 1987

86. Kang YG, Martin DJ, Marquez J et al: Intraoperative changes in blood coagulation and thromboelastographic monitoring in liver transplantation. Anesth Analg 64:888, 1985

87. Kang Y: Liver transplantation. In Firestone LL (ed): Anesthesia and Organ Transplantation, pp 59–86. Boston, Little, Brown and Co, 1991

88. Aggarwal S, Kang Y, Freeman JA et al: Postreperfusion syndrome: Cardiovascular collapse following hepatic reperfusion during liver transplantation. Transplant Proc 19(Suppl 3):54, 1987

89. Haberer JP, Schoeffler P, Coudere E et al: Fentanyl pharmacokinetics in anaesthetized patients with cirrhosis. Br J Anaesth 54:1267, 1982

90. Rosenberg PH, Oikkonen MP, Orko RH et al: A transplanted liver rapidly begins to metabolize enflurane in humans. Anesth Analg 63:1131, 1984

91. Marquez J, Martin D, Virji MA et al: Cardiovascular depression secondary to citrate intoxication during hepatic transplantation in man. Anesthesiology 65:457, 1986

92. Lewis JH, Bontempo FA, Awad SA et al: Liver transplantation: Intraoperative changes in coagulation factors in 100 first transplants. Hepatology 9:710, 1989

93. Kang Y, Aggarwal S, Pasculle R et al: Clinical evaluation of autotransfusion during liver transplantation. Anesth Analg 72:94, 1991a

94. Shaw BW, Martin DJ, Marquez JM et al: Venous bypass in clinical liver transplantation. Ann Surg 200:524, 1984

95. Griffith BP, Shaw BW, Hardesty RL et al: Veno-venous bypass without systemic anticoagulation for transplantation of the human liver. Surg Gynecol Obstet 160:270, 1985

96. Wall WJ, Grant DR, Duff JH et al: Blood transfusion requirement and renal function in patients undergoing liver transplantation without venous bypass. Transplant Proc 19(Suppl 3):17, 1987

97. Khoury GF, Mann ME, Porot MJ et al: Air embolism associated with veno-venous bypass during orthotopic liver transplantation. Anesthesiol 67:848, 1987

98. Paulsen AW, Whitten CW, Ramsay MAE et al: Considerations for anesthetic management during veno-venous bypass in adult hepatic transplantation. Anesth Analg 68:489, 1989

99. Martin TJ, Kang Y, Marquez JM et al: Ionization and hemodynamic effects of calcium chloride and calcium gluconate in the absence of hepatic function. Anesthesiology 73:62, 1990

100. Martin DJ, Marquez JM, Kang YG et al: Liver transplantation: Hemodynamic and electrolyte changes seen immediately following revascularization (abstract). Anesth Analg 63:246, 1984

101. Prager MC, Gregory GA, Ascher NL et al: Massive venous air embolism during orthotopic liver transplantation. Anesthesiology 72:198, 1990

102. Ellis JE, Lichtor JL, Feinstein SB et al: Right heart dysfunction, pulmonary embolism and paradoxical embolization during liver transplantation. Anesth Analg 68:777, 1989

103. Navalgund AA, Kang Y, Sarner JB et al: Massive pulmonary thromboembolism during liver transplantation. Anesth Analg 67:400, 1988

104. Iwatsuki S, Popovtzer MM, Corman JL et al: Recovery from "hepatorenal syndrome" after orthotopic liver transplantation. N Engl J Med 289:1155, 1973

105. Ontell SJ, Makowka L, Ove P et al: Improved hepatic function in the 24-hour preserved rat liver with UW-lactobionate solution and SRI 63-441. Gastroenterology 95:1617, 1988

106. Shaw BW, Gordon JRD, Iwatsuki S et al: Retransplantation of the liver. Semin Liver Dis 5:394, 1985

107. Starzl TE, Demetris AJ (eds): Candidacy, original disease, and outcome. In: Liver Transplantation, pp 119–130. Chicago, Yearbook Publishers, 1990

108. Evans RW, Manninen DL, Overcast TD et al: The National Heart Transplantation Study: Final Report. Seattle, Battelle Human Affairs Research Centers, Health Care Financing Administration (HCFA) Publ, 1984

109. Kriett JM, Kaye MP: The registry of the International Society for Heart Transplantation: Seventh Official Report—1991. J Heart Lung Transp 10:491, 1991

110. Hunt SA, Gamberg P, Stinson EB et al: The Stanford experience: Survival and renal function in the pre-Sandimmune era compared to the Sandimmune era. Transplant Pro 22(Suppl 1):1, 1990

111. Clark NJ, Martin RD: Anesthetic considerations for patients undergoing cardiac transplantation. J Cardiothorac Anesth 2:519, 1988

112. Caine N, O'Brien V: Quality of life and psychological aspects of heart transplantation. In Wallwork J (ed): Heart and Heart-Lung Transplantation, pp 389–422. Philadelphia, WB Saunders, 1989

113. Massie BM, Conway M: Survival of patients with congestive heart failure: Past, present, future prospects. Circulation 75(IV):11, 1987

114. Braunwald E: Heart failure: Pathophysiology and treatment. Am Heart J 3:486, 1981

115. Cohn JN, Levine TB, Oliveri MT et al: Plasma norepinephrine as a guide to prognosis in patients with chronic congestive heart failure. N Engl J Med 311:819, 1984

116. Hardesty RL, Griffith BP, Trento A et al: Mortally ill patients and excellent survival following cardiac transplantation. Ann Thorac Surg 41:126, 1986

117. Griffith BP, Hardesty RL, Kormos RL et al: Temporary use of the Jarvik-7 total artificial heart before transplantation. New Engl J Med 316:130, 1987

118. Menkis AH, McKenzie FN, Novick RJ et al: Special considerations for heart transplantation in congenital heart disease. J Heart Transplant 9:602, 1990

119. Badellino M, Nairns B, Fucci P et al: Influence of diabetes mellitus on the course of cardiac transplantation. J Am Coll Cardiol 11:103A, 1988

120. Addonizio LJ, Gersony WM, Robbins RC et al: Elevated pulmonary vascular resistance and cardiac transplantation. Circulation 76(Suppl V):52, 1987

121. Dummer JS: Infectious complications of transplantation. In Thompson ME (ed): Cardiac Transplantation, pp 163–178. Philadelphia, FA Davis, 1990

122. Stein KL, Darby JM, Grenvik A: Intensive care of the cardiac transplant recipient. J Cardiothorac Anesth 2:543, 1988

123. Copeland JG: Heart transplantation. Mod Tech Surg Cardiothorac Surg 66:1, 1984

124. Guerraty A, Alivizatos P, Warner M et al: Successful orthotopic canine heart transplantation after 24 hours in vitro preservation. J Thorac Cardiovasc Surg 82:531, 1981

125. Mendez-Picon GJ, Goldman MH, Wolfgang TC et al: Long-distance procurement and transportation of human hearts for transplantation. Heart Transplant 1:63, 1981

126. Watson DC, Reitz BA, Baumgartner WA et al: Distant heart procurement for transplantation. Surgery 86:56, 1979

127. Gilbert EM, Krueger SK, Murray JL et al: Echocardiographic evaluation of potential cardiac transplant donors. J Thorac Cardiovasc Surg 95:1003, 1988

128. Walsh TR, Syttendorf J, Dummer S et al: The value of protective isolation procedure in cardiac allograft recipients. Ann Thorac Surg 47:539, 1989

129. Ozinsky J: Cardiac transplantation. S Afr Med J 41:1268, 1967

130. Keats AS, Strong JM, Girigis KZ et al: Observations during anesthesia for cardiac homotransplantation in ten patients. Anesthesiology 30:192, 1969

131. Harrison GA, Bailey RJ, Thomson PG: A heart transplantation. Med J Austra 1:670, 1969

132. Fernando NA, Keenan RL, Boyan CP: Anesthetic experience with cardiac transplantation. J Thorac Cardiovasc Surg 75: 531, 1978

133. Grebenik CR, Robinson PN: Anaesthesia for surgery in a patient with a transplanted heart. Br J Anaesth 58:1199, 1986

134. Demas K, Wyner J, Mihm FG et al: Anaesthesia for heart transplantation. Br J Anaesth 58:1357, 1986

135. Waterman PM, Bjerke R: Rapid-sequence induction technique in patients with severe ventricular dysfunction. J Cardiothorac Anes 2:602, 1988

136. Borow KM, Neumann A, Arensman FW et al: Cardiac and peripheral vascular responses to adrenoceptor stimulation and blockade after cardiac transplantation. J Am Coll Cardiol 14:1229, 1989

137. Armitage JM, Hardesty RL, Griffith BP: Prostaglandin E₁: An effective treatment of right heart failure after orthotopic heart transplantation. J Heart Transpl 6:348, 1987

138. Bethune DW, Hardy I, Kneeshaw J et al: Anaesthesia and cardiopulmonary bypass for cardiac transplantation. In Wallwork J (ed): Heart and Heart-Lung Transplantation, pp 145–153. Philadelphia, WB Saunders, 1989

139. Bhatia SJS, Kirshenbaum M, Shemin RJ et al: Time course of resolution of pulmonary hypertension and right ventricular remodeling after orthotopic cardiac transplantation. Circulation 76:819, 1987

140. Fonger JD, Borkon AM, Baumgartner WA et al: Acute right heart failure following heart transplantation: Improvement with PGE1 and right ventricular assist. J Heart Transpl 5:317, 1986

141. Renlund DG, Bristow MR, Lee HR et al: Medical aspects of cardiac transplantation. J Cardiothorac Anesth 2:500, 1988

142. Cassella ES, Humphrey LS: Bronchospasm after cardiopulmonary bypass in a heart-lung transplant recipient. Anesthesiology 69:135, 1988

143. Griffith BP, Hardesty RL, Trento A et al: Asynchronous rejection of heart and lungs following cardiopulmonary transplantation. Ann Surg 40:488, 1985

144. Theodore J, Lewiston N: Lung transplantation comes of age. N Engl J Med 322:772, 1990

145. Trulock EP, Cooper JD, Kaiser LR et al: The Washington University-Barnes Hospital experience with lung transplantation. JAMA 266:1943, 1991

146. Miyoshi S, Trulock EP, Schaefers HJ et al: Cardiopulmonary exercise testing after single and double lung transplantation. Chest 97:1130, 1990

147. Griffith BP, Zenati M: The pulmonary donor. Clin Chest Med 11:217, 1990

148. Todd TR, Goldberg M, Koshal A et al: Separate extraction of cardiac and pulmonary grafts from a single organ donor. Ann Thorac Surg 46:356, 1988

149. Conacher ID: Isolated lung transplantation: A review of problems and guide to anesthesia. Br J Anaesth 61:468, 1988

150. Conacher ID, McNally B, Choudhry AK et al: Anaesthesia for isolated lung transplantation. Br J Anaesth 60:588, 1988

151. Gayes JM, Giron L, Nissen MD et al: Anesthetic considerations for patients undergoing double-lung transplantation. J Cardiothorac Anesth 4:486, 1990

152. Thomas BJ, Siegel LC: Anesthetic and postoperative management of single-lung transplantation. J Cardiothorac Vasc Anesth 5:266, 1991

153. Morgan E, Lima O, Goldberg M et al: Improved bronchial healing in canine left lung reimplantation using omental pedicle wrap. J Thorac Cardiovasc Surg 85:134, 1983

154. Dubois P, Choiniere L, Cooper JD: Bronchial omentopexy in canine lung allotransplantation. Ann Thorac Surg 38:211, 1984

155. Schaefers H-J, Waxman MB, Patterson GA et al: Cardiac innervation after double lung transplantation. J Thorac Cardiovasc Surg 99:22, 1990

156. Bierman MI, Stein KL, Stuart RS et al: Critical care management of lung transplant recipients. J Intensive Care Med 6:135, 1991

157. Smiley RM, Navedo AT, Kirby T et al: Postoperative independent lung ventilation in a single-lung transplant recipient. Anesthesiology 74:1144, 1991

158. Dauber JH, Paradis IL, Dummer JS: Infectious complications in pulmonary allograft recipients. Clin Chest Med 11:291, 1990

159. Burke CM, Theodore J, Dawkins KD et al: Post-transplant obliterative bronchiolitis and other late lung sequelae in human heart-lung transplantation. Chest 86:824, 1984

160. National Diabetes Data Group: Diabetes in America: NIH publication no. 85-1467. Washington, DC, U.S. Department of Health and Human Services, August 1985

161. Sutherland DER, Gillingham K, Moudry-Munns KC: Registry report on clinical pancreas transplantation. Transplant Proc 23:55, 1991

162. Sutherland DER, Dunn DL, Goetz FC et al: A 10-year experience with 290 pancreas transplants at a single institution. Ann Surg 210:274, 1989

163. Bilous RW, Mauer SM, Sutherland DER et al: The effects of pancreas transplantation on the glomerular structure of renal allografts in patients with insulin-dependent diabetes. N Engl J Med 321:80, 1989

164. Sollinger HW, Cook K, Kamps D et al: Clinical and experimental experience with pancreaticocystostomy for exocrine pancreatic drainage in pancreas transplantation. Transplant Proc 16:749, 1984

165. Tzakis AG, Ricordi C, Alejandro R et al: Pancreatic islet transplantation after upper abdominal exenteration and liver replacement. Lancet 336:402, 1990

166. Starzl TE, Rowe MI, Todo S et al: Transplantation of multiple abdominal viscera. JAMA 261:1449, 1989

167. Grant D: Intestinal transplantation: Current status. Transplant Proc 21:2869, 1989

168. Tzakis AG, Todo S, Madariaga J et al: Upper abdominal exenteration in transplantation for extensive malignancies of the upper abdomen: An update. Transplantation 51:727, 1991

169. DeWolf A: Multiviscera and pancreas transplantation. In Firestone LL (ed): Anesthesia and Organ Transplantation, pp 111–136. Boston, Little, Brown and Co, 1991

170. Deltz E, Muller-Hermelink HK, Ulrichs K et al: Development of graft-versus-host reaction in various target organs after small intestine transplantation. Transplant Proc 13:1215, 1981

171. Report of special task force. Guidelines for the determination of brain death in children. Pediatrics 80:298, 1988

172. Freeman JM, Ferry PC: New brain death guidelines in children—Further confusion (editorial). Pediatrics 80:301, 1988

173. Broelsch CE, Emond JC, Thistlethwaite JR et al: Liver transplantation, including the concept of reduced-size liver transplants in children. Ann Surg 208:410, 1988

174. Busuttil RW: Living-related liver donation. Con. Transplant Proc 22:1489, 1990

175. Starnes V: Heart, heart-lung, and lung transplantation in the first year of life. Ann Thorac Surg (in press), 1992

176. Ho M, Jaffe R, Miller G et al: The frequency of E-B virus infection and associated lymphoproliferative syndrome after transplantation. Transplantation 45:719, 1988

177. Penn I: The changing pattern of posttransplant malignancies. Transplant Proc 23:1101, 1991

178. Turcotte JG, Campbell DA, Dafoe DC et al: Pediatric renal transplantation, pp 349–360. In Cerelli GJ (ed): Organ Transplantation and Replacement. Philadelphia, JB Lippincott, 1988

179. Fine RN, Ettenger RB: Renal transplantation in children. In Morris PJ (ed): Kidney Transplantation: Principles and Practice, pp 635–691. Philadelphia, WB Saunders, 1988

180. Warady B, Kriley M, Farrell S et al: Growth and development of infants with end-stage renal disease receiving long-term peritoneal dialysis. J Pediatr 112:714, 1988

181. McGraw ME, Haka-Ikse K: Neurologic developmental sequelae of chronic renal failure in infancy. J Pediatr 106:579, 1985

182. Ingelfinger J, Grupe W, Harmon W et al: Growth acceleration following renal transplantation in children less than 7 years of age. Pediatrics 68:255, 1981

183. Fennell K, Rasbury W, Fennell E et al: Effects of kidney transplantation on cognitive performance in a pediatric population. Pediatrics 74:273, 1984

184. Chavers BM, Matas AJ, Nevins TE et al: Results of pediatric kidney transplantation at the University of Minnesota. In P Terasaki (ed): Clinical Transplants, pp 253–266. UCLA Tissue Typing Laboratory, Los Angeles, 1989

185. Van Meurs IP, Terasaki PI, Cecka JM et al: A report from the UNOS scientific renal transplant registry. Transplant Proc 23:53, 1991

186. Najarian J, So SK, Simmons RL et al: The outcome of 304 primary renal transplants in children (1968–1985). Ann Surg 204:246, 1986

187. Gordon RD, Bismuth H: Liver transplant registry report. Transplant Proc 23:58, 1991

188. Lichtor JL, Emond J, Chung MR et al: Pediatric orthotopic liver transplantation: Multifactorial predictions of blood loss. Anesthesiology 68:607, 1988

189. Salt A, Barnes AP, Mowat R et al: Five years' experience of liver transplantation in children. Transplant Proc 22:1514, 1991

190. Bismuth H, Houssin D: Reduced-size orthotopic liver graft in hepatic transplantation in children. Surgery 95:367, 1984

191. Kriett JM, Kaye MP: The registry of the International Society for Heart Transplantation: Seventh official report, 1990. J Heart Transplant 9:323, 1990

192. Pahl E, Fricker FJ, Armitage J et al: Coronary arteriosclerosis in pediatric heart transplant survivors: Limitation of long term survival. J Pediatr 116:177, 1990

193. Starnes V, Oyer P, Bernstein D et al: Heart and heart-lung transplantation in the first year of life. J Heart Lung Transplant 10:162, 1991

194. Bailey L, Kahan B, Nehlsen-Cannarella S: The neonatal immune system: Window of opportunity? J Heart Lung Transpl 10:828, 1991

195. Kaye MP: Intrathoracic transplantation. Transplant Proc 23:51, 1991

196. Smyth RL, Scott JP, Whitehead G et al: Heart-lung transplantation in children. Transplant Proc 22:1470, 1990

197. Gryzan S, Paradis IL, Zeevi A et al: Unexpectedly high incidence of Pneumocystis carinii infection after lung-heart transplantation: Implications for lung defense and allograft survival. Am Rev Respir Dis 137:1268, 1988

198. Stratta RJ, Armbrust MJ, Oh CS et al: Withdrawal of steroid immunosuppression in renal transplant recipients. Transplantation 45:323, 1988

199. Leapman SB, Vidne BA, Butt KM et al: Elective and emergency surgery in renal transplant patients. Ann Surg 183:262, 1976

200. Dretchen KL, Morgenroth VH, Standaert FG et al: Azathioprine: Effects on neuromuscular transmission. Anesthesiology 45:604, 1986

201. Hunt SA, Gamberg P, Stinson EB et al: The Stanford experience: Survival and renal function in the pre-Sandimmune era compared to the Sandimmune era. Transpl Proc 22(Supp 1):1, 1990

202. Erice A, Jordin MC, Chace BA: Gancyclovir treatment of cytomegalovirus disease in transplant recipients and other immunocompromised hosts. J Amer Med Assoc 257:3082, 1987

203. Glenn J: Cytomegalovirus infections following renal transplantation. Rev Infect Dis 3:1151, 1981

204. Weir MR, Irwin BC, Maters AW et al: Incidence of cytomegalovirus disease in cyclosporine-treated renal transplant recipi-

ents based on donor/recipient pretransplant immunity. Transplantation 43:187, 1987

205. Hanto DW, Simmons RL, Najarian JS: Epstein-Barr virus-induced lymphoproliferative diseases in renal allograft recipients. J Heart Transplant 3:121, 1984

206. Nalesnik MA, Locker J, Jaffe R et al: Clonal characteristics of posttransplant lymphoproliferative disorders. Transplant Proc 20:280, 1988

207. Cirella VN, Pantuck CB, Lee YJ et al: Effects of cyclosporine on anesthetic action. Anesth Analg 66:703, 1987

208. Firestone LL, Martin T, Liu P et al: The effect of cyclosporine on the potencies of general anesthetics. Anesth Analg 70:S105, 1990

209. Crosby E, Robblee JA: Cyclosporine-pancuronium interaction in a patient with a renal allograft. Can J Anaesth 35:300, 1988

210. Bakkaloglu M, Hamilton DNH, MacPherson SG et al: Morbidity and mortality in renal transplant patients after incidental surgery. Br J Surg 65:228, 1978

211. Mehta MU, Venkataramanan R, Burckart GJ et al: Antipyrine kinetics in liver disease and liver transplantation. Clin Pharmacol Ther 39:372, 1986

212. Steed DL, Brown B, Reilly JJ et al: General surgical complications in heart and heart-lung transplantation. Surgery 98:739, 1985

213. Colon R, Frazier OH, Kahan BD et al: Complications in cardiac transplant patients requiring general surgery. Surgery 103:32, 1988

214. DiSesa VJ, Kirkman RL, Tilney NL et al: Management of general surgical complications following cardiac transplantation. Arch Surg 124:539, 1989

215. Jones MT, Menkis AH, Kostuk WJ et al: Management of general surgical problems after cardiac transplantation. Canad J Surgery 31:259, 1988

216. Isono SS, Woolson ST, Schurman DJ: Total joint arthroplasty for steroid-induced osteonecrosis in cardiac transplant patients. Clin Ortho 217:201, 1987

217. Camann WR, Goldman GA, Johnson MD et al: Cesarean delivery in a patient with a transplanted heart. Anesthesiology 71:618, 1989

218. Kanter SF, Samuels SI: Anesthesia for major operations on patients who have transplanted hearts. A review of 29 cases. Anesthesiology 46:65, 1977

219. Eisenkraft JB, Dimich I, Sachdev VP: Anesthesia for major noncardiac surgery in a patient with a transplanted heart. Mt Sinai J Med 48:116, 1981

220. Bricker SRW, Sugden JC: Anaesthesia for surgery in a patient with a transplanted heart. Br J Anaesth 40:210, 1985

221. Grebenik CR, Robinson PN: Cardiac transplantation at Harefield. Anaesthesia 40:131, 1985

222. Samuels SI, Wyner J: Anaesthesia for surgery in a patient with a transplanted heart. Br J Anaesth 58:1199, 1986

223. McKeown DW, Armstrong IR: Anaesthesia for surgery in a patient with a transplanted heart. Br J Anaesth 58:1200, 1986

224. Camann WR, Goldman GA, Johnson MD et al: Cesarean delivery in a patient with a transplanted heart. Anesthesiology 71:618, 1989

225. Rowan RA, Billingham ME: Myocardial innervation in long-term heart transplant survivors: A quantitative ultrastructural survey. J Heart Transplant 7:448, 1988

226. Kaye MP: Denervation and reinnervation of the heart. In Randall WC (ed): Nervous Control of Cardiovascular Function, pp 278–306. New York, Oxford University Press, 1984

227. Dong E, Hurley EJ, Lower RR et al: Performance of the heart two years after autotransplantation. Surgery 56:270, 1964

228. Johnson TH, Kubo SH, McGinn AL et al: Physiologic importance of sympathetic reinnervation after cardiac transplantation (abstract). J Heart Transplant 10:178, 1991

228a. Wilson RF, Christensen BV, Olivari MT et al: Evidence for structural sympathetic reinnervation after orthotopic cardiac transplantation in humans. Circulation 83:1210, 1991

229. Pope SE, Stinson EB, Daughters GT et al: Exercise response of the denervated heart in long-term cardiac transplant recipients. Am J Cardiol 46:213, 1980

230. Mason JW, Harrison DC: Electrophysiology and electropharmacology of the transplanted human heart. In Narula OS (ed): Cardiac Arrhythmias: Electrophysiology, Diagnosis and Management, pp 66–81. Baltimore, Williams & Wilkins, 1979

231. Kavanagh T, Yacoub MH, Mertens DJ et al: Cardiorespiratory responses to exercise training after orthotopic cardiac transplantation. Circulation 77:162, 1988

232. Stinson EB, Griepp RB, Clark DA et al: Cardiac transplantation in man. VIII. Survival and function. J Thorac Cardiovasc Surg 60:303, 1970

233. Verani MS, George SE, Leon CA et al: Systolic and diastolic ventricular performance at rest and during exercise in heart transplant recipients. J Heart Transplant 7:145, 1988

234. Higgins CB, Vatner SF, Braunwald E: Parasympathetic control of the heart. Pharmacol Rev 25:119, 1973

235. Cannom DS, Graham AF, Harrison DC: Electrophysiologic studies in the denervated transplanted human heart: Response to atrial pacing and atropine. Circ Res 32:268, 1973

236. Firestone LL: Autonomic influence on cardiac performance: Lessons from the transplanted (denervated) heart. Int Anesthesiol Clin 27:283, 1988

237. Uretsky BF: Physiology of the transplanted heart. In Thompson ME (ed): Cardiac Transplantation, pp 21–56. Philadelphia, FA Davis, 1990

238. Hunt SA, Stinson EB: Accelerated atherosclerosis in the cardiac allograft. In Wallwork J (ed): Heart and Heart-Lung Transplantation, pp 359–367. Philadelphia, WB Saunders, 1989

239. Stark RP, McGinn AL, Wilson RF: Chest pain in cardiac-transplant recipients. N Engl J Med 324:1791, 1991

240. Goodman DJ, Rossen RM, Cannom DS et al: Effect of digoxin on A-V conduction: Studies in patients with and without autonomic innervation. Circulation 51:251, 1975

241. Bhatia SJS, Kirshenbaum JM, Shemin RJ et al: Time course of resolution of pulmonary hypertension and right ventricular remodeling after orthotopic cardiac transplantation. Circulation 76:819, 1987

242. Borow KM, Neumann A, Arensman FW et al: Cardiac and peripheral vascular responses to adrenoceptor stimulation and blockade after cardiac transplantation. J Am Coll Cardiol 14:1229, 1989

243. Baumgartner WA, Augustine S, Borkon AM et al: Present expectations in cardiac transplantation. Ann Thorac Surg 43:585, 1987

244. Baumgartner WA, Williams GM, Fraser CD et al: Cardiopulmonary bypass with profound hypothermia. An optimal preservation method for multiorgan procurement. Transplantation 47:123, 1989

245. Pierson RN, Reemtsma K, Rose EA: Cardiac xenografting. In Baumgartner WA, Reitz BA, Achuff SC (eds): Heart and Heart-Lung Transplantation, pp 303–312. Philadelphia, WB Saunders, 1990

VI

POSTANESTHESIA AND CONSULTANT PRACTICE

56

Roger S. Mecca

Postoperative Recovery

Individualized, problem-oriented patient assessment is essential to ensure optimal postoperative recovery with minimum risk, inconvenience, and expense. Facility design, staffing, and equipment requirements for a state-of-the-art postanesthesia care unit (PACU) are reviewed elsewhere.[1,2]

ADMISSION CRITERIA

The level of postoperative observation that a patient needs should be assessed before the patient is transferred from the operating room. The need for postoperative care is determined by the severity of underlying illness, the duration and complexity of the anesthetic and surgical procedures, and the potential for postoperative complications, regardless of whether surgery is performed on an ambulatory or an inpatient basis. Patients undergoing superficial procedures under local infiltration or peripheral regional anesthetics (i.e., digital or field blocks) can usually recover safely in less intensive settings, even when mild sedation is employed. Whenever doubt exists concerning a patient's ability to recover safely in an unmonitored setting, the patient should be admitted to the PACU.

Every patient admitted to the PACU should have heart rate, systemic blood pressure, and ventilatory rate and character recorded initially and at intervals that vary with clinical condition. (I prefer assessment every 5 minutes for the first 15 minutes and every 15 minutes thereafter as a minimum.) Axillary or oral temperature should be documented at least on admission and discharge, and more frequently if appropriate. Rectal or esophageal determinations can be employed when accurate assessment of core temperature is important. Qualitative assessment of level of consciousness, skin color, and airway patency is essential. In my opinion, routine postoperative laboratory testing should be avoided. Diagnostic tests should be individually ordered for specific indications, based on clinical presentation.[3]

Every patient admitted to the PACU should be monitored with a pulse oximeter and a single-lead, continuous electrocardiogram (ECG). Patients needing mechanical ventilation or those at risk of compromised ventilatory function should be monitored with capnography or arterial blood gas determinations as appropriate. It is still debatable whether all patients need continuous capnographic monitoring during the postoperative period.[4] All invasive intraoperative monitors should be utilized during recovery, so equipment necessary for transduced measurement of central venous, systemic arterial, pulmonary arterial, and intracranial pressures must be available.

On admission, anesthesiology personnel should manage the patient until PACU staff have secured admission vital signs (at least heart rate and rhythm, blood pressure, and ventilatory rate). A succinct clinical report should be prepared that includes sufficient information to allow rapid evaluation and intervention for postoperative complications (Table 56-1). A standardized format printed on the PACU record can be a useful tool to ensure transfer of pertinent data. Plans to achieve specific therapeutic end points during recovery and means of contacting the responsible anesthesiologist should be clearly outlined. Responsibility must not be turned over to PACU personnel until the patient's airway, ventilatory, and hemodynamic status is appropriate. Function of equipment, intravenous (iv) catheters, and monitoring devices must be checked just prior to leaving the patient.

POSTOPERATIVE PAIN MANAGEMENT

Achieving optimal relief of surgical pain with minimal side-effects is a primary goal in PACU care. Incisional pain can be effectively treated with intermittent iv administration of long-acting opiates such as morphine or meperidine, although shorter acting agents are useful in ambulatory settings. Because peak effect evolves rapidly, iv administration allows titration to a desired level of analgesia with assessment of incremental respiratory or cardiovascular depression. Sufficient control of pain is the clinical end point, even if large doses of opioids are necessary in tolerant patients who are suffering chronic pain syndromes or who abuse opioids or alcohol. The disadvantages of intramuscular administration include the requirement for larger doses, a delayed onset of action, unpredictable uptake in hypothermic patients, and unnecessary tissue trauma. Oral and transdermal analgesics have little role in immediate postoperative recovery, but can be useful for ambulatory patients in a predischarge recovery setting. Rectal administration of analgesics is appropriate in selected pediatric patients. In my

TABLE 56-1. Components of a PACU Admission Report

1. *Preoperative History*
   Medication allergies or reactions
   Pertinent earlier surgical procedures
   Underlying medical illness
   Chronic medications
   Acute problems (ischemia, acid-base status, dehydration)
   Premedications
   NPO status

2. *Intraoperative Factors*
   Surgical procedure
   Type of anesthetic
   Relaxant/reversal status
   Time and amount of opioids administered
   Type and amount of intravenous fluids administered
   Estimated blood loss
   Urine output
   Unexpected surgical or anesthetic events
   Intraoperative vital sign ranges
   Intraoperative laboratory findings
   Drugs given (*e.g.,* steroids, diuretics, antibiotics, vasoactive
     medications)

3. *Assessment and Report of Current Status*
   Airway patency
   Ventilatory adequacy
   Level of consciousness
   Heart rate and heart rhythm
   Endotracheal tube position
   Systemic pressure
   Intravascular volume status
   Function of invasive monitors
   Size and location of intravenous catheters
   Anesthetic equipment (*e.g.,* epidural catheters)
   Overall impression

4. *Postoperative Instructions*
   Expected airway and ventilatory status
   Acceptable vital sign ranges
   Acceptable urine output and blood loss
   Surgical instructions (positioning, wound care)
   Anticipated cardiovascular problems
   Orders for therapeutic interventions
   Diagnostic tests to be secured
   Therapeutic goals and end points prior to discharge
   Location of responsible physician

opinion, nonopioid analgesics offer little advantage over opioids for PACU applications. The use of clonidine and ketorolac tromethamine as analgesic agents has interesting potential.[5-7]

In addition to improving patient comfort, relief of pain reduces sympathetic nervous system (SNS) response and helps to control postoperative hypertension, tachycardia, and agitation. However, analgesia coupled with direct or histamine-induced vasodilation from opioids can precipitate hypotension in patients relying on SNS activity to support cardiovascular homeostasis. Hypovolemic patients are at especially high risk for hypotension after the elimination of painful stimuli. A normotensive or hypotensive patient who complains of severe postoperative pain must be carefully assessed prior to administration of analgesics, especially if tachycardia is also present. Similarly, sedation caused by elimination of pain can combine with the direct depressant effects of analgesics to precipitate hypoventilation, with consequent respiratory acidemia and hypoxemia.

Fear, anxiety, confusion, or disorientation often accompany postoperative pain, especially during emergence from general anesthesia. Incremental titration of an iv sedative such as diazepam or midazolam can attenuate this psychogenic component of postoperative discomfort. It is important to differentiate between the requirements for analgesia and for sedation. Although highly touted, the sedative properties of opiates are relatively weak compared to those of more specific sedative medications. Similarly, the analgesic effects of most sedatives are very poor.

Whenever possible, one should use relatively innocuous interventions such as repositioning, extubation of the trachea, Foley catheter removal, or plain reassurance to eliminate or minimize discomfort. To avoid masking symptoms of an unrelated condition or surgical complication, the clinician should ascertain that the nature and degree of the patient's pain are appropriate for the operative procedure and the anesthetic technique before administering analgesics or sedatives.[8] For a given surgical procedure, the degree of postoperative pain can vary among different anesthetic techniques, perhaps related to the way in which intraoperative pain is processed by the central nervous system (CNS). The wide divergence that sometimes appears between cognitive appreciation of postoperative pain and SNS response is probably related to psychological, cultural, and cardiovascular variations among individuals. Some patients perceive severe pain without evidence of autonomic nervous system activity, while others may develop severe hypertension, tachycardia, and even cardiac dysrhythmias with minimal complaint of discomfort. The CNS effects of hypoxemia, respiratory acidemia, or cerebral hypoperfusion often mimic the signs of postoperative pain, especially in patients emerging from general anesthesia. Administration of parenteral analgesics or sedatives can acutely worsen underlying hypoventilation, airway obstruction, or hypotension, causing sudden deterioration and arrest. Evaluating the level of arousal and orientation, along with the cardiovascular and pulmonary status, usually identifies such patients.

Several analgesic modalities are available that allow provision of postoperative pain relief beyond the PACU interval. Intravenous opioid loading in the PACU is a key element for smooth transition to postoperative patient-controlled analgesia. Whether a patient should assume control of iv opioid titration before or after discharge from the PACU is a matter of program design and individual preference. Whoever assumes responsibility for regulating postoperative patient-controlled analgesia must also have knowledge of and input into operative and PACU opioid regimens.

Injection of opioids into the epidural or subarachnoid space during anesthesia or in the PACU can yield prolonged postoperative analgesia in selected patients.[9-11] Both immediate and delayed ventilatory depression can occur, probably related to vascular uptake and caudal spread in cerebrospinal fluid, respectively, so the use of epidural or intrathecal opioids mandates careful ventilatory monitoring. The efficacy and safety of adding vasoconstrictors, potentiators, or local anesthetics for extended postoperative management remain to be clearly demonstrated. Postinjection nausea and pruritus are bothersome side-effects of both patient-controlled analgesics and spinal opioids. The addition of clonidine may enhance analgesia and decrease the risk of side-effects from epidural opiates.[5,12-14]

In selected patients, placement of long-acting regional analgesic blocks can effectively reduce postoperative pain, improve postoperative ventilatory function, and control SNS activity. Unilateral percutaneous intercostal blocks can markedly reduce analgesic requirements after thoracic or high abdominal incision or injury (thoracotomy, cholecystectomy, chest tube placement, gastrostomy, multiple rib fractures), though beneficial effects on postoperative pulmonary function are questionable.[15-17] An analgesic interscalene block can yield almost complete relief with only moderate motor impairment after painful shoulder and upper extremity procedures. In patients with morbid obesity or severe chronic obstructive pulmonary disease, injection of local anesthetic through an indwelling epidural catheter can assist in weaning from mechanical ventilation after major abdominal surgery.[18] Caudal analgesia is very effective in children who have undergone inguinal or genital procedures. Intraoperative infiltration of local anesthetic into joints, soft tissues, or incisions also decreases the intensity of postoperative pain. Control of conversation and input of positive suggestion during surgery might have some influence on analgesic requirement and recovery course.[19,20] Other modalities for pain relief, such as transcutaneous nerve stimulation, "white noise," acupuncture, and hypnosis, seem to have relatively limited immediate postoperative utility.

Expansion of the anesthesiologist's role in providing analgesia farther into the postoperative period increases the need for careful planning. Therapies like patient-controlled analgesia, spinal opiates, and postoperative regional analgesic blocks are effective for prolonged periods and mandate anticipation of risk beyond the PACU. One should commit to an extended postoperative course of pain therapy prior to induction of surgical anesthesia, and orient the anesthetic and PACU care with that course of therapy in mind. If an extended therapy proves inadequate, great caution should be used before adding a second innovative modality. In the interest of minimizing the complexity and risk of therapy after discharge from the PACU, it is usually wiser to rely on evaluation by experienced floor personnel and timed intramuscular analgesic administration.

DISCHARGE CRITERIA

Prior to discharge, a patient should be sufficiently oriented to assess his or her own physical condition and summon assistance if necessary. Airway reflexes and motor function must be sufficient to preclude aspiration of vomitus or secretions. Ventilation and oxygenation should be acceptable, with sufficient functional reserve to cover minor deterioration in unmonitored settings. Systemic blood pressure, heart rate, and indices of intravascular volume and peripheral perfusion need to be relatively constant for at least one-half hour. Cessation of shivering is necessary prior to discharge, although warming to normal body temperature is not an absolute requirement. An acceptable level of analgesia must be achieved before transfer. Patients should be observed for a minimum of 20–30 minutes after the last dose of iv opioid or sedative has been given, in order to reliably assess peak effects. Longer periods of observation may be prudent after reinforcement of regional anesthetic techniques. Patients should be observed for 15–20 minutes after discontinuation of supplemental oxygen to detect unexpected hypoxemia. Likely adverse surgical sequelae (e.g., bleeding, severe edema, vascular compromise, pneumothorax) and acute complications of underlying conditions like coronary artery disease, diabetes, hypertension, or asthma should be assessed prior to discharge. The results of postoperative diagnostic tests should be reviewed.

If these generic criteria cannot be met, postponement of discharge or transfer to a specialized unit for appropriate care and monitoring is advisable. Fixed discharge criteria must be used with great caution in the PACU setting, since variability among patients is tremendous. Scoring systems that attempt to quantify physical status might be useful to ensure thorough assessment but cannot replace individual evaluation.[21,22] Numerical thresholds for vital signs or blood test results do not replace assessment of specific values with respect to a given patient's condition. Ideally, each patient should be individually evaluated for discharge by an anesthesiologist using a consistent set of general criteria (Table 56-2). The type and severity of the underlying disease, the anesthetic and recovery course, and postoperative destination should be carefully considered. Assessment of ambulatory patients must be particularly meticulous, given the low level of care and observation available outside the medical facility (see Chapter 50).

CARDIOVASCULAR COMPLICATIONS

Postoperative Hypotension

Systemic hypotension is a common postoperative complication that can cause hypoperfusion and inadequate delivery of oxygen and substrates to organ systems. Consequent tissue hypoxia promotes inefficient anaerobic metabolism and accumulation of lactic acid. (Unexplained metabolic acidemia is a reliable indicator of inadequate systemic perfusion.) Autoregulation in vital organs helps maintain adequate blood flow when systemic perfusion pressure is reduced. During hypotension, the autonomic nervous system preferentially diverts blood flow to the brain, heart, and kidneys, so that symptoms of hypotension referable to these organs (disorientation, nausea, loss of consciousness, angina pectoris, reduced urine output) indicate a critical failure of compensatory mechanisms. Complications of hypotension include ischemia or infarction of the myocardium, cerebrum, renal tubules, spinal cord, or bowel. Reduced venous flow velocities increase the risk of deep vein thrombosis and subsequent pulmonary embolism. Decreased hepatic oxygen delivery might change metabolic pathways for drugs, causing accumulation of toxic metabolites and hepatic damage. The systemic blood pressure at which the risk of complications increases depends in part on the preoperative blood pressure.[23] Minimum tolerable pressures are higher in patients with arteriosclerotic disease, fixed stenotic vascular lesions, chronic hypertension, increased intracranial pressure, renal failure, or conditions that interfere with autoregulation.

Spurious Hypotension

Blood pressure cuffs that are too large yield falsely low values. The cuff width should equal approximately two-thirds the arm circumference. An arterial catheter transducer system that is improperly zeroed, poorly calibrated, or excessively damped by air bubbles or catheter obstruction also yields artificially low readings. Intense arterial constriction in hypothermic patients or those receiving alpha-adrenergic receptor agonist medications can result in radial or brachial blood pressure readings that are lower than central aortic pressure. Ruling out spurious hypotension avoids the risks of unnecessary treatment and serious iatrogenic hypertension.

TABLE 56-2. Guidelines for Discharge Evaluation from a PACU	

General condition	Oriented to time, place, and surgical procedure
	Responds to verbal input and follows simple instructions
	Acceptable color without cyanosis, splotchiness, or paleness
	Adequate muscular strength and mobility for minimal self-care
	Absence or control of specific acute surgical complications
	(*e.g.,* bleeding, edema, neurologic weakness, diminished pulses)
	Suitable control of nausea and emesis
	Destination unit appropriate for patient's status
Systemic blood pressure	Within ±20% of resting preoperative value
Heart rate and rhythm	Relatively constant for at least 30 minutes
	Resolution of any new dysrhythmia
	Acceptable intravascular volume status
	Any suspicion of myocardial ischemia rectified
Ventilation and oxygenation	Ventilatory rate greater than 10, less than 30 breaths·min^{-1}
	Forced vital capacity approximately twice tidal volume
	Adequate ability to cough and clear secretions
	Qualitatively acceptable work of breathing
Airway maintainance	Protective reflexes (swallow, gag) intact
	Absence of stridor, retraction, or partial obstruction
	No further need for artificial airway support
Control of pain	Ability to localize and identify intensity of surgical pain
	Adequate analgesia, at least 15 minutes since last opioid
	Safe, appropriate orders for postdischarge analgesics
Renal function	Urine output >30 ml·h^{-1} (catheterized patients)
	Appropriate color and appearance of urine, evaluation of hematuria
	Follow-up orders *in re* output if spontaneous voiding has not
	occurred
Metabolic/laboratory	Acceptable hematocrit level in view of hydration, blood loss, and
	potential for future losses
	Suitable control of blood glucose
	Appropriate electrolyte homeostasis
	Evaluation of chest radiograph, ECG, and other tests as appropriate
Ambulatory patients	Ability to ambulate without dizziness, hypotension, or support
	Suitable control of nausea and vomiting after ambulation

Not all criteria will be satisfied by every patient, especially if discharge is to a critical care unit. Clinical judgment must always supersede established guidelines if the patient's condition is less than optimal in a given area. Whenever doubt exists about diagnosis or patient safety, discharge should be delayed.

Hypovolemia

A reduction in circulating intravascular volume ("absolute" hypovolemia) decreases ventricular filling and cardiac output. Compensatory tachycardia, increased systemic vascular resistance (SVR), and venoconstriction mediated by the SNS can usually maintain blood pressure despite a 15–20% loss of intravascular volume, but greater deficits usually cause hypotension.

Failure to adequately replace preoperative fluid deficit, evaporative losses during surgery, and blood loss frequently causes postoperative hypovolemia. Ongoing hemorrhage, sweating, insensible losses, and "third-space losses" (exudation of fluid into tissues) in the PACU will exacerbate postoperative hypovolemia. Blood loss is sometimes occult, as with hemorrhage into muscle after trauma or orthopaedic procedures, retroperitoneal bleeding, or diffuse oozing related to acute coagulopathy (disseminated intravascular coagulation, residual anticoagulation, dilutional coagulopathy, or thrombocytopenia).[24] Third-space losses can continue for 24–48 hours after surgery and can be massive during accumulation of ascites, high-permeability pulmonary edema, or anaphylaxis. If intraoperative hypothermia has caused venoconstriction, a relatively low intravascular volume might be sufficient to maintain cardiac output on PACU admission, but an increase in venous capacity with rewarming can cause profound hypovolemia and hypotension.[25]

Often, a "normal" intravascular volume is inadequate to maintain postoperative blood pressure (relative hypovolemia). Spinal or epidural anesthesia increases venous capacitance by interfering with SNS regulation of venous tone. Sympathectomy also prevents the constriction of veins in response to hemorrhage, the discontinuation of pressors, and positional changes. Sudden decreases in endogenous SNS activity caused by removal of stimulation (extubation of the trachea, relief of pain) or vasovagal responses can also increase venous capacity, as can medications that mimic alpha-adrenergic receptor blockade (droperidol, chlorpromazine), release histamine (curare, morphine), or directly dilate veins (nitrates, furosemide). Rapid administration of blood, fresh frozen plasma, low molecular weight dextrans, or platelets sometimes causes venodilation, probably secondary to histamine release.

Positive intrathoracic pressure from mechanical ventilation or tension pneumothorax can compress thoracic veins and impede venous return, as can inferior vena caval compression in patients with a gravid uterus or increased intraabdominal pressure from large tumors or tense ascites. Acute pericardial tamponade also impedes ventricular filling and causes postoperative hypotension from relative hypovolemia.

On admission to the PACU, a patient's intravascular volume must be assessed in terms of preoperative fluid status, type and duration of surgery, estimated blood loss, intraoperative fluid replacement, and hemostasis. Monitoring the urine output as an index of intravascular volume can be misleading. Surgery and anesthesia interfere with renal concentrating ability, while osmotic diuresis caused by glycosuria can generate the false belief that intravascular volume is adequate. If intravascular volume status is uncertain, invasive evaluation with central venous or pulmonary arterial catheterization is indicated. Systolic blood pressure variation with positive pressure ventilation can also provide a useful index of intravascular volume.[26]

Ventricular Dysfunction

Postoperative hypotension caused by ventricular dysfunction usually occurs in patients with impaired baseline ventricular contractility. Such patients usually need high left ventricular end-diastolic pressure (LVEDP) and elevated SNS activity to maintain cardiac output. In patients with poor ventricular dynamics, excessive fluid administration is a common cause of ventricular dilation, decreased cardiac output, and hypotension, often complicated by pulmonary edema and hypoxemia. Overhydration may not be evident, especially in patients recovering from spinal or epidural anesthestics. If sympathetic blockade was treated only with fluid administration, ventricular filling pressures can be normal during early recovery, despite moderate hypervolemia. When the SNS blockade resolves, a characteristically high level of SNS outflow causes venous constriction and mobilizes large volumes of fluid to the central circulation, precipitating ventricular failure in vulnerable patients.

Other factors can accentuate ventricular dysfunction and cause hypotension. Recovering patients may still exhibit significant alveolar partial pressures of inhalational anesthetics that reduce ventricular contractility and decrease SNS outflow. The resulting myocardial depression may cause hypotension or limit ability to increase cardiac output in response to hypotension from other causes. The administration of beta receptor blocking drugs can attenuate catecholamine enhancement of myocardial contractility, but usually causes hypotension only in patients with severe myocardial disease who rely on maximal SNS activity for cardiovascular stability. Toxic local anesthetic blood levels from intravascular injection or uptake in highly vascular tissues might cause severe myocardial depression and hypotension during postoperative regional analgesic techniques. Although metabolic or respiratory acidemia initially elicits profound SNS activity and augmented contractility, very low pH levels interfere with catecholamine-receptor interaction and depress cerebral SNS outflow, dramatically decreasing ventricular performance. Low ionized calcium levels caused by dilution, chelation by citrate preservatives in banked blood, or acute respiratory or metabolic alkalemia can also decrease ventricular contractility, although clinical impact is usually minor. Right ventricular dysfunction caused by pulmonary thromboembolism or air embolism often presents with systemic hypotension.

Myocardial Ischemia

Postoperative myocardial ischemia or infarction is often initiated by intraoperative hypotension or tachycardia in high risk patients.[27] In the PACU, a decrease in diastolic filling

time during tachycardia caused by pain, hypotension, acidemia, anxiety, or medications can precipitate ischemia, as can an inadequate aortic diastolic blood pressure. Increased myocardial oxygen consumption secondary to shivering or severe hypertension, and elevation of ventricular wall tension secondary to overhydration or increased SNS activity can also initiate ischemia, even with adequate aortic diastolic pressure. Severe hypoxemia secondary to pulmonary dysfunction or hypoventilation will generate ischemia independent of coronary perfusion.

Often, postoperative ischemia does not generate typical signs and symptoms.[28] Chest pain may be hidden by the analgesic effects of residual anesthetics or opioids and by competing painful stimuli from surgical incisions or gastric distention. Signs of hypoperfusion or ventricular dysfunction are also elusive. Many cases of postoperative ischemia are truly silent. The incidence of ischemic dysrhythmia is difficult to determine, given the high incidence of benign postoperative dysrhythmias.

Hypotension secondary to ischemic ventricular dysfunction can quickly progress to irreversible infarction. Close evaluation of hemodynamic responses to fluid challenge, ST segment and T wave morphology on the ECG, and pulmonary artery pressures can sometimes uncover ischemia before hypotension occurs (Fig. 56-1), although the diagnostic value of these indices varies. Aggressive monitoring of patients at risk, control of precipitating factors, and timely therapy are important measures that will decrease the morbidity from intraoperative and postoperative myocardial ischemia.[29,30]

Cardiac Dysrhythmia

Pre-existing myocardial disease or rhythm disturbances increase the risk of postoperative hypotension caused by a cardiac dysrhythmia (see Cardiac Dysrhythmias in the Postoperative Period, below). Sinus or nodal bradycardia can decrease cardiac output and blood pressure, as can slow ventricular rhythms associated with complete heart block. Tachydysrhythmias (e.g., paroxysmal atrial tachycardia, atrial fibrillation or flutter, fast ventricular tachycardia) that generate ventricular rates greater than 140–150 beats·min^{-1} might not allow adequate diastolic intervals for ventricular filling, markedly decreasing stroke volume, cardiac output, and systemic blood pressure. Ventricular fibrillation, asystole, or electromechanical dissociation cause obvious, life-threatening reductions in output.

Postoperative cardiac rhythm disturbances caused by wide swings in autonomic nervous system activity place patients with valvular abnormalities at particular risk of hypotension. An increased heart rate in patients with aortic stenosis reduces the systolic ejection time, promoting increased LVEDP, ventricular dilation, and hypotension. Tachycardia in patients with mitral stenosis impedes ventricular filling, markedly increasing left atrial pressure and decreasing cardiac output and systemic pressure. Augmented contractility or an increased heart rate causes similar problems with hypertrophic subaortic stenosis. In patients with mitral regurgitation, an increased SVR will compromise cardiac output and systemic pressure by increasing regurgitant fraction.

Decreased Systemic Vascular Resistance

Postoperative hypotension associated with regional anesthesia, alpha-adrenergic receptor blocking drugs, vasoactive blood components, and warming is caused by decreased

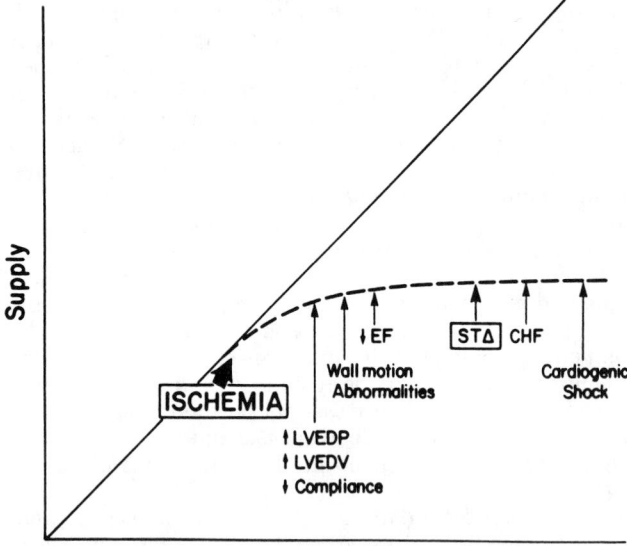

Figure 56-1. Physiologic consequences of myocardial ischemia. Note that changes in ventricular pressure and compliance may precede electrocardiographic changes (ST segment). (LVEDP = left ventricular end-diastolic pressure, LVEDV = left ventricular end-diastolic volume, EF = ejection fraction, STΔ = ST segment change, CHF = congestive heart failure.) (Reproduced with permission from Barash PG: Monitoring myocardial oxygen balance: Physiologic basis and clinical application. In Barash PG, Deutsch S, Tinker J [eds]: Refresher Courses in Anesthesiology, vol 13, p 21. Philadelphia, JB Lippincott, 1985.)

SVR as well as by reduced venous return. Severe systemic acidemia decreases SVR through a direct vasodilatory effect and by interfering with the action of catecholamines on alpha receptors. Antihypertensive medications like hydralazine and nitroprusside can cause profound hypotension in hypovolemic patients by interfering with arteriolar constriction. Systemic sepsis can interfere with arteriolar constriction, generating a high output, low resistance hypotension. (In end-stage sepsis, myocardial depression is usually superimposed on very low SVR.)

Postoperative hypotension can also be caused by surgical or anesthetic interference with baroreceptor function,[31,32] or by intracranial pathology.[33] Rarely, postoperative hypotension occurs as a late manifestation of acute steroid deficiency if the adrenal axis has been suppressed by prolonged administration of exogenous steroids. Hypotension secondary to steroid deficiency is often preceded by lethargy, fever, somnolence or nausea accompanied by hyponatremia, hyperkalemia, and hypoglycemia. The response to administration of supplemental steroids is often dramatic.

Treatment of Postoperative Hypotension

Generally, a 20–30% reduction in systemic arterial systolic pressure from chronic preoperative levels or symptoms of vital organ hypoperfusion are indications for intervention. In patients at high risk for complications of hypotension, acceptable limits for pressure and heart rate should be defined on admission to the PACU.

If hypotension occurs, the pressure determination should be quickly validated. Palpation of carotid or femoral pulses and auscultation of heart sounds are useful qualitative indicators of central blood pressure. Supplemental oxygen should be administered, and the iv infusion rate should be increased to maximum because hypovolemia is by far the most common etiology. If hypotension is spurious or caused by a reduced SVR or ischemia, the amount of fluid infused while these diagnoses are established will usually be inconsequential. Trendelenburg positioning might also be helpful. Cardiac rate and rhythm and breath sounds should be checked. Recent drug administration should be noted, and infusions that might cause vasodilation should be stopped. A 12-lead ECG, arterial blood gas determinations, and a chest radiography might be indicated. If pulses or ventilation are absent, cardiopulmonary resuscitation with endotracheal intubation must be instituted immediately.

Definitive therapy for postoperative hypotension should be directed toward the specific abnormality reducing systemic blood pressure, with repeated reassessment of the diagnosis. Simple maneuvers such as reducing airway pressure, placing pregnant patients in a lateral tilt position, or supine positioning of patients with orthostatic changes should be used when appropriate. Infusion of crystalloid solutions is usually sufficient to treat hypovolemia, although plasma expanders or blood facilitate more rapid volume expansion. Sympathomimetic pressors that increase SVR and venous return can be used judiciously to maintain systemic pressure until sufficient volume can be infused. Increased venous capacity or obstruction to venous return can be treated with an alpha-adrenergic drug such as phenylephrine in conjunction with fluid therapy. Ephedrine is effective but less desirable, since increased heart rate and contractility are usually unnecessary. Tension pneumothorax must be immediately evacuated.

If fluid administration (300–500 ml) does not improve hypotension, myocardial dysfunction should be considered. For dysfunction not related to ischemia, drugs that augment contractility (dopamine, ephedrine, calcium chloride, digoxin) in conjunction with systemic vasodilators often restore cardiac output and systemic pressure. If hypotension is caused by ischemia, resolution of the ischemia usually restores baseline myocardial function. Support of aortic diastolic pressure with an alpha receptor agonist such as phenylephrine and reduction of LVEDP with nitroglycerin can be useful to maximize the coronary artery pressure gradient.[34] Control of heart rate with analgesics for pain, sedatives for anxiety, or beta receptor blockers is essential. Making an accurate diagnosis is critical, because therapy for ischemia can worsen hypotension caused by hypovolemia, decreased SVR, or nonischemic ventricular dysfunction. Hypotension caused by ventricular dysfunction is an indication for pulmonary artery catheterization to measure cardiac output (for estimation of SVR) and pulmonary capillary wedge pressure (indicative of LVEDP).

If hypotension occurs coincident with severe metabolic acidemia, bicarbonate should be given iv while the cause is remedied. Severe hypoxemia or respiratory acidemia mandates tracheal intubation and mechanical ventilation with supplemental oxygen. Sinus bradycardia unrelated to hypoxemia usually responds to iv administration of atropine, glycopyrrolate, or ephedrine. Refractory bradycardia caused by sinus node disease or complete heart block must be managed with iv administration of epinephrine or isoproterenol, or with artificial cardiac pacing. Digitalization or calcium channel blockade reduces the ventricular rate from acute onset atrial fibrillation, whereas paroxysmal atrial tachycardia often disappears with maneuvers or drugs that change cardiac conduction rates. If hypotension from a tachydysrhythmia is severe, immediate low-energy direct current cardioversion (50 joules) is indicated.

Hypotension caused by a low SVR in the setting of a high cardiac output is treated with an alpha-adrenergic agent. Sympathectomy from regional anesthesia usually responds to low levels of alpha stimulation. However, during advanced sepsis or catecholamine depletion, norepinephrine infusions may be required to restore SVR. If decreased SVR is caused by acidemia, correction of pH is necessary before pressor therapy will be effective.

Postoperative Hypertension

A moderate elevation in systemic blood pressure is common in the immediate postoperative period.[35] However, significant hypertension increases the risk of morbidity and should be aggressively evaluated and treated. Hypertension can increase postoperative hemorrhage and third-space losses from either arterial or venous sources. Disruption of major vascular suture lines is possible. High ventricular intracavitary pressures can cause ventricular dilation or myocardial fiber stretch, leading to cardiac dysrhythmias, while an increase in myocardial wall tension might precipitate ischemia. Increased intracranial pressure, cerebral edema, intracranial hemorrhage, or elevated intraocular pressure can also occur.

An inappropriately small blood pressure cuff will yield erroneously high readings, especially in obese patients. An improperly zeroed or calibrated transducer, or a pressure transducing system with an excessive amount of resonance and electronic "overshoot," can grossly overestimate systolic pressure. Overshoot does not significantly change the accuracy of diastolic readings if calibration and zeroing have been done correctly.

Patients with pre-existing hypertension often have exaggerated postoperative blood pressure responses. Noncompliant arteriosclerotic vasculature, elevated peripheral vascular tone mediated by the renin-angiotensin system, or high levels of baseline endogenous SNS activity can all be contributory, as can pre-eclampsia.

Enhanced SNS activity is a frequent cause of postoperative hypertension. Peripheral arteriolar and venous constriction mediated by alpha-adrenergic stimulation increases SVR and venous return, respectively, whereas increased beta$_1$ receptor stimulation increases ventricular contractility and heart rate. SNS outflow most often reflects an appropriate response to noxious stimuli or adverse physiologic conditions (Table 56-3). SNS activity might also be nonphysiologic (e.g., enzyme inhibition, administration of exogenous sympathomimetics, pheochromocytoma, drug interactions). Expansion of intravascular volume can increase cardiac output and blood pressure in spite of compensatory decreases in SVR and heart rate, especially if hypothermia causes coincident vasoconstriction. However, hypervolemia and hypothermia are usually more contributory than causative in the evolution of postoperative hypertension. Abnormal baroreceptor function after carotid endarterectomy can also generate significant postoperative hypertension.[36] Cerebral vascular accidents, hypoxic encephalopathy, increased intracranial pressure, or severe osmotic changes can interfere with central SNS regulation, causing autonomic dysfunction and severe hypertension.[33]

General indications for the treatment of postoperative hypertension include a systolic or diastolic pressure greater than 20–30% above resting blood pressure, signs or symptoms of complications (e.g., headache, bleeding, ocular changes, angina, or ST segment depression), or an unusual risk of morbidity (e.g., increased intracranial pressure, open

TABLE 56-3. Factors That Increase Postoperative Cardiac Sympathetic Influence

Factors Increasing Sympathetic Activity

Noxious stimuli
  Pain, anxiety, carinal stimulation, full bladder, endotracheal intubation
Adverse physiologic conditions
  Hypercarbia/acidosis, hypoxemia, hypotension, hypoglycemia, congestive heart failure, increased intracranial pressure, myocardial ischemia
Medications
  Beta-mimetic pressors
    ephedrine, isoproterenol, epinephrine
  Dopamine, dobutamine
  Bronchodilators
    terbutaline, aminophylline
  Anesthetics
    ketamine, isoflurane
  Antihypertensives
    Hydralazine, nitroprusside

Factors Decreasing Parasympathetic Activity

Medications
  Parasympatholytics
    Atropine, glycopyrrolate
  Relaxants
    Pancuronium, gallamine

eye injury, mitral regurgitation). Pressure should be reduced to near preoperative baseline levels, since "normal" systemic pressures may promote hypoperfusion of vital organs in patients with chronic hypertensive disease. Treatment should first be directed toward causes of increased SNS activity by administering analgesics for pain or sedatives for anxiety, correcting acidemia or hypoxemia, and ensuring ability to void. If hypertension persists, iv administration of antihypertensive medications might be necessary, avoiding the uptake problems characteristic of oral or intramuscular routes. A combination of iv hydralazine and propranolol for rate control is useful for short-term pressure control, as are iv labetolol,[37] iv esmolol,[38] or iv nicardipine.[39] Intravenous alpha-methyldopa yields longer lasting control and can easily be switched to an oral regimen. Potent iv vasodilators (nitroprusside, nitroglycerin, trimethaphan) should be reserved to treat refractory or profound hypertension. Of these, nitroprusside seems most effective for systemic pressure control.

Cardiac Dysrhythmias in the Postoperative Period

Asymptomatic ECG Abnormalities

After general anesthesia, many patients exhibit ECG changes indicative of abnormal myocardial physiology without signs or symptoms of actual cardiac pathology (see Chapter 29).[40] Changes occur in axis, intraventricular conduction, P and T wave morphology, and ST segments, but most resolve spontaneously within 3–6 hours. ECG changes most likely reflect the electrophysiologic effects of inhalation anesthetics, autonomic nervous system imbalance, mild electrolyte abnormalities, and hypothermia.[41] Whenever ECG changes indicative of ischemia appear, it is still important to optimize factors governing myocardial oxygen

Factors Increasing Parasympathetic Activity

Vagal reflexes
  Carotid sinus massage, Valsalva maneuver, gagging, rectal exam,
    increased ocular pressure, bladder distention, pharyngeal
    stimulation
Parasympathomimetic medications
  Acetylcholinesterase inhibitors
    Neostigmine, edrophonium
  Alpha-adrenergic drugs
    Neosynephrine, norepinephrine
  Opioids
    Morphine, fentanyl
  Succinylcholine

Factors Decreasing Sympathetic Activity

High spinal or epidural anesthesia
Withdrawal of stimulus, extubation, emptying bladder
Severe acidemia/hypoxemia
Sympatholytic medications
  Beta-receptor blockers (propranolol)
  Opioids/sedatives/general anesthetics
  Ganglionic blockers
  Local anesthetics

supply and demand and to follow up with repeated ECGs, enzyme determinations, and prolonged monitoring if appropriate.

Bradycardia

Any factor that increases parasympathetic nervous system activity or decreases SNS influence reduces spontaneous depolarization rates in supraventricular pacemakers and promotes sinus bradycardia in the postoperative period (Table 56-4). "Sick sinus syndrome," sinoatrial nodal ischemia, or severe hypoxemia can also reduce sinus rate. In most patients, sinus bradycardia does not cause hypotension until the rate falls below 40–45 beats·min^{-1}. Therapy involves elimination of factors causing autonomic nervous system imbalance or restoration of sympathetic or peripheral nervous system tone to normal. Bradycardia caused by excess peripheral nervous system activity usually responds to muscarinic blocking drugs such as atropine or glycopyrrolate. If decreased SNS activity is the cause, administration of a beta-mimetic drug such as ephedrine can be effective.

Emergence of a dominant pacemaker located in either the lower atrioventricular (AV) node or the bundle of His is also usually caused by postoperative autonomic imbalance. Increased parasympathetic nervous system activity sometimes seems to slow a dominant sinus node pacemaker more than other suppressed pacemaker cells, allowing a slower focus to emerge. Various anesthetic drugs promote emergence of nodal rhythms intraoperatively (e.g., halothane and pancuronium). Factors that stop sinus impulses from reaching the ventricle (sinoatrial nodal exit block or AV nodal block) also cause the appearance of nodal rhythms. Nodal rhythms are benign unless a low ventricular rate reduces cardiac output and blood pressure. Lack of coordinated atrial contraction can in itself decrease cardiac output by 10–15%. If hypotension occurs, administration of atropine or beta-mimetic medications can restore the sinoatrial node as the dominant pacemaker. However, these measures might only increase nodal rate, especially if the nodal rhythm oc-

curs during general anesthesia. Such dysrhythmias can be difficult to convert, requiring support of blood pressure until spontaneous resolution occurs.

Idioventricular bradycardia almost always indicates life-threatening heart block, hypoxemia, acidemia, or myocardial ischemia. Seldom will a slow idioventricular rhythm generate adequate cardiac output to sustain blood pressure. Emergency treatment hinges on the immediate assessment and elimination of underlying conditions while supporting the patient. If acute third-degree AV nodal block occurs secondary to digitalis toxicity or ischemia, atropine might improve AV nodal conduction enough to allow supraventricular impulses to reach the ventricles. Atropine will not increase the depolarization rates of ventricular pacemakers, since they lack parasympathetic nervous system innervation. The addition of epinephrine, isoproterenol, or cardiac pacing may be necessary to accelerate the ventricular rate.

Tachycardia

Sinus tachycardia is undoubtedly the most common rhythm change encountered during the postoperative period and is nearly always associated with a normal, physiologic increase in SNS influence (see Table 56-3). Sinus tachycardia is usually harmless, but it can decrease diastolic filling time and precipitate acute myocardial ischemia in patients with coronary artery disease.[28] Sinus tachycardia seldom interferes with ventricular filling, but output can be severely compromised in patients with stenotic valvular lesions. Tachycardia can also exacerbate hypertension. Identification of an underlying stimulus is important, for tachycardia might herald a serious condition such as acidemia, hypoxemia, or malignant hyperthermia. Postoperative sinus tachycardia is best treated by controlling its underlying cause. Administration of analgesics for postoperative pain, iv fluids to counteract hypovolemia or hypotension, sedatives to calm anxiety, or catheterization to relieve a full bladder are usually sufficient. Tachycardia caused by sympathomimetic drugs resolves as serum drug levels fall. If SNS activity is beyond control or if tachycardia presents a threat to well-being, beta blockade is useful to control rate. Digoxin is ineffective to control sinus tachycardia unless ventricular failure is the underlying cause.

Sudden onset atrial fibrillation can generate ventricular rates in excess of 150 beats·min^{-1} and might appear on the ECG as a fast, nearly regular supraventricular tachycardia. Patients recovering from thoracic surgical procedures or those with atrial dilation from mitral valvular disease or pulmonary emboli have a higher incidence of postoperative fibrillation. Untreated atrial fibrillation with a fast ventricular rate can cause significant hypotension or myocardial ischemia. Treatment includes administration of digoxin or calcium channel blockers to decrease the number of impulses that can traverse the AV node per minute. If hemodynamic compromise is too serious to wait for drugs to decrease ventricular rate, direct current cardioversion might convert fibrillation back to sinus rhythm.

Atrial flutter is relatively rare in postoperative patients. Rapid ventricular rate is the major clinical manifestation, but ventricular response is more regular, reflecting a fraction of atrial rate. Treatment is directed toward decreasing the ventricular rate and regularizing atrial electrical activity. Paroxysmal atrial tachycardias (PATs) are usually caused by circus re-entry in a loop of conduction tissue, although 10–15% are caused by discrete, rapidly firing islands of atrial cells. Emergence of PATs during recovery is relatively uncommon, probably because residual anesthetic medications depress conduction. When PAT does occur, the excessive ventricular rate can interfere with ventricular filling between beats, compromising cardiac output. The treatment of PAT involves slowing the conduction velocities of cardiac impulses to interrupt re-entrant synchrony, allowing a dominant pacemaker to re-emerge at a slower rate. Often PATs can be "broken" by increasing parasympathetic nervous system influence on the heart (see Table 56-4). Digoxin or calcium channel blockers can also be useful. PATs caused by a rapidly firing atrial pacemaker focus may slow with beta blockade or other interventions that decrease spontaneous depolarization rates.[42]

Postoperative ventricular tachycardia or fibrillation almost always reflects severe myocardial ischemia, systemic acidemia, or hypoxemia, although re-entrant ventricular tachycardia does occur. Cardiopulmonary resuscitation, controlled ventilation and oxygenation, manipulation of serum pH, cardioversion, and beta-mimetic medications may be useful to restore a synchronized rhythm.

Premature Contractions. An aberrant impulse arising in the atrium, AV node, or upper bundle of His usually generates an atrial premature contraction (APC), manifested by an early but otherwise normal QRS complex on the ECG that often is not preceded by a P wave. APCs in postoperative patients usually appear during periods of increased SNS activity, are almost always benign, and seldom result in hemodynamic compromise. Control of stimuli causing increased SNS activity is usually sufficient to eliminate these ectopic impulses (see Table 56-3).

The appearance of large-amplitude, wide, bizarre complexes on the ECG is quite common in postoperative patients. Peculiar QRS complexes are often categorically labeled premature ventricular complexes (PVCs), implying origination of an impulse peripherally in ventricular conducting tissue. Actually, the majority of these complexes

are caused by other electrophysiologic mechanisms which seldom indicate serious physiologic abnormality.[42] ECG complexes generated by actual PVCs usually occur at varying intervals from a previous normal QRS. Also, the interval between previous and subsequent normal QRS complexes is often twice the normal interval between sinus complexes (compensatory pause; Fig. 56-2A). In postoperative patients, spontaneous depolarization in ventricular conducting tissue is usually associated with either excessive parasympathetic or sympathetic nervous system influence. Increased parasympathetic nervous system influence reduces spontaneous depolarization rates in supraventricular pacemakers, allowing the emergence of ventricular escape beats. Ventricular escape beats are best treated by accelerating supraventricular pacemaker rates with vagolytic or sympathomimetic medications. An increase in SNS activity accelerates spontaneous depolarization rates in ventricular automatic cells, allowing depolarization between supraventricular impulses. Increased SNS activity also promotes emergence of parasystolic foci. Treatment hinges on analyzing and eliminating autonomic nervous system imbalance, although beta receptor blockade can also be effective. Failure to eliminate ventricular depolarizations with control of autonomic nervous system imbalance may implicate myocardial ischemia, causing nonphysiologic depolarization.[43] However, mechanical stimulation from central catheters, stretch of myocardial fibers during hypertension or ventricular dilation, digitalis toxicity, and electrolyte disturbances might also be responsible. The iv administration of antidysrhythmics such as lidocaine, procainamide, and bretylium can be useful to control automaticity in ischemic ventricular conducting tissue and muscle.

If a supraventricular impulse enters the ventricular conduction system before all pathways have recovered excitability, asynchronous ventricular depolarization generates wide, high-amplitude ECG complexes that are difficult to

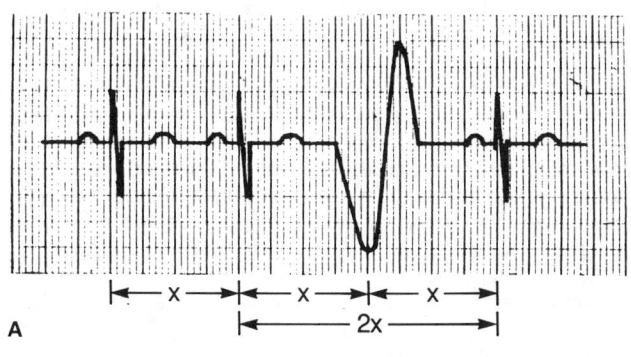

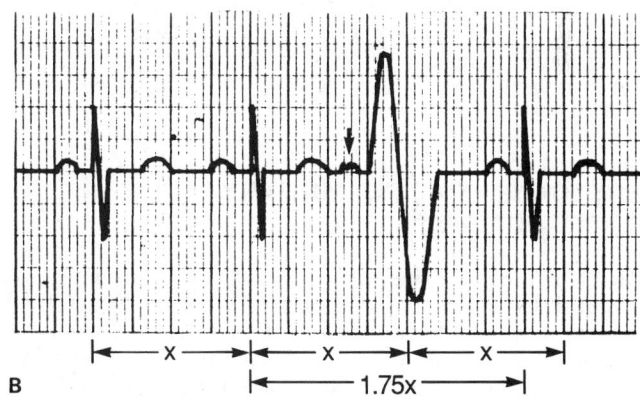

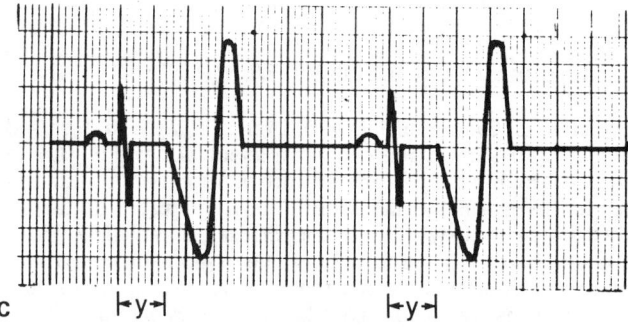

Figure 56-2. Premature ventricular complexes. (*A*) Actual ventricular depolarization. Note wide, high-amplitude configuration, reverse initial deflection, and compensatory pause between previous and subsequent normal QRS (x = normal R-R interval, $2x$ = full compensatory pause). (*B*) Aberrantly conducted atrial premature depolarization. Note initial deflection and general configuration similar to normal QRS, presence of abnormal preceding P wave (*arrow*), and noncompensatory pause between previous and subsequent normal QRS (x = normal R-R interval, $2x$ = full compensatory pause, $1.75x$ = noncompensatory pause). (*C*) Re-entry with fixed coupling. Note uniform configuration of abnormal QRS and fixed interval (y) between preceding normal QRS and abnormal complex.

distinguish from true PVCs. These aberrantly conducted, premature supraventricular depolarizations are sometimes preceded by a P wave that may not resemble dominant P waves. The interval between a previous and a subsequent normal QRS is usually less than twice a normal interval (noncompensatory pause; Fig. 56-2B). Also, the aberrant QRS often resembles normal complexes in general shape, being merely wider and higher in amplitude. Increased SNS activity is usually responsible for generating premature supraventricular impulses with aberrant conduction. However, delayed recovery of excitability in conducting tissues caused by chronic disease, general anesthetics, electrolyte abnormalities, or ischemia also favors aberrant conduction.

If a sinus impulse is delayed in one ventricular conduction pathway long enough to encounter tissue that has recovered excitability, the impulse can depolarize this tissue a second time and spread throughout the entire heart.[44] This "re-entrant" depolarization generates a wide, high-amplitude complex very similar to a true PVC. Re-entrant ECG complexes are usually uniform in configuration, manifest full compensatory pauses, follow a preceding normal complex by a constant interval (fixed coupling), and often appear in a bigeminal pattern (Fig. 56-2C). Many diseases, medications, and environmental influences can create viable re-entrant loops. Postoperative re-entry is often related to increased SNS activity, especially in conjunction with inhalational anesthetics such as halothane.

A high percentage of abnormal ventricular complexes encountered in postoperative patients represent aberrantly conducted supraventricular complexes or re-entrant dysrhythmias rather than actual PVCs. Differentiation is important, because aberrant conduction and re-entry are almost always benign and seldom require treatment. If aberrantly conducted impulses are so frequent that cardiac output is compromised, control of autonomic nervous system imbalance can be effective in restoring a regular rhythm. Cardiac antidysrhythmics are usually unnecessary, although beta receptor blockade might be useful. Treatment of re-entrant impulses should be based on elimination of factors that cause conduction delay or nonuniform recovery of excitability, and on control of SNS activity. Administration of antidysrhythmic medication is seldom indicated and often ineffective.

POSTOPERATIVE PULMONARY DYSFUNCTION

Postoperative pulmonary dysfunction can be caused by mechanical, hemodynamic, and pharmacologic influences related to surgery and anesthesia.[45,46] Considering ventilation, arterial oxygenation, and maintenance of airway patency and protection as separate pulmonary functions facilitates identification of factors causing postoperative dysfunction and simplifies the selection of appropriate treatment.

Inadequate Postoperative Ventilation

Effective alveolar ventilation delivers fresh gas to perfused alveoli and should remove a sufficient volume of carbon dioxide to match peripheral carbon dioxide production, maintaining a constant serum $Paco_2$ and pH. Ventilation distributed to airways and nonperfused alveoli (i.e., dead space ventilation) cannot participate in gas exchange. Alveolar ventilation is primarily regulated by medullary centers that are sensitive to pericellular pH in cerebrospinal fluid (CSF). When hypercarbia causes CSF acidosis, the neural output to muscles of ventilation increases ventilatory rate and tidal volume, increasing both total and effective alveolar ventilation. A consequent reduction in $Paco_2$ resolves acidemia. This negative feedback loop facilitates maintenance of a constant $Paco_2$. Peripheral chemoreceptors in carotid bodies can also increase minute ventilation if the carotid Pao_2 falls, protecting against hypoxemia caused by hypoventilation. Respiratory rate, depth, and pattern are modulated by various neural elements (e.g., slow-adapting parenchymal stretch receptors, chest wall mechanoreceptors, J receptors). Volitional or subconscious cortical input can override more physiologic regulation mechanisms.[47,48]

Clinically, an elevation in $Paco_2$ does not necessarily indicate that ventilation is inadequate. One should suspect inadequate postoperative ventilation when (1) respiratory acidemia occurs coincident with tachypnea, anxiety, dyspnea, labored ventilation, or increased SNS activity, (2) hypercarbia reduces the arterial pH below 7.25, even in the absence of symptoms, or (3) a progressive increase in $Paco_2$ is noted with an appropriate decrease in arterial pH.

Inadequate Respiratory Drive

In the immediate postoperative period, the residual effects of iv or inhalational anesthetics blunt the ventilatory responses to both hypercarbia and hypoxemia.[49-52] Medullary centers that regulate SNS activity are also affected, so that responses to acidemia and hypoxemia such as hypertension, tachycardia, cardiac dysrhythmia, and agitation are blunted. The lack of SNS response to acidemia will often conceal inadequate ventilation.

In the PACU, some degree of respiratory acidemia is expected and acceptable. The evolution of serious hypoventilation and hypercarbia often begins insidiously during transfer from the operating room.[53] Ventilatory depression caused by medications administered during surgery is most profound on admission to the PACU and wanes thereafter, but if iv opioid is given just prior to admission, the peak depressant effect can occur in the PACU. The time of administration, amount, and route of all respiratory depressant medications the patient has received must be clearly documented. Certain neuroleptic or opiate anesthetic techniques might produce biphasic, delayed respiratory depression and hypoventilation.[54-56] Sedatives can also directly depress ventilation, synergistically augment depression from opiates and anesthetics, or ablate the conscious will to ventilate (sometimes a significant component of ventilatory drive).[57-59] A cautious balance must be struck between an acceptable degree of pain or agitation and an acceptable level of postoperative ventilatory depression. If ventilatory depression from opioids is excessive, titration of iv naloxone or nalmefene[60] will reverse respiratory depression without affecting analgesia. Administration of doxapram, a central respiratory stimulant, has also been shown to improve hypoventilation in postoperative patients,[61] though its routine use probably is not advisable.

Other factors affect postoperative ventilatory drive. The abrupt diminution of a noxious stimulus (e.g., extubation of the trachea, administration of a postoperative regional analgesic block) can upset an existing balance between the depressant effects of medication and the excitatory effects of stimuli, promoting airway obstruction or hypoventilation. Pain relief after administration of iv opioids potentiates direct ventilatory depression from the medication. Intracranial hemorrhage or edema after posterior fossa craniotomy often initially manifests with apnea,[33] while bilateral damage to the carotid bodies (as might occur after bilateral carotid endarterectomy) can ablate peripheral hypoxic drive.[31,62] Chronic respiratory acidemia (as seen with carbon dioxide retention in chronic obstructive pulmonary disease) alters CNS sensitivity to pH changes. Although such patients are at theoretical risk of hypoventilation after administration of supplemental oxygen, this problem rarely appears in the PACU. Patients suffering from abnormal carbon dioxide/pH responses associated with morbid obesity, chronic upper airway obstruction, or sleep apnea disorders are often sensitive to respiratory depressants and at increased risk of inadequate postoperative ventilation. After anesthesia, preterm infants are at increased risk for apnea, which depends on postconceptual age[63,64] and preoperative anemia.[65] Although the type of anesthetic administered may influence the incidence of postoperative apnea and bradycardia,[66] all preterm infants should be appropriately monitored for at least 12 hours after surgery.

Increased Airway Resistance

High resistance to gas flow through the airways increases the work of breathing and carbon dioxide production. If inspiratory muscles cannot generate sufficient pressure gradients along airways to overcome resistance, effective alveolar ventilation can be so reduced that progressive respiratory acidemia and ventilatory failure occur.

In the PACU, increased airway resistance is commonly caused by upper airway obstruction in the pharynx (posterior tongue displacement, soft-tissue collapse), the larynx (laryngospasm, laryngeal edema), or large airways (extrinsic compression from hematoma or tumor, tracheal stenosis). Immediate relief of obstruction is essential. If the airway is clear of vomitus or foreign bodies, simple airway maneuvers such as jaw lift, mandible elevation, lateral positioning, or placement of an artificial oropharyngeal or nasopharyngeal airway will usually relieve pharyngeal obstruction by the tongue or soft tissues. (If gag reflexes are functional, a nasopharyngeal airway might be better tolerated.) Improving the patient's level of consciousness can be equally useful. During emergence, stimulation of pharyngeal tissues or vocal cords by secretions or foreign matter can generate tight vocal cord apposition by laryngeal constrictor muscles, termed laryngospasm. Most episodes of laryngospasm can be overcome with 100% oxygen under gentle positive pressure in the oropharynx. If laryngospasm is prolonged and severe, a very small dose of succinylcholine (e.g., 0.1 mg·kg^{-1}) yields sufficient relaxation to allow ventilation of the lungs. Edema of the vocal cords, glottis, or tracheal mucosa after extubation of the trachea, bronchoscopy, or airway surgery sometimes reduces upper airway caliber and increases resistance, especially in children. However, complete obstruction from edema is rare, and airway compromise is often ameliorated by nebulized racemic epinephrine inhaled in oxygen.

Acute extrinsic upper airway compression (as seen with an expanding neck hematoma) should be relieved whenever possible. If the airway is compromised by a relatively fixed obstruction (e.g., epiglottitis, retropharyngeal abscess, or encroaching tumors), emergency tracheal intubation might be necessary. Airway manipulation under such circumstances is fraught with danger. Even minor trauma from intubation attempts can easily convert a marginal airway into a total obstruction. Administration of sedatives to facilitate laryngoscopy and tracheal intubation can promote further hypoventilation and worsen obstruction by compromising the patient's volitional efforts to maintain the airway. Use of muscle relaxants eliminates spontaneous ventilation and

ablates muscular tone necessary to keep the airway patent. An acute airway emergency can be precipitated if tracheal intubation and face mask ventilation are impossible to accomplish after paralysis. Given these risks, equipment and personnel necessary for emergency cricothyroidotomy (Fig. 56-3) or tracheostomy and positive pressure ventilation should be readily available. Cricothyroidotomy using a 14-gauge iv catheter permits oxygenation and marginal ventilation until the airway can be secured (Fig. 56-4), especially if jet ventilation with 100% oxygen is employed.[67]

Reduction of cross-sectional area in small airways generates a marked increase in overall airway resistance because airway resistance varies inversely with the 4th power of the airway radius during laminar air flow and with the 5th power during turbulent air flow. In the PACU, pharyngeal or tracheal stimulation from secretions, suctioning, aspiration, or endotracheal intubation often triggers a reflex constriction of bronchial smooth muscle, especially as the bronchodilatory effects of inhalational anesthetics wane. Histamine release precipitated by medication or allergic reactions can also increase airway smooth muscle tone. Decreased airway caliber may be caused by diffuse bronchospasm or airway wall edema in asthmatics or smokers with reactive airway disease. Decreased radial airway traction can also reduce airway cross-sectional area in patients with chronic obstructive pulmonary disease, as can decreased lung volume secondary to obesity, surgical manipulation, excessive lung water, or hypoexpansion from splinting against a painful incision. When ventilatory requirements are increased by warming, hyperthermia, or an increased work of breathing, high flow rates through small airways will convert normal, low-resistance laminar flow to chaotic, high-resistance turbulent flow.

In postoperative patients, increased airway resistance does not always present with audible turbulent air flow (wheezing), because flow might be so impeded that no sound is produced. The generation of a forced vital capacity expiration is useful to unmask high airway resistance. (Resistance is usually highest during expiration because intermediate-diameter airways are compressed by positive intrathoracic pressure.) The signs of increased small airway resistance can mimic those of decreased pulmonary compliance. Spontaneously breathing patients exhibit an increased

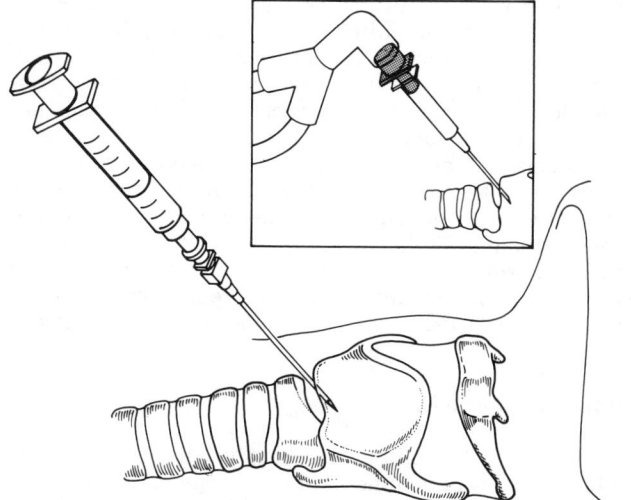

Figure 56-3. Cricothyroidotomy using large-bore (14-gauge) intravenous catheter attached to syringe.

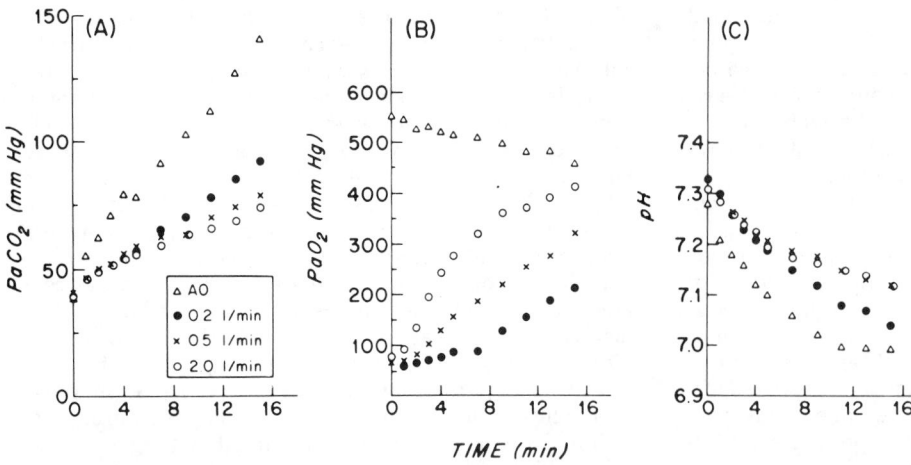

Figure 56-4. The effects of apneic oxygenation (Ao) and oxygen flow at 0.2, 0.5, and 2.0 l·min⁻¹ through a small-bore tracheal catheter in an anesthetized canine preparation. Pao_2 was well maintained (Ao) and improved with low flow oxygen. Despite marked changes in $Paco_2$ and pH, no dog exhibited signs of circulatory instability. (Reproduced with permission from Slutsky AS, Watson J, Leith DE et al: Tracheal insufflation of oxygen [TRIO] at low flow rates sustains life for several hours. Anesthesiology 63:278, 1985.)

work of breathing with either condition, as evidenced by accessory muscle recruitment and labored ventilation, while mechanically ventilated patients exhibit an elevation in the peak inspiratory pressure needed for delivery of a given tidal volume.

The treatment of high small airway resistance should be directed toward an underlying etiology. Laryngeal or airway stimulation should be eliminated if possible. Administration of isoetharine or metaproterenol nebulized in oxygen resolves postoperative bronchospasm in most cases with minimal tachycardia or agitation. Intramuscular or sublingual terbutaline can be added when necessary. If effective ventilation is still compromised or unduly labored, an aminophylline loading dose and maintenance infusion should be administered. However, if bronchospasm is life-threatening, an iv epinephrine infusion usually yields profound bronchodilation while allowing blood levels of epinephrine to be rapidly reduced if unwanted side-effects appear. An occasional patient with bronchospasm resistant to beta₂-sympathomimetic medication may benefit from a trial of a parasympatholytic medication such as atropine.[68]

Increased small airway resistance caused by mechanical factors (e.g., loss of lung volume, retained secretions, pulmonary edema) usually does not resolve with bronchodilators. Restoration of lung volume with incentive spirometry or deep tidal ventilation increases external radial traction on small airways and decreases overall resistance. A reduction in left ventricular filling pressures and improvement in left ventricular function can be beneficial if high airway resistance is caused by increased lung water. Sometimes a reduction in pulmonary microvascular filtration pressure does little to ameliorate symptoms acutely, because airway wall edema and interstitial fluid accumulation require time to resolve. After an acute exacerbation of long-standing bronchospasm, a patient will sometimes seem resistant to bronchodilators. Prolonged contraction of airway smooth muscle causes venous and lymphatic obstruction in airway walls. The consequent edema and reduction of airway cross-sectional area persist even after the smooth muscle relaxes.

Decreased Compliance

Factors that reduce pulmonary compliance (i.e., the change in lung/chest wall volume per unit change in transthoracic pressure) will increase the work of breathing. In the extreme, low compliance can cause progressive respiratory muscle fatigue and respiratory acidemia, as well as signifi-

cant loss of lung volume and hypoxemia from ventilation-perfusion (V/Q) mismatching.[69,70] Postoperative pulmonary compliance depends to a degree on preoperative status. Obesity decreases pulmonary compliance,[71,72] especially in supine or lateral positions when adipose tissues compress the thoracic cage. Increased intra-abdominal pressure caused by abdominal fat impedes diaphragmatic excursion, leading to a reduction in functional residual capacity (FRC), closure of small airways, and collapse of distal lung tissue. Re-expansion of atelectatic parenchyma and airways requires increased energy expenditure. Analogous reductions in compliance are encountered in patients with large intra-abdominal tumors, ascites, bowel obstruction, intra-abdominal hemorrhage, and intrauterine pregnancies.[73] Pulmonary contusion, atelectasis, consolidation, or hemorrhage secondary to thoracic or upper abdominal trauma interfere with lung expansion and accentuate the work of breathing. Restrictive lung diseases, musculoskeletal abnormalities, pneumonias, intrathoracic tumors or aneurysms, and massive cardiomegaly can also cause marked decreases in baseline pulmonary compliance.[74] Patients with hydrostatic pulmonary edema (caused by fluid overload, left ventricular failure, or mitral valve dysfunction) or high permeability pulmonary edema (caused by sepsis, aspiration, or other causes of adult respiratory distress syndrome) often exhibit a serious reduction in compliance that leads to ventilatory failure. Interstitial fluid and blood volume increase the lung's weight and inertia, making expansion more difficult, while accumulation of fluid or secretions in air spaces interferes with the effectiveness of pulmonary surfactant in minimizing surface tension.

Numerous intraoperative factors can cause atelectasis or reduce compliance, including accumulation of gas in the stomach or bowel, intra-abdominal manipulation or fluid accumulation, main-stem tracheal intubation, excessive airway suctioning, and hemothorax or tension pneumothorax. In the lateral position, mediastinal compression and interstitial fluid accumulation lower compliance in the dependent lung. Chest or abdominal dressings can reduce pulmonary compliance, as can severe cellulitis or extensive scar tissue on the thoracic or upper abdominal walls.

In the PACU, therapy to improve compliance and decrease the work of breathing should be aimed at resolving causative problems and restoring lung volume. Allowing patients to recover in a semisitting position (rather than supine or full sitting position) can improve ventilatory dynamics and decrease the work of breathing.[75,76] Incentive spirometry and chest physiotherapy are useful,[77,78] as are positive end-expiratory pressure (PEEP) or continuous positive airway pressure (CPAP).[79] However, in patients with severe chronic obstructive pulmonary disease and highly compliant lungs, positive airway pressure can force the rib cage and diaphragms toward the limits of their respective excursions, accentuating muscular effort required to achieve further increases in thoracic volume during inspiration. This hyperexpansion reduces spontaneous effective minute alveolar ventilation or interferes with weaning from mechanical ventilation.

Neuromuscular and Skeletal Problems

Postoperative hypoventilation is sometimes caused by incomplete reversal of intraoperative neuromuscular relaxation. Inadequate reversal may be secondary to insufficient dosage or the gradual onset of anticholinesterase effect, especially if hypothermia limits access of the drug to neuromuscular junctions. Marginal reversal can be more dangerous than near total paralysis. A gasping, agitated patient exhibiting dyscoordinate movements and airway obstruction is readily identified. However, a somnolent patient with marginal neuromuscular function exhibiting only mild stridor and abdominal rocking motions is more easily overlooked. Insidious hypoventilation with progressive respiratory acidemia or regurgitation with aspiration may occur well into the recovery period, when patients may be less closely observed.

Patients with preoperative neuromuscular abnormalities such as myasthenia gravis, Eaton-Lambert syndrome, periodic paralysis, or a variety of muscular dystrophies can exhibit exaggerated or prolonged responses to administration of muscular relaxants. Even without relaxant administration, such patients can exhibit postoperative ventilatory insufficiency from inadequate neuromuscular reserve.[80] Certain medications potentiate neuromuscular relaxants or interfere with reversal (e.g., antibiotics, furosemide, propranolol), as do hypocalcemia or hypermagnesemia.[81] The duration of paralysis after administration of succinylcholine can be markedly increased in patients with atypical pseudocholinesterase.

The strength and coordination of diaphragmatic contraction are probably compromised in some postoperative patients, forcing more reliance on intercostal muscles to overcome decreased compliance or to meet increased ventilatory demands.[82] Administration of morphine may compromise intercostal function as well, further compounding ventilatory inadequacy.[83] Postoperative diaphragmatic fatigue may improve with aminophylline infusion.[84]

Thoracic spinal or epidural blockade interferes with external intercostal muscle function and reduces ventilatory ability, especially in patients with chronic obstructive pulmonary disease. Damage to phrenic nerves from regional anesthetics, trauma, or thoracic and neck operations will "paralyze" one or both diaphragms. Adequate ventilation can be maintained with only one functional diaphragm, while marginal ventilation can often be maintained by external intercostal muscles alone. However, in a patient with underlying lung disease, increased work of breathing, or increased ventilatory demands, a nonfunctional diaphragm significantly impedes ventilation.[85] Patients with abnormal motor neuron function (e.g., Guillain-Barré syndrome, cervical spinal cord trauma) can certainly exhibit postoperative ventilatory insufficiency.[86] Severe kyphosis or scoliosis can markedly reduce ventilatory capacity. Multiple rib fractures that allow paradoxical inward movement of the chest wall during inspiration can impede thoracic cavity expansion to

such a degree that ventilatory failure supervenes. Loss of compliance from pulmonary contusion underlying such a flail segment is probably of greater significance with respect to ventilatory impairment.[87]

Several simple bedside tests can be useful to assess mechanical ability to ventilate. Forced vital capacity greater than 10–12 ml·kg^{-1} and inspiratory pressure more negative than −25 cm H_2O usually indicate adequate strength of ventilatory muscles to sustain ventilation. Failure on these tests does not necessarily indicate the need for assisted ventilation of the lungs, as many patients with chronic lung diseases cannot meet these criteria preoperatively. Ability to hold the head elevated from a supine position usually indicates sufficient muscular recovery to ensure functional airway protective reflexes.[88] (Often patients will be resistant to lifting the head because of abdominal incisional discomfort, but will sustain a head lift if assisted into position.) Hand-grip, pedal extension, and other maneuvers are less reliable indicators. Observation of expiratory time yields a qualitative assessment of airway resistance.

Occasionally, a clinical picture of postoperative ventilatory insufficiency appears when ventilation is adequate. Voluntary limitation of chest cavity expansion in response to pain from an upper abdominal or thoracic incision will sometimes generate a labored, rapid, shallow breathing pattern characteristic of inadequate ventilation. However, the impact of incisional pain on measurable pulmonary function is limited,[89] and seldom does hypercarbia or respiratory acidemia appear. This ventilatory pattern usually regularizes with repositioning or analgesic administration. Ventilation with small tidal volumes in response to thoracic restriction or reduced compliance generates afferent input from pulmonary stretch receptors. Dyspnea, labored breathing, and accessory muscle recruitment can occur in spite of appropriate minute ventilation. (This also occurs during mechanical ventilation with low inspired volumes.) Achieving a large, "satisfying" lung expansion often relieves these symptoms. Finally, hyperventilation necessary to compensate for metabolic acidemia may require a level of ventilation beyond that which a patient can easily generate. Tachypnea and labored ventilation are easily mistaken for primary ventilatory insufficiency, especially if one evaluates only arterial pH and ignores the low Pa_{CO_2}.

Increased Dead Space

Ventilation to air spaces that are not perfused (e.g., dead space ventilation) cannot remove carbon dioxide. Similarly, ventilation of alveoli with high V/Q ratios is less effective in removing carbon dioxide. If dead space volume increases without a change in tidal volume, the fraction of each breath wasted in dead space (VD/VT) increases. A reduction in tidal volume also increases VD/VT. If VD/VT is large, greater demand for effective alveolar ventilation will require a proportionally larger increase in total minute ventilation. Many conditions that increase dead space also interfere with ventilatory mechanics, thus severely compromising ventilatory reserve. Patients with large dead space volume are therefore at greater risk for postoperative ventilatory failure. If the postoperative VD/VT fraction is between 0.55 and 0.60 (normal, approximately 0.30), a patient will usually need mechanical assistance to maintain adequate effective alveolar ventilation. If the ratio is greater than 0.60–0.65, conventional volume ventilation often cannot deliver adequate ventilation. High-frequency ventilation may facilitate carbon dioxide removal at higher VD/VT ratios.

Postoperative hypercarbia and respiratory acidemia are

occasionally caused by an acute increase in dead space. Upper airway dead space is reduced by approximately 75% after endotracheal intubation, and almost eliminated by tracheostomy. However, excessive tubing volume, inappropriate connections, or valve reversal in breathing circuits can increase anatomic dead space, promoting rebreathing of expired gas rich in carbon dioxide. Increases in anatomic dead space can also occur if airway volume is expanded after application of PEEP or CPAP, especially in patients with high pulmonary compliance. Dead space volume may appear to be increased if expiration is interrupted by a subsequent inspiration before spent alveolar gas is completely exhaled. Consequent "gas trapping" and carbon dioxide retention occur if improper inspiratory to expiratory time ratios or excessive ventilatory rates are used during mechanical ventilation, especially when high airway resistance lengthens the time required for complete expiration.

Pulmonary embolization with air, thrombus, cellular debris, or foreign matter can generate significant V/Q mismatching in the lung, creating an increase in physiologic dead space. The impact of high V/Q units on carbon dioxide excretion is often masked by large increases in minute ventilation mediated by hypoxic drive or reflex responses to emboli.[90] Capnographic real-time evaluation of end-expired Pco_2 is useful to detect pulmonary embolization. Pulmonary hypotension can also change V/Q matching and increase V_D/V_T.[91] Irreversible increases in physiologic dead space occur postoperatively whenever a pathologic process disrupts or destroys pulmonary microvasculature. For example, elevation of V_D/V_T is often encountered in adult respiratory distress syndrome related to sepsis, massive transfusion, severe hypotension, trauma, or hypoxemia. Increased dead space usually causes progressive difficulty in maintaining adequate levels of mechanical ventilation several days into a postoperative ICU course.

Increased Carbon Dioxide Production

Total body carbon dioxide production varies directly with metabolic rate, body temperature, and substrate availability. During anesthesia, carbon dioxide production can fall by 20–40% of normal (approximately 2.3 $ml \cdot kg^{-1} \cdot min^{-1}$) as hypothermia lowers metabolic activity and neuromuscular relaxation reduces tonic muscle contraction. In the postoperative period, warming returns metabolic rate, oxygen consumption, and carbon dioxide production toward normal. Shivering, an increased work of breathing, infection, SNS activity, or rapid carbohydrate metabolism during iv hyperalimentation can markedly accelerate carbon dioxide production.[92] Even mild postoperative augmentation of carbon dioxide production can precipitate respiratory acidemia and ventilatory failure if decreased compliance, increased airway resistance, or residual neuromuscular paralysis interfere with ventilatory ability. More pronounced increases in carbon dioxide production can generate ventilatory insufficiency even with normal ventilatory capacity. An episode of malignant hyperthermia will generate carbon dioxide production many times greater than normal, which will rapidly exceed ventilatory reserve and cause a severe respiratory acidemia.[93]

There are few indications for manipulation of carbon dioxide production in the PACU, with the exception of adjusting hyperalimentation or treating malignant hyperthermia. However, if increased dead space precludes mechanical delivery of adequate alveolar ventilation, deliberate hypothermia and paralysis can be employed to reduce carbon dioxide production in the hope that the increased V_D/V_T ratio is partially reversible.

Inadequate Postoperative Oxygenation

Systemic arterial Po_2 is still the most reliable index to assess the efficiency of pulmonary oxygen transfer from alveolar gas to pulmonary venous blood. Noninvasive analysis of arterial hemoglobin saturation (pulse oximetry) monitors the adequacy of arterial oxygenation, but yields less information on alveolar-arterial gradients. Saturation is also affected by hemoglobin dissociation curve shifts.[6] Evaluation of metabolic acidemia, mixed venous oxygen content, or venous hemoglobin saturation yields better insight into peripheral oxygen delivery and utilization than into pulmonary oxygen transfer. Adequate systemic arterial oxygenation does not guarantee that arterial perfusion pressure, cardiac output, and distribution of systemic blood flow are sufficient to maintain tissue oxygenation. Marked tissue ischemia can occur with normal pulmonary oxygenation in the presence of peripheral shunts, sepsis, severe hypotension or anemia, hemoglobin dissociation abnormalities, and poisoning with carbon monoxide, arsenic, or cyanide.

In the PACU, there is little benefit in elevating the Pao_2 above 100–110 mm Hg, because the hemoglobin is fully saturated and the additional amount of dissolved oxygen at higher Pao_2 is negligible. Each patient should be individually evaluated when defining an "acceptable" lower limit for Pao_2 or an acceptable alveolar-arterial oxygen gradient (i.e., Pao_2 at a given fraction of inspired oxygen [Fio_2]). One must also assess the risk of interventions needed to maintain the Pao_2. Reducing the Pao_2 to below 70 mm Hg may cause significant arterial hemoglobin desaturation, although tissue oxygen delivery can be maintained at lower levels. I prefer to maintain Pao_2 between 80 and 100 mm Hg (saturation greater than 93–95%) to ensure adequate peripheral oxygen delivery while minimizing therapeutic intervention. In routine cases requiring postoperative mechanical ventilation, if the Pao_2 is above 80 mm Hg with 40% inspired oxygen and 5 cm H_2O PEEP or CPAP, patients can usually sustain peripheral oxygenation after tracheal extubation.

Distribution of Ventilation

Ventilation-perfusion mismatch caused by loss of lung volume and ventilation in dependent parenchyma is probably the most common cause of postoperative arterial hypoxemia. A reduction in FRC decreases the radial traction on airways, causing small airway collapse, distal atelectasis, and V/Q mismatch that can progressively worsen for 24–36 hours after surgery. Decreased ventilation to dependent lung is particularly damaging because gravity directs a significant proportion of pulmonary blood flow to dependent areas.[94-96]

Certain patients are at increased risk for reduction of FRC during and after surgery. Older patients usually exhibit some degree of airway closure at end-expiration. Chronic obstructive pulmonary disease promotes more severe airway closure, which can be markedly exacerbated by even small reductions in FRC.[97] Obesity and increased intraabdominal pressure limit diaphragmatic excursion and decrease lung volume. Patients with low pulmonary compliance caused by increased lung water, atelectasis, pleural effusions, gastric distention, or restrictive disorders are also at increased risk. Retraction, packing, and manipulation

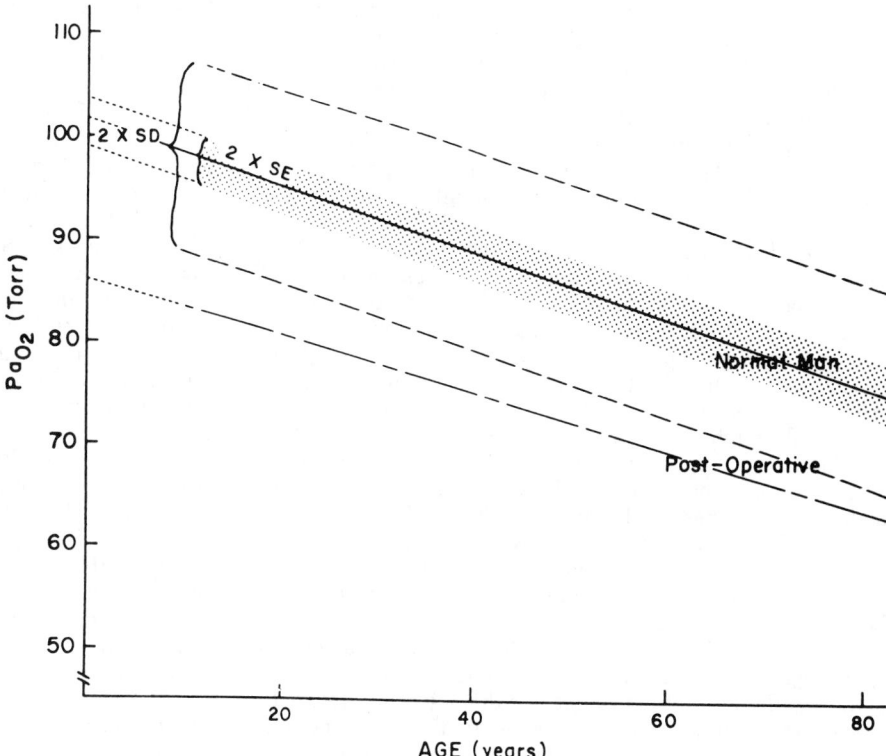

Figure 56-5. The influence of age on PaO$_2$. For any given age the PaO$_2$ is lower in the postoperative period. The *dashed line* indicates range of normal individual values; the *shaded area* indicates the range of normal mean values. (Reproduced with permission from Marshall BE, Wyche MQ Jr: Hypoxemia during and after anesthesia. Anesthesiology 37:178, 1972.)

during upper abdominal surgery reduce FRC, as does external abdominal compression from leaning surgical assistants. Prone, lithotomy or Trendelenburg positions are disadvantageous, especially in obese patients (Figs. 56-5 and 56-6).[98]

A significant reduction in FRC and profound V/Q mismatching frequently occur during intrathoracic surgery, especially when endobronchial intubation and one-lung anesthesia are employed in a laterally positioned patient. Direct surgical compression, the weight of unsupported mediastinal contents, and pressure from abdominal contents forcing the paralyzed dependent diaphragm into the chest cavity all reduce dependent lung volume.[99,100] Augmentation of blood flow to the dependent lung worsens intrapulmonary shunting, especially when anesthetic agents interfere with hypoxic pulmonary vasoconstriction.[101] Interstitial fluid accumulation caused by gravity and lymphatic obstruction accentuates V/Q mismatching. (This "down lung syndrome" often appears as unilateral pulmonary edema on a postoperative chest X-ray film.)

Acute postoperative pulmonary edema, though rare, does occur in the PACU, even in patients without predisposing disease states.[102] Accumulation of fluid in air spaces caused by overhydration, ventricular dysfunction, or increased capillary permeability interferes with both diffusion of oxygen and V/Q matching. Pneumothorax or hemothorax, pulmonary blebs, pulmonary contusion, or intrapulmonary hemorrhage also upset V/Q matching and promote hypoxemia. Retention of secretions, bronchospasm, and airway wall edema or inflammation promote hypoventilation of distal air spaces, as will obstruction of larger airways by foreign body aspiration, main-stem intubation, or external compression by tumor or vascular abnormalities. Right upper lobe

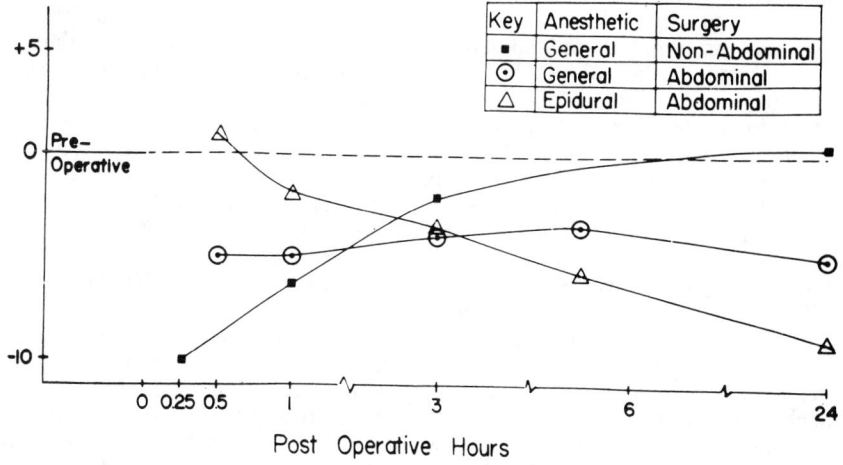

Key	Anesthetic	Surgery
■	General	Non-Abdominal
⊙	General	Abdominal
△	Epidural	Abdominal

Figure 56-6. Effect of anesthetic technique on early and late hypoxemia. General anesthesia administered for nonabdominal procedures has maximal decrease in PaO$_2$ upon emergence, and returns to normal within 3 hours. In contrast, general anesthesia for abdominal surgery is followed by similar early changes, but PaO$_2$ does not return to baseline value within 3 hours. Regional anesthesia for abdominal operations results in a late decrease in PaO$_2$. (Reproduced with permission from Marshall BE, Wyche MQ Jr: Hypoxemia during and after anesthesia. Anesthesiology 37:178, 1972.)

collapse caused by partial right main-stem intubation is a frequently overlooked cause of significant postoperative hypoxemia. Also, strong inspiratory efforts against an obstructed airway can both decrease FRC and promote hydrostatic pulmonary edema.[103]

In the PACU, conservative measures aimed at restoring lung volume often produce marked and lasting improvement in arterial oxygenation. Obese patients should recover in a semisitting position whenever possible to reduce the pressure of abdominal contents on the diaphragms. Deep tidal ventilation, vigorous cough, chest physiotherapy, and appropriate suctioning will help mobilize secretions and accustom a patient to minor incisional discomfort during deep inspiration. Application of incentive spirometry can be particularly helpful to maintain FRC. Some authorities advocate intermittent positive pressure breathing techniques, although their effectiveness is questionable.[104,105]

Adequate postoperative analgesia is pivotal to ensuring restoration and maintenance of FRC, especially with upper abdominal or chest wall incisions. Pain with ventilatory motion encourages rapid, shallow breathing, which may provide adequate minute ventilation but does little to restore lung volume and maintain expansion. Analgesia can be provided with parenteral or epidural opioids, or with selected regional anesthetic techniques. Intercostal blocks relieve pain from thoracotomy and cholecystectomy incisions, while continuous lumbar or thoracic epidural techniques are effective for upper abdominal incisions. Continuous regional analgesia can be helpful in weaning patients with limited pulmonary reserve from ventilatory support.[15,18,106]

Because of the high risk of hypoxemia in the immediate postanesthetic period, all patients, including those who have had surgery under regional anesthesia, should receive supplemental oxygen during transfer and initial recovery unless oxygen is waived by an anesthesiologist for specific medical reasons.[53,107-109] The use of supplemental oxygen in the PACU does not preclude the development of postoperative hypoxemia.[110] Neither careful clinical observation nor assessment of cognitive function accurately screens for hypoxemia, so monitoring by oximetry is essential during and especially after supplemental oxygen administration.[111-113] Hypoxemia is also a significant problem in children, especially those with perioperative upper respiratory infections or chronic adenotonsillar hypertrophy.[114-118] Alternative delivery methods are available to administer supplemental oxygen to children who will not tolerate face masks or nasal prongs.[119] The routine use of humidification probably is of little benefit unless endotracheal intubation bypasses natural humidification.

Administration of supplemental oxygen often improves Pao_2 to some degree, although the effect of a given Fio_2 is highly variable. The actual inspired concentration is difficult to assess with commonly used face masks, tents, or nasal prongs, since ambient gas is entrained with each inspiration.[120] In addition, if hypoxemia is caused by shunting, supplemental oxygen should have a negligible effect on Pao_2. (Shunted blood is not exposed to increased Fio_2, whereas blood passing ventilated alveoli is already fully saturated.) However, if hypoxemia is caused by low V/Q units, increasing Fio_2 to marginally ventilated air spaces can improve saturation in passing blood. Supplemental oxygen does not rectify underlying problems causing poor V/Q matching, but the risk of administration is negligible. An Fio_2 greater than 0.8 may promote resorption atelectasis as inert nitrogen in poorly ventilated alveoli is replaced with oxygen. The inspiration of 100% oxygen for 24–36 hours can generate early signs of pulmonary oxygen toxicity, characterized by alveolar epithelial degeneration and evolution of capillary leak pulmonary edema.[121] The development of oxygen toxicity is accelerated in patients undergoing hyperbaric oxygen therapy. The administration of supplemental oxygen might accelerate pulmonary damage associated with bleomycin therapy,[122] although doubt exists concerning actual risk.[123,124] Alveolar Po_2 should probably be maintained as near to room air values as possible in patients exposed to bleomycin, with monitoring of Pao_2 or oxygen saturation.

If loss of lung volume is significant, CPAP is very effective for restoring and maintaining FRC in the postoperative period. CPAP (5–7 cm H_2O) can be delivered effectively by face mask for several hours to maintain Pao_2 within acceptable limits until factors promoting loss of lung volume resolve.[125] However, if arterial hypoxemia is severe or if patient acceptance of mask CPAP is poor, endotracheal intubation is usually required. Intubation of the trachea for delivery of CPAP does not indicate a need for positive pressure ventilation. Ventilatory requirements should be assessed independently, considering $Paco_2$, arterial pH, and work of breathing, because the institution of positive pressure ventilation increases the risk of cardiovascular compromise.[126] In most patients, 5–10 cm H_2O of CPAP or PEEP is sufficient to restore lung volume and Pao_2 without pressure transmission to thoracic veins, which would cause hypotension or an increase in intracranial pressure.[127] The risk of barotrauma is minimal, even when positive airway pressure is administered as PEEP with positive pressure ventilation. If improvement in Pao_2 is not achieved with 5–10 cm H_2O positive pressure, the etiology of the low Pao_2 should be re-evaluated, for higher positive pressure is seldom helpful in routine postoperative settings. In an occasional patient with severe pulmonary pathology (e.g., adult respiratory distress syndrome, severe pulmonary contusion), higher levels of pressure may yield improvement in both oxygenation and compliance. However, pressures greater than 10–15 cm H_2O are more transmitted to thoracic veins and are probably associated with higher peak pressures and an increased incidence of barotrauma.[128-130] In addition, high positive pressure can increase vascular resistance in more compliant portions of lung and actually divert blood toward poorly ventilated areas, worsening V/Q matching. This phenomenon is rare at more conservative levels of positive pressure.

Endotracheal intubation eliminates a patient's expiratory resistance and "physiologic PEEP" (2–5 cm H_2O), which is very useful in maintaining lung volume during spontaneous ventilation. Exposing an intubated trachea to ambient airway pressure in the postoperative period can cause a gradual, progressive reduction in FRC, significant V/Q mismatch, and arterial hypoxemia. Generally, a patient whose trachea is intubated should exhale against some degree of CPAP. Young, slender patients left intubated without positive pressure for short periods (0.5–1 hour) are usually able to spontaneously restore any reduction in FRC after extubation.

Distribution of Perfusion

The distribution of pulmonary blood flow is primarily determined by mechanical factors (pulmonary arterial and venous pressures, arteriolar and capillary resistance), which in turn are affected by gravity, airway pressure, lung volume, and cardiovascular dynamics. The distribution of blood flow is modulated by hypoxic pulmonary vasoconstriction, which diverts flow away from air spaces that are poorly ventilated and exhibit low alveolar P_{O_2}. Poor distribution of pulmonary perfusion also interferes with V/Q matching and postoperative oxygenation.

In the PACU, SNS response to pain, agitation, hypoxemia, or acidemia increases cardiac output and pulmonary vascular resistance, elevating pulmonary artery pressure. Increased pulmonary artery pressure can increase blood flow to less dependent areas of lung and through the bronchial circulation and pulmonary arteriovenous anastomoses, interfering with V/Q matching. Recruitment of pulmonary vessels can interfere with the overall effectiveness of hypoxic pulmonary vasoconstriction in regulating localized distribution of blood flow.[131] All of these changes can reduce arterial oxygenation. Elevated pulmonary venous pressures caused by hypervolemia or left ventricular dysfunction necessitate an increase in pulmonary arterial pressures to maintain output.

A significant reduction in pulmonary artery pressure may also change V/Q matching. Pulmonary artery pressure can decrease to a point that perfusion to uppermost parenchyma is compromised. If loss of dependent lung volume simultaneously causes redistribution of fresh ventilation to nondependent lung, regional V/Q mismatch results. Also, the effectiveness of hypoxic pulmonary vasoconstriction depends on differences in flow resistance among areas of the vascular bed, and varies with pulmonary artery pressure in a bimodal fashion.[132] Position changes affect oxygenation by changing the distribution of blood flow, especially when gravity directs flow to areas with reduced ventilation. Placing a patient with severe unilateral ventilatory abnormality (e.g., pneumonitis, main-stem intubation) lateral with the poorly ventilated lung dependent can cause serious reductions in Pa_{O_2}, while placing the unventilated lung in a nondependent position can improve V/Q matching and arterial oxygenation. Great caution should be exercised when placing a diseased lung in a nondependent, "up" position, for drainage of purulent or obstructing material to the unaffected dependent lung might create a more global problem. Position can also affect oxygenation by changing venous return and filling pressures.

Pulmonary vascular resistance and distribution of blood flow can also be increased by positive airway pressure changes in lung volume either above or below FRC.[133] Positive pressure lung inflation can increase resistance in both intra-alveolar and extra-alveolar vessels, whereas spontaneous "negative pressure" inspiration probably decreases extra-alveolar vascular resistance. A reduction in dependent lung volume can decrease capillary transmural pressure gradients and may promote an increase in dependent vascular resistance. The resulting decreases in blood flow could cause an improvement in V/Q matching, because ventilation is also decreased in the dependent lung. However, redistribution of blood flow to nondependent lung might also worsen matching. The net effects of changes in lung volume on V/Q matching are difficult to predict.

Postoperative V/Q matching is affected by various medications. Inhalational anesthetics or sympathomimetics can markedly alter pulmonary arterial and venous pressure and can change the distribution of pulmonary blood flow.[134] Anesthetic drugs may also affect pulmonary vascular tone directly. Nitrous oxide, ketamine, and pentazocine may cause pulmonary vascular constriction, whereas pentolinium, phentolamine, and nitroprusside appear to cause pulmonary vasodilation. Inhalational anesthetics and nitroprusside also significantly impair hypoxic pulmonary vasoconstriction,[135] at least partially explaining a well-documented increase in alveolar-arterial oxygen gradient associated with general anesthesia. (Changes in lung volume and distribution of ventilation probably also contribute.) The effects of anesthetics on hypoxic pulmonary vasoconstriction persist well into recovery. Other ancillary medications such as antihypertensives and beta-mimetic drugs also probably interfere with V/Q matching and oxygenation.

Several other factors are suspected to interfere with postoperative V/Q matching. Circulating endotoxin can impair hypoxic pulmonary vasoconstriction, contributing to difficulties encountered in maintaining Pa_{O_2} in patients with systemic sepsis.[136] Patients with cirrhosis of the liver often exhibit poor V/Q matching and arterial hypoxemia,[137] perhaps caused by circulating humoral substances related to inappropriate hepatic metabolism. An increased $F_{I_{O_2}}$ has also been shown to interfere with V/Q matching in patients with acute lung disease. Whether this is due to interference with hypoxic pulmonary vasoconstriction or to resorption atelectasis is unclear.

Few therapeutic interventions are useful to improve V/Q matching by changing pulmonary blood flow. With respect to cardiovascular dynamics, maintenance of pulmonary artery pressure within acceptable limits will probably optimize V/Q matching. Positioning a patient to avoid placing severely diseased lung tissue in a dependent location occasionally improves oxygenation. Although eliminating beta-mimetic or vasodilatory medications may improve Pa_{O_2}, the therapeutic benefit of the medication usually outweighs the drawbacks of impaired hypoxic pulmonary vasoconstriction. In short, V/Q abnormalities are more easily resolved by improving the distribution of ventilation than by manipulating perfusion.

Inadequate Alveolar P_{O_2}

Occasionally, postoperative hypoxemia is caused by a global reduction in the alveolar partial pressure of oxygen (Pa_{O_2}), usually due to a ventilatory problem that interferes with delivery of fresh gas to alveoli. Whenever uptake of oxygen from alveoli exceeds delivery of oxygen, Pa_{O_2} and arterial oxygenation decreases. Many factors interfere with postoperative ventilation, causing variable degrees of respiratory acidemia. However, hypoventilation must be severe for hypoxemia to appear based solely on a reduction in oxygen delivery.

Hypoxemia can occur when severe hypoventilation is caused by respiratory center depression from excessive opioid administration. Significant arterial desaturation can also occur during periodic apnea or obstruction,[138] or because opiates and residual anesthetic levels interfere with hypoxic respiratory drive. Although rare, apnea caused by supplemental oxygen administered to patients with severe chronic obstructive pulmonary disease represents another example of hypoxemia related to hypoventilation. (Death in such circumstances is probably related more to progressive respiratory acidemia than to hypoxemia.)

Complete airway obstruction caused by foreign bodies, soft-tissue edema, or laryngospasm rapidly depletes alveolar oxygen, as do severe increases in airway resistance that preclude effective ventilation. However, partial obstruction or moderate increases in airway resistance do not usually interfere with ventilation enough to reduce Pa_{O_2}, especially in postoperative patients receiving supplemental oxygen. Increasing the oxygen content in the FRC to safeguard against hypoxemia from hypoventilation or airway obstruction is an excellent rationale for providing supplemental oxygen in the postoperative period.

Occasionally, excessive concentrations of a second gas in alveoli can reduce P_{AO_2} to a point that clinically significant hypoxemia occurs. For example, when relatively insoluble nitrous oxide is discontinued at the end of a general anesthetic, a very rapid outpouring of nitrous oxide from pulmonary arterial blood into alveoli causes volume displacement of alveolar gas.[139] High alveolar partial pressures of nitrous oxide can lower P_{AO_2} to dangerous levels, especially if a patient is hypoventilating or breathing ambient air. The danger of this "diffusion hypoxia" can be minimized by administration of 100% oxygen during emergence to dilute alveolar nitrous oxide and maintain P_{AO_2} within acceptable limits. Volume displacement of oxygen by carbon dioxide can also occur if severe hypoventilation markedly elevates P_{CO_2} in a patient breathing ambient air, although severe respiratory acidemia is usually more significant than hypoxemia.

Reduced Mixed Venous Po2

Systemic mixed venous partial pressure of oxygen (P_{vo_2}) is affected by arterial oxygen content, cardiac output, and tissue oxygen extraction. If Pao_2 decreases or tissue extraction increases, P_{vo_2} may fall, depending on the proportional contributions of different tissue beds. Venous blood with low P_{vo_2} that is shunted or distributed to low V/Q units causes a larger decrease in Pao_2 than if P_{vo_2} were normal. A reduction in P_{vo_2} therefore amplifies the impact of shunt or V/Q mismatch on Pao_2. A reduction in P_{vo_2} also necessitates extraction of larger volumes of oxygen from alveolar gas in order to saturate hemoglobin. Increased extraction might gradually reduce Pao_2 if hypoventilation or airway obstruction reduces the delivery of fresh gas. Supplemental oxygen will attenuate the exaggerated impact of low V/Q units on Pao_2 and offset the reduction in Pao_2 caused by increased alveolar extraction. Very low P_{vo_2} can also increase the risk of resorption atelectasis in poorly ventilated alveoli. In the PACU, shivering, infection, or hypermetabolism can significantly increase peripheral oxygen extraction and lower P_{vo_2}. A reduction in cardiac output and/or systemic blood pressure caused by hypovolemia, myocardial depression, or arteriolar dilation can also lower P_{vo_2} by decreasing tissue oxygen delivery. However, the actual impact of a reduced P_{vo_2} is usually small, if recovering patients at risk for V/Q mismatching are placed on supplemental oxygen.

Aspiration

When upper airway reflexes are ineffective during induction of anesthesia or recovery, aspiration can generate postoperative pulmonary morbidity of varying severity, depending on the type and volume of the aspirate. Although aspiration of gastric contents is most widely feared, surgical patients are also at risk for other aspiration syndromes.

Aspiration of clear oral secretions during induction of anesthesia, face mask ventilation of the lungs, or extubation of the trachea is undoubtedly common and of relatively minor significance. Cough, mild tracheal irritation, and transient laryngospasm are usual sequelae, although chronic or large-volume aspiration might predispose to small airway obstruction, infection, or pulmonary edema. Aspiration of blood secondary to trauma, epistaxis, or surgical manipulations in the oropharynx or large airways often generates frightening changes on the chest radiograph that are far

out of proportion with clinical symptoms. Aspirated "sterile" blood causes minor airway obstruction but is rapidly cleared from air spaces by resorption and phagocytotic processes. Massive blood aspiration severely impedes gas exchange and causes pulmonary hemochromatosis from iron accumulation in phagocytic cells. Accumulation of fibrinous material in air spaces can also occur. Secondary infection is always a threat, especially if bits of tissue, purulent matter, or foreign bodies are also aspirated.

Aspiration of solid foreign matter (unswallowed food, small objects, pieces of teeth or dental appliances) can cause persistent cough, diffuse reflex bronchospasm, airway obstruction with distal atelectasis, and pneumonia. Unless airway obstruction is massive and life-threatening, complications are often localized to a small portion of lung and are easily treated with antibiotics and supportive pulmonary care once the foreign matter has been expelled or removed by bronchoscopy. Secondary thermal, chemical, or traumatic airway injury from aspiration of hot, caustic, or sharp objects can cause more significant damage and may require later surgical intervention.[140]

Aspiration of acidic gastric contents during vomiting or regurgitation causes a serious chemical pneumonitis characterized initially by diffuse bronchospasm, hypoxemia, and atelectasis. The subsequent airway epithelial degeneration, interstitial and alveolar edema, and hemorrhage into air spaces rapidly progress to adult respiratory distress syndrome with high permeability pulmonary edema. Destruction and sloughing of Type I and II pneumocytes, decreased surfactant activity, accumulation of fibrinous exudates, hyaline membrane formation, and destruction of parenchyma with atelectasis or emphysematous changes can all occur after severe aspiration, leading to V/Q mismatching and marked reductions in compliance. Occlusion or destruction of pulmonary microvasculature is often evident, causing increased pulmonary vascular resistance, pulmonary arterial pressure, and V_D/V_T. The severity and eventual resolution of pathologic changes depend on both the volume and the pH of the aspirate.[141] The morbidity sharply increases when the pH of the aspirate is below 2.0–2.5. Aspiration of fluid with a pH greater than 2.5 is less damaging but still interferes with surfactant activity and disrupts cellular function through osmotic or chemical interactions.[142] Morbidity also increases with acid aspirate volumes greater than 0.4–1.0 $ml \cdot kg^{-1}$. The presence of partially digested food in aspirate worsens and prolongs aspiration pneumonitis. Food particles cause mechanical airway obstruction and serve as a nidus for secondary bacterial infection. Aspirated vegetable matter is particularly resistant to phagocytosis and causes a chronic granulomatous process resembling that caused by miliary tuberculosis.[143]

The risk of aspiration is particularly high in surgical patients, so a high degree of caution is necessary.[144] Interference with protective airway reflexes by muscle relaxants and central depressant medications (inhalational anesthetics, barbiturates, opiates) is the greatest risk factor for perioperative aspiration. Recovery of sufficient neuromuscular function to sustain spontaneous ventilation does not necessarily indicate that airway protection is restored.[145] Airway trauma, laryngeal nerve blocks, or complications of regional anesthetic placement (seizure, high spinal, cervical plexus involvement) also seriously compromise airway reflexes.

Large volumes of intragastric food and fluid in patients requiring emergency surgery increases the risk of aspiration. Delayed gastric emptying caused by ileus, bowel obstruction, pain, anxiety, opioid administration, salt depletion, or peristaltic abnormalities accentuate gastric accumulation. Pregnant or morbidly obese patients have increased gastric volume and acidity, as well as interference with gastroesophageal sphincter function secondary to mechanical displacement.[146] Hiatal hernia, achalasia, esophageal diverticuli or tumors, amyotrophic lateral sclerosis, and other abnormalities affecting gastroesophageal function or swallowing also increase the risk of regurgitation and aspiration.

Preventing aspiration is critical, because the effectiveness of therapy is limited. A traditional recommendation is that surgery should be delayed for at least 8–12 hours to allow gastric emptying in patients considered to have a full stomach, even if a regional anesthetic technique is planned. In patients at risk for acid aspiration, administration of nonparticulate antacids such as sodium citrate will increase the pH of existing gastric fluid without producing an excessive increase in volume. Particulate antacids should be avoided because subsequent aspiration of the medication can cause chronic granulomatous reactions.[147] Administration of H_2 receptor blockers (cimetidine or ranitidine) reduces the rate of accumulation and increases the pH of subsequent secretions. The addition of metoclopramide increases gastroesophageal sphincter tone and accelerates gastric emptying.[148,149] The introduction of a nasogastric tube for gastric emptying is often ineffective in removing particulate matter and may interfere with gastroesophageal sphincter integrity.

The induction of general anesthesia in patients at risk for regurgitation and aspiration requires endotracheal intubation using an oral rapid sequence technique (oxygenation, cricoid pressure, obtundation, rapid paralysis without fasciculation, and oral intubation) or an awake oral or nasal approach. Wide-bore suction devices should always be available during any anesthetic induction. Once tracheal intubation has been achieved, every effort should be made to empty gastric contents. The presence of an endotracheal tube does not preclude aspiration of acidic fluid around an inflated cuff.[150] Frequent pharyngeal suctioning helps guard against silent aspiration. One should avoid cuff deflation in intubated patients because the rigid tube holds the vocal cords open, increasing the risk of serious aspiration. If deflation is necessary, the time should be minimized.

The risk of aspiration persists in the PACU. The incidence of postoperative nausea and emesis is significant, especially with accumulation of gas in the stomach. Hypotension, hypoxemia, acidemia, or other serious postoperative complications can also cause both emesis and obtundation, increasing the risk of serious aspiration. During emergence from general anesthesia, the function and integration of protective reflexes are often marginal. Persisting effects of laryngeal nerve blocks, topical local anesthetics, or other intraoperative interventions used to reduce airway irritability will decrease postoperative airway protection. Residual neuromuscular paralysis reduces the patient's ability to generate laryngospasm or cough. The trachea of patients at high risk of aspiration should not be extubated until complete restoration of airway reflexes is ensured. Care must be exercised to completely suction the pharynx and extubate the trachea at end-inspiration or with positive airway pressure to avoid aspiration of material trapped below the vocal cords but above an inflated endotracheal tube cuff.

Anatomic distortion can mechanically interfere with airway protection and clearance in patients with mandibular fractures or soft-tissue trauma. Mandibular fixation makes expulsion of vomitus, blood, or secretions from the mouth almost impossible, so equipment for immediate release of fixation should be at hand throughout the postoperative period. Patients recovering with mandibular fixation should demonstrate cognitive and physical ability to clear the airway before the trachea is extubated. Careful observation is essential after tracheal extubation because airway reflexes can be temporarily ineffective after prolonged intubation.

In any patient, the appearance of gastric secretions in the pharynx mandates immediate lateral head positioning (assuming cervical spine integrity), clearance by suction, and endotracheal intubation if airway reflexes are absent or compromised. (Although the Trendelenburg position may promote regurgitation, head-down positioning aids in clearance of secretions once regurgitation or vomiting has occurred. Head elevation should be avoided in obtunded patients, for it establishes a gravitational gradient from pharynx to lung and makes airway management difficult.) After tracheal intubation, suctioning the trachea through the endotracheal tube prior to instituting positive pressure ventilation is critical to avoid widely disseminating aspirated material to distal airways. Instillation of saline or alkalotic solutions is not recommended. Assessment of the pH in a tracheal aspirate is of little use because buffering is almost immediate. Determination of the pH in a pharyngeal aspirate is more reliable but of little practical value.

Suspicion of intraoperative or postoperative aspiration mandates careful observation over 24–48 hours for development of aspiration pneumonitis. Such observation includes serial temperature checks, white blood cell counts with differential, serial chest x-ray films, and blood gas determinations or pulmonary function testing if appropriate. Fluffy infiltrates may appear on the chest x-ray film immediately or within 24 hours of an event. Hypoxemia can develop quickly or evolve insidiously as lung pathology progresses. Aggressive chest physiotherapy, incentive spirometry, and reinstitution of medications used to treat pre-existing pulmonary conditions will minimize the loss of lung volume, V/Q mismatching, and infection secondary to aspiration. If the likelihood of significant aspiration is small, follow-up may be done on an outpatient basis, assuming hypoxia, cough, wheezing, or chest x-ray abnormalities do not appear within 4–6 hours after the event.[151] However, the patient must be given explicit instructions to contact a medical facility at the first appearance of malaise, fever, cough, or other symptoms indicative of pneumonitis.

If significant aspiration causes hypoxemia, increased airway resistance, consolidation, or pulmonary edema, institution of support with supplemental oxygen, PEEP or CPAP, and mechanical ventilation is often necessary. The criteria for selection of therapy are similar to those for treatment of ARDS. Pulmonary edema is usually secondary to increased capillary permeability and should not be treated with diuretics to decrease intravascular volume unless high filling pressures or hypervolemia exist. In fact, hypovolemia from fluid losses into the lung after aspiration can necessitate aggressive fluid management. Although still controversial, the administration of high-dose steroids probably yields little real benefit or improvement of long-term outcome after aspiration. Because bacterial infection is not necessarily a component of aspiration pneumonitis, prophylactic antibiotic administration merely promotes colonization by resistant organisms. If evidence of secondary bacterial infection appears, specific antibiotic therapy should be instituted, based on sputum samples obtained for Gram stain and culture. If culture results cannot be obtained or are equivocal, broad-spectrum antibiotics should be chosen, with coverage for gram-negative rods and anaerobes, including *Bacteroides fragilis*.[152,153]

POSTOPERATIVE RENAL COMPLICATIONS

Monitoring Renal Function

Evaluation of renal function in the PACU is important to reduce postoperative morbidity, especially in patients with marginal cardiovascular status or underlying renal disease. The ability to void spontaneously should be routinely recorded for all recovering patients, because the sympatholytic or parasympathomimetic effects of regional anesthetics or opioids interfere with sphincter relaxation and promote urine retention. Patients with indwelling catheters should have urine output recorded hourly. Using urine output as an index of intravascular volume status or renal viability can be misleading because surgical and anesthetic factors cause osmotic diuresis or interfere with renal regulatory mechanisms in postoperative patients.

Postoperative analysis of urine character can yield valuable information concerning renal tubular function.[154] Urine color is relatively useless for estimating renal concentrating ability but can signal hematuria, hemoglobinuria, or pyuria. Urine osmolarity (affected by the number of particles in solution) is a more reliable index of tubular function than is specific gravity, which varies with molecular weight. An osmolarity greater than 450 $mOsm \cdot l^{-1}$ indicates a reasonable tubular concentrating ability. (Inorganic fluoride ions released during metabolism of potent inhalational anesthetics such as enflurane will cause a transient, reversible decrease in maximum concentrating ability.) A urine sodium concentration far below or a urine potassium concentration above serum concentrations also indicates renal tubular viability. Osmolarity and electrolyte values close to those in serum may indicate poor tubular function related to acute tubular necrosis. Evaluation of urine pH is also useful, as acidification or alkalinization of urine requires intact tubular function.

Oliguria

Oliguria (<0.5 $ml \cdot kg^{-1} \cdot h^{-1}$) occurs frequently during recovery, usually reflecting an appropriate kidney response to perceived hypovolemia or systemic hypotension. However, a decreased urine output occasionally indicates a critical abnormality of renal function. The acceptable degree and duration of oliguria vary with the patient's underlying renal status, the surgical procedure, and the anticipated postoperative course. Oliguria in patients who have experienced surgical manipulations or intraoperative events that might jeopardize renal function (possible ureteral ligature, aortic cross-clamping, severe hypotension, massive transfusion) must be aggressively evaluated. When assessing low urine output in uncatheterized patients, the urge to void, bladder fullness, and interval since last voiding should be checked to differentiate between inability to void and oliguria. Catheterization is sometimes necessary. Indwelling urinary catheters should be checked for patency, since obstruction from kinking, blood clots, or debris mimics oliguria, as can positions such as the Trendelenburg position that force the catheter tip above the urine level in the bladder.

Ensuring that systemic pressure is adequate for renal perfusion (based on preoperative pressures) is critical in an oliguric patient. To assess whether oliguria represents a renal response to hypovolemia, a 300–500 ml iv crystalloid bolus should be given after urine is sent for electrolyte and osmolarity determinations, even if intraoperative fluid replacement seems adequate. If output does not improve after fluid infusion, one might consider a larger bolus or a diagnostic trial of 5 mg of furosemide. Furosemide interferes with tubular resorption and increases urine output if oliguria is caused by retention of fluid by the kidneys. Patients on chronic diuretic therapy who might require diuretic effect to maintain brisk postoperative urine output will also usually respond to a furosemide challenge.

The persistence of oliguria despite an adequate perfusion pressure, hydration, and a small furosemide challenge increases the possibility of acute tubular necrosis, renal artery or vein occlusion, ureteral obstruction, or inappropriate antidiuretic hormone secretion. Preoperative administration of desmopressin for hematologic purposes seldom has any significant effect on postoperative urinary output. Cystoscopy, intravenous pyelography, angiography, or radionuclide scintigraphy may help clarify renal status, whereas pulmonary artery catheterization can clarify cardiovascular function. Administration of osmotic or loop diuretics and low-dose dopamine or dobutamine is probably useful to attenuate renal damage.[155,156]

Polyuria

Profuse postoperative urine output is a common occurrence, usually related to generous intraoperative fluid administration. However, sustained polyuria ($>4–5$ $ml \cdot kg^{-1} \cdot h^{-1}$) can indicate abnormal regulation of water clearance, especially if urinary losses compromise intravascular volume and systemic blood pressure.

Osmotic diuresis caused by hyperglycemia and glycosuria is a frequent cause of postoperative polyuria. Output can be massive if glucose-containing crystalloid solutions are used to replace urinary losses. The diagnosis is made by urine and serum glucose determination. Therapy other than glucose restriction is unnecessary because the process is self-limited. Polyuria might also reflect the persistent effects of intraoperative diuretic administration. Polyuria related to diabetes insipidus can occur secondary to intracranial surgery, pituitary ablation, head trauma, increased intracranial pressure, or inadvertent omission of preoperative vasopressin administration. The diagnosis is made by comparing urine and serum electrolytes and osmolarity. Diagnostic or therapeutic administration of vasopressin can also be useful.[33] The possibility of high output renal failure should also be considered.

METABOLIC COMPLICATIONS

Postoperative Acid-Base Disorders

The categorization of postoperative acid-base disorders into discrete primary and compensatory abnormalities is often difficult because the rapid evolution of pathophysiology often generates two or more primary disorders. Appropriate hemodynamic, ventilatory, and metabolic support will usually restore postoperative acid-base homeostasis.

Respiratory Acidemia

Respiratory acidemia is frequently encountered in the PACU because inhalational anesthetic agents, narcotics, and sedative medications promote hypoventilation by decreasing CNS sensitivity to pH. In awake, spontaneously breathing PACU patients receiving adequate postoperative analgesia, hypercarbia and acidemia are usually mild ($Paco_2$ of

45–50 mm Hg). However, without supplemental ventilation or reversal of ventilatory depression, anesthetized or deeply sedated patients can suffer serious acidemia. Compensation for acute respiratory acidemia is limited because the kidneys require many hours to generate a compensatory metabolic alkalosis.

Some postoperative patients are unable to sustain adequate ventilation in spite of an appropriate CNS drive to ventilate. Residual neuromuscular paralysis, increased airway resistance, or decreased pulmonary compliance can severely impede ventilation and generate progressive respiratory acidemia, especially if dead space is increased. Elevated carbon dioxide production caused by shivering, fever, hyperalimentation, or malignant hyperthermia will amplify the problem.[92,93]

Respiratory acidemia causes agitation, confusion, ventilatory dissatisfaction, and tachypnea. Hypertension, tachycardia, and dysrhythmias secondary to increased SNS activity can increase the risk of myocardial ischemia, postoperative bleeding, or cerebrovascular accident. (Respiratory acidemia caused by CNS depression often produces less intense signs of SNS activity because central autonomic responses are also depressed.) At very low pH, the interaction of catecholamines with adrenergic receptors becomes ineffective, and heart rate and blood pressure can decrease precipitously. Respiratory acidemia also increases cerebral blood flow and intracranial pressure in patients with head injury, intracranial tumor, or cerebral edema.

Therapy is directed toward correcting the imbalance between carbon dioxide production and effective alveolar ventilation. Arousal, reversal of opioids or neuromuscular relaxants, relief of airway obstruction, or improvement of ventilatory mechanics and airway resistance are useful measures. If spontaneous ventilation cannot maintain carbon dioxide elimination, tracheal intubation and mechanical ventilation are necessary. Reducing carbon dioxide production by eliminating high glucose loads or controlling fever, shivering, and the work of breathing may be helpful, but extreme measures such as core cooling or paralysis are seldom appropriate in the PACU setting.

Metabolic Acidemia

The differential diagnosis of acute metabolic acidemia is relatively straightforward. Patients suffering from renal failure, renal tubular acidosis, or small bowel drainage are usually identified by history and exhibit a preoperative metabolic acidemia. An overdose of phenformin, aspirin, or methanol can also increase metabolic acid, but such cases are rare. Postoperative metabolic acidemia is occasionally caused by ketoacidosis is severe diabetics. Serum glucose levels are usually elevated, and ketones are detectable in blood or urine.

Once a pre-existing metabolic problem and ketoacidosis are excluded, postoperative metabolic acidemia almost always represents lactic acid accumulation secondary to insufficient delivery or utilization of oxygen in peripheral tissues. Hypotension leading to peripheral hypoperfusion is often caused by low cardiac output (hypovolemia, cardiac failure, dysrhythmia) or decreased SVR (sepsis, catecholamine depletion, sympathectomy). Intense arteriolar constriction from severe hypothermia or inappropriate pressor administration can reduce perfusion to tissues, as can inappropriate distribution of blood flow. Hypoxemia, decreased oxygen-carrying capacity of blood (severe anemia, carbon monoxide poisoning), interference with release of oxygen from hemoglobin (alkalemia, hypothermia), or inability to utilize oxygen in the mitochondria (cyanide or arsenic poisoning) may also generate lactic acidemia.

In a spontaneously breathing patient with an intact ventilatory drive, generation of a respiratory alkalosis to compensate for postoperative metabolic acidemia is rapid, but anesthetic agents interfere with ventilatory response.[157] The sympathetic response to acute metabolic acidemia is often somewhat milder than the response to respiratory acidemia because hydrogen and bicarbonate ions cross the blood-brain barrier with more difficulty than carbon dioxide.

Therapy should be directed toward the condition causing the accumulation of metabolic acid. Ketoacidosis is treated with iv insulin, potassium, and sometimes glucose. If lactic acidemia is mild and conditions causing lactate accumulation are improving, acidemia will resolve spontaneously through acid metabolism and renal excretion of hydrogen ions. Improvement of cardiac output or systemic blood pressure can reduce lactic acid production, as can rewarming. If acidemia is severe or progressive, iv administration of bicarbonate or a suitable substitute is useful to maintain the pH near normal.

Respiratory Alkalemia

Excessive operative pain or anxiety during emergence from anesthesia commonly causes hyperventilation and acute respiratory alkalemia in the PACU. Pain from clumsy attempts at arterial blood gas sampling can generate a spurious alkalemia. Excessive mechanical ventilation frequently causes postoperative respiratory alkalemia, especially when hypothermia or paralysis decreases carbon dioxide production. Pathologic causes of "central" hyperventilation include sepsis, cerebrovascular accident, or paradoxical CNS acidosis (an imbalance of bicarbonate concentration across the blood-brain barrier caused by prolonged mechanical hyperventilation).

Acute respiratory alkalemia can generate confusion or dizziness, atrial dysrhythmias, or mild cardiac conduction abnormalities. If the alkalemia is severe, a reduction in serum ionized calcium ion concentration can precipitate muscle fasciculation or hypocalcemic tetany. In patients with cerebrovascular disease, alkalemia can decrease cerebral blood flow, causing hypoperfusion and even stroke. Very high pH levels will directly depress cardiovascular, CNS, and catecholamine receptor function.

Metabolic compensation for acute respiratory alkalemia is very limited, again because renal time constants for bicarbonate excretion are large. The addition of carbon dioxide to inspired gases or rebreathing of exhaled carbon dioxide have little clinical application in the PACU. The correction of respiratory alkalemia necessitates reducing the effective alveolar ventilation, usually by administration of analgesics and sedatives to control pain and anxiety.

Metabolic Alkalemia

Metabolic alkalemia is rare in PACU patients unless alkalemia from prolonged vomiting, gastric suctioning, dehydration, or administration of alkaline substances or potassium-wasting diuretics existed prior to surgery. Excessive intraoperative bicarbonate administration will cause postoperative metabolic alkalemia, but alkalemia caused by large infusions of sodium lactate or citrate in blood products usually does not appear within the first 24 hours.

Respiratory compensation for metabolic alkalemia through retention of carbon dioxide is rapid but somewhat limited since hypoventilation beyond a certain point causes hypoxemia. Hydration and correction of hypochloremia and hypokalemia are important to allow the kidney to excrete excess bicarbonate. An iv hydrochloric acid drip is seldom necessary but can be effectively utilized through a central venous catheter to treat severe, life-threatening metabolic alkalemia.

Glucose Disorders

Repeated accurate serum glucose determination is far superior to urine glucose measurement for managing blood sugar abnormalities. However, urine glucose concentration can help assess osmotic diuretic effects and estimate renal transport (Tm) by comparison with serum levels.

Hyperglycemia

Glucose infusions and the stress response commonly elevate serum glucose levels in patients recovering from surgery.[158] In diabetic patients, hyperglycemia may indicate severe insulin deficiency and evolution of diabetic ketoacidosis. Moderate hyperglycemia (200–300 mg·dl^{-1}) usually resolves without treatment and probably has no significant effect on wound healing. Higher glucose levels cause glycosuria and osmotic diuresis and interfere with the accuracy of serum electrolyte determinations. Severe hyperglycemia can increase serum osmolality to a point that cerebral disequilibrium and "hyperosmolar coma" supervene. Treatment includes titration of iv regular insulin (in small incremental doses or by continuous infusion), allowing careful titration of blood glucose without the delay to peak effect associated with longer acting insulins or the potential uptake problems associated with subcutaneous administration. Potassium replacement and monitoring of serial blood glucose levels are essential.

Hypoglycemia

Hypoglycemia in the PACU can be caused by excessive or inadvertent insulin administration or by endogenous insulin secretion. Serious postoperative hypoglycemia is rare and easily treated by the iv administration of 50% dextrose followed by glucose infusion. Sedation or excessive SNS activity may mask signs and symptoms of hypoglycemia during recovery.

Electrolyte Disorders

Hyponatremia

Postoperative hyponatremia occurs if excess free water is inadvertently infused during surgery or if large amounts of sodium-free irrigating solution have been absorbed *via* prostatic venous sinuses during transurethral prostatic resection. Accumulation of serum glycine or its metabolite, ammonia, might exacerbate symptoms.[159-161] Free water retention can also be caused by inappropriate antidiuretic hormone secretion, prolonged induction of labor with oxytocin, and respiratory uptake of nebulized droplets. Symptoms include nausea, agitation, disorientation, and visual disturbances. Severe hyponatremia causes unconsciousness, decreased effectiveness of airway reflexes, and CNS irritability that can progress to grand mal seizures. Therapy includes infusion of normal saline and iv administration of furosemide to promote renal wasting of free water in excess

of sodium. Administration of hypertonic saline may be necessary to replace a calculated sodium deficit when hyponatremia is severe, but careful monitoring of serum sodium concentration and osmolality is essential.

Hypokalemia

Though usually inconsequential, postoperative hypokalemia can generate serious dysrhythmias, especially in patients taking digitalis preparations. A significant potassium deficit from chronic diuretic administration, prolonged nasogastric suctioning, or vomiting often underlies hypokalemia.[162] Intraoperative urinary and hemorrhagic losses, dilution during massive volume replacement, or insulin therapy often generate potassium deficits that can worsen acutely during an acute respiratory alkalemia. Hypokalemic patients should be closely observed during periods of excess SNS activity, and during infusion of calcium, insulin, or beta-mimetic medications.[163] The addition of supplemental potassium to iv fluids will usually restore an acceptable serum concentration, but infusion of concentrated solutions through a central catheter may be necessary in selected cases.

Hyperkalemia

Serious postoperative hyperkalemia can occur after inadvertent excessive potassium administration, or in patients with chronic renal failure or malignant hyperthermia.[162] Acute acidemia will exacerbate postoperative hyperkalemia.[164] Administration of succinylcholine for tracheal intubation in the PACU might increase serum potassium to dangerous levels in patients with burns, multiple trauma, or neurologic injuries. Treatment with iv insulin and glucose is efficacious in acutely lowering serum potassium level, while iv calcium can temporarily counter myocardial effects. Beta-mimetic medications might also have some role. Whenever a laboratory specimen reveals an unusually high serum potassium level with no apparent cause, one should suspect spurious hyperkalemia caused by a hemolyzed specimen or sampling near an iv line carrying potassium or banked blood.

Hypocalcemia

Massive fluid replacement or underlying parathyroid disease will cause a reduction in total body and ionized calcium, although symptomatic postoperative hypocalcemia seldom occurs. A further reduction in the critical ionized fraction by metabolic or respiratory alkalemia may cause myocardial conduction and contractility abnormalities, decreased vascular tone, or tetany. The administration of calcium chloride to hypocalcemic patients can improve cardiovascular dynamics and the response to iv fluid administration. Transfusion of blood containing chelating agents rarely causes symptomatic hypocalcemia, so routine administration of calcium is not warranted.

MISCELLANEOUS COMPLICATIONS

Nausea and Vomiting

Nausea and vomiting are common problems during emergence from general anesthesia, although the incidence varies dramatically with the patient's age, the surgical procedure, and the anesthetic technique and duration.[165-168]

Aside from unpleasantness for the patient and staff, vomiting poses genuine medical risks. Patients are at risk of aspirating gastric contents, especially if airway reflexes are marginal or after surgical procedures requiring postoperative oral fixation. Increased intra-abdominal pressure can jeopardize abdominal or inguinal suture lines, while an elevated central venous pressure might increase morbidity after ocular, tympanic, or intracranial procedures. SNS responses during emesis elevate heart rate and systemic blood pressure, increasing the risk of myocardial ischemia or dysrhythmias. Movement during vomiting accentuates the autonomic response by worsening postoperative pain. Gagging and retching can also elicit a parasympathetic response with consequent bradycardia and hypotension. Finally, postoperative vomiting often delays discharge or necessitates overnight admission of ambulatory patients, reducing the efficiency of services and patient satisfaction with anesthetic care.

A history of postoperative emesis or motion sickness predisposes to postoperative nausea. Starvation, the direct effects of anesthetics on chemotactic centers, autonomic imbalance, and postoperative pain all probably increase the incidence of postoperative nausea and vomiting.[169] Conditions that affect the gastroesophageal junction (obesity, hiatal hernia) may also increase the likelihood of emesis in the PACU. The risk of nausea is higher following surgical procedures involving extraocular muscle or middle ear manipulation, peritoneal or intestinal irritation, and testicular traction.[170,171] Swallowed blood or secretions promotes postoperative vomiting, as does accumulation of gas in the stomach from difficult face mask ventilation, nitrous oxide diffusion, or esophageal intubation. Undergoing a general anesthetic near menses increases the incidence of vomiting in women,[172] perhaps related to an increase in circulating E_2 estrogen levels.[173]

Regional anesthesia is associated with a lower incidence of postoperative vomiting than general anesthesia, although this difference probably narrows if parenteral narcotics are needed to control postoperative pain once a regional block has resolved. Some investigators have noted a decrease in postoperative vomiting when nitrous oxide is excluded from an anesthetic,[174,175] although this finding is still controversial.[176-178] The incidence of nausea does not appear to differ whether halothane, enflurane, or isoflurane is utilized for inhalational anesthesia.[179] However, barbiturate induction seems less offensive than ketamine or etomidate inductions, while induction with propofol may have a lower incidence still.[180] The administration of opioid analgesics probably increases the incidence of postoperative nausea when compared with "pure" inhalational techniques,[181,182] especially in ambulatory surgical patients. The administration of neostigmine for reversal of neuromuscular relaxants, or of physostigmine to counteract sedation, also increases the incidence of postoperative nausea.[183,184] Meperidine seems to generate a higher incidence of postoperative nausea than morphine. Using small doses of the shorter acting narcotics (e.g., fentanyl, 1–1.5 $\mu g \cdot kg^{-1}$; alfentanil, 6–8 $\mu g \cdot kg^{-1}$) in ambulatory patients may partially circumvent this problem. Supplementation with nonopioid analgesics may also decrease the incidence of nausea.

Several interventions have been evaluated for the prevention of postoperative nausea. Avoiding gastric distention and providing adequate postoperative analgesia are important, as is limiting postoperative vestibular stimulation by minimizing brisk head motion. Evacuation of stomach contents with an orogastric tube may decrease the incidence of postoperative emesis, although the routine use of this measure is questionable.[185,186] The antiemetic effect of iv droperidol has been extensively evaluated.[170,187-191] A majority of studies show that perioperative iv administration of droperidol decreases the incidence and severity of postoperative nausea, although the efficacy varies with different procedures and individual patients. If the total dosage is kept below 1–2 $\mu g \cdot kg^{-1}$ or 1.25 mg total dose in adults, droperidol should not prolong recovery time or cause excessive sedation. Giving additional droperidol iv for breakthrough nausea in the PACU is also effective, although sedation may delay the discharge of ambulatory patients. Droperidol has alpha-adrenergic blocking properties that can precipitate hypotension in hypovolemic patients. Transient extrapyramidal side-effects are infrequent and usually inconsequential.[192]

Administration of iv metoclopramide, alone or in combination with droperidol, probably decreases the incidence of postoperative vomiting without prolonging recovery time.[188,193-195] Whether metoclopramide merely affects gastric volume and emptying or has a central antiemetic action is unclear, but its use has been implicated in causing dysphoria.[196] Using iv scopolamine as an antiemetic causes unacceptable psychogenic reactions during recovery. Although transdermal scopolamine may have some benefit as a prophylactic agent, its low efficacy and its tendency to cause visual disturbances make it a poor substitute for other agents.[197-199] Ephedrine has been suggested to treat postoperative nausea related to ambulation or motion,[200,201] although its efficacy has been questioned.[202] Dimenhydrinate may also be effective for postoperative nausea.[203] Ondansetron, a new serotonin receptor blocker, may also prove to be an effective antiemetic for postoperative nausea, but its effectiveness compared with that of droperidol still needs to be established.[204,205] Acupuncture stimulation or acupressure may reduce the incidence of postoperative vomiting.[206]

Prior to instituting treatment, it is always important to consider more serious causes of nausea and emesis such as hypotension, increased intracranial pressure, hypoxemia, hypoglycemia, or gastric bleeding.

Incidental Trauma

Anesthetized patients are at risk for incidental trauma from positioning, equipment, and nonsurgical manipulations. Corneal injury from drying or inadvertent eye contact during face mask ventilation or intubation causes tearing, decreased visual acuity, pain, and photophobia in the PACU. Fluoroscein staining is useful for diagnosis. Abrasion usually heals spontaneously within 72 hours without permanent scarring, but severe injury can cause cataract formation and impair vision. Treatment with artificial tears and eye closure is primarily symptomatic.[207]

Laryngoscopy, indwelling airways, or biting frequently generate soft-tissue trauma in the mouth. Lip, tongue, or gum abrasions heal quickly and require only an icepack for treatment, but penetrating injuries caused by entrapment of tissue between teeth and the laryngoscope blade or airway may require treatment with topical antibiotics. After a traumatic or difficult tracheal intubation, the possibility of upper airway edema or hematoma must be considered prior to extubation. Airway edema may improve after administration of nebulized racemic epinephrine. A dental consultation should be obtained if loosened or broken teeth or dental appliances are discovered, and the patient should be evaluated later for signs of aspiration such as fever and cough.

Sore throat and hoarseness after endotracheal intubation

occur in 20–50% of patients, depending on the degree of trauma incurred during laryngoscopy and oropharyngeal suctioning, the duration of tracheal intubation, and the type of tube.[208-211] Mucosal irritation often manifests with a sensation of unquenchable dryness in mouth and throat. The use of local anesthetic ointments to lubricate endotracheal tubes probably does not appreciably decrease the incidence of this problem and may cause additional irritation to tracheal mucosa.[212] Topical viscous lidocaine attenuates irritation from indwelling nasogastric tubes during recovery, but the risk of aspiration secondary to interference with reflexes must be balanced against benefit. The severity of postintubation laryngeal edema or tracheitis in children depends on age, intubation trauma, the duration of intubation, and coughing or positioning with an endotracheal tube in place.[213] Though most children recover with only cool mist therapy, administration of racemic epinephrine will significantly improve upper airway obstruction. Some authorities recommend administration of dexamethasone. Other traumatic complications of laryngoscopy and tracheal or esophageal intubation include hypoglossal, lingual, or recurrent laryngeal nerve damage, vocal cord evulsion, desquamation of laryngeal or tracheal mucosa, airway wall edema or ulceration, and tracheal perforation.[214,215] Some patients experience sore throat without tracheal intubation, caused by drying from unhumidified gases or trauma from oral airways and suctioning.

Compression injuries caused by improper positioning during general or regional anesthesia can generate serious long-term complications.[216] The clinician should carefully evaluate any complaint of pain, numbness, or weakness from a postoperative patient, for peripheral nerve compression against hard surfaces may cause sensory and motor deficits, as may stretch injuries from inadvertent hyperextension of an extremity.[217,218] Whenever pressure-related bruising or skin breakdown is noted, underlying nerve damage is also possible. Spinal cord injury during positioning for intubation of the trachea can occur, as can accumulation of compressive hematomas or nerve injury after placement of regional anesthetics. Retinal arterial or venous occlusion from ocular compression causes postoperative visual disturbances ranging from loss of acuity to permanent blindness. During long surgical procedures, ischemia and necrosis of soft tissue can occur, especially if pressure points are improperly padded. Prolonged scalp pressure may cause localized alopecia. Entrapment of breasts, genitalia, ears, skin folds, and other superficial soft tissues may cause necrosis, especially during lateral or prone positioning. Regional ischemia secondary to arterial pressure occlusion is possible, though rare. Excess intraoperative joint or muscle extension causes postoperative pain, stiffness, backache, and even joint instability if severe. Thermal, electrical, or chemical burns caused by cautery equipment, preparatory solutions, adhesives, or other substances occasionally occur. Extravasation of iv medications into tissues may cause severe sloughing or localized chemical neuropathy.

Each patient admitted to the PACU should be carefully evaluated for likely traumatic complications. Incidental injury also occurs in the PACU, especially with thrashing or disorientation during emergence. Dangers include bruising caused by contact with bed rails, hematoma or drug extravasation caused by dislocation of indwelling catheters, damage to dental appliances caused by biting on rigid airways, and corneal injury caused by rigid disposable face masks. The discovery or suspicion of a complication necessitates careful documentation, notification of primary physicians responsible for extended postoperative care, consultation with appropriate subspecialists, and assiduous follow-up.

Therapy for most incidental traumatic complications is supportive.

Skeletal Muscle Pain

Postoperative muscle pain is variable in degree and undoubtedly caused by a variety of intraoperative factors. Prolonged lack of motion or unusual muscle stretch during positioning often contribute to muscle stiffness and aching in the PACU. The administration of succinylcholine has been implicated in causing postoperative myalgias, perhaps related to fasciculation during depolarizing blockade.[219-221] Administration of a subparalyzing dose of nondepolarizing relaxant may reduce the incidence or severity of postoperative myalgia,[222] although this tactic is still controversial. Pretreatment with a "self-taming" dose of succinylcholine does not appear to have a protective effect. Acute myalgia also occurs with somewhat lower frequency after the administration of other relaxants and in patients receiving no relaxant whatsoever. Some patients complain of delayed-onset "muscle fatigue" that appears days after surgery and resolves spontaneously. The incidence, etiology, and importance of this problem are unclear.

Hypothermia and Shivering

Many patients undergoing surgery exhibit postoperative hypothermia. During general anesthesia, the temperature at which the body begins to actively regulate temperature (i.e., the thermoregulatory threshold) is decreased by approximately 2.5°C.[223] Core temperature falls as heat is lost through radiation and convection from the skin and surgical wound, and through evaporation during prepping and airway humidification of dry gases. Cooling is accelerated by low ambient temperatures and cold iv fluids. Once temperature reaches the thermoregulatory threshold, an adult patient's ability to maintain temperature is severely compromised. Paralysis and anesthesia impair shivering, and nonshivering thermogenesis is relatively ineffective in adults. Peripheral thermoregulatory vasoconstriction decreases heat loss[224] but is less effective in anesthetized patients. The amount or rate of heat loss is approximately the same during general and regional anesthesia, but patients receiving regional anesthetics rewarm more slowly because residual vasodilation and paralysis of striated musculature interfere with heat generation and retention. Elderly, cachectic, traumatized, or burned patients are prone to serious reduction of core body temperature. Infants are at increased risk of intraoperative hypothermia because their body mass is relatively small compared with surface area. Hypothermic patients often exhibit increased SNS activity, elevated peripheral vascular resistance, decreased venous capacitance, and hypertension in the PACU.

Hypothermia can increase the risk of postoperative morbidity.[225] Hypoperfusion of peripheral tissues promotes tissue hypoxia and metabolic acidemia, and jeopardizes the viability of marginal tissue grafts. Vasoconstriction can decrease the diagnostic reliability of pulse oximetry, intra-arterial pressure monitoring, and peripheral nerve stimulation. The avidity of hemoglobin for oxygen increases because hypothermia affects both pH and oxygen dissociation, contributing to poor oxygenation of hypothermic tissues. Reduced perfusion and decreased drug biotransformation might increase the duration of action of neuromuscular relaxants, sedatives, or hypnotics. The MAC of inhalational anesthetics decreases approximately 5–7% per 1°C decrease in core temperature, accentuating sedation from residual alveolar partial pressures in the PACU. Moderate hyperglycemia is common, and mild coagulopathy can occur secondary to visceral sequestration of platelets, decreased platelet function, and reduced activity of clotting factors. Severe hypothermia interferes with cardiac rhythm generation and impulse conduction. PR, QRS, or QT intervals can lengthen, and J waves can appear on the ECG. The danger of ectopic impulse generation and dysrhythmia during mechanical stimulation of the myocardium is increased. Spontaneous ventricular fibrillation can occur if temperature falls below 28°C.

During emergence from general anesthesia, hypothalamic regulating mechanisms increase metabolic activity and generate shivering in order to increase endogenous heat production. Postoperative shivering is uncomfortable, increases the risk of incidental trauma, and makes routine postoperative care more difficult to deliver. Severe shivering can increase peripheral oxygen consumption and carbon dioxide production by 200–300%, requiring augmented cardiac output and minute ventilation. Myocardial ischemia or ventilatory failure can supervene in patients with coronary artery disease or limited ventilatory reserve. The intensity of postoperative shivering is sometimes accentuated by inhalational anesthetic–related tremor, which has both clonic and tonic components.[226] The clonic component may be related to lack of cortical influence on spinal cord reflexes but is triggered by hypothermia,[227] while the tonic component probably reflects normal shivering. The administration of morphine, meperidine, droperidol, chlorpromazine, magnesium sulfate, or methylphenidate has been advocated to suppress shivering if dangerous cardiopulmonary stress occurs.[228-230] Withholding reversal of intraoperative neuromuscular relaxants in intubated, ventilated patients can also attenuate postoperative shivering, although rewarming time is increased. The wisdom of administering additional relaxants during recovery just to eliminate shivering is questionable.

Covering the patient's body and head surfaces and warming of ambient air, iv fluids, and irrigating solutions during surgery is useful to maintain body temperature. The use of surface or radiant warmers or heated humidification of inspired gases will also help. Most patients suffer an intraoperative reduction of core temperature of less than 2° to 3°C and spontaneously rewarm during routine recovery, although moderate shivering often occurs. Patients undergoing prolonged, major surgical procedures with significant fluid replacement can arrive in the PACU with marked hypothermia. Temperature below 35°C is an indication for assisted rewarming using radiant lighting,[231] heating blankets, forced air,[232] reflective coverings, or heated nebulization of inspired gas for intubated patients.[233] All hypothermic patients should receive supplemental oxygen. As the temperature rises, patients must be carefully observed for hypotension related to increasing venous capacitance and for "posthypothermic" hyperthermia. The resolution of metabolic acidemia usually accompanies rewarming, although bicarbonate administration may be needed after prolonged hypothermia.

Hyperthermia

Elevation of core body temperature above normal is relatively uncommon in the PACU. Occasionally, a patient will be admitted with self-limited hyperthermia secondary to close draping and aggressive heat preservation in the operating room. Acute postoperative fever is often caused by exacerbation of an existing infection by the surgical procedure (e.g., resection of infected tonsils or appendix, abscess drainage, urinary tract manipulation) or by emergence of an unrelated, previously asymptomatic condition (e.g., influenza, sinusitis, otitis, upper respiratory or urinary tract infection). Atelectasis and mild pneumonitis secondary to intraoperative loss of lung volume or retention of secretions is another frequent cause. Unrecognized intraoperative aspiration will also sometimes present with fever. An elevated temperature is a frequent manifestation of a drug or transfusion reaction, so one should carefully assess the medications and blood products a patient has received, especially those which bear a temporal relationship to the onset of fever. The intraoperative administration of muscarinic blocking agents like atropine can interfere with a patient's ability to cool and can contribute to postoperative fever. Certainly fever will occur during an episode of malignant hyperthermia, but other signs such as muscle rigidity, dysrhythmia, extremes of ventilation, and acidemia will usually establish the diagnosis before marked temperature elevation occurs. One must also consider other rare causes of hypermetabolism like thyroid storm.

Therapy for fever in the PACU setting is generally supportive. Ambient cooling, aggressive chest physiotherapy, incentive spirometry, and appropriate administration of antipyretics is usually sufficient. If a drug or transfusion reaction is suspected, the offending medication or blood product should be withheld. The primary physician responsible for the patient's long-term care should be notified to ensure that persisting fever does not signal a serious underlying complication and that therapeutic measures are continued beyond the PACU. Therapy for malignant hyperthermia or thyroid storm is well described elsewhere.

Persistent Sedation

The evaluation and treatment of prolonged unconsciousness after anesthesia requires an organized approach. The level of preoperative responsiveness must be assessed to rule out the possibility of unrecognized intoxication with drugs or alcohol, or pre-existing mental dysfunction. The time of administration and the amount of all preoperative and intraoperative sedative medications should be noted, and unusual intraoperative events should be reviewed. When an obtunded patient is examined in the PACU, assessment of level of consciousness should include a firm tactile stimulus, which is often more effective than verbal stimulation to elicit arousal. The rate and character of spontaneous ventilation can help indicate residual anesthesia depth. The diagnostic value of pupillary size and response is questionable. Evaluation of heart rate, rhythm, and systemic blood pressure can indicate the adequacy of cerebral perfusion and the prevailing level of autonomic tone.

Residual sedation from anesthetic medications is the most frequent cause of somnolence in the PACU.[234] Prolonged unconsciousness from inhalational anesthetics is more likely after long surgical procedures, in obese patients, or when high inspired concentrations are continued through the end of surgery to facilitate a "deep" extubation. Sedation caused by intraoperative narcotic or sedative administration is generally dose related. Long-acting sedatives used for premedication or intraoperative sedation (e.g., pentobarbital, hydroxyzine, promethazine, droperidol, lorazepam, scopolamine) contribute to postoperative somnolence. Even in patients who are susceptible to sedation, a response to stimulus should be obtainable within 60–90 minutes after a reasonably conducted anesthesia. If unconsciousness persists, low-dose iv naloxone (0.04-mg increments every 2 minutes, up to 0.2 mg) can be administered to reverse a potential sedative effect of intraoperative opioids. With careful titration of naloxone, respiratory depression and sedation can be reversed without precipitating dangerous reversal of analgesia. Unless a patient has received a massive narcotic overdose, 0.2 mg of iv naloxone will generate an increase in ventilatory rate and arousal if unconsciousness is related to residual opioids effect. The iv administration of physostigmine (1.25 mg) will sometimes counteract sedation caused by inhalational anesthetics and other sedative medications.[235] If a response is not obtained after administration of naloxone and physostigmine, it is still possible that a preoperative overdose with depressant oral drugs is responsible for prolonged sedation. Administration of flumazenil, a new competitive benzodiazepine antagonist, may prove useful to reverse sedation from midazolam and diazepam,[236-238] although its duration of action is relatively short compared with the sedative effects of the benzodiazepines.

Profound residual neuromuscular paralysis might mimic unconsciousness in the PACU by precluding a visible response to stimuli. This could occur after gross overdosage, if reversal agents are omitted, or in patients with unrecognized neuromuscular disease or phase II blockade caused by excessive succinylcholine administration or pseudocholinesterase deficiency. Observation of purposeful motion, spontaneous ventilation, reflex activity, or other evidence of neuromuscular function eliminates residual paralysis as an explanation for unresponsiveness.

Once the residual effects of anesthetic agents or neuromuscular relaxants have been eliminated, other causes of postoperative unresponsiveness should be considered. Patients who were exhausted before surgery often are difficult to arouse after anesthesia. This is especially true when normal sleep patterns are interrupted in children who have undergone emergency surgery at night. A patient may be feigning unresponsiveness. Hypothermia below 33°C can impair consciousness and accentuate the potency and duration of depressant medications. At core temperatures below 30°C, fixed dilation of pupils, absence of reflexes, and progressive evolution of coma can occur. Evaluation of serum glucose levels will eliminate severe hypoglycemia or hyperglycemic, hyperosmolar coma as causes. The suspicion that unresponsiveness may be caused by hypoglycemia is an indication for an immediate empirical trial of iv 50% dextrose. Iatrogenic hyposmolar states such as acute hyponatremia should be ruled out with evaluation of serum electrolyte concentrations and osmolarity. Arterial blood gas analysis will reveal whether severe hypercarbia and carbon dioxide narcosis or unrecognized hypoxemia underlie the coma.

If the diagnosis remains elusive, a thorough, carefully documented neurologic evaluation should be performed in consultation with a neurologist. Occasionally, unresponsiveness in the PACU represents subclinical grand mal seizures secondary to delirium tremens or an underlying seizure disorder. CNS depression secondary to iv local anesthetic toxicity or inadvertent subarachnoid injections can mimic postoperative coma.[239] Untoward intraoperative events such as severe hypotension, dysrhythmias, hypoxemia, or hypercarbia must be considered as potential causes of cerebral anoxia during surgery. The possibility of unrecognized head trauma and increasing intracranial pressure must be considered in injured patients. Intraoperative cerebral thromboembolism is another possibility, especially in patients recovering from cardiac, proximal major vascular, or invasive neck surgery,[240] or in those who have undergone internal jugular, subclavian, or intra-arterial cannulation. Patients with a history of atrial fibrillation, hemodynamically significant carotid bruits, or hypercoagulable states are also at increased risk of thromboembolism.[241] Paradoxical air embolism through a right-to-left intracardiac shunt, or intracerebral hemorrhage secondary to intraoperative hypertension, can also cause postoperative cerebrovascular accidents.[242] Postoperative cerebrovascular accidents in other patients are rare and usually occur later in the postoperative course.[243] Increased intracranial pressure from bleeding or edema must also be considered in patients recovering from intracranial surgery.

Altered Mental Status

On occasion, a recovering patient will exhibit inappropriate mental reactions ranging from lethargy and confusion through extreme disorientation and physical combativeness. Aside from the disturbance and upset these reactions cause to staff and other patients in the PACU, there are real risks associated with this problem. Forceful, thrashing movements of combative patients can jeopardize suture lines, orthopaedic fixations, vascular grafts, drains, tracheal tubes, and indwelling vascular catheters. The risk of incidental trauma increases, including the possibility of contusion or fracture from contact with equipment or side rails, corneal abrasion from dislodged oxygen apparatus, and sprains from violent struggling against restraints. Least appreciated is the risk of injury to PACU staff struggling to contain a combative patient. Agitated patients also manifest high levels of SNS tone with consequent tachycardia and hypertension, which can cause serious medical complications.

An adverse psychological response to emergence from general anesthesia is probably the most frequent cause of emergence reactions. For a short period after consciousness is regained, many patients appear unable to process and react to sensory input appropriately. This lack of integration presents in different ways. Many patients exhibit somnolence, slight disorientation, and sluggish mental reactions that gradually clear, while others experience wide emotional swings such as uncontrollable weeping during emergence. On occasion, a patient will exhibit escalating combativeness in response to positioning and restraint.

It is difficult to predict accurately which patients will have emergence reactions. Extreme emergence reactions are more prevalent in children and young adults, while recovery of cognitive functions may be slower in the elderly.[244] Anxiety in young children is undoubtedly heightened by separation from the parents. Patients exhibiting personality aberrations preoperatively will generally exhibit those same aberrations during emergence. Individuals with mental retardation, clinically evident psychiatric disorders, organic brain dysfunctions, or hostile interactions preoperatively also have a higher frequency of emergence problems. Ethnic, cultural, and psychological differences among patients undoubtedly play some role.[245,246] A language barrier can accentuate an emergence reaction because reassuring input from PACU staff might not be understood. Inability to speak, owing to oral fixation or endotracheal intubation, can generate frustration or fear, which will exaggerate emergence reactions. The incidence of stormy emergence is probably higher after procedures such as breast or testicular biopsies, which are charged with anxiety and emotional significance.

Patients premedicated with long-acting sedatives or those taking psychogenic medications can exhibit clouded sensorium and disorientation in the PACU. Acute preoperative intoxication or postoperative withdrawal can elicit bizarre emergence behavior in patients who abuse alcohol, opioids, cocaine, or other drugs. Disorientation, paranoia, and combativeness have been well described after use of parenteral scopolamine as a premedication or antiemetic. Scopolamine-induced disorientation can be treated with iv physostigmine. Patients receiving long-term preoperative meperidine therapy or atropine premedication can also exhibit anticholinergic-induced postoperative delirium.[247,248] Ketamine can cause postoperative dysphoria and hallucination, although acute reactions are rare. The use of etomidate for induction contributes to restlessness.[249]

Surgical pain amplifies confusion, agitation, and aggressive behavior during emergence, so every effort should be made to ensure adequate postoperative analgesia early in the PACU course. Urinary bladder distention or gastric distention by entrapped gas also generates marked discomfort and agitation in an emerging patient, as do tight dressings, painful phlebotomy, or poor positioning. Discomfort from endotracheal or nasogastric tubes, urinary catheters, or infiltrated vascular catheters can be equally troublesome. Attending personnel should always check for unrecognized sources of pain such as corneal abrasion, entrapment of sensitive body parts, or small pieces of equipment left beneath a patient.

Nausea and dizziness are very distressing to an emerging patient, as is severe pruritus caused by medication reactions. Some patients will struggle vigorously during emergence to move up from a supine position into a more comfortable semisitting position. This is common in obese patients or in those with gastroesophageal reflux or pulmonary congestion. Inability to move can generate significant agitation during emergence. Patients will often fight vigorously against physical restraint until the restraint is relaxed. Even if ventilation is adequate, inadequate recovery from neuromuscular relaxation causes severe agitation during emergence and will elicit violent, uncoordinated motions that make a patient appear disoriented and combative. Lack of strength, a peculiar flapping nature of voluntary motion, and quantitative electrical nerve stimulation are helpful in the diagnosis.

Confusion, delirium, or combativeness after anesthesia can also indicate serious respiratory dysfunction. Moderate hypoxemia often manifests clinically with clouded mentation, disorientation, and agitation which is difficult to distinguish from that caused by pain in an emerging patient. Respiratory acidemia caused by airway obstruction or poor ventilatory mechanics also elicits profound agitation. (Hypercarbia caused by ventilatory center depression generates less agitation because higher CNS functions are also depressed.) Hypercarbia without coincident acidemia is generally asymptomatic unless mild carbon dioxide narcosis causes somnolence and disorientation.

Limitation of inspiratory volume by tight chest dressings, increased intra-abdominal pressure, gastric distention, or splinting gradually causes a vague dissatisfaction with lung inflation similar to air hunger. This problem is also seen in patients receiving postoperative mechanical ventilation with low delivered volumes, and is probably mediated by stretch receptors that monitor changes in lung volume. Inability to generate a forceful cough or to clear secretions can cause distress, as can an increase in the work of breathing due to high airway resistance or partial upper airway obstruction. Engorgement of pulmonary vasculature with early interstitial pulmonary edema elicits symptoms of chest fullness and air hunger well before airway flooding occurs. Agitation caused by such problems can be profound even when ventilation and oxygenation are adequate by arterial blood gas analysis.

When cardiac output or systemic pressure is inadequate to maintain peripheral perfusion, lactic acidemia can cause anxiousness and mild disorientation. If systemic blood pressure falls so low that cerebral perfusion is not maintained, a patient can exhibit lethargy, disorientation, agitation, and combativeness. This is a medical emergency that requires aggressive restoration of cardiac output or peripheral vascular resistance. Administration of sedative or analgesic medications for a mistaken diagnosis of anxiety or pain might generate a catastrophic cardiopulmonary collapse in such a patient. Several metabolic abnormalities interfere with lucidity in the PACU. Acute hyponatremia after transurethral prostatic resection is one example of a hypo-osmolar state that markedly clouds the sensorium, but acute cerebral fluid shifts should also be considered in dialysis patients and after acute repletion of severe dehydration or massive fluid infusion. Acute hyperosmolarity secondary to hyperglycemia from excessive glucose infusion or insufficient insulin can cloud consciousness during recovery. Although uncommon, severe hypoglycemia will cause significant agitation or markedly diminished responsiveness.

Once these reversible causes of delirium or agitation are eliminated, the possibility of a primary neurologic problem must be considered as an etiology. Acute cerebral embolism, hemorrhage, or infarct sometimes manifest with disorientation, inability to vocalize, or a reduced level of consciousness.[250] Unrecognized seizure activity can mimic agitation and combativeness, or the patient can appear disoriented and somnolent during the postictal phase. One should suspect seizures in patients with epilepsy, head trauma, chronic alcohol intoxication, or cocaine abuse.

Therapy for altered mental status in the PACU is essentially supportive. Waiting 10–15 minutes for the depth of residual anesthesia to lighten is usually sufficient treatment for emergence reactions. Verbal reassurance that surgery is completed and that the patient is doing well can be invaluable. Using the patient's and surgeon's name frequently and stressing the time and location are also helpful. When practical, it is often useful to allow a patient to determine his or her own position. Adequate analgesia should be provided to minimize whatever contribution postoperative pain is making to the patient's agitation. A small dose of parenteral sedative will sometimes relieve fear or anxiety and smooth the emergence. Identifying whether a patient is reacting to pain or to anxiety is important when choosing which medication to employ, for opioids are relatively poor sedatives, while benzodiazepines and barbiturates are ineffective analgesics. Physical restraint should be used only as a last resort and when a patient's physical safety is in jeopardy. No matter how bizarre the patient's complaints may seem, there is usually an element of reality to them.

If aggressive evaluation reveals that altered mental status is a symptom of a physiologic abnormality (e.g., hypoxemia, acidemia, hypoglycemia, hypotension), sedative or analgesic medications should not be administered. Rather, the underlying problem causing the physiologic abnormality should be treated and the patient's mental status reassessed.

REFERENCES

1. Finch JS: Equipment and monitoring. In Israel JS, Dekornfeld TJ (eds): Recovery Room Care, p 25. Chicago, Year Book Medical Publishers, 1987

2. DeFranco M: Planning the physical structure of the PACU. In Frost EAM (ed): Post Anesthesia Care Unit, p 187. St Louis, CV Mosby Co, 1990

3. Cooper MH, Primrose JN: The value of postoperative chest radiology after major abdominal surgery. Anaesthesia 44:306, 1989

4. Turner KE, Sandler AN, Vosu HA et al: Noninvasive monitoring of carbon dioxide in nonintubated patients: Comparison of $Paco_2$ versus $Etco_2$ and $Paco_2$ versus $Tcco_2$. Anesth Analg 68:S296, 1989

5. Bonnet F, Boico O, Rostaing S et al: Clonidine induced analgesia in postoperative patients: Epidural versus intramuscular administration. Anesthesiology 72:423, 1990

6. Segal IS, Jarvis DA, Duncan SR et al: Perioperative use of transdermal clonidine as an adjunctive agent. Anesth Analg 68:S79, 1989

7. Bernard JM, Lechevalier T, Pinaud M et al: Postoperative analgesia by IV clonidine. Anesthesiology 71:A154, 1989

8. Henderson JJ, Parbrook GD: Influence of anaesthetic technique on postoperative pain. Br J Anaesth 48:587, 1976

9. Chrubasik J, Wiemers K: Continuous-plus-on-demand epidural infusion of morphine for postoperative pain relief by means of a small, externally worn infusion device. Anesthesiology 62:263, 1985

10. Cuschieri RJ, Morran CG, Howie JC et al: Postoperative pain and pulmonary complications: Comparison of three analgesic regimens. Br J Surg 72:495, 1985

11. Cousins MJ, Mather LE: Intrathecal and epidural administration of opioids. Anesthesiology 61:276, 1984

12. Bonnet F, Boico O, Rostaing S et al: Extradural clonidine analgesia in postoperative patients. Br J Anaesth 63:465, 1989

13. Motsch J, Graber E, Ludwig K: Addition of clonidine enhances postoperative analgesia from epidural morphine: A double blind study. Anesthesiology 73:1067, 1990

14. Mendez R, Eisenbach JC, Kashtan K: Epidural clonidine analgesia after cesarean section. Anesthesiology 73:848, 1990

15. Toledo-Pereyra LH, DeMeester TR: Prospective randomized evaluation of intrathoracic intercostal nerve block with Dupicaine on postoperative ventilatory function. Ann Thorac Surg 27:203, 1979

16. Ross WB, Tweedle JH, Leong YP et al: Intercostal blockade and pulmonary function after cholecystectomy. Surgery 105:166, 1989

17. Miguel R, Hubbell D: Postoperative pain management and pulmonary function after thoracotomy: A prospective randomized study. Anesthesiology 73:A777, 1990

18. Pflug AE, Murphy TM, Butler SH: The effects of postoperative peridural analgesia in pulmonary therapy and pulmonary complication. Anesthesiology 41:8, 1974

19. Evans C, Richardson PH: Improved recovery and reduced postoperative stay after therapeutic suggestions during general anaesthesia. Lancet 4:491, 1988

20. Boeke S, Bonke B, Bouwhuis-Hoogerwerf ML et al: Effects of sounds presented during general anaesthesia on postoperative course. Br J Anaesth 60:697, 1988

21. Aldrete JA, Kroulik D: A postanaesthetic recovery score. Anesth Analg 49:924, 1970

22. Steward DJ: A simplified scoring system for the postoperative recovery room. Can Anaesth Soc J 22:111, 1975

23. Lindrop MJ: Complications and morbidity of controlled hypotension. Br J Anaesth 47:799, 1975

24. Ellison N: Diagnosis and management of bleeding disorders. Anesthesiology 47:171, 1977

25. Ivanov J, Weisel RD, Mickleborough LL et al: Rewarming hypovolemia after aortocoronary bypass surgery. Crit Care Med 12:1049, 1984

26. Vrillon M, BeBret F, Vrints J: Systolic blood pressure variation in postoperative ventilated patients: A sensitive indicator of low preload states. Anesthesiology 73:A243, 1990

27. Mangano DT: Perioperative cardiac morbidity. Anesthesiology 72:153, 1990

28. Wong MG, Wellington MS, London MJ et al: Prolonged postoperative myocardial ischemia in high risk patients undergoing non-cardiac surgery. Anesthesiology 69:A57, 1988

29. Slogoff S, Keats AS: Does perioperative myocardial ischemia lead to postoperative myocardial infarction? Anesthesiology 62:107, 1985

30. Becker RC, Underwood DA: Myocardial infarction in patients undergoing noncardiac surgery. Cleve Clin J Med 54:25, 1987

31. Wade JG, Larson CP Jr, Hickey RF: Effect of carotid endarterectomy on carotid chemoreceptor and baroreceptor function in man. N Engl J Med 282:823, 1977

32. Bove EL, Fry WJ, Gross WS, et al: Hypotension and hypertension as consequences of baroreceptor dysfunction following carotid endarterectomy. Surgery 86:633, 1979

33. Marsh ML, Marshall LF, Shapiro HM: Neurosurgical intensive care. Anesthesiology 47:149, 1977

34. Myers RW: Effects of nitroglycerine and nitroglycerine-methoxamine during acute myocardial ischemia in dogs with pre-existing multivessel coronary occlusive disease. Circulation 51:632, 1975

35. Gal TJ, Cooperman LH: Hypertension in the immediate postoperative period. Br J Anaesth 47:70, 1975

36. Satiani B, Vasko JS, Zarins CK: Hypertension following carotid endarterectomy. Arch Surg 117:1073, 1982

37. Leslie JB, Kalayjian RW, Sirgo MA et al: Intravenous labetalol for treatment of postoperative hypertension. Anesthesiology 67:413, 1987

38. Kataria BK, Bubois MY, Gadde PL et al: Evaluation of intravenous esmolol for treatment of postoperative hypertension. Anesth Analg 70:S192, 1990

39. IV Nicardipine Study Group: Efficacy and safety of intravenous nicardipine in the control of postoperative hypertension. Chest 99:393, 1991

40. Breslow MJ, Miller CF, Parker SD et al: Changes in T-wave morphology following anesthesia and surgery: A common recovery room phenomenon. Anesthesiology. 64:398, 1986

41. Atlee JL, Bosnjak ZJ: Mechanisms for cardiac dysrhythmias during anesthesia. Anesthesiology 347, 1990

42. Pratila MG, Pratila V: Anesthetic agents and cardiac electromechanical activity. Anesthesiology 49:338, 1978

43. Cranefield PF, Wit AL, Hoffman BF: Genesis of cardiac arrhythmias. Circulation 47:408, 1973

44. Wit AL, Rosen MR, Hofman BF: Electrophysiology and pharmacology of cardiac arrhythmias: II. Relationship of normal and abnormal electrical activity of cardiac fibers to genesis of arrhythmias. B Reentry. Am Heart J 88:664, 1974

45. Beard K, Jick H, Walker AM: Adverse respiratory events occurring in the recovery room after general anesthesia. Anesthesiology 64:269, 1986

46. Hewlett AM, Branthwaite MA: Postoperative pulmonary function. Br J Anaesth 47:102, 1975

47. Mitchell RA, Berger AJ: Neural regulation of respiration. Am Rev Respir Dis 111:206, 1975

48. Shea SA, Walter J, Pelley K et al: The effect of visual and auditory stimuli upon resting ventilation in man. Respir Physiol 68:345, 1987

49. Harper MH, Hickey RF, Cromwell TH: The magnitude and duration of respiratory depression produced by fentanyl and fentanyl plus droperidol in man. J Pharm Exp Ther 199:464, 1976

50. Jordan C: Assessment of the effects of drugs on respiration. Br J Anaesth 54:763, 1982

51. Hudson HE, Harber PI, Smith TC: Respiratory depression from alkalosis and opioid interaction in man. Anesthesiology 40:543, 1974

52. Knill RL, Gelb AW: Ventilatory responses to hypoxia and hypercarbia during halothane sedation and anesthesia in man. Anesthesiology 49:244, 1978

53. Sybert DA, Block FE, McDonald JS: Oxygenation and ventilation during transport to recovery room. Anesthesiology 71:A442, 1989

54. Becker LD, Paulson BA, Miller RD: Biphasic respiratory depression after fentanyl-droperidol or fentanyl alone used to supplement nitrous oxide anesthesia. Anesthesiology 44:291, 1976

55. Krane BD, Kreutz JM, Johnson DL et al: Alfentanil and delayed respiratory depression: Case studies and review. Anesth Analg 70:557, 1990

56. Clark NJ, Meuleman T, Liu WS et al: Comparison of sufenta-

nil-N$_2$O and fentanyl-N$_2$O in patients without cardiac disease undergoing general surgery. Anesthesiology 66:130, 1987

57. Fink BR: Influence of cerebral activity in wakefulness on regulation of breathing. J Appl Physiol 16:15, 1961

58. Alexander CM, Gross JB: Sedative doses of midazolam depress hypoxic ventilatory responses in humans. Anesth Analg 67: 377, 1988

59. Bailey PL, Pace NL, Ashburn MA: Frequent hypoxemia and sedation with midazolam and fentanyl. Anesthesiology 73: 826, 1990

60. Radvanyi T, Marin F, Bikhazi GB et al: Antagonism of the postoperative respiratory depression caused by large doses of morphine. Anesthesiology 73:A1173, 1990

61. Gupta PK, Dundee JW: Post operative pain relief with morphine combined with doxapram and naloxone. Anaesthesia 29:33, 1974

62. Lugliani R, Whipp BJ, Seard C: Effect of bilateral carotid body resection on ventilatory control at rest and during exercise in man. N Engl J Med 285:1105, 1971

63. Kurth CD, Spitzer AR, Broennle AM et al: Postoperative apnea in preterm infants. Anesthesiology 66:483, 1987

64. Kurth CD, LeBard SE, Downes JJ: Association of airway obstruction, hypoxemia, and postoperative apnea in preterm infants. Anesthesiology 73:A1131, 1990

65. Welborn LG, Hannallah RS, Higgins T et al: Does anemia increase the risk of postoperative apnea in former preterm infants? Anesthesiology 73:A1091, 1990

66. Welborn LG, Rice LJ, Hannallah RS et al: Postoperative apnea in former preterm infants: Prospective comparison of spinal and general anesthetics. Anesthesiology 72:838, 1990

67. Slutsky AS, Watson J, Leith DE et al: Tracheal insufflation of oxygen (TRIO) at low flow rates sustains life for several hours. Anesthesiology 63:278, 1985

68. Ingram RA, Wellman JS, McFadden ER: Relative contributions of large and small airways to flow limitation in normal subjects before and after atropine and isoproterenol. J Clin Invest 59:696, 1977

69. Aldrich TK: Respiratory muscle fatigue. Clin Chest Med 9:225, 1988

70. Aubier M, Banzett RB, Bellamare F et al: Respiratory muscle fatigue: Report of the Respiratory Muscle Fatigue Workshop Group. Am Rev Respir Dis 142:474, 1990

71. Hedenstierna G, Santesson J: Breathing mechanics, deadspace and gas exchange in the extremely obese. Acta Anaesthesiol Scand 20:248, 1976

72. Paul DR, Hoyt JL, Boutros AR: Cardiovascular and respiratory changes in response to change of posture in the very obese. Anesthesiology 45:73, 1976

73. Weinberg JSE, Weiss ST, Cohen WR et al: Pregnancy and the lung. Am Rev Respir Dis 121:559, 1980

74. Bergofsky EH: Respiratory failure in disorders of the thoracic cage. Can Med Assoc J 119:643, 1979

75. Crosbie WJ, Sim DT: The effect of postural modification on some aspects of pulmonary function following surgery of the upper abdomen. Physiotherapy 72:487, 1988

76. Melendez JA, Alagesan R, Weissman C et al: Effect of postural changes on post thoracotomy respiratory muscle mechanics during incentive spirometry. Anesthesiology 73:A1176, 1990

77. Ohmura A, Katagiri J: Chest wall vibration increases lung volumes and diaphragm displacement in healthy volunteers and patients after upper abdominal surgery. Anesthesiology 71: A215, 1989

78. Chuter TAM, Weissman C, Mathews DM et al: Abdominal breathing maneuvers increase diaphragmatic motion after surgery. Anesthesiology 71:A1114, 1989

79. Katz JA, Marks JD: Inspiratory work with and without continuous positive airway pressure in patients with acute respiratory failure. Anesthesiology 63:598, 1985

80. d'Empaire G, Hoaglin DC, Perlo VP et al: Effect of prethymectomy plasma exchange on postoperative respiratory function in myasthenia gravis. J Thorac Cardiovasc Surg 89: 592, 1985

81. Burkett L, Bikhazi GB, Thomas KC: Mutual potentiation of the neuromuscular effects of antibiotics and relaxants. Anesth Analg 58:107, 1976

82. Ford GT, Whitelaw WA, Rosenal TW et al: Diaphragm function after upper abdominal surgery in humans. Am Rev Respir Dis 127:43, 1983

83. Rigg RA, Rondi P: Changes in rib cage and diaphragm contribution in ventilation after morphine. Anesthesiology 55:507, 1981

84. Dureuil B, Desmonts JM, Mankikian B et al: Effects of aminophylline on diaphragmatic dysfunction after upper abdominal surgery. Anesthesiology 62:242, 1985

85. Loh L, Hughes JMB, Newson Davis J: The regional distribution of ventilation and perfusion in paralysis of the diaphragm. Am Rev Respir Dis 119:121, 1979

86. Troyer AD, Heilporn A: Respiratory mechanics in quadriplegia: The respiratory function of the intercostal muscles. Am Rev Respir Dis 122:591, 1980

87. Richardson JD, Adams L, Flint LM: Selective management of flail chest and pulmonary contusion. Ann Surg 128:481, 1982

88. Pavlin EG, Holle RH, Schoene RB: Recovery of airway protection compared with ventilation in humans after paralysis with curare. Anesthesiology 70:381, 1989

89. Sprung J, Cheng EY, Rodarte JR: Mechanism producing respiratory insufficiency after upper abdominal surgery: Pain vs. diaphragm dysfunction (human and dog study). Anesth Analg 70:S388, 1990

90. Moser KM: Pulmonary embolism. Am Rev Respir Dis 115:829, 1977

91. Khambatta HJ, Stone JG, Matteo RS: Effect of sodium nitroprusside-induced hypotension on pulmonary deadspace. Br J Anaesth 54:1197, 1982

92. Askanazi J, Mordenstraum J, Rosenbaum SH et al: Nutrition for the patient with respiratory failure. Anesthesiology 54:373, 1981

93. Steward DJ: Malignant hyperthermia: The acute crisis. In Britt BA (ed): Malignant Hyperthermia. Int Anesthesiol Clin 17(4): 1, 1979

94. Meyers JR, Lambeck L, O'Kane H: Changes in functional residual capacity of the lung after operation. Arch Surg 110:576, 1975

95. Craig DB: Postoperative recovery of pulmonary function. Anesth Analg 60:46, 1981

96. Tokics L, Hedenstierna G, Strandberg A et al: Lung collapse and gas exchange during general anesthesia: Effects of spontaneous breathing, muscle paralysis, and positive end expiratory pressure. Anesthesiology 66:157, 1987

97. Rehder K, Marsh HM, Rodarte JR: Airway closure. Anesthesiology 47:40, 1977

98. Parfrey PS, Harte PJ, Quinlan JP: Pulmonary function in the early postoperative period. Br J Surg 64:384, 1977

99. Larsson A, Malmkvist G, Werner O: Variations in lung volume and compliance during pulmonary surgery. Br J Anaesth 59: 585, 1987

100. Kerr JH, Crampton Smith AC, Prys-Roberts C: Observations during endobronchial anaesthesia: II. Oxygenation. Br J Anaesth 46:84, 1974

101. Benumof JL: One lung ventilation and hypoxic pulmonary vasoconstriction. Anesth Analg 64:821, 1985

102. Warner MA, Wever BA, Warner ME: Etiologies and incidence of acute pulmonary emphysema in the immediate perioperative period. Anesth Analg 70:S421, 1990

103. Jackson FN, Rowland V, Corssen G: Laryngospasm induced pulmonary edema. Chest 78:819, 1980

104. Inverson LIG, Ecker RR, Fox HE et al: A comparative study of IPPB, the incentive spirometer, and blow bottles: The prevention of atelectasis following cardiac surgery. Ann Thorac Surg 25:197, 1978

105. Craven JL, Evans GA, Davenport PJ et al: The evaluation of the incentive spirometer in the management of postoperative pulmonary complications. Br J Surg 61:793, 1974

106. Spence AA, Smith G: Postoperative analgesia and lung function: A comparison of morphine with extradural block. Br J Anaesth 43:144, 1971

107. Hudes ET, Marans HJ, Hirano GM et al: Recovery room oxygenation: A comparison of nasal catheters and 40 percent oxygen masks. Can J Anaesth 36:20, 1989

108. Zvara MJ, Labaille T, Benlabed M et al: Does significant post-

operative arterial desaturation occur with regional anesthesia? Anesthesiology 71:A898, 1989

109. Tait AR, Kyff JV, Crider B et al: Postoperative arterial oxygen saturation: Up in a puff of smoke? Anesth Analg 86:284, 1989

110. Moller JT, Wittrup M, Johansen SH: Hypoxemia in the postanesthesia care unit: An observer study. Anesthesiology 73:890, 1990

111. Russell GB, Graybeal JM: Persistent occurrence of postoperative arterial oxygen desaturations despite oxygen therapy. Anesthesiology 73:A540, 1990

112. Daley MD, Colmenares ME, Sandler AN et al: Continuous pulse oximetry in the post anesthesia care unit. Anesth Analg 70:S77, 1990

113. Kimovec MA, Grutsch JF, Napcil JA: Incidence of postoperative hypoxemia prior to recovery room discharge. Anesthesiology 71:A373, 1989

114. Tomkins DP, Gaukroger PB, Bentley MW: Hypoxia in children following general anaesthesia. Anaesth Intens Care 16:177, 1988

115. Kataria PK, Harnik EV, Mitchard R et al: Postoperative arterial oxygen saturation in the pediatric population during transportation. Anesth Analg 67:280, 1988

116. Pullerits J, Burrows FA, Roy WL: Arterial desaturation in healthy children during transfer to the recovery room. Can J Anaesth 34:470, 1987

117. Pandit UA, Levy L, Randel GI et al: Perioperative respiratory complications in children with upper respiratory infection. Anesthesiology 71:A1011, 1989

118. McGowan FX, Kenna MA, Kleinman CS et al: Hypoxemia and pulmonary hypertension in children with adenotonsillar hypertrophy. Anesthesiology 71:A1010, 1989

119. Amar D, Winikoff S, Hollinger IB et al: An alternative oxygen delivery system to infants and children in the post anesthesia care unit. Anesth Analg 86:S9, 1989

120. Gibson RL, Comer PB, Beckman RW: Actual tracheal oxygen concentrations with commonly used oxygen equipment. Anesthesiology 44:71, 1976

121. Klein J: Normobaric pulmonary oxygen toxicity: Anesth Analg 70:195, 1990

122. LaMantia KR, Glick JH, Marshall BE: Supplemental oxygen does not cause respiratory failure in bleomycin treated patients. Anesthesiology 60:65, 1984

123. Goldiner PG, Carlon GC, Cvifkovic E: Factors influencing postoperative morbidity and mortality in patients treated with bleomycin. Br J Med 1:1664, 1978

124. Blom-Muilwijk MC, Vriesendorp R, Veninga TS et al: Pulmonary toxicity after treatment with bleomycin or in combination with hyperoxia: Studies in the rat. Br J Anaesth 60:91, 1988

125. Greenbaum DM, Millen JE, Eross B: Continuous positive airway pressure without tracheal intubation in spontaneously breathing patients. Chest 69:615, 1976

126. Jardin F, Delorme G, Hardy A et al: Reevaluation of hemodynamic consequences of positive pressure ventilation: Emphasis on cyclic right ventricular afterloading by mechanical lung inflation. Anesthesiology 72:966, 1990

127. Quist J, Pontoppidan H, Wilson R: Hemodynamic responses to PEEP. Anesthesiology 42:45, 1975

128. Cullen DJ, Caldera DL: The incidence of ventilator-induced pulmonary barotrauma in critically ill patients. Anesthesiology 50:185, 1979

129. Huseby JS, Pavlin EG, Butler J: Effect of PEEP on intracranial pressure. J Appl Physiol 44:225, 1978

130. Haake R, Schlichtig R, Ulstad DR et al: Barotrauma: Pathophysiology, risk factors, and prevention. Chest 91:608, 1987

131. Benumof JL, Wahrenbrock EH: Blunted hypoxic pulmonary vasoconstriction by increasing lung vascular pressure. J Appl Physiol 38:846, 1975

132. Marshall C, Kim SD, Marshall BE: The influence of vascular pressure on hypoxic pulmonary vasoconstriction. Anesthesiology 73:A1139, 1990

133. Roos A, Thomas LJ, Nagel EL: Pulmonary vascular resistance as determined by lung inflation and vascular pressures. J Appl Physiol 16:77, 1961

134. Mathers J, Benumof JL, Wahrenrock EA: General anesthetics

and regional hypoxic pulmonary vasoconstriction. Anesthesiology 46:111, 1977

135. Benumof JL: Hypoxic pulmonary vasoconstriction and sodium nitroprusside perfusion. Anesthesiology 50:481, 1979

136. Reeves JT, Grover RF: Blockade of acute hypoxic pulmonary hypertension by endotoxin. J Appl Physiol 36:328, 1974

137. Daoud FS, Reeves JT, Schaefer JW: Failure of hypoxic pulmonary vasoconstriction in patients with liver cirrhosis. J Clin Invest 51:1076, 1972

138. Catley DM, Thornton C, Jordan C et al: Pronounced episodic oxygen desaturation in the postoperative period: Its association with ventilatory pattern and analgesic regimen. Anesthesiology 63:20, 1985

139. Fink BR, Carpenter SL, Holaday DA: Diffusion anoxia during recovery from nitrous oxide/oxygen anesthesia. Fed Proc 13:354, 1954

140. Bartlett JG, Gorbach SL: The triple threat of aspiration pneumonia. Chest 68:560, 1975

141. Greenfield LJ, Singleton RP, McCaffree DR: Pulmonary effects of experimental graded aspiration of hydrochloric acid. Ann Surg 170:74, 1969

142. Schwartz DJ, Wynne JW, Gibbs CP: The pulmonary consequences of aspiration of gastric contents at pH values greater than 2.5. Am Rev Respir Dis 121:119, 1980

143. Vidyarthi SC: Diffuse miliary granulomatosis of the lungs due to aspirated vegetable cells. Arch Pathol 83:215, 1967

144. Laxmaiah M, Colliver JA, Marrero TC et al: Assessment of age related acid aspiration risk factors in pediatric, adult and geriatric patients. Anesth Analg 64:11, 1985

145. Stanec A, Nuesa W, Akturk A et al: Recovery of respiratory muscle function in surgical outpatients. Anesthesiology 73:A878, 1990

146. James CF, Gibbs CP, Banner T: Postpartum perioperative risk of aspiration pneumonia. Anesthesiology 61:756, 1984

147. Gibbs CP, Schwartz DJ, Wynne JW: Antacid pulmonary aspiration in the dog. Anesthesiology 51:380, 1979

148. Solanki DR, Suresh M, Ethridge HC: The effects of intravenous cimetidine and metoclopramide on gastric volume and pH. Anesth Analg 63:599, 1984

149. Manchikanti L, Colliver J, Marrero T et al: Ranitidine and metoclopramide for prophylaxis of aspiration pneumonitis in elective surgery. Anesth Analg 63:903, 1984

150. Petring OU, Adelhoj B, Jensen BN et al: Prevention of silent aspiration due to leaks around cuffs of endotracheal tubes. Anesth Analg 65:777, 1986

151. Wever JG, Warner MA, Warner ME: Perioperative pulmonary aspiration: Incidence and risk factors. Anesthesiology 73:A1017, 1990

152. Bynum LJ, Pierce AK: Pulmonary aspiration of gastric contents. Am Rev Respir Dis 114:1129, 1976

153. Bartlett JG, Gorbach SL, Finegold S: The bacteriology of aspiration pneumonia. Am J Med 56:202, 1974

154. Berns AS, Linas SL, Miller TR: Urinary diagnostic indices in acute renal failure. Kidney Int 10:495, 1976

155. Levinsky NG, Bernard DB, Johnson TA: Mannitol and loop diuretics in acute renal failure. In Brenner BM, Lazarus JM (eds): Acute Renal Failure, p 462. Philadelphia, WB Saunders, 1983

156. Hilberman M, Maseda J, Stinson EB et al: The diuretic properties of dopamine in patients after open heart operation. Anesthesiology 61:489, 1984

157. Knill RL, Clement JL: Ventilatory responses to acute metabolic acidemia in humans awake, sedated, and anesthetized with halothane. Anesthesiology 62:745, 1985

158. Doze VA, White PF: Effects of fluid therapy on serum glucose levels in fasted outpatients. Anesthesiology 66:223, 1987

159. Roesch RP, Stoelting RK, Lingeman JE: Ammonia toxicity resulting from glycine absorption during a transurethral resection of the prostate. Anesthesiology 58:577, 1983

160. Wang JM-L, Creel DJ, Wong KC: Transurethral resection of the prostate, serum glycine levels, and ocular evoked potentials. Anesthesiology 70:36, 1989

161. Alexander JP, Polland A, Gillespie IA: Glycine and transurethral resection. Anaesthesia 41:1189, 1986

162. Kliger AS, Hayslett JB: Disorders of potassium balance. In

Brenner BM, Stein JH (eds): Acid Base and Potassium Homeostasis, p 168. New York, Churchill Livingstone, 1978

163. Brown MJ, Brown DC, Murphy MB: Hypokalemia from beta-2 receptor stimulation by circulating epinephrine. N Engl J Med 309:1414, 1983

164. Scribner BH, Fremont-Smith K, Burnell JM: The effect of acute respiratory acidosis on the internal equilibrium of potassium. J Clin Invest 34:1278, 1975

165. Patel RI, Hannallah RS: Anesthetic complications following pediatric ambulatory surgery: A three year study. Anesthesiology 69:1009, 1988

166. Palazzo MG, Strunin L: Anesthesia and emesis: I. Etiology. Can Anaesth Soc J 31:178, 1984

167. Palazzo MG, Strunin L: Anesthesia and emesis: II. Prevention and management. Can Anaesth Soc J 31:407, 1984

168. Hines RL, Barash PG, Dubow H et al: Ambulatory surgical complications in the postoperative period: We can't just walk away. Anesth Analg 86:S122, 1989

169. Anderson R, Crohg K: Pain as a major cause of postoperative nausea. Can Anaesth Soc J 23:366, 1976

170. Lerman J, Eustis S, Smith DR: Effect of droperidol pretreatment on postanesthetic vomiting in children undergoing strabismus surgery. Anesthesiology 65:322, 1986

171. Caldamone AA, Rabinowitz R: Outpatient orchiopexy. J Urol 127:286, 1982

172. Lindblad T, Beattie WS, Buckley DN et al: Menstruation increases risk of post-operative emesis. Anesthesiology 73:A17, 1990

173. Beattie WS, Forrest JB, Bucley DN et al: Nausea and vomiting correlates with estrogen levels and dose response for droperidol. Anesthesiology 71:A957, 1989

174. Lonie DS, Harper NJN: Nitrous oxide anaesthesia and vomiting. Anaesthesia 41:703, 1986

175. Melnick BM, Johnson LS: Effects of eliminating nitrous oxide in outpatient anesthesia. Anesthesiology 67:982, 1987

176. Muir JJ, Warner MA, Offord KP et al: Role of nitrous oxide and other factors in postoperative nausea and vomiting: A randomized and blinded prospective study. Anesthesiology 66:513, 1987

177. Sengupta P, Plantevin OM: Nitrous oxide and day-case laparoscopy: Effects on nausea, vomiting and return to normal activity. Br J Anaesth 60:570, 1988

178. Hovorka J, Korttila K, Erkola O: Nitrous oxide does not increase nausea and vomiting following gynaecological laparoscopy. Can J Anaesth 36:145, 1989

179. Carter JA, Dye AM, Cooper GM: Recovery after day-case anaesthesia: The effect of different inhalational anaesthetic agents. Anaesthesia 40:545, 1985

180. Marais ML, Maher MW, Wetchler BV et al: Reduced demands on recovery room resources with propofol (Diprivan) compared to thiopental-isoflurane. Anesthesiol Rev 16:29, 1989

181. Hunt TM, Plantevin OM, Gilbert JR: Morbidity in gynaecological day-case surgery: A comparison of two anaesthetic techniques. Br J Anaesth 51:785, 1979

182. Sanders RS, Sinclair ME, Sear JW: Alfentanil in short procedures: A comparison with halothane using etomidate or methohexitone for induction of anesthesia. Anaesthesia 39:1202, 1984

183. King MJ, Milazkiewicz R, Carli F et al: Influence of neostigmine on postoperative vomiting. Br J Anaesth 61:403, 1988

184. Toro-matos A, Rendon-Platas AM, Avil-Valez E et al: Physostigmine antagonizes ketamine. Anesth Analg 59:644, 1980

185. McCarroll SM, Mori S, Bras PJ et al: The effect of gastric intubation and removal of gastric contents on the incidence of postoperative nausea and vomiting. Anesth Analg 70:S262, 1990

186. Kraynack BJ, Bates MF, Gintautas J et al: Antiemetic efficacy of ranitidine, metoclopramide, and gastric suctioning in outpatient laparoscopy. Anesth Analg 70:S218, 1990

187. Eustis S, Lerman J, Smith D: Droperidol pretreatment in children undergoing strabismus repair: The minimal effective dose. Can Anaesth Soc J 33:S115, 1986

188. Pandit SK, Kothary SP, Pandit UA et al: Dose-response study of droperidol and metoclopramide as antiemetics for outpatient anesthesia. Anesth Analg 68:798, 1989

189. Williams JJ, Goldberg ME, Boerner TF et al: A comparison of three methods to reduce nausea and vomiting after alfentanil anesthesia in outpatients. Anesth Analg 68:S311, 1989

190. Jorgensen NH, Coyle JP: Effect of intravenous droperidol upon nausea and vomiting using alfentanil anesthesia. Anesth Analg 68:S139, 1989

191. Grunwald Z, Scheiner MS, Pamess J et al: Droperidol decreases vomiting after tonsillectomy and adenoidectomy in children. Anesth Analg 70:S138, 1990

192. Melnick BM: Extrapyramidal reactions to low-dose droperidol. Anesthesiology 69:424, 1988

193. Cohen SE, Woods WA, Wyner J: Antiemetic efficacy of droperidol and metoclopramide. Anesthesiology 60:67, 1984

194. Doze VA, Shafer A, White PF: Nausea and vomiting after outpatient anesthesia: Effectiveness of droperidol alone and in combination with metoclopramide. Anesth Analg 66:S41, 1987

195. Broadman LM, Ceruzzi W, Patane PS: Metoclopramide reduces the incidence of vomiting following strabismus surgery in children. Anesthesiology 72:245, 1990

196. Horton BF, Chadwick D: Metoclopramide may cause dysphoria. Anesthesiology 73:A38, 1990

197. Uppington J, Dunnet J, Blogg CE: Transdermal hyoscine and postoperative nausea and vomiting. Anaesthesia 41:16, 1986

198. Tigerstedt I, Salmela L, Aromaa U: Double-blind comparison of transdermal scopolamine, droperidol and placebo against postoperative nausea and vomiting. Acta Anaesthesiol Scand 32:454, 1988

199. Bailey PL, Streisand JB, Pace NL et al: Transdermal scopolamine reduces nausea and vomiting after outpatient laparoscopy. Anesthesiology 72:977, 1989

200. Rothenberg D, Parnass S, Newman L et al: Ephedrine minimizes postoperative nausea and vomiting in outpatients. Anesthesiology 71:A322, 1989

201. Rothenberg DM, Parnass SM, Litwack K et al: Efficacy of ephedrine in the prevention of postoperative nausea and vomiting. Anesth Analg 72:58, 1991

202. Poler SM, White PF: Does ephedrine decrease nausea and vomiting after outpatient anesthesia? Anesthesiology 71:A995, 1989

203. Bidwai AV, Meulman T, Thatte WP et al: Prevention of postoperative nausea with dimenhydrate (Dramamine) and droperidol (Inapsine). Anesth Analg 68:S25, 1989

204. Bodner M, Poler SM, White PF: Initial evaluation of ondansetron: A novel antiemetic. Anesthesiology 73:A328, 1990

205. Wetchler BV, Sung YF, Duncalf D et al: Ondansetron decreases emetic symptoms following outpatient laparoscopy. Anesthesiology 73:A36, 1990

206. Dundee JW, Ghaly RG, McKinney MS: P6 acupuncture antiemesis comparison of invasive and noninvasive techniques. Anesthesiology 71:A130, 1989

207. Batra KY, Bali ML: Corneal abrasion during general anesthesia. Anesth Analg 56:363, 1977

208. Monroe MC, Gravenstein N, Saga-Rumley SA: Postoperative sore throat: Effect of oropharyngeal airway. Anesthesiology 71:A951, 1989

209. Jensen PJ: Sore throat after operation: Influence of tracheal intubation, intracuff pressure, and type of cuff. Br J Anaesth 54:453, 1982

210. Loeser EA, Stanley TH, Jordan W et al: Postoperative sore throat: Influence of tracheal tube lubrication versus cuff design. Can Anaesth Soc J 27:156, 1980

211. Stout DM, Bishop MJ, Dwersteg JF et al: Correlation of endotracheal tube size with sore throat and hoarseness following general anesthesia. Anesthesiology 67:419, 1987

212. Stock MC, Downs JB: Lubrication of tracheal tubes to prevent sore throat from intubation. Anesthesiology 57:418, 1982

213. Koka BV, Jeon IS, Andre JM et al: Post intubation croup in children. Anesth Analg 56:501, 1977

214. Keane WM, Denneny JC, Rowe LD et al: Complications of intubation. Ann Otol Rhinol Laryngol 91:584, 1982

215. Friedman M, Toriumi DM: Esophageal stethoscope: Another possible cause of vocal cord paralysis. Arch Otolaryngol Head Neck Surg 115:95, 1989

216. Dornette WHL: Compression neuropathies: Medical aspects

and legal implications. In Hindman BJ (ed): Neurological and Psychological Complications of Surgery and Anesthesia, p 201. Boston, Little, Brown & Co, 1986

217. Alvine FG, Schurrer ME: Postoperative ulnar nerve palsy: Are there predisposing factors? J Bone Joint Surg 69A:255, 1987

218. Kroll DA, Caplan RA, Ward RJ et al: Perioperative nerve injuries. Anesthesiology 71:A929, 1989

219. O'Sullivan EP, Williams NE, Calvey TN: Differential effects of neuromuscular blocking agents on suxamethonium induced fasciculations and myalgia. Br J Anaesth 60:367, 1988

220. Manchikanti L, Grow JB, Colliver JA et al: Atracurium pretreatment for succinylcholine induced fasciculations and postoperative myalgia. Anesth Analg 64:1010, 1985

221. Trepanier CA, Brousseau C, Lacerte L: Myalgia in outpatient surgery: Comparison of atracurium and succinylcholine. Can J Anaesth 35:255, 1988

222. Pace NL: Prevention of succinylcholine myalgias: A meta-analysis. Anesth Analg 70:477, 1990

223. Sessler DI, Olofsson CI, Rubinstein EH et al: The thermoregulatory threshold in humans during halothane anesthesia. Anesthesiology 68:836, 1988

224. Sessler DI, Moayeri A, Stoen R et al: Thermoregulatory vasoconstriction decreases cutaneous heat loss. Anesthesiology 73:656, 1990

225. Slotman GJ, Jed EH, Burchard KW: Adverse effects of hypothermia in postoperative patients. Am J Surg 149:495, 1985

226. Sessler DI, Israel D, Pozos RS et al: Spontaneous post-anesthetic tremor does not resemble thermoregulatory shivering. Anesthesiology 68:843, 1988

227. Sessler DI, Rubinstein EH: Hypothermia triggers spontaneous postanesthetic tremor. Anesthesiology 73:A173, 1990

228. Claybon LE, Hirsch RA: Meperidine arrests postanesthetic shivering. Anesthesiology 59:S180, 1983

229. Rodriguez JL, Weissman JC, Damask MC et al: Physiologic requirements during rewarming: Suppression of the shivering response. Crit Care Med 11:490, 1983

230. MacIntyre PE, Pavlin EG, Dwersteg JF: Effect of meperidine on oxygen consumption, carbon dioxide production, and respiratory gas exchange in post anesthesia shivering. Anesth Analg 66:751, 1987

231. Lipton JM, Schroeder T, Banish P et al: Control of postanesthetic shivering by localized regulated radiant heat. Anesth Analg 70:S243, 1990

232. Lennon RL, Hosking MP, Conover MA et al: Evaluation of a forced air system for warming hypothermic postoperative patients. Anesth Analg 70:424, 1990

233. Saunders PR, McCarroll SM, Harris J: Does heated humidified oxygen in the recovery room aid warming of the hypothermic patient? Anesthesiology 71:A185, 1989

234. Denlinger JK: Prolonged emergence and failure to regain consciousness. In Orkin FK, Cooperman LH (eds): Complications in Anesthesiology, p 368. Philadelphia, JB Lippincott, 1983

235. Bourke DL, Rosenberg M, Allen PD: Physostigmine: Effectiveness as an antagonist of respiratory depression and psychomotor effects caused by morphine or diazepam. Anesthesiology 61:523, 1984

236. Jensen S, Knudsen L, Kirkegaard L et al: Flumazenil used for antagonizing the central effects of midazolam and diazepam in outpatients. Acta Anaesthesiol Scand 33:26, 1989

237. Ghoneim MM, Dembo JB, Block RI: Time course of antagonism of sedative and amnesic effects of diazepam by flumazenil. Anesthesiology 70:899, 1989

238. Fragen RJ, Katz JA, Dunn KL: Flumazenil reversal of midazolam sedation in the elderly. Anesth Analg 70:S113, 1990

239. Douglass JH, Ross JD, Bruce DL: Delayed awakening due to lidocaine overdose. J Clin Anesth 2:126, 1989

240. Skillman JJ: Neurologic complications of cardiovascular surgery: I. Procedures involving the carotid arteries and abdominal aorta. In Hindman BJ (ed): Neurological and Psychological Complications of Surgery and Anesthesia, p 135. Boston, Little, Brown & Co, 1986

241. Gutierrez IZ, Barone DL, Makula PA et al: The risk of perioperative stroke in patients with asymptomatic carotid bruits undergoing peripheral vascular surgery. Am Surg 53:487, 1987

242. Hindman BJ: Perioperative stroke: The noncardiac surgical patient. In Hindman BJ (ed): Neurological and Psychological Complications of Surgery and Anesthesia, p 101. Boston, Little, Brown & Co, 1986

243. Larsen SF, Zaric D, Boysen G: Postoperative cerebrovascular accidents in general surgery. Acta Anaesthesiol Scand 32:698, 1988

244. Chung F, Seyone C, Dyck B et al: Age related cognitive recovery after general anesthesia. Anesth Analg 71:217, 1990

245. Taenzer P, Melzack R, Jeans ME: Influence of psychological factors in postoperative pain, mood, and analgesic requirements. Pain 24:331, 1986

246. Jamison RN, Parris WC, Maxson WS: Psychological factors influencing recovery from outpatient surgery. Behav Res Ther 25:31, 1987

247. Eisendrath SJ, Goldman B, Douglas J et al: Meperidine induced delirium. Am J Psychiatry 144:1062, 1987

248. Hammon K, Demartino BK: Postoperative delirium secondary to atropine premedication. Anesth progress 32:107, 1985

249. Heath PJ, Kennedy DJ, Ogg TW et al: Which intravenous induction agent for day surgery? A comparison of propofol, thiopentone, methohexitone, and etomidate. Anaesthesia 43:365, 1988

250. Oliver SB, Cucchiara RF, Warner MA et al: Unexpected focal neurologic deficit on emergence from anesthesia: A report of three cases. Anesthesiology 67:823, 1987

57

Timothy R. Lubenow   Anthony D. Ivankovich
Robert J. McCarthy

Management of Acute Postoperative Pain

Acute postoperative pain is a complex physiologic reaction to tissue injury, visceral distention, or disease. It is a manifestation of autonomic, psychological, and behavior responses that result in an unpleasant, unwanted sensory and emotional experience. Patients often perceive postoperative pain as one of the more ominous aspects of undergoing surgery. Historically, the treatment of postoperative pain has been given a low priority by both surgeons and anesthesiologists. As a result, patients previously accepted pain as a requisite part of the postoperative experience.

With the development of an expanding awareness of the epidemiology and pathophysiology of pain, more attention is being focused on the management of pain in an effort to improve quality of care and reduce morbidity. The natural progression of this focus is the formation of a postoperative analgesic service or acute pain service, involving a group of individuals who specialize in pain management and who apply an ever-increasing number of modalities to control postoperative pain. This chapter reviews the pathophysiology of pain, examines some pharmacologic considerations, and compares the use of oral, parenteral, and central neuraxial analgesics. Peripheral nerve blocks that have application for postoperative pain relief are highlighted, as are some nonpharmacologic therapies. Incorporation of this knowledge into clinical practice is the basis and the rationale for the formation of a postoperative analgesic service.

FUNDAMENTAL CONCEPTS

Nociception

Nociception refers to the detection, transduction, and transmission of noxious stimuli. Stimuli generated from thermal, mechanical, or chemical tissue damage may activate nociceptors, which are free nerve endings. Nociceptors can be further classified into exteroceptors, which receive stimuli from skin surfaces, and interoceptors, which are located in the walls of viscera or deeper body structures. In addition to nociceptors, the skin is richly innervated by specialized somatosensory receptors that are sensitive to other forms of stimulation (Table 57-1). Each sensory unit includes an end-organ receptor, accompanying axon, dorsal root gan-

glion, and axon terminals in the spinal cord.[1] In contrast to other special somatosensory receptors, nociceptors exhibit high-response thresholds and persistent discharge to suprathreshold stimuli without rapid adaptation and are associated with small receptive fields and small afferent nerve fiber endings.[2]

Peripheral Nerve Afferent Fibers

Nerve fibers were first described according to their type of covering and the presence or absence of myelination. Neural fibers may be covered with neurolemma, or myelin, or both. Speed of conduction is determined by fiber size and the presence or absence of myelination. Small, unmyelinated fibers transmit at a slower speed than larger myelinated afferent fibers.[1]

With the invention of the oscilloscope, Erlanger and Gasser were able to describe a more functional classification of peripheral nerve fibers.[3] Nerve fibers were categorized into three groups (A, B, and C), depending on size, degree of myelination, rapidity of conduction, and distribution of fibers. A refinement of this classification is the functional subdivision of the Class A fibers into the subtypes of alpha, beta, gamma, and delta.[4]

Class A. These neurons, composed of large myelinated fibers, exhibit a low threshold for activation, conduct impulses at a speed of 5–100 m·sec^{-1}, and measure 1–20 μm in diameter. Class A delta fibers mediate pain sensation, whereas Class A alpha fibers transmit motor and proprioceptive impulses. Class A beta and A gamma fibers are responsible for cutaneous touch and pressure as well as regulation of muscle spindle reflexes.

Class B. These neurons constitute the medium-sized myelinated fibers with a conduction velocity ranging from 3–14 m·sec^{-1} and a diameter less than 3 μm. They have a higher threshold (lower excitability) than Class A fibers but a lower threshold than Class C fibers. The postganglionic sympathetic and visceral afferents belong to this group.

Class C. These fibers are unmyelinated or thinly myelinated and have conduction velocities in the range of 0.5–2 m·sec^{-1}. This class is composed of preganglionic autonomic

TABLE 57-1. Somatosensory Receptors

Receptor	Sensation Perceived
Nerve fibers on hair follicles	Touch
Merkel's disks	Touch
Meissner's corpuscles	Touch
Free nerve endings (nociceptors)	Pain
Krause's end bulbs	Cold
Ruffini's endings	Heat
Pacinian corpuscles	Pressure
Golgi-Mazzoni endings	Pressure

fibers and pain fibers. Approximately 50–80% of C fibers modulate nociceptive stimuli.

An additional classification of afferent muscle nerve fibers used by neurophysiologists divides the large myelinated fibers into three functional groups (Ia, Ib, II), placing the thinly myelinated (III) and unmyelinated fibers (IV) into separate groups. The muscle afferents of Erlanger and Gasser's Class A alpha fibers are subdivided into two groups, Ia and Ib. Fibers from the annulospiral endings of the muscle spindles compose the Ia Group, whereas Group Ib fibers emanate from the Golgi tendon organs. Group II consists of the tactile and proprioceptive fibers of Classes A beta and A gamma, respectively, whereas the primary nociceptive nerve fibers of Classes A delta and C are equivalent to Groups III and IV, respectively, within this classification.[5]

Spinal Cord and Brain Pathways

The peripheral afferent neuron, termed the first-order neuron, has its cell body located in the dorsal root ganglion and sends axonal projections into the dorsal horn and other areas of the spinal cord. At this point, a synapse occurs with a second-order afferent neuron, which can be categorized, depending on the afferent input they receive, as nociceptive-specific (NS) or wide-dynamic-range (WDR) neurons. Nociceptive-specific neurons process afferent impulses only from nociceptive afferent fibers, while A beta, A delta, and C fibers communicate with WDR neurons. In the dorsal horn, further synaptic connections occur between first-order neurons and regulatory internuncial neurons. First-order neurons also communicate with the cell bodies of the sympathetic nervous system and ventral motor nuclei, either directly or through the internuncial neurons.[6] The cell body of the second-order neuron lies in the dorsal horn, and axonal projections of this neuron cross to the contralateral hemisphere of the spinal cord (Fig. 57-1). This second-order afferent neuron ascends from that level in the lateral spinothalamic tract to synapse in the thalamus. Along the way this neuron divides and sends axonal branches that synapse in the regions of the reticular formation, nucleus raphe magnus, periaqueductal gray, and other areas in the brain stem. In the thalamus, the second-order neuron synapses with a third-order afferent neuron, which sends axonal projections into the sensory cortex.

Modulation of Nociception

Even though nociceptors and the afferent sensory neural pathways detect and transmit noxious stimuli reliably, modification occurs at several levels in the pathway prior

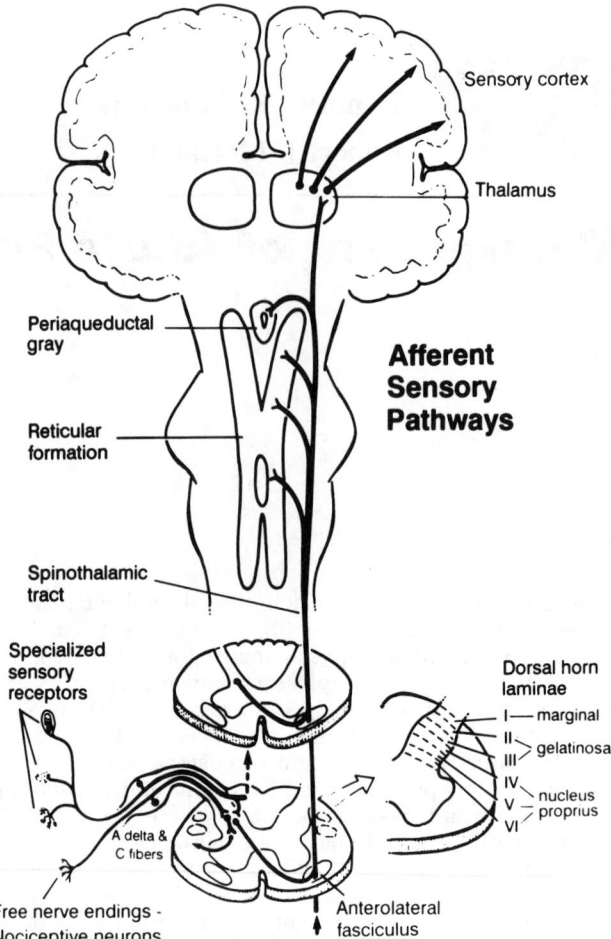

Figure 57-1. Afferent sensory pathways for detection and transmission of nociceptive impulses.

to perception of the signal at the cortical levels. Modulation can occur either in the periphery or at any point where synaptic transmission occurs.

Peripheral

Peripheral modulation occurs either by the liberation or by the elimination of certain allogenic substances in the vicinity of the nociceptor. Allogenic mediators—such as potassium and hydrogen ions, lactic acid, serotonin, bradykinin, histamine, and the prostaglandins—sensitize and excite nociceptors and act as mediators of inflammation. This effect can occur either directly or indirectly because of alterations in the peripheral microcirculation. Aspirin and nonsteroidal anti-inflammatory drugs exert an analgesic effect by inhibiting prostaglandin synthesis and reducing prostaglandin E_1- and E_2-mediated sensitization of nociceptors in the periphery.

Spinal

Modulation in the spinal cord results from the action of neurotransmitter substances in the dorsal horn or from spinal reflexes, which convey efferent impulses back to the peripheral nociceptive field. The excitatory amino acids L-glutamate and aspartate in particular, and several neuropeptides, including vasoactive intestinal peptide, cholecystokinin, gastrin-releasing peptide, angiotensin II, and calcitonin gene-related peptide, are found in central terminals of the first-order neurons and have been shown to modulate transmission of nociceptive afferent signals.[7] Substance P, which is found in the synaptic vesicle of unmyelinated C fibers, is also an important neurotransmitter that can enhance or aggravate pain.[8,9] Inhibitory substances involved in the regulation of afferent impulses in the dorsal horn include the enkephalins, beta-endorphins, and norepinephrine. Somatostatin, a neuropeptide found in cells that do not contain substance P, may represent another inhibitory neuropeptide involved in afferent modulation.[9,10]

Afferent modulating mechanisms at the spinal level may also involve spinal reflexes in which afferent signals directly evoke somatic and/or sympathetic efferent impulses. These impulses discharge in the area of the efferent nociceptive signal. For example, skeletal muscle spasm in an injured area is part of a somatic efferent reflex that is induced as a result of nociceptive afferent signals. Increased skeletal muscle tone initiates more nociceptive signals in a positive feedback loop system from the muscles (Fig. 57-2). In addition, spinal reflexes may involve the discharge of efferent sympathetic signals evoked from the nociceptive impulse (Fig. 57-2). Efferent sympathetic signals emanate from cell bodies located in the intermediolateral column of the spinal cord. These cell bodies receive internuncial projections from the dorsal horn of the gray matter. This sympathetic reflex produces smooth muscle spasm, vasoconstriction, and liberation of norepinephrine in the vicinity of the wound, thereby generating more pain. This may be attributed to changes in the microcirculation and local chemical environment. Release of norepinephrine has been shown to produce or augment pain following injury.[11]

Supraspinal

Brain Stem. Descending inhibitory tracts at the brain stem level originate from cell bodies located in the region of the periaqueductal gray, reticular formation, and nucleus raphe magnus. These inhibitory tracts descend into the dorsolateral fasciculus and synapse in the dorsal horn. Neurotransmitters act presynaptically on the first-order neuron and postsynaptically on the second-order neuron of the spinothalamic tract or on the internuncial neuron pool. Internuncial neurons can be inhibitory in nature and can regulate synaptic transmission between primary and secondary afferent neurons in the dorsal horn. At least two groups of nerve fibers have been identified as participants in this inhibitory modulation. One group of fibers involves the opioid system and contains the neurotransmitters beta-endorphin and enkephalins as well as other neuropeptides. Several studies have demonstrated that analgesia is produced during electrical stimulation of the periaqueductal gray and that this effect is blocked by naloxone.[12,13,14] These opioid projections from the nucleus raphe magnus and reticular formation interface presynaptically with the first-order afferent neurons. Neurotransmitters released from these projections hyperpolarize Class A delta and C fibers, which serves to negate or shunt out the depolarizing current that approaches the terminal end plate, thereby diminishing the release of neurotransmitters such as substance P (Fig. 57-3).[15] In addition to this presynaptic modulation, studies have shown that exogenously applied opioids will inhibit L-glutamate–evoked discharge of dorsal horn neurons, suggesting that opioids exert a direct postsynaptic effect.[16,17] In summary, opioids modulate transmission of afferent impulses in the dorsal horn presynaptically at the level of the first-order neuron. The enkephalinergic transmitter that is released from the descending inhibitory pathways hyperpolarizes the afferent terminals to block neurotransmitter release. Evidence also exists suggesting that opioids exert a direct inhibitory effect on the postsynaptic membrane potential (see Fig. 57-3).

In addition to the opioid descending inhibitory pathway, an alpha adrenergic pathway has been identified that also originates from locations in the periaqueductal gray and reticular formation. Stimulation of these pathways inhibits synaptic transmission in the dorsal horn similar to the inhibition produced by the opioid system. It has been demonstrated that electrical stimulation of these pathways and intracerebral injections of alpha$_2$-agonists can inhibit spinal nociceptive reflexes and that this effect can be antagonized by intrathecally administered alpha$_2$-adrenergic antagonists.[18,19] Further evidence of the alpha-adrenergic pathway stems from the observation that the intrathecal administration of alpha$_2$-adrenergic agonists produces analgesia, implying that alpha$_2$ adrenoreceptors are responsible for this antinociceptive effect.[20,21] These alpha-adrenergic fibers descend into the dorsolateral fasciculus, in a manner similar to that of the opioid fibers, and synapse in the substantia gelatinosa region of the dorsal horn. Norepinephrine is released from these nerve terminals and produces hyperpolarization of the first-order neurons, internuncial neurons, and wide dynamic range neurons in the spinothalamic tract. In addition, there are some alpha$_2$ adrenoreceptor projections into the ventral gray matter area of the motor nuclei.

The opioid and the alpha$_2$ receptors share a common mechanism of action. At the cellular level, these receptors

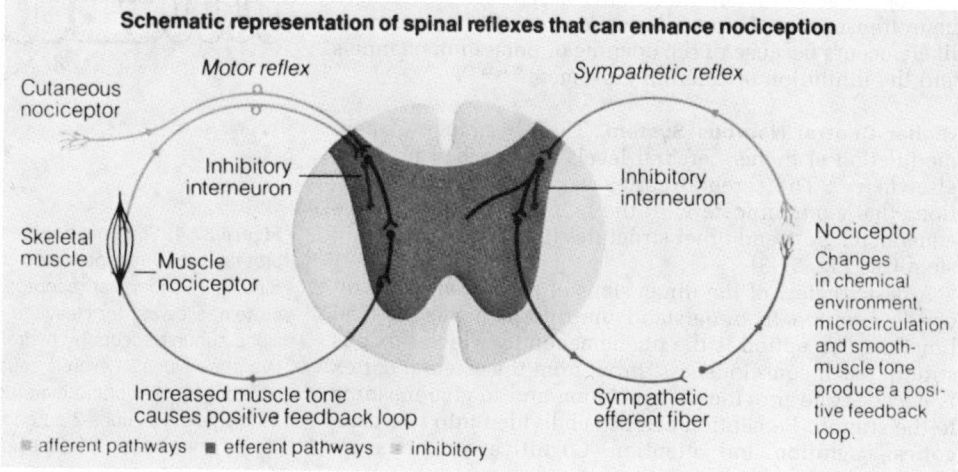

Figure 57-2. Schematic representation of spinal reflexes involved in pain modulation. (Reprinted with permission from Bonica JJ, Liebeskind JC, Albe-Fessard DG [eds]: Advances in Pain Research and Therapy, pp 3–32. New York, Raven Press, 1979.)

Schematic representation of spinal reflexes that can enhance nociception

Motor reflex

Sympathetic reflex

Cutaneous nociceptor

Inhibitory interneuron

Inhibitory interneuron

Skeletal muscle

Muscle nociceptor

Nociceptor

Changes in chemical environment, microcirculation and smooth-muscle tone produce a positive feedback loop

Increased muscle tone causes positive feedback loop

Sympathetic efferent fiber

afferent pathways   efferent pathways   inhibitory

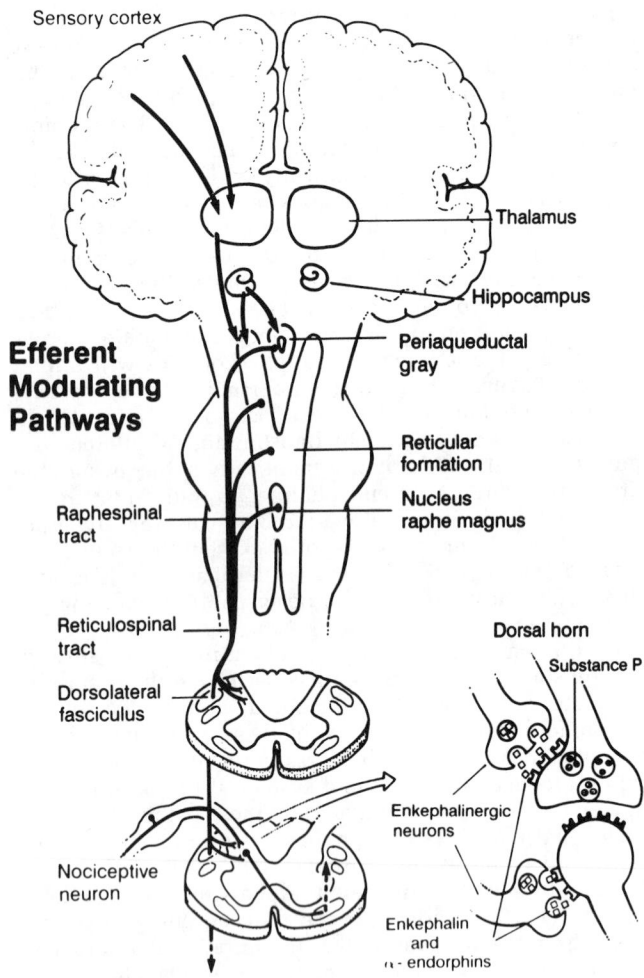

Figure 57-3. Efferent pathways involved in nociceptive regulation.

those abilities that recognize, discriminate, memorize, or judge afferent information that stems from external stimuli. Therefore, cognitive modulation of pain involves the patient's ability to relate a painful experience to another event. For example, pain experienced in a pleasant environment elicits less pain response than pain experienced in a setting of depression. The other area of perception is attention. Attention operates on the premise that only a fixed number of afferent stimuli can reach cortical centers. If a patient in pain concentrates on a separate and unrelated image, it is possible to reduce the effect of a painful sensation. This is achieved because the patient is focused on something else. The positive impact on pain from biofeedback or hypnosis also operates on this principle.

PATHOPHYSIOLOGY OF PAIN

Components of Surgical Stress

Perhaps the most compelling reason to search for more effective methods of analgesia is the realization that approximately 75% of hospitalized patients, despite receiving routine intermittent on-demand opioid analgesics, remain in moderate to severe pain.[27,28] In addition to the purely humanitarian aspects of providing postoperative analgesia is our growing understanding of the deleterious effects of post-

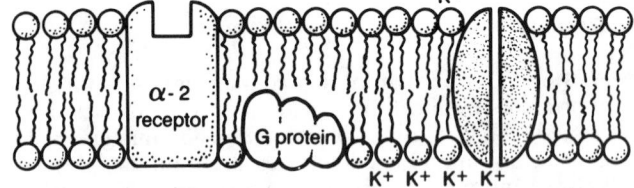

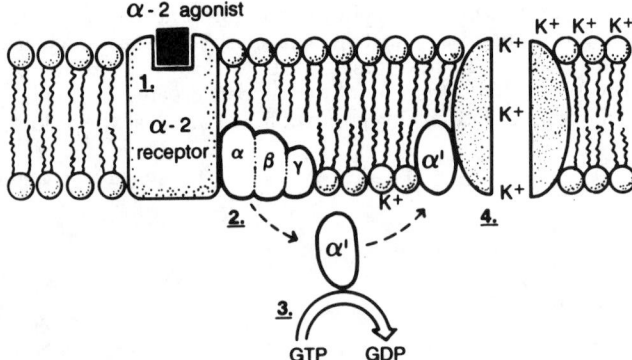

Figure 57-4. Schematic representation of cellular mechanisms of G protein–linked receptor, depicted as an alpha$_2$-adrenergic receptor. Binding of agonist at receptor causes conformational change in G protein, allowing for cleavage of the alpha subunit. Activation of the alpha subunit occurs by hydrolysis of guanosine triphosphate to active state alpha', which is capable of increasing K$^+$ movement and resulting in membrane hyperpolarization. (Adapted with permission from Maze M: Alpha-2 adrenoceptor agonists: Defining the role in clinical anesthesia. Anesthesiology 74:581, 1991.)

appear to belong to a family of receptors that are coupled with a G protein (Fig. 57-4).[22,23] The G protein exerts its membrane function through a secondary messenger protein capable of converting guanosine triphosphate to guanosine diphosphate. When the receptor is occupied, the alpha subunit of the G protein releases from the beta and gamma subunits and modulates cellular functions such as ion exchange, adenyl cyclase, and phospholipase C activity. Hyperpolarization of the nerve results in decreased transmission of the action potential and decreased release of stored neurotransmitter. Hyperpolarization of the nerve most likely occurs because of the opening of potassium channels and the inhibition of calcium movement.[23-25]

Higher Central Nervous System. The physiology of pain modulation at higher cerebral levels is described in detail elsewhere.[26] The cerebral cortex has several interconnections that communicate with the reticular formation, periaqueductal gray, and other structures in the brain and brain stem (see Fig. 57-3).

A basic review of the dimensions of perceptual psychology is required to understand the role of higher cortical function. Perception is the phenomenon by which noxious stimuli reach consciousness. Input from the cerebral cortex is necessary to provide interpretation and to give meaning to the stimuli. Perception can be subdivided into two categories: cognition and attention. Cognitive functions are

TABLE 57-2. Adverse Physiologic Sequelae of Pain

Organ System	Clinical Effect
Respiratory	
Increased skeletal muscle tension	Hypoxemia
Decreased total lung compliance	Hypercapnia
	Ventilation-perfusion abnormality
	Atelectasis
	Pneumonitis
Endocrine	
Increased adrenocorticotropic hormone	Protein catabolism
Increased cortisol	Lipolysis
Increased glucagon	Hyperglycemia
Increased epinephrine	
Decreased insulin	
Decreased testosterone	Decreased protein anabolism
Decreased insulin	
Increased aldosterone	Salt and water retention
Increased antidiuretic hormone	
Increased cortisol	Congestive heart failure
Increased catecholamines	Vasoconstriction
Increased angiotensin II	Increased myocardial contractility
	Increased heart rate
Cardiovascular	
Increased myocardial work (mediated *via* catecholamines, angiotensin II)	Dysrhythmias
	Angina
	Myocardial infarction
	Congestive heart failure
Immunologic	
Lymphopenia	Decreased immune function
Depression of reticuloendothelial system	
Leukocytosis	
Reduced killer T-cell cytotoxicity	
Coagulation Effects	
Increased platelet adhesiveness	Increased incidence of thromboembolic phenomena
Diminished fibrinolysis	
Activation of coagulation cascade	
Gastrointestinal	
Increased sphincter tone	Ileus
Decreased smooth muscle tone	
Genitourinary	
Increased sphincter tone	Urinary retention
Decreased smooth muscle tone	

operative pain on specific organ systems and our concern with the general well-being of the convalescing patient (Table 57-2).

Endocrine

Numerous hormones are released in response to pain and in turn have myriad biochemical effects. In addition to the rise in catabolically active hormones such as catecholamines, cortisol, angiotensin II, and antidiuretic hormone, stress causes an increase in the adrenocorticotropic hormone, growth hormone, and glucagon.[29-31] The stress response results in lower levels of anabolic hormones, such as testosterone and insulin. Epinephrine, cortisol, and glu-

cagon produce hyperglycemia by promoting insulin resistance and increases in gluconeogenesis. They induce protein catabolism and lipolysis to provide substrates for gluconeogenesis. The stress response causes a negative nitrogen balance postoperatively. Aldosterone, cortisol, and antidiuretic hormone influence water and electrolyte reabsorption by promoting Na^+ and water retention while expending potassium. This contributes to increases in the extravascular fluid compartment both peripherally and within the pulmonary parenchymal tissue. Finally, catecholamines sensitize peripheral nociceptive endings, which serve to propagate more intense pain and may contribute to a vicious pain-catecholamine release-pain cycle.[32,33]

Cardiovascular

The cardiovascular effects of pain are initiated by the release of catecholamines from sympathetic nerve endings and the adrenal medulla, of aldosterone and cortisol from the adrenal cortex, and of antidiuretic hormone from the hypothalamus, and by activation of the renin-angiotensin system. These hormones have direct effects on the myocardium or vasculature, and they augment salt and water retention, which places a greater burden on the cardiovascular system.

Angiotensin II causes generalized vasoconstriction, whereas catecholamines increase heart rate, myocardial contractility, and systemic vascular resistance. The sympathoadrenal release of catecholamines and the effects of angiotensin II may result in hypertension, tachycardia, and dysrhythmias and consequently may lead to myocardial ischemia in susceptible patients. Salt and water retention secondary to aldosterone, cortisol, and antidiuretic hormone, in combination with the previously described effects of catecholamines and angiotensin II, can precipitate congestive heart failure in patients with limited cardiac reserve. Although it may be difficult to quantitate the influence of pain with its accompanying neuroendocrine stress response on postoperative cardiovascular complications, it is probably more important than previously recognized.

Respiratory

Increases in extracellular lung water may contribute to ventilation-perfusion abnormalities. For surgical procedures performed on the thorax and abdomen, pain-induced reflex increases in skeletal muscle tension may lead to decreased total lung compliance, splinting, and hypoventilation. These changes then promote atelectasis, contribute to further ventilation-perfusion abnormalities, and result in hypoxemia. In major surgical procedures or in high-risk patients, these respiratory effects of pain may lead to a significant reduction in functional residual capacity ranging from 25–50% of preoperative values.[34,35] Hypoxemia typically stimulates increases in minute ventilation. Although tachypnea and hypocapnia are common initially, prolonged increases in the work of breathing may result in hypercapnic respiratory failure. Pulmonary consolidation and pneumonitis may occur because of hypoventilation and further aggravate the clinical scenario.

Gastrointestinal

Studies have shown that pain-induced sympathetic hyperactivity may cause reflex inhibition of gastrointestinal function. This promotes postoperative ileus, which contributes to postoperative nausea, vomiting, and discomfort.[36-38]

Genitourinary

An increase in sympathetic activity responses to pain causes reflex inhibition of most visceral smooth muscle, including urinary bladder tone. This results in urinary retention with subsequent urinary tract infections and related complications.

Immunologic

The pain-related stress response results in lymphopenia, leukocytosis, and depression of the reticuloendothelial system.[39,40] In addition, some anesthetic agents reduce chemotaxis of neutrophils and may be one factor involved in the reduction of monocyte activity.[41,42] These effects can lower resistance to pathogens and may be key factors in the development of perioperative infectious complications. In patients with neoplasms in whom surgical manipulation of the tumor causes release of tumor cells, the postoperative stress response can reduce the cytotoxicity of killer T cells. Increases in catecholamines, glucocorticoids, and prostaglandins in response to stress all may contribute to the altered immunologic response and allow metastatic spread of the neoplasm.[43]

Coagulation

Stress-related alterations in blood viscosity, platelet function, fibrinolysis, and coagulation pathways have been described.[44-49] These stress-mediated effects include increased platelet adhesiveness, diminished fibrinolysis, and promotion of a hypercoagulable state. When these effects are coupled with the microcirculatory effects of catecholamines as well as immobilization of the patient in the postoperative period, thromboembolic events are more likely to occur.

General Well-Being

Pain increases skeletal muscle tone in the area of the surgical field. This postoperative impairment of muscle function may lead to physical immobility and a delayed return to normal function. Poorly controlled pain also contributes to insomnia, anxiety, and a feeling of helplessness. These psychological factors, coupled with the immobilization that occurs because of the increased skeletal muscle tone, create a perioperative atmosphere that has been feared by most patients.

Magnitude of Stress Response

Small peripheral surgical procedures performed with the use of local anesthesia produce minimal or no physiologic changes. The more extensive the surgical procedure, the greater the magnitude of an adverse physiologic response. In general, intrathoracic and intra-abdominal procedures elicit a greater neuroendocrine stress response than do procedures performed on an extremity. Intracranial procedures involve smaller changes because of the relatively small surgical field and the absence of pain receptors in the brain.

From the previous discussion, it is apparent that the physiologic changes that occur postoperatively are not homeostatic mechanisms but are reproducible adverse responses to the stress of surgery and anesthesia. The net result is myriad adverse physiologic events that can contribute to or be responsible for postsurgical morbidity and mortality.

Influence of Anesthesia on the Surgical Stress Response

General Anesthesia

It has been demonstrated that general anesthesia, either with intravenous or inhalational anesthetics, does not effectively attenuate the neuroendocrine stress response.[50] One exception to this assertion is the administration of high-dose opioid anesthesia. Extremely high doses of certain opioids can inhibit some aspects of the stress response, but lower doses of opioids generally are unable to hinder the neuroendocrine effects of stress.[51-53] In a dose response study, investigators noted that fentanyl, in doses of 10 and 30 μg·kg^{-1}, was not adequate to suppress the surgical stress response but 50 μg·kg^{-1} of fentanyl was effective.[54] High doses of inhalational agents (1.5 MAC) may suppress the catecholamine response intraoperatively but do not diminish the catecholamine response that develops postoperatively.

Regional Anesthesia and Analgesia

Regional anesthesia and analgesia have been shown to reduce catecholamine and other stress hormone responses during the perioperative period for certain surgical procedures.[55-59] The finding that regional anesthesia and analgesia can ablate the neuroendocrine stress responses is not universal. Other studies have demonstrated that central neuroaxial techniques have no significant influence on cortisol release.[60,61] The differing results may be related to the level of the afferent neural blockade. The other confounding variable in these studies is the region of the body where the surgical procedure was performed. In studies where regional anesthesia did not have an influence on the cortisol response, surgery was performed in the upper abdomen, whereas in most studies that demonstrate inhibition, surgery was performed on a lower extremity or the lower abdomen. Sensory blocks below L1 generally have no effect on cortisol response. In order to prevent a cortisol response to surgery, all afferent pathways from the surgical site must be blocked.[62]

Besides reducing the neuroendocrine stress response, regional anesthesia can reduce myocardial work and oxygen consumption by reducing heart rate, arterial pressure, and left ventricular contractility.[63,64] Left ventricular ejection fraction is not significantly affected by epidural anesthesia in normal patients, whereas patients with chronic stable angina experience a modest but significant improvement in left ventricular ejection fraction and left ventricular wall motion provided that volume loading is limited.[65,66] In patients with unstable angina that is refractory to treatment with nitrates, beta blockers, and Ca^{2+} antagonists, thoracic epidural analgesia alleviates chest pain without changing coronary perfusion pressure, cardiac output, or systemic vascular resistance.[67] A reduction in infarct size in experimental models of acute coronary occlusion has also been demonstrated.[63]

Vital capacity and functional residual capacity can be restored to near preoperative levels with epidural local anesthetic blockade.[68] This is associated with a reduction in the spontaneous work of breathing, requirements for mechanical ventilation, and facilitation of chest physiotherapy.[68] These factors all play an important role in preventing unwanted respiratory complications postoperatively. Epidural opioid analgesia has also been demonstrated to improve pulmonary function postoperatively compared with parenteral opioids.[35,69]

In patients undergoing total hip replacements, epidural anesthesia reduces the incidence of deep venous thrombosis and pulmonary embolism.[49] Epidural anesthesia and analgesia can also reduce the degree of postoperative hypercoagulability in vascular surgery patients.[70] The reduced incidence of thromboischemic phenomena from these studies may be related to an inhibitory effect on platelet aggregation as well as to improvements in lower limb blood flow.[71,72] Another salutary effect of epidural anesthesia and analgesia is improved fibrinolytic function.[73]

The most significant evidence regarding the beneficial effects of regional anesthesia and analgesia is found in clinical outcome studies that compare general anesthesia and intramuscular opioids with general anesthesia and epidural analgesia for postoperative pain relief. These studies demonstrated that epidural analgesia can improve pulmonary function postoperatively[35] as well as reduce cardiovascular, infectious, and overall morbidity and mortality[59,74] at lower total hospital cost.[59] Major respiratory and cardiovascular complications occurring in the postoperative period may be a consequence of surgical pain and the stress responses. Anesthetic management that blunts this response can have a positive impact on patient care. It is likely that the advantages attributed to the use of regional anesthesia and analgesia are a result of extending suppression of the surgical stress response to pain into the postoperative period.

PHARMACOLOGY OF POSTOPERATIVE PAIN MANAGEMENT

Agents administered orally for postoperative pain management can be grouped by their mechanism of effect as opioid or nonopioid analgesics.

Nonopioid Analgesics

Mechanisms of Analgesic Effects

Aspirin, acetaminophen, and the nonsteroidal anti-inflammatory drugs (NSAIDs) are the principal nonopioid analgesics used to treat minor or moderate acute postoperative pain (Table 57-3). Although these compounds represent diverse chemical entities, their common mechanism of action is inhibition of prostaglandin-mediated amplification of chemical and mechanical irritants on the sensory pathways. Whereas sensitization or intensification of painful stimuli is mediated by the prostaglandins and lowers the threshold for further activation of the nociceptors, the prostaglandins directly evoke little painful response.[75]

The majority of these agents modulate prostaglandin synthesis through inhibition of the action of the enzyme cyclo-oxygenase, which is one of the first steps in the conversion of arachidonic acid into prostaglandins.[76] By reducing prostaglandin synthesis, cyclo-oxygenase inhibitors block the nociceptive response to endogenous mediators of inflammation such as bradykinin, acetylcholine, and serotonin.[77] Although the exact mechanism for the participation of endogenous substances such as prostaglandins in the generation and transduction of nociceptive stimuli is unknown, the effect is greatest in tissues that have been subjected to trauma and inflammation.[78] The prostaglandins represent a diverse group of compounds that mediate many cellular and subcellular functions. The order of the sensitizing or hyper-

algesic effect that is generally observed with this group is $PGE_1>PGE_2>PGF_{s\alpha}$, whereas PGA_1, PGB_2, and PGI_2 exhibit little sensitizing effect.[77]

Although mediation of the peripheral inflammatory response is an important component of pain modulation by this group of agents, inhibition of central mechanisms of hyperalgesia is likely.[79] Acetaminophen and ketorolac are cyclo-oxygenase inhibitors that have potent antipyretic and analgesic properties. They are equipotent to aspirin in inhibiting prostaglandin synthesis in the central nervous system but much less potent in inhibiting prostaglandin synthesis at peripheral sites. The site of activity of these agents may be a result of pharmacokinetic factors such as drug distribution, but more likely it reflects differences in these enzyme systems throughout the body. The peripheral actions of cyclo-oxygenase inhibition on platelet function, chemotaxis, and vascular responses to inflammation may be undesirable in the postoperative patient but very desirable in the patient with rheumatoid arthritis. Understanding these factors is important when selecting an agent for postoperative analgesia.

Since all the compounds in this group do not block cyclo-oxygenase, the membrane stabilization theory has also been postulated for these agents.[80] Membrane stabilization could account for decreased prostaglandin release seen at concentrations that are lower than those needed for effective cyclo-oxygenase inhibition. This theory is supported by the correlation of analgesic potency with the octanol/water partition coefficient within this group.[80] Corticosteroids, tricyclic antidepressants, and local anesthetics are also considered to possess membrane-stabilizing effects. This might explain the beneficial effects that have been reported with their use in acute pain management.

Absorption/Biotransformation/Elimination

Following oral administration, nonopioid analgesics are rapidly and completely absorbed. Food generally delays absorption but does not affect absolute bioavailability. Intramuscular absorption of ketorolac is complete and occurs within 50 minutes of administration.[81] With the exception of acetaminophen, protein binding for this group is >80%. Displacement of other highly protein-bound drugs, such as warfarin, may occur when these agents are administered concurrently. Biotransformation by liver enzyme systems and renal excretion of conjugated metabolites are the primary modes of elimination of these agents. Caution must be exercised in patients with renal and liver dysfunction.

Adverse Effects

Gastrointestinal discomfort and central nervous system disturbances are the most common adverse effects of short-term therapy with nonopioid analgesics. Nausea, vomiting, dyspepsia, heartburn, and epigastric discomfort occur in 5–25% of patients receiving aspirin, and in 3–9% of patients receiving NSAIDs. Dizziness, headache, and drowsiness occur in about 1–9% of patients receiving NSAIDs. Prolonged bleeding is a result of the action of these agents on prostaglandin synthesis in platelets. This effect is generally reversible with the NSAIDs 24 to 48 hours after discontinuing therapy. It is much more prolonged after discontinuation of aspirin because of the irreversible acetylation of the platelet surface. Although this effect persists for the life of the platelet, clinical prolongation of bleeding time is thought to be reversed in about 1 week. More severe adverse effects include an exacerbation of bronchospasm and rhini-

TABLE 57-3. Pharmacokinetic Parameters/Maximum Dosage Recommendations of Nonopioid Analgesics

	Route	Time to Peak Levels (hr)	Half-Life (hr)	Analgesic Actions (hr) Onset	Analgesic Actions (hr) Duration	Maximum Recommended Daily Dose (mg)
Salicylates						
Aspirin/sodium salicylate	po	0.5–2	2–3[1]	0.5–1	2–4	3600
Diflunisal (Dolobid)	po	2–3	8–12	1–2	8–12	2000
Propionic Acids						
Fenoprofen (Nalfon, various)	po	1–2	2–3	1	4–6	3200
Flurbiprofen (Ansaid)	po	1.5	5.7	—	—	300
Ibuprofen (Motrin, Rufen, various)	po	1–2	1.8–2.5	0.5	4–6	3200
Ketoprofen (Orudis)	po	0.5–2	2.4	0.5	4–6	300
Naproxen (Naprosyn)	po	2–4	12–15	1	4–7	1500
Naproxen Sodium (Anaprox)	po	1–2	12–13	1	4–7	1375
Indoles						
Indomethacin (Indocin, various)	po	1–2	4.5	0.5	4–6	200
Indomethacin (Indocin SR, sustained release)	po	2–4	4.5–6	0.5	4–6	150
Sulindac (Clinoril, various)	po	2–4	7.8 (16.4)[2]	—	—	400
Tolmetin (Tolectin)	po	0.5–1	1–1.5	—	—	2000
Ketorolac (Torodol)	im	1	4–6[6] 5–9[7]	0.5–1	4–6	120[8]
Fenamates						
Meclofenamate (Melcomen, various)	po	0.5–1	2 (3.3)[3]	0.5–1	4–6	400
Mefenamic acid (Ponstel)	po	2–4	2–4	1	4–6	1000
Oxicans						
Piroxicam (Feldene)	po	3–5	30–86	1	48–72	20
Phenylacetic Acids						
Diclofenac sodium (Voltaren)	po	2–3	2	1	4–6	200
Pyrazolidinediones						
Phenylbutazone (Butazolidin, various)	po	2	50–100	—	—	400
p-Aminophenols						
Acetaminophen (Tylenol, Datril, various)	po	0.5–1	1–4	0.5	2–4	1200
Phenacetin[4]	po	1 1–2[5]	— —	— —	— —	2400 —

[1] Half-life of aspirin dose-dependent.
[2] Half-life of active sulfide metabolite.
[3] Half-life with multiple dosing.
[4] 75–80% of phenacetin converted to acetaminophen.
[5] Time to peak acetaminophen levels.
[6] Half-life in healthy adults.
[7] Half-life in renal failure.
[8] Daily recommended dose for first day of therapy, 150 mg.

tis induced by aspirin as well as by other NSAIDs in patients with a history of nasal polyps, asthma, and rhinitis. Ulceration and bleeding of the gastrointestinal mucosa can occur owing to direct irritation by the drug. This effect, coupled with the inhibition of prostaglandin-mediated bicarbonate and mucus secretion, allows for further erosion of the tissue. Patients with diabetes or gastric or peptic ulcers are at higher risk for gastrointestinal bleeding, ulceration, and even perforation. Misoprostol, a synthetic PGE_2, can be used to increase bicarbonate and mucus production in high-risk patients. An acute renal insufficiency syndrome—hyperkalemia and peripheral edema—can be precipitated in elderly patients, those with congestive heart failure or renal or hepatic dysfunction or patients on diuretic therapy. This is a result of the blockade of prostaglandin-mediated effects on renal blood flow.[82] Proteinuria, interstitial nephritis, and papillary necrosis have been reported, but the mechanism of their association with prostaglandin inhibition is less clear. Acetaminophen is generally free of adverse effects in dosages used for acute pain management.

Clinical Uses

Unlike the opioid analgesics, the mechanisms of analgesia with the nonopioid analgesics are not specifically involved in interrupting the transmission of the nociceptive stimulus. This transmission depends in large part on the central and peripheral inflammatory responses to tissue injury. This property can serve to enhance the analgesic effect when these agents are combined with opioids, such as the use of acetaminophen with various forms of codeine and its congeners. Based on their pharmacologic mechanisms, it is not surprising to find that the analgesic effect of nonopioid agents is confined to somewhat narrow therapeutic ranges above which there is little increase in analgesia but a considerable increase in toxicity. To reduce the postoperative amplification of the nociceptive response to tissue injury, the most efficacious use of these agents would be prior to surgery. This is because the effect of PGE_2 can last for many hours and the sensitizing effects of circulating prostaglandins are not reversed by cyclo-oxygenase inhibitors.[77] There also appears to be a greater value when using these agents in procedures involving musculoskeletal, post-traumatic, and inflammatory pain and in conditions such as dysmenorrhea, renal colic, and biliary obstruction, in which prostaglandins are known to be involved in the pathogenesis of the pain.[80]

Opioid Analgesics

Mechanism of Analgesic Effects

Morphine and related compounds act as agonists, producing their biologic effects by interacting with stereoselective and saturable membrane-bound receptors that are nonuniformly distributed throughout the central nervous system. Researchers using binding studies have identified the major sites of opioid activity in the central nervous system to include the periaqueductal and periventricular gray, nucleus reticularis gigantocellularis, medial thalamus, mesencephalic reticular formation, lateral hypothalamus, raphe nuclei, and spinal cord.[83] The endogenous neuromodulating peptides of the enkephalin and beta-endorphin classes also bind to this family of receptors, which are collectively referred to as the opioid receptors. The unique properties of the individual agents of this group are a result of their specific receptor activity and affinity. Currently, five distinct types of opioid receptors have been identified (mu, μ; kappa, κ; delta, δ; sigma, σ; and epsilon, ϵ) and subtypes of mu, kappa, and sigma have also been proposed. The cellular mechanisms of these interactions have been discussed previously in this chapter. In addition to their effect on the opioid receptor, agents such as fentanyl, sufentanil, and meperidine in high concentrations can produce weak local anesthetic effects on the nerve fibers.[24]

Affinity and activity of the agent at four of these receptor groups, mu, delta, kappa, and sigma, have been shown to be responsible for the pharmacologic effects of the opiates (Table 57-4).[84] The enkephalins and opiates have affinity and activity at the mu_1 receptor, which mediates supraspinal analgesia, prolactin release, and euphoria. Mu_2 receptors that are opiate-selective appear to mediate respiratory depression and physical dependence. Delta and kappa receptors are at least partially responsible for spinal analgesia.

Miosis and sedation are a result of kappa receptor activity, whereas sigma activity can produce dysphoria and hallucinations. Pure opioid agonists (Table 57-5) have affinity and at least moderate activity at the mu_1, mu_2, delta, and kappa receptors, which explains their central and spinal analgesic effect as well as their dose-related side-effects and addictive potential. The differences in potency and side-effects among agents in this class are a result of receptor selectivity, affinity, and lipophilicity of the agent.

The pharmacologic properties of the mixed agonist-antagonist analgesics are also a result of their affinity for the opioid receptor subclasses. Unlike the pure agonist, however, not all of these agents produce an agonist effect when they interact with the receptor. There are two distinct groupings of the agonist-antagonist agents based on their receptor affinity and activity. The first of these groups is characterized by high mu receptor affinity with activity less than or similar to that of morphine. Agents in this category include buprenorphine and dezocine. The second group of agonist-antagonist analgesics processes only moderate affinity without activity at the mu receptor, high affinity with at least moderate activity at the kappa receptor, and at least moderate affinity and some activity at the sigma receptor. This group includes pentazocine, butorphanol, and nalbuphine and accounts for the highly sedative effects and potential for psychomimetic reactions seen with these drugs. Additionally, because of the affinity of both of these classes at the mu receptor with activity less than that of the pure agonists, all of these agents have the potential for reversing the effect of an agonist, including precipitation of withdrawal symptoms.

Absorption/Biotransformation/Elimination. Although opioid analgesics are well absorbed from the gastrointestinal tract, differences in analgesic equivalence between oral and parenteral doses are a result of a significant first-pass metabolism by the liver. Codeine, oxycodone, and hydrocodone do not undergo extensive first-pass metabolism owing to the methoxy substitution of the phenolic component of the phenanthrene ring, and they have greater oral to parenteral equivalency than morphine. Parenteral administration results in a more rapid onset of effect compared with oral and rectal administration. Distribution is dependent upon the lipophilicity of the agent; smaller amounts of the more hydrophobic morphine reach the brain as opposed to more lipophilic agents such as methadone, meperidine, and codeine. Biotransformation followed by renal elimination of conjugated metabolites is the primary mode of elimination. Active metabolites of morphine (morphine-6-glucuronide), codeine (morphine), meperidine (normeperidine), and propoxyphene (norpropoxyphene) add to their primary pharmacologic effect as well as to the toxicity of these agents. Renal elimination is primarily by glomerular filtration, with a small fraction of drug excreted in the feces.

Adverse Effects. With short-term, moderate-dose therapy, central nervous system and gastrointestinal side-effects predominate. Sedation, dizziness, lightheadedness, miosis, nausea, vomiting, and constipation are extensions of the pharmacologic actions of these agents and occur in dose-dependent fashion. Tolerance to the sedative and other central nervous system effects develops rapidly over the first few days of therapy or after an increase in dosage. Constipation is a result of decreased peristalsis of the bowel and decreased secretory actions of the stomach, biliary tract, and pancreas. Spasm of the sphincter of Oddi can increase pressure in the common bile and contribute to epigastric distress. This effect can persist for up to 24 hours after a single

TABLE 57-4. Pharmacology of Opioid Receptors

Receptor	Mu — Mu$_1$	Mu$_2$	Delta		Kappa		Sigma	
Effect								
Analgesia	Supraspinal		Spinal		Spinal			
Affect	Euphoria	Sedation			Sedation		Dysphoria/ hallucinations	
Pupil	Miosis				Miosis		Mydriasis	
Respiration		Depression	Depression				Tachypnea	
Gastrointestinal	Nausea/ vomiting	Constipation	Nausea/vomiting					
Genitourinary	Urinary/ retention		Urinary/retention		Diuresis			
Temperature	Increase							
Other	Pruritus		Pruritus Physical depen- dence					
Tolerance	Yes		Yes		Little			
Cross-tolerance	Delta		Mu		No			
Binding Properties	Affinity	Activity	Affinity	Activity	Affinity	Activity	Affinity	Activity
Agonists								
Morphine	+ + +	+ + +	+ +	+ +	+	+		
Meperidine	+ +	+ +	+ +	+ +	+	+		
Fentanyl	+ + + +	+ + + +	+	+				
Agonist-Antagonists								
Pentazocine	+ +	0			+ + +	+ + +	+ + +	+ + +
Nalbuphine	+ +	0			+ + +	+ + +	+ +	+
Butorphanol	+ +	0			+ + +	+ +	+ +	+ +
Buprenorphine	+ + +	+			+ +			
Dezocine	+ + +	+	+ +	+	+	+		

Key: affinity: + + + + very high, + + + high, + + moderate, + low
    activity: 0 no activity, + low activity, + + moderate activity, + + + high activity, + + + + very high activity.

Adapted with permission from Benedetti C, Butler SH: Systemic analgesics. In Bonica JJ (ed): The Management of Pain, vol II, 2nd ed, pp 1640–1675. Philadelphia, Lea & Febiger, 1990.

therapeutic dose of an opioid. Low doses of naloxone and vasodilating agents have been used to relieve this discomfort. Biliary colic tends to occur more often in patients after morphine administration than after meperidine administration despite the similar rise in biliary pressure seen with both these agents. The agonist-antagonists tend to produce less of a rise in biliary pressure than the pure agonist. Stool softeners and laxatives are warranted in patients with severe constipation. Urinary retention may also result from the increase in sphincter tone and release of antidiuretic hormone secondary to opioid administration. Physical dependence and analgesic tolerance are not generally a problem when used short term but may be troublesome after chronic opioid therapy. Respiratory depression, apnea, cardiac arrest, circulatory collapse, coma, and death can occur after high intravenous doses.

Clinical Uses

Opioids remain the primary pharmacologic therapeutic agents for moderate to severe postoperative pain. Analgesia is achieved by blunting the central response to noxious stimuli without loss of consciousness or affecting tactile, visual, or auditory sensation. Dose-limiting side-effects such as nausea, vomiting, constipation, urinary retention, and respiratory depression can be overcome by proper selection of the agent and route of administration. Sedation and euphoria may be desired in the immediate postoperative period. Analgesic potency is not necessarily an advantage because at equianalgesic doses there are parallel increases in side-effects. Agonist-antagonists can be effective analgesics in the postoperative period and have a ceiling effect for respiratory depression. Unfortunately, dose escalations with these agents may also produce a ceiling for their analgesic effects while increasing their sedative and dysphoric properties.

Unlike the NSAIDs, opioid analgesics do not interfere with healing processes or inhibit platelet function. Traditional therapeutic regimes that utilized on-demand administration are being replaced with continuous or around-the-clock orders as the benefits of a reduced stress response in the postoperative period are becoming more apparent. As the patient's analgesic requirements diminish, the transition from parenteral to oral therapy is more empirical and generally involves replacing the opioid with an opioid/NSAID combination such as acetaminophen with codeine. Codeine, hydrocodone, and oxycodone are limited in their analgesic potency because of their high incidence of side-effects at equianalgesic doses as compared with morphine or meperidine and are best utilized for minor to moderate pain.

TABLE 57-5. Pharmacokinetic Parameters/Maximum Dosage Recommendations for Oral and Parenteral Opioid Analgesics

	Dosage		Half-Life (h)	Analgesic Action (h)			Equivalency Ratio	Comment
	Route	mg		Onset	Peak	Duration		
AGONISTS								
Naturally Occurring Alkaloids								
Morphine (Various)	iv	2.5–15	2–3.5	—	0.125	—	—	Rapid onset, peak respiratory depression 10 minutes
	im	10–15		0.3	0.5–1.5	3–4	1	
	po	30–60		0.5–1	1–2	4	6	Equivalence to im dose decreases with repeated dosing
Codeine (Various)	im	15–60	3	0.25–0.5	1–5	4–6	12	im route has little advantage compared with im morphine
	po	15–60		0.25–1	0.5–2	3–4	20	Oral potency due to low first-pass effect
Partially Synthetic Derivatives of Morphine								
Hydromorphone (Dilaudid, various)	im	1–4	2–3	0.3–0.5	1	2–3	0.2	Potent analgesic but short duration limits usefulness
	po	1–4		0.5–1	1	3–4	0.6	Well absorbed from gastrointestinal tract
Oxymorphone (Numorphan)	im	1–1.5	2–3	0.5	1	2–3	0.1	
Hydrocodone (Vicodin)	po	5–7.5	3.3–4.5	—	—	3–8	—	Similar to codeine, preparations contain acetaminophen
Oxycodone (Percodan)	po	5	2–3	0.5	1–2	3–6	3	Short-acting, preparations contain acetaminophen
Synthetic Compounds								
Morphans								
Levorphanol (Levo-Dromoran)	im	2–3	12–16	1	2	4–6	0.2	Drug accumulation precludes usefulness
	po	2–4		1.5	2	4–6	0.4	Well absorbed after oral administration
Phenylheptylamines								
Methadone (Dolophine)	im	2.5–10	15–30	0.25	0.5–1	4–6	1	Used more widely in Europe
	po	2.5–10		0.5–1	1.5–2	4–8	1	
Propoxyphene HCl (Darvon, various)	po	32–65	3–4	0.25–1	1–2	3–6	30	Weak opioid, optical enantiomer of methadone
Propoxyphene Napsylate (Darvon N)	po	50–100					100	Delayed absorption compared with hydrochloride salt
Phenylpiperidines								
Meperidine (Demerol, various)	im	50–100	3–4	0.12–0.5	1	2–4	10	Short duration of effect. One-tenth as potent as morphine.
	po	50–100		0.5–1	1–2	2–3	20	Active metabolite normeperidine accumulates in renal failure and has a half-life of 12–16
MIXED AGONIST-ANTAGONIST								
Buprenorphine (Buprenex)	im	0.3–0.6	2–3	0.12	1	6–8	0.04	High mu affinity, may precipitate withdrawal
	iv	.03–.2*						Decreased onset and duration compared with im route
Butorphanol (Stadol)	im	2–4	2.5–3.5	0.1–0.2	0.5–1	3–4	0.2	May precipitate withdrawal
Dezocine (Dalgan)	im	5–20	2.5	0.25–0.5	0.5–1.5	2–4	1	Potency similar to that of morphine
	iv	5–10		0.25				
Nalbuphine (Nubain)	im	10–20	5	0.25	1	3–6	1	May precipitate withdrawal
	iv	1–5*						Onset 2–3 minutes
Pentazocine (Talwin)	im	30–60	2–3	0.12–0.5	1–3	3–6	6	Used primarily for cancer pain
	po	50				4–7	18	

*Intravenous route generally used for antagonist properties.

Adapted with permission from Intrurrsi CE, Foley KM: Narcotic analgesics in the management of pain. In Kuhar M, Pasternak G (eds): Analgesics, Neurochemical, Behavioral, and Clinical Preservatives, pp 257–288. New York, Raven Press, 1984.

METHODS OF ANALGESIA

Pain relief may involve pharmacologic use of analgesics by various routes of administration or nonpharmacologic application of mechanical, electrical, or psychological techniques. In any patient, the optimal combinations of these techniques are dependent on the type and degree of pain, the patient's perception of the pain, and the underlying medical, social, and environmental conditions in which the pain is managed. In this section oral and parenteral routes of analgesic delivery are described first, followed by regional analgesic techniques. Nonpharmacologic methods of acute pain management are discussed last.

Routes of Analgesic Delivery

Oral

Oral analgesics are generally considered less than optimal for moderate to severe acute postoperative pain management because of their lack of titratability, prolonged time to peak effect, and long duration of effect and because they require patients to have a functioning gastrointestinal system. Traditionally, hospitalized patients have received systematically administered opioids and then have been switched to oral analgesics when the need for rapid adjustments in the level of analgesia has diminished. Both nonopioid and opioid analgesic agents are available for oral administration alone or in combination. With the increased number and complexity of surgical procedures being performed in the outpatient setting, there is a growing need to find efficacious regimens of analgesia for moderate to severe acute postoperative pain in this subset of patients. Although newer methods of drug delivery such as transdermal or transmucosal administration may be of some value, it is likely that oral analgesics will be the mainstay of therapy.[84a]

Parenteral

Parenteral administration of opioid analgesics remains the primary pharmacologic route for the treatment of moderate to severe postoperative pain. Advances in microprocessor technology and newer therapeutic agents have played a role in refining methods of delivery and reducing side-effects of parenterally administered agents.

Intramuscular. Intramuscular administration of postoperative analgesics produces a more rapid onset and time to peak effect than oral administration. It is also simple to administer analgesics by this route because no special infusion device is needed. However, pain at the injection site, patient apprehensiveness of needle sticks, the potential for delayed respiratory depression, and wide variability in drug serum concentrations limit the viability of this route. Absorption from intramuscular sites is dependent on the lipophilicity of the agent and blood flow in the area of the injection. Following intramuscular injections of morphine or meperidine, plasma concentrations may vary as much as three- to fivefold, and time to peak concentration may vary from 4–108 minutes among patients.[85,86] On the other hand, there is much less variability in the minimum analgesic plasma concentration for any patient.[87] Small changes in plasma concentrations (10–20%) for a patient may represent a spectrum of effects from inadequate analgesia to complete pain relief.[88]

The relationship between plasma concentrations, effect, and time is depicted in Figure 57-5. Plasma concentrations following intramuscular administration of high doses of an opioid analgesic such as morphine at long dosing intervals establish a cyclic pattern of sedation, analgesia, and finally inadequate analgesia. When morphine is administered by this route on a 3- or 4-hour basis, plasma concentrations will exceed or meet analgesic requirements for only about 35% of the dosing interval because of the delayed absorption and narrow therapeutic window.[85] This situation is exacerbated by the dynamic nature of analgesic requirements. Newer methods of delivery such as patient-controlled analgesia and continuous epidural infusions circumvent many of the problems of intramuscular administration and may provide more effective analgesia with fewer side-effects by maintaining tighter control of plasma levels.

Most opioids can be administered by the intramuscular route; however, only one NSAID, ketorolac, is currently

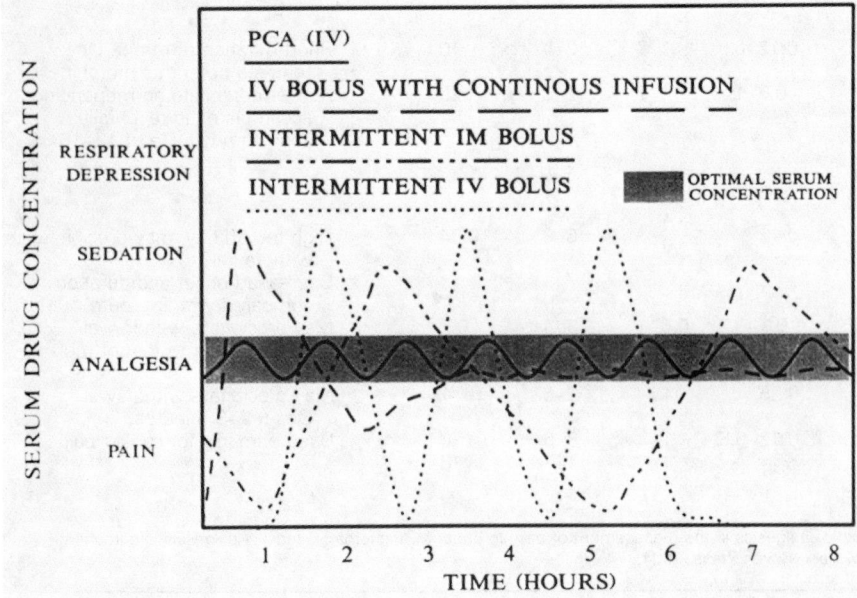

Figure 57-5. Relationship between serum drug concentration, pharmacologic effect, and method of administration. (Reprinted with permission from Tuman KJ, McCarthy RJ, Ivankovich AD: Pain control in the postoperative cardiac surgery patient. Hosp Formulary 23:580, 1988.)

available for intramuscular injection to manage postoperative pain. Ketorolac is a potent analgesic with limited anti-inflammatory properties and only moderate effects on platelet function. Limited clinical trials in patients with moderate to severe pain undergoing general, gynecologic, or orthopedic surgeries have demonstrated efficacy of this agent equal to that of moderate doses of opioids and NSAIDs.[89] When an intravenous preparation becomes available, combinations of ketorolac and opioids may represent a significant therapeutic alternative compared with single-agent therapies.

Intravenous. Intermittent iv bolus infusions of opioids are feasible in situations such as an intensive care unit where close continuous monitoring of the patient is available. With a small iv bolus, the time delay for analgesic effect and the variability in plasma concentrations that is seen with im administration can be minimized. Rapid redistribution of the drug will shorten the duration of effect after a single iv administration compared with im injections. The personnel needed to supervise frequent administration of boluses and monitoring of the fluctuations seen in plasma concentrations has led to the use of continuous iv infusions.

Continuous iv infusions offer the advantages of maintaining nearly constant plasma drug concentrations and reducing the peak-and-valley effect inherent in intermittent injections. Without the use of an initial bolus loading injection, continuous infusion techniques are inadequate because of the long time required for the drug to reach steady state (4–5 half-lives). Initiating therapy with a loading dose eliminates this problem but still does not allow for rapid dosage adjustments as analgesic requirements change.

Patient-Controlled Analgesia. By combining the advantages of a continuous infusion with the flexibility of interposing low bolus doses as analgesic requirements vary, patient-controlled analgesia (PCA) would appear to be the answer for many patients' analgesic needs. This method has evolved not only out of the needs for improved drug delivery but also because of advances in computer technology. Early PCA devices permitted a patient to titrate analgesic needs by delivering a low bolus dose of an opioid such as

morphine sulfate when the patient activated a switch. Limits could be placed on the number of activations per unit time the patient was allowed and the minimum time that would have to elapse between activations (lockout interval). Refinements of this system permit administration of a continuous background infusion superimposed on patient-controlled boluses. These new devices also allow the system to record a profile of the drug administration, including number and time of bolus delivery, number of activations that did not result in drug delivery, and total amounts of the agent that were administered per unit time.

Compared with traditional methods of on-demand analgesic delivery, PCA has been shown to provide superior analgesia, with less total drug use, less sedation, fewer nocturnal sleep disturbances, and a more rapid return to physical activity.[90] Most patients tend to determine a level of pain at which they feel comfortable and taper their dosage requirements as they convalesce.[91] In addition, patient acceptance of PCA is high, since patients feel that they have significant control over their therapy.

One limitation to PCA therapy is the selection of agents currently available for use in the PCA devices (Table 57-6). Ideally, a drug administered by a PCA should be highly efficacious, have a rapid onset of action and a moderate duration of effect, should not accumulate or change pharmacokinetic properties with repeated administration, and should have a large therapeutic window. Morphine and meperidine, the drugs most widely prescribed by this route, are far from ideal, and limitations imposed by the pharmacology of the agonist-antagonist group has made their use in these devices disappointing.

Other problems encountered with PCA therapy are primarily a result of operator or mechanical errors.[92] Because patients titrate their own therapy, they must be capable of understanding the concepts of the device, be able to activate the trigger, and be willing to participate. This often makes the use of PCA devices in pediatric and in older and more debilitated patients difficult.

Optimum results from PCA therapy can only be obtained when the patient's analgesic needs can be met within the prescribed parameters set on the device. The patient's age, surgical procedure, need for a continuous background infu-

TABLE 57-6. Guidelines Regarding the Bolus Doses, Lockout Intervals, and Continuous Infusions for Various Parenteral Analgesics When Using a PCA System

Drug	Bolus Dose (mg)	Lockout Interval (min)	Continuous Infusion (mg·hr^{-1})
Agonists			
Fentanyl citrate	0.015–0.05	3–10	0.02–0.1
Hydromorphone hydrochloride	0.10–0.5	5–15	0.2–0.5
Meperidine hydrochloride	5–15	5–15	5–40
Methadone hydrochloride	0.50–3.0	10–20	—
Morphine sulfate	0.50–3.0*	5–20	1–10
Oxymorphone hydrochloride	0.20–0.8	5–15	0.1–1
Sufentanil citrate	0.003–0.015	3–10	0.004–0.03
Agonist-Antagonists			
Buprenorphine hydrochloride	0.03–0.2	10–20	—
Nalbuphine hydrochloride	1–5	5–15	1–8
Pentazocine hydrochloride	5–30	5–15	6–40

*For pediatric dosing, see text.

sion, number and amount of boluses allowed, and total analgesic requirements are considered. Anesthesiologists must incorporate some flexibility into protocols for ordering PCA therapy to account for the variability produced by these factors.

Central Neuraxial Analgesia

The technique of spinal analgesia was described by Bier and Tuffler in 1898 and that of sacral epidural analgesia by Sicard and Cathelin in 1901. In 1949, a major advance in the application of central neuraxial analgesia was the description by Cleland of the use of a continuous catheter epidural for postoperative analgesia.[93] Analgesia was maintained for 1–5 days postoperatively by administering intermittent bolus doses of a local anesthetic. Although effective analgesia was obtained, a significant sympathetic block accompanied the analgesia, and all patients required at least one dose of a vasopressor. Additional shortcomings of this technique, as with any intermittent dosing regimen, were the fluctuating levels of analgesia that occur as the effect of the bolus begins to wear off, and the medical staff required to reinject the patient every several hours.

Because of the shortcomings of intermittent dosing, the continuous infusion of local anesthetics along the central neuraxis was subsequently recommended as an alternative to the intermittent bolus technique. The continuous infusion of local anesthetics simplified maintenance of analgesia, but the use of local anesthetics in concentrations sufficient to produce pain relief usually resulted in sensory and occasional motor blockade. These are unwanted effects in the postoperative period because sensory and motor blockade prohibit ambulation, an important factor in postoperative convalescence.

Although it has long been recognized that application of local anesthetic agents along the spinal canal could provide effective analgesia, the demonstration that opioids could produce analgesia by this route has been responsible for the explosive growth of the practice of central neuraxial analgesia that has evolved during the past decade. The increased interest in this route of administration has also been a direct result of the shortcomings of intramuscular and intravenous therapies. By interrupting pain pathways at the level of communication between the first- and second-order neurons, a method for providing effective analgesia without the associated central nervous system depression and cyclical nature of pain associated with other parenteral routes of administration can be achieved.

Intrathecal. The intrathecal administration of opioids has the advantage of providing long-lasting analgesia after a single injection. The onset of analgesic effect following the intrathecal administration of an opioid is directly proportional to the lipid solubility of the agent, whereas the duration of the effect is longer with more hydrophilic compounds. Morphine, for example, has been shown to produce peak analgesic effects in 20–60 minutes that last for 2–12 hours when doses ranging from 0.25 mg–4 mg were administered intrathecally to adults.[94,95] In routine clinical practice, 0.25 mg–1 mg morphine can be expected to provide effective analgesia, whereas doses in the range of 0.25 mg–0.5 mg generally maintain analgesic efficacy while minimizing the potential for respiratory depression.[94]

Intrathecal bolus injections share many of the problems of other intermittent techniques: lack of titratability and extensive time requirements for monitoring and reinjection. In addition, the potential for infection, a greater risk of respiratory depression owing to rostral spread of the drug, and a higher incidence of side-effects make this technique less desirable than epidural administration (Table 57-7). Widespread clinical experience has shown that continuous epidural infusions may be preferable to intrathecal techniques when using central neuraxial analgesia. The practical aspects of having a catheter in the intrathecal space for a prolonged period of time and reports of cauda equina syndrome following continuous spinal anesthesia may be additional advantages of the continuous epidural technique.[96]

Epidural Analgesia. Epidural administration of opioids and local anesthetics has evolved in parallel with intrathecal techniques. As noted above, the advantages of epidural administration of agents such as opioids and local anesthetics include the reduced incidence of side-effects and a diminished propensity for opioid-induced respiratory depression when compared with the intrathecal route. When an agent is placed in the epidural space, it must first cross the dura before it can reach the spinal cord. Besides the physical barrier presented by the dura, the epidural space is highly vascularized, and a significant redistribution of drug to the systemic circulation occurs. The epidural space also contains fat, connective tissues, a lymphatic network, and the dorsal and ventral roots of the spinal nerves, all of which can serve as a repository for lipophilic agents.

The influence of these factors can be demonstrated by an examination of the pharmacokinetics of epidurally administered hydrophilic (morphine)[97] and lipophilic (fentanyl)[98] opioids. Ten milligrams of morphine, given either intrave-

TABLE 57-7. Complications of the Use of Neuraxial Opioids

Complication	Reported Incidence (%)*		Treatment
	Spinal	*Epidural*	
Respiratory depression	5–7	0.1–2	Support ventilation; naloxone
Pruritus	60	1–100	Antihistamine; naloxone
Nausea and vomiting	20–30	20–30	Antiemetic; transdermal scopolamine; naloxone
Urinary retention	50	15–25	Catheterize; naloxone

* Reported incidences vary widely, appear to be related to dose, and are higher with spinal than with epidural administration.

Reprinted with permission from Ready LB: Regional analgesia with intraspinal opioids. In Bonica JJ (ed): The Management of Pain, vol II, p 1976. Philadelphia, Lea & Febiger, 1990.

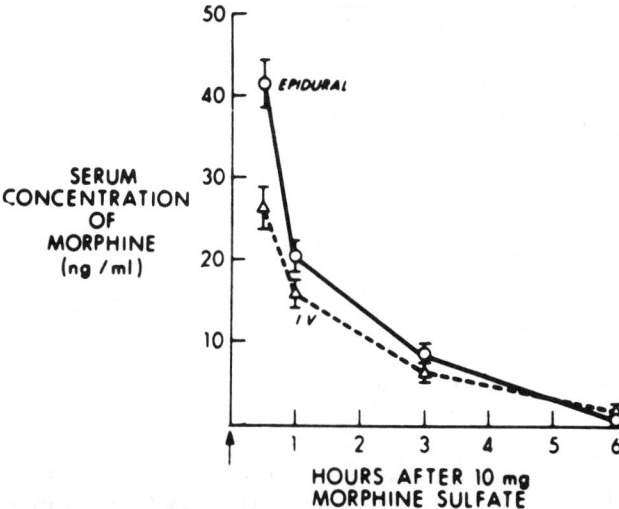

Figure 57-6. Serum concentration of morphine (mean ± SEM) after intravenous and lumbar epidural administration of 10 mg of morphine sulfate in 10 subjects; triangles, intravenous, circles, epidural. (Reprinted with permission from Bromage PR, Camporesi EM, Durant PAC, Nielsen CH: Nonrespiratory side effects of epidural morphine. Anesth Analg 61:490, 1982.)

nously or epidurally, produce peak serum levels and decay curves that are nearly identical (Fig. 57-6). Whereas the duration of pain relief from intravenous administration is short-lived (1–2 hours), the epidural morphine can provide 12 or more hours of analgesia. This indicates that although much of an epidural dose is absorbed into the systemic circulation, a small fraction of the morphine dose (about 2–10%) diffuses across the dura to bind spinal opiate receptors and produce pain relief. In contrast, when epidural fentanyl, 200 μg, is given in a similar manner, peak serum levels are only approximately 50% of those following a similar im injection.[98] However, serum levels of fentanyl 24 hours after a continuous rate infusion are similar to those obtained from a similar iv infusion.[99] This implies that with the initial bolus of fentanyl, redistribution of the drug to lipophilic sites such as those found in the epidural space is occurring and that these sites become saturated with continuous administration. Therefore, only a small fraction of a typically administered epidural dose is necessary to provide pain relief at the spinal level.

Since the diffusion of drugs across the dura is both concentration- and time-dependent, it is necessary to administer significantly larger amounts of drugs than those necessary to effectively saturate spinal opiate receptors. These higher doses are more likely to produce unwanted side-effects from systemic and rostral distribution of the drug, but fewer than those associated with equianalgesic intrathecal doses. When these factors are considered, the margin of therapeutic safety and the decrease in side-effects with epidural administration make this route preferred for postoperative analgesia.

Intermittent epidural bolus doses of morphine sulfate (up to 15 mg over 24 hours) have been utilized for postsurgical analgesia.[100] Although this method of administration provides excellent analgesia for up to 12 hours, side-effects associated with these bolus doses limits the widespread application of this technique. An intermittent bolus technique also has the disadvantage of limiting the number of usable

narcotics to the longer-acting opioids (e.g., morphine and hydromorphone).

In an effort to mitigate the frequency and severity of opioid-induced side-effects associated with bolus techniques, El-Baz et al described the use of a continuous infusion of epidural morphine.[101] The study indicated that a continuous morphine infusion (100 μg·h⁻¹) provided equivalent analgesia and fewer side-effects than epidural boluses of either bupivacaine (0.5%) or morphine (5 mg) (Fig. 57-7 and Table 57-8). Subsequent studies documented that continuous epidural infusions of opioids provide effective analgesia while reducing the side-effects associated with bolus administration.[102-105]

Because the laws of mass action apply to diffusion of drugs out of the epidural space to their sites of action, several hours are often required to provide adequate analgesia when using continuous infusions alone. Our experience has shown that it may take as long as 3–4 hours to provide effective analgesia with epidural infusions administered at a continuous rate. This delayed onset of effective analgesia can readily be overcome by adjusting the infusion rate to provide the equivalent of a small (5–10 ml) bolus of the epidural solution over 5–15 minutes prior to beginning the maintenance infusion. This allows an adequate concentration of the analgesic drug(s) to be present at their site(s) of action in a shorter period of time.

In addition to a reduction in adverse effects, another advantage of a continuous epidural infusion over an epidural bolus injection is the ability to titrate the level of the analgesia (Table 57-9). Although morphine is described as providing 12 hours of pain relief after a single epidural bolus, wide variability has been reported in the duration of effective analgesia (4–24 hours) depending on the site and extent of surgical trauma and age of the patient.[35,100,106] Because of this variability, it becomes difficult to titrate uniform levels of analgesia. A continuous infusion provides easier analgesic titration, particularly when shorter-acting narcotics such as fentanyl are employed. Fentanyl has an onset of action

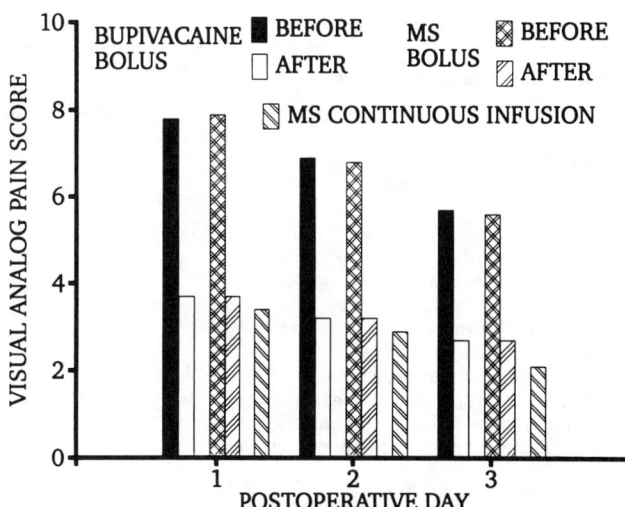

Figure 57-7. Analgesic effectiveness of continuous morphine epidural infusion compared with epidural bolus doses of morphine sulfate or bupivacaine. See text for details. (Adapted with permission from El-Baz NM, Faber LP, Jensik RJ: Continuous epidural infusion of morphine for treatment of pain after thoracic surgery. A new technique. Anesth Analg 63:757, 1984.)

TABLE 57-8. Postoperative Epidural Analgesia

Route	Group A (Bupivacaine 25 mg/5 ml, 0.5%) Epidural Bolus	Group B (Morphine 5 mg) Epidural Bolus	Group C (Morphine 100 $\mu g \cdot h^{-1}$) Epidural Infusion
Urinary retention	30 (100%)	30 (100%)	2 (7%)
Hypotension	7 (23%)	0	0
Weakness of hands	12 (40%)	0	0
Pruritus	0	12 (40%)	1 (3%)
Depressed consciousness	0	8 (27%)	0

Adapted with permission from El-Baz NM, Faber LP, Jensik RJ: Continuous epidural infusion of morphine for treatment of pain after thoracic surgery. A new technique. Anesth Analg 63:757, 1984.

within 4–5 minutes and a peak effect within 20 minutes.[107,108] Because of the rapid onset, it becomes much easier to adjust dosage, observe the desired effect, and titrate to an optimal analgesic level. Morphine, on the other hand, has an onset time of 30 minutes with a time to peak effect ranging from 60–90 minutes.

Initiation and Maintenance of Therapy. Based on the above considerations, achievement of optimal results with a continuous epidural analgesia technique requires appropriate perioperative planning and assessment. This strategy includes identifying patients who may benefit from epidural analgesia and scheduling the epidural catheter placement as part of the anesthetic plan. At the authors' institution, epidural catheters are generally placed while the patient is in the holding area prior to being taken to the operating room. This practice allows the anesthesiologist to administer a test dose of local anesthetic while the patient is still awake. The application of bolus administration followed by a continuous infusion mandates that the test dose be administered to an awake patient. This facilitates diagnosis of intrathecal, intravascular, or subdural catheter placement and allows confirmation of segmental epidural analgesia when the test dose of local anesthetic is administered. This practice also allows the continuous epidural infusion to be started intraoperatively. Solutions of morphine (0.1 mg·ml^{-1}), with bupivacaine (1 mg·ml^{-1}), or fentanyl (10 μg·ml^{-1}) with bupivacaine (1 mg·ml^{-1}) are the most commonly used. The infusion is begun intraoperatively at a rate of 4–6 ml·h^{-1}, augmenting the general anesthetic and providing sufficient time to achieve good analgesia and smooth emergence. If the surgical procedure is expected to exceed 3–4 hours, sufficient solution should be infused into the epidural space to achieve analgesia upon the patient's awakening. If the procedure is to be of short duration (1–2 hours), a 5- to 10-ml bolus of the epidural solution may be given as a rapid infusion as described above, to hasten the onset of analgesia. As an alternative, the patient may be

TABLE 57-9. Comparison of Epidural Administration Techniques

Advantages	Disadvantages
Continuous Epidural Infusions	
1. Less rostral spread so side-effects are minimized.	1. Need for sophisticated infusion device.
2. Provides continuous analgesia avoiding the peaks and valleys seen with intermittent bolus.	
3. Allows for concomitant use of dilute local anesthetic solutions.	
4. Allows the use of shorter-acting opiates such as fentanyl or sufentanil.	
5. Less potential risk of contamination from injection, since the catheter system has fewer breaks in sterile technique.	
6. Simple and easy maintenance. Removes the need for anesthesia personnel to administer injections to patients periodically.	
Intermittent Epidural Bolus	
1. Simple (provided that resident or nursing staff accepts the responsibility of epidural catheter injections).	1. Limited number of suitable opioids.
2. No need for infusion devices.	2. Higher incidence of side-effects.
	3. Extra effort to inject catheter every 8–12 hours.
	4. Excludes the use of local anesthetics.
	5. More difficult to titrate dose.

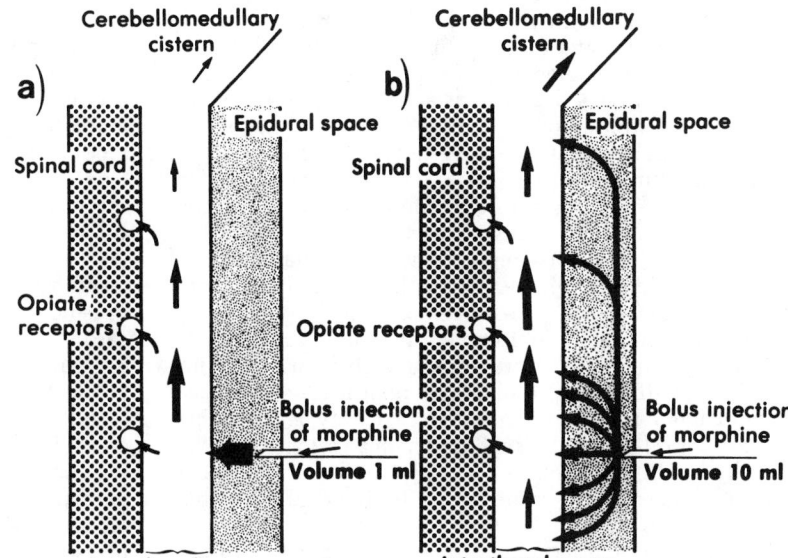

Figure 57-8. Rostral spread of central neuraxial morphine: *a*, in low injection volumes of 1 ml after dura penetration in the intrathecal space, and *b*, in high injection volumes of 10 ml in the intrathecal and epidural spaces. (Reprinted with permission from Chrubasik J: Investigations on respiratory depression. In Chrubasik J: Spinal Infusions of Opiates and Somatostatin, pp 19–25. Oberursel, FRG, Verlag Hygeineplan GmBh, 1985.)

given an epidural bolus of 0.5% bupivacaine combined with either fentanyl (50–100 μg) or morphine (2–5 mg).

Placement of Epidural Catheter. Hydrophilic compounds such as morphine, when injected epidurally, result in cerebrospinal fluid concentrations of the drug that allow it to follow the rostral spread of the cerebrospinal fluid and saturate the entire length of the spinal cord (Fig. 57-8).[109] Because of this property, epidural morphine may be infused at a lower lumbar level and still provide analgesia for surgical procedures performed on the upper abdomen and thorax. Lipophilic agents such as fentanyl tend to provide more of a segmental analgesic effect. This may be due in part to the lipophilic compounds binding of lipid structures in the spinal canal, such as epidural fat and the lipid spinal cord. This segmental nature of analgesia mandates the need to place an epidural catheter in a position to cover the dermatomes included in the surgical field. Suggested spinal segments that need to be blocked correspond to the dermatomes in the surgical field. A general guideline for such blocks in the various types of surgery is as follows: thoracic surgery—upper to lower thoracic; upper abdominal and re-

nal surgery—low thoracic to high lumbar; orthopedic procedures of the lower extremities and lower abdominal and gynecologic surgery—lumbar region. Alternatively, catheter placement should be approximately at the dermatomal level that corresponds to a point intersecting the upper one third and lower two thirds of the surgical incision. In general, it has been the authors' observation that most anesthesiologists tend to place the epidural catheter at a level lower than necessary to cover the expected dermatome when they are using epidural fentanyl, resulting in increased infusion requirements that may lead to an increase in side-effects.

Selection of Analgesics. The differences among the opioids used for epidural analgesia relate to their duration of action and propensity to produce side-effects. The duration of pain relief is longer with hydrophilic agents such as morphine than with the more lipid-soluble hydromorphone or fentanyl (Table 57-10). Lipophilic compounds such as fentanyl and sufentanil and to a lesser extent hydromorphone partition into the spinal cord and lipid structures in the epidural space more than hydrophilic agents, which remain in the

TABLE 57-10. Epidural Opioids: Latency and Duration of Postoperative Analgesia

Agent	Bolus Dose	Analgesic Effect			Continuous Infusion	
		Onset (min)	Peak (min)	Duration (h)	Concentration	Rate (ml·h⁻¹)
Meperidine	30–100 mg	5–10	12–30	4–6	—	—
Morphine	5 mg	23.5±6	30–60	12–24	0.01%	1–6
Methadone	5 mg	12.5±2	17±3	7.2±4.6	—	—
Hydromorphone	1 mg	13±4	23±8	11.4±5.5	0.005%	6–8
Fentanyl	100 μg	4–10	20	2.6±5.7	0.001%	4–12
Diamorphine	5 mg	5	9–15	12.4±6.5	—	—
Sufentanil	30–50 μg	7.3±5.6	26.5±8.1	3.9±6.9	0.0001%	10
Alfentanil	15 μg·kg⁻¹	15		1–2	—	—

Adapted with permission from Cousins MJ, Mather LE: Intrathecal and epidural administration of opioids. Anesthesiology 61:276, 1984.

cerebrospinal fluid to a greater extent. Higher cerebrospinal fluid concentrations of hydrophilic drugs permit rostral ascension, extending the level of analgesia and producing a higher incidence of some side-effects.

The relatively long duration of action of epidural or intrathecal morphine allows it to be used effectively as an intermittent bolus given every 12 hours, whereas because of a shorter duration of analgesia, fentanyl is better suited for continuous epidural infusions. Morphine can be used as a continuous epidural infusion and has been associated with reduced side-effects compared with epidural bolus injections.[101] Hydromorphone, which has a lipid solubility between that of morphine and fentanyl, is 7–10 times as potent as morphine. Intermittent epidural bolus administration of hydromorphone provides effective analgesia for 7–12 hours with a reduced incidence of pruritus and nausea as compared to morphine.[110] Therefore, it may be preferable to use lipophilic opioids such as fentanyl rather than the more hydrophilic morphine to produce a more segmental level of analgesia and to decrease the incidence of side-effects.

Studies have reported obtaining effective analgesia from the concomitant use of morphine-bupivacaine and fentanyl-bupivacaine continuous epidural infusions, combinations that are designed to take advantage of the desirable properties of both local anesthetics and opioids. The rationale for these combinations is to benefit from the synergy between opioids and concentrations of bupivacaine that provide analgesia without motor blockade. This synergy, which has been demonstrated in animal and clinical studies,[111,112] may be a result of blockade of afferent impulses at two different sites in the spinal cord. Opioids produce analgesia by binding to opiate receptors in the substantia gelatinosia, whereas local anesthetics block transmission of afferent impulses at the nerve roots and dorsal root ganglia. Another rationale for these combinations is to reduce dosage of the individual agents with concomitant reduction in the incidence and severity of side-effects. Despite wide acceptance of these combinations, the clinical value of the synergistic action of bupivacaine 0.1% and fentanyl 0.01% in orthopedic procedures of the knee has recently been questioned.[113]

Epidural sufentanil has been described for postoperative pain relief and for relief of labor pain.[114-116] Sufentanil can be given in bolus doses ranging from 30–70 µg with an expected duration of analgesic action of about 4–6 hours.[117] Doses of 50 µg or greater are more likely to be associated with respiratory depression, and observation of patients who are given such dosages in a monitored setting should be instituted.[116,117] In the authors' institution, epidural sufentanil (30 µg) with epidural local anesthetic has been used for surgery for several years without any cases of clinically significant respiratory depression, and the authors believe this to be the optimal dose. Continuous infusions of sufentanil (10 µg·h^{-1}) combined with bupivacaine (0.1–0.125%) have also been described.[114,115]

Butorphanol, a mixed agonist-antagonist, has been proposed as an alternative to morphine because it provides effective analgesia, has reduced side-effects, and has a ceiling for respiratory depression.[118,119] Butorphanol has been used alone or combined with morphine or local anesthetics, but because of a short duration of action (2–3 hours), it is probably best utilized as a continuous infusion when given alone or combined with a longer-acting opioid and administered as a single bolus. When compared with the agonists, pruritus is reduced with butorphanol, but an increased incidence of somnolence limits the usefulness of this agent.[120,121]

The alpha$_2$ agonists represent an old class of medications that are finding a new use in anesthesiology. The alpha$_2$ agonists provide intraspinal analgesia by their effect on alpha$_2$ receptors in the dorsal horn of the spinal cord. They modulate pain relief in a fashion similar to that of opioids. One important distinction is that they appear to produce minimal respiratory depression compared with opioids.[122] Clonidine has been the most widely used agent for epidural analgesia to date. It provides analgesia in a dose-dependent fashion when given as a single bolus.[123,124] Epidural clonidine has been associated with hypotension and with bradycardia, which are thought to be caused by inhibition of preganglionic sympathetic fibers. This is most prevalent at lower doses, whereas increased doses appear to normalize blood pressure because of systemic vasoconstriction that overrides the central hypotensive effect. The most promising use of epidural clonidine may be in combination with narcotics to produce synergy and minimize side-effects. Effective analgesia without a significant reduction in blood pressure has been reported with a combination of clonidine and morphine.[125] Newer alpha$_2$ agonists that may be introduced into clinical practice include dexmetotomidine and tizanidine. Dexmetotomidine is a pure alpha$_2$ agonist with a very high alpha$_2$ to alpha$_1$ selectivity (1600) compared with clonidine (ratio of 200).[126] Tizanidine, an analogue of clonidine, produces analgesia in a manner similar to clonidine but has minimal cardiovascular effects.[127] Clinical trials are currently defining the role these agents will have in acute postoperative pain management.

Management of Inadequate Analgesia. Although epidural analgesia is generally effective, patients may occasionally experience inadequate pain relief. An algorithm designed to evaluate and correct the cause(s) of inadequate analgesia is presented in Figure 57-9. Once the integrity of the catheter system is determined, a bolus of the epidural infusion

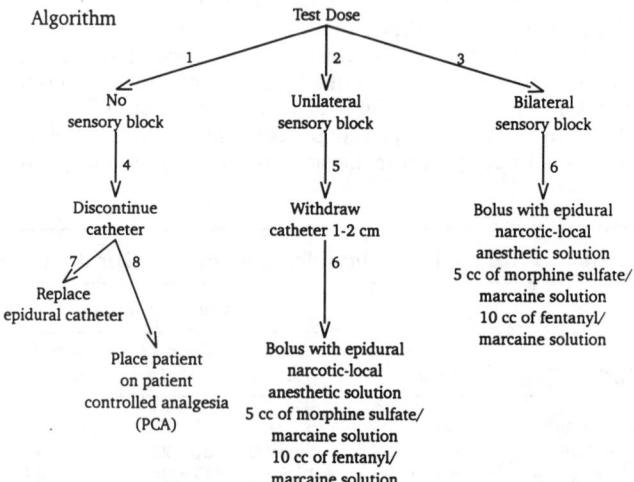

Figure 57-9. Test dose algorithm for inadequate analgesia utilizing 2% lidocaine with epinephrine 1:200,000 (5 ml for lumbar catheters; 3 ml for thoracic catheters) is given by anesthesia personnel. (Reprinted with permission from Lubenow TR, Ivankovich AD: Organization of an acute pain management service. In Stoelting RK, Barash PG, Gallagher TJ [eds]: Advances in Anesthesia, pp 1–28. Chicago, Mosby Year Book, 1991.)

is administered and the patient is assessed after a short interval (30–60 minutes). If analgesia remains inadequate, a test dose of a local anesthetic solution, such as 2% lidocaine with 1:200,000 epinephrine, can be given to confirm correct epidural catheter placement. The test dose generally yields one of three results. If bilateral sensory block occurs in a few segmental dermatomes, correct catheter placement is confirmed. In this case, insufficient volume of infusion mixture was the likely cause of inadequate analgesia, and increasing the rate of infusion may produce effective analgesia. A unilateral sensory block is most likely indicative of the anesthesiologist placing the catheter tip too far into the epidural space, with migration through the neuroforamina laterally. The catheter can be withdrawn 1–2 cm and the test dose repeated. Finally, lack of any sensory block indicates that the epidural catheter is no longer in the epidural space. In this situation the catheter is removed and the patient is given the option of having another epidural catheter placed or switching to PCA therapy.

Safety Considerations. Serious complications that can occur with a continuous epidural technique include accidental intrathecal administration of drug, infection-related problems, epidural hematoma, and respiratory depression. In order to decrease the incidence of these complications, the authors propose the following guidelines:

1. Use a low concentration of local anesthetics (e.g., 0.1% bupivacaine) in combination with an opioid analgesic to allow subarachnoid catheter migration to be identified early because of the progressive levels of sensory blockade produced.
2. Examine catheter insertion sites daily, monitoring temperature curves, and periodically evaluate for signs of meningism. If any findings consistent with infection are present, the catheter is removed and cultures performed. In the authors' experience of more than 7000 cases of postoperative epidural analgesia, no cases of epidural abscess or significant subcutaneous infections have been encountered. In a small number of patients, infections limited to the cutaneous structures have developed and have been resolved with conservative therapy.
3. Place the epidural catheter in patients requiring anticoagulation at least 1 hour prior to heparinization. The risk of epidural hematoma formation following catheter placement in anticoagulated patients is controversial. The authors agree with the observation of others that if epidural catheters are placed at least 1 hour before heparinization, the incidence of epidural hemorrhage is not clinically significant.[128-130] Likewise, epidural catheters may be inserted safely in patients who are to receive warfarin postoperatively as long as their coagulation status is normal at the time of catheter insertion.
4. Monitor the respiratory rates and level of sedation every hour for the first 24 hours of the epidural infusion and every 4 hours thereafter. Concern for the occurrence of potentially catastrophic respiratory depression is the primary reason that some institutions limit the use of epidural opioids to patients in an intensive or postanesthesia care setting. Unfortunately, this practice severely limits the number of patients who can benefit from epidural analgesia. Patients should have their respiratory rate and level of sedation observed once an hour for the first 24 hours. Apnea moni-

tors can be used to supplement direct observation but should not replace direct patient observation. Patients who may be at a higher risk for respiratory compromise include the elderly and those with debilitating diseases. In the authors' institution, an apnea monitor is required for the first 24 hours when bolus doses of morphine 2 mg or greater are given as loading doses.

An additional safeguard may be employed to diminish the risk of respiratory depression caused by the inadvertent bolus of the epidural solution. This is a volume-limiting device (e.g., Buretrol chamber) placed in line between the infusion bag and the volumetric pump. Alternatively, a low maximum infusion rate pump (Pain Management Provider Pump, Abbott Laboratories, North Chicago, IL) can be employed.

By using these guidelines, the authors have encountered only six instances of respiratory depression (respiratory rates of 6–8 breaths per minute) and no instances of apnea in over 7000 patients receiving continuous epidural opioid infusions over the past several years. A similar incidence of respiratory depression (0.09%) has been reported from studies done on over 14,000 patients receiving epidural opioids in Sweden.[131]

In summary, a continuous infusion technique simplifies maintenance of epidural analgesia and allows greater analgesic titratability than an epidural bolus injection. Proper patient selection, catheter placement, and methods to identify and treat inadequate analgesia are an important aspect of postoperative pain management. Patient safety is paramount. Guidelines should be established to provide for prevention and early diagnosis and treatment of complications.

Caudal. Caudal nerve blocks play a minor role in acute postoperative pain management in adults. Since they are technically more difficult to perform in adults than other efficacious forms of lumbar epidural blocks, they are utilized less frequently in adults than in the pediatric population. Continuous caudal analgesia for postoperative pain has a limited utility because of the difficulty of securing a catheter, but it may have a role in select patients such as those who have had extensive lumbar or thoracic spine surgery. In those unusual situations where continuous caudal analgesia is employed, the standard solutions that are used for lumbar epidural analgesia may be utilized, although infusion rates may need to be higher than those used with a lumbar epidural infusion.

Pediatric ("kiddie") caudals have become popular for intraoperative supplementation and postoperative pain relief. Palpation of the sacral hiatus is much easier in the pediatric population, and a distinct pop can be heard as the needle pierces the sacrococcygeal membrane. A short 22- or 23-gauge needle should be utilized; the block is generally performed with the child in the lateral position. Following needle insertion, needle aspiration should be performed to avoid inadvertent injection into the intrathecal or vascular space. Volumes of local anesthetic ranging from 0.75–1 ml·kg^{-1} of body weight of 0.25% bupivacaine should provide analgesia to the T10 level, which is sufficient for procedures in the groin and lower extremities.[132,133] Even though bupivacaine generally provides 4 to 6 hours of effective pain relief, several studies have demonstrated that children receiving caudal nerve blocks at the time of surgery exhibit better pain relief and utilize significantly fewer supplemental opioids during the first 12 postoperative hours.[133,134]

As with other combined regional and general techniques,

a relatively lighter plane of general anesthesia is required to maintain adequate surgical anesthesia when this block is instituted prior to the surgical incision, and this may represent an advantage over the use of a caudal block placed at the conclusion of the procedure. Blocks placed prior to surgical incisions also allow the patient to awaken more quickly and to benefit from a smoother emergence from general anesthesia.

Peripheral Nerve Blocks

General Considerations. Peripheral application of local anesthetics to block nociceptive neural transmission can be a useful adjunct in the treatment of acute postoperative pain. Although peripheral neural blocks are simple to perform and have an historical record of safety, the relatively short duration of analgesia and the selective nature of these blocks preclude their general application to all patient populations. With proper selection of the patient and the local anesthetic, the pain relief afforded by regional nerve blocks may be superior to that achievable with systemic narcotics.

Mechanism of Action of Local Anesthetics. The electrophysiology of local anesthetics has been described in detail elsewhere.[135-137] Local anesthetics produce their neuronal blocking effect by diffusing across the nerve membrane and inhibiting sodium channels, thereby preventing the normal influx of sodium ions that is necessary for depolarization and nerve transmission. Thus, the membrane is left in its normal polarized state, and neither local miniature end plate potentials nor action potentials are generated.

Local Infiltration. Local infiltration, the instillation of local anesthetics in the vicinity of the surgical incision, is a simple technique for providing postoperative analgesia for the first several hours after a minor surgical procedure. Needle aspiration prior to injection should be performed to avoid intravascular injection or perforation of deep vascular structures. Even when blood has not been aspirated prior to injection, it is still possible for local anesthetic to be delivered intravascularly during a local infiltration. In addition to intravascular injection, exceeding recommended total volume and dosages of local anesthetic is another factor that can be responsible for untoward reactions.

The primary advantages of the local infiltration technique are simplicity and the ability to block afferent nerve activity in the area of the incision without affecting the general sensorium. A major disadvantage is the limited duration of analgesia, which usually lasts only several hours. The most commonly used local anesthetic for this procedure is bupivacaine because of its longer duration of effect compared with most other local anesthetics. Ropivacaine, a new local anesthetic, may be useful for this type of block because of its long duration of effect.

A special type of local infiltration is the intra-articular injection of local anesthetics following arthroscopic procedures. This technique decreases postoperative discomfort and facilitates recuperation following surgery.[138,139] Bupivacaine is the most commonly used local anesthetic, with doses of 100 mg providing effective analgesia while maintaining serum levels below toxic levels.[138,140]

Intercostal. Intercostal blocks are useful for providing analgesia after operations of the thorax and upper abdomen. A 22- or 25-gauge needle is advanced at the mid- or postaxillary line until a rib is contacted. The needle is then walked off the inferior border and advanced 1 mm. When per-

forming intercostal blocks for large thoracic incisions, it is important to identify the sensory dermatomes supplying the surgical incision so that each can be blocked. Dermatomes that supply the area where thoracostomy drainage tubes may be inserted should also be blocked. When abdominal incisions are large and lie in or extend across the midline, a large volume of local anesthetic is needed for optimal pain relief. Providing adequate analgesia for these types of incisions generally requires the use of multiple bilateral intercostal blocks. In general, postoperative pain management for abdominal surgery is better carried out with continuous epidural infusion of opioids or with opioid and local anesthetic solutions. An additional problem with intercostal blocks is the potential for pneumothorax and respiratory compromise. Bupivacaine or bupivacaine with epinephrine is recommended for postsurgical pain relief with an intercostal nerve block. Intercostal blocks should be performed in the midaxillary or posterior axillary line. The site of the injection must be proximal or more posterior to the area of incision. This may occasionally present technical difficulties because the ribs tend to project more anteriorly as they approach the posterior midline. Adequate analgesia for a surgical incision generally requires application of local anesthetic to a minimum of two intercostal segments, and optimal analgesia usually requires that a minimum of three segments be blocked.

An alternative to the injection of local anesthetic on the intercostal nerve is the use of a cryoprobe, which is designed to produce local intercostal nerve freezing (cryoanalgesia).[141] This technique has been reported to produce reversible nerve disruption while preserving intraneural and peridural connective tissues. For optimal results, the cryoprobe should be applied on the intercostal nerve from within the chest by piercing the parietal pleura, and two to three levels above and below the incision should be blocked. Two to three weeks following cryoanalgesia nerve function and structure begin to recover, with complete recovery occurring within 1 to 3 months. Advantages reported with this technique include a low incidence of neuritis or neuroma formation. Because of the extended period of postoperative analgesia, this technique is advantageous when the postoperative analgesic requirement is expected to last for a prolonged time, such as in the patient with chest trauma or significantly limited respiratory function.[142]

Ilioinguinal. An ilioinguinal nerve block is useful for pain relief following inguinal or femoral herniorrhaphy, appendectomy, or procedures involving the scrotum. A simple technique to perform ilioinguinal nerve block involves palpation of the anterior superior iliac spine.[143] Following this, locate a position two finger breadths medial and two finger breadths superior until an imaginary line drawn from the anterosuperior iliac spine to the umbilicus is reached. At this point, a 22-gauge 8.75-cm spinal needle is advanced perpendicular to the skin. The needle is advanced slowly and bounced every several millimeters until a paraesthesia is elicited. This is indicative of needle contact with the fascia immediately outside the external oblique muscle pierced by the ilioinguinal nerve on its way to more superficial structures. Once the needle is in this location, 10–15 ml of local anesthetic is injected after aspiration. The needle is then withdrawn by several centimeters and redirected laterally until the tip reaches the medial edge of the anterior superior iliac spine. An additional 10–15 ml of local anesthetic solution is then injected. Complications of ilioinguinal nerve blocks include hemorrhage and hematoma at the injection site. Occasionally numbness in the distribution of the lateral femoral cutaneous nerve can be demonstrated. Ilioinguinal nerve blocks are useful for acute postoperative analgesia after outpatient procedures such as inguinal herniorrhaphy.

Penile. A penile nerve block performed with .25% bupivacaine can provide effective analgesia following circumcision or orchidopexy. Two techniques are described for performing this block. One involves injecting half of the volume of local anesthetic at the 10:00 o'clock position at the base of the penis with the remainder at the 2:00 o'clock position.[144] An alternative involves placing the local anesthetic in a ring of the subcutaneous tissue 360 degrees around the base of the penis.[145] Epinephrine-containing local anesthetic should not be utilized for penile blocks because of the risk of vasoconstriction and ischemic necrosis of the skin.

Brachial Plexus. Continuous postoperative brachial plexus analgesia has been previously described using catheters placed via the infraclavicular, supraclavicular, axillary, or interscalene approach.[146-149] A catheter-over-needle technique utilizing an 18-gauge 5-cm Teflon-coated intravenous catheter threaded over a 22-gauge 8.75-cm spinal needle is one method.[149] A nerve stimulator is essential to elicit paresthesias and to identify when the neurovascular bundle is contacted. Another method for catheter placement utilizes the Seldinger technique. With this technique the needle is placed with the aid of a nerve stimulator, and after paresthesias are elicited, a guidewire is passed through the needle. Sterile "alligator" clips connected to the nerve stimulator can then be placed on the guidewire after the needle has been removed to confirm that the guidewire is still contacting the brachial plexus. A 20-gauge catheter is passed over the guidewire, which is then removed. For rapid sequential confirmation of correct catheter placement, the guidewire can be reinserted through the catheter at any time and a nerve stimulator used to determine if paresthesia can be elicited.

Postoperative brachial plexus analgesia has been described using bupivacaine 0.25% at rates ranging from 6–10 ml·h^{-1}. When infusion rates are maintained in this range, it is unlikely that serum levels will become toxic. It has been the authors' experience and that of others (personal communication, April 19, 1990, Prithvi Raj), that serum levels always remain far below toxic levels when using these dosing parameters. Use of this regimen does not preclude the use of any commonly used doses and volumes of local anesthetics currently recommended for surgical anesthesia with brachial plexus blockade. One disadvantage to this technique is postoperative catheter migration. The authors' experience has shown that the infraclavicular and interscalene approaches may be better suited to continuous postoperative analgesia of the upper extremity because there tends to be less catheter migration when compared with the axillary approach.

Intrapleural. Intrapleural regional analgesia has been described using the percutaneous placement of a catheter in the thoracic cage between the visceral and parietal pleurae.[150] The procedure is generally performed with the patient in the lateral decubitus position. An intercostal space between the fifth and tenth ribs is usually chosen, and a 17-gauge Touhy needle is inserted in the posterior axillary line over the superior aspect of the rib. A saline-lubricated glass syringe filled with 3–4 ml of air is attached to the needle, and the syringe and needle unit is advanced with

the needle bevel directed in a cephalad direction. Once the pleural space is entered, the negative interpleural pressure draws the syringe plunger down in a manner analogous to the hanging drop technique of Gutierrez used for locating the epidural space. An epidural catheter may then be advanced 6 cm into the pleural space in a rapid fashion to prevent the development of a clinically significant pneumothorax. If patients are on mechanical ventilation, positive pressure ventilation should be interrupted while the needle and catheter are being inserted in order to prevent injury to the pulmonary parenchyma. When patients are breathing spontaneously, the needle and catheter procedure should be performed during end exhalation.

Local anesthetics placed in the pleural cavity diffuse across the parietal pleura to the intercostal neurovascular bundle, producing a unilateral intercostal nerve block at multiple levels. To achieve a more extensive block, two catheters may have to be placed in the interpleural space.[151] Interpleural analgesia utilizing intermittent boluses of local anesthetic may be used to provide postoperative analgesia after upper abdominal surgical procedures, such as open cholecystectomy with subcostal incisions.[152] Effective postoperative pain relief requires intermittent intrapleural injections every 6 hours with approximately 20 ml of 0.25–0.5% bupivacaine. Similar to what occurs during other intermittent bolus techniques, peaks and valleys in interpleural analgesia occur when sequential doses are separated by hours.

Intrapleural analgesia for post-thoracotomy pain has been examined by several authors and has been found to be less effective for post-thoracotomy pain than after other procedures in which the pleura is intact and there are no pleural drainage tubes to divert the local anesthetic from its site of action.[152,153] Certain intercostal incisions, particularly those used for anterior thoracotomies, require that pleural drainage tubes be clamped for a short time after each intermittent local anesthetic injection to allow the local anesthetic to cross the parietal pleura and provide effective analgesia.[154] Intermittent clamping of the pleural drainage tube following injection of the local anesthetic may not be tolerated in patients with a moderate or large air leak from the pulmonary parenchyma after thoracotomy. The risk of pneumothorax and the problems of fluctuating levels of analgesia with intermittent dosing of interpleural catheters suggest that other techniques, such as continuous thoracic epidural analgesia, may be preferable after thoracotomy when there is an anterior intercostal incision.

Other Modalities

Transcutaneous Electrical Nerve Stimulation

Although transcutaneous electrical stimulation (TENS) was initially prescribed for relief of chronic pain, its use has been extended to control postoperative pain. TENS is a simple, conservative technique that utilizes electrical stimulation of the skin to provide pain relief. Two or four electropads are placed on the skin adjacent to the skin incision. These pads are then connected to a battery-operated pulse generator with varying modes, frequencies, and strengths of stimulation. Current strength can be varied from 100–200 mA. The mechanism by which TENS produces pain relief is thought to involve the release of endogenous endorphins by the electrical stimulation of afferent cutaneous nerves. The endogenous endorphin release has an inhibitory effect on the dorsal horn and augments the descending inhibitory modulating pathways. Partial reversal by naloxone of the analgesia produced by TENS supports this hypothesis.[155] The degree of pain relief that patients experience is variable, ranging from satisfactory to negligible in many instances. With the introduction of other more effective techniques (e.g., epidural narcotics, PCA) the application of TENS for postoperative pain relief is now less common.

Psychological Interventions for Postoperative Analgesia

The use of various analgesic techniques involving nerve blocks and of opioids applied to the central neuraxis as well as administered via intravenous infusions has produced dramatic changes in the management of pain. Nevertheless, it is sometimes necessary to augment these techniques with various psychological interventions. Psychological interventions are employed widely in the treatment of chronic pain, and the role of these behavioral strategies is now being defined for the management of acute pain. This often involves approaching the treatment of pain on a cognitive basis and utilizing interventions such as distraction or imagery that attempt to focus attention away from the painful event. Other more simple methods consist of educating patients about their surroundings, disease state, treatment plans, and the hospital environment in an effort to reduce fear and anxiety about unknown events or situations in the perioperative period. Despite the banality of this approach, it is a frequently overlooked element when dealing with patients who often are unfamiliar with the hospital environment. Other psychological interventions that may be effective are relaxation techniques such as deep breathing exercises or muscle relaxation training, which have been shown to reduce anxiety and muscle tension.[156,157]

ORGANIZATION OF A POSTOPERATIVE ANALGESIA SERVICE

With the increasing number and complexity of modalities for treating postoperative pain, it is logical that an organized, systematic approach involving all members of the health care team has evolved in the form of the postoperative analgesia service. The anesthesiologist is uniquely qualified to lead this team because of his or her knowledge of the neurophysiology, pathophysiology, pharmacology, and anatomic pathways involved in the modulation of acute pain. Furthermore, with the postoperative analgesia service under the direction of the anesthesiologist, continuity of pain care management is enhanced because the anesthesiologist is routinely involved in the preoperative assessment, intraoperative management, and postoperative follow-up of surgical patients. Since anesthesiologists are the logical choice for managing the postoperative analgesia service, it is desirable that each department of anesthesiology assume responsibility for organizing and maintaining efficient operation of the service.

When initiating a postoperative analgesia service, it is essential that the department of anesthesiology have one or more members who will take on the position of director or codirector. This ensures that at least one person will be responsible for communication with the pharmacy, nursing and surgical departments, development of policy and procedural protocols, and departmental representation when issues concerning postoperative pain management arise.

The delivery of central neuraxial opioid analgesia requires cooperation among the anesthesiology, nursing, surgery, and pharmacy staffs. Success of such an interdisciplinary program for postoperative analgesia often requires

significant flexibility to satisfy the needs of all the parties concerned. This flexibility is most important in areas such as the use of epidural analgesia after major vascular surgery, where case management strategies are controversial. Each institution must identify the approach that is practical and most beneficial for its patients after considering available resources and important data such as that found in outcome studies. With these considerations, protocols that reflect individual practice patterns can be effectively developed. These protocols should include written policy and procedure manuals for nursing staff (see Appendices A and B) as well as preprinted epidural analgesia orders (see Appendix C). Postoperative pain relief has generated intense interest and fostered the interest and introduction of several new analgesic modalities (e.g., epidural opioids, PCA, interpleural analgesia). Although these techniques have been shown to provide better pain relief than conventional intermuscular administration of opioids, the complexity of these modalities requires the use of an organized approach to maximize efficacy while minimizing potentially adverse effects.

When formulating the strategy for development and initiation of an epidural analgesia service, consideration must be given to the choice of continuous infusion techniques, intermittent bolus regimens, or combinations of these methods. In addition, with the use of PCA devices, similar protocols outlining the initial parameters for starting therapy should be established to facilitate effective use when these devices are prescribed (see Appendix D).

The basic goals of the postoperative analgesia service are (1) administering and monitoring postoperative analgesia, and (2) identifying and managing complications or side-effects of postoperative analgesic techniques. Implicit in these goals is the inclusion of an active quality assurance program directed at maintaining high-quality patient care while minimizing complications. When the postoperative analgesia service is managed by anesthesiologists, quality assurance monitoring can be applied to the heterogeneous surgical population so that the goals of pain management can be refined for the individual patient. This is much more difficult to achieve when particular surgical services are charged with the management of postoperative pain. Nonetheless, successful implementation of these principles requires the cooperation and involvement of health care providers outside of the department of anesthesiology, such as surgeons, nurses, and pharmacy personnel.

The foundation of an effective postoperative analgesia service is based on education of all members of the interdisciplinary health care team. This educational process must begin within the department of anesthesiology and be directed by those physicians with special qualifications in pain management and regional anesthesia. A corollary of this educational process is the use of a standardized approach to the initiation of pain management, which may include choices among fixed medication protocols, algorithms to identify and treat inadequate analgesia, and preprinted postoperative orders. The use of such methods increases efficiency, serves as a guideline for health care providers involved with the postoperative analgesia service, and gives the postoperative analgesia service team the flexibility to individualize therapy. This approach also facilitates the education of ancillary personnel, such as nursing staff, necessary to the functioning of the service.

Ideally, all members of each anesthesia department should become well versed in the basic principles necessary for the day-to-day operation of the postoperative analgesia service. Although its management usually is the responsibility of a limited number of anesthesia personnel, education of all members of the department ensures the smooth operation of the service when those key individuals are not available after hours or on weekends. While patients receiving postoperative analgesia should be seen on a regular basis by the anesthesiologist, it may be necessary for nurse clinicians or anesthesiology residents to assist in performing these functions if the service is very large. It is the responsibility of the anesthesiologist to educate these individuals in the principles of pain management. Nurse clinicians often have excellent rapport with other nursing staff and can act as effective liaisons. In addition, nurse clinicians can facilitate the operation of the postoperative analgesia service by performing tasks such as charting daily progress notes, inspecting epidural catheter sites, removing epidural catheters when therapy is discontinued, notifying the anesthesiologist of any problems pertaining to pain management, and collecting patient data to facilitate quality assurance. The participation of anesthesiology residents in the postoperative analgesia service allows them to gain knowledge and expertise in this new area of patient involvement by anesthesiologists. Depending on the size of the surgical population and the scope of the service, additional support may be required from clinical pharmacologists, nurse anesthetists, or other physicians. Developing this solid foundation is an important consideration when establishing a postoperative analgesia service.

In addition to 24-hour-a-day support from the anesthesia department, a successful postoperative analgesia service requires the cooperation and education of nursing staff so that they are responsive to the needs of the patients. In-service training of hospital nurses requires instruction in the principles of analgesic techniques, including appropriate aspects of neuroanatomy, neuropharmacology, side-effects and their treatment, monitoring skills, analgesia assessment, and the technical aspects of the operation of PCA and epidural infusion devices. This instruction should be conducted under the supervision of the anesthesiologist in charge of the postoperative analgesia service but may also involve a clinical nurse specialist trained by the department of anesthesia, who may assist in solving nursing problems related to the operation of the service. To minimize dosing and medication errors and to improve patient comfort by early treatment of inadequate analgesia and complications such as pruritus, nurses must understand the use of the standardized protocols.

Another key aspect to the initiation of a postoperative analgesia service is the identification of patient populations that are most likely to benefit from improved postoperative pain management. Patients undergoing thoracic and upper abdominal procedures, major orthopedic operations such as hip surgery, and high-risk vascular surgical procedures are examples of groups in whom effective postoperative pain management will produce the most rewarding results. It is often useful to consider a pilot program using PCA and/or epidural analgesia when surgeons are doubtful or hesitant about the efficacy of these methods. After the utility of the postoperative analgesia service has been demonstrated to surgeons, referring physicians, and others, the service can expand logically to patient populations in which improved analgesia will be obvious but in which the effects on outcome may be more subtle. Initiation of the service in any subset of patients also requires the education of surgical staff regarding (1) the advantages to their practice of being able to offer patients surgery with less postoperative discomfort, and (2) the potential differences in outcome when using certain methods of postoperative analgesia. At the authors' institution, the development of an effective postoper-

ative analgesia service has prompted the surgeons to extol the benefits of the service to their patients: improved convalescence and decreased postoperative discomfort. Despite the lack of large-scale, randomized studies to demonstrate that improved postoperative analgesia (especially the use of epidural analgesia in high-risk patients) is definitively associated with improved outcomes (such as shorter, less expensive hospital stays, with fewer major complications), there is more than enough evidence currently in the literature to support a major change in practice. Surgeons must understand that their patients will receive attentive care and that an essential element of the postoperative analgesia service is the maintenance of a cooperative spirit among disciplines.

Once the appropriate subsets of patients and their surgeons have been identified and educated, the physicians in charge of initiating the postoperative analgesia service must make plans for the provision of the capital resources necessary to operate the service. Plans must be made regarding types of equipment needed for continuous and/or patient-controlled intravenous or epidural analgesia, whether such devices are to be rented or purchased, types of monitoring equipment deemed necessary, any pharmacy-related factors necessary to prepare solutions of drugs for administration, and the printing of standard orders for the postoperative management of pain and treatment of complications. Decisions regarding funding sources for these capital expenses often must involve discussions with hospital administrators. In the present medical-economic climate, hospital administrators may be opposed to the purchase of new equipment if old methods appear to be functional. It is important to educate administrators who are reluctant to support the concept of a postoperative analgesia service about the potential benefits to some patients in terms of shorter, less complicated, less expensive hospital stays. Not only can the service be cost-effective, but sometimes it can be used by hospital administrators as a marketing tool to attract surgical patients. Preprinted order forms usually require approval from the hospital's medical records/forms department. Job descriptions and resources are necessary to define and fund support staff such as nurse clinicians, psychologists, or clinical pharmacologists. Thus, a significant degree of planning, effort, and commitment is necessary to initiate a properly functioning postoperative analgesia service. When such efforts are expended, the establishment of such a service allows the anesthesiologist to play an important new role in the postoperative period and to provide a valuable service to patients.

SPECIAL CONSIDERATIONS IN PEDIATRIC ACUTE PAIN MANAGEMENT

Acute pain management in the pediatric patient provides a unique challenge to the anesthesiologist. It is often more difficult to evaluate pain intensity in children because the expression of pain is manifested over a broad emotional spectrum. For instance, some children withdraw and become nonverbal with the onset of pain, whereas others become emotionally labile, with crying, screaming, and violent behavior. Psychological distress is often compounded in children by separation from their parents and the lack of an appropriate understanding of their disease and its treatment. Furthermore, depending on age, lack of cognitive development makes it more difficult to communicate relevant concepts to children. In view of these difficulties, a useful monitor of analgesic efficacy in children is behavior obser-

TABLE 57-11. Pharmacologic Considerations for Pediatric Patients

Drug	Dose (Age > 3 mo)	Interval (h)	Route	Comments
Nonopioid				
Acetaminophen	5–15 mg·kg^{-1}	4–6	po	Overdose may cause hepatotoxicity
	20 mg·kg^{-1}	4–6	R	
Ibuprofen	8 mg·kg^{-1}	6	po	
Naproxen	5 mg·kg^{-1}	8–12	po	
Opioid				
Codeine	0.5–1 mg·kg^{-1}	4–6	po	Most commonly combined with acetaminophen
Oxycodone	0.005–0.15 mg·kg^{-1}	4–6	po	Similar to codeine
Meperidine	1–1.5 mg·kg^{-1}	3–4	im	May cause less constipation, ileus
	0.8–1 mg·kg^{-1}	2–3	iv	and urinary retention than morphine
Morphine*	0.1–0.15 mg·kg^{-1}	3–4	im	
	0.08–0.1 mg·kg^{-1}	2	iv	
	0.05–0.06 mg·kg^{-1}·h^{-1}		iv	Continuous infusion
	50 µg·kg^{-1}	12–24	epi	Abdominal surgery
	120–150 µg·kg^{-1}	12–24	epi	Thoracic surgery
	50–100 µg·kg^{-1}	12–24	caudal	Diluted in equal volume of normal saline
Fentanyl	1–1.5 µg·kg^{-1}	1–2	iv	Minimum age 1 yr
	2–4 µg·kg^{-1}·h^{-1}		iv	Continuous infusion

*Epi = epidural (L3–L5); caudal = S4–S5.

vation. Some behavior such as crying can be easily understood, but social withdrawal and the inability to be distracted often indicate that a young patient has distressing pain.

The selection and dosing of analgesic agents also requires special attention in the pediatric patient (Table 57-11). Neonates and infants, because of immature hepatic function and reduced plasma proteins and plasma protein-binding capacity, exhibit a higher fraction of free drug in the central compartment. This effect is offset to some degree by the higher total body water, extracellular fluid, and larger blood volume in this group compared with adults. Increased susceptibility to the respiratory depressant component of opioids may be a result of the increased fraction of cardiac output to the developing brain, or reduced metabolic pathways leading to accumulation of opioids and their metabolites. Morphine exhibits an increase in half-life and respiratory depressant effect in infants less than 1 month old owing to immature glucuronidation pathways. The half-lives of meperidine and fentanyl are similarly increased during the first 3 months of life. The pharmacokinetics of local anesthetics exhibit a similar pattern of development in neonates and infants. Free fractions of local anesthetics approach those seen in adults by 6 months of age (Table 57-12).[158]

Oral Analgesics

Nonopioid

Nonsteroidal anti-inflammatory drugs are useful oral drugs for acute postoperative pain management in the pediatric population. Ibuprofen can be administered at 6- to 8-hour intervals in doses of 8 mg·kg^{-1}.[159] Contraindications to the

TABLE 57-12. Maximum Local Anesthetic Dosages in Infants and Children

Agent	Infant Dose (mg·kg^{-1}): Age	Child Dose (mg·kg^{-1})
Lidocaine (plain)	5:from birth on	5
Lidocaine (epinephrine)	7:from birth on	7
Mepivacaine	4:<6 mo	5
Bupivacaine (plain)	2:<3 mo	3
Bupivacaine (epinephrine)	2:<3 mo	4
Chloroprocaine (plain)	4:<6 mo	8
Chloroprocaine (epinephrine)	5:<6 mo	10

Reprinted with permission from Vetter TR: Acute pediatric pain management. In Stoelting RK, Barash PG, Gallagher TJ (eds): Advances in Anesthesia, vol 8, pp 29–54. Chicago, Mosby Year Book, 1991.

use of nonsteroidal anti-inflammatory drugs in the pediatric population are similar to those in adults. The most frequently encountered adverse effects are gastrointestinal. Platelet function alteration can occur, but this is usually not a significant clinical problem after short-term administration in the postoperative period. Acetaminophen has fewer side-effects than ibuprofen and can be administered in doses of 5–15 mg·kg^{-1} orally or 20 mg·kg^{-1} rectally every 4–6 hours.[159]

Opioid

Codeine in combination with acetaminophen is a commonly used oral preparation for moderate postoperative pain in the pediatric population. The recommended oral dosage range is 0.5–1 mg·kg^{-1} every 4–6 hours.[159]

Patient-Controlled Analgesia

PCA is an opioid delivery system that has been used with increasing frequency to treat acute postoperative pain in children. Morphine sulfate given as a loading dose of 0.1–0.2 mg·kg^{-1} administered as small incremental boluses of 10–30 μg·kg^{-1} can be used to initiate PCA therapy. After this, maintenance doses of morphine sulfate, 0.01–0.015 mg·kg^{-1}, given every 6–10 minutes with a 4-hour limit of 0.25 mg·kg^{-1} are appropriate. Incorporation of a continuous infusion of 0.01–0.015 mg·kg^{-1}·h^{-1} into the regimen may be beneficial.[160] Meperidine in maintenance doses of 0.15–0.20 mg·kg^{-1} with a 4-hour limit of 2–3 mg·kg^{-1} has been used and may be associated with fewer side-effects than morphine.[158]

Epidural Opioids

Like other methods of pain control, the use of epidural opioids has not been extensively studied in the pediatric population. Lumbar epidural analgesia has been utilized for young patients undergoing abdominal, urologic, or orthopedic procedures.[158] Since lumbar epidural catheters may be more difficult to place in the pediatric patient than in adults, an alternative is to perform a "kiddie caudal" with a mixture of local anesthetic and opioid for postoperative analgesia. Morphine is the preferable drug for single injection techniques and can be administered as a 0.05 mg·kg^{-1} bolus, in volumes appropriate for the age and weight of the child.[161] Additional information on caudal analgesia is reported in earlier sections of this chapter.

RELATIONSHIP BETWEEN ACUTE AND CHRONIC PAIN

For an individual patient, the development of a chronic pain syndrome may simply be the extension of inadequately treated acute pain following trauma or surgery. Differentiation between acute and chronic pain is important in clinical practice because therapy is generally vastly different. It is generally agreed that pain persisting longer than 6 months can be viewed as chronic pain. Acute pain management techniques are usually not effective and may add to the problems when applied to chronic pain. For instance, systemic opioids for long-term use are often associated with the development of tolerance and, occasionally, drug dependency. Chronic pain is not simply the extension of acute

pain as an isolated entity but involves multiple other factors such as altered mechanisms of nociceptive modulation and amplification of neural responses that account for the differences in clinical presentation and, more important, in choice of therapeutic modality.

SUMMARY

Postoperative pain management requires continued input to refine, explore, and open new avenues to further improve current techniques. Increasing interest in postoperative pain management over the past decade has fostered a new subspecialty in anesthesiology. With the currently available techniques, a postoperative analgesia service has several modalities with which to effectively combat postoperative pain. This chapter has reviewed the physiology of nociception and the production of acute postoperative pain as well as compared and contrasted various methods for analgesia. In addition, the rationale behind the development of a team of individuals aimed at managing postoperative pain has been addressed. It will be exciting to see how this new subspecialty and the interest it generates will foster further discoveries in the treatment of acute pain.

REFERENCES

1. Bonica JJ: The anatomical basis of pain. In Bonica JJ (ed): The Management of Pain, pp 27–61. Philadelphia, Lea & Febiger, 1972
2. Chapman CR, Bonica JJ: Acute pain. In Current Concepts, pp 4–16. Kalamazoo, The Upjohn Company, 1983
3. Erlanger J, Gasser HS: The compound nature of the action current of nerve as disclosed by cathode ray oscillograph. Am J Physiol 70:624, 1924
4. de Jong RH: Function and diameter of nerve fiber. In de Jong RH (ed): Physiology and Pharmacology of Local Anesthesia, pp 97–102. Springfield, Charles C Thomas, 1970
5. Guyton AC: Sensory receptors; neuronal circuits for processing information. In Guyton AC (ed): Textbook of Physiology, 8th ed, pp 495–506. Philadelphia, WB Saunders, 1991
6. Kerr FWL: The structured basis of pain: Circulatory and pathway. In NG LWY, Bonica JJ (eds): Pain Discomfort and Humanitarian Care, pp 49–60. New York, Elsevier, 1980
7. Synder SH: Peptide neurotransmitters with possible involvement in pain perception, pp 233–244. In Bonica, JJ (ed): Pain. New York, Raven Press, 1980
8. Henry JL: Effects of substance P on functionally identified units in cat spinal cord. Brain Res 114:439, 1976
9. Jessel TM, Mudge AW, Leeman SE, Yaksh TL: Release of substance P and somatostatin in vivo from primary different terminal in mammalian spinal cord. Neurosci Abst 5:611, 1979
10. Randic M, Miletic V: Depressant actions of methionine-enkephalin and somatostatin in cat dorsal horn neurons activated by noxious stimuli. Brain Res 152:196, 1978
11. Nathan PW: Involvement of the sympathetic nervous system in pain, pp 311–324. In Kosterlitz HW, Tereniries LY (eds): Pain and Society. Weinheim, Germany, Verlag Chemie Gm-Bh, 1980
12. Richardson DE, Akil H: Pain reduction by electrical brain stimulation in man. Part I: Acute administration in periaqueductal and periventricular sites. J Neurosurg 47:178, 1977
13. Adams JE: Naloxone reversal of analgesia produced by brain stimulation in the human. Pain 2:161, 1976
14. Hosobuchi Y, Adams JE, Linchitz R: Pain relief by electrical stimulation of central grey matter in humans and its reversal by naloxone. Science 197:183, 1977
15. Yaksh TL: Multiple opioid receptor systems in brain and spinal cord: Part 2. Eur J Anesthesiol 1:201, 1984
16. Zieglgansberger W, Bayerl H: The mechanism of inhibition of

neuronal activity by opiates in the spinal cord of cat. Brain Res 115:111, 1976

17. Zieglgansberger W, Tulloch IF: The effects of methionine and leucine-enkephalin on spinal neurones of the cat. Brain Res 167:53, 1979

18. Camarata PJ, Yaksh TL: Characterization of the spinal adrenergic receptors mediating the spinal effects produced by microinjection of morphine into the periaqueductal gray. Brain Res 336:133, 1985

19. Yaksh TL: Direct evidence that spinal serotonin and noradrenaline terminals mediate the spinal actinociceptive effects of morphine in the periaqueductal gray. Brain Res 160:180, 1979

20. Kuraishi Y, Harada Y, Takagi H: Noradrenaline regulation of pain-transmission in the spinal cord mediated by alpha-adrenoreceptors. Brain Res 174:333, 1979

21. Reddy SV, Maderdrut JL, Yaksh TL: Spinal cord pharmacology of adrenergic agonist mediated antinociception. J Pharmacol Exp Ther 213:525, 1980

22. North RA, Williams JL, Surprenant A, Christie MJ: Mu and delta receptors belong to a family of receptors that are coupled to potassium channels. Proc Natl Acad Sci USA 84:5487, 1987

23. Maze M, Tranquilli W: Alpha-2 adrenoreceptor agonists: Defining the role in clinical anesthesia. Anesthesiology 74:581, 1991

24. Sabbe MB, Yaksh TL: Pharmacology of spinal opioids. J Pain Symptom Manag 5:191, 1990

25. North RA, Yoshimura M: The action of noradrenaline on neurons of the rat substantia gelatinosa in vitro. J Physiol (Lond) 349:43, 1984

26. Chapman CR, Bonica JJ: Acute pain. In Current Concepts, pp 16–18. Kalamazoo, The Upjohn Company, 1983

27. Marks RM, Sachar EJ: Undertreatment of medical inpatients with narcotic analgesics. Ann Intern Med 78:173, 1973

28. Cohen FL: Postsurgical pain relief—patient's status and nurse's medication choices. Pain 9:265, 1980

29. Moran WH Jr, Zimmerman B: Mechanisms of antidiuretic hormone (ADH) control of importance to the surgical patient. Surgery 62:639, 1967

30. Hagen C, Brandt MR, Kehlet H: Prolactin, LH, FSH, GH and cortisol response to surgery and the effect of epidural analgesia. Acta Endocrinol 94:151, 1980

31. Halter JB, Pflug AE, Porte D Jr: Mechanism of plasma catecholamine increases during surgical stress in man. J Clin Endocrinol Metab 45:936, 1977

32. Levin JD, Coderne JS, Basbaum AI: The peripheral nervous system and the inflammatory process. In Dubner R, Gebhart GF, Bond MR (eds): Proceedings of the Vth World Congress on Pain, pp 33–44. Amsterdam, Elsevier Science Publishers, 1988

33. Wall PD, Gutnick M: Ongoing activity in peripheral nerves: The physiology and pharmacokinetics of impulses originating from a neuroma. Exp Neurol 43:580, 1974

34. Spence AA: Pulmonary changes after surgery. Reg Anesth 7(suppl):S119, 1982

35. Rawal N, Sjostrand U, Christoffersson E et al: Comparison of intramuscular and epidural morphine for postoperative analgesia in the grossly obese: Influence on postoperative ambulation and pulmonary function. Anesth Analg 63:583, 1984

36. Bing HI: Viscerocutaneous and cutaneovisceral thoracic reflexes. Acta Med Scand 89:57, 1936

37. Donovan IA, Alexander-Williams J: Postoperative gastric retention and delayed gastric emptying. Surg Clin North Am 56:1413, 1976

38. Gelman S, Feigenberg Z, Dintzman M, Levy E: Electroenterography after cholecystectomy. The role of high epidural analgesia. Arch Surg 112:580, 1977

39. Gann D: Endocrine and metabolic responses to injury. In Schwartz S, Shire GT, Spencer F, Storer E (eds): Principles of Surgery, pp 1–64. New York, McGraw Hill, 1979

40. Munster AM, Eurenius K, Mortensen RF, Mason AD Jr: Ability of splenic lymphocytes from injured rats to induce a graft versus host reaction. Transplantation 14:106, 1972

41. Kehlet H, Wandall J, Hjortso NC: Influence of anesthesia and surgery on immunocompetence. Reg Anesth 7(suppl):S68, 1982

42. Hole A: Effect of general anesthesia and epidural anesthesia on some monocyte and lymphocyte functions during and after surgery. Reg Anesth 7(suppl):S75, 1982

43. Pollock RE, Lotzoua E, Stanford SD: Mechanism of surgical stress impairment of human perioperative natural killer cell cytotoxicity. Arch Surg 126:338, 1991

44. Schneider RA: The relation of stress to clotting time, relative viscosity and certain other biophysical alterations of the blood in the normotensive and hypertensive subject. Res Publ Assoc Res Nerv Ment Dis 29:818, 1950

45. Dreyfuss F: Coagulation time of the blood, level of blood eosinophils and thrombocytes under emotional stress. J Psychosom Res 1:252, 1956

46. Tuman KJ, Spiess BD, McCarthy RJ, Ivankovich AD: The effect of progressive blood loss on coagulation as measured by thromboelastography. Anesth Analg 66:856, 1987

47. Garcia-Frade LJ, Landin L, Avello AG et al: Changes in fibrinolysis in the intensive care patient. Thromb Res 47:593, 1987

48. Tofler GH, Brezinski D, Schafer AI et al: Concurrent morning increase in platelet aggregability and the risk of myocardial infarction and sudden cardiac death. N Engl J Med 316:1514, 1987

49. Modig J, Hjelmstedt A, Sahlstedt B, Maripuu E: Comparative influences of epidural and general anaesthesia on deep venous thrombosis and pulmonary embolism after total hip replacement. Acta Chir Scand 147:125, 1981

50. Oyama T: Influence of anesthesia on the endocrine system. In Stoeckel H, Oyama T (eds): Endocrinology in anaesthesia and surgery, pp 39–51. New York, Springer Verlag, 1980

51. Hall GM, Young C, Holdcroft A, Alaghband Zahed J: Substrate mobilization during surgery. A comparison between halothane and fentanyl anaesthesia. Anaesthesia 33:924, 1978

52. Haxholdt OS, Kehlet H, Dyrberg V: Effects of fentanyl on the cortisol and hyperglycemic response to abdominal surgery. Acta Anaesthesiol Scand 25:434, 1981

53. Cooper GM, Paterson JL, Ward ID, Hall GM: Fentanyl and the metabolic response to gastric surgery. Anaesthesia 36:667, 1981

54. Roizen MF, Horrigan RW, Frazer BM: Anesthetic doses blocking adrenergic (stress) and cardiovascular response to incision—MAC BAR. Anesthesiology 54:390, 1981

55. Rem J, Brandt MR, Kehlet H: Prevention of postoperative lymphopenia and agranulocytosis by epidural anesthesia. Lancet 1:283, 1980

56. Hagen C, Brandt MR, Kehlet H: Prolactin LH, FSH, GH and cortisol response to surgery and the effect of epidural analgesia. Acta Endocrinol 94:151, 1980

57. Pflug AE, Halter JB: Effect of spinal anesthesia on adrenergic tone and the neuroendocrine response to surgical stress in humans. Anesthesiology 55:120, 1981

58. Engquist A, Brandt MR, Fernandes A, Kehlet H: The blocking effect of epidural analgesia on the adrenocorticoid and hyperglycemic response to surgery. Acta Anaesthesiol Scand 21:330, 1977

59. Yeager MP, Glass DD, Neff RK, Brinck-Johnsen T: Epidural anesthesia and analgesia in high-risk surgical patients. Anesthesiology 66:729, 1987

60. Bromage PR, Shibata HR, Willoughby HW: Influence of prolonged epidural blockade on blood sugar and cortisol responses to operations on the upper part of the abdomen and thorax. Surg Gynecol Obstet 132:1051, 1971

61. Traynor C, Paterson JL, Ward ID et al: Effects of extradural anesthesia and vagal blockade on the metabolic and endocrine response to upper abdominal surgery. Br J Anaesth 54:319, 1982

62. Cosgrove DO, Jenkins JS: The effect of epidural anaesthesia on the pituitary-adrenal response to surgery. Clin Sci Mol Med 46:403, 1974

63. Vik-Mo H, Ottesen S, Renck H: Cardiac effects of thoracic epidural analgesia before and during acute coronary artery occlusion in open-chest dogs. Scand J Clin Lab Invest 38:737, 1978

64. Blomberg S, Emanuelsson H, Ricksten SE: Thoracic epidural anesthesia and central hemodynamics in patients with unstable angina pectoris. Anesth Analg 69:558, 1989

65. Baron JF, Coriat P, Mundler O et al: Left ventricular global and regional function during lumbar epidural anesthesia in patients with and without angina pectoris. Influence of volume loading. Anesthesiology 66:621, 1987

66. Saada M, Duval AM, Bonnet F et al: Abnormalities in myocardial segmental wall motion during lumbar epidural anesthesia. Anesthesiology 71:26, 1989

67. Bloomberg S, Curelaru I, Emanuelsson H et al: Thoracic epidural anaesthesia in patients with unstable angina pectoris. Eur Heart J 10:437, 1989

68. Bryan-Brown CW: Development of pain management in critical care. In Cousins MJ, Phillips GD (eds): Acute Pain Management, Clinics in Critical Care Medicine, pp 1–20. New York, Churchill Livingstone, 1986

69. Shulman M, Sandler AN, Bradley JW et al: Postthoracotomy pain and pulmonary function following epidural and systemic morphine. Anesthesiology 61:569, 1984

70. Tuman KJ, McCarthy RJ, Spiess BD et al: Epidural anesthesia and analgesia decreases postoperative hypercoagulability in high-risk vascular patients. Anesth Analg 70:414, 1990

71. Henry CP, Odoom JA, Ten-Cate JW et al: Effects of extradural bupivacaine on the haemostatic system. Br J Anaesth 58:301, 1986

72. Modig J, Malmberg P, Karlstrom G: Effect of epidural versus general anaesthesia on calf blood flow. Acta Anaesthesiol Scand 24:305, 1980

73. Modig J, Borg T, Bagge L, Saldeen T: Role of extradural and of general anesthesia in fibrinolysis and coagulation after total hip replacement. Br J Anaesth 55:625, 1983

74. Tuman KJ, McCarthy RJ, March R et al: Effects of epidural anesthesia and analgesia on coagulation and outcome after major vascular surgery. Anesth Analg 73:696, 1991.

75. Ferreira SH, Moncada S, Vane JR: Prostaglandins and the mechanisms of analgesia produced by aspirin-like drugs. Br J Pharmacol 49:86, 1973

76. Vane JR: Inhibition of prostaglandin synthesis as a mechanism of action for aspirin-like drugs. Nature [New Biol] 231:232, 1971

77. Bonica JJ: Biochemistry and modulation of nociception and pain. In Bonica JJ (ed): The Management of Pain, vol I, pp 95–121. Philadelphia, Lea & Febiger, 1990

78. Ferreira SH: Prostaglandins hyperalgesia and the control of inflammatory pain. In Bonta IL, Bray MA, Parnham MJ (eds): Handbook of Inflammation, vol 5: The Pharmacology of Inflammation, pp 108–116. New York, Elsevier, 1985

79. Ferreira SH: Prostaglandins: Peripheral and central analgesia. In Bonica JJ, Lindblom U, Iggo S (eds): Advances in Pain Research and Therapy, vol 5, pp 627–634. New York, Raven Press, 1983

80. Lee VC: Non-narcotic modalities for the management of acute pain. Anesth Clin North Am 7:101, 1989

81. Jung D, Mroszczak E, Bynum L: Pharmacokinetics of ketorolac tromethamine in humans after intravenous, intramuscular and oral administration. Eur J Clin Pharmacol 35:423, 1988

82. Carmichael J, Shankel SW: Effects of nonsteroidal anti-inflammatory drugs on prostaglandin and renal function. Am J Med 78:992, 1985

83. Fredrickson RC: Endogenous opioids and related disorders, pp 9–68. In Kuhnar M, Pasternak G (eds): Analgesics: Neurochemical, Behavioral, and Clinical Perspectives. New York, Raven Press, 1984

84. Pasternak GW: Multiple morphine and enkephalin receptors: Biochemical and pharmacologic aspects. In Kelly DD (ed): Stress-Induced Analgesia, pp 130–140. New York, Annals of the New York Academy of Sciences, 1986

84a. Stanley TH, Hague B, Mock DL et al: Oral transmucosal fentanyl citrate (lollipop) premedication in human volunteers. Anesth Analg 69:21, 1989

85. Rigg JR, Browne RA, Davis C et al: Variation in the disposition of morphine after administration in surgical patients. Br J Anaesth 50:1125, 1978

86. Austin KL, Stapelton JVC, Mather LE: Multiple intramuscular injections: A major source of variability in analgesic response to meperidine. Pain 8:47, 1980

87. Gourlay GK, Kowalski SR, Plummer JL et al: Fentanyl blood concentration-analgesic response relationship in the treatment of postoperative pain. Anesth Analg 67:329, 1988

88. Edwards DJ, Svensson CK, Visco JP, Lalka D: Clinical pharmacokinetics of pethidine:1982. Clin Pharmacokinet 7:421, 1982

89. Buckley MM, Brogden RN: Ketorolac. A review of its pharmacodynamic and pharmacokinetic properties, and therapeutic potential. Drugs 39:86, 1990

90. Egbert AM, Parks LH, Short LM, Burnett ML: Randomized trial of postoperative patient-controlled analgesia vs intramuscular narcotics in frail elderly men. Arch Intern Med 150:1897, 1990

91. Bennett RL, Batenhorst RL, Graves DA et al: Morphine titration in postoperative laparotomy patients using patient-controlled analgesia. Curr Ther Res 66:81, 1982

92. White PF: Mishaps with patient-controlled analgesia. Anesthesiology 66:81, 1987

93. Cleland JG: Continuous peridural caudal analgesia in surgery and early ambulation. NW Med J 48:26, 1949

94. Abboud TK, Dror A, Mosaad P et al: Mini-dose intrathecal morphine for the relief of post-cesarean section pain: Safety, efficacy and ventilatory responses to carbon dioxide. Anesth Analg 67:137, 1988

95. Aun C, Thomas D, St. John-Jones L et al: Intrathecal morphine in cardiac surgery. Eur J Anaesthesiol 2:419, 1985

96. Rigler ML, Drasner K, Krejcie TC et al: Cauda equina syndrome after spinal anesthesia. Anesth Analg 72:275, 1991

97. Bromage PR, Camporesi EM, Durant PAC, Neilsen CH: Non-respiratory side effects of epidural morphine. Anesth Analg 61:490, 1982

98. Negre I, Gueneron JP, Ecoffey C et al: Ventilatory response to carbon dioxide after intramuscular and epidural fentanyl. Anesth Analg 66:707, 1987

99. Loper KA, Ready LB, Downey M et al: Epidural and intravenous fentanyl infusions are clinically equivalent after knee surgery. Anesth Analg 70:72, 1990

100. Bromage PR, Camporesi E, Chestnut D: Epidural narcotics for postoperative analgesia. Anesth Analg 59:473, 1980

101. El-Baz NM, Faber LP, Jensik RJ: Continuous epidural infusion of morphine for treatment of pain after thoracic surgery. A new technique. Anesth Analg 63:757, 1984

102. Chestnut DH, Owen CL, Bates JN et al: Continuous infusion epidural analgesia during labor: A randomized double-blind comparison of 0.0625% bupivacaine/0.0002% fentanyl versus 0.125% bupivacaine. Anesthesiology 68:754, 1988

103. Cullen ML, Staren ED, el-Ganzouri A et al: Continuous thoracic epidural analgesia after major abdominal operations: A randomized prospective double-blind study. Surgery 98:718, 1985

104. Fischer RL, Lubenow TR, Liceaga A et al: Comparison of continuous epidural infusion of fentanyl-bupivacaine and morphine-bupivacaine in the management of postoperative pain. Anesth Analg 67:559, 1988

105. Logas WG, el-Baz N, el-Ganzouri A et al: Continuous thoracic epidural analgesia for prospective pain relief following thoracotomy: A randomized prospective study. Anesthesiology 67:787, 1987

106. Cohen SE, Woods WA: The role of epidural morphine in the postcesarean patient: Efficacy and effects on bonding. Anesthesiology 58:500, 1983

107. Cousins MJ, Mather LE: Intrathecal and epidural administration of opioids. Anesthesiology 61:276, 1984

108. Rutter DV, Skewes DG, Morgan M: Extradural opioids for postoperative analgesia. A double blind comparison of pethidine, fentanyl and morphine. Br J Anaesth 53:915, 1981

109. Chrubasik J: Investigations on respiratory depression. In Chrubasik J: Spinal infusions of opiates and somatostatin, pp 19–25. Oberursel, FRG, Verlag Hygieneplan GmBh, 1985

110. Shulman MS, Wakerlin G, Yamaguchi L, Brodsky JB: Experience with epidural hydromorphone for post-thoracotomy pain relief. Anesth Analg 66:1331, 1987

111. Akerman B, Arwenstrom E, Post C: Local anesthetic potentiates spinal morphine antinociception. Anesth Analg 67:943, 1988

112. Hjorts NC, Lund C, Mogensen T et al: Epidural morphine improves pain relief and maintains sensory analgesia during

continuous epidural bupivacaine after abdominal surgery. Anesth Analg 65:1033, 1986

113. Badner NH, Reimer EJ, Komar WE, Moote CA: Low-dose bupivacaine does not improve postoperative epidural fentanyl analgesia in orthopedic patients. Anesth Analg 72:237, 1991

114. Phillips G: Continuous infusion epidural analgesia in labor: The effect of adding sufentanil to 0.125% bupivacaine. Anesth Analg 67:462, 1988

115. Lubenow TR, Fischer RL, Besser TP et al: Comparison of continuous epidural infusions of sufentanil-bupivacaine with morphine-bupivacaine. Anesthesiology 3A:397, 1988

116. Rosseel PM, van den Broek WG, Boer EC, Prakash O: Epidural sufentanil for intra- and postoperative analgesia in thoracic surgery: A comparative study with intravenous sufentanil. Acta Anaesthesiol Scand 32:193, 1988

117. Van der Auwera D, Verborgh C, Camu F: Analgesic and cardiorespiratory effects of epidural sufentanil and morphine in humans. Anesth Analg 66:999, 1987

118. Abboud TK, Afrasiabi A, Zhu J et al: Bupivacaine/butorphanol/epinephrine for epidural anesthesia in obstetrics: Maternal and neonatal effects. Reg Anesth 14:219, 1989

119. Lawhorn CD, McNitt JD, Fibuch EE et al: Epidural morphine with butorphanol for postoperative analgesia after cesarean delivery. Anesth Analg 72:53, 1991

120. Abboud TK, Moore M, Zhu J et al: Epidural butorphanol or morphine for the relief of post cesarean section pain: Ventilatory response to carbon dioxide. Anesth Analg 66:887, 1987

121. Lubenow TR, Durrani Z, Ivankovich AD: Evaluation of continuous epidural fentanyl/butorphanol infusion for postoperative pain. Anesthesiology 73:A800, 1990

122. Bailey RL, Sperry RJ, Johnson GK et al: Respiratory effects of clonidine alone and combined with morphine, in humans. Anesthesiology 74:43, 1991

123. Eisenach JC, Lysaks Z, Viscomi CM: Epidural clonidine following surgery: Phase I. Anesthesiology 71:640, 1989

124. Eisenach JL, Rauch RL, Buzzanell C, Lysak SZ: Epidural clonidine for intractable cancer pain: Phase I. Anesthesiology 71:647, 1989

125. Motsch J, Graber E, Ludwig K: Addition of clonidine enhances postoperative analgesia from epidural morphine: A double-blind study. Anesthesiology 73:1067, 1990

126. Nagasaka H, Yaksh TL: Pharmacology of intrathecal adrenergic agonists: Cardiovascular and nociceptive reflexes in halothane-anesthetized rats. Anesthesiology 73:1198, 1990

127. McCarthy RJ, Kroin JS, Lubenow TR et al: Effect of intrathecal tizanidine on antinociception and blood pressure in the rat. Pain 40:333, 1990

128. Rao TL, El-Etr AA: Anticoagulation following placement of epidural and subarachnoid catheters: An evaluation of neurologic sequelae. Anesthesiology 56:618, 1981

129. Odoom JA, Sih IL: Epidural analgesia and anticoagulant therapy: Experience with one thousand cases of continuous epidurals. Anaesthesia 38:254, 1983

130. Mathews ET, Abrams LD: Intrathecal morphine in open heart surgery (letter). Lancet 2:543, 1980

131. Rawal N, Arner S, Gustafsson LL, Allvin R: Present state of extradural and intrathecal opioid analgesia in Sweden. A nationwide followup survey. Br J Anaesth 59:791, 1987

132. Wolf AR, Valley RD, Fear DW et al: Bupivacaine for caudal analgesia in infants and children: The optimum effective concentration. Anesthesiology 69:102, 1988

133. Dalens B, Hasnaoui A: Caudal anesthesia in pediatric surgery: Success rate and adverse effects in 750 consecutive patients. Anesth Analg 68:83, 1989

134. Chauvet P, Lefeuvre M, Chelma C et al: Caudal block in the surgical repair of vesico-renal reflux. Agressologie 3:32, 1990

135. de Jong RH: Genesis of resting and action potential. In de Jong RH: Physiology and pharmacology of local anesthesia, pp 27–45. Springfield, Charles C Thomas, 1970

136. Carpenter R, Mackey D: Local anesthetics. In Barash P, Stoelting RK, Cullen BF (eds): Clinical Anesthesia, pp 371–403. Philadelphia, JB Lippincott, 1989

137. Butterworth JF 4th, Strichartz GR: Molecular mechanisms of local anesthesia: A review. Anesthesiology 72:711, 1990

138. Katz JA, Kaeding CS, Hill JR, Henthorn TK: The pharmacokinetics of bupivacaine when injected intraarticularly after knee arthroscopy. Anesth Analg 67:872, 1988

139. Henderson RC, Campion ER, DeMasi RA, Taft TN: Postarthroscopy analgesia with bupivacaine. A prospective randomized, blinded evaluation. Am J Sports Med 18:614, 1990

140. Kaeding CC, Hill JA, Katz J, Benson L: Bupivacaine use after knee arthroscopy: Pharmacokinetics and pain control study. Arthroscopy 6:33, 1990

141. Katz J, Nelson W, Forest R et al: Cryoanalgesia for postthoracotomy pain. Lancet 1:512, 1980

142. Benumof JL: Management of postoperative pain. In Benumof JL: Anesthesia for Thoracic Surgery, pp 467–476. Philadelphia, WB Saunders, 1987

143. Moore DC: Regional block. In Moore DC: A Handbook for Use in the Clinical Practice of Medicine and Surgery, pp 169–170. Springfield, Charles C Thomas, 1981

144. Goulding FJ: Penile block for postoperative pain relief in penile surgery. J Urol 126:337, 1981

145. Elder PR: Post circumcision pain. A prospective evaluation of subcutaneous ring block of the penis. Reg Anesth 9:48, 1984

146. Ansbro FP: A method of continuous brachial plexus block. Am J Surg 71:716, 1946

147. DeKrey JA, Schroeder F, Buechler DR: Continuous brachial plexus. Anesthesiology 30:332, 1969

148. Manriquez RG, Pallares V: Continuous brachial plexus block for prolonged sympathectomy and control of pain. Anesth Analg 57:128, 1978

149. Rosenblatt R, Pepitone-Rockwell F, McKillop MJ: Continuous axillary analgesia for traumatic hand injury. Anesthesiology 51:565, 1979

150. Reiestad F, Stromskag KE: Intrapleural catheter in the management of postoperative pain: A preliminary report. Reg Anesth 11:89, 1986

151. Ferrante FM, Chan VW, Arthur GR, Rocco AG: Intrapleural analgesia after thoracotomy. Anesth Analg 72:105, 1991

152. Stromskag KE, Reiestad F, Holmqvist EL, Ogenstad S: Intrapleural administration of 0.25%, 0.375%, 0.5% bupivacaine with epinephrine after cholecystectomy. Anesth Analg 67:430, 1988

153. Rosenberg PH, Scheinin BM, Lepantalo MJ, Lindfors O: Continuous intrapleural infusion of bupivacaine for analgesia after thoracotomy. Anesth Analg 67:811, 1987

154. Kambam JR, Hammon J, Parris WC, Lupinetti FM: Intrapleural analgesia for post-thoracotomy pain and blood levels of bupivacaine following intrapleural injection. Can J Anaesth 36:106, 1989

155. Chapman CR, Benedetti C: Analgesia following transcutaneous electrical stimulation and its partial reversal by a narcotic antagonist. Life Sci 21:1645, 1977

156. Bonica JJ, Chapman CR: Acute pain. In Current Concepts, pp 33–38. Kalamazoo, The Upjohn Company 1983

157. Clum GA, Luscomb RL, Scott L: Relaxation training and cognitive redirection strategies in the treatment of acute pain. Pain 12:175, 1982

158. Vetter TR: Acute pediatric pain management. In Stoelting RK, Barash PG, Gallagher TJ (eds): Advances in Anesthesia, vol 8, pp 29–54. Chicago, Mosby Year Book, 1991

159. Berde CB: Pediatric postoperative pain management. Pediatr Clin North Am 36:921, 1989

160. Lubenow TR, Ivankovich AD: Patient-controlled analgesia for postoperative pain. Crit Care Nurs Clin North Am 3:35, 1991

161. Tyler D, Krane E: Postoperative pain management in children. Anesth Clin North Am 7:155, 1989

APPENDIX A
POLICY AND PROCEDURES FOR INITIATION AND NURSING CARE OF PATIENTS WITH POSTOPERATIVE EPIDURAL ANALGESIA

I. Purpose
   A. To list guidelines for the initiating and monitoring of patients receiving postoperative epidural anal-

gesia and to provide quality assurance and patient safety.

II. Candidates
   A. Postsurgical patients who have no previous history of allergy to the ordered analgesics.
   B. Patients who do not have any contraindications to the placement of an epidural catheter (e.g., sepsis, severe coagulopathy, circulatory hypovolemia, head injury).

III. Equipment
   A. Infusion pump.
   B. Cassette tubing.
   C. Epidural catheter tray.
   D. Micropore tape.
   E. Tegaderm dressing.
   F. 4×4 gauze.
   G. Apnea monitor (if required—see below).
   H. Naloxone 0.4 mg·ml^{-1}—two ampules.
   I. 3-ml syringes with needles.
   J. Alcohol wipes.
   K. Epidural solution.
      1. Fentanyl citrate 0.001%/bupivacaine HCl 0.1% —150 ml
      2. Morphine sulfate 0.01%/bupivacaine HCl 0.1% —150 ml

IV. Treatment initiation and guidelines
   A. Placement of epidural catheter is performed by the anesthesiologist.
   B. Epidural order sheet must be completed by the anesthesiologist.
      1. Anesthesiologist's written order for epidural solution should include the name and amount of fluid, rate of infusion, name and dosage of any medications added, and supplemental intravenous/intramuscular pain medications as required.
   C. Epidural solution must be administered *via* designated infusion pump.
   D. Baseline blood pressure and respiratory rate must be documented before initiating epidural infusion.
   E. Blood pressure, heart rate, level of consciousness, and temperature are to be monitored every 4 hours for the first 24 hours of the epidural infusion.
   F. Respiratory monitoring.
      1. An apnea monitor is required for patients who received an epidural bolus of morphine sulfate 2 mg or greater. Patients may receive an epidural bolus of fentanyl, 50–150 μg, without the routine use of an apnea monitor.
      2. Respiratory rate to be monitored every 1 hour for the first 24 hours of the epidural infusion.
         a. Naloxone, syringe, and needle are to be available at the bedside at all times.
   G. The epidural solution bag and volumetric pump cassette are not changed unless otherwise ordered.

V. Nursing responsibilities
   A. Record vital signs (blood pressure, level of consciousness, ambulation, temperature) every 4 hours for first 24 hours of epidural infusion, then as ordered.
   B. Record respiratory rate every hour for the first 24 hours of the epidural infusion and every 4 hours thereafter.
      1. If the respiratory rate falls below 8 breaths per minute, notify the postoperative analgesia service and administer naloxone as ordered.
   C. Record all analgesic medications administered on the medication record.
   D. Use the Visual Analogue Scale to record patient's subjective level of pain with vital signs on flow sheet.
      1. Scale for pain: 0–10, with 0 = no pain and 10 = worst pain ever.
   E. Assess epidural catheter integrity and check dressing for wetness every shift and as needed.
      1. Reinforce with dry 4×4 gauze if dressing is wet.
      2. Cover with clear plastic tape.
      3. Notify postoperative analgesia service if excessive wetness or integrity of catheter is in question.
         a. If epidural catheter becomes dislodged or disconnected.
            (1. Notify postoperative analgesia service.
            (2. If catheter is disconnected, cover end of catheter with 4×4 gauze (do not reconnect).
            (3. If catheter becomes dislodged, keep for inspection by anesthesiologist.
   F. Assess and document signs and symptoms of side-effects.
      1. Pruritus with and without rash.
      2. Nausea and/or vomiting.
      3. Paresthesia, numbness, motor weakness.
      4. Headache.
      5. Back ache.
      6. Signs of infection around catheter site.
      7. Urinary retention.
   G. Record any prescribed treatment administered for side-effects or supplemental analgesics on patient care record.

VI. Postoperative analgesia service responsibilities
   A. See patients daily and chart progress notes documenting adequacy of pain relief and the occurrence of side-effects or problems associated with epidural use. Adjust therapy or institute test dose algorithm if current protocol is associated with inadequate analgesia, side-effects, or complications. Collect and maintain data for review by anesthesiologist on a weekly basis.
   B. Organize and conduct in-service training of hospital nursing staff.
   C. Review epidural medication record to ensure adequate documentation of use and disposal of medications.
   D. Evaluate and make recommendations regarding new equipment for epidural analgesia.
   E. Analyze data, identify problems, propose changes if any, and evaluate changes for quality assurance purposes.

VII. Pharmacy responsibilities
   A. Keep daily log of all patients receiving epidural analgesia with type of solution and amount dispensed.
   B. Generate computer printout of all patients started on epidural analgesia in the last 24 hours. Printout should be available in pharmacy at 8 A.M., Monday through Saturday. Patients started on epidural analgesia on Saturday or Sunday will be on the Monday morning printout. This list will be picked up by the postoperative analgesia service personnel to aid in identifying those patients started on epidural analgesia.

C. Collaborate with postoperative analgesia service personnel in quality assurance matters.

VIII. Termination

A. Epidural infusions ordinarily will be terminated by the postoperative analgesia service in conjunction with the primary surgical service using guidelines established for the type of surgical procedure and patients' analgesic requirements.

IX. Questions/Problems

A. Any questions or problems regarding epidural drip or catheter are referred to the postoperative analgesia service between 8:00 A.M. and 4:30 P.M. or the anesthesiologist on call after 4:00 P.M. and on weekends.

APPENDIX B
PATIENT-CONTROLLED ANALGESIA (PCA) SERVICE PROTOCOL FOR POSTSURGICAL PAIN RELIEF

I. Purpose

A. To list guidelines to follow when PCA is ordered and to provide quality assurance and patient safety.

II. Candidates

A. Postsurgical patients who have no previous history of allergy to the ordered analgesics.

B. Mentally alert patients who understand basic instructions and are physically capable of operating the PCA infusion device.

III. Treatment initiation

A. Treatment may be initiated by any surgical service as well as by anesthesia personnel. PCA treatment initiated by surgical services must conform to the guidelines listed below.

IV. Postoperative PCA guidelines

A. The physician's order for PCA must include the following:
1. Drug (only morphine and meperidine are available for routine use for postsurgical pain. Fentanyl and other drugs may be used only with the approval of the postoperative analgesia service physician or anesthesiologist-on-call when the service is not available).
2. Loading dose (if patient has pain when PCA is ordered).
3. Maintenance infusion (if desired).
4. Incremental or maintenance dose.
5. Lockout interval.
6. Four-hour limit.
7. Mode of operation—PCA.

B. Recommended starting parameters
1. Loading dose, morphine 1–4 mg, meperidine 10–40 mg.
2. Maintenance dose, morphine 1 mg, meperidine 10 mg.
3. Lockout interval, 6–10 minutes.
4. Four-hour limit, morphine 20 mg, meperidine 200 mg.
5. Mode of operation—PCA.

V. Surgical staff responsibilities

A. Initiate preprinted order sheet.
B. Evaluate adequacy of therapy.
C. Contact postoperative analgesia service personnel if pain relief is inadequate or patient has requirements for more complex PCA dosing.
D. Monitor for complications.

VI. Nursing responsibilities

A. Obtain and ensure prompt delivery of PCA morphine/meperidine vials from pharmacy to nursing units.
B. Verify proper and patent iv line.
C. Monitor and record vital signs per orders.
D. Reinforce patient teaching on use of PCA, if needed.
E. Assess pain level and effectiveness of PCA.
F. Change PCA tubing every 48 hours.
G. Document accurate dosage of narcotic used or wasted in separate PCA medication sheets (two signatures needed for drug wasted).
H. Verify that PCA is programmed to deliver dosage as ordered.
I. Check the PCA flow sheet, the pump readout, and the labeled syringe at the nurses' change of shift. The amount of drug administered in the previous 8 hours will be recorded on the PCA medication sheet.
J. Notify postoperative analgesia service personnel and primary surgical service if the patient experiences side-effects, complications, or inadequate analgesia.
K. Assess and document signs and symptoms of side-effects.
  a. Pruritus with or without rash.
  b. Nausea and/or vomiting.
  c. Sedation/decreased mentation.
  d. Decreased respiration.
  e. Ileus/constipation.
  f. Signs of infection or infiltration around catheter site.
  g. Urinary retention.
L. Record any prescribed treatment administered for side-effects or supplemental analgesics on patient care record.

VII. Postoperative analgesia service responsibilities

A. Instruct patients on the use of PCA when ordered by anesthesia and provide additional teaching if PCA is ordered by surgical service.
B. See patients daily and chart progress notes documenting adequacy of pain relief and the occurrence of side effects or problems associated with PCA use. Adjust therapy or substitute with a new protocol if current therapy is associated with inadequate analgesia, side-effects, or complications. Collect and maintain data for review by anesthesiologist on a weekly basis.
C. Organize and conduct in-service training of hospital nursing staff.
D. Review epidural medication record to ensure adequate documentation of use and disposal of medications.
E. Evaluate and make recommendations regarding new equipment for epidural analgesia.
F. Analyze data, identify problems, propose changes if any, and evaluate changes for quality assurance purposes.

VIII. Pharmacy Responsibilities

A. Keep daily log of all patients receiving PCA with type of solution and amount dispensed.
B. Generate computer printout of all patients started on epidural analgesia in the last 24 hours. Printout

should be available in pharmacy at 8 A.M., Monday through Saturday. Patients started on PCA on Saturday or Sunday will be on the Monday morning printout. This list will be picked up by the postoperative analgesia service personnel to aid in identifying those patients started on epidural analgesia.

    C. Collaborate with PAS personnel in quality assurance matters.

IX. Termination

    A. Epidural infusions ordinarily will be terminated by the postoperative analgesia service in conjunction with the primary surgical service using guidelines established for the type of surgical procedure and patients' analgesic requirements.

X. Questions/Problems

    A. Any questions or problems regarding epidural drip or catheter are referred to the postoperative analgesia service between 8:00 A.M. and 4:30 P.M. or the anesthesiologist on call after 4:00 P.M. and on weekends.

APPENDIX C
POSTOPERATIVE EPIDURAL ANALGESIA ORDER SHEET

(PLEASE CIRCLE ORDERS TO BE IMPLEMENTED AND COMPLETE BLANKS WHERE APPROPRIATE)
(DATE AND TIME FOR EACH PROCEDURE ARE TO BE NOTED)

1. Admit to PAR or SIT.*
2. Routine PAR or SIT vital signs.
3. Discharge from PAR per anesthesia care team.
4. On floor:
    a. Intravenous line per service or 1 l D5LR% TKO* #1.
    b. Vital signs every 4 hours.
    c. Tape two ampules of naloxone with syringe and needle at bedside.
    d. Monitor for respiratory depression.
        (1. Apnea monitor _____ hours during bed rest.
        (2. Respiratory rate every hour for the first 24 hours, then every 4 hours thereafter.
        (3. If respiratory rate less than 8 breaths per minute, give .4 mg naloxone intravenously immediately and call postoperative analgesia service.
5. Epidural solution (circle one).
    a. Morphine sulfate, 15 mg, with bupivacaine, 150 mg in 150 ml normal saline, rate _____ ml·hr^{-1} as needed for pain for 72 hours.
    b. Fentanyl, 1500 μg, with bupivacaine, 150 mg in 150 ml normal saline, rate _____ ml·hr^{-1} as needed for pain for 72 hours.

    c. Sufentanil, 500 μg, with bupivacaine, 500 mg in 500 ml normal saline, rate 8–10 ml·hr^{-1} as needed for pain.
6. Supplemental medications.
    a. Morphine sulfate, 2 mg intravenously, intramuscularly, or subcutaneously every 2–4 hours, as needed for pain.
    b. Metoclopramide, 10 mg intramuscularly, every 4–6 hours as needed for nausea.
    c. Diphenhydramine, 25–50 mg orally, intravenously, or intramuscularly, every 4–6 hours as needed for pruritus.
    d. If pruritus is unresponsive to two doses of diphenhydramine, give naloxone, .080 mg intravenous push (dilute one ampule naloxone with 4 ml normal saline in 5-ml syringe, give 1 ml of mixture. May repeat once every 5 minutes).
7. Nursing staff on floor should call postoperative analgesia service if any problems arise or catheter needs to be discontinued. Call anesthesia on-call pain center resident after 4:30 P.M. and on weekends.
8. All other preoperative orders, medications, and diet per service with the exception of narcotics.

Signed _____, M.D.† Date _____

Key: *PAR = postoperative analgesia service; SIT = surgical intensive therapy unit; 1 l D5LR% = 1 liter of 5% dextrose in lactated Ringer's solution; TKO = to keep open.

    †Signature and title required with each order.

APPENDIX D
POSTOPERATIVE PATIENT-CONTROLLED ANALGESIA ORDER SHEET

_____

Medication: Morphine sulfate 30 mg per 30 ml prefilled syringe
             Loading dose = 2 mg
             Maintenance dose = 1 mg
             Lockout interval = 6 minutes
             4-hour time limit at 20 mg*

Disregard all other narcotic orders during patient-controlled analgesia use.

Physician signature _____

    *If analgesia is inadequate, 4-hour limit may be increased to 30 mg.

58

Stephen E. Abram
J. David Haddox

Chronic Pain Management

Pain should be considered chronic not when it has reached a certain duration, but when it has extracted a substantial toll on the individual in terms of functional loss, psychological distress, and social and vocational dysfunction. Such a toll may be minimal in a patient with a focus of nociceptor activation that has gone on for many years, or it may be profound in another individual several weeks after a minor injury. Patients being treated for ongoing painful conditions must be assessed medically to determine the physical reasons for activation of the pain projection system, but they also must be evaluated to determine the underlying cultural and psychological background on which the painful condition is superimposed. One must also be aware of the social, vocational, and psychological consequences that result from the painful condition. Treatment decisions should be based on the relative severity of each of these components.

PAIN PATHWAYS AND MECHANISMS

Pain is most often experienced as a result of injury. Its survival value to an organism is based on the fact that it is initiated by tissue injury or by stimuli that threaten damage[1] and that it produces sufficient arousal and distress that it is unlikely to be ignored. It is tempting to envision pain as a straightforward receptive system, with transducers that respond to intense, tissue-threatening stimuli and neurons that project to areas of the brain capable of processing pain information. Unfortunately, such a view of pain perception fails to explain the tremendous variation in pain sensitivity between individuals or the dramatic shifts in sensitivity that can occur in a single individual. It also fails to explain chronic pain that is experienced without any noxious stimulation. Oversimplified anatomic concepts also predispose to simplistic therapeutic interventions, such as neurectomy or rhizotomy, that may aggravate rather than relieve pain.

In reality, the nociceptive system is highly complex and highly adaptable. Sensitivity of most of its components can be reset by a variety of physiological conditions. Injury to neural elements may result in loss of ability to perceive pain or may cause spontaneous pain or heightened pain sensitivity.

An understanding of acute pain perception requires a knowledge of the physiology of receptors that respond to tissue-threatening stimuli, the anatomy of peripheral and central nervous system pathways that are activated by noxious stimulation, and the mechanisms by which various components of the pain projection system can be sensitized or suppressed. Mechanisms of chronic pain are even more complex. Chronic injury may lead to marked alterations in nociceptor sensitivity or to spontaneous firing of peripheral or central pain projection fibers. To further complicate matters, a variety of psychological and behavioral alterations frequently occur in patients with long-standing pain. This section provides an overview of the anatomic pathways, the physiological modulating mechanisms, and the pathologic alterations that are important to the perception of pain.

ANATOMIC PATHWAYS

Nociceptors

The existence of receptors that respond exclusively to intense, potentially tissue-damaging stimuli is now well accepted. Cutaneous nociceptors have been extensively studied and are now fairly well characterized. Receptors responsive to intense stimuli have been studied in deep somatic structures, but considerably less is known about their response characteristics and function. Still less is known about the physiology of visceral pain.

Cutaneous Nociceptors

There are several different types of cutaneous nociceptors, which are characterized by the fiber type involved (thinly myelinated and unmyelinated) and by the types of stimuli to which they respond. High threshold mechanoreceptors have thinly myelinated axons (A-delta) and respond only to intense mechanical stimuli. C-polymodal nociceptors have unmyelinated (C) fibers and respond to intense mechanical or thermal stimuli and to a variety of chemical irritants.[1] There are both C and A fibers that respond to noxious mechanical and noxious heat stimuli. There are termed C-fiber mechano-heat nociceptors and A-fiber mechano-heat nociceptors.[2]

High threshold mechanoreceptor axons conduct mainly in the A-delta range, although velocities into the A-beta range have been recorded.[3] They respond to strong pressure applied to several discrete points within a receptive field that can cover 1 cm[2] or more of skin. High threshold mechanoreceptors do not ordinarily respond to noxious heating of the skin, but may become responsive to heating following a period of sensitization by high temperatures.[4] The receptors of high threshold mechanoreceptors have been recently described through electron microscopy studies.[5] Fine myelinated fibers were shown to send nonmyelinated processes into the epidermis, terminating near keratinocytes in the basal layer. Myelinated mechanical nociceptors are generally believed to subserve fast, well-localized, pricking pain.

C-polymodal nociceptor units respond with slow adaptation to strong pressure. They respond rapidly to noxious heat and are excited by a range of irritant chemicals.[3] Receptive fields may be over 1 cm wide in primates.[6] Firing frequency increases in a roughly linear fashion as skin temperature is increased within the noxious range (Fig. 58-1). Some units demonstrate sensitization by prior strong heating of the receptive field. Heat sensitization is probably related to release of several peptides and amines from local tissues.[3]

Small myelinated axons that respond to noxious heat, strong pressure, and chemical irritation have been found in humans[7] and nonhuman primates.[8] These rapidly conducting polymodal nociceptors may be responsible for rapid reactions to intense heating of the skin. Some fibers have been described that appear to be insensitive or poorly responsive to strong mechanical stimuli. These units have been termed thermal nociceptors, but are probably best characterized as polymodal units that occupy the most insensitive end of the mechanical sensitivity range.[3] Likewise, some C fibers have been found that respond to strong pressure, but not heat.[9] It is not clear whether these structures represent a separate group from the C-polymodal nociceptors.

Nociceptors in Other Somatic Structures

A large number of A-delta and C fibers may be found in muscle, fascia, and tendon that are poorly responsive to normal stretching or contraction and are probably nociceptive in function. Many of the C fibers are responsive to chemical irritants, heat, and strong pressure.[3] A few respond to strong contraction and to ischemia, whereas others fire in response to muscle stretching.[10] Some A-delta fibers in muscle have relatively low sensitivity to mechanical stimuli, responding best to chemicals, such as bradykinin. Others, which tend to be arranged near muscle–tendon junctions, respond to local pressure, stretch, and contractions.[3]

It is obvious from clinical experience that joints are well endowed with nociceptors. Small myelinated and unmyelinated fibers terminate in free nerve endings in joints, and A-delta fibers form a widespread plexus in capsules, fatpads, and ligaments.[11] Some of the A-delta axons respond to noxious stimuli.[12] Moncada et al[13] have reported generalized nociceptive responses to intracapsular bradykinin injections in anesthetized dogs. The responses were enhanced by prostaglandin injection.

Corneal sensitivity serves a primarily protective function, and most stimuli to corneal epithelium are sensed as pain. Innervation is mainly from A-delta fibers, with fine terminals devoid of Schwann cell covering.[3] These fibers have response characteristics similar to C-polymodal nociceptors. Tooth pulp afferents respond to a variety of chemical stimuli, strong heating, cooling, and pressure. Electrical

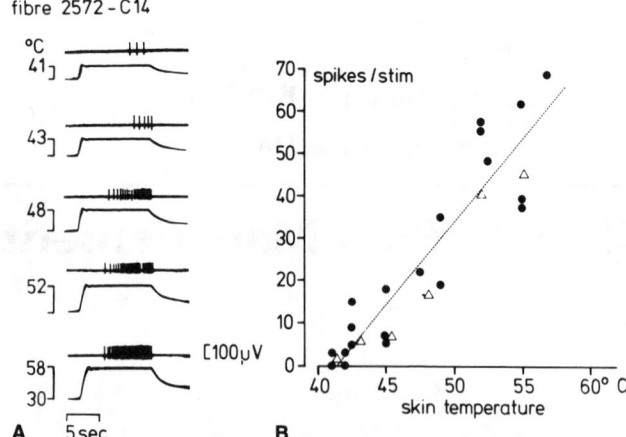

Figure 58-1. Discharges from a single C nociceptor during radiant heat stimulation of the skin. (*A*) Specimen records on various degrees of heating. Time course of skin temperature displayed below. (*B*) Relationship between the surface temperature of the skin and the total number of spikes/stimulus (*solid circles*) and the averaged number of spikes during the last 4 seconds of any stimulus, respectively (*open triangles*). (Reprinted with permission from Zimmermann M, Handwerker HO: Total afferent inflow and dorsal horn activity upon radiant heat stimulation of the cat's footpad. In Advances in Neurology, vol. 4. New York, Raven Press, 1974.)

stimulation produces almost exclusively painful sensations.[3]

Visceral Pain Receptors

Because of the infrequency with which visceral structures are exposed to potentially damaging events, it would not seem efficient to provide these structures with receptors designed solely to detect intense stimuli in the environment. Although severe pain of visceral origin is a common clinical phenomenon, there is little evidence that specialized pain receptors exist in visceral structures. Many damaging stimuli, such as cutting, burning, or clamping, produce no pain when applied to visceral structures. On the other hand, inflammation, ischemia, mesenteric stretching, or dilation or spasm of hollow viscera may produce severe pain. These stimuli are usually associated with pathologic processes, and the pain they induce may serve a survival function by promoting immobility.

For almost all intrathoracic, intra-abdominal, and pelvic viscera, pain perception is a function of visceral afferent (sometimes termed sympathetic afferent) fibers.[3] These neurons accompany sympathetic efferent axons in the sympathetic chain and intra-abdominal and intrathoracic plexuses, but most, like other afferent fibers, have their cell bodies in the dorsal root ganglia and synapse with dorsal horn neurons.

Pain Perception in the Gut

It has been widely accepted that nociceptive-specific fibers do not exist in the gut.[14] Pain is thought to result from intense activation of afferent fibers that serve other functions, such as stretch receptors. High frequency activation of these visceral afferents in turn activates dorsal horn pain projection neurons, producing pain perceived within cutaneous referral sites. This referred pain is probably the result of viscerosomatic convergence, the phenomenon of a single spinothalamic tract neuron that can be activated by visceral or somatic stimuli.[15] Another type of convergence, reported by Bahr et al,[16] is based on the existence of afferent neurons with two sensory branches, one visceral (sympathetic afferent) and one somatic (Fig. 58-2). It is not possible to locate the site of a painful stimulus to the gut with any accuracy, because stimulation of widely distant sites can give rise to the same referred sensations.[17]

Cardiac Pain

The phenomenon of cardiac pain, or at least the behavioral manifestations of pain, in response to intracoronary injection of bradykinin,[18] strongly suggests the presence of a nociceptor. Cardiac afferent fibers, conducting in the C and A-delta range, have been shown to fire at high rates in response to coronary occlusion or to intracoronary bradykinin.[19] However, to designate these nerves as nociceptors, they should respond only to noxious stimuli and should exhibit no background discharge.[20] Malliani[19] has shown that these putative nociceptors are tonically active, demonstrate mechanosensitivity, and respond to normal hemodynamic events. It is likely that cardiac afferents that are responsive to tissue-threatening stimuli have physiological functions under normal circumstances, but give rise to volleys of activity that can cause poorly localized pain referred to somatic structures. Viscerosomatic convergence probably occurs with these fibers.

Other Visceral Structures

Pain from the upper portions of the esophagus is most likely caused by activation of vagal afferents.[3] Heartburn pain may be a vagally mediated phenomenon, but little study of the activation of pain by acids in the esophagus has been carried out.

Distension of the renal pelvis or ureters is known to produce pain, but few studies have characterized afferent responses from the urinary tract. Pain of urethral origin is probably transmitted via sacral nerve roots rather than through sympathetic afferents.

Little is known about pain of hepatic origin. Stretching of the bile ducts and gallbladder activates two populations of afferent fibers, one responding to small changes in pressure and the other responding only to high pressures (>25 mm Hg).[21] The high threshold stretch receptors may have a nociceptive function.

Peptides and Excitatory Amino Acids Involved in Nociception

Painful cutaneous stimulation results in local vasodilation that is independent of central mechanisms and does not require activation of dorsal horn neurons. There is now abundant evidence that substance P, an 11 amino acid peptide, plays a role in producing local vasodilation as well as transmission of nociceptive impulses. It is thought to have a role in the function of the nociceptor's transducer mechanism. In response to axonal transmission centrally, substance P is released in the dorsal horn, serving as a sensory neurotransmitter or neuromodulator, facilitating activation of spinothalamic and other pain projection neurons. Ana-

tomically, substance P axons are not simple structures that connect a few receptors to a synapse in the dorsal horn. It appears that there is branching near the cutaneous end that sends fibers to nearby blood vessels, mast cells, hair follicles, and sweat glands.[22] More centrally, but distal to the dorsal root ganglion, further branching occurs. These more central collaterals are thought to go via rami communicans to the paravertebral sympathetic chain and ganglia and to visceral structures[22] (Fig. 58-2).

Following relatively mild painful stimulation, activation of a simple orthodromic mechanism may be the only pathway involved. When stimulation is intense, antidromic activation of cutaneous branches occurs, with release of substance P, causing vasodilation and release of histamine from mast cells. High intensity activation of substance P containing nociceptors may also antidromically activate branches to the sympathetic chain and viscera, causing postganglionic sympathetic discharge and perhaps alterations in visceral function. Thus, such a network could cause dramatic changes in vasomotor, autonomic, and visceral function independent of any spinal cord effect of sensory stimulation. Visceral branches of substance P containing neurons may be activated to high firing rates by distension, spasm, ischemia, or inflammation. Intense activation of the visceral branch may, in turn, cause antidromic activation of the cutaneous branch of the axon, producing cutaneous vasodilation and histamine release, as well as pain perception within that cutaneous distribution.

The activation of ascending pain projection systems is not a simple mechanism involving the release of a specific neurotransmitter that in turn activates the second-order neuron. It is well known that prolonged volleys of nociceptor activity, particularly if C fibers are involved, can produce a hyperalgesic state, in which allodynia becomes a predominant feature. It is now evident that the release of certain peptides or excitatory amino acids contributes to the sensitization of spinothalamic pain projection systems. The characterization of such mechanisms might then lead to the development of clinically useful receptor antagonists capable of reversing such hyperalgesic states.

Many small primary afferents contain substance P, which is known to be a primary sensory transmitter of acute nociception in the mammalian spinal cord.[23] However, there are several other peptides, such as calcitonin gene-related peptide, somatostatin, vasoactive intestinal polypeptide, and bombesin.[24] In addition, it has been noted that several excitatory amino acids, most notably glutamate, are released by small primary afferents.[25] The effects of glutamate on the N-methyl-D-aspartate (NMDA) receptor are probably responsible for certain pathological states, such as allodynia following nerve injury or prolonged C fiber inputs.[26] Excitatory amino acids have been shown to coexist with substance P in small dorsal root ganglion cells[27] and may be coreleased from primary afferent neurons, each substance modulating the effect of the other. NMDA receptor agonists administered intrathecally are capable of producing pain behavior and secondary hyperalgesia,[28] and NMDA receptor antagonists are capable of reversing the central sensitization induced by high threshold primary afferent inputs.[29]

Nociceptor Sensitization

As a result of inflammation or repeated tissue injury, nociceptors may be sensitized, becoming responsive to innocuous stimuli. It is generally believed that this peripherally induced hyperalgesic state is mediated by several endoge-

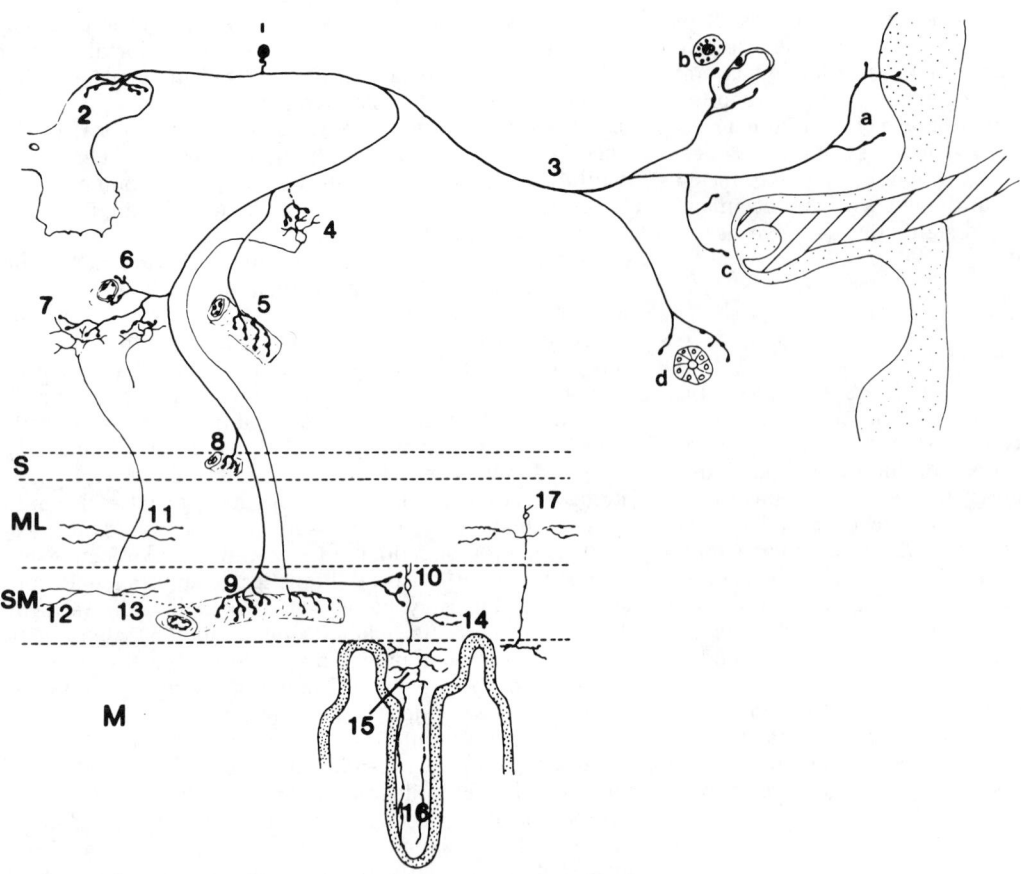

Figure 58-2. Proposed organization of the distribution of substance P (SP)-containing fibers innervating the skin and the alimentary tract and its blood vessels. Tentative or putative nerve connections are indicated by broken lines. Sensory SP immunoreactive neurones of dorsal root ganglia, here presented as a single cell (1), send their central processes into laminae I and II of the spinal cord (2) and their peripheral processes pass either to the somatic territory including the skin (3) or toward the visceral territory. In the skin, SP immunoreactive fibers terminate as free endings (a) in the dermis and deepest stratum of the epidermis. In the dermis, SP-containing fibers are closely associated with blood vessels and mast cells (b) that are involved in histamine release, with hair follicles (c), and with sweat glands (d). Peripheral processor SP-containing fibers enter the visceral territory by passing, through rami communicans, through the paravertebral sympathetic ganglia, where SP immunoreactive collaterals may be given off. The postganglionic territory of these ganglia includes the major blood vessels of the region, which receive also an SP immunoreactive innervation at this level (5). The SP immunoreactive fibers pass on, by way of splanchnic nerves, through the prevertebral ganglia (6, 7), where there is evidence that collaterals of the SP immunoreactive sensory fibers form the basis of the intraganglionic varicose SP immunoreactive nerve works (7). The postganglionic territory of the prevertebral ganglia includes the myenteric and submucous plexuses of the alimentary tract (11, 12) and to some extent the intramural blood vessels (13). The SP immunoreactive enteric sensory fibers pass from the prevertebral ganglia to the gut, supplying SP immunoreactive nerve networks to its blood vessels, including mesenteric and serosal (8) vessels and the submucosa (9), and contributing large boutons to the submucous plexus (10). Intrinsic SP immunoreactive neurons in the myenteric (17) and submucous plexuses (10) provide dense SP immunoreactive meshworks of fine caliber locally throughout the plexuses and in the muscle coats (14, 17) and in the mucosa form pericryptal (15) and subepithelial villous (16), and SP immunoreactive networks, including SP immunoreactive nerve strands in the muscularis mucosae. (s = serosa, ML = muscular layer, SM = submucosa, M = mucosa.) (Reprinted with permission from Cuello AC, Matthews MR: Peptides in peripheral sensory nerve fibers. In Melzack R, Wall PD [eds]: Textbook of Pain, p 77. Edinburgh, Churchill Livingstone, 1984.)

nous chemical substances. Two vasoactive amines, 5-hydroxytryptamine and histamine, and a widely distributed peptide, bradykinin, have been shown to lower nociceptor thresholds and to produce spontaneous pain under certain circumstances.[30]

Prostaglandins are complex fatty acids, whose precursors are found in cell membranes. They are released in response to noxious stimuli. They do not themselves produce pain, but markedly potentiate the algesic action of bradykinin, and probably act as sensitizers of nociceptors. They are formed from cell membrane phospholipids in a stepwise fashion. Cell membrane phospholipids are acted on by phospholipase A_2 to form arachidonic acid, which is transformed by cyclo-oxygenase to form cyclic endoperoxides. Cyclic endoperoxides are transformed to prostacyclin or to prostaglandin E_2 and F_{2a}. Prostacyclin potentiates bradykinin or histamine-induced edema, while prostaglandin E_2 potentiates pain induced by those substances.[30] Corticosteroids exert at least part of their anti-inflammatory action by inhibition of phospholipase A_2, while aspirin and other nonsteroidal anti-inflammatory drugs are cyclo-oxygenase inhibitors.

The lipoxygenase pathway is the alternate pathway for arachidonic acid metabolism. The lipoxygenase enzymes convert arachidonic acid to hydroperoxy derivatives (HPETEs and HETEs) and 5-s-hydroperoxy derivatives (5-H-PETE), which are enzymatically converted to active leukotrienes.[2] The effects of leukotrienes and other lipoxygenase products on pain and inflammation are not well understood. Their levels in the tissues are increased following mechanical or thermal trauma, and they appear to have a role in the production of tissue edema and circulatory and respiratory dysfunction.[31] Leukotrienes also have been implicated in the development of hyperalgesia that is dependent on the presence of polymorphonuclear leukocytes.[2]

Dorsal Horn Mechanisms

The spinal dorsal horn and its analogue in the medulla are exceedingly complex sensory processing areas. They contain the central terminals of peripheral afferent fibers, projection neurons of spinothalamic and other ascending tracts, local neurons that activate or inhibit projection neurons, and axon terminals of descending brainstem fibers.

As nerve roots approach the dorsal horn, segregation of fibers according to size takes place, with large myelinated afferents becoming arranged medially, and small, unmyelinated and thinly myelinated fibers arranged laterally. Most large myelinated fibers enter the cord medial to the dorsal horn. Many of these axons bifurcate, sending one branch rostrally in the dorsal columns. The other branch enters deeper layers of the dorsal horn, sending terminals into laminae IV and V and extensive arborizations into the substantia gelatinosa (laminae II and III) (Fig. 58-3).

Most unmyelinated or thinly myelinated afferents pass directly through the outer layer of lamina I, where they synapse with marginal layer cells and send a few branches into the underlying substantia gelatinosa. Some axons pass ventrally through these outer layers to terminate in laminae V and X.[32]

There are two groups of cells in the dorsal horn that respond to noxious stimulation in the periphery. One group, located mainly in lamina I, responds exclusively to noxious stimulation.[33] Most of these cells, termed nociceptive specific, have relatively limited receptive fields, confined to some fraction of a dermatome. The second group of cells,

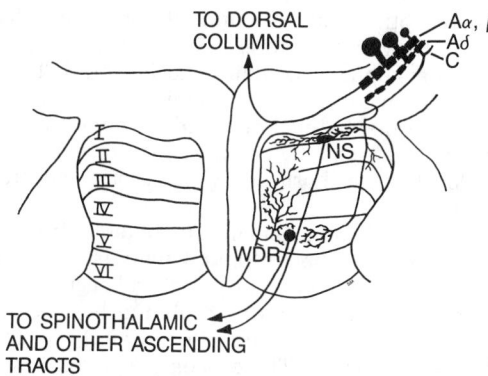

Figure 58-3. Simplified scheme of sensory input to the dorsal horn. Large non-nociceptive afferents (A alpha, beta) enter through the medial aspect of the dorsal root, send a branch cephalad in the dorsal columns and a branch ventrally to enter the deeper layers of the dorsal horn. They synapse with wide dynamic range (WDR) neurons, lamina V, and send extensive arborizations into the substantia gelatinosa (laminae II and III). A-delta mechanical nociceptors, arranged more laterally in the dorsal root, enter the dorsal horn directly through lamina I, synapse with nociceptive-specific (NS) neurons in lamina I and WDR neurons in lamina V. C-polymodal nociceptors also enter through the lateral aspect of the dorsal root directly into lamina I, where they synapse with NS neurons. Both A-delta and C fibers send a few arborizations into the substantia gelatinosa.

termed wide dynamic range neurons, can be activated by either tactile or noxious stimuli. Most of these cells are located in lamina V. They have large, complex receptive fields that often have a central area of responsiveness to either noxious or tactile stimulation, surrounded by an area of responsiveness only to noxious stimulation. Stimulation just outside the entire receptive field may produce inhibition.[34] It is generally accepted that wide dynamic range neurons contribute to pain perception and that their selective activation is sufficient to cause pain.[34] It is likely that many of the neurons in laminae I and V that respond to noxious stimuli are spinothalamic tract (STT) neurons.

There are several systems capable of suppressing activity in STT neurons. There is substantial evidence that both descending and segmental neuronal inputs can inhibit activation of nociceptive specific and wide dynamic range neurons. The amino acids glycine and gamma-aminobutyric acid (GABA) are known to be inhibitors of synaptic transmission, and there is some speculation that they are important mediators of segmental inhibition of nociception.[35] There are two known GABA recognition sites, $GABA_A$, for which muscimol is an agonist,[36] and $GABA_B$, for which baclofen is an agonist.[37] $GABA_B$, but not $GABA_A$ agonists, provide analgesic effects at doses that do not block motor activity.[36,37] Unlike the analgesic effect of spinal opiates and α-adrenergic substances, $GABA_B$ agonism does not appear to act through blockade of substance P release.[38] Spinally administered benzodiazepines, such as midazolam, appear to produce analgesia in animals[39] and inhibit sympathetic response to noxious stimuli.[40]

Two pentapeptides, leucine enkephalin and methionine enkephalin, appear to be important spinal cord inhibitors of nociception. STT neurons in laminae I and V receive input from enkephalin-containing cells in the dorsal horn. It has been proposed that enkephalins are released in proximity to primary afferent terminals in the dorsal horn, activating presynaptic opiate receptors that prevent release of substance P. However, the presence of direct synaptic contact between enkephalin-containing cells and STT neurons suggests that their inhibitory mechanism is, at least in part, postsynaptic. Enkephalins are found in highest concentrations in laminae I and II, but are also present in deeper laminae. Most dorsal horn enkephalins originate from intrinsic neurons.

It is not clear whether dorsal horn enkephalins function in a tonic fashion or whether their activity is stimulated for the most part by descending or peripheral segmental activity. If there is significant tonic inhibition by enkephalins, then administration of naloxone should markedly increase activity in STT neurons. There is only equivocal evidence for such disinhibition.[34] Release of enkephalins in response to descending neural activity has not been well documented. There is, however, evidence of enkephalin release in response to segmental activity.[41]

Both 5-hydroxytryptamine (serotonin, 5HT) and norepinephrine produce analgesia when injected intrathecally, and their antagonists (methysergide for 5HT, phentolamine and phenoxybenzamine for norepinephrine) attenuate the analgesia produced by certain pharmacologic interventions.[34] It is likely that both of these neurotransmitters are involved in descending control mechanisms that originate in the midbrain and medulla.

Adenosine receptors appear to play a role in the modulation of nociceptive transmission in the dorsal horn.[42] There are two receptor subtypes, A_1, which inhibits adenylcyclase activity, and A_2, which stimulates it.[43] Adenosine receptors may play a role in the analgesia provided by transcutaneous electrical stimulation, as it has been demonstrated that dorsal horn inhibition induced by high frequency stimulation is blocked by methylxanthines, which antagonize adenosine receptor activity.[44,45] The adenosine receptor may also play a role in the mediation of analgesia induced by spinally administered opiates.[46] Adenosine agonists have been shown to reduce the tactile hyperesthesia induced by low-dose spinal strychnine, a glycine receptor antagonist,[47] and may prove to be effective in certain hyperalgesic states.

In summary, the dorsal horn functions as a relay center for nociceptive and other sensory activity. The degree of activation of ascending pain projection systems depends on the degree of activation of segmental and descending inhibitory neurons in the dorsal horn, the pre-existing concentration of excitatory neurotransmitters, the intensity of the noxious stimulus, and the degree of sensitization of nociceptors in the periphery.

Ascending Pathways

The spinothalamic tract (STT) has been considered for many years to be the most important pathway transmitting nociceptive stimuli to the brain. Although it is important to normal perception of pain, it is by no means the only pathway with that function. The ability of patients to perceive pain following spinothalamic tractotomy provides evidence that other pathways are involved.

Many of the neurons in laminae I and V that respond to noxious stimulation are probably cells of origin of the STT. The majority of STT fibers cross near their level of origin. There are thought to be two functionally distinct divisions of the STT: the neospinothalamic tract, whose fibers tend to be more lateral, and the paleospinothalamic tract, located in the medial portion of the pathway. The phylogenetically newer neospinothalamic tract projects to posterior nuclei of the thalamus, such as the ventral posterolateral nucleus, and is thought to be involved with discriminative functions, e.g., location, intensity, and duration of noxious stimulation.[48] The paleospinothalamic tract projects to medial thalamic nuclei, and its activation is probably associated with autonomic and unpleasant emotional aspects of pain. This older portion of the STT is likely to be important in pain associated with denervation dysesthesia. Stimulation of the thalamic projections of the paleospinothalamic tract in patients with denervation dysesthesia reproduces the burning pain these patients experience spontaneously.[49]

The spinoreticular tract is likely to play a role in pain perception. Its cells of origin are unknown. It is thought to produce arousal associated with pain perception and probably contributes to neural activity underlying motivational, affective, and autonomic responses to pain.[50] The spinomesencephalic tract projects to the midbrain reticular formation. It probably evokes nondiscriminative painful sensations and may be important in the activation of descending antinociceptive pathways.[50]

Following bilateral spinothalamic tractotomy, it is still possible for patients to perceive pain from peripheral stimulation. There must necessarily be pathways in the dorsal portions of the spinal cord that are capable of producing pain perception. The spinocervical tract is a likely candidate for such a function. It is located in the dorsolateral funiculus. Its fibers ascend uncrossed to the lateral cervical nucleus, which serves as a relay, sending fibers to the contralateral thalamus.[50] There is also evidence that some fibers in the dorsal columns are responsive to noxious stimuli.

The distinction between ascending pathways is not entirely clear-cut. For instance, some spinothalamic neurons projecting to the ventrobasal portion of the thalamus also send collaterals to the periaqueductal gray and midbrain reticular formation. Therefore, some spinothalamic fibers are also spinomesencephalic. Similarly, collateralization exists between spinothalamic and spinoreticular fibers.[50]

Descending Control

In the early 1970s several reports showed that electrical stimulation of the periaqueductal gray area of the midbrain could produce widespread analgesia in animals and humans.[34] The periaqueductal gray area was later found to have high concentrations of endogenous opiates and to be rich in opiate receptors. Microinjection of small quantities of morphine into that area could also produce generalized analgesia.[51] Anatomic connections from the periaqueductal gray area to the nucleus raphe magnus and to the medullary reticular formation were subsequently described. From the nucleus raphe magnus, serotoninergic fibers descend via the dorsolateral funiculus to spinal cord dorsal horn cells. It is not clear whether serotoninergic fibers produce a direct, postsynaptic inhibition of STT neurons or whether they act by activation of inhibitory neurons that release enkephalins or GABA.[52]

There are also adrenergic fibers that descend in the dorsolateral funiculus that are thought to be inhibitors of pain. The cells of origin of these descending adrenergic pathways has not been firmly localized, but it is generally believed that they lie in the locus ceruleus and parabrachial regions of the medulla.[51] The role of adrenergic pathways in producing analgesia is complex. There is substantial evidence for analgesic effects of adrenergic agonists in the spinal cord, but adrenergic agents applied to some areas of the medulla tend to facilitate nociceptive transmission.[52]

Multiple environmental factors appear to be able to activate descending pain-control mechanisms. Nociceptive inputs and various types of stress can produce generalized increases in pain threshold. Anxiety, depression, and emotional distress can reduce pain threshold. The descending control mechanisms described may respond to such factors.

Deafferentation Pain

The preceding discussions have concentrated on mechanisms of pain perception in normal individuals. When damage to the nervous system occurs, pathologic changes occur in the peripheral and central nervous system that can give rise to pain in the absence of potentially tissue-injuring stimuli.[53] Deafferentation pain may result from peripheral nerve injury, spinal cord lesions, or lesions in the brain. The common factor in all of these situations is spontaneous activity or heightened sensitivity of neurons in the pain projection system.

Spontaneous discharge of injured peripheral nerves was demonstrated by Wall and Gutnick,[54] who reported spontaneous neural activity originating from experimentally induced neuromas. It was later demonstrated that sympathetic stimulation or norepinephrine infusion could increase such abnormal firing.[55,56] Devor[57] proposed that sodium and calcium channel proteins and adrenergic receptor proteins are transported to abnormal areas of nerve membrane (neuroma sprouts, demyelinated segments). Spontaneous depolarization takes place at these areas and is enhanced by stimulation of the alpha receptors.

Another possible mechanism for chronic pain following peripheral nerve lesions involves the short-circuiting of action potentials (ephaptic transmission, cross-talk) across demyelinated segments. Several possible types of interaction might exist. Demyelination of large afferent fibers could cause activation of nociceptors at the site of injury in response to stimulation of mechanoreceptors by non-noxious stimuli. Injury of motor fibers could cause nociceptor activation in response to motoneuron activation. Loss of Schwann cell protection of postganglionic sympathetics could produce nociceptor firing in response to sympathetic discharge. While there is some anatomic evidence that focal loss of myelin or Schwann sheath occurs following nerve injury, little physiologic evidence for ephaptic transmission has been reported.

In addition to impulse generation originating from the site of injury, there is considerable evidence that impulse generation occurs at points of membrane instability proximal to the injury. Wall and Devor[58] reported spontaneous discharge originating from dorsal root ganglia in sciatic nerve-sectioned rats. They proposed that the dorsal root ganglia impulses could contribute to pain after peripheral nerve injury.

Intact peripheral nerve pathways are essential for normal function of pain projection neurons and inhibitory interneurons in the dorsal horn. Following loss of peripheral nerve activity, there may be an increase in sensitivity or onset of spontaneous activity in STT neurons. It has been postulated that disruption of large afferents, which send extensive arborizations into the substantia gelatinosa, decreases the activity of inhibitory neurons in those areas.

Spontaneous activity or heightened sensitivity of neurons is thought to occur at more central locations within the pain projection system as well. Thalamic cells may undergo such changes following cord injury or some cerebrovascular accidents. Sensitization of central neurons may also occur some time after peripheral nerve injuries.

Sympathetically Maintained Pain

There are several mechanisms by which the sympathetic nervous system influences the perception of pain. Interactions between sympathetic outflow and spontaneous depolarization of injured nerve segments has already been discussed. Following trauma, surgery, and certain illnesses, a syndrome of pain, hyperalgesia, autonomic dysfunction, and dystrophy, usually referred to as reflex sympathetic dystrophy (RSD), can occur. A common explanation is that there is interference with the normal regulatory function of the sympathetics to the affected area induced by pain or injury. Periods of heightened sympathetic activity result in vasoconstriction, ischemia, changes in interstitial environment, and, perhaps, release of prostaglandins, bradykinin, and other pain-sensitizing substances. This explanation is highly simplistic and fails to account for the fact that early in the course of RSD the affected limb is usually warm and erythematous. In addition, enhanced sensitivity of nociceptors in RSD patients is not generally demonstrable. There may be central dysregulation of autonomic function in these patients, however. Experimental evidence for interference with sympathetic regulatory function following injury was provided by Blumberg and Janig,[59] who demonstrated loss of the normal reciprocity between skin and muscle vasoconstrictors following peripheral nerve lesions in animals. Skin vasoconstrictors are normally under the influence of hypothalamic centers. They are important in thermoregulation, and tend to be inhibited by stimuli that activate muscle vasoconstrictors, which are under medullary control. Following peroneal nerve lesions, skin vasoconstrictors tend to respond like muscle vasoconstrictors and appear to be under medullary control[59] (Fig. 58-4).

Another possible interaction between sympathetic activity and pain perception involves ephaptic transmission, or "cross-talk," between different fiber types at injured nerve segments. Segmental loss of myelin or Schwann cell protection of axons could lead to depolarization of nociceptor fibers by efferent sympathetic transmission. While such segmental demyelination has been demonstrated anatomically, physiologic evidence for the phenomenon is scant.

Another proposal is the direct sensitization of nociceptor nerve endings by sympathetic nerve terminals. Again, there is little evidence that such nociceptor sensitization occurs. There is, however, considerable evidence that sympathetic fibers are in direct contact with mechanoreceptors and that sympathetic activity can sensitize mechanosensitive afferents.[60] Roberts[60] has proposed that a combination of sensitization of mechanoreceptors plus disinhibition of wide dynamic range neurons could occur in certain post-traumatic states. Such a situation would lead to high frequency firing of spinothalamic tract neurons and pain perception in response to non-noxious mechanical stimulation (Fig. 58-5).

PSYCHOLOGICAL MECHANISMS

Any discussion of chronic pain is not complete without some consideration of the psychological factors that are related to pain. In 1986, the International Association for the

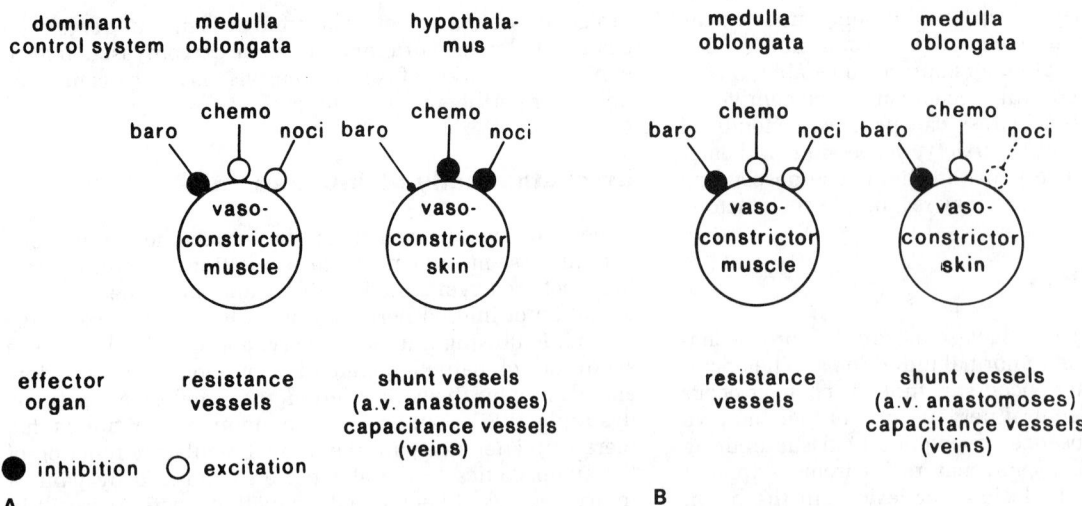

Figure 58-4. Reflex patterns in postganglionic vasoconstrictor neurons supplying skeletal muscle and skin under normal conditions (*A*) and after chronic nerve lesions (*B*). The patterns are simplifications and represent the (most common) pure cases. The term "dominant control system" indicates the brain structure that controls the respective vasoconstrictor system predominantly (but not, of course, exclusively). It is proposed that the cutaneous vasoconstrictor system is under predominant control of the medulla oblongata. Note the uniformity of the reflex patterns in *B*. (Reprinted with permission from Janig W: The sympathetic nervous system in pain: Physiology and pathophysiology. In Stanton-Hicks M (ed): Pain and the Sympathetic Nervous System, p 17. Boston, Kluwer Academic Publishers, 1990.)

Study of Pain published a taxonomy of pain-related terms in an effort to promote uniformity of usage and enhance accurate reporting of clinical and experimental phenomena.[61] Pain was defined as "an unpleasant sensory and emotional experience associated with actual or potential tissue damage, or described in terms of such damage." The salient features of that definition are that (1) pain is unpleasant, which is no surprise to most, (2) that it may have a sensory component, also not surprising, (3) that is has an emotional component, which distinguishes it from other sensory experiences such as touch, pressure, and vibration, and, most importantly, and (4) that pain is an experience and, as such, is subjective, personal, private, and can only be verified by report of the individual suspected of suffering from pain. This last point cannot be overemphasized. While much of what a physician does when dealing with pain patients is objectively verifiable by monitors, touch, or direct vision, these clinical tools only allow us to make inferences about another's suffering. The gold standard for determining if a patient is in pain is to ask the patient if he or she hurts. Other observations may aid in formulating a diagnostic impression, but only the patient can tell you if he or she has pain.

Psychological mechanisms can contribute to the pain experience in two general ways. A direct influence is exemplified by a situation in which psychological factors are entirely the cause of a report of pain. An example of this is psychogenic pain, which is considered to be quite rare. The psychological construct that is invoked to explain this involves the production of a perception of pain as a result of purely psychological factors, such as the need to suffer, as a means of assuaging guilt, or as a way to resolve some other intrapsychic conflict. This type of condition does exist, but is frequently overdiagnosed. In fact, the likelihood of diagnosing psychogenic pain is inversely proportional to the skill and expertise of the physician examining the patient. The histories of these patients present no clear patterns or

similarities, making a neat diagnostic algorithm impossible. Dramatic presentations or, conversely, apparent indifference, are not pathognomonic.[62]

Other direct psychological influences are found in the somatization disorders. These are a group of psychiatric disorders that are typified by a preoccupation with bodily function or symptoms.[63] Hypochondriasis is a condition in which the individual is preoccupied with the notion that he or she is sick, despite continual reassurance from physicians. The exact psychological mechanism is not well understood, but this condition should be treated by a psychologist or psychiatrist. In suspecting this diagnosis, it is wise to remember that the term arose from patients describing pain below the right costal margin (hypochondriac) at a time when cholecystitis was not recognized as a bona fide medical entity. Patients with fears or convictions that they are ill do, on occasion, turn out to be right,[64] so a careful history and physical examination coupled with performance of clearly indicated tests is advisable.

Somatization disorder is characterized by an onset of physical symptoms before the age of 30 years and includes at least 12 (for men) or 14 (for women) out of 37 symptoms involving various organ systems. These symptoms are of sufficient severity to cause the individual to seek medical attention, to take medicines, or to otherwise alter his or her lifestyle. These patients typically have undergone extensive investigations, usually from multiple physicians, all of which have yielded negative, equivocal, or conflicting results. Frequent surgeries, usually of an exploratory nature, are a common historical feature. These features are superimposed on any genuine somatic diseases suffered by the person, presenting a very complex clinical picture. The mechanism for this disorder is not proved, but it is suspected that these persons come from families in which little credence or attention is given to display of emotion, yet care and attention are provided in response to physical symptoms. Thus, the theory goes, the patient learns that the exhibition

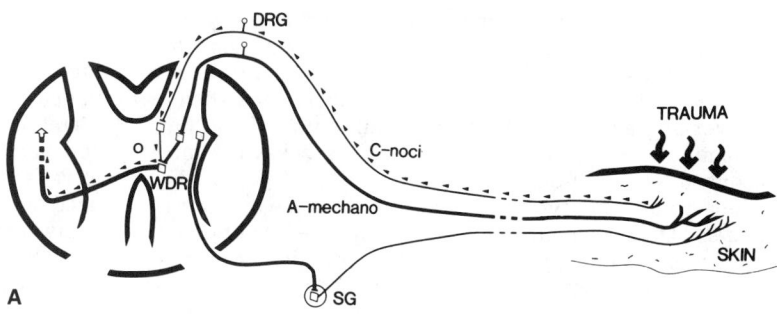

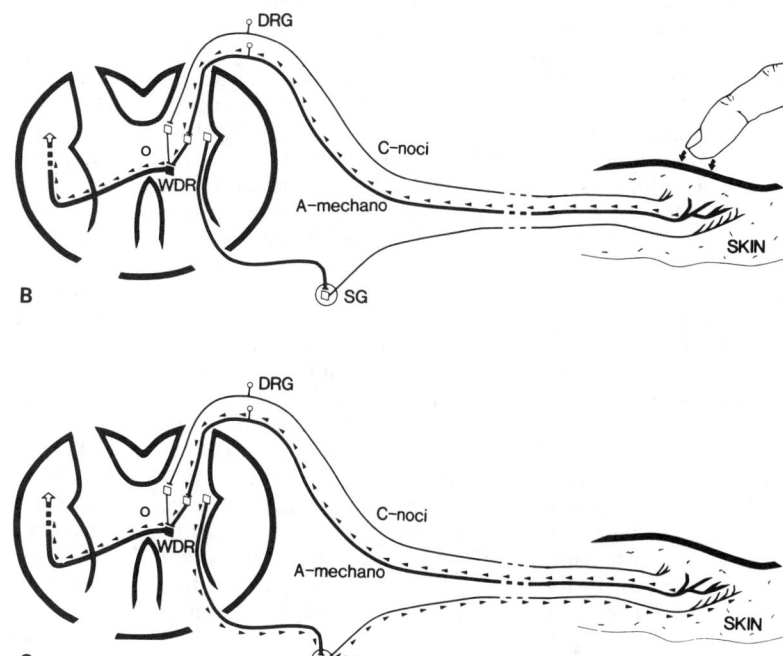

Figure 58-5. Schematic diagram of physiologic model. (*A*) The immediate response to cutaneous trauma. Action potentials in C nociceptors propagate through the dorsal root ganglion (DRG) to the spinal cord where they activate and sensitize wide dynamic range (WDR) neurons whose axons ascend to higher centers. (*B*) The WDR neurons remain sensitized and now respond to activity in large diameter A-mechanoreceptors that are activated by light touch. This state produces allodynia. (*C*) The same sensitized WDR neurons respond again to A-mechanoreceptor activity, but this activity is initiated by sympathetic efferent actions on the sensory receptor, in the absence of cutaneous stimulation. This phase represents sympathetically maintained pain. Although spinal interneurons are shown to be interposed in the pain pathway, this is just one of many possible arrangements. (Reprinted with permission from Roberts WJ: A hypothesis on the physiological basis for causalgia and related pains. Pain 24:297, 1986.)

of a physical symptom results in attention to the patient's needs. This *modus operandi* becomes ingrained on a subconscious level and then becomes part of the person's psychic constitution. This condition is not nearly so rare as psychogenic pain and, therefore, is likely to be seen with some frequency by a physician treating patients presenting with pain.

Factitious disorders (Munchausen's syndrome) present with reporting of symptoms and the intentional creation of signs that are intended to lead a physician to suspect a medical or surgical disorder. Patients have been known to instrument their urethra to cause hematuria and complain of flank pain or to use tourniquets to induce edema of the limb. The motivation for this behavior appears to be to occupy the role of a patient. The reasons for this goal are poorly understood.

Another similar condition is malingering, which is differentiated only by motivation. In this case, the motivation to assume the role of a patient is driven by the wish to avoid some other alternative that the individual feels is distasteful, such as military service or apprehension by the police, or to achieve financial gain. Fortunately, these charades are usually transparent to the astute physician. The incidence of this disorder in pain clinics is probably quite low.

Indirect psychological effects that influence the pain ex-

perience are common in chronic pain syndromes. At its most basic level, the presence of an ongoing nociceptive process that is not well relieved and produces continual suffering is bound to have some psychological sequelae that will color the whole pain experience. Such secondary effects as sleep deprivation, fatigue, irritability, and anger are commonly observed.[65]

The issue of depression and pain has been discussed by several authors.[62,66,67] It is not surprising that most patients with chronic pain are likely to show signs of depression. It is difficult at times, however, to clarify the distinction between a set of depressive features that are reactive to having chronic pain and an episode of major depression because there can be so much overlap in symptoms.[67] The *Diagnostic and Statistical Manual of Mental Diseases*[63] includes many somatic and related symptoms in its criteria for diagnosing major depression. Most chronic pain patients will have several of these, but the genesis of the symptom (e.g., insomnia) may be due to the pain itself rather than depression. It is clear, however, that a negative affective state such as depression serves to enhance the suffering of a person with chronic pain.

Another indirect influence is that of pain behavior. Pilowsky *et al*[68,69] have described the concept of illness behavior as it applies to pain patients. Simply stated, an illness is the individual's reaction or response to a disease. Illness behaviors arise from the patient's underlying physical condition and may consist of active behaviors, such as taking pills and visiting physicians, or passive behaviors, such as not working and lying down or sitting much of the day. In many chronic pain patients the illness behaviors must become a focus of treatment.

Behaviors of any type are subject to influence by operant factors.[70] Operant conditioning states that the likelihood of a behavior being expressed in a given situation can be altered by the consequences of the behavior. In chronic pain, for example, pain behavior (moaning) may be unwittingly reinforced by a spouse (showing attention), resulting in an increased frequency of the behavioral expression in the presence of the spouse. This is an example of positive reinforcement. By rewarding the behavior, its frequency is increased. The term secondary gain is often used to describe the type of paradigm wherein the individual, despite suffering with pain, does receive some benefit from it. Negative reinforcement increases the frequency of the behavior by removing a noxious condition from the environment in response to the behavior. Avoiding taking the garbage out by complaining of back pain is an example. Punishment, or the provision of undesirable consequences in response to a behavior, and extinction, the provision of no consequences, lead to decreased frequency of a behavior.

Cognitive factors also influence a pain experience.[71] The belief that a person has about the meaning of his or her pain can substantially alter the actual perception of the pain. An important issue in this regard is the perceived degree of control over the pain. Using this fact, it is common practice for dentists to tell patients to raise their finger if anything hurts during the procedure. This granting of control allows patients to tolerate procedures with greater comfort. Contrast this with a patient suffering from poorly controlled cancer. Here, every time a pain is experienced, it reminds the patient of the cancer and the likelihood of an imminent and probably painful death.

MANAGEMENT OF COMMON CHRONIC PAIN SYNDROMES

It is beyond the scope of this chapter to consider the entire spectrum of long-term pain problems. Instead, the medical management of several painful conditions that are likely to respond to regional analgesic techniques or other modalities that anesthesiologists are likely to use are discussed. In addition, this section presents, in general terms, the use of some pharmacologic agents that are useful in certain pain syndromes and gives a brief overview of the psychological principles that are important in managing chronic pain.

Lumbosacral Radiculopathy

The increasing acceptance of the use of epidural steroid injections for managing lumbosacral radiculopathy in recent years has encouraged many anesthesiologists to become involved with pain management outside of the operating suite. Since many patients referred with low back pain do not respond to epidurals, many anesthesiologists began to seek other methods of dealing with the difficult and complex back pain patients referred to them. In addition to development of other interventional modalities, physical and psychological modalities have been incorporated into many former nerve block clinics.

After Mixter and Barr[72] reported on the relationship between sciatica and lumbar disk protrusion in 1934, surgical intervention became the accepted treatment for lumbosacral radiculopathy. Unfortunately, it took nearly 20 years for the literature to reflect the fact that outcomes from laminectomy and nerve root decompression were not entirely satisfactory. Even after disappointing results were published, laminectomy has continued to be performed frequently and, in many cases indiscriminately. One study published in 1952[73] and another published in 1963[74] reported that long-term success after surgery for sciatica was achieved in fewer than one third of patients. Subsequent studies indicate that more than 75% of patients with acute lumbosacral radiculopathy who are treated nonsurgically will experience complete or nearly complete pain relief.[75-77]

Mechanical nerve root compression was originally presumed to be the cause of pain in discogenic radiculopathy. The lack of uniform success with surgical decompression and the fact that many asymptomatic patients demonstrate substantial disk protrusion on myelography[78] or on subsequent postmortem examination[79] suggests that other mechanisms must be operative as well. Following a period of mechanical nerve root compression, an acute inflammatory process may ensue, leading to intraneural accumulation of serum proteins and fluid, raised intraneural pressure, ischemia, and axonal degeneration.[80] It has also been proposed, on the basis of animal experimentation, that intense inflammation of the nerve root may result from exposure to degenerating glycoprotein material from the nucleus pulposus.[81]

It has been proposed that epidural or subarachnoid injection of corticosteroids provides beneficial effects by reducing the inflammation initiated by either mechanical or chemical insult to the nerve root.[82] The earliest use of epidural steroids was published by Lievre et al[83] in 1957, who reported good to excellent results in 50% of patients following injection of cortisone acetate plus radiographic dye. Most subsequent series of epidural steroid injections used a combination of local anesthetic and insoluble steroids. In order to determine whether local anesthetic alone provided benefit for patients with sciatica, Coomes[84] compared patients receiving bed rest plus epidural injections of procaine with patients treated with bed rest alone. He found that patients treated with procaine became ambulatory in 11 days, while it took the noninjected patients an average of 31 days to regain ambulation. Swerdlow and Sayle-Creer,[85] in a nonrandomized study, found consistently better results among chronic pain patients treated with epidural lidocaine and methylprednisolone than for patients treated with caudal saline or lidocaine injections. There was no difference in success rates among the three treatment groups for patients with acute or recurrent sciatica. Winnie et al[86] compared patients treated with epidural methylprednisolone with patients treated with local anesthetic combined with the steroid. Success was close to 100% in both groups, suggesting that the steroid, rather than the local anesthetic, was providing the benefit.

Unfortunately, few controlled studies of the efficacy of epidural steroid injections have been published. Dilke et al[87] reported that patients treated with epidural steroids had a lower incidence of severe pain, were less likely to take analgesics, and were more likely to have returned to work than patients treated with placebo. Breivik et al,[88] in a randomized, cross-over designed study, reported that patients treated with caudal steroid plus bupivacaine had an initial success rate of 56%, whereas only 26% of patients treated with bupivacaine alone responded to initial therapy. They also noted that 73% of patients who failed to respond to bupivacaine improved when crossed over to steroid treatment. A few studies failed to document that epidural steroid injections were more effective than epidural local anesthetics alone. Two such studies[89,90] compared results 24 to 48 hours after injection, before response to steroids is usually seen, and one of the studies employed injections at the L3–4 level, well above the usual level of radiculopathy.[90]

Few studies have assessed long-term responses to epidural steroid injections. One of the few studies to do so compared the long-range responses of patients whose initial response to epidural steroid injections was favorable with patients who were considered treatment failures.[91] After 6 months patients in the initial success group were significantly more likely to rate their pain level lower and were significantly less likely to be unemployed as a result of their pain when compared with initial failure patients. However, there was no difference in subsequent analgesic use between success and failure patients.

The L5 and S1 nerve roots are most commonly affected by disk disease, partly because disk degeneration is more likely at the L4–5 and L5–S1 levels and partly because those roots pass through a narrow lateral bony recess as they exit the spinal canal, a circumstance that increases the likelihood of root compression.[92] Tears of the annulus fibrosus usually cause pain referred to the upper, lateral portion of the buttock. Symptoms of lumbosacral radiculopathy consist of varying degrees of low back pain, pain radiating a varying distance into the lower extremity, and, in more severe cases, motor and sensory loss consistent with damage to the affected root. Typical signs and symptoms are listed in Table 58-1.

If bowel and bladder dysfunction are present, indicative of a large midline disk, prompt surgical intervention may be indicated. Otherwise, initial treatment of acute discogenic radiculopathy consists of short periods (a few days) of immobilization and mild analgesics. Most patients are able to tolerate the pain reasonably well when placed on bed rest. If severe pain persists after reasonable trials of conservative management, epidural steroids may be used.

Triamcinolone diacetate or methylprednisolone acetate are the most commonly used preparations. Injection should be performed as close to the affected nerve root as possible. Placing the patient in the lateral position with the involved side down may increase the amount of steroid reaching the affected root. Addition of a small volume (3 to 4 ml) of local anesthetic will produce considerable analgesia if it reaches the affected nerve root, confirming proper drug placement. In occasional patients, particularly those with S1 pathology, the drug will not spread adequately to the affected root. Placement of the epidural laterally in the L5–S1 interspace or caudal injection will sometimes result in better drug access to the injured nerve. Reassessment should be carried out 1 to 2 weeks after the initial treatment. If the patient has little or no pain at the time of the return visit, there is no point in repeating the injection. If symptoms are improved, but some pain is still present, it is likely that a repeat injection will produce further improvement. A third block can be performed 1 to 2 weeks later if some symptoms persist. There is some controversy regarding the advisability of repeating injections when no benefit is evident at the end of 1 to 2 weeks. The authors' experience is that few patients obtain relief from subsequent injections if the first epidural was of no help at all.

Intrathecal steroid injection has been advocated for patients who obtain minimal or no benefit from epidural steroids. A study that evaluated response of such patients to intrathecal injections of methylprednisolone acetate or triamcinolone diacetate failed to demonstrate any benefit to intrathecal steroids in patients who were totally unresponsive to epidural steroid injections.[93] Patients who had experienced partial improvement from epidural injections were likely to experience some further improvement from intrathecal injections. However, the study was terminated early because of the fairly high incidence of symptoms consistent with aseptic meningitis that appeared in the first 48 hours after intrathecal injection. While there is little evidence to suggest that intrathecal steroid injections pose a substantial risk of permanent neurologic damage, many practitioners are reluctant to use the technique because of the theoretical risk of injecting the preservatives these drugs contain intrathecally.

Patients with chronic radicular low back pain are much less likely to benefit from epidural steroid injections than are patients with more acute symptoms. Abram and Anderson[94] reported in a retrospective study that patients with long-standing symptoms were much less likely to experience even transient relief from epidural steroid injections. Similar findings were seen in a subsequent prospective study.[91] Patients who had undergone previous back surgery also had a much lower success rate. Several mechanisms may lead to chronic radicular pain that is unresponsive to steroid injections. Spontaneous activity or ephaptic transmission may occur from the injured, demyelinated root. Scarring of the root, with replacement of neural elements with fibrous tissue, causes inelasticity of the nerve. The nerve root can no longer stretch with leg motion, and chronic mechanical irritation ensues.[80] Loss of large afferent

---

TABLE 58-1. Pain Distribution and Physical Signs Associated With Acute Disk Herniation

Level of Herniation	Pain Distribution	Numbness	Weakness	Reflex Changes
L3–4 disk (L4 root)	Low back, buttock, lateral thigh, anterior calf, ankle, and occasionally big toe	Lower anterior thigh and patella	Mild (quadriceps)	Diminished (knee jerk)
L4–5 disk (L5 root)	Low back, buttock, lateral thigh, and calf, big toe	Lateral calf, web space of first and second toe	Foot (dorsiflexion)	None
L5–S1 disk (S1 root)	Low back, buttock, posterior thigh, and calf	Posterior calf, lateral heel, and foot	Foot (plantar flexion)	Diminished or absent (ankle jerk)

Reprinted with permission from Abram SE: Management of pain. In Cottrell JE, Turndorf H (eds): Anesthesia and Neurosurgery, p 496. St Louis, CV Mosby, 1986.

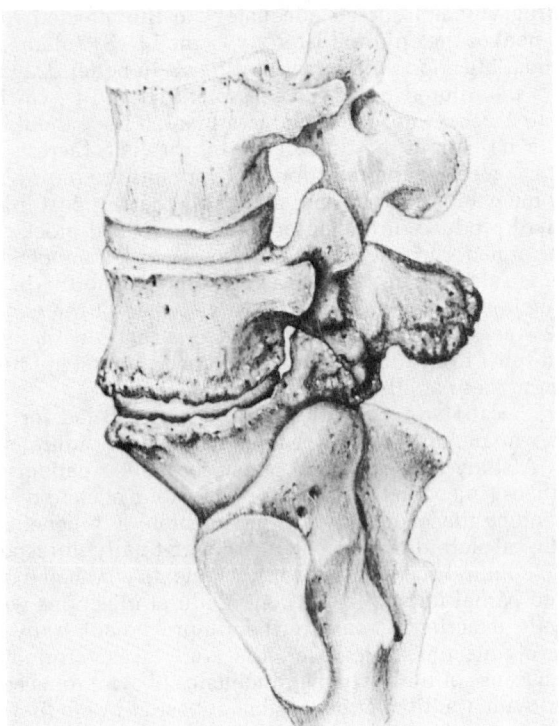

Figure 58-6. Stenosis of the L5–S1 intervertebral foramen and central canal secondary to degenerative changes. (Reprinted with permission from Finneson BE: Low Back Pain, 2nd ed, p 306. Philadelphia, JB Lippincott, 1980.)

fibers may lead to disruption of dorsal horn gating mechanisms and disinhibition of spinothalamic projection cells. Loss of disk height following herniation can lead to narrowing of intervertebral foramina, with subsequent root irritation laterally, or may cause redundancy and buckling of the posterior longitudinal ligament, which can effectively narrow the spinal canal. Loss of disk height can also produce facet joint subluxation and degeneration, producing pain from the joint itself and osteophyte formation, which can narrow foramina or the central canal. Injury to the vertebral plate, the cartilagenous portion of the vertebral body adjacent to the disk, often accompanies disk disease and may lead to osteophytic growth into the central canal[95] (Fig. 58-6).

With increasing duration of symptoms, the emphasis of therapy should be shifted away from medical types of intervention (injections, analgesic medications, surgery) and toward rehabilitation and psychological approaches. Programs that teach patients new ways of coping with pain, reduce dependency on chemical substances, and actively work to develop strength, range of motion, and physical conditioning are more likely to be of benefit to patients with chronic low back pain.

Lumbosacral Arthropathies

Degeneration and inflammation of the lumbar facet joints and sacroiliac joints can produce low back pain that is often difficult to distinguish from radicular pain. Both conditions may cause pain that radiates to the lower extremities. Computed tomographic scanning is a fairly reliable method of demonstrating pathology in these joints.[96,97] Bone scans,

particularly single photon emission computed tomography (SPECT) scanning, may also be useful diagnostically.

When facet arthropathy is the suspected cause of low back pain, the diagnosis can be confirmed by injection of local anesthetic into the facet joint. The procedure can be done easily under fluoroscopic control. The patient is placed prone and the affected side is tilted upward until the joint space is visualized (Fig. 58-7). Proper needle placement can be confirmed by injection of 0.5 to 1 ml of contrast. The injection should transiently reproduce the patient's pain, and the dye will outline the extent of the capsule. Occasionally, herniation of the capsule into the foramen, which can produce radiculopathy, can be documented. Injection of 1 ml of local anesthetic should produce dramatic relief of arthropathic pain. Injection of a small volume of insoluble corticosteroid into an affected joint will produce analgesia lasting 6 months or longer in about one third of patients who experience relief from the local anesthetic.[96] Nonsteroidal anti-inflammatory drugs may be of some benefit. Resistant cases have been treated with radiofrequency coagulation of the nerves supplying the facet joints, but long-term success is generally low with that technique. More recently, cold lesioning (cryoanalgesia) of the facet nerves has been reported to be helpful. Long-term follow-up data are not yet available, however.

When sacroiliac pathology is demonstrated, injection of the joint with local anesthetic will help confirm the diagnosis. One of the authors, using a technique similar to that described by Bonica,[98] found that 25 of 35 patients with suspected sacroiliac disease had pain relief from local anesthetic injection of the joint. After injection of triamcinolone diacetate, 7 of 20 patients who were followed long-term experienced at least 6 months of moderate to complete pain relief (unpublished data).

Myofascial Pain

The myofascial syndrome is an extremely common cause of somatic pain. It is associated with marked tenderness of discrete points (trigger points) within affected muscles, pain

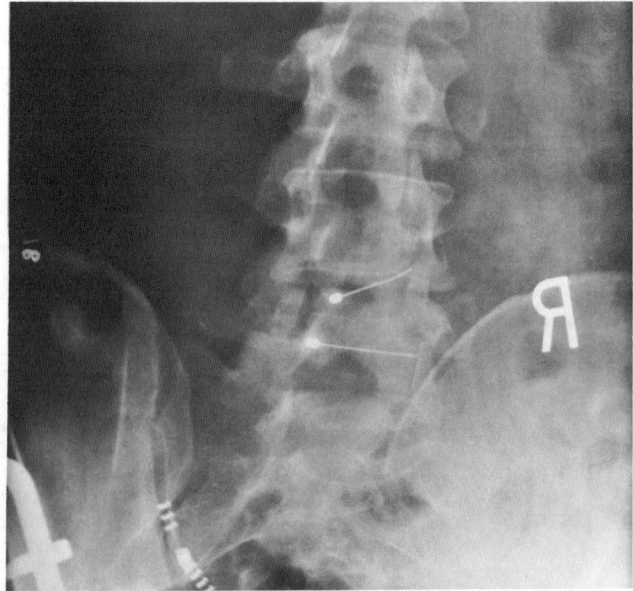

Figure 58-7. Right L4–5 and L5–S1 facet injections. Note slight bending of needle at the L4–5 level, which is typical when needle lies within the joint space.

that is referred to areas some distance from the trigger point, and the appearance of tight, ropy bands of muscle. Autonomic changes, such as vasoconstriction and skin conductivity changes may occur some distance from the affected muscle.[99] Biopsies of trigger points have been reported to show little or no change or to show degenerative changes, the severity of which corresponds to the intensity of the symptoms.[99] Although the pathophysiology of the condition has not been clearly defined, Travell and Simons[99] propose the following explanation: acute muscle strain causes disruption of sarcoplasmic reticulum and release of calcium, which in turn produces sustained or repeated contraction and fatigue. Blood flow becomes inadequate for the degree of metabolic activity occurring locally. Adenosine triphosphate becomes depleted, preventing release of myosin from actin, causing sarcomeres to become rigid and affected muscles to become taut. Nociceptor-sensitizing substances, such as prostaglandins, bradykinin, and serotonin, are released from platelets and mast cells, causing increased firing of muscle nociceptors.

Many of the commonly affected muscles, the sites of their trigger points, and their zones of referred pain have been mapped out.[100] The scapulocostal syndrome, one of the most common patterns of myofascial pain, is characterized by a trigger point located just medial and superior to the upper portion of the scapula and pain that can radiate to the occipital region, shoulder, medial aspect of the arm, or anterior chest wall.[101] Myofascial pain involving gluteal muscles produces pain referred into the posterior thigh and calf, mimicking S1 radulopathy. Myofascial pain involving the piriformis muscle, which overlies the sciatic nerve, can produce sciatic irritation and, occasionally, hypoesthesia, again resembling radiculopathy.

The most important aspect of treatment for myofascial pain is to regain muscle length and elasticity. This is best done by maneuvers that gently stretch affected muscles. Because of the sensitization of muscle afferents, appropriate physical therapeutic maneuvers are often painful and may reinitiate muscle contraction. Therapy aimed at reducing muscle pain and sensitivity should therefore be employed before stretching exercises. Trigger point injection, infiltration of local anesthetic directly into the trigger point, is a valuable initial therapy. Pain relief following injection confirms the diagnosis of myofascial syndrome, and a series of several injections performed daily or every several days can markedly reduce muscle sensitivity. Fairly vigorous therapy can be carried out during the analgesic period after each injection. Ultrasound therapy applied over the affected muscle may also produce periods of analgesia.

Trigger point injections and ultrasound require the participation of trained personnel, precluding their use on a frequent regular basis (e.g., several times per day). Several treatment modalities can be used by the patient alone or with the help of family members. Transcutaneous electrical nerve stimulation (TENS), applied directly over the trigger points, may produce analgesia during stimulation and often for some time afterward. Stimulation should be carried out for 20 to 30 minutes prior to stretching exercises. Some patients who do not respond to the usual high frequency TENS may benefit from a brief period (about 5 to 10 minutes) of low frequency (2 to 4 Hz) high intensity TENS. The current should be high enough to cause muscle contraction and mild discomfort. Vapocoolant spray (e.g., fluorimethane) sprayed over the affected muscle may produce transient analgesia sufficient to facilitate physical therapy. Massage of the affected muscle with ice may also be of some benefit.

It is the belief of many physicians that myofascial pain often develops in patients whose response to stress is increased muscle tone. Surface measurement of electromyography in such patients will often demonstrate extremely high activity at rest. Electromyographic biofeedback is a useful added therapy for such patients and appears to be helpful in preventing future painful episodes for patients with recurrent problems.

Sympathetically Mediated Pain

There is a spectrum of disorders of the limb that are characterized by pain, sensory and motor abnormalities, autonomic dysfunction, and dystrophic changes. This is a heterogeneous group of disorders with respect to clinical presentation, underlying mechanisms, and response to treatment. The diversity of clinical presentations and the disagreement on underlying pathophysiologic mechanisms have resulted in a confusing array of terms used to describe these conditions. Presently, the term reflex sympathetic dystrophy (RSD) is used most widely. A special interest group for the study of RSD was recently organized under the auspices of the International Association for the Study of Pain. That group adopted the following operational definition of RSD:

> RSD is a descriptive term meaning a complex disorder or group of disorders that may develop as a consequence of trauma affecting the limbs, with or without obvious nerve lesion. RSD may also develop after visceral diseases, and central nervous system lesions or, rarely, without an obvious antecedent event. It consists of pain and related sensory abnormalities, abnormal blood flow and sweating, abnormalities in the motor system and changes in structure of both superficial and deep tissues (trophic changes). It is not necessary that all components are present. It is agreed that the name "RSD" is used in a descriptive sense and not to imply specific underlying mechanisms.

The following discussion uses the term RSD according to the previous definition. The term causalgia refers to conditions that fit the previous description that are associated with major nerve trunk injury.

Reflex Sympathetic Dystrophy

Common antecedents to the development of RSD include crush injuries, lacerations, fractures, sprains, and burns.[102] Many postoperative cases occur after surgery involving the median nerve distribution, such as carpal tunnel release or palmar fasciectomy.[102] The syndrome occasionally occurs after cerebrovascular accident or myocardial infarction. The pain is usually burning in quality and is often accompanied by diffuse tenderness and pain on light touch. The hand or foot are commonly the major sites of pain. The pain and hyperalgesia often spread beyond the original sites of pain.

Autonomic dysfunction is manifested as changes in skin temperature, cyanosis, edema, and hyperhydrosis. Early in the course of the disease, the skin may be warm and erythematous, with occasional to frequent bouts of intense vasoconstriction. As the process becomes more chronic, the involved extremity is usually cool and pale or cyanotic. The vascular phase of bone scanning often demonstrates differences in flow between the normal and the affected extremity. Thermography or local measurement of skin temperature using surface thermistors is also useful in documenting differences in regional blood flow.

Dystrophic changes become increasingly evident with time if the condition is untreated. Skin of the affected area becomes smooth and glossy. Bone demineralization takes place to a much greater extent than would be expected on the basis of reduced activity. Joints in the affected extremity become stiff and painful as a result of synovial edema, hyperplasia, fibrosis, and perivascular inflammation.[103]

Local anesthetic blockade of the sympathetic chain is useful diagnostically, particularly when only a portion of the spectrum of possible symptoms are present. Cervicothoracic sympathetic block is usually carried out by injection of local anesthetic on the anterior tubercle of C6 or on the transverse process of C7. Lumbar sympathetic block is performed by injecting local anesthetic at the anterolateral aspect of the L2 vertebral body. Once the diagnosis is confirmed, treatment consists of a series of local anesthetic sympathetic blocks. If lumbar sympathetic block is technically difficult or is particularly painful to the patient, repeated or continuous lumbar epidural blockade can be used instead. Injections are generally continued until symptoms are minimal. Three to seven blocks are usually sufficient, but the series may occasionally be longer. Physical therapy, consisting of desensitizing techniques and active or active-assisted range of motion, is usually indicated and should be carried out immediately after each sympathetic block. Vigorous passive range of motion and heavy weights should be avoided, as they may retrigger RSD symptoms.

Patients whose condition is diagnosed and treated early are very likely to respond to sympathetic blocks. Success rates of 90% or more have been reported.[104,105] In one of a very few studies of outcome for RSD, Wang et al[106] reported that, at 3-year follow-up, 65% of patients treated with sympathetic blockade were considered to have satisfactory results, whereas only 41% of patients who did not receive blocks were doing well. Patients treated with sympathetic blockade within 1 month of the onset of symptoms had a success rate of 87%, whereas the long-term success for patients treated 6 months to a year after the onset of symptoms was 50%.

Hannington-Kiff[107] described an alternative technique for producing temporary sympathetic blockade using intravenous regional injection of guanethidine. The technique has been shown to be as effective as local anesthetic blockade in some reports[108,109] and has the advantage of being safer in anticoagulated patients. No reports have yet shown the technique to be superior to local anesthetic blocks. The author treated 32 RSD patients with one to four intravenous guanethidine blocks. Most of the patients had experienced symptoms for at least 6 months, and all had gotten only transient relief (up to 48 hours) from local anesthetic sympathetic blocks. Most patients in the series experienced 1 to several days of relief from the guanethidine blocks, but only three patients had relief for 3 months or more (unpublished data). A major limitation to the use of intravenous regional guanethidine is the fact that the injectable preparation is not approved by the Food and Drug Administration for use in the United States at the time of this writing. Intravenous regional bretyllium has been used in a similar fashion, but there are no well-controlled studies to date documenting lasting benefit.

The use of systemic sympathetic blocking drugs is occasionally useful clinically. Prazosin and phenoxybenzamine, both alpha-adrenergic blocking agents, provide partial symptomatic relief in some patients, particularly those patients exhibiting signs of vasoconstriction. Intravenous phentolamine, given in small incremental doses up to 30 mg maximum, is helpful in predicting response to oral alpha-adrenergic blockers. Oral and transdermal clonidine

are also occasionally useful. Other systemic medications that have been used with variable success include calcium channel blockers, tricyclic antidepressants, and anticonvulsants. None of these medications have been thoroughly and systematically studied for RSD, and their use is based on empirical trials and anecdotal reports.

Kozin et al[110] reported substantial benefit from treatment of RSD with a brief course of high-dose corticosteroids. Their success rate was 82%, which is particularly impressive since many of their patients had experienced long-term symptoms. Unfortunately, their criteria for diagnosing RSD were somewhat vague and did not include response to sympathetic block, allodynia, hyperpathia, or burning pain. Side-effects from high-dose systemic steroids are often troublesome. An alternative treatment is the intravenous regional injection of soluble steroids in the affected limb.[111] TENS is often a useful adjunctive treatment for RSD. Increased skin temperature during stimulation has been documented in patients who experience pain relief following treatment,[112] and TENS has been reported to provide substantial clinical benefit when used as the sole therapy for RSD.[113]

Patients with long-standing symptoms of RSD, who develop dystrophic changes and, frequently, the behavioral and psychological profiles typical of chronic pain patients, are extremely resistant to the types of intervention described previously. Surgical or neurolytic sympathectomy has been suggested as a treatment for RSD patients who respond only transiently to sympathetic blocks.[105] It is the authors' experience, however, that most patients with chronic RSD get no relief or only a few days to weeks of benefit from sympathetic ablation. Therapy instead should be directed toward extinguishing pain behavior, increasing strength and mobility, and developing coping strategies.

Causalgia

The term causalgia (Greek, meaning burning pain) has been used interchangeably with RSD and a variety of other terms that denote pain syndromes with autonomic findings. More recently, causalgia has been used to indicate a specific syndrome of burning pain and autonomic dysfunction associated with major nerve trunk injury.[105] Most cases of causalgia are caused by gunshot wounds. Rapid, violent deformation of the nerve seems to play a major pathophysiologic role. Most cases involve partial injury to the brachial plexus, median nerve, or tibial division of the sciatic nerve proximal to the elbow or knee. Pain often begins immediately after injury and may spread to involve previously unaffected areas. There is usually severe burning pain, allodynia, and hyperpathia, often accompanied by deep shooting, crushing, or stabbing pains. The pain is aggravated by movement or any physical stimulation, such as light touch or pressure. Stimuli that increase sympathetic activity, such as a loud noise, a flash of light, or anxiety, often increase the severity of the pain. Pain may persist for many years in inadequately treated patients.[114] There is usually evidence of reduced sympathetic activity in the affected extremity, which is generally warm, dry, and venodilated. Vasoconstriction, hyperhydrosis, cyanosis, and edema are occasionally seen. Dystrophic changes of skin, bone, and joints, similar to those encountered in RSD patients, often begin early.

Reports on the therapy of causalgia from the early 1900s described surgical destruction of peripheral nerves, which was uniformly unsuccessful. Narcotic analgesics were likewise ineffective. In 1930, Spurling[115] published encouraging results of treatment with sympathetic ganglionectomy.

Since then, numerous reports have documented the efficacy of such treatment. Mayfield[116] reported complete relief of symptoms in 91% of 105 causalgia victims treated with surgical sympathectomy. Bonica,[105] in a review of over 500 cases, found that over 80% of patients responded to sympathectomy.

More recently, less invasive therapy has been undertaken in the management of causalgia. Neurolytic lumbar sympathetic block has been proposed as an alternative to surgical lumbar sympathectomy and has been shown to produce long-term sympathetic denervation in the large majority of patients.[117] Aggressive treatment with local anesthetic sympathetic blockade has met with some success. Bonica[105] reported success in 10 of 17 causalgia patients managed with frequent local anesthetic blocks. The authors have treated three patients with early, severe causalgia who responded dramatically to continuous infusion lumbar epidural blockade or continuous infusion brachial plexus block that was maintained for 5 to 7 days (unreported findings).

PHARMACOLOGIC ADJUNCTS FOR CHRONIC PAIN

The use of opiates in the treatment of chronic pain not associated with malignancies is controversial. Concerns about inducing tolerance and dependency and suppression of endogenous pain control mechanisms are the main deterrents to their long-term use. Additionally, it is the belief of most experts that a large number of patients with chronic pain syndromes are not responsive to opiates. Although opiates are the mainstay of treatment of pain from malignancies, there is a void in the pharmacopeia available to treat chronic nonmalignant pain syndromes.

Years of clinical experience, treatment of coexisting affective and other disorders, and serendipity have given rise to the understanding that drugs generally used in the fields of psychiatry and neurology have a place in treating some patients suffering from chronic pain syndromes. These drugs and some of their characteristics are briefly reviewed.

Since the observation of Paoli et al[118] that imipramine was useful in the treatment of some chronic pain conditions, much clinical experience with the antidepressants has accumulated. This expanding class of drugs has many members that are referred to as tricyclic antidepressants, most of which share common properties. Recent years have seen the addition of tetracyclics, triazopyridine derivatives, and other new chemical compounds to this functional group. Current thinking would suggest that all of these drugs, regardless of structure, exert at least part of their action through blockade of presynaptic reuptake of serotonin or norepinephrine or both.[119] The differences between members of the antidepressant group reside mainly in their potency and side-effect profiles. No conclusive data exist to suggest superiority of one drug over another in any given pain condition.

The clinically relevant benefits to be expected from judicious use of these drugs in patients with chronic pain syndromes are normalization of sleep patterns, reduction in anxiety and depression (if present), and reduction of the patient's perception of pain. The effect on sleep is thought to be due to some direct sedation provided by these drugs, as well as enhancement of serotoninergic effects. The improvement in sleep patterns provided by these drugs usually occurs very early in the course of treatment and does not share the typical 1 to 2 week lag time commonly observed before the onset of antidepressant effects. These drugs do provide some suppression of rapid eye movement sleep, so abrupt cessation can be associated with rapid eye movement rebound in the form of restless sleep, with excessively vivid and pervasive dreams. Some of the newer drugs, such as buproprion and fluoxetine, are better given in the morning, since they appear to energize the patient and are generally not well tolerated at night.[120,121]

The common side-effects of the tricyclics include the antimuscarinic effects of xerostomia, impaired visual accommodation, urinary retention, and constipation. Antihistaminic effects occur via blockade of both H_1 and H_2 receptors and include sedation and an increase in gastric pH.[122] Orthostatic hypotension is mediated through the blockade of peripheral alpha$_1$ adrenergic receptors. Cardiac conduction effects mimic the actions of quinidine, but in general are of little clinical relevance, except in the case of overdosage. The lethal potential of these drugs in overdose is substantial, especially when doses exceed 2000 mg of amitriptyline or the equivalent.[123]

Most studies of efficacy of these drugs in pain syndromes are open and are not controlled for placebo effects or for the presence of depression. Since the first double-blind placebo-controlled study by Watson et al in 1982,[124] several well-designed studies have been conducted. Watson et al studied the effects of gradually increasing doses of amitriptyline in patients suffering from postherpetic neuralgia. After 3 weeks, 16 of 24 patients had obtained good to excellent relief, with doses below the norm for treatment of depression and with no change in a standard psychometric instrument assessing the presence and severity of depression. Getto et al[125] reviewed 24 studies and found 19 to report some degree of benefit. Four double-blind placebo studies with a combined enrollment of 107 subjects yielded a 68% response rate with the active drug, as compared with a 13% response with placebo. Studies of a double-blind placebo crossover design included 140 subjects in five reports and revealed an aggregate response rate of 61%.

Major tranquilizers, also known as antipsychotics or neuroleptics, have been employed to treat some painful syndromes. These drugs, while falling into several distinct chemical classes, all have the blockade of dopamine receptors as their major action. None of these drugs, however, are highly selective about where they block dopaminergic transmission, which accounts for much of the side-effect profile of this class. Blockade of dopamine receptors in the mesolimbic system is thought to be responsible for antipsychotic action. When dopamine receptors are blocked in the nigrostriatal pathways, however, extrapyramidal side-effects occur, the most easily recognized of which is a drug-induced parkinsonian syndrome, characterized by mask facies, festinating gait, cogwheel rigidity, and bradykinesia. Oculogyric crisis is a term that describes an acute dystonic reaction in which the body is involuntarily contorted into bizarre postures. Akathisia, a syndrome characterized by extreme restlessness, agitation, and a pronounced feeling of ill being, is seen frequently after the administration of potent neuroleptics, including droperidol, to young adults. A late complication of the use of these drugs is the potential for the development of tardive dyskinesia, which is an involuntary movement disorder typified by choreoathetoid movements of skeletal muscle groups, such as lip smacking, tongue darting, or truncal instability.

The antipsychotics have common side-effect profiles that include sedation, antihistaminic effects (some are chemically based on an antihistamine structure), α_1-adrenergic receptor blockade, and antimuscarinic effects. As a general rule, the less potent a drug in this class is, the more likely it is to have the previously mentioned effects.

The mechanism of action of these drugs in pain syndromes is essentially unknown. Studies of their efficacy are almost entirely anecdotal. Emergence of side-effects can be a serious limitation, especially in the young adult and the very old patient. Most reports have discussed their utility in treating neuropathic pains, such as neuropathies and neuralgias. Several authors have suggested that they work best in combination with an antidepressant.[126,127] Others have argued that the literature provides no scientific support for their use in treating pain.[128]

Another class of agents said to have some efficacy in the treatment of chronic pain syndromes are the anticonvulsants. Unlike the antidepressants and neuroleptics, the pharmacology of this group varies from drug to drug.[129] The members of this class said to have some benefit in pain patients are phenytoin, valproic acid, carbamazepine, and clonazepam. The first three variously affect either sodium, potassium, or calcium flux across the neuronal membrane, while clonazepam is a benzodiazepine and works via the benzodiazepine-GABA-chloride channel receptor complex.

The side-effect profiles of these drugs are also variable, with nausea and ataxia being commonly seen with any of them. Phenytoin can cause vitamin D and K and folate deficiencies, hirsutism, and gingival hyperplasia. Valproic acid use is associated with hepatic enzyme elevations, rare but occasionally fatal hepatic necrosis in children, and significant gastrointestinal effects that can be somewhat ameliorated by prescription of the enteric coated form of the drug. Carbamazepine can cause clinically a significant decrease in any of the blood elements selectively or can induce pancytopenia. Clonazepam is occasionally associated with disinhibition, leading to hostility and aggression or emotional lability.

Unlike the other drugs discussed, there exists some basic science that would suggest some specific analgesic action for the anticonvulsants. Most of this work has been done with experimental neuromas.[130] Neuromas are known to spontaneously generate action potentials, fire vigorously after minimal stimulation, and exhibit after-discharge, which is firing after stimulus removal. Treating animals with some of this class tends to make the neuroma behave closer to normal. These drugs have found their greatest utility in treating neuropathic pain states, i.e., pain that is generated from diseased nerves themselves, rather than nociceptive signals that are transmitted from other tissue across neural pathways.

In summary, the neuropsychiatric drugs have found some usefulness as aids in the management of patients suffering from chronic pain syndromes. They are not magical cures and have significant potential for side-effects, some of which are serious. They must be judiciously prescribed as one part of a comprehensive pain management plan by a practitioner who is well versed in their use.

PSYCHOLOGICAL TREATMENTS FOR CHRONIC PAIN

Psychological input into the diagnosis and treatment of chronic pain has become an accepted part of any comprehensive team approach to the management of this class of patients. Since the psychological influences on pain experiences are myriad, the regular consultation of a specialist in behavioral medicine is invaluable. In addition to helping to understand some of the psychological influences mentioned earlier, the psychologist has at his or her disposal a number of specific techniques that prove useful as part of a multidisciplinary treatment plan for chronic pain management.

Psychodynamic approaches to the patient in chronic pain are typified by an attempt to understand the patient in terms of personality structure, biologic drives, social contexts, wishes, and expectations.[131] This leads to a psychodynamic formulation that posits a relationship between any or all of these factors and the presenting problem. Therapy is usually done on an individual basis and is aimed at establishing a therapeutic alliance with the patient, providing an interpretation of relevant symptoms, leading the individual to new levels of understanding about the derivation of their symptoms, and enhancing symptom resolution through the patient–therapist relationship, with termination of that relationship as the ultimate goal. To engage in this sort of approach requires a knowledge of fundamental psychoanalytic and therapeutic principles, training in the particulars of psychotherapy with chronic pain patients, and the time to engage in weekly or more frequent sessions with the patient for months to years of therapy. Clearly, this is out of the realm of expertise or desire of most anesthesiologists and is typically so labor intensive that it is not practical for many psychologists. In general, a very small proportion of patients in a given clinic population would be either amenable or appropriate to involvement in this style of therapy.

Much more common is the use of cognitive therapies. This group of strategies focuses on the cognitive or thought processes that are found in chronic pain patients. Often the thinking style of an individual has a great deal of effect on how he or she copes with pain. As mentioned earlier, the meaning of the pain experience can greatly influence the suffering. A classic example of this is the often quoted observation by Beecher[132] that injured soldiers on the battle front in the Second World War often complained of pain far less than would be expected from the severity of their wounds. When they were safely behind the lines, however, they would complain just as loudly as anyone else when multiple venipunctures or other mildly painful procedures were required, disproving the notion that these people were stoic by nature. Beecher[132] reasoned that the meaning of the pain was making the difference in that a significant injury meant that one would be taken back home and, therefore, would survive the war. A common clinical example in a pain clinic would be the individual who is convinced that he or she cannot cope with a flare-up of pain. Such an individual will frequently think catastrophic thoughts such as "If this pain gets real bad, I don't know what I'll do!" These thoughts can become the focus of treatment and can, with motivation and practice on the part of the patient, be changed to more adaptive thoughts. This in time will give the individual some degree of control over the situation and will prevent him or her from engaging in self-defeating destructive thought patterns. Coping ability is thereby improved.[133]

Behavioral therapies involve efforts to reshape behaviors, rather than the sensory or emotional conditions that underlie them. This is a direct outgrowth of the work of Fordyce et al,[134] who adapted B. F. Skinner's operant model of behavior to the human pain patient. As previously discussed, this model states that behaviors can be cued by certain stimuli and can be modified by conditions that follow the emission of the behavior. Taking this antecedent-behavior-consequence paradigm view of pain behaviors such as limping, groaning, seeking dependence on others, taking inappropriate analgesics, etc., Fordyce and colleagues imposed strict control on the environment into which the chronic pain patient was placed. No reinforcement of pain behaviors was forthcoming from the staff (extinction) and positive reinforcement for wellness behaviors was instituted. This resulted in a significant decrease in pain behaviors. A critique of this method was that only the behaviors were decreased, but Fordyce et al argue that many patients state that after a largely behavioral treatment program they perceive less pain.[135] The principles of behavior modification extend to the staff of a pain clinic, the patient's workplace, and the home, in that solicitous responses from a spouse in response to pain behaviors by the patient may sabotage an otherwise intact and appropriate treatment plan.

Biofeedback is the providing of information to an individual about bodily functions that are commonly held to be inaccessible to the conscious mind.[136] Commonly used devices measure surface electromyographic activity, temperature, or electrodermal activity. When feedback from these systems is provided, a patient can frequently be taught to control those functions at will. Originally, the logical assumption was made that teaching an individual to reduce muscle tone in a specific muscle would reduce the pain by the mechanism of muscle relaxation. While the outcome is generally that which is expected, the mechanism is not universally accepted to be reduction in muscle tone, leading to decreased activation of muscle nociceptive afferent neurons. The same statement can be made for the other modes of biofeedback. This does not, however, detract from the usefulness of the techniques, and they remain a valuable psychological intervention for some patients.

Numerous strategies have evolved for the induction of a state of relaxation in chronic pain. The theory is that relaxation induces both positive mental and physical changes in the individual that promote a sense of well being, decrease muscle tone, and enhance coping. Jacobson[137] developed the first standardized approach to relaxation using the progressive contraction and relaxation of muscle groups in an ascending sequence from feet to head. There have been numerous procedures since then that can be learned to induce relaxation. These techniques rely on conscious manipulation of the body to induce a relaxed state, not merely getting comfortable on the couch and propping up one's feet. Benson[138] studied the physiologic concomitants of a relaxed state and found commonalities to the conditions induced by a variety of methods. These included a decrease in sympathetic tone, regularity in respiratory pattern, decreased skeletal muscle tone, and a feeling of well being. He termed this physiologic pattern the relaxation response and postulated that the means of achieving it was unimportant and, in fact, developed a very simple and straightforward induction method. This and similar techniques find great applicability to chronic pain patients, especially those with muscular involvement such as myofascial pain syndromes.

Hypnosis has long been used to help alleviate surgical and other acute pains. It has some utility in the chronic pain population as well.[139] In order for an individual to become hypnotized, several conditions must exist: (1) an ability to concentrate, (2) a belief in the process, and (3) some motivation for the process to ensue. The trance state is thought to be a naturally occurring phenomenon in most people, although there is great variability in the population with regard to frequency and ease of occurrence. Trance state can be defined as an altered state of awareness characterized by extremely focused attention, relaxation, and responsiveness to suggestion. It is thought by most modern practitioners that the hypnotist does not hypnotize the subject, but rather facilitates entry into trance by directing and guiding the individual's attention. The use of hyp-

nosis can, in the properly selected individual, be a useful adjunct to therapy of chronic pain. It has found particular utility in the treatment of patients with cancer pain, possibly because these patients are so profoundly motivated. The mechanism of analgesia associated with hypnosis is unclear, but it does not appear to be due to endogenous opiates or to be solely due to placebo effect.[140]

Group therapy, supportive therapy, education, and family therapy are other types of psychological interventions that have utility in the management of chronic pain patients. A skilled practitioner of behavioral medicine will aid the anesthesiologist in the diagnosis, conceptualization, and treatment of patients presenting with chronic pain by selecting evaluation and therapeutic strategies that are tailored to each individual's presentation.

CANCER PAIN

In assessing patients with malignant disease who seek treatment for pain, it is essential to determine the specific site and mechanism of their pain. It is not enough to make a diagnosis of cancer pain. The entire range of acute and chronic pain mechanisms is encountered among patients with malignancy. It is also essential to know the stage of the patient's malignant disease. The approach to a given pain for a terminal patient may vary greatly from the approach to the same type of pain in a patient whose cancer is curable.

It is useful to determine whether the patient's pain is acute or chronic, and whether it is related to tumor progression, therapeutic intervention, or as is occasionally the case, factors unrelated to the patient's malignant disease (arthritis, herniated disk, etc.).[141] It is also useful to know whether the patient has a history of chronic pain or drug abuse predating the onset of malignant disease.[142] Pain caused by tumor progression can result from compression or infiltration of peripheral nerves, nerve root, or spinal cord, infiltration of bone and soft tissue, obstruction or distension of visceral structures, and vascular occlusion. Surgical intervention may lead to scar pain, neuroma formation, sympathetic dystrophy, and venous or lymphatic obstruction. Chemotherapy may be associated with peripheral neuropathies. Therapy with steroids can cause aseptic bony necrosis or rheumatoid-like symptoms when therapy is withdrawn. Herpes zoster is associated with agents that suppress immune function. Radiation therapy sometimes results in esophagitis, plexopathy and myelopathy, and bone necrosis.[142]

There is a substantial range of therapeutic options available to the cancer patient. A major consideration in approaching the patient with severe pain is when to institute a particular modality. It is generally advisable to consider less invasive, lower risk options initially, progressing to procedures that are more invasive, more painful to perform, and carry a higher risk of complications only when the more benign procedures are ineffective. Occasionally, it is prudent to select a more invasive procedure early in the course of management if it is thought that it will provide the patient maximum comfort or if the patient's pain level has progressed to a crisis state.

Pharmacologic Therapy

The use of oral analgesic agents is the mainstay of treatment for cancer pain. Adequate analgesia can be achieved in the large majority of patients with cancer-related pain if sound pharmacologic principles are employed. Several guidelines are essential to cancer pain management:

1. Use agents appropriate for the nature and severity of the patient's pain. Weaker opioids such as codeine may be adequate for mild-to-moderate pain. For severe pain, potent agents such as morphine, hydromorphone, or methadone should be employed. Agonist–antagonist agents such as pentazocine have a ceiling effect on their analgesic efficacy and are generally effective only for relatively mild pain. Meperidine is a poor drug for repetitive dosing, since accumulation of its metabolite normeperidine can cause central nervous system stimulation manifested as anxiety, tremors, or seizures.[143] Be aware of the oral bioavailability of the drug used. The oral dose of morphine, for instance, is about three times the parenteral dose. When peripheral nociceptive processes are involved (such as bony or soft tissue invasion), the addition of nonsteroidal anti-inflammatory drugs may be very helpful.

2. Use adequate doses. The dose of opioid analgesic should be escalated until satisfactory analgesia occurs (usually the case) or until problematic side-effects occur. The potent agonists, e.g., morphine, do not usually have a ceiling on analgesic effect. The dose required varies tremendously. It is not unusual for cancer patients to require 100–200 mg of oral morphine or more every 3 to 4 hours. As patients become tolerant or as tumor spreads, dose requirements increase.

3. Maintain steady blood and tissue levels of analgesic. All analgesics should be given by the clock. As-needed administration invariably results in periods of inadequate relief. The time interval for administration should be consistent with the duration of action of the drug. When possible, use long-acting agents. Methadone, whose plasma half-life is 24–36 hours, can be given twice a day, avoiding the need for nighttime awakening for analgesic administration. Morphine is available in a time-release form that can be administered twice a day. Transdermal fentanyl provides prolonged, steady release that achieves fairly constant blood levels.

4. Consider the use of adjuvant drugs. Tricyclic antidepressants are frequently beneficial for postherpetic neuralgia, may be helpful for some patients with other types of neuralgic pain or denervation dysesthesia, and can be very effective for treating concomitant depression. Some anticonvulsants may be beneficial for neuralgic pain. Phenothiazines or butyrophenones have been shown to reduce symptoms of nausea, agitation, and pain when used in conjunction with narcotic analgesics.[144] Corticosteroids should be considered for increased intracranial pressure, cord compression, severe bone pain, or pain from liver metastases. Calcitonin is effective in some patients with bone pain.

5. Anticipate and promptly treat side-effects. Constipation, which may become a major problem, occurs in most patients on opiates. Prophylactic management is essential. Nausea is a common opiate side-effect and concomitant administration of antiemetics may be necessary. Respiratory depression in tolerant patients is generally mild and can usually be managed with verbal stimulation and close observation. When severe, it should be treated with small incremental doses of intravenous naloxone (e.g., 0.05–0.1 mg) until the respiratory rate increases to an acceptable range. Large doses precipitate withdrawal, reverse much of the patient's analgesia, and initiate vomiting.

Patients who are unable to take analgesics orally can often be satisfactorily managed with parenteral opiate administration. Some patients who do not achieve satisfactory analgesia with oral drugs may have adequate control with parenteral agents, possibly because enteric absorption is poor. When the parenteral route is chosen, a constant infusion technique is usually superior to intermittent intramuscular injections. Many cancer patients have long-term venous access ports for chemotherapy that can be used for narcotic infusion.

When beginning opiate infusions, it is generally prudent to begin with a relatively low-dose bolus injection and a modest infusion rate. If analgesia is inadequate after 1–2 hours, a small bolus is repeated and the infusion rate is increased. The process is repeated until the infusion rate is adequate. An alternate, less labor intensive method is to use a patient-controlled analgesia device.[145] Once the daily narcotic requirement is established, the patient can be switched to a portable, battery powered constant infusion device or portable patient-controlled analgesia. When venous access is not available, portable external infusion devices can be used to deliver opiates subcutaneously through a "butterfly" type needle.[146] The infusion site is changed every few days or when soreness occurs. When large doses are required, the use of a concentrated preparation of hydromorphone (10 mg·ml^{-1}) allows for longer intervals between refilling the portable infusion pump and reduces the mass of fluid injected.

Transdermal fentanyl offers an alternative to parenteral opioids for patients who are unable to take medications orally. It is available in four dosage forms, which deliver 25, 50, 75, or 100 µg of fentanyl per hour. The continuous use of the 100 µg·h^{-1} form offers roughly the same analgesia as 360 mg of oral morphine or 60 mg of parenteral morphine per 24 hours. If higher delivery rates are required, multiple patches can be used simultaneously.

Intraspinal Opioids

Some cancer patients do not achieve satisfactory analgesia with systemic opiates without pushing the doses to the point of marked sedation or confusion. Less conventional methods of opiate administration may be effective for some of these patients. The discovery of spinal cord opiate receptors led to speculation regarding the feasibility of intraspinal administration of opioids. In 1979 Wang et al[147] reported profound analgesia lasting up to 24 hours after intrathecal injection of 0.5–1 mg of morphine in eight patients with cancer pain. Since then, the chronic administration of epidural opioids for the treatment of cancer pain has come into fairly widespread use.

Most experience with chronic intraspinal opioids administration has been with morphine, probably because it has a long duration, allowing bolus as well as continuous administration, and because it has been approved by the Food and Drug Administration for intraspinal use. Wang et al[147] reported essentially no side-effects or complications in their initial series of cancer patients treated with intrathecal morphine. Subsequent use of intraspinal opioids in patients who had not previously been on systemic opioids, e.g., postoperative patients and volunteers, was associated with nausea and vomiting, urinary retention, pruritus, and respiratory depression. As more experience with cancer patients accumulated, it became evident that these problems were, indeed, uncommon in this population, probably because the patients had been on systemic opioids chronically and had become tolerant to these side-effects.

Intraspinal opioids have been chronically administered by both the epidural and intrathecal routes. Intrathecal administration has the advantage of allowing use of much lower doses, potentially minimizing systemic side-effects, but carries the risks of cerebrospinal fluid leak, headache, meningitis, and arachnoiditis. With either epidural or intrathecal administration, the drug may be administered as a bolus, by infusion *via* an external pump, or by infusion *via* a totally implanted pump.

Percutaneous placement of an epidural catheter followed by bolus administration of opioid constitutes the simplest method of administration. The principal drawback of this technique is the risk of infection, which may spread to the epidural space. Such a technique is useful as a temporary measure to evaluate efficacy of epidural narcotics and is a reasonable method of administration for patients whose life expectancy is very short. The simple expedience of tunneling the catheter subcutaneously to the flank minimizes the risk of epidural infection and allows the patient access to the catheter exit site to facilitate dressing changes.

The decision to use an external pump is based on pharmacokinetic, technical, and financial considerations. There is some evidence that lower doses of morphine can be employed when using a continuous infusion. Coombs et al[148] were able to provide good analgesia for a group of cancer pain patients using a mean dose of 2 mg·day^{-1} initially and 6.6 mg·day^{-1} at the end of 12 weeks. Reports of studies that use bolus injection describe much higher daily doses. Bolus injection produces much higher peak cerebrospinal fluid levels,[149,150] which may predispose to more cephalad migration of the drug. Another advantage to continuous infusion techniques is the lower incidence of catheter occlusion. Inability to inject is a fairly common problem with bolus injection technique. When an obstructed catheter is removed, it is common to find fibrin material in the lumen. The use of large-bore silicone rubber catheters should minimize that possibility, however. Patients with epidural metastases may have severe pain with bolus injection, but tolerate continuous infusion quite well. Perhaps the biggest drawback to continuous infusion techniques is the expense. Portable pumps cost up to several thousand dollars, and the use of implantable systems adds several thousand dollars in additional physician and operating room expenses.

The totally implantable infusion pump is the most elegant, and expensive, drug delivery system. The Infusaid pump is a freon-driven device with a 50-ml, percutaneously filled drug chamber and a constant infusion rate.[151] Pumps with a 2–3 ml·day^{-1} flow rate will run for 15–20 days between refills. Daily dose is adjusted by changing the morphine concentration. A separate drug injection septum allows injection directly into the catheter, bypassing the drug chamber. The technique is most appropriate for patients with a relatively long life expectancy (months rather than weeks). Medtronic produces an electronically driven, externally programmable implanted pump that allows variations in rate plus the administration of intermittent bolus injections.

Perhaps the most frustrating problem associated with intraspinal opioid administration is the development of marked resistance or tolerance to the medication. While most patients develop tolerance slowly and to a limited degree, some demonstrate rapid escalation of doses. Woods and Cohen[152] reported a patient who had been on 280 mg of morphine intravenously and 90 mg of methadone orally per day who was initially comfortable on 5 mg of epidural morphine per day. However, by the fifth day of epidural morphine administration, the dose had increased to 7–10 mg·h^{-1} (Fig. 58-8). Greenberg et al[153] reported a patient who initially experienced 17 hours relief from 1 mg of intrathecal

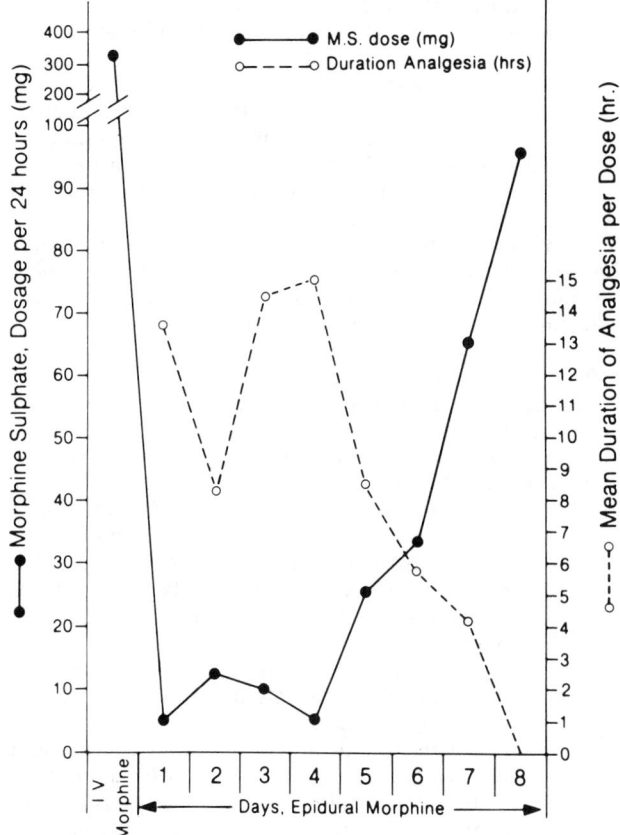

Figure 58-8. Daily dose of morphine (oral and intravenous) and duration of analgesia produced by epidural morphine (2.5 to 15 mg). After the fifth day, even the large dose of morphine produced only a few hours of analgesia. (Reprinted with permission from Woods WA, Cohen SE: High-dose epidural morphine in a terminally ill patient. Anesthesiology 56:311, 1982.)

morphine, who, after several weeks, required an intrathecal infusion of 96 mg·day^{-1} plus modest oral doses of levorphanol. One of the authors (SA) has treated a patient who required 60 mg of epidural morphine four times a day plus an intravenous morphine infusion of 300 mg·h^{-1}.

Various efforts to overcome the massive tolerance occasionally seen with intraspinal opioids have been undertaken. Limited trials of the alpha$_2$-agonist clonidine injected epidurally and intrathecally have proved at least temporarily effective.[154] There is some evidence that patients who are highly tolerant to mu-receptor agonists (morphine, fentanyl, meperidine) may experience good relief from intraspinal delta-receptor agonists, e.g., D-Ala-D-Leuenkephalin.[155] However, it now appears that tolerance to delta agonists also develops rapidly, and there is some cross-tolerance between mu- and delta-receptor agonists. Another approach is to provide several days of analgesia with intraspinal local anesthetics, allowing the opiate receptors to again become sensitive to their ligands, or to use combinations of opiates and dilute local anesthetics. The combined use of these agents makes sense, as the local anesthetic, even at sub-blocking concentrations, can reduce the maximum firing rates of nociceptor fibers, and the opiate reduces the sensitivity of wide dynamic range and nociceptive specific neurons in the dorsal horn to activation by nociceptors. Other substances that may have promise in either reversing tolerance or producing analgesia when injected intraspinally are GABA agonists, e.g., baclofen, NMDA antagonists, serotonin agonists, or adenosine agonists.

One potential problem that can arise when instituting treatment with intraspinal opioids is the occurrence of withdrawal symptoms, particularly if the total daily opioid dose is reduced sharply.[156] Withdrawal symptoms can be minimized by the use of oral clonidine or maintenance doses of oral methadone or time-release morphine.

Following is a suggested technique for the percutaneous administration of epidural opioids. It is simple, inexpensive, and effective. We have had no serious infections with the technique and very few superficial abscesses.

I. Temporary prognostic catheter
  A. Place percutaneous epidural catheter
    1. Low lumbar region
    2. Secure with self-adherent sterile dressing
  B. Dose adjustment
    1. Begin with 5-mg morphine bolus for patients on low-to-moderate systemic opioid doses
    2. Start with 10 mg or 5–10% of the daily systemic morphine equivalent for patients on high doses
    3. Add incremental doses (2–5 mg) if no analgesia within 2 hours
    4. When analgesic dose is reached, allow pain to begin to return to determine duration; adjust dosing according to duration
    5. If the technique provides good analgesia and no significant side-effects, consider permanent catheter placement. If adequate analgesia is not achieved, try infusion of 0.125% bupivacaine plus 1–3 mg·h^{-1} of morphine (if a difficult placement is anticipated, plan to tunnel the initial catheter)

II. Placement of permanent catheter
  A. Inject temporary catheter with morphine and remove just prior to procedure to ensure patient comfort. If local anesthetic used with temporary catheter, allow to wear off
  B. Start iv, hydrate with crystalloid
  C. Place patient in lateral position with side up that catheter will be tunneled to
  D. Prep
    1. Administer intravenous antibiotic prophylactically (e.g., cephalosporin)
    2. Surgical antiseptic preparation of skin and draping, as for any surgical procedure—include back and flank
    3. Surgical scrub, gown, gloves, mask for operator
  E. Place epidural catheter percutaneously
    1. Mid-to-high lumbar level, above site of temporary catheter; if use of local anesthetic is anticipated, stay near painful segments
    2. Thread catheter cephalad 5–6 cm
    3. Withdraw epidural needle slightly (a few millimeters); do not remove
    4. Attach luer adapter to catheter. Inject test dose local anesthetic (4 ml of 1% lidocaine with epinephrine 1:200,000). If no reaction, inject 10 ml of 1% lidocaine
    5. When segmental analgesia is achieved, make a small incision at needle entry site (use subcutaneous lidocaine if necessary), incorporating needle into incision
    6. Make a small skin incision in lateral abdominal wall and pass catheter passer from anterior incision to incision at needle site

    7. Remove epidural needle and pass catheter through catheter passer to flank
    8. Suture catheter to supraspinal ligament or to subcutaneous tissues at incision in back and suture incision
    9. Place silver-impregnated cuff around catheter subcutaneous at catheter exit site
    10. Apply sterile self-adherent dressing (Op-Site or Tegaderm) to incision and catheter exit site
    11. Place bacterial filter on luer adapter. Tape small plastic bag to abdominal wall and place external portion of catheter and filter in bag

III. Patient instruction
  A. Patient and family should be instructed in catheter injection technique, principles of sterile technique, and technique for dressing change. Provide patient with written, illustrated instruction manual
  B. Set up frequent follow-up visits for suture removal, inspection of exit site, analgesic needs. As patient becomes more debilitated, much interaction can be done by phone; some house calls by physician may be needed

IV. Precautions
  A. Ensure that patients do not have coagulopathy. Disseminated intravascular coagulopathy (DIC) is extremely common with certain tumors, e.g., prostatic cancer
  B. Make sure patients do not have intraspinal tumor at level of proposed catheter placement
  C. Avoid the technique if there is systemic or local bacterial infection
  D. Make sure there are adequate resources in patient's home. Patient or family must be capable of injecting. If that is a problem, external infusion pump may be preferable. Involve visiting nurses

Hogan et al[157] reported on a series of patients treated with a protocol similar to that listed previously. Sixteen consecutive patients treated with epidural opioids were selected for such therapy out of 1205 oncology service patients. There were 13 lumbar, 1 thoracic, and 1 cervical epidural. Mean duration of catheter placement was 35 days (range, 6 to 965). Six patients had adequate analgesia with morphine alone. Ten patients had adequate analgesia with a combination of morphine and bupivacaine, but in two cases treatment was discontinued because motor block was unacceptable to the patients. There were four subcutaneous infections, two of which required catheter removal (silver impregnated cuffs were not used in that series). There were no epidural infections. One epidural hematoma occurred, which began 11 days after catheter removal and required laminectomy. That patient had developed DIC in conjunction with a prostatic tumor several weeks after the initial catheter placement. Other problems included dislodgement of catheter, pain on injection, and leak of solution out of the epidural space. In a series reported by Plummer et al[158] using subcutaneous ports rather than percutaneous catheters, all of the same problems were encountered with the exception of catheter dislodgement.

Non-Neurolytic Nerve Blocks

The anesthesiologist is often called on to perform neurodestructive nerve blocks to control intractable pain from advanced malignancy. These procedures carry a significant risk of paresis, bowel and bladder dysfunction, and painful neuritis. There are several conditions encountered in patients with cancer that are likely to respond to less dangerous nerve block procedures. RSD occurs fairly often in cancer patients. Severe burning pain following surgery, particularly if accompanied by any symptoms of autonomic dysfunction, should arouse suspicion. Occasionally tumor invasion of soft tissues may trigger RSD. Sympathetic blocks should be performed diagnostically if the diagnosis is entertained, and blocks should be repeated if there is substantial improvement in symptoms.

Myofascial pain is common among cancer patients. It is often associated with bony infiltration, neural compression, or visceral pain. Local anesthetic injections of trigger points may be surprisingly effective. Fluorimethane spray of trigger points combined with gentle stretching of affected muscles can be very helpful. TENS is also very likely to be of benefit.

Tumor compression of nerve roots, brachial or femoral plexus, or peripheral nerves sometimes responds dramatically to perineural injection of insoluble steroids. The authors have found that pain relief can be achieved for up to 1 month in many instances. When radicular pain is caused by epidural tumor spread, epidural injections of triamcinolone diacetate are likely to be of benefit. Tumor compression of the brachial plexus may respond to brachial plexus block with a combination of depo steroid and local anesthetic. The interscalene, supraclavicular, infraclavicular, or axillary approaches may all be used, the choice depending on the site of pathology. Femoral plexopathy can be treated with a paravertebral approach (psoas compartment block) to the femoral plexus, again using triamcinolone diacetate and local anesthetic. Steroid local anesthetic blocks of peripheral nerves that are irritated or compressed by tumor are occasionally beneficial, particularly if they are performed reasonably soon after the onset of pain. Patients with severe neurogenic pain should be warned that if the injections are successful in producing pain relief, they are likely to be left with some numbness, not from the injections, but from the already present neural pathology.

Acute herpes zoster is a relatively common and often debilitating source of pain in patients with malignancy. There is some evidence that local anesthetic blockade of sympathetic fibers, using either paravertebral sympathetic blocks or epidurals, will promptly relieve pain, may shorten the acute phase of the illness, and may reduce the incidence of postherpetic neuralgia.[159] Even if the overall course of the illness is not dramatically affected, patients are usually extremely grateful for any respite from the severe pain associated with this condition.

Occasionally patients with severe cancer pain are refractory to any opioid intervention. These patients may progress to psychological decompensation without reasonably prompt intervention. The use of continuous infusion local anesthetic blockade may be the best answer for patients who reach such a crisis. Continuous epidurals with dilute local anesthetics can be performed at any level of the neuraxis. When upper thoracic or cervical approaches are used, close monitoring of blood pressure and respiratory function is necessary.

Neurolytic Blocks

There is a much greater willingness among anesthesiologists to perform neurolytic blocks for terminal cancer patients with pain than for patients with nonmalignant causes of pain. Reluctance to use neurolytic blocks for noncancer

pain is certainly justified. The extent and duration of analgesia from neurodestructive procedures is limited by regrowth of axons and development of central pain mechanisms (denervation dysesthesia). While neurolytic blocks can produce dramatic relief for some cancer pain patients, there are some serious potential drawbacks to the technique, and overzealous use of neurodestructive procedures should be avoided.

The principal disadvantage of neurolytic blocks is the inability to precisely control the spread of the destructive agents. Loss of motor function and inability to control bowel or bladder function following neurolysis can be devastating to a patient and will greatly impair the quality of remaining life. The expected analgesia may not always result from destruction of the intended neural structures, even when prognostic local anesthetic blocks have been performed. If central nervous system mechanisms play a major role in a patient's pain, neurolysis is unlikely to be of benefit. In some cases, tumor progression rapidly produces pain beyond the confines of the block. With the advent of improved methods of cancer therapy, more patients survive well beyond the efficacy of the block. Overall, the incidence of fair to good results following neurolytic blockade is estimated at 50-60%.[160]

Alcohol and phenol are the agents most commonly used for prolonged interruption of neural function. There is relatively little difference in overall efficacy between these agents, but there are major differences in the initial responses. Phenol produces no pain on injection, has an initial anesthetic effect, and takes about 15 minutes to exert its neurolytic effect. Alcohol causes significant pain on injection and produces neurolysis promptly. When used for intrathecal neurolysis, alcohol is hypobaric, while phenol in glycerine, the usual intrathecal preparation, is hyperbaric.

Intrathecal neurolysis with small volumes of alcohol or phenol requires careful positioning to place the affected sensory root uppermost (for alcohol) or in the most dependent position (for phenol). In such a way, only the involved sensory roots are affected. Patient movement during or shortly after injection can produce spread of drug to the cord, other dermatomes, or motor roots. Papo and Visca[161] published results in a large series of patients who underwent phenol rhizotomy. They reported good results (pain free until death) in 40% of 290 patients and fair results (reduced analgesic requirements or temporary complete relief) in 35%. Patients whose pain was localized to sacral dermatomes had the best results, while patients with pain in the upper thoracic area or upper or lower extremities had poor analgesia and more frequent complications. Swerdlow[162] reviewed 13 reports of the results of phenol and alcohol rhizotomies and found good relief of pain in about 60% of patients. In reviewing results on his own patients, he found that analgesia lasted less than 2 months in half the patients and less than 1 month in 25% of patients. Complications lasting longer than a week occurred in 15% of patients.

Patients with severe, localized perineal pain are very likely to experience relief with intrathecal blocks with phenol in glycerine. One of the authors uses 7% phenol in glycerine, injected in 0.25-ml increments up to a maximum of 2 ml, with the patient in the sitting position. This treatment is limited to patients who have undergone fecal and urinary diversion procedures.

Bladder pain and spasm have been successfully treated with trans-sacral phenol injections.[163] If blocks are confined to one or two roots, there is little risk of disrupting bladder function. There are several reports of gasserian ganglion alcohol injection for severe facial pain.[164] Unfortunately most of these reports constitute a description of the procedure, and few data about efficacy are available.

Celiac plexus block for pain associated with upper abdominal malignancy is the most successful and rewarding of the neurolytic blocks. Thompson et al[165] reported that 94% of 97 patients who underwent celiac plexus block for pain of upper abdominal cancer had good-to-excellent pain relief. Injections were performed with 50 ml of 50% alcohol. Survival from the cancer ranged from 2 days to 14 months. Fourteen patients required repeat injections for recurrent pain. Ten patients experienced transient orthostatic hypotension, and one patient had partial motor loss in one leg.

The classical technique for percutaneous injection of the celiac plexus involves bilateral placement of block needles just anterior to the body of L1 and posterior to the aorta and diaphragmatic crura.[166] Recently, techniques have been described that involve more anterior positioning of the needle tip with computed tomographic assistance so that it lies anterior to the diaphragmatic crura.[167,168] The injected solution can be seen to spread more anteriorly, surrounding the aorta. There is much less tendency of the injected solution to spread posteriorly to the paravertebral nerve roots or sympathetic chain, minimizing risk of paresis or orthostatic hypotension. Ischia et al,[168] using such a technique, reported 93% success in relieving pain in 28 patients with cancer pain. Similar placement can be achieved with the use of biplane fluoroscopy. Five-inch 22-gauge needles are advanced from both sides at a point 7 cm from the midline, at the lower border of the 12th rib toward the midpoint of the L1 vertebral body, and advanced under anteroposterior fluroscopy until they are just past the lateral border of the body. Under lateral fluoroscopy, the right-sided needle is advanced 1 cm beyond the anterior border of the body. It will probably lie between the aorta and vena cava. The left-sided needle is advanced the same distance, but will usually enter the aorta at this point. If so, it is advanced through the aorta until negative aspiration occurs. Half the total alcohol dose is then injected through each needle.

Since celiac ganglion neurolysis is highly effective and carries a relatively low incidence of complications, it may be reasonable to consider its implementation early in the course of the patient's pain. When tumor becomes more widespread late in the course of the disease, it becomes more difficult to completely block the appropriate visceral afferent fibers with neurolytic solution. Systemic or epidural narcotics may be a better choice in advanced disease.

Other Modes of Therapy

There are a number of therapeutic options that are relatively specific for the type of malignancy one is dealing with. When dealing with tumors that are extremely radiosensitive, radiation therapy is often the most effective form of intervention. If chemotherapeutic options are available, they may provide analgesia through reduction of tumor mass. Pain caused by hormonally sensitive tumors may be best treated by appropriate manipulation of the patient's hormonal environment. Surgical debulking of a large tumor will sometimes relieve pain of obstruction or abdominal distension. Stabilization of an isolated pathologic fracture can be an extremely effective pain-relieving procedure. Certain neurosurgical procedures, such as spinal cord stimulation, cordotomy, or hypophysectomy may afford months of profound relief in certain types of cases. Some patients benefit considerably from psychological interventions such as hypnosis or other cognitive strategies. With the complexity

of the disease processes involved with cancer-related pain and the number of pain mechanisms and therapeutic interventions that are possible, it is essential that the full range of medical and behavioral science disciplines be made available to this group of patients.

ORGANIZATION OF A PAIN CLINIC

The successful management of the entire range of pain problems encountered in clinical practice requires an extensive array of physician specialties, diagnostic facilities, therapeutic modalities, nonphysician health care professionals, research capabilities, and office support staff. Ideally, each patient should have access to the full range of facilities and professional expertise. In order to support such staff and facilities, a pain treatment center must have a considerable and diverse case load. Obviously, our ideal pain clinic must be located in a large metropolitan area or at a substantial tertiary care center. Unfortunately, the need for effective pain management is not confined to larger population centers, and modifications of the ideal approach must be accepted where more extensive facilities cannot be supported. This section describes the relatively new multidisciplinary approach to pain management and discusses some alternative organizational plans that may be more appropriate for smaller medical centers and for specific conditions.

In 1985, the number of pain facilities in the United States was estimated at over 400.[169] That number has undoubtedly increased substantially since then. Pain treatment centers are generally categorized as multidisciplinary (implying ability to manage a diverse group of disorders using a wide range of modalities), syndrome-oriented, or modality-oriented clinics. The multidisciplinary clinic is the ideal pain management facility defined in the previous paragraph. The syndrome-oriented clinic is organized to treat a specific type of pain problem, such as low back pain, headache, or facial pain. The most successful of the syndrome-oriented clinics are organized in a multidisciplinary fashion. They have the advantage of needing fewer specialists and may function with more limited physical facilities than the diverse multidisciplinary clinic. A physician staffing a syndrome-oriented clinic will have a better chance of developing an in-depth understanding of the entire range of problems he or she is likely to encounter. Modality-oriented clinics are organized around a single type of treatment, such as nerve blocks, biofeedback, acupuncture, or hypnosis. In order for such clinics to function in a productive fashion, the referring physician must be aware of the clinic's capability and must know which patients are likely to benefit from the treatment offered. The practitioner operating such a clinic must confine his or her efforts to patients with a high likelihood of responding to their therapy and must coordinate the treatment with other appropriate therapeutic interventions.

A fourth type of organization that does not fit clearly into any of the previously described categories is seen rather commonly. It is organized around a small group of specialists who have a fairly wide understanding of the pain conditions they encounter, but are limited to a restricted range of modalities that are directly provided in the clinic. Such a clinic functions effectively, however, by using consultation mechanisms within their medical center. Perhaps the best title for such a clinic is "oligodisciplinary." A typical composition might be an anesthesiologist, a clinical psychologist or psychiatrist, a physical therapist, and a nurse. While a substantial percentage of referrals may be successfully managed by such a team, consultation by other disciplines will invariably be needed for some patients, and patients with certain conditions (e.g., headache) might be better managed by a clinic with a somewhat different composition. The composition of a pain clinic is determined by the interest, expertise, and availability for pain clinic practice of the health care professionals in that community.

The Multidisciplinary Model

Setting

Both inpatient and outpatient facilities have a role in chronic pain management. Initial screening and most therapy can be adequately managed on an outpatient basis. Inpatient treatment should be used for very chronic patients who require drug detoxification, intensive behavior modification, which may require total removal from the home environment, or invasive therapeutic interventions.

The outpatient facility should have examination rooms adequately stocked with appropriate physical diagnosis equipment and examining tables. Treatment rooms should be equipped with operating room type tables, adequate lighting, patient monitoring equipment (blood pressure, electrocardiogram, pulse oximetry, skin temperature), intravenous equipment, and resuscitation drugs and equipment (including defibrillator and "crash cart"). Adequate storage facilities for nerve block equipment, TENS equipment, linen and gowns, and resuscitation drugs and equipment must be furnished. Oxygen, suction, adequate counter space, and a sink are needed in each treatment room. Separate recovery facilities will allow more rapid turnover of treatment areas.

The clinic area should have pleasant waiting facilities and should provide patients with space for filling out questionnaires and psychological testing instruments and for viewing educational materials. A quiet treatment area is needed for biofeedback training and other cognitive strategies and for psychiatric interviews and treatment. Clinic staff should have office space and conference facilities that are physically separated from patient reception, waiting, and treatment areas. View boxes and appropriate audiovisual equipment should be available in the conference areas. Office staff should have space within the clinic for reception, patient files, and transcription facilities.

Ideally, inpatient facilities for chronic pain patients should be separated from conventional medical, surgical, psychiatric, or rehabilitation floors. It is important that pain clinic inpatients not think of their problems in conventional medical model terms. They should be provided with facilities where they can meet and socialize during nontherapy times. Extensive exercise and physical therapy equipment and space must be provided. Space for group and individual psychotherapy and for educational sessions should be available. A nursing station, with around-the-clock staffing, is required for detoxification protocols, for administration of maintenance nonanalgesic drugs, and for monitoring of medical problems that may arise during periods of increasing physical activity.

Staffing

The composition of the pain clinic staff will depend on the interest and availability of personnel with chronic pain management skills and the needs of the population served. The director must be a physician, as a wide variety of medical problems will be encountered among clinic patients. According to a 1979 Pain Clinic/Center Directory, published by the American Society of Anesthesiologists, anesthesiologists served as directors of 61% of 251 pain clinics listed.[170] Regardless of specialty, the director should have a broad range of knowledge and experience with chronic pain management. At least one integral member of the team should specialize in behavioral sciences. There are advantages to having both psychiatry and clinical psychology directly involved with the clinic. Psychologists generally have expertise and interest in psychometrics, cognitive strategies, behavior modification protocols, and group therapy, while psychiatrists are needed for assessment and therapy of major psychiatric disorders that are often seen in the pain clinic population. Obviously, there is some overlap in the interests and abilities of these practitioners.

The composition of the remainder of the physician staff depends on the emphasis and philosophy of the clinic. If the goals are predominantly rehabilitative, a physiatrist will be an essential member. If a large number of relatively acute problems are encountered, anesthesiologists and orthopedic surgeons should be heavily involved. For cancer pain patients, anesthesiology, radiation therapy, and oncology staff should be involved. If a large number of headache patients are seen, a neurologist should be an active member. For facial pain, neurology and dentistry specialists should be included on the staff. Services of specialties that are not members of the pain clinic team should be available, in a timely fashion, on a consultation basis.

Services that should be available on a regular and continuing basis are physical therapy, nursing, pharmacy, social services, dietetics, vocational services, occupational therapy, and exercise physiology. Diagnostic radiology and laboratory services must be readily accessible. Reception and secretarial services should be dedicated to pain clinic rather than shared with other services.

Admission Criteria

The characteristics of the patients admitted to the pain clinic will depend on the emphasis and philosophy of the clinic staff. Treatment outcomes will be greatly influenced by the type of patients admitted, and some centers may admit as few as one third of their referrals in an effort to maintain high success rates. While there has been increased public awareness of the value of multidisciplinary pain management, third party payers, particularly government-funded programs, are often reluctant to cover the cost of comprehensive pain management programs, and many centers must limit admissions to patients with adequate health insurance.

In order to maximize benefit to the patients evaluated by the pain clinic, certain guidelines should be followed strictly. (1) All patients must be referred by a physician. Patients referred by lawyers or insurance representatives are almost invariably being sent to collect information that may be helpful to the patient's case or the insurance company's case. Referrals from an emergency room or walk-in clinic are inappropriate. Patients from these facilities are inadequately worked up and often present with problems that are better managed by other types of clinics. (2) Referring physicians must send enough historical, physical examination, and laboratory data prior to the first visit to provide a reasonable working diagnosis and to rule out conditions that require specific medical or surgical intervention. Patients with an inadequate data base should be referred to an appropriate diagnostic service or sent back to the referring physician for further workup. The pain clinic should not be the initial facility to evaluate the patient's condition. (3) Referred patients should have an understanding of the purpose of the referral and of the nature of the proposed pain clinic treatment. Patient brochures, provided by referring physicians or sent directly to the patient, are helpful in providing such information. It is useful to describe explicitly clinic policy on narcotic prescriptions in order to discourage drug-seeking behavior at the time of the initial visit.

The Initial Visit

An extensive pain questionnaire is an extremely valuable tool in evaluation of the pain patient and should be completed before the physician's history and physical. It should ask about the onset, duration, location, and intensity of the pain, associated symptoms, previous treatment, and analgesic and other medications. A pain diagram (anterior, posterior, right, and left lateral human body drawings on which the patient shades in the painful areas) and pain intensity scales should be included. Other questions should inquire about effects of the pain on sleep, employment, social, recreational, and sexual activity and interpersonal relationships. Financial consequences of the painful condition (compensation for injuries, present income sources, pending litigation) should be explored.

Psychological testing is generally carried out on the first visit. It is helpful for detecting psychopathology that may initiate or aggravate pain complaints and for determining the psychological impact of chronic pain and illness. Several types of testing instruments have proved useful for assessing pain patients. The State-Trait Anxiety Inventory is a self-administered test that evaluates the patient's level of anxiety or distress. Very high scores correlate with suicidal intent. Several depression scales have been used for pain clinic populations. The McGill Pain Questionnaire is a checklist of words describing the patient's symptoms. Certain pain problems, e.g., radiculopathy, are typically associated with particular descriptors. Selection of descriptors not typical of that condition might raise doubts concerning the diagnosis. Selection of a large number of descriptors or of predominantly affective descriptors would suggest a strong psychological component to that patient's pain. The Dartmouth Questionnaire combines the McGill checklist with an assessment of the effect of pain on the patient's daily activity. It asks the patients to compare the way they feel now to the way they felt before their pain started.

A personality assessment is often a part of the initial psychological screening procedure. The Minnesota Multiphasic Personality Inventory has been widely used in pain clinics, but has several drawbacks. It is lengthy, often taking over an hour to complete, and has a number of questions that patients find insulting or objectionable. Investigators have found relatively little qualitative difference in results between patients with acute pain and those with chronic pain. The SCL 90 is a computer-scored personality inventory that pain clinic patients find more palatable.

A psychologist's behavioral assessment, looking for the character and frequency of verbal complaints and evaluating nonverbal complaints (moaning, grimacing, posturing) is a helpful addition to psychological testing. A psychological interview helps assess the degree of psychological distress associated with the patient's pain.

On the first visit, the patient is assigned to a physician, sometimes termed "pain manager," who will be primarily responsible for making decisions regarding that patient's care. While that physician will not necessarily directly provide most of the patient's care, he or she will direct the diagnostic and therapeutic intervention. In a teaching institution a resident or fellow may act as a patient's pain manager, consulting with staff physicians prior to making decisions regarding that patient's care. The pain manager usually conducts the initial history and physical examination.

The history should complement the pain questionnaire. In addition to a detailed history of the pain complaint, a complete history and review of systems should be carried out. The social, psychological, and vocational aspects of the history are particularly important in these patients. A complete physical examination should be carried out. Major emphasis should be placed on the painful area. Maneuvers to test neurologic function, including procedures for evaluating radicular or peripheral nerve sensitivity, are done routinely. A systematic search for myofascial trigger points should be carried out. Evaluation of autonomic function (skin color, temperature, moisture, edema) and peripheral pulses are important components of the evaluation. Range of motion must be evaluated. When motion of a joint is limited, it should be noted whether limitation is secondary to pain or to mechanical conditions.

Attempts at measurement of the patient's pain may be carried out on the first visit. A 10-cm long visual analogue scale with two anchors, one at either end (no pain, worst pain imaginable), is commonly used. The patient is instructed to make a mark on the line that corresponds to the level of pain. The visual analogue scale has been shown to be reliable and valid and is useful in assessing the degree of improvement following intervention. The ischemic tourniquet test was developed for evaluating efficacy of analgesic medications, but has been adapted for pain clinic use. Following mild exercise of an upper extremity under ischemic conditions, time elapsed until pain begins (pain threshold) is determined. The tourniquet remains inflated, and time to patient request to terminate the ischemia (pain tolerance) is measured. The patient is also asked to acknowledge the point in time when the ischemic pain equals the clinical pain. If the clinical pain is perceived as mild, it will be close to the threshold. If it is severe it should be close to the tolerance time.

If, following the first day's evaluation, the pain manager determines that the patient's pain is fairly straightforward and that a particular course of treatment is warranted, that treatment would be initiated at that time. If further evaluation is needed, the appropriate evaluations are scheduled. The patient may be asked to keep a pain diary, noting times of the day that the pain is most severe, when analgesics are taken, and what physical activities are done.

Subsequent Visits

Once the assessment is complete, members of the pain team meet to discuss the patient and to decide on treatment options. Once a course of therapy is decided on, it is discussed with the patient and the patient's family. Often family members will be given important roles in the patient's rehabilitation. At this time the patient should be made aware of what the goals of therapy will be. If physical or medical interventions are planned, what is the chance that they will reduce the patient's pain? If treatment is aimed at developing coping skills, reducing analgesic use, and increasing physical activity, those goals should be made clear and should be acceptable to the patient before treatment is started.

When treatment consists of progressive increases in activity, giving up pain behaviors, and decreasing medication use, goals should be spelled out in writing. It is particularly useful to list behaviors or activities that will not be tolerated by the treatment team, such as requesting replacement of medications that were "lost" or "stolen" or "accidentally flushed down the toilet." These expectations of the patient can be expressed as a written contract, with notice that flagrant disregard for contractural obligations will result in dismissal from the program.

When physical modalities such as nerve blocks, TENS, or physical therapy are employed, it is important to document the degree of analgesia achieved by the procedure and to follow the patient's progress from one visit to the next. Immediate changes can be assessed with visual analogue scales and with objective changes in range of motion or tenderness. Changes occurring over days to weeks can be assessed with visual analogue scales and with pain diaries or activity scales. When treatment is behavioral or operant, pain diaries and activity levels are much more important assessment tools than are subjective pain ratings.

The Modality-Oriented Clinic

Many anesthesia departments and individual practitioners have organized pain clinics, whose function is based on the use of nerve blocks for the management of difficult pain problems. It is well established that certain regional anesthetic techniques can provide dramatic benefit for certain intractable pain problems, most of which are relatively acute, such as RSD, sciatica, and some types of cancer pain. Nerve blocks also serve important diagnostic functions, such as differentiation between somatic and visceral pain, and are of prognostic use. However, the usefulness of nerve blocks in the management of chronic pain is not as clear-cut. While regional block techniques may be useful adjuncts in managing chronic pain,[171] success rates of nerve blocks used as the sole modality in treating noncancer pain of long duration are very low.[171]

For a modality-oriented clinic to serve a worthwhile function, it is extremely important that the director be aware of the limitations of the modality employed. When therapeutic techniques are used for conditions that are unlikely to respond, the added costs, risks, and frustrations to the patient are considerable. When procedures are performed unnecessarily on a large scale, insurance carriers become reluctant to reimburse for those services, even when used appropriately.

For physicians who staff modality-oriented clinics, frequent referrals of patients who are unlikely to respond to the modality offered become a major source of frustration. In order to better serve the population of referred patients, those physicians may choose one of two options. The first option is to expand the clinic services to include modalities that many referred patients require. The addition of psychological services, pharmacologic management (including drug detoxification), and physical therapy, for instance, can markedly increase the range of patients who can be successfully managed in a nerve block clinic. The second option involves integration with other pain management facilities. If a psychology-rehabilitation medicine pain program is already in existence in the community, patients who need the services of such a program can be evaluated and treated by that facility simultaneously. Establishment of a common data base between various separate components of the pain program will minimize referral delays and reduce duplication of services. Anesthesia services can be integrated with

rehabilitation and psychological services in a productive way. For instance, nerve blocks or trigger point injections can be scheduled prior to physical therapy sessions that are ordinarily painful to the patient.

Cancer Pain Service

The concept of an interdisciplinary approach to cancer pain management is belatedly finding application in many centers. The need for a team approach is most critical in this field. The severity of the pain, the complexity of the medical care needed, and the desperation of the patient and the family do not permit a leisurely approach to the cancer pain patient. Sequential use of consultants results in inexcusable delays in starting appropriate therapy. A modality-oriented approach will leave the majority of patients with grossly suboptimal care.

The oncologist is usually (and appropriately) the central physician member of the cancer pain team. The oncologist's familiarity with the course of the disease, the definitive and palliative chemotherapeutic management, and management of nonpain complications is essential to rational patient care. Most oncologists are reasonably skilled in conventional pharmacologic approaches to cancer pain (the use of oral and parenteral narcotics, non-narcotic analgesics, psychotropics, steroids, etc.). The radiation oncologist is a critical member of the team. The appropriate use of radiation in the palliation of certain cancer pain problems can greatly reduce the use of depressant medications and high-risk procedures. Anesthesiology is another critical discipline. The advent of intraspinal opioids has greatly strengthened the anesthesiologist's armamentarium. Neuroablative techniques can be performed with neurolytic agents, with less trauma than most neurosurgical procedures. Local anesthetic block techniques can sometimes provide lasting relief, and continuous blocks can provide periods of respite from crisis situations when prolonged, severe pain has caused a state of desperation. Psychological services are essential. While the psychological contributions to pain in cancer differ to some extent from those associated with noncancer pain, they are nevertheless exceedingly important, and the services of a psychiatrist or psychologist who is familiar with the psychodynamics of cancer pain are very important. Neurosurgery consultation is certainly not needed on all patients with cancer pain, but neuroablation or central nervous system stimulation may be the best option for some patients. Therefore, the neurosurgeon must be available for consultation in a timely fashion.

Without the services of a skilled oncology nurse, any cancer pain management program is sure to fail. Without the nurse's input, recognition of problems may not occur. The nurse must provide feedback to the physician when treatment is inadequate or when side-effects are becoming intolerable. The nurse must be resilient and able to adapt to new or innovative treatment protocols. The nurse's role as interface between patient and physician is nowhere more critical than in cancer pain management. With the increasing complexity of analgesic techniques, it is essential that the pharmacist be intimately involved with the cancer pain team. The use of infusion pumps for drug administration requires the pharmacist's familiarity with a variety of systems. Maintenance of analgesic infusions outside the hospital setting requires close cooperation of pharmacy and visiting nurse programs.

Most new cancer pain problems are encountered in an inpatient setting. They occur in two different settings. The first setting involves patients who are receiving definitive treatment for their cancer. It is often not clear whether these patients are curable. Patients and their oncologists may wish to use their pain symptoms as a measure of treatment success and do not always seek major intervention for pain control. Such motives are occasionally taken to extremes, however, and patients may be deprived of appropriate analgesic management. The second setting involves the terminal patient. These patients may be in the hospital or hospice specifically for management of intractable pain. It is critical that their pain be addressed promptly and as aggressively as the situation warrants. Humanitarian considerations must be kept in mind, however. It may be far more humane, for instance, to push narcotic analgesics to the point of marked sedation to relieve pain than to risk loss of bowel or bladder function in a near terminal patient. Such ethical questions are common in this setting and often need to be discussed with the patient and the family.

The format of the cancer pain management may vary greatly, but certain elements are necessary: (1) input by the needed services listed previously, (2) prompt and frequent staffing conferences on new pain problems by members of those services, (3) prompt institution of measures decided on by the team, and (4) quick recognition of treatment inadequacy or side-effects and institution of alternative measures. Ward rounds on patients selected by the oncology nurse as having significant pain problems serves as a very useful tool. A relatively small nucleus of the pain team may be involved in initial rounds, with other members being called in as needed. Less frequent staffing involving the entire team should be carried out for the most difficult patients.

REFERENCES

1. Burgess PR, Perl ER: Cutaneous mechanoreceptors and nociceptors. In Iggo A (ed): Handbook of Sensory Physiology, vol 2, p 29. Berlin, Springer Verlag, 1973
2. Raja SN, Meyer RA, Campbell JN: Peripheral mechanisms of somatic pain. Anesthesiology 68:571, 1988
3. Lynn B: The detection of injury and tissue damage. In Melzack R, Wall PD (eds): Textbook of Pain, p 19. New York, Churchill Livingstone, 1984
4. Campbell JN, Meyer RA, LaMotte RH: Sensitization of myelinated nociceptive afferents that innervate the monkey hand. Neurophysiology 42:1669, 1979
5. Kruger L, Perl ER, Sedivic MJ: Fine structure of myelinated mechanical nociceptor endings in cat hairy skin. J Comp Neurol 198:137, 1981
6. Torebjork HE: Afferent C units responding to mechanical, thermal and chemical stimuli in human non-glabrous skin. Acta Physiol Scand 92:374, 1974
7. Adriaensen H, Gybels J, Handwerker HO et al: Latencies of chemically evoked discharges in human nociceptors and the concurrent subjective sensations. Neurosci Lett 20:55, 1980
8. Georgopoulos AP: Functional properties of primary afferent units probably related to pain mechanisms in primate glabrous skin. J Neurophysiol 39:71, 1976
9. Bessou P, Perl E: Response of cutaneous sensory units with unmyelinated fibers to noxious stimuli. J Neurophysiol 32:1025, 1969
10. Kniffki K-D, Mense S, Schmidt RE: Muscle receptors with fine afferent fibers which may evoke circulatory reflexes. Circ Res 48:I25, 1981
11. Freeman MAR, Wyke B: The innervation of the knee joint. An anatomical and histological study of the cat. J Anat 101:505, 1967
12. Burgess PR, Clark FJ: Characteristics of knee joint receptors in the cat. J Physiol 203:317, 1969
13. Moncada S, Ferreira SH, Vane JR: Inhibition of prostaglandin biosynthesis as the mechanism of analgesia of aspirin-like drugs in the dog knee joint. Eur J Pharmacol 31:250, 1975
14. Kendall GPN: Visceral pain. Br J Surg 72(suppl):s4, 1985
15. Milne RJ, Foreman RD, Giesler GJ et al: Viscerosomatic convergence onto primate spinothalamic neurones: An explanation for referral of pelvic visceral pain. In Bonica JJ (ed): Advances in Pain Research and Therapy, vol 5, p 131. New York, Raven Press, 1983
16. Bahr R, Blumberg H, Janig W: Do dichotomizing afferent fibers exist which supply visceral organs as well as somatic structures? Neurosci Lett 24:25, 1981
17. Moriarty KJ, Dawson AM: Functional abdominal pain: Further evidence that the whole gut is affected. Br Med J 284:1670, 1982
18. Guzman F, Braun C, Lim RKS: Visceral pain and the pseudoaffective response to intra-arterial injection of bradykinin and other algesic agents. Arch Int Pharmacodyn 136:353, 1962
19. Malliani A: Cardiovascular sympathetic afferent fibers. Rev Physiol Biochem Pharmacol 94:11, 1982
20. Perl ER: Is pain a specific sensation? J Psychiatr Res 8:273, 1971
21. Cervero F: Afferent nerve activity evoked by natural stimulation of the biliary system in the ferret. Pain 13:137, 1982
22. Cuello AC, Matthews MR: Peptides in peripheral sensory nerve fibers. In Melzack R, Wall PD (eds): Textbook of Pain, p 65. New York, Churchill Livingstone, 1984
23. Murray CW, Cowan A, Larson AA: Neurokinin and NMDA antagonists (but not a kainic acid antagonist) are antinociceptive in the mouse formalin model. Pain 44:179, 1991
24. Yaksh TL, Almone LD: The central pharmacology of pain transmission. In Wall PD, Melzack R (eds): Textbook of Pain, p 181. Edinburgh, Churchill Livingstone, 1989
25. Johnson JL: The excitant amino acids glutamic and aspartic acid as transmitter candidates in the vertebrate nervous system. Prog Neurobiol 10:155, 1978
26. Robinson MB, Coyle JT: Glutamate and related acidic excitatory neurotransmitters: From basic science to clinical application. FASEB J 1:446, 1987
27. Battaglia G, Rustioni A: Co-existence of glutamate and substance P in dorsal root ganglion neurons of the rat and monkey. J Comp Neurol 277:302, 1988
28. Aanonsen LM, Wilcox GL: Nociceptive action of excitatory amino acids in the mouse: Efficacy of spinally administered opioids, phencyclidine and sigma agonists. J Pharmacol Exp Ther 243:9, 1987
29. Woolf CJ, Thompson SWN: The induction and maintenance of central sensitization is dependent on N-methyl-D-aspartic acid receptor activation: implications for the treatment of post-injury pain hypersensitivity states. Pain 44:293, 1991
30. Terenius L: Biochemical mediators in pain. Triangle 20:19, 1981
31. Denzlinger C, Rapp S, Hagman W, Keppler D: Leukotrienes as mediators in tissue trauma. Science 230:330, 1985
32. Light AR, Perl ER: Spinal termination of functionally identified primary afferent neurons with slowly conducting myelinated fibers. J Comp Neurol 168:133, 1979
33. Wall PD: The dorsal horn. In Melzack R, Wall PD (eds): Textbook of Pain, p 80. New York, Churchill Livingstone, 1984
34. Dubner R, Bennett GJ: Spinal and trigeminal mechanisms of nociception. Ann Rev Neurosci 6:381, 1983
35. Duggan AW: Transmitters involved in central processing of nociceptive information. Anaesth Intensive Care 10:133, 1982
36. Aanonsen LM, Wilcox GL: Muscimol, gamma-aminobutyric acid A receptors and excitatory amino acids in the mouse spinal cord. J Pharmacol Exp Ther 248:1034, 1988
37. Hwang AS, Wilcox GL: Baclofen, gamma-aminobutyric acid B receptors and substance P in the mouse spinal cord. J Pharmacol Exp Ther 248:1026, 1988
38. Sawynok J, Kato N, Havlicek B et al: Lack of effect of baclofen on substance P and somatostatin release from the spinal cord in vitro. Naunyn Schmiederbergs Arch Pharmacol 319:78, 1982

39. Goodchild CS, Serrao JM: Intrathecal midazolam in the rat: Evidence for spinally-mediated analgesia. Br J Anaesth 59: 1563, 1987

40. Niv D, Whitwam JG, Loh L: Depression of nociceptive sympathetic reflexes by intrathecal administration of midazolam. Br J Anaesth 55:541, 1983

41. Yaksh TL, Elde RP: Factors governing release of methionine enkephalin like immunoreactivity from mesencephalon and spinal cord of the cat in vivo. J Neurophysiol 46:1056, 1981

42. Sawynok J, Sweeney MI, White TD: Classification of adenosine receptors mediating antinociception in the rat spinal cord. Br J Pharmacol 88:923, 1986

43. Van Calker P, Muller M, Hemprecht B: Adenosine regulates via two different types of receptors the accumulation of cAMP in cultured brain cells. J Neurochem 33:999, 1979

44. Daly JW, Bruno RF, Snyder SH: Adenosine receptors in the central nervous system: Relationship to the central action of methylxanthines. Life Sci 28:2083, 1981

45. Salter MW, Henry JL: Evidence that adenosine mediates the depression of spinal dorsal horn neurons induced by peripheral vibration in the cat. Neuroscience 22:631, 1987

46. Sweeney MI, White TD, Sawynok J: Involvement of adenosine in the spinal antinociceptive effects of morphine and noradrenaline. J Pharmacol Exp Ther 243:657, 1987

47. Sosnowski M, Yaksh TL: The role of spinal adenosine receptors in modulating the hyperesthesia produced by spinal glycine receptor antagonism. Anesth Analg 69:587, 1989

48. Yaksh TL, Hammond DL: Peripheral and central substrates involved in the rostrad transmission of nociceptive information. Pain 13:1, 1982

49. Tasker RR: Deafferentation. In Melzack R, Wall PD (eds): Textbook of Pain, p 119. New York, Churchill Livingstone, 1984

50. Willis WD: The origin and destination of pathways involved in pain transmission. In Melzack R, Wall PD (eds): Textbook of Pain, p 88. New York, Churchill Livingstone, 1984

51. Fields HL: Brainstem mechanisms of pain modulation. In Kruger L, Liebeskind JC (eds): Advances in Pain Research and Therapy, vol. 6, p 241. New York, Raven Press, 1984

52. Basbaum AI, Fields HL: Endogenous pain control systems: Brainstem spinal pathways and endorphin circuitry. Ann Rev Neurosci 7:309, 1984

53. Basbaum AI: Cytochemical studies of neural circuitry underlying pain and pain control. Acta Neurochir (Wien) 38 (suppl):5, 1987

54. Wall PD, Gutnick M: Ongoing activity in peripheral nerves: The physiology and pharmacology of impulses originating from a neuroma. Exp Neurol 43:580, 1974

55. Blumberg H, Janig W: Discharge pattern of afferent fibers from a neuroma. Pain 20:335, 1984

56. Devor M, Janig W: Activation of myelinated afferents ending in neuroma by stimulation of the sympathetic supply in the rat. Neurosci Lett 24:43, 1981

57. Devor M: Nerve pathophysiology and mechanisms of pain in causalgia. J Auton Nerve Syst 7:371, 1983

58. Wall PD, Devor M: Sensory afferent impulses originate from dorsal root ganglia as well as from the periphery in normal and nerve injured rats. Pain 17:321, 1983

59. Blumberg H, Janig W: Changes in vasoconstrictor neurons supplying cat hindlimb following chronic nerve lesions: A model for studying mechanisms of reflex sympathetic dystrophy? J Auton Nerve Syst 7:399, 1983

60. Roberts WJ: A hypothesis on the physiological basis for causalgia and related pains. Pain 24:297, 1986

61. Merskey H: Pain terms: A list with definitions and notes on usage. Pain 6:249, 1979

62. Engel GL: "Psychogenic" pain and the pain-prone patient. Am J Med 26:899, 1959

63. Williams JBW (ed): Diagnostic and Statistical Manual of Mental Disorders, 3rd ed. Washington, DC, American Psychiatric Association, 1987

64. Hall RCW, Popkin MK, DeVaul RA et al: Physical illness presenting as psychiatric disease. Arch Gen Psychiatry 35:1315, 1978

65. Haddox JD: Psychological aspects of pain. In Abram SE, Haddox JD, Kettler RE (eds): The Pain Clinic Manual, p 31. Philadelphia, Lippincott, 1990

66. Blumer D, Heilbronn M: Chronic pain as a variant of depressive disease—the pain-prone disorder. J Nerv Ment Dis 170:381, 1982

67. Turk DC, Rudy TE, Steig RL: Chronic Pain and Depression. Pain Management 1:18, 1987

68. Pilowsky I, Spence ND: Pain and illness behaviour: A comparative study. J Psychosom Res 20:131, 1976

69. Pilowsky I, Chapman CR, Bonica JJ: Pain, depression and illness behavior in a pain clinic population. Pain 4:183, 1977

70. Skinner BF: Science and Human Behavior. New York, The Macmillan Company, 1953

71. Turk DC, Meichenbaum D, Genest M: Pain and Behavioral Medicine: A Cognitive-Behavioral Perspective. New York, Guilford Press, 1985

72. Mixter WJ, Barr JS: Rupture of the intervertebral disc with involvement of the spinal cord. N Engl J Med 211:210, 1934

73. Aitken AP: Rupture of the intervertebral disc in injury: Further observations and results. Am J Surg 84:261, 1952

74. Hirsch C, Nachemson A: The reliability of lumbar disc surgery. Clin Orthop 29:189, 1963

75. Hakelius A: Prognosis in sciatica. Acta Orthop Scand 129 (suppl):1, 1970

76. Green LN: Dexamethosone in the management of symptoms due to herniated lumbar disc. J Neurol Neurosurg Psychiatry 38:1211, 1975

77. Friedenberg ZB, Shoemaker RC: The results of non-operative treatment of ruptured lumbar discs. Am J Surg 88:933, 1954

78. Hitzelberger WE, Witten RM: Abnormal myelograms in asymptomatic patients. J Neurosurg 28:204, 1968

79. McRae DL: Asymptomatic intervertebral disc protrusions. Acta Radiol (Stockh) 46:9, 1956

80. Murphy RW: Nerve roots and spinal nerves in degenerative disc disease. Clin Orthop 129:46, 1977

81. Marshall LL, Trethwie ER: Chemical irritation of nerve roots in disc prolapse. Lancet 2:230, 1973

82. Benzon HT: Epidural steroid injections for low back pain and lumbosacral radiculopathy. Pain 24:277, 1986

83. Lievre JA, Block-Michael H, Attali P: L'injection transsacrée. Etude Clinique et Radiologique. Bull Soc Med 73:1110, 1957

84. Coomes EN: A comparison between epidural anesthesia and bedrest in sciatica. Br Med J 1:20, 1961

85. Swerdlow M, Sayle-Creer W: A study of extradural medication in the relief of the lumbosciatic syndrome. Anaesthesia 25:341, 1970

86. Winnie AP, Hartman JT, Myers HL et al: Pain clinic II: Intradural and extradural corticosteroids for sciatica. Anesth Analg 51:990, 1972

87. Dilke TFW, Burry HC, Grahame R: Extradural corticosteroid injection in management of lumbar root compression. Br Med J 2:635, 1973

88. Breivik H, Hesia PE, Molnar I et al: Treatment of chronic low back pain and sciatica: Comparison of caudal epidural steroid injections of bupivacaine and methylprednisolone with bupivacaine followed by saline. In Bonica JJ, Albe-Fessard D (eds): Advances in Pain Research and Therapy, vol. 1, p 927. New York, Raven Press, 1976

89. Snoek W, Weber H, Jorgensen B: Double blind evaluation of extradural methylprednisolone for herniated lumbar discs. Acta Orthop Scand 48:635, 1977

90. Cuckler JM, Bernini PA, Wiesel SW et al: The use of epidural steroids in the treatment of lumbar radicular pain. J Bone Joint Surg 67A:63, 1985

91. Abram SE, Hopwood MB: What factors contribute to outcome with lumbar epidural steroids. In Bond MR, Charlton JE, Woolf CJ (eds): Proceedings of the VIth World Congress on Pain, 491. Amsterdam, Elsevier, 1991

92. Finneson BE: Low Back Pain. Philadelphia, Lippincott, 1973

93. Abram SE: Subarachnoid corticosteroid injection following inadequate response to epidural steroids for sciatica. Anesth Analg 57:313, 1978

94. Abram SE, Anderson RA: Using a pain questionnaire to predict response to steroid epidurals. Reg Anesth 5:11, 1980

95. Keim HA, Kirkaldy-Willis WH: Low back pain. Clin Symp 32:2, 1980

96. Carrera GF: Lumbar facet joint injection in low back pain and sciatica. Radiology 137:665, 1980

97. Carrera GF, Foley WD, Kozin F et al: CT of sacroiliitis. Am J Radiol 136:41, 1981

98. Bonica JJ: The Management of Pain, p 1200. Philadelphia, Lea & Febiger, 1953

99. Travell JG, Simons DG: Myofascial Pain and Dysfunction. Baltimore, Williams & Wilkins, 1983

100. Travell JG, Rinzler SH: The myofascial genesis of pain. Postgrad Med 11:425, 1952

101. Berges PV: Myofascial pain syndromes. Postgrad Med 53:161, 1953

102. Kleinert HE, Cole NM, Wayne L et al: Post-traumatic sympathetic dystrophy. Orthop Clin North Am 4:917, 1973

103. Genant NK, Kozin F, Bekerman C et al: The reflex sympathetic dystrophy syndrome. Radiology 117:21, 1975

104. Carron H, Weller RM: Treatment of post-traumatic sympathetic dystrophy. In Advances in Neurology, vol. 4, p 485. New York, Raven Press, 1974

105. Bonica JJ: Causalgia and other reflex sympathetic dystrophies. In Bonica JJ, Albe-Fessard D (eds): Advances in Pain Research and Therapy, vol. 1, p 141. New York, Raven Press, 1979

106. Wang JK, Johnson KA, Ilstrup DM: Sympathetic blocks for reflex sympathetic dystrophy. Pain 23:13, 1985

107. Hannington-Kiff JG: Intravenous regional sympathetic block with guanethidine. Lancet 1:1019, 1974

108. Boneli S, Conoscente F, Movilia PG et al: Regional intravenous guanethidine vs. stellate block in reflex sympathetic dystrophies: A randomized trial. Pain 16:297, 1983

109. Eriksen S: Duration of sympathetic blockade. Anaesthesia 36:768, 1981

110. Kozin F, Ryan LM, Carrera GF et al: The reflex sympathetic dystrophy syndrome (RSDS) III. Scintigraphic studies, further evidence for the therapeutic efficacy of systemic corticosteroids, and proposed diagnostic criteria. Am J Med 70:23, 1981

111. Poplawski ZJ, Wiley AM, Murray JF: Post-traumatic dystrophy of the extremities. J Bone Joint Surg [Am] 65:642, 1983

112. Abram SE, Asiddao CB, Reynolds AC: Increased skin temperature during transcutaneous electrical stimulation. Anesth Analg 59:22, 1980

113. Stilz RJ, Carron H, Sanders DB: Reflex sympathetic dystrophy in a 6 year old: Successful treatment by transcutaneous nerve stimulation. Anesth Analg 56:438, 1977

114. Abram SE, Lightfoot R: Treatment of long-standing causalgia with prazosin. Reg Anesth 6:79, 1981

115. Spurling RG: Causalgia of the upper extremity: Treatment by dorsal sympathetic ganglionectomy. Arch Neurol Psychiatry 23:784, 1930

116. Mayfield FH: Causalgia. Springfield, IL, Charles C. Thomas, 1951

117. Boas RS, Hatangdi VS, Richards EG: Lumbar sympathectomy—a percutaneous technique. In Bonica JJ, Albe-Fessard D (eds): Advances in Pain Research and Therapy, vol. 1, p 485. New York, Raven Press, 1976

118. Paoli F, Darcourt G, Corsa P: Note preliminare sur l'action de l'imipramine dans les etats douloureaux. Rev Neurol 102:503, 1960

119. Aronoff GM, Wagner JM, Spangler AS: Chemical interventions for pain. J Consult Clin Psychol 54:769, 1986

120. Weintraub M, Evans P: Buproprion: A chemically and pharmacologically unique antidepressant. Hosp Form 24:254, 1989

121. Wernicke JF: The side effect profile and safety of fluoxetine. J Clin Psychiatry 46:59, 1989

122. Mangla JC, Pereira M: Tricyclic antidepressants in the treatment of peptic ulcer disease. Arch Intern Med 142:273, 1982

123. Frommer DA, Kulig KW, Marx JA et al: Tricyclic antidepressant overdose. JAMA 257:521, 1987

124. Watson CP, Evans RS, Reed K et al: Amitriptyline versus placebo in postherpetic neuralgia. Neurology 32:671, 1982

125. Getto CJ, Sorkness CA, Howell T: Antidepressants and chronic nonmalignant pain: A review. Journal of Pain and Symptom Management 2:9, 1987

126. Mendel CM, Klein RF, Chappell DA et al: A trial of amitriptyline and fluphenazine in the treatment of painful diabetic neuropathy. JAMA 255:637, 1986

127. Clarke IMC: Amitriptyline and perphenazine (Triptafen DA) in chronic pain. Anaesthesia 36:210, 1981

128. McGee JL, Alexander MR: Phenothiazine analgesia—fact or fantasy? Am J Hosp Pharm 36:633, 1979

129. Rall TW, Schleifer LS: Drugs effective in the therapy of the epilepsies. In Gilman AG, Goodman LS, Rall TW (eds): The Pharmacological Basis of Therapeutics, p 446. New York, Macmillan, 1985

130. Burchiel KJ: Carbamezepine inhibits spontaneous activity in experimental neuromas. Exp Neurol 102:249, 1988

131. Pilowski I: Psychotherapy in persistent pain: Psycho-social assessment and intervention. In Lynch NT, Vasudevan SV (eds): Persistent Pain. Boston, Kluwer Academic Publishers, 1988

132. Beecher HK: The Measurement of Subjective Responses: Quantitative Effects of Drugs. New York, Oxford University Press, 1959

133. Taylor ML: Psychological treatment of chronic pain. In Abram SE, Haddox JD, Kettler RE (eds): The Pain Clinic Manual, p 225. Philadelphia, Lippincott, 1990

134. Fordyce WE, Fowler RS, Lehman JF et al: Operant conditioning in the treatment of chronic clinical pain. Arch Phys Med Rehab 54:399, 1973

135. Fordyce WE, Roberts AH, Sternbach RA: The behavioral management of chronic pain: A response to critics. Pain 22:113, 1985

136. Fields HL: Pain, p 325. New York, McGraw-Hill, 1987

137. Jacobson E: Progressive Relaxation. Chicago, University of Chicago Press, 1929

138. Benson H: The Relaxation Response. New York, William Morrow Co., 1975

139. Hilgard ER: Hypnosis and pain. In Sternbach RA (ed): The Psychology of Pain, 2nd ed, p 197. New York, Raven Press, 1986

140. Evans FJ: Placebo mechanisms. In Advances in Neurology, vol. 4, p 289. New York, Raven Press, 1974

141. Foley KM: The treatment of pain in the patient with cancer. CA 36:194, 1986

142. Payne R, Foley KM: Recent advances in cancer pain management. Cancer Treat Rep 68:173, 1984

143. Kaiko RF, Foley KM, Grabinski PY et al: Central nervous system excitatory effects of meperidine in cancer patients. Ann Neurol 13:180, 1983

144. Walsh TD, Saunders CM: Heroin and morphine in advanced cancer. N Engl J Med 31:599, 1984

145. Baumann TJ, Batenhorst RL, Graves DA et al: Patient-controlled analgesia in the terminally ill cancer patient. Drug Intell Clin Pharm 20:297, 1986

146. Miser AW, Davis DM, Hughes CS et al: Continuous subcutaneous infusions of morphine in children with cancer. Am J Dis Child 137:383, 1983

147. Wang JK, Nauss LA, Thomas JE: Pain relief by intrathecally applied morphine in man. Anesthesiology 50:149, 1979

148. Coombs DW, Saunders RL, Gaylor MS et al: Relief of continuous chronic pain by intraspinal narcotics infusion via an implanted reservoir. JAMA 250:2336, 1983

149. Jorgensen BC, Andersen HB, Engquist A: CSF and plasma morphine after epidural and intrathecal application. Anesthesiology 55:714, 1981

150. Coombs DW, Fratkin JD, Meier FA et al: Neuropathologic lesions and CSF morphine concentrations during chronic continuous intraspinal morphine infusion. A clinical and postmortem study. Pain 22:337, 1985

151. Coombs DW, Saunders RL, Gaylor M et al: Epidural narcotic infusion reservoir: Implantation technique and efficacy. Anesthesiology 56:469, 1982

152. Woods WA, Cohen SE: High-dose epidural morphine in a terminally ill patient. Anesthesiology 56:311, 1982

153. Greenberg HS, Taren J, Ensminger WD *et al*: Benefit from and tolerance to continuous intrathecal infusion of morphine for intractable cancer pain. J Neurosurg 57:360, 1982

154. Coombs DW, Saunders RL, Lachance D *et al*: Intrathecal morphine tolerance: Use of intrathecal clonidine, DADLE and intraventricular morphine. Anesthesiology 62:358, 1985

155. Moulin DE, Max MB, Kaiko RF *et al*: The analgesic efficacy of D-Ala-D-Leu-enkephalin in cancer patients with chronic pain. Pain 23:213, 1985

156. Messahel FM, Tomlin PJ: Narcotic withdrawal syndrome after intrathecal administration of morphine. Br Med J 283:471, 1981

157. Hogan Q, Haddox JD, Abram SE *et al*: Epidural opiates for the management of cancer pain. Pain 42:271, 1991

158. Plummer JL, Cherry DA, Cousins MJ *et al*: Long-term spinal administration of morphine in cancer and non-cancer pain: A retrospective study. Pain 44:215, 1991

159. Tenicela R, Lovasik D, Eaglstein W: Treatment of herpes zoster with sympathetic blocks. Clin J Pain 1:63, 1985

160. Swerdlow M: Relief of Intractable Pain. Amsterdam, Excerpta Medica, 1974

161. Papo I, Visca A: Phenol subarachnoid rhizotomy for the treatment of cancer pain: A personal account of 290 cases. In Bonica JJ, Ventafridda V (eds): Advances in Pain Research and Therapy, vol. 2, p 339. New York, Raven Press, 1979

162. Swerdlow M: Subarachnoid and extradural neurolytic blocks. In Bonica JJ, Ventafridda V (eds): Advances in Pain Research and Therapy, vol. 2, p 325. New York, Raven Press, 1979

163. Simon DL, Carron H, Rowlingson JC: Treatment of bladder pain with transsacral nerve block. Anesth Analg 61:46, 1982

164. Madrid JL, Bonica JJ: Cranial nerve blocks. In Bonica JJ, Venta-Fridda V (eds): Advances in Pain Research and Therapy, vol. 2, p 347. New York, Raven Press, 1979

165. Thompson GE, Moore DC, Bridenbaugh LD *et al*: Abdominal pain and alcohol celiac plexus nerve block. Anesth Analg 56:1, 1977

166. Moore DC: Regional Block. Springfield, IL, Charles C Thomas, 1975

167. Singler RC: An improved technique for alcohol neurolysis of the celiac plexus. Anesthesiology 56:137, 1982

168. Ischia S, Luzzani A, Ischia A *et al*: A new approach to the neurolytic block of the celiac plexus: The transaortic technique. Pain 16:333, 1983

169. Kroening RJ: Pain clinics structure and function. Seminars in Anesthesia 4:231, 1985

170. Moya F, Mayne GE: Organization of a pain clinic. In Raj PP (ed): Practical Management of Pain, p 20. Chicago, Year Book Medical, 1986

171. Abram SE, Anderson RA, Maitra d'Cruze AM: Factors predicting short-term outcome of nerve blocks in the management of chronic pain. Pain 10:323, 1981

59

Morris Brown

ICU—Critical Care

Critical care medicine is now a clearly recognized specialty of the practice of medicine. It is a multidisciplinary specialty based in the intensive care unit, with its primary concern being care of the patient with a critical illness. Critical care medicine crosses traditional departmental and specialty lines and requires a physician whose knowledge is broad, involving all aspects of management of the critically ill patient.[1]

HISTORY OF CRITICAL CARE MEDICINE

The Society of Critical Care Medicine (SCCM), founded in 1970, was the first formal organization established in the United States to represent physicians and ancillary personnel devoted to the care of critically ill patients. In 1977, the American Board of Medical Specialties allowed recognition for physicians with expertise in critical care medicine. Thereafter, the American Board of Anesthesiology (ABA) received approval to issue a certificate of special qualifications in critical care medicine to its diplomates. Anesthesiologists were the first specialists to be issued certificates of special qualifications in critical care medicine by virtue of an examination administered in September 1986. Since that time, the American Boards of Internal Medicine, Pediatrics, and Surgery have offered examinations for their diplomates. The American Society of Critical Care Anesthesiologists (ASCCA) was formed to organize anesthesiologists interested in the practice of critical care medicine. The ASCCA maintains liaison with the American Society of Anesthesiologists (ASA) and the SCCM.

ANESTHESIOLOGISTS AND CRITICAL CARE MEDICINE

Critical care medicine has always been an integral part of the practice of anesthesiology. Anesthesiologists have been intimately involved, indeed instrumental, in the development of critical care medicine as a specialty. Many consider the practice of operating room anesthesiology the practice of critical care medicine limited to the operative period. The anesthesiologist is involved daily with rapid alterations in physiologic status that require prompt recognition and early intervention—the hallmarks of critical care medicine. By virtue of training, experience, competence, and interest, the anesthesiologist brings skills and knowledge that uniquely qualify him or her to care for critically ill patients. This expertise has been recognized by the ABA, which included critical care medicine in its definition of anesthesiology, and by the ASA, which included critical care medicine in its standards of practice. Further, training in critical care medicine is an integral part of the curriculum for residents in anesthesiology. Advanced training in this specialty following completion of residency training is required to be eligible to receive a certificate of special qualifications in critical care medicine by the ABA. Recommendations for the content of fellowship training programs in critical care medicine as well as recommendations for the qualifications of a director of these programs have been developed by a task force on guidelines from the SCCM.[2,3]

HISTORY OF INTENSIVE CARE UNITS

Intensive care units (ICUs) have been in existence for over 30 years.[4,5] They evolved from postanesthesia care units and surgical recovery rooms. The earliest ICUs developed in this country were multidisciplinary medical-surgical units.[6] In the 1960s there was a proliferation of cardiac care units when lifesaving detection and treatment of cardiac dysrhythmias were noted.[7] This led to the proliferation of other organ-specific intensive care units, such as respiratory, neurologic, and cardiothoracic ICUs. However, it appears that interdisciplinary ICUs have both patient care and economic advantages over segregated departmental or specialty organ-oriented units.[8] Certainly, staffing is easier and the ability to share resources is a distinct advantage. However, some units such as neonatal ICUs, burn units, and spinal cord centers may justify special designation established on a regional basis.[9] Current estimates indicate that 60% of hospitals with intensive care facilities have only one identifiable ICU. If coronary units are excluded, 82% of hospitals with intensive care facilities have only a single unit.

The numbers of ICU beds required for an institution vary between 3 and 25% of the total hospital beds, with an average of 12% for major adult and general hospitals.[10] In children's hospitals the percent of special care beds averages over 23% and may be as high as 46%. Currently, ICU beds constitute 7–8% of all hospital beds.[11] The number of beds required for any institution varies, depending on the patient population served. It appears, however, that with changes in the political climate and only the very sickest of patients being admitted to the hospital, there will be a need in the future for more critical care beds and fewer beds for elective admissions.

COST AND OUTCOME OF INTENSIVE CARE

There is increasing concern about the cost of medical care, especially associated with critical illness. ICU beds are growing at approximately 6% annually, whereas other beds are closing.[12] ICU care consumes 20% of total hospital charges. In addition, because of the intensity and stress placed on the personnel working in ICUs, there is a disproportionally high loss of personnel from these areas.[13] It has been estimated that the annual turnover of nurses from critical care units approaches 50%, and it is common not to be able to use all resources because of inadequate staffing.[14]

It is still uncertain whether ICU care decreases patient morbidity and mortality. Reports in the literature are conflicting. Several early studies demonstrated a significant benefit of ICU care when specialty units were reviewed.[15-18] For example, in a review of coronary ICUs, a reduction in mortality was noted and attributed to these units.[19] Similarly, the national burn information exchange noted a reduction in mortality and in the length of hospitalization in burned patients due to improvement in the critical care aspects of burn management.[17] Likewise, other studies have shown a reduction in mortality in noncardiac surgical patients, trauma patients, and other selected surgical groups after the introduction of a surgical ICU teaching service and computer-based approach to patient monitoring and therapy.[20] However, these studies and many in the literature have used historical controls. Unfortunately, this does not consider differences in treatment modalities and other factors that may have contributed to the change in morbidity and mortality. Indeed, several studies have failed to show any benefit from hospitalization in critical care units.[21-22] More carefully designed, rigorously controlled trials are necessary to assess the true efficacy of ICUs.

PATIENT ASSESSMENT SYSTEMS

Because intensive care is so expensive and consumes so many resources, several attempts have been made to develop methods to predict patient outcome. In this way patient care could be optimized by limiting admission to only those patients who would benefit from intensive care and withholding or removing therapy from patients who would not. This clearly would be a means of significantly reducing medical costs and providing optimal use of available resources. Unfortunately, the systems introduced to assess the severity of illness of patients and their need for intensive care as well as to predict outcome have met with limited success.

Illness severity scoring systems have been devised on an anatomic, therapeutic, and physiologic basis.[23] The Clinical Classification System was introduced as a means to assess severity of illness along with a therapeutic intervention scoring system to measure the amount of therapy given.[24] The therapeutic intervention scoring system serves as an indirect measure of illness severity, with the greater number of interventions occurring with sicker patients. The clinical

classification system, along with the therapeutic intervention scoring system has been used to assist in appropriate use of facilities, to provide information on nurse staffing ratios, and to relate costs to extent of care given in both the adult and pediatric populations. In addition, it was an attempt to be able to compare treatment and outcome in different ICUs.[24-27] This system, however, has been criticized because of its limited utility in comparing patients who may have been treated by different standards of critical care in different institutions.

The acute physiology and chronic health evaluation (APACHE) system relates the severity of a patient's illness to the degree of physiologic derangement of a series of physiologic measurements. With an assigned weight given to each measurement, it is then possible to assess preadmission health status and probability of survival.[28] It also has been used to compare patient populations in different institutions.[29,30] Attempts to simplify the APACHE system resulted in the simplified acute physiology score and APACHE II.[31,32] The APACHE III study currently in progress attempts to improve the scoring system as well as the evaluation of the progress of care and the application of a predictive system for individual patients. The physiologic stability index is an adaptation of the APACHE system for use in the pediatric population.[33] Other scoring systems have been developed for patients following trauma,[34] myocardial infarction,[35] adult respiratory insufficiency,[36] shock,[37] and neonatal resuscitation.[38] Unfortunately, to date none of these systems can unequivocally predict outcome or benefit from intensive care.

CENTRAL NERVOUS SYSTEM

Assessment and treatment of critically ill patients with central nervous system disorders require a thorough knowledge of cerebral blood flow and metabolism as well as of cerebral pharmacology, neurophysiology, and pathophysiology.

Determinants of Cerebral Blood Flow

Control of cerebral perfusion is essential in maintaining neurologic function in pathologic states. Cerebral blood flow is regulated by intracerebral and extracerebral factors. Intracerebral blood flow regulation is controlled by chemical and metabolic influences, including hydrogen ion concentration, cyclo-oxygenase, products of phospholipid membrane metabolism, and adenosine. In addition, neurogenic and myogenic components contribute to the regulation of cerebral blood flow.[39]

The extracerebral determinants of blood flow include the arterial partial pressure of carbon dioxide ($Paco_2$) and oxygen (Pao_2), arterial blood pressure, venous blood pressure, and pharmacologic effects of drugs. There is a linear correlation between cerebral blood flow and $Paco_2$ with progressive hypercarbia. Similarly, there is a marked reduction in cerebral blood flow during hypocarbia through a pH-mediated change in arteriolar tone that results in vasoconstriction and reduced intracranial pressure (ICP).[40,41] Taken to extremes, hypocarbia provides no additional benefit and may be detrimental.[42] Therefore, current recommendations suggest maintaining $Paco_2$ between 25 mm Hg and 30 mm Hg. However, prolonged hypocarbia is ineffective because cerebrospinal fluid bicarbonate adapts to the change in $Paco_2$. Therefore, the long-term value of hyperventilation of the lungs for reducing ICP is offset by the normalization of cerebrospinal fluid pH, which occurs in 6 hours.[43]

Arterial oxygenation has a lesser effect on cerebral blood flow than does carbon dioxide. When the PaO_2 falls below 50 mm Hg, cerebral vasodilation and an increase in cerebral blood flow result, which may exacerbate intracranial hypertension.[44] Hyperoxia generally results in very small changes in cerebral blood flow until PaO_2 exceeds 300 mm Hg.

Autoregulation

Autoregulation, the ability of the brain to maintain cerebral blood flow constant despite alterations in mean arterial pressure, is functional over a mean arterial pressure range of 50–150 mm Hg. At levels below 50 mm Hg, symptoms of cerebral ischemia may appear. If the upper limit of autoregulation is exceeded, cerebral blood flow increases, which may result in cerebral edema. It is important to note that the autoregulatory curve may be shifted in the presence of chronic hypertension, intracranial tumors, head trauma, and shock states, which render the brain more susceptible to ischemic effects.[45]

Intracranial Pressure Monitoring

ICP can normally range up to 15 mm Hg, and beyond that point any increase in ICP can result in a decrease in cerebral perfusion pressure. Once cerebral perfusion pressure falls below 40–60 mm Hg, ischemic injury to nerve cells may occur. There is a close correlation between clinical outcome and the level of ICP elevation after acute injury.[46] Aggressive treatment of elevated ICP in the ICU is essential. The symptoms associated with increased ICP are variable, although they generally reflect effects of compression of structures around the tentorial opening. If left untreated, raised ICP leads to global cerebral ischemia, coma, and death.

Continuous monitoring of ICP can be accomplished through a ventriculostomy, a subdural bolt, or an epidural transducer (see Chapter 32).[47] Advantages and disadvantages of each technique are outlined in Table 59-1. The intraventricular catheter is inserted through a burr hole through the coronal suture. It provides an accurate and reliable reading of ICP as well as allowing withdrawing cerebrospinal fluid for pressure control and culture. Disadvantages of this technique include the necessity of passing through brain tissue in order to introduce the catheter into the ventricle. This may be very difficult when the brain is distorted from trauma and edema. Further, the risk of infection is greatest with this technique as compared with the others. Indeed, positive cerebrospinal fluid culture results have been reported in approximately 9% of patients monitored with intraventricular catheters.[48] The possibility of infection is reduced if catheterization is limited to 3 days and prophylactic antibiotics are administered.

The subarachnoid bolt is a less invasive means of monitoring ICP. This device is inserted into the skull after the dura and arachnoid have been opened. It is easily inserted, does not require penetration of brain tissue, and can be done at the bedside. As with all invasive procedures, insertion of a subarachnoid bolt carries the risk of infection.

The epidural transducer used to monitor ICP is placed between the inner table of the skull and the dura. This device is easy to place and monitors pressures exerted by the cerebrospinal fluid and brain on the dura. Although this technique carries little risk of infection, its accuracy and reliability for monitoring ICP are questionable.[47]

Control of Elevated Intracranial Pressure

Treatment of increased ICP is generally recommended when levels exceed 20 mm Hg. Certainly, treatment may be indicated at a lower pressure if evidence of impaired cerebral perfusion is present. Modalities available to treat increased ICP include diuretics and fluid restriction, hyperosmotic agents, hyperventilation of the lungs, corticosteroids, barbiturates, positioning, and removal of cerebrospinal fluid.

Once surgically correctable causes of increased ICP have been eliminated, treatment should be initiated with hyperventilation to maintain $PaCO_2$ between 25 and 30 mm Hg. Additional measures include drainage of cerebrospinal fluid if an intraventricular catheter has been placed and elevation of the head to 30 degrees, which encourages venous drainage from the brain and hence lowers ICP. Mannitol may be added in an attempt to remove brain water. This osmotic agent helps draw water from the tissues because of the transient increase in plasma osmolarity. The onset of action following intravenous administration of mannitol is 30 minutes, with a maximum lowering of ICP occurring within 1–2 hours and lasting 6 hours. Diuretics such as furosemide may also be used to lower ICP and are especially useful in patients with increased intravascular volume. Corticosteroids are effective in lowering ICP owing to localized cerebral edema surrounding intracranial tumors. Dexamethasone is the most commonly used steroid preparation and generally causes improvement in neurologic status within 12–36 hours of therapy. Barbiturate administration can also assist in lowering ICP by a dose-related reduction in cerebral metabolic oxygen requirement as well as by decreasing cerebral blood volume. Some authors suggest barbiturate coma for cerebral protection in patients with elevated ICP.[49-51]

Fluid and electrolyte abnormalities including hyponatremia, hypokalemia, and hypochloremia with fluid retention are common accompaniments of central nervous system disease. Other complications include acute respiratory failure, gastrointestinal bleeding, hypertension, cardiac dysrhythmias, and disseminated intravascular coagulation.[52] These related complications must be recognized and treated if they occur.

Seizures

The etiology of a seizure generally depends on the age of the patient and the type of seizure.[53] Young children frequently present with seizures associated with febrile illness. In adolescent and young adults, head trauma is a major cause of focal seizure disorders, whereas generalized seizures tend to be associated with drug or alcohol withdrawal in this age

TABLE 59-1. Techniques of Direct Intracranial Pressure Monitoring

ICP Monitor	Advantage	Disadvantage
Ventriculostomy	Very accurate Access to cerebro-spinal fluid for pressure control and culture	Must pass through brain tissue Infection
Subarachnoid bolt	Easily performed Bedside procedure	Infection Less accurate
Epidural transducer	Easy to place Little risk of infection	Questionable accuracy and reliability

group. Brain tumors are the most common cause of seizures in patients between 30 and 50 years of age, and over 50 years of age cerebrovascular disease is the most common cause of focal or generalized seizure disorders.[52] The initial evaluation of the patient with a seizure consists of insuring adequate ventilation and perfusion as well as stopping the seizure. A full history and examination must be obtained. It is important to differentiate the kind of seizure in order to aid in determining the etiology. Treatment is directed at eliminating the cause and suppressing the seizure.[53] Certainly, metabolic disturbances such as hypoglycemia or hypocalcemia should be sought and corrected. Structural brain lesions must be removed. Most seizure disorders are amenable to anticonvulsant medication.[54] However, neurosurgical treatment should be considered if a structural lesion causes recurrent seizures and removal of that lesion and nearby affected brain tissue will make them easier to control or eliminate them entirely. In addition, neurosurgical ablation of epileptogenic foci may prove a valuable treatment modality.

Central Nervous System Trauma

Head injuries are a significant cause of morbidity and mortality, with over 2 million injuries causing brain damage yearly. In order to quantitate the severity of head injury, an objective clinical scale was developed. The Glasgow Coma Scale evaluates motor response, verbal response, and eye opening (Table 59-2).[55] It provides an estimate of the severity of neurologic dysfunction and predicts an 85% mortality within 24 hours after injury.[56] Evoked potentials are another means of assessing prognosis in patients following head injury. The accuracy of evoked potentials is greater than that of clinical observation and ICP measurements. Somatosensory evoked potentials are the most useful and can predict death or a vegetative state in approximately 90% of patients if they are bilaterally absent.[57]

Any patient who presents with severe head injury should have the airway protected and secured, ventilation and blood pressure stabilized, and attention given to life-threatening noncranial injuries followed by a full neurologic evaluation. As with any head injury, the possibility of cervical spine injury should be considered and the cervical spine should be immobilized until full evaluation is possible. Surgically treatable causes of increased ICP should be sought, including epidural or subdural hematoma and intracerebral hemorrhage. Aggressive surgical intervention may dramatically improve outcome.[58,59] If, however, there are no surgically treatable lesions found on computed tomographic scan, attention should be directed toward reducing increased ICP.[60] Direct intracranial pressure monitoring should be considered.[61] Hypoxia, hyperthermia, hypercarbia, malpositioning of the endotracheal tube, and high mean airway pressures may exacerbate the intracranial hypertension. Persistent elevation of ICP despite conservative therapy generally portends a poor prognosis. Fluid and electrolytes should be monitored closely. Anticonvulsants and prophylaxis to prevent gastrointestinal bleeding are generally administered.

It must be remembered that patients who sustain head trauma have other associated problems. Indeed, medical complications generally dominate the intermediate term intensive care of head trauma patients. Fluid and electrolyte balance can be a major problem following head injury.[62] Indeed, over half of the patients who have persistent coma develop abnormalities of fluid and electrolyte balance. It is important to monitor serum osmolarity and sodium concentrations because treatment of intracranial hypertension may cause marked alterations in these parameters. Coagulation parameters must also be monitored, since disseminated intravascular coagulation may accompany head trauma in 5–10% of cases.[63]

CARDIOVASCULAR SYSTEM

Cardiogenic Shock

Cardiogenic shock is a syndrome that results directly from severely impaired left ventricular pump function. This may result from end-stage cardiac disease or as a catastrophic complication of acute myocardial infarction. With improvement in cardiac dysrhythmia monitoring and treatment, cardiogenic shock has emerged as the most common cause of death among patients in coronary care units. Indeed, cardiogenic shock occurs in 10–15% of patients who suffer an acute myocardial infarction.[64] Mortality remains high despite advances in hemodynamic monitoring and newer pharmacologic drugs. Cardiogenic shock, like hypovolemic or septic shock, manifests as inadequate oxygen delivery to tissues, with failure of mitochondrial oxidative metabolism and accumulation of lactic acid. Inadequate organ perfusion in cardiogenic shock is caused by a marked reduction in the quantity of contracting myocardium. The initial insult leads to a decrease in arterial pressure with a resultant decrease in coronary blood flow. This fall in coronary perfusion pressure further compromises myocardial function, leading to progressive circulatory deterioration. The clinical consequences of the decrease in myocardial contractility manifest as either circulatory insufficiency (forward failure) or circulatory congestion (backward failure).

Typical signs and symptoms of patients in cardiogenic shock include restlessness and mental confusion; the skin is cool, moist, and cyanotic. Peripheral pulses are usually weak and rapid, and arterial blood pressure is decreased. However, shock can occur without severe hypotension, a relatively late indicator of inadequate reflex vasoconstriction. Nonetheless, the syndrome is usually defined by a systolic arterial pressure less than 80 mm Hg, with a cardiac index of less than 2 $l \cdot min^{-1} \cdot m^{-2}$ and an increase in left ventricular end-diastolic pressure or pulmonary capillary wedge pressure greater than 18 mm Hg.[65]

TABLE 59-2. Glasgow Coma Scale

Parameter	Response	Score
Eye opening	Spontaneously	4
	To verbal command	3
	To pain	2
	No response	1
Motor response	Obeys verbal command	6
	Localizes pain	5
	Flexion-withdrawal	4
	Decorticate rigidity	3
	Decerebrate rigidity	2
	No response	1
Verbal response	Oriented and converses	5
	Disoriented and converses	4
	Inappropriate words	3
	Incomprehensible sounds	2
	No response	1

Because prognosis is poor and mortality is high, close monitoring and early aggressive intervention are essential for successful outcome. Certainly, any patient in shock should have continuous monitoring of arterial pressure and left ventricular filling pressures. Measurement of central venous pressure alone is inadequate and may actually be misleading because it often fails to reliably reflect left ventricular pressures.[66] Close monitoring of urinary output is important, as it gives an indication of renal artery perfusion and provides a monitor of the progress of treatment.

Successful treatment of cardiogenic shock depends on early restoration of adequate tissue perfusion to meet metabolic demands. To achieve this goal, initial resuscitation and general supportive measures should be instituted immediately. Specific pharmacologic therapy to maintain adequate blood pressure, cardiac output, and oxygenation should be initiated. Consideration should then be given to mechanical cardiac assist devices or cardiac surgical intervention, including transplantation and implantation of an artificial heart.[67]

Drugs with positive inotropic properties improve the contractile performance of the failing heart. Sympathomimetic amines are potent positive inotropic drugs that exert their effects through action on alpha- and beta-adrenergic receptors. Isoproterenol is rarely used in the treatment of shock. Although it increases contractility, it does so at an increase in myocardial oxygen consumption and reduction of coronary perfusion pressure. Norepinephrine is a combined alpha and beta agent, with alpha properties generally dominant, causing intensive vasoconstriction. It can be useful in raising blood pressure, but the increase in afterload causes a marked increase in myocardial oxygen consumption. Dopamine has been used successfully as a positive inotropic drug with varying effects at different dosage ranges.[68,69] At low doses the drug has positive chronotropic and inotropic effects, but at higher doses vasoconstriction occurs through an alpha-mediated response. Dobutamine is a synthetic, sympathomimetic amine with positive inotropic effects without the chronotropic or peripheral vasoconstrictive properties of dopamine.[70] It therefore should be used in patients without profound hypotension. Dopamine and dobutamine may also be used in combination.[71] Amrinone is a newer inotropic drug that causes a dose-dependent increase in cardiac output while reducing systemic vascular resistance and left ventricular filling pressures. In addition, it increases renal blood flow and improves renal function.[72] Other new phosphodiesterase inhibitors such as milrinone, enoximone, and piroximone are currently under investigation.

Mechanical circulatory assist devices, most commonly the intra-aortic balloon pump, have gained widespread clinical use since first introduced by Moulopoulus in 1962.[73] The balloon pump assist device results in a reduction in myocardial oxygen consumption and therefore myocardial ischemia. In addition, by decreasing left ventricular volume and pressure and augmenting coronary perfusion, there is a positive balance established between myocardial oxygen demand and supply. The intra-aortic balloon pump has been shown in experimental models to improve hemodynamics,[74] augment myocardial perfusion, enhance impaired contractile function,[75-77] and potentially limit infarct size.[78-79] Indeed, it has been shown that an increase in coronary blood flow is seen in patients in cardiogenic shock.[80] Unfortunately, although myocardial ischemia is relieved and heart failure lessened in most patients with intra-aortic balloon pump assist, long-term survival has not been established. In recent clinical experience, intra-aortic balloon

pumping alone was associated with an overall survival rate of less than 30% when used in patients with cardiogenic shock. The addition of emergency cardiac surgical revascularization has improved survival rates.[81]

Although intra-aortic balloon pumping is generally a simple and relatively safe procedure, serious complications occur in 10% of patients.[82] Complications include aortic and arterial trauma, vascular insufficiency in the catheterized limb distal to the insertion site, infection, embolic phenomena, balloon rupture with gas embolization, and thrombocytopenia. With newer assist devices on the horizon[83] and the success of percutaneous transluminal coronary angioplasty, temporary assistance may provide support until definitive therapy can be undertaken.

With refractory cardiogenic shock, heart transplantation should be considered. The 1-year survival for heart transplant recipients exceeds 80%, with a 5-year survival of 50–60%.[67] Certainly, surgical approaches should be explored when cardiogenic shock cannot otherwise be managed.

Cardiac Tamponade

The accumulation of fluid or blood in the pericardial space resulting in a fall in cardiac output due to insufficient inflow of blood to the ventricles results in tamponade. The amount of fluid necessary to cause pericardial tamponade is variable, depending on the rapidity of accumulation. Rapid accumulation of as little as 250 ml can result in tamponade, whereas over 1000 ml can accumulate slowly in the pericardial space without tamponade. The most common cause of tamponade is blood in the pericardial space following cardiac surgery, trauma, tuberculosis, or tumor. However, other etiologies include acute viral or idiopathic pericarditis, postradiation pericarditis, and renal failure. Clinical manifestations of tamponade include dyspnea, jugular venous distention, and low arterial blood pressure with very distant heart sounds. Electrical alternans may be seen on the electrocardiogram and distention of the jugular veins on inspiration (Kussmaul's sign) may also be noted. Another finding suggestive of pericardial tamponade is a paradoxical occurrence of greater than 10 mm Hg inspiratory decrease in systolic arterial pressure. Equalization of pulmonary artery wedge, right atrial, right ventricular, and pulmonary artery diastolic pressures with low cardiac output may also be seen.

Treatment of cardiac tamponade must be initiated immediately because pericardiocentesis may be lifesaving. A small catheter advanced over a needle inserted in the pericardial space allows drainage of pericardial fluid and return of cardiac function.

Pulmonary Embolism

Pulmonary embolism is a leading cause of morbidity and mortality in the United States. It has been estimated that pulmonary embolism accounts for over 50,000 deaths annually, although most pulmonary emboli are nonfatal. The vast majority of pulmonary emboli arise in the deep venous system of the lower extremities. The three primary etiologic factors in the development of deep vein thrombosis and subsequent pulmonary embolism are venous stasis, abnormalities of the vessel wall, and alterations in blood coagulation.[84]

Pulmonary embolism should be suspected in any patient

with sudden onset of unexplained dyspnea in association with venous thrombosis.[85] Other symptoms may include substernal chest pain, syncope, cardiac dysrhythmias, worsening of congestive heart failure, or sudden worsening of chronic obstructive lung disease. Pleuritic chest pain and hemoptysis may be present, but only when pulmonary infarction has occurred. Physical examination may be remarkably normal. Rales or wheezing may be noted on auscultation of the lungs. A pleural friction rub or effusion may be present if infarction has occurred. Findings on auscultation of the heart may include tachycardia, right ventricular gallop, wide splitting of the second heart sound, or systolic ejection murmur in the pulmonic area.

Laboratory studies may assist with the diagnosis of pulmonary embolism.[85,86] The electrocardiogram is generally normal aside from tachycardia. However, there may be evidence of right axis deviation, tall peaked P waves, or ST-T wave changes consistent with right ventricular strain. Chest x-ray film findings may be very subtle. Indeed, a normal chest x-ray film does not exclude the possibility of pulmonary embolism and is a common finding. Arterial blood gases associated with pulmonary embolism generally reveal arterial hypoxemia with hypocapnia and respiratory alkalosis. However, normal arterial blood gas analysis does not exclude the possibility of thromboembolic disease.

The diagnosis of pulmonary embolism can be confirmed by radioisotope-tagged and microaggregated albumin perfusion scan along with a xenon ventilation scan. The definitive diagnosis, however, is with pulmonary angiography, which is the only means for providing anatomic information about the pulmonary vasculature.[86] Heparin administration is the initial treatment of pulmonary thromboembolism. Fibrinolytic agents also have been used to dissolve venous thrombi in the pulmonary vasculature. Surgical therapy with formal thoracotomy and thrombectomy produces uniformly poor results.

Thrombolytic Therapy

Streptokinase, urokinase, and tissue plasminogen activator are pharmacologic activators used to accelerate fibrinolysis in patients with massive pulmonary emboli, acute arterial and coronary thrombi, and peripheral venous thrombi. Streptokinase is an indirect activator that forms a complex with plasminogen and initiates fibrinolysis. Urokinase, like tissue plasminogen activator, can directly convert plasminogen to plasmin. Tissue plasminogen activator peripherally activates plasminogen when it is absorbed to fibrin clots.[87] The major complication of fibrinolytic therapy is hemorrhage caused by hypofibrinogenemia and intense systemic fibrinolysis. Therefore, fibrinolytic therapy is not recommended for patients with recent surgery, indwelling cannulas, a history of neurologic lesions, or gastrointestinal bleeding. Indications for fibrinolytic therapy include massive pulmonary emboli, acute peripheral arterial embolism, and extensive iliofemoral thrombophlebitis. The fibrinolysis begins immediately after vascular injury, although clot lysis and vessel recannulation may not be complete for 7–10 days.[88] Fibrinolytic therapy has also gained widespread clinical use in treatment of intracoronary lytic therapy to restore arterial patency and reduce myocardial damage during acute coronary occlusion.[89–91] Indeed, in a recent study, patients with suspected acute anterior or inferior myocardial infarctions had lower early mortality when treated with streptokinase.[90] In particular, tissue plasminogen activator has been used successfully with improved left ventricular

function.[92] Additionally, tissue plasminogen activator can lyse fibrin clots without causing systemic fibrinolysis and bleeding. In a recent review of the effectiveness of tissue-type plasminogen activator and anisoylated plasminogen streptokinase activator complex, short-term mortality in acute myocardial infarction was shown to be significantly reduced by both agents.[91]

RESPIRATORY SYSTEM

Acute Respiratory Failure

Acute respiratory failure in the critically ill patient is often synonymous with the adult respiratory distress syndrome. This is a descriptive term applied to many acute diffuse infiltrative lung lesions with diverse etiology. However, severely diminished lung compliance, refractory hypoxemia, and diffuse radiographic abnormalities are common denominators. Regardless of the initiating event, this form of acute respiratory failure is associated with increased lung water. This type of pulmonary edema is associated with relatively normal cardiac function and "leaky" pulmonary capillaries and has been termed *high permeability pulmonary edema*.[93] The precise incidence of adult respiratory distress syndrome is difficult to determine, although it appears to be increasing.[94] One third of adult deaths from shock and trauma following severe injury result from progressive respiratory failure.[95] Although adult respiratory distress syndrom may be precipitated by many different causes (Table 59-3), the resulting clinical syndrome is the same. The mortality rate remains higher than 50% despite current supportive therapy and treatment modalities.[94,96]

Pathophysiology

Following injury to the lung with damage of the alveolar capillary membrane, there is an increased permeability of the capillary endothelium and alveolar epithelium, with leakage of plasma and erythrocytes into the interstitial and alveolar spaces. In addition, there is proliferation of Type II pneumocytes, which probably aid in the restoration of the integrity of the capillary-endothelial lining.[97]

Although platelet aggregation occurs, the major alterations in lung function relate to leukoaggregation on endothelial surfaces.[98] Indeed, bronchoalveolar lavage fluid from patients with adult respiratory distress syndrome contains an accumulation of neutrophils and leukocyte elastase.[99] These cells release mediators of inflammation such as leukotrienes, thromboxanes, and prostaglandins. These leukoagglutinins are caused by activation of complete factor C5a.[100] Thus, complement activation, a frequent accompaniment of trauma, sepsis, and other predisposing clinical insults, may explain the leukoaggregates commonly found in

---

TABLE 59-3. Conditions Associated with Adult Respiratory Distress Syndrome

Shock	Fat or air embolism
Aspiration	Burns
Sepsis	Drug ingestion
Trauma	Uremia
Pancreatitis	Massive blood transfusion
Head injury	Cardiopulmonary bypass
Radiation of thorax	Drowning

the lungs of patients with adult respiratory distress syndrome.[101] With release of toxic oxygen radicals and lysosomal proteases, these aggregated neutrophils damage the endothelial cells by destruction of structural protein and promotion of local inflammatory reactions.[96]

In addition to leukoaggregates, microemboli are commonly found in patients with adult respiratory distress syndrome at autopsy.[102] Indeed, platelet and coagulation abnormalities have been implicated in the pathogenesis of the syndrome. Trauma, sepsis, and other predisposing conditions can activate the coagulation system, either by release of thromboplastin from soft tissue injury or through complement activation of the coagulation cascade. This results in platelet adhesiveness and aggregation which, along with the generation of fibrin, produce microemboli that are washed into the pulmonary vasculature.[103] These defects have been clearly demonstrated by wedge angiography and correlated with the severity of lung injury.[104]

Clinical Manifestations

Patients may be asymptomatic immediately following insult. The earliest signs are frequently tachypnea followed by dyspnea. Arterial blood gas analysis generally reveals a respiratory alkalosis caused by hyperventilation and mild hypoxemia. At this time, administration of supplementation oxygen frequently improves arterial oxygenation. As the disease progresses, however, hypoxemia cannot be corrected by increasing inspired oxygen concentrations because hypoxemia is the result of right-to-left shunting of blood through collapsed or fluid-filled alveoli. Mechanical ventilatory support with positive airway pressure therapy is then required to maintain adequate oxygenation.[105]

Treatment

Certainly, early recognition and prompt initiation of therapy are essential. The cornerstone of therapy is to ensure adequate tissue oxygenation. An indwelling arterial cannula is useful to monitor arterial blood pressure and allow access for measurement of arterial blood gases and other laboratory values. A pulmonary artery catheter aids immeasurably in optimizing fluid management. A Foley catheter is important to ensure close and accurate measurement of urine output. Bronchial hygiene is an important aspect of the management of these patients. Antibiotics should be used only if evidence of infection is present, and treatment should be guided by the results of cultures and antibiotic sensitivity testing. Prophylactic antibiotics are not indicated and may cause a drug-resistant infection. The use of high-dose corticosteroids in the treatment of adult respiratory distress syndrome remains controversial despite their widespread clinical use. Theoretical advantages of steroids include inhibition of complement-induced granulocyte aggregation, disaggregation of neutrophils, and limitation of the increase in lung microvascular permeability. However, a recent prospective double-blind, placebo-controlled trial of methylprednisolone therapy found no difference in mortality.[106]

Fluid management in patients with adult respiratory distress syndrome presents a clinical dilemma. Fluid is constantly lost through the alveolar capillary membrane into the lung parenchyma. Yet, adequate circulatory volume is essential to restore the perfusion important in reversal of lung damage. Therefore, it is crucial that fluid administration be judicious. It is best guided by the use of a balloon-tipped, flow-directed pulmonary artery catheter. Diuretics and vasoactive agents can be used to maximize tissue oxygen delivery. Fluid replacement with crystalloid or colloid solution remains controversial.[107,108] Regardless of the choice, meticulous attention must be given to fluid balance.

If adequate oxygenation cannot be maintained with an increased inspired oxygen concentration, mechanical ventilatory support should be instituted. The supportive benefits of positive end-expiratory pressure (PEEP) therapy are well documented.[109] The clinical goals include improvement in arterial oxygenation, decrease in the work of breathing, and improvement in ventilation-perfusion inequality. With diffuse lung injury, PEEP improves functional residual capacity, compliance, and arterial oxygenation. In addition, PEEP decreases shunting, dead space ventilation, and venous admixture. This allows adequate arterial oxygenation with a lower inspired oxygen concentration.[81]

Several criteria have been applied in attempting to define the clinical end point for PEEP therapy.[110] Indices used include arterial oxygen tension, alveolar-arterial oxygen gradient, shunt fraction, compliance, and oxygen delivery.[111,112] The usual clinical approach is to increase PEEP in increments of 3 cm H_2O to 5 cm H_2O and obtain appropriate measurements. Certainly, the optimal PEEP level chosen for any individual must fulfill the oxygenation as well as hemodynamic needs of that patient.[113] The appropriate level depends on the degree of hypoxemia, the type of lung disorder, the functional residual capacity of the lungs, the presence of pre-existing pulmonary disease, lung compliance, the state of hydration, and the status of left ventricular function.

Although PEEP therapy is an integral part of the treatment of acute respiratory failure, it causes complex hemodynamic effects. Changes in airway pressure can be anticipated to impact on the heart and great vessels within the thorax. Potential adverse effects of PEEP include impaired venous return,[114] decreased ventricular filling,[115] increased pulmonary vascular resistance,[116] interference with subendocardial blood flow,[117] reduced left ventricular afterload, and altered configuration and compliance of the right and left ventricles.[118] In addition to hemodynamic alterations, PEEP may cause interstitial emphysema, pneumothorax, and pneumomediastinum.[119] Other effects of PEEP therapy include changes in ICP,[120] alterations in renal function,[121] and abnormalities in hepatic and gastrointestinal function.[122,123]

Research on adult respiratory distress syndrome has emphasized the mechanism of lung injury in the hope of identifying a marker that would facilitate its early recognition. Current investigation is directed at altering the pathogenic sequence of increased alveolar capillary permeability and destruction of pulmonary structure.[124,125] Some experimental therapeutic interventions, including anticoagulation, extracorporeal membrane oxygenation[126] cyclo-oxygenase inhibitors, oxygen free radical scavenger therapy, anti-endotoxin antibody therapy, and prostaglandin E therapy, have not yet proved to be of definite benefit to patients with adult respiratory distress syndrome and await further prospective, controlled clinical trials.

Mechanical Ventilation

Types of Ventilators

There are three kinds of mechanical ventilators. The simplest mechanical ventilators are those that substitute for diaphragmatic function, such as the pneumobelt or rocking bed. These devices have limited utility and are used only in patients with neuromuscular disease and normal lung function. A second kind of mechanical ventilator is the intermittent negative pressure ventilator. These devices artificially produce a negative extrathoracic pressure during inspiration to substitute for the pleural and airway pressures normally produced by contraction of the respiratory muscles. Examples of this form of mechanical ventilation include the chest cuirass and iron lung. These devices are best suited for patients with respiratory muscle dysfunction and normal lungs.

The third kind of mechanical ventilator, and the one most commonly used today, is the intermittent positive-pressure ventilator. In this system, gas is directed under positive airway pressure into the lungs. The major advantages of intermittent positive-pressure ventilation are the ability to ventilate the lungs adequately despite increased airway resistance or decreased lung compliance, patient accessibility, and access for bronchial hygiene. The mean airway pressure is positive with intermittent positive-pressure ventilation, so that venous return is compromised and cardiac performance may be impaired.[127] Most of the positive pressure ventilators in common clinical use today are volume ventilators that deliver a preset volume to the patient's lungs. Cycling of standard ventilators occurs whenever a certain volume or pressure is reached or at a preset time interval. When positive PEEP is added to intermittent positive-pressure ventilation, it is called continuous positive pressure ventilation.

In recent years, mechanical ventilators have become very sophisticated and complex.[128] The current microprocessor-based new generation of mechanical ventilators is a logical extension of earlier counterparts. The newest generation of adult mechanical ventilators offers more modes of ventilation, intrinsic microprocessors, computer-compatible monitoring or control, and extensive patient data monitoring and collection in a highly versatile and flexible ventilating device.[129] The microprocessor control, in addition, reduces the number of moving components, enhances data management, and allows upgrading or addition of new features with only a change in software. However, many of the new methods of ventilation available must await the results of rigorously controlled, objective, double-blind, randomized studies. The most common ventilatory modes available today with standard positive pressure ventilators are controlled-mode ventilation, assist controlled-mode ventilation, and intermittent or synchronized intermittent mandatory ventilation. Newer ventilatory modalities include pressure support ventilation, high-frequency ventilation, extended mandatory minute ventilation, airway pressure release ventilation, pressure control ventilation, and pressure control inverse ratio ventilation. (Fig. 59-1).

Controlled Mechanical Ventilation. Controlled mechanical ventilation of the lungs is the oldest mode of intermittent positive-pressure ventilation. The ventilator obligatorily delivers a gas at a preset rate and volume independent of patient effort or response. The patient is unable to alter or influence any portion of the ventilatory cycle. Thus, a patient with an intact ventilatory drive often must be hyper-

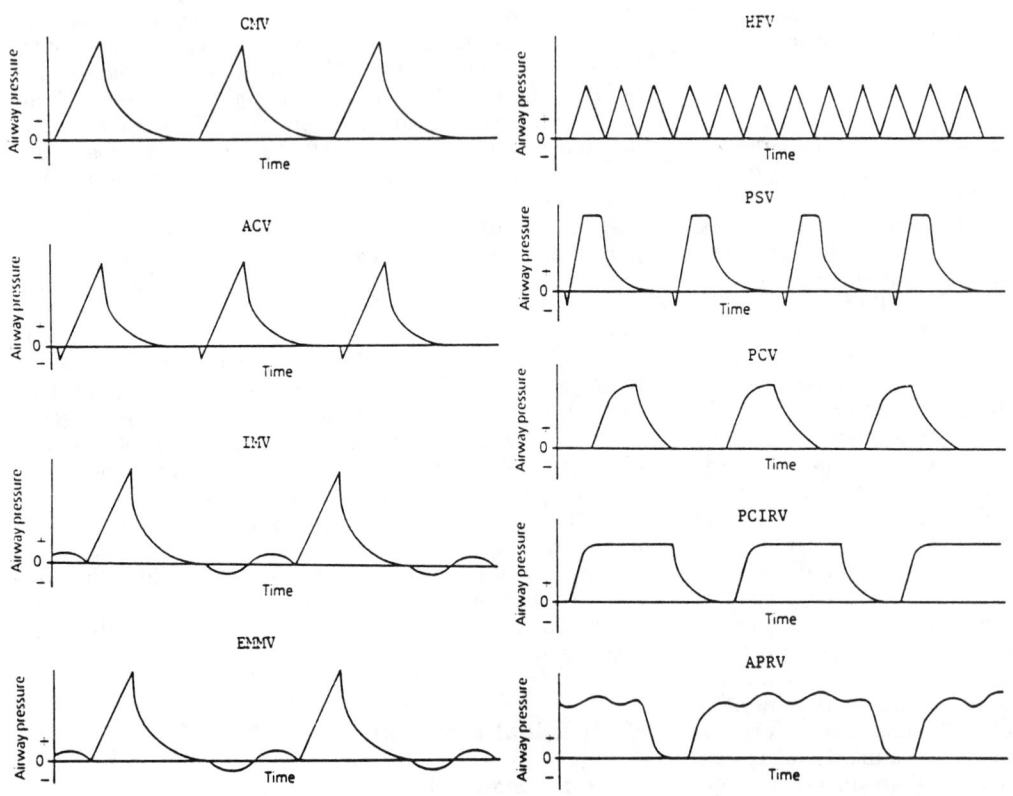

Figure 59-1. Airway pressure waveforms. (CMV = controlled mechanical ventilation; ACV = assist control ventilation; IMV = intermittent mandatory ventilation; EMMV = extended mandatory minute ventilation; HFV = high-frequency ventilation; PSV = pressure support ventilation; PCV = pressure control ventilation; PCIRV = pressure control inverse ratio ventilation; APRV = airway pressure release ventilation.)

ventilated or given sedatives or muscle relaxants to diminish the tendency to breathe asynchronously with the ventilator. In addition, mean airway pressure is highest with this form of intermittent positive-pressure ventilation.[130]

Assist Control Ventilation. Assist mechanical ventilation, or assist control, is an intermittent positive-pressure ventilation mode in which the patient creates a sub-baseline pressure in the inspiratory limb of the ventilator circuit that triggers the ventilator to deliver a predetermined tidal volume. If the patient's ventilatory rate falls below a preset level, the machine automatically enters the control mode.[130]

Intermittent Mandatory Ventilation. Intermittent mandatory ventilation is a mode of intermittent positive-pressure ventilation in which the ventilator delivers a preset volume at a specified interval while also providing a continuous flow of gas for spontaneous ventilation. The patient spontaneously breathes gas with the same temperature, humidity, and oxygen concentration as the ventilator provides while the ventilator delivers a preset tidal volume at predetermined intervals through a parallel ventilatory circuit.

Synchronized Intermittent Mandatory Ventilation. Synchronized intermittent mandatory ventilation is a mode using a combination of assist control with a mechanism and circuitry that allows for independent spontaneous ventilation. In this mode the patient may spontaneously breathe through the circuit, while at a predetermined interval the spontaneous breath is assisted by the machine. Therefore, a positive pressure breath is always in synchrony with the patient's spontaneous ventilatory pattern. In this system a pressure-sensing device is located near the patient's airway that detects the initiation of a spontaneous breath; this activates the ventilator or the demand flow device. The major disadvantage of the demand flow system is the delay in providing adequate gas flow, which can result in increased work of breathing.

Pressure Support Ventilation. Pressure support ventilation is a form of ventilation that aids normal breathing with a predetermined level of positive airway pressure. Pressure support ventilation is similar to intermittent positive-pressure ventilation but differs in that airway pressure is held constant throughout the inspiratory period. Pressure support ventilation differs from conventional volume-cycled ventilation in that the clinician selects only the inspiratory pressure. The patient controls ventilatory timing and interacts with the delivered pressure to determine the inspiratory flow and tidal volume. The unique waveforms of pressure and flow produced by pressure support ventilation may have an advantage by providing better support of spontaneous tidal volume and by decreasing the overall work of breathing.[131] The objective of pressure support ventilation is to increase the patient's spontaneous tidal volume by delivering airway pressure to achieve volumes equal to 10 ml·kg^{-1} to 12 ml·kg^{-1}. Pressure support ventilation may also decrease airway resistance by increasing air flow during inspiration and thereby decrease the work of breathing and delay muscle fatigue. Indeed, the literature suggests that pressure support ventilation can reduce ventilatory workload, prevent diaphragmatic fatigue, compensate for the additional work of breathing caused by poorly functioning demand valves and undersized endotracheal tubes, improve patient-ventilator synchrony, and facilitate weaning.[132-138] Unfortunately, to date there are few clinical studies docu-

menting the efficacy of this new ventilatory mode, although theoretical advantages and safety of the mode in appropriately monitored patients support its use. Further studies are required to better evaluate the complex process of ventilatory reflexes and muscle conditioning during mechanical ventilation in order to fully establish the proper role of pressure support ventilation.

Extended Mandatory Minute Ventilation. Extended mandatory minute ventilation provides a preset minute volume of gas either from a positive pressure breath or from spontaneous breathing. The clinician determines the minimal accepted minute volume and selects the appropriate rate and volume. As the patient's ability to spontaneously breathe improves, less assisted ventilation is provided.[139] Application of extended mandatory minute ventilation may enhance the weaning process by encouraging spontaneous breathing and enabling the patient to adjust to short-term changes in oxygen demand.[140] Extended mandatory minute ventilation may also prove useful in tailoring tidal volume and respiratory rate more closely to meet patient needs. It may encourage patients who have become ventilator-dependent to use their respiratory muscles.

Airway Pressure Release Ventilation. Airway pressure release ventilation was designed to augment ventilation for those patients with decreased lung compliance.[141,142] The system is designed to provide alveolar ventilation as an adjunct to continuous positive airway pressure by intermittent and transient release of positive pressure, followed by restoration of pressure back to the continuous positive airway pressure level. The duration and frequency of continuous positive airway pressure release provide whatever level of ventilation is required. Because the peak airway pressure during airway pressure release ventilation equals the level of continuous positive airway pressure, cardiovascular depression, barotrauma, and ventilation-perfusion mismatch associated with conventional forms of ventilatory support may be expected to decrease. Theoretical advantages of airway pressure release ventilation over conventional positive pressure ventilatory techniques include its lower peak and mean airway pressures, improved arterial oxygenation, and smaller physiologic dead space ventilation.[142] These advantages may lead to less depression of cardiac function as well as a decreased incidence of barotrauma. It differs from the inverse inspiratory to expiratory ratio (I:E) ventilation in that with airway pressure release ventilation, the patient breathes in an unrestricted manner during all parts of the ventilatory cycle. In contradistinction, an inverse I:E ratio requires skeletal muscle paralysis, sedation, or hyperventilation because no gas flow is available for spontaneous breathing during mechanical inspiration. Certainly, further study is necessary to better define the role of airway pressure release ventilation.

High-Frequency Ventilation. High-frequency ventilation was originally used as a technique to provide adequate oxygenation and alveolar ventilation for rigid bronchoscopy and laryngeal surgery.[143] Since that time, the literature is replete with clinical applications of high-frequency ventilation. It is important to note that there are several different modalities to provide high-frequency ventilation. These ventilatory modes include high-frequency positive-pressure ventilation,[144] high-frequency jet ventilation,[145] high-frequency flow interrupters,[146] and high-frequency oscillation.[147] Several reviews of high-frequency ventilation are available.[148-152] The common characteristic of all forms of high-frequency ventilation is ventilation at low tidal volumes (less than dead space) with high rates (60–3000 breaths·min^{-1}). These systems enhance diffusive transport, minimize bulk transport, and improve intrapulmonary gas distribution. Problems described with high-frequency ventilation include inadequate humidification, barotrauma, necrotizing tracheobronchitis, hepatocellular injury, bronchospasm, and inadequate monitoring capabilities.[152] Thus, although high-frequency ventilation is effective in maintaining pulmonary gas exchange at lower mean airway pressures, its precise role is yet to be determined.

Pressure Control Ventilation. Pressure control ventilation is a patient or time-triggered, pressure-limited, time-cycled mode of ventilatory support. It is characterized by a rapid rise to peak pressure afforded by a decelerating inspiratory flow pattern. A pressure-controlled breath can be delivered in intermittent mandatory ventilation or assist mechanical ventilation instead of volume-oriented breaths, or in conjunction with pressure support ventilation. The potential advantage of pressure control ventilation is that because flow rate is geared to reach peak inspiratory pressure quickly, flow will exceed patient demand and, therefore, improve patient-ventilator synchrony and decrease the work of breathing. Further, pressure control ventilation might potentially improve distribution of gas within the lung by using the decelerating flow pattern and square wave air pressure pattern. The major disadvantage of pressure control ventilation is that tidal volume varies as compliance and resistance of the airways change.

Pressure Control Inverse Ratio Ventilation. Pressure control inverse ratio ventilation is a time-triggered, pressure-limited, time-cycled mode of ventilation characterized by a decelerating inspiratory flow pattern, square wave air pressure pattern, and inspiratory-to-expiratory ratio of greater than or equal to 1:1. The potential advantage of this mode of ventilation is the recruitment of collapsed alveoli by prolonged inspiratory times, which allow alveolar units with slow time constants to fill. This improves both oxygenation and ventilation. Potential hazards include the development of auto-PEEP and consequent high airway pressures. Further prospective randomized controlled trials are necessary to determine the benefits to patients from the use of pressure control inverse ratio ventilation.

Have all the advances in technology and new ventilatory modalities had an impact on the outcome of critically ill patients in the ICU? Clearly, for select patient populations, ventilatory support has improved survival. For example, in the infant respiratory distress syndrome, this has been accomplished by the use of continuous positive airway pressure.[153] Outcome has been similarly affected in patients with neuromuscular paralysis by the use of simple mechanical ventilation. However, despite all the newer ventilatory modalities available, little impact has been made on many other patient groups. The adult form of adult respiratory distress syndrome has not shown the documentable increase in survival obtained in infant respiratory distress syndrome. Further, in patients with multiple organ system failure, including respiratory failure requiring mechanical support, outcome is determined more by the underlying cause than by the technique of mechanical ventilatory support. Despite an increasingly sophisticated array of mechanical support devices and detailed physiologic methodologies for augmenting support, little or no further increment

of survival has been demonstrated in patients whose lungs are commonly ventilated with underlying sepsis and multiple organ failure. Certainly, ventilatory support has a place in effecting outcome in critical illness, although newer ventilatory techniques and technology must await further evaluation.

Cystic Fibrosis

Cystic fibrosis is an inherited multisystem disorder characterized by abnormalities in exocrine gland function. The most common cause of morbidity and mortality in patients with cystic fibrosis is pulmonary dysfunction.[154] Pancreatic dysfunction is also a common accompaniment, as is hepatobiliary and genitourinary disease. The median survival time for patients with cystic fibrosis is about 20 years. However, with improvements in diagnosis and treatment, many patients survive through the third and fourth decades of life.

All levels of the respiratory tract can be involved with cystic fibrosis. Nasal polyposis, sinusitis, and lower respiratory tract disease are common findings in these patients. The common denominator is the alteration in mucus secretion. These patients have large amounts of secretion that predispose them to bacterial pneumonia, particularly with *Pseudomonas aeruginosa*.

Other organ systems involved with cystic fibrosis include the gastrointestinal and genitourinary systems and the sweat glands.[155] Pancreatic insufficiency leading to protein and fat malabsorption is common, and recurrent pancreatitis may occur. Hepatobiliary disease is common in older patients with chronic cholestasis, inflammation, fibrosis, and even cirrhosis. Extrahepatic disease of the biliary system and abnormalities of the genitourinary tract are also common.

Abnormality in sweat gland function is the most reliable diagnostic test for cystic fibrosis. Examination of sweat of patients with cystic fibrosis reveals elevations of sodium, potassium, and chloride levels.[156] This increase in electrolyte content results from a failure of reabsorption in the sweat duct.

Treatment of patients with cystic fibrosis is primarily directed at the respiratory system. Every attempt must be made to increase mechanical drainage and clear secretions with chest physiotherapy and exercise programs. Control of bacterial infection with antibiotic therapy is essential. Bronchodilators should be used to reverse any bronchospastic component of the lung disease. Fluid management and general supportive measures are essential to successful treatment.[157]

RENAL SYSTEM

Acute Renal Failure

Acute renal failure is impairment of the normal homeostatic functions of the kidney resulting in retention of nitrogenous wastes. It is a common problem occurring in 5% of all hospitalized patients.[158] It is particularly problematic in critically ill patients, in whom the incidence of acute renal failure is approximately 23%.[159] Despite advances in understanding the disease process, mortality remains high.[158-160] Sixty percent of all cases of acute renal failure are related to surgery or trauma. The most common cause is renal ischemia with sepsis, hypovolemic shock, and nephrotoxic agents as major etiologic factors. The site of interference with renal function may be prerenal, renal, or postrenal.

Prerenal Causes

Prerenal causes of acute renal failure result from hypoperfusion of the kidneys, most commonly from extracellular fluid volume contraction. Reduced renal perfusion results from decreased effective circulating volume due to hypovolemia or redistribution of circulating volume. Reduction in cardiac output can also result in prerenal failure because of inadequate perfusion of the kidneys. This may result from primary myocardial disease, valvular heart disease, constrictive pericarditis, or cardiac tamponade. Decreased perfusion of the kidneys may also result from vascular disease of both large and small vessels. Certainly, bilateral renal artery stenosis can cause prerenal azotemia. However, although most prerenal causes of renal failure are accompanied by hypotension, renal artery stenosis is usually associated with hypertension.

Intrinsic Renal Causes

Intrinsic renal causes of acute renal failure can be divided by the component of the kidney most affected i.e., the glomeruli, blood vessels, and the tubulointerstitial region. Glomerular diseases account for 5–10% of all cases of acute renal failure[161] and may be caused by direct immunologically mediated injury or decreased renal perfusion. Vascular disease can result in intrinsic renal failure primarily caused by either thromboembolic injury or systemic diseases.

Acute tubular necrosis is the most common cause of acute renal failure in critically ill patients and accounts for over 75% of the renal causes of kidney failure. The two major causes of acute tubular necrosis are ischemia and nephrotoxins.[162] Renal ischemia is the most common cause of acute renal failure and may be caused by a variety of clinical conditions, including volume depletion, shock, and operations that interrupt the renal circulation. It appears that prostaglandins play an important role in maintaining renal perfusion; therefore patients taking drugs that inhibit prostaglandin synthesis may be predisposed to renal injury with hypoperfusion.

Nephrotoxic agents may also cause acute tubular necrosis. Categories of toxins include antibiotics, contrast material, anesthetic drugs, heavy metals, and organic solvents. In the past heavy metals, organic solvents, and glycols were a common cause of acute renal failure. However, today aminoglycosides have supplanted them as the major nephrotoxic cause of acute renal failure.[163] All aminoglycosides have nephrotoxic potential. Clinical nephrotoxicity, defined as a decrease in glomerular filtration rate, occurs in 5–25% of patients receiving aminoglycosides. The toxicity of these antibiotics is enhanced by advanced age, pre-existing renal dysfunction, concomitant administration of other nephrotoxic agents, and hypotension. Renal toxicity can also occur with antibiotics other than aminoglycosides, including cephalosporins, penicillins, and amphotericin B.

Toxic acute renal failure associated with the use of radiocontrast media is the second most common cause of nephrotoxic acute tubular necrosis. Patients particularly at risk for radiocontrast-induced renal failure include those with diabetes mellitus, the elderly, and those with pre-existing renal insufficiency. Dehydration compounds the risk in susceptible patients.

Methoxyflurane is the most common of the anesthetic drugs described to precipitate acute renal failure. Anesthetic-induced nephrotoxicity is generally attributable to fluoride toxicity. Because toxicity results from high free fluoride levels in the plasma, prolonged duration of anesthesia and pre-existing renal dysfunction appear to put patients at risk for methoxyflurane nephrotoxicity.[160] Several common chemotherapeutic drugs can also cause acute tubular necrosis, including cisplatin and high-dose methotrexate.[160] Adequate extracellular fluid volume expansion and concomitant use of diuretics may significantly lessen nephrotoxic effects of cisplatin, and alkalinization of the urine may decrease toxicity of high-dose methotrexate. Rhabdomyolysis has become an important cause of acute renal failure described in association with crush injuries, extensive burns, muscle inflammation, and a variety of settings in which muscle blood flow and metabolism are disturbed or muscle energy production is increased. The toxic effect of myoglobin causes acute tubular necrosis with rhabdomyolysis, just as hemoglobin is the toxic pigment in acute tubular necrosis associated with hemolysis from mismatched blood.

An increasing number of drugs have been associated with acute interstitial nephritis and subsequent acute renal failure.[164] The most common cause of acute interstitial nephritis is an acute drug-induced hypersensitivity reaction. Drugs commonly implicated include beta-lactam antibiotics (especially methicillin), nonsteroidal anti-inflammatory agents, and diuretics. Acute interstitial nephritis is associated with an increased eosinophil count in blood and urine.

Postrenal Causes

Postrenal causes of acute renal failure may be asymptomatic and must be considered in any patient with renal failure. This form of acute deterioration of renal function is often reversible and occurs in up to 10% of patients with decreasing renal function.[165] Obstruction to urine flow may occur at any level from the kidney to the bladder. Ureteral obstruction from calculi, clots, tumor, stricture, retroperitoneal fibrosis, or malignancy may cause ureteral obstruction, whereas bladder tumors or a neurogenic bladder can result in obstruction at the level of the bladder. Urethral obstruction can be caused by prostate disorders, urethral stricture, cervical carcinoma, or meatal stenosis. In most cases of possible obstruction, a combination of a flat abdominal film, renal scan, and ultrasonogram can supply as much information as excretory urography with much less risk.[165] However, if the clinical history is suggestive of obstruction, even if the noninvasive studies are negative, cystoscopy and retrograde pyelography should be considered.

Oliguric *Versus* Nonoliguric Acute Renal Failure

In the past acute renal failure was often defined by oliguria, the production of less than 400 ml·day^{-1} of urine. However, nonoliguric acute renal failure is now recognized as a distinct clinical entity with a more favorable prognosis.[166] Hospitalization time, complications, and mortality are less in nonoliguric patients. Drugs that increase solute excretion, such as mannitol and furosemide, may have the capacity to convert oliguric acute renal failure to the nonoliguric type. Some authors suggest that high doses of intravenous furosemide be given to attenuate the course of acute renal failure, whereas others claim that furosemide responders simply may have less severe renal impairment. The results are still controversial, and the efficacy of furosemide may depend on its administration in the initiation phase of acute renal failure. Nonetheless, after prerenal and postrenal factors contributing to azotemia have been corrected, a trial of furosemide 2–10 mg·kg^{-1} can be given in an attempt to convert an incipient oliguric renal failure to a nonoliguric state with restoration of blood volume if diuresis ensues.[165]

Urinary Indices

Urine sediment is almost never normal in acute renal failure.[167] A chemical profile of the urine aids immeasurably in assessing the cause of acute renal failure. In prerenal azotemia, tubular function remains relatively intact, and sodium and water resorption results. There is an increase in sodium loss in the urine in patients with acute tubular necrosis because tubular function is impaired (Table 59-4).[168] In acute oliguric renal failure, daily increases of blood urea nitrogen and serum creatinine average 10 mg·dl^{-1} to 20 mg·dl^{-1}, and 0.5 mg·dl^{-1} to 1 mg·dl^{-1}, respectively. If creatinine is elevated out of proportion to the blood urea nitrogen it suggests that rhabdomyolysis may be the etiology of acute renal failure. The rapid rise in serum creatinine levels with rhabdomyolysis is attributable to the release of creatine from skeletal muscle; creatine is converted by nonenzymatic hydrolysis to creatinine.[169]

Complications of Acute Renal Failure

Hyponatremia, edema, and pulmonary congestion can occur with oliguric acute renal failure as a result of salt and water overload. In addition, serum potassium concentration may rise because of the decreased elimination of potassium associated with acute renal failure. The usual rate of increase in serum potassium in the noncatabolic, oliguric patient is 0 mEq to 0.5 mEq 24 hr^{-1}. If potassium increases at a greater rate, other contributing factors should be sought and treated. Other electrolyte abnormalities present in acute renal failure include hyperphosphatemia, hypocalcemia, and mild hypermagnesemia. These abnormalities must be monitored closely and treated accordingly.

Because the kidneys can no longer eliminate the daily production of nonvolatile acid, there is a daily decrease of 1 mEq–2 mEq in plasma bicarbonate levels, with a resultant anion gap metabolic acidosis. Still other complications include anemia, platelet abnormalities, and altered host defenses leading to an increased incidence of infection. Gastrointestinal complications include nausea, vomiting, and, most commonly, gastrointestinal hemorrhage that occurs in 10–30% of patients.

Treatment

Mortality rates of patients with acute renal failure vary from 30–60%. However, if acute renal failure follows surgery or trauma, the mortality may be as high as 70%. The first step in the management of acute renal failure is to exclude remedial causes. Specifically, identification and correction of prerenal and postrenal factors are essential. The treatment of acute renal failure includes diuresis and control of the extracellular fluid volume, treatment of hyperkalemia and acidosis, prophylaxis against infection and gastrointestinal

TABLE 59-4. Diagnostic Urinary Indices

Parameter	Prerenal	Renal
Urinary osmolality	>500 mOsm	<350 mOsm
Urine/plasma creatinine	>30	<20
Urine sodium concentration	<20 mEq·l^{-1}	>40 mEq·l^{-1}
Fractional excretion of sodium	<1%	>2%
Renal failure index	<1%	>2%

bleeding, nutritional support, and dialysis. Since the prognosis is better with polyuria than with anuria, efforts should be made to produce and maintain a polyuric state. Intake and output must be monitored closely.

Conservative therapy is frequently ineffective for critically ill patients with acute renal failure; therefore some form of dialytic therapy is usually indicated. The absolute indications for dialysis include symptomatic uremia, development of resistant hyperkalemia, severe acidemia or fluid overload not responsive to conservative therapy, and pericarditis. In addition, many advocate maintaining a blood urea nitrogen level less than 100 mg·dl^{-1} and a creatinine level less than 8 mg·dl^{-1}. Inadequate nutrition has been recognized as a reason for dialysis. Both hemodialysis and peritoneal dialysis have been used to manage acute renal failure, and survival data are similar.[170] Each method has unique advantages and disadvantages.

Recently, several modifications of hemodialysis have been applied to patients with acute renal failure. These include slow continuous ultrafiltration with intermittent hemodialysis, continuous arteriovenous hemodialysis, and continuous arteriovenous hemofiltration. All of these methods provide excellent hemodynamic stability. Access to blood is obtained either by percutaneous cannulation of the femoral artery and vein or by way of an arteriovenous shunt. No blood pump is used in this system because blood is driven by the patient's own arterial pressure. In continuous arterial venous hemofiltration, large amounts of ultrafiltrate are removed through a porous filter with the ultrafiltrate replaced by sterile intravenous fluid.[171] In slow continuous ultrafiltration, much smaller volumes of ultrafiltrate are removed to correct any extracellular fluid volume expansion. However, intermittent dialysis is required to control uremia, hyperkalemia, and acidemia.[172] With continuous arterial venous hemodialysis, dialysate flows through the dialysate compartment at approximately 20 ml·min^{-1}, which is sufficient to achieve a low, steady-state blood urea nitrogen and creatinine levels.[173] Unfortunately, the various improvements in resuscitative techniques and technical advances in dialytic therapy have not reduced the mortality of acute renal failure.

Hepatorenal Syndrome

Acute renal failure in the presence of severe advanced liver disease in the absence of clinical, laboratory, or anatomic evidence of other causes of renal dysfunction is known as hepatorenal syndrome. It is usually an oliguric form of renal failure with low urinary sodium concentrations. The picture appears similar to that of a prerenal azotemia; however, it occurs in the setting of advanced liver disease. The precise mechanism for the renal failure is unknown. Currently, there is no effective treatment for hepatorenal syndrome.

INFECTIOUS DISEASES

Nosocomial Infections

Advances in technology and the use of a greater number of monitoring devices and therapeutic interventions have led to an increased number of infections. Indeed, hospital-acquired infections have emerged as the leading cause of death in most critical care units. These infections are often polymicrobial, involve multiple resistant strains of bacteria, and do not respond to simple therapy. The incidence of nosocomial infections in ICUs is commonly 40–50%, many of which are preventable.[174] The cost implications of prolonged hospitalization and treatment of infection are apparent.[175]

The major determinants of the incidence and outcome of nosocomial infections include patient age, underlying disease, integrity of mucosal and integumentary surfaces, and the status of the immunologic defenses. Common sources of hospital-acquired infections in critically ill patients include the urinary tract, surgical wounds, pneumonia, intravascular devices, and sinusitis. Immunocompromised patients with a deficiency in any of the multifaceted host defenses are particularly prone to these infections and to other unusual infections. In particular, patients with acquired immunodeficiency syndrome commonly present with opportunistic infections caused by viruses, bacteria, parasites, and fungi. These patients invariably die despite transiently effective antimicrobial therapy and current attempts at immune reconstitution.[176]

Urinary Tract Infections

Urinary tract infections account for approximately 40% of hospital-acquired infections.[177] Because most critically ill patients have an indwelling Foley catheter, it is not surprising that the urinary tract is a common source of infection. It is the most common site resulting in gram-negative bacteremia. The urinary tract should be considered a possible source of infection if the patient has bacteriuria and a clinical picture consistent with infection.

Wound Infections

Most surgical wound infections are caused by the introduction of bacteria directly into the tissue at the time of operation. They account for 10% of all infections in postsurgical ICU patients.[178] Wounds should be observed for any signs of infection, and any purulent material should be sampled and sent for Gram's stain and culture. Most wound infections are evident 3–7 days following surgical intervention. Wounds infected within 24 hours are generally fulminant infections caused by *Clostridium* or beta-hemolytic streptococci. Later surgical wound infections are generally caused by gram-negative bacilli, anaerobic bacteria, and staphylococci. The administration of prophylactic antibiotics has aided immeasurably in reducing the postoperative wound infection rate.

Pneumonia

The most serious complication among hospital-acquired infections is lower respiratory tract infection. Hospital-acquired pneumonia occurs in up to 15% of ICU patients and is the leading cause of mortality in this group.[179] The major organisms causing pneumonia in the critically ill patient population are gram-negative bacilli and *Staphylococcus aureus*.[180] The diagnosis of pneumonia in critically ill patients who are maintained on mechanical ventilatory support can be difficult.[179] Physical examination by itself is not an adequate screening procedure.[181,182] Bacterial colonization of the upper airway is common[183,184] and may not reflect lower respiratory tract disease.[185,186] Nosocomial pneumonia is generally diagnosed by signs and symptoms of infection with bacteriologic verification in addition to a new pulmonary infiltrate that is unchanged by physical therapy. Unfortunately, Gram's stain and culture of aspirated material through the endotracheal tube may not be reliable indicators of true lower respiratory tract infection.[187,188] Antibody coating and quantitative cultures have not significantly improved diagnostic efficacy. Protected brush catheter bronchoscopy has recently been advocated as an effective adjunct to the diagnosis of pneumonia for patients maintained on mechanical ventilatory support.[189]

Intravascular Devices

With advances in technology and invasive monitoring, intravascular device-related bacteremia has become a common problem accounting for over 25,000 cases of bacteremia annually.[190] Contamination of intravascular devices may occur anywhere along the line from the infusate bottle to the skin entry site. Predisposition to intravascular device-related bacteremia is determined by both patient and hospital factors. The patient-related factors generally reflect the severity of underlying disease. Hospital-related factors are more controlled and include the type of catheter, the site of insertion, the technique of placement, and the duration of cannulation.[191] Recommendations for prevention of intravascular device–related infections should be based on the Centers for Disease Control guidelines.[192]

Intra-abdominal Infections

Abdominal infections generally occur in patients who have undergone prior intra-abdominal procedures. Risk factors for infection include prolonged operative time, use of foreign substances, inadequate drainage, presence of devitalized tissue, hematoma formation, and fecal contamination at the time of surgery.[193] Acalculous cholecystitis is another potential etiology of abdominal infection in the postoperative period. Stress ulceration with significant gastrointestinal bleeding and perforation, or perforation due to mechanical causes, such as nasogastric drainage, can result in intra-abdominal infection in the absence of prior surgical intervention. The diagnosis of intra-abdominal infection relies primarily on physical examination with adjunctive radiologic evaluation including computed tomographic scan, ultra-sonography, and abdominal roentgenograms.

Sinusitis

One of the recognized complications of nasotracheal intubation is the development of sinusitis. Nosocomial sinusitis accounts for 5% of all nosocomial infections in the critically ill patient population.[194] However, this infection is frequently difficult to diagnose and often goes unrecognized. Patients may present with fever and leukocytosis but with few other signs or symptoms of overt infection. Fewer than half of the patients have purulent nasal drainage. The diagnosis of sinusitis relies on x-ray films of the paranasal sinuses. Unfortunately, these are frequently of suboptimal quality because they are taken in the critical care unit with a portable apparatus. However, if opacification of the sinuses is present or an air-fluid level is noted and aspiration reveals purulent material, the endotracheal tube should be removed and replaced using the oral route along with initiation of antibiotic therapy. Patients generally respond well and rarely require surgical drainage.

Central Nervous System Infections

Nosocomial central nervous system infections are uncommon in critically ill patients unless there are predisposing conditions such as neurosurgical procedures or central nervous system trauma. All pyogenic infections of the cranial contents originate either by hematogenous spread or extension from contiguous sites. Acute meningitis is a medical emergency that requires high level diagnostic and therapeutic skills because it has a significant mortality rate. Patients frequently present with headache, stiff neck, seizures, and altered mental status. In order to differentiate bacterial meningitis from an aseptic meningitis syndrome, analysis of the cerebrospinal fluid is necessary. All febrile patients with lethargy, headache, or confusion of sudden onset, even if only low-grade temperature is present, should be subjected to a lumbar puncture.

Brain abscess has occurred with a constant incidence even with the introduction of broad-spectrum antibiotic coverage. It is associated with a high morbidity and mortality. The most common age of patients for a brain abscess to occur is between 30 and 40 years of age, and it is frequently associated with sinusitis or otitis. Streptococci are the most common etiologic organisms. Treatment is both medical and surgical, with anaerobic antibiotic coverage and surgical drainage. Although mortality has improved, there is still a significant incidence of neurologic residual, primarily seizure disorders.

Fungal Infections

With the use of broad-spectrum antibiotic therapy, organ transplantation, prosthetic cardiac valves, and immunosuppression from neoplasm, transplants, burns, and drugs, there has been an increased incidence of fungal infections. Clinical manifestations range from thrush to disseminated candidiasis. Organs involved with systemic disease include the kidneys, brain, myocardium, and eyes. The hallmark, pathologically, is diffuse microabscesses with a combined suppurative and granulomatous reaction. The diagnosis of candidemia may be difficult because serum antibodies have been uniformly disappointing and culture results are often negative. Although not all patients with candidemia require antifungal therapy, if treatment is indicated, amphotericin B is the drug of choice.

Sepsis Syndrome

The definition of the sepsis syndrome is based on easily acquired clinical data that can be applied to a broad population of patients. The clinical evidence is based on a high index of suspicion and does not require confirmation with positive blood cultures or cultures of material from a closed space. Indeed, the sepsis syndrome can be defined in terms of the systemic response to infection expressed as tachycardia, fever or hypothermia, tachypnea, and evidence of inadequate organ perfusion. That is, the systemic response is what differentiates sepsis from simple infection or bacter-

---

TABLE 59-5. Clinical Features of the Sepsis Syndrome

Clinical evidence of infection
Hypothermia/hyperthermia
Impaired organ function or evidence of inadequate perfusion:
   Altered mentation
   Hypoxemia
   Elevated plasma lactate level
   Oliguria

---

emia. The object of such a broad definition is to facilitate early recognition and prompt institution of therapeutic interventions.

Sepsis has been estimated to occur in 1 out of 100 hospitalized patients in the United States. Although its precise incidence is unknown, it has been estimated that up to 500,000 cases of sepsis occur each year in the United States. When the sepsis syndrome is accompanied by hypotension that is unresponsive to fluid therapy, it is often referred to as septic shock. Shock develops in approximately 40% of patients with sepsis. The increased survival of immunocompromised patients, those receiving organ transplants, and those with malignancy and inflammatory disease as well as the use of invasive medical devices and procedures has increased the incidence of sepsis.

The two primary criteria for the diagnosis of the sepsis syndrome are (1) clinical evidence of infection such as tachycardia, tachypnea, and hyperthermia or hypothermia, and (2) evidence of altered organ perfusion or organ system dysfunction, such as alterations in mental status, arterial hypoxemia, elevated plasma lactate levels, or oliguria (Table 59-5).

The sepsis syndrome can be identified as a systemic manifestation of presumed sepsis. In a recent study of patients with the sepsis syndrome, the mortality rate was nearly 30% of the 382 patients enrolled.[195] Only 45% of these patients had positive blood cultures, and almost 64% either had shock on entry into the study or developed shock after entry. The adult respiratory distress syndrome developed in 25% of these patients. Although the traditional definitions of sepsis (requiring positive blood or closed-space cultures) and of shock were not met by the condition of the majority of patients, the overall mortality rate was significant and similar to that reported by several investigators in patients with sepsis. The incidence of adult respiratory distress syndrome was also similar to that of previously published reports. Clearly, the sepsis syndrome has a clinically significant morbidity and mortality rate. Progression from the sepsis syndrome to the associated clinical sequelae of septic shock and adult respiratory distress syndrome may be prevented by intervention at the onset of the sepsis syndrome. Identification and clinical evaluation of the criteria for the sepsis syndrome may demonstrate an appropriate point for evaluating therapeutic interventions.

Septic Shock

Septic shock is a form of circulatory shock that usually develops as a complication of an overwhelming infection. As with any form of shock, it is a state in which the supply of blood to the tissues of the body is inadequate to meet the body's metabolic demands. It has been estimated that over 300,000 gram-negative bacteremias occur in the United

States each year. When bacteremia is caused by gram-negative bacteria, shock intervenes in up to 40% of these patients with a 40–90% mortality.[196] *Escherichia coli* is the most common causative organism, followed by *Klebsiella*, *Enterobacter*, *Proteus*, *Pseudomonas*, and *Serratia*. As is evident from the causative agents, the sites of infection are usually the urinary, intestinal, biliary, and female genital tracts. Predominantly males over 40 years of age and females between 20 and 45 years of age are affected.[197] Nonspecific predisposing afflictions are quite common, including diabetes mellitus, cirrhosis of the liver, burns, neoplasms, and drug therapy, including chemotherapy and steroids.

Unfortunately, it has become very commonplace to label septic shock as gram-negative shock or endotoxin shock. It appears that gram-negative bacillary endotoxin is only one of the potential culprits in the pathogenesis of the clinical manifestations of the shock syndrome. Indeed, it has been extremely difficult to clinically differentiate between gram-positive and gram-negative infection.[198] The gram-negative bacilli have a complex, three-layered cell wall structure. The lipopolysaccharide component of the outermost layer has been of particular interest because of its association with endotoxin properties.[199,200]

Endotoxin is a complex molecule consisting of an outer core of repetitive sugar moieties, an O-antigen–specific side chain conferring serologic specificity, and an inner core linked to a structure termed lipid A.[201] Endotoxin and other bacterial products activate cell membrane phospholipases to liberate arachidonic acid and initiate synthesis and release of leukotrienes, prostaglandin, and thromboxanes.[202] It is these inflammatory mediators that primarily influence vasomotor tone, microvascular permeability, leukoaggregation, and the aggregation of platelets. Bacterial endotoxin can trigger a cascade of enzymatic processes, which leads to the release of vasoactive kinins, kallikreins in particular.[203] The microorganisms activate the classic complement pathway, whereas endotoxin activates the alternate pathway. Complement activation, leukotriene generation, and the direct effect of endotoxin on neutrophils lead to accumulation of inflammatory cells in the lung. This has been proposed as the underlying mechanism for initiation of acute respiratory distress syndrome, which is a common accompaniment of septic shock.[204] In addition, activation of the intrinsic coagulation cascade *via* a direct effect on Hageman factor leads to activation of the fibrinolytic system and possibly to disseminated intravascular coagulation, which may accompany the shock syndrome.

Hemodynamic alterations in septic shock generally take two forms.[195,200,205-207] Early in shock, the patient may have an increase in cardiac output, vasodilation, decrease in systemic vascular resistance, decrease in central venous pressure, and an increase in stroke volume. As shock progresses, the predominant picture is one of vasoconstriction with an increase in systemic vascular resistance and a decrease in cardiac output, central venous pressure, and stroke volume.

Organ systems involved in septic shock include the cardiac, renal, respiratory, and hematologic systems. Cardiac failure may develop in the setting of sepsis, primarily related to a myocardial depressant factor.[208] Disseminated intravascular coagulation is not uncommon in septic shock. The pathogenesis probably involves the activation of the intrinsic clotting system by Hageman factor leading to activation of kallikrein. This, in turn, activates the potent vasodilator, bradykinin, which promotes pooling of blood in peripheral tissues as well as increases in capillary permeability and localized tissue damage. Respiratory failure is probably the most important cause of death in patients with shock. Septic shock is an important cause of acute respiratory distress syndrome and severe respiratory failure.[204] The kidneys are also target organs in septic shock, with resultant acute renal failure. Oliguria occurs early and probably results from inadequate renal perfusion.

Clinically, gram-negative bacteremia usually begins abruptly with chills, fever, nausea, vomiting, diarrhea, and prostration. When septic shock develops, there is in addition tachycardia, tachypnea, hypotension, cool pale extremities with peripheral cyanosis, mental obtundation, and oliguria.

Laboratory data vary greatly and depend on both the cause and extent of the shock syndrome. There is usually leukocytosis. However, the white blood cell count may be normal or even depressed. Serum bicarbonate is usually low and blood lactate level elevated. Electrolyte pattern may vary considerably, although there is a tendency to hyponatremia and hypochloremia.

Treatment of septic shock is directed at two primary therapeutic goals: (1) rapid reversal of perfusion failure, and (2) identification and control of infection. Certainly, every effort should be made to identify the cause of infection. However, treatment must be initiated early if it is to be successful. Indeed, antibiotic therapy should be initiated immediately and not await blood culture results. Early aggressive intervention, including antibiotics, fluid resuscitation, vasoactive drug support, mechanical ventilatory support, and surgical drainage of any infected site, is essential for successful treatment. Surgical drainage of closed space infections is mandatory, and a vigorous search for the infectious site is indicated in all patients.

Fluid resuscitation is the mainstay of treatment of septic shock. The fluid of choice for volume repletion remains controversial.[209] Regardless of the fluid infused, however, it appears that survival can be improved if stroke volume or cardiac output improves in response to fluid challenge. If volume resuscitation and other supportive measures are inadequate in restoring perfusion, vasoactive drug support may be indicated. Because in the low flow state of hypodynamic septic shock peripheral vascular resistances increase, drugs with predominantly alpha-adrenergic effects should be avoided. Dopamine and dobutamine have been used successfully in treating septic shock. These drugs have predominantly beta-adrenergic effects and result in an increase in cardiac output due to an increase in both contractility and heart rate. It is also important to maintain urine flow in an attempt to prevent renal failure. Urine output should ideally be kept higher than $30 \text{ ml} \cdot \text{hr}^{-1}$–$40 \text{ ml} \cdot \text{hr}^{-1}$, with fluid resuscitation and if necessary diuretic therapy.

Corticosteroids have been advocated in the past as adjunctive therapy to the treatment of septic shock.[210-212] However, more recent studies suggest that the use of high-dose corticosteroids provides no benefit in the treatment of severe sepsis and septic shock and is no longer recommended.[213,214] Efforts are now being directed at developing techniques to facilitate early diagnosis of the septic syndrome, to identify markers of causative organisms, and to discover more promising pharmacologic or immunologic drugs to reduce the still unacceptably high mortality from systemic sepsis. Because bacteremia and septic shock are associated with the release of endotoxin into the circulation, immunotherapy with human polyclonal antiserum or plasma directed against endotoxin core determinants has been shown in trials to reduce mortality in patients with gram-negative bacteremia[215] and to protect high-risk surgical patients from septic shock.[216]

HA-IA is a human monoclonal IgM antibody that binds to the lipid A domain of endotoxin and is produced by the stable heteromyeloma cell line A6(H4C5) developed by Teng et al.[217] Several recent studies have demonstrated that adjunctive therapy with HA-IA in the human monoclonal antibody against endotoxin reduces mortality significantly in patients with sepsis and gram-negative bacteremia.[218]

Other areas of active investigation for the treatment of septic shock include high-dose naloxone,[219] prostaglandin E₁,[220] anticomplement (C5) antibodies,[221] ibuprofen,[222] indomethacin,[223] and antiserum directed against cachectin.[224]

NUTRITION

Adequate nutrition is essential to replace the nutrients used to meet the energy needs of tissues and to repair tissues being catabolized. In the critically ill or injured patient, nutrition is an essential part of treatment (see Chapter 12).[225,227] For patients undergoing surgical procedures, malnutrition is well documented to be a risk factor, and perioperative nutritional support can reduce complications, mortality, morbidity, and length of hospital stay.[228,229]

Nutritional Assessment

Assessment of nutrition is the first step in ensuring adequate support for the critically ill patient. Adequacy of nutrition can be assessed by anthropomorphic measurements, delayed cutaneous hypersensitivity to several antigens, and laboratory measurements reflecting severe protein and calorie malnutrition.[230-233] Nitrogen balance is an important measure of nutritional status. The relationship between urea nitrogen excretion and metabolic rate is attributable to the obligatory oxidation of body cell mass that occurs with stress and starvation. Therefore, the extent of hypermetabolism can be predicted from a simple clinical determination of urea nitrogen collected in a timed urine specimen.

Estimation of Energy Requirement

The Harris-Benedict equation derived from indirect calorimetry measurements provides a reasonable estimate of basal caloric requirements (Table 59-6). Basal energy expenditure calculated in this manner correlates well with values obtained by contemporary techniques of continuous expired air analysis.[234] The goal of nutritional support in nondepleted postoperative patients is to prevent excessive loss of lean tissue, whereas in nutritionally depleted patients it is restoration of lean tissue with concomitant restoration of fat reserves.[235] Calculated basal energy needs should be increased by 30% with sepsis.

Enteral *Versus* Parenteral Nutrition

The gastrointestinal tract is the route of choice for nutritional supplementation whenever possible.[236] There are a variety of commercially available enteral feeding formulas. With near normal proteolytic and lipolytic activity in the gastrointestinal tract, meal replacement formulas can be used. These formulas are polymeric mixtures containing proteins, fats, and carbohydrates in high molecular weight forms. The lactose content is generally low, and fat content represents approximately 30% of the calories. Elemental

TABLE 59-6. Harris-Benedict Equations for Estimation of Basal Energy Expenditure (BEE)

Female: BEE = 655 + (9.6 × Wt) + (1.8 × Ht) − (4.7 × age)
Male: BEE = 66 + (13.7 × Wt) + (5 × Ht) − (6.8 × age)

Wt = weight in kilograms; Ht = height in centimeters; age = age in years.

diets use amino acids as the nitrogen source and usually contain little fat and no lactose. These diets also have a low viscosity that make them particularly useful for infusion through needle catheter jejunostomy tubes. Feeding modules are concentrated sources of one nutrient that can yield a small volume, high caloric mixture when added to a formula diet. This is particularly useful for patients on fluid restriction. A continuous-drip infusion of enteral feedings through a feeding tube is the preferred technique. The most common complication of enteral feedings is diarrhea. Other potential hazards include malpositioning of the feeding tube, hyperglycemia, and abnormalities in liver function tests.

When the enteral route is unavailable or provides inadequate intake for the depleted patient, parenteral nutrition support should be undertaken. Certainly, critically ill patients who are hypercatabolic, nutritionally depleted, or have multiple organ system failure should have total parenteral nutrition administered through a central line.

It is important that adequate calories be supplied to critically ill patients, and distribution of calories provided as carbohydrates, fats, and protein is equally important. Historically, caloric requirements for total parenteral nutrition were given primarily as carbohydrates, which has a respiratory quotient of 1, resulting in a large increase in carbon dioxide production and oxygen consumption. In recent years an appreciation has been gained that fat emulsions supply essential fatty acids in a concentrated source of calories.[237] Because fat emulsions are oxidized with a respiratory quotient of 0.7, carbon dioxide production and ventilatory requirements are reduced.[238]

Although nutritional support has been shown to improve wound healing, decrease morbidity and mortality, and assist in immunocompetence, many complications have been described. Technical complications relate primarily to insertion of the central venous catheter used for access.[239] Other complications of hyperalimentation include sepsis, metabolic abnormalities, electrolyte disturbances, acid-base disorders, hepatic dysfunction, hypercalcemia and pancreatitis, metabolic bone disease, and fluid overload.[240]

DISORDERS OF COAGULATION

There are three essentials for a normal clotting mechanism: (1) vascular integrity, (2) normal platelet function, and (3) normal coagulation factors. The initial step in normal coagulation is compensatory reduction in intravascular pressure of the severed ends of blood vessels, followed by platelets covering the damaged surfaces. They accumulate at the site to ultimately form a hemostatic plug. The coagulation cascade is then activated with the formation of fibrin. Two distinct pathways operate to form thrombin, which then converts fibrinogen into fibrin. The intrinsic pathway produces thrombin from factors present only in the plasma, whereas the extrinsic pathway uses extraplasma tissue factors as well as plasma factors. The final step in the normal coagulation scheme is removal of the fibrin and platelet clot by the fibrinolytic system. The end result of the activation of these pathways is the conversion of plasminogen into plasmin, which cleaves both fibrinogen and fibrin. There is an ongoing equilibrium between the activation of the coagulation system and the activation of the fibrinolytic system.

Disorders in the coagulation system lead either to bleeding or to thrombosis. Clinical evaluation of disorders of coagulation is based on history, physical examination, and laboratory studies. A history of abnormal bleeding or evidence of bleeding on physical examination may assist in making a definitive diagnosis. Laboratory screening tests for hemostatic profile are essential.[241] Such a profile of test should include a platelet count, bleeding time, prothrombin time, partial thromboplastin time, and review of the peripheral blood smear. The prothrombin time is a measure of the efficiency of thrombin formation by the extrinsic pathway. Abnormalities in the prothrombin time can be caused by absence or impairment of any coagulation factor in the intrinsic or extrinsic clotting system. The partial thromboplastin time is used to assess the efficiency of the intrinsic clotting system. Prolongation of the partial thromboplastin time generally represents deficiency or inhibition of Factors I, II, V, VIII, IX, X, XI, or XII. Qualitative abnormalities in platelets are manifested by prolongation of the bleeding time. If platelet function is intact, bleeding abnormalities usually do not occur unless the platelet count is below 100,000·mm³.

Disorders of hemostasis in critically ill patients are generally complex and represent multiple acquired deficiencies. Indeed, in most critically ill patients a bleeding disorder is only one manifestation of a complex series of failing organ system interactions. Common acquired deficiencies of hemostasis include disseminated intravascular coagulation, liver disease, vitamin K deficiency, anticoagulants, and massive blood transfusion.

Disseminated Intravascular Coagulation

Disseminated intravascular coagulation is a syndrome and not a primary disease state that reflects severe underlying pathology. The coagulation cascade is activated, resulting in the deposition of small thrombi and emboli throughout the microvasculature. This phase is then followed by secondary fibrinolysis. Repetition of this cycle leads to depletion of coagulation proteins and platelets and the antihemostatic effects of fibrin degradation products. Clinical manifestations of disseminated intravascular coagulation can result in thrombosis or hemorrhage. Most commonly bleeding is manifest from multiple sites, including venipuncture sites, nasogastric tubes, urinary catheters, or endotracheal tubes. Laboratory manifestations of disseminated intravascular coagulation include thrombocytopenia, hypofibrinogenemia, and prolongation of the prothrombin time. Abnormalities of these indicators confirm disseminated intravascular coagulation. If all are not abnormal, additional studies including partial thromboplastin time, thrombin time, and fibrin degradation products should be ordered.[241] In addition, review of the peripheral smear may reveal a microangiopathic hemolytic anemia from cell trapping and damage within fibrin thrombi.

The treatment of disseminated intravascular coagulation is the treatment of the underlying cause. Some authors have suggested the use of heparin as supportive therapy in order to reduce thrombin generation and prevent further consumption of clotting proteins until the underlying disease process could be controlled.[242] Although it remains controversial, current recommendations do not support the use of routine heparin therapy but rather the administration of fresh frozen plasma and cryoprecipitate to replace depleted clotting factors and of platelet concentrates to correct thrombocytopenia.[243]

An unusual cause of bleeding can result from defects in the fibrinolytic system. Patients with alpha₂ plasmin inhibitor deficiency, cirrhosis of the liver, or malignancy may develop diffuse bleeding from primary fibrinolysis rather than disseminated intravascular coagulation. Laboratory data reveals relatively normal prothrombin time and partial thromboplastin time with a normal platelet count and a disproportionally low fibrinogen level. Patients with clearly established primary fibrinolysis should receive epsilon aminocaproic acid and not heparin. However, if concomitant disseminated intravascular coagulation is suspected, epsilon aminocaproic acid should be avoided because it can cause massive, often fatal thrombosis.

POISONING

Despite preventive health programs and increased public awareness, poisoning remains a common and serious medical problem. Accidental poisonings account for approximately 5000 deaths per year, with suicides by chemical agents causing an additional 6000 deaths per year.[244] Poisoning is of particular importance in the pediatric population. As many as 2 million children in the United States accidentally swallow toxic material and approximately one ingestion out of 1000 is fatal. However, poisoning is by no means a problem limited to children. One half of all poisoned patients are over the age of 20.

The causative agents in poisoning vary with age. Children less than 5 years of age tend to ingest household products, whereas older patients are more likely to choose drugs. Aspirin accounts for 25% of all ingestions and is reported as the most common medicine involved in poisoning.

Prompt recognition and early intervention are essential to the successful treatment of poisoning. The diagnosis of poisoning can be very difficult to make because the toxic effects of many agents are nonspecific. Certainly, a high index of suspicion must be maintained when confronted with a patient presenting with seizures, coma, psychosis, acute renal or hepatic insufficiency, or bone marrow depression. However, most poisoning syndromes manifest nonspecific symptoms. Similarly, it is uncommon for the physical examination to show characteristic toxic effects of chemical substances.

Identification of the toxic agent should be attempted in every case of poisoning. Gastric fluid, urine, and blood samples should be sent to the laboratory to screen for possible poisons. Modalities available to identify the offending agents include thin-layer chromatography, gas-liquid chromatography, high-performance liquid chromatography, and spectrometry. Patients poisoned with drugs frequently take more than one agent, which can lead to drug interactions and difficulty in interpreting test results.

Treatment

Treatment of poisoning should not await toxicologic determinations. Supportive care should begin immediately, including the essentials of basic cardiopulmonary support. In addition, symptomatic treatment of neurologic, renal, and hepatic dysfunction is mandatory. Attention should then be directed to minimizing absorption of the poison. For ingested poisons this means prevention of absorption from the gastrointestinal tract by lavage, emetics, and adsorbents such as charcoal. Cathartics generally have no role in treating poisoning.[245]

Attempts should also be made to hasten elimination of absorbed poisons. Techniques available to increase elimination of poisons include diuresis, dialysis, chelation, hemoperfusion, exchange transfusion, and antibodies. Glomerular filtration and dialysis are generally effective only with substances found in plasma water and not protein-bound poisons. Hemoperfusion is most effective if used immediately after ingestion of the poison. Exchange transfusion may be especially useful in small children in whom hemoperfusion may be technically difficult. Antibodies can also be used as a high-affinity adsorbent in the patient's bloodstream to hasten elimination.

Common Poisons

Application of the principles used for the management of acute poisonings can be exemplified by several common agents.

Acetaminophen

This aspirin substitute is a frequent cause of poisoning. Clinical manifestations are generally nonspecific. Patients may initially present with pallor, lethargy, nausea, vomiting, and diaphoresis. Hepatotoxicity may become evident 1 to 2 days after ingestion and can be fatal. Liver damage results when the normal metabolic pathways become saturated so that an increased fraction of drug is inactivated by the cytochrome P-450 system, glutathione stores are depleted, and the reactive intermediates bind to liver macromolecules. Treatment of acetaminophen intoxication is initiated by induction of emesis or gastric lavage followed by administration of activated charcoal. Attention is next directed toward increasing sulfhydryl donors such as glutathione to allow greater binding of the toxic acetaminophen metabolites and therefore reduce liver damage. Early administration of n-acetylcystine can significantly reduce the incidence of acetaminophen-induced hepatotoxicity.[246]

Alcohols

Although the low molecular weight alcohols—methanol, ethanol, ethylene glycol, and isopropanol—are relatively weak poisons, the result of their metabolism can be fatal. Ethanol depresses ventilation, decreases myocardial contractility, predisposes to hypothermia, and causes hypoglycemia, especially in children. Although there is no antidote to ethanol and no way to hasten its metabolism, it is readily removed by hemodialysis.[247] However, usually critical care support with assisted ventilation of the lungs suffices in the treatment of ethanol intoxication. It is as important to treat associated illnesses in the patient with an ethanol overdose as it is to support the patient for the effects of the drug poisoning.

Methanol and ethylene glycol poisonings are common yet frequently undetected. It is important to detect poisoning with these agents early because the metabolites are potent poisons and may lead to irreversible toxicity if they go unrecognized.[248,249] Methanol is present in windshield washer

antifreeze and solvents and in organic synthetic processes, whereas ethylene glycol is the major component in automotive antifreeze and is found in various organic solvents and cosmetics. Treatment of methanol and ethylene glycol poisoning is systemic alkalinization to decrease ocular and renal toxicity followed by hemodialysis to accelerate elimination of the alcohols and their metabolites.

Carbon Monoxide

Carbon monoxide (CO) is a colorless, odorless, tasteless, nonirritating gas produced by the incomplete combustion of carbonaceous material. It is the major cause of death in patients exposed to smoke inhalation from fires. CO is responsible for approximately 3500 accidental and suicidal deaths per year in the United States. It exerts its toxic effects through tissue hypoxia.[250] The hemoglobin molecule has an affinity for carbon monoxide that is over 200 times greater than its affinity for oxygen. The combination of CO with hemoglobin forms carboxyhemoglobin, which is incapable of carrying oxygen. It also interferes with the release of oxygen from oxyhemoglobin, which decreases the amount of oxygen available to the tissues. In addition, because the rate of dissociation of CO from hemoglobin is extremely low, carboxyhemoglobin produces an acute decrease in blood oxygen content that is not readily reversed. The amount of carboxyhemoglobin present in blood depends on the concentration of CO in the inspired air and on the time of exposure.[251]

Symptoms depend on the amount of carboxyhemoglobin present and the patient's activity level, tissue oxygen demands, and hemoglobin concentration. Exposure to low concentrations of CO causes irritability, altered visual and motor skills, headache, nausea, vomiting, and predisposition to angina pectoris. Severe poisoning may result in seizures, coma, respiratory failure, and death. The classic cherry red color of the skin and mucous membranes of patients with CO poisoning results from the bright red cast of carboxyhemoglobin. However, in patients with severe poisoning, cyanosis may predominate over the cherry red color.

Treatment of CO poisoning is to remove the offending agent and provide a high oxygen enriched environment. The half-time of CO elimination can be shortened from 4 hours to 40 minutes by hyperventilation of the lungs with 100% oxygen. Ventilation may require mechanical support. Other treatment modalities include hyperbaric oxygen, transfusion therapy, and diuretics and steroids for the treatment of complicating cerebral edema.[250]

LEGAL AND ETHICAL ISSUES

Brain Death

Brain death is defined as the irreversible cessation of all functions of the entire brain.[252] This clinical definition is confirmed by autopsy studies revealing destruction of the entire brain in both the cerebral hemispheres and the brain stem. The primary insult leads to brain edema with increases in ICP. In the vast majority of brain death cases, the ICP exceeds systolic blood pressure within 12–24 hours. Currently, most states recognize brain death as sufficient criteria for declaration of death. There have been many definitions offered of brain death. However, the broadly held consensus opinion was reflected in *Defining Death*, a report issued in 1981 by the President's Commission for the Study of Ethical Problems in Medicine and Biomedical and

Behavioral Research.[253] In response to a congressional mandate, the commission recommended a statute, The Uniformed Determination of Death Act (UDDA), which has become the most widely accepted legal formulation of the standards for determining human death. In addition, it also provided an update formulation of the medical criteria for applying the standard.[254] Representatives of the American Bar Association, American Medical Association, National Conference of Commissioners on Uniform State Laws, and the Academy of the American Encephalographers Society agreed on the UDDA definition as follows: An individual who has sustained either (1) irreversible cessation of circulatory and respiratory functions, or (2) irreversible cessation of all functions or the entire brain, including the brain stem, is dead. A determination of death must be made in accordance with accepted medical standards. These guidelines are now widely accepted by physicians and hospitals for clinical decision making. This formulation of brain death is based on a clinical diagnosis with certain preconditions and confirmatory tests.[255,256]

With advances in technology and medical capability, even seemingly clear-cut definitions, such as death, become complex and difficult to translate into law and policy. Indeed, for many years courts were slow to modify the common law definition of death, i.e., cessation of all vital functions including respiration and circulation, in order to accept the determination of death based on irreversible cessation of all functions of the brain. The most common and familiar criteria for the diagnosis of whole brain death are the Harvard criteria published in 1968[257] by an Ad Hoc Committee of the Harvard Medical School. Tests generally used to determine brain death rely on response to stimuli, the presence of reflexes and spontaneous movements, and the electroencephalogram. There must be no evidence of hypothermia or drugs that depress brain function. The findings must persist over 24 hours. These Harvard criteria are now widely accepted by the medical profession and can be recognized legally as defining death in many states.

Indeed, organ transplantation was a major impetus for focusing public attention on the need to update standards for determining death, even though only approximately 15% of patients who are declared brain dead become organ donors. A special standard only for organ donors would fail to address the overwhelming majority of comatose ventilator-supported cases. This could create a separate standard of death for donors that could lead to abuse and confusion.[258] Thus, along with the clinical diagnosis, confirmatory tests are generally required and can be dependent on normal function or intracranial blood flow.

Do Not Resuscitate Orders

Few areas in clinical medicine generate as much controversy and debate as does the decision to withdraw or withhold treatment of critically ill patients.[259-261] Certainly, the opinion in the Joseph Saikewicz case issued by the Massachusetts Supreme Judicial Court in November 1977 was the most controversial judicial decision in the health law field in recent years.[262] In this case a profoundly retarded institutionalized 67-year-old man with acute myeloblastic monocytic leukemia was appointed a guardian and the court was asked to decide if treatment should be undertaken. It was understood that treatment would be painful and carry potential hazards with very little hope for recovery. The County Probate Court recommended withholding therapy and the Supreme Court affirmed this order. However, the

Supreme Court further stated that the decision to withhold or withdraw the life-support measures in a terminally ill, incompetent patient was not within the jurisdiction of any hospital committee or panel, but rather the ultimate decision-making responsibility rested with the courts. Justice Paul J. Liacos, the author of the Saikewicz decision, offered a different approach to do not resuscitate (DNR) orders when he suggested they present a case for physician discretion, and that the principles of Saikewicz are inapplicable.[263]

In a subsequent court opinion, in the matter of Dinnerstein, the legality of DNR orders was addressed. In this case, the patient was a 67-year-old woman with Alzheimer's disease, a massive stroke, and left hemiparesis. She was left in a persistent vegetative state, immobile, speechless, unable to swallow without choking, and barely able to cough. The patient's physician recommended no resuscitation in the event of cardiopulmonary arrest and the patient's family concurred. Because of the legal uncertainty surrounding "no code" orders, the physician, hospital, and family asked the court to rule about the legality of the order. The Massachusetts Appeal Court held that a DNR order in these circumstances was lawful and advance judicial approval was not necessary to write such orders. Resuscitation was not "a treatment offering hope of restoration to normal integrated functioning cognitive existence. Attempts to apply resuscitation if successful will do nothing to cure or relieve the illness, which will have brought the patient to the threshold of death."[264] A second Massachusetts case upholding DNR orders involved a 5-month-old infant abandoned at birth who suffered from profound congenital cardiopulmonary disease with little hope of survival. The patient's physician recommended a DNR order be entered on the patient's medical chart, but the guardian, the Department of Social Services, refused to consent. In this case the Massachusetts Supreme Judicial Court found that a full resuscitation effort would not serve the child's interest and that the child would reject full resuscitation if were competent to decide.[265]

The right to reject resuscitative or any lifesaving medical treatment was best outlined in the Karen Ann Quinlan case.[266] The court stated that the constitutional right to privacy encompasses the freedom of the terminally ill but competent individual to decline medical treatment when such treatment will only prolong suffering needlessly and denigrate the quality of life. In a recent report the Council on Ethical and Judicial Affairs of the American Medical Association outlined the guidelines for the appropriate use of Do Not Resuscitate Orders.[267]

In this report the Council recommended that (1) efforts should be made to resuscitate patients who suffer cardiac or respiratory arrest except when circumstances indicate that administration of cardiopulmonary resuscitation would be futile or not in accord with the desires or best interests of the patient; (2) if a patient is incapable of rendering the decision regarding the use of cardiopulmonary resuscitation, a decision may be made by a surrogate decision maker based on the previously expressed preferences of the patient, or if such preferences are unknown, in accordance with the patient's best interest.

The practice of critical care medicine frequently requires decisions regarding the level of care to be provided to patients. These decisions are generally made in highly stressful situations and carry significant medical, legal, psychological, ethical, and economic ramifications. They are very complex, emotional, and controversial areas that must be confronted when treating critically ill patients.

Should families dictate medical therapy? Is withdrawing therapy different than withholding it? What are the legal ramifications of these kinds of decisions? There is a fine line distinguishing prolonging life and prolonging the dying process. There are many complex and difficult issues confronting the critical care practitioner that still await further clarification.

REFERENCES

1. Grenvik A, Leonard JJ, Arens JR et al: Critical care medicine. Certification as a multidisciplinary subspecialty. Crit Care Med 9:2, 1981
2. Bekes CE, Greenbaum DM, Fein A et al: Recommendations for program content for fellowship training in critical care medicine. Crit Care Med 15:971, 1987
3. Bekes CE, Greenbaum DM, Fein A et al: Recommendations for the qualifications of a director of a fellowship training program in critical care medicine. Crit Care Med 15:977, 1987
4. Sadove MS, Kritchmer HE, Wyant GM et al: An ideal recovery room. Modern Hosp 76:88, 1951
5. Ibsen B: The anesthetist's viewpoints on treatment of respiratory complications in polymyelitis during the epidemic in Copenhagen. Proc R Soc Med 47:72, 1954
6. Safar P, DeKornfeld T, Pearson J et al: Intensive care unit. Anaesthesia 16:275, 1961
7. American Heart Association: Coronary care unit (1) and (2). A specialized intensive care unit for acute myocardial infarction. Mod Concepts Cardiovasc Dis 34:23, 1965
8. Safar P, Grenvik A: Critical care medicine, organizing and staffing intensive care units. Chest 59:535, 1971
9. Safar P, Grenvik A: Organization and physician education in critical care medicine. Anesthesiology 47:82, 1977
10. Weil MH, Shubin H: Symposium on care of the critically ill. Mod Med 39:83, 1971
11. Greenbaum DM: Standards for critical care medicine. In Shoemaker WC, Thompson WL, Holbrook PR (eds): Textbook of Critical Care Medicine, p 1004. Philadelphia, WB Saunders, 1984
12. Lave JR, Knaus WA: The economics of intensive care units. In Abramson NS, Grenvik A (eds): Medicolegal Aspects of Critical Care, p 87. Gaithersberg, Maryland, Aspen, 1986
13. Greenbaum DM: Physician manpower in critical care medicine. Crit Care Med 10:407, 1986
14. Wagner KD: Exodus of the ICU nurse: The cause is the cure. Focus on AACN 9:4, 1982
15. Rogers RM, Weiler C, Ruppenthal B: Impact of the respiratory intensive care unit in survival of patients with acute respiratory failure. Chest 77:501, 1972
16. Klaus AP, Sarachek NS, Greenberg D et al: Evaluating coronary care units. Am Heart J 79:471, 1970
17. Feller I, Tholen D, Cornell RG: Improvements in burn care, 1965–1979. JAMA 244:2074, 1980
18. Sinclair JC, Torrance GW, Boyle MH et al: Evaluation of neonatal intensive care programs. N Engl J Med 305:489, 1981
19. Stern MP: The recent decline in ischemic heart disease mortality. Ann Intern Med 91:630, 1979
20. Siegel JH, Cerra FB, Moody EA et al: The effect on survival of critically ill and injured patients of an ICU teaching service organized about a computer-based physiologic CARE system. J Trauma 20:558, 1980
21. Mather HJ, Morgan DC, Pearson NG et al: Myocardial infarction: A comparison between home and hospital care for patients. Br Med J 1:925, 1976
22. Hill JD, Hampton JR, Mitchell JRA: A randomized trial of home-versus-hospital management for patients with suspected myocardial infarction. Lancet 2:837, 1978
23. Baldock GJ, Marshal C: Illness severity scoring in the general intensive care unit. Intensive Care World 4:54, 1987
24. Cullen DJ, Civetta JM, Briggs BA et al: Therapeutic intervention scoring system: A method for quantitative comparison of patient care. Crit Care Med 2:57, 1974
25. Cullen DJ: Results and costs of intensive care. Anesthesiology 47:203, 1977
26. Rothstein P, Johnson P: Pediatric intensive care: Factors that influence outcome. Crit Care Med 10:34, 1982
27. Yeh TS, Pollack MM, Holbrook PR et al: Assessment of pediatric intensive care—application of the therapeutic intervention scoring system. Crit Care Med 10:497, 1982
28. Knaus WA, Zimmerman JE, Wagner DP et al: APACHE— Acute physiology and chronic health evaluation: A physiologically based system. Crit Care Med 9:591, 1981
29. Draper EA, Wagner DP, Knaus WA: The use of intensive care: A comparison of a university and community hospital. Health Care Financing Rev 3:49, 1981
30. Wagner DP, Knaus WA, Draper EA: Statistical validation of a severity of illness measure. Am J Public Health 73:878, 1983
31. LeGall JR, Loirat P, Alperovitch A et al: A simplified acute physiology score for ICU patients. Crit Care Med 12:975, 1984
32. Knaus WA, Draper EA, Wagner DP et al: APACHE II: A severity of disease classification system. Crit Care Med 13:818, 1985
33. Pollack MM, Yeh TS, Ruttiman VE et al: Development of the physiologic stability index (PSI) for use in critically ill infants and children. Pediatr Res 16:187A, 1982
34. Champion HR, Sacco WJ, Lesper RL et al: An anatomic index of injury severity. J Trauma 20:197, 1980
35. Mulley AG, Thibault GE, Hughes RA et al: The course of patients with suspected myocardial infarction. N Engl J Med 302:943, 1980
36. Bartlett RH, Gazzaniga AB, Wilson AF et al: Mortality prediction in adult respiratory insufficiency. Chest 67:680, 1975
37. Ledingham IM, Cowan BN, Burns HJ: Prognosis in severe shock. Br Heart J 284:443, 1982
38. Apgar V: A proposal for a new method of evaluation of the newborn infant. Anesth Analg 32:260, 1953
39. Siesjo BK: Cerebral circulation and metabolism. J Neurosurg 60:883, 1984
40. Michenfelder JD, Theye RA: The effect of profound hypocapnia and dilutional anemia on canine cerebral metabolism and blood flow. Anesthesiology 31:449, 1969
41. Harp JR, Wollman H: Cerebral metabolic effects of hyperventilation and deliberate hypotension. Br J Anaesth 45:256, 1973
42. Sounsen SC: Theoretical considerations on the potential hazards of hyperventilation during anesthesia. Acta Anaesthesiol Scand 67(suppl):106, 1978
43. Plum F, Siesjo BK: Recent advances in CSF physiology. Anesthesiology 42:708, 1975
44. Cohen PJ, Alexander SC, Smith TC et al: Effects of hypoxia and normocarbia on cerebral blood flow and metabolism in man. J Appl Physiol 23:183, 1967
45. Defalque RJ, Musunuru VS: Disease of the nervous system. In Stoelting RK, Dierdorf SF (eds): Anesthesia and Coexisting Disease, p 239. New York, Churchill-Livingstone, 1983
46. Miller JD, Becker DP, Ward JD et al: Significance of intracranial hypertension in severe blood injury. J Neurosurg 47:503, 1977
47. Zierski J: Extradural, ventricular, and subdural pressure recording: Comparative clinical study. In Shulman K, Marmarou A, Miller JD et al (eds): Intracranial pressure IV, p 371. Berlin, Springer-Verlag, 1980
48. Mayball CG, Archer NH, Lamb VA et al: Ventriculostomy-related infections: A prospective epidemiologic study. N Engl J Med 310:553, 1984
49. Marshall LF, Smith RW, Shapiro HM: Outcome with aggressive treatment in severe head injuries: Acute and chronic barbiturate administration in the management of head injury, Part II. J Neurosurg 50:26, 1979
50. Rockoff M, Marshall L, Shapiro H: High dose barbiturate therapy in humans: A clinical review of 60 patients. Ann Neurol 6:194, 1979
51. Woodcock J, Ropper AH, Kennedy SK: High dose barbiturates in non-traumatic brain swelling: ICP reduction and effect on outcome. Stroke 13:785, 1982
52. Ropper AH: Trauma on the head and spinal cord. In Braunwald E, Isselbacher KJ, Peterdorf RG et al (eds): Harrison's Principles of Internal Medicine, p 1960. New York, McGraw-Hill, 1987

53. Engel J Jr, Troupin AS, Crandall PH et al: Recent developments in the diagnosis and treatment of epilepsy. Ann Intern Med 97:584, 1982

54. Leppik IE: Drug treatment of epilepsy. In Johnson RT (ed): Current Therapy in Neurologic Disease, p 41. Philadelphia, BC Decker, 1986

55. Jennett B, Teasdale G: Aspects of coma after severe head injury. Lancet 1:878, 1977

56. Jennett B, Teasdale G, Braakman R et al: Predicting outcome in individual patients after head injury. Lancet 1:1081, 1976

57. Narayan RK, Greenberg RP, Miller JD et al: Improved confidence of outcome prediction in severe head injury. A comparative analysis of the clinical examination, multimodality evoked potentials, CT scanning, and intracranial pressure. J Neurosurg 54:751, 1981

58. Miller JD, Becker DP, Ward JD et al: The outcome of severe head injury with early diagnosis and intensive management. J Neurosurg 47:491, 1977

59. Marshall LF, Smith RW, Shapiro HM: The outcome with aggressive treatment in severe head injuries. J Neurosurg 48:679, 1978

60. Marshall LF, Shapiro HM: Examination by computerized axial tomography. Int Anesthesiol Clin 17:391, 1979

61. Narayan RK, Greenberg RP, Miller JD et al: Intracranial pressure: To monitor or not to monitor? J Neurosurg 56:650, 1982

62. Kern KB, Meislin HW: Diabetes insipidus: Occurrence after minor head trauma. J Trauma 24:69, 1984

63. Ropper AH, Kennedy SK, Zervas NT (eds): Neurological and Neurosurgical Intensive Care. Baltimore, University Park Press, 1983

64. Thompson JA, Ayres SM, Hess ML: Cardiogenic shock: Causes, diagnosis and management. J Crit Ill 2:22, 1987

65. Pasternak RC, Braunwald E, Alpert JS: Acute myocardial infarction. In Braunwald E, Isselbacher KJ, Peterdorf RG et al (eds): Harrison's Principles of Internal Medicine. New York, McGraw-Hill, 1987

66. Forrester JS, Diamond G, Chatterjee K: Medical therapy for acute myocardial infarction by application of hemodynamic subsets. N Engl J Med 295:1356, 1976

67. Schroeder JS, Hunt S: Cardiac transplantation. JAMA 258:3142, 1987

68. Goldberg LI: Cardiovascular and renal effects of dopamine: Potential clinical applications. Pharmacol Rev 24:1, 1972

69. Mueller HS, Evan R, Ayres SM: Effect of dopamine on hemodynamics and myocardial metabolism in shock following acute myocardial infarction in man. Circulation 27:271, 1978

70. Bourdarias JP, Dubourg O, Gveret P et al: Inotropic agents in the treatment of cardiogenic shock. Pharmacol Ther 22:53, 1983

71. Richard C, Ricome JL, Rimailho A et al: Combined hemodynamic effects of dopamine and dobutamine in cardiogenic shock. Circulation 67:620, 1983

72. Bennotti JR, Grossman W, Braunwald E et al: Effects of amrinone on myocardial energy metabolism and hemodynamics in patients with severe congestive heart failure due to coronary artery disease. Circulation 62:28, 1980

73. Moulopoulus SD, Topaz S, Kolff WJ: Diastolic balloon pumping with carbon dioxide in the aorta—a mechanical assistance to the failing circulation. Am Heart J 63:669, 1962

74. Buckley MJ, Craver JM, Gold HK et al: Intra-aortic balloon pump assist for cardiogenic shock after cardiopulmonary bypass. Circulation 48(suppl 3):90, 1973

75. Gill CC, Wechsler AS, Newman GE et al: Augmentation and redistribution of myocardial blood flow during acute ischemia by intraaortic balloon pumping. Ann Thorac Surg 16:455, 1973

76. Limet RR, Freola M, Glick G et al: Effects of intraaortic balloon counterpulsation (IABCP) on the distribution of coronary blood flow in experimental ischemic left ventricular failure. J Cardiovasc Surg 22:305, 1971

77. Saini VK, Hood WB Jr, Hechtman HB et al: Nutrient myocardial blood flow in experimental myocardial ischemia. Circulation 52:1086, 1975

78. Maroko PR, Bernstein EF, Libby P et al: Effects of intraaortic balloon counterpulsation on the severity of myocardial isch-

emic injury following acute coronary occlusion. Circulation 45:1150, 1972

79. Roberts AJ, Alonso DR, Combes JR et al: Role of delayed intraaortic balloon pumping in treatment of experimental myocardial infarction. Am J Cardiol 41:1202, 1978

80. Mueller HS, Evan R, Ayres SM et al: Effect of isoproterenol, 1-neopinephrine, and intraaortic counterpulsation on hemodynamics and myocardial metabolism in shock following acute myocardial infarction. Circulation 45:335, 1972

81. Brown, M: Immediate postresuscitation care: Part I. Emergency Med Clin North Am 3:671, 1983

82. Amsterdam EA, Awan NA, Lee G et al: Intra-aortic balloon counterpulsation: Rationale, application and results. Cardiovasc Clin 11:79, 1981

83. Ream AK, Portner PM: Cardiovascular assist devices and the artificial heart. In Ream AK, Fogdall RP (eds): Acute Cardiovascular Management: Anesthesia and Intensive Care, p 852. Philadelphia, JB Lippincott, 1982

84. Goldhaber SZ (ed): Pulmonary Embolism and Deep Venous Thrombosis. Philadelphia, WB Saunders, 1985

85. Bell WR, Simon TL: Current status of pulmonary thromboembolic disease: Pathophysiology, diagnosis, prevention and treatment. Am Heart J 103:239, 1982

86. Hull RD, Raskob GE, Hirsh J: The diagnosis of clinically suspected pulmonary embolism: Practical approaches. Chest 89:417S, 1986

87. Sobel BE: Pharmacologic thrombolysis: Tissue-type plasminogen activator. Circulation 76:39, 1987

88. Laffel GL, Braunwald E: Thrombolytic therapy: A new strategy for the treatment of acute myocardial infarction. N Engl J Med 311:710, 1984

89. The TIMI study group: The thrombolysis in myocardial infarction (TIMI) trial: Phase I findings. N Engl J Med 312:932, 1985

90. Midgette AS, O'Connor GT, Baron JA, Bell J: Effects of Intravenous streptokinase on early mortality in patients with suspected acute myocardial infarction. Ann Intern Med 113:961, 1990

91. Held PH, Teo KK, Yusuf S: Effects of tissue-type plasminogen activator and anisoylated plasminogen streptokinase activator complex on mortality in acute myocardial infarction. Circulation 82:1668, 1990

92. Guerci AD, Gerstenblith G, Brinker JA et al: A randomized trial of intravenous tissue plasminogen activator for acute myocardial infarction with subsequent randomization to elective coronary angioplasty. N Engl J Med 317:1613, 1987

93. Robin ED: Permeability pulmonary edema. In Fishman AP, Renkin EM (eds): Pulmonary Edema. Bethesda, American Physiologic Society, 1979

94. Hudson LD: Adult respiratory distress syndrome. Semin Respir Med 2:99, 1981

95. Michaelis LL: Pulmonary changes in shock and trauma. Review course, general surgery. Cook County Graduate School of Medicine, 1982

96. Shapiro BA, Cane RD: Acute lung injury and positive end expiratory pressure. Anesth Clin North Am 5:797, 1987

97. Demling RH: The pathogenesis of respiratory failure after trauma and sepsis. Surg Clin North Am 60:1373, 1980

98. Rinaldo JE, Rogers RM: Adult respiratory distress syndrome—Changing concepts of lung injury and repair. N Engl J Med 306:900, 1982

99. Lee CT, Fein AM, Lippmann M et al: Elastolytic activity in pulmonary lavage fluid from patients with adult respiratory distress syndrome. N Engl J Med 304:192, 1981

100. Hammerschmidt D, White JG, Craddock PR: Corticosteroids inhibit complement-induced granulocyte aggregation. J Clin Invest 63:798, 1979

101. Hammerschmidt D, Hudson LD, Weaver LJ et al: Association of complement activation and elevated plasma C5a with adult respiratory distress syndrome—pathophysiological relevance and possible prognostic value. Lancet 1:947, 1980

102. Bone RC, Francis PB, Pierce AK: Intravascular coagulation associated with adult respiratory distress syndrome. Am J Med 61:585, 1976

103. Blaisdell FW, Lim RC, Stallone RJ: The mechanism of pulmo-

nary damage following traumatic shock. Surg Gynecol Obstet 130:15, 1970

104. Greene R, Zapol W, Snider M et al: Early bedside detection of pulmonary vascular occlusion during acute respiratory failure. Am Rev Respir Dis 124:593, 1981

105. Shapiro BA, Crane RD, Harrison RA: Positive end-expiratory pressure therapy in adults with special reference to acute lung injury: A review of the literature and suggested clinical correlations. Crit Care Med 12:127, 1984

106. Bernard GR, Luce JM, Sprung CL et al: High dose corticosteroids in patients with the adult respiratory distress syndrome. N Engl J Med 317:1565, 1987

107. Vergilio RW, Rice CL, Smith DE et al: Crystalloid vs colloid resuscitation: Is one better? Surgery 85:129, 1979

108. Lowe RJ, Moss GS, Jilek J et al: Crystalloid vs colloid in the etiology of pulmonary failure after trauma: A randomized trial in man. Surgery 81:676, 1977

109. Brown M: Immediate post-resuscitative care: Part I. Emerg Med Clin North Am 1:671, 1983

110. Mathru M: The therapeutic application of positive end-expiratory pressure. Anesth Clin North Am 5:789, 1987

111. Gallagher TJ, Civetta JM, Kirby RR: Terminology update: Optimal PEEP. Crit Care Med 6:323, 1978

112. Suter PM, Fairley HB, Isenberg MD: Optimum end-expiratory airway pressure in patients with acute pulmonary failure. N Engl J Med 292:284, 1975

113. Marini JJ: Hemodynamic assessment and management of patients with respiratory failure. Clin Crit Care Med 14:179, 1988

114. Qvist J, Pontoppidan H, Wilson RS et al: Hemodynamic responses to mechanical ventilation with PEEP: The effect of hypervolemia. Anesthesiology 26:754, 1975

115. Jarden F, Farcot JC, Boisante L et al: Influence of positive end-expiratory pressure on left ventricular performance. N Engl J Med 304:387, 1981

116. Roos A, Thomas LJ Jr, Nagel EL et al: Pulmonary vascular resistance as determined by lung inflation and vascular pressure. J Appl Physiol 16:77, 1961

117. Buda AJ, Pinsky MR, Ingels NB Jr, et al: Effect of intrathoracic pressure on left ventricular performance. N Engl J Med 301:453, 1979

118. Rowbotham JL, Lixfeld W, Holland L et al: The effects of positive end-expiratory pressure on right and left ventricular performance. Am Rev Respir Dis 121:677, 1980

119. Hillman KM: Pulmonary barotrauma. Clin Anesthesiol 3:877, 1985

120. Luce JM, Huseby J, Kirk W et al: Mechanism by which positive-end expiratory pressure increases cerebrospinal fluid pressure in dogs. J Appl Physiol 52:231, 1982

121. Annat G, Viale JP, Xuan BB et al: Effect of PEEP ventilation on renal function, plasma renin, aldosterone, neurophysins, urinary ADH and prostaglandins. Anesthesiology 136:141, 1983

122. Beyer J, Beckenlechner P, Messmer K: The influence of PEEP ventilation on organ blood flow and peripheral oxygen delivery. Int Care Med 8:75, 1982

123. Brendenberg CE, Paskanik A, Fromm D: Portal hemodynamics in dogs during mechanical ventilation with postive end-expiratory pressure. Surgery 90:817, 1981

124. Petty TL: Adult respiratory distress syndrome. Semin Respir Med 3:219, 1982

125. Niedermyer ME, Brigham KL: Prospects for therapeutic interventions in acute respiratory failure. Respir Ther 14:15, 1984

126. Zapol WM, Snider MT, Schneider RC: Extracorporeal membrane oxygenation for acute respiratory distress syndrome. Am J Med 61:585, 1976

127. Luce JM: The cardiovascular complications of mechanical ventilation and positive end-expiratory pressure. JAMA 252:807, 1984

128. Brown M, Smith PC: Special requirements of perioperative airway pressure support. In Shapiro BA, Cane RD (eds): Anesthesiol Clin North Am 126:857, 1987

129. Spearman CB, Sanders HG: The new generation of mechanical ventilators. Resp Care 32:403, 1987

130. Cane RD, Shapiro BA: Mechanical ventilatory support. JAMA 254:87, 1985

131. MacIntyre NR: Respiratory function during pressure support ventilation. Chest 89:677, 1986

132. Banner MJ, Kirby RR: Pressure support ventilation. Crit Care Med 14:665, 1986

133. Branson RD, Campbell RS, Davis K Jr et al: Altering flowrate during maximum pressure support ventilation (PSV_{max}): Effects on cardiorespiratory function. Respir Care 35:1056, 1990

134. Brochard L, Pluskwa F, Lemaire F: Improved efficiency of spontaneous breathing with inspiratory pressure support. Am Rev Respir Dis 136:411, 1987

135. Fiastro JF, Habib MP, Quan SF: Pressure support compensation for inspiratory work due to endotracheal tubes and demand continuous positive airway pressure. Chest 93:499, 1988

136. Hurst JM, Branson RD, David K Jr, Barrett RR: Cardiopulmonary effects of pressure support ventilation. Arch Surg 124:1067, 1989

137. Tokioka H, Saito S, Kosaka F: Effects of pressure support ventilation on breathing patterns and respiratory work. Intensive Care Med 15:491, 1989

138. Kacmarek RM: Inspiratory pressure support: Does it make a clinical difference? Intensive Care Med 15:337, 1989

139. Hewlett AM, Platt AS, Terry G: Mandatory minute volume: A new concept in weaning from mechanical ventilation. Anesthesia 32:163, 1977

140. Willatts SM: Alternatives for mechanical ventilation. Intensive Care Med 11:51, 1985

141. Downs JB, Stock MC: Editorial: Airway pressure release ventilation: A new concept in ventilatory support. Crit Care Med 15:459, 1987

142. Stock MC, Downs JB: Airway pressure release ventilation: A new approach to ventilatory support during acute lung injury. Resp Care 32:517, 1987

143. Eng UB, Eriksson I, Sjostrand U: High frequency positive pressure ventilation: A review based upon its use during bronchoscopy and for laryngoscopy and microlaryngeal surgery under general anesthesia. Anesth Analg 59:594, 1980

144. Sjostrand U: High-frequency positive-pressure ventilation (HFPPV): A review. Crit Care Med 8:345, 1980

145. Gallagher J: Clinical use of high-frequency jet ventilation in intensive care. In Carlon GC, Howland WS (eds): High Frequency Ventilation in Intensive Care and During Surgery, p 159. New York, Marcel Dekker, 1985

146. Gettinger A, Glass DD: High frequency positive pressure ventilation use in neonatal and adult intensive care. In Carlon GG, Howland WS (eds): High Frequency Ventilation in Intensive Care and During Surgery, p 63. New York, Marcel Dekker, 1985

147. Kolton M: A review of high frequency oscillation. Can Anaesth Soc J 31:416, 1984

148. Drazen JM, Kamm RD, Slutsky AS: High-frequency ventilation. Physiol Rev 64:505, 1984

149. Froese AB: High-frequency ventilation: A critical assessment. In Shoemaker WC (eds): Critical Care: State of the Art, vol 5, (A)1. Fullerton, CA, Society of Critical Care Medicine, 1984

150. Froese AB, Bryan AC: State of the art: High frequency ventilation. Am Rev Respir Dis 135:1363, 1987

151. Smith RB: Ventilation at high respiratory frequencies. Anaesthesia 37:1011, 1982

152. McCullock PR, Froese AB: High frequency ventilation. In Shapiro BA, Cane RD (eds): Positive Airway Pressure Therapy: PPV and PEEP, vol 5, p 873. Philadelphia, WB Saunders, 1987

153. Gregory GA, Kitterman JA, Phibbs RH et al: Treatment of the idiopathic respiratory distress syndrome with continuous positive airway pressure. N Engl J Med 284:1333, 1971

154. Matthews LW, Dearborn DG, Tucker AS: Cystic fibrosis. In Fishman AP (ed): Pulmonary Diseases and Disorders, p 600. New York, McGraw-Hill, 1980

155. Park RW, Grand RJ: Gastrointestinal manifestations of cystic fibrosis: A review. Gastroenterology 81:1143, 1981

156. Shwachman H, Mahmoodian A, Neff RK et al: The sweat test: Sodium and chloride values. J Pediatr 98:576, 1981

157. Davis PB: Cystic fibrosis. Semin Resp Med 6:243, 1985

158. Hou SH, Bushinsky DA, Wish JB et al: Hospital-acquired renal insufficiency: A prospective study. Am J Med 74:243, 1983

159. Wilkins RG, Faragher EB: Acute renal failure in an intensive care unit. Incidence, prediction, and outcome. Anaesthesia 38:628, 1983

160. Brenner BM, Lazarus JM (eds): Acute Renal Failure. Philadelphia, WB Saunders, 1983

161. Glassock RJ, Adler SG, Ward HJ: Primary glomerular disease—rapidly progressive glomerulonephitis. In Brenner BM, Rector FL (eds): The Kidney, p 939. Philadelphia, WB Saunders, 1986

162. Jindal K, Goldstein MB: Acute renal failure in critically ill patients. J Crit Illness 2:13, 1987

163. Cronin RE: Aminoglycoside nephrotoxicity: Pathogenesis and prevention. Clin Nephrol 11:251, 1979

164. Linton AL, Clark WF, Driedger AA et al: Acute interstitial nephritis due to drugs. Ann Intern Med 93:735, 1980

165. Schrier RW: Acute renal failure: Pathogenesis diagnosis and management. Hosp Pract 93:112, 1981

166. Anderson RJ, Lines SL, Burns AS et al: Non-oliguric acute renal failure. N Engl J Med 296:1134, 1977

167. Miller TR, Anderson RJ, Linas SL et al: Urinary diagnostic indices in acute renal failure—prospective study. Ann Intern Med 89:47, 1978

168. Goldstein MB: Acute renal failure. Med Clin North Am 61:1325, 1983

169. Bastl CP, Rudnick MR, Narins RG: Diagnostic approaches to acute renal failure. In Brenner BM, Stein JH (eds): Acute Renal Failure, p 17. New York, Churchill-Livingstone, 1980

170. Kleinknecht D, Jungers P, Chanard J et al: Uremic and nonuremic complications of acute renal failure: Evaluation of early and frequent dialysis on prognosis. Kidney Int 1:190, 1972

171. Kramer P: Continuous arteriovenous hemofiltration of physiologic and effective kidney replacement therapy. Contrib Nephrol 44:236, 1985

172. Paganini EP, O'Hara P, Nakamoto S: Slow continuous ultrafiltration in hemodialysis-resistant oliguric acute renal failure patients. Trans Am Soc Artif Intern Organs 30:173, 1984

173. Geronemus R, Schneider N: Continuous arteriovenous hemodialysis: A new modality for the treatment of acute renal failure. Trans Am Soc Artif Intern Organs 30:610, 1984

174. Farber BF: Nosocomial infections: An introduction. In Farber BF (ed): Infection Control in Intensive Care, p 1. New York, Churchill-Livingstone, 1987

175. Farber BF: Reimbursement for nosocomial infections under prospective payment plan: The future or decline of infection control. Infect Control 5:425, 1984

176. Fauci AS, Lane HC: The acquired immunodeficiency syndrome: An update. Ann Intern Med 102:800, 1985

177. Centers for Disease Control: Nosocomial infection surveillance. 1983. In CDC Surveillance Summaries 33 (No. 2ss):9ss, 1984

178. de Jongh CA, Caplan ES, Schimpff SC: Infections in the critical care patient. In Shoemaker WC, Thompson WL, Holbrook PR (eds): Textbook of Critical Care, p 505. Philadelphia, WB Saunders, 1984

179. Lambert RS, Geroge RB: Diagnosing nosocomial pneumonia in mechanically ventilated patients. J Crit Illness 2:57, 1987

180. Sanford JP, Pierce AK: Lower respiratory tract infections, p 255. In Bennett J, Brachtman P (eds): Hospital Infections. Boston, Little Brown & Co, 1979

181. Jay SJ: Nosocomial infections. Med Clin North Am 67:1251, 1984

182. Bell R, Coalson JJ, Smith JD et al: Multiple organ system failure and infection in adult respiratory distress syndrome. Ann Intern Med 99:293, 1983

183. Johanson WG Jr, Pierce AK, Sanford JP: Changing pharyngeal bacterial flora of hospitalized patients. N Engl J Med 281:1137, 1969

184. Johanson WG Jr, Higuchi JH, Chadhuri TR et al: Bacterial adherence to epithelial cells in bacillary colonization of the upper respiratory tract. Am Rev Respir Dis 121:55, 1980

185. Andrews CP, Coalson JJ, Smith JD et al: Diagnosis of nosocomial bacterial pneumonia in acute diffuse lung injury. Chest 80:254, 1981

186. Berger R, Arango L: Etiologic diagnosis of bacterial nosocomial pneumonia in seriously ill patients. Crit Care Med 13:833, 1985

187. Guckian JC, Christensen WD: Quantitative culture and Gram stain of sputum in pneumonia. Am Rev Respir Dis 118:997, 1978

188. Barrett-Connor E: The nonvalue of sputum culture in the diagnosis of pneumococcal pneumonia. Am Rev Respir Dis 103:845, 1971

189. Baughman RP, Thorpe JE, Staneck J et al: Use of the protected specimen brush in patients with endotracheal or tracheostomy tubes. Chest 91:233, 1987

190. Henderson DK: Bacteremia due to percutaneous intravascular devices. In Mandell GL, Douglas RG, Bennett JE (eds): Principle and Practice of Infectious Diseases. New York, p 1612. John Wiley, 1985

191. Maki DG: Infections associated with intravascular lines. In Remington JA, Swartz MA (eds): Current Topics in Infectious Diseases, vol 3, p 309. New York, McGraw-Hill, 1982

192. Centers for Disease Control Working Groups: Guidelines for prevention of intravascular infections. In Guidelines for the Prevention and Control of Nosocomial Infections. VSDHHS-PHS, 1981

193. Nichols RL, Smith JW, Klein DB et al: Risk of infection after penetrating abdominal trauma. N Engl J Med 311:1065, 1984

194. Caplan ES, Hoyt NJ: Nosocomial sinusitis. JAMA 647:639, 1982

195. Bone RC, Fisher CJ Jr, Clemmer TP: Sepsis syndrome: A valid clinical entity. Crit Care Med 17:389, 1989

196. Parker MM, Parrillo JE: Septic shock: Hemodynamics and pathogenesis. JAMA 250:3324, 1983

197. Kreger BE, Craven DE, Carling PC et al: Gram-negative bacteremia: III. Reassessment of etiology, epidemiology, and ecology in 612 patients. Am J Med 68:332, 1980

198. Wiles JB, Cerra FB, Siegel JH et al: The systemic septic response: Does the organism matter? Crit Care Med 8:55, 1980

199. McCabe WR, Treadwell TL, DeMaria A Jr: Pathophysiology of bacteremia. Am J Med 75:225, 1983

200. Root RK, Sande MM: Septic Shock. New York, Churchill-Livingstone, 1985

201. Shine KI: Aspects of the management of shock. Ann Intern Med 93:723, 1980

202. Bernton EW, Long JB, Holaday JW et al: Opioids and neuropeptides: Mechanisms in circulatory shock. Fed Proc 44:290, 1985

203. O'Donnell TF Jr, Clowes GH Jr, Talamo RC et al: Kinin activation in the blood of patients with sepsis. Surg Gynecol Obstet 539, 1976

204. Raffin TA: Novel approaches to ARDS and sepsis. In Chernon B, Shoemaker WC (eds): Critical Care State of Art, vol 7, p 247. Fullerton, CA, Society of Critical Care Medicine, 1986

205. Sibbald WJ, Driedger AA: Specific organ function/dysfunction in sepsis and septic shock: Cardiovascular. In Sibbald WJ, Sprung CL (eds): Perspectives on sepsis and septic shock, p 125. Fullerton, CA, Society of Critical Care Medicine, 1986

206. Goldfarb RD: Cardiac mechanical performance in circulatory shock: A critical review of methods and results. Circ Shock 9:633, 1982

207. Hess ML, Hastills A, Greenfield LJ: Spectrum of cardiovascular function during gram-negative sepsis. Prog Cardiovasc Dis 23:279, 1981

208. Lefer A: Blood-borne humoral factors in the pathophysiology of circulatory shock. Circ Res 33:129, 1973

209. Demling RH: Colloid or crytalloid resuscitation in sepsis. In Sibbald WJ, Sprung CL (eds): Perspectives on Sepsis and Septic Shock, p 275. Fullerton, California, Society of Critical Care Medicine, 1986

210. Sprung CL, Caralis PV, Marcial EH et al: The effects of high-dose corticosteroids in patients with septic shock. N Engl J Med 311:1137, 1984

211. Sheagren JN: Septic shock and corticosteroids. N Engl J Med 305:456, 1981

212. Shumer W: Steroids in the treatment of clinical septic shock. Ann Surg 184:333, 1976

213. Bone RC, Fisher CJ Jr, Clemmer TP: A controlled clinical trial

of high-dose methylprednisolone in the treatment of severe sepsis and septic shock. N Engl J Med 317:653, 1987

214. Henshaw L, Peduzzi P, Young E et al: Effect of high-dose glucocorticoid therapy on mortality in patients with clinical signs of systemic sepsis. N Engl J Med 317:659, 1987

215. Ziegler EJ, McCutchan JA, Fiere J et al: Treatment of gram-negative bacteremia and shock with human antiserum to a mutant *Escherichia coli* N Engl J Med 307:1225, 1982

216. Baumgartner J-D, Glauser MP, McCutchan JA et al: Prevention of gram-negative shock and death in surgical patients by antibody to endotoxin core glycolipid. Lancet 2:59, 1985

217. Teng NNH, Kaplan HS, Herbert JM et al: Protection against gram-negative bacteremia and endotoxemia with human monoclonal IgM antibodies. Proc Natl Acad Sci USA 82:1790, 1985

218. Ziegler EJ, Fisher CJ, Sprung CL et al: Treatment of gram-negative bacteremia and septic shock with HA-IA human monoclonal antibody against endotoxin. N Engl J Med 324:429, 1991

219. Holaday JW, Faden AL: Naloxone reversal of endotoxin hypotension suggests role of endorphins in shock. Nature 275:450, 1978

220. Holcroft SW, Vassar MJ, Wever CJ: Prostaglandin E1 and survival in patients with adult respiratory distress syndrome. Ann Surg 203:371, 1986

221. Stevens JH, O'Hanley P, Shapiro JM et al: Effects of anti-C5a antibodies on the adult respiratory distress syndrome in septic primates. J Clin Invest 77(6):1812, 1986

222. Jacobs ER, Soulsby ME, Bone RC et al: Ibuprofen in canine endotoxin shock. J Clin Invest 70:536, 1982

223. Fletcher JR, Ramwell PW: Modification by aspirin and indomethacin, of the hemodynamic and prostaglandin releasing effects of E. coli in the dog. Br J Pharmacol 61:175, 1977

224. Beutler B, Milsark IW, Cerami AC: Passive immunization against cachectin/tumor necrosis factor protects mice from lethal effects of endotoxin. Science 229:869, 1985

225. Luce JM: Pathogenesis and management of septic shock. Chest 91:883, 1987

225. Moldawar LL, Bistrian BR, Sobrado J et al: Muscle proteolysis in sepsis trauma. N Engl J Med 309:494, 1983

226. Lundholm KG: Nutritional problems in trauma. Acta Chir Scand 522(suppl):183, 1985

227. Cuthbertson DP: Post-traumatic metabolism: A multidisciplinary challenge. Surg Clin North Am 58:1045, 1978

228. Corman LC: The relationship between nutrition, infection and immunity. Med Clin North Am 69:519, 1985

229. Blackburn GL, Maini BS, Pierce EC: Nutrition in the critically ill patient. Anesthesiology 17:101, 1977

230. Blackburn GL, Bistrian BR, Maini BS et al: Nutritional and metabolic assessment of the hosptalized patient. JPEN 1:11, 1977

231. Bistrian BR, Blackburn GL, Sherman M et al: Therapeutic index of nutritional depletion in hospitalized patients. Surg Gynecol Obstet 141:512, 1975

232. Shetty PS, Watrasiewicz KE, Jung RT et al: Rapid turnover transport proteins: An index of subclinical protein-energy malnutrition. Lancet 2:230, 1979

233. Ingenbleck Y, Van Den Schrieck HG, De Nayer P et al: The role of retinol-binding protein in protein-calorie malnutrition. Metabolism 24:633, 1975

234. Long CL, Schaffel N, Geiger JW et al: Metabolic response to injury and illness: Estimation of energy and protein needs from indirect calorimetry and nitrogen balance. JPEN 3:452, 1979

235. Elevyn DH: Nutritional requirements of adult surgical patients. Crit Care Med 8:9, 1980

236. Cerra FB: Nutrition in the critically ill: Modern metabolic support in the intensive care unit. In Chernon B, Shoemaker WC (eds): Critical Care State of the Art, vol 7, p 1. Fullerton, CA, Society of Critical Care Medicine, 1986

237. Wretlind A: Current status of intralipid and other fat emulsions. In Meng HC, Wilmore DW (eds): Fat Emulsions in Parenteral Nutrition, p 109. Chicago, American Medical Association, 1976

238. Askanazi J, Nordenstrom J, Rosenbaum SH et al: Nutrition for the patient with respiratory failure: Glucose vs fat. Anesthesiology 54:373, 1981

239. Ryan JA Jr, Abel RM, Abbott WM et al: Catheter complications in total parenteral nutrition: A prospective study of 200 consecutive patients. N Engl J Med 290:757, 1974

240. Michel L, Serrano A, Malt RA: Nutrition support of hospitalized patients. N Engl J Med 304:1147, 1981

241. Giddings JC, Peake IR: Laboratory support in the diagnosis of coagulation disorders. Clin Haematol 14:571, 1985

242. Lasch HG, Heene DH: Heparin therapy of DIC. Thromb Haemost 33:105, 1974

243. Mant MJ, King EG: Severe acute disseminated intravascular coagulation: A reappraisal of its pathophysiology, clinical significance and therapy based on 47 patients. Am J Med 67:557, 1979

244. Friedman PA: Poisoning and its management. In Wilson J, Braunwald E, Isselbachee K et al: Harrison's Principles of Internal Medicine, p 883. New York, McGraw-Hill Book Company, 1987

245. Powell SH, Van De Graaff WB, Thompson WI et al: Charcoals, emetics, and cathartics in care of poisoned patients. Crit Care Med 8:233, 1980

246. Rumack BH, Peterson RG: Acetaminophen overdose: Incidence, diagnosis and management in 416 patients. Pediatrics 62(suppl):898, 1978

247. Levy R, Elo T, Hanenson IB: Intravenous fructose treatment of acute alcohol intoxication: Effects on alcohol metabolism. Arch Intern Med 137:1175, 1977

248. DaRosa R, Henning RJ, Sunshine I et al: Acute ethylene glycol poisoning. Crit Care Med 12:1003, 1984

249. Kaplan K: Methyl alcohol poisoning. Am J Med Sci 244:170, 1982

250. Dolan MC: Carbon monoxide poisoning. Can Med Assoc J 133:392, 1985

251. Turino GM: Effect of carbon monoxide on the cardiorespiratory system. Circulation 63:253A, 1981

252. Black PM: Brain death (2 parts). N Engl J Med 299:338, 1978

253. President's Commmission for the Study of Ethical Problems in Medicine and Biomedical and Behavioral Research: Defining Death. Washington DC: US Government Printing Office, 1981

254. President's Commission for the Study of Ethical Problems in Medicine and Biomedical and Behavioral Research: Guidelines for the determination of death. JAMA 246:2184, 1981

255. Black PM: Brain death in the intensive care unit. J Intensive Care Med 2:177, 1987

256. Powner DJ: The diagnosis of brain death in the adult patient. J Intensive Care Med 2:181, 1987

257. Ad Hoc Committee of Harvard Medical School: A definition of irreversible coma. JAMA 205:337, 1968

258. Cranford RE: Brain death and the persistent vegetative state. In Doudera AE, Petus JD (eds): Legal and Ethical Aspects of Treating Critically and Terminally Ill Patients, p 63. Ann Arbor, AUPHA Press, 1982

259. Ruark JE, Raffin TA: Initiating and withdrawing life support: Principles and practice in adult medicine. N Engl J Med 318:25, 1988

260. Tomlinson T, Brody H: Ethics and communication in do-not-resuscitate orders. N Engl J Med 318:43, 1988

261. American Thoracic Society Bioethics Task Force: Withholding and withdrawing life-sustaining treatment. Ann Internal Med 115:479, 1991

262. Curran WJ: The Saikewicz decision. N Engl J Med 298:499, 1978

263. Liacos PJ: Dilemma of dying. In Doudera AE, Peters JD (eds): Legal and Ethical Aspects of Treating Critically and Terminally Ill Patients, p 149. Ann Arbor, AUPHA Press, 1982

264. In the matter of Shirley Dinnerstein, 380 NE 2d 134 (Mass App Ct 1978)

265. Custody of A Minor 385 Mass 697, 434 NE 2d 601 (1982)

266. In the matter of Karen Quinlan, 70 NJ 10, 355 A 2d 647, 1976

267. Council on Ethical and Judicial Affairs, American Medical Association: Guidelines for the Appropriate Use of Do-Not-Resuscitate Orders. JAMA 265:4, 1991

60

Alan Jay Schwartz
Frederick W. Campbell

Cardiopulmonary Resuscitation

HISTORY OF CARDIOPULMONARY RESUSCITATION

Cardiopulmonary resuscitation (CPR) seems synonymous with the growth of modern medicine. Development of CPR, however, is not a recent "dramatic achievement . . . comparable to the conquest of Mt. Everest."[1] The currently accepted CPR procedures evolved over years of slow, stepwise progress, and many concepts initially relegated to obscurity were rediscovered and applied to clinical practice.

The earliest reference to CPR is found in the biblical story of creation, where God created Adam ". . . and breathed into his nostrils the breath of life."[2] Use of an artificial airway was suggested by Vesalius, and tracheal intubation was popularized at the end of the 18th century. A connection between use of an airway and mouth-to-mouth rescue breathing was not made until the late 19th and early 20th centuries.[3-7] In 1744, the surgeon William Tossach reported successful mouth-to-mouth ventilation for a victim who had suffered cardiac arrest.[8] Clinicians, however, used other methods of resuscitation such as barrel rolling and bellows insufflation of the lungs, and mouth-to-mouth ventilation did not become popular. Interestingly, laboratory physiologists often used rescue breathing as early as the 1850s.[6]

Use of mouth-to-mouth rescue breathing in the clinical setting did not become a possibility until the 1940s. Ralph Waters taught his students that the active rescue breathing technique should be considered in emergency care of the arrest victim.[6] Subsequently, David Cooper in the U.S. Army was faced with solving the problem of life support for soldiers poisoned with nerve gas.[5,6] The accepted but remarkably ineffective method for artificial ventilation commonly employed during those days was the Schafer prone-pressure method. Compression of the lower portion of the thoracic cage posteriorly was thought to effect pulmonary gas exchange. Cooper and his colleagues proved that a modification of the gas mask could be used effectively for mask-to-mask ventilation.[6] Pulmonary gas exchange was analyzed and data provided to show that the use of exhaled air from the rescuer could benefit a nonbreathing victim.[9] James Elam combined the data of clinical effectiveness and respiratory physiology and began to popularize the mouth-to-mouth technique with the help of Gordon.[10-12] Safar, an anesthesiologist, made the final contribution to the adoption of the active rescue breathing technique by making everyone aware of the fact that airway patency was much easier to establish with the new technique and almost impossible with the older, passive resuscitation methods.[13] The anesthesiologist was needed to make the connection between what was known about the effectiveness of mouth-to-mouth rescue breathing and the fact that an open airway was essential for any breathing technique. Thus, from Tossach's report in 1744 to Safar's contribution in 1960, more than 200 years elapsed before the modern rescue breathing technique was defined.

Development of the technique for producing artificial circulation and defibrillation has also required an extended time.[14] In the late 1800s and early 1900s, laboratory animals were resuscitated by chest massage.[15] In 1899 Prevost and Battelli reported that electrical countershock stopped ventricular fibrillation.[16] As public utility companies developed in the early 1900s, more and more accidental electrocutions were reported. Under the sponsorship of the Consolidated Edison Electric Company, a major research effort was launched in the 1920s at the Rockefeller Institute and Johns Hopkins University to solve the electrocution problem. The modern defibrillator is a direct result of this effort.[14]

In 1947 the first success at human open-chest defibrillation was reported,[17] and a few years later Kouwenhoven developed a closed-chest defibrillation device.[18] Recognition of the need for a portable defibrillator spurred the development of the direct current (DC) defibrillator. By the late 1950s, a portable defibrillator was available that was effective without damaging the heart and did not require an open chest for delivery of current.

In 1954, during the development of the defibrillator, Guy Knickerbocker, who was working with Kouwenhoven, observed that when defibrillator paddles were applied to the chest cage of experimental animals, the external chest pressure resulted in a rise in blood pressure.[19] This led to the rediscovery of the effective production of artificial cardiac output by external chest compression, a technique described first in the 1920s.[14] As the 1960s began, closed-chest cardiac compression, artificial mouth-to-mouth rescue breathing, and the portable DC defibrillator, three essential ingredients for modern-day CPR, were clinically available. It would take another 10 to 15 years of application and discussion before the development of standard CPR protocols using these techniques and equipment.

THE NEED FOR CARDIOPULMONARY RESUSCITATION

The American Heart Association (AHA) CPR program was initiated to treat the major complications of coronary artery disease, myocardial infarction, and lethal cardiac dysrhythmias. In the United States, cardiovascular disease affects an estimated 63.4 million individuals.[20] The number of patients in the United States with the clinical diagnosis of coronary artery disease is 4.8 million. Deaths due to diseases of the heart numbered 986,370 in 1984, 540,400 of which were attributed to ischemic disease. Of the leading causes of death, diseases of the heart rank first, accounting for 54.8%.[20]

More than one-half of the deaths attributed to ischemic heart disease occur outside a hospital setting within the first several hours after the onset of symptoms. Patients with chest pain often deny or ignore the presence of a serious problem. This delays the initiation of measures that might prevent more lethal events resulting from the ischemic heart disease.

The AHA developed its program to cope with those otherwise healthy individuals in whom coronary artery disease may produce sudden lethal cardiac dysrhythmias or an acute myocardial infarction with heart failure or dysrhythmias as later sequelae. The AHA reasoned that many of these people should not die under these circumstances. The goal of the program is to educate the public to (1) recognize the disease process and symptoms; (2) seek help immediately; and (3) provide resuscitation, at the scene, to victims without respiration or cardiac output.

Several studies have documented the success of this approach.[21-23] Teaching basic resuscitative procedures to the lay public, who then apply these techniques to victims in the community within a short time (4 minutes or less) after a cardiac arrest, and adding to this the provision of more advanced CPR within yet another brief interval (a total elapsed time of 8–10 minutes), results in approximately 40% overall survival.[24] Delay in either the basic or advanced life-support maneuvers results in a significant decrease in survival.

The same basic and advanced life-support system can and should be applied in all situations requiring life support. Many trauma and stroke victims are not salvageable, but some may experience full recovery if given the chance provided by the basic and advanced CPR life-support measures.

Life support provided as CPR is a specific application of intensive care medicine. Mobile intensive care, a concept and technique introduced in the late 1960s, is CPR provided in the field setting where cardiac arrest so often occurs.[25] Highly developed community-based health care delivery systems have been established in many locations throughout the country with clearly documented success.[23,24]

A key CPR concept is that cardiac arrest most often occurs in the community and, therefore, requires response from and within the community. In its 1980 CPR standards, the AHA emphasized this point, stating ". . . it is clear that the community deserves to be recognized as the ultimate coronary care (or life support) unit."[26]

CARDIOPULMONARY RESUSCITATION: THE PROBLEM AND ITS SOLUTION

Deficiency of oxygen delivery is the source of all cardiopulmonary arrests, irrespective of the initial cause. Basic cardiac life support (BCLS) solves the problem by providing temporary oxygen delivery, *i.e.*, oxygen delivery to the lungs with rescue breathing and oxygen transport from the lungs to the body tissues with cardiac compression (Table 60-1, Fig. 60-1A).[27] Long-term survival depends on the return of spontaneous oxygenation on the part of the arrest victim. Only when patients can ventilate and perfuse their own tissues with oxygenated blood is successful resuscitation achieved.

Advanced cardiac life support (ACLS) provides the necessary supportive maneuvers such that patients can maintain their own adequate cardiac output.[27] The prerequisites for spontaneous oxygen delivery (cardiac output) by the patient include a relatively normal cardiac rate, rhythm, and contractility and relatively normal vascular volume and tone. The recommended components of ACLS (Table 60-1, Fig. 60-1B) directly or in a supportive manner contribute to the return and continuation of spontaneous cardiac output.

TABLE 60-1. Component Parts of Cardiopulmonary Resuscitation

BCLS: Temporary Oxygen Delivery to the Cardiac Arrest Victim by a Rescuer

Diagnoses

1. Stupor or coma
2. Presence of breathing
3. Presence of circulation

Therapy

1. Rescue breathing
2. Artificial circulation

ACLS: Therapy Directed Toward Re-establishment of Spontaneous Oxygen Delivery by the Victim

Diagnoses

1. Dysrhythmias
2. Cardiovascular instability
3. Acid-base derangements

Therapy

1. Cardioversion/defibrillation
2. Intravascular access/monitoring/volume replacement
3. Pharmacologic therapy for hemodynamic/acid-base derangements

PRLS: Definition of the Primary Cause of the Cardiac Arrest and Maintenance of What Has Been Salvaged During BCLS-ACLS

Diagnoses

1. Cause of the cardiac arrest
2. Consequences of the cardiac arrest

Therapy

1. General intensive care
2. Specific intensive care—pulmonary/cardiovascular/renal/metabolic/brain resuscitation

BCLS = basic cardiac life support; ACLS = advanced cardiac life support; PRLS = postresuscitation life support.

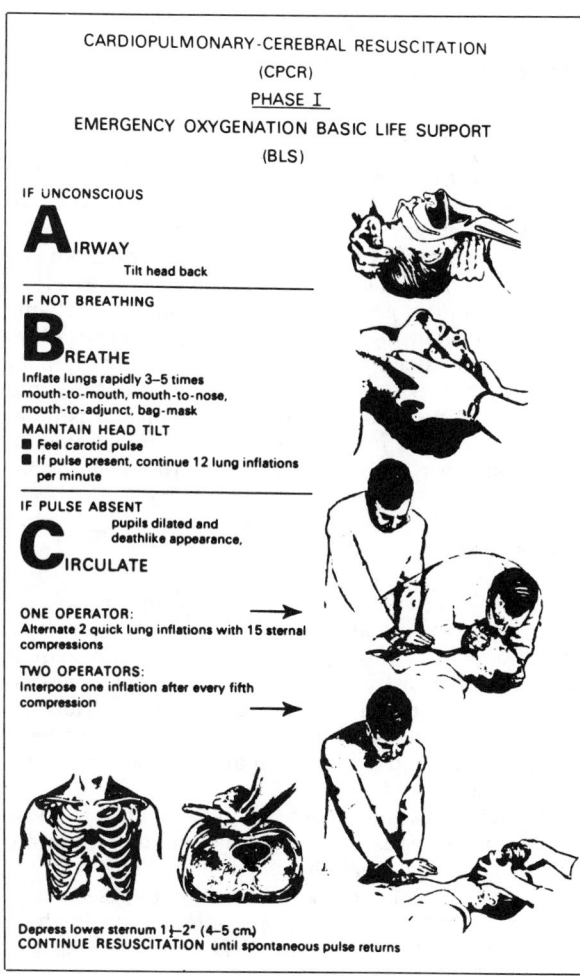

A

CARDIOPULMONARY-CEREBRAL RESUSCITATION
(CPCR)
PHASE I
EMERGENCY OXYGENATION BASIC LIFE SUPPORT
(BLS)

IF UNCONSCIOUS

AIRWAY
Tilt head back

IF NOT BREATHING

BREATHE
Inflate lungs rapidly 3–5 times
mouth-to-mouth, mouth-to-nose,
mouth-to-adjunct, bag-mask
MAINTAIN HEAD TILT
■ Feel carotid pulse
■ If pulse present, continue 12 lung inflations
per minute

IF PULSE ABSENT
pupils dilated and
deathlike appearance,

CIRCULATE

ONE OPERATOR:
Alternate 2 quick lung inflations with 15 sternal
compressions

TWO OPERATORS:
Interpose one inflation after every fifth
compression

Depress lower sternum 1½–2" (4–5 cm)
CONTINUE RESUSCITATION until spontaneous pulse returns

B

CARDIOPULMONARY-CEREBRAL RESUSCITATION
(CPCR)
PHASE II
ESTABLISHMENT OF NORMAL ARTERIAL OXYGEN TRANSPORT
(RESTART SPONTANEOUS CIRCULATION)
ADVANCED LIFE SUPPORT
(ALS)

DO NOT INTERRUPT CARDIAC COMPRESSIONS AND LUNG VENTILATION
INTUBATE TRACHEA WHEN POSSIBLE

DRUGS AND FLUIDS, I.V. LIFELINE
EPINEPHRINE
0 5–1 0 mg I V repeat larger dose as necessary

SODIUM BICARBONATE
1 mEq/kg I V
Repeat dose every 10 minutes until pulse returns.
Monitor and normalize arterial pH

I V FLUIDS as indicated

E K G. Ventricular fibrillation? Asystole? Bizarre complexes?

FIBRILLATION TREATMENT
EXTERNAL DEFIBRILLATION
D C 100–400 W/sec
Repeat shock as necessary
LIDOCAINE
1–2 mg/kg I V if necessary
IF ASYSTOLE
repeat step D calcium and vasopressors as needed
CONTINUE RESUSCITATION until good pulse
is maintained

D C 100–400 W sec

C

CARDIOPULMONARY-CEREBRAL RESUSCITATION
(CPCR)
PHASE III
POST-RESUSCITATIVE LIFE SUPPORT
(PLS)

GAUGING
Determine and treat cause of demise
Determine salvageability

HUMAN MENTATION-- **C**EREBRAL RESUSCITATION
Support perfusion pressure, xygenation, ventilation
If arrest > 5 min , coma > 5 min after reperfusion
---clinical trials (e g , thiopental)

INTENSIVE CARE

$PaCO_2$ 25-35   Art , CV, (PA) catheters
PaO_2>100   Temp Control, EKG
pHa 7 3-7 6   (Curarization)

ICP (osmotherapy, hypothermia)
Suppress convulsions
Steroid, Dextrose 5-10%, electrol., IV Fluids, alimentation
Hct , plasma COP, serum osm
Outcome

Figure 60-1. (A) Basic life support: emergency oxygenation, a temporizing measure provided by a rescuer or rescuers. (B) Advanced life support: techniques to aid restoration of spontaneous oxygen delivery by the cardiac arrest victim. (C) Postresuscitative life support: critical care therapies to support and maintain the resuscitated victim with particular emphasis on the cause of the cardiopulmonary arrest, its treatment and prevention, and the post-CPR cardiopulmonary, neurologic, and renal status. (Reproduced with permission from Safar P: Cardiopulmonary-cerebral resuscitation including emergency airway control. In Schwartz GR, Safar P, Stone JH et al [eds]: Principles and Practice of Emergency Medicine, p 177. Philadelphia, WB Saunders, 1978.)

If spontaneous oxygen delivery by the victim can be re-established, the CPR effort is termed a short-term success. To maintain this status, the post–resuscitative life support (PRLS) phase of CPR must be activated[27] (Table 60-1, Fig. 60-1C). Airway, hemodynamic, and pharmacologic supportive therapy is employed where indicated to allow the victim to continue adequate spontaneous oxygen delivery and not revert to another cardiac arrest state. Brain resuscitation is a specific and vital part of this PRLS phase that is designed to salvage as much normally functioning central nervous system tissue as possible. A major task during PRLS is determining the underlying malady that resulted in the cardiac arrest and correcting it. Only through PRLS intensive care and monitoring can long-term survival result from a CPR effort.

BASIC LIFE SUPPORT (EMERGENCY OXYGENATION)

The temporary delivery of oxygen to vital tissues is accomplished by providing effective airway management, ventilation, and artificial circulation (Table 60-2). Supportive equipment and drugs, e.g., ventilating devices, oxygen, and epinephrine, which enhance oxygen delivery during basic life support should be used when available.

Airway Management During Cardiopulmonary Resuscitation

Obstruction of the hypopharynx by the epiglottis and base of the tongue is the most common cause of airway obstruction in the unconscious individual. With depression of consciousness, relaxation of the head and neck muscles supporting the mandible, tongue, and epiglottis occurs. The epiglottis and base of the tongue fall against the posterior pharyngeal wall in the hypopharynx, obstructing the airway and prohibiting gas flow into the trachea. In 80 anesthetized, spontaneously breathing adults, Safar found an unobstructed airway in only 10% with the head in a neutral position and airway unsupported.[28] Airway obstruction can occur regardless of whether the subject is prone, lateral, or supine in position. Although gravity aids drainage of liquid from the pharynx of a lateral or prone individual, it does not ensure airway patency.[29]

Manual Airway Opening

The cardinal ingredient of manual airway opening techniques is anterior displacement of the mandible, which elevates the epiglottis and base of tongue from the posterior pharyngeal wall. This can be accomplished by lifting the mentum of the mandible with the fingers of one hand, the chin-lift maneuver (Fig. 60-2). When more effort is required to relieve airway obstruction, the mandible can be pushed forward by the fingers of both hands behind the angles of the jaw, which is called the jaw thrust (Fig. 60-3). Cervical hyperextension is often employed with mandibular displacement to augment airway opening; however, when used alone, it is comparatively ineffective, providing an open airway in fewer than 50% of obstructed persons.[28,30] If the patient has dentures, they should be left in place to help maintain a normal facial contour facilitating adequate lip or mask seal for ventilation.

Adjuncts to Airway Opening

Pharyngeal Airways

When airway obstruction persists despite maximal mandibular displacement, insertion of an oropharyngeal or nasopharyngeal airway may be helpful. These airways hold the epiglottis and base of the tongue off the posterior pharyngeal wall. The oropharyngeal airway is generally the more effective of the two but is not tolerated by responsive patients and may induce vomiting. Additionally, improper insertion or use of an undersized oral airway can exacerbate upper airway obstruction by pushing the tongue backward into the posterior pharynx. The nasopharyngeal airway is more likely to be accepted by responsive subjects. Proper mandibular displacement must be maintained during use of both pharyngeal airways.

Tracheal Intubation

When a patient's altered consciousness is not quickly reversible and airway opening is required for hours or days, measures should be taken to protect the airway from aspiration of regurgitated gastric contents as well as prevent gastric inflation during positive pressure ventilation. Tracheal intubation reliably accomplishes these goals and also allows tracheal suctioning and provides an alternative drug delivery route during resuscitation.

Attempts at tracheal intubation should not delay oxygenation of the unconscious or arrested patient and are rarely the first airway management efforts initiated. Ventilation by bag and mask with manual airway opening or insertion of a pharyngeal airway should precede attempts at tracheal intubation. The technique of tracheal intubation is described in Chapter 26.

Esophageal Obturator Airway

The esophageal obturator airway is an uncommonly used airway opening device but one with which anesthetists must be familiar if complications related to its use and removal are to be avoided (Fig. 60-4). Although the technique of esophageal obturator airway insertion is easily learned because laryngoscopy and glottic visualization are not required, adequate ventilation with the device often is not achieved by many rescuers.[31] The esophageal obturator airway is regarded as an alternative to tracheal intubation when the rescuer cannot intubate the trachea or equipment for tracheal intubation is not available.

The anesthetist is most likely to encounter the esophageal obturator airway in place in a patient with cardiac arrest transported to a medical facility. It is desirable to replace the esophageal obturator airway with a tracheal airway in order to ensure effective ventilation and oxygenation. However, passive regurgitation of gastric contents must be assumed to follow deflation of the esophageal cuff and obturator removal. It should be removed, therefore, only after the patient has awakened and regained protective airway reflexes or after the airway has been secured with a cuffed endotracheal tube. After preoxygenation and ventilation using the esophageal obturator airway, the mask is detached from the obturator, which is left in place during tracheal intubation to prevent regurgitation and aspiration. Laryngoscopy can be performed easily with the esophageal airway moved to the left side of the mouth. Once tracheal airway position is confirmed and the tracheal cuff is inflated, the esophageal cuff may be deflated and the obturator removed.

TABLE 60-2. American Heart Association Basic Life Support Sequences for Adults, Children, and Infants

	Objectives	Actions Adult (over 8 yrs.)	Child (1 to 8 yrs.)	Infant (under 1 yr.)
A. Airway	1. Assessment: Determine unresponsiveness	Tap or gently shake shoulder.		
		Say, "Are you okay?"		Observe
	2. Get help.	Call out "Help!"		
	3. Position the victim.	Turn on back as a unit, supporting head and neck if necessary. (4–10 seconds)		
	4. Open the airway.	Head-tilt/chin-lift		
B. Breathing	5. Assessment: Determine breathlessness.	Maintain open airway. Place ear over mouth, observing chest. Look, listen, feel for breathing. (3–5 seconds)		
	6. Give 2 rescue breaths.	Maintain open airway.		
		Seal mouth to mouth		mouth to nose/mouth
		Give 2 rescue breaths, 1 to 1½ seconds each. Observe chest rise. Allow lung deflation between breaths.		
	7. Option for obstructed airway	a. Reposition victim's head. Try again to give rescue breaths.		
		b. Activate the EMS system.		
		c. Give 6–10 subdiaphragmatic abdominal thrusts (the Heimlich maneuver).		Give 4 back blows.
				Give 4 chest thrusts.
		d. Tongue–jaw lift and finger sweep	Tongue–jaw lift, but finger sweep only if you see a foreign object.	
		If unsuccessful, repeat a, c, and d until successful.		
C. Circulation	8. Assessment: Determine pulselessness.	Feel for carotid pulse with one hand; maintain head-tilt with the other. (5–10 seconds)		Feel for brachial pulse; keep head-tilt.
	9. Activate EMS system.	If someone responded to call for help, send them to activate the EMS system.		
	Begin chest compressions: 10. Landmark check	Run middle finger along bottom edge of rib cage to notch at center (tip of sternum).		Imagine a line drawn between the nipples.
	11. Hand position	Place index finger next to finger on notch:		Place 2-3 fingers on sternum, 1 finger's width below line. Depress ½–1 in.
		Two hands next to index finger. Depress 1½–2 in.	Heel of one hand next to index finger. Depress 1–1½ in.	
	12. Compression rate	80–100 per minute		At least 100 per minute
CPR Cycles	13. Compressions to breaths.	2 breaths to every 15 compressions.	1 breath to every 5 compressions.	
	14. Number of cycles.	4 (52–73 seconds)	10 (60–87 seconds)	10 (45 seconds or less)
	15. Reassessment.	Feel for carotid pulse. (5 seconds)		Feel for brachial pulse.
		If no pulse, resume CPR, starting with 2 breaths.	If no pulse, resume CPR, starting with 1 breath.	
Option for entrance of 2nd rescuer: "I know CPR. Can I help?"	1st rescuer ends CPR.	End cycle with 2 rescue breaths.	End cycle with 1 rescue breath.	
	2nd rescuer checks pulse (5 seconds).	Feel for carotid pulse.		Feel for brachial pulse.
	If no pulse, 2nd rescuer begins CPR.	Begin one-rescuer CPR, starting with 2 breaths.	Begin one-rescuer CPR, starting with 1 breath.	
	1st rescuer monitors 2nd rescuer.	Watch for chest rise and fall during rescue breathing; check pulse during chest compressions.		
Option for pulse return	If no breathing, give rescue breaths.	1 breath every 5 seconds	1 breath every 4 seconds	1 breath every 3 seconds

Reproduced with permission from Albarran-Sotelo R, Flint LS (eds): Instructor's Manual for Basic Life Support. Dallas, American Heart Association, 1987.

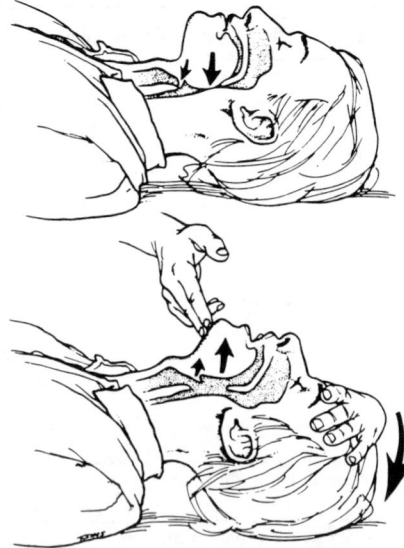

Figure 60-2. Airway obstruction and the chin-lift airway opening maneuver. The fingers of one hand lift the jaw anteriorly, grasping the mentum or ramus of the mandible. This elevates the epiglottis and lifts the base of the tongue from the posterior pharyngeal wall. Care must be taken not to compress the soft tissue under the chin, thereby obstructing the airway. The rescuer's other hand is used to extend the victim's head or operate manually powered ventilating devices. (Reproduced with permission from Albarran-Sotelo R, Flint LS [eds]: Instructor's Manual for Basic Life Support. Dallas, American Heart Association, 1987.)

Treatment of Airway Obstruction Caused by a Foreign Body

Airway obstruction, ventilatory insufficiency, and hypoxemia may result from aspiration of an occlusive foreign body into the hypopharynx, glottis, or trachea. Foreign body

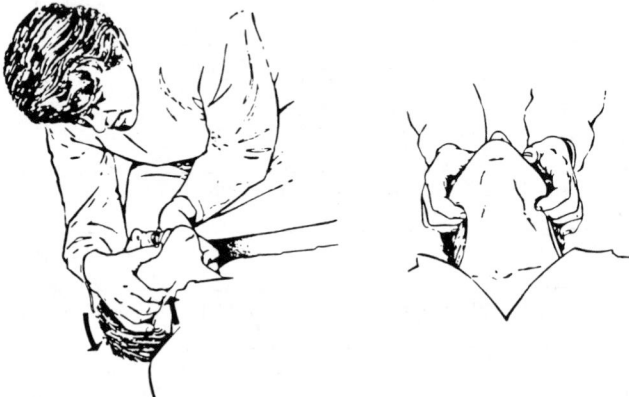

Figure 60-3. Two-handed jaw thrust maneuver. The mandible is pulled forward by the fingers of both hands behind the angles of the jaw. This maneuver is often effective when the one-handed chin lift has not opened the airway. Simultaneous extension of the head augments airway opening. A second person is needed to operate manual ventilating devices. The jaw thrust without cervical extension generally provides a patent airway in patients with suspected cervical spine injury. (Reproduced with permission from Safar P, Bircher NG: Cardiopulmonary Cerebral Resuscitation, 3rd ed. London, WB Saunders Co Ltd, 1988.)

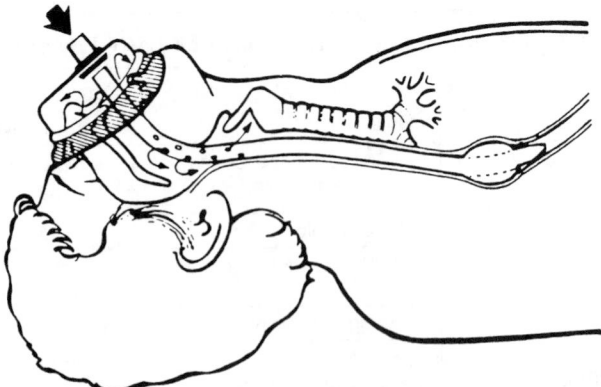

Figure 60-4. Structure and function of the esophageal obturator airway (EOA). The EOA is a 9.5-mm inside diameter tube with multiple air outlets along its proximal portion and a 30-cc inflatable cuff just proximal to its occluded distal tip. The proximal end of the tube snaps into a face mask and is inserted blindly into the esophagus of the unconscious subject with the mask in place on the obturator. The EOA is inserted maximally so that the mask seats properly on the face and ensures a sealed external airway. The cuff rests in the distal esophagus below the level of the carina in the adult patient. After inflation of the esophageal cuff, ventilation is provided by attaching any ventilating device to the proximal end of the obturator. Since the esophagus is occluded, inspiratory gas flow passes through the multiple openings of the EOA in the hypopharynx into the trachea. If it is properly positioned, the esophageal balloon precludes air entry into the stomach and the mask prevents air leak from the mouth and nose. Adequate ventilation is often not achieved by many rescuers because of a retrograde air leak from the mouth and nose owing to difficulty obtaining a good mask fit and obstruction of the air ports by the base of the tongue when the mandible is not held in a displaced position. Tracheal intubation therefore is the preferred method for provision of airway patency and protection during CPR. (Reproduced with permission from Safar P, Bircher NG: Cardiopulmonary Cerebral Resuscitation, 3rd ed. London, WB Saunders Co Ltd, 1988.)

airway obstruction in adults usually occurs while eating and is associated with elevated blood alcohol levels, poor dentition, dentures, and ingestion of large, poorly chewed pieces of food. In addition to food, children can choke on a variety of small foreign objects while playing.

Early recognition of foreign body airway obstruction is essential so the appropriate therapeutic maneuvers can be applied (Table 60-3). Differential diagnosis of this emergency from other conditions that cause acute respiratory distress is important.

The management of airway obstruction following foreign body aspiration varies with the degree of obstruction and gas exchange that results. It is crucial to distinguish partial airway obstruction with adequate air exchange from both partial obstruction with ineffective gas exchange and complete airway obstruction. The former is recognized when the conscious choking victim can speak and generate an effective cough despite some respiratory distress. As long as adequate oxygenation continues, a rescuer should not interfere with the subject's own efforts to expel the foreign object. Artificial cough techniques produce less expulsive pressure and flow than natural coughs, and there is a grave risk that an artificial cough will move the object to a more critical position in the airway, converting a partial obstruc-

TABLE 60-3. American Heart Association Treatment Sequences for Foreign Body Airway Obstruction in Adults, Children, and Infants

	Objectives	Actions Adult (over 8 yrs.)	Child (1 to 8 yrs.)	Infant (under 1 yr.)
Conscious Victim	1. Assessment: Determine airway obstruction.	Ask, "Are you choking?" Determine if victim can cough or speak.		Observe breathing difficulty.
	2. Act to relieve obstruction.	Perform subdiaphragmatic abdominal thrusts (Heimlich maneuver).		Give 4 back blows.
				Give 4 chest thrusts.
	Be persistent.	Repeat Step 2 until obstruction is relieved or victim becomes unconscious.		
Victim Who Becomes Unconscious	3. Position the victim; call for help.	Turn on back as a unit, supporting head and neck, face up, arms by sides. Call out, "Help!" If others come, activate EMS.		
	4. Check for foreign body.	Perform tongue–jaw lift and finger sweep.	Perform tongue–jaw lift. Remove foreign object only if you actually see it.	
	5. Give rescue breaths.	Open the airway with head-tilt/chin-lift. Try to give rescue breaths.		
	6. Act to relieve obstruction.	Perform subdiaphragmatic abdominal thrusts (Heimlich maneuver).		Give 4 back blows.
				Give 4 chest thrusts.
	7. Check for foreign body.	Perform tongue–jaw lift and finger sweep.	Perform tongue–jaw lift. Remove foreign object only if you actually see it.	
	8. Try again to give rescue breaths.	Open the airway with head-tilt/chin-lift. Try to give rescue breaths.		
	9. Be persistent.	Repeat Steps 6–8 until obstruction is relieved.		
Unconscious Victim	1. Assessment: Determine unresponsiveness.	Tap or gently shake shoulder. Shout. "Are you okay?"		Tap or gently shake shoulder.
	2. Call for help; position the victim.	Turn on back as a unit, supporting head and neck, face up, arms by sides. Call out, "Help!" If others come, activate EMS.		
	3. Open the airway.	Head-tilt/chin-lift		Head-tilt/chin-lift, but do not tilt too far.
	4. Assessment: Determine breathlessness	Maintain an open airway. Ear over mouth; observe chest. Look, listen, feel for breathing. (3–5 seconds)		
	5. Give rescue breaths.	Make mouth-to-mouth seal.		Make mouth-to-nose-and-mouth seal.
		Try to give rescue breaths.		
	6. Try again to give rescue breaths.	Reposition head. Try rescue breaths again.		
	7. Activate the EMS system.	If someone responded to the call for help, that person should activate the EMS system.		
	8. Act to relieve obstruction.	Perform subdiaphragmatic abdominal thrusts (Heimlich maneuver).		Give 4 back blows.
				Give 4 chest thrusts.
	9. Check for foreign body.	Perform tongue–jaw lift and finger sweep.	Perform tongue–jaw lift. Remove foreign object only if you actually see it.	
	10. Rescue breaths.	Open the airway with head-tilt/chin-lift. Try again to give rescue breaths.		
	11. Be persistent.	Repeat Steps 8–10 until obstruction is relieved.		

Reproduced with permission from Albarran-Sotelo R, Flint LS (eds): Intructor's Manual for Basic Life Support. Dallas, American Heart Association, 1987.

tion with adequate gas exchange to a complete obstruction without gas exchange. Gordon et al demonstrated that manual thrusts in unconscious individuals, i.e., Heimlich maneuvers, produce one fourth to one fifth of the airway pressure produced by a normal cough starting from resting lung volume (functional residual capacity) in the same subjects when awake.[32]

The conscious individual with partial airway obstruction should be permitted to assume whatever body position he or she perceives to be the most comfortable. This will most likely be a forward-leaning sitting position. Supplemental oxygen, if available, and continued observation for deterioration of gas exchange should be provided.

Complete airway obstruction and partial obstruction with poor air exchange are characterized by inability to speak and an absent or weak cough. In the unconscious person whose aspiration and collapse were not witnessed, foreign body airway obstruction is suspected upon observing paradoxical spontaneous respiratory efforts and chest wall retractions or noting inability to ventilate the lungs despite several attempts to open the airway manually or with supportive equipment if available.

Artificial Cough Techniques

In 1974, Heimlich introduced a simple manual method for relieving airway obstruction, the abdominal thrust. He theorized that since aspiration of a foreign body occurred during inspiration, air is trapped in the lungs behind the obstruction.[33] With rapid inward and upward compression of the victim's epigastrium, the diaphragm is forced cephalad, compressing the trapped air volume. The rapid increase in airway pressure and air flow generated should move the foreign body from its obstructing position in the airway. Chest thrusts, manual thrusts applied to the middle or lower chest, compress the intrathoracic air volume directly and produce airway pressures and flows comparable to those achieved with abdominal thrusts (Table 60-4).

Early recommendations for clearing foreign body airway obstructions included the use of back blows and were based on laboratory (e.g., Table 60-4) and clinical data obtained during comparison of the various methods of producing an artificial cough. Combinations of back blows and abdominal or chest thrusts were more effective in clearing pieces of meat from airways of anesthetized animals than was either maneuver used alone.[32] In a clinical report of 386 trials of various maneuvers, alone and in combination, successes and failures were attributed to each of the methods.[34] When used alone, back blows were effective in 20% of trials; abdominal thrusts, 44%; chest thrusts, 36%; and finger probes, 17%. When used in combination with other maneuvers, back blows were successful in 49% of trials; abdominal thrusts, 79%; chest thrusts, 64%; and finger probes, 58%. Each method was sometimes given credit for success after another method had failed. It was concluded that a combination of maneuvers was more likely to be effective than any single maneuver.

Subsequently, Day et al used an accelerometer to measure the inertial forces generated in the airways of subjects receiving back blows.[35] When struck on the back, the head and neck of the subjects were propelled in a cephalad direction. It was inferred that, as a consequence, a foreign object in the airway might actually be impacted farther into the airway rather than expelled by back blows. Transmission of inertial forces directly to the foreign body as well as to the head and neck and the degree to which the expulsive intrathoracic pressure would counteract the potentially harmful cervical inertial forces were not studied. Thus, the theoretical basis supporting the efficacy of back blows is unsettled.

Manual thrusts are currently recommended for relief of foreign body airway obstruction in the adult and child over 1 year of age. This is based on the undisputed theoretical and clinical observations supporting the effectiveness of the Heimlich maneuver and its variation, the chest thrust (Fig. 60-5).

Series of chest thrusts and back blows, in combination, are recommended for children less than 1 year of age with foreign body obstruction. When back blows are administered to an infant whose head and torso are supported by the opposite hand or thigh of the rescuer, intrathoracic pressure rises most likely as a result of both the direct blow and the compression of the thorax in a manner physiologically analogous to the chest thrust. The inertial forces propelling the head and neck in a cephalad direction are probably minimized when the infant's head and torso are restrained.

As the conscious choking victim becomes asphyxiated and unconscious, glottic muscle relaxation occurs, and maneuvers that were previously ineffective may dislodge the object. With relaxation it may also become possible to ventilate around the obstruction with slow forceful breaths and to remove the obstructing object with a finger sweep of the posterior pharynx administered in conjunction with a tongue–jaw lift maneuver (Fig. 60-6). Complications have been reported following use of each airway clearing maneuver. Manual thrusts have resulted in rupture of the stomach, esophageal laceration, regurgitation, fractured ribs, retinal detachment, and abdominal aortic rupture. Hazards resulting from finger probes include pharyngeal abrasion, regurgitation, and impacting a foreign body deeper into the airway.

Direct Laryngoscopy

Direct laryngoscopy and instrumentation of the airway to extract the obstructing body may be employed by rescuers who are proficient in their application, i.e., anesthetists. Once the subject is unconscious, direct visualization can be accomplished with a laryngoscope, tongue blade, or spoon and a flashlight. A forceps or clamp may then be used with visualization to grasp and extract the object. Blind grasping attempts in the posterior pharynx using forceps or clamps should be avoided.

Cricothyrotomy and Transtracheal Ventilation

Percutaneous cricothyrotomy and transtracheal catheter ventilation may allow institution of ventilation and oxygenation when the necessary equipment and expertise are available and foreign body airway obstruction is not relieved

TABLE 60-4. Comparison of Artificial Cough Techniques in Anesthetized, Apneic Adults*

Techniques and Victim Position (Rescuer at Victim's Side)	Partial Airway Obstruction† Peak Flow Rate (l·min⁻¹)	Complete Obstruction‡ Peak Airway Pressure (mm Hg)
Normal Cough		
From end exhalation	108	72
From end inspiration	162	115
Artificial Cough		
Back Blows		
Sitting	12	35
Lateral horizontal	11	30
Abdominal Thrusts		
Sitting	120	15
Supine	132	12
Chest Thrusts		
Sitting	132	19
External Cardiac Compression	120	17

*Mean values for six human volunteers. Normal cough measurements were made prior to induction of general anesthesia.

†Airway pressure not reported.

‡No air flow when airway completely obstructed.

Modified with permission from Gordon AS, Belton MK, Ridolpho PF: Emergency management of foreign body airway obstruction. In Safar P, Elam JO (eds): Advances in Cardiopulmonary Resuscitation, p 43. New York, Springer Verlag, 1977.

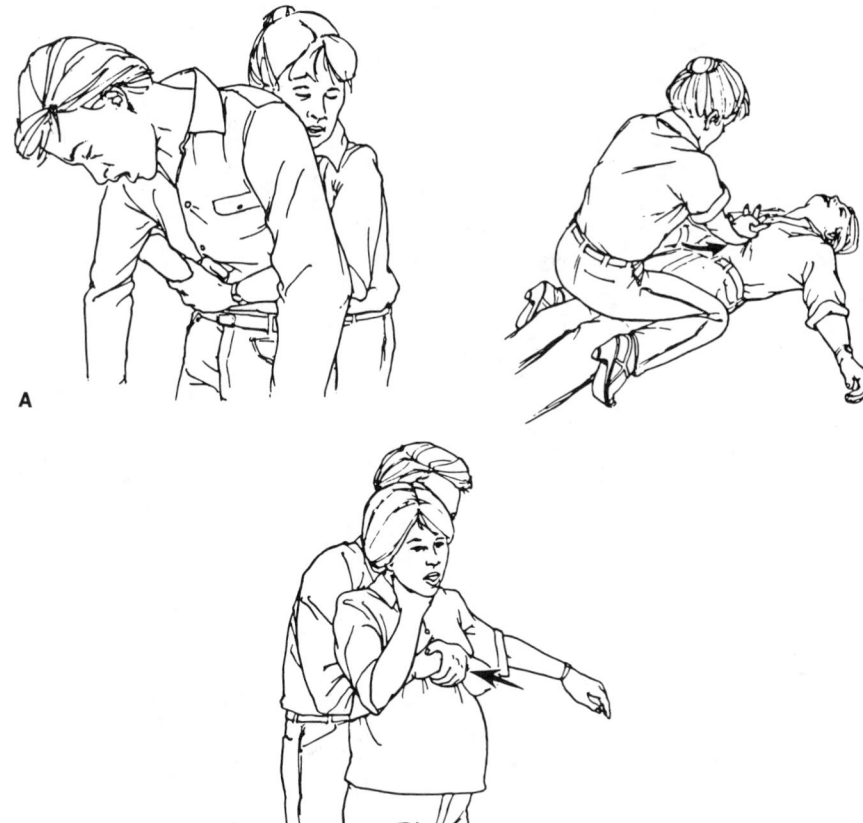

Figure 60-5. Manual thrust artificial cough techniques. (*A*) Abdominal thrust (Heimlich maneuver). Rapid inward and upward compression of the choking victim's epigastrium forces the diaphragm in a cephalad direction, compressing the air volume trapped in the lungs below the obstruction. The rapid increase in airway pressure and air flow generated should move the foreign body from its position in the airway. (*B*) Chest thrust. Rapid manual thrusts applied to the lower chest produce rises in airway pressure and air flows similar to those produced by abdominal thrusts. In certain persons (infants, obese victims, and pregnant women) chest thrusts will be more effective and cause fewer complications than abdominal thrusts. (Reproduced with permission from Albarran-Sotelo R, Flint LS [eds]: Instructor's Manual for Basic Life Support. Dallas, American Heart Association, 1987.)

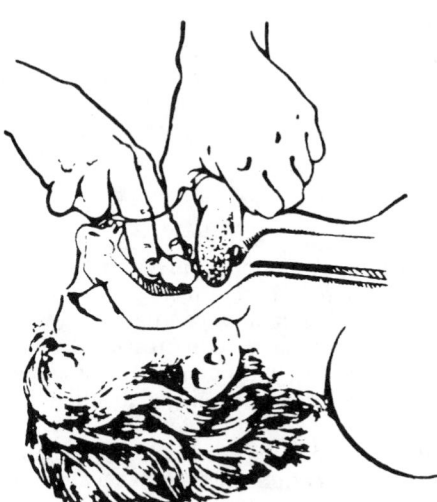

Figure 60-6. Tongue-jaw lift maneuver and finger sweep of the hypopharynx. Firmly grasping the victim's mandible and tongue between the thumb and fingers of one hand, the rescuer pulls this block of tissue anteriorly, thereby dislodging supraglottic foreign bodies or, at least, providing more space in the hypopharynx for the finger sweep. Caution must be exerted during blind probing of the pharynx to avoid impaction of an object deeper into the airway. Because this risk is greatest in the small mouths of infants and children, finger sweeps of the posterior pharynx are not recommended in these age groups unless the foreign object is visualized. (Reproduced with permission from Safar P, Bircher NG: Cardiopulmonary Cerebral Resuscitation, 3rd ed. London, WB Saunders Co Ltd, 1988.)

by simpler measures. The technique is also useful in other situations of uncorrectable airway obstruction and impossible tracheal intubation: maxillofacial and laryngeal trauma, epiglottitis, airway burns, and angioneurotic edema. Subsequent tracheostomy, controlled tracheal intubation, or endoscopic examination may be performed while transtracheal catheter ventilation continues.

Transtracheal catheter ventilation is provided by a high-flow oxygen source and specialized ventilation system through a large-bore intravenous cannula inserted into the airway through the cricothyroid membrane (Fig. 60-7). Transtracheal catheter ventilation may also be accomplished with simplified equipment by using an ordinary wall oxygen flow meter set at the flood or flush position (approximately 30 l·min^{-1}) and a piece of standard oxygen tubing with a side hole cut near its distal end. This end is connected *via* a stopcock, or other connector, to the transtracheal cannula. Lung inflation occurs when the side hole in the tubing is occluded by the rescuer's thumb, and exhalation occurs passively when the thumb is removed.

If effective ventilation and oxygenation are to be achieved, insertion of a transtracheal cannula of adequate size and use of an appropriate ventilating device are mandatory. A 12-, 14-, or 16-gauge intravenous catheter (2 inches in length) can be used to provide ventilation in adults and children in conjunction with high-flow jet oxygen ventilation systems. A bag-valve device coupled to a 15-mm tracheal tube connector attached to the intravenous catheter does not permit effective ventilation.[36,37] Satisfactory ventilation and oxygenation with bag-valve devices or anesthesia ventilating systems can only be achieved provided that a 3.0-mm internal diameter or larger transtracheal cannula is

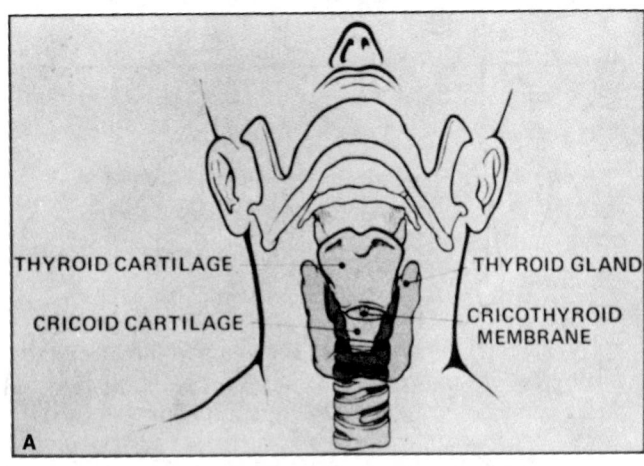

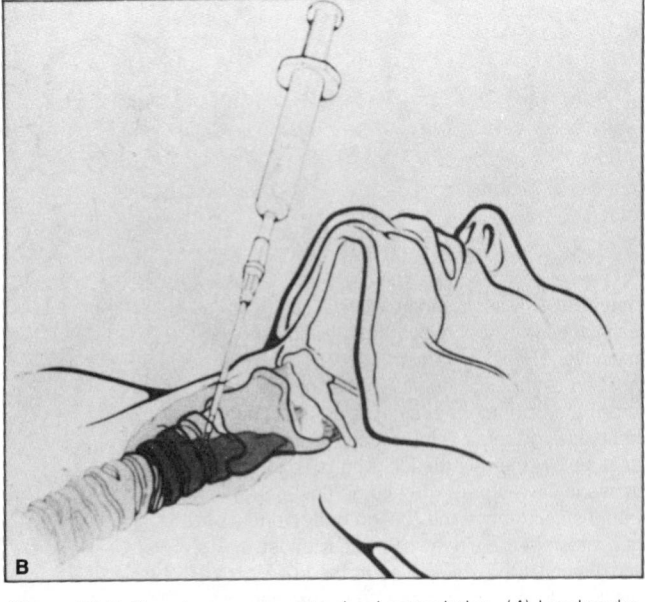

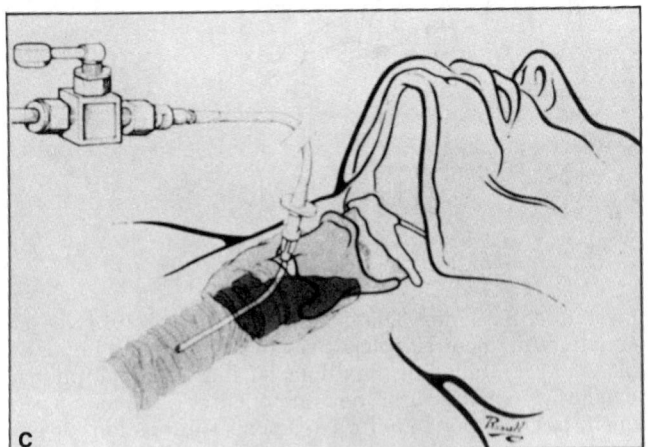

Figure 60-7. Percutaneous transtracheal cannulation. (*A*) Landmarks for the cricothyroid membrane. This membrane is felt as a horizontal indentation on the anterior surface of the neck in the midline between the thyroid and cricoid cartilages. The subcutaneous tissue overlying the cricothyroid membrane is relatively avascular, and the trachea lies immediately posterior to the membrane. (*B*) Tracheal cannulation. The intravenous catheter assembly is passed through the cricothyroid membrane. Aspiration of air signifies tracheal entry. The catheter is advanced into the trachea. (*C*) Catheter connected to the ventilating system. The cannula is connected by a length of intravenous extension tubing to a hand-operated release valve. The release valve is, in turn, connected by tubing to a source that delivers 100% oxygen at 50 psi. The source may be a wall oxygen outlet, an oxygen tank with a pressure-reducing valve, or an anesthetic machine. Inspiration is initiated by depressing the hand-operated release valve. (Reproduced with permission from the Textbook of Advanced Cardiac Life Support, 2nd ed. Dallas, American Heart Association, 1987.)

used.[38] Cannulation devices (3.5 mm and larger internal diameter) for percutaneous cricothyrotomy are available commercially.

Once cricothyrotomy is performed and the catheter is connected to the ventilating device, a jet of oxygen is introduced into the trachea. Lung inflation occurs despite a retrograde air leak. When the patient's chest is visibly inflated, inspiration is stopped and exhalation occurs passively through the upper airway if open. Effective ventilation and arterial oxygenation are readily achieved by transtracheal catheter ventilation in adults and children without severe parenchymal lung disease or upper airway obstruction. Complete obstruction in or above the glottis prevents exhalation from occurring during transtracheal catheter ventilation and may produce dangerously high airway pressures. In this situation, the transtracheal cannula permits apneic oxygenation of patients with native circulation by insufflation of oxygen to meet basal metabolic requirements. Although marked hypercarbia develops, arterial oxygenation is maintained while tracheostomy is performed. In cases of partial airway obstruction, slow ventilation rates and low inspiration to exhalation time (I:E) ratios must be used to allow for complete passive exhalation through the upper

airway between breaths and to prevent overinflation of the lungs.[39] Some hypercarbia will result.

Adequate oxygenation and ventilation have been provided during external chest compression in arrested animals for periods up to 30 minutes by transtracheal catheter ventilation[40] and by high-flow oxygen insufflation *via* transtracheal catheter.[41]

Pneumothorax and subcutaneous and mediastinal emphysema are complications of transtracheal catheter ventilation.

Artificial Ventilation

When apnea or hypoventilation is recognized and the airway is opened, ventilation and oxygenation must be initiated (Table 60-5). The usefulness of mouth-to-mouth ventilation is related to rescuers' ability to institute the procedure quickly without the use of special equipment and to deliver normal tidal volumes. Mouth-to-nose and mouth-to-stoma ventilation are alternatives to the mouth-to-mouth technique, respectively, when it is impossible to ventilate the victim *via* the mouth (e.g., the rescuer is unable to establish

TABLE 60-5. Artificial Ventilation Rates

Patient Age Group	Ventilation Rate (breaths·min^{-1})
Adult (>8 yr)	12–16
Child (1–8 yr)	16–20
Infant (<1yr)	20–24

Tidal volumes, 10–15 ml·kg^{-1}, should produce observable chest expansion. 100% oxygen should be administered as soon as possible.

a tight lip seal around the mouth) or when the victim has a tracheostomy.

Mouth-to-Mask Ventilation

Increasing concern about transmission of infection between patient and rescuer is leading to substitution of mouth-to-mask ventilation for mouth-to-mouth techniques and to the incorporation of filters and nonrebreathing valves in these portable devices to protect rescuer and patient from exhaled droplets (Fig. 60-8).

Exhaled air ventilation techniques provide an F_{IO_2} of 0.15–0.18 and, therefore, an alveolar oxygen tension (P_{AO_2}) of less than 80 mm Hg. The arterial oxygen tension (Pa_{O_2}) is considerably less as a result of CPR factors such as reduced cardiac output and increased intrapulmonary shunting contributing to an increased alveolar-arterial oxygen difference. In anesthetized adults, exhaled air ventilation performed with recommended tidal volumes and ventilatory rates is also associated with mild hypercarbia.[41a] Hence, use of ventilating devices that provide a high F_{IO_2} and allow increased ventilation should be instituted as soon as available.

Manually Powered Ventilators

Manually powered self-inflating resuscitators, e.g., the bag-valve device, and anesthesia ventilating systems permit the administration of a high F_{IO_2} and effective ventilation when used by skilled providers. These devices may be used to provide ventilation in conjunction with a mask, esophageal obturator airway, or endotracheal tube. The F_{IO_2} delivered by a simple resuscitation bag (Fig. 60-9) is limited to 0.4–0.6 (oxygen inflow 10–15 l·min^{-1}) because bag inflation exceeds the oxygen inflow rate, necessitating entrainment of room air and dilution of the bag's oxygen mixture. A higher inspired oxygen concentration can be delivered with bag-

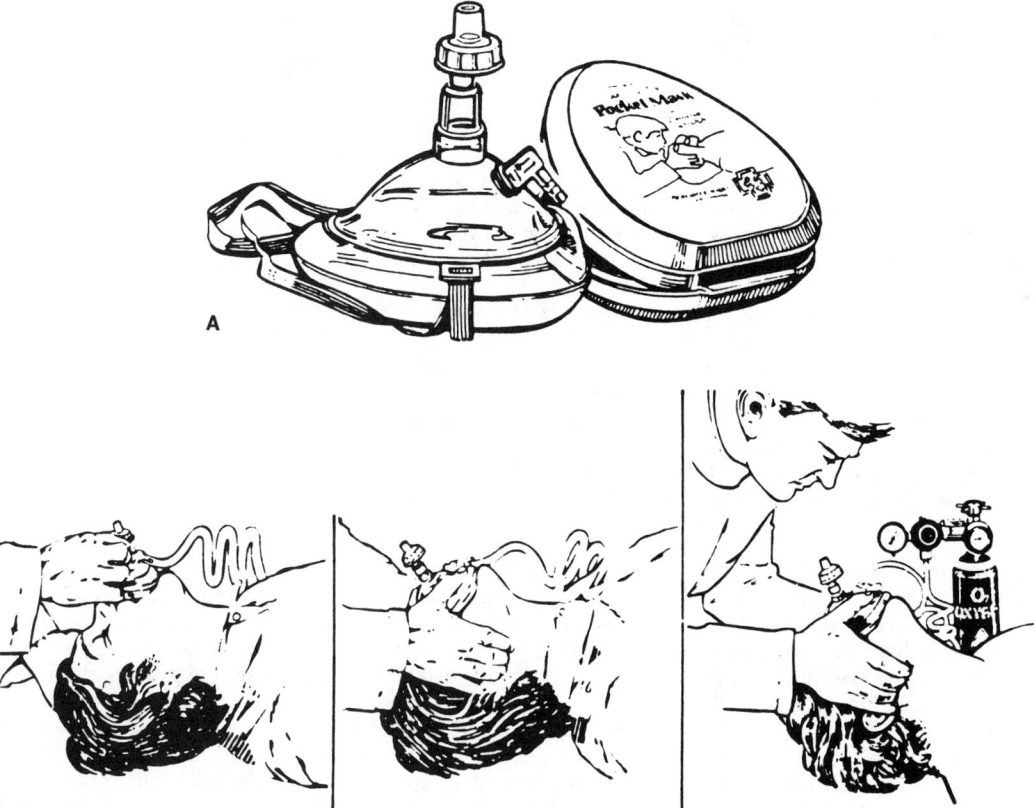

Figure 60-8. (A) Portable ventilating face mask with nonrebreathing valve and oxygen inlet. (B) Mouth-to-mask exhaled air ventilation. Mouth-to-mask exhaled air ventilation is most effectively accomplished when the mask is applied to the face by the rescuer's thumbs and thenar eminences, and the airway is opened with the jaw thrust technique. Many providers achieve ventilation with this apparatus more easily than with bag and mask because exhaled air breaths provide larger tidal volumes to overcome mask leaks and both hands are used for airway control and mask fit. Many portable emergency ventilating masks for mouth-to-mask ventilation include oxygen inlet ports for oxygen supplementation. (Reproduced with permission from Safar P, Bircher NG: Cardiopulmonary Cerebral Resuscitation, 3rd ed. London, WB Saunders Co Ltd, 1988.)

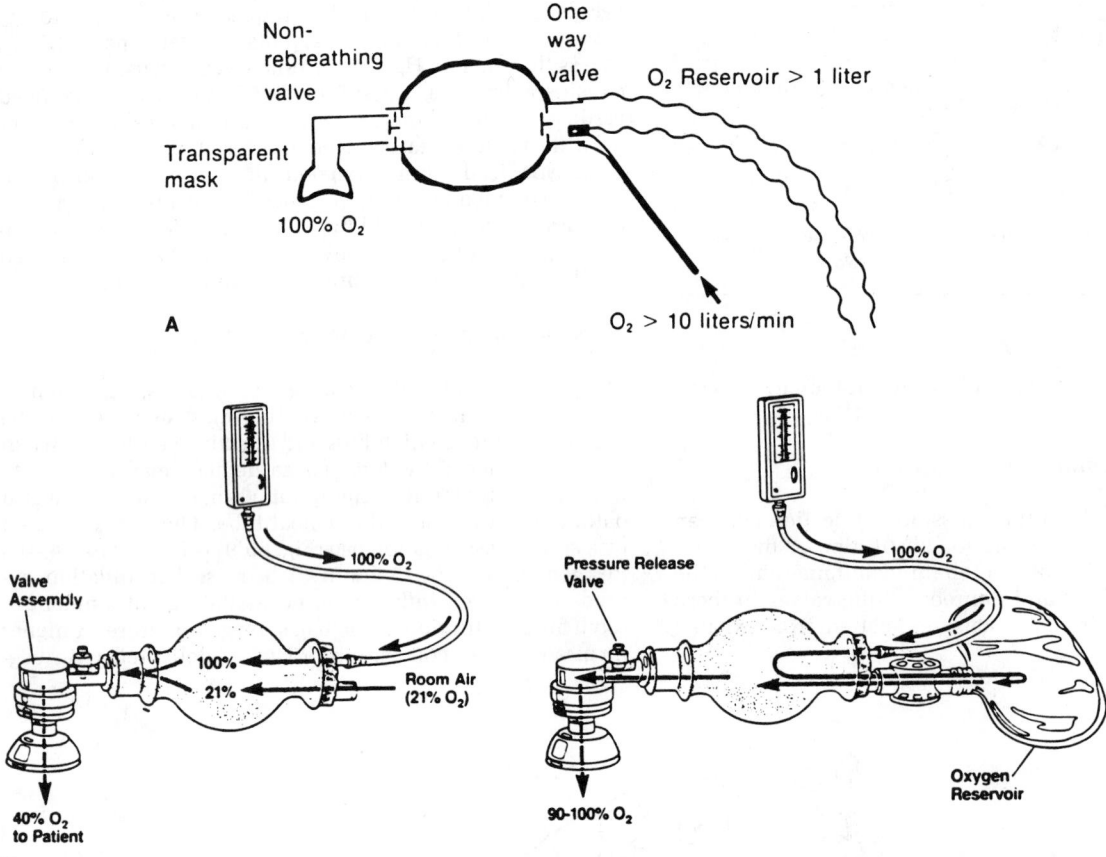

Figure 60-9. Manually powered self-inflating resuscitator (bag-valve device). (*A*) Bag-valve devices consist of a hand-powered, self-inflating bag with inflow and nonrebreathing valves. On bag compression the intake valve closes, stopping oxygen and air inflow, and the nonrebreathing valve opens, permitting delivery of the bag's gas mixture to the patient. During exhalation, the recoil of the bag causes reinflation with oxygen and air *via* the opened intake valve. The nonrebreathing valve directs the patient's exhaled gases to the atmosphere and prevents re-entry into the bag. (Reproduced with permission from Safar P, Bircher NG: Cardiopulmonary Cerebral Resuscitation, 3rd ed. London, WB Saunders Co Ltd, 1988.) (*B*) Effect of an attached oxygen reservoir on delivered F_{IO_2}. An attached reservoir at the intake valve accumulates oxygen while the valve is closed during inspiration. When bag reinflation occurs, oxygen enters the ventilating bag from the oxygen source and from the reservoir, thereby minimizing the volume of room air entrained and increasing the oxygen concentration in the bag. (Reproduced with permission from Chamedies L (ed): Textbook of Pediatric Advanced Life Support. Dallas, American Heart Association, 1988.)

valve devices fitted with an oxygen reservoir. With oxygen inflow rates of 10 and 15 $l \cdot min^{-1}$, inspired oxygen concentrations of 75% and 90% or greater are delivered. Pop-off valves are not desirable features on these devices (neonatal bag-valve devices are an exception) because inflation pressures required for ventilation during CPR may exceed those that open the pop-off mechanism.

Anesthesia ventilating systems, e.g., Jackson-Rees or Mapleson D breathing circuits, administer an F_{IO_2} of 1.0 when supplied by an oxygen source, but oxygen inflow rates must be properly set to minimize rebreathing of exhaled gas and over- or underinflation of the bag. Rebreathing is minimized when the oxygen inflow is set to a rate (liters/minute) at least two times the delivered minute ventilation.

The efficacy of bag-valve device and anesthesia ventilating system ventilation when used in conjunction with a mask is most often related to the operator's skill. Inadequate ventilation due to mask leakage, airway obstruction, and gastric distention are the common problems.

Gastric inflation occurs during positive pressure exhaled air or bag and mask ventilation when inspiratory airway pressure exceeds esophageal opening pressure, approximately 15 cm H_2O. High pharyngeal pressures are likely to result from ventilation using excessive tidal volumes or rapid inspiratory flow rates, especially in the presence of airway obstruction. Distention of the stomach may be minimized during exhaled air or bag-and-mask ventilation by application of cricoid pressure (Sellick's maneuver) by a second rescuer, using slow inspiratory flow rates (administer each breath over a 1.0–1.5 second inspiratory time), avoiding unnecessary continuous positive airway pressure or positive end-expiratory pressure, limiting tidal volume to that producing observable chest expansion, and correcting airway obstruction. As soon as tracheal intubation is accomplished, gastric inflation is prevented and the preceding admonitions may be violated. The stomach should be decompressed by oro- or nasogastric tube insertion only after the trachea is protected by tracheal intubation.

Oxygen-Powered Ventilators

Chest compression prematurely terminates inspiration provided by pressure-cycled mechanical ventilators. Volume-cycled machines may not be able to deliver adequate tidal volumes if the pressure limits are set too low. Manually triggered, oxygen-powered ventilating devices that provide instantaneous oxygen flow rates of 100 l·min^{-1} or more may be used during CPR to overcome the problems associated with the other types of mechanical ventilators. These devices are time-cycled and enable one to rapidly interpose breaths between compressions, inflating the lungs with 100% oxygen for as long as the control button or lever is depressed or until the airway pressure rises to 50 cm H_2O. Chest excursion is observed during inflation to avoid over-inflation. Gastric distention may develop when rapid inspiratory flow rates are delivered to a partially obstructed airway; therefore, use of these ventilation devices with the esophageal obturator airway or endotracheal airway is preferred.

Monitoring Artificial Ventilation

The efficacy of ventilation and arterial oxygenation must be assessed throughout resuscitation, and failure to achieve these goals should prompt rapid trouble shooting and corrective measures (Table 60-6).

Artificial Circulation

External Chest Compression

An absent central pulse is the indication for initiating artificial circulation by external chest compression. Pulselessness is determined by palpating the carotid or femoral artery, as these central pulses persist when more peripheral pulses are no longer palpable. A central pulse is generally not palpable when the systolic blood pressure is less than 50 mm Hg; peripheral pulses are lost below 70 mm Hg. Patients in shock with marked peripheral vasoconstriction

---

TABLE 60-6. Monitoring and Trouble Shooting Artificial Ventilation

Assessment

Chest excursion
Breath sounds
Exhaled air flow and condensate
Pulmonary compliance
Oximetry
Capnometry
Arterial blood gas analysis

Trouble Shooting

Uncorrected airway obstruction
Mouth-to-mouth or mask leak
Low tidal volume
Malfunctioning ventilatory device
Insufficient oxygen inflow
Mainstem bronchus intubation
Esophageal intubation
Occluded tracheal tube
Pneumothorax
Severe gastric distention

---

and absent peripheral pulses are best treated with measures such as fluids and drugs that augment the native circulation.

Circulation of unoxygenated blood will not sustain cerebral or myocardial viability, and sternal compression alone produces minimal ventilation. Chest compression must always be accompanied by effective airway management and oxygenation.

External chest compression can produce systolic blood pressures of 100 mm Hg and higher but diastolic pressures of not more than 10–40 mm Hg.[42-44] Carotid artery blood flow is generally less than one third of normal.[44-47] As a result of the low aortic diastolic pressures, myocardial perfusion during closed chest compression seldom exceeds 5–10% of normal levels.[43,47-49] Although these blood flows will temporarily sustain cerebral viability, prompt restoration of native circulation and coronary perfusion by advanced cardiac life support techniques is critical for survival.

Elements of compression technique are essential for effective externally produced artificial circulation. Inadequate sternal displacement and improper hand position are the most common reasons for poor external artificial circulation. The depth achieved by chest compression must exceed a threshold value in order to produce blood flow.[50] Above this threshold blood flow is linearly related to compression depth. Improper hand position during compression is not only less effective but increases the incidence of complications. These complications include rib and sternal fractures, costochondral separation, blunt traumatic injuries to intrathoracic and intra-abdominal organs, and pneumothorax.

The importance of correct ratio of compression to relaxation time in each compression cycle has been demonstrated using a computer-driven chest compression device for patients with cardiac arrest undergoing CPR.[51] During chest compression at a constant rate of 60 compressions per minute, increasing compression duration from 40% of cycle length to 50 and 60% increased Doppler measured carotid or femoral blood flow velocities by 34% and 85%. If a compression duration of 60% of cycle length was maintained, flow velocity and arterial pressure were not significantly different at compression rates of 40, 60, or 80 compressions per minute. In a later animal model in which cerebral and myocardial perfusion were measured using radiolabeled microspheres, the same relationship between compression duration and vital organ blood flow was observed.[52] If the optimal rate of chest compression is the rate that most easily brings compression duration to 50% of the cycle length, this rate is 80 compressions per minute or greater.[53] At this rate, natural body movement during compression and release of the chest bring systolic duration near 50%.

Efforts to discover more effective external chest compression techniques have led to the understanding that two mechanisms are responsible for generation of blood flow during CPR. A cardiac pump mechanism occurs when the ventricles are compressed between the sternum and vertebral column, thereby ejecting blood into the aorta and pulmonary artery in a manner analogous to that of open chest cardiac massage. Blood flow produced by direct cardiac compression is directly related to compression rate, as stroke volume is fixed by ventricular geometry in the presence of an unlimited venous return.[54]

A thoracic pump mechanism resulting from phasic increases in intrathoracic pressure created by rhythmic chest compression has also been documented.[44,55] Blood flow resulting from this mechanism occurs because the elevated intrathoracic pressure generated during artificial systole is transmitted to the extrathoracic arteries although not to the extrathoracic veins (owing to anatomic and functional valves at the thoracic inlet).[56] This unequal transmission of intrathoracic pressure elevations to the extrathoracic arteries and veins produces an extrathoracic arteriovenous (carotid artery–jugular vein) pressure gradient that generates blood flow during artificial systole. When chest compression is released, intrathoracic pressure decreases below venous pressure, and blood from the extrathoracic venous system flows into the chest. Thoracic pump blood flow is directly related to the magnitude of the rise in intrathoracic pressure produced by sternal depression and the duration over which the increased pressure is maintained.

An array of alternative techniques to improve blood flow and oxygen delivery during closed chest compression have been proposed. These techniques aim to increase compression rate (high-impulse CPR[54]) or augment the rise in intrathoracic pressure generated during compression. Intrathoracic pressure rise during sternal compression may be enhanced by (1) pressurizing the airway during compression (simultaneous compression-ventilation CPR),[44,46,47,57] (2) binding the abdomen to restrict diaphragmatic motion during compression,[46,58] (3) circumferential compression of the thorax (pneumatic vest CPR),[43] and (4) combinations of these modalities.

Interposed abdominal compression CPR is another alternative to conventional CPR in which an additional rescuer compresses the abdomen during the diastolic interval between chest compressions.[59-61] This produces diastolic augmentation of blood flow in a manner similar to intra-aortic balloon counterpulsation.

Survival from cardiopulmonary resuscitation is directly related to coronary perfusion pressure produced during chest compression.[62-66] Each of the investigational CPR modalities that augment intrathoracic pressure have been shown to improve one or more hemodynamic parameters (arterial blood pressure; aortic, carotid, or cerebral blood flow) compared to conventional closed-chest compression. Coronary perfusion pressure and myocardial blood flow, however, are not enhanced by simultaneous compression-ventilation CPR[42,46,47,67,68] or continuous abdominal binding during CPR.[68,69] Studies of coronary perfusion during pneumatic vest CPR report improved myocardial perfusion (measured by radiolabeled microsphere technique)[43] or no difference in coronary perfusion pressure[67,68] when compared with conventional CPR. Failure to enhance myocardial perfusion may occur because the augmented aortic pressure does not persist into the diastolic phase when coronary flow takes place, or the intrathoracic pressure generated during artificial systole is also transmitted to the intracardiac chambers and maintained into diastole, thus diminishing the pressure gradient driving blood across the coronary circulation.

Coronary blood flow during external artificial circulation is improved by increasing compression rate. High impulse manual chest compression, 150 per minute, produced superior coronary perfusion pressure and aortic blood flow when compared with manual chest compression at 60 per minute[70,71] and simultaneous compression-ventilation CPR and pneumatic vest CPR techniques at 60 per minute.[72] Coronary blood flow measured by electromagnetic flow probe is enhanced by increasing compression rate from 60 to 120 compressions per minute during manual[70] and pneumatic vest CPR[73] (Fig. 60-10).

Few comparable studies analyzing outcome from CPR have been accomplished using alternative methods of external artificial circulation. In one report, pneumatic vest CPR produced better 24-hour survival and neurologic function

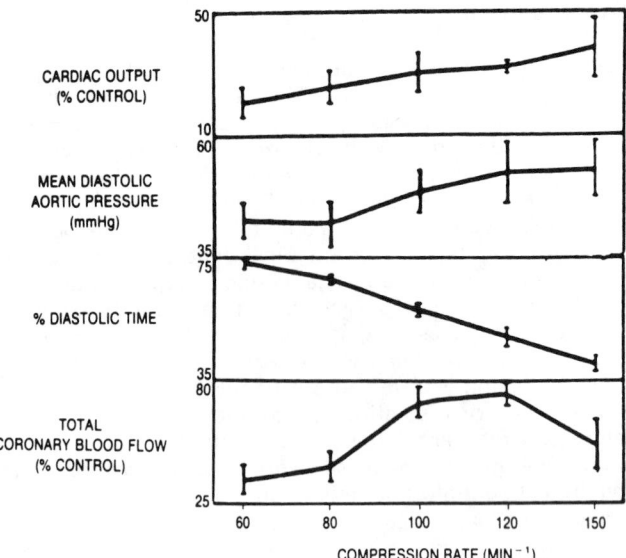

Figure 60-10. Influence of compression rate on hemodynamics during manually performed closed-chest compression in instrumented dogs. Increasing compression frequency from 60–150 compressions per minute produced proportional elevations of cardiac output and increases in aortic blood pressure. Coronary perfusion pressure rose over the range of compression rates studied, but myocardial blood flow decreased when compression was performed at 150 compressions per minute. At this rapid compression rate, the period of artificial diastole during which coronary perfusion occurs is reduced to a degree compromising myocardial blood flow despite the adequate perfusion pressure. (Reproduced with permission from Wolfe JA, Maier GW, Newton JR et al: Physiologic determinants of coronary blood flow during external cardiac massage. J Thorac Cardiovasc Surg 95:523–532, 1988.)

in animals when compared with conventional CPR,[43] whereas no differences were measured in another comparison of conventional CPR, simultaneous compression-ventilation CPR, and pneumatic vest CPR.[67] In a comparative trial during prehospital resuscitation of humans with cardiac arrest, simultaneous compression-ventilation CPR resulted in a survival rate inferior to that produced by conventional CPR.[74] Improved 24-hour survival after manual CPR was produced by use of a faster compression rate, 150 versus 60 compressions per minute, in a canine model.[71]

The cardiac pump and thoracic pump theories are not mutually exclusive, and both may explain aspects of the generation of blood flow during external chest compression.[56,75] Which one is predominant in a particular patient may depend on patient-related factors (heart size, anteroposterior chest diameter, thoracic compliance, and duration of cardiac arrest) and technique-related variables (manual *versus* mechanical compression and compression duration and depth). Observations of improved hemodynamics produced by rapid compression rates are consistent with both theories. Improved blood flow and pressure occur as a result of the direct compression rate effect on cardiac output (cardiac pump) and increase in the compression:relaxation ratio of each compression cycle (thoracic pump).

The effectiveness of artificial circulation is enhanced when supportive equipment and intravenous epinephrine are employed to maximize cardiac output and perfusion pressures produced with closed chest compression.

Adjuncts for Artificial Circulation

Cardiac Back Board. Cardiac output is produced when the relatively immovable objects (sternum and spine) squeeze the movable objects (heart and lungs) in sandwich-like fashion. To ensure that the bony structures effectively squeeze the soft tissues, the spine must be anchored. If the spine is not fixed in position, compression of the sternum toward the vertebrae results in displacement of the entire thoracic cage rather than compression of the intrathoracic contents. This commonly occurs when chest compression is being performed on a patient lying on a soft mattress. Inability to perform cardiac compression on a victim in water is also accounted for in this way. A more rigid foundation under the spine is required to anchor and limit its displacement. Such a rigid surface is always available by placing the patient on a walking surface such as the floor. A back board serves the same purpose and obviates the need to move the victim out of bed onto the floor. Ideally, the board is made of material rigid enough to serve as a resistive surface on which to compress the chest. A bed board should be located in all areas where life-support equipment is available. Modern-day design of dental chairs and other similar medical devices must take into account the potential need to perform cardiac compression and should be manufactured with materials adequate for producing a rigid back rest.

Oxygen-Powered Mechanical Compression Device. The ultimate in adjuncts for cardiac compression is the mechanical chest compression device consisting of a back board and oxygen-powered plunger. Cardiac compression can be regulated without fatigue by a rescuer who need only monitor correct position of the plunger and adequacy of sternal motion. The "thumper," as it is often called, will consistently provide cardiac compression as long as there is sufficient gas supply. Although the gas-driven compression devices permit longer periods of CPR when used in some transport settings, e.g., air transport rescue, the oxygen tank size (oxygen quantity) is limited and, therefore, time is a factor. Extremes in temperature also alter gas-powered mechanical compressors by changing gas volumes and pressures as well as gas valve function.

Integral in the design of the oxygen-driven mechanical chest compressor is a volume-cycled ventilator delivering 100% oxygen. The use of a volume-cycled ventilator rather than the ideal CPR time-cycled ventilator derives from the limited amount of oxygen that may be available. When a volume-cycled ventilator with a low oxygen flow rate of approximately 40–60 l·min^{-1} is used, a longer time is required to produce adequate tidal volumes. Cardiac compression must be stopped long enough to permit ventilation of the lungs with this type of ventilator. Because oxygen serves as the driving force for both the compressor and ventilator, the oxygen flow rate for the ventilating portion of the device must be limited so as not to deplete the gas source.

Open-Chest Cardiac Compression. Historically, open-chest cardiac compression was the first method used to provide cardiac output during cardiac arrest. Kouwenhoven's report of the effectiveness of closed-chest cardiac compression, however, obviated the need to continue the more complicated and dangerous open-chest method. Although closed-chest compression has replaced direct cardiac compression during CPR, it is apparent that direct cardiac massage produces superior arterial blood pressure, cardiac output, and coronary perfusion compared with external compression.[45,63,76,77] If open-chest CPR is delayed 20 minutes or

more, outcome is not improved despite the superior hemodynamics. In a report of patients with out-of-hospital cardiac arrest, open-chest CPR failed to improve survival when applied after 30 minutes of arrest time and external cardial compression.[78]

Although early thoracotomy and direct cardiac compression have been recommended by some in instances of unsuccessful resuscitation employing external CPR,[79] it is impractical for use on most patients with out-of-hospital arrest and is inappropriate for unskilled rescuers. The results of early open-chest CPR are unstudied. There are, however, indications for open-chest cardiac compression in a hospital setting (Table 60-7), including:

1. Cardiac arrest occurring in the operating room during intrathoracic procedures.
2. Cardiac arrest associated with penetrating or blunt injuries to the chest where thoracotomy may allow control of hemorrhage or eliminate the underlying pathology. Flail chest may preclude effective thoracic compression.
3. Cardiac tamponade.
4. Cardiac arrest associated with major mediastinal shifts, e.g., tension pneumothorax, massive pleural effusion, or the postpneumonectomy patient.
5. Anatomic deformities of the chest, e.g., severe kyphoscoliosis and severely emphysematous, barrel-chested patients with inelastic chest walls that preclude adequate thoracic compression.
6. In the patient who cannot assume the supine position, e.g., patients undergoing neurosurgical procedures in an upright position.
7. Massive air embolism where thoracotomy allows needle aspiration of the air from the heart under direct vision.
8. Massive pulmonary embolism where thoracotomy allows direct access to the obstructing embolus.
9. Cardiac arrest associated with exsanguination below the diaphragm, e.g., ruptured abdominal aortic aneurysm—thoracotomy facilitates clamping of the aorta proximal to the diaphragm before instituting cardiac compression.
10. Refractory ventricular fibrillation in a victim of hypothermic cardiac arrest—pericardial lavage with warm

---

TABLE 60-7. Indications for Thoracotomy and Direct Cardiac Compression

Operating room
  Thorax or upper abdomen already open
Conditions prohibit effective artificial circulation by closed chest
    compression
  Severe anatomic thoracic cage abnormalities
  Flail chest
  Cardiac tamponade
  Tension pneumothorax
  Major mediastinal shift, e.g., postpneumonectomy, massive
    pleural effusion
Cause of arrest is defined and treated by thoracotomy or peri-
    cardiotomy
  Cardiac tamponade
  Tension pneumothorax
  Penetrating chest surgery
  Infradiaphragmatic exsanguination
  Hypothermia
  Thromboembolic and air embolism

saline may warm the heart to a temperature permitting defibrillation.

Cardiopulmonary Bypass. Emergency cardiopulmonary bypass has been employed in canine models of cardiac arrest without thoracotomy using the femoral artery and vein for access to the circulation. When instituted after 12 minutes of cardiac arrest in place of BCLS and ACLS[80,81] or following 30 minutes of cardiac arrest and external chest compression,[82] cardiopulmonary bypass improved immediate resuscitability and short-term survival when compared with conventional resuscitation techniques. Neurologic outcome was not consistently improved in all studies. Emergent cardiopulmonary bypass is useful for the rapid rewarming of victims of hypothermic cardiac arrest.

Drug Therapy During Artificial Circulation

Initial pharmacologic therapy during CPR is directed at correction of hypoxemia, attenuation of acidemia, and elevation of coronary and cerebral perfusion pressures during chest compression. Oxygen and epinephrine, when combined with artificial ventilation and circulation, serve these purposes and are the mainstays of drug therapy during CPR (Table 60-8). Once a diagnosis of the cause of arrest is known, other drugs with actions directed at the mechanism of cardiac arrest are also used to restore native circulation (see the section on Advanced Cardiac Life Support).

Epinephrine

Epinephrine, an endogenous catecholamine with $alpha_{1,2}$ and $beta_{1,2}$ adrenergic actions, is widely accepted as the first cardiovascular stimulant to be administered during cardiac arrest, including those situations in which a specific diagnosis is unknown.[83] Administration of the drug increases cerebral and coronary perfusion pressures and blood flow during artificial circulation. The improved hemodynamics are associated with greater rates of successful resuscitation in models of ventricular fibrillation[84,85] and asystole.[86-89]

The relative benefits of alpha and beta agonists during CPR have been studied in a number of resuscitation models. Results of drug studies in asphyxiated dogs in asystole or electromechanical dissociation, where resumption of spontaneous circulation was the end point, strongly support the efficacy of alpha-adrenergic stimulation.[85-89] Epinephrine, phenylephrine, metaraminol, and methoxamine were equally effective. Beta receptor stimulation by isoproterenol or dobutamine had little or no beneficial effect. When myocardial blood flow was assessed in a fibrillating heart supported by cardiopulmonary bypass, alpha-adrenergic effects resulted in improved intramyocardial blood flow.[90] Thus, it is epinephrine's $alpha_1$ and $alpha_2$ adrenergic effects and not the beta-adrenergic actions that are responsible for the return of spontaneous circulation from asystolic cardiac arrest and that make the fibrillating myocardium more susceptible to defibrillation. The improved perfusion and oxygenation of vital organs results from epinephrine's ability to produce peripheral vasoconstriction to elevate aortic blood pressure and limit blood flow to nonvital tissues.[91,92]

Pure alpha-adrenergic agonists may have a theoretical advantage over epinephrine during CPR because the desired vascular effects may be obtained without a concomitant increase in myocardial oxygen consumption.[93] Although phenylephrine and methoxamine, drugs with almost solely $alpha_1$ activity, have been shown to be as effective as epinephrine in the restoration of circulation in earlier models of arrest,[84-89] equivalent or improved vital organ perfusion during CPR and frequency of resuscitation relative to that produced by epinephrine have not been consistently demonstrated in recent studies with these alpha agonists.[94-101] Norepinephrine, an $alpha_{1,2}$, $beta_{1,2}$ drug with less $beta_2$ activity than epinephrine, has produced hemodynamics, myocardial oxygen delivery:consumption ratios, and defibrillation rates similar or superior to those resulting from epinephrine in recently reported models.[102-105] Improved long-term clinical outcome has not yet, however, been related to the use of any alpha agonist in place of epinephrine during CPR. The use of alpha-adrenergic agonists as alternatives to epinephrine must await more complete evaluation of their efficacy and definition of their dose-response relationships.

The optimal dose of epinephrine to enhance coronary and cerebral perfusion during closed chest compression is unknown. The early reports of epinephrine's efficacy described the administration of 1 mg to dogs with approximate average weights of 10 kg.[86,87] Most current studies of epinephrine in animal models of cardiac arrest use dosages greater on a milligram per kilogram basis than the recommended human dose of 1 mg for adults (or approximately $10-15 \mu g \cdot kg^{-1}$). Experimental and clinical data suggest that

---

TABLE 60-8. Basic Life-Support Pharmacology

Drug	Indication	Bolus Dose*	Remarks
Oxygen	All cardiac arrests	F_{IO_2} = 1.0	Never withhold; support ventilation as required Select ventilating device to deliver highest F_{IO_2} Verify oxygenation by examination, oximetry, blood gas analysis
Epinephrine	All cardiac arrests	0.5–1.0 mg (children 10 $\mu g \cdot kg^{-1}$) Repeat every 5 minutes Consider higher doses in refractory arrest	Prefilled syringes 1:10,000 = 100 $\mu g \cdot ml^{-1}$ (10 ml = 1 mg) Beneficial effect results from alpha-adrenergic action: increases perfusion pressure during CPR

*Drugs are administered by bolus dose only to patients in cardiac arrest.

improvements in aortic diastolic blood pressure[106-108] and myocardial blood flow[109] are directly related to epinephrine dose. A ceiling dose may exist, above which further increases in the administered dose of epinephrine do not result in greater improvements in hemodynamics. Epinephrine, 15 $\mu g \cdot kg^{-1}$, given to dogs in cardiac arrest did not increase aortic diastolic blood pressure but doses greater than or equal to 45 $\mu g \cdot kg^{-1}$ produced sustained elevations in aortic diastolic pressure.[106] Myocardial blood flow during CPR was significantly improved in arrested swine treated with epinephrine, 200 $\mu g \cdot kg^{-1}$, in contrast to those receiving 20 $\mu g \cdot kg^{-1}$. No further improvement was seen when the epinephrine dose was increased to 2 $mg \cdot kg^{-1}$.[109] Two studies conducted during prolonged adult human resuscitation have demonstrated that epinephrine doses of 5 mg[107] and 200 $\mu g \cdot kg^{-1}$[108] significantly raised coronary perfusion pressure, whereas the conventional dose did not. Although improved rates of immediate resuscitation have been associated with the use of "high-dose epinephrine" in some instances of cardiac arrest,[110] higher rates of long-term survival, i.e., hospital discharge, have not been achieved. At present, no dose-response investigations or outcome trials have been performed in humans to confirm the efficacy or guide the selection of increased epinephrine doses. Further studies may indicate that the proper epinephrine dose, or selection of an alternative vasopressor, will be guided by the cause and the duration of arrest.[83]

Ideally, when cardiac output is low, epinephrine should be administered via the central venous route to ensure delivery. Effective chest compression can circulate drugs from a peripheral venous access site, although the circulation time is delayed. Three other routes may be used. If intravenous access is delayed, epinephrine can be instilled directly into the endotracheal tube. Peak plasma drug concentration and onset of pressor effect are achieved at a rate comparable to that of peripheral intravenous injection.[111] Plasma drug levels are sustained following endotracheal administration, reflecting gradual intravascular absorption from the airway. When equal doses of drug are administered by endotracheal or intravenous routes to anesthetized animals with spontaneous circulation, there is a two- to threefold increase in the pressor response to the intravenous route compared with the endotracheal route.[112] In a comparison of the two routes of administration during CPR in a model of cardiac arrest, the median effective endotracheal dose was ten times the effective dose given intravenously.[111] Endotracheally administered epinephrine, 10 $\mu g \cdot kg^{-1}$, did not increase plasma epinephrine levels significantly in an arrested animal model.[113] Significant elevation of plasma catecholamine levels was observed after tracheal administration of epinephrine, 100 $\mu g \cdot kg^{-1}$. Epinephrine, 1 mg, given endotracheally to humans in cardiac arrest did not produce a measurable rise in arterial epinephrine concentrations.[114] Intravenous administration resulted in more than a threefold increase. Although it is evident from these findings that a dose higher than that injected intravenously is required to achieve an equivalent hemodynamic action, the dose to be administered via the endotracheal tube has not been established.

Drugs to be given to the adult via the endotracheal tube may be diluted if necessary to achieve an injectate volume of at least 10 ml. This will enhance drug effect by reducing droplet formation in the tracheal tube and promoting peripheral intrapulmonary dispersion. Hyperventilation after endotracheal injection also promotes drug distribution throughout the lung. Other resuscitation medications may also be delivered via the endotracheal tube provided that

excessive volume (e.g., sodium bicarbonate) or irritating agents (e.g., calcium chloride) that may result in an aspiration syndrome are avoided.

Intraosseous administration of fluids and drugs, including epinephrine, can be used temporarily in pediatric patients when intravenous access cannot be achieved. The anterior surface of the tibia below the tibial tuberosity is pierced with an 18-gauge or larger needle. Gravity-driven or pressurized infusion systems attached to the needle are used to flush the drug into the marrow cavity. The rates of onset and dose-response obtained via the intraosseous route are comparable to those obtained with peripheral venous injection.

When an intravenous, endotracheal, or intraosseous route is not available, intracardiac injection may be the only remaining alternative. Although direct intracardiac injection has been used, often with success, blind transthoracic intracardiac injection is currently recommended as the least desirable route owing to the availability of other safer techniques of drug administration and the recognition of the complications associated with its use: myocardial and coronary vessel laceration, pneumohemopericardium, pneumothorax, and intramyocardial injection.

Acid-Base Therapy

The acidemia occurring in the patient suffering cardiopulmonary arrest is the result of combined respiratory and metabolic acidosis due, respectively, to apnea and ischemia-induced anaerobic metabolism. Reduction of intracellular pH leads to significant depression of myocardial contractility,[115,116] a lowered threshold for the induction of ventricular fibrillation,[117] and increased energy dose requirements for defibrillation in the presence of lidocaine therapy.[118] Myocardial and vasomotor responsiveness to low doses of catecholamines is inhibited during respiratory and metabolic acidemia,[119] but whether pH-related effects occur at the higher catecholamine doses used during CPR is unclear.[120,121]

The actions of acute acidosis occurring in the first several minutes following cardiopulmonary arrest that are detrimental to resuscitation are the result of carbon dioxide retention.[122,123] This occurs because carbon dioxide accumulates at a rate faster than lactic acid early after arrest and carbon dioxide diffuses into cells, decreasing intracellular pH more rapidly than extracellular hydrogen ions can alter cellular acid-base balance.[116] Correction of the acidosis is accomplished, therefore, primarily by ventilation with 100% oxygen, most easily achieved via endotracheal tube, and effective artificial circulation in order to eliminate carbon dioxide from the tissues and lungs.

The degree of acidemia caused by hypercarbia during CPR is underestimated by arterial blood gas analysis.[124] During cardiac arrest, a progressive venoarterial gradient of pH and Pco_2 between arterial and mixed venous blood develops, and an abrupt decrease in end-tidal exhaled CO_2 occurs. Accumulation of CO_2 in mixed venous blood, and therefore in systemic tissues, results from and is indicative of decreased CO_2 clearance from the lungs. During CPR, venous hypercarbia occurs because the low cardiac output and pulmonary blood flow generated by external chest compression fail to deliver CO_2 to the lungs at a rate commensurate with its production. On the other hand, arterial blood gases reflect the ventilation of the pulmonary blood flow that is delivered to the arterial circulation.

The central venous acidemia has important implications. Intracellular pH is decreased immediately by increases in extracellular CO_2. Carbon dioxide diffuses rapidly across cell membranes in contrast to delayed diffusion of hydrogen and bicarbonate ions. VonPlanta et al have demonstrated the existence of venoarterial CO_2 and pH gradients across the coronary circulation and severe intramyocardial respiratory acidosis in a porcine model of cardiac arrest.[122] Any measure further elevating extracellular CO_2 potentially exacerbates intracellular acidosis and resulting cellular dysfunction.

Neutralization of lactate and other metabolic acids by administration of sodium bicarbonate buffer has been a mainstay of resuscitation but without scientific evidence to substantiate this practice. Current information demonstrates that while bicarbonate administration during metabolic acidosis can normalize arterial pH, intracellular acidosis is not improved[66] and outcome from resuscitation is not altered.[65,66,125] In part, this may be attributable to CO_2 generation during bicarbonate-induced acid neutralization: $H^+ + HCO_3^- = H_2CO_3 = H_2O + CO_2$. When liberated in the extracellular space of perfused tissues, the CO_2 moves rapidly into cells, exacerbating the intracellular hypercarbic acidosis. A paradoxical acidosis results: arterial blood is normal or alkalotic, whereas tissues and venous blood are acidotic. This is supported by the demonstration of early depression and late augmentation of myocardial contractility after intracoronary bicarbonate infusion.[126] The early action was attributed to intracellular respiratory acidosis resulting from increased levels of intramyocardial CO_2, and the late effect was attributed to equilibration of bicarbonate ion across cell membranes. A similar phenomenon of arterial alkalemia and cerebrospinal fluid acidosis during cardiac resuscitation has been observed.[127]

Experience with non–CO_2-liberating buffers that avoid the drawback of paradoxical respiratory acidosis indicates that their administration also fails to correct tissue intracellular acidosis.[125] This may be explained by inadequate drug delivery to body tissues as a result of the low systemic and myocardial perfusion produced during CPR.

Thus, despite the importance of totally correcting the acidosis that occurs during cardiopulmonary arrest, no available modalities exist to accomplish this. Efforts to improve acid-base status must aim to increase tissue perfusion and pulmonary blood flow during CPR. Severe uncorrectable acidosis may be avoided if definitive therapy is administered promptly and successfully restores native circulation and ventilation.

Monitoring Artificial Circulation

Indices of cardiac output and blood pressure produced during CPR would be useful guides to adjusting therapy, including chest compression rate and depth, epinephrine dose, or need for alternative artificial circulation techniques, e.g., direct cardiac massage. Palpation of a central pulse during chest compressions has served this purpose; however, this pressure impulse provides little information about blood flow and oxygen delivery.

Measurement of exhaled end-tidal carbon dioxide tension during CPR may provide an index of cardiac output and predict outcome from resuscitation. During low blood flow states including CPR, in the presence of a constant level of adequate ventilation, end-tidal CO_2 tension reflects the rate of CO_2 delivery to the lungs and is directly related to pulmonary blood flow, i.e., cardiac output.[128,129] In animals[129] and humans[130,131] undergoing CPR with closed-chest compression, higher exhaled end-tidal CO_2 values are observed in eventual survivors than in nonsurvivors. Measurement of

end-tidal CO_2 tensions less than 10–15 mm Hg obtained after tracheal intubation during closed-chest compression and ventilation carries a poor prognosis for survival.

ADVANCED CARDIAC LIFE SUPPORT

The most effective therapeutic approach to cardiopulmonary arrest is immediate application of the definitive treatment that restores native circulation and ventilation (oxygenation). Basic life-support measures should not delay the initiation of specific therapy when it is immediately available. The specific electrical, pharmacologic, or other special therapies provided are selected on the basis of the cause of arrest.

Recognition of Dysrhythmias

Cardiac arrest may result from marked derangements in heart rate, cardiac rhythm, venous blood return to the heart, or myocardial contractile function. Acute disturbances in heart rate and cardiac rhythm are the most common immediate causes of cardiac arrest and may occur primarily (e.g., sudden cardiac death) or secondarily (e.g., due to hypoxemia resulting from respiratory arrest). The rapid recognition and treatment of cardiac rhythm disturbances are central to the process of resuscitation. Early detection and correction of prodromal dysrhythmias may prevent the development of life-threatening or lethal rhythm disturbances. Electrocardiogram (ECG) monitoring, in addition to oxygen therapy and vascular access, should be established in all patients with respiratory distress, hypotension, or symptoms of myocardial ischemia.

In instances of acute cardiac arrest in the absence of established ECG monitoring, the heart rate and rhythm can be determined most rapidly using defibrillator chest paddles that incorporate "quick look" ECG electrodes. Rapid ECG monitoring permits differentiation of ventricular fibrillation and ventricular tachycardia from asystole and electromechanical dissociation. After applying the "quick look" paddles to the patient's chest, the rhythm is displayed on the defibrillator oscilloscope, and in the presence of ventricular tachycardia or fibrillation, the unit can be charged and definitive electrical therapy administered immediately.

During prolonged resuscitation it is desirable to place stick-on or strap-on ECG electrodes that allow uninterrupted chest compression. Limb placement of the ECG electrodes will not interfere with subsequent defibrillation attempts or central venous access.

Ventricular Fibrillation and Tachycardia

Ventricular fibrillation is a lethal dysrhythmia that generates no cardiac output and results in pulselessness. Ventricular tachycardia is a life-threatening dysrhythmia that generally produces inadequate cardiac output and hypotension. When the rate of ventricular contraction during ventricular tachycardia is extremely rapid, pulselessness may result because ventricular filling is prohibited. Ventricular tachycardia is an unstable rhythm that may degenerate to ventricular fibrillation. Ventricular fibrillation and pulseless ventricular tachycardia are the most common mechanisms of sudden cardiac death. Electrical cardioversion is the only effective therapy for these rhythm disturbances and is, therefore, the mainstay of advanced cardiac life support.

TABLE 60-9. Determining Origin of Wide Complex Tachycardias*

	Ventricular Tachycardia	Supraventricular Tachycardia
Clues from previous ECG in sinus rhythm	Old infarction	Delta waves Short P-R interval Right or left bundle-branch block
Clues from ECG in the tachycardia	Atrioventricular dissociation Capture beats Fusion beats QRS >0.14 sec Left axis deviation, *e.g.*, right bundle-branch block pattern	

*With the exception of atrioventricular dissociation, capture and fusion beats during the tachycardia (which are diagnostic of ventricular tachycardia), these clues are merely suggestive of the origin of the tachycardia. When in doubt, treat as ventricular tachycardia.

Ventricular tachycardia may be differentiated from other tachydysrhythmias with a wide QRS complex (Table 60-9). Their prognosis and drug therapy differ. The other wide complex tachycardias include supraventricular tachycardia with aberrant conduction (e.g., due to pre-existing bundle-branch block) and supraventricular tachycardia with ventricular activation *via* an accessory pathway (e.g., Wolff-Parkinson-White syndrome). In a series of patients with stable wide complex tachycardia, ventricular tachycardia was observed most commonly, documented, and accounted for 85% of the dysrhythmias.[132] For the ACLS provider, the diagnosis of the wide complex tachycardia's supraventricular or ventricular origin is often a luxury afforded only in the case of a hemodynamically stable patient. Unstable tachydysrhythmias are treated emergently with electrical cardioversion regardless of their origin.

Torsades de pointes is a polymorphic ventricular tachycardia characterized by a changing ECG axis and amplitude. This rhythm disturbance occurs in patients with prolonged Q-T intervals, including Type 1A antidysrhythmic-induced Q-T prolongation, phenothiazine and tricyclic antidepressant toxicity, and congenital long Q-T syndrome. This form of ventricular tachycardia is usually unstable and requires cardioversion. Recurrence of this dysrhythmia is prevented by discontinuing the responsible drug, correcting associated electrolyte abnormalities, and infusion of lidocaine or bretylium. If the postcardioversion heart rate is slow, pacing is used to prevent recurrence.

Defibrillation and Cardioversion

Restoration of cardiac output requires the resumption of a relatively normal electrical impulse pattern in the heart. Pharmacologic therapy may be used to restore normal electrical impulse pattern but often requires a significant amount of time for an effect to occur. Many dysrhythmias alter hemodynamic stability in such a drastic fashion that they require more rapid intervention. Electrical therapy using a defibrillator is often the only practical therapy available to treat these rhythm disturbances[133] (Fig. 60-11).

The defibrillator delivers electrical current to the heart. This current uniformly depolarizes the myocardium, which subsequently repolarizes in a coordinated fashion. Electrical current administered to the heart, however, may result in myocardial cell damage.[134,135] Minimizing the electrical current administered minimizes myocardial destruction.[136] Dispersion of the current over a greater area by use of larger defibrillator paddles[137] and less frequent delivery of repetitive shocks with greater recovery time between shocks also reduce the amount of myocardial damage.

The ideal defibrillation dose is not known even though many factors have been outlined that affect defibrillation success.[138-142] Study of the dose needed for defibrillation on a $watt \cdot s^{-1} \cdot kg^{-1}$ basis has failed to clearly demonstrate a dose-weight relationship or a need for high-dose defibrillators. Several important factors apart from dose have been identified as crucial in defibrillation success. The more rapidly defibrillation therapy is administered after the onset of cardiac arrest, the better the outcome (Fig. 60-12). A critical mass of myocardial tissue must be defibrillated to be successful. Supraventricular rhythms and ventricular fibrillation are more responsive to defibrillation than idioventricular rhythms or asystole.

Reduction of transthoracic impedance to electrical current flow enhances defibrillation success (Table 60-10). Transthoracic impedance or resistance to current flow is reduced by use of electrically conductive interface materials linking the defibrillator paddles with the chest wall. Saline-soaked gauze pads and electrode paste or gel increase chest wall conductance. Alcohol-soaked pads risk burns and fire with the application of electrical therapy and should be strictly avoided.

Chest wall and cardiac resistances to current flow are reduced with repetitive shocks.[143] Experimental studies have demonstrated that although the first defibrillation may be ineffective, subsequent shocks at the exact same dose may be successful because of better current flow. Effective defibrillation occurs best when the electrical shock is delivered during the expiratory phase of the respiratory cycle—less air is in the lungs during expiration. Because air is a poor conductor of electrical current flow, the smaller air barrier between the paddles and heart during end-expiration results in better success with defibrillation.

The recommended procedure (see Fig. 60-11) for defibrillation includes BCLS measures that are continuously provided for all victims of cardiac arrest while a defibrillator is brought to the scene. The defibrillator should have an integral ECG monitor. Defibrillator paddles capable of "quicklook" ECG monitoring are very desirable. Because

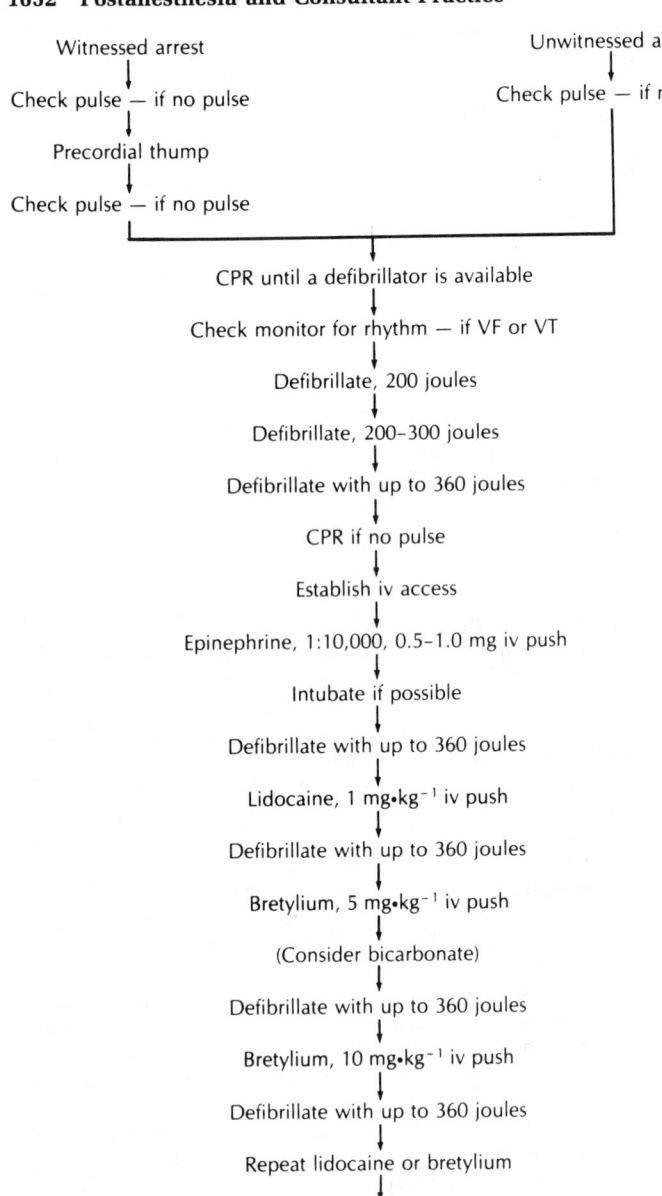

Witnessed arrest

↓

Check pulse — if no pulse

↓

Precordial thump

↓

Check pulse — if no pulse

Unwitnessed arrest

↓

Check pulse — if no pulse

CPR until a defibrillator is available

↓

Check monitor for rhythm — if VF or VT

↓

Defibrillate, 200 joules

↓

Defibrillate, 200–300 joules

↓

Defibrillate with up to 360 joules

↓

CPR if no pulse

↓

Establish iv access

↓

Epinephrine, 1:10,000, 0.5–1.0 mg iv push

↓

Intubate if possible

↓

Defibrillate with up to 360 joules

↓

Lidocaine, 1 mg·kg^{-1} iv push

↓

Defibrillate with up to 360 joules

↓

Bretylium, 5 mg·kg^{-1} iv push

↓

(Consider bicarbonate)

↓

Defibrillate with up to 360 joules

↓

Bretylium, 10 mg·kg^{-1} iv push

↓

Defibrillate with up to 360 joules

↓

Repeat lidocaine or bretylium

↓

Defibrillate with up to 360 joules

Figure 60-11. AHA treatment algorithm for cardiac arrest caused by ventricular fibrillation (and pulseless ventricular tachycardia). The AHA algorithm, as well as the others reproduced in this chapter, were developed to teach a fundamental and generic treatment plan for a broad range of patients. Some patients may require care not specified herein. This algorithm should not be construed as prohibiting such flexibility. Flow of algorithm presumes that ventricular fibrillation (or ventricular tachycardia) is continuing. (a) Check pulse and rhythm after each shock. If ventricular fibrillation (or ventricular tachycardia) recurs after transiently converting (rather than persists without converting), use the energy level that has previously been successful for subsequent defibrillation. Lidocaine should be administered, or the dose repeated, to prevent recurrence of ventricular fibrillation (or ventricular tachycardia). (b) Epinephrine should be repeated every 5 minutes. The drug may be given *via* endotracheal tube in the absence of an iv line. Use of epinephrine prior to lidocaine in treatment of ventricular fibrillation (or pulseless ventricular tachycardia) refractory to defibrillation is empirical. The order in which epinephrine and lidocaine are administered does not affect outcome.[133a] (c) If tracheal intubation can be performed simultaneously with other maneuvers, the earlier it is accomplished the better. However, defibrillation is more important initially if the patient can be ventilated without intubation. (d) Alternatively, lidocaine may be repeated. (e) The value of sodium bicarbonate (dose titrated to neutralize base deficit calculated from arterial blood gas analysis) is questionable during cardiac resuscitation, and it is not recommended as routine therapy. Continuing arrest refractory to therapy necessitates further history taking, physical examination, laboratory studies, and review of resuscitation technique to detect and correct underlying causes of refractory arrest and flaws in CPR delivery. Once ventricular fibrillation or tachycardia is terminated, begin a continuous infusion of lidocaine, or the antidysrhythmic drug that facilitated cardioversion, in order to suppress recurrence of the rhythm disturbance. (Reproduced with permission from the Textbook of Advanced Cardiac Life Support, 2nd ed. Dallas, American Heart Association, 1987.)

asystole or some other dysrhythmias without a pulse may not be treated best by defibrillation, it is desirable to diagnose the cardiac rhythm before an electrical shock is delivered. The diagnosis of asystole must be made cautiously. Low-voltage ventricular fibrillation may masquerade as asystole. An additional reason for an apparent asystolic ECG tracing is inaccurately low calibration of the monitor oscilloscope. These two circumstances must be kept in mind to avoid withholding electrical shock therapy when the true but unrecognized rhythm is ventricular fibrillation.

When the diagnosis of ventricular fibrillation is made, the paddles are applied to the chest with adequate electrode-gel interface and the defibrillator capacitor is charged. An appropriate initial dose for the average adult patient is 200 watt·s^{-1} (joules). Ideally, the operator who is holding the paddles should be able to operate and discharge the device without the need for additional personnel. This eliminates potential miscommunication and incorrect charging and discharging of the paddles, with resultant complication to the patient or injury to the rescuers.

The ECG must be re-evaluated immediately after the initial defibrillation. If an organized rhythm is apparent, hemodynamic status should be assessed by feeling for the pulse and measuring blood pressure. If ventricular fibrillation persists, the paddles should be recharged immediately to a dose of 200–300 joules and discharged in the same way as before. If after the second electrical defibrillation the rhythm disturbance and pulselessness persist, a third electrical discharge at 360 joules is administered. If this is still unsuccessful and the patient remains pulseless, other ACLS measures must be instituted (see Fig. 60-11).

Pulselessness may be associated with rhythm disturbances other than ventricular fibrillation, e.g., supraventricular and ventricular tachycardias. Defibrillation is used only for ventricular fibrillation. Other rhythms are cardioverted (in synchronized fashion). Ventricular fibrillation can be precipitated by delivering an electrical shock to a supraventricular or ventricular tachycardia during the late systolic period of vulnerability immediately prior to the appearance of the T wave. The defibrillator discharge can be synchro-

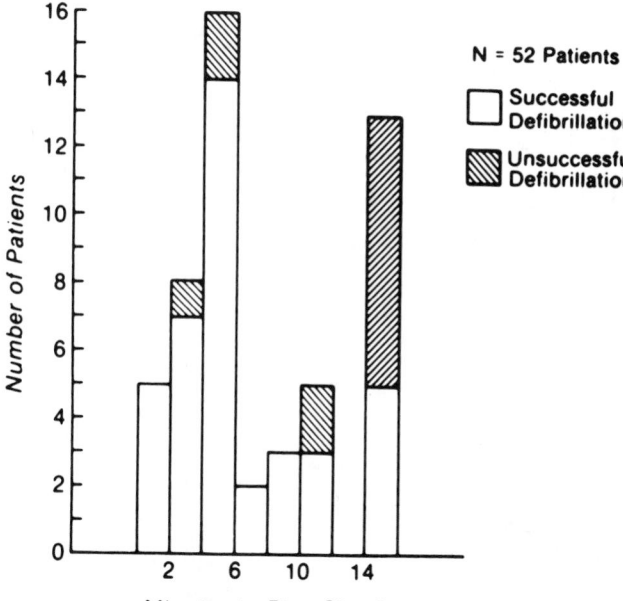

Figure 60-12. The relationship of the delay before the first defibrillating dose and the success of defibrillation shows the beneficial effect of rapid defibrillation therapy on resuscitation. (Reproduced with permission from Kerber RE, Sarnat W: Factors influencing the success of ventricular defibrillation in man. Circulation 60:226, 1979.)

nized to the ECG (the QRS deflection can be sensed and discharge of the paddles timed accordingly) to avoid delivery of electrical shock at this vulnerable time.

In situations in which a defibrillator does not have an ECG monitor, the device is used as a defibrillator, irrespective of the dysrhythmia, and if ventricular fibrillation is unintentionally produced when another rhythm is being treated, it is then defibrillated.

Hemodynamic consequences of rhythm disturbances other than ventricular fibrillation vary. If blood pressure and perfusion are adequately maintained, drug therapy may be more appropriate than cardioversion, or if electrical therapy is selected, it will be provided as a controlled elective procedure (Fig. 60-13). If blood pressure and perfusion are diminished, the choice of drugs or cardioversion and the rapidity of treatment depend on the magnitude of organ

---

TABLE 60-10. Factors Decreasing Transthoracic Resistance to Cardioversion Current

Proper paddle size*
Electroconductive gel, paste, or pads†
Correct paddle position‡
Firm pressure on paddles
Exhalation of air from lungs
Repetitive shocks

---

* Paddles should be as wide in diameter as possible and permit complete electrode contact with chest surface.

† Saline-soaked gauze sponges are an acceptable alternative. Do not use alcohol swabs.

‡ The heart must lie between the paddles. In the standard paddle position, one paddle is placed on the upper right thorax below the clavicle and the other paddle is placed lateral to the apex of the heart on the lower left chest at the midaxillary line.

---

compromise. If blood pressure and perfusion are absent, emergency electrical therapy is indicated. Dose for synchronized cardioversion is decided based on the hemodynamic status described (see Fig. 60-13 and Table 60-11).

Internal defibrillation is provided when the chest cage or pericardiac sac is open and internal defibrillation paddles are available. Lower energy is required when the paddles are placed directly on the heart. The dose for internal defibrillation is the same as for elective external cardioversion, i.e., one tenth to one fifth the dose used for external defibrillation.

Precordial Thump

The precordial thump consists of a single sharp blow delivered to the midportion of the sternum with the fist from a height of 20–30 cm above the patient's chest.[144a] The role of the precordial thump in CPR continues to be a controversial matter. There is clinical experimental evidence that one precordial thump can convert sudden ventricular tachycardia to normal sinus rhythm. In early phases of complete heart block with ventricular asystole, repetitive thumping (fist pacing) may produce a QRS complex and cardiac contraction, which may serve to maintain perfusion until drug therapy or a pacemaker is available. It is questionable, however, whether the electrical current produced in the heart by the precordial thump is of sufficient magnitude to terminate ventricular fibrillation. Indeed, the thump applied to a patient in any rhythm other than ventricular fibrillation may unexpectedly induce ventricular fibrillation.

The thump cannot be expected to generate cardiac contraction in anoxic asystole or to cardiovert a long-standing ventricular fibrillation. A single thump delivered quickly in the witnessed cardiac arrest situation will not significantly delay the institution of subsequent BCLS and ACLS (see Fig. 60-11). The precordial thump is not recommended in pediatric patients.

Intravenous Therapy

Drug and fluid administration, blood sampling, and cardiovascular monitoring all require placement of intravascular catheters. Intravenous and in some instances intra-arterial and pulmonary artery cannulation are essential in the precardiac arrest and postcardiac arrest periods.

In the acute cardiac arrest setting, it may not be possible to adhere to rigid aseptic technique when inserting catheters. Nosocomial infections are a real threat. Any attempts to observe sterile precautions and reduce the number of local or systemic bacteremias produced are worthwhile. In the postarrest period, invasive devices introduced during the acute arrest should be evaluated with respect to need for replacement or for treatment of potential infection.

The hollow steel needle and its variant, the butterfly needle, can be used during resuscitation if they are already in place when a cardiac arrest occurs. As soon as possible a needle should be replaced with some form of plastic catheter.

Intravenous catheters can be placed in peripheral or central veins. A catheter placed in a peripheral vein is acceptable for administration of fluids or drugs during CPR. Drugs given via these peripheral catheters will circulate and be effective, although the circulation time may be slower during cardiac compression than during normal cardiac output. It is inappropriate to withhold indicated medications for

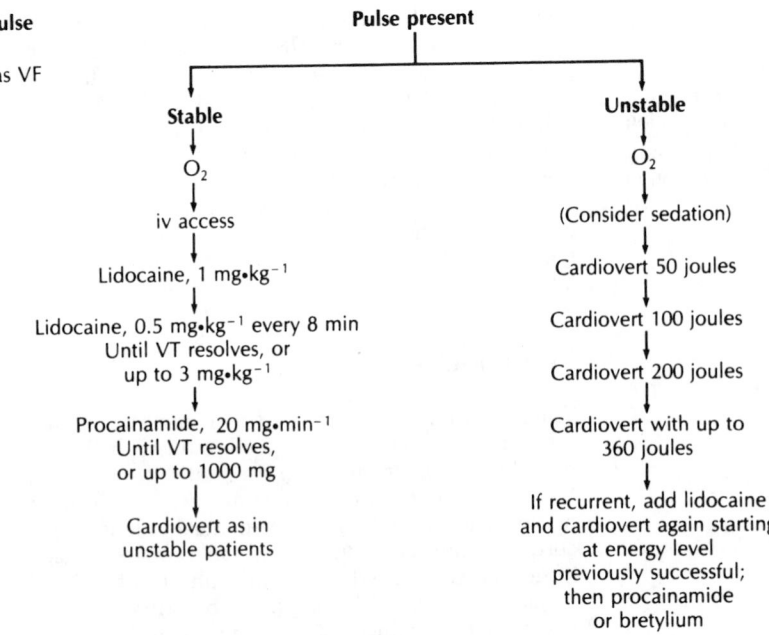

Figure 60-13. AHA treatment algorithm for ventricular tachycardia with a pulse. Flow of algorithm presumes that ventricular tachycardia is continuing. (a) If patient becomes unstable at any time, move to "Unstable" arm of algorithm. (b) Unstable patients are recognized by signs of stupor, hypotension, pulmonary edema, or symptoms of angina or dyspnea. (c) Sedation, administered by cautious titration, may be considered for patients with mild signs and symptoms of hemodynamic compromise. Sedation is associated with risks of regurgitation and aspiration, hypotension, hypoventilation, and postcardioversion somnolence and is not indicated in the presence of coma, pulmonary edema, or severe hypotension. (d) If coma, pulmonary edema, or severe hypotension indicative of severe hemodynamic compromise is present, unsynchronized cardioversion may be provided to avoid delay associated with synchronization. (e) Precordial thump may induce ventricular fibrillation and is not recommended. (f) If coma, pulmonary edema, or severe hypotension is present, use lidocaine, followed if necessary by bretylium. In all other patients, recommended drug order is lidocaine, procainamide, and then bretylium. Once ventricular tachycardia is terminated, begin a continuous infusion of lidocaine, or the antidysrhythmic drug that facilitated cardioversion, in order to suppress recurrence of the rhythm disturbance. (Reproduced with permission from the Textbook of Advanced Cardiac Life Support, 2nd ed. Dallas, American Heart Association, 1987.)

administration through an as yet unestablished central catheter when a peripheral catheter is operational. Central venous catheters are the preferred route for drug therapy during CPR, as this better guarantees that drugs will reach and potentially affect the heart, brain, and kidneys. The preferred site for central venous cannulation is that most familiar to the operator.

The femoral vein has been suggested as the preferred central venous route during CPR because establishing a catheter in this area does not interfere with airway management and cardiac compression. It may be difficult to identify the femoral vein if a femoral arterial pulse is not palpable. The infection potential in the femoral region must always be kept in mind. The internal jugular, subclavian, and supraclavicular venous routes for central catheter placement are effective but require knowledge of the cervical and thoracic anatomy.

TABLE 60-11. Recommended Initial Energy Dose for Emergent Cardioversion*

Dysrhythmia	Energy Dose (joules)	Synchronized or Unsynchronized†
Ventricular fibrillation	200	Unsynchronized
Ventricular tachycardia	50	Synchronized
Paroxysmal supraventricular tachycardia	75	Synchronized
Atrial fibrillation	100	Synchronized
Atrial flutter	25	Synchronized

*Any dysrhythmias producing pulselessness is cardioverted like ventricular fibrillation.

†Unsynchronized cardioversion should be administered to hemodynamically unstable patients if synchronization process will cause delay in therapy.

Cannulation of these veins often requires a pause in BCLS.

When intravenous catheters are employed, either a minimal amount of fluid is given to keep the lumen patent for drug administration or large amounts of fluid are given to resuscitate intravascular volume. Choice of fluid depends on the cause of the cardiac arrest. Salt-containing solutions are avoided in myocardial infarction situations, whereas salt-containing solutions and other volume expanders are used in hypovolemic settings.

Drug Therapy for Ventricular Tachydysrhythmias

In addition to epinephrine, antidysrhythmic agents are administered during cardiac arrest caused by tachydysrhythmias in order to promote sustained cardioversion (Table 60-12). These drugs act by suppressing ectopic impulse formation in irritable myocardium, permitting normal cardiac pacemakers to initiate conduction upon cardioversion before the dysrhythmia recurs.

Lidocaine and bretylium tosylate are equally effective during resuscitation from ventricular fibrillation and pulseless ventricular tachycardia.[144,145] Lidocaine is the preferred drug because of its faster onset of peak effect. The pharmacokinetics of lidocaine in patients in cardiac arrest are not well described, but animal data suggest that high plasma drug levels are achieved and maintained because volume of drug distribution and rate of clearance are diminished as a result of the low cardiac output seen during CPR.[146] In cardiac arrest, therefore, lidocaine should be given by intermittent intravenous bolus only and excessive doses should be avoided. Procainamide is not used during cardiac arrest and CPR because the drug's vasodilating actions compromise blood pressure generated during chest compression.

Pharmacologic cardioversion of stable ventricular tachycardia not requiring rapid electrical cardioversion is achieved by titration of procainamide or lidocaine (see Fig. 60-13).

TABLE 60-12. Advanced Cardiac Life-Support Pharmacology

Drug	Indication	Bolus Dose*	Infusion Rate	Remarks
Chronotropes				
Atropine sulfate	Asystole	1.0 mg iv or ET		Total dose 2 mg (children 1.0 mg)
	Bradycardia, heart block	0.3–1.0 mg iv or ET (children 0.01–0.03 mg·kg^{-1})		Dose selected by degree of hemodynamic compromise
				Beware of tachydysrhythmias, myocardial ischemia
Isoproterenol	Atropine-refractory bradycardia, heart block		2–20 μg·min^{-1}; titrate to effect (children 0.1–0.5 μg·kg^{-1} ·min^{-1})	Do not use during CPR, reduces perfusion pressure
				Beware of tachydysrhythmias, myocardial ischemia
Antidysrhythmics				
Lidocaine	Cardiac arrest– ventricular fibrillation, tachycardia	1.0 mg·kg^{-1} iv or ET Repeat 0.5 mg·kg^{-1} every 5 minutes to total dose 3 mg·kg^{-1}		
	Ventricular ectopy, stable ventricular tachycardia	1.0 mg·kg^{-1} iv Repeat 0.5 mg·kg^{-1} every 5 minutes to total dose 3.0 mg·kg^{-1}, OR use loading infusion	Loading infusion: 15 mg·min^{-1} to total dose 3 mg·kg^{-1} Maintenance infusion: 2–4 mg·min^{-1} (children 30–50 μg·kg^{-1}·min^{-1})	Central nervous system toxicity at plasma levels > 9 μg·ml^{-1} Reduce dose in patients with congestive heart failure, hepatic disease, advanced age
Procainamide	Ventricular ectopy, stable ventricular tachycardia		Loading infusion: 20–50 mg·min^{-1} to total dose 15 mg·kg^{-1} or toxicity Maintenance infusion: 1–4 mg·min^{-1}	Toxicity: hypotension, atrioventricular block, QRS widening (>50%) Reduce dose in patients with congestive heart failure, renal failure Check blood levels
Bretylium tosylate	Cardiac arrest- ventricular fibrillation, tachycardia	5 mg·kg^{-1} iv or ET; Repeat 10 mg·kg^{-1} every 15 minutes to total dose 30 mg·kg^{-1}		Peak therapeutic effect delayed 10–15 minutes after injection
	Stable ventricular tachycardia	5–10 mg·kg^{-1} iv over 10 minutes; repeat in 1–2 hr, then infusion	Maintenance infusion: 1–2 mg·min^{-1}	Side-effects: postural hypotension, nausea/ vomiting Use with caution in digitalis toxicity

(continued)

TABLE 60-12. Advanced Cardiac Life-Support Pharmacology (continued)

Drug	Indication	Bolus Dose*	Infusion Rate	Remarks
Adenosine	Re-entrant atrioventricular node tachycardia	6 mg iv; repeat 12 mg every 2 minutes twice (children, 50-100-200 $\mu g \cdot kg^{-1}$)		Inject rapidly; metabolized in <1 minute Beware of transient heart block
Verapamil	Re-entrant atrioventricular node tachycardia; atrial fibrillation, flutter; MAT	0.075–0.15 $mg \cdot kg^{-1}$ iv (max 10 mg) Repeat in 15 minutes as necessary		Beware of hypotension Use with caution in congestive heart failure, atrioventricular block, hypotension, presence of beta blockade Not recommended for WPW with pre-excitation
Esmolol	Re-entrant atrioventricular node tachycardia; atrial fibrillation, flutter; MAT; sinus tachycardia; ventricular ectopy	0.1–0.5 $mg \cdot kg^{-1}$ iv	25–200 $\mu g \cdot kg^{-1} \cdot min^{-1}$ Titrate to effect	Beware of heart failure, bronchospasm Not recommended for WPW with pre-excitation
Propranolol	Re-entrant atrioventricular node tachycardia; atrial fibrillation, flutter; MAT; sinus tachycardia; ventricular ectopy	0.1–1.0 mg iv; Titrate cautiously to total dose 0.1 $mg \cdot kg^{-1}$		Beware of heart failure, bronchospasm Not recommended for WPW with pre-excitation
Inotropes				
Dopamine	Hypotension, low cardiac output, atropine-refractory bradycardia		Initial rate 2–5 $\mu g \cdot kg^{-1} \cdot min^{-1}$ Titrate to effect	Dopaminergic 2–5 $\mu g \cdot kg^{-1} \cdot min^{-1}$ Beta-adrenergic 5–10 $\mu g \cdot kg^{-1} \cdot min^{-1}$ Alpha-adrenergic effect predominates >20 $\mu g \cdot kg^{-1} \cdot min^{-1}$ Beware of tachydysrhythmias, myocardial ischemia
Dobutamine	Hypotension, low cardiac output, atropine-refractory bradycardia		Initial rate 2–5 $\mu g \cdot kg^{-1} \cdot min^{-1}$ Titrate to effect	Beware of tachydysrhythmias, myocardial ischemia
Epinephrine	All cardiac arrests	0.5–1.0 mg iv or ET (children 10 $\mu g \cdot kg^{-1}$); Repeat every 5 minutes Consider higher doses in refractory arrest		See BLS pharmacology, Table 60-8
	Hypotension, low cardiac output, atropine-refractory bradycardia		Initial rate 2–4 $\mu g \cdot min^{-1}$ (children 0.1 $\mu g \cdot kg^{-1} \cdot min^{-1}$) Titrate to effect	Beta-adrenergic 1–2 $\mu g \cdot kg^{-1}$ Alpha-adrenergic effect predominates >12 $\mu g \cdot min^{-1}$ Beware of tachydysrhythmias, myocardial ischemia
Calcium chloride (CaCl$_2$)	Hypotension, low cardiac output	5–10 $mg \cdot kg^{-1}$ iv; Repeat every 10 minutes as necessary		Useful in hypocalcemia, hyperkalemia CaCl$_2$ preferred to calcium gluconate because higher, more predictable ionized calcium levels result
Amrinone	Low cardiac output	Loading dose 0.75 $mg \cdot kg^{-1}$ iv over 5 minutes	5–10 $\mu g \cdot kg^{-1} \cdot min^{-1}$	Beware of hypotension due to vasodilation
Vasopressors				
Norepinephrine	Hypotension		Initial rate 0.1–0.5 $\mu g \cdot kg^{-1} \cdot min^{-1}$ Titrate to effect	Central route preferable

(continued)

TABLE 60-12. Advanced Cardiac Life-Support Pharmacology (continued)

Drug	Indication	Bolus Dose*	Infusion Rate	Remarks
Phenylephrine	Hypotension	50–200 μg iv	Initial rate 100–200 μg·min^{-1} Titrate to effect	
Methoxamine	Hypotension	1–5 mg iv		
Vasodilators				
Sodium nitro-prusside	Low cardiac output, pulmonary edema		Initial rate 0.25–0.5 μg·kg^{-1}·min^{-1} Titrate to effect	Beware of cyanide toxicity at infusion rates > 8–10 μg·kg^{-1}·min^{-1} Beware of hypotension
Trimethaphan	Low cardiac output, pulmonary edema	1–2 mg iv	Initial rate 1–2 mg·min^{-1} Titrate to effect	Beware of hypotension
Nitroglycerin	Myocardial ischemia pulmonary edema	50–100 μg iv	Initial rate 0.25–0.5 μg·kg^{-1}·min^{-1} Titrate to effect	Beware of hypotension
Morphine sulfate	Myocardial ischemia pulmonary edema	2–5 mg iv		Beware of hypotension; respiratory depression

*Drugs are administered by bolus dose only to patients in cardiac arrest.

Abbreviations: BLS = basic life support, ET = endotracheal route, MAT = multifocal atrial tachycardia, WPW = Wolff-Parkinson-White syndrome.

Ventricular Ectopy

Premature ventricular beats are a common electrocardiographic finding and may not signal a risk of more serious dysrhythmia. The need to treat ventricular ectopy is debatable.[147,148] A stable pattern of ventricular ectopy requires no therapy. New ventricular ectopy requires, most important, a look for an inciting cause. Pharmacologic suppression of frequent and multifocal ectopy and of nonsustained ventricular tachycardia is becoming less common when continuous ECG surveillance and immediate defibrillation are available.

Suppressive therapy (Fig. 60-14) is indicated upon observing an increasing pattern of ectopy, including frequent or multifocal premature complexes or ventricular tachycardia in the absence of an immediate resuscitation capacity. Continuous infusion of antidysrhythmic therapy is also indicated for at least 24 hours following resuscitation from ventricular fibrillation or tachycardia.

Supraventricular Tachycardia

Supraventricular tachycardias are often hemodynamically stable, permitting pharmacologic therapy. Treatment is guided by the specific supraventricular tachycardia present (Fig. 60-15). Cardiovascular instability during supraventricular tachycardia may occur in patients with underlying ischemic or stenotic valvular heart disease and requires urgent synchronized cardioversion.

Drug treatment of supraventricular tachycardia in patients with accessory pathways (e.g., Wolff-Parkinson-White syndrome) differs according to the path of atrioventricular conduction. When atrioventricular conduction occurs through the atrioventricular node (manifest by normal QRS width and configuration on ECG during the dysrhythmia), drugs that slow atrioventricular node conduction may be used. These include adenosine, verapamil, beta-adrenergic antagonists, and digoxin. When ventricular activation occurs *via* the accessory pathway (usually during atrial fibril-lation or flutter and manifest by a wide QRS complex on the ECG during the dysrhythmia), drugs that slow the rate of atrioventricular node conduction can paradoxically accelerate these tachycardias, resulting in cardiac arrest.[149] Procainamide and lidocaine are the drugs of choice for slowing supraventricular tachycardia with ventricular activation occurring *via* an accessory pathway.

Maneuvers that increase vagal tone, e.g., carotid sinus massage, slow the rate of atrioventricular node conduction and may terminate supraventricular tachycardia caused by a re-entrant circuit in the atrioventricular node. These maneuvers may also help to distinguish re-entrant supraventricular tachycardia, sinus tachycardia, and atrial flutter. Re-entrant supraventricular tachycardia is either converted by the maneuver or nothing happens. In contrast, in sinus tachycardia and atrial flutter, transient slowing of the rhythm often allows tell-tale atrial activity to become apparent.

Adenosine, an adenosine receptor agonist, is the drug of choice for re-entrant supraventricular tachycardia.[150,151] Adenosine and verapamil are equally effective in terminating this rhythm disturbance, with an incidence of successful conversion approaching 90%. However, use of verapamil, a calcium channel blocker, is associated with a higher incidence of hemodynamic side-effects. Hypotension results from the drug's vasodilating and negative inotropic actions. Pretreatment with calcium chloride, 1 g iv, over 5–10 minutes prior to verapamil administration, has been shown to reduce the hypotensive effect without diminishing the drug's antidysrhythmic action.[152]

Adenosine must be injected rapidly *via* a free-flowing intravenous line in order to deliver the dose to the heart because of the drug's rapid clearance from the circulation. Adenosine's side-effects—heart block, flushing, and dyspnea—are transient, usually lasting less than a minute owing to the drug's metabolism by circulating adenosine deaminase and rapid transport into cells. The drug is not effective in the treatment of rapid atrial fibrillation or flutter because adenosine's slowing of atrioventricular node conduction is only transient. After a brief period of slowed

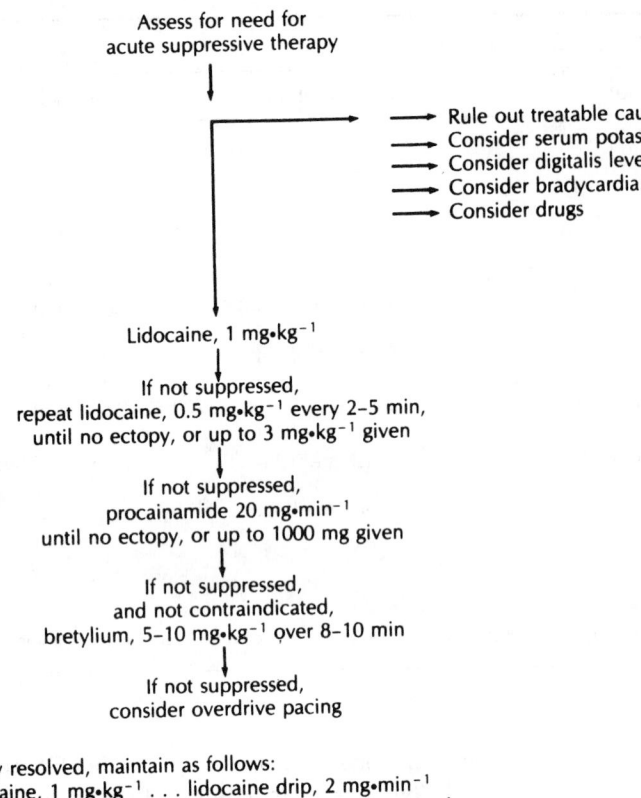

Assess for need for
acute suppressive therapy

→ Rule out treatable cause
→ Consider serum potassium
→ Consider digitalis level
→ Consider bradycardia
→ Consider drugs

Lidocaine, 1 mg·kg⁻¹

If not suppressed,
repeat lidocaine, 0.5 mg·kg⁻¹ every 2–5 min,
until no ectopy, or up to 3 mg·kg⁻¹ given

If not suppressed,
procainamide 20 mg·min⁻¹
until no ectopy, or up to 1000 mg given

If not suppressed,
and not contraindicated,
bretylium, 5–10 mg·kg⁻¹ over 8–10 min

If not suppressed,
consider overdrive pacing

Once ectopy resolved, maintain as follows:
  After lidocaine, 1 mg·kg⁻¹ . . . lidocaine drip, 2 mg·min⁻¹
  After lidocaine, 1–2 mg·kg⁻¹ . . . lidocaine drip, 3 mg·min⁻¹
  After lidocaine, 2–3 mg·kg⁻¹ . . . lidocaine drip, 4 mg·min⁻¹
  After procainamide . . . procainamide drip, 1–4 mg·min⁻¹ (check blood level)
  After bretylium . . . bretylium drip, 2 mg·min⁻¹

Figure 60-14. AHA treatment algorithm for the suppression of ventricular ectopy. As an alternative to the intermittent bolus technique, lidocaine therapy may be initiated with a loading infusion at a rate of 15 mg·min⁻¹ until the ectopy resolves or a total loading dose of 3 mg·kg⁻¹ has been given. The dose is reduced by 50% for patients with heart failure, hepatic dysfunction, and advanced age. Procainamide administration is guided by blood pressure and electrocardiogram monitoring. The drug exerts negative inotropic and vasodilating actions, which produce hypotension. Adverse electrocardiographic effects include widening of the QRS complex by 50% of its original duration and lengthening of the P-R and Q-T intervals. Bretylium tosylate is more effective in the treatment of ventricular fibrillation than in suppression of ventricular ectopy. The usefulness of the drug is limited by its side-effects, postural hypotension, and nausea. The degree of nausea and vomiting is related to the rate of drug administration. (Reproduced with permission from the Textbook of Advanced Cardiac Life Support, 2nd ed. Dallas, American Heart Association, 1987.)

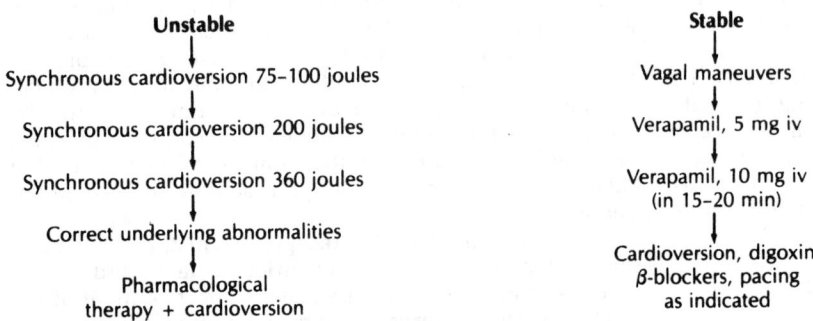

Unstable

Synchronous cardioversion 75–100 joules

Synchronous cardioversion 200 joules

Synchronous cardioversion 360 joules

Correct underlying abnormalities

Pharmacological
therapy + cardioversion

Stable

Vagal maneuvers

Verapamil, 5 mg iv

Verapamil, 10 mg iv
(in 15–20 min)

Cardioversion, digoxin,
β-blockers, pacing
as indicated

If conversion occurs but paroxysmal supraventricular tachycardia (PSVT) recurs, repeated electrical cardioversion is *not* indicated. Sedation should be used as time permits.

Figure 60-15. AHA treatment of algorithm for paroxysmal supraventricular tachycardia (PSVT) (re-entrant atrioventricular node tachycardia). For treatment of patients with atrial fibrillation or flutter, multifocal atrial tachycardia, and those with Wolff-Parkinson-White syndrome, see text. Flow of algorithm presumes supraventricular tachycardia is continuing. Unstable patients are recognized by signs of stupor, hypotension, pulmonary edema, or symptoms of angina or dyspnea. Energy doses for synchronized cardioversion of supraventricular tachycardias other than PSVT are listed in Table 6-11. Adenosine, rather than verapamil, is the drug of choice for re-entrant atrioventricular node tachycardias. If an initial dose of 6 mg, injected rapidly, is unsuccessful, the drug is repeated twice, in a dose of 12 mg, at 2-minute intervals. If the dysrhythmia persists, verapamil may be used. Lower doses of verapamil should be used for elderly, anesthetized, or unstable patients. Verapamil-induced hypotension is treated with a vasopressor. Esmolol, a beta-adrenergic antagonist with rapid onset and brief duration of action, may be a useful adjunct in the termination of supraventricular tachycardia. Esmolol and verapamil should not be administered in close temporal proximity. (Reproduced with permission from the Textbook of Advanced Cardiac Life Support, 2nd ed. Dallas, American Heart Association, 1987.)

atrioventricular conduction, the rapid ventricular rate recurs.

Initial drug therapy of rapid atrial fibrillation or flutter aims to provide sustained slowing of atrioventricular node conduction to reduce the rate of ventricular response. The drug used is determined by the patient's blood pressure, presence of underlying pulmonary disease or myocardial dysfunction, previous digoxin therapy, and clinical urgency. Once the ventricular response rate has slowed, procainamide or quinidine may be administered to stabilize the atrial tissue and convert the rhythm to sinus rhythm provided that the onset of atrial fibrillation was recent and atrial mural thrombi are unlikely.

Multifocal atrial tachycardia may be mistaken for atrial fibrillation because it is also an irregularly irregular rhythm. Multifocal atrial tachycardia is distinguished from atrial fibrillation by the presence of discrete P waves of three or more different morphologies. This dysrhythmia is most often seen in the setting of underlying pulmonary or cardiac disease. It is refractory to digoxin and best treated by correcting the underlying cause, e.g., hypoxemia, hypercarbia, theophylline excess, or volume overload. Verapamil, in low doses, is cautiously titrated when drug therapy is needed to control the ventricular rate.

Asystole

Asystole is a lethal dysrhythmia commonly observed after prolonged cardiac arrest initiated by other rhythm disturbances, e.g., ventricular fibrillation. Mortality from asystole, therefore, is extremely high. Resuscitation from asystole is more likely when ventricular standstill results from sudden complete heart block in the atrioventricular node. In the latter instance, atrioventricular node conduction may be restored by correcting the inciting cause (e.g., surgical traction reflex, drug toxicity, hyperkalemia, hypoxemia, inferior wall myocardial ischemia) or treatment with atropine or beta$_1$-adrenergic agonists.

Cardiac pacing fails to produce ventricular depolarization and resuscitation from asystole when initiated minutes or more after cardiac arrest.[153,154] Cardiac contraction may be stimulated by cardiac pacing in instances of acute ventricular standstill if the pacemaker is activated immediately after cardiac arrest. This is most likely to occur when a hospitalized patient is known to be at risk for development of complete heart block (e.g., new conduction defect during anterior myocardial infarction, pulmonary artery catheterization in the presence of a pre-existing left bundle-branch block, or emergency surgery for a patient with syncope and trifascicular block on ECG) and the pacemaker has been prophylactically applied.

In the absence of effective electrical therapy, treatment of asystole consists of measures that provide oxygen to the heart to restore spontaneous impulse formation and ventricular depolarization. Ventilation with oxygen and artificial circulation augmented by epinephrine are the mainstays of this therapy (Fig. 60-16). Isoproterenol, dobutamine, or other drugs with predominantly beta-adrenergic actions are not indicated in cardiac arrest caused by asystole because coronary perfusion during CPR is diminished by beta-adrenergic–mediated vasodilation.

Atropine may be effective in treating ventricular standstill caused by complete heart block in the atrioventricular node. In other instances of cardiac arrest owing to asystole, atropine may improve the likelihood of immediate resuscitation but has not been shown to increase the frequency of survival to hospital discharge.[155,156]

If rhythm is unclear and possibly ventricular fibrillation, defibrillate as for VF. If asystole is present

↓

Continue CPR

↓

Establish iv access

↓

Epinephrine, 1:10,000, 0.5–1.0 mg iv push

↓

Intubate when possible

↓

Atropine, 1.0 mg iv push (repeated in 5 min)

↓

(Consider bicarbonate)

↓

Consider pacing

Figure 60-16. AHA treatment algorithm for cardiac arrest caused by asystole. For witnessed ventricular standstill in the presence of a rapidly applied external pacemaker, cardiac pacing should be provided as initial therapy. (a) Asystole should be confirmed checking two electrocardiographic leads, paddle or electrocardiographic lead contact and cable connections, and oscilloscope gain adjustment to avoid withholding proper therapy of ventricular fibrillation mistaken for asystole. Because fine ventricular fibrillation can appear similar to asystole but be terminated by defibrillation, the rhythm should be defibrillated if it is possibly ventricular fibrillation. (b) Epinephrine should be repeated every 5 minutes. The drug may be given *via* endotracheal tube in the absence of an iv line. (c) If tracheal intubation can be performed simultaneously with other maneuvers, the earlier it is accomplished the better. However, CPR and epinephrine are more important initially if the patient can be ventilated without intubation. (d) Value of sodium bicarbonate (dose titrated to neutralize base deficit calculated from arterial blood gas analysis) is questionable during cardiac resuscitation, and it is not recommended as routine therapy. Continuing arrest refractory to therapy necessitates further history taking, physical examination, laboratory studies, and review of resuscitation technique to detect and correct underlying causes of refractory arrest and flaws in CPR delivery. (Reproduced with permission from the Textbook of Advanced Cardiac Life Support, 2nd ed. Dallas, American Heart Association, 1987.)

Calcium chloride, previously used for treatment of cardiac standstill, has no beneficial effect in asystole[157,158] except in those cases caused by hyperkalemia or toxicity of a calcium channel blocking agent.

Bradycardias and Heart Block

Complete or third-degree heart block is a life-threatening dysrhythmia that may result in hypotension if the rate of the escape pacemaker is slow. The significance of complete heart block depends on the level at which the atrioventricular block occurs. When it occurs at the level of the atrioventricular node, a junctional escape pacemaker with a rate of 40–60 beats per minute will initiate ventricular depolarization. Because the site of origin of this pacemaker is above the bifurcation of the bundle of His, ventricular depolarization occurs in normal sequence, resulting in a normal QRS complex. This type of block is usually transient and has a favorable prognosis. Infranodal complete heart block, on the other hand, usually indicates extensive conduction system disease. The escape pacemaker initiating ventricular depolarization in situations of infranodal complete heart block produces a wide QRS complex and has an inherent firing rate of less than 40 beats per minute. This is not a stable pacemaker, and the rhythm may degenerate to asystole or

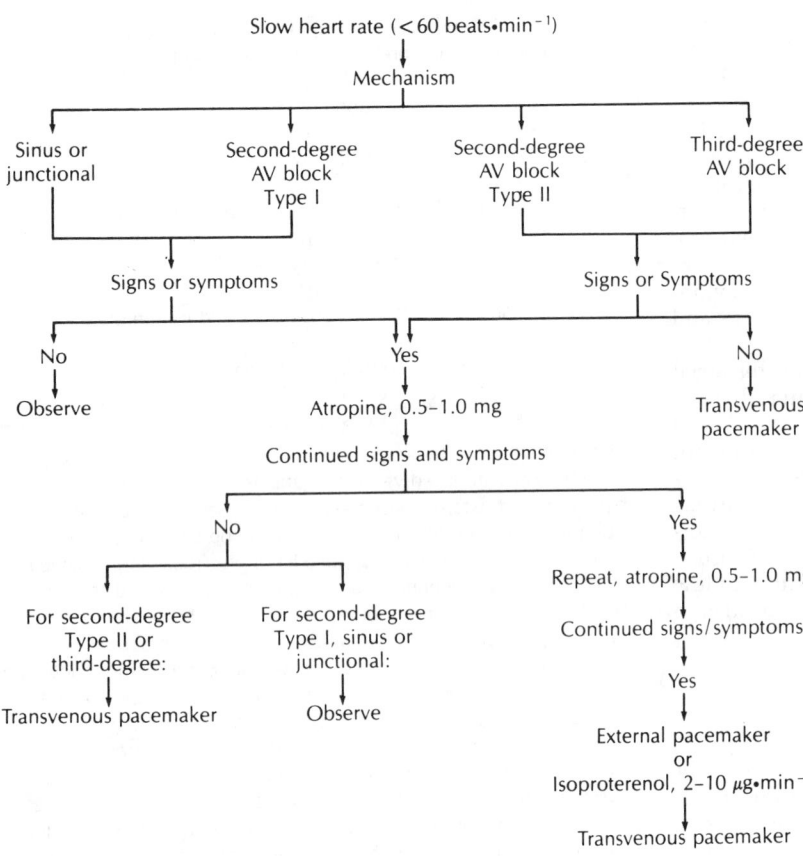

Figure 60-17. AHA treatment algorithm for bradycardias and heart block. A-V = atrioventricular. (a) Need for treatment is based on the site of conduction block and the patient's degree of hemodynamic compromise. (b) Signs: Hypotension, altered sensorium, pulmonary edema, ventricular escape complexes on ECG. Symptoms: Angina or dyspnea. (c) Temporizing therapy prior to transvenous pacemaker insertion. External transcutaneous pacing is the preferred method of rapidly increasing heart rate of atropine-refractory bradycardias with heart block until a transvenous pacemaker is inserted. In the absence of an external pacemaker, a titrated infusion of a beta-adrenergic agonist is used to temporarily accelerate heart rate. Dopamine or epinephrine may be preferable to isoproterenol because the combined alpha- and beta-adrenergic actions elevate perfusion pressure as well as heart rate. (Reproduced with permission from the Textbook of Advanced Cardiac Life Support, 2nd ed. Dallas, American Heart Association, 1987.)

ventricular fibrillation. Mobitz II second-degree heart block is a prodromal dysrhythmia occurring at the level of the His bundle or below. Progression to complete heart block should be anticipated. On the other hand, Mobitz I second-degree heart block (Wenckebach phenomenon) is usually a transient conduction block occurring in the atrioventricular node that infrequently progresses to complete heart block.

Atropine is effective first-line drug therapy when bradycardia or heart block arises in the sinus or atrioventricular node (Fig. 60-17). Second- and third-degree heart blocks occurring below the atrioventricular node are generally refractory to atropine because of the paucity of muscarinic receptors in His-Purkinje tissue. Sympathomimetic drugs, beta-adrenergic agonists (including isoproterenol, dobutamine, dopamine, and epinephrine) and external cardiac pacing may be used to increase ventricular rate temporarily in these situations until transvenous pacing is established.

Cardiac Pacing

Bradydysrhythmias and asystole are associated with diminished or absent cardiac output. Rhythmic electrical stimulation of the heart with a pacing catheter is indicated in these situations to restore a more normal heart rate and perfusion. Prophylactic insertion of pacing catheters is also indicated in certain instances of myocardial infarction likely to be associated with bradycardia and heart block. Occasionally, a pacing catheter is used to override a tachycardia. Overdrive pacing, a paced rate more rapid than the dysrhythmia, may control impulse generation and allow subsequent slowing of the rate with elimination of the dysrhythmia.

External thoracic pacing devices are occasionally used; however, the most reliable method for cardiac pacing is use of an internal pacing electrode. A central venous insertion route is required through which a pacing catheter is positioned in the right side of the heart, i.e., right atrium, coronary sinus, or right ventricle. Heart block, in which conduction of the electrical impulse from atrium to ventricle is absent, requires placement of the electrode in the right ventricle. A pacing catheter or other catheter with pacing capability, such as pacing pulmonary artery catheter, may be used. A pulse generator is connected to the properly positioned pacing electrode. Amperage, rate, and fixed versus demand pacing mode are set according to the rhythm disturbance and its consequences on the hemodynamics of the patient.

Electromechanical Dissociation

The presence of an organized ECG rhythm does not assure circulation. A patient with an organized ECG pattern but no pulse has electromechanical dissociation. Electromechanical dissociation may be a terminal phenomenon, the result of extensive myocardial damage; it may also be produced by conditions that interfere with venous return to the heart (tension pneumothorax, cardiac tamponade, massive pulmonary thrombotic or air embolus, hypovolemia, anaphylactic shock) or markedly depress cardiac inotropy (myocardial ischemia, hypocalcemia, anesthetic overdose). In the presence of electromechanical dissociation, a high index of suspicion of these conditions is crucial because prompt intervention may restore cardiac output and be lifesaving.

Pericardiocentesis

The pericardial sac is a relatively fixed space containing the heart and a small amount of pericardial fluid. Blood added to the pericardial fluid can be accommodated up to the compliance limits of the pericardial sac. When the contents of the sac (cardiac volume, pericardial fluid, and blood) exceed this limit, increased pressure within the sac results. A traumatic cardiac injury allows blood to enter the pericardial space and compress the heart. Diminished diastolic filling and cardiac output result from increased volume and pressure within the sac. A slow accumulation of pericardial fluid is compensated for, and 800–1200 ml may be tolerated with minimal impairment of cardiac output. Rapid accumulation of pericardial fluid, however, is poorly tolerated, and as little as 150–300 ml may cause cardiac compression and marked hypotension. The process is rapidly reversible by acute removal of pericardial fluid.

Subxyphoid insertion of a spinal needle, guided by attachment to and monitoring of the ECG, allows safe withdrawal of pericardial fluid. After the acute removal of fluid and stabilization of the hemodynamic status, it may be desirable to insert a continuously draining pericardial catheter or create an open pericardial window for drainage. The major disadvantage of pericardiocentesis is that associated with transthoracic needle insertion into the heart.

Decompression of a Tension Pneumothorax

Air can accumulate within the pleural space as a result of pulmonary rupture and air leak from the lung or a break in the integrity of the thoracic wall and air leak from the atmosphere into the chest. Excessive air accumulation results in pressurization of the hemithorax. This tension pneumothorax not only compromises alveolar gas exchange but by its mediastinal shift compromises venous return to the heart and ultimately cardiac output.

Emergency treatment of a tension pneumothorax requires converting it to an open, simple pneumothorax. A large-bore needle or catheter over needle is inserted into the second or third intercostal space in the anterior chest wall. Insertion at the midclavicular line and no further medially avoids internal mammary artery puncture. Insertion of the needle over the top of the rib avoids intercostal artery puncture. A gush of air indicates that tension has been relieved and hemodynamic stability should rapidly return. Intravenous extension tubing can be attached to the needle or catheter, and an underwater seal provided with a cup partly filled with water. Subsequently, a standard chest tube can be inserted electively.

Drug Therapy for Electromechanical Dissociation

In the absence of a reversible cause of electromechanical dissociation, treatment consists of CPR, oxygen, and epinephrine to provide myocardial oxygen delivery and thereby restore inotropic function (Fig. 60-18). If bradycardia is present with electromechanical dissociation, atropine and cardiac pacing may be used to increase heart rate and cardiac output. The efficacy of calcium chloride is questionable in most instances of electromechanical dissociation.[159-161] Calcium chloride increases cardiac inotropy in patients with low ionized blood calcium levels and may be beneficial when electromechanical dissociation occurs in the setting of confirmed or suspected hypocalcemia.

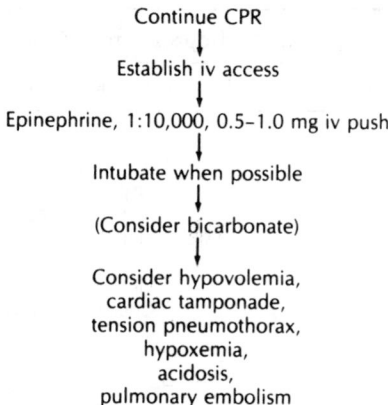

Continue CPR
↓
Establish iv access
↓
Epinephrine, 1:10,000, 0.5–1.0 mg iv push
↓
Intubate when possible
↓
(Consider bicarbonate)
↓
Consider hypovolemia,
cardiac tamponade,
tension pneumothorax,
hypoxemia,
acidosis,
pulmonary embolism

Figure 60-18. AHA treatment algorithm for cardiac arrest caused by electromechanical dissociation (EMD). Reversible causes of EMD (listed at bottom of algorithm) should be considered immediately upon recognition of the condition and specific therapy provided before or simultaneously with drug administration and intubation. (a) Epinephrine should be repeated every 5 minutes. The drug may be given *via* endotracheal tube in the absence of an iv line. (b) If tracheal intubation can be performed simultaneously with other maneuvers, the earlier it is accomplished the better. However, CPR and epinephrine are more important initially if the patient can be ventilated without intubation. (c) Value of sodium bicarbonate (dose titrated to neutralize base deficit calculated from arterial blood gas analysis) is questionable during cardiac resuscitation, and it is not recommended as routine therapy. Continuing arrest refractory to therapy necessitates further history taking, physical examination, laboratory studies, and review of resuscitation technique to detect and correct underlying causes of refractory arrest and flaws in CPR delivery. (Reproduced with permission from the Textbook of Advanced Cardiac Life Support, 2nd ed. Dallas, American Heart Association, 1987.)

SPECIAL SITUATIONS IN CARDIOPULMONARY RESUSCITATION

Cardiopulmonary arrest may occur as a result of noncardiac injuries and conditions that superimpose pathophysiologic and therapeutic concerns on those discussed above. In these situations, basic and advanced cardiac life support, as indicated, must be provided simultaneously with rapid correction of the primary insult (Table 60-13). In several situations, *e.g.*, exsanguination arrest, correction of the primary problem is prerequisite to artificial oxygen delivery and restoration of native circulation. Refractory cardiac arrest requires thorough evaluation (Table 60-14).

PEDIATRIC CARDIOPULMONARY RESUSCITATION

The principles of resuscitation delineated for adult patients apply as well to pediatric patients. The causes of cardiopulmonary arrest may be quite different in the pediatric population, but oxygen deficit as a result of an oxygen delivery problem remains the common denominator for all cardiac arrests.[162] Airway management, production of effective cardiac output, stabilization of cardiovascular parameters, and continued postresuscitative evaluation and support are the fundamental elements of pediatric CPR.

TABLE 60-13. Special Cardiopulmonary Resuscitation Situations

Cause of Arrest	Pathophysiology	Treatment
Trauma	Arrest due to massive blunt head and visceral injury, uncorrectable Reversible arrest caused by exsanguination, tension pneumothorax, cardiac tamponade airway obstruction (due to loss of consciousness or airway injury) Associated cervical injuries, hypothermia	1. Basic life support with cervical spine precautions for airway opening 2. Rapid primary survey for reversible causes of arrest and specific treatment 3. See Exsanguination, below 4. Consider thoracotomy for direct cardiac massage, treatment of pneumothorax and tamponade, clamping of aorta or pulmonary hilum
Exsanguination	Respiratory and cardiac arrest due to loss of cerebral and myocardial perfusion Chest compression ineffective in absence of venous return	1. Control hemorrhage 2. Restore blood volume via ≥2 large iv catheters with crystalloid solutions and O-negative blood 3. Basic life support and ACLS as indicated; ACLS not effective until artificial circulation achieved
Electrocution	Primary apnea followed by secondary cardiac arrest due to hypoxemia, or Primary ventricular fibrillation or asystolic cardiac arrest Associated burns, muscle destruction, myoglobinuria, bone fractures	1. Do not become a second victim! 2. Artificial ventilation as soon as possible 3. Chest compression and ACLS as indicated
Near-drowning	Submersion-induced asphyxiation followed by secondary cardiac arrest due to hypoxemia Full stomach due to swallowed water Pulmonary edema Hypothermia possible	1. Do not become a second victim! 2. Artificial ventilation as soon as possible; start mouth-to-mouth ventilation in water 3. Do not attempt to expel gastric water 4. Chest compression and ACLS as indicated
Hypothermia	Bradycardia, dysrhythmias, myocardial depression, coma, when T < 28°C Cardiac arrest due to ventricular fibrillation or asystole Refractory to drugs, defibrillation, pacing until warmed Metabolic acidosis Diuresis	1. ECG monitoring 2. Dry patient 3. Core warming; iv fluids, heated inspired gas, warm lavage of pericardium, body cavities, and viscera, cardiopulmonary bypass 4. BLS and ACLS as indicated
Carbon monoxide (CO) poisoning	Displacement of O_2 from hemoglobin, myoglobin, cytochrome binding sites by CO Airway obstruction due to unconsciousness, ventilatory depression Seizures Myocardial depression, dysrhythmias	1. BLS and ACLS as indicated 2. Ventilation with oxygen: CO elimination half-life 1.5 hours in 100% O_2 at 1 atm; 0.5 hours in 100% O_2 at 3 atm

There are specific anatomic, physiologic, and pathophysiologic variations in the pediatric population that must be recognized. An understanding of how these variants impact on the fundamental processes of CPR is essential for appropriate tailoring of CPR to pediatric patients.

The first minutes of life are a transition period from intrauterine to extrauterine existence when oxygen deficit may be present and oxygen delivery impaired. Airway obstruction from blood or meconium, respiratory depression from maternally administered and placentally transferred sedatives, hypovolemia, acidosis from marginal placental blood supply during labor and delivery, and congenital anomalies are some of the common causes of a depressed newborn in need of resuscitation. Use of the Apgar score to evaluate the adequacy of oxygenation in the newborn and resuscitation therapy is described in Chapters 46 and 47. This discussion is therefore confined to non-newborn pediatric CPR.

Basic Cardiopulmonary Resuscitation for Pediatric Resuscitation (Table 60-15)

Mouth (of rescuer) to mouth and nose (of infant or small child) or mouth (of larger child), and bag-valve–mask or endotracheal methods of ventilation may be used. Oxygen supplementation is essential. Oxygen-powered ventilating devices are not recommended in pediatric resuscitation because dangerously high airway pressure may be generated, potentially damaging the lungs. An esophageal obturator airway for pediatric use does not exist.

Cardiac compression for the infant is provided either by (1) the method whereby the rescuer's hands encircle the thorax, allowing the fingers to serve as the back board and the thumbs as the piston on the sternum; or (2) the standard method of having the rescuer positioned at the infant's side,

TABLE 60-14. Trouble Shooting: Looking for Correctable Causes of Refractory Arrest

Underlying Factors

Drug/anesthetic toxicity or overdose	Hypovolemia
Hypoxemia/hypercarbia	Tension pneumothorax
Hyper-/hypokalemia, -magnesemia, -calcemia	Cardiac tamponade
Acidemia/alkalemia	Embolism (air, thrombus)
Hypo-/hyperthermia	Pulmonary aspiration

Flaws in CPR Technique

Uncorrected airway obstruction	iv disconnected, infiltrated
Insufficient tidal volume	Correct drug(s) not given
Malfunctioning ventilating device	Incorrect drug dose
Insufficient oxygen inflow	Defibrillator, pacemaker not functioning
Mainstem bronchus intubation	Paddles not connected
Esophageal intubation	Paddle size too small
Occluded tracheal tube	No electroconductive interface
Severe gastric distention	Poor paddle position
Improper hand position during CPR	Insufficient paddle pressure
Inadequate sternal displacement	Defibrillator synchronized in presence of ventricular fibrillation
Compression rate too slow/fast	Residual air in lungs

placing two fingers on the sternum. Body structures are in relatively the same position in the infant and small child as in the adult; therefore, the compression point over the ventricles is located 1 fingerbreadth below the midsternum.[163] Compression of the lower sternum in the infant can result in liver laceration and fatal hemorrhage. It might be wise to loosen the diaper of an infant receiving cardiac compression, as this will allow better diaphragmatic descent with cardiac compression and minimize trauma to intraabdominal contents. The normal infant heart rate (approximately 100 beats·min^{-1}) is faster than the adult's and cardiac compression should, therefore, be more rapid.

Advanced Cardiopulmonary Resuscitation for Pediatric Resuscitation

Most newborn and pediatric cardiopulmonary arrests are the result of an airway and ventilation problem, and the resultant hypoxia is the prime concern of therapy (Table 60-16). Additional therapy directed at the cardiovascular problems of hypovolemia; poor cardiac contraction, rate, or rhythm; and acidosis may also have to be treated.

Vascular access, essential in pediatric resuscitation, is accomplished using a peripheral or central venous route. The same routes, techniques, and precautions observed in adults apply to the insertion of venous catheters in pediatric patients, but equipment specific for children should be employed. When intravenous access is absent, intraosseous injection into the anterior tibial bone marrow is used.

Drug therapy for pediatric resuscitation is fundamentally the same as for adults (Tables 60-17, 60-18, and 60-19). Oxygen, bicarbonate, and epinephrine are the mainstays of therapy. Bicarbonate is administered to infants in a 1:1 dilution to reduce the toxicity of the solution and minimize the chances of resultant intracranial hemorrhage.

Defibrillation is less commonly needed in pediatric resuscitation, since atherosclerotic cardiovascular disease is not present. Ventricular fibrillation and ventricular tachycardia are less commonly seen because ventilatory problems, which are usually the cause of pediatric cardiopulmonary arrests, produce hypoxia that often results in asystole. Congenital cardiac lesions do result in dysrhythmias that may require defibrillation or cardioversion. It is most desirable in pediatric patients to monitor the ECG and make the correct diagnosis to determine if pulselessness is the result of a rhythm disturbance amenable to defibrillation or cardioversion.

If electrical therapy is indicated in children, the same basic principles apply as in the adult therapy. Particular attention should be paid to proper paddle size so that the largest paddle surface making full contact with the thoracic wall is utilized. To avoid myocardial damage and postshock dysrhythmias, the recommended dose for pediatric defibrillation is 2 J·kg^{-1}.[164] The dose, if unsuccessful, is doubled until effective.

The postresuscitative care of infants and children requires the same intensive/critical care facilities are outlined for adults. It may be necessary to transport a resuscitated and stabilized child to a pediatric referral center that can provide pediatric intensive care for postresuscitative treatment.

POSTRESUSCITATION LIFE SUPPORT

After resuscitation, the patient is transferred to an intensive care environment where an evaluation is initiated to determine the degree of cerebral, cardiovascular, pulmonary, and renal function that has been salvaged as well as the primary underlying cause of the cardiopulmonary arrest. If a primary contributing condition can be identified, prompt definitive treatment may prevent recurrence of arrest and promote return to prearrest cardiopulmonary function. Coronary thrombolytic therapy to dissolve an acute coronary thrombus responsible for myocardial ischemia and cardiac arrest, for example, must be initiated within 4 hours of thrombus formation to restore perfusion and salvage ischemic myocardium.

Stabilization and support of cardiovascular function are achieved with general and specific intensive care measures

TABLE 60-15. Basic Life Support Performance Sheet for Infant Cardiopulmonary Resuscitation

Name _____ Date _____

Step	Objective	Critical Performance	S	U
1. **A**IRWAY	Assessment: Determine unresponsiveness.	Tap or gently shake shoulder.		
	Call for help.	Call out "Help!"		
	Position the infant.	Turn on back as unit, supporting head and neck.		
		Place on firm, hard surface.		
	Open the airway.	Use head-tilt/chin-lift maneuver to sniffing or neutral position.		
		Do not overextend the head.		
2. **B**REATHING	Assessment: Determine breathlessness.	Maintain open airway.		
		Ear over mouth, observe chest: look, listen, feel for breathing (3–5 sec).		
	Ventilate twice.	Maintain open airway.		
		Make tight seal on infant's mouth and nose with rescuer's mouth.		
		Ventilate 2 times at 1–1.5 sec/inspiration.		
		Observe chest rise.		
		Allow deflation between breaths.		
3. **C**IRCULATION	Assessment: Determine pulselessness.	Feel for brachial pulse (5–10 sec).		
		Maintain head-tilt with other hand.		
	Activate EMS system.	If someone responded to call for help, send him/her to activate EMS system.		
		Total time, Step 1—Activate EMS system: 15–35 sec.		
	Begin chest compressions.	Imagine line between nipples (intermammary line).		
		Place 2–3 fingers on sternum, 1 finger's width below intermammary line.		
		Equal compression–relaxation.		
		Compress vertically, ½ to 1 inches.		
		Keep fingers on sternum during upstroke.		
		Complete chest relaxation on upstroke.		
		Say any helpful mnemonic.		
		Compression rate: at least 100/min (5 in 3 sec or less).		
4. Compression/Ventilation Cycles	Do 10 cycles of 5 compressions and 1 ventilation.	Proper compression/ventilation ratio: 5 compressions to 1 slow ventilation per cycle.		
		Pause for ventilation.		
		Observe chest rise: 1–1.5 sec/inspiration; 10 cycles/45 sec or less.		
5. Reassessment	Determine pulselessness.	Feel for brachial pulse (5 sec).* If there is no pulse, go to Step 6.		
6. Continue CPR	Ventilate once.	Ventilate 1 time.		
		Observe chest rise: 1–1.5 sec/inspiration.		
	Resume compression/ventilation cycles.	Feel for brachial pulse every few minutes.		

*If pulse is present, open airway and check for spontaneous breathing, (a) If breathing is present, maintain open airway and monitor breathing and pulse, (b) if breathing is absent, perform rescue breathing at 20 times/min and monitor pulse.

Instructor _____ Check: Satisfactory _____ Unsatisfactory _____

TABLE 60-16. Equipment Guidelines According to Age and Weight

Equipment	Age (50th Percentile Weight)					
	Premie (1–2.5 kg)	Neonate (2.5–4.0 kg)	6 Months (7.0 kg)	1–2 Years (10–12 kg)	5 Years (16–18 kg)	8–10 Years (24–30 kg)
Airway—oral	Infant (00)	Infant/small (0)	Small (1)	Small (2)	Medium (3)	Medium/large (4/5)
Breathing						
Self-inflating bag	Infant	Infant	Child	Child	Child	Child/adult
O$_2$ ventilation mask	Premature	Newborn	Infant/child	Child	Child	Small adult
Endotracheal tube	2.5–3.0 (uncuffed)	3.0–3.5 (uncuffed)	3.5–4.0 (uncuffed)	4.0–4.5 (uncuffed)	5.0–5.5 (uncuffed)	5.5–6.5 (cuffed)
Laryngoscope blade	0 (straight)	1 (straight)	1 (straight)	1–2 (straight)	2 (straight or curved)	2–3 (straight or curved)
Suction/stylet (F)	6–8/6	8/6	8–10/6	10/6	14/14	14/14
Circulation						
BP cuff	Newborn	Newborn	Infant	Child	Child	Child/adult
Venous access						
Angiocath	22–24	22–24	22–24	20–22	18–20	16–20
Butterfly needle	25	23–25	23–25	23	20–23	18–21
Intracath	—	—	19	19	16	14
Arm board	6″	6″	6″–8″	8″	8″–15″	15″
Orogastric tube (F)	5	5–8	8	10	10–12	14–18
Chest tube (F)	10–14	12–18	14–20	14–24	20–32	28–38

From Chamedies L (ed): Textbook of Pediatric Advanced Life Support. Reproduced with permission of the American Heart Association, Dallas, 1988.

TABLE 60-17. Resuscitation Medications, by Weight and Age, for Infants and Children 0–10 Years

Age	50th Percentile Weight (kg)	Epinephrine		Atropine		Bicarbonate*	
		mg	ml†	mg	ml†	mEq	ml†
Newborn	3.0	0.03	0.3	0.1	1.0	3.0	6.0
1 Month	4.0	0.04	0.4	0.1	1.0	4.0	8.0
3 Months	5.5	0.055	0.55	0.11	1.1	5.5	11.0
6 Months	7.0	0.07	0.7	0.14	1.4	7.0	7.0
1 Year	10.0	0.10	1.0	0.20	2.0	10.0	10.0
2 Years	12.0	0.12	1.2	0.24	2.4	12.0	12.0
3 Years	14.0	0.14	1.4	0.28	2.8	14.0	14.0
4 Years	16.0	0.16	1.6	0.32	3.2	16.0	16.0
5 Years	18.0	0.18	1.8	0.36	3.6	18.0	18.0
6 Years	20.0	0.20	2.0	0.40	4.0	20.0	20.0
7 Years	22.0	0.22	2.2	0.44	4.4	22.0	22.0
8 Years	25.0	0.25	2.5	0.50	5.0	25.0	25.0
9 Years	28.0	0.28	2.8	0.56	5.6	28.0	28.0
10 Years	34.0	0.34	3.4	0.68	6.8	34.0	34.0

*The use of bicarbonate in cardiac arrest is controversial (see text). Good ventilation must be established before bicarbonate is used.

†Volume (ml) is based on the following concentrations:
epinephrine: 1:10,000 (0.1 mg·ml^{-1})
atropine: 0.1 mg·ml^{-1}
bicarbonate: ≤3 months = 4.2% solution (0.5 mEq·ml^{-1})
>3 months = 8.4% solution (1 mEq·ml^{-1})

From Chamedies L (ed): Textbook of Pediatric Advanced Life Support. Reproduced with permission of the American Heart Association, Dallas, 1988.

TABLE 60-18. Drugs for Pediatric Cardiopulmonary Resuscitation

Drug	Dose	How Supplied*
Epinephrine hydrochloride	0.01 mg·kg^{-1} 0.1 ml·kg^{-1}	1:10,000 (0.1 mg·ml^{-1})
Sodium bicarbonate	1 mEq·kg^{-1} 1 ml·kg^{-1}	1 mEq·ml^{-1} (8.4% solution)
Atropine sulfate	0.02 mg·kg^{-1} 0.2 ml·kg^{-1}	0.1 mg·ml^{-1}
Calcium chloride	20 mg·kg^{-1} (0.2 ml·kg^{-1})	100 mg·ml^{-1} (10% solution)
Glucose	0.5–1.0 gm·kg^{-1}	0.5 g·ml^{-1} D$_{50}$W
Lidocaine hydrochloride	1 mg·kg^{-1}	10 mg·ml^{-1} (1%) 20 mg·ml^{-1} (2%)
Bretylium tosylate	5 mg·kg^{-1}	50 mg·ml^{-1}
Infusions		
Epinephrine infusion	0.1–1.0 μg·kg^{-1}·min^{-1}	1 mg·ml^{-1} 1:1000
Dopamine hydrochloride infusion	2–20 μg·kg^{-1}·min^{-1}	40 mg·ml^{-1}
Dobutamine infusion	5–20 μg·kg^{-1}·min^{-1}	250 mg·vial^{-1} lysophilized
Isoproterenol infusion	0.1–1.0 μg·kg^{-1}·min^{-1}	1 mg·5 ml^{-1}
Lidocaine infusion	20–50 μg·kg^{-1}·min^{-1}	40 mg·ml^{-1} (4%)

*For iv push medications, preparation listed is form available in prefilled syringes.

From Chamedies L (ed): Textbook of Pediatric Advanced Life Support. Reproduced with permission of the American Heart Association, Dallas, 1988.

appropriate for management of the patient's hemodynamic and neurologic condition. The patient who is awake and breathing spontaneously after successful resuscitation should be continuously monitored in an intensive care environment for recurrence of cardiac arrest, have an intravenous line established and receive supplemental oxygen and appropriate diagnostic investigation for underlying causes of the arrest. A continuous prophylactic antidysrhythmic infusion, most commonly lidocaine, is indicated for 24 hours following resuscitation from ventricular fibrillation and ventricular tachycardia to reduce the likelihood of reappearance of the dysrhythmia.

The subject who remains unresponsive, apneic, and has cardiovascular instability after resuscitation is likely to have hypoxia-related multiple organ failure and requires stabilization of cardiorespiratory function and support of the postischemic central nervous system. In addition to continuous ECG surveillance and antidysrhythmic infusion, cardiovascular therapy may include invasive hemodynamic monitoring to guide the treatment of cardiogenic shock. Tracheal intubation and controlled ventilation will be necessary until responsiveness, airway reflexes, and pulmonary function recover. Renal, gastrointestinal, and metabolic intensive care are other elements of the postresuscitation life support. Specific discussion of intensive care management can be found in Chapter 59. Although postresuscitative care of the central

nervous system cannot alter the primary ischemic-anoxic insult, it can modify the degree of secondary injury occurring with reperfusion. Support of the brain entails general measures that maintain cerebral oxygen delivery and control cerebral metabolic rate. Restoring homeostasis of vital extracranial organ systems is essential to provide the postischemic brain opportunity for recovery. Continued hypotension, hypoxemia, and acidemia following resuscitation merely potentiate reperfusion injury to the brain. Animals that experience normotension after resuscitation from complete ischemia have a better neurologic outcome than animals that are hypotensive following arrest.[165,166] In fact, a brief period of hypertension may be of value, but severe prolonged hypertension is associated with a poor neurologic outcome.[166]

Hyperthermia and seizures increase cerebral metabolic rate, thereby elevating oxygen consumption and promoting cerebral edema. Normothermia, or mild hypothermia to reduce cerebral metabolic rate, should be maintained with the aid of temperature monitoring and external cooling, if necessary. Shivering should be controlled with the use of neuromuscular blockade, as this increases ventilation and oxygenation needs.

Hyperglycemia at the time of cerebral ischemic insult in dogs[167] and humans[168,169] is related to a less favorable neurologic outcome when compared with those who are normo-

TABLE 60-19. Infusion Medications,* by Weight and Age, for Infants and Children 0–10 Years

Add 0.6 mg (3 ml)† of isoproterenol
0.6 mg (0.6 ml)† of epinephrine **to** 100 ml of diluent
60.0 mg (1.5 ml)† of dopamine
60.0 mg (2.4 ml)† of dobutamine

Infuse at 1 ml·kg^{-1}·h^{-1} or according to following table in order

To give 0.1 µg·kg^{-1}·min^{-1} isoproterenol
0.1 µg·kg^{-1}·min^{-1} epinephrine
10 µg·kg^{-1}·min^{-1} dopamine
10 µg·kg^{-1}·min^{-1} dobutamine

Age	50th Percentile Weight (kg)	Infusion Rate (ml·h^{-1})
Newborn	3	3.0
1 Month	4	4.0
3 Months	5.5	5.5
6 Months	7.0	7.0
1 Year	10.0	10.0
2 Years	12.0	12.0
3 Years	14.0	14.0
4 Years	16.0	16.0
5 Years	18.0	18.0
6 Years	20.0	20.0
7 Years	22.0	22.0
8 Years	25.0	25.0
9 Years	28.0	28.0
10 Years	34.0	34.0

*These are starting doses. Adjust concentration to dose and fluid tolerance.
†Based on the following concentrations:
  isoproterenol: 0.2 mg·ml^{-1}
  epinephrine: 1:1000 (1 mg·ml^{-1})
  dopamine: 40 mg·ml^{-1}
  dobutamine: 25 mg·ml^{-1}

From Chamedies L (ed): Textbook of Pediatric Advanced Life Support. Reproduced with permission of the American Heart Association, Dallas, 1988.

glycemic. Elevated blood glucose levels may contribute to development of a more severe intracellular lactic acidosis during ischemia. Whether it is prudent to limit infusion of dextrose-containing solutions or monitor blood glucose levels following resuscitation from cardiac arrest is uncertain.

Investigations of specific therapeutic modalities including hyperventilation,[170] immobilization with neuromuscular blockade,[171] and hemodilution and anticoagulation[172] have failed to identify measures that favorably alter neurologic outcome from global cerebral ischemic injury. Reduction of cerebral metabolic rate and amelioration of neurologic injury by moderate and high doses of barbiturates have not been consistently produced in animal models of global cerebral ischemia.[173] In a multi-institutional study of high-dose barbiturates after cardiac arrest in humans, no improvement in outcome as a result of barbiturate treatment was observed.[174] Anticonvulsants, including barbiturates, however, in conjunction with electroencephalographic monitoring, may be beneficial following resuscitation from cardiac arrest. Suppression of abnormal electroencephalographic patterns by thiopental in an animal model of cardiac arrest reduced mortality following global cerebral ischemia.[175]

Slow calcium channel blocking drugs, intended to reduce cerebrovascular resistance and improve blood flow, have produced conflicting results in animal models of cerebral resuscitation from global ischemia. Nimodipine treatment after resuscitation from out-of-hospital cardiac arrest in humans did not improve survival compared with patients receiving a placebo.[176]

Corticosteroids are effective in reducing cerebral edema associated with intracranial mass lesions; however, there is no evidence that they reduce neuronal injury or improve neurologic outcome after cardiac arrest.

Modalities that retard free radical generation during reperfusion following ischemia, including desferoxamine, superoxide dismutase, and mannitol, are under investigation.

MEDICOLEGAL CONSIDERATIONS

Over the last 15 years, CPR has developed into an effective set of sophisticated medical techniques that often results in survival from cardiac arrest. This fact raises many medicolegal questions with regard to the delivery of CPR, e.g., the provider's responsibility to provide CPR, the standard of care, definitions of death, termination of CPR, "do not resuscitate" orders, and discontinuation of life-support systems. Consideration of all of these issues directs the provision of the best of CPR available against provision of reasonable care in light of an individual's medical status and psychological desires.[177]

Once physicians begin the treatment of a patient, they have an implied contractual responsibility to complete such care. A similar situation exists in an emergency facility such as a life-support unit or hospital emergency room. Physicians working in such units must provide CPR in the patient's best interest, even when the patient is unable to request treatment and establish a normal physician–patient relationship. At present in the United States (in distinction to some European countries), there is no legal obligation for a physician to provide CPR to an unknown victim on the street so long as the physician is not acting as a part of a mobile life-support unit. The moral and ethical reasons to initiate CPR in the field are compelling, but no legal obligation to respond exists in the United States for the physician, paramedical person, or lay person. It must be recognized, however, that if field delivery of CPR is initiated by the "good samaritan" (physician or nonphysician), then the victim cannot be abandoned and the care must be performed up to the level of expertise of the rescuer. Many states have "good samaritan" statutes to protect those who render such aid.

The standard of care for CPR is defined in a rather uniform manner throughout the United States. The AHA CPR protocols are one acceptable standard of care, although not the only to be applied to the definition. The implied standard of care for CPR within the confines of a hospital requires that a cardiac arrest team be defined and readily available to render immediate resuscitative efforts.

One of the major issues that is still not totally resolved is that of an acceptable definition of death. Until this concern is addressed, it is difficult to make rational decisions about the timing of or even the need for CPR in any of its phases. The traditional definition of death had been based on the absence of cardiovascular function: if the heart stopped and was refractory to return of function, death was present. A more recent perspective on death focuses on the brain. Criteria for brain death have been established, the most famous being the Harvard Criteria. Both medical and legal sanctions have been given to the concept of brain death. The definition of death by criteria for absence of both cardiac and brain viability is required for CPR decisions. On the one hand, CPR is begun and often maintained because of the probability of brain viability or even the lack of proof of brain death. On the other hand, CPR may be terminated because it is obvious that cardiovascular unresponsiveness is present and brain viability is in jeopardy.

Decisions to begin or end CPR must consider cardiac and brain function and responsiveness to therapy.[178,179] In general, CPR is initiated in all instances where brain viability is assumed and no other overriding consideration (e.g., patient's desire not to be resuscitated) precludes this action. It must be remembered that a prospective diagnosis of irreversible brain damage is almost impossible to make. Many cases have been reported where neurologic recovery occurred months after the initial insult. Additionally, hypothermia or medications may depress central nervous system function and mimic brain death that is not truly present. CPR is often begun to evaluate cardiovascular responsiveness. Often, it is only by a trial of CPR that the heart can be diagnosed as irreversibly damaged and unresponsive to further therapy. A major difficulty in deciding brain and cardiac viability is deciding when the cardiac arrest occurred. Many cardiopulmonary disasters occur totally unwitnessed. It is virtually impossible to determine the length of time of absent oxygen delivery when a rescuer arrives at the scene of the arrest or the patient is delivered to a life-support facility. "Dead on arrival" (DOA) diagnosis is clearly harder to make accurately than was once thought.

In the past several years the personal wish of individuals not to be resuscitated has been a major legal issue. A number of court cases have upheld the desires of mentally competent adults who believe that they have terminal illness and, therefore, do not want CPR, a technique designed for prevention or treatment of sudden, unexpected death. "Do not resuscitate" orders are less clear, however, when a mentally incompetent patient is involved. Under these circumstances as well as in situations where life-support systems might be discontinued, if brain death is documented, CPR and other life-support methods can be stopped. When strict brain death criteria cannot be met, however, each case should be decided on its own merits with the assistance of the courts.

All who may be involved with CPR or life-support procedures should be aware of the medicolegal ramifications of their actions or lack of action so that reasonable care may be provided to all who require it and excessive care or excessive lack of care can be avoided.

ROLE OF THE ANESTHESIOLOGIST IN CARDIOPULMONARY RESUSCITATION

The professional responsibilities of an anesthesiologist include CPR. The American Board of Anesthesiology in its *Booklet of Information*, and the U.S. Department of Labor in its definition of the specialty of anesthesiology, i.e., its job description, cite, as tasks of the anesthesiologist, clinical care in and teaching of life support and cardiac and pulmonary resuscitation. In addition, CPR research and administrative functions are often delegated to the anesthesiologist.

The practice of operating room anesthesia and critical care medicine gives the anesthesiologist considerable expertise in acute life-support practices. A deficiency may exist with anesthesiologists and physicians in general, however, in their field delivery of CPR. Anesthesiologists have been shown to lack CPR knowledge and skill,[180,181] which can be easily corrected through continuing education. As important members of the team delivering CPR, anesthesiologists must remain current with accepted CPR practice.

Teaching CPR is an important activity for the anesthesiologist. Guiding a student through procedures of tracheal intubation or concepts of pharmacologic intervention can be best accomplished by the anesthesiologist. Rewards for the anesthesiologist CPR tutor include knowledge that the student becomes competent; the anesthesiologist becomes a respected educator at the medical school or hospital; and a future anesthesiologist may have been recruited.

The administrative duties of the anesthesiologist include review of CPR equipment and its function and establishment of anesthesia response to and collaboration with the total CPR and emergency medical service effort within the community.

CPR research is an activity anesthesiologists have participated in throughout the years. Only by continued investigative effort can basic science rationale be uncovered for the clinical practice of CPR.

REFERENCES

1. Comroe JH, Dripps RD: Ben Franklin and open heart surgery. Circ Res 35:661, 1974
2. Resen Z, Davidson JT: Respiratory resuscitation in ancient Hebrew sources. Anesth Analg 51:502, 1972

3. Vesalius A: De humani corporis fabrica, libu system, Bosel, Oporinus, 1543, 661

4. Dill DB: Background on manual artificial respiration and mouth-to-mouth resuscitation. Physiologist 23:33, 1980

5. Gordon AS: Background on cardiopulmonary resuscitation. Physiologist 23:35, 1980

6. Cooper DY: Mouth-to-mouth resuscitation: Influence of alcohol on revival of an old technique. Life Sci 16:487, 1975

7. Comroe JH: ". . . In comes the good air." Part II, mouth-to-mouth method. Am Rev Respir Dis 119:1025, 1979

8. Tossach W: Medical Essays and Observations. Edinburgh, 1744

9. Elam JO, Brown ES, Elder JD: Artificial respiration by mouth-to-mouth method. A study of respiratory gas exchange of paralyzed patients ventilated by operator's expired air. N Engl J Med 250:749, 1954

10. Elam JO, Green DG: Mission accomplished: Successful mouth-to-mouth resuscitation. Anesth Analg 40:578, 1961

11. Gordon AS, Frye CW, Gittelson L et al: Mouth-to-mouth versus manual artificial respiration for children and adults. JAMA 172:320, 1960

12. Gordon AS: The principles and practice of heart-lung resuscitation. Acta Anaesthesiol Scand 9 (suppl): 134, 1961

13. Safar P: Ventilatory efficacy of mouth-to-mouth artificial respiration: Airway obstruction during manual and mouth-to-mouth artificial respiration. JAMA 172:335, 1960

14. Kouwenhoven WB, Langworth OR: Cardiopulmonary resuscitation. JAMA 226:877, 1973

15. Jude JR, Kouwenhoven WB, Knickerbocker GG: Cardiac arrest. JAMA 178:1063, 1961

16. Prevost J, Battelli F: La mort par les courants electrique. J Gen Physiol 1:1085, 1899

17. Beck CS, Pritchard WH, Feil HS: Ventricular fibrillation of long duration abolished by electric shock. JAMA 135:985, 1947

18. Kouwenhoven WB, Milnor WR, Knickerbocker GG et al: Closed chest defibrillation. Surgery 42:550, 1957

19. Kouwenhoven WB, Jude JR, Knickerbocker GG: Closed chest cardiac massage. JAMA 173:1064, 1960

20. Heart Facts: 1987. American Heart Association (55-005-K). Dallas, Texas, 1986

21. Lemire JG, Johnson AL: Is cardiac resuscitation worthwhile? A decade of experience. N Engl J Med 286:970, 1972

22. Copley DP, Mantle JA, Rogers WJ et al: Improved outcome for prehospital cardiopulmonary collapse with resuscitation by bystanders. Circulation 56:901, 1977

23. Eisenberg MS, Hallstrom A, Bergner L: Long-term survival after out-of-hospital cardiac arrest. N Engl J Med 306:1340, 1982

24. Eisenberg M, Bergner L, Hallstrom A: Paramedic programs and out-of-hospital cardiac arrest: 1. Factors associated with successful resuscitation. Am J Public Health 69:30, 1979

25. Pantridge JF, Geddes JS: A mobile intensive-care unit in the management of myocardial infarction. Lancet 2:271, 1967

26. Standards and guidelines for cardiopulmonary resuscitation (CPR) and emergency cardiac care (ECC). JAMA 244:453, 1980

27. Safar P: Cardiopulmonary-cerebral resuscitation including emergency airway control. In Schwartz GR, Safar P, Stone JH et al (eds): Principles and Practice of Emergency Medicine, Philadelphia, WB Saunders, 1978

28. Safar P, Escarraga LA, Chang F: Upper airway obstruction in the unconscious patient. J Appl Physiol 14:760, 1959

29. Safar P: Failure of manual respiration. J Appl Physiol 14:84, 1959

30. Guildner CW: Resuscitation-opening the airway: A comparative study of techniques for opening an airway obstructed by the tongue. J Am Coll Emerg Phys 5:588, 1976

31. Smith JP, Bodai BI, Seifkin A et al: The esophageal obturator airway: A review. JAMA 250:1081, 1983

32. Gordon AS, Belton MK, Ridolpho PF: Emergency management of foreign body airway obstruction, In Safar P, Elam JO (eds): Advances in Cardiopulmonary Resuscitation, p 39. New York, Springer Verlag, 1977

33. Heimlich HJ, Hoffman KA, Canestri FR: Food-choking and drowning deaths prevented by external subdiaphragmatic compression: Physiological basis. Ann Thorac Surg 20:188, 1975

34. Redding JS: The choking controversy: Critique of evidence of the Heimlich maneuver. Crit Care Med 7:475, 1979

35. Day RL, Crelin ES, DuBois AB: Choking: The Heimlich abdominal thrust vs back blows: An approach to measurement of inertial and aerodynamic forces. Pediatrics 70:113, 1982

36. Yealy DM, Stewart RD: Translaryngeal cannula ventilation: continuing misconceptions (letter). Anesthesiology 67:445, 1987

37. Zornow MH, Thomas TC, Scheller MS: The efficacy of three different methods of transtracheal ventilation. Can Soc Anaesth J 36:624, 1989

38. Neff CC, Pfister RC, Van Sonnenberg E: Percutaneous transtracheal ventilation: Experimental and practical aspects. J Trauma 23:84, 1983

39. Stothert JC Jr, Stout MJ, Lewis LM, Keltner RM Jr: High pressure percutaneous transtracheal ventilation: The use of large gauge intravenous type catheters in the totally obstructed airway. AM J Emerg Med 8:184, 1990

40. Dunlap LB: A modified simple device for the emergency administration of percutaneous transtracheal ventilation. J Am Coll Emerg Phys 7:42, 1978

41. Branditz FK, Kern KB, Campbell SC: Continuous transtracheal oxygen delivery during cardiopulmonary resuscitation: An alternative method of ventilation in a canine model. Chest 95:441, 1989

41a. Harris LC, Kirimli B, Safar P: Ventilation-cardiac compression rates and ratios in cardiopulmonary resuscitation. Anesthesiology 28:806, 1967

42. Niemann JT, Rosborough JP, Ung S et al: Coronary perfusion pressure during experimental cardiopulmonary resuscitation. Ann Emerg Med 11:127, 1982

43. Halperin HR, Guerci AD, Chandra N et al: Vest inflation without simultaneous ventilation during cardiac arrest in dogs: Improved survival from prolonged cardiopulmonary resuscitation. Circulation 74:1407, 1986

44. Chandra N, Weisfeldt ML, Tsitlik J et al: Augmentation of carotid flow during cardiopulmonary resuscitation by ventilation at high airway pressure simultaneous with chest compression. Am J Cardiol 48:1053, 1981

45. DelGuercio LR, Feins NR, Cohn JD et al: Comparison of blood flow during external and internal cardiac massage in man. Circulation 31:I171, 1965

46. Koehler RC, Chandra N, Guerci AD et al: Augmentation of cerebral perfusion by simultaneous chest compression and lung inflation with abdominal binding after cardiac arrest in dogs. Circulation 67:266, 1983

47. Luce JM, Ross BK, O'Quin RJ et al: Regional blood flow during cardiopulmonary resuscitation in dogs using simultaneous and nonsimultaneous compression and ventilation. Circulation 67:258, 1983

48. Ditchey RV, Winkler JV, Rhodes CA: Relative lack of coronary blood flow during closed-chest resuscitation in dogs. Circulation 66:297, 1982

49. Bellamy RF, DeGuzman LR, Pedersen DC: Coronary blood flow during cardiopulmonary resuscitation in swine. Circulation 69:174, 1984

50. Babbs CF, Voorhees WD, Fitzgerald KR et al: Relationship of blood pressure and flow during CPR to chest compression amplitude: Evidence for an effective compression threshold. Ann Emerg Med 19:527, 1983

51. Taylor GJ, Tucker WM, Green HL et al: Importance of prolonged compression during cardiopulmonary resuscitation in man. N Engl J Med 296:1515, 1977

52. Halperin HR, Tsitlik JE, Guerci AD et al: Determinants of blood flow to vital organs during cardiopulmonary resuscitation in dogs. Circulation 73:539, 1986

53. Weisfeldt ML, Halperin HR: Cardiopulmonary resuscitation: Beyond cardiac massage. Circulation 74:443, 1986

54. Maier GW, Tyson GS, Olsen CO et al: The physiology of external massage: High impulse cardiopulmonary resuscitation. Circulation 70:86, 1984

55. Rudikoff MT, Maughan WL, Effron M et al: Mechanisms of

blood flow during cardiopulmonary resuscitation. Circulation 61:345, 1980

56. Paradis NA, Martin TB, Goetting MG et al: Simultaneous aortic, jugular bulb, and right atrial pressures during cardiopulmonary resuscitation in humans: Insights into mechanisms. Circulation 80:361, 1989

57. Chandra N, Rudikoff M, Weisfeldt ML: Simultaneous chest compression and ventilation at high airway pressure during cardiopulmonary resuscitation. Lancet i:175, 1980

58. Niemann JR, Rosborough JP, Ung S et al: Hemodynamic effects of continuous abdominal binding during cardiac arrest and resuscitation. Am J Cardiol 53:269, 1984

59. Ralston SH, Babbs CF, Niebauer MJ: Cardiopulmonary resuscitation with interposed abdominal compression in dogs. Anesth Analg 61:645, 1982

60. Voorhees WD, Niebauer MJ, Babbs CF: Improved oxygen delivery during cardiopulmonary resuscitation with interposed abdominal compressions. Ann Emerg Med 12:128, 1983

61. Ward KR, Sullivan RJ, Zelenak RR, Summer WR: A comparison of interposed abdominal compression CPR and standard CPR by monitoring end-tidal P_{CO_2}. Ann Emerg Med 18:831, 1989

62. Niemann JT, Criley JM, Rosborough JP et al: Predictive indices of successful cardiac resuscitation after prolonged arrest and experimental cardiopulmonary resuscitation. Ann Emerg Med 14:521, 1985

63. Sanders AB, Kern KB, Atlas M et al: Importance of the duration of inadequate coronary perfusion pressure on resuscitation from cardiac arrest. J Am Coll Cardiol 6:113, 1985

64. Paradis NA, Martin GB, Rivers EP et al: Coronary perfusion pressure and the return of spontaneous circulation in human cardiopulmonary resuscitation. JAMA 263:1106, 1990

65. Guerci AD, Chandra N, Johnson E et al: Failure of sodium bicarbonate to improve resuscitation from ventricular fibrillation in dogs. Circulation 74 (suppl IV):IV75, 1986

66. Kette F, Weil MH, vonPlanta M et al: Buffer agents do not reverse intramyocardial acidosis during cardiac resuscitation. Circulation 81:1660, 1990

67. Kern KB, Carter AB, Showen RL et al: Comparison of mechanical techniques of cardiopulmonary resuscitation: Survival and neurologic outcome in dogs. Am J Emerg Med 5:190, 1987

68. Swenson RD, Weaver WD, Niskanen RA et al: Hemodynamics in humans during conventional and experimental methods of cardiopulmonary resuscitation. Circulation 78:630, 1988

69. Bircher N, Safar P, Steward R: A comparison of standard, MAST-augmented, and open-chest CPR in dogs: A preliminary investigation. Crit Care Med 8:147, 1980

70. Wolfe JA, Maier GW, Newton JR Jr et al: Physiologic determinants of coronary blood flow during external cardiac massage. J Thorac Cardiovasc Surg 95:523, 1988

71. Feneley MP, Maier GW, Kern KB et al: Influence of compression rate on initial success of resuscitation and 24 hour survival after prolonged manual cardiopulmonary resuscitation in dogs. Circulation 77:240, 1988

72. Newton JR Jr, Glower BB, Wolfe JA et al: A physiologic comparison of external cardiac massage techniques. J Thorac Cardiovasc Surg 95:892, 1988

73. Ben-Haim SO, Shoftie R, Ostrow B, Dinnar U: Effect of vest cardiopulmonary resuscitation rate on cardiac output and coronary blood flow. Crit Care Med 17:768, 1989

74. Krischer JP, Fine EG, Weisfeldt ML et al: Comparison of prehospital conventional and simultaneous compression-ventilation cardiopulmonary resuscitation. Crit Care Med 17:1263, 1989

75. Beattie C, Guerci AD, Hall T et al: Mechanisms of blood flow during pneumatic vest cardiopulmonary resuscitation. J Appl Physiol 70:454, 1991

76. Weiser FM, Adler LN, Kuhn LA: Hemodynamic effects of closed and open chest cardiac resuscitation in normal dogs and those with acute myocardial infarction. Am J Cardiol 10:555, 1962

77. Bircher N, Safar P: Comparison of standard and "new" closed-chest CPR and open chest CPR in dogs. Crit Care Med 9:384, 1981

78. Geehr EC, Lewis FR, Auerbach PS: Failure of open-heart mas-

sage to improve survival after prehospital nontraumatic cardiac arrest (letter). N Engl J Med 314:1189, 1986

79. Bircher N, Safar P: Open-chest CPR: An old method whose time has returned. Am J Emerg Med 2:568, 1984

80. Pretto E, Safar P, Saito R et al: Cardiopulmonary bypass after prolonged cardiac arrest in dogs. Ann Emerg Med 16:611, 1987

81. Martin GB, Nowak RM, Carden DL et al: Cardiopulmonary bypass vs CPR as treatment for prolonged canine cardiopulmonary arrest. Ann Emerg Med 16:628, 1987

82. Levine R, Gorayeb M, Safar P et al: Emergency cardiopulmonary bypass after cardiac arrest and prolonged closed-chest CPR in dogs. Ann Emerg Med 16:620, 1987

83. Paradis NA, Koscove EM: Epinephrine in cardiac arrest: A critical review. Ann Emerg Med 19:1288, 1990

84. Redding JS, Pearson JW: Resuscitation from ventricular fibrillation. JAMA 203:255, 1968

85. Otto CW, Yakaitis RW, Redding JS et al: Comparison of dopamine, dobutamine, and epinephrine in CPR. Crit Care Med 9:640, 1981

86. Pearson JW, Redding JS: Epinephrine in cardiac resuscitation. Am Heart J 66:210, 1963

87. Redding JS, Pearson JW: Evaluation of drugs for cardiac resuscitation. Anesthesiology 24:203, 1963

88. Yakaitis RW, Otto CW, Blitt CD: Relative importance of alpha and beta adrenergic receptors during resuscitation. Crit Care Med 7:293, 1979

89. Otto CW, Yakaitis RW, Blitt CD: Mechanism of action of epinephrine in resuscitation from asphyxial arrest. Crit Care Med 9:321, 1981

90. Livesay JJ, Follette DM, Fey KM et al: Optimizing myocardial supply/demand with alpha-adrenergic drugs during cardiopulmonary resuscitation. J Thorac Cardiovasc Surg 76:244, 1978

91. Michael JR, Guerci AD, Koehler RC et al: Mechanisms by which epinephrine augments cerebral and myocardial perfusion during cardiopulmonary resuscitation in dogs. Circulation 69:822, 1984

92. Koehler RC, Michael JR, Guerci AD et al: Beneficial effect of epinephrine infusion on cerebral and myocardial blood flows during CPR. Ann Emerg Med 14:744, 1985

93. Ditchey RV, Lindenfeld J: Failure of epinephrine to improve the balance between myocardial oxygen supply and demand during closed-chest resuscitation in dogs. Circulation 78:382, 1988

94. Brilliman J, Sanders A, Otto CW et al: Comparison of epinephrine and phenylephrine for resuscitation and neurologic outcome of cardiac arrest in dogs. Ann Emerg Med 16:11, 1987

95. Brown CG, Werman HA et al: The effect of high-dose phenylephrine versus epinephrine on regional cerebral blood flow during CPR. Ann Emerg Med 16:743, 1987

96. Schleien CL, Koehler RC, Gervais H et al: Organ blood flow and somatosensory-evoked potentials during and after cardiopulmonary resuscitation with epinephrine or phenylephrine. Circulation 79:1332, 1989

97. Brown CG, Katz SE, Werman HA et al: The effect of epinephrine versus methoxamine on regional myocardial blood flow and defibrillation rates following prolonged cardiorespiratory arrest in a swine model. Am J Emerg Med 5:362, 1987

98. Brown CG, Taylor RB, Werman HA et al: Myocardial oxygen delivery/consumption during cardiopulmonary resuscitation: A comparison of epinephrine and phenylephrine. Ann Emerg Med 17:302, 1988

99. Roberts D, Landolfi K, Dobson K, Light RB: The effects of methoxamine and epinephrine on survival and regional distribution of cardiac output in dogs with prolonged ventricular fibrillation. Chest 98:999, 1990

100. Turner LM, Parsons M, Luetkemeyer RC et al: A comparison of epinephrine and methoxamine for resuscitation from electromechanical dissociation in human beings. Ann Emerg Med 17:443, 1988

101. Olsen DW, Thakur R, Stueven HA et al: Randomized study of epinephrine versus methoxamine in pre-hospital ventricular fibrillation. Ann Emerg Med 18:250, 1989

102. Robinson LA, Brown CG, Jenkins J et al: Effect of norepineph-

rine *versus* epinephrine on myocardial hemodynamics during CPR. Ann Emerg Med 18:336, 1989

103. Brown CG, Robinson LA, Jenkins J et al: The effect of norepinephrine *versus* epinephrine on regional cerebral blood flow during cardiopulmonary resuscitation. Am J Emerg Med 7:278, 1989

104. Lindner KH, Ahnefeld FW: Comparison of epinephrine and norepinephrine in the treatment of asphyxial or fibrillatory cardiac arrest in a porcine model. Crit Care Med 17:437, 1989

105. Lindner KH, Ahnefeld FW, Schuermann W, Bowdler IM: Epinephrine and norepinephrine in cardiopulmonary resuscitation: Effects on myocardial oxygen delivery and consumption. Chest 97:1458, 1990

106. Kosnik JW, Jackson RE, Keats S et al: Dose-related response of centrally administered epinephrine on the change in aortic diastolic pressure during closed-chest massage in dogs. Ann Emerg Med 14:204, 1985

107. Gonzelez ER, Ornato JP, Garnett AR et al: Dose-dependent vasopressor response to epinephrine during CPR in human beings. Ann Emerg Med 18:920, 1989

108. Paradis NA, Martin GB, Rosenberg J et al: The effect of standard and high-dose epinephrine on coronary perfusion pressure during prolonged cardiopulmonary resuscitation. JAMA 265:1139, 1991

109. Brown CG, Werman HA, Davis EA et al: The effects of graded doses of epinephrine on regional myocardial blood flow during cardiopulmonary resuscitation in swine. Circulation 75:491, 1987

110. Martin C, Callaham M: High dose epinephrine improves the return of spontaneous circulation rates in human victims of cardiac arrest. Ann Emerg Med 20:722, 1991

111. Ralston SH, Tacker WA, Showen L et al: Endotracheal versus intravenous epinephrine during electromechanical dissociation with CPR in dogs. Ann Emerg Med 14:1044, 1985

112. Roberts JR, Greenberg MI, Knaub M et al: Comparison of the pharmacological effects of epinephrine administered by the intravenous and endotracheal routes. J Am Coll Emerg Phys 7:260, 1978

113. Crespo CG, Schoffstall JM, Fuhs LR, Spivey WH: Comparison of two doses of endotracheal epinephrine in a cardiac arrest model. Ann Emerg Med 20:230, 1991

114. Quinton DN, O'Byrne G, Aitkenhead AR: Comparison of endotracheal and peripheral intravenous adrenaline in cardiac arrest: Is the endotracheal route reliable? Lancet 1:828, 1987

115. Cingolani HE, Faulkner SL, Mattiazzi AR et al: Depression of human myocardial contractility with "respiratory" and "metabolic" acidosis. Surgery 77:427, 1975

116. Weisfeldt ML, Bishop RL, Green HL: Effects of pH and Pco_2 on performance of ischemic myocardium. In Roy PE, Rona G (eds): Recent Advances in Studies on Cardiac Structure and Metabolism, 10:355–364, Baltimore, University Park Press, 1975

117. Gerst PH, Fleming WH, Malm JR: Increased susceptibility of the heart to ventricular fibrillation during metabolic acidosis. Circ Res 19:63, 1966

118. Echt DS, Cato EL, Coxe BR: pH-dependent effects of lidocaine on defibrillation energy requirements in dogs. Circulation 80:1003, 1989

119. Houle DB, Weil MH, Brown EB et al: Influence of respiratory acidosis on ECG and pressor response to epinephrine, norepinephrine, and metaraminol. Proc Soc Exp Biol Med 94:561, 1957

120. Anderson MN, Border JR, Mouritzen CV: Acidosis, catecholamines, and cardiovascular dynamics: When does acidosis require correction? Ann Surg 166:344, 1967

121. Houle DB, Weil MH, Brown EB, Campbell GS: Influence of respiratory acidosis on ECG and pressor response to epinephrine, norepinephrine, and metaraminol. Proc Soc Exp Biol Med 94:561, 1957

122. vonPlanta M, Weil MH, Gazmuri RJ et al: Myocardial acidosis associated with CO_2 production during cardiac arrest and resuscitation. Circulation 80:684, 1989

123. Jaffe AS: New and old paradoxes: Acidosis and cardiopulmonary resuscitation. Circulation 80:1079, 1989

124. Weil MH, Rackow EC, Trevino R et al: Difference in acid-base state between venous and arterial blood during cardiopulmonary resuscitation. N Engl J Med 315:153, 1986

125. Gazmuri RJ, vonPlanta M, Weil MH, Rackow EC: Cardiac effects of carbon dioxide-consuming and carbon dioxide-generating buffers during cardiopulmonary resuscitation. J Am Coll Cardiol 15:482, 1990

126. Clancy RL, Cingolini HE, Taylor RR et al: Influence of sodium bicarbonate on myocardial performance. Am J Physiol 212:917, 1967

127. Berenyi KG, Wolk M, Killip T: Cerebrospinal fluid acidosis complicating therapy of experimental cardiopulmonary arrest. Circulation 52:319, 1975

128. Ornato JP, Garnett AR, Glauser FL: Relationship between cardiac output and the end-tidal carbon dioxide tension. Ann Emerg Med 19:1104, 1990

129. Gudipati CV, Weil MH, Bisera J et al: Expired carbon dioxide: A non-invasive monitor of cardiopulmonary resuscitation. Circulation 77:234, 1988

130. Sanders AB, Kern KB, Otto CW et al: End-tidal carbon dioxide monitoring during cardiopulmonary resuscitation: A prognostic indicator for survival. JAMA 262:1347, 1989

131. Callaham M, Barton C: Prediction of outcome of cardiopulmonary resuscitation from end-tidal carbon dioxide concentration. Crit Care Med 18:358, 1990

132. Steinman RT, Herrera C, Schuger CD, Lehmann MH: QRS tachycardia in the conscious adult: Ventricular tachycardia is the most frequent cause. JAMA 261:1013, 1989

133. Cobb LA, Hallstrom AP: Community-based cardiopulmonary resuscitation: What have we learned? Ann NY Acad Sci 382:330, 1982

133a. Weaver WD, Fahrenbruch CE, Johnson DD et al: Effect of epinephrine and lidocaine therapy outcome after cardiac arrest due to ventricular fibrillation: Circulation 82:2027, 1990

134. Dahl CF, Ewy GA, Warner ED et al: Myocardial necrosis from direct current countershock. Circulation 50:956, 1974

135. Warner ED, Dahl C, Ewy GA: Myocardial injury from transthoracic defibrillator countershock. Arch Pathol Lab Med 99:55, 1975

136. Weaver WD, Cobb LA, Copass MK et al: Ventricular defibrillation: A comparative trial using 175-J and 320-J shocks. N Engl J Med 207:1101, 1982

137. Thomas ED, Ewy GA, Dahl CF et al: Effectiveness of direct current defibrillation: Role of paddle electrode size. Am Heart J 93:463, 1977

138. Adgey AA: Electrical energy requirements for ventricular defibrillation. Br Heart J 40:1197, 1978

139. Crampton JA, Crampton RS, Sipes JN et al: Energy levels and patient weight in ventricular defibrillation. JAMA 242:1380, 1979

140. Gasch JA, Crampton RS, Cherwek ML et al: Determinants of ventricular defibrillation in adults. Circulation 60:231, 1979

141. Lown B, Crampton RS, DeSilva RA et al: The energy for ventricular fibrillation—too little or too much? N Engl J Med 298:1252, 1978

142. Kerber RE, Jensen SR, Gascho JA et al: Determinants of defibrillation: Prospective analysis of 183 patients. Am J Cardiol 52:739, 1983

143. Dahl CF, Ewy GA, Ewy MD et al: Transthoracic impedance to direct current discharge: Effect of repeated countershocks. Med Instrum 10:151, 1976

144. Haynes RE, Chinn TL, Copass MK et al: Comparison of bretylium tosylate and lidocaine in management of out-of-hospital ventricular fibrillation: A randomized clinical trial. Am J Cardiol 48:353, 1981

144a. Pennington JE, Taylor J, Lown B: Chest thump for reverting ventricular tachycardia. N Engl J Med 283:1192, 1970

145. Olson DW, Thompson BM, Darin JL et al: A randomized comparison study of bretylium tosylate and lidocaine in resuscitation of patients from out-of-hospital ventricular fibrillation in a paramedic system. Ann Emerg Med 13:807, 1984

146. Chow MMS, Ronfeld RA, Hamilton RA et al: Effect of external cardiopulmonary resuscitation on lidocaine pharmacokinetics in dogs. J Pharmacol Exp Ther 224:531, 1983

147. Kimball JT, Killip T: Aggressive treatment of arrhythmias in

acute myocardial infarction: Procedures and results. Prog Cardiovasc Dis 10:483, 1968

148. Lie KI, Wellens HJ, Downar E *et al:* Observations on patients with primary ventricular fibrillation complicating acute myocardial infarction. Circulation 52:755, 1975

149. McGovern BA, Garan H, Ruskin JN: Precipitation of cardiac arrest by verapamil in patients with Wolff-Parkinson-White syndrome. Ann Intern Med 104:791, 1986

150. Garratt C, Linker N, Griffith M *et al:* Comparisons of adenosine and verapamil for termination for paroxysmal junctional tachycardia. Am J Cardiol 64:310, 1989

151. Rankin AC, McGovern BA: Adenosine or verapamil for the acute treatment of supraventricular tachycardia? (editorial). Ann Intern Med 114:513, 1991

152. Schoen MD, Parker RB, Hoon TJ *et al:* Evaluation of the pharmacokinetics and electrocardiographic effects of intravenous calcium chloride pre-treatment in normal subjects. Am J Cardiol 67:300, 1991

153. Hedges JR, Syberud SA, Dalsey WC *et al:* Pre-hospital trial of emergency transcutaneous cardiac pacing. Circulation 76:1337, 1987

154. Barthell E, Troiano P, Olson D *et al:* Pre-hospital external cardiac pacing: A prospective, controlled clinical trial. Ann Emerg Med 17:1221, 1988

155. Stueven HA, Tonsfeldt DJ, Thompson BM *et al:* Atropine in asystole: Human studies. Ann Emerg Med 13:815, 1984

156. Iseri LT, Humphrey SB, Siner EJ: Pre-hospital bradysystolic cardiac arrest. Ann Intern Med 88:741, 1978

157. Stueven HA, Thompson BM, Aprahamian C *et al:* Calcium chloride: Reassessment of use in asystole. Ann Emerg Med 13:820, 1984

158. Stueven HA, Thompson BM, Aprahamian C *et al:* Lack of effectiveness of calcium chloride in refractory asystole. Ann Emerg Med 14:630, 1985

159. Stueven HA, Thompson BM, Aprahamian C *et al:* Use of calcium in pre-hospital cardiac arrest. Ann Emerg Med 12:136, 1983

160. Harrison EE, Amey BD: Use of calcium in electromechanical dissociation. Ann Emerg Med 13:844, 1984

161. Stueven HA, Thompson B, Aprahamian C *et al:* The effectiveness of calcium chloride in refractory electromechanical dissociation. Ann Emerg Med 4:626, 1985

162. Torphy DE, Minter MG, Thompson BM: Cardiorespiratory arrest and resuscitation of children. Am J Dis Child 138:1099, 1984

163. Orlowski JP: Optimal position for external cardiac massage in infants and children. Crit Care Med 12:224, 1984

164. Chamedies L (ed): Textbook of Pediatric Advanced Life Support. Dallas, American Heart Association, 1988

165. Fischer EG, Ames A: Studies on mechanisms of impairment of cerebral circulation following ischemia: Effects of hemodilution and perfusion pressure. Stroke 3:538, 1972

166. Bleyaert AL, Sands PA, Safar P *et al:* Augmentation of postischemic brain damage by severe intermittent hypertension. Crit Care Med 8:41, 1980

167. D'Alecy LG, Lundy ER, Karton KJ *et al:* Dextrose-containing intravenous fluid impairs outcome and increases death after eight minutes of cardiac arrest and resuscitation in dogs. Surgery 100:505, 1986

168. Longstreth WT Jr, Inui TS: High blood glucose level on hospital admission and poor neurological recovery after cardiac arrest. Ann Neurol 15:59, 1984

169. Pulsinelli WA *et al:* Increased damage after ischemic stroke in patients with hyperglycemia with or without established diabetes mellitus. Am J Med 74:540, 1983

170. Safer P, Nemoto EM: Brain resuscitation. Acta Anaesth Scand 70:60, 1978

171. Gisvold SE, Safar P, Rao G *et al:* Prolonged immobilization and controlled ventilation do not improve outcome after global brain ischemia in monkeys. Crit Care Med 12:171, 1984

172. Bleyaert A, Safar P, Nemoto E *et al:* Effect of postcirculatory arrest life-support on neurological recovery in monkeys. Crit Care Med 8:153, 1980

173. Gisvold SE, Safar P, Hendricks HHL *et al:* Thiopental treatment after global brain ischemia in pigtailed monkeys. Anesthesiology 60:88, 1984

174. Brain Resuscitation Clinical Trial I Study Group: Randomized clinical study of thiopental loading in comatose survivors of cardiac arrest. N Engl J Med 314:397, 1986

175. Todd MM, Chadwick HS, Shapiro HM *et al:* The neurological effects of thiopental therapy following experimental cardiac arrest in cats. Anesthesiology 57:76, 1982

176. Roine RO, Caste M, Kinnunen A *et al:* Nimodipine after resuscitation from out-of-hospital ventricular fibrillation: A placebo-controlled, double-blind, randomized trial. JAMA 264:3171, 1990

177. American Heart Association: Textbook of Advanced Cardiac Life Support (70-1004 [CP]), p 271. Dallas, 1987

178. Ruark JE, Raffin TA *et al:* Initiating and withdrawing life support. N Engl J Med 318:25, 1988

179. Tomlinson T, Brody H: Ethics and communication in do-not-resuscitate orders. N Engl J Med 318:43, 1988

180. Schwartz AJ, Orkin FK, Ellison N: Anesthesiologists' training and knowledge of basic life support. Anesthesiology 50:191, 1979

181. Schwartz AJ, Ellison N, Ominsky AJ *et al:* Advanced CPR—Student, teacher, administrator, researcher (editorial). Anesth Analg 61:629, 1982

INDEX

Page numbers followed by t and f indicate tables and figures, respectively.